SECOND EDITION

The New Aird's COMPANION IN SURGICAL STUDIES

'Surgery is learnt by apprenticeship and not from textbooks, not even from one profusely illustrated. The surgical student's illustration is the living patient and his blackboard is the operation wound. Yet to make the most of his clinical opportunities, the student must have ready and rapid access to the ever growing canon of established surgical fact; he should be aware of the surgical conquests of the past, the tactics of the present and the strategy of the immediate future. When he examines a patient he should be armed already with a vicarious experience gained from reading and should be able to distinguish between the symptoms and signs which illustrate, and those which contradict, the observations of his clinical predecessors.'

Ian Aird,
Companion in Surgical Studies;
Ch. 1, p. 1, first edition 1949.

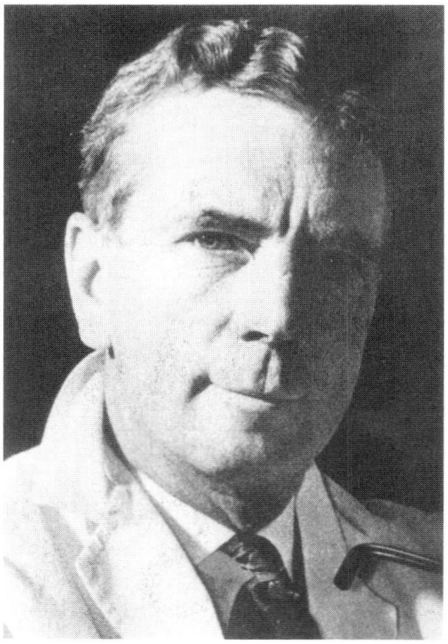

SECOND EDITION

The New Aird's COMPANION IN SURGICAL STUDIES

Edited by

Kevin G Burnand MS FRCS
Professor of Surgery
St. Thomas' Hospital
London
UK

Anthony E Young MA MChir FRCS
Consultant Surgeon
Surgical Directorate
St. Thomas' Hospital
London
UK

CHURCHILL LIVINGSTONE

LONDON EDINBURGH NEW YORK PHILADELPHIA SYDNEY TORONTO 1998

CHURCHILL LIVINGSTONE
A division of Harcourt Brace & Co Limited

First published 1992
Reprinted 1997
Second Edition 1998

ISBN 0 443 05326X

British Library Cataloguing in Publication Data
A catalogue record for this book is available from the British Library.

Library of Congress Cataloging in Publication Data
A catalog record for this book is available from the Library of Congress.

Medical knowledge is constantly changing. As new information becomes available, changes in treatment, procedures, equipment and the use of drugs become necessary. The editors/authors/contributors and the publishers have, as far as it is possible, taken care to ensure that the information given in the text is accurate and up to date. However, readers are strongly advised to confirm that the information, especially with regard to drug usage, complies with latest legislation and standards of practice.

The publisher's policy is to use **paper manufactured from sustainable forests**

Printed and bound in Great Britain by Bath Press

Contents

Contributors

Eric G Anderson MB, MSc FRCS(Ed and Glas) F Ch S (Hon)
Consultant Orthopaedic Surgeon, Western Infirmary, Glasgow, UK

Roger M Atkins MA DM FRCS
Consultant Orthopaedic Surgeon, Bristol Royal Infirmary; Clinical Reader In Orthopaedic Surgery, University of Bristol, Bristol, UK

L C Bainbridge MB ChB FRCS
Consultant Hand Surgeon, Pulvertaft Hand Centre, Derbyshire Royal Infirmary, Derby, UK

John Bancewicz BSc (Hons) ChM FRCS (Glasg and Eng)
Reader in Surgery, University of Manchester, Manchester; Honorary Consultant Surgeon, Hope Hospital, Salford, UK

A A B Barros D'Sa MD FRCS FRCS(Ed)
Consultant Vascular Surgeon, Royal Victoria Hospital, Belfast, UK

Irving S Benjamin BSc (Hons) MD FRCS(Glasg and Eng)
Professor of Surgery and Honorary Consultant Surgeon, King's College School of Medicine and Dentistry, King's College Hospital, London, UK

Frank E Boulton BSc MD FRCPath
Lead Physician and Consultant in Transfusion Medicine, National Blood Service, Southampton, UK

Jonathan A Britto BSc MB FRCS
Craniofacial Fellow, Craniofacial Centre, Great Ormond Street Hospital For Children, London, UK

Peter Bullock FRCS MRCP
Consultant Neurosurgeon, King's College Hospital and Honorary Consultant, Guy's and St Thomas' Hospital Trust, London, UK

Frank D Burke MB BS FRCS
Director of The Pulvertaft Hand Centre, Derbyshire Royal Infirmary; Professor of Hand Surgery To The Medical Sciences Department, University of Derby, Derbyshire Royal Infirmary, Derby, UK

K G Burnand MS FRCS
Professor of Surgery, UMDS St Thomas' Hospital, London, UK

Ken Callum MS FRCS
Consultant Surgeon, Derbyshire Royal Infirmary, Derby, UK

John Clarke MB BS FRCS
Consultant Plastic Surgeon, Queen Mary's University Hospital, London, UK,

H. Brendan Devlin CBE MA MD MCh FRCS
Director of Surgical Epidemiology, Royal College of Surgeons of England, Honorary Consultant Surgeon, North Tees General Hospital, Stockton-on-Tees, UK

J Michael Dixon BSc (Hons) MB ChB MD FRCSEd FRCSEng
Honorary Senior Lecturer in Surgery, University of Edinburgh; Consultant Surgeon, Edinburgh Breast Unit, West General Hospital, Edinburgh, UK

David P Drake MA FRCS DCH
Consultant Paediatric Surgeon, Great Ormond Street Hospital for Children, London, UK

Roger J H Emery MS FRCS (Ed)
Consultant Orthopaedic Surgeon, St Mary's Hospital, London, UK

Susannah J Eykyn FRCP FRCS FRCPath
Professor of Clinical Microbiology, UMDS, St Thomas' Hospital, London, UK

John R Farndon BSc MD FRCS
Professor of Surgery, University of Bristol; Honorary Consultant Surgeon, United Bristol Healthcare Trust, Bristol, UK

Lesley A Fenton MB BS MRCPath
Consultant Histopathologist, Dewsbury and District Hospital, Dewsbury, West Yorkshire, UK

Oliver M Fenton MB BS FRCS
Consultant Plastic Surgeon, Pinderfields Hospital, Wakefield, West Yorkshire, UK

J W L Fielding MD FRCS
Consultant Surgeon, Queen Elizabeth Hospital, Edgbaston, Birmingham, UK

Christopher G Fowler FRCP FRCS (Urol)
Consultant Urological Surgeon, The Royal Hospitals NHS Trust; Senior Lecturer in Urology, St Bartholomew's and The Royal London School of Medicine and Dentistry, London, UK

D T Gault MB ChB FRCS
Consultant Plastic Surgeon, Mount Vernon Hospital and Middlesex Hillingdon Hospital, Middlesex, UK

Peter Goldstraw FRCS
Consultant Thoracic Surgeon, Director of Surgery, The Royal Brompton Hospital, London, UK

Paul J Gregg MD FRCS
Professor of Orthopaedic Surgery, University of Newcastle Upon Tyne and Freeman Hospital NHS Trust, Newcastle on Tyne, UK

Hany M Hafez MB BS FRCS
Specialist Registrar, St Mary's, London, UK

John R W Hardy BSc MD FRCS
Consultant Orthopaedic Surgeon, Southmead General Hospital; Senior Lecturer, University of Bristol, Bristol, UK

Fred Heatley MB BChir FRCS
Professor of Orthopaedic Surgery, UMDS, Consultant Orthopaedic Surgeon, Guy's & St Thomas' Hospitals Trust, London, UK

Edward R Howard MS FRCS(Eng and Edin)
Professor of Hepato-biliary Surgery and Consultant Surgeon, King's College Hospital, London, UK

K Hussain MB BS BDS FDSRCS(Eng) FRCS(Eng)
Consultant Oral & Maxillofacial Surgeon to Guy's Hospital, London and Queen Mary's Hospital, Sidcup, Kent, UK

Barry Jackson MS FRCS
Consultant Surgeon, St Thomas' Hospital, London, UK

David N James MB BS FRCA
Consultant Anaesthetist, St Thomas' Hospital, London, UK

Martin Henry Jourdan BSC PhD MS FRCS
Consultant Surgeon and Reader in Surgery, Guy's and St Thomas' Hospitals, London, UK

Douglas M Justins MB BS FRCA
Consultant in Pain Management and Anaethesia, St Thomas' Hospital, London, UK

Andrew N Kingsnorth BSc MBBS MS FRCS
Professor of Surgery and Honorary Consultant Surgeon, Derriford Hospital, Plymouth, UK

Roger S Kirby MA MD FRCS (Urol) FEBU
Consultant Urologist, St George's Hospital, London, UK

Jonathan Lucas FRCS (Orth)
Clinical Orthopaedic Lecturer
United Medical and Dental Schools of Guy's and St Thomas', London, UK

Valerie J Lund MS FRCS FRCSEd
Honorary Consultant ENT Surgeon, Royal National Throat, Nose, and Ear Hospital and Moorfields Eye Hospital; Professor of Rhinology, Institute of Laryngology and Otology, University College London, London, UK

Malcolm F Macnicol MBChB BSc (Hons) FRCS MCh FRCSEd (Orth)
Consultant Orthopaedic Surgeon and Senior Orthopaedic Lecturer, Royal Hospital For Sick Children and Princess Margaret Rose Orthopaedic Hospital, W Edinburgh, UK

Robert E Mansel MS FRCS
Professor of Surgery, University of Wales, College of Medicine, Cardiff, UK

Robert Mason BSc ChM MD FRCS
Consultant Gastrointestinal Surgeon, Guy's Hospital and St Thomas' Hospitals, London, UK

Mark McGurk MD FRCS DLO FDS RCS
Professor of Maxillofacial Surgery, UMDS, Guy's and St Thomas' Hospital Trust, London, UK

Paul McMaster MA MB ChM FRCS FICS
Consultant Hepatobiliary and Transplant Surgeon, Queen Elizabeth Hospital, Edgbaston, Birmingham, UK

Raducu Mihai MD
University Assistant, Department of Endocrinology, Carol Davila University, Bucharest, Romania;
Research Fellow, University of Bristol, Bristol, UK

Neil Mortensen MA MB ChB MD FRCS
Consultant Colorectal Surgeon, John Radcliffe Hospital, Oxford; Clinical Reader in Colorectal Surgery, University of Oxford, Oxford, UK

John A Murie MA BSc MD FRCS
Consultant Vascular Surgeon, Royal Infirmary of Edinburgh NHS Trust; Honorary Senior Lecturer in Surgery, University of Edinburgh, Edinburgh, UK

James E Nicholl
Orthopaedic Snr Registrar, Guy's & Thomas' Hospitals Trust, London, UK

R J Nicholls MChir FRCS (Eng) FRCS (Glasg)
Consultant Surgeon, St Mark's Hospital, Harrow, UK

John Northover MS FRCS
Consultant Surgeon, St Mark's Hospital, Harrow, UK

David Nunn FRCS FRCSEd ORTH
Consultant Orthopaedic Surgeon, Guy's and St Thomas' Hospitals Trust, London, UK

Alec Fitzgerald O'Connor MB ChB FRCS
Consultant Otolaryngologist, Guy's and St Thomas' Hospital; Consultant Neurotologist, The London Hospital, London, UK

John K O'Dowd MB BS FRCS FRCSOrth
Consultant Spinal Surgeon, Frimley Park Hospital, Surrey; Honoroary Consultant Orthopaedic Surgeon, St Thomas' Hospital, London, UK

W J Owen BSc MS FRCS
Consultant Surgeon, Guy's and St Thomas' Hospital, London, UK

S Papagrigoriadis MD
Lecturer in Surgery, King's College School of Medicine and Dentistry, UK

Simon Paterson-Brown MS MPhil FRCS
Consultant General Surgeon, Edinburgh Royal Infirmary, Edinburgh, UK

Anthony L G Peel MA MChir FRCS
Consultant Surgeon, North Tees General Hospital, Stockton-on-Tees, UK

Brian J Rowlands MD FRCS FACS
Professor of Surgery, Queens University of Belfast, Belfast; Consultant Surgeon, Royal Group Hospitals Trust, Belfast, Northern Ireland, UK

Robert W Ruckley MB ChB FRCS
Consultant ENT Surgeon, Darlington Memorial Hospital, Darlington, UK

R C G Russell MS FRCS
Consultant Surgeon, The Middlesex Hospital, London, UK

John H Scurr BSc MB BS FRCS
Senior Lecturer, Consultant Surgeon, University College and Middlesex Hospitals, London, UK

Neeraj K Sharma MS Dip (Urol) FRCS (Urol)
Consultant Urologist, Royal Oldham Hospital, Oldham, UK

John S Shilling MB FRCS FCOphth
Consultant Ophthalmic Surgeon, St Thomas' Hospital and Greenwich District Hospital, London, UK

M A Smith FRCS
Consultant Orthopaedic Surgeon, Guy's & St Thomas' Hospitals, London, UK

P J Smith MB BS, FRCS
Consultant Plastic and Hand Surgeon, Mount Vernon Hospital, The Hospital for Sick Children, London, UK

Michael C Stacey DS FRACS
Associate Professor of Surgery, Fremantle Hospital, Fremantle, Western Australia

Peter T Taylor Ma MChir FRCS
Consultant Surgeon, Guy's and St Thomas' Hospitals, London, UK

Adrian R Timothy MB FRCP FRCR
Consultant Clinical Oncologist, Guy's and St Thomas' Cancer Centre, St Thomas' Hospital, London, UK

R C Tiptaft BSc FRCS
Consultant Urologist, Director of Stone Surgery, Lithotripter Centre, St Thomas' Hospital, London, UK

David A Tolley MB BS FRCS (Eng) FRCS(ED)
Consultant Urological Surgeon and Director of the Scottish Lithotripter Centre, Western General Hospital, Edinburgh; Honorary Senior Lecturer, University of Edinburgh, Edinburgh, UK

Tom Treasure MD MS FRCS
Professor of Cardiothoracic Surgery, St George's Hospital Medical School; Consultant Cardiothoracic Surgeon, St George's Hospital, London, UK

David Tweedle MB ChB FRCS FRCS(Ed) ChM
Consultant General Surgeon, University Hospital of South Manchester and The Christie Hospital, Manchester, UK

D M A Wallace MB BS FRCS
Consultant Urologist, University of Birmingham NHS Trust, Birmingham, UK

Malcolm H Wheeler MD FRCS
Professor of Endocrine Surgery, Consultant Surgeon, University Hospital of Wales, Cardiff, UK

Norman S Williams MS FRCS
Professor and Director of Surgery, St Bartholomew's and The Royal London School of Medicine and Dentistry, The Royal London Hospital, London, UK

John H N Wolfe MB BS MS FRCS
Consultant Vascular Surgeon, St Mary's Hospital, London, UK

Richard F M Wood MD FRCS
Professor of Surgery, University of Sheffield, Northern General Hospital, Sheffield, UK

Anthony E Young MA MChir FRCS
Consultant Surgeon, St Thomas' Hospital, London, UK

Preface

This is the fourth edition of a book whose first editions appeared in 1949 and in 1957 and which began a new life under our joint editorship in 1992. The first two editions were unusual in that they had but a single author; our subsequent editions are unashamedly multi-author works. We have, nevertheless, continued to choose authors who are clinically and academically active and who teach. We are grateful for the enthusiasm and knowledge with which they have imbued their contributions. We hope that our editing has ensured that Airdís declared style of direct and simple writing has been retained, together with his intention that the book should not be a dry textbook but a companion during the clinical studies of the postgraduate surgical trainee, and a ready reference for the trained surgeon needing to expand his knowledge of the general or the particular. For this reason, we have continued the habit of extensive referencing.

This edition differs from the third in that orthopaedics is now included for completeness and to allow trainees to reduce the number of books to which they refer.

We are grateful not only to our authors for their patience with our editorial criticisms but also to Lizzie Payne and to Deborah Russell and Nora Naughton, for their skill and energy in distilling a book which we hope will be friendly as well as helpful. We would also like to thank the Lecturers and Registrars at the Department of Surgery, St Thomas' Hospital for their help with reading the page proofs.

London 1998

AEY
KGB

Ian Aird: Historical note

Ian Aird was born in Edinburgh in 1902. He showed early brilliance in school and later in university there, where he studied medicine. He went on to postgraduate medical studies in Paris, Vienna and St Louis, USA, before returning as Assistant Surgeon to the Royal Hospital for Sick Children in Edinburgh.

It was at this time, in the early 1930s, that what was later to be the Companion first began to take embryonic shape. To accompany his lectures to postgraduate students for their examination for the Edinburgh Fellowship, he prepared sets of duplicated lecture notes. These notes, treasured by past students, proved of such value that copies changed hands for substantial sums of money.

After war service in the Royal Army Medical Corps in North Africa, he returned to Edinburgh, and then in 1947 moved to London as Professor of Surgery at London University's Postgraduate Medical School, Hammersmith Hospital. He held his post until his death by his own hand in 1962.

Those 15 years saw a prodigious research and educational output from him as he put his department and particularly its research unit at the leading edge of world surgical progress.

An outstanding communicator, he was particularly concerned with the international dissemination of surgical knowledge. He lectured and examined widely on every continent except Antarctica.

He published a constant stream of articles in the medical journals of many countries. But his teaching reached its pinnacle and its widest audience in his Companion in Surgical Studies.

1992 Margaret Aird

1 An introduction to the history of surgery

B. T. Jackson

It is common for surgical textbooks, monographs and articles to begin with a brief historical introduction. Why should this be so? Why should the student, whether undergraduate or postgraduate, be expected to learn history in addition to core facts, current beliefs and future trends? In short, what is the justification for this chapter? There is no simple answer. For many, the desire to know the origins of the subject, the wish to enquire into what has gone before and the enthusiasm to discover how current knowledge has been derived is intrinsic to learning and understanding. It has been suggested that those who cannot remember the past are condemned to repeat it,[1] an observation that will ring especially true to all who have embarked on a research project or reviewed the literature for a clinical paper or presentation. For some, historical vignettes simply leaven the hard work of learning and aid the memory, and it is not unknown for a smattering of historical knowledge to help in passing examinations! For all, it is desirable to know how surgery, as part of medicine as a whole, has influenced the various societies in which it has been practised and, conversely, how technical, cultural and economic changes within society have had an impact upon surgeons and surgery.

In a few pages this chapter can offer only a glimpse into surgical history although it may stimulate the reader to seek more detailed information from the references which include selected well-referenced review articles as well as numerous primary sources. The chapter may therefore be used as a basis for further historical enquiry or simply read as an overview of the subject. Biographical details have largely been avoided and many famous names are missing. Instead, important ideas and key developments in surgery are described, especially those of the last hundred years. It is during this time that surgery as we know it today has evolved, even though the sum of modern knowledge has been acquired by the accumulation of observations made over 2000 years or more.

EARLY HISTORY

The craft of surgery is as old as mankind. It is reasonable to believe that the drainage of abscesses, the dressing of wounds and the staunching of haemorrhage were practised by early humans although our knowledge of prehistoric surgery is largely conjectural. The setting of fractures may also have been performed but there is no firm evidence of this. The one operation that is known with certainty to have been carried out by neolithic man is trephination of the skull.[2] Hundreds of skulls with trephine holes, some multiple, have been discovered in Europe and America and from the evidence of callus formation it is known that many individuals survived. The indication for the operation, which is thought to have been performed with a sharpened flint, was probably to release supposed evil spirits from the skull of those with headache, vertigo, epilepsy or similar disorders. Other operations that may have been performed before written or pictorial records began are amputation of limbs and digits, and circumcision.[3]

The ancient east

Firm knowledge of early surgery relies on documentary evidence, of which there is a large amount regarding the practice of surgery in ancient Egypt, Babylon and India. For example, the Edwin Smith papyrus, discovered in Luxor in 1862, is over 45 metres in length and contains descriptions of injuries, wounds, fractures, dislocations and tumours.[4] Forty-eight surgical case histories are given and these detail physical examination, diagnosis, prognosis and treatment. It is the oldest known surgical text, having been compiled about 1700 BC.

The well-known code of Hammurabi, one of the earliest kings of Babylon, is engraved on a 2.5 metres tall pillar of polished black stone and may be seen in the Louvre.[5] It records various laws relating to medicine and surgery of the time: 'if a physician shall make a severe wound with a bronze lancet and kill him [the patient] or shall open an eye socket with a bronze lancet and destroy the eye, his hand shall be cut off'. If the patient was cured, or the eye preserved, the physician received 10 shekels of silver!

Ancient Hindu surgery was well-advanced by the time of Susruta in the fifth century AD.[6] He advocated dissection of dead bodies, described the manual skills necessary for surgery and suggested practising incisions on water melons and cucumbers. He described over a hundred surgical instruments and many operations including amputation, lithotomy, tonsillectomy and operations for anal fistulae. In the treatment of perforating wounds of the abdomen he advised that any protrusion of the intestines should be

REFERENCES

1. Santayana G The Life of Reason, vol 1 1905
2. Parry T W Br Med J 1923; 1: 457
3. Bishop W J The Early History of Surgery. Hale, London 1960
4. Breasted J H The Edwin Smith Surgical Papyrus. University Press, Chicago 1930
5. Majno G The Healing Hand: Man and Wound in the Ancient World. Harvard University Press, Cambridge, Massachusetts 1975
6. Prakash U B S Surg Gynecol Obstet 1978; 146: 263

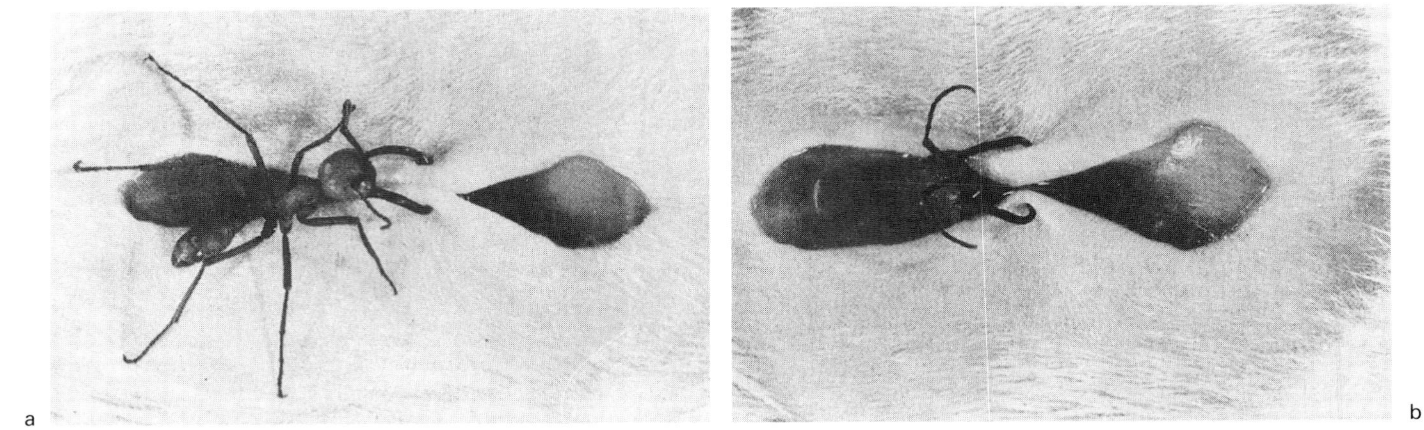

Fig. 1.1 (a) The jaws of a dead South American soldier ant *Eciton burchelli* holding together the edges of a skin wound in a dead rat in a laboratory experiment. (b) The body of the ant has been removed. Reproduced with permission from The Healing Hand. Majno G Harvard University Press, Cambridge, Massachusetts 1975.

washed with milk, lubricated with butter and reintroduced into the abdomen. If the intestine was perforated, the defect should be closed by applying black ants, of which the powerful jaws acted like pincers and held the edges of the wound in apposition.[7] The body of the ant was then removed (Fig. 1.1). Perhaps the best known operation practised in India at that time was rhinoplasty. This was performed to reconstruct a nose that had been amputated either in battle or as a punishment. The principles of rotating a skin flap used by these early Indian surgeons are still used by surgeons today.

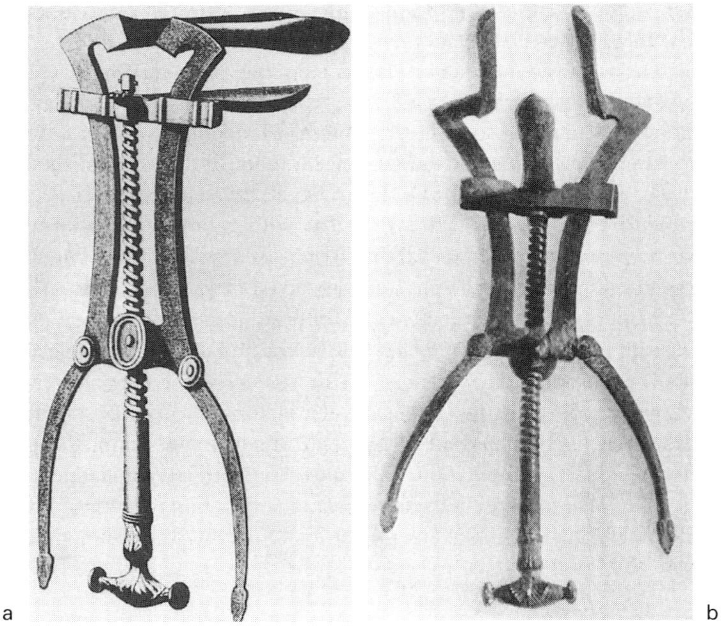

Fig. 1.2 (a) A vaginal speculum from AD 79 excavated at Pompeii, showing one of the earliest known applications of the screw; about one-third actual size (23 cm). Reproduced from Vulpes B *Illustrazione di tutti gli instrument chirurgici scaveti in Ércolano e in Pompeii*. Stamperia Reale, Naples 1847. (b) Photograph of the same speculum showing the remarkable state of preservation after nearly 2000 years. Reproduced from Milne J S Surgical Instruments in Greek and Roman Times. Clarendon Press, Oxford 1907.

Greeks and Romans

Most of the operations performed by Greek and Roman surgeons of classical times had been known and practised for centuries and few technical innovations were made. Their main contribution was to lay the scientific foundation of the profession by separating medicine from magic and basing clinical practice upon the study of anatomy and physiology. The importance of making a diagnosis only after taking a careful history and making an adequate physical examination was recognized; case histories were recorded and the literature of surgery came into being. The two best known names are Hippocrates, who practised around 400 BC, and Celsus, who practised in AD 30.[8]

The Hippocratic writings, many of which were not written by Hippocrates himself but by pupils and followers, cover many surgical problems such as fractures, dislocations, head injuries and rectal and anal disorders. Celsus, a cultured Roman, wrote an eight-volume medical treatise, of which the last two volumes were on surgery. He suggested that a surgeon should be young, have a strong and steady hand, be ambidextrous, have clear vision and not be moved by the cries of his patient. Celsus is still remembered by medical students today for his description of the four cardinal features of inflammation, *rubor*, *tumor*, *calor et dolor*, to which a hundred years later Galen added loss of function. Many surgical instruments from the time of Celsus were found in the ruins of Pompeii and are now preserved in the National Archaeological Museum in Naples (Fig. 1.2).

The Middle Ages

After the fall of the Roman Empire there was very little progress in the art or science of medicine until the advent of the Renaissance nearly 1000 years later. There was no study of anatomy or

REFERENCES

7. Gudger E W JAMA 1925; 84: 1861
8. Garrison F H An Introduction to the History of Medicine, 4th edn. Saunders, Philadelphia 1929

physiology; dissection was prohibited by the Church; there were no medical schools in western Europe; the practice of surgery fell into the hands of the uneducated; the itinerant operator for hernia, stone and cataract flourished. The use of the ligature to control haemorrhage, widely practised by the Greeks, was virtually abandoned and the use of the red-hot cautery and the application of boiling oil to wounds became standard practice.

The 11th and 12th centuries, however, saw the establishment of the great universities of western Europe, among which were Salerno, Paris, Bologna, Montpellier, Padua, Oxford and Cambridge. Medical schools were present in these universities but little attention was paid to the teaching of surgery which was considered an inferior discipline when compared with internal medicine. The physician was a learned graduate while the surgeon, with few exceptions, was an ill-educated artisan. Theodoric of Bologna, who lived around 1250, was such an exception.[9] He wrote a textbook of surgery in which he stressed the use of simple wound dressings. He maintained that pus was not always laudable and described the use of soporific sponges to induce sleep during operations. These sponges, which were used by several surgeons of the Middle Ages, were soaked in a decoction of herbs such as mandragora and are the forerunners of modern anaesthetic agents. Other noteworthy names of this period are Lanfranc of Milan, the author of an important surgical textbook that was widely read and which was translated into English some 200 years later; William of Saliceto, also an Italian, who wrote that surgeons should be reflective, quiet and have a downcast countenance, thus giving an impression of wisdom; and Guy de Chauliac of France who wrote the definitive *Chirurgia Magna* in which he gave a history of surgery, described many instruments and operations, insisted on the importance of anatomy, opposed quacks, and suggested that a good surgeon should be courteous, sober, pious, merciful, not greedy of gain and with a sense of his own dignity.[10]

The Renaissance

During the 200 years or so of the Renaissance there were profound changes in the theory and practice of surgery, both of which had remained more or less static since classical times. The new wave of scholasticism that occurred at this time, the revival of ancient classical culture, the burgeoning of scientific enquiry and the freedom from restriction imposed by the Church had its origin in Italy, especially Florence, and spread throughout Europe. It was in Italy too that artists such as Donatello, Michelangelo, Raphael and Leonardo da Vinci were among the first to take up the scientific study of human anatomy, a key advance necessary for the progression of surgery. All of these artists, especially Leonardo da Vinci, engaged in dissection of the human body, a practice that had been non-existent since the ancient dissections of a thousand years earlier. Although there had been sporadic anatomical demonstrations in Italian medical schools since the early 14th century, their main purpose was to help memorize the writings of a thousand years earlier. The professor sat in a raised chair and read from an inaccurate manuscript while a demonstrator pointed out the organ to the audience. When there were discrepancies between text and demonstration the professor explained that the human body had changed since Galen's time! A transformation occurred with the publication in 1543 of *De humani corporis fabrica* by Andreas Vesalius of Padua, then a 28-year-old surgeon and anatomist.[11] This folio-sized book, illustrated by a pupil of Titian, is the foundation of modern topographical human anatomy and one of the most important books in the history of science (Fig. 1.3). In the same year the astronomer Copernicus, who was also qualified in medicine, suggested for the first time that the sun rather than the earth was the centre of the planetary system in *De revolutionibus orbium coelestium*, another book that is an accepted landmark in the history of ideas. The introduction of printing from movable type by Gutenberg in Germany a hundred years earlier and the ability to reproduce woodcuts not only made these two great books possible but also had a profound influence on the diffusion of learning generally as well as the spread of surgical knowledge.

Another factor that had a major influence on the development of surgery at this time was the introduction of gunpowder and the resultant change in the nature and surgery of war wounds, best exemplified by the writings of Ambroise Paré of France, one of the greatest military surgeons of all time.[12] A one-time barber's apprentice who was unschooled in Latin, Paré reintroduced ligation of blood vessels to stop haemorrhage after amputation and abandoned the use of cautery and boiling oil. A man of courage, compassion and humility, he became surgeon to four kings of France. He wrote voluminously and his books reached a wide audience because they were written in the vernacular rather than in Latin. His famous aphorism 'I dressed the wound but God healed it' gives a measure of his sound common sense.

In England, Thomas Gale wrote the first surgical textbook in the English language in 1563[13] (Fig. 1.4), although some years earlier an English translation of a German text had been published (Fig. 1.5). William Clowes wrote on gunshot wounds in 1588,[14] the year of the great Armada, and John Woodall advocated lemon juice as a cure for scurvy in 1617, some 300 years before the discovery of vitamin C.[15] Quackery still abounded with sowgelders, tinkers and cobblers keen to perform surgical operations if the patient was fool enough, or desperate enough, to pay. In order to improve surgical standards, Henry VIII assented to the union of barbers and surgeons and in 1540 the Barber–Surgeon's Company was founded; this was the forerunner of the Royal College of Surgeons of England.[16] The Company laid down strict rules both for barbers and for surgeons and imposed fines on unlicensed surgical practitioners in London. The bodies of four executed criminals were dissected each year in Barber–Surgeon's Hall and an examination

REFERENCES

9. Edwards H Proc R Soc Med 1976; 69: 553
10. Ogden M S (ed) The Cyrurgie of Guy de Chauliac. Early English Text Society, London 1971
11. Simeone F A Am J Surg 1984; 147: 432
12. Bagwell C E Surg Gynecol Obstet 1981; 152: 350
13. Gale T Certaine Workes of Chirurgerie. Hall, London 1563. Reproduced in facsimile by De Capo Press, New York 1971
14. Poynter F N L Selected Writings of William Clowes 1544–1604. Harvey & Blythe, London 1948
15. Appleby J H Med Hist 1981; 25: 51
16. Dobson J, Walker R M Barbers and Barber–Surgeons of London. Blackwell, Oxford 1979

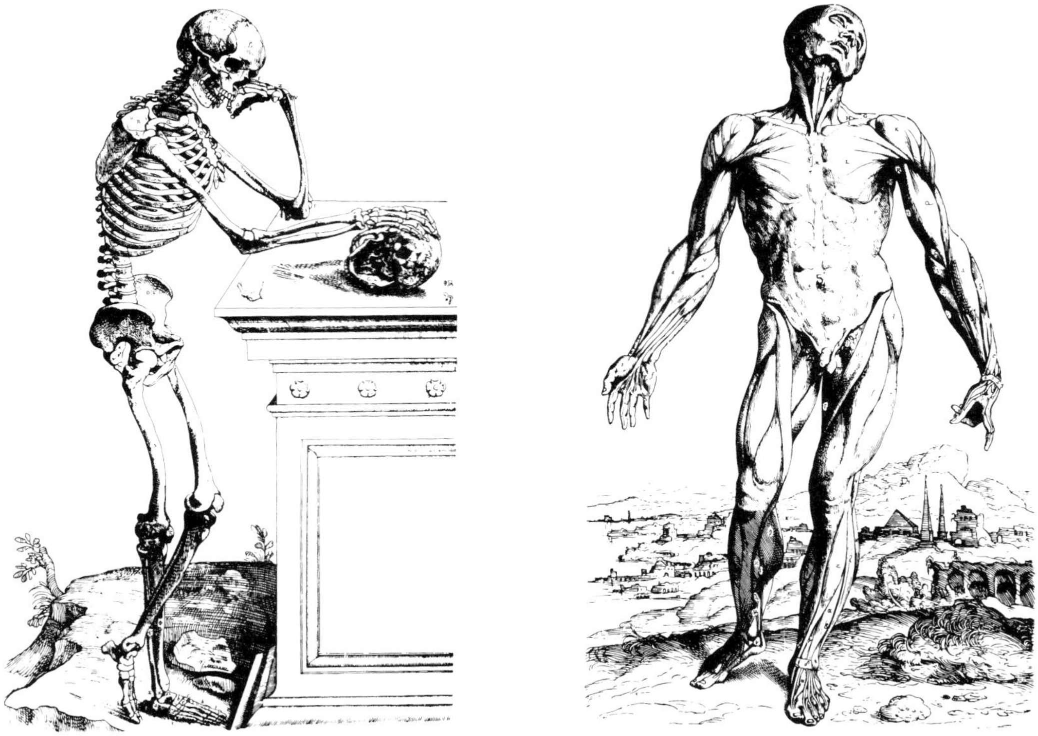

a b

Fig. 1.3 Two plates from Vesalius's *De humani corporis fabrica* 1543. (**a**) A plate from the osteology series. Note the hyoid on the left and two of the ossicles on the right of the separate skull. Although this depiction of the skeleton is far more accurate than any earlier anatomical illustration, some errors of proportion are present. (**b**) One of the 16 plates from the myology series. These were designed for the use of artists and sculptors as well as physicians. The background is real and has been identified as being just outside Padua.

was introduced for surgeons at the end of their apprenticeship. This represented the start of formal surgical education.

The 17th and 18th centuries

The 250 years after the Renaissance were marked by the consolidation and refinement of techniques and knowledge rather than by spectacular advances. For example, the use of skin flaps in amputation was introduced in 1679 by a naval surgeon from Plymouth[17] and this technique gradually became more widely used, although in military practice the old circular method remained in favour, when the raw stump was allowed to heal by secondary intention. The use of the cautery diminished, and ligature of blood vessels became more widely practised, although not by all surgeons. Several factors militated against change. As the surgeon often operated alone the application of ligatures to 20 or 30 bleeding vessels in an amputation stump took time, and without an assistant to control the bleeding it was much easier and quicker to sear the flesh with a cautery. Possibly the greatest hindrance to change however, then as now, was an inborn reluctance of many surgeons to alter established practice.

Harvey's publication of *De motu cordis* in 1628 provided a major impetus to the understanding of circulatory physiology, although this work had no immediate impact on the practice of surgery.[18] Before this time, blood had been thought to ebb and flow through the heart but Harvey observed that the venous, aortic and pulmonary valves only allowed blood to flow in one direction. He reasoned that the blood must circulate through the body even though the capillaries were unknown to him and were not discovered until after his death.

Early attempts at blood transfusion, first in dogs and sheep and then between animals and humans, took place in Oxford and Paris in the mid 17th century.[19] Samuel Pepys makes reference to these experiments in his diary for 1667 when he writes of meeting a 32-year-old Bachelor of Divinity at Cambridge who had been transfused with the blood of a sheep by Fellows of the Royal Society and paid 20 shillings for the experience. Pepys, who had an interest in medical matters and who had himself undergone a lithotomy for vesical calculus, comments that the patient was 'cracked a little in his head, though he speaks very reasonably and very well'.[20]

Lithotomy was perhaps the elective operation most often performed at this time.[21] Vesical calculus was common and exceptionally painful owing to the associated cystitis and trigonitis. For this reason many patients submitted themselves to the ordeal of the operation and, although most survived, many were left with a urinary fistula. The operation of the 'apparatus minor' had been

REFERENCES

17. Poynter F N L (ed) The Journal of James Yonge (1647–1721) Plymouth Surgeon. Longmans, London 1963
18. Keynes G The Life of William Harvey. Clarendon Press, Oxford 1966
19. Farr A D Med Hist 1980; 24: 143
20. Latham R (ed) The Shorter Pepys. Bell and Hyman, London 1986
21. Ellis H A History of Bladder Stone. Blackwell, Oxford 1969

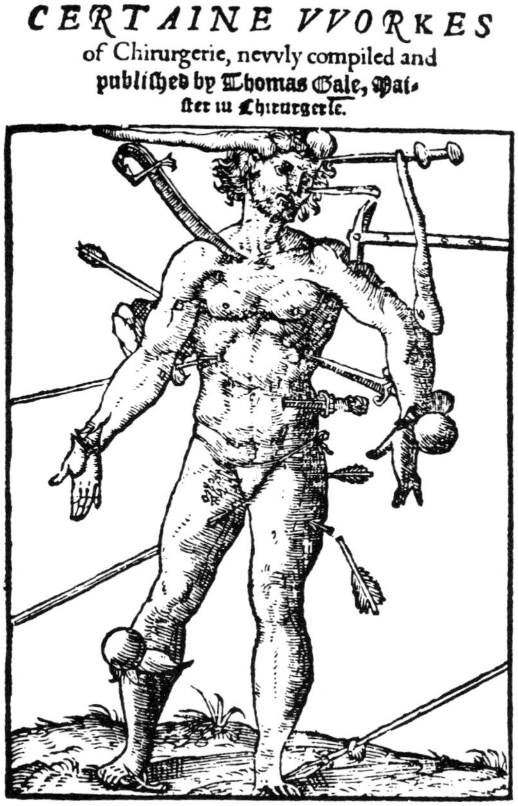

Fig. 1.4 The title page of Gale's *Certaine Workes of Chirurgerie* (Hall, London 1563), the first book on surgery written in English. It comprises four parts and contains several illustrations of surgical instruments. The wound man of the title page is seen in many early printed medical books and depicts the injuries that may have confronted a surgeon of the time.

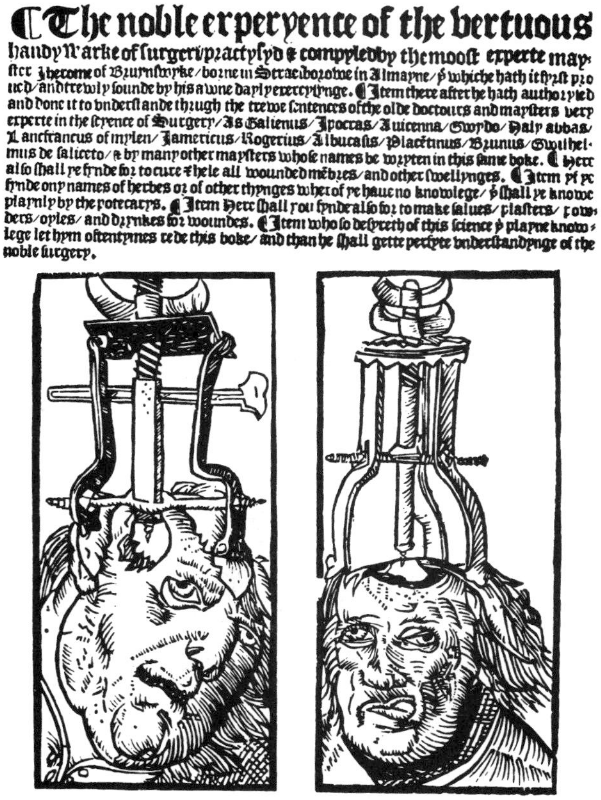

Fig. 1.5 The title page of the English translation of *Das Buch der Cirurgie* by Hieronymous Brunschwig 1525. The translator is unknown. Originally published in Strasburg in 1497, the English version is notable for its many dramatic woodcut illustrations. The text is mainly concerned with military surgery.

used for centuries. The bladder was incised through the midline of the perineum while a finger in the rectum pushed the stone on to the perineum. A blunt hook was then used to extract the stone.

In the late 16th century a new technique was introduced using the 'apparatus major', comprising a staff in the urethra, a series of instruments to dilate the incision and large stone-holding forceps to extract the calculus. This operation, which took up to an hour to perform, often damaged the prostate and bladder neck, causing severe haemorrhage, impotence and urinary fistula. An itinerant unqualified Frenchman, Jacques Beaulieu, better known as Frère Jacques, introduced the lateral approach to the bladder, thus avoiding the prostate and bladder neck and giving better access with less tissue trauma and a reduced morbidity. He is said to have performed the operation some 4500 times before he died in 1714. The lateral operation was taken up by William Cheselden of London, the author of the foremost anatomical textbook of the time, and so refined by him by practice on cadavers that the operation could be performed in a minute or less.[22] In 1740, Cheselden published his results in 213 patients cut publicly in front of an audience.[23] 105 were under the age of 10 years. Of the first 50 only three died; of the second 50, three; of the third 50, eight; and of the last 63, six. Cheselden explained that the reason so few died in the early part of the series was because at that time only good-risk patients came forward for the operation. Later, when the good results became known, poor-risk patients volunteered. This account is a noteworthy early example of honest surgical audit.

Many well-known names in the history of surgery date from the 18th century with John Hunter being arguably the most famous and certainly the most important.[24] He was a man with an original mind, astonishing industry and a colourful character. Hunter was the first surgeon to apply experimental method to surgery, especially with his work on inflammation and ligature of arteries in cases of aneurysm. He brought the study of pathology and physiology to surgery, which previously had been based almost exclusively on anatomy. He dissected animals as well as humans, examined diseased parts as well as normal anatomy and built up a vast collection of specimens of comparative anatomy and pathology that forms the basis of the Hunterian Museum in the Royal College of Surgeons of England. He influenced the development of surgery for decades after his death, not only by his writings but also through the work of his pupils, many of whom became the leading surgeons of the day.

REFERENCES

22. Cope Z William Cheselden. Livingstone, Edinburgh 1953
23. Cheselden W The Anatomy of the Human Body, 5th edn. Bowyer, London 1740
24. Qvist G John Hunter 1728–1793. Heinemann, London 1981

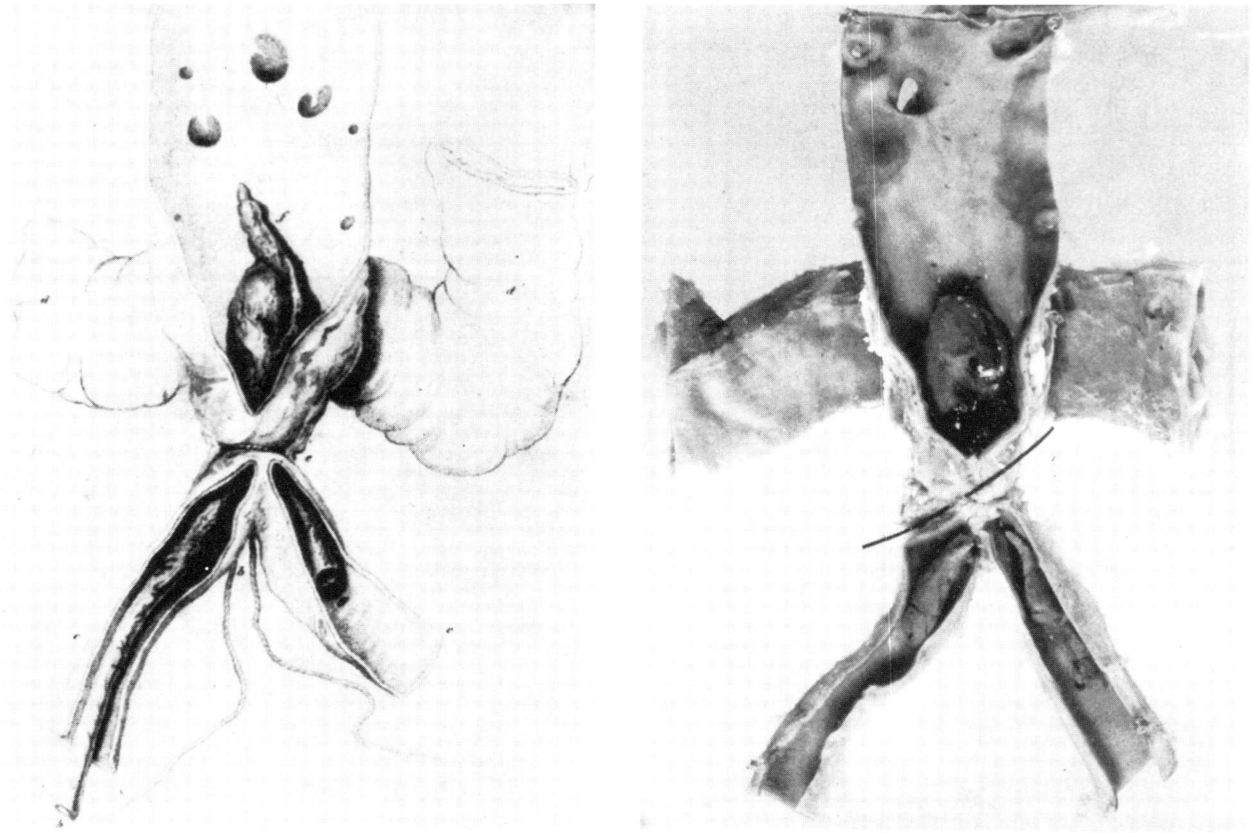

a b

Fig. 1.6 **(a)** A plate from *Surgical Essays* by Astley Cooper and Benjamin Travers 1818, in which Astley Cooper reported the first ligation of the human aorta. The operation was performed by Cooper in Guy's Hospital in 1817 on a 38-year-old man with a ruptured aneurysm extending from the left common iliac artery to the femoral artery. The patient survived 40 h. **(b)** The original specimen now preserved in the Astley Cooper pathological collection at St Thomas's Hospital, London.

One of Hunter's best known pupils was Sir Astley Cooper, who wrote classic texts on hernias, dislocation and fractures of joints, diseases of the testis and breast, and on the anatomy of the thymus gland.[25] He was the first surgeon to ligate the aorta for iliac aneurysm (Fig. 1.6), the first to perform a through-hip amputation, and one of the last great surgeons who felt the necessity to dissect the human body on a regular daily basis. He stated: 'if I laid my head upon my pillow at night without having dissected something that day I should think I had lost that day'. Unfortunately the supply of cadavers for such dissections was limited to the bodies of executed criminals and this shortage of material led to the rise of the 'body snatcher' or 'resurrectionist' who dug up freshly buried bodies at night from churchyard graves.[26] Cooper was a noted patron of these body snatchers and allegedly paid well. However, when the notorious Burke and Hare murders in Scotland started to supply the surgeon's dissecting room, public outcry led to the introduction of the Anatomy Act of 1832 in Great Britain and Ireland and this regularized the supply of bodies for anatomical study.[27]

ANAESTHESIA AND ANTISEPSIS

The introduction of general anaesthesia in 1846[28] in the USA and the expounding of the principles of antisepsis by Lister in Scotland in 1867[29] were two of the most fundamental advances in the history of surgery and transformed the image of the profession. In the early 19th century, operations were infrequently performed because they were dangerous, painful, and had a high complication rate.[30] Although we can read of the triumphs of a few great surgeons, we read little of their disasters or the poor results of many lesser surgeons. Sepsis was almost universal. The surgeon had to operate rapidly to minimize shock and reduce excessive haemorrhage. Operations took place only once a week at most hospitals, when two or three operations would be performed before a large audience. For example, in 1831 a surgeon at Guy's Hospital in London excised a tumour weighing 56 lb (25 kg) in front of an audience of 680 onlookers. The death of the patient was ascribed by *The Lancet* to prolonged exposure in an atmosphere so poisoned by human exhalations that many onlookers were pale as death and near to fainting.[31]

REFERENCES

25. Brock R C The Life and Work of Astley Cooper. Livingstone, Edinburgh 1952
26. Ball J M The Sack-'em-up Men: An Account of the Rise and Fall of the Modern Resurrectionists. Oliver and Boyd, Edinburgh 1928
27. Richardson R Death, Dissection and the Destitute. Routledge & Kegan Paul, London 1987
28. Bigelow H J Boston Med Surg J 1846; 35: 309
29. Lister J Lancet 1867; i: 326
30. Jackson B T Guy's Hosp Rep 1971; 120: 229
31. Leading Article Lancet 1830–1831; ii: 83

The range of operative procedures was limited: tuberculosis, aneurysms, surface tumours, cataracts and abscesses accounted for most of the operations. Contrary to popular belief, a major amputation was unusual. Mortality was high, sometimes amounting to 60% for more extensive procedures. The surgeon needed to be a man of special demeanour and courage and to have great physical strength in order to reduce dislocations, set fractures and operate with great speed on the conscious patient. Surgery was universally considered to be of lower status than medicine, and physicians and surgeons did not rank equal in the eyes of society or each other. By the end of the 19th century, however, this picture had changed profoundly.

Anaesthesia

The early history of anaesthesia is long and convoluted and has been admirably described elsewhere.[32] Soporific sponges soaked in herbs were used by the ancients to deaden pain, as were alcohol and opium. Morphine, named after Morpheus, the god of dreams, was discovered in 1805.[33] Humphrey Davy, later of chemistry fame, discovered the anaesthetic properties of nitrous oxide in 1799 and in the following year suggested that this gas might be used with advantage in surgical operations,[34] but his suggestion was not followed up. Instead, nitrous oxide was used as 'laughing gas' to enliven parties and dull lectures.

Inhalational anaesthesia was probably first used for an operation some 40 years later when in 1842 an American medical student, William Clark, administered ether to enable a tooth to be painlessly extracted. In the same year, Crawford Long of Georgia removed a small cyst from the neck of a patient under the influence of ether. Neither of these events was written up at the time, however, and the wider introduction of anaesthesia had to wait a little longer.

Horace Wells, a dentist, used nitrous oxide to extract teeth in 1844, but the credit for the true realization of the importance of inhalational ether as an anaesthetic agent is now generally credited to William Morton, another dentist who, on 16 October 1846 in Boston, administered ether to a young man named Gilbert Abbott while John Collins Warren, surgeon at the Massachusetts General Hospital, removed a vascular malformation from his neck. Several more painless operations were performed in Boston in the next few days and a month later the discovery was published.[28] Within another month the news had crossed the Atlantic and Robert Liston performed an above-knee amputation under ether anaesthetic at University College Hospital, London on 21 December 1846.[35] By February 1847, *The Lancet* and other journals were reporting operations performed under ether from all parts of Britain, and most European centres were also using the technique. Chloroform, introduced by James Young Simpson of Edinburgh in the same year,[36] rapidly superseded ether as the most widely used anaesthetic. Within a short time painful surgery had become obsolete and speed of operating was no longer the hallmark of the master surgeon. Despite the rapid spread of the technique, however, anaesthesia was slow to develop as a specialty. For years it was considered sufficient for the house surgeon or even a medical student to give the anaesthetic and most hospitals did not appoint a consultant anaesthetist until well into the 20th century.

Local anaesthesia began with topical cocaine which was first isolated from the coca leaf in 1860[37] but not clinically used for some 20 years afterwards;[38] endotracheal anaesthesia was introduced in the late 19th century;[39] intravenous anaesthesia in 1932 using hexobarbitone;[40] and relaxant anaesthesia as recently as 1942 using curare.[41] These developments made many major operations possible, not merely painfree, and were the direct result of increasing interaction between physiology, pharmacology, technology and medicine—associations that have led to many other important developments in modern surgery.

The rapid acceptance of anaesthesia perhaps stemmed in part from the general trend towards humanitarianism that was taking place in the mid 19th century. Reforms in public health, education, the prisons, the almshouses and the drive against drunkenness all had their origin in the wish to improve the human condition. Florence Nightingale, the founder of the modern nursing profession, was largely inspired by the desire to improve the lot of the common soldier after seeing at first hand the appalling conditions under which soldiers lived and fought during the Crimean war.[42]

Antisepsis

Anaesthesia was speedily accepted; the greater advance of antisepsis and the germ theory of infection had a more difficult and lengthy gestation. Before Lister, surgeons and patients alike accepted that almost all wounds became septic and visible pus was called 'laudable', for if the wound was draining freely, infection was less likely to loculate and cause septicaemia. The cause of the sepsis was unknown. As early as 1546 Fracastoro of Verona, now better known for his naming and recognition of syphilis, had postulated the presence in the air of invisible particles that carried disease.[43] As there was no objective evidence that such particles existed his theory was not accepted. The development of microscopy in the 17th century[44] enabled micro-organisms to be seen, but it still took some time for these to be accepted as the cause of infection, largely because of the theory of spontaneous generation which postulated that the micro-organisms present in diseased and necrotic tissue had arisen de novo. Another unhelpful

REFERENCES

32. Duncum B M The Development of Inhalational Anaesthesia. Oxford University Press, London 1947
33. Sertürner F W A J Pharm (Lpz) 1805; 14: 47
34. Davy H Researches, Chemical and Philosophical, chiefly concerning Nitrous Oxide. Johnson, London 1800. Reprinted Butterworths, London 1972
35. Cock F W Am J Surg (Anaesthesia suppl) 1915; 29: 98
36. Simpson J Y Lancet 1847; ii: 549
37. Nieman A Ueber eine neue organische Base in den Cocablättern. Huth, Göttingen, 1860
38. Halsted W S NY Med J 1885; 42: 294
39. Macewen W Br Med J 1880; 2: 122
40. Weese H, Scharpff W Dtsch Med Wochenschr 1932; 58: 1205
41. Griffith H R, Johnson G E Anesthesiology 1942; 3: 418
42. Goldie S M (ed) Florence Nightingale in the Crimean War 1854–56. Manchester University Press, Manchester 1987
43. Meade R H An Introduction to the History of General Surgery. Saunders, Philadelphia 1968
44. Clay R S, Court T H The History of the Microscope. Griffiths, London 1932

but common belief was that miasma, a poisonous invisible gas generated from sewage, caused infection.[45]

Although several far-sighted individuals—most now forgotten—had earlier suggested that infection was transmissible and that handwashing and cleanliness were effective methods for preventing its spread, it was the obstetrician, Ignaz Semelweiss, working in Vienna, who popularized these ideas.[46] In 1846, the same year that general anaesthesia was discovered, Semelweiss noted that there was a higher incidence of puerperal fever in the ward where medical students examined patients without washing their hands than in another ward where midwives, who had a higher standard of personal hygiene, attended the patient. In the following year, he observed that the post-mortem appearance of one of his colleagues who died after cutting his finger during a necropsy was similar to that of the cadaver his colleagues had been examining. Semelweiss realized that a transmissible agent was responsible for the infection and instituted a rigorous policy of handwashing in calcium chloride solution, after which the maternal mortality dropped from 10% to 1.2% within a year. Regrettably, his views were not accepted by the majority of his colleagues; he met with strong personal criticism, became mentally ill and died at the age of 47.

Joseph Lister, later Lord Lister, the first surgical peer, held the chair of surgery in Glasgow when he began his work on the use of carbolic acid in the prevention of infection. He had already published original scientific papers on inflammation, the intrinsic muscles of the eye and coagulation of the blood.[47] He was influenced in his research by the work of Louis Pasteur, published in the early 1860s, which showed that putrefaction and fermentation were caused by micro-organisms carried in the air and on dust.[48] Lister reasoned that sepsis might be prevented if these micro-organisms could be killed. After preliminary experiments with other chemicals, Lister learned that in Carlisle the obnoxious smell of sewage had been notably reduced by treatment with carbolic acid and that an outbreak of typhoid in the city had rapidly subsided at the same time. He therefore tried out carbolic acid as a topical dressing in patients with compound fractures of the leg, a condition that hitherto had usually been treated by amputation. Lister published his results in *The Lancet* in 1867[29] (Fig. 1.7). Eleven patients were described: nine did well, one needed amputation and one died. Lister followed up this first report with numerous lectures and further publications, continually refining the technical details of his method. He applied the antiseptic principle to many other operations with equal success and also showed that catgut, if sterilized in carbolic acid, could be safely used as a ligature.[49] He was a perfectionist and it is generally believed that it was his scrupulous attention to detail that enabled his results to be better than some of his detractors. One of his famous aphorisms was 'success depends upon attention to detail'.

The acceptance of Lister's work was not universal. Some surgeons quickly became converts to his teaching (Fig. 1.8), while others were sceptical.[50] By and large, his British contemporaries were slow to adapt while overseas surgeons, especially those in Germany, were rapid converts to the antiseptic principle. The reasons for hesitation were several: the method relied on great attention to detail and therefore was slow; carbolic acid was unpleasant, causing irritation to the wounds and carboluria if

ON A

NEW METHOD OF TREATING COMPOUND FRACTURE, ABSCESS, ETC.

WITH OBSERVATIONS ON THE CONDITIONS OF SUPPURATION.

BY JOSEPH LISTER, ESQ., F.R.S.,

PROFESSOR OF SURGERY IN THE UNIVERSITY OF GLASGOW.

PART I.

ON COMPOUND FRACTURE.

THE frequency of disastrous consequences in compound fracture, contrasted with the complete immunity from danger to life or limb in simple fracture, is one of the most striking as well as melancholy facts in surgical practice.

If we inquire how it is that an external wound communicating with the seat of fracture leads to such grave results, we cannot but conclude that it is by inducing, through access of the atmosphere, decomposition of the blood which is effused in greater or less amount around the fragments and among the interstices of the tissues, and, losing by putrefaction its natural bland character, and assuming the properties of an acrid irritant, occasions both local and general disturbance.

a

[MARCH 16, 1867. 327

lieve, of improper management; but subsequent trials have more than realised my most sanguine anticipations.

Carbolic acid* proved in various ways well adapted for the purpose. It exercises a local sedative influence upon the sensory nerves; and hence is not only almost painless in its immediate action on a raw surface, but speedily renders a wound previously painful entirely free from uneasiness. When employed in compound fracture its caustic properties are mitigated so as to be unobjectionable by admixture with the blood, with which it forms a tenacious mass that hardens into a dense crust, which long retains its antiseptic virtue, and has also other advantages, as will appear from the following cases, which I will relate in the order of their occurrence, premising that, as the treatment has been gradually improved, the earlier ones are not to be taken as patterns.

CASE 1.—James G——, aged eleven years, was admitted into the Glasgow Royal Infirmary on August 12th, 1865, with compound fracture of the left leg, caused by the wheel of an empty cart passing over the limb a little below its middle. The wound, which was about an inch and a half long, and three-quarters of an inch broad, was close to, but not exactly over, the line of fracture of the tibia. A probe, however, could be passed beneath the integument over the seat of fracture and for some inches beyond it. Very little blood had been extravasated into the tissues.

b

Fig. 1.7 **(a)** The beginning of Lister's historic article in *The Lancet* of 16 March 1867 in which he introduced the theory of antisepsis. **(b)** The first reference in the article to carbolic acid and details of the injury of the first patient to be treated by the new method. Arguably the most important patient of the 19th century, young James Greenlees made an uncomplicated infection-free recovery from a condition that normally necessitated amputation.

contact was prolonged; the method was expensive and, probably most importantly, there was a failure by many surgeons to understand fully the theory of infection. Those who claimed to use Lister's methods often used carbolic dressings that had fallen on the floor, or which had been in contact with their dirty apron, thereby showing a lack of understanding of the principles involved.

Over a period of 20 years, however, Lister's contributions became widely accepted and antisepsis gradually gave way to asepsis, a technique particularly associated with the name of von

REFERENCES

45. Wangensteen O H, Wangensteen S D The Rise of Surgery from Empiric Craft to Scientific Discipline. Dawson, Folkestone 1978
46. Wheeler E S Am J Surg 1974; 127: 573
47. Lister J The Collected Papers of Joseph, Baron Lister. Clarendon Press, Oxford 1909
48. Guthrie D Lord Lister, his Life and Doctrine. Livingstone, Edinburgh 1949
49. Lister J Lancet 1869; i: 451
50. Leading Article Lancet 1882; i: 1088

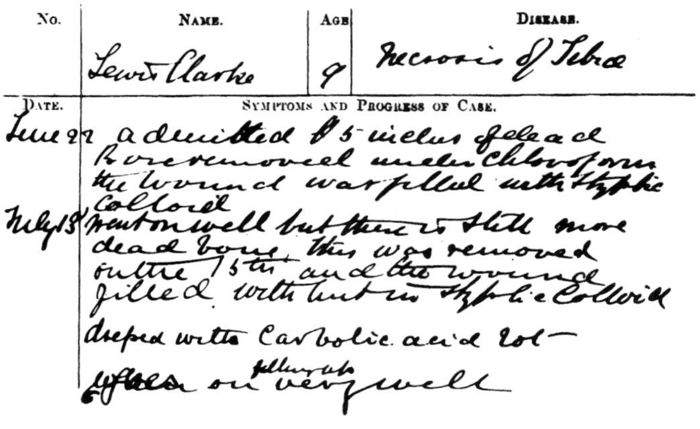

No.	Name.	Age	Disease.
	Lewis Clarke	9	Necrosis of Tibia

Date. Symptoms and Progress of Case.

June 27 admitted 1⁵ inches of dead bone removed under Chloroform the wound was filled with styptic Colloid

July 18 went on well but there is still more dead bone, this was removed on the 15th and the wound filled with lint in styptic Colloid

dressed with Carbolic acid lot-

goes on very well

Fig. 1.8 An extract dated 13 July [1867] from the case book of Thomas Kendall, surgeon in King's Lynn, Norfolk, describing the use of carbolic acid dressings some 4 months after Lister's paper had been published. Kendall is believed to be one of the first converts to Lister's antiseptic method. Reproduced with permission from Ann R Coll Surg Eng 1974; 54: 189.

Bergmann of Berlin, who introduced steam sterilization of gowns and dressings in the 1880s and who tried to make the operating theatre germ-free.[51] The introduction of rubber surgical gloves is popularly credited to William Halsted of Baltimore who, in 1889, arranged for the Goodyear Rubber Company to make gloves with gauntlets for his scrub nurse whose hands were allergic to the mercurial hand rinse.[52] In fact, rubber gloves were being used in the operating theatre by a number of others before this time.[53] Gauze face-masks were probably first worn by Berger in Paris in 1897.[54] By the turn of the century, operating theatres were designed according to aseptic principles with easily washable walls and floors, absence of awkward angles, a reduced spectator area, running water, sterilizers and filtered air ventilation[55] (Fig. 1.9). A new range of operations could be performed, made possible by the reduced risk of infection. Lister lived to declare open some of these new theatres; when he died in 1912 he was internationally famous.

THE POST-LISTERIAN ERA

The general acceptance of asepsis marks a watershed in the history of surgery. The several thousand years of surgical knowledge before Lister can be summarized reasonably easily, but the hundred years after Lister have encompassed such an explosion of knowledge and scientific advance that greater selection and condensation of the developments become inevitable. By the turn of the 19th century the practice of surgery had been transformed, not only by Lister, but also by developments in other scientific disciplines. Most of today's standard operations in abdominal surgery were regularly performed, while operations on the brain, the lungs and the heart had all been recorded. Elective hernia repair was starting to replace the truss. Electric lighting not only gave better illumination in the operating theatre but also enabled inspection of body cavities through primitive endoscopes such as the electric cystoscope, an instrument introduced by Nitze[56] (Fig. 1.10). Diagnostic imaging had begun with the discovery of X-rays by Röntgen in 1895[57] and therapeutic radiology was introduced soon afterwards, first for benign skin conditions[58] and subsequently in the treatment of cancer.[59] Microscopy had been used to study and classify the resected surgical specimens and the science of bacteriology was in its infancy. Publicity for these advances had been aided by the increased speed of transmission of scientific information: telegraphy was widely used, scientific journals were

REFERENCES

51. von Bergmann E Ther Mh 1887; 1: 41
52. Halsted W S Johns Hopkins Hosp Rep 1890–1891; 2: 308
53. Miller J M Surgery 1982; 92: 541
54. Berger P Bull Soc Chirurgiens Paris 1899; 25: 187
55. Wangensteen O H, Wangensteen S D Surgery 1975; 77: 403
56. Nitze M Wien Med Wochenschr 1879; 29: 649
57. Röntgen W C S B phys-med Ges Würzburg 1895; 132. English translation Nature 1896; 53: 274
58. Freund L Wien Klin Wochenschr 1897; 10: 73
59. Lazarus-Barlow W S Br Med J 1909; 1: 1465

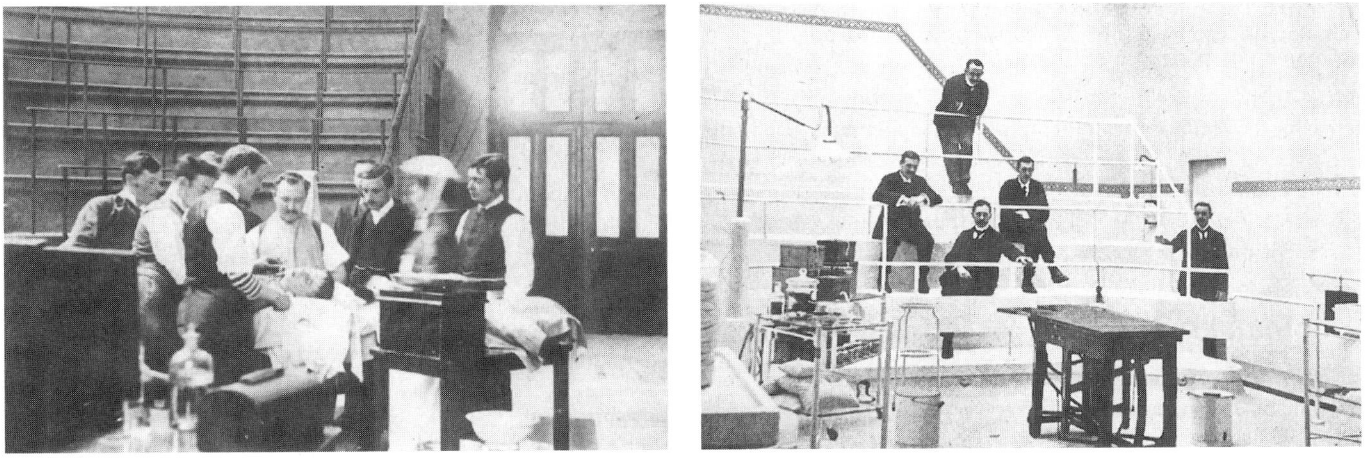

a b

Fig. 1.9 The operating theatre of St Thomas's Hospital, London before and after the acceptance of Lister's teachings. (a) In the 1880s: the doors opened directly on to the main hospital corridor and the wooden spectator standings could accommodate 200 visitors. Wooden beams supported the roof 13.5 m above the floor and the lighting was by gas. The theatre was regularly used by medical students for entertainment! **(b)** The same theatre in 1901 after conversion to incorporate the principles of asepsis. It was declared open by Lister himself. The floor and walls were tiled, the small spectator area was made of white marble and positive pressure ventilation was present throughout. Note that the wooden operating table had not yet been upgraded. Reproduced with permission from St Thomas's Hosp Gazette 1978; 76: 8.

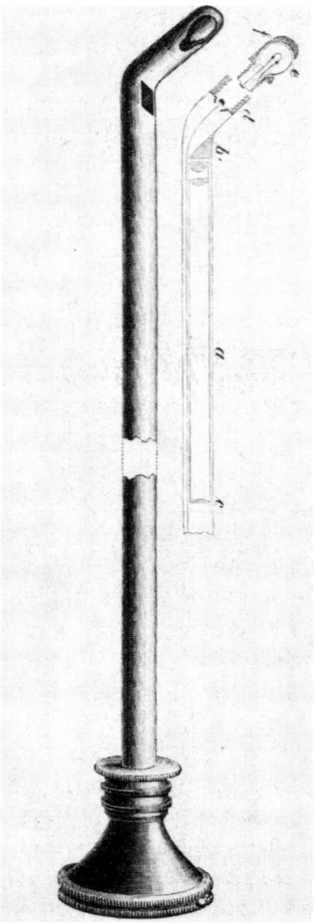

Fig. 1.10 Max Nitze of Berlin demonstrated the forerunner of the modern cystoscope at a meeting in Dresden. The illumination was by means of an incandescent platinum loop which required a cumbersome cooling system. This was soon replaced by a small carbon filament bulb which gave a much improved view of the bladder. Earlier instruments had been illuminated by reflected light, usually from a candle, down a silvered hollow tube. This illustration from Nitze's book on cystoscopy is designed to show the electrical features of his instrument rather than the cystoscope itself. Reproduced from Nitze M *Lehrbuch der Kystoskopie*. Bergmann, Wiesbaden, 1889.

increasing in number, photography was applied to medicine (Fig. 1.11), and the age of steam enabled easy travel for surgeons to visit clinics and colleagues in different countries. The years between 1870 and 1900 have been called 'the exciting years', with the some justification.[60]

Abdominal surgery

Various operations on the contents of the abdominal cavity were occasionally reported before the last quarter of the 19th century, but only colostomy and ovariotomy were performed with any regularity. Littré of Paris was the first to suggest elective colostomy after he performed a necropsy on an infant with congenital anal atresia in 1710,[61] but the operation was not carried out successfully until 1793.[62] The patient, a neonate of 3 days with an imperforate anus, lived for 45 years. During the next 50 years colostomy was

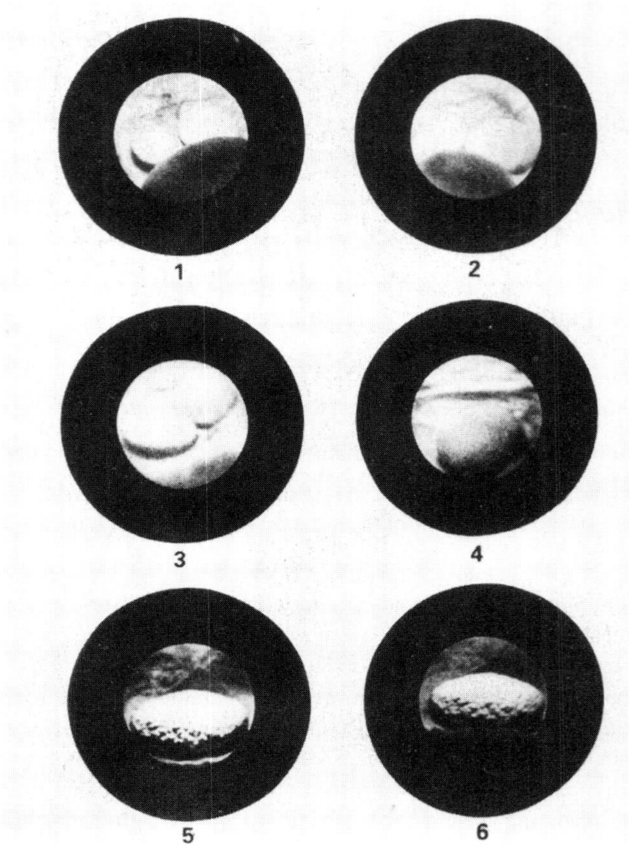

Fig. 1.11 Photography was utilized in the teaching of clinical medicine from the early 1850s but did not have widespread use in surgical books and articles until towards the end of the century; most Victorian publications were illustrated by wood or steel engravings. These photographs of stones in the human urinary bladder are from an early atlas of endoscopy and were the first published photographs taken through a cystoscope. Reproduced from Nitze M *Kystophotographischer Atlas*. Bergmann, Wiesbaden, 1894.

performed through a transperitoneal approach by a number of surgeons, notably in France, but with few survivors. Most of these early operations were for anal atresia rather than for obstructing carcinoma of the rectum or colon. In 1839 Amussat of Paris reviewed the literature and, not unexpectedly, found that most of the deaths resulted from peritonitis.[63] This led him to devise an extraperitoneal colostomy fashioned in the lumbar region, an operation he performed successfully on several occasions. Amussat's lumbar approach soon became the standard technique and was practised for the next 40 years until transperitoneal operations became safe with the introduction of antisepsis. From 1880 onwards, there is virtually no reference to a lumbar colostomy in the surgical literature.

REFERENCES

60. Cartwright F F The Development of Modern Surgery. Barker, London 1967
61. Dinnick T Br J Surg 1934; 22: 142
62. Duret C Rec Périod Soc Med Paris 1798; 4: 45
63. Amussat J Z Mémoire sur la Possibilité d'établir un Anus artificiel dans la Région lombaire sans pénétrer dans le Péritoine. Baillière, Paris 1839

a

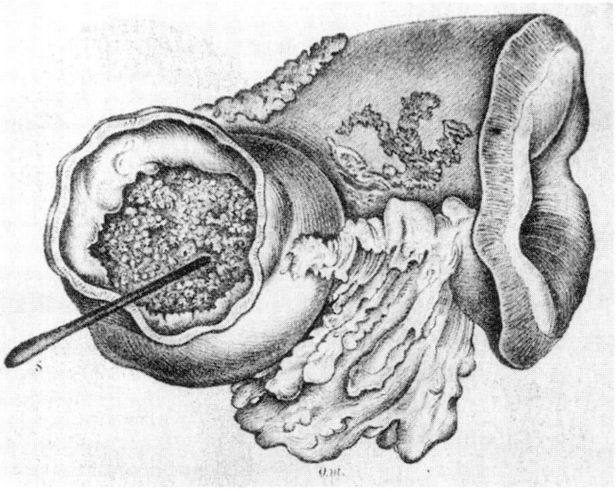

b

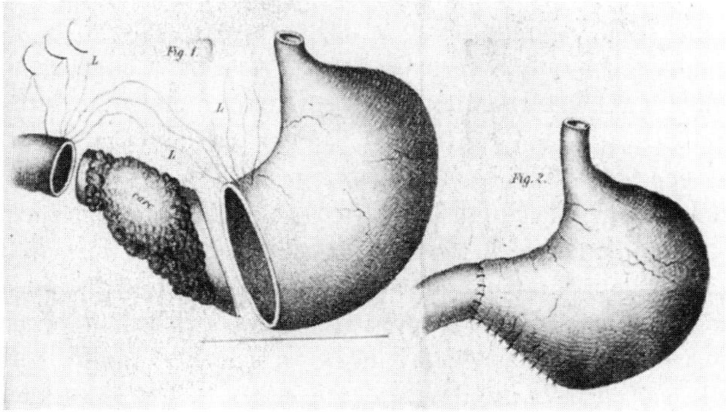

Fig. 1.12 The first successful partial gastrectomy. This was performed by Billroth on 29th January 1881 on a 43-year-old woman with pyloric stenosis caused by a carcinoma. (**a**) The resected specimen showing the carcinoma almost totally obstructing the antrum. A probe passes through the lumen. (**b**) The method of reconstruction. Sixty-four carbolized silk sutures were used, most being serosa to serosa as described by Lembert but a few including the mucosa. No drain was inserted but carbolic acid-soaked swabs were used throughout. The operation lasted 1½ hours. Wine enemas were given during the first 2 weeks after operation but by 3 weeks the patient was able to eat a cutlet and a beefsteak. Sadly, the patient died of recurrent disease 4 months later. Reproduced from Billroth T Clinical Surgery translated by Dent C T. The New Sydenham Society, London 1881.

Ovariotomy, now called ovarian cystectomy, was first performed by a general practitioner surgeon named Ephraim McDowell of Kentucky in 1809.[64] A giant cyst weighing over 3 kg was removed after preliminary incision and drainage of nearly 7 kg of gelatinous content. The operation took 25 minutes, during which time the patient sang hymns and recited psalms to boost her morale. Amazingly, she lived for 32 years after her ordeal. McDowell performed this operation successfully on several more patients and can fairly claim to be the first person to perform a successful elective laparotomy. As a result of McDowell's success, several other surgeons performed this operation both in the USA and Europe, leading to a review by Atlee in 1851 of 222 published cases.[65] In the UK the most notable ovariotomist was Thomas Spencer Wells. His results, published in 1880,[66] showed that his operative mortality dropped dramatically after the adoption of Lister's techniques. In his first 500 cases there was a 25.4% mortality; in the next 300 a mortality of 25.6% and in his final 100, when antisepsis had been introduced, a mortality of 11%. Spencer Wells is now best known for his artery forceps, the final design of which he introduced in 1879.[67]

A large number of surgeons contributed to the rapid development of abdominal surgery during the last three decades of the 19th century. One name, Theodore Billroth must be singled out since, by common consent, he is regarded as the father of abdominal surgery.[68] A graduate of Berlin university, Billroth was not only an outstanding innovator in surgery but also a man of culture and a musician of special ability. A pianist and violinist, he played chamber music with Brahms, who became a close friend and who dedicated two of his string quartets to him. Appointed Professor of Surgery in Vienna in 1867, Billroth established himself as an outstanding teacher and practical surgeon with many notable achievements, all meticulously recorded. His voluminous writings, with emphasis on surgical statistics, contributed to his fame. Although in 1872 he was the first to perform total resection of the oesophagus[69] and 2 years later the first to perform a total laryngectomy,[70] he is best known for the first successful partial gastrectomy for cancer of the pylorus, which he performed in 1881[71] (Fig. 1.12). Surgeons from Europe and the USA visited him in Vienna and through them he was instrumental in influencing gastrointestinal surgery throughout the world. Paradoxically, he was not an early advocate of Lister's methods and at first resisted their introduction on his unit, although he later adopted them enthusiastically.

Surgery of the gallbladder was developing alongside surgery of the stomach and intestine. Although gallstones had been recognized since ancient times, it was not until the 18th century that surgeons suggested their removal to treat cholecystitis although, so far as is known, no attempts at this procedure were made. In 1867 a little-known surgeon in Indianapolis, John Bobbs, was the first to perform a cholecystotomy and remove gallstones,[72] although it must be recorded that during the same operation he was also the first surgeon known to leave a stone behind! Nevertheless, the patient lived virtually symptom-free for a further 46 years[73] (Fig. 1.13). The first successful cholecystectomy was performed 15 years later, in 1882, by Carl Langenbuch of Berlin.[74]

Severe pain in the right iliac fossa was for years known as 'iliac passion' and was thought to be caused by typhoid ulceration;[75] the first elective appendicectomy was almost certainly that performed in 1880 by Lawson Tait of Birmingham but not recorded until 10

REFERENCES

64. Ellis H Famous Operations. Harval, Pennsylvania 1984
65. Atlee W L Trans Am Med Assoc 1851; 4: 286
66. Leading Article Br Med J 1880; 1: 931
67. Wells T S Br Med J 1879; 1: 926
68. Rutledge R H Surgery 1979; 86: 672
69. Billroth T Arch Klin Chir 1872; 13: 65
70. Gussenbauer C Arch Klin Chir Berl 1874; 17: 343
71. Billroth T Wien Med Wochenschr 1881; 31: 161. English translation in Hurwitz A, Degenshein G A (eds) Milestones in Modern Surgery. Hoeber, New York 1958
72. Bobbs J S Trans Med Soc Indiana 1868; 18: 68
73. Sparkman R S Surgery 1967; 61: 965
74. Langenbuch C J A Berl Klin Wochenschr 1882; 19: 725. English translation Gastroenterology 1983; 85: 1430
75. Cope Z A History of the Acute Abdomen. Oxford University Press, London 1965

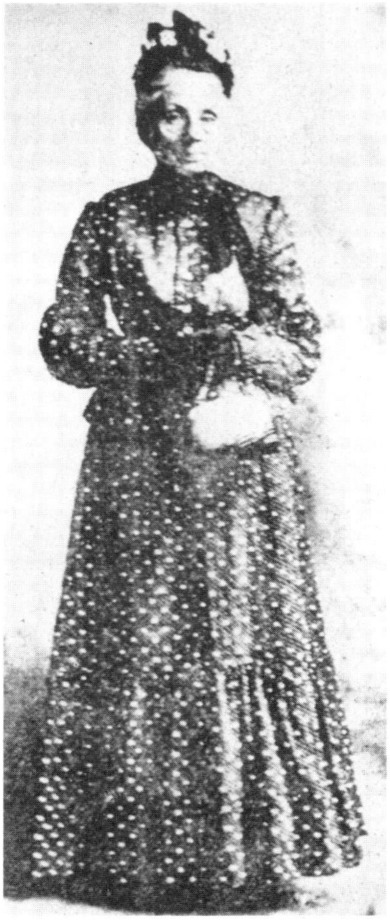

Fig. 1.13 Mary Wiggins Burnsworth aged 68. In 1867, 38 years before this photograph was taken, Mrs Burnsworth was the first patient to undergo cholecystotomy and removal of gallstones. About 50 stones were removed but one was left behind and was the cause of occasional abdominal discomfort in succeeding years. The operation was performed under chloroform anaesthesia by John Bobbs and was carried out on the third floor of a local drug store in Indianapolis. It was not performed again for another 11 years. Mrs Burnsworth died in 1913 age 77. Reproduced with permission from Surgery 1967; 61: 965.

years later;[76] the masterly writings of the pathologist, Reginald Fitz of Harvard, in 1886 classified the pathology of appendicitis, a name he coined, and finally distinguished it unequivocally from inflammation of the caecum.[77] Important as these historical details are, it is for another reason that acute appendicitis holds a special place in the history of surgery. Despite the enormous advance in the range of operations and the techniques employed, surgery in the early 20th century was still generally looked upon with fear and trepidation by the public and not without misgiving by many surgeons. The mortality rate was still high for major operations and it needed something more than surgical ingenuity to alter public attitude and for surgery to gain widespread acceptance. In the UK this change came about in 1902 with the drainage of an appendix abscess by Frederick Treves of the London Hospital. The patient was King Edward VII and the operation took place 2 days before his intended coronation.[78] The publicity that this operation received probably did more to promote the advance of surgery and to increase the esteem of the surgeon in the mind of patients than any of the far more dramatic events of the previous three decades; public confidence was gained.

Anastomoses, sutures and staples

An early problem in the development of gastrointestinal surgery was to devise a satisfactory method of suturing so as to lessen the likelihood of anastomotic leakage. Intestinal anastomosis, usually using waxed silk sutures, had been performed sporadically in earlier times in cases of intestinal obstruction, although most of the patients died. Several surgeons in the early 19th century experimented with anastomotic techniques in dogs but found that the anastomoses often failed to heal. The cause of this failure is now difficult to establish, though it may have been the result of ischaemia, the inaccurate placement of sutures or the unsuitable material used. Antoine Lembert described his well-known sero-muscular technique as early as 1826.[79] As gastric and intestinal operations became routine there was renewed interest in surgical technique and many different methods of anastomosis were described, some involving the placement of up to 200 sutures. Various mechanical splinting devices were introduced,[80] such as decalcified bone plates, rawhide plates, catgut rings, silver plates and the famous Murphy button which worked on the principle of a male and female half being inserted into the open ends to be anastomosed, snapped together by means of a spring, and the serosa lightly closed over the device[81] (Fig. 1.14). A few days later it became detached as a result of pressure necrosis and was passed per rectum. In the late 20th century a similar device made of biofragmentable material was introduced[82] and mechanical aids for anastomosis in the form of surgical staplers were again to become popular.

A vast assortment of suture and ligature material has been used by surgeons past and present.[83] Two thousand years ago horsehair, cotton, animal sinews, strips of leather and fibres from the bark of trees were used. Galen refers to the use of catgut and other Roman authors suggested human hair. Silk has been used for a thousand years or more. During this century surgeons and suture makers have sought the ideal suture material, which should combine such qualities as high tensile strength, ease of handling and knotting, lack of tissue drag, absence of tissue reaction, ease of sterilization and predictability of absorption rate. A succession of synthetic materials, both absorbable and non-absorbable, has been introduced in recent years, each one supposedly better than the last.

Catgut has withstood the test of time longer than most. Made from the submucosa of sheep's intestine, it is thought to derive its

REFERENCES

76. Tait R L Birmingham Med Rev 1890; 27: 27
77. Fitz R H Trans Assoc Am Physicians 1886; 1: 107
78. Trombley S Sir Frederick Treves: The Extra-Ordinary Edwardian. Routledge, London 1989
79. Lembert A Repert gén Anat Physiol Pathol 1826; 2: 100
80. Ravitch M M South Med J 1982; 75: 1520
81. Murphy J B Med Rec (NY) 1892; 42: 665
82. Hardy T G, Pace W G, Maney J W, Katz A R, Kaganov K L Dis Colon Rectum 1985; 28: 484
83. Goldenberg I S Surgery 1959; 46: 908

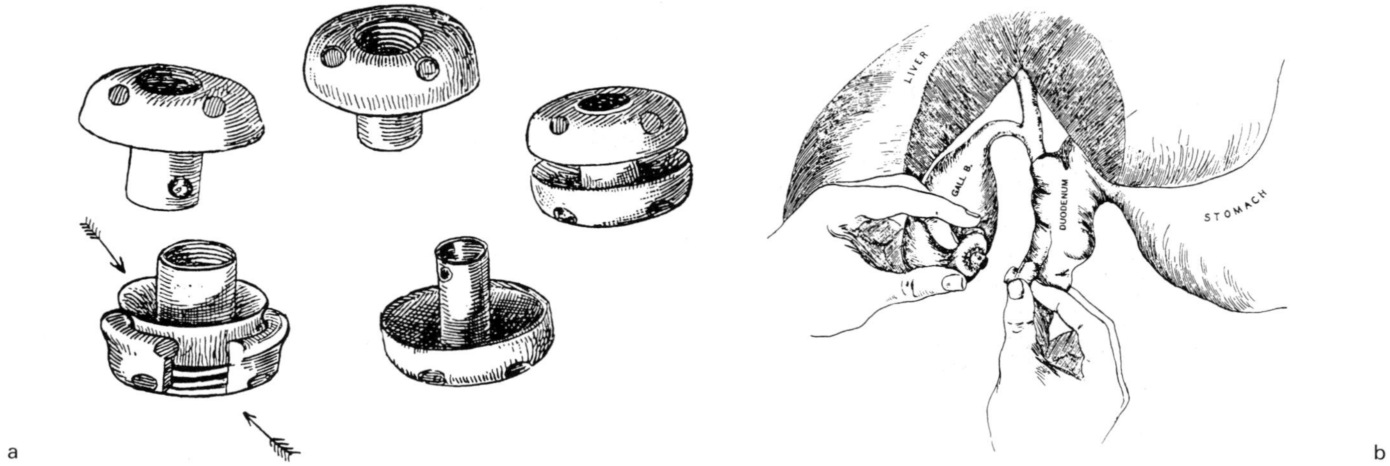

Fig. 1.14 (**a**) The Murphy anastomotic button shown open and assembled. (**b**) The button in use during a cholecystoduodenostomy. This technique was popular for many years for all types of intestinal anastomosis despite some cases of intestinal obstruction caused by impaction of the device in the ileum. Reproduced from Murphy J B Med Rec (NY) 1892; 42: 665.

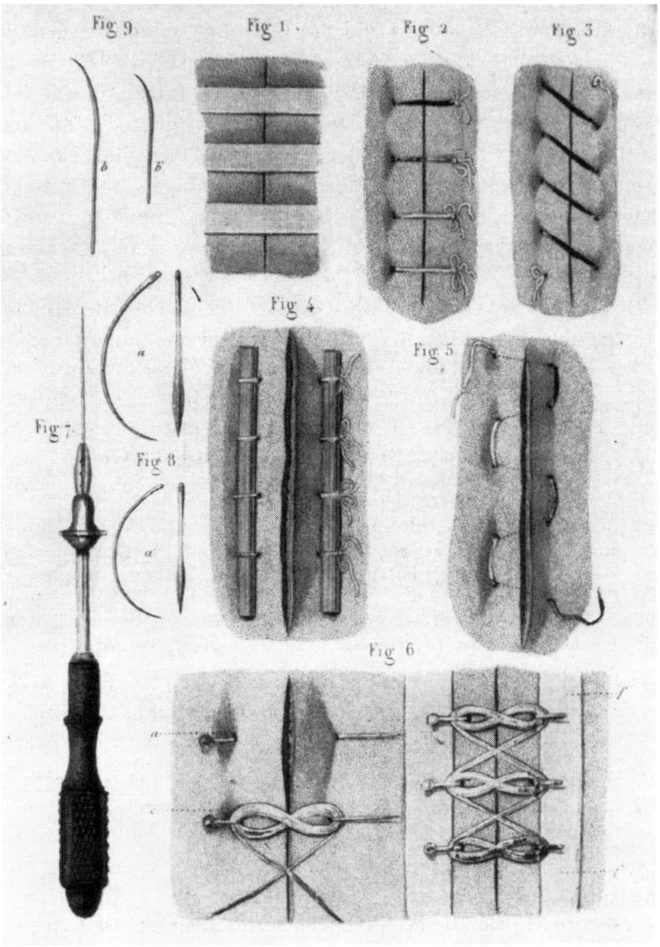

Fig. 1.15 Methods of skin approximation used in the mid 19th century. Note that adhesive plaster strips were used as an alternative to sutures. The instrument is an early design of needleholder. Reproduced from Bernard C, Huette C Illustrated Manual of Operative Surgery and Surgical Anatomy translated by Van Buren W, Isaacs C, New York 1857.

name from a corruption of the term 'kitgut', the string used on a small fiddle, known as a kit and played by Italian dancing masters. Intermittently used through the centuries, it became especially popular after Lister first described its sterilization with carbolic acid and then showed that treatment with chromic acid would delay its absorption and thus make it safe for intestinal anastomosis.[84] The problem of spore contamination of catgut lasted long after Lister, however, and was not eliminated until the 1930s.

Just as there are some surgeons today who avoid cutaneous sutures and close the skin with strips of adhesive plaster, so there were similar advocates in the past (Fig. 1.15) In 1808 Samuel Young vigorously decried the stitching of skin wounds and advocated adhesive strapping in a monograph devoted to the subject.[85]

Wire sutures of gold were used in the 16th century while silver wire was used extensively in the 19th century, especially by Sims in the repair of vesicovaginal fistula.[86] In the 1930s wires made of annealed iron, aluminium and bronze were available but met with little favour. Stainless steel, although used in the manufacture of some instruments from 1918, was not used as a suture material until the 1950s. The eyeless atraumatic needle with the suture material attached to the end of the needle also dates from this time.

Although first used by Hültl in Budapest in 1908[87,88] and refined by von Petz in 1924[89] and Friedrich in 1934,[90] it is only in the past few years that stapling instruments have become popular. This was stimulated by the development of modern instruments by Russian technologists in the 1950s and 1960s. Successive models were

REFERENCES

84. Lister J Trans Clin Soc London 1881; 14: xliii
85. Young S An Attempt at a Systematic Reform of the Modern Practice of Adhesion Especially in Relation to the Use and Abuse of the Thread Suture. Matthews and Leigh, London 1808
86. Sims J M Am J Med Sci 1852; 23: 59
87. Hültl H Pester Med-Chir Presse 1909; 45: 108
88. Robicsek F Surg Gynecol Obstet 1980; 150: 579
89. von Petz A Zentralbl Chir 1924; 51: 179
90. Friedrich H Zentralbl Chir 1934; 61: 504

perfected and marketed by the Scientific and Research Institute for Experimental Surgical Apparatus and Instruments, established in Moscow. Initially introduced for making end-to-end anastomoses of blood vessels without any narrowing, they were subsequently refined to enable side-to-side and tangential vascular anastomoses. Instruments for gastrointestinal stapling soon followed and were taken up by instrument makers in other parts of the world, notably the USA.[91]

In the past three decades there have been sporadic attempts to obviate the need for both sutures and staples by substituting fast-acting cyanoacrylate adhesives. These have been used on blood vessels, intestine and skin. The first account of an anastomosis effected by glue was in 1960.[92]

PHYSIOLOGY AND SURGERY

Until the introduction of antisepsis the successful practice of surgery largely depended on a sound knowledge of anatomy. This was now complemented by advances in physiology, a science that developed rapidly in the 19th century. So many advances were made, and from so many different countries, that only a few examples of particular surgical importance can be mentioned. William Beaumont, an army surgeon in the USA, made important contributions to gastric physiology in the 1820s when he analysed the gastric juice of Alexis St Martin, a patient who had developed a gastrocutaneous fistula after a gunshot wound to the abdomen.[93] Some years later the German physiologist Rudolph Heidenhain designed an experimental gastric pouch that was to be widely used for the study of gastric function by surgical physiologists of later generations. Claude Bernard, working in Paris, developed the concept of the *milieu intérieur* in 1859 and made important contributions to the understanding of exocrine pancreatic function, glycogenesis and the vasomotor system.[94] Bernard was also joint author of a successful textbook of operative surgery,[95] suggesting that he was aware of the importance of physiology to the surgeon (Fig. 1.15). In 1877 the Russian Nicholas Eck described his method of anastomosing the portal vein to the inferior vena cava,[96] the first recorded successful anastomosis between blood vessels. However, Rudolph Virchow arguably eclipsed all of these famous names. Although now remembered by surgeons mainly for his eponymous supraclavicular lymph node enlargement and the triad of factors predisposing to vascular thrombosis, Virchow's major importance lies in his being the founder of cellular pathology.[97] He showed that cells were essential components of all living tissues and that each cell had a physiological function. This concept allowed the development of histopathology and enabled surgeons to understand better such fundamental problems as inflammation and wound healing. He also clarified the nature of embolism, was the first to observe and define leucocytosis, founded an influential medical journal which is still published today (*Virchows Archiv*) and became a distinguished politician, spending some 13 years as a member of the German parliament.[98]

In the early part of the 20th century an understanding of shock was gradually unravelled, notably by Crile[99] and by Blalock,[100] and the concept of homeostasis was introduced.[101] In the 1950s, Francis Moore in Boston contributed greatly to the realization that metabolism was important in the management of the surgical patient[102] and this work laid the foundation for the subsequent development of total parenteral nutrition.[103]

Neurosurgery

The beginnings of neurosurgery depended greatly on advances in physiology. Apart from trephination, elective surgery on the brain and spinal cord could not develop until accurate anatomical localization of the diseased area could be obtained. This advance depended upon the meticulous correlation of neurological physical signs with subsequent post-mortem studies of the underlying disease and, more especially, on physiological experiments in animals when various areas of the brain were electrically stimulated and the resulting systemic effect observed. By the 1870s these studies had advanced sufficiently for there to appear several publications detailing the physiological anatomy of the brain.[104]

Applying this knowledge, William Macewen of Glasgow was able accurately to diagnose, localize and remove a meningioma from the left frontal lobe of a 14-year-old girl.[105] This operation, performed in 1879, was the first successful excision of a cerebral tumour. Victor Horsley of London was the first to remove successfully an accurately localized tumour of the spinal cord.[106] Enormous interest was generated by these reports and during the decade 1886–1896 more than 500 different surgeons reported operations on the brain, but few were as successful as Macewen or Horsley. Tumours were enucleated roughly with the fingers and haemorrhage from both the brain and the skull was difficult to control, with the result that the mortality was high, probably averaging around 40%.

It was Harvey Cushing of Boston who recognized the need for careful and gentle handling of tissues and the importance of

REFERENCES

91. Steichen F M, Ravitch M M Curr Probl Surg 1982; 19: 4
92. Nathan H S, Nachlas M M, Soloman R D, Halpern D, Seligman A M Ann Surg 1960; 152: 648
93. Beaumont W Experiments and Observations on the Gastric Juice and the Physiology of Digestion. Allen, Plattsburgh 1833
94. Franklin K J A Short History of Physiology, 2nd edn. Staples Press, London 1949
95. Goldwyn R M Plast Reconstr Surg 1986; 78: 115
96. Eck N V Voyenno Med J 1877; 130: 2. English translation in Surg Gynecol Obstet 1953; 96: 375
97. Virchow R L K Die Cellularpathologie. Hirschwald, Berlin 1858. English translation by Chance F Cellular Pathology. Churchill, London 1860
98. Ackerknecht E H Rudolf Virchow: Doctor, Statesman, Anthropologist. University of Wisconsin Press, Madison 1953
99. Crile G W An Experimental and Clinical Research into Certain Problems Relating to Surgical Operations. J B Lippincott, Philadelphia 1901
100. Blalock A Arch Surg (Chicago) 1927; 15: 762
101. Cannon W B Physiol Rev 1929; 9: 399
102. Moore F D Metabolic Care of the Surgical Patient. W B Saunders, Philadelphia 1959
103. Dudrick S J, Wilmore D W, Vars H M, Rhoads J E Surgery 1968; 64: 138
104. Walker A E (ed) A History of Neurological Surgery. Williams & Wilkins, Baltimore 1951
105. Macewen W Glasg Med J 1879; 12: 210
106. Gowers W R, Horsley V Med Chir Trans 1888; 71: 377

ensuring haemostasis—two fundamental concepts in the prevention of shock, which extended far beyond neurosurgery. Cushing introduced silver clips to control bleeding of cerebral vessels.[107] and stressed that speed in operating was of itself no virtue. His results justified his slow and bloodless techniques for in 1915 he was able to publish a series of 130 excisions of brain tumours with a mortality of only 8%,[108] by far the best results of the time. Although a primitive electrocautery had been used in surgical operations some years earlier,[109] in the mid 1920s Cushing encouraged W. T. Bovie, a physicist, to develop the forerunner of modern electrocautery and introduced the technique into clinical practice, thus reducing blood loss even more.[110] This was perhaps the first application of physics leading to advances in operative technique. Cushing's syndrome was described in 1932.[111]

Further developments in neurosurgery depended on advances in radiology with the introduction of air ventriculography in 1918[112] followed in later years by pneumoencephalography,[113] myelography[114] and cerebral arteriography[115] (Fig. 1.16). Electroencephalography was introduced in 1929.[116] A forerunner of modern techniques for imaging brain tumours was the intravenous injection of fluoroscein labelled with radioactive iodine.[117] This enabled the shape and limits of a tumour to be observed. Computed tomography[118] and magnetic resonance[119] are recent innovations which have largely superseded earlier imaging methods.

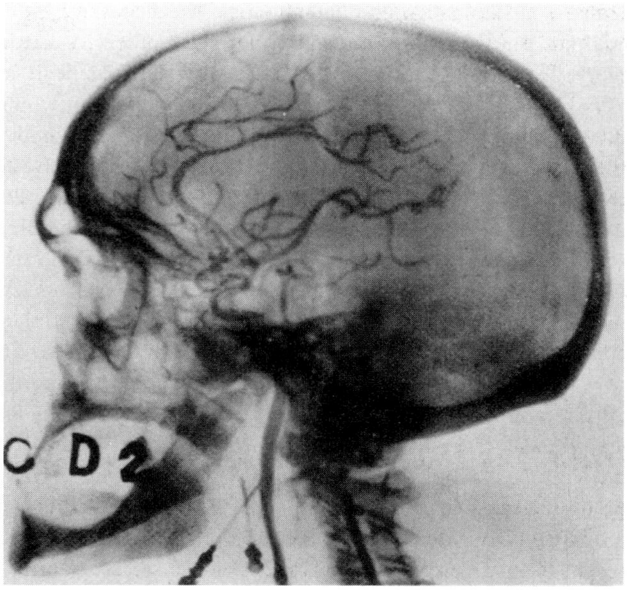

Fig. 1.16 Carotid arteriography was introduced by Egas Moniz of Portugal in 1927 as a means of localizing cerebral tumours. He practised the technique in animals and human cadavers before obtaining his first images in the living patient. Nine years later he introduced the operation of prefrontal leucotomy and in 1949 was awarded a Nobel prize for his contributions to medicine. This illustration from his first paper on arteriography shows a carotid arteriogram in a cadaver head obtained using a 30% solution of sodium iodide. Reproduced from Rev Neurol (Paris) 1927; 34: 72.

Thoracic surgery

An understanding of physiology was essential before elective operations on the thoracic contents could be undertaken, for if the pleural cavity was opened the lung collapsed, causing respiratory distress. Early attempts at overcoming this problem were made at the beginning of the 20th century with the development of endotracheal insufflation anaesthesia.[120] By 1910, primitive positive pressure anaesthetic apparatus was in use for operations on pulmonary tuberculosis, but there were still difficulties with the risk of over-distension of the lung and also with the build-up of carbon dioxide. A soda-lime absorber was first devised in 1915 but was not widely applied in clinical practice until 10 years later. Some years earlier, Ferdinand Sauerbruch, working in the department of Mikulicz in Breslau, had ingeniously tried a different approach. He devised a large negative pressure operation chamber which accommodated the patient and the entire surgical team; the patient's head projected to the exterior through a snugly fitting collar, thus allowing atmospheric pressure to inflate the lung.[121] Not surprisingly, the practical difficulties of performing operations in these circumstances limited its acceptance. Sauerbruch also utilized physiological knowledge when in 1913 he was one of the first to describe section of the phrenic nerve in order to paralyse the diaphragm and so rest the lung in pulmonary tuberculosis.[122]

The surgery of tuberculosis and bronchiectasis accounted for almost all early thoracic operations. Although the first successful lobectomy for carcinoma of the bronchus was performed in 1912,[123] operations for cancer of the lung were not widely practised until the 1930s. The first successful pneumonectomy for carcinoma was performed by Evarts Graham of Washington in 1933.[124] The mortality and morbidity of lung resection remained high until the problems of postoperative sepsis and leakage from the transected bronchial stump were reduced by the introduction of antibiotics in the 1940s.

Cardiac surgery

The development of cardiac surgery provides another example of the interdependence and interaction of many different fields of technology and science leading to surgical advance. Physiology, radiology, haematology, perfusion techniques, engineering, physics,

REFERENCES

107. Cushing H Ann Surg 1911; 54: 1
108. Cushing H JAMA 1915; 64: 189
109. Clark W L J Adv Ther 1911; 29: 169
110. Cushing H, Bovie W T Surg Gynecol Obstet 1928; 47: 751
111. Cushing H Bull Johns Hopkins Hosp 1932; 50: 137
112. Dandy W E Ann Surg 1918; 68: 5
113. Dandy W E Ann Surg 1919; 70: 397
114. Sicard J A, Forestier J Rev Neurol (Paris) 1921; 28: 1264
115. Egas Moniz Rev Neurol (Paris) 1927; 34: 72. English translation J Neurosurg 1964; 21: 15
116. Berger H Arch Psychiatr Nervenk 1929; 87: 527
117. Moore G E, Peyton W T, French L A, Walker W W J Neurosurg 1948; 5: 392
118. Ambrose J, Hounsfield G Br J Radiol 1973; 46: 148, 1016
119. Hinshaw W S, Bottomley P A, Holland G N Nature 1977; 270: 722
120. Meade R H A History of Thoracic Surgery. Thomas, Springfield, Illinois 1960
121. Sauerbruch F Verh Dtsch Ges Chir 1904; 32: 105
122. Sauerbruch F München Med Wochenschr 1913; 60: 625
123. Davies H M Br J Surg 1913; 1: 228
124. Graham E A, Singer J J JAMA 1933; 101: 1371

chemistry, mathematics and immunology are just some of the disciplines that have contributed to the development of cardiac surgery. Until the Second World War surgery of the heart had largely been confined to the suturing of stab and gunshot wounds and resection of the pericardium.[125] The occasional attempt at valve surgery had also been made. In 1923, Elliot Cutler of Boston performed the first successful mitral valvotomy when he used a tenotomy knife introduced blindly through the left ventricle.[126] Two years later Souttar, working in London, performed the same operation by introducing his finger through the left atrium and dilating the stenosed valve.[127] Both operations were on children and both patients survived, but conservative medical opinion of the time was critical of such bold and innovative operations and they were rarely repeated. The next major advance was 13 years later when a patent ductus arteriosus was successfully ligated.[128] In 1944, Crafoord of Stockholm excised a coarctation of the aorta and reunited the cut ends by direct suture.[129] This operation utilized suturing techniques that had first been used in peripheral vascular surgery some 40 years earlier, in 1902, when Alexis Carrel of Lyons described an end-to-end everting technique of anastomosing blood vessels.[130] Carrel, who subsequently worked closely with Charles Guthrie in Chicago, published numerous papers on experimental vascular surgery, including the transplantation of vessels and organs in animals. He was awarded the Nobel prize for medicine in 1912, and was the second surgeon to have been given this distinction—Theodor Kocher of Berne had been the first in 1909.

Another major advance in closed cardiac surgery was the systemic pulmonary bypass operation introduced by Blalock and Taussig in 1945 in cases of Fallot's tetralogy.[131] Many regard this operation as the beginning of modern heart surgery as it showed that cyanotic congenital heart disease, previously nearly always fatal, could be cured.

Until 1952, all cardiac surgery was performed on the closed heart. The first open heart operation was closure of an atrial septal defect carried out with the patient rendered hypothermic by surface cooling of the body to 30°C.[132] This allowed some 6–10 minutes of safe circulatory arrest. At the end of the decade, profound hypothermia was introduced[133] whereby the patient was cooled to 10–15°C, giving safe circulatory arrest for up to 60 minutes, but this technique did not gain wide appeal. Extracorporeal circulation, allowing surgery on the dry heart, had been an ideal for many years and research had been carried out into such techniques since the 1930s.[134] During the 1950s and 1960s, several different heart–lung machines were devised, each using a different design of oxygenator.[135] These enabled more complex procedures to be carried out with relative safety, such as the first successful human mitral valve replacement which was reported in 1961.[136] Remarkably the first aortic valve replacement was performed a decade earlier, before the advent of cardiac bypass, when in 1952 Hufnagel of Washington successfully inserted a plastic ball valve of his own design into the descending aorta of a 30-year-old woman with aortic incompetence.[137]

In recent years, operations on the coronary circulation have become a major part of cardiac surgery. Coronary endarterectomy was introduced in 1957[138] but this was superseded within a few years by coronary artery bypass grafting, first performed in 1962 but not reported until several years later.[139] The first long-term survivor of this operation was reported by De Bakey's team in 1973.[140] Also in the 1970s, percutaneous transluminal coronary balloon angioplasty was introduced as a method of dilating atherosclerotic plaques in patients with angina.[141] The success of these techniques depended on the accurate preoperative localization of the stenoses by coronary arteriography, a procedure first used clinically in the early 1950s[142] and refined a few years later by Sones,[143] who was the first to cannulate selectively the coronary vessels.

Peripheral vascular surgery

Simple ligation of peripheral arteries proximal and distal to an aneurysm had been practised for centuries but reconstructive peripheral vascular surgery did not develop until the 1950s. Although Carrel had devised a satisfactory technique for vascular anastomosis at the turn of the century,[130] further advancement could not be made until accurate localization of atheromatous plaques within blood vessels was possible, until blood coagulation could be reliably controlled and until satisfactory arterial substitutes had been introduced. These three advances were made over a period of some two decades.

Arteriography originated almost simultaneously in Germany[144] and the USA[145] in the early 1920s. In 1927 Egas Moniz of Portugal introduced carotid arteriography[115] (Fig. 1.16) and 2 years later R. dos Santos, also of Portugal, performed translumbar aortography;[146] radiology of the vascular system then advanced steadily. Seldinger introduced his technique of catheter angiography in 1953.[147]

Although heparin had been purified in 1918,[148] it did not come into general clinical use for several years. By the end of the Second World War, however, safe anticoagulation of patients was possible

REFERENCES

125. Johnson S L The History of Cardiac Surgery 1896–1955. Johns Hopkins Press, Baltimore 1970
126. Cutler E C, Levine S A Boston Med Surg J 1923; 188: 1023
127. Souttar H S Br Med J 1925; 2: 603
128. Gross R E, Hubbard J P JAMA 1939; 112: 729
129. Crafoord C, Nylin G J Thorac Surg 1945; 14: 347
130. Carrel A Lyon Méd 1902; 98: 859
131. Blalock A, Taussig H B JAMA 1945; 128: 189
132. Lewis F J, Taufic M Surgery 1953; 33: 52
133. Drew C E, Anderson I M Lancet 1959; i: 748
134. Gibson J H J Lab Clin Med 1939; 24: 1192
135. DeWall R A, Grage T B, Mcfee A S, Chiechi M A Surgery 1961; 50: 931, 1962; 51: 251
136. Starr A, Edwards M L Ann Surg 1961; 154: 726
137. Hufnagel C A, Harvey W P, Rabil P J, McDermott T F Surgery 1954; 35: 673
138. Bailey C P, May A, Lemmon W M JAMA 1957; 164: 641
139. Sabiston D C Jr Johns Hopkins Med J 1974; 134: 314
140. Garrett H E, Dennis E W, De Bakey M E JAMA 1973; 223: 792
141. Grüntzig A Lancet 1978; i: 263
142. DiGuglielmo L, Guttadauro M Acta Radiol (Stockh) 1951; Suppl 97, 5
143. Sones F M, Shirey E K, Proudfit W L and Westcott R N Circulation 1959; 20: 773
144. Berberich J, Hirsch S Klin Wochenschr 1923; 2: 2226
145. Brooks B JAMA 1924; 82: 1016
146. dos Santos R, Lamas A, Caldas J Bull Soc Med Chir Paris 1929; 55: 587
147. Seldinger S Acta Radiol 1953; 39: 368
148. Howell W H, Holt L E Am J Physiol 1918–1919; 47: 328

and contrast radiology enabled accurate assessment of atherosclerotic plaques. The first superficial femoral thromboendarterectomy was performed by J. C. dos Santos in 1947[149] and this new technique soon became used to remove atheromatous plaques in other vessels, culminating in the carotid arteries in 1953.[150]

It soon became apparent that endarterectomy was not a satisfactory treatment for all arterial lesions and this realization led to much research into the replacement of arteries using homografts[151] as well as methods of preservation using freeze-drying techniques.[152] The first abdominal aortic aneurysm to be resected, by Dubost in Paris in 1951, was replaced by an arterial homograft.[153] Despite the early good results, however, the long-term outcome of arterial homografting was unsatisfactory because of aneurysm formation, and synthetic arterial grafts were soon developed. Originally made of cloth, synthetic grafts were used first in dogs[154] and 2 years later in humans.[155] Materials subsequently evaluated include nylon, Ivalon, Marlex, Dacron and Teflon.[156] Velour surface grafts were introduced in 1970.[157] The use of reversed autogenous vein for bypassing atherosclerotic small-calibre arteries was first reported in France in 1949[158] and this technique became steadily more widely used during the subsequent decade.

Bypass grafting was not without complications and a new approach to the treatment of stenosed arteries began in 1964 when transluminal dilatation of the femoral artery was reported using graded dilators made of Teflon.[159] Grüntzig, working in Zurich, refined this technique by introducing the balloon catheter,[160] an innovation which led to modern angioplasty techniques.

The surgery of arterial embolism was revolutionized by the introduction of a narrow-gauge balloon catheter by Fogarty in 1963,[161] a device that was subsequently adapted for use in the treatment of venous thrombosis and the retrieval of stones in the common bile duct.

In recent years, the introduction of the operating microscope and the manufacture of ultrafine suture materials have enabled the development of microvascular anastomoses whereby severed digits and limbs can be replanted. This procedure was first successfully performed in a human in 1962 when a 12-year-old boy sustained a traumatic amputation of the right arm below the shoulder. It was successfully replanted at the Massachussets General Hospital in Boston.[162]

SURGERY AND WAR

Advances in surgery have regularly been made during times of war. For example, the management of trauma and the treatment of shock have been heavily influenced by the knowledge gained during two world wars and in later conflicts. The specialty of plastic surgery as now understood began during World War I with the work of Harold Gillies, a New Zealander, who introduced new techniques of facial reconstruction using bone grafts and soft tissue tube pedicle grafts.[163] During World War II another New Zealander, Archibald McIndoe, made important contributions with his work on the treatment and rehabilitation of severely burned aircrew.[164] Two major advances particularly associated with war, and which have had widespread surgical application, have been the use of blood transfusion and the introduction of antibiotics.

Blood transfusion

Early experiments in the transfusion of blood took place in the 17th century. Richard Lower is generally credited with the first successful attempt when he transfused blood from one mastiff to another in Oxford in 1666.[165] In the following year, Jean Denis from Paris reported the successful transfusion of 9 oz (252 ml) of lamb's blood into the vein of a 15-year-old youth.[166] Several other transfusions from animals to humans were reported but the procedure rapidly fell into disrepute owing to the severe reactions and occasional death that resulted. All these early attempts were in cases of disease rather than in the treatment of severe blood loss.

Interest in transfusion was not revived until the 19th century when James Blundell, a lecturer in physiology and midwifery at Guy's and St Thomas's Hospitals in London, described in 1819 the transfusion of 12–14 oz (336–392 ml) of blood collected from several donors into a patient moribund from gastric outlet obstruction.[167] This is the first authenticated record of transfusion of blood from human to human. Although this patient died soon afterwards, Blundell recorded several other human transfusions with a success rate of 40%.

There were a number of other successful transfusions performed in the 19th century, notably by Aveling,[168] the main indication being post-partum haemorrhage. Throughout the 19th century the main use of transfusion was in the practice of obstetrics but the results were poor because of the practical difficulties of transfusion, as well as the frequent untoward reactions. The transfusion apparatus was crude and cumbersome (Fig. 1.17), and the donor blood often clotted within it while the transfusion was taking place, a factor which paradoxically may well have been beneficial as it prevented an over-infusion of incompatible blood taking place. In order to overcome this problem Crile, working in Cleveland in 1907, reported a technique of direct transfusion from the radial artery of the donor to an elbow vein of the recipient through a

REFERENCES

149. dos Santos J C Mém Acad Chir (Paris) 1947; 73: 409
150. Strully K J, Hurwitt E S, Blankenberg H W J Neurosurg 1953; 10: 474
151. Gross R E, Bill A H, Poerce E C Surg Gynecol Obstet 1949; 88: 689
152. Deterling R A, Coleman C C, Parshley M S Surgery 1951; 19: 419
153. Dubost C, Allary M, Oeconomos N Arch Surg 1952; 65: 405
154. Voorhees A B, Jaretzki A, Blakemore A H Ann Surg 1952; 135: 332
155. Blakemore A H, Voorhees A B Ann Surg 1954; 140: 324
156. Harrison J H Am J Surg 1958; 95: 16
157. Lindenauer S M, Lavanway J M, Fry W J Gurr Top Surg Res 1970; 2: 491
158. Kunlin J Arch Mal Coeur 1949; 42: 371
159. Dotter C T, Judkins M P Circulation 1964; 30: 654
160. Grüntzig A Fortschr Röntgenst 1976; 124: 80
161. Fogarty T J, Cranley J J, Krause R J, Strasser R J, Strasser E S, Hafner C D Surg Gynecol Obstet 1963; 116: 241
162. Malt R A, McKhann C F JAMA 1964; 189: 716
163. Gillies H D Plastic Surgery of the Face. Oxford University Press, London 1920
164. McIndoe A H Postgrad Med 1949; 6: 187
165. Maluf N S R J Hist Med 1954; 9: 59
166. Denis J Philos Trans 1667; 2: 489
167. Blundell J Med Chir Trans 1819; 10: 296
168. Aveling J H Obstet J Gt Brit 1873; 1: 289

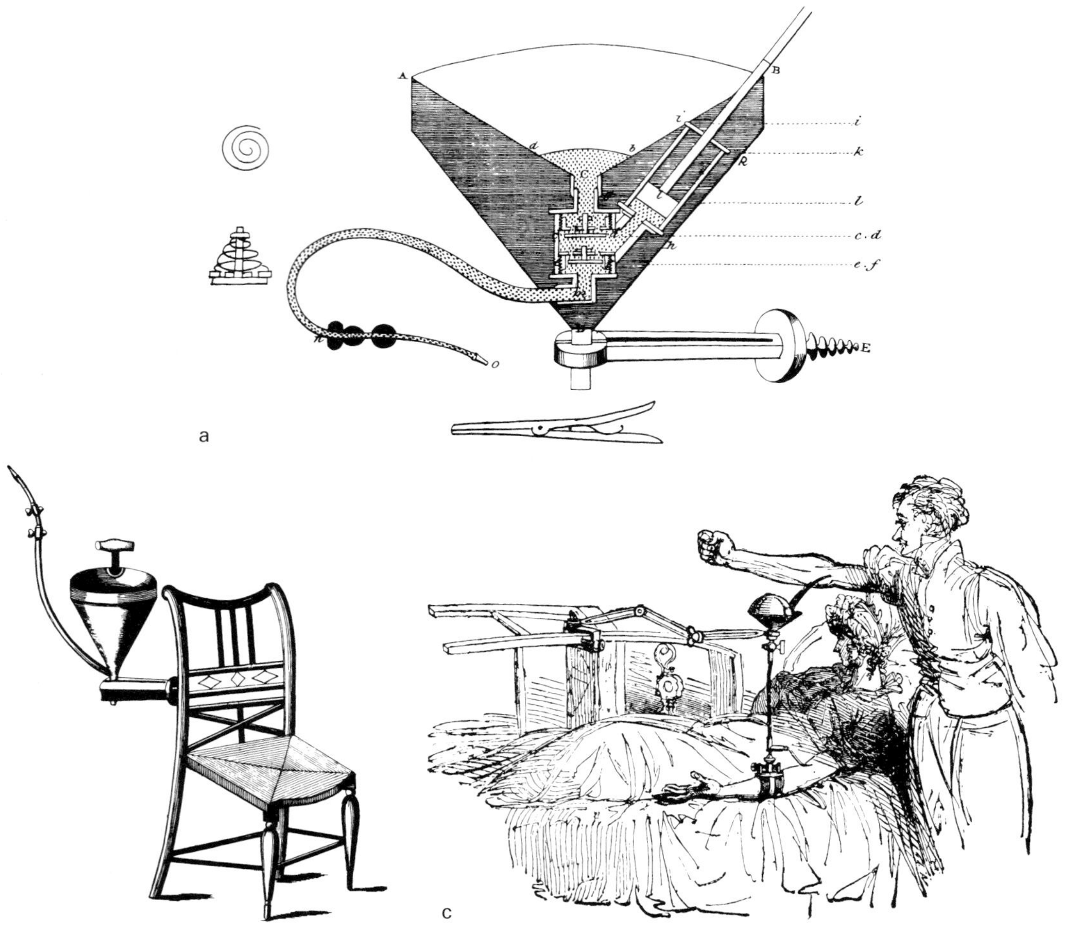

a

b

c

Fig. 1.17 Blood transfusion apparatus used by James Blundell, lecturer in physiology and midwifery at Guy's and St Thomas's Hospitals, London, the first person to transfuse blood from human to human. (**a**) Blundell's 'impellor'. The outer (shaded) compartment was filled with warm water. The donor's blood flowed into the funnel-shaped part above and the action of the pump forced the blood along a tube by means of two oppositely acting spring valves to the cannula inserted in the recipient's vein. (**b**) When in use the impellor was screwed to the back of a chair to give it stability. The blood donor sat on the chair while blood was flowing from his arm into the funnel. Reproduced from Blundell J Researches Physiological and Pathological. Cox, London 1824. (**c**) Blundell's 'gravitator' superseded his impellor. There were fewer moving parts and the blood flowed by gravity. Again the apparatus was fixed to a chair but this time the donor had to stand while he watched his blood gushing into the funnel. Reproduced from Blundell J Lancet 1828–1829; ii: 321.

silver tube.[169] This method did not gain wide acceptance because it was not possible to determine the amount of blood transfused and also because of the arterial damage sustained by the donor. The problem of clotting was not overcome until 1914 when, more or less simultaneously, Agote in Buenos Aires,[170] Hustin in Belgium[171] and Lewisohn in the USA[172] discovered that sodium citrate mixed with the donor blood was an effective anticoagulant and was not toxic to the recipient. Subsequent major advances in the history of anticoagulation included the purification of heparin in 1918[148] and its early use in humans in 1936,[173] the first clinical use of dicoumarol in 1941[174] and the introduction of warfarin (named after the Wisconsin Alumni Research Foundation) in the 1950s.[175]

Death and illness after transfusion were common in the 19th century and were then wrongly attributed to the accidental infusion of air bubbles into the recipient. Karl Landsteiner discovered agglutinins and isoagglutinins in blood in 1901[176]—an advance for which he was later awarded a Nobel prize—and within a few years the ABO grouping had been formalized and cross-matching could be performed before transfusion. Despite the under-standing of blood groups and the effective means of anticoagulation, blood transfusion was used infrequently until towards the end of the First World War. Even then, battle casualties were more often treated with intravenous saline, and blood transfusion was only used as a desperate life-saving measure.

During the two decades after the First World War, however, enormous advances were made in the design of transfusion apparatus as well as in the discovery of many minor blood groups. It

REFERENCES

169. Crile G W Ann Surg 1907; 46: 329
170. Agote L An Inst Mod Clin Med (B Aires) 1914–1915; 1: 24
171. Hustin A Bull Soc R Sci Med Brux 1914; 72: 104
172. Lewisohn R Med Rec (NY) 1915; 87: 141
173. Hedenius P, Wilander O Acta Med Scand 1936; 88: 443
174. Butt H R, Allen E V, Bollman L L Proc Mayo Clin 1941; 16: 388
175. Link K P Circulation 1959; 19: 97
176. Landsteiner K Wien Klin Wochenschr 1901; 14: 1132

was about this time also that experiments into blood preservation were made that enabled the establishment of blood banks.[177] At the beginning of the Second World War the rhesus system was discovered[178] and blood increasingly began to be transfused on a large scale to injured civilians and service personnel. During this war it was realized that large volumes of blood could be safely transfused to an individual patient, thus paving the way for the advances in surgical techniques made in the post-war years.

Antibiotics

Topical antiseptics of varying types were in widespread use at the beginning of the 20th century. The first systemic antiseptic, an arsenical named Salvarsan, was introduced by Ehrlich[179] and became widely used against spirochaetal infections, especially during the First World War. Ehrlich called this drug his 'magic bullet'. In 1935 Domagk discovered Prontosil,[180] a drug that killed streptococci in mice; its active constituent was soon afterwards found to be sulphanilamide. This, the first of the sulphonamides, could be given orally or parenterally, and was of special value in the treatment of gonorrhoea. Within a few years numerous other sulphonamides were synthesized that were active against a range of different organisms; they were widely used in the early part of World War II.[181]

Disappointment with the results of sulphonamide treatment of war wounds led to intensified research into a more potent chemotherapeutic agent by Florey and Chain in Oxford. These workers had already started to study the mould *Penicillium notatum*, the bactericidal effect of which had been described in 1929 by Alexander Fleming of St Mary's Hospital, London.[182] A year earlier, Fleming had noticed by chance that *Penicillium* mould, which had contaminated a culture plate, killed staphylococci and in a series of laboratory experiments using a filtrate of the mould he showed that other pathogenic organisms were also killed. He named the filtrate penicillin. Although Fleming suggested that his findings might have clinical application, this potential was not appreciated at the time.

Florey and Chain produced a crude extract of penicillin in 1940 and showed that it was active in vivo.[183] In the following year the drug was given to six human patients, the first being a policeman with septicaemia arising from an infected cut on his face. When the small supply of penicillin available ran out the treatment was interrupted while the drug was recovered from the patient's urine for reinjection. Even though the first patient died, an exceedingly favourable therapeutic response was obtained overall.[184] By 1943 sufficient quantities of the new drug had been produced to allow its use under the strict control of doctors of the allied forces. Other antibiotics were quickly developed, including streptomycin in 1943,[185] a drug which within a year was shown to be active against tuberculosis,[186] and chloramphenicol in 1947.[187]

ORGAN TRANSPLANTATION

Transplantation of the cornea was successfully performed in animals in the early 19th century[188] and in humans from 1906.[189] The cornea was a special case, however, and early attempts using other tissues were failures. For example, John Hunter grafted human teeth into a cock's comb and the spur of a young cock into the comb of a hen without success,[190] and several workers, including Victor Horsley, unsuccessfully transplanted human thyroid in patients with myxoedema.[191] Baronio of Milan published his experiments on free skin grafting in sheep in 1804[192] and was the first to show that, while autografts from the same animal took successfully, allografts from another were rejected.

Transplantation of organs with revascularization began to be practised in experimental animals soon after a reliable technique for vascular anastomosis had been devised by Alexis Carrel at the turn of the century.[130] Carrel himself, working with Guthrie first in Chicago and later in New York, transplanted kidney, heart, lung, thyroid and ovary in dogs but in every instance the organ was rejected.[193,194] The explanation for this rejection, and for the similar lack of success in other early experiments, remained obscure until the pioneer work of P. B. Medawar during the Second World War. In a series of classic experiments, Medawar showed that the rejection of grafts in both humans[195] and animals[196] was an immunological phenomenon. This realization led to extensive research into immunosuppression. Some years later, Medawar himself was one of the earliest workers to devise a clinically useful method of immunosuppression when he demonstrated that cortisone therapy significantly prolonged the survival of skin grafts in rabbits.[197]

Renal transplantation

The kidney was the organ most used for experimental study during the early years of research into transplantation biology because of its paired nature and the ease of removal and replacement with a single arterial and venous anastomosis. Later, the development by Kolff of the first efficient dialysis machine[198] was also important in making renal transplantation possible (Fig. 1.18). Ullmann, in Vienna in 1902, is believed to have performed the first renal

REFERENCES

177. Fantus B JAMA 1937; 109: 128
178. Landsteiner K, Wiener A S Proc Soc Exp Biol NY 1940; 43: 223
179. Ehrlich P, Hata S Die Experimentelle Chemotherapie der Spirillosen. Springer, Berlin 1910
180. Domagk G Dtsch Med Wochenschr 1935; 61: 250
181. Lockwood J S Surg Gynecol Obstet 1941; 72: 307
182. Fleming A Br J Exp Pathol 1929; 10: 226
183. Chain E, Florey H W, Gardner A D et al Lancet 1940; ii: 226
184. Abraham E P, Chain E, Fletcher C M et al Lancet 1941; ii: 177
185. Waksman S J Bacteriol 1943; 46: 229
186. Hinshaw H C, Feldman W H Proc Mayo Clin 1945; 20: 313
187. Smadel J E, Jackson E B Science 1947; 106: 418
188. Bigger S L Dublin J Med Sci 1837; 11: 408
189. Zirm E K v Graefes Arch Ophthalmol 1906; 64: 580
190. Dobson J John Hunter. Livingstone, Edinburgh 1969
191. Paget S Sir Victor Horsley. A Study of his Life and Work. Constable, London 1919
192. Baronio G Degli innesti Animali del Genio. Milan 1804. English translation On Grafting in Animals. Sax J B Boston 1985
193. Carrel A, Guthrie C C Am Med 1905; 10: 1101
194. Carrel A, Guthrie C C JAMA 1908; 51: 1662
195. Gibson T, Medawar P B J Anat 1943; 77: 299
196. Medawar P B J Anat 1944; 78: 178
197. Billingham R E, Krohn P L, Medawar P B Br Med J 1951; 1: 1157
198. Kolff W J, Berk H T J, Welle M, Ley A J W, Dijk E C, Noordwijk J Acta Med Scand 1944; 117: 121

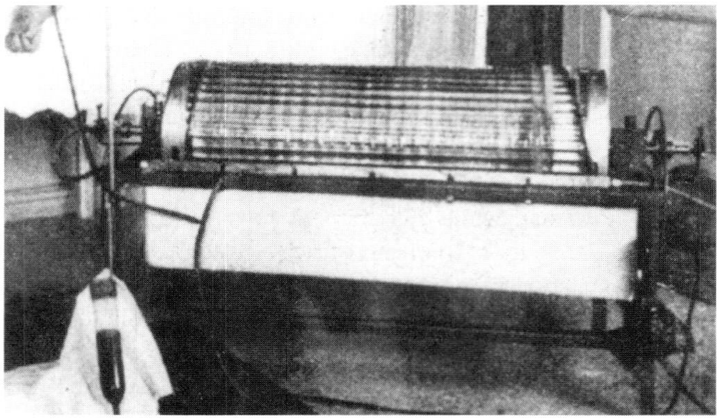

Fig. 1.18 The Kolff artificial kidney. A cellophane tube 30 m long is wound spirally around a revolving ridged aluminium cylinder which is partially immersed in a tank of warm, dialysing liquid. The heparinized blood within the cellophane tank sinks to the lowermost point and passes from left to right as the cylinder rotates, thus covering the cylinder with a thin film. The dialysing area is about 20 000 cm² — the same as the human glomeruli. Reproduced with permission from Kolff W J, Berk H T J, Welle M, Ley A J W, Dijk E C, Noordwijk J Acta Med Scand 1944; 117: 121.

transplantation in animals,[199] but Carrel and Guthrie's work is better known.[193] Soon after this, Jaboulay, Carrel's teacher in Lyons, carried out the first recorded kidney transplant to humans using animals as donors.[200] He transplanted a pig kidney to the arm of one patient and a goat kidney to the thigh of another. A few years later, in 1909, Unger in Berlin attempted a monkey-to-human transplant in a young girl with renal failure.[201]

The first human renal allograft was in 1936 by Voronoy in the Ukraine in a patient with mercury poisoning[202] but this, like all of the few other human transplants performed around this time, was a failure. In the early 1950s two groups, one in Paris and the other in Boston, simultaneously restarted human kidney allografts. The French surgeons used no immunosuppression[203] but Hume and his colleagues in Boston reported nine human renal transplants, of which four functioned between 37 and 180 days with the use of low-dose steroids for immunosuppression.[204] Although hardly a success, these results gave impetus to further human studies and fully successful transplants, first between identical twins[205] and then between unrelated subjects using cadaveric donor kidneys,[206] were reported within a few years.

During the 1960s, three major developments changed the course of clinical transplantation. First, the understanding of tissue typing;[207] second, improved methods of obtaining vascular access were devised, thus enabling regular haemodialysis;[208,209] third, and most importantly, better methods of immunosuppression were introduced. Whole-body irradiation had earlier been shown to be useful but had a high incidence of severe toxic effects[210] and 6-mercaptopurine was only moderately effective.[211] After its introduction in 1961,[212] azathioprine quickly became the mainstay of treatment, usually used in combination with other drugs. A more powerful immunosuppressant was not discovered until 1976 when Borel introduced cyclosporin A.[213] In the early 1980s antilymphocyte globulin and antithymocyte globulin became increasingly used if conventional immunosuppression failed,[214] and monoclonal antibodies are now being evaluated.[215]

Liver transplantation

In a brief communication published in 1955,[216] C. S. Welch of New York was the first to report liver transplantation. He transplanted an auxiliary liver into the abdomen of a dog leaving the original liver in place. The following year, together with his research team, he described 49 such canine auxiliary liver transplants.[217] Many different workers performed hundreds of animal experiments before the first human liver transplant was attempted by Starzl in Denver in 1963 on a 3-year-old child with biliary atresia.[218] This was unsuccessful. Sporadic further attempts were made in humans before the first successful liver transplant was performed, again by Starzl, in 1967.[219] By this time immunosuppressive techniques had improved considerably and the patient, an 18-month-old child with a hepatoma, survived 13 months before dying of metastatic disease.

Heart, lung and pancreatic transplantation

Transplantation of the heart and lungs dates back to Carrel and Guthrie who performed canine heart and lung transplants with survival of the graft for several hours.[193] Important work was carried out during the 1940s by Demikhov of the Soviet Union who performed 250 heterotopic and 67 orthotopic canine heart–lung transplants with some animals surviving for several days; his work was not translated into English until 1962.[220] It was in the USA that the now standard technique of orthotopic cardiac transplantation was developed in painstaking animal experiments by Shumway and his team,[221] although Barnard in Cape Town was the first to

REFERENCES

199. Ullmann E Wien Klin Wochenschr 1902; 15: 281
200. Jaboulay M Lyon Méd 1906; 107: 575
201. Unger E Berl Klin Wochenschr 1909; 1: 1057
202. Voronoy Y Y El Siglo Med 1936; 97: 296
203. Küss R, Teinturier J, Milliez P Mem Acad Chir 1951; 77: 755
204. Hume D M, Merrill J P, Miller B F, Thorn G W J Clin Invest 1955; 34: 327
205. Merrill J P, Murray J E, Harrison J H, Guild W R JAMA 1956; 160: 277
206. Merrill J P, Murray J E, Takacs F J, Hager E B, Wilson R E Dammin G J JAMA 1963; 185: 347
207. Dausset J Immunogenetics 1980; 10: 1
208. Quinton W E, Dillard D H, Scribner B H Trans Am Soc Artif Intern Organs 1960; 6: 104
209. Brescia M J, Cimino J E, Appel K, Harwich B J N Engl J Med 1966; 275: 1089
210. Murray J E, Merrill J P, Dammin G J et al Surgery 1980; 48: 272
211. Schwarz R, Damshek W Nature 1959; 183: 1682
212. Calne R Y, Murray J E S Forum 1961; 12: 118
213. Borel J F, Feurer C, Gubler H U, Stähelin H Ag Actions 1976; 6: 468
214. Cosimi A B Transplant Proc 1980; 13: 462
215. Cosimi A B Antilymphocyte globulin and monoclonal antibodies. In: Morris P J (ed) Kidney Transplantation, 3rd edn. Saunders, Philadelphia 1988
216. Welch C S Transplant Bull 1955; 2: 54
217. Goodrich E O, Welch H F, Nelson J A, Beecher T S, Welch C S Surgery 1956; 39: 244
218. Starzl T E, Marchioro T L, von Kaulla K N, Hermann G, Brittain R S, Waddell W R Surg Gynecol Obstet 1963; 117: 659
219. Starzl T E, Groth C G, Brettschneider L et al Ann Surg 1968; 168: 392
220. Demikhov V P Experimental Transplantation of Vital Organs. Translated by Haigh B Consultants Bureau, New York 1962

carry out a human heart transplant.[222] The patient was a 54-year-old dentist who lived for 17 days after the operation.

Isolated lung transplantation in a human was first reported in 1963[223] and combined heart–lung transplantation in 1969[224]—both these operations were performed in the USA. Around this time, too, the first human pancreatic transplant was reported.[225]

SURGERY IN THE LATE 20TH CENTURY

The past two decades have witnessed the beginning of a major change in the practice of surgery. Although the disease processes facing the surgeon are largely the same as in Lister's time, the expectations of the surgeon and patient with regard to treatment and outcome have changed dramatically. The post-Listerian era during which ever greater and more complex open operations were devised and perfected is now being superseded by a new epoch in which there is an increasing trend towards less invasive, less mutilating and thereby less painful treatments. The introduction of histamine H_2-receptor antagonists in the treatment of peptic ulcer,[226] extracorporeal shock-wave lithotripsy in the treatment of renal stones[227] and gallstones,[228] balloon dilatation of pyloric stenosis[229] and ultrasonically guided percutaneous drainage of abscesses[230] are just a few examples of where the application of modern technology has begun to obviate the need for open surgical operation. This concept of minimally invasive surgery is well-illustrated by recent developments in therapeutic endoscopy.

Endoscopy

Throughout its history, endoscopy has been largely dependent on advances in optical technology. In 1806, Bozzini demonstrated the first primitive endoscope in Vienna.[231] The instrument comprised a silver cylinder containing a wax candle, the light of which was reflected along the cylinder by a concave mirror. The instrument was warmed, lubricated and inserted into various body cavities but the very poor illumination prevented its widespread adoption. Improved designs, but still lit by candles, were hardly an improvement.[232] In 1853 Desormeaux in Paris devised, and several years later described,[233] an instrument with polished tube, lenses and mirrors illuminated by a lamp burning a mixture of alcohol and turpentine. He named it an endoscope. This had greater appeal but it was the invention of the carbon filament lamp by Edison that allowed Nitze to introduce, in 1879,[56] an electric lighted cystoscope that for the first time provided satisfactory illumination of the interior of a body cavity (Fig. 1.10).

In the field of gastroenterology, the first attempts at gastroscopy were made by Kussmaul in 1868[234] but again the poor illumination precluded the technique from general use. Even after the introduction of electric bulbs the illumination remained poor for many years to the continued use of proximal lighting sources for both gastroscopy and sigmoidoscopy (Fig. 1.19). It was not until the 1920s that gastroscopy became an established diagnostic technique, largely owing to the work of Schindler[235] who, a few years later, was the first to use a semi-flexible instrument.[236] Around this time too, arthroscopy had its inception.[237]

The development of fibreoptics in the 1950s revolutionized the delivery of light and also enabled the transmission of ultra-clear images through flexible instruments. Hopkins, working in England, developed the forerunner of the modern flexible fibrescope[238] and 3 years later, in 1957, Hirschowitz in the USA passed a much-improved version into the stomach of a young woman in Ann Arbor.[239] This, the first flexible gastroscopy, was the beginning of modern diagnostic fibrendoscopy; its application to other areas of the body such as in ureteroscopy,[240] choledochoscopy[241] and

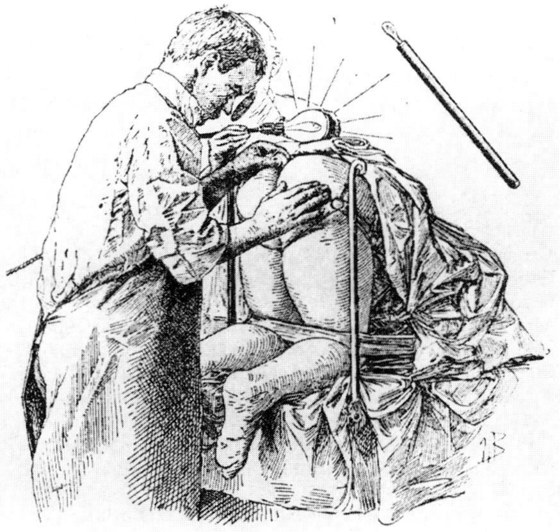

Fig. 1.19 The technique of sigmoidoscopy using reflected electric light, popularized by Kelly at the beginning of the 20th century. Distal lighted instruments that allowed much-improved views were later introduced by Strauss in Germany and by J. P. Lockhart-Mummery in England. Reproduced with permission from Kelly H A Ann Surg 1895; 21: 468.

REFERENCES

221. Shumway N E, Lower R R, Stofer R C Transplantation of the heart. In: Advances in Surgery. Year Book Medical Publishers, Chicago 1966
222. Barnard C S Afr Med 1967; 41: 1271
223. Hardy J D, Webb W R, Dalton M L, Walker G R JAMA 1963; 186: 1065
224. Cooley D A, Bloodwell R D, Hallman G L, Nora J J, Harrison G M, Leachman R D Ann Thorac Surg 1969; 8: 30
225. Kelly W D, Lillehei R C, Merkel F K, Idezuki Y, Goetz F C Surgery 1967; 61: 827
226. Wyllie J H, Hesselbo T, Black J W Lancet 1972; ii: 1117
227. Chaussy C, Brendel W, Schmidt E Lancet 1980; ii: 1265
228. Sauerbruch T, Delius M, Paumgartner G et al N Engl J Med 1986; 314: 818
229. Benjamin S B, Cattau E L, Glass R L Gastrointest Endosc 1982; 28: 253
230. Smith E H, Bartrum R J AJR 1974; 122: 308
231. Bozzini P J Pract Heilk 1806; 24: 107 English translation Urology 1974; 3: 119
232. Ségalas P S Rev Med Fr Étrang 1827; 1: 157
233. Desormeaux A J De l'endoscope et de ses applications. Baillière, Paris 1865
234. Kussmaul A Dtsch Arch Klin Med 1869; 6: 456
235. Schindler R Arch VerdauKr 1922; 30: 133
236. Schindler R Münch Med Wochenschr 1932; 79: 1268
237. Bircher E Zentralbl Chir 1921; 48: 1460
238. Hopkins H H, Kapany N S Nature 1954; 173: 39
239. Hirschowitz B I, Curtiss L E, Peters C W, Pollard H M Gastroenterology 1958; 35: 50
240. Marshall V F J Urol 1964; 91: 110

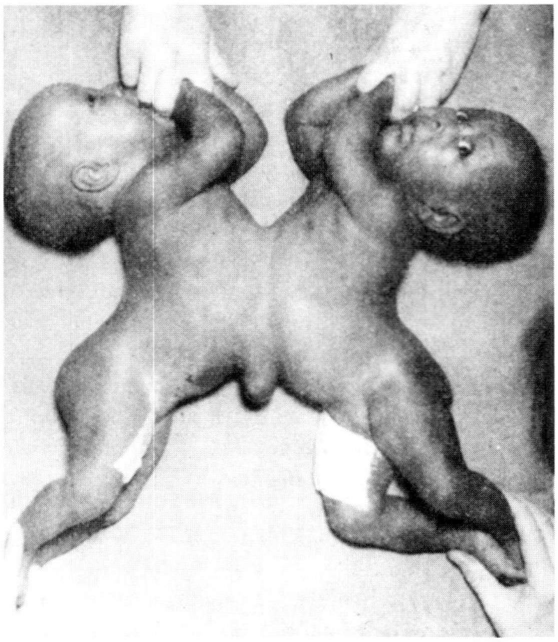

Fig. 1.20 The conjoined twins of Kano. These twins were born in Kano, Nigeria and shared a common liver and peritoneal cavity. They were separated by Ian Aird at the Hammersmith Hospital, London in November 1953, in an operation which received widespread publicity. It was the first surgical separation of conjoined twins who shared a liver. There are many examples of conjoined twins in history, the most famous being the brothers Chang and Eng who were born in Siam in 1811, who emigrated to the USA, became exhibits in Barnum's circus, married English sisters, fathered 19 children between them and lived as farmers in later life. Unseparated, they died at the age of 63 within an hour of each other. Reproduced with permission from Aird I Br Med J 1954; 1: 831.

arterioscopy[242] followed rapidly. Endoscopic retrograde cholangiopancreatography was first reported in 1968.[243]

The next decade saw the emergence of therapeutic endoscopy as technical advances enabled instruments of increasingly sophisticated design to be passed alongside the fibreoptic bundle. Endoscopic dilatation of oesophageal strictures in the USA,[244] endoscopic biliary sphincterotomy simultaneously in Germany[245] and Japan[246] and endoscopic percutaneous nephrolithotomy also in the USA[247] were introduced in the early 1970s. Each of these techniques became rapidly accepted and refined as improved instrumentation became available. In 1973, the passage of a laser beam down an endoscope was first reported[248] and within a year or so laser endoscopy was being used therapeutically to control upper gastrointestinal haemorrhage.[249] At the end of the decade endoscopic biliary stenting was introduced[250]—yet another technique which has reduced the need for open surgical operation.

Minimal-access surgery

To a varying extent over the past 10 years, traditional practice in almost all surgical specialties has been transformed by advances in camera technology that enable the transmission of high-definition magnified images of endoscopic views to a television screen. Aided by an ever-increasing range of specially designed endoscopic instruments, minimal-access operations are now widely performed.

Surgical research

The high point of open operative surgery has now passed. Alternative, less invasive methods of treatment are steadily being introduced and operations common until recently, such as vagotomy procedures for peptic ulcer, are now rarely performed. Change in surgical practice is not new however. Gastrorrhaphy, nephropexy, splanchnicectomy and cardio-omentopexy were operations often performed in the years between the two world wars; today they are historical curiosities. This continually changing scene is, in large measure, the outcome of research, a discipline without which surgery would stagnate. A multiplicity of different sciences now interact within the broad title of surgical research including genetics, immunology, physiology, biochemistry, radiology, pharmacology and engineering. Surgical research has flourished and expanded greatly, especially in recent years, having been stimulated by the founding of surgical research societies in the UK and elsewhere, an ever-increasing trend towards specialization, particularly in the USA, and the development of academic surgical departments throughout the world. First written in 1926,[251] the far-sighted words of Lord Moynihan are even more true today: 'surgery in days to come will be advanced by men [and women] trained in the methods and imbued with the spirit of experimental research, though it will no doubt continue to be practised to their profit by those who are merely craftsmen'. Ian Aird, the progenitor of this *Companion*, was one such surgeon who eschewed the rewards of private surgical practice in order to pursue research and advance scientific knowledge. He made important contributions to surgical pathology with the discovery of the relationship between blood groups and carcinoma of the stomach[252] and peptic ulcer[253] and became a public figure when he separated the conjoined twins of Kano in 1953[254] (Fig. 1.20).

The history of surgery has been a story of steady but uneven progress, with the advances of the 20th century being outstanding. It seems reasonable to suggest that the scientific training of young surgeons today, if combined with an intellectual curiosity and the facility for interdisciplinary collaboration, will ensure surgical advances in the 21st century and thereby a continued and ever-evolving history.

REFERENCES

241. Shore J M, Lippman H N Lancet 1965; i: 1200
242. Greenstone S M, Shore J M, Heringman E C, Massell T B Arch Surg 1966; 93: 811
243. McCune W S, Shorb P E, Moscovitz H Ann Surg 1968; 167: 752
244. Lilly J O, McCaffery T D Am J Dig Dis 1971; 16: 1137
245. Classen M, Demling L Dtsch Med Wochenschr 1974; 99: 496
246. Kawai K, Akasaka Y, Murakami K, Tada M, Kohli Y, Nakajima M Gastrointest Endosc 1974; 20: 148
247. Bissada N K, Meachum K R, Redman J F J Urol 1974; 112: 414
248. Nath G, Gorisch W, Kreitmair A, Keifhaber P Endoscopy 1973; 5: 213
249. Frümorgen P, Bodem F, Reidenbach H D, Kaduk B, Demling L Gastrointest Endosc 1976; 23: 73
250. Soehendra N, Reijnders-Frederix V Dtsch Med Wochenschr 1979; 104: 106
251. Moynihan B Lancet 1926; ii: 789
252. Aird I, Bentall H H, Roberts J A F Br Med J 1953; 1: 799
253. Aird I, Bentall H H, Mehigan J, Roberts J A F Br Med J 1954; 2: 315
254. Aird I Br Med J 1954; 1: 831

2 Fluid and nutrient replacement

D. Tweedle

FLUID AND ELECTROLYTE REPLACEMENT

Water is the major component of the human body comprising more than half of the total body weight.[1] In a healthy individual various hormonal systems conserve water and electrolytes and control the distribution and volume of these substances within intracellular and extracellular spaces. This fluid environment allows transport of essential substances to cells and excretion of unwanted waste products. Disorders of fluid and electrolyte balance may be a reflection of abnormal homeostasis (e.g. hypercalcaemia as a result of hyperparathyroidism) or the failure to achieve a correct balance because of an abnormal intake or loss (e.g. hypokalaemia as a result of pyloric stenosis). In some patients the concentration of an electrolyte may be normal, but the total body content is abnormally high or low, in others there may be a normal total body content but an abnormal concentration as the result of hypovolaemia or hypervolaemia. Occasionally, there may be a combination of both abnormalities. The measured extracellular concentration of an electrolyte may be a very poor reflection of the total body content, particularly when an intracellular electrolyte such as potassium is measured in an extracellular fluid (Fig. 2.4). Alterations in both the total quantity and the concentration of an electrolyte can produce severe clinical effects.

FLUID COMPARTMENTS

Total body water depends on the patient's sex, age and bodily composition. In a young male adult the total body water is about 60% of body weight (45 litres) but it constitutes only about half of the body weight in young females who usually have more fat and less muscle. Above the age of 60 the total body water in men falls to about 50% because of a fall in muscle mass. Total body water is divided into two major fluid spaces (Fig. 2.1), the intracellular fluid and the extracellular fluid. In healthy adults, approximately 30 litres is intracellular and 15 litres is extracellular.[1] Extracellular fluid can be subdivided into intravascular (3 litres) and interstitial fluid (12 litres). These two compartments within the extracellular fluid differ in their protein content (particularly albumin) but otherwise the composition of the extracellular fluid is very similar throughout the body, particularly in its electrolyte content (Table 2.1). This is in contrast to the intracellular fluid whose electrolyte composition shows greater variation depending upon the tissue of origin. Intracellular concentrations of electrolytes cannot be measured as easily or as accurately as extracellular concentrations.

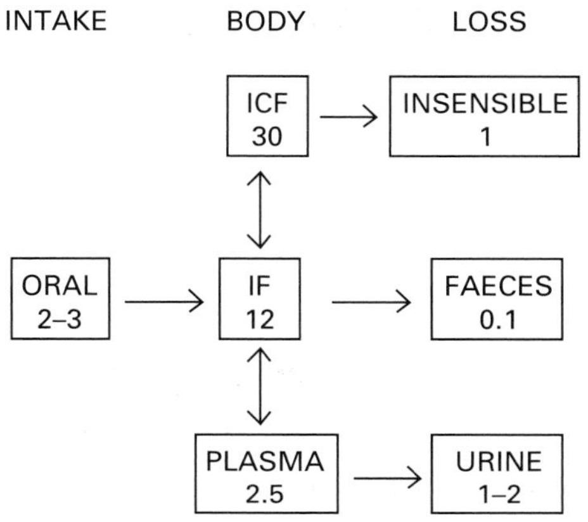

Fig. 2.1 Daily water balance (litres).

The intracellular fluid contains 98% of the body's potassium and magnesium but only a small quantity of sodium (Table 2.1). The major intracellular anions are phosphate, sulphate, bicarbonate and protein. Sodium is actively extruded from the cell. It is within the intracellular fluid that all synthetic processes and energy transferences occur with consumption of oxygen and production of carbon dioxide (the correct scientific meaning of respiration). The composition of the intracellular fluid can only be ascertained by sophisticated equipment, usually by in vitro measurements. The predominant cation in the extracellular fluid is sodium and the predominant anion is chloride, probably reflecting the origin of man and other animals from creatures living in the sea. This extracellular

Table 2.1 Electrolyte concentrations (mmol/l)

	Extracellular fluid	*Intracellular fluid*
Sodium	140	10
Potassium	3.8	150
Calcium*	2.3	1
Magnesium	0.9	12
Chloride	100	3
Bicarbonate	28	10
Phosphate	1.0	100
Sulphate	0.8	10

*Total (protein bound and ionic)

REFERENCE

1. Moore F D, Olsen K H et al The Body Cell Mass and its Supporting Environment. Saunders, Philadelphia 1963

fluid provides a medium for transport of nutrients to and waste products away from cells.

Within the extracellular fluid, the major difference between plasma and interstitial fluid is in the content of plasma protein and particularly of albumin. Without the oncotic affect of albumin, the interstitial fluid compartment increases dramatically and the body becomes waterlogged. The interchange of water and other substances at the capillary interface (Fig. 2.2) is determined by differences in hydrostatic pressure at the arterial and venous end of the capillaries and the osmotic counteraction of albumin.[2] This flow may be as great as 80 000 litres daily.[3]

The overall distribution of fluid and electrolytes within the body is controlled by hormonal mechanisms. If the plasma osmolarity becomes too high (above 290 mmol/l) this is detected by osmoreceptors in the hypothalamus and antidiuretic hormone is secreted which increases the permeability of the collecting tubules[4] and thereby reduces the amount of water excreted by the kidneys. If the extracellular concentration of sodium falls too low, renin is secreted by the granular cells of the afferent glomerular arteriole. Renin converts angiotensinogen, a circulating globulin in the plasma, into angiotensin I. Within the lung and other tissues angiotensin I is converted by another enzyme to angiotensin II. Angiotensin II produces peripheral vasoconstriction, thereby maintaining blood pressure in a patient with an inadequate extracellular volume, and also stimulates the secretion of aldosterone by the adrenal cortex. Aldosterone increases reabsorption of sodium in the renal tubules effectively increasing the extracellular fluid volume. If this volume becomes too high, natriuretic hormone is secreted from the cardiac atrium.[5] This peptide inhibits reabsorption of sodium in the distal tubule and counteracts the vasoconstrictive effects of angiotensin II.

Water

The daily water balance of a healthy 70 kg male in a temperate climate is shown in Figure 2.1. In these circumstances the balance of the 45 litres of water is a consequence of fluctuation in intake and output of only 1.5–3 litres each day. In healthy individuals, the oral intake of water is usually determined by social factors and by thirst. The latter is usually a reflection of the need to keep pace with daily losses. Oxidation of ingested food supplies about 0.3 l/d.

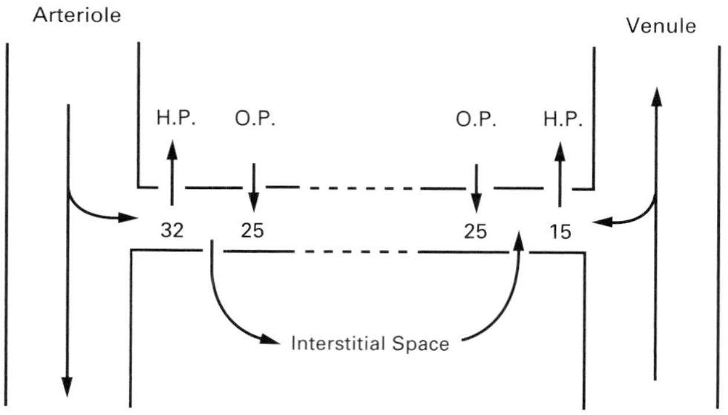

Fig. 2.2 The influence of hydrostatic pressure (H.P.) and oncotic pressure (O.P.) upon movement of fluid in the interstitial space (figures shown are in mmHg, for kPa divide by 7.52).

The average volume and electrolyte content of daily intestinal secretions is shown in Table 2.2 and it can be seen that 8 litres a day is usually secreted and almost totally reabsorbed. It is apparent from these figures why the loss of just one day's gastrointestinal secretion has such a profound effect upon fluid balance, being much greater than either the normal daily intake or loss. Insensible loss from sweat and humidification of inspired air in the lungs is usually about 1 l/d. An unacclimatized individual in a tropical climate can lose several litres by this route. Obese patients have a greater surface area and lose proportionately more water through sweating. The loss through the lungs is much greater in patients with tracheostomies and their inspired gases should always be humidified. The insensible loss is also greatly increased in all patients with fever, the loss increasing by 10% for each 1°C increase in temperature.[6] In health less than 100 ml is usually lost in the faeces but huge losses may be fatal in those with severe infective diarrhoea as occurs in cholera. The urinary loss of water is usually rigidly controlled by the hormonal mechanisms discussed above. Excessive loss may reflect renal disease and the much rarer endocrine disturbances discussed below.

Measured effects of water depletion and excess are usually apparent from the electrolyte concentration and the volume of the plasma and urine as shown in Table 2.3. In patients with water excess, the urine often contains larger quantities of sodium than might be expected because aldosterone secretion is reduced by the expansion in the plasma volume.

Sodium

The daily sodium balance of a healthy 70 kg male in a temperate climate is shown in Figure 2.3. In addition to these quantities, it should be remembered that about 70% of the 2000 mmol of sodium contained in bone is freely diffusible with the extracellular fluid and constitutes an important homeostatic mechanism. Sweat is hypertonic and in temperate climates the insensible loss of sodium is insignificant. In unacclimatized patients the loss can be much greater and sodium depletion can occur if sweat is replaced by water alone. In the acclimatized patient, however, the concentration of sodium in the sweat is less than 10 mmol/l.[7] Like water, it is apparent from Table 2.1 that the loss of one day's gastrointestinal secretion of sodium has a far greater effect than the loss of a normal daily intake or any variation in urinary output. The faecal loss of sodium is usually insignificant but large losses can occur in patients with infective diarrhoea. Within the body, the loss of sodium is usually accompanied by loss of water in the same proportion to that in extracellular fluid but sodium excess and depletion can occur and the effects are shown in Table 2.4.

REFERENCES

2. Starling E H J Physiol 1896; 19: 312
3. Guyton A C, Taylor A E, Granger H J Circulatory Physiology II. Dynamics and Control of Body Fluid. Saunders, Springfield Illinois 1975
4. Robertson G L, Mahr E A et al J Clin Invest 1973; 52: 2340–2352
5. Bukalew V M, Gruber K A Ann Rev Physiol 1984; 46: 343–358
6. Shelley M P Br J Hosp Med 1988; 39: 506–518
7. Tinckler L F Br Med J 1966; i: 1263–1267

Table 2.2 The daily volume and electrolyte content of the intestinal secretions

Secretion	*Volume (litres)*	*Na^+ (mmol/l)*	*K^+ (mmol/l)*	*Cl^- (mmol/l)*	*HCO_3^- (mmol/l)*
Saliva	1.5	15	30	10	30
Gastric	2.0	50	15	120	—
Small bowel	3.0	140	10	100	30
Bile	0.6	140	5	100	35
Pancreatic	0.7	140	5	70	100
Total	7.8	725	112	764	226

Table 2.3 Effects of water depletion and excess

	Water depletion	*Water excess*
Plasma	Packed cell volume ↑ Sodium concentration ↓	Packed cell volume ↓ Sodium concentration — normal
Urine	Volume ↓ Sodium concentration ↓	Volume ↑ Sodium concentration ↑

Sodium depletion is a frequent consequence of gastrointestinal disease because of the large daily quantities secreted into the gastrointestinal tract (Table 2.2). This may be lost by vomiting, diarrhoea, through fistulae and by temporary or permanent loss into the peritoneal cavity. Large quantities are also lost in patients with burns (see Chapter 6). Chronic loss of sodium may be caused by inappropriate use of diuretics and very occasionally by hypoaldosteronism which occurs in Addison's disease (see Chapter 35). The signs of sodium depletion usually become apparent when there has been a loss of approximately 4 litres of saline. Initially, the kidneys excrete dilute urine until extracellular osmolarity is restored with a subsequent reduction in the extracellular volume unless there is salt-losing nephritis. The sodium concentration of the urine falls rapidly. At first the plasma proteins maintain the plasma oncotic pressure and the reduction in the extracellular fluid compartment is mainly in the interstitial compartment. When sodium depletion is established, plasma oncotic pressure falls and so does plasma volume producing an increase in packed cell volume. The signs and symptoms of early water and sodium depletion are compared in Table 2.5.

Excessive retention of sodium in the body can occur as the result of chronic congestive cardiac failure, renal disease, the metabolic response to injury, hepatic failure, primary aldosteronism (Conn's syndrome) and steroid therapy, but in surgical practice the most common cause is probably excessive infusion of intravenous saline. The concentration of plasma sodium is a poor indicator of the total body content because a corresponding quantity of water is usually retained by the kidney so that the osmolarity is restored. Consequently, the plasma concentration of sodium is usually normal but the packed cell volume is decreased. Oedema only becomes apparent when the average patient has at least 4 litres of excess saline in the body. The urine volume is increased and the concentration of urinary sodium is high.

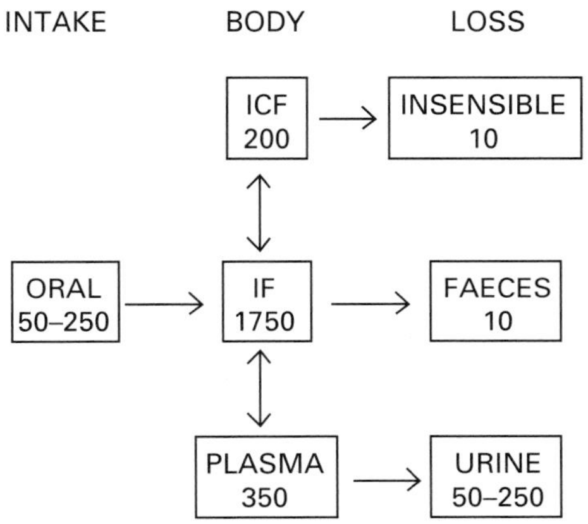

Fig. 2.3 Daily sodium balance (mmol).

Table 2.4 Effects of sodium depletion and excess

	Sodium depletion	*Sodium excess*
Plasma	Packed cell volume ↑ Sodium concentration ↓	Packed cell volume ↓ Sodium concentration — normal
Urine	Volume ↓ Sodium concentration ↓	Volume ↑ Sodium concentration ↑

Potassium

The daily potassium balance of a healthy 70 kg male is shown in Figure 2.4 and should be compared with that of sodium in Figure 2.3. 98% of total body potassium is within cells and it is readily apparent why the 10–15 mmol contained in 3 litres of plasma is such a poor reflection of the intracellular concentration. The disparity between intracellular and extracellular concentrations and quantities is even greater than that pertaining to sodium (Table 2.1). From Table 2.2 it is apparent that loss of one day's intestinal secretion is much less than that of sodium, but as the quantity of potassium in the extracellular compartment is so small, the percentage loss within

Table 2.5 Early symptoms and signs of water and sodium depletion

	Water depletion	*Sodium depletion*
Thirst	Present	Absent
Venous filling	Normal	Reduced
Orbit	Normal	Sunken
Skin turgor	Normal	Reduced

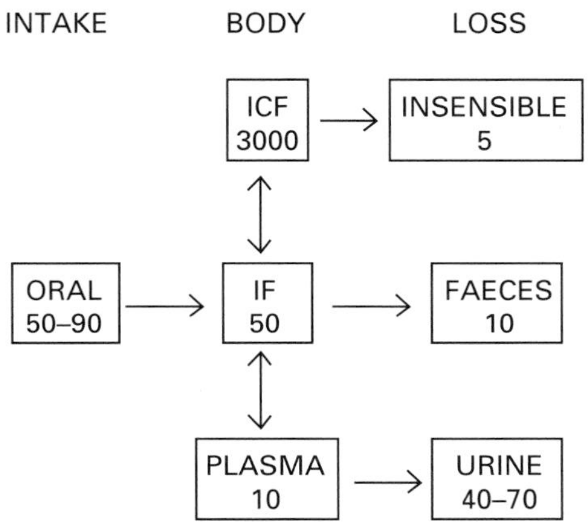

Fig. 2.4 Daily potassium balance (mmol).

the extracellular fluid is much greater. The daily loss of potassium from intestinal secretions is about twice the total quantity in the extracellular fluid but the daily loss of sodium is only about one third. The quantity of potassium normally lost in the faeces is very small.

Large quantities of potassium can be lost in patients with inflammatory bowel disease such as ulcerative colitis or infective diarrhoea. The loss of potassium in saliva and gastric juice in patients with pyloric obstruction may also produce hypokalaemia. Huge quantities of potassium may be lost from the secretion of a villous adenoma at any site in the gastrointestinal tract, but most commonly in the rectum (see Chapter 30). Potassium depletion may also occur in patients with renal disease, in Cushing's syndrome (see Chapter 35) and in patients taking diuretics or steroids. One of the most common causes of potassium depletion is iatrogenic following intravenous infusion of potassium-free solutions. The extracellular concentration of potassium has profound effects upon neuromuscular conductivity, and hypokalaemia is associated with lethargy and fatigue. Neuromuscular weakness and intestinal atony develop when the concentration falls to 2.5 mmol/l. Changes occur on the electrocardiogram with depression of the ST segment, a small T wave and the appearance of a U wave.

Hyperkalaemia affects renal function and paradoxically the urine may contain large quantities of potassium. It may occur in acute or chronic renal failure from any cause and as a consequence of Addison's disease (see Chapter 35). In surgical practice hyperkalaemia may be the result of simple contraction of extracellular volume in dehydrated patients, as a consequence of too rapid intravenous administration, following massive blood transfusion and following haemolysis of red blood cells as can occur after crush injuries (see Chapter 7), extensive burns (see Chapter 6) and transfusion of incompatible blood (see Chapter 3). There are few clinical signs: estimation of the serum potassium concentration is vital if hyperkalaemia is suspected. The electrocardiogram shows diminution or absence of the P wave, abnormal QRS complexes and peaked T waves. Eventually ventricular fibrillation and cardiac arrest may occur.

Calcium

The daily calcium balance of a healthy 70 kg male is shown in Figure 2.5. In addition to the 70 mmol of calcium within the intracellular and extracellular fluid, there exists about 27 000 mmol of calcium in bone, but this is contained in hydroxyapatite, a complex salt, and isotopic studies have shown that only 125 mmol is freely exchangeable from this source. Extracellular calcium occurs in three forms:

a. As non-ionized protein bound calcium—50%.
b. As divalent cations—45%.
c. As calcium anion complexes—5%.

The degree of ionization increases inversely with pH. It is ionized calcium that affects coagulation, calcification, neuromuscular conductivity and other physiological functions. The total plasma calcium in a healthy adult is within the range of 2.5–2.8 mmol/l. When the total calcium concentration is low because of hypoproteinaemia, the ionic calcium concentration may be normal without any physiological disturbance. As total serum calcium concentration fluctuates according to the quantity of serum protein and, in particular, with the concentration of plasma albumin, if the ionic calcium cannot be measured a more accurate reflection of the physiological effect is to calculate the corrected serum calcium from the formula:

$$\text{corrected calcium (mmol/l)} = \text{measured calcium} + (40 - \text{albumin concentration}) \times 0.02$$

Calcium homeostasis is regulated by three hormones. Parathormone acts directly on bone and kidney, promoting calcium resorption and inhibiting phosphate resorption in the distal tubule. It also increases formation of 1,25-dihydroxyvitamin D in the proximal convoluted tubule.[8] In turn, 1,25-dihydroxyvitamin D stimulates absorption of calcium and phosphate from the intestine. Calcitonin inhibits absorption of calcium from bone when the serum calcium concentration becomes too high (see Chapter 19).

Calcium depletion may present as hypocalcaemia or as metabolic bone disease. Hypocalcaemia may produce tetany which, in its latent form, can be elicited by Trousseau's and Chvostek's tests, but neuromuscular conductivity is affected by the relative concentrations of six ions. Hypertonia may be produced by low extracellular concentrations of calcium and magnesium or high concentrations of sodium and potassium ions and by high concentrations of hydroxyl and low concentrations of hydrogen ions as occurs in alkalosis. The converse changes may produce paralysis and hypotonia. Hypocalcaemia often accompanies osteomalacia but in osteoporosis the serum calcium concentration is usually normal. Hypocalcaemia may occur in acute pancreatitis as a result of saponification of fat within the peritoneal cavity and from hypoalbuminaemia. It may also occur in chronic pancreatitis as a result of increased faecal excretion associated with steatorrhoea (see Chapter 33). It may also be the result of an inadequate intake of vitamin D and a consequence of hypoparathyroidism following thyroidectomy (see Chapter 19).

REFERENCE

8. Galenite L, MacAuley S et al Lancet 1972; i: 985–987

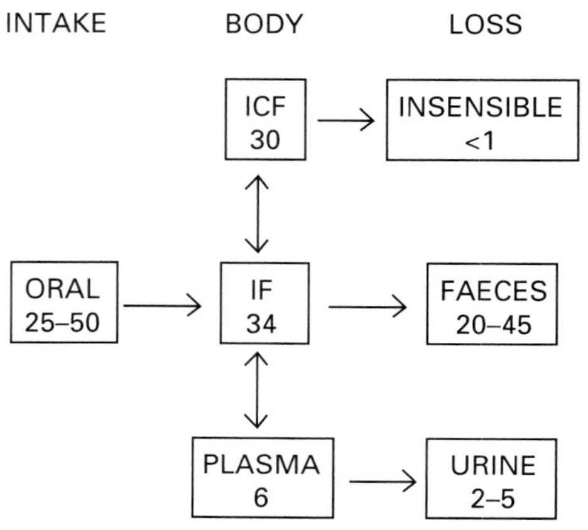

Fig. 2.5 Daily calcium balance (mmol).

In addition to hypotonia, hypercalcaemia is associated with anorexia, vomiting, constipation and mental disturbances. It may be produced by hyperparathyroidism, osteolytic metastases, immobilization or the excessive intake of vitamin D, or by sarcoidosis (see Chapter 19).

Magnesium

The daily magnesium balance of a healthy 70 kg male is shown in Figure 2.6. Like potassium, the vast majority of freely available magnesium ions is in the intracellular compartment. Like calcium, there is a large reserve available in bone of approximately 500 mmol, but like calcium only a small quantity is freely available, the majority being bound into complex salts. Like calcium, the daily turnover within the gastrointestinal tract is very high when compared with the quantity in the extracellular fluid and, like calcium, about one third of the ions in plasma are bound to proteins. The control of magnesium homeostasis is uncertain but parathormone appears to have similar effects to those exerted upon calcium.

The effects of hypermagnesaemia and hypomagnesaemia mimic those of similar changes in calcium concentration. Thus hypomagnesaemia is usually asymptomatic but may produce tetany and paroxysmal tachycardia. Hypomagnesaemia may occur in patients who have large intestinal loses from colitis and steatorrhoea and in those with intestinal malabsorption or following extensive resection. It may also occur in patients who are fed intravenously for long periods with magnesium-free solutions. Hypermagnesaemia is associated with lethargy and muscular flaccidity. The ECG may show prolonged PR and QT intervals with peaked T waves. The commonest cause of hypermagnesaemia is renal failure. It may also occur in hyperparathyroidism, following excessive infusion and, rarely, following excessive purgation with magnesium sulphate.[9,10]

Chloride

The daily chloride balance of a healthy 70 kg male is shown in Figure 2.7 and the distribution is very similar to that of sodium (Fig. 2.2). The metabolism of chloride is governed mainly by that

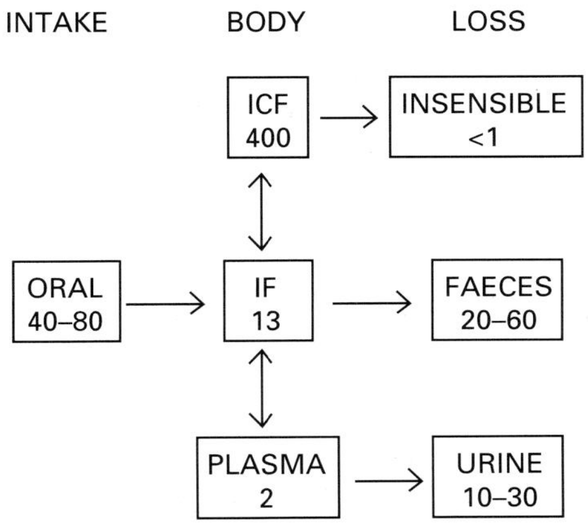

Fig. 2.6 Daily magnesium balance (mmol).

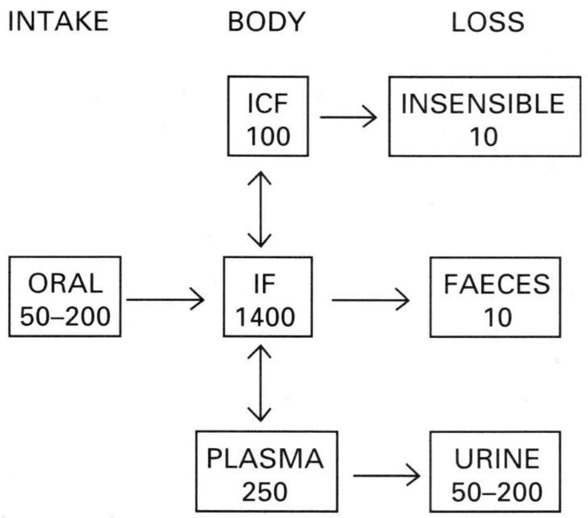

Fig. 2.7 Daily chloride balance (mmol).

of sodium, chloride being retained to preserve electroneutrality, but chloride can be reabsorbed in the kidney independently of sodium for acid–base homeostasis. Insensible loss of chloride is usually small in temperate climates, but accompanying sodium it may be considerable in unacclimatized individuals in hot climates. Like sodium, the loss of one day's gastrointestinal secretion (Table 2.2) can be profound. The most common cause of hypochloraemia is overhydration. Although the concentration may be low, the total body content may be increased as may occur in oedematous patients. Hypochloraemia is common in pyloric stenosis, when chloride ions are lost in the same quantity as the combined loss of hydrogen and sodium ions. As there is a greater loss of chloride ions when compared with hydrogen ions, a metabolic alkalosis develops. Hyperchloraemia may occur in patients with renal disease and following uretero-colic anastomosis (see Chapter 37).

Bicarbonate

The daily bicarbonate balance of a healthy 70 kg male is shown in Figure 2.8. Although this is the second major anion of the extracellular fluid, unlike other ions in the body there is virtually no oral intake, the ions being produced by the combination of water and carbon dioxide:

$$H_2O + CO_2 \rightleftharpoons H^+ + HCO_3^-$$

13 000 mmol of bicarbonate can be produced daily, but an equivalent quantity of hydrogen ions are produced and there is a limit to the amount of these that can be excreted by the urine. Bicarbonate can be lost in biliary and pancreatic secretions (Table 2.2) producing a metabolic acidosis. Ingestion of bicarbonate is usually minimal but occasional dyspeptic patients ingest excessive quantities. Excess bicarbonate is easily excreted by the kidneys or by combination with hydrogen ions with ultimate excretion of carbon dioxide through the lungs.

REFERENCES

9. Mordes J P, Wacker W E C Pharmacol Rev 1978; 29: 273–281
10. Randall R E, Cohen E D et al Ann Intern Med 1964; 61: 73–80

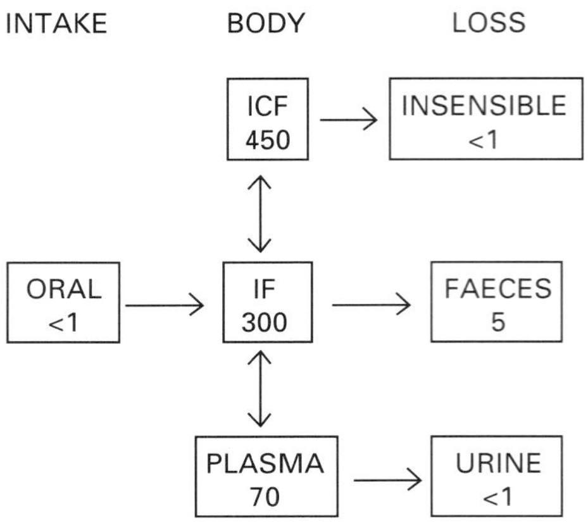

Fig. 2.8 Daily bicarbonate balance (mmol).

Phosphorus

The daily inorganic phosphorus balance of a healthy 70 kg male is shown in Figure 2.9. Within the normal range of extracellular pH, 80% of phosphorus ions are divalent and 20% are monovalent. Phosphate is predominantly intracellular and, like calcium, a large quantity is contained in hydroxyapatite in bone. Also like calcium, large quantities are ingested daily and excreted in the faeces, but when compared with the quantities contained in the body, the loss of one day's intake or faecal loss is of little importance. The product of the concentrations of calcium and phosphorus in the plasma is constant, an increase of one producing a decrease in the other. Absorption of phosphorus is decreased by parathormone (see Chapter 19). Hypophosphataemia increases the affinity of haemoglobin for oxygen, producing tissue hypoxia.[11] The usual cause is infusion of large quantities of glucose for intravenous feeding. Phosphate deficiency may also occur as a chronic phenomenon as a result of inadequate intake, particularly in alcoholics, and as a result of vitamin D deficiency and malabsorption in patients with steatorrhoea. Excessive renal excretion may produce hypophosphataemia in patients with hyperparathyroidism (see Chapter 19). Hyperphosphataemia is usually secondary to hypocalcaemia and is most common in patients with renal failure. There are no obvious symptoms.

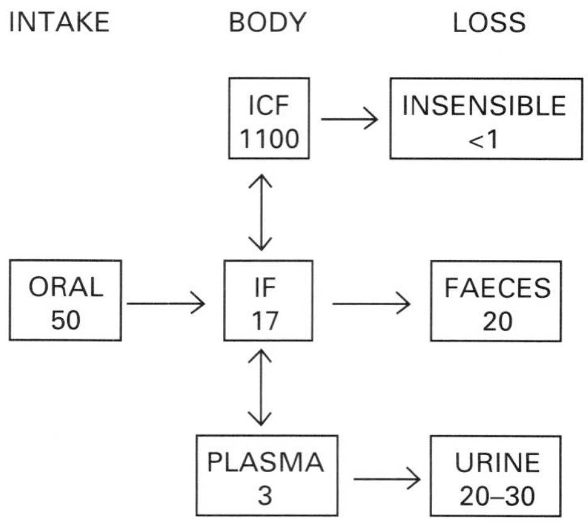

Fig. 2.9 Daily phosphorus balance (mmol).

FLUID AND ELECTROLYTE DISORDERS

Some of the conditions which may produce disturbances of homeostasis of individual components of fluid and electrolyte balance are enumerated above. The overall consequences of the common disease processes encountered in surgical practice are discussed below. When considering how these abnormalities arose and how they might be treated, it is helpful to record the massive volumes of fluid and quantities of electrolytes that flow through the regulating systems of the body each day: daily cardiac output averages 7200 l/d; flow across the capillary endothelium is about 80 000 l/d; healthy kidneys filter about 180 l/d from 800 litres of plasma; and healthy lungs can excrete carbon dioxide equivalent to 13 000 mmol of hydrogen each day.

Preoperative patients

Many patients in an increasingly aged surgical population are suffering from medical conditions unconnected with their surgical pathology. These conditions may produce abnormalities of fluid and electrolyte homeostasis. The most common causes are severe cardiovascular and renal disease and diabetes. Others have disturbances induced by their surgical pathology: of these patients, the great majority are suffering from gastrointestinal or endocrinological disorders.

Gastrointestinal disease

In health almost all the electrolytes within gastrointestinal secretions (Table 2.2) are reabsorbed. In patients with gastrointestinal disease they may be lost by vomiting, therapeutic aspiration, fistulae or diarrhoea. Electrolytes may also be temporarily lost internally from translocation into the gastrointestinal lumen or peritoneal cavity. This is termed 'third space loss', the intracellular and extracellular spaces being the first and second spaces. The site of the problems within the gastrointestinal tract determines the electrolyte composition of the secretions lost.

Oropharyngeal and oesophageal lesions usually allow the passage of fluid but ingestion of nutrients is often inadequate. In some patients, there may be insufficient fluid intake as a consequence of apathy or pain.[12]

Pyloric obstruction may be caused by peptic ulceration, benign or malignant disease (see Chapter 28). Gastric juice is dilute hydrochloric acid with some sodium and potassium chloride, the secretion of acid being less in patients with malignant disease. There is a metabolic alkalosis and a compensatory respiratory acidosis. Although there is a metabolic alkalosis, the patients often have an acid urine because hydrogen ions are exchanged for sodium ions in the renal tubule to conserve sodium.[13] Ultimately, potassium ions are also exchanged for sodium ions in the kidney and hypokalaemia develops. Patients require infusion of isotonic saline with added potassium chloride.

REFERENCES

11. Travis S F et al N Engl J Med 1971; 285: 763–771
12. Tweedle D E F et al Res Clin Forums 1979; 1: 59
13. LeQuesne L P Surg Gynaecol Obstet 1961; 113: 1–12

High intestinal obstruction distal to the papilla of Vater produces rapid loss of gastric, biliary, pancreatic, duodenal and jejunal solutions. The bowel above the obstruction loses its power of absorption.[14] The surgeon must balance the need for fluid restoration and the requirement for surgical relief of obstruction. In most patients, preoperative restoration of extracellular loss with isotonic saline containing potassium and bicarbonate is the sensible approach, to be followed by laparotomy some hours later. When there is the possibility of strangulation, blood volume should be restored with a plasma expander such as gelatin, starch or dextran before undertaking urgent laparotomy (see Chapter 27).

High intestinal fistulae produce similar but more chronic losses to those produced by high intestinal obstruction. Pancreatic fistulae are associated with losses of bicarbonate (see Chapter 33). Too hasty surgical intervention in patients with high intestinal fistulae is associated with a high mortality. Many of these patients are severely malnourished and require nutritional repletion before undergoing surgery. Many simple entero-cutaneous fistulae, especially those with a direct communication between gut and skin without an intervening abscess cavity, will close spontaneously if the patient is fed intravenously and gastrointestinal secretion is suppressed by somatostatin.[15,16] Ignoring nutritional requirements, these patients require intravenous isotonic saline with potassium and bicarbonate ions according to the secretions lost.

Low intestinal obstruction does not usually produce major disturbances until the later stages as fluid and electrolytes may still be absorbed in the small bowel (see chapter 29). After some days the distal obstruction produces some degree of obstruction in the small bowel but the disturbance is never as severe as obstruction arising de novo in the small intestine. These patients require intravenous isotonic saline.

Low intestinal fistulae usually produce little disturbance and many of these patients do not require intravenous replacement.

Inflammatory bowel disease from acute infections such as cholera may produce fatal loss of fluid and electrolytes. It was the treatment of cholera by intravenous infusions of saline that first established the importance of fluid replacement in gastrointestinal disease.[17] Other chronic inflammatory conditions such as ulcerative colitis and Crohn's disease (see Chapter 29) are associated with severe malnourishment and the loss of large quantities of potassium and magnesium.

Villous adenoma is an uncommon tumour which may occur throughout the gastrointestinal tract[18] but is most common in the rectum (see Chapter 30). In the majority of patients the losses of sodium and potassium in the mucus secreted by the adenoma are not great enough to produce systemic disturbance but in some patients up to 3 litres of mucus per day may be lost containing 160 mmol/l of sodium and 120 mmol/l of potassium. In these patients there may be neuromuscular weakness and they require rapid potassium repletion.

Endocrine disorders

The anterior pituitary gland secretes corticotrophin (ACTH) which in turn stimulates the suprarenal cortex to secrete glucocorticoids and to a lesser extent mineralocorticoids. Cushing's disease (see below under suprarenal glands) may follow excessive secretion by benign or malignant tumours of the anterior pituitary gland. Conversely, adrenocortical deficiency may be caused by destruction of the anterior pituitary by tumours, irradiation or surgery.

The posterior pituitary gland secretes antidiuretic hormone (ADH or vasopressin) whose function is described above. Lack of antidiuretic hormone results in diabetes insipidus—usually a consequence of a craniopharyngioma or its treatment by irradiation or surgery. Patients have a hypertonic plasma (> 290 mosmol/l), hypernatraemia (> 150 mmol/l) but excrete large volumes of hypotonic urine (< 150 mosmol/l) daily. Treatment is by intramuscular injections of pitressin tannate or pituitrin snuff.

The suprarenal glands secrete aldosterone and cortisol (see Chapter 35). As described above, aldosterone conserves sodium ions at the expense of hydrogen and potassium ions in the kidney. Primary aldosteronism (Conn's syndrome) is usually caused by an adenoma of the adrenal cortex and less commonly by a carcinoma or hyperplasia (see Chapter 35). Secondary aldosteronism is more common, particularly in patients with hepatic or congestive cardiac failure. The loss of potassium and hydrogen ions produces a hypokalaemic alkalosis with hypernatraemia. The opposite disturbances may occur as a consequence of hypoaldosteronism from suprarenal failure.

Cortisol has profound effects upon substrate metabolism and has similar but weaker effects to those of aldosterone upon sodium, potassium and hydrogen ions. Unlike aldosterone, it stimulates the excretion of water. Excessive secretion of cortisol produces Cushing's syndrome with profound effects upon fluid and electrolyte homeostasis (see Chapter 35). In most patients, the concentration of the electrolytes is normal but the total body potassium content is reduced causing neuromuscular weakness. The total body calcium content is reduced with osteoporosis. In severe cases there is hypokalaemia and alkalosis. The syndrome may be the result of excessive corticotrophin release (see under anterior pituitary) or less commonly may result from ectopic corticotrophin such as secreted by an oat cell carcinoma of the bronchus (see Chapter 22) or by benign or malignant tumours of the suprarenal gland (see Chapter 35). Primary suprarenal failure may be from disease of the glands (Addison's disease) or a consequence of surgical removal. Secondary suprarenal failure may be a consequence of primary failure of the anterior pituitary gland. Excessive quantities of sodium and chloride ions are lost in the urine and there is hyponatraemia and hypochloraemia. Patients require treatment with cortisol and may require infusion of colloids and saline.

Calcitonin is secreted by the parafollicular cells (C cells) of the thyroid gland, lowering the serum concentration of calcium by reducing resorption of calcium from bone (see Chapter 19). It is

REFERENCES

14. Sheilds R Br J Surg 1965; 52: 774–779
15. Tweedle D E F Zeitschrift fur Gastroenterologie 1980; 16: 68–73
16. Nubiola-Calonge P, Badia J M, Sancho J et al Lancet 1987; 2: 672–674
17. Latta T Lancet 1831–2; ii: 243
18. Birzgalis A R, Tweedle D E F J Roy Coll Surg Edinb 1993; 38: 170–174

often released in excessive quantities in patients with medullary carcinoma of the thyroid.

The parathyroid gland secretes parathormone which controls the serum concentration of calcium and phosphorus as described above. Primary hyperparathyroidism is most commonly caused by an adenoma but may be the result of hyperplasia or carcinoma of the parathyroid glands (see Chapter 19). Secondary hyperparathyroidism may occur when there is persistent hypocalcaemia, usually in patients with chronic renal failure. In some patients this response to hypocalcaemia becomes autonomous and primary hyperparathyroidism develops. Some refer to this as tertiary hyperparathyroidism. The hypercalcaemia results in anorexia, constipation, hypertonia and mental depression. Later there is nephrocalcinosis, and renal failure may modify the biochemical findings. The treatment is surgical. Hypoparathyroidism is usually a transient phenomenon following operations upon the parathyroid and thyroid glands resulting in hypocalcaemia and hypomagnesaemia (see Chapter 19). Treatment is by intravenous and oral supplements until normal parathyroid function is restored.

The pancreas gland may be secondarily responsible for disturbances of fluid and electrolyte balance. In diabetes mellitus, the polyuria may be associated with a loss of sodium and potassium. There is usually dehydration caused by an osmotic diuresis from the glycosuria. This dehydration may be compounded by vomiting with further loss of potassium. In the absence of insulin, glucose utilization is depressed and large quantities of fat are utilized for energy. Keto-acids are formed and the serum bicarbonate concentration falls. The metabolic acidosis stimulates the exchange of extracellular hydrogen ions for intracellular potassium ions. Treatment is predominantly with isotonic saline to correct the dehydration, and insulin to restore the normal metabolism. Restoration of normal metabolism and renal function usually results in rapid correction of the acidosis, but if the serum bicarbonate concentration is less than 10 mmol/l or if the pH is less than 7.1 then sodium bicarbonate should be infused. The concentration of potassium in the serum varies greatly, reflecting exchange of potassium for hydrogen ions at the cellular interface, the contraction of the extracellular volume and the altered renal dynamics. The extracellular potassium concentration can fall dramatically and repeated estimations are required to monitor replacement therapy.

Postoperative patients

Major changes occur in metabolism following operations or injury.[19] These changes in metabolism are generalized and not confined to the injured tissue. They are a consequence of increases in the secretion of catabolic hormones, cortisol, glucagon and catecholamines[20–22] and a failure of insulin secretion in response to hyperglycaemia.[23] Changes in fluid and electrolyte metabolism after injury may be secondary to changes in substrate metabolism induced by the changes in the secretion of hormones.

Water

Following operation or injury there is retention of water as the result of the secretion of antidiuretic hormone.[24] The quantity of water retained is greater than is appropriate for the retention of sodium, and a concentrated urine may be excreted in the presence of a hypotonic plasma indicating that the secretion of antidiuretic hormone is not a secondary phenomenon as a consequence of the increased postoperative secretion of aldosterone (see below).

Sodium

Following operation or injury there is increased secretion of aldosterone[25] so that the urinary excretion of sodium falls to less than 25 mmol/d. The maximum retention of sodium occurs about the third or fourth day after injury but water retention is maximal on the first and second postoperative day.

Potassium

On the first day after injury or operation the urinary excretion of potassium increases to 100 mmol/d and usually begins to fall about the third day. Thus the maximal excretion of potassium and conservation of sodium are not coincidental and, in particular, potassium excretion cannot be entirely the result of the increased secretion of aldosterone (see above). The maximal increase in potassium excretion does not coincide with the maximal increase in the excretion of nitrogen as a consequence of post-traumatic protein catabolism. Furthermore, the potassium: nitrogen ratio in muscle is 2.5–3 mmol/g and the increased excretion of potassium and nitrogen after injury is at a ratio of 5–15 mmol/g. This 'differential intracellular depletion' should be compared with the 'balance depletion' with a normal potassium: nitrogen ratio that occurs during starvation.[26]

Postoperative fluid and electrolyte therapy

Most surgeons consider that this alteration in post-traumatic metabolism is inevitable and may be a homeostatic mechanism inherited from our animal predecessors. Retention of water and sodium were noted to be little influenced by postoperative infusion of up to 4 litres of saline.[27] Consequently, in the majority of patients postoperative intravenous infusion is usually restricted to 2 litres of water and 80 mmol of sodium daily in uncomplicated cases. However, following major injury or surgery there is evidence that many patients receive inadequate fluid replacement, particularly during operation, with resultant increased morbidity and mortality.[28] In the first 48 hours potassium is lost from the cells

REFERENCES

19. Cuthbertson D F Lancet 1942; i: 433
20. Dudley H A F, Robson J S, Smith M, Stewart C P Metabolism 1959; 8: 895–903
21. Walker W F Proc Roy Soc Med 1965; 58: 1015–1017
22. Meguid M M, Brennan M F Lancet 1974; i: 319
23. Allison S P, Prowse K, Chamberlain M J Lancet 1967; i: 478–481
24. Cline T M, Cole J W, Holden W D Surg Gynaecol Obstet 1953; 96: 674–676
25. Zimmerman B Surg Clin N Am 1965; 45: 299–315
26. Moore F D, Ball M R In: The Metabolic Response to Injury. Thomas, Springfield Illinois 1952 p 361
27. LeQuesne L P, Lewis A A G Lancet 1953; i: 153–158
28. Shoemaker W C, Appel P L, Kram H B, Waxman K, Tai-Shion L Chest 1988; 94: 1176–1186

but there is usually a normal or increased extracellular concentration so that potassium infusion at this time is unnecessary. By the third postoperative day, hypokalaemia may be evident and 50 mmol/d should be given. In most patients there is no requirement to give any other electrolytes in the postoperative period.

General therapy

As emphasized at the beginning of this section on fluid and electrolyte disorders, the body's homeostatic mechanisms are remarkably effective and in many patients restore normality with a little help. Thus, alkalosis caused by pyloric stenosis is corrected rapidly by the kidneys if the extracellular volume is restored by infusion of isotonic saline. The loss of potassium may however require replacement. The content of commonly used replacement solutions is shown in Table 2.6.

Glucose

Isotonic (5%) solutions of D-glucose (dextrose) provide water. The oxidation of the glucose produces 32 g of water. Thus infusion of 1 litre of isotonic glucose provides 1032 ml of water. Thirst usually indicates a deficit of at least 1.5 litres of water to restore normality in addition to the requirements for the coming day.

Electrolytes

Isotonic saline (0.9%) is the most commonly used solution for replacement of extracellular fluid. Hypertonic solutions are sometimes infused in patients with hyponatraemia. Most of these patients have excessive total body sodium content and the major proportion of this excess is in the interstitial space. The infused sodium usually rapidly diffuses into the interstitial space through the capillary membranes and many patients are made worse by such treatment. The chloride content of isotonic saline is greater than the normal extracellular concentration but the excess ions are usually excreted easily by the kidneys. Some clinicians prefer to restore extracellular volume by the use of Hartmann's solution in which the chloride concentration is similar to plasma and the required anion concentration is achieved by adding lactate. Ringer's lactate, which is modified Hartmann's solution, also contains chloride and lactate ions but a lower concentration of sodium and some potassium and calcium when compared with the standard Hartmann's solution. This solution comes closest to normal extracellular electrolyte content and hypokalaemia is less likely to develop. As deficiencies of electrolytes other than sodium, potassium and chloride are uncommon in surgical patients, solutions containing just these ions are the most popular and two are in common use, one being hypertonic. In patients who have lost large quantities of potassium, additional potassium chloride may be added to intravenous solutions. The concentration should not exceed 80 mmol/l and the infusion should not exceed 20 mmol/h. 150 mmol/d can be given if the plasma concentration does not exceed 3 mmol/l. The plasma concentration should be measured daily. Patients with diabetic acidosis and those being fed intravenously with hypertonic solutions of glucose require large quantities of potassium as the infused insulin stimulates cellular uptake.[29] Infusion of potassium should stop when the serum concentration reaches 5 mmol/l.

The concentration of ionized calcium falls following the removal of parathyroid tumours and sometimes following thyroidectomy resulting in tetany. This can be treated initially by infusion of a 10% solution of calcium gluconate (see Chapter 9). 100 ml may be required in the first 24 hours and the serum concentration should be monitored. Oral replacement is begun at the same time and restoration of homeostasis by increased secretion from the remaining glands usually occurs spontaneously within 2 weeks. Hypocalcaemia in patients with acute pancreatitis is predominantly the result of hypoalbuminaemia (see Chapter 33). It is usually symptomless and does not require treatment: normocalcaemia is restored as the albumin concentration improves. Hypomagnesaemia is rare but may occur in severely debilitated patients undergoing prolonged intravenous feeding with magnesium-free solutions. Magnesium chloride is usually prepared in the pharmacy as a molar solution. Its addition to other electrolyte and intravenous feeding solutions may result in the precipitation of complex salts and it is best to infuse 20 mmol/d by slow infusion in isotonic glucose solutions. Like hypokalaemia, hypophosphataemia may follow the infusion of large quantities of glucose and insulin. Severe hypophosphataemia prevents release of oxygen from erythrocytes.[30] During intravenous feeding, 15 mmol of inorganic phosphorus should be given with each 100 g (556 mmol) of glucose as KH_2PO_4, K_2HPO_4 or a mixture of the two.

In surgical patients with metabolic acidosis, the restoration of renal function by the re-expansion of extracellular volume is usually sufficient to achieve acid–base homeostasis unless the pH has fallen

REFERENCES

29. Hinton P, Allison S P, Littlejohn S, Lloyd J Lancet 1971; I: 767
30. Travis S F, Sugarman H J, Ruberg R L et al N Engl J Med 1971; 285: 763–768

Table 2.6 The content of intravenous replacement solutions (mmol/l)

Solution	*Glucose*	*Na*	*K*	*Ca*	*NH_4*	*Cl*	*HCO_3*	*Lactate*	*mosm/l*
D-glucose 5% (isotonic)	278	—	—	—	—	—	—	—	278
Sodium chloride 0.9% (isotonic)	—	154	—	—	—	154	—	—	308
Hartmann's solution	—	154	—	—	—	103	—	51	308
Ringer's lactate* (modified Hartmann's)	—	131	5	2	—	111	—	29	280
Sodium chloride 0.9% and potassium chloride 0.3%	150	40	—	—	190	—	—	380	—
Sodium bicarbonate 1.4% (1/6 molar)	—	167	—	—	—	—	167	—	334
Ammonium chloride 0.9% (1/6 molar)	—	—	—	—	167	167	—	—	334

*The original solution also contained a small quantity of magnesium to 7.1. It may be treated by the infusion of sodium bicarbonate and in severe lactic acidosis as much as 2500 mmol/d have been given. An 8.4% (molar) solution contains 1 mmol/ml of bicarbonate. Lactate ions are converted by a healthy liver into a similar number of bicarbonate ions and solutions containing lactate have no advantage over solutions of bicarbonate. In a healthy liver ammonium ions are converted to urea, releasing hydrogen and chloride ions, and this mechanism may be used in the treatment of alkalosis but, again in surgical patients, there is rarely a need for acidifying solutions, particularly if the plasma bicarbonate concentration does not reach 30 ml/l. Solutions of arginine hydrochloride act in a similar manner.

ACIDOSIS AND ALKALOSIS

An acid is a substance which donates hydrogen ions (protons), and a base accepts hydrogen ions. A strong acid gives up hydrogen ions readily and a strong base accepts hydrogen ions avidly. Hydrogen ion concentrations are very small and the acidity or alkalinity of a substance is expressed as pH, the negative logarithm of the hydrogen ion concentration, i.e. $1/\log [H^+]$. Acidaemia and alkalaemia are states in which the blood pH is abnormally low or high. The normal range is 7.35–7.45, which is equivalent to 45–35 nmolH^+/l body water. The range of viability is 6.8–7.7, which is equivalent to 160–20 nmolH^+/l body water. Extracellular and intracellular pH may differ considerably because hydrogen ions cannot cross cell membranes easily. Acidosis and alkalosis are terms used to denote pathological processes that have a tendency to produce acidaemia and alkalaemia respectively. Like other ions, the concentration of hydrogen ions in body tissues is dependent upon production, transport and elimination. The tendency for acidosis or alkalosis to produce acidaemia and alkalaemia in the body is greatly diminished by the existence of buffers which will be described in detail below.

HYDROGEN ION PRODUCTION

Each day about 30–80 mmol of hydrogen ions are produced from ingested food.[31] In a normal mixed diet oxidation of proteins produces small quantities of mineral (sulphuric and phosphoric) and organic (keto and uric) acids which are often referred to as non-respiratory acids. Complete oxidation of carbohydrate produces water and carbon dioxide, both of which are excreted without any influence upon acid–base balance. Under hypoxic conditions, cellular metabolism via the tricarboxylic acid cycle (Krebs cycle) ceases and pyruvic acid is converted to lactic acid. This is a common cause of metabolic acidosis in surgical patients. Similarly, incomplete oxidation of fats leads to the production of aceto-acetic and β-hydroxybutyric acids. In addition there is a potential daily production of 15 000 mmol of hydrogen ions in the form of carbon dioxide which is normally excreted by the lungs. If this pulmonary excretion is inadequate then carbon dioxide combines with water in the presence of the enzyme carbonic anhydrase, producing carbonic acid and potentially huge quantities of hydrogen ions:

$$CO_2 + H_2O \Leftrightarrow H_2CO_3 \Leftrightarrow H^+ + HCO_3^-$$

HYDROGEN ION EXCRETION

Renal excretion

The kidney regulates hydrogen ion excretion by several mechanisms. The renal tubule cells contain the enzyme carbonic anhydrase which allows the production of hydrogen and bicarbonate ions as described above. The bicarbonate ions can be reabsorbed into the plasma and the hydrogen ions are excreted in the urine. Every minute approximately 3 mmol of bicarbonate ions are filtered by the kidneys, but virtually all (more than 4000 mmol/d) is reabsorbed. The tubular cells also contain the enzyme glutaminase which breaks down the amino acid glutamine with the production of ammonia (NH_3), which is also produced by the oxidation of the amino acids glycine, alanine, leucine and aspartic acid. Ammonia accepts hydrogen ions to form ammonium ions (NH_4^+) which are exchanged for sodium ions in the tubular urine. Similarly, monohydrogen phosphate (HPO_4^{--}) accepts hydrogen ions and is excreted as dihydrogen phosphate ($H_2PO_4^-$). Hydrogen ions may also be exchanged directly with sodium ions in the renal tubules. Under physiological conditions, body metabolism produces excess hydrogen ions and these mechanisms assist hydrogen ion excretion without excessive changes in urine pH (see under Buffers, below). Normal urine pH is 5.5–6.5 and the urinary excretion of hydrogen ions is about 20–30 mmol/d. Disturbances of metabolism usually produce an even greater acidosis but, in uncommon alkalotic states, the mechanisms can work in reverse.

Pulmonary excretion

Carbon dioxide produced by cellular metabolism is converted to carbonic acid under the influence of carbonic anhydrase. Carbonic acid is transported to the lungs where the process is reversed and carbon dioxide is excreted. The potential acidosis that can be caused by failure of this homeostatic mechanism is much greater than that which results from failure of the renal mechanisms of acid–base homeostasis.

BUFFERS

In the reaction:

$$HB \Leftrightarrow H^+ + B^-$$

B^- is the conjugate base of the acid HB and HB is the conjugate acid of the base B^-.

The buffers in the body are weak acids in the presence of salts of strong conjugate bases. The bases temporarily combine with hydrogen ions to form weak acids which are transported to the

REFERENCES

31. Krück F Klin Wschr 1958; 36: 946

kidneys or lungs where the reaction is reversed, allowing hydrogen ions to be excreted by the kidneys and carbon dioxide by the lungs. The temporary combination with hydrogen ions to produce a weak acid produces a minimal alteration in extracellular pH. There are a number of buffers in the body but in the extracellular fluid the most important is the bicarbonate–carbonic acid system alluded to under hydrogen ion production.

$$H^+ + HCO_3^- \Leftrightarrow H_2CO_3 \Leftrightarrow H_2O + CO_2$$

Carbonic acid (H_2CO_3) is a weak acid which dissociates incompletely to hydrogen and bicarbonate (HCO_3^-) ions. At pH 7.4 the ratio of HCO_3^- to H_2CO_3 is 20:1. Extracellular hydrogen ion concentration is maintained predominantly by this buffer because of the potential for carbonic acid to dissociate also to water and carbon dioxide which can be excreted by the lungs. However, the hydrogen that is being buffered in this reaction requires similar quantities of bicarbonate ion. Bicarbonate ions are reabsorbed from the distal renal tubule so that it can be argued that hydrogen ion excretion is ultimately limited by the kidneys.

The next most important buffer system is the haemoglobin system:

$$H^+ + Hb^- \Leftrightarrow HHb$$

Reduced haemoglobin is a better buffer than oxyhaemoglobin. Thus venous blood, which must carry more hydrogen ions and carbon dioxide from the tissues, has a greater buffering capacity than arterial blood. Plasma proteins are also buffers but their buffering capacity is only about one sixth that of haemoglobin. Phosphoric acid, as described above, also contributes to the buffering capacity of the blood and extracellular fluid. Proteins and organic and inorganic phosphates are probably the principal intracellular buffers but, in routine practice, they cannot be measured. Thus, as with measurements of extracellular concentrations of ions, measurement of the acid–base status of the extracellular fluid may give a poor picture of the acid–base status within the cells. Indeed, it is theoretically possible for intracellular alkalosis to exist in the presence of extracellular acidosis.

CLINICAL DISORDERS

These are usually denoted by their primary origin from respiratory or metabolic causes. The latter are sometimes referred to as 'non-respiratory'.

Respiratory acidaemia

This is a consequence of carbon dioxide retention with an arterial concentration greater than 6.0 kPa; the common causes are shown in Table 2.7. There is an increase in pCO_2 and a fall in pH (Table 2.12). Ultimately there is renal compensation when the plasma bicarbonate concentration increases and an acid urine is excreted so that the pH can be restored to near normal. The increase in arterial concentration of carbon dioxide stimulates the respiratory centre, and tachypnoea is a feature in patients whose respiration is not depressed by drugs or cerebral injury. There is usually peripheral vasodilatation. There may be impaired consciousness with involuntary twitching. In severe cases the patient becomes delirious and passes into a coma.

Table 2.7 Causes of respiratory acidosis

Respiratory depression
Head injury, coma, cerebral tumours, cerebrovascular accidents
Drugs—opiates, anaesthetics, sedatives
Abdominal distension
Impaired gaseous exchange
Impaired muscular activity—poliomyelitis, polyneuritis, myasthenia gravis, thoracic injury
Obstructive airway disease—asthma, tracheal compression, bronchitis, bronchial tumours
Alveolar disease—pneumonia, adult respiratory distress syndrome, pulmonary fibrosis

Metabolic acidaemia (non-respiratory acidaemia)

This is a consequence of increased production or inadequate excretion of hydrogen ions or of an excessive loss of base. The causes are shown in Table 2.8 and, as discussed above, the most common cause is hypoxia and sepsis which results in incomplete oxidation of substrates in the tricarboxylic acid cycle. In established acidaemia renal excretion of hydrogen ions may reach 700 mmol/d, the lowest urinary pH being 4.6, when all the phosphate buffer is present as dihydrogen phosphate. Plasma pH and bicarbonate concentrations fall (Table 2.12). The fall in extracellular pH stimulates brainstem chemoreceptors and the lungs attempt to compensate by hyperventilation to increase the excretion of carbon dioxide to restore pH to normal. When acidaemia is mild there are few symptoms but the patient may complain of lethargy, nausea and loss of appetite. When severe, cardiac output is reduced with hypotension in spite of vasoconstriction. The increased hydrogen ion concentration stimulates the respiratory centre so that the patient breathes deeply and frequently; the so-called 'air hunger' or Kussmaul respiration. Ultimately there may be impaired consciousness and coma.

Respiratory alkalaemia

This is produced by a reduction in the arterial concentration of carbon dioxide lower than 4.7 kPa (Table 2.11). Ultimately there is

Table 2.8 Causes of metabolic acidosis

Excessive production of hydrogen ions
Uncontrolled diabetes mellitus
Lactic acidosis
Septicaemia
Starvation
Impaired excretion of hydrogen ions
Renal failure (acute or chronic)
Adrenal insufficiency
Excessive loss of base
Intestinal, biliary and pancreatic fistulae
Diarrhoea
Uretero-colic anastomosis

Table 2.9 Causes of respiratory alkalosis

Stimulation of respiratory centre
High altitude
Pneumonia, pneumothorax, pulmonary embolism, adult respiratory distress syndrome
Fever
Head injury
Salicylate poisoning
Increased alveolar gaseous exchange
Anxiety, pain, hysteria
IPPV

a compensatory decrease in plasma bicarbonate concentration. The causes are shown in Table 2.9. It should be noted that some causes are common to both respiratory acidaemia and respiratory alkalaemia. Thus, adult respiratory distress syndrome can produce an acidosis by its interference with gaseous exchange within the alveoli but can also produce an alkalosis from its stimulant effect upon ventilation. The majority of patients who are tachypnoeic are breathing more rapidly to excrete excessive quantities of carbon dioxide to compensate for metabolic acidosis. The major symptoms are increased excitability of the peripheral and central nervous systems because of a fall in hydrogen ion concentration. Patients may develop frank or latent tetany, demonstrable by a positive Chvostek's or Trousseau's sign.

Metabolic alkalaemia (non-respiratory alkalaemia)

This is the result of excessive loss of hydrogen ions or retention of base. The plasma pH and bicarbonate concentrations are both increased. The increase in extracellular pH reduces the stimulation for ventilation via the brainstem chemoreceptors, but the compensatory production of a respiratory acidosis with an increase in pCO_2 is not usually very marked. The causes are shown in Table 2.10. In surgical practice vomiting or nasogastric aspiration of acidic gastric juice is the most important and common cause. Potassium is also lost when gastrointestinal loss is prolonged, and severe and hypokalaemic alkalosis occurs. There may then be paradoxical excretion of an acid urine when hydrogen ions are exchanged for potassium ions in the renal tubules in an attempt to preserve extracellular potassium concentration. Excessive intake of antacids such as aluminium hydroxide and sodium bicarbonate in patients with peptic ulceration used to be a potent cause of alkalosis, particularly when there was consequent pyloric stenosis and vomiting of acid. The milk–alkali syndrome is now uncommon because acid suppression is usually induced by proton-pump inhibitors and H_2 antagonists. Clinically, metabolic alkalaemia produces few signs or symptoms but, like respiratory alkalaemia, there may be increased irritability of the peripheral and central nervous systems as the result of the reduction in hydrogen in concentration. The patient may complain of numbness and paraesthesiae and there may be latent and frank tetany. Unlike respiratory alkalaemia, it usually results in slow shallow respirations because of depression of the respiratory centre by the reduced hydrogen ion concentration. An alkaline pH shifts the oxygen dissociation curve to the left, interfering with oxygen release in the tissues.

Table 2.10 Causes of metabolic alkalosis

Excessive loss of hydrogen ions
Vomiting, nasogastric aspiration, gastric fistula
Diuretic therapy, Cushing's syndrome, primary aldosteronism
Hypokalaemia
Excessive intake of base
Antacids

DIAGNOSIS

The many causes of acid–base disturbance are shown in Tables 2.7–2.10 and are discussed above. In some patients the cause is very evident, in others less so. A careful clinical history and examination should indicate whether the primary disturbance is metabolic or respiratory. In clinical practice the majority of patients present a mixed picture because secondary changes are present to compensate for the primary disturbance. Thus, in metabolic disturbances alterations in respiratory rate partially compensate for changes in pH by reducing or increasing carbon dioxide excretion. Similarly, if there is a primary respiratory disturbance, alterations in the renal tubular excretion and reabsorption of bicarbonate produce some degree of compensation. In all these situations compensation is never complete. The diagnosis is usually confirmed biochemically by measurements of arterial pH, bicarbonate concentration and pO_2 and pCO_2. When arterial blood is sent for these analyses, a measurement of the amount of bicarbonate buffer in the extracellular fluid, the so-called base excess, is computed.[32] If there is too little, then there is a base deficit. The normal values for these measurements are shown in Table 2.11 and the changes observed in the uncompensated and compensated disturbances are shown in Table 2.12.[33] The majority of patients demonstrate compensation. In primary metabolic disturbances, the major change is in the bicarbonate concentration, and in respiratory disturbances the major change is in the pCO_2 concentration. Analysis of the urine should always be performed. Urine is usually acid but in patients with acidaemia the pH is usually less than 6. In alkalaemia the pH is usually greater than 7.4, but in patients with pyloric stenosis there may be a paradoxical acid urine due to hypokalaemia as described above. The urine may also reveal underlying pathology producing the acid–base disturbance such as unsuspected diabetes or renal diseases.

Calculation of the anion gap may help to differentiate various causes of metabolic acidaemia. Within the extracellular fluid there must be electroneutrality and the sum of the anions must be the same as the cations. In routine laboratory estimations only the concentrations of sodium, potassium, chloride and bicarbonate are measured. In normal individuals sodium and potassium account for more than 95% of the cations but chloride and bicarbonate ions account for a considerably lower proportion of total anion content. There is an apparent gap in the total anion content which represents protein (particularly albumin), organic acids, phosphate and

REFERENCES

32. Astrup P, Siggard-Andersen O Advanc Clin Chem 1963; 6: 1
33. Lyons J H Jr, Moore F D Surgery 1966; 60: 93

Table 2.11 Arterial acid–base measurements—normal values

pH	7.35–7.45
pO_2 (kPa)	10.7–16.0
pCO_2 (kPa)	4.7–6.0
HCO_3 (mmol/l)	22–26
Base excess (mmol/l)	–2 – +2
Anion gap (mmol)	10–14

Table 2.12 Acid–base measurements—clinical disturbances

	Uncompensated			*Compensated*		
Primary disturbance	*pH*	*pCO_2*	*HCO_3^-*	*pH*	*pCO_2*	*HCO_3^-*
Metabolic acidaemia	↓↓	Normal	↓↓	↓	↓	↓
Respiratory acidaemia	↓↓	↑↑	Normal	↓	↑↑	↓
Metabolic alkalaemia	↑↑	Normal	↑↑	↑	↑	↑
Respiratory alkalaemia	↑↑	↓↓	Normal	↑	↓↓	↓

sulphate anions.[34] Changes in the extracellular concentration of potassium ions are relatively small, so that the anion gap (AG) can be calculated by:

$$AG = [Na^+] - ([CL^-] + [HCO_3^-])$$

The normal range is 10–14 mmol/l. Increased anion gap is due to an increase in the organic anions discussed above and occurs in starvation, diabetic acidosis, lactic acidosis, alcoholic poisoning and renal failure. Metabolic acidaemia with a normal anion gap is usually associated with loss of plasma bicarbonate due to diarrhoea, fistulae or renal tubular acidosis. Although bicarbonate ions are lost there is retention of a similar quantity of chloride so there is no change in the anion gap.

TREATMENT

As emphasized above under the treatment of electrolyte disturbances, effective treatment of the primary patho-logy often enables the body's normal physiological mechanisms to restore normality. If the acid–base disturbance is severe then direct treatment to correct this disturbance is required.

Metabolic acidaemia

The requirement is for bicarbonate, and the quantity can be calculated[35] from the equation:

$$\text{Base deficit (mmol/l)} \times 0.3 \text{ body weight (kg)} = \text{mmol sodium bicarbonate}$$

In most patients, the calculated amount of bicarbonate should be infused over a minimum of 4 hours as more rapid infusion may produce tetany. Simultaneous rehydration often improves the acidaemia by normal physiological processes described above. Thus in a few patients the calculated amount may prove to be too much and the patient may be rendered alkalotic.

Sodium bicarbonate solutions are usually available in two strengths: 8.4% contains 1 mmol bicarbonate/ml and 2.54% contains 0.3 mmol/ml so that a 70 kg patient with a base deficit of 10 mmol/l requires $10 \times 0.3 \times 70 = 210$ ml of 8.4% sodium bicarbonate or 200/0.3 (700) ml of 2.54% sodium bicarbonate. The choice of solution is determined by other clinical factors. The molar solution of bicarbonate may tend to induce a hyperosmolar state as each mmol of bicarbonate is accompanied by a mmol of sodium, but patients with cardiac failure may not be able to withstand the rapid infusion of the 0.3 molar solution in quantities required to restore acid–base balance. Alkali may also be given as sodium lactate solution, the lactate ion ultimately being oxidized to pyruvate. Lactate infusion is obviously contraindicated in patients with lactic acidosis. Whichever solution is chosen, infusion of alkaline solutions may be dangerous in patients with coexistent hypokalaemia as the cardiac effects of the hypokalaemia are potentiated and cardiac arrest may occur. In severe metabolic acidosis, up to 200 mmol of bicarbonate may be given in 2 hours but in most patients 500 mmol/d is sufficient. Patients with severe acidosis require regular monitoring and treatment in an intensive therapy unit. Biochemical analysis of acid–base status should be performed hourly until a satisfactory state is achieved.

Respiratory acidaemia

In patients with acute respiratory acidaemia the requirement is to improve either mechanical ventilation or intrapulmonary gas exchange or both. In the majority of surgical patients this entails intermittent positive pressure ventilation in an intensive care unit (Chapter 5). In some patients it is sufficient to administer oxygen in the ward by means of a face-mask, but there is a potential danger in a small group of patients with severe chronic obstructive airway disease in whom there may be pre-existing chronic retention of carbon dioxide. In these patients the respiratory centre becomes unresponsive to alterations in arterial carbon dioxide concentrations and is stimulated by a decrease in arterial oxygen concentration. Inhalation of oxygen may remove this anoxic stimulus, with fatal consequences.

Metabolic alkalaemia

It is rarely necessary to treat metabolic alkalosis unless there is frank tetany. If renal function is adequate it is unusual to develop a base deficit greater than 5 mmol/l. Rapid, temporary improvement can be achieved by increasing the arterial carbon dioxide concentration by rebreathing into a bag. If considered necessary, arginine hydrochloride can be infused. The requirement is calculated in a similar manner to that for sodium bicarbonate in metabolic acidosis:

$$\text{Base excess (mmol/l)} \times 0.3 \text{ body weight (kg)} = \text{mmol arginine hydrochloride}$$

REFERENCES

34. Nairns R G, Emmett M Clinical use of the anion gap. Medicine 1997; 56: 38–54
35. Mellemgaard K, Astrup P J Clin Lab Invest 1960; 12: 187–199

A molar solution of arginine hydrochloride contains 20 g/100 ml.

Respiratory alkalaemia

If the patient exhibits frank tetany then rapid and temporary treatment in a conscious patient can be instituted by rebreathing into a bag. Severe cases caused by anxiety or hysteria may require treatment with sedatives, but care must be taken not to depress respiration.

ENTERAL AND PARENTERAL NUTRITION

Homeostasis

The daily energy requirement of a healthy 70 kg male who has a sedentary occupation is about 7.5 MJ. This may be provided by protein and carbohydrates like glucose which provide 17 kJ/g, and fats which provide 39 kJ/g.

Protein only supplies energy after it has been oxidized and cannot then be utilized as a synthetic source of essential body components. Every day protein is lost from the body in the form of secretions, by desquamation of skin and mucosa and following breakdown and oxidation. Sometimes it is used for gluconeogenesis. Approximately 70 g of protein is required daily to replace this loss. Proteins are complex molecules built from many amino acids.[36] There are about 300 amino acids in nature, but human proteins are made from 21 amino acids shown in Table 2.13. The first 10 amino acids cannot be synthesized in a healthy individual and must be included in the diet. They are usually termed 'essential amino acids'. The other amino acids can be synthesized in the healthy body by amination or transamination but this may not be possible in patients with severe sepsis[37] or injury.[38]

Carbohydrate is mainly ingested in the form of starch with smaller quantities of monosaccharides such as glucose and fructose. Whatever the source, the majority of carbohydrate from food reaches peripheral organs as glucose, and its utilization requires the action of insulin. Any glucose produced in excess of the body's immediate requirements is stored initially as glycogen in the liver and muscles; when these stores are replete, further excess is deposited as triglyceride in fat depots.

The other major source of energy in the diet is fat, which has a very high energy content. Fats are esters of fatty acids and glycerol (triglycerides). Glycerol is common to all fats but the fatty acids show considerable variation and may be divided into short, medium or long chain fatty acids according to the length of their carbon chain (Table 2.14). Some, such as stearic acid, are completely saturated with hydrogen, but others, such as linoleic and linolenic, are unsaturated with double-bond carbon linkages. Animals are unable to synthesize fatty acids such as linoleic and linolenic acid which have double-bond carbon linkages proximal to the ninth carbon atom in the chain. Fatty acids that cannot be synthesized by man must be included in the diet and are termed 'essential fatty acids'.[39] Structural fat contained in cell membranes and in the grey matter of the brain is composed predominantly of polyunsaturated, long chain (18–22 carbon atoms) fatty acids.

Table 2.13 Amino acids found in human protein

*Essential**	*Non-essential**
Isoleucine	Alanine
Leucine	Aspartic acid
Lysine	Citrulline
Histidine	Cysteine/cystine
Threonine	Glutamic acid/glutamine
Methionine	Glycine
Tyrosine	Ornithine
Arginine	Proline
Valine	Serine
Phenylalanine	Tryptophane

*see text

Table 2.14 Fatty acids in ingested triglycerides

	Carbon chain length	*Examples*
Short chain	Less than 6	Butyric acid (4 C)
Medium chain	6–12	Caprylic acid (8 C)
		Capric acid (10 C)
Long chain	More than 12	Palmitic acid (16 C)
		Stearic acid (18 C)

Depot fat within the cells of the subcutaneous fat and omentum is composed predominantly of saturated fatty acids of varying chain lengths.

Malnutrition

Malnutrition implies that nourishment is consistently less than requirements. This deficiency may be highly specific or general. The latter is often referred to as protein–energy malnutrition, but this term has no exact definition. Severe malnutrition has always been endemic and epidemic in parts of Africa: the terms kwashiorkor and marasmus originate from here. The association between malnutrition and an increased susceptibility to infection has also long been appreciated and in developing countries is responsible for much morbidity and a high mortality. Less severe malnutrition has also been identified in hospital patients in the USA[40] and in the United Kingdom,[41] where it remains an important problem.[42] It is more common in long stay patients and in those with malignant disease and those who have had major abdominal operations. The contribution of malnutrition to morbidity and mortality in these patients is far less easy to quantify.

Starvation

When Benedict[43] investigated the effects of starvation in a healthy male volunteer, he found that as the subject lost weight there was a

REFERENCES

36. Rose W C Fed Proc 1949; 8: 546
37. Groves A C, Woolf L I, Allardyce B D Surg Forum 1974; 25: 54
38. Dale G, Young G, Latner A L, Goode A W, Tweedle D E F, Johnson I D A Surgery 1977; 81: 295
39. Burr G O, Burr M M J Biol Chem 1930; 86: 587
40. Bistrian B R, Blackburn G L et al JAMA 1974; 230: 858–860
41. Hill G L, Blackett R L, Pickford L et al Lancet 1977; i: 689–692
42. McWhirter J P, Pennington C R Br Med J 1994; 308: 945–948
43. Benedict F G A Study of Prolonged Fasting. Carnegie Institute of Washington, Washington 1915

concomitant decrease in oxygen consumption, respiratory quotient and the urinary excretion of nitrogen (reflecting protein breakdown). This was associated with an increase in the urinary excretion of β-hydroxybutyrate and aceto-acetate formed by the oxidation of fatty acids. These changes are indicative of a diminution in the contribution of protein and an increase in the contribution of fat to the metabolic fuel. Subsequent studies using more sophisticated methods have confirmed these findings and demonstrated the mechanisms involved.[44–46] Tissues such as the brain and the bone marrow which normally prefer glucose as a substrate respond to starvation by increased utilization of ketone bodies. Cahill[44] has estimated that after a few days of starvation the total daily glucose requirement falls to 80 g/d, produced mainly by gluconeogenesis from protein in both the liver and kidney. Thus protein breakdown is reduced from 75 g/d in early starvation to 20 g/d in late starvation. The quantity of fat that is burnt increases from 160 g/d to only 180 g/d because total energy requirement is reduced in prolonged starvation.

Post-traumatic metabolism

The response to injury differs quantitatively and qualitatively when compared with simple starvation alone. Following injury there is a fall in the secretion of the anabolic hormone insulin and an increase in the secretion of the catabolic hormones cortisol, glucagon and the catechol amines.[47–50] It is probably the effect of the catabolic hormones which is of greater importance because gluconeogenesis from starvation is inhibited by the infusion of small quantities of glucose but, after injury, infusion of even large quantities of glucose with insulin does not have a major effect upon intermediary metabolism.

Following injury there is an increased expenditure of energy.[51,52] The increase is usually modest except in patients with burns and sepsis (Table 2.15), and in the great majority of patients undergoing uncomplicated operations there is very little change in total energy requirements. This response to injury is reduced in patients who are nutritionally impoverished before injury, but it is also known that morbidity and mortality is particularly severe in these patients[53] and this has been subsequently confirmed.[54]

Table 2.15 Protein and energy loss in health, starvation and injury

	Protein loss		*Energy loss*	
	g N/d	*g/d*	*MJ/d*	*kcal/d*
Health	11	70	7.5	1800
Early starvation	9	55	6.7	1600
Late starvation	7	45	5.2	1250
Cholecystectomy	12	75	7.5	1800
Pancreatectomy	16	100	8.4	2000
Oesophago-gastrectomy	14	90	8.4	2000
Small bowel fistula (without sepsis)	20	125	8.0	1900
Ulcerative colitis (severe)	30	190	9.0	2150
Peritonitis	18	110	9.0	2150
Typhoid fever	30	190	10.5	2500
Burns				
0–25%	20	125	11.3	2700
25–50%	25	155	13.2	3150
50–75%	30	190	15.1	3600
Respiratory failure and sepsis	18	110	11.7	2800
Renal failure and sepsis	20	125	11.7	2800
Simple fracture	14	90	8.8	2100

Nutritional assessment

The confirmation that morbidity and mortality were related to nutritional impoverishment stimulated considerable investigation to identify those patients at risk more precisely and at an earlier stage. In addition to estimations of skeletal muscle protein, which can be derived from measurements of arm circumference and subcutaneous fat using skin fold calipers,[55] others have emphasized the importance of so-called visceral proteins.[56] Much effort was spent attempting to identify an individual substance which would act as an independent index of malnutrition. Traditionally, albumen has been used as such an index and it can be useful if it is estimated over a period of weeks. However, it has a biological half-life of about 2–3 weeks and its concentration in the blood is affected by changes in hydration. Other proteins such as transferrin, prealbumin and retinol binding protein have shorter half-lives (8 days, 2 days and 12 hours respectively) and are more sensitive indicators of subclinical protein depletion.[57] Even when hypoproteinaemia is identified, it must be remembered that there are many causes. In one patient it may reflect simple inadequacy of normal intake while in another it can be the result of lack of synthesis within a diseased liver. A third category is patients with excessive loss of protein from the renal or gastrointestinal tract. The consequences of the same depletion of skeletal and visceral proteins in each of these patients may be quite different. In an attempt to obtain a more balanced assessment of nutritional depletion throughout the body, others have combined individual indices and calculated an overall index.[58] This has also proved to be too insensitive for everyday use in identifying patients who required nutritional support but these indices are of value in categorizing the severity of malnutrition within groups of patients who are entered into clinical trials. For many years clinicians had relied upon a careful clinical examination to assess nutritional status, noting reduced tissue turgor, muscle wasting (particularly of the interossei and intercostal muscles), a weak grip, sunken eyes and mental apathy. A careful clinical assessment by an experienced clinician has been shown to be as accurate in identifying malnutrition and its consequences as the numerous indices discussed above.[59]

REFERENCES

44. Cahill G F, Herrera M G, Morgan A P et al J Clin Invest 1966; 45: 1751
45. Owen O E, Morgan A P, Kemp H G, Sullivan J M, Herrera M G, Cahill G F Jr J Clin Invest 1967; 46: 1589
46. Cahill G F N Engl J Med 1970; 282: 668
47. Dudley H A F, Robson J S, Smith M, Stewart C P Metabolism 1959; 8: 895
48. Walker W F, Zileil M S, Reutter F W, Shoemaker W C, Moore F D Am J Physiol 1959; 197: 773
49. Wilmore D W, Lindsey C A, Moylan J A, Faloona G R, Pruitt B A Jr, Unger R H Lancet 1974; 1: 73
50. Allison S P, Hinton P, Chamberlain M J Lancet 1968; 2: 1113
51. Kinney J M, Duke J H, Long C L, Gump F E J Clin Pathol 1970; 234(suppl.): 65
52. Tweedle D E F, Johnson I D A Br J Surg 1971; 58: 771
53. Studley H O JAMA 1936; 106: 458
54. Bistrian B R, Blackburn G L, Hallowell E, Heddle R JAMA 1974; 230: 858–860
55. Frisancho A R Am J Clin Nutr 1974; 27: 1052–1058
56. Bistrian B R, Blackburn G L Fed Proc 1974; 33: 691
57. Young G A, Hill G L Am J Clin Nutr 1981; 34: 166–172
58. Hobbiss J H, Buxton A, Gallagher P, Roberts C, Tweedle D E F Clin Nutr 1984; 3 (4): 227–230
59. Jeejeebhoy K N Curr Opin Gastroenterol 1988; 4: 306–314

NUTRITION IN DISEASE

Immunocompetence

It has been known for many years that malnutrition results in impaired immune function.[60] Cell mediated immunity is affected earlier and to a greater extent than humoral immunity. As specific tests of immune function were developed, it became evident that both T and B lymphocyte function were impaired and there was a generalized lymphopenia in malnourished patents.[61] Delayed cutaneous hypersensitivity is frequently found in malnourished patients.[62] This phenomenon is often associated with increased morbidity and mortality. Some of the specific deficiencies in immunocompetence, including cutaneous hypersensitivity, can be restored by nutritional repletion,[63,64] associated with an improved clinical outcome. However, alterations in immunocompetence may also have been due to sepsis or the effects of the underlying disease which were treated concomitantly.

Hepatic disease

The majority of protein synthesis in the body occurs in the liver; as a consequence, patients with liver disease are frequently hypoproteinaemic. Unfortunately, these patients are intolerant of protein and inappropriate ingestion or infusion may cause hepatic encephalopathy. It has been suggested that this encephalopathy is mainly a consequence of alteration in the concentrations of the neurotransmitters dopamine and noradrenaline and their replacement by false neurotransmitters such as octopamine and phenylethanolamine from alterations in the concentrations of individual amino acids.[65] The aromatic amino acids tyrosine, phenylalanine and tryptophane are important precursors in the synthesis of neurotransmitters. In patients and experimental animals with hepatic encephalopathy there is decreased hepatic clearance of these aromatic amino acids with an increased concentration in the plasma. Hepatic breakdown of insulin is also decreased and it is believed that the increased concentration of this hormone in the periphery produces increased catabolism of the branches chain amino acids valine, leucine and isoleucine in skeletal muscle. It is believed that the alteration in the ratio of the aromatic amino acids and the branched chain amino acids in the plasma induces the formation of false neurotransmitters.[66] It has subsequently been demonstrated that hepatic encephalopathy can be improved by infusions of amino acid solutions containing large quantities of branched chain amino acids and very small quantities of aromatic amino acids.[67] Unfortunately, although manipulation of plasma amino acid concentrations is a useful adjunct in patients with hepatic disease, particularly in the acute phase, it has no influence upon the progress of the hepatic pathology and the ultimate clinical outcome (see Chapter 31).

Renal failure

More than half of patients undergoing haemodialysis or chronic ambulatory peritoneal dialysis are severely malnourished.[68] The great majority are hypoalbuminaemic; morbidity and the need for admission to hospital are related to deficient protein metabolism. Patients with acute or chronic renal failure require a normal intake of protein but unfortunately retain the nitrogenous end-products of protein metabolism (urea, creatinine and uric acid). When attempts were made to reduce the production of nitrogenous waste by diets low in protein and high in carbohydrate which were designed to reduce the requirement for gluconeogenesis from protein, it was found that protein catabolism still occurred at rates in excess of 100 g/d and the patient's muscle mass wasted at an alarming rate.[69] Urea can be used as a source of nitrogen in the synthesis of non-essential amino acids: in the pre-dialysis era this mechanism was used in the treatment of patients with chronic renal failure, patients being given minimum daily requirements of essential amino acids with a high carbohydrate intake—the Giordano–Giovannetti diet.[70,71] A similar approach uses parenteral infusion of solutions containing essential amino acids and glucose in patients with acute renal failure, with improved survival.[72] In countries where dialysis is readily available, these therapeutic diets are of little importance. It should not be forgotten, however, that between 9 and 12 g of amino acids are removed by 4 hours of haemodialysis.[73] Even greater amounts may be lost during peritoneal dialysis.

Malignant disease

The cachexia associated with cancer is the result of a reduction in all body proteins (visceral and skeletal) and the fat stores. This cachexia can occur in patients who have tumours that do not involve the gastrointestinal tract. Such patients often lose the sensation of taste and are anorexic. Their resting energy expenditure is sometimes slightly increased but it is apparent that this cachexia cannot be explained on the simple basis of either decreased intake or increased energy expenditure. It has been postulated that tumours may directly affect intermediary metabolism, and much effort has been spent in attempting to identify the substances responsible.[74] Nearly half of adult cancer patients in hospital have lost 10% of their body weight and a quarter have lost 20% or more. Several studies have shown that preoperative weight loss of 15% or more is associated with higher postoperative morbidity and mortality in a

REFERENCES

60. Cannon P R Protein Metabolism 1945; 128: 360
61. Chandra R K Br Med Bull 1981; 37: 89–94
62. Twomey P, Ziegler D, Rombeau J L JPEN 1982; 6: 50–57
63. Law D K, Dudrick S J, Abdou N I Ann Intern Med 1973; 79: 545
64. Haffejee A A, Anghorn I B, Brain P P, Duursma J, Baker L W Br J Surg 1978; 65: 480
65. Fischer J E, Baldessarini R J Lancet 1971; 2: 75
66. Fischer J E, Funovics J M, Aguirre A et al Surgery 1975; 78: 276
67. Fischer J E, Rosen H M, Ebeid A M, James J H, Keane J M, Soeters P B Surgery 1976; 80: 77
68. Markmann P Clin Nephrol 1988; 29: 75
69. Lee H A, Sharpstone P, Ames A C Postgrad Med J 1967; 43: 81
70. Giordano C J Lab Clin Med 1963; 62: 231
71. Giovannetti S, Maggiore Q Lancet 1964; 1: 1000
72. Abel R M, Beck C H, Abbott W M, Ryan J A, Barnett G O & Fischer J E N Engl J Med 1973; 288: 695
73. Kopple J D, Jones M, Fukuda S et al Amino acid and protein metabolism in renal failure. Am J Clin Nutr 1978; 31: 1532–1540
74. Editorial: Cancer cachexia Lancet 1984; 1: 833–834

variety of gastrointestinal tumours.[53,75,76] There is debate concern-ing the merits of preoperative nutritional restoration and delayed surgical intervention.[76–79] There is no evidence that, in the majority of patients, nutritional therapy has any influence upon clinical outcome.[80] A few severely malnourished patients may not survive major resections and in these patients it may be worthwhile to delay operation until nutritional repletion has been completed.

Patient selection

There are few patients in whom the indication for nutritional support is absolute. Nutritional support is required in any patient who is unable to ingest enough food to satisfy normal requirements, particularly resting energy expenditure, if a period of starvation is likely to be detrimental. The majority of these patients have gastrointestinal disease. Some patients with burns or severe sepsis are unable to eat sufficient food to satisfy their greatly increased resting energy requirements. The details in Table 2.16 are taken from a 2-year survey of gastroenterological practice in a teaching hospital.[81] The number of patients requiring nutritional support in a general surgical practice in a district general hospital will be considerably less. This table also shows the relative use of enteral and intravenous routes of nutritional support.

ROUTES OF NUTRITIONAL SUPPORT

Enteral feeding

Utilization of substrates is always more efficient when these are given enterally rather than parenterally (intravenously). Nutrients infused into the gastrointestinal tract also have an important trophic effect upon the mucosa and may be given in the immediate postoperative period.[82] Furthermore, the enteral route is safer, avoiding potentially life-threatening complications that may occur with parenteral nutrition.[83] If the gastrointestinal tract is intact, the simplest method of delivering nutrients to its lumen is to ask the patient to drink or eat them. Many severely ill patients are anorexic, particularly those with malignant disease. Some have obstruction in the upper part of the gastrointestinal tract, but even these may be able to swallow partially liquidized food or liquid nutrients. 'Sip feeding' throughout the day may allow sufficient nutrients to be taken. Nutrients must be given by some form of tube if the patient is unable for some reason or other to ingest sufficient nutrients but the gastrointestinal function is otherwise adequate.

Naso-enteral feeding

The standard Ryle's tubes used for nasogastric aspiration after operation harden on contact with digestive juices and are unsuitable for naso-enteral feeding. Naso-enteral tubes should be made of pliable polyurethane or Silastic and may be coated with a special lubricant that maintains a slippery surface. Even then irritation of the nasopharynx or distal oesophagus is common. Fine-bore tubes with an internal diameter of 1 mm have been developed but not all enteral nutrient solutions can be infused through them.[84] These tubes should be radiopaque or have a radiopaque marker at the distal end so that this can be identified. The development of better systems for gastrostomy and jejunostomy,[85] particularly when performed percutaneously, has greatly reduced the requirements for naso-enteral feeding.

Insertion

The patient must be able to breathe adequately through one nostril before the tube is inserted and should be allowed to feel the pliability of the tube to be inserted. The patient is sat upright and the lubricated tube is inserted gently in a horizontal plane (not upwards) into the nasopharynx. The tube should then be pushed gently and rotated as the patient swallows. Some patients prefer to

REFERENCES

75. Mullen J L, Buzby G P, Matthews D C, Smale B F, Rosato E F Ann Surg 1980; 192: 604–613
76. Müller J M, Brenner U, Dienst C, Pilchmaier H Lancet 1982; i: 68–71
77. Moghissi K, Hornshaw J, Teasdale P F, Dawes E A Brit J Surg 1977; 64: 125–839
78. Holter A R, Fischer H E J Surg Res 1977; 23: 31–34
79. Heatley R V, Williams R H P, Lewis M H Postgrad Med J 1979; 55: 541–545
80. Daly J M, Redmond H P, Lieberman M D, Jardines L Surg Clin N Am 1991; 71, 3: 523–536
81. Tweedle D E F In: Metabolic Care. Churchill Livingstone, Edinburgh 1982 p 166
82. Carr C S, Ling K D E, Boulos P, Singer M Brit Med J 1996; 312: 869–871
83. Souba W W Brit Med J 1996; 321: 684
84. Jones B M Gut 1986; 27: S1, 47–50
85. Ponsky J L, Gauderer M W L, Stellato T A Arch Surg 1983; 118: 913–914

Table 2.16 The site of disease and route of infusion in patients requiring nutritional support

Site	*Total*	*Benign*	*Malignant*	*Enteral*	*Parenteral*	*Total**	*%*
Oesophagus	56	47	9	5	2	7	12.5
Stomach	114	64	50	5	5	10	8.8
Duodenum	96	95	1	1	6	6	6.3
Biliary system	200	191	9	3	8	8	4.0
Pancreas	87	62	25	9	17	19	21.8
Large bowel	277	232	45	5	1	6	2.2
	830	691	139	28	39	57	6.9

*Some patients received nutritional support by enteral and parental routes

swallow the tube with sips of water sucked through a straw. The tube should have external markings: insertion of 50 cm is usually sufficient for infusion into the stomach, but approximately 75 cm is required to reach the duodenum. Occasionally, a fine-bore naso-enteral tube may be inadvertently inserted into the trachea without any reaction from a conscious patient. A small quantity of air should be introduced using a syringe and the patient's abdomen auscultated to ensure that the tube is in the gut. Gastrointestinal fluid may be aspirated for further confirmation. Metal markers on the distal end of some tubes allow radiological confirmation that the tube is within the abdominal cavity before beginning infusion. If a tube cannot be passed through an oesophageal stricture, the stricture can be dilated and a fine-bore tube can be inserted alongside an endoscope.[86] The distal end of the tube is drawn into the biopsy channel of the distal end of the endoscope with biopsy forceps and when the endoscope has been passed into the stomach, the distal tip of the feeding tube is released before the endoscope is withdrawn. Naso-enteral tubes can also be inserted at laparotomy.

Percutaneous tube feeding

All patients experience some discomfort within the nasopharynx when naso-enteral tubes are used. A tube of larger diameter may be brought out through the oropharynx just below the angle of the jaw: this technique of cervical pharyngostomy is often used by surgeons operating on the head and neck.[87] and produces remarkably little irritation within the pharynx. A gastrostomy or jejunostomy requires the creation of an unnatural opening between the gastrointestinal tract and the abdominal wall and the presence of a tube in the peritoneal cavity (although the length of the tube within the peritoneal cavity should be reduced to an absolute minimum by suturing the opening in the abdominal wall to the site of insertion into the intestine). In the past the incidence of complications associated with surgically constructed gastrostomies and jejunostomies was considerable.[88] Complications included peritonitis, volvulus, intestinal obstruction, haemorrhage and failure of spontaneous closure when the tubes were removed. It used to be possible to insert tubes only under general or local anaesthesia in the operating theatre. This is no longer necessary and such tubes can be inserted by combined percutaneous and endoscopic or radiological techniques with minimum sedation. Commercial systems have been developed which are easily inserted and associated with fewer complications compared with traditional surgical methods.[89] Major complications occur less commonly following radiological gastrostomy (6%) than following endoscopic gastrostomy (9.5%) or surgical gastrostomy (20%).[90]

Enteral feeds

There are now probably more than 100 commercially available enteral diets available throughout the world.[91] The majority are polymeric diets in which the protein is provided as whole protein. The most common source is a hydrolysate of casein. The fat is often a mixture of long chain and medium chain triglycerides and the carbohydrate is usually a hydrolysate of starch. Some patients with gastrointestinal disease are unable to digest and absorb these nutrients and require peptides and free amino acids and energy provided predominantly as hydrolysed starch with a small quantity of medium chain triglycerides. These predigested or chemically defined elemental diets may be further modified according to the disease from which the patient is suffering (see above). All these diets should contain the necessary electrolytes, minerals and vitamins.

Infusion

Many patients suffer abdominal discomfort, distension and diarrhoea if full strength nutrients are infused on the first day at the required rate of intake. Ideally the infusion should begin with water at a slow rate (50 ml/h). Following this a similar rate of infusion of diluted nutrients should be given at increasing strengths until full strength nutrients are given on about the third day. Alternatively, full strength nutrients can be infused at a greatly reduced rate on the first day and the quantity progressively increased. Infusion should be constant during day and night: the incidence of diarrhoea and other complications is then greatly reduced when compared with bolus infusion.[92] A constant infusion is best maintained by the use of an infusion pump which can be carried with the source of nutrients on a small carrying frame suspended from the shoulder, allowing the patient full mobility. If diarrhoea does occur, it will usually respond to a temporary reduction in the rate of infusion and the addition of 30 mg codeine phosphate syrup 4 hourly. A common cause of diarrhoea in these patients is the concomitant prescription of antibiotics. Lactose intolerance is rare in Europe but more common in Asia.[93] Excessive quantities of medium chain triglycerides within the nutrient solution may also produce diarrhoea.[94] Hyperglycaemia may occur during enteral feeding but is far less common and severe than that seen after parenteral feeding.[95] With the constant, slow infusion of modern commercially manufactured nutrient solutions, the incidence of all these side-effects is greatly reduced. The greatest drawback associated with naso-enteral feeding is spontaneous regurgitation of the tube by the patient. If this occurs when the patient is sleeping in a supine position, there is a danger of continued infusion into the oropharynx with aspiration pneumonia.[96]

REFERENCES

86. Atkinson M, Walford S, Allison S P Lancet 1979; ii: 829
87. Graham W P III, Royster H P Surg Gynaecol Obstet 1967; 125: 127–128
88. Delaney H M, Carnevale N, Garvey J W, Moss C M Ann Surg 1977; 186: 165
89. Moran B J, Taylor M B, Johnson C D Br J Surg 1990; 77: 858–862
90. Wollman B, D'Agostino H B, Walus-Wigle J R, Easter D W, Beale A Radiology 1995; 197: 699–704
91. Silk D B A Gut 1986; 27: S1, 40–46
92. Tweedle D E F, Skidmore F D, Gleave E N, Knass D A, Gowland E Res Clin Forums 1979; 1: 59
93. Neale G Proc R Soc Med 1968; 61: 1099–1117
94. Simoons F J Am J Dig Dis 1969; 14: 819
95. Woolfson A M J, Ricketts C R, Hardy S M, Sauor J N, Pollard B J, Allison S P Postgrad Med J 1976; 52: 678–682
96. Jones B J M, Payne S, Silk D B A Lancet 1980; 1: 1057

Parenteral feeding

The technique of intravenous feeding began before the First World War, with the infusion of casein hydrolysate.[97] The initial solutions were not particularly hypertonic and could be infused into a peripheral vein. It soon became apparent that insufficient fats and carbohydrate were being given so that the infused proteins were being used for energy rather than for synthesis. In North America infusion of adequate quantities of non-protein energy was achieved by the use of highly concentrated solutions of glucose[98] which were infused into central veins to avoid thrombosis of peripheral veins. Fat emulsions were developed in Sweden; these are less concentrated and can be infused peripherally.[99] Nevertheless, intravenous feeding with adequate quantities of amino acids, glucose, fat, minerals and vitamins necessitates the infusion of hypertonic solutions and the majority of patients receiving parenteral nutritional support are fed through a central catheter.

Central venous catheterization

Catheters for intravenous feeding are usually made of non-thrombogenic polytetrafluoroethylene (PTFE) or siliconized rubber (Silastic).[100] Some catheters have a small, external cuff of Dacron which can be placed subcutaneously close to the exit site from the skin. As well as preventing movement this cuff may also prevent migration of organisms along a subcutaneous tunnel. The catheters can be inserted through veins draining into the superior or inferior vena cava. Contrary to common belief, the incidence of complications following insertion of catheters into the inferior vena cava via the long saphenous vein is no greater than when the superior vena cava is catheterized.[101] The superior vena cava can be used, however, following direct percutaneous puncture of the external and internal jugular and subclavian veins (the most commonly used site). Infusion via these sites is usually less cumbersome. Insertion of a central venous catheter should be performed using an aseptic technique. Ideally, the tip of the catheter should just reach the right atrium where the nutrients mix with the large volume of blood returning to the heart. This should be confirmed by a radiograph before the infusion is begun. The veins in the neck are in close apposition to many important structures, and before attempting to catheterize them it is necessary to be familiar with their anatomy (Fig. 2.10).

The physical complications of intravenous feeding include phlebitis, thrombosis, pneumothorax and haemothorax, air embolism and arterial damage, and are mainly a consequence of poor technique. The major consequence of intravenous feeding through central venous catheters is septicaemia. The majority of septic complications are avoidable and numerous studies have demonstrated that septic complications are far less common when the catheter is cared for by appropriately trained nutrition nurses and patients.[102] Most authorities, but not all, consider that the incidence of sepsis is less with cuffed catheters inserted along a subcutaneous tunnel. The majority of catheter related sepsis is due to infection with *Staph. epidermidis* and *Staph. aureus*. Haematogenous spread from gastrointestinal sites also occurs and it is sometimes difficult to determine whether the catheter is responsible for the bacteraemia and should be removed. If simultaneous samples of blood are taken from the catheter and a peripheral vein, and the colony count in the catheter blood is five times greater than in the peripheral blood, then primary catheter related sepsis is likely.[103]

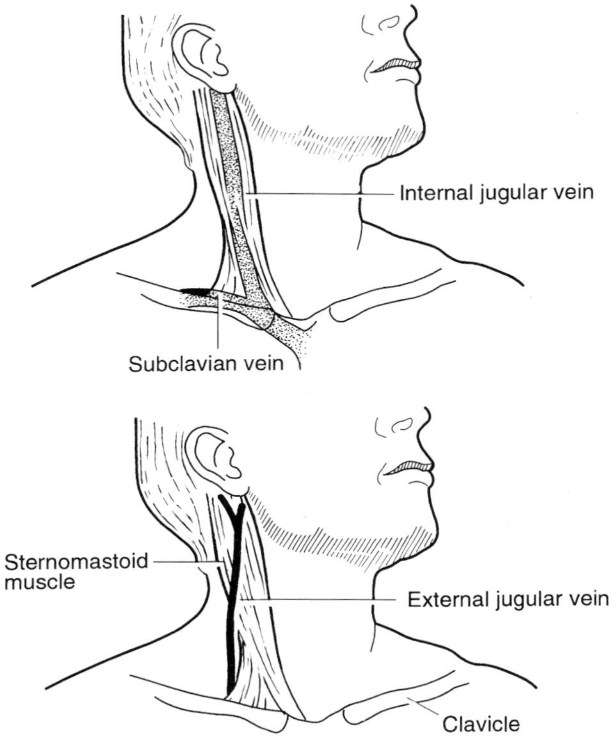

Fig. 2.10 The superficial landmarks of the great veins of the chest and neck.

Parenteral nutrients

The protein solutions available after the Second World War were hydrolysates of naturally occurring proteins. The amino acid content of those solutions reflected that of the protein from which they were made. The hydrolysis was incomplete and as much as 30% of the protein content was in the form of peptides whose utilization varied. These solutions were replaced with synthetic solutions which contained only amino acids. Initially the composition of these solutions reflected ease of manufacture rather than clinical need, and excessive amounts of some amino acids were

REFERENCES

97. Elman R, Weiner D O JAMA 1939; 112L: 796–802
98. Dudrick S J, Wilmore D W, Vars H M et al Surgery 1968; 64: 134–142
99. Hallberg D, Schuberth O, Wretlind A Nutritio et Dieta 1966; 8: 245–281
100. Tweedle D E F Metabolic Care. Churchill Livingstone, Edinburgh 1982 p 178
101. Rich A J Clin Nutr 1990; 9: 127–130
102. Keohane P P, Jones B J, Attrill H H, Cribb A, Northover J, Frost P, Silk D B A Lancet 1983; 2: 1388–1390
103. Mosca R, Curtas S, Forbes B, Meguid M M Surgery 1987; 102: 718–723

simply excreted in the urine.[104] The difficulties in manufacturing stable solutions with an amino acid profile that is appropriate for intravenous requirements in man have been overcome and all solutions now meet these requirements. Specific solutions that have been tailored to suit a specific clinical condition such as hepatic or renal failure have also been devised.[67,72,105]

Glucose is the natural source of carbohydrate energy in man and the majority of carbohydrates derived from food reach the peripheral organs as glucose. When large quantities of glucose are infused it is necessary to provide insulin, consequently there have been many attempts to substitute other carbohydrates in the belief that they do not require insulin. Fructose, sorbitol and xylitol have all had their advocates. Ultimately all these substrates are converted into glucose and, like glucose, their final metabolic pathway is oxidation within the tricarboxylic acid cycle. Following their infusion the concentration of blood glucose rises at the same rate as after an infusion of glucose, thus all these substrates require insulin for complete oxidation. Unfortunately, unlike glucose, the initial steps in their breakdown may be rapid and uncontrolled, producing fatal lactic acidosis,[106] and their use is to be discouraged. Ideally about half the non-protein energy requirements should be given in the form of glucose. Insulin requirements vary from patient to patient: in the severely ill patient on the Intensive Care Unit, hourly blood glucose estimations may be required. The majority of patients require one unit of insulin for 4 g of glucose. A scale for maintaining the concentration of blood glucose at 6–11 mmol/l in a patient given 400 g of glucose per day is shown in Table 2.17.

Table 2.17 Insulin requirements during intravenous feeding (start at 4 iu/h)

Blood glucose (mmol/l)	*Insulin (iu/h)*
0–3	None
3–5	Reduce by 2
5–7	Reduce by 1
7–11	Same as previously
11–15	Increase by 2
> 15	Increase by 4

Long chain fatty acids predominate in the fat emulsions used for intravenous feeding, replicating the normal oral intake. The concentration of the essential fatty acids in these emulsions is ample to prevent deficiency. The great advantage of fat emulsions as a source of energy lies in their low initial solute load, shown in Table 2.18. Complete utilization of either fat or carbohydrate substrate results in the excretion of the hydrogen atoms as water and the carbon atoms as carbon dioxide without any change in osmolarity. Fat emulsions should contribute approximately half of the non-protein energy requirements.

Table 2.18 The energy and solute content of intravenous carbohydrate and fat solutions (1 litre)

Substrate	*Energy content (MJ)*	*(kcal)*	*Solute load (mosmol)*
Intralipid® 10%	239	1000	280
Glucose 30%	272	1140	2100
Intralipid® 20%	478	2000	330
Glucose 50%	455	1900	3800

Metabolic complications

Hyperglycaemia and hypoglycaemia. The rapid infusion of highly concentrated solutions of glucose (i.e. 50%) without adequate quantities of insulin can cause fatal hyperglycaemic hyperosmolar coma as the renal excretion of glucose requires water, resulting in dehydration from the ensuing osmotic diuresis. Rapid infusion of isotonic or hypotonic electrolyte solutions and insulin restores normality. Hypoglycaemia is uncommon but may follow the rapid cessation of an infusion of highly concentrated solutions of carbohydrates if further oral or intravenous glucose is not started.

Electrolyte disturbances. The majority of patients fed intravenously receive their daily nutrients in a large plastic bag which has been made up in the Pharmacy. The electrolyte content of these solutions should also be tailored to the clinical requirements. A variety of electrolyte disturbances may occur if insufficient attention is paid to this requirement. Perhaps the most common of these is hypokalaemia as a result of potassium entering cells with glucose under the influence of insulin.

Trace element deficiency. It became apparent that some elements were required in trace quantities in the human diet in patients who were being fed intravenously for prolonged periods without any oral intake of food. Deficiencies of iron, zinc, copper, manganese and iodine have all been identified in patients undergoing prolonged intravenous feeding.[107] Such deficiency usually takes several weeks or months to develop and the majority of patients can ingest the small quantities required to prevent this.

Vitamin deficiencies. Overt deficiency of vitamins is a rare occurrence during intravenous feeding as there are many commercially available mixtures of water- and fat-soluble vitamins that can be added to intravenous nutrients.

Hepatic dysfunction. Many patients fed intravenously for prolonged periods have evidence of hepatic dysfunction demonstrated by an elevation of the serum concentrations of bilirubin, alkaline phosphatase and transaminases.[108] These changes have been observed following parenteral and enteral nutrition in patients who had previously normal hepatic function and had not undergone anaesthesia, operation or radiation. These patients had no evidence of sepsis and were not suffering from malignant disease. The cause remains obscure. Liver biopsies show changes which are similar to those seen in drug-induced cholestasis, but no permanent damage to the liver has been identified and the serological changes return to normal following cessation of parenteral or enteral infusion.

REFERENCES

104. Tweedle D E F, Spivey J, Johnston I D A Metabolism 1972; 22: 173
105. Silk D B A Gut 1986; S1, 103–110
106. Cohen R D, Woods H F Clinical and biochemical aspects of lactic acidosis. Blackwell Scientific Publications, Oxford 1976 p 194
107. Phillips G D, Gararys V P JPEN 1981; 5: 11–14
108. Tweedle D E F, Skidmore F D, Gleave E N, Knass D A, Gowland E Res Clin Forums 1979; 1: 59

3 Blood: haemostasis and transfusion

F. E. Boulton

The arrest of bleeding and the replenishment of blood is a challenge to surgeons and haematologists alike and has generated much recent literature.[1] Many middle-aged practitioners in the UK will recall the declaration by Richard Gordon's fictional Sir Lancelot Spratt about blood being the surgeon's natural enemy.

HAEMOSTASIS

Haemostasis is a general term describing all the activities of blood and related tissues which are directed towards the control of haemorrhage including endothelial, vascular, hepatic, lymphatic and myeloid cells. A natural corollary is the maintenance of fluidity of blood within the circulation by means of the endogenous anticoagulants and fibrinolysins (Fig. 3.1). Central to haemostasis is the interaction between platelets and the plasma clotting factors.

Platelets[2]

Platelets are formed from the cytoplasm of megakaryocytes. These are derived from myeloid stem cells differentiating through megakaryoblasts. The platelet count in blood is normally $300 \pm 150 \times 10^9$/l. Resting platelets are biconvex discs with mean volumes of about 8.5 fl. Although they do not have nuclei, they possess mitochondria, unlike red cells, and metabolize aerobically. Cytoplasmic granules store amines such as adrenaline, adenosine diphosphate and serotonin (5-hydroxytryptamine) and other haemostatic proteins such as platelet factor 4 (an antiheparin), β-thromboglobulin, von Willebrand factor, fibrinogen, clotting factor V and tissue factor pathway inhibitor. Acute haemorrhage or inflammation leads to higher platelet counts by increasing the production of the specific growth factor *thrombopoietin*.[3] This acts on megakaryoblasts, giving rise to bigger megakaryocytes and a generation of fresh platelets.

Glycoproteins in the platelet membrane are receptors for platelet activation and aggregation. Glycoprotein Ib binds collagen, and thrombin; glycoprotein IIb/IIIa binds fibrinogen; and both glycoproteins bind von Willebrand factor.[4–6] Von Willebrand

REFERENCES

1. Lake C L, Moore R A (eds) Blood. Hemostasis, Transfusion, and Alternatives in the Perioperative Period. Raven Press, New York, 1995
2. Crawford N, Scrutton M C In: Bloom A L, Forbes C D, Thomas D P, Tuddenham E G D (eds) Haemostasis and Thrombosis. Churchill Livingstone, Edinburgh 1994 pp 89–114
3. Nishihira H, Toyoda Y, Miyazaki H, Kigasawa H, Ohsaki E Br J Haematol 1996; 92: 23–28
4. Shullek J, Jordan J, Montgomery R R J Clin Invest 1984; 73: 421–428
5. Peerschke E I B Semin Hematol 1985; 22: 241–259
6. Ruggieri Z M, DeMarco L, Gatti L, Bader R, Montgomery R R J Clin Invest 1982; 72: 1–12

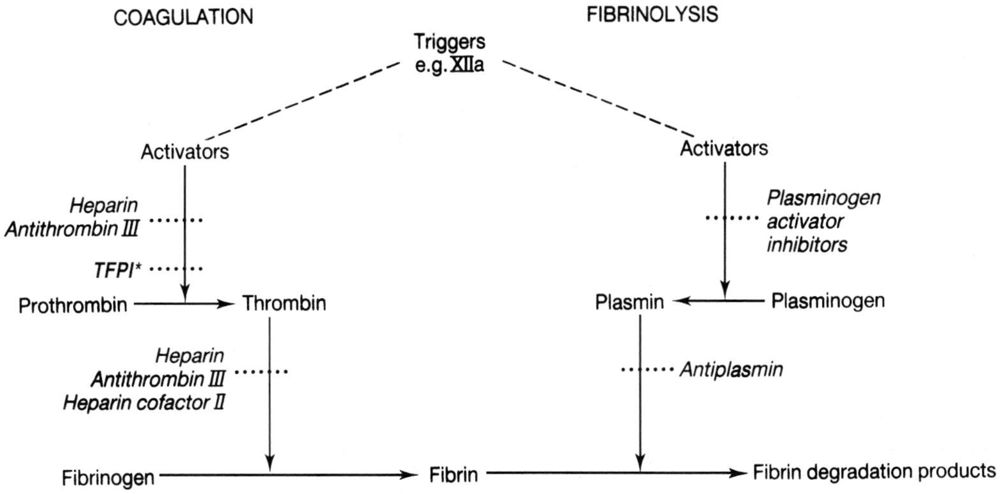

Fig. 3.1 Inter-relation of coagulation and fibrinolysis. Solid arrows represent forward reactions. Dotted lines represent the site of action of enzyme inhibitors, noted in adjacent *italics*. *tissue factor pathway inhibitor

factor causes activated platelets to adhere to each other and to subendothelial collagen exposed by endothelial damage. During activation the granules discharge and the membrane turns inside out, exposing the inner lipids which provide a thromboplastic substrate (platelet factor 3). Derivatives of the membrane phospholipids — prostaglandins such as thromboxane[7] (Fig. 3.2) and platelet activating factor — also cause platelet aggregation. The discharged granular contents enhance platelet aggregation; thus an amorphous mass of irreversibly aggregated platelets (the haemostatic plug) is produced. Actin in the platelet cytoplasm causes retraction and consolidation of the plug after some minutes.

Platelet activation is summarized in Table 3.1. Platelets are activated through many mechanisms; this explains why individual antiplatelet drugs are generally disappointing when used singly for preventing thrombosis.

Coagulation (Fig. 3.3)

The illustrative principle of the 'amplifying cascade of coagulation', conceived in the early 1950s, has stood the test of time not only as a teaching aid but also as a rational guide for choosing appropriate clotting tests. However, new understanding at the molecular and genetic level has advanced our concepts. This was predicted by the proponents of the cascade in 1962.[8] The new schemes—such as that of Broze[9]— are directed mostly at the initiating processes, and are based on a more integrated concept of the extrinsic and the intrinsic systems.

In vivo, coagulation is initiated by the activation of factors VII and XII following local injury or exposure of subendothelium. In the presence of calcium ions, tissue factor and platelet factor 3 provide 'thromboplastic' phospholipid surfaces which strongly adsorb the vitamin K-dependent proenzymes (factors VII, IX, X and II) (Fig. 3.4). Factors V and VIII bind to phospholipid surfaces directly. The enzymes and their substrates are therefore brought together and eventually release thrombin (Fig. 3.5). The term 'prothrombinase' is preferred over 'thromboplastin' or 'thrombokinase'; it does not describe a single enzyme moiety in the usual sense, but rather an activity which is generated in blood during clotting. Thrombin in turn acts on local fibrinogen to form fibrin, the structure of which is further strengthened by cross-linking peptide bonds formed through the agency of activated factor XIII. It also induces a negative feedback by activating protein C (see later and Fig. 3.6).

Virtually all the enzymes of haemostasis—procoagulant or anticoagulant, whether dependent on vitamin K for their formation or not—belong to the group of so-called serine proteases. These lyse peptide bonds after basic amino acids, especially arginine, and have a serine residue at the heart of the active site.

Tissue factor

Tissue factor is a transmembranous protein present in fibroblasts and macrophages. Most of the single peptide chain of 263 amino acids, which is coded from a gene on the short arm of chromosome 9, projects outside the cell where complex carbohydrates are bound to it. It has structural affinities to the cytokine/interferon receptors, and

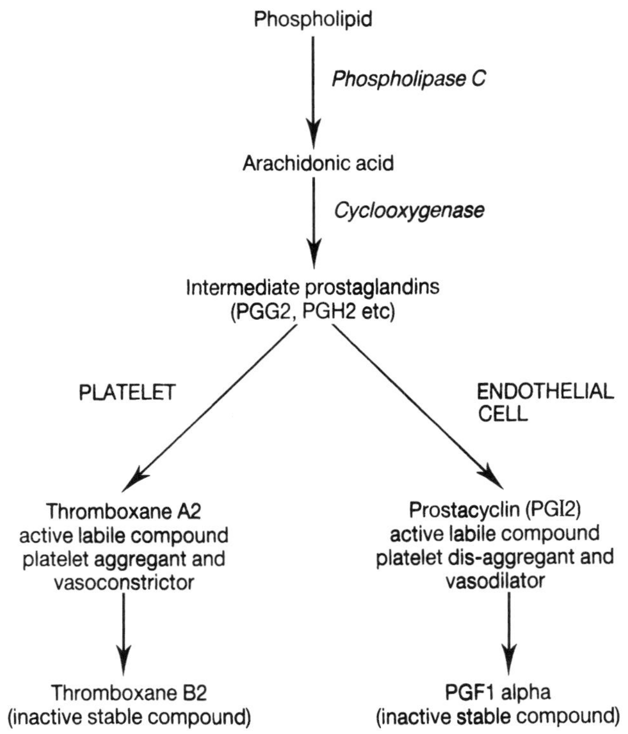

Fig. 3.2 The derivation of platelet thromboxane and endothelial prostacyclin from membrane phospholipid and arachidonic acid through the prostaglandin pathway.

the overall mass is about 50 000 daltons (50 kDa). The fully functional factor is combined with lipids, optimally a ratio of 2:1 phosphatidyl choline to phosphatidyl serine. In this state it binds factor VII and initiates proteolysis of the proenzyme factors IX and X.

Plasma factors

There follows an account of the factors most frequently associated with the best-understood inherited disorders of haemostasis: factors VIII, IX, X, prothrombin and fibrinogen. Deficiencies have however, been described for all factors — and indeed were usually the means by which they were first identified.

Factor VIII and von Willebrand factor[10,11]

These distinct substances are described together because their function and behaviour are intimately linked.

REFERENCES

7. Mayes P A In: Harper H A, Rodwell V W, Mayes P A (eds) Review of Physiological Chemistry, 17th edn. Lange Medical Publications 1979 Los Altos, California
8. Biggs R, MacFarlane R G. Human Blood Coagulation, 3rd edn. Blackwell Scientific Publications, Oxford 1962
9. Broze G J In: Haemostasis and thrombosis. Bloom A L, Forbes C D, Thomas D P, Tuddenham E G D (eds) Churchill Livingstone, Edinburgh 1994 pp 349–377
10. Bithell T C In: Lee G R, Bithell T C, Foerster J, Athens J W, Lukens J N (eds) Wintrobe's Clinical Hematology 9th edn Lea & Febiger, Philadelphia 1993 p 566
11. O'Brien D P, Tuddenham E G D In: Bloom A L, Forbes C D, Thomas D P, Tuddenham E G D Haemostasis and Thrombosis. Churchill Livingstone, Edinburgh 1994 p 333

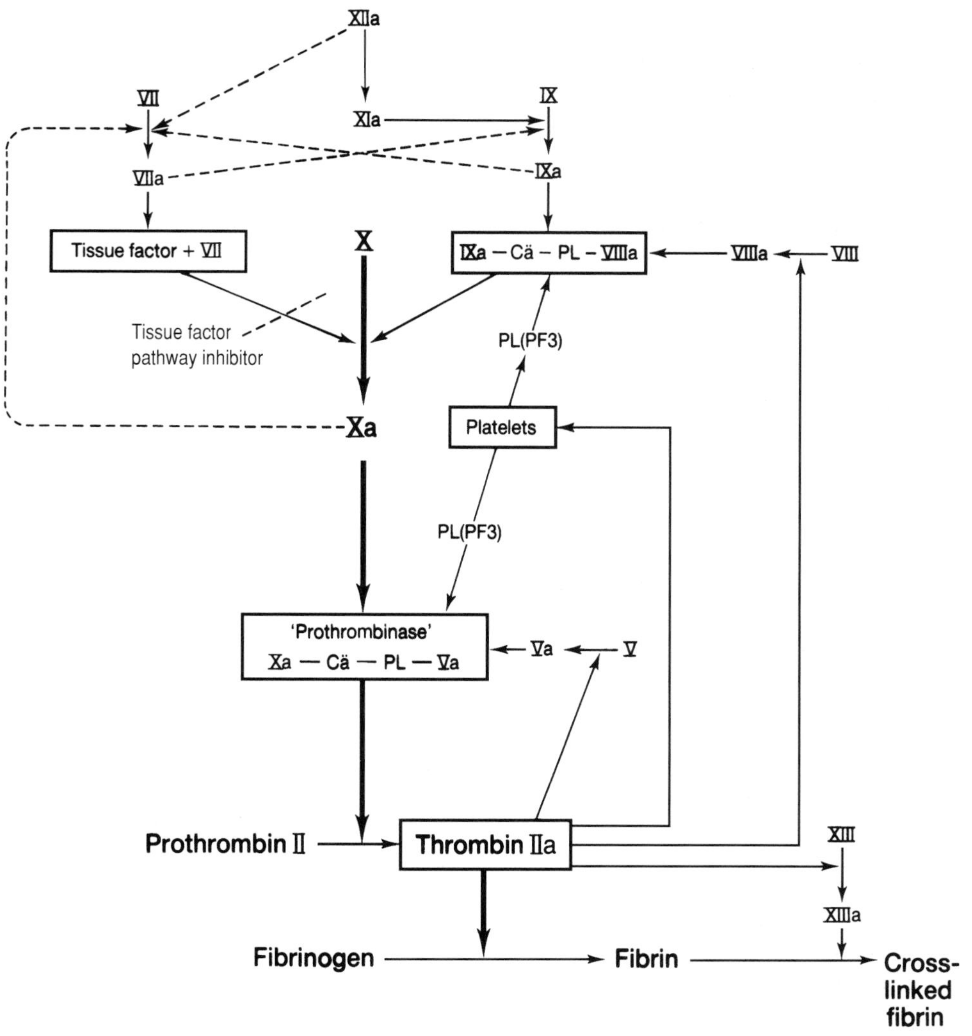

Fig. 3.3 The main features of the coagulation cascade.

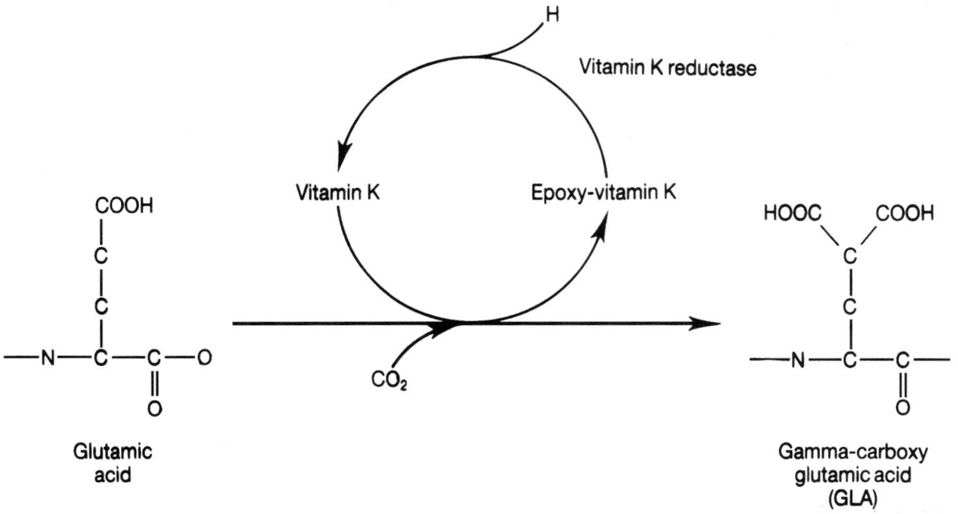

Fig. 3.4 Mode of action of vitamin K in the synthesis of prothrombin, and factors VII, IX, X, and proteins S and C from their precursor proteins in the hepatocyte.

Table 3.1 Platelet activation and sequelae

Event	*Time scale*	*Consequence*
Initial stimulus, e.g. collagen, adenosine diphosphate, thrombin	Seconds	Shape changes—spherical with protrusions. Membrane activation with prostaglandin and thromboxane production
Reversible aggregation	1–2 minutes	Secretion of amines, e.g. 5-hydroxytryptamine (with capillary vasoconstriction) and von Willebrand factor. Further membrane activity exposing platelet factor with subsequent clot promotion
Irreversible aggregation via von Willebrand factor and fibrin(ogen), producing the haemostatic plug	2–5 minutes	Further secretion of proteins, e.g. platelet factor 4, fibrinogen and factor V. Clot formation
Clot retraction	5–20 minutes	Consolidation of haemostatic plug. Fibrin cross-linking

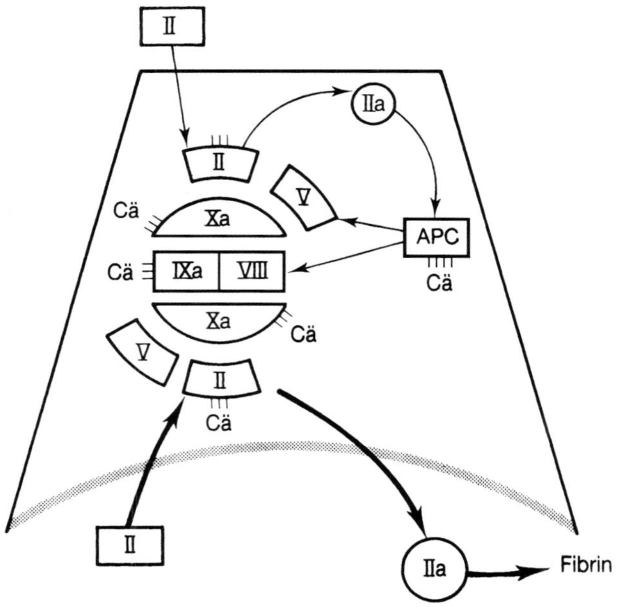

Fig. 3.5 Diagrammatic representation of the formation and release of thrombin (IIa) from the phospholipid surface on which the plasma coagulation factors are concentrated. From the IXa–VIII complex represented centrally, absorbed factor X becomes activated to Xa which, with factor V, enables the conversion of adsorbed prothrombin to free thrombin. Also represented is the formation of activated protein C (APC) and its inhibitory influence on clotting via inactivation of factors V and VIII. Calcium-dependent binding is shown by ≡Cä.

Procoagulant factor VIII (anti-haemophilic factor), factor VIIIc, or factor VIII[11–14]

This is missing or defective in people with haemophilia A. The 'native' human protein is a glycosylated chain of 2332 amino acids, arranged in a pattern of domains—sequences of several hundred amino acids which are generally (but not exactly) repeated within the molecule.[11] Factor V has a strikingly similar overall structure.

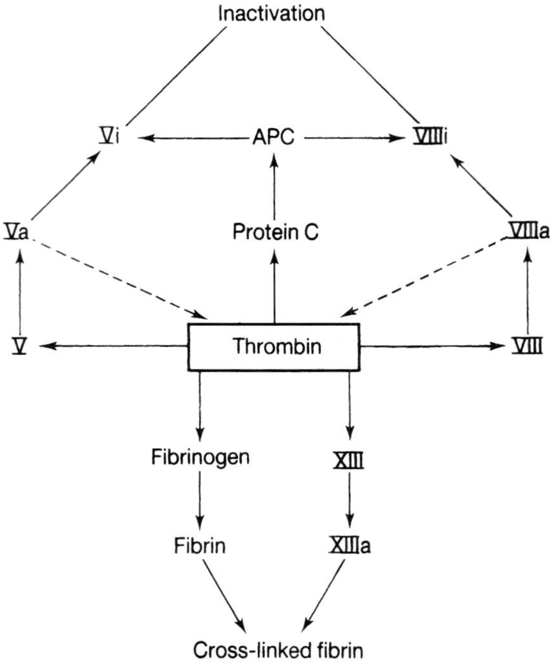

Fig. 3.6 Plasma protein substrates of thrombin. Factors Va and VIIIa enhance thrombin production but are inhibited indirectly by thrombin through the generation of activated protein C (APC). Thrombin also reinforces the fibrin clot through the generation of XIIIa which allows the formation of cross-linked fibrin. Thrombin is also a powerful platelet-activator.

While in the hepatocyte, the single chain is split into a heavy and a light chain bridged by heavy metal ions and secreted as such into the plasma. Thrombin proteolysis activates this into a heterotrimer; and further proteolysis by protein C[13] (see later) leads to irreversible inactivation. Less discriminatory proteolysis by plasmin destroys factor VIII dimer directly. The activation and inactivation of factor V follow a closely analogous pattern.[13,14] After the production of VIII dimer from VIII monomer within the hepatocyte, physiological activation by thrombin produces a heterotrimer of activated Factor VIII (VIIIa). This then becomes physiologically inactivated by protein C to produce VIIIi. These physiological events take place within the plasma or on the thrombus. VIII dimer is also inactivated within the plasma or on the thrombus by plasmin.

Although the factor VIII protein can be assayed immunologically, the international unit (iu) of clotting activity, based on the factor VII activity in 1 ml of normal plasma, is preferred. In both men and women this ranges from 0.5 to 1.5 iu/ml plasma, rises slowly with age and considerably during adrenergic stimulation. Its activity is also increased by vitamin K antagonists through a decrease in protein C.[15]

....

REFERENCES

12. Kane W H, Davie E W Blood 1988; 71: 535–555
13. Fulcher C A, Gardiner J E, Griffin J H, Zimmerman T S. Blood 1984; 63: 486–489
14. Pittman D D, Marquette K A, Kaufman R J Blood 1994; 84: 4124–4225
15. Kellett H A, Sawers J S A, Boulton F E, Cholerton S, Park B K, Toft A D Q J Med 1986; 58: 43–51

von Willebrand factor (formerly factor VIII-related antigen)

This has two functions: to assist the aggregation of platelets to each other and to damaged subendothelium; and to carry and stabilize plasma factor VIII. There follows an account of the factors most frequently associated with the best understood inherited disorders of haemostatis; factors VIII, IX, X, prothrombin and fibrinogen. However, deficiencies have been described for all factors – and indeed were usually the means by which they were first identified.

Von Willebrand factor is highly mutable, as shown by the many abnormal forms causing lack of von Willebrand factor activity resulting in a bleeding state—von Willebrand disease.

The factor VIIIc–von Willebrand factor complex

Virtually all of the factor VIII is bound via specific molecular sites to von Willebrand factor; but von Willebrand factor circulates in excess within plasma and most is unbound. The complex is easily disrupted by heparin.

Von Willebrand factor stabilizes the factor VIII, and protects it from activated protein C. Pure factor VIII infused into people with severe von Willebrand disease disappears much more quickly than in haemophilics; however infusion of normal von Willebrand factor—with or without factor VIII—into people with classical von Willebrand disease is followed by a prolonged rise in factor VIII activity, although the von Willebrand factor activity declines quickly. This was thought to indicate de novo synthesis but is more probably because of the stabilizing effect of the infused von Willebrand factor reducing the tumour of factor VIII.

Factor IX (Christmas factor) and factor X[16]

Factor IX is also coded on the X chromosome, although not closely linked to the factor VIII locus. Inherited deficiency of factor IX was reported in two separate papers in 1952; one from the USA[17] and one from the UK in a Canadian boy surnamed 'Christmas'; the fact that this was reported in the Christmas issue of the British Medical Journal in 1952[18] is coincidental. As one of the prothrombin complex subclass of serine proteases it has about 12 residues of the unique gammacarboxyglutamic acid (gla) among the first 30 or so amino acids at the aminoterminus of the molecule. These are sited so as to bind strongly to calcium ions and thence to the phospholipid surface of the procoagulant complex (see Fig. 3.4 and ref 18a).

Factor IX molecules are single chains of 415 amino acids with one intrachain disulphide bond. This factor is activated through proteolysis by factor XI and/or the tissue factor and factor VII complex. The factor IXa which results is a lighter two-chain molecule with one interchain disulphide bond; it forms part of the procoagulant complex bound to the phospholipid (thromboplastic) surface, where it proteolyses and activates factor X.

Factor X molecules are also initially single chains of similar size to factor IX, but the inactive circulating form is a dimer of a light chain which carries the gla residues and a heavy chain which carries the serine-based active centre. This is only revealed after proteolysis removes a portion of the heavy chain.

Prothrombin (factor II)[19]

This is the penultimate protein of the classical cascade. It was Morawitz's realization in 1905 that prothrombin is the circulating inactive precursor of a protease which forms fibrin which founded the modern concepts of blood coagulation.

Prothrombin provides the bulk of the circulating vitamin K-dependent prothrombin complex. It has a chain of 581 amino acids and shares with factor IX (and factors VII and X) the characteristic gla residues (Fig. 3.4) through which it is adsorbed on to activated phospholipid surfaces during clotting. Under the influence of factor Xa in the prothrombinase, the activated protein thrombin is detached from the prothrombinase surface into the local environs, so that it can act on its plasma substrates, principally fibrinogen (Fig. 3.6).

Fibrinogen[20]

Although fibrinogen is completely coded from one gene, its molecules are synthesized as hexamers formed by pairs of three types of chain, designated Aα, Bβ, and γ, each of 70, 60, and 50 kDa respectively. The whole molecule, $A\alpha_2B\beta_2\gamma_2$, is 360 kDa. There is a total of 29 disulphide bonds between the chains. About 3–5% of each chain is glycosylated. This increases in liver disease—part of the cause of the dysfibrinogenaemia (along with increased fibrin degradation products—see later). More than 250 genetic variant dysfibrinogens have been described.

Each molecule is symmetrical and long—about 23 × 9 nm. Each half is joined at the amino end by a disulphide 'knot' between the Bβ and the γ chains. In the first stage of fibrin formation, thrombin releases the fibrinopeptides A and B from each Aα and Bβ chain, leaving the remaining 93% of the molecule as fibrin monomer or $(\alpha\beta\gamma)_2$. Through the action of activated factor XIII (sic), fibrin monomer is transformed into insoluble fibrin by peptide bonds cross-linking γ-chains of different monomers. Factor XIIIa is produced from factor XIII by thrombin (Figs 3.6 and 3.7).

Clottable fibrinogen assays show normal concentra-tions of 1.5–4.0 g/l plasma. Some 75% of fibrinogen circulates in the plasma; the rest is mainly in the lymph. Being an acute-phase reactant, it increases in inflammatory and febrile states. It leaks into extravascular spaces when capillary endothelium is damaged. Fibrinogen stays in the circulation for about 5 days; there is a

REFERENCES

16. Reiner A P, Davie E W In: Bloom A L, Forbes C D, Thomas D P, Tuddenham E G D (eds) Haemostasis and Thrombosis. Churchill Livingstone, Edinburgh 1994 pp 309–331
17. Aggeler P M, White S G, Glendening M B, Page E W, Leake T B, Bates G Proc Soc Exp Biol Med 1952; 79: 692–694
18. Biggs R, Douglas A S, MacFarlane R G et al Br Med J 1952; 2: 1378–1382

18a. Gallop P M, Lian J B, Hauschka P V N Engl J Med 1980; 302: 1460–1466

19. Jackson C M. In: Bloom A L, Forbes C D, Thomas D P, Tuddenham E G D (eds) Haemostasis and Thrombosis. Churchill Livingstone, Edinburgh 1994 pp 397–438
20. Bithell T C. In: Lee G R, Bithell T C, Foerster J, Athens J W, Lukens J N (eds) Wintrobe's Clinical Hematology, 9th edn Lea & Febiger, Philadelphia 1993 p 566

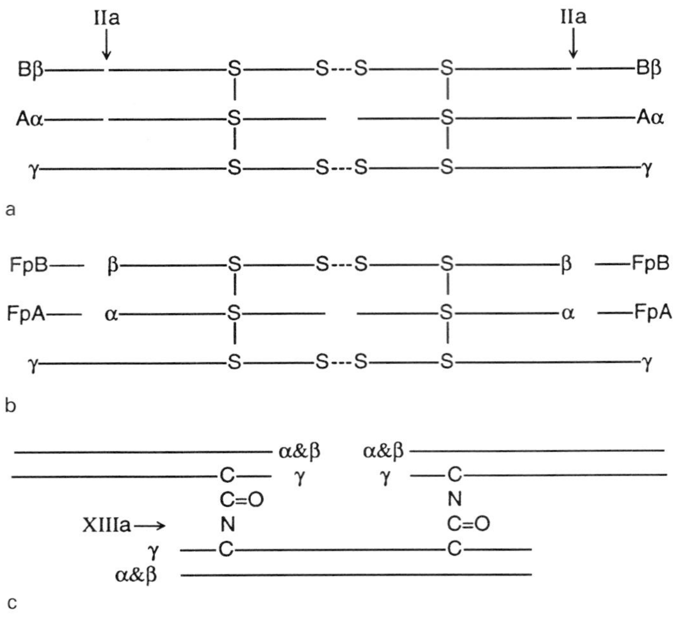

Fig. 3.7 Representation of the molecules of fibrinogen and of fibrin monomer. (**a**) Fibrinogen showing signs of proteolytic activation by thrombin (IIa); (**b**) fibrin monomer after release of fibrinopeptides A and B; (**c**) cross-linked fibrin, formed by factor XIIIa creating peptide bonds between γ-chains.

constant slow catabolism by traces of plasmin, so that there are also traces of the fibrinogen degradation products in the normal plasma.

Epidemiological studies show that fibrinogen levels in healthy adults are influenced by smoking, obesity and birth weight.[21] Humphries et al[22] claim that populations prone to coronary thrombosis have significantly higher plasma fibrinogen concentrations.

Natural anticoagulation and fibrinolysis

(Fig. 3.8)

The ability to control bleeding from a blood vessel without precipitating widespread thrombosis involves not only the controlled formation of the clot but also the ability to confine the clot to the injured area by anticoagulation. This begins early; an important protein—tissue factor pathway inhibitor[11]—inhibits tissue factor. This has 276 amino acids in a single chain, with three domains. It is stored in endothelium from which it is released by heparin; and 90% of the circulating tissue factor pathway inhibitor is bound to plasma lipoproteins which are also probably affected by heparin. A slightly different form is synthesized in megakaryocytes and stored in platelets.

Once formed, thrombin is rapidly inactivated by adsorption on to freshly formed fibrin; any remaining thrombin is neutralized by endothelial uptake and by heparans in the presence of antithrombin III.

The role of protein C; activated protein C resistance and factor V Leiden[23]

Thrombin activates proteins C and S (vitamin K-dependent gla-containing serine proteases in plasma produced by hepatocytes) with the assistance of thrombomodulin secreted by endothelial cells. Activated protein C inactivates factors Va and VIIIa (see above

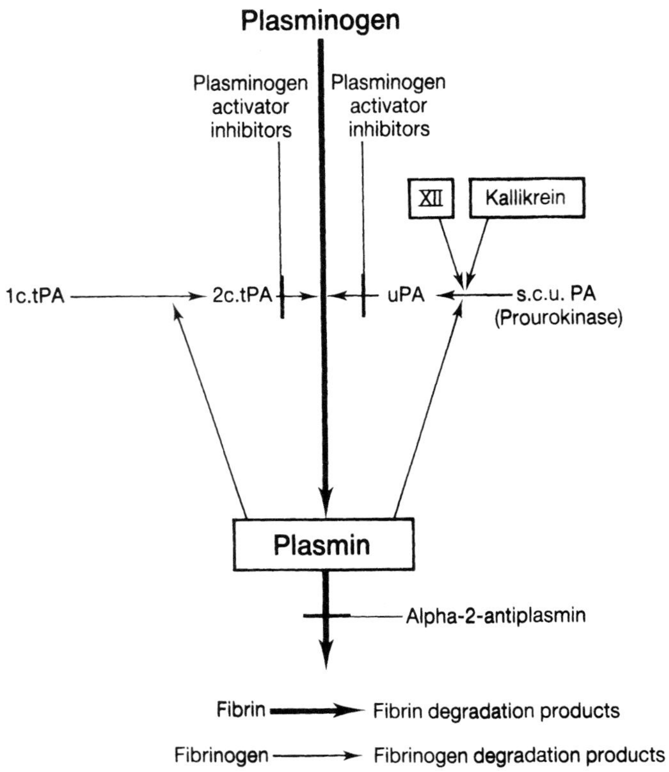

Fig. 3.8 The formation of plasmin from plasminogen. These reactions are enhanced on a fibrin surface. 2c.tPA = Two-chain tissue plasminogen activator; uPA = urinary plasminogen activator (identical to heavy-molecular-weight urokinase); s.c.u. PA = single-chain urinary plasminogen activator. Inhibitory action is shown by boxes. Main forward reactions are indicated by heavy arrows.

Fulcher[13] and Fig. 3.6) and also boosts fibrinolysis. A common genetic variant of factor V, found in up to 7% of normal people, has relative resistance to inactivation by activated protein C. This variant (factor V Leiden) results from the arginine at position 506 in normal factor V being replaced by glutamine, which removes a cleavage site for the activated protein C. The homozygous state, which is present in 0.09–0.5% of the population, predisposes to recurrent thromboses. Hence, the clinicopathological state of activated protein C resistance is not caused by defective protein C, but by a variant of factor V which persists to promote coagulation.

Circulating plasma contains tissue plasminogen activator,[24] prourokinase[25] and plasminogen[26]—all serine proteases which are adsorbed on to freshly forming fibrin. Plasmin, formed by the

REFERENCES

21. Martyn C N, Meade T W, Stirling Y, Barker D J P Br J Haematol 1995; 89: 142–146
22. Humphries S E, Cook M, Dubowitz M et al Lancet 1987; i: 1452–1455
23. Greengard J S, Eichinger S, Griffin J H, Bauer K A. N Eng J Med 1994; 331: 1559–1562
24. Walter P B In: Davidson J F, Donati M B, Coccheri S (eds) 1985 Progress in Fibrinolysis VII. Churchill Livingstone, Edinburgh
25. Gurevich V, Pannell R, Louie S, Kelley P, Suddith R L, Greenlee R J Clin Invest 1984; 73: 1731–1739
26. Collen D, Lijnen H R In: Collen D, Lijnen H R, Verstraete M (eds) Thrombolysis. Churchill Livingstone, Edinburgh 1985

proteolytic action of tissue plasminogen activator and prourokinase on plasminogen, degrades fibrin into degradation products. Traces of plasmin can leak into plasma and degrade other proteins such as fibrinogen, but are neutralized by α_2-antiplasmin.[27] The plasmin–α_2 antiplasmin complexes can then be adsorbed on to fibrin. Tissue plasminogen activator and prourokinase are similarly restrained by plasminogen activator inhibitors.[28] Streptokinase complexed with plasminogen also has a high affinity for fibrin and releases plasmin locally, thereby assisting rapid lysis of freshly formed thrombus.

Endothelial cell–platelet interaction

Listed below are some of the activities of the endothelial cells which promote the maintenance of the fluidity of blood by anticoagulation, fibrinolysis and vasodilation; or the cessation of blood flow by coagulation and inhibiting fibrinolysis.

1. *Anticoagulation*
   a. Directly, by synthesizing antithrombin III. Also by binding glycosaminoglycans (heparans) which release tissue factor pathway inhibitor (inhibitor factor VIIa and Xa). Heparan–antithrombin III complexes also neutralize thrombin.
   b. Indirectly, by secreting and binding thrombomodulin, a co-factor in the thrombin-induced activation of protein C which inactivates factors V and VIII.
2. *Fibrinolysis*
   a. Directly, by synthesizing and secreting tissue plasminogen activator.
   b. Indirectly, by activating factor XII with heparan (see Fig. 3.1).
3. *Coagulation*
   a. Directly, by synthesizing and secreting von Willebrand factor.
   b. Indirectly, by activating factor XII with heparan (see point 2b above and Fig. 3.2).
4. *Antifibrinolysis*
   Directly, by synthesizing and secreting plasminogen activator inhibitor type 1.
5. *Vasodilatation*
   Directly, by synthesizing endothelial-derived relaxant factor and prostacyclin. Endothelial-derived relaxant factor is nitrous oxide; prostacyclin also inhibits platelet aggregation by thromboxane A_2.

Platelets interact with endothelial cells at several points. Platelet factor 4 inhibits endothelial-bound heparan; vasoactive amines secreted by platelets increase endothelial permeability as well as inducing capillary vasoconstriction; thromboxane secreted by activated platelets also induces vasoconstriction. In turn, several endothelial activities influence platelets: endothelial secretion of von Willebrand factor allows platelets to adhere to the subendothelium, and endothelial secretion of prostacyclin inhibits thromboxane-induced platelet aggregation and induces vasodilation.

The prostaglandins thromboxane and prostacyclin are mutually antagonistic products of arachidonic acid metabolism formed from the oxidation of platelet and endothelial membrane phospholipids. Their synthesis is summarized in Figure 3.2. Although the cyclo-oxygenase in the synthetic pathways in both cells is inhibited by aspirin, the effect on the non-nucleated platelet is more severe as cyclo-oxygenase cannot be regenerated. Thus, aspirin is more effectively anti-platelet in doses up to 600 mg daily.[29] The balance between normal thromboxane and prostacyclin production illustrates a fine-tuning mechanism of homeostasis. Platelets do not however, adhere to undamaged endothelium deprived of prostacyclin.

Veins and arteries differ in their susceptibilities to thrombus formation, and venous and arterial thrombi are structurally distinct. Venous thrombi are predominantly composed of fibrin with enmeshed cells while arterial thrombi consist predominantly of layers of platelets. Although Virchow's triad of determinant factors can generally be considered to hold true (blood flow, blood constituents, and vessel wall; see Chapter 11), the single most important determinant for venous thrombi is probably the presence of traces of thrombin, while for arteries it is damaged endothelium.

The bleeding time

Duke's description of the cessation of haemorrhage from a standardized skin incision (originally the ear lobe) established the role of platelets in haemostasis.[30] It measures not only platelet aggregability, but also vasoconstriction in response to the vasoactive amines, particularly 5-hydroxytryptamine. The bleeding time,[31] remains the best in vivo test of platelet and capillary function, but lacks precision and cannot be quantified. In a patient with normally functioning platelets, it does have a relationship to reduced platelet numbers, and this was used to predict the efficacy of platelet infusions.[32] It is also of modest use in monitoring the effect of factor VIII in the treatment of von Willebrand's disease. It does not, however, reliably indicate the amount of bleeding which can be expected from major surgical incisions and is not a good indicator of the need for platelet therapy.[33]

Laboratory tests of clotting

When taken into a glass tube, normal venous blood has an intrinsic tendency to clot within 5–10 minutes depending on the temperature and the type of glass. This is the whole blood clotting time as described by Lee and White.[34] Clotting occurs in seconds. if homogenates or extracts of brain, kidney or placenta are added. This extrinsic tissue factor bypasses the slower intrinsic factors accelerating the activation of clotting factor VII. A refinement is

REFERENCES

27. Wiman B, Collen D J Biol Chem 1979; 254: 9291–9297
28. Wun T C, Capuano A Blood 1987; 69: 1354–1362
29. Preston F E, Whipps S, Jackson C A et al N Engl J Med 1981; 304: 76–79
30. Duke W W Arch Intern Med 1912; 10: 445
31. Ivy A C, Nelson D, Bucher G J Lab Clin Med 1940; 26: 1812
32. Slichter S J, Harker L A Br J Haematol 1976; 34: 403–419
33. De Caterina R, Lanza M, Manca G, Strata G B, Maffei S, Salvatore L Blood 1994; 84: 3363–3370
34. Lee R I, White P D, Amer J Med 1913; 145: 495

the activated clotting time, in which 2 ml of unanticoagulated venous blood is placed into a glass tube with kaolin particles to stimulate initiation of clotting, and then incubated at 37°C. Clotting normally occurs within 2 minutes. Portable equipment for doing activated clotting time tests outside the laboratory is now well-established and reliable.

Tests using citrated blood

Nine volumes of venous blood (i.e. 5 volumes of plasma) are added to 1 volume of 3.2% sodium citrate. Allowance should be made for patients with very abnormal haematocrits. After centrifugation the cell-free plasma is used for testing while fresh.

Prothrombin time

This test is unchanged in principle from that described by Quick.[35] It is now used most commonly to monitor the effects of therapy with warfarin or similar vitamin K antagonists. It is also a useful test of liver function, and is an important test of haemostatic integrity. It is not very sensitive to heparin. It is the time taken for plasma to clot after adding thromboplastin (usually homogenized rabbit brain) and calcium chloride. The result is expressed as a ratio (the prothrombin time ratio of the patients to a control plasma clotting time); the control is normally 12–15 seconds.

Thromboplastins from different manufacturers can give different results with plasma that is low in clotting factors. This lack of standardization used to be overcome by using the international reference thromboplastin,[36] but this is now unavailable. Laboratories may however calculate what the prothrombin time would have been by referring to calibration tables. This international normalized ratio can differ significantly from the actual test result, but the standardized approach greatly improves the control of warfarin.[37] Standardization is further improved by the provision of whole thromboplastin from DNA-derived recombinant tissue factor combined with specific phospholipids, the reliability of which has been confirmed.[38]

The international normalized ratio is abnormal if it is greater than 1.3. This may be caused by low levels not only of prothrombin, but also of any other protein in the extrinsic system, i.e. factor VII, X or V, either singly or in combination. Factor VII is the most sensitive to lack of vitamin K.

Activated partial thromboplastin time (or kaolin cephalin clotting time)

This test is virtually unchanged since first described in 1953[39] as the one-stage procedure which formed the basis for assays of intrinsic clotting factors. It is most commonly used in screening for haemostatic integrity, although it is prolonged in liver failure. It reflects the antithrombotic effect of warfarin therapy more sensitively than the international normalized ratio, but is susceptible to greater variation. It is the best test for monitoring heparin therapy.[40] The partial thromboplastin is a procoagulant phospholipid such as cephalin which is added to citrated plasma prior to calcification. This substitutes for platelet factor 3. Clotting is initiated through factor XII by the kaolin, and normally occurs in 30–45 seconds. Abnormal times are more than 6 seconds longer than the control but can be corrected by adding fresh normal plasma if there is a defect in the intrinsic system or common pathway. Lack of correction indicates the presence of an inhibitor.

Thrombin time, reptilase time and fibrinogen estimations

Plasma will clot directly on the addition of thrombin or reptilase (Batroxobin). The amount added is adjusted to give normal times of 12–15 seconds for the thrombin time and 18–22 seconds for the reptilase time. These reagents are commonly used to check for defibrination and fibrinolysis; the thrombin time may be used to check heparin therapy. The thrombin is usually of bovine origin: very occasionally, it may be antagonized by antibodies in the patient's plasma resulting from the use of bovine thrombin as a haemostat in previous surgery (personal observation). Reptilase is extracted from the venom of the snake Bothrops atrox and initiates formation of fibrin by releasing only fibrinopeptide A, e.g. no fibrinopeptide B, from fibrinogen. Prolongation of either clotting time by more than 2 seconds is abnormal and indicates defibrination and fibrin degradation products, or dysfibrinogenaemia. The reptilase time is particularly sensitive to fibrin degeneration products generated early. A prolonged thrombin time with a normal reptilase time indicates the presence of heparin. Dysfibrinogenaemia may result from rare inherited abnormalities, and from severe liver disease.

Fibrin/fibrinogen degradation products

When fibrinogen or fibrin is degraded by plasmin, a series of successively smaller fragments (X, Y, D and E) result. The earlier fragments (X and Y) are strong antagonists of thrombin (and reptilase), thus prolonging the thrombin time. Fibrin degradation products are detectable immunologically, and the widely used Wellco-Thrombo test (Wellcome, Beckenham) utilizes latex particles coated with antibodies which aggregate in the presence of fibrinogen or fibrin degradation products. The test is made more specific by using serum diluted to give the highest titre which causes agglutination. It is very sensitive but of low specificity. The presence of fibrin degradation products is not diagnostic of disseminated intravascular coagulation as increases are also found after parturition, surgery (such as exploratory laparotomy) and septicaemia without the consumption of clotting factors characteristic

REFERENCES

35. Quick A J J Biol Chem 1935; 109: 73
36. Thomson I M, Darby K V, Poller L Thromb Haemost 1986; 55: 379–382
37. Poller L Br Med 1987; 1: 1184
38. Tripodi A, Chantarangkul V, Braga M et al Thromb Haemost 1994; 72: 261–267
39. Langdell R D, Wagner R H, Brinkhous K M J Lab Clin Med 1953; 41: 637
40. Basu D, Gallus A S, Hirsh J, Cade J N Engl J Med 1972; 287: 324–327

of disseminated intravascular coagulation. Specific detection of fibrin degradation is offered by a monoclonal antibody which detects a neoantigen formed by a dimer of two D fragments.[41] However, the presence of fibrin degradation products is generally more cheaply determined by the thrombin time.

Tests of clot lysis potential

These are usually only required when monitoring therapy, such as streptokinase, or when investigating causes of defibrination. The usual test is the euglobulin clot lysis time,[8] in which a cold-acid precipitate of plasma (the euglobulin) is clotted by thrombin and its spontaneous lysis time measured; the normal range is between 90 and 120 minutes. The production and characteristics of the euglobulin are altered in the presence of heparin, so that when conducted on plasma from heparinized patients the results are unreliable.

Specific immunological assays of plasminogen, tissue plasminogen activator, prourokinase and the plasminogen activator inhibitors are now available and are replacing the euglobulin test, which is a global assay of fibrinolysis.

Automated tests

Recent developments in electronic technology have resulted in several devices which promise to provide a reliable and rapid bedside testing system on very small samples. For example, the international normalized ratio, activated partial thromboplastin time and many other clotting and lytic tests can be reliably conducted by applying a drop of citrated blood (one for each test) to a specially prepared slot on a test card. The system also offers a high degree of security of patient identification.[42] It is, of course, essential to maintain high-quality standards by regular monitoring of test performance.

Platelet tests

The platelet count is an essential part of the clotting screen, as is assessing the appearance of platelets on a standard blood smear. Tests of platelet aggregation are more appropriate for investigating congenital bleeding disorders; but the infrequently conducted prothrombin consumption index,[8] which is a global test of coagulation, can indicate how well the platelets are functioning. Normally, less than 20% of the prothrombin remains in the serum at 1 hour; consumption (adsorption on to fibrin) is defective if there is more than 25%. If the platelet count and plasma clotting tests are normal but the prothrombin consumption index is high, a platelet abnormality is likely. This picture is not uncommon after cardiac bypass, where it may indicate the need for platelet therapy, or in disorders such as renal failure or myeloma where platelet function is inhibited.

Interpretation of clotting screens

Isolated prolongation of either the international normalized ratio or the activated partial thromboplastin time indicates a specific protein deficiency (factor VII deficiency for the former, and factor VIII or factor IX deficiency for the latter). Prolongation of both tests with a normal thrombin time indicates a deficiency of factors X, V or II, or a more general deficiency as the result of liver failure or warfarin therapy. Antiprothrombinase antibodies, such as systemic lupus erythematosus inhibitor,[43] and antibodies to factor VIII, cause a prolonged activated partial thromboplastin time which cannot be corrected by adding normal plasma.

Investigation of patients with a history of bleeding disorder

In many cases the history is clear, with repeated bleeding episodes following trauma or minor surgery. A family history affecting males only is characteristic of about two-thirds of all cases of haemophilia. A recent uneventful dental extraction goes a long way to exclude a significant bleeding tendency.

Patients with a history suggestive of von Willebrand's disease and a normal platelet count should have a bleeding time (which is usually prolonged) and a clotting screen including an activated partial thromboplastin time and factor VIII assay. Patients with a prolonged bleeding time and normal clotting factors are likely to have a specific platelet defect. A normal activated partial thromboplastin time may however be found in people with mildly low levels of factors VIII, IX, XI or XII (down to about 30%). As the activities—particularly of factor VIII and fibrinogen—are liable to adrenergic boosts, repeated screens and assays taken when the patient is more relaxed may be necessary to demonstrate mild deficiencies.

The most common platelet defect is caused by recent ingestion of aspirin or similar non-steroidal anti-inflammatory drug, and this must always be excluded. In the absence of such drugs an error of platelet function is likely, either acquired, for example, through blood dyscrasias or degranulation in an extracorporeal circulation, or inborn. This may be revealed by platelet aggregometry and electron microscopy, although Glanzmann's syndrome has abnormally large platelets in the blood film.[44] Hereditary capillary fragility was formerly cited as a cause of a bleeding tendency with mild to moderate prolongation of the bleeding time, normal tests of coagulation and normal platelet count and morphology. These probably do not exist outside such obvious clinical entities as the Ehlers–Danlos syndrome, which is an inborn defect of collagen formation. Several cases of hereditary capillary fragility are probably due either to von Willebrand's disease or to a heterogeneous group of inherited disorders of platelet function with defective α or

REFERENCES

41. Whitaker A N, Masci P, Rowbotham P et al Applications of plasma assays of cross-linked fibrin degradation products (XLFDP) in the diagnosis of thromboembolic disease. Thromb Haemost 1987; 58: 231
42. Medical Devices Agency Evaluation Reports 96/07 and 96/08. HMSO 1996
43. Green D In: Bloom A L, Thomas D P (eds) Haemostasis and Thrombosis. Churchill Livingstone, Edinburgh 1987
44. Bithell T C In: Lee G R, Bithell T C, Foerster J, Athens J W, Lukens J N (eds) Wintrobe's Clinical Hematology, 9th edn. Lea & Febiger, Philadelphia 1993 p 1397

β granules. Surgical bleeding in such cases may be alleviated by platelet concentrates, cryoprecipitate or desmopressin.

BLOOD TRANSFUSION

Blood donation

In the UK the collection of all blood used for preparing therapeutic products is organized under the statutory authority of the National Blood Transfusion Services, which operate according to Guidelines[45] drawn up by senior doctors and scientists of the Services. Prior to donation, all attenders are required to answer questions regarding their personal health. First-time donors have a personal interview. All sign an undertaking that they do not participate in high-risk behaviour for transmission of human immunodeficiency virus (HIV) or hepatitis virus. A fingerprick sample is taken for estimating blood haemoglobin (more than 125 g/l for women and 135 g/l for men).

During collection, the donor lies comfortably recumbent. A pressure cuff is applied and blood is collected, sometimes under local anaesthesia, from an antecubital vein after careful cleaning of the overlying skin. Microbial contamination cannot be eliminated because skin cannot be sterilized, but it is reduced so that any surviving micro-organisms are eliminated by the powerful antiseptic qualities of the opsonins and white cells in freshly shed blood. Within 12 minutes 450 ml of venous blood is taken into a plastic pack containing 63 ml of a precisely formulated anticoagulant–preservative solution based on citrate supplemented with phosphate, dextrose and usually adenine. This allows blood to be stored for up to 35 days at 4°C with no more than 25% loss of red cell viability. The minimum interval between donations is 12 weeks, though donors are usually called 4–6-monthly.

Users of blood should be aware that there is a degree of donor morbidity, although it is low. In one study[46] there was a rate of one hospital referral among 198 119 donors, mostly those attending for the first time. The most frequent event was a severe vasovagal attack (sometimes leading to further injury), although angina, arterial puncture and phlebitis also occurred.

Donation testing prior to banking

Blood grouping

Twenty-three systems of blood group antigens (and five collections and two series) are currently described.[47] Although our knowledge is now extending into molecular genetics, only a few are regarded as being of potential clinical significance. Each donation is tested for ABO, full Rh CDE phenotype and red cell antibodies. Recognition of the importance of a few immunogens such as Rh c, K (Kell), Duffy (Fy), and Kidd (Jk) is increasing, especially in women of childbearing age. Blood packs are increasingly labelled with fuller phenotype information, offering better guidance to hospital blood banks.

Microbiological screening

Currently in the UK, this includes the hepatitis B surface antigen, and antibodies to syphilis, HIV types 1 and 2, and to the hepatitis C virus. It is policy to trace all donors confirmed positive for any of these markers for advice and, where appropriate, counselling. Screening for antibodies to human T lymphotrophic virus I is not yet being conducted, although it is under discussion.[48]

A few cases of transfusion-transmitted hepatitis B still occur each year through carriers with undetectable hepatitis B surface antigen. Some can be detected by tests for antibodies to viral core proteins (anti-core), usually a marker of immunity. The judicious use of such tests could extend the screening procedure.

Transmission of syphilis is well-recognized but very rare. The spirochaete only survives in stored blood for a few days. People with a history of clinical syphilis—and yaws and pinta—are permanently banned from donation. The antibody markers used (Venereal Disease Research Laboratory, Treponema pallidum haemagglutinin) are not specific and, although quite sensitive, may miss recently infected people.

Testing for HIV antigens, or for genes by nucleic acid amplification is under investigation. The rates of transfusion-transmitted HIV varies widely throughout the world,[49] although in the UK since 1985 there have been only 1.02 cases/million (in contrast with 3.61/million in the USA). The current risk of HIV transmission to recipients in the UK is estimated to be of the order of one in 2 million. These are from infected donations which are missed by the enzyme-linked immunosorbent assay test, nearly always because the donation was collected during the 21-days so-called window period after infection but before detectable antibody formation. The incidence is substantially higher in parts of North America.[50] So far in the UK, only persons attending donor sessions have been found to carry HIV 2.

More than 90% of people reacting positively with previous tests for surrogate markers for non-A non-B hepatitis were later confirmed as having antibody to hepatitis C virus. Screening for hepatitis C virus antibodies started in 1991, and these are currently found in about 1 donor per 15 000 in the UK[51,52]—a dramatic reduction reflecting a successful strategy in excluding donations at risk. The most common risk factor (apart from blood transfusion before 1991) is a history of recreational injections, and goes back to the 'flower power' era of the late 1960s. Such attenders should be excluded by the current more rigorous personal interview. Sexual transmission was thought to be uncommon, but some studies in Europe show that up to 5% of the sexual contacts of people with chronic hepatitis C are positive.

REFERENCES

45. Guidelines for the Blood Transfusion Service, 3rd edn. HMSO, London 1996
46. Popovsky M A, Whitaker B, Arnold N L Transfusion 1995; 35: 734–737
47. Daniels G. Human Blood Groups. Blackwell Science, Oxford 1995
48. Pagliuca A, Pawson R, Mufti G J Br Med J 1995; 311: 1313–1314
49. Franceschi S, Dal Maso L, La Vecchia C Br Med J 1995; 311: 1534–1536
50. Lackritz E M, Satten G A, Aberle-Grasse J et al N Eng J Med 1995; 333: 1721–1726
51. Alter H I, Purcell R H, Shih J W et al N Engl J Med 1989; 321: 1494–1500
52. Vrielink H, Zaaijer H L, Reesink H W, Borst-Loef J, Cuypers H T M, Lelie P N Vox Sang 1995; 69: 257–258

A study of recipients infected with hepatitis C virus by blood[53] and referred to a tertiary centre (which may therefore have selected for more seriously affected recipients) has shown that the intervals from transfusion to chronic persistent hepatitis, chronic active hepatitis, cirrhosis and hepatocellular carcinoma increase, with a mean of 10.9, 11.2, 20.6 and 28.3 years respectively. In another unpublished study by Alter, the outcome for every 100 patients infected was: 15 resolved, 68 got a stable disorder and 17 developed cirrhosis, of whom 4 died either of liver failure or hepatocellular carcinoma. Infection with hepatitis C virus, especially in the early stages, is amenable to therapy with interferons.

Surrogate tests for hepatitis have proved difficult to abandon, and have largely become a cost–benefit argument.[54] Nevertheless, further viruses undoubtedly remain to be discovered; current alphabetical nomenclature of identified viruses has reached 'HGV'.

Some organisms of high prevalence in the community, such as parvovirus, cytomegalovirus and Epstein–Barr virus, are also transmitted by blood transfusion. There is however no need to exclude previously infected donors who are well, although transmission of cytomegalovirus to vulnerable recipients, such as premature babies and immunosuppressed individuals, must be avoided by selecting sero-negative donations or depleting the leucocyte content. Parvovirus B19[55] usually causes non-specific malaise, although it can produce erythema infectiosum in children and arthritis in adults; and marrow aplasia in non-immune recipients of blood collected from viraemic but symptomless donors. It is difficult to exclude such donors from the general blood supply. Human T lymphotrophic virus I and II are rare in the UK but commoner among Afro-Caribbean and Japanese communities. Nucleic and amplification tests will soon enhance the detection of most micro-organisms.

Chagas disease (Trypanosoma cruzi) can be transmitted in rural parts of South America and people who have exposed themselves to such infections are not acceptable as donors unless they are negative for T. cruzi antibodies. Similarly, people with a history of malaria can donate providing they have no malarial antibody.

Processing into blood products (Fig. 3.8)

Virtually all blood is processed within hours of collection, with either some plasma or platelets or both removed for therapeutic use. Most of the separated plasma is further fractionated into therapeutic clotting factor concentrates, albumin and immunoglobulins.

Red cell products

The primary red cell products are:

1. Whole blood (rarely used now, except in paediatric formulations).
2. Red cell concentrates, prepared by removing 200 ± 20 ml of plasma for fractionation, leaving the haematocrit of the residue at about 70%. It is difficult to produce this to a consistent standard. Red cell viability is not compromised, but red cell concentrates with higher haematocrits are too viscous for easy transfusion.
3. Red cell concentrates—supplemented. All the available plasma has been removed, the cells being supplemented in 100 ml of a crystalloid nutritive optimal additive solution.[57–59] The average haematocrit is close to 60%, with a narrow range, and the products have better consistency and flow characteristics than standard red cell concentrates. The diluents are crystalloid solutions, usually of saline, glucose, adenine and mannitol; some formulations have additional nutrients. They can extend the shelf-life of the red cells. Unless the buffy coat is removed however from the whole blood, the non-red cellular elements can form an agglutinum;[60] this is preventable by adding citrate to the diluents,[61] although in practice the agglutinum seems not to cause any problems.

Packs designed for paediatric use are available in which every donation is partitioned into several packs, each of which may contain less than 100 ml of red cell product. This allows either each child requiring top-up transfusions to get blood from a more limited number of donors (although this requires blood to be used throughout its 35-day shelf-life), or for several patients to benefit from one donation within a few days of collection.

For a few patients such as those sensitive to foreign plasma proteins, red cell preparations can be washed (through successive changes of crystalloid solutions). The shelf-life of these transfusions is only 24 hours. Red cells can also be frozen under conditions which allow their recovery. When thawed they are washed so that leucocyte and plasma contamination are minimized. Blood of rare types, can be stored frozen and there are several international stocks.

Platelet concentrates[33]

Although Slichter and Harker[32] reported that up to 85% of platelets could be recovered in platelet concentrates from single donations, these yields can rarely be attained routinely. Standard concentrates usually contain little more than 6×10^{11} platelets suspended in 60 ml plasma. Plastic packs with special plasticizers[61] are used for storage; these allow efficient gaseous exchange and therefore sustained oxidative metabolism in the platelets while they are in

REFERENCES

53. Tong M J, El-Farra N S, Reikes A R, Co R L N Engl J Med 1995; 332: 1463–1466
54. Dodd R Y, Reesink H W Vox Sang 1995; 69: 280–281
55. Tsujimura M, Matsushita K, Shiraki H, Sato H, Okochi K, Maeda Y Vox Sang 1995; 69: 206–212
56. Hogman C F, Akerblom O, Hedblund K et al Vox Sang 1983; 45: 217–223
57. Lovric V A, Prince B, Bryant J Vox Sang 1977; 33: 346–352
58. Heaton A, Miripol J et al Br J Haematol 1984; 57: 467–478
59. Robertson M, Boulton F E, Doughty R et al Vox Sang 1985; 49: 259–266
60. Napier J A F, Ashford P R, Hayward M M Vox Sang 1985; 49: 315–318
61. Rock G, Sherring V A, Tittley P Transfusion 1984; 24: 147–152

the packs, enabling storage for up to 5 days at 22°C.[62] Platelets cannot be stored at any other temperature. Longer storage is not allowed as bacterial contamination from donor skin[63] can proliferate, causing severe septic reactions.[64] Five separate platelet concentrates, usually pooled prior to transfusion, constitute an adult therapeutic dose. The platelet count should rise by about 0.1 $\times 10^9$/l of blood per kilogram body weight of the recipient for each platelet concentrate, or 25 $\times 10^9$/l for each adult therapeutic dose, given to a 60 kg adult (doubled in asplenic patients), with a return to baseline within 3 days.

Standard platelet concentrates contain traces of red cells (up to 1.0×10^9) and also at least 10% of the donated leucocytes (up to 0.2 $\times 10^9$ per unit). This can cause pyrexia in patients receiving repeated platelet concentrates, and transmit cellular viruses such as cytomegalovirus and human T lymphotrophic virus I. Some of the pyrogenic material derives from the contents of the leucocytes leaking into the suspension.[65] Sepsis from the platelet concentrates should not be forgotten as blood products which are not stored at 4°C are poor at self-sterilization.

In recent years platelet demand has increased, particularly for supporting patients with chemotherapeutically induced marrow aplasia. Developments such as buffy coat-derived platelets have helped meet the need, and reduced pyrogenic reactions. The 'bottom and top'[66] approach has been widely adopted in the UK (see Fig. 3.9). The platelet-rich buffy coat of whole blood collected into standard citrate phosphate dextrose anticoagulant—along with about 30 ml of red cells and 50 ml of plasma—is retained after removing the red cells into optimal additive solutions and taking the plasma into a separate pack. Four ABO-compatible buffy coats are pooled, mixed and lightly spun; the supernatant platelet-rich plasma is taken off and is available as one adult therapeutic dose. Platelets produced in this way may have fewer than 5×10^6 (5 million) leucocytes and more than 250×10^9 platelets—sufficient to meet the criterion of leucocyte-depleted products indicated when trying to avoid the complications of cytomegalovirus carriage, or of leucocyte alloimmunization which results from sensitization to class I and class II human leucocyte antigens carried on contaminating 'passenger' white cells. Although only Class I human leucocyte antigens are present on platelets, the development of anti-class I antibodies in the patient's plasma diminishes the recovery of donor platelets in the circulation, sometimes making such patients very markedly refractory to treatment. Sensitized recipients recover better when given human leucocyte antigen class I-compatible platelet concentrates. This usually requires collection from selected donors by automated apheresis procedures. Additive solutions can also be used to improve the quality of platelet concentrates[67,68] and increase the yield of plasma. Storage beyond 5 days is, however, not licensed because of the risk of bacterial contamination and proliferation mentioned previously.

Plasma and cryoprecipitate

The freshly separated plasma is rapidly frozen to –30°C or even colder: a proportion is retained for clinical use as frozen fresh plasma or as cryoprecipitate, and the rest is sent for fractionation. Freshly separated plasma can be stored at 4°C; and plasma may be separated from the cells up to 5 days after expiry. These practices are not common in the UK, but do yield a product (single donor plasma) which has previously helped in the management of surgical bleeding exacerbated by hypoprothrombinaemia. Although the proteins of the prothrombin complex are intact in liquid-stored plasma, factor V and factor VIII are labile. Factor VIII activity is reduced by half after 24 hours at 20°C.[69] It should also be noted that the sodium content of fresh plasma is high— about 170 mmol/l—whereas time-expired plasma will have a lower sodium and a higher potassium content. Cryoprecipitate is prepared from fresh frozen plasma by careful thawing at 4°C, which allows a gelatinous precipitate, rich in factor VIII, von Willebrand's factor, fibrinogen and fibronectin, to be retained after re-centrifugation. The volume of the product is 10–30 ml and it contains all the other coagulation factors found in fresh frozen plasma.[70] For adults, 5–10 donations are usually pooled prior to transfusion. Investigations are currently under way to improve the safety of fresh frozen plasma and cryoprecipitate by treatments such as solvent-detergent or ultraviolet light to inactivate viruses, but these are not yet licensed.[71]

Changes in blood on storage

Although more than 75% of the red cells are still viable at expiry (35 days), platelets and granulocytes are dead by 2 days' storage of whole blood or red cell concentrates at 4°C. Many lymphocytes are also dead, but some T and B memory cells survive.

Although red cell viability is maintained, membrane rigidity increases; and the glycolytic intermediate 2,3-diphosphoglycerate, characteristic of circulating red cells, becomes depleted by 10 days of storage, causing increased oxygen avidity. These changes revert to normal within hours of transfusion. Post-transfusion jaundice is not uncommon in adults receiving several units of viable blood. Three units of red cells, each of which gives approximately 80% recovery in the circulation, means that up to 100 ml of the cells are non-viable, forming about 1250 mg of bilirubin. If even a tenth of the theoretical peak of serum bilirubin were to be reached in the following 24 hours, the level would be more than 4 mg/dl or 70 μmol/l.

REFERENCES

62. Turner V S, Mitchell S G, Kang S K, Hawker R J Vox Sang 1995; 69: 195–200
63. Anderson K C, Lew M A, Gorgone B C, Martel J, Leamy C B, Sullivan B Am J Med 1986; 81: 405–411
64. Chiu E K W, Yuen K Y, Lie A K W et al. Transfusion 1994; 34: 950–954
65. Ferrara J L M Transfusion 1995; 35: 89–90
66. Hogman C F, Eriksson L, Hedlund K, Wallvik J Vox Sang 1988; 55: 211–217
67. Adams G A, Swenson S D, Rock G Vox Sang 1987; 52: 305–312
68. Holme S, Heaton W A, Courtright M Br J Haematol 1987; 66: 233–238
69. Prowse C V, Waterston Y G et al Vox Sang 1987; 52: 257–264
70. Pool J D, Shannon A E N Engl J Med 1965; 273: 1443–1447
71. Williamson L M, Allain J P Vox Sang 1995; 69: 159–165

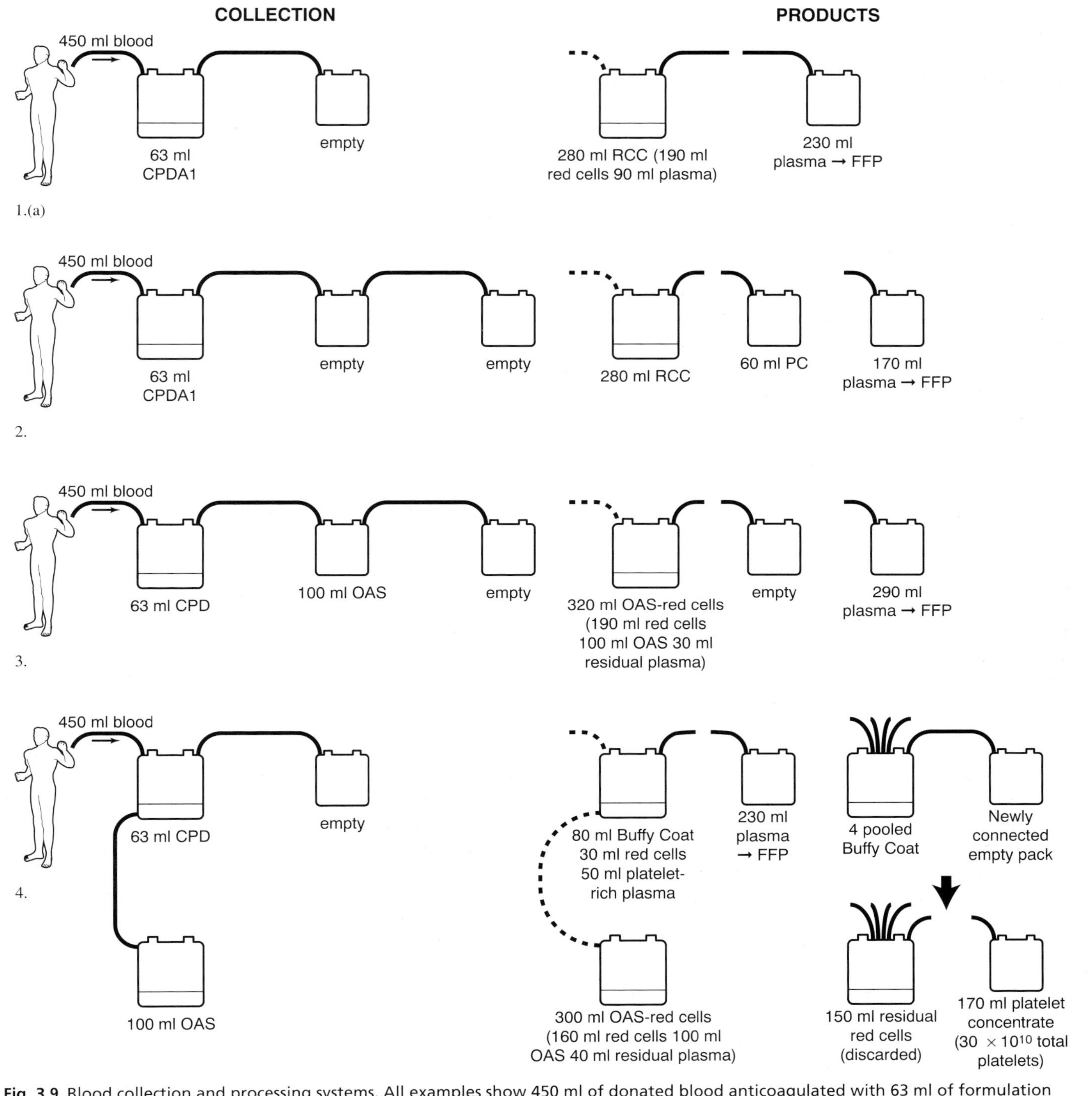

Fig. 3.9 Blood collection and processing systems. All examples show 450 ml of donated blood anticoagulated with 63 ml of formulation citrate phosphate dextrose adenine. **1a,b** Double-bag systems, giving fresh frozen plasma (FFP) and red cells. **2** Triple-bag system, giving FFP and platelets. **3** Triple-bag (optimal additive system; OAS) giving plasma. **4** Bottom-and-top (BAT) system in which, after centrifugation, the red cells are deposited straight into OAS, the plasma for FFP taken into an empty pack, and the residual 80 ml buffy coat used for preparing platelets (see text). The dashed line attached to the primary red cell packs after processing represents the segmented donor line, the contents of which are available for pre-transfusion compatibility testing. CPDA1 = Citrate phosphate dextrose adenine solution; CPD = citrate phosphate dextrose; RCC = red cell concentrates; PC = plasma concentrate.

In plasma the labile clotting factors V and VIII decline, and potassium rises to 25 mmol, by expiry. Microaggregates of dead cells and platelets surrounded by fibrin begin to accumulate after 7 days. In most clinical situations these are of little relevance, although it became customary for many anaesthetists to use microaggregate filters routinely. This expensive policy was not always applied rationally; for example, filters are ineffective for blood less than 7 days old. Some febrile transfusion reactions associated with older blood may however be reduced by the judicious use of filters,[72] although the pyrogenic effects of cytokines released from dying white cells cannot be filtered out.

The term 'fresh blood' defies a precise description. It is logistically difficult for modern services to provide blood safe for transfusion within 24 hours of donation, let alone the 2 hours or so which might justify its use. There is no doubt that very fresh blood is an excellent haemostat but haemostasis is equally well-provided by platelet concentrates with less risk of circulatory overload and viral contamination. When 'fresh' blood is used for neonatal transfusion it may be up to 5 days old, as the red cells at this stage have not yet become depleted of the glycolytic intermediates, or rigid; and the potassium content of the donor plasma is still low.

PRODUCT LIABILITY

It should be realized that the blood transfusion services of the UK are now obliged under British and European Community law[73] to ensure that all products issued for patient use are of the highest standard. This liability, which enhances the concept of professional responsibility, extends to the clinician who orders the actual transfusion. Similar laws apply internationally.

Pre-transfusion testing (cross-matching)

Blood grouping

The visible direct agglutination of red cells by specific and potent sera allows the group of the blood to be determined. Until recently, with the exception of certain animal and plant-derived lectins, all such sera were of human donor origin. High-quality anti-ABO and anti-RhD reagents are now available as monoclonal antibodies.[74,75]

Compatibility testing

The rate of adverse immune reactions after transfusing blood selected only for ABO-compatibility, which would include group O blood being transfused to non-group O patients, is less than 1%. Such reactions can however be very severe, and are easily avoided by selection of blood after more specific tests. Conceptually, the most satisfactory procedure involves exposing the donor red cells to the patient's serum and observing for haemolysis or agglutination. This became known as the cross-match (although the 'cross' became redundant when the reciprocal act of exposing the patient's cells to the donor plasma was abandoned). The sensitivity of this test can be enhanced by additional steps such as the Coombs' antiglobulin test, which has been used for 50 years.[76] This agglutinates cells which have reacted with, but not been directly agglutinated by, the immune globulin (complement components and/or immunoglobulins). Coombs' antiglobulin reagent is antibody raised in animals to human immune globulins.

By the mid 1970s a number of tests of increasing complexity had been developed, involving diverse temperatures and additives such as enzymes and enhancing solutions in order to ensure that no antibody of possible significance was present in the patient's serum. Transfusionists then began to rationalize pre-transfusion testing by using more selective techniques, avoiding cold incubations, and using panels of prepared red cell suspensions to detect and identify any antibodies of realistic clinical significance in the patient's serum.[77] Procedures conducted in advance of planned surgery, such as the 'group, screen and save serum' allow compatible blood to be provided from stocks when required. The most reliable techniques are still based on the antiglobulin (Coombs') test, which in practice most often equates with clinical significance. In an emergency, blood for patients with no antibodies detectable on the screen can be provided securely within 15 minutes.

A system for electronic cross-matching has been advocated, particularly in the USA where it is already in use.[78] Blood is selected for patients of known group and negative antibody screen by matching the patient's records with that of the donation. A high level of confidence is required which can only be given by a comprehensive system of computerization.

When antibodies of potential clinical significance are discovered, blood negative for the offending antigen should be selected. Panels of donors of unusual or rare blood types are regularly maintained; but in emergencies, a decision must sometimes be taken before such blood becomes available, and although colloid support can delay the need to transfuse red cells, it may be necessary to select the least incompatible blood. A particularly difficult situation arises in patients with autoimmune haemolysis and a positive direct antiglobulin (Coombs') test, as this indicates the presence of antibodies reacting not only against the patient's own red cells, but also against transfused cells. The patient's serum may additionally contain alloantibodies which could increase the reaction against transfused cells. If there is time these should be excluded by special laboratory techniques. Patients should not be denied blood transfusion on the basis of an in vitro incompatibility, as this may not be reflected absolutely in vivo. High-dose corticosteroids are indicated.

REFERENCES

72. Helton M R, Huang S T, Floyd D M, McGowan E I Transfusion 1987; 27: 279–280
73. The Consumer Protection Act. Inst Med Lab Sci Gaz 1988; April: 201–202
74. McGowan A, Todd A, Chirnside A et al Vox Sang 1989; 56: 122–138
75. Jones J Vox Sang 1995; 69: 236–241
76. Coombs R R A, Mourant A E, Race R R Br J Exp Pathol 1945; 26: 255
77. Boulton F E, Bruce M, Lloyd E Clin Lab Haematol 1987; 9: 333–341
78. Marsh W L, Reid M E, Kuriyan M, Marsh N J A handbook of clinical and laboratory practices in the tranfusion of red blood cells. Virginia Moneta Med Press 1993

Blood transfusion ordering policies

Reducing the amount of cross-matched blood that is not used reduces the traffic of blood through the blood bank and maximizes the available stock. Systems which allow a unit to be matched for more than one person at the same time are very difficult to operate. It is far better to maintain stocks and issue only when there is a reasonable certainty of use. As many operations do not require blood, and as a 'group, screen and save' policy allows a rapid delivery of compatible blood when required, the problems of storing a designated pack of blood in the theatre or ward holding area can be avoided. This has allowed the adoption of protocols for junior medical staff which can substantially reduce the amount of blood ordered without compromising patient care.[79–81] Details vary according to local circumstances.

Overuse of group O blood

It is a remarkable observation that at any one time in the UK, the proportion of blood of group O held within the National Blood Authority stocks is significantly lower than the proportion of people with blood of group O in the general population (46%). At times the proportion in stock was less than half—23%. The stocks of group O Rh D-negative blood were at times in even more extreme imbalance—there should be nearly 8% in stock. The corollaries are that there are more donors of group O on the national panels and more blood of group O is collected, and that stocks of group AB blood are often high relative to the frequency of this group in the population (3%); indeed this also applies to blood of group B.

Group O RhD-negative blood is often regarded (inappropriately) as the universal donor type, and held in reserve refrigerators or emergency rooms—sometimes with little provision for adequate records of storage conditions or withdrawal procedures. Some of these holding areas are in relatively remote areas of hospital premises and this encourages waste. These patterns result from systems which require significant quantities of group O blood to be available without much prospect of it being used. This may apply not only to emergency cover but sometimes more routinely where group O blood is selected for patients of group B or even AB. Even though the problems of transfusing ABO-incompatible plasma with red cells of group O are slight— and even more slight when supplemented red cell concentrate is used—the given blood should be ABO-identical with the patient's ABO group whenever possible. This would enhance the availability of group O blood when it is really needed.

Administration of blood[82]

Obsessional care should be taken to identify the correct patient who is to receive the blood. One British study[83] estimated that 1 in 6000 blood samples from patients about to undergo transfusion had been taken from another patient; most incidents were identified through inconsistency with previous records which, given the population frequencies, indicates that this figure is an underestimate. The same study also estimated that 1 in 29 000 wrong units were submitted for transfusion, either through sampling error, or error of identifying the recipient or the pack. Such errors have been successfully avoided by a system of additional unique identification of the recipient and supplying the blood in a combination-locked plastic overwrap.[84]

Blood should always be administered through a giving set with an in-line filter which has been primed with saline or dextrose saline. Solutions containing calcium—Ringer lactate and Haemaccel, for example—should be washed through thoroughly. Microaggregate filters are not routinely required. Giving sets should be replaced every 24 hours and phlebitis may be reduced by changing the drip site every 2 or 3 days. Unless acute blood loss is being replaced, each pack of blood should be infused over 4 hours, although up to 8 hours is acceptable if the cardiovascular reserve is limited. Longer periods encourage bacterial growth and decrease red cell viability. Air embolism is now rarely a problem as the blood is supplied in collapsible plastic packs, but as albumin solutions are usually supplied in bottles it is important to ensure that the line is watched and that positive air pressure is not used to enhance flow.

Effects of blood transfusion

One donor-unit of blood contains about 190 ml of red cells. Transfusion of a fully viable and serologically compatible unit will raise the venous blood haematocrit of a 60 kg adult by about 4.5% (0.045), and the haemoglobin concentration by about 14 g/l (1.4 g/dl or 10% in the old parlance). These recoveries are somewhat lower for buffy coat-derived red cells and for washed cells because of losses during production. In the absence of further blood loss or destruction after transfusion, the red cells will senesce normally over the next 120 days. Although transfusion is usually uneventful, pulse, blood pressure and temperature should be recorded throughout. The rapid transfusion of several units of cold blood may be undesirable, especially if delivered through a central line, but warming blood should be conducted very carefully. Blood is best warmed by feeding an extended giving set through a carefully controlled heat exchanger. Warming blood packs directly is wrong, and any unused blood so warmed should be discarded.

Adverse effects

Improperly stored blood (too long, too warm, too cold, or inadvertent freezing) will cause storage lesions, giving suboptimal

REFERENCES

79. Friedman B A, Oberman H A, Chadwick A R, Kingdon K I Transfusion 1976; 16: 380–387
80. Penney G C, Moores H M, Boulton F E Br J Obstet Gynaecol 1982; 89: 100–105
81. Napier J A F, Biffen A H, Lay D Br Med J 1985; 291: 799
82. McClelland D B L (ed) Handbook of Transfusion Medicine. UK Blood Transfusion Services. HMSO, London 1989
83. McClelland D B L, Phillips P Br Med J 1994; 308: 1205–1206
84. Mercuriali F, Inghilleri G, Colotti M T et al Vox Sang 1996; 70: 16–20

responses and early haemolysis. Profound jaundice may mimic hepatitis, and poor recovery of cells in the circulation may suggest an immune destruction. But even properly stored blood can cause adverse reactions, of which there are two main causes—immune-mediated phenomena and infections.

Infectious causes

Viral transmission in blood is much reduced by current donor selection and microbiological screening, but bacterial infection is often overlooked as a cause of problems. Serious morbidity from bacterial contamination is more common than transfusion transmitted HIV in the UK. With platelet concentrates, where the common organisms are skin contaminants such as coagulase-negative staphylococci, as many as 2% may be contaminated,[85] although a more accepted figure is 1 in 2000 units of single platelet concentrates, or 1 in 350 pooled units.[86] Such high rates indicate the need for a pre-release monitoring system;[87] unfortunately no suitable one is yet available, although it is under development.[88] The organisms have to survive storage at 4°C in red cell preparations, even though they may flourish better at higher temperatures, which may be reached when the bags are in transit. Such organisms are often Gram-negative bacilli such as Pseudomonas[89], Yersinia spp or Serratia spp.[90] These are unlikely skin contaminants, which suggests that they gain access to the contents of the blood pack after collection, during processing, transport or storage. Yersinia enterocolitica may be carried in donor granulocytes.

The symptoms of acute bacterial infection are often dramatic, although they may be obscured in recipients of platelets by problems caused by the accompanying non-infective pyrogens. The clinical reaction to contaminated cells, which is actually caused by bacterial endotoxins, is rapid, with profound hypotension, shock and disseminated intravascular coagulation compounded by bleeding and renal failure. In surgical patients under anaesthesia the first sign is often excessive bleeding from small vessels. Conscious patients may develop acute gastrointestinal symptoms with cramps and vomiting. Only patients inherently fit prior to transfusion are likely to survive. High-dose antibiotics, corticosteroids and transfusion of blood products must be started at once. ABO-incompatibility must be excluded by rechecking the groups of the blood residues, and the presence of bacteria sought by direct microscopy and Gram stain. Attempts should be made to culture the bacteria from the patient's blood, taking account of any antibiotic therapy. This may have to be at post-mortem, on many occasions.

Immune-related phenomena

All the elements of blood are capable of immunizing recipients, even plasma proteins and transfused immunoglobulins. Occasional patients, particularly those who have had previous transfusions or pregnancies, may react adversely by developing a low-grade pyrexia, urticaria, severe rigors, bronchospasm or angioedema. These reactions are usually the result of antibodies in the patient's serum against donor white cells, although angioedema may reflect sensitization to infused plasma protein. The reverse—antibodies in the donor plasma reacting with the patient's white cells—is well-established as a cause of 'acute transfusion-related lung injury,'[91] a serious complication resulting in acute oedema of the lungs which may require a period of artificial ventilation as well as vigorous diuresis and corticosteroids.

The less dramatic shivering symptoms of immune reactions not related to red cells are particularly unpleasant for patients receiving frequent transfusions. They may be controlled by antipyretics such as paracetamol (aspirin is not indicated because of its antiplatelet activity). The routine use of chlorpheniramine, 10 mg, and hydrocortisone, 100 mg, is no longer recommended. Antihistamines cannot counter infusions of cytokines; and repeated hydrocortisone produces Cushing's syndrome (see Chapter 19). The severity of reactions can be reduced or eliminated by using blood from which most of the leucocytes have been removed. This can be partly achieved by using microaggregate filters on centrifuged blood in which the microaggregates are coalesced,[72] but is better achieved by purpose-designed leucocyte depletion filters, or even better by removing the bulk of leucocytes during processing of the blood, as this avoids the 'cytokine shower'.[65]

Immune haemolysis of transfused red cells may still occur in spite of improved compatibility testing, but acute reactions are very rare if the identification procedures are conducted correctly.[83] When a patient experiences an adverse response, the infusion should be slowed down or stopped. The urine output should be monitored for haemoglobinuria and oliguria. Although traces of ABO-incompatible red cells (less than 0.5 ml) in platelet concentrates are most unlikely to provoke severe reactions, part transfused packs of red cell preparations (less than 100 ml) can produce anaphylactic shock, gastrointestinal symptoms and renal failure, and require active resuscitation. Donations associated with such reactions should be returned for further investigations, with 10 ml clotted and 5 ml ethylenediaminetetraacetic acid blood from the patient. If a further transfusion is still required, it should be closely observed; if not required immediately, time should be allowed for further red cell serological tests to be completed.

Delayed haemolytic reactions occur when a patient who has previously been sensitized to a red cell antigen, but in whom the antibody titres have become undetectable serologically, is exposed to the same antigen again. At first, the transfused cells are unaffected; but when, usually after a few days, the secondary response produces high titres of specific antibody, the cells are haemolysed resulting in jaundice and sometimes transient renal impairment.

REFERENCES

85. Goldman M, Blajchman M A Transfusion Med Rev 1991; 5: 73–83
86. Chiu E K W, Yuen K Y, Lie A K W et al Transfusion 1994; 34: 950–954
87. Blajchman M A Transfusion 1994; 34: 940–942
88. Krisher K K, Whyburn D R, Koepnick F E J Clin Microbiol 1993; 31: 793–797
89. Scott J, Boulton F E, Govan J R W, Miles R, McClelland D B L, Prowse C V Vox Sang 1987; 54: 201–204
90. Personal observation Boulton F E Transfusion Med 1997; 7 Suppl 1: 13
91. Mollison P L, Engelfriet C P, Contreras M Blood Transfusion in Clinical Medicine, 9th edn. Blackwell Scientific Publications, Oxford 1993 pp 681–682

The destruction of 200 ml of red cells releases 240 mg of iron and 2.5 g of bilirubin. The antibodies involved are usually those best detected by the Coombs' antiglobulin test (Rh, Fy, Jk, K, etc).

Post-transfusion purpura

This unusual complication is how recognized more frequently.[92] Recipients are usually multiparous women who receive a perioperative transfusion some years after their last pregnancy. Five to ten days later a thrombocytopenic purpura develops, and the serum contains strongly active alloantibodies to platelets which cross-react with the patient's own platelets. Severely affected patients usually respond favourably to high doses of intravenous gammaglobulin (0.4 g/kg over 2–3 days) or to plasma exchange (2.5 litres daily for 3 or more days).[93,94]

Non-specific immunomodulative effects and transfusions during surgical treatment for cancers[95–97]

For some time a programme of blood transfusion—usually as red cell concentrates—prior to renal transplantation has been used to reduce rejection (see Chapter 8). The mechanism is obscure, and indeed the validity of the observations has been questioned.[98] Furthermore, graft-versus-host disease has been transmitted to immunosuppressed patients by viable lymphocytes.[99]

There has been increasing concern on whether blood, or more specifically the 'passenger' leucocytes, may have a deleterious effect on the survival of patients if transfused during surgical resection of cancer. In 1995, Vamvakas[97] analysed 60 studies published in the English language from 1985 to 1994 on the effects of transfusion in six types of surgical cancers (colorectal, breast, head and neck, lung, prostate and stomach). Study sizes varied from 58 to 1000 cases; most were retrospective. It was difficult to identify confounding factors, such as whether an apparently adverse effect of the blood might be because it was more often used for people with more advanced disease, or because of suppression of the immunosurveillance of neoplastic tissues. There was however no demonstrable adverse effect of transfusion in breast cancer (eight studies). In colorectal cancer, 28 studies, of which since 1990 five out of 10 were prospective also failed to show benefit. The issue can only be clarified by trials comparing non-leucocyte-depleted blood with blood containing less than one million leucocytes in each donated unit. A few studies even show a slight benefit of transfusion of non-leucodepleted blood. There are similar concerns in relation to predisposition to post-operative infection.[101] Removal of leukocytes during blood processing is likely to become more common.

The use of high-dose aprotinin

The infusion of very large doses of aprotinin, a general inhibitor of peptidases which has structural affinities to tissue factor pathway inhibitor, has been shown to reduce blood requirements in cardiovascular surgery quite dramatically.[101] The mechanism may involve reducing intraoperative fibrinolysis; whether this approach is ultimately safe and can be used more generally is not yet known.

Autologous transfusion programmes[102–104]

Concern about blood safety in the wake of HIV has led to increased use of preoperative donation, where patients deposit two or more units of their own blood in the few weeks prior to surgery. Preoperative autologous donation has become routine in some British hospitals for many years; suitable patients must be selected, their operations must be documented and performed expeditiously. These schemes have not generally thrived because of cost and perceived inconvenience. Nevertheless, preoperative autologous donation is suitable for many patients and is likely to become more attractive. Various techniques of cell salvage offer an alternative, ranging from simple but rather cumbersome systems in which heparinized blood shed into clean wounds is aspirated directly into a container bag and reinfused, to the expensively elaborate manufactured but effective cell savers.

At a consensus conference in October 1995,[104] an independent panel of medical and non-medical experts drew up a statement for the UK which highlighted the appropriateness of autologous blood being collected either in the weeks preoperatively or perioperatively. Preoperative autologous donation was deemed especially useful in orthopaedic surgery, although there is an apparent, but not necessarily real, disadvantage from being committed to a specific operative date. The technique of acute normovolaemic haemodilution, in which certain patients have blood removed and simultaneously replaced with crystalloid or colloid solutions while they are being prepared in the anaesthetic room, was discussed in some depth by the conference but did not gain approval from the panel on grounds of danger (for example, silent myocardial infarction) and rather poor actual reduction of blood losses.

Some indications for blood transfusion

Red cell preparations

Wherever possible red cell concentrates or suspended red cell concentrates should be used.

REFERENCES

92. Walker W, Yap P L, Kilpatrick D C et al Blut 1988; 57: 323–325
93. Hamblin T J, Naorose Abidi D M, Nee P A et al Vox Sang 1984; 49–164
94. Berney S I, Metcalfe P, Wathen N C, Waters A H Br J Haematol 1985; 61: 627–632
95. Blumberg N, Agarwal M M, Chuang C Br Med J 1985; 290: 1037–1039
96. Singh S K, Margnet R I, de Bruin R W F Br J Surg 1988; 75: 377–379
97. Vamvakas E C Transfusion 1995; 35: 760–768
98. Editorial. Time to abandon pre-transplant blood transfusion? Lancet 1988; 1: 567–568
99. Sheehan T, McLaren K M, Salter D, Ludlam C A Br J Haematol 1988; 69: 571–572
100. Jensen L S, Kissmeyer-Nielsen P, Wolff B et al. Lancet 1996; 348: 841–845
101. Royston D, Taylor K M, Bidstrup B P, Sapsford R N Lancet 1987, ii: 1289–1291
102. Voak D, on behalf of the Autologous Transfusion Working Party of the British Committee for Standards in Haematology. Autologous Transfusion. Transfusion Med 1993; 3: 307–316
103. Tawes R L, Spence R K Semin Vasc Surg 1994; 7: 65–130
104. Christie B Br Med J 1995; 311: 971

Preoperative chronic anaemia

In order to avoid even the minimal risk of transmitting a viral infection, transfusion prior to non-urgent surgery should not be given to persons with chronic iron deficiency of known cause. A course of iron should be prescribed. If the anaemia is the result of chronic severe blood loss, particularly when an underlying malignancy is suspected, it may not be reasonable to wait for iron therapy to take effect. Even then, however, transfusion is often unnecessary unless the haemoglobin level is reduced to less than 90 g/l in adults. Deficiency of vitamin B_{12} or folic acid of known causes, or combined haematinic deficiency, should similarly receive specific therapy rather than transfusion unless surgery is urgent.

Intraoperative transfusion

This depends on the vital signs being monitored by the anaesthetist. An adult may withstand a loss of up to 1 litre of blood without ill effect. Fluid replacement, if necessary with artificial colloid, may suffice. Unless there is an episode of brisk bleeding, red cell concentrates should be used. For certain procedures, e.g. vascular surgery, it is probably beneficial for the patient's postoperative replacement of red cells to be less than the amount lost. Flow is improved as viscosity is lowered and thrombosis may become less likely.

Surgical procedures of an hour or more are associated with alterations in platelet number and function in addition to a lengthening of clotting times.[105] The effects of intra- and postoperative hypothermia have to be considered, as alterations in platelet function[106] and coagulation factors[107] may be a complication. Even the hypothermia which often occurs in operations such as total hip replacement, has been associated with increased transfusion requirements.[108] Although this detailed study found no differences in the in vitro pattern of changes in platelet function or coagulation during mild hypothermia (35.0°C at the end of 85 minutes surgery). The introduction of the extracorporeal circulation and of profound hypothermia for cardiac surgery was accompanied by an extra demand for blood products, though these have now been largely refined, and are referred to briefly in the section on the Sanguis study (see below).

Postoperative anaemia

Transfusion is not indicated if surgery has been completed successfully and blood loss is not a problem. Iron therapy, although slower to take effect, is safer and preferred. There is no evidence that anaemia delays healing.

The Sanguis study[109]

This major European collaborative study on the safe and good use (of blood) in surgery was conducted in 1990 and 1991, and involved 158 surgical units in 43 teaching hospitals in 10 countries including Greece and the UK. A total of 8126 cases undergoing first-time procedures were studied; four procedures requiring regular blood replacement (hemicolectomy, coronary artery bypass graft, abdominal aorta aneurysmectomy and total hip replacement) and two requiring only occasional replacement (cholecystectomy and transurethral prostatectomy) were selected.

The study's findings are important. They reveal a wide variation in surgical transfusion practice, even within the same country. The transfusion trigger—for example, of preoperative haematocrit—varied widely, as did the proportion of patients and the amount of blood transfused. For coronary artery bypass grafting, where the numbers of patients receiving blood per hospital ranged from 17 to 100%, one hospital used very little blood or artificial colloid during or after surgery, whereas others required at least two units of red cells per case, often accompanied by plasma and/or artificial colloid. The amount transfused correlated only broadly with length of surgery and even with recorded blood loss. One British hospital used a high proportion of whole blood; and in others, the total amount of blood given correlated positively with colloid use—i.e. more blood product, more colloid. In some, platelets were used prophylactically. Yet for each hospital the average haematocrit of patients on discharge was similar throughout—0.33.

Similarly, in elective abdominal aortic aneurysmectomy, some hospitals used a lot of colloid (sometimes using human albumin and fresh frozen plasma and artificial colloid) as well as red cells. Indeed, the range of use of any one of these three materials was 0–100%; and while some hospitals were more sparing of allogeneic blood, there was also a marked disparity in the use of autologous blood.

The value of this study is that awareness of such dramatic variations should encourage a better analysis and therefore understanding of different clinical practices. On the face of it, there seems little justification for a lack of standardization, which would not be tolerated in, for instance, prescribing practice. The morbidity of the donation process alone[47] should make practitioners conscious of the need to conserve blood usage.

Sickle-cell disease and β-thalassaemia major

Patients with compensated sickle-cell anaemia often have a haemoglobin level of about 80 g/l; nevertheless, transfusion is not indicated.[110] Crises such as splenic sequestration in children or haemolytic or aplastic crisis may however require transfusion.[108]

REFERENCES

105. Schmied H, Kurtz A, Sessler D I, Kozek S, Reiter A Lancet 1996; 347: 289–292
106. Michelson A D, MacGregor H, Barnard M R et al Thrombos Haemost 1994; 71: 633–640
107. Rohrer M, Natale A. Crit Care Med 1992; 20: 1402–1405
108. Lee A, Thomas P, Cupidore L, Serjeant B, Serjeant G. Improved survival in homozygous sickle cell disease: lessons from a cohort study. Br Med J 1995; 311: 1600–1602
109. Sirchia G, Giovanetti A M, McClelland D B L, Fracchia G N Safe and Good Use of Blood in Surgery (SANGUIS). Use of Blood and Artificial Colloids in 43 European Hospitals. European Commission, Luxembourg 1994
110. Huntsman R C Sickle-cell Anemia and Thalassemia—A Primer for Health Care Professionals. Canadian Sickle Cell Society, St John's, Newfoundland 1987

Prior to surgery, exchange transfusion may be beneficial in order to reduce the number of the patient's cells to less than 20%. This may be achieved by a single blood volume replacement. The selection of blood may be difficult for patients who have been transfused previously, especially if they are in an ethnic minority, as unusual antibodies may be present. Any blood given is best fresh (less than 7 days old) and should not, of course, be from a donor with sickle trait. Patients doubly heterozygous for haemoglobins S and C, or S and D, may not be anaemic but do pose special problems with surgery and anaesthesia. Major surgery, for example, cardiovascular operations, may require preoperative exchange transfusion. Good hydration and oxygenation are also essential.

The thalassaemia syndromes, on the other hand, require a very different approach. People with β-thalassaemia minor (heterozygotes) have a mild anaemia which is microcytic but does not respond to iron therapy; indeed, unless coexisting iron deficiency is demonstrated, iron is contraindicated as it risks causing siderosis. However, people with β-thalassaemia major have a severe anaemia from a few months after birth which is incompatible with life without regular transfusion. Inadequate blood tranfusion result in gross bony distortion through marrow overgrowth. A regular hypertransfusion regimen is now advocated, but the challenge is to reduce transfusion-induced siderosis by chelating agents, the best of which—Desferal—has to be given parenterally.[111] The search for oral chelators has produced deferiprone which, however, has some toxic potential and is still on trial.[112] After some years, it is usually necessary to remove the spleen which inevitably becomes hypersplenic, causing increased transfusion requirements.[113] This is also necessary for many patients with thalassaemia intermedia, a group of thalassaemics with a miscellaneous genetic background, some of whom have Hb H disease, a form of α-thalassaemia in which only one out of the usual four α genes is functional.

Platelet therapy

In the UK currently up to 90% of platelets are used for supporting patients with malignancies who are undergoing treatment to ablate their bone marrow. The remaining use is mostly surgical, occasionally for people with known disorders of platelet function undergoing otherwise minor procedures such as dental extraction, or more usually supporting major surgery—planned or urgent—during which there is a high loss of blood. The prophylactic administration of platelet concentrates is however rarely indicated during surgery.[114] In cardiac surgery, even the most modern extracorporeal circuits damage platelets and some degree of thrombocytopenia and dysfunction can be expected. In uncomplicated situations, spontaneous recovery of megakaryocyte function makes platelet transfusion unnecessary, but prolonged surgery and complications with heparin reversal can be helped by platelet infusion. In patients who are sensitive to protamine (such as diabetics who were formerly treated with protamine-zinc insulin), heparin reversal can be safely achieved by the platelet factor 4 content of platelet concentrates.[115] Platelets should be used when indicated by specific tests for disseminated intravascular coagulation and in the management of large blood losses. Patients with resistant idiopathic thrombocytopenic purpura and thrombocytopenia undergoing splenectomy should receive their platelets immediately after the splenic pedicle has been clamped (see Chapter 34).

Clinical use of fresh frozen plasma and cryoprecipitate

Fresh frozen plasma has been grossly overused.[116,117] The only absolute indications are as a replacement in plasma exchange in rare cases of thrombotic thrombocytopenia, and in disseminated intravascular coagulation where supplementation with cryoprecipitate may also be indicated. Although its use as a source of factor VIII or von Willebrand factor has largely declined in western Europe and the USA, cryoprecipitate is effective for treating some people with platelet storage pool deficiency[118] or uraemia.[119] The main indication for fresh frozen plasma now is in acquired depletion of plasma fibrinogen, as in disseminated intravascular coagulation.

Plasma fractionation products

The main products that can be derived from plasma are albumin, factor VIII, immunoglobulin and various forms of concentrate of factor IX, with or without factors II, X and sometimes VII. All these preparations are treated to prevent viral contamination.

Albumin

This is available as a physiological solution containing 4.5–5% albumin or as a salt-poor concentrate of 20%. The sodium content is 130–150 mmol; the potassium content is usually low—less than 2 mmol; traces of citrate may be present, and stabilizers such as caprylic acid are added to enable pasteurization. Recombinant albumin is under development.

REFERENCES

111. Giardini C, Galimberti M, Lucarelli G et al Br J Haematol 1995; 89: 868–873
112. Olivieri N F, Brittenham G M, Matsui D et al Iron-chelation therapy with oral deferiprone in patients with thalassemia major. N Eng J Med 1995; 332: 918–922
113. Lukens J N In: Lee G R, Bithell T C, Foerster J, Athens J W, Lukens J N (eds) Wintrobe's Clinical Hematology, 9th edn. Lea & Febiger, Philadelphia 1993 p 1102
114. National Institutes of Health Consensus Development Conference. Statement on Platelet Transfusion Therapy. Bethesda, MD 1986
115. Walker W S, Reid K G, Hider C F, Davidson I A et al Successful cardiopulmonary bypass in diabetics with anaphylactoid reactions to protamine. British Heart Journal 1984; 52: 112–114
116. Tullis J L on behalf of the Consensus Development Panel: National Institutes of Health. Fresh-frozen plasma. Indications and risks. JAMA 1985; 253: 551–553
117. Oberman H A In: Garratty G (ed) Current Concepts in Transfusion Therapy. American Association of Blood Banks, Arlington, Virginia 1985
118. Gerritsen S W, Akkerman I W N, Sixma J I. Br J Haematol 1978; 40: 153–160
119. Janson P A, Jubelirer S J, Weinstein M J, Deykin D. N Engl J Med 1980; 303: 1318–1322

Indications

Five per cent albumin is used as a plasma volume expander for acute blood loss or thermal injury, and as a replacement fluid in plasma exchange. Although albumin has an extremely good record of safety from transmitted viruses, there is no convincing evidence that it is better than synthetic colloids for volume replacement, nor is there clear evidence for maintaining the serum albumin level above a certain level in patients in intensive care units.[120] Controversy persists over whether crystalloid or colloid is better in the treatment of acute hypovolaemia and shock.[121] Pulmonary compliance is impaired by excessive use of albumin, and massive use of crystalloids is safe in the absence of renal impairment. Albumin is more expensive than the artificial colloids, hydroxyethyl starch or modified gelatins, and should not be used to dilute red cell concentrates, or be given in conjunction with them to maintain fluid input. Twenty per cent albumin solutions can be used in the short term to treat the hypoproteinaemic oedema of protein-losing enteropathies or nephropathies. It can also be given to patients with poor oral intake from dysphagia or excessive loss from gastrointestinal fistulae (see Chapter 2). It may also be useful in persistent shock as the result of sepsis. Care should be taken that the oncotically induced increase in plasma volume does not overload the heart. Salt-poor albumin cannot be regarded as a nutrient or a source of essential amino acids.

Surgery in patients with haemophilias A and B, and von Willebrand disease

Clinical presentation

Haemophilia is the most notorious of the inherited disorders of haemostasis, affecting 1 in 10 000 males in its severe form. Its sex-linked pattern of inheritance was well-described in the 19th century and summarized by Bulloch and Fildes in 1911.[122] In the same year, Addis[123] came very close to establishing its pathogenesis when he found that small amounts of normal plasma (from which he was unable to exclude platelets) corrected the long clotting time of haemophilic plasma. He inferred that haemophilic prothrombin had an 'anatomical defect' which retarded its conversion to thrombin. In 1936 Patek and Stetson[124] confirmed that a substance present in normal cell-free plasma shortened the clotting time of haemophilic blood. This was soon called anti-haemophilic globulin and later factor VIII, but its role was recognized only dimly until the 1950s, when factor VIII was first clearly distinguished from factor IX (Christmas factor).[17,18] Crude therapeutic concentrates were first prepared from plasma shortly after this.[125]

Clinical haemophilia may be mild (activities of factor VIII range from about 15% to 50%), moderate (2–15%) or severe (below 2%). Genetic mutations are common; although a few 'hot-spot' mutations may occur in unrelated individuals, most families have their own mutation. Gene deletions are associated with total absence of the factor and severe disease, and while some mis-sense mutations can produce an abnormal severely defective factor VIII protein, other families with milder clinical states have a subnormal protein which may express good antigenic levels but which is only partly procoagulant. The degree of clinical severity runs true in families, but may vary between individuals with apparently similar reductions of factor VIII activity. Clinically, the bleeding tends to occur into muscles and joints, although it can occur anywhere. Soft-tissue abscesses such as quinsy can swell alarmingly with sudden haematoma formation, although spontaneous cerebral haemorrhage is unusual.

Factor IX deficiency—Christmas disease or haemophilia B—is clinically indistinguishable from factor VIII deficiency, and has an identical family pattern. There are severe and milder presentations, as in factor VIII deficiency. To this day we do not know what form affected Queen Victoria's descendants, although factor VIII deficiency is four times more common in her family.

Both disorders are quite distinct from the more common classical von Willebrand's disease in which there is a long bleeding time and moderately reduced factor VIII (0.2 iu/ml). Specific assays of van Willebrand factor-induced platelet aggregation have been developed. The bleeding tendency is more the result of defective platelet activity than the low factor VIII clotting activity and shows a more mucosal pattern, with epistaxes and menorrhagia being a problem. Subcutaneous easy bruising is also a feature (to be excluded when investigating child abuse). A recent clinicopathological classification[126] distinguished between quantitative (type 1) and qualitative defects (type 2) of von Willebrand factor. The rare homozygotes and mixed heterozygotes (type 3) have no detectable von Willebrand factor and bleed more than haemophiliacs.

Therapeutic concentrates—factor VIII

The earliest concentrates were processed from fresh human plasma, and from bovine and porcine plasma, as these have five- to 10-fold the human activity. These were very impure, and the von Willebrand factor the animal materials caused thrombocytopenia. Purer porcine materials are still available for patients who are highly refractory to modern preparations of human factor VIII.

Cryoprecipitation was discovered in 1965 as a convenient means of concentrating factor VIII and fibrinogen from plasma[71] and provided a dramatic improvement in the case of haemophiliacs. Not only could it be given directly, but it helped produce a standardized product from many thousands of pooled donations. The resulting intermediate-purity preparations came as freeze-dried powder in vials containing 200–500 iu, which were then reconstituted in water. These preparations were, however, still very impure, containing significant quantities of immunoglobulins, including anti-A and anti-B, which sensitized the cells of patients of group A or B when given in large doses; and also of partly

REFERENCES

120. Soni N Br Med J 1995; 310: 885–886
121. Moss G S In: Collins J A (ed) Massive Transfusion in Surgery and Trauma. Alan Liss, New York 1982
122. Bulloch W, Fildes P. Treasury of Human Inheritance, parts V and VI. University of London, Francis Galton Laboratory for National Eugenics. Dulau 1911
123. Addis T J J Pathol Bacteriol 1911; 15: 427–452
124. Patek A J, Stetson R P. J Clin Invest 1936; 15: 531–542
125. Kekwick R A, Wolf P Lancet 1957; i: 647
126. Sadler J W, Gralnick H R Blood 1994; 84: 676–679

denatured fibrinogen which paradoxically interfered with normal fibrin formation. Many patients experienced adverse responses (fever, urticaria, etc.) which could usually be managed with antihistamines.

No methods of inactivating donor-transmitted viruses, which were inevitably present in such materials, were developed until the mid-1980s. As a result, in the UK by 1985 about 1200 people with haemophilia and 100 with Christmas disease became infected with HIV and virtually all became infected with hepatitis B and C. In the USA and some European countries which were wholly dependent on commercial manufacturers, more than 80% of haemophilics became infected with HIV. Whereas for most, hepatitis B was an acute self-limiting disease (although a few became carriers), hepatitis C has a much greater propensity for chronic disease, especially in those also infected with HIV. All newly diagnosed haemophilics should now be vaccinated against hepatitis B as an extra precaution.

In the last decade the goal has been safety as well as efficacy. This has been achieved by virus inactivation procedures, such as solvent detergent or heating in the presence of thermoprotectants, which allow clotting activity to be retained. As yet, methods of inactivating viruses in plasma and cryoprecipitate are not yet licensed although they are under development.[72] Hence, although cryoprecipitate can be very effective for treating von Willebrand's disease and haemophilia A, its use cannot now be recommended. Another drawback is the lack of precision of factor VIII content in each pack, as well as its impurity and the inconvenience of its presentation (frozen), which make it less suitable for home therapy. Indeed, one rare hazard with cryoprecipitate is the tranfusion-related acute lung injury, which can be life-threatening.

Recombinant DNA techniques are now available for the pharmaceutical synthesis of human factor VIII. These will undoubtedly become the products of choice in the near future,[128] although highly purified and virally inactivated plasma-derived factor VIII is likely to be available for some time. An unexpected development with highly purified factor VIII—both recombinant and plasma-derived—has however been a high incidence of immune inhibitor production[129] which, however, is spurious.

Factor IX concentrates

Factor IX concentrates derived from human plasma have been available for many years. These are produced in vials containing 200–500 iu of freeze-dried material to be reconstituted in water; they also contain large amounts of factors II and X, and some preparations also contain factor VII. They are used to treat bleeding associated with Christmas disease, and also in hypoprothrombinaemic states which may result from warfarin overdose or liver disease. They are often preferred to fresh frozen plasma, especially in patients with heart failure. Slight activation of the factors during manufacture can produce unacceptably thrombogenic products, especially when given in large doses such as 200 iu/kg, which can cause disseminated intravascular coagulation.[130] In recent years, much purer preparations of plasma-derived factor IX have become available with negligible quantities of the other vitamin K factors and virtually no potential for thrombogenesis.[131]

Calculation of dosages

Over 90% of factor VIII of whatever source is recovered in the plasma after intravenous infusion, and activity declines with an overall half-life of about 12 hours. A dose of 500 iu given to a 60 kg haemophilic with a plasma volume of 2.5 litres will raise the factor VIII activity by about 20%, which is often enough to abort a small bleed. Major surgery requires factor VIII activity to be maintained at more than 0.5 iu/ml plasma (50%) during the perioperative period, and at more than 0.25 iu/ml throughout the recovery period of 2 or 3 weeks.[132] This requires two infusions of 10–30 iu/kg per day, and close monitoring by specific assays. Orthopaedic procedures usually need immobilization throughout this period, but after general surgery normal mobilization should be encouraged. A patient may require more than 40 000 units of factor VIII for one surgical episode. The treatment of Christmas disease is similar to the treatment of haemophilia, although only about half the factor IX is recovered in the circulation; the half-life is longer—15–24 hours—which means it only needs to be given once a day.

People with von Willebrand's disease respond to intermediate-purity factor VIII preparations as these contain von Willebrand's factor. Purer concentrates without factor VIII are under development and will be effective through stabilizing the patient's own factor VIII and increasing this activity. The von Willebrand's factor however requires to be given at least once each day for severe injury or after surgery, whatever the factor VIII activity. Monitoring by a specific assay is possible but a good guide can be obtained by measuring the bleeding time, although this is not a test which should be performed very often.

Alternative agents

Mild haemophiliacs and patients with von Willebrand's disease with basal levels of factor VIII greater than 0.05 iu/ml (5%) may respond to intravenous desmopressin. This is an analogue of vasopressin, initially licensed for treating patients with diabetes insipidus:[133] 0.3 μg/kg is infused over 20 minutes. Desmopressin is thought to act by releasing platelet-activating factor from monocytes which causes von Willebrand's factor and factor VIII to be released from the endothelium.[134] As tissue plasminogen activator is also released,[135] reversal of the increased fibrinolysis with

REFERENCES

128. Tuddenham E G D, Laffan M Br Med J 1995; 311: 465–466
129. Colvin B T, Hay C R M, Hill F G H, Preston F E Br J Haematol 1995; 89: 908–910.
130. Littlewood I D, Dawes J, Smith J K et al Br J Haematol 1987; 65: 463–468
131. Poon M-C, Aledort L M, Anderle K, Kunschak M, Morfini M and the factor IX study group Transfusion 1995; 35: 319–323
132. Duthie R B, Malthews J M, Rizza C R, Steel W M. The Management of Musculoskeletal Problems in the Haemophilias. Blackwell Scientific Publications, Oxford 1972
133. Mannucci P M, Ruggeri Z M, Pareti F et al 1-Deamino-8-d-arginine vasopressin. Lancet 1977; i: 869–872
134. Hashemi S, Aye M T, Trudel E, Couture C, Palmer D S Transfusion Med 1996; 6: 96
135. Editorial DDAVP in haemophilia and von Willebrand's disease. Lancet 1983; ii: 774

500 mg tranexamic acid t.d.s. is advisable, particularly for procedures such as dental clearance. Haemostasis also requires meticulous attention to surgical technique and the judicious use of antibiotics. Antifibrinolytics are not indicated for internal surgery.

Unfortunately, the response to desmopressin declines with daily use, so it cannot provide prolonged cover after major surgery and infusions of specific factors may become necessary. Desmopressin has also been advocated in the control of bleeding in uraemia[136] and after cardiovascular surgery.[137]

Congenital platelet disorders do not usually cause severe problems, but surgery in such patients requires special haemostatic precautions. As with haemophiliacs, dental surgery can generally be managed well with care and tranexamic acid 500 mg t.d.s. for 7 days. Platelet concentrates may also be required, particularly if extensive surgery is being conducted, but may be followed by platelet antibody formation.

Treatment of patients with immune inhibitors

Alloantibodies to factor VIII may arise. In some cases these are of high titre and make clinical management very difficult. Cytotoxic immunosuppression is generally of little value. Tolerance to factor VIII antibodies may be achieved by daily doses of factor VIII. However, very resistant patients may need alternatives such as factor VIII inhibitor bypassing activity, porcine factor VIII, or even repeated plasma exchange[138] to lower antibody titres. Factor VIII inhibitor bypassing activity is found in slightly activated prothrombin complex in which the factor VIIa is probably the most active component. Indeed, recombinant factor VII, which is still very expensive, has been used very successfully. Inhibitors to factor VIII or von Willebrand's factor may also arise spontaneously in non-haemophiliacs.

Immunoglobulins

Preparations of immunoglobulins (containing immunoglobulin G only) are available for intramuscular or intravenous administration. The intramuscular route is suitable when small quantities are required, but patients needing high doses, such as hypogammaglobulinaemics, or those requiring therapy for the immune platelet disorders, need intravenous administration. This requires the removal of IgG aggregates which, although of no consequence in the intramuscular preparations, can cause profound reactions when given intravenously.

The management of massive bleeding during or after surgery

Massive bleeding may be regarded as the loss of the whole blood volume (70 ml/kg body weight) within 24 hours or less. A steady loss of this amount does not cause serious problems if volume replacement is maintained, and special haemostatic support need not be necessary in previously healthy patients who can mobilize platelets and coagulation proteins. A complete blood exchange reduces the platelet count to 35–40%[139] but platelet therapy is not justified unless bleeding is accompanied by significant thrombocytopenia. Intermittent hypovolaemic shock, hepatic impairment and sepsis may each cause clotting factor insufficiency or consumption coagulopathy, but fresh frozen plasma and cryoprecipitate are not indicated unless the international normalized ratio and the activated partial thromboplastin time are high, and the fibrinogen level low. Testing may take 30 minutes or more and it is therefore sensible to start coagulation monitoring early.

Generalized bleeding throughout the surgical field indicates significant thrombocytopenia, clotting factor insufficiency or excessive fibrinolysis. These are also signs of transfusion-transmitted bacterial infection or ABO incompatibility. Disseminated intravascular coagulation results from the release of thromboplastic material into the circulation (e.g. amniotic fluid, placental fragments, marrow fat embolus, severely damaged soft tissue and severe head injury) and may all be characterized by profound defibrination and complete thrombocytopenia: blood samples will not clot. Less severe depletion may result from consumption at the site of surgery or injury.

Heparin therapy is contraindicated unless the cause of the disseminated intravascular coagulation is well-established and known still to be operating. The cause of the disseminated intravascular coagulation must if possible be eradicated and sepsis treated vigorously. Blood product support with platelet concentrates, cryoprecipitate and red cell preparations is vital. Circulatory overload can be reduced by omitting fresh frozen plasma. Antifibrinolytics are contraindicated. The citrate content of blood products can cause hypocalcaemia when infusion is rapid, but not enough to interfere with haemostasis; calcium (gluconate or chloride) is not indicated unless there are definite signs of hypocalcaemia, for example on electrocardiography.

The use of 'fibrin glue' (fibrin sealant)[140]

This can be a very useful topical haemostat, especially in cardiovascular and neurosurgery. Fibrinogen-rich cryoprecipitate and thrombin (usually of bovine origin) are delivered together over the site and clotting occurs rapidly, helping to secure haemostasis. The cryoprecipitate can be prepared from the patient's own blood, collected in advance. Cadaver–derived patches of dura mater are not to be used because of the risk of transmitting prion diseases. Bovine thrombin is under a similar constraint.

REFERENCES

136. Manucci P, Renuzzi G, Pusineri F et al Deamino-8-d-arginine vasopressin shortens the bleeding time in uremia. N Engl J Med 1983; 303: 8–12
137. Salzman E W, Weinstein M J, Weintraub R M et al N Engl J Med 1986; 314: 1402–1406
138. Colvin B T Role of plasma exchange in the management of patients with factor VIII inhibitors. Ric Clin Lab 1983; 13: 85
139. Noe D A, Graham S M, Luff R, Sohmer P Transfusion 1982; 22: 392–395
140. Brennan M. Fibrin glue. Blood Rev 1991; 5: 240–244

4 Surgical infections and the use of antibiotics

S. J. Eykyn

This chapter will consider the pathogenesis and epidemiology of infection, concentrating especially on infections likely to be encountered in surgical practice and their prevention, and the therapeutic and prophylactic use of antibiotics. The old terminology of pyogenic and non-pyogenic infections will not be used; the differentiation is in any case a somewhat arbitrary one depending on whether the organism produces a suppurative response. Some bacteria such as *Staphylococcus aureus* are obviously pyogenic, while others such as *Clostridium tetani* are clearly non-pyogenic, but numerous other pathogenic bacteria cannot be readily assigned to these groups.

PATHOGENESIS OF INFECTION[1]

Bacteria vary in their pathogenicity, that is, their capacity to produce disease: the most pathogenic or virulent microbes, as for example, *Streptococcus pyogenes*, can and do cause infection, which is sometimes very severe, in a previously healthy immunocompetent host. Other bacteria, such as *Pseudomonas aeruginosa*, are much less virulent and are virtually incapable of causing infection in a patient with normal host defences; they are opportunists.

Bacteria produce disease by direct invasion or by the production of toxins, but although some infections may result from a single pathogenic mechanism, in most both mechanisms are involved. Invasiveness depends on microbial factors that damage the host or actively promote the spread of infection, often referred to as aggressins; these include extracellular enzymes such as hyaluronidase, phospholipase, coagulase, leucocidins and haemolysins. The distinction between aggressins and exotoxins (see below) is not absolute: for instance the phospholipase (lecithinase) produced by *Cl. perfringens* that is largely responsible for the tissue destruction in clostridial gas gangrene can be regarded as a potent exotoxin. Invasiveness also depends on the ability of the bacterium to resist phagocytosis by virtue of cell surface factors such as capsules or various components of its cell wall.

Bacterial toxins are broadly divided into those that are secreted by multiplying bacteria (exotoxins) and those that are associated with the bacterial cell wall and are released after its death (endotoxins).

Most exotoxins are produced by Gram-positive bacteria, although they can be produced by both Gram-positive and Gram-negative organisms. They are proteins, some of which are enzymes. When released at a local site of infection they can cause cell and tissue damage, but they may also enter the blood stream and produce generalized toxic effects. Certain potent exotoxins act systemically at sites remote from the original bacterial infection, as for example that of *Corynebacterium diphtheriae* which acts on the heart and peripheral nerves, that of *Cl. tetani* which acts on the central nervous system, and the erythrogenic toxin of *Str. pyogenes* that causes the generalized erythematous rash of scarlet fever. The enterotoxins are an important group of exotoxins produced by certain Gram-negative intestinal pathogens, including *Vibrio cholerae*, and certain strains of *Shigella dysenteriae*, and *Escherichia coli*; these toxins act locally on the intestinal epithelium.

Endotoxins are complex lipopolysaccharides derived from the outer membrane of Gram-negative bacteria; they are not actively secreted by living bacteria, but are released only after the death and disintegration of bacteria. The range of biological properties of endotoxin is extensive and its mode of action is complicated. Endotoxins affect the vascular system: they produce the clinical state of septic shock, often referred to as endotoxic shock, as well as triggering the coagulation enzyme cascade resulting in disseminated vascular coagulation; they are also pyrogenic. Many—perhaps most—of the actions of lipopolysaccharide result from the stimulation of cytokine release from macrophages and other cells. Despite all these toxic effects, it is likely that some of the cellular responses to lipopolysaccharide might actually *benefit* the host by assisting in the recognition and destruction of bacteria.

MANIFESTATIONS OF INFECTION

Not all encounters with pathogenic bacteria result in the clinical signs of infection, and quite often the pathogen is eliminated without causing any clinical lesion. It may be possible to detect such subclinical infection by the demonstration of specific antibodies in the serum or of specific tissue hypersensitivity.

When a pathogen gives rise to the clinical signs of infection in the host, these may be manifested in a variety of ways.

Localized infection

Perhaps the commonest example of this is the staphylococcal furuncle or boil. The organisms breach the host defences and multiply in the tissues, provoking an inflammatory reaction which

REFERENCE

1. Mims C A, Dimmock N J, Nash A, Stephen J Mims' Pathogenesis of Infectious Disease, 4th edn. Academic Press, London 1995

is characterized by vascular dilation and increased vascular permeability with extravasation of plasma and leucocytes into the tissues. The leucocytes are initially neutrophil polymorphonuclear cells and later mononuclear cells. This produces the classical signs of inflammation: heat, redness (caused by vasodilation), swelling (vasodilation, cell and fluid exudate) and pain (distension of tissues, presence of pain mediators) described long ago by Celsus. Local inflammation may result in the formation of pus which consists of bacteria, both living and dead, polymorphs and damaged host cells. A collection of pus is referred to as an abscess, and abscesses can occur at a wide variety of sites. The inflammatory response also involves dilation of the lymphatic capillaries which take up the bacteria and inflammatory fluids and transport them to local lymph nodes where organisms are phagocytosed by the macrophages lining the lymph sinuses and the local immune response is activated. The lymph nodes become swollen and tender with lymphadenitis as the blood vessels dilate and distend with inflammatory cells and exudate. Most organisms are filtered out and inactivated in lymph nodes but some are able to spread through the lymphatic system and into the blood stream (see below).

Damage at sites distant from the local site of invasion

As has already been mentioned, some bacteria, by virtue of their exotoxins, produce damage at sites remote from those of the initial site of invasion.

Spreading infection

In certain infections, particularly, those caused by *Str. pyogenes* and some anaerobic bacteria, organisms spread through the surrounding connective tissue by the action of the enzyme hyaluronidase, and cause a diffuse inflammation known as cellulitis.

Bacteraemia, septicaemia and pyaemia

Bacteria commonly enter the blood stream and this is known as bacteraemia. They may gain access to the blood from local foci of infection, either directly, or via the lymphatic system. They may also enter from sites with a normal flora as a result of various physical insults such as chewing, tooth-brushing, dental extraction and urethral catheterization. In many cases the invading organisms are rapidly cleared from the blood and the bacteraemia is a silent and transient affair. The signs of septicaemia with fever and rigors may develop if large numbers of bacteria persist in the blood. As a result of bacteraemia, whether transient or persistent—probably more usually the latter—metastatic blood-borne infection may arise in any body tissue. Some bacteria have a specific affinity or tropism for certain sites. Unfortunately in the clinical context, the terms 'bacteraemia' and 'septicaemia' tend to be used interchangeably; to compound the confusion they are sometimes used to describe a clinical condition irrespective of whether a causative organism is isolated from the blood or not. This is particularly true where shock occurs. The suggestion that septicaemia can be distinguished from bacteraemia by the demonstration of multiplying bacteria in the blood is impractical.

The following simple guidelines to terminology are offered:

1. *Bacteraemia*: the presence of bacteria in the blood as shown by their recovery from the blood on culture; a significant positive blood culture. Bacteraemia may or may not be symptomatic in the patient, and does not of itself imply a need for specific treatment.
2. *Septicaemia*: a clinical term for a severe febrile illness caused by bacteria, often with rigors and sometimes with profound toxaemia and shock. Septicaemia will usually, but not always, be associated with a demonstrable, and persistent, bacteraemia; it requires specific treatment.
3. *Pyaemia*: a term now seldom used, and best avoided, to describe a septicaemia with metastatic infection.

Chronic infection

When the host's defences fail to eliminate a pathogen, this may result in persistent active disease. Sometimes the initial encounter with the pathogen is symptomless, but the infection remains latent, only to be re-activated later when the host immunity changes.

EPIDEMIOLOGY OF INFECTION

Although in the individual patient with infection it is not always possible to determine the source or mode of acquisition of the microbe, in general, bacterial disease is either endogenous or exogenous.

Endogenous infection

Sometimes referred to as autogenous infection, this is acquired from the individual's own commensal microbes. Endogenous infections are common after trauma, surgery and instrumentation, and in conditions of lowered local or general resistance. The commensal flora, whilst always present at certain sites, is not of consistent composition, but rather is constantly changing; it is dramatically altered by antibiotics, particularly broad-spectrum agents. As so many commensal organisms are potential pathogens, knowledge of the nature and whereabouts of the commensal flora is crucial to the understanding of much human infection. The skin and mucous membranes have a rich commensal flora, and this flora is predominantly anaerobic on the mucous membranes. The major bacterial species found as commensal flora at various sites are as follows:[2]

1. *Skin*: the skin has a rich resident microbial flora;[3] it is not evenly distributed. The main organisms found are the coagulase-negative staphylococci, usually referred to, inaccurately if conveniently, as *Staphylococcus epidermidis*. Numerous individual species of coagulase-negative staphylococci are now recognized but their taxonomy is of little interest or concern to the surgeon. Micrococci and

REFERENCES

2. Skinner F A, Carr J G (eds) The Normal Microbial Flora of Man. Academic Press, London 1974
3. Noble W C Microbiology of Human Skin, 2nd edn. Lloyd-Luke, London 1981

coryneforms, including the anaerobic coryneforms, the propionibacteria, are also common. Anaerobic cocci are found at sites with large numbers of sebaceous glands, such as the axilla and perineum. In many people *Staph. aureus* is found as normal skin flora, particularly in the nose, axilla, perineum and toewebs. The carriage rate of *Staph. aureus* is variously reported, and not all carriers carry the organism permanently. Around 30% of people are permanent carriers of *Staph. aureus*. Coliforms are sometimes found on the skin, particularly in moist areas such as the axilla and groin.

2. *Respiratory tract*: although the lower respiratory tract is sterile, the mouth and nasopharynx are heavily colonized. The gingival margin and dental plaque consist almost entirely of bacteria. The nasal flora is that of the skin. The oropharyngeal flora consists of several species of viridans streptococci, coryneforms and various neisseria, including occasionally *Neisseria meningitidis*, as well as small numbers of pneumococci and *Haemophilus influenzae*. *Str. pyogenes* is rarely found as part of the normal oropharyngeal commensal flora. There is a rich anaerobic flora that includes *Porphyromonas asaccharolyticus*, *Prevotella* spp., fusobacteria, spirochaetes and anaerobic cocci. The microaerophilic *Actinomyces* spp. are also found.
3. *Gastrointestinal tract*: few organisms are found in the healthy stomach, although where there is blood or necrotic tumour tissue, bacteria are found in profusion. The small intestine has a scanty commensal flora, somewhat similar to that of the oropharynx. The large intestine bears a vast microbial load which consists predominantly of anaerobic bacteria. Very many anaerobic species are found, but the commonest include *Bacteroides* spp. of the *fragilis* group, and these outnumber *B. fragilis* itself, bifidobacteria, which are rarely pathogenic, and the clostridia. There are also significant numbers of aerobes such as *E. coli* and *Enterococcus*, previously called *Streptococcus, faecalis*.
4. *Genital tract*: the normal vagina is heavily colonized with lactobacilli, but small numbers of *Gardnerella vaginalis* and anaerobes (although not the *fragilis* group of *Bacteroides*) are also sometimes found. The urethra in both sexes is colonized with coagulase-negative staphylococci, coryneforms and occasional anaerobes.

Exogenous infection

This is acquired from a source outside the patient, mostly from other people, but also from animal and environmental sources.

Human sources

These include patients with overt clinical infections and those with inapparent or subclinical infections as well as carriers of pathogenic organisms. Organisms may be transmitted from one person to another by direct contact, by the faecal—oral route, by the respiratory tract through inhalation, by sexual intercourse or transplacentally. In practice, transfer of organisms from one patient to another, usually by their attendants' hands, though sometimes by other routes, is referred to as cross-infection.

Animal sources

Animals are an important source of human infections, which are called zoonoses. Organisms may be acquired from sick or apparently healthy animals; they are transmitted in a variety of ways including direct contact with the animal and, most importantly, by ingestion of contaminated meat or animal products such as milk and cheese.

Environmental sources

These include soil and water. Even in hospital practice contaminated water can pose an infection hazard to patients. Many outbreaks of infection have resulted from solutions contaminated with water-loving microbes, usually *Ps. aeruginosa* or other *Pseudomonas* spp. Legionellae such as *Legionella pneumophila*, which is the usual pathogen in Legionnaire's disease, can also contaminate water, and contaminated droplets from cooling systems and shower heads have usually been implicated in their transmission. This has occurred both in hospitals and in the community.

Many patients with infection who are seen by surgeons have acquired their infection in the community, whether by an endogenous or exogenous route. Such infections may arise spontaneously or in association with trauma. Although community-acquired infections can be extremely severe— indeed, on occasions lethal— they are seldom caused by antibiotic-resistant microbes. Hospital-acquired nosocomial infection is largely iatrogenic and has reached alarming proportions, particularly in intensive therapy and neonatal units. Whilst hospital-acquired infections can be caused by bacteria similar to those found in the community, they are also caused by highly resistant organisms, the latter usually reflecting antibiotic use, or rather abuse. In this chapter the infections that present to surgeons are considered in the following groups:

1. Infections arising in the community.
2. Hospital-acquired, nosocomial, infections.
3. Certain specific infections.

There is some overlap between these groups. With increasing day surgery and shorter inpatient stays, patients are likely to present to their general practitioners or accident and emergency departments with infections, particularly wound infections, that have been acquired in hospital.

INFECTIONS ARISING IN THE COMMUNITY

Many of the infections described in this section are those that are likely to be seen in accident and emergency departments.

Skin and soft tissue infections

These occur at a variety of sites and are common. Many arise as a result of minor trauma, itself a frequent occurrence, that allows ingress of usually commensal organisms, frequently *Staph. aureus* or *Str. pyogenes*, and sometimes both. Some of these infections are also caused by anaerobic bacteria.

Boils or furuncles

These result from infection of hair follicles with *Staph. aureus*; although they may affect any hair-bearing area, they are most common on the face, neck, axilla and buttocks. Boils tend to be recurrent, sometimes over a period of months. Systemic antibiotics are not indicated; they do not affect resolution. Individual boils that are large and painful should be incised. Recurrent boils are best tackled by eradication of the inevitable carriage of *Staph. aureus* by applying an antiseptic such as chlorhexidine, an antibiotic such as mupirocin or neomycin or a combination of these, such as Naseptin, to the nose, and using an antiseptic soap. In recalcitrant cases of recurrent boils the temptation to prescribe systemic antibiotics—usually flucloxacillin—is overwhelming, but there is no evidence of their efficacy.

Carbuncle

A carbuncle is an extensive infection of the hair follicles caused by *Staph. aureus*; it involves adjacent follicles and the subcutaneous tissues. Multiple draining sinuses develop. These infections are uncommon and usually occur in diabetics. Systemic flucloxacillin should be given in addition to surgical incision when required.

Styes

Styes are infections of the eyelash follicles with *Staph. aureus*. They do not require antibiotics, either systemic or local.

Cellulitis

Cellulitis is an acute spreading infection of the skin and subcutaneous tissues. Although numerous microbes can produce cellulitis, by far the commonest cause is *Str. pyogenes*. The term 'erysipelas', which literally means red skin, is sometimes used to describe streptococcal cellulitis at any site, but is more often reserved for streptococcal cellulitis of the face, a condition seldom seen now which is usually unilateral, but occasionally bilateral. In facial erysipelas the erythema is sharply demarcated, and there is marked oedema and systemic upset (Fig. 4.1a and b). Much more frequently encountered is streptococcal cellulitis of the limbs, when minor trauma or skin lesions commonly precede the infection. The degree of systemic disturbance varies.

In some cases of streptococcal cellulitis, there is no detectable local lesion from which to recover the causative organism, and a streptococcal aetiology must be presumed, or confirmed by a raised serum ASO titre. In others *Str. pyogenes* can be grown from a minor initiating skin lesion. There may be blistering of the skin and serous discharge and this too can sometimes yield *Str. pyogenes*. Blood cultures are seldom positive.

Streptococcal cellulitis should be treated with penicillin, and in most cases this is best given initially intravenously. The clinical response is often slow (Fig. 4.1c). Patients with lymphoedema often suffer from repeated attacks of streptococcal cellulitis (see Chapter 2). Tinea pedis (athlete's foot) is common in lymphoedema, and the cracks that this causes in the skin may allow bacteria to enter the subcutaneous tissue. Prophylactic penicillin or erythromycin may be worth trying, but appropriate treatment of the concomitant tinea pedis with terbinafine may help prevent reinfection.

The increase in *Str. pyogenes* infections that has occurred in many countries since the middle 1980s is typical of the well-recognized epidemic cycles of infection with this organism.[4] This recent

REFERENCE

4. Stevens D L Pediatr Infect Dis J 1994; 13: 561–566

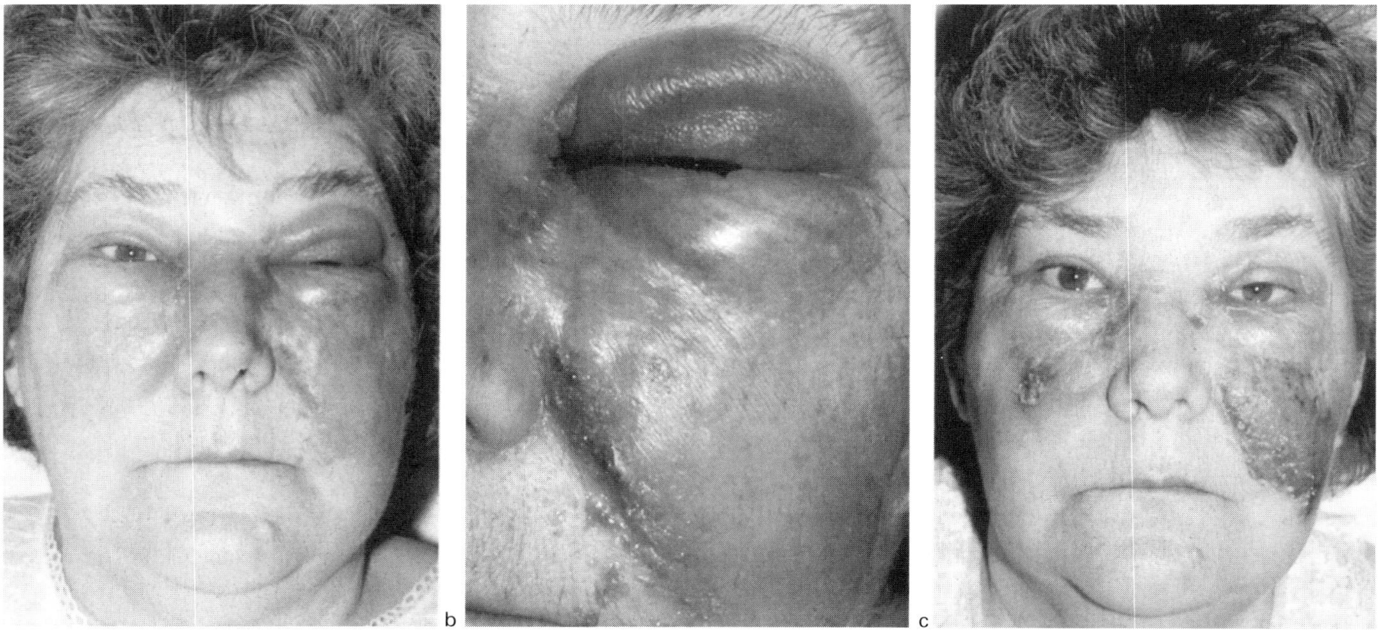

Fig. 4.1 Bilateral erysipelas (*Streptococcus pyogenes*). **(a)** and **(b)** Patient on admission to hospital; **(c)** patient after 5 days' treatment with intravenous penicillin. Note that the response to antibiotic was slow.

overall increase in streptococcal infections has been paralled by an increase in severe infections; one such infection in particular has excited intense media attention in the UK and has been dubbed the 'flesh-eater'—acute streptococcal necrotizing fasciitis and gangrene.[5] *Str. pyogenes* is not the only cause of necrotizing fasciitis; indeed, it is one of the more uncommon causes, but it is probably one of the most severe varieties of this infection.

Streptococcal necrotizing fasciitis

Despite the impression that may have been gained from the UK media, streptococcal necrotizing fasciitis is not a new disease; in fact it was probably first described by Hippocrates as a complication of erysipelas. Meleney[6] seems to have been the first to attribute it to the 'hemolytic streptococcus' and, interestingly, his classic paper described cases seen whilst he was working in China at the time of a known streptococcal epidemic. It is more common in men and follows a minor, often unnoticed injury. It usually affects the limbs but may affect other parts of the body, including the penis and scrotum (see Chapter 40). The patient is ill with fever and rigors and the affected part becomes swollen, hot, red and tender, and then anaesthetic. Blisters and bullae appear within a day or two and then frank gangrene. At the end of the last century, Fournier described the spontaneous development of scrotal gangrene in previously healthy young men, all of whom recovered.[7] No bacteriological studies were reported but no foul-smelling discharge was described (see below) and, as suggested by Meleney, these cases of what has come to be known as Fournier's gangrene were almost certainly caused by *Str. pyogenes* (see Chapter 40).

In severe streptococcal infections, including necrotizing fasciitis, blood cultures are usually positive and some patients have a generalized rash, multisystem failure and shock—the syndrome of streptococcal toxic shock. The mortality is higher if this is present.

Synergistic anaerobic cellulitis and necrotizing fasciitis

These infections are more common than streptococcal necrotizing fasciitis and they usually have a less acute clinical presentation. They can be confused with streptococcal infection and also, as there is often gas in the tissues, with clostridial gas gangrene (see later), but the patient with the latter is always desperately ill. Although generally referred to as 'anaerobic', these infections are mixed infections caused by a combination of anaerobic and aerobic bacteria; the species of organisms isolated varies with the site of the infection. This is usually the foot or leg in patients, often diabetics, with vascular insufficiency. It may however occur at other sites, including the perineum and scrotum (Fig. 4.2a and b) when it is usually referred to as Fournier's gangrene (see above); such cases are common in diabetics and alcoholics and usually result from anorectal sepsis or disorders of the lower genitourinary tract such as urethral strictures.[8] The discharge is always foul and this was reported 70 years ago[9,10] when bacteriological confirmation of the predicted anaerobic aetiology was unavailable.

REFERENCES

5. Cartwright K, Logan M, McNulty C et al Epidemiol Infect 1995; 115: 387–397
6. Meleney F L Arch Surg 1924; 9: 317–364
7. Fournier J A Sem Med 1883; 56: 345–347
8. Clayton M D, Fowler J E, Sharifi R, Pearl R K Surg Gynecol Obstet 1990; 170: 49–55
9. Randall A J Urol 1929; 4: 219–235
10. Gibson T E J Urol 1930; 23: 125–153

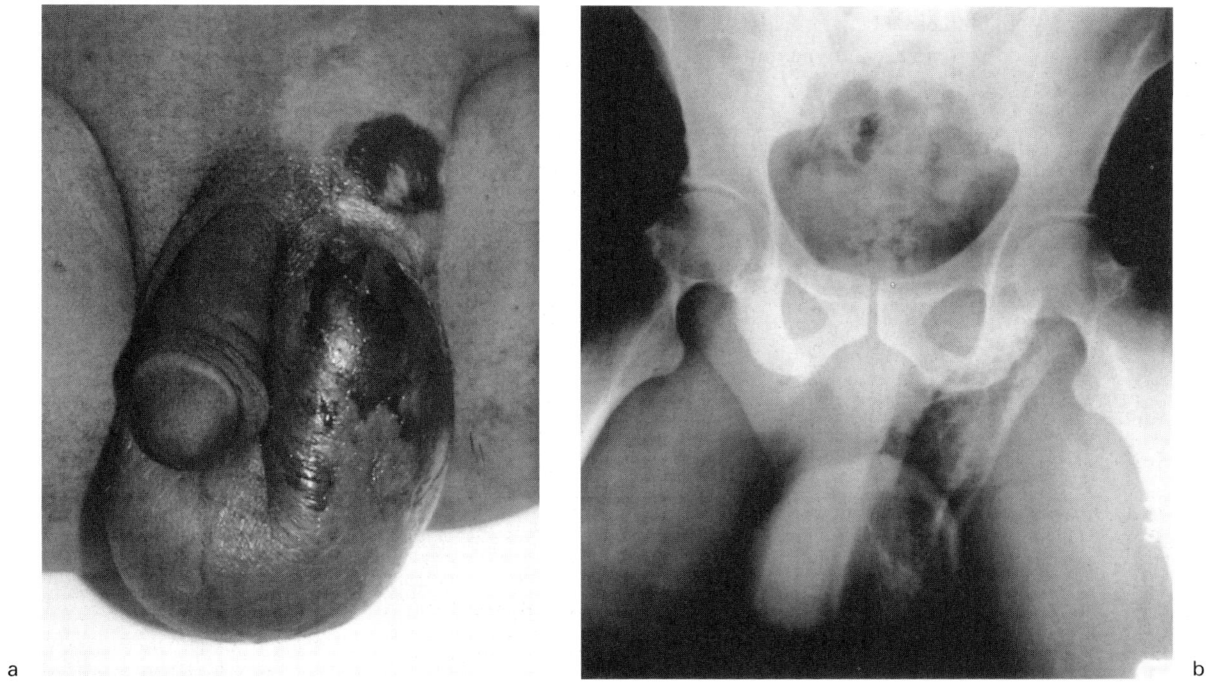

Fig. 4.2 Fournier's gangrene. Synergistic necrotizing fasciitis in a previously undiagnosed diabetic. **(a)** Clinical picture; **(b)** X-ray: there is gas in the scrotum.

These necrotizing anaerobic infections often arise spontaneously, particularly when they involve the abdomen, buttock or perineum, but they may also arise in association with intra-abdominal or other sepsis and after surgery at a variety of sites. Meleney reported on the 'chronic gangrene of the skin' that followed various abdominal operations;[11] he attributed this to a 'microaerophilic non-haemolytic streptococcus'—almost certainly one of the *Str. milleri* group which are so commonly isolated with anaerobes—and *Staph. aureus*, although other bacteria were cultured from some of his cases. Anaerobic cultures were not mentioned. These eponymous descriptions of Meleney's and Fournier's gangrenes are probably now best consigned to history. It is preferable to define the causative organisms in such cases.

Whatever the microbes isolated and whatever the site of the infection, the treatment of these necrotizing infections is surgical. Antibiotics appropriate for the pathogen should be given for a few days, but unless the affected tissue is adequately excised and debrided, the infection will progress.

Paronychia

Paronychia is a common acute infection of the nailfold of the finger and less often of the toe, when it is usually associated with ingrowing toenails. Although the usual pathogen is *Staph. aureus*, *Str. pyogenes* is also common, and a range of other microbes is found. One-third of paronychias yield anaerobes on culture, almost always with aerobes.[12] The anaerobes are the oropharyngeal commensals. These infections tend to be more chronic than those caused by aerobic bacteria alone. Even more chronic are paronychias caused by yeasts, usually *Candida albicans*. Once pus has formed, only surgical drainage cures the condition and antibiotics are not indicated, but at the early cellulitic stage of these infections antibiotics may sometimes be beneficial. In the absence of definitive bacteriology co-amoxiclav (Augmentin) or erythromycin is suitable.

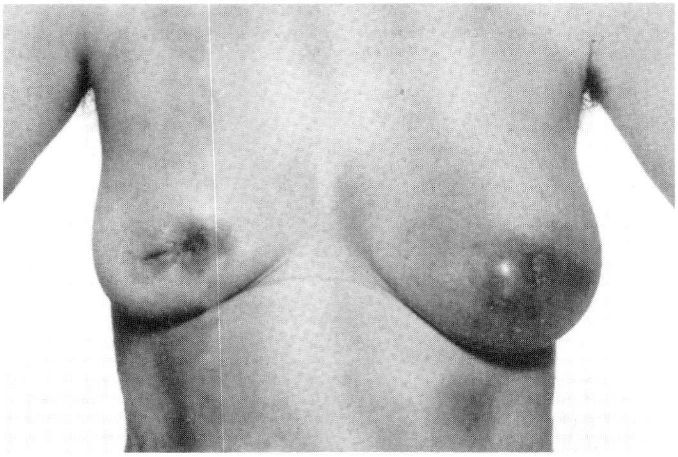

Fig. 4.3 Breast abscess. An acute non-lactational abscess in the left breast. A previous abscess has left an inverted nipple and a sinus at the edge of the areola. These are typical appearances.

Abscesses and other inflammatory conditions affecting the soft tissues

Many subcutaneous abscesses are caused by *Staph. aureus*, and some of these are essentially boils. Like boils, they can be recurrent, particularly those of the axilla and buttock. In other abscesses, and in particular those in regions rich in apocrine glands, the underlying pathology is that of apocrine blockage and infection is secondary to this. Such infections are almost always caused by anaerobes. Their hallmark is chronicity and recurrence. Infections of sebaceous cysts are also largely anaerobic. At certain sites, such as for example the perirectal area, an associated fistula will determine the abscess flora (see Chapter 30). In general, abscesses require drainage, and those with underlying apocrine blockage require attention to this. Antibiotics are rarely helpful.

Certain common subcutaneous abscesses will be considered in more detail.

Axillary abscess

Axillary abscesses account for about a sixth of all cutaneous abscesses, and although about two-thirds are caused by *Staph. aureus*, at least a quarter are caused by mixed anaerobes.[13] Anaerobic abscesses often have small satellite lesions adjacent to the main abscess which provide a useful clue to their aetiology. Many patients with anaerobic axillary abscesses have frank or incipient hidradenitis suppurativa manifested by sinuses, induration and scarring as well as intermittent putrid discharge from acute flare-ups of the condition. For years this infection was attributed to *Staph. aureus*, even though the foul discharge is so typical of anaerobes. The anaerobes are most frequently *Porph. asaccharolyticus* and anaerobic cocci. Antibiotics offer little, though they are sometimes prescribed for months on end; these unfortunate patients need surgical excision. The disease, which is primarily one of pilosebaceous obstruction, is often bilateral and may also affect the groin and other apocrine-rich areas.

Breast abscess

Although breast abscesses, like axillary abscesses, are still usually assumed to be staphylococcal in origin, these too are sometimes anaerobic. Puerperal breast abscesses, now uncommon, are nearly always caused by *Staph. aureus*, whereas those in the non-puerperal woman are as likely to be anaerobic as to be staphylococcal.[14] The clinical picture of an anaerobic abscess is distinct: they are subareolar and nearly always associated with an inverted nipple (Fig. 4.3). There may be an associated discharge. The underlying pathology is duct blockage and the infection is secondary to this. The anaerobes are usually *Prevotella* spp. and anaerobic cocci. In some cases a vaginal source seems probable. Whereas

REFERENCES

11. Meleney F L Surg Gynecol Obstet 1933; 56: 847–867
12. Whitehead S M, Eykyn S J, Phillips I Br J Surg 1981; 68: 420–422
13. Leach R D, Eykyn S J, Phillips I, Corrin B, Taylor E A Br Med J 1979; 2: 5–7
14. Leach R D, Eykyn S J, Phillips I, Corrin B Lancet 1979; i: 35–37

staphylococcal abscesses are satisfactorily treated by drainage and antibiotics are usually unnecessary, anaerobic abscesses require surgical attention to the duct abnormality, and unless this is carried out the abscess will recur, sometimes over years, because of a mamillary fistula (see Chapter 25).

Pilonidal abscess

This results from infection of a pre-existing pilonidal sinus. Most pilonidal abscesses are anaerobic infections; the anaerobes are most commonly *Porph. asaccharolyticus* and anaerobic cocci, but *Bacteroides* spp. of the *fragilis* group are found in about a third of cases. The treatment of a pilonidal abscess is surgical; antibiotics are not indicated.

Anorectal abscess

These are common and their aetiology and microbiology vary.[15] Certain perianal abscesses result from infections of hair follicles and are thus essentially boils caused by *Staph. aureus*; others arise in sebaceous or apocrine glands and are caused by anaerobes often with skin organisms, the *Str. milleri* group and, rarely, coliforms. The anaerobes are predominantly *Porph. asaccharolyticus* and anaerobic cocci; they do not include *Bacteroides* spp. of the *fragilis* group. Possibly the largest group of anorectal abscesses are those that arise from infected anal glands, from which infection spreads through muscle, creating a fistula-in-ano, to the ischiorectal or perianal tissues. These abscesses, not surprisingly, yield colonic microbes, that is to say gut-specific *Bacteroides* spp. of the *fragilis* group and coliforms, as well as the *Str. milleri* group. Anorectal abscesses require drainage; an associated fistula needs laying open or the abscess will recur. The microbiology results obtained from culture of the pus from anorectal abscesses can act as a useful indicator of the presence of a fistula as this may not be apparent at the initial drainage operation (see Chapter 30).

Infections secondary to trauma

Although infection secondary to injury of the skin or soft tissues is usually caused by *Staph. aureus* or *Str. pyogenes* or both, particular mention must be made of infections associated with bites, for both animal and human bites have a high incidence of infection which is often severe. The usual clinical concern is of the risk of tetanus which must be almost unknown after bites, but these infections are caused by the commensal flora of the mouth.

Infections from animal bites

Most infections are from dog bites, but occasionally other animals may be responsible; cats tend to scratch rather than bite but such wounds can become infected in a similar way to bites. Rabies is not a consideration in the UK, but of course may be elsewhere. Dog bites and cat scratches commonly become infected with *Pasteurella multocida*, but various other organisms are found including many anaerobes, as the canine and feline mouth, in common with the human mouth, has an anaerobic commensal flora. Particular mention must be made of the organism *Capnocytophaga canimorsus* (previously known as DF: dysgonic fermenter-2) that can cause a severe, sometimes fatal, multisystem septicaemic illness after a dog bite or scratch.[16,17] These infections are more common in the asplenic or otherwise immunocompromised host, but can occur in apparently immunocompetent individuals. Patients with infected bites should begiven antibiotics in addition to whatever debridement is needed. Amoxycillin plus metronidazole, co-amoxiclav (Augmentin) or erythromycin are all suitable; it seems wise to give prophylactic antibiotics to patients with uninfected bites even though they will not necessarily prevent infection occurring.

Infections from human bites

These most commonly involve the hand; the pathogens are the oral commensals, predominantly anaerobes, and there is sometimes marked tissue damage. Similar infections follow fist injuries. These hand infections may involve joints. There is also the additional possibility of acquiring hepatitis B or even human immunodeficiency virus (HIV) by this means. Numerous organisms are isolated, including the *Str. milleri* group, *Haemophilus* spp., *Eikenella corrodens* as well as *Fusobacterium* spp., and other oral anaerobes. The fusobacteria have long been considered of particular importance, and Meleney, writing in 1933,[11] referred to the 'fusospirochaetal infection of the skin' that followed human bites or wounds contaminated with mouth secretions. The same prophylactic antibiotics, as for animal bites should be given in addition to the necessary irrigation and debridement.

Infected leg ulcers

Leg ulcers, for which there are a number of underlying causes, are frequently colonized with bacteria (see Chapter 11). Of these, *Staph. aureus* is most often isolated but many other bacteria are found, including coliforms, *Ps. aeruginosa* and anaerobes, the latter undoubtedly accounting for the foul smell of some ulcers, and perhaps predisposed to by the occlusive dressings that are often used to encourage healing. Leg ulcers are sometimes associated with frank cellulitis and in such cases *Str. pyogenes* may be isolated; much more commonly there is associated erythema around the ulcer margin and, if streptococci are grown, they are more likely to be those of Lancefield's groups B, C or G, and are usually colonizing the surface of the ulcer. Patients with leg ulcers are frequently subjected to courses of antibiotics; unfortunately there is no evidence that these do any good, and they result in colonization of the ulcer with different but more resistant organisms. There seems to be little purpose in culturing leg ulcers unless they are associated with a true cellulitis.

REFERENCES

15. Whitehead S M, Leach R D, Eykyn S J, Phillips I Br J Surg 1982; 69: 166–168
16. Butler T, Weaver R E, Ramani V et al Ann Intern Med 1977; 86: 1–5
17. Brenner D J, Hollis D G, Fanning G R, Weaver R E J Clin Microbiol 1989; 27: 231–235

Infections associated with the gastrointestinal tract

These include the acute intestinal infections, acute inflammation associated with another abnormality of the gut such as obstruction or trauma, mesenteric adenitis and peritonitis. The pathogens which are associated with these conditions are briefly considered.

Intestinal infections

An ever-increasing variety of infectious agents are now recognized as intestinal pathogens. Only those likely to be of relevance to surgeons are described here. Some of these infections are referred to as 'food-poisoning', and others as 'dysentery'—terms that readily confuse. Many infectious agents are transmitted by food or water or by the oral–faecal route, but not all cause an intestinal upset, like, for example, *Listeria monocytogenes*. The major importance of intestinal infections to the surgeon is that they may be confused with inflammatory bowel disease and they may mimic—or in some cases probably even cause—acute appendicitis. Most, indeed probably all, bacterial intestinal infections can occasionally be followed by a reactive arthritis. The importance of culturing stools from all patients with diarrhoea cannot be overemphasized. There is an increasing tendency to rely on the sigmoidoscope rather than the laboratory.

Salmonella[18]

The genus of *Salmonella* is most conveniently divided into the enteric fever salmonellas, *S. typhi* and *S. paratyphi* (A, B and C), that are exclusively human pathogens, and the non-enteric fever or food-poisoning salmonellas, an enormous number of species that are acquired from animals. In the UK the commonest of these is *S. enteritidis*, the current scourge of the poultry industry which superseded *S. typhimurium* over a decade ago. The enteric fever salmonellas, although acquired by ingestion, do not primarily cause diarrhoea and vomiting, though intestinal ulceration with haemorrhage may occur late in the disease, but rather a septicaemic illness that usually presents as a pyrexia of unknown origin; such infections are uncommon in the UK and are usually imported.

Disease caused by the food-poisoning salmonellas is common. Although often described as gastroenteritis, it may also involve the colon, with ulceration, and is best termed an enterocolitis. These salmonellas occasionally cause invasive, that is bacteraemic infection, sometimes with localization in various organs or tissues. Pre-existing disease with necrotic or scarred tissue favours localization of blood-borne organisms, as do diseases of the haematopoietic system. A choleraic type of diarrhoea with massive fluid loss sometimes occurs in patients who have had a previous gastrectomy or in those with achlorhydria.

Whilst antibiotics, and in particular chloramphenicol, have long been used to treat enteric fever, that is typhoid or paratyphoid and invasive or bacteraemic disease caused by food-poisoning salmonellas, until quite recently it was generally held that antibiotics were of no value in salmonella enterocolitis. They had no effect on the clinical course of the disease and could actually prolong excretion of the salmonella. However, the quinolone antibiotics, in particular ciprofloxacin, have proved effective in salmonella enterocolitis, both in alleviating symptoms and in eradicating carriage of the salmonella. They are also effective in the treatment of enteric fever and invasive salmonellosis.

Campylobacter[19]

The major human pathogen is *Campylobacter jejuni* and, like salmonellosis, campylobacteriosis is a zoonotic disease. Campylobacters were not recognized as human intestinal pathogens until the late 1970s, and until then the appropriate culture medium for their isolation from stools was not set up in laboratories,[20] they are now the commonest reported bacterial cause of gastrointestinal disease, exceeding salmonellas and shigellas. The disease is similar to salmonellosis, but campylobacters are perhaps even more likely to cause an acute colitis, readily confused with inflammatory bowel diseases such as ulcerative colitis. Bacteraemia is much less common than in salmonellosis and prolonged excretion is rare. In many cases, the infection is self-limiting, but for severe disease antibiotics, conventionally erythromycin, should be given, even though the evidence for their efficacy is mostly anecdotal. Erythromycin therapy results in the rapid elimination of campylobacters from the stool. Ciprofloxacin can also be used but whereas resistance of campylobacters to erythromycin is rare, some 5–8% of campylobacters are now resistant to ciprofloxacin.

Helicobacter pylori (formerly *Campylobacter pyloridis/pylori*)[21]

This organism, originally isolated from endoscopic biopsy specimens of human gastric mucosa, warrants a brief mention here, as although its pathogenic role is quite different from that of true campylobacters, it was previously classified as a campylobacter. *H. pylori* is associated with chronic gastritis, but most infected persons are symptomless. It is also a marker of high risk for duodenal ulcer, and of the likelihood of ulcer relapse after treatment. The correlation with gastric ulcer is less strong. *H. pylori* is sensitive in vitro to a wide range of antibiotics, metronidazole-resistant strains occur. It is also sensitive to bismuth, but the ideal regimen for its treatment remains to be defined. Triple regimens of two antibiotics plus bismuth, omeprazole or ranitidine, given for 1 or 2 weeks, produce higher eradication rates than dual therapy (usually an antibiotic plus omeprazole for 2 weeks) but compliance may be a problem.

REFERENCES

18. Miller S I, Hohmann E L, Pegues D A In: Mandell G L, Bennett J E, Dolin R (eds) Principles and Practice of Infectious Diseases, 4th edn. Churchill Livingstone, New York 1995 pp 2013–2033
19. Blaser M J In: Mandell G L, Bennett J E, Dolin R (eds) Principles and Practice of Infectious Diseases, 4th edn. Churchill Livingstone, New York 1995 pp 1948–1956
20. Skirrow M Br Med J 1977; ii: 9–11
21. Blaser M J In: Mandell G L, Bennett J E, Dolin R (eds) Principles and Practice of Infectious Diseases, 4th edn. Churchill Livingstone, New York 1995 pp 1956–1964

Shigella[22]

The enterocolitis caused by shigellas is often referred to as bacillary dysentery. It is the most communicable of all the bacterial diarrhoeas, as less than 200 bacteria can produce the disease in healthy adults.[23] Unlike salmonellosis and campylobacteriosis, it is an infection acquired from humans, not a zoonosis. Bacteraemia is rare, as is prolonged carriage. The commonest shigellas indigenous to the UK are *Shigella sonnei* and certain strains of *Sh. flexneri*, but other more virulent species are sometimes imported from abroad; *Sh. sonnei* and *Sh. flexneri* are not of course restricted to the UK.

Antibiotic sensitivities of shigellas vary, and they readily become resistant after treatment. It has thus been conventional to reserve antibiotics for the more severely ill patients. Ampicillin (amoxycillin), tetracyclines and co-trimoxazole have been recommended in the past but strains are sometimes resistant. Ciprofloxacin is also effective, both at producing amelioration of symptoms and in the rapid elimination of the organism. Shigellas are usually sensitive to the quinolones.

Other organisms

Although salmonellas, campylobacters and shigellas are the commonest bacterial causes of enterocolitis, a number of other agents, bacterial, viral and parasitic, can affect the gut causing various syndromes. Amongst these are enterotoxigenic *Escherichia coli*; *Vibrio cholerae*; certain viruses; *Giardia lamblia* and *Cryptosporidium parvum* that affect the proximal small bowel and produce watery diarrhoea; invasive strains of *E. coli*; *Aeromonas hydrophila* and *Entamoeba histolytica* that affect the colon, and *Yersinia* spp. that produce several syndromes.

Cl. difficile-associated colitis (pseudomembranous colitis)[24]

In addition to the infections described above, another important, largely iatrogenic, disease must be briefly mentioned, that of *Clostridium difficile* colitis, perhaps more likely to arise in hospital than outside, but nevertheless most conveniently considered here. This is sometimes referred to as pseudomembranous colitis and the infection in its most florid form is characterized by a pseudomembrane often recognizable on sigmoidoscopy. The disease of pseudomembranous enterocolitis was originally described in the pre-antibiotic era, typically occurring after abdominal surgery but reported cases over the past two decades have been almost exclusively associated with antibiotic administration, especially those with broad-spectrum activity, including anti-anaerobe activity.

The disease is caused by the cytotoxin of *Cl. difficile*, an organism occasionally found as part of the normal adult intestinal flora, and in many healthy newborn infants. Very many antibiotics, both oral and parenteral, have been associated with this infection, and it may appear several weeks after the causative antibiotics have been discontinued; *Cl. difficile* may also be transmitted in hospitals. The disease really came into prominence in the late 1970s when its cause was described. It was then most commonly associated with clindamycin and lincomycin, antibiotics widely used at that time for the treatment and prophylaxis of anaerobic infections, especially in abdominal surgery. It subsequently became clear that cases also followed treatment with ampicillin and the cephalosporins. Most antibiotics used in humans have been implicated; it has even, paradoxically, been reported after metronidazole, an antibiotic used to treat the disease!

The diagnosis can readily be confirmed by the demonstration of the toxin in the stool. Causative antibiotics should be stopped and the more severe cases treated with either oral vancomycin or oral metronidazole. The initial treatment of *Cl. difficile* colitis is usually successful but 15–20% of patients relapse, sometimes repeatedly, and cytotoxin is again detected in the stools. Some novel remedies have been used successfully in these patients when the above conventional methods have failed; they include the rectal infusion of homologous faeces,[25] lactobacilli[26] and brewer's yeast.[27]

Acute inflammation associated with abnormality or obstruction of the gut

In these conditions the bacterial infection is secondary; the commonest examples are acute appendicitis and acute diverticulitis (see Chapter 27). The causative bacteria are the colonic commensals, and in the absence of previous antibiotic treatment, consist of *E. coli*, enterococci, the *Str. milleri* group and the *fragilis* group of *Bacteroides*. Whilst the place of antibiotics in acute appendicitis is as prophylaxis, to prevent subsequent wound infection (see section on prophylactic use of antibiotics, below), antibiotics are given as part of the initial non-operative treatment of acute diverticulitis (see Chapter 30). There are many possible regimens, but in light of the polymicrobial nature of these infections, a broad-spectrum antibiotic is required. The combination of metronidazole plus cefuroxime is widely used.

Mesenteric adenitis

This condition mimics acute appendicitis in its clinical presentation. Whilst in the pre antibiotic era *Str. pyogenes* was a common cause, today the most frequently reported pathogen is *Yersinia*—usually *Y. enterocolitica*, less commonly *Y. pseudotuberculosis*—sometimes acquired from an animal source. The disease usually occurs in young children and adolescents. Although the histology of resected nodes may suggest the diagnosis, it is confirmed by serology. Stool cultures are rarely positive. In most cases the disease is self-limiting and antibiotics are not required.

REFERENCES

22. DuPont H L In: Mandell G L, Bennett J E, Dolin R (eds) Principles and Practice of Infectious Diseases, 4th edn. Churchill Livingstone, New York 1995 pp 2033–2039
23. DuPont H L, Levine M M, Hornick R B et al J Infect Dis 1989; 159: 1126
24. Guerrant R L In: Mandell G L, Bennett J E, Dolin R (eds). Principles and Practice of Infectious Diseases, 4th edn. Churchill Livingstone, New York 1995 pp 992–995
25. Schwan A, Sjölin S, Trottestam U Lancet 1983; ii: 845
26. Gorbach S L, Chang T-W, Goldin B Lancet 1987; ii: 1519
27. Schellenberg D, Bonington A, Champion C, Lancaster R, Webb S, Main J Lancet 1994; 343: 171–172

Peritonitis

Infective peritonitis may be primary or, much more commonly, secondary to some intra-abdominal process.

Primary peritonitis[28]

The spontaneous primary peritonitis of childhood that was seen in the pre-antibiotic era seems to have largely disappeared; the infection, usually caused by *Str. pneumoniae* or *Str. pyogenes*, reached the peritoneum via the blood stream, presumably from a remote inapparent focus of infection in the respiratory tract or perhaps in the female from the genital tract. Primary peritonitis is now most commonly seen in cirrhotic patients, and the usual pathogen is *E. coli*. Tuberculous peritonitis is considered elsewhere in this chapter. The antibiotic treatment of primary peritonitis depends on the causative pathogen.

Secondary peritonitis

This results from a wide variety of intra-abdominal processes including acute appendicitis, acute diverticulitis, tubo-ovarian infection and perforation of intra-abdominal viscera. The infection is polymicrobial and broad-spectrum antibiotics are required.

Hepatobiliary infections

Acute cholecystitis

Almost all cases occur in association with gallstones (see Chapter 32). The pathogens are colonic aerobes, predominantly *E. coli*, but also other coliforms and enterococci. The organisms can sometimes be recovered from the blood, as well as from the bile and the gallstones. The *E. coli* are increasingly resistant to ampicillin (amoxycillin), and preferred antibiotics include cefuroxime and co-amoxiclav (Augmentin).

Acute cholangitis

The pathogens are similar to those found in cholecystitis, but anaerobes are likely to be involved in those patients who have had previous biliary–intestinal anastomoses. Bacteraemia is common. Antibiotic treatment should encompass colonic anaerobes. Thus either cefuroxime plus metronidazole or co-amoxiclav (Augmentin) is suitable.

Infections of the liver

A variety of agents can infect the liver including bacteria, viruses, protozoa and helminths. The viral hepatitis most likely to concern the surgeon is hepatitis B: not only can this infection be acquired from a patient but surgeons who are hepatitis B-positive have also infected patients during operations. With the availability of an effective vaccine this should no longer happen. Amoebic and hydatid infections of the liver are considered separately.

Liver abscess

Pyogenic liver abscess is uncommon. The source of the infection is most often biliary disease with ascending cholangitis. Infection may also arise from diverticulitis or inflammatory bowel disease via the portal vein, by direct spread from a contiguous infection, and very rarely via the hepatic artery in septicaemia. The commonest pathogens are the *Str. milleri* group, but anaerobes, particularly fusobacteria, are sometimes found, as are coliforms.[29] In the older literature there were frequent reports of sterile liver abscesses, undoubtedly because of inadequate culture techniques. The *Str. milleri* group are readily mistaken for an anaerobic streptococcus and previous reports of anaerobic streptococci in liver abscesses were probably actually the *Str. milleri* group. Why *Str. milleri*, and particularly those of Lancefield's group F, has this predilection for the liver remains unexplained.

Blood cultures are frequently positive in patients with liver abscesses; sometimes the pathogen is isolated from the blood before the diagnosis has been considered. The isolation of *Str. milleri* from the blood of a patient with a febrile illness and abnormal liver function tests should immediately raise the possibility of a liver abscess. It must be stressed however that there are other causes of *Str. milleri* bacteraemia. The treatment of pyogenic liver abscess is essentially drainage, now increasingly performed by radiologists, and antibiotics are secondary to this. Penicillin remains the antibiotic of choice for *Str. milleri*. Other antibiotics will be required for other pathogens.

Urinary tract infections

These may be confined to the bladder or involve the kidney, and very occasionally abscesses may occur in or adjacent to the kidney. Bladder infections are frequently referred to as cystitis, but the term is also widely used, particularly by patients, to denote symptoms of dysuria and frequency, and these may or may not be associated with detectable bacteriuria. Various terms have been coined for 'cystitis' with negative urine cultures; these include the urethral syndrome and abacterial cystitis. Bacteriuria, that is, bacteria in the urine, may occur in the absence of symptoms, and this is generally referred to as asymptomatic bacteriuria. Urinary tract infections involving the kidney (upper tract infections) are much more severe than those confined to the bladder and usually produce marked systemic disturbance as well as loin pain (see Chapter 36). This is acute pyelonephritis and the causative pathogen can sometimes be recovered from the blood as well as from the urine. Urinary infection, particularly in women, may occur in the presence of an entirely normal urinary tract, or may be secondary to some underlying abnormality.

REFERENCES

28. Levison M E, Bush L M In: Mandell G L, Bennett J E, Dolin R (eds) Principles and Practice of Infectious Diseases, 4th edn. Churchill Livingstone, New York 1995 pp 708–710
29. Moore-Gillon J C, Eykyn S J, Phillips I Br Med J 1981; 283: 819–821

Interpretation of laboratory results

Much emphasis has been placed on the number of bacteria required to diagnose urinary tract infection on culture of a midstream specimen, and an almost mystical significance has been attached to the figure of 10^5 bacteria/ml.[30] In many cases, symptomatic urinary infection is characterized by large numbers of bacteria in a midstream urine, often well over 10^5; accurate counting is in any case seldom done, and most laboratories report somewhat approximate counts. In some cases, fewer bacteria are present, but in pure growth and in the presence of symptoms they must be assumed to be significant. Interestingly, in a recent epidemic of multiresistant *E. coli* serogroup 015 urinary infection, low bacterial counts were frequently seen despite severe symptoms.[31]

White blood cells (pus cells) are almost invariably found in the urine in urinary tract infection; most laboratories report an approximate estimate rather than an exact count. Red blood cells too may be found in cystitis.

Bladder infection (cystitis)

Bladder infection is markedly more common in the female. The pathogen is almost invariably *E. coli* of bowel origin, although some 15% of infections are caused by organisms other than *E. coli*; these include *Staph. saprophyticus* particularly in young women, *Proteus mirabilis*, *Klebsiella* spp. and *Ent. (Str.) faecalis*. About 40% of *E. coli* are now resistant to ampicillin (amoxycillin) and an increasing number are also resistant to trimethoprim. Hence blind treatment with these drugs may occasionally fail, but laboratory reports of resistance do not always equate with clinical failure, and ampicillin (amoxycillin) and trimethoprim still remain useful antibiotics for urinary tract infections. Sulphonamides must now be considered obsolete, and co-trimoxazole should not be used; its sulphonamide component (sulphamethoxazole) is responsible for most of its side-effects and for most pathogens it confers no additional advantage over trimethoprim. Co-amoxiclav (Augmentin), oral cephalosporins and ciprofloxacin are other useful antibiotics; nitrofurantoin, effective against most organisms other than *Proteus*, often produces nausea. As symptomatic relief rapidly follows (usually) the first dose of antibiotic, and patients seldom finish the courses of drugs prescribed, short courses, even single doses, have much to commend them.

In some 40% of women with dysuria and frequency, no urinary pathogen can be demonstrated, even though in many cases there is a response to antibiotics. There are many possible causes, including urethritis and vaginal infections, but sometimes low counts of urinary pathogens in pure growth are reported as contaminants by laboratories and they may be relevant.

Acute pyelonephritis

This is much less common than cystitis but, like cystitis, occurs predominantly in the female. The causative organisms are the same as those responsible for cystitis. In some cases oral antibiotics are appropriate, but when there is nausea and vomiting or severe systemic disturbance parenteral antibiotics should be given; cefuroxime, co-amoxiclav (Augmentin) or gentamicin are reliable first choices before sensitivities are known.

Recurrent urinary tract infections

These may involve the same organism in repeated episodes, defined as relapse, or different organisms, which implies reinfection. Reinfections are much more common than relapsing infections, but the latter are usually the result of an underlying abnormality and are unlikely to resolve until this is remedied. It thus follows that investigation of patients with relapsing infection is more rewarding than that of those with reinfection. Many patients with recurrent infections tend to be prescribed long-term antibiotics; this should only be done as a last resort and continually monitored.

Asymptomatic bacteriuria

The chance finding of bacteriuria in the absence of any symptoms of urinary tract infection is common, particularly in the elderly. There is scant evidence that exhibiting antibiotics to such patients is of any value.

Perinephric abscess and intrarenal abscess

Both are uncommon. A perinephric abscess usually arises by direct extension of infection from the kidney; it is seldom haematogenous in origin. The causative organisms are the coliforms that cause acute pyelonephritis; any antibiotic treatment is secondary to drainage.

An intrarenal abscess is an infection (usually with *Staph. aureus*) of the renal parenchyma, for which the term 'renal carbuncle' has been used. Such infections result from bacteraemia and may extend into the perinephric area. Drainage will usually be required in addition to appropriate antibiotic therapy.

If these abscesses communicate with the renal pelvis the causative organism can be cultured from the urine and blood cultures may be positive.

Infections of the genital tract

Many, though not all, infections of the genital skin and mucous membranes are sexually transmitted and thus the concern of the genitourinary physician rather than the surgeon and it is not proposed to address them in this chapter. Only those conditions of relevance to surgeons will be considered.

Infections of the female genital tract

Vaginal discharge

Since this is such a common female complaint, and since reports of cultures of high vaginal swabs are sometimes confusing, mention

REFERENCES

30. Kass E H Arch Intern Med 1957; 100: 709–714
31. Phillips I, Eykyn S J, King A et al Lancet 1988; i: 1038–1041

will be made of its aetiology. Many cases are attributable to *Candida* spp. or *Trichomonas vaginalis* and present no problems with laboratory diagnosis or treatment. *N. gonorrhoeae* seldom causes vaginal discharge. Bacterial vaginosis, sometimes called anaerobic vaginosis, is one of the commonest causes of vaginal discharge. It is characterized by a foul odour (and this is the patient's main complaint) and is caused by anaerobic organisms together with *G. vaginalis*.

Pelvic inflammatory disease

This may be acute or chronic. Acute cases are gonococcal with *N. gonorrhoeae* readily recovered from a cervical swab, but most cases, and especially the chronic cases, present diagnostic difficulty since there is seldom material available for culture and their aetiology must remain speculative rather than proven. Most are probably polymicrobial, though predominantly anaerobic, but aerobic vaginal commensal organisms such as group B streptococci are also found. *C. trachomatis* and the genital mycoplasmas may also be relevant.

It is conventional to treat acute pelvic inflammatory disease with an antibiotic or combination of agents active against gonococci and anaerobes, and ampicillin (amoxycillin) and metronidazole are widely used, usually to good effect in acute infections. The antibiotic management of chronic infections is far more difficult. Many agents are used including those such as tetracycline with antichlamydial activity, but no single regimen can be recommended with any confidence.

Infections of the male genital tract

Balanitis

This common infection can be caused by *Candida* spp., *Trichomonas vaginalis*, herpes simplex or pyogenic streptococci, but erosive disease, usually with an associated foul discharge is caused by anaerobes (see Chapter 39).

Prostatitis (see Chapter 38)

Various symptoms referable to the lower urogenital tract and perineum are described under the general heading of prostatitis; such complaints are very common, but the term 'prostatitis' requires definition as it is not a homogenous entity.[25] A distinction must be made between the minority of patients who have associated bacteriuria and the majority who do not. Four groups of patients can be defined:

1. *Acute bacterial prostatitis*: a rare but severe infection with pyuria, bacteriuria and often bacteraemia, usually caused by *E. coli*.[32] There is a rapid response to antibiotic treatment whether or not the drug used penetrates prostatic tissue. Occasionally acute bacterial prostatitis progresses to abscess formation and anaerobes are often isolated from prostatic abscesses, usually with coliforms.[33] It may also result in chronic bacterial prostatitis.
2. *Chronic bacterial prostatitis*: this is characterized by recurrent symptomatic urinary infections, always with the same organism, which is usually *E. coli*, but occasionally other coliforms, *Ps. aeruginosa* or enterococci. Long-term suppressive antibiotics such as trimethoprim or ciprofloxacin, which achieve good levels in prostatic tissue, usually effect a symptomatic if not a bacteriological cure; remarkably, the pathogens do not seem to become resistant to the antibiotic given for long-term suppression.
3. *Abacterial (or non-bacterial) prostatitis*: this is not only much more common than chronic bacterial prostatitis, it is infinitely more difficult to treat effectively as the cause is unknown. Even though some patients complain of dysuria and frequency, bacteriuria is not found. Its aetiology remains obscure; indeed, it is far from clear that it is an infection. The prostatic secretions contain pus cells, but whether the urethral commensals that can be recovered on culture have any role in the disease is unknown. Not surprisingly, treatment is unsatisfactory and all that can be said is that antibiotics help some patients sometimes.
4. *Prostatosis/prostatodynia*: This condition is probably as common as abacterial prostatitis and with similar symptoms and no bacteruria. The prostatic secretions do not contain pus cells. A therapeutically frustrating condition for patient and doctor alike, there is no convincing evidence that it has anything to do with bacteria.

Epididymo-orchitis

Sexually transmitted infections with *Neisseria gonorrhoeae*, or more often *Chlamydia trachomatis*, are the usual cause in younger men, but in older men epididymo-orchitis is usually caused by urinary pathogens such as *E. coli* and is associated with urinary tract infection. In many cases the pathogen remains unknown as the urine is sterile.[34]

Scrotal abscess

This may result from a previous episode of acute epididymo-orchitis, when the pathogen is generally *E. coli*;[35] it may also complicate scrotal or urethral surgery. Some two-thirds of cases arise spontaneously and many are recurrent. The predominant pathogens are anaerobes, though in many cases aerobes too are isolated. The infection is probably secondary to blocked apocrine glands, and interestingly is more common in black men, whose skin contains more apocrine glands than that of white men. The anaerobes are predominantly *Porph. asaccharolyticus*, *Prevotella* spp. and anaerobic cocci. The treatment of scrotal abscess consists of drainage, but where there is associated cellulitis metronidazole may offer additional benefit.

REFERENCES

32. Bruce A W, Fox M Br J Urol 1960; 32: 302–305
33. Weinberger M, Cytron S, Servadio C, Block C, Rosenfeld J B, Pitlik S D Rev Infect Dis 1988; 10: 239–249
34. Berger R E In: Holmes K K, Mardh P A, Sparling P F (eds) Sexually Transmitted Diseases. McGraw Hill, New York 1990; pp 641–651
35. Whitehead S M, Leach R D, Eykyn S J, Phillips I Br J Surg 1982; 69: 729–730

Respiratory tract infections

Infections of the upper respiratory tract and associated structures

Str. pyogenes remains an important pathogen in tonsillitis and peritonsillar abscesses or quinsy; it may also cause acute otitis media and acute sinusitis, but *Str. pneumoniae* and *Haemophilus influenzae* are probably more common. Ampicillin/amoxycillin, co-amoxiclav (Augmentin) or erythromycin are appropriate antibiotics for treatment. Anaerobes are important pathogens in chronic sinusitis, including the occasional resultant orbital cellulitis, chronic otitis media and mastoiditis, but in these conditions it is drainage or cleaning that is required rather than antibiotics. Anaerobes may also be involved in peritonsillar abscesses. *Ps. aeruginosa* is commonly found in chronic middle-ear disease, not surprisingly in view of its well-known predilection for moist cavities. Although gentamicin eardrops are frequently used, it is aural toilet that is needed. *Ps. aeruginosa* is a common cause of chronic sinus infection and resultant lung infections in patients with HIV infection.

Anaerobes, of either odontogenic or pharyngeal origin, are major pathogens, together with upper respiratory aerobes, in the relatively rare but potentially very serious infections that involve the fascial compartments of the neck, sometimes extending to the mediastinum. The term 'Ludwig's angina' is used for those infections arising from the floor of the mouth that spread to involve the sublingual and submandibular spaces (see Chapter 13). Successful management of these dangerous infections requires surgical drainage by a faciomaxillary surgeon and debridement and maintenance of the airway and antibiotics (ampicillin/amoxycillin plus metronidazole) are secondary to this.

Infections of the lower respiratory tract

Patients with community-acquired pneumonia, usually caused by *Str. pneumoniae*, are unlikely to present to surgeons; the frequently encountered acute exacerbations of chronic bronchitis are sometimes associated with *Haemophilus influenzae* in the sputum, or at least may respond to antibiotics with activity against this organism.

Lung abscess and empyema[36]

As empyema (frank pus in the pleural cavity) results from lung infection, if not from a detectable abscess, and as the pathogens in lung abscess and empyema are similar, they will be considered together. In some cases there is an underlying tumour, but in many it is a primary infection (see Chapter 22).

Although a lung abscess can result from bronchial obstruction, pneumonia, infected pulmonary infarcts, transdiaphragmatic spread of infection or haematogenous infection, in most cases the relevant causative factor is aspiration from the oropharynx, and there are many reasons why this occurs. In light of this aetiology it is not surprising that anaerobes are important pathogens in lung abscess, particularly *Porph. asaccharolyticus*, *Prevotella* spp., anaerobic cocci and fusobacteria. Aerobes generally accompany the anaerobes and overall the commonest aerobes isolated are the *Str. milleri* group, though many others may be found. Occasionally only a single species of bacteria is responsible for a lung abscess or empyema and when this occurs it is usually one of the *Str. milleri* group, *Str. pneumoniae*, *Staph. aureus* or a fusobacteria. The treatment of both lung abscess and empyema is drainage, and until this is achieved the patient will not improve whatever antibiotics are given. Although antibiotics—amoxycillin and metronidazole are a useful combination—help the resolution of lung abscesses, they confer no benefit in the treatment of empyema (see Chapter 22).

Infection of bone and joint

Osteomyelitis

Osteomyelitis may arise as a result of haematogenous invasion, by direct spread from an adjacent infection or as a result of vascular insufficiency (see Chapter 42). Whereas haematogenous infections usually involve a single pathogen, other bone infections are generally mixed infections; they are also chronic and recurrent. In children, usually boys, haematogenous osteomyelitis involves the long bones, but in adults the most common site is the lumbar spine. Over the last decade long-bone osteomyelitis in children has become very uncommon and is now rarely seen, whereas vertebral osteomyelitis has become more common or perhaps is increasingly recognized. It is particularly common in the elderly, in whom misdiagnosis is frequent. Overall the commonest pathogen is *Staph. aureus*, but when the infection originates in the urinary tract then coliforms are responsible. Antibiotic treatment depends on the pathogen and definitive surgery is often required.

Chronic osteomyelitis

This always requires surgery to remove dead bone and unless this is done the infection will persist whatever antibiotics are given (see Chapter 42). Whether antibiotics offer any additional benefit once curative surgery has been undertaken is questionable but they tend to be given for weeks or months.

Septic arthritis

Septic arthritis is a haematogenous infection that sometimes arises as an extension from infected bone, and sometimes as a direct infection of the synovial space (see Chapter 42). The infection usually involves a single joint, most often the knee, but may be multifocal, particularly in patients with underlying joint disease. In the very young child the commonest pathogen until recently was *H. influenzae*, but with the advent of Hib vaccine this infection has virtually disappeared. Most cases, whatever the patient's age, are caused by *Staph. aureus*, but a variety of organisms can cause the infection, including both *N. gonorrhoeae* and *N. meningitidis*. Diabetes, rheumatoid arthritis, osteoarthritis and other joint diseases predispose to the infection and the causative pathogen is also usually readily detected on a Gram-stained smear of pus

REFERENCE

36. Neild J E, Eykyn S J, Phillips I Q J Med 1985; 57: 875–882

aspirated from the infected joint. Treatment involves drainage, joint washouts, which sometimes require to be repeated, and antibiotics as for osteomyelitis.

The reactive arthritis that may result from infection with a variety of gastrointestinal pathogens is often labelled 'septic arthritis'. In these cases the joint aspirate is often turbid and contains pus cells but never the frank pus that usually characterizes pyogenic septic arthritis. Organisms are not detected on a Gram-stained smear or grown on culture, and antibiotics have no effect on the course of the disease.

Infective endocarditis

The virtual disappearance of rheumatic fever in the UK has not resulted in a decreased incidence of infective endocarditis. Different populations are now at risk, including patients with degenerative valves and prosthetic valves (see Chapter 23). Patients with a congenital abnormality such as a bicuspid aortic valve, ventricular septal defect or mitral leaflet prolapse are also at risk. Apart from intravenous drug abusers, in whom the predominant pathogen is *Staph. aureus*, and early-onset infection of prosthetic valves, in which the main pathogens are coagulase-negative staphylococci, the causative organisms in most cases of infective endocarditis are still the various viridans streptococci acquired from the teeth or gums. Staphylococci are also common, and *Staph. aureus* will attack both previously normal and abnormal valves and is a very destructive microbe. The incidence of native valve infection with coagulase-negative staphylococci (mostly *S. epidermidis*) is increasing, though the reasons for this are unclear.[37]

HOSPITAL-ACQUIRED OR NOSOCOMIAL INFECTIONS

Whilst many patients are admitted to hospital with infection, others acquire infection during their stay. Such nosocomial infections cause considerable morbidity, even mortality, and are increasingly the subject of litigation. Some, but not all, are preventable. The need for surveillance and routine collection of data is constantly stressed and although this has not been shown to affect infection rates per se, the presence of infection control personnel on wards may well do so. Whether this is cost-effective is another issue. Infections acquired in hospital may be caused by the patient's endogenous organisms or by exogenous bacteria. There is no doubt that the most important vehicle for the transfer of bacteria is the hands of medical and nursing staff. The increase in invasive devices and procedures, particularly in vulnerable patients such as the premature newborn and those in intensive therapy units, has seen a parallel increase in nosocomial infection. The most important nosocomial infections are considered below.

Postoperative wound infection[38]

Every surgical wound inevitably carries a risk—albeit usually a very small risk—of infection. In clean surgery where no contaminated site except the skin is encountered, the infection rate should be below 2%. The pathogen is usually *Staph. aureus*, most probably of endogenous origin. Such infections vary from a minor stitch abscess to cellulitis and frank pus and occasionally septicaemia. Few UK surgeons are aware of their individual infection rates for clean operations, yet this could provide a most useful measure of antiseptic as well as surgical technique. Very occasionally postoperative infection is caused by *Str. pyogenes*; such infections tend to be very severe and present early in the postoperative period, often with rigors and misleading symptoms such as vomiting and diarrhoea. Whilst the streptococcus may have been acquired endogenously, it may also have come from an exogenous source—a person—and enquiries should always be instituted as a matter of urgency if such an infection occurs.

The more contaminated the operative site, the greater the risk of postoperative infection. The commensal flora of human mucous membranes is predominantly anaerobic, hence most infections after operations at these sites are caused by anaerobic bacteria. An obvious example is operations on the gastrointestinal tract. These infections are actually mixed infections of anaerobes and aerobes. The advent of appropriate prophylactic antibiotics directed against the anaerobes has seen a significant reduction in the incidence of postoperative wound infections, but they still sometimes occur, and serve as a reminder of the importance of intact intestinal anastomoses and adequate bowel preparation (see Chapter 30).

Infection of intravenous access sites

All intravenous access devices can become infected, sometimes after a surprisingly short time in situ. These infections are usually limited to the site of insertion, but they may also give rise to septicaemia. The predominant pathogen for many years was *Staph. aureus*, but now the coagulase-negative staphylococci, usually *Staph. epidermidis*, are as common as *Staph. aureus*. Other organisms, including many Gram-negative aerobes—though curiously, seldom *E. coli*—and yeasts are also sometimes isolated.

These infections usually arise as a result of previous colonization at the exit site, but other routes of infection include hub contamination, especially for coagulase-negative staphylococci, secondary seeding of the access site from a bacteraemia arising at a distant site and infected infusion fluid. Infected infusion fluid is now very rare, if it occurs at all.

Once infection becomes established it is difficult to eradicate. Infections with *Staph. aureus* are often severe and attempts to suppress them with antibiotics while leaving the device in situ usually fail. With coagulase-negative staphylococcal infections, it may be possible to suppress the infection while leaving the device in situ, and vancomycin is the antibiotic that is most often appropriate as many strains acquired in hospital are multiresistant.

Once the infected device is removed, the infection generally resolves, often without antibiotics; but in some cases, there may be signs of continuing infection, often with persistent positive blood cultures, the result of infected thrombophlebitis, for which antibiotics are required.

REFERENCES

37. Etienne J, Eykyn S J Br Heart J 1990; 64: 381–384
38. Cruse P J E, Foord R Surg Clin North Am 1980; 60: 27–40

Prevention of these infections can only be achieved by scrupulous attention to antisepsis, not only at the time of insertion of the cannula or catheter but also thereafter. Those hospitals which have designated staff to care specifically for indwelling lines have achieved low rates of infection Prophylactic antibiotics are no substitute for asepsis and should not be used.

Urinary tract infection

The commonest nosocomial infection is that of the urinary tract, though it must be noted that many of these 'infections' are really colonization rather than infection and reflect a malfunctioning bladder as well as the inevitable urethral catheter. Although in the short term it should be possible to prevent catheter-associated urinary infection, in the long term such infection becomes virtually inevitable. Many of the bacteria involved are multiresistant coliforms or pseudomonads, some of which have been acquired by cross-infection, often transferred from one patient to another on their attendants' hands. Such organisms initially colonize the perineum and urethra around the catheter, and then reach the bladder via the outside of the catheter. Bladder organisms are unlikely to be acquired from the drainage bag by retrograde spread up the catheter.

Most patients with catheter-associated bacteriuria remain symptomless, and antibiotic treatment achieves little except the substitution of one microbe by another which is resistant to whatever drug was last used. Problems arise in such patients with instrumentation or other urethral manipulation, including sometimes catheter changes or bladder washouts, when there is a significant risk of bacteraemia, occasionally even with septic shock. Appropriate prophylactic antibiotics can often prevent this.

Respiratory tract infection

Hospital-acquired respiratory tract infections usually follow general anaesthesia or ventilation; they also occur in comatose or semicomatose patients. Many of these infections are difficult, if not impossible, to prevent. They result from aspiration of oropharyngeal contents compounded by collapse and stasis. Postoperative respiratory tract infection can be caused by *Str. pneumoniae* and *H. influenzae*, both organisms characteristic of the normal commensal flora, but this tends to occur in patients in previous good health who are admitted for elective operations. In patients with chronic chest disease—often the recipients of numerous antibiotics —and in sick patients in hospital, the normal commensal oropharyngeal flora becomes replaced by coliforms and other microbes more characteristic of the colon than the throat. It is these organisms that are usually responsible for any subsequent pneumonia.

Antibiotics cannot prevent postoperative respiratory tract infection; physiotherapy is the key not only to the prevention but also to the management of many of these infections. If antibiotics are needed, their choice should be guided by the sensitivities of the organisms isolated. Unfortunately, in many patients with hospital-acquired pneumonia, and particularly in those on ventilators, the organisms persist in the respiratory secretions despite apparently adequate treatment with an appropriate antibiotic. This may be partly explained by the notoriously poor penetration of many antibiotics into the sputum, but other factors must also be involved.

Septicaemia from instrumentation

The dangers of urethral instrumentation or catheterization in the presence of a urinary infection have already been mentioned. Septicaemia can sometimes occur, particularly after urethral dilatation, in the absence of a detectable urinary infection, presumably from urethral bacteria. Endoscopic procedures are increasingly carried out on the biliary tract, frequently through infected bile, and septicaemia may follow.

CERTAIN SPECIFIC INFECTIONS OF RELEVANCE TO SURGEONS

Tuberculosis

Tuberculosis is a chronic infection characterized by granuloma formation caused by *Mycobacterium tuberculosis*, and occasionally by *M. bovis*. Other atypical mycobacteria can also cause human disease, some of which mimics that caused by *M. tuberculosis*, especially in the lung. Mycobacteria can cause disease in virtually every organ in the body and the manifestations at various sites are considered in other chapters. This section addresses laboratory diagnosis and the principles of treatment. The Mantoux or Heaf tests are of limited use in the diagnosis of tuberculosis as a positive result is not necessarily diagnostic, nor does a negative one exclude the presence of disease. It is important to recover the causative microbe.

Any fluid or tissue—and it is pointless to send a swab—can be submitted to the laboratory for the detection and isolation of mycobacteria. The stains used for their detection are either the Ziehl–Neelsen using light microscopy, or auramine using fluorescence microscopy; the latter is more sensitive. Very small numbers of bacilli may escape detection on these stains and thus a laboratory report of a negative smear does not exclude the diagnosis. Small numbers of bacilli are usual in extrapulmonary sites. Culture, which requires special media, is much slower than for pyogenic bacteria and the speed of growth is also determined by the number of organisms present. Specimens containing large numbers of mycobacteria will sometimes grow in 7–10 days, whereas those with few organisms may take several weeks. The atypical mycobacteria vary from the so-called rapid-growers to those that take as long, or even longer, to grow than *M. tuberculosis*. Once a mycobacterium has been grown, definitive identification and sensitivity testing can be undertaken. New laboratory techniques have enabled these investigations to yield results much more quickly than in the past—a distinct advantage in management of the patient. Nevertheless, compared with the pyogenic bacteria, the laboratory diagnosis of tuberculosis is usually slow, and treatment is often started before culture results are available either on the basis of a positive smear result or in its absence, on strong clinical indications. As tuberculosis requires lengthy and specific treatment, speculative trials of anti-tuberculous treatment should if possible be avoided.

Tuberculosis is treated in two phases: an initial phase using at least three drugs, usually isoniazid, rifampicin and pyrazinamide, in a combination tablet for 2 months to reduce the population of viable bacteria as rapidly as possible, and to prevent the emergence of resistance; and a continuation phase of a further 4 months' treatment, usually with isoniazid and rifampicin in a combination tablet. Primary resistance to these drugs is unusual, but if it is found then other drugs must be substituted and their choice governed by laboratory testing. As a result of carefully conducted trials, the length of treatment for pulmonary disease has become progressively shorter (see Chapter 22) over the past two decades, with 6 months now being the norm. For sites other than the lung there have been few trials to determine the optimum length of treatment but this should certainly not be less than that for pulmonary disease. Supervision of long-term treatment is essential to ensure compliance, and any contacts of patients with tuberculosis should be screened.

Tuberculosis and infection with atypical mycobacteria, particularly the *M. avium* complex, are common in patients with HIV infection: *M. tuberculosis* may not only be present in large numbers in infected secretions, it may also be multiresistant. Such patients present a formidable infection risk.

Tetanus

Tetanus is now a rare disease in the western world; many of the few reported cases in the UK occur in elderly gardeners.[39] The disease has been reported as a complication of surgery, both elective and emergency, particularly cholecystectomy, and in American intravenous drug abusers. Neonatal tetanus remains a major public health problem in developing countries.

Tetanus is caused by the potent neurotoxin, tetanospasmin, of the anaerobic spore-forming bacillus *Clostridium tetani*. This organism is widespread in the soil but is also found in the faeces of humans and animals. Spores are usually introduced into the body by puncture wounds and in the presence of a suitable environment revert to the vegetative forms of the organism and elaborate tetanus toxin, which is then spread by the blood or lymphatics to the central nervous system. The incubation period varies from a few days to several weeks, but the average onset is within 14 days. Although the disease may be localized to the site of injury with persistent contractions of muscles, much more often it is generalized with painful spasms involving the muscles of the face producing trismus or lockjaw, and those of the neck and spine (Fig. 4.4). The diagnosis must be made clinically, as *Cl. tetani* is seldom detected in specimens from the initiating wound either on Gram-stained smear or culture. Thus in an infection in which the clinical diagnosis can be difficult, since tetanus can be confused with several medical conditions such as tetany, meningitis and epilepsy, the laboratory is of no help to the clinician.

The treatment of tetanus principally consists of sedation to control spasms and assisted ventilation. The wound should be drained or debrided; penicillin, active against *Cl. tetani*, is conventionally given to destroy any remaining bacilli. Human tetanus-immunoglobulin is sometimes given intramuscularly, intravenously or intrathecally. Tetanus immunoglobulin was reported to be significantly more effective administered intrathecally than intramuscularly in early tetanus. The equine antitoxin serum should be avoided.

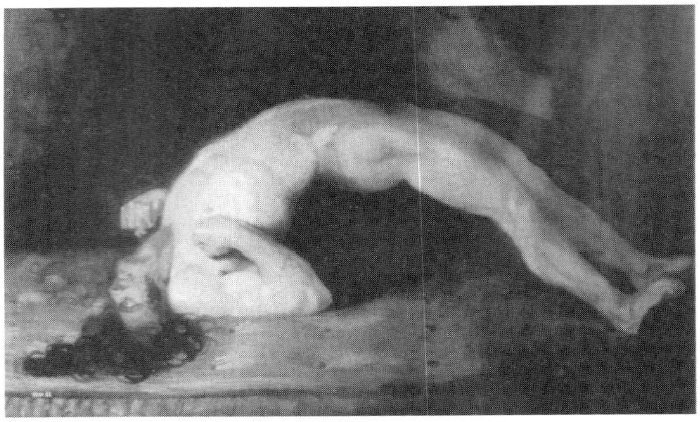

Fig. 4.4 Sir Charles Bell's portrait of opisthotonos in a soldier suffering tetanus from a wound sustained at the Battle of Corunna (1809). The painting hangs in the Royal College of Surgeons in Edinburgh.

The demise of tetanus in the western world can be attributed to effective prophylaxis by active immunization of infants with tetanus toxoid and 10-yearly booster doses thereafter. Passive immunization with tetanus immunoglobulin can be given to non-immune persons with dirty penetrating wounds, together with appropriate attention to the wound and prophylactic penicillin. Contrary to popular belief, toxoid will not provide immediate protection from tetanus in a non-immune person.

Gas gangrene: clostridial cellulitis, fasciitis and myonecrosis

Gas gangrene is rarely seen in UK hospital practice; when it does occur it usually results from trauma or occurs following surgery such as amputation of the lower leg for vascular insufficiency (Fig. 4.5) or operations on the alimentary tract. In the past it was seen after back-street abortions. It sometimes arises spontaneously. When the infection involves the legs, it is readily confused by the inexperienced with the much more common but much less severe condition of non-clostridial synergistic bacterial gangrene caused by multiple anaerobic and aerobic species, also characterized by necrosis and gas formation and common in diabetics.

Clostridial gas gangrene is produced by the α-toxin of *Cl. perfringens* (*welchii*). It is occasionally also caused by other clostridial species, including *Cl. septicum*, *Cl. bifermentans*, *Cl. novyi* and possibly others. These organisms are normal commensals of the gastrointestinal and female genital tract, and thus gas gangrene is an endogenous infection. The incubation period is usually only about 24–48 hours and the disease is characterized by the acute onset of pain and swelling with profound systemic

REFERENCE

39. Bleck T P. In: Mandell G L, Bennett J E, Dolin R (eds.) The Principles and Practice of Infectious Diseases, 4th edn. Churchill Livingstone, New York 1995 pp 2173–2178

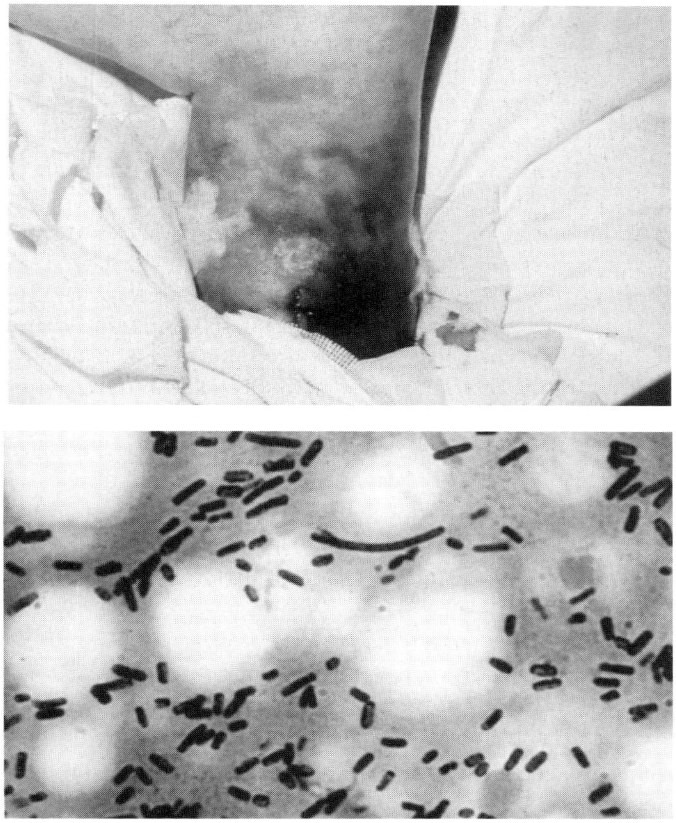

a

b

Fig. 4.5 Gas gangrene (*Clostridium perfringens*). (**a**) Stump 36 hours after a below-knee amputation for vascular insufficiency; (**b**) Gram-stained film of exudate from the wound showing no pus but large numbers of Gram-positive bacilli.

disturbance and shock. There is obvious crepitus, a bluish discoloration of the skin often with bullous formation and usually a watery discharge with an unpleasant sweetish odour, quite different from the putrid smell of other anaerobic infections. A Gram-stained smear of this material will readily confirm what is essentially a clinical diagnosis by demonstrating large numbers of Gram-positive bacilli and a virtual absence of pus cells.

The treatment of gas gangrene is early and extensive debridement of all affected tissues, and will often involve amputation. Penicillin should be given to destroy any remaining clostridia, but antibiotics are of secondary importance to surgery. Gas gangrene antitoxin which is of equine origin is of no benefit and should not be given. The use of hyperbaric oxygen has never been subjected to a controlled trial, though it is sometimes advocated. It seems reasonable to use it if it is readily available.

Actinomycosis

Actinomycosis is a chronic infection that may involve almost any site in the body, but the most common types are cervicofacial, accounting for about half of the cases (Fig. 4.6), abdominal, thoracic and female genital tract.[40] The causative organism is most usually the Gram-positive filamentous microaerophilic bacterium *Actinomyces israelii*, often inaccurately described as a fungus. Sometimes other actinomycetes such as *Propionibacterium* (previously *Arachnia*) *propionica* are responsible and frequently other organisms, both aerobes and anaerobes, are found in association with the actinomycete. Yellowish granules—the so-called sulphur granules —are found in the discharge or other material submitted to the laboratory and crushing these demonstrate the tangled filaments of actinomyces; Gram-positive branching filaments can also usually be seen in smears of pus even without obvious sulphur granules. Culture is slow and it may take a week or more to grow the organism.

REFERENCE

40. Russo T A In: Mandell G L, Bennett J E, Dolin R (eds) The Principles and Practice of Infectious Diseases, 4th edn. Churchill Livingstone, New York 1995 pp 2280–2288

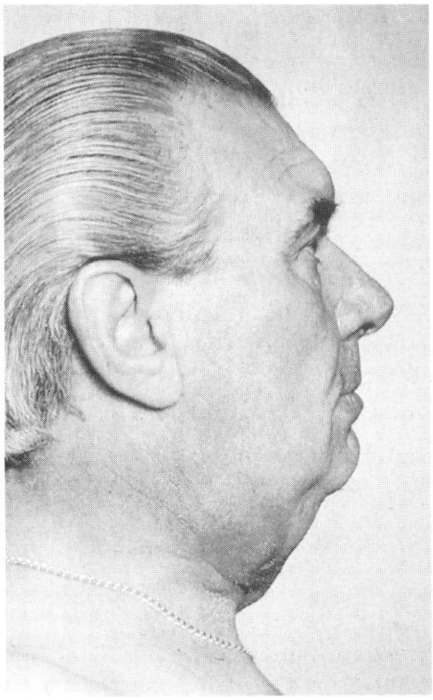

a

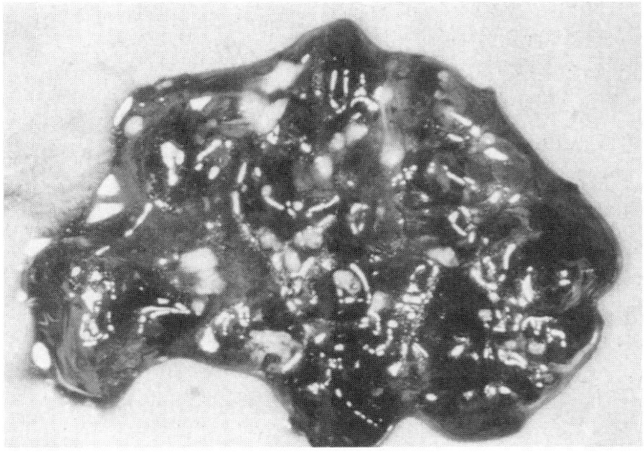

b

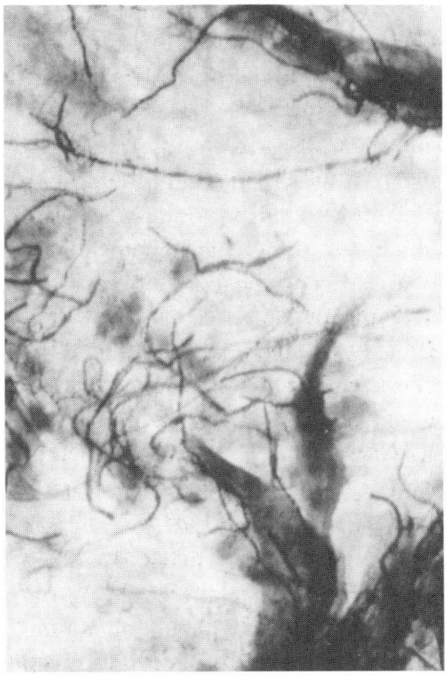

c

Fig. 4.6 Cervicofacial actinomycosis from underlying chronic dental infection. (**a**) Patient; (**b**) material drained showing sulphur granules; (**c**) Gram stain of crushed granules showing Gram-positive branching filaments.

Actinomyces form part of the normal flora of the mouth, lower gastrointestinal tract and female genital tract and actinomycosis is thus an endogenous infection. The clinical manifestations vary according to the site of infection.

Cervicofacial actinomycosis

This usually presents as a chronic enlarging, generally painless mass in the parotid or submandibular region. It is indurated and woody and, as the disease progresses, draining sinuses form that may discharge sulphur granules. In most patients there is obvious dental disease, and this is the usual source of their infection. Attention to this as well as drainage of the actinomycotic lesion is required. It is not unknown for the mass to be drained by a general surgeon who fails to look in the mouth and a second anaesthetic is then sometimes required to deal with the dental disease!

Abdominal and pelvic actinomycosis

Unless this presents, as it occasionally does, with a woody mass in the right iliac fossa secondary to appendiceal disease, there is likely to be considerable diagnostic delay. The infection is readily confused with carcinoma of the colon or other bowel pathology, such as Crohn's disease. Many patients have had previous surgery for inflammatory bowel disease. Any pus (or sulphur granules) that is drained should be submitted to the laboratory, but in practice the diagnosis is often first suggested by the histopathologist to whom the excised 'carcinoma' is sent. Pelvic actinomycosis has been reported in association with intrauterine contraceptive device use[41] and with cervical cerclage.[42] Actinomyces-like organisms are sometimes detected on cervical smears by cytologists, but these organisms may be carried by healthy women and in the absence of pelvic symptoms should be ignored.

The treatment of actinomycosis requires appropriate drainage or excisional surgery together with antibiotics. Actinomyces are very sensitive to penicillin and this is the antibiotic of choice; however, as already mentioned, in many cases other bacteria, particularly anaerobes, are also found, and it is therefore advisable to give metronidazole as well, or to use an antibiotic such as co-amoxiclav (Augmentin) that offers activity against actinomyces and anaerobes. In the past prolonged intravenous therapy with penicillin was recommended, but in most cases this is unnecessary and intravenous antibiotics can be given for about a week, after which oral drugs can be substituted for a further 2–4 weeks. In many cases of cervicofacial disease, all antibiotic treatment can be taken orally. Each case warrants individual assessment before blanket recommendations are applied.

Hydatid disease

Humans are an accidental intermediate host in the lifecycle of the small dog tapeworm *Echinococcus granulosus*; the normal intermediate host is the sheep. Humans in close contact with dogs, usually sheepdogs, ingest the eggs of the tapeworm that are shed in the dog's faeces and contaminate their fur. The emergent embryo eventually passes through the intestinal wall into the portal and lymphatic systems and thence usually to the liver, although other organs may be involved (see Chapter 31). The embryo then develops into a hydatid cyst. Many cysts are symptomless, and are discovered by chance, sometimes at autopsy, but others expand, sometimes become infected and thus give rise to symptoms. In the UK, apart from a few foci in Wales, hydatid disease is likely to be seen in immigrants from Cyprus and the Middle East. Hydatid cysts can be very long-lived and are sometimes detected in middle-aged or elderly patients who acquired their infection in childhood. The importance of an accurate geographical history cannot be overemphasized when considering a diagnosis of hydatid disease.

Diagnosis, other than the unexpected finding of hydatid at surgery, is made serologically or by typical appearances on computed tomography and ultrasound scan of the liver. Diagnostic aspirations of 'liver cysts' detected on scans should not be undertaken until the results of hydatid serology are known if there is any likelihood of hydatid disease as dissemination of the infection may occur. Symptomless hydatid cysts discovered by chance seldom require treatment. Symptomatic disease is treated by surgery where this is feasible and albendazole, started where possible before the operation.

ANTIMICROBIAL CHEMOTHERAPY

Although antibiotics have already been recommended for individual infections and bacteria, the general principles governing the rational use of this group of drugs will be outlined. Antibiotics, and particularly intravenous antibiotics, account for a sizeable part of the pharmacy budget, yet audit both in the UK and elsewhere has repeatedly shown that their use is often inappropriate. Not only is such use uneconomic, but in common with all groups of drugs, antibiotics produce unwanted side-effects, and many encourage the overgrowth of resistant organisms.

General principles of treatment

When bacterial infection is suspected, antibiotics are often prescribed as soon as the relevant specimens have been sent for culture. Information on the causative pathogen and its sensitivity is not usually available for 24–48 hours and most initial prescribing must of necessity be by informed guesswork. If the site of the infection is known, the prescription should be based on the usual sensitivity patterns of common microbes at that site; this information should be readily available from the microbiology laboratory. A single agent can often be chosen. When infection is suspected but its site is unknown, then the therapeutic net must be widened. The initial antibiotic regimen should always be re-assessed, and if necessary changed, when laboratory results become available.

When patients become 'septic' whilst in hospital, relevant microbiological results are sometimes already available and these

REFERENCES

41. Henderson S Obstet Gynecol 1973; 41: 726–732
42. Chappate O A, Eykyn S J, Kenney A J Obstet Gynaecol 1993; 13: 292–293

should be consulted before antibiotics are selected. An obvious example is the patient who becomes unwell, perhaps with a rigor or hypotension within hours of urological instrumentation; a recent laboratory report of infected urine may already be available. This should determine the choice of antibiotic.

The isolation of a microbe is seldom in itself an absolute indication for prescribing an antibiotic. Although, for example, the isolation of *Str. pyogenes* is virtually synonymous with the need for antibiotic treatment, this is not the case for most other organisms. Nowhere is this more true than for catheter specimens of urine; these are usually infected, yet the patient seldom needs—but often gets—an antibiotic. The urge to treat what is, in effect, a laboratory report should be resisted. Many clinicians become unnerved by laboratory reports of microbes, particularly those with unfamiliar names, and turn immediately to antibiotic treatment. Such practice may actually do harm.

Route of administration

This is determined by the severity of the infection and the condition of the patient: oral antibiotics are seldom appropriate in severely ill patients; absorption is too slow and unreliable. Nor are they suitable for patients who are vomiting. The route of administration is also determined by the pharmacokinetics of the antibiotic: if the drug is not absorbed, it must be given by injection to achieve a systemic effect.

Oral administration

The manufacturer's guidelines, such as administration before food or otherwise, should be followed. Although 6-hourly dosing is feasible in hospital practice, it is unlikely to meet with compliance in the community. There is a cogent argument for preferring oral agents that can be given once or twice daily. When two antibiotics are prescribed, as for example flucloxacillin plus fusidic acid for staphylococcal bone infection, they should whenever possible be given at the same dose interval.

Parenteral administration

Many parenteral antibiotics can be given either intramuscularly or intravenously: the intravenous route is most usual in hospital practice. Repeated intramuscular injections are painful and should be avoided. Intravenous antibiotics are usually administered by intermittent bolus injection, but continuous infusion is sometimes used. There is no evidence that either method is superior, but bolus injection is probably more reliable. The length of time over which a bolus injection should be administered varies and the manufacturer's instructions should always be consulted. Parenteral antibiotics are always more expensive than oral, and as soon as the patient's condition allows, a change to oral administration should be made.

Length of treatment

Patients are constantly encouraged to finish the course of antibiotics but in practice it is likely that many do not comply with these instructions and few, if any, come to any harm by so doing. Many antibiotics are prescribed for too long, yet the length of treatment for the majority of infections is unknown and many estimates are based on anecdote. Certain infections, such as for example tuberculosis, require several months of specific therapy; infections of bone, joint or heart valves require several weeks of treatment, though exactly how many is debatable, but many common infections can be treated satisfactorily with only a few days of antibiotic and some, such as lower urinary tract infection, with just a single dose. A more critical approach to the length of treatment is needed; many side-effects could be avoided and money saved.

Combinations of antibiotics

These are indicated to provide broad-spectrum cover for a wide variety of microbes, to prevent resistance emerging during treatment or, and only occasionally, to achieve bactericidal synergy. Despite the fact that certain combinations of antibiotics are antagonistic in a test-tube, there is no evidence that this test-tube antagonism is important in clinical practice. Drugs that show test-tube synergy is only relevant in the treatment of enterococcal endocarditis.

The use of broad-spectrum combinations of two, three or even more antibiotics should seldom be necessary for more than a few days; when the pathogen is known, the regimen should be changed or stopped if the infection has already been treated. Prolonged courses of combinations of antibiotics have become all too common, particularly in intensive therapy units; such practice is seldom justified and results in colonization with resistant bacteria or yeasts.

Choice of antibiotic

For most infections, there are many possible effective regimens and this may lead to clinical confusion. Surgeons are advised to seek advice from a competent clinical microbiologist before changing their antibiotic policy.

When patients have impaired renal or hepatic function, antibiotics excreted by the kidney or metabolized by the liver will accumulate; dose modification is required, and certain agents should be avoided altogether. Most problems occur with the aminoglycosides, especially gentamicin, and if these antibiotics are prescribed, regular monitoring of the serum concentration is essential in every patient.

Prophylactic use of antibiotics in surgery[43]

General principles

Ever since antibiotics became available, they have been used to prevent infection in surgical practice. Much of this use has been uncritical, owing more to dogmatic anecdote than informed evaluation. Audits of antibiotic use in the UK and elsewhere have

REFERENCE

43. Keighley M R B, Burdon D W Antimicrobial Prophylaxis in Surgery. Pitman, London 1979

revealed that 25–50% of all antibiotics prescribed are for prophylaxis, and that the prophylactic use of antibiotics is much more often inappropriate than is the therapeutic use. Although the antibiotics prescribed are usually active against the expected microbes, the timing is often irrational: the principal error is the use of prolonged courses, sometimes lasting many days or even weeks postoperatively. The past 20 years have seen the publication of numerous papers on the efficacy of prophylactic antibiotics in surgery, and the overwhelming message from the few well-designed trials is that, where prophylaxis is justified, it should be short; often a single dose will suffice.

If rational antibiotic prophylaxis is to be given, information must be available on the likely pathogens that occur after various procedures, and on their antibiotic sensitivity patterns. No single regimen will be appropriate for all types of surgery. Given the numbers of antibiotics now available, it is possible to devise an almost infinite number of permutations and combinations for use in surgical prophylaxis. Such temptations should be resisted.

Most prophylactic antibiotics used in surgery are given to prevent postoperative wound infection, and not to prevent other infectious sequelae of the operation, such as respiratory or urinary tract infections. Occasionally the aim is to prevent septicaemia, for example, during instrumentation of sites that are colonized or infected with microbes.

The objective of most antibiotic prophylaxis is to achieve a high tissue level of an appropriate agent at the operative site at the time of surgery, hence the preference for intravenous antibiotics administered at the induction of anaesthesia. This is more reliable than administration with premedication because the interval between the latter and surgery often varies. It should never be forgotten that antibiotics can never compensate for clumsy operating and hypoxic conditions. The use of short-term, even single-dose regimens has been advocated, but when overt infection or faecal spillage is encountered at surgery, antibiotics are usually given for several days or longer; this is not prophylaxis, it is treatment, and the concepts should not be confused.

Specific procedures for which prophylactic antibiotics are justified will be considered and suitable regimens suggested. These recommendations are well-tried, safe and cheaper than many alternatives; they are not of course the only possibilities. These guidelines are not intended to be comprehensive.

Gastrointestinal surgery

The incidence of wound infection and the causative organisms vary with the type of surgery and the condition for which it was performed. Prophylaxis is not indicated for highly selective vagotomy even though this is now rare, because the gastrointestinal tract is not entered. Should it occur, wound infection is caused by *Staph. aureus*, the result of inadequate aseptic technique. The incidence of wound infection increases markedly when the stomach and oesophagus contain large numbers of organisms, including those more usually found in the colon; this occurs when there is decreased motility and acidity—mechanisms that normally restrict the growth of bacteria—in a bleeding duodenal ulcer, gastric ulcer pyloric obstruction or gastro-oesophageal cancer. In these cases, the incidence of wound infection without prophylactic antibiotics approaches that of elective colorectal surgery.

Anastomotic dehiscence is also an important cause of infection after gastrointestinal surgery. Prophylactic antibiotics cannot prevent this; they are given to prevent wound infection. A widely used regimen is one to three doses of cefuroxime plus metronidazole. Co-amoxiclav (Augmentin) is an alternative that has the advantage of being a single agent, but there is little published evidence of its efficacy. Many other regimens are possible.

Biliary tract surgery

The incidence of wound infection after biliary tract surgery varies with the type of operation and the underlying condition for which it was performed. Infection is more common when the bile is infected at the time of the operation. Wound infection that occurs in the presence of sterile bile is usually caused by *Staph. aureus*, and cannot be prevented by prophylactic antibiotics. In contrast, wound infection in the pres-ence of bactibilia is usually caused by the biliary bacteria; these are predominantly coliforms, especially *E. coli*, though enterococci and the *Str. milleri* group are also found. Bactibilia is likely in patients over 70 years, those who have had previous biliary surgery, those with a history of jaundice or who are jaundiced at operation, those in whom the common bile duct is obstructed by stones and those who have had recent surgery for acute cholecystitis (see Chapter 31). All these patients probably warrant prophylaxis. It has been suggested that selective prophylaxis can be based on a Gram-stained film of an operative specimen of bile, but this is impractical. No antibiotic regimen has proved superior in practice, and many of the published trials are of defective design. Although enterococci are sometimes found in bile, they seldom prove major pathogens, and cephalosporins, for example cefuroxime (one to three doses), antibiotics that are inactive against enterococci, are widely used. Co-amoxiclav (Augmentin) is an alternative that encompasses activity against enterococci, but published trials in which it has been used are few.

Endoscopic retrograde cholangiopancreatography

When an endoscopic retrograde cholangiopancreatography is performed in the presence of infected bile, there is a risk of subsequent septicaemia sometimes with shock, and intravenous antibiotics should be given immediately before the procedure. Unfortunately, septic shock occasionally occurs despite appropriate prophylaxis. As the microbial status of the bile is generally unknown, it is probably wise to give prophylaxis to all patients having such a procedure. Although most documented cases of septicaemia are with coliforms, enterococci have also been implicated and cover should encompass both groups of bacteria. A single-dose regimen such as gentamicin (maximum dose for weight) plus either amoxycillin or co-amoxiclav (Augmentin) is appropriate.

Elective colorectal surgery (see Chapter 30)

Postoperative wound infection after elective colorectal surgery is dramatically reduced by prophylactic antibiotics. It has long ceased to be ethical to undertake prophylactic trials using a placebo in this type of surgery, though there were several in the early 1970s. The colonic flora consists predominantly of anaerobes, especially those of the *B. fragilis* group, but also of aerobes such as *E. coli* and enterococci. In this type of surgery, although there is no debate about the efficacy of prophylaxis, it remains unproven whether prophylaxis against the anaerobes alone using, for example, metronidazole is sufficient. Nevertheless most authorities recommend a regimen directed against both aerobes and anaerobes.

Two approaches have been used for prophylaxis—either *pre*-operative, usually non-absorbable antibiotics to reduce the bacterial load in the colon, or *per*operative systemic antibiotics to achieve a high tissue concentration. The latter are now almost universally used, although both methods are effective and neither has been proved to be superior in practice. Metronidazole remains the most effective agent for anaerobes despite many years of clinical use; if it is used then another drug is needed for the aerobes. Antibiotics such as co-amoxiclav (Augmentin), though theoretically suitable, have been subjected to few critical trials. Cephalosporins are widely used and are preferred to gentamicin or other aminoglycosides as the dosing with the latter is so often inadequate for fear of toxicity. Cefuroxime and metronidazole (one to three doses) are widely used in combination. Adequate preparation of the bowel before surgery is also important, and no antibiotic regimen can hope to prevent infection in the face of anastomotic dehiscence.

Appendicectomy (see Chapter 27)

Although infection or even peritonitis is apparent before surgery in some patients undergoing appendicectomy, this is not always the case, and while the risk of postoperative wound infection is greater when the appendix is infected than when it is normal, there is a cogent argument for giving metronidazole to all patients undergoing appendicectomy. If the appendix is found to be abnormal at surgery, metronidazole with or without cefuroxime can be continued for a few days. A metronidazole suppository provides cheap and effective prophylaxis provided sufficient time (at least 2 and preferably 4 hours) is allowed for its absorption.

Cardiothoracic surgery

Pulmonary resection

Antibiotics, though widely used, have not been shown to prevent wound infection after pulmonary resection. When infection does occur, it is likely to be caused by *Staph. aureus*. Prophylactic antibiotics are not recommended.

Cardiac surgery

Although many published trials of prophylactic regimens in cardiac surgery do not show a definite benefit from prophylaxis, a useful meta-analysis[44] has done so. In any event prophylaxis is always given, both for valve surgery and coronary artery bypass grafts. Operative contamination may result not only in wound infection, but also, though very rarely, in endocarditis. The predominant pathogens are staphylococci, both *Staph. aureus* and coagulase-negative staphylococci. Infection with *Staph. aureus* is the more dramatic. Sternal wound infection is also caused by Gram-negative bacilli, usually acquired as a result of inadequate antisepsis of the groin, hence prophylaxis tends to be directed against both types of bacteria. No regimen has been proved to be superior and many are used. Many hospital-acquired strains of coagulase-negative staphylococci are now multiply-resistant, and this includes resistance to flucloxacillin. The only reliable drugs for these resistant staphylococci are vancomycin or teicoplanin. Cephalosporins are widely used, but whilst they are active against *Staph. aureus* and throughout MRSA most Gram-negative bacilli, they are not active against many coagulase-negative staphylococci. No prophylaxis should be given for more than 48 hours, nor should it be forgotten that scrupulous antisepsis and careful technique will do more to prevent wound infection than antibiotics.

Vascular surgery

A wide variety of organisms is responsible for wound infection in vascular surgery, but the risk is much greater for infrainguinal procedures and aortic reconstruction than for brachiocephalic procedures.[45] Prophylactic antibiotics should not be given for brachiocephalic procedures; if these become infected it is likely to be with *Staph. aureus*, and such infection reflects a failure of antiseptic technique. Operations on the aorta and legs are most likely to become infected with coliforms and perhaps very occasionally with anaerobes acquired from the groin and seldom with *Staph. aureus*. But as with *Staph. aureus* infections, this is also the result of antiseptic failure. Nevertheless, the few published trials suggest that antibiotics—in most cases cephalosporins—are of benefit, and they are generally used. Cefuroxime or co-amoxiclav (Augmentin) is suggested, and one to three doses are sufficient.

Orthopaedic surgery

Joint replacement

The Medical Research Council ultraclean air trial in the 1970s demonstrated that prophylactic antibiotics were as effective as ultraclean air at reducing postoperative infection.[46] It has since been shown that antibiotic cement (usually containing gentamicin) is as effective as systemic antibiotics. Whilst the major pathogen is *Staph. aureus*, coagulase-negative staphylococci and coliforms are also found. Cephalosporins are usually given for 24 hours and gentamicin cement is widely used. There is no justification for prophylaxis for patients with joint prostheses undergoing dental procedures.

REFERENCES

44. Kreter B, Woods M J Thorac Cardiovasc Surg 1992; 104: 590–599
45. Winslet M C, Obeid M L. Eur J Vasc Surg 1993; 7: 638–641
46. Norden C W Rev Infect Dis 1991; 13 (suppl 10): 842–846

Open fractures[47]

The severity of the fracture and the degree of damage to the surrounding soft tissue is the most important determinant of infection. Available data support the early use of antibiotics with activity against *Staph. aureus*, but whether Gram-negative cover confers additional benefit is unknown. Both flucloxacillin and cephalosporins are given.

Open reduction of closed fractures

Until recently no trial had demonstrated the efficacy of prophylactic antibiotics for the open reduction of closed fractures but antibiotics were often given. A large multicentre Dutch study has now shown that a single preoperative dose of the long-acting cephalosporin ceftriaxone substantially reduces the incidence of wound infection.[48]

Leg amputation

Amputation of an ischaemic leg, from whatever cause, carries a small but significant risk of postoperative clostridial gas gangrene. The organism involved is *Cl. perfringens* (*welchii*) from the patient's own bowel flora. Prophylaxis is usually with benzyl penicillin (one to three doses). Patients allergic to penicillin can be given metronidazole.

Urological surgery

Septicaemia and septic shock are most likely to occur when instrumentation is performed in the presence of infected urine and may also occur after transrectal biopsy of the prostate. If the sensitivity of the urinary pathogen is available, then this should determine the choice of prophylaxis; if not, then a single dose of gentamicin (maximum dose for weight) is recommended.

Endocarditis

No antibiotic regimen has been shown to prevent endocarditis but it is known that this infection may follow dental procedures, genitourinary surgery or instrumentation and obstetric and gynaecological procedures, and it has become accepted practice to give prophylactic antibiotics to patients with abnormal or prosthetic heart valves undergoing these procedures. The *British National Formulary* gives the recommendations of the Working Party of the British Society for Antimicrobial Chemotherapy and should be consulted before prophylactic regimens are devised for patients.

Splenectomy

Asplenic patients are at increased risk of infection, sometimes overwhelming infection, with capsulate bacteria, particularly *Str. pneumoniae*, but also *N. meningitidis* and *H. influenzae*. The risk is lifelong but highest in the first 2 years after splenectomy and in those with malignant disease. Hospitals should have a policy for splenectomized patients and a card to give them. All asplenic patients should have an explanation of the risk and be provided with a supply of antibiotics to take if they get any febrile illness. Pneumococcal, meningococcal and Hib vaccines should be given, preferably before the splenectomy, but in traumatic splenectomies as soon as possible thereafter. Prophylactic penicillin can be given but in many case cases compliance will be poor and it is unrealistic to expect that it will be taken for life.

CONTROL OF HOSPITAL INFECTION

Infection poses a continual threat to a patient in hospital: not only can an individual become infected in many different ways and at many different sites, but also bacteria that are sometimes multiresistant can be transferred from one patient to others (cross-infection) and outbreaks can result.[49] Much of this infection is preventable. This section cannot hope to be comprehensive, but briefly addresses the organization of infection control within a hospital, cross-infection, outbreaks, theatre hygiene and HIV infection and the surgeon.

Organization of infection control

Every hospital has an infection control officer who should be a medically qualified microbiologist, and it is to this individual that any problem should be referred by surgeons. There is also a control of infection committee. Its members include the infection control officer, a senior clinician relevant to the problem, the infection control nurse, a senior nurse and others as appropriate to the circumstances. Although in some hospitals such a committee meets regularly, this may not be necessary provided that it can be convened when problems arise. As the recommendations of such committees are sometimes unpopular, particularly with surgeons, the chair should be someone whose authority is respected within the hospital. Hospitals are also required to have infection control policies which should be widely available and user-friendly.

Many laboratories can now provide information on isolates from different sites over defined periods for each specialty or ward, although this does not necessarily equate with the infection rate. This requires a clinical assessment of the patient, which is clearly impossible on a large scale. Routine laboratory surveillance is of limited use. Clusters of similar organisms may be picked up by the laboratory, but more often it is the clinician who turns to the microbiologist for help, having identified a problem.

Cross-infection

This is the spread of an organism from one person to another. The organism may cause clinical infection or just colonize a site; the

REFERENCES

47. Dellinger E P. Rev Infect Dis 1991; 13 (suppl 10): 847–857
48. Boxima H, Broekhuizen T, Patka P, Oosting H Lancet 1996; 347: 1133–1137
49. Ayliffe G A J, Lowbury E J L, Geddes A M, Williams J D Control of Hospital Infection: A Practical Handbook, 3rd edn. Chapman & Hall Medical, London 1992

latter is more common. In hospital, organisms are most often transferred from one patient to another, but staff are also involved, sometimes as a source of the organism, but more often as the means by which the microbe is transferred from one patient to another. The single most important measure in the control of cross-infection is handwashing, for the hands of staff represent one of the main routes of spread of organisms. Rapid decontamination of the hands can be achieved by the application of alcoholic chlorhexidine gluconate with emollients (Hibisol), and it is useful to keep this near any patient posing an infection risk to remind those who examine or undertake procedures on that patient to use it.

Many different bacteria can be involved in cross-infection, but the most common problems on surgical wards are with *Staph. aureus*, particularly the epidemic strains of methicillin-resistant—often also multiresistant—staphylococci, MRSA multiresistant coliforms such as *Klebsiella, Serratia* and *Acinetobacter* and *Str. pyogenes*. Some hospitals are also afflicted with vancomycin-resistant enterococci (VRE). Before concluding that cross-infection has occurred, the microbiologist should ensure, by the appropriate typing method, that the strains isolated are the same. Similar antibiotic sensitivity patterns may or may not be indicative of the same type of organism; for example, many strains of *Staph. aureus* are resistant only to penicillin, but they are not all the same; many different phage types are found. In most cases, isolation of the patient and attention to handwashing will suffice. Antibiotics and antiseptic preparations may be indicated depending on the nature of the bacteria and the site of the infection or colonization: microbiological advice should always be sought.

Outbreaks of infection

The term 'outbreak' is used to describe a number of cases of infection or colonization with the same organism. Outbreaks can arise as a result of cross-infection (see above) but also from a common source of an organism that is transmitted to several people without person-to-person spread occurring. There are many examples of common-source outbreaks in hospital, some of the more extreme of which have been the subject of government inquiries—salmonella food poisoning at Stanley Royd and legionnaire's disease at Stafford, for example.

Common-source outbreaks specific to surgical practice originate in the operating theatre or on the ward. There are many examples, but perhaps the most common include postoperative wound infection, virtually always acquired in the theatre or recovery, and the contamination of solutions. These can vary from disinfectant solutions used for a multitude of purposes to eyedrops and contamination occurs with pseudomonads or other environmental bacteria. Such outbreaks necessitate a search for the source of the organism so that the appropriate action can be taken to prevent further cases, and the nature of the organism will determine which direction this should take. A cluster of postoperative wound infections with the same *Staph. aureus* in patients operated on by the same team warrants an investigation of all members of the team for staphylococcal lesions and usually nasal swabbing. In contrast, a cluster of infections with *Pseudomonas* would immediately suggest a watery source.

Theatre hygiene

Staff in the operating theatre

No one should be in the operating theatre with a septic skin lesion or a severe sore throat: there is a real risk of transmission of *Staph. aureus* and *Str. pyogenes*. Boils and paronychia, often considered to be of trivial importance by their owners, can be the source of postoperative wound sepsis.

Specific clothing should always be worn in the operating theatre, and this should not be worn elsewhere in the hospital. Unnecessary people should not enter the theatre: the greater the number of people in an operating theatre, the greater the number of skin bacteria that are liberated into the air. This air-borne dispersal of skin bacteria is of particular relevance to implant surgery.

Cleaning and ventilation of the operating theatre

The physical environment of the theatre is of minor importance as a source of infection, and excessive cleaning of the walls and ceilings is unnecessary: two to four times a year is adequate. Cleaning should be with detergent, reserving disinfectant for spillage of body fluids. A plenum ventilation system by which clean air is pumped into the cleanest area of the operating suite is adequate for routine surgery. Routine bacteriological monitoring should not be performed; it is more useful to measure air flows at regular intervals. For implant surgery, such as joint replacement operations, a laminar flow ultraclean air system or occlusive clothing may confer some advantage in infection control, but at considerable cost, and postoperative wound infec-tion rates have been similar using conventional ventila-tion systems and prophylactic antibiotics. The technical skill of the surgeon remains a major determinant of outcome.

Skin disinfection

Hands of operating team

An antiseptic soap or detergent such as 4% chlorhexidine gluconate, or povidone-iodine surgical scrub should be used for some 2 minutes and well rinsed off to remove bacteria from the hands. Sterile gloves further reduce the likelihood of inoculation of bacteria into the wound, provided the gloves remain intact.

Preoperative disinfection of patient's skin

For most operations, a single application of chlorhexidine or povidone-iodine with or without 70% alcohol is recommended. For high-risk operations performed through the heavily contaminated skin of the groin, such as for example coronary artery bypass grafts and aortofemoral surgery, repeated applications of antiseptic are advised, both on the ward for bathing and in the theatre. When Gram-negative bacteria infect a sternal wound, this can only reflect inadequate skin disinfection. Interestingly, shaving the operative site increases the rate of wound infection in all types of surgery, particularly if it is done several days before the operation. Mechanical clippers are preferred for removing hair. Depilatory creams often cause skin irritation and are expensive.

HIV and the surgeon[50]

The potential risk of HIV infection in health care workers has been recognized since the discovery of the virus in 1983. Whilst all body fluids from HIV-positive patients must be assumed to be infective, the major risk is from blood or blood-containing body fluids, either from incorrect handling of sharps or by contamination of damaged skin or mucous membranes. Most of the documented cases of HIV seroconversion in health care workers have occurred after needle-stick injuries or cuts with sharp objects. The risk of occupational transmission of HIV is related to the depth of the injury, amount of contaminating and the concentration of the virus in the fluid. Rapidly changing new agents are being recommended as prophylaxis. A national scheme for the reporting of incidents involving potential HIV contamination and the provision of up-to-date advice on prophylactic treatment for HIV is run by the Communicable Disease Surveillance Centre of the Public Health Laboratory Service at Colindale.

The following patients should be considered as HIV risks: those known to be HIV-positive, homosexual or bisexual males, injecting drug abusers, haemophiliacs who have received untreated blood products, sexual partners of the above groups and children of seropositive mothers.

Not unexpectedly, some surgeons would like to introduce HIV testing for patients on whom they are to operate. This requires the prior consent of the patient; it should not be forgotten that such tests, even though negative, may compromise insurance policies. Furthermore, seroconversion may take 3 months or more after exposure, thus a single negative test may not exclude the infection.

Surgical procedures on HIV-positive or high-risk patients should only be undertaken if absolutely necessary for the diagnosis and management of the patient. That is not to say that HIV patients should be denied essential investigations. Precautions should be taken as for Hepatitis B.

REFERENCE

50. Henderson D K In: Mandell G L, Bennett J E, Dolin R (eds) Principles and Practice of Infectious Diseases, 4th edn. Churchill Livingstone, New York 1995 pp 2632–2656

5 Anaesthesia and analgesia

David N. James, Douglas M. Justins

ANAESTHESIA

A BRIEF HISTORY

The first successful public demonstration of general anaesthesia occurred in 1846 when W T G Morton administered ether to a patient having a tumour removed from his jaw at Massachusetts General Hospital.[1] The news spread rapidly in a world where pain and brutality accompanied every surgical operation and within 2 months ether had been used in England and Scotland. At University College Hospital Robert Liston, University of London Professor of Surgery, performed an above-knee amputation on an anaesthetized patient. This operation was a grand public success and Liston commented: 'This Yankee dodge beats mesmerism hollow'.

Innovation and experimentation followed as anaesthesia was introduced into clinical practice. James Young Simpson in Edinburgh and John Snow in London popularized the use of chloroform and in 1853 Snow administered chloroform to Queen Victoria during the birth of her eighth child and gained enthusiastic Royal approval for anaesthesia.

Deaths were soon reported during anaesthesia, particularly with chloroform, and it was apparent that the alleviation of surgical pain would not be achieved casually or without risk.

Ether, chloroform and nitrous oxide were to remain the mainstays of general anaesthesia for almost the next 100 years. Other inhalational agents such as cyclopropane were introduced whilst innovative anaesthetists including Sir Ivan Magill developed and refined techniques including tracheal intubation. These innovations were often made in response to surgical requirements and in turn by making anaesthesia safer created opportunities for further surgical advances.

During this long period when general anaesthesia was solely dependent upon inhalational agents, regional anaesthesia enjoyed widespread popularity and was often used for major surgery. Regional anaesthesia dates from 1884 when Carl Koller in Vienna first used cocaine to produce topical anaesthesia of the eye. In 1898 August Bier performed the first successful clinical spinal anaesthetic and by 1904 when procaine was synthesized regional anaesthesia had begun to blossom.

The modern era of general anaesthesia was ushered in by the introduction of the intravenous induction agent, thiopentone, in 1934 and the muscle relaxant, curare, in 1942. Muscle relaxation represented a major advance in anaesthesia and allowed the development of artificial ventilation techniques which were further improved during the polio epidemic in the early 1950s. Extracorporeal bypass for open heart surgery was first used in 1953.

Further pharmacological and technical refinements have created an aura of safety and security surrounding anaesthesia but the need for constant care and vigilance on the part of the anaesthetist remains, as does the need for close communication and cooperation between surgeon and anaesthetist.

PREPARATION FOR ANAESTHESIA AND SURGERY

Surgery and anaesthesia are inexorably linked, a fact attested to by accumulating data collected since the original report of the Confidential Enquiry into Perioperative Deaths (CEPOD) in 1987 and all subsequent National Enquiry into Perioperative Deaths (NCEPOD) reports.[2] Clearly, the minimization of morbidity and mortality for individual patients requires close cooperation between the surgeon and the anaesthetist and an appreciation of the requirements of each by the other.

Modern techniques can provide surgical anaesthesia for patients in virtually any physical condition, albeit with differing degrees of risk of an adverse outcome. The dilemma is not whether the patient is 'fit for anaesthesia' but, more often, whether the patient's condition can be improved preoperatively so that he or she is as fit as is possible and thereby maximizing the chances of a good outcome. The delay needed to optimize the patient's condition may be only an hour or so when fluid resuscitation is required, but may be longer when more complex medical conditions such as cardiac failure, hypertension or anaemia require correction.

Poor assessment and preparation for anaesthesia, most especially for emergency surgery, are major contributors to perioperative mortality. The surgeon must make a precise and realistic assessment of the degree of urgency of the operation and allow time for adequate patient preparation and resuscitation.[2]

When an operation is planned and there are doubts about the patient's fitness, the anaesthetist should be consulted as early as possible, the surgical staff pointing out what they perceive to be

REFERENCES

1. Bryn Thomas K The Development of Anaesthetic Apparatus. Blackwell, Oxford 1975
2. Buck N, Devlin H B, Lunn J N The Report of the Confidential Enquiry into Perioperative Deaths. Nuffield Provincial Hospitals Trust/King's Fund, London 1987

Table 5.1 ASA physical status classification

ASA 1	A normal healthy patient
ASA 2	A patient with a mild systemic disease (e.g. mild diabetes mellitus, controlled hypertension)
ASA 3	A patient with a severe systemic disease that limits activity (e.g. stable angina, obstructive pulmonary disease)
ASA 4	A patient with severe systemic disease that is a constant threat to life (e.g. unstable angina, heart failure)
ASA 5	A moribund patient not expected to survive 24 hours (e.g. ruptured aneurysm, head injury with rising intracranial pressure)

The letter 'E' is added if the operation is an emergency

potential problems. Anaesthetic clinics exist in some hospitals so that patients can be assessed when the operation is first planned.[3] The American Society of Anesthesiologists has produced a physical status grading system which attempts to quantify the risks of anaesthetizing patients in varying clinical conditions (Table 5.1).[4] This is by no means a perfect system but it has stood the test of time and it must be emphasized that 'physical status' is not synonymous with risk.[5]

FACTORS THAT MAY HAVE AN INFLUENCE ON THE CHOICE AND CONDUCT OF ANAESTHESIA

The surgical condition

The surgical condition which necessitates the operation may have significant anaesthetic implications. In emergency surgery the effects of massive haemorrhage make induction of anaesthesia in the hypovolaemic patient very hazardous. Injured patients require careful examination to exclude head injury, spinal injury, and pneumothorax in particular as anaesthesia can worsen the outcome of these conditions unless they are recognized preoperatively. Delayed gastric emptying caused by pain and a recent meal in emergency cases make regurgitation and aspiration a real danger. Other problems may be created, by fluid and electrolyte abnormalities in patients with peritonitis or by hypothermia in elderly patients or infants.

Elective operations can also present difficulties but these can be evaluated in comparative leisure. Head and neck tumours, particularly of the larynx and thyroid, may make tracheal intubation difficult and require specialized equipment. Alternative techniques such as regional anaesthesia may have to be considered.[6] Tumours elsewhere may secrete active substances, and preoperative control is part of the preparation. This applies particularly to phaeochromocytomas (see Chapter 35) and carcinoid tumours. Most endocrine gland surgery is now performed with any hypersecretion well controlled and replacement therapy provided for hyposecretion, but anaesthesia in uncontrolled disease such as thyrotoxicosis is still dangerous (see Chapter 18).

A tumour that has caused obstructive jaundice may have deranged blood clotting and will also predispose to the development of postoperative renal failure (see Chapter 34). A patient scheduled for a splenectomy may have thrombocytopenia from hypersplenism and require platelet transfusion (see Chapter 3).

A number of surgical conditions predispose the patient to regurgitation. A pharyngeal pouch or oesophageal tumour may trap food and patients with a hiatus hernia or achalasia will be at great risk of pulmonary aspiration. The full-blown picture of pulmonary acid aspiration syndrome can follow aspiration of as little as 25 ml of gastric fluid with a pH below 3.6. In any patient at risk of acid aspiration attempts should be made to raise the gastric pH, to empty the stomach physically or pharmacologically and, most importantly, to prevent reflux of stomach contents by using properly applied cricoid pressure as part of a rapid-sequence induction.

Surgical procedure

Any special peroperative and postoperative requirements must be discussed with the anaesthetist as early as possible. For example, during major corrective spinal surgery it is sometimes desirable to waken the patient briefly in the middle of the operation to exclude spinal cord damage (see Chapter 46).[7] Surgeons differ in their desire for muscle relaxation during hernia repair and in their need for controlled hypotension in a wide range of operations. The prone position also has significant anaesthetic implications.

In most cases the operation removes the offending part or repairs the damage, returning the patient to a normal state. This is not, however, always the case. Total excision of an endocrine gland requires postoperative replace-ment therapy. Total pancreatectomy requires postoperative insulin. Major faciomaxillary surgery can conclude with the patient's jaws wired firmly together so anaesthetic techniques that produce rapid recovery are required to guarantee a safe, unobstructed airway immediately postoperatively.[8]

Postoperative vomiting is undesirable in all cases but following ophthalmic or middle ear surgery it may be particularly dangerous so emetic drugs such as the opiodes are best avoided.

Previous anaesthetics

A history of previous uneventful anaesthesia is usually encouraging although the anaesthetic chart may reveal problems of which the patient has no knowledge. The patient may be unaware that intubation was difficult during a previous anaesthetic. Patients often mention nausea and vomiting as a complication of previous anaesthesia, although the real culprit may have been the postoperative analgesia or the actual operation (e.g. middle ear surgery).

The interval since the last anaesthetic is of crucial interest if repeat exposure to halothane is to be avoided. Current guidelines recommend an interval of at least 3 months between exposures to halothane to reduce the likelihood of causing jaundice but opinion is divided on this issue.[9,10]

REFERENCES

3. Burn J M B Lancet 1974; ii: 886–888
4. American Society of Anesthesiologists. Anesthesiology 1963; 24: 111
5. Lunn J N. Anaesthesia 1990; 45: 1
6. Saxe A W, Brown E, Hamburger S W Surgery 1988; 103: 415–420
7. Schofield N McC In: Loach A B (ed) Anaesthesia for Orthopaedic Patients. Edward Arnold, London 1983
8. Thurlow A C In: Wylie D, Churchill-Davidson H (eds) A Practice of Anaesthesia. Lloyd Luke, London 1984

An adverse reaction to an anaesthetic drug may have occurred during a previous anaesthetic and re-exposure of the patient to that drug is extremely hazardous.

Familial problems such as plasmacholinesterase deficiency,[11] or susceptibility to malignant hyperpyrexia[12] may have complicated previous anaesthetics given to the patient or family.

Patient's medical condition

The commonest reason for postponing an operation is the discovery of uncontrolled or previously undiagnosed medical illness. Hypertension, cardiac arrhythmias and cardiac failure are the conditions most frequently missed. Previously undiagnosed anaemia, uncontrolled respiratory disease and unsuspected diabetes are also common reasons for postponement. Postponement is always undesirable and wasteful of medical resources but is ultimately in the best interests of the patient, particularly if the surgery is not urgent. The preoperative visit is not the right time for these conditions to be unearthed for the first time and great effort should be made to detect these potential problems at an earlier stage.[13]

Diseases with anaesthetic implications can be found throughout all the body systems and some of the more important conditions are detailed in the section that follows.

Cardiovascular system

The relative contribution of various cardiovascular signs and symptoms has been analysed in the Multifactorial Cardiac Risk Index[14] and this has demonstrated that the most dangerous are a history of myocardial infarction within the preceding 6 months, the presence of a third heart sound or jugular venous distension, or an electrocardiogram with rhythm changes or more than 5 premature ventricular beats per minute. Age, the patient's general fitness, the site and urgency of the operation can exaggerate the risk of these cardiac factors (Table 5.2). The high-risk periods for patients with cardiac disease are during induction of anaesthesia and tracheal intubation, and again during postoperative recovery.

Anaesthesia and surgery performed within 3 months of a myocardial infarct carry a 40% risk of perioperative reinfarction and this has a very high mortality.[15] By 6 months after the infarction the risk has returned to acceptable levels so any surgery (unless it is life-saving) should be postponed for that period. When surgery is unavoidable during this period of increased risk perioperative invasive cardiovascular monitoring and postoperative intensive care are essential.

Ischaemic heart disease in the absence of recent infarction can still pose problems. These patients are often smokers with associated respiratory disease which adds to their risk. Ischaemic heart disease is the most common cause of congestive cardiac failure and this must be treated vigorously before anaesthesia.

Cardiac arrhythmias also require thorough preoperative assessment and control. Surgical conditions associated with electrolyte disturbances, notably serum potassium, may predispose to arrhythmias. The various types of heart block are of particular anaesthetic importance. First-degree bifascicular heart block (sometimes called trifascicular block) and Mobitz type II second-degree heart block can be very dangerous if unrecognized. More severe degrees of heart block may require preoperative pacing.

Internal pacemakers may also create problems, especially if electrocoagulation diathermy is used. Different types of pacemaker are affected to differing degrees, although most modern pacemakers are relatively safe with diathermy. Diathermy should however be avoided if there is any doubt.[16]

The relationship between preoperative hypertension and perioperative morbidity is well recognized but imprecise. It may be the association of hypertension with other cardiac risk factors such as coronary artery disease and heart failure that is important but patients with uncontrolled hypertension invariably have very labile blood pressure during anaesthesia.[15,17] A diastolic pressure of 100 mmHg is usually considered the upper limit for elective surgery after taking account of the patient's age and any coexisting cardiac disease. Hypertension caused by a phaeochromocytoma should be controlled preoperatively. Anti-hypertensive drug therapy should not be stopped preoperatively although some drugs, such as β-blockers and calcium channel blockers, can interact with anaesthetic agents.

The significance of particular cardiovascular pathology varies considerably, but certainly unrecognized aortic stenosis is associated with sudden death. Antibiotic cover is generally considered advisable in all patients with diseased or prosthetic valves as prophylaxis against infective endocarditis. Advice as to which antibiotic is appropriate should be given by the hospital microbiologist.[18]

Regional anaesthetic techniques are often very useful in patients with cardiovascular disease, although the hypotension produced by the sympathetic blockade which accompanies spinal

Table 5.2 The Goldman cardiac risk index

Criteria	*Points*
Cardiac failure (third heart sound, gallop rhythm, raised jugular venous pressure)	11
Myocardial infarction in previous 6 months	10
Rhythm other than sinus or premature atrial contractions	7
Five premature ventricular contractions/minute at any time preoperatively	7
Age > 70 years	5
Emergency	4
Important valvular aortic stenosis	3
Abnormal blood gases, electrolytes, bed-ridden, or chronic liver disease	3
Operation: intraperitoneal, intrathoracic, aortic	3
Total	53

REFERENCES

9. Blogg C E Br Med J 1986; 292: 1691–1692
10. Brown B R Jr, Gandolfi A J Br J Anaesth 1987; 59: 14–23
11. Donati F, Bevan D R Clin Anaesthesiol 1985; 3: 371–385
12. Ellis F R, Heffron J J A In: Atkinson R A, Adams A P (eds) Recent Advances in Anaesthesia and Analgesia, vol 15. Churchill Livingstone, Edinburgh 1985
13. Whelan E, Gordon H L Ann R Coll Surg Engl 1987; 69: 296
14. Goldman L, Caldera D L et al N Engl J Med 1977; 297: 845–850
15. Foster E D, Davis K B et al Ann Thorac Surg 1986; 41: 42–50
16. Bloomfield P, Bowler G M R Anaesthesia 1989; 44: 42
17. Goldman L, Caldera D L Anesthesiology 1979; 50: 285–292
18. Simmons N A, Cawson R A et al Lancet 1986; i: 1267

or epidural anaesthesia may be very dangerous in certain patients, including those with untreated hypertension, low or fixed cardiac output states or severe valvular disease.

Respiratory disease

The common cold, asthma and chronic bronchitis are the three common preoperative respiratory problems that confront the anaesthetist.

Upper respiratory tract infection is associated with increased per- and postoperative risks of airway and pulmonary complications, as a result of increased mucus secretion, bronchospasm, ventilation–perfusion mismatch and the possibility of lower respiratory tract infection which will impair gas exchange even further.[19,20] Anaesthesia does not benefit the common cold and elective surgery should almost always be postponed.

Asthma and anaesthesia are a potentially lethal combination and asthmatic patients must be managed very carefully perioperatively. The severity of disease should be objectively assessed by preoperative lung function testing, and factors that could precipitate bronchospasm should be avoided. The drugs given and airway manipulations that occur during anaesthesia can trigger a savage attack of bronchospasm. Surgery should always be postponed until optimal control is established and where possible the anaesthetic must avoid histamine-releasing drugs such as suxamethonium. The patient's normal asthma therapy should be continued during the perioperative period and postoperative physiotherapy is required.

Patients with chronic obstructive airways disease present a number of anaesthetic problems.[21] They may have abnormal respiratory control and be hypersensitive to sedative and analgesic drugs. During anaesthesia any bronchoconstrictive component of the disease may become active so that gas-trapping and progressive hyperinflation occur in the face of pre-existing ventilation–perfusion mismatch. Serious abnormalities of gas exchange then develop. Any active infection should be treated preoperatively with antibiotics and physiotherapy; elective surgery should be performed during quiescent phases of the illness. Excessive bronchial mucus secretion is by definition a feature of chronic bronchitis and perioperative attention to clearance of these secretions is vital. Smoking should be stopped well in advance of the planned surgery.[22]

Cigarette smoking in any patient is associated with increased postoperative morbidity of the respiratory system. These changes include excess sputum production, irritable airways which predispose to coughing and bronchospasm, increased closing volumes, increased ventilation–perfusion mismatch, and increased circulating levels of carboxyhaemoglobin, which all contribute to postoperative hypoxaemia. Smokers are also at increased risk of developing postoperative chest infections. Smoking should be stopped 6 weeks preoperatively to make a significant impact on postoperative respiratory morbidity but abstinence for as little as 12 h improves the available oxygen.[23]

Many other less common pulmonary or chest wall diseases can cause anaesthetic worries: these include the restrictive lung diseases (e.g. fibrosing alveolitis), restrictive chest wall disease (e.g. kyphoscoliosis), pleural effusions, bronchopleural fistulae, bronchiectasis, lobar emphysema, bullae, cysts and pneumothoraces. A pneumothorax can expand rapidly during anaesthesia, especially if positive pressure ventilation is used, and a tension pneumothorax can develop. A chest drain should be inserted preoperatively in all cases or if possible surgery should be postponed.

When a pneumonectomy is planned careful selection criteria must be applied to ensure that the patient will retain sufficient lung function postoperatively (see Chapter 22). Criteria include lung function tests, blood gas analysis and exercise tolerance.[24]

Regional anaesthesia is often considered the anaesthetic technique of choice for many operations in patients with severe respiratory disease and these techniques can often be utilized to provide superb postoperative analgesia minimizing the effects that pain has on respiratory function.[25] Patients with severely impaired lung function who are having general anaesthesia for major surgery may require elective ventilation postoperatively with controlled oxygen therapy.

Liver disease

The patient with pre-existing hepatic disease presents a number of potential anaesthetic problems. Liver disease may impair drug metabolism, especially the elimination of opioids and benzodiazepines. Impaired vitamin K absorption and reduced clotting factor synthesis creates abnormal coagulation and preoperative vitamin K and peroperative fresh frozen plasma is usually given to these patients. Hypoalbuminaemia may also be corrected preoperatively. Patients with jaundice (especially obstructive jaundice) are at particular risk of developing postoperative renal failure, the so-called 'hepatorenal syndrome'. Multiple aetiological factors may be responsible for this and the inevitable fall in peroperative hepatic blood flow, irrespective of the anaesthetic technique, may further aggravate matters.[26] Hypovolaemia and hypotension cause additional insult. This complication is best avoided by adequate preoperative hydration, correction of hypoalbuminaemia, close monitoring of urine output and avoidance of hypotension. Postoperative liver problems are discussed later in this chapter.

Renal disease

Surgery is a fairly common event in the lives of many patients with chronic renal failure. These patients are invariably anaemic as a

REFERENCES

19. Dueck R, Young I et al Anesthesiology 1980; 52: 113–125
20. Empey D W, Laitinen L A et al Am Rev Respir Dis 1976; 113: 131–139
21. Milledge J S, Nunn J F Br Med J 1975; 3: 670–673
22. Gracey D R, Divertie M B, Didier E P Chest 1979; 76: 123–129
23. Jones R M, Rosen M, Seymour L Anaesthesia 1987; 42: 1–2
24. Gothard J W W, Branthwaite M A Anaesthesia for Thoracic Surgery. Blackwell, Oxford 1982 pp 8–27
25. Charlton J E In: Wildsmith J A W, Armitage E N (eds) Principles and Practice of Regional Anaesthesia. Churchill Livingstone, Edinburgh 1987
26. Walton B In: Taylor T H, Major E (eds) Hazards and Complications of Anaesthesia. Churchill Livingstone, Edinburgh 1987

result of impaired erythropoiesis, although this is often well compensated for by increased cardiac output, a shift to the right of the oxyhaemoglobin dissociation curve and increased 2,3-diphosphoglyceric acid. Little reserve however remains for additional oxygen carriage. With the advent of synthetic exogenous erythropoietin treatment, anaemia is slowly becoming less prevalent.

Hyperkalaemia is a potentially dangerous problem unless the patient has recently been dialysed. Opinions vary but in general it would seem prudent to avoid non-urgent surgery in patients with renal failure if the serum potassium is greater than 6.5 mmol/l. Urgent short-term control of an elevated potassium can be obtained with a glucose and insulin infusion or a calcium ion exchange resin given orally.[27] Hyper- or hyponatraemia may also occur. Fluid overload may cause congestive cardiac failure and hypertension is a common finding. These patients are prone to cardiac arrhythmias and myocardial function may already be compromised by coronary artery disease or a uraemic pericardial effusion.[28] Diabetes mellitus and hypertension may coexist.

These patients are often very sensitive to drugs and in particular to those medications that depend totally or partially on renal excretion. They appear to be particularly sensitive to the opioid drugs. General anaesthesia requires great care and attention to detail in patients with chronic renal failure and regional anaesthesia has much to commend it, providing coagulation is normal.

Central nervous system disease

Anaesthesia for patients with neurological disease or with an acute head injury can pose a number of unique problems for the anaesthetist (see Chapter 16). Many anaesthetic drugs, most especially the inhalational agents, increase cerebral blood flow and thereby raise intracranial pressure which can aggravate the effect of a space-occupying lesion or extend areas of existing damage.[29] Stress-free tracheal intubation, muscular relaxation and intermittent positive pressure ventilation are essential for all patients with head injury who require general anaesthesia. Hyperventilation, drainage of cerebrospinal fluid, hyperosmolar osmotic agents (e.g. mannitol), steroids and diuretics can all be used to reduce raised intracranial pressure. Patients with intracranial space-occupying lesions are at risk of developing deteriorating cerebral function if they are given any drugs that depress consciousness and reduce respiratory drive, e.g. hypnotic agents such as benzodiazepines and opioids. The temptation to sedate a head injured patient who is confused and aggressive should be strongly avoided even for the purposes of cerebral imaging procedures. The assistance of an anaesthetist should be sought so that general anaesthesia with control of the airway and breathing can be instituted. The patient either has an appropriate anaesthetic or nothing at all!

Airway and breathing difficulties and associated extracranial injuries may accompany head injury. Fractures of the cervical spine are particularly worrying and the head must be carefully fixed and supported during anaesthesia to avoid additional spinal cord damage. Spinal cord injury, even if unassociated with head injury, produces immediate and long-term changes in the pulmonary and cardiovascular systems and in autonomic reflex activity.[30]

Numerous relatively uncommon neurological diseases have implications for anaesthesia. Patients with myasthenia gravis who present for operation may require postoperative ventilation because of respiratory failure which develops as a result of muscle weakness (myasthenia itself or a cholinergic crisis) or as a result of their marked sensitivity to muscle relaxants.[31] Carcinoma of the bronchus can also be associated with a myasthenic syndrome, as can thyroid or adrenal disease, or high-dose steroid therapy.

Patients with multiple sclerosis may also be taking steroids but, apart from an unproven concept that regional anaesthesia is best avoided in case the technique is incriminated if the disease progresses, these patients present no particular anaesthetic problems.

Regional anaesthesia is also probably best avoided in porphyria in case residual neurological weakness is attributed to the technique. Anaesthetic drugs which may trigger acute porphyria include thiopentone, etomidate, methohexitone, lignocaine and enflurane.[32]

Haematological diseases

Anaemia is one of the most common reasons for unexpected postponement of operation; a haemoglobin of 10 g/dl is the limit that is conventionally accepted for elective surgery, although it is difficult to obtain evidence that surgery and anaesthesia below this level are harmful. Patients with coronary artery disease and cardiac failure may be most at risk from anaemia as the excessive demands on the myocardium caused by surgical stress may render it ischaemic or unable to raise the cardiac output to meet the additional demands. The major concern in anaemic patients is the reduced oxygen-carrying capacity of the blood, which may be disguised by the compensating mechanisms. Unless the indication for operation is urgent the cause of the anaemia should be identified preoperatively and appropriate therapy prescribed.

Polycythaemia carries an increased risk of haemorrhage and thrombosis and should be treated vigorously before operation. Venesection and haemodilution may be necessary if emergency surgery is indicated.

Sickle cell disease in the homozygous form, when the HbS fraction may be 90%, renders general anaesthesia hazardous. The cells may sickle at a partial pressure of oxygen of about 5.5 kPa and preoperative exchange transfusion may be indicated if the haemoglobin is low and major surgery is in prospect. Hypoxia, hypotension, hypothermia, acidaemia and hypovolaemia must be avoided during anaesthesia; regional anaesthesia should be used wherever possible. Sickle trait, when for example HbS concentration may be 40%, does not represent the same threat as the homozygous

REFERENCES

27. Beven D R In: Taylor T H, Major E (eds) Hazards and Complications of Anaesthesia. Churchill Livingstone, Edinburgh 1987
28. Lazarus J M Kidney Int 1980; 18: 783–796
29. Shapiro H M Surg Clin North Am 1975; 55: 1913
30. Fraser A, Edmonds-Seal J Anaesthesia 1982; 37: 1084–1098
31. O'Shea P J In: Taylor T H, Major E (eds) Hazards and Complications of Anaesthesia. Churchill Livingstone, Edinburgh 1987
32. Jackson S H In: Katz J, Berumof J, Kadis L B (eds) Anesthesia and Uncommon Diseases, 2nd edn. W B Saunders, Philadelphia 1981 pp 1–67

disease, as long as adequate oxygenation is ensured and dehydration avoided. The use of a tourniquet is best avoided.[33]

Disorders of blood coagulation are described in Chapter 3. Haemophiliac patients may have human immunodeficiency virus and hepatitis infection and additional precautions must be taken with all procedures in these patients.

Endocrine disorders

Pharmacological methods usually allow preoperative control of endocrine dysfunction which smooths the course of the anaesthetic.

Uncontrolled hyperthyroidism can cause cardiac irritability and arrhythmias, congestive cardiac failure, increased sensitivity to neuromuscular blockers and thyrotoxic crisis (tachycardia, hypotension, hyperpyrexia). Hypothyroidism can produce cardiomyopathy and congestive cardiac failure. An enlarged gland can produce airway obstruction preoperatively, and postoperative problems may follow recurrent laryngeal nerve trauma, haematoma or tracheal collapse. The recently introduced laryngeal mask may be particularly useful in patients with preoperative airway obstruction[34] or regional techniques may have to be considered.[6]

Acute stridor may be one of the manifestations of hypocalcaemia following parathyroid surgery and preoperative hypercalcaemia can cause cardiovascular problems.

Cushing's syndrome provides many potential anaesthetic problems including diabetes mellitus, obesity, vascular fragility, hypertension, osteoporosis, hypocalcaemia and polycythaemia.

Anaesthesia for the patient with a phaeochromocytoma requires long and careful preparation to dampen the effects of the excess catecholamine secretion which can cause severe cardiovascular problems including hypertension, arrhythmias and cardiac failure. Preoperative preparation usually includes an α-adrenoreceptor blocker such as phenoxybenzamine and a β-adrenoreceptor blocker if tachycardia remains a prominent symptom; both drugs are administered until the hypertension is controlled and the peripheral circulation is normal.[35]

Carcinoid tumours may cause problems following release of histamine, serotonin or bradykinin. Hypertension, hypotension and bronchospasm are the commonest manifestations. H_1-receptor and H_2-receptor antagonists, corticosteroids, serotonin inhibitors, aprotinin and somatostatin have all been used to control excess secretion.[36]

The perioperative management of patients with diabetes mellitus has been much simplified by the development of methods that allow rapid blood sugar estimation. This facility means that instantaneous adjustments can be made in insulin therapy to maintain the blood sugar in the range of 4–8 mmol/l peroperatively and to prevent the development of dehydration and ketoacidosis.[37] Diabetics who are well controlled on diet alone or with oral hypoglycaemic therapy generally pose few problems. Chlorpropamide has a half-life of 36 h so it should be stopped 2 days before operation, whereas other hypoglycaemic agents are omitted on the day of operation to avoid hypoglycaemia during the period of perioperative starvation. Patients who are poorly controlled on oral hypoglycaemic therapy should be changed to insulin for the perioperative period. Insulin-dependent diabetics undergoing any operation other than minor surgery are best managed using an infusion of glucose with or without potassium, depending on the serum potassium concentration. The insulin is given on a sliding scale according to the blood glucose measurements, which can be checked regularly throughout the whole perioperative period.

Miscellaneous conditions

Many other conditions should be drawn to the anaesthetist's attention preoperatively. Alcoholism and drug addiction create problems of drug tolerance and have increased risks of hepatitis and human immunodeficiency virus infection. Homosexuals for the same reasons now represent a serious anaesthetic hazard.[38] Patients at the extremes of age and pregnant women require very careful anaesthetic administration, as do patients with most chronic illnesses. For example, patients with rheumatoid arthritis may have an unstable cervical spine and myocardial disease and a patient with ankylosing spondylitis may be very difficult to tracheally intubate.[39] Even religion becomes significant if the patient is a Jehovah's Witness who refuses blood transfusion, though with adequate preparation even cardiac surgery can be performed on these patients. Damage to teeth is a common complication of anaesthesia so careful examination of the dental state should be made preoperatively.

Drug therapy

The drug history should be specifically enquired for in all patients. Although the possibilities for drug interaction are vast, very few drugs need to be stopped preoperatively. Anti-hypertensive drugs in particular should be continued to avoid the problems of rebound hypertension. Awareness of the patient's medication allows suitable anaesthetic modifications to be made.

Oestrogen containing oral contraceptives pose a problem as the risk of thromboembolic episodes may be increased following major surgery. If they are discontinued for 4 weeks preoperatively, however, this creates the risk of an unwanted pregnancy. It is probably best to continue treatment and, if the patient has no other risk factors for deep vein thrombosis, it may not even be necessary to use routine thromboprophylaxis.[40]

The most important drug interactions are perhaps those associated with monoamine oxidase inhibitor antidepressants, notably when drugs such as the pethidine-like analgesics and indirectly acting sympathomimetic agents are used.

PREMEDICATION

Traditional dogma holds that premedication must be given before every anaesthetic yet many of the arguments used to justify this are

REFERENCES

33. Davies S C, Hewitt P E Br J Hosp Med 1984; 31: 440
34. Brain A I J, McGhee T D Anaesthesia 1985; 40: 356
35. Desmonts J M, Marty J Br J Anaesth 1984; 56: 781
36. Oates J A N Engl J Med 1986; 315: 702–704
37. Thompson J, Husband D J et al Br J Surg 1986; 73: 301–304
38. Sim A J W, Dudley H A F Br Med J 1988; 296: 80
39. Sinclair J R, Mason R A Anaesthesia 1984; 39: 3–11
40. Sue-Ling H, Hughes L E Br Med J 1988; 296: 447

illogical with modern anaesthetic techniques. Premedication is meant to encompass some or all of the following aims: to reduce anxiety, produce amnesia and provide analgesia; to allow smooth induction of anaesthesia and to reduce salivation and vagal activity. Common regimens combine either an opioid or a phenothiazine with an anticholinergic drug; however drowsiness alone does not necessarily relieve anxiety—benzodiazepines specific are anxiolytics. The administration of a potent opioid analgesic preoperatively can cause nausea, respiratory depression and confusion. Opioids can now be easily administered at the time of induction. Modern inhalational agents used after an intravenous induction do not usually produce the excess salivation and heightened vagal activity which characterized some of the older agents. A significant exception to this is in paediatric anaesthesia where most experts would still consider anticholinergic premedication (atropine) essential in the very young.[41]

Wide variations exist between different anaesthetists with regard to their premedication practice but current opinion suggests that standard premedication schemes applied routinely to all patients are illogical. Premedication should be tailored to suit the needs of each individual patient. Many anaesthetists now avoid injections altogether and prescribe just a simple anxiolytic tablet such as temazepam 10–20 mg given 1½ hours preoperatively. Additional specific drugs may be added as necessary and include antacid, antihistamine, antithrombotic drugs, antibiotics, insulin, hydrocortisone and bronchodilators. A reassuring preoperative visit from a sympathetic anaesthetist and a full understanding of what is planned can often do more to allay a patient's fears than any amount of drugs.

SELECTION OF GENERAL ANAESTHETIC TECHNIQUE

The large range of available drugs and techniques creates numerous options for the anaesthetist but there are really only two fundamental questions that need to be considered: firstly whether the patient should have his or her trachea intubated, and secondly whether muscle relaxation and artificial ventilation should be used.

The choice of technique is dictated by a number of factors including the nature of the planned operation, the patient's condition, and the skill, experience and specific requirements of the surgeon. In addition the physiological and pharmacological effects of the various anaesthetic agents should be considered as well as the skill and experience of the anaesthetist and the facilities of the operating theatre and recovery room. Day-care surgery has additional specific requirements.[42]

The decisions are often simple; for example, patients having ear, nose and throat surgery almost always warrant tracheal intubation or use of a laryngeal mask airway; all intra-abdominal, thoracic, cardiac and intracranial surgery requires relaxation and therefore mechanical ventilation. Tracheal intubation can be used to ensure a patent airway when access to the patient is restricted, or to protect the airway when the surgical procedure is likely to cause airway obstruction. It also provides airway protection when the patient has a full stomach and the danger of regurgitation exists. Tracheal intubation is the rule when mechanical ventilation of the paralysed patient is contemplated. Sometimes a spontaneously breathing patient needs to be intubated because of a 'difficult airway'. Other patients have to be tracheally intubated because they require muscle relaxants as part of a balanced anaesthetic technique, even though relaxation is not actually required for the surgical access. Long orthopaedic operations are examples of where this is desirable. The use of a balanced anaesthetic technique usually gives a much speedier postoperative recovery. Finally, tracheal intubation and ventilation may be used to ensure unimpaired oxygenation and ventilation in any infirm patient irrespective of the proposed surgical procedure.

Tracheal intubation and ventilation add to anaesthetic complexity and these techniques may generate their own complications. Failure to achieve tracheal intubation, aspiration of gastric contents whilst attempting intubation and unrecognized oesophageal intubation are regular contributors to anaesthetic-related mortality.[43] Failure to maintain adequate ventilation of a paralysed patient, following inadvertent disconnection, is another serious mishap. Relatively minor problems such as pharyngeal or dental trauma can occur during intubation.

Mechanical ventilation can decrease cardiac output and cause changes in acid–base homeostasis. Hypocarbia may also result from over zealous intermittent positive pressure ventilation and this can cause a marked reduction in cerebral blood flow. This may be useful in neurosurgery because of the resultant reduction in intracranial pressure, but if cerebral circulation is already compromised a fall in cerebral perfusion is potentially harmful.

Once the decision is made regarding intubation and ventilation the anaesthetist will then evaluate which drugs to use with regard to the patient's condition and the surgical requirements. For example, for an atopic individual with asthma it is prudent to avoid histamine-releasing drugs such as thiopentone and suxamethonium. During a myringoplasty the surgeon may wish to avoid the diffusion of nitrous oxide into the middle ear. Every anaesthetic has to be formulated to suit each individual case and although techniques and styles of anaesthesia may vary widely between individual anaesthetists in different hospitals, all are ultimately designed with the object of allowing the surgeon to operate with maximum ease whilst avoiding any pain, distress or harm to the patient.

GENERAL ANAESTHESIA

Many theories have been advanced to explain the action of anaesthetic agents on the brain. Current opinion supports the view that by inducing molecular and conformational changes in the cell membrane they produce alterations in the ionic balance and electrophysiology of the neurones.[44] General anaesthesia implies reversible loss of consciousness and this can be produced by either

REFERENCES

41. Sumner E, Facer E Clin Anaesthesiol 1986; 4: 577–600
42. Knight R F Clin Anaesthesiol 1986; 4: 509–526
43. Wilson M E In: Atkinson R S, Adams A P (eds) Recent Advances in Anaesthesia and Analgesia, vol 15. Churchill Livingstone, Edinburgh 1985
44. Wardley-Smith B, Halsey M J In: Kaufman L (ed) Anaesthesia Review, vol 2. Churchill Livingstone, Edinburgh 1984

intravenous or inhalational agents. The commonest techniques utilize both routes—an intravenous induction and maintenance with a gas or volatile agent. Variations upon the theme are common and, for example in paediatrics, many anaesthetists favour inhalational induction instead of injection, thereby avoiding the use of needles in young children.

Maintenance of anaesthesia just using an inhalational agent is certainly the simplest technique for maintaining unconsciousness but this cannot be relied upon to produce analgesia or muscle relaxation unless very deep planes of anaesthesia are approached. Rather than using a single agent for all purposes the concept of balanced anaesthesia has been developed which utilizes intravenous injections of specific muscle relaxants and analgesic drugs in addition to the inhaled anaesthetic. The amount of each drug needed is thereby reduced by using combinations. Mechanical ventilation becomes necessary once muscle relaxants or potent respiratory-depressant opioids are used.

Inhalational anaesthetic agents

Nitrous oxide was first prepared by Priestley in 1772 and its anaesthetic properties were first demonstrated by Sir Humphrey Davy in 1800, but some 60 years elapsed before the gas gained widespread clinical acceptance. Although some authorities have voiced serious misgivings about the toxicity and safety of nitrous oxide, the gas is the foundation of virtually every general anaesthetic administered in the UK.[45] Nitrous oxide is a relatively potent analgesic but a weak anaesthetic so that if used with oxygen the risk of awareness by the patient exists during the operation.

The analgesic action of nitrous oxide may be used to good effect to manage acute pain with a 50:50 mixture of oxygen and nitrous oxide; this mixture is widely used in obstetrics. A rapidly reversible inhalational analgesic is an attractive proposition in intensive care, but long-term administration of nitrous oxide interferes with folate metabolism and produces bone marrow depression. Surgeons become aware of nitrous oxide during anaesthesia when the gas diffuses into various closed body cavities and causes an increase in pressure or volume; for example, the bowel may become distended by the gas, the pressure of a pneumothorax may be increased or a tympanoplasty may be disrupted.

A large number of vapours have been used as anaesthetic agents but some, such as chloroform and methoxyflurane, have proved too toxic to remain in use. Others such as diethyl ether are rarely used in the UK now despite widespread safe usage in developing countries. Other agents such as trichloroethylene have disappeared in the face of competition from halothane and the other more recent additions to the volatile anaesthetic library.[46,47]

Halothane was first used clinically in 1956 in Manchester.[48] It is a potent halogenated hydrocarbon volatile anaesthetic vapour, but a poor analgesic. Two other halogenated methyl ethyl ethers, enflurane and isoflurane, currently enjoy widespread popularity, while two newer agents, desflurane and sevoflurane, are becoming more widely available. All five of these agents cause respiratory depression to some degree. Halothane is an effective bronchodilator and produces marked cardiovascular effects. It is a direct myocardial depressant and causes peripheral vasodilatation, depression of the vasomotor centre and sympathetic ganglion blockade; it also predisposes to cardiac arrhythmias, especially when exogenous catecholamines (e.g. adrenaline) are used. Enflurane, isoflurane, desflurane and sevoflurane have less depressant action on the myocardium but all produce reversible falls in arterial pressure. Arrhythmias are uncommon with all of them, but if adrenaline is infiltrated at the site of operation the total dose should not exceed 4 μg/kg. All five agents produce rises in cerebral blood flow and intracranial pressure although isoflurane, desflurane and sevoflurane are the least problematic. Enflurane may produce epileptiform changes in the electroencephalogram and is contraindicated when patients have epilepsy.

The renal blood flow and glomerular filtration rate are reduced, as is hepatic blood flow. Halothane and perhaps enflurane can cause jaundice in some patients. This is a hepatocellular jaundice which is thought to be caused by an immune reaction involving hypersensitivity to biotransformation metabolites. This appears to be most likely following repeat administration in obese middle-aged women.[25]

Halothane may occasionally cause malignant hyperpyrexia.[49]

Intravenous agents

Inhalational anaesthetics are potent drugs which are fairly quickly reversible but they do require complex vaporizers, for safe administration and they cause theatre pollution unless adequate scavenging is installed. Intravenous drugs can be easily administered and do not cause pollution but often their effects are less readily reversed. Thiopentone, introduced in 1934, is still the yardstick by which other induction agents are measured. An ultrashort-acting barbiturate, it causes rapid depression of the cerebral cortex and reticular activating system before its sedative action is terminated by redistribution of the drug away from the brain. Ultimately the drug is metabolized, principally by the liver, but this is a much slower process and is not responsible for the brevity of its initial action.

As well as depressing cerebration, thiopentone also depresses respiration and the circulation. Myocardial contractility is reduced and cardiac output falls, whilst pooling of blood occurs in the dilated systemic capacitance vessels, thereby limiting venous return. The normal individual can usually compensate but patients with cardiac disease, hypertension or untreated hypovolaemia may suffer disastrous falls in blood pressure. Thiopentone is a very potent drug and must be used with great caution.[50]

Thiopentone also suffers from other shortcomings. It is not analgesic; extravascular or inadvertent intra-arterial injection can cause tissue necrosis; thrombophlebitis may occur; metabolites

REFERENCES

45. Nunn J F Br J Anaesth 1987; 59: 3–13
46. White D C In: Kaufman L (ed) Anaesthesia Review, vol 3. Churchill Livingstone, Edinburgh 1985
47. Cashman J N Recent Advances in Anaesthesia 1994; 18: 21–38
48. Johnstone M Br J Anaesthesia 1956; 28: 392
49. Ellis F R, Heffron J J A In: Atkinson R S, Adairns A P (eds) Recent Advances in Anaesthesia and Analgesia, vol 15. Churchill Livingstone, Edinburgh 1985 p 173
50. Sear J W Br J Anaesth 1987; 59: 24–45

may cause prolonged cerebral effects and rare but serious anaphylactic reactions can occur. Thiopentone is contraindicated in patients with porphyria. It must be used with extreme care in patients with cardiac or respiratory disease and in very ill or debilitated patients.

Methohexitone is another barbiturate; some anaesthetists prefer it to thiopentone because its more rapid total body plasma clearance may result in speedier recovery.

Etomidate is a carboxylated imidazole and has the advantage of great cardiovascular stability and freedom from histamine release on induction. This is unlike most other intravenous induction agents, so it may be selected in shocked patients or in those with proven drug hypersensitivity or asthma.

Ketamine is a phencyclidine derivative which possesses unique properties as an induction agent. It is a useful analgesic, causes a rise in blood pressure and does not depress respiration. Administration may be by either intravenous or intramuscular injection and it may be used as the sole agent for a minor operation, especially in children. Ketamine is an excellent emergency drug for use in the rescue and treatment of injured patients a long way from hospital.[51] Emergence hallucinations limit the usefulness of the drug as a routine induction agent in adults.

Propofol is the most recent intravenous induction agent to be introduced into anaesthetic practice. Recovery is very rapid, although after a couple of hours this is indistinguishable from thiopentone. Pain on injection and respiratory depression have been reported but the drug is currently very popular, especially for outpatient anaesthesia.

Other drugs given for intravenous induction include the benzodiazepines and droperidol. Midazolam has been used by itself for induction in cardiovascular surgery and in the elderly. The antegrade amnesia and anxiolytic effect of the benzodiazepines can be very useful but prolonged drowsiness and weakness can be a disadvantage. Droperidol, a butyrophenone related to the major tranquillizer haloperidol, produces neurolepsis and can be used with an opioid analgesic to supplement general anaesthesia or very frequently in small doses (e.g. 1.0 mg) solely for its prolonged anti-emetic effect.

Other drugs that can be given at induction include the muscle relaxants and analgesics.

Muscle relaxants

Although Sir Walter Raleigh wrote about South American arrow poison in 1596, the naturally occurring substance curare was not introduced into clinical practice until 1942. Tubocurarine is a non-depolarizing competitive neuromuscular blocker which is now rarely used since, at least eight other major muscle relaxants have been introduced into clinical service since 1942. These include pancuronium, atracurium and vecuronium, which are most commonly used at the present time, as well as mivacurium and rocuronium.

During this time only one depolarizing blocker, suxamethonium, has enjoyed wide usage. Suxamethonium has a rapid onset and brief duration of action; the non-depolarizing relaxants have a variable speed of onset and a much longer duration of action. Artificial ventilation becomes essential to maintain adequate pulmonary gas exchange whenever a neuromuscular blocking agent is administered. This may be accomplished by a mask for a short period, but ultimately in most cases by passage of an endotracheal tube.

The action of suxamethonium terminates spontaneously but the non-depolarizing blockers require reversal with an anticholinesterase such as neostigmine. Atracurium and mivacurium are exceptions, as the former undergoes Hoffman degradation and non-specific ester hydrolysis and the latter is hydrolysed by plasma cholinesterase, so that the action of these drugs terminates without reversal by neostigmine. Atracurium is probably the agent of choice in chronic renal failure although vecuronium is safe as well.

Prolonged apnoea may follow the use of either group of agents. Absence or deficiency of plasma cholinesterase produces prolonged apnoea following suxamethonium. Adequate ventilation must be maintained until full neuromuscular function returns, which may take several hours. The patient and near relatives should be screened for the presence of abnormal plasma cholinesterase and issued with warning bracelets if this condition is diagnosed.

The duration of a non-depolarizing block may be influenced by a number of factors. These include abnormalities such as myasthenia gravis, collagen disease, renal failure, hypokalaemia, hypothermia and acidosis. Drug interactions may occur with substances such as the aminoglycoside antibiotics, antidysrhythmic agents, benzodiazepines and lithium and magnesium.[52]

The non-depolarizing relaxants have variable cardiovascular effects and this may influence the choice of agent. Curare is a ganglion blocker and commonly causes hypotension, whereas vecuronium, pancuronium, mivacurium and rocuronium all have minimal cardiovascular effects. Atracurium and curare can both cause histamine release.

Suxamethonium, although widely used, is a far from perfect drug yet it is the only agent that produces rapid, certain, brief paralysis. Amongst its many disadvantages are muscle pains, hyperkalaemia, raised intraocular pressure, potential malignant hyperpyrexia and true anaphylactic reactions.

Neostigmine is a cholinesterase inhibitor which produces an increase of acetylcholine at the neuromuscular junction and thus overcomes the competitive blockade of the non-depolarizing blockers, but acetylcholine accumulates at other receptors as well and dangerous bradycardia can result unless an anticholinergic such as atropine or glycopyrrolate is administered at the same time. There is some evidence that neostigmine administration may predispose to disruption of bowel anastomoses.[53]

Analgesics

The induction agents, inhalational agents and neuromuscular blockers produce unconsciousness and paralysis but do not suppress nociceptive input so that the patient still exhibits reflex

REFERENCES

51. Stoddart J C Trauma and the Anaesthetist. Baillière Tindall, London 1984
52. Hunter J M Br J Anaesth 1987; 59: 46–60
53. Kaufman L In: Kaufman L (ed) Anaesthesia Review, vol 1. Churchill Livingstone, Edinburgh 1982

autonomic and somatic responses to a surgical stimulus. The latter responses are not synonymous with the patient being 'awake'!

The analgesic effect of an opioid administered as a premedication hopefully extends into the operative period, but where no opioid premedication has been given, or when major surgery is planned, intravenous injection of an opioid usually accompanies induction.

The drugs used vary from morphine, and pethidine, which have a relatively prolonged action, to the short-acting opioids primarily designed for perioperative use such as fentanyl, alfentanil, phenoperidine, sufentanyl and more recently remifentanyl. Whichever opioid is chosen, the major side-effect remains respiratory depression. These drugs also contribute to postoperative nausea and vomiting and inhibit gastrointestinal peristalsis. In very high doses (e.g. 25 μg/kg) fentanyl attenuates the endocrine metabolic response to surgery.[54]

Naloxone is a specific opioid antagonist and reverses opioid-induced respiratory depression but it is important to realize that the half-life of the drug is relatively short and respiratory depression may reappear if only a single bolus is given. An initial dose of 0.1–0.4 mg should be given intravenously with great care as administration of naloxone has occasionally been associated with sudden cardiovascular collapse.

Controlled hypotension

Deliberate hypotension can be used to reduce blood loss during surgery.[55] The blood pressure can be lowered by specific agents such as the direct-acting vasodilators (e.g. sodium nitroprusside). Hypotension is also a frequent side-effect of many anaesthetic techniques; as long as control is retained, this can be used to surgical advantage. Spinal and epidural blocks may be associated with reduced peroperative blood loss. Halothane, enflurane, isoflurane, desflurane, and sevoflurane are all capable of producing marked hypotension when used alone, but they are frequently used in lower concentrations in a balanced technique. Intermittent positive pressure ventilation with a muscle relaxant such as curare can produce pronounced hypotension. A further reduction in bleeding may be achieved by judicious use of posture, particularly in head and neck operations. The judicious use of β-blockers or the combined α- and β-blocker labetalol may also aid smooth control of blood pressure.[56,57] These techniques are potentially lethal when applied without thought. Cerebral and myocardial ischaemia are the main consequences of poor technique. Deliberate hypotension should only be employed when the indications are clear-cut and both surgeon and anaesthetist are familiar with the technique. Accurate continuous monitoring of blood pressure and tissue oxygenation must be available. Indications for controlled hypotension include the following: neurosurgery, microsurgery, plastic surgery, operations where massive haemorrhage is anticipated and when blood transfusion is unavailable or unacceptable (e.g. Jehovah's Witness).

Contraindications include hypovolaemia, coronary artery disease, cardiac failure, uncontrolled hypertension, cerebrovascular disease, pregnancy and old age. Problems may arise if organ perfusion is already compromised by obstructive arterial disease. Autoregulation of cerebral blood flow may be disturbed. Head-up posture during extreme hypotension may be disastrous. Rebound hypertension following cessation of the procedure has to be countered.[55]

The same drugs and techniques used in controlled hypotension may be used to control swings in blood pressure in phaeochromocytoma and cardiac surgery and in the recovery room.

Day-case surgery

The expansion of day-case surgery is creating new problems for anaesthetic services.[41] Areas of concern include the preoperative assessment of the patients and the selection of anaesthetic techniques that allow optimal short- and long-term recovery. Regional anaesthetic techniques can be very useful in outpatient surgery.

As much preoperative assessment as possible should be performed before the day of surgery. Rigorous criteria must be used to exclude patients with potentially hazardous medical conditions.[58] Modern general anaesthetic agents can provide remarkably quick recovery times but patients must be escorted home and warned to rest and avoid driving for 24 h.

COMPLICATIONS OF ANAESTHESIA

Intraoperative problems

The provision of adequate anaesthesia, analgesia and cerebral oxygenation are the primary peroperative objectives.

Depth of anaesthesia

Awareness during anaesthesia occurs most commonly during techniques which use muscle relaxants and mechanical ventilation when insufficient supplementary agent is administered to ensure the patient is unconscious as well as paralysed.[59] Nitrous oxide alone is not a reliable anaesthetic. The problem is most common in obstetric and emergency surgery. Light anaesthesia can be avoided by carefully monitoring the vital signs especially heart rate, blood pressure and pupil size and by judicious use of supplementary drugs such as the inhalational agents. The possibility of awareness and the implications of possible subliminal acoustic input during anaesthesia mean that all theatre staff should avoid any personal comments about the patient. Regional anaesthetic techniques may occasionally fail to produce a totally effective block; further local infiltration or light general anaesthesia may be a necessary supplement.

REFERENCES

54. Kehlet H In: Cousins M J, Phillips G D (eds) Acute Pain Management. Churchill Livingstone, London 1986
55. Enderby G E H (ed) Hypotensive Anaesthesia. Churchill Livingstone, Edinburgh 1985
56. Utting J E Br J Anaesth 1987; 59: 877–890
57. McDowall D G Br J Anaesth 1985; 57: 110–119
58. Cooper G In: Taylor T H, Major E (eds) Hazards and Complications of Anaesthesia. Churchill Livingstone, Edinburgh 1987 p 401
59. Aitkenhead A R In: Taylor T H, Major E (eds) Hazards and Complications of Anaesthesia. Churchill Livingstone, Edinburgh 1987 p 280

Oxygenation

Adequate pulmonary gas exchange may fail because of airway obstruction, respiratory failure or failure of the equipment.

Obstruction can occur at any level of the respiratory pathway or externally in the anaesthetic circuit. Upper airway obstruction can usually be overcome with an oro- or nasopharyngeal airway. Obstruction at the glottis by, for example, a foreign body, vomiting, oedema or laryngeal spasm can be much more serious. Laryngeal spasm may be precipitated by painful surgical stimuli, especially during perineal operations, and a dangerous situation can evolve very rapidly unless the airway can be re-established. The coughing and exaggerated respiratory effort which accompanies laryngeal spasm is likely to precipitate regurgitation and if the patient remains in the lithotomy position serious pulmonary aspiration may occur. The surgeon should be prepared to lower the patient's legs and help turn him or her into a lateral position.

Emergency tracheostomy is rarely required but midline cricothyroid puncture with a large intravenous cannula has been suggested as a first aid measure in extreme cases. Acute epiglottitis is a medical emergency and a surgeon must be present in case intubation fails and tracheostomy is urgently required.

Difficulty with intubation is encountered for many reasons which range from anaesthetist inexperience to anatomical abnormalities of the patient. Danger for the patient arises not through the failure of the anaesthetist to succeed in intubation but only if the anaesthetist fails to provide adequate oxygenation during the period in which intubation is being attempted. The same rules apply at a cardiac arrest where the need to intubate is often given preference over the absolutely vital provision of oxygen, which can be easily achieved with a mask in most cases.

Inadvertent oesophageal intubation, particularly following difficulty in visualizing the larynx, is an unfortunately common cause of serious anaesthetic accidents. If any doubt exists about the position of the tube in a cyanosed patient the anaesthetist must remove the tube and provide oxygen by mask as the first step. Further management can then be assessed in a live patient! Vital factors in the management of the difficult airway or failure to intubate are the availability of experienced help for the anaesthetist and of access to a range of special equipment such as fibreoptic laryngoscopes and nasal tracheal tubes.

Table 5.3 Summary of the standards of monitoring: Association of Anaesthetists of Great Britain and Ireland

1. Anaesthetist should be continuously present and make an adequate record.
2. Monitoring should start before induction and continue until recovery is complete.
3. The anaesthetic machine should be monitored by an oxygen analyser with alarms and a disconnection alarm.
4. Continuous monitoring of ventilation and circulation is essential. This should be by clinical observation supplemented by monitoring devices.
5. Frequency of blood pressure and pulse rate measurements should be appropriate to the state of the patient.
6. A peripheral nerve stimulator should be available when muscle relaxants are employed.
7. Long and complicated operations and sick patients may require additional monitoring.
8. Adequate monitoring is required during brief operations, and during procedures under local anaesthetic and sedation.
9. Appropriate monitoring should be used during transport of a patient.
10. Adequate instruction concerning monitoring should be given to the recovery ward staff, and appropriate monitors should be available.

Bronchospasm, either in a known asthmatic or in response to drugs or airway manipulation, can be very serious and requires rapid intervention. The diagnosis of bronchospasm should only be made after the anaesthetist has confirmed that the anaesthetic circuit and the airway are patent and that the tracheal tube is not in the oesophagus. An incorrect diagnosis in these circumstances has been fatal.

Peroperative respiratory failure is usually caused by drugs such as the barbiturates or opioids. Assisted ventilation is essential until the effect has waned or has been reversed. Sudden peroperative respiratory failure may indicate the presence of a pneumothorax. Any surgery near the pleura requires vigilance for this possibility and a chest drain inserted should a pneumothorax develop.

Cardiac problems

Arrhythmias usually result from the anaesthetic agents or pre-existing cardiac disease but are often linked to a surgical stimulus in a lightly anaesthetized patient.

Hypotension may be caused by a primary cardiac problem, by a drug response or by hypovolaemia. Hypertension may be caused by a surgical stimulus, inadequate ventilation, the release of pathological vasoactive substances or may be the result of pre-existing hypertension.

Cardiac arrest during anaesthesia may occur as a result of pre-existing myocardial disease, respiratory failure, a drug effect or from hypovolaemia. The arrest is usually preceded by an arrhythmia or severe hypotension. Despite the advanced equipment available in the operating theatre, the standard resuscitation principles still apply under these circumstances and failure to institute them prejudices the outcome. To the basic tenet of airway, breathing and circulation (ABC) might be added *communication* between anaesthetist and surgeon. External cardiac massage should be performed while the patient is ventilated with pure oxygen whilst other management strategies are being considered.

Monitoring

A whole new range of sophisticated non-invasive monitors can provide a wealth of information during operations. Pulse oximetry provides evidence of inadequate tissue oxygenation. Oximetry monitoring can be extended into the postoperative period when patients are often at greatest risk.

Intensive perioperative monitoring has been popular for many years in the USA and it is now becoming justifiably popular throughout the world. Minimal standards have now been defined for differing types of surgery and these recommendations carry considerable medicolegal importance (Table 5.3).[60,61]

REFERENCES

60. Hanning C D Br J Anaesth 1987; 59: 1201
61. Association of Anaesthetists of Great Britain and Ireland. Recommendations for the Standard of Monitoring During Anaesthesia and Recovery, London 1988

Blood loss

Increased bleeding during an operation may be from surgical, anaesthetic or other causes. The anaesthetic causes are usually related to respiratory obstruction or hypoventilation producing hypercapnia, anything which raises the intrathoracic pressure and increases of venous pressure. Hypertension and tachycardia can also increase the risk of haemorrhage.

Posture or an overloaded or inefficient circulation can increase venous pressure. A hyperdynamic circulation also increases bleeding, as does any systemic disease that interferes with coagulation. This includes haemophilia, liver failure, disseminated intravascular coagulation, massive or incompatible blood transfusion, concurrent anticoagulant or aspirin therapy.

Hiccup

Hiccup may occur intraoperatively following stimulation of sensory nerves in the phrenic or vagal territories. Control is sometimes difficult but often deepening the anaesthesia or giving a large dose of muscle relaxant will solve the problem.

Hypothermia

Temperature control is often neglected as the patient lies semi-naked, paralysed, in a cool environment, with the intestine exposed and with cool dry gases being used for ventilation. Precautions against hypothermia should be routine; these include a warming mattress, convective warm-air devices, a blood warmer and humidification of gases.[62] Hypothermia is most likely in infants and the elderly, and the risk continues into the postoperative period. Hypothermia impairs the normal function of a number of different organs.

Malignant hyperpyrexia

This is an autosomal dominant inherited condition which produces cyanosis, rash, muscle rigidity, hypercapnia, arrhythmia and eventually hyperpyrexia leading to cardiac arrest.[63] Drugs which can trigger malignant hyperpyrexia include all the inhalational anaesthetic agents, suxamethonium, tubocurarine and gallamine as well as the amide local anaesthetics. A number of surgical conditions are associated with a higher incidence of the syndrome and these include strabismus, ptosis, hernia, kyphoscoliosis and cleft palate.[49] Immediate treatment should include withdrawal of anaesthetic agents, administration of 100% oxygen, cooling, acid–base control, infusion of glucose and insulin, and intravenous injection of dantrolene which is a direct acting muscle relaxant that acts directly on muscle metabolism.[64]

Sweating

Sweating peroperatively can merely be a manifestation of high anxiety or inadequate anaesthesia, or it may reflect a high ambient temperature or overheated patient, hypercapnia or shock.

Position of patient

Other sequelae of anaesthesia result from damage inflicted during anaesthesia, or from prolonged pressure on vulnerable sites such as nerves and eyes. The position of the patient may expose unprotected sites to damage, but more importantly it can affect cardiorespiratory performance. The Trendelenburg and prone positions can seriously impair respiration, especially in the obese. The head-up position, particularly the sitting posture, may predispose to air embolism and elevation of the head is also dangerous if controlled hypotension is being used.

Contrary to the still widely held belief, the head-down position may be positively harmful in shock states when it can further reduce arterial pressure and cerebral blood flow and increase the risk of cerebral oedema. In these cases elevation of the legs is all that is required.

Drug interactions

The polypharmacy of many present-day anaesthetics is far removed from the simplicity of an open ether anaesthetic and there is great potential for significant drug inter-action.[65] The interaction may affect the pharmacokinetics (uptake, distribution, metabolism and elimination) or the pharmacodynamics (tissue and organ response) of the drugs. Anaesthetic drugs may interact even before administration (suxamethonium and thiopentone should not be mixed together) or after administration (halothane will potentiate the hypotensive effect of curare). Adrenaline, administered peroperatively by the surgeon as a vasoconstrictor, will potentiate the arrhythmic effect of halothane. Anaesthetic agents may also interact with drugs acting on the cardiovascular, autonomic and central nervous systems.

Adverse drug reactions

Drugs used in anaesthesia are usually very potent and often possess very narrow safety margins. Administration of an overdose is the most frequent cause of problems but even in normal dosage unwanted pharmacological effects may occur. For example, thiopentone almost invariably causes hypotension and respiratory depression; the opioids produce respiratory depression and also nausea and vomiting. Following overdose these unwanted effects predominate. Sometimes adverse effects follow administration of an inappropriate drug to specifically susceptible individuals such as those suffering from, or prone to, porphyria, malignant hyperpyrexia, plasma deficiency and glucose-6-phosphate dehydrogenase deficiency. Adverse drug reactions may occur when the agent is administered into the wrong place. Extravascular injection of thiopentone can cause local tissue damage; inadvertent

REFERENCES

62. Holdcroft A Body Temperature Control. Baillière Tindall, London 1980 p 120
63. Allan G C Current Opinion in Anaesthesiology 1996; 9(3): 271
64. Kolb M E et al Anesthesiology 1982; 56: 254–262
65. Halsey M J Br J Anaesth 1987; 59: 112–123

intravascular injection of local anaesthetics can produce serious cerebral or cardiovascular toxicity.

Immunologically mediated reactions can also occur, on the first exposure to the drug or as a hypersensitivity reaction following re-exposure.[66] Classical anaphylactic reactions manifesting as hypotension and bronchospasm may occur as a response to the drug or the carrier solvent. Anaesthetists should be alert to the possibility of this in an individual who suffers from atopy or has shown adverse reaction on previous exposure.[67,68] Established guidelines for the management of anaphylaxis occurring under anaesthesia have been published.[69] The unexplained jaundice which may follow halothane anaesthesia is thought to have an immunological basis.

Postoperative problems

Delayed recovery

A distinction should be made between depression produced by centrally acting drugs and muscle weakness produced by prolonged neuromuscular blockade. In more cases cerebral hypoxia or hypoperfusion may have occurred; this can only be assessed when the patient is fully recovered. Known or unsuspected diseases such as diabetes or hypothyroidism can also cause prolonged unconsciousness.

Respiratory complications

Upper airway obstruction is the most common postoperative problem yet it should be easily prevented and is generally easily treated. In simple terms, noisy breathing is obstructed breathing and it usually only requires chin-lift and jaw-thrust or an oropharyngeal airway to eliminate the problem. More difficult to manage are causes such as laryngeal spasm, laryngeal oedema, tracheomalacia or recurrent laryngeal nerve paresis.[70] Retained throat packs represent a readily avoidable cause of obstruction. Compression of the trachea by a haematoma developing after thyroid, carotid or cervical spine surgery is normally treated by evacuation of the clot but intubation is often also necessary to bypass the attendant laryngeal oedema.

Delayed recovery from anaesthesia can also contribute to postoperative respiratory difficulty and this can be exaggerated in the face of pre-existing neuromuscular disease or electrolyte abnormalities. Incomplete reversal of muscle relaxant should be diagnosed by the anaesthetist with a peripheral nerve stimulator who reveals an absent or reduced twitch response.

Continuing postoperative respiratory failure can occur because of more specific cardiorespiratory abnormalities; these include all the causes of the adult respiratory distress syndrome and pulmonary oedema.[71] The most common causes of this syndrome include aspiration of gastric contents, pneumonia and the combination of trauma, blood loss, hypotension and massive transfusion. Emboli, whether air, amniotic fluid, fat, thrombotic or from stored blood microaggregates, can produce respiratory embarrassment of wide-ranging severity.

Pain, abdominal distension, inability to cough and persistent drowsiness can lead to inefficient ventilation, sputum retention and atelectasis. Early postoperative hypoxaemia is most common in the obese, the elderly, smokers and those with pre-existing cardiorespiratory disease. Oxygen therapy, using a mask, is provided for the majority of patients in the initial recovery period. This is meant to provide a safety cushion against the effects of postoperative hypoxaemia. When respiratory failure occurs or threatens then mechanical ventilation via a tracheal tube is indicated whilst the cause of the failure is treated. Respiratory depression is usually indicated by a reduction in rate, tidal volume and PaO_2, and an increase in $PaCO_2$. Early intervention is indicated in such cases, rather than waiting until respiratory or cardiac arrest is imminent. Proper recovery facilities with constant nursing surveillance are essential to allow early detection of incipient respiratory failure. Mechanical ventilation can be accomplished in the recovery ward for short periods using simple ventilators, but if long-term ventilation becomes necessary or major complications have occurred then transfer to a properly equipped intensive care or high-dependency unit is indicated.

Cardiovascular complications

Postoperative hypertension is usually the result of unrelieved pain, pre-existing hypertension, or hypoventilation. Hypotension occurs most commonly because of hypovolaemia as a consequence of either inadequate blood or fluid replacement in the face of continued blood loss. It may also be caused by drugs and in some cases by hypoadrenalism. Arrhythmias may occur in a patient with existing cardiac disease, or as the result of electrolyte abnormalities, and these may also result in hypotension.

Vascular complications

The vascular complications which may develop after operation include phlebitis, thrombosis and infection related to intravascular lines. Vigorous antibiotic therapy may be necessary after removal of the offending intravenous cannula but prevention by strict attention to asepsis should be the aim in every patient. Venous emboli can occur and arterial lines create the additional problem of arterial damage and distal emboli.

Renal dysfunction

Anaesthesia produces a reduction in urine volume and solute excretion but more major changes result from the stress of surgery.

REFERENCES

66. Watkins J Br J Anaesth 1987; 59: 104–111
67. Clarke R S J, Fee J H, Dundee J W In: Watkins J, Ward A M (eds) Adverse Responses to Intravenous Drugs. Academic Press, London 1978 p 41
68. Simpson P J In: Kaufman L (ed) Anaesthesia Review, vol 5. Churchill Livingstone, Edinburgh 1988
69. Association of Anaesthetists. Anaphylactic Reactions Associated with Anaesthesia, London 1990.
70. Marshall A In: Taylor T H, Major E (eds) Hazards and Complications of Anaesthesia. Churchill Livingstone, Edinburgh 1987 p 15
71. Barrowcliffe M, Jones J G In: Kaufman L (ed) Anaesthesia Review, vol 5. Churchill Livingstone, Edinburgh 1988 p 182

The aetiology of these changes is multifactorial. The preoperative patient is anxious and starved, so has enhanced production of antidiuretic hormone and sympathetic stimulation.[72] Anaesthetic agents reduce renal blood flow and glomerular filtration rate, and intermittent positive pressure ventilation, hypotension, hypoxia and hypocapnia also adversely affect renal function. The preservation of adequate renal function peroperatively depends on the maintenance of normovolaemia, the avoidance of hypotension and if necessary by fluid loading, low-dose dopamine infusion, use of loop diuretics or intravenous mannitol. Jaundice, sepsis and major muscle trauma (rhabdomyolysis) also contribute to postoperative renal failure and in these patients it is particularly important to maintain renal function. Intravenous mannitol, for example, can be given to jaundiced patients preoperatively.

Hepatic dysfunction

Although rather unfortunately labelled as 'halothane hepatitis', postoperative jaundice has been reported following the use of virtually all agents and techniques. Following major surgery some 70% of patients develop liver function abnormalities although in the majority this is only a mild transient disturbance. The most common changes may reflect a preoperative reduction in hepatic blood flow in combination with transient hypoxia or hypotension. Haemolysis of transfused blood can result in an increased bilirubin load.

Slightly more severe changes in liver function might suggest a direct drug effect, and very high levels would point to cholelithiasis or malignant obstruction. The problem of halothane jaundice is mentioned briefly elsewhere.

Immunological sequelae

Postoperative liver damage may have an immunological basis and, not surprisingly, anaesthesia can have other wide-ranging immunological effects.[68] This has implications for the surgeon because marked changes can occur in non-specific immune mechanisms and in cellular responses to infection and malignancy.

Other problems

Other problems which may hinder postoperative recovery include nausea and vomiting,[73] hypothermia, shivering, sore throat and the discomfort of various indwelling tubes such as a urinary catheter and nasogastric tubes.

REGIONAL ANAESTHESIA

The techniques and drugs used in regional anaesthesia have been refined and now offer an attractive alternative to general anaesthesia in many instances.[74] It is often illogical to anaesthetize the whole body and brain to perform an operation on a single limb. Local anaesthetic techniques avoid the risks and problems of general anaesthesia and many of the undesirable postoperative consequences. The airway remains unthreatened and cardiorespiratory depression is avoided. The regional block can provide profound analgesia and muscle relaxation in the operative field and this analgesia usually extends into the postoperative period. Regional techniques provide the best single method of protection from the stress response to surgery.[54]

There are, however, disadvantages of regional anaesthesia. The local anaesthetic drugs can cause serious toxic reactions if dose schedules are ignored or the drug is administered into the wrong place, especially if an inadvertent intravascular injection is given. Hypotension is a frequent accompaniment of epidural and spinal blocks and inadvertent intrathecal injection during an epidural block may result in a very high spinal block with serious cardiorespiratory embarrassment. Peripheral nerve or plexus blocks may be associated with damage to the nerves themselves, or to adjacent structures such as the pleura. It may be worrying for the patient if numbness and muscle weakness are prolonged into the postoperative period.

The performance of regional blocks may be more time-consuming than general anaesthesia and operating lists have to be arranged accordingly. Even in the most expert hands some blocks result in incomplete analgesia and single-bolus techniques run the risk of becoming ineffective before the operation has been completed. Catheter techniques can usually avoid this problem. The preservation of consciousness during the operation, a potentially attractive feature to some, is unacceptable to many other patients so some sort of sedation, or even very light general anaesthesia, is often necessary.

The factors that govern the selection of regional anaesthesia include all those that influence the choice of the general anaesthetic technique. The patient's condition may strongly favour a regional technique. For example, this may simplify control of a diabetic having surgery, or it may offer a safe form of postoperative analgesia for a patient with chronic respiratory disease.

Other factors are very specific contraindications to regional anaesthesia and these include refusal of consent by the patient, local sepsis at the site of a proposed block, anticoagulant therapy or a coagulation defect and some cases of peripheral neurological disease. In contrast patients who have had a bad experience from general anaesthesia or those who have sensitivity to anaesthetic drugs often readily accept regional anaesthesia.

The performance of regional blocks requires considerable skill and experience and these techniques should not be regarded as anaesthetic short-cuts. The blocks must be performed using a good aseptic technique and with drugs and equipment for resuscitation immediately available. Deaths have been caused by attempts at regional anaesthesia performed by untrained doctors in inappropriate circumstances.[75]

Local anaesthetic drugs

These belong to two groups, either esters (procaine) or amides (lignocaine, bupivacaine). These agents produce temporary

REFERENCES

72. Beven D R Renal Function in Anaesthesia and Surgery. Academic Press, London 1979
73. Editorial Lancet 1989; i: 651
74. Wildsmith J A W, Armitage E N (eds) Principles and Practice of Regional Anaesthesia. Churchill Livingstone, Edinburgh 1987
75. Reynolds F Anaesthesia 1984; 39: 105

blockade of neural transmission by impeding the passage of sodium ions through the axon membrane sodium channels during depolarization.[76]

Regional anaesthetic techniques

Local infiltration is the simplest and most widely used technique and allows performance of major operations like emergency caesarean section.[77] Blockade of single or multiple nerves can produce a wide field of analgesia anywhere from the scalp to the toes. For example, ilioinguinal and genitofemoral nerve blocks can be used for inguinal herniorrhaphy (Fig. 5.1; see Chapter 26).[78] Brachial plexus blocks are very useful for upper limb surgery (Fig. 5.2; see Chapter 43). A number of approaches to the brachial plexus have been described and the selection of technique is governed by the proposed site of operation as different approaches tend to block different parts of the plexus.[79] Intravenous regional anaesthesia (so-called Bier's block) can produce excellent operating conditions in a limb but serious local anaesthetic toxicity can follow premature tourniquet deflation. Preservative-free prilocaine is the agent of choice and bupivacaine should never be used for this technique because it is highly cardiotoxic.[71]

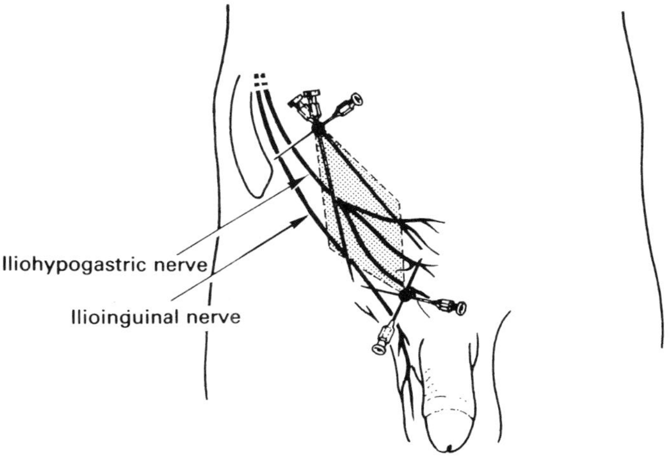

Fig 5.1 Technique for local anaesthesia in inguinal hernia repair.

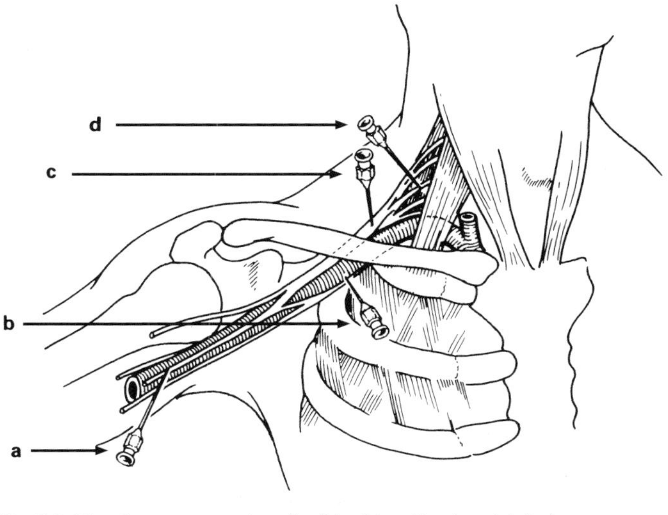

Fig 5.2 The four approaches for blocking the brachial plexus. (**a**) Axillary; (**b**) infraclavicular; (**c**) supraclavicular; (**d**) interscalene.

Epidural and spinal injections block nerve roots and usually produce a very widespread area of analgesia. The extent of the block is determined by the height to which the injected solution spreads along the spinal cord (Fig. 5.3). A block to the level of T10 is suitable for total hip replacement but an analgesic level of T5 is needed for abdominal surgery.

ANALGESIA: THE MANAGEMENT OF POSTOPERATIVE PAIN

Introduction

Pain relief following surgical interventions is sometimes inadequate, causes unnecessary suffering, and improvements in management are still required. These facts were first highlighted nearly fifty years ago.[80–83]

REFERENCES

76. Arthur G R, Wildsmith J A W, Tucker G T In: Wildsmith J A W, Armitage E N (eds) Principles and Practice of Regional Anaesthesia. Churchill Livingstone, Edinburgh 1987 p 22
77. Gordh T In: Eriksson E (ed) Illustrated Handbook in Local Anaesthesia. Lloyd Luke, London 1979
78. Littlewood D G In: Wildsmith J A W, Armitage E N (eds) Principles and Practice of Regional Anaesthesia. Churchill Livingstone, Edinburgh 1987 p 132
79. Hughes T J, Desgrand D A In: Wildsmith J A W, Armitage E N (eds) Principles and Practice of Regional Anaesthesia. Churchill Livingstone, Edinburgh 1987

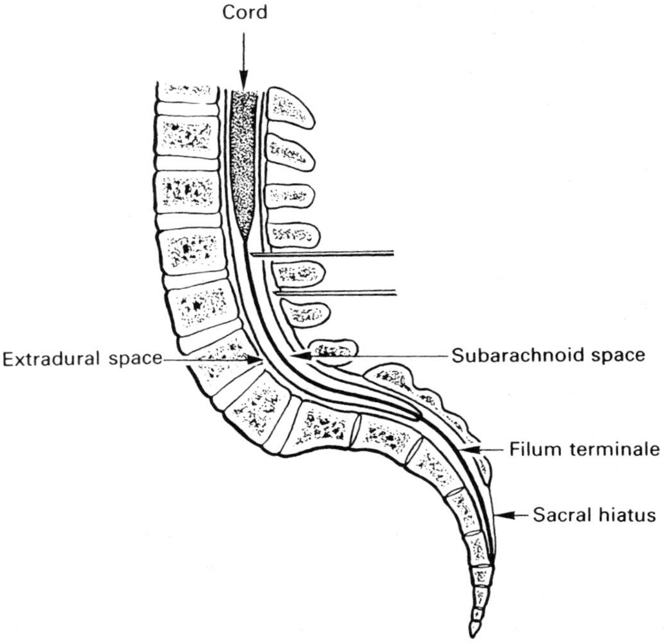

Fig 5.3 Diagrammatic representation of the lumbar and sacral regions of the spine showing needle placements in the subarachnoid and epidural space.

The reason for this state of affairs is not callous indifference on the part of clinical staff, but rather a lack of training coupled with the perpetuation of a number of widely held misconceptions about pain and pain management. These include:

a. An exaggerated fear about the side-effects of analgesic drugs.
b. The notion that postoperative pain causes only transient discomfort.
c. An idea that patients do not suffer permanent damage from poorly controlled postoperative pain.
d. A belief that good pain relief obscures clinical signs of surgical complications.
e. An assumption that the continued use of opioids will lead to addiction.
f. Erroneous methods of opioid dose prediction (often based on patients' weight or the contents of one ampoule!) and the dosing interval.
g. Intractable ward routine and dogma.

Apart from the humanitarian requirement for clinicians to provide good postoperative pain relief for the patients in their care, social pressures and consumer demand have heightened awareness of the problem. The public is becoming increasingly aware that good pain relief following surgery is possible and that severe post-operative pain is not inevitable.[84–86] An impetus to achieving better pain relief after surgery has also come from a number of official organizations and governmental bodies.[80,87–90] Effective post-operative analgesia is not, however, free from potential complications, so that any attempt to provide effective postoperative analgesia whilst ensuring patient safety will inevitably incur additional economic costs.[91]

Definition of pain

The International Association for the Study of Pain defines pain as: 'an unpleasant sensory and emotional experience associated with actual or potential tissue damage or described in terms of such damage'.[93] This definition of pain emphasizes that pain may exist where no discernible tissue damage is present. This is not to say that such pain is imaginary and any less distressing for the individual concerned, but appreciation of this fact may allow other avenues of treatment to be explored. Pain perception is a property of the sensory nervous system. It is stimulus specific and reproducible between and within individual subjects. Pain tolerance, on the other hand, is a very individual experience that varies greatly in both severity and nature between patients. It is pain tolerance that is of concern to clinicians. The pain tolerance of individual patients is affected by the interaction of a number of components. These include:

a. The site, nature and duration of surgery (probably the most important factor).[94]
b. Continued activity of the original pathology and the development of complications.
c. Other trappings of postoperative care such as nasogastric tubes, urethral catheters, intravenous cannulae, infusions, transfusions and drain sites, which may cause significant discomfort.
d. Pre-existing psychological factors such as previous painful experiences, cultural background, the nature of the clinical diagnosis and prognosis, behavioural factors (coping mechanisms), and affective responses (anxiety and depression).
e. The psychological, physiological and pharmacological preparation of the patient.
f. The quality of postoperative care.

Classification of pain

Pain can be classified as being:

(i) Nociceptive (somatic and visceral).
(ii) Neuropathic or neurogenic.[95]
(iii) Psychogenic.[96]

Nociceptive pain is normally the result of ongoing activation of physiologically normal nerve fibres and pain pathways. Pain that is variously described as neurogenic or neuropathic can be regarded as 'pathological pain' and is associated with abnormality, injury or disease in the nervous system. Neuropathic pain states include mononeuropathies (e.g. intercostal neuralgia), polyneuropathies (e.g. diabetes mellitus), deafferentation (e.g. brachial plexus avulsion, central post-stroke pain), and sympathetically maintained pain. A small group of people exist whose pain is the result of or associated with psychological factors, but this is not to say that their pain is any less real than that of a person with nociceptive pain of definable origin.

Pain may also be conveniently classified as acute and non-acute (chronic) in nature. Acute pain is almost exclusively nociceptive. Chronic pain may have nociceptive, neurogenic/neuropathic, and psychogenic components. It is acute nociceptive pain that occurs in the postoperative period, although the existence of the chronic pain state has to be borne in mind for two reasons: patients with continuing chronic pain occasionally need operations and their postoperative analgesia can pose significant problems; more

REFERENCES

80. Royal College of Surgeons and College of Anaesthetists Working Party on Pain After Surgery. Pain After Surgery. Royal College of Surgeons, London 1990
81. Owen H et al Pain 1990; 41: 303–308
82. Editorial BMJ 1978; 2: 215
83. Papper E et al Surgery 1952; 32: 107–109
84. Allis S Time International 1992; 140: 79–81
85. Clark I Lancet 1993; 341: 27
86. Rosenbaum S, Barash P Anesthesia and Analgesia 1989; 69: 555–557
87. Faculty of Anaesthetists and Royal Australasian College of Surgeons. Melbourne 1991
88. Ready L B, Edwards W T Y. Management of Acute Pain. IASP Publications, Seattle 1992
89. US Department of Health and Human Services, Agency for Health Care Policy and Research No. 92–0032. AHCPR Publications, Rockville MD 1992
90. Ready L B et al Anesthesiology 1995; 82: 1071–1081
91. Rawal N, Berggren L Pain 1994; 57: 117–123
92. Zolte N Ann R Coll Surg 1986; 68: 209–210
93. International Association for the Study of Pain Subcommittee on Taxonomy Pain 1986 (suppl 3); S217
94. Parkhouse J et al Br J Anaesth 1961; 33: 345
95. Woolfe C J Br J Anaesthesia 1989; 63: 139–146
96. Mersky H, Bogduk N Classification of Chronic Pain, 2nd edn. IASP Press, Seattle 1994

importantly, however, unrelieved nociceptive pain may give rise to a pathological, chronic pain condition.[97]

Pathophysiology of pain

A detailed description of the complex physiology and pathophysiology of acute pain is beyond the scope of this chapter so a synopsis of the important principles is provided and the reader is advised to consult specialized monographs for more information.

Surgery is responsible for local tissue damage which causes: (i) the local release of algesic (pain producing) substances (e.g. prostaglandins, histamine, serotonin, bradykinin, substance P), and (ii) the generation of noxious (nociceptive) stimuli that are transduced by nociceptors and transmitted by A-delta and C nerve fibres to the spinal cord (neuraxis). Further transmission is determined by complex modulating influences in the dorsal horn of the spinal cord. Some impulses pass to the ventral horn to provoke segmental reflex responses. Other impulses are transmitted to higher centres via the spinothalamic and spinoreticular tracts where they induce suprasegmental and cortical responses. These modulating influences at the spinal cord level were first postulated by Melzack and Wall in 1965 in their 'gate control theory of pain'.[98] Since then the immense complexities of the neurophysiology of nociception have become partially revealed. The transduction of a peripheral nociceptive stimulus into the consciously perceived experience of pain involves a very complex, plastic system which uses a large number of excitatory, facilitatory and inhibitory neurotransmitters and receptor types and subtypes. Briefly, it appears that pain impulses can: (i) alter the functional configuration of the pain-modulating systems of the dorsal horn of the spinal cord and ultimately increase the sensitivity of the components of the pain pathway to further painful stimuli (central sensitization), and (ii) bring about the release of inflammatory mediators that increase the sensitivity of peripheral nociceptors (peripheral sensitization).

The plasticity of the pain-responsive components of the nervous system may have clinical implications for the relief of postoperative pain. This is based on an as yet unproven theory that the effectiveness of the analgesia at the time of the nociceptive barrage on the nervous system (i.e. surgical trauma) may affect the subsequent intensity and duration of postoperative pain experienced by the patient.[95,99–101] This concept has been termed 'pre-emptive analgesia' or 'pain prophylaxis'. Studies have demonstrated that a decrease in the postoperative analgesia requirements may follow the use of opioid premedication, local anaesthesia of peripheral nerves, spinal and epidural blockade, and the use of non-steroidal anti-inflammatory drugs prior to surgery.[102–103] This theory is not universally accepted.[104,105]

Measurement of pain

Pain severity may be measured by subjective (patient rated) and objective (observer rated) methods.

Objective assessment of pain severity by observing a patient's behaviour and vital signs is notoriously unreliable—the observer tends to under-rate the severity of the pain. This method should not be used unless the patient is unable to communicate. A patient reporting his or her own pain is the most reliable means of measuring pain severity and its response to treatment. Unfortunately, using this method, patients tend to under-report the presence of considerable pain.[106] In adults the three most widely used measures are the visual analogue scale, the verbal numerical rating scale and the categorical rating scale.

The visual analogue scale (VAS) uses a drawn 10 cm line with end-points labelled 'no pain' (at the left-hand end) and 'worst pain imaginable' (at the right-hand end). The patient is asked to mark a point on the line that best represents his or her current pain, the distance from the 'no pain' end-point is measured and this value equals that patient's visual analogue scale score at that time. This method is not perfect in that it is more time-consuming than other methods and patients may not be able to cooperate in the immediate postoperative period. It has the advantage that the end-points can be worded in any language. Visual analogue scoring can also be used to measure other variables such as nausea and vomiting and patient satisfaction.

The verbal numerical rating scale (VNRS) is similar to the visual analogue scale. The patient is asked to imagine that '0 equals no pain' and '10 equals the worst pain imaginable', then give a number between that which represents their pain severity at that time. Problems arise where there is a language barrier or the patient has difficulty understanding the concept, but no equipment is needed.

A major problem with both these systems is defining the score at which the patient is actually 'comfortable'. There may be large inter-patient variability on this point and different patients may be 'comfortable' at higher pain scores than others. So titration of analgesia against isolated scores may be more applicable if the patient's comfort is also taken into account. It is worth noting that these two scoring systems correlate well.

A number of categorical rating scales (CRS) exist of varying complexity; all use words to rate pain severity. One which is frequently used rates the present pain as: none, mild, moderate, severe, very severe, and worst pain imaginable.

Complete relief of pain at all times is not normally possible, practical or safe. A realistic aim of treatment is for patient comfort at rest and ideally on movement and coughing. Pain should always be assessed on coughing, deep breathing, or movement (dynamic or incident pain) and not simply at rest (static pain). It should be assessed at regular intervals during the postoperative period and the frequency of these assessments should be increased if the patient's pain is poorly controlled or if further painful stimuli are anticipated. Pain scores should be measured routinely, and recorded on the 'vital signs' chart located at the end of the patient's bed.

REFERENCES

97. Cousins M Regional Anesthesia 1989; 14: 162–179
98. Melzack R, Wall P D Science 1965; 150: 971–979
99. Wall P D Pain 1988; 33: 289–290
100. McQuay H et al Anaesthesia 1990; 45: 101–102
101. Katz J et al Anesthesiology 1992; 77: 439–446
102. Tverskoy M et al Anesthesia and Analgesia 1990; 70: 29
103. Bugedo G et al Regional Anaesthesia 1990; 15: 130
104. Dierking G et al Br J Anaesth 1992; 68: 334–348
105. Dahl J et al Br J Anaesth 1992; 69: 4–8
106. Wilder-Smith C, Schuler L Pain 1992; 212: 689–691

The benefits of postoperative analgesia

Pain is associated with both a 'stress response' and a desire to avoid further pain. These may be mechanisms of survival but are themselves associated with morbidity. Pain has widespread effects, the extent of which is related to both the severity of the painful insult and the site of origin of the pain. Effective analgesia can lessen the degree of organ system dysfunction and may have a positive effect on the patient's outcome.

Respiratory effects

Poorly controlled postoperative pain associated with surgery involving the upper abdomen and thorax may cause chest and abdominal wall splinting secondary to a reflex increase in skeletal muscle tone and spasm[107] as well as diaphragmatic dysfunction.[108] This, coupled with any diaphragmatic splinting which occurs secondary to bowel distension, may lead to a reduction in respiratory tidal volume, vital capacity, functional residual capacity and alveolar ventilation. Atelectasis, hypoxaemia and respiratory failure may follow. It has been shown that the analgesia provided by epidural and other regional techniques may prevent or reduce chest complications.[109–120]

Cardiovascular effects

Pain is frequently associated with stimulation of the sympathetic nervous system, which in turn may result in tachycardia, hypertension and increased systemic vascular resistance. These effects in turn may be associated with increased cardiac work and hence an increased myocardial oxygen demand and possibly a decreased myocardial oxygen supply. In patients suffering from significant coronary arterial disease this chain of events may precipitate myocardial ischaemia, infarction or cardiac failure. Furthermore, the myocardial effects of pain may be exacerbated by any co-existing hypoxaemia.[121] Effective epidural analgesia following major surgery can reduce these problems.[122–128]

Thromboembolism effects

Effective postoperative analgesia may allow earlier postoperative mobilization, which in turn may reduce the occurrence of venous thromboembolic problems. It has been shown that intraoperative epidural anaesthesia prolonged into the postoperative period using a combination of low-dose local anaesthetic and opioid by infusion reduces the risk of both venous and arterial thromboembolic complications. This may be related to effects on thrombogenesis, fibrinolysis and blood flow.[129–133]

Gastrointestinal and genitourinary effects

The increased autonomic nervous activity induced by uncontrolled pain may influence the smooth muscle and sphincter function of the gut and urinary bladder. The reduction in gastrointestinal smooth muscle activity may encourage postoperative ileus, which may be prolonged if parenteral or epidural opioids are used. This may not be the case if epidural local anaesthetic is used alone or with opioids.[134–138] Postoperative urinary retention may also be related to pain-induced autonomic stimulation.[139]

Neuro-endocrine and metabolic effects

Poorly controlled postoperative pain may contribute to the neuroendocrine 'stress response' associated with surgery. Sodium and water are retained secondary to increased secretion of antidiuretic hormone and aldosterone, and there is increased catabolism, demonstrated by increased blood concentrations of glucose, free fatty acids, ketones and lactate, in response to increased circulating levels of cortisol, adrenaline, growth hormone and glucagon. Additionally, a state of decreased anabolism occurs as a result of reduced anabolic hormone secretion of insulin and testosterone. The metabolic rate and total body oxygen consumption increase and a negative nitrogen balance develops.[120,140,141]

Effects on immunological function and infection

Immunological dysfunction appears to be less marked when epidural anaesthesia and analgesia is used rather than general anaesthesia with conventional analgesia.[142–144] High-risk surgical

REFERENCES

107. Duggan J, Drummond G Anesthesia and Analgesia 1987; 66: 852
108. Ford B et al Am Rev Resp Dis 1983; 127: 431
109. Spence A, Smith G Br J Anaesth 1971; 43: 144–148
110. Pflug A et al Anesthesiology 1974; 41: 8–17
111. Rawal N et al Anesthesia and Analgesia 1984; 63: 583–592
112. Hendolin H et al Acta Anaesthesiologica Scandinavica 1987; 31: 645–651
113. Buckley D et al Anesthesiology 1990; 73: A764
114. Wahba R Can J Anaesth 1991; 38: 384–400
115. Pansard J et al Anesthesiology 1993; 78: 63–71
116. Booke M et al Anesthesia and Analgesia 1995; 80: S49
117. de Leon-Casasola O et al Regional Anesthesia 1994; 19: 307–315
118. Moiniche S et al Regional Anaesthesia 1994; 19: 352–356
119. Yeager M et al Anesthesiology 1987; 66: 729–736
120. Richardson J et al J Cardiovasc Surg 1994; 35: 219–228
121. Gill N et al Br J Anaesth 1992; 68: 471–473
122. Reiz S, Ostman G Regional Anaesthesia 1982; 7 (suppl): 8–18
123. Breslow M et al JAMA 1989; 261: 3577–3581
124. Beattie W et al Anesthesiology 1990; 73: A71
125. Blonberg S et al Anesthesiology 1990; 73: 840–847
126. de Leon Casasola O Regional Anaesthesia 1993; 18: 66
127. Stenseth R et al Anesthesia and Analgesia 1993; 77: 463–468
128. Kirno K et al Anesthesia and Analgesia 1994; 79: 1075–1081
129. Modig J et al Anesthesiology 1980; 53: S34
130. Modig J et al Anesthesia and Analgesia 1983; 62: 174–180
131. Tuman K et al. Anesthesia and Analgesia 1991; 73: 696–704.
132. Rosenfeld B et al Anesthesiology 1993; 79: 435–443
133. Christopherson R et al Anesthesiology 1993; 79: 422–434
134. Ahn H et al Br J Surg 1988; 75: 1176–1178
135. Worsley M et al Br J Anaesth 1988; 60: 836–840
136. Thoren T et al Acta Anaesthestheiologica Scanandinavica 1989; 33: 181–185
137. Wattwill M et al Anesthesia and Analgesia 1989; 68: 353–358
138. de Leon Casasola O et al Anesthesia and Analgesia 1993; 76: S73
139. Tammela T et al Scand J Urol Nephrol 1986; 20: 197–201
140. Stenseth R et al Acta Anaesth Scand 1994; 38: 834–839
141. Kehlet H Regional Anesthesia 1994; 19: 369–377
142. Hole A et al Acta Anaesth Scand 1982; 26: 301–307
143. Ryhanen P et al Gynecol Obst Invest 1985; 19: 139–142
144. Tonnesen E and Wahlgreen C Brit J Anaesth 1988; 60: 500–507

patients who received prolonged postoperative epidural analgesia had far fewer septic complications[119] than similar patients receiving general anaesthesia and standard analgesia.

Psychological effects

Poorly controlled postoperative pain can cause sleep disturbance and affective dysfunction (anxiety and depression). This in turn can affect the patient's pain tolerance and thereby create a vicious cycle of increasing psychological disturbance.[141,145]

Persistent post-surgical pain

Surgical operations may initiate pain that continues long after the patient has left hospital. The various persistent pain syndromes that occur may result from the interaction of nociceptive pain (from the continued stimulation of nociceptors), neuropathic/neurogenic pain (resulting from peripheral and central sensitization developing in the perioperative period), and psychological factors. Some of the contributory factors that have been identified are:

(i) a genetic predisposition to neuroma formation
(ii) the duration and severity of pain before and after surgery
(iii) surgical technique
(iv) the patient's age.[146,147]

Persistent pain following different types of surgery is more common than is generally appreciated[145] and is especially well documented after thoracotomy.[145,148,149] Two groups of researchers have demonstrated that preoperative and perioperative epidural blocks can prevent the development of post-amputation pain.[150,151]

Economic effects

Clear economic advantages have been demonstrated when conventional postoperative analgesia is compared with 'balanced' multimodal analgesia, incorporating the epidural route, in groups of high-risk surgical patients. These accrue from more rapid immediate recovery from surgery and anaesthesia, reduced need for intensive care, and shorter hospital stay.[117–119,141,152–154]

Patient outcome

Adequate postoperative analgesia may reduce postoperative complications and shorten the hospital stay for high-risk surgical patients,[117,119,120,133,141,155,156] although the influence of anaesthesia and analgesia on surgical outcome is controversial.[158] Good postoperative analgesia renders patients less tired, both mentally and physically, and more motivated to take part in postoperative rehabilitation.[118,141,154]

A number of harmful physiological and psychological effects may ensue if acute pain is under-treated. Good analgesia allows earlier physical exercise, respiratory training and enteral feeding.[117,141]

Methods of treating postoperative pain

After any operation occasionally patients require little or no analgesia. Most patients need some analgesia in fairly predictable doses. The drugs available to treat postoperative pain are still extracts of poppy (morphine) and willow bark (aspirin), albeit chemical refinements of these natural substances. More sophisticated methods for analgesic delivery are now widely available (e.g. patient controlled analgesia and epidural infusions) and the benefits of drug combinations are being realised. Patients must be carefully monitored and supervised when invasive techniques and potentially lethal drugs are employed.

Systemic opioids

Opioids are drugs which act as agonists to the opioid receptors (μ, κ and δ). They may be naturally occurring compounds like morphine, synthetic like pethidine, or semi-synthetic like diamorphine. The term opiate refers to the naturally occurring opioids, and the term narcotic should be avoided. Opioid receptors are located in the brain, spinal cord, and peripherally.[158] Opioid drugs may be administered by almost any route. Opioids of rapid onset may be given intravenously and the dose titrated directly against the severity of the pain. Most opioids are strong μ-opioid receptor agonists and are capable of relieving all acute pain. All opioides cause depression of respiration, nausea and vomiting, delayed gastric emptying, and tolerance phenomena. The partial μ-opioid receptor agonists also cause respiratory depression equivalent to their analgesic effects, but with continued use this side-effect and dependence become less and they are less liable to be abused. Some are antagonists at the μ-opioid receptor and agonists at the κ-opioid receptor (called agonist-antagonist drugs). κ receptor stimulation is not capable of achieving the same degree of analgesia as μ receptor stimulation. Opioids remain the mainstay of postoperative analgesia although the requirements may be reduced by concurrent use of other analgesic drugs. Morphine remains the principal strong opioid for postoperative pain relief and all other compounds are still compared with it.

Analgesic doses of an appropriate opioid may be administered by a number of routes, including: oral, rectal, sublingual, transdermal, intramuscular, subcutaneous and intravenous; the last two as either bolus injection or continuous infusion.

Traditionally the intramuscular route has been used to treat postoperative pain because of its simplicity and widespread

REFERENCES

145. Cousins M. In: Wall P D, Melzack R (eds) Textbook of Pain, 4th edn. Churchill Livingstone, Philadelphia pp 375–385
146. Woolf C, Chong M-S Anesthesia and Analgesia 1993; 77: 329–331
147. Kehlet H Brit J Anaesth 1989; 63: 189–195
148. Kalso E et al Acta Anaesth Scand 1992; 36: 96–100
149. Richardson J, Sabanathan S International Monitor on Regional Anaesthesia 1993; 5: 36
150. Bach S et al Pain 1988; 33: 297–301
151. Jahangiri P et al Annals of the Royal Colllege of Surgeons of England 1994; 67: 324–326
152. Bellamy C et al Anesthesiology 1989; 71: A686
153. Walmsley P et al Anesthesiology 1989; 71: A684
154. Moiniche S et al Acta Anaesth Scand 1994; 38: 328–335
155. Rawal N et al Anesthesia and Analgesia 1984; 63: 583–592
156. Wasylak J et al Can J Anaesth 1990; 37: 726–731
157. Covino B G Acta Chir Scand 1989; 550
158. Stein C et al N Engl J Med 1991; 325: 1123–1126

applicability, the dose of drug being given on a *pro re nata* (as necessary) basis. This method of postoperative analgesia is frequently unsatisfactory for many reasons, the most obvious being that administration of a *standard dose* of opioid ignores the wide variability in opioid requirements of individual patients. This occurs because of the highly variable pharmacokinetic handling of, and pharmacodynamic response to opioids by individual patients.[159,160] Unfortunately the phrase 'prn' is often interpreted as 'give as infrequently as possible'. There is little flexibility with this method and frequently the postoperative analgesia it provides is inadequate.

There is little scientific justification for the calculation of intramuscular analgesic doses based on body weight or surface area[161] and the intramuscular route is not necessarily as safe as is often believed. Episodes of hypoxaemia from respiratory depression may be more severe than with the newer methods of opioid delivery.[162,163] If the intramuscular route is to be more effectively used as a delivery system, given its unpredictability, frequent patient assessment is needed with adjustments of dose and frequency to achieve optimal pain relief.

Intravenous opioid infusions can avoid wide swings in plasma concentration and permit easy, quick titration of the drug to the analgesic requirements of individual patients. Patients must be regularly monitored if life threatening respiratory complications are to be avoided.[164]

Inability to swallow may limit the use of oral opioids in the immediate postoperative period but the oral route can be successfully used when gastric and small bowel function return to normal. Transdermal drug delivery is becoming popular in some hospitals but there is no place for this method of drug delivery in postoperative pain management at present[165] as the peak analgesic action of transdermal fentanyl may be delayed for 15 hours, with an effective half-life of 21 h.[166] It has been shown that opioids do alter the clinical signs of patients with acute abdominal pain in proportion to the dose given, but they do not alter the diagnosis.[92]

Patient controlled analgesia

Patient controlled analgesia is the self administration of small doses of, usually, intravenous opioids by the patient in response to the pain severity (a negative feedback system). This method is designed to overcome the variability of the pharmacokinetics and pharmacodynamics of opioid drugs in individual patients. The danger of the system is related mainly to third person intervention (e.g. clinical staff and relatives) rather than equipment malfunction or incorrect prescribing, although these have been reported. Most patient controlled analgesia devices consist of a microprocessor-controlled syringe pump, triggered by depressing a button. A preset amount of opioid as a bolus dose is then delivered into an intravenous line. If the device does not have dedicated intravenous access, and has to be incorporated into an existing intravenous line the following precautions should be taken:

a. A one-way valve should be incorporated into the system to prevent retrograde passage of the opioid drug up the drip-set, allowing a potentially large bolus of opioid to be administered.
b. It should be attached as close to the venepuncture site as possible to minimize the dead space.
c. The reservoir should be placed below the level of the patient to prevent any siphoning of the drug into the patient.

A timer prevents further bolus doses being delivered until a specified period has elapsed (lockout period). The prescriber sets the bolus dose and the lockout period and may additionally set an overall dose limit for a longer period of time, usually a 4 hour total dose limit. Some devices can deliver a continuous background infusion, although it is better to avoid this when constant surveillance is not available. If a continuous infusion is added to patient controlled analgesia it offers no advantage over patient controlled analgesia alone. The total number of demands and the total amount of drug used are similar.[167]

Patient controlled analgesia does not cause more respiratory depression and hypoxaemia than standard p.r.n. intramuscular opioid regimens.[168] Patient controlled analgesia with opioids has a good safety record but cases of respiratory depression have been reported, usually when the patient is very old or hypovolaemic, or when large bolus doses are given with an additional background infusion. The quality of the analgesia is generally regarded as superior to that achieved by intramuscular opioids and this is often achieved with a lower overall dose and increased patient and staff satisfaction. The satisfaction with this method is related to a perception of patient autonomy, elimination of time delays in providing analgesia, avoidance of painful intramuscular injections, and increased ease of nursing.

All the standard opioid drugs have been used for intravenous patient controlled analgesic although morphine remains the most popular. The patient controlled pump should be available as soon as possible after the operation, preceded by the administration of a loading dose of the drug to be used, ideally titrated to achieve optimum analgesic effect by the anaesthetist giving the anaesthetic. The patient should only be discharged from the recovery ward when the pain is controlled and only side-effects are minimal. Respiratory depression and over-sedation must be avoided, while nausea, vomiting and pruritus may require symptomatic relief.

Patient controlled opioids may also be administered by the subcutaneous route using the same equipment but with a more concentrated solution of the drug to minimize the volume required.

The efficacy of the analgesia depends on the dose of drug given and the lockout period. Too low a dose may result in poor pain control and loss of confidence by the patient and ward staff; too high a dose produces unacceptable side-effects.[169] Too long a

REFERENCES

159. Austin K et al Anesthesiology 1980; 53: 460
160. Austin K et al Pain 1980; 8: 47
161. Belville J et al JAMA 1971; 217: 1835
162. Catley D et al Anesthesiology 1985; 63: 20
163. Brose W, Cohn S Anesthesiology 1989; 70: 948
164. Catling J et al BMJ 1980; 281: 478
165. Caplan J et al JAMA 1989; 261: 1036
166. Holley F, Van Steenis C Brit J Anaesth 1988; 60: 608–613
167. Owen H et al Anaesthesia 1990; 45: 619–622
168. Wheatley R et al Brit J Anaesth 1990; 64: 267–275
169. Semple P et al Anaesthesia 1992; 47: 399–401

lockout period results in poor pain control while too short a period may lead to overdosage.

Regional anaesthetic techniques

Local anaesthetic drugs can completely control acute pain both at rest and on movement. Regional anaesthetic techniques used for surgery may be continued into the postoperative period. A complete description of all these techniques is not possible and the following serve as examples.

Infiltration of local anaesthetic into the operative wound is simple to perform and cannulae can be left in the wound to allow prolonged wound analgesia. This is particularly helpful after upper abdominal surgery.[170] A single injection of 0.25% bupivacaine into an inguinal hernia incision can produce effective postoperative pain relief[171] whilst repeated injections of a 0.5% solution of this agent subcutaneously can provide lasting pain relief.[172] These methods are only effective for superficial somatic pain; they do not work for visceral pain.

Long-acting local anaesthetic agents used for intraoperative nerve or plexus blockade can still be effective in the postoperative period. An interscalene brachial plexus block used for shoulder surgery can be effective for 12–24 hours and intercostal nerve blocks for 6–12 hours after thoracic and upper abdominal surgery.[173] Local anaesthetic agents infused via intercostal and paravertebral catheters are also an effective means of providing analgesia following upper abdominal and thoracic surgery.[174–176] Local anaesthetic agents infused through catheters placed into the axillary[177,178] and femoral sheaths[179] and in the vicinity of the lumbar plexus[180] and sciatic nerve[181] provide effective postoperative analgesia and prolonged sympathetic blockade. Intrapleural local analgesia has been used to produce pain relief after upper abdominal and thoracic surgery. This technique can cause pneumothorax and paralysis of the muscles of respiration, especially when a bilateral technique is used.[182]

Spinal subarachnoid local anaesthesia can provide postoperative analgesia for several hours if long-acting local anaesthetic agents are used. Continuous epidural anaesthesia through an indwelling catheter is a very versatile technique for postoperative analgesia. Many different combinations and concentrations of local anaesthetics, opioids and other drugs are used for this purpose, the idea being to minimize the dose of each and achieve high-quality analgesia with minimal motor and sympathetic nerve blockade.

The main side-effects of local anaesthetic agents are:

a. Toxic effects of large doses of these agents.
b. Hypotension related to sympathetic blockade.
c. Motor weakness.
d. The potential to mask pain as an important clinical sign.

An example of the latter would be its ability to mask compartment syndrome in the lower limbs; this does not appear to be the case when opioids are used alone for postoperative pain relief.[183]

Epidural opioids may cause respiratory depression, although this may be delayed for some hours. It is usually responsive to intravenous naloxone in standard doses. Epidural opioids can also cause pruritus that usually responds to intravenous antihistamines and naloxone in standard doses. Urinary retention is also not uncommon and may require bladder catheterization. Nausea and vomiting can also occur and is treated with conventional anti-emetics.

Intra-articular analgesia

Opioids, local anaesthetic agents and non-steroidal anti-inflammatory agents injected into the joint space following arthroscopic knee surgery may be effective.

Non-opioid analgesics

Non-steroidal anti-inflammatory drugs

These drugs inhibit cyclo-oxygenase, interfering with prostaglandin formation. Prostaglandins appear to increase the algesic effect of bradykinin and histamine. These drugs are widely used for postoperative analgesia,[184] usually in combination with opioid drugs as their analgesic potency is not enough to control severe postoperative pain alone. They appear to improve the quality of postoperative analgesia whilst having an 'opioid sparing' effect.[147,185] The analgesic potency of these drugs must be considered separately to their anti-inflammatory potency.[186] Parenteral preparations of these agents are now available (e.g. ketorolac and diclofenac) making them more attractive for use in the perioperative period. The advantages of using these agents used with opioids include a reduction in opioid side-effects, absence of addiction or tolerance and less sedation.

Non-steroidal anti-inflammatory drugs may adversely affect patient outcome, although evidence for this is scant. The major side-effects of these agents are leukotriene-induced bronchoconstriction, gastric erosions which are uncommon with short-term postoperative use, interference with primary haemostasis although a significant increase in operative blood loss is largely unproven, and renal dysfunction from sodium and water retention and a fall in renal plasma flow.[187]

Nitrous oxide

This still has a useful role especially for short acutely painful procedures such as dressing changes and superficial wound

REFERENCES

170. Watson D et al Brit J Anaesth 1991; 67: 656P
171. Ryan J et al Am J Surg 1984; 148: 313–316
172. Hashemi K, Middleton M Ann R Coll Surg Engl 1983; 65: 38
173. Moore D BJA 1975; 47: 284
174. Hashimi H et al Surg Gyne Obstet 1991; 173: 116–118
175. Sabanathan S et al Ann Thorac Surg 1988; 46: 425–426
176. Sabanathan S et al Brit J Surg 1990; 77: 221–225
177. Selander D Acta Anaesth Scand 1977; 21: 324–329
178. Audenaert S et al Anesthesiology 1991; 74: 368–370
179. Rosenblatt R Anesthesia and Analgesia 1980; 59: 631
180. Brands E, Callanan V Anaesth Int Care 1978; 6: 256
181. Smith G et al Anaesthesia 1984; 39: 55
182. Stromskag K et al Anesthesia and Analgesia 1988; 67: 430–434
183. Montgomery C, Ready L Anesthesiology 1991; 75: 541
184. Dahl J, Kehlet H Brit J Anaesth 1991; 66: 703–712
185. McCormack K, Brune K Drugs 1991; 41: 533–547
186. Harris K Brit J Anaesth 1992; 69: 233–235
187. Dahl J et al BJA 1990; 64: 518

debridement.[188,189] It has rapid onset and cessation of action and is usually administered as 'Entonox', a 50:50 mixture of nitrous oxide and oxygen.

Cryoanalgesia

Cooling peripheral nerves to temperatures between –5 and –20°C causes disintegration of axons and myelin sheath whilst preserving the perineurium and epineurium. Nerve conduction is disrupted for several weeks[190,191] and recovery depends on the rate of nerve regeneration and the distance of the damage from the end-organ. Intercostal cryoanalgesia has been used after thoracotomy[192] and this reduces post-thoracotomy pain and analgesia requirements. A significant number of patients treated in this way have suffered a persistent dysaesthetic neuropathic pain in the longer term.[193,194]

Coping mechanisms

Psychological factors may have a profound bearing on the tolerance of acute pain. Identical injuries can engender very different responses in different people, who will have differing analgesic requirements. Acute pain is definitely affected by the 'psychological state' of the patient. Preoperative anxiety is common,[195] and this appears to affect postoperative pain, analgesic requirements and complications. Psychological interventions, such as behavioural and cognitive modification, have been used in adult and paediatric patients.[196] Simpler methods have also been shown to reduce perioperative anxiety, including giving adequate amounts of information and reassurance.[197] The use of distraction and imagery may also be effective.[198]

Stimulation analgesia

The benefits of these various techniques are uncertain and other methods are at present more effective. Acupuncture and electro-acupuncture can produce effective postoperative analgesia but the effect is neither consistent[199] nor sustained.[200]

Transcutaneous electrical nerve stimulation (TENS) used post-operatively has a variable response, although it is simple, non-invasive and free of side-effects.[201,202] The mechanism of action is not known.[203]

The placebo effect

This term is often used to imply that the pain is imaginary. In reality this is probably the result of the activation of the body's own analgesic systems that modulate pain at either the spinal cord or at higher centres. The existence of such a mechanism is to be utilized.[204]

Balanced analgesia[185]

Balanced analgesia describes the additive or synergistic properties of different analgesic drugs or techniques used in combination. This allows the minimum dose of each agent to be used, limiting the side-effects of each agent and improving patient safety.

At present the ideal combination of analgesic drugs for the management of postoperative pain probably consists of neural blockade with a local anaesthetic agent in combination with an opioid, and a non-opioid analgesic agent (such as a non-steroidal anti-inflammatory drug) begun preoperatively and continued for as long as possible after operation.[120,205] This regimen should provide pain control throughout the perioperative period.[98,146,206]

Acute pain services

Effective and safe postoperative pain management seems most likely to succeed if it is delivered by a separate service. The first formal acute pain service was established in Seattle in 1986, although the concept itself is much older. This service is usually run by anaesthetists but this is unimportant provided the clinicians involved are familiar with the analgesic drugs used and have skills in the regional analgesic techniques necessary for the relief of severe postoperative pain. Many publications have appeared describing the establishment of such a service[89,90,207–213] which appears to ensure patients' safety.[214–217]

Postoperative pain relief in children

The widespread belief that the nervous system of neonates and infants is insufficiently developed to feel pain in the same way that older children and adults do, has led to poor pain management in this age group. Owing to their inability to communicate the

REFERENCES

188. Baskett P et al BMJ 1971; 1: 509
189. Kripke B et al Crit Care Med 1983; 11: 105
190. Katz J et al Lancet 1980; 1: 512
191. Maiwand M BMJ 1981; 282: 1749
192. Glynn C et al Thorax 1980; 35: 325
193. Müller L et al Ann Thorac Surg 1989; 48: 15
194. Katz J Ann Thorac Surg 1989; 48: 5
195. Norris W, Baird W Brit J Anaesth 1967; 39: 503–509
196. Wilson J et al J Human Stress 1982; 8: 13–23
197. Egbert L et al N Engl J Med 1964; 270: 825–827
198. Reading D Social Science and medicine 1979; I3A: 641–654
199. Leong D, Chernow B Inter Anesth Clin 1988; 26(3): 213–217
200. Christiansen P et al Br J Anaesth 1989; 62: 258–262
201. Rooney S-M et al Anesthesia and Analgesia 1983; 62: 1010–1012
202. McCallum P et al Br J Anaesth 1988; 61: 308–312
203. Melzack R Pain 1975; 1: 357
204. Wall P In: Melzack R, Wall P D (eds). Textbook of Pain 3rd ed. The placebo and placeo response pp 1297–1308
205. Richmond C et al Lancet 1993; 342: 73–76
206. Brevik H Current Opinions in Anaesthesiology 1994; 5: 458–461
207. Editorial Anaesthesia and Intensive Care 1976; 4: 95
208. Ready L et al Anesthesiology 1988; 68: 100–106
209. Macintyre P et al Med J Austr 1991; 153: 417–421
210. Wheatley R et al Brit J Anaesth 1991; 67: 353–359
211. Gould H et al BMJ 1992; 305: 1187–1193
212. Schug S, Haridas A Austr N Zealand J Surg 1993; 63: 8–13
213. Brevick H Pain Digest 1993; 3: 27–30
214. Dawson P et al Anaesth Int Care 1991; 19: 569–591
215. Kelt H, Dahl J et al Anesthesia and Analgesia 1993; 77: 1048–1056
216. Kvalsvik O, Gisvold S Acta Anaesth Scand 1993; 37(suppl 100): 226
217. Steude G et al Anesthesia and Analgesia 1995; 80: S473

assessment of pain in infants and neonates is difficult.[218,219] Recently pain management in the very young has become more interventional and more closely monitored.[220] The normal response of healthy neonates and infants to painful stimuli is non-purposeful movement of all limbs accompanied by crying and grimacing. More painful stimuli seem to generate louder and more distressed cries with non-verbal signs of agitation and distress.[221] Simply cuddling a baby may reduce anxiety and sensitivity to painful stimuli. Opioids appear to cause more respiratory depression in the neonates. The elimination of these drugs is more variable and generally more prolonged than in older age groups. If opioids are used in spontaneously breathing neonates close monitoring with apnoea alarms and pulse oximetry is essential. The need for opioids can be reduced by the use of local anaesthetic agents administered regionally or spinally. The hypotension caused by neuraxial analgesia in neonates is less common than in adults. Caudal epidural block is easy to perform and is used frequently for perineal and lower abdominal surgery, and in small children a catheter may be threaded as far as the thoracic region from this entry site. Paracetamol and non-steroidal anti-inflammatory agents (such as diclofenac and ibuprofen) are used to reduce or remove the need for opioids postoperatively. Intravenous patient controlled analgesia has been used successfully in children as young as four years, but continuous intravenous infusions appear to be better tolerated. If intermittent intramuscular analgesia is required a cannula can be placed in a muscle before the end of anaesthetic, so avoiding the need for repeated painful injections.

Chronic and cancer pain

The definition of pain given previously[103] encompasses a broad range of conditions and it lends credence to the patient whose complaint of pain is made in the absence of any obvious pathological cause. Even if the pain has a more central or perhaps psychological origin, it is none the less completely real to the patient and therefore warrants treatment.[222] The effects of unrelieved acute pain are mainly physiological, whereas those of unrelieved chronic pain are mainly psychosocial with depression, disability and dependence upon others in many cases. Eventually the psychological and behavioural changes induced by the pain can become self-sustaining and represent a disease entity in themselves. These changes represent an extreme end of the spectrum in patients with chronic pain.

The causes of chronic pain can be considered in simple terms as tissue damage (e.g. chronic pancreatitis, rheumatoid arthritis), nerve damage (e.g. post-herpetic neuralgia, post-stroke pain) and as pains that have a predominant psychological component. Many conditions, for example back pain and cancer pain, may represent a combination of more than one of these categories.

Assessment and management of patients with intractable pain is best carried out in a pain relief clinic where the expertise of various medical specialists can be blended with that of psychologists, physiotherapists and others to devise an optimal plan of treatment. Anaesthetists were originally involved in chronic pain management because of their skills with needles and they continue to play a pivotal role in the modern pain relief clinic.

Treatment options

Drugs

Complex or inappropriate drug therapy can be harmful to the patient with chronic pain and rationalization of medication should be an early aim of treatment. The drugs used in chronic pain management include analgesics, ranging from aspirin to morphine, as well as a wide range of adjuvant or supplementary drugs which include antidepressants, anticonvulsants and steroids. Specific pain syndromes sometimes have indications for specific drug therapy such as carbamazepine for trigeminal neuralgia. A full understanding of pain mechanisms and neuropharmacology often reveals that opioid drugs are very unlikely to be effective in many forms of chronic pain and this is frequently borne out in clinical practice.

The use of opioids for chronic non-malignant pain where life expectancy is long requires careful thought, but no such constraints apply to patients with cancer pain and these powerful drugs should be used as early as necessary in adequate dosage.[223] The problems of tolerance and physiological dependence can be managed if and when they occur. The threat of true psychological dependence is never a problem in patients with cancer pain and it is cruel to deny these patients adequate pain relief because of this theoretical risk. There is no place for intramuscular injections of opioids in the management of cancer pain. A simple analgesic ladder should be used starting with oral non-steroidal anti-inflammatory drugs, then codeine-like drugs and finally morphine or diamorphine should be given by mouth, or if this is impractical by subcutaneous infusion. The drugs should be given at a regular time to ensure that the pain is prevented rather than subdued each time it returns. The side-effects of constipation and nausea often require treatment. These simple analgesic regimens can control the pain in the majority of patients. If the drugs fail or the side-effects are too great, alternative drugs, routes of administration or neuroablative methods must be considered, though the need for this is very rare.

Nerve blocks

Nerve blocks and other injection therapy are still appropriate in some conditions. Injections may be of local anaesthetics, steroids or neurolytic agents.[224] Enthusiasm for neuroablative procedures has waned. The complexity of pain transmission pathways is such that the initially appealing concept of cutting or destroying nerves to obtain pain relief is founded on gross oversimplification and in fact neuroablative procedures often aggravate matters by creating additional problems such as anaesthesia dolorosa or neuralgia.

REFERENCES

218. McGrath P Pain 1987; 31: 147–176
219. McGrath P Pain 1990; 41: 253–254
220. Lloyd-Thomas A Brit J Anaesth 1990; 64: 85–104
221. Grunau R et al Pain 1990; 42: 295–305
222. Wall P D, Melzack R (eds) Textbook of Pain, 2nd edn. Churchill Livingstone, Edinburgh 1989
223. Twycross R G Cancer Surv 1988; 7: 29–54
224. Charlton J E In: Swerdlow M (ed) The Therapy of Pain. MTP Press, Lancaster 1986

Somatic nerve blocks can be useful in cancer pain, and epidural steroid injection benefits certain patients with back pain.[225]

Sympathetic nerve blocks are sometimes effective in treating causalgia, reflex sympathetic dystrophy, ischaemic rest pain and chronic abdominal pain.[226] Lumbar sympathetic blockade can alleviate rest pain in the absence of tissue necrosis and coeliac plexus block can relieve the pain of carcinoma of the pancreas in up to 80% of cases.[227] These blocks should not be performed without adequate assessment and a full understanding by the patient of what is planned and what risks are involved. Major neurolytic blocks demand a meticulous technique and the use of an image intensifier with the injection of contrast medium to ensure that the injected neurolytic solution does not spread beyond the desired target site.

Neurosurgery

Neurosurgical operations for chronic pain relief are now performed less frequently because of poor results and a fuller understanding of pain mechanisms. Cutting nerves for benign pain is seldom, if ever, indicated. A neuroma will form wherever a nerve is cut and the axonal sprouts of this neuroma can generate a barrage of nociceptive signals so that pain, hyperaesthesia and other neuralgic symptoms develop, leaving the patient in a worse condition. Excising a pain-generating neuroma appears tempting but this often merely moves the problem more proximally.

Selective destruction has been performed in the dorsal root entry zone of the spinal cord using a radiofrequency 'lesion generator' which produces coagulation damage that is occasionally beneficial.[223]

Neuroablative methods find their widest application in patients with cancer. Anterolateral spinothalamic tractotomy can be performed via a small, high cervical laminectomy or percutaneously with the radiofrequency 'lesion generator'. This technique is usually simply described as a cordotomy and it can produce pain relief when properly performed for well localized unilateral intractable cancer pain.[228]

Stimulation techniques

Acupuncture and transcutaneous electrical nerve stimulation are claimed to act by stimulation of endogenous pain inhibitory systems, but although very successful in some patients these methods fail in others with seemingly similar clinical pictures.

Implantation of electrodes in the epidural space can be used to provide spinal cord stimulation. This complicated and expensive neurosurgical procedure has been claimed to be helpful in many otherwise intractable conditions such as arachnoiditis, lower limb ischaemia and intractable angina. The place of this treatment has not yet been fully established.

Other therapies

Physical therapies such as manipulation, exercise, massage and aromatherapy may help some patients with chronic pain and certainly exercise therapy can be a vital part of a rehabilitation programme.

Psychological therapies can be invaluable in helping patients whose pain has a significant psychological component. Psychologists can also teach coping skills and relaxation therapy to most patients. Cognitive-behavioural pain management programmes employ the skills of clinical psychologists, occupational and physiotherapists to achieve the best possible level of physical and emotional function within the confines of the continuing pain. Pain reduction is not the aim of such programmes, although this may follow functional improvement. Patients learn how to cope better with their pain.[229]

Surgical patients with chronic pain

A surgeon confronted by a patient with intractable pain for which no operation is indicated should not be tempted to dismiss the patient with the accusation that 'it is all in your head' nor state that the patient 'will just have to learn to live with the pain'. Yet another 'exploratory operation' creates new damage and new scars and is often counterproductive if there is no definite indication so, if no other specific therapy is appropriate, the patient should be referred to a pain clinic where symptomatic relief may be provided and where any psychological or behavioural issues which are clouding the picture can be addressed.[230]

REFERENCES

225. Benzon H T Pain 1986; 24: 277–296
226. Rubin A P In: Wildsmith J A W, Armitage E N (eds) Principles and Practice of Regional Anaesthesia. Churchill Livingstone, Edinburgh 1987 p 185
227. Brown D L, Moore D C J Pain Symptom Manage 1988; 3: 206
228. Thomas D G T. Sheehy J J Neurol Neurosurg Psychiatr 1982; 45: 949
229. Lipton S In: Wall P D, Melzack R (eds) Textbook of Pain. Churchill Livingstone, Edinburgh 1984
230. Sternbach R A (ed) The Psychology of Pain, 2nd edn. Raven Press, New York 1986

6 Burns

J. A. Clarke

HISTORY

The great Dupuytren made an early and lasting contribution to burn care. He first described the well-known gastrointestinal haemorrhage in burned patients, recommended baths, described six degrees of burn wound depth, four phases of the burn illness—irritation, inflammation, suppuration and exhaustion—and in 1828 published the first analysis comparing age, sex surface area and mortality. In 1833 Sir George Ballingall of Edinburgh described the natural history of burned patients, noting deaths from febrile crises at 10–12 days and later deaths at 3–6 weeks, with patients 'exhausted by the profuse discharge of matter from the suppurating surface'.

Treatment continued to be by purgation and blood letting. Lisfranc introduced wet dressings of sodium and calcium chloride in 1835, and Passavant saline baths in 1858. Parascandolo resuscitated burns with intravenous saline in 1901 and Underhill, investigating burn blister fluid and changes in haemoglobin and haematocrit levels in 1921, declared burn shock to be caused by protein loss. The Coconut Grove disaster in Boston, USA encouraged further research and Cope & Moore in 1942 suggested that fluid was sequestered within both burned and unburned areas and that shock was not entirely the result of external losses.

In 1952 Everett Evans, relating likely fluid requirements to the surface area burned, suggested a burn shock formula that remains the basis for many of the current regimens. Pollock in 1870 was the first surgeon to skin graft a burn. He used the patient's own skin, the skin of a black person and his own skin, observing the delayed rejection of the allografts at 8 weeks.

Wallace reintroduced the method of burn wound exposure in 1949,[1] whereby the wound was left without any topical application or dressing. Many thought, and still think, that this form of treatment is simple neglect. Numerous topical antiseptics and antibacterials have been used to try and limit burn wound sepsis but none have been entirely effective. Aggressive surgical excision and grafting before sepsis can occur have been advocated by many but remain difficult to achieve.[2] An excellent historical review of the development of burn treatment has been published by Shedd.[3]

DEFINITION

A burn is a coagulative destruction of the surface layers of the body. This damage is usually caused by heat but, by convention, injuries from chemicals or irradiation are included.

INCIDENCE

In the UK each year there are about 600 deaths from burns, 150 000 burn injuries and 12 000 hospital admissions. Domestic burns and scalds account for 6% of the casualties attending accident and emergency departments and over half of these occur in young children. The overall incidence of large yet survivable burns appears to be falling, although the number of burns seen in the elderly is increasing.

PREVENTION

Legal measures to introduce flame-retarding materials, particularly for nightwear, have made tremendous differences to the pattern of burn injuries in the UK where clothing burns in children are now rare. Legislation concerning the use of fireguards, the design of paraffin heaters and the transport and storage of flammable materials has been very effective. Little can be done to legislate against poverty, alcoholism, drug addiction, epilepsy, old age and social disadvantage—factors that are found so frequently in those with burns.

DEPTH

It is most sensible to classify burns according to the depth of tissue that has been injured, yet there is no uniformly accepted classification of depth. It is useful to consider burns as being superficial, dermal or deep, and subdivide dermal burns into superficial dermal and deep dermal burns (Fig. 6.1):

1. Superficial burns.
2a. Superficial dermal burns.
2b. Deep dermal burns.
3. Deep or full-thickness burns.

Superficial burns re-epithelialize rapidly from remaining basal cells and leave no scarring.

Superficial dermal burns are re-surfaced from regenerating epithelium derived from the deeper undamaged hair follicles, sweat and sebaceous glands. Healing takes between 10 and 14 days and is usually accompanied by little or no scarring.

REFERENCES

1. Wallace A B Br J Plast Surg 1949; 1: 232–244
2. Constable J D Burns 1994; 20: 316–324
3. Shedd D P Surgery 1958; 43: 1024–1035

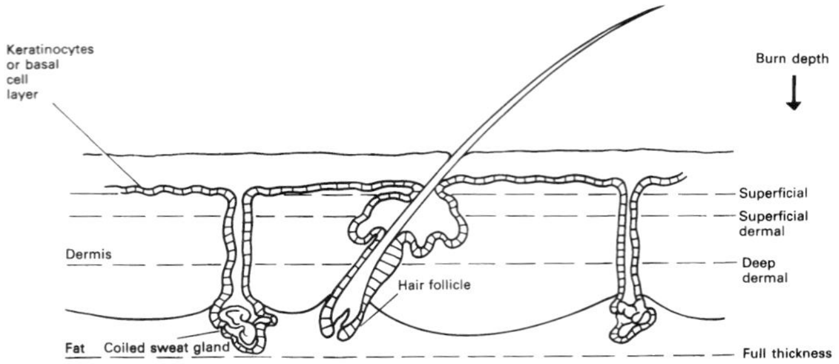

Fig 6.1 Burn depth. Note that basal cells are the source of new epithelium and that the bases of the hair follicles and sweat glands extend *below* the dermis.

Deep dermal burns heal more slowly, taking 3–4 weeks, and scarring is inevitable as there is a conflict between the processes of inflammation, collagenous repair and spontaneous re-epithelialization.

Deep or full-thickness burns coagulate and destroy all layers of the skin; no regeneration of the skin can occur and the wound must heal by contraction of granulation tissue and ingrowth of peripheral epithelium.

Although most tissue damage occurs at the moment of burning, desiccation of the wound probably leads to an increase in depth, and bacterial infection causes further dermal loss, inflammation and delay or inhibition of epithelial regeneration.

The diagnosis of depth is not always easy and most burns are of mixed depth. Superficial burns are red, blistered, blanch on pressure and are very painful when pricked with a needle. Superficial dermal burns are pink, blister, blanch less briskly on pressure, and are painful to pinprick. Deep dermal burns have a creamy base, have blistered, do not blanch and are analgesic although not anaesthetic to pinprick. Deep burns are discoloured, do not blister and are painless and numb.[4]

AREA

Wallace's rule of nines—9% for the head, 9% for an arm, 18% for a leg and 36% for the trunk—is easy to recall and accurate enough for adults.[5] The Lund & Browder[6] modification takes into account the different proportions of a child, with the head being relatively larger and the limbs smaller. In practice it helps to measure the number of palmfuls burned, as the palmar surface of the patient's hand is about 1% of his or her body surface area (Fig. 6.2).

Mortality is related to burn size and Bull & Fisher's table of chances of survival can help the surgeon to give a reliable prognosis (Table 6.1).[7]

PATHOPHYSIOLOGY

Tissue necrosis is directly related to temperature and duration.[8] Boiling water in contact with the skin for a tenth of a second causes a superficial burn, and for 1 second a full-thickness burn. A fall into bath water of 75°C results in partial-thickness skin loss after 1 second and full-thickness loss by 10 seconds. Pain and rapid withdrawal are seen at 43.5°C with tissue damage occurring at temperatures above 48°C.[9]

LUND AND BROWDER CHARTS

IGNORE SIMPLE ERYTHEMA

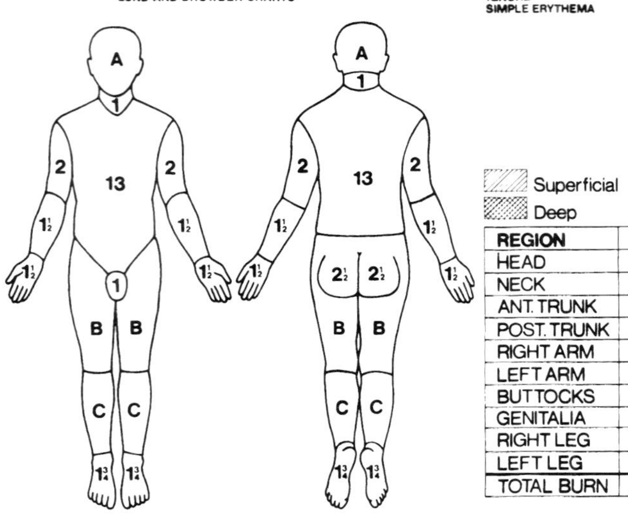

REGION	%
HEAD	
NECK	
ANT. TRUNK	
POST. TRUNK	
RIGHT ARM	
LEFT ARM	
BUTTOCKS	
GENITALIA	
RIGHT LEG	
LEFT LEG	
TOTAL BURN	

RELATIVE PERCENTAGE OF BODY SURFACE AREA AFFECTED BY GROWTH

AREA	AGE 0	1	5	10	15	ADULT
A = ½ OF HEAD	9½	8½	6½	5½	4½	3½
B = ½ OF ONE THIGH	2¾	3¼	4	4½	4½	4¾
C = ½ OF ONE LEG	2½	2½	2¾	3	3¼	3½

Fig 6.2 Surface area chart for estimating severity of burn wounds. By permission of Smith & Nephew Ltd.

Heat causing tissue damage leads to a marked increase in capillary permeability which is inevitable and unalterable but temporary. It is maximal at 8 hours, usually returning to normal at 36–48 hours. Proteins up to a molecular weight of 350 kDa escape into the tissue leading to oedema, and the fluid loss that results is roughly proportional to the area damaged. With injuries in excess of 30% of the body surface area, a generalized increase in capillary permeability is seen in most body tissues. Platelets and polymorphonuclear leuocytes adhere to the damaged intima, increasing the resistance to flow, and erythrocytes are damaged when passing through affected capillaries. The early inexorable loss of protein and fluid causes circulatory collapse unless treated promptly.

Increased metabolism and oxygen consumption, nitrogen loss and wasting of energy through heat and water losses all have prolonged effects. The immediate rise in cortisol triggers protein catabolism and mobilization of gluconeogenic precursors, and in major burns both impaired insulin release and insulin resistance are seen. Following shortly afterwards but lasting much longer, catecholamines and glucagon increase oxygen consumption and heat production by breaking down protein and fat.[10] A massive catabolic drive (autocannibalism) leads to the breakdown of protein to provide the carbohydrate intermediaries that are essential for the

REFERENCES

4. Jackson D M Br J Plast Surg 1953; 40: 588–596
5. Kyle M J, Wallace A B Br J Plast Surg 1951; 3: 194–204
6. Lund C L, Browder N C, Surg Gynecol Obst 1944; 79: 352–354
7. Bull J P, Fisher A J Ann Surg 1954; 139: 169–274
8. Moritz A R, Henriques F C Am J Pathol 1947; 23: 695–720
9. Lawrence J C, Bull J P J Inst Mech Eng 1976; 5: 61–63
10. Arturson G J Burn Care Rehabil 1985; 6: 129–146

Table 6.1 Grid of approximate mortality probabilities (1965–70) for various combinations of age and area of burn. (Reproduced, with permission, from Bull (1971) Lancet 2, 1133–1134.)

Body area burned (%)	*Age (years)* 0–4	5–9	10–14	15–19	20–24	25–29	30–34	35–39	40–44	45–49	50–54	55–59	60–64	65–69	70–74	75–79	80+
93+	1	1	1	1	1	1	1	1	1	1	1	1	1	1	1	1	1
88–92	.9	.9	.9	.9	1	1	1	1	1	1	1	1	1	1	1	1	1
83–87	.9	.9	.9	.9	.9	.9	1	1	1	1	1	1	1	1	1	1	1
78–82	.8	.8	.8	.8	.9	.9	.9	.9	1	1	1	1	1	1	1	1	1
73–77	.7	.7	.8	.8	.8	.8	.9	.9	.9	1	1	1	1	1	1	1	1
68–72	.6	.6	.7	.7	.7	.8	.8	.8	.9	.9	.9	1	1	1	1	1	1
63–67	.5	.5	.6	.6	.6	.7	.7	.8	.8	.9	.9	1	1	1	1	1	1
58–62	.4	.4	.4	.5	.5	.6	.6	.7	.7	.8	.9	.9	1	1	1	1	1
53–57	.3	.3	.3	.4	.4	.5	.5	.6	.7	.7	.8	.9	1	1	1	1	1
48–52	.2	.2	.3	.3	.3	.3	.4	.5	.6	.6	.7	.8	.9	1	1	1	1
43–47	.2	.2	.2	.2	.2	.3	.3	.4	.4	.5	.6	.7	.8	1	1	1	1
38–42	.1	.1	.1	.1	.2	.2	.2	.3	.3	.4	.5	.6	.8	.9	1	1	1
33–37	.1	.1	.1	.1	.1	.1	.2	.2	.3	.3	.4	.5	.7	.8	.9	1	1
28–32	0	0	0	0	.1	.1	.1	.1	.2	.2	.3	.4	.6	.7	.9	1	1
23–27	0	0	0	0	0	0	.1	.1	.1	.2	.2	.3	.4	.6	.7	.9	1
18–22	0	0	0	0	0	0	0	.1	.1	.1	.1	.2	.3	.4	.6	.8	.9
13–17	0	0	0	0	0	0	0	0	0	.1	.1	.1	.2	.3	.5	.6	.7
8–12	0	0	0	0	0	0	0	0	0	0	.1	.1	.1	.2	.3	.5	.5
3–7	0	0	0	0	0	0	0	0	0	0	0	0	.1	.1	.2	.3	.4
0–2	0	0	0	0	0	0	0	0	0	0	0	0	0	.1	.1	.2	.2

oxidation of body fat.[11] This demand for energy is prolonged. Although energy losses by radiation and water evaporation can be modified by the local environmental conditions, septic complications, should they occur, further increase energy needs. Cold stress, temperature falls during surgery, pain and anxiety must be minimized wherever possible.

Infection is responsible for at least half the burn deaths. Colonization by endogenous organisms is seen within a week and the warm moist wound is an ideal culture medium for bacterial growth. The damage to the local circulation impairs the already weakened humoral and cellular defences. Reduced phagocytic activity and sluggish chemotaxis encourage invasive infection, and poor clearance of bacteria by the reticuloendothelial system worsens the situation.[12] The specific responses against antigens are similarly impaired. Immediate loss of immunoglobulins is usually transient, but bacterial endotoxins and peptides from damaged tissue act as immunosuppressive substances, impairing T lymphocyte and macrophage activity. Under such conditions opportunist yeasts and Gram-negative organisms thrive.[13] It is likely that organisms from the lumen of the bowel can translocate into the portal circula-tion and thence to the burn wound.[14] Selective decontamination of the gut has not proved helpful in burns as it fails to control methicillin-resistant strains of *Staphylococcus aureus* and *Acinetobacter* spp., but early enteral feeding with protein will reduce the likelihood of such translocation (see Chapter 2).

MANAGEMENT

First aid

Immediate immersion in cold water is the only effective form of first aid treatment, having both a quenching and analgesic effect. Emergency dressings of a plastic bag or plastic wrap for small areas, and wet dressings for larger areas, are useful and relieve pain. Such dressings should be quick to put on and both quick and painless to take off. No topical creams should be applied as a temporary first aid dressing.

Small burns

The great majority of burns can be treated on a simple outpatient basis. Small burns, of less than 5% body surface area, should have their blisters emptied but not removed. A simple Vaseline gauze layer is placed on the burn, covered with several thicknesses of real cotton gauze with an absorbent layer of real cotton wool, with everything held in place with a firm bandage. The dressing should be generous, should cover the wound thoroughly and should not slip. Repeated dressing changes will introduce bacteria and encourage infection and, by tearing off the new epithelium, will delay healing. The wound can be left undisturbed for 10 days, and if healing is not complete at 14 days, a skin graft should be seriously considered.

Larger burns

Resuscitation

Correction of fluid loss in small burns can be achieved orally using salt-containing fluids. Administration of large volumes of water will lead to hyponatraemia and water intoxication is a potentially serious complication, especially in children. Dioralyte, as used for the replacement of electrolyte loss in diarrhoea, is especially useful in children and, for adults, Moyer's solution (4 g NaCl plus 1.5 g

REFERENCES

11. Jahoor F, Desai M, Herndon D N, Wolfe R R Metabolism 1988; 37: 330–337
12. Heggers J P, Heggers P, Robson M C J Am Med Technol 1982; 44: 99–102
13. Pruitt B A, McManus A T Am J Med 1984; 76: 146–153
14. Deitch E A, Berg R J Burn Care Rehabil 1987; 8: 475–482

$NaHCO_3$ per litre of tap water) or a 1 g tablet of NaCl every hour together with 250 ml water has been recommended for mass casualties.

Burns involving greater than 10% of the body surface area in children, or greater than 15% of the body surface area in adults, require intravenous fluid resuscitation and with areas greater than 30% a rapid infusion is essential.

Many types of fluid regimens have been described and their adherents continue to engage in excited controversy. The principles involved have been elucidated by Settle.[15]

1. A fluid containing salt and water is required for 48 hours after the burn.
2. The total volume is between 2 and 4 ml/kg/% body surface area burn and should contain 0.5 mmol sodium/kg/% burn.
3. The total volume required can be reduced by the addition of colloid or by using hypertonic saline solutions.
4. Water loss through the burn wound varies according to the environment but when nursed in conventional dressings, metabolic water requirements are of the order of 1.5–2 ml/kg/per h, with a minimum of 30 ml/hour for infants.
5. Care must be taken to avoid overprovision of water with the development of hyponatraemia.

A burn resuscitation formula is only a guide to the average amount of fluid that is commonly required. It tends to be unreliable in the young, the elderly, in massive burns, multiple injuries and, when dealing with serious associated medical problems, formulae are of little help. The adequacy of fluid resuscitation must be monitored at frequent and regular intervals with rates of infusion altered appropriately. Monitoring is best kept as simple as possible and should include examination of the peripheral circulation, skin colour and warmth, pulse rate, blood pressure, core and peripheral temperature. Four-hourly haemoglobin and haematocrit levels and hourly readings of urinary output are extremely valuable. Invasive techniques are best avoided as venous access must be safeguarded, and central venous pressure readings are of no help or guidance in uncomplicated burns. Infusion rates aimed at maintaining a normal central venous pressure are very likely to lead to a significant fluid overload, particularly with colloid free solutions.

In general, one-half of the total volume required should be given in the first 12 hours after the burn. Metabolic water (50 ml/kg per 24 h) is given orally whenever possible.

Examples

In the Muir & Barclay plasma formula,[16] the 36 hours after the burn are divided into periods—three of 4 hours, two of 6 hours and one of 12 hours. The calculated volume of plasma is given in each individual period, according to the formula: 0.5 ml/kg/% burn period for plasma, or 0.65 ml/kg/% burn period for albumin (purified protein fraction is 98% albumin).

The Parkland formula[17] employs lactated Ringer's solution 4 ml/kg/% burn, half of which is given in the first 8 hours, and half in the next 16 hours. In the second 24 hours the volume required is 2 litres of 5% dextrose plus colloid (0.5 ml × % burn × kg). The large volumes of crystalloid cause widespread oedema, a paralytic ileus and often pulmonary overloading, but is argued that delaying colloid for 24 hours limits wasteful protein losses through inevitably leaking capillaries.

The Monafo formula[18] reduces the volumes of fluid administered by giving hyperosmolar solutions containing Na 300 mmol/l + lactate 200 mmol/l + Cl 100 mmol/l. About 3–3.5 ml/%/kg is required in 48 hours. Biochemical monitoring must be frequent and precise but it is claimed that oedema and lung problems are avoided.

Choice of formula[19]

Whichever formula is chosen depends upon prejudice and locally available resources. Crystalloids are cheap but plasma is very expensive and hard to obtain. Alternative colloids include large-molecular-weight dextrans and hetastarch, but the polygelines are excreted too rapidly to be reliable. A formula should be easy to understand and regular use will lead to increasing familiarity and confidence.

Blood transfusion

In deep burns 1 unit of blood should be given for every 10% deep burn but this does not need to be administered until the end of the 48-hour 'shock phase'. Increased fragility of the red cells is persistent with a decrease in their survival time. Furthermore, blood is lost steadily at dressing changes, operations and even repeated investigations, and attempts should be made to keep the haemoglobin levels above 10 g/dl.

COMPLICATIONS

Massive burns

In massive deep burns of greater than 80% body surface area, there is considerable breakdown of red cells with ensuing haemoglobinuria, large potassium loads and disseminated intravascular coagulation. Myocardial depressant factors limit cardiac output and it is unlikely that anything can be done to influence the outcome in such circumstances.

Deep burns

Myonecrosis with myoglobinuria can be expected in high-tension electrical burns, deep crushing burns and in any very deep burn that results in charring. Treatment should be directed at maintaining a high urinary output with a pH of about 6.5. Large volumes of fluid are required, with careful monitoring of the central venous pressure and serum potassium. Excision of the dead

REFERENCES

15. Settle J A D Proc R Soc Med 1982; 75 (suppl 1): 7–11
16. Muir I F K, Barclay T L Burns and their Treatment. Lloyd Luke, London 1962
17. Baxter C R, Parkland C Clin Plast Surg 1974; 1: 693–703
18. Monafo W W, Halverson J D, Schectman K Surgery 1984; 95: 129–135
19. Demling R H Surg Clin North Am 1987; 67: 15–22

tissue with generous decompression through fasciotomies of the surrounding tissue must be urgently performed.

Children

Children under 9 months of age lack the ability to concentrate urine fully and an output of 1.5 ml/kg per h should be maintained if possible. Inappropriate excretion of antidiuretic hormone can be a problem.[20] The early depletion of glycogen leads to rapid hypoglycaemia.

Hypovolaemia

Failure to respond to apparently adequate resuscitation is likely to be the result of myocardial depression, increased peripheral resistance and right ventricular dilation. Inotropes and the careful administration of blood and colloid will usually correct the situation, but plasma exchange has been recommended.[21]

Hypernatraemia

Unreplaced water losses through the eschar may result in dehydration with hypernatraemia and this is a particular problem in patients nursed on an air-fluidized bed. A surprising amount of intravenous dextrose water solution may be required to correct the situation.

Hyponatraemia

Water intoxication may have very serious effects in small children, with the development of cerebral oedema and convulsions, or burn encephalopathy, where neurological damage may become permanent.[22] This is usually the result of resuscitation with inappropriate volumes of hypotonic fluids, and may be seen after even very small burns in young children.[23] Therefore wherever possible metabolic requirements should be given orally.

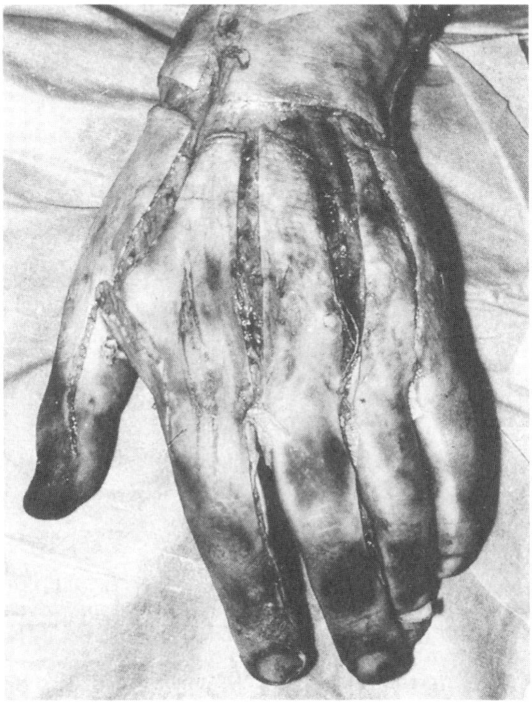

Fig 6.3 Escharotomy.

Gastrointestinal haemorrhage

Ileus can be avoided by the use of colloids, and early feeding, particularly with milk, has dramatically decreased stress ulceration and bleeding. H_2-antagonists are not routinely prescribed, but are valuable when feeding is delayed. Ulceration of the stomach and the upper small intestine is commonly found at post-mortem in those who have died from their burns.[24] Septic complications can be accompanied by steady or even massive gastrointestinal haemorrhage and surgery in these circumstances is extremely hazardous. Locating the site of haemorrhage is difficult as ulceration is often diffuse and superficial. Vagotomy and pyloroplasty is the most simple procedure but the incidence of recurrent bleeding is high. Partial or total gastrectomy should be reserved for patients with chronic or recurrent ulceration, but the operative mortality is significant.[25] Perforation of a stress ulcer in burns is thankfully very rare.[26]

Circumferential burns

Deep circumferential burns of the limbs or trunk produce a tourniquet effect as they dry, and therefore should be generously incised before the circulation or ventilation is impaired.[27] The escharotomy can be done at the bedside as deep burns are anaesthetic (Fig. 6.3). Incisions should be made on both sides of a limb, on the ulnar border of the fingers, and in a chequerboard fashion on the chest. Blood loss is considerable and blood transfusions, cautery, running sutures and firm dressings are usually required. Fasciotomies are rarely needed, although in very deep burns with charring and in most extensive electrical burns, a wide fasciotomy may limit muscle loss.

Burn diabetes

A pseudodiabetic, non-ketotic, hyperosmolar state is occasionally seen when there has been an overprovision of carbohydrate calories (see Chapter 2). Clinically there is marked dehydration from hyperglycaemia and glycosuria, but no keto-acids are found in the urine.[28] Treatment is by stopping the overfeeding, correcting water and electrolyte loss, and forcing glucose and potassium back into the cells with insulin.

REFERENCES

20. Crum R L, Dominic W et al Arch Surg 1990; 125: 1065–1070
21. Schnarrs R H, Cline C W et al J Burn Care Rehabil 1986; 7: 230–233
22. McManus W F, Hunt J L, Pruitt B A J Trauma 1974; 14: 396–401
23. Antoo A, Volpe J, Crawford J Pediatrics 1972; 50: 609–616
24. Curling T B, Trans R Med Clin Soc Lond 1842; 25: 260–281
25. Kirksey T D, Pruitt B A Am J Surg 1968 116: 627–633
26. McConnell C M, Hummel R P Burns 1981; 7: 203–207
27. Pruitt B A, Dowling J A, Moncrief J A Arch Surg 1968; 96: 502–507
28. Warden G D, Wilmore D, Rogers P, Mason A D, Pruitt B A Arch Surg 1972; 106: 420–425

Renal failure

Oliguria, seen as a falling volume of concentrated urine, usually indicates that fluid replacement therapy is inadequate and responds to a colloid challenge. Acute renal failure, although nowadays uncommon, is characterized by an inability to concentrate the urine. A reduction in urinary urea excretion and urine osmolality are diagnostic. Acute renal failure occurs when resuscitation has been delayed or when large amounts of haemoglobin or myoglobin have been released in very deep burns. A mannitol-induced diuresis is worth trying cautiously whilst monitoring the central venous pressure, but help from a renal physician with early haemodialysis is usually required.[29] Renal failure may be precipitated by septicaemia and nephrotoxic drugs, particularly amphotericin.

Septic thrombophlebitis and pulmonary embolus

The cannulation of peripheral veins, often through a cut-down, may lead to a purulent phlebitis with recurrent bacteraemias or septicaemias. Milking along the line of the vessel yields pus, and the infected vein should be removed through a long overlying skin incision which is not closed.[30] Massive pulmonary embolus is surprisingly very rare in burned patients, but septic microemboli associated with central vein cannulation are becoming more common. Long lines should be avoided and all intravascular cannulae must be re-sited every 72 hours to prevent septic thrombophlebitis developing.

Toxic shock syndrome

This alarming syndrome is seen rarely following small scalds in very young children. The onset is sudden with vomiting and diarrhoea and a temperature greater than 40°C, a diffuse macular rash which later desquamates, tachypnoea, oliguria, irritability, convulsions and coma. Typically developing on the third or fourth day, the signs are usually associated with a fall in the haemoglobin and white cell count. Toxic shock syndrome appears to be due to a toxin produced by *Staphylococcus aureus* phage type 29/52. Treatment must be prompt with control of temperature by vasodilatation, reduction of cerebral oedema, if necessary by hyperventilation, and the administration of whole blood, immunoglobulins and antibiotics.[31]

Burn wound colonization

For a short period after the injury the burn is sterile but inevitable contamination occurs within 48 hours if no topical antibacterial is used. The source of bacteria is frequently endogenous, but failure to control colonization, even with the most fastidious wound care, is a common and discouraging experience.

The burn wound is ideally suited to bacterial growth and it is often of enormous size. Colonization starts around hair follicles and soon extends below the eschar. It is common to find 10^3–10^5 bacteria per gram of eschar.[32] The bacteria are in a privileged position: they are isolated from topical antibacterials as these, with the exception of mafenide, do not penetrate well. Systemic antibiotics do not diffuse through necrotic tissue and have little effect on colony counts. Regular bacterial surveillance of the wound, nose and throat is essential.

Invasive infection

Invasive infection is often diagnosed in retrospect and a mixed growth of organisms is common. Greater than 10^6 organisms per gram of tissue increases the likelihood of invasive infection. Deterioration of the burn wound with an inflammatory flare, odour, areas of focal necrosis or obvious purulence are indications that significant burn wound sepsis has developed and that appropriate systemic antibiotics are urgently required.[33]

Staphylococcal invasion tends to be of rapid onset with a high fever, leucocytosis, disorientation, ileus and hypovolaemia.

Pseudomonal sepsis is usually more insidious with a subnormal temperature and a very low white cell and platelet count. Ecthyma gangrenosum, a virulent pseudomonal invasion of burned and occasionally unburned tissue with extensive vascular infarcts, carries a grave prognosis. *Acinetobacter* and *Streptococcus faecalis* infections are becoming more common and are difficult to treat as the organisms are frequently resistant to most commonly prescribed antibiotics. Colonization of the throat or wound with Lancefield group A, C and G haemolytic streptococci are clear indications for antibiotic therapy, as are invasive sepsis and septicaemia from these organisms.

Routine and regular bacterial sampling of the burn wound will suggest an appropriate antibiotic, yet these must be used sparingly. A narrow-spectrum bactericidal antibiotic, given in very high dosage, should be selected to treat the most likely organism. The addition of a second antibiotic may be considered after 24 hours, but broad-spectrum multi-agent therapy will result in superinfection and the rapid emergence of resistant strains. Systemic antibiotics must be accompanied by a thorough cleaning of the burn wound, if possible under a general anaesthetic, with daily or twice-daily changes of the dressing.[34]

Hypercatabolism

It is now appreciated that the body can destroy itself in trying to meet the enormous and persistent energy demands of the burn wound. Pain, cold stress, anaesthesia and infection all increase nutritional requirements and in most burns of more than 20% body surface area, supplementary feeding through a fine-bore nasogastric tube is necessary. The enteral route has definite advantages (see Chapter 2) and intravenous feeding should be avoided in view of the increased risk of septic complications. An aggressive feeding policy prevents weight loss and encourages the rapid healing of donor sites. It helps to combat infection and improves

REFERENCES

29. Hauben D J Burns 1988; 14: 113–114
30. Stein J M, Pruitt B A, N Engl J Med 1970; 282: 1452–1455
31. Cole R P, Shakespeare P G Burns 1990; 16: 221–224
32. McManus W F, Goodwin C W, Mason A D, Pruitt B A J Trauma 1981; 21: 3133–3138
33. Parks D H, Linares H, Thompson P D Surg Gynecol Obstet 1981; 153: 374–376
34. Robson M C Crit Care Clin 1988; 4: 281–298

Table 6.2 Average nutritional requirements in burned patients

Patients	*Calories*
Adults with burns of >20% body surface area	25 kcal/kg + 40 kcal/% burn
Children < 8 years	60 kcal/kg + 35 kcal/% burn
Protein	
3 g/kg + 1 g% burn	

tolerance to operations by diminishing morbidity and mortality, allowing earlier discharge from hospital.[35] There is experimental evidence that the presence of protein within the lumen of the gut helps maintain mucosal integrity and avoid bacterial translocation. Early feeding also eradicates the problem of stress ulceration, and it is therefore recommended that feeding starts as soon as possible.[36]

Numerous formulations of ready digested feeds are commercially available. An excellent alternative is the 35-egg-a-day diet introduced by Hirschowitz et al.[37] Cheap, sterile, easily obtainable and universally acceptable, the tedium of such a diet is relieved by the ingenuity of the nursing staff. Others manage with large amounts of dairy products, with a constant supply of cold milk at the bedside and persistent encouragement.

The actual nutritional requirements have been investigated by many[38,39] and average amounts are given in Table 6.2.

Sensible scheduling of operative procedures and dressing changes helps to keep the periods of perioperative starvation to a minimum. It is also important to avoid excess carbohydrate calories to minimize the risk of hyperosmosis, and the ratio of non-protein calories per gram of nitrogen should be kept to 100 or 120:1. Very high carbohydrate provision leads to the massive production of carbon dioxide, which places an exhausting load on the effort of respiration and sometimes ventilatory support is required.

Supplemental iron and vitamins are required throughout the hospital stay and zinc supplements are recommended in extensive burns in a dose of 20 mg zinc sulphate/kg per day.

Intravenous feeding is necessary during septic episodes and to cover periods when frequent operations are indicated. Access lines should be replaced at least every 72 hours.

MANAGEMENT OF THE BURN WOUND

Partial-thickness burns

Wounds that are likely to heal spontaneously need to be protected from bacterial colonization and this may be achieved by exposure in a warm, dry atmosphere which encourages a dry eschar to form (Fig. 6.4). The essential requirement is a dry wound as this is inhospitable to bacteria. If a moist surface still persists after 3 or 4 days, bacterial growth will progress and the wound must be dressed. The Qatari method of exposure, with daily baths in half normal saline, can produce excellent results with a remarkable recovery of the epithelium and surprisingly little hypertrophic scar.[40]

The alternative to exposure is treatment in dressings. Large wounds become rapidly contaminated and some antibacterial dressing is needed. Nearly all topical agents cause maceration, delay the spontaneous separation of the eschar and fail to sterilize the wound. At best they keep the bacterial inoculum down to reasonable levels.

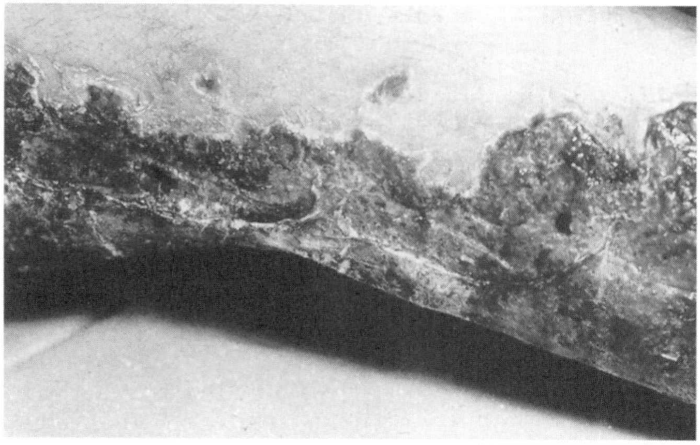

Fig 6.4 Exposed wound: dry eschar on leg, with no inflammation and no sign of infection.

Deep dermal burns and those of mixed depth

(Figs 6.5 and 6.6)

These burns are commonly treated conservatively. After 2 weeks the partial-thickness elements will have healed and under a general anaesthetic remaining areas can be shaved down with a skin graft knife and immediately grafted. Janzekovic[41] introduced a more aggressive approach, and this has now been adopted widely. On the third or fourth post-burn day, before there is significant bacterial contamination, all burned areas are shaved down to a healthy bleeding layer. The undoubted advantages are preservation of dermis with better cosmetic and functional results, less loss of skin grafts from sepsis and a more rapid rehabilitation. The technique requires considerable care and experience and can result in heavy blood loss. When practised on large areas it is hazardous and meticulous excision of all tissues of doubtful viability, careful graft application and attention to dressings are critical.[42]

Full-thickness burns

There is clearly no point in waiting for full-thickness burns to heal spontaneously and they should be excised and closed with a skin graft as soon as it is practicable. Excision down to deep fascia helps to diminish blood loss and permits better graft adherence, although at the expense of a marked long-term cosmetic deformity.

A conservative approach in the elderly and infirm is sometimes reasonable, with a policy of active mobilization and daily dressings

REFERENCES

35. Alexander J W, MacMillan B G et al Beneficial effects of aggressive protein feeding in severely burned children. Ann Surg 1980; 192: 505–517
36. Henley M Burns 1989; 15: 351–361
37. Hirschowitz J W, Brook J G, Kaufmann T, Titelman U, Mahler D Br J Plast Surg 1975 28: 185–188
38. Pasulka P S, Wachtel T L Surg Clin North Am 1987; 67: 109–131
39. Curreri P W J Trauma 1990; 30 (suppl): S20–S23
40. Al-Baker A, El-Ekiabi S, Ghanem A, Al-Ggoul A Burns 1984; 10: 355–362
41. Janzekovic Z J Trauma 1970; 10: 1103–1108
42. Burke J F, Bondoc C C, Quinby W C J Trauma 1974; 14: 389–395

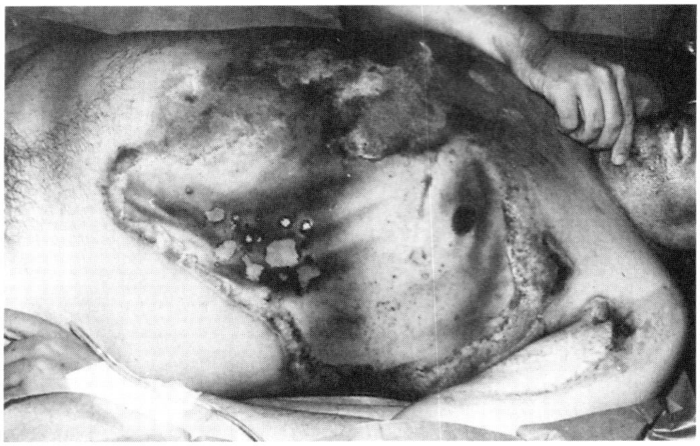

Fig 6.5 Deep burn: a flame with smoke staining over the left flank, with no blistering and analgesia to pinprick.

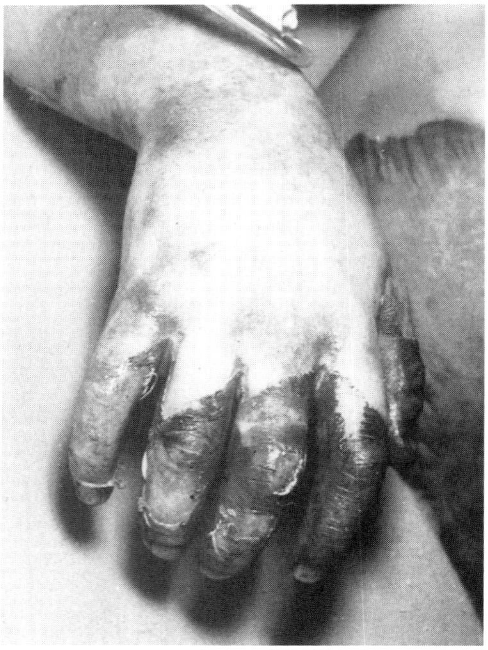

Fig 6.6 Deep dermal burn: blister removed showing white base.

until there is spontaneous separation of the eschar. Delayed thin split-skin grafting is then carried out on the prepared granulation tissue and the trauma of surgical excision and blood loss is avoided.[43]

Topical applications

Silver sulphadiazine[44] is a widely used topical antibiotic; it is a cream which is comfortable to apply and remove, with a good spectrum against Gram-negative organisms. Silver nitrate (0.5%) soaks[45] are very useful when started before the onset of infection, although not popular because they cause inconvenient staining, require frequent dressing change and result in chloride loss. Mafenide,[46] although never widely used because of pain and carbonic anhydrase inhibition, penetrates the eschar deeply and can be applied as a cream or a solution. Povidone-iodine and

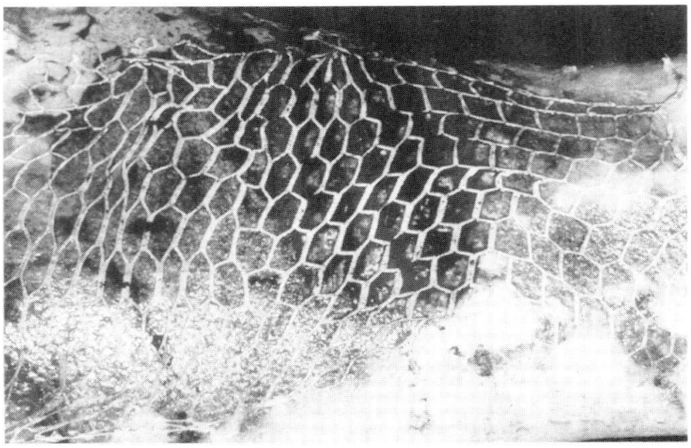

Fig 6.7 Mesh graft.

chlorhexidine have their advocates but are not widely used on large burns. Cerium sulphadiazine[47] has the effect of tanning the wound; a layer of calcium precipitates in the eschar delaying spontaneous separation by minimizing sepsis. It is very useful in the treatment of deep dermal and deep burns, and allows a more leisurely approach to burn wound excision.

Wet dressings of phenoxytol or hypochlorite[48] are of great benefit in dealing with areas of graft loss from infection. They need to be changed very frequently and must be accompanied by surgical excision of necrotic tissue. Nitrofurazone-impregnated dressings[49] encourage a neo-eschar to form and keep the wound dry whilst still having a good antibacterial spectrum. Hydrocortisone/oxytetracycline ointment is invaluable for controlling areas of exuberant granulation tissue.

WOUND CLOSURE

Skin grafts should be thin to allow early healing of the donor sites and thus early cropping. Meshed grafts expanded 1:1.5, 1:3 or even 1:6 will take on oozing or infected wounds, and are very helpful when large areas have to be covered (Fig. 6.7). They need to be covered with greasy or medicated dressings so that they do not dry out. Sheet grafts should be placed on the hands and face to provide the best cosmetic result.

In extensive burns critical areas such as the hands, the flexor surfaces of the elbows, knees and neck should be excised and grafted as early as possible. Similarly, areas where grafts are most likely to take, such as the chest, abdomen, forearms and thighs,

REFERENCES

43. Cadier M A, Shakespeare P G Burns 1995; 21: 200–204
44. Fox C L Arch Surg 1968; 96: 184–188
45. Moyer C A, Brentano L, Gravens D F, Margraf H W, Monafo W W Arch Surg 1965; 90: 812–867
46. Kucan J O, Smoot E C J Burn Care Rehabil 1993; 14: 158–163
47. Boeckx W, Blondeel Ph N, Vandersteen K, De Wolf-Peeters C, Schmitz A Burns 1992; 18: 456–462
48. Heggars J P, Zazy J A, et al J Burn Care Rehabil 1991; 12: 420–424
49. Moncrief J A Clin Plast Surg 1974; 1: 563–576

should receive priority. Blood loss following the excision of large areas of burnt tissue will be rapid, often dramatic, and often difficult to control, although diathermy and sutures are useful. Early blood replacement with large volumes of warmed blood is important, together with intravenous calcium and cryoprecipitate.

Allograft skin has been used as a temporary wound cover for many years. Burke et al[50] immunosuppressed their patients and were able to prolong allograft take with outstanding results in children. Immunosuppression of the graft using ultraviolet light has also extended allograft survival from 20 to 80 days. The Chinese have placed large sheets of allograft on the excised burn before seeding them with tiny transplants of autograft skin. The autoepidermis invades the allodermis and complete wound closure occurs before there is widespread rejection.[51] A further and very useful variation, introduced by Alexander and colleagues,[52] is to cover widely expanded (6 : 1) autograft with less widely expanded allograft. Wound closure is achieved as the sandwich adheres and is rapidly revascularized. The autograft, being protected by the allograft, spreads quickly and replaces the allograft layer without the process of graft rejection developing. Particular caution must be taken with the selection of allograft donors as it is possible to transmit human immunodeficiency virus to the graft recipient.[53] Allograft skin should therefore be reserved for life-threatening burns and the donor chosen from a close member of the family, or skin obtained from a reputable skin bank.

The ability to grow keratinocytes in the tissue culture laboratory has led to their use in burns. However, such thin layers of epidermal cells are naturally delicate, take very poorly and do not prevent alarming contraction of the wound.[54] Until some way of incorporating keratinocytes with an artificial or synthetic dermis has been developed and found to be reliable, these tissue culture methods will not be of practical value.[55] Enthusiasm for biological dressings, for example amnion and pigskin, has been tempered by experience, and their only real uses are in the relief of pain in superficial burns, keeping granulation tissue clean and ready for grafting. Banked allograft and glycerol-treated skin[56] are widely used and are of particular value in protecting the interstices of widely expanded meshed graft.

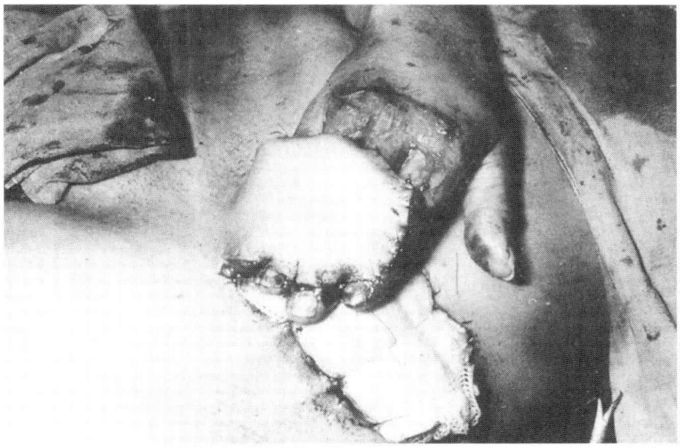

Fig 6.8 Groin flap used on hand to cover exposed tendons. A hot press injury.

Many artificial skins and temporary burn wound dressings have been described, from polyurethane foam to potato skins. They may be of value in cleaning a burn wound in preparation for grafting, or in maintaining the wound in a state of readiness for grafting. Their adherence is the important factor in keeping the number of bacteria down, as is the frequency of the dressing changes.

Skin graft donor sites

Thin skin grafts should be used in burned patients as they take well and their donor site heal within 2 weeks and can be recropped 1 week later. In the largest burns the scalp is an excellent source of skin; thin grafts will not be hair-bearing and the donor site heals very quickly and comfortably. Usual sites for skin graft harvesting are the thighs, abdomen and the back. They are traditionally dressed with tulle gras, cotton gauze and an absorbent layer of wool, and are ideally left until they can be soaked off in a bath after 2 weeks. Vapour-permeable dressings are excellent for dressing smaller areas.

BURNS OF SPECIAL AREAS

Hands

Superficial and dermal burns of the hand are best treated by placing them in a plastic bag which contains silver sulphadiazine or a similar antiseptic. Pain is immediately relieved and elevation and early movements diminish oedema. The bags need to be changed daily.[57] Deep dermal burns respond well to early tangential excision at day 3 or 4.[58] An experienced surgeon can shave the burn under a tourniquet and immediate cover with a thin split-skin graft allows rapid return of function with little or no hypertrophic scarring.

Superficial burns can be left for 14 days, but if not healed by then they should be grafted. Deep burns need a more aggressive approach. Some shortening of the finger will be inevitable if the finger nails have come away as there has usually been deep damage to the vascular pedicle. Exposed tendons and joints need to be covered with a pedicled flap of skin (Fig. 6.8) or fascia, and the joints should be immobilized with Kirschner wires.[59] All hand burns that are grafted need to be immobilized with the wrist at 45° in dorsiflexion, the fingers in full extension and the metacarpophalangeal joints at 90° of flexion. The thumb web should be fully abducted (Fig. 6.9).

REFERENCES

50. Burke J F, Bondoc C C, Quinby W C J Trauma 1974; 14: 389–395
51. Chih-Chun Y, Tsi-Siang S, Te-An C, Wei-Shia H, Shou-Yen K, Yen-Fei C Burns 1980; 6: 141–145
52. Alexander J W, Macmillan B W, Law E, Kittur D S J Trauma 1981; 21: 433–441
53. Clarke J A Lancet 1987; 1: 983
54. Eldad A, Burt A, Clarke J A Burns 1987; 13: 173–180
55. Sheridan R L, Tompkins R G J Trauma 1995; 38: 48–50
56. Kreis R W, Vloemans R F P M et al J Trauma 1989; 29: 51–54
57. Syke P J, Bailey B N Burns 1975; 2: 162–168
58. Hunt J L, Sato R, Baxter C R Ann Surg 1979; 189: 147–151
59. Nuchtern J G, Engrav L H, Nakamura C T R, Dutcher K A, Heimbach D M, Vedder N B J Burn Care Rehabil 1995; 16: 36–42

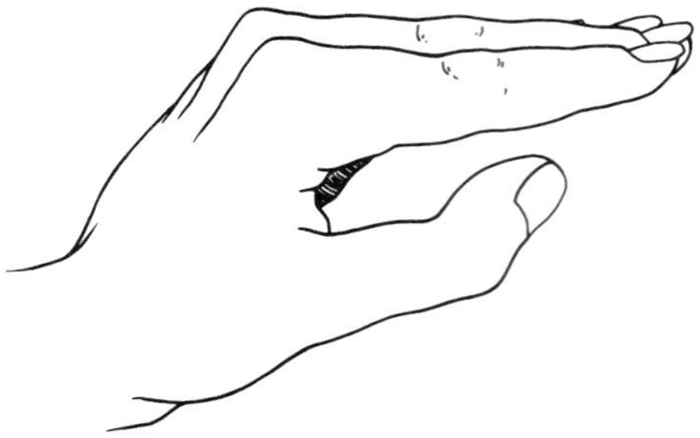

Fig 6.9 Hand position: 45° flexion at wrist, 90° flexion at metacarpophalangeal joint, with full extension at the fingers.

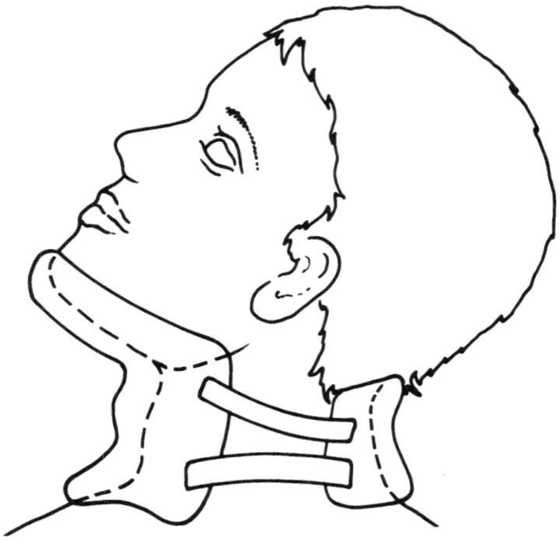

Fig 6.10 Collar to hold neck in extension in the treatment of burns of the neck.

Face

Many burns of the face heal well as the skin and its adnexae are thick and well-vascularized. Deeper burns, although they heal spontaneously, may develop severe hypertrophic scarring. The eyes, nostrils and ears should be kept as clean as possible and free from crusts and loose scabs. Early excision and grafting can give good results, as can light shaving and cover with allograft skin. Sheet skin grafts should be applied to cover cosmetically important sites. One sheet is used to cover the whole cheek, another to cover the whole nose, with the graft margins lying between the anatomical planes. Pressure over burned ears must be avoided and signs of suppurative perichondritis—pain, loss of the definition of the sulcus behind the ear and swelling of the ear itself—demand surgical drainage and removal of damaged cartilage.

Neck

Burns involving the anterior neck should be treated by removing the pillow from beneath the patient's head, and replacing it behind the shoulders to maintain hyperextension of the neck (Fig. 6.10). Grafting is carried out early and followed by prolonged splintage. Failure to re-surface the neck quickly results in rapid contracture and increasing difficulty for the anaesthetist. Two sheets of skin should be used, one to re-surface the horizontal area beneath the chin and the other to replace the vertical area of the neck.

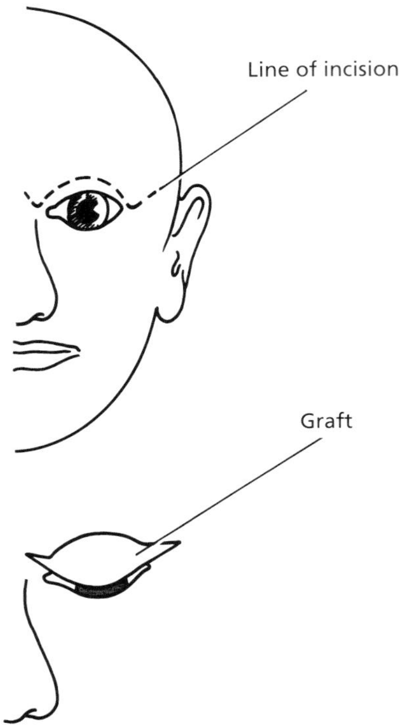

Fig 6.11 Incision and split-skin grafting to correct ectropion of upper eyelid.

Burns involving the eyelids

Flame burns and flash burns rarely damage the cornea, but with deep burns of the lids there can be early loss of corneal cover: exposure keratitis as a severe problem (see Chapter 15). There is no place for a tarsorrhaphy in the treatment of such burns as the sutures cut through the lid margins. At the first sign of an inability to cover the cornea, an incision should be made into the burn near the lash margin of the upper lid (Fig. 6.11). Dissection is continued superficially beneath the eschar, accompanied by downwards traction, until complete release of the lid is achieved. The incision will have to extend beyond the medial and lateral canthi and the defect needs to be closed with a thin skin graft, and splinted with a stent. It may be necessary to repeat the incision and grafting before the tendency to contract has ceased.[60]

Ectropion of the lower lid (see Chapter 15) is uncomfortable but does not place the eye at risk from exposure keratitis. It is corrected by a lash margin incision, again extending beyond the canthi, but is closed with a thick partial-thickness skin graft or post auricular Wolfe graft.[61]

Burns associated with fractures, or exposed bone

Every effort should be made to immobilize limb fractures as soon as possible after the burn. Intramedullary nailing and internal

REFERENCES

60. Schofield A L Br J Plast Surg 1954; 7: 67–91
61. Converse J M, Smith B Plast Reconstr Surg 1959; 23: 21–26

fixation can be done safely and without great risk of infection if performed within 24 hours of injury. External fixation carries an obvious, but in practice minor, increase in the risk of pin track infection, yet allows the patient to be nursed comfortably, making dressing changes and skin grafting relatively straightforward.[62] Where the skull is exposed, excision of the outer table usually reveals a vascular bed capable of supporting a skin graft, but smaller areas of exposed and dead bone should be covered with a local or distant skin or a muscle flap, encouraging revascularization and slow replacement of the bone.

Heterotopic calcification

Periarticular bone formation can develop in patients with extensive burns but its cause remains unknown. It is seen most frequently in extensive burns, particularly where there has been a prolonged period of immobilization, but occasionally occurs in areas that were not burned. The joint most commonly involved is the elbow where the olecranon fossa becomes obliterated, blocking extension. Anterior joint deposits may occur in more severe cases and similar changes are seen around the hip, but the shoulder is rarely involved. Physiotherapy worsens the condition if passive movements are allowed beyond the painfree limit. Treatment is limited to encouraging active exercises and excision of the bone when it is radiologically mature. Early surgical intervention, when the calcification is of toothpaste consistency, is followed by early recurrence. Formal surgical excision many months after the wounds have healed, followed by vigorous physiotherapy, produces a very worthwhile improvement.[63]

Hypertrophic scarring

Many burns, especially those that have taken longer than 3 weeks to heal, leave the patient with thick livid hypertrophic scars. They are frequently confused with keloid scars but they always fade spontaneously, in contrast with true keloids. The scars are hard, red and very itchy, and are best treated with custom-made elastic pressure garments, worn 24 hours a day, until the symptoms are relieved and the scars start to fade. It is common for children to wear such garments for 18–24 months as their scars are often particularly florid.[64] Such therapy helps to control the itching and lessens the need for secondary surgery, but must be supervised regularly and is of course expensive. Hypertrophic scars in some areas such as the neck and axilla prove difficult to control and early surgery is often required to allow room for normal growth.

Livid hypertrophic scarring of the face is best managed with a close-fitting, custom-made, transparent flexible mask, moulded from a plaster cast. Such masks are worn continuously, except at meal times, and will control itching almost immediately.[65]

Burn contractures

Ideally, surgery to relieve contractures should wait until the scar tissue is mature, pale, soft and tissue-papery. The contractures are caused by a tissue deficit which is usually much larger than first appreciated. Skin has therefore to be introduced as either a free graft of thick split skin or as a flap. Grafts will contract and need to be splinted for months. Thick flaps of adjacent skin and fatty tissue can be raised at fascial level and transposed across the line of the contracture. Such flaps do not contract, do not have to be splinted and are to be preferred. The reconstructive surgery of burned patients is prolonged and multi-staged, and is best carried out in specialist centres.

INHALATIONAL INJURIES

Nowadays the commonest cause of early death after burn injuries is the damage done to the lungs by the toxic products of incomplete combustion. Hydrogen cyanide from polyurethanes induces rapid tissue hypoxia, and hydrochloric acid from polyvinyl chloride and aldehydes from wood are very irritant when absorbed on to soot particles. Reactions within bronchioles and alveoli cause direct chemical damage. Carbon monoxide, which binds 250 times more avidly than oxygen with haemoglobin, leads to rapid deprivation of tissue oxygen. 0.1% Carbon monoxide in the inspired air binds with 60% of the available haemoglobin. Severe headache develops early followed by irritablility, confusion and convulsions.[66,67] High concentrations of carbon dioxide at the scene of the fire stimulate hyperventilation which, together with paroxysmal coughing, accelerates hypoxia and the inhalation of noxious gases.

Little thermal damage occurs to the bronchial tree below the carina except following the inhalation of superheated steam when heat damage can extend down to the terminal bronchioli and alveoli. The irritation and chemical damage of the respiratory tract cause intense bronchospasm, bronchorrhoea and sputum trapping; epithelium can slough off and separate as a cast, and there is often massive hyperaemia of the whole respiratory tract. Chemical damage to the alveoli, with exposure of the alveolar basement membrane and a widespread increase in capillary permeability, leads to a loss of protein-rich fluid into the lung tissues. Chemotactic factors trap neutrophils, releasing proteolytic enzymes which increase alveolar damage. A picture of progressive pulmonary failure, arteriovenous shunting, interstitial oedema and hypercarbia develops.[68] Several clinical presentations are seen.

1. Acute pulmonary insufficiency of early and rapid onset, which is usually fatal.
2. Oedema of the upper airways with deep burns of the face and chest.
3. Pulmonary oedema presenting at 24–72 hours.
4. Limited respiratory excursion caused by circumferential deep burns of the chest.
5. Bronchopneumonia at 5–7 days.

REFERENCES

62. Curtis M J, Clarke J A Injury 1989; 20: 333–336
63. Evans E B Clin Orthop 1991; 263: 94–101
64. Ward R S, J Burn Care Rehabil 1991; 12: 257–262
65. Powell B W E M, Haylock C, Clarke J A Br J Plast Surg 1985; 38: 561–566
66. Kinsella J Burns 1988; 14: 269–279
67. Boutros A R, Hoyt J L Crit Care Med 1976; 4: 144–147
68. Herndon D N, Barrow R E et al Burns 1988; 14: 349–356

6. Power failure, or chest wall fatigue, where the massive carbon dioxide load from serious infection or the overgenerous supply of replacement carbohydrates leads to an inability to cope with a greatly increased minute volume.

Diagnosis and treatment

A history of being trapped in an enclosed space should arouse suspicion of inhalational burns; fibreoptic bronchoscopy, chest X-ray and blood gas estimations may confirm lung damage.

The head end of the bed should be raised by 30° to minimize cerebral effects and to avoid an increase in intrathoracic pressure, which adversely affects cardiac output. Humidified gases are essential to keep secretions moist and lavage with small amounts of saline, regular tracheal suction and physiotherapy helps to remove mucus. It is wise to increase inspired oxygen levels to 100% immediately before and after suction. Increased restlessness following adequate resuscitation usually indicates hypoxia, which can usually be confirmed by a Pulse oximeter. Arterial blood gases should be monitored and any bronchospasm treated with salbutamol, given intravenously or as an insufflation. Falling carbon dioxide levels followed by falling oxygen levels indicate the need for ventilatory support, and prompt endotracheal intubation, thorough bronchial toilet and physiotherapy are vital. The inspired oxygen tension should be kept as low as feasible to avoid toxicity and artificial ventilation should be discontinued as rapidly as practicable. There is no evidence that prophylactic antibiotic therapy is useful, yet the spread of organisms contaminating the burn surface into the lung can occur within 24 hours. The mortality from endotracheal intubation, and even more from tracheostomy, is significant.[69]

ELECTRICAL BURNS

An electrical current is the flow of electrons, amperage is the rate of this flow and voltage is the driving force, which can be direct or alternating. The damage done to tissues is influenced by their resistance (measured in ohms), the voltage applied, the time of the exposure and the cross-sectional area of the tissues through which the current passed. The skin resistance of the palm may be 1 000 000 ohms/cm^2; of dry skin 5000 ohms/cm^2, and of wet skin 1000 ohms/cm^2. Skin and bone offer the most resistance with the current thus flowing electively through muscles, nerves and blood vessels.[70] In high-tension injuries of greater than 1000 volts there is charring at the point of entry, an explosive wound at the point of exit and usually gross muscle damage in between. Massive amounts of heat are generated with thrombosis of the smaller nutrient vessels, whereas larger vessels with high flow rates tend to survive. Such damaged tissues may take hours to cool.

Alternating domestic currents may cause tetanic spasms, trapping the victim against the source and even causing muscle ruptures or fractures. Current passing across the chest can cause fatal disturbances of cardiac conduction and rhythm, yet conversely it may arc, jumping externally from one surface to another, with enough energy to vaporize tissue.

Early or late spinal cord injuries can occur in which motor signs are often more marked than sensory loss, although peripheral nerves appear to withstand both direct and alternating currents well and a surprising amount of spontaneous recovery can be anticipated. Perforation of viscera and the late development of cataracts have also been described.

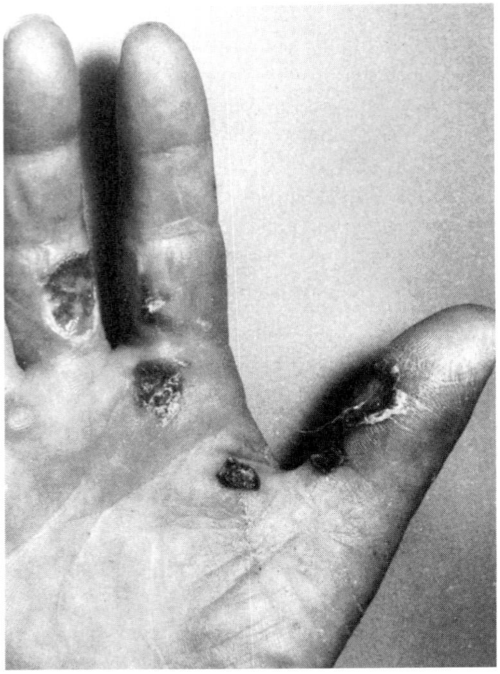

Fig 6.12 Small punctate electrical burns.

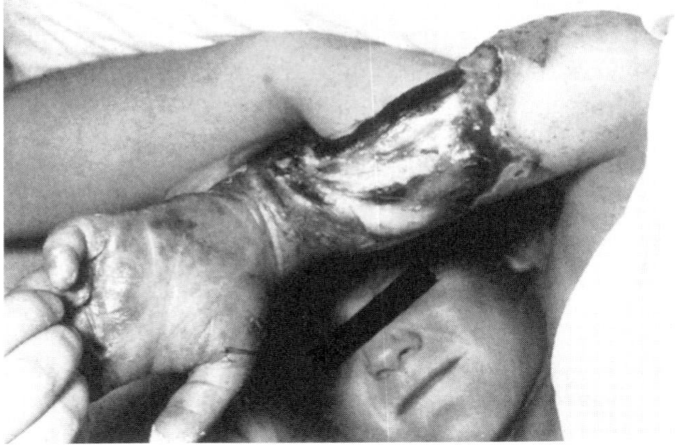

Fig 6.13 Electrical burn. Amputation is required.

Electrical injuries are always deep and slow to heal. Small punctate hand burns (Fig. 6.12) of less than 2 cm diameter may be covered with zinc oxide tape which is changed daily by the patient. Normal movements are maintained and healing is without complications. Larger hand burns require early excision with cover of exposed structures with a flap (Fig. 6.13). Where the contact point overlies muscle, a small skin defect may mask more extensive muscular damage, and in high-tension injuries this is usually massive. Large fluid volumes are required to correct losses of

REFERENCES

69. Rue L W, Cioffi W G, et al Arch Surg 1993; 128: 772–780
70. Bingham H Clin Plast Surg 1986; 13: 75–85

plasma and red cells, and to maintain a high urinary output, thereby eradicating haemoglobin and myoglobin pigments. Acidosis should be corrected with bicarbonate: an alkaline urine is produced by these pigments, and urine alkalinity is not therefore a reliable guide for monitoring treatment. Escharotomies and fasciotomies need to be carried out urgently to decompress tissues, and excisions of dead or doubtful tissue should be repeated frequently. Flap repair to cover exposed tendons, bones and neurovascular structures offers the only hope of salvage, and revascularization of the hand can be achieved using microvascular techniques. An aggressive approach is usually rewarding as serious wound infection and gross scarring complicate delay. Secondary haemorrhage does occur after electrical injuries, although it is very unusual in uncomplicated thermal burns.

Flash burns

The flash from an electric arc has a temperature of about 4000°C and lasts a tenth of a second. It causes superficial burns unless clothing is ignited and no electricity passes through the body, although the victim may be thrown some distance. The speed of the blink reflex protects the cornea.

Lightning injuries

The spectrum of lightning injuries varies from fatal cardiac, cerebral or visceral injuries to transitory superficial marking of the skin. Two-thirds of the victims survive. Some 95% of lightning injuries result from a negatively charged downward flash to earth followed by a positively charged return flash from earth, and multiple flashes can occur. The course of the current will be influenced by atmospheric humidity, wet clothes, local contacts to earth and neighbouring conductors. Direct entry through the body or spread over the surface of the skin (a flashover) are the most frequent types seen. The characteristic, transitory, fern-like or fractal pattern may be caused by a secondary positive flashover from an adjacent object.[71]

The clinical presentation is varied. The major cause of death is from cardiac asystole, ventricular fibrillation or apnoea. Cardiopulmonary massage is worth continuing for up to 1 hour as fixed dilated pupils in these injuries do not always indicate irreversible cerebral damage. Cutaneous burns tend to be relatively small and superficial, but a paralytic ileus is frequent and may take several days to correct itself. Cataracts may develop after some years.

CHEMICAL BURNS

Acid and alkali burns

Acid burns cause tissue damage by coagulative necrosis (Fig. 6.14). Their action is rapid and relatively short-lived, whereas alkali burns are much more penetrating, and their effects are more prolonged (Fig. 6.15). Lavage with water restores the pH of acid burns to normal within 30 minutes, but in alkaline burns the pH remains raised for many hours. First aid treatment is therefore vital and consists of simply immersing the affected part under running water. No time should be spent in searching for a chemical antidote as this leads to delay and the exothermic chemical reaction adds thermal damage to the underlying chemical injury.[72]

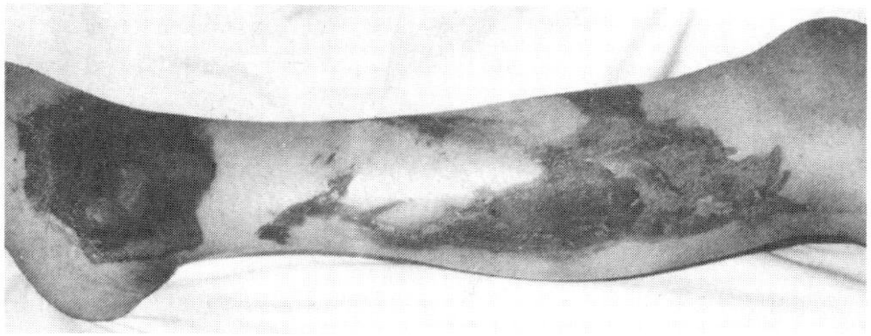

Fig 6.14 Acid burn: coagulative necrosis.

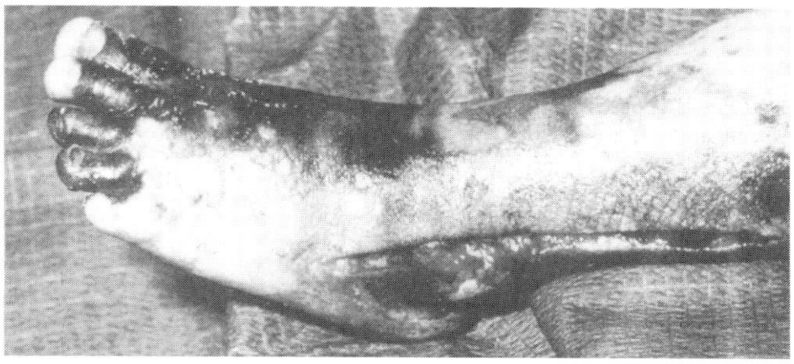

Fig 6.15 Alkali burn: colliquative necrosis.

Insensibility to pinprick indicates that the burn is deep and it should therefore be excised and grafted. Where first aid was delayed, particularly with alkali burns, the slough should be excised down to an apparently healthy level, the wound dressed and re-inspected, and if necessary re-excised 48 hours later.[73]

Hydrofluoric acid burns

Hydrofluoric acid, widely used in the electronics and chemical industries, is very corrosive and toxic.[74] The fluoride ion penetrates the skin, causing intense pain and progressive damage which may even extend down to bone. Treatment is again by thorough irrigation followed by calcium gluconate ointment repeatedly rubbed into the affected areas. Injections of subcutaneous calcium gluconate have been recommended, but it is possible that this might in turn cause further tissue damage.

Cement burns

Cement is mainly calcium oxide with a small amount of free lime. Calcium hydroxide produced after hydration can cause superficial or deep dermal burns when applied to the skin for several hours. The injuries are seen most commonly with ready mixed concrete where the pH is often between 11 and 13. The burns usually involve the legs and are best shaved down to a healthy bleeding level and covered with a thin split-skin graft, otherwise healing will be prolonged.[75]

REFERENCES

71. ten Duis H J, Klasen H J, Nijsten M W N Burns 1987; 13: 141–146
72. Saydari R, Abston S, Desai M H, Herdon D N J Burn Care Rehabil 1986; 7: 404–408
73. Sawney C P, Kaushish R Burns 1989; 15: 132–135
74. Sheridan R L, Ryan C M, Quinby W C, Blair J, Tompkins R G Burns 1995; 21: 62–64
75. Wilson G R, Davidson P M Burns 1985; 12: 139–145

7 Principles in the management of major trauma

Brian J. Rowlands   Aires A. B. Barros D'Sa

INTRODUCTION

Once confined to the battlefield, major trauma has now become commonplace in most modern societies. The increasing prevalence of serious physical injury over the last three decades coincides with rapid technological advances, the proliferation of motor vehicles and the growth of vast industrialized conurbations. Endemic criminal violence, sustained terrorism and indiscriminate assault on a civil population by sophisticated weaponry and explosive devices add to the problem in some well recognized locations.

Major trauma is an important cause of mortality and permanent disability in the younger population, and has obvious economic implications in terms of provision of medical services and lost working days. While education and legislation contribute to prevention, adequate staffing and facilities must be provided in order to save life, limit disability and rehabilitate the injured. A heightened awareness of the problem is reflected by a greater interest in the clinical management of trauma and research into improving treatment. This has in turn aroused the interest of government and has caught the attention of the media, by highlighting the lack of adequate organization of emergency medical services into a comprehensive system.

Terms used to describe major trauma include 'multiple injuries', 'critical trauma', 'multitrauma' or 'polytrauma', all of which cover the infinite permutations of injuries that can occur in the individual patient. By definition, major trauma is severe and complex, with injuries to one or more body cavities and two or more extremities which together may endanger life. Death occurring soon after injury is from respiratory, circulatory and neurological failure, but in those who survive the initial stages sepsis and multiple organ dysfunction and failure are the major causes of mortality.[1–3]

Improvements in the outcome of victims of major trauma are attributable to a variety of factors: increasing knowledge of the pathophysiology of trauma, rapid rescue by well equipped ambulances and helicopters, implementation of triage, energetic resuscitation at the scene and en route to designated trauma centres by a trained team of medical, nursing and ancillary personnel, the advent of computerized tomography and magnetic resonance imaging in delineating injury to specific organs, early definitive surgery, precise monitoring and intensive care, prophylactic mechanical ventilation, prevention of sepsis, nutritional support and rehabilitation.

HISTORY (see Chapter 1)

In ancient civilizations in Egypt and Greece and thereafter in the early Christian era, physicians like Celsus, Galen and others were principally concerned with the control of life-threatening haemorrhage and the simple treatment of wounds. Little progress was made for a millennium and a half, until Ambroise Pare ligated bleeding vessels and cleansed rather than cauterized battle wounds. In the early 19th century, Baron Jean Larrey, chief surgeon to Napoleon Bonaparte, introduced new concepts which still persist: firstly, the ambulance volant or flying hospital which significantly reduced the time between injury and treatment, and secondly, a casualty treatment area close to the front line with graded levels of surgical care.

The mechanization of societies in the wake of the Industrial Revolution caused the types of accidents and injuries which still occur today. By the end of the 19th century the discoveries of bacteria, mechanisms of infection, antisepsis, anaesthesia and blood grouping techniques had quite fortuitously prepared the combatants in World War I to deal with the unprecedented volume of major trauma. Despite these advances, the conservative management of open fractures of the femur had a mortality rate of 80%, dropping dramatically to 10% when formal wound excision and the Thomas splint were introduced. In addition, an understanding of the pathophysiology of shock and the life-saving value of plasma transfusion were signal advances that were largely nullified by a prolonged evacuation time of 12–18 hours, resulting in a mortality of 8.5%. Based on his wartime experience, Lorenz Bohler, father of modern accident surgery, established a hospital in Vienna which was famed for its organization and innovative surgical techniques in treating patients with occupational injuries.

In World War II, the provision of facilities for the primary care of the injured behind the battlelines, by staff responsible for eventual evacuation, lowered the mortality rate to 5.8%, despite an evacuation time of 6–12 hours. In 1941, the Queen's Hospital in Birmingham, under the directorship of William Gissane, became the first British accident hospital dedicated to the management of

REFERENCES

1. Baue A E Arch Surg 1975; 110: 779
2. Fry D E In: Carter D, Polk H C (eds) Trauma, vol 1. Butterworths, London 1981
3. Olerud S, Aligower M World J Surg 1983; 7: 143

industrial injuries and air-raid casualties. Despite the deserved worldwide reputation of this hospital for its contributions to the pathophysiology, treatment and prevention of major injury, little effort was made to open similar centres elsewhere in the country and this hospital has now closed. During the Korean conflict, various factors led to a reduction in the mortality rate to 2.4%: a shortened evacuation time of 2–4 hours, transportation by helicopter, volume fluid replacement in resuscitation of haemorrhagic shock and routine antibiotic prophylaxis. The type of warfare in Vietnam resulted in a greater loss of life, but the mortality rate remained unchanged at 2.6% for those admitted within 3 hours and 1.7% for those seen in less than 65 minutes. Once more this improvement was attributable to evacuation by air, perioperative volume replacement and an organized system of optional transfer to first-, second- or third-echelon stations of trauma care.[4] A new development described as the 'systems approach' was introduced in the regional care of major trauma at the Maryland Institute for Emergency Medical Services in Baltimore[5] and at the Cook County Hospital, Chicago.[6] The concurrent successes observed at these hospitals and in Vietnam were a product of swift helicopter evacuation and treatment by qualified personnel using modern equipment for monitoring and support and applying structured protocols which have since served as excellent models for trauma centres elsewhere.

A better understanding of the metabolic response to trauma[7–9] and an enlightened approach to the value of nutritional support in the surgical patient[10] represented further progress, especially as it became apparent that protein malnutrition was a key feature of multiple organ dysfunction. Mechanical ventilators tuned to the requirements of the critically injured patient, incorporating the benefits of positive end-expiratory pressure, were developed.[11] The introduction of the Glasgow Coma Scale,[12] the application of non-invasive computerized tomographic scanning[13] and mechanical ventilation[14] represented three major advances in the management of patients with central nervous system injury. The practice of diagnostic peritoneal lavage, especially in the unconscious patient, has permitted the more accurate diagnosis of abdominal injuries, avoiding unnecessary laparotomy in many patients.[15] Osteosynthesis of major fractures, a milestone in the management of bone injuries, has alleviated prolonged pain and shortened the period of immobility, thereby minimizing pulmonary complications and reducing the need for continued ventilation with its attendant complications.[16]

The technological advances of the last two decades have facilitated the management, monitoring and survival of patients but have also brought with them the problem of sepsis and the dilemma of continuing support in the presence of irreversible brain damage. This has highlighted the importance of frequent, careful physical examination rather than placing undue reliance on electronic and similar data.[17] Pioneers confronted by the complexities of emergency management of the critically injured advocated the need for a 'systems approach' to trauma care in designated centres where multidisciplinary trauma teams could receive sufficient experience to become proficient in delivering the best possible care.[18] Specific tasks allocated to each member of the team during the resuscitation and assessment of the injured patient in a structured and organized manner were formalized relatively recently with the inception of strict protocols of management and a variety of injury severity scoring systems which continue to evolve.[19–23]

EPIDEMIOLOGY

Injury and mortality to individuals on the roads, in the home and in industry are either ignored by governments and professional bodies or obscured by the preoccupation of the media with wars and dramatic disasters.[24,25] The incidence of major trauma should be kept in perspective. In the 11 years of the Vietnam War, 43 000 American soldiers died in battle while in the USA 25 times that number died from accidents and 10 times that number died from road traffic accidents. In the USA, trauma is responsible for 150 000 deaths and 10–17 million disabilities each year. Approximately 380 000 cases of disability are permanent, including 80 000 from brain and spinal cord injury. This gives a ratio of 1 death and 2 permanently disabled victims for every 40 less severely injured cases.[26,27] Between the ages of 1 and 44 years trauma is the greatest killer, and among teenagers and young adults it accounts for three quarters of all mortality. Of 68 million injuries annually, 2 million require hospital admission and account for 22 million bed-days; that is, more than the number of bed-days needed to deal with all heart disease, and four times as many bed-days as required for cancer patients. Accidents on the road, in the home and at work drain the US economy in medical expenses, wage losses, insurance payments and damage to property by a figure of 75–100 billion dollars a year. Paradoxically, research into trauma receives less than 2% of the total health research budget.

Reliable and relevant information on injuries in the UK is hard to obtain and fragmented. In a prospective study in the UK undertaken in 1976[28] the mortality and morbidity figures were similar to those reported from the USA. Deaths from accidents in the UK

REFERENCES

4. Shires T, Cohn D et al Arch Surg 1964; 88: 688
5. Boyd D R, Cowley R A World J Surg 1983; 7: 150
6. Lowe R J, Baker R J J Trauma 1973; 13: 285
7. Moore F D, Ball M R The Metabolic Response to Surgery. Charles C Thomas, Springfield 1952
8. Cuthbertson D P Br J Surg 1970; 57: 718
9. Johnston I D A Br J Anaesth 1973; 45: 252
10. Dudrick S J, Wilmore D W et al Surgery 1968; 64: 134
11. Ashbaugh D G, Petty J L et al J Thorac Cardiovasc Surg 1969; 57: 31
12. Teasdale G, Jennett B Lancet 1974; ii: 81
13. French B N, Dublin A B Surg Neurol 1977; 7: 171
14. Gordon E Acta Anaesthesiol Scand 1971; 15: 208
15. Fischer R P, Beverlin B C et al Am J Surg 1978; 136: 701
16. Tscherne H, Oestern H J, Sturm J World J Surg 1983; 7: 80
17. London P S World J Surg 1983; 7: 167
18. Eastman A B, Lewis F R et al Am J Surg 1987; 154: 79
19. Baker S P, O'Neill B et al J Trauma 1974; 14: 187
20. Champion H R, Sacco W J et al J Trauma 1989; 29: 623
21. Champion H R, Copes W S et al J Trauma 1990; 30: 1356
22. Knaus W A Draper E A et al Crit Care Med 1985; 13: 818
23. Champion H R World J Surg 1993; 7: 4
24. Road accidents in 1987 Br Med J 1988; 296: 1201
25. Report of the Working Party on the Management of Patients with Major Injuries. Royal College of Surgeons of England, London 1988
26. Trunkey D D Sci Am 1983; 249: 28
27. Injury in America. Committee on Trauma Research, National Research Council and the Institute of Medicine. National Academic Press, Washington DC 1985

number 14 500 a year, and 545 000 patients are discharged from hospitals following injury; road traffic accident victims alone account for 850 000 bed-nights in hospital. In men and in a large number of women under 35 years, accidental injuries and their sequelae are the principal reason for hospital admission or death; the mortality rate exceeds the combined figure for heart disease and cancer (Fig. 7.1). The cost to the British economy of road traffic accidents alone in 1985 was £2.8 billion.[29] The price in economic terms paid by society, as estimated by the World Health Organization, is approximately 1% of the gross national product of a country.

Although the establishment of accident and emergency medicine as a specialty in the UK over the last 20 years has been a success, it has also highlighted deficiencies in management, particularly in those services associated with transfer from one hospital to another.[30] A retrospective study[31] on 1000 deaths from injury in 11 coroners' districts in England and Wales included 514 patients admitted alive. A total of 335 died from injury to the central nervous system (7% of which were judged by independent assessors to be preventable) and 175 died from other injuries, 43% of which were considered preventable (Fig. 7.2). Of the preventable deaths, one third died within 4 hours and a further third by the end of the first week, mainly from acute hypoxia or haemorrhage—largely as a consequence of misdiagnosis, failure to act and delayed or inadequate surgery (Fig. 7.3). A retrospective review of deaths from road traffic accidents in Northern Ireland emphasized the need for improved prehospital care by skilled staff. This study emphasized that some patients with cerebral injuries and intrathoracic haemorrhage who died at the scene or en route to hospital could have been saved if optimally managed.[32]

The development of emergency medicine as a specialty in the USA gained impetus when studies in the San Francisco Bay area showed that the management of surgically salvageable major trauma in some poorly equipped hospitals was responsible for a preventable mortality rate of up to 73%. As a result, five centres in Orange County, Southern California, were designated for admission of major injuries, dramatically reducing the preventable mortality rate from 73% to 4%.[33] Further studies corroborated the rewards of concentrating a sufficient number of major injury cases in well equipped centres with trained senior staff.[34–36] The momentum generated by these studies was reflected in the deliberations of the Committee on Trauma of the American College of Surgeons which produced four successive reports over a decade (1977–1986) examining the hospital and prehospital resources required for optimal care of the injured patient.[37] The excellence and organization of the German model of delivering a nationwide trauma service would be difficult to reproduce in other countries. The quality is reflected in the ambulance and air rescue services, the network of trauma centres staffed round-the-clock by trained and experienced medical and ancillary staff, the well run intensive care units and a strong rehabilitation programme.

MECHANISMS OF INJURY

Penetrating injury

Sharp objects such as knives, splinters of glass, shards of metal, bullets, shrapnel and fragments from a variety of explosive devices account for most penetrating injuries. A stabbing severs tissues quite cleanly causing minimal injury outside the track of the blade. In contrast, the wounding force of a bullet is considerable and is

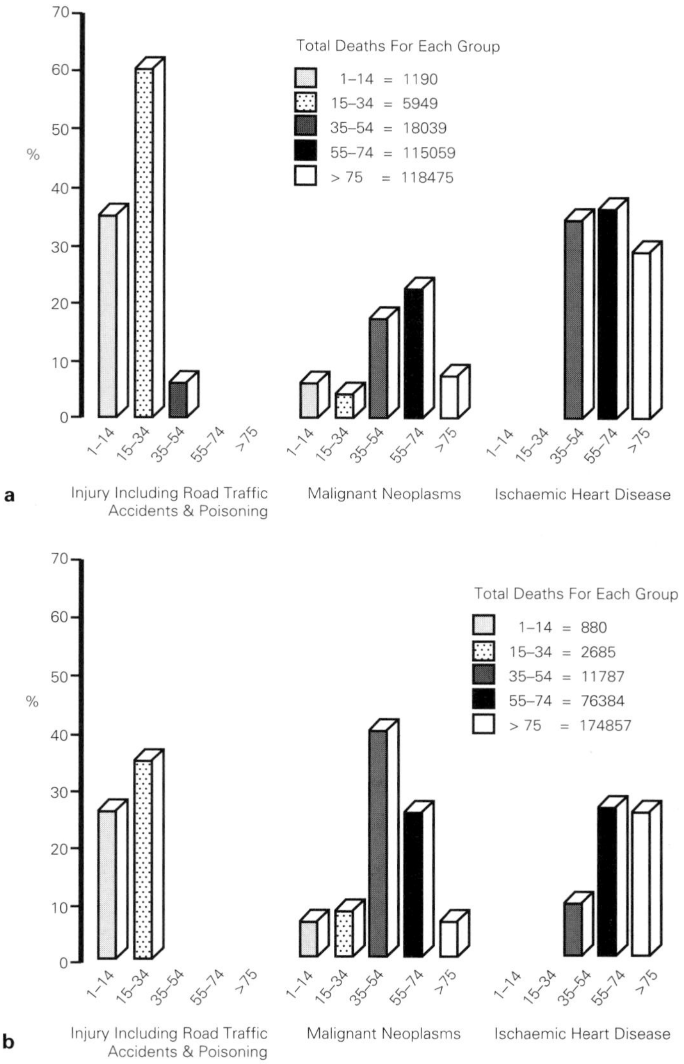

Fig. 7.1 Mortality by age group from injury, cancer and heart disease in England in 1987: **(a)** males; **(b)** females. From Report of the Working Party on the Management of Patients with Major Injuries.[25]

REFERENCES

28. Hoffmann E Ann R Coll Surg 1976; 58: 233
29. Accidents in the UK. Lancet 1988; 840
30. Buck N, Devlin H B, Lunn J N (eds) Report of the Confidential Enquiry into Perioperative Deaths. Nuffield Provincial Hospitals Trust and the Kings Fund, London 1987
31. Anderson I D, Woodford M et al Br Med J 1988; 296: 1305
32. Gilroy D Injury 1985; 16: 241
33. Cales R H Ann Emerg Med 1984; 13: 1
34. West J G, Cales R H, Gazzaniga A B Arch Surg 1983; 118: 740
35. Kreis D J, Plasencia G et al J Trauma 1986; 26: 649
36. Shackford S R, Hollingford-Frilund P et al J Trauma 1986; 26: 812
37. Committee on Trauma of the American College of Surgeons Bull Am Coll Surg 1986; 71: 4

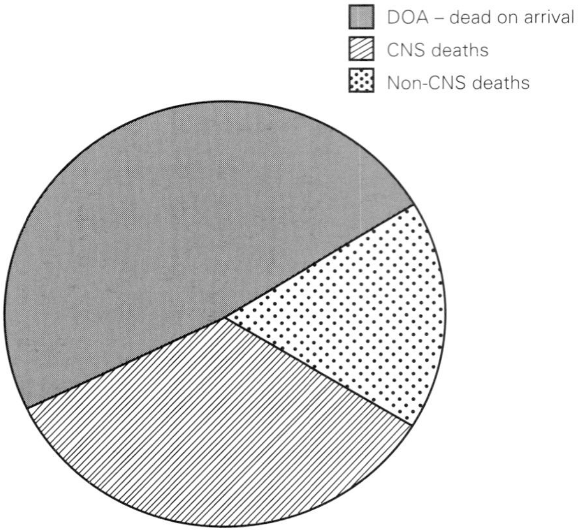

Fig. 7.2 Cause of death in 1000 cases of trauma death. From Anderson et al.[31]

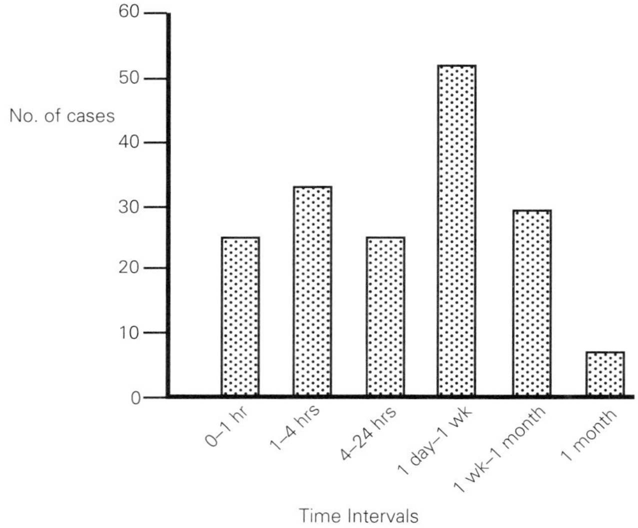

Fig. 7.3 Time interval to death of preventable deaths. From Anderson et al.[31]

related to its mass, the muzzle velocity and the distance travelled.[38,39] A low-velocity bullet moving at speeds up to 304 m/s (1000 f/s) disrupts only those tissues lying in its path, whereas the temporary cavitational effect of a high-velocity bullet travelling at speeds in excess of 762 m/s (2500 f/s) causes traumatic displacement and destruction of tissues at right angles to its track. If bone is struck, dissipating some of the energy, the resulting fragments of bone behave as secondary missiles, wreaking havoc on the soft tissues. In addition, the process of cavitation sucks in fragments of clothing and skin along with dirt and organisms so predisposing the wound to infection. The wounding potential of a shotgun blast is related to the bore (calibre), the choke (constriction of muzzle outlet), the shot size and the proximity of the target.[40] When discharged at close range the concentration of pellets imparts maximum kinetic energy, comparable to that of some high-velocity weapons, causing immense damage which is not always apparent on external inspection; the tissues are contaminated by wadding and pellets which carry in debris from the surface, skin and clothing (Fig. 7.4). In the UK 'assaults' are still much more common than gunshot wounds[41] (Table 7.1).

Blast injury

Bomb explosions are no longer confined to theatres of war and, tragically, innocent populations are killed and maimed by bombs ranging from small-charge anti-personnel devices to vehicles packed with over 1000 kg of explosives.[42,43] Survivors of large bomb explosions sustain a multiplicity of injuries with widespread destruction of all body tissues caused initially by the blast wave, which spreads faster than the speed of sound (Fig. 7.5), and also by the impact of flying fragments, secondary missiles and falling masonry. The decay of the blast wave is shown in Figure 7.6 and the damage it can cause in Table 7.2.

Blunt injury

Road accidents, the main source of blunt trauma, generally cause multiple injuries. These involve the craniocervical axis (50%), the abdomen (25%), the chest (20%) and the extremities. As more than one area may be affected, mortality and morbidity are high. Apart from direct injury from impact, indirect damage may ensue as a result of the intense shearing forces generated by the sudden violent angulation and fracture of long bones, or the avulsing forces which bring about dislocation of joints such as the knee.[44] The legal requirement to use seat-belts in motor vehicles dramatically lowered the incidence of injuries and fatalities in the UK and elsewhere, but the understandable support for these devices should be tempered by an awareness that the seat-belt is occasionally responsible for blunt trauma to the abdomen.[45]

Deceleration injury

The deceleration forces on impact which occur in road accidents, air crashes or falls from a great height cause damage to less robust tissues and to the sites where relatively mobile anatomical structures are anchored. The junction of the cranium and cervical spine, the brain itself, the main bronchus, the isthmus of the thoracic aorta, the vascular pedicle of the kidney and transverse mesocolon are most vulnerable.[46] Many of these injuries are not immediately apparent and can be missed or remain unsuspected before surfacing later when the patient is in a critical condition.

REFERENCES

38. Barach E, Tomlanovich M et al J Trauma 1986; 26: 225
39. Barach E, Tomlanovech M et al J Trauma 1986; 26: 374
40. Roberts R M, String S T Surgery 1984; 96: 902
41. Hocking M A J Roy Soc Med 1989; 82: 281
42. Barros D'Sa A A B Ann R Coll Surg Engl 1982; 64: 37
43. Barros D'Sa A A B Injury 1982; 14: 51
44. Lefrac B A Arch Surg 1976; 111: 1021
45. Huelke D F, Mendelsohn R A, States J D J Trauma 1978; 18: 533
46. Sandblom P Surg Clin North Am 1973; 53: 1191

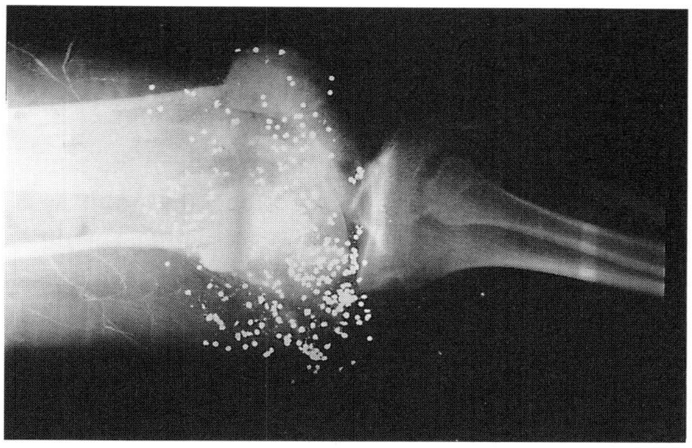

Fig. 7.4 Shotgun injury to the knee.

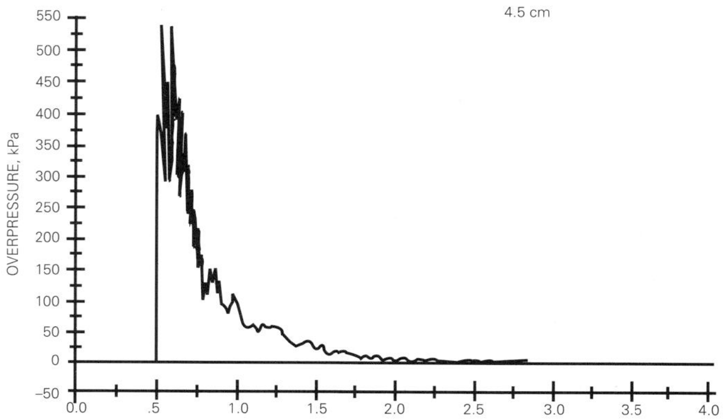

Fig. 7.5 The form of a blast wave (6.9 psi = 1 kPa).

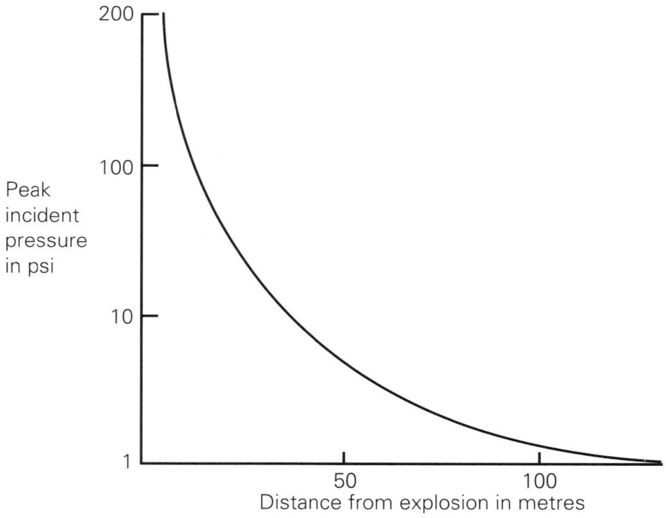

Fig. 7.6 Decay of blast wave following explosion (50 lb of TNT).

Table 7.1 Type of attack

	No.	*%**
Punched with fists	194	46
Kicked	74	17
Miscellaneous weapons	72	17
Knifed	66	15
Miscellaneous (no weapon)	38	9
Bottled†	37	9
Manhandled	23	5
Unknown	23	5
Human bite	9	2

* Many patients sustained more than one type of assault hence the figures total more than 100%
† Bottled = attack with broken glass

Crush injury

This clinical picture sometimes occurs in industrial, mining, farming, train and road traffic accidents, as well as in natural disasters such as earthquakes. The initial injury caused by falling masonry is compounded by sustained compression of a part of the body under the weight of the rubble. The consequent ischaemia and muscle necrosis accelerate the progression of the 'crush syndrome' as myoglobin and other breakdown products that are released block the renal tubules and cause acute tubular necrosis, particularly when the renal blood flow is decreased due to hypervolaemia. Once anuria has developed in these cases, even renal dialysis may not alter the bleak prognosis.

Miscellaneous

Other less common causes of major trauma include radiation, electricity, extremes of heat and cold, chemical fumes and barotrauma.

Table 7.2 Relative effects of various overpressures lasting for 4 ms

Overpressure (psi)	*Effect*
1	Damage to ordinary structures—flying glass and debris
2	Slight chance of perforation of tympanic membrane
15	50% chance of perforation of tympanic membrane
40	Serious damage to reinforced concrete structures
70	50% chance of severe pulmonary damage
130	50% mortality

PATHOPHYSIOLOGY

The initial effects of the injury are continuous, and a trimodal distribution of death is observed when the death rate is plotted against time. This is represented by three peaks which give significance to the underlying pathophysiological sequelae of injury (Fig. 7.7). The first peak is of 'immediate deaths' occurring within minutes of injury and resulting from lacerations of the brain, the brainstem and upper spinal cord, the heart, the aorta and the great vessels. Only a small fraction of these victims can be saved. The second peak of 'early deaths', occurring within the first 2–3 hours after injury, results from hypoxia and external haemorrhage or from bleeding into the cranium, chest, abdomen or limbs. During this 'golden hour' many potentially operable conditions may be

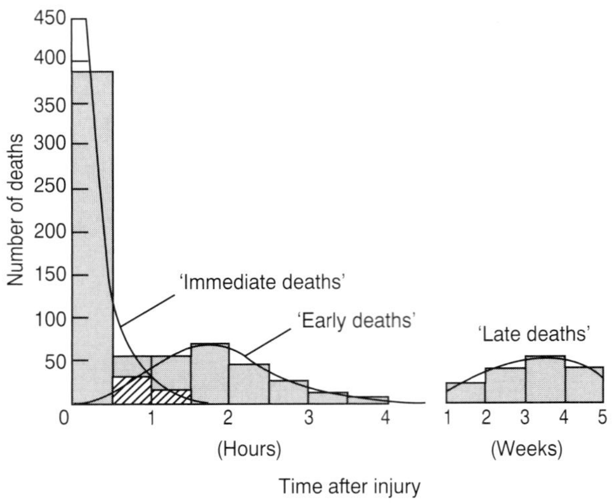

Fig. 7.7 Trimodal distribution of deaths following trauma plotted as a function after injury showing the three peaks of immediate, early and late mortality in a sample of 862 deaths over a 2-year period at the San Francisco General Hospital.[26]

successfully treated. The third peak of 'late deaths' is from pulmonary embolism, overwhelming sepsis and multiple organ dysfunction and failure. These late deaths may be related to inadequacies of resuscitation and management immediately after injury or arise from complications associated with injury and its management.

Neuroendocrine response to injury

The circulatory and metabolic responses to injury are affected by nervous and humoral factors which mediate through complex and incompletely understood neuroendocrine reflexes. These systemic reflexes are initiated by precise afferent neural stimuli to various areas within the central nervous system where they are integrated and modulated, generating efferent signals which set in motion a range of neural and humoral responses aimed at countering the damaging effect of the injury (Fig. 7.8). Injury to the brain and spinal cord obviously compromises these reflexes.

The early response to trauma is stimulated by pain in the conscious patient and the 'fight or flight' defence reaction. The afferent impulses originate partly in injured tissue from nociceptors stimulated by a variety of vasoactive substances, and partly from baroreceptors excited by poorly filled arteries and atria. These impulses are transmitted to the autonomic centres in the central nervous system, resulting in a generalized sympathetic discharge aimed at maintaining tissue perfusion and supporting circulating blood volume.[47] The injured tissues, not generally affected by vasoconstriction, go on releasing local tissue factors such as prostaglandins, leukotrienes, histamine, serotonin and bradykinin which activate further afferent impulses. All the afferent signals from the site of injury and cardiovascular receptors are modulated by neural and endocrine influences in the ascending columns of the spinal cord and medullary centres, integrating with an input from the brainstem to induce analgesia. The continuing effects of injury introduce other stimuli such as hypoxia, hypercapnia, acidosis and reduced core body temperature which alter the efferent response. Despite a fall in core temperature, presumably caused by impaired thermoregulation, the increasing gradient of temperature to the periphery reflects the relative adequacy of peripheral perfusion.[48,49]

The efferent responses to injury commence in the pituitary and in the autonomic centres of the brainstem: the pituitary releases either mediating hormones or hormones which act directly on effector organs, while the sympathetic nervous system acts directly on the vascular system and indirectly on the adrenal medulla leading to catecholamine release. Plasma concentrations of adrenaline, noradrenaline and dopamine have been shown to correlate well with Injury Severity Scores.[50,51] In the acute phase adrenaline plays a role in restoring blood pressure, but mainly acts in mobilizing body glycogen stores to release large amounts of energy-yielding substrates. The nociceptive signals arriving in the medulla travel to the hypothalamus where corticotrophin-releasing factor is secreted, acting on the anterior pituitary to release adrenocorticotrophin, a hormone which stimulates immediate production and release of cortisol.[52] Rises in the plasma cortisol are proportionate to the severity of the injury but reach a ceiling which is refractory to greater injury. Glucocorticoids ensure the restoration of plasma volume by bringing about fluid shifts from the extravascular space and also influence metabolism and the immune response.[53,54] Arginine vasopressin is secreted by the hypothalamus and posterior lobe of the pituitary, controlling water excretion by the kidney and maintaining blood pressure. Under hypothalamic control circulating levels of growth hormone and prolactin also fulfil a metabolic role. The release of beta-endorphins, various opiate peptides and encephalins provides endogenous sources of analgesia which may in future be manipulated to beneficial effect.[55]

Noradrenaline released by the sympathetic nerves is far more influential than adrenal catecholamines[56] in producing vasoconstriction, hypoperfusion, reduced transcapillary exchange, accumulation of metabolites, red cell aggregation, cellular hypoxia and acidosis.[57] These changes stimulate coagulation and platelet activity, as well as thromboplastic activity. The resulting hypercoagulable state can be reversed by immediate resuscitation unless endotoxins have been released causing protein digestion, microcirculatory collapse and irreversible organ failure. While the responses to injury are geared towards restoration of blood volume, it is possible that altered transmembrane potentials may

REFERENCES

47. Gann D S, Lilly M P In: Wilder R J (ed) Multiple Trauma. Karger, Basel 1984
48. Little R A, Stoner H B Br J Surg 1981; 68: 221
49. Ledingham R McA, Finlay W E I, Little K In: Carter D, Polk H C (eds) Trauma, vol 1. Butterworths, London 1981
50. Davies C L, Newman R J et al J Trauma 1984; 24: 99
51. Frayn K N, Little R A et al Circ Shock 1985; 16: 229
52. Gann D S, Ward D G, Carlson D E Recent Prog Horm Res 1978; 34: 357
53. Barton R N, Little R A J Endocrinol 1978; 76: 293
54. Barton R N, Passingham B J J Endocrinol 1980; 86: 363
55. Morley J E Metabolism 1981; 30: 195
56. Chien S Phys Rev 1967; 47: 214
57. Messmer K World J Surg 1983; 7: 26

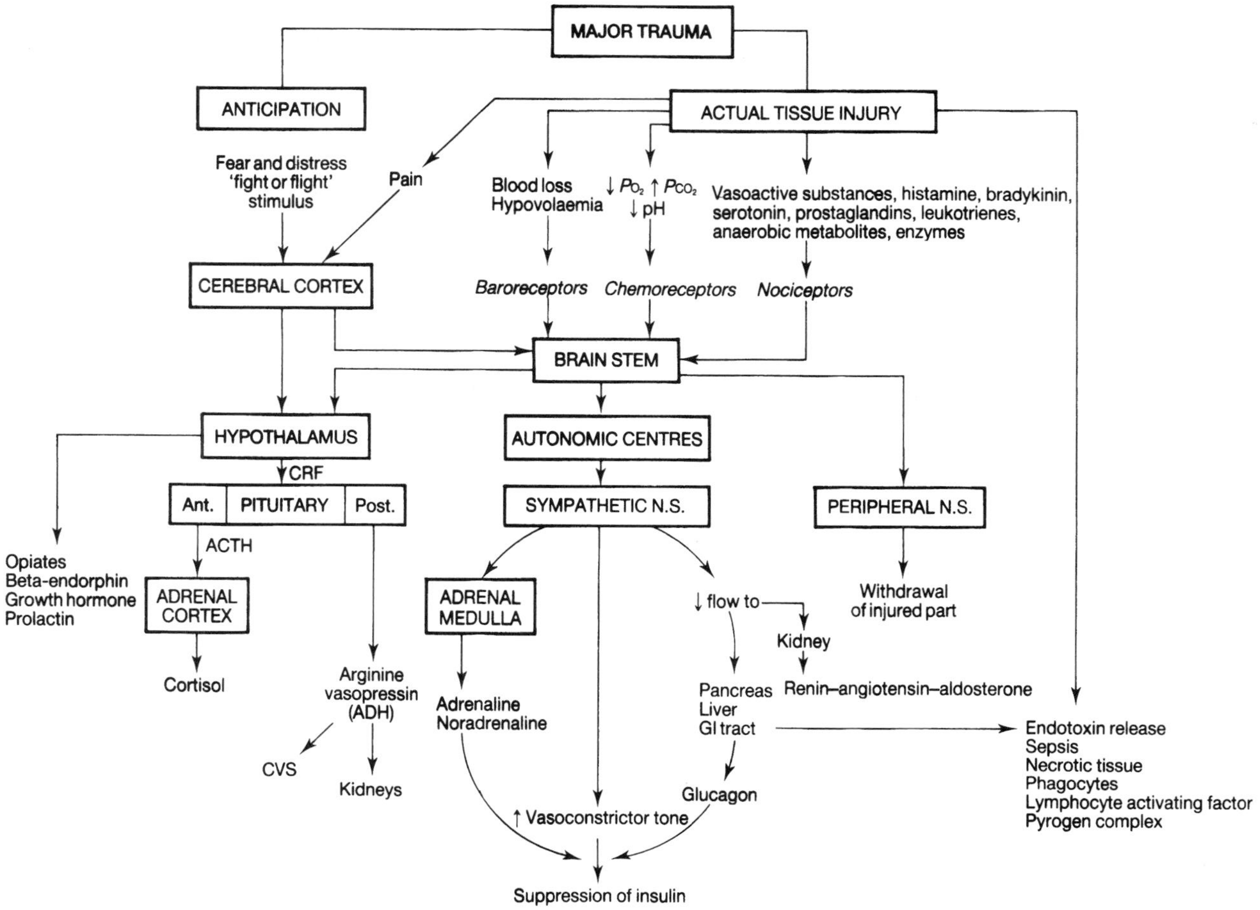

Fig. 7.8 Neuroendocrine response to injury illustrating the primary afferent pathways activated by major trauma and the efferent nervous and humoral pathways which lead to catecholamine and cortisol release and to other effects. CRF = corticotrophin-releasing factor; ACTH = adrenocorticotrophic hormone; ADH = antidiuretic hormone; CVS = cardiovascular system; GI = gastrointestinal. Modified from Gann & Lilly.[47]

herald irreversible circulatory failure when the amount of haemorrhage exceeds a quarter of the blood volume.

The increase in autonomic sympathetic outflow stimulates other humoral mechanisms such as the renin–angiotensin–aldosterone, glucagon and insulin systems. Plasma insulin concentrations fall in proportion to the severity of the injury, partly antagonized by the production of glucagon and catecholamines and partly from accelerated degradation of insulin. Insulin resistance characterizes the acute phase, but later large quantities of insulin are required to achieve the same uptake of glucose.[58] Insulin is important in carbohydrate metabolism but it also has a major part to play in the metabolism of fat and protein. As the ratio of insulin to glucagon rises, normal metabolic function such as glycogen production and protein synthesis begins to resume in liver and muscle, though insulin resistance may persist as the result of a sustained elevation of catecholamines and glucocorticoids.

Metabolic response

Half a century has elapsed since Cuthbertson[59] postulated the existence of a brief 'ebb' phase, followed by a longer 'flow' phase which characterized the depression and resurgence of metabolism and vitality after injury. He also included within the 'ebb' phase a 'necrobiotic' phase representing the state of irreversible shock and progressive failure of oxygen transport which heralds death.[60] More recently Cerra has described the interrelationship between hypermetabolism and organ failure and the important role of toxins, bacteria, cytokines and immunological dysfunction in the development of defects of oxygenation and perfusion of major organs.[61] These metabolic responses to trauma are mainly mediated by the hormones adrenaline, cortisol, glucagon and insulin. Survivors pass through a biphasic metabolic response beginning with the acute phase of approximately 1–3 days' duration, followed by the adaptive or convalescent phase which lasts a few weeks before there is a return to normality. The acute phase is characterized by protein catabolism, gluconeogenesis, glycogenolysis

REFERENCES

58. Irving M H, Stoner H B In: Carter C, Polk H C (eds) Trauma, vol 1. Butterworths, London 1981
59. Cuthbertson D P Lancet 1942; i: 233
60. Cuthbertson D P In: Porter R, Knight J (eds) Trauma. Elsevier, London 1970
61. Cerra F B Surgery 1987; 101: 1

and increased oxidation of fat from lipolysis. Proteolysis of muscle, which is the main endogenous source of protein, is increased, leading to greater amounts of circulating free amino acids which are used for synthesis and as energy fuel substrates.[62] Muscle mass diminishes as a result of reduced synthesis and greater breakdown, while the liver continues to produce an excess of proteins, plasma levels of which reflect intravascular volume changes rather than the metabolic state. Concentrations of branched-chain amino acids in plasma and muscle increase and, along with carbohydrates, these govern the amounts of glutamine or alanine released from muscle to be converted in the liver into glucose, releasing nitrogen in the form of urea. Nitrogen losses are considerable, reaching 20 g/day and even 40 g/day, depending on the patient's size and the available pool of protein. Accompanying losses of phosphorus, potassium, magnesium and zinc occur, though these elements are simultaneously being absorbed to enhance protein synthesis.[63]

Respiratory failure

Respiratory failure may follow assorted injuries: direct injury to the chest, spinal cord injury with respiratory muscle paralysis, head injury and damage to the respiratory centres, direct injury to the epithelium of the respiratory tract by burns or chemicals.[64] In addition, other sites of injury involving extensive tissue damage, blood loss and hypotension may lead to a post-traumatic adult respiratory distress syndrome variously described as 'adult hyaline membrane disease', 'shock lung', 'traumatic wet lung' and 'white lung syndrome'.[65] A number of factors enhance respiratory failure. These include sepsis (particularly if Gram-negative), systemic shock, aspiration of gastric contents, an acute central nervous system event, pneumonia, pulmonary embolism, fat embolism and disseminated intravascular coagulopathy. Therapeutic intervention such as narcotic overdosage, excessive volume replacement, oxygen toxicity and mechanical hyperventilation may aggravate the condition.

Injury to the endothelium of the pulmonary microvasculature allows leakage of protein-rich fluid into the interstitial space and across the alveolar membrane. Simultaneous vasoconstriction results in impaired diffusion and arterial hypoxaemia. Increased permeability is probably induced by leukotrienes, platelet-activating factor and free oxygen radicals, while the various vasoactive substances released at the site of tissue injury contribute to pulmonary vasoconstriction. Arteriovenous shunting occurs in areas of affected lung so that increasing concentrations of inspired oxygen are required to maintain tissue oxygen supply as the ventilation–perfusion ratio rises. The inactivation of alveolar surfactant contributes to atelectasis. As adult respiratory distress syndrome develops, blood pressure and cardiac output fall compounding the impairment of tissue perfusion and oxygenation.

The first clinical phase of respiratory failure occurs between 12 and 48 hours after injury and is marked by tachypnoea, dyspnoea and hyperventilatory respiratory alkalosis, before any clinical signs or radiological evidence of lung damage are present. In the second phase mild hypoxia, intercostal retraction caused by reduced pulmonary compliance and minor chest signs appear, accompanied by diffuse pulmonary infiltrates on chest radiograph involving all lobes but typically sparing the costophrenic angles. As compliance decreases, the physiological dead space increases, inflation pressure rises and arterial oxygenation can only be maintained by mechanical ventilation and positive end-expiratory pressure. Death is inevitable if the condition remains untreated, but with optimal therapy half those affected survive.

Renal failure

The hypovolaemia which commonly complicates major trauma impairs renal perfusion. Aldosterone release enhances sodium reabsorption and antidiuretic hormone release which concentrates the urine, resulting in oliguria with low sodium and high potassium levels. Trauma to the base of the brain may result in diabetes insipidus with polyuria, further compromising renal function. Urinary obstruction or urethral damage from pelvic fracture (see Chapter 52) occasionally causes post-renal failure. Tubular necrosis may be a consequence of ischaemia, myoglobinuria, sepsis and the toxic effects of drugs and antibiotics such as the aminoglycosides and cephalosporins. When renal failure follows major injury the mortality often exceeds 50% despite the use of haemodialysis and haemofiltration.[66]

Hepatic failure

Prolonged hypotension, hypoxia and reduced cardiac output in the immediate post-injury period inevitably impair hepatic function. Drugs, sepsis, massive transfusion and inappropriate nutritional support may compound the liver damage. Hepatic dysfunction may be represented simply by elevation of liver enzymes, hyperbilirubinaemia and reduced albumin levels, or it may progress to florid jaundice and even coma, after which recovery is unlikely.[67]

Stress ulceration

Major trauma may be complicated by acute gastrointestinal bleeding in association with head injury, shock and sepsis. The pathophysiology of stress ulceration remains unexplained but several predisposing factors have been implicated, including relative mucosal ischaemia caused by the sympathetic reflex response and catecholamine release, lack of oral alimentation, altered mucus barrier function in the stomach and back-diffusion of gastric acid. This complication is less common nowadays because of better general management and support for trauma victims.

REFERENCES

62. Blackburn G L, Maini B S, Pierce E C Anaesthesiology 1977; 47: 181
63. Schmitz J E, Ahnefeld F W, Burri C World J Surg 1993; 7: 132
64. Petty T L Intensive and Rehabilitative Respiratory Care. Lea & Febiger, Philadelphia 1982
65. Said S I, Butler P M In: Wilder R J (ed) Multiple Trauma. Karger, Basel 1984
66. Belzberg H, Cornwell E E et al Surg Clin N Amer 1996; 76: 971
67. Fry D E, Pearlstein L, Fulton R L Arch Surg 1980; 115: 136

Infection

Mortality following major trauma is consistently attributed to multiple organ dysfunction and failure despite the most heroic therapeutic efforts. Elegant studies by Fry[2] have shown that the incidence of pulmonary, renal and hepatic failure, and gastrointestinal stress bleeding was similar in each of the four organ systems following splenectomy, abdominal abscess and *Bacteroides* sepsis. Disturbances of other essential systems result in metabolic substrate disequilibrium, neurological dysfunction, disseminated intravascular coagulation, and immunological failure. Uncontrolled sepsis is the one common denominator which appears to be of central importance in the development of multiple organ dysfunction and failure. Frequently, a precise source of sepsis cannot be defined and a prolonged period of hypoperfusion may be the initiating event in multiple system organ failure. Although early mortality rates following major trauma have fallen, late mortality accounts for up to 78% of all deaths and is almost entirely attributable to sepsis, mainly of the chest and abdomen. Previous malnutrition, addiction to alcohol, steroid therapy and diabetes render the injured patient particularly susceptible to infection.

Infections begin by inoculation of organisms from the wounding agent. Contamination of the wound occurs from the environment and the resident flora of the skin or gastrointestinal tract. Release of organisms from the bowel into the peritoneal cavity following penetrating injury or bowel surgery leads to peritonitis and paralytic ileus, which in turn facilitate further transmigration of bacteria into the peritoneal cavity. Perforation of the gastrointestinal tract results in polymicrobial contamination, mainly by aerobic *Escherichia coli* and *Bacteroides fragilis*, which leads to peritonitis and abscess formation if left untreated.[68]

In the oral cavity, endogenous flora are a mixture of aerobic and anaerobic bacteria (predominantly the latter) and evidence exists that the aerobic Gram-negative bacilli 'colonize' the oropharynx and upper gastrointestinal tract before causing infection. The protective commensals, principally anaerobic flora, must be maintained, especially when broad-spectrum antibiotics are being administered.[69] The pathogens chiefly associated with infections in compound fractures are *Staphylococcus aureus*, *S. epidermidis* and *E. coli*; the incidence of osteomyelitis is closely related to the severity of soft tissue trauma. In head injuries where a tear of the meninges and leakage of cerebrospinal fluid is complicated by meningitis, *Streptococcus pneumoniae* and Gram-negative bacteria are the most frequently observed pathogens.

Casualties of major trauma have a higher incidence of nosocomial or hospital-acquired infections (approximately 30%) than any other group of surgical patients. Apart from being responsible for the complications and deaths of patients suffering from major trauma, nosocomial infections prolong hospital stay and add to the costs of treatment. The management of major trauma in intensive care units is profoundly undermined by sepsis, especially of the respiratory tract, predominantly by endogenous aerobic Gram-negative bacilli including *Pseudomonas aeruginosa*, *Enterobacter*, *Klebsiella* and *E. coli*. Bacterial colonization is facilitated by the presence of invasive monitoring and treatment devices such as urinary catheters, monitoring lines, endotracheal tubes, ventilators and humidifiers, nasogastric tubes, chest and wound drains and screws from external bone fixators. It is also encouraged by lapses in aseptic technique and by cross-infection with organisms which are highly resistant to broad-spectrum antibiotics in a host with severely compromised natural defences.[70–72]

Defective host defences are caused by failure of the T cell or cell-mediated response, a failure of B cell or humoral response and the development of certain substances which inhibit the normal phagocyte chemotactic reaction.[73,74] Failure to respond to macrophage-processed antigen is described as anergy, an indicator of immunological incompetence which is accentuated by the presence of established sepsis. Undrained abscesses and intraperitoneal sepsis induce anergy and lead to septicaemia with its high mortality even when aggressively treated.

When necrotic tissue and pus persist, an endogenous pyrogen complex (endogenous pyrogen complexed with leucocyte endogenous mediating factor and lymphocyte-activating factor) is released which stimulates phagocytosis.[75] This causes pyrexia and an intensification of the catabolic aspect of the neuroendocrine response. Increased muscle protein breakdown and protein synthesis occur in the viscera and white cell production and systemic antibacterial activity are also elevated.[76,77] As a consequence of increased protein synthesis, the gut mucosa and liver are stimulated to prevent entry of gut bacteria and endotoxins. Plasma proteins synthesized in the liver are released for breakdown to amino acids to be utilized in the tissues, or alternatively they are returned to the liver for resynthesis. These processes result in increased metabolic rate, raised oxygen consumption, and depletion of energy substrate reserves, with the generation of more heat. A raised cardiac output is required to dissipate the excess heat.[78]

This hypermetabolic state precipitated by major trauma and sepsis results in raised levels of insulin and glucagon, the latter enhancing hepatic gluconeogenesis for energy production at the expense of lean body mass. Eventually these demands can only be met by augmented external support. Untreated sepsis, fever, cardiopulmonary failure, the enforced supine position, and a continuing negative nitrogen balance in association with altered muscle mitochondrial function all lead to multiple organ dysfunction and failure.[77] This condition is declared by stress ulceration, biochemical signs of hepatic failure and lethargy progressing to coma, and high oxygen delivery with limited oxygen extraction (demonstrable by increased mixed venous oxygen levels). The plasma contains increased amounts of lactate, pyruvate, glucagon,

REFERENCES

68. Rowlands B J, Ericsson C D et al J Trauma 1987; 27: 250
69. Stoutenbeek C P, van Saene H K F, Zandstra D F J Antimicrob Chemother 1987; 19: 513
70. Stoutenbeek C P, van Saene H K F, Miranda D R Int Care Med 1984; 10: 185
71. Ledingham I McA, Alcock S R, Eastaway A T Lancet 1988; i: 785
72. Leading article Lancet 1988; i: 803
73. Christou N V, McLean A P H, Meakins J L J Trauma 1980; 20: 833
74. MacLean L D World J Surg 1983; 7: 119
75. Powanda M, Beisel W Am J Clin Nutr 1982; 35: 762
76. Cuthbertson D P Injury 1980; 11: 175
77. Hassett J, Border J R World J Surg 1983; 7: 125

glucose and triglycerides. A terminal complex of irreversible cardiopulmonary failure, renal failure and clotting disorders may develop.

TRAUMA SEVERITY SCORING

A more analytical approach to the management of major trauma has been provided by the development of trauma severity scoring methods. These enable the emergency medical team to predict survival, to assess the results of different treatment regimens and to compare the performances of individual trauma centres.[79,80]

The Abbreviated Injury Scale was used to grade injuries in non-fatal road traffic accidents on a 0–5 scale in five anatomical areas (Table 7.3), but this method failed to take account of multiple injuries.[81] The Injury Severity Score, an improvement on the Abbreviated Injury Scale, grades injuries at death or discharge on a 1–5 scale in six anatomical regions of the body and takes the sum of the squares of the three highest values, the maximum score being 75. The Injury Severity Score is a useful predictor of the mortality rate, the length of time before death or discharge and the degree of residual disability. Although the Injury Severity Score lacks vital data such as age and individual risk factors related to the patient, it provided an excellent method of studying different courses of management in patients with multiple injuries. For example, it demonstrated that early operative stabilization of fractures was safe, with less chance of dying from sepsis, and that early fixation also reduced the duration of prophylactic ventilation and the risk of adult respiratory distress syndrome.[82]

The process of triage involves an assessment of the severity of the injuries at the scene of the accident or on admission to hospital, correlating it with the probability of survival. The Glasgow Coma Scale (see Chapter 6) assesses brain function on the basis of three behavioural responses: eye-opening, best motor response and best verbal response (Table 7.4). The Glasgow Coma Scale score has been shown to correlate well with outcome.[83] The Triage Index was developed by combining the Glasgow Coma Scale with four other physiological measurements: respiratory rate and effort, systolic blood pressure and capillary refill time. This provides the Trauma Score, ranging from 1 with the worst prognosis to 16 with the best. This system proved to be very sensitive with a high predictive index of survival, particularly in patients with penetrating injuries, and was a useful instrument in field triage to select referral of appropriate cases. The Revised Trauma Score (Table 7.5) combines the Glasgow Coma Scale with the systolic blood pressure and the respiratory rate, each measurement receiving an appropriately coded value which is then weighted by an assigned figure based on the regression analysis of over 26 000 patients from the Major Trauma Outcome Study.[84] The Revised Trauma Score has been found to be more accurate than the old Trauma Score in field triage. The combination of the Revised Trauma Score with the Injury Severity Score formed the basis of the TRISS method[21] which is useful for audit purposes and for predicting outcome. When the patient's age is used to weight the TRISS formula, giving zero for 54 years or less, and 1 for 55 years or more, then an even more accurate probability of survival can be calculated and unexpected deaths and survivors are identified (Fig. 7.9).

Table 7.3 Examples of injuries scored by abbreviated injury scale

Injury	*Score*
Shoulder pain (no injury specified)	0
Wrist sprain	1 (Minor)
Closed undisplaced tibial fracture	2 (Moderate)
Head injury—unconscious on admission but for less than one hour thereafter, no neurological deficit	3 (Serious)
Major liver laceration, no loss of tissue	4 (Severe)
Incomplete transection of the thoracic aorta	5 (Critical)
Laceration of the brainstem	6 (Fatal)

Table 7.4 Glasgow Coma Scale

	Score
Eyes open:	
Spontaneously	4
To speech	3
To pain	2
Never	1
Best motor response:	
Obeys commands	6
Localizes pain	5
Flexion withdrawal	4
Decerebrate flexion	3
Decerebrate extension	2
No response	1
Best verbal response:	
Orientated	5
Confused	4
Inappropriate words	3
Incomprehensible sounds	2
Silent	1

MANAGEMENT

In ensuring adequate care of the victims of major trauma, consideration must be given to the access to care, prehospital care, hospital care and rehabilitation. Other areas that need to be addressed include prevention, disaster medical care, education and research.[85]

Prevention

The prevention of major trauma must be based on reliable data and research into the epidemiology of its causes and mechanisms. Possible avenues to achieve this goal include education of potential

REFERENCES

78. Wilmore D W, Aulick L H et al Ann Surg 1977; 186: 444
79. Champion H R, Sacco W J et al World J Surg 1983; 7: 4
80. Moore E E, Cogbill T H et al Surg Clin N Amer 1995; 75: 293
81. Rowlands B J, Blair P H B In: Taylor E W (ed) Infection in Surgical Practice. Oxford Medical, Oxford 1992
82. Goris R J A World J Surg 1983; 7: 12
83. Jennett B, Teasdale G, Braakman R Lancet 1976; i: 1031
84. Rowlands B J In: Russell R C G (ed) Recent Advances in Surgery 13. Churchill Livingstone, London 1988
85. Trunkey D D Br J Surg 1988; 75: 937

Table 7.5 Revised trauma score

	Coded value	x weight	= score
Respiratory rate (breaths/min):			
10–29	4		
> 29	3		
6–9	2	0.2908	
1–5	1		
0	0		
Systolic blood pressure (mmHg):			
> 89	4		
76–89	3	0.7326	
50–75	2		
1–49	1		
0	0		
Glasgow coma scale:			
13–15	4		
9–12	3	0.9368	
6–8	2		
4–5	1		
3	0		
	Total = revised trauma score:		

A Glasgow Coma Scale	*B* Systolic blood pressure	*C* Respiratory rate	*Points*	*Probability of survival*
13–15	>89	10–29	4	0.995
9–12	76–89	> 29	3	0.969
6–8	50–75	6–9	2	0.879
4–5	1–49	1–5	1	0.766

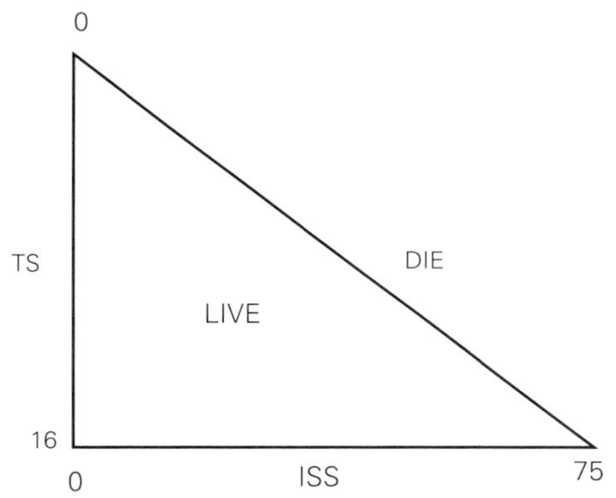

Fig. 7.9 Trauma audit with 'TRISS'. The number of survivors in one hospital can be compared to the expected number derived from a set of patients with equivalent injuries whose outcomes have been predicted by a norm derived from the baseline population data. Measuring injury with TRISS allows accurate identification of the trauma case mix in a district. TS = Trauma Score; ISS = Injury Severity Score.

victims supported by legislation to enforce changes in their behaviour, and modifications in design and engineering to improve the quality of the product and the environment to protect the individual. Seat-belt legislation significantly reduced the incidence of road deaths, and the drinking and driving campaign in the UK also appears to be showing similar benefits.[86] Several social issues in the USA, such as alcohol consumption, the use of narcotic drugs, the uncontrolled availability of guns and the use of seat-belts and motorcycle safety helmets, are not being seriously addressed, when in fact most of the deaths and disabilities from major trauma are linked to these factors.[87]

Trauma centres

The nature of major trauma in a country ought to dictate the type of service which should be provided. An abundance of penetrating trauma in the US and the frequency of high-speed accidents on West German roads catalysed the evolution of appropriate trauma services. Similarly, in Northern Ireland, the surgical services of the Royal Victoria Hospital have responded to the sudden outbreak of major penetrating trauma and recurrent disasters.

Elsewhere in the UK the incidence of penetrating trauma has been negligible, but the management of cases of multiple injury resulting from road traffic accidents has, in general, suffered from a lack of training and facilities. The inability of many hospitals to cope with major injuries and the recognition that death has resulted from potentially treatable conditions such as airway obstruction and hypovolaemia has quite rightly caused disquiet.[25] Preliminary reports on two prospective studies, one of which uses the TRISS index method of trauma audit, indicate that rapid transfer, skilled resuscitation, delineation of intracranial damage by computerized tomographic scanning followed by early and definitive surgery have contributed to improved survival, while deficiencies in this approach have led to the deaths of patients who might have been expected to survive.[25]

A trauma centre should drain a geographical area which is large enough to provide sufficient numbers of patients to allow the

REFERENCES

86. Strategies for accident prevention. DHSS report of a colloquium of medical royal colleges of the UK. HMSO, London 1988
87. Trunkey D D Surgery 1982; 92: 123
88. Loft H S, Bunker J P, Enthoven A C N Engl J Med 1979; 301: 1364

trauma team to develop expertise and refine their techniques of management. In certain high-risk surgical procedures, such as cardiac and vascular surgery, it has been shown that the outcome is related to the number of operations performed by a surgeon, and an absolute minimum of 50 per year should be undertaken.[88] An equivalent figure in the management of major trauma is required in order to discourage the dilution of experience in poorly staffed hospitals with limited facilities.

An American report[37] on trauma services proposed the designation of levels I, II and III hospitals, the last being community hospitals of a kind not found in the UK. A recent British report has advocated the setting up of two levels of trauma centres, for which improved resources will be required.[25] A level II trauma centre (equivalent to a District General Hospital) run by a consultant in accident and emergency medicine would receive patients with an Injury Severity Score of 20 or less, and as most patients will have sustained musculoskeletal injuries the centre should be linked to a good orthopaedic service. A level I trauma centre serving approximately 2 million people would receive either directly or by inter-hospital transfer patients with life-threatening injuries to the trunk and head in addition to those with multiple musculoskeletal injuries.[25] The level I centre directed by a surgeon with appropriate training in trauma management would provide a 24-hour service, ideally run by three teams of consultants or senior registrars in surgery, anaesthesia and radiology, and appropriately trained nursing and paramedical staff equipped with a full range of diagnostic facilities, operating theatres and an intensive care unit. The director would depend on an accident and emergency colleague to deal with a variety of associated medical problems including myocardial infarction, hypoglycaemia and psychiatric problems and would be supported by specialists in neurosurgery, ophthalmology, otolaryngology and cardiothoracic, orthopaedic, vascular, paediatric and, if possible, plastic and maxillofacial surgery.[25] Ideally, the training of a director demands first-hand experience in busy trauma centres, attendance at Advanced Trauma Life Support courses, operative skills in some of the important specialities related to trauma, such as orthopaedic, thoracic, plastic, vascular and neurosurgery, exposure to intensive care, regular audit and quality control.

A trauma team must be immediately available in that 'golden hour' to save life. A non-designated but otherwise adequate emergency department dependent on 'on-call' senior staff or untrained junior staff may result in more patients dying. In a retrospective assessment of emergency care of those with Injury Severity Scores exceeding 16 attending one centre, the treatment of 42% of patients was comparable in quality to the best achievable elsewhere; in the remaining 58% a variety of errors in diagnosis, investigation and treatment were related to the inexperience of junior staff who were unsupervised outside normal working hours, when the most severely injured patients were admitted.[89] In response to these findings, junior staff were phased out, the Revised Trauma Score was introduced as a tool for triage and a senior trauma team was set up to guide and supervise the management of patients with a score below 12. An independent audit of performance 5 years later using similar criteria showed that errors in management had dropped to 26%; an overall improvement of over 50%. An emergency team functions effectively if the doctor in charge has defined priorities and adheres to standardized management protocols so that essential steps are not omitted.

The trauma centre and especially the resuscitation area must be kept in a state of constant readiness, maintaining efficient radio and telephone contact with prehospital services either by sending out medical support or by transmitting advice. This is particularly important in the management of major accidents and disasters involving public transport, industry or criminal explosions, where coordination with the emergency services as well as the public is required.[90,91] The prehospital care teams must select the correct patients to evacuate to level I and level II centres. The severity of the injury and the time and distance involved require field triage, for which a scheme has been recommended (Fig. 7.10).

Prehospital care

Prehospital care requires a rapid response from ambulance staff, paramedics and doctors equipped to provide first aid and to arrange rapid transport of patients to hospital. In the UK this service varies from a complete dependence on ambulance staff (some of whom have received extended training in active resuscitation) to schemes provided by general practitioners.[25] In contrast, prehospital care in West Germany is provided by hospital doctors and in the USA by trained paramedics. Inevitably, 5% of patients, representing 50% of the mortality from trauma, die within the first 10 minutes of injury from rapid exsanguination, massive head injury, cord transection or major airway disruption.[92] As 80% of patients are stable, this leaves a group of 10–15% of potentially salvageable cases who die from airway obstruction, cerebral and cord injury, haemorrhage or pneumothorax.

The most useful skill to have available at the scene of the injury is endotracheal intubation which protects the airway and permits ventilation. The use of an oesophageal obturator airway has been shown to be ineffective in as many as 70% of patients.[92] Cardiopulmonary resuscitation by non-medical personnel requires special training. External bleeding can be easily controlled by manual compression or by a pad and bandage but, if internal bleeding is suspected, a delay in inserting an inadequate intravenous infusion is counterproductive when balanced against blood lost over time. On the other hand, early volume replacement is imperative if the patient cannot be easily extricated, especially in a major accident occurring some distance from a hospital.

The spinal cord must be protected by log-rolling the victim on to a firm stretcher and immobilizing the head between sandbags. Spinal cord damage usually occurs at the time of impact, but the fear of causing injury to the cord from a possible cervical fracture should not prevent effective management of life-threatening

REFERENCES

89. Dearden C H, Rutherford W H Injury 1985; 16: 249
90. Rutherford W H, Illingworth R N et al Accident and Emergency Medicine, 2nd edn. Churchill Livingstone, Edinburgh 1989
91. Rowlands B J Injury 1990; 21: 61
92. Lewis F R In: Trunkey D D, Lewis F R (eds) Current Therapy of Trauma 1984–1985. Decker & Mosby, Philadelphia 1984

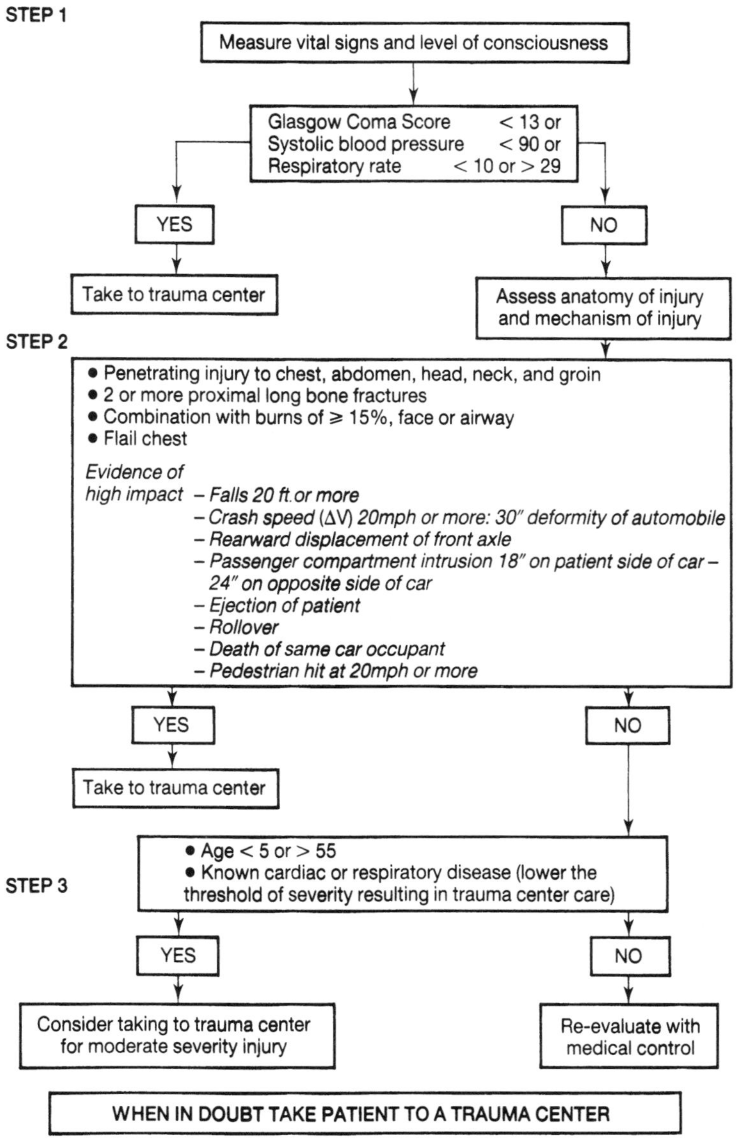

Fig. 7.10 A triage decision scheme recommended by the Committee on Trauma of the American College of Surgeons.[37]

airway obstruction.[92] Fractures of the extremities are immobilized by inflatable or rigid splints which contribute to resuscitation by reducing pain and soft tissue injury and improving distal blood flow.

Resuscitation

Rapid treatment is vital to the survival of the 5% of patients with life-threatening injuries causing airway obstruction, tension pneumothorax, torrential bleeding, cardiac tamponade and cervical spine injuries. Next in priority are injuries to the chest, abdomen, brain and spinal cord. The first few minutes of encounter between patient and doctor often dictate success or failure. Delayed resuscitation and failure to diagnose the true extent of injuries account for a substantial proportion of preventable deaths. Information from ambulance staff, relatives and bystanders as to whether the victim was a pedestrian, driver or passenger and if he or she was wearing a seat-belt is helpful. Details of the deceleration forces on impact, the nature of the wounding agent, the amount of blood lost, the presence of pre-existing cardiac disease, diabetes, respiratory disease and regular medication can be obtained while resuscitation is being undertaken. Alcohol intoxication confers major disadvantages: disorientation and aggression limit cooperation; neurological, respiratory and cardiac functions are depressed; vasodilatation causes hypothermia and platelet function is impaired.

Resuscitation is aimed at ensuring an adequate airway, breathing and circulation (i.e. the ABCs), which are the key to preservation of life.[93] The team effort is directed at simultaneous resuscitation, assessment of all injuries and initial management. One doctor, aided if necessary by others, secures an airway, provides ventilation, excludes a sucking chest wound, flail chest or pneumothorax, inserts a chest drain if indicated and determines vital signs and electrocardiograph activity. Simultaneously, a second doctor and assistants look for signs of haemorrhage externally or into body cavities, set up one or more intravenous lines, send off blood samples and commence energetic volume replacement. The next stage involves rapid physical assessment, immobilization of fractures and insertion of a urethral catheter, nasogastric tube and one or more central venous lines. The resuscitation area should be well equipped with an oxygen source, suction devices, pressure lines, electrocardiograph leads and electric outlets to facilitate assessment and management of the injured patient.

Immediate surgery may be necessary but if the patient is stable, constant vigilance is required for signs of recurrent hypovolaemia. The surgeon undertakes a rapid but comprehensive examination of the fully undressed patient, beginning at the top and moving down, not forgetting the neck, axillae, back and perineum. Distraction by a dramatic injury may mean that another inconspicuous but vital injury is missed. Intelligent appraisal of wounds may permit the prediction of the track of a wounding knife or missile, while the presence of a large exit wound suggests a high-velocity bullet injury. Monitoring is maintained while rapid radiological investigations are undertaken to evaluate the cervical spine, chest and pelvis prior to more specific radiological assessment of obvious injuries.

Only after this full examination should pain be relieved, partially arresting the neuroendocrine response to trauma and improving tissue perfusion. A 2 mg intravenous bolus of morphine sulphate is effective, short-acting and repeatable while intramuscular and subcutaneous injections are ineffective when given into underperfused tissues. Heavy sedation using narcotics depresses respiration, obscures pupillary and abdominal signs and eliminates restlessness which may provide vital evidence of hypoxia. Antibiotic treatment is commenced after successful resuscitation.

Airway and ventilation

Hypoxia aggravates the effects of haemorrhage and hypovolaemia and potentiates damage from a head injury. The first priority is to establish a patent airway by removing dentures, broken teeth, food, vomitus and blood, either digitally or by a high-flow low-volume sucker. Tachypnoea and cyanosis, stridor and the reflex use of accessory muscles of respiration suggest upper respiratory tract obstruction. It is always worth remembering that in the anaemic patient hypoxia may not manifest itself by cyanosis.

An oropharyngeal tube is inserted if pharyngolaryngeal reflexes are present. The tongue is pulled forward and 100% oxygen is given via a face-mask. Endotracheal intubation with a low-pressure cuffed tube is undertaken if these reflexes are absent. The correct placement of the endotracheal tube is confirmed by inflating the lungs and listening for breath sounds. Tracheal and bronchial toilet is carried out before the patient is connected to a ventilator. The presence of an expanding neck haematoma or the possibility of tracheal injury also necessitates the insertion of an endotracheal tube to secure an airway. Inflation of the cuff prevents extravasation of blood into the lungs. A skilled anaesthetist duly aware of the dangers can usually achieve intubation without hyperextending the neck, if an unconscious patient with a possible cervical spine fracture has to be intubated. When an anaesthetist is not available, and only if time permits, the neck may be stabilized by sandbags or less effectively by a collar before intubation is attempted. A flexible bronchoscope is then used to facilitate endotracheal intubation or the nasotracheal route is employed. Intubation of the apnoeic patient to overcome hypoxia and hypercapnia is essential. It is also life-saving in the patient with a head injury who is breathing inadequately but is conscious enough to resist. When uncertainty exists as to the likelihood of aspiration following regurgitation or active vomiting, rapid sequence induction and endotracheal intubation become vital, maintaining cricoid pressure and relaxing it only after the cuff has been inflated.

In maxillofacial injuries which cause obstruction of the nose and mouth, or if the airway at and above the level of the larynx is damaged, a cricothyroidotomy giving direct access to the trachea buys time (see Chapter 20). A small transverse incision over the cricothyroid membrane avoids thyroid tissue and allows the insertion of a small-gauge tracheostomy tube with minimal bleeding. Alternatively, one or two number 14 gauge needles can be pushed through the membrane and connected to an oxygen supply or a high-pressure jet ventilator to minimize aspiration. Injury to the larynx is rare and may occur in association with a cervical spine fracture at C6/7. An emergency tracheostomy is often required to correct hypoxia.

If respiratory distress persists despite intubation and assisted ventilation, a tension pneumothorax must be considered; if unrelieved, this can cause circulatory failure simply by drastically reducing the cardiac preload. When a pneumothorax is suspected, and if fatality is to be averted, a precautionary chest drain should be inserted into one or both sides before placing the patient on a ventilator. Tension pneumothorax in the presence of surgical emphysema may be caused by a major air leak from a bronchial tear. Equally, lung contusion from a crush injury may be responsible. Losing no time for radiological confirmation, a wide-bore intravenous cannula inserted through the second intercostal space in the mid clavicular line relieves tension prior to the insertion of a definitive chest drain through the fifth intercostal space in the mid axillary line (see Chapter 22). This allows the lung to re-expand, and evacuates any blood in the pleural cavity. The source of bleeding is usually the intercostal or internal mammary vessels though it can occasionally come from a pulmonary vessel at the hilum. A thoracotomy is indicated if there is immediate blood loss of 1500 cc or continuing blood loss in excess of 250 ml/h. A bronchial tear demands emergency bronchoscopy to confirm its presence prior to operative repair. The effects of all the measures taken to improve pulmonary function in major trauma are monitored by serial estimations of arterial blood gases. The desirability of continued ventilatory support is kept under constant review.

REFERENCE

93. Advanced Trauma Life Support for Physicians Manual, 5th edn. American College of Surgeons 1993

One simple procedure which can protect respiratory function is the insertion of a nasogastric tube. A patient with a head injury, a combined thoraco-abdominal injury or under the influence of alcohol loses the reflexes that protect the airway, a situation calling for immediate stomach evacuation if the serious and frequently fatal problem of massive pulmonary aspiration is to be averted. Regardless of how much time has elapsed since injury, it must be assumed that the stomach has failed to empty, simply as the result of pain, fear and distress. In the supine patient aspirated stomach contents may obstruct the airway, particularly the wider and more vertical right main stem bronchus, while liquid aspirate tends to gravitate to the right upper lobe or superior segment of the right lower lobe. A wide-bore nasogastric tube is passed and all the stomach contents aspirated prior to leaving the tube to drain freely into a collecting bag.

Circulation

Bleeding wounds are controlled initially by digital compression and then by a firm pad and pressure bandage; if this fails, a vascular clamp is preferable to a blindly applied haemostat which may damage the vessel and adjacent nerves. A tourniquet is undesirable except following traumatic amputation because, if its presence is forgotten, permanent vascular and nerve damage may ensue with subsequent limb loss.

The blood pressure is a traditional but insensitive measure in early shock as it may be maintained in a healthy young adult even after a loss of 15–20% of intravascular volume, dropping to 60–80 mmHg systolic after a 30% volume loss, and falling precipitously thereafter. This exponential behaviour of blood pressure which suddenly 'crashes' must be understood, particularly as such an event is sometimes mistakenly attributed to sudden bleeding from a large vessel. The pulse rate, skin perfusion and urinary output are more useful indicators of hypovolaemia. In elderly patients, dependence on the blood pressure and urine output is inadvisable as the presence of impaired renal function, diabetes and myocardial disease invalidate these indicators.

Replenishment of circulating volume is the major objective after severe trauma: special consideration must be given to the large third space losses in intestinal and retroperitoneal injuries where the soft tissues act as a physiological sponge. Large-bore intravenous cannulae are inserted, by cutdown if necessary. After major blood loss, the internal jugular and subclavian veins may be particularly collapsed. Leg veins normally avoided in abdominal injury are ideal for access on the rare occasion when superior vena cava injury is suspected.

Both crystalloid and colloid fluids have been used successfully but debate continues on the choice of fluid to be given. The proponents of a balanced salt solution are supported by the knowledge that a functional deficit of extracellular fluid requires replacement.[94] Raised filtration pressure, lowered colloid osmotic pressure and increased capillary permeability following major trauma and shock, however, favour the development of pulmonary oedema, and over-zealous crystalloid administration may encourage the development of adult respiratory distress syndrome. Initially, volume expansion is more quickly achieved with colloid rather than crystalloid, but eventually the two fluids will equilibrate in the extravascular space.[95] Natural colloid solutions such as human albumin are expensive and should be reserved for patients who are hypovolaemic but with significant hypoproteinaemia. Artificial colloids such as Haemaccel, a gelatin cross-linked with hexamethylene di-isocyanate, are quite suitable and may be infused into one line, with Hartmann's solution, for example, being administered through another. These fluids may lower the haematocrit to unacceptably low levels and it is unwise to use them to replace major blood losses. One replacement scheme is shown in Figure 7.11.

There is no substitute for fresh blood in severe haemorrhage. Transfusions of cross-matched, warmed and microfiltered blood should be commenced at the earliest opportunity (see Chapter 3), aimed at maintaining a haematocrit of 30–35%. Banked blood is

REFERENCES

94. Bhatia K N, Turner W W, Giesecke A H In: Wilder R J (ed) Multiple Trauma. Karger, Basel 1984
95. Shoemaker W C, Hauser C J Crit Care Med 1979; 7: 117

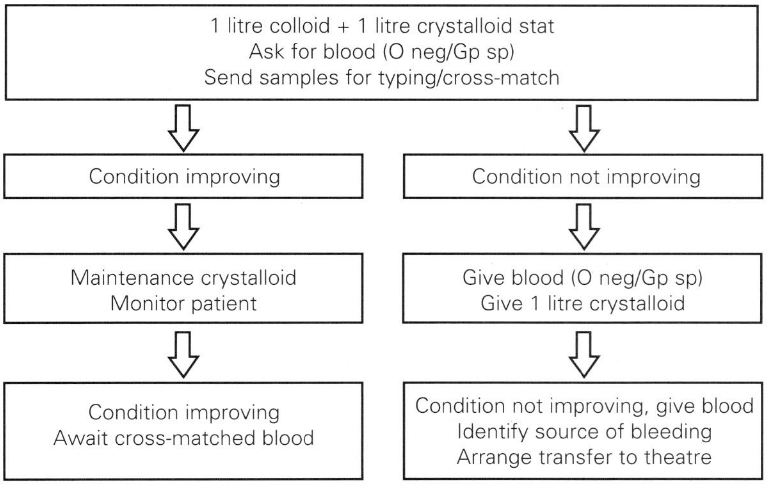

Fig. 7.11 Fluid replacement regimen for an adult with signs of established shock.

cold, low in pH, clotting factors and platelet activity, and high in potassium. Red cell concentrates and fresh frozen plasma can be used as an alternative if fresh blood is not available although platelet transfusions are also then required. Estimations of the haematocrit, platelet count and coagulation screening determine further requirements. A policy of numbering each new bag of fluid or blood is very helpful in keeping track of volume replacement. Serious unquantifiable hidden losses of blood into the pleural and peritoneal cavities from visceral or major vessel injury or into the soft tissues and retroperitoneum following fractures of the femur and pelvis cause profound hypovolaemic shock. Exsanguination on this scale may warrant immediate surgery rather than protracted unrewarding resuscitation. The heart may fail as a consequence of tension pneumothorax, cardiac tamponade, myocardial ischaemia, myocardial contusion or even coronary occlusion. The rare instance of combined hemiparesis and myocardial ischaemia caused by air embolism from a lacerated lung has also been described.[96]

Following major trauma the classical features of cardiac tamponade, namely pulsus paradoxus, falling arterial pressure, elevated venous pressure and muffled heart sounds, are not always apparent. Patients with wounds near the mediastinum who continue to remain hypotensive despite an elevated central venous pressure should be assumed to have cardiac tamponade until proved otherwise. Traditionally, pericardiocentesis is performed by directing a needle from the left xiphocostal space at an angle of 45° pointing to the left shoulder. A large needle could conceivably damage a coronary artery, but a successful pericardial tap of 20 ml of blood can bring about dramatic improvement in cardiac output. A more effective technique involves the prompt creation of a small pericardial window under local or light general anaesthesia. A short sub-xiphoid incision is made in the linea alba and digital exploration is continued down to the pericardial sac which is then incised and entered. If inexperienced in this technique, the surgeon should perform an emergency thoracotomy through the fourth or fifth anterior interspace. A longitudinal pericardiotomy is then made to allow the evacuation of clot; bleeding can normally be controlled by a couple of sutures in the myocardium.

A cardiac contusion may be the consequence of an injury to the chest wall and is sometimes associated with a flail chest or sternal fractures.[97,98] Evidence of cardiac damage can be obtained by ST segment and T wave changes on serial electrocardiography, by measurement of myocardial isoenzymes and by radionuclide scanning. Whether pump failure is the result of a contusion or a coronary artery occlusion may not be clear in the older patient but in either circumstance cardiac performance is monitored and special care taken with general anaesthesia.

Emergency thoracotomy in a properly equipped and staffed operating theatre is warranted if the patient is obviously moribund or in a state of recent or incipient cardiac arrest from hypovolaemic shock due to penetrating chest or abdominal trauma. This aggressive stance is both accepted and justified in patients who are near death with cardiac wounds, and has been rewarded by 40% survival in one series.[99] Emergency thoracotomy permits immediate relief of cardiac tamponade, control of the bleeding site and effective cardiac massage.[100] The placement of a clamp across the descending thoracic aorta affords the patient with a tense haemoperitoneum dying from major abdominal trauma a last chance of survival. This procedure at one stroke reduces the rate of blood loss, substantially improves coronary and cerebral perfusion, and at laparotomy allows evacuation and easy inspection instead of a final exsanguination before proximal control can be obtained. The value of this technique in salvaging one fifth of obviously moribund patients with injuries to the aorta and its branches cannot be ignored.[101] These procedures are rewarding if undertaken by trained personnel accustomed to working in a trauma centre with a purpose-built operating room close at hand. Emergency thoracotomy or laparotomy should *not* be performed in the resuscitation room where equipment, lighting and assistance is suboptimal. Rapid transportation of the patient to a well equipped operating room gives the best chance for survival.

Reassessment

Resuscitation may appear to restore the stability of the patient as judged by frequent observations of vital signs and electrocardiograph recordings, but the haemodynamic situation is often in a state of flux and a sudden decline is always possible. By this stage the patient should have:

- A central venous line, both for infusion and measurement of pressure, especially in response to a 'fluid challenge'.
- An arterial line for systemic arterial pressure measurement and sampling for gas analysis.
- A urinary catheter to estimate hourly urine output.

In certain head injuries, intracranial pressure measurement is essential and time may be found to insert an intraventricular cannula.

A more detailed examination surveying individual body areas, organs and systems becomes possible if the patient's condition remains stable (Table 7.6). This secondary assessment or survey provides the clinical basis for organizing further radiographs (Figs 7.12–7.14) or other specific investigations (Fig. 7.15) which are helpful before planning operations. Any tendency to indulge in unnecessary investigation may be counterproductive and this particularly applies when numerous casualties require simultaneous assessment and treatment. A patient in hypovolaemic shock with peritoneal signs needs a laparotomy rather than the refinements of a computerized tomography scan, peritoneal lavage or angiography; the tendency to document excessively rather than to intervene speedily may prove fatal and must be balanced against the minimal morbidity of the occasional negative laparotomy.[92] A reliable record must, however, be kept of all findings, impressions, resuscitative procedures and investigations for continuity of care in the operating theatre, intensive care unit and the ward. Documentation will necessarily be brief but it should be complete.

REFERENCES

96. Shaftan G W World J Surg 1983; 7: 19
97. Liedtke A J, DeMuth W E Am Heart J 1973; 86: 687
98. Jones J W, Hewitt R L, Drapanas T Ann Surg 1975; 181: 567
99. Feliciano D V, Carmel G, Bitondo P A C Ann Surg 1984; 199: 717
100. Asensio J A, Stewart B M et al Surg Clin N Amer 1996; 76: 685
101. Baker C C, Thomas A N, Trunkey D D J Trauma 1980; 20: 848

Table 7.6 Check-list for secondary survey

Head	
	All of scalp
	Facial skeleton
	Eyes, ears, nose, mouth
	Glasgow Coma Scale
	Limb movements and reflexes
	(CT scan)
Neck	
	Cervical spine
	Trachea
	Neck veins
	Cervical spine radiograph
Chest	
	Bruising
	Movement, percussion, auscultation
	Chest radiograph
Abdomen	
	Bruising
	Tenderness
	Auscultation
	Rectal examination
	Pelvic radiograph
	(Peritoneal lavage)
	(Ultrasound)
Back	
	Bruising
	Interspinous gap
	Saddle area sensation
	Anal tone
Limbs	
	Look, feel, move
	Pulses

Procedures in brackets performed only if indicated

Head injuries

Once the patient has been resuscitated, scalp wounds and suspected open depressed fractures are covered with sterile dressings. Bleeding or cerebrospinal fluid leaks from the ear and nose are noted. Observations of the patient's mental state, degree of confusion and agitation are made and the level of consciousness is assessed as determined by the Glasgow Coma Scale which influences surgical intervention and remains as a useful record for medicolegal purposes. Cranial nerve examination provides important clues to brainstem injury. A full neurological examination to exclude lateralizing signs may be compromised by injuries to the limbs but should be performed if possible (see Chapter 16). Hypotension in a multiply injured patient who is not obviously bleeding should not, as a rule, be attributed to a closed head injury, except in instances where a spinal cord injury has resulted in paraplegia and a loss of sympathetic tone (see Chapter 46).

The possibility of an expanding extradural haematoma must be excluded if the level of consciousness falls in a patient with multiple injuries despite energetic correction of hypoxia and hypovolaemia (see Chapter 16). Evacuation of an extradural haematoma can be a life-saving manoeuvre but coincident exsanguinating mortal wounds of the chest and abdomen must be given first priority.

Computerized tomographic scanning has transformed neurosurgical practice in defining damage from depressed fractures and in delineating extradural, subdural or intracerebral haematomas and their effects on the brain. Skull radiographs display fractures, foreign bodies and intracranial air (Fig. 7.12a) but provide no information on the extent of intracranial damage.

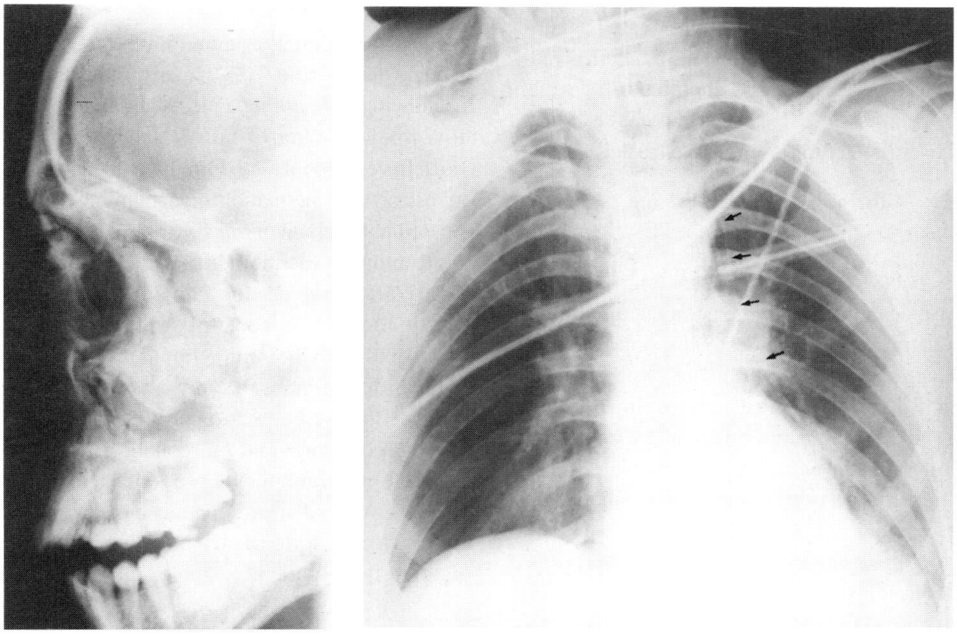

a b

Fig. 7.12 Multiply injured patient with trauma to head, face, eye, chest, abdomen and limbs. (**a**) Lateral radiograph of anterior head and face shows fracture of frontonasal process, aerocele in frontal area, disruption of orbit and elements of a Le Fort III fracture of mid-third of face. (**b**) Chest radiograph shows surgical emphysema especially in the neck and pneumomediastinum and displacement of the pleura (arrows) caused by a bronchial tear.

Facial injuries

When an airway has been secured, haemorrhage must be stemmed. Lacerations of the scalp and face can only be partly controlled by compression, and losses should be taken into account when assessing the volume replacement that will be required. Continuing haemorrhage from the nasopharynx can be brought under control by inserting a no. 20 Foley catheter through one of the nostrils, inflating the balloon and applying traction to the catheter or by packing the postnasal space and pharynx once the airway is secured (see Chapter 20).[92] An ophthalmological opinion is required if there is any suspicion of injury to the eye (see Chapter 15).

The bones of the face are then examined externally and intraorally, palpating the supraorbital margins, the zygomata, maxillae and mandible to identify fractures (see Chapter 13). The signs looked for are malocclusion, open-bite deformity, mobility of the upper jaw and hard palate and anaesthesia in the distribution of the intraorbital nerve. Amongst the numerous permutations of the Le Fort grades of fractures involving the bones of the middle third of the face is the classical dish-face deformity seen in the Le Fort II and III fractures (Fig. 7.12a). The facial bone structure has the capacity to absorb the force of impact in a deceleration injury and by crumpling inwards protects the brain from fatal trauma. Other fractures involving the zygoma and 'blowout' fractures of the orbit are associated with displacement of the globe of the eye. Strong muscular attachments of the mandible ensure that when it fractures the patient displays obvious deformity and inability to close the mouth; numbness of the lower lip may be noted (see Chapter 13). Multiple mandibular fractures may affect both sides and frequently involve the necks of the condyles. Bilateral fractures at the angles of the mandible allow the body carrying the tongue to fall back and occlude the airway, a situation of utmost importance in the unconscious patient.

Being associated with lacerations of the mouth and face, many facial fractures must be regarded as compound and treated accordingly. The maxillofacial surgeon will be interested in detailed radiographs of the facial bones (see Chapter 13), the quality of which improves as the gross oedema subsides. He or she may have to wait, in any case, while other life-threatening injuries are treated first.

Neck injuries

Simple inspection of the neck may provide clues: engorged neck veins may be a sign of cardiac tamponade or tension pneumothorax, the latter confirmed by a tracheal deviation to the opposite side; surgical emphysema indicates a tear of the bronchus or occasionally of the oesophagus (Fig. 7.12b). The most serious injury to be excluded is a fracture of the cervical spine: if pain and local tenderness are present the fracture must be assumed to be unstable and the neck immobilized by sandbags or a rigid collar. In the unconscious patient, fracture of the cervical spine should be presumed until proved otherwise by the appropriate radiographs. Paraplegia may not be evident in the unconscious patient if transection of the cord has already occurred, except indirectly by a rapid pulse and hypotension, which are poor indicators in the multiply injured patient. Skull traction must be applied as soon as other life-saving surgery has been undertaken, after which the patient can be safely log-rolled, a necessary manoeuvre in the routine care of the paraplegic. A high cord lesion associated with respiratory distress demands careful endotracheal intubation.

The neck radiographs must include the most commonly injured vertebrae C6 and C7, often missed in routine radiological examination. Fracture dislocations of the facetal joints occur in hyperflexion injury and are extremely unstable. In contrast, a fall on the head generally results in stable compression fractures of the vertebrae though some fragments may impinge on the cord. Hyperextension injuries tend to occur in the older patient with established cervical spondylosis. Later CT scanning may allow a more confident diagnosis if doubt still exists after plain radiographs.

Chest injuries (see Chapter 22)

The chest will already have been examined in some detail while life-saving procedures are being undertaken. Radiological investigations can be extremely helpful if the patient's condition allows a safe interval before definitive surgery is required. Indications for immediate surgery in patients with closed thoracic injuries are a major air leak, continuing haemorrhage and a ruptured diaphragm. Penetrating injuries, with a dangerous predicted track and the likelihood of a coexisting intra-abdominal injury, should also lead to surgical intervention. The chest and abdomen must be considered as one contiguous cavity as apparent intrathoracic injuries are frequently associated with damage to abdominal viscera. Plain chest radiographs must be examined thoroughly for useful diagnostic clues. The adequacy of apical and sump drains in evacuating air and blood is assessed by repeated films. Surgical emphysema is usually present in relation to penetrating injury but if located in the mediastinum and neck may indicate tear of the bronchus or oesophagus (Fig. 7.12b). A flail ribcage with a fractured sternum following a steering-wheel injury raises the possibility of myocardial contusion. Cardiac tamponade whether caused by blunt or penetrating trauma may be recognized by the flask-shaped cardiac outline (Fig. 7.13). In crush injuries there may be evidence of shadowing of the lung fields. Pulmonary oedema may be observed following aspiration of gastric contents or if excessive crystalloid solutions have been infused. Finally, evidence of diaphragmatic elevation or a tear with herniation of abdominal viscera is a diagnosis often missed in deceleration injury.

Rupture of the thoracic aortic isthmus should be suspected if in a deceleration injury the first and second ribs are fractured, particularly if this is associated with superior mediastinal widening. High quality radiographs show additional features of aortic rupture such as distortion of the aortic contour, apical 'capping' or obliteration of the medial left upper lung field, opacification of the space between the aorta and pulmonary artery, tracheal shift to the left, multiple rib fractures, depression of the left main bronchus, and displacement of a radiopaque nasogastric tube to the right (Fig. 7.14). Urgent aortography[102] is the most accurate diagnostic investigation if the patient is stable. This usually demonstrates a rather

REFERENCE

102. Symbas P N Trauma to the Heart and Great Vessels. Grune & Stratton, New York 1978

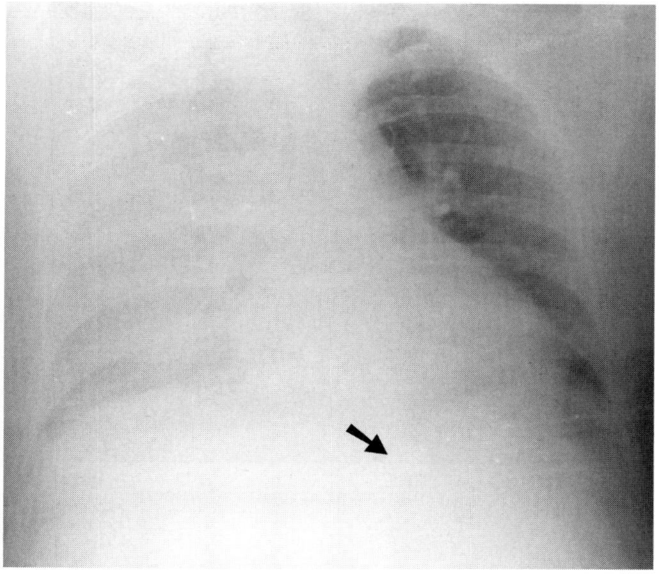

Fig. 7.13 Chest radiograph of victim who survived attempted assassination by several gunshot wounds presenting with signs of cardiac tamponade and shock. Classical features of haemopericardium and right haemothorax caused by bullet (arrow) which had penetrated liver, right lung, intrathoracic and subdiaphragmatic vena cava and right ventricle.

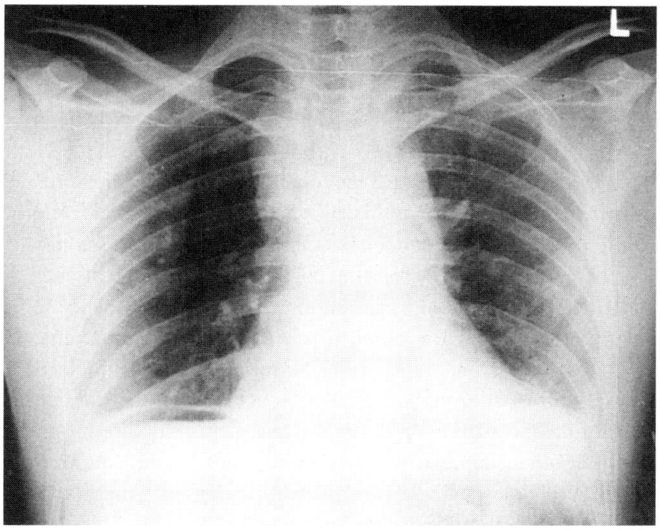

Fig. 7.14 Chest radiograph of patient who suffered sudden deceleration injury of the isthmus of the thoracic aorta showing widening of superior mediastinum, opacification between aorta and pulmonary artery and loss of clarity of left upper lung field ('apical capping'). Aortic injury suspected only after laparotomy for visceral injuries which accounts for air under the diaphragm.

vertical descending arch, intimal tears and pseudoaneurysm formation (Fig. 7.15). A computerized tomographic scan now usually confirms the diagnosis without resort to arteriography. Immediate surgery may be wiser if the evidence is convincing as patients have been known to die before reaching the operating theatre and have even arrested during induction of anaesthesia.[103]

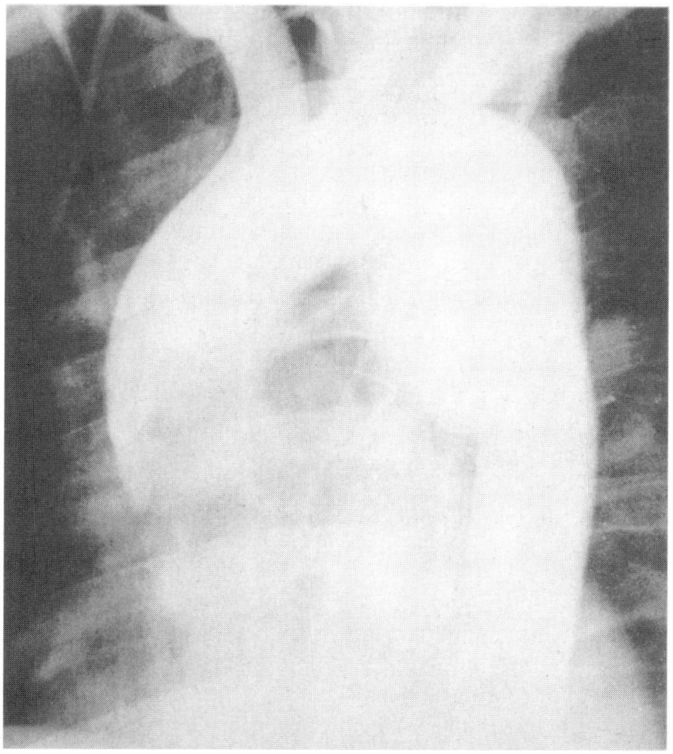

Fig. 7.15 Aortogram showing isthmic rupture of the thoracic aorta resulting in false aneurysm formation. At operation haematoma extended from the root of the thoracic aorta down to the mid descending aorta. The femoral artery and left atrium were cannulated for bypass, the aorta was cross-clamped proximal and distal to the rupture, and after excising the edges a Dacron graft was successfully interposed.

Abdominal injuries (see Chapter 27)

The abdominal cavity extends from the level of the nipple line above to that of the gluteal crease below and therefore the intrathoracic and intrapelvic extensions of the abdomen must be kept in mind. The onus is on the surgeon to regard any wound of the torso, whether by knife or bullet, as potentially involving both the chest and the abdomen and a careful search is required when an exit wound cannot be found. Exploration of a knife wound with a gloved finger to check if the peritoneal cavity has been breached cannot be relied upon.

In closed injuries the location of bruises, abrasions and the characteristic patterned bruise caused by a seat-belt, tyre mark or other object which points to crush injury may assist in predicting damage to an organ or major vessel. It is worth emphasizing that free blood or urine in the peritoneal cavity may not abolish bowel sounds even when a hollow viscus has perforated. Generalized tenderness with rebound tenderness indicates the presence of blood or visceral contents in the peritoneal cavity. Haemorrhage into the peritoneal cavity or major vessel trunk injury has to be assumed if the patient's abdomen is distending and the patient is unconscious and

REFERENCE

103. Plume S, DeWeese J A Arch Surg 1979; 114: 240

unresponsive to resuscitation. Immediate laparotomy is necessary instead of resorting to futile investigations as the situation becomes rapidly irretrievable.

Plain radiographs of the abdomen are of limited value in decision-making but if available may be used to advantage. Free air in the decubitus position suggests perforation, and the retroperitoneal position of the duodenum and descending colon should be remembered where air may be trapped in small quantities. Rib fractures of the lower thoracic cage on the right and left may be associated with damage to the liver and spleen respectively. In the latter case, elevation of the diaphragm and displacement of the gastric air bubble towards the midline may be present. Kidney damage should be suspected if there is evidence of anterior abdominal wall injury associated with fractures of the transverse processes of lumbar vertebrae and if the psoas outline is lost.

The two most valuable investigative tools when the clinical findings are equivocal, or when head injury or cord damage make physical signs unreliable, are computerized tomography and peritoneal lavage. These are only justifiable when the patient is in a stable condition. Computerized tomographic scanning is useful in defining injury to the liver, spleen, kidneys, pancreas, duodenum and major vessel trunks (Fig. 7.16). Aortography may also be used to define injuries to major vessels.

If the pelvis is intact, significant haematuria demands intravenous urography which either demonstrates extravasation at the site of a major rupture of the kidney or non-opacification of the kidney due to disruption of the renal artery, in which case angiography is indicated (see Chapter 10).

Peritoneal lavage has an accuracy as high as 98% in diagnosing intraperitoneal bleeding or soiling from a ruptured viscus, and is particularly informative in the unconscious, inebriated or paraplegic patient. It should not be considered as an alternative to sound clinical judgement but as a means of reinforcing opinions for or against laparotomy. It is particularly valuable in establishing intra-abdominal injury in penetrating wounds of the chest and back, but false-positive results do occur in association with retroperitoneal injuries such as rupture of the diaphragm, lacerations of the pancreas and duodenum and perforations of small bowel.[15] Peritoneal lavage may illuminate the confusing picture of abdominal stab wounds where significant internal injuries are discovered in a third of patients without suspicious physical signs and, conversely, no injuries are found in 15% of patients with striking clinical signs. The technique requires the insertion of a dialysis cannula or a 14 F multi-fenestrated catheter via a small subumbilical incision, made under local anaesthetic, through which 1 litre of isotonic saline is allowed to run in and equilibrate with peritoneal contents. A decision to undertake laparotomy is made if the effluent comprising at least half the infusate contains a red blood cell count of 50 000–100 000/ml or a white cell count of over 500/ml (Table 7.7).[104] Great care must be taken to avoid causing bleeding during insertion of the catheter.

Pelvic injuries

Blunt pelvic trauma follows road traffic accidents and crush injuries and presents with massive invisible retroperitoneal bleeding and shock, often complicated by damage to the bladder and urethra (see Chapter 37). Penetrating trauma in this region may also involve the large and small bowel and iliac vessels. Serious pelvic injuries involve compression of the pelvic ring with fractures of the pubic rami or disruption of the symphysis anteriorly and fracture dislocations of the sacroiliac joint posteriorly. When the victim is run over a severe diastasis or 'open oyster shell' injury results. The other serious injury in this area is that of central dislocation of the hip joint caused by sudden deceleration and compression.

When the deformity of the pelvis is not visible it may be confirmed by palpation. Examination should include inspection of the urethral meatus for blood, the scrotum for haematoma, the vagina for lacerations, and rectal examination for sphincter tone, the position of the prostate and presence of blood. Radiographs will define the extent of injury to the pelvis but urethrography should exclude damage to the membranous urethra and cystography via a Foley catheter will identify rupture of the bladder in both open and closed injuries (see Chapter 37).

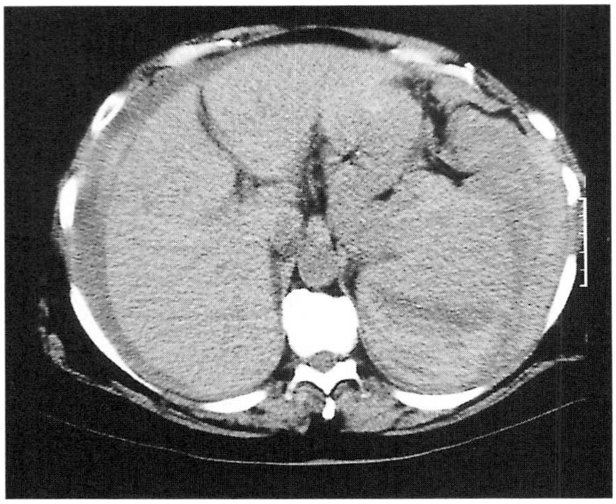

Fig. 7.16 CT scan of a patient with a ruptured spleen.

Table 7.7
Criteria for positive peritoneal lavage following infusion of 1 litre of normal saline

Red blood cell count	> 50 000/ml
White blood cell count	> 500/ml
Bile	Present
Bacteria	Present on Gram stain
Vegetable fibre	Present

Thoracolumbar spine injuries (see Chapter 46)

Sudden deceleration, as in a road accident or a fall from a height, usually results in major injury to organs and viscera in the chest and abdomen which may distract the examiner from noticing a serious spinal injury. A thorough peripheral neurological examination is therefore always required. Sensation, including that of the

REFERENCE

104. Rowlands B J In: Taylor I (ed) Progress in Surgery, vol. 3. Churchill Livingstone, Edinburgh 1988

perianal area, motor function and reflexes including anal sphincter tone and the bulbocavernosus reflex should be checked repeatedly over the next few hours. Careful log-rolling of the patient while applying traction along the axis of the body allows inspection of the back for bruises and wounds, and palpation for tenderness over the spinous processes, for a 'step-off' or gibbus indicating collapse, or for adjacent paravertebral spasm.

The patient is moved to a firm trolley for plain radiography and computerized tomographic scans which provide finer anatomical detail. The wedge compression fracture of a vertebral body from hyperflexion at the thoracolumbar junction is very painful but usually stable. Equally stable are vertical compression fractures, though the fragments of a burst vertebra may be displaced posteriorly to compress the cord or nerve roots. Unstable fractures are classically the flexion and rotation injuries at the thoracolumbar junction and of the posterior structures of the vertebra. Severe trauma may lead to a further type of unstable injury, usually above T10, in which the vertebra may be displaced laterally or anteroposteriorly, almost invariably associated with complete paraplegia. The 'Chance fracture' is a horizontal splitting of the neural arch and vertebral body caused by flexion distraction forces as following a seat-belt injury. These injuries require the attention of an orthopaedic surgeon experienced in managing spinal injuries.

Limb injuries

Attention will already have been paid to bleeding wounds. Apart from bruises and lacerations any obvious deformities and instability thought to be the result of fractures or fracture dislocations must be documented. Dislocations of all the major joints of upper and lower limbs, particularly at the knee, may be associated with serious neurovascular injury—a situation demanding a formal assessment of the peripheral pulses aided by Doppler ultrasound and a peripheral nervous system examination as well. Antibiotics should be administered immediately to all patients with compound fractures. Fractures and dislocations must be clearly defined by biplanar X-ray films and, if a vascular injury is suspected, early blind exploration or formal angiography should be undertaken immediately to reduce the ischaemic period between injury and restoration of flow. Temporary intraluminal shunts (Fig. 7.17) can be rapidly inserted at the start of surgery to bridge severed arteries and veins before a formal repair is begun,[105,106] although an alternative is to perform the vascular repair before stabilizing the skeleton and dealing with soft tissue injuries.

Anaesthesia

Anaesthetists possess the required expertise to establish an airway and maintain and control ventilation, but trauma teams should also have this training. It is important to know of any medications or addiction to drugs such as lysergic acid diethylamide (LSD), amphetamines, marijuana and alcohol which interact with anaesthetics. Anaesthetic agents cannot entirely be relied upon to maintain haemodynamic stability in patients who are in hypovolaemic shock. The chosen agent should provide smooth induction, adequate analgesia and amnesia, and minimal cardiovascular

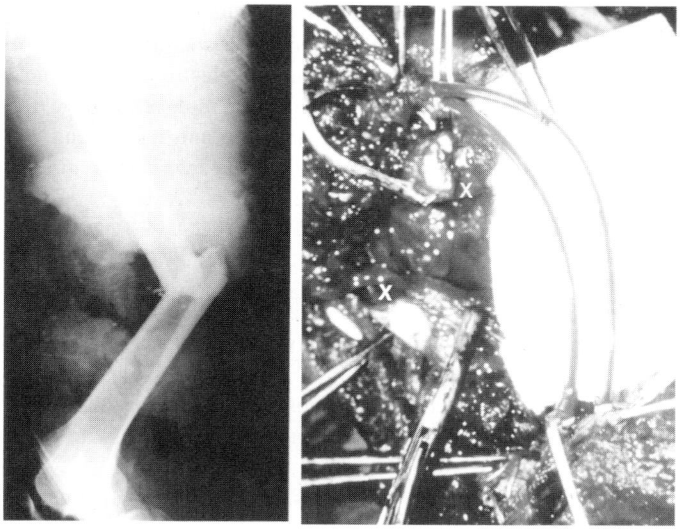

a b

Fig. 7.17 Blunt and penetrating injury to passenger in car crash. **(a)** Radiograph shows virtual dismemberment (note defect in soft tissues) at right mid femoral level, the only structures in continuity being fascia lata, lateral hamstrings and a bruised sciatic nerve. **(b)** Javid shunt in transected artery perfusing distal limb and another in severed vein draining it. Both ends (XX) are aligned prior to fixation followed by reconstruction of femoral artery and two large veins; fasciotomy was not required and limb function recovered completely 2 years later.

depression. It is therefore vital that systemic arterial pressure, central venous pressure and cardiac activity are monitored accurately and continuously at this stage. Anaesthetic agents may not be tolerated in patients with chest injuries, and thoracotomy may have to be commenced using oxygen and muscle relaxants, adding other drugs as the patient's condition improves. In the event of a major bronchial fracture a double-lumen endotracheal tube is inserted, ventilating one lung as a temporary expedient. When the globe of the eye is injured, further damage and possible loss is avoided by keeping the intraocular pressure down, particularly during anaesthetic induction.

The internal jugular vein rather than an arm vein should be cannulated for infusion and pressure measurements in an emergency, and certainly if the upper limbs are injured. This allows the surgeons free access to proceed swiftly with the operation. The left atrial filling pressure can be measured by direct catheterization if a thoracotomy has been done. Hypothermia in the major trauma patient is a serious problem from exposure at time of injury, cold infusions, and intraoperative heat loss. As the core temperature falls, myocardial perfusion worsens, arrhythmias occur, coagulation deficiencies follow and blood sample analysis becomes less reliable. Hypothermia can be corrected by using warmed humidified air, warmed blood and intravenous fluids and a warming

REFERENCES

105. Barros D'Sa A A B In: Greenhalgh R M, Jameson C W, Nicolaides A N (eds) Limb Salvage and Amputation for Vascular Disease. Saunders, London 1988
106. Barros D'Sa A A B Eur J Vasc Surg 1989; 3: 471

blanket. During surgery, the anaesthetist forewarns the intensive care unit; when the operation is over, he or she ensures that the patient is as stable as possible. A portable electronic mechanical ventilator and monitoring equipment are employed during the transfer, and on arrival at the intensive care unit monitoring and respiratory support are continued whilst the operating team discuss the patient with the staff of the unit.

Drugs

Steroids may protect the microvasculature from injury and on this basis methylprednisolone has been given for the first 24–48 hours but such practice is not customary.[107] Postoperative pain from rib fractures may be relieved by intercostal nerve blocks and, similarly, analgesia in upper limb injuries can be attained by brachial plexus blocks (see Chapter 5).

As volume replacement continues, an inotropic agent such as dopamine, carefully administered, is sometimes of value if cardiac output is depressed. In doses of 1–5 μg/kg per minute, dopamine is mildly inotropic, its main action being on dopaminergic receptors, thereby improving renal and mesenteric blood flow. In doses of 5–10 μg/kg per minute the β-adrenergic effects supervene, whereas in high doses of more than 20 μg/kg per minute the α-receptors are stimulated to cause arteriolar vasoconstriction.[108] It must be remembered, however, that hypovolaemia has to be corrected and that high-dose dopamine mainly provides post-load cardiac support. Care must be taken to ensure that the advantages of using dopamine are not compromised by acidosis, arrhythmias and renal failure. Dobutamine is an effective inotropic agent when myocardial function is suboptimal, e.g. hypotension in respiratory failure, but unlike dopamine it does not improve renal or mesenteric blood flow.

Patients with myocardial contusions, myocardial ischaemia or septicaemia may develop severe peripheral vasoconstriction which burdens the left ventricle. Vasodilators such as sodium nitroprusside given very cautiously are titrated against response, watching for a dangerous drop in blood pressure which can be counteracted by vasopressors and volume expanders. Such drugs are used when volume replacement is adequate and blood loss has been corrected.

Adrenaline is a powerful myocardial stimulant and is reserved for the patient in extremis who fails to respond to conventional therapy. Digitalis is only of value in a previously healthy victim of major trauma and may be dangerous if used acutely in the unstable patient. Calcium chloride has a valuable inotropic function and is given as an infusion under electrocardiographic control which will detect signs of irritability and arrhythmia. Lignocaine may have a useful role in treating arrhythmias associated with contusion of the myocardium or underlying myocardial ischaemia and, once again, must be administered under electrocardiographic monitoring.

Monitoring and intensive care

The purpose of monitoring a patient is to obtain accurate regular data on the effects of trauma, to assess the response of treatment and to detect signs of deterioration. Data is recorded precisely on a flow chart to illustrate the progress of the patient. In order to assist in the monitoring of patients in intensive care an elaborate variety of clinical indices and severity scales have been developed based on clinical information and laboratory investigations. The first sequence of observations, based mainly on circulatory measurements, is used to guide further action.

When mechanical ventilation has been instituted its performance must be monitored to avoid the complications of sepsis, tracheal erosion and barotrauma from delivering large tidal volumes. Increments in tidal volume rather than increases in respiratory rate are required to overcome the loss of pulmonary compliance following trauma in order to achieve adequate alveolar ventilation. Raising the fraction of inspired oxygen from a baseline of 40% becomes dangerous and, if the inspired oxygen has to be maintained beyond 70% for prolonged periods, oxygen toxicity may cause interstitial pulmonary fibrosis. For this reason, if the fraction of inspired oxygen exceeds 50%, positive end-expiratory pressure maintained at 5–10 cmH_2O is preferred as this improves the ventilation–perfusion ratio, minimizing shunting and enhancing oxygenation. Positive end-expiratory pressure is particularly valuable in cases of lung contusion, especially if associated with massive blood transfusion or sepsis. The anaesthetist must remain alert to its dangers, which are a reduction in venous return and cardiac output if the patient is still hypovolaemic, and it also carries the risk of tension pneumothorax.

During ventilation the rate, minute volume, inspired oxygen concentration and peak airway pressure must all be controlled. The response is assessed by arterial sampling or by automated analysis, noting the partial pressure of oxygen and carbon dioxide, and the acid–base excess, which are employed to adjust the delivery of ventilatory support. Weaning the patient off the ventilator is much easier if intermittent mandatory ventilation has been employed. This enables a weakened patient to breathe spontaneously in between assisted respirations and gradually to resume independent respiration.

Central venous pressure monitoring is vital to avoid under-replacement of fluid losses and to gauge myocardial function during rapid massive infusions. This is especially relevant in elderly patients with myocardial disease or in those with myocardial contusions, cardiac tamponade or tension pneumothoraces, all of which lead to heart failure. It has been suggested that the central venous pressure ought to be maintained above 10 cmH_2O during resuscitation and at a higher level if mechanical ventilation is required.[109]

Systemic arterial pressure measurement is more accurate than Doppler ultrasound techniques, and this observation in association with heart rate may assist in the estimation of volume deficit. An arterial pressure line is also essential to monitor inotropic drugs or vasopressors. After a negative Allen's test, the radial artery is cannulated, alternative sites being the dorsalis pedis or brachial artery.

REFERENCES

107. Luce J M, Pierson D J Sem Resp Med 1981; 2: 151
108. Civetta J M Intensive Care Therapeutics. Appleton-Century-Crofts, New York 1980
109. Border J R, Bone L In: Kinney J M et al (eds) Manual of Surgical Intensive Care. Saunders, Philadelphia 1977

The routine use of the balloon-tipped flow-directed Swan–Ganz catheter in intensive care units is of particular importance in the management of an unstable patient with complex injuries, especially in the presence of coexisting heart disease.[110] This device is rarely needed in the early management of the injured patient when the central venous pressure provides essential information simply and quickly. The Swan–Ganz catheter is inserted via the right internal jugular vein and advanced through the right heart into the pulmonary artery where characteristic tracings confirm correct positioning. The pulmonary artery pressure is measured, as is the pulmonary capillary wedge pressure which correlates well with left atrial pressure, providing a good indicator of left ventricular end-diastolic pressure. A Swan–Ganz catheter is ideal for monitoring safe volume replacement in an injured patient who also has a compromised myocardium. In the young trauma victim, a pulmonary capillary wedge pressure below 12–18 mmHg indicates inadequate volume replacement. The pulmonary catheter is the route by which the mixed venous oxygen content, which is the best indicator of oxygen delivery and utilization, can be estimated. In addition the Swan–Ganz catheter can be used to measure the right atrial pressure and the cardiac output by means of a thermistor.

The earlier the measurements of cardiac output are undertaken following major trauma the more accurately they assist in resuscitation. The measurement of atrial pressure guides volume replacement and determines the need for inotropic support of the myocardium. The balloon must always be deflated when measurements are not being made as it can damage the tricuspid valve and pulmonary artery, causing thrombosis and pulmonary infarction. The insertion and use of the catheter requires experience and considerable expertise.

Following major trauma, a urinary output of approximately 0.5–1.0 ml/kg per hour ought to be maintained in the first 48 hours. More useful measurements of renal function are provided by the ratio of urinary to plasma osmolality and the urine sodium concentration. An osmolality ratio of more than 1.2 associated with a urinary sodium of less than 20 mmol/l in an oliguric patient is indicative of inadequate perfusion, while a ratio of less than 1.2 when the urinary sodium is more than 40 mmol/l suggests inadequate renal function.

Continuing blood losses must be accurately recorded. Periodic haemoglobin and haematocrit estimations may indicate haemodilution. Once a reasonable state of stability has been achieved a coagulation profile and a platelet count must be checked and deficiencies corrected. Other routine estimations should include a white cell count and differential, urea, creatinine and electrolytes, biochemical screening, protein and albumin concentrations. Lactic dehydrogenase, isoenzyme and α_1-antitrypsin concentrations are indicators of the severity of trauma.

Prevention and treatment of infection

While impaired ventilation and haemorrhage contribute to early death, sepsis represents the second most important cause of late mortality. The prevention and control of infection is a challenge which severely tests the capabilities of trauma teams in intensive care units. So far, the only worthwhile immunizations are tetanus toxoid and the use of polyvalent pneumococcal vaccine in splenectomized patients. Immune enhancement of host defences by immunomodulation and specific replacement of opsonic proteins may help in the prevention of serious sepsis but there is little clinical evidence of the efficacy of these techniques.

Strict asepsis and antisepsis must be maintained, both in the operating theatre and in the intensive care unit. Care must be taken in hand-washing, glove usage, and preparation of the skin for insertion of lines and catheters. As invasive procedures provide entry for infection they must be based on need rather than routine habit, and every tube and catheter must be considered at each ward round and removed at the earliest possible opportunity.

Devitalized and necrotic tissue must be excised, foreign bodies removed and the wound thoroughly irrigated and cleansed of contaminants. Infected tissues must be debrided, abscesses drained immediately and an occult infection pursued until it is discovered if generalized sepsis and progression to multiple organ failure are to be arrested. Gentle handling of tissues, care in the use of retractors and clamps, avoidance of wound dehydration, the use of inert unbraided sutures, attention to haemostasis, and minimal use of coagulation diathermy contribute significantly to the prevention of infection. Contaminated wounds may be left open for 3–5 days, and after inspection delayed primary suture is undertaken.

Prophylactic antibiotics are required for open injuries, compound fractures and joint and tendon injuries, penetrating trauma of the gastrointestinal and respiratory tracts, and when prostheses have to be implanted. Perforation of an abdominal viscus results in polymicrobial (both aerobic and anaerobic) bacterial infection. Experimental studies have supported the use of antibiotics active against most anaerobes and in preventing abscess forma-tion and septicaemia. The most commonly recommended regimen has in the past been an aminoglycoside and clindamycin, a combination perfectly adequate to combat all pathogens with the possible exception of enterococci, which can be covered by adding penicillin or ampicillin, if it is thought relevant.[111] Difficulties in maintaining adequate therapeutic levels of gentamicin in patients with an unstable circulation or renal failure increase the risks of nephrotoxicity and damage to the audiovestibular apparatus.[112] The risk of clindamycin-induced pseudomembranous colitis has strengthened the preference for metronidazole. First-generation cephalosporins were promising, but the development of increasingly resistant bacterial strains combined with their nephrotoxicity—especially when they were given with frusemide—has led to the use of safer, less toxic and more effective third-generation cephalosporins such as cefotaxime. Antibiotic therapy for abdominal trauma should not be extended beyond 72 hours after injury.[68]

Penicillin is extremely effective in dealing with the mixed flora of bacteria likely to cause infection after injuries involving the oral cavity. This may be supplemented by metronidazole if resistant

REFERENCES

110. Swan H J C, Ganz W Surg Clin North Am 1975; 55: 501
111. Ericsson C D, Rowlands B J In: Miller T A (ed) Physiological Basis of Modern Surgical Care. Mosby, St Louis 1988
112. Reed R L Surg Clin N Amer 1991; 71: 765

anaerobes are responsible for persistent infection. A combination of flucloxacillin with or without gentamicin significantly reduces infection after compound fracture but must be combined with a thorough debridement of the wound. The possibility of clostridial infection is high in severe open fractures accompanied by extensive soft tissue destruction, or after traumatic amputations, and a regimen of an aminoglycoside plus a penicillinase-resistant penicillin such as flucloxacillin, in addition to penicillin G, is recommenced. The efficacy of antibiotics in preventing meningitis after head injuries with cerebrospinal fluid leaks has never been proven, but penicillin or cefotaxime or even rifampicin for a period of 3 days is recommended. A reduction in the level of consciousness may indicate the development of meningeal sepsis.

The diagnosis of sepsis in the injured patient is based on the presence of pyrexia, rigors, hypotension, increased oxygen consumption, leucocytosis or hyperfibrinogenaemia. Positive blood cultures and Gram stain of the drainage fluid, sputum, urine and effluent confirm the presence of micro-organisms.

Nosocomial infections of the lower respiratory tract have been treated in the past by a combination of an aminoglycoside and a semisynthetic penicillin such as piperacillin, but currently cefuroxime or cefotaxime is preferred, and for late *Pseudomonas* infections cefrazidine or ciprofloxacin may be more appropriate. Debate continues about the value of selective decontamination of the digestive tract which aims to prevent colonization with aerobic Gram-negative bacilli and to preserve the commensal anaerobic flora. Application of this policy was responsible for a striking reduction of infection rates from 81 to 16% in major trauma patients.[70] Various regimens have been employed, the most promising of which is SPEAR (selective parenteral and enteral antisepsis regimen) embracing selective decontamination of the digestive tract (oral polymyxin E, tobramycin and amphotericin B), systemic cefotaxime and microbiological monitoring.[113] A recent meta-analysis of randomized controlled trials of selective digestive decontamination has shown a good reduction of nosocomial infection, especially of the respiratory tract, but no effect on mortality.[114] The regimen has not been associated with the development of bacterial resistance but careful microbiological surveillance must be maintained.

Nutritional support

The injured patient who recovers without complications can obviously resume a normal diet. However, the major trauma patient who develops a sustained ileus, prolonged sepsis, especially if associated with retained necrotic tissue and abscesses, or large sequestered retroperitoneal haematomas, needs energetic nutritional support. Exceptional losses through fever, wound drainage, and aspirate from nasogastric tubes also need extra compensation. One or more of these problems may arise in the individual patient and a suitable plan for long-term intravenous nutrition may have to be devised (see Chapter 2). At the same time, abscesses must be drained and necrotic tissues excised if a downward catabolic trend and multiple organ dysfunction and failure are to be averted.

The objectives of intensive nutritional support are to conserve protein, maintain the energy balance and administer fluids, electrolytes and other essential dietary requirements. Clinical indicators of progress include the mid-arm circumference and skinfold thickness, the creatinine–height index and the basal energy expenditure which can be calculated using the Harris–Benedict equation based on age, sex, weight and height. Estimations of the serum albumin, urinary nitrogen and creatinine, and more recently of the lymphocyte count and serum transferrin level, as well as delayed hypersensitivity skin tests, may provide additional information. Nutritional support should be started within 48 hours of major trauma, gradually stepping up intake to cover losses. It is continued through the convalescent phase which may last many weeks depending on the severity of the trauma, the extent of the surgery, the presence of sepsis and the duration of gastrointestinal dysfunction. It may not be possible or desirable to achieve a positive nitrogen balance in the trauma patient despite optimal nutritional support and a number of strategies are now recognized to enhance recovery from catabolic illness.[115]

A nasogastric small-calibre Silastic weighted feeding tube delivers nutrition beyond the pylorus if the gastrointestinal tract is functioning, so avoiding accumulation in the stomach and the attendant risks of vomiting and aspiration (see Chapter 2). The opportunity may be taken to insert a feeding jejunostomy tube if a laparotomy is required for an abdominal injury. A large tube permits the delivery of a higher nutrient density to the gastrointestinal tract. Enteral nutrition has been shown to be superior to parenteral nutrition in maintaining nutritional status and reducing complications in trauma patients who require nutritional support (see Chapter 2).[116,117]

Renal support

Signs of impending renal failure must be recognized quickly and corrective action taken. Hypovolaemia as a cause of oliguria is indicated by a low sodium concentration in urine. The diagnosis is confirmed by an increased urinary output in response to a fluid challenge. Such a challenge can be hazardous in the absence of a Swan–Ganz catheter if myocardial disease or a cardiac contusion is present. Polyuric syndromes caused by glycosuria, post-traumatic diabetes insipidus and sepsis can also result in hypovolaemia and acute tubular necrosis. In the anuric patient, peritoneal dialysis is quite effective if the abdomen is intact, but if it is breached the only alternative is haemodialysis. Continuous haemofiltration allows a more sustained correction of uraemia under better haemodynamic control. Significant hyperkalaemia associated with renal failure may be temporarily controlled by a glucose and insulin infusion, by sodium bicarbonate and polystyrene sulphonate (kayexalate) given either orally or as retention enemas. Systemic calcium chloride may also be used. Myoglobinaemia, which may be prevented

REFERENCES

113. Blair P H B, Rowlands B J et al Surgery 1991; 110: 303
114. Selective Decontamination of the Digestive Tract Trialists Collaborative Group. Br Med J 1993; 307: 525
115. Wilmore D W N Engl J Med 1991; 325: 695
116. Kudsk K A, Groce M A et al Ann Surg 1992; 215: 503
117. Moore F A, Feliciano D V et al Ann Surg 1992; 216: 172

initially by excision of devitalized muscle, also threatens renal function. Mannitol infusions facilitate myoglobin excretion, providing there has been adequate volume replacement, but eventually dialysis may be required. Aminoglycosides must be withdrawn and dialysis may be used to expedite their removal from the circulation.

Organ donation

Inevitably victims of major trauma die in intensive care units and before they do so they become potential organ and tissue transplant donors; the most suitable are those who suffer head injury which results in brain death. The process of obtaining consent from a potential donor requires delicacy, sensitivity and close collaboration amongst relatives and medical staff (see Chapter 8). Precise criteria exist for each organ, taking into account the age of the patient, the past and present medical history, the mechanism of injury, clinical and biochemical evidence of organ function, the blood and tissue type, the complications of treatment and the warm ischaemia time. The cornea tolerates 12 hours and the kidney 1 hour of warm ischaemia, but for the heart/lung, liver and pancreas the time is shorter.

Rehabilitation

The patient's body and mind must be sustained in the best possible shape through the prolonged illness and recovery which follow major trauma. He or she must then be prepared for a return to the outside world. Initially, the best contribution is good surgical care, energetic nursing and efficient physiotherapy. Effective pain relief facilitates passive movement and allows the patient to cooperate in graded active exercises to improve breathing and limb mobility. Isometric exercises to increase muscle strength and isotonic exercises to widen the range of movement are taught along with reinforcement techniques which help to prevent muscle wasting. Later programmes include hydrotherapy, electrical stimulation, gymnasium and circuit training.

An early assessment of functional disability is important so that the goals of rehabilitation can be clearly defined and the patient regularly reminded of them. Supervision should be continued on an outpatient basis under the care of a team which has liaised with the patient in hospital. This rehabilitation team consists of physiotherapists, occupational and speech therapists, social workers, community health personnel, voluntary organizations and, of course, the close family of the victim. The after-effects of brain damage, paraplegia, limb loss, loss of a hand, impaired nerve function or bladder control result in varying degrees of dependence. It is the responsibility of the team as a whole to supervise, guide, encourage and instil optimism. By allaying doubts, reducing anxiety and contending with emotional lability, the patient and the relatives are gradually motivated and gain in confidence. Despite all efforts, a permanent disability may remain and the victim must be helped to come to terms with it. This may become even more difficult if the patient is old or lives alone and if previous disease such as rheumatoid arthritis or social and economic handicaps exist.

8 Transplantation

P. McMaster R. F. M. Wood

Transplantation is now firmly established as the major form of treatment for patients with end-stage renal failure and programmes for heart, heart–lung, liver and pancreas transplantation are achieving increasing success rates. Rapid progress in clinical transplantation is a result of an expanding knowledge of the immunological mechanisms of rejection and the ability to manipulate the immune response using powerful immunosuppressive drugs.

Organ transplantation became a practical possibility through the pioneering experimental work of Alexis Carrel in the early years of this century. Carrel left his native France to work in the USA and, in collaboration with Charles Guthrie, established a technique for transplanting the kidney in the cat and the dog using sutured vascular anastomoses.[1,2] Although Carrel & Guthrie recorded the failure of allografted organs to achieve good long-term function, more than 30 years elapsed before there was any real understanding of the mechanism of rejection. Gibson & Medawar, in a paper published in 1943[3] deduced that the failure of a second set of skin allografts in a patient with severe burns was due to an active immune process. Returning to the experimental laboratory, Medawar established that stimulation of the recipient immune system by donor antigen caused the development of lymphocytes capable of invading and destroying grafted tissue.[4,5] Mitchison[6] then demonstrated that sensitized lymphoid cells from an animal which had rejected a graft could be used passively to transfer transplant immunity. Cell transfer produced accelerated rejection of a graft in a previously unsensitized recipient.[6] The publication of these results led to the search for therapeutic agents which would suppress the immune reaction and prevent graft rejection. Azathioprine, a derivative of the anti-cancer drug 6-mercaptopurine, emerged as the most potent immunosuppressive agent.[7] The combination of azathioprine with prednisolone formed the drug regimen which allowed the establishment of clinical renal transplant programmes in the late 1960s.

TISSUE TYPING AND THE HUMAN MAJOR HISTOCOMPATIBILITY COMPLEX

Glycoprotein molecules on the surface of all somatic cells act as self-markers which are responsible for triggering the immune reaction leading to allograft rejection. These molecules were originally detected on leukocytes and therefore named human leukocyte antigens—they are now universally referred to as HLA antigens. These histocompatibility antigens are genetically controlled by loci on the short arm of chromosome 6 which make up the major

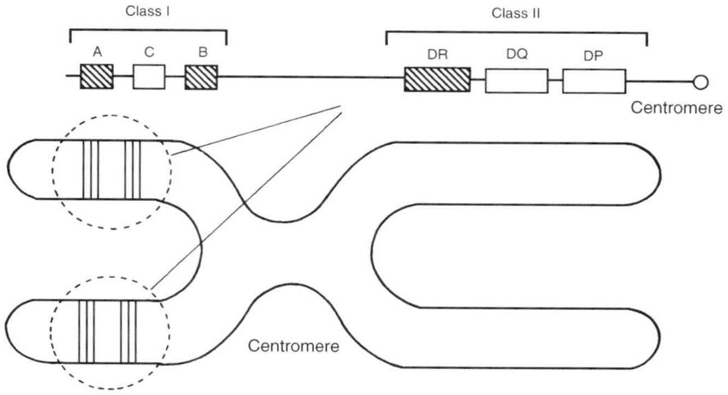

Fig. 8.1 The loci which make up the major histocompatibility complex on the short arm of chromosome 6. Tissue-typing techniques detect the cell surface molecules controlled by the A, B and DR loci.

histocompatibility complex (Fig. 8.1). The important antigens in transplantation are the class I products HLA-A, B and C antigens, and the class II products HLA-D region antigens. Foreign class I and class II antigens are capable of stimulating the recipient immune system and triggering lymphocyte sensitization, as described below (Fig. 8.2).

Tissue typing

For most organ transplants, and particularly for renal allografts, tissue matching improves the chances of long-term graft survival. Matching is carried out using a plate with multiple wells, each containing an antiserum to a known HLA specificity. Lymphocytes from the individual under test are plated out into the wells, together with complement. After incubation the wells are scanned for evidence of cell killing as the result of complement-mediated damage following antibody binding to a specific target antigen. The tissue type is recorded by analysis of the pattern of response. Donor–recipient matching is carried out for the HLA-A,

REFERENCES

1. Carrel A, Guthrie C C Science 1905; 22: 473
2. Carrel A, Guthrie C C Science 1906; 23: 394
3. Gibson T, Medawar P B J Anat 1943; 77: 299
4. Medawar P B J Anat 1944; 78: 176
5. Medawar P B J Anat 1945; 79: 157
6. Mitchison N A Nature 1953; 171: 267
7. Calne R Y, Alexandre G P J, Murray J E Ann NY Acad Sci 1962; 99: 743–761

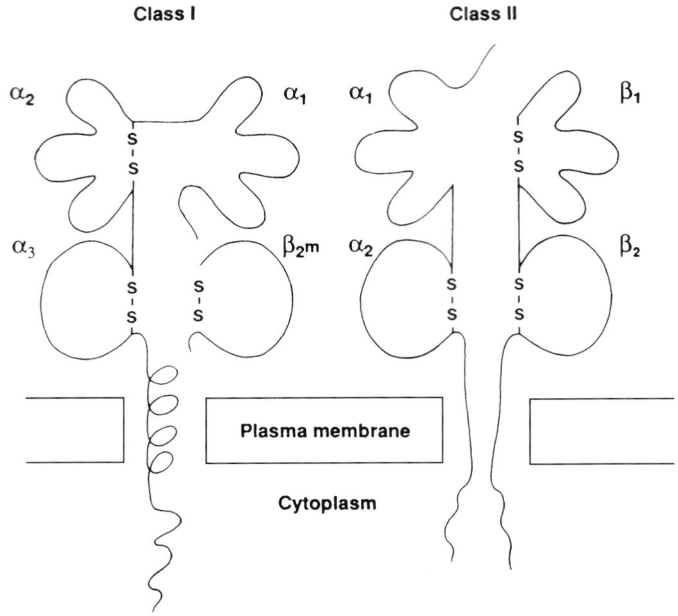

Fig. 8.2 The cell surface glycoprotein molecules controlled by major histocompatibility complex genes. The class I products (controlled by the A and B loci) are composed of three globular domains α_1, α_2 and α_3. The α_3 domain is closely associated with a non-major histocompatibility complex encoded peptide β_2-microglobulin. The class II products (controlled by the D region genes) are composed of two peptide strands—an α chain with two domains α_1 and α_2 and a shorter β chain again with two domains, β_1 and β_2. As illustrated, both class I and class II antigens traverse the plasma membrane of the cell.

B (class I) and DR (class II) loci. There are some 18 A locus determinants and more than 40 B locus determinants and good matching for class I antigens can only be achieved with a large pool of potential recipients. Matching for DR, where there are only 20 determinants, can be achieved more readily and evidence suggests that DR matching has a more important influence on allograft survival than matching for the A and B loci.[8,9] With the introduction of molecular biology it is now possible to perform genetic typing of HLA determinants.

HYPERACUTE REJECTION

Previous exposure to foreign HLA antigens can result in the formation of circulating cytotoxic antibodies in the blood of the potential transplant recipient. These antibodies may form following blood transfusion, as a result of pregnancy (against fetal antigens of paternal origin) or against mismatched determinants in a previous failed graft. Transplantation of a graft bearing mismatched antigens to which the recipient has cytotoxic antibodies risks the development of hyperacute rejection. Following revascularization of the graft the recipient's antibodies can become fixed to class I determinants on the vascular endothelium of the donor, resulting in endothelial cell destruction and activation of the coagulation system. Platelets adhere to the damaged areas, blocking the microcirculation of the graft.

Hyperacute rejection is an irreversible process and it is therefore vital to avoid the reaction by careful preoperative cross-matching techniques. A fresh serum sample and serum samples collected from the recipient during the year preceding the transplant should all give a negative reaction when tested with lymphocytes from a prospective donor. In clinical transplantation the risk of hyperacute rejection is a major concern in renal programmes, although it has also been described following cardiac transplantation. The liver, despite expressing HLA-A and B antigens on the endothelium, is much less susceptible to hyperacute rejection.

THE MECHANISM OF ACUTE REJECTION

In all forms of organ transplantation it is the formation of sensitized lymphoid cells causing acute rejection which poses the greatest threat to the survival of the graft. The initial phase in the sensitization process is the presentation of donor antigen to T (thymus-derived) lymphocytes of the recipient. There are two possible means by which this initial sensitization can be achieved. Recipient macrophages may take up antigenic fragments washed out into the circulation following revascularization of the graft. Alternatively, non-sensitized lymphocytes may come into contact with the so-called passenger leucocytes or dendritic cells of the donor which strongly express class II antigens on their surface. It is probable that both these mechanisms are involved in antigen presentation. For transformation into activated blast cells the T lymphocytes need, in addition to antigen, stimulation by a second signal in the form of a soluble mediator—interleukin 1, secreted by the recipient macrophages. Presence of accessory signals at the surface of the dendritic cell (B7, CAM-1, LFA3) is also required in order to fully activate recipient T cells. If the situation was not controlled by immunosuppression the T lymphoblasts would rapidly proliferate and invade the graft.

These activated T cells secrete a number of effector molecules, known as lymphokines. Of these the most important is interleukin 2, which causes clonal expansion of the T cell population with the generation of cytotoxic T lymphocytes. The cytotoxic cell is able to cause direct cell killing of its target without the involvement of complement. In addition, sensitized T cells can secrete additional factors, for example, macrophage activation factor (also known as interferon γ), leukocyte migration inhibition factor and chemotactic factors. These soluble agents probably augment the inflammatory reaction within the graft by involving recipient populations, such as polymorphs and macrophages, which are not specifically sensitized to graft antigen.

Although T lymphocyte sensitization is undoubtedly the main mechanism of graft rejection, stimulation of antibody-secreting B lymphocytes also occurs. Histologically antibody-mediated rejection is thought to be characterized by prominent vascular damage with fibrinoid necrosis of arterioles.

Understanding of the mechanisms of acute rejection and the complex cell–cell interactions involved comes from both animal

REFERENCES

8. Albrechtsen D, Moen T, Thorsby E Transplant Proc 1983; 15: 1120–1123
9. D'Ardenne A J, Dunnill M S ??? et al J Clin Pathol 1986; 39: 144–151

experimentation and studies on material from human transplants obtained by fine-needle aspiration biopsy[10,11] and Tru-cut biopsy.[12] Precise identification of the cells infiltrating the graft has been achieved by the use of monoclonal antibodies able to identify both individual cell types in the white cell series[13] and activation markers such as the interleukin 2 receptor.[14]

CHRONIC REJECTION

In addition to hyperacute rejection caused by cytotoxic antibodies and cell-mediated acute rejection, organ grafts are subject to chronic rejection. This can be defined as slow but progressive deterioration in graft function over a period of weeks or months. In many cases chronic rejection is the end-result of acute rejection damage with the development of interstitial fibrosis. However, in some cases the process is due to the effects of non-cytotoxic antibodies which bind to antigenic determinants on the vascular endothelium of the graft, stimulating intimal hyperplasia and hence a gradual reduction in the blood supply. Cytokines can also play a role.

IMMUNOREGULATORY MECHANISMS

Acute rejection phenomena occur in the early weeks after transplantation and after that time the risk of rejection recedes. There is no doubt that immunoregulation occurs, although the precise mechanisms are relatively poorly understood. From animal experimentation and in vitro human studies there is evidence that suppressor T cells develop which are capable of subverting the cytotoxic T cell population.[15] In addition, anti-idiotypic antibodies may form which effectively switch off the reactive sites on the T cell. So far it has not proved possible to regulate these suppressor phenomena in any controlled way. However, blood transfusion prior to transplantation has been shown to induce a degree of immune suppression with a significant improvement in graft survival.[16] The reasons for the transfusion effect have not been defined but most centres now pursue a policy of deliberate transfusion. On average, 3 units of blood is given to previously non-transfused individuals before they are placed on the transplant waiting list. This modest amount of blood does not usually excite a cytotoxic antibody response, which would cause cross-matching problems.

IMMUNOSUPPRESSION

The immunosuppressive cocktail of azathioprine and prednisolone was developed in the 1960s and although modifications, such as the use of low-dose prednisolone from the time of transplantation,[17] reduced transplant morbidity the search for new and more specific immunosuppressive drugs proved frustrating. Antilymphocyte globulin has been a popular addition to conventional immunosuppression used either as adjunctive initial therapy[18] or as a treatment for rejection.[19] However, although improved graft survival may be achieved, the use of antilymphocyte globulin is associated with an increased risk of viral and fungal infection and malignancies (lymphoma). Numerous chemical agents have been tested for immunosuppressive activity but although several, such as the imidazoles,[20] have shown promising results in experimental animals, it is only since the discovery of cyclosporin that there has been a real breakthrough capable of creating a significant improvement in the results of transplantation.

Cyclosporin, FK506

Cyclosporin has now become the main ingredient of immunosuppressive protocols, replacing azathioprine and prednisolone as standard therapy. The drug is a metabolite of the soil fungus *Tolypocladium inflatum* Gams and has specific activity against T lymphocytes.[21] Cyclosporin does not interfere with antigen or interleukin binding to the T cell surface but appears to act by inhibiting calmodulin activity. Calmodulin is a calcium-dependent regulator protein involved in many intracellular metabolic processes. It has been shown that the cyclosporin–calmodulin interaction blocks the increases in cyclic guanosine monophosphate associated with T cell proliferation and lymphokine production (mainly interleukin 2). Therefore, cyclosporin effectively prevents the generation of a population of cytotoxic effector cells capable of attacking the graft.

Cyclosporin has relatively little effect on B lymphocytes, macrophages and polymorphs and its use has resulted in a dramatic reduction in the incidence of infection associated with previous immunosuppressive regimens. Despite its undoubted benefits, cyclosporin has some major side-effects and drug interactions which can pose problems in clinical practice. Nephrotoxicity is the most important and difficult problem. This has been shown to occur not only in renal allograft recipients but also in patients with heart, liver and bone marrow grafts. Patients with high drug levels are also at risk of hepatotoxicity. Cyclosporin is now used in an initial dose of 10–12 mg/kg/per day, rapidly tapering to maintenance levels of 5–6 mg/kg/per day. Although initially used as a single agent, most centres now use cyclosporin in combination with low-dose prednisolone (15–20 mg/day).

FK506, a macrocyclic lactone derived from a fungus, was discovered in Japan 7 years ago. It is a very potent immunosuppressive agent that has the same mechanism of action as cyclosporin (blocking of interleukin 2 production by T cells); FK506 also shares a similar toxicity profile.

REFERENCES

10. Hayry P, Von Willebrand E et al Immunol Rev 1984; 77: 85–142
11. Wood R F M, Bolton E M et al Lancet 1982; ii: 278
12. McWhinnie D L, Thompson J F et al Transplantation 1986; 42: 352–358
13. Bolton E M, Thompson J F et al Transplantation 1983; 36: 728–731
14. Robb R J, Greene W C, Rusk C M J Exp Med 1984; 160: 1126–1146
15. Wang H B, Heacock E H et al J Immunol 1982; 128: 1382–1385
16. Opelz G, Terasaki P I Transplantation 1980; 29: 153–158
17. McGeown M G, Kennedy J A et al Lancet 1977; ii: 648–651
18. Sheil A G R, Kelly G E et al Lancet 1971; i: 359–363
19. Hoitsma A J, van Lier H J et al Transplantation 1985; 39: 274–279
20. Miller J J, Salaman J R In: Salaman J R (ed) Immunosuppressive Therapy. MTP Press, Lancaster 1981
21. Hess A D, Tutschka P J, Santos G W In: White D J G (ed) Cyclosporin A. Elsevier Biomedical Press, Amsterdam 1982

Table 8.1 A regimen for triple therapy with cyclosporin, azathioprine and prednisolone

Drug	At operation	Initial postoperative dose	Maintenance therapy
Cyclosporin	2 mg/kg intravenously 24 h	8 mg/kg per day orally	Adjust oral dose to maintain cyclosporin trough level within 25% of bottom of normal range
Azathioprine	—	1.5 mg/kg per day orally	1.5 mg/kg per day orally
Prednisolone	0.5 g intravenously over 2 h	20 mg/day orally	10 mg/day orally

Azathioprine and prednisolone

The azathioprine dosage is regulated to maintain the total white cell count between 4000 and 6000/mm^3. In general this usually means a maintenance dose of around 1.5–2.5 mg/kg/per day. Long-term steroid therapy can produce deleterious side-effects, for example Cushingoid facies, diabetes, hypertension, fragile skin and avascular necrosis of bone. These complications can be reduced by giving low-dose steroids (20 mg prednisolone per day) from the time of transplantation and giving the drug on an alternate-day basis in the maintenance phase after transplantation.

Alternative forms of immunosuppression

Radiotherapy, whether directly to the graft or to suppress the bone marrow, has largely been abandoned in organ grafting. A few centres have reported success with total lymphoid irradiation as a pretransplant preparation for high-risk patients with previous failed grafts who are unable to have dialysis treatment.[24]

Thoracic duct drainage, to deplete the patient of lymphocytes, was one of the techniques employed in the early stages of transplantation but has been abandoned now that powerful immunosuppressive drugs have become available.

Monoclonal antibodies to human T lymphocytes have proved an effective means of reversing acute rejection.[25] Unfortunately, the development of antibodies to the mouse immunoglobulin of the monoclonal reagent and immune modulation, the disappearance of receptor antigens from the T cell surface without the induction of cytotoxicity, tend to limit the effectiveness of current therapy.[26]

RENAL TRANSPLANTATION

The transplant donor

The majority of kidneys transplanted come from cadaver donors, although most programmes are prepared to consider transplants from living related donors. The ideal living related transplant is from an HLA-identical sibling; in this case the risks of rejection are minimal. Since the introduction of cyclosporin, excellent results have also been achieved in 'one-haplo-type' matched transplants, where the donor and recipient have half of their total major histocompatibility complex antigens in common. These are mainly parent-to-child transplants but one-haplo-type matching can also be a means of achieving transplantation between non-HLA-identical siblings.

Most cadaver donors are patients in intensive care units with irreversible structural brain damage who have been declared brain-dead following tests of brainstem function.[27] Since the acceptance of the brain death criteria it has become standard practice to start the organ retrieval procedure while ventilation and circulation are maintained.

The kidneys are usually removed using an en bloc technique, taking segments of aorta and vena cava above and below the renal vessels. This ensures that if there are multiple renal arteries these can be included in a Carrel patch of aorta for subsequent anastomosis to the external iliac artery. There are no collateral connections on the arterial side of the renal circulation and failure to revascularize a polar artery will result in an area of infarction in the donor kidney. Of itself this is not of particular importance, but it is vital that lower polar vessels are connected as they will frequently be a major source of blood supply to the pelvis and ureter of the graft. As a further protection of its blood supply, the loose connective tissue around the ureter should be dissected in continuity.

Renal preservation

Whether the graft will function immediately after transplantation is related to the degree of ischaemic injury to which it has been subjected. The *warm ischaemic time* is the time during which the kidney remains at body temperature without a blood supply. After a period of 20 minutes of warm ischaemia it is almost inevitable that there will be a period of acute tubular necrosis with oliguria or anuria until the graft recovers. Warm ischaemic intervals in excess of 45 minutes are associated with a risk of cortical necrosis, from which recovery of function is impossible. Following harvesting of the kidney it is flushed with a cold preservation solution to clear the organ of blood and rapidly reduce the core temperature to 4°C. At this temperature cellular metabolism is slow and using solutions such as hyperosmolar citrate[28] the deterioration of the tubular cells during storage can be minimized. If the kidney has been removed from a 'heart-beating' cadaver, the dissection can be virtually completed before switching off the ventilator and clamping the aorta and vena cava. The warm ischaemic time can therefore be

REFERENCES

22. Hess A D, Colombani P M, Esa A In: Williams G M, Bardick J F, Solez K (eds) Kidney Transplant Rejection. Marcel Dekker, New York 1986
23. Jones R M, Murie J A et al Br J Surg 1988; 75: 4
24. Najarian J S, Sutherland D E R et al Transplant Proc 1981, 13: 417–424
25. Ortho Multicentre Transplant Study Group N Engl J Med 1985; 313: 337–342
26. Norman D, Barry J et al Transplant Proc 1985; 17: 39
27. Pallis C In: Morris P J (ed) Kidney Transplantation, Principles and Practice, 3rd edn. W B Saunders, Philadelphia 1988
28. Marshall V C, Jablonski P, Scott D F In: Morris P J (ed) Kidney Transplantation, Principles and Practice, 3rd edn. W B Saunders, Philadelphia 1988

reduced to the 2 or 3 minutes required to complete the removal of the organs and their transfer to a tray of sterile ice on a separate table to carry out the perfusion.

As an alternative the kidneys can be perfused in situ using a large volume of perfusate introduced via a double-balloon catheter in the aorta, venting blood and perfusate via a suction catheter in the inferior vena cava. This system is the preferred technique when the liver or pancreas is being harvested in addition to the kidneys.

Once the kidneys have been cooled and perfused the aorta and vena cava can be split, taking care to ensure that polar arteries are preserved with the aortic patch. Each kidney is placed in the innermost of a series of three sterile polythene bags with a little of the cold preservation solution. Once sealed the bags are placed in an insulated transit box and surrounded by crushed ice. If the warm ischaemic time is less than 5 minutes the kidney should be capable of withstanding a cold ischaemic time of up to 48 hours and still have a good chance of immediate function on revascularization.

Recipient selection and preoperative preparation

There are now virtually no patients who develop renal failure who cannot be considered for a renal transplant. The increased susceptibility of patients over the age of 50 to infective complications has been reduced following the introduction of cyclosporin. Transplantation rather than dialysis is now the preferred treatment for children with end-stage renal disease. Lack of bladder function is an undoubted problem but kidneys can be successfully transplanted with ureteric drainage into an ileal loop.[29] Patients with incipient left ventricular failure, although a high-risk group, will frequently show an improvement in cardiac function following a successful renal graft.

The selection of the most appropriate recipient for a given donor kidney is based on ABO blood group compatibility and HLA matching. Using national and international organ-matching schemes it is theoretically possible to achieve either complete AB and DR matching or have only one mismatch between the A and B loci in more than 60% of cases. Analysis of more than 2000 kidney transplants performed in the UK between 1979 and 1984 demonstrates that these beneficially matched grafts had survival rates in excess of 80% at 1 year—a more than 10% improvement on all other match grades.[30] However, the pressure to use kidneys locally for high-priority cases makes it difficult to implement a policy in which all organs harvested are offered for beneficially matched recipients.

Before proceeding with the transplant a negative cytotoxic cross-match is essential to ensure that the potential recipient does not have circulating antibodies which might precipitate hyperacute rejection.

The transplant operation

The iliac fossa was selected as the site for renal transplantation by the groups in Boston and Paris who performed the first successful cases in the 1950s. The essential features of the procedure have remained unchanged ever since. The kidney is transplanted

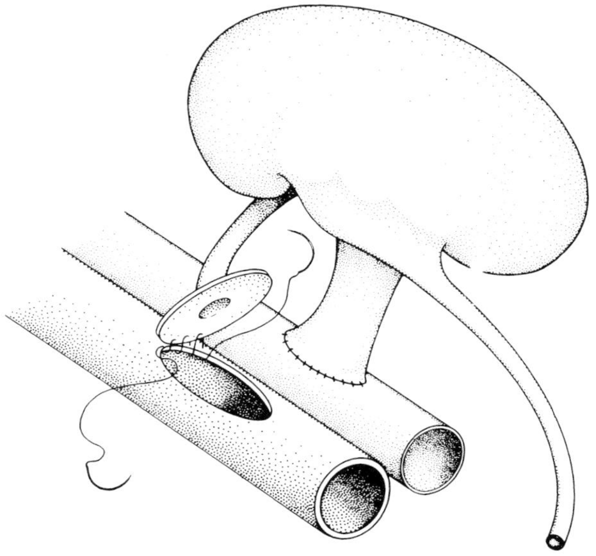

Fig. 8.3 The vascular anastomoses in a renal transplant. The renal vein is anastomosed end-to-side to the external iliac vein. The illustration shows the method of anastomosis of the Carrel patch of aorta around the donor renal artery to the recipient external iliac artery.

extraperitoneally in the iliac fossa, anastomosing the renal artery to either the internal iliac artery (end-to-end) or the external iliac artery (end-to-side) and joining the renal vein end-to-side to the external iliac vein. In this position only a short length of ureter is required to reach the bladder.

A curved inguinal incision is used dividing the external oblique aponeurosis in the line of its fibres and dividing the internal oblique muscle in the line of the wound. The transversalis fascia can then be incised allowing the peritoneum to be mobilized away from the floor of the iliac fossa. In the male the spermatic cord can usually be preserved but access to the bladder is facilitated by dividing the inferior epigastric vessels. In mobilizing the iliac vessels it is essential that any lymphatic trunks divided should be carefully ligated. Divided lymphatic trunks which have not been tied off may produce a collection of lymph around the kidney, compressing the ureter and causing hydronephrosis. The development of a lymphocele can cause difficult postoperative problems.[31]

The arterial and venous anastomoses are carried out using standard vascular techniques with 5/0 monofilament nylon sutures (Fig. 8.3). Many renal patients have impaired coagulation and it is usually unnecessary to employ systemic heparinization during the 25–30 minutes required for the completion of the anastomoses. Following the release of the clamps the kidney should rapidly become pink and firm with immediate urine production. To encourage a diuresis the central venous pressure should be maintained in excess of 10 cm of water and frusemide, mannitol or dopamine can also be given. There are a number of ureteric

REFERENCES

29. MacGregor P, Novick A C et al J Urol 1986; 135: 686–688
30. Gilks W R, Bradley B A, Gore S M Lancet 1986; i: 509
31. Schweizer R T, Cho S I et al Arch Surg 1972; 104: 42–45

implantation techniques but many surgeons prefer to use a submucosal tunnel to reduce the risk of reflux and ascending infection in the graft.

Complications

Technical

Early arterial and venous occlusion are uncommon problems but all large series encounter late renal artery stenosis with an incidence ranging from 5 to 25%. Classically this is heralded by increasing blood pressure and the presence of a bruit over the graft. Surgical correction of renal artery stenosis is hazardous. A review of 180 cases found that while 76% benefited there was a 3% mortality rate and a 12% incidence of graft loss.[32] Although good results have been reported following percutaneous transluminal angioplasty it appears that long-term success is only achieved in a third of cases.[33]

A urinary leak in the early postoperative period can occur if the catheter becomes blocked. This is a particular problem in patients with small, contracted bladders. Necrosis of the lower end of the ureter is relatively rare and tends to present insidiously with suprapubic tenderness and a gradual reduction in urine output 5–10 days after transplantation. In some circumstances it may be possible to reimplant the transplant ureter. However, if necrosis is extensive it will be necessary to use the patient's own ureter or a bladder flap to rescue the situation. Late ureteric stenosis is one of the differential diagnoses in patients with a gradual reduction in renal function. The resulting hydronephrosis is readily detected on ultrasound scanning. The stenosis is frequently localized to the lower end of the ureter and reimplantation is not unduly difficult.

Recurrence of the original renal disease can be a problem, particularly in patients with mesangiocapillary type II glomerular nephritis, immunoglobulin A nephropathy and malignant focal glomerulosclerosis.[34] Oxalosis has previously been considered to be a contraindication to transplantation due to the rapid deposition of oxalate in the transplanted kidney. However, acceptable graft survival rates can be achieved in this unfavourable situation by ensuring a massive diuresis and using daily dialysis to reduce oxalate load in the immediate postoperative period.[35]

Infection remains one of the major causes of morbidity following transplantation, although there has been a reduction in the incidence of all types of infection since the introduction of cyclosporin. A wide variety of infections with bacteria, viruses, fungi and protozoa have been reported in transplant recipients.[36] The use of prophylactic antibiotics at the time of transplantation has undoubtedly been helpful but it is still essential to be vigilant for infective complications in the early postoperative period.

Treatment for acute rejection episodes

The standard method of treating acute rejection episodes is to use bolus doses of 0.5 g intravenous methylprednisolone, given as a 3-day course and repeated if necessary after an interval of 5 days if there is no evidence of a response. Alternatively one can use antilymphocyte globulin or monoclonal antibodies.

Results

Over the past 20 years improvements in survival in both dialysis and transplant patients have resulted in an expansion in the provision of treatment for end-stage renal failure. In Europe in 1990 more than 200 patients per million of population (pmp) had a functioning transplant or were receiving some form of dialysis. This figure will continue to rise as the criteria for treatment of irreversible kidney disease are widened. A steady state with around 300–350 pmp on end-stage renal failure programmes will probably not be achieved until the early years of the 21st century. The proportion of patients with a successfully functioning graft has steadily increased. In the UK, in the 15–44-years age group, over 60% of patients have been grafted and most of the remaining 40% are on a transplant waiting list.

Survival after cadaver transplantation

Collected statistics for cadaver transplantation in Europe comparing individuals transplanted in 1970–1974 and 1980–1984 are shown in Tables 8.2 and 8.3. Patient survival rates increased by over 20% and graft survival rates by more than 15%. As cyclosporin was

Table 8.2 Patient survival after first cadaver graft (collected figures for Europe from the European Dialysis and Transplant Association)

Year of first graft	Survival at	
	2 years	4 years
1980–1984		
Age 15–44 years	91%	86%
Age 45–64 years	81%	71%
1970–1974		
Age 15–44 years	72%	64%
Age 45–64 years	55%	45%

Age given is age at time of transplantation. From Brunner F P, Broyers M et al Nephrol Dial Transplant 1988; 2: 109–122

Table 8.3 Graft survival after first cadaver graft (collected figures for Europe from the European Dialysis and Transplant Association)

Year of first graft	Survival at	
	2 years	4 years
1980–1984		
Age 15–44 years	63%	54%
Age 45–64 years	61%	50%
1970–1974		
Age 15–44 years	47%	40%
Age 45–64 years	39%	31%

Age given is age at time of transplantation. From Brunner F P, Broyers M et al Nephrol Dial Transplant 1988; 2: 109–122

REFERENCES

32. Lohr J W, MacDougall M L et al Am J Kidney Dis 1986; 7: 363–367
33. Reisfeld D, Matas A J et al Transplant Proc 1989; 21: 1955–1956
34. Cameron J S Transplantation 1982; 34: 237–245
35. Watts R W E, Morgan S H et al Transplantation 1988; 45: 1143–1145
36. Cohen J, Hopkin J, Kurtz J In: Morris P J (ed) Kidney Transplantation, Principles and Practice, 3rd edn W B Saunders, Philadelphia 1988

only introduced on a commercial basis in 1983 a further significant improvement in these figures can be expected during the next decade.

There has been a dramatic fall in the incidence of opportunistic infection in transplant patients and most units now have patient survival figures of around 95% at 1 year. These statistics are all the more impressive as many more high-risk individuals with heart disease and diabetes are being grafted and patients over the age of 60 are now routinely considered for transplantation.

The influence of tissue matching and blood transfusion on the outcome of transplantation

Tissue matching remains an important determinant of graft survival, even in the cyclosporin era. Matching for the DR locus is particularly important and, as mentioned earlier, the best results are obtained in beneficially matched kidneys where there are no mismatches at the DR locus and only one mismatch in the four determinants at the A and B loci. However, for many patients with rare tissue types there is little prospect of receiving a beneficially matched kidney.

Large population studies have allowed the frequency of individual antigens within the population to be calculated. On this basis an individual match prognosis index can be calculated. This will give an indication of the time a patient might have to wait to receive a well-matched graft. This information can help in making a sensible decision about the degree of mismatching it would be reasonable to accept in an individual to minimize the time spent on the waiting list. Conversely the index will indicate patients with common tissue types where there may be an excellent chance of receiving a beneficially matched graft within a year on the waiting list. In this situation the individual should not be offered a kidney with only a moderate degree of match.

Tissue matching

Tissue matching is of particular importance in patients with cytotoxic antibodies and those receiving second transplants. Figure 8.4 shows percentage graft survival related to tissue matching in sensitized patients who have antibodies which will react with cells from more than 50% of the normal population. By 2 years, graft survival is 25% better in those receiving a perfectly matched kidney compared to individuals were there is a 5- or 6-antigen mismatch. The figures are essentially similar after second transplantation, with better than 80% survival in well-matched grafts compared with around 60% survival in the poorest-match grades. Third and fourth transplants are possible but technically difficult. Where previous grafts have failed because of rejection most patients will be found to have developed high levels of cytotoxic antibodies, which make it difficult to find a cross-match-negative donor. In situations where it was possible to proceed with transplantation the European figures for 1980–1984 show a 1-year graft survival rate of 52%, falling to 35% at 4 years.[37]

During the azathioprine and prednisolone era blood transfusion was demonstrated to have a potent beneficial effect on the results of cadaver transplantation. However, the picture has changed

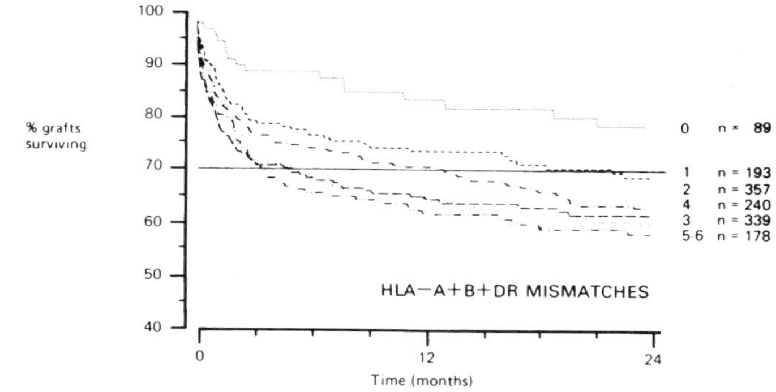

Fig. 8.4 The influence of tissue matching on graft survival in sensitized patients with more than 50% antibody reactivity. The results are stratified on the basis of 0–6 mismatches. At 2 years, graft survival in patients with no mismatches was 25% better than in those receiving poorly matched kidneys. (Figures from the International Collaborative Transplant Study, by kind permission of Dr G. Opelz.)

considerably since the introduction of cyclosporin. Recent figures from the collaborative transplant study in Heidelberg, with information from more than 300 centres, demonstrate that in cases transplanted in 1984–1985 the transfusion effect is barely perceptible (Opelz 1989, personal communication; Fig. 8.5).

Living related transplantation

Cadaver kidneys remain in short supply and living related donation continues to form a significant component of most transplant programmes. Recipients of kidneys from HLA-identical siblings can expect an excellent outcome, with graft survival in excess of 90% at 5 years. Living related transplantation can also be considered in one-haplotype matches, where the donor and recipient have half their major histocompatibility complex antigens in common, for example, parents and children and two-thirds of non-identical siblings. The overall statistics for patient and graft survival following live-donor transplantation in Europe are shown in Table 8.4. With azathioprine and prednisolone immunosuppression, results in these one-haplotype transplants can be improved by donor-specific blood transfusion.[38] However, as in cadaver transplantation, it is likely that there will be a reduced transfusion effect with cyclosporin immunosuppression.

Conclusions

Transplantation has become established as the major means of replacement therapy for patients with end-stage renal failure. The indications for operation have widened, with treatment being offered to the paediatric age group and to patients in their 60s. Transplantation is now associated with better rehabilitation and lower morbidity and mortality rates than either haemodialysis or continuous ambulatory peritoneal dialysis. Despite the economic

REFERENCES

37. Brunner F P, Broyer M et al Nephrol Dial Transplant 1988; 2: 109–122
38. Salvatierra O, Vincenti F et al Ann Surg 1980; 192: 543–552

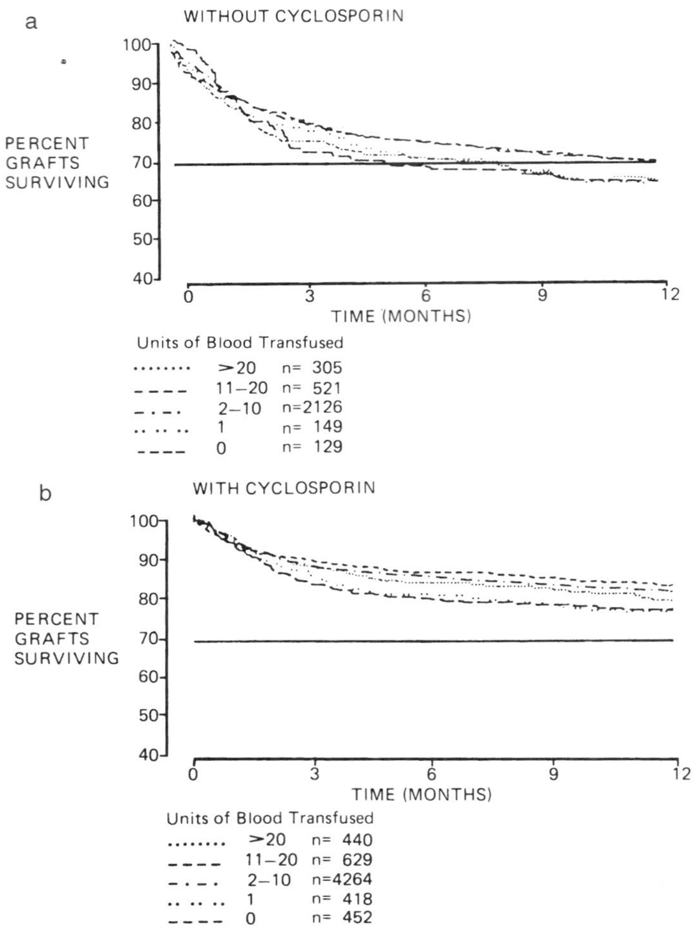

Fig. 8.5 Statistics from patients transplanted in 1984–1985 showing that with both (a) conventional immunosuppression and (b) cyclosporin the transfusion effect is barely perceptible. (Figures from the International Collaborative Transplant Study, by kind permission of Dr G. Opelz.)

advantages of kidney grafting, units throughout the world are hampered by a chronic shortage of suitable organs. For donor referral rates to improve, public education programmes will have to be combined with a greater awareness among health care professionals of the enormous benefits of successful transplantation.

PANCREATIC TRANSPLANTATION

With the introduction of insulin into clinical practice in the 1920s by Banting and Best, the immediate diabetic deaths due to ketoacidosis became largely preventable.[39] However, by the late 1930s it became clear that this did not resolve the whole syndrome of diabetic disease; patients were still dying with microangiopathic complications. Diabetic patients are 25 times more prone to blindness, five times more prone to peripheral gangrene and amputation, and are 17 times more likely to develop major kidney disease. These major difficulties result in a reduction of the diabetic patient's life expectation by nearly one-third, and in the USA insulin-dependent diabetes is now the fifth most common cause of death.[40]

Table 8.4 Patient and graft survival after living related transplantation in Europe: grafts performed 1980–1984 (figures from the European Dialysis and Transplant Association)

Year of first graft	Survival at	
	2 years	4 years
1980–1984		
Age 15–44 years	95%	92%
Age 45–64 years	95%	89%
1970–1974		
Age 15–44 years	78%	63%
Age 45–64 years	77%	70%

Age given is age at time of transplantation. From Brunner F P, Broyers M et al Nephrol Dial Transplant 1988; 2: 109–122

Table 8.5 Experimental studies demonstrating stabilization or resolution of diabetic microangiopathic complications following pancreas transplantation

Complications prevented	Study	Year
Kidney	Maeur[45]	1974
	Federlin 8 Bretzel[46]	1984
	Orloff et al[47]	1986
Eyes	Krupin et al[48]	1979
Neuropathy	Orloff et al[49]	1975

The treatment of diabetic nephropathy, producing kidney failure, also continues to increase. While in 1976 6% of dialysis patients in the USA were diabetic, just a decade later that figure had risen to 25%.[41] The uraemic diabetic patient presents a formidable clinical management problem because of the occular, cardiovascular, neurological and psychological complications of diabetes.[42]

The concept of pancreatic transplantation was initially explored over 90 years ago in an effort not just to stabilize the carbohydrate control but also to delay or prevent the microangiopathic complications leading to so much morbidity. By the end of 1994 more than 6000 grafts had been performed. The rationale behind kidney and pancreas transplantation was first, to resolve the clinical syndrome of diabetes and improve the patient's quality of life, and second, to improve carbohydrate control and delay or prevent microvascular complications.[43] Increasing evidence suggests that the control of carbohydrate homeostasis has a marked influence on microvascular complications and that even quite marked diabetic renal damage will improve if optimal carbohydrate control is obtained[44] (Table 8.5).

Technique of pancreatic grafting

Islets of Langerhans implantation

Ideally the islets of Langerhans, the active component of insulin release, would be the only cells transferred from donor to recipient, and in small animal models this is a viable proposition, with

REFERENCES

39. Bliss M The Discovery of Insulin. Paul Harris, Edinburgh 1983
40. Carter Center of Emory University. Diabet Care 1985; 8: 391–406
41. Brunette P Diabet Nephropath 1985; 4: 103
42. Friedman E A Diabet Nephropath 1983; 2: 3
43. Williams P W Br Med J 1984; 2: 1303
44. The DCCT Research Trial Group N Engl J Med 1993; 329

Table 8.6 Islet encapsulation

Model (donor; recipient)	n	Normoglycaemia	Histology
Rat (Wistar; Lewis)	113	1–2 years	Good
Rat (rat; mouse)	?	100 days	
Pig islets; rats	?	50 days	
Dry allografts	22	80.0 ± 6.6	57.6 ± 7.1 (regraft)

rejection prevented by immunosuppressive agents such as cyclosporin A. However, in larger animals and humans the purity of islets and their viability after extraction are much less satisfactory, and attempts at islet transplantation in humans have yielded little success.[50] Attempts at cellular microincapsulation of islets within a polyisoprene-alginate membrane have been introduced[51] in an effort to reduce the immunological damage. These megaislets or clusters can, in animal models, be success-fully transferred without immunological destruction[52] and current studies in humans are under way. However, fibrosis around the capsule may prove to be a limiting factor of this technique.

Pancreatic vascularized graft

An alternative approach to islet grafting is the implantation of a segment of the pancreas or the whole pancreatic organ itself, first undertaken by Lillihei in the late 1960s.[53] At first only patients with the most advanced complications were considered, but now increasingly unstable diabetic patients with impending or frank renal failure are considered for pancreatic grafting. Careful evaluation, including coronary artery assessment, is needed because of the multiple complications so often encountered in these patients. Investigations usually include electrocardiogram and ultrasound stress electrocardiogram and coronary angiography to assess the extent of coronary artery disease. These are done with increased frequency. Baseline studies of the eyes and of peripheral nerves should also be done.

Surgical technique

Pancreatic grafts are obtained from cadaveric donors at the same time as removal of the kidneys and livers. Dissection of the coeliac axis and splenic artery is followed by perfusion of all the abdominal organs followed by removal of the pancreas. One of the difficulties of segmental or whole-organ pancreatic implantation is the need to provide a drainage system for the exocrine acinar tissue of the graft. The development of the ingenious method of ductal injection with neoprene—a latex polymer glue—by Dubernard et al in 1978[54] reawakened interest in pancreatic transplantation (Fig. 8.6a). However, this technique resulted in progressive fibrosis and sclerosis of the acinar tissue, leaving a scarred gland in the long term. Operative techniques have been developed which drain the pancreas into the bladder (Fig. 8.6b). The acute infective complications when the pancreas is drained into the bladder appear less than when drained into the intestine, making this the current optimal choice for pancreatic ductal drainage. If this fails because of leakage, the transplant may be rescued by intestinal drainage. The pancreas graft is placed intraperitoneally as this location is better able to manage episodes of pancreatitis.

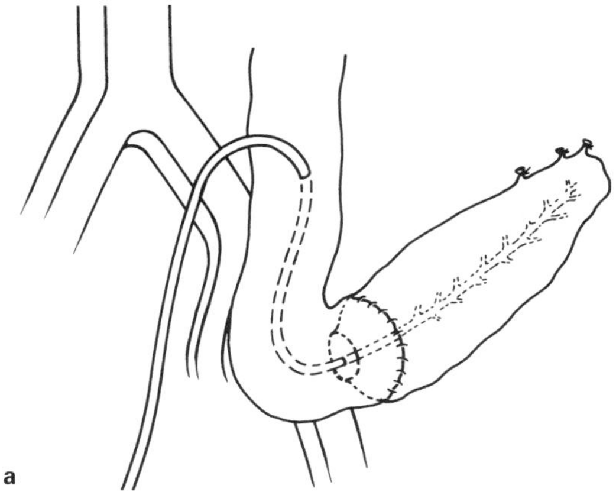

a

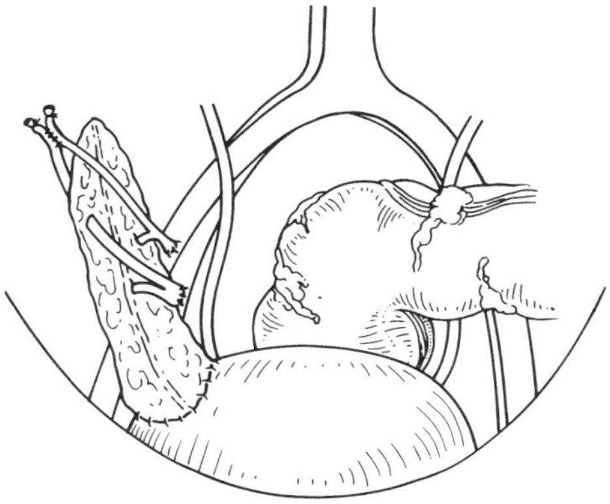

b

Fig. 8.6 (a,b) Transplantation techniques allowing drainage of pancreatic duct into the bladder or intestine.

Results of transplantation

Reports from the International Registry show that the developing techniques have become increasingly safe.[55] One-year patient and graft survival rates after bladder-drained kidney–pancreas transplant are now 91% and 76% respectively (Fig. 8.7). With more stringent selection criteria for both donors and recipients, it is possible to achieve better results (graft survival > 85%). One-year survival after pancreas transplantation alone remains lower

REFERENCES

45. Mauer S M Diabetes 1974; 23: 748–753
46. Federlin K F, Bretzel R G World J Surg 1984; 8: 169–178
47. Orloff M J, Yamanaka N et al Diabetes 1986; 35: 347–354
48. Krupin T, Waltman S R et al Invest Ophthalmol Visual 1979; 18: 1185–1196
49. Orloff M J, Lee S et al Ann Surg 1975; 182: 198–206
50. Kendall D M, Robertson R P Diabetes Metabolism 1996; 22: 157–163
51. O'Shea G M, Sun A M Diabetes 1986; 35: 445–446
52. Sun A M, O'Shea, Goosen M F Appl Biochem Biotechnol 1984; 10: 87–99
53. Lillihei R C, Simmons R L et al Ann Surg 1970; 172: 405–436
54. Dubernard J M, Traeger J, Neyra P Surgery 1978; 84: 633–639
55. Gruessner A, Sutherland D E R In: Cecka and Terasaki (ed) Clinical Transplants 1996; 47–67
56. Sollinger H W, Geffner S R Surg Clin North Am 1994; 74(5): 1183–1195

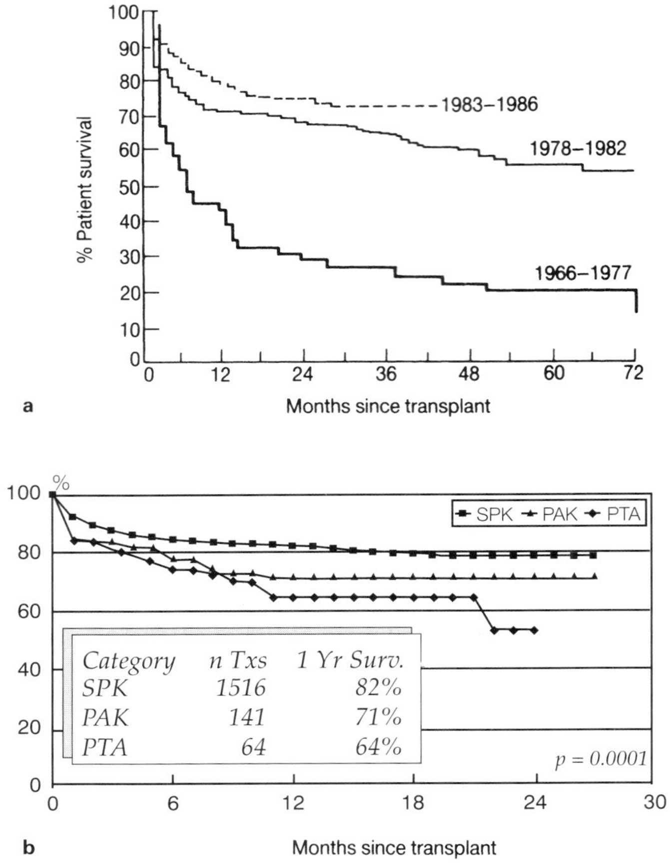

Fig 8.7 International Pancreas Transplantation Register data for patient and pancreatic graft survival (12 months) by era showing a slow but definite improvement in results. **(a)** Patient survival. 1966–1977; n = 64; 40% survival; $P < 0.001$. 1978–1982; n = 201; 72% survival; $P < 0.001$. 1983–1986: n = 646; 79% survival; $P = 0.012$. **(b)** USA Pancreas Graft Function by Category 1994–1996. This graph analyzes cases for the three major recipient categories: simultaneous pancreas kidney transplants (SPK); pancreas after kidney transplants (PAK); and pancreas transplants alone (PTA). An improvement in GSRs (graft survivals rates), compared to the 1987–96 data, could be shown over the analyzed time period for all categories: for 1994–96, SPK (n = 1516), PAK (n = 141) and PTA (n = 64) pancreas GSRs at 1 year were 81%, 71% and 64% respectively. Kidney GSR for 1994–96 SPK cases was 88% at 1 year.

(around 60%) than when in combination with the kidney.[56] While the clinical syndrome of diabetes mellitus, namely glycosuria, polyuria and polydipsia, is resolved by implantation of a pancreatic graft, the long-term impact on microvascular complications is less certain.[55] Improvement in nerve conduction studies has been clearly demonstrated with stabilization of the retina, and transplant biopsies of kidney grafts in these same patients have not shown typical development of diabetic glomerulobasal membrane thickening, as would have been expected.

LIVER TRANSPLANTATION

In the 30 years since the first attempts at liver transplantation in humans,[57] this procedure has progressed to become of major benefit to patients with advanced liver disease. Over 2000 liver grafts are performed in Europe alone each year and the development of newer surgical techniques, combined with the introduction of cyclosporin A, has led to a significant improvement in overall success rates.[58]

Table 8.7 Diseases treatable by hepatic replacement

Children	Adults
Cirrhosis due to:	Primary biliary cirrhosis
Biliary atresia	Chronic active hepatitis
Congenital hepatic cirrhosis	Sclerosing cholangitis
Congenital hepatic fibrosis	Secondary biliary cirrhosis
Metabolic disorders	*Metabolic disorders*
Glycogen storage disease	Haemochromatosis
α_1-Antitrypsin deficiency	Wilson's disease
Tyrosinaemia and galactosaemia	Budd–Chiari syndrome
Byler's disease and sea-blue histiocyte syndrome	Primary hepatocellular carcinoma

Current patient selection

While primary hepatocellular carcinoma might appear at first sight to be the most obvious indication for liver replacement, recurrent cancer is the rule rather than the exception. Cholangiocarcinoma is now a contraindication. For the most part, patients considered for liver transplantation will be developing major hepatic decompensation due to advanced parenchymatous liver disease (Table 8.7). Alcoholic liver disease, one of the major causes of adult cirrhosis, is not usually considered a prime indication for liver replacement. However, patients with alcoholic liver disease who have clearly desisted from drinking for 6 or more months and are active participants in Alcoholics Anonymous have proved to be acceptable or even good candidates for transplantation.

Again, developments in the field of acute liver failure have suggested that this is a growing indication for hepatic replacement, although the time interval between onset of fulminant non-A, non-B hepatitis and death may be relatively short.

Children

By far the most important indication in children is following a failed correction of biliary atresia, a condition affecting 1 per 8000 live births in western countries[59] and, while in a third of these children satisfactory binary drainage can be achieved by a Kasai-type procedure,[60] for the most part advanced cirrhosis and decompensation will occur. Such children are best not treated by re-intervention but should be urgently considered for hepatic replacement.

Children suffering from primary metabolic disorders or inborn errors of metabolism which do eventually lead to complete liver destruction are also considered for replacement when cirrhosis and portal hypertension develop.

REFERENCES

57. Starzl T E Experience in Hepatic Transplantation. W B Saunders, Philadelphia 1969
58. Levy M F, Goldstein R M et al. Clin Transplant 1993; 14: 161–173
59. Balistrei W F J Pediatrics 1985; 106: 171
60. Kasai M Progr Pediatr Surg 1974; 6: 6

Surgical technique

Of all the organ transplant procedures currently undertaken, liver transplantation affords the most major technical problems. Not only is the liver a complex biochemical structure with multiple vascular anatomical relationships, but it also seems particularly susceptible to ischaemic damage.

While up to 60 minutes of warm ischaemia can be tolerated in some clinical situations, this has rarely been associated with satisfactory function when a period of cold preservation is also required.[61] Therefore meticulous surgical technique in organ harvesting and preservation is required to ensure rapid cooling to below 4°C and, even so, implantation of the liver will normally be required in less than 12 hours.

The recipient is prepared for the removal of the diseased liver and subsequent implantation (Fig. 8.8). This complex procedure may be undertaken using venous bypass from the lower inferior vena cava and portal vein to the superior cava to avoid diminished cardiac return during the phase at which the liver is being exchanged.

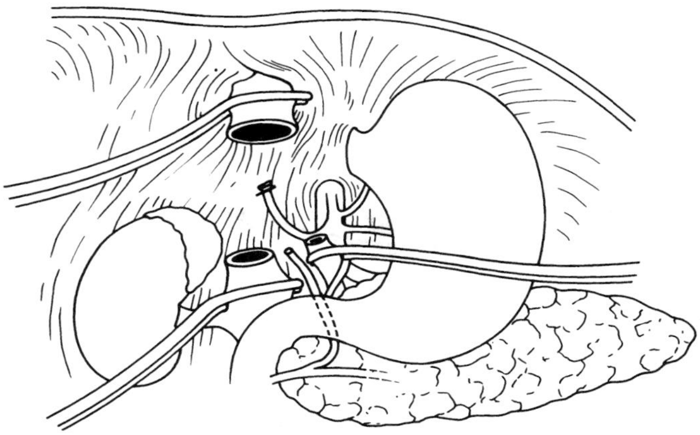

Fig. 8.8 Recipient following hepatectomy.

Postoperative management

The grafted liver must function immediately otherwise a consumptive coagulopathy will occur, leading to death within 24 hours from overwhelming haemorrhage. During this phase, while haemodynamic stability is being re-established, patients are normally ventilated with meticulous monitoring of cardiac output and renal function and immunosuppression is started to diminish the risk of major hepatic rejection. Intravenous cyclosporin A 5 mg/kg body weight with steroids (200 mg hydrocortisone intravenously daily) will usually be continued until intestinal absorption can occur, when patients are transferred to oral preparations. The liver transplant patient's absorption of cyclosporin and its excretion when hepatic dysfunction occurs vary considerably, and careful monitoring and management of cyclosporin are needed to avoid both toxicity and a failure of immunosuppression. The same considerations apply to FK506.

Diagnosis of hepatic rejection has proved much more difficult than that of other organs such as the kidney. The patient may develop liver dysfunction because of a combination of reasons which include ischaemia, infection, biliary obstruction or cytomegalovirus infection, and these all need to be excluded before the diagnosis of rejection can be confirmed, usually on liver biopsy. In approximately 10% of patients the graft fails with progressive deterioration in function and, under these circumstances, retransplantation may be the only hope of saving the patient.

Results of liver grafting

As in any surgical endeavour, the results of liver transplantation will be largely dependent on the selection criteria. Patients in the final agonal stages of their disease can often not be offered liver replacement because of the high morbidity and mortality but almost all adult patients below the age of 60 with terminal liver disease should be considered. Some centres report an 85% 1-year survival with over 75% still alive and well after 5 years.[62,63] In the absence of transplantation, these patients' survival is usually measured in months.

REFERENCES

61. Shaw B W, Gordon R D et al Transplant Proc 1985; 17: 264
62. European FK506 Liver Study Group: Lancet 1994; 344: 423–428
63. Goldstein R M Recent Developments in Transplant Medicine. Glerricine, Illinois 1996

9 The skin, skin tumours and plastic surgery

Jonathan A. Britto Leslie Fenton Oliver M. Fenton

INTRODUCTION

The aim of plastic surgery is to restore form and function to different parts of the body. Improvements in the understanding of applied anatomy and physiology in the last two decades have resulted in major advances in reconstructive and aesthetic surgery. Tumour resection and regional reconstruction, the treatment of congenital defects of the head and neck, trunk, hand and genital area, and the management of the consequences of trauma and infection are all now within the remit of the plastic surgeon. The accurate diagnosis of skin lesions is as important as it is gratifying, and it is vital to be able to recognize the difference between benign and malignant lesions. This chapter describes the structure and function of skin, those skin and subcutaneous lesions often referred for a surgical opinion, and the management of difficult scars and wounds. The major developments of historical importance to plastic surgical practice, current principles of surgical reconstruction, and a short section on aesthetic surgery are also included.

FUNCTIONAL ANATOMY OF THE SKIN

A worldwide industry has developed to find new ways to clean, adorn, nourish and rejuvenate the skin in its capacity as an external face to the world, but skin is more than just a covering for the body. It is a complex organ, acting as a physical barrier to infection and noxious substances, and as an immunological barrier by its immunoglobulin content. It also protects against ultraviolet sunlight, and provides an important means of interaction with the environment and other people by subtle sensory perception, crudely divided for testing purposes into fine touch, pain, temperature and vibration.

The skin is a homeostatic organ, controlling body temperature by the regulation of flow through cutaneous capillary beds and by eccrine sweat gland perfusion. It also has a regulatory role in salt and water control. As a closed keratinized surface it limits the uncontrolled egress of body fluid, and saline sweat production by the eccrine glands is controlled by neuro-endocrine mechanisms. Skin has an endocrine function which is essential in vitamin D synthesis. The initial step in the pathway is dependent upon ultraviolet light, which converts dihydrocholesterol in the skin to vitamin D3. This undergoes sequential hydroxylation in the liver and kidney to potent vitamin D.

Skin in different areas of the body shows a wide variation in structure and function. The skin of the back is ten times thicker than the skin of the eyelid, and the hairless skin of the palm of the hand, with its profuse ridges and sweat glands, is in sharp contrast to the sebaceous and hairy skin of the scalp. The basic structure is however similar, if not identical, throughout the body (Fig. 9.1).

Epidermis

The epidermis is a stratified keratinized squamous epithelium, and constitutes the external surface of the skin. It consists of four distinct layers: the basal cell layer (stratum basale), the prickle cell layer (stratum spinosum), the granular cell layer (stratum granulare) and the keratin layer (stratum corneum) which vary in appearance in different areas of the body. The skin appendages (hair follicles, sebaceous glands, sweat glands and nails) are all derived from epidermis. Keratinocytes, which are the dominant cell type, develop from basal cells and show a progressive increase in keratin content with loss of their nuclei, so that the most superficial keratin layer itself consists of flat dead cells that are lost through desquamation following washing and other activities. There are at least two populations of keratinocytes: epidermal keratinocytes that form the stratified squamous epithelium of the skin, and adnexal keratinocytes that form the adnexal or appendage components.[1]

Clear cells

In addition to keratinocytes, the epidermis contains three types of clear cells: melanocytes, Langerhans cells and Merkel cells.

Melanocytes

Melanocytes are round clear cells, derived from neuroectoderm, in the basal cell layer of the epidermis, and comprise about one tenth of the cell population. The number of melanocytes in white and black races is the same, but in darker skin and in freckles more melanin is produced by each cell. Melanocytes supply the surrounding keratinocytes with melanin through their dendritic processes. The pigmented keratinocytes serve to protect the underlying basal cell layer from the effects of ultraviolet radiation, which is reflected in the very low incidence of melanoma in black

REFERENCE

1. McGregor I A, McGregor F M Cancer of the Face and Mouth. Churchill Livingstone, Edinburgh 1986 p 56

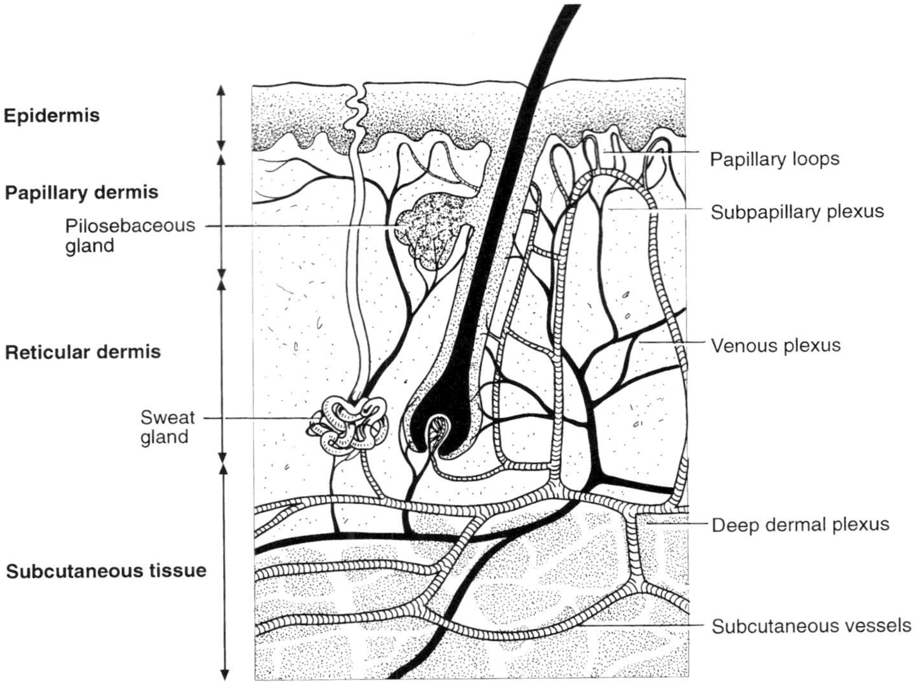

Fig. 9.1 The structure of the skin, showing the blood supply and appendages.

races, and the increasing incidence in whites exposed to excessive sunlight.

Langerhans cells

These cells are found in the suprabasal layers of the epidermis. They are also clear cells with dendritic processes and are present in similar numbers to melanocytes. They can be differentiated from melanocytes by histochemical stains and the presence of tennis racquet-shaped granules in the cytoplasm on electron microscopy. They are thought to be derived from the monocyte/macrophage cell series in the bone marrow and their function in immunosurveillance of the skin is to process antigens, either viral or neoplastic, and present them in a form that is recognized by T lymphocytes. They probably play a part in contact sensitization and in graft-versus-host disease of the skin, and they are increased in mycosis fungoides.

Merkel cells

Merkel cells are present in small numbers in the basal layer of the epidermis. They cannot be identified by routine histological staining but can be seen with silver stains. They are thought to be epithelial neuro-endocrine cells which act with peripheral nerve endings as slowly adapting mechanoreceptors and are responsible for tactile stereognosis.

Epidermal appendages

Hair

Hair of the adult scalp goes through a cycle of growth: anagen, a stage of active growth which lasts 3 years; catagen, a stage of regression lasting 3 weeks; and telogen, a resting period lasting 3 months. In the anagen stage the hair follicle has a bulb-like base surrounding a connective tissue dermal hair papilla. The cells of the hair bulb develop into the inner root sheath and the hair shaft. The outer root sheath is produced by invagination of the epidermis and resembles the superficial epidermis in its upper portion. In its lower portion, below the level of entry of the sebaceous duct which opens into every hair follicle, the outer root sheath is covered by an inner root sheath and does not keratinize. The hair follicle is surrounded by a vascular fibrous tissue sheath separated from the external root sheath by a basement membrane. The erector pili muscle is inserted into the fibrous sheath. The hair shaft consists, from the outside in, of a cuticle of overlapping cells, a cortex consisting of cells which, as they grow upwards, lose their nuclei and keratinize, and an inner medulla which is only partially keratinized.

Hair colour is determined by the quantity of melanin produced by melanocytes present in the basal layer of the hair bulb. In humans the hair serves a decorative and to a small degree protective function but the cells of the hair follicle are of enormous importance as a source of epidermal regeneration following superficial traumatic skin loss, such as occurs in dermal burns (see Chapter 6) and the donor sites of skin grafts (see below).

Sebaceous glands

Sebaceous glands secrete a protective coating of mixed lipids known as sebum into the hair follicle via the sebaceous duct. In some areas of the body these glands are not associated with hairs, such as on the labia minora, the areola of the breast and as Montgomery's tubercles around the nipple (see Chapter 25).

The Meibomian glands of the eyelids are modified sebaceous glands (see Chapter 15).

Sebaceous glands are composed of one or more lobules that are connected to a hair follicle by an excretory duct lined by squamous epithelium. Sebaceous glands are holocrine glands whose secretions are formed by disintegration of the cells adjacent to the lumen.

Eccrine sweat glands

Eccrine glands produce sweat which is similar in composition to plasma; they have a primary heat-regulating function, although sweating also occurs in response to mental stress. Eccrine glands are present in greatest numbers on the soles of the feet and palms of the hands but occur everywhere on the body except the lips, the nail beds, the labia minora and the glans of the penis.

The secretory part of the gland lies in the lower part of the dermis at the junction with the subcutaneous fat, and is composed of a single layer of cells forming a tubular gland with a discontinuous outer layer of myoepithelial cells which aid secretion by their contractile ability. The gland leads into an intradermal duct through which it reaches the skin surface via the intraepidermal eccrine duct, which has a spiral course.

Apocrine sweat glands

Apocrine glands are found in only a few sites: in the axillae, in the anogenital region, in the breast, in a modified form in the external auditory meatus as ceruminous glands, and in the eyelid as Moll's glands. They become functional at puberty and, in animals at least, act as scent glands. The secretory portion of the gland lies in the subcutaneous fat and is made up of a single layer of secretory cells surrounded by myoepithelial cells like an eccrine gland. The cells have eosinophilic cytoplasm and secretion of cell contents is by formation of a cap of cytoplasm at the apex of the cell, which is detached, or decapitated, into the lumen of the gland which is large.

Nails

The nail is a tough plate of keratinized cells that originate from the germinal matrix under the nail fold (Fig. 9.2). The distal portion of the germinal matrix is visible as the pale lunula, to which the nail plate is only loosely adherent. Thereafter, the nail plate is firmly adherent to the underlying nail bed, so that an injury to the finger tip frequently leaves the nail attached to the nail bed, but avulses it out of the nail fold. Nails grow at approximately 0.1 mm a day, although the rate of growth varies with age, site, season, nutrition and disease. Nails support the finger pulp and are important in initiating pinch, especially where small objects are involved.

Dermis

The dermis is a network of collagenous and elastic fibres embedded in ground substance that contains the vascular, neural and cellular elements that support the overlying epidermis. It is divided into two layers, the more superficial papillary dermis and the deeper reticular dermis. The papillary dermis is a narrow band occurring between and immediately under the rete ridges of the epidermis, and comprises fine collagen and elastic fibres which are loosely and irregularly arranged. The reticular dermis is responsible for the thickness of the skin, and the collagen and elastic fibres are organized in thick bundles that lie parallel to the surface of the skin. They produce the lines of skin cleavage, or relaxed skin tension lines (RSTLs), as demonstrated by Langer.[2]

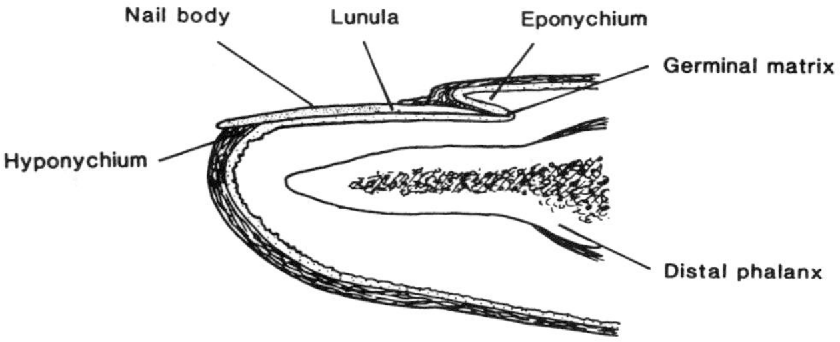

Fig. 9.2 The structure of the nail and nail fold.

The primary dermal cell type is the fibroblast, which generates collagen into the matrix in the ground substance. Collagen turnover is constant, and is greater under tension or mechanical stress. Fibroblasts also generate elastin, and these proteins form a matrix embedded in ground substance, which consists of glycosaminoglycans and proteoglycans.

The vascular network of the dermis is comprised of a subdermal plexus feeding a more superficial papillary plexus just deep to the epidermis. Veins have a similar arrangement, but include a third, mid-dermal, plexus. The subdermal fatty tissue is a discrete layer of the integument distinct from perineural or perivascular fat and is comprised of fat lobules separated by fibrous septa running from the dermis superficially to the deep fascia. Cutaneous nerves and vessels pass in these septa, but the capillary supply to the fat cells lies within each lobule.[3]

Inflow to the subdermal plexus is from vessels originating beneath the deep fascia and running through the subdermal fat. These vessels pass almost vertically to supply a narrow area of skin, or are angulated longitudinally and in concert with the cutaneous nerves, giving branches to supply a larger skin area. They may be reinforced by anastomoses with branches from other similar vertically orientated subfascial vessels, and may course either through muscles or around them.[3]

The epidermis has no blood supply and, like cartilage, is nourished by diffusion. The neural component comprises sensory and autonomic nerves as free nerve endings and special end-organs. The special end-organs are Pacinian corpuscles detecting pressure and vibration, Meissner's corpuscles and Merkel cell hair discs which both appreciate touch sensation.

Unlike the epidermis, which is replaced by mitosis from the basal layer of the pilosebaceous units, the dermis does not regen-

REFERENCES

2. Gibson T Br J Plast Surg 1978; 31(1): 1–2
3. Cormack G C, Lamberty B G H The Arterial Anatomy of Skin Flaps, 2nd edn. Churchill Livingstone, Edinburgh 1994 pp 16–19

erate. In cases of partial-thickness skin loss, such as burns or skin graft donor sites, the quality of the resultant scar is directly dependent on the amount of dermis that remains (see below).

The subdermal integument—fascia

The deep fascia consists of two different types: that of the trunk, covering muscle and relatively distensible; and that of the limbs, covering muscle and forming compartments that are relatively indistensible. The deep fascia of the limbs prevents bowstringing of tendons, is continuous with joint capsules, and gives rise to muscular attachments. It therefore has a well developed blood supply in the form of fascial plexuses which are exploited in the designing of fasciocutaneous flaps of the limbs.

THE MANAGEMENT OF WOUNDS

CHRONIC WOUNDS

A knowledge of wound care is a fundamental part of plastic surgery training. A wound constitutes a break in the epithelial integrity of the skin. Wounds can be usefully divided clinically into clean, dirty, infected, partial thickness or full thickness, those with a defined edge or ill defined edge, and those with or without skin loss. The myriad aetiology of wounds results in a wide range of clinical presentation and biological behaviour. This range in the character of wounds renders clinical trials of wound care difficult to design with scientific objectivity, and has resulted in a broad range of 'wound' products and clinical therapies. In addition, the explosion in knowledge of the basic science of wound healing has ushered in a range of biological growth factors and chemical wound manipulations which are of dubious clinical benefit. Given the multiple molecular mechanisms involved, it is unlikely that any single successful therapy to accelerate wound healing will be developed.

Certain phenomena are known to be detrimental to the outcome of wound care. Wounds heal better in a protected, warm, moist and oxygenated environment. Adequate nutritional substrates must be present for tissue healing.

Oxygenation

Fibroblasts are oxygen sensitive and will not generate collagen synthesis at tissue oxygen tensions of less than 40 mmHg. Hyperoxygenation improves collagen synthesis, which is directly proportional to the tensile strength of the wound. Oxygenation also improves host defence mechanisms against microbial infection and wound re-epithelialization rates.[4] Hypoxia has been reported to be the most common cause of wound infection and failure to heal. The oxygen tension in the healing wound is affected by many variables: the oxygen fraction in inspired air, the oxygen–haemoglobin saturation dynamics in red cells of adequate number and function, and the efficiency of the circulatory system and microcirculation. Any of these mechanisms may be malfunctioning in the susceptible patient.

Steroid therapy

Steroids inhibit the action of wound macrophages, which are essential to all stages of wound healing although they are particularly involved in the demolition and organization phases. Fibroblast function and collagen synthesis are also compromised by steroids, as are myofibroblast mediated wound contraction and the process of angiogenesis.[4] Non-steroidal anti-inflammatory agents at therapeutic doses have also been shown to reduce collagen synthesis significantly via the prostaglandin pathway.

Vitamins, zinc and wound healing

Oral vitamin A therapy stimulates collagen deposition and increases wound breaking strength, and topical therapy accelerates re-epithelialization. The mechanisms are unclear. The benefits of vitamin C have long been accepted and can be summarized as: accelerating maturation of fibroblasts, contributing to the higher structure of the extracellular matrix, and contributing to angiogenesis. Whereas deficiency can be clinically debilitating, dietary loading does not boost supranormal healing.[4] Vitamin E increases the breaking strength of preoperatively irradiated wounds and neutralizes lipid peroxidation, limiting levels of free radical and thus oxidative tissue damage. Studies differ regarding its effect on collagen synthesis.[4]

Zinc is a ubiquitous component of enzyme systems of great importance to the physiology of wound healing. Low zinc levels contribute to reduction in fibroblast and epithelial proliferation, but investigators differ over the value of dietary loading in non-deficiency states.

Smoking

As a potent vasoconstrictor, nicotine reduces perfusion and oxygenation to wounds. The carbon monoxide component of cigarette smoke causes carboxyhaemoglobin levels to rise, and further reduces oxygen carriage to the tissues. Patients should be advised to cease smoking at least six weeks before reconstructive procedures.

Age

Wound tensile strengths and closure rates decrease with age. This may be a function of reduced cellular division and metabolic activity or increased susceptibility to insult. These factors may be synergistic.

Denervation

Denervated skin ulcerates faster and heals more slowly than sensate skin.

Infection

An infected wound stimulates an inflammatory response which is aimed at demolition and bacteriolysis rather than regeneration and

REFERENCE

4. Rohrich R J, Robinson J B Select Read Plast Surg 1992; 7(1): 1–42

repair. Angiogenesis, granulation and epithelialization are impaired by this catabolic response, made worse by infection.

Chemotherapy and radiotherapy

Chemotherapeutic agents usually decrease fibroblast activity and reduce wound contraction.[5] It has been recommended that adjuvant systemic chemotherapy should not commence until two weeks after an operation. Acute radiation injury is characterized by a vasculitis, intravascular stasis, and small vessel occlusion. In addition, direct irreversible fibroblast damage has been reported; this also compromises wound healing.

Diabetes mellitus

Small vessel occlusion is no longer considered the only problem in diabetes mellitus as the larger vessels may also develop arteriosclerosis. Denervation injury also contributes to poor healing, which is further compromised by an increased incidence of infection.

PRESSURE NECROSIS

Pressure sores are a significant cause of morbidity, lengthy hospital stay, and increased cost to health services, estimated at £150 million per year in Great Britain.[6] They are caused by prolonged weight bearing and mechanical shear forces on the soft tissue over bony prominences, with resultant increase in the pressure across small blood vessels, reduced tissue perfusion and ischaemic necrosis.[7]

The prevalence of pressure necrosis in the UK hospital population is 7–8%,[8] with 70% of sores occurring in patients over 70 years of age. Immobility is the primary contributing factor, and prolonged bed rest from cardiopulmonary disease, bone and joint problems, trauma or neurological disease increases patient susceptibility. Approximately 80% of paraplegics develop a pressure sore.[8] Tissue damage is thought to occur when uninterrupted pressures of greater than 9.3 kPa are sustained[9] but in healthy sitting people an inverse relationship occurs between tissue pressure and duration of tolerance.[10] It is therefore those patients who are unable to change position that are most at risk—this includes those patients undergoing long operative procedures, with implications for patient positioning especially when there is prolonged iatrogenic hypotension in theatre. Early reports indicated that shearing forces are of major importance and that patients positioned at 45° develop worse sacral necrosis than patients lying flat.[11] These forces result in tearing of the vessels and connective tissue laminae of the subcutaneous fat, with subsequent thrombosis and haematoma. Tissue maceration from sweating and incontinence also reduces tissue integrity.

The most common sites for pressure sores are the sacrum (43%), greater trochanter (12%), heel (11%), lateral malleolus (6%), and ischial tuberosity (5%)[6] (Fig. 9.3). Occipital sores are also quite common in the bed ridden. The American National Pressure Ulcer Advisory Panel classification is the most common classification system in current use:

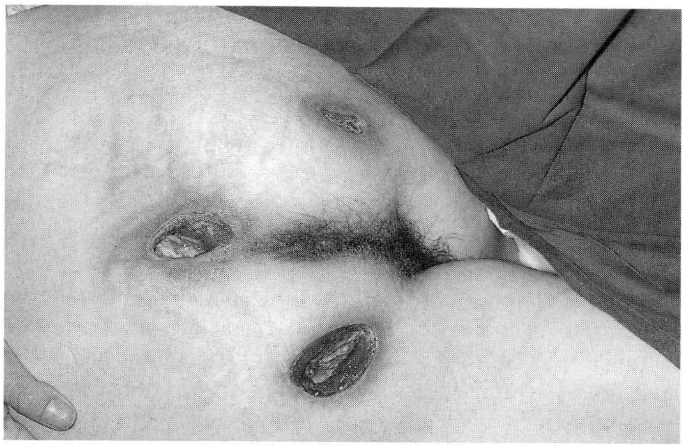

Fig. 9.3 Sacral and bilateral ischial pressure sores.

Stage 1	Erythema that will not blanch—indicates extravasated blood from cutaneous capillary beds.
Stage 2	Partial thickness skin loss—a shallow abrasion wound.
Stage 3	Full thickness skin loss with fat at the base of the wound.
Stage 4	Extensive soft tissue loss through deep fascia, often with underlying muscle necrosis.

This classification system contradicts a theoretical aetiology of pressure sores, that the final common pathway of damage is ischaemic, and that muscle and fat are more poorly tolerant of ischaemia than the fascia or skin. When pressure sores occur in sites where muscle covers bone, such as the sacrum and trochanters, the muscle damage may precede any visible cutaneous signs.

Laser Doppler scanning shows that there is less cutaneous blood flow over the sacral area compared to the gluteal area when controlled pressure is applied.[12] An ischaemia–reperfusion injury may also result from continuous small changes in blood flow, and net increases in tissue pressure reduce venous and lymphatic outflow and thus clearance of toxic metabolites. Furthermore, the factors which are known to slow wound healing also contribute to the risk and severity of pressure necrosis.

Repeated laser duplex fluximetry and measurement of serum creatinine phosphokinase levels may indicate the onset of pressure necrosis but have yet to replace clinical vigilance. Prophylactic clinical care—which includes frequent turning (2–4-hourly), skin inspection, massage and toiletting—and the use of specially designed aids, mattresses and cushions to even pressure gradients have reduced the risk of pressure sores.[6] A variety of high cost

REFERENCES

5. Rockwell W B, Cohen I K, Erhlich H P Plast Reconstr Surg 1989; 84: 827–83
6. Vohra R K, McCollum C N Br Med J 1994; 309: 853–857
7. Reuler I B, Coonery T J Ann Intern Med 1981; 94: 661–666
8. Dealey C J Adv Nurs 1991; 16: 663–670
9. Kosiak M Arch Phys Med Rehabil 1961; 42: 19–29
10. Barbanel J C Prosthetics and Orthotics Int 1991; 15: 225–231
11. Reichel S M JAMA 1958; 166: 762–763
12. Schubert V, Fragrell B Clin Physiol 1989; 9: 535–545

air-fluidized, alternating air, static air, and water mattresses are available, and demand evaluation by well designed clinical trials. Air- and gel-filled cushions are used in wheelchairs to reduce the incidence of ischial sores, where a high body weight to dependent area ratio necessarily occurs.

When preventative care fails, the options for management are both conservative and surgical. The principles are: to improve tissue perfusion and oxygenation; to relieve pressure; to optimize wound healing by treating infection as it arises; and to provide optimal nutritional support. There is no place for prophylactic antibiotics. There is a need for scientific and clinical evaluation of the wide variety of topical dressings, agents from inorganic chemicals to enzymes and growth factors, and the use of hyperbaric oxygen, vacuum assist machines, hydrotherapy, ultrasound and electrotherapy. The broad spectrum of clinical wounds encountered in practice brings a challenge to trial design—most results are anecdotal and open to misinterpretation.

Surgical options for wound closure include a variety of fascial and composite muscle-containing flaps for each site. The principles of reconstruction are to choose the simplest appropriate procedure as these patients may have compromised primary healing, and to appreciate that the procedure may be palliative rather than curative. Large flaps should be used that can be rerotated in case of pressure sore recurrence, and which do not preclude the use of other flaps in the area (Figs 9.4 and 9.5). The cavity produced by the debridement of a pressure sore must be filled by perfused tissue, usually muscle, to introduce a blood supply and encourage healing. It is a misconception that muscle flaps provide 'padding' over a pressure point, as muscle is more vulnerable to ischaemia than the overlying skin. Scars that result from these operations should not be placed over pressure points as they are liable to repeated dehiscence. Where possible, muscle tone and skin sensation should be preserved and the postoperative care of the patient directed towards minimizing the risk of recurrence. Recurrence of pressure necrosis is depressingly common unless the aetiological factors can be corrected. The bony 'pressure point' is seldom, if ever, removed as this merely transfers pressure to another site.

a

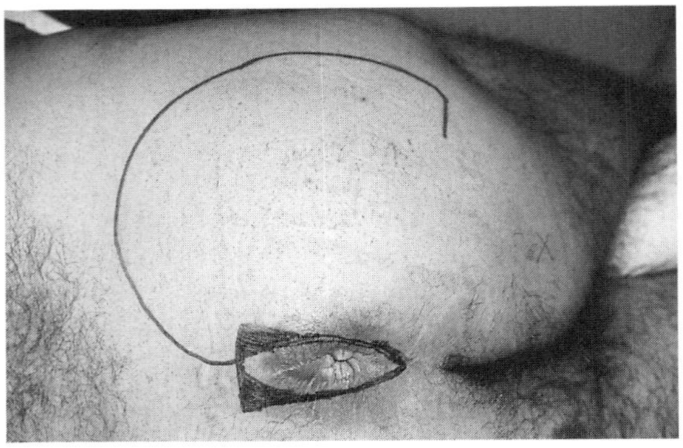

b

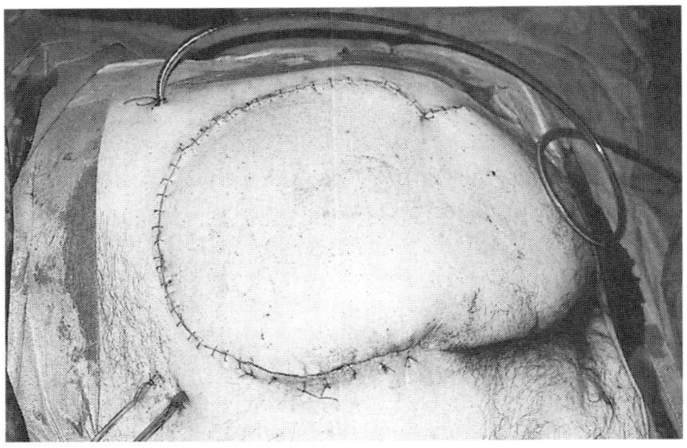

Fig. 9.4 Gluteal rotation flap for sacral pressure sore: (**a**) before; (**b**) after.

EXTRAVASATION INJURY

The leakage of cytotoxic drugs, parenteral nutrition, ionic solutions and even 5% dextrose from a cannula or vein into the surrounding tissues can cause skin necrosis, and may precipitate scarring and atrophy around tendons, vessels, nerves and joints. The injury is proportional to the toxicity of the agent and analogous to a subcutaneous chemical burn with a wide zone of injury. Quick referral of this common problem, which has a 4.5% risk in parenteral cytotoxic therapy,[13] and prompt action can save much morbidity. These injuries are justifiably considered plastic surgical emergencies (Fig. 9.6).

Delay in treatment usually results in increasingly serious outcome. This includes fixed extension at the wrist and digital amputation[14] in the neonatal intensive care setting. Treatment has varied from aggressive early surgical debridement and grafting[15] to a more conservative expectant approach using ice and elevation.[16] The damage is caused by the acidity and hypertonicity of the infused solution. Cytotoxic agents also impede the potential for wound healing and may become incorporated into the local cells and surrounding tissue, increasing the risk of late ulceration.[14] Vasoconstriction may potentiate an ischaemic necrosis.[17,18] Calcium and potassium infusions, in addition to their acidity and hypertonicity, may cause direct cellular damage by protein precipitation.[19] Infusion of the injurious agent should be stopped as quickly as possible to minimize the zone of damage and conserve healthy tissue.

A technique for subcutaneous washout has been described in an attempt to treat all types of fresh extravasation injury in adults and children.[14,20] The injured area is subcutaneously injected with up to 1500 units of hyaluronidase to dissolve the connective tissue matrix and allow perfused fluids to pass freely through the subcutaneous tissue. Peripheral incisions are made around the 'clock face' of the injury and the subcutaneous tissue of the damaged area is perfused with up to 500 ml of normal saline using an atraumatic cannula. The washout fluid can be tested for decreasing

REFERENCES

13. Wang J J, Cortes E, Sinks L F, Holland J F Cancer 1971; 28: 837–843
14. Gault D T Br J Plast Surg 1993; 46: 91–96
15. Linder R M, Upton J, Osteen R J Hand Surgery 1983; 8A: 32–38
16. Larson D L Plast Reconstr Surg 1985; 75: 397–402
17. Lewis G B H, Hecker J F Anaesth Intensive Care 1984; 12: 27–32
18. Larson D L Clin Plast Surg 1990; 17(3): 509–518
19. Dufresne R G Cutis 1987; 39: 197–198
20. Davies J, Gault D T, Buchdahl R Arch Dis Child 1994; 70: F50–51

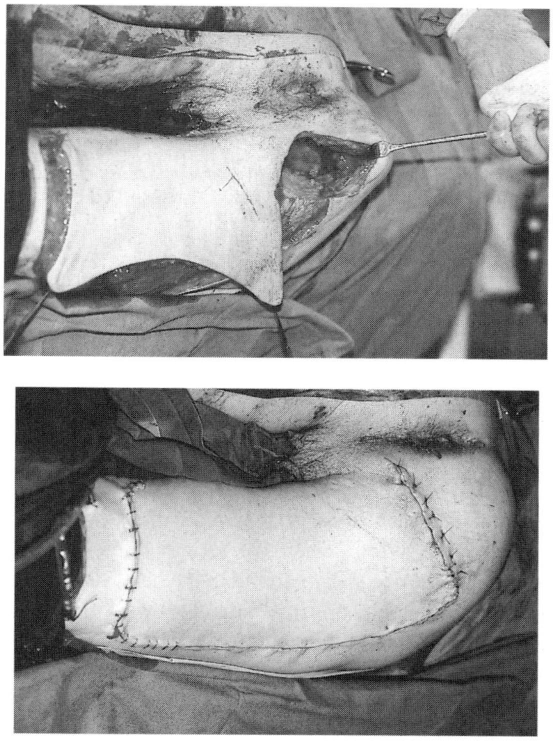

a

b

Fig. 9.5 Posterior thigh flap for ischial pressure sore: (**a**) before; (**b**) after.

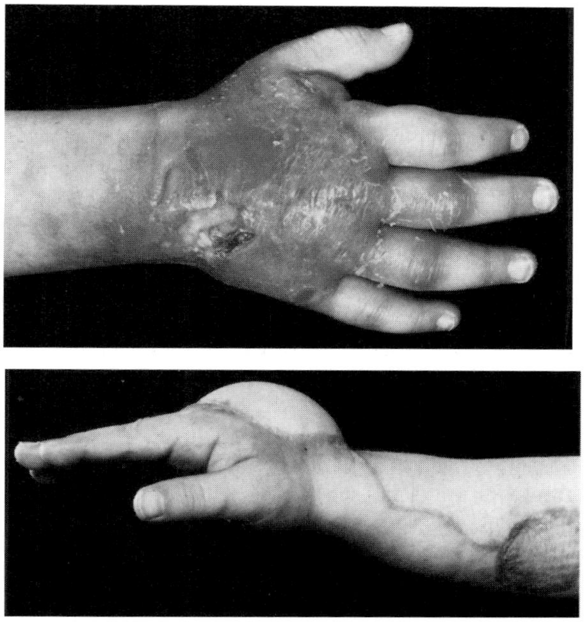

a

b

Fig. 9.6 (**a**) Untreated extravasation injury on dorsum of right hand, showing extensive subcutaneous extravasated fluid and skin damage. (**b**) Excised and debrided wound, defect reconstructed with islanded forearm flap.

concentrations of toxin. The procedure may require general anaesthesia, and prophylactic antibiotics are recommended. For larger areas, liposuction may be combined with saline flushout to achieve a more effective tissue penetration.

SKIN LESIONS

Skin lesions may present in a variety of shapes, textures and colours. The same skin tumour may have a very different presentation in different individuals, or in different body sites of the same individual. It is therefore important to have a common language and set of descriptive terms applied to these lesions, both to facilitate communication between clinicians, and to reduce confusion and anxiety for the patient. For a brief definition of common terms see Table 9.1.

BENIGN SKIN LESIONS

Seborrhoeic keratosis

Synonyms: basal cell papilloma, seborrhoeic wart

These very common skin blemishes occur after middle age and present as single or multiple, round or oval, slightly greasy lesions that have a very characteristic 'stuck-on' appearance. They may have a varying degree of pigmentation from light brown to black and the surface varies from velvety to warty (Fig. 9.7). They most commonly develop on the face and trunk but can occur anywhere on the body. Multiple seborrhoeic keratoses have been associated with internal malignancy (the Leser–Trélat sign).

There is great variation in the histological appearance of these lesions but all are characterized by hyperkeratosis, acanthosis and papillomatosis. The acanthotic part of the epidermis is composed of cells with a basaloid appearance. Occasionally squamous 'eddies' are seen mixed with the basal cells, and this constitutes the irritated seborrhoeic keratosis, a histological variant.

Differential diagnosis

These are the benign skin lesions most commonly confused with malignant melanoma but the characteristic appearances usually allow the correct clinical diagnosis to be made.

Treatment

The keratosis normally lies wholly above the level of the surrounding normal epidermis, thus allowing it to be treated by superficial shaving or cautery without leaving visible scarring. Although both squamous and basal cell carcinomas have been reported as arising in a seborrhoeic keratosis, this is exceptional and they can be treated as benign lesions.

Stucco keratoses

Stucco keratoses are very common warty lesions and usually occur on the dorsum of the extremities in the middle-aged to elderly. They are small, flat, roughened areas with a grey or light brown colouration. They can easily be removed by shaving or abrasion. Histologically they appear to be a variant of hyperkeratotic seborrhoeic keratosis.[21]

REFERENCE

21. Willoughby C, Soter N A Arch Dermatol 1972; 105: 859

Table 9.1 Terminology

Cyst	A tumour that contains fluid
Hamartoma	An overgrowth of one or more cell types that are normal constituents of the organ in which they arise. The commonest examples are haemangiomas, lymphangiomas (see Chapter 10) and neurofibromas
Macule	A flat impalpable lesion, e.g. a port wine stain
Naevus	A lesion present from birth, composed of mature structures normally found in the skin but present in excess or in an abnormal disposition. This type of lesion is also referred to as a hamartoma. The term 'naevus' is also used to describe lesions composed of naevus cells as in melanocytic or pigmented naevi
Papilloma	A benign overgrowth of epithelial tissue
Papule	A small elevated lesion
Plaque	An elevated area, usually larger than 2 cm across
Pustule	A raised lesion that contains pus
Tumour	Literally, a swelling. Commonly but inaccurately used to mean a malignant swelling
Ulcer	An area of dissolution of an epithelial surface
Vesicle	A small blister

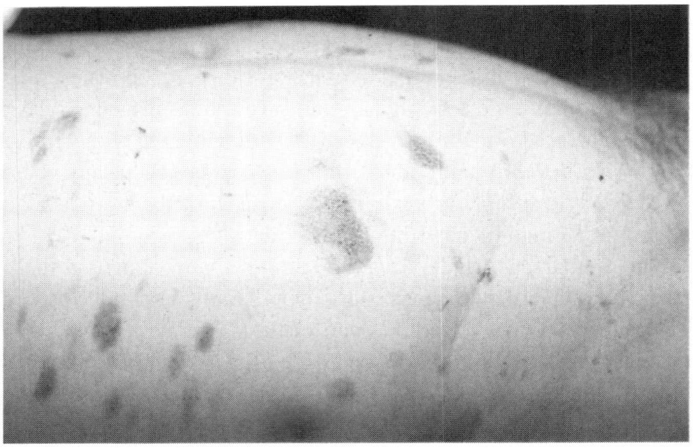

Fig. 9.7 A seborrhoeic keratosis.

Skin tags

Synonyms: fibroepithelial papilloma, achrochordon, fibroma molle, soft fibromas

These are very common benign skin tumours which tend to occur after the first decade and become more frequent with increasing age. In their most common form, they present as discrete multiple tags around the neck and axilla. They are also found as solitary, fleshy papillomas on the trunk, although they may occur anywhere. They consist of a vascular, loose connective tissue core covered by papillomatous squamous epithelium.

They are easily treated by simple excision using a pair of sharp scissors under a local anaesthetic, although occasionally a single suture is needed to control bleeding from the feeding vessel.

Linear epidermal naevus

Synonyms: verrucous naevus, naevus hystrix, naevus unius lateris

These light brown warty naevi may be present at birth or appear shortly thereafter. They have a variable clinical presentation which ranges from small linear warts measuring less than 1 cm to multiple parallel hyperkeratotic papillomas which almost give the impression that they have been poured on to the body (Fig. 9.8). They may occur in a localized area or may have a bilateral symmetrical distribution, when the term ichthyosis hystrix has been used. They are commonly found in the head and neck area but may occur anywhere. Extensive warty growths are part of the epidermal naevus syndrome that includes skeletal and central nervous system abnormalities.[22]

Hyperkeratosis and papillomatosis is seen on histological examination. The linear epidermal naevus extends deeply into the dermis with elongation of the rete ridges below the level of the surrounding epidermis. This distinguishes it both histologically and clinically from a seborrhoeic keratosis where the growth of the tumour is largely upward, producing a sharp demarcation between the lower border of the tumour and normal underlying dermis. This allows seborrhoeic keratoses to be shaved with complete resolution and no scarring, whereas linear epidermal naevae must be surgically excised. They look deceptively superficial but almost always recur when shaved or treated by electrodissection. This form of treatment is often used, however, and may be repeated when the naevus regrows. For large and unsightly lesions excision is necessary for permanent cure.[23] Malignant transformation to both squamous cell and basal cell carcinoma has been described.

Differential diagnosis

Large linear epidermal naevi are quite characteristic because of their 'streaming' appearance, and the clinical history differentiates them from viral warts and seborrhoeic keratoses.

Keratoacanthoma

Synonym: molluscum sebaceum

Keratoacanthomas are rapidly growing (6–8 weeks), solitary skin tumours which can be mistaken, both clinically and histologically,

REFERENCES

22. Su W P D Am J Dermatopathol 1982; 4: 161–170
23. Solomon L M, Fretzin D F, Dewald R L Arch Dermatol 1968; 97: 273–285

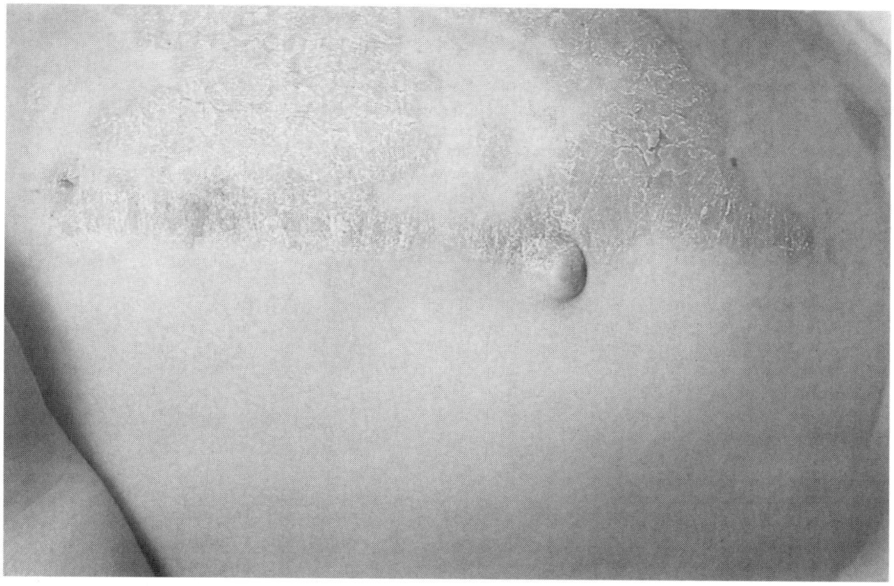

Fig. 9.8 A linear epidermal naevus.

for well differentiated squamous cell carcinomas. The aetiology is unknown, but they occur on sun-exposed parts of the body, more frequently in males than females, and present as a dome-shaped lesion measuring up to 2.5 cm in diameter with a central keratin-filled crater (Fig. 9.9). They involute in approximately 6 months if untreated, leaving only a depressed scar behind. When there is doubt as to the nature of the tumour a complete excision biopsy is preferred, because the histological diagnosis depends more on the architecture than on the cytological features. If the keratoacanthoma cannot be entirely excised, an elliptical biopsy should be taken through the centre of the lesion, including both lateral margins.

Histologically, the tumour consists of a keratin-filled crater surrounded by a cup-shaped swelling with overhanging edges, composed of keratinized, well differentiated squamous epithelium. The lower border of the tumour extends into the dermis but is usually rounded and clearly demarcated from the surrounding dermis. Cytologically, the tumour can look alarming, with cellular atypia and prominent mitotic activity. Sometimes it may not be possible to distinguish keratoacanthomas from well differentiated squamous carcinomas, and in the elderly patient they should be regarded with great suspicion and excised completely with an adequate margin.[24]

CYSTS

Epidermal cysts and trichilemmal cysts

Synonyms: sebaceous cysts, wens, pilar cysts, epidermoid cysts

Both these cysts are referred to as 'sebaceous cysts' by the majority of clinicians, and it is unlikely that the name will pass from common usage. Neither, however, is derived from sebaceous glands, and although they are clinically indistinguishable they can be separated histologically.[25]

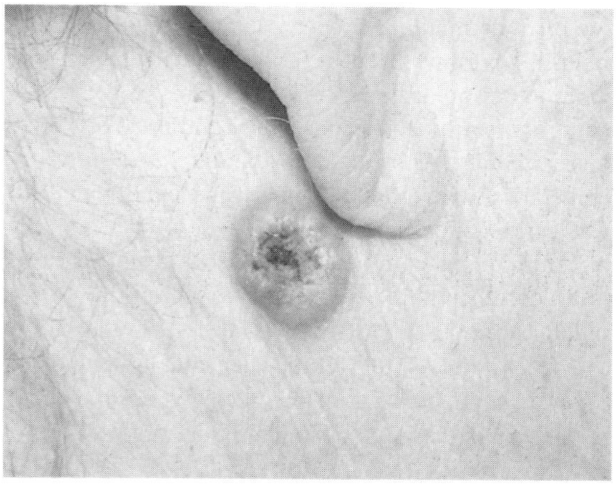

Fig. 9.9 A keratoacanthoma.

Epidermal cysts

These cysts are usually solitary and may occur at any age and in almost any site; they are most common however on the face, trunk, neck, extremities and scalp, in descending order (Fig. 9.10). They are thought to arise from the infundibular portion of hair follicles. An identical cyst occurs from traumatic implantation of epidermis and is called an implantation or inclusion dermoid cyst.[26]

These cysts can be of almost any size and present as a round, smooth, firm to soft swelling which is attached to the skin. A punctum is normally present near the apex of the cyst which may exhibit a plastic deformation which helps to distinguish it from a

REFERENCES

24. Rook A, Whimster I W Br J Dermatol 1979; 100: 41–47
25. Lever W F, Schaumberg-Lever G Histopathology of the Skin. J B Lippincott, Philadelphia 1990 p 535
26. McGavran M H, Binnington B Arch Dermatol 1968; 94: 499–508

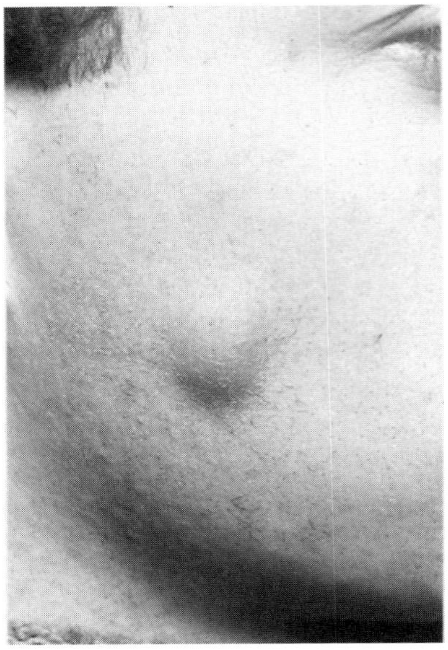

Fig. 9.10 A sebaceous cyst.

lipoma. Sebaceous cysts can become infected with subsequent discharge of foul-smelling, cheesy contents. Multiple cysts occur in Gardner's syndrome in association with intestinal polyposis, desmoid tumours and osteomas.[27]

The cyst is filled by keratinous debris and lined by keratinizing squamous epithelium with a distinct granular layer. It may rupture, releasing keratinous material into the dermis and causing a foreign-body giant cell reaction.

Treatment requires complete removal of the entire cyst and its contents. Recurrence is likely if even a small portion of the cyst lining is left behind. For this reason, the cyst should be removed intact with an ellipse of skin over the apex containing the punctum. To remove a cyst intact is a good technical exercise in making use of tissue planes and learning to handle tissues gently.

Trichilemmal cysts

Trichilemmal cysts are not as common as epidermal cysts, and 90% occur on the scalp (Fig. 9.11). They are often multiple, with only 30% occurring as a single lesion. This type of cyst has a genetic predisposition with an autosomal dominant mode of inheritance.[28]

Trichilemmal cysts are lined by epithelial cells with palisading of the outer cell layer which surrounds inner layers of pale, swollen cells that undergo abrupt keratinization. This differs from the keratinization of the lining cells of epidermal cysts (these have an intervening granular layer which is a normal component of epidermis), and supports the view that trichilemmal cysts are derived from hair follicle epithelium rather than epidermis.[29,30]

There may also be calcification of the cyst contents which is not seen in epidermal cysts. Sometimes there may be proliferation of the cyst lining epithelium resembling that seen in a pilar tumour, or proliferating trichilemmal cyst, which may represent a transition between these two lesions.

The proliferating trichilemmal cyst or tumour is usually solitary and, like the trichilemmal cyst, also occurs on the scalp in 90% of

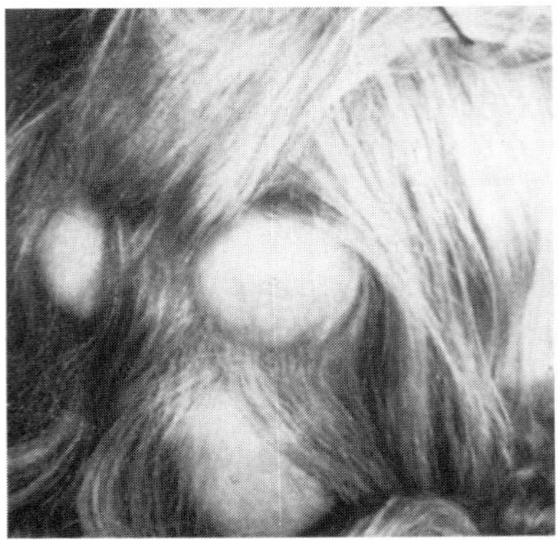

Fig. 9.11 Multiple epidermal/trichilemmal cysts.

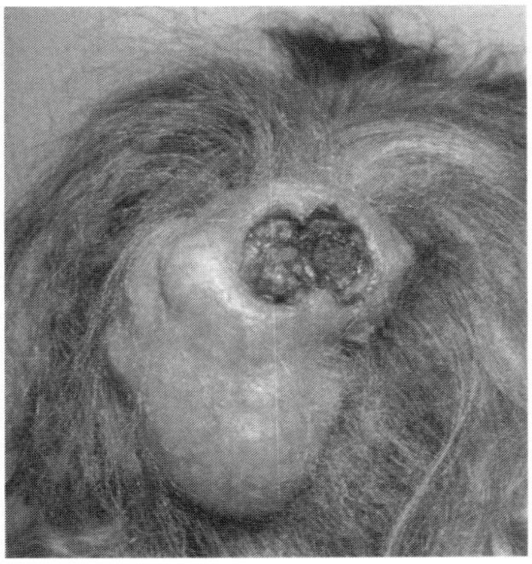

Fig. 9.12 A Pott's peculiar tumour.

cases. The tumour may reach a very large size and ulcerate, and may resemble a squamous carcinoma both clinically and histologically, when it is called a Pott's peculiar tumour (Fig. 9.12). The tumour nearly always behaves in a benign manner, although it may recur after excision. Very rarely metastases have been reported in tumours that have undergone malignant transformation and grown rapidly.[31] Treatment is as for epidermal cysts.

Dermoid cysts

These are congenital subcutaneous cysts and are the result of the developmental inclusion of epidermis along lines of fusion. The cyst is lined by stratified squamous epithelium but, unlike the epidermal cyst, the wall also contains functioning epidermal appendages such as hair follicles, sweat and sebaceous glands.

REFERENCES

27. Lever W F, Schaumberg-Lever G Histopathology of the Skin. J B Lippincott, Philadelphia 1990 p 670
28. Lever W F, Schaumberg-Lever G Histopathology of the Skin. J B Lippincott, Philadelphia 1990 p 537
29. Pinkus H Arch Dermatol 1969; 99: 544–555
30. Leppard B J, Sanderson K V Br J Dermatol 1976; 94: 379–390
31. Lever W F, Schaumberg-Lever G Histopathology of the Skin. J B Lippincott, Philadelphia 1990 p 590

Common sites are the lateral and medial ends of the eyebrow (when they are called external and internal angular dermoid cysts—Fig. 9.13), the midline of the nose (called nasal dermoid cysts), sublingually, and the midline of the neck, perineum and sacrum. Treatment consists of complete excision but great care must be taken to establish the extent of the cyst. An external angular dermoid frequently creates a bony depression and it rarely penetrates down to the dura. A nasal dermoid may present as a deceptively small superficial pit that is the only visible part of an extensive cyst that passes between the nasal bones towards the sphenoid sinus in a dumb-bell fashion. Skull radiographs and a computerized tomography scan may be indicated. These are not cysts that should be excised by an inexperienced surgeon under local anaesthetic.

Milia

Milia are small, white, superficial spots that can occur in large numbers on the face, and are an almost normal feature of newborn babies. Like epidermal cysts, they are derived from hair follicles. Secondary milial cysts (keratocysts) are frequently seen after dermabrasion or skin grafting. Treatment is by incision of the cyst with a needle or scalpel, and expression of the contents.

SKIN APPENDAGE TUMOURS

Skin appendage tumours are uncommon and most are benign. They arise from the adnexal structures of the skin and therefore can show variable differentiation towards hair follicle, sebaceous, eccrine or apocrine structures.[32]

Hair follicle tumours

Only the most common are described.

Trichofolliculoma

Trichofolliculomas are slow-growing, solitary dome-shaped nodules, often with a central umbilication from which white hairs may protrude. They are skin-coloured and usually measure 0.5 cm in diameter at the time of presentation. Histologically they consist of a dilated central hair follicle lined by keratinizing squamous epithelium, continuous with the surface epidermis. The central cyst is surrounded by epithelial extensions showing varying degrees of attempted pilar formation with some containing birefringent hair fragments.[33] The most important differential diagnosis is basal cell carcinoma. Simple excision is curative.

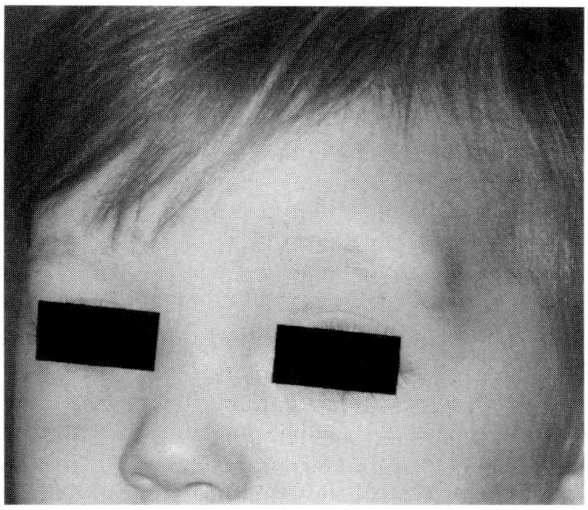

Fig. 9.13 An external angular dermoid cyst.

Trichoepithelioma

Synonym: epithelioma adenoides cysticum

These may be solitary or multiple tumours, in the latter case being associated with an autosomal dominant inheritance. The first lesions usually appear in the first two decades of life and, in the case of multiple tumours, these appear synchronously and increase in number into adult life. The most common site is on the face, around the nose, forehead and upper lip. The lesions are flesh-coloured, firm nodules and papules which may be confluent, with a translucent surface and occasional telangiectasia. They are usually half a centimetre in diameter but can measure up to 2.5 cm.[34] Solitary trichoepitheliomas also occur on the face but are not inherited and appear in early adult life. They may be confused with basal cell carcinomas and with sebaceous cysts.[35] Treatment is by simple excision, although this may be difficult in the case of multiple and confluent trichoepitheliomas; these lesions are best treated by diathermy excision or shaving, which may need to be repeated.

Pilomatrixoma

Synonym: calcifying epithelioma of Malherbe

Pilomatrixomas arise on the head, neck and upper extremities, predominantly in the first two decades of life. They present as firm red-to-white subepidermal nodules and may measure several centimetres in diameter with a normal overlying epidermis (Fig. 9.14). The white appearance is caused by visible calcification, which occurs in most cases and gives the lesion a granular feel.

The tumour has a distinctive histological appearance being made up of two types of cell, the round or oval basophilic cell and the more eosinophilic shadow cells which have lost their nuclei and are keratinized. The basophilic cells are usually arranged around the periphery of the tumour and merge into, or in other areas change abruptly into, the shadow cells. Most of these tumours contain calcium, and ossification occurs in up to 20%.[36] Treatment is by simple excision. Invasive growth has been reported in those lesions that recur.[37]

REFERENCES

32. Headington J T Am J Pathol 1976; 85: 479–514
33. Gray H R, Helwig E B Arch Dermatol 1962; 86: 619
34. Gray H R, Helwig E B Arch Dermatol 1963; 87: 102
35. Zeligman I Arch Dermatol 1960; 82: 35
36. Forbis R Jr, Helwig E B Arch Dermatol 1961; 83: 606
37. Wood M G, Parhizgar B, Beerman H Arch Dermatol 1984; 120(6): 770–773

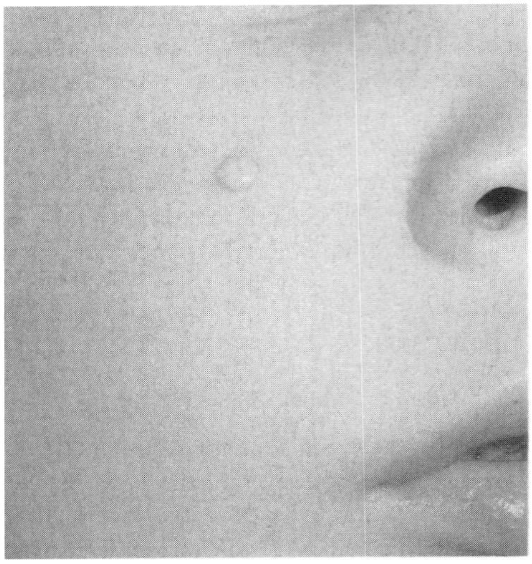

Fig. 9.14 A pilomatrixoma.

Trichilemmoma

Trichilemmomas may present as solitary tumours or as multiple lesions in Cowden's disease.[38] Solitary lesions are quite common and present as small pink or brownish papules on the face, usually after the third decade. They are frequently mistaken for basal cell carcinoma clinically, and may be difficult to distinguish from a verruca vulgaris both clinically and histologically as a result of their epidermal type of keratinization and marked granular layer. Some tumour cells may appear clear owing to their glycogen content.[38]

Cowden's disease has an autosomal dominant inheritance and presents as multiple trichilemmomas on the face around the nose, mouth and ears and on the lips, gingiva and tongue. It is a multiple hamartoma syndrome, usually associated with fibrous hamartomas of the gastrointestinal tract, breast and thyroid, and it is associated with breast cancer and other visceral malignancies.[39]

Sebaceous tumours

These include sebaceous adenoma, basal cell carcinoma with sebaceous differentiation and sebaceous carcinoma. There are two other important conditions that may cause confusion with these neoplasms (the naevus sebaceus of Jadassohn and senile sebaceous hyperplasia.

Naevus sebaceus of Jadassohn

This is also referred to as an organoid naevus. It is a true naevus because it involves the whole skin organ and more than one adnexa. It occurs on the head and neck, the scalp being the most common site. The lesion is usually present at birth as a well circumscribed, hairless, papillomatous area. At puberty the lesion becomes verrucous and nodular as a result of hyperplasia of sebaceous glands and also sometimes apocrine glands. It then takes on the familiar appearance of a soft, warty, papillomatous naevus (Fig. 9.15). A third stage of development occurs in up to 20% of cases when other tumours arise in the naevus. These can be benign

a

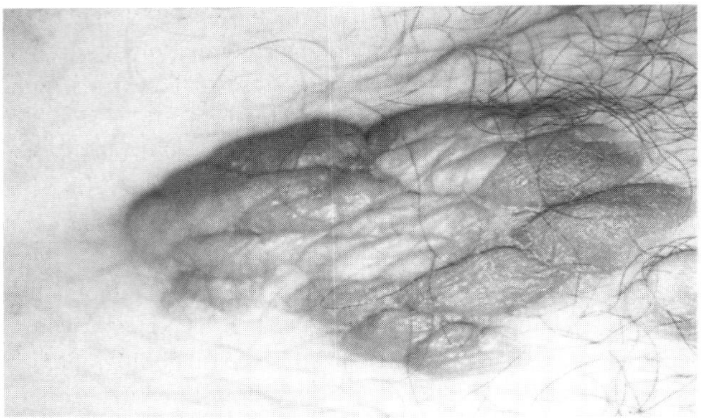

b

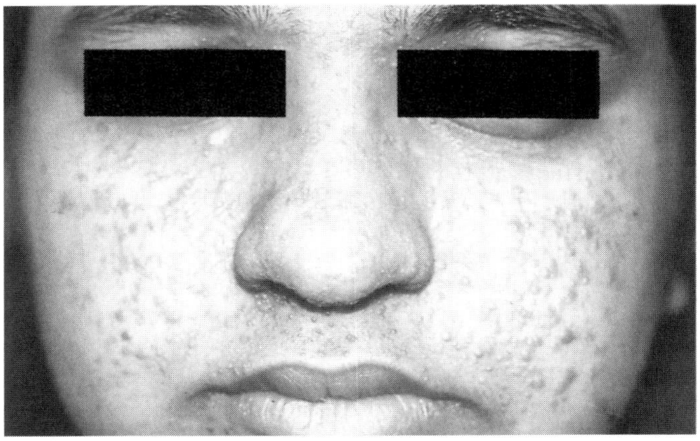

Fig. 9.15 (**a**) A naevus sebaceus of Jadassohn; (**b**) multiple sebaceous adenomas in a case of tuberose sclerosis.

tumours such as syringocystadenoma papilliferum, syringoma, trichilemmoma and proliferating trichilemmal cysts. Basal cell carcinomata develop in adult life in approximately 10% of cases, and basaloid cell proliferations are often seen histologically; the latter may represent incomplete hair follicle development rather than true basal cell carcinoma. Squamous carcinoma may also very occasionally develop in these naevi, and other adnexal carcinomas have been described.[40]

Histologically, the lesion is easily mistaken in childhood, but after puberty the large numbers of sebaceous glands and papillomatous hyperplasia of the epidermis are diagnostic. Extensive involvement may overlap with linear epidermal naevus, and be associated with neurocutaneous syndromes. Treatment is by excision, which in larger lesions may necessitate the use of a skin graft or flap.

Senile sebaceous hyperplasia

This is a fairly common lesion, predominantly of middle-aged to elderly males, occurring on the forehead or cheeks as solitary or

REFERENCES

38. Brownstein M H, Shapiro L Arch Dermatol 1973; 107: 866–869
39. Brownstein M H, Mehregan A H Br J Dermatol 1979; 100: 667–673
40. Mehregan A H, Pinkus H Arch Dermatol 1965; 91: 574

multiple soft yellowish papules, often with a central depression. It may be confused with basal cell carcinoma.

The lesion is composed of a single wide sebaceous duct surrounded by numerous grape-like lobules opening into the duct to form one large sebaceous gland. It is probably a hamartoma rather than the hyperplasia found in rhinophyma. Treatment is by excision, electrocautery or cryosurgery.

Sebaceous adenoma

Sebaceous adenomas are rare solitary, smooth, firm tumours often found on the face and scalp in middle age and measuring less than one centimetre in diameter.

Multiple sebaceous adenomas have been described in association with the Muir–Torre syndrome, in which visceral malignancies are associated with sebaceous lesions and sometimes keratoacanthomas. There is a genetic predisposition in some cases, in which there is often an association with other carcinomas. Cancer of the colon is the most common coexisting malignancy, followed by other tumours, all usually of low-grade malignancy.[41] Histologically, the adenoma is a well circumscribed, slightly elevated, multilobular tumour made up of small generative cells at the periphery of the lobule; surrounding cells show increasing sebaceous differentiation towards the centre of the lobule. Treatment is by excision.

Sweat gland tumours

Eccrine poroma

The eccrine poroma is a common benign tumour in adults and is usually found on the plantar surface of the feet or palms of the hands, but can develop in other sites. They are usually solitary, sessile or slightly pedunculated, reddish-pink nodules measuring less than 2 cm (Fig. 9.16). They can be confused clinically with granuloma pyogenicum if they have a vascular surface appearance, but more often look like naevi or even an amelanotic malignant melanoma.

Histologically the tumour is composed of well circumscribed islands of small cells lying in the lower border of the epidermis and extending into the dermis to form coalescing sheets or strands of cells. The cells are cuboidal, being smaller than the surrounding epithelial cells. They appear sharply demarcated from the surrounding normal epidermis and dermis.[42] Malignant eccrine poromas are very rare. Treatment is by simple excision.

Eccrine spiradenoma

The eccrine spiradenoma is a solitary and often painful tumour and may therefore be confused with a glomus tumour. It occurs as a subcutaneous, firm, skin-coloured small nodule in young adults anywhere on the body. Histologically it is an extremely cellular tumour with two cell types forming sharply demarcated dermal lobules. Small cells with dark nuclei surround cells with larger pale nuclei. The cellularity of the spiradenoma combined with the scanty cytoplasm around the cells may cause an erroneous diagnosis of malignancy. Malignant transformation has been reported but is very rare.[43] Treatment is by complete excision.

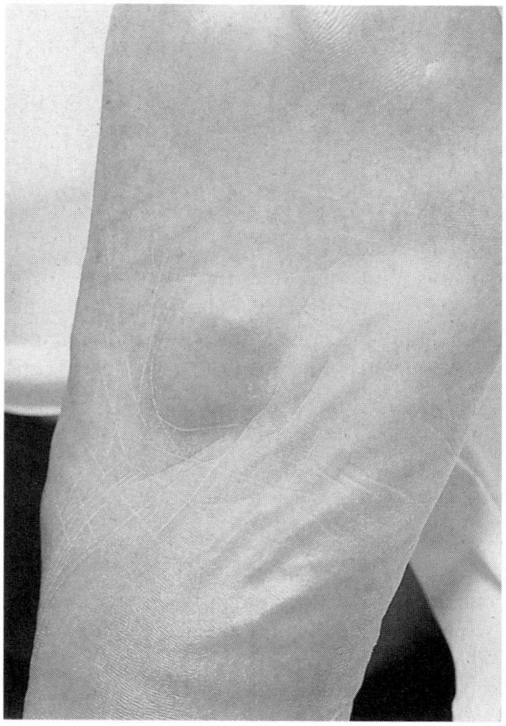

Fig. 9.16 An eccrine poroma.

Eccrine acrospiroma

Synonyms: clear cell hidradenoma, nodular hidradenoma, solid cystic hidradenoma

These are nodules or cystic dermal nodules that occur anywhere on the body of adults. They usually measure 1–2 cm across and have a red or bluish colour. They may be tender and can be covered by intact skin or they may ulcerate. A clear cell hidradenoma is composed of two cell types: one polyhedral with a rounded nucleus, and the other round with clear cytoplasm. These form well circumscribed lobular masses in the dermis and subcutaneous fat. Malignant clear cell hidradenomas are rare but can metastasize and cause death. Treatment is by excision.

Syringoma

Syringomas are usually multiple but may also occur as single small, 1–2 mm, flesh-coloured or yellowish papules around the lower eyelids and cheeks of women. They appear at puberty or in later life. They are rarely associated with cicatricial alopecia when they are present on the scalp in large numbers.

Histologically, the tumour is composed of numerous duct-like structures together with strands of basaloid cells in a fibrous stroma. The more superficial ducts may be cystic and filled with

REFERENCES

41. Torre D Arch Dermatol 1968; 98: 549–555
42. Pinkus H, Rogin J R, Goldman P Arch Dermatol 1956; 74: 511
43. Lever W F, Schaumberg-Lever G Histopathology of the Skin. J B Lippincott, Philadelphia 1990 p 537

keratin. They can be mistaken histologically for a basal cell carcinoma or trichoepithelioma. Treatment is by cryotherapy, electrodesiccation or excision.

Chondroid syringoma

Synonym: mixed tumour of the skin

These are benign intradermal nodules measuring up to 3 cm in diameter arising on the head and neck. Histologically the tumour has both epithelial and mesenchymal elements with tubular, sometimes branching lumina set in a mucoid or cartilaginous stroma. It is benign but malignant transformation can occur. Treatment is by excision.

Cylindroma

Synonym: turban tumour

Cylindromas occur either as solitary or multiple smooth, pink nodules on the head and scalp. Multiple tumours are inherited as a genetic dominant and may form coalescing clusters on the scalp, the so-called turban tumour. They arise in adult life and grow slowly. These tumours are associated with multiple trichoepitheliomas which have the same pattern of inheritance.

Histologically, cylindromas have a distinctive appearance, being composed of islands of epithelial cells fitting together like a jigsaw and surrounded by a pink hyaline sheath and a thin rim of collagen. The cells may show peripheral palisading. It is uncertain whether they are derived from eccrine or apocrine glands.[44] Malignant transformation of both solitary and multiple tumours has been reported. Treatment is by excision; an extensive area may require resurfacing with skin grafts or flaps.

Sweat gland carcinomas may arise from the tumours described above and have a high incidence of metastatic growth.

Apocrine tumours

Tumours derived from apocrine cells are rare.

Apocrine hidrocystoma

Synonym: apocrine cystadenoma

This tumour develops as a small, translucent, cystic nodule which may contain brown fluid. It usually occurs on the face in adults and has a bluish hue which may cause it to be confused with a blue naevus or even a melanoma. Histological examination shows one or several cystic spaces lined by secretory cells often in a papillary configuration with apocrine decapitation secretion. Treatment is by excision.

Syringocystadenoma papilliferum

Syringocystadenoma papilliferum is usually present at birth or arises in early childhood. It consists of one or several verrucous nodules in a linear arrangement on the scalp or face. The tumour may arise at puberty in a pre-existing naevus sebaceus. It is composed of papillary projections into cystic spaces which open on to the epidermal surface. The papillae are covered by squamous epithelium near the skin surface but deeper in the dermis they are covered by glandular epithelium and plasma cells are present. In approximately one third of cases there is an associated naevus sebaceus and in 10% there is a basal cell carcinoma; because of this association with basal cell carcinoma the lesion should be completely excised together with any surrounding naevus sebaceus.

Hidradenoma papilliferum

This tumour occurs exclusively in women on the labia and perineal region. It presents as a small nodule covered by normal skin. Histologically the lesion is a well circumscribed cystic dermal nodule with papillary projections covered by columnar cells showing apocrine secretion. Treatment is by excision.

Rhinophyma

This condition is caused by an overgrowth of the sebaceous glands of the nose, which produces an enlargement of the skin and subcutaneous tissues but spares the nasal cartilages and bone (Fig. 9.17). It predominates after the fifth decade and is 12 times more common in men than in women. Despite literary allusions, it has no association with alcohol and probably represents a severe degree of acne rosacea. Malignant transformation into both squamous and basal cell carcinoma has been reported, but is very rare.[45]

The most common and effective treatment is surgical planing of the nose until the base of the sebaceous glands is reached, from which re-epithelialization can occur. This can be achieved with a scalpel, a skin graft knife, laser, electrocautery or cryotherapy. It is a sensible precaution to take the first layer of the nose as a skin graft to resurface any inadvertent full-thickness defects. The resulting wound may then be left exposed to form a crust, or a light non-adherent dressing can be applied.[46]

HIDRADENITIS SUPPURATIVA, ACNE CONGLOBATA, PERIFOLLICULITIS CAPITIS

All three conditions represent chronic and recurrent deep-seated cutaneous infections. Their cause is unknown, but it seems unlikely that they are a primary bacterial infection, as many of the abscesses are sterile on culture and steroids may produce regression of the disease. Staphylococcal, streptococcal and anaerobic bacteria have been isolated, but these may represent commensal organisms. It has been suggested that these conditions are the result of an antigen–antibody reaction with blockage of follicular secretions and subsequent abscess formation.[47] Hidradenitis affects the

REFERENCES

44. Cotton D W K, Braye S G Br J Dermatol 1984; 111: 53–61
45. Acker D W, Helwig E B Arch Dermatol 1967; 95: 250–254
46. McCarthy J G Plastic Surgery. W B Saunders, London 1990 pp 1987–1990
47. Dvorak V C, Root R K, MacGregor R R Arch Dermatol 1977; 113: 450–453

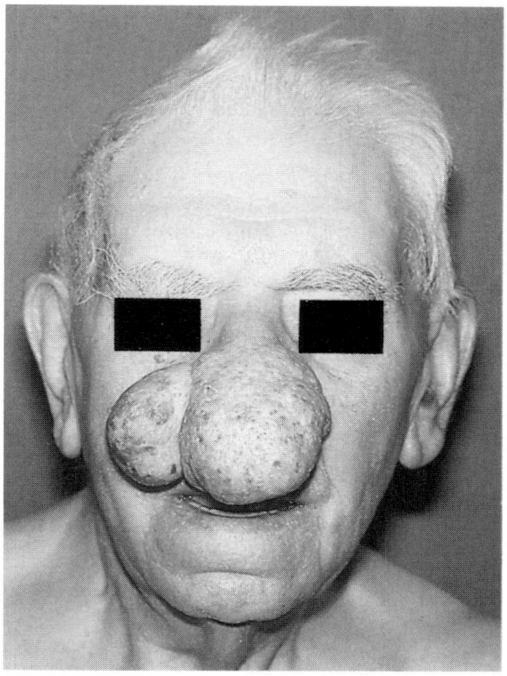

Fig. 9.17 A rhinophyma.

axillae (Fig. 9.18) and the perineum and occurs most frequently in overweight women; acne conglobata affects the back, buttocks and chest, and occurs in either sex; perifolliculitis capitis affects the scalp. The severity of the disease varies from the occasional well localized abscess that responds to incision and antibiotics to widespread watering-can sinuses that require radical excision and skin grafting.

Mild hidradenitis suppurativa can often be managed by prescribing long-term metronidazole or tinidazole. More severe and recurrent disease requires excision; primary closure can be achieved where the disease is well localized, but the patient must be warned that recurrence is possible. Extensive disease requires excision of the whole hair-bearing area and replacement with a skin graft or a local skin flap, but even then there may be recurrence, especially in the perineum. Although it has been suggested that these defects can be left to heal secondarily,[48] as in other areas of the body this does not seem to offer any advantage over meshed skin grafting.

MISCELLANEOUS CONDITIONS

Hamartoma

Hamartomas are not true tumours but represent an overgrowth of one or more cell types that are normal constituents, but arranged in an irregular fashion, of the organ in which they arise. The most common examples are haemangiomas, lymphangiomas, lipomas and neurofibromas.

Haemangioma

Haemangiomas are discussed in Chapter 10.

Pyogenic granuloma

This lesion is neither pyogenic nor a granuloma. It is a benign, solitary, rapidly growing capillary haemangioma that may be sessile or pedunculated and usually measures less than 1 cm across. The surface may be smooth or ulcerated and the nodule is bright red and friable and bleeds readily (Fig. 9.19). It commonly occurs on the face or hands of children and young adults, and on the gums and lips of pregnant women. Although they were thought at one time to occur after trauma, there is usually no history of a previous injury.

Histologically, they resemble capillary haemangiomas. Regression is uncommon, except in those that arise in pregnancy, and they are treated by curettage with diathermy of the base. Recurrence with satellite nodules has been described, especially on the backs of children.[49] Any recurrent or refractory granuloma should be sent for histological confirmation to exclude a malignant haemangioendothelioma or an amelanotic melanoma.

REFERENCES

48. Morgan W P, Harding K G et al Br J Surg 1980; 67: 277–280
49. Warner J, Jones E W E Br J Dermatol 1968; 80: 218–227

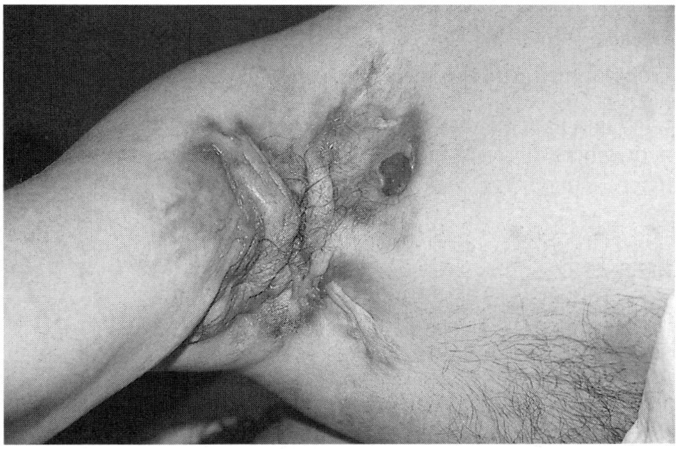

Fig. 9.18 Hidradenitis suppurativa.

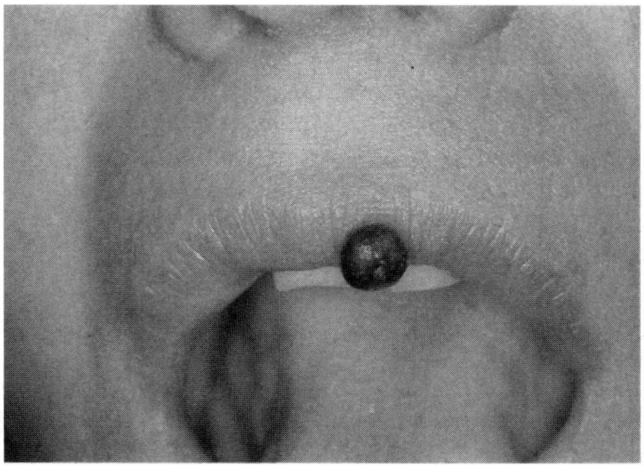

Fig. 9.19 A pyogenic granuloma.

Lymphangioma

The classification of lymphangiomas is complex. The clinical varieties are:

1. Cystic (cystic hygroma).
2. Solid or diffuse.
3. Cutaneous (lymphangioma circumscriptum).
4. Mixed vascular and lymphatic hamartoma (lymphohaemangioma).

These may occur as distinct clinical types, or as combinations.

Histologically, all lymphangiomas consist of abnormal lymphatic vessels producing cystic spaces of variable size, lined with a single layer of endothelium. The surrounding connective tissue may be loose or dense, with varying amounts of fibrosis and lymphocytic infiltration. Red blood cells may be present either from haemorrhage or because of vascular connections. The lymphatic vessels frequently extend into the surrounding tissues.[50]

The majority of lymphangiomas are present at birth, and grow with the child. Only cystic hygromas regress. Rapid growth over the course of a few hours is not uncommon, usually as a result of haemorrhage into the cystic cavities or infection. On occasion this may cause respiratory obstruction, requiring urgent decompression.

Cystic hygroma presents at birth as a soft, fluctuant swelling in the supraclavicular area that brilliantly transilluminates (Fig. 9.20). The overlying skin is normal. Frequently, solid areas can be felt within the loculated mass. Regression of the loculated areas is the rule by the time the child is 4 years old, with or without the injection of sclerosant materials.[51] Surgical resection in this area may damage the facial nerve, and in most cases a 'watch-and-wait' policy should be pursued in early childhood. Persistence into adolescence may be treated by attempts at aspiration and injection of sclerosing agents. Surgical excision may be attempted if these methods fail but this is technically demanding and is often incomplete. Surgery should only be undertaken by surgeons with experience of the condition.[52]

Solid or diffuse lymphangiomas (Fig. 9.21) and lymphohaemangiomas can involve any area of the body, and are usually present at birth. Growth usually occurs at the same rate as the rest of the body, but may be associated with local overgrowth of surrounding soft tissues and bone, especially in the face and neck. The diffuse nature of the lesion makes complete surgical excision difficult and local recurrence and regrowth are common.

Cutaneous lymphangioma (Fig. 9.22) presents as small multiple transparent or red vesicles of skin and mucosa that may be present at birth but more often develop later in childhood. They can occur in isolation or in combination with solid lymphangiomas and lymphohaemangiomas. Painful infection and bleeding occur, and these complications, together with the cosmetic disfigurement caused by the vesicles, are reasons for surgical treatment. Whimster[53] has shown that the vesicles are caused by 'lymph bladders' or cisterns situated in the dermis injecting fluid into the overlying skin. Extensive superficial lesions can be controlled by periodic point diathermy. Excision requires removal of a wide area of subcutaneous tissue beneath the ellipse of skin containing the vesicles. Complete excision is often difficult and recurrence is common.[54]

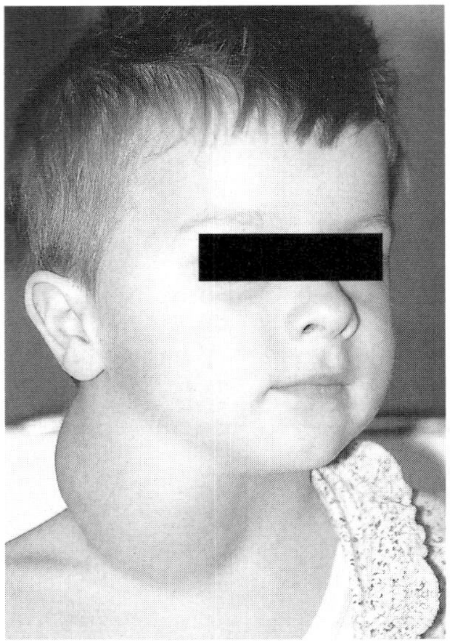

Fig. 9.20 A cystic hygroma.

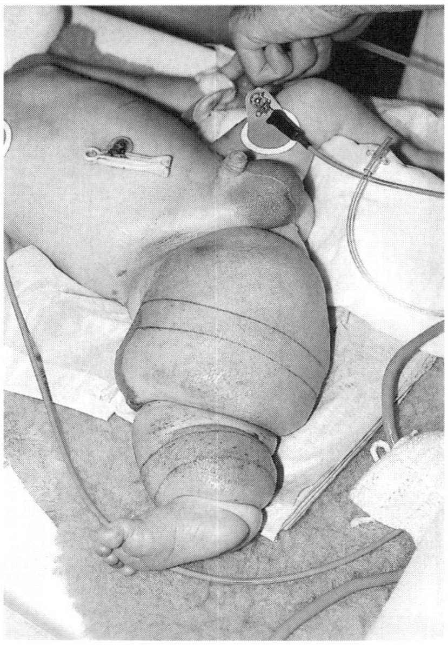

Fig. 9.21 A solid or diffuse lymphangioma.

Lipoma and liposarcoma

Lipomas are very common tumours that can occur anywhere in the body where there are fat cells, although the subcutaneous layer is most common. They can be single or multiple, and can reach quite

REFERENCES

50. Lever W F, Schaumberg-Lever G Histopathology of the Skin. J B Lippincott, Philadelphia 1990 pp 549–551
51. Broomhead I W Br J Plast Surg 1964; 17: 225
52. Lindsay W K In: Mustarde J, Jackson I (eds) Plastic Surgery in Infancy and Childhood. Churchill Livingstone, Edinburgh 1988 p 448
53. Whimster I W Br J Dermatol 1976; 94: 473–486
54. Browse N L, Whimster I et al Br J Surg 1986; 73: 585–588

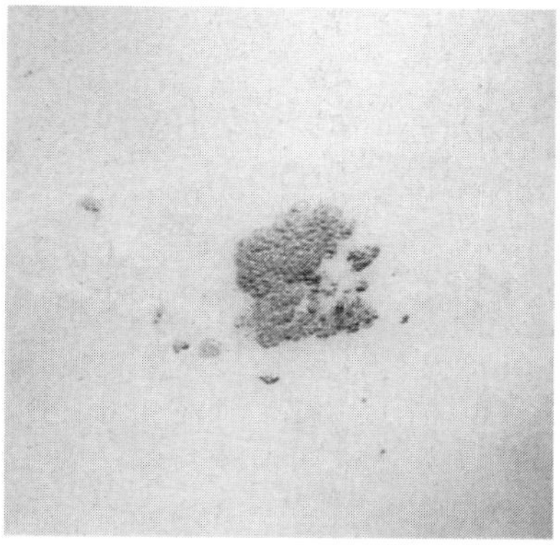

Fig. 9.22 A lymphangioma circumscriptum.

enormous proportions. The neck and trunk are particular sites of predilection (Fig. 9.23).

Lipomas are mobile, subcutaneous nodules of varying size and are usually fairly soft to palpation. They may characteristically have a lobular feel, and gentle pressure over the edge of the tumour causes it to slip beneath the fingers. Unlike epidermoid cysts, they do not indent. Most are solitary and are found on the back, neck, forearms and buttocks. Multiple lipomas are common, usually on the arms and trunk; these can occasionally be painful, when the condition is termed adiposa dolorosa or Dercum's disease.[55]

Lipomas are composed of mature fat cells. A variant known as an angiolipoma occurs around the age of puberty and is often painful; in addition to the fat cells, angiolipomas have a prominent vascular component. A further variant is the hibernoma, which presents as a benign solitary swelling on the back of children or adults and comprises brown fat cells similar to those found in hibernating animals.[56]

Lipomas are excised for cosmetic and diagnostic reasons. Recently they have been removed very successfully with suction lipolysis through a small, remote incision.[57] Malignant change in lipomas does not appear to occur. Liposarcomas arise de novo, not from pre-existing lipomas, and they are usually large, occur in an older age group and tend to arise in the deeper tissues of the lower extremities.

Neurofibroma

This is a benign tumour derived from peripheral nerve elements and can occur as solitary or multiple lumps. Multiple tumours are usually associated with von Recklinghausen's disease, which has an autosomal dominant mode of inheritance with a positive family history in half the cases, and is usually associated with café-au-lait spots on the skin (Fig. 9.24). Six or more café-au-lait spots greater than 1.5 cm in diameter make the diagnosis of von Recklinghausen's disease almost certain, but one third of cases have no spots.[58] Other occasional associated features are scoliosis, intracranial anomalies and mental retardation.

Clinically, neurofibromas present as soft pedunculated nodules or, if they arise from deeper nerves, they can result in diffuse enlargement of the peripheral nerve with involvement of the skin (plexiform neurofibroma; Fig. 9.25), which can result in severe deformity. The spinal cord and cranial nerves may be compressed, and the surrounding bone destroyed. Neurofibromas are not encapsulated and are composed of spindle cells with elongated serpentine nuclei. Malignant transformation of neurofibromas tends to occur only in von Recklinghausen's disease and the incidence is approximately 5–13%. The nerves involved are large nerve trunks of the neck or extremities, and the prognosis is poor.[59]

Treatment of large or multiple tumours is by excision and presents enormous difficulties, especially in the head and neck, because of the very diffuse nature of the neurofibroma and the difficulty in controlling bleeding. Local regrowth is common.

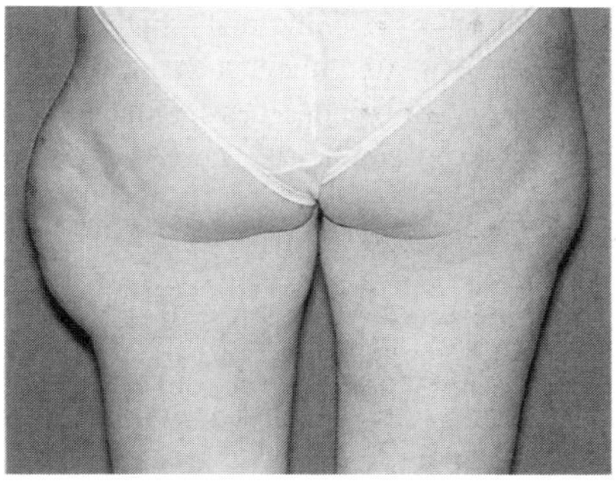

Fig. 9.23 A lipoma.

REFERENCES

55. Blomstrand R, Juhlin L Acta Dermatol Venereol 1971; 51: 243–250
56. Lever W F, Schaumberg-Lever G Histopathology of the Skin. J B Lippincott, Philadelphia 1990 p 722
57. Illouz Y-G Body Sculpturing Lipoplasty. Churchill Livingstone, Edinburgh 1989 p 373
58. Griffith B H, McKinney P Plast Reconstr Surg 1972; 49: 647–653
59. Sordillo P P, Helson L Cancer 1981; 47: 2503–2509

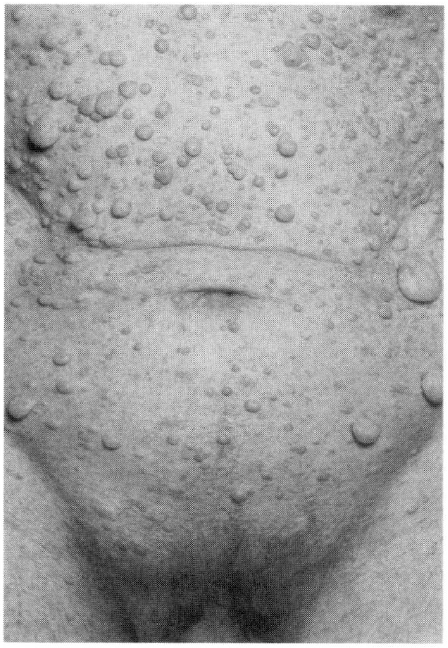

Fig. 9.24 Multiple neurofibromas (von Recklinghausen's disease).

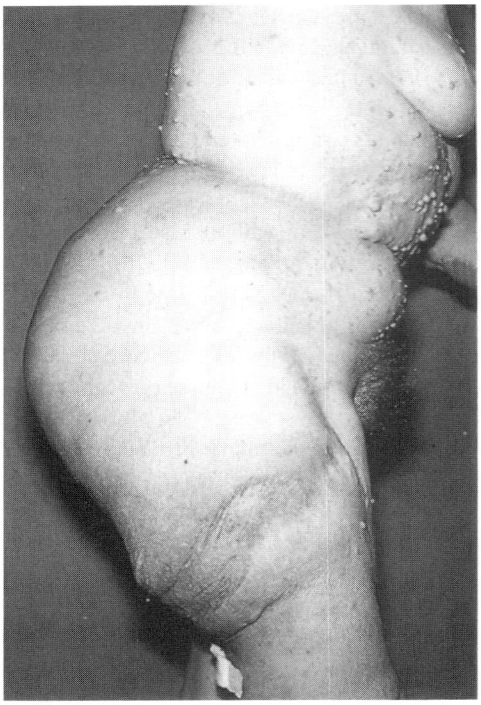

Fig. 9.25 A plexiform neurofibroma.

Viral warts (verruca vulgaris)

These common lesions usually occur on the hands, fingers and the soles of the feet (Fig. 9.26), especially in teenagers. The behaviour and transmission of warts are enigmatic but they commonly occur in areas of repetitive skin trauma, such as occurs in nail-biting, and over pressure spots. In immunosuppressed patients they can be multiple and recurrent.

Warts are the result of infection of the squamous epithelium of the skin by human papillomavirus (HPV), of which there are over 40 recognized types. The types causing the common hand warts are HPV 1, 2 and 4. They present as small hyperkeratotic papillomatous lesions, frequently multiple and occurring in groups (Fig. 9.27). Microscopically, there is papillomatosis, acanthosis, hyper- and parakeratosis, with inpointing of the rete ridges. Viral inclusions are frequently seen within the wart.

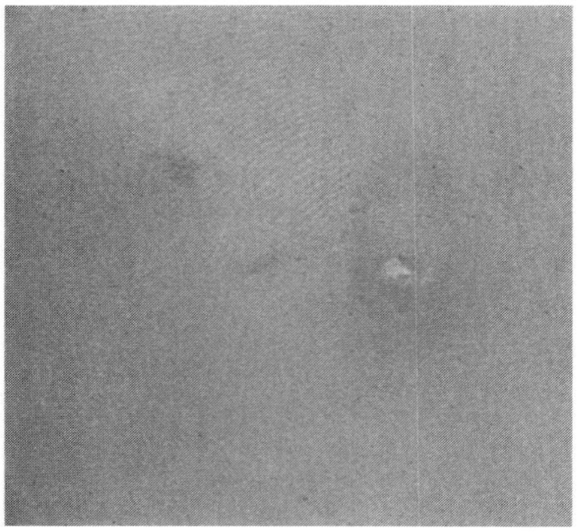

Fig. 9.26 A verruca.

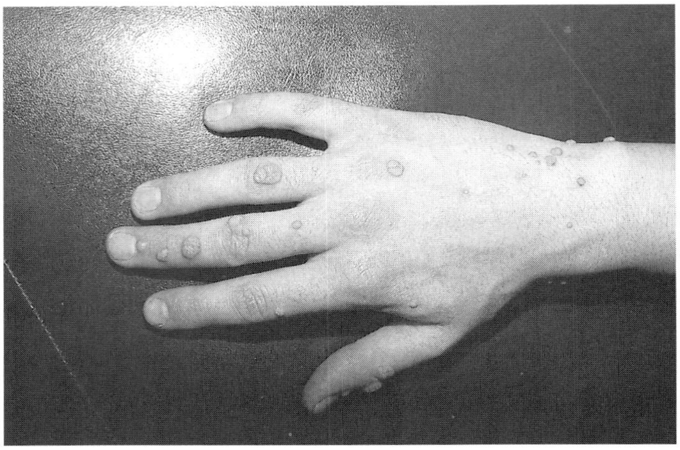

Fig. 9.27 Warts on the hand.

Viral warts often undergo spontaneous regression, an event that is thought to be T cell mediated and which makes comparisons of different methods of treatment difficult. Simple measures include the local application of keratolytics such as salicylic acid or cytotoxics like podophyllin. Cryotherapy may also be used, while more resistant warts can usually be eradicated by curettage and diathermy of the base or by intralesional injection of bleomycin.[60] In immunosuppressed and elderly patients there is evidence that viral warts can undergo malignant transformation to squamous cell carcinoma (Fig. 9.28).[61]

Condylomata acuminata are identical lesions which occur in the anogenital region and are sexually transmitted. They can reach a large size, presenting as cauliflower-like masses. HPV 6 and 11 have been isolated in these lesions, although HPV 16 and 18 are found more frequently in those with additional dysplasia and malignant change. In women these viruses are strongly associated with cervical dysplasia and neoplasia.[62]

Molluscum contagiosum

These are virally induced lesions, molluscum being a member of the poxvirus group. The warts are common in young children and occur on the face and trunk as a result of direct contact. Clinically, the lesions are smooth, pale, firm nodules about 2–5 mm in diameter, with a central depression (Fig. 9.29). They can be single or multiple. They are more common in immunosuppressed individuals. They have a symmetrical cup-shaped downgrowth of lobules of epidermis, packed full of eosinophilic or basophilic intracytoplasmic inclusions, growing in size until they reach the surface.[63]

Molluscum contagiosum undergoes spontaneous regression but can easily be treated by curettage. There is no association with malignancy.

REFERENCES

60. Bunney M H, Nolan M W Br J Dermatol 1984; 110: 197–207
61. Barr B B, Benton E C Lancet 1989; i: 124–129
62. Editorial Lancet 1985; 12: 1045–1046
63. McKee P H Pathology of the Skin. J B Lippincott, Philadelphia 1989 pp 4–16

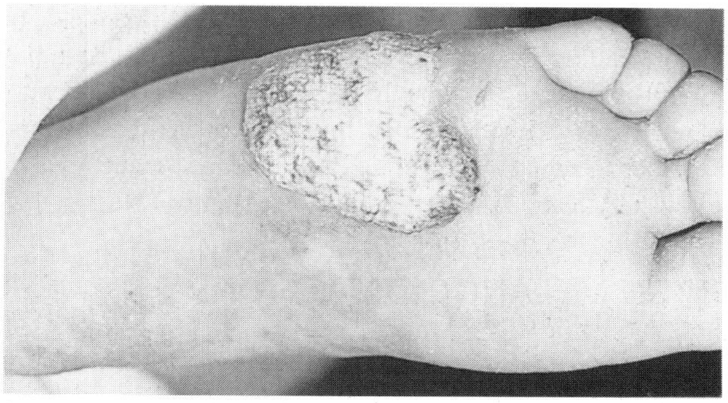

Fig. 9.28 Carcinoma cuniculatum.

Juvenile xanthogranuloma

This usually presents in early infancy as a small, solitary, yellowish-red nodule, often on the face (Fig. 9.30). It is composed of fat-laden histiocytes, and excision is curative.[64]

Dermatofibroma

Synonyms: fibrous histiocytoma, sclerosing haemangioma, fibroma durum

Dermatofibromas are extremely common small, often pigmented, firm nodules that can occur anywhere (Fig. 9.31), but are most frequently found on the legs of young to middle-aged women. They are usually a pink or light brown but may vary in colour from red to yellow or black, and may therefore be confused with malignant melanoma or basal cell carcinoma. The very firm woody feel is characteristic. There is often a past history of minor trauma or an insect bite, and this led to a belief that these were not true tumours, but were reactive. The histogenesis has been further confused by their variable histological appearance; some tumours are cellular, being composed largely of histiocytes, and others are fibrous, being composed of fibroblasts and collagen. Yet others have a predominantly angiomatous component. The failure of dermatofibromas to resolve spontaneously makes it very likely that they are true tumours, and recent work has shown that dermal fibroblasts are the likely stem cell.[65] Treatment is by simple excision.

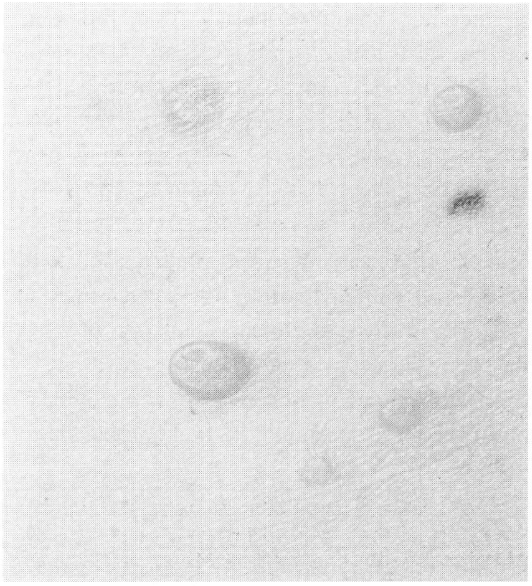

Fig. 9.29 Molluscum contagiosum.

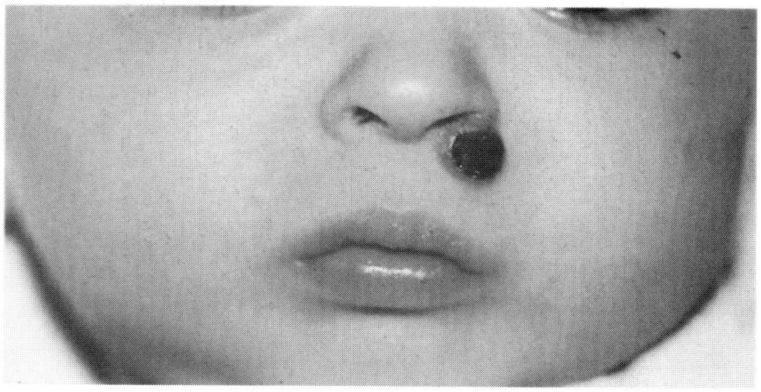

Fig. 9.30 A juvenile xanthogranuloma.

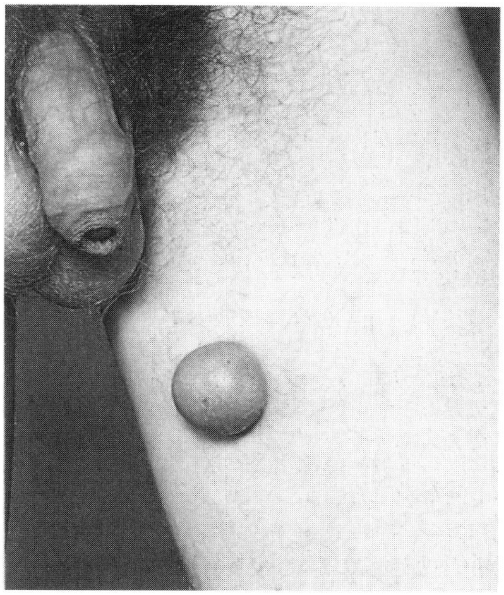

Fig. 9.31 A dermatofibroma.

Xanthoma

Xanthomata are formed by collections of lipid-laden macrophages which occur in the dermis or around tendons and have a yellowish colour. They occur typically in patients with primary or secondary hyperlipidaemic states.

Xanthelasmata are yellow plaques on the eyelids (Fig. 9.32); two thirds of patients have normal serum lipid levels. Treatment is by excision, which is easily performed under local anaesthetic by snipping the xanthelasmata off in a horizontal direction with a sharp pair of scissors. More diffuse areas may respond well to chemical peel using trichloracetic acid.

REFERENCES

64. Lever W F, Schaumberg-Lever G Histopathology of the Skin. J B Lippincott, Philadelphia 1990 pp 442–444
65. Cerio R, Spaull J et al Br J Dermatol 1989; 120: 197–206

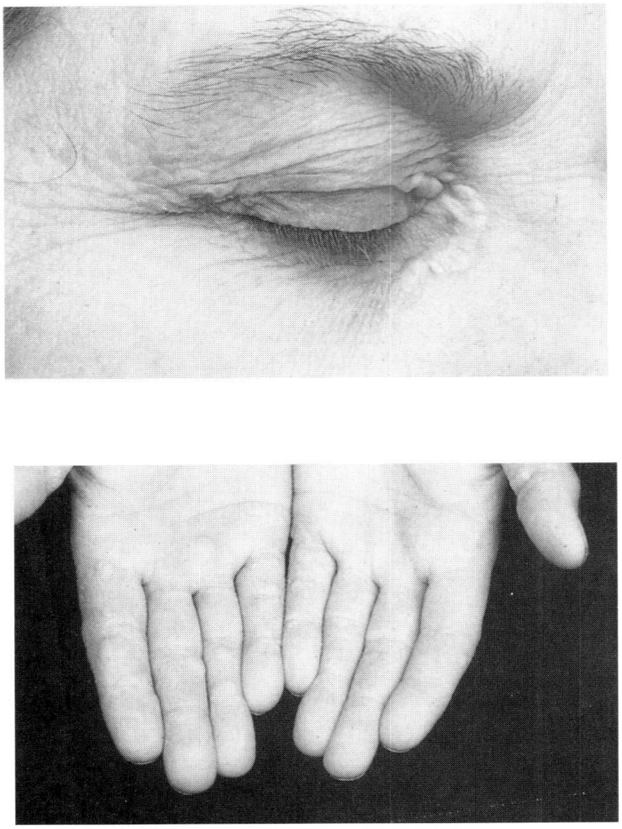

a

b

Fig. 9.32 Xanthelasmata.

Atypical fibroxanthoma

Atypical fibroxanthoma presents as a noduloulcerative lesion on sun-damaged skin of the head and neck of elderly patients. It is not clear whether it is a neoplastic or inflammatory lesion, but it is believed to be fibrohistiocytic in origin and is the cutaneous variant of a malignant fibrous histiocytoma. It has been reported to follow treatment with radiotherapy and is also recorded as occurring on the trunk and arms of younger individuals.

The epidermis is usually ulcerated, and within the dermis there is a well circumscribed cellular lesion, composed of large bizarre cells with hyperchromatic nuclei, atypical mitoses and pleomorphic-looking giant cells, all lying in a haphazard arrangement. Histologically, spindle cell malignant melanoma and spindle cell squamous carcinoma must be excluded by using S100 and cytokeratin stains: these do not react in atypical fibroxanthoma.

Atypical fibroxanthoma is invariably benign. If the lesion recurs or metastasizes, the diagnosis must be reviewed as it is almost always a malignant fibrous histiocytoma (q.v.).[66]

Granular cell tumour (granular cell myoblastoma)

This tumour was once thought to originate from muscle but is now known to be derived from Schwann cells. It is usually found in the tongue (40%), lip (see Chapter 13), skin and subcutaneous tissue, but can occur anywhere. It presents as a solitary, painless, firm, discrete swelling less than 3 cm in diameter. Multiple tumours occur in 10% of cases. Although it is benign, there is a tendency for local recurrence if it is not adequately excised. Malignant granular cell tumours account for 3% of all cases, and can frequently appear histologically bland in spite of clinically malignant behaviour.[67]

BENIGN MELANOCYTIC LESIONS

Freckles

These are common lightly pigmented macules which are related to exposure to sunlight and are more common in individuals with red hair and blue eyes. Histologically, the architecture of the epidermis is normal with no increase in melanocytes. There is, however, an increase in basal pigment.

Solar lentigo

These are benign pigmented macules that occur in the sun-damaged skin of the elderly and are therefore common on the face and dorsum of the hands. They vary in size, but can reach 1–2 cm in diameter and may coalesce. Microscopically, there is solar damage to collagen, hyperkeratosis and an increase in melanocytes and pigment along the basal layer. There is, however, no cellular atypia.

Naevi—lentigo simplex, junctional, compound, intradermal and blue naevus

Histologically, melanocytic naevi are proliferative collections of melanocytes, which in normal skin are scattered along the basal layer of the epidermis between the keratinocyte population. Melanocytic naevi can be congenital or acquired; most are of the acquired variety, and appear to have a well established natural history, with the various stages recognized both clinically and histologically as lentigo simplex, junctional naevus, compound naevus and intradermal naevus (Fig. 9.33).

Clinically, flat naevi tend to be a lentigo or a junctional naevus. Slightly elevated naevi tend to be compound, and papular or papillomatous naevi are usually intradermal. Acquired naevi first appear in childhood and adolescence, mature through middle age, and decrease in number thereafter.

Lentigo simplex

These appear as pigmented macules, often jet-black in colour and measuring less than 5 mm in diameter. They occur in infancy and early childhood. Histologically, there is an elongation of rete ridges and a proliferation of melanocytes along the basal layer in a linear fashion. Melanin pigment is abundant, accounting for the clinical appearance. These lesions may be seen around the oral and buccal mucosa in the

REFERENCES

66. Leong A S, Milios J Histopathology 1987; 11: 463–475
67. Lever W F, Schaumberg-Lever G Histopathology of the Skin. J B Lippincott, Philadelphia 1990 pp 746–749

Simple naevus: proliferation of melanocytes replaces the basal layer

a

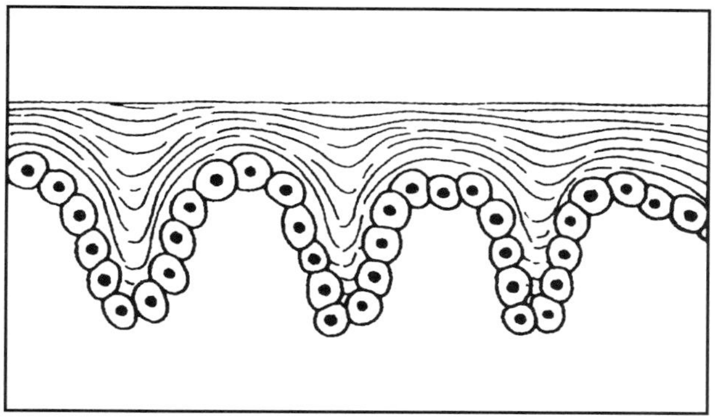

Junctional naevus: further proliferation results in nodular masses of melanocytes projecting into dermis (junctional change)

b

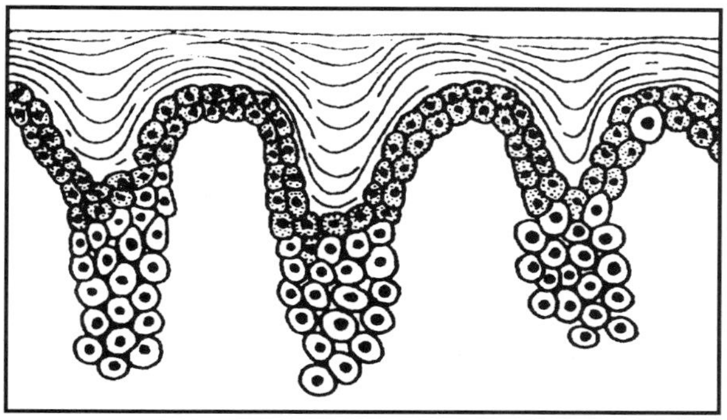

Intradermal naevus (no junctional change): junctional activity ceases. Packets of adult naevus cells in dermis

c

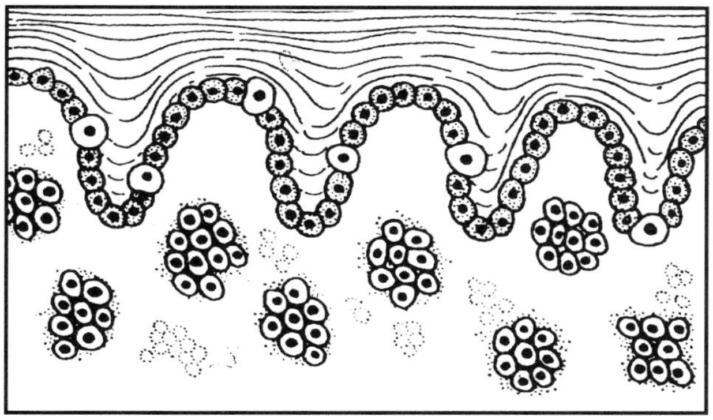

Compound naevus (junction and intradermal): some of the nodules of melanocytes become detached and become nature naevus cells in the dermis

d

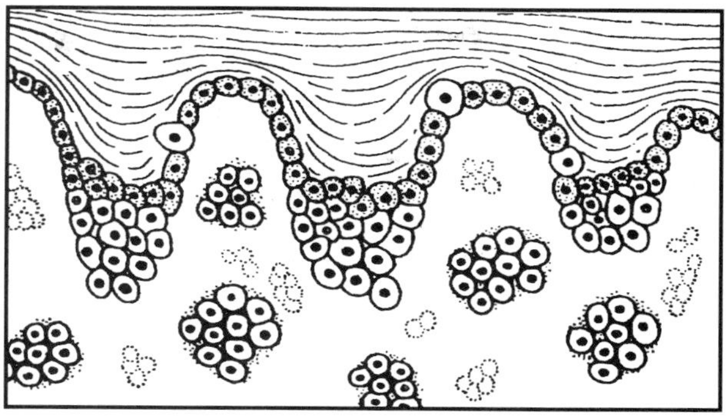

Blue naevus: occasionally melanocytes in transit from neural crest become arrested in the dermis

e

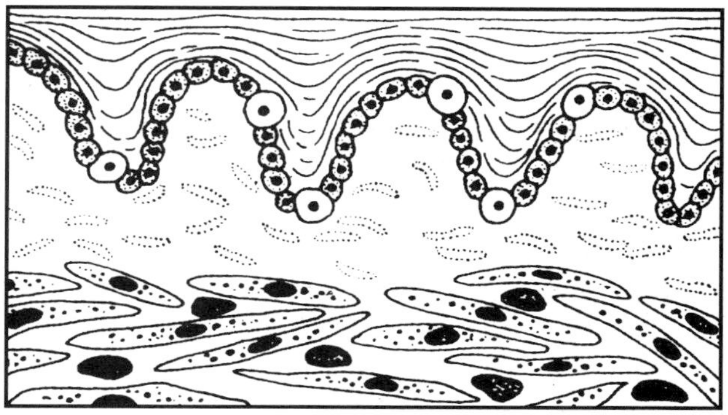

Fig. 9.33 (**a**) Simple; (**b**) junctional; (**c**) intradermal; (**d**) compound and (**e**) blue naevi.

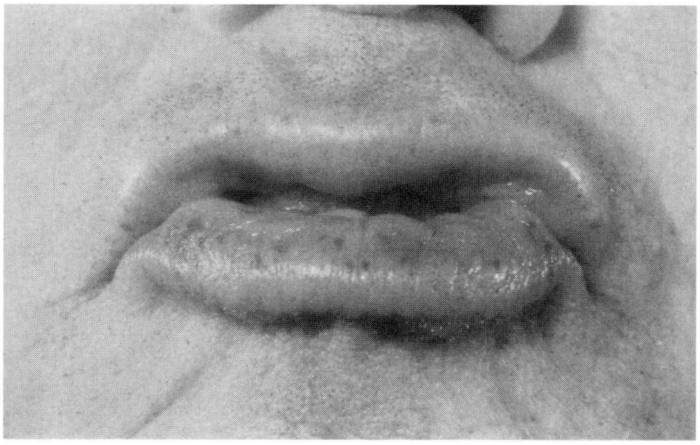

Fig. 9.34 Peutz–Jeghers syndrome.

Peutz (Jeghers syndrome, which is an inherited autosomal dominant condition (Fig. 9.34). The patients have multiple hamartomatous polyps throughout the gastrointestinal tract (see Chapter 29).

Junctional naevi

This is the stage after lentigo simplex in the development of naevi. Clinically, the lesions are still macular and are a little larger but rarely exceed 7 mm. They are less deeply pigmented than the lentigo simplex, and are usually a homogenous brown-black colour. Histologically, there is again proliferation of melanocytes at the basal layer, but they now form clusters or nests of cells, and are restricted to the tips of the rete pegs. New melanocytic lesions in adults with abundant junctional activity should be carefully studied by the pathologist to rule out malignancy.

Compound naevi

There is maturation of the junctional naevi during childhood and adolescence; clinically these lesions become pale brown and papular. Histologically, there is still a junctional component but in addition naevus cells, alone and in groups, drop down from the proliferating nests into the dermis.

Intradermal naevi

By the end of the third decade, most naevi are of the intradermal type, and appear as flesh-coloured papules with little pigment. Clinically, they are common as the occasional pigmented, hairy mole on the face of the middle-aged. Histologically, all the melanocytic nests are confined to the dermis with no proliferation seen at the basal layer of the epidermis.

All of these naevi—lentigo simplex, junctional, compound and intradermal—are biologically benign. Several studies have suggested however that the presence of excessive numbers of benign naevi on the skin constitutes a risk factor for cutaneous melanoma.[68] Also, patients with melanoma frequently give a history of having a 'mole' present at the site of their melanoma for many years. Histologically, evidence of pre-existing naevi is present in approximately 20% of malignant melanomas.[69]

Pseudomelanoma

Pseudomelanoma occurs in young adults a few weeks after a partial surgical shave excision of an intradermal naevus. Clinically, it presents as stippled pigmentation within a scar; histologically, there is residual intradermal naevus and a striking intraepidermal melanocytic change closely resembling that of a superficial spreading malignant melanoma.

Spitz naevus (juvenile melanoma)

Spitz naevi are a variant of benign melanocytic lesions and have distinctive clinical and histological features; their recognition is important as they can be mistaken histologically for a malignant melanoma. They usually occur in children and young adults under 30 years of age, although they have been reported in older individuals.[70] They are slightly more common in women. Spitz naevi can occur in any area of the body, but have a predilection for the head and neck area and lower limbs, and present as a single, pink, dome-shaped symmetrical nodule less than 1 cm in diameter (Fig. 9.35).

Histologically, one of the most important features is the symmetry of the lesion on low-power examination. The melanocytic cells are plump, epithelioid in type and lie in an oedematous and vascular stroma. The overlying epidermis usually exhibits hyperplasia. Pigment deposition is not prominent. The most important differential diagnosis is that of malignant melanoma and this is usually only a problem in the naevi which do not show the classic features. Worrying histological features include marked nuclear atypia, lack of maturation at the deep aspect of the naevus, atypical mitoses, and lack of symmetry on low-power examination.[71] Spitz naevi are benign, only needing local excision, often as an excision biopsy to exclude melanoma. Complete regression can also occur.

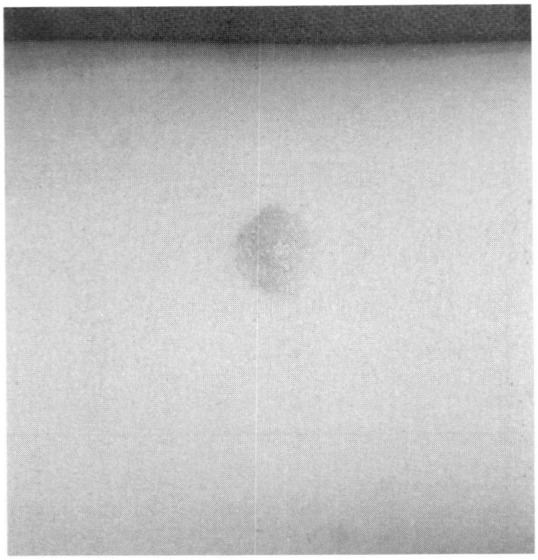

Fig. 9.35 A Spitz naevus.

Halo naevi

Halo naevi are benign pigmented naevi surrounded by an area of depigmentation (Fig. 9.36). They may be solitary or multiple, and the presence of the halo does not represent a sinister change in a mole. They occur most commonly on the back of young adults, and are caused by invasion of the naevus by lymphoid cells that destroy the melanocytes, initially in the adjacent skin, but ultimately in the naevus itself. The reasons for this are not known, but the mechanism appears to be that the naevus cells produce an antigen that stimulates an antibody in the surrounding lymphocytes.[72] The area of depigmentation may persist for years, but repigmentation occurs in almost all cases. No treatment is required unless there are other features of the mole that suggest malignant change. Regression and depigmentation may also occur around a malignant melanoma.[73]

Blue naevi

Blue naevi are benign melanocytic lesions that are recognized clinically by their slate-blue colour. There are two types: the common and the cellular blue naevus.

The common blue naevus occurs relatively frequently and is more common in women than in men. Its incidence is maximal in

REFERENCES

68. English J, Swerdlow A J et al Br Med J 1987; 294: 152
69. English D R, Armstrong B K Br Med J Clin Res 1988; 296: 1285–1288
70. Weedon D, Little J H Cancer 1977; 40: 217–225
71. Spitz S Am J Pathol 1948; 24: 591–609
72. Lever W F, Schaumberg-Lever G Histopathology of the Skin. J B Lippincott, Philadelphia 1990 p 764
73. Shapiro L, Kopf A W Arch Dermatol 1965; 92: 64–68

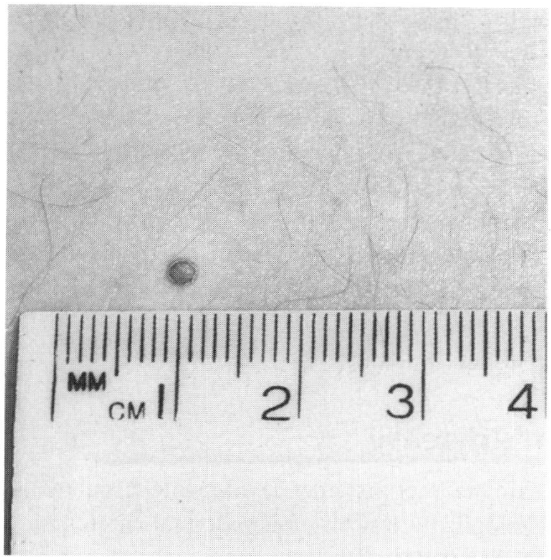

Fig. 9.36 A halo naevus.

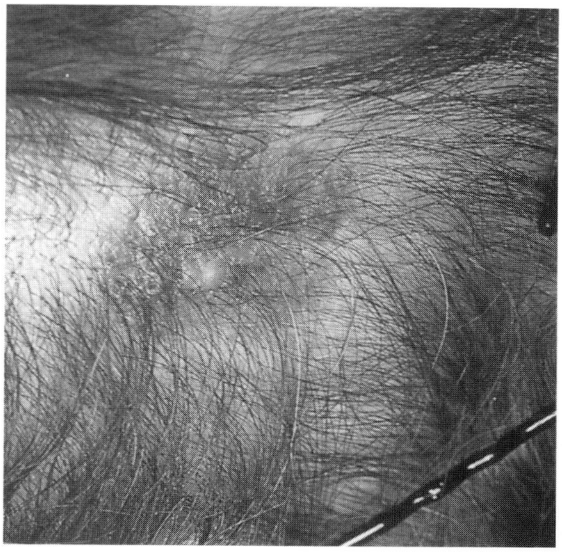

Fig. 9.37 A benign mole (compound or blue naevus).

the fourth decade. They are seen most often on the scalp and face and dorsum of the hands and feet. Macroscopically, they are dome-shaped blue-black lesions measuring up to 1 cm (Fig. 9.37). The common blue naevus comprises a dermal collection of spindle melanocytes with abundant melanin pigment lying free and also within dendritic cells. A histological variant of the common blue naevus is the combined naevus which has similar features, but in addition has an overlying junctional component.

The cellular blue naevus is uncommon and occurs most often in women. More than half are located in the sacrococcygeal area and buttocks.[74] Clinically, they present as painful and sometimes ulcerated blue-black lesions 2 cm or more in size. Histologically, they comprise a dermal cellular population of epithelioid and spindle cells arranged in sheets, with heavy deposition of melanin pigment and extending into the deep dermis and occasionally into subcutaneous fat (see Fig. 9.33e).

Both types of blue naevus are biologically benign. Less than 1% undergo malignant transformation[75] which can be recognized histologically by the presence of necrosis, cellular pleomorphism and mitoses.

Congenital naevi

Congenital melanocytic naevi can be single or multiple, are present at birth and are frequently greater than 1.5 cm across (Fig. 9.38). They show enormous variation in size, degree and uniformity of pigmentation, regularity of their border and the presence of hair. Growth is compatible with the normal growth of the child. Giant pigmented naevi, which may be called giant hairy naevi or bathing trunk naevi, have no agreed definition but the term should probably be reserved for naevi that are at least 20 cm in diameter.[76] Some also have a distinct dermatomal distribution, occurring in a bathing trunk, vest-like or stocking arrangement (Fig. 9.39). Clinically, they may be flat, pale brown and virtually hairless, or lumpy, pitch-black and hairy or anything in between. Multiple smaller naevi are frequently present on the rest of the body and may continue to appear throughout childhood. Giant naevi of the neck or scalp may be associated with intracranial involvement, which can present with epilepsy, and the subsequent development of malignant melanoma.[77]

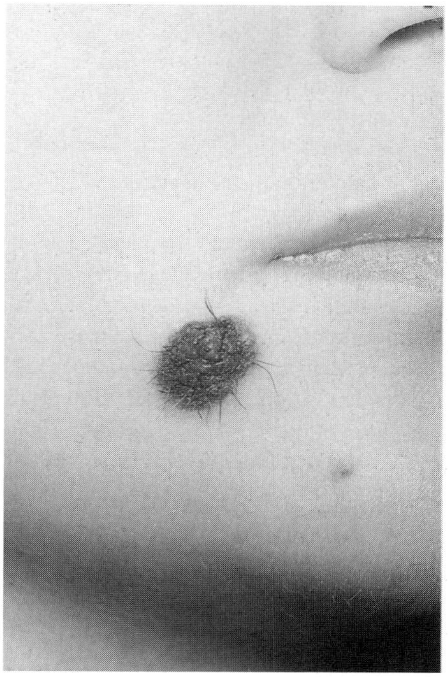

Fig. 9.38 A congenital naevus.

Histologically, they can be compound or intradermal, similar to the acquired naevi, but there are subtle differences. The epidermis is frequently abnormal, being hyperkeratotic, acanthotic and exhibiting papillomatosis. Within the dermis the melanocytes

REFERENCES

74. Rodriguez H A, Ackerman L V Cancer 1968; 21: 393–405
75. Mishima Y Arch Dermatol 1970; 101: 104–110
76. Kopf A W, Bart R S et al J Am Acad Dermatol 1979; 1: 123–130
77. Slaughter J C, Hardman J M et al Arch Pathol 1969; 88: 298–304

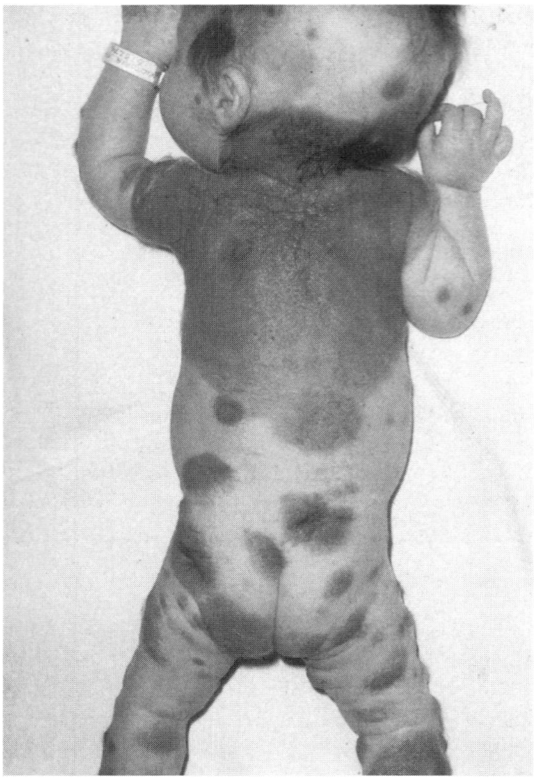

Fig. 9.39 A giant pigmented hairy naevus.

occur in sheets with no nesting and frequently extend into subcutaneous fat and surrounding appendages. They may even infiltrate into the walls of small vessels.

Malignant melanoma may develop in these large pigmented naevi, mostly before the age of 15 years, and carries a particularly poor prognosis. The lifetime risk for developing malignant melanoma in these patients has been variously estimated at between 1 and 42%, but is probably nearer to 8%.[78,79]

Treatment of giant naevi is very difficult. Shaving the naevus in the first few weeks of life can be effective in some children, probably where the melanocytes are superficial. When the naevus is predominantly intradermal, shaving is ineffective and recurrence inevitable. Total excision and skin grafting produces a very poor cosmetic result, with some pigment recurring in both the graft and the donor sites; it is also a painful and protracted procedure for the child.[80] Some naevi are small enough to be removed using tissue expansion, and serial expansion is the treatment of choice for most of these naevi.[81] Lasers have been used for treatment, but the long-term benefits are yet to be evaluated, and it is not clear what effect newer therapies might have on later malignant potential.

PREMALIGNANT SKIN LESIONS

Actinic keratosis

Synonyms: senile keratosis, solar keratosis

Actinic keratoses commonly occur on the sun-exposed sites of the face and dorsum of the hands of elderly people. They are scaly erythematous or greyish lesions which are usually multiple (Fig. 9.40) and represent in situ squamous cell carcinomata. Microscopically, there is hyperkeratosis and focal parakeratosis, with irregular acanthosis and variable dysplasia of the epidermis. There is associated solar damage to dermal collagen. Untreated, approximately a quarter will progress to an invasive squamous carcinoma after a number of years. Treatment is by shaving the affected skin, by cryotherapy or by topical application of the cytotoxic agent, 5-fluorouracil. It has been suggested that retinoic acid, used for treating acne, may also be of benefit in reversing the damaging effects of sunlight.[82]

Bowen's disease

This is a skin disorder that may develop into a squamous cell carcinoma; histologically it is an intraepidermal carcinoma. It presents as a single irregular reddish-brown enlarging plaque which may be ulcerated or crusted and can occur on any part of the body but particularly on the trunk (Fig. 9.41). Bowen's disease of the glans penis is called erythroplasia of Queyrat (see Chapter 39; Fig. 9.42). There may be an association between Bowen's disease and the development of an internal malignancy, usually 5–7 years later, particularly if it occurs in an area that has never been exposed to the sun.[83] Microscopically, there is loss of the rete pegs and full-thickness dysplasia of the epidermis. Unlike solar keratosis, sun damage to dermal collagen is unusual. A small percentage progress to invasive squamous cell carcinoma.[84] Treatment is by excision with at least a 0.5 cm margin; a skin graft may then be required to close the defect.

REFERENCES

78. Lever W F, Schaumberg-Lever G Histopathology of the Skin. J B Lippincott, Philadelphia 1990 p 537
79. Quaba A A, Wallace A F Plast Reconstr Surg 1986; 78: 174–181
80. Miller C J, Becker D W Jr Br J Plast Surg 1979; 32: 124–126
81. Fenton O M Br Med J 1987; 295: 684–685
82. Kligman A M J Am Acad Dermatol 1989; 21: 650–654
83. Andersen S L, Nielsen A et al Arch Dermatol 1973; 108: 367–370
84. Lever W F, Schaumberg-Lever G Histopathology of the Skin. J B Lippincott, Philadelphia 1990 pp 549–551

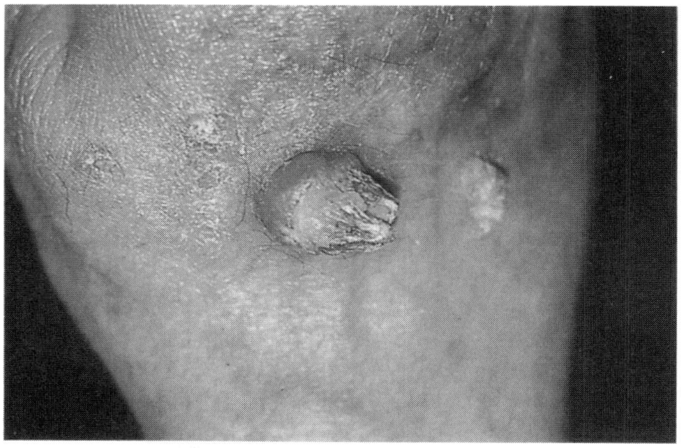

Fig. 9.40 Areas of actinic keratosis with a squamous cell carcinoma.

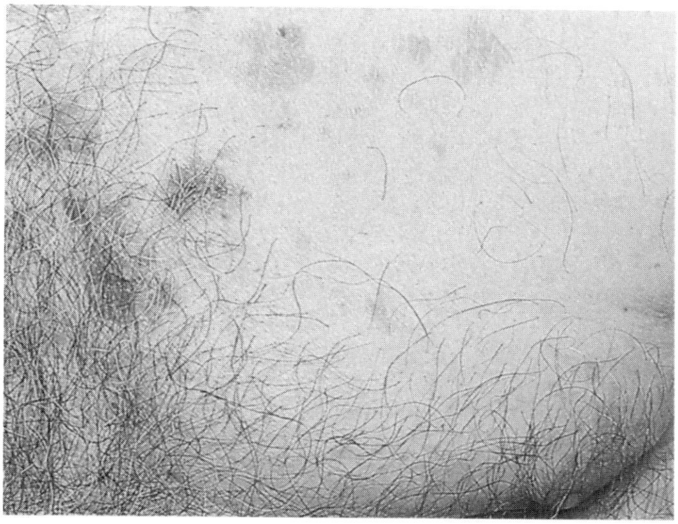

Fig. 9.41 Bowen's disease.

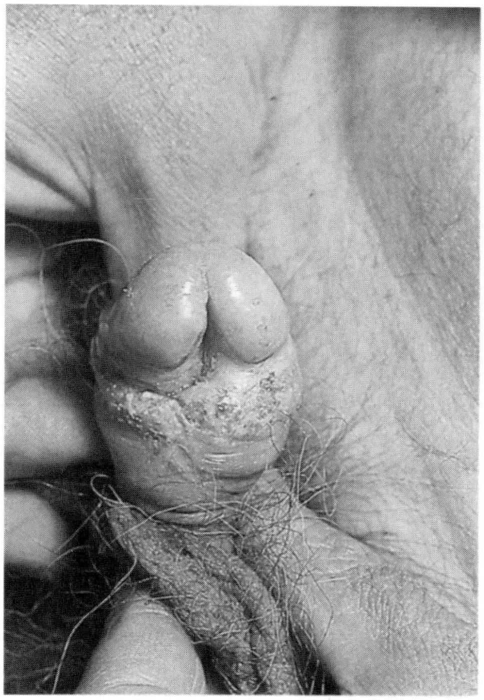

Fig. 9.42 Erythroplasia of Queyrat.

Leucoplakia

Leucoplakia is a clinical description of a white patch that occurs on the vermilion border of the lips, the oral mucosa or the vulva, that will not rub off and is not due to any other specific disease entity, e.g. lichen planus, *Candida albicans* infection. It is the visible end-result of thickening and maceration of the keratinized squamous epithelium of the mucosa. 80% of cases are benign and are caused by external irritation, whether mechanical from teeth and dentures, noxious from tobacco and betel nuts, or radiation from sunlight. The remaining 20% show varying degrees of dysplastic change, and 3% of these already have invasive carcinoma.[85] Between 7 and 13% of cases ultimately develop a carcinoma,[86] and this occurs more frequently in leucoplakia of the floor of the mouth (68%) than in the buccal mucosa (4%).[87] As it is impossible to detect the development of carcinoma by clinical examination, it is necessary to biopsy any area of leucoplakia that persists for more than a few weeks after the suspected cause has been removed (see Chapter 13).

The term erythroplakia describes red patches on the oral mucosa, with or without leucoplakia, that always demonstrate in situ or invasive carcinoma.

Lentigo maligna (Hutchinson's melanotic freckle)

This is a relatively common melanocytic lesion with the potential for invasive growth, occurring on sun-damaged skin, particularly on the face and occasionally on the dorsum of the hands or forearm. Lentigo maligna presents clinically as a flat pigmented, brown-to-black naevus with an irregular outline, which gradually enlarges over the years (Fig. 9.43). It particularly affects those in their fifth to seventh decades.

Histologically, the epidermis is atrophic and there is marked solar damage to dermal collagen. An abnormal proliferation of atypical melanocytes occurs along the dermoepidermal junction and extends down into the hair follicles. There is no dermal invasion, and the lesion represents the 'carcinoma in situ' stage of malignant melanoma.

REFERENCES

85. Waldron C A, Shafer W G Cancer 1975; 36: 1386–1392
86. Pindborg J J Am J Dermatopathol 1980; 2: 277–278
87. Lever W F, Schaumberg-Lever G Histopathology of the Skin. J B Lippincott, Philadelphia 1990 p 546

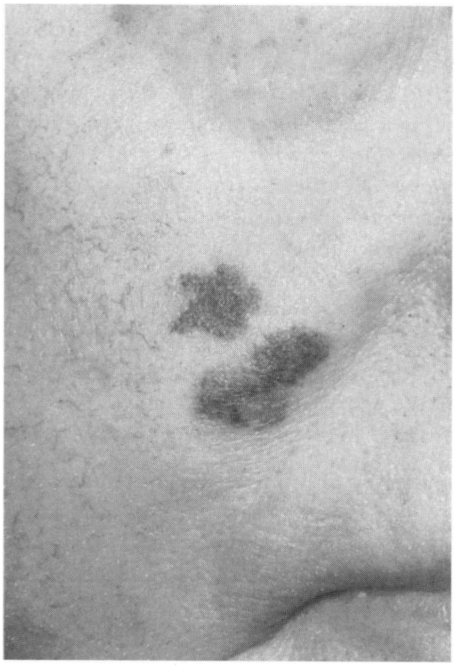

Fig. 9.43 A Hutchinson's freckle (lentigo maligna).

After 10–30 years, the lentigo maligna transforms into a malignant melanoma, detected clinically by the development of a black or tan nodule within the flat lesion, and detected histologically by the spread of the atypical melanocytic cells from the dermoepidermal junction into the dermis.[88]

MALIGNANT SKIN TUMOURS

Basal cell carcinoma

Synonym: rodent ulcer

Basal cell carcinomas are the most common skin malignancy and usually occur on hair-bearing skin of elderly people, most commonly on sun-exposed areas and particularly around the eye. They can be single or multiple. Excessive sun exposure, particularly ultraviolet light in the UVB range, predisposes to their development. There is also an increased incidence in smokers, in patients with xeroderma pigmentosum, and as a late feature of naevus sebaceus (q.v) or of radiotherapy scars.

Basal cell carcinomas commonly present as a small, waxy nodule which is frequently covered with surface telangiectasia. The waxy or pearly appearance is more apparent on lightly stretching the skin.

Several different clinical types are recognized:

1. *Nodular or noduloulcerative*. This is the most common type. It usually has a clearly defined margin. As it enlarges, central ulceration occurs, resulting in a rolled edge (Fig. 9.44).
2. *Cystic*. This has a cystic appearance, both clinically and histologically (Fig. 9.45).
3. *Pigmented*. The pigmentation is from melanin, and can cause confusion with malignant melanoma (Fig. 9.46).
4. *Morpheic or sclerosing*. The tumour is flat or even depressed with a poorly defined edge, and skin ulceration occurs late. The lack of a clearly defined border and the infiltrative nature often results in incomplete excision.
5. *Cicatricial (field-fire, bush-fire)*. This presents as multiple, superficial erythematous lesions interspersed with pale atrophic 'burnt-out' areas (Fig. 9.47).
6. *Superficial*. Superficial basal cell carcinomas occur on the trunk and present as reddened scaly patches which increase in size. They should not be confused with Bowen's disease.
7. *Multiple basal cell carcinomas*. These can occur both in susceptible individuals with sun-damaged skin and as an inherited condition. The naevoid basal cell epithelioma syndrome, or Gorlin's syndrome (Fig. 9.48), is autosomal dominant and presents in early adult life with multiple basal cell carcinomas, keratocysts of the jaw, skeletal abnormalities and palmar and plantar pits.[89]

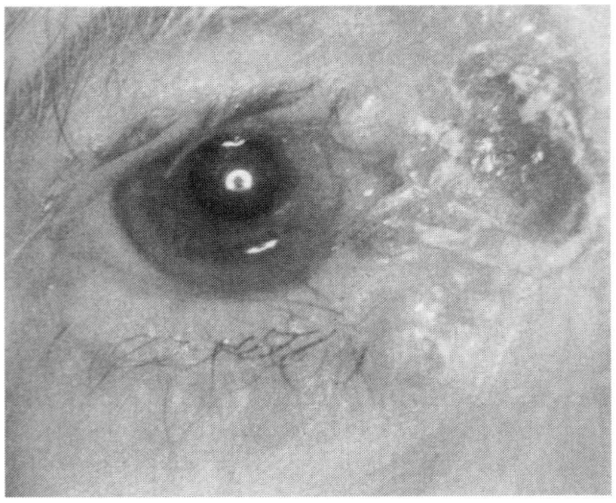

Fig. 9.44 A noduloulcerative basal cell carcinoma.

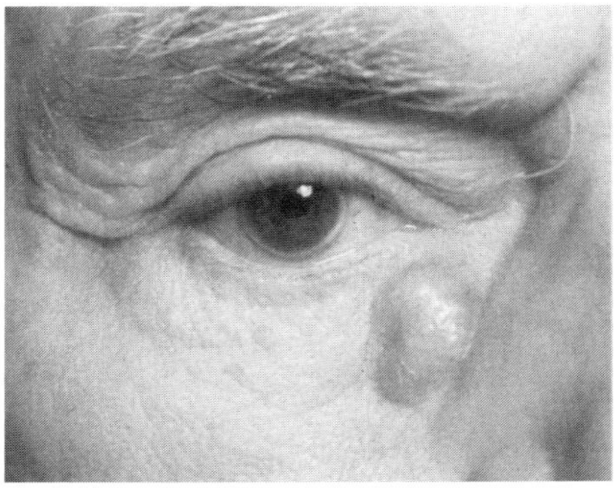

Fig. 9.45 A cystic type of basal cell carcinoma.

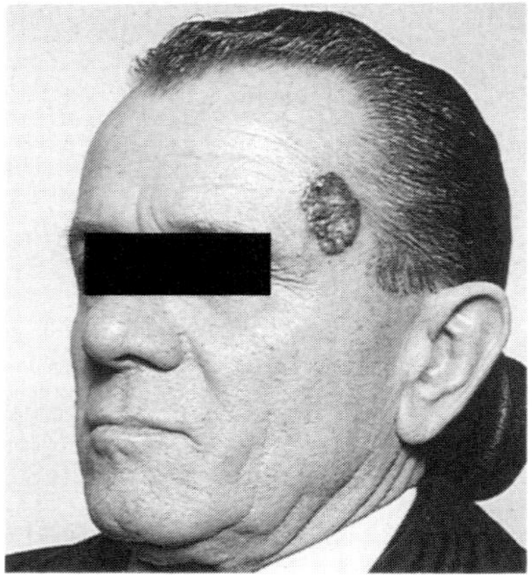

Fig. 9.46 A pigmented basal cell carcinoma.

Microscopically, basal cell carcinomas have several patterns but all consist of nests and islands of basaloid cells in the dermis, similar to those seen in the basal layer of the epidermis. There is peripheral palisading in the nests of cells and there is a high mitotic rate. The epidermis is frequently ulcerated. Areas of squamous differentiation may be seen, but the tumour has the overall architecture and behaviour of a basal cell carcinoma.

Basal cell carcinomas are only locally invasive, although they can be quite destructive depending on their location (Fig. 9.49). Metastasis does occur, but is extremely rare.[90] Treatment is by local excision. For discrete nodular tumours the excision margin need not exceed half a centimetre, but poorly defined or indurated tumours require a wider margin of excision, especially at the inner canthus of the eye, nasolabial fold, nasal floor and the ear. Some of

REFERENCES

88. Weinstock M A, Sober A J Br J Dermatol 1987; 116: 303–310
89. Gorlin R J, Sedano H O Birth Defects 1971; 8: 140–148
90. Farmer E R, Helwig E B Cancer 1980; 46: 748–757

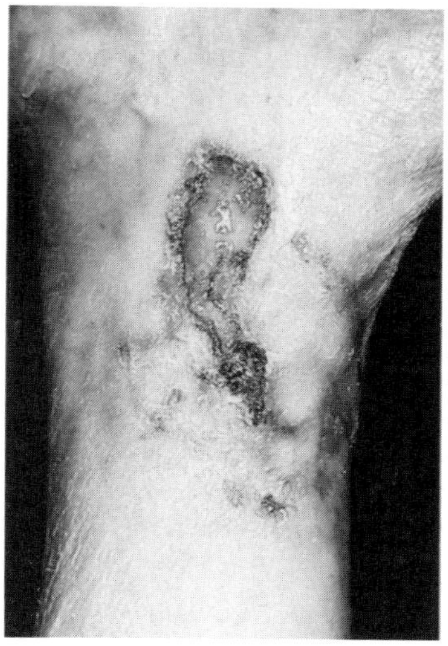

Fig. 9.47 A bush-fire type of basal cell carcinoma.

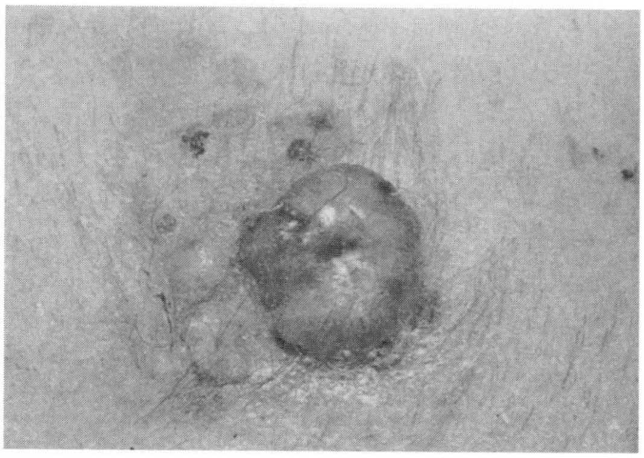

Fig. 9.48 A naevoid basal cell epithelioma (Gorlin's syndrome).

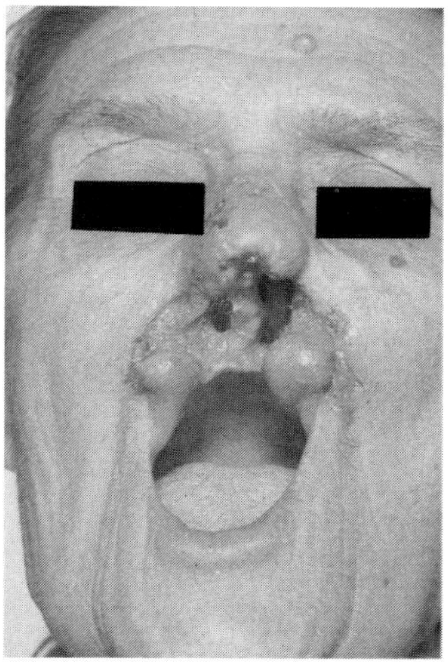

Fig. 9.49 A destructive basal cell carcinoma that has completely destroyed the nose.

these tumours may require confirmation that margins are clear by intraoperative reporting of marginal frozen sections by an informed pathologist to ensure adequate clearance.

Excellent results can also be obtained with radiotherapy, Mohs' surgery, which is staged chemosurgery with frequent histological assesment of margins,[91] and electrodesiccation. The choice of technique is dependent on the site and extent of the lesion and the experience of the surgeon. The cure rate for locally treated primary lesions is between 95 and 99%.[91,92] Recurrent lesions require wider resection and have a significantly higher recurrence rate themselves.[93]

Squamous cell carcinoma

Synonyms: epidermoid carcinoma, epithelioma

Squamous cell carcinomas are the second most common cutaneous malignancy. They arise from the keratinizing cell layer of the epidermis. They may develop in a pre-existing actinic keratosis, in an area of Bowen's disease or may arise de novo. Immunosuppressed patients may develop multiple squamous cell carcinomas. Malignant transformation of viral warts has been described (see below) and HPV 5 and 8 have been isolated from these tumours. The principal predisposing factors are sun exposure, radiation, certain chemicals, chronic sinuses and chronic cutaneous ulceration such as in Marjolin's ulcer (squamous carcinoma in chronic venous ulcers) and long-standing unhealed burn wounds. Epitheliomas are most commonly found on the face and dorsum of the hand, especially on the external ear, nose and lower lip in the elderly.[94]

They present as enlarging keratotic nodules with a heaped-up border. Central ulceration occurs as the tumour enlarges (Fig. 9.50). A well differentiated lesion may present as a keratin horn. Suspicious lesions should be biopsied, as squamous cell carcinomas are commonly mistaken for keratoacanthoma (see p. 198), basal cell carcinoma, amelanotic melanoma and adnexal tumours.

Microscopically, there are long irregular tongues of dysplastic-looking squamous epithelium arising from the epidermis or ulcer base which extend into the deep dermis and subcutaneous fat in a haphazard fashion. The adjacent epidermis usually shows evidence of intraepidermal carcinoma. The tumour may be well differentiated with keratin production, moderately differentiated or poorly differentiated, where the spindle cell morphology has to be differentiated from melanoma, atypical fibroxanthoma and cylindroma.

Untreated squamous carcinomas are locally destructive and may metastasize to local lymph nodes. Treatment is as for basal cell carcinoma, although a wider excision margin is indicated for less well differentiated lesions. Prophylactic node dissection is not thought to be of benefit except for large anaplastic tumours in patients under 50 years of age.[94] The local recurrence rate for squamous cell carcinomata is twice that of basal cell carcinomata; metastasis to regional nodes occurs in 5–10%, but is very low in

REFERENCES

91. Mohs F E Arch Dermatol 1976; 112: 211–215
92. Binns J H, Sherriff H M et al Br J Plast Surg 1975; 28: 133–134
93. Menn H, Robins P et al Arch Dermatol 1971; 103: 628–631
94. Paletta F X Clin Plast Surg 1980; 7: 313–336

a

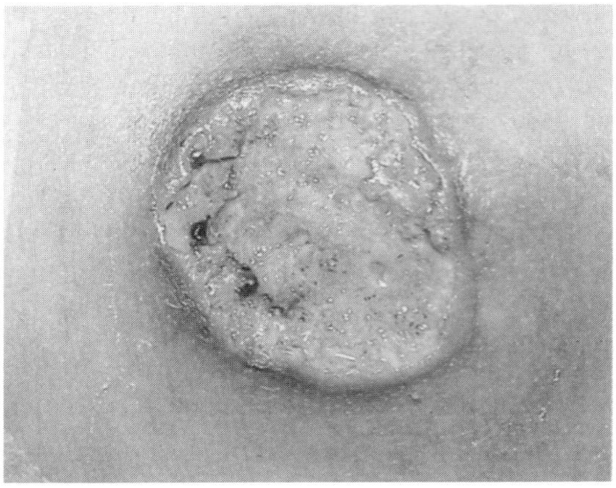

b

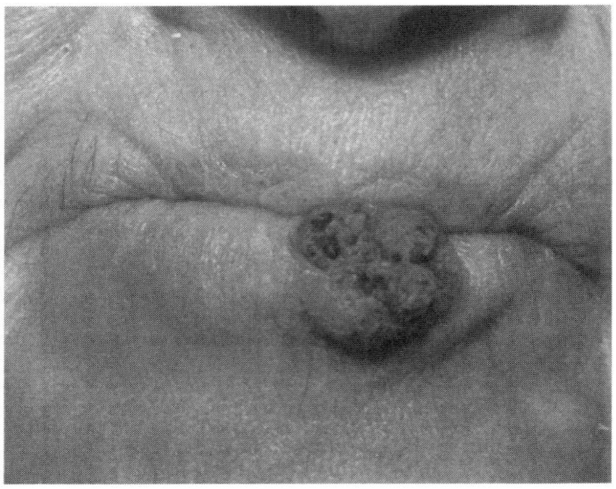

Fig. 9.50 (**a**) A squamous cell carcinoma; (**b**) a squamous cell carcinoma of the lip.

those tumours arising in sun-damaged skin (0.5%),[95] and is highest in tumours that arise in mucosal surfaces, irradiated areas and the edges of ulcers and sinuses (20%).[96] Local recurrence is treated in a similar manner to recurrent basal cell carcinoma. Regional node spread is treated by surgical block dissection, or radiotherapy, or both. This reduces local recurrence and long-term mortality.

Dysplastic naevus syndrome (B–K mole syndrome; FAMM syndrome)

Dysplastic naevi are melanocytic lesions with distinctive clinical and histopathological features, and the use of the term should be restricted to naevi with both of these components. Recognition of dysplastic naevi is important as they are considered to be precursors of malignant melanoma.

Following Clark's report[97] on two families (B and K) with a family history of malignant melanoma and multiple dysplastic moles, much controversy has arisen over the relationship of dysplastic naevi, family history and melanoma. There is certainly a markedly increased risk of developing malignant melanoma in those patients who have dysplastic naevi and a family history of melanoma,[98] although there is no proven increased risk of melanoma in patients with solitary dysplastic naevi without a family history.[99] All patients with dysplastic naevi should avoid excessive sunlight. As with all malignant melanomas, tumours may arise in normal skin rather than in a pre-existing naevus.[100]

The naevi tend to occur on the trunk, have an irregular, ill defined border, are usually greater than 5 mm in diameter and have a variegated colour of tan through to dark brown on a pink background (Fig. 9.51). Surrounding erythema is common. Histologically, the dysplastic naevus is a junctional or compound naevus, with lentiginous or epithelioid hyperplasia and cytological atypia with hyperchromatic nuclei.

The lifetime risk for the development of melanoma from dysplastic naevi is in the order of 20% in patients with no family history of melanoma.[101] In the familial syndrome, where at least two members have had a malignant melanoma, the actuarial lifetime risk of developing melanoma for a family member who has cutaneous dysplastic naevi is close to 100%. The majority of dysplastic naevi do not undergo malignant transformation; environmental factors such as sunlight may be important in their natural history. Patients with dysplastic naevi should be examined carefully, over the whole of the body surface, and a family history obtained. Whole-body photographs have been used to quantify changes in individual moles and to detect new lesions.[101]

Malignant melanoma

Malignant melanoma, a tumour first described in 1787 by John Hunter,[102] is an important though relatively uncommon tumour in the UK, with an approximate incidence of 6 per 100 000 of the population per year.[103]

REFERENCES

95. Lund H Z Arch Dermatol 1965; 92: 635
96. Martin H, Strong E et al Cancer 1970; 25: 61–71
97. Clark W H Jr, Reimer R R et al Arch Dermatol 1978; 114: 732–738
98. Greene M H, Clark W H Jr et al N Engl J Med 1985; 312: 91–97
99. Welkovich B, Schmoeckel C et al Arch Dermatol 1987; 123: 1280
100. Elder D E Pathology 1985; 17: 291–297
101. Cook M G, Fallowfield E Histopathology 1990; 16: 2935
102. Bodenham D C Ann R Coll Surg Engl 1968; 43: 218–239
103. MacKie R M et al Lancet 1985; ii: 859–863

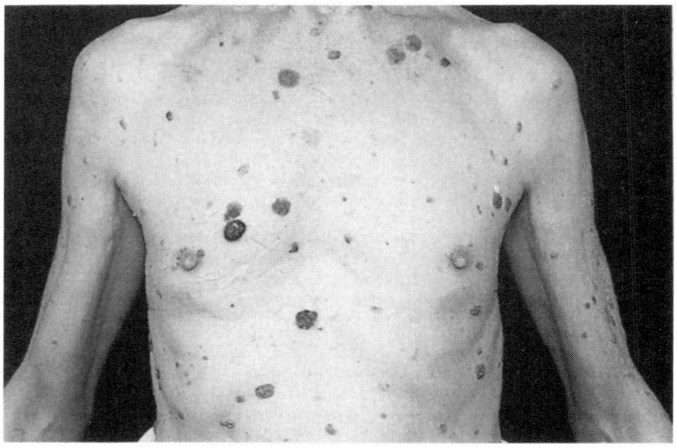

Fig. 9.51 The dysplastic naevus syndrome.

The worldwide incidence varies considerably, with the highest risk being in Queensland, Australia, where it is in the order of 33 per 100 000 per year.[104,105] The incidence in black populations is very much lower, being approximately 0.6 per 100 000. Results of several large studies in different countries, including the UK, have revealed an alarming increase in the incidence in the last few years.[104,106,107] One third of the patients are under 40 at the time of diagnosis, and melanoma is now the most common cancer in young adults aged between 20 and 39. It also accounts for most of the deaths from cutaneous malignancy. It is fortunate that increased awareness, earlier diagnosis, and more streamlined intervention have combined to significantly increase 5-year survival rates in all groups of patients in recent decades.[108]

In the UK, the incidence is higher in women than in men, although this sex difference is reversed elsewhere in the world.[109] Melanoma can occur at any site on the skin's surface but has a predilection for the legs of young women and the trunk of middle-aged men, reflecting social patterns of sun exposure.[110]

Melanoma can also occur outside the skin, for example in the nasal cavities, the eye and the gastrointestinal tract. The tumour occurs at any age: young women in their 20s and 30s are particularly affected. Approximately 90% of malignant melanomas arise in otherwise normal skin and only 10% develop in a pre-existing naevus.[111]

Malignant melanoma is extremely rare in children, but when it does occur it almost always develops in a large congenital pigmented naevus. In the elderly, it presents as lentigo maligna melanoma (see p. 000). Malignant melanomas are therefore known to develop in dysplastic naevi, large congenital naevi and lentigo maligna. These features and some of the defining tenets of the behaviour of melanoma were described in 1820 and 1857 by William Norris.[112,113]

The development of malignant melanoma has been strongly associated with exposure to ultraviolet light. Epidemiological studies show a complex association of melanoma with sun exposure.[114,115] The highest incidences are in fair-skinned people living near the equator. Those with red hair and a fair complexion who burn easily in sunlight are most at risk.[114,116]

The condition appears to be initiated by an episode of severe burning rather than constant exposure, and blistering sunburn during childhood and adolescence is associated with an increased incidence of later melanoma.[117] It also appears that the skin is most sensitive to the effects of the sun below the age of 10 years.[118] Trauma has also been suggested as a cause but this has not been substantiated. Other risk factors include: a previous melanoma, which increases the risk of a second primary three and a half times; more than 20 benign pigmented naevi, which increases the risk three times; and family history in first degree relatives, which increases the risk one and a half times.[118] Xeroderma pigmentosum, a familial condition associated with the failure of DNA transcription, carries a large risk.

The diagnosis of malignant melanoma is usually not difficult. A rapid increase in the size of a mole, ulceration, bleeding, irregularity of its outline, marked variation in colour, and itching all arouse suspicion. The appearance of pigmented satellite lesions also lends suspicion of malignancy to a pigmented lesion. Excision biopsy should be performed if there is doubt about a 'mole' that has undergone any sort of change. The lesions most commonly mistaken for melanoma include pigmented basal cell carcinomas, pigmented seborrhoeic keratoses, dermatofibromas and thrombosed haemangiomas. When excisional biopsy might result in a poor scar in a lesion that has yet to be histologically identified, incisional biopsy of the most suspicious area may be performed without compromising prognosis, though in the knowledge that sampling error may yield a false negative result.[119]

Pathology

Histologically, a malignant melanoma usually consists of nests and groups of melanocytes which are cytologically malignant and are invading the epidermis with destruction leading to incipient or actual ulceration. The malignant cells infiltrate into the deeper parts of the dermis and sometimes into the subcutaneous fat. Invasion of vascular channels is occasionally seen and is another feature supporting malignant transformation. The histological diagnosis can be very difficult in 'early' melanomas, when pathologists often disagree. Under these circumstances it is better to treat these patients as if they have a malignant melanoma and widely re-excise the surrounds.

Significant advances were made in the understanding of malignant melanoma when Clark et al in 1969[120] introduced their concept of levels of invasion and related them to prognosis (Fig. 9.52). In 1970, Breslow[121] described the thickness of the primary tumour measured in millimetres and illustrated a direct correspondence to clinical outcome (Fig. 9.53). Although both Clark level and Breslow thickness are recorded on the pathology report (Table 9.2), Breslow thickness has been shown to be a better indicator of prognosis, as there is a wide range of thicknesses in the reticular dermis in different body sites.

Four types of melanoma are recognized by the nature of their intraepidermal component. The gross histological feature of greatest prognostic importance in invasive melanomas is that of

REFERENCES

104. Little J H, Holt J et al Med J Aust 1980; 1: 66–69
105. Schreiber M M, Bozzo P D et al Arch Dermatol 1981; 117: 6–11
106. Osterlind A, Moller Jensen O In: Gallagher R P (ed) Epidemiology of Malignant Melanoma. Springer-Verlag, Berlin 1985
107. Cosman B, Heddle S B Plast Reconstr Surg 1976; 57: 50–56
108. Boring C C, Squires T S, Tong T A Cancer Journal for Clinicians 1993; 43(1): 7–26
109. Lee J A H, Storer B E et al Lancet 1980; ii: 1337–1339
110. Lee J A H Epidemiol Rev 1982; 4: 110–136
111. Crucioli V, Stilwell J J Cutan Pathol 1982; 9: 396–404
112. Norris W Edin Med Surg J 1820; 15: 562
113. Norris W Eight Cases of Melanosis with Pathological and Therapeutical Remarks on that Disease. Longman, London 1857
114. Elder D E J Invest Dermatol 1989; 92: 297
115. Koh H K, Kligler B E, Lew R A Photochem Photobiol 1990; 51: 765–779
116. Crombie I K Br J Cancer 1979; 40: 185
117. Lew R A et al J Dermatol Surg Oncol 1983; 9: 981
118. Anderson R G Select Read Plast Surg 1992; 7: 1–35
119. Lees V C, Briggs J C Br J Surg 1991; 78: 1108
120. Clark W H Jr, From Li et al Cancer Res 1969; 29: 705–727
121. Breslow A Ann Surg 1970; 172: 902–908

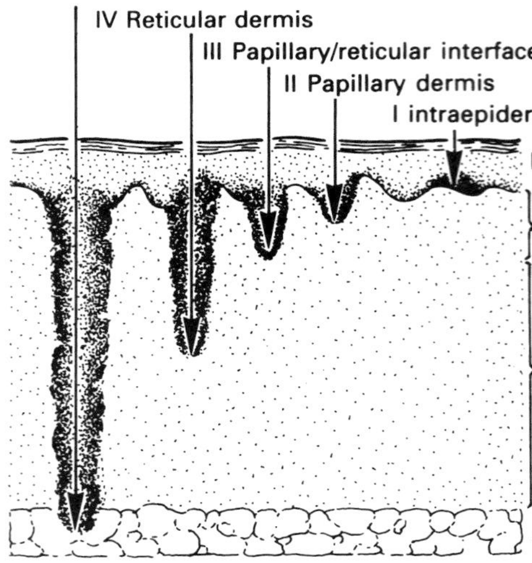

Fig. 9.52 Clark's level of melanoma invasion.

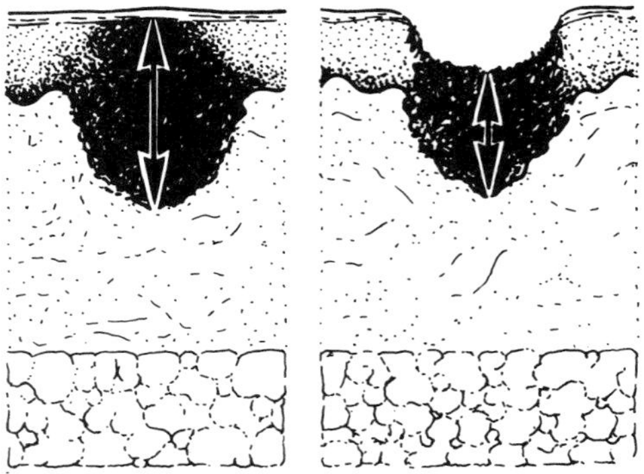

Fig. 9.53 Breslow's thickness of malignant melanoma.

Table 9.2 Staging and clinical prognosis of malignant melanoma

		Prognosis
Clark's level		*5-year survival*
I	epidermis only	98%
II	invades papillary dermis	96%
III	fills papillary dermis	94%
IV	invades reticular dermis	78%
V	subcutaneous tissue invasion	44%
Breslow thickness		*10-year survival*
< 0.76 mm		92%
> 3 mm		50%
> 4 mm		30%
Lymph node involvement		8-year survival < 40%

From Anderson[118]

horizontal and vertical growth phases. A predominantly vertical growth results in deeper penetration of the dermis and confers a poorer prognosis.

Superficial spreading melanoma

This is the most common type of malignant melanoma (70%);[122] its incidence is increasing worldwide, probably as a result of increased sun exposure associated with improved travel and leisure facilities. It occurs in both covered and uncovered areas, often on the back in men and on the legs in women, though it can occur anywhere on the body after puberty.[120] The presence of horizontal or pagetoid spread in the epidermis at the margin of the melanoma gives rise to a red, white and blue appearance which is characteristic (Fig. 9.54). The horizontal growth phase is predominant and the prognosis is usually good.

Nodular melanoma

This type often develops on the trunk and is frequently raised, polypoidal and ulcerated (Fig. 9.55). Histologically, there is no recognizable intraepidermal component at the margin of the tumour mass, all of the cells being in the vertical growth phase. This type of melanoma has a significantly worse prognosis than other forms, and accounts for 15–30% of reported melanomas.[122]

Lentigo maligna melanoma

This arises on a background of lentigo maligna and therefore almost always on sun-damaged skin of the face or the dorsum of the hands in elderly people[123] (Fig. 9.56). Histologically, there are features of lentigo maligna (see above) with gross sun damage to the dermal collagen. Additionally, there are islands of malignant melanocytic cells within the dermis. The intraepidermal component is that of lentiginous proliferation of the atypical melanocytes continuous along the basal layer in a similar fashion to that seen in lentigo maligna. The epidermis is atrophic.

Acral lentiginous melanoma

This type of melanoma is the least common, occurring on hairless skin, particularly in the subungual regions and soles and palms of the hands and feet (Fig. 9.57).[124] It is the most common type of melanoma in South East Asia and in black races, though the reported increased incidence in blacks over whites may reflect the much lower incidence of general cutaneous melanoma in the black population.[125,126]

Histologically, the intraepidermal component is that of a lentiginous proliferation of atypical or malignant cells at the margin of the tumour. In contrast to lentigo maligna, the epidermis is hyperplastic.

Miscellaneous types

Amelanotic melanoma. This is malignant melanoma with no visible pigmentation (Fig. 9.58) and carries a poor prognosis—either from a delay in diagnosis or aggressive behaviour, or both.

REFERENCES

122. McGovern V J, Mihm M C Jr et al Cancer 1973; 32: 1446–1457
123. McGovern V J, Shaw H M et al Histopathology 1980; 4: 235–242
124. Krementz E T, Feed R J et al Ann Surg 1982; 195: 632–645
125. Reintgen D S, McCarty J M Jr et al JAMA 1982; 248: 1856–1859
126. Stevens M G, Liff J M, Weiss N S Int J Cancer 1990; 45: 691

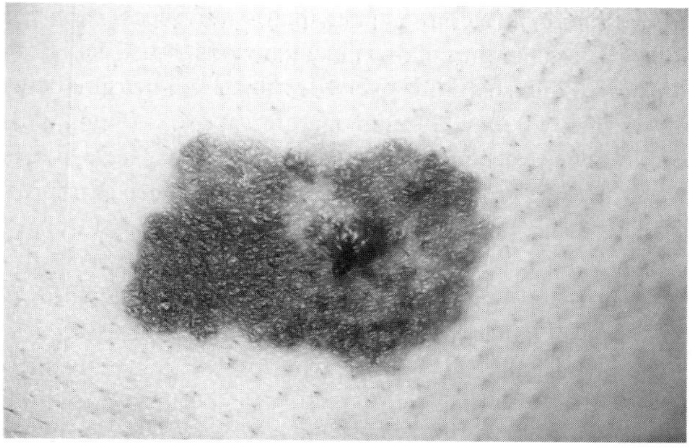

Fig. 9.54 A superficial spreading melanoma.

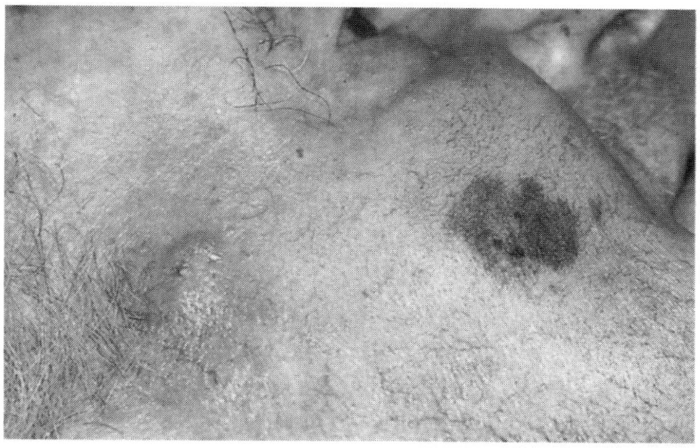

Fig. 9.56 Lentigo maligna.

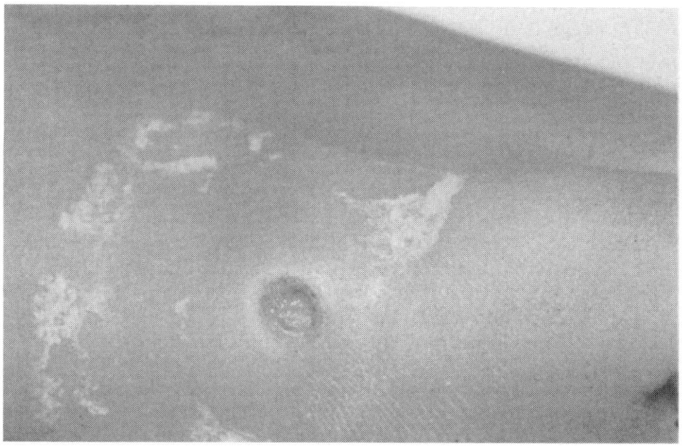

Fig. 9.58 An amelanotic malignant melanoma.

Secondary melanoma without a primary lesion identified. This accounts for about 4% of metastatic melanoma. It may represent an extreme example of regression in the primary, or primary melanoma in a non-cutaneous location.[127] Satellite secondaries are quite common in the skin around the primary melanoma.

Desmoplastic melanoma. This frequently arises in a recurrent melanoma or lentigo maligna melanoma. It is usually not pigmented and may grow to a large size. The prognosis is poor.

Malignant blue naevus. This shows no involvement of the junctional layer of the epidermis and may arise in a pre-existing benign blue naevus. Long-term survival has been reported, despite metastatic spread.[128,129]

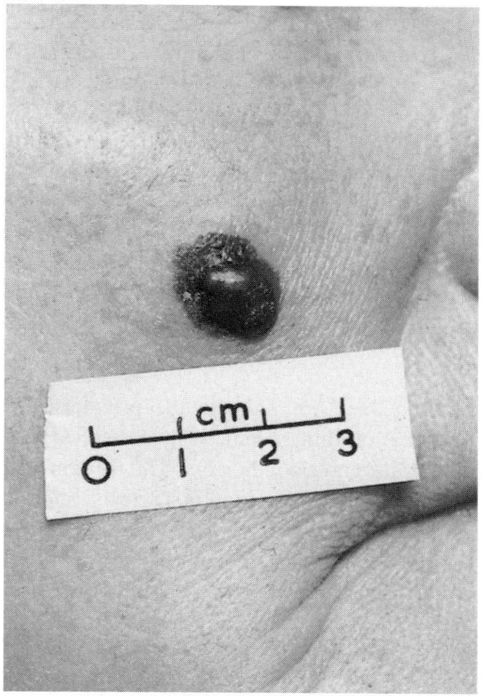

Fig. 9.55 A nodular malignant melanoma.

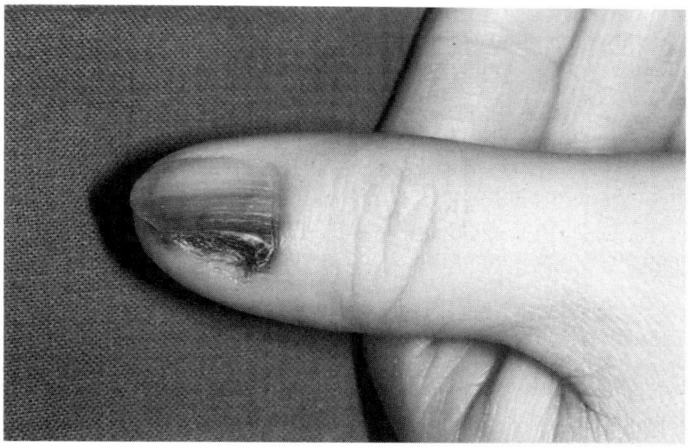

Fig. 9.57 An acral lentiginous melanoma.

Clinical staging

A updated 4-stage system has been developed to stage melanomas clinically and provide a more accurate prognosis[130] (Table 9.3).

REFERENCES

127. Park G T et al JAMA 1961; 176(1): 55–56
128. Merkow L P, Burt R C et al Cancer 1969; 24: 888–896
129. Dorsey C S, Montgomery H J Invest Dermatol 1954; 22: 225
130. Beahrs O H, Myers M H Manual for Staging of Cancer. Am Joint Comm Cancer/Lippincott, Philadelphia 1983 p 117

Table 9.3 Clinical staging system for malignant melanoma

Clinical stage	*Histopathological stage*
IA	< 0.75 mm or Clark level II
IB	0.75–1.5 mm or Clark level III
IIA	1.5–4.0 mm or Clark level IV
IIB	> 4.0 mm or Clark level V
III	Lymph node metastasis in one regional drainage area, or > 5 in transit metastases
IV	Advanced regional metastasis or distant metastasis

From Beahrs & Myers[130]

Prognosis

Thickness alone does not indicate the prognosis in individual cases, as 5–10% of thin melanomas metastasize. There are a number of other prognostic indicators. The median age of patients with stage I disease at presentation is 45 years, and older patients tend to have thicker lesions than younger ones.[131] Women have a better overall prognosis, with a greater incidence of limb extremity melanomas and lower frequency of ulceration.[131] A poor prognosis is associated with trunk (especially back), scalp, hand and foot primary sites. This may relate to diagnostic delay and, on the trunk, multiple potential sites of lymph node metastasis.[132] Melanomas arising on the upper back, posterolateral arms, posterior neck and posterior scalp were said to have a poorer prognosis than those at other sites.[133] This has however been disputed.[134] Apart from growth phase and thickness, several histological features confer a poor prognosis. An ulcerated tumour has a worse prognosis than a tumour of equal stage that has not ulcerated.[135] Depigmentation and tumour regression, creating a pale halo around the lesion with increased vascularity, fibrosis, and evidence of macrophages containing melanin, may or may not influence prognosis: the evidence is contradictory.[136,137] Aneuploidy and high mitotic index indicate a high tumour grade and a worse prognosis.[138]

Treatment

Surgical excision remains the treatment of choice, with combinations of surgery, radiotherapy, chemotherapy and newer therapies being reserved for palliation. Local recurrence and distant spread can still occur despite an adequate margin of excision, and this reflects the biological unpredictability and heterogeneity of the tumour.

William Sampson Handley was to establish surgical principles of wide excision and regional lymphadenectomy, based upon observations from a single autopsy, that held sway for 50 years.[139] The original concept of an extensive margin of excision down to or including deep fascia, with elective regional lymph node dissection, has now been replaced by less aggressive ablation based on numerous studies relating the thickness of the tumour to prognosis.[140,141]

Diagnostic biopsy, if positive for melanoma, should be followed by definitive excision. Delay of 3 weeks before definitive excision does not worsen the outcome.[142] Definitive excision should include a margin of grossly normal tissue, which, up to a certain limit, should be increased proportional to the Breslow depth of the tumour. The risk of local recurrence is related to the depth of tumour invasion[143] rather than width of excision per se —wide excision margins of 3–5 cm are no longer justified. Lesions less than 0.76 mm should be excised with a 1 cm margin; between 0.76 mm and 1.0 mm, a 2 cm margin; above 1.0 mm, a 3 cm margin. Wider excisions, even in thick tumours, have not been shown to have any effect in reducing local recurrence or improving survival[141] despite the observation that rates of local recurrence and development of satellites can be up to 20% for tumours greater than 4 mm thick.[144] Excision should be performed down to deep fascia where practicable; the evidence that deep fascial excision increases metastatic risk is contradictory.[145,146] Local recurrence may be significantly delayed; when it occurs, local excision and close follow-up are necessary.[147]

The median time to nodal metastasis for patients with thin and intermediate lesions is 1.3 years.[148] Where there is clinical suspicion of regional node metastasis, lymph node biopsy or fine-needle aspiration may be performed; for frankly palpable nodes, therapeutic block dissection is carried out. Surgical lymphadenectomy is the only potential cure for nodal metastatic disease. Areas where lymph drainage is unpredictable, as on the trunk, head and neck, provide clinical concern and require frequent surveillance. In these cases, lymphoscintigraphy or PET scanning may provide indications for the need for block dissection of neck nodes.

The role of elective prophylactic node dissection remains controversial. It may be undertaken immediately or delayed for over a month. Non-randomized trials have shown a improvement in 5- and 10-year survival after elective node dissection in patients with tumours between 1.5 and 4 mm thick.[131,149] The high morbidity of the procedure outweighs its benefit in patients with thin melanomas < 0.76 mm, or with thick melanomas (> 4 mm) where disseminated micrometastasis is likely at presentation (70%). There is no benefit in areas where there are multiple pathways of lymph drainage, e.g. the back or the trunk.

These results have not yet been confirmed by randomized trial,[150] although Veronesi has reported results of a prospective trial

REFERENCES

131. Balch C M, Soong S J et al In: Balch C M, Milton G W (eds) Cutaneous Melanoma. J B Lippincott, Philadelphia 1985
132. Rogers G S, Kopf A W et al Arch Dermatol 1983; 119: 644–649
133. Day C L Jr, Mihm M C et al Ann Surg 1982; 195: 30–34
134. Cascinelli N, Vaglini M et al Cancer 1986; 57: 441–444
135. Balch C M, Wilkerson J A Cancer 1980; 45: 3012–3017
136. McGovern V J, Shaw H M, Milton G S Histopathology 1983; 7: 673
137. Grommett M A, Epstein W L, Blois M S Cancer 1978; 42: 2282
138. Salman S M, Rogers G S J Dermatol Surg Oncol 1990; 16: 413
139. Handley W S Lancet 1907; 1: 927, 996
140. Heenan P J, Weeramanthri T et al Aust NZ J Surg 1985; 55: 229–234
141. Zeitels J, La Rossa D et al Plast Reconstr Surg 1988; 81: 688
142. Landthaler M, Braun Falco O et al Cancer 1989; 64: 1612–1616
143. Schultz S, Kane M et al Surg Gynaecol Obstet 1990; 171: 393–397
144. Balch C M et al Cancer 1979; 43: 883
145. Olson G Cancer 1964; 17: 1159
146. Kenady D E, Brown B W, McBride C M Surgery 1982; 92: 615
147. Griffiths R W, Briggs J C Br J Plast Surg 1984; 37: 507
148. Balch C M et al Ann Surg 1981; 193: 377
149. Balch C M, Soong S J et al Ann Surg 1982; 196: 677–684
150. Meyer K L, Kenady D E Surg Gynecol Obstet 1985; 160: 379–386

indicating that elective nodal dissection gave no additional benefit over close follow-up and therapeutic nodal dissection when indicated.[151] Similarly, a recent review of elective axillary block dissection in melanoma patients showed minimal differences in 5-year survival for the two groups of patients having clinically negative, but histologically either positive or negative nodes. The morbidity in this series appeared to outweigh any possible benefit. The 5-year survival for patients with palpable nodes in this series was significantly reduced.[152]

Therapeutic nodal dissection en bloc for palpable nodes may increase survival, but the prognosis remains poor (see Table 9.2). Overall survival is thought to decrease with the number of nodes found to be positive at operation.[153]

In susceptible patients, distant metastases to lung, liver, bone, brain and intestine develop a median of 3 years after initial presentation of a cutaneous melanoma. In patients presenting with nodal disease, distant metastases present within a mean of a year.[118] The most common causes of death are pulmonary failure and intracerebral haemorrhage. Palliation may be obtained by selective radiotherapy, chemotherapy and surgery.

Adjuvant therapies

Adjuvant therapies for metastatic melanoma are in constant development and subject to clinical trial. No current option is sufficiently effective to be accepted for routine prophylactic use. A definite indication for trial is symptomatic metastatic spread where surgery alone can provide no benefit.

Melanomas are not very radiosensitive, though radiotherapy may provide palliation in cases of nerve compression.[154] Factors affecting outcome are tumour bulk and the radiation dose and frequency. Radiotherapy has proved to be beneficial in combination with intralesional BCG therapy.[155] Systemic chemotherapy is toxic and provides minimally prolonged survival, which may be improved by co-adjuvant tamoxifen therapy. Isolated limb perfusion with melphalan after nodal dissection may be used in patients with multiple local recurrence or 'in transit' recurrences deposited along lymphatic pathways, with improved long-term survival.[156] Isolated limb perfusion and heat therapy have also been combined, with encouraging results.[157] Immunotherapies for melanoma include the use of vaccines to raise an anti-melanoma antibody response,[158] monoclonal antibody therapy,[158] and the use of various cytokine interferons, either systemically or delivered by suitably transfected tumourophilic lymphocytes.[158] These developing therapies are currently under evaluation.

The control of melanoma depends on avoidance of the aetiological factors and recognition of those at risk with early detection through public education campaigns. This has partially succeeded, with an increase in the number of lesions removed when under 1.5 mm.[103]

Other malignant skin tumours

Merkel cell carcinoma (trabecular carcinoma)

This rare but highly aggressive tumour is believed to be derived from the Merkel cell population which are primitive neuroendocrine cells in the skin.[159] These tumours occur in the elderly, in the seventh to eighth decade, with a slight female preponderance. They tend to occur in sun-exposed sites, particularly the head and neck and limbs, and present as an enlarging firm painless nodule. The overlying epidermis is usually not ulcerated and may be violaceous in colour.

Histologically, the lesion is quite distinctive and consists of an ill defined dermal nodule made up of cords and trabeculae of medium-sized cells with very little cytoplasm, with a high mitotic and apoptotic rate. Foci of squamous or eccrine differentiation may also be present. The diagnosis is one of exclusion, with malignant lymphoma and metastatic small cell carcinoma being the two conditions which require differentiation. Immunohistochemistry is very helpful in excluding a lymphoma, but a metastatic small cell carcinoma often needs to be excluded clinically.

The prognosis is poor with a local recurrence developing in 36% and metastasis in 28%. Approximately half of patients are dead within 2 years.[160,161]

Paget's disease

Mammary and extramammary Paget's disease are two distinct entities in which the epidermis is infiltrated by adenocarcinoma cells. Paget's disease of the breast is discussed in Chapter 25.

Extramammary Paget's disease occurs in the genital and perianal region, predominantly in women. It has also been described in the axilla, and therefore occurs where apocrine glands are situated. It can occur in association with a mucin-secreting carcinoma of the rectum or endocervix. In the majority of cases, unlike the disease in the breast, an underlying carcinoma is not found.

Clinically, it presents as an eczematous, red velvety area, with oozing and crusting. It is intensely pruritic. Histologically, there is infiltration of the epidermis by Paget's cells, singly and in groups. The Paget cells are large, pale cells with abundant cytoplasm and a large nucleus. Malignant melanoma has to be excluded, and this can be achieved by performing an S100 stain which is negative in Paget's cells and positive in melanoma.

Treatment is by surgical excision, but local recurrence is common because the margins of the tumour are very difficult to define and Paget's disease is often multifocal. The prognosis is good when Paget's disease is not associated with a tumour, but poor when it is.[162]

REFERENCES

151. Veronesi U et al N Engl J Med 1977; 297: 627
152. Karakousis C P et al Am J Surg 1991; 162: 202
153. Bevilacqua R G et al Ann Surg 1990; 212: 125
154. Herbert S H et al Cancer 1991; 67: 2472
155. Plesnicar S, Rudolf Z Cancer 1982; 50: 1100
156. McBride C M, Sugerbaker E V, Hickey R C Ann Surg 1975; 182: 316
157. Ghussen F, Kruger I, Smalley R V, Groth W World J Surg 1989; 13: 598–602
158. Oratz R, Bystryn J C Dermatol Clin 1991; 9(4): 669
159. Warner T F C S, Umo H et al Cancer 1983; 52: 238–245
160. Sibley R K, Dehner L P et al Am J Surg Pathol 1985; 9: 95–108
161. Raaf J H, Urmacher C et al Cancer 1986; 57: 178–182
162. Jones R E Jr, Austin C et al Am J Dermatopathol 1979; 1: 101–132

Sebaceous carcinoma

This is a rare malignant tumour arising from sebaceous glands of the skin. It chiefly occurs in the fifth and sixth decades, with women affected more often than men. It develops on the eyelids, where it has its origin from Meibomian glands, but also arises elsewhere on the head and neck.[163] It presents as a nodule with a red-yellow discoloration that increases in size and may ulcerate (Fig. 9.59). Histologically, the tumour consists of lobules of undifferentiated cells in the dermis; some of the cells have foamy cytoplasm, suggesting a sebaceous origin. Pagetoid spread of the tumour cells in the epidermis occurs in the eyelid tumours. Stains for fat are positive, confirming the diagnosis.[164] Treatment is by local excision.

SOFT TISSUE SARCOMAS

A sarcoma is a malignant tumour arising from or differentiating towards a tissue of mesenchymal origin. Sarcomas may thus arise anywhere in the body, though this account is restricted to those which may affect the skin and subcutaneous tissues. Numerous histological variants of these tumours exist; they have a range of biological behaviour from indolent growth and local recurrence to rapid growth, invasion and dissemination. Sarcomas are fortunately rare: only 1500 new cases are seen in the UK each year, and collected individual experience outside a specialist centre is unlikely. Nevertheless, growing clinicopathological experience married to the application of molecular biology techniques has improved the management and prognostic accuracy relating to these tumours.[165]

The clinical picture is an essential component of the eventual diagnosis, as many of these tumours display age, site and gender predominance: cutaneous angiosarcomas occur in the elderly, liposarcomas and malignant histiocytomas are tumours of adults; embryonal rhabdomyosarcoma is a tumour of children. Synovial sarcoma is commonly a tumour of the lower limb in young adult males, whereas epithelioid sarcoma occurs in the upper limb in the same patient group.

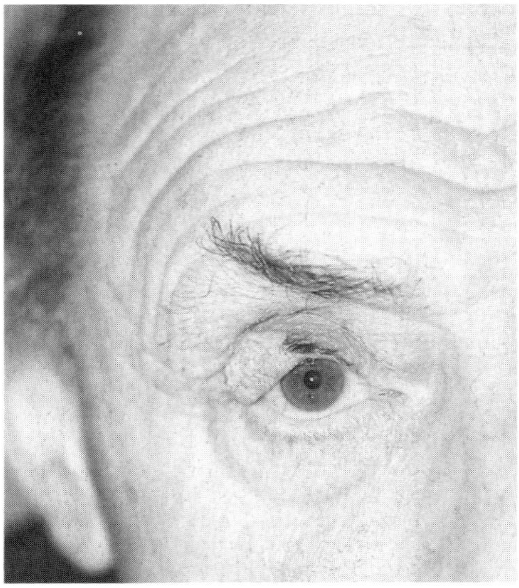

Fig. 9.59 A sebaceous carcinoma.

The speed of growth and the plane or depth of origin of the tumours also give important clues to the diagnosis, though high-grade sarcomas may have been present as a mass for years before presenting with a rapid growth phase. Deeper tumours are more aggressive than superficial ones such as dermatofibrosarcoma protuberans, though the clinician should be aware that the exceptions—angiosarcomas, malignant fibrous histiocytomas and epithelioid sarcomas—prove the rule.

For further details of clinical evaluation, pathology and classification and treatment of sarcomas, see Chapter 54.

Fibrosarcomas

These tumours produce collagen fibres and may contain differentiated fibroblasts. Accurate diagnosis is made on immunohistochemistry and electron microscopy: a diagnosis of nerve sheath tumour or synovial sarcoma may be made in error and conveys a worse prognosis. Low-grade fibrosarcomas are relatively benign.

Dermatofibrosarcoma protuberans

This is commonly encountered as a dermal, multinodular, plaque-like growth. The tumour is usually firm and non-tender, with a purple, red or yellow hue. The overlying epidermis is usually firm, smooth and shiny (Fig. 9.60). Dermatofibrosarcoma protuberans is infiltrative and recurs if not widely excised, but has a very low rate of metastasis.[166] It shows spindle cell differentiation in a cartwheel pattern. Aggressive sarcomatous change follows multiple recurrences, thus the tumour demands careful diagnosis and wide local excision on the first occasion.

Leiomyosarcoma

This occurs in the skin and is less commonly diagnosed in the deeper tissues. The diagnosis is aided by immunohistochemical analysis for smooth muscle antibodies.

Malignant peripheral nerve sheath tumours

The sarcomas of nerve and nerve sheath are currently classified as the malignant peripheral nerve sheath tumours (MPNST), and the Schwann cell is the most common pattern of differentiation. Not all tumours are associated with the defined nerve trunks of neurofibromata, though patients with neurofibromatosis have a 4% incidence of malignant change.[167] Histologically, ultrastructurally, and chemically these tumours are extremely variable; the outcome is not easily predictable for these patients though it is generally worse for those with neurofibromatosis.

REFERENCES

163. Rao N A, Hidayat A A et al Human Pathol 1982; 13: 113–122
164. Graham R M, McKee P H et al Clin Exp Dermatol 1984; 9: 466–471
165. Fisher C Br J Plast Surg 1996; 49: 27–33
166. Kahn L B, Saxe N et al Arch Dermatol 1978; 114: 599–601
167. Ricardi V N Engl J Med 1981; 305: 1617–1626

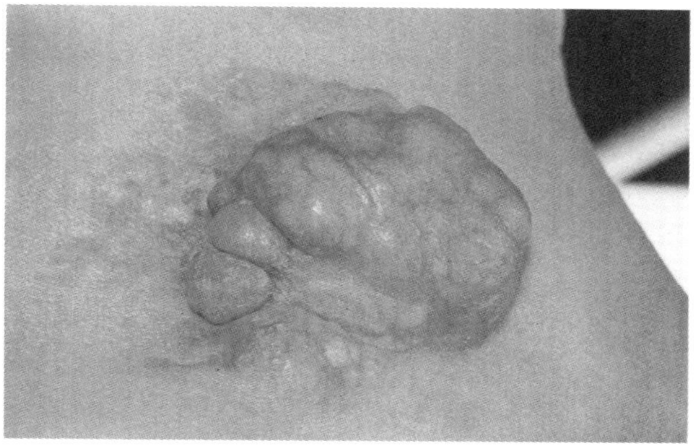

Fig. 9.60 A dermatofibrosarcoma protuberans.

The leiomyosarcomas, synovial sarcomas and malignant peripheral nerve sheath tumours are histologically heterogeneous, variably graded and of variable prognosis.

Epithelioid sarcoma

This presents as an ulcerating nodule on the upper limb. The tumours are slow-growing, painless, intradermal or subcutaneous nodules which are often multiple. The diagnosis is almost always made histologically (aided by cytokeratin immunostaining), rather than clinically, which results in the primary excision margins often being inadequate. The tumour spreads insidiously along tendons, nerves and fascial planes, and early nodal involvement is common. Treatment is by early wide excision, which frequently necessitates amputation. The local recurrence rate even after adequate surgery is approximately 75%; metastases develop in approximately 30–50%, with lymph nodes and lungs being the most frequent initial site of occurrence.[168]

Kaposi's sarcoma

Kaposi's sarcoma may be a difficult histological diagnosis: when the spindle cells predominate it resembles a fibrosarcoma; the anaplastic or pleomorphic variants resemble an angiosarcoma. It may be well circumscribed or diffuse, with interposed dilated blood vessels and intercellular channels creating a sieve-like appearance. The tumour may be situated immediately below the epidermis, sometimes ulcerating through it, or more deeply in the dermis at the level of the sweat glands.

There are four clinical presentations.[169] The classical European lesion described by Kaposi in 1872[170] appears in the elderly as a painless red or brown nodule, usually on the leg or foot, growing slowly and eventually ulcerating. The subcutaneous lymph nodes may be involved in a few cases.[171] In 10% the viscera are involved: the gastrointestinal tract, liver and lungs are most often affected.[172] The endemic form was described in tropical Africa in the 1960s. It presents initially as nodules in the extremities which may be present for months or years before medical help is sought (Fig. 9.61). It metastasizes and infiltrates locally, though in children the endemic form may affect lymph nodes primarily, as the lymphadenopathic variant.[173]

The third, allograft-associated, type of Kaposi's sarcoma is seen in immunosuppressed patients, particularly kidney transplant recipients.[174] The fourth type, the epidemic form of Kaposi's sarcoma, was described in the 1980s, particularly in homosexual men, and was associated with the outbreak of the acquired immune deficiency syndrome (AIDS).[175,176] In immunosuppressed patients, Kaposi's sarcoma resembles a combination of the nodular classical type and the lymphadenopathic endemic form; the Kaposi lesions are more widely distributed, often involving the mucous membranes of the mouth, anus and gastrointestinal tract. The skin lesions in this form differ from classical Kaposi's sarcoma because of their small size and extensive distribution. The rate of progression varies, from indolent tumours present for many years to rapidly progressive disease with widespread involvement of many organs.

Angiosarcoma

This is a highly malignant tumour of vascular origin and is rare in the skin. It occurs in the face and scalp of the elderly and has a very

REFERENCES

168. Chase D R, Enzinger F M Am J Surg Pathol 1985; 9: 241–263
169. Ziegler J L, Templeton A C et al Semin Oncol 1984; 11: 47–52
170. Kaposi M Arch Dermatol Syph (Berl) 1872; 4: 265–278
171. Amazon K, Rywlin A M Am J Dermatopathol 1979; 1: 173–176
172. Temim P, Stahl A et al Br J Dermatol 1961; 73: 303–309
173. Taylor J F, Templeton A C et al Int J Cancer 1971; 8: 122–135
174. Harwood A R, Osoba D et al Am J Med 1979; 67: 759–765
175. Friedman-Kein A E, Laubenstein L J et al Ann Intern Med 1982; 96: 693–700
176. Gottlieb G J, Ackerman A B Human Pathol 1982; 13: 882–892

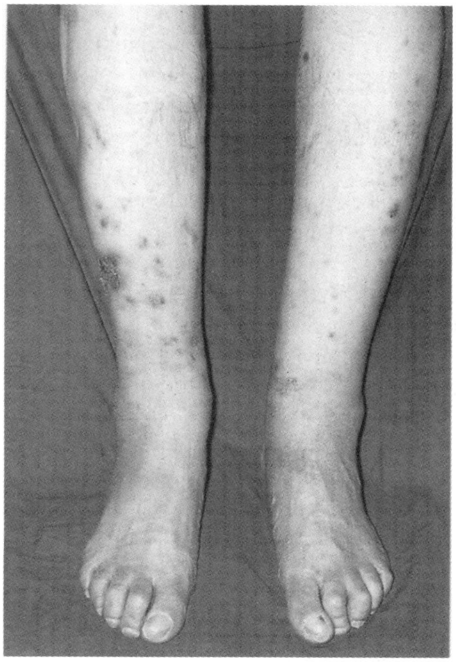

Fig. 9.61 Kaposi's sarcoma.

poor prognosis, with death from local destruction.[177] The clinical diagnosis is usually delayed, as angiosarcoma presents as a variety of bruise-like lesions, cellulitis, haemorrhagic plaques or nodules that bleed easily with trauma or ulcerate. The plaques and nodules enlarge locally, but by this stage the lesion already extends much further than is clinically apparent, which results in inadequate surgical excision.

Lymphangiosarcoma often develops in limbs with chronic lymphoedema (Fig. 9.62), which may be either primary or secondary. The best-known example occurs in the oedematous limb following radical mastectomy for breast carcinoma, and is known as the Stewart–Treves syndrome.[178] The microscopic appearance consists of irregular anastomosing channels lined by large atypical endothelial cells with mitoses, within the dermis. At the margin of the lesion, which is irregular, endothelial cells can be seen insinuating between the collagen bundles.

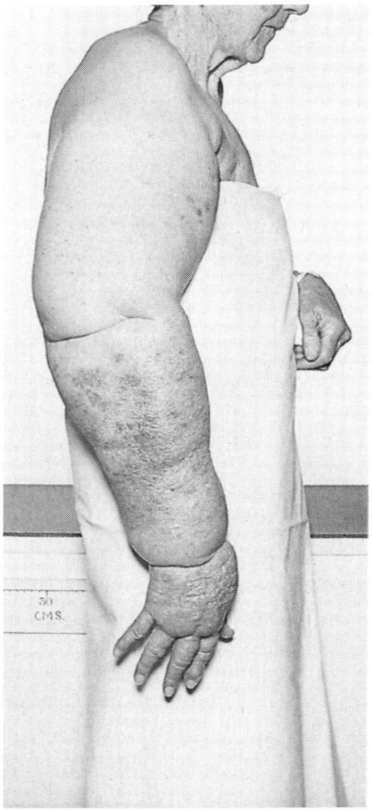

Fig. 9.62 A lymphangiosarcoma.

CUTANEOUS MALIGNANT LYMPHOMA

The skin may be infiltrated by leukaemic cells and by malignant lymphocytes in non-Hodgkin's lymphoma. Skin infiltration may even precede the onset of systemic disease. Involvement of the skin by Hodgkin's disease usually occurs late in the course of the illness and presents as a plaque, nodule or ulcer. Microscopically there is a heavy lymphoid infiltrate and occasional Reed–Sternberg cells are seen.

Non-Hodgkin's lymphomas can be either of B cell or, more commonly, of T cell type. 5% of B cell lymphomas arise in the skin. Clinically, they present as a smooth nodule or plaque of variable colour which slowly enlarges (Fig. 9.63). Microscopically, there is a heavy lymphoid infiltrate within the dermis which extends into subcutaneous fat. The epidermis is not involved and there is a narrow band of uninvolved dermis deep to the epidermis, known as the Grenz zone. Immunohistochemistry confirms the presence of B cells producing immunoglobulin with only one of the light chains, kappa or lambda (light chain restriction).

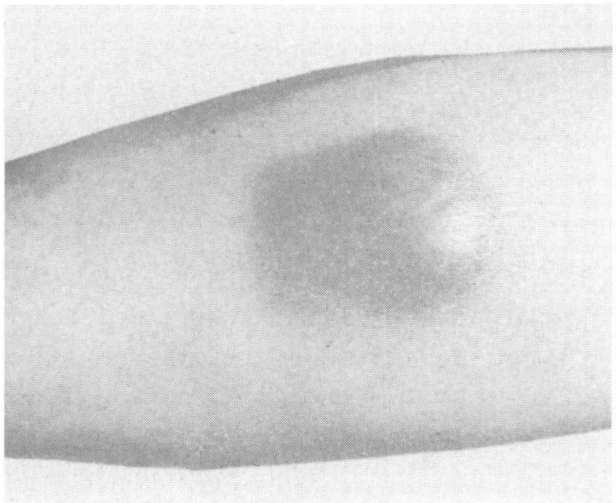

Fig. 9.63 A cutaneous T cell lymphoma.

T cell lymphomas encompass adult T cell lymphoma, mycosis fungoides and Sezary syndrome, and often have cutaneous involvement.

Mycosis fungoides is a T cell lymphoma which presents in the skin. It has been suggested that the incidence may be higher in industrial areas and in individuals exposed to certain industrial chemicals.[179] It occurs in late middle age and in the elderly, and presents as an area of localized eczema or as a plaque within the skin.

The Sezary syndrome presents with generalized exfoliative erythroderma, lymphadenopathy and involvement of the peripheral blood. The diagnosis can be difficult in the early stages as the histological features are rather non-specific. There is usually a mild perivascular mononuclear cell infiltrate with occasional atypical cells, some of which infiltrate the epidermis. Later, there is a heavier polymorphic inflammatory cell infiltrate with occasional large atypical cells with hyperconvoluted nuclei. At a later stage the overlying skin may ulcerate. Immunohistochemistry can be helpful in the early stages by showing abnormal T cell markers or a loss of expression of one or more of the normal T cell marker range.

The prognosis of all cutaneous lymphomas and leukaemias is dependent on the grade and stage of disease. Ultimately they spread to the lymph nodes, when the outlook is poor. Surgical biopsy is required to make a diagnosis but treatment is by radiation and cytotoxic chemotherapy.

REFERENCES

177. Girard C, Johnson W C et al Cancer 1970; 26: 868–883
178. Stewart F W, Treves N Cancer 1948; 1: 64–81
179. Slater D N J Pathol 1987; 153: 5–19

CUTANEOUS METASTASES

Cutaneous metastases almost always occur at a late stage, and thus carry a poor prognosis. They occasionally arise from a silent internal malignancy. The deposit may be single or multiple and is often umbilicated (Figs 9.64–66). The most common primary sites are the bronchus or oesophagus in men and the breast or ovaries in women. Metastases occur in all areas of the skin, but the chest wall is the most common site, especially when the primary is a carcinoma of the breast.

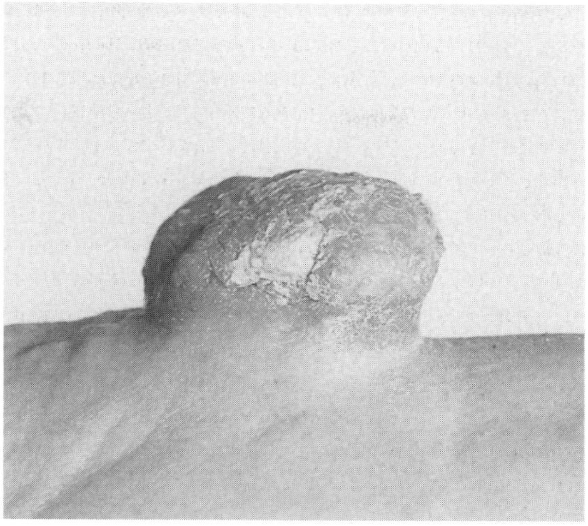

Fig. 9.64 A cutaneous secondary deposit from a carcinoma of the bronchus.

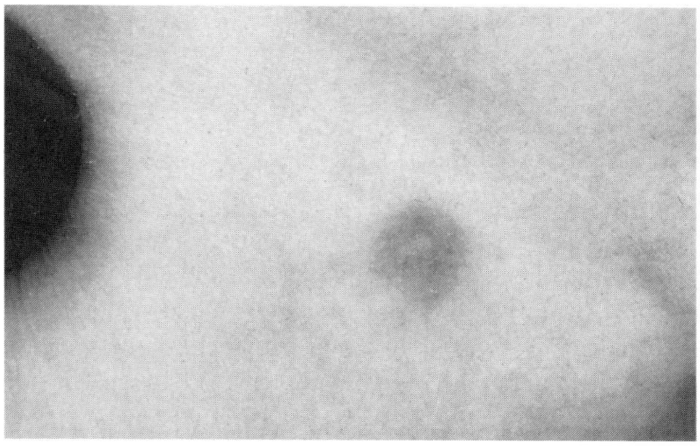

Fig. 9.65 A skin secondary from a carcinoma of the colon.

TECHNIQUES IN PLASTIC SURGERY

Scars and scar revision

Optimal healing after surgical skin closure is helped by a favourable genetic background, scar orientation, nutrition, oxygenation and surgical technique, with minimal inflammation. The aim is a thin, flat, non-pigmented, aesthetic scar that compromises neither structure nor function. Some fundamental principles apply. Wounds must be adequately debrided with removal of all foreign bodies. Haemostasis must be secure and haematomas avoided. Tissues should be handled gently and never crushed. The skin closure should not be under tension, and should be made with an everted edge. Incisions should be placed parallel to natural relaxed skin tension lines and natural folds in the skin wherever possible, and sutures should be correctly chosen and placed. Non-dissolving sutures must be removed early and the wound supported with Steristrips and dressings as appropriate.

Relaxed skin tension lines in the face are lines of facial expression. In cases of doubt, pinching the skin allows the natural wrinkles to be seen and the vector of tension becomes apparent. Scars should be parallel to these lines, which are usually perpendicular to the vector of muscle contraction. Unsatisfactory scars can be revised and improved, but both surgeon and patient must be realistic about the aims and likely outcome of such revisional procedures. Satisfactory scars are those that cannot be improved, however displeasing the social or aesthetic considerations may

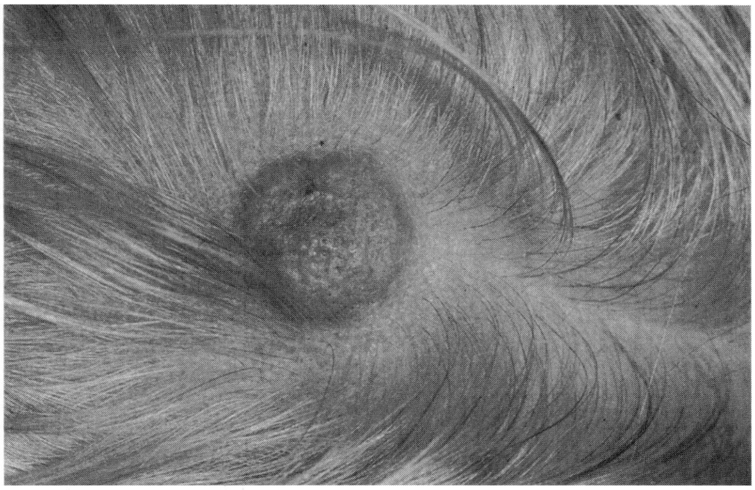

Fig. 9.66 An umbilicated cutaneous secondary from a carcinoma of the breast.

be.[180] Most scars within tension lines are aesthetic and satisfactory, many scars crossing tension lines are not. The oldest scar revision technique is elliptical excision and direct closure, but the technique which is most widely used is the Z-plasty, described in the early 1900s.[181,182] Other scars may benefit from a W-plasty.[183]

Both of these techniques break up the linear anti-tension-line scar into smaller components at oblique angles parallel to the relaxed skin tension lines, though the net scar length is longer. The Z-plasty is a double transposition flap. The increase in scar length is geometrically predictable and results from the 'borrowing' of tissue adjacent to the scar to divide it into smaller components, reducing its deformity. This borrowing of neighbouring skin to increase scar length and decrease tension is of great value in reducing contracture and its functional sequelae[184] (Fig. 9.67).

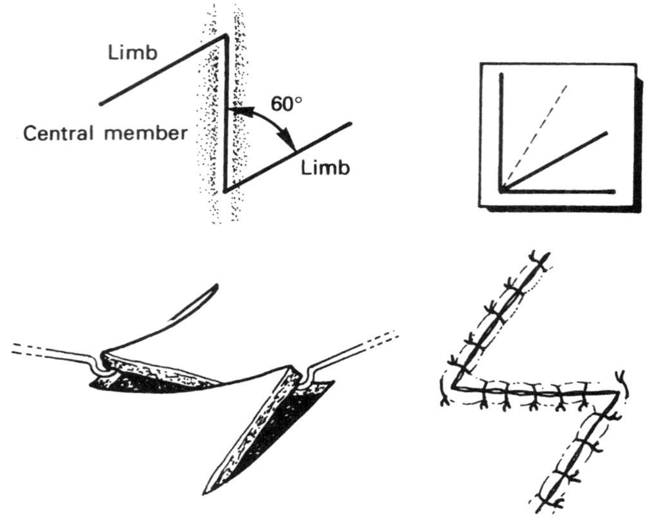

Fig. 9.67 A Z-plasty for taking the stress off a scar.

Hypertrophic scar and keloid

A scar is the natural consequence of the body's attempt to repair an area of epithelial loss, whether it be from a surgical incision, mechanical trauma or a burn. There is an enormous individual variation in the degree of scar formation and it is still not clear why some people scar badly and others scar well. Keloid scars were originally described in the Smith Surgical papyrus (2500 BC), but first given a name in 1806 by Jean Louis Alibert to describe an 'overhealing' phenomenon.[185]

The term 'keloid' is often misappropriated for all bad scars, making the true incidence difficult to define, though 6.2% has been quoted for a rural African community.[186] Much work has been done to elucidate the aetiology and pathogenesis of scar hypertrophy and keloid, but the aetiology remains unknown. The predisposition of pigmented races to aggressive keloid scarring has been attributed to abnormal melanocyte physiology, which is consistent with the observation that areas of low melanocyte density, such as the palms or the soles of the feet, have a low incidence of abnormal scarring even in pigmented races. It is not known why there is an age predisposition (see Table 9.4) but the higher incidence in younger people may reflect skin of greater youthful turgor associated with a higher rate of collagen synthesis.

Fetal tissue heals with minimal scarring,[187,188] and the potential for minimal scar carries into the early neonatal period. Wounds associated with infection, trauma, burns or tension have a greater incidence of both scar hypertrophy and keloid, though the high incidence of keloid associated with scars around the ear reflects none of these variables directly.

Under the light microscope, the two are indistinguishable, each demonstrating dense swirling collagen fibrils and a dense epidermal cell layer containing many fibroblasts and much mucinous ground substance. Under the scanning electron microscope, the collagen arrangement of keloids is more irregular with a reduction in interfibrillar distance compared to that seen in hypertrophic

REFERENCES

180. Borges A F Clin Plast Surg 1977; 4 (2): 223–237
181. Marino H Br J Plast Surg 1959; 12: 34–42
182. McGregor I A Br J Plast Surg 1966; 19: 82–87
183. Borges A F Br J Plast Surg 1959; 12: 29–33
184. McGregor I A, McGregor A Fundamental Techniques in Plastic Surgery, 16th edn. Churchill Livingstone, Edinburgh 1995
185. Alibert J L M Descriptions des Maladies de la Peau Observees á l'Hôpital Saint Louest et Expositions des Meileures. Methodes suives pour leurs Traitement. Barois l'Aine et Fils, Paris 1806 p 113
186. Oluwasanmi J O Clin Plast Surg 1974; 1: 179–195
187. Rowsell A R Br J Plast Surg 1984; 37: 635
188. Seibert J W, Burd A R et al Plast Reconstr Surg 1990; 85: 495–502

Table 9.4 Clinical characteristics of abnormal scars

	Keloid scar	*Hypertrophic scar*
Genetic predisposition	Significant Occur only in humans	Less well established Occur only in humans
Aetiology	Unknown	Unknown
Age	Puberty to 30 years	Any, but most common 8–20 years
Gender	Females > males	No predisposition
Race	Blacks and Hispanic races	No predilection
Appearance	Outgrows its scar margins, tumour-like proliferation	Remains confined to scar
Location	Earlobes, deltoid region, mandible, neck, chest	Across flexor surfaces
Clinical course	Appears months after injury and continues to grow	Appears soon after injury and regresses spontaneously
Treatment	May recur aggressively following surgery and adjuvant therapy	Responds to treatment regimens

From Rockwell et al[5]

scarring. Discrete collagen bundles do not occur, the fibres are haphazardly arranged and are not orientated parallel to the epithelial surface as in a normal scar.[189,190]

There are also biochemical differences. Proline hydroxylase activity correlates well with the rate of collagen synthesis, and it has been shown that its activity is higher in keloids than hypertrophic or normal scars, where the rate does not differ greatly from normal unscarred skin. Collagenase activity has been reported to be greater in both keloid and hypertrophic scars, seeming to indicate that total collagen turnover is increased, though these findings have been disputed.[191] The many enzyme and collagen synthesis and analysis studies, however, have not yet defined better methods of management. Relative hypoxia has been observed and mooted to be an aetiological factor in hypertrophic scar,[192] possibly causing increased but compromised fibroblast activity.

Immunological differences exist amongst patients with hypertrophic or keloid scars, though in interpreting the studies it must be noted that abnormal areas may lie adjacent to normal scar in the same individual. In keloid scars, IgG levels are increased when compared to normal scar[193] whereas there is no HLA association. Antinuclear antibodies to keloid fibroblasts have been found,[194] as have selectively increased serum levels of C3 and IgM.[195] The response of fibroblasts to epidermal growth factor and transforming growth factor β is being studied.

Some of the clinical differences between hypertrophic and keloid scarring are noted in Table 9.4 (see also Figs 9.68–70).

Treatment of keloid and hypertrophic scar

Treatment methods include conservative, surgical, radiation and chemotherapeutic approaches. The futility of surgical revision alone is apparent[196] and recurrence has been reported at 55%, irrespective of depth of excision.[197] Surgical revision is therefore usually combined with adjuvant radiotherapy, pharmacological or mechanical approaches. Wound closure is by direct suturing, local Z-plasty or skin grafting to avoid excessive tension. Full thickness skin grafts with primary closure of the donor site result in less donor site morbidity where a skin graft is deemed unavoidable.[198] Shaving of the keloid flush with normal skin and split skin grafting has been proposed but has not become popular.

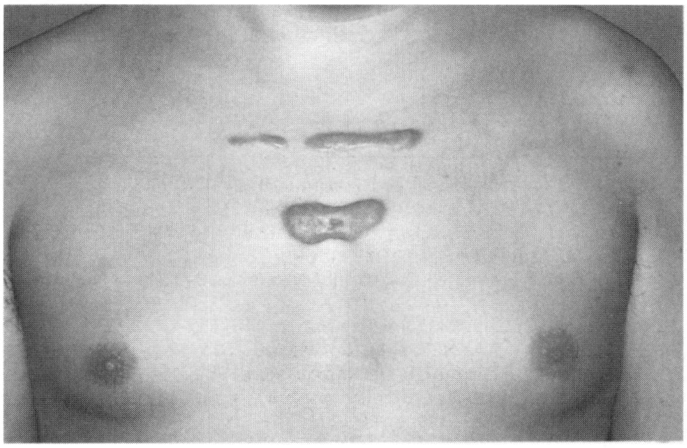

Fig. 9.68 A keloid scar.

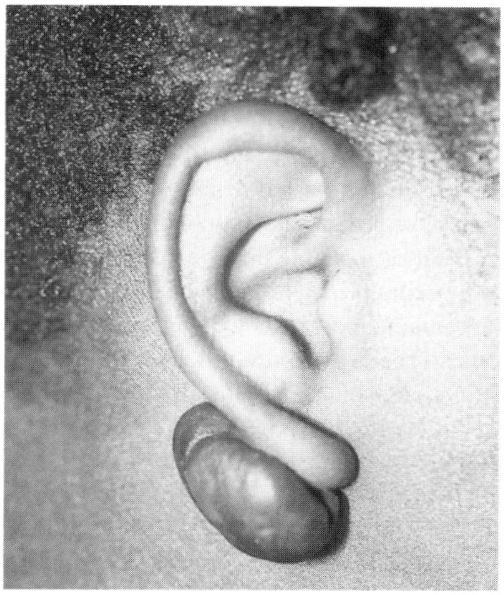

Fig. 9.69 A keloid in the earlobe following piercing.

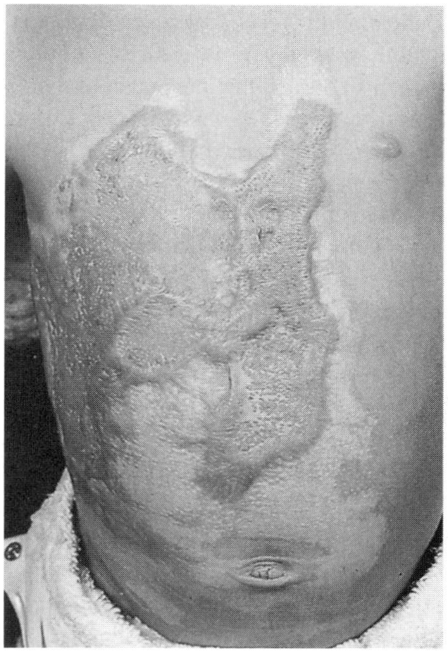

Fig. 9.70 A hypertrophic scar.

REFERENCES

189. Knapp T R, Daniels J R, Kaplan E N Am J Pathol 1977; 86: 47–70
190. Kischer C W Scanning Microsc (Pt 1) 1984; 423
191. Cohen I K, Keiser H R, Sjoerdsma A Surg Forum 1971; 22: 488–489
192. Sloan D F, Brown R D, Wells C H, Hilton J G Plast Reconstr Surg 1978; 61: 431
193. Cohen I K, McCoy B J, Mohanakumar T, Deigelmann R F Plast Reconstr Surg 1979; 63: 689–695
194. de Limpens A M, Cormane R H Aesthet Plast Surg 1982; 6: 149
195. Bloch E F, Hall M G, Denson M J, Slay-Solomon V Plast Reconstr Surg 1984; 73: 448–451
196. Da Costa J C Modern Surgery. W B Saunders, Philadelphia 1903
197. Cosman B, Wolff M Plast Reconstr Surg 1972; 50: 163–166
198. Brown L A, Pierce H E J Dermatol Surg Oncol 1986; 12: 51

The beneficial effects of mechanical pressure have been documented[199] and studies show decreased nodule formation, decreased cellularity and increased interstitial space with decreasing numbers of myofibroblasts over time.[200] The effect of pressure therapy has been attributed to relative hypoxia, also mooted as an aetiology of scar hypertrophy, and to reduced delivery of α_2-microglobulin—a collagenase inhibitor.[200] Correctly applied pressure therapy should be unrelenting, uniform, and maintained day and night for up to a year.[201] Failure occurs principally at sites of mobility where pressure cannot be maintained[202] though difficult sites, such as the earlobe, have also been successfully treated.[203] Pressure therapy is used both as treatment and prophylaxis. Silicone gel has also been reported to provide effective topical therapy[204] though its mechanism is unclear.

Radiation therapy has been used to treat keloids since 1906, and its use before and after surgery was reported by Gillies.[205] There is no clear consensus over the timing or dose of postoperative irradiation and the variation in response rates quoted makes comparison difficult.[206] Success rates of 88% have been reported; the time between excision and radiation was thought not to influence the result in 47 patients followed for between 6 months to 9 years.[207] The length of follow-up clearly influences interpretation of these results. It has been suggested that the potential morbidity of radiotherapy only justifies its use for scars resistant to surgery, pressure and steroid therapy.[208] Primary radiotherapy in the absence of surgery has not found favour for reasons of variable success and poorer cosmetic outcome.

Many pharmacological manipulations have been attempted, including vitamin E, the enzymes pepsin and hyaluronidase, and snake venom! Triamcinolone intralesional injection is the current mainstay of therapy,[206,209] and is thought to effect a decrease in normal collagen turnover. An intradermal solution of triamcinolone and lignocaine is injected into the scar, using an insulin syringe with a fixed needle, until the scar becomes white. This is a painful procedure and children may require a general anaesthetic. The patient is reviewed after 6 weeks and, if there has been some improvement, the injection may be repeated. The area should be carefully inspected to make sure there are no steroid-related skin changes, characterized by a thinning of the skin, depigmentation and the formation of multiple telangiectasia. Treatment should not be repeated if there has been no improvement in the scar.

Further therapies under investigation include laser surgery with carbon dioxide or argon beam, oral colchicine, ultrasound, topical retinoic acid and topical chemotherapy. None has yet found widespread clinical acceptance.

RECONSTRUCTIVE PLASTIC SURGERY

PRINCIPLES OF REGIONAL RECONSTRUCTION

The simplest techniques of wound closure are direct approximation in an ellipse, or methods which use lateral tissue excess such as the Z-plasty or local tissue flaps. Where local tissue cannot provide adequate structure, function or cosmesis, distant tissue must be imported in the form of distant flaps or grafts. A graft is any tissue, be it skin, nerve, vessel, bone or cartilage, that is transferred without a blood supply. Its survival therefore becomes dependent upon its acquiring a blood supply from a healthy donor bed within a limited period of time. It follows that only small or thin tissues can be transferred and that grafts must be placed into a healthy environment if they are to 'take'.

Flaps comprise tissue transferred with an intact blood supply and can therefore be of any size appropriate to the size of the defect. They can be transferred into a potentially unhealthy area where a graft would not take, such as irradiated postmastectomy skin or an open tibial fracture. Flaps often contain more than one type of tissue, and are called 'composite' flaps (e.g. fascia, fat and skin in fasciocutaneous flaps). The intact vascular pedicle used to be a limiting factor determining the distance over which the tissue transfer could take place. Vascularized tissue can now also be transferred by division of the vascular pedicle and microvascular re-anastomosis to a vessel in the recipient site. In strict terminology this is transfer of a composite vascularized graft, but this is more usually known as a 'free flap'. The different terms relating to tissue transfer are summarized in Table 9.5.

The concept of a 'reconstructive ladder' has evolved, where the surgeon plans and rejects theoretical reconstructions of increasing complexity until a suitable candidate reconstruction is selected from the possible options. In practice, a variety of techniques are usually possible, and the choice depends on the relative benefits of each to provide the best structural, functional and cosmetic outcome for the patient. The potential for complications and donor site morbidity are important considerations. The chosen method should combine the simplest procedure that provides the best possible functional and aesthetic result with the minimum donor site morbidity.

Skin grafts

Where wound closure is required but cannot be achieved without tension, a skin graft may be used (Fig. 9.71). This may be of split skin or full thickness skin with direct closure of the donor site, which is usually an area of relative laxity. Autografts are transferred within the same animal. Allografts are carried out between animals of the same species; xenografts are carried out between animals of different species, e.g. porcine skin used as a temporary cover for burn wounds (see Chapter 6).

Although successful skin grafting had been reported in the early 1800s, Reverdin[210] in Paris is credited with the first significant use

REFERENCES

199. Larson D L, Abston S et al J Trauma 1971; 11: 807–823
200. Baur P S, Larson D L et al J Trauma 1976; 16: 958–967
201. Davies D M Br Med J 1985; 290: 1056–1058
202. Rose M P, Deitch E A Burns Include Therm Inj 1985; 12: 58
203. Brent B Ann Plast Surg 1978; 1: 579–581
204. Quinn K J, Evans J H, Courtney J M, Gaylor J D S Burns 1985; 12: 102–108
205. Levitt W M, Gillies H Lancet 1942; 1: 440–442
206. Lawrence W T Ann Plast Surg 1991; 27: 164–178
207. Enhamre A, Hammar H Dermatologica 1983; 167: 90–93
208. Nicholai J P, Bos M Y, Bronkhorst F B, Smale C E Aesthet Plast. Surg 1987; 11: 29–32
209. Maguire H C JAMA 1965; 192: 325–326
210. Reverdin J L Bull Soc Imperiale Chir Paris 1869; 10

Table 9.5 Definitions of terms relating to tissue transfer

Graft	A tissue, or composite of tissues, taken from one body site (donor site) and transferred to a new (recipient) site, independent of a blood supply. The graft must gain vascularity from the recipient site bed.
Flap	A flap is comprised of tissue(s) transferred from one site of the body to another, whilst maintaining a continuous blood supply through a vascular pedicle. For the various types of flaps see text.
Pivot point	All transposition and rotation flaps rotate around a fixed point in transferring from a donor to a recipient site. This limits the potential movement of the flap, and is therefore important in planning a flap.
Island flap	A composite or free flap can be raised on a narrow single arterial pedicle for ease of transfer and to gain mobility. Such a flap is said to be 'islanded' upon the named vessel.
'Free flap'	Tissue that contains an arterial pedicle and an outflow vein, or veins, wholly detached from one body site, the donor site, and transferred to a new recipient site, where the blood supply is re-established by microvascular anastomosis.
Axial/random pattern flaps	A random pattern flap has no predictable arterial or venous anatomy, and must therefore have a wide base and short length to ensure perfusion throughout. An axial pattern flap is planned upon the predicted territory of one or several arteries and veins.
'Reverse flow' flap	A flap based upon 'reverse flow' up an artery that has been proximally severed and included in the flap, perfused by back flow via collateral branches from another arterial territory. Flaps may also be raised on a vein but are perfused initially only by relatively de-oxygenated venous blood until they gain a new vasculature in their recipient site ('parasitic' blood supply).
Neurovascular flap	A flap containing nerves allowing skin sensation or muscle tone.

of skin grafts in 1869. The use of sheet grafts was introduced by Ollier in 1872,[211] and Thiersch in 1874.[212] The reported use of full thickness skin grafts soon followed.[213–216] Subsequent advances in harvesting skin grafts were made with the introduction of guarded skin graft knives (Humby), drum dermatomes (Padgett and Hood) and mechanical dermatomes (Brown, Davis).

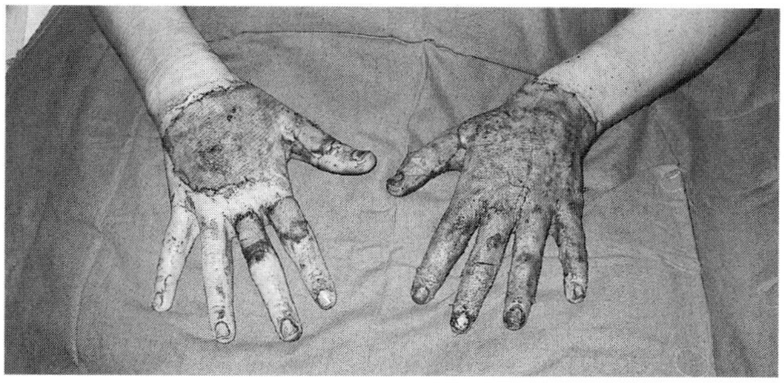

a

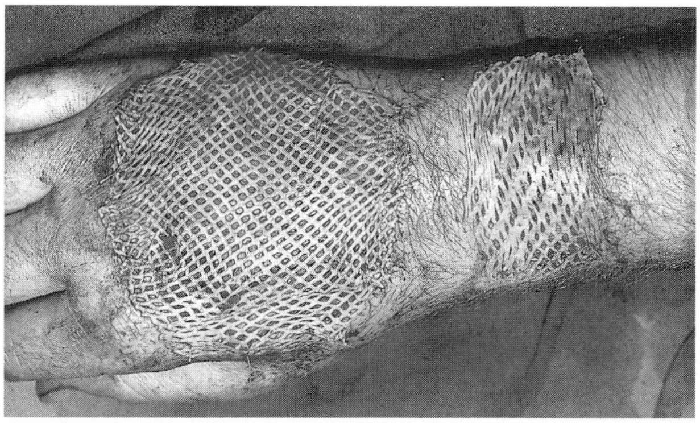

b

Fig. 9.71 (a) Sheet grafts on the dorsum of both hands. Courtesy of Mr A Phipps. **(b)** A meshed skin graft on the dorsum of the hand. Courtesy of Mr A Phipps.

Skin grafts always contain the entire thickness of the epidermis and a portion of the underlying dermis. The epidermis regenerates from hair follicles (Fig. 9.72), sebaceous glands and sweat glands within the dermis, which itself does not regenerate. The quality of a skin graft, or a donor site, is determined by the thickness of the dermis at that site. A thin split-skin graft donor site should re-epithelialize within about 10 days, with little or no residual scarring. A further skin graft can then be harvested from this site; this is frequently necessary in treating major burns (see Chapter 6). Conversely, a thick split-skin graft removes the majority of the dermis from the donor site, which then re-epithelializes slowly and is likely to form a hypertrophic scar. A thin split-skin graft, transferred to a healthy recipient site, rapidly establishes a blood supply but, because of the lack of dermis, the quality of the graft is poor and it has a tendency to contract. A thick skin graft establishes a blood supply more slowly but produces a superior end-result with less tendency to contract. Thick grafts can also develop 'ghosting'—loss of the surface of the graft, which then re-epithelializes from its adnexal structures in much the same way as the donor site.

Graft 'take'

Skin graft 'take' is a complex process. On a healthy recipient site, the graft sticks within seconds and establishes a new blood supply in 24–48 h. It is secure by 7 days. Initial adherence is produced by fibrin which is formed from extravasated plasma fibrinogen; later incorporation parallels vascular ingrowth.[217] This function of fibrin

REFERENCES

211. Ollier L Bull Acad Med 1872; 1: 243
212. Thiersch C Arch Klin Chir 1874; 17: 318
213. Pollock G C Lancet 1870; ii: 669
214. Lawson G Lancet 1870; ii: 708
215. LeFort L Bull Soc Chir Paris 1872; 1: 39
216. Wolfe J R Med Times Gazette 1876; 1: 608
217. Kelton P L Select Read Plas Surg 1992; 7(2): 1–25

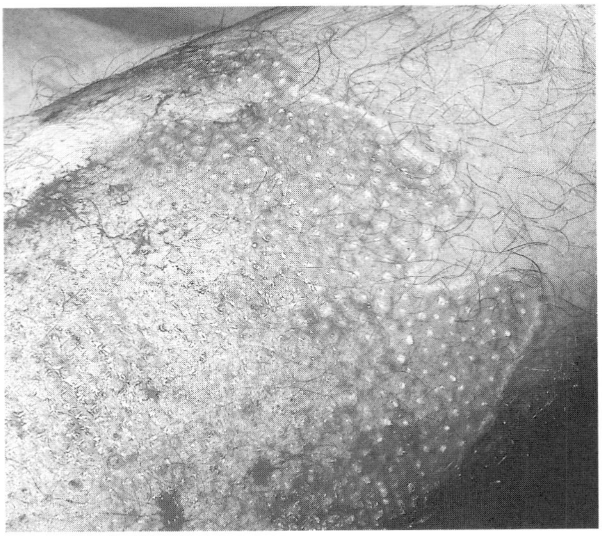

Fig. 9.72 Healing islands of epithelium around hair follicles.

has been harnessed clinically with the development of fibrin glue to fix grafts of all types.[218,219]

Until it is established, the graft survives by 'imbibition' of plasma, which is drawn up into the capillary bed of the graft. It is clear that this process can keep the graft alive until new capillary ingrowth occurs, which is a function of the vascularity and perfusion of the recipient bed. During the first few days after grafting there is great epithelial activity with an increased mitotic rate. The epithelial thickness rapidly increases and desquamation occurs. This process is less florid in full thickness grafts.[220] The ribonucleic acid content and enzymic activity also increase after about 4 days, paralleling the epithelial events.[221] The dermal component does not regenerate, and fibroblasts seen in skin graft biopsies are thought to migrate into the graft after the third day.[222] Collagen turnover approaches normal levels at 10–14 days,[217] with 85% being replaced after 5 months[223]—a turnover rate double that of normal skin. Elastin fibres have also regenerated at about one month, after initial breakdown.[224] A fine neovasculature connects the graft to capillary buds in the bed by 48 hours.[225] This may be by new ingrowth of independent vessels or by revascularization of graft vessels.[217] Lymphatic patency is established by the fifth or sixth day after grafting.[226] Sensation also returns with good 2-point discrimination as nerves enter the graft from the edge and bed of the recipient site, but full recovery takes months or years.[227]

The quality and match of a skin graft depends not only on whether it is partial-thickness or full thickness, but also on whether the donor skin has a good colour and texture match to the recipient area. Initially all grafts are white, but they revascularize to a blanchable blush over 3–4 days. A thick split graft taken from the thigh is always a poor colour and texture match for the face, whereas a full thickness postauricular Wolfe graft is an excellent match for the cheek and lower eyelid (Fig. 9.73). The choice of the skin graft and the choice of the donor site therefore depend on aesthetic and functional considerations as well as the size of the area to be covered and the state of the recipient bed.

All grafts contract after harvesting, known as primary contracture, and then again after insetting to the recipient bed, which is called secondary contracture. Thin grafts contract more than thick ones but the mechanisms by which the dermis appears to inhibit the normal wound contractile process are unclear.[228–230] Thick full-thickness skin grafts die after 3–4 days in storage, whereas after cold storage thin split-thickness skin grafts may take on a well vascularized bed up to 14 days after storage.

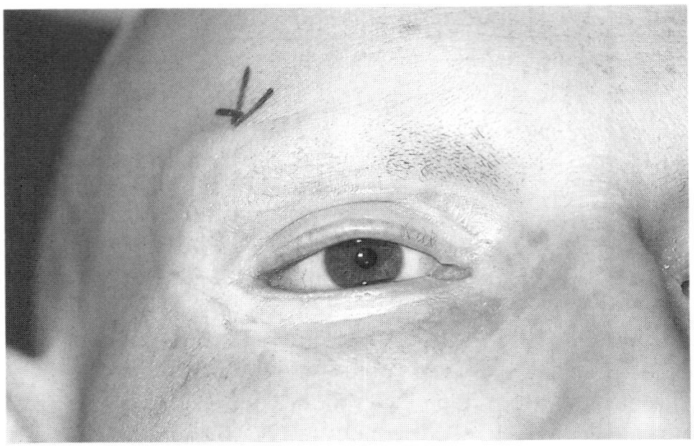

Fig. 9.73 A Wolfe graft in a case of morphea to achieve lid closure.

Requirements for skin graft take

For a skin graft to take, it is necessary for the recipient bed to have a healthy blood supply. This can be either on a freshly denuded bed, provided by the excision of a skin tumour, or healthy granulation tissue. Skin grafts do not take over exposed cortical bone without periosteum, tendon without peritenon, cartilage without perichondrium, unhealthy or necrotic tissue, or irradiated tissue. They do, however, take on most other tissues including fat, pericardium and even brain. They also take on cancellous bone and the bone of the orbit and palate.

Once a healthy bed has been prepared, new skin graft can be applied and must then be held immobile to allow a circulation to become established. It is obvious that haematoma, seroma or pus must not be allowed to build up beneath the skin graft as this separates it from the underlying bed. The skin graft can either be held in place with a dressing sutured or stapled down to the wound edges, or can be left exposed to allow any pockets of serum that develop to be let out.

Many skin grafts are now meshed, by passing them through a mesher that makes multiple symmetrical perforations (see

REFERENCES

218. Stuart J D, Moran R F, Kenney J G Ann Plast Surg 1990; 24: 52
219. Saltz R et al Plast Reconstr Surg 1991; 88: 1005–1015
220. Medawar P B J Anat 1944; 78: 157
221. Scothorne R J, Tough J S Br J Plast Surg 1952; 5: 161
222. Converse J M, Ballantyne D L Plast Reconstr Surg 1962; 30: 415
223. Rudolph R, Klein L Surg Forum 1971; 22: 489
224. Hinshaw J R, Miller E R Arch Surg 1965; 91: 658
225. Converse J M et al Br J Plast Surg 1975; 28: 274
226. McGregor I A, Conway H Transplant Bull 1956; 3: 46
227. Waris T et al Br J Plast Surg 1989; 42: 576
228. Corps B V M Br J Plast Surg 1969; 22: 125
229. Rudolph R et al Surg Forum 1977; 28: 524
230. Brown D, Garner W, Young V L South Med J 1990; 83: 789

Fig. 9.71b).[231] Meshing allows the graft to expand and cover a larger area than would be possible with an unmeshed sheet graft, thus conserving donor site. It also allows any serum or haematoma to escape through the interstices, reducing graft separation. Insetting a meshed graft into body contours is also easier than with a comparable sheet graft, and the interstices present more edges from which epithelialization can ensue. The expansion of the meshed graft depends on the size of the hole; in large burns a wide mesh is used to allow as much expansion as possible to cover the largest possible area. A major disadvantage of meshed skin grafts is that the final scar appearance is patterned, because the interstices heal by epithelialization alone, and contain no dermis. Other techniques for expansion of split-skin graft include intermingling allograft and autograft with wide expansion ratios[232] and intermingling allograft from relatives with patient autograft.[233]

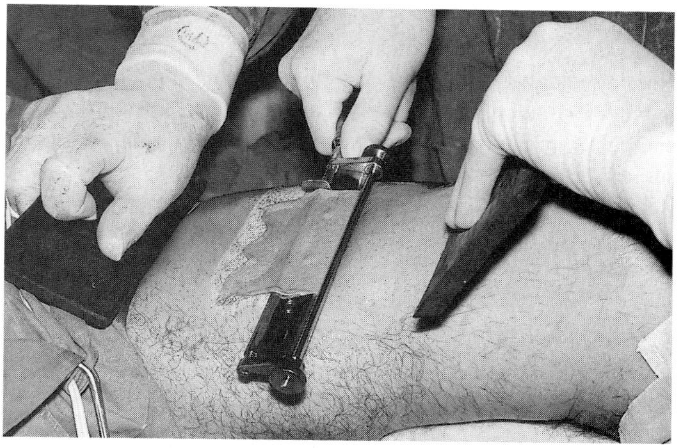

Fig. 9.74 A skin graft being taken with a hand knife.

Harvesting of skin grafts

Skin grafts can be harvested using a variety of hand-held electric or gas-powered dermatomes. The most common hand-held skin graft knives are the Watson and Braithwaite modifications of the Humby knife (Fig. 9.74). In Europe and the USA, most skin grafts are taken with an electric or gas-powered dermatome which has a great advantage over a hand knife, producing a skin graft of very even thickness from almost any site, with minimal expertise.

Donor sites

The choice of the donor site depends on the size of the area to be resurfaced and aesthetic considerations of both the recipient site and donor site. Where a very large area of skin has to be resurfaced, all available skin is pressed into donor site service, including the scalp and the sole of the foot. The best colour and texture match is obtained if the skin graft is taken from a site immediately adjacent to the defect. In general, a site is selected that can be readily concealed. Common donor sites are the thigh, the buttock and the inner arm. Less common sites are the lower leg and the trunk. The medial thigh is a reasonable donor site and is capable of providing a large sheet of skin while remaining relatively inconspicuous. Where the surface area of the defect permits, it is even better to use the buttock, especially in the young. It is often preferable to use an electric dermatome as this leaves a better scar.

In the elderly, the skin throughout the body is very thin and the best donor sites are the lateral thigh or back, as these are the sites where the dermis remains thickest. In spite of this, it is often good practice to expand the skin graft by meshing and then return half of it to the donor site as an 'over-graft' to partially close the wound.[234]

Care of the donor site

The donor site heals by epithelialization from the pilosebaceous units and to a lesser extent from sweat glands. The thinner the skin graft, the more of these adnexal structures remain, and the faster is the healing process. In a thin split-skin graft, the donor site can be expected to heal in 7–10 days, whereas a thicker graft may take up to 2 weeks. Modern dressing materials promote quicker healing with less discomfort. The most common of these materials are calcium and sodium alginate, hydrocolloid and hydrophilic dressings and various synthetic membranes.

Nerve grafts[235]

Nerve can be transferred either as a free non-vascularized graft or as a vascularized transfer. The most common donor sites are the sural nerve in the leg and the medial cutaneous nerve of the forearm. Both of these are sensory nerves but the long-term sensory deficit is negligible (see Chapter 44). The most common uses for nerve grafts are in replacing the facial nerve, either as an interposition graft or as a cross-facial nerve graft. They are also used as cable grafts for the major nerves of the upper limb, and in brachial plexus injuries. The rate of axonal growth down a nerve graft is approximately 1 mm a day, but this varies enormously with age and conditions. The longer the graft, the worse the axonal growth becomes, so that grafts longer than 10 cm show poor nerve regeneration at the distal end. Vascularized nerve grafts probably fare better than non-vascularized grafts in these situations.[236]

Bone grafts[235]

Bone can also be transferred as a non-vascularized graft or a vascularized 'free flap'; vascularized bone is better and may promote bony union in relatively avascular areas.[237] Cancellous bone is preferred as bone graft material as it establishes a blood

REFERENCES

231. Davison P M, Batchelor A G, Lewis Smith P A Br J Plast Surg 1986; 39: 462
232. Yeh F L, Yu G S et al J Burn Care Rehabil 1990; 11: 221–223
233. Phipps A R, Clarke J A Br J Plast Surg 1991; 44: 608–611
234. Rees T D, Casson P R Plast Reconstr Surg 1966; 38: 522
235. McCarthy J (ed) Plastic Surgery, vol 1. W B Saunders, London 1990 pp 630–697
236. Breidenbach W C, Terzis J K Ann Plast Surg 1987; 18: 137–146
237. Cutting C B, McCarthy J G et al Plast Reconstr Surg 1984; 74: 603–610

supply more rapidly than cortical bone. Cortical bone has, however, been used successfully in well vascularized areas.[238] Non-vascularized bone grafts are commonly used in the treatment of bony non-union, as alveolar grafts in the management of cleft lip and palate, in nasal and craniofacial reconstructions and in spinal surgery. The most common donor sites are a rib or the iliac crest. Recently, and especially in craniofacial surgery, cranial bone has been used as it is a readily accessible donor site with a concealed scar, and there seems to be less absorption of the graft.[239]

FLAPS

Definition and development

A flap is comprised of tissue, or tissues, transferred from one site of the body to another whilst maintaining a continuous blood supply through a vascular pedicle. Large amounts of composite tissue can be transferred on one or more pedicles to areas where a graft would not take or would be inadequate for reconstruction.

The biggest advance in plastic and reconstructive surgery this century has been the identification and utilization of the regional blood supply of skin. Until the early 1970s, most skin flaps were raised on a random blood supply—no thought was given to including a specific artery and vein within the flap. This 'random pattern' flap was raised with a length-to-width ratio of 1:1, as longer flaps did not have a reliable circulation, except in the well vascularized areas of the head and neck. Although the length-to-width rule was later shown to be fallacious,[240] this presumed limitation on the size of a flap led to the extensive use of the tube pedicle, which was essentially two random pattern flaps joined at their ends as a strap, which was then tubed to obliterate the raw surface. The tube pedicle was the chief tool of reconstructive surgery from its invention in 1917[241,242] until its replacement in the early 1970s by 'axial pattern' flaps. The concept of axiality was a great advance, as this allowed flaps to be raised with an increased length to breadth ratio. These flaps can be designed to cover a greater distance, with a narrower pedicle and advantageous 'pivot point' (see Table 9.5). The tube pedicle, whilst acknowledged to be a significant advance in reconstructive surgery, is now largely of historical interest only.

Anatomists and surgeons had independently described the segmental nature of the blood supply of the skin in the late 1800s[243] but it was not until 1973[244] that the distinction between random and axial pattern flaps became appreciated.

All areas of the integument have a segmental blood supply from perforating vessels which enter through the deep fascia, where this is present, from the underlying muscle or intermuscular septum. The understanding of this led to a rapid increase in the discovery of not only cutaneous axial pattern flaps, but also composite musculocutaneous, fasciocutaneous and bony composite flaps.

Axial pattern flaps are based on a named artery and vein. Isolated examples of this type of flap had been described in the plastic surgery literature throughout the 1900s,[245–250] but the dominance of the tube pedicle flap delayed their usage. Most early axial pattern flaps were purely cutaneous and had an intact skin bridge, but it was soon apparent that this type of flap could survive isolated on the vessels alone as an 'island' of skin, which made the flap more mobile. The development of microvascular surgery allowed free flaps to be transferred with immediate anastomosis to vessels at the donor site (see Table 9.6).

Classification of flaps

Flaps can be classified according to their blood supply, the method of transfer and the incorporated tissues (Fig. 9.75). All flaps are random or axial, local or distant, and can contain any tissue that is capable of transfer, including omentum and bowel. Axial flaps can be pedicled, islanded, or transferred 'free' with a microvascular anastomosis. Flaps may also contain nerves, tendons or even joints. This allows the surgeon to tailor a flap to suit the requirements of the reconstruction, for example reconstruction of the ramus of the mandible with skin cover and intraoral lining produced by a single flap.

Indications for flap reconstruction

Flaps are used in situations where grafts will not take, or where the aim is to reconstruct with tissue that is 'like for like' (bone, joint, tendon, nerve, epithelial lining, etc.), and which provides optimal structure, function and cosmesis. Flaps are also used to import a blood supply to areas of doubtful viability, such as in the reconstruction of pressure sores or after complex trauma.

There is now a vast choice of flaps for each reconstruction. Donor site morbidity has become an important consideration when planning surgery. A free radial forearm flap is often used for intraoral reconstruction in head and neck cancer, but leaves an unsightly donor site defect in a young girl. A scapular flap is better hidden, with the scar placed within the bra line, or alternatively a fascial or muscle flap can be harvested through a very short skin incision.

All flaps require careful planning; the defect should be created before the flap is raised so that one can be certain that it can be covered without tension or kinking of the vascular supply. The presence of scars which may compromise the circulation should be taken into account. When the viability of a flap is in doubt, a delayed transfer may be advisable—the flap is incised or undermined, but the actual transfer is delayed for 1–2 weeks to get the flap used to surviving on the blood supply from its base.[252]

REFERENCES

238. Piggot T A, Logan A M Br J Plast Surg 1983; 36: 9–15
239. Zins J E, Whitaker L A Plast Reconstr Surg 1983; 72: 778
240. Milton S H Br J Surg 1970; 57: 502
241. Gillies H D NY Med J 1920; 3: 1
242. Filitov V P 1917 Translated Surg Clin North Am 1959; 39: 277
243. Manchot C Die Hautarterien des Menschlichen Korpers. F C W Vogel, Leipzig 1889
244. McGregor I A, Morgan G Br J Plast Surg 1973; 26: 202
245. Tansini I Gazz Med Ital 1906; 57: 141
246. Esser J Artery Flaps. De Vos van Kleef, Antwerp 1929
247. Webster J P Surg Clin North Am 1937; 17: 145
248. Shaw D T, Payne R L Surg Gynecol Obstet 1946; 83: 205
249. Owens N Plast Reconstr Surg 1955; 15: 369
250. Bakamjian V Y Plast Reconstr Surg 1965; 36: 173
251. Hodges P L Select Read Plast Surg 1992; 7(3): 1–31
252. Myers M B, Cherry G W Plast Reconstr Surg 1969; 44: 52

Table 9.6 Milestones in the modern evolution of surgical flaps

Date/surgeon	*Milestone*
1814 Carpue; 1818 von Graefe	Forehead flap rhinoplasty, pedicled random pattern flaps
Late 19C, early 20C Mutter, Gersuny, Trotter, Volkmann, Deiffenbach, Morax, Syndacker	Random pattern cutaneous flaps
1906 Tansini	Latissimus dorsi muscle flap for breast reconstruction
1907 Syndacker, 1908 Morax	Platysma flaps
1917 Filatov, Ganser, Gillies, Aymard	First tube pedicled flaps; observations of the value of delay
1919 Davis	Observations on pedicled flaps, review of Manchot's work describing vascular territories
1921 Blair	Delay phenomenon in non-pedicled flaps
1936 Salmon	Arterial anatomy of skin flaps (long unrecognized thereafter)
1942 Converse, 1946 Kazanjian	Median forehead flap
1946 Shaw & Payne	Hypogastric flap (tubed)
1955 Owens	Compound sternomastoid skin flap
1963 Bakamjian	Deltopectoral flap
1972 McGregor & Jackson	Groin flap
1950s and 1960s Conley, DesPrez, Egerton, Wilson, Wookey, Zovikian	Empiric development of head and neck and trunk flaps
1973 McGregor & Morgan	Formalization of 'axial' and 'random pattern' flaps; arterial anatomic territories and importance of 'dynamic' arterial territories
1967 Wilson	Arterial anatomy and angiotomes
1973 Behan & Wilson	Angiotomes and 'prop' arteries defined
1968 Ger	Muscle flaps rediscovered
1970s Atlanta, Georgia: McCraw, Furlow, Vasconez, Mathes, Nahai, Maxwell, Orticochea, Serafin	Muscle and musculocutaneous local and free flaps
1963 Goldwyn et al	First experimental free tissue transfer
1963 in Shanghai	Successfully replanted hand (Chen 1982)
1965 Komatsu & Tamai	First complete thumb replant
1967 Cobbett	First toe thumb transfer
1971 Antia & Buch 1972 McLean & Buncke; Harii et al 1973 Taylor & Daniel; O'Brien	First English literature reports of human free tissue transfer
1976 Radovan	Expanded flaps
1981 Ponten	Fasciocutaneous flaps
1987 Taylor & Palmer	Angiosomes

After Cormack & Lamberty[3] and Hodges[251]

Types of flap in common use

Local flaps

All local flaps use local tissue laxity to provide wound closure 'borrowing from Peter to pay Paul'.

Advancement. This is the simplest type of flap. The skin is undermined and advanced to cover the defect. Direct closure of an elliptical defect is, in effect, the advancement of opposing flaps to allow the skin edges to be primarily sutured.

V–Y and Y–V flaps. These are advancement flaps that mobilize skin on a subdermal pedicle containing blood vessels. The skin is mobilized by selective undermining and is retained in its new position by careful suturing to take up the tension (Fig. 9.76). The donor site is directly closed.

Transposition. A flap of skin is transposed to cover an adjacent defect, leaving a secondary defect. The pivot point of the flap is the base of the flap furthest from the defect and dictates the distance the flap will reach (Fig. 9.77). A Z-plasty is a type of transposition flap (see Fig. 9.67).

Bilobed. This is a transposition flap where a secondary, smaller flap is also raised to fill the primary donor defect (Fig. 9.78) and the secondary donor defect is directly closed.

Rhomboid. The defect is designed (excised) in a rhomboid shape, and an equivalent rhomboid of adjacent skin is transposed to cover it, such that it is possible to close the secondary defect in the direction of greatest skin laxity (Fig. 9.79). There are four possible geometric flaps for each defect, though only two optimal clinical choices to place the resultant scar in relaxed skin tension lines.[253]

Rotation. This is a semi-circle of skin that rotates to fill an adjacent defect, usually allowing primary closure of the donor defect. Many such flaps combine elements of transposition and rotation. Local skin flaps are particularly useful in the head, face and neck where there is a greater capillary density in the dermis than elsewhere (Fig. 9.80).[254]

Distant flaps

Distant tissue can be imported as pedicled or free flaps. Pedicled flaps can be 'islanded', where the skin paddle is entirely detached

REFERENCES

253. Borges A F Plast Reconstr Surg 1978; 62(4): 542–545
254. Pasyk K A et al Plast Reconstr Surg 1989; 83: 939

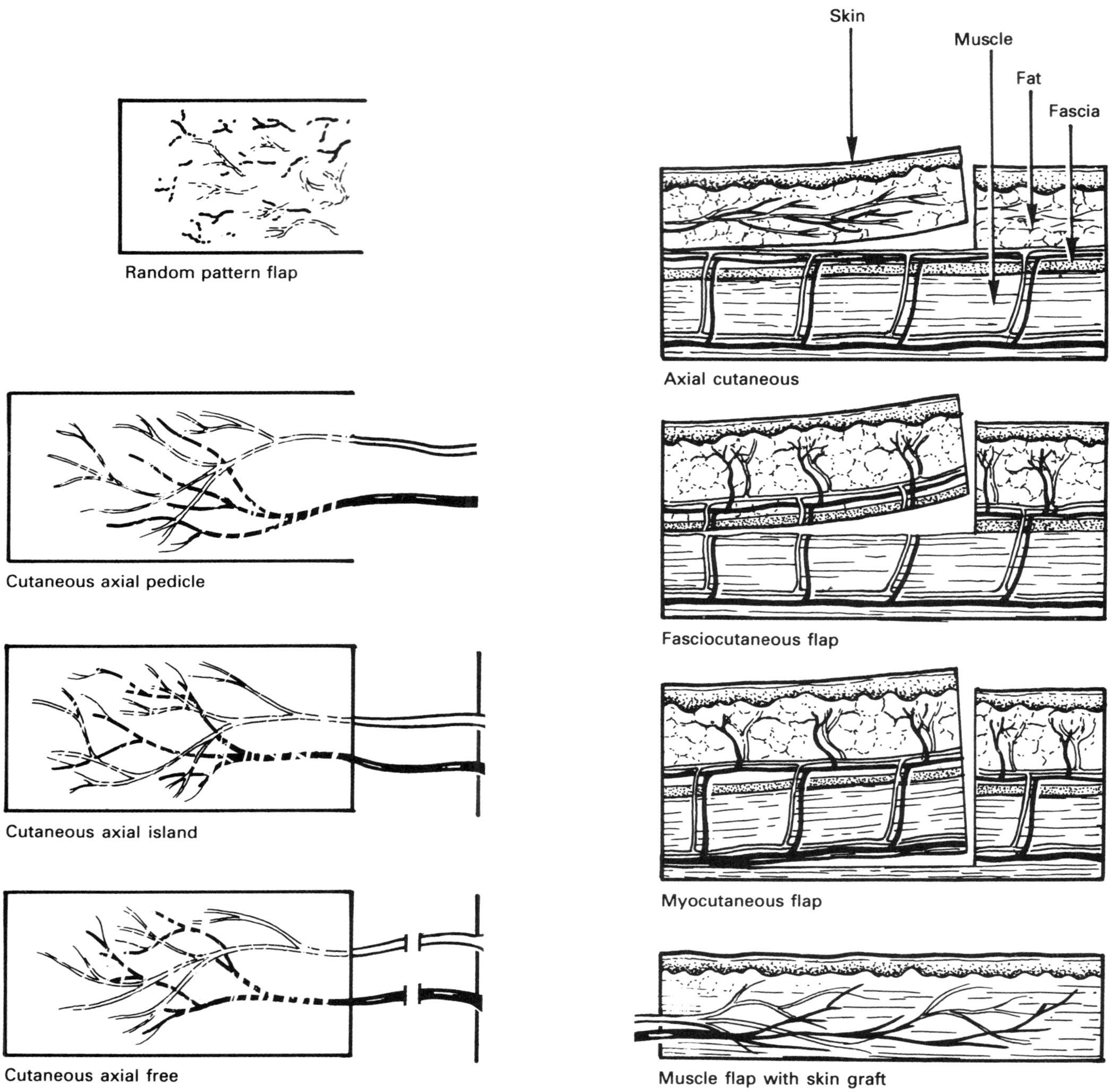

Fig. 9.75 Random and axial flaps: random flaps have a random vascular supply based on the subdermal vascular plexus. Axial flaps have a known vascular supply based on a named artery and vein. This makes them much safer and more versatile. Axial flaps may be raised as skin and fat only; skin, fat and fascia; skin, fat, fascia and muscle, depending on the blood supply to the skin. They may also be fascia or muscle only, which can then be grafted.

from the surrounding skin except for a subcutaneous vascular pedicle, allowing greater mobility (Fig. 9.81).

Although the 'reconstructive ladder' escalates through theoretical reconstructions of increasing complexity—skin graft, local flap, distant flap, composite flaps, island flaps versus pedicled flaps, free tissue transfer, composite neurovascular free tissue transfer—all the options are now commonly performed by suitably experienced teams. Reconstruction with composite free tissue transfer is the treatment of choice if it gives a better functional and cosmetic result with a more tolerable donor site deficit than skin grafting. The ladder is thus used as a 'surgical sieve' of available options, which are considered for their suitability in individual patients.

Axial pattern skin flaps

These flaps are based on arteries and accompanying veins which run in the subcutaneous fat, superficial to the deep fascia and parallel to the skin surface. Such end arteries are confined to

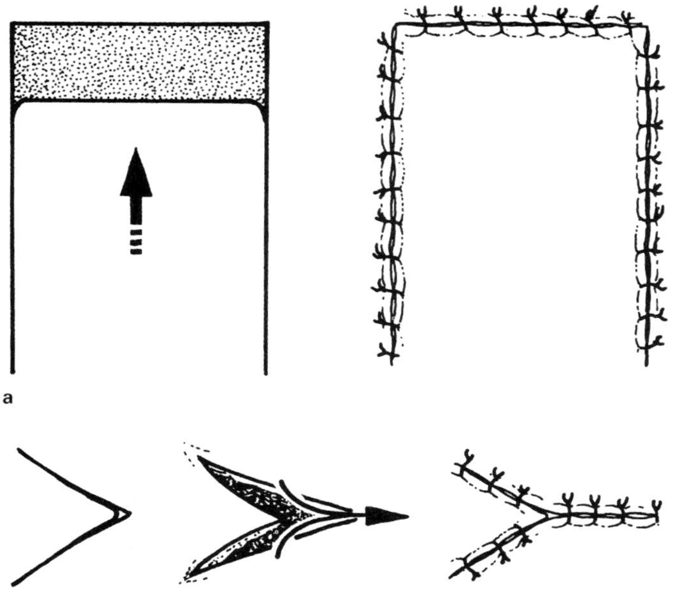

Fig. 9.76 (**a**) An advancement flap; (**b**) a V–Y plasty advancement.

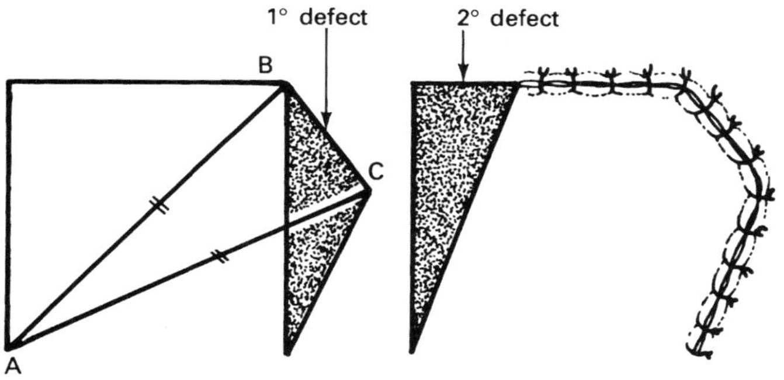

Fig. 9.77 A transposition flap.

certain areas of the anatomy, and are not connected deeply by perforators to the fascial or muscular systems, allowing large mobile skin islands to be raised upon them (see Table 9.7). The territories that they easily perfuse, based on cadaveric injection studies, are termed their 'anatomic' territories.[3]

Dynamic and potential territories

In addition to the arterial territories predicted by cadaveric perfusion studies, each artery has a 'dynamic' territory that it will perfuse through collateral vessels if their perfusion pressure from an alternative source falls. This 'dynamic' territory can be exploited by ligating a neighbouring high pressure trunk. An example is the forehead flap based on the superficial temporal artery; this can perfuse the territories of the ligated ipsilateral and contralateral supraorbital and supratrochlear arteries and that of its contralateral namesake—a dynamic territory of four anatomic territories—to provide a much larger flap.

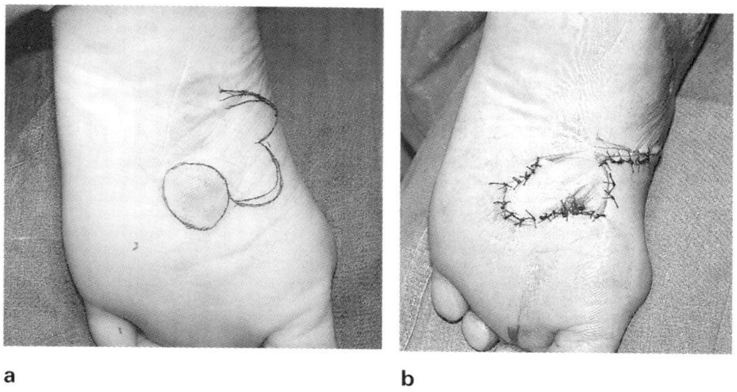

Fig. 9.78 A bilobed flap used to resurface a defect on the sole of the foot (see Fig. 9.16).

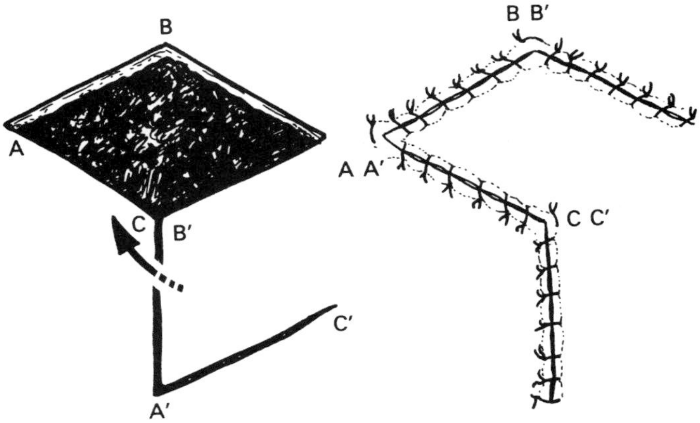

Fig. 9.79 A rhomboid flap.

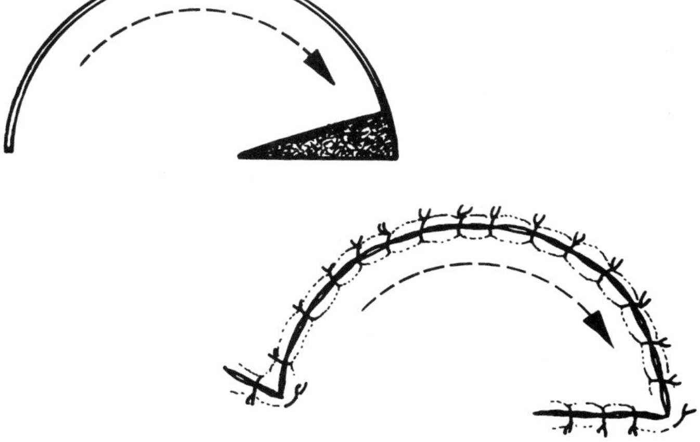

Fig. 9.80 A scalp rotation flap.

A further 'potential' territory is also available. This is most easily demonstrated by clinical experience, and cannot be plotted by knowledge of the anatomy alone. The 'potential territory' consists of the area supplied by both the 'anatomic' and 'dynamic' territories, plus a variable area of tissue beyond, perfused by vessels of a random pattern.[3]

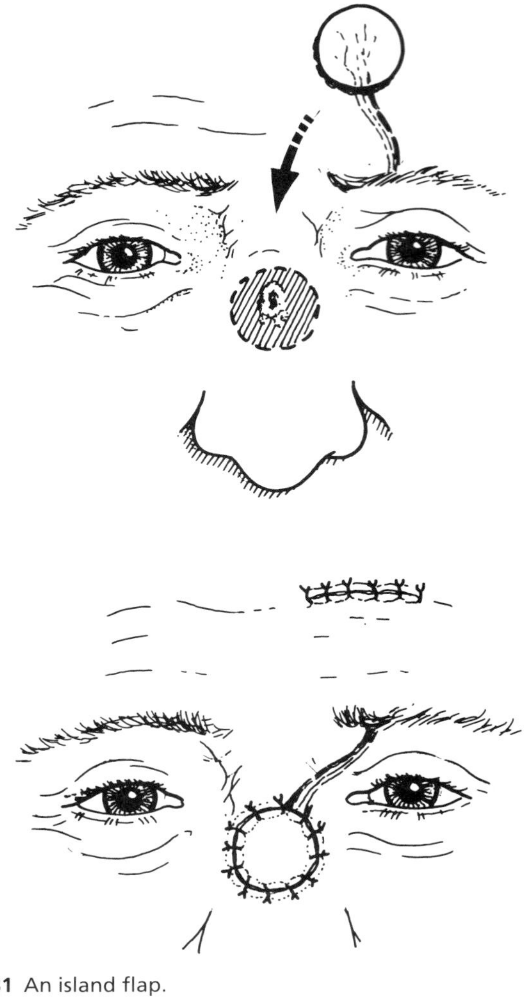

Fig. 9.81 An island flap.

Table 9.7 Axial pattern flaps and the vessels on which they are based

Direct cutaneous vessel	*Clinical surgical flap*
Superficial temporal artery	Forehead flap
Supratrochlear and supraorbital artery	Median forehead flap
Posterior auricular artery	Postauricular flap
Internal thoracic artery—2nd/3rd intercostal perforators	Deltopectoral flap
Superficial circumflex iliac artery	Groin flap
Superficial inferior epigastric artery	Hypogastric flap
Dorsalis pedis artery	Dorsalis pedis flap

Musculocutaneous flaps

These are composite flaps containing skin, subcutaneous fat, fascia and muscle based on one or more perforating branches to the skin from vessels primarily supplying muscle. These perforating vessels pierce the deep fascia and ramify in the subcutaneous tissues (see Fig. 9.75). Musculocutaneous flaps were described in the literature as early as 1906,[245] and isolated descriptions appeared intermittently in the literature.[255,256] More recently, Ger rediscovered their potential and described the use of muscle flaps with skin grafts to cover difficult lower limb defects and pressure sores.[257]

The current plethora of musculocutaneous flaps were mostly described in the 1970s following the understanding of the axial flap principle.[244] All or part of the muscle may be detached from its origin, its insertion, or both, and transferred with a paddle of overlying skin as a local, distant or free flap. The blood supply to the muscles of the body varies,[258,259] making some muscles more suitable than others for use as musculocutaneous or muscle flaps, but there are few, if any, muscles that have not been used in reconstructive surgery (Table 9.8). Increasing anatomical knowledge has allowed selective raising of muscle flaps to leave innervated, perfused mucle bellies behind to minimize donor deficit, e.g. the latissimus dorsi flap, or include them in the flap, e.g. the neurovascular gracilis for facial reanimation surgery. Similarly, combination muscle flaps may be raised together, e.g. the latissimus dorsi with the serratus anterior, or tensor fasciae latae with gluteus medius. Muscle flaps are useful to fill dead space with well vascularized tissue, and provide the possibility of motor function.

The muscles of the body have been classified into five groups (see Table 9.9), some of which are interchangeable, depending upon their clinical context.[3,258]

Several important features of the applied anatomy of muscle flaps must be considered in flap planning. It is important to know whether the muscle is to be raised with skin, and the quantity and mobility of the available skin paddle. Skin is most commonly used as a waterproof lining or surface cover, and is also valuable postoperatively to monitor perfusion of the whole composite flap by its capillary refill. The pedicle length, and variability and reliability of the possible alternative pedicles, are important to plan the mobility or arc of rotation of the flap. Similarly the suitability of the pedicle for microanastomosis must be considered if free flap transfer is an alternative. The nerve supply and function is an important consideration, either to protect in the donor deficit, or to utilize in the flap. Increasingly, donor site morbidity is a key consideration in the choice of flap design.

Fasciocutaneous and adipofascial flaps

Although the value of taking the deep fascia with a skin flap to improve its blood supply had been suggested in 1920,[260,261] the role of the fascial perforating blood vessels in enhancing the surviving length of skin flaps was not appreciated until 1981.[262] Fascial, adipofascial and fasciocutaneous flaps have less bulk than equivalent musculocutaneous flaps, which is advantageous in certain situations, e.g. inside the mouth or on the dorsum of the hand.

The fasciocutaneous system incorporates vessels passing to the skin along fascial septa, between, rather than through muscle bellies, to fan out in the deep fascial plexus—predominantly its superficial surface. These plexuses in turn send superficial

REFERENCES

255. Hueston J T, McConchie H A Aust NZ J Surg 1968; 38: 61–63
256. Olivari N Br J Plast Surg 1976; 29: 126–128
257. Ger R Surgery 1968; 63: 757
258. Mathes S J, Nahai F Plast Reconstr Surg 1981; 67: 177–187
259. Mathes S J, Nahai F Clinical Applications for Muscle and Musculocutaneous Flaps. CV Mosby, St Louis 1982
260. Esser J Berlin Klin Wochenschr 1918; 55: 1197
261. Gillies H D NY Med J 1920; 3: 1

Table 9.8 Commonly used flaps

Cutaneous and fasciocutaneous flaps	*Muscle and myocutaneous flaps*	*Specialized parts and organs*
Scalp, forehead	Trapezius	Bones
Temporal fascia	Pectoralis major	Rib—alone, with serratus anterior, with latissimus dorsi
Supraclavicular	Pectoralis minor	Sternum with pectoralis major
Deltopectoral	Serratus anterior	Humerus with lateral arm
Scapular, parascapular	Latissimus dorsi	Scapula with trapezius (spine) or scapular flap (medial border)
Deltoid	External oblique	Radius with radial forearm
Axillary	Internal oblique	Radius with ulnar forearm
Lateral arm	Superior rectus abdominis	Iliac crest with groin flap
Medial arm	Inferior rectus abdominis	Fibula with or without skin
Radial forearm (Chinese)	Superior gluteus maximus	Toe transfers
Ulnar forearm	Inferior gluteus maximus	Pulp transfers
Groin, hypogastric	Gracilis	Nail bed transfers
Medial thigh	Tensor fasciae latae	Joint transfers
Anterior thigh	Rectus femoris	Vascularized nerve
Lateral thigh	Gastrocnemius	Testes
Posterior thigh		Small bowel
Anterior tibial		Large bowel
Posterior tibial		Omentum
Saphenous		
Sural		
Dorsalis pedis		
Sole of foot		

Table 9.9 Classification of the vascular anatomy of muscles

Group	*Vascularity*	*Examples*
Type I	One vascular pedicle	Gastrocnemius; tensor fasciae latae; vastus intermedius
Type II	Dominant vascular pedicle at muscle attachment; smaller pedicles to muscle belly	Biceps femoris, semitendinosus, rectus femoris, vastus lateralis, gracilis, soleus, peroneus longus and brevis, brachioradialis, trapezius, platysma, sternomastoid, temporalis
Type III	Two vascular pedicles	Gluteus maximus, rectus abdominis serratus anterior, orbicularis oris
Type IV	Multiple equal pedicles	Vastus medialis, sartorius, flexor digitorum longus, flexor hallucis longus; extensor digitorum longus, extensor hallucis longus, tibialis anterior
Type V	Dominant vascular pedicle, plus minor segmental pedicles	Pectoralis major, latissimus dorsi

branches to the skin, thus allowing the fascia to be raised as an adipofascial or fasciocutaneous flap. Initial length to breadth ratios of 2.5:1 were achieved in the notoriously difficult area below the knee (Fig. 9.82),[262] dramatically improving choice in the management of both upper and lower limb defects.

There are several important features to consider in planning these flaps. The size and presence of an axial vessel to the fascial plexus must be considered in pedicled or free flap planning. The contribution of perforators to the plexus, and whether they can be sacrificed must be appreciated before the flap is raised. Donor site morbidity is also an important consideration.

Microvascular surgery and free tissue transfer

An operating microscope has been used in otolaryngology and ophthalmology for decades, but after the pioneering work of Carel[263] and Guthrie[264] in the early 1900s microvascular and microneural surgery did not resume until the 1960s. Successful replantation of severed limbs and digits[265,266] was followed in 1969 by the first elective transfer of a toe to replace an amputated thumb.[267] Improving equipment and techniques coincided with the recognition of axial pattern flaps, and the first successful free skin flap transfer occurred in 1973.[268]

Initially, free flap transfer was considered a complex and time-consuming procedure, only used where other methods were not available and often occupying a whole day in the operating theatre. Free flaps were felt to be less reliable than conventional flaps, and a great deal of time and ingenuity were put into devices that monitored the flap postoperatively[269] to allow early intervention in case of failure. Increasing experience has demonstrated that microvascular transfer of flaps need take little longer than conventional transfer, and that flap survival is often better than conventional pedicle transfer. Use of free flaps is now routine in reconstructive surgery.

Indications

Free flap transfers have many advantages over conventional flaps, often making them the procedure of choice in quite simple

REFERENCES

262. Ponten B Br J Plast Surg 1981; 34: 215
263. Carel A Lyon Med 1902; 98: 859
264. Guthrie C Blood Vessel Surgery and its Application. University of Pittsburgh Press, Pittsburgh 1912
265. Malt R A, McKhann C JAMA 1964; 189: 716
266. Komatsu S, Tamai S Plast Reconstr Surg 1965; 42: 374
267. Cobbett J R J Bone Joint Surg 1969; 51: 677–699
268. Daniel R K, Taylor G I Plast Reconstr Surg 1973; 52: 111–117
269. Jones B M Plast Reconstr Surg 1984; 73: 843–850

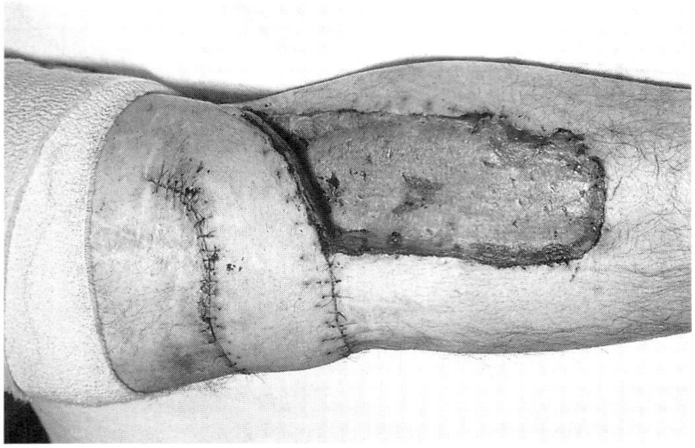

Fig. 9.82 A fasciocutaneous flap used to cover a defect of the upper tibia (note a length-to-width ratio in excess of 3:1).

situations. Microvascular transfer of a flap allows the flap to be exactly tailored to fit the size and requirements of the defect, without the constraints of a pedicle. It allows a single-stage reconstruction that can dramatically shorten hospital stay, negating the cost of increased operating time. A wide choice of possible donor sites allows the surgeon to use an appropriate flap for a better aesthetic result that causes the minimum donor defect. A free flap may bring in an improved blood supply to an unhealthy or ischaemic area, e.g. irradiated tissues. Free flaps have a 95% success rate,[270] and can be moved to almost any area of the body and taken from almost anywhere. Free tissue transfer does, however, require an increased operating time (although this is becoming shorter) and the need for specialized equipment and training.

Types of free flaps

Any tissue that can be isolated on a vascular pedicle can be transferred by microvascular techniques. Some of the more common flaps and tissues are listed in Table 9.8. The list is by no means comprehensive, but includes those flaps that are used most often and which fulfil the majority of reconstructive needs. A healthy free flap should be pink, show normal refilling of the capillaries on digital pressure, have a nominal tissue tension, be at the same temperature as the adjacent tissues, and show normal bleeding in response to a pinprick. Some healthy free flaps with very good venous drainage may be pale and apparently flaccid, and the most reliable test of their patency is to stab the flap with a pin, although not over the vascular pedicle, and watch for bleeding. Venous failure produces a very pink flap with rapid capillary refilling and marked swelling and congestion. The colour changes to purple to blue to black, and immediate surgical intervention is required at the pink to purple stage to re-perform the venous anastomosis, as a delay of even 30 minutes can mean the difference between flap salvage and failure.

The next major advance in plastic and reconstructive surgery is likely to be the safe suppression of allograft tissue rejection that will allow reconstruction of complex areas of the body using tissue transplantation.

TISSUE EXPANSION

The principle of tissue expansion has been apparent throughout human history. Pregnancy, obesity, lymphoedema and a variety of other physiological and pathological conditions cause stretching of the skin that all too often produces a permanent redundancy that may require surgical removal. It required a leap of imagination to turn a surgical problem to surgical advantage. In 1976, Radovan presented skin expansion as a new technique for the reconstructive surgeon.[271] The technique involves localized stretching of skin using an inflatable silicone implant, which is surgically placed underneath normal skin adjacent to a defect or area that is to be excised (Fig. 9.83). Over a few weeks, the implant is inflated through a remote valve using injections of normal saline. Once sufficient skin has been generated, the implant is removed, the lesion is excised and the resulting defect is covered utilizing the excess skin produced by the expander. In effect, a skin flap has been preformed at an ideal site to allow reconstruction of the defect.

Radovan subsequently discovered that a similar method had been used by Neumann in 1957[272] and that others had been working independently on the same lines.[273,274] Radovan, however, brought the technique into popular use, now employed successfully in all areas of reconstructive surgery. In many areas of the body the skin has specific characteristics which cannot be matched by skin grafts or distant skin flaps. The best example is the hair-bearing scalp—extensive loss of hair, whether from trauma or natural processes, may leave a defect that is difficult to replace (Fig. 9.84), and in the past such patients were condemned to wear a wig. Tissue expansion allows the use of adjacent matching skin that has all the characteristics appropriate to that site. Apart from hair-bearing properties, these also include colour, texture, thickness and sensation.

There are other advantages of tissue expansion over conventional techniques. There is no donor defect, as occurs with skin

REFERENCES

270. Shaw W W In: Furnas P (ed) Frontiers of Microsurgery. C V Mosby, St Louis 1983
271. Radovan C Am Soc Plast Reconstr Surg Forum. Boston, Mass, September 30th 1976
272. Neuman C G Plast Reconstr Surg 1957; 19: 124–129
273. Austad E D, Rose G L Plast Reconstr Surg 1982; 70: 588–594
274. Lapin R, Daniel D et al Breast 1980; 6: 20–26

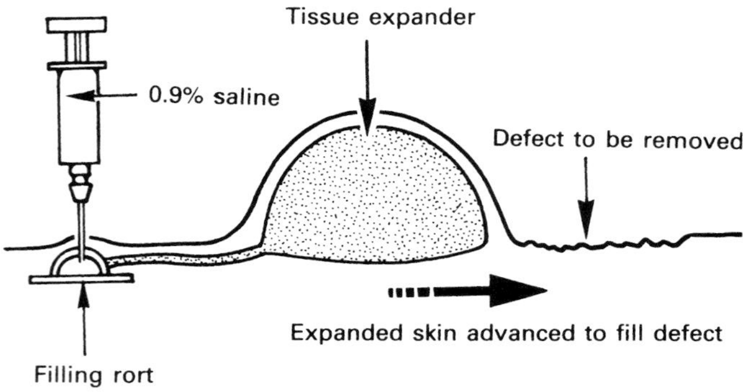

Fig. 9.83 The technique of tissue expansion.

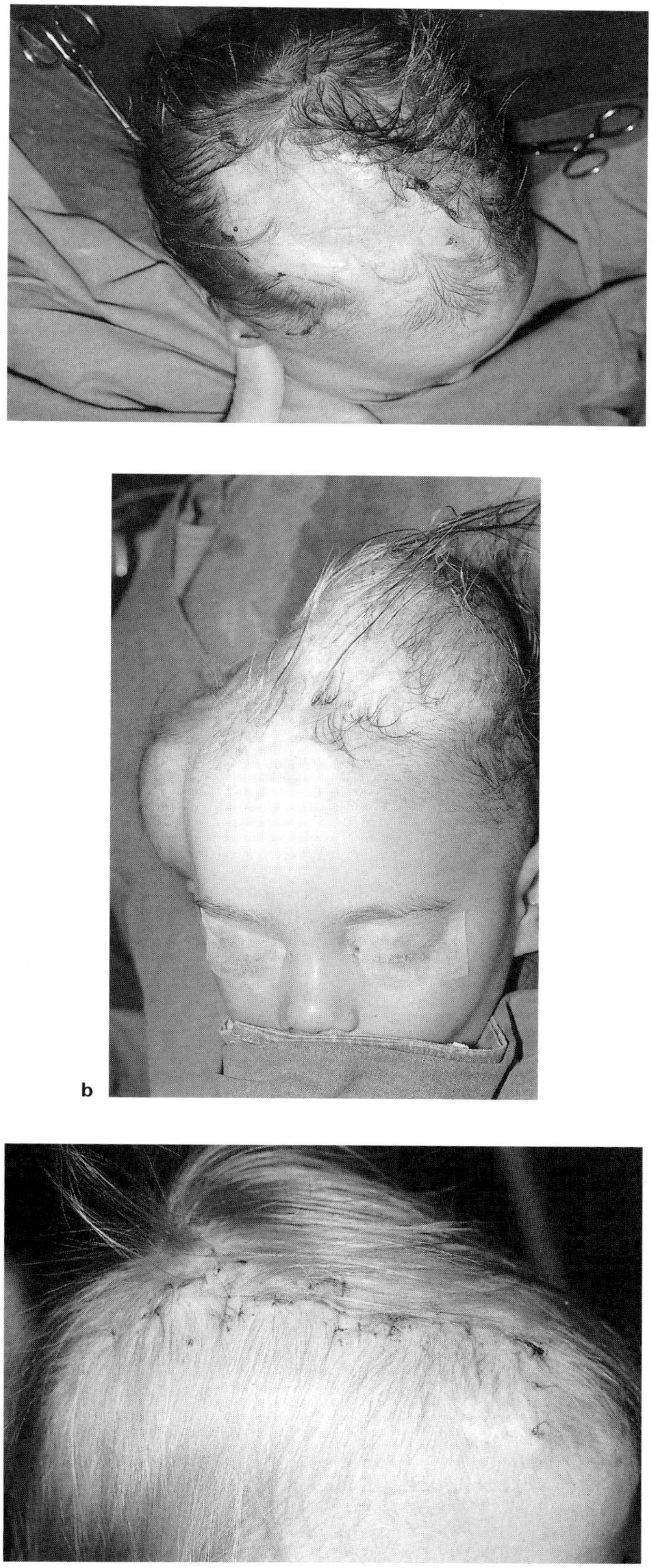

Fig. 9.84 Tissue expanders used to close a scalp defect caused by a burn. (a) Scalp defect; (b) expanded tissue; (c) closed defect.

grafts and distant flaps. The expanded skin has an increased vascularity,[275,276] which helps in the design of safe skin flaps and may promote the revascularization of bone grafts placed beneath. Epidermal thickness remains the same as unexpanded skin, but the dermis becomes progressively thinner.[277,278] This dermal thinning is compensated for by the thickness of the highly vascularized[279] capsule surrounding the implant, so that there is little overall thinning of the flap that is then used for reconstruction. The dermis eventually returns to normal, but hair follicles and other adnexal structures become separated in expanded skin. Their morphology remains normal and the separation that occurs in scalp expansion is rarely of any clinical importance.

The effect on other structures is less clear. It is known that expanded muscle undergoes some atrophic changes, but this does not invariably seem to affect muscle function severely. It has been used to advantage by some clinicians[280] and opens up the possibility of tailoring innervated muscles for reconstruction, such as in facial palsy. The effect on nerves, tendons and other structures is currently being investigated. The benefits of being able to fashion tailor-made muscle, tendon and nerve units are enormous.

There are several disadvantages that may make the technique unsuitable for individual cases. Time is required to inflate the balloon—between 3 and 25 weeks[281] depending on site, age of the patient and the amount of skin required. During this time, the patient has to attend the hospital at least twice a week to have the expander inflated, on each occasion by a percutaneous injection, which can be traumatic for some children. This is an expensive proposition for patients who live a long way from the hospital, or who have other social or economic commitments. There is also the problem of the appearance of the expander during this time. Many patients prefer to remain indoors between hospital visits, because of embarrassment.

The complication rate can be as high as 40%.[279] The most common complications are infection, haematoma, exposure of the expander or tubing (either through the incision or by erosion through the skin) and implant failure causing a leak and deflation. In practice, the vast majority of these complications do not affect the final result, and can be controlled by conservative measures while inflation continues.

There seem to be very few areas of the body that cannot be expanded, given careful planning and the correct type of expander. It has yet to be determined how often the same area of skin can be expanded. The theoretical advantages this offers for resurfacing large areas of the body, such as in burns scarring or to replace giant hairy naevi, are immense. Tissue expansion has been used to treat

REFERENCES

275. Cherry G W, Austad E et al Plast Reconstr Surg 1983; 72: 680–687
276. Sasaki G H, Krizek T J Plast Surg Res Council. Durham, North Carolina, May 19th 1983
277. Austad E D, Pasyk K et al Plast Reconstr Surg 1982; 70: 704–710
278. Pasyk K A, Austad E Plast Reconstr Surg 1984; 74: 493–507
279. Manders E K, Schenden M et al Plast Reconstr Surg 1982; 70: 37–47
280. Radovan C Plast Reconstr Surg 1984; 74: 482–492
281. Leonard A G, Small J O Br J Plast Surg 1986; 39: 42–56

traumatic hair loss and male-pattern baldness, in scar and tattoo removal, in ear and nasal reconstruction, in syndactyly, in facial reconstruction, for port wine stains and giant pigmented naevi—in fact, anywhere where there is a defect to be covered. Expanders are even available which allow primary cleft palate closure or alveolar ridge restoration in the edentulous patient to allow dentures to be fitted. The future use of expanders is likely to be limited only by the surgeon's imagination and implant design.

AESTHETIC SURGERY

There is no clear boundary that separates aesthetic or cosmetic surgery from reconstructive surgery, and patients seeking such surgery can have physical and psychological difficulties that are as severe as those of patients presenting for reconstructive surgery. The existence of aesthetic surgery is dependent on preconceptions of 'normal' that vary from society to society, and the desire of individuals to fit into the normal group. This need by the majority of individuals to be accepted blends imperceptibly with the desire of other individuals to remain young. A child is often made aware of his prominent ears or repaired cleft lip from the first day of school; adults may view a receding hairline or varicose veins with dread. In assessing the suitability of a patient for aesthetic surgery, the surgeon must have an idea of what represents 'normal', but more importantly must assess the effect that the abnormality is having on the patient, and whether surgery will be truly beneficial. The history should include a comprehensive social history and a psychological evaluation of the patient's suitability and expectations. Where there is any doubt, formal psychological evaluation should be requested.

It is usual for 'normal' people to be unsympathetic towards friends or relatives wishing to have aesthetic surgery, as this wish is often derided as a weakness of character or a whim rather than a permanent inability to accept their appearance. This blemish frequently becomes a dominating factor in the patient's life, and life can be transformed if it can be permanently corrected.[282,283]

Blepharoplasty and face lift

Indications

These procedures are amongst the most hazardous and time consuming in aesthetic surgery, and are outside the scope of this book. The normal indications are to improve the ageing face but other indications include descent of the eyelids sufficient to obscure normal vision, static correction of facial palsy, congenital craniofacial conditions, and removal of excessive skin in neurofibromatosis and vascular tumours.

Blepharoplasty, or eyelid reduction, involves removal of excess eyelid skin and fat through an upper eyelid crease and lower subciliary or transconjunctival incisions (Fig. 9.85). The most common complications are haematomas and the excision of too much skin on the lower lids giving rise to an ectropion that can be very difficult to correct (see Chapter 15).

A face lift is carried out through the incision shown in Figure 9.86 or a close variant. The skin is undermined as shown, pulled up and back, and excess skin is excised at the hair-bearing areas, where the weight of the face lift is taken. Remaining skin is then trimmed off without tension in front of and behind the ears. The most common complications are haematoma formation, skin loss, especially behind the ears in covert smokers, infection, and damage to the branches of the facial nerve that supply the forehead and lower lip. There are many variations on both blepharoplasty and face lift in approach and execution, and interested readers are referred to the listed texts.[284–286]

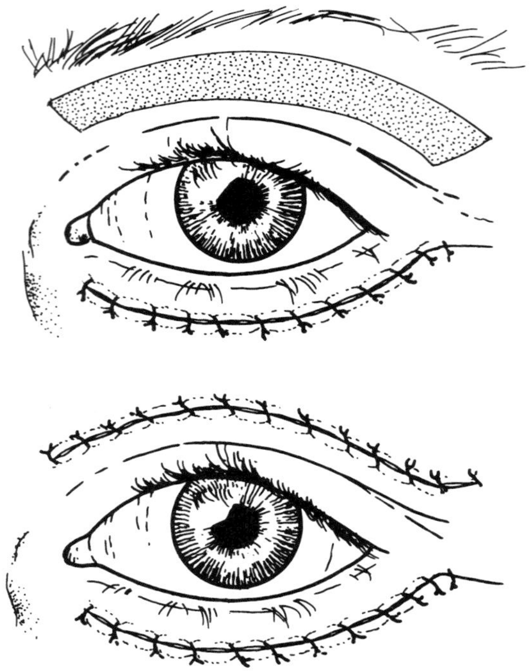

Fig. 9.85 Blepharoplasty showing the eyelid crease and subciliary incisions.

Rhinoplasty

Indications

The nose can be abnormal in size or shape following injury or as the result of an inherited familial or racial characteristic. After injury it is common for there to be breathing difficulties from a deviated nasal septum (Fig. 9.87), which can be corrected at the same time as the external appearance, by a septorhinoplasty. Patients may present with breathing difficulties or a painful nose, especially where spectacles rub; however, the most common reason for presentation is dissatisfaction with the appearance.

REFERENCES

282. Reich J In: Smith J, Aston S (eds) Grabb & Smith's Plastic Surgery, 4th edn, Little Brown, Boston 1991
283. Reich J Plast Reconstr Surg 1975; 55: 5–13
284. Regnault P, Daniel R K Aesthetic Plastic Surgery. Little Brown, Boston 1984
285. McCarthy J G (ed) Plastic Surgery. W B Saunders, Philadelphia 1990
286. Smith J, Aston S (eds) Grabb & Smith's Plastic Surgery. Little Brown, Boston 1991

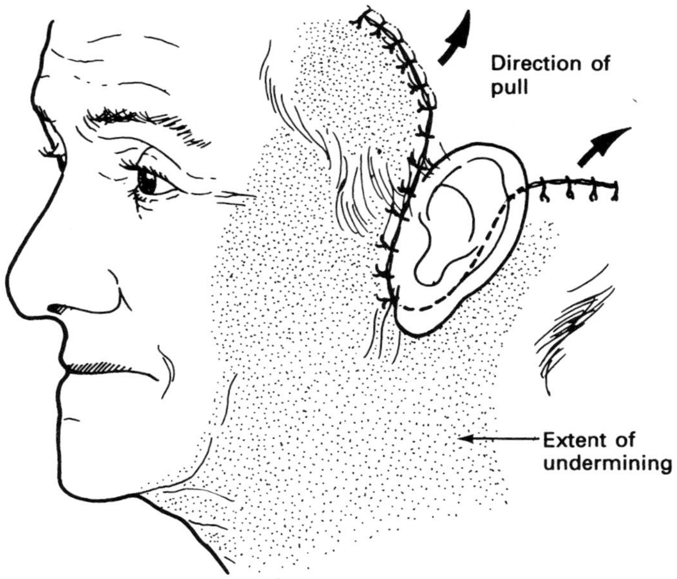

Fig. 9.86 The incisions and extent of undermining for a face lift.

Assessment

The nose is examined for deviation, abnormal width or length, a nasal hump or depression, abnormal tip prominence or bulk, and the presence of scars. A nasal speculum is used to examine the septum for deviation or perforations and obstruction caused by prominent turbinates. A clear distinction must be made between abnormalities of the bony skeleton and those of the cartilaginous skeleton. Correcting bony abnormalities is usually easier than correcting cartilaginous abnormalities, as cartilage is elastic and has a tendency to return to its preoperative state. Patients must be made aware that correcting the cartilaginous deviation may be difficult, and that some mild distortion may persist after the operation. It is not possible to convert a large and bulbous nose into a petite nose without resorting to external scars or removing so much of the supporting skeleton that nasal collapse occurs.

Procedure

In the UK, the operation is usually carried out under a general anaesthetic, whereas in the USA it is carried out under local anaesthetic with heavy sedation. Through an intranasal incision, the bony hump is removed with an osteotome, saw or a rasp, or a

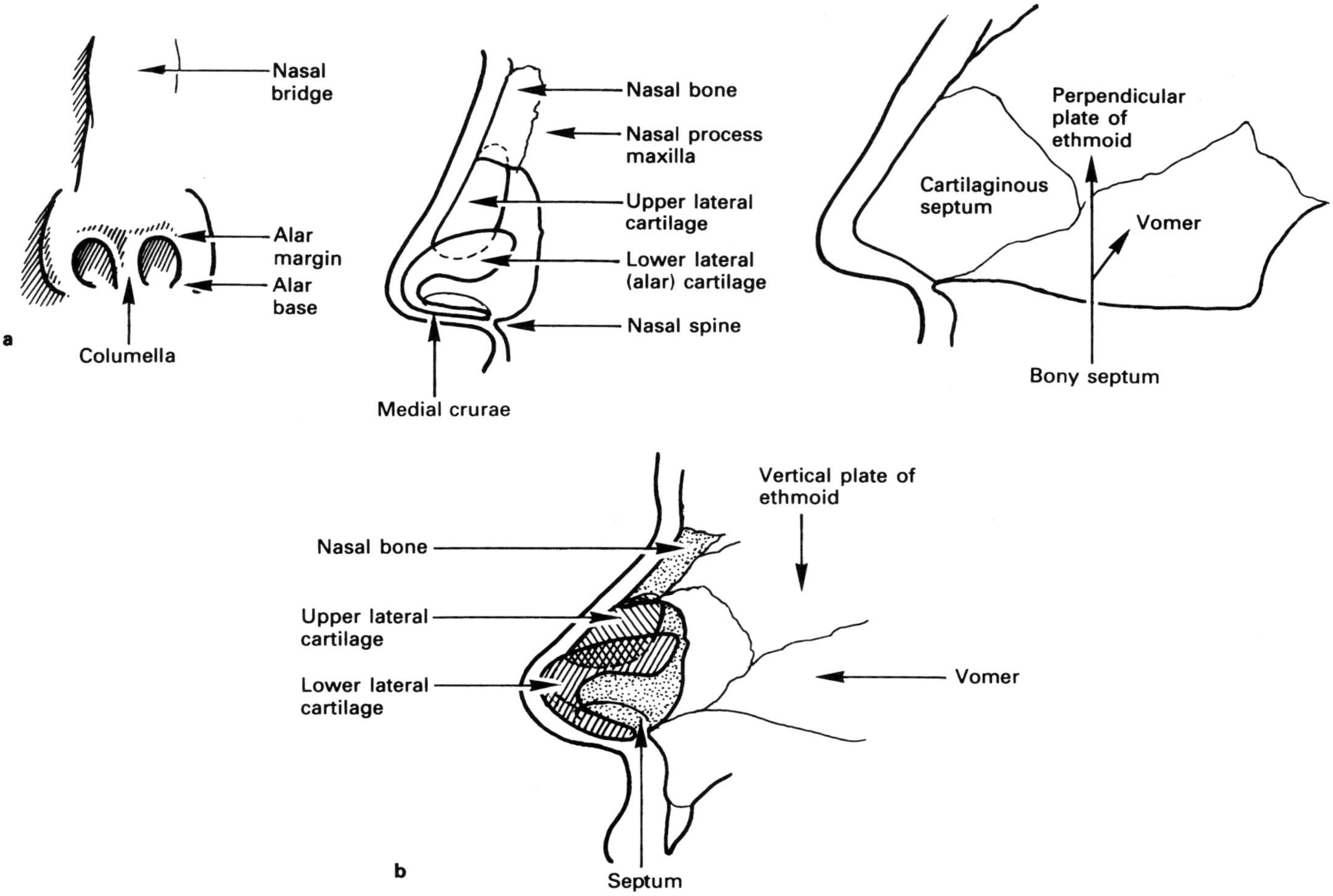

Fig. 9.87 Nasal anatomy.

combination of the three. This reduces the nasal bridge to a flat plateau which is corrected by carrying out lateral osteotomies on the nasal processes of the maxilla to allow the remaining bony skeleton to be infractured and narrowed. The cartilaginous septum is then reduced in both height and length, as necessary, using a knife or special cartilage scissors. Finally, the nasal tip is reduced by mobilizing and trimming the upper and lower alar cartilages. Great care must be taken not to remove so much cartilage that the tip support is lost. This produces a 'pinched' appearance over subsequent years. A plaster of Paris or similar splint is applied over the bridge to give support for about 10 days. Difficult noses may be best treated by an 'open' approach, particularly if there has been previous surgery. A transverse incision is made through the columella and the skin is reflected to allow direct vision of all the nasal structures.

Deficient noses can be augmented using silicone or porous synthetic prostheses, bovine cartilage, or autologous bone, cartilage, fascia or dermis. Synthetic prostheses can become infected, necessitating their removal. Autografts need a donor site, add to operating time, and can be prone to resorption or warping. Infection is rare and the most serious complication is bleeding. This usually settles with sedation and sitting the patient upright.

Correction of prominent ears

Indications

This is usually carried out in childhood because of teasing, but adults may request treatment when parents have previously disapproved of surgery. If at all possible, the operation should be deferred until 7 years of age, as the ear cartilage is still soft and actively growing before this time. There are two main types of prominent ear, and they are treated with different procedures. Scaphoconchal ears show a failure of formation of the normal scaphoconchal fold, giving the ear a smooth 'shell' appearance. Conchal ears show an abnormal depth and angle of the concha itself, so that the ear sticks out from the side of the head but retains a normal fold. The two types are often mixed (Fig. 9.88).

Procedure

The operation may be carried out under local or general anaesthesia, depending on the age and temperament of the patient. An incision is made in the postauricular sulcus, and the cartilage exposed. A scaphoconchal deformity is corrected by making an incision along the length of the cartilage at the site of the desired fold, and then exposing the anterior surface of the cartilage. The cartilage is then scored on the anterior surface along the line of the new fold, releasing the tension that exists in the elastic cartilage of the ear so that the intact posterior surface causes the cartilage to curl into the desired position. Conchal ears are treated by excising the excess conchal depth and closing the resultant cartilaginous defect with buried absorbable sutures to pull the ear into a normal position. In ears with both deformities, these two procedures may be combined. Complications include infection, bleeding and skin necrosis if the bandage has been applied too tightly.

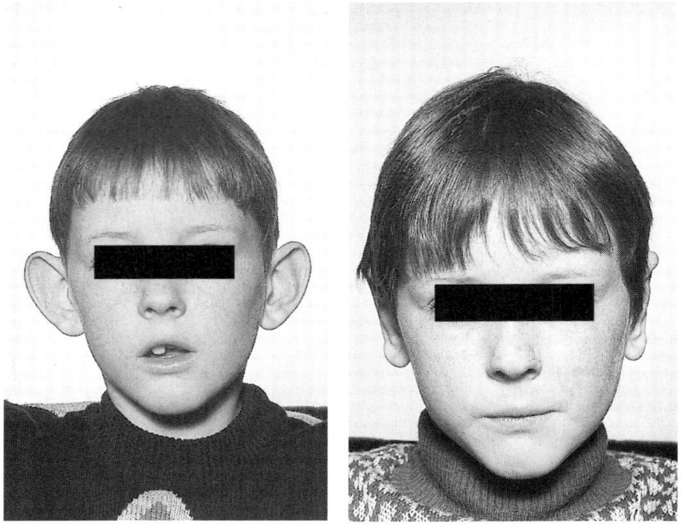

a b

Fig. 9.88 (**a**) Before and (**b**) after pinnaplasty.

Body contour surgery

Reduction mammoplasty

Most patients request a breast reduction for physical reasons rather than appearance. The most common complaints are backache, neckache, bra straps cutting in, intertrigo, difficulty in buying bras and clothes that fit, physical problems with running or exercise, and sexual harassment. The patient must be aware that there will be visible scars on the breast, that nipple sensation may be lost and that subsequent breast-feeding may not be possible. The size and symmetry of the breasts and the proportion of breast tissue to excess skin is noted, as this can affect the type of operation that is performed.

There are numerous different operations for breast reduction, but they can be classified into four main types (Fig. 9.89). Lateralizing operations remove tissue from the inferior and lateral parts of the breast and result in a scar that runs from the new areolar position inferiorly and laterally. Vertical operations remove tissue from all four quadrants of the breast and result in an inverted T scar, which, in combination with the scar around the areola, produces the appearance of an anchor. Both of these procedures have in common the need to preserve the blood supply to the nipple on a dermal pedicle or dermal bridge. In very large breasts, the length of this pedicle may be such that it threatens the viability of the nipple and the bulk of the pedicle may compromise the desired size of the breast. In this situation, the third type of reduction may be necessary, consisting of a T-shaped reduction of the breast with a free nipple graft. The advantage of this procedure is that the size and shape of the breast can be tailored without compromises caused by the need to preserve a pedicle. The nipple graft may fail to take, however, and can become flat. The amount of tissue removed from each breast should be weighed to ensure a symmetrical result. The patient should be warned about the nature of the scars, possible loss of both tactile and erogenous nipple sensation, loss of ability to breast-feed and possible partial or total loss of the

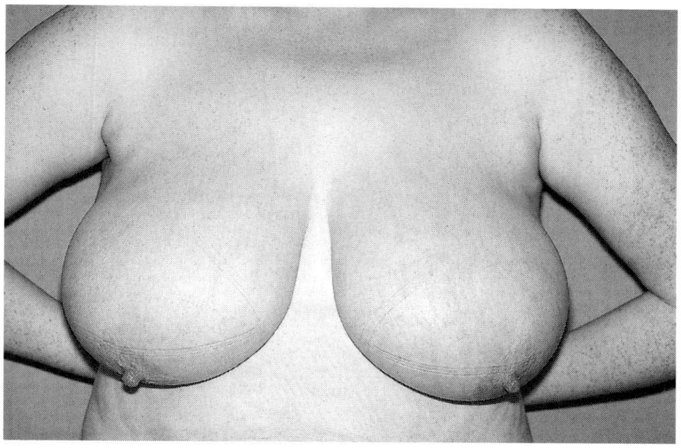

a

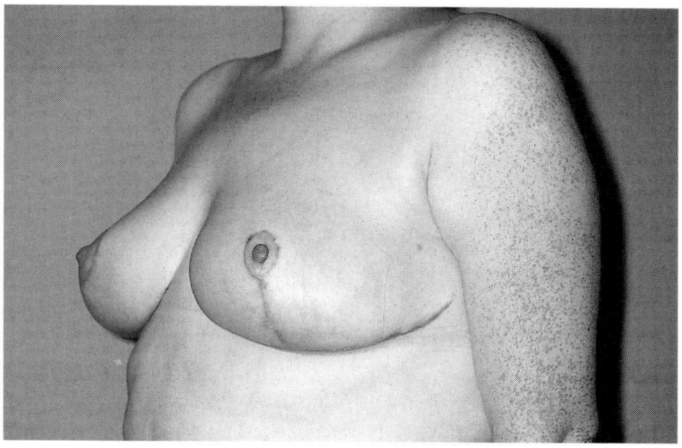

b

Fig. 9.89 (**a**) Before and (**b**) after reduction mammoplasty.

nipple. Wound infection, dehiscence and haematoma formation are also possible.

Augmentation mammoplasty

Indications

Patients present for breast augmentation because they are flat chested or have small breasts. Some women have a loss of breast tissue following pregnancy and breast-feeding, whilst others may have breast asymmetry. Poland's syndrome, hypoplasia or aplasia of the breast, in association with hypoplasia or absence of the muscles of the chest wall and brachysyndactyly of the hand, is a rare problem and reason for referral for augmentation or reconstruction. These patients have usually withstood years of teasing from friends, family and the family physician. The improvement in self confidence produced by augmentation can be gratifying as the patient's body image is restored.[287]

Assessment

A thorough social and psychological history is taken, and a psychiatric opinion should be sought where the breasts are considered to be within 'normal' limits. The operation should be for the patient rather than for a spouse. The size of implant to be used will largely be determined by the amount of available skin. It is not possible to put a very large implant into a completely flat chest, and conversely a ptotic breast requires a large implant to take up the excess skin.

Procedure

The implants themselves are made of a pliable silicone envelope containing silicone gel. Some surgeons prefer to use an inflatable implant containing saline instead of gel, but these do have the disadvantage of occasional spontaneous deflation.

Implants used to have a smooth outer layer and 40% developed a firm outer capsule, associated with symptoms from mild discomfort to severe pain and requiring removal of the implant. The latest generation of implants have a rough outer coating that reduces the rate of capsular contracture to 2%.[288] There has been much controversy over the safety of silicone prostheses, and the term 'silicone disease' has been introduced to describe the purported detrimental effects of silicone. At present there is no evidence that 'silicone disease' has any scientific basis, and there is good evidence that silicone bears no association to the incidence of breast cancer or any autoimmune disease.[289,290] The Chief Medical Officer in the UK has found no reason to restrict the use or sale of silicone gel implants in this country.

Breast implants can be inserted through a submammary, axillary, circumareolar or transareolar approach (Fig. 9.90). In Britain the submammary and axillary approaches are favoured. The latest generation of implants are placed in a subglandular plane, in the layer of loose areolar tissue that separates the breast from the underlying pectoralis muscle, in a pocket sufficiently large that the implant is not constricted. The pocket is created by blunt dissection to minimize bleeding, and the implant is manipulated through the small (5 cm) incision in much the same way as reducing a hernia. The patient may be given a single intravenous dose of prophylactic antibiotic such as cefuroxime and the implant cavity may be irrigated with a bactericidal solution of the surgeon's choice. The wounds are closed in layers. The main complication used to be the development of a firm capsule around the implant but modern implants now produce a soft and impalpable implant in 98% of cases. Infection and haematoma formation can occur but are uncommon. However, most implants are radiopaque and interfere with mammography, and special radiography techniques are required to overcome this.[291]

REFERENCES

287. Hetter G P Plast Reconstr Surg 1979; 64: 151
288. Vogt P A Contemp Surg Sept 1990
289. Dunn K W, Hall P N, Khoo C T Br J Plast Surg 1992; 45(4): 315–321
290. Park A J, Black R J, Watson A C Br J Surg 1993; 80(9): 1097–1100
291. Gumucio C A Pin P, Young V L et al Plast Reconstr Surg 1989; 84: 772–778

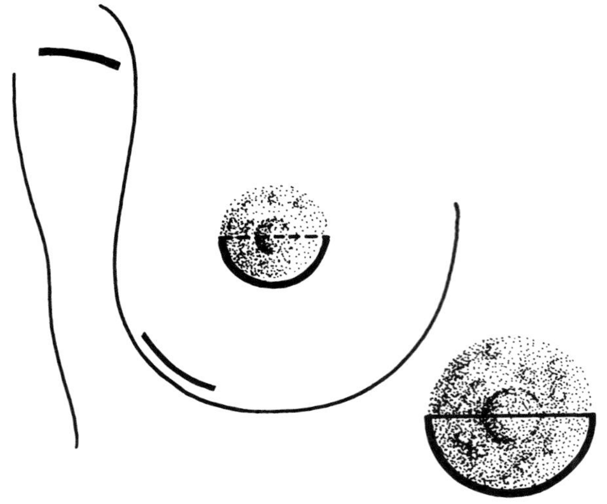

Fig. 9.90 Augmentation mammoplasty. Note the transverse axillary incision, short submammary incision on the breast, not in the breast fold, circumareolar incision halfway around the areola, and a transareolar incision bisecting the areola and nipple.

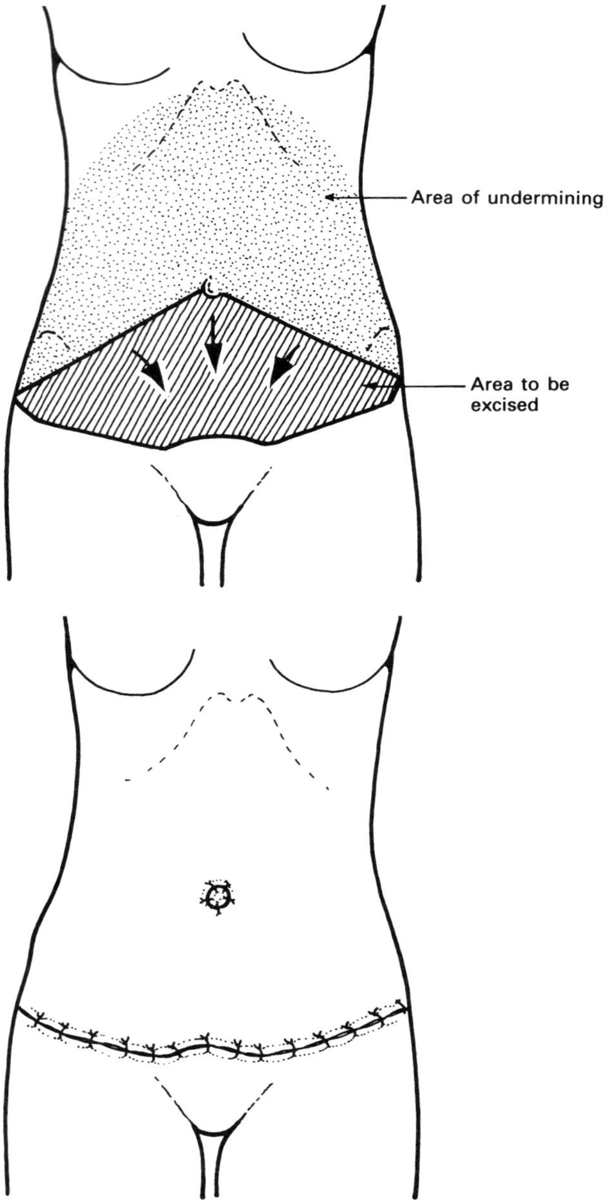

Fig. 9.91 Standard abdominoplasty showing the area of undermining and the area to be excised.

Abdominoplasty (apronectomy)

Abdominoplasty is usually carried out in multiparous women in whom pregnancy has permanently stretched the skin and weakened the abdominal fascia, creating redundant skin folds and a lax anterior abdominal wall. This may or may not be associated with prominent stretch marks and the presence of unsightly or tethered scars from previous caesarean sections. It is wise to defer abdominoplasty until no further pregnancies are envisaged. The history should concentrate on the enforced changes in lifestyle, such as not taking children to the swimming baths, not going on holiday, a change in the style of clothes, and any alteration in sexuality. The patient is examined standing up and the amount of redundant skin is assessed. In most cases, it is possible to remove all the skin inferior to the umbilicus; however, in moderate cases it may be sufficient to remove a smaller ellipse without distorting the umbilicus, often in combination with liposuction. The patient is then examined lying down and is asked to lift her head off the couch to assess the strength of the abdominal muscles and to check for divarication of the rectus abdominis muscles. The presence of any abdominal scars should be noted as transverse or oblique scars may interfere with the blood supply of the abdominal skin.

Procedure

A low transverse abdominal incision is made, skirting the pubic hair (Fig. 9.91). The skin is completely mobilized up to the costal margin, but the umbilicus is left attached to the anterior abdominal wall. Any laxity of the abdominal fascia and divarication of the rectus abdominis muscle is corrected by plicating the fascia in the midline with several layers of heavy non-absorbable monofilament sutures. The abdominal skin is then pulled down until the site of the umbilicus reaches the lower wound edge, and the surplus skin is resected and discarded. A new opening is made for the umbilicus, which is pulled through and sutured in place before the wound is closed over suction drains. In less severe cases, a mini-abdominoplasty may be carried out, mobilizing only the lower abdominal skin through a much shorter incision, leaving the umbilicus in place. The siting of the incision deliberately conceals the scar beneath the 'bikini line'. In patients who have lost a great deal of weight and have folds of redundant skin it may be necessary to combine a low abdominal incision with a full-length vertical incision to remove all redundant skin without producing dog-ears. The degree of undermining of the skin means that any infection can spread rapidly and have severe consequences. Complications are increased in the obese because of the relatively poor blood supply of fat. There may be some temporary numbness of the abdominal skin; sensation returns within 6 months.

Liposuction

Indications

Fat suction has proved to be remarkably effective in removing localized fat deposits since its introduction in 1977.[292] Lipomas and localized fat dystrophies over the hips, buttocks, thighs, knees and ankles are particularly amenable to liposuction as it is very difficult to treat these by dieting. Once fat has been removed by liposuction, it will not recur as the fat cells have been permanently removed. Liposuction is also useful to treat gynaecomastia, where this is predominantly fat rather than a prominent breast disc, and to reduce excessively bulky skin flaps. It is used as an adjunctive procedure in face lifts, abdominoplasty and upper arm reduction. It is not indicated for generalized obesity. The technique relies on the skin retracting and redraping over the areas where fat has been removed. Patients of any age who have loose skin are poor candidates, unless they accept that surgical skin reduction with a resulting scar may also be necessary. Liposuction is not an effective procedure for correcting the peau d'orange appearance of cellulite, although the recent introduction of very superficial liposculpture may be effective for this condition.

The patient's motivation, previous attempts at dieting and expectations from surgery should be assessed, and the usual social and psychological evaluations performed. The patient should be examined standing and lying to define the localized fat deposits, and the skin tension and elasticity is assessed to determine whether skin resection is necessary.

Procedure

The procedure involves blunt suction of the deeper layers of the fat using specially designed cannulae attached to high vacuum suction equipment. Suction pumps are increasingly being replaced by suction syringes that use finer cannulae and obviate the need for bulky and heavy tubing (Fig. 9.92). An additional benefit is that they make no noise. Suction syringes allow a safer, controlled dissection in the superficial layers of the fat under the dermis. Large volumes of saline containing bupivacaine and adrenaline are infiltrated, to provide hydrodissection, haemostasis, analgesia and an even removal of fat.

The cannulae are inserted through a remote stab incision, and the smallest possible cannula should be used as this reduces the risk of uneven fat removal. The fat is removed through a series of tunnels so that the intervening blood vessels and nerves are preserved and no large cavities are produced that encourage haematoma or infection (Fig. 9.93). The fat seen through the transparent suction tubing should be yellow and contain no blood

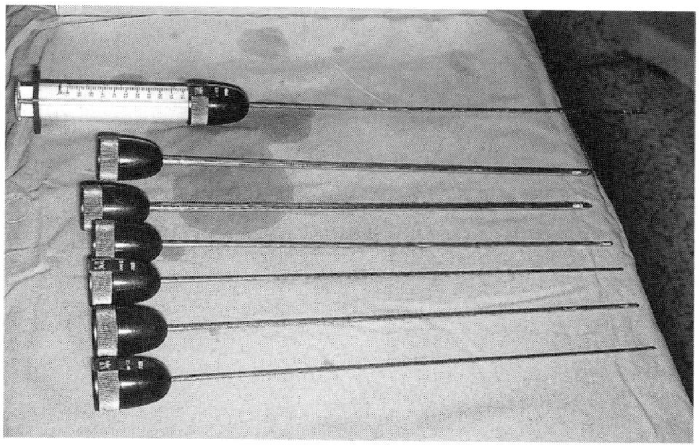

Fig. 9.92 Tulip liposculpture cannulae.

REFERENCE

292. Illouz Y G Plast Reconstr Surg 1983; 72: 591–597

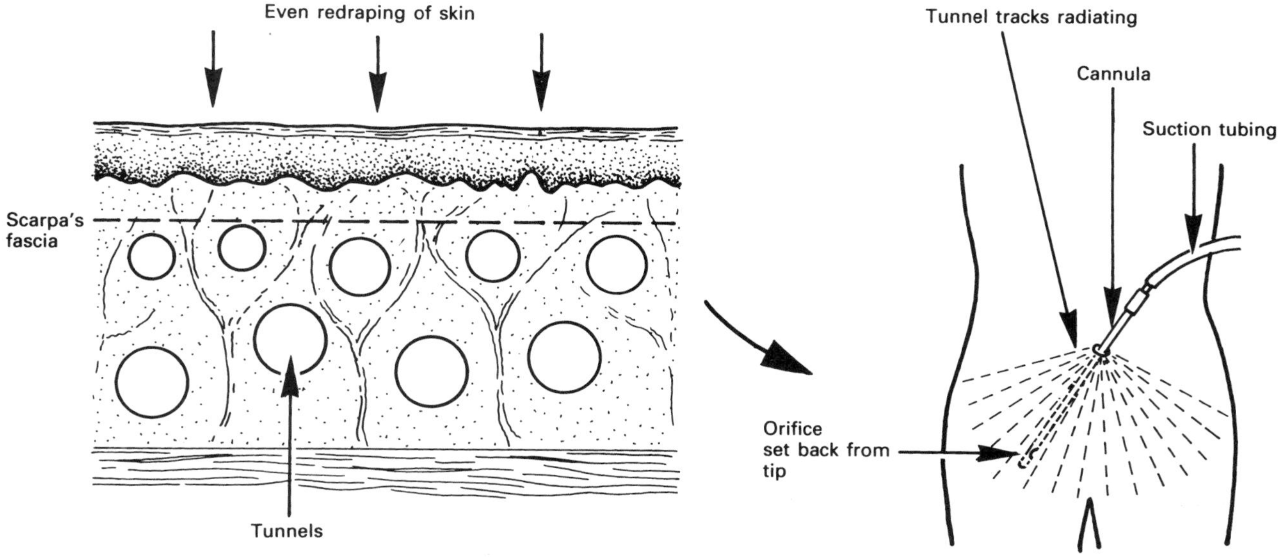

Fig. 9.93 The technique of liposuction; the tunnels should be made through the fat, preserving the vessels.

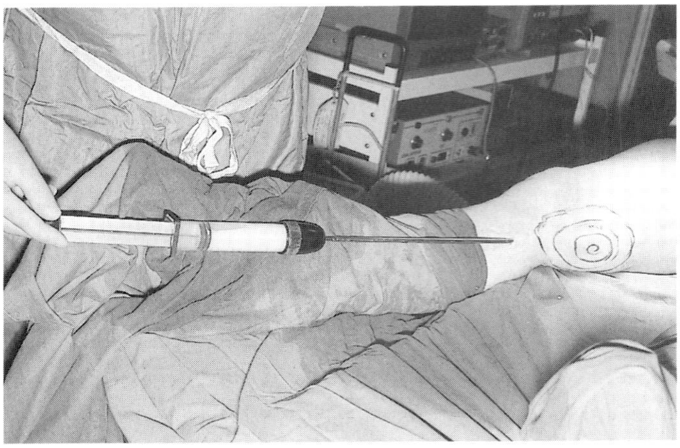

Fig. 9.94 Liposculpture. Note the absence of blood in the aspirate using the 'wet' technique.

(Fig. 9.94). When blood starts to appear, the cannula should be removed from that tunnel and a further tunnel created. The adoption of a crossing tunnel arrangement reduces the likelihood of surface irregularities. It is important to avoid removing the superficial fat adjacent to the skin as this can produce surface rippling effects. The area is strapped for 1 week to flatten the skin while it redrapes. Drains are not necessary.[293] Serious complications are very uncommon; the most frequent problem is an uneven removal of fat, necessitating a further procedure 6–12 months later. Temporary numbness and marked bruising can occur, but severe infection and skin loss is very rare.

REFERENCE

293. Illouz Y G Body Sculpturing by Lipoplasty. Churchill Livingstone, Edinburgh 1989

10 The arteries

K. G. Burnand P. T. Taylor J. A. Murie K. Callum

INTRODUCTION

Although a number of diseases affect arteries, atherosclerosis is responsible for nearly 90% of all arterial disease occurring in the western world.[1] The prevalence of atherosclerosis in Africa, the Indian subcontinent and the Far East is much lower,[2] while arteritis, although still relatively rare, is more common in India and the Far East.[3] Vasospastic diseases which are accentuated by a cold climate appear to be increasing in incidence,[4] but syphilitic arteritis has almost disappeared since the advent of antibiotics.

The prevalence of arterial injury has risen proportionally with the increase in road traffic accidents,[5] operative surgery and interventional radiology, but armed insurrection and wars[6] are still responsible for sudden surges in the frequency of serious vascular injury. In the USA over the last 20 years, there has been a large increase in the number of vascular injuries in civilians caused by knife and gunshot wounds.[7] This type of trauma remains relatively rare in Europe, but its incidence is slowly increasing.

True arterial tumours are extremely rare; the development of the acquired immune deficiency syndrome has led to an epidemic of Kaposi's sarcoma though there is dispute whether this is a true tumour.[8] The majority of angiomata are hereditary malformations and should therefore be classified as hamartomas rather than tumours.

Aneurysmal disease of arteries appears to be increasing,[9] but the incidence of arterial emboli appears to be falling in parallel with a decline in rheumatic heart disease.[10] This may also be related to the increased prescribing of warfarin to patients in atrial fibrillation.[11]

Heredity, diet, racial and environmental factors all influence the prevalence of arterial disease, and fluctuations in these factors in various parts of the world are probably responsible for the differing proportions of arterial pathology that are found in individual countries.

The symptoms caused by arterial disease are dependent on the vessels that are affected, but there are many pathophysiological outcomes, symptoms and signs that are common to all arterial diseases. These are discussed first, before the individual pathological processes are described in detail in the subsequent sections. Coronary arterial disease will be mentioned in this chapter where it is relevant but is described in detail in Chapter 23.

PATHOPHYSIOLOGY OF ARTERIAL DISEASE

Disease in the arterial wall can lead to narrowing or dilatation of the vessel lumen: both outcomes can result from the same pathological process (e.g. atheroma) and can even develop simultaneously at different sites in the same individual. Three main territories are affected:

1. Cardiac.
2. Cerebrovascular.
3. Aorta and limbs.

Visceral and mesenteric involvement is less common and that of the upper limb is very rare.

Arterial stenosis

A reduction in the cross-sectional area of the arterial lumen has little consequence at first as flow is governed by Poiseuilles's law,[12] which states that flow is proportional to the radius of the vessel to the power four and inversely proportional to the length of the vessel and the viscosity of the blood. Therefore the radius of the vessel wall has to be considerably reduced before there is any reduction in flow.

Blood flow in normal arteries is smooth and laminar, but wall abnormalities set up eddy currents and these alter shear forces which accentuate any arterial damage. A haemodynamically significant stenosis, which is one which will cause appreciable changes in pressure and flow, does not occur until the cross-sectional area has been decreased by 75% (equivalent to a diameter reduction of at least 50%).[13] Stenoses of this magnitude do not allow an increase in blood flow when distal vasodilatation is caused by increased demand, and the tissues supplied by the artery are therefore deprived of oxygen.[14] An oxygen debt then develops, leading to anaerobic metabolism and accumulation of unwanted

REFERENCES

1. Robertson W B Pathol Microbiol 1967; 30: 810
2. McGill H C Lab Invest 1968; 18: 465
3. Tejada C, Strong J P et al Lab Invest 1968; 18: 509
4. Olsen N, Nielsen S L Scand J Clin Lab Invest 1978; 37: 761
5. Trunkey D D Sci Am 1983; 249: 28
6. Rich N M, Baugh J H, Hughes C W J Trauma 1970; 10: 359
7. Rich N M In: Bongard F S, Wilson S E, Perry M O (eds) Vascular Injuries in Surgical Practice. Prentice Hall, London pp 1–31
8. Durack D T N Engl J Med 1981; 305: 1465
9. Collin J Br J Surg 1987; 74: 332
10. Abbott W M, Maloney R D et al Am Surg 1982; 143: 460
11. Petersen P et al Lancet 1989; 1: 175
12. Poiseuille J L M Acad Sci 1840; 11: 961
13. Sumner D S In: Rutherford R B (ed) Vascular Surgery, 4th edn. W B Saunders, London 1995 pp 18–25
14. May A G, Van De Berg L et al Surgery 1963; 54: 250

metabolites.[15] This process results in symptoms of angina in ischaemic heart muscle (Chapter 23) and intermittent claudication in the lower limbs.

The exact mechanism for the development of the pain of claudication remains obscure, but may be related to anoxia, acidosis and the accumulation of metabolites. Sol Cohen[16] suggested that claudication was the result of 'defective terminal circulation interfering with the insulation of nerve fibres, permitting the overflow of efferent sympathetic stimuli to neighbouring sensory fibres'. Lewis and his associates[17] related the onset of claudication to accumulation of substance P within the muscles; this eventually stimulates local pain endings. Little new has been added to these theories in recent years.

Intermittent claudication is a cramp-like pain which is the result of muscle ischaemia caused by arterial stenosis or occlusion. The muscle group affected depends upon the site of the arterial occlusion. The muscles of the thigh and buttock are the site of claudication if there is a stenosis or occlusion of the aorta or the iliac vessels; in men this may be associated with impotence. Claudication pain is, however, most commonly felt in the large muscles of the posterior calf where it is often the result of a stenosis or occlusion of the superficial femoral artery. Occasionally it affects the muscles of the upper limb, and very rarely the small muscles of the foot. The pain can rarely occur in the jaw muscles of patients with Takayasu's disease.

The upper limb can occasionally be affected in patients with severe stenoses or occlusions of the subclavian, axillary or brachial vessels, but it is much less frequent than lower limb claudication because of the reduced incidence of arterial disease in the upper limbs and the presence of good collateral pathways. Rarely, it can affect women who have previously undergone radiotherapy for carcinoma of the breast.

Claudication pain increases with exercise and is relieved completely by rest. The distance at which the pain develops (the claudication distance) may vary from day to day, often depending upon the ambient temperature, but shortens if the disease extends or the vessel occludes. It is usually worse on walking up hills and better when walking on the level or downhill. Claudication pain can be categorized into a series of grades depending on the severity of the symptoms,[18] but the distance to the onset of the pain and the maximum distance that can be achieved by the patient (by walking through the pain) is simpler to comprehend and can be objectively measured on a treadmill.

Stenosis of the extracranial vessels is most commonly found at the junction of the common, internal and external carotid arteries.[19] Stenotic disease of one carotid bifurcation rarely produces symptoms as the result of reduced blood flow. Symptoms may occur, however, if there is a severe stenosis or a total occlusion of the opposite carotid or if the circle of Willis is incomplete. Symptoms from a unilateral stenosis are invariably the result of platelet emboli breaking loose from the diseased arterial wall causing transient ischaemic attacks which recover within 24 hours, episodes of fleeting blindness usually lasting a few minutes (amaurosis fugax) or completed strokes where the neurological deficit lasts longer than 24 hours (cerebral infarcts). Stenoses in the vertebrobasilar system may give rise to loss of consciousness and vertigo on sudden changes of posture or after rapid neck movements. Occasionally severe carotid stenosis may follow neck irradiation for lymphomas or carcinoma of the thyroid gland.

A severe stenosis of one renal artery was shown experimentally by Goldblatt et al[20] to promote the release of renin which acts on angiotensinogen, a plasma globulin proenzyme, to produce angiotensin which acts directly on the arterial wall, resulting in generalized arteriolar contraction and hypertension. Renal artery stenosis is an important treatable cause of hypertension and is also responsible for a number of patients presenting with chronic renal failure.

Stenoses of the coeliac and mesenteric vessels can produce severe abdominal pain after meals. This is called 'intestinal angina' and must be differentiated from other more common causes of severe indigestion. Patients usually stop eating to avoid the pain and may rapidly lose weight. They literally have a 'fear' of food.

'Arterial impotence' is the result of an inability to increase blood flow through the helicine arteries of the penis. Arterial influx must exceed venous drainage in order to produce and maintain tumescence.[21] Closure of the arteriovenous fistulae within the erectile tissue may be unable to compensate for poor arterial inflow[22] (see Chapter 39).

Acute arterial occlusion

Stenotic disease of the arterial wall may progress until the lumen is completely obliterated, but much more commonly an acute thrombosis is the eventual cause of arterial occlusion. Atheromatous plaque within the arterial wall may fissure and rupture, allowing blood to enter the plaque and red cells and fibrin to accumulate within the arterial wall.[23] This occludes the lumen and usually results in propagated thrombosis extending as far as the next major collateral branch and occasionally beyond. Acute arterial occlusions may also be produced by emboli, thrombosis of an aneurysm, arterial dissection, external compression, ligation and trauma. Rarely, massive trauma may disrupt the artery but more commonly intimal tears can result from fractures of bones adjacent to arteries, particularly the brachial artery in supracondylar fractures of the humerus in children and the popliteal artery in fractures around the knee caused by hyperextension injuries in adults (Fig. 10.1).

Both the speed of the occlusion and the available collateral circulation determine the subsequent symptoms. When the occlusion is gradual and the collaterals good, the symptoms may be minimal or equivalent to those already described for arterial stenosis, but if the occlusion is sudden and the collateral circulation poor, then symptoms of acute ischaemia and tissue infarction rapidly develop.

REFERENCES

15. Burton A C Physiology and Biophysics of the Circulation.Year Book, Chicago 1972
16. Cohen S Postgrad Med J 1946; 22: 1
17. Lewis T, Pickering G W, Rothschild P Heart 1929; 15: 359
18. Fontaine R, Kieny R et al J Cardiovasc Surg 1964; 4: 463
19. Fields W S, Sharkey P C et al Neurology 1960; 10: 431
20. Goldblatt H, Lynch J et al J Exp Med 1934; 59: 347
21. Virag R, Bouilly D, Frydman D Lancet 1985; i: 181
22. Michal V, Simana J et al J Physiol Biochem 1983; 32: 497
23. Davis M J, Thomas A C Br Heart J 1985; 53: 363

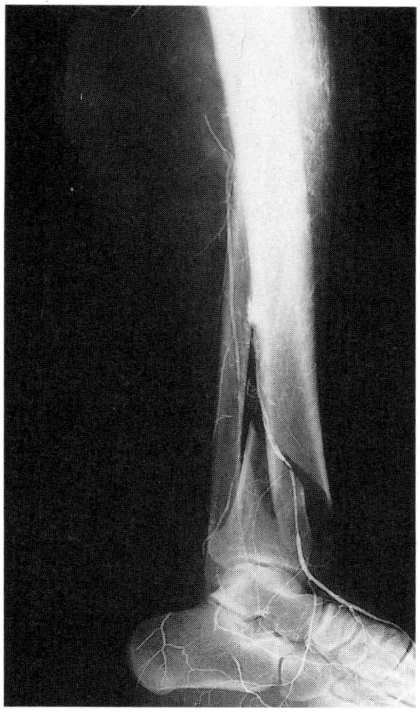

Fig. 10.1 Fractured tibia showing disruption of tibial vessels.

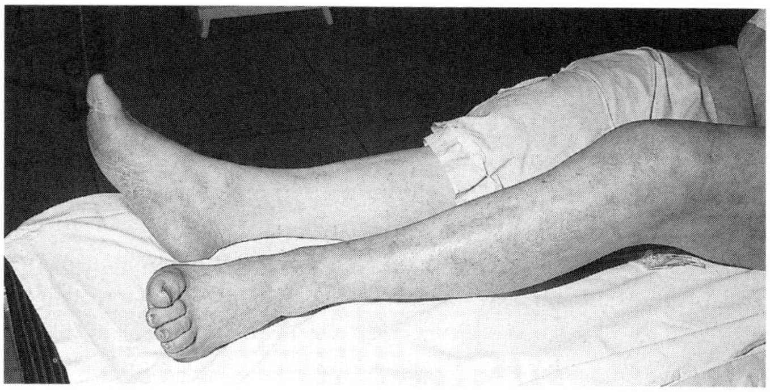

Fig. 10.2 Leg (left) with acute ischaemia showing mottling and marble-like appearances.

Coronary arteries

An acute occlusion of one of the coronary vessels can be symptomless but frequently produces a myocardial infarct, a cardiac arrhythmia or cardiac arrest (see Chapter 23).

Aorta, iliac and lower limb arteries

Acute occlusion of the aorta and iliac vessels is rare but may occur if an aneurysm thromboses, or if acute thrombosis supervenes on atheromatous disease. A saddle embolus may lodge at the aortic bifurcation and occlude both iliac arteries.[24] When an acute aortic occlusion does occur the patient first complains of sudden severe pain in both lower limbs, which are noted to be pale and cold. The pallor may persist and deepen in a cold environment, but if the surroundings are warm and the limbs dependent, pallor is soon replaced by cyanosis which can affect the abdomen to the level of the umbilicus. If the condition is left untreated for some hours, white patches (Bier spots)[25] appear amongst the blue or purple background, and these then coalesce to produce a mottled appearance; streaking by pigment-stained venules completes the similarity to marble (Fig. 10.2). This state may take some days to develop and is reversible in its early stages. Blood blisters indicating cutaneous damage may also appear, and these easily brush off to leave superficial oozing ulcers. The limbs continue to cool centripetally and may later become oedematous.

Pain is often severe and of a 'bursting' nature, though it may occasionally be mild, amounting only to numbness and paraesthesia. When the blood supply is restored after some delay, neuritic pain may persist with hypersensitivity to both painful and thermal stimuli. Nerve and muscle function rapidly ceases if ischaemia persists, with nerve conduction disappearing between 15 and 30 min and permanent muscle damage developing within a few hours. The limbs may become anaesthetic at the same time, and this anaesthesia has a 'stocking' type distribution.[25]

Although skin tolerates periods of ischaemia up to 48 h reasonably well, nerve and muscle recovery is much more variable and is usually incomplete. The muscles of the anterior compartment of the lower leg are invariably the most severely affected with the extensor hallucis longus muscle often the last to recover. The muscles of the plantar compartment recover poorly if at all, and the skin of the sole may remain anaesthetic even after the rest of the leg has returned to normal.[25] Human striated muscle virtually never regenerates after a period of severe ischaemia; it is replaced by fibrous tissue which causes severe contracture.[26]

At an advanced stage of acute ischaemia, revascularization of the limb is hazardous, as toxic metabolites, myoglobin and large quantities of potassium[27] may be released into the circulation causing sudden death from cardiac arrhythmia, renal failure, respiratory distress syndrome or general toxaemia.[28] A history of ischaemia extending beyond 24 hours, associated with anaesthesia, muscle tenderness and swelling, should alert the clinician to this risk, and any attempt at revascularization must then be carefully considered and accompanied by the judicious use of extensive fasciotomies.[29] Amputation may be safer in these circumstances.

An identical picture can be produced in a single limb by an acute embolus lodging or thrombosis occurring at the superficial femoral and profunda femoris bifurcation.[30] Acute occlusions below this point rarely cause such a florid picture because of the better collateral channels which are available. An acute thrombosis of a popliteal aneurysm, when the crural vessels have already been occluded by distal emboli, is an exception to this rule, and is an important cause of severe acute ischaemia of the calf and foot.[31,32] A combination of an acute proximal thrombosis with prior disease

REFERENCES

24. Johnson N M, Gaspar M R et al Arch Surg 1974; 108: 792
25. Lewis T Vascular Disorders of the Limbs. Macmillan, London 1944
26. Von Volkman R, Von Pitha, Bilroth H (eds) In: Handbuch der allgemeinen und specielsen Chirurgie, vol 2. Stuttgart 1872
27. Haimovici H Contemp Surg 1980; 17: 33
28. Haimovici H Surgery 1979; 85: 461
29. Carter A B, Richards R L, Zachary R B Lancet 1949; ii: 298
30. Blaisdell W F, Steele M, Allen R E Surgery 1978; 84: 222
31. Hara M, Thompson B W Arch Surg 1966; 92: 504
32. Gifford R W, Hines E A, Janes J M Surgery 1953; 33: 294

of the crural or popliteal vessels from any cause also produces acute ischaemic changes.

Extracranial vessels

An acute occlusion of either the common or internal carotid artery may be well tolerated because an adequate circle of Willis is capable of supplying the opposite hemisphere from a patent vertebral or contralateral carotid artery.[33] A carotid occlusion usually results in cerebral infarction and a major stroke if the circle of Willis is congenitally incomplete or diseased,[34,35] or if there are additional stenoses or occlusions in the other extracranial vessels (Fig. 10.3). This presents as a sudden onset of monoplegia or hemiplegia, which may be accompanied by dysphasia, dysarthria, visual disturbance, cognitive loss or emotional lability. Recovery depends upon the size of the initial infarct and the adequacy of the collateral circulation.[33] Cerebral infarcts can also follow occlusions of the brachiocephalic trunk[36] and the vertebrobasilar vessels,[37] but most strokes that are not the result of a carotid occlusion are caused by an intracerebral haemorrhage,[38] or by a thrombosis of or an embolism into one of the intracerebral vessels.[39]

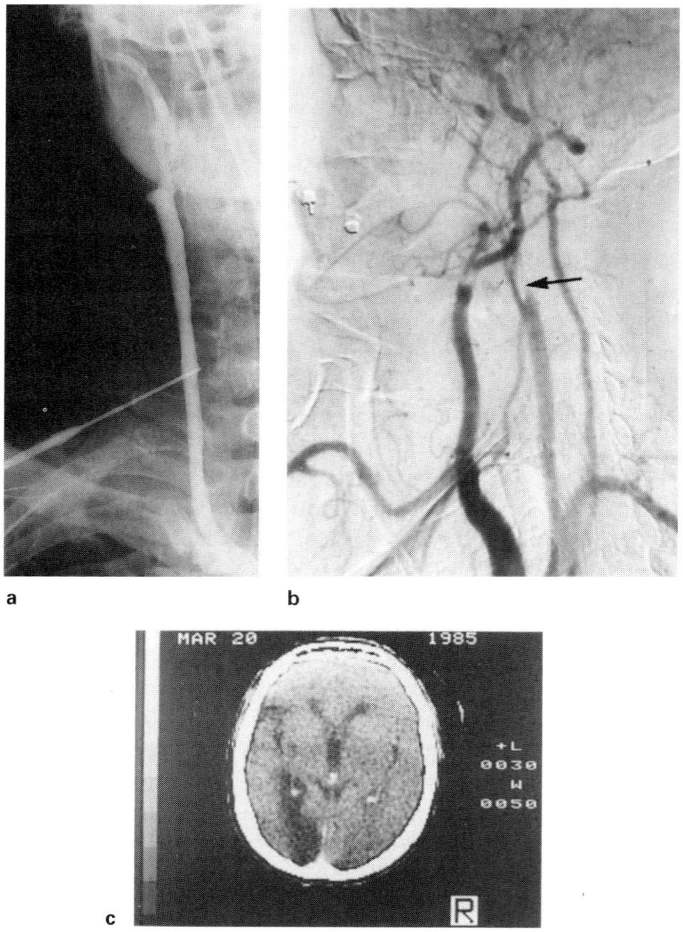

Fig. 10.3 **(a)** An occluded carotid artery. **(b)** An arch aortogram showing an occluded left internal carotid artery. This resulted in the cerebral infarct shown on the computerized tomography scan of the brain **(c)**.

Upper limb arteries

Sudden occlusion of the subclavian, axillary or brachial arteries may result from thrombosis or embolism. Occasionally occlusion of an aneurysm related to a cervical rib or from an arteritis in the vessel wall may be responsible. Atherosclerotic occlusions of the upper limb are uncommon, but they can give rise to ischaemic pain on exercise, subclavian steal syndrome and even acute ischaemia of the upper limb.

The subclavian steal syndrome occurs when a block in the first part of the subclavian artery leads to the stealing of blood from the circle of Willis by retrograde flow down the vertebral artery, which acts as a collateral to the arm during muscular exercise[40–42] (Fig. 10.4). This is a rare disorder which produces multiple and diverse symptoms during muscular work involving the affected arm. These symptoms include visual disturbance, vertigo, ataxia, syncope, motor and sensory deficits, dysarthria and dysphasia. Some still doubt the existence of the syndrome.

Acute ischaemia of the upper limb is identical in presentation and appearance to that of the lower limb.

Visceral vessels

The three anterior abdominal aortic branches—the coeliac, the superior and inferior mesenteric vessels—may all occlude acutely as a result of thrombosis, embolism, a dissecting aneurysm or vasculitis. There is normally a good collateral circulation between all three visceral arteries, and patients may remain symptomless despite occlusions of all three major vessels. An acute embolus or thrombosis lodging at the origin of the superior mesenteric artery with propagating thrombus extending into the smaller vessels usually produces a mesenteric infarct, without severe disease in the other vessels, as this is an end artery.[43,44]

The infarcted bowel is at first pale but then becomes oedematous and suffused before rapidly discolouring and turning dark blue as the stagnant blood in its extensive vascular bed becomes deoxygenated and the anaerobic and putrefactive organisms begin to multiply. Initially the mucosa ulcerates but as the ischaemia progresses it necroses and separates. The serosal surface becomes dull and eventually black with the cessation of peristaltic movement. No pulsation can be felt in the mesenteric blood vessels.

REFERENCES

33. Fields W S, Bruetman M E, Weibel J Monographs In the Surgical Sciences. Williams & Wilkins, Baltimore 1965
34. McCormick W F In: Structure and Function of Nervous Tissue. Academic Press, New York 1969
35. Toole J F, Patel A N Cerebrovascular Disorders. McGraw-Hill, New York 1967
36. Crawford E S, De Bakey M E et al Surgery 1969; 65: 17
37. Loeb C, Meyer J S Strokes due to Vertebro-basilar Disease. Charles C Thomas, Springfield Illinois 1965
38. Imparato A M J Vasc Surg 1985; 2: 626
39. Sandercock P A G, Molyneaux A, Warlow C P Br Med J 1985; 43: 74
40. Editorial N Engl J Med 1961; 265: 912
41. Gonzales L, Weintraub R A et al Radiology 1964; 82: 211
42. Reivich M, Holling H E et al N Engl J Med 1961; 265: 878
43. Chiene J J Anat Physiol 1869; 3: 65
44. Marston A Gut 1967; 8: 203

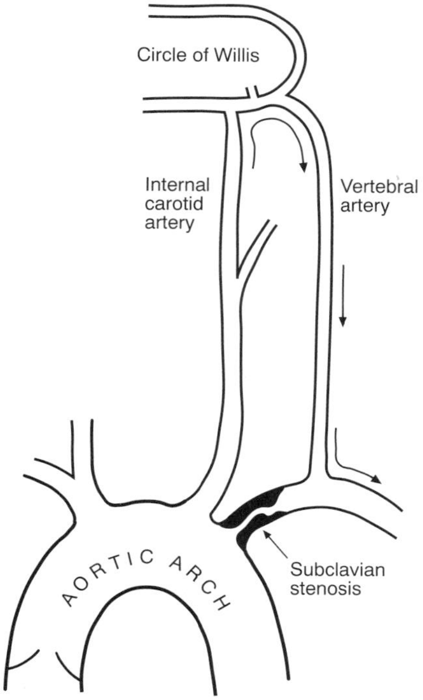

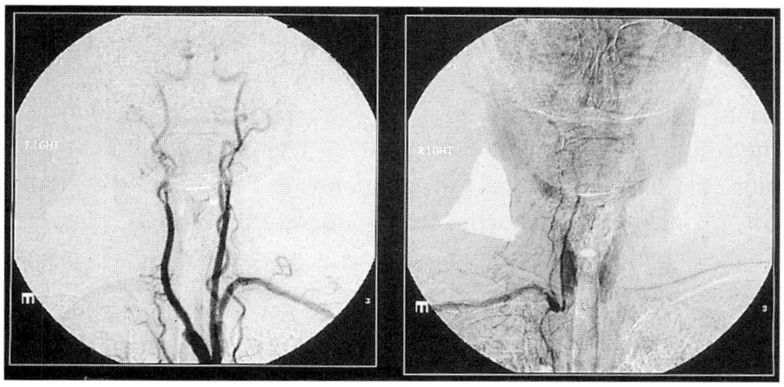

Fig. 10.4 The subclavian steal syndrome. (**a**) Diagrammatic representation of flow; (**b**) intravenous digital subtraction angiography showing late filling of (right) subclavian artery via the vertebral artery.

Patients with mesenteric infarction complain of persistent, severe and generalized abdominal pain. The severity of the pain is often matched by a paucity of physical signs. The patients rapidly become toxic and shocked and die from the consequences of septic shock if left untreated.

Miscellaneous arteries

The arterial supply of the kidneys, spleen and liver can become acutely occluded by one of the common pathological processes described above. Splenic infarcts are commonly associated with sickle cell anaemia or hypersplenism and can result in a decrease in size of an enlarged spleen which is often referred to as autosplenectomy.[45] The liver, like the lungs, receives a dual blood supply and therefore rarely infarcts, even when the hepatic artery is accidentally or deliberately ligated or embolized to treat metastatic tumours (Chapter 31).

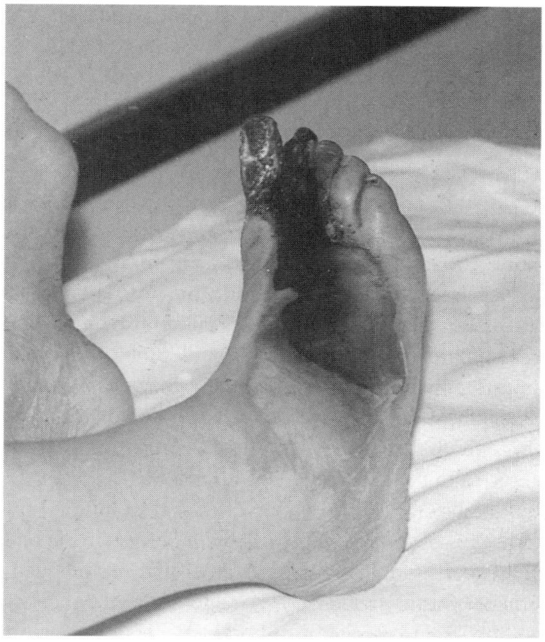

Fig. 10.5 A limb with an area of wet gangrene.

Gangrene

Gangrene is characterized by irreversible tissue necrosis, often associated with putrefaction, and may follow an acute occlusion of the blood supply to an organ or extremity. Gangrene occurs most commonly in the lower limb but the upper limb and intestine may also be affected.

Gangrene has two forms—wet and dry—but gradations occur, from the water-logged gangrene of rapidly extending infection to the mummification of gradual arterial occlusion. Dry gangrene is discussed with chronic occlusive vascular disease in the subsequent section.

Wet gangrene follows an acute arterial occlusion that is left untreated, particularly if the limb is oedematous or has defective venous drainage. Wet gangrene occurs if the arterial occlusion is sufficiently sudden to prevent the loss by evaporation of the normal tissue fluid. Micro-organisms secondarily invade the moist gangrenous tissue which provides an excellent medium for bacterial growth. Wet arterial gangrene has to be differentiated from infected clostridial or non-clostridial gas gangrene (see Chapter 4). Antibiotic chemotherapy often fails to prevent infection because the drugs cannot reach the ischaemic tissues. Antibiotics may, however, be useful in preventing the spread of organisms to healthy tissues and in encouraging demarcation.[46,47]

Wet gangrene has a dusky appearance, often intermingled with the erythema of inflammation, which has an ill defined and spreading edge (Fig. 10.5). The skin may blister and the digits soon

REFERENCES

45. Bowdler A J Clin Haematol 1983; 12: 467
46. Frier J, Daniel D, Davis C Rev Inf Dis 1979; 1: 210
47. Shaffer J O Surgery 1947; 21: 692

become insensitive and immobile because of ischaemic changes in the nerves and muscles of the limb. Gas bubbles may form within the tissues causing crepitus (surgical emphysema); if left untreated the limb gives off a characteristic putrefying stench.

Chronic occlusion

When a severe arterial stenosis predates an acute arterial occlusion, pre-existing collateral channels usually ensure that the symptoms of acute ischaemia and wet gangrene do not develop. In some instances where there are very good collateral pathways, patients may even remain free of symptoms, and should gangrene occur the changes are often minimal. In many instances, however, the eventual occlusion leads to a sudden but rapid deterioration in symptoms, which then usually improve as collateral channels open up in response to the new ischaemic stimulus.

Acute on chronic occlusions invariably develop on top of pre-existing disease of the arterial wall, and atherosclerosis or arteritis is usually responsible. Rupture of an atheromatous plaque with the development of intraplaque haemorrhage is still the most common cause of the final arterial thrombotic occlusion,[23] but gradual thickening of the subintimal layer with platelet deposition may also account for some of the more chronic occlusions.[48] Rupture of an atheromatous plaque may shower emboli into the distal circulation causing occlusion of the digital arteries. This gives rise to the 'blue toe syndrome', or if the upper limb is affected, the 'blue finger syndrome'.[49] When the emboli are more extensive and produce widespread ischaemic areas, the changes are often called 'trashfoot'.

Coronary arteries

A chronic coronary artery occlusion often leads to a myocardial infarct but may produce angina or remain symptomless. This is discussed in more detail in Chapter 23.

Aortoiliac and lower limb vessels

A chronic aortoiliac occlusion often presents with new or deteriorating claudication which is usually experienced in both thighs and buttocks as well as in the lower leg and calf. Erectile impotence and muscle wasting are additional features of Leriche's syndrome.[50] A single common iliac occlusion may cause unilateral buttock claudication, while an external iliac occlusion usually produces unilateral thigh claudication. An acute or chronic aortoiliac occlusion almost never causes rest pain or dry gangrene of the feet, unless there are additional stenoses or occlusions of the distal vessels.[51] Atherosclerosis is, of course, a generalized disease and other stenoses and occlusions are quite common.

The external iliac and the common femoral arteries may also become chronically occluded, and the profunda femoris artery is often narrowed or occluded at its origin, though this vessel is usually disease-free in some part of its course.[52]

The most common site of stenosis in the lower limb is in the superficial femoral artery as it passes through the adductor canal.[51] This artery may later occlude, while the popliteal artery, particularly in its lower third, is often comparatively disease-free (Fig. 10.6). Individual crural vessels, the pedal arches, the metatarsal and digital arteries may all become chronically occluded as the result of mural disease (Fig. 10.7). The more distal the occlusion, the less the prospect of collateral pathways and the greater the likelihood of ischaemic rest pain, ulceration and gangrene. Diabetic patients, in particular, commonly have disease of multiple segments which often affects the arteries distal to the popliteal trifurcation.[53]

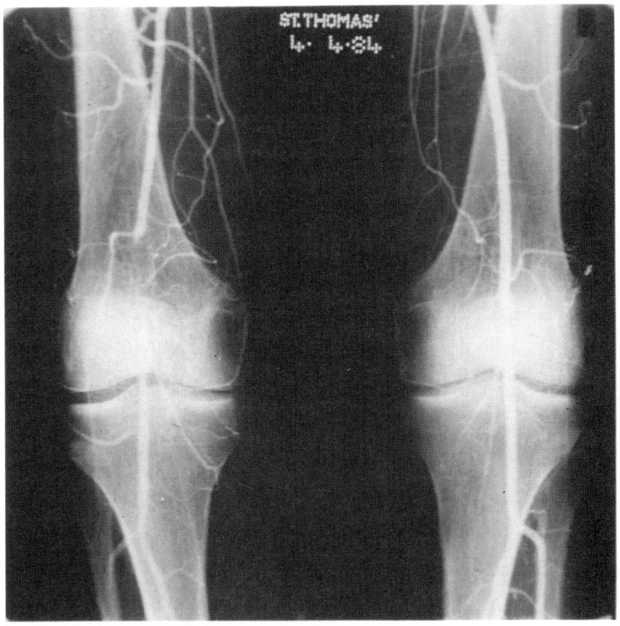

Fig. 10.6 An aortogram showing an occluded upper popliteal artery on the right with a relatively spared (normal) lower popliteal artery.

Critical limb ischaemia

This has been defined as rest pain, ulceration or gangrene associated with a Doppler pressure at the ankle of less than 50 mmHg or at the toe of 20 mmHg in patients who are not diabetic.[54] Tissue necrosis will almost inevitably ensue in limbs with critical ischaemia if the circulation cannot be improved.

Rest pain

Rest pain is usually experienced in the dorsum of the foot and the toes, being worse at night. The pain is dull and severe and usually

REFERENCES

48. Wolfe N The Pathology of Atherosclerosis. Butterworths, London 1982
49. Karmody A M, Powers S R et al Arch Surg 1976; 111: 1263–1268
50. Leriche R Presse Med 1940; 48: 601
51. Dibble J H The Pathology of Limb Ischaemia. Oliver and Boyd, Edinburgh 1966
52. Beales J S M, Adcock F A et al Br J Radiol 1971; 44: 854
53. Conrad M C Circulation 1967; 36: 83–91
54. European Working Group on Critical Limb Ischaemia. Eur J Vasc Surg 1992; (suppl A): 1–32

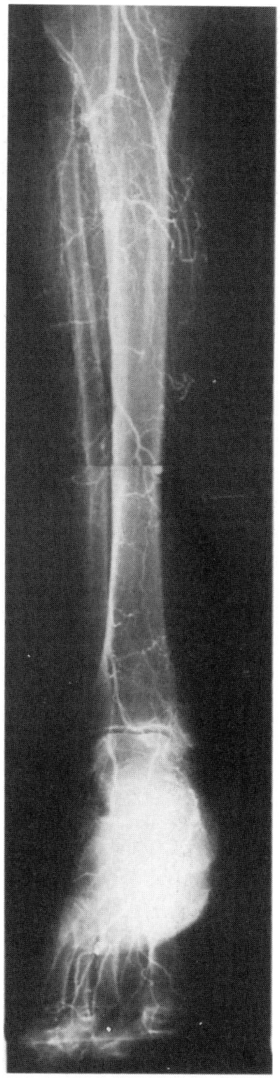

Fig. 10.7 An arteriogram showing atherosclerotic occlusions of the crural vessels. A bypass was made to the peroneal artery and the plantar arch.

requires opiate analgesia for symptomatic relief. The patient wakes up with a painful cold foot which is relieved by hanging the foot over the side of the bed or by walking around. Placing the leg in a dependent position allows gravity to improve the blood flow, and exercise also increases the blood flow to the limb. Patients may even take to sleeping in a chair to avoid the pain associated with elevation of the legs. The pain comes on at night because of the reduction in cardiac output that accompanies sleep with a decrease in blood pressure and an increase in peripheral vasodilatation. Although the exact mechanism of rest pain remains obscure, a reduced blood supply to peripheral nerves and an accumulation of metabolites have both been implicated.[55]

Dry gangrene

Nutritional changes vary in extent from dry necrosis of the skin of the fingertips or toes (as in Raynaud's disease or scleroderma) to gangrene of one or more limbs. Sometimes the first sign of arterial

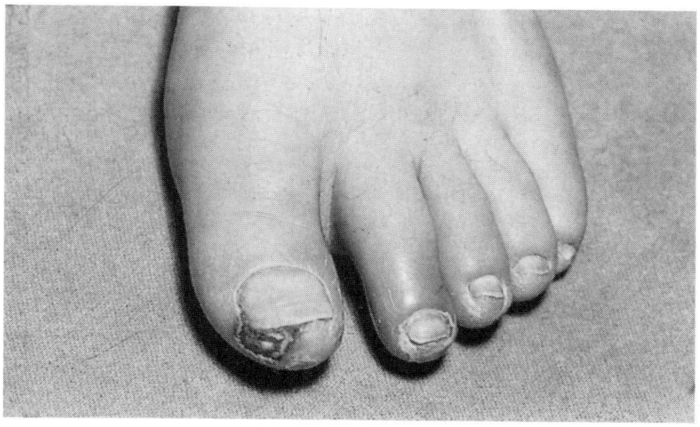

Fig. 10.8 An ischaemic nailfold.

insufficiency is a nailfold infection in, for example, a patient with thromboangiitis obliterans (Fig. 10.8). Ulceration of the legs which fails to heal (Fig. 10.9) or tiny fissures in the skin of the feet may be early signs of incipient gangrene. Dry gangrene develops from the gradual interruption of the supply of tissues, free from oedema, liberally drained by open veins, exposed to evaporation and remaining uninfected. An area of skin, often at the tip of a digit or at a point of contact between two adjacent toes, becomes dark and blackens. This area is often small at first but may then extend for a varying distance. Sensation is lost, and the gangrenous part becomes shrunken and wrinkled. This process of tissue death extends until a level is reached where an adequate blood supply remains. The vessels at this level dilate and signs of mild inflammation arise to produce a barrier of granulation tissue—the line of demarcation between living and dead tissue (Fig. 10.10).

When the process is allowed to proceed uninterrupted, the gangrenous extremity separates, and as the superficial tissues are dried by evaporation to a more proximal level than the deep tissues, the resultant stump is conical with an apex of exposed bone which may later separate as a sequestrum, before being covered by epithelium.

It is rarely possible or practical to await this process of autoamputation when gangrene extends into the forefoot or above the level of the heel (Fig. 10.11) and surgical ablation is invariably required to relieve pain and provide a functional myoplastic stump.

Extracranial vessels

Chronic occlusion of the common carotid, external and internal carotid vessels is the normal progression of severe stenosis in these vessels. The vertebral and basilar arteries may also occlude, as may the main brachiocephalic/innominate trunk. Chronic occlusions of individual vessels may be symptomless in the presence of a well formed circle of Willis, or may be associated with transient ischaemic attacks, progressive dementia, blindness and cerebral infarction.[56]

REFERENCES

55. Lewis T Arch Intern Med 1932; 49: 413
56. Mitchell J R A, Schwartz C J Arterial Disease. Blackwell, Oxford 1965

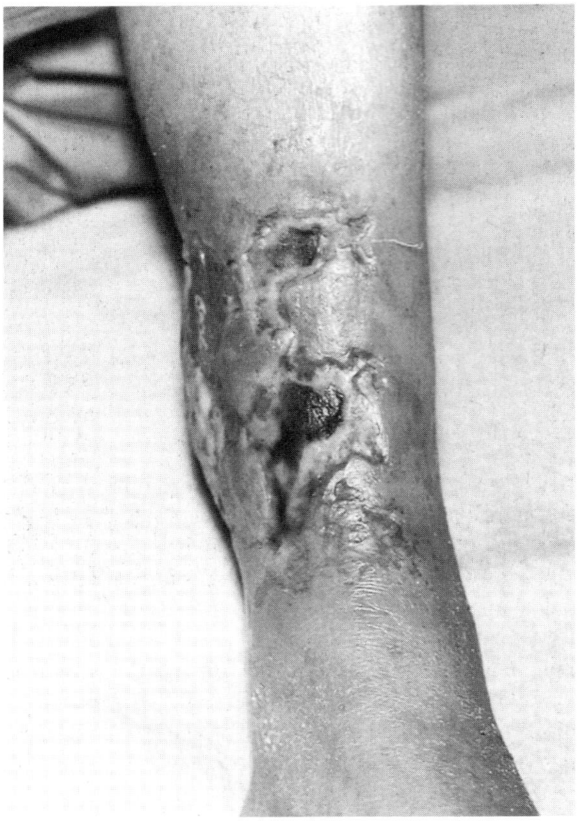

Fig. 10.9 An ischaemic ulcer.

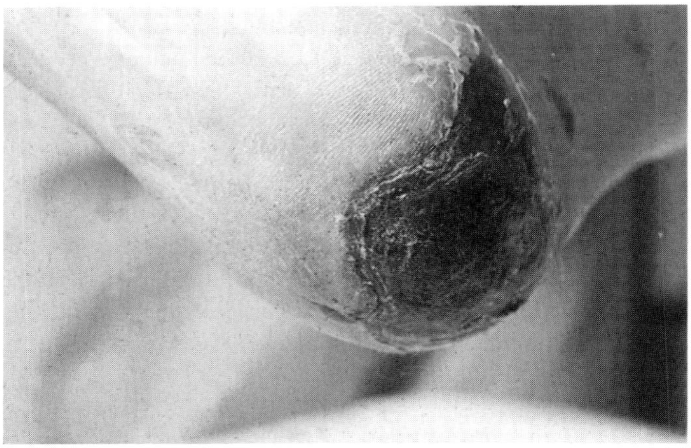

Fig. 10.10 A clear line of demarcation between living and dead tissue.

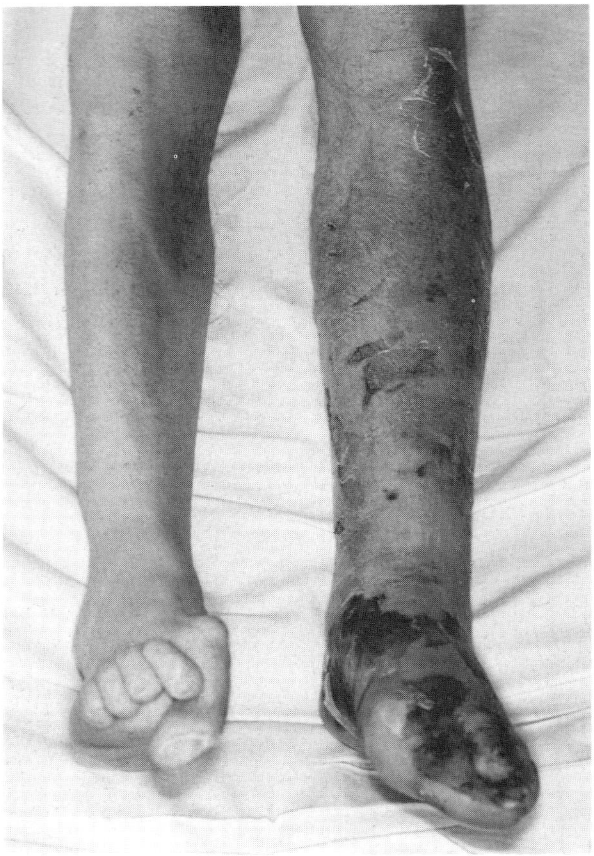

Fig. 10.11 Extensive gangrene involving the foot and lower leg. The heel could not have been preserved even if the limb had been successfully revascularized.

Transient ischaemic attacks are reversible episodes of focal cerebral malfunction which recover within 24 hours.[57] The majority of these abate within a few minutes or a couple of hours, although minor neurological signs may persist for longer. The majority of transient ischaemic attacks are the result of platelet clumps breaking off from ulcerated plaques in the extracerebral vessels and embolizing into the cerebral or retinal vessels where they lodge temporarily, occluding the blood supply, before subsequently breaking up.[58–60] Transient ischaemic attacks can occur in patients with occluded cerebral vessels, and it is still debatable whether these are the result of platelet emboli arising from the proximal end of an occluded vessel, or whether they represent true cerebral hypoperfusion as the result of critically reduced blood flow.[61] Evidence has shown that cerebral hypoperfusion certainly does exist,[62,63] while the former hypothesis remains speculative. Hypoperfusional transient ischaemic attacks tend to follow exertion or vasodilatation (e.g. following a glass or two of whisky) and may occur many times a day.[64] They usually affect patients who have often not sustained a full cerebral infarct with one or more occluded extracranial vessels (i.e. both carotids and one vertebral).

The majority of major extracerebral arterial occlusions cause cerebral infarction. The infarct originally appears as an area of hyperaemic congested brain which rapidly becomes oedematous. The oedema may extend out into the surrounding normal brain

REFERENCES

57. Fisher C M Neurol Pschiatry 1951; 65: 356
58. Harrison M G H, Marshall J Br Med J 1975; 1: 616
59. Hollenhorst R W JAMA 1961; 178: 23
60. Zukowski A J, Nicolaides A N et al J Vasc Surg 1984; 1: 782
61. Barnett H J M, Peerless S J, Kaufman J C E Stroke 1978; 9: 448
62. Gibbs J M, Wise R J S et al Lancet 1984; i: 310
63. Ackerman R H, Correia J A, Alpert N M Arch Neurol 1981; 38: 537
64. Kistler J P, Roppr A H, Heros R C N Engl J Med 1984; 311: 27

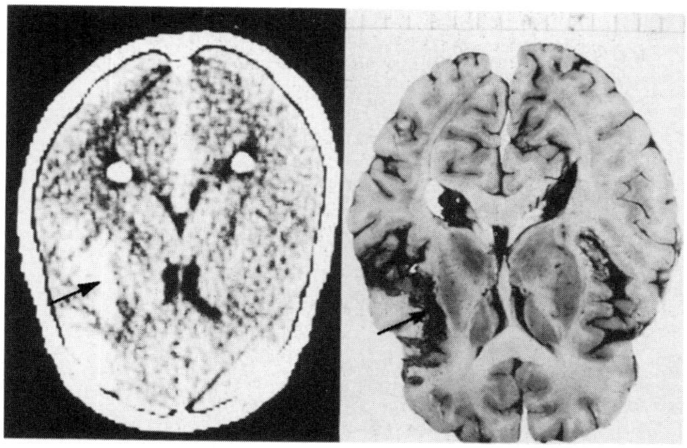

a b

Fig. 10.12 A computerized tomographic scan (**a**) showing a liquefied cerebral infarct; (**b**) the corresponding post-mortem section of the brain.

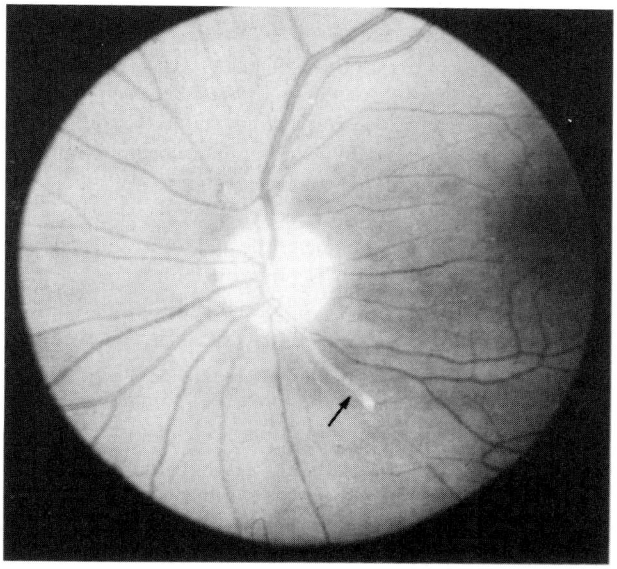

Fig. 10.13 A cholesterol embolus occluding a branch of the retinal artery.

causing raised intracranial pressure, tentorial herniation and eventually coning of the brainstem. The infarct then becomes softened and pulpy, containing a white emulsion which consists of fatty globules, the remains of cells and fibres, containing many phagocytes. Later the infarct may liquefy and even calcify before being replaced by scar tissue, although a central cystic area can persist (Fig. 10.12).

A platelet or cholesterol embolus arising from disease in the wall of the aorta, the brachiocephalic artery or the carotid vessels may cause transient blindness (amaurosis fugax),[65] or permanent loss of vision if the retinal artery or one of its major branches remains occluded. Fundoscopy may show emboli within the retinal vessels (Fig. 10.13) or may show pale areas of retinal infarction (Fig. 10.14). Visual field examination usually shows areas of field loss.

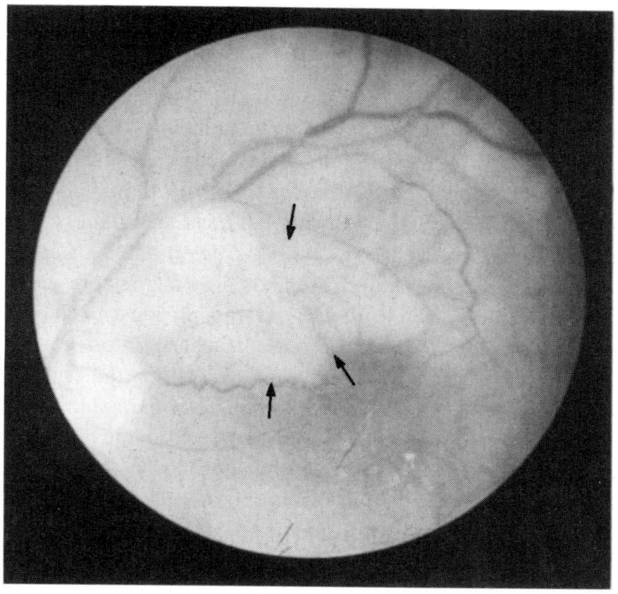

Fig. 10.14 A retinal infarct.

Progressive dementia is a rare but important consequence of chronic occlusive and embolic disease of the extracranial and intracerebral vessels. It is less common than other forms of dementia such as Alzheimer's disease but must be considered in all patients presenting with presenile dementia.[66] Loss of the superficial temporal or carotid pulse, poor pulsation seen in the retinal vessels, extracranial or postorbital bruits, and evidence of ischaemic vascular disease elsewhere should all alert the clinician to the possibility of a vascular cause for the dementia.

Visceral vessels

Chronic occlusions of one of the visceral vessels may, like a severe stenosis, pass unnoticed providing the other major vessels are free of disease. An acute occlusion of the superior mesenteric artery usually causes mesenteric infarction because collateral channels, although present, may not be able to dilate sufficiently swiftly to overcome the acute reduction in blood flow.[44]

Symptoms of intestinal angina and mesenteric infarction invariably follow a major visceral occlusion if there is stenotic or occlusive disease in the other two vessels.[67] A poor marginal artery in association with a chronic reduction in mesenteric blood flow can lead to ischaemic colitis which presents with persistent and sometimes blood-stained diarrhoea, abdominal pain and weight loss[68] (see Chapter 27).

Chronic stenosis of a single renal artery causes hypertension and a decrease in renal size. Bilateral stenoses also result in hypertension, a decrease in renal size and eventually a progressive deterioration in renal function resulting in renal failure.

REFERENCES

65. Marshall J, Meadows S Brain 1968; 91: 419
66. Liston E H, La Rue A Biol Psychiatry 1983; 18: 1451
67. Dick A P, Graff R et al Gut 1967; 8: 206
68. Marston A, Pheils M T et al Gut 1966; 7: 1

CLINICAL HISTORY OF ARTERIAL DISEASE

The name, sex and age of the patient together with his or her occupation are essential. The initial symptoms, the time of their first presentation and any subsequent change must be documented. For example, if the complaint is of intermittent claudication of the lower limb, the time of onset, the site of the pain, the exact distance at which it develops, the maximum walking distance and the time taken for the pain to pass off must be determined. In addition progression and regression of symptoms from first presentation should be carefully noted. Direct questioning must exclude rest pain, and evidence of vascular disease in other territories must be carefully sought in all patients presenting with symptoms of an arterial nature. The effect of the symptoms on the patient's daily life, work and hobbies must also be assessed from the history, and all patients with vascular symptoms must be closely questioned on their tobacco habits. A family history of vascular disease may be important in vasospastic disorders and atherosclerosis, and the patient's occupation may provide useful pointers as, for example, regular usage of vibrating tools may induce vasospasticity in the digital vessels. A history of significant trauma, however long ago, must not be overlooked, neither should a history of frostbite. A detailed history of drug intake and allergy may be important, and the patient's previous and present general health may also provide useful and relevant information. A past history of rheumatic fever, atrial fibrillation, diabetes, syphilis, rheumatoid arthritis and ergot intake may also provide important clues to the diagnosis of the underlying arterial disorder.

THE PHYSICAL SIGNS OF ARTERIAL DISEASE

Many of the physical signs associated with arterial disease have already been discussed in the description of the pathophysiology of arterial disease but they are summarized here for the sake of completeness. The lower limbs will be used as examples of the physical signs associated with peripheral arterial disease.

1. The temperature of the limb should be assessed and compared with the opposite side. Relative coolness indicates a significant reduction in blood flow while frigidity follows an acute occlusion with poor collaterals.

2. Colour changes in the skin range from pallor, through normal skin colour, to cyanosis and rubor. These changes may remain constant, vary with position or undergo cyclical changes in vasospastic disease. Intense pallor is usually seen in the early stages of an acute arterial obstruction with poor collaterals. At a later stage the limb becomes cyanotic before gangrene develops. Chronic ischaemia is often associated with cyanosis and rubor, as accumulated metabolites attempt to stimulate capillary vasodilatation, but the poor blood flow results in desaturation of the stagnant blood. Buerger's test exploits the response of ischaemic tissues to elevation. Buerger's angle of circulatory insufficiency is the angle at which a limb is held to produce pallor.[69] This test is very inaccurate but can be used to compare a normal and an abnormal limb if both limbs are elevated to 60° for 2 min.[70] Pallor is then obvious on the sole of the ischaemic foot. The time taken for each limb to become pallid is observed. The veins in the elevated ischaemic limb may become empty causing venous guttering, and if the legs are then placed in a dependent position, the ischaemic limb shows a delayed but pronounced hyperaemic response.

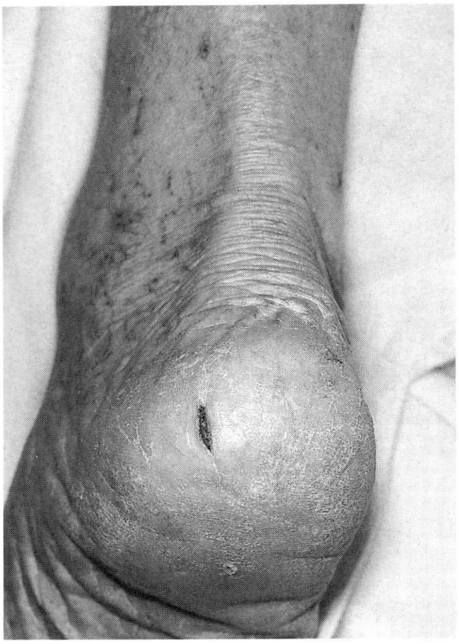

Fig. 10.15 An ischaemic crack over the heel.

3. Evidence of early ischaemic change is seen in rapidly growing tissues. The nails become brittle and short, and hair growth is said to be poor (although it is often difficult to detect marked differences in hair growth between normal and abnormal limbs).

4. In advanced chronic ischaemia cracks may develop over the heel (Fig. 10.15); the pulp spaces may become infected and ulceration may appear over the pressure points and between the toes. Eventually frank gangrene is seen in the distal tissues (Figs 10.8–11, 10.16).

5. In acute ischaemia the leg is pallid and rapidly becomes swollen over the muscle compartment. Later the muscles become tender as neuromuscular weakness and finally paralysis develops. This is associated with loss of sensation in the skin to light touch and pain. Such a neurosensory deficit indicates severe ischaemia.

6. The presence and extent of any gangrene should be carefully inspected and recorded, and the existence of a clear line of demarcation noted (Figs 10.10, 10.11). Ischaemic ulceration can occur anywhere, on the toes, foot or around the ankle. Ischaemic ulcers do not have any distinguishing signs. They have sloping terraced edges. They are not surrounded by lipodermatosclerosis but usually have a slough covered surface and poor pale granulation tissue in their base. Multiple showers of tiny emboli have the characteristic features already described (Fig. 10.17). Their appearance should lead to a careful search for a proximal aneurysm or an ulcerated plaque.

REFERENCES

69. Buerger L Circulatory Disturbances of the Extremities. W B Saunders, Philadelphia 1924
70. Insall R L, Davies R J, Prout W G J R Soc Med 1989; 82: 729

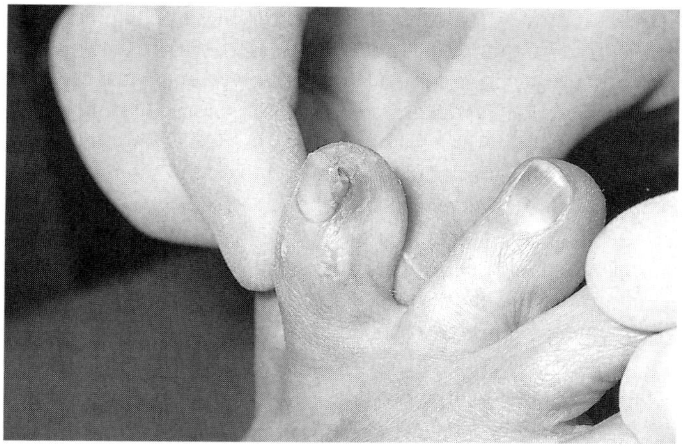

Fig. 10.16 Ischaemic ulceration appearing between the toes.

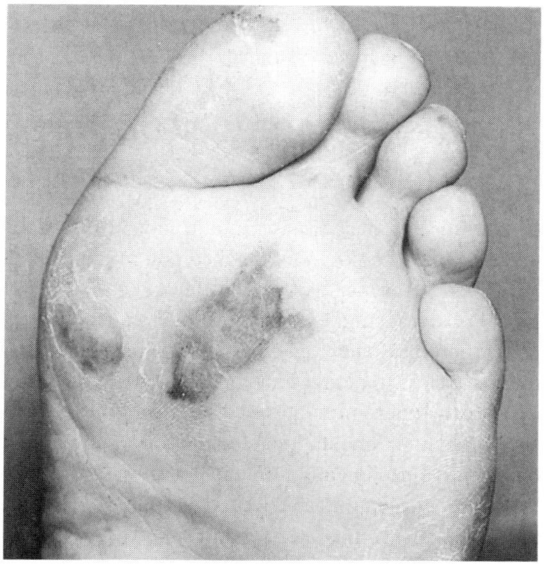

Fig. 10.17 The appearance produced by showers of platelet emboli lodging in the capillaries of the feet.

7. Absence of arterial pulsation indicates arterial occlusion which may be assumed to lie below the lowest palpable and above the highest impalpable pulse. Large collateral vessels may maintain a reduced distal pulse even when the main artery is occluded. In the lower limbs the aortic pulse, both femoral, popliteal, posterior tibial and dorsalis pedis pulses must be palpated and recorded as present, diminished, absent or enlarged. Although a complicated grading system has been proposed to gauge pulse volume,[71] the use of these four simple descriptions is probably more valuable. It is important to remember that anatomical variations can exist: the dorsalis pedis is absent from its normal position in 14% of the population and the peroneal artery replaces the posterior tibial artery in 5%.[72] The astute clinician will also feel for the peroneal trunk as it lies in front of the lateral malleolus.

A true expansile pulsation must be distinguished from transmitted pulsation, and the upper and lower extent of any aneurysm must be determined. When an aneurysm is found, all other aneurysmal sites must be carefully palpated to exclude the presence of multiple aneurysms. An aneurysm in the popliteal fossa is easily missed by the conventional method of palpation. It may be better felt if the knee is hyperextended by one hand, pushing the artery onto the flexed fingers of the other hand.

8. All the arteries that supply the lower limbs must be carefully auscultated to detect bruits or machinery murmurs. It is important to listen over the aorta, the iliac vessels, the common femoral arteries and the superficial femoral artery in the adductor canal and the popliteal artery as these are the common sites of arterial stenoses.

9. In patients suspected of having vascular disease, all the other major vessels must be examined by palpation and auscultation. The superficial temporal artery pulse should be felt in front of the external auditory meatus, and middle cerebral bruits may be heard through the closed upper eyelid. Carotid pulsation and carotid bruits may be felt and auscultated at the anterior border of the sternomastoid behind and below the angle of the jaw. Subclavian and vertebral bruits are listened for in the supraclavicular fossa. All bruits heard over the vessels of the head and neck can be transmitted from cardiac murmurs, and it is therefore important to auscultate over the precordium to exclude this possibility. In the upper limb the brachial, radial and ulnar pulses should be palpated and the blood pressure taken in both antecubital fossae. The presence of a cardiac irregularity is noted when the pulses are examined, and any abnormality of the jugular venous pressure must also be recorded.

10. The heart and lungs must be fully examined (Chapters 22 and 23) as abnormal findings may support a particular diagnosis and influence management. A general examination of the patient should enable anaemia, polycythaemia, xanthomata, xanthelasmata, arcus senilis and other major pathology to be detected (Fig. 10.18).

11. A full neurological examination including fundoscopy must be carried out if the patient complains of transient ischaemic attacks, amaurosis fugax, vertebrobasilar insufficiency or completed strokes. It is also essential if a cervical bruit is found on routine examination.

12. There are few physical signs of chronic mesenteric ischaemia apart from the doubtful relevance of an abdominal bruit. Some patients however present with vague abdominal pains associated with cachexia from a large decrease in body weight. Even when an acute mesenteric infarct develops there may be little in the way of physical signs, the patient complaining of severe abdominal pain out of proportion to the findings on clinical examination. Patients subsequently develop signs of acute peritonitis with generalized tenderness, rebound tenderness, guarding, rigidity and absent bowel sounds. Eventually, abdominal distension and septic shock supervene (see Chapter 29).

13. Machinery murmurs may be heard over arteriovenous fistulae, or over their major feeding vessels. The neck veins may be elevated if a fistula is causing cardiac embarrassment, and a left ventricular heave may be detected on palpation of the precordium.

REFERENCES

71. Adachi B Das Arteriensystem. Arf Maruzen, I Paner: Kyoto 1920
72. Ludbrook J, Clark A M, McKenzie J K Br Med J 1962; 1: 1724

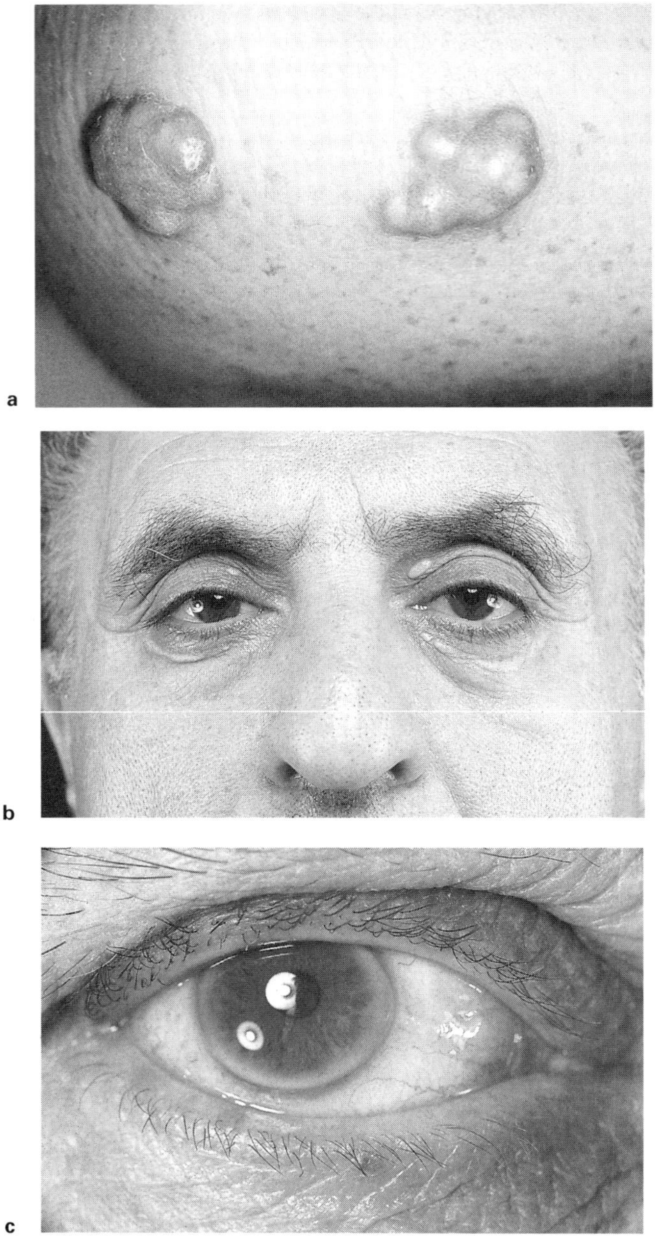

Fig. 10.18 Examples of (a) xanthomata, (b) xanthelasmata and (c) arcus senilis.

An indication of the amount of the circulatory embarrassment produced by arteriovenous fistulae within the limbs can be obtained by Branham's test[73,74] in which the pulse rate is recorded for 1 min before a pneumatic tourniquet is placed around the root of the affected limb and inflated above systolic pressure to occlude arterial inflow. The pulse rate is then retaken. A marked fall in the pulse rate indicates a large left-to-right shunt and potential cardiac embarrassment. Occasionally an abdominal aortic aneurysm may rupture into the inferior vena cava. The classical signs are lower limb oedema and cyanosis, a machinery murmur on abdominal auscultation and marked elevation of the jugular venous pressure.

14. Patients with vasospastic disease may have their symptoms provoked by exposure to cold. The integrity of the palmar arch can be assessed by Allen's test.[75] In this test digital compression is applied over the ulnar and radial arteries at the wrist, while the patient is instructed to make a fist repeatedly to empty the capillary circulation of the hand. Partial or complete palmar flushing is seen when the pressure over one of the vessels is released. The continuity of the palmar arch and its dependent vessels of supply can be deduced if this test is repeated for the other feeding vessel.

15. Thoracic outlet syndrome may cause occlusion of the subclavian artery. This syndrome is most commonly associated with a cervical rib but can be caused by a tight band, bony exostoses or hypertrophied muscle. The radial pulse, which is palpable when the arm is at rest by the side, will fade or disappear when the arm is abducted and externally rotated to 90°, and exercise of the hand in this position rapidly causes ischaemic pain associated with pallor. This test is not specific and can be positive in normal individuals.

16. Popliteal entrapment syndrome occurs when the popliteal artery passes beneath the medial head of gastrocnemius. Normal pedal pulses are present at rest but become impalpable on plantar flexion of the ankle against resistance.

THE INVESTIGATION OF VASCULAR DISEASE

Blood and urine tests

All patients with vascular disease should have a full blood count which includes the haemoglobin, packed cell volume, differential white blood cell count, platelet estimation and a blood film where necessary. Polycythaemia is an important cause of peripheral vascular symptoms, and anaemia may make symptoms of ischaemia worse. Leukaemia and thrombocythaemia can lead to thrombosis of the microcirculation.

The erythrocyte sedimentation rate or blood viscosity andC-reactive protein are elevated in autoimmune conditions such as collagen diseases, including rheumatoid arteritis and other disorders such as Buerger's disease or inflammatory aneurysms. The urea, electrolytes and creatinine give an estimate of renal function and may be abnormal if patients have been on long-term diuretic treatment.

Elevated serum cholesterol and fasting triglyceride concentrations are important risk factors which can be treated with dietary and pharmacological manipulation to prevent rapid progression of atherosclerotic disease. Family screening and counselling can be performed in patients with inherited hyperlipidaemias.[76]

The urine should be tested for sugar and a random blood glucose measured in order to exclude diabetes. A glucose tolerance test is indicated if the screening tests are equivocal or if diabetes is suspected.

Serum autoantibodies may be raised in the collagen diseases, and blood should be screened for antinuclear factor, anti-DNA, Rose–Waaler and latex agglutination, antinuclear cytoplasmic antibody (ANCA), immunoglobulins and complement (C3, C4) in

REFERENCES

73. Branham H H J Surg 1890; 3: 250
74. Nicoladoni C Arch Klin Chir 1875; 18: 252
75. Allen E V Am J Med Sci 1929; 178: 237
76. Lewis B T The Hyperlipidaemias: Clinical and Laboratory Practice. Blackwell, Oxford 1976

patients suspected of having a vasculitis or inflammatory arteritis.

A coagulation screen comprising the prothrombin time (measuring the activity of the extrinsic system), the activated partial thromboplastin time (for the intrinsic system) and the thrombin time may be helpful, particularly in patients with liver disease and in those having major surgery. The clotting time provides a measure of the overall coagulation ability. Young patients who present with arterial occlusion, and patients who thrombose bypass grafts when no technical reason is apparent should have a thrombophilia screen which includes protein C and S estimation,[77] antithrombin III levels[78] and antiphospholipid antibodies (also known as anticardiolipin antibodies or lupus anticoagulant).[79] Activated protein C should also now be measured as this is the most common form of thrombophilia.[80,81] Other tests such as platelet aggregation tests,[82] thrombomodulin assay[83] and the thromboelastograph[84] have not yet found their way into the routine assessment of arterial disorders.

Cardiorespiratory investigations

A chest radiograph and electrocardiogram are essential in patients with atheromatous peripheral vascular disease. The chest radiograph allows an assessment of cardiac size and chamber dilatation to be made, and detects significant pulmonary pathology such as carcinoma of the bronchus, which is an important concomitant condition in heavy smokers with severe atherosclerosis. Peak expiratory flow rate is a useful test of respiratory function, and spirometry and arterial blood gases may be measured in some patients with asthma or chronic obstructive airways disease.

The electrocardiograph diagnoses arrhythmias and may also provide evidence of myocardial ischaemia. An exercise electrocardiograph may uncover ischaemic changes which are not present at rest.

An echocardiogram is useful in confirming the diagnosis of cardiac valvular disease, and in showing thrombus in an atrial appendage or attached to the wall of the left ventricle.[85] The transoesophageal route is more sensitive than a transthoracic echocardiograph in detecting abnormalities of the heart and great vessels.[86] Echocardiography before and after exercise may detect abnormalities of wall motion secondary to reversible coronary ischaemia. Thallium scanning before and after vasodilatation with dipyridamole also defines areas of cardiac ischaemia.[87] Thallium is taken up into healthy myocardium, but infarction produces 'cold spots'. A cold spot which appears after dipyridamole suggests an area of reversible ischaemia. Coronary catheterization and angiography may be necessary in patients with severe angina and in those who have positive stress tests. Positron emission tomography is very good at assessing cardiac ischaemia but is very expensive and available at few hospitals.

Intravenous pyelography[88,89] and barium contrast[68] studies may be helpful in assessing patients suspected of renal vascular disease or mesenteric occlusions. Small ischaemic kidneys may be seen on the renogram phase of the pyelogram with delay in the appearance of contrast which often appears to be very concentrated. Reduced function can be confirmed by an isotopic renogram.[90] Thumbprinting or ischaemic strictures may occasionally be seen in patients with ischaemic colitis (see Chapter 30), but at present there are no satisfactory tests for detecting intestinal ischaemia other than arteriography, and even then the anatomical appearances do not always relate to the pathophysiology of the condition.[91–93]

Specific vascular investigations

Doppler ultrasound pressure measurement

Ultrasound probes emit and receive continuous high-frequency sound waves through two crystals. When the emitted sound strikes a moving object such as the red cell, it is reflected back. This is detected by the probe as an increase or decrease in frequency depending on the direction of movement of the object. This is known as the Doppler shift or Doppler effect. This Doppler shift is perceived as a change in the pitch of a siren or train whistle as an ambulance or train passes an observer. The increase in frequency is proportional to the velocity of the moving particle. This increased frequency is detected audibly as an increase in pitch, and can be recorded and quantified by its spectral wave form.[94] The peak of the spectral trace is related to the highest velocity in the lumen—usually found in the centre of the vessel. When the lumen is narrowed, the velocity must increase to maintain flow, and this is reflected by an increase in the spectral wave form. The stenosis produces local turbulence with a wide variation in velocities at any one point, and this causes a spectral broadening. The normal wave form is triphasic with a sharp upstroke related to acceleration, a downstroke from deceleration, reversal of flow and a small component representing forward flow. The wave form distal to a stenosis may become bi- or uniphasic (Fig. 10.19).

The Doppler probe should be held at 45–60° to the skin overlying the vessel and an acoustic gel used to obliterate air from the interface to ensure good coupling. The probe can be used in combination with a sphygmomanometer cuff to measure the pressure in peripheral arteries,[95] which is very useful if the pulse is impalpable or weak. When the cuff of the sphygmomanometer is inflated above the systolic pressure, the lumen of the vessel is occluded by the external compressive force, blood flow ceases and the sound disappears. As the tourniquet is released flow and sound return,

REFERENCES

77. Atkinson S D, Leclerc J R In: Leclerc J R (ed) Venous Thrombo-embolic Disorders. Lea and Febiger, Beckenham 1991 pp 29–32
78. Egeborg O Thromb Diath Haemorrh 1965; 13: 516
79. Boey L M, Colaco C B et al Br Med J 1983; 287: 1021
80. Dahlback B Haemostatis 1994; 24: 139
81. Koster T, Rosendaal FR, de Ronde H et al Lancet 1993; 342: 1503
82. Emmons P R, Mitchell J R A Lancet 1965; i: 71
83. Ludlam C A, Cash J D In: Semer G G, Prentice C R M (eds) Haemostasis and Thrombosis. Academic Press, London 1978
84. Heather B, Jennings S, Greenhalgh R M Br J Surg 1980; 67: 63
85. Nishide M, Irino T et al Stroke 1983; 14: 541
86. Lagattolla N R, Burnand K G, Stewart A Br J Surg 1995; 82: 16651
87. Boucher C A, Brewster D C et al N Engl J Med 1985; 312: 389
88. Maxwell M H, Lupu A N J Urol 1968; 100: 395
89. Stamey J C, Fry W J Arch Surg 1977; 112: 1291
90. Maxwell M H, Lupu A N, Taplin E V J Urol 1968; 100: 376
91. Derrick J R, Pollard H S, Moore R M Ann Surg 1959; 149: 684
92. Harward T R S, Smith S, Seeger M D J Vasc Surg 1993; 17: 738
93. Marston A World J Surg 1979; 3: 495
94. Strandness D E Cardiovasc Surg 1970; 11: 192

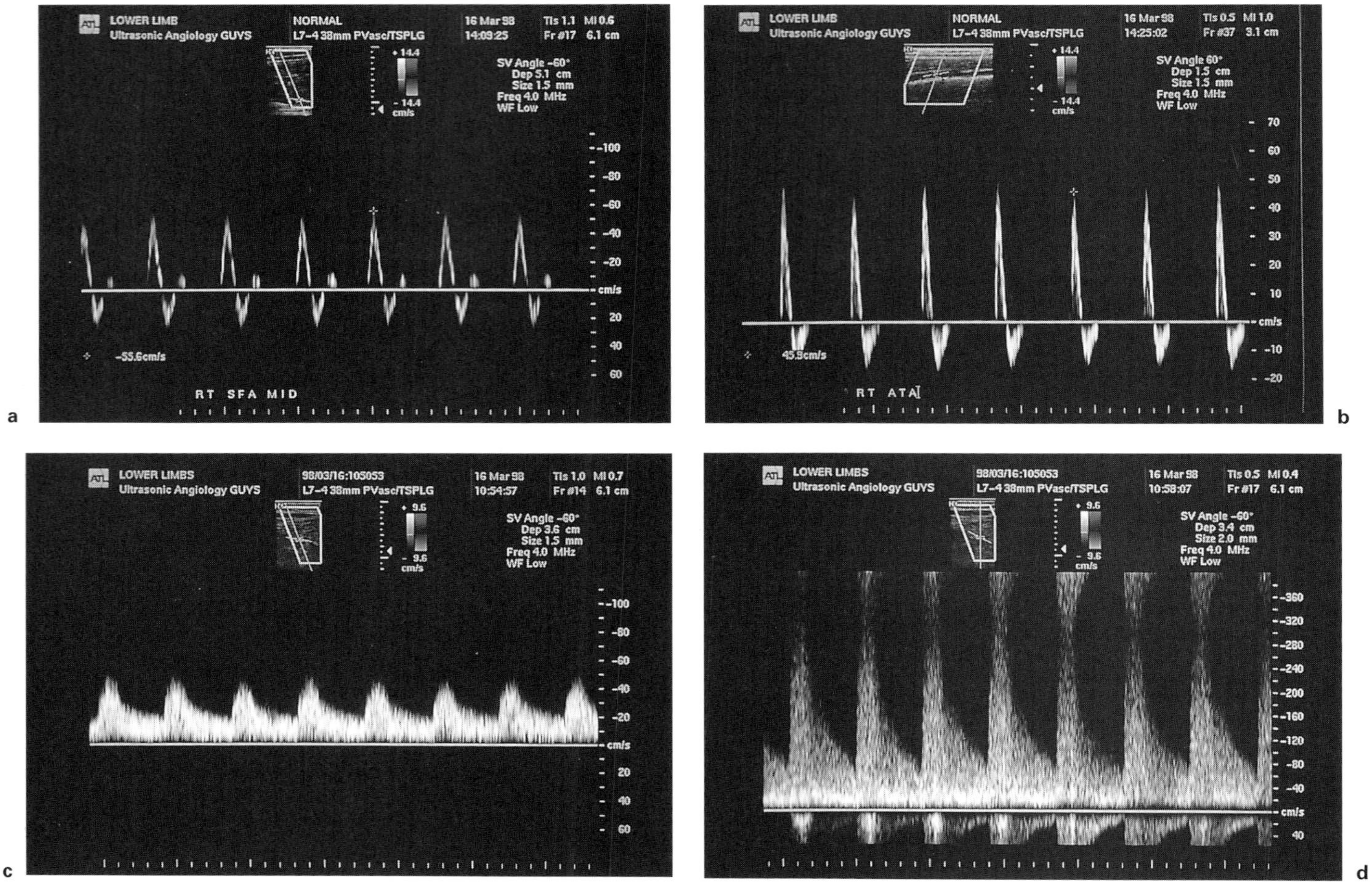

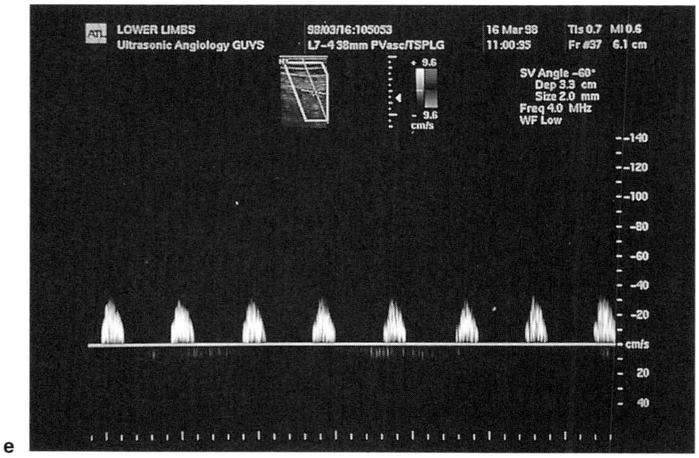

Fig. 10.19 (a) Normal triphasic waveform: forward systolic flow with sharp well defined peak, reversed flow component in diastole and small forward flow due to elastic recoil of arteries consistent with normal flow in high resistance peripheral arteries. **(b)** Biphasic waveform: forward systolic flow with reversed flow in diastole without the third phase of forward flow. **(c)** Monophasic waveform with continuous forward diastolic flow which shows spectral broadening compared with (a), consistent with low resistance flow e.g. internal carotid artery or renal artery. **(d)** Very high velocity with spectral broadening consistent with a significant stenosis. **(e)** Monophasic damped low velocity waveform with no diastolic flow consistent with waveforms found distal to an occlusion, or in a vessel with very low flow.

and this pressure is recorded. By comparing the pressure in the dorsalis pedis, peroneal and posterior tibial arteries at the ankle with the normal brachial systolic pressure measured by the same technique, a Doppler index is obtained—the ankle:brachial pressure index (ABPI). In normal vessels this index is close to unity.[95] In moderate occlusive disease the index is between 0.5 and 0.9, and in severe disease with rest pain or gangrene it is less than 0.4. Absolute pressures may give a more accurate picture. The pressure is normally above 50 mmHg in at least one ankle vessel in moderate disease, and below this level in all vessels if the limb is critically ischaemic.[96] This index is usually reliably reproducible and can be used to follow patients over time and assess the results of revascularization procedures.

Doppler pressures are incongruously high in patients with heavily calcified peripheral vessels because these arteries resist compression by the tourniquet and the Doppler signal persists. For this reason pressure measurements in patients with diabetes and/or renal failure are unreliable.[97] Pulses below 75–85 mmHg are usually impalpable, therefore the combination of an impalpable

REFERENCES

95. Yao J S T, Hobbs J T, Irvine W T Br J Surg 1969; 56: 676
96. Jamieson C W Br J Surg 1982; 69(suppl 2): 52
97. Quin R O, Evans D H, Bell P R F J Cardiovasc Surg 1975; 16: 586

pulse with a high Doppler pressure (greater than 120 mmHg) is diagnostic of incompressible arteries.

A treadmill with both adjustable speed and gradient provides an objective and reproducible assessment of the claudication distance.[98] It may help to differentiate pain on walking caused by arterial disease from other causes such as spinal claudication. A fall in Doppler pressure of more than 15 mmHg after exercise (3 minutes of walking at 4 km/hour on a 10° slope) can identify patients with stenotic arterial disease.[99,100] The routine use of exercise testing, however, adds little to the information given by the resting ankle brachial pressure index.

A number of methods have been used to assess the sonogram wave form in greater detail in attempt to separate the relative importance of proximal and distal stenoses and occlusions when both problems coexist in the same patient. Pulsatility index, principal component analysis, damping factor and transfer factor are some of the techniques that have been used to analyse the Doppler wave form.[101–103] None of these measurements, however, has shown a perfect correlation with the findings of biplanar arteriography.[104]

In some patients with severe critical ischaemia, the Doppler probe may not be sensitive enough to detect flow at the ankle. The signal can be augmented by inflating a pneumatic cuff around the calf, a technique called pulse-generated run-off. This may detect patent distal arteries which are not detected on Doppler examination or on arteriography.[105] Dopplers measured with the legs dependent will often detect ‘flow’ if the vessels are patent and this technique has reduced the need for the pulse-generated technique.

Doppler mapping

This technique of individual insonation of the digital vessels has been used to assess vasospastic disease in the hand.[106] The more severe the vasospasm, the fewer the number and lengths of vessel that can be insonated.

B-mode ultrasound imaging

The simple Doppler probe uses continuous wave ultrasound signals which cannot give anatomical information. Pulsed ultrasound probes send out short bursts of ultrasound waves: this allows the depth to be calculated by noting the time for the signal to return to the transducer. A two-dimensional image is built up based on the reflection of ultrasound waves from changes in tissue density. The grey scale is related to the strength of the returning signal. The signal is very strong and is represented as white if all the sound waves are returned to the probe. When no signal is detected the area is black. Intermediate signal strength is depicted as varying shades of grey. Abdominal B-mode ultrasound scanning[107,108] is an excellent technique for identifying and measuring the dimensions of infrarenal abdominal aortic aneurysms. The most accurate measurement is the antero–posterior diameter. Difficulties may arise when there is a poor acoustic window, often present in obese patients and in those with a large amount of bowel gas. Ultrasound can be used as a screening technique for abdominal aortic aneurysms in men aged 65–80 years. A randomized controlled study showed that screening significantly decreased the incidence of rupture and mortality when compared to an unscreened control group.[109,110]

Duplex ultrasound scanning

The combination of pulsed Doppler and B-mode imaging is known as duplex imaging. The direction of flow is depicted by a change in colour (colour flow imaging), with flow directed towards the probe seen as one colour and flow away as another (usually red and blue). The velocity of flow can also be encoded in colour, making areas of high velocity readily identifiable. The addition of colour renders the vessel and areas of disease easier to visualize and therefore decreases the time taken to perform the study. This makes duplex scanning of the peripheral arteries a viable alternative to contrast radiology. Power Doppler detects the amplitude of the signal and therefore encodes for velocity of flow but not for direction. It is particularly useful for determining the presence of flow before an impending occlusion.[111] It has the disadvantage that it increases the number of artefacts. There are now a number of ultrasound contrast agents which enhance the acoustic backscatter from moving blood and may improve its definition.[112] Duplex scanning has now become established as the first investigation for many patients with arterial disease. Its value in assessing carotid stenoses is well established.[113] The excellent images now obtained have been used to characterize the morphology of atheromatous plaques at the carotid bifurcation.[112] This may allow the identification of high risk plaques which require treatment from those which have a low risk of causing ischaemic neurological events.

Duplex can also be used to measure stenoses in native arteries and in arterial bypass grafts.[114–117] Localized changes in peak systolic velocity with a ratio greater than 2 suggest that the stenosis is haemodynamically significant, i.e.equivalent to a 75% reduction in cross-sectional area or 50% diameter reduction (Fig. 10.20). The identification of grafts with significant stenoses is important as remedial measures (angioplasty or vein patching) may maintain graft patency.[118] Although the circumstantial evidence is strong for the efficacy of graft surveillance programmes using duplex, no scanning randomized controlled study has yet been published.

REFERENCES

98. Clyne C A C, Tripolitis A, Jamieson C W Surg Gynecol Obstet 1979; 149: 727
99. Lainge S P Br Med J 1980; 1: 13
100. Yao J S T Br J Surg 1970; 57: 761
101. Woodcock J P, Gosling R G, Fitzgerald D E Br J Surg 1972; 59: 226
102. Strandness D E J Vasc Surg 1985; 2: 341
103. Skidmore R, Woodcock J P Ultrasound Med Biol 1980; 6: 7
104. Campbell W B, Cole S L A et al Br J Surg 1984; 71: 302
105. Beard et al Br J Surg 1970; 57: 761
106. O'Reilly M J G, Dodds A J et al Br J Surg 1979; 66: 712
107. Axelbaum S, Schellinger D et al Am J R 1976; 127: 75
108. Leopold G R Radiology 1970; 96: 9
109. Scott R A P et al Br J Surg 1995; 82: 1066
110. Rubin J M et al Radiology 1995 197: 183
111. Fobbe F et al Radiology 1992; 185(P): 142
112. Strandness D E In: Greenhalgh R M (ed) Vascular Imaging for Surgeons. W B Saunders, London 1995 pp 41–50
113. Nicholls S C, Phillips D J et al J Vasc Surg 1985; 2: 375
114. Edwards J M et al J Vasc Surg 1991; 13: 69
115. Van der Heijden F H W M et al Eur J Vasc Surg 1994; 7: 71
116. Bandyk D et al J Vasc Surg 1989; 9: 286
117. Brewster DC et al Arch Surg 1983 118: 1043–1047
118. Ramaswami G et al Eur J Vasc Surg 1994; 8: 214

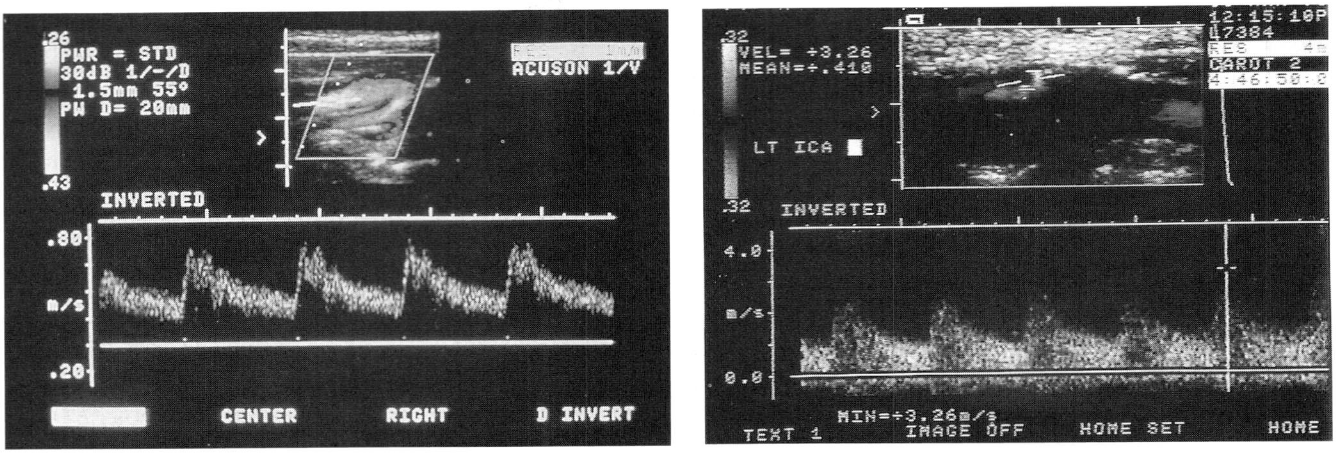

a b

Fig. 10.20 Doppler scans indicative of (**a**) normal carotid arteries and (**b**) a tight stenosis.

Duplex scanning has also been used to guide and monitor percutaneous transluminal angioplasty of lower limb arteries.[118]

Intravascular ultrasound

An ultrasound catheter is inserted into the lumen of the vessel over a guidewire, and a series of cross-sectional scans are recorded as it is pulled back.[119] These scans can now be combined to produce a three-dimensional image of the inside of the artery which can be rotated to view all aspects. This technique may be very useful following balloon angioplasty and after the placement of stents and stent grafts.

Contrast arteriography

Non-invasive tests are now able to diagnose the extent of arterial disease with considerable accuracy. The role of diagnostic contrast arteriography has therefore diminished. Some clinicians use non-invasive tests such as Doppler and duplex alone to assess the vessels before intervention.[120,121] The majority of surgeons and radiologists still however use contrast radiography to visualize arterial stenoses or occlusions before treatment. There are a number of different techniques for obtaining arteriograms and these are now described with an account of their relative advantages and disadvantages, indications and contraindications.[122]

Direct needle puncture

This was first described by Dos Santos et al in 1929.[123] A hollow needle is inserted directly into the arterial lumen upstream of the area of interest. A bolus of radiopaque contrast medium is injected directly into the lumen of the vessel and a rapid series of radiographs is taken of the vessels downstream of the injection site. Any direct puncture into an artery carries the risk of local damage, wall dissection, haemorrhage, false aneurysm formation, thrombosis and embolism.[124] Any injection of contrast can produce allergic and anaphylactic reactions[125] but this risk is reduced by using an iso-osmolar contrast medium.[126]

Translumbar aortography is reported to have a mortality of between 0.1 and 1%,[127] and is now rarely used. A similar order of risk is reported for carotid arteriography.[128] Direct puncture arteriography is contraindicated in patients with a bleeding tendency which cannot be corrected (including those being anticoagulated), and in patients with a known allergy to contrast medium. This technique, although useful in the operating theatre, has been superseded by the Seldinger technique.

Seldinger retrograde arteriography

The Seldinger technique uses a small plastic cannula which is inserted into the artery over a flexible guidewire placed in the vessel through a hollow needle.[129] This allows a catheter to be passed both retrogradely into a proximal vessel and antegradely into a distal vessel. The femoral artery is the most commonly used access site. The advent of guidable and steerable catheters[130] has permitted retrograde insertion of these catheters into the root of the aorta. Views of the aortic arch and great vessels can be obtained from an unselective arch injection. Selective studies can be performed when a catheter is inserted into the origins or even passed up the individual great vessels for more detailed images. Selective carotid angiograms can provide information about the circle of Willis, but the risk of stroke is higher than for arch injections.[131–134] Retrograde insertion to the level of the renal arteries

REFERENCES

119. Gerritsen G P et al J Vasc Surg 1993; 18: 31
120. Shearman C P, Gywnn B R et al Br Med J 1986; 293: 1086
121. Moore W S et al Ann Surg 1988; 208: 91
122. Irvine A, Burnand K G, Lea Thomas M Curr Prac in Surg 1996; 8: 72
123. Dos Santos R, Lamas A C, Caldas J P Arteriographie des Membres et de L'Aorte Abdominale. Masson, Paris 1931
124. McAffee J G Radiology 1957; 68: 825
125. Prendergrass H P, Hodes P J, Tondreau R L AJR 1955; 74: 262
126. Alment T, Aspelin P, Levin B Invest Radiol 1975; 10: 519
127. Szilagyi E D, Smith R F et al Arch Surg 1977; 112: 399
128. Hass W, Fields W et al JAMA 1968; 203: 159
129. Seldinger S I Acta Radiol 1953; 39: 368
130. Neiman H L, Brand T D, Greenberg M Arch Surg 1981; 116: 821

allows an assessment to be made of renal artery stenoses in hypertensive patients with peripheral vascular disease. A catheter inserted to this level also produces good views of the infrarenal aorta and the iliac, femoral and popliteal arteries. It is conventional to pass the catheter up the normal femoral artery or 'least diseased' side. Retrograde insertion to the level of the iliac vessel can be performed by insertion of the catheter into the ipsilateral femoral artery when proximal disease is not suspected and no views of the other leg are required. The contrast medium then passes down the single limb giving good views of the distal vasculature in the leg and the foot. Antegrade femoral puncture is rarely required for diagnostic purposes, but is useful when angioplasty of distal stenoses is being contemplated, especially if these cannot be reached via the iliac bifurcation from puncture of the contralateral femoral artery or the arm.

It is possible to damage the vessel wall by the Seldinger technique, but general anaesthesia is avoided, as is direct puncture of a very large vessel with its attendant risks. It is often more difficult to insert contrast medium as swiftly through a catheter as through a large-bore needle and the image of the vessel containing the catheter is distorted by its presence.[135]

Digital subtraction arteriography

This has now become the preferred radiological method for imaging arteries and can be performed with contrast injected into either the veins or the arteries. Images are taken of the field of interest and these are digitized. Contrast medium is then injected into the circulation and further views taken. The control images can be subtracted from those taken after contrast, giving high quality images of the arteries.[136] The patient must not move, and poor images are obtained if involuntary movement takes place, particularly in the abdomen, when bowel peristalsis can cause gas artefacts. If intravenous contrast is used, this passes through the right heart and pulmonary circulation before reaching the left heart and the peripheral arteries. The patient must have good cardiac function as a large volume of contrast medium has to be used in intravenous studies. The technique is contraindicated in patients with poor cardiac output and also in patients with renal failure.[137] The hazards of direct arterial puncture are avoided by the intravenous technique, although of course those of contrast sensitivity remain.

The advantages of seeing the vessels without background interference from bone together with the low volume of contrast that is required for intra-arterial injection have established digital subtraction angiography as the technique of choice.

Both intravenous and intra-arterial digital angiography are particularly useful for imaging the carotid vessels,[136] the aortic arch, and the thoracic and abdominal aorta.[138] Other arteries which require intra-arterial delivery of contrast are the intracerebral vessels, the renal and visceral arteries and the coronary vessels.

Abdominal greyscale ultrasound scanning[107,108] and CT scanning[139] are excellent methods of imaging and sizing aortic aneurysms; CT is particularly useful in determining the extent of the aneurysm, the possibility of a controlled rupture[140] or the presence of periaortic fibrosis[141] (Fig. 10.21). The recent development of spiral CT scanning has allowed rapid acquisition of data as the patient moves continuously through the scanner. This allows much thinner slices to be reconstructed in three dimensions, so allowing identification of the relationship of the neck of an abdominal aortic aneurysm to the renal and visceral vessels in almost all cases.[142]

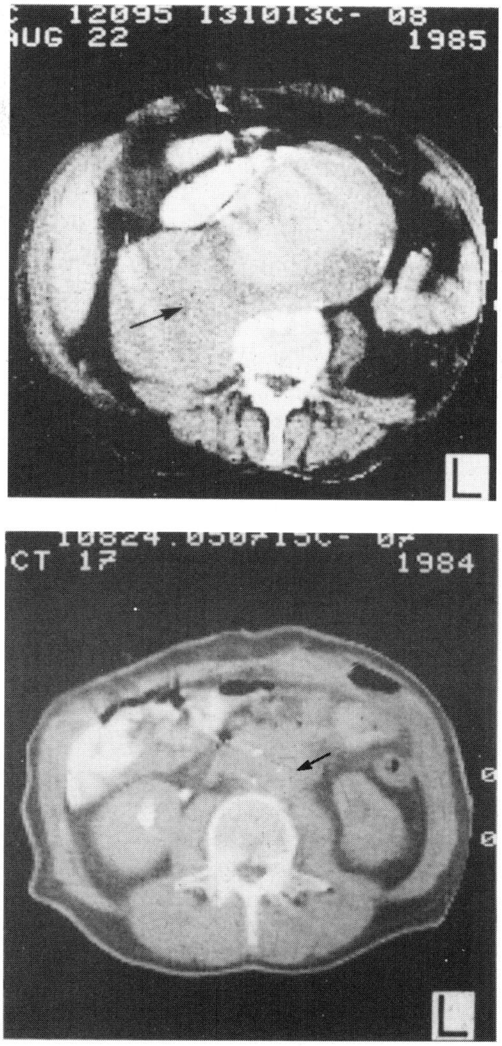

a

b

Fig. 10.21 (**a**) Computerized tomographic scan showing a controlled rupture of an aortic aneurysm (arrowed). (**b**) Computerized tomographic scan showing the features of an inflammatory aneurysm. A soft tissue mass outside the wall is seen (arrowed).

REFERENCES

131. Faught E, Trader S D, Hanna G R Neurology 1979; 29: 4
132. Oivercrona H Neuroradiology 1977; 14: 175
133. McIver J et al Br J Radiol 1987; 60: 117
134. Hankey G J, Warlow C P, Sellar R J Stroke 1990; 21: 209
135. Shaw P J, Reidy J F, Salari M R Br Med J 1983; 286: 604
136. Chilcote W A, Modie M T et al Radiology 1981; 139: 287
137. Dawson P Clin Radiol 1988; 39: 474
138. Buonocore E, Meany T F et al Radiology 1981; 139: 281
139. Leopold G R, Goldbergr L D, Bernstein E F Surgery 1972; 73: 939
140. Senepati A, Hurst A E et al J Cardiovasc Surg 1986; 27: 719
141. Baskerville P A, Blakeney C G et al Br J Surg 1983; 70: 381
142. Rubin G D, Dake M D et al Radiology 1993; 186: 147

Magnetic resonance imaging (MRI) provides a non-invasive method of assessing aortic aneurysms and has the ability to image vessels in the coronal plane. One disadvantage of MRI is that turbulence can result in signal loss, but this can be overcome by the infusion of gadolinium which allows good images of arterial pathology to be taken.[143] It also has the advantage that an angiogram can be obtained from the acquisition of the magnetic data (magnetic resonance angiography; Fig. 10.22).[144] This may at some stage abolish the need for contrast arteriography.

CT, MRI and ultrasound scanning may be used to investigate aneurysms at other sites, and CT and MRI can determine the extent of a congenital vascular anomaly[145–147] (Fig. 10.23). Magnetic resonance and computerized tomographic scans of the brain delineate areas of infarction[148] and generalized cerebral atrophy.[149] MRI may be a more accurate method of detecting inflammatory aneurysms than CT scanning.

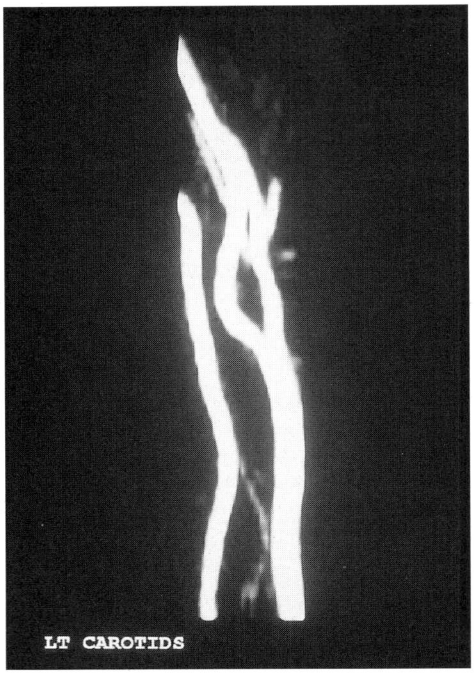

Fig. 10.22 Magnetic resonance angiography of the left carotid vessels.

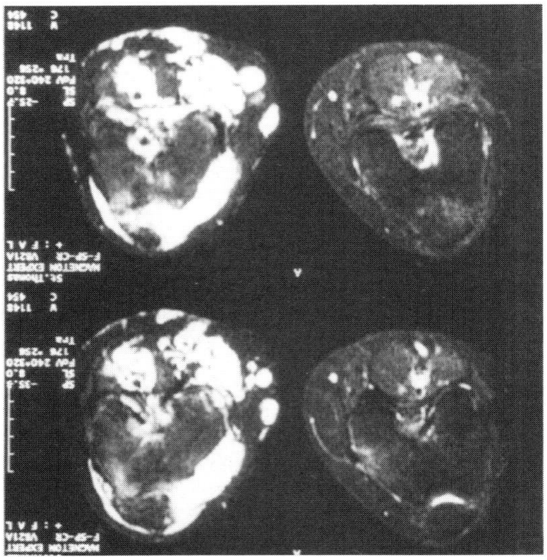
Fig. 10.23 Magnetic resonance scan of a congenital vascular anomaly.

Cerebral vascular disease

Patients who are thought to have cerebral vascular disease may require computerized tomography and magnetic resonance scans of the brain. Positron emission tomography of the brain,[150,151] or xenon clearance with and without inhalation of carbon dioxide,[152] provides an estimation of the cerebral vascular reserve where cerebral hypoperfusion is suspected, although these tests are largely research tools at present. Middle cerebral Doppler velocity before and after inhalation of carbon dioxide is a less expensive alternative.[153]

Renal vascular disease

Ultrasound has become the first line investigation for renal disease. Not only can it detect abnormalities in morphology, but with the addition of pulse Doppler, colour Doppler and power Doppler, the renal vasculature can now be assessed.[154] Spiral CT angiography with 3D reconstruction can provide excellent images of the renal arteries (Fig. 10.24)[155] as can magnetic resonance angiography.[156] Intra-arterial digital subtraction angiography still remains the best form of imaging.[157]

Gastrointestinal tract blood vessels

Duplex Doppler assessment of the visceral arteries can be undertaken in starved patients. The coeliac axis and the superior mesenteric arteries can be visualized but only the proximal part of the inferior mesenteric artery can be seen.[92] Arteriography remains the best method of detecting disease in the visceral arteries at present, but the anatomical appearances do not always relate to the extent of the bowel ischaemia.[91,93]

Barium contrast[68] studies may be helpful in assessing patients with suspected mesenteric arterial ischaemia. Thumb-printing or

REFERENCES

143. Prince M R Radiology 1994; 191: 155
144. Anderson C M, Edelman R R, Turski P A (eds) Clinical Magnetic Resonance Angiography. Raven Press, New York 1993
145. Christenson J J, Gunterberg B Br J Surg 1985; 72: 748
146. Rutherford R D, Whitehill T A, Davis K J Vasc Surg 1988; 8: 64
147. Avigdor M, Saks F F R et al Radiology 1995; 194: 908
148. Oxford Community Stroke Project Br Med J 1983; 287: 713
149. Bradshaw J R, Thompson J L G, Campbell M J Br Med J 1983; 286: 277
150. Wise R J S, Bernandi S et al Brain 1983; 106: 197
151. Brown M M, Wade J P H et al J Neurol Neurosurg Psychiatry 1986; 49: 899
152. Norving B, Nilssons B, Risberg J Stroke 1982; 13: 155
153. Bishop C C R, Powell S et al Stroke 1986; 17: 913
154. Scoutt L M, Taylor K J W In: Taylor K J W, Burns P N, Wells P N T (eds) Clinical Applications of Doppler Ultrasound. Raven Press, New York 1995 pp 155–178
155. Rubin G D, Dake M D et al Radiology 1994; 190: 181
156. Debatin S F, Spritzer C E et al Am J Roentgenol 157: 981
157. Kim D, Porter D H et al Angiology 1991; 42: 345

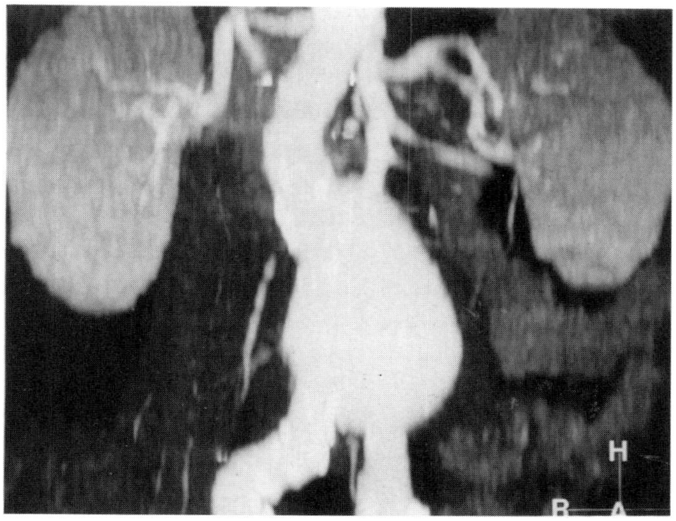

Fig. 10.24 Spiral CT angiography with 3D reconstruction to show renal arteries.

ischaemic strictures may occasionally be seen in patients with ischaemic colitis. Colonic biopsy may confirm evidence of ischaemia, which can also be detected by sigmoid tonometry.[158]

Other techniques

Plethysmography by a variety of different techniques[159,160] and isotopic clearance studies[161–163] have been used to measure regional blood flow, but are still largely research tools and have not found a definite place in clinical diagnosis at present. Pneumo-oculo-plethysmography was used to assess significant carotid stenosis, but this investigation is now obsolete.[164,165]

A transcutaneous oxygen electrode can be used to determine the flux of oxygen across the skin: this is dependent on blood flow and oxygenation of arterial blood. Absolute oxygen levels, arm:leg ratios and the percentage of oxygen fall on exercise have been used to assess patients with claudication or critical leg ischaemia,[166,167] and transcutaneous oxygen readings may be of help in deciding on the level of amputation.[168,169]

Intravenous guanethidine retained in the limb by a sphygmomanometer cuff may abolish vasospasm: this test in combination with local anaesthetic symptomatic ganglion block (described in Chapter 5) may be used to confirm the diagnosis of vasospastic disease and assess the likely effect of treatment.[170]

CONGENITAL ARTERIAL DISORDERS

Arteriovenous fistulae

These are found in many tissues at many sites but are most commonly found in the head, the neck and the extremities.[171] Congenital arteriovenous fistulae may be localized or diffuse, and may be between large (macrofistulae) or small vessels (microfistulae). They may on occasions form arteriovenous aneurysms. Congenital (arteriovenous) fistulae are uncommon and their incidence is probably less than 1 per million live births.[172] Although they are present from birth, they often increase in size during puberty or pregnancy.[173]

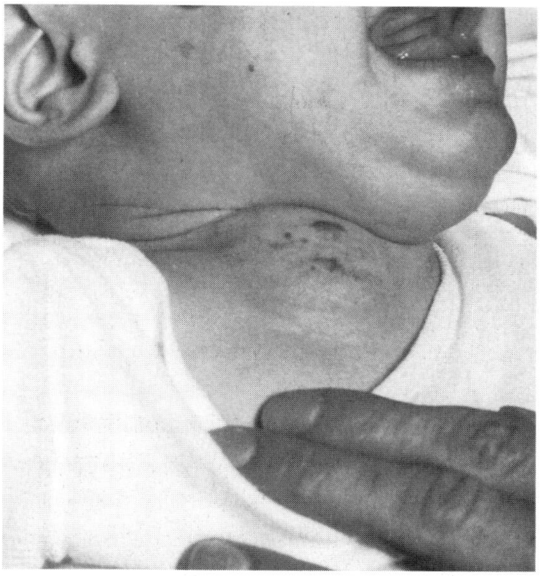

Fig. 10.25 An arteriovenous malformation presenting as a localized pulsatile swelling. Dilated vessels can be seen in the overlying skin.

Localized fistulae (cirsoid aneurysms)

These arise in the head and neck, often in the scalp from the superficial temporal vessels, but are also frequently found in the limbs. They appear as a soft warm pulsatile swelling which is often covered by dilated cutaneous vessels in the overlying skin or mucous membrane (Fig. 10.25). Patients often complain because the lesion is unsightly; it may enlarge, and as it does so it can cause aching pain. The overlying mucous membrane or skin may ulcerate and this can give rise to repeated and frightening haemorrhages. Platelets are occasionally sequestrated by these anomalies, but heart failure is an unusual complication. The small arteries, veins and even the capillaries are dilated and produce a swelling which is like a bag of pulsating worms. There is often a palpable

REFERENCES

158. Soong C V, Halliday M I et al Br J Surg 1993; 80: 521
159. Sumner D S, Strandness D E Surgery 1969; 65: 763
160. Van De Water J M, Don Ochowski J R et al Surgery 1971; 70: 954
161. Kety S S Am J Med Sci 1948; 215: 352
162. Lassen N A, Kampp M Scand J Clin Lab Invest 1965; 17: 447
163. Gutajar C L, Brown N J G, Marston A Br J Surg 1971; 58: 532
164. Gee W, Smith C A et al Med Invest 1974; 8: 244
165. Hauser C J, Shoemaker W C Ann Surg 1983; 197: 337
166. Franzeck H K, Talke P et al Am Surg 1984; 147: 510
167. Gannon M X, Goldman M et al J Cardiovasc Surg 1986; 27: 450
168. Mustapha N M, Redhead R G, Jain S K Surg Gynecol Obstet 1983; 156: 282
169. Radcliffe D A, Clyne C A C, Chant A D B Br J Surg 1984; 71: 219
170. Hannington-Kiff J G Lancet 1974; i: 1019
171. Szilagyi D E, Elliott J P et al Surgery 1965; 57: 61
172. Mulliken J B, Young A E Vascular Birthmarks. W B Saunders, Philadelphia 1978
173. Fontaine R Lyon Chir 1967; 62: 3332

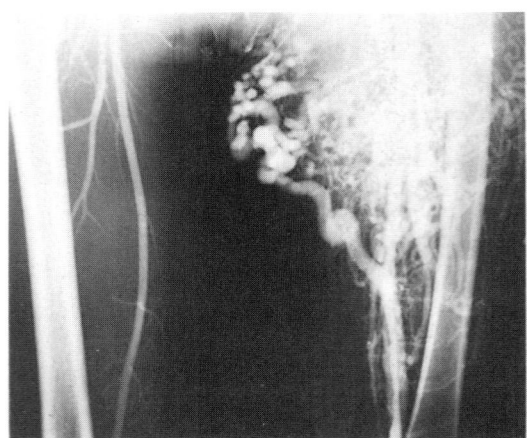

Fig. 10.26 An arteriogram showing massive venous filling from an arteriovenous fistula.

thrill over the swelling and a machinery murmur can be heard on auscultation. Pressure over the main feeding vessel that abolishes the pulsation may cause a bradycardia if the fistula is large (Branham's test).

Selective arteriography (Fig. 10.26), MR angiography and CT scanning establish the extent and connections of a cirsoid aneurysm, which can easily be distinguished from a pure venous angioma by its physical signs. A highly vascular secondary deposit (e.g. a thyroid carcinoma) must be considered in the differential diagnosis of a pulsatile mass of late onset and an acquired traumatic arteriovenous fistula must also be differentiated from the congenital variety.

When a cirsoid aneurysm develops during pregnancy it should be treated expectantly, as should all small localized fistulae that are not enlarging or causing symptoms. Lesions that enlarge in pregnancy commonly regress after delivery.[173] If they are expanding or producing symptoms the risks of treatment have to be weighed against the improvement that can be expected and the final cosmetic result that can be achieved in each individual patient.

Treatment can be by therapeutic embolization[174,175] or by occlusion of the feeding vessel combined with excision of the mass.[176] The risks of inadvertent cerebral embolization during therapeutic embolization of arteriovenous fistulae in the head and neck mean that this treatment must be carried out by a very experienced radiologist using great care,[177–179] and many anomalies in this situation are best treated by surgical excision.

In the limbs the risk of inadvertent misplaced embolism is less but digital gangrene is not unknown. Blood clot, gelfoam, skeletal muscle, lead shot, alginates and tungsten coils have all been used to occlude feeding vessels with varying success.[180–183] Improvements are often temporary and repeated embolization may be required at regular intervals.[184] Simple ligation of feeding vessels is always ineffective, and this abolishes a potentially useful site of access for future therapeutic embolization. Any attempt at surgical obliteration of the feeding vessels must if possible be followed by an immediate attempt to excise the whole abnormality.

In the past, efforts have been made to obliterate these fistulae by direct injections of sclerosant solutions including alcohol.[185] This technique has not proved effective and has been abandoned.

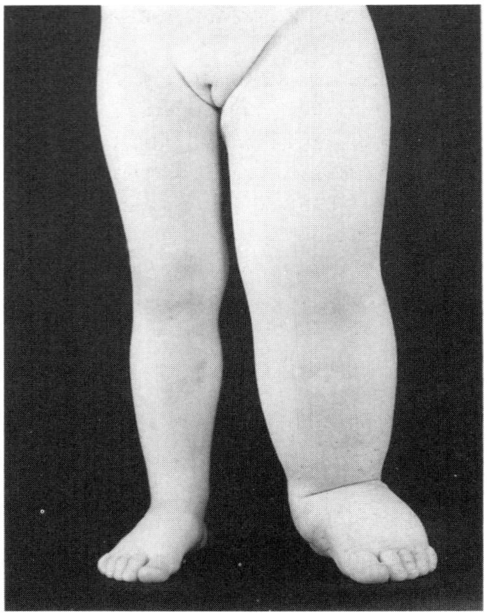

Fig. 10.27 A limb with Parkes-Weber syndrome.

Multiple arteriovenous fistulae (Parkes-Weber syndrome)[186]

Multiple arteriovenous fistulae usually present with an overall increase in the size of a limb (the common site of occurrence). The limb is often deformed, covered with dilated veins and may later develop severe lipodermatosclerosis and intractable ulceration (Fig. 10.27). Multiple arteriovenous fistulae often eventually cause high-output cardiac failure[187] and may occasionally cause severe thrombocytopenia.[188] The limb is usually hot and is increased in width as well as length with an overgrowth of bone. Bruits and thrills may be audible or palpable but they are not always present. A tourniquet inflated around the root of the limb usually causes slowing of the pulse (Branham–Nicoladoni sign).

The condition needs to be distinguished from Klippel–Trenaunay syndrome where there is bony and soft tissue overgrowth associated with a venous malformation, primitive varicose veins and a capillary naevus, but no arteriovenous fistulae are present. Local

REFERENCES

174. Stanley R J, Cubillo E Radiology 1975; 115: 609
175. Natali J, Merland J J J Cardiovasc Surg 1976; 17: 465
176. Biller H F, Krepski Y P, Som P M Otolaryngol Head Neck Surg 1982; 90: 37
177. Devine K D Plast Reconstr Surg 1959; 23: 273
178. Castaenda-Zuniga W R, Tadavarthy S M et al Radiology 1981; 141: 238
179. Rappaport I, Yim D Arch Otolaryngol 1973; 97: 350
180. Dotter D T, Goldman M D, Rosch J Radiology 1975; 114: 227
181. Gianturco C, Anderson J H, Wallace S J Roentgenol 1975; 124: 428
182. Hemingway A P, Allison D J Radiology 1988; 166: 669
183. Djin R, Cophignon J et al Neuroradiol 1973; 6: 20
184. Barth K H, Stranberg J D, White R I Invest Radiol 1977; 12: 273
185. Morgan J F, Schow C E J Oral Surg 1974; 32: 363
186. Parkes-Weber F Br J Dermatol 1907; 19: 231
187. Reid M R Bull Johns Hopkins Hosp 1920; 31: 43
188. Kasabach H H, Merritt K K Am J Dis Child 1940; 59: 1063

gigantism and lymphoedema must also be considered in the differential diagnosis.[189]

The increase in cutaneous temperature and local blood flow can be confirmed by thermography or plethysmography; arteriography shows the characteristic appearance of rapid blushing through the abnormal communications with early arrival of the dye in the veins (Fig. 10.28). It is often impossible to visualize individual fistulae unless they are very large.

In early life the condition is probably best treated expectantly, unless severe deformity or evidence of cardiac overload develops. It is usually impossible to embolize or excise all the fistulae, but if they are derived from a single peripheral artery, embolism may be attempted.

Where microfistulae are present throughout a limb an attempt can be made to inject microspheres of a known diameter into the feeding vessels in the hope that these will preferentially enter and occlude large numbers of fistulae because of their increased blood flow.[190] This technique may be repeated on many occasions but does carry the risk of causing distal ischaemia and has not proved very effective in the long term.

It is occasionally worthwhile inserting orthopaedic staples across the epiphysis of the limb in an attempt to slow down bone growth.[191] If this fails, a shoe-raise for the heel of the opposite foot may level the stance and prevent pelvic tilting. Graduated elastic stockings reduce superficial venous hypertension, compress dilated surface veins and may prevent or delay the development of lipodermatosclerosis and ulceration.

After childhood an attempt may be made to ligate all the branches of the feeding artery under tourniquet control. This process of deafferentation or skeletonization, originally described by Malan & Puglionise[192] and popularized by Cotton & Sykes,[193] is an effective method of treating fistulae derived from a single artery and allows the main sites of communication to be ablated. It too carries the risk of producing distal ischaemia and is followed by a high incidence of recurrence. It may therefore be preferable to carry out repeated selective embolization of the main sites of fistulation. This treatment is usually required at regular intervals throughout life as new fistulae are constantly developing. The cardiac output must also be regularly monitored.

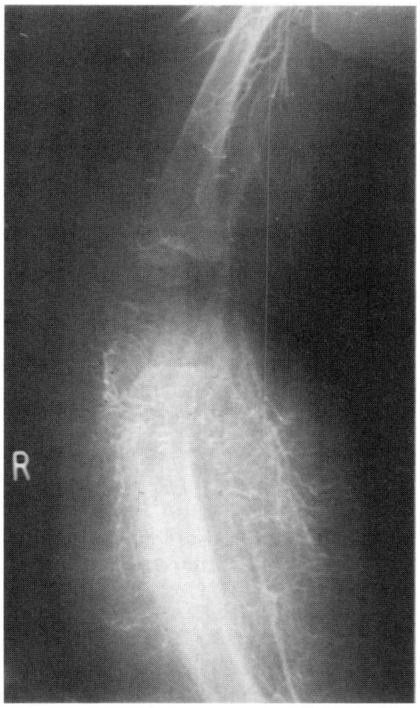

Fig. 10.28 An arteriogram of a limb with multiple arteriovenous fistulae. Many abnormal vascular channels are seen with early filling of the veins.

Ablation of the affected part is the final option if pain, deformity or cardiac failure become serious problems. This may require radical amputation of abnormal limbs with the prospect of poor mobility. This option should be reserved for severe complications when all other methods of treatment have failed.[194]

There are a number of other syndromes where congenital arteriovenous fistulae extend throughout organs such as the brain, liver or the intestine.[195,196] These can cause compression of surrounding tissues, recurrent haemorrhage, congestive cardiac failure or platelet consumption. The same principles apply to their management as those already discussed above. Other congenital malformations commonly coexist. Acquired arteriovenous fistulae are discussed in the section on arterial injury.

Vascular malformations

Most malformations display arterial, venous and lymphatic elements in some part of their structure. Those malformations that are predominantly venous (venous angioma) or lymphatic (lymphangioma circumscriptum) are discussed in other chapters, but all other vascular malformations are discussed here.

Vascular malformations have in the past been called angiomas, to which the prefixes haem-, lymph-, capillary or cavernous are then applied. The term 'angioma' is however a misnomer because the lesion is not a true tumour of blood vessels but a malformation or hamartoma. These malformations are thought to develop as an abnormal proliferation of the embryonic vascular network.[197] It has been suggested that angiogenic[198] and hormonal factors may be responsible for their development, which might explain why they are found more commonly in the female sex.[199] All angiomata may ulcerate and induce hyperkeratosis in the overlying stratum corneum. They rarely if ever undergo malignant change.

Capillary malformations

These lesions account for two thirds of all vascular malformations and include naevi, port wine stains, telangiectasis and spider naevi.

REFERENCES

189. Robertson D J Ann R Coll Surg Engl 1956; 18: 73
190. Berenstein A M, Kricheff I Radiology 1979; 132: 631
191. Blount W P, Clarke G R J Bone Joint Surg 1949; 319: 464
192. Malan E, Puglionise A J Cardiovasc Surg 1965; 6: 255
193. Cotton L T, Sykes B J Proc R Soc Med 1969; 62: 245
194. Masbet N W Br J Surg 1953; 41: 659
195. Sturec W A Trans Clin Soc London 1879; 12: 162
196. Parkes-Weber F Proc R Soc Med 1929; 22: 431
197. Ribbert V A Arch Pathol Anat 1898; 151: 381
198. Folkman J, Haundschild C Nature 1980; 288: 551
199. Rosen S, Smoller B R J Am Dermatol 1987; 17: 164

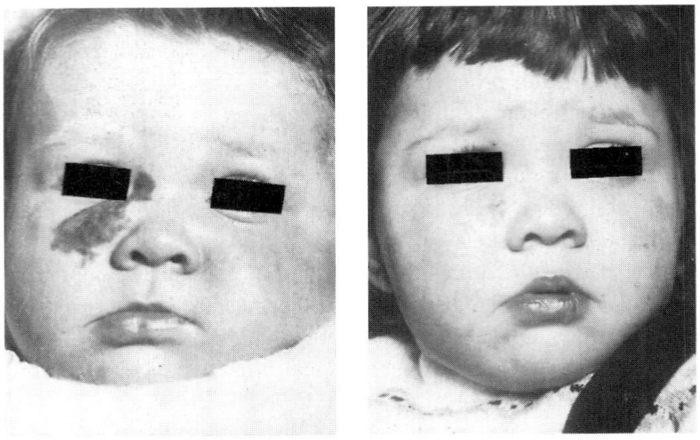

Fig. 10.29 (**a**) A cutaneous naevus on the face; (**b**) its resolution.

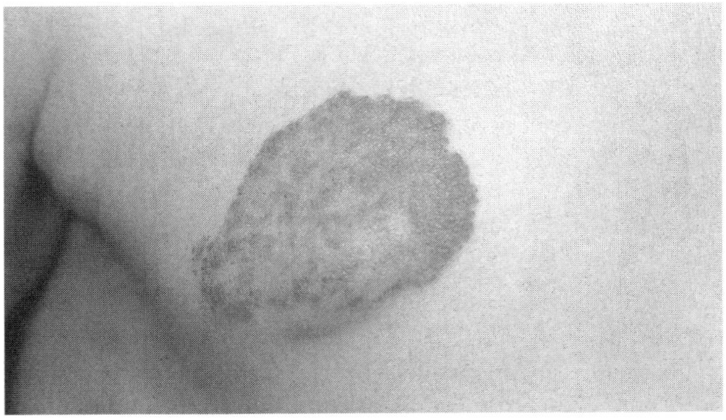

Fig. 10.30 A strawberry naevus.

Their incidence is between 1 and 2.6%.[200] Half occur as a single lesion, and 20% of affected infants have more than one malformation.[201]

Cutaneous naevi

Naevus flammeus neonatorum (salmon patch). This is a pink or red network of small capillaries without much cellular proliferation, radiating from a central punctum which is formed by an artery in the subcutis which supplies the tumour.[202] It can occur anywhere on the skin surface but most commonly arises on the face; it appears as a salmon-coloured patch which lies flush with the skin surface unless there is an overlying cutaneous proliferation (Fig. 10.29). Naevi may be multiple and their size can vary enormously but they are usually unilateral and rarely transgress the median plane.[203] They can arise on mucous membranes and in the central nervous system where they occasionally appear as small red spongy tumours embedded in the walls of cysts.

Strawberry patch. This is another descriptive term given to certain naevi which appear bright red, lobulated and raised above the surface (Fig. 10.30). This naevus often develops external extensions which separate from the tumour at first but later fuse with the main haemangioma; this variety commonly ulcerates.

Telangiectasis. This is simply a dilatation of normal capillaries rather than a vascular malformation. They arise after skin irradiation and certain syndromes are recognized where multiple

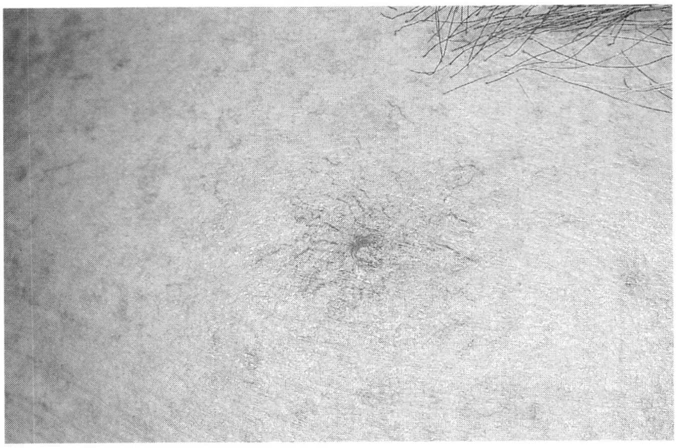

Fig. 10.31 A spider naevus.

telangiectases are associated with gastrointestinal haemorrhage, epistaxis, haematuria and even intracerebral haemorrhage.[204–206]

Spider naevus (naevus araneus). This is a form of telangiectasis which occurs over the upper torso, head and neck in adults, often in association with liver insufficiency or pregnancy (Fig. 10.31).[207] The presence of more than five spider naevi is regarded as pathological (see Chapter 9).

Hereditary haemorrhagic telangiectasia (Rendu–Osler–Weber syndrome).[204–206] This is inherited as a Mendelian dominant, with incomplete penetrance.[208] It is a rare disease with an incidence of 1–2 per 100 000. Tiny capillary haemangiomas scattered over mucous membranes and sometimes the skin may give rise to overt and occult haemorrhage presenting as haematemesis, haematuria, melaena or iron-deficiency anaemia.

Campbell de Morgan's spot. This is a uniformly red capillary naevus that is usually 2–3 mm in diameter. It often develops on the trunk in middle age. It is of no clinical significance.[209]

Port-wine stain (naevus vinosus). This is a purple-blue naevus of skin which commonly arises on the face and may involve the lips and mucous membrane of the mouth. These naevi also arise on the limbs in association with Klippel–Trenaunay syndrome (Fig. 10.32; see Chapter 11).

Clinical features

All vascular naevi appear to contain blood vessels and empty on compression, although often incompletely. A glass slide can be

REFERENCES

200. Pratt A G Arch Dermatol 1967; 67: 302
201. Margileth A M, Musezes M JAMA 1965; 194: 523
202. Pack G T, Miller T R Angiology 1980; 1: 408
203. Bowers R E, Graham E A, Tomlinson K M Arch Dermatol 1960; 82: 667
204. Rendu M Bull Soc Med Hosp-Paris 1896; 13: 731
205. Osler W Bull Johns Hopkins Hosp 1901; 12: 333
206. Parkes-Weber F Lancet 1907; ii: 160
207. Barter R H, Letterman E S, Schurter M Surg Gynecol Obstet 1963; 87: 628
208. Schnyder U W Arch Dermatol 1955; 200: 483
209. Bean W B Vascular Spiders and Related Lesions of the Skin. Charles C Thomas, Springfield Illinois 1958

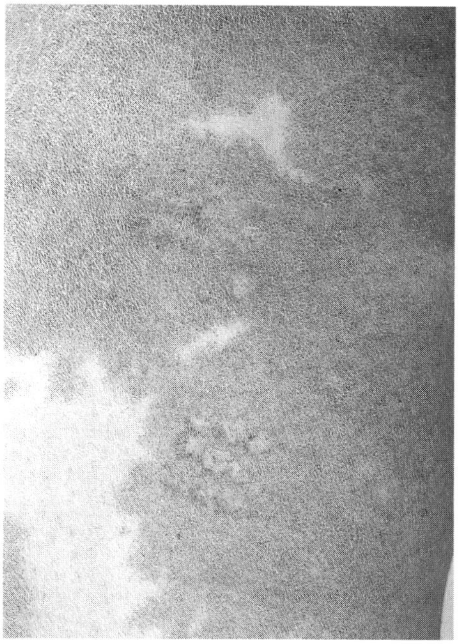

Fig. 10.32 A port wine stain.

used to demonstrate the sign of emptying. Doubts about the diagnosis can be clarified by biopsy.

Management

The presence of other conditions, such as the Klippel–Trenaunay syndrome and Rendu–Osler–Weber syndrome, must be considered. The majority of capillary naevi do not require treatment unless they are causing symptoms. Camouflage paint produces acceptable cosmesis in many instances.[210] Carbon dioxide snow (cryotherapy)[211] and laser photocoagulation[212] have been used to destroy capillary naevi and are effective methods of treatment although time-consuming and expensive. The red-blue discoloration of the naevus is often exchanged for white scar tissue unless these treatments are carefully applied.[212] Radiotherapy, electrolysis, thermocautery, sclerotherapy, surgical excision and skin grafting have also been used with variable success.[185,213–215] Tattooing has also been tried[216] but camouflage paints are usually preferable. Corticosteroids may reduce the size of large angiomas and restore platelet counts to normal.[217]

Cavernous haemangioma (strawberry patch)

This occurs in the subcutaneous tissue of the skin or beneath mucous membranes and becomes apparent as a bluish slightly elevated patch a few weeks after birth. Cavernous haemangiomata can also arise in the liver and other internal organs. They consist of dilated blood spaces with thin walls supported by a tenuous stroma.

60% of these malformations undergo spontaneous resolution by the age of 3 and some may then organize and calcify. The overlying skin may occasionally break down and ulcerate (Fig. 10.33). These haemangiomata may also occasionally cause thrombocytopenia and cutaneous bleeding.

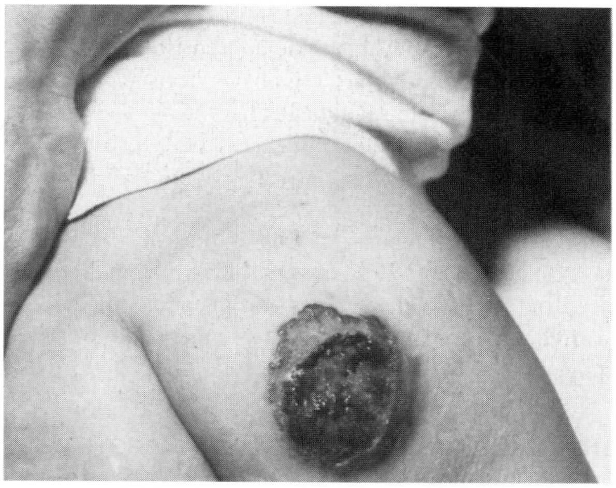

Fig. 10.33 Ulceration over a cavernous haemangioma.

When spontaneous resolution does not occur, the malformation usually requires excision and some form of plastic repair if treatment is justified on cosmetic grounds.[214,215] Repeated diathermy coagulation and cryotherapy[211,215] have also been tried but the recurrence rate is high.

Mixed naevi

These have a combination of capillary and cavernous elements, often with diffuse endothelial proliferation compressing the dilated capillary channels. These naevi also have a high incidence of spontaneous regression but they may occasionally ulcerate and become infected. Excision with reconstruction or radiotherapy are the two main techniques that have been used in treatment.[213,214,218] The complications that can follow radiotherapy favour surgical excision where this is possible.

Cystic disease of the arterial wall

Although this condition is grouped with congenital disorders of the arteries it is debatable if it is truly congenital. The diagnosis is usually made when the vessel occludes, which is almost always in early adult life.[219,220] Claudication or acute ischaemia developing in a young adult suggests the possibility of an arterial cyst, but it must be differentiated from an entrapment syndrome, an embolus or

REFERENCES

210. Cosman B Lasers Surg Med 1980; 1: 133
211. Blaisdell J H N Engl J Med 1936; 215: 485
212. Adams S J, Swain C P et al Br J Dermatol 1987; 117: 487
213. Park W C, Phillips R JAMA 1970; 212: 1496
214. Weber T R, West K W, Cohen M J Vasc Surg 1984; 1: 423
215. Matthews D N Plast Reconstr Surg 1968; 41: 528
216. Grabb W C, MacCallum M S, Tan N G Plast Reconstr Surg 1977; 59: 667
217. Brown S H, Neerhout R C, Fonkalsrud E W Surgery 1972; 71: 168
218. Sealy R, Barry L et al Proc R Soc Med 1989; 82: 198
219. Ejrup B, Hierton T Acta Chir Scand 1954; 108: 217
220. Bliss B P Am Heart J 1964; 68: 838

premature atherosclerosis. The cyst is filled with mucopolysaccharide and forms in the layers of the arterial wall; it has a similar structure to a ganglion.[221] Cysts have been most commonly reported to occur in the popliteal artery.[220,222] The diagnosis is by arteriography and duplex ultrasound or CT scanning of the popliteal fossa.

Treatment is by deroofing or excising the cyst if possible[221] and extracting distal thrombosis, if this is present, with a Fogarty balloon catheter. The abnormal vessel wall must be resected and replaced by a vein graft or prosthetic material[223] if deroofing is impossible. Excision of the cyst with a primary end-to-end arterial anastomosis is rarely possible.[223]

Congenital entrapment syndromes

The most common sites of arterial entrapment are at the thoracic outlet, often by a cervical rib, and in the popliteal fossa by an abnormal attachment of the popliteus or gastrocnemius muscles. Other rarer causes of entrapment include the anterior tibial syndrome, vertebral artery compression and coeliac axis compression.

Thoracic outlet syndrome

A cervical rib can definitely compress, occlude and damage the subclavian artery, but a fibrous band situated in the position of a cervical rib or muscular hypertrophy are more contentious causes of compression at the thoracic outlet. As the diagnosis is difficult to refute—or for that matter to prove—many patients in certain parts of the world have undergone thoracic outlet decompression on fairly nebulous grounds, often perhaps for disease in the cervical spine.

Cervical rib

This occurs in 0.4% of the population, with 70% having bilateral cervical ribs,[224,225] but it is only symptomatic in approximately 60%. Of the patients with symptoms, neurological manifestations of cervical rib outweigh vascular complications by approximately 20 to 1.[226] The cervical rib was first resected by Coote in London in 1861,[227] some 40 years before Bramwell[228] suggested that a normal first rib could compress the brachial plexus.

Patients with symptomatic cervical ribs complain of cramping pain in the arm and hand which may become pallid, cyanosed or oedematous during use. Paraesthesiae, weakness and numbness commonly coexist as a result of compression of the T1 nerve root, but vascular symptoms do occasionally occur in isolation. A cervical rib can cause secondary vasospasm which may progress to fingertip necrosis and even digital gangrene. Emboli from a subclavian false aneurysm are usually the cause of patchy necrosis and gangrene of the hand and digits. Acute thrombosis of the subclavian artery is unusual but can cause extensive ischaemia of the upper limb. Patients occasionally present because they have noticed a mass or pulsation in the neck. Obstruction to the venous return from the arm may also occur in isolation or in association with neuritic or vascular symptoms. Venous symptoms consist of engorgement, oedema, cyanosis and discomfort during exercise,

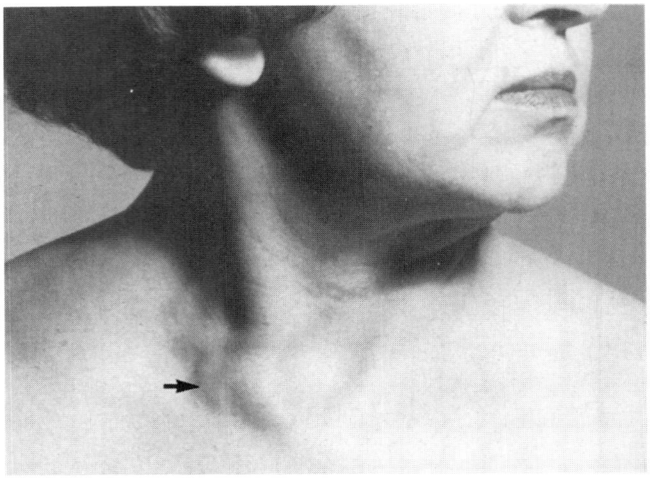

Fig. 10.34 A visible cervical rib (arrowed) causing a swelling above the clavicle.

but the first sign is often an acute axillary venous thrombosis (see Chapter 11).

The signs of a cervical rib fall into four distinct categories: local signs from the rib and artery; signs of venous obstruction or occlusion; neurological signs in the upper limb; and least common but most serious, signs of arterial spasm or ischaemia, usually affecting the fingers and hand. In a thin person it may be possible to observe and palpate a bony swelling in the supraclavicular fossa above the clavicle (Fig. 10.34). The subclavian pulse may be palpable above the bony mass, or it may simply appear more prominent. A truly expansile pulsation usually signifies a traumatic false aneurysm. This is uncommon and must be carefully distinguished from a 'prominent' pulsation. A bruit may be heard over the artery in the supraclavicular fossa and this may vary in differing degrees of abduction of the arm. Patients exceptionally develop a Horner's syndrome.

Signs of venous obstruction are most obvious during periods of increased flow, such as exercise. The subcutaneous veins of the arm become distended and may remain so even during arm elevation. The hand and arm may be cyanosed and there may be mild swelling which is apparent as pitting oedema on the dorsum of the hand. These signs all become more obvious if the axillary vein thromboses, when collateral veins develop in the skin over the anterior shoulder and the scapula (see Chapter 11).

The neurological signs are the result of T1 root compression as this loops over the cervical rib. There is weakness and wasting of the small muscles of the hand and anaesthesia over the T1 and occasionally C8 dermatomes.

REFERENCES

221. Lewis G J T, Douglas D M et al Br Med J 1967; 3: 411
222. Flanigan D P, Burnham S J et al Ann Surg 1979; 189: 165
223. Tracey G D, Ludbrook J, Rundle F F J Vasc Surg 1969; 3: 10
224. Young H A, Hardy D G Br J Hosp Med 1983; 1: 487
225. Lewis M R, Dale W A Surg Digest 1973; 1: 7
226. Pollack E W Surg Gynecol Obstet 1980; 150: 97
227. Coote H Lancet 1861; i: 360
228. Bramwell F Rev Neurol Psychiatry 1903; 1: 236

The radial and ulnar pulses are usually present and of normal volume, but they may be reduced in amplitude or obliterated in certain positions of the shoulder joint. These positions include: the position of attention with the shoulder pressed down; when the shoulder is braced backwards; when the shoulder is abducted against resistance; when it is abducted or adducted and extended backwards; and when the neck is hyperextended.[229–231] Unfortunately all these manoeuvres can reduce the pulse of a normal individual, and it is therefore important not to attach too much significance to these signs.[232,233]

The vascular symptoms and signs of a cervical rib are almost always unilateral but they tend to progress after they have developed; areas of necrosis, patchy gangrene and eventually more extensive gangrene can appear if the arterial compression is left untreated (Fig. 10.35). An acute thrombosis of the subclavian artery leads to massive ischaemia of the upper limb, but this is unusual because of the excellent potential for a collateral circulation.

Mechanism of symptoms. A number of mechanisms for the symptoms of cervical rib or thoracic outlet compression have been postulated. It has been suggested that the artery is compressed between the rib and the scalenus anterior,[234] between the rib and the clavicle (costoclavicular compression),[235,236] between a band arising from the rib and the clavicle, between the two heads of scalenus medius or between the converging heads of the median nerve.[237,238] At one stage it was even suggested that the symptoms were not the result of direct pressure on the artery, but of symptomatic paralysis[239] or irritation[240] from damage to the periarterial sympathetic plexus or nerve fibres in the T1 cord. Aird (1st edition) pointed out that continued sympathetic irritation always ended in paralysis, making this mechanism unlikely. These theories do not explain why subclavian aneurysms and digital gangrene develop.

Thoracic outlet syndrome may follow fracture of the clavicle, which causes distortion. It may also be caused by fibrous bands coming off a large transverse process of the seventh cervical vertebra, or by a rudimentary cervical rib, or even by hypertrophy of the scalene muscles which may be found in body builders, champion swimmers or gymnasts. An abnormality of the first rib, which may include congenital enlargement, fracture or a tumour, is a rare cause of symptoms.[241] The axillary vein may occasionally be compressed by the phrenic nerve or by an accessory pectoral muscle.[242]

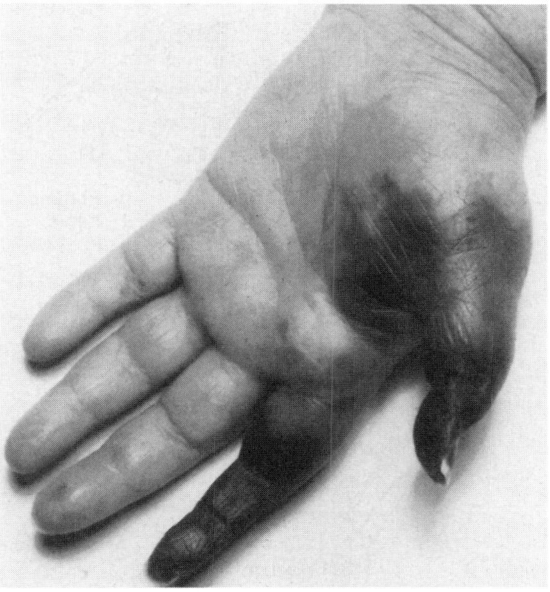

Fig. 10.35 A gangrenous hand caused by a thrombosed subclavian artery.

The thoracic outlet syndrome is a condition that is often overdiagnosed and the neurological symptoms must be carefully differentiated from those of cervical spondylosis, cervical disc protrusions and spinal cord tumours, syringomyelia, a Pancoast's tumour, osteoarthritis of the shoulder, supraspinatus tendonitis, ulnar neuritis and carpal tunnel syndrome. Impaired conduction velocity down the ulnar nerve on electromyography may help to confirm the diagnosis,[243] but this is not always present and is not essential for diagnosis. Venous symptoms must be differentiated from an axillary vein thrombosis, which many now consider to occur only in patients with thoracic outlet syndrome.[244] The arterial symptoms of a cervical rib must be differentiated from atherosclerotic disease of the subclavian artery, Takayasu's disease, Buerger's disease and both primary and secondary vasospastic disorders. The presence of a cervical rib or a large transverse process of the seventh cervical vertebra on plain radiographs of the thoracic inlet (Fig. 10.36) provides some support for the diagnosis, and at the same time radiographs of the cervical spine and shoulder should be obtained to exclude some of the other conditions from which the outlet syndrome must be differentiated. Axillary phlebograms and arteriograms with the arms in different degrees of abduction may show a marked kink in the artery or vein (Fig. 10.37), and this also provides support for the diagnosis.[245] At a later stage, these investigations may show evidence of a thrombosis in the axillary vein or artery and sometimes signs of multiple emboli within the small vessels of the hand. Occasionally a localized aneurysm related to the rib is demonstrated (Fig. 10.38).

Management of outlet syndrome. The final decision to decompress the thoracic outlet is a clinical one if all these investigations remain inconclusive. When the diagnosis remains in doubt, it is better to err towards caution and try to improve posture and strengthen the trapezius muscle with a course of exercises, reserving decompression for persistent or deteriorating symptoms.

REFERENCES

229. Adson A W Surg Gynecol Obstet 1947; 85: 687
230. Adson A W, Coffey J R Ann Surg 1927; 85: 839
231. Wright I S Am J Heart 1945; 29: 1
232. Eden K C Br J Surg 1939; 27: 11
233. Warrens A N, Heaton J M Ann R Coll Surg Engl 1987; 69: 203
234. Murphy J B Surg Gynecol Obstet 1906; 3: 574
235. Telford E D, Mottershead S Br Med J 1947; 1: 325
236. Telford E D, Mottershead S J Bone Joint Surg 1948; 30: 249
237. Todd T W J Anat Physiol 1911; 45: 293
238. Todd T W Anat Anz 1912; 47: 250
239. Leriche R Bull Mem Soc Nat Chir 1935; 61: 1292
240. Telford E D, Stopford J S B Br J Surg 1931; 18: 557
241. Coote H Med Times Gaz 1861; 2: 108
242. Boontje A H Br J Surg 1979; 66: 331
243. Urshel H C, Paulson D L, McNamara J J Ann Surg 1968; 6: 1
244. Stevenson I M, Parry E W J Cardiovasc Surg 1975; 16: 580
245. Lang E K Radiology 1965; 84: 296

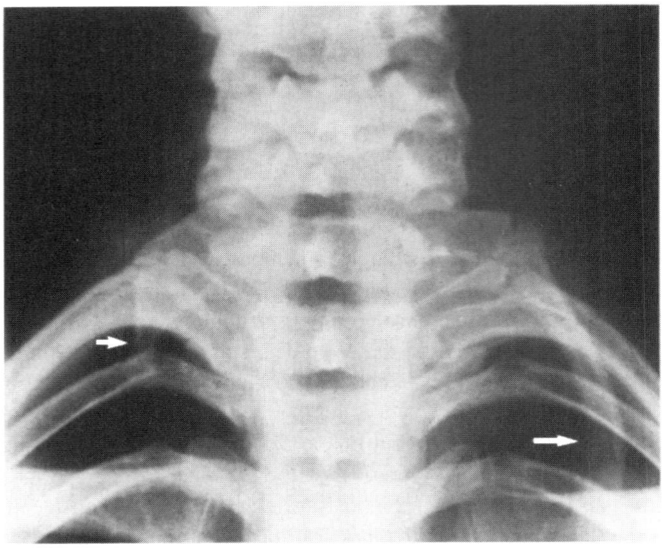

Fig. 10.36 A plain radiograph of the thoracic inlet showing cervical ribs (arrowed).

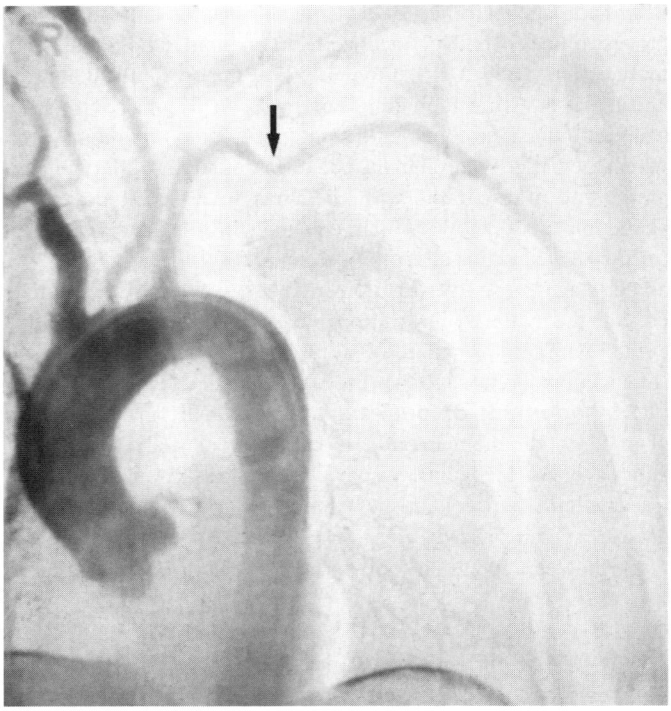

Fig. 10.37 An arch aortogram showing a kink in the subclavian artery caused by a fascial band.

Patients must be warned that decompression does not always relieve symptoms, and can cause the complications of Horner's syndrome or brachial neuritis. A neurologist's opinion is always helpful to rule out other causes of symptoms that the surgeon may have overlooked.

Decompression of the thoracic outlet: resection of a cervical rib. The operation can be performed through a supraclavicular approach. The clavicular fibres of sternomastoid and the omohyoid muscle are divided (Fig. 10.39). The phrenic nerve is retracted off

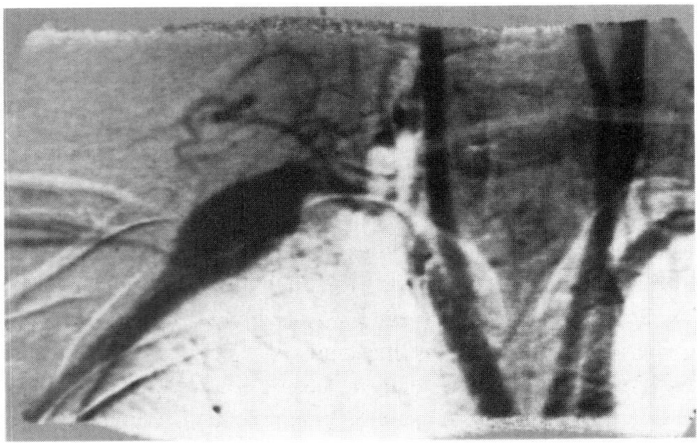

Fig. 10.38 A digital subtraction angiogram showing a subclavian aneurysm caused by a cervical rib.

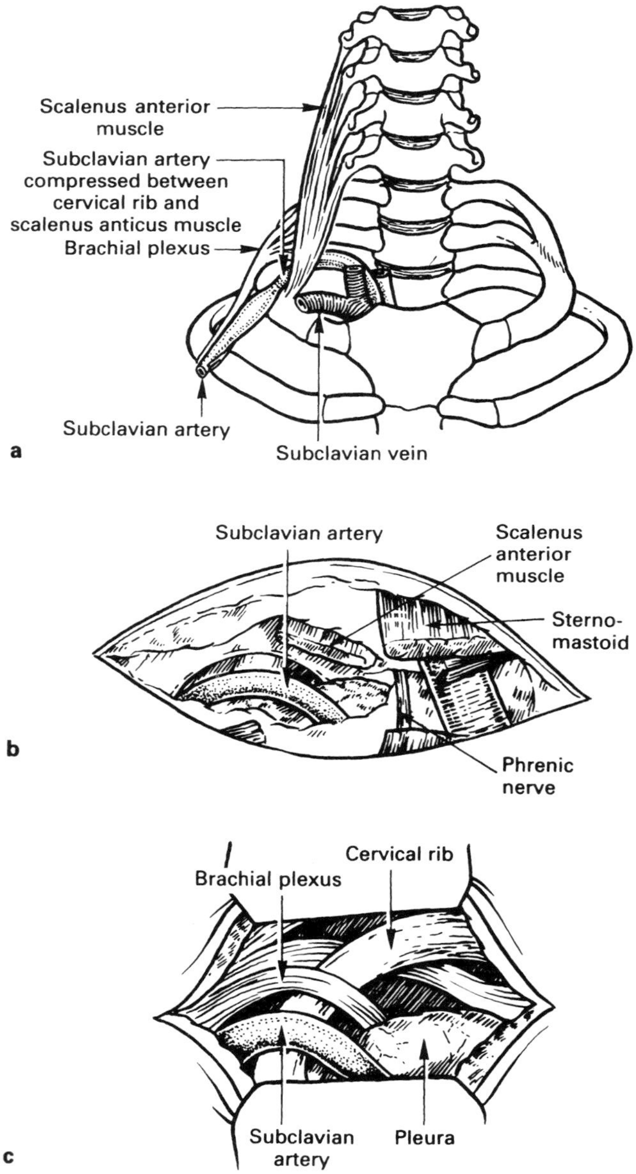

Fig. 10.39 Resection of a cervical rib (cervical approach).

the anterior surface of the scalenus anterior before this muscle is divided. The subclavian artery, which lies directly behind the muscle, is dissected free from its sheath and is retracted upwards or downwards before the pleurocervical fascia (Sibson's fascia) is divided. The pleura is exposed and reflected off the inner surface of the first rib. A cervical rib is then felt as a bony spur directed towards the upper surface of the first rib. The T1 nerve root is located, passing up over the neck of the first rib and looping over the cervical rib as it passes laterally to form the brachial plexus (Fig. 10.39). A cervical rib often passes between the nerve trunks of the brachial plexus as it is traced upwards and backwards towards its articulation with the transverse process and body of the seventh cervical vertebra. The rib can then be removed by bone-nibblers or simply divided as close to the vertebral articulation as possible.

When a subclavian aneurysm is present, its limits must be defined and the vessel isolated, before it is cross-clamped and the aneurysm resected. It is extremely unusual for there to be enough arterial length to allow an end-to-end anastomosis to be made, and the resected aneurysm is normally replaced by a segment of long saphenous vein or a prosthetic graft. Embolectomy, thrombectomy, thrombolysis, and occasionally bypass surgery are required for ischaemic complications, when the results are much more unpredictable.

Roos[246] prefers to decompress the thoracic outlet by entering the chest through a transverse incision placed in the axilla; after collapsing the lung he resects the first rib under direct vision (Fig. 10.40). This approach does not allow cervical ribs to be seen but is favoured by Roos for patients with outlet syndromes who do not have cervical ribs. The first rib can also be resected from above using a supra- and infraclavicular approach.

The results of surgery are good[247] in patients with a true outlet syndrome, but ribs can re-form if the periosteum is left intact. Complications include pneumothorax, Horner's syndrome, and damage to the brachial plexus and subclavian artery. Patients can die from major vascular injuries and the hand may have to be amputated if ischaemia cannot be reversed.

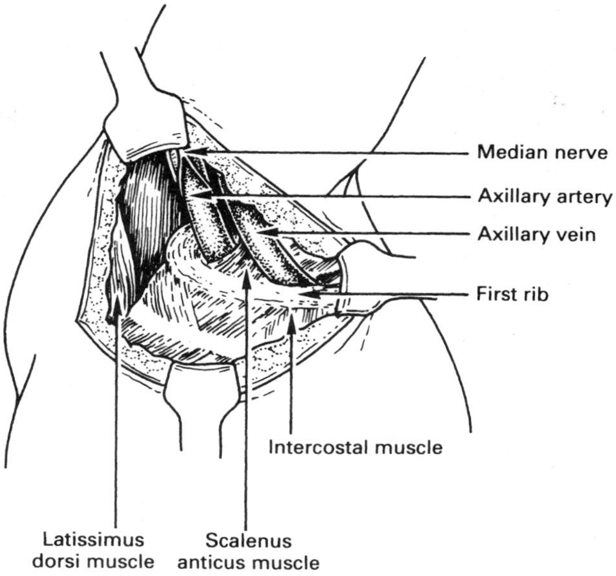

Fig. 10.40 The axillary approach used to resect the first rib.

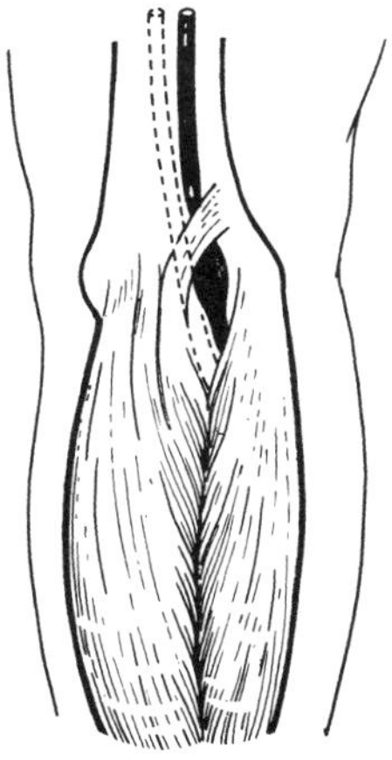

Fig. 10.41 Popliteal entrapment by a third head of the gastrocnemius muscle.

Popliteal entrapment

The popliteal artery may pass medially around the anatomically normal medial head of the gastrocnemius muscle,[248] or may pass beneath an aberrant band arising from any of the muscles in the popliteal fossa[249] (Fig. 10.41). A number of other variations have been described but all are rare. Contraction of the fibres of these muscles can occlude the artery and cut off the blood supply to the calf, causing claudication. Eventually the repeated occlusion or the constant trauma of muscle contraction can damage the arterial wall and result in intimal thickening, plaque formation, fibrosis and thrombosis. This often occurs after a particularly violent episode of exercise.[250]

The condition should be suspected in a young and often physically fit subject (usually male) who complains of claudication on exercise. Contraction of the calf muscles against resistance often causes the foot pulses to disappear.[251] Popliteal entrapment must be differentiated from popliteal cystic disease, premature atherosclerosis, arteritis, chronic compartment syndrome and embolism.

Duplex scanning at rest and during muscle contraction may confirm cessation of blood flow. Arteriography often shows a medial deviation in the artery as it crosses the popliteal fossa (Fig. 10.42),[252] and CT or MR scan at knee level shows muscle passing either side of the vessel.[253] Magnetic resonance scanning also provides very good images of this anomaly.

Division of the muscle belly is all that is required if the vessel has not occluded, but thrombectomy and replacement of the damaged vessel is necessary if thrombosis has occurred. Muscle

REFERENCES

246. Roos D B Surgery 1982; 92: 1077
247. Lepanto M, Lindgren K-A et al Br J Surg 1989; 76: 1255
248. Stuart T P A J Anat Physiol 1879; 13: 162
249. Insua J A, Young J R, Humphries A W Arch Surg 1970; 101: 771
250. Madigan R R, McCampbell B R J Bone Joint Surg 1981; 64: 1490
251. Harris J D, Jepson R P Surgery 1971; 69: 246
252. Barabas A P, Macfarlane R Br J Hosp Med 1985; 1: 304
253. Muller N, Morris D C, Nichols D M Radiology 1984; 151: 157

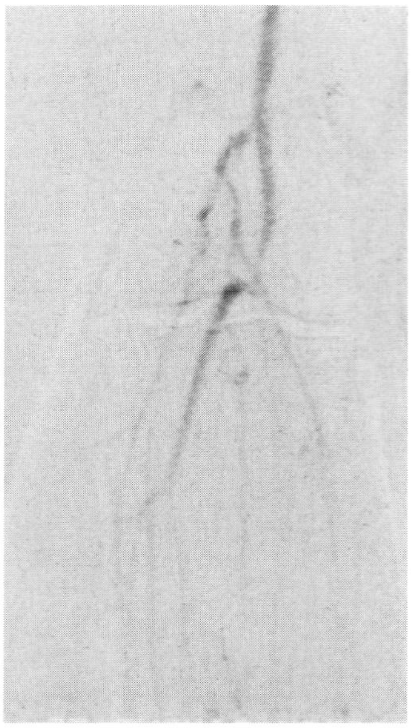

Fig. 10.42 An arteriogram showing medial deviation of the popliteal artery as a result of entrapment by an aberrant muscle.

division is curative,[252] but if the vessel has thrombosed the end result is less predictable. The opposite popliteal fossa must be carefully examined: muscle division should be undertaken prophylactically if there are signs of compression.

ARTERIAL INJURY

Arterial injuries may be either open or closed and can be caused by direct damage by a missile, a stabbing weapon or a piece of shrapnel; alternatively, they may be caused indirectly by a bony injury which secondarily impinges upon or lacerates the vessel wall.[254–256] A significant proportion of all arterial injuries are now the result of medical, surgical or radiological intervention, and these iatrogenic injuries are increasing every year.[257–260] Arteries may also be damaged by extremes of temperature and inadvertent injections of noxious agents.

The injured artery may be contused, punctured, lacerated or partially divided; the intima may be damaged, or the vessel may be completely divided with separation of the ends (Fig. 10.43). These injuries result in haemorrhage, spasm, occlusion, thrombosis, dissection or the development of false aneurysms and arteriovenous fistulae.

Arterial haemorrhage

This may be primary, secondary or reactionary, and can be either concealed or revealed, depending upon whether the injury is open or closed. Most lacerations or missile injuries which partially or completely sever an artery result in a visible haemorrhage which is bright red and pulsatile. Both sharp arterial transections and crushing tearing injuries of the vessels cause arterial spasm; this, combined with the hypotension caused by blood loss and rapid platelet deposition, quickly leads to a reduction in, or cessation of bleeding. Bleeding may be prolonged if there is a lateral tear in the

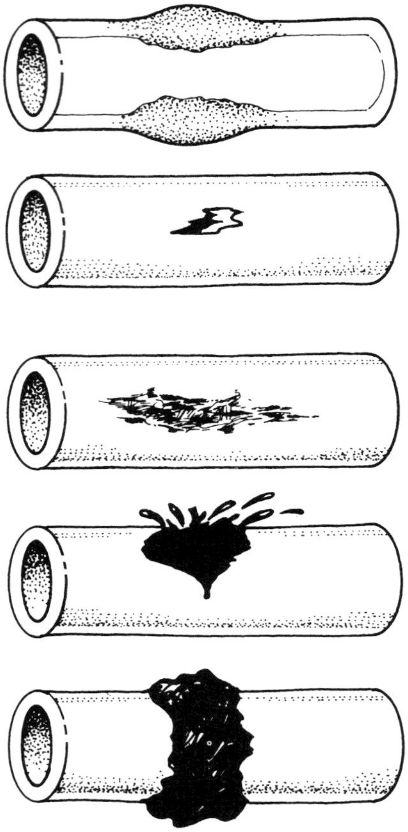

Fig. 10.43 The different types of arterial injury.

artery or the laceration is held open. When the blood pressure recovers, muscle spasm may wear off and platelet thrombi are expelled, resulting in a reactionary haemorrhage. A secondary haemorrhage can occur if infection erodes the arterial wall; this is usually between 7 and 10 days after the initial injury.

Arteries may also be torn or damaged and bleed internally. The profunda femoris or one of its perforating arteries, for example, is commonly torn by a fracture of the shaft of the femur, producing a massive haematoma in the thigh without overt signs of haemorrhage (see Chapter 47). Concealed bleeding may occasionally cause such a rise in the intercompartmental pressure that it occludes arterial inflow and leads to ischaemic necrosis.

The first-aid management of arterial haemorrhage is to apply external pressure directly over the bleeding point or at one of the well recognized compression points along the proximal course of the damaged artery where it crosses a bony prominence and external compression is capable of producing occlusion. A tourniquet should only be used if haemorrhage cannot be controlled by

REFERENCES

254. Klingen Smith W, Olis P, Martinez H Am J Surg 1965; 110: 849
255. Koostra E, Schipper J J et al Surg Gynecol Obstet 1976; 142: 339
256. Makin G S, Howard J M, Green R L Surgery 1966; 59: 203
257. Bouhoutsos J, Morris T Br Med J 1973; 3: 396
258. Slaney G, Ashton F Postgrad Med J 1971; 47: 257
259. Thomas W E G, Baird R N Injury 1983; 15: 30
260. McMillan I, Murie J A Br J Surg 1984; 71: 832

pressure and then its application must be carefully monitored as the risk of distal ischaemia and metabolic derangement following release is considerable. The application of a tourniquet in theatre may on occasion make the subsequent exploration and arterial reconstruction much easier. Artery forceps (haemostats) should not be used in the accident and emergency department to control bleeding arteries in the depths of wounds unless patients are in extremis and arteries that are bleeding cannot be controlled by the measures described above. Local pressure followed by resuscitation should normally proceed to rapid exploration under general anaesthesia. There is no place for arteriography or other investigations if arterial haemorrhage is massive, but an appropriate quantity of blood must be sent for cross-matching before the patient is taken to theatre. Plain radiographs and arteriography can be obtained if the patient is stable and there is no overt external bleeding. This will confirm the sites of injury and detect bony damage and foreign body fragments such as shrapnel.

At operation, after proximal and distal control of the bleeding vessel has been achieved, the artery is repaired, extending the skin wound as necessary. Few arteries should be ligated if they can be repaired, although individual vessels in the forearm and calf can usually be tied off with safety. Once a suitable length of normal artery has been exposed above and below the site of the injury, the patient should be given systemic heparin (5000 u, with smaller doses in children or small patients and larger quantities in large or obese subjects) before arterial occluding clamps are applied on either side of the injured segment.

Arteriography should be carried out on the operating table using a fine needle or catheter inserted directly into the vessel, with films wrapped in sterile towels placed beneath the injured part if the extent of the arterial damage is not apparent from external inspection, or if it is suspected that a distal vessel is occluded by thrombus. Alternatively a C arm with digital subtraction facilities is an excellent alternative providing the patient is on a radiotranslucent table. The artery should be opened and the lumen inspected if there is any evidence of intimal damage or distal propagation of thrombus shown on the arteriogram. The damaged portion of the vessel must be resected and a Fogarty catheter passed distally to remove propagated thrombus. A completion arteriogram should be obtained to ensure that all the distal thrombus has been removed after a repair of the artery has been effected.

Arterial repair may be by simple suture, lateral continuous suture, patch repair, end-to-end anastomosis or interposition grafting (Fig. 10.44). The type of injury determines the type of repair. A small puncture wound commonly occurring after radiological or cardiac catheterization can usually be closed by one or two simple sutures placed in the axis of the vessel to avoid narrowing. A linear laceration or a small branch avulsed from the side of the vessel can usually be closed by a single continuous suture provided that arterial wall has not been lost, and provided that the lumen will not be narrowed by this type of repair. A patch should be inserted to repair any defect where there is a risk of stenosis. Vein is usually the material of choice for the patch but prosthetic material (Dacron or polytetrafluoroethylene) can be used when a suitably thick-walled vein is not available providing there is no risk of infection.

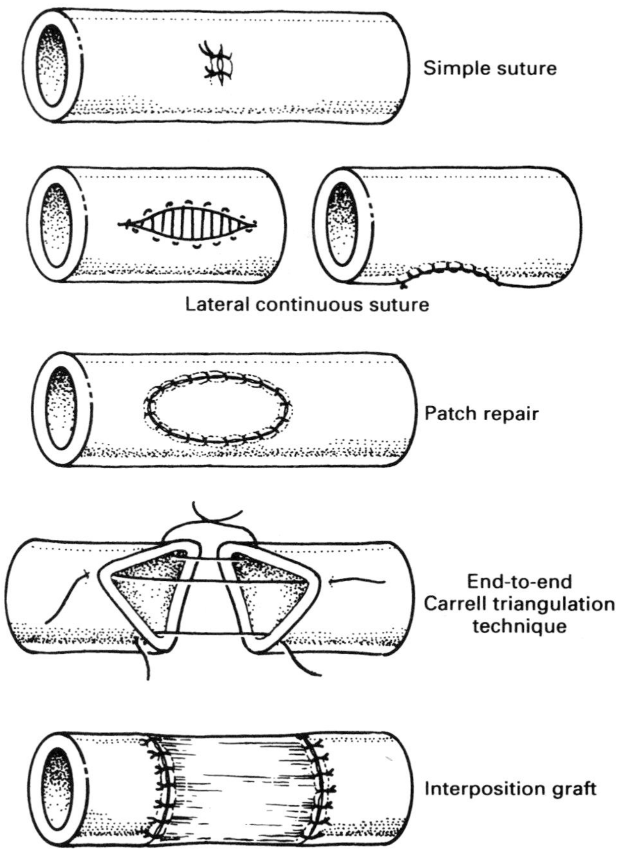

Fig. 10.44 Methods of repairing arterial injuries.

Occasionally it is possible to mobilize a sufficient length of artery to excise the damaged arterial wall and carry out an end-to-end anastomosis. This is possible when the vessel has been neatly transected but should not be attempted if the anastomosis has to be made under tension, or if a damaged segment of vessel must be retained in order to allow a satisfactory anastomosis to be made. An end-to-end anastomosis may be made using a double-ended suture or by the triangulation method of Carrel (Fig. 10.44).[261]

An interposition graft of vein or prosthetic material should be used to replace any segment of severely damaged vessel if excision and end-to-end anastomosis are not possible (Fig. 10.44). Long saphenous vein is usually the material that is chosen for this purpose in patients with arterial damage in the limbs, but this vein must not be taken from a limb with a concomitant venous injury because this may sacrifice an important collateral.[262] The long or short saphenous vein of the contralateral undamaged limb or the cephalic vein is used instead. The internal and external jugular veins and the brachial veins provide useful alternatives if arteries of the calibre of the iliac, carotid or subclavian arteries have been damaged.[263] Alternatively the cephalic or saphenous veins can be

REFERENCES

261. Carrel A Lyon Med 1902; 98: 859
262. Barros D'Sa A Ann R Coll Surg Engl 1982; 64: 37
263. Thompson B W, Read R C, Casali R E Am J Surg 1975; 130: 733

fashioned into a larger calibre panel composite or compilation graft[264]. Prosthetic materials can be used to replace major vessels if vein is unavailable or unsuitable but should not be used in contaminated wounds because of the dangers of graft infection. An indwelling shunt of the Javid or Pruitt type can be used to maintain the arterial inflow and venous outflow while other injuries are being repaired.[262] Many now prefer to perform the vascular repairs first and stabilize bones or repair nerves and soft tissue later.[265] The internal iliac artery can be used as a free graft if the arterial injury is within the abdomen.

Arterial spasm

It is now recognized that post-traumatic arterial spasm is a dangerous diagnosis to make, as it is often associated with intimal damage and intraluminal thrombosis which can only be excluded by arteriography or exploration. Traumatic spasm certainly does occur, but should only be diagnosed in retrospect after arteriography has shown typical appearances or arteriotomy fails to demonstrate intimal damage.

Arterial spasm is often the only visible sign of a severe arterial injury, with wall contusion and intimal damage underlying the area of spasm.[266] Urgent arteriography should be carried out when a patient presents with a cold extremity following a direct or crushing injury, especially if this is associated with a bone fracture such as supracondylar fracture of the humerus, and the distal pulses are impalpable or cannot be detected with a Doppler ultrasound probe. Surgical exploration is indicated if the artery is locally stenosed or occluded on arteriogram. When the vessel has been exposed and the haemorrhage controlled, areas of arterial contusion or persistent spasm should be investigated by intraoperative arteriography, or alternatively the luminal surface can be directly inspected through an appropriately sited arteriotomy.

Intramuscular or intraluminal injections of papaverine and careful division of the adventitia may alleviate the stenosis[267,268] if the arteriogram confirms smooth spasm of the wall. This can be confirmed by repeating the arteriography. Persistent spasm is an indication for inspection of the luminal surface. Damaged arterial wall is dealt with by the methods described above.

Arterial occlusion

This follows severe wall contusion with mural thrombus or intimal tears and also occurs when the vessel has been completely transected. The symptoms and signs are those of arterial haemorrhage combined with evidence of an acute arterial occlusion. Arteriography is helpful to determine the upper limit of the occlusion but rarely shows the distal arterial tree because the collateral pathways have not yet had time to develop. When an occluded artery is exposed it appears swollen, discoloured and solid, and is either non-pulsatile or feebly pulsatile. The vessel lumen is explored through an arteriotomy which is begun above the damaged segment and extended through the injured portion of the vessel. Distal thrombus is removed by a Fogarty catheter before the damaged artery is repaired or excised. When the vessel has been completely divided, the two ends of the transected artery are mobilized and occluded by clamps before continuity is restored by end-to-end anastomosis or interposition grafting.

Limbs that have sustained acute arterial occlusions should have early and adequate fasciotomies made to prevent massive rises in compartment pressure[269] when the period of acute ischaemia has been considerable (more than 3 or 4 h), or when there has been any associated venous injury. Postoperatively, distal pulses must be monitored by regular clinical examination, supplemented if necessary by Doppler ultrasound pressure measurement. Disappearance of pulsation is a late indication for re-exploration of the vessel. Patients should be given systemic antibiotics in order to try to prevent secondary infection. Tissues that are not viable must be excised but it is important to achieve soft tissue cover of all arterial suture lines.[270]

Arterial dissection

This is the consequence of an intimal tear with arterial blood entering the media, and it becomes clinically apparent when the vessel occludes.[271] The dissection rarely extends for any great distance down the vessel because the media is normal and not weakened from cystic median necrosis. Arteriography usually shows a smoothly narrowed vessel with contrast outlining the origin of the dissection. The damaged segment of artery must be excised and replaced.

Traumatic or false aneurysm (pulsating haematoma)

A laceration through part of an arterial wall results in a local haematoma which may eventually be contained by the surrounding normal tissues. Fibrous tissue develops around this haematoma and this then contracts to give a false sac containing thrombus which remains in continuity with the vessel lumen. Continued arterial pulsation erodes the wall of a false aneurysm, increasing the cavity in the haematoma.[272]

There is often a history of considerable primary haemorrhage from a small wound and there may be signs of marked swelling and local oedema.[273] Distal pulsation is usually maintained but a local bruit may precede the appearance of the expansile pulsation. Surrounding structures are compressed as the aneurysm expands, and limb oedema, deep vein thrombosis and nerve damage causing pain may all complicate its development. It is extremely rare for the artery to occlude, however, and treatment rarely needs to be

REFERENCES

264. Livingston R H, Wilson R I Br Med J 1975; 1: 667
265. Radonic V, Baric D, Petricevic A et al Br J Surg 1995; 82: 777
266. Kinmonth J B Br Med J 1952; 1: 59
267. Kinmonth J B, Hadfield G L et al Br J Surg 1956; 44: 164
268. Barros D'Sa A Vasa-Supplementum 1991; 33: 66
269. Patman R D, Thompson J E Arch Surg 1970; 101: 663
270. Ledgerwood A, Lucas C E Am J Surg 1973; 125: 690
271. Zelenock G B, Kazmers A et al Arch Surg 1982; 117: 425
272. Patterson-Ross J Br Med J 1946; 1: 1
273. Blackwood M Postgrad Med J 1946; 22: 75

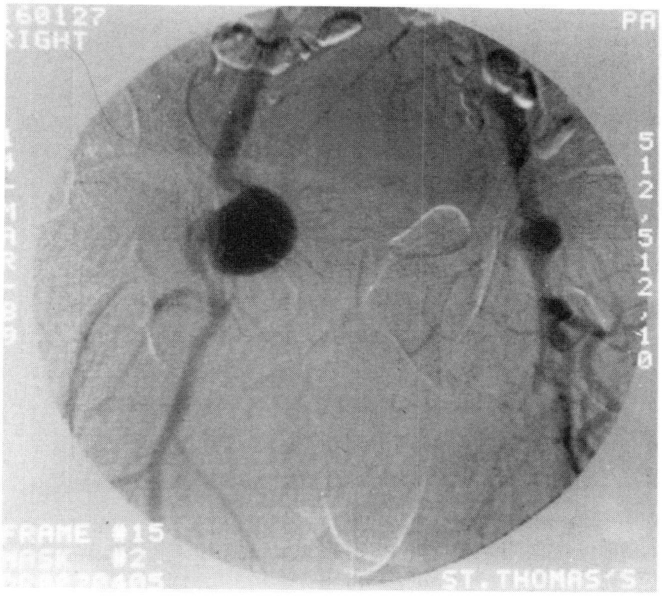

Fig. 10.45 A digital subtraction arteriogram showing a false aneurysm.

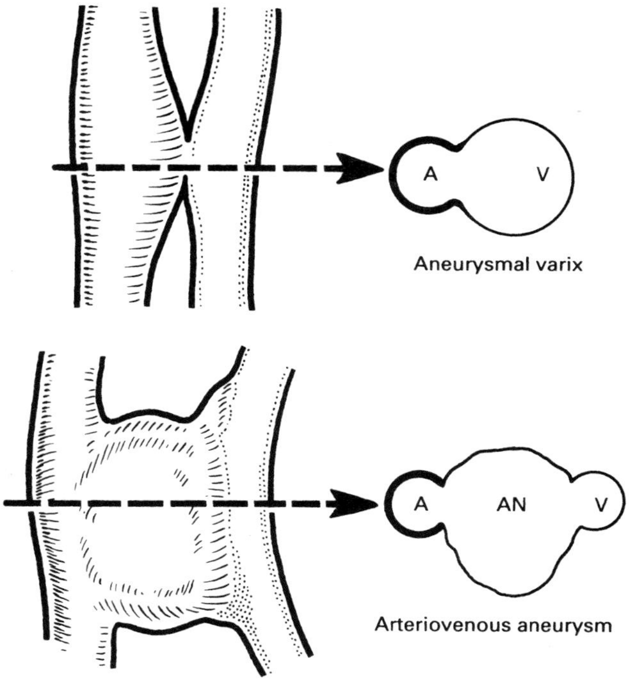

Fig. 10.46 Different types of arteriovenous fistula.

urgent unless there is danger of skin necrosis or sepsis developing over the sac. At first it may be difficult to decide whether there is just a local haematoma lying over the vessel with transmitted pulsation. Re-examination over a period of days invariably dispels doubt, but a colour duplex scan usually confirms the presence of a false aneurysm, and if it is found early and the defect is small it may be possible to occlude the site of the leak using the duplex scanner probe to provide precise pressure.[274,275] This causes some aneurysms to rethrombose and obliterate. Digital or conventional arteriography[276] usually confirms the presence and exact location of a false aneurysm (Fig. 10.45) which can be repaired electively when compression fails. Arteriography also demonstrates the state of the distal arterial tree. When the vessels proximal and distal to the aneurysm have been displayed and controlled, the sac is opened and the arterial defect is closed. When all the vessels entering the false sac cannot be easily controlled before it is opened, troublesome back-bleeding can be prevented by inserting Fogarty catheters into the relevant branches and inflating the balloons until the bleeding ceases.[277] Closure with simple sutures often suffices if the defect is small, but if it is large, a patch or interposition graft may be required.[262,278] There is almost no place today for arterial ligation in the treatment of false aneurysm unless access to the sac is extremely difficult. The results of surgical repair are very good: providing the false aneurysm is tackled before it becomes too large or complications have developed, repairs carry a low morbidity and mortality[278,279] and can normally be carried out without compromising arterial patency. The development of covered stents may make this the easiest method of obliterating false aneurysms in future, especially if the patient is old and unfit and the aneurysm is in an inaccessible site.[280] The undistended stent is inserted over a guidewire, positioned across the neck of the false sac and expanded to occlude the opening.

Traumatic arteriovenous fistula

This usually develops when there is a simultaneous partial laceration of a vein and artery, lying in close apposition with both vessels opening into a common haematoma cavity (an arteriovenous aneurysm). Occasionally the vessels communicate directly, with complete or partial redirection of arterial blood into the vein (an aneurysmal varix). Sometimes a second injury of the arterial wall may produce a false aneurysm in the artery in addition to the arteriovenous aneurysm, and rarely the proximal end of the divided artery appears to join the distal end of the divided vein (Fig. 10.46). Arteriovenous fistulae do not form immediately after wounding, usually taking some days to develop. The patient may notice a thrill or even become aware of a buzzing noise if the fistula is situated in the head or neck. Fistulae usually follow an open wound but may also follow a closed injury which may be trivial; they can occasionally occur after mass ligation of an artery and its adjoining vein.[281] A traumatic fistula may develop between two insignificant peripheral vessels or may involve vessels as large as the aorta and inferior

REFERENCES

274. Agrawal S K, Pinheiro L J Am Coll Cardiol 1992; 20: 610
275. Hajarizadeh H, La Rosa C R J Vasc Surg 1995; 22: 425
276. Picus D, Totty W G AJR 1984; 142: 567
277. Gaspar M R, Barker W (eds) Major Problems in Clinical Surgery, Peripheral Vascular Arterial Disease. Saunders, Philadelphia 1981
278. McMillan I, Murie J A Br J Surg 1984; 71: 832
279. Elkin D C, Shumacker H B Surgery in World War II. Vascular Surgery. Government Print Office, Washington DC 1955
280. Parodi J C J Vasc Surg 1995; 21: 549
281. Holman E Arteriovenous Aneurysm. Abnormal Communications Between the Arterial and Venous Circulations. Macmillan, New York 1937

vena cava. Many are now caused by needles or catheters inserted by cardiologists or radiologists as part of investigations or treatment.

The symptoms and signs are initially similar to those of a traumatic aneurysm although the swelling is often less and the thrill or bruit is predominant. Later the adjoining veins around the fistula dilate and may form a plexiform pulsating mass. A machinery murmur is heard loudest over the fistula, but it is usually transmitted for some distance in all directions. The murmur is usually loudest in systole and can be abolished by direct pressure over the fistula.

When the fistula is large, it may at first cause a fall in both the systolic and diastolic pressure, an increase in heart rate and raised venous pressure both proximal and distal to the fistula.[281] The cardiac output increases as a result of the increased venous return, and the venous oxygen content also rises. The arterial blood flow beyond the fistula is reduced and rarely this may cause gangrene. As the patient acclimatizes to the fistula, the circulating blood volume increases, both the systolic and diastolic pressure rise and the pulse rate returns to normal.[281] The adjoining vessels continue to enlarge if the fistula is not repaired at this stage and may even develop atherosclerosis and phlebosclerosis. The heart then begins to dilate and may eventually fail.[281] When the fistula is situated in a limb, this may hypertrophy and lengthen,[282,283] and the chronic venous hypertension may lead to lipodermatosclerosis and venous ulceration. Most of these effects are reversed when the fistula is closed. Bacterial endocarditis is a rare but potentially lethal complication.[284]

Confirmation of the effect

Confirmation of the effect of the fistula on cardiac output is demonstrated by the bradycardic reaction of Branham and Nicoladoni.[73,74] The pulse rate is recorded for a minute before the fistula is occluded. It is then measured for a further minute and a marked fall in pulse rate in the second period is indicative of a sizeable left-to-right shunt with cardiac compensation. The fistula can be safely treated by ligation if the distal vessels still pulsate when the fistula is occluded (the Henle–Coenen sign),[285,286] but in practice surgical correction should always aim to separate the vessels and close the defect.

Before operation arteriography should be obtained to delineate the site of the fistula and confirm the presence of a normal distal arterial tree (Fig. 10.47).[287] It is occasionally helpful to measure the cardiac output and pulmonary oxygen saturation. A small fistula which can be held occluded by pressure from a duplex probe may occasionally close spontaneously.[288] If this fails, the choice lies between inserting a covered stent over the defect[280] or direct operative closure. A large fistula in an unfit patient is ideal for stenting, whereas a small peripheral fistula in a fit young patient should be corrected by operation.

At operation the artery and the vein should be controlled above and below the point of connection; after systemic heparin has been given the vessel can be occluded by clamps and separated. The defect in both the artery and the vein should be directly closed if possible.[289–292] Occasionally, in for instance a large aortocaval fistula, it may be difficult to obtain direct access to the fistula;

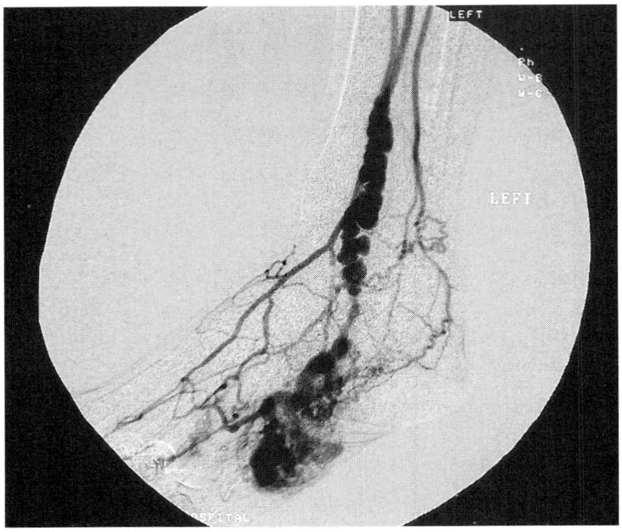

Fig. 10.47 An angiogram showing an AV fistula.

under these circumstances it may be preferable to open the artery and close the fistula from within the lumen.[293] A covered stent placed over the defect is then an attractive alternative. The draining veins should not be ligated if possible as symptoms of defective venous drainage may develop in the future. Closure of the fistula almost instantly cures cardiac failure which may have needed intensive treatment before the operation. Most traumatic arteriovenous fistulae can be corrected surgically without great risk to life or limb provided the patient is fit for anaesthesia and the operation is carried out by an experienced vascular surgeon.[287,289]

Iatrogenic arterial injuries

Ligation

In any operation sudden life-threatening haemorrhage may require rapid surgical control, and the application of haemostatic artery forceps and ligatures forms part of all operations. There are no undesirable consequences providing the tissues supplied by the occluded vessels have an alternative means of blood supply or are being removed as part of the operation, but from time to time a major vessel is inadvertently ligated. This must be recognized

REFERENCES

282. Robertson D J Ann R Coll Surg Engl 1956; 18: 73
283. Luke J C Can Med Assoc J 1940; 42: 341
284. Reinhoff W H, Hamman L Ann Surg 1935; 102: 905
285. Henle A R Zbl Chir 1914; 41: 92
286. Coenen H Zbl Chir 1913; 40: 191
287. Szilagi D E, Elliott J P et al 1965; 57: 61
288. Feld R, Patton G M N, Carabasi A J Vasc Surg 1992; 16: 832
289. Seeley S F, Hughes C W et al Am J Surg 1952; 83: 471
290. Panayiotopoulos Y P, Taylor P R Eur J Vasc Endovasc Surg 1995; 10: 114
291. Perry M O Management of Acute Vascular Injuries. Williams & Wilkins, Baltimore 1981
292. Rich N, Spencer F Vascular Trauma. W B Saunders, Philadelphia 1978
293. McClelland R M, Canizaro P C, Shires G T Major Prob Clin Surg 1971; 3: 146

immediately and appropriate steps taken to restore blood flow. This may simply entail removal of the ligature, but if the arterial wall has been devitalized by its application the damaged vessel must be resected. The principles of vascular repair of an injured artery have already been described. There is almost never a good reason for not restoring arterial inflow and relying instead on collateral pathways to develop.

External compression from plasters, bandages and splints

Plasters, bandages and splints may produce arterial occlusion in two ways:

1. The edge of the splint or plaster cast may compress an area of skin and occlude the underlying vessels.
2. The plaster or bandage is applied too tightly, occluding the veins, causing oedema and raising the tension beneath the external occlusion until the arteries eventually become obstructed.

This complication should be entirely preventable if the digits of all limbs encased in plasters or tight dressings are regularly inspected and by responding to all complaints of excessive pain by releasing dressings, splitting plasters and inspecting encased limbs. Cold digits and absent distal pulsation are late signs.

Iatrogenic arterial puncture damage

Radiologists and cardiologists are regularly required to perform arterial punctures for contrast arteriography and cardiac investigation, and doctors of all specialties sample arterial blood for gas and pH analysis. Any arterial puncture carries the risks already described of dissection, haemorrhage, thrombosis, false aneurysm and arteriovenous fistula formation. These risks must be recognized and are minimized by careful technique and adequate external pressure applied for an appropriate period (2–5 min) over all arterial puncture sites. Punctures into the external iliac artery above the inguinal ligament or into the profunda femoris artery are more difficult to control. Careful monitoring should detect developing complications which can be rapidly corrected by the appropriate surgical manoeuvres.

Intra-arterial injection of drugs and chemicals

A number of compounds, given intravenously with complete safety, have disastrous consequences if injected into an artery. Short-acting barbiturates for anaesthesia,[294–296] sodium tetradecyl sulphate as a vein sclerosant[297] and quinine given for malaria[298] are examples of drugs which can be safely injected into veins but severely damage arteries. Drug abusers may inadvertently self-administer barbiturates or benzodiazepines into arteries with disastrous consequences.[299] As arteries often lie in close proximity to veins these complications are well recognized. They may be prevented if bright red pulsatile blood is noted to enter the barrel of the syringe; even when the injection has begun, disaster may still be averted if further injection is immediately abandoned when the patient complains of severe limb pain.[297]

The limb may be lost from gangrene or severely compromised by the development of a Volkmann's contracture if a toxic compound is inadvertently injected into a peripheral artery before it is recognized. Limbs that recover may later develop Raynaud's phenomenon.

In many patients who receive an inadvertent arterial injection there is a congenital arterial anomaly. In 10% there is a high bifurcation of the brachial artery with the ulnar artery passing superficial to the common flexor origin and so presenting more readily to the needle.[300] The antecubital fossa should not be used for thiopentone injections, and a pause should always be made after a small quantity of barbiturate has been injected to discover if this is painful. The vessel thromboses because of acute intimal damage, perhaps as a result of the release of noradrenaline or the high pH of thiopentone,[301] and the thrombosis rapidly extends into all the major tributaries. The moment this disaster is recognized the syringe should be removed from the needle and an injection of heparin given through the same needle. An intravenous infusion of dextran may be started and the patient should be continued on systemic anticoagulants.[297] Alternatively a prostacycline infusion may be tried.

A stellate ganglion block, a lumbar sympathectomy or a local periarterial sympathetic block may abolish arterial spasm while external cooling may help to prevent tissue loss. Urgent arteriography may indicate the need for thrombectomy if these measures fail to improve the circulation, although the results of this desperate surgery are often poor. A significant proportion of these injuries end in amputation and litigation.[302]

Ergot poisoning

This is now rare but is discussed in more detail on page 294.

Environmental arterial injury

Frostbite

This affects high-altitude mountaineers and those who are exposed in cold climates without adequate protection. The dangers of cold weather and suggestions for withstanding its effects are recorded in ancient Aryan and Assyrian texts.[303] Hippocrates and Galen also recognized the signs of cold injury[303] and suggested methods to protect against its development. Xenophon[304] recorded that during the retreat of the Greek soldiers from Persia 'they left behind

REFERENCES

294. Cohen S M Lancet 1948; ii: 361
295. Lundy J S Clinical Anaesthesia. Saunders, Philadelphia 1942
296. Kinmonth J B, Shepherd R C Br Med J 1959; 2: 914
297. MacGowan W A L, Holland P D J et al Br J Surg 1972; 59: 103
298. Genevrier M Soc Med Nil Franc 1921; 15: 169
299. Wright C B, Lamoy R E, Hobson R W Surgery 1976; 79: 425
300. Aird I (ed) Companion in Surgical Studies, 2nd edn. Livingstone, Edinburgh 1957
301. Burn J H Br Med J 1960; 2: 414
302. Macgowan W A L J Roy Soc Med 1985; 78: 136
303. Schechter D C, Sarot I A Surgery 1968; 63: 527
304. Xenophon Anabasis, vol IV. Bristol Classic Press, 1981

soldiers who had lost their eyesight because of snow blindness and also those whose toes rotted off because of the cold'. He suggested that it was beneficial to keep moving and to take sandals off at night. He noted 'that the straps cut into the feet' of those who went to sleep wearing their sandals. Matters were made worse when new uncured leather was used to make replacements for sandals that had worn out. Larrey, Napoleon's surgeon in the Polish campaign, provided a classical description of the ravages of frostbite,[305] and cold injury still caused many casualties in World War II despite the improvements in protective clothing; it proved a particular hazard in high-altitude aerial combat.[306] Even in the Falklands conflict cold injury proved a major problem.[307]

Response to freezing

The first signs of cold injury appear in the extremities at tissue temperatures of 15°C.[308,309] The fingers and toes redden because of a relative oxygen surplus: oxygen consumption is less than demand. At 10°C the skin is red and hypersensitive, and digital movements become clumsy. Below 10°C the skin becomes pink and painful; at lower temperatures the vessels become permanently contracted and the tissues appear cold and white (Stray's sign).[310] At 2.5°C ice crystals form in the tissues, which become anaesthetic and immobile, sometimes with scattered areas of cyanosis. Even at this stage recovery can occur because cells have the capacity to supercool beyond their freezing point without solidifying. Tissue destruction occurs between –4 and –10°C, and true freezing may not develop until a temperature of –20°C is reached.[311]

When water is transformed to ice the osmolality of the extracellular space increases, leading to diffusion of water from the intracellular space. Protein denaturation, pH changes, cellular dehydration, rupture of cell membranes and destruction of cellular enzymes are all caused by freezing. Long periods of oxygen lack at this temperature are well tolerated because the cellular metabolism becomes suspended. The cold, which is amplified by wind chill,[312] stimulates the autonomic nervous system causing vasoconstriction. The slowing of the blood flow leads to haemoconcentration, increasing viscosity, causing capillary sludging and further reducing the blood supply of the frozen part. Eventually thrombosis leads to ischaemia and gangrene. It is a moot point whether direct tissue injury or thrombosis of the arterioles and capillaries is responsible for tissue necrosis. Initially there is discomfort and local blanching but this usually disappears as sensation is lost. Numbness and tingling give way to a wooden feeling. The affected person is often unaware of the blanching, which is most common on the ear and face, and an appreciation of the potential risks by colleagues may be valuable.[313]

Recovery

Pain and swelling are common as the tissues rewarm. Arteriolar spasm relaxes and the capillaries dilate, allowing plasma to circulate. Blisters develop as fluid leaks out of damaged capillaries and the skin changes to a dull red colour as cellular metabolism restarts. Diagnosis is rarely difficult. A Doppler probe may be used to assess the patency of the small vessels.

Prophylaxis

This is always preferable to treating the established condition, which is essentially incurable. In wartime cold exposure often cannot be avoided and great care must then be taken of both hands and feet. Insulated boots and gloves are now standard issue in arctic conditions, and tight shoes and straps must be avoided. Warm hats with ear-flaps are also valuable[313] while emollients are useless. Depression, misery and lack of exertion all encourage frostbite, and a positive attitude and enforced exercise may delay and avoid its development.

Treatment

There is disagreement over whether rewarming should be slow or rapid[305–316] but frozen extremities should probably be left exposed in a cool moist environment or gently heated in warm water at a temperature not exceeding 60°C. Rapid rewarming in a whirlpool bath at 37–40°C now appears to be the most popular method of treatment.[317] The whole body should be gently warmed before the extremity is heated. Blisters should be left alone unless they reach massive proportions, when their contents may be aspirated through a sterile needle. Topical applications of Flamazine or other antibiotics may prevent secondary infection if the skin separates, and systemic antibiotics are given for established infection. Thrombosis may be reversed by full doses of heparin administered by the intravenous or subcutaneous routes, although the evidence for its effectiveness is fairly weak.[318] Dextran may improve tissue survival by preventing capillary sludging[318] but carries an increased risk of bleeding, especially if used in combination with heparin. The place of sympathectomy is disputed but it is probably beneficial,[319,320] and temporary stellate ganglion or brachial plexus block has never been tested in a controlled trial. Phenoxybenzamine and hyperbaric oxygen has also been advocated on an anecdotal basis. Good results have also been achieved using a topical thromboxane inhibitor (*Aloe vera*) in combination with aspirin used as a systemic antiprostaglandin agent, but this regimen was assessed in a consecutive series of patients without a

REFERENCES

305. Dunning M W F Br J Surg 1964; 51: 883
306. Simeone F A Arch Surg 1960; 80: 396
307. Oakley E H Ergonomics 1984; 27: 631
308. Meryman H T Physiol Rev 1957; 37: 233
309. Kulka J P Angiology 1961; 12: 491
310. Stray L Publ Norw Acad Sci 1943; 3
311. Schumaker H B, Lempke R E Surgery 1951; 30: 873
312. Wilson O, Goldman R J Appl Physiol 1970; 29: 658
313. Lehmusicallio E, Lindholm H et al Brit Med J 1995; 311:1661
314. Green R Lancet 1942; ii: 695
315. Schumaker H B, Lempke R E Surgery 1951; 30: 873
316. Mills W J In: Viereck E (ed) Proceedings of the Symposia on Arctic Medicine and Biology in Frostbite. Arctic Aero Medical Laboratory, Fort Wainwright Alaska 1964
317. Mills W J Out in the Cold. E M Books, New York 1979
318. Mundth E D In: Viereck (ed) Proceedings of the Symposia on Arctic Medicine and Biology in Frostbite. Arctic Aero Medical Laboratory, Fort Wainwright Alaska 1964
319. Isaacson N H, Harrel J B Surgery 1953; 33: 810
320. Schumaker H B, Kilman J W Arch Surg 1964; 89: 575

control group.[321] Preliminary reports suggest that thrombolysis may be helpful[322] but treatment with a prostaglandin analogue (ilioprost) may be preferable.[323] Local amputations of necrotic digits should be carried out when a clear line of demarcation has developed,[324] although sometimes pain or the onset of infection may necessitate an earlier intervention. Amputation should be delayed as long as possible—between 30 and 90 days after freezing appears to be ideal. Fasciotomies may be required if there is evidence of a compartment syndrome. Split-skin grafts may be used to provide skin cover but more complex reconstructions using plastic surgical techniques may be required to retain digit length and provide a functional hand (see Chapter 45).

When recovery is underway active movements should be encouraged by a physiotherapist. Severe cold must always be avoided after an episode of frostbite, because of increased susceptibility to further damage and an often exaggerated response of the affected limbs to cold and heat.[325] Causalgia and Raynaud's syndrome are late complications which can follow severe frostbite.[325] Hyperhidrosis may also be a problem during recovery.

It is often difficult to judge the extent of the final tissue loss at an early stage but a knowledge of the conditions and the length of the exposure may allow a sensible estimation to be made.[326]

Immersion foot (trench foot, shelter foot)

These conditions have long been familiar to mariners. Shannon, marooned in the Arctic for 7 days in 1832, lost 30 of his company of 49 men from trench foot, and Shackleton and his comrades were also affected by it on their passages from Elephant Island to South Georgia. Some of the British marines and paratroopers in the Falkland Island campaign who 'yomped' their way across the cold wet terrain fell victims to trench foot[327] and more recently it has been highlighted as a problem for the homeless.[328] It is often seen in survivors of shipwrecks in cold waters and in those who sleep outside in cold and wet environments wearing tight constricting footwear. As the sea freezes at –1.9°C and the tissues only freeze at –2.5°C, exposure to unfrozen sea is not capable of freezing tissues, but the wet increases the conduction of cold and heat losses, preventing the supercooling which protects against frostbite.[329,330] In addition, injury by water absorption in the stratum corneum of the skin of the feet is thought to be important.[328] The extremities become numb during the period of exposure and victims feel as though they are walking on cotton wool. Pain is unusual but cramp may occur; after a few days the feet swell, producing a feeling of constriction in shod feet. The skin at this stage turns red, then pale, then yellow, blue and eventually black (Fig. 10.48).

When the limbs are removed from this environment and released from their constraining footwear, they at first remain cold, swollen, discoloured, numb and powerless. The pedal pulses are usually impalpable and gangrene may develop. When this does not occur the limb usually becomes hyperaemic and swollen and this is accompanied by pain and paraesthesia. The small muscles of the affected feet and hands become weak and wasted. The skin blisters and may ulcerate. Even at this stage—which often lasts 6–10 weeks—gangrene may still develop. The normal temperature

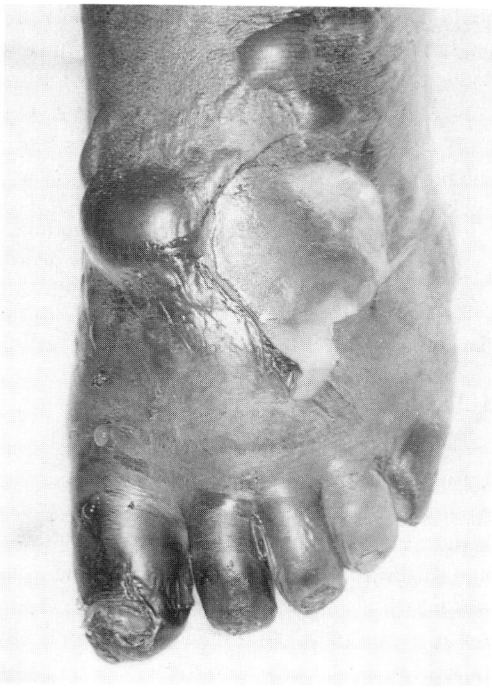

Fig. 10.48 A trench foot.

gradient is often lost with the affected skin feeling warm or warmer than the skin of the groins and axillae. The extremities usually redden with dependence and blanch with elevation. Shooting pains are common, occurring at night and brought on by warmth, dependence, exercise or cold. Glove-and-stocking anaesthesia may develop in the affected skin, but often has a variable and irregular upper limit. Hair may fall out and nails may be shed, and patients often feel unwell with a low fever, weight loss and tachycardia.

Eventually most limbs recover completely but patients with severe initial damage may develop hyperaesthetic smooth shining hairless skin, pigmentation, telangiectases, hypersensitivity to extremes of temperature, and wasted and pointed digits with stiff joints.[329,331]

Treatment

When first seen or rescued, the patient should have their boots and clothes cut away and should then be gently warmed while the extremities are protected from heat, though not over-cooled.[332] The

REFERENCES

321. McCauley R C, Hing D N et al J Trauma 1983; 23: 143
322. Skolnick A A JAMA 1992; 267: 2008
323. Groechenig E Lancet 1994; 34: 1152
324. Minor T M, Shumaker H B Surgery 1967; 61: 562
325. Blair J R, Schatzkir, Orr K D JAMA 1957; 163: 1203
326. Knize D M, Weatherley-White R C A et al J Trauma 1969; 9: 749
327. Marsh A R J Roy Soc Med 1983; 76: 972
328. Wrenn K Arch Int Med 1991; 151: 785
329. Ungley C C, Blackwood W Lancet 194; ii: 447
330. White J C, Scoville W B N Engl J Med 1945; 232: 415
331. Whayne T F, De Bakey M E Office of the Surgeon General, Department of the Army 1958
332. Learmonth J R, Wingley C C Proc R Soc Med 1943; 36: 515

patient should be placed in a draught from an open window or an electric fan, but the skin should be kept dry. The value of sympathectomy at an early stage is disputed.[314,315] Ice packs may provide symptomatic relief during the hyperaemic phase, and patients should be kept in bed until the swelling has disappeared and walking is painless. Smoking is prohibited, and sympathectomy may be valuable during recovery if vasospasm proves problematic.[315] Prostaglandin infusions may also be beneficial.[323] Local amputation may be required at this stage to remove necrotic digits. It is best to delay amputation as long as possible to avoid unnecessarily excising potentially recoverable tissue.

ATHEROSCLEROSIS

Atherosclerosis is a focal intimal accumulation consisting of lipids and fibrous tissue (collagen and elastin) associated with smooth muscle proliferation, found mainly in large and medium-sized arteries.[333] It develops as a plaque or series of plaques beneath the endothelium—called atheroma from the Greek word meaning gruel or porridge.

Pathology

The fatty streak is the earliest change: it has been seen in the large and medium-sized arteries of both children and adults.[333] It is simply a collection of lipid, usually forming as a longitudinal streak beneath the aortic endothelium. It is not known if this streak lesion is capable of regressing or extending to form the more advanced gelatinous plaque.[334] The latter is thought to develop into the fully mature fibrolipid plaque which has a cholesterol lipid-rich base covered by a fibrous cap, surrounded by proliferating smooth muscle cells.

Lipids are first seen in the vessel wall within macrophages which then coalesce before becoming surrounded by smooth muscle cells. These macrophages have been shown to originate from blood monocytes.[335,336] The accumulation of lipid in the arterial wall may disrupt the overlying endothelium, exposing the subendothelial tissues. This encourages platelet adherence with the release of thromboxane, which further stimulates the accumulation of platelets, and the release of platelet-derived growth factor, which may be responsible for the smooth muscle proliferation.[337] The initial problem is thought to be endothelial dysfunction caused by biochemical and haemodynamic stresses.[338] Oxidation of low density lipoprotein cholesterol stimulates leucocyte adhesion and the production of the monocyte chemo-attractant protein,[339] which sets off the chain of events described.

The mature plaque accumulating in the arterial wall narrows the vessel lumen and prevents blood flow from increasing during periods of maximum demand. Plaques which erode through the endothelial lining present a roughened ulcerated surface which is highly thrombogenic. Platelets adhere to these ulcers and accumulate, projecting into the lumen.[340] Platelet accumulation produces a further reduction in blood flow and encourages thrombosis. Large clumps of platelets and even cholesterol break off and embolize distally to obstruct the peripheral circulation and produce small infarcts. Mature plaques may fissure and rupture, allowing blood to track into the wall, resulting in rapid swelling of the plaque which then occludes the vessel and leads to distal thrombosis.[341–344] Some plaques appear to weaken the vessel wall, allowing aneurysms to develop,[345] while dystrophic calcification can occur in atheroma at any site.[346] Whether atheroma is really responsible for aneurysm development is still open to dispute, as proteolytic degeneration and remodelling appears to be more important.

The cause of atheroma is still not known but a number of theories have been put forward in an effort to explain its development. In view of the lipid nature of the plaque it was originally proposed that cholesterol, cholesterol esters and other triglycerides were imbibed or absorbed through the endothelium where they accumulated within the intima.[347] An active transport mechanism for lipid absorption has been postulated as this process takes place across a concentration gradient.[348] As cholesterol and triglycerides are almost insoluble in aqueous solutions they are transported in the blood in water-soluble molecules called lipoproteins. Epidemiological studies have shown that elevated lipoprotein concentrations in the blood, especially of the low density lipoproteins, are associated with an increased risk of atherosclerotic disease.[349–351] Lipoproteins can be subdivided into five classes by their density characteristics on ultracentrifugation.[352,353] These five classes are chylomicrons; very low density lipoproteins; low density lipoproteins; intermediate density lipoproteins; and high density lipoproteins. The plasma cholesterol concentration correlates with the level of low density lipoproteins in the blood,[354] and the plasma triglyceride level is reflected by the chylomicrons and very low density lipoprotein concentration. High density lipoproteins vary independently of cholesterol and triglycerides, and high levels of these compounds appear to be beneficial because they prevent low density lipoproteins from entering the vessel wall.[355]

REFERENCES

333. Mitchell J R A, Schwartz C J Arterial Disease. Blackwell, Oxford 1965
334. Woolf N Pathology of Atherosclerosis. Butterworths, London 1982
335. Gerrity R G Am J Pathol 1981; 103: 181
336. Gerrity R G Am J Pathol 1981; 103: 191
337. Harker L A, Ross R, Glomset J Ann NY Acad Sci 1976; 275: 321
338. Dzau V J Am Heart J 1994; 128: 1300
339. Ross R Nature 1993; 330: 1431
340. Genton E, Barnett H J M et al Stroke 1977; 8: 150
341. Davies M J, Thomas A C Br Heart J 1985; 53: 363
342. Constantides P J Atheroscl Res 1966; 6: 1
343. Sanders M Pharmac Ther 1994; 61: 109
344. Davies M J Brit Med Bull 1994; 50: 789
345. Greenhalgh R M, Laing S, Taylor G W J Cardiovasc Surg 1981; 21: 559
346. Astrup T, Hendriksen E Exp Cell Res 1954; 6: 151
347. Virchow R Phlogose und Thrombose Im Gefass-system. Gesammelte Abhandlungen zur Wissenschaftlichen Medizin. Meidinger, Frankfurt 1856
348. Dayton S, Hashimoto S Circ Res 1966; 19: 1041
349. Gofman J W, Lindgren F T et al J Gerontol 1951; 6: 105
350. Gordon T, Kannel W B et al Arch Int Med 1981; 141: 1128
351. Miller G J, Miller N E Lancet 1975; i: 16
352. Havel R J, Eder H A, Bragdon J H J Clin Invest 1955; 34: 1345
353. Lewis B The Lipoproteins of Plasma in the Hyperlipidaemias; Clinical and Laboratory Practice. Blackwell, Oxford 1976
354. Brown M S, Faust J R, Goldstein J L J Clin Invest 1975; 55: 783
355. Carew T E, Koschinsky T et al Lancet 1976; i: 1315

Experimental animals fed a diet high in cholesterol and animal fat develop similar lesions to human atheroma.[356,357] In these models mucopolysaccharide accumulates within the intima before lipid deposition occurs, suggesting that the high levels of cholesterol and low density lipoprotein may cause chemical damage to the endothelium and stimulate atheroma formation.[358] Human endothelial cells grown in tissue culture have been shown to have a surface receptor which is capable of recognizing and binding low density lipoproteins, which are then absorbed and transported to the lysozymes where hydrolysis occurs.[359] The cholesterol ester core of low density lipoprotein is hydrolysed to release free cholesterol and fatty acids into the cell cytoplasm.

The imbibition of lipid does not explain the focal nature of atheromatous disease; Rokitansky[360] and Duguid[361,362] suggested that mural thrombi were encrusted by endothelium and incorporated into the vessel wall at many sites in the arterial tree. These intimal thrombi were then thought to be replaced with lipid to form atheromatous plaque. This theory explains the presence of fibrin and other constituents of the blood that are seen in and around many atheromatous deposits. Evidence of widespread intravascular thrombosis has, however, never been confirmed.

Russel Ross suggested that traumatic intimal damage may lead to platelet adherence with release of mitogens into the vessel wall which stimulate smooth muscle cell proliferation.[363] These smooth muscle cells may migrate into the intima and metaplase to form cells which are thought to encourage the deposition of lipid.

Mechanical damage from shear stress, hypertension, arterial bending and muscle or tendon trauma, and chemical damage from hyperlipidaemia, adrenaline and nicotine, have all been implicated as causes of intimal damage.[334] There is little firm evidence that structural intimal damage occurs, but endothelial permeability may be increased and this may allow fibrinogen and lipoproteins to enter the vessel wall.

The recognition that atheroma occurs near bifurcations and that blood flow is not uniform throughout the arterial tree has led to the investigation of mechanical factors as aetiological agents in atherogenesis. It was originally thought that high shear stresses, which are a function of the velocity of blood flow, the viscosity of blood and the radius of the vessel wall, might disrupt the endothelium.[364,365] Experimental studies in animal models fed atherogenic diets, however, showed that plaques developed in segments of low shear stress, like the iliac artery ostia, and similar sites are affected in humans.[366] It seems possible that low levels of shear stress reduce the transport of atherogenic-promoting substances away from the wall and encourage their accumulation in or on the vessel wall.[367] Low shear stress may also interfere with endothelial metabolism.

Atheroma depositing in the carotid bifurcation, a common site for the disease, may be influenced by the flow patterns of blood passing through the carotid sinus, which by its bulbous shape encourages flow separation.[368] This is responsible for a low shear velocity along the posterior wall with a reversal of axial flow and the development of vortical patterns in the formed elements of the blood. This again allows particles to have a longer time in contact with the endothelium, increasing the chance of adhesion and absorption. The development of early plaques may also encourage turbulence, seen as random patterns in the passage of blood particles, which may stimulate or encourage further deposition on the wall.

Atheroma is only found in the pulmonary arteries of patients with pulmonary hypertension and in vessels above a coarctation which have a raised blood pressure, implying that raised blood pressure may encourage atherogenesis.[369] There is however no evidence of increased coronary artery disease in patients with mild or moderate hypertension.[370]

Cigarette smoking, obesity, lack of physical exercise, anxiety and personality disorders, diabetes, renal failure and dietary fat intake have all been incriminated as risk factors in the development of atherogenesis, and there are others, including the hardness of the drinking water, diminished thyroid function and various forms of hyperlipidaemia, that may also play a part.[334,371,372] The aetiology of this complex disease appears to be multifactorial, even though Benditt & Benditt[373] suggested that the whole process was the result of a monoclonal proliferation of smooth muscle cells. They found that all the smooth muscle cells within an atheromatous plaque have the same chromosomal pattern, and may have arisen from a single cell, perhaps stimulated by the local release of growth factors. It is possible that reduced production of nitric oxide may be implicated in the genesis of atheroma.

Clinical features and treatment

Obliterative atherosclerosis produces symptoms as the result of a reduced blood supply to the tissues in the distribution of the arteries affected by the disease. It must not be forgotten that this is a generalized disease and it often produces simultaneous symptoms in several different sites. Most of the presentations have already been discussed, but the symptoms, signs, investigation and treatment of stenosing atherosclerosis will now be summarized for each commonly affected vessel.

REFERENCES

356. Anitschkow N N In: Cowdry E V (ed) Experimental Atherosclerosis in Animals—a Summary of the Problem. Macmillan, New York 1933
357. Constantinides P Experimental Atherosclerosis. Elsevier, Amsterdam 1965
358. Taylor C B, Cox G E et al Arch Pathol 1962; 74: 16
359. Brown M S, Ho Y K, Goldstein J L Ann NY Acad Sci 1976; 275: 224
360. Rokitansky C Handbuch der Pathologischen Anatomie, vol 2. Bradmuller & Seidel, Vienna 1844
361. Duguid J B J Pathol Bacteriol 1946; 58: 207
362. Duguid J B J Pathol Bacteriol 1946; 60: 57
363. Ross R, Glomset J A N Engl J Med 1976; 295: 369
364. Fry D L Circ Res 1968; 22: 165
365. Reidy M A, Bowyer D E Atherosclerosis 1977; 26: 181
366. Zarins C K, Trylor K E, Lundell M I Proceedings of Specialist Workshop in the Role of Fluid Mechanics in Atherosclerosis 1978
367. Caro C, Fitzgerald J M, Schroter R C Nature 1969; 223; 1159
368. Zarins C K, Giddens D P, Bharadvaj B K Circ Res 1983; 53: 502
369. Dustan H P In: Paoletti R, Gotto A M (eds) Atherosclerosis Reviews, vol 2. Raven Press, New York 1977
370. MRC Working Party Br Med J 1988; 296: 1565
371. McGill H C Adv Exp Med Biol 1977; 104: 273
372. Ross R, Harker L Science 1976; 193: 1094
373. Benditt E P, Benditt J M Proc Natl Acad Sci USA 1973; 70: 1753

Intracranial atherosclerosis

Originally atherosclerosis was thought to often affect the intracerebral vessels, where it was held to be the major cause of cerebral thrombosis and cerebral infarction. In the 1950s however, Fisher[374] recognized that atherosclerotic plaques were commonly present in the carotid bifurcations of patients dying of stroke, and subsequent post-mortem surveys confirmed that the carotid bifurcation was the site of predilection for atheroma in the arteries of the head and neck.[333] The pendulum has, however, swung too far, and it seems to have been forgotten that atherosclerosis can and does involve the intracranial carotid arteries, the basilar artery, and all the cerebral arteries, including those that make up the circle of Willis. Patients with disease in the intracranial vessels can present with transient ischaemic attacks, strokes and progressive dementia. These symptoms have to be differentiated from those of extracranial atherosclerosis which causes reduced cerebral perfusion and acts as a source of platelet emboli.

Other conditions which need to be considered in the differential diagnosis of stroke and transient ischaemic attacks include cerebral tumours, cerebral haemorrhage, hypertensive encephalopathy, migraine, demyelinating disease, cardiac arrhythmias, sickle cell disease, systemic lupus erythematosus, polycythaemia and Alzheimer's disease, which may all have similar neurological presentations.[375] Referral to a neurologist and investigation with CT or magnetic resonance scanning may be necessary to exclude these disorders.[376,377]

Patients with transient ischaemic attacks or progressive dementia with a carotid or cerebral bruit should have a duplex Doppler assessment of the extracranial vessels supplemented by intravenous digital subtraction angiography or magnetic resonance angiography.[378,379] Intra-arterial arteriography is necessary to confirm a diagnosis of intracerebral atherosclerosis with certainty but carries the risk of precipitating a stroke.[380] At present there is no surgical procedure that is capable of curing diffuse intracerebral disease that has caused dementia, or localized disease that has resulted in cerebral infarction. Aspirin and dipyridamole may reduce platelet embolization[381] but do not improve cerebral perfusion. Extracranial–intracranial bypass has been shown to improve cerebral perfusion, although there is no evidence that it extends life.[382,383] Omental pedicle grafts applied to the cerebral surface have not gained widespread acceptance.[384]

Internal carotid artery atherosclerosis

Atheroma in the carotid arteries is usually localized to the carotid bifurcation.[333,334,385] Unfortunately the majority of patients still present for the first time with completed strokes.[376] Many patients, however, have transient ischaemic attacks which are usually hemispheric affecting the contralateral limbs, or develop amaurosis fugax in the ipsilateral eye.[386] These symptoms are usually the result of repeated microemboli derived from carotid plaque, consisting of either platelet aggregates or cholesterol intraplaque debris after ulceration of the plaque. True cerebral hypoperfusion is rare unless extensive stenoses or occlusions are present in the other cerebral vessels, or there is a poorly formed circle of Willis.[387]

The superficial temporal pulse is impalpable if the common carotid artery is occluded. A bruit is heard in 80% of patients with some degree of carotid stenosis, although bruits are often not heard in patients with severe stenoses.[388–390] Bruits may also be picked up on routine examination of symptomless patients.

A neurological examination may confirm evidence of an upper motor neurone lesion if cerebral infarction has occurred. Retinal examination may disclose evidence of cholesterol emboli or retinal infarction (Figs 10.13 and 10.14).

Migraine, epilepsy and Stokes–Adams attacks must be differentiated from transient ischaemic attacks, and another source of emboli must also be considered. The heart and the aortic arch are the two most common alternative sources of emboli, and transoesophageal echocardiography may be useful if a cardiac cause is suspected.[391] Space-occupying cerebral lesions, intracerebral arterial disease and hypertensive encephalopathy may also present with similar symptoms.[377] Takayasu's disease, fibromuscular hyperplasia, carotid aneurysms and carotid kinking are other rare causes of transient ischaemic attacks.[392,393]

Most patients with transient ischaemic attacks without evidence of a cardiac cause should have the carotid bifurcation imaged by duplex ultrasound scanning; vessels proximal to the bifurcation may be assessed conveniently by intravenous digital subtraction angiography.[379,394] Intravenous or intra-arterial digital subtraction angiography (possibly with selective injection of the individual extracranial vessels) should be considered if duplex scanning is equivocal or the duplex and intravenous angiogram produce conflicting results. Conventional intra-arterial arteriography has about a 2% risk of stroke,[395] and even digital subtraction techniques are not free from major complications.[396] There has therefore been a trend in recent years to rely on ultrasonographic evidence alone if a satisfactory duplex scan is obtained by an experienced operator. The introduction of magnetic resonance angiography may avoid

REFERENCES

374. Fisher C M Arch Neurol Psychiatry 1957; 72: 187
375. Reinmuth O M In: Tyler H R, Dawson D (eds) Current Neurology. Houghton Mifflin, New York 1975
376. Oxfordshire Community Stroke Project Br Med J 1983; 287: 713
377. Allen C M J R Soc Med 1984; 77: 878
378. Turnipseed W D, Sakett J F et al Arch Surg 1981; 116: 470
379. Horrocks M Br J Med 1986; 2: 53
380. Eisenberg R C, Bank W O, Hedgecock M W Neurology NY 1980; 30: 895
381. Canadian Cooperative Study Group N Engl J Med 1978; 299: 53
382. EC/IC Bypass Study Group N Engl J Med 1985; 313: 1191
383. Bishop C C R, Burnand K G et al Br J Surg 1987; 74: 802
384. Ni M S et al Chin Med J 1983; 96: 787
385. Hutchinson E C, Yates P O Lancet 1957; i: 2
386. Ross Russell R W Lancet 1961; ii: 422
387. Fields M S, Bruetman M E, Weibel J Collateral Circulation of the Brain. Williams & Wilkins, New York 1965
388. Kistler J P, Ropper A H, Heros R C N Engl J Med 1984; 311: 27
389. Baird R N Br J Surg 1983; 70: 83
390. Murie J A, Sheldon C D, Quin R O Br J Surg 1984; 71: 50
391. De Bono D P, Warlow C P Lancet 1981; i: 343
392. Volmar J, Nadjafi A F, Stalker L G Br J Surg 1976; 63: 847
393. Wylie E J, Binkely F M, Palubinskas A J Am J Surg 1966; 112: 149
394. Hartnell G C Br J Hosp Med 1986; 2: 433
395. Leow K, Murie J A Br J Surg 1988; 75: 428
396. Turner W H, Murie J A Br J Surg 1989; 76: 1247

these complications and provide satisfactory images.[397] Many still favour a combination of duplex scanning and intravenous digital subtraction angiography at present. CT and magnetic resonance imaging detect space-occupying cerebral lesions and infarcts. Positron emission tomography, magnetic resonance spectroscopy, measurement of cerebral blood flow using radioactive xenon, and transcranial Doppler ultrasonography,[398] with and without inhalation of carbon dioxide, are techniques which may be useful for assessing the cerebral reserve in patients with cerebral hypoperfusion.

Patients with carotid territory transient ischaemic attacks or amaurosis fugax related to an internal carotid artery found to have a significant stenosis of 70% or more (by diameter) should be offered carotid endarterectomy.[399–401] Surgery should take place as soon after diagnosis as practically possible as the benefits are reduced if there is a delay of more than six months from the onset of symptoms. Patients with lesser degrees of stenosis should be treated with antiplatelet agents and only operated upon if their medication fails to arrest symptoms. It has been suggested that certain features of the atheromatous plaque, other than the degree of stenosis, may render it particularly liable to cause embolism. Duplex scanning may indicate plaque friability[402] and identify those at particular risk of stroke.[402,403] Patients with an occluded carotid artery can usually be treated conservatively. In the rare instance of continuing symptoms from proven hypoperfusion, extracranial–intracranial bypass may still have a place to relieve symptoms.[383] Percutaneous transluminal balloon angioplasty of carotid stenosis has been carried out successfully in several centres but its place in the overall management of carotid disease is not yet clear.[404] Carotid angioplasty with or without stenting should only be carried out within the confines of a clinical trial at present.

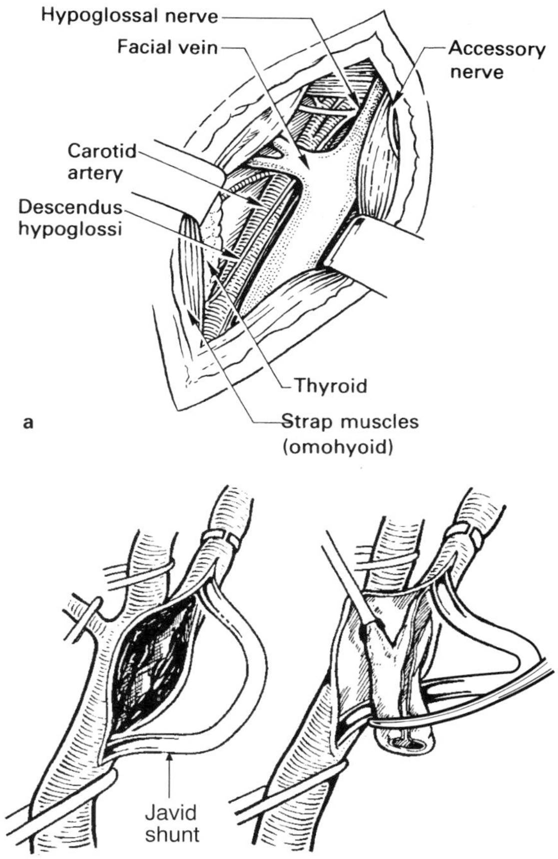

Fig. 10.49 Carotid endarterectomy.

Carotid endarterectomy

The carotid artery is approached through an incision along the anterior border of the sternomastoid. The internal jugular vein is mobilized posteriorly after the common facial vein has been ligated and divided (Fig. 10.49a). The common, internal and external carotid arteries are then dissected free, taking care to preserve and protect the vagus and the hypoglossal nerves. The carotid sinus nerve is blocked with local anaesthetic to prevent excessive variations in blood pressure which may occur during dissection. When the upper and lower limits of the diseased arterial segment have been defined, systemic heparin is given and the vessels are clamped. An arteriotomy in the common carotid artery is continued cephalad through the narrowed internal carotid ostium and as far as normal vessel. When an intraluminal shunt of the Javid or Pruitt type[405–407] is to be used, it is inserted at this stage to allow continuation of cerebral perfusion via the operated internal carotid vessel (Fig. 10.49b). The plane between the plaque and the residual arterial wall is developed and the full extent of the plaque is removed, taking care to avoid leaving residual disease or an intimal flap at the upper end of the endarterectomy. When a smooth intraluminal surface has been achieved, the arteriotomy is closed with a continuous monofilament suture. Before completion of the suture line arterial clamps are re-applied and the shunt removed. The use of a patch of vein or prosthetic material to prevent narrowing of the lumen during closure of the arteriotomy has been widely advocated.[408] This technique is particularly attractive for vessels of narrow calibre, especially in women when it may prevent late re-stenosis.[409] When a vein patch is used, saphenous vein should be taken from the upper end near the sapheno-femoral junction as the lower part of the vein is prone to rupture.[410] The width of the vein patch is the subject of controversy[411] but it should not be too wide.

REFERENCES

397. Murie J A, John T G, Morris P J Br J Surg 1994; 81: 827
398. Padayachee T S, Gosling R G et al Br J Surg 1987; 174: 260
399. European Carotid Surgery Trialists' Collaborative Group. Lancet 1991; 337: 1235
400. Mayberg M R, Wilson S E et al for the Veteran's Affairs Cooperative Studies Program 309 Trialist Group JAMA 1991; 266: 3289
401. North American Symptomatic Carotid Endarterectomy Trial Collaborators N Engl J Med 1991; 325: 445
402. European Carotid Plaque Study Group Eur J Vasc Surg 1995; 10: 23
403. Cave E M, Pugh N D et al Eur J Vasc Surg 1995; 10: 77
404. McGuinness C, Burnand K G Br J Surg 1996; 83: 1171
405. Javid H, Julian O C et al World J Surg 1979; 3: 167
406. Pruitt C Contemp Surg 1983; 23: 1
407. Thompson J E JAMA 1957; 202: 1046
408. Eikelboom B C, Ackerstaff R G A et al J Vasc Surg 1988; 7: 240
409. Hertzer N R, Beven E G et al Ann Surg 1987; 206: 628
410. John T G, Bradbury A W, Ruckley C V Br J Surg 1993; 80: 852
411. Katz M M, Jones G T et al J Cardiovasc Surg 1987; 28: 2

The number of surgeons who never use a shunt during this operation has dwindled. Most either shunt routinely or selectively although the basis of selection for shunting varies. A shunt should be used if there is severe contralateral disease or a low pressure in the carotid after it has been clamped (a stump pressure of below 50 mmHg).[412,413] The operation can be carried out under local anaesthesia[414] and a shunt inserted if the patient starts to develop ischaemic symptoms or signs. Electroencephalography can be used to monitor cerebral function during general anaesthesia.[415,416] The introduction of transcranial Doppler ultrasonography to monitor flow in the middle cerebral artery throughout, may indicate the need to insert a shunt if the signal disappears. When the vessel is clamped[417] light-reflective cerebral oximetry may also be used to assess cerebral perfusion. In this technique near infrared light is transmitted to the brain through the scalp, and spectroscopy is performed on the reflected wave. A marked reduction of cerebral oxygenation indicates the need for a shunt.[418]

Patients with fibromuscular hyperplasia, recognized by the string-of-beads appearance on angiography[419] (Fig. 10.50), may be best treated by angioplasty with or without stenting.[420]

Kinked carotid arteries are best left untouched unless patients are having severe recurrent transient ischaemic attacks for which no other cause is evident.[421] Methods of operative correction generally involve division, resection and re-anastomosis of the artery.

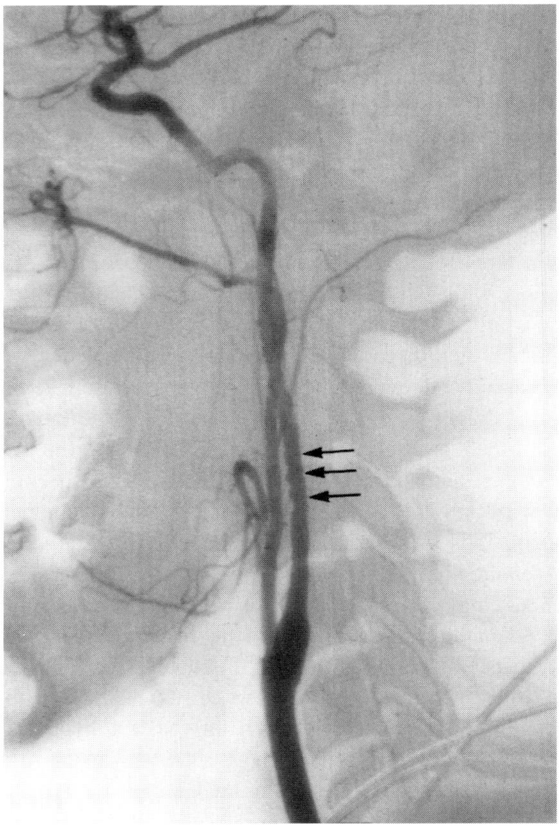

Fig. 10.50 An arteriogram showing the appearances of fibromuscular hyperplasia of the carotid artery.

Results

Three major prospective randomized trials have recently confirmed the value of carotid endarterectomy.[399–401] Patients with carotid territory transient ischaemic attacks, amaurosis fugax or a mild stroke, with a 70% or greater (diameter) stenosis, should be offered carotid endarterectomy. Those with a stenosis of less than 70% are less likely to benefit from surgery although the trials of this subgroup are still continuing. Patients with ulcerated plaques who are continuing to have symptoms on antiplatelet agents should also be offered surgery although there are no studies to support this. The degree of benefit for those in whom operation is indicated is substantial: a sixfold reduction in stroke at three years compared with best medical management.[399] It should not be forgotten, however, that good surgical results depend upon good operative technique. Carotid endarterectomy has a mortality of 1–2% in experienced hands with a stroke risk of 1–2%[422–424] but these figures are doubled if less experienced surgeons operate.[425,426]

At present, there is little justification for operating on patients who have progressing or completed strokes. The indications for operation in those with a symptomless carotid stenosis are not yet clear. Two multicentre randomized studies, the asymptomatic carotid atherosclerosis study (ACAS),[427] and its European counterpart, the asymptomatic carotid surgery trial (ACST),[428] have been established. The former has already reported, indicating that in certain well defined circumstances a tight stenotic lesion merits surgical correction. The symptomatic trials demonstrate that four carotid endarterectomies are required to prevent one stroke per year, while the ACAS asymptomatic data suggest that nearly 20 operations are needed in symptomless patients to prevent one stroke every 5 years.[429] The ACST trial continues and may help resolve this dilemma.

A number of patients develop recurrent stenosis of the endarterectomized vessel. In the early months this is usually the result of myointimal hyperplasia[430] and is often symptomless unless it is severe and bilateral. The role of aspirin and vein patching in preventing the complication has not yet been established.[431,432] After several years atheroma can recur and may give

REFERENCES

412. Moore W S, Hall A D Arch Surg 1969; 99: 702
413. Hays R J, Levinson S A, Wylie E J Surgery 1972; 72: 953
414. Connolly J E, Kwaan J H M, Stemmer E A Ann Surg 1977; 186: 334
415. Baker J D, Gluecklich B et al Stroke 1976; 78: 787
416. Callow A D Am J Surg 1980; 140: 181
417. Gaunt M E, Martin P J et al Br J Surg 1994; 81: 1435
418. Williams I M, Picton A et al Br J Surg 1994; 81: 1291
419. Wylie E J, Binkley F M, Palubinskas A J Am J Surg 1966; 112: 149
420. Morris G C, Carson W P et al Surgery 1971; 69: 498
421. Riser M M, Geraud J, Ducoudray J Rev Neurol 1951; 85: 145
422. Browse N L, Ross-Russell R W Br J Surg 1984; 71: 53
423. Hertzer N J Vasc Surg 1988; 7: 611
424. Sundt T M, Sharbrough F W et al Ann Surg 1986; 203: 196
425. Prioleau W H, Aiken A F, Hairston P Ann Surg 1977; 185: 678
426. Cafferata H T, Gainey M D J Cardiovasc Surg 1986; 27: 557
427. Executive Committee for the Asymptomatic Carotid Atherosclerosis Study JAMA 1995; 273: 1421
428. Warlaw C Lancet 1995; 345: 1254
429. Irvine C D, Baird R N, Lamont P M, Davies A H Br Med J 1995; 311: 1113
430. Cossman D, Callow A D et al Arch Surg 1978; 113: 275
431. Callow A D Arch Surg 1982; 117: 1082
432. Hertzer N R, Bevan E G et al Ann Surg 1987; 206: 628

rise to new symptoms. Re-operations are often difficult and as a consequence more hazardous for the patient. Repeat endarterectomy with a vein patch may be possible, but resection and vein interposition is often preferable, especially if myointimal hyperplasia is the cause.[433]

Vertebrobasilar atherosclerosis

Patients with vertebrobasilar insufficiency usually present with vertigo, faintness, giddiness or loss of consciousness which is often brought on by changes in posture. Cerebellar symptoms and occipital visual disturbances can also occur.[434] There is a considerable overlap between the symptoms of carotid and basilar ischaemia, and differentiation may be difficult.

There may be few signs, though a bruit may be audible over the course of the vertebral artery and nystagmus may be present.[435] Vertebrobasilar insufficiency must be differentiated from cervical spondylosis, migraine and other conditions which cause brainstem compression or infiltration.[436]

Many patients with mild symptoms can be treated by advice to avoid rapid changes in posture, and prescription of antihistamines to prevent vertigo and nausea. Operative endarterectomy of the lower end of the vertebral artery has been performed for disabling symptoms associated with a localized stenosis,[437] and more radical bypasses are now being suggested for relief of symptoms. These procedures have still not been tested in good controlled clinical trials and their value has therefore not been established.

Aortic arch, innominate and common carotid atherosclerosis

These vessels are much less commonly affected by atheroma than the carotid bifurcation or the vertebrobasilar arteries and they are therefore a rarer source of ischaemic attacks and stroke. Takayasu's disease does, however, cause significant stenosis in these vessels. Surgical treatment is rarely indicated unless symptoms are the result of hypoperfusion or persist despite antiplatelet treatment. Often carotid–carotid bypass in the neck or another extra-anatomical bypass is possible, with a lower mortality than major thoracocervical procedures.[438,439]

Subclavian, axillary and brachial atherosclerosis and the subclavian steal syndrome

Atherosclerosis rarely produces symptoms in the vessels supplying the upper limbs. It is often stated that this is because the collateral pathways are so extensive that ischaemic symptoms do not develop, but atheroma less frequently affects these vessels. Upper limb claudication and digital gangrene can occur, and if the occlusion or stenosis is in the proximal part of the subclavian artery patients may experience vertebrobasilar symptoms when they exercise the affected limb.[385,440] This is the result of a reversal of flow in the vertebral artery on the side of the stenosis, which acts as a collateral to supply blood to the ischaemic arm 'stealing' blood from the circle of Willis and cerebral vessels (Fig. 10.4a). Many doubt the existence of this syndrome, which is often associated with carotid stenoses. The finding of diminished pulses at the wrist

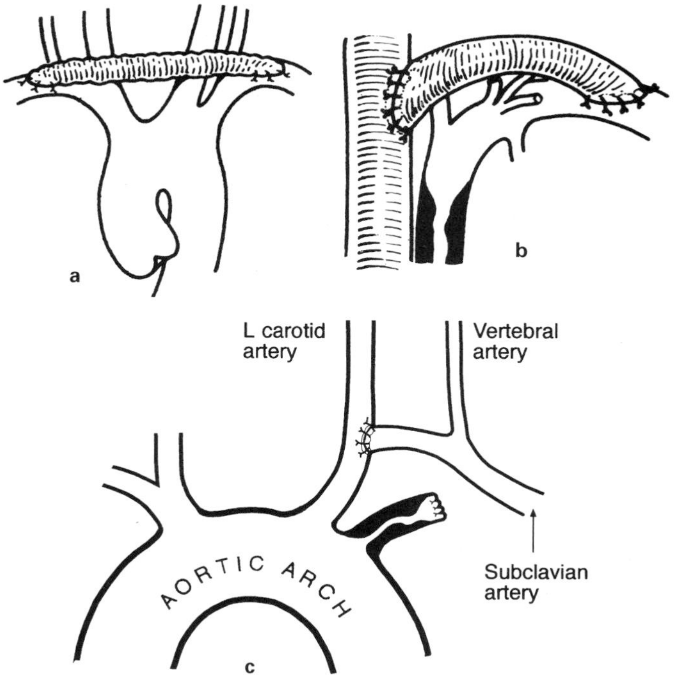

Fig. 10.51 (**a**) Subclavian–subclavian bypass; (**b**) carotid–subclavian bypass; (**c**) subclavian–carotid anastomosis.

or a reduced blood pressure in the affected arm supports the diagnosis if the patient gives a good history of arm claudication, or symptoms consistent with a subclavian steal, especially if a supraclavicular bruit is heard. Other causes of subclavian obstruction include arteritis, embolism and cervical ribs.

Duplex ultrasound scanning showing reversed flow in the vertebral artery enhanced by exercise confirms the diagnosis.[441] Arteriography, by catheter or digital subtraction equipment, should be used to confirm the diagnosis before reconstruction is contemplated. Reconstruction of the subclavian artery can be by subclavian–subclavian bypass (Fig. 10.51a), by carotid–subclavian bypass or by carotid–axillary bypass[442,443] using vein or prosthetic material (Fig. 10.51b). Others[444] have preferred division of the subclavian artery with end-to-side anastomosis of the vessel to the carotid artery, and have claimed better results (Fig. 10.51c). One study comparing transposition with bypass showed improved patency in patients treated by transposition.[445] Angioplasty with or

REFERENCES

433. Lattimer C, Burnand KG Br J Surg; In Press
434. Millikan C H Circulation 1965; 32: 438
435. Loeb C, Meyer J S Strokes Due to Vertebro-basilar Disease. Charles C Thomas, Springfield Illinois 1965
436. Brain W R, Northfield D, Wilkinson M Brain 1952; 75: 187
437. Edwards W H, Mulherin J L Surgery 1980; 87: 20
438. Crawford E S, De Bakey M E et al Surgery 1969; 65: 17
439. Thevenet A Med Hyg 1980; 38: 4154
440. Reivich M H, Helling H E et al N Engl J Med 1961; 265: 878
441. Berguer R, Higgins R, Nelson R N Engl J Med 1980; 302: 1349
442. Forester J E, Ghosh S K et al Surgery 1972; 71: 136
443. Jacobsen J H, Mozersky D J et al Arch Surg 1983; 166: 24
444. Edwards W H, Wright R S Ann Surg 1972; 175: 975
445. Kretschmer G, Teleky B, Marosi L J Cardiovasc Surg 1991; 32: 334

without stent insertion is often selected as best first line treatment for subclavian stenoses. There have not been any controlled trials comparing these treatments with surgery at this site.

A long vein bypass must be taken from a healthy artery above the occlusion to an unaffected segment beyond if the axillary or brachial artery is occluded, tunnelling the bypass through the thoracic outlet. These bypasses are often difficult to perform and tend to occlude early, perhaps because of kinking and occlusion during shoulder movement.

External carotid atherosclerosis

A stenosis of the origin of the external carotid artery is usually treated at the same time as bifurcation disease. External carotid endarterectomy[446] is only justified as an isolated procedure if the patient develops eye symptoms on the side of an internal carotid occlusion,[447] when there is an associated tight external carotid stenosis. External carotid endarterectomy can also be performed as a prelude to extracranial–intracranial bypass.

Atherosclerosis of the thoracic aorta

Although atheroma is quite commonly found in this vessel it rarely causes a stenosis or occlusion, and only produces symptoms if embolism or aneurysmal dilatation occurs.

Atherosclerosis of the abdominal aorta, the renal arteries and the iliac vessels

The abdominal aorta and iliac bifurcations are common sites for atheroma to develop, and the trunks of the aorta and iliac vessels are often affected by more diffuse disease which may extend into the renal arteries. In some patients the disease appears to be localized to the aortoiliac segment, while others have much more diffuse disease involving all the vessels of the lower limb.[333,448]

Rest pain or gangrene does not usually occur if the atheroma is confined to the aorta and iliac vessels because the collateral circulation is normally adequate; even if these vessels are totally occluded patients only complain of intermittent claudication providing the other vessels in the limb are not occluded or stenosed. Patients with aortoiliac disease usually develop buttock and thigh claudication and may lose the ability to achieve penile erection—a syndrome that Leriche & Morel felt was the result of a hypoplastic aorta.[449] When severe distal disease is already present, rest pain and gangrene usually supervene when the aortoiliac segment occludes. Patients occasionally present with symptoms of distal emboli in their feet (Fig. 10.17).

It is important to differentiate aortic claudication from disease of the spinal cord[450,451] (see Chapter 46). Absent or weak femoral pulses are always present in patients with severe aortoiliac disease, and appropriately sited bruits may be heard over critical stenoses.

There is often only a marginal reduction in the resting Doppler pressure index, but this is invariably accentuated by exercise. The Doppler wave form of the femoral pulse may show characteristic features and help to determine the major site of disease.[452] Intravenous digital subtraction arteriography or intra-arterial contrast aortography confirms the diagnosis and displays the distal arterial tree (Fig. 10.52). Duplex ultrasound may now provide enough information although bowel gas may make aortoiliac visualization difficult unless special measures are taken.

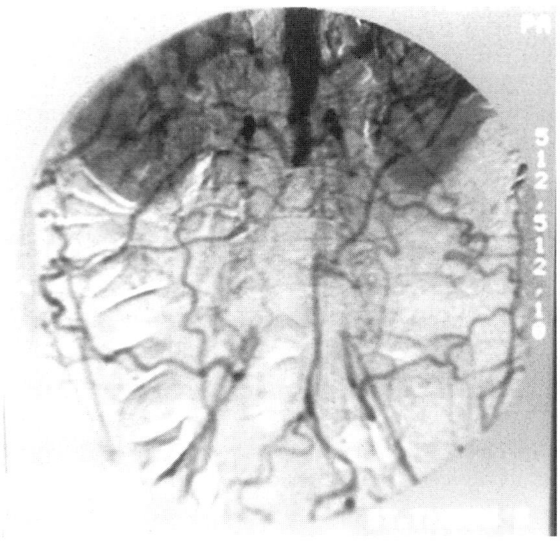

Fig. 10.52 An intravenous digital subtraction arteriogram demonstrating an aortoiliac occlusion.

A reasonable period should be allowed from the onset of symptoms for collaterals to develop as symptoms may improve; all claudicants should be encouraged to stop smoking. Intervention is clearly indicated in patients with rest pain or early gangrene, and may be requested by patients if the claudication pain is interfering with their work or hobbies. This is a reasonable request and should be acceded to providing the patients are otherwise fit and well.

Reconstruction for atherosclerosis of the aortoiliac segment[453–455]

Single stenoses of the iliac vessels can now be treated very adequately with balloon angioplasty (percutaneous transluminal angioplasty) with good long-term results.[456] More extensive stenoses or occlusions may also be treated by balloon angioplasty although extensive or recurrent lesions usually require endovascular stenting.[457] Angioplasty is much simpler than surgery, with

REFERENCES

446. Karmody A M, Shah D M et al Am J Surg 1978; 136: 176
447. Jackson B B Am J Surg 1967; 113: 375
448. Aston N, Lea Thomas M, Burnand K G Eur J Cardiovasc Surg 1991; (in press)
449. Leriche R, Morel A Ann Surg 1948; 127: 193
450. Blau J N, Logue V Lancet 1961; i: 1081
451. Snyder E N, Mulfinger G L, Lambret R W Am J Surg 1975; 130: 172
452. Woodcock J P, Gosling R G, Fitzgerald D E Br J Surg 1972; 59: 226
453. Szilagyi D E, Smith R F et al Ann Surg 1975; 162: 453
454. Cockett F B, Maurice B A Br Med J 1963; 40: 153
455. Jamieson C W Surgical Management of Vascular Disease. Heinemann, London 1982
456. van Andel G J, van Erp W F M Radiology 1985; 156: 321
457. Gunther R W, Vorwerk D AJR 1991; 156: 389

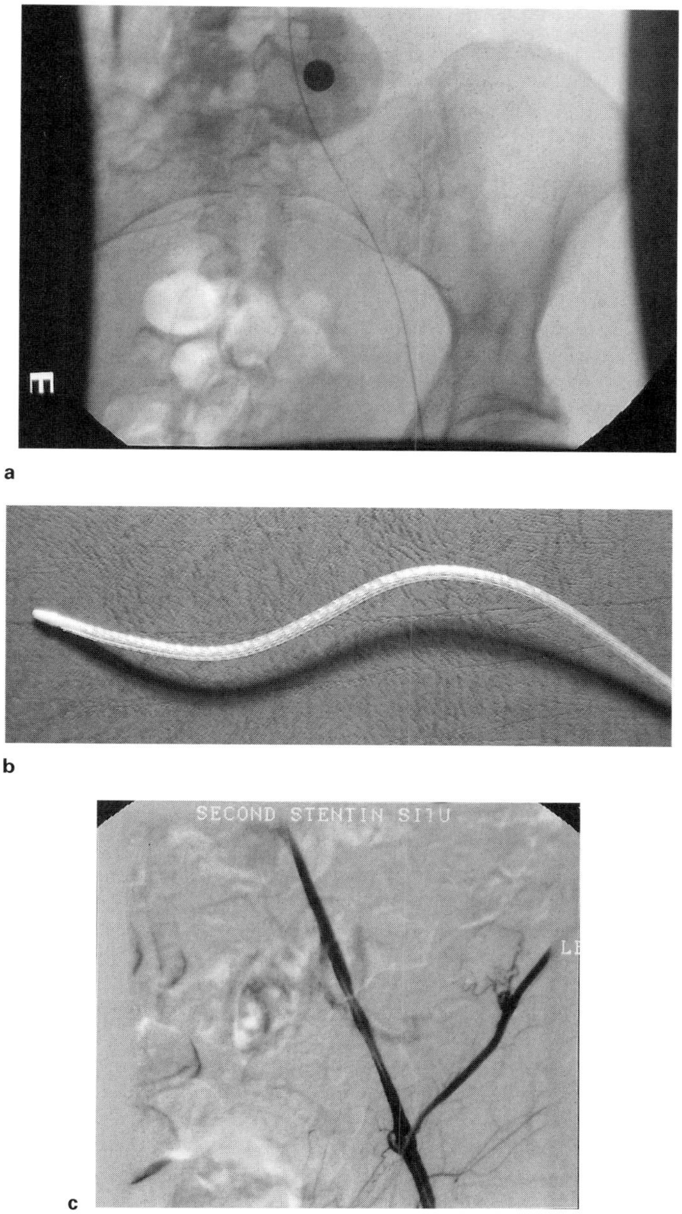

a b c

Fig. 10.53 Stent grafts in iliac arteries: (a) plain radiograph of stent graft in iliac artery; (b) undistended wall stent; (c) arteriogram of expanded wall stent.

lower morbidity and mortality and a much shorter hospital stay. The long-term patency following dilatation of the iliac vessels is in excess of 80%, making aortoiliac endarterectomy a rare operation as the majority of the lesions previously treated by endarterectomy can now be satisfactorily treated by angioplasty followed by placement of an intraluminal stent if there is residual narrowing or dissection. Long occlusions are best treated by primary stenting.[458,459] The number of angioplasties performed has increased enormously[460] and surgery tends to be reserved for failed passage of the guidewire. Intraluminal stents are made of strong flexible metal or nitrinol and are inserted over the guidewire before being 'expanded' across the stenosis or occlusion by balloon dilation (Fig. 10.53).

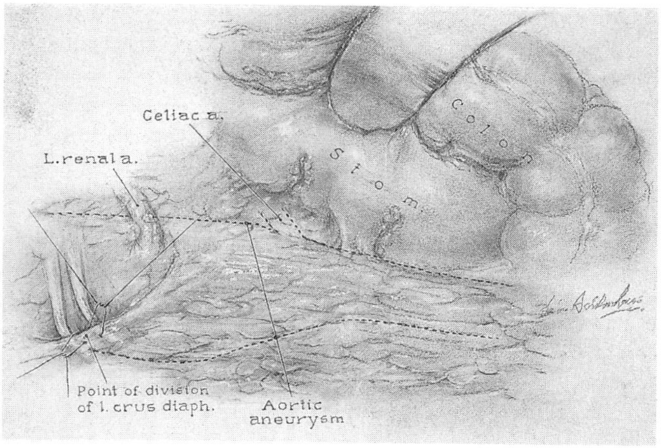

Fig. 10.54 Retroperitoneal approach to aorta. Courtesy of M. Williams.

Localized aortoiliac occlusions in young patients can be treated by endarterectomy. Arteriotomies are made through the distal and proximal limits of the disease and the endarterectomy plane developed.[455] Closed Volmar ring strippers can be pushed up the iliac arteries from below, but aortic atheroma must be removed by open endarterectomy.[461] A bifurcated Dacron bypass graft is the best means of improving the blood supply to the lower limbs if the disease is more extensive. This is the operation of choice where the whole aorta and iliac system is occluded up to the renal arteries.[453,461] The trunk of the prosthesis can be sewn end-to-end to the divided aorta, suturing off the distal aortic lumen, or end-to-side on to the anterior surface of the aorta. Debate continues as to which of these two options is preferable.[462] Whatever technique is used, the graft should be sutured to the most normal piece of aorta, which is usually at or just below the renal arteries.

Surgeons differ in their approach to the abdominal aorta (Fig. 10.54), some using long transverse abdominal incisions, others choosing long midline or paramedian incisions, while oblique incisions with an extraperitoneal approach extending behind or through the pleural cavity may be used, especially if the suprarenal aorta is to be exposed. When a transperitoneal approach is used the small intestine can be packed away inside the abdomen or exteriorized in a plastic bag. The aorta is reached by mobilizing the fourth part of the duodenum to the right and dividing the posterior peritoneum vertically over the front of the aorta. The periaortic fat and lymph glands must also be divided in order to expose the anterior surface of the aorta. The whole procedure is facilitated by a large self-retaining retractor like the Buckwalter or the Omnitract, both of which fix to the operating table.

The whole aorta must be dissected free if an endarterectomy is to be performed, but this is not necessary for bypass procedures when a short segment of undiseased subrenal aorta is mobilized

REFERENCES

458. Palmaz J C, Garcia O J et al Radiology 1990; 174: 969
459. Becker G J, Palmaz J C et al Radiology 1990; 176: 31
460. Pell J P, Whyman M R, Ruckley C V Br J Surg 1994; 81: 832
461. Szilagyi D E, Smith R F, Whitney D G Arch Surg 1964; 89: 827
462. Brewster D C, Darling R C Surgery 1978; 84: 739

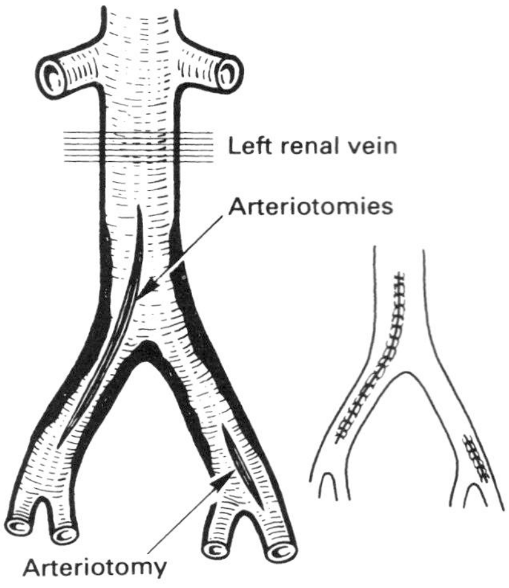

Fig. 10.55 Aortoiliac endarterectomy.

and snared. Before an endarterectomy can be performed the lumbar vessels must be defined and ligated or individually occluded, and both iliac vessels must be followed down until a normal segment of artery is displayed. If this is beyond the bifurcation of the external and internal iliac arteries, a bypass is usually preferable. Arteriotomies are made through the distal and proximal limits of the disease into normal artery, and the endarterectomy plane is developed.

The incisions used for this purpose are shown in Figure 10.55. On completion of the endarterectomy the arteriotomies are closed by simple suture providing the lumen is adequate; prosthetic patches must be used if the vessel would be narrowed by a direct closure. The distal limbs of a bifurcated graft can be anastomosed end-to-side to the iliac vessels or passed down in a retroperitoneal tunnel behind the inguinal ligament and anastomosed end-to-side to the common, superficial or profunda femoris vessels (Fig. 10.56). This anastomosis should extend into an undiseased portion of the profunda artery if the superficial femoral artery is occluded, and some surgeons routinely bypass to the profunda.[463]

When the aortic occlusion extends up to the renal artery orifices, the segment of aorta immediately beneath these vessels is dissected free and snared. A vertical incision is made in the prepared segment of vessel before clamps are applied, and the surgeon's thumb is pressed back on the pulsating portion of the vessel at the level of the renal arteries and gently but firmly squeezed down to extrude the thrombus by compressing it like toothpaste between the thumb and the vertebral column. The atherothrombotic plug is expelled from the vessel and is followed by a rapid gush of blood. Bleeding is controlled by finger pressure, while a clamp is applied across the aorta between the arteriotomy and the renal arteries.[464,465] The graft limbs can be anastomosed to the iliac vessels but are usually tunnelled retroperitoneally and anastomosed end-to-side to the common or profunda femoris arteries which are exposed through oblique or vertical groin incisions.

The suprarenal aorta and the renal arteries may be dissected out if there is extensive atheroma extending into and narrowing the renal vessels. An extensive endarterectomy of this whole segment can then be carried out through an appropriately sited arteriotomy.[466]

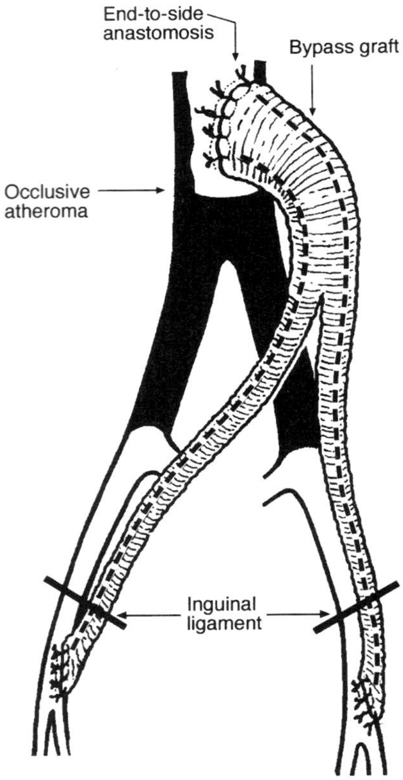

Fig. 10.56 An aortofemoral bypass in place.

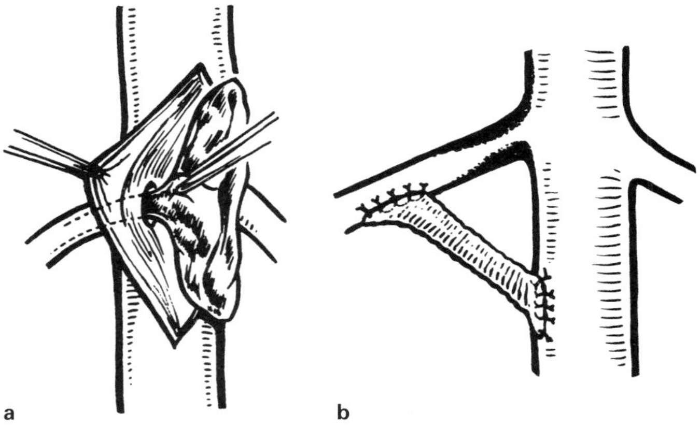

Fig. 10.57 Techniques for revascularizing the renal arteries.

It is rarely necessary to begin the bypass above the renal vessels. Side grafts of vein or prosthetic material can be taken off the main stem to revascularize the renal arteries if necessary (Fig. 10.57). On most occasions it is better to ignore mild or moderate concomitant stenotic disease of the renal vessels and simply treat hypertension with drugs as there is little evidence that

REFERENCES

463. Malone J M, Goldstone J, Moore W S Ann Surg 1978; 188: 817
464. Barker W F, Cannon J A Am J Surg 1959; 25: 912
465. Starrett R W, Stoney R J Surgery 1974; 76: 890
466. Stoney P J In: Rutherford R B (ed) Vascular Surgery. W B Saunders, Philadelphia 1977

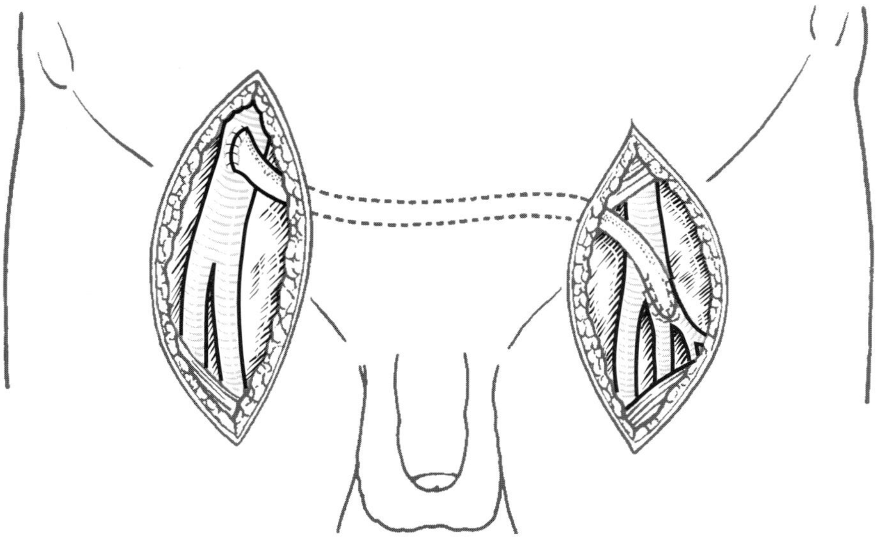

Fig. 10.58 Techniques for dealing with a single iliac artery occlusion: femorofemoral bypass.

renal revascularization cures hypertension although it may prevent renal failure[467,46]

Disease in a single external iliac artery can be treated by endarterectomy, by iliofemoral or aortofemoral bypass, or by femorofemoral cross-over grafts, providing the vessels of the opposite limb are undiseased (Fig. 10.58). There are advantages and disadvantages to each of these procedures.[454,455,469–471] They have largely been eclipsed by the development of angioplasty and stenting (see above).

External iliac endarterectomy may be performed with Volmar strippers from below taking great care to avoid loose distal plaque. Patches of vein or Dacron must be used to close the arteriotomies if there is any risk of narrowing. The vertical incision made over the femoral artery can be extended up over the abdomen as an alternative means of exposing the iliac vessels. This gives excellent access to the whole of the external iliac artery but the inguinal ligament has to be divided and resutured. This increases the risk of a subsequent prevascular hernia. An oblique muscle cutting extraperitoneal approach can be used to bypass this segment with Dacron or polytetrafluoroethylene anastomosed end-to-side above and below the diseased segment, the prosthesis being blindly tunnelled retroperitoneally beneath the inguinal ligament.

In a cross-over femorofemoral graft the external iliac or femoral vessels of the normal side are exposed and a tunnel is made in the subcutaneous fat above the pubis, though some make the tunnel behind the rectus abdominis muscles.[472] A tube of Dacron, polytetrafluoroethylene or, if infection is considered a risk, a reversed saphenous vein is sutured end-to-side to the donor vessels and to the common femoral or profunda femoris artery of the opposite side below the level of the obstruction.

In old or unfit patients an axillobifemoral graft may be used to bypass an occluded aorta.[473–475] A bifurcated Dacron or polytetrafluoroethylene graft is tunnelled subcutaneously and anastomosed end-to-side to the axillary and femoral arteries (Fig. 10.59). The graft may be strengthened by an external support[476,477] to prevent occlusion during flexure. The axillary artery is approached by

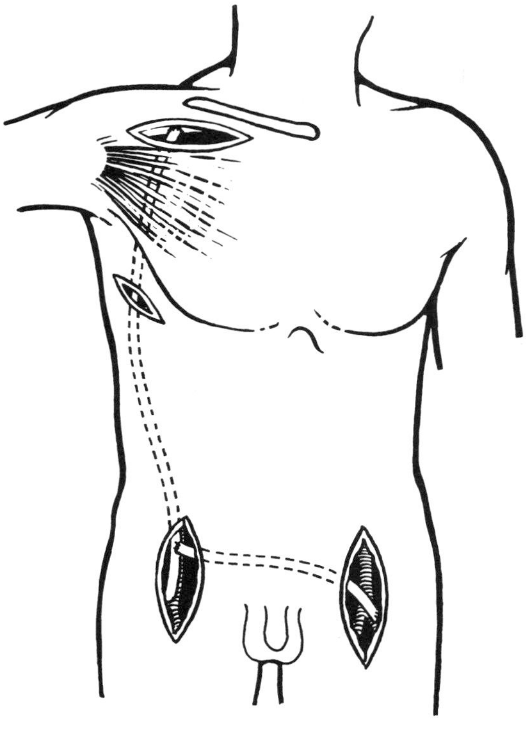

Fig. 10.59 The technique for performing an axillobifemoral graft.

REFERENCES

467. Kaufman J J Trans Am Assoc Genitourin Surg 1973; 65: 12
468. Simon N M, Del Greco F Circulation 1964; 29: 376
469. Laufman H Surg Clin North Am 1960; 40: 153
470. Brief D K, Brener F J et al Arch Surg 1975; 110: 1294
471. Helsby R, Moosa A R Br J Surg 1975; 62: 596
472. Tyson R R, Reichel F A Surgery 1972; 72: 401
473. Louw J H Lancet 1963; ii: 1401
474. Blaisdell F W, Hall A D Surgery 1963; 54: 563
475. Mannick J A, Nabseth D C N Engl J Med 1968; 278: 461
476. Ray L I, O'Connor J B et al Am J Surg 1979; 138: 117
477. Kenny D A, Sauvage L R et al Surgery 1982; 931: 946

splitting the pectoralis major muscle below the clavicle and dividing pectoralis minor. The graft is tunnelled subcutaneously and anastomosed end-to-side to the femoral vessels exposed through two groin incisions.

Results of reconstruction of the aortoiliac segment

Aortoiliac and aortofemoral Dacron grafts have a 90–95% 5-year patency providing there is a good distal arterial tree.[453,455,462,478,479] The patency of endarterectomy is probably not quite as good.[454,461,462] Cross-over bypass grafts have a 5-year patency of approximately 70–80%[470,471,480] and axillofemoral grafts have a lower patency of about 60–70%.[474–476,481] Angioplasty of single iliac stenoses has a 7-year patency of 90%[456] and the results of stenting may improve the results of dilating longer stenoses and occlusions.

Complications

Aortic operations have an operative mortality of 2–5%.[455,462,478,479] Patients die from chest infection, myocardial infarction and pulmonary embolism. Careful preoperative cardiac assessment combined with fastidious intraoperative monitoring to reduce cardiac work to a minimum may further reduce this mortality. Graft infection and aorto graft–enteric fistulae are the major post-operative disasters which usually necessitate graft removal and an extra-anatomical reconstruction, using axillobifemoral grafts[482] or tunnelling a bypass through the obturator foramen. More recently composite vein grafts have been used to replace the aorta.[483] Graft infection and graft–enteric fistulae have a high mortality of around 50%.[484] Other late problems include false aneurysm formation[485,486] and graft thrombosis; these require re-anastomosis, extra-anatomical bypass, graft thrombectomy and procedures to improve the outflow of the graft.[487]

Atherosclerosis of the femoropopliteal, profunda femoris and crural arteries

The most common site of atheromatous plaque is in the superficial femoral artery, as it passes through the adductor canal.[488] Patients complain of intermittent claudication if this vessel is severely stenosed or occluded, providing that the aortoiliac and crural vessels are not also diseased. Rest pain and gangrene are liable to ensue when there are additional occlusions in other arteries. Diffuse atheroma can involve the whole of the superficial femoral artery, and occlusions up to the origin of the profunda femoris are common.[448]

The profunda femoris artery is often relatively disease free, although posterior plaque in the common femoral artery extending into the profunda origin may narrow or occlude its proximal portion. There are however many exceptions to this adage, and on occasion disease may spread for a considerable distance down the profunda femoris artery and even involve its muscular branches. Combined occlusions in the profunda and superficial femoral arteries are more likely to cause rest pain and gangrene.

The infragenicular segment of the popliteal artery is another site that is often spared from significant disease, but there are also many exceptions to this observation, and the entire popliteal artery and trifurcation, including the origins of the crural vessels, are often occluded.[448] This situation is invariably associated with severe claudication, rest pain or gangrene.

It is now recognized that atherosclerosis can cause stenoses and occlusions of all the crural vessels and even involve the dorsalis pedis artery and the plantar vessels of the foot.[448] A widely patent plantar arch may affect the outcome of bypasses to the crural vessels,[489] although this observation is still disputed.[490]

Atheromatous disease in the vessels of the lower limb may lead to embolism and thrombosis which may in turn cause occlusions of the digital vessels. Peripheral arterial revascularization should rarely be attempted if there is extensive gangrene spreading on to the forefoot (Fig. 10.11), especially if the heel cannot be preserved by a conservative amputation. Reconstruction is also rarely justified to allow a major amputation to be performed at a lower level (e.g. below rather than above the knee), although there are occasional exceptions to this rule. The absolute indication for peripheral reconstruction (below the groin) of the arteries of the lower limb is rest pain or early gangrene (critical ischaemia), providing that there is a suitable vessel in the distal part of the limb that is capable of accepting a bypass.

Investigation

Attempts were originally made to define critical limb ischaemia according to the ankle systolic pressure. Further evidence showed that arbitrary blood pressure measurements are of little clinical relevance[491] and no definition of chronic limb ischaemia can predict which diabetics will require amputation.[492] The suitability of a vessel in the distal part of the limb to accept a bypass is usually determined by arteriography, but Doppler mapping, Doppler scanning and intraoperative arteriography have also been used to assess the run-off[493]. The technique of pulse-generated Doppler run-off was first described 10 years ago[494,495] and is probably better at detecting vessels communicating with the pedal arch than arteriography[496] although dependent Doppler has been found to be equally effective.[496] Digital subtraction angiography with multiple

REFERENCES

478. Crawford E S, Bamberger R A Surgery 1981; 90: 1055
479. Taylor G W, Calo A R Br Med J 1962; 1: 507
480. Dick L S, Brief D R et al Arch Surg 1980; 115: 1359
481. Burrell M J, Wheeler J R et al Ann Surg 1982; 195: 6796
482. Trout H H, Kozloff L, Giordano J M Ann Surg 1984; 199: 669
483. Van-Det R J, Brands L C Surgery 1981; 89: 543
484. Perdue G D, Smith R B et al Surgery 1980; 192: 237
485. Szilagy D E, Smith F R, Elliott J P Surgery 1975; 178: 808
486. Benhamou D E, Kieffer E et al J Cardiovasc Surg 1984; 25: 118
487. Bergan J J, Yao J S T Reoperative Arterial Surgery. Grune & Stratton, Orlando 1986
488. Watt J K Br Med J 1965; 2: 1455
489. Dardik H, Ibrahim I M et al Surg Gynecol Obstet 1981; 152: 645
490. Ascer E, Veith F J et al J Vasc Surg 1984; 1: 817
491. Thompson M M, Sayer R D Eur J Vasc Surg 1993; 7: 420
492. Tyrell M R, Wolfe J H N Br J Surg 1993; 80: 177
493. Shearman C P, Gywnn B R et al Br Med J 1986; 293: 1086
494. Beard J D, Lee R E et al J Vasc Surg 1986; 4: 588
495. Beard J D, Scott D J A et al Br J Surg 1988; 75: 361
496. Currie I C, Baird R N, Lamont P M Br J Surg 1994; 81: 1448

exposures provides detailed views of all the vessels below the knee.[497] It is important to assess the amount of disease in the aortoiliac segment because the inflow influences the patency of a distal bypass. Intra-arterial pressure measurements at rest and after administration of papaverine provide functional information about the inflow but are rarely used clinically.[498] Duplex scanning, assessing the peak systolic velocity above and below a stenosis, may be a better method of assessing haemodynamically significant stenoses than simply feeling the femoral pulse.[499]

Management

Conservative measures

Arterial reconstruction is not essential in patients presenting with claudication, and a period of conservative management is almost always indicated before surgery is considered.[500] Patients should always be advised to stop smoking[501] and to try to walk through the pain to encourage the development of collateral vessels.[502] Any polycythaemia or anaemia should be corrected,[503] and coincidental diabetes should be treated. β-blockers should be discontinued as these may cause a diminution of the claudication distance,[504] although other studies[505] refute this. Any cardiac irregularities should be treated or controlled if possible. Vasodilating drugs are of little value and any improvement achieved in the claudication distance is almost always marginal.[506,507] On theoretical grounds it is unlikely that these drugs can improve much on nature, as ischaemic tissue is the most powerful vasodilatory stimulus that is known. Therapeutic haemodilution has proved equally ineffective, and many other drugs, including haemorrheological agents, antiplatelet drugs, fibrinolytic stimulants and anticoagulants, have also been tried without success.[508] Achilles tenotomy, selective crushing of the nerves supplying the calf muscles and raising the heels of shoes have also been abandoned.[509] Exercise programmes have been shown to be as effective as angioplasty in improving the claudication distance.[510,511]

Indications for revascularization and selection of the procedure

Angioplasty and operations for claudication may be considered when symptoms are seriously interfering with the patient's occupation or enjoyment of life, providing that they have been present for six months or more so that there has been time for collaterals to develop and maximum spontaneous improvement to occur.[512] Patients should also have given up smoking and be reasonably fit. These rules may perhaps be relaxed a little where clinical features such as weak distal pulses with mid thigh arterial bruits and reduced post exercise Doppler ankle systolic pressures suggest stenoses suitable for treatment by angioplasty.[513] The long-term outcome remains poor if patients continue to smoke. Colour duplex scanning may also be very helpful in selecting suitable patients for angioplasty,[514] but arteriography is still usually required to get a detailed picture of the distal arterial tree.

Patients with rest pain or digital ischaemia rarely have isolated superficial femoral occlusions. They usually have associated aorto-iliac disease, a diseased profunda femoris artery, crural vessel obstruction or distal occlusions within the pedal vessels.

Lumbar sympathectomy may help patients with mild rest pain, although it is probably most effective in treating symptoms of coldness, numbness and tingling. As it increases skin blood flow, sympathectomy may aid the healing of superficial ulcers, but it is ineffective once there is frank gangrene and it is doubtful if sympathectomy ever saves a limb from amputation. Phenol ablation of the sympathetic chain by percutaneous injection is now the preferred technique.

An associated stenosis of the aortoiliac segment may require angioplasty, stenting, endarterectomy or bypass in combination with a femoropopliteal bypass.[515]

The saphenous vein should be assessed preoperatively with either saphenous phlebography[516,517] or colour duplex scanning[518] which has the advantage that the site of branches can be marked on the skin. Prosthetic material (polytetrafluoroethylene or human umbilical vein) may be used to bypass occlusions in the limb vessels in patients with arterial ischaemia if the saphenous vein is unsuitable or has been previously removed. Prosthetic grafts are more prone to occlude than vein.[519] Improved results have been reported when a cuff of vein is interposed between the distal end of the graft and the recipient arteries.[520–522] The short saphenous vein, the cephalic and basilic veins[523,524] and even the femoral vein have been used as an alternative to prosthetics.[525] Long endarterectomies of the superficial femoral artery are also possible,[454] but are not

REFERENCES

497. Aston N, Lea Thomas M, Burnand K G J Cardiovasc Surg 1991; 32: 360
498. Baker A R, Macpherson D S, Bell P R F Eur J Surg 1987; 1: 273
499. Legemate D A, Teeuwen C, Eikelboom B C Br J Surg 1991; 78: 1003
500. Charlesworth D Br J Hosp Med 1986; 2: 361
501. Juergens J L, Barker N W, Hines E A Circulation 1960; 21: 188
502. Larsen D A, Lassen N A Lancet 1966; ii: 1093
503. Barabas A P Br J Hosp Med 1980; 23: 289
504. Bogaert M G, Clement D L Eur Heart J 1983; 4: 203
505. Radack K, Deck C Arch Intern Med 1991; 151: 1769
506. Boobis L H, Bell P F R Br J Surg 1985; 69(suppl 17): 23
507. Coffman J D N Engl J Med 1979; 300: 713
508. Ruckley C V Br Med J 1986; 292: 970
509. Anonymous Br Med J 1976; 2: 1165
510. Creasy T S, McMillan P J, Fletcher E W L Eur J Vasc Surg 1990; 4: 135
511. Lungren F, Dahllof A et al 1989; 209: 346
512. Quick C R G, Cotton L T Br J Surg 1982; 69(suppl 24): 26
513. Nicholson M L, Byrne R L, Callum K G Eur J Vasc Surg 1993; 7: 59
514. London N J M, Nydahl S In: Greenhalgh R M (ed) Vascular Imaging for Surgeons. W B Saunders, London 1995 p 321
515. Wake P, Mansfield A O Br J Hosp Med 1980; 120: 129
516. Sapala J A, Szilagyi E Surg Gynecol Obstet 1975; 140: 265
517. Senapati A, Burnand K G et al Ann R Coll Surg Engl 1985; 72: 183
518. Davies A H, Magee T R Eur J Vasc Surg 1991; 5: 633
519. Szilagyi D E J Cardiovasc Surg 1982; 23: 183
520. Miller J H, Foreman R K Aust N Z J Surg 1984; 54: 283
521. Taylor R S, McFarland R J, Cox M I Eur J Vasc Surg 1987; 1: 335
522. Tyrell M R, Wolfe J H N Br J Surg 1991; 78: 1016
523. Campbell D R, Hoar C S, Gibbons G W Ann Surg 1979; 190: 740
524. Harris R W, Andros G et al Ann Surg 1984; 200: 785
525. Schulman M L, Badhey M R Arch Surg 1981; 116: 1141

as reliable as a good quality, long saphenous vein of satisfactory diameter (4 mm or greater).

Amputation is the final option for both acute and chronic ischaemic disease of the lower extremities if revascularization procedures are impossible or ineffective. There is now a little evidence that the number of patients coming to amputation is decreasing.[526]

Femoropopliteal vein bypass grafting[527–529]

The popliteal artery is explored first if the distal run-off is questionable, or an on-table arteriogram can be obtained to determine the state of the run-off if external examination of the distal vessels suggests that they are severely diseased; otherwise the long saphenous vein is usually dissected out, either through a long incision placed over the vein or through a series of short incisions. The vein is either reversed or anastomosed in situ.

The tributaries of the long saphenous vein are ligated and divided for an appropriate distance to allow the vein to be used as a reversed bypass graft. Alternatively it can be left in situ if this is the preferred operation, when the tributaries are ligated or clipped in continuity. The common femoral, profunda femoris and superficial femoral artery are dissected free and isolated through the upper end of the incision used to mobilize the vein. The upper end of the reversed vein is normally anastomosed to the common femoral artery and the lower end is anastomosed to the popliteal artery, either above or below the knee depending on the condition of the vessel (Fig. 10.60). The vein can be placed subcutaneously or tunnelled through the adductor muscles to the popliteal fossa. The popliteal artery is either dissected out above the knee, if this segment of artery is patent and relatively free of disease, or alternatively the infrageniculate portion of the vessel, which is often less severely diseased, is dissected free from its accompanying veins. The suprageniculate popliteal artery is approached by mobilizing the sartorius along either its anterior or posterior border. The infrageniculate popliteal artery is found by incising the deep fascia longitudinally just behind the posteromedial border of the tibia. The space between the medial head of the gastrocnemius and the tibia is then opened and retracted. The popliteal artery is found behind the popliteal vein.

A new passage is made, using a special tunnelling instrument if the reversed vein is to be used, passing from the popliteal fossa, through the adductor magnus and the subsartorial canal, up into the femoral triangle. The carefully prepared vein is then positioned in this channel, and end-to-side anastomoses are made to the common femoral artery in the groin and the chosen segment of the popliteal artery behind the knee.

For in situ grafting, which is the method of choice in crural and pedal anastomoses,[529] the long saphenous vein is left in its anatomical position; after the major tributaries have been ligated the upper end is freed, mobilized and detached from the femoral vein, which is oversewn. The cusps of the most proximal saphenous valve are excised through the open end of the vein which is then anastomosed end-to-side to the femoral artery. After the arterial clamps have been released blood is allowed to distend the upper end of the vein as far as the first competent valve. A valvulotome is then

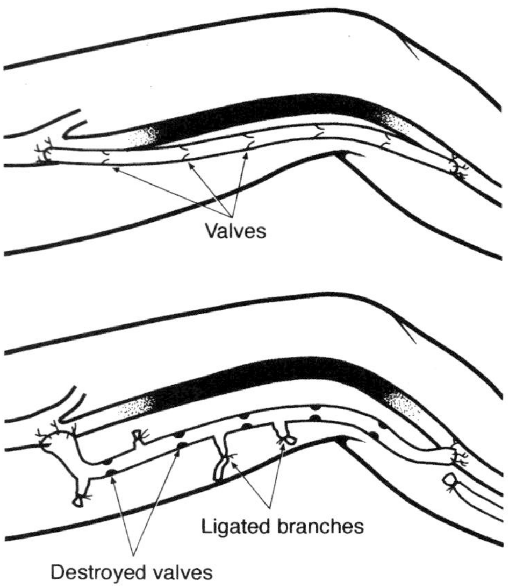

Fig. 10.60 The techniques of femoropopliteal vein bypass grafting: (**a**) reversed; (**b**) in situ.

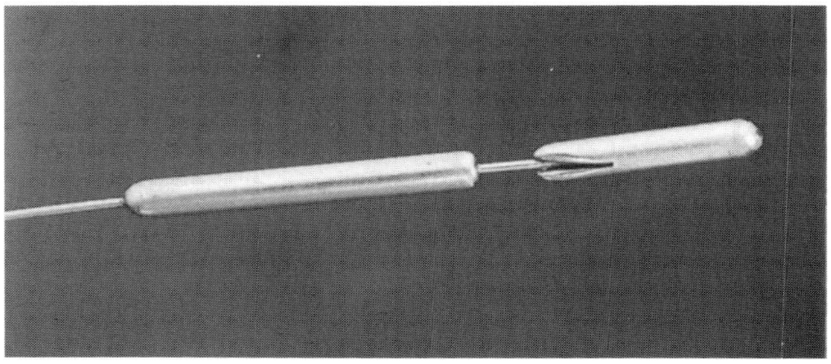

Fig. 10.61 Hallís valvulotome used for excising the saphenous valves during in situ vein bypass grafting.

passed up the vein through its divided lower end to the upper anastomosis and this is then gently withdrawn, engaging the valves one by one before being gently pulled through them. This avulses the cusps and renders each valve incompetent. A number of different valvulotomes have been devised for this operation; the most popular are Hall's strippers (Fig. 10.61), although Cartier's and Leather & Karmody's instruments have their advocates.[529,530]

A good flow of arterial blood should be obtained from the cut end of the divided vein when the valvulotome is delivered from the distal venotomy. The valvulotome should be inserted and pulled down a second time if the flow remains poor. Small diameter valvulotomes may be followed by progressively larger instruments although care must be taken not to damage the intima by inserting oversized valvulotomes. Persistently poor blood flow from the

REFERENCES

526. Department of Health and Social Security and Office of Population Censuses and Surveys Hospital Inpatient Enquiry (1974–1984). HMSO, London
527. Gardham J R C, Marston A Br J Hosp Med 1975; 679
528. Burnand K G, Browse N L In: Greenhalgh R M (ed) Vascular Surgical Techniques. Butterworths, London 1989
529. Leather R P, Powers S R, Karmody A M Surgery 1979; 86: 453
530. Hall K V Surgery 1962; 51: 492

divided distal vessel suggests the presence of a large unligated tributary, and further examination of the vein by on-table angiography or angioscopy may confirm its presence. When a good flow has been achieved the distal anastomosis is performed.

Alternatives

A prosthetic graft can be used if the vein is known to have been stripped out in the past, or is judged to be inadequate on preoperative saphenography[517] or duplex scanning,[518] or is found to be poor or absent at operation. Alternatively a composite graft can be made from arm veins, the short saphenous vein, or a segment of undamaged long saphenous vein.[531] The long saphenous vein from the opposite limb may be used if this is of adequate quality. Prosthetic grafts can be of Dacron which may be externally supported,[477] polytetrafluoroethylene[532,533] or glutaraldehyde tanned human or animal umbilical veins,[534] which have to be externally supported to prevent aneurysm formation. The anastomosis between the prosthetic and lower vessel may be made via a Miller cuff,[520] a Taylor patch[521] or a St Mary's boot[522] (Fig. 10.62).

A long endarterectomy can be performed using a Volmar's ring stripper to core out the atheroma.[454,455,535] An endarterectomy may also be carried out through a long open incision into the artery but a vein graft is then usually required to prevent stenosis during closure. After endarterectomy the luminal surface should be inspected by arteriography or with an angioscope[535,536] to ensure that it is smooth. In future the rough luminal surface may be lined by a smooth prosthesis.

Angioplasty now provides a credible alternative to vein bypass grafting, and the use of the subintimal route and stenting may continue to improve results.[537] Patients considered for femoropopliteal angioplasty should also be considered appropriate for surgical bypass which may be urgently required if complications develop.

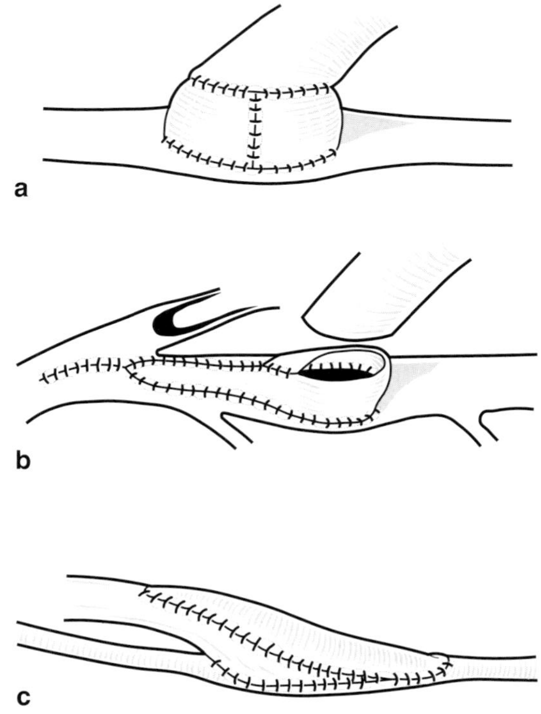

Fig. 10.62 A CT scan showing an aortic aneurysm. a= Miller cuff; b = St Mary's boot; c = Taylor patch.

Femorocrural and pedal grafts

Long saphenous vein, preferably using the in situ technique, is again the material of choice for these bypasses. Prosthetic bypasses to these small vessels are much less satisfactory, but improved results have been reported using vein cuffs,[520] patches[521] or boots[522] via which the PTFE grafts are anastomosed to the distal vessels. The anterior and posterior tibial arteries and the peroneal vessels can all be easily exposed in the lower part of the calf. The posterior tibial artery passes down behind the soleal arch and lies on the muscles on the posterior surface of the tibia almost directly beneath the long saphenous vein. The anterior tibial artery lies deep in the anterior compartment almost on the interosseous membrane and continues down as the dorsalis pedis artery over the front of the ankle between the tendons of the anterior compartment. The peroneal artery lies deep to the fibula and can be easily reached by resecting the middle third of this bone, or with more difficulty by burrowing across the posterior compartment of the calf from the medial side. The technique for femorodistal or crural bypass is otherwise identical to femoropopliteal grafting, although postoperative on-table arteriography is required to ensure a correctly performed anastomosis (Fig. 10.63). Many surgeons use magnifying loops to allow them to place their sutures with greater accuracy because of the small size of the vessels.

When the distal run-off is poor, anastomosis to more than one crural vessel may improve graft patency[531] and some surgeons have made an arteriovenous anastomosis at the distal end to prevent grafts occluding by decreasing the peripheral resistance,[534] although at present there is no evidence that this improves patency.[538]

Angioplasty

Transluminal balloon dilatation of the distal vessels is effective for stenotic lesions but has proved less successful in occlusive disease,[539,540] although some good results have been obtained with low-profile catheters and steerable guidewires.[541] A guidewire is passed through the stenosis or occlusion under radiographic control, and coaxial plastic balloon catheters are distended within the diseased segment to dilate the stenosis. It is not fully understood how the compressed atheroma 'disappears' but it is split by

REFERENCES

531. Edwards W S, Gerety E et al Surgery 1976; 80: 722
532. Campbell C D, Brooks D H et al Surgery 1979; 85: 177
533. Veith F J, Moss C M et al JAMA 1978; 240: 1867
534. Dardik H, Dardik I Ann Surg 1976; 183: 252
535. Volmar J F, Storz L W Surg Clin North Am 1974; 54: 111
536. Itoh T, Hori M Surgery 1983; 93: 391
537. Varty I C, Nydahl P, Butterworth P Br J Surg 1996; 83: 953
538. Harris P L, Campbell H Br J Surg 1983; 70: 377
539. Cumberland D Clin Radiol 1983; 70: 377
540. Gruntzig A Lancet 1978; i: 263
541. Schwarten D E, Cutcliff W B Radiology 1988; 169: 71

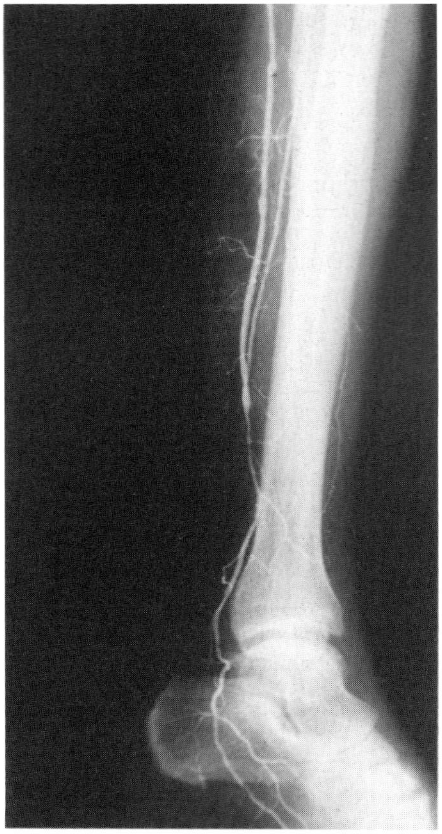

Fig. 10.63 An operative arteriogram showing a femoroposterior tibial vein graft that remained patent 2 years later.

the dilating process into a number of longitudinal fissures. The vessel itself is also dilated. The procedure may be regularly repeated, but it can cause vessel rupture, dissection and thrombosis, especially in inexperienced hands. It is more effective in the aortoiliac segment than in the distal vasculature and is better for treating stenotic than occlusive disease although this tenet is now being challenged[537] by use of the subintimal technique and greater application of stents.

Profundaplasty

Profundaplasty,[542,543] which is widening of the profunda orifice (Fig. 10.65), or extended deep femoral angioplasty[544] are now rarely considered to be effective on their own and are usually combined with an aortic graft or some form of femoropopliteal or distal bypass.

Combination disease (aortoiliac and femorocrural disease)

There is a small group of patients in whom an aortoiliac occlusion exists in association with severe profunda disease and a superficial femoral occlusion, where adequate outflow from an aortic graft can only be achieved by a synchronously performed aortic procedure and femoropopliteal bypass. In a number of patients it is difficult to determine whether apparently mild aortic disease will

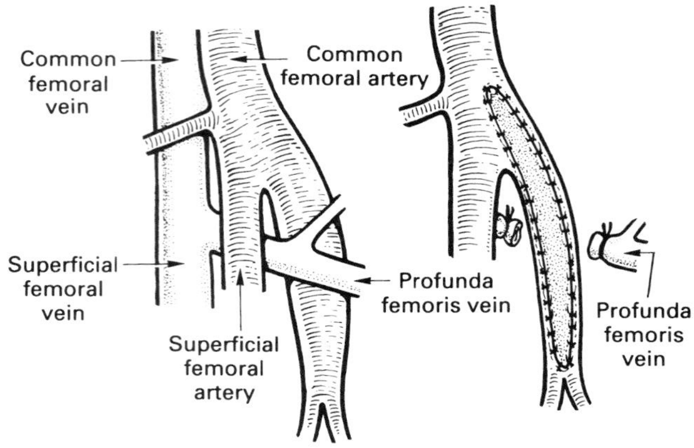

Fig. 10.65 Diagram of profundaplasty or extended deep femoral angioplasty.

reduce the patency of a femorodistal bypass. A proximal bypass should take precedence; angiography can be performed in cases of doubt and may be carried out in theatre at the time of the distal bypass. Many of these patients can now be treated by preoperative or intraoperative iliac angioplasty and stenting combined with a distal vein bypass graft.

Postoperative care

Fibrous strictures develop in 20–30% of vein grafts in the first 12 months after operation.[545,546] For this reason vein graft surveillance programmes have been advocated[547] although conflicting results have questioned their value. Colour duplex scanning is probably the most cost effective technique although intravenous digital subtraction angiography is more reliable.[546] Rather surprisingly, these stenoses are not usually related to vascular clamp sites, tributaries or residual valve cusps.[548] A trial of in situ versus reversed femoropopliteal vein grafts showed no difference in the short term nor in longer term results up to 6 years.[549] The main advantage of the in situ technique is that the smaller lower end of the vein more closely matches the distal artery, and most surgeons choose this technique for anastomoses to the crural vessels.

Results

Femoropopliteal bypass grafts performed for intermittent claudication have a cumulative patency of between 60 and 80% at 5 years and 30–40% at 10 years.[550–552] Prosthetics, endarterectomies and

REFERENCES

542. Hill D A, Jamieson C W Br J Surg 1977; 64: 359
543. Martin P, Bouhoutsos J Br J Surg 1977; 64: 194
544. Berguer R, Cotton L, Sabri S Br Med J 1973; 1: 469
545. Grigg M J, Nicolaides A N, Wolfe J H N Br J Surg 1988; 75: 737
546. Moody A P, de Cossart L M, Harris P L Eur J Vasc Surg 1990; 4: 117
547. Harris P L Br J Surg 1992; 79: 97
548. Moody A P, Edwards P R, Harris P L Eur J Vasc Surg 1992; 6: 509
549. Moody A P, Edwards P R, Harris P L Br J Surg 1992; 79: 750
550. Grimley R P, Obeid M L et al Br J Surg 1979; 66: 723
551. Darling R C, Linton R R, Razzuk M A Surgery 1967; 61: 31
552. DeWeese J A, Robb C G Surgery 1977; 82: 775

angioplasties have not achieved the same patency to date, being between 20 and 30% worse than vein.[550–556] Graft patency is even worse in patients with digital gangrene and critical ischaemia and is significantly reduced in single crural vessel bypasses when compared to popliteal bypasses.[557,558] Graft failure does not always equate with limb loss, which must remain the final arbiter in determining graft success.[559] Regular graft surveillance followed by intervention with angioplasty or further surgery appears to have improved (secondary) graft patency to 80% at 5 years[560] although as stated above this is still debated.

ISCHAEMIA OF THE GASTROINTESTINAL TRACT

The coeliac axis, superior and inferior mesenteric arteries, with branches from the internal iliac artery, supply the whole of the gastrointestinal tract with blood. Because of the many connections between the branches of these arteries, single or even multiple occlusions within the main vessels are often well tolerated, providing they are of gradual onset.[561,562] Only an acute occlusion of the superior mesenteric artery is usually capable of producing small bowel infarction.

Atherosclerotic aortic disease may gradually narrow the orifices of all the visceral vessels, and may on occasion cause an acute thrombosis.[563] Emboli can impact within the visceral arteries and this aetiology accounts for at least 25% of all acute mesenteric occlusions.[563–565] Mesenteric venous thrombosis is another important cause of acute mesenteric ischaemia,[563–565] and low cardiac output can cause bowel ischaemia without there being any occlusions of the mesenteric vessels.[566,567] It has been reported that the coeliac artery can be compressed by the median arcuate ligament of the diaphragm, causing the coeliac axis compression syndrome, although some doubt its existence.[568–570] Chronic mesenteric ischaemia is almost invariably caused by atherosclerotic disease involving the aorta or the trunks of the major visceral vessels, although Buerger's disease, other forms of vasculitis, aortic dissection, fibromuscular hyperplasia and external compression are occasionally responsible.

Clinical features

Acute mesenteric ischaemia is described in Chapter 27. Chronic mesenteric ischaemia usually presents with severe postprandial pain which develops soon after food is taken and lasts for several hours. This pain, which has been called intestinal angina,[571,572] is usually felt in the epigastrium. There is often a genuine fear of food because of the pain that it will produce. Weight loss is usually marked, and if the inferior mesenteric artery is occluded, diarrhoea and rectal bleeding predominate.[573] An abdominal bruit is the only physical sign which may be present: this is heard in 75% of patients with this condition.[574] It is not diagnostic, and other much more common causes of chronic abdominal pain must be excluded by endoscopy, ultrasound and endoscopic retrograde cholangiopancreatography. The differential diagnosis includes peptic ulcer disease, chronic cholecystitis, chronic pancreatitis, irritable bowel syndrome and obscure slow-growing intra-abdominal tumours.

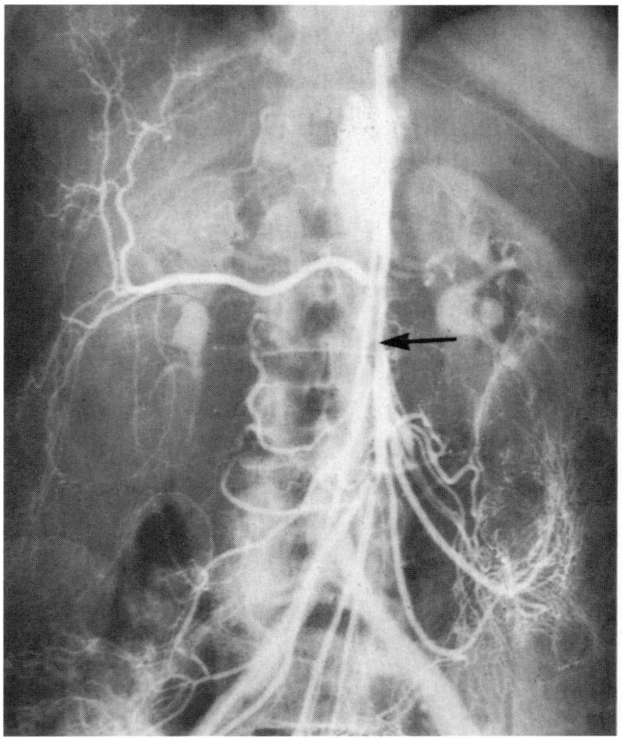

Fig. 10.65 An aortogram showing narrowing of the superior mesenteric artery near its origin and occlusion of the inferior mesenteric artery.

Investigations

Duplex scanning of the visceral arteries can be performed but the investigation of choice at present remains angiography. Lateral aortography may show stenosis or occlusion of one or more of the major vessels[575] (Fig. 10.65). Thumb-printing or pseudopolyposis

REFERENCES

553. Veith F J, Gupta S K et al J Vasc Surg 1986; 3: 104
554. Anderson L I, Nielson O M, Buchardt-Hansen M D Surgery 1985; 97: 294
555. Cannon J A, Barker W F, Kawakami I G Surgery 1958; 43: 76
556. Bergan J J, Veith F J et al Surgery 1982; 92: 921
557. Kacoyanis G P, Whittemore A D et al Arch Surg 1981; 116: 1529
558. Harris P L, Cave-Bingley D J, McSweeney L Br J Surg 1985; 72: 317
559. Dardik H, Kahn M et al Surgery 1982; 91: 64
560. Moody P, Gould D A, Harris P L Eur J Vasc Surg 1990; 4: 1117
561. Horsbourgh A Br J Hosp Med 1980; 113: 118
562. Carrucci J J Am J Surg 1953; 85: 47
563. Jackson B B Occlusion of the Superior Mesenteric Artery. Thomas, Springfield, Illinois 1963
564. Windsor C W O Ann Roy Coll Surg Engl 1977; 59: 50
565. Trotter L B C Embolus and Thrombosis of the Mesenteric Vessels. Cambridge University Press, Cambridge 1913
566. Berger R L, Byrne J J Surg Gynecol Obstet 1961; 112: 529
567. Britt L G, Cheek R C Ann Surg 1969; 169: 704
568. Anonymous Br Med J 1970; 1: 317
569. Drapanas T, Bron K M Ann Surg 1966; 164: 1085
570. Edwards A J, Hamilton J D et al Br Med J 1970; 1: 342
571. Schnitzler F Wien Med Wochenschr 1901; 11: 506
572. Warburg E Munchen Med Wochenschr 1905; 52: 1174
573. Marcuson R W Br J Hosp Med 1974; 203
574. Stoney R J, Wylie E J Ann Surg 1966; 164: 174
575. Dick A P, Graff R et al Gut 1967; 8: 206

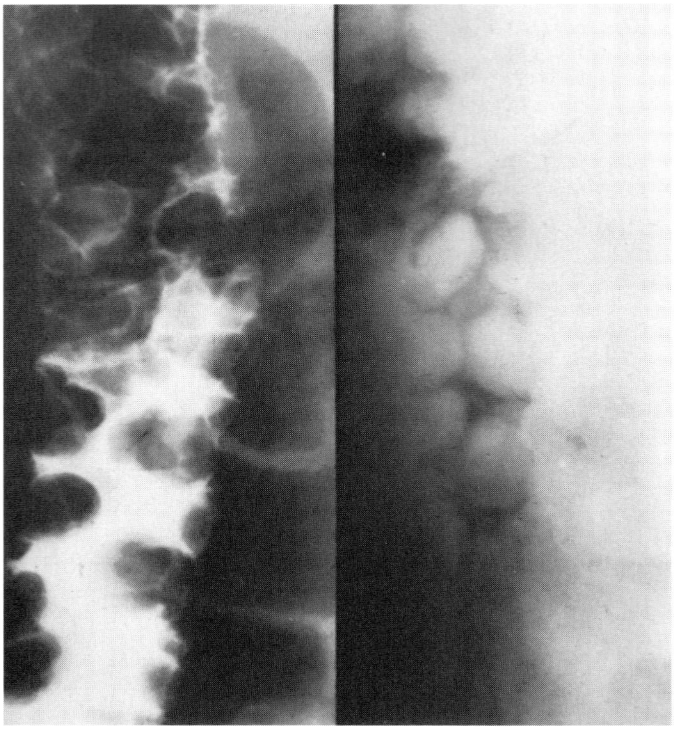

Fig. 10.66 A barium enema examination showing thumb-printing, which is characteristic of ischaemic colitis.

of the colonic mucosa may be seen in patients with ischaemic colitis on barium enema[576,577] (Fig. 10.66). Gastroduodenal biopsy may demonstrate the features of ischaemia on histological examination.[578] Evidence of malabsorption may be provided by a Shilling test,[579,580] a d-xylose test, faecal fat estimation or chromium-labelled albumin. The diagnosis rests on a high index of suspicion combined with appropriate arteriographic findings.

Treatment

If the superior mesenteric artery is narrowed, revascularization can be performed by a vein bypass graft from the aorta,[581,582] endarterectomy[583,584], which is technically difficult, or a side-to-side anastomosis between the ileocolic and right common iliac arteries.[585] Operative treatment carries not inconsiderable risks (10% mortality at least), but can produce good results in selected patients,[582,584] with 90% or more being symptom-free after surgery.

A reduction in blood flow to the colon often preferentially damages the mucosa causing mucosal sloughing.[586] A similar picture may be seen with clostridial infection.[587,588] Patients with full-thickness gangrene of the small or large bowel require resection, but patients at an earlier stage of ischaemic colitis may be best treated at first with intravenous fluids and broad-spectrum antibiotics.[573]

RENOVASCULAR HYPERTENSION

Renal artery stenosis

Renal artery stenosis is a well recognized cause of hypertension, but more recently it has also been demonstrated to be an important cause of renal failure. Hypertension is a condition in which there is permanent elevation of both the systolic and diastolic pressure; if the diastolic pressure is persistently above 95 or 100 mmHg some form of treatment is required. In most patients with hypertension no cause is found and the hypertension is therefore called 'essential'. A number of causes for hypertension are, however, recognized and include Cushing's syndrome, Conn's syndrome, phaeochromocytomas, coarctation of the aorta and renovascular disease. Renovascular hypertension and renal failure is discussed here.

Pathophysiology

Hypertension

Goldblatt et al[589] showed that partial compression of one renal artery by a clamp produced experimental hypertension. This effect persisted when the kidney was transplanted to another site, indicating that it was independent of any nervous mechanism. The experimental hypertension was abolished by the removal of the clamped kidney. This renovascular hypertension was later shown to be caused by release of renin from the juxtaglomerular apparatus into the renal venous blood. The renin converts angiotensinogen, a circulating protein, into the pressor angiotensin I which is itself rapidly converted to the even more potent angiotensin II.[590–592] When this substance is infused into a peripheral vein it produces a substantial rise in both the systolic and diastolic pressure. Between 2 and 7% of all patients with hypertension have a renovascular cause[593,594] although some have suggested that this figure is an overestimate.[595] After the age of 50, identification of renovascular disease is probably unnecessary unless the hypertension is severe and uncontrollable by drugs.[596]

Renal failure

Acute renal failure can be caused by atherosclerotic renovascular disease, and is often precipitated by the use of angiotensin converting enzyme (ACE) inhibitors.[597] In a prospective study

REFERENCES

576. Boley S J, Schwartz S et al Surg Gynecol Obstet 1963; 116: 53
577. Lea Thomas M Clin Gastroenterol 1972; 1: 581
578. Watt J K Br Med J 1968; 3: 231
579. Fry W J, Kraft R O Surg Gynecol Obstet 1963; 117: 417
580. Webb W R, Hardy J D Ann Intern Med 1962; 57: 289
581. Mikkelsen W P Am J Surg 1957; 94: 262
582. Bergan J J Surg Clin North Am 1967; 47: 109
583. Shaw R S, Maynard E P N Engl J Med 1958; 258: 874
584. Stoney R J, Ehrenfeld W K, Wylie E J Ann Surg 1977; 186: 468
585. Mavor G E, Lyall A D et al Br J Surg 1962; 50: 219
586. Marston A, Pheils M T et al Gut 1966; 7: 1
587. Killingback M J, Lloyd-Williams K Br J Surg 1961; 49: 175
588. Tate G T, Thompson H, Willis A T Br J Surg 1965; 52: 194
589. Goldblatt H, Lynch et al J Exp Med 1934; 59: 347
590. Page I H, Helmer O H J Exp Med 1940; 71: 29
591. Braun-Menedez E, Fasciolo J C et al Rev Soc Argent Biol 1939; 15: 420
592. Lentz K E, Skeggs L T et al J Exp Med 1956; 103: 183
593. Sutton D Postgrad Med J 1966; 42: 183
594. Dean R H, Kieffer R W et al Arch Surg 1981; 116: 1408
595. Tucher R M, Labarthe D R Mayo Clin Proc 1977; 52: 549
596. Shapiro A P, Perez-Stable F et al Am J Med 1969; 47: 175
597. Kalra P S et al Quart J Med 1990; 282: 1013

performed on patients taken on to a dialysis programme, angiography performed when there was evidence of atherosclerotic disease elsewhere showed that in 14% the renal failure was the result of atherosclerotic renal vascular disease.[598] A recent prospective study has shown that 5% of patients presenting with a greater than 60% stenosis of the renal artery progressed to arterial occlusion within 1 year and 11% at 2 years.[599] This study also showed that progression from less than 60% stenosis to greater than 60% stenosis or occlusion occurred in 23% at 1 year, and in 42% at 2 years. Another prospective duplex study has shown that 19% of patients with greater than 60% stenosis of the renal artery lose 1 cm or more in length of the kidney in the next 12 months. No change in renal dimensions was found if the stenosis was less than 60%.[600]

Aetiology

Hypertension

Atherosclerotic disease accounts for approximately two thirds of all cases of renovascular hypertension, and fibromuscular hyperplasia accounts for most of the rest.[601–603] Polycystic kidneys, pyelonephritis and hydronephrosis are other conditions that can cause renal hypertension, and vascular malformation, aortic dissections, various forms of arteritis and emboli are rare causes of renovascular hypertension.[604]

Renal failure

Acute occlusion of the renal artery can lead to death of the kidney. The pathological events occurring in gradual occlusion are more complex and are still not fully understood. A severe stenosis of 80–85% will cause a reduction in flow below the critical perfusion pressure.[605] Eventually there is loss of renal parenchyma resulting in a decrease in renal length and the onset of renal failure.

Diagnosis and investigation

The diagnosis of renovascular hypertension must be suspected in young males if there is a relatively sudden onset of symptoms (headaches, giddiness, epistaxis, visual disturbances or dyspnoea), especially if there is evidence of an abdominal bruit, or casts of red and white cells are found within the urine.[604,606] A family history of arterial disease, an early age at onset and drug resistance are other pointers to a possible renal cause. Patients presenting with chronic renal failure who have atheromatous disease elsewhere should be suspected of having a renal artery stenosis. Some patients with renal artery stenosis present with pulmonary oedema which is completely reversible by revascularizing the kidney.[607]

An ultrasound scan may reveal loss of renal length and thinning of the renal cortex in patients with renal failure. Duplex ultrasound scanning can be used to detect renal artery stenosis although the renal artery can be difficult to visualize.[608] An intravenous pyelogram may confirm renal disease.

The nephrogram is delayed and the contrast appears to be more concentrated in a smaller kidney if it is ischaemic.[609] The serum creatinine is often raised and the creatinine clearance is reduced.[610] Isotope renography shows an ischaemic pattern with delayed

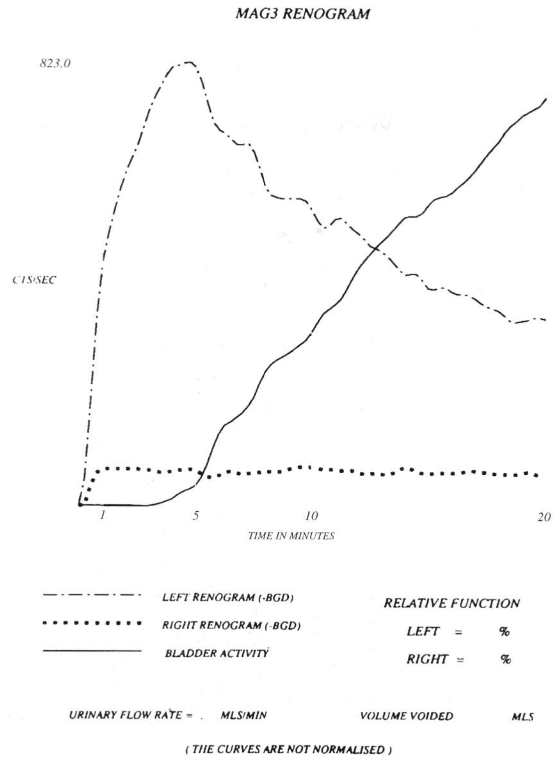

Fig. 10.67 An isotope renogram showing delayed uptake and secretion characteristic of ischaemia.

uptake and secretion (Fig. 10.67).[611] Isotope renography before and after the administration of captopril is a sensitive technique for displaying renal artery stenosis, which is unmasked by the captopril. Selective ureteric catheterization should confirm a low sodium excretion on the side of the stenosis,[612] and selective venous catheterization should demonstrate elevation of renin in the appropriate renal vein.[613–616] A renal vein renin ratio of 1.5 is highly suggestive of the diagnosis,[617] but before this is measured all antihypertensive treatment must be stopped. False positive and

REFERENCES

598. Scoble J E et al Clin Nephrol 1989; 31: 119
599. Zierler R E et al J Vasc Surg 1994; 19: 250
600. Guzman R P et al Hypertension 1994; 23: 346
601. McCormack L J, Poutasse E F et al Am Heart J 1966; 72: 188
602. McCormack L J Med Clin North Am 1961; 45: 247
603. Harrison E G, McCormack L J Proc Mayo Clin 1971; 46: 161
604. Page I H, McCubbin J W Renal Hypertension. Year Book, Chicago 1968
605. May A G et al Surgery 1963; 53: 513
606. Foster J H, Oates J A et al Surgery 1966; 60: 240
607. Messina L M et al J Vasc Surg 1992; 15: 73
608. Hoffman U et al Kidney Int 1991; 39: 1232
609. Maxwell M H, Gonick H C et al N Engl J Med 1964; 270: 213
610. Howard J E, Connor T B Am J Surg 1964; 107: 58
611. Winter C C J Urol 1957; 78: 107
612. Stamey T A Postgrad Med J 1961; 40: 347
613. Judson W E, Helmer O Hypertension 1965; 13: 79
614. Amsterdam E A, Couch N P et al Am J Med 1969; 47: 860
615. Cohen E L, Rovner D R, Conn J W JAMA 1966; 197: 973
616. Kaufman J J, Lupu A N et al J Urol 1970; 103: 702
617. Dean R H, Foster J H Surgery 1973; 74: 926

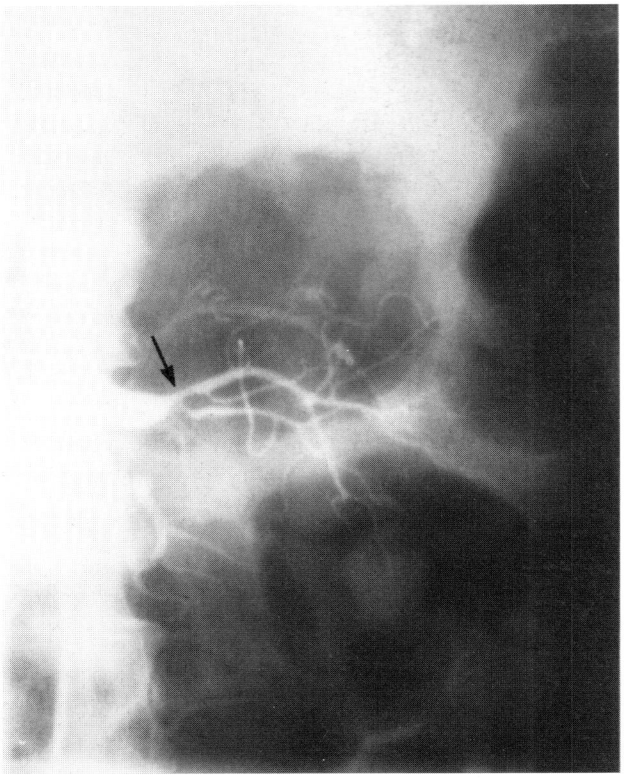

Fig. 10.68 A selective arteriogram showing a stenosis near the origin of the renal artery.

negative results do occur, but this investigation is the most sensitive diagnostic test and should be repeated if necessary. Arteriography by digital subtraction or by selective catheterization[618,619] confirms the renal artery stenosis (Fig. 10.68).

Management

Many patients who are elderly and have well preserved renal function are best treated by antihypertensive medication.[620] Surgery is contraindicated in elderly patients with extensive bilateral disease who have serious concomitant pathology.[621] In the young or middle-aged, an attempt should be made to treat a symptomatic vascular stenosis. Percutaneous transluminal angioplasty is a simple manoeuvre which is particularly effective in treating isolated short stenoses in the main trunk of the renal artery, especially in patients with fibromuscular hyperplasia.[622,623] An endovascular stent can be inserted if this technique fails or if the stenosis is mainly at the ostium of the renal artery. Although early results have been encouraging, long-term follow-up studies are necessary to compare stenting with the proven benefit of surgery.[624]

Aortorenal vein bypass is probably the treatment of choice (Fig. 10.57b). Saphenous vein, hypogastric artery and synthetic material have all been used for this purpose.[625–627] A bypass from the splenic or hepatic arteries is a useful alternative when the aorta is severely diseased but does not require replacement. The San Francisco surgeons[628] have championed extensive aortorenal endarterectomy in patients with severe aortorenal atheroma and this approach is very useful if there is extensive coexistent aortic

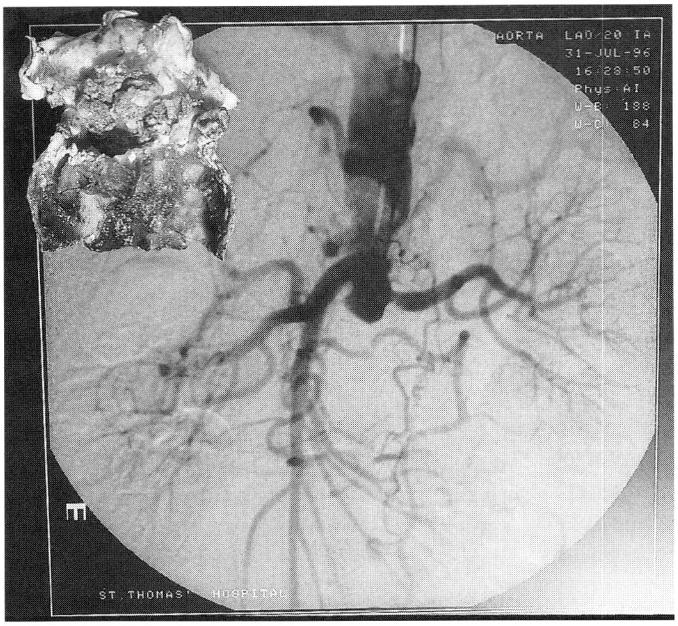

Fig. 10.70 Angiogram showing suprarenal plaque. The excised plaque is shown top left.

disease above the renal arteries extending into the superior mesenteric or coeliac arteries (Fig. 10.69).

The kidney should be cooled and removed if the stenosis extends into its hilum, particularly in patients with fibromuscular hyperplasia.[629,630] Careful surgical repair can then be performed on the bench using vein grafts to widen the renal branches before the kidney is reimplanted, usually onto the internal iliac artery and common iliac vein. The ureter is then reimplanted into the bladder.

Nephrectomy is indicated if the kidney function is poor and there is little remaining cortex, providing that the function of the other kidney is normal. It is also indicated if reconstruction is considered impossible or dangerous.[631,632]

Results

Transluminal angioplasty has an early success of about 90% in patients with fibromuscular hyperplasia but it is usually poorly

REFERENCES

618. Sutton D, Brunton F J, Starer R Clin Radiol 1962; 78: 879
619. Gomes A S, Pais S O, Barbaric Z L Am J Radiol 1983; 140: 779
620. Whelton A K, Harris A P et al Johns Hopkins Med J 1981; 149: 213
621. Hallet J W, Fowl R, O'Brien P C J Vasc Surg 1987; 5: 622
622. Gruntzig A, Vetter W et al Lancet 1978; i: 801
623. Tegtmeyer C J, Kofler T J, Ayers C A AJR 1984; 142: 17
624. Raynaud A C et al J Vasc Intervent Radiol 1994; 5: 849
625. Morris G C, Debakey M E et al Surg Gynecol Obstet 1966; 122: 1255
626. Kaufman J J, Maloney P J J Urol 1967; 98: 140
627. Dean R H, Krueger T C et al J Vasc Surg 1984; 1: 234
628. Wylie E J, Perloff D L, Stoney R L Ann Surg 1969; 170: 416
629. Ota K, Mori S et al Arch Surg 1967; 94: 370
630. Belzer F O, Salvatierra O Ann Surg 1975; 182: 456
631. Smith H W Am Med 1948; 4: 724
632. Brown J J, Owen K et al Br Med J 1960; 2: 327

maintained with nearly half the patients requiring a further dilatation within 2 or 3 years.[623,633] This treatment is less successful in atherosclerotic disease. Surgical bypass is also effective in lowering the blood pressure to normal in 90% of patients with fibromuscular hyperplasia but is less effective in atherosclerotic disease, producing an improvement in blood pressure control in about 50–60% without preserving renal function.[627,634]

DIABETIC ISCHAEMIA

Diabetes is a common disease which affects approximately 5% of the population. The Framingham study showed that diabetic patients were three to four times more likely to have intermittent claudication than those without diabetes.[635,636] This was true of both insulin dependent diabetes and maturity onset diabetes, and was also related to smoking. The natural history of peripheral vascular disease is worse in diabetic patients, with an increase in both mortality and limb loss.[637] This may be related to abnormalities in serum lipids and lipoproteins,[638] to an increase in platelet aggregation[639] and to a prothrombotic tendency.[640]

Diabetes can affect the foot because of three interrelated factors: neuropathy, infection and ischaemia. The neuropathy can affect both somatic and autonomic nerves.[641] Absence of pain allows mechanical damage to the foot from tight shoes, penetrating injuries and nail cutting to pass unnoticed. Loss of temperature sensation can result in similar thermal injuries from bathing in hot water and keeping the feet too close to a hot water bottle, fire or radiator. Damage to motor fibres causes wasting and weakness of the intrinsic muscles of the feet resulting in a cavus deformity, claw toes, abnormal weight distribution and callus formation.[642] Degeneration of the sudomotor axons results in loss of sweating causing dry skin, cracks, fissures and ulceration. Neuropathic ulceration results from the alteration of weight distribution which produces callosities and subkeratotic haematomas. This causes tissue necrosis below the callus which may ulcerate and encourage infection. Neuropathic ulcers are painless, surrounded by callus, usually circular and punched out. They may be very deep, extending to the bone. They usually develop beneath the metatarsal heads and the tips of the toes, but may also occur over the dorsal interphalangeal joints of clawed toes and over both malleoli where they rub against footwear. Pedal pulses are usually easily palpable.

Infection in diabetic patients occurs because of an impaired immune response. The polymorph leucocyte has a reduced activity, particularly against *Staph. aureus* and *E. coli*.[643] Wound healing is also impaired[644] which makes minor injuries slow to heal. Non-clostridial gas-forming organisms quite commonly invade diabetic feet and produce gas in the tissues. Crepitus is present and a characteristic putrifying stench is apparent. Plain radiographs show the free gas in the tissues.

Ischaemia is the result of both large and small vessel disease, although the importance of the latter may have been overemphasized. Large vessel atherosclerosis presents at an earlier age and is more severe in diabetic patients compared with non-diabetic controls.[645] The proximal vessels are usually spared, with the majority of the disease affecting the arteries below the knee.[646] Occlusions are more likely to occur at multiple levels and to be bilateral.[647]

The blood flow through diabetic feet is often greater than in equivalent atherosclerotic patients without diabetes;[648] this may be the result of arteriovenous shunting. The basement membrane of the capillaries is thickened[649] and more permeable although the significance of this is disputed. Crural arterial occlusion is the most important cause of digital and pedal gangrene, although secondary infection is quite common. The ulceration associated with ischaemia has no surrounding callus, and frequently affects the first and fifth metatarsal heads and the toes. There is usually a preceding history of intermittent claudication and rest pain.

A full blood count, blood glucose, and blood glycosylated haemoglobin should be obtained. Swabs should be taken from the ulcers for bacterial culture and sensitivity to antibiotics. Plain radiograph of the foot may confirm osteomyelitis or septic arthritis although evidence of bone destruction is often late. Calcification of the digital vessels and the presence of gas in the tissues may also be shown. Doppler pressures are usually misleading as calcification in the walls of the crural arteries prevents their compression by the sphygmomanometer cuff. Duplex examination may identify arterial occlusions and stenoses but may also be hampered by calcification in the vessels. Intra-arterial digital subtraction angiography should be performed whenever ischaemia is suspected.

The diabetic foot is best managed by a special team consisting of a diabetic physician, a vascular surgeon, an orthopaedic surgeon, a diabetic nurse, a chiropodist, a physiotherapist, an orthotist and a limb fitter. All diabetics, especially those with claudication or neuropathy, should be encouraged to inspect their feet every night: a mirror is useful to see the sole of the foot. Progression of early skin damage may be avoided by bed rest and antibiotics.

Established neuropathic ulceration is treated by removing the callus, eradicating infection and reducing weight bearing forces. All patients should be prescribed broad-spectrum antibiotics until healing is complete. Infections are usually caused by a number of different bacterial species including Gram-positive, Gram-negative, enteric and anaerobic organisms. The most common are staphylococci, enterococci, enterobacteria and anaerobes such as

REFERENCES

633. Ramsay L E, Waller P C Br Med J 1990; 300: 569
634. Bergentz S-E, Berqvist D, Weibull H Br J Surg 1989; 76: 429
635. Garcia et al Diabetes 1980; 29: 105
636. Kannel W B, McGee D L Circulation 1979; 59: 8
637. Shadt D C et al JAMA 1961; 175: 937
638. Stout R W Lancet 1987; i: 1077
639. Mustard J F, Packham M A New Engl Med J 1984; 311: 665
640. Fuller J H et al Br Med J 1979; 2: 964
641. Watkins P J Br Med J 1982; 285: 493
642. Delbridge L et al Br J Surg 1985; 72: 1
643. Rayfield E J et al Am J Med 1982; 72: 439
644. Goodson W H, Hunt T K Surg Gyn Obstet 1979; 149: 600
645. Kannel W B, McGee K L cited above; Beach K W, Strandness D E Diabetes 1980; 29: 882
646. Bendick et al Progression of atherosclerosis in diabetics surgery 1983; 93: 834
647. Royster T S et al Surg Gyn Obstet 1976; 143: 949
648. Rayman G et al Br Med J 1986; 292: 87
649. Vracko R, Strandness D E Circulation 1967; 35: 690

Peptostreptococcus and *Bacteroides*.[650] The patient should be admitted to hospital for bed rest and limb elevation if cellulitis is present. Blood cultures should be performed before intravenous antibiotic therapy is begun. An insulin infusion and sliding scale may be required to control the blood glucose. Any associated cardiac failure should be treated. When healing has been achieved, patients should be advised on footwear, chiropody, smoking, obesity and diabetic control. Surgical debridement of dead tissue and infected bone should be performed and all pockets of pus should be drained.

Distal atherosclerotic arterial disease should be treated by angioplasty or bypass surgery. The distal nature of the disease in diabetic patients means that the superficial femoral and the popliteal arteries can be used as the donor vessel.[651] Bypasses are usually made to the crural arteries near the ankle. Sympathectomy is usually ineffective in diabetic patients who are already auto-sympathectomized,[652] and the results of prostaglandin infusion are also poor. Trophic ulcers of the sole of the foot may heal if the limb is enclosed in a below-knee plaster with a rocker.[653] Recurrence may be prevented by excising the metatarsal heads.[654]

In every ischaemic diabetic foot it is important to determine the extent of the ischaemia, neuropathy and infection before deciding on the best method of treatment. A gangrenous digit in a warm foot with impaired proprioception and deep pain but normal foot pulses can be treated by digital, transmetatarsal or ray amputation with a reasonable chance of success.[654–657] A cold foot with absent pulses must be investigated by arteriography with a view to simultaneous reconstruction and amputation if possible.[658]

ARTERIAL DILATATION

Generalized dilatation of the whole arterial tree is known as arteriomegaly. A vessel which has increased in size to less than twice its normal diameter is said to be 'ectatic'. An arterial aneurysm is defined as a localized or segmental pathological dilatation to more than twice the diameter of the normal vessel.

Arteriomegaly is an ill understood condition in which many vessels become dilated. Patients with this condition are liable to develop multiple aneurysms.[659,660] It was recently suggested that multiple aneurysms and arteriomegaly, which are endemic in certain strains of mice, are associated with copper deficiency,[661,662] but this has not been confirmed and further studies are required to define the aetiology of this condition. Proteolytic degeneration and remodeling are now thought to be important in the aetiology, and the role of atheroma as a causative agent is disputed.

ANEURYSMS

Aneurysms are classified into true and false, depending on the involvement of the arterial wall in the aneurysmal process. In true aneurysms the dilatation involves all layers of the arterial wall; in false aneurysms the wall of the vessel has been breached and the aneurysmal sac is made up of surrounding structures that have been compressed by the escaping blood. A false aneurysm usually starts as a pulsating haematoma. The blood that escapes from a partially divided artery normally thromboses, but eventually the pulsation beating through the defect in the wall may excavate a cavity in the haematoma. The surrounding tissues are eroded by the continuing pulsation as the aneurysm expands.

Sometimes a nearby artery and vein are damaged by the same injury with both vessels opening into the one haematoma cavity. The same process of haematoma cavitation can then occur with the aneurysmal sac communicating with both the artery and vein to give an arteriovenous aneurysm. This type of aneurysm is also found as a developmental abnormality. If the arterial flow is directly diverted into the vein, this distends and becomes an aneurysmal varix.

True aneurysms are subdivided into fusiform (spindle-shaped enlargement of the whole luminal circumference) or saccular (when only a small segment of arterial wall balloons outwards as a rounded bulbous mass).

Atherosclerosis is said to be the most common cause of true aneurysms, but the reason for dilatation developing in some individuals while stenosing disease occurs in the majority remains obscure. It has been suggested that the lipoprotein profile may differ[663] or that the amounts of elastin in the wall may influence development.[664,665] A genetic or familial predisposition has also been established.[666] Syphilis is an unusual cause of aneurysms today, but used to produce mainly saccular aneurysms occurring in any vessel. Marfan's and Ehlers–Danlos syndromes and pseudoxanthoma elasticum are rare collagen diseases associated with the development of saccular or dissecting aneurysms. Congenital aneurysms found on the circle of Willis are called 'berry' aneurysms; it is not known how or why they develop. Aortic dissections should not be classified as aneurysms (see Chapter 23).

Mycotic aneurysms develop when a vegetative endocarditis or an infected embolus lodges in the systemic circulation. This usually occurs at a bifurcation, allowing the contained organisms to proliferate and weaken the arterial wall.

Clinical features

Arteriomegaly is usually symptomless until aneurysmal dilatation occurs at specific sites. Aneurysms often cause no symptoms but

REFERENCES

650. Wheat L J et al Arch Intern Med 1987; 4: 475
651. Veith F J et al Surgery 1981; 90: 980
652. DaValle M J et al Surg Gyn Obstet 1981; 152: 784
653. Pollard J P, Le Quesne L P Br Med J 1983; 286: 436
654. Singer A Arch Surg 1976; 111: 964
655. Turnbull A R, Chester J F Ann R Coll Surg Engl 1988; 50: 329
656. McKittrick L S, McKittrick J B, Risley T S Ann Surg 1949; 130: 826
657. Sizer J S, Wheelock F C Surgery 1972; 72: 980
658. Wheelock F C N Engl J Med 1961; 264: 316
659. Leriche R Presse Med 1943; 51: 554
660. Lea Thomas M Br J Surg 1971; 58: 690
661. Andrews E J, White W J, Bullock L P Am J Pathol 1975; 78: 199
662. Tilson M D Arch Surg 1982; 117: 1212
663. De Palma R G In: Bergan J J, Yao J S T (eds) Aneurysms, Diagnosis and Treatment. Grune & Stratton, New York 1982
664. Busuttil R W, Cardenas A In: Bergan J J, Yao J S T (eds) Aneurysms, Diagnosis and Treatment. Grune & Stratton, New York 1982
665. Powell J T, Campa J et al Br J Surg 1985; 72: 401
666. Clifton M A Br J Surg 1977; 64: 765

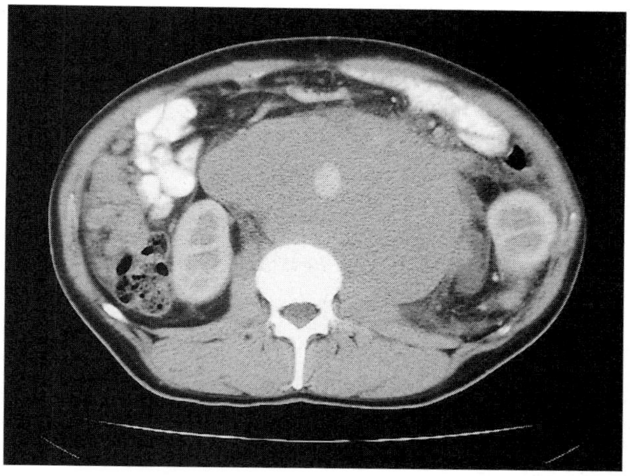

Fig. 10.70 Aorta surrounded by a mass of lymphematous lymph nodes.

the abnormally large pulsation may occasionally be noticed by the patient or found by a doctor during routine examination. Aneurysms may compress and erode surrounding structures (including nerves, intestine and bone), and they may rupture causing haemorrhage into serous cavities, hollow viscera or on to the skin surface. Intraluminal thrombus may embolize distally, and rarely the whole aneurysm may thrombose. The expansile pulse of an aneurysmal artery must be differentiated from the transmitted pulse of a mass overlying a vessel. An expansile pulse expands in two planes, while a transmitted pulse is only felt in one. Occasionally a highly vascular tumour may prove difficult to differentiate from an aneurysm. Also, a mass of retroperitoneal nodes plastered around the aorta may feel like an aneurysm (Fig. 10.70). Aneurysms are most frequently found in the abdominal aorta, the iliac vessels and the femoral and popliteal arteries.

Management

Modern techniques have rendered obsolete the proximal ligation of Hunter (above a popliteal aneurysm),[667] the distal ligation of Bradsor[668] (for an innominate aneurysm) and a combination of proximal and distal ligation without reconstruction. Endoaneurysmorrhaphy,[669] which consists of closure of a saccular aneurysm from within the neck, is also now rarely practised, and wrapping[670–672] and intra-aneurysmal wiring[673] have all given way to the technique of resection and reconstruction. There is at present considerable interest in the use of endovascular stented grafts for lining and treating aneurysms. The long-term results of endovascular repair are not yet available and controlled trials of this new treatment against standard operation are required before they are widely accepted.[674]

Aneurysms of individual vessels

Thoracic aorta

Thoracic aneurysms are much less common than abdominal aortic aneurysms.[675] A true aneurysm of the thoracic aorta needs to be differentiated from an unfolded aorta, an aortic dissection and, occasionally, a mediastinal tumour, especially if it presents a shadow on a chest radiograph (Fig. 10.71). CT scanning, magnetic resonance imaging and trans-oesophageal ultrasound may establish that a true dilatation of aorta is present and exclude the double lumen seen in a dissecting aneurysm[676,677] (see Chapter 23). Thoracic aneurysms may also present with back pain from bone erosion, dysphagia and stridor as the result of compression of the oesophagus and trachea respectively. They may also occasionally rupture, causing severe shortness of breath and shock.[678,679]

Symptomless thoracic aneurysms in elderly patients are probably better left alone, but a large expanding or symptomatic aneurysm in a young fit patient should be resected if possible.[680] The risk of producing a paraplegia by interrupting the blood supply of the spinal cord, which is provided by the arteries of Adamkiewicz, may be reduced by reimplanting these vessels if they have been accurately located preoperatively.[681] Patients with ruptured thoracic aneurysms rarely reach the operating room.

In an elective case the upper and lower limits of the aneurysm are controlled and a Dacron prosthesis is inserted end-to-end with the normal artery above and below the dilatation. Major side branches are reimplanted.[682,683] If a thoracic aneurysm extends into the abdomen the inlay technique described by Crawford[675] (Fig. 10.72) has replaced the side branch relantation technique described by De Bakey[684] (Fig. 10.73). Endovascular stent grafts have been used with some success in treating localized thoracic aneurysms.[685]

Thoracoabdominal aneurysms

There are four types of thoracoabdominal aneurysm: these are shown in Figure 10.74. Type II is the most extensive and treatment has the highest risk in this category. Thoracoabdominal aneurysms should only be operated upon if the patient is fit and there is evidence of continued expansion. The Crawford technique of

REFERENCES

667. Hunter J A Treatise on the Blood, Inflammation and Gunshot Wounds. In: Palmer J F (ed) The Works of John Hunter. Longman, London 1837 p 601
668. Deschamps F In: Observations on Aneurysm. Sydenham Society, London 1844
669. Matas R Ann Surg 1903; 37: 161
670. Benson E A Ann R Coll Surg Engl 1977; 59: 65
671. Robicsek F, Daugherty H K et al J Cardiovasc Surg 1976; 17: 195
672. Bos J C, Biemanis R G M J Cardiovasc Surg 1988; 29: 522
673. Power D A, Colt G H Lancet 1903; ii: 808
674. Yusuf S W, Hopkinson B R In: Greenhalgh R M, Fowkes F G R (eds) Trials and Tribulations of Vascular Surgery. W B Saunders, 1996 pp 193-202
675. Crawford E S Ann Surg 1974; 179: 763
676. Bresnihan E R, Keates P G Clin Radiol 1980; 31: 105
677. Moncado R, Salinas M et al Lancet 1981; i: 238
678. Bickerstaff L K, Hollier L et al Surgery 1982; 92: 1103
679. McNamara J J, Aessler V M Ann Thorac Surg 1978; 26: 468
680. Connolly J E JAMA 1962; 179: 615
681. Connolly J E, Zuber W F et al Ann Surg 1970; 172: 909
682. De Bakey M E, Crawford E S et al Ann Surg 1965; 162: 650
683. Ergin M A, Griepp R B World J Surg 1980; 4: 535
684. De Bakey M A, Cooley D A et al J Thorac Surg 1958; 36: 393
685. Semba C P, Dake M D In: Chuter T A M, Donayre C E, White R A (eds) Endovascular prostheses. Little Brown, Boston 1995

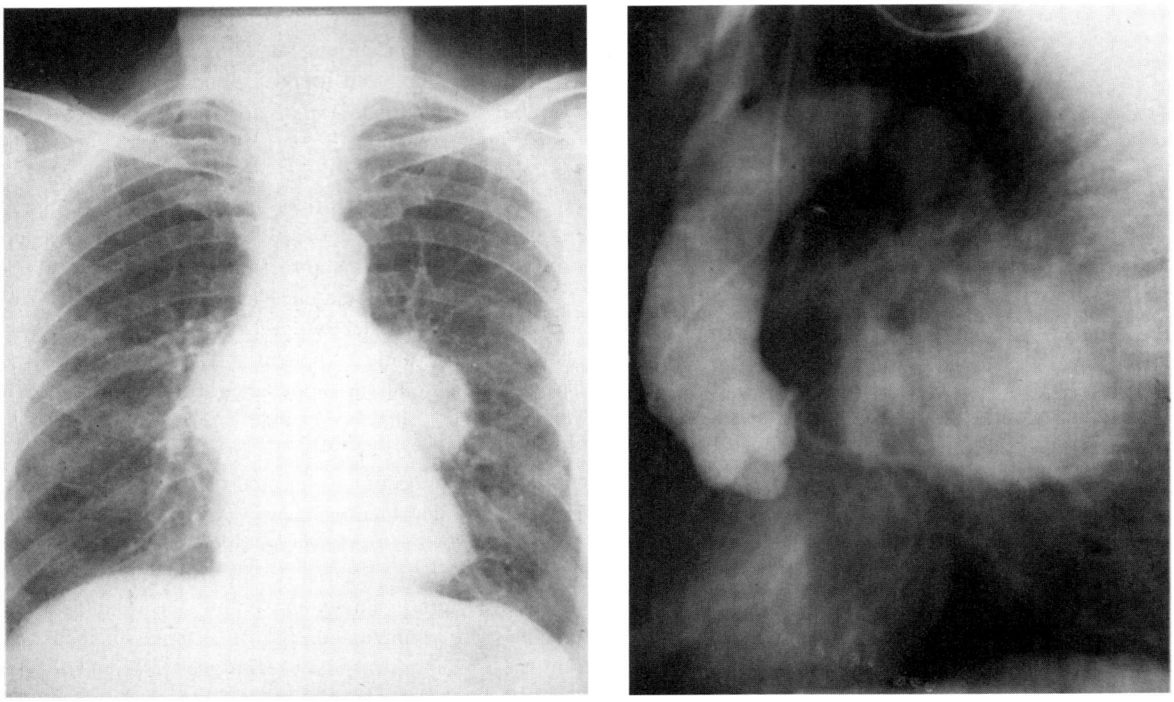

Fig. 10.71 (**a**) A chest radiograph showing a soft tissue mass that was subsequently shown (**b**) to be a thoracic aneurysm on arteriography.

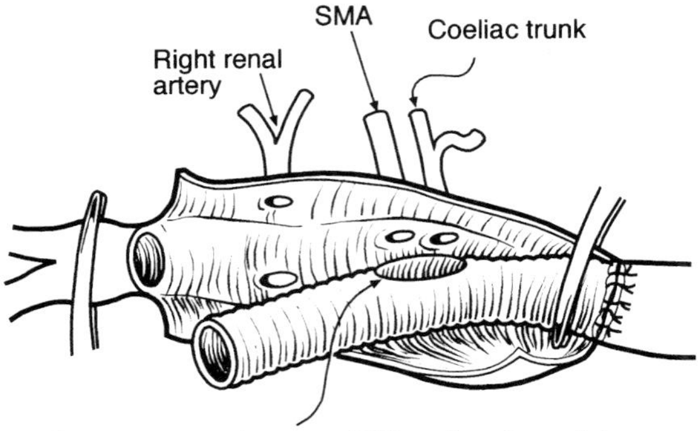

Fig. 10.72 The Crawford technique for repairing thoracoabdominal aneurysms.

'clamp and go' has mostly been replaced by the more controlled conditions provided by aortofemoral bypass. The inlay technique of Crawford is, however, still favoured. The risk of paraplegia remains high. Some surgeons use continuous drainage of cerebrospinal fluid in order to increase the perfusion pressure during aortic cross-clamping, to reduce the risk of paraplegia. A prospective randomized trial showed no benefit from this technique.[686] The risk of paraplegia remains high at 10–20% even in expert hands and there is considerable mortality (10–50%). Renal failure is also a common complication following surgical repair of thoracoabdominal aneurysms, and is predictive of a poor long-term outcome.[687] The largest experience of thoracoabdominal aneurysm surgery was by Stanley Crawford, and his excellent results are summarized in Table 10.1.

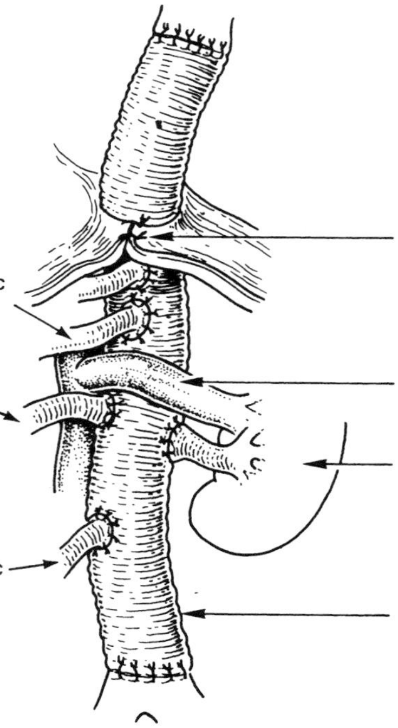

Fig. 10.73 The De Bakey technique for repairing thoracoabdominal aneurysms. Each artery is anastomosed to a Dacron side branch sutured on to the main graft.

REFERENCES

686. Crawford E S et al J Vasc Surg 1991; 13: 36
687. Svensson et al J Vasc Surg 1989; 10: 230

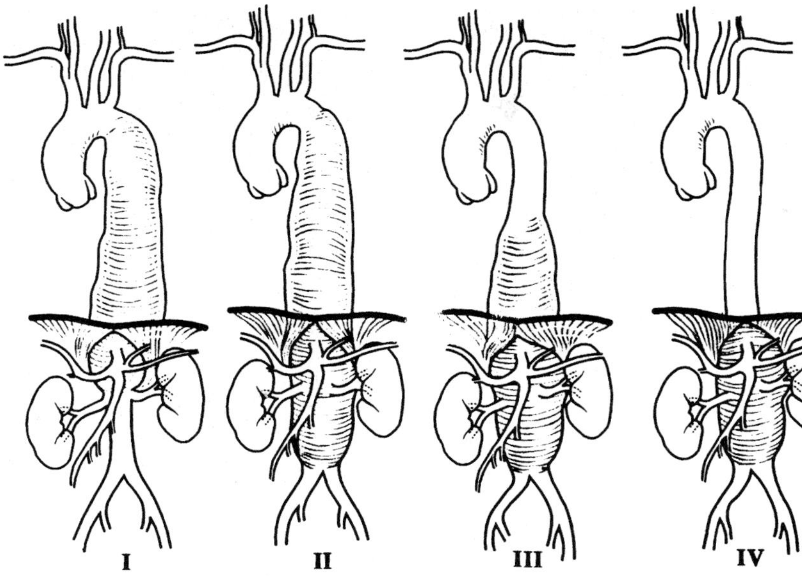

Fig. 10.74 The Crawford classification of thoracoabdominal aneurysms.

Table 10.1 Results of surgical treatment of thoracoabdominal aortic aneurysms

Extent	*No. of patients*	*Deaths (%)*	*Paraplegia (%)*	*Haemodialysis (%)*
I	270	23 (9)	38 (14)	20 (7)
II	353	36 (10)	102 (29)	34 (10)
III	285	25 (9)	16 (6)	28 (10)
IV	285	19 (7)	10 (4)	24 (8)
Total	1193	103 (9%)	166 (14%)	106 (9%)

Abdominal aortic aneurysms

The abdominal aorta is the most frequent site of aneurysms and abdominal aortic aneurysms are found in 2% of all post mortems.[688–691] The incidence of abdominal aortic aneurysm appears to be genuinely increasing in a number of countries, and in some the condition appears to be reaching epidemic proportions.[692–695] The dilation usually begins below the renal arteries and extends to the aortic bifurcation or below. Aortic aneurysms are often associated with aneurysms of the iliac, femoral and popliteal arteries, especially when they occur in patients with generalized arteriomegaly.[696] Only 1–2% of abdominal aneurysms are associated with aneurysmal dilatation extending above the renal arteries (see above).

Aortic aneurysms are often found on routine medical examination when a central abdominal pulsatile mass is discovered during abdominal palpation. They also cause severe abdominal pain and shock when they rupture; many patients develop symptoms of chronic back pain as the result of pressure on the lumbar vertebrae, which may be eroded.[697–699] Thrombosis, distal embolization and rupture into the intestine or vena cava are rare complications.[700,701]

The incidence of abdominal aneurysm appears to be greatest in elderly (above the age of 60) male hypertensives who smoke. The value of ultrasound screening to detect unsuspected abdominal aortic aneurysms in selected at-risk or high-risk populations has been assessed in a randomized controlled study. This showed that there was little benefit in screening women. In men aged 65–80 years, screening decreased the incidence of rupture by 55% compared with an unscreened group, and reduced death from rupture by 42%.[702]

Patients who present electively must be fully examined to determine their general fitness for surgery and the state of their distal vasculature. Aortic dilatation can be confirmed by plain radiograph (Fig. 10.75), ultrasound scanning (Fig. 10.76) or CT scanning (Fig. 10.77). Magnetic resonance imaging can also be used to assess the dimensions of an aortic aneurysm.[703] All these scans allow a more accurate assessment of the width and extent of the aneurysm.[704–706] Ultrasound is the least expensive but spiral CT gives a more accurate size estimation and has the advantage that the renal arteries and periaortic structures can usually be clearly seen. Arteriography is obtained if involvement of the renal arteries is suspected, or the state of the distal vascular tree is in doubt

REFERENCES

688. Da Gama A D J Cardiovasc Surg 1984; 25: 505
689. Lie M, Grimsgaard C et al J Cardiovasc Surg 1988; 29: 418
690. Turk K A D Proc Roy Soc Med 1965; 58: 869
691. Darling R C, Messina R et al Circulation 1977; 56 (suppl): 161
692. Castieden W M, Mercer J C et al Br J Surg 1985; 72: 109
693. Collin J Br J Hosp Med 1988; 64: 67
694. Fowkes F G R, MacIntyre C C A, Ruckley C V Br J Med 1989; 298: 33
695. Hopkins N F G Br Med J 1987; 294: 790
696. Crawford E S, Cohen E S Arch Surg 1982; 117: 1393
697. Osler W Lancet 1905; ii: 1089
698. Gleidman M L, Ayers W B, Vestal B L Ann Surg 1957; 146: 207
699. Fielding J W L, Black J et al Br Med J 1981; 283: 355
700. Lehman E P Ann Surg 1938; 108: 694
701. Reckless J P D, McColl I, Taylor G W Br J Surg 1972; 59: 461
702. Scott R A P et al Br J Surg 1995; 82: 1066
703. Kaufman J A et al JVIR 1994; 5: 489
704. Robicsek F Surgery 1981; 89: 275
705. Gomes M N, Hufnagel C A J Cardiovasc Surg 1979; 2: 511
706. Young A E, Lea Thomas M, Wright C H Br Med 1980; 1: 765

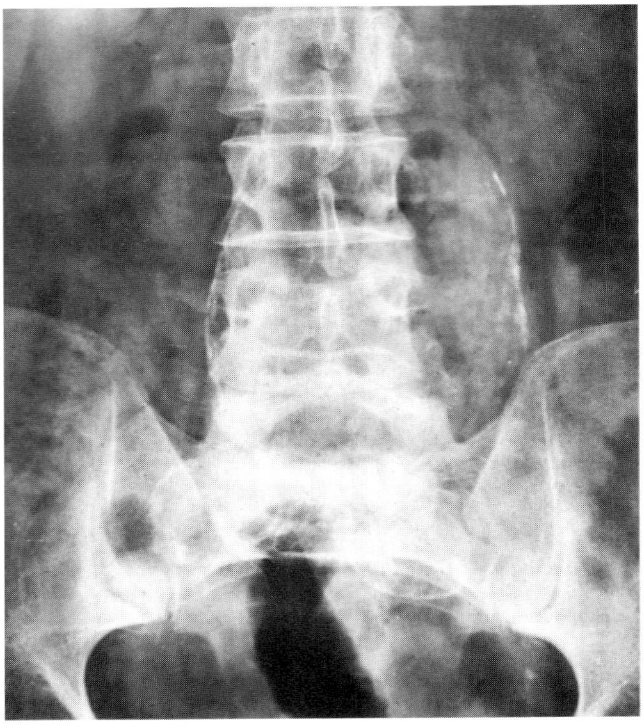

Fig. 10.75 A plain abdominal radiograph of an abdominal aortic aneurysm, showing calcification in the wall and a soft tissue mass.

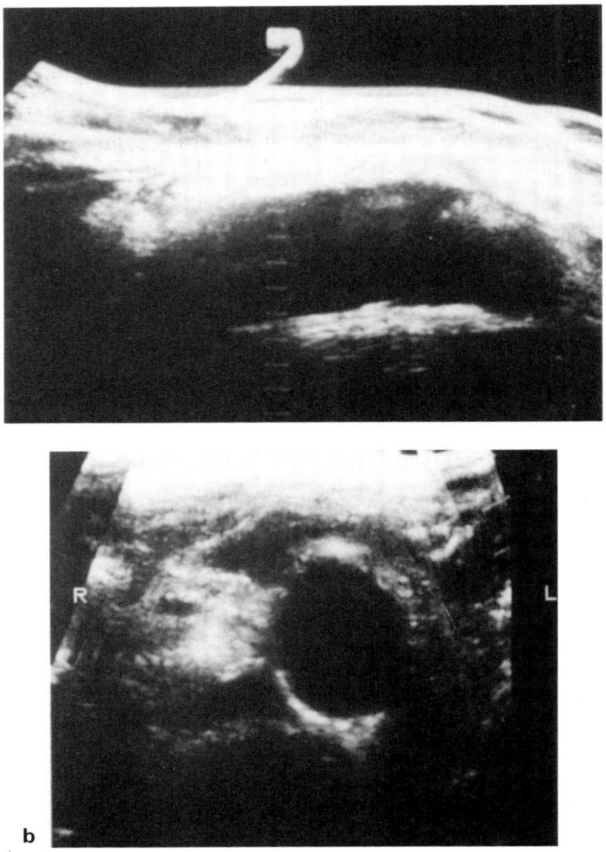

Fig. 10.76 An ultrasound scan of an abdominal aortic aneurysm. (**a**) longitudinal; (**b**) transverse.

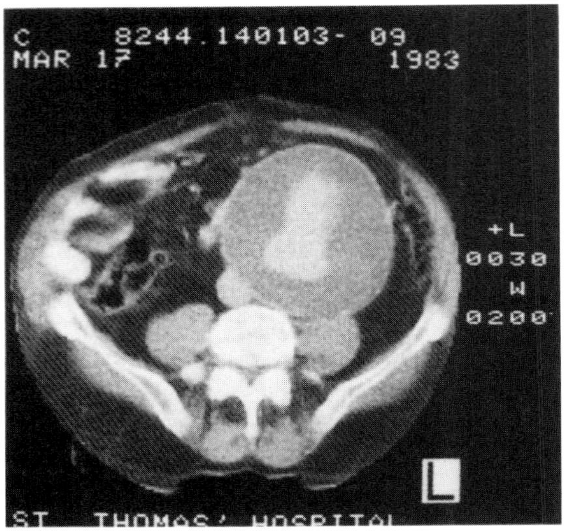

Fig. 10.77 A computerized tomographic scan showing a large aortic aneurysm.

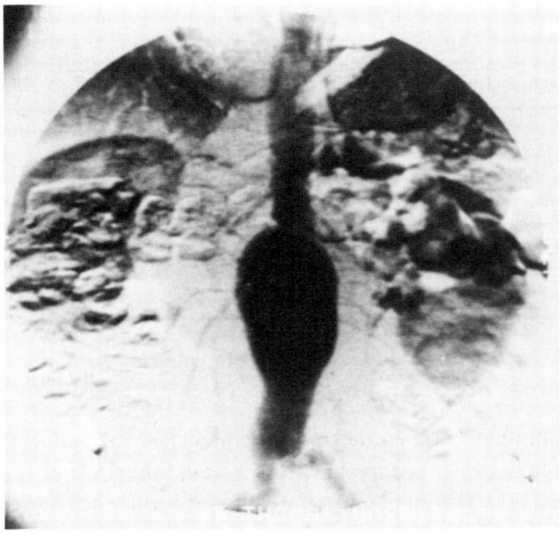

Fig. 10.78 A digital subtraction arteriogram showing the extent of an abdominal aneurysm.

(Fig. 10.78).[707] An elevated erythrocyte sedimentation rate should arouse suspicion of inflammatory change,[708] which can be confirmed by CT or MRI scan (see Fig. 10.21).[709] The aetiology of inflammatory aneurysms (periaortic fibrosis) is not known, but surgery is invariably difficult and can be deferred until a course of steroids has reduced the size of the inflammatory mass.[709] There is an association between an inflammatory aneurysm and retroperitoneal fibrosis. The ureters may have to be lysed at the time of aneurysm surgery, although insertion of lighted double J stents can also be used to ensure patency of the ureter.[710]

REFERENCES

707. Brewster D C, Retana A et al N Engl J Med 1975; 292: 822
708. Walker D I, Bloor K et al Br J Surg 1972; 59: 609
709. Baskerville P A, Blakeney C G et al Br J Surg 1983; 70: 381
710. Bainbridge E T, Woodward D A K J Cardiovasc Surg 1982; 23: 365

Most patients who are found to have a 6 cm diameter aneurysm (i.e. 2 cm greater than 4 cm, which is twice the normal aortic diameter) should be offered surgical repair providing they are reasonably fit and can be expected to survive the operation. The risk of smaller aneurysms (between 4 and 5 cm) rupturing is much less. Aneurysms that are greater than 7 or 8 cm are very liable to rupture and such patients should be offered early operations.[711] The growth rate of aneurysms is unpredictable but may be monitored by serial ultrasound examinations.[712] Trials are in progress to determine whether small aneurysms (less than 5.5 cm) are best treated expectantly or should be electively repaired.[713] The UK Small Aneurysm Trial has randomized patients with aortic aneurysms of between 4 and 5.5 cm in diameter into groups receiving either conservative surveillance with regular duplex ultrasound or surgical repair. This trial is also designed to assess the natural history of small aneurysms of 3–4 cm in diameter.

Elective aortic aneurysm repair[714–717]

The aorta is approached as described on page 300. The neck of the aneurysm is defined and controlled and the iliac arteries are dissected free and controlled. After heparin has been given and clamps have been applied a tube graft is inlayed into the aorta if the iliac arteries are not diseased.[718,719] The lumbar arteries and inferior mesenteric artery are sewn off if they back bleed. Aortoiliac or femoral bypass is required if the iliac arteries are aneurysmal or occluded. At least one internal iliac artery must be revascularized to avoid colonic or buttock ischaemia.

Endovascularly placed stent grafts

The first report of the successful endoluminal repair of an abdominal aortic aneurysm was by Parodi et al.[720] Since then other types of stent graft have been developed.[721] Measurement of the length and the diameter of the neck of the aortic aneurysm is extremely important, as each graft must fit perfectly and is therefore usually slightly oversized. The diameter is measured by spiral CT scan, and the length by performing angiography with a catheter marked at 1 cm intervals. Less than 5% of aortic aneurysms are suitable for tube grafts. The limiting factor is usually the absence of a sufficiently long distal neck, although a short proximal neck may also be important. The proximal neck must be at least 1.5 cm long, and the distal neck 1 cm long to achieve good fixation. The presence of thrombus at the site of stent fixation is a contraindication to endoluminal repair, as a leak will develop in time. The use of a bifurcated stent graft allows more aneurysms (up to 40%) to be treated, as the absence of a distal aortic neck is not important.[721] There is evidence that the haemodynamic insult to the patient is much less with endovascular repair than with open surgery[722] although the incidence of microembolization to the legs is greater.[723] Aneurysms which are excluded from the circulation usually decrease in size, but there is good evidence that in patients with significant endoluminal leaks the aneurysm continues to expand and is at continued risk of rupture.[724] The place of stent grafting in aneurysm repair is yet to be established and will require controlled trials to be carried out in the future.

Ruptured abdominal aortic aneurysm

Patients with ruptured abdominal aneurysms present as emergencies with severe abdominal pain and shock. The pain commonly radiates to the back, and patients often collapse with the onset of pain. The finding of a tender pulsatile central mass on examination of the abdomen clinches the diagnosis, but hypotension may render the mass impalpable, and signs of hypovolaemia may predominate. Mesenteric thrombosis, myocardial infarction, acute pancreatitis, perforated peptic ulcer, ureteric calculus and mesenteric volvulus are other diagnoses which must be considered.[725,726] Dilatation of the femoral or popliteal arteries corroborates the diagnosis. Abdominal radiographs often show calcification in the wall of the aneurysm and the psoas shadow may be lost.

CT scanning may confirm a localized haematoma in patients with pain and no signs of shock (Fig. 10.21a) but this investigation may be falsely negative and is only indicated if the patient is in a stable condition.[707,727,728] An electrocardiogram and chest radiograph may be helpful as part of the initial assessment but urgent surgery should not be delayed by over-investigation, and once the diagnosis has been made the aim should be to get the patient to theatre as quickly as possible.

10 or 12 units of blood should be urgently cross-matched, but grouped uncross-matched blood can be given before cross-matched blood is available. It is unwise to resuscitate the patient over-vigorously until the aorta has been cross-clamped because a reactionary haemorrhage may prove fatal as the blood pressure rises. Patients with severe hypotension and hypovolaemia must however receive blood or plasma expanders to produce a recordable blood pressure. It is important to stress again that over-vigorous resuscitation must be avoided. Application of gravity suits is advocated by some surgeons[729] but their removal in theatre can be difficult and there is no clear evidence that they are beneficial. A urinary catheter and a number of intravenous lines should be inserted, one of which should be a central line. The patient should have a crash induction of anaesthesia in theatre, having

REFERENCES

711. Darling R C Am J Surg 1970; 179: 397
712. Bernstein E F, Dilley R B et al Surgery 1976; 80: 765
713. The UK Small Aneurysm Trial participants. Eur J Vasc Endovasc Surg 1995; 9: 42
714. Martin P Br Surg 1961; 18: 530
715. Creech O Ann Surg 1966; 164: 935
716. Du Bost C, Allary M, Oeconomos N A Mem Acad Chir (Paris) 1951; 77: 381
717. Estes J E Circulation 1950; 2: 258
718. Orr W McC, Davis M Br J Surg 1974; 61: 847
719. Makin G S Ann Roy Coll Surg Engl 1983; 65: 309
720. Parodi J C, Palmaz J C, Barone H D Ann Vasc Surg 1991; 5: 491
721. Jusuf S W et al Lancet 1994; 344: 650
722. Baxendale B et al Br J Anaesth 1995; 74: 138
723. Thompson M et al Br J Surg 1996; 83: 565
724. Parodi J C J Vasc Surg 1995; 21: 549
725. Walker E M, Hopkinson B R, Makin G S Ann R Coll Surg Engl 1983; 65: 311
726. Gardham J R C Br J Hosp Med 1982; 40: 47
727. Senapati A, Hurst P A E et al J Cardiovasc Surg 1986; 27: 719
728. Greatorex R A, Dixon A K et al Br Med J 1988; 297: 284
729. Jenkins A McL, Ruckley C V, Nolan B Br J Surg 1986; 73: 395

already been prepared and draped, with the surgeon poised to open the abdomen the moment that anaesthesia is established.

The abdomen is swiftly entered through a long midline incision, the diagnosis is confirmed, and the aneurysm neck is rapidly controlled by the application of a clamp. Many different approaches have been described to isolate the neck of the aneurysm in order to apply the clamp; using two suckers, a direct approach through the haematoma after exteriorizing the bowel is usually straightforward. The haematoma often facilitates the dissection. If difficulties arise with severe, uncontrolled bleeding, a clamp may be applied to the suprarenal aorta below the diaphragm for a short period, or alternatively a large Foley catheter on an introducer can be inserted through the rupture and the balloon blown up in the upper aorta to control haemorrhage.[730,731] It is even possible to insert a Fogarty catheter into the aorta above the aneurysm via a cutdown in a peripheral artery before the aneurysm is opened.[732] The right colon and duodenum can be mobilized to the left if access to the neck of the aneurysm is difficult. The aorta is then approached from the right side, avoiding the haematoma. Once the haemorrhage has been controlled vigorous resuscitation restores blood volume, blood pressure and urine output, which may be further stimulated by mannitol, diuretics and dopamine, although there is little evidence that these urinary stimulants have any effect other than to please the surgeon and anaesthetist!

Repair of a leaking aneurysm then proceeds using identical techniques to those employed for elective repair (Fig. 10.79). Occasionally the neck of the aneurysm is so poor that sutures cut out, and under these exceptional circumstances the aorta can be closed off with a suture, balloon or even an orthopaedic staple before an axillobifemoral graft is used to restore blood flow to the legs.[733,734]

Results. The mortality for elective aortic aneurysm repair should be less than 5%[735–737] and a 2–4% mortality has been achieved in some selected series.[738–741] Many patients with aortic aneurysms that rupture fail to reach hospital,[742,743] when sudden death is often ascribed to other causes, but of those reaching hospital, mortality should be less than 50% and a 32% mortality has been achieved.[729] Death is commonly the result of renal failure, uncontrolled bleeding, myocardial infarction, respiratory and multisystem organ failure.

Complications of surgery. As with aortic grafts for occlusive disease graft infection may lead to septicaemia, sinus formation or aortic graft–enteric fistula, which requires removal of the graft and restoration of the distal blood flow by an axillobifemoral graft.[744,745] This should be suspected in patients presenting with an upper gastrointestinal bleed who have previously had an aortic aneurysm repair. Prophylactic antibiotics and careful wrapping of the graft by the aneurysm sac or omentum may reduce the incidence of this complication. Early graft occlusions are rare in patients with aneurysms.

False aneurysms usually develop after groin anastomoses, and require re-operation, excision of the false sac and re-anastomosis.[746] This complication usually develops several years after the initial operation. Myocardial infarction, deep vein thrombosis, pulmonary embolism, chest infection, stroke and multisystem organ failure are all recognized complications following elective and emergency surgery on aneurysms.

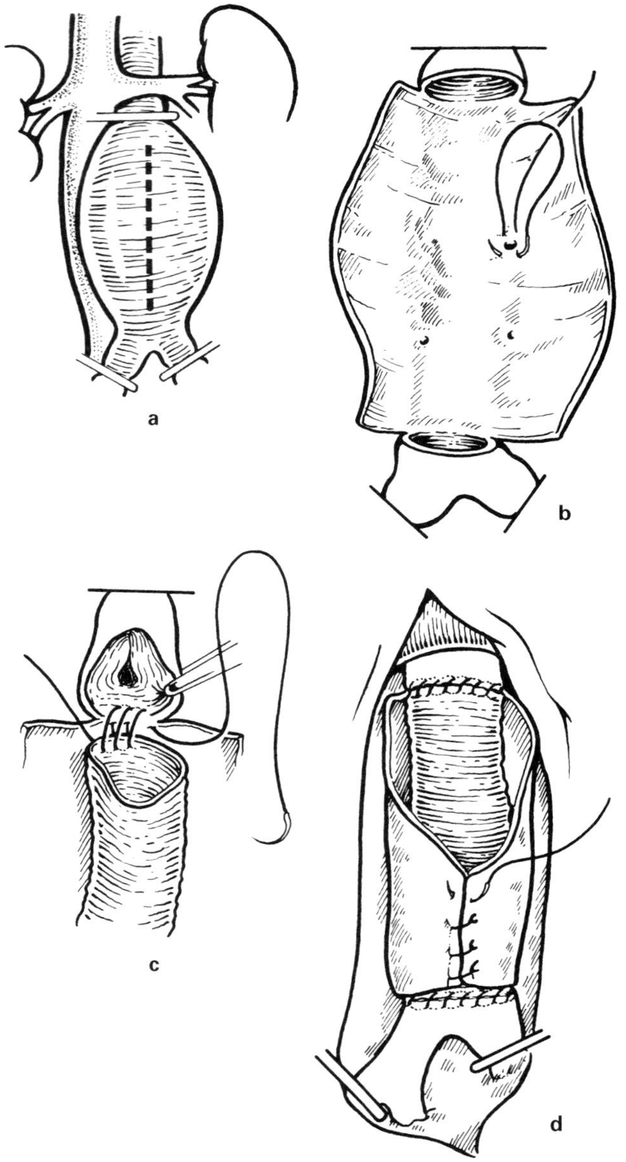

Fig. 10.79 The technique for repairing an abdominal aortic aneurysm.

REFERENCES

730. Wyatt A P Ann Roy Coll Surg Engl 1976; 58: 52
731. Hesse F, Kletsch K A Ann Surg 1962; 155: 320
732. Hyde G L, Sullivan D M Surg Gyn Obstet 1982; 154: 197
733. Berguer R, Scheider J, Wilner H I Surgery 1978; 83: 425
734. Karmody A M, Leather R P et al Surgery 1983; 94: 591
735. Fielding J W L, Black J et al Br Med J 1981; 283: 355
736. Berridge D, Chamberlain J et al Brit J Surg 1995; 82: 906
737. Kazmers A, Jacob L et al J Vasc Surg 1996; 23: 191
738. Soreide O, Lillestol J et al Surgery 1982; 91: 188
739. Campbell W B, Collin J, Morris P J Ann R Coll Surg Engl 1986; 68: 275
740. Whittemore A D, Clowes A W et al Ann Surg 1980; 192: 414
741. Mutirangura P, Stonebridge P A et al Br J Surg 1989; 76: 1251
742. Armour R H Br Med J 1977; ii: 1055
743. Dent A, Kent S J S, Young T W Br J Surg 1986; 73: 318
744. O'Brien T, Collin J Br J Surg 1992; 79: 1262
745. Hannon R J, Wolfe J H, Mansfied A O Br J Surg 1996; 83: 654
746. Szilagyi D E, Smith R F et al Surgery 1975; 78: 800

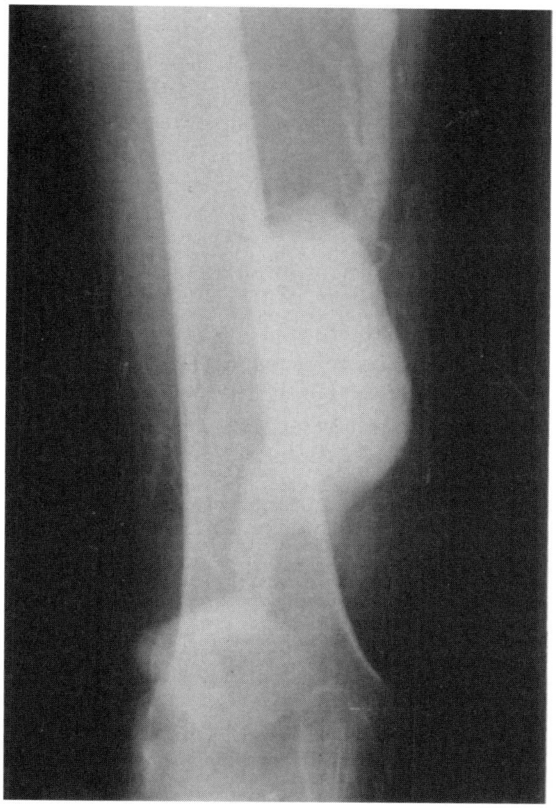

Fig. 10.80 An arteriogram showing a popliteal aneurysm.

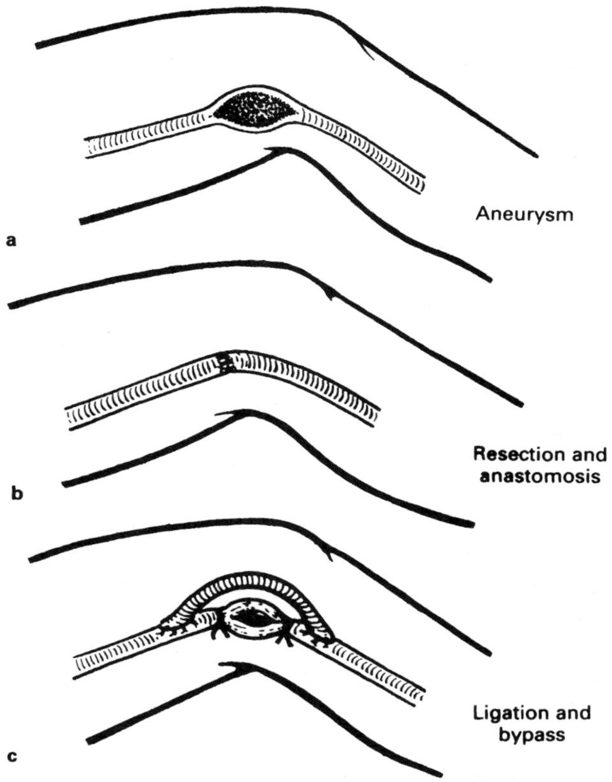

Fig. 10.81 The techniques used to repair a popliteal aneurysm.

Femoral artery aneurysms

Aneurysms of the femoral artery are usually part of a generalized arterial dilatation, although isolated aneurysms of the common femoral vessels are recognized.[747] The majority are symptomless; they rarely rupture but they may be a source of distal emboli and they occasionally thrombose. A pulsatile swelling in the femoral triangle must be differentiated from other masses in this region. Confirmation of an expansile mass makes other diagnoses unlikely. Repair is by insertion of a prosthetic graft or reversed saphenous vein (though this is rarely of sufficient size) between the external iliac artery and the superficial femoral artery, incorporating the profunda artery orifice if possible in the distal anastomosis. The profunda artery may be separately anastomosed to the graft if it cannot be retained on the lower patch. Aneurysms of the profunda femoris artery are rare but do occur.[748] They can usually be safely ligated but can be resected and replaced if necessary.

Popliteal artery aneurysms

This is the second most common site of aneurysms, accounting for 70% of all peripheral aneurysms.[749,750] Popliteal aneurysms occasionally present as large pulsatile masses noticed by the patient or physician, but are much more commonly diagnosed when the patient presents with peripheral ischaemia from embolization of contained thrombus or when the aneurysm itself thromboses.[751,752] They used to be an occupational hazard of cavalrymen and postboys but are now invariably 'atherosclerotic' in aetiology and are often part of arteriomegaly with multiple sites of aneurysmal dilatation. The diagnosis can be confirmed by arteriography, ultrasound or CT scan (Fig. 10.80),[753] and femoral arteriography is also helpful to assess the patency of the crural vessels.[754] A symptomatic popliteal aneurysm should be treated by resection and replacement by a vein bypass graft (Fig. 10.81) to avoid the considerable risk of gangrene and limb loss.[752,754] It is important to open the sac and ligate all the geniculate branches to avoid continued aneurysmal dilation. The approach is otherwise similar to a femoropopliteal vein bypass graft. In an acutely ischaemic limb, infusions of streptokinase or tissue plasminogen activator should be given to lyse the thrombus before the aneurysm is repaired.[755,756] There is still controversy over the management of symptomless popliteal aneurysms. Some suggest that all should be repaired to prevent the disastrous consequences of thrombosis,[757]

REFERENCES

747. Cutler B S, Darling R C Surgery 1973; 74: 764
748. Symes J M, Eadie D G J Cardiovasc Surg 1973; 14: 220
749. Linton R R Surgery 1949; 26: 41
750. McCollum C H, De Bakey M E, Myhre M O Cardiovasc Res 1983; 21: 93
751. Downing R, Grimley R P et al J Roy Soc Med 1985; 78: 440
752. Guvendik L, Bloor K, Charlesworth D Br J Surg 1980; 67: 294
753. Davis R P, Neiman M L et al Arch Surg 1977; 112: 55
754. Graham A R, Lord R S A et al Aust NZ J Surg 1983; 53: 99
755. Ramesh S, Michaels J A, Galland R B Br J Surg 1993; 80: 1531
756. Elsey J K, Rosenthal D Am Surg 1994; 60: 942
757. Halliday A W et al Ann Roy Coll Surg Engl 1991; 73: 771

while others argue that surgery carries risks which may outweigh the natural history of the disease, and recommend conservative management until thrombosis occurs.[758]

Innominate and extracranial carotid arteries

Many so-called aneurysms in these sites are produced by tortuous, kinked and atherosclerotic vessels. These are called 'student's aneurysms'. True aneurysms do rarely occur and may require resection and replacement,[759,760] especially if they are a source of emboli.

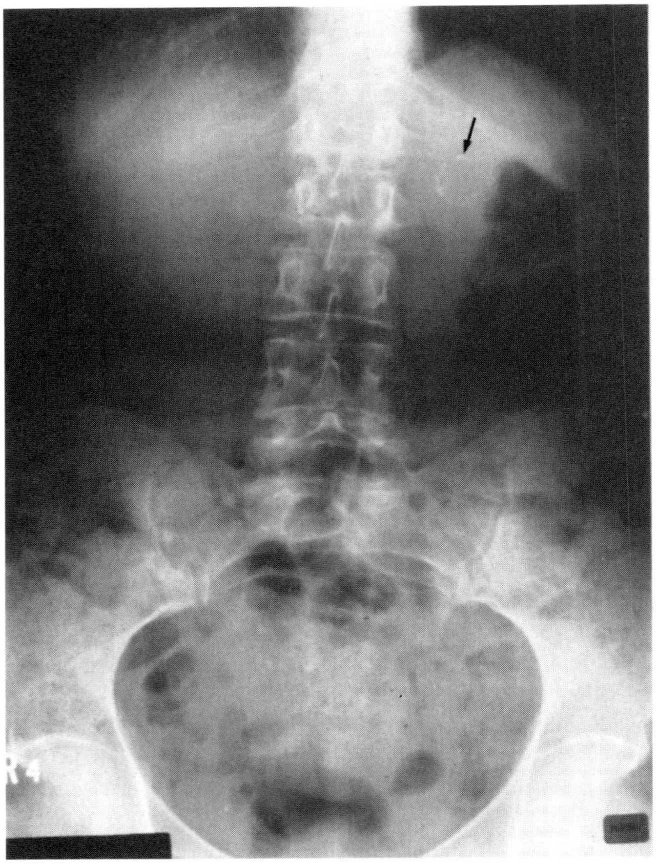

a

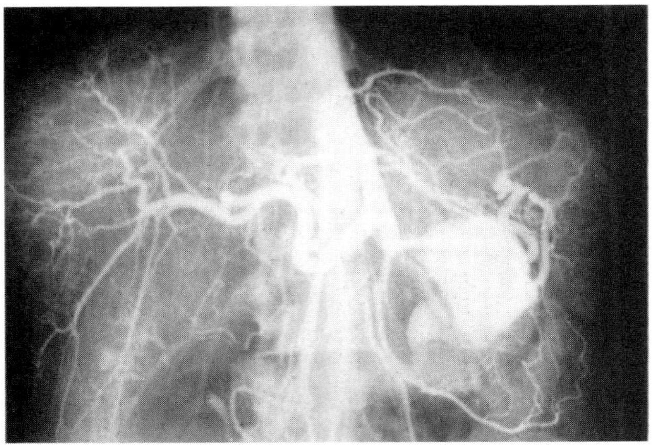

b

Fig. 10.82 **(a)** A ring of calcification in the wall of a splenic artery aneurysm. **(b)** An arteriogram of a splenic artery aneurysm.

Subclavian and axillary arteries

Subclavian aneurysms used to develop in dock labourers and coal heavers but mechanization has almost abolished this particular occupational hazard; aneurysms of these vessels are now usually found in relation to a cervical rib as a poststenotic dilatation. Axillary aneurysms used to occur in patients using crutches but are rarely seen today.

Radial arteries

Radial artery aneurysms are usually traumatic or iatrogenic false aneurysms and are most commonly seen after insertion of radial artery catheters. They can be treated by proximal and distal ligation if the Allen test is normal, or the artery can be reconstructed using vein if the vascularity of the hand is in doubt.

Splenic, hepatic, mesenteric and renal artery

Aneurysm of the splenic artery is the second most common intra-abdominal aneurysm (0.01–0.08%), affecting women four times as commonly as men, principally during the childbearing years.[761] They are normally symptomless unless they rupture. This is the only important complication and it occurs in a quarter of all cases. Rupture is most likely in the third trimester of pregnancy.[762] Portal hypertension and pancreatitis are both thought to predispose to splenic aneurysm formation. The chance finding of a ring of calcification in the epigastrium or left hypochondrium on plain abdominal radiograph (Fig. 10.82) may allow the diagnosis to be made before rupture. Operation is indicated for aneurysms greater than 3 cm in diameter and in pregnant patients.[763] Aneurysms can be excised and the artery reconstituted by end-to-end anastomosis or interposition graft. If reconstruction is difficult or impossible, ligation on either side of the aneurysm does not always presage splenectomy.[764] Splenic artery aneurysms have also been induced to thrombose by percutaneous embolization.[765]

Hepatic artery aneurysms,[766] which are one third as common as splenic aneurysms, commonly present when they rupture into the biliary system or the peritoneal cavity.[767] Intrabiliary rupture produces abdominal pain, gastrointestinal bleeding and jaundice. Excision of the aneurysm and, if possible, reconstruction of the artery by a vein graft is required for large extrahepatic aneurysms, although aberrant anatomy or good collaterals may make reconstruction unnecessary.[768] Intrahepatic aneurysms are best treated by therapeutic embolization.[769]

REFERENCES

758. Hands L J, Collin J Br J Surg 1991; 78: 996
759. Kauup H A, Haid S P et al Surgery 1972; 72: 946
760. Rhodes E L, Stanley J C et al Arch Surg 1976; 111: 339
761. Stanley J C, Fry W J Surgery 1974; 76: 898
762. McFarlane J, Thorbjarnarson B Am J Obstet Gynecol 1966; 95: 1024
763. Trastek V F, Bairolero P C et al Surgery 1982; 91: 694
764. Green D R, Gorey T F et al J Roy Soc Med 1988; 81: 387
765. Probst P, Castaneda-Zuniga W R et al Diagnostic Radiol 1978; 128: 619
766. Shaw J F L Br J Hosp Med 1982; 1: 404
767. Deterling R A J Cardiovasc Surg 1971; 12: 309

Coeliac (Fig. 10.83) and mesenteric artery aneurysms usually present with non-specific abdominal pain which may or may not be associated with a mobile pulsatile mass. They are often mycotic and may be related to pancreatitis. Surgical resection and reconstruction are required but the collateral circulation is often good enough to maintain viability if the aneurysm is ligated.[767,770] More recently, these aneurysms have been treated by therapeutic embolization.

Renal artery aneurysms are rare, and are often associated with hypertension. They are usually saccular and found at the bifurcation of the renal arteries.[771] They are commonly the result of medial necrosis but atherosclerosis and fibromuscular hyperplasia may also be causative factors. Rupture is unusual, but can occur in pregnancy; these aneurysms normally present as a chance finding during the investigation of hypertension. They can usually be safely ignored, but occasionally large aneurysms require excision, cold perfusion, bench surgery and reimplantation of the kidney into the pelvis.

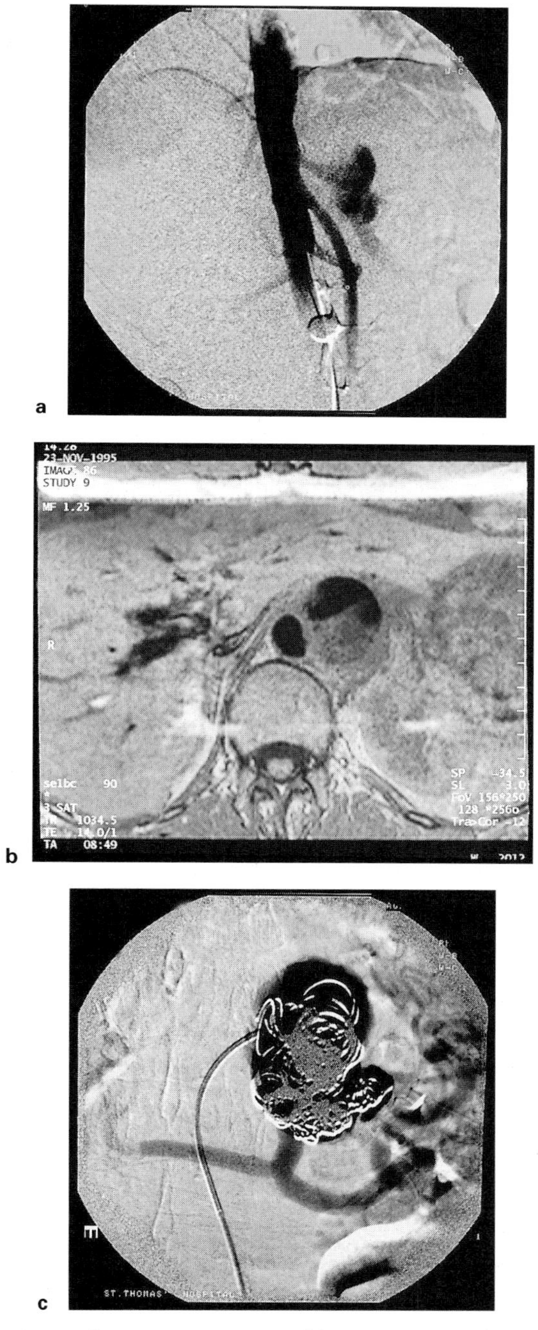

Fig. 10.83 Coeliac artery aneurysm: (**a**) arteriogram; (**b**) MR scan; (**c**) with coils inserted.

Aneurysms of the intracerebral arteries are discussed in Chapter 16.

ARTERIAL EMBOLISM AND ACUTE THROMBOTIC ISCHAEMIA

An embolus is the passage of matter from one part of the circulation to another through a vascular lumen.[772] The common site of origin of arterial emboli is the myocardium, the most frequent cause being thrombus in the atrial appendage secondary to atrial fibrillation.[773,774]

Mural thrombus on a myocardial infarct is another important source of embolism. Endocarditis on a rheumatic heart valve is now rare, but acute bacterial endocarditis after intravenous drug abuse with unsterile needles is an important source of peripheral emboli. Occasionally emboli may derive from prosthetic cardiac valves. Small emboli may also originate from mural arterial disease anywhere within the vascular tree — so-called 'artery-to-artery' emboli. Thrombus within an aneurysm may become dislodged, as may platelet aggregates or cholesterol debris from the surface of an atherosclerotic plaque. The former, like cardiac emboli, may occlude major vessels, while the latter usually produce small distal infarcts or temporary ischaemia, e.g. the blue toe syndrome. Cholesterol emboli are now a well recognized complication of balloon angioplasty and endovascular stenting.

Tumour emboli and paradoxical emboli are rare causes of arterial embolization. Tumour emboli are almost always microscopic but large macroscopic tumour emboli may occasionally be encountered[775] and left atrial myxoma is a well recognized but rare source of peripheral embolism.[776] Paradoxical embolism occurs when a venous embolism, derived from a deep vein thrombosis, passes into the systemic arterial circulation via a large congenital communication between the right and left heart circulation.[777] Very rarely a bullet may pass through the arterial circulation,[778] and other foreign bodies, such as intravenous catheters or disrupted prosthetic cardiac valves, may also embolize.

REFERENCES

768. Dwight R W, Ratcliffe J W Surgery 1952; 31: 915
769. Kadir S, Athanasoulis C A et al Radiology 1980; 134: 335
770. De Bakey M E, Cooley D A Ann Surg 1953; 19: 202
771. Stanley J C, Rhodes E L et al Arch Surg 1975; 110: 1327
772. Virchow R Die Cellular Pathologic. Verlag von August Hirschwald, Berlin 1859
773. Baxter-Smith D, Ashton F, Slaney G J Cardiovasc Surg 1988; 28: 453
774. Lusby R J, Wylie E J World J Surg 1983; 7: 340
775. Till A S, Fairburn E A Br J Surg 1947; 35: 86
776. Mercier A L, Suggon M G et al Am J Cardiol 1978; 41: 437
777. Thompson T, Evans W Q J Med 1930; 23: 135
778. Cooper F W, Harris M H, Kahn J W Ann Surg 1948; 127: 1

Emboli usually lodge at the bifurcation of the aorta or in the femoral, popliteal, brachial or carotid arteries; they may also lodge in branches of the aorta. The effects of embolism depend on the site of obstruction, the level of occlusion, the potential for collateral formation and the speed of collateral development.[779]

Small emboli of platelet aggregates or cholesterol debris arising from the arch of the aorta and extracranial vessels are the most frequent cause of amaurosis fugax and transient ischaemic attacks. In the upper limb small peripheral emboli may arise from a subclavian aneurysm complicating a cervical rib. These may cause distal vasospasm and secondary Raynaud's syndrome or even small areas of digital gangrene in the tips of the fingers.[780]

Distal emboli may also affect the lower limbs; they may arise from aortic atherosclerosis and aortic, femoral and popliteal aneurysms.[781,782] These cause vasospasm and occlusion of the distal vessels, leading to claudication, rest pain and eventually frank gangrene. Cutaneous gangrene secondary to small peripheral emboli has a characteristic appearance, with showers of dark spots appearing at multiple sites in the foot (Fig. 10.17). This appearance is almost pathognomonic of peripheral emboli but must be differentiated from polycythaemia or a platelet abnormality.

An embolus of vegetations arising on a heart valve with bacterial endocarditis may lodge at an arterial bifurcation where it can erode the arterial wall and produce a mycotic aneurysm.[783,784] The incidence of this complication has declined with the reduced incidence of bacterial endocarditis and the advent of effective antibiotics. Air embolism is a rare condition that may cause cerebral infarction and cardiac arrest. Fat embolism may complicate the recovery of patients with multiple fractures (see Chapter 7). The fat globules that enter the circulation usually impact in the brain and lungs, causing hypoxia and confusion. It is not appropriate to discuss amniotic emboli here as they are almost exclusively a gynaecological problem.

Clinical features

Large emboli present with symptoms of acute arterial occlusion beyond the point of obstruction. It must be noted, however, that embolism is no longer the most common cause of acute lower limb ischaemia in western nations; that distinction now belongs to acute thrombosis on pre-existing atheroma.[785] It is often difficult to distinguish between the two pathologies on clinical grounds.[774,786] When there is a potential embolic source and there is no history of claudication or other evidence of significant atherosclerosis, an embolism is the most likely cause. Most patients, however, present a diagnostic challenge with some blurring of the classical picture. It is then helpful to obtain an angiogram, which is preferable to blind exploration. It not only assists diagnosis, but also provides access for thrombolysis.[787] Other causes of acute arterial occlusion that must be considered include an aortic dissection and a thrombosed aneurysm, the latter especially at the popliteal site. Acute traumatic occlusions and occlusions secondary to arteritis rarely cause diagnostic difficulty. Acute occlusions can also be caused by arterial entrapment and congenital abnormalities of the arterial wall, such as cysts.

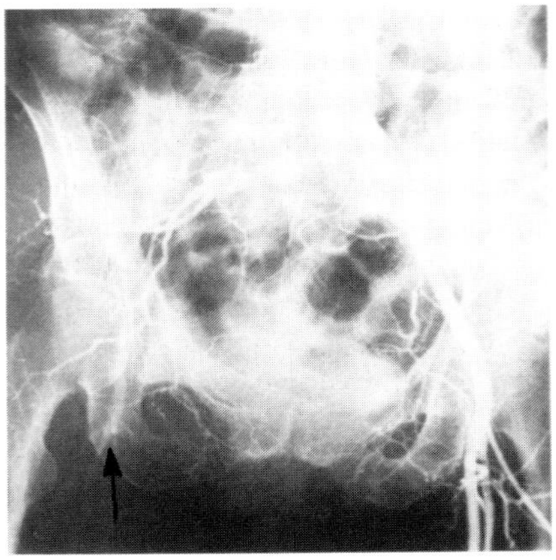

Fig. 10.84 An arteriogram showing an occlusion of the right femoral artery with a sharp cut-off indicative of an embolic occlusion.

Investigations

Angiography usually shows an occlusion with a sharp cut-off at the upper end (Fig. 10.84),[788] and there may be evidence of occlusion in other vessels, suggesting fragmentation or multiple emboli.[789] Collaterals are usually poor unless there is coexisting atherosclerosis, when even angiography may fail to distinguish the two conditions. An electrocardiogram and chest radiograph, along with a full blood count and urea and electrolyte estimation, should be obtained before operation. Trans-oesophageal echocardiography is the best way of demonstrating residual thrombus within the heart. It also delineates valvular disease and anatomical abnormalities such as a patent ductus or an atrial septal defect.[790] This investigation is usually obtained after the presence of an embolus has been confirmed, when it will influence the strategy for preventing recurrent emboli.

Management

In a few patients the embolus passes into a small peripheral vessel and disintegrates, causing minimal symptoms which quickly resolve. Under these circumstances it is only necessary to determine the source of embolus and prevent recurrence, usually by anticoagulation with warfarin. In the majority of patients persistence of acute ischaemia demands more active management by operative embolectomy or catheter-directed intra-arterial thrombolysis.[787]

REFERENCES

779. Longland C J Ann R Coll Surg Engl 1953; 13: 161
780. Gunning A J, Pickering G W, Robb-Smith A H T Q J Med 1964; 33: 133
781. Crane C Arch Surg 1967; 94: 96
782. Hara M, Thompson B W Arch Surg 1966; 92: 504
783. Anderson C B, Butcher H R, Ballinger W F Arch Surg 1974; 109: 712
784. Baird R N Eur J Vasc Surg 1989; 3: 95
785. Mills J L, Porter J M Ann Vasc Surg 1991; 5: 96
786. Blaisdell F W, Steele M, Allen R E Surgery 1978; 84: 822
787. Braithwaite B D, Earnshaw J J Br J Surg 1994; 81:1705
788. Galbraith K, Collin J et al Ann R Coll Surg Engl 1985; 67: 30
789. Elliott J P, Hageman J H et al Surgery 1980; 88: 833
790. Lagattolla N, Burnand K G, Stewart A Br J Surg 1995; 82: 1651

It is wise to commence full anticoagulation with intravenous heparin once acute ischaemia has been diagnosed. This measure is essential to prevent thrombust propagation in the relatively static columns of blood distal and proximal to the site of arterial occlusion. Surgeons should also remember not to devote all their attention to the peripheral problem; patients with emboli are systemically unwell, usually from a cardiac cause. It is the central, not the peripheral problem which mainly accounts for the mortality rate of up to 30%, associated with major arterial embolism to the lower limbs,[791,792] and it is wise to involve a physician or cardiologist at an early stage of management.

Surgical embolectomy

The operation may be performed under local, regional or general anaesthesia, depending on the patient's fitness. An anaesthetist should be present throughout the proceedings to monitor the patient, even when local anaesthetic is used. If a saddle embolus has lodged at the aortic bifurcation, both common femoral arteries are exposed through vertical or oblique groin incisions and controlled. The deep and superficial femoral arteries are also exposed and encircled with slings. An arteriotomy is made without the application of clamps if no pulsation is felt in the vessels. Thrombus may be encountered in the lumen, or a small amount of back bleeding from collaterals may occur. This is easily controlled by temporary application of clamps or by traction on the slings. A Fogarty balloon catheter[793] of Fr gauge 4 or 5 is passed up from both groins into the abdominal aorta. The balloon is inflated and the catheter withdrawn (Fig. 10.85a). This should extrude the embolus from the arteriotomy and establish downflow. A Fr gauge 3 or 4 catheter is then used to clear any fragmented embolus or propagated thrombus from the distal femoral vessels (Fig. 10.85b). When the distal vessels have been cleared there should be adequate backflow. A peroperative angiogram should be obtained at this point to ensure that all distal emboli have been removed. Anticoagulation may need to be continued in the long term, depending on the cause of the embolism; in such circumstances warfarin is substituted for heparin.[794]

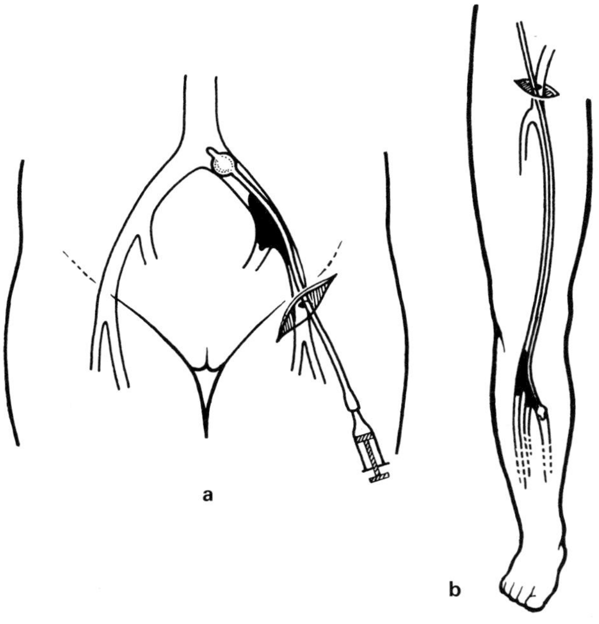

Fig. 10.85 The technique of embolectomy.

Variations

The aorta may have to be explored if satisfactory inflow cannot be established. When the catheter will not pass proximally with ease the probable cause is atherosclerosis; if it passes easily but no blood flow is obtained on withdrawal the probability of aortoiliac dissection should be considered.

Poor backflow despite the easy passage of the catheter distally to the ankle may indicate residual thrombus in the tibial vessels. This can be confirmed by peroperative angiography. Further passage of the catheter may complete the removal of distal emboli or thrombus. If not, the tibial vessels may be individually swept by a small Fogarty catheter inserted via an arteriotomy in the infrageniculate popliteal artery. Peroperative thrombolysis via the common femoral arteriotomy is another option. This is performed by injecting a lytic solution into the vessels and allowing a suitable time for clot dissolution. Although early reports of the use of streptokinase were disappointing,[795] recent studies using streptokinase (100 000 units in 100 ml of normal saline infused over 30 minutes) or urokinase have been more encouraging.[796–798] Tissue plasminogen activator may also be effective.[799,800]

The popliteal artery may have to be explored if poor backflow is still obtained or the operative arteriogram shows that there is residual thrombus within the crural vessels. Further passage of balloon catheters into the crural arteries should enable complete removal of distal emboli, but occasionally these vessels need to be exposed at the ankle. Arteriotomies in the popliteal artery and distal vessels need to be carefully closed with vein patches.

Thrombosis in the microcirculation may be suspected if adequate revascularization is not achieved despite good inflow to the groin and clear distal vessels. This may result in limb loss. Occlusive atheromatous disease is present if the Fogarty catheter will not pass to the ankle; in this situation a bypass graft, from the common femoral to the popliteal artery or crural vessel, may be beneficial. An operative arteriogram may indicate the potential value of a vein bypass graft to the distal vessels.

REFERENCES

791. Murie J A, Mathieson M J Cardiovasc Surg 1987; 28: 516
792. Connett M C, Murray D H, Wenneker W W Am J Surg 1984; 148: 14
793. Fogarty T J, Cranley J J et al Surg Gynecol Obstet 1963; 116: 241
794. Holm J, Schersten T Acta Chir Scand 1972; 138: 683
795. Cohen L H, Kaplin M, Bernhard V M Arch Surg 1986; 121: 708
796. Comerota A J, White J V, Grosh J D Surg Gyn Obstet 1989; 169: 283
797. Parent N E, Bernhard V M, Pabst T S et al J Vasc Surg 1989; 9: 153
798. Beard J D, Nyamekye I et al Br J Surg 1993; 80: 21
799. Ad Hoc Committee on Clinical Research J Vasc Surg 1992; 15: 886
800. Andaz S, Shields D A, Scurr J H, Coleridge Smith P D Eur J Vasc Surg 1993; 7: 595

Emboli can also be removed from the femoral, popliteal and brachial bifurcations using the same techniques. Mesenteric emboli can be removed by balloon catheter (see Chapter 29). It is rarely practical to remove cerebral emboli.

Thrombolysis

Streptokinase, urokinase and tissue plasminogen activator can be infused directly into an embolus or thrombus developing at a site of pre-existing atheroma via a small calibre catheter inserted percutaneously.[787] The most common route is via the common femoral artery in the groin, the catheter being advanced distally if the occlusion is in the leg vessels or proximally over the aortic bifurcation to the contralateral side if the iliac vessels are occluded. Fibrinolysis is also now used to remove emboli, but it is particularly useful for acute ischaemia secondary to thrombosis. In either case it can only be used if the state of the limb allows, i.e. if sensation and motor power have not been lost. If, on the other hand, the neurological deficit is marked, operation should be undertaken as there is inadequate time for lysis to be effective before irreversible ischaemic change occurs. Other contraindications to lysis include conditions with a risk of haemorrhage, a stroke within the preceding two months, and major surgery within the preceding few days. Many dosage and time regimens have been described,[800] and time to lysis can be reduced by using a spray catheter and injector programmed to deliver the lytic solution in pulses, the so-called pulse-spray technique.[801,802] Using such modern systems a mean time to lysis of less than an hour has been achieved in some cases (more usually 2 to 3 hours) but, since lysis cannot be guaranteed, surgery may still be preferable if the situation is critical. Lysis of iliac thrombus can be dangerous as it can cause major problems if it migrates into the distal limb vessels.

It should be appreciated that the technique of intra-arterial thrombolysis is evolving, and no established technique has yet been developed. Angiographic patency can be achieved in up to 90% of selected cases, but the clinical results are not as good in that a fair proportion of arteries re-occlude.[800] Although the delivery of the lytic agent directly into the embolus or thrombus aims to prevent widespread systemic lysis, the technique is nevertheless associated with significant bleeding complications and its use should at present be restricted to vascular surgical units with experienced interventional radiological and surgical staff. Nevertheless the recent controlled trial by Ouriel et al[803] in patients with acute peripheral ischaemia showed that thrombolytic therapy produced fewer complications and significantly reduced mortality when compared to immediate surgical revascularization. The limb salvage rate was similar in the two groups.

Complications and results of surgery

The mortality associated with surgical embolectomy remains depressingly high at between 10 and 20%.[786,788,790,791] This is largely the result of the poor general condition of the patients, especially those with emboli arising from mural thrombus on a myocardial infarct. A significant proportion of patients who present after a prolonged period of acute ischaemia develop severe metabolic problems after revascularization. This is usually the result of large amounts of potassium, myoglobin and other toxic metabolites being released back into the systemic circulation following the restoration of the blood supply.[804] Cardiac arrest and renal failure may ensue. Glucose and insulin, mannitol and haemodialysis may be helpful in overcoming some of these complications.[805] Restoration of blood flow may also cause compartment syndromes: fasciotomies should be performed if this complication is considered probable and are essential if it occurs. Ischaemic contractures (e.g. Volkmann's) may develop if there is a delay in restoring the blood supply in the face of severe ischaemia. Amputation may be necessary if the limb remains ischaemic after all reasonable attempts at revascularization. It should be noted, however, that delayed embolectomy can be carried out successfully up to a few weeks after the acute event, providing irreversible ischaemia has not developed and the embolus has not become too adherent to the arterial wall.[806]

ARTERIAL VASOSPASM (VASOMOTOR DISEASE)

Arterial spasm may be either a primary vasomotor malfunction or may be secondary to another pathological process affecting the vessel wall. A number of primary vasomotor disturbances are recognized by the appearances they produce but their aetiology still remains largely conjectural. These disorders include Raynaud's disease, acrocyanosis, erythrocyanosis frigida and erythromelalgia. The vasospasm of the first three conditions is precipitated by cold, while arterial vasodilatation in erythromelalgia appears to be related to venous congestion, warmth or pressure.[807] The primary vasospastic disorders cause considerable misery in cold climates, where numb and painful digits may progress to ulceration and even frank necrosis and gangrene during winter months.

Vasomotor changes can follow division of peripheral nerves and are common after poliomyelitis. Paralysed limbs may become cold, oedematous and cyanotic. Sympathectomy is beneficial if severe chilblains or cutaneous necrosis develop.[808]

Collagen diseases, repeated trauma, nerve damage, obliterative vascular disease, vessel entrapment syndromes, certain drugs and poisons may all cause secondary vasospasm and must be differentiated from a primary disorder.[809] Collagen diseases in particular give rise to severe vasospasm in the small arteries of the hand, foot,

REFERENCES

801. Yusuf S W, Whitaker S C et al Eur J Vasc Endovasc Surg 1995; 10: 136
802. Yusuf S W, Whitaker S C, Grepson R H S et al Br J Surg 1995; 82: 338
803. Ouriel K, Shortell C K, DeWeese J A J Vasc Surg 1994; 19: 1021
804. Haimovichi H Surgery 1979; 85: 461
805. London P S J Hosp Med 1968; 1: 312
806. Ammann J, Seiler H, Vogt B Br J Surg 1976; 63: 73, 76
807. Lewis T Clin Sci 1933; 211: 175
808. Kinmonth J B, Rob C G, Simeone F A Vascular Surgery. Arnold, London 1962
809. Rivers S P, Porter J M In: Bergan J J (ed) Arterial Surgery. Churchill Livingstone, Edinburgh 1984

toes and fingers, with a greater incidence of digital necrosis and gangrene than is found in the primary vasospastic disorders.

Arterial spasm may complicate intraluminal thrombosis or embolism, and spasm of the coronary vessels is thought to be one cause of sudden death in the absence of an occluding thrombus. It is also an important cause of morbidity after inadvertent intra-arterial injection of noxious substances including thiopentone, other barbiturates, venous sclerosants, quinine and hypertonic solutions. Spasm also occurs after poisoning by arsenic, heavy metals and ergot.

Raynaud's phenomenon (or syndrome) and Raynaud's disease

Maurice Raynaud published his thesis on local asphyxia and gangrene of the extremities in 1862.[810] He described a set of symptoms in a series of patients, and this collection of symptoms came to be called Raynaud's disease. In 1946 Lewis[811] suggested that the term 'Raynaud's disease' should be reserved for those patients with typical symptoms of intermittent digital vasospasm in whom no cause could be found, while Raynaud's 'phenomenon' or 'syndrome' should be applied to patients with an established cause.[812] It has been suggested that most patients thought to have primary Raynaud's disease actually have some autoimmune abnormality and the term may become obsolete as new causes for the phenomenon are established.[813] Despite this there are some individuals whose digital vessels appear to be extremely sensitive to cold, and in whom no systemic or local abnormality can be found; for this reason it may be helpful to retain the term 'Raynaud's disease'. The episodic digital ischaemia is provoked by emotion,[814,815] trauma,[816] hormones,[817] and drugs[818] in addition to the normal cold trigger.

Raynaud described three classic phases: local syncope or blanching of the digits from digital arterial spasm; local asphyxia or cyanosis, when the fingers become swollen, blue and painful from stagnant anoxia; recovery or reactive hyperaemia when the fingers become red and tingling as the accumulation of vasoactive metabolites causes vasodilatation and again allows the blood to circulate.[811] These attacks are episodic and can occur in either the fingers or toes, in response to cold or emotional stimuli. Many attacks do not pass through all the colour changes described above, with either blanching or cyanosis predominating and the hyperaemic phase often being dimly perceived. The spectrum of attacks ranges from mild episodic pallor and paraesthesiae to constant pain, ulceration and frank necrosis (Fig. 10.86). Table 10.2 lists some of the many diseases which have been associated with Raynaud's colour changes.

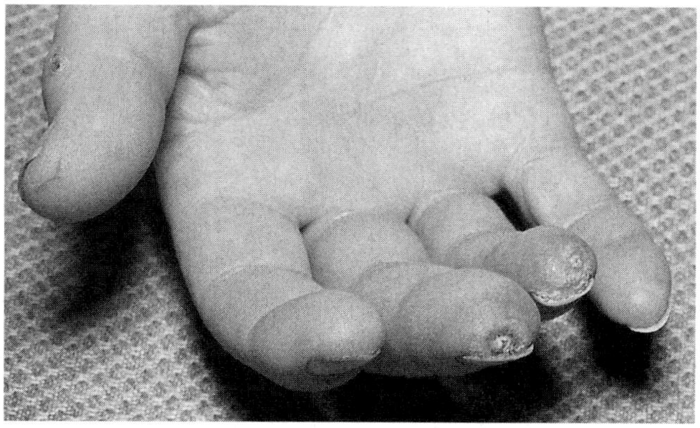

Fig. 10.86 Raynaud's disease with necrosis of fingertips.

Table 10.2 Secondary Raynaud's phenomenon

Connective tissue disorders
Systemic sclerosis (scleroderma)
Systemic lupus erythematosus
Dermatomyositis
Polyarteritis nodosa
Rheumatoid arthritis
Sjögren's syndrome
Arterial disease
Atherosclerosis
Buerger's disease (thromboangiitis obliterans)
Embolism from cervical rib
Trauma
Vibration-induced white finger
Sequel to frostbite
Blood disorders
Cold agglutinins
Cryoglobulinaemia
Hyperviscosity (polycythaemia)
Drugs
Oral contraceptives
β-blockers

Pathophysiology

A fixed obstruction of the small vessels may predispose to Raynaud's phenomenon without any increase in vasomotor activity, as a normal response to a cold challenge may cause temporary closure of the already diseased small vessels; a proximal occlusion may produce a similar effect by reducing the distal pressure and flow. In patients with normal vessels there is evidence that there is some fault in the α-receptors of the vascular smooth muscle.[819] This local fault must be an abnormality either of smooth muscle contraction or of arterial wall elasticity.[820] Much work has centred on associated haemorrheological faults: hyperviscosity, platelet dysfunction, hyperfibrinogenaemia, cold agglutinins and cryoglobulins have all been incriminated as a cause of vasospasm in some patients.[821–825]

REFERENCES

810. Raynaud M On Local Asphyxia and Symmetrical Gangrene of the Extremities. New Sydenham Society, London 1888
811. Lewis T Vascular Disorders of the Limbs. Macmillan, London 1946
812. Allen E V, Brown G E Am J Med Sci 1932; 183: 187
813. Anderson C J, Bardana E J et al Clin Res 1980; 28: 76
814. Fox R H Proc R Soc Med 1968; 61: 785
815. Freedman R R, Ianni P Br Med J 1983; 287: 1499
816. Loriga G In: Occupation and Health Encyclopaedia of Hygiene, Pathology and Social Welfare, vol 2. International Labour Office, London 1934
817. Eastcott H H Br Med J 1976; ii: 477
818. Marshal A J, Robert L J C, Barritt D W Br Med J 1976; i: 1498
819. Jamieson G G, Ludbrook J, Wilson A Circulation 1971; 44: 254
820. Sumner D S, Strandness D E Ann Surg 1972; 175: 294

Clinical features

60–90% of all sufferers from Raynaud's phenomenon are women. The majority are teenagers or young adults at onset.[826] The prevalence of this condition is said to range from 5 to 20%,[827,828] but the criteria accepted for diagnosis are fairly non-specific and are influenced by the ambient temperature. Environmental factors obviously affect the prevalence of the condition, with half of the food-processing employees exposed to intermittent hot and cold conditions being affected[829] and a similar proportion of those who constantly use vibrating tools.[830–832] The diagnosis is usually made from the clinical history of the attacks, but some use digital plethysmography and cold provocation tests as a means of confirmation.[833–835] Doppler mapping after cold stimulation may be a useful method of quantifying the severity of attacks.[836,837] Unilateral disease suggests a local organic cause such as a thoracic outlet syndrome or disease of the arterial wall, but unilateral vasospasm is also recognized.

The fingers of patients with Raynaud's syndrome often appear red or reddish-blue between attacks; the skin is usually dry and the nails brittle. Trophic changes develop in the finger pulps of more advanced cases, with chronic paronychia, ulceration and gangrene (Fig. 10.87). The wrist pulses are normally present; their absence suggests that the Raynaud's syndrome is secondary to disease of the large vessels. The neck must be examined to exclude cervical ribs, aneurysms and bruits. Digital pulses may be insonated with Doppler ultrasound and the pattern of occlusion after cold provocation can be recorded.[836,837] Arteriography is indicated if proximal atherosclerosis or digital occlusions are suspected. Plethysmography reveals low flow,[838] and thermography shows a temperature gradient developing between the hand and the fingers during body cooling and rewarming.[839]

Raynaud's phenomenon must be distinguished from acrocyanosis and other vasospastic disorders, including the normal cold response. Once a diagnosis of Raynaud's phenomenon is made, a battery of tests is indicated to exclude a possible cause. A full blood count and measurements of urea and electrolytes, erythrocyte sedimentation rate, cryoglobulins, antinuclear factor, rheumatoid antibodies, anti-mitochondrial and anti-thyroid antibodies should all be obtained.[840,841] When there is a history of dysphagia, a barium swallow may confirm the disordered peristalsis which is found in patients with scleroderma.

Management

Patients must be advised to keep warm, and avoid going out in ice and snow without gloves. Some may be able to move to a warm climate, and if this opportunity is available it should be taken. Cigarette smoking should be abandoned, and β-blockers[815] and ergot-containing drugs[841] should be avoided. Heated gloves may be helpful in reducing the number of attacks in winter.[842]

Numerous vasodilatory drugs such as inositol nicotinate, thymoxamine and naftidrofuryl oxalate have been tried and may help some patients.[843] Reserpine in a dose of 0.25 or 0.5 mg has a proven effect,[833,834] but can cause depression and other unpleasant side-effects. It, like guanethidine, can be used intravenously; reserpine has also been given intra-arterially.[843,844] Methyldopa and prazosin have also been used with some success[845,846] and more recently calcium-blocking agents like nifedipine have gained in popularity.[847,848] The 5-hydroxytryptamine antagonist ketanserin has also been used to treat Raynaud's disease.[849] Prostacyclin and prostaglandin E1, orally or by intravenous infusion, have been used to good effect, especially in patients with digital gangrene.[850–852] Repeated plasmapheresis has helped some severely affected patients,[853,854] but its place in management of this condition is not fully established. The anabolic steroid stanozolol which enhances fibrinolysis reduces the severity and frequency of attacks in some patients but its value is unpredictable.[855] Oxypentifylline, another agent which reduces blood viscosity, may also be helpful[856] and transdermal glyceryltrinitrate and prostaglandin analogues have been found to be of some benefit.[857–859]

Many patients with Raynaud's disease can achieve a satisfactory quality of life with minimal symptoms by cold avoidance, tobacco abstinence, and using warm or heated gloves in the winter months and vasodilatory drugs during severe attacks. A few however develop severe irreversible ischaemia of the digits and

REFERENCES

821. Goyle K G, Dormandy J A Lancet 1976; i: 1317
822. Perzanowski A, Mysliwiec M Wlad Lek 1972; 25: 771
823. Ellis H A, Stanworth D R J Clin Pathol 1961; 14: 179
824. Hutchinson J H, Howell R A Ann Intern Med 1953; 39: 350
825. Jarrett P E M, Morland M, Browse N L Br Med J 1978; 2: 523
826. Olsen N, Nielsen S C Scand J Clin Lab Invest 1978; 37: 761
827. Heslop J, Coggon D, Acheson E D J R Coll Gen Pract 1983; 33: 95
828. Holling H E Peripheral Vascular Disease; Diagnosis and Management. Lippincott, Philadelphia 1972
829. Mackiewisz A, Piskortz A J Cardiovasc Surg 1977; 18: 151
830. Loriga G In: Occupation and Health Encyclopaedia of Hygiene, Pathology and Social Welfare, vol 2. International Labour Office, London 1934
831. Agate J N, Druett H A Br J Indust Med 1947; 4: 141
832. Taylor W The Vibration Syndrome. Academic Press, London 1974
833. Krakenbuhl B, Nielsen S L, Lassen N A Scand J Clin Lab Invest 1977; 37: 71
834. Peacock J H Clin Sci 1960; 19: 505
835. Rosch J, Porter J M, Gralion B J Circulation 1977; 55: 807
836. Yao J S T, Gourmos G et al Surg Gyn Obstet 1972; 135: 373
837. O'Reilly M J G et al Br Med J 1979; 1: 1113
838. Coffman J D, Cohen S A New Engl J Med 1971; 285: 259
839. Charles C R, Carmick E S Arch Dermatol 1970; 101: 331
840. Porter J M, Rivers S P et al Am J Surg 1981; 142: 183
841. Henry L G, Blackwood J S et al Arch Surg 1975; 110: 929
842. Kempson G E, Coggon D, Acheson E D Br Med J 1983; 286: 268
843. Coffman J D New Engl J Med 1979; 300: 713
844. McFayden I J, Housley E, MacPherson A I S Arch Intern Med 1973; 132: 526
845. Varadi D P, Lawrence A M Arch Intern Med 1969; 124: 13
846. Taylor L M, Baur G M, Porter J M Ann Surg 1981; 193: 453
847. Kahan A, Weber S et al Ann Intern Med 1980; 94: 546
848. Smith C D, McKendry R J L Lancet 1982; ii: 1299
849. Stranden E, Roald O K, Krohg K Br Med J 1982; 285: 1069
850. Pardy B J, Lewis J D, Eastcott H H G Surgery 1980; 88: 826
851. Clifford P C, Martin M F R et al Br Med J 1980; 28: 1031
852. Belch J J F, Newman P et al Lancet 1983; i: 313
853. Talpos G, White J M et al Lancet 1978; i: 416
854. Dodds A J, O'Reilly M J G et al Br Med J 1979; 2: 1186
855. Jarrett P E M, Morland M, Browse N L Br Med J 1978; 2: 523
856. Roath S Br Med J 1986; 293: 88
857. Franks A G Lancet 1982; i: 76
858. Fischer M, Reinhold B et al Z Kardiol 1985; 74: 298
859. Dunger D B, Dillon M J et al Lancet 1985; ii: 50

require more drastic measures. Regular prostacyclin or prostaglandin analogue infusions at 4–8-weekly intervals may tide some patients through severe winters, and others should be considered for cervical sympathectomy.[860] This operation usually produces a dramatic early benefit, but this is invariably short-lived and after a year or two there is usually only a marginal improvement.[861,862] Recent developments in minimally invasive therapy have established the endoscopic transthoracic approach for cervical sympathectomy.

Prognosis

Raynaud's phenomenon is at present an incurable disorder which may be alleviated by a number of treatments, outlined above. Severe ischaemia of the fingertips may have to be treated by amputation in a small proportion of patients (usually those with collagen diseases such as scleroderma, which invariably have a more severe course).

Those with occupational Raynaud's phenomenon should be encouraged to change jobs. Aird (1st edition) emphasized the importance of vibration-induced 'white finger' (occupational Raynaud's phenomenon) in cold riveters and suggested that Sorbo pads in the gloves or on the handles of machines might help, together with a change to soft riveting every few months.

Acrocyanosis

This is a generalized cyanosis of the hands which follows exposure to cold and principally affects women. It is bilateral and symmetrical; although its intensity may vary, it is often associated with sluggish and awkward finger movements and a loss of sensation.[811] As the attacks subside, the hands become warm, red, swollen and painful. Between attacks the hands remain cold and the palms feel sweaty.

In contrast to the digital artery spasm found in Raynaud's disease, the spasm of acrocyanosis occurs in the smaller arteries and arterioles, thus slowing the circulation through the capillary bed.[863] The stagnant anoxia that develops encourages the accumulation of metabolites which cause the capillaries to dilate, increasing stagnation and producing the typical cold, blue cyanotic appearance.

Cold avoidance is the mainstay of treatment, and the benefits of vasodilators and sympathectomy are usually marginal.

Erythrocyanosis frigida

This disorder, sometimes known as Bazin's disease,[808] affects healthy young women of stout build, with fat and often hairless legs. As in acrocyanosis, the capillaries dilate while the arterioles remain constricted. In cold weather the legs develop dusky reddish-purple blotches in the skin of the calf just above the ankles. The skin over the triceps may also be affected, but is rarely a cause of complaint. In severe cases the skin of the lower half of the leg is purple, especially on its posterior aspect. The affected area blanches with pressure but rapidly refills on release, and is tender to friction, warmth and touch. Induration and nodularity are often palpable within the subcutaneous fat, and the skin overlying these 'chilblains' often feels cold to the touch.[864] These areas may break down and ulcerate and they then have to be differentiated from other types of cutaneous leg ulcers. In severe long-standing cases the whole limb develops a solid and persistent oedema. Histology of the nodules shows areas of fat necrosis with occasional giant cells, which is why the condition was originally thought of as a form of cutaneous tuberculosis.[865]

Yet again patients should be advised to protect themselves from the cold. Vasodilators and sympathectomy may be helpful in healing chilblains in the most severely affected cases.[864] Weight loss is also advised.

Erythromelalgia

This condition is characterized by redness of the extremities, which is often associated with burning pain.[807,866] The erythema and pain are accentuated by dependence, and even by the pressure of bed coverings or shoes. The pain may be eased by elevating and cooling the limbs. Erythromelalgia is a rare disorder which affects women more than men, and it is usually worse in the summer months.

It was originally thought to be a centrally mediated vasomotor neurosis, but Aird (1st edition) suggested that it was an inappropriate inflammatory response occurring within the skin of susceptible individuals, provoked by stimuli which were normally subliminal. The cause appears to be neurochemical with an inappropriate release of vasodilator substances which dilate the capillaries and stimulate pain endings. Serotonin (5-hydroxytryptamine) accumulation within the tissues may be responsible for the condition. Little has been added to this hypothesis in 20 years. It has even been suggested that erythromelalgia is related to vitamin deficiency: vitamin B thymoxamine has been used in its treatment, with some anecdotal success.

Erythromelalgia must be differentiated from polycythaemia, pernicious anaemia, Buerger's disease, gout, systemic lupus erythematosus, rheumatoid arthritis, venous insufficiency and peripheral neuritis. It may not be a distinct disorder.[807]

Treatment is empirical. Cooling may be helpful but is often unpredictable. Lumbar sympathectomy has helped some patients but others have been made worse,[808] and a local anaesthetic injection which allows the effect of sympathectomy to be evaluated should be tried first. Many patients are best treated by reassurance, combined with analgesic and psychotropic drugs where necessary. Aspirin, ergotamine and methysergide have also been used to treat the condition,[867,868] and the 5-hydroxytryptamine blocker ketanserin may also be worth trying. Nerve section has been used to relieve pain in patients with severe symptoms.

REFERENCES

860. Baddeley R M Br J Surg 1965; 52: 426
861. Gifford R W, Hines E A, Craig W M Circulation 1958; 17: 5
862. Johnson E N M, Summerly R, Birnstingl M Br Med J 1965; 962
863. Stern E S Br J Dermatol 1937; 49: 100
864. Lynn R B Surg Gynecol Obstet 1954; 99: 720
865. McGovern T, Wright I S Am Heart J 1941; 22: 583
866. Weir Mitchell S W Am J Med Sci 1878; 76: 2
867. Catchpole B N Lancet 1964; i: 909
868. Muhlbacher W Munch Med Wochenschr 1935; 82: 1242

Livedo reticularis

This is another rare vasospastic disorder in which cyanotic blotchy mottling of the skin, especially of the lower extremity, develops the appearance of an irregular network. Recently this change has been linked to systemic lupus erythematosus and the anticardiolipin antibody.[869] The cutaneous changes are produced by spasm of the arterioles and dilatation of the capillaries and venules, causing local stagnation. The meshwork appearance may be the result of the anatomy of the cutaneous circulation, with the pale areas representing the sites of arterial inflow and the cyanotic lacework the sluggish peripheral capillaries and venules.[870] Histological examination of the arterioles shows proliferation of the intima with a perivascular infiltration of inflammatory cells.

Apart from its bizarre appearances, the major reason for seeking advice is the development of cutaneous ulceration which is often indolent and resistant to treatment. Three categories of livedo are recognized:[871] cutaneous marmirato (only appearing on exposure to cold); idiopathic (persistent changes), and symptomatic (associated with polyarteritis nodosa, syphilis and systemic lupus erythematosus).

Patients should be advised to avoid cold, and occasionally lumbar sympathectomy or prostaglandin infusions may help to heal ulceration.

Ergotism

A diet of rye contaminated by *Claviceps purpurea* causes dry gangrene of the extremities if ingested for long periods.[872] Chronic migraine sufferers may also overdose with ergotamine tartrate.[873] There is a rapid response to withdrawal of the drug, providing gangrene has not become established. The chronic intake of ergot produces spasm of the small vessels and eventually intimal proliferation. Captopril, which inhibits angiotensin conversion, may be of specific benefit in reversing ergotamine-induced ischaemia.[874]

Hyperhidrosis

This is excessive sweating which is unrelated to heat but often stimulated by anxiety. It especially affects the palms of the hands and the soles of the feet though the whole body, especially the axillae and groins, may be involved.

It is debatable whether hyperhidrosis is a true vasomotor abnormality, but Aird (1st edition) classified it as such. It is no longer true to say that it is more common in men than women: the reverse is true.[875] It is a social stigma which discourages physical contact. It also interferes with writing, and although ledgers are now a thing of the past, Uriah Heep is the archetypical hyperhidrosis patient. The feet may also be affected, but are rarely considered as important as the hands. The axillae are another common site for hyperhidrosis, leaving unsightly damp patches on the armpits of shirts, blouses and dresses.[876]

Hyperhidrosis erythematosus traumatica is a rare occupational form of the condition in which excessive sweating occurs in skin which is in contact with a vibrating surface, especially a capstan lathe.[877] Symptoms disappear when the stimulus is removed. Hyperhidrosis can also occur on the face of patients with syringomyelia and in those with Frey's syndrome. The cause of the condition is not known but thyrotoxicosis must always be excluded.[878]

Treatment

Regular painting with aluminium hexachloride solution may reduce axillary hyperhidrosis[879] but many patients request a permanent cure. Good results are obtained by excising the hair-bearing area of the axillary skin, and this is the treatment of choice for axillary hyperhidrosis.[880] Cervical sympathectomy is an effective way of abolishing excessive palmar sweating, and lumbar sympathectomy alleviates its plantar counterpart.[881] Cervical sympathectomy may be performed by the cervical,[882] transaxillary[883] or thoracoscopic route,[884] depending upon surgical preference. Total sympathectomy may produce annoying postural hypotension, and in addition excessive sweating around the midriff may be annoying.[885] This procedure is, if possible, best avoided. Cervical or thoracoscopic sympathectomy provides excellent and long-lasting relief of symptoms.[886]

THE VASCULITIDES

These are a group of diseases in which inflammatory cells (principally lymphocytes, plasma cells and histiocytes) invade the arterial wall causing swelling and obstruction. A number of different patterns are seen with varying outcomes.

Thromboangiitis obliterans (Buerger's disease)[887]

This disease, originally called endarteritis by von Winiwarter,[888] almost exclusively affects young men in their 20s or 30s who are

REFERENCES

869. Harris E N, Gharavi A E, Hughes G R V Clin Rheum Dis 1985; 11: 591
870. Barker N M, Hines E A, Craig W M C K Am Heart J 1941; 21: 592
871. Williams C M, Goodman H JAMA 1925; 85: 955
872. Merhoff G C, Porter J M Ann Surg 1974; 180: 773
873. Von Storch T J JAMA 1938; 111: 293
874. Zimran A, Ofek B, Herschko C Br Med J 1984; 288: 364
875. Ellis J J Roy Coll Med 1982; 75: 555
876. Shelley W B, Hurley H J Br J Dermatol 1966; 78: 127
877. Davies J Br J Indust Med 1951; 8: 95
878. Ellis H Br J Hosp Med 1972; 1: 641
879. Scholes K T, Crow K D et al Br Med J 1978; 2: 84
880. Ellis H Am J Surg 1976; 45: 546
881. Gillespie J A Br J Hosp Med 1975; 418
882. Telford E D Br J Surg 1935; 23: 448
883. Atkins H J B Lancet 1949; ii: 1152
884. Hederman W P In: Greenhalgh R M (ed) Vascular and Endovascular Surgical Techniques. W B Saunders, London pp 281–284
885. White J C, Smitchwick R H The Autonomic Nervous System. Kimpton, London 1946
886. Greenhalgh R M, Rosengarten D S, Martin P Br Med J 1971; 1: 332
887. Buerger L Am J Med Sci 1908; 136: 567
888. Winiwarter Von F Arch Klin Chir 1879; 23: 203

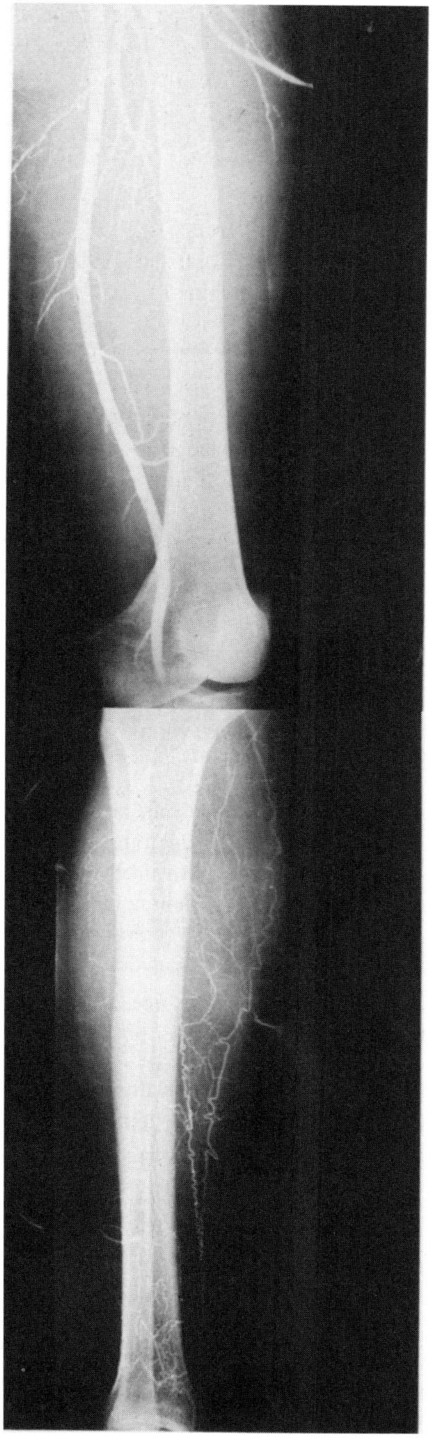

Fig. 10.87 An arteriogram showing the typical features of Buerger's disease. Multiple peripheral arterial occlusions are bypassed by 'corkscrew' collaterals.

tobacco addicts. Although it was first described in American Jews,[887] it is now recognized in all races and appears to be particularly common in Arabs, Indians and Chinese.[889,890] Some have cast doubt on the existence of the condition,[891] regarding it as a variant of accelerated atherosclerosis, but most now regard it as a separate disorder.[892,893]

Pathology

The distal (medium-sized) arteries of the lower limb become progressively obliterated, and these changes are also found in similar-sized arteries in the upper limb. Histology of the vessels shows a transmural round cell infiltration which is associated with intimal proliferation.[890] Luminal thrombosis is common. The accompanying veins and nerves may also become involved in the inflammatory process and recurrent superficial venous thrombosis is quite common. Collagen is laid down around the vessels, encasing them in a thick fibrous coat. The vasculitis may rarely involve the intra-abdominal vessels, including the mesenteric and renal arteries,[894,895] and may even occasionally affect the cerebral and coronary vessels.[896]

Clinical features

Patients usually present with chronic paronychias, poorly healing ulcers or digital gangrene.[897] These symptoms may have been preceded by a history of claudication. Superficial and deep vein thrombosis may be the first manifestation of Buerger's disease in a few patients, and erythema nodosum is occasionally one of the presenting complaints.

In the lower limbs the popliteal pulse is usually preserved, but the pedal pulses are often missing. The thickened vessels may themselves be palpable and tender.[892] Buerger's disease must be differentiated from early-onset atherosclerosis, diabetic arterial disease, thrombocythaemia, polycythaemia, recurrent embolism from the heart or an aneurysm, thrombophlebitis migrans, rheumatoid arteritis, homocysteinaemia and Behçet's disease. Arteriography shows a characteristic pattern of normal proximal vessels and distal occlusions with many 'corkscrew' collaterals[898–900] (Fig. 10.87). Biopsy of an occluded vessel may provide histological confirmation of the diagnosis.[893,901] Circulating antibodies to collagen are present in the blood of 45% of patients with Buerger's disease,[902] who often test positive for human leucocyte antigen B5.[903]

Management

Patients must be encouraged, bullied or cajoled to stop smoking. The risks of ignoring this advice must be clearly explained.[904]

REFERENCES

889. Goodman R M, Ewan B et al Am J Med 1965; 39: 601
890. Shionoya S Pathol Microbial 1975; 43: 163
891. Wessler S, Ming S et al New Engl J Med 1960; 262: 1149
892. McPherson J R, Juergens J L, Gifford R W Ann Intern Med 1963; 59: 288
893. McKusick V A, Harris W S et al JAMA 1962; 181: 5
894. Richards R L Br Med J 1953; 1: 478
895. Kinmonth J B Lancet 1948; ii: 717
896. Inada K, Katsumara T Angiology 1972; 23: 668
897. Ohta T, Shionoya S Br J Surg 1988; 75: 259
898. Szylagyi D E, Derusso F J, Elliot J P Arch Surg 1964; 88: 824
899. Suzuki S, Mine H et al Clin Radiol 1982; 33: 235
900. McKusick V A, Ottensen O E, Goodman R M Bull Johns Hopkins Hosp 1962; 110: 145
901. Shionoya S, Ban I et al Surgery 1974; 75: 695
902. Adar R, Papa M Z N Engl J Med 1984; 308: 113
903. McLoughlin G, Helsby R et al Br Med J 1976; ii: 1165

Progressive ischaemia leads first to digital and then more major amputations of all limbs.[892,895] Sympathectomy often relieves rest pain and allows nailfold infection and small incipient patches of gangrene to heal.[897,905] It is particularly valuable in Buerger's disease, perhaps because there is an important element of arterial spasm in the affected vessels. Surgical rather than chemical sympathectomy is often preferred to ensure complete and permanent nerve section.

Lumbar sympathectomy

The lumbar sympathetic chain is approached through a transverse incision at the level of the umbilicus on the side to be denervated. The oblique muscles of the abdominal wall are split or divided in the line of the incision until the peritoneum is exposed. This is freed off the deep surface of the transversus abdominis muscle by blunt dissection and retracted medially to allow the retroperitoneal space to be entered. The front of the psoas is displayed, and the groove between the medial border of psoas, the lumbar vertebrae and the aorta on the left or the vena cava on the right is defined. The lumbar sympathetic chain can usually be palpated as a firm cord punctuated by a number of swellings lying in the fibrofatty tissue of this groove on the front of the vertebrae. The chain is defined and picked up on a nerve hook, before it is dissected down to the pelvic brim and up to the crura of the diaphragm. All the rami that join the ganglia are divided. The first, second and third lumbar ganglia are resected. The wound is closed in layers with suction drainage.

Alternative treatments and progress

Apart from sympathectomy, there is little that avoids digital ablation, which is reserved for dead and devitalized tissue or bone. Bypass surgery is usually impossible and fruitless, although it has been successful.[906] Antibiotics, foot care, prostaglandins[907] and analgesics may all be tried in an attempt to tide patients over periods of acute ischaemia until collaterals develop. Many patients who cannot abandon smoking end up with one or more major amputations.

Takayasu's disease (pulseless disease)

In 1908 Takayasu[908] reported that young Japanese women developed a disease in which they lost pulses in one or more branches of the aortic arch. It is now recognized that this disease occurs in occidentals as well as Orientals, and in men as well as women.[909,910] Many patients seen in the west have a Turkish and Middle Eastern ancestry. The symptoms depend on which vessel is affected but disease in the carotid and subclavian arteries can cause transient ischaemic attacks, blindness, stroke or arm claudication, and ischaemia.[911] Aortic disease must be differentiated from coarctation and produces similar symptoms. The aortic arch and its branches, the descending, thoracic and the abdominal aorta can all be affected. The arteritis gives rise to local pain and is often accompanied by pyrexia, malaise and an elevated sedimentation rate in the acute stage. Arteriography demonstrates a smooth tapering stenosis (Fig. 10.88) or total occlusion.

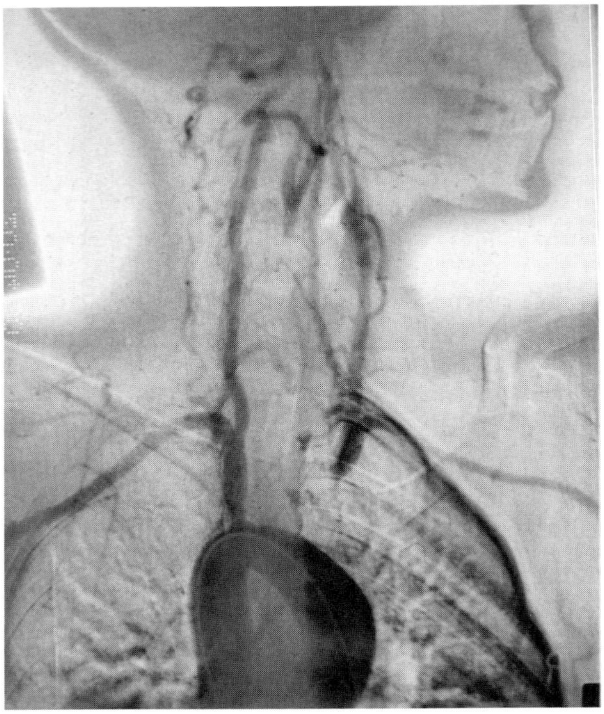

Fig. 10.88 An arch arteriogram showing changes consistent with Takayasu's disease.

Surgical bypass to normal vessels beyond the limits of the disease is required for ischaemic symptoms,[912,913] and has rewarding results.[914] The disease tends to burn itself out with time, and the place of steroids in reducing inflammation remains unproven.[915] The same is true of azathioprine and cyclosporin. Five-year survival from the time of diagnosis ranges from 60 to 80%.[916,917]

Temporal arteritis

This condition, first described by Jonathan Hutchinson in 1889,[918] is usually seen after the age of 60, and is twice as common in women as men.[919] The arteritis usually starts with malaise, fever and myalgia, which often persist for several months. A frontoparietal headache then develops and the skin over the affected area

REFERENCES

904. Hill G L Br J Surg 1974; 61: 476
905. Kunlin J, Lengua F et al J Cardiovasc Surg 1973; 1: 21
906. Shionoya S, Ban I et al Br J Surg 1976; 63: 841
907. Szczeklik A, Cryglewski R J et al Thromb Res 1980; 191
908. Takayasu M Acta Soc Ophthalmol 1908; 12: 554
909. Schire V, Asherton R A Q J Med 1964; 33: 439
910. Caccamise W E, Whitman J F Am Heart J 1952; 44: 629
911. Lupi-Herrera E, Sanchez-Torres G et al Am Heart J 1977; 93: 94
912. Crawford E S, De Bakey M E et al J Thorac Cardiovasc Surg 1962; 43: 38
913. Thompson B W, Read R C, Campbell G S Arch Surg 1969; 98: 607
914. Fraga A, Mintz G et al Arthritis Rheum 1976; 15: 617
915. Robbs J V, Human R R et al Vasc Surg 1986; 3: 605
916. Ishikawa I C Circulation 1970; 57: 27
917. Urban-Waern A, Anderson P, Hemmingsson A Angiology 1983; 17: 311
918. Hutchinson J Arch Surg (Lond) 1889; 1: 323
919. Huston K A, Hunder G G et al Ann Intern Med 1978; 88: 162

is tender to touch and sometimes red.[920] The superficial temporal artery may be visible, thickened and tender, with absent pulsation. Visual loss occurs in between one third and one half of all cases; if this is left untreated it becomes permanent.[921] Retinoscopy is initially normal, but at a later stage ischaemic papillopathy develops and there may be evidence of occlusion of the central retinal artery or its branches.[921] Ophthalmoplegia also occurs. There may be an associated arteritis in the peripheral vessels causing, for example, brachial artery occlusion.

The diagnosis is usually made by taking a segment of the superficial temporal artery for biopsy under local anaesthetic, through an incision placed directly over the vessel. Histology shows a florid intimal thickening, a round cell infiltration through all coats of the arterial wall which is associated with destruction of the internal elastic lamina, and the presence of a few giant cells.[919,920] Treatment is by systemic steroids, which should begin immediately in large doses (60 mg prednisone a day) but can then be reduced at a later stage.[922] Steroids reduce the incidence of blindness.[923] Some 40% of biopsies do not show any of the characteristic histological features;[924] if the diagnosis is strongly suspected on clinical grounds, treatment with steroids should be started without delay. Azathioprine may also be used to treat patients with this condition and has an important steroid-sparing role.[925]

VASCULAR TUMOURS

Angiomas have been discussed and are properly considered as malformations (hamartomas) rather than as benign tumours.

Glomus tumour (angiomyoneuroma, glomangioma)

This is the only true benign tumour of blood vessels. It is a small painful tumour originally described by Wood in 1829.[926] The glomus tumour lies in the skin but may grow into the deeper layers, although its greatest diameter is seldom more than a few millimetres. The largest on record measured 2.5 × 3.6 cm.[927] It usually has a well marked capsule, especially on the deep surface of the tumour. Histologically the tumour consists of a tangled mass of blood vessels lined by a layer of flattened or swollen endothelial cells on a supporting fibrous stroma, surrounded by epithelial cells and smooth muscle fibres: the latter being well differentiated or taking the form of muscle fibrils within the epithelial cells.[928,929] The epithelioid glomus cells, which have well defined outlines, have short contractile fibrils within their cytoplasm; the glomus cells often lie both inside and outside the muscular layer of the vessel wall and are mixed up with myelinated and non-myelinated nerve fibres. The haemangiopericytoma first described by Stout & Murray[930] is a similar type of tumour but is not as painful or as vascular. The cutaneous myoma arising from the erector pili may also occasionally be mistaken for a glomus tumour.[931]

Clinical features

Glomus tumours usually occur in the extremities: two thirds are in the upper limb but some arise on the trunk.[932] Half develop in the digits, one third in a subungual position. Tumours tend to develop on the fingers and toes in women, while in men they are usually more centrally placed. The peak incidence is in the 20s. Less than 2% are painless. Most tumours give rise to exquisite pain which is burning, throbbing or bursting in nature, occurring in paroxysms which are brought on by pressure, heat or cold,[928,932,933] although the pain can arise spontaneously. Relief is often sought by the application of heat or cold, and a bandage or glove is occasionally worn for protection. The pain may be localized or so diffuse that the tiny trigger spot cannot be located. The nail is often left uncut by the patient if the tumour is subungual; sudden unexpected trauma can cause fainting. Occasionally relief is obtained by gentle pressure to empty the tumour, rendering it colourless and painless for several hours.[934] The pain is so disproportionate to the size of the tumour that a psychoneurosis may be suspected. The pain may be precisely located by stroking the affected area with a pinhead. The pain pathways are not clearly understood as pain is not abolished by blocking both the sympathetic and somatic nerves. The affected extremity may occasionally become flushed and warm, or pallid, cold and sweaty. Most tumours are blue or purplish in colour; few are red. The colour may change with alteration in the position of the limb or compression of the feeding and draining vessels. The colour of a subungual tumour does not show through the nail, making it difficult to detect, and many of the superficial cutaneous tumours are impalpable and invisible because the overlying skin is often thick and wrinkled. The nail overlying a subungual tumour is often thickened, unduly convex and longitudinally striated from retarded growth. The bone of the underlying phalanx may be eroded, excavated or rarefied and the affected extremity is usually warmer than its fellow of the opposite side. During an attack of pain the whole extremity may become cool and sweaty, and a unilateral Horner's syndrome may even develop.

Treatment is by surgical excision. A wide margin of tissue must be taken around the possible site of an invisible, impalpable tumour to ensure its satisfactory removal.[935]

Angiosarcoma

This tumour affects young men and women and usually develops in the skin and soft tissues of the extremities. Rapid growth produces a bulky, painful, hot tumour, which is liable to bleed.[936] A

REFERENCES

920. Meadows S P Proc R Soc Med 1966; 59: 329
921. Graham E, Holland A et al Br Med J 198; 282: 269
922. Hunder G G, Sheps S G et al Ann Intern Med 1975; 82: 613
923. Bengisson B A, Malmvall B E Acta Med Scand 1982; (suppl 658)
924. Allsop C J, Gallagher P J Am J Surg Pathol 1981; 5: 317
925. Desilva M, Hazelman B L Ann Rheum Dis 1986; 445: 136
926. Wood W Trans Med Chir Soc Edin 1829; 3: 317
927. Grant R T Heart 1930; 15: 281
928. Masson P Lyon Chir 1924; 21: 257
929. Lendrum A D, Mackey W A Br Med J 1939; 2: 676
930. Stout A P, Murray M R Ann Surg 1942; 116: 26
931. Beaton L E, Davis L Q Bull Northwest Univ Med School 1941; 15: 245
932. Mullis W F, Rosato F E et al Surg Gynecol Obstet 1972; 135: 705
933. Love J G Minn Med 1949; 32: 275
934. Mason M L, Weil A Surg Gynecol Obstet 1934; 58: 807
935. Strahan J, Bailie H W C Br J Surg 1972; 59: 91

special variety affects the nasal cavity. Death is usually the result of lung metastases. Although angiosarcomas are radiosensitive and respond to chemotherapy, radical amputation is still advised.

A number of subtypes are recognised:

1. A haemangioendothelioma arises in bone[937] and may also affect the spleen.

2. Angiosarcomata may occasionally develop in a long-standing developmental angioma. This is a rare condition but should be considered if a long-standing angioma suddenly increases in size or becomes painful. Surgical excision for biopsy is then indicated.

3. Angiosarcomas can arise in the liver, causing massive hepatic enlargement and ascites.[938] These tumours occur in children and young adults and must be differentiated from other liver tumours, such as hepatoblastomas (see Chapter 31). The prognosis is poor.

4. Angiosarcomas can arise in chronically lymphoedematous limbs, although lymphangiosarcoma is the more usual lesion.[939]

Kaposi's multiple haemangiosarcoma[940]

The incidence of this 'tumour' has increased dramatically with the advent of acquired immune deficiency syndrome.[941] Until the 1980s this was a rare tumour, predominantly affecting young Mediterranean men between their teens and 40s.[942] It was also reported to be common in Bantus and in other African nationalities.[943] It usually starts in the skin of the lower extremity or the penis. A bluish-red well demarcated macule appears first and grows. Other macules then appear close by and these enlarge to fuse with the first macule, becoming elevated as they grow (Fig. 9.61). The other lower limb is often affected at the same time and the lesion spreads up the leg and on to the lower part of the trunk.[942,944] The nodules are painless, apart from those on the penis or the soles of the feet. Spread is usually by the blood stream to the liver and lungs.[945] This diagnosis should be suspected in all homosexuals or haemophiliacs who develop suggestive skin lesions. The diagnosis is confirmed by biopsy[946] and by testing the blood for antibodies to the human immunodeficiency virus.[947] Histologically the blood spaces within the tumour are surrounded by anaplastic fibroblasts with nuclear atypia and multiple mitotic patterns.

Treatment is by a combination of cytotoxic chemotherapeutic agents and superficial irradiation.[948] In some patients a good initial response is obtained but eventually all tumours recur and death is inevitable.

Carotid body tumours (chemodectomas)

The carotid body is situated at the carotid bifurcation and contains numerous sinusoidal capillaries which allow the blood to come in close contact with the glomus cells that form its main structure. These cells are thought to originate from paraganglionic cells derived from neural crest.[949,950] They are richly supplied by afferent nerve endings (chemoreceptors) and are sensitive to changes in the oxygen, carbon dioxide content and pH of the perfusing blood. They stimulate the cardiovascular and respiratory centres to alter heart rate and sympathetic tone to maintain homeostasis. Chemoreceptors are also found in the aortic arch, the internal jugular vein, the middle ear, the ganglion nodosum of the vagus nerve and the retroperitoneum around the abdominal aorta in the organ of Zuckerkandl.[951]

Pathology

Tumours of the carotid body are rare but well recognized. Just over 200 cases had been reported by 1943,[952] and 546 by 1960;[953] the Cleveland clinic reported a total experience of 41 cases in 54 years,[954] and chemodectomas represented 0.03% of all tumours on the Christie Hospital tumour register.[955] Chemodectomas at other sites are rarer still. These tumours have an equal sex distribution and occur over a wide age range, with a median in the fifth decade.[956] They can be familial, and a third of the familial tumours are reported to be bilateral. 10% of non-familial tumours are bilateral.[957] Chronic hypoxia is thought to be a causal factor and there is a high incidence of carotid body tumours in Peru and Mexico City.[958]

Chemodectomas are ovoid tumours arising in the carotid bifurcation, distorting and encasing the carotid vessels. Hutchinson called them 'potato tumours' because he thought a potato could be likened to their macroscopic appearance on transection,[959] but they usually appear more reddish-brown and are highly vascular, making them easily compressible. The tumour cells are polygonal or spindle-shaped, and the neoplastic cell masses are enclosed in a box-like framework of fine connective tissue with an extensive sinusoidal blood supply. The microscopic appearances are unhelpful in predicting malignant behaviour,[960] but local invasion and lymphatic or blood-borne metastases occur in between 2.5 and 50% of cases,[961,962] though some regard all tumours as malign.[963] Left untreated, about 5–10% develop metastases within 10 years.[964]

REFERENCES

936. Willis A T Pathology of Tumours. Butterworths, London 1945
937. Stout A P Ann Surg 1943; 118: 445
938. Pollard S, Millward-Sadier G H J Clin Pathol 1974; 27: 214
939. Stewart F W, Treves N Cancer 1948; 1: 64
940. Kaposi M Arch Dermatol Syph 1872; 4: 265
941. Sonnabend J, Wilkins S S, Purtilo T JAMA 1983; 249: 2370
942. McCarthy W D, Pack G T Surg Gynecol Obstet 1950; 91: 465
943. Rothman S Arch Dermatol 1962; 85: 311
944. Ziegler J L et al Semin Oncol 1984; 11: 47
945. Davis J N Y J Med 1968; 68: 2067
946. Willis A T Pathology of Tumours. Butterworths, London 1945
947. Pinching A J Clin Exp Immunol 1984; 56: 1
948. Volberding P Semin Oncol 1984; 11: 60
949. Kohn A Arch Mike Anat 1903; 263: 268
950. Mulligan R M Syllabus of Human Neoplasms. Lea & Febiger, Philadelphia 1950
951. Glenner G G, Grimley P M Tumours of the Extradrenal Paraganglion System (including Chemodectomas). Atlas of Tumour Pathology. Armed Forces Institute of Pathology, Washington DC 1974
952. Kinmonth J B, Lockhart K T St Thomas' Gaz 1943; 41: 4
953. Dallachy R, Simpson I C J Laryngol Otol 1960; 74: 217
954. Lees C D, Levine H L et al Am J Surg 1981; 142: 362
955. Jackson A W, Koshiba R Proc R Soc Med 1974; 67: 267
956. Mitchell D C, Clyne C A C Br J Surg 1985; 72: 903
957. Rush B F Ann Surg 1963; 157: 633
958. Farr H W Cancer J Clin 1980; 30: 260
959. Hutchinson J Illus Med News 1888; 1: 50
960. Pryse-Davis J, Dawson I M Cancer 1964; 17: 185

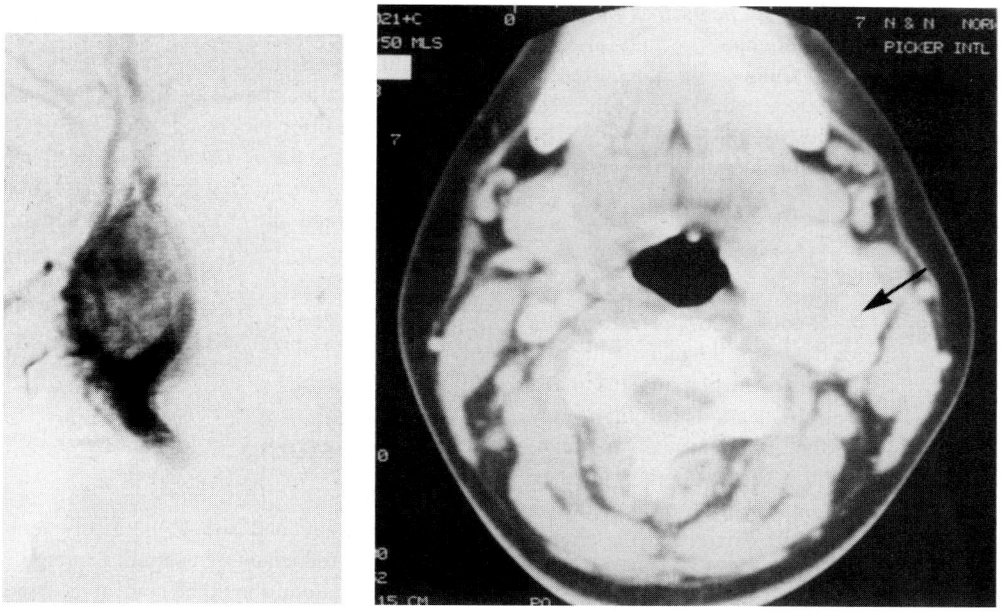

a b

Fig. 10.89 **(a)** A carotid body tumour causing splaying of the carotid bifurcation; the vascularity of the tumour can be seen. **(b)** Computerized tomography scan of the neck also shows the tumour.

Clinical features

Patients present with solitary or bilateral lumps just in front of and deep to the anterior border of the sternomastoid muscle. The mass is closely related to the carotid pulse, usually at the level of the hyoid bone.[965] The carotid pulse is transmitted by the tumour but on occasions the tumour is so vascular that it appears to be truly expansile. The tumour may decrease in size with compression and in 20% there is a thrill or an audible bruit over a highly vascular tumour.[966] The mass can be shown to move laterally but not vertically, and this movement displaces the carotid pulse. A carotid body tumour must be differentiated from a branchial cyst, a neurofibroma and an enlarged lymph node. A third are incorrectly diagnosed on clinical examination. Further dissection should be abandoned without a biopsy being taken if a tumour is found unexpectedly at operation.[965] Re-exploration can then be carried out by an experienced vascular surgeon after appropriate investigation.

Investigations

Carotid arteriography by catheter, needle[963,967] or intravenous digital subtraction arteriography[968] shows a splayed carotid bifurcation containing a highly vascular tumour (Fig. 10.89a). Duplex ultrasonography[969] and CT scanning[968] (Fig. 10.89b) are alternative means of diagnosis but neither gives any information on the cerebral circulation or the potential collaterals. MR angiography also provides detailed images.

Management

Carotid body tumours enlarge slowly but inexorably if left untreated and may eventually obstruct the carotid vessels. There is a greater risk of malignancy as their size increases, and the larger the tumour the more difficult the operation. The carotid bifurcation is exposed as for a carotid endarterectomy. The vessels are isolated above and below the tumour and taped. The tumour is then dissected off the vessels in the subadventitial plane,[970,971] using careful sharp dissection and meticulous haemostasis, with underrunning of large branches and diathermy of the smaller feeding vessels. There is usually a plane of cleavage along the posterior border of the internal carotid artery. The external carotid artery can be ligated and divided if necessary to provide better access. A shunt and interposition vein graft can be used if the internal carotid artery has to be sacrificed during removal of the tumour.[972]

Results and complications

Surgical treatment is the method of choice in patients under the age of 50, but in older patients a 'watch' policy may be adopted. The small risk of hemiplegia (1–2%) and the greater risk of nerve palsy, which varies between 12 and 40%, must be explained to the patient before operation; some will then decline surgery.[968] Radiotherapy

REFERENCES

961. Harrington S W, Clagett O T, Dockerty M B Ann Surg 1941; 114: 820
962. Whinster W T, Massen A F Cancer 1970; 26: 239
963. Dent T L, Thompson N W, Fry W Y Surgery 1976; 80: 365
964. Shamblin W R, Remine W H et al Am J Surg 1971; 122: 732
965. Browse N L Br Med J 1982; 284: 1507
966. Wilson R Surgery 1966; 59: 483
967. Lees C D, Levine H E et al Am J Surg 1971; 122: 732
968. McPherson G A D, Halliday A W, Mansfield A O Br J Surg 1989; 76: 33
969. Dickinson P H, Griffin S M et al Br J Surg 1986; 72: 14
970. Gordon-Taylor G Br J Surg 1940; 28: 163
971. Vanasperen D C, Boer F R S et al Br J Surg 1981; 68: 433
972. Javid H, Chawla S K et al Arch Surg 1976; 111: 344

has been shown to be effective and this may be used as the treatment of choice in elderly, high-risk patients.[956] It may also be employed to treat patients with residual tumour or local recurrence. Preoperative embolization has been advocated to reduce the size and vascularity of large tumours but few use this technique.[971] The mortality of the operation has declined considerably in recent years and should be in the order of 1 to 2%.[965,966,968,969]

Glomus jugulare tumour

This is a rare tumour arising in the jugular bulb, presenting as a lump situated between the posterior border of the mandibular and the mastoid processes.[951,968,973,974] Apart from noticing the mass, patients may complain of buzzing in the head. This tumour may easily be mistaken for a carotid body tumour (it is usually too high) or a parotid neoplasm (it is usually too deep). Glomus jugulare tumours may arise in the vagus, glossopharyngeal or hypoglossal nerves and can extend up into the middle ear or into the cranial cavity. Excision may be followed by palsies of the 10th, 11th, and 12th nerves. Radiotherapy is an alternative method of treatment.

MISCELLANEOUS CONDITIONS

Radiation arteritis

This follows high doses of irradiation applied near major arteries. The carotid and iliac arteries are often affected because irradiation to the neck and pelvis is the usual treatment for cervical lymphomas and pelvic tumours.[975] Damage to the vasa vasorum leads to intimal thickening, transmural fibrosis and eventually to arterial occlusion. Occluded segments can be treated by bypass to healthy vessels.

Ainhum (dactylolysis spontanea)

This is a rare condition affecting black races.[976] Digital gangrene develops in a single digit, usually the fifth toe, which mummifies and either separates or is amputated. The aetiology of this condition is obscure but it appears to be self-limiting. A local vasculitis is suspected.

Carotid sinus syndrome

The baroreceptors of the carotid sinus normally maintain a constant blood pressure by means of reflex changes in the heart and peripheral blood vessels.[977] Pathological instability or hypersensitivity of the carotid sinus may cause episodes of bradycardia or asystole, transient falls in blood pressure, or syncopal attacks.[978,979] These attacks may be initiated by sudden turning of the head or follow undue pressure on the neck. Attacks can be reproduced by pressure over the sinus and, if troublesome, may be abolished by sectioning the carotid sinus nerve.[980,981]

Leiomyomas and leiomyosarcomas

Leiomyomas and leiomyosarcomas are extremely rare in arteries. They are much more common in veins (see Chapter 11).

AMPUTATION

Successful revascularization procedures in the lower limb may allow limited digital or transmetatarsal amputations which inevitably fail if the blood supply of the foot cannot be improved. Every effort should be made to obtain a successful below-knee amputation in patients in whom reconstruction is impossible, and through-knee and above-knee amputation should be regarded as inferior options to be avoided whenever possible.[982] There are a few exceptions: for example when the patient has severe arthritis of the knee, a marked fixed flexion deformity or when the limb to be amputated is paralysed from a stroke so that a prosthesis is unlikely to be used.

The ideal stump

This should heal by first intention; the scar should not have to transmit pressure and should be freely mobile; the soft tissue should not be redundant, but should fit snugly over a well rounded bone end; the stump should be conical in shape and free from pain. The joints above the stump should be fully mobile.[983]

After treatment

The stump should be inspected at 5–7 days if the postoperative course is uncomplicated, but the dressings may be taken down earlier if infection or poor healing is suspected. Patients should start to carry out exercises to strengthen the upper limb muscles as soon as possible; these should ideally begin before surgery.[984] The amputation stump can be mobilized and strengthened by exercises from 24 to 48 h after operation, but weight bearing should not start until 5 or 6 days have passed, and the fashion of immediate application of a temporary prosthesis in theatre with very early weight bearing has now been largely abandoned.[985] If the stump is satisfactory by 5 or 6 days, then the pneumatic post-amputation mobility (PAM) aid[986] (Fig. 10.90) can be applied to the stump to allow relatively early mobilization. This apparatus consists of an inflatable bag inside a metal frame which is attached to a pylon. The pneumatic bag is inflated to act as a socket and this allows early walking practice without the necessity for casting a formal socket. Less emphasis is now placed on bandaging, and more on the early use of the pneumatic mobility aid.

REFERENCES

973. Alford B R, Guildford F R Laryngoscope 1962; 72: 765
974. Taylor D M, Alford B R, Greenberg S D Arch Otolaryngol 1965; 82: 5
975. Lawson J A J Cardiovasc Surg 1985; 26: 151
976. Hircherson D C Ann Surg 1950; 132: 312
977. Waller A Proc R Soc Med 1862; 11: 302
978. Weiss S, Baker J P Medicine(Balt) 1933; 12: 297
979. Hutchinson E C, Stock J P P Lancet 1960; ii: 445
980. Eascott H H G Arterial Surgery. Pitman, London 1969
981. Capps F C W, Detakats G J Clin Invest 1938; 17: 385
982. McCollum P T, Spence V A, Walker W F Br J Surg 1988; 75: 1193
983. Brodie I A O D Br J Hosp Med 1970; 4: 596
984. Anonymous Br Med J 1981; 283: 684
985. Vitali M, Readhead R G Ann R Coll Surg Engl 1967; 40: 251
986. Little J M, Gosling L, Weeks A Med J Aust 1972; 1: 1300

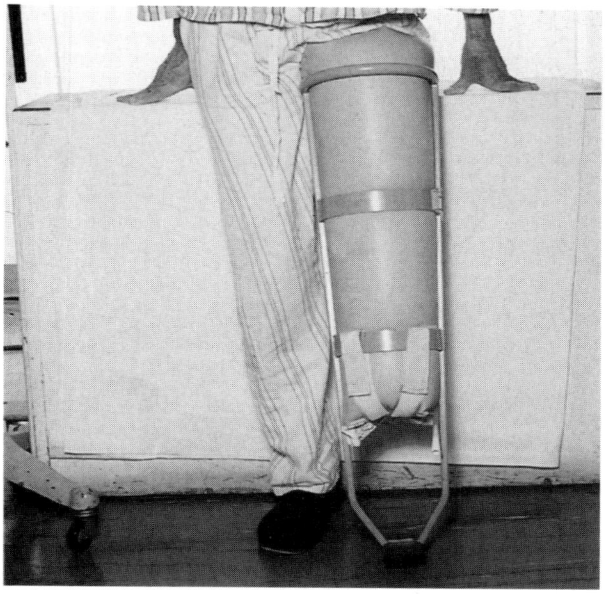

Fig. 10.90 The pneumatic post-amputation mobility (PAM) aid.

Early measurement and assessment of the stump by a prosthetist allows prompt fitting of the definitive limb. The development of lightweight (carbon-fibre) modular prostheses[987] has reduced production time and increased mobility. It is hoped that administrative changes in the amputation service around the world will continue to improve the speed of obtaining prostheses.[988]

Complications

1. *Haematoma formation*. This should be avoided by careful haemostasis and the provision of adequate drainage. Should it occur formal evacuation is required.

2. *Infection*. This cannot be completely avoided, especially if there is infected gangrene in the amputated tissues. Avoidance of haematomas is important. A swab should be taken if possible two or more days prior to operation so that appropriate antibiotics can be given. Penicillin and metronidazole are effective against clostridia and other anaerobes.[989] Formal drainage is occasionally required and healing often then takes place by secondary intention.

3. *Ischaemic necrosis*. This is the most common complication after amputations performed for ischaemia and is the result of poor technique. Haematomas, suturing under tension and incorrect selection of the level of amputation with persisting ischaemia of the skin flaps are usually responsible.[990]

4. *Osteomyelitis*. This is relatively unusual since the advent of antibiotics. If it occurs it may necessitate re-amputation at a higher level.[991]

5. *Spurs and osteophytes*. These only require treatment if they cause pain. Treatment usually consists of revision of the amputation to a higher level.

6. *Ulceration of the stump*. This can be the result of infection and ischaemia, or pressure and friction from the prosthesis. This usually requires refashioning of the stump or recasting the socket.

7. *Scar*. An adherent or uncomfortable scar may require refashioning.

8. *Stump neuroma*. This is usually the result of a failure to cut back the nerves far enough. A thick bulbous neuroma forms on the transected nerve; this is exquisitely painful when compressed by a prosthesis. Shooting pain is produced by localized pressure. Local anaesthetic infiltration usually abolishes the pain and confirms the diagnosis. The pain may also be helped by repeated percussion or application of a mechanical vibrator.[992] Transcutaneous electrical nerve stimulation may also prove effective (see Chapter 5). The definitive treatment is to section the nerve at a higher level, but the neuroma may still recur.

9. *Phantom limb*. This curious phenomenon is experienced by most amputees to some extent.[993] In some the painful sensation derived from a non-existent limb becomes unbearable and disrupts their life, making treatment imperative. Antidepressant tablets, tranquillizers, hypnotherapy and acupuncture have all been tried with some success, but carbamazepine (Tegretol) and nerve division appear to be of greater value.[994] The phantom limb pain is thought to be caused by persistence of the sensory cortex, and is often most severe in the fingers and toes, which have the largest cortical representation. In most cases it quickly fades, but may persist as 'telescoping', with the feeling that the foot is attached to the thigh, or the hand to the upper arm when the patient goes to scratch the non-existent digit. It is a strange fact that if several fingers are amputated, only the first is affected by phantom feelings, and if multiple amputations are required, only the first ever causes a phantom.[995] Local and repeated percussion with a patella hammer over a painful spot may occasionally alleviate a painful phantom. Prior insertion of epidural anaesthesia often avoids the subsequent development of phantom limb.[996]

10. *Causalgia*. This is an intractable burning type of pain thought to result from sympathetic fibres growing down systemic nerves. It is often associated with a smooth red shiny skin. Guanethidine blocks or sympathectomy may bring relief.[997]

11. *Jactitation*. This unexplained sudden 'jumping' of the leg may result from a neuroma or from a psychogenic cause.

12. *Aneurysms and arteriovenous fistulae*. These are rare complications that may occasionally require treatment.

13. *Fixed flexion deformity*. This develops if patients with rest pain or gangrene are left in severe pain for some time before coming to amputation. The hip and knee are flexed in an effort to provide relief; if this position is maintained for long periods,

REFERENCES

987. Foorte J, Lawrence R B, Davies R M International Rehab Med 1984; 6: 72
988. McColl I Review of Artificial Limb and Appliance Centre Service: The Report of an Independent Working Party. DHSS, London 1986
989. Haynes I G, Middleton M D Ann Roy Coll Surg Eng 1981; 63: 342
990. Jamieson C W, Hill D Br J Surg 1981; 63: 693
991. Desai Y, Robbs J V, Keenan J P Br J Surg 1986; 73: 392
992. Richie Russell W M R Med J 1949; 1: 1024
993. Weir-Mitchell S Injuries of Nerves and Their Consequences. Lippincott, Philadelphia 1872
994. Sherman R A, Tippens J K Orthopaedics 1982; 5: 1595
995. Sunderland S Nerves and Nerve Injuries. Livingstone, Edinburgh 1968
996. Bach S, Noreng M, Tjellden N Pain 1988; 33: 297
997. Glynn C J, Basedow R W, Walsh J A Br J Anaesth 1981; 53: 1297

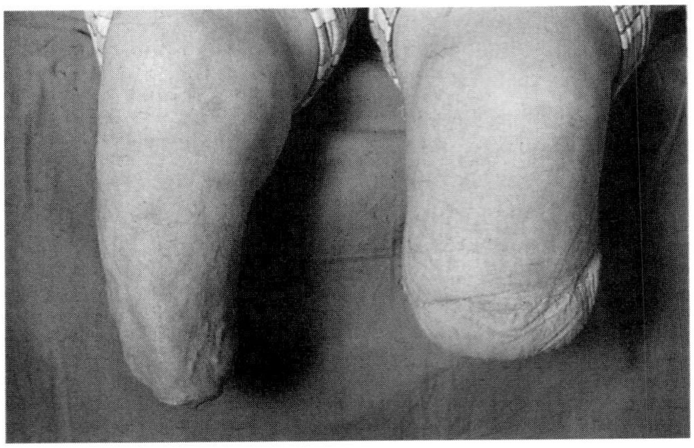

Fig. 10.91 A poor below-knee stump caused by muscle retraction on the right leg; a good stump on the left leg.

contractures may develop. This complication is best avoided by regular active movements. Physiotherapy may help, or manipulation under anaesthesia may be necessary, and even this may not be successful when the contracture is long-standing. Amputation at a higher level is then required.

14. *Muscle herniation.* The muscles may slip off the bone leaving it uncovered and ruining the shape of the stump, which may no longer fit its socket (Fig. 10.91). Refashioning is required.

15. *Non-union.* This may occur between the patella and the end of the femur after a Stokes–Gritti amputation.[998] The stump should be refashioned to an above-knee amputation if this happens.

16. *Disruption of the amputation stump* following falls is a major problem that often leads to refashioning to a higher level.

Guillotine amputation[999]

This method of amputation is used when healing cannot be guaranteed in the presence of severe tissue trauma or infection. It aims to remove all the dead and potentially dangerous tissue. Flaps are raised and the tissues are divided down the bone which is then transected. The flaps are left open with the end of the stump being covered by sterile dressings. The operation can be performed in a field hospital during war-time, allowing definitive surgery to be carried out in a more formal setting 3–5 days later when further excision of any necrotic tissue is undertaken before the flaps are sutured.

Amputations at specific sites

The toes

Toe amputations are carried out through racket-shaped incisions with the bone being divided through the shaft of the phalanx or through the neck of the underlying metacarpal bone. Although it is tempting to amputate through a joint, this leaves avascular cartilage beneath the suture which may cause poor healing.[1000] The dorsal and ventral tendons are divided at the same level as the bone, and the digital vessels are ligated. Individual toes cannot be successfully amputated for ischaemia unless the blood supply has been improved. Infective diabetic gangrene of individual toes responds well to digital amputation in the presence of a good blood supply.

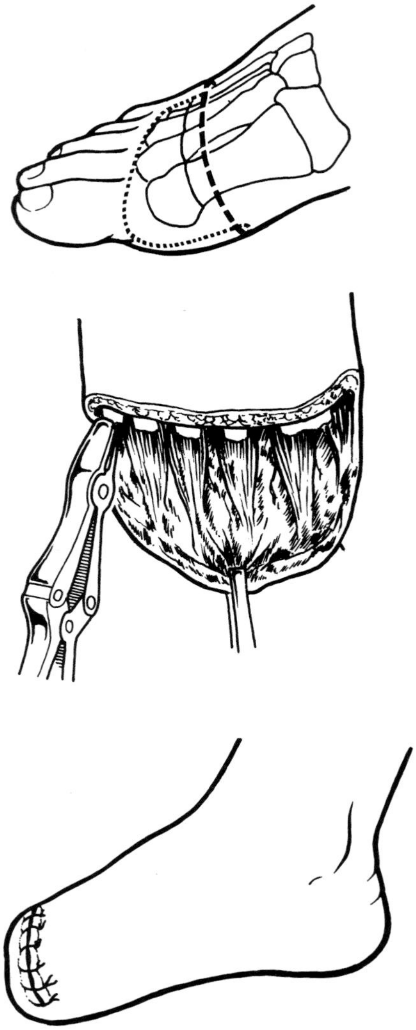

a

b

c

Fig. 10.92 The transmetatarsal amputation.

The foot

A transmetatarsal amputation can be used in diabetic patients who have gangrene of the forefoot, or in patients with many toes that remain irreversibly ischaemic after a successful revascularization. The patient is provided with a good stump and walking is usually excellent. The only prosthesis that is required is a shoe-filler.[1000] The amputation is made at the level of the metatarsal necks; a long plantar flap is used to close the defect as this skin has the best blood supply (Fig. 10.92). The bones may be individually divided by a vibrating saw or a Gigli saw. Chopart's and Lisfranc's amputations,[1001–1003] which are made through the tarsal bones, are rarely performed because the heel tends to develop equinovarus with

REFERENCES

998. Martin P, Wickham J Lancet 1962; ii: 16
999. McIntyre K E et al Arch Surg 1984; 119: 450
1000. Robinson K Br J Hosp Med 1976; 629
1001. Chopart F, Desault P J Traite des Maladies Chirurgicales et des Operations qui leur Conviennent. Vulier, Paris 1795

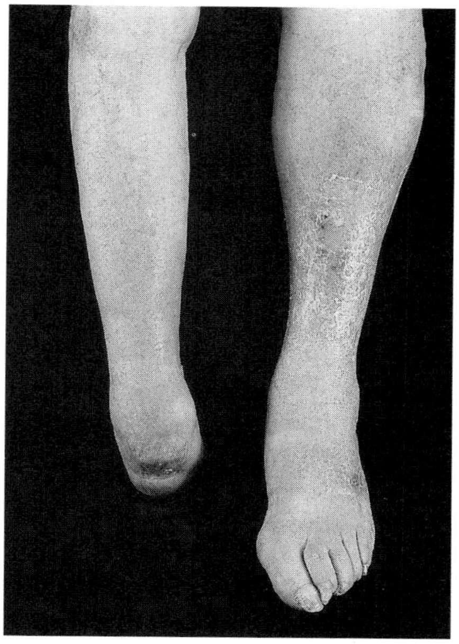

Fig. 10.93 Chopart's amputation of the right foot.

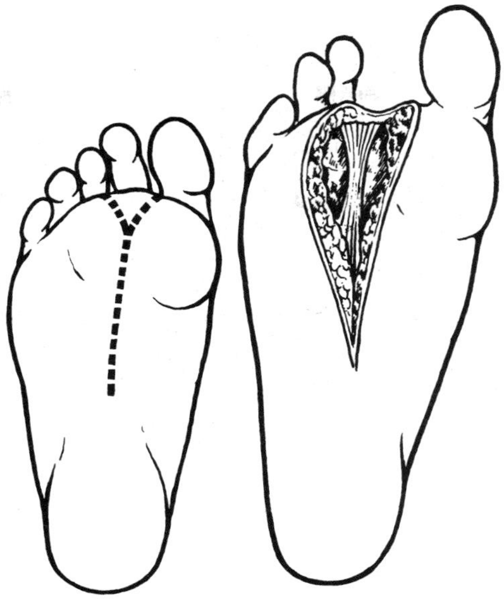

Fig. 10.94 A ray amputation for diabetic gangrene.

inversion, restricting subsequent mobility. Nevertheless some patients have maintained good mobility for many years on this type of stump, and they are slowly coming back into fashion (Fig. 10.93).

Individual rays consisting of one or more toes with their related metatarsal from the medial, lateral or central part of the forefoot can be excised. This amputation is useful in diabetic gangrene with infection spreading back along the line of the toe and its metatarsal, and heals up well by secondary intention (Fig. 10.94).

The heel (Syme's amputation)[1004]

This amputation is still popular with some orthopaedic surgeons but is rarely performed for ischaemia, and is not favoured by the limb fitters. Although it is classed as an end-bearing stump, few such stumps continue to weightbear, and any prosthesis used does not have enough room for ankle or sole springs. Most prosthetists feel the patient is better served by a good below-knee amputation.[1005] Aird (1st edition) pointed out that many of these amputations carried out in World War I developed painful stump ulcers. The prosthesis required is ugly and the operation is technically difficult and requires considerable expertise before success is consistently achieved. Patients can, however, walk without a prosthesis while at home, having the advantage of what the Germans call 'earth-feeling'.

In the classical Syme's amputation, the bones are divided just above the ankle with the malleoli being sawn off and a bulky heel fashioned over the divided bone. The details of the operation can be found in textbooks of operative surgery.[1006] The approach has been modified[1007] to divide the bone slightly higher (2 cm above the joint space) and Figure 10.95 shows the skin incision and the general technique with the modification. The incision joins the two malleoli anteriorly and drops vertically down to encircle the heel just in front of its prominence. A third of of Syme's amputations are subsequently revised to a higher level because of poor healing, ulceration or poor function.[1008]

Below-knee amputation

This is the level of amputation that most surgeons try to achieve in patients who require a major amputation for severe ischaemia of the lower limb. It has been shown that 80% of patients with ischaemic gangrene can have a successful amputation at this level.[1009] There is some evidence that failed arterial reconstruction leads to a high level of amputation[1010] although more recent work seems to refute this.[1011]

A number of tests, including Doppler ankle pressures, oximetry, isotope clearance, arteriography, thermography and plethysmography,[1012–1021] have been used in an effort to determine

REFERENCES

1002. Lisfranc J Nouvelle Method Operatoire Pour L'Amputation Partielle du Pied: Son Articulation Tarso-metafarsienne: Methode Precedes des Nombreuses Modifications qu'a Susbies Cette de Chopart. Gambon, Paris 1815
1003. Murdoch G, Donovan R G Amputation Surgery and Lower Limb Prosthetics. Blackwell, Oxford 1988
1004. Syme J Monthly J Med Sci 1843; 3: 93
1005. Callum K G In Clinical Problems in Vascular Surgery. Edward Arnold, London 1994 p 83
1006. Fiddian N J Amputations in General Surgical Operations. Churchill Livingstone, London 1987 p 416
1007. Harris R I Can J Surg 1964; 7: 53
1008. Aird I A Companion in Surgical Studies. E & S Livingstone, Edinburgh 1958
1009. McCollum P T, Spence V A, Walker W A Br J Surg 1988; 75: 1193
1010. Evans W E, Hayes J P, Vermilion B D Am J Surg 1990; 160: 217
1011. Cook T A, Davies A H, Horrocks M, Baird R N Eur J Vasc Surg 1992; 6: 599
1012. Barnes R W, Thornhill B et al Arch Surg 1981; 116: 80
1013. Welch G H, Lieberman D P et al Br J Surg 1985; 72: 888

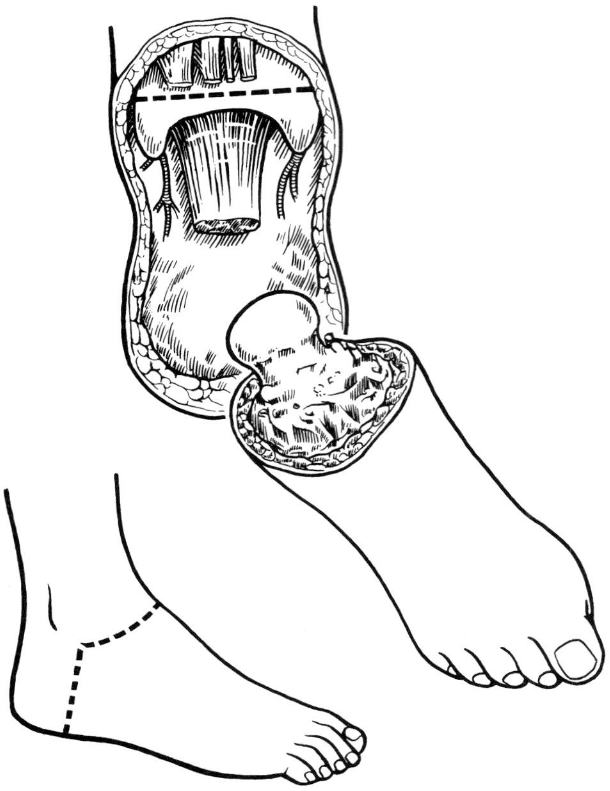

Fig. 10.95 The technique of Syme's amputation.

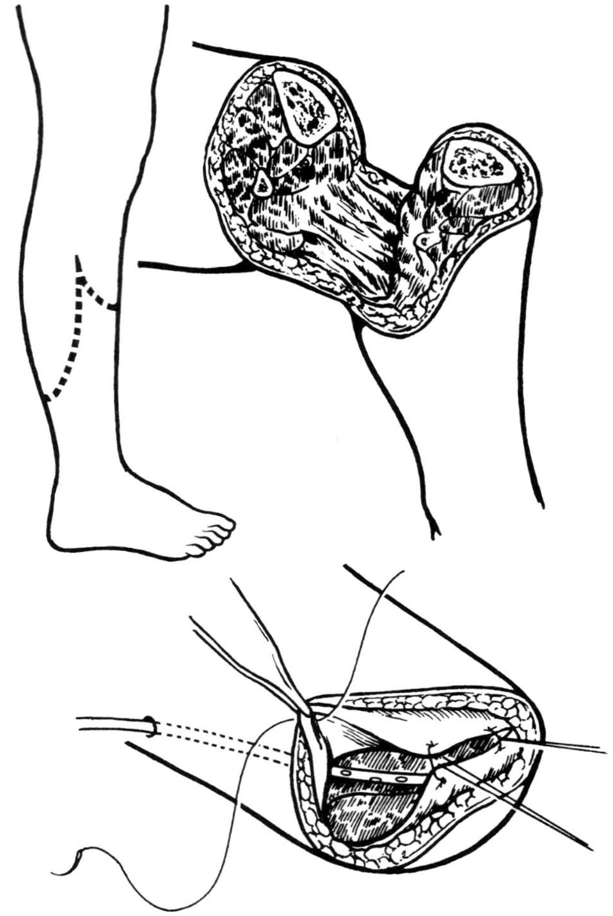

Fig. 10.96 The technique of below-knee amputation (Burgess) with a long posterior flap.

the likely success of amputation at this level. The proponents of oximetry and thermography make reasonable claims for their value, but they are not in standard clinical practice around the world, and sound clinical judgement combined with inspection of flap bleeding is probably the best guide to success.[1022] Although this was stated over 20 years ago it is probably still true.

The two methods that are now commonly used to perform this operation are the long posterior flap of Burgess[1023] and the skew flap of Kingsley Robinson et al.[1024] Early studies suggested that healing might be better with a skew-flap operation,[1025] but when the two techniques were evaluated in a controlled clinical trial there was little difference in the healing rate.[1026] A subsequent study also showed no difference in the healing rate, but did show earlier limb fitting and mobilization with skew flaps;[1027] this was thought to be because it is easier to get a nicely rounded stump with the skew-flap operation.

The Burgess technique uses a long posterior flap which employs the posterior calf muscles to cover the transected bones. The incision extends from the medial border of the tibia horizontally across the front of the leg to the lateral border of the leg, approximately 15 cm below the tibial tuberosity. Another method of arriving at the correct level of amputation is to measure 1 inch below the tibial tubercle for every foot of the patient's height (i.e. 5 inches for a 5-foot individual and 6 inches for a 6-foot individual). This leaves a reasonable stump to fit in a prosthesis without leaving it too long, which can make subsequent limb fitting difficult. The incision then extends vertically down the leg on either side and joins across the calf just above the origin of the Achilles tendon (Fig. 10.96). If the posterior flap is too long, this can be trimmed later when the muscles are thinned.

Details of the operative technique can be found in textbooks of operative surgery.[1028] The important points are that the end of

REFERENCES

1014. Burgess E M, Matsen F A et al J Bone Joint Surg 1982; 64: 378
1015. Mustapha N M, Redhead R G et al Surg Gynecol Obstet 1983; 156: 582
1016. Malone J M, Leal J M et al J Surg Res 1981; 30: 449
1017. McCollum P T, Spence V A, Walker W F Br J Surg 1985; 72: 310
1018. Spence V A, Walker W F J Surg Res 1984; 36: 278
1019. McCollum P T, Spence V A, Walker W F Prosth Orthop Int 1985; 9: 100
1020. Siegel M E, Giargiana F A et al A J R 1973; 118: 814
1021. Baddeley R, Fulford J C Br J Surg 1964; 51: 658
1022. Browse N L Scand Clin Lab Invest 1973; 128 (suppl): 249
1023. Burgess E M Clin Orthop 1967; 37: 17
1024. Robinson K P, Hoile R, Coddington T Br J Surg 1982; 69: 554
1025. Harrison J D, Southworth S, Callum K Br J Surg 1987; 74: 930
1026. Ruckley C V, Prescott R J In: Greenhalgh R M (ed) Limb Salvage and Amputation for Vascular Disease. W B Saunders, London 1988
1027. Reynolds J, Callum K G Br J Surg 1991; 78: 370
1028. McCollum C N In: Greenhalgh R M (ed) Vascular Surgical Techniques. W B Saunders, London 1989 p 340

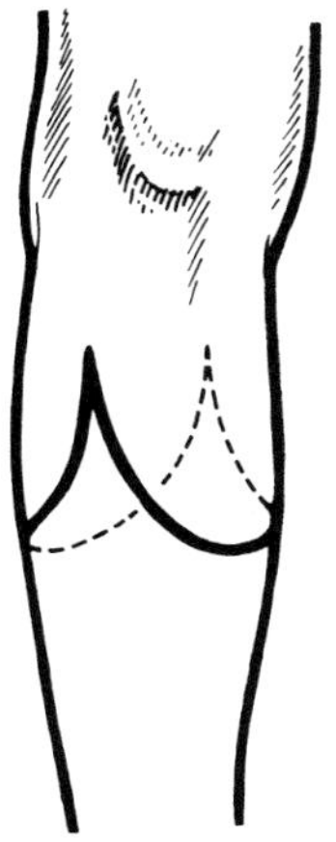

Fig. 10.97 The technique of below-knee amputation using a skew flap (Robinson).

the tibia must be carefully bevelled and the calf muscles thinned to prevent a bulky musculocutaneous flap. The skin is carefully approximated with very gentle non-absorbable sutures or a subcuticular suture and adhesive tapes.

In the skew-flap procedure, the skin flaps are raised as shown in Figure 10.97 and the final suture line runs obliquely anteroposteriorly. Otherwise the technique is similar to the Burgess operation.

Through-knee amputation

Equal lateral flaps are normally used for this amputation, which is not popular in ischaemic disease as it heals poorly.[1029] Even if primary healing is obtained, it leaves a large bulbous stump which makes it difficult to fit a prosthesis. It has the advantage that it is quick to perform and relatively atraumatic. The stump is end-bearing.

Supracondylar (Gritti–Stokes) amputation[1030]

This leaves a longer stump than the standard above-knee amputation, which may be an advantage in a bilateral amputee who wishes to change position in bed or on a chair when a prosthesis is not being worn. Because of the length of the stump it is difficult to fit an internal knee mechanism in the prosthesis and this has made this amputation unpopular with the prosthetists.[1031]

The skin flaps are shown in Figure 10.98. The knee joint is entered by deepening the anterior incision through the patella tendon and the joint capsule, before the knee is disarticulated by dividing the capsule above the meniscus and sectioning the cruciate ligaments. The vessels which are found behind the bone are ligated and divided. The nerves are pulled down and transected. The anterior flap and patella are turned upwards and the femur is divided immediately above the condyles before the articular surface of the patella is removed with a saw. The patella is then wired to the end of the femur or carefully fixed with non-absorbable sutures. There is less tendency for the patella to dislocate off the femur if the transected femur is angled slightly backwards.[1031] There is some evidence that mobility with a prothesis is better after a Gritti–Stokes than after an above-knee amputation.

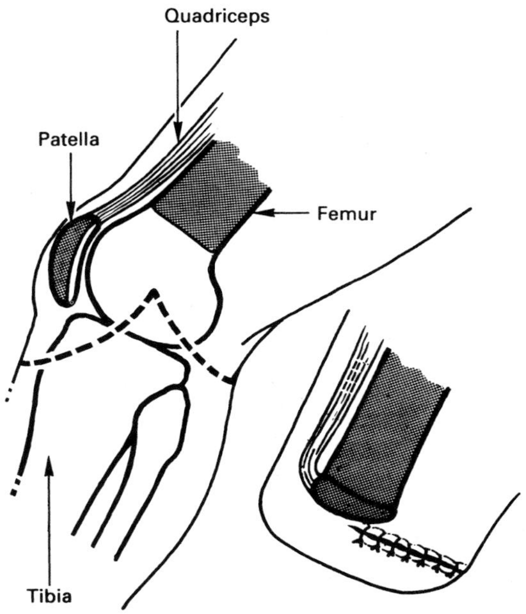

Fig. 10.98 The technique of Gritti–Stokes amputation.

Above-knee amputation

In this amputation equal anterior and posterior semicircular flaps are cut with their upper limit at the level of the bone section, which is ideally 25–30 cm below the tip of the greater trochanter. Enough room must be left for a knee mechanism to fit beneath the stump (usually 12 cm up from the knee joint). The divided vasti and quadriceps must be sutured over the end of the conically bevelled bone to provide a well shaped myoplastic stump.[1032] The muscles may be sutured to the bone end[1033] (a myodesis), but this refinement is almost certainly unnecessary.

Disarticulation of the hip[1034]

This is hardly ever required for vascular disease and is now mainly performed to eradicate soft tissue and bony tumours in the upper thigh (see Chapter 54). A long posterior flap is used to cover the defect (Fig. 10.99). The femoral vessels are carefully ligated, the capsule of the joint is divided and the head of the femur is dislocated forwards before the round ligament is divided. The obturator and gluteal vessels are then ligated and divided and the sciatic nerve is cut back.

Hindquarter amputation

This amputation was devised to treat bony and soft tissue tumours in the pelvic bones, the upper femur and the soft tissues of the

REFERENCES

1029. Chilvers A S, Briggs J et al Br J Surg 1971; 58: 824
1030. Gritti R Ann Univ Med (Milano) 1857; 161: 5
1031. Doran J, Hopkinson B R, Makin G S Br J Surg 1978; 65: 135
1032. Dederich R Ann R Coll Surg Engl 1967; 40: 222
1033. Robinson K P Br J Hosp Med 1976; 629: 631
1034. Boyd H B Surg Gyn Obstet 1947; 84: 346

upper thigh and buttock (Chapter 54). It has also been used for severe traumatic injuries in this region causing unreconstructable damage to the blood supply. It was first performed by Billroth in 1891 (whose patient did not survive),[1035] and later by Girard whose patient lived.[1036] Gordon-Taylor[1037,1038] popularized the operation in the UK and was its chief exponent, but it is now relatively rarely performed.

Amputations of the fingers

See Chapter 45.

Amputations in the upper limbs[1039]

These can be made through the forearm or arm above the elbow. A stump of 15 cm from the tip of the olecranon is ideal, and above the elbow 19 cm from the acromion to the cut end of humerus is preferred. These stumps should not be less than 10 and 7.5 cm respectively. Amputations through the arm are occasionally required for ischaemia, but the majority are required for trauma, vascular malformation, infection or tumours. The shoulder joint may be disarticulated, and a forequarter amputation is occasionally required for malignancy.

Other indications for amputation

Between 80 and 90% of all amputations are now carried out for ischaemic arterial disease, including Buerger's disease, diabetic vasculitis, emboli and trauma.[1033] Rare indications include arteriovenous fistulae, gas gangrene, septic arthritis, osteomyelitis (now rare), intractable venous ulceration, congenital deformities, malignancy and painful paralysed limbs.

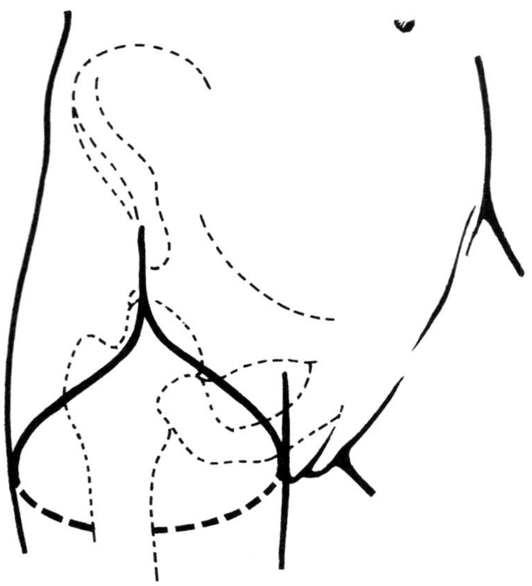

Fig. 10.99 The technique of hip disarticulation.

REFERENCES

1035. Savairiaud cited by Gordon-Taylor G, Wiles P Br J Surg 1935; 22: 695
1036. Girard C Congres Franc Chir 1895; 9: 823
1037. Gordon-Taylor G, Wiles P Br J Surg 1935; 22: 671
1038. Gordon-Taylor G Br J Surg 1940; 27: 643
1039. London P S Br J Hosp Med 1970; 4: 590

11 The veins

K. G. Burnand J. H. Scurr M. Stacey

The veins of the lower limb including those of the pelvis and abdomen are much more commonly the subject of disease and disorder than are the veins of the head and neck, the upper limb and the thorax. This may relate to the special demands placed on the veins in the lower half of the body, to continue to function and overcome the influence of gravity that has resulted from the adoption of the erect stance. The presence of large saccular veins within the powerful posterior muscles of the calf provides an accessory pumping mechanism or peripheral heart capable of augmenting venous return against the hydrostatic gradient. The 'calf-pump', in combination with unidirectional valves which are present within the venous lumen to prevent retrograde blood flow, enhances venous return from the lower extremities during exercise.[1] This mechanism prevents the development of high superficial venous pressures which over-distend the subcutaneous veins and interfere with capillary flow and exchange. Chronic disorders of the veins of the lower extremities are usually the result of valve malfunction which interferes with the action of the calf muscle pump. Veins provide the capacitance required for changing degrees of circulatory filling because of their ability to distend and empty rapidly without altering their resistance to flow.[2] Veins can undergo large changes in volume with little change in transmural pressure. The proper functioning of the venous system also requires that it must accommodate an enormous variation in the rates of flow at different sites at any one time, and at the same site at different times. Thrombus formation is a major problem throughout the venous system and this risk is exacerbated by low blood flow.

CONGENITAL DISORDERS OF THE VEINS

Veins develop from an intercommunicating network of blood 'islands' which coalesce and differentiate into a number of dominant pathways as flow becomes established.[3] Not surprisingly this complex process fails on occasions and congenital venous anomalies are quite common. The major veins of the lower limb, abdomen and thorax develop from pairs of anterior, posterior, superior and subcardinal veins. These vessels interconnect and coalesce in a complex manner and the iliac veins, inferior and superior vena cavae and the azygos veins are formed by the development of dominant flow pathways through certain sectors of this network (Fig. 11.1). Normally the right common cardinal vein, which is formed by the coalescence of the anterior and posterior cardinal veins behind the heart, achieves dominance, with the inferior vena cava having a complex derivation from four rudimentary veins (Fig. 11.1). This leads to some bizarre malformations including paired venae cavae, multiple cross-connecting vessels, total agenesis and a retroaortic left renal vein.[3–5] In the limbs, rotation and regression of the original axial veins can fail to occur, resulting in a persistent lateral vein which may be associated with agenesis of all or part of the main venous channels.[6] Most venous anomalies can be classified as aplasias, hypoplasias, reduplications or persistence of vestigial vessels. They may coexist with other anomalies in the cardiovascular or skeletal systems.[7] Agenesis of venous valves and structure defects in the composition of the vein wall can also occur.

Aplasia and hypoplasia

The total absence of a vein or segment of vein usually occurs in vessels with a complex development (e.g. the inferior vena cava). This anomaly may be extensive, or localized with a 'membrane' crossing the lumen,[8] and it may be incomplete resulting in narrow or hypoplastic veins.[7] Aplastic or hypoplastic segments of vein interfere with the venous return and patients present with symptoms of venous engorgement, swelling and discomfort. Abnormal collaterals are usually present (Fig. 11.1b). The defect can be delineated by phlebography; venous bypass surgery is occasionally indicated if symptoms cannot be adequately controlled by external compression.

Reduplication

This is a common anomaly; double venae cavae, renal veins, superficial femoral and saphenous veins are not unusual.[7] They do not require treatment.

REFERENCES

1. Ludbrook J Aspects of Venous Function in the Lower Limbs. Thomas, Illinois 1966
2. Shepherd J T, Vanhoutte P M Veins and their Control. Saunders, Philadelphia 1975
3. Langman J Medical Embryology, 4th edn. Williams & Wilkins, Baltimore 1981
4. Hirsch D M, Chan K JAMA 1963; 185: 729
5. May R, Nissl R In: May R (ed) Surgery of the Veins of the Leg and Pelvis. Thieme, Stuttgart 1979
6. Servelle M, Babillot J Phlebologic 1980; 33: 31
7. Browse N L, Burnand K G, Lea Thomas M Diseases of the Veins. Arnold, London 1988
8. Sen P K, Kinare S G et al J Cardiovasc Surg 1987; 8: 344

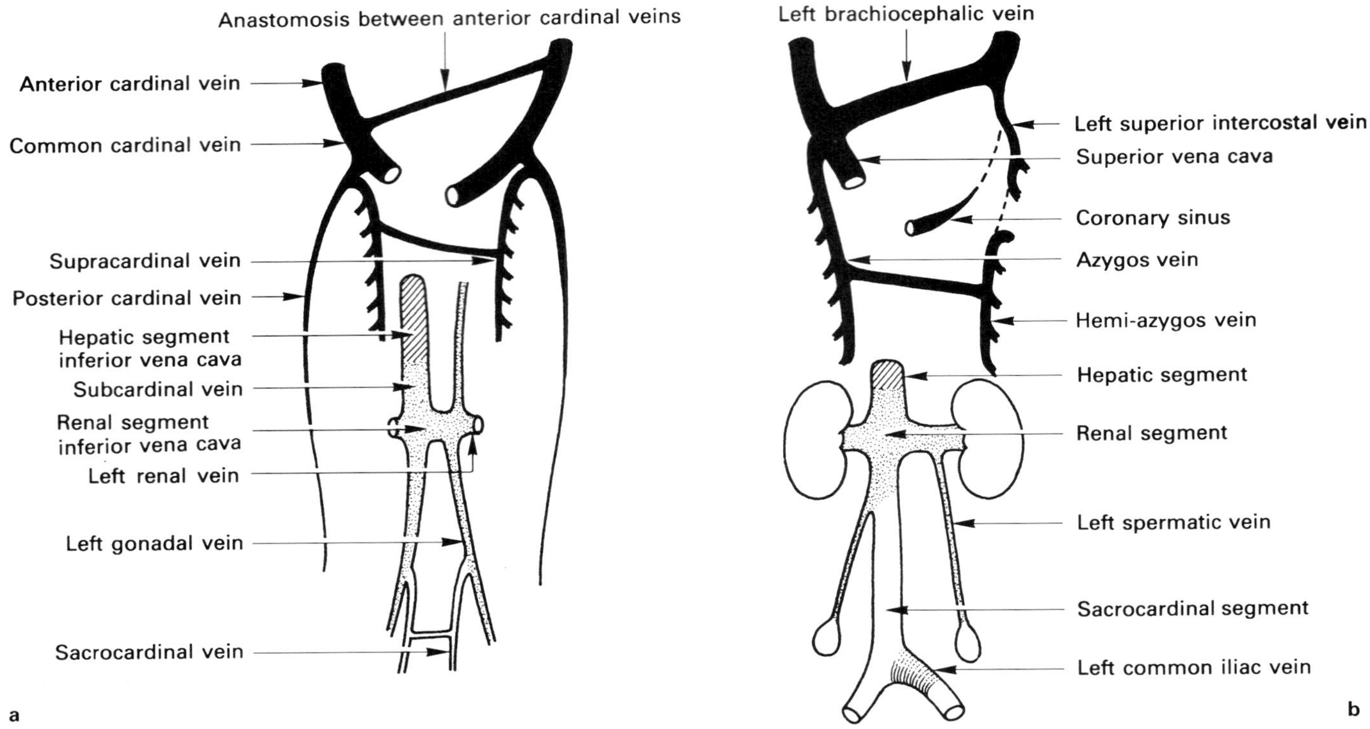

Fig. 11.1 Development of the venous pathways from the lower limb: (**a**) embryonic veins; (**b**) final appearance showing deviation from originals.

Persistence of vestigial vessels (venous 'angiomas')

This malformation may result in a reduplication but more commonly presents as a confluent mass of anomalous veins usually but erroneously referred to as a venous angioma. Venous angiomas vary from small localized collections of abnormal surface veins to an extensive network which can extend deeply into the soft tissues, bones and joints.[9] Most angiomas are first noticed as a variable swelling often situated beneath a cluster of dilated veins within the skin, or seen as bluish discoloration through the skin (Fig. 11.2). Deep angiomas may not cause a swelling and present with local pain or with episodes of haemorrhage or thrombosis. Angiomatous swellings are compressible and collapse when raised above the level of the heart. Venous angiomas must be differentiated from capillary haemangiomata, multiple arteriovenous fistulae and lymphangiomata (see Chapters 10 and 12). Occasionally a venous angioma may be mistaken for a soft tissue sarcoma or an abscess if it is complicated by thrombosis or haemorrhage. The extent and nature of the angioma can be determined by CT scanning of the limb but a STIR sequence of magnetic resonance provides even better information (Fig. 11.3).[10]

Venous angiomas are often difficult to excise completely, yet this remains the best form of treatment.[11] Sclerotherapy rarely helps and embolization is ineffective. The extent of the lesion determines the prospect of surgical success. Tissue defects left after excision can be covered by split-skin grafts, pedicle flaps or even vascularized free flaps.[12]

Partial removal with oversewing of residual angiomatous tissue usually produces an improvement even in more extensive lesions. It is, however, vital to avoid damaging nerves or major arteries and it is often preferable to leave some of the angioma and carry out a further excision on a later occasion than to produce unnecessary complications by an over-ambitious initial operation. Excision of angiomas from limbs is easier if the limb is exsanguinated and the operation is performed after a tourniquet has been applied.

Valve abnormalities

Total venous valvular agenesis is extremely rare with fewer than 50 cases having been reported.[13] Kistner reported a group of patients in Hawaii with 'floppy' edges of their valve cusps which invert and allow venous reflux. This has now been confirmed by others. Kistner developed an operation for tightening up venous valves which has now been modified by a number of other surgeons using a variety of open and closed techniques, some using angioscopy to visualize the suturing and confirm valve competency.[14] If valvular agenesis is confined to the lower limb veins, a

REFERENCES

9. Arland R Phlebologie 1980; 33: 547
10. Sacks A, Irvine A, Burnand K G Radiology 1995
11. Christenson J T, Gunterberg B Br J Surg 1985; 7: 748
12. Multiken J B, Young A E Vascular Birthmarks. Saunders, Philadelphia 1989
13. Lodin A, Lindvall N, Gentele H Acta Chir Scand 1958; 116: 256
14. Kistner R L Arch Surg 1975; 110: 1336

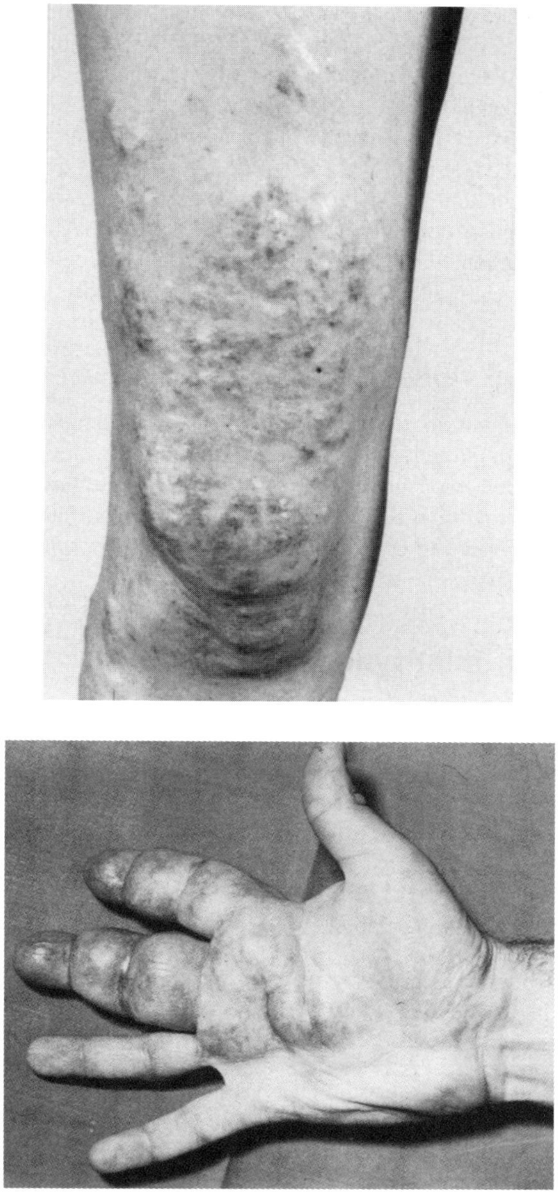

a

b

Fig. 11.2 Venous angioma: (**a**) on the leg; (**b**) on the hand.

brachial valve may be transplanted into the femoral popliteal vein. Enthusiastic early reports have often not been fulfilled by good long-term results and the benefits of these operations are still debated.[15]

Vein wall abnormalities

Relatives of patients with varicose veins have been shown to have defects in the collagen and mucopolysaccharide content of their vein walls.

The Klippel–Trenaunay syndrome

This syndrome was first described by Klippel & Trenaunay in 1900[16] as the combination of a cutaneous naevus, varicose veins

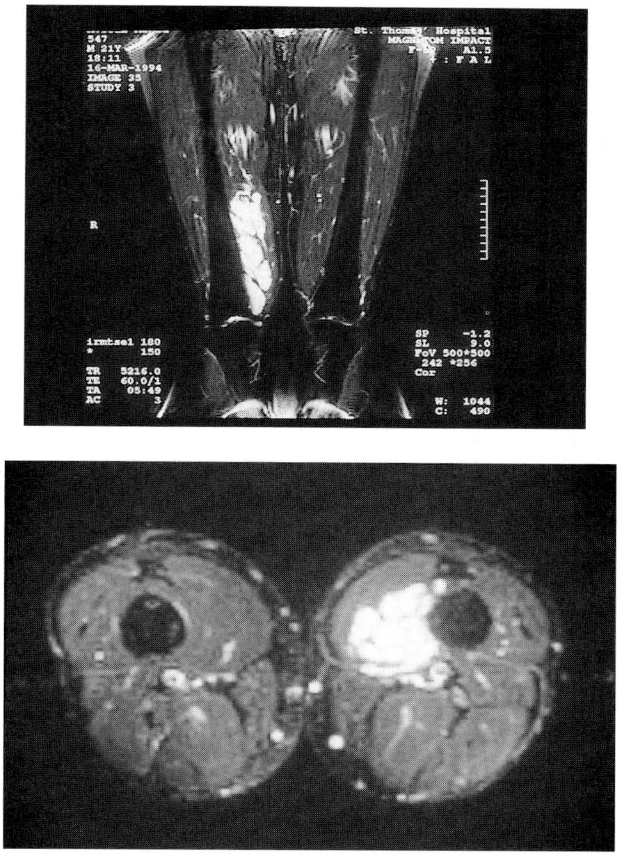

a

b

Fig. 11.3 Venous angioma shown by MRI scan using STIR sequence: (**a**) transverse cut; (**b**) vertical cut.

with bone and soft tissue deformity affecting one or more limbs. The condition must be differentiated from Parkes-Weber syndrome, in which there are multiple arteriovenous fistulae which also cause limb hypertrophy. The Klippel–Trenaunay syndrome is a diffuse mesodermal abnormality often associated with lymphatic and other congenital abnormalities. The naevus, limb hypertrophy and visible veins present at birth or develop in childhood. The naevus is variable in extent, usually pale purple, affecting part or all of the limb and extending on to the trunk in many instances. It characteristically has a metameric distribution (Fig. 11.4). The varicose veins are often extensive and unsightly. They are usually situated over the lateral surface of the limb and connect with a persistent primitive lateral limb vein (Fig. 11.4) which has failed to regress.[16] Approximately a quarter of the patients with this syndrome have pelvic venous anomalies which may give rise to rectal bleeding or haematuria.[17] Aplasia of the deep veins is present in 5% or 10% of patients and this, together

REFERENCES

15. Perrin M, Calvignac J L, Hiltbrand B, Bayon J M Phlebology 1995; suppl 1: 968
16. Klippel M, Trenaunay P Arch Gen Med (Paris) 1900; 185: 641
17. Baskerville P A, Ackroyd J S et al Br J Surg 1985; 72: 232

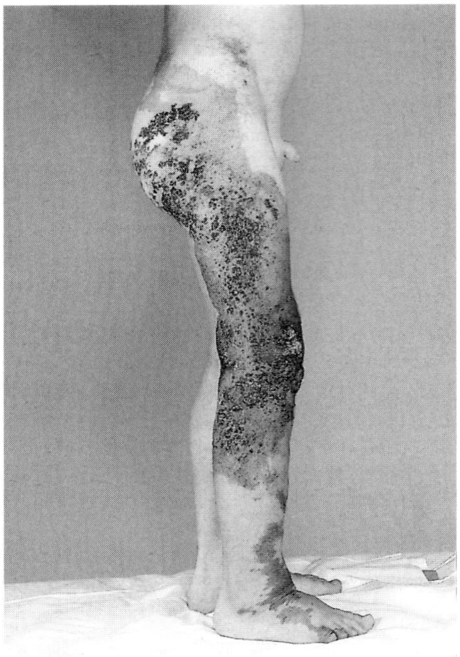

Fig. 11.4 Klippel–Trenaunay syndrome.

with lymphatic obliteration, is responsible for the limb swelling and ankle oedema that is often present.[18]

There is an increased incidence of deep vein thrombosis and pulmonary embolism in patients with the Klippel–Trenaunay syndrome and there may be an associated abnormality of Protein C. Lipodermatosclerosis and ulceration of the skin of the calf are however relatively rare. Bone hypertrophy and limb lengthening may lead to an abnormal gait which in turn may cause joint problems and lumbar backache.[19] The soft tissues may also be hypertrophic.[20] Associated congenital abnormalities include spina bifida, syndactyly, coxa vara, digital agenesis, atresia of the ear canal and clinodactyly. Klippel–Trenaunay syndrome can usually be distinguished from Parkes-Weber syndrome on clinical examination, but if this proves difficult blood flow estimation and arteriography are diagnostic.[17] Bipedal ascending phlebography is the only certain method of confirming deep venous agenesis, although duplex scanning is an alternative and should always be carried out before any surgery is undertaken on the superficial veins.

Most patients should be advised to wear elastic support which relieves aching and swelling and may prevent the development of lipodermatosclerosis and ulceration. Surgical eradication of the superficial veins should only be advised if the deep veins are normal, if the patient has never had a deep vein thrombosis, and if the symptoms are not relieved by stockings. Sites of superficial to deep communication should be disconnected and surface varices can be 'stripped out' or avulsed.[17] Some recurrence is inevitable and eradication of surface varices is rarely complete, so patients should be advised to continue with elastic support even after successful surgery. The naevus may be disguised by camouflage cream if it is disfiguring, although extensive laser photocoagulation is an alternative.

Gigantism of the toes and forefoot may be treated by local amputations but more extensive limb ablations are almost never required.[17] Excessive limb growth may be controlled by epiphyseal stapling or epiphysiolysis,[21] but these procedures are often ineffective and a heel raise for the opposite limb may be all that is required.

Although limbs with the Klippel–Trenaunay syndrome will always remain deformed, elastic compression usually provides good palliation. Patients having surgery should receive heparin prophylaxis to reduce the risk of deep vein thrombosis.

Popliteal vein entrapment

This is similar to the equivalent arterial entrapment. Patients present with intermittent swelling and discomfort which comes on during exercise, or they may present with an acute thrombosis.[22] When the condition is diagnosed before thrombosis has occurred the entrapment can be treated by dividing the abnormal muscle, which is usually one head of the gastrocnemius.

Thoracic inlet syndrome

The axillary vein may be compressed at its entry through the thoracic inlet, in a similar manner to the subclavian artery and the T1 nerve root.[23] Obstruction to the venous return is the most common cause of an axillary vein thrombosis. If there is radiological evidence of compression,[24] outlet decompression by resection of a cervical or the first rib may prevent thrombosis and relieve symptoms. Roos[25] carries this out through an axillary approach with special instrumentation but the results are difficult to assess.

Cystic degeneration of the vein wall

Cystic degeneration of the vein wall has similarities with cystic change in the arterial wall. The cysts contain transparent gelatinous material which is identical to the contents of a ganglion.[26] Patients present with a mass related to the vein, or signs of venous obstruction and thrombosis. The cyst may be visible on CT scanning or ultrasound imaging as a swelling compressing the vessel wall, and it can also occasionally be seen on phlebography as a smooth filling defect protruding into the vein lumen. The cyst may be deroofed and the contents expelled or the affected segment of vein can be resected and replaced with a short vein graft.[7,27]

REFERENCES

18. Young A E Birth defects: original article series 1978; 14: 289
19. Vollmar J, Vogt K Chirurgie 1976; 47: 205
20. Van Der Molen H R Soc Franc Phleb 1968; 2: 187
21. Blount W P, Clark G R J Bone Joint Surg 1949; 31A
22. Rich N M, Hughes C W Am J Surg 1967; 113: 696
23. McLeer R S, Kesterson J E et al Ann Surg 1951; 133: 588
24. Dunant J H Int Angiol 1984; 3: 157
25. Roos D B Surg 1982; 92: 1077
26. Mentha C Presse Med 1963; 71: 2205
27. Fyfe N C M, Sillocks P B, Browse N L J Cardiovasc Surg 1980; 21: 703

VENOUS INJURY

Any injury to soft tissue or bone is associated with some damage to small and medium-sized veins, but haemorrhage or occlusion of these vessels can usually be safely ignored although a haematoma often develops and may occasionally require drainage. When similar veins are damaged during operations they can be safely ligated, but injuries to the large axial veins of the limbs, pelvis and abdomen cannot be ignored, nor can these vessels be safely ligated as this results in acute or chronic venous obstruction.

Many major venous injuries unfortunately still pass unnoticed and only come to light when the post-thrombotic syndrome develops some time later. It is therefore impossible to provide an accurate figure for the incidence of major venous injury, although a number of large series of vascular injuries during war or civil unrest have been reported.[28–32] These reports have shown that in war there is a high incidence of arterial injury in the limbs, particularly in the leg, and that concomitant venous injury is common (Table 11.1). The rising incidence of violence and automobile accidents in recent years has been mirrored by an increasing risk of major venous injury in civilian life.[32–36]

Method and type of injury

Veins may be injured in one of five ways: they can be incised, lacerated (torn), contused, stretched or divided (Fig. 11.5). A number of external forces are responsible for these injuries. These include stab wounds, bullet wounds and bomb fragments (shrapnel) which can produce incisions, lacerations, contusions or transections of the vein wall. Blows or crushing injuries which fail to disrupt the vein wall can produce contusions or intimal damage, both of which may lead to secondary thrombosis. Veins lying close to fractures or dislocations may be over-stretched, disrupting one or more layers of the vein wall and usually leading to thrombosis.

Iatrogenic venous injuries are now an important cause of vein damage.[35] Large veins can be inadvertently damaged at operation, especially during difficult arterial surgery (e.g. abdominal aneurysms). Veins can also be damaged by direct puncture when a catheter or needle is inserted for monitoring or nutrition and during cardiac or radiological investigations. Toxic substances injected into the veins in error may also cause intimal damage and thrombosis.[38]

Symptoms, signs and investigations

A venous injury produces either concealed or revealed haemorrhage. The latter is seen as dark blood which wells up out of the wound. Concealed blood loss may only be recognized when symptoms of hypovolaemic shock develop. There may also be signs of venous obstruction in the affected part with congested vessels, cyanosis and oedema. Evidence of a post-thrombotic limb may develop later. Investigations are irrelevant if the patient is actively bleeding, and adequate resuscitation should be followed by operation and venous repair. Phlebography may be helpful when late signs of venous obstruction or thrombosis develop.

Table 11.1 Incidence of combined arterial and venous injuries in the Vietnam War

Artery injured	*Number of arterial injuries*	*Number of concomitant venous injuries (%)*
Axillary	59	20 (33.8)
Brachial	283	54 (19.0)
Iliac	26	11 (42.3)
Common femoral	46	17 (36.9)
Superficial femoral	305	139 (45.5)
Popliteal	217	116 (53.5)
Total	936	357 (37.9)

From Rich et al[37]

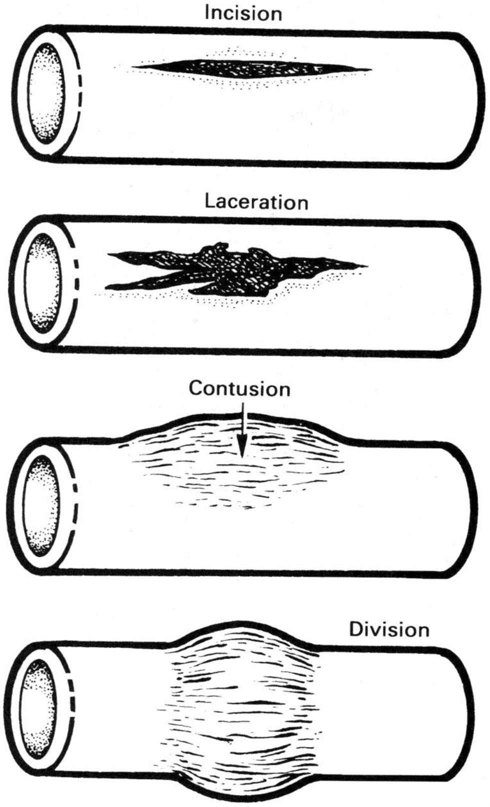

Fig. 11.5 Types of venous injury. From Browse et al[183] with kind permission.

Management

Pressure and elevation are effective first aid treatment, but the patient should be quickly transferred to hospital, where resuscitation and cross-matching of blood should precede operative exploration of the wound under general anaesthesia. Skin wounds are

REFERENCES

28. De Bakey M E, Simeone F A Ann Surg 1946; 123: 534
29. Hughes C W Surg Gynecol Obstet 1954; 99: 91
30. Rich N M J Cardiovasc Surg 1970; 11: 368
31. Livingstone R H, Wilson R Br Med J 1975; 1: 667
32. Schramek A, Hashmonai M Br J Surg 1977; 64: 644
33. Gaspar M R, Treiman R L Am J Surg 1960; 100: 171
34. Drapanas T, Hewitt R L et al Ann Surg 1970; 172: 351
35. Vollmar J In: May R (ed) Surgery of the Veins of the Leg and Pelvis. Thieme, Stuttgart 1979
36. Nypaver T J, Schuler J J, McDonnell P et al Vasc Surg 1992; 16: 762

extended as necessary to visualize the bleeding point or points, and suction helps to display the anatomy. Haemorrhage from a large vein can usually be controlled by finger pressure on either side of the laceration which allows the vein wall to be dissected out and inspected. Fogarty catheters can be inserted through the venous defect if control cannot be achieved and their insertion helps to control blood loss.

Once the vein has been dissected free, a small laceration can be closed by a simple or continuous suture while a more complicated venous injury may require administration of systemic heparin before cross-clamping and repair by vein patch or interposition graft[34] (Fig. 11.6). If blood loss is the equivalent of 6 units or more, heparin administration is not necessary as the patient already has a coagulopathy. Once the bleeding has been controlled the wound must be inspected to exclude any associated injuries to other important structures such as accompanying arteries and nerves. The continuity of major veins should be restored at an early stage, before other structures are repaired. This is especially important if the associated artery is also damaged. Autogenous vein is the material of choice for venous reconstruction, but this should not be taken from the injured extremity as all veins may act as useful collaterals should the graft fail. When a segment of vein wall has been lost, a vein patch must be used to prevent narrowing[35,39] (Fig. 11.6). An interposition vein graft may be made up as a composite to provide the desired diameter to replace a damaged or transected vessel. The long and short saphenous, the cephalic, brachial and internal jugular veins can all be used for this purpose. These veins can be split open and sewn spirally[40] or as a series of panels[41] to produce a graft of appropriate diameter (Fig. 11.7). Distal thrombus can be expelled by applying a tight bandage from the foot up the limb.

Heparin should normally be administered for several days after a vein repair, although its value in preventing thrombosis has been questioned.[42] A flow-enhancing distal arteriovenous fistula or pneumatic compression leggings may also reduce the risk of a perioperative or postoperative thrombosis.[43,44] Fasciotomies should be performed if there has been extensive venous damage or associated arterial damage. The wound should be drained and the patient put on broad-spectrum antibiotics if there has been severe contamination. Under these circumstances delayed primary suture of the skin wound is advisable. If delayed closure of the skin wound is to be employed, the damaged vein should not be left exposed but an effort must be made to cover it with viable muscle. Blood loss from large veins can be prevented by isolating the injury with an intraluminal shunt[45] which also provides an ideal environment for venous repair (Fig. 11.8). Patients who sustain blunt trauma to the abdomen and pelvis with associated pelvic fractures may have significant venous injury. Blind exploration of the patient can cause death from uncontrollable haemorrhage. The absence of continuing bleeding after initial resuscitation is an indication to adopt a conservative approach. CT scanning will help to exclude intraperitoneal blood. Phlebography can then be performed to identify trauma to the vena cava, common iliac or external iliac veins. Injury to these veins may require direct operative intervention and repair.

REFERENCES

37. Rich N M, Baugh J H, Hughes C W J Trauma 1970; 10: 359
38. MacGowan W A L, Holland P D J et al Br J Surg 1972; 59: 103
39. Rich N M, Hughes G W, Baugh J H Ann Surg 1970; 171: 724
40. Hobson R W, Yeager R A et al Am J Surg 1983; 146: 220
41. O'Reilly N J H, Hood J M et al Br J Surg 1980; 67: 337
42. Hobson R W, Groom R D, Rich N M Ann Surg 1973; 178: 773
43. Hobson R W, Lee B C et al Surg Gynecol Obstet 1984; 159: 284
44. Bryant M E, Lazenby W D, Howard J M Arch Surg 1958; 76: 289
45. Matto K L Surgery 1982; 91: 497

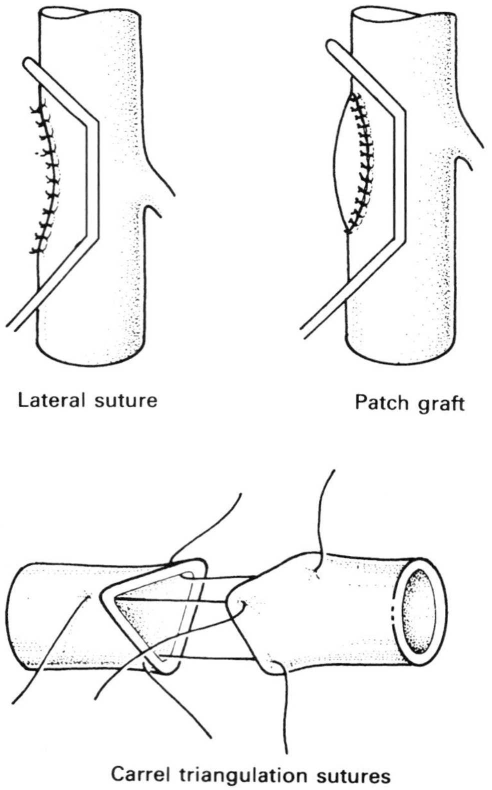

Fig. 11.6 Methods of repairing venous injury. From Browse et al[183] with kind permission.

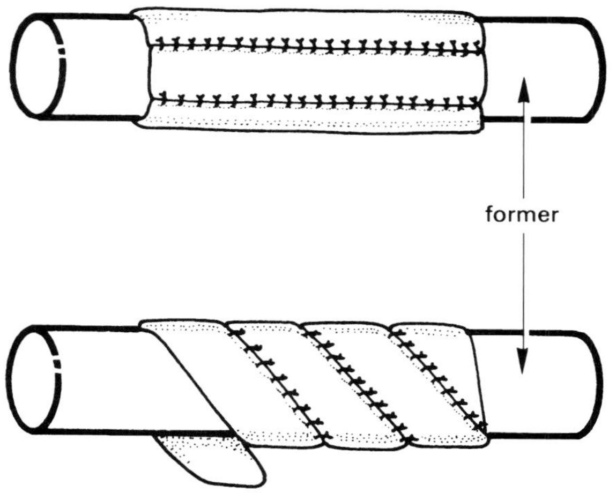

Fig. 11.7 Methods of producing a composite venous graft. From Browse et al[183] with kind permission.

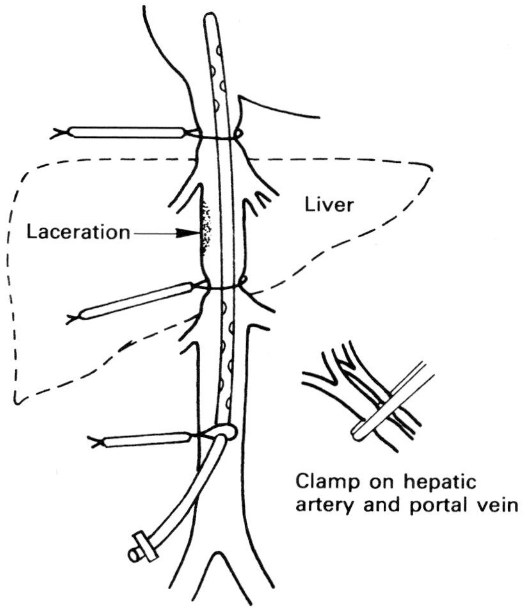

Fig. 11.8 Insertion of an intraluminal shunt which allows venous repair to be carried out in a bloodless field.

Results

The simultaneous repair of damaged veins and arteries has been shown to increase the prospects of limb survival.[31] Ligation of large veins is known to predispose to chronic venous insufficiency, but the long-term patency rates of vein repair have not been well documented. Between 30 and 70% of repairs have been claimed to be successful.[40]

Complications

Major venous injuries may be complicated by the development of arteriovenous fistulae, air embolism, deep vein thrombosis, pulmonary embolism, post-thrombotic limb, secondary infection and haemorrhage.[35,39]

VARICOSE VEINS

A varicose vein is a vein that is tortuous and dilated, and varicose veins are invariably associated with valvular incompetence. The prevalence of this condition in Europe and the USA has been shown by a number of large surveys to be about 2% with a slightly higher incidence in women than men, which increases with age.[46–49]

Pathology

Varicose veins may be defined as primary if the cause is not known or they may be secondary to other conditions which include post-thrombotic damage, pregnancy, pelvic tumours and congenital disorders such as the Klippel–Trenaunay syndrome.

The influence of heredity on the development of varicose veins has been clearly demonstrated[49–51] but the role of valvular damage versus a wall defect is still debated.[52,53] There is anatomical evidence that venous dilatation occurs below rather than above valves.[54] The collagen and mucopolysaccharide content of the vein wall is abnormal in patients with established varicosities and in their relatives before varicose veins have developed.[55] These findings are in favour of an inherited abnormality of the vein wall causing secondary valvular incompetence.[53] Congenital valvular agenesis is an extremely rare but well documented cause of varicose veins.[56] However, in situ vein bypass grafts in which all the valves have been deliberately destroyed do not become varicose or aneurysmal.

Varicose veins only affect humans and the erect stance appears to be relevant. Hormonal and haemodynamic factors are probably not of primary importance but may encourage varicosis. The concept that all varicose veins are secondary to incompetence of the communicating veins is no longer tenable. Other factors which have been thought to predispose to varicose veins include age, the female sex, parity,[57] occupation[58] and clothing.[59] It has even been suggested that varicosities are the result of faulty bowel habit causing faecal masses to interfere with the venous return from the lower limb.[60] The sedentary position for defecation adopted by western societies does not appear to be important![49]

Histological studies of varicose veins have shown that there is a considerable increase in the fibrous tissue within the vein wall which breaks up the smooth muscle and extends into all coats of the vein wall.[53] The valve sinuses are at first over-stretched causing the valves to atrophy. Varicosities usually occur in the tributaries of the saphenous vein rather than the main trunks, although the saphenous veins can occasionally develop some abnormal sacculation.[54]

Symptoms

Unsightliness or disfigurement of the legs is one of the main reasons why patients with varicose veins, particularly women, present for treatment. Varicose veins can also cause discomfort which is characteristically an ache felt in or over the veins, usually worse after prolonged standing or at the end of the day. The pain does not appear to be related to the size of the varicosities.[61] Pain and tenderness of the varicosities can be a prominent feature in women just before and during their period. Night cramps, ankle

REFERENCES

46. Borschberg E The Prevalence of Varicose Veins of the Lower Extremity. Karger, Basle 1967
47. Widmer L K Peripheral Venous Disorders. Prevalence and Socio-medical Importance. Hans Huber, Berne 1978
48. National Health Survey 1935–1936 US Dept of Health Education and Welfare, Washington DC 1938
49. Callum M Br J Surg 1994; 81: 167
50. Virchow R Cellular Pathology. Churchill, London 1860
51. Gundersen J, Hauge M Angiology 1969; 20: 346
52. Ludbrook J Lancet 1963; ii: 1289
53. Rose S S, Ahmed A J Cardiovasc Surg 1986; 27: 534
54. Cotton L Br J Surg 1961; 48: 589
55. Svejcar J, Prerovsky I et al Clin Sci 1963; 24: 325
56. Lindvall N, Lodin A Acta Chir Scand 1962; 124: 310
57. Foote R R Varicose Veins. Butterworths, London 1954
58. Lake M, Pratt G H, Wright I S JAMA 1942; 119: 696
59. Mekky S, Schilling R S F, Walford J Br Med J 1969; 2: 591
60. Burkitt D P Br Med J 1972; 2: 556
61. Browse N L, Burnand K G, Lea Thomas M Diseases of the Veins. Amold, London 1988

swelling and 'restless legs' are other common complaints. Varicose veins have an increased tendency to develop superficial thrombophlebitis, and they occasionally rupture spontaneously and bleed dramatically. Varicose veins are infrequently associated with lipodermatosclerosis (pigmentation, induration and inflammation in the calf skin) and this can be complicated by venous ulceration.

Examination

The patient should be examined standing on a low stool or platform in a well lit and warm room with the lower limbs fully exposed from groin to toes. The distribution of all the major subcutaneous varicosities on both aspects of the limb should be carefully recorded on outline diagrams of the leg.[62] An attempt should be made to determine which major tributaries have become varicose and any unusual channels should also be recorded (e.g. a large lateral vein in the Klippel–Trenaunay syndrome). Careful inspection may reveal a saphena varix or a dilated short saphenous termination. The presence of an ankle flare, indicative of venous hypertension, or dilated calf blowouts is suggestive of incompetent calf communicating veins (Fig. 11.9).[63] Any skin change around the ankle, especially lipodermatosclerosis, ulceration and eczema, indicates the possibility of post-thrombotic damage, which is further supported by findings of groin or abdominal collaterals.

Some varicose veins are more easily felt than seen and it is advisable to lightly run a hand over the course of both the long and the short saphenous territories.[61] Ankle oedema and a temperature difference between the limbs may also be detected by this type of palpation, which will often pick up thickening in the gaiter skin which may be the first sign of lipodermatosclerosis. A cough impulse should be examined for over the saphenofemoral junction and over any large varices further down the limb.[19,64] If a thrill is felt, the upper valves of the long saphenous vein must be incompetent. Valvular incompetence can also be assessed by percussing over a varix and finding an impulse passing up and down a dilated and valveless vein. Although it has been suggested that palpation over the medial calf may detect fascial defects where incompetent communicating veins pierce the deep fascia,[65] this test has been shown to be hopelessly inaccurate.[66] The use of a 'sliding finger' to control reflux through incompetent perforating veins has been championed by some[67] but others have found this test to be equally ineffective for localizing the communicating veins. An arteriovenous fistula is suspected if a bruit is heard over a localized collection of varices.

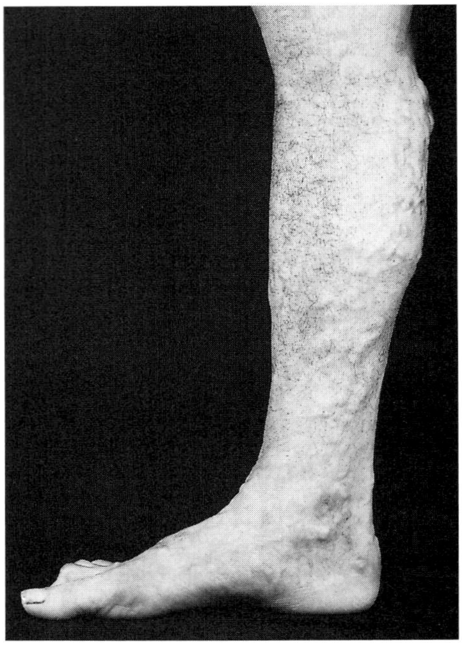

Fig. 11.9 A limb showing signs of calf blowouts and ankle flare.

Tourniquet tests

The Brodie–Trendelenburg test[68,69] consists of the application of a single tourniquet around the upper thigh after all the surface veins have been emptied by elevation of the limb and gentle massage.[57,61,62] Long saphenous incompetence is confirmed if the varicosities remain empty when the patient stands erect (Fig. 11.10). The varicosities rapidly refill from above when the tourniquet is released. If the varices do not remain empty when the patient stands erect the test should be repeated with the tourniquet placed just above the knee. Control at this level indicates the presence of an incompetent mid thigh perforating vein. A tourniquet which controls the varices when placed below the knee is indicative of short saphenous incompetence. Calf tourniquets and multiple tourniquets applied at intervals along the leg have been used to try to determine the position of incompetent calf communicating veins, but these tests are extremely difficult to interpret and often inaccurate. In Perthes' walking test,[70] a single tourniquet is applied around the thigh or knee in combination with heel-raising or walking. The patient has long or short saphenous incompetence with normal calf communicating veins and deep veins if the surface veins empty. This test is useful as an overall assessment of the competence of the deep and communicating veins.

Diagnosis

The majority of varicose veins can be assessed from the history and a careful clinical examination supplemented by the tourniquet tests,[57,61,62] but in some patients the history or physical signs will not convince the clinician that varicose veins are responsible for the symptoms and additional tests to exclude disease of the hips, knees, spine, peripheral vessels or nervous system are helpful.

REFERENCES

62. Dodd H J, Cockett F B The Pathology and Surgery of the Veins of the Lower Limb. Churchill Livingstone, Edinburgh 1976
63. Cockett F B Br Med J 1953; 2: 1399
64. Chevrier L Arch Gen Chir 1908; 2: 44
65. Fegan W G Varicose Veins: Compression Sclerotherapy. Heinemann, London 1967
66. O'Donnell T F, Burnand K G et al Arch Surg 1977; 112: 31
67. Hobbs J Arch Surg 1974; 109: 793
68. Brodie B Lectures Illustrative of Various Subjects in Pathology and Surgery. Longmans, London 1846
69. Trendelenburg F Klin Chir 1891; 7: 195
70. Perthes G Dtsch Med Wochenschr 1895; 21: 253

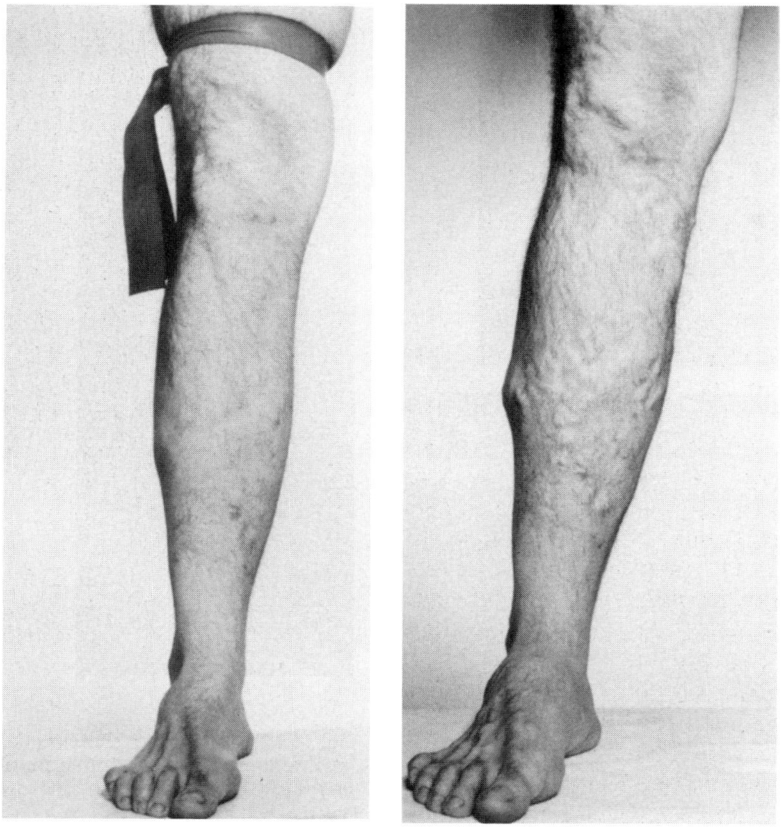

a b

Fig. 11.10 The Brodie–Trendelenburg tourniquet test. (**a**) The varicose tributaries of the long saphenous vein are kept empty by the tourniquet and (**b**) fill on release.

Occasionally there will be concern that the varicose veins are secondary to another cause, or it will not be possible to determine the extent and connections of the varicosities from the clinical examination. Further investigations are then necessary.

Doppler ultrasound testing of venous reflux in the long saphenous, short saphenous[71] and calf communicating veins[72] has been used with some success. This investigation is valuable in detecting saphenous reflux but is less helpful in locating incompetent calf communicating veins.[66] The long and short saphenous terminations are located using a cough impulse and calf compression. The presence of a bidirectional signal on calf compression (forward and backward flow) or retrograde flow on valvular or tourniquet release indicates trunk vein incompetence. The head of the saphenopopliteal junction can be variable; Doppler ultrasound can locate this junction and therefore direct the site of incision in the popliteal fossa if surgery is to be undertaken.

Duplex ultrasound which determines the presence of retrograde flow in a defined vein has revolutionized the assessment of long and short saphenous incompetence in patients where clinical examination or simple Doppler[73] has failed to establish a clear diagnosis. Duplex may also be valuable in determining incompetence in the communicating (Fig. 11.11) and deep veins although it is not completely accurate in these veins where phlebography still has a place.[74]

Bipedal ascending phlebography, injecting non-ionic contrast media into foot veins with ankle tourniquets to direct the contrast into the deep system, is still the most accurate method of detecting post-thrombotic damage[75] and also confirms the presence of many incompetent calf communicating veins.[76] Direct injection of similar contrast media into surface veins (varicography) outlines the extent and connections of varicosities and is particularly useful if the clinical tests are equivocal or if the patient has had previous operations for varicose veins (Fig. 11.12).[77–79]

Venous pressure recordings taken from a foot vein during exercise,[80] foot volumetry[81] and other plethysmographic tests[82] all assess the function of the calf-pump, which is dependent upon the competence of the deep and communicating veins, but these tests give little information of diagnostic value and are still primarily research tools.

REFERENCES

71. Hoare M C, Royle J P Aust N Z J Surg 1984; 54: 49
72. Miner S S, Foote A V Br J Surg 1974; 61: 653
73. Coleridge-Smith P D, Scurr J H Curr Prac Surg 1995; 7: 182
74. De Maeseneer M G et al Cardiovasc Surg 1993; 1: 686
75. Baker S, Burnand K G, Sommerville K M et al 1993; 341: 400
76. Burnand K G, O'Donnell T F et al Lancet 1976; i: 936
77. Corbett C R, McIrvine A J et al Ann R Coll Surg Engl 1984; 66: 412
78. Bradbury A W, Stonebridge P A, Callum M J et al Br J Surg 1994; 81: 373
79. Bradbury A W, Stonebridge P A, Ruckley C V Br J Surg 1993; 80: 849
80. Bjordal R I Acta Chir Scand 1972; 138: 251
81. Norgren L Acta Chir Scand 1973; (suppl) 444
82. Norris C S, Beyrau A, Barnes R W Surgery 1983; 94: 758

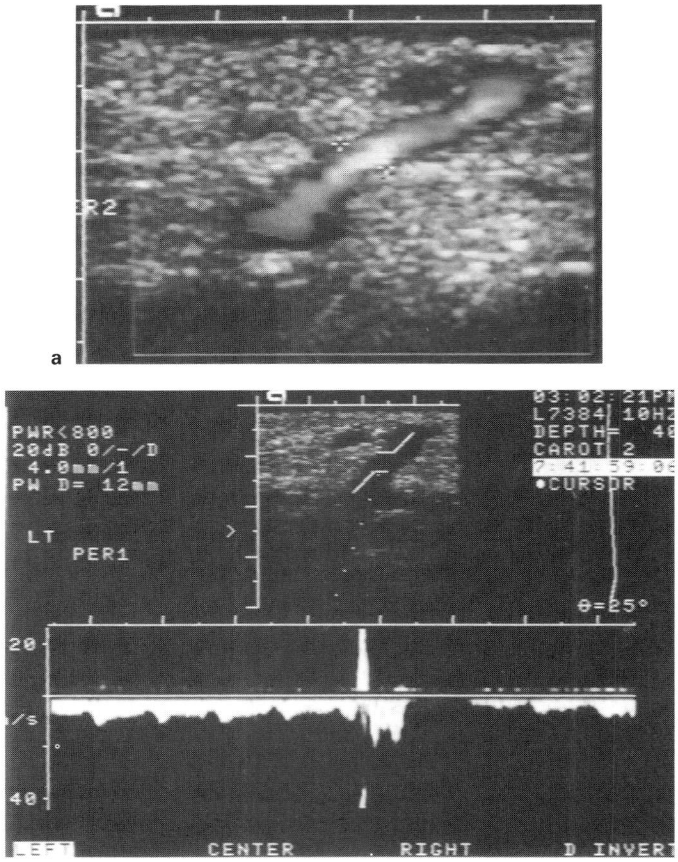

a

b

Fig. 11.11 Duplex scan showing incompetent calf communicating veins.

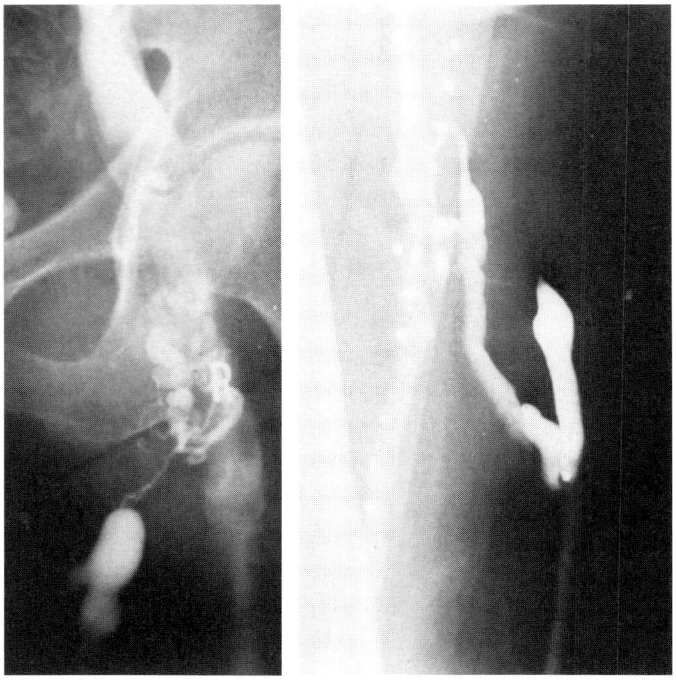

a b

Fig. 11.12 Varicograms showing: (a) groin recurrences; (b) an incompetent hunterian communicating vein, connecting to previously ligated long saphenous vein.

Management

When patients with varicose veins have been fully assessed, they should be placed in one of several categories:

1. Definite long or short saphenous varicosities with a single saphenous vein incompetence or a combination of both long and short saphenous incompetence, which is often more difficult to diagnose and may require Doppler, duplex or varicography to confirm the diagnosis.
2. A combination of saphenous incompetence and incompetence of communicating veins in the calf or thigh.
3. Isolated calf communicating vein incompetence (rare).
4. Minor tributary vein incompetence without evidence of saphenous or communicating vein incompetence.

The venous system requires a more detailed evaluation if there is suspicion of post-thrombotic damage or when skin changes are present in the gaiter region of the calf.

Treatment

Patients with minor cosmetic varicosities or visible veins can be treated by reassurance or elastic support stockings. Patients with clear evidence of long or short saphenous incompetence or a combination of the two, almost always associated with branch vein varicosities, should have the saphenofemoral or saphenopopliteal junction surgically ligated if their symptoms justify intervention. This should be combined with stripping of the incompetent long saphenous vein to the knee or the incompetent short saphenous vein to the ankle and avulsion of all the varicose tributaries. These operations have been shown by Hobbs[83] to have a lower incidence of recurrence than sclerotherapy when major saphenous incompetence is present.

The saphenous veins must be disconnected flush with the femoral and popliteal veins and all the tributaries near their termination must be ligated and divided to prevent recurrence.[57,61–63] The value of vein stripping has been debated and is still being examined in clinical trials[84–86] but it prevents the possibility of reconnection and removes some of the communicating veins as well as disconnecting the venous tributaries from the main channels (Fig. 11.13).

The saphenofemoral junction is approached with the patient lying flat with legs abducted and elevated. An oblique incision is made 2 cm below and lateral to the public tubercle and the long saphenous vein is found passing up through the subcutaneous fat. It is traced to its termination with the femoral vein as it dips down through the cribriform fascia and fossa ovale. The superficial inferior epigastric vein, the superficial external and deep external pudendal veins and the superficial external iliac veins usually join the long saphenous vein near its termination (Fig. 11.14). These

REFERENCES

83. Hobbs J T Br J Surg 1968; 55: 777
84. Sarin S, Scurr J H, Coleridge-Smith P D Br J Surg 1992; 79: 889
85. Bergan J J Cardiovasc Surg 1993; 1: 624
86. Woodyer A B, Dormandy J A Phlebol 1996; 1: 221

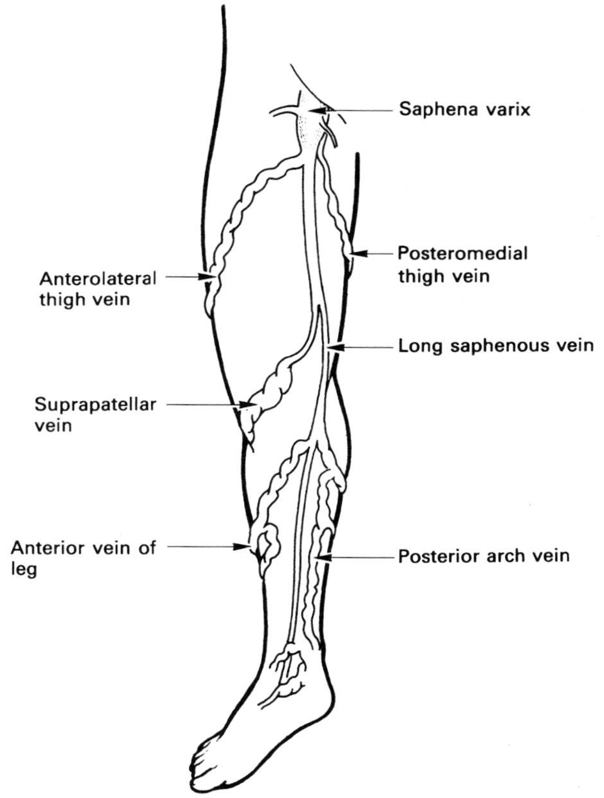

Fig. 11.13 The major tributaries that join the long saphenous vein in its course up the leg.

tributaries must be carefully ligated and divided. When the saphenofemoral junction has been defined the vein is divided and ligated, before a flexible intraluminal stripper is passed down the vein to knee level or just below. The stripper is recovered through

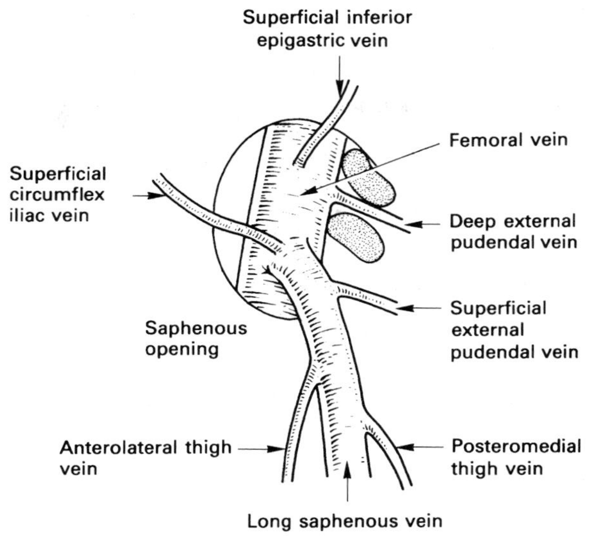

Fig. 11.14 The tributaries that enter the long saphenous vein near its termination.

a small incision placed over its tip and the vein is avulsed by steady downward traction on the distal end. An additional stripper may be passed up from a separate incision made over the vein near the knee or at the ankle (Fig. 11.15) if the stripper will not pass down the vein. Pin stripping, developed by Oesch,[87] invaginates the vein and may reduce the postoperative bleeding but this has not really been confirmed by controlled trials.[88,89]

REFERENCES

87. Oesch A Phlebol 1993; 4: 171
88. Coleridge-Smith P D, Butler C M, Sommerville K M, Scurr J H Phlebol 1995; 1: 493
89. Tyrell M R, Rocker N, Maisey N et al Phlebol 1995; 1: 451

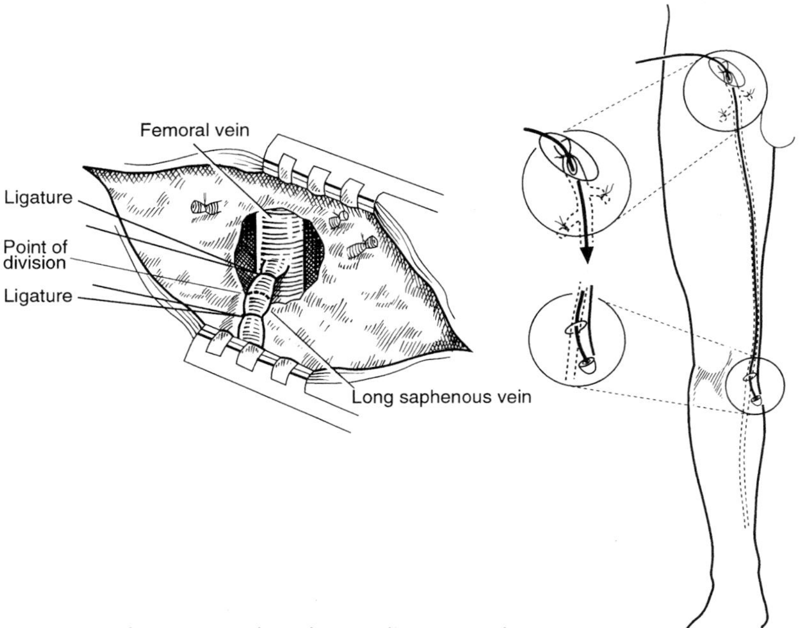

Fig. 11.15 High saphenous ligation and stripping of the long saphenous vein.

The short saphenous vein is approached with the patient lying prone. An incision is made at the ankle and the vein is dissected off the sural nerve. The vein is ligated and the stripper is inserted through a venotomy and passed up towards the knee where it can be felt to 'kick' and pass deeply at the level of the saphenopopliteal junction. The short saphenous termination is more accurately located by on-table phlebography or preoperative duplex scanning or varicography.[90,91] An appropriately sited transverse incision is then made over the saphenopopliteal junction and the short saphenous vein containing the stripper is located lying beneath the deep fascia (Fig. 11.16) before being traced to its T-junction with the popliteal vein. The short saphenous vein is then disconnected, its stump is ligated and the distal vein is stripped out. Many surgeons simply ligate the short saphenous vein without stripping it.

Branch varicosities are avulsed through multiple minute incisions placed directly over the varicosities at appropriate intervals of about 5–10 cm[92] (Fig. 11.17). The veins are teased out using specially designed hooks or mosquito forceps and the whole process may be easier and relatively bloodless if a tourniquet is used to exsanguinate the limb. Incompetent communicating veins are ligated through short incisions placed in Langer's lines if they can be located preoperatively. Otherwise a long vertical calf incision, described by Linton[93] and Cockett,[63] is made over the medial border of the leg just behind the posterior border of the tibia extending from the medial malleolus to just above the middle of the calf, to explore the calf communicating veins if skin changes are present. After the skin, subcutaneous tissue and deep fascia have been divided all the veins which cross the deep fascia in the medial compartment of the leg are defined, ligated and divided (Fig. 11.18). Recently a minimally invasive approach has been developed using a specially designed telescope inserted beneath the deep fascia through a small incision in the upper calf,[94,95] to ligate and divide the incompetent calf communicating veins. Early results are encouraging but further studies are required to confirm efficiency. The major advantage of this operation is that in patients with established lipodermatosclerosis incision through the affected area can be avoided.

Patients with minor branch varicosities who demand treatment, or those who develop tributary recurrences after correctly performed saphenous surgery, are best managed by injection sclerotherapy; there are still some who will treat all varicosities by this technique. Introduced originally by Tavel[96] and improved by Tournay in France[97] and Fegan in Ireland,[98] sclerotherapy has been shown to be an effective method of eradicating varicose veins providing major saphenous incompetence is not present or following surgical ligation of the saphenofemoral or saphenopopliteal junction.[83] Sodium tetradecyl sulphate 1%, a detergent, is one agent commonly used to inject empty veins which are compressed and bandaged for a period of 3–6 weeks. The period of bandaging is now disputed,[99] and a compromise of 3 weeks seems appropriate. Injections can be repeated on many occasions until all the varices have been eradicated. Extravasation of sclerosant and inadvertent intra-arterial injections[100] are disasters that can be avoided by careful technique. Some mild skin staining is an unwanted side-effect of successful sclerosis in a few patients. Nevertheless toxic sclerosants are being evaluated and sclerotherapy using duplex scanning to define venous

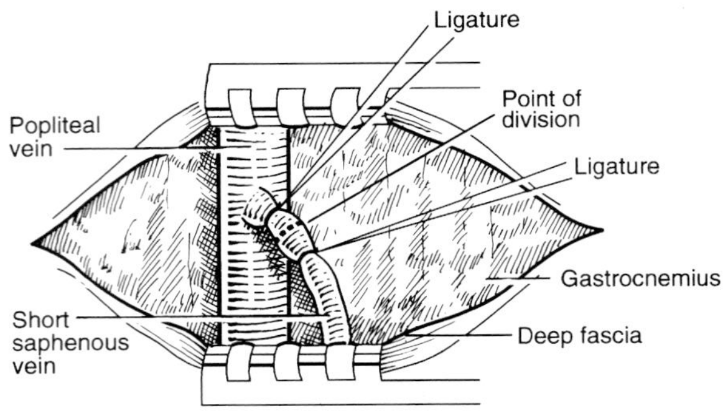

Fig. 11.16 The popliteal dissection for short saphenous incompetence.

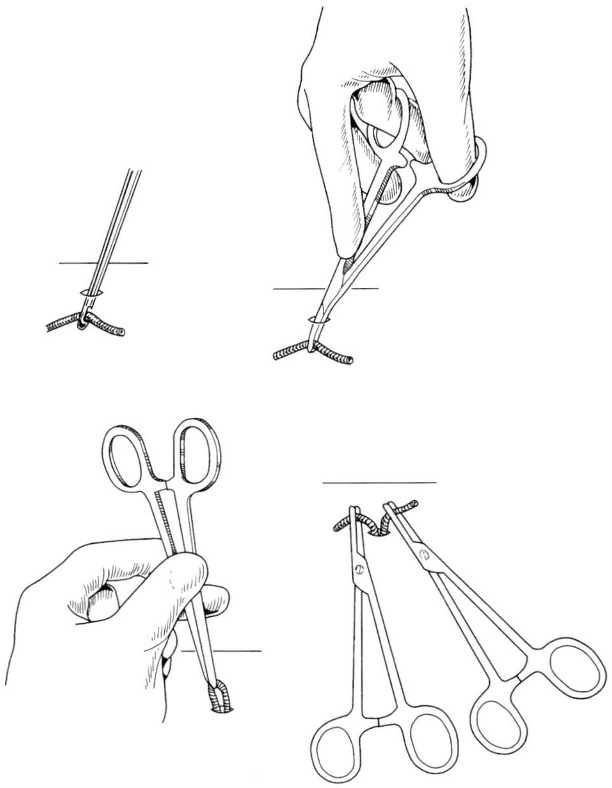

Fig. 11.17 Avulsion of varicose tributaries.

incompetence and confirm obliteration may improve results. It is not known if this approach is cost effective.

REFERENCES

90. Hobbs J T Br Med J 1980; 2: 1528
91. Burnand K G Phlebologie 1983; 1: 269
92. Rivlin S Br J Surg 1975; 62: 413
93. Linton R R Ann Surg 1938; 107: 582
94. Gloviczki M D, Robert A, Camria M D et al J Vasc Surg 1996; 23 (3): 517
95. Hauer G, Borkun J, Wigger I et al Surg Endosc 1988; 2: 5
96. Tavel E Dtsch Z Chir 1912; 116: 735
97. Tournay R Bull Med Paris 1931; 45: 73
98. Fegan W G Lancet 1963; ii: 109
99. Fraser I A, Perry E P et al Br J Surg 1985; 72: 488
100. MacGowan W A L J R Soc Med 1985; 78: 136

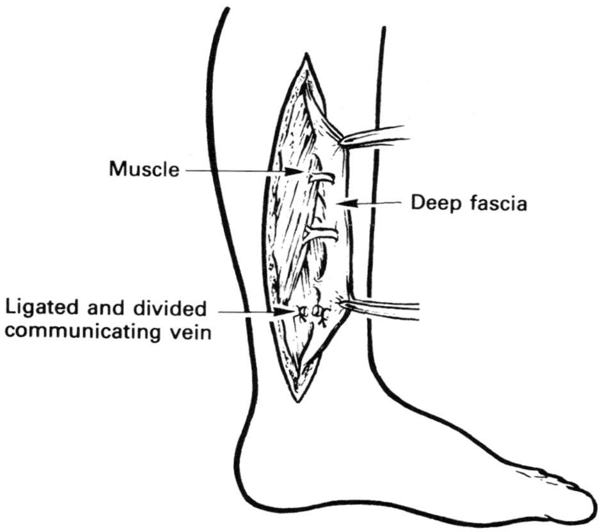

Fig. 11.18 Ligation of incompetent calf communicating veins.

Results

Varicosity can always develop in superficial veins that were not treated initially, because at the time they were not affected. Despite this, very good results have been reported for both surgery[92] and sclerotherapy,[98] although there are no series that have been subjected to independent scrutiny. About two thirds of patients never demand further treatment, although a third of these develop some new veins.

Recurrences

Patients should be warned that varicose veins can recur. Inadequate or incorrect surgery requires re-operation. This surgery is difficult and has a greater risk of complications.[61,62] Groin recurrences are most common, and after their presence has been confirmed by varicography (Fig. 11.12), the saphenofemoral junction should be approached over the front of the femoral artery. The stump of the long saphenous vein is ligated and any tributaries entering this segment of the femoral vein are disconnected.

VENOUS LIPODERMATOSCLEROSIS

Skin changes develop in the gaiter skin around the ankle of only a few patients with primary varicose veins while in most they occur some years after a deep vein thrombosis. The skin and subcutaneous tissues become indurated, tender and inflamed in the gaiter area of the calf[61,62] (Fig. 11.19). The skin becomes pigmented with both melanin and haemosiderin. These skin changes are invariably associated with incompetence of the ankle communicating veins and dilated capillaries beneath the malleolus (an ankle flare).[63] When these changes are present they precede and coincide with the development of venous ulceration (Fig. 11.11).

VENOUS ULCERATION

Ulceration may develop spontaneously but more commonly a minor injury breaks the continuity of skin already damaged by

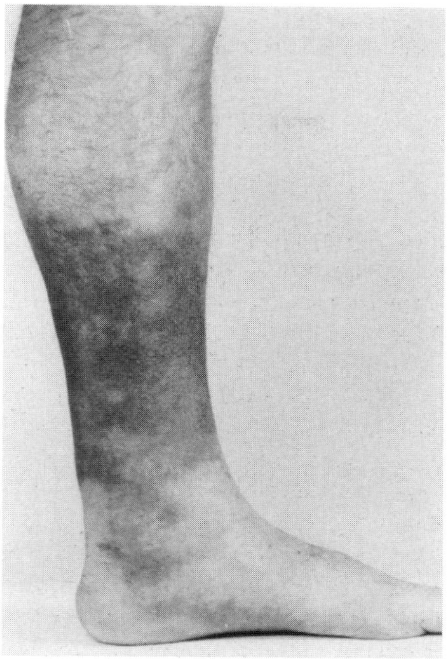

Fig. 11.19 The changes of lipodermatosclerosis.

lipodermatosclerosis. The factors involved in the genesis of ulcers include a high venous pressure, pericapillary fibrin deposition, white cell activation and trapping and increased production of free radicals.[101–105] The exact mechanism is still not known and remains the subject of much research. A number of surveys have shown that the prevalence of venous ulceration is around 0.3%[106,107] although this may represent an underestimate.[108,109] Between a half and a third occur in limbs that have sustained a previous deep vein thrombosis.

Venous ulcers are terraced simple ulcers with gently sloping edges (Fig. 11.20). The granulations in their base vary with the state of healing of the ulcer. These appear red and velvety if the ulcer is uninfected and healing well; white and fibrous if it is long-standing and stationary; and yellow and offensive if it is infected and enlarging. Venous ulcers invariably occur within an area of lipodermatosclerosis in the gaiter skin, but are not always associated with visible varicose veins. When present, the nature of the superficial venous incompetence must be carefully determined by clinical examination and special investigations. Venous ulcers

REFERENCES

101. Burnand K G, Whimster I, Clemenson G et al Br J Surg 1981; 68: 297
102. Browse N L, Burnand K G Lancet 1982; 2: 243
103. Burnand K G, Whimster I, Naidoo A, Browse N L Br Med J 1982; 285: 1071
104. Thomas P R S, Nash G B, Dormandy J A Br Med J 1988; 296: 1693
105. Coleridge-Smith P D, Thomas P, Scurr J H, Dormandy J A Br Med J 1988; 296: 1726
106. Callum M J, Ruckley C V, Harper D R, Dale J J Br Med J 1985; 290: 1855
107. Edwards A T, MChir Thesis 1997, University of Wales
108. Nelzen O, Bergqvist D, Lindhagen A Br J Surg 1996; 83: 255
109. Baker S R, Stacey M C, Jopp-McKay A G et al Br J Surg 1991; 78: 864

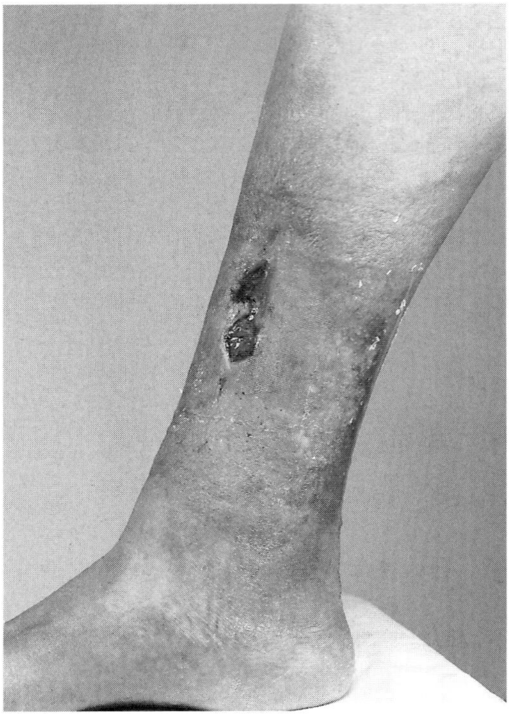

Fig. 11.20 A venous ulcer.

must be differentiated from ischaemic ulcers (Fig. 11.21a), traumatic ulcers, vasculitic ulcers (e.g. rheumatoid or scleroderma) (Fig. 11.21b) and neoplastic ulcers (basal cell or squamous cell carcinomas) (Fig. 11.21c,d). Other rare causes of leg ulceration include neuropathic damage (e.g. diabetes) (Fig. 11.21e) syphilis, tuberculosis, pyoderma gangrenosum (Fig. 11.21f), necrobiosis lipoidica, arteriovenous fistulae, blood dyscrasias (Fig. 11.21g) and artefactual damage (Fig. 11.21h).[110,111]

The peripheral pulses must always be palpated and if they cannot be felt Doppler ultrasound pressures must be measured. Microbiological swabs should be taken and cultured for aerobes and anaerobes and a full blood count and erythrocyte sedimentation rate obtained. Autoantibodies should be measured if there is a suspicion of vasculitis and serological tests should be performed for syphilis if the cause of the ulcer remains obscure. The urine and blood should be tested for sugar, and if there are any signs of neuropathy (e.g. loss of deep pain and proprioception) an electromyogram may be helpful. When an ulcer fails to heal, a biopsy must be taken and this should be done at once if

REFERENCES

110. Dodd H, Cockett F B The Pathology and Surgery of the Veins of the Lower Limb. Churchill Livingstone, Edinburgh 1976
111. Browse N L, Burnand K G, Lea Thomas M Diseases of the Veins. Arnold, London 1988

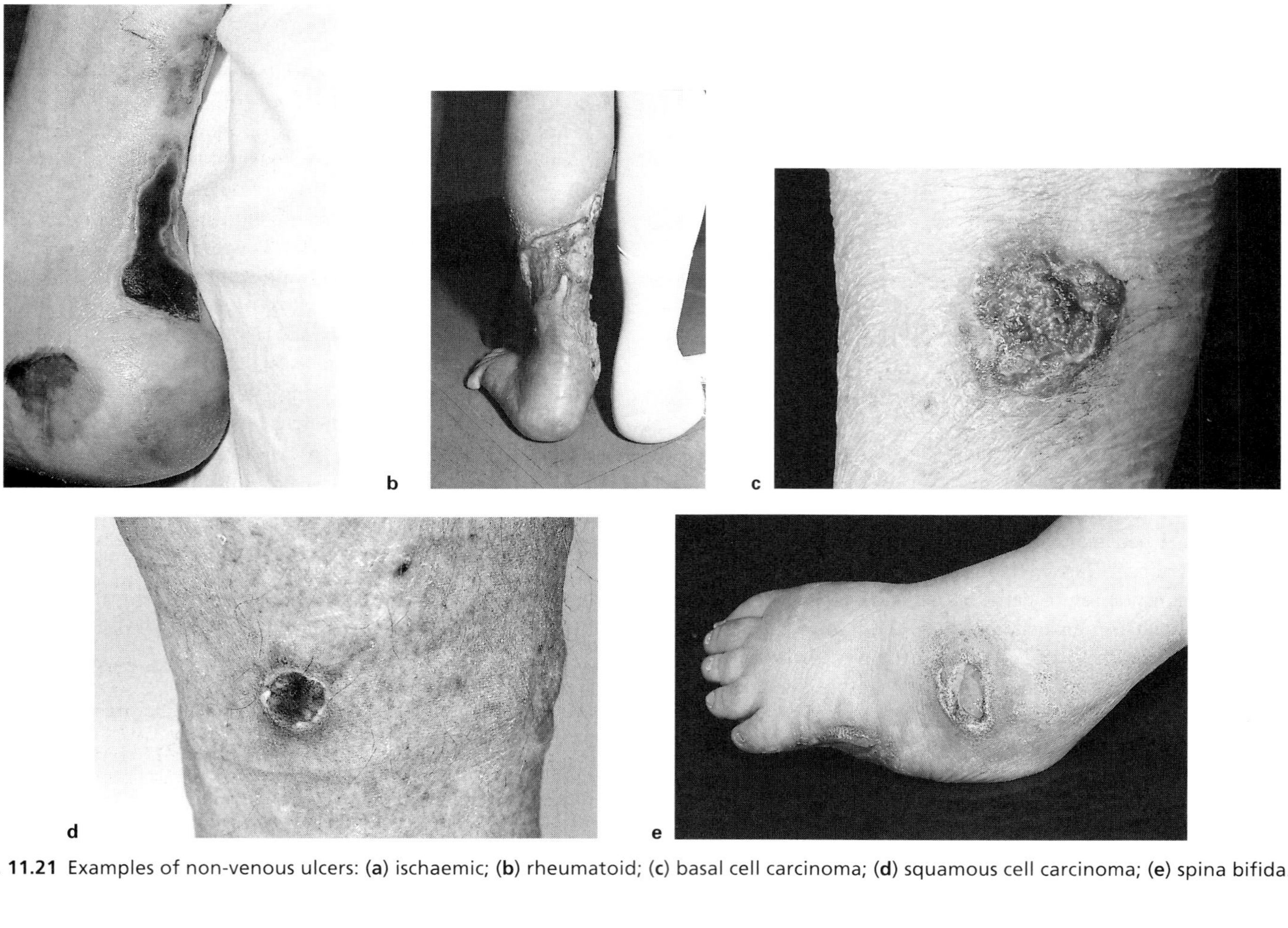

a b c d e

Fig. 11.21 Examples of non-venous ulcers: (**a**) ischaemic; (**b**) rheumatoid; (**c**) basal cell carcinoma; (**d**) squamous cell carcinoma; (**e**) spina bifida.

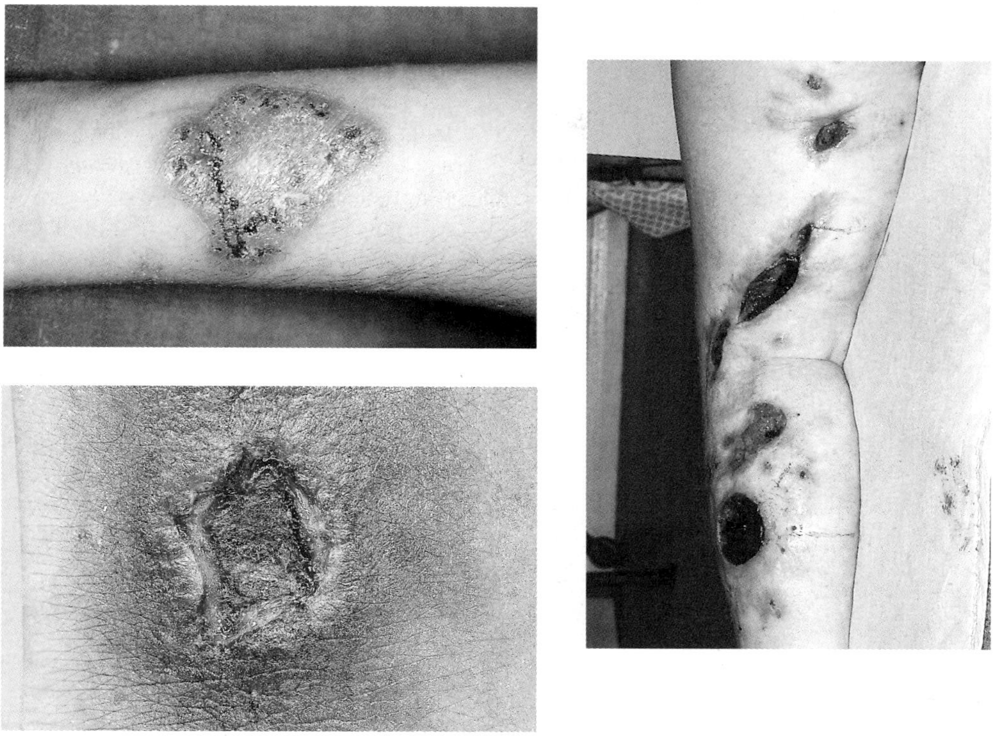

f g h

Fig. 11.21 (continued) Examples of non-venous ulcers: (**f**) pyoderma gangrenosum; (**g**) sickle; (**h**) self inflicted.

there is any suspicion of malignancy (elevated and overhanging edge) which can develop in a long-standing venous ulcer (Marjolin's ulcer).[112]

Management

Most ulcers which are considered on initial assessment to be venous are treated conservatively at first. This treatment consists of occlusive dressings covered by compression bandages or stockings, worn from the foot to the knee. Many different types of dressings and bandages have been used but provision of adequate compression over the calf-pump is probably more important than the type of dressing, although a number of studies have compared the efficacy of different dressings and compression regimens in promoting ulcer healing.[113,114]

Dry, non-adherent dressings or paste bandages, both covered by elasticated bandages, are the most popular methods of achieving compression (Fig. 11.22). The ulcer is gently cleaned once a week and the dressing and bandages are carefully reapplied. More frequent changes of dressings and bandages may be required if there is copious exudate from the ulcer. The area of ulceration should be measured at each attendance and, providing the ulcer is closing, conservative treatment may be continued.

Between 50% and 70% of ulcers are healed at three months and 80–90% by 12 months. Operative management is indicated if the ulcer remains static or if it enlarges. This consists of excising the ulcer base back to healthy tissue and applying pinch grafts,[115] mesh grafts or postage-stamp split-skin grafts to the ulcer base.[116] There is no evidence that antibiotics, antiseptics or local applications speed ulcer healing and they may delay healing. When the ulcer has healed the patient should be investigated by duplex Doppler, venous pressure measurements (or an equivalent test of calf-pump function) and phlebography. When the venous abnormality has been clearly defined this should be corrected if possible. Saphenous surgery and communicating vein ligation are successful in preventing re-ulceration in patients with normal deep veins but have not proved effective in post-thrombotic limbs. The relative value of saphenous and communicating vein surgery is disputed and awaits new randomized clinical studies.[117] Permanent use of graduated elastic support stockings, stimulation of fibrinolysis and reduction of viscosity by drugs,[118] venous reconstruction[119] and valvular transplantation[120] have all been used in post-thrombotic limbs in an attempt to prevent re-ulceration,[111] (Fig. 11.23) but few good control trials have yet been published. Permanent elastic hosiery should be prescribed for all those who have had a venous ulcer and patients should be

REFERENCES

112. Marjolin J N Ulcere diet de med practique, 2nd edn. Paris 1846.
113. Burnand K G, Northeast A D R et al Br J Surg 1989; 76: 1332
114. Blair S D, Wright D D I et al Br Med J 1988; 297: 1159
115. Poskitt K R, James A J et al Br Med J 1987; 294: 674
116. Chilvers A S, Freeman G K Lancet 1969; ii: 1087
117. Burnand K G, O'Donnell T F et al Lancet 1976; 1: 936
118. Burnand K G, Pattison M, Browse N L In: Davidson J F, Bachman F et al (eds) Progress in Fibrinolysis, vol 6. Churchill Livingstone, Edinburgh 1983
119. Bergan J J, Yao J S T et al J Vasc Surg 1986; 3: 174
120. Taheri S A, Lazar L et al Surgery 1982; 91: 28

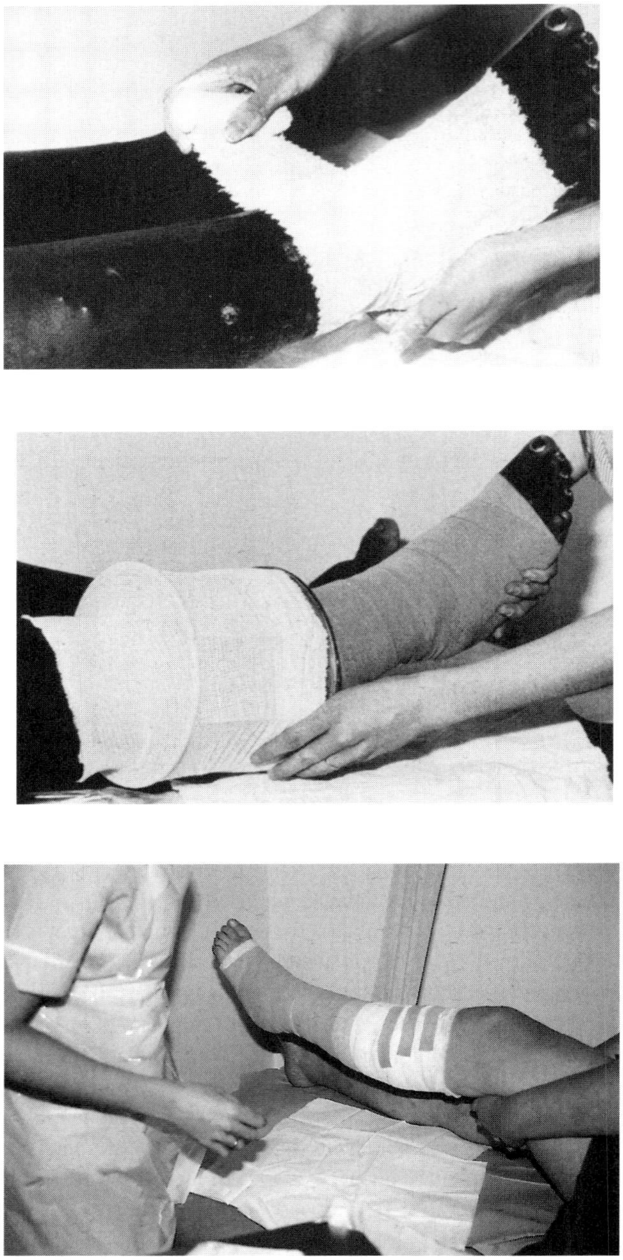

a

b

c

Fig. 11.22 **(a,b)** A paste bandage being applied to an ulcerated limb. **(c)** Application of a four-layer bandage.

warned to take care of their legs as there is always the possibility of re-ulceration, especially after minor trauma.[121]

DEEP VEIN THROMBOSIS

A thrombosis is a semi-solid mass, formed from blood constituents, which develops within the blood stream. Venous thrombosis is a common condition which can arise in the deep and superficial veins of the lower limb and in the veins of the pelvis. It may also occur in the veins of the upper limb in association with thoracic inlet syndrome or iatrogenic trauma.

Incidence/prevalence

98% of all venous thrombi arise in the deep veins of the legs and pelvis and 2% develop at other sites.[122] The true incidence of venous thrombosis in the general population is not known, although clinical and phlebographic studies in patients from a defined population presenting with symptoms in Scandinavia suggest that the incidence is approximately 0.5%.[123] 30% of all patients over the age of 40 undergoing major surgical operations develop a deep vein thrombosis if no prophylaxis is used.[124] After major hip surgery, the incidence was 60%,[125] and after major gynaecological surgery, 20–30%.[126] Deep vein thrombosis is not confined to surgical patients, the incidence in medical patients after myocardial infarction and cerebrovascular accidents is 20%.[127] The incidence of deep vein thrombosis in patients under the age of 40 having major surgery is less than 5%, but in patients over the age of 80, particularly with a past history of venous thrombosis, the incidence approaches 100%. Prophylactic measures have now reduced all these figures.

Aetiology

An interaction between the vessel wall, platelets and the coagulation system modified by the fibrinolytic system is responsible for the development of thrombosis. In 1856 Virchow[128] described three factors which he felt were important in the development of deep vein thrombosis. These factors, known as Virchow's triad, are stasis, vein wall damage and increased coagulation of blood. Alterations in the coagulation system, which include congenital deficiencies or acquired abnormalities, increase the risk of venous thrombosis. The importance of antithrombin III, the lupus anticoagulant, heparin co-factor, protein C, α_2-macroglobulin, protein S and α_1-antitrypsin and activated protein C resistance is now recognized.[129,130] Abnormalities within the fibrinolytic system may also be of importance. Subtle changes in the structure and function of the endothelium may encourage white cells and platelets to adhere to the wall and thrombus to accumulate.[131] The initial thrombus is encouraged to propagate if this is combined with stasis or hypercoagulability. Increasing age, pregnancy, coexisting malignancy, a past history of venous thrombosis or pulmonary embolism, obesity, administration of oestrogens and varicose veins are all associated with an increased risk of deep vein thrombosis.[132] The risk factors for deep vein thrombosis are listed in Table 11.2.

REFERENCES

121. Browse N L Br Med J 1983; 286: 1920
122. Gibbs N M Br J Surg 1957; 191: 15
123. Bergqvist D, Lindblad N Br J Surg 1985; 72: 105
124. Carr K, Nicolaides V V et al Lancet 1972; i: 540
125. Hull R, Hirsch J et al Thromb Res 1979; 15: 227
126. Clark-Pearson D L, Synan I S et al Obst Gynaecol 1984; 63: 92
127. Nicolaides A M, Kakkar V V et al Br Med J 1971; 1: 132
128. Virchow R R Cellular Pathology. Churchill, London 1860
129. Melissari E, Bonte G, Lindo V S et al Blood Coagulation and Fibrinolysis 1992; 3(6): 749
130. Weston-Smith S, Revell P, Savidge G F Br J Hosp Med 1989; 41: 368
131. Stewart G R, Rithchie W G M, Lynch P E Am J Pathol 1974. Cited in: Nicolaides A N (ed) Thromboembolism. MTP, Lancaster, 1975
132. Nicolaides A N, Gordon-Smith I In: Nicolaides A N (ed) Thromboembolism. MTP, Lancaster 1975

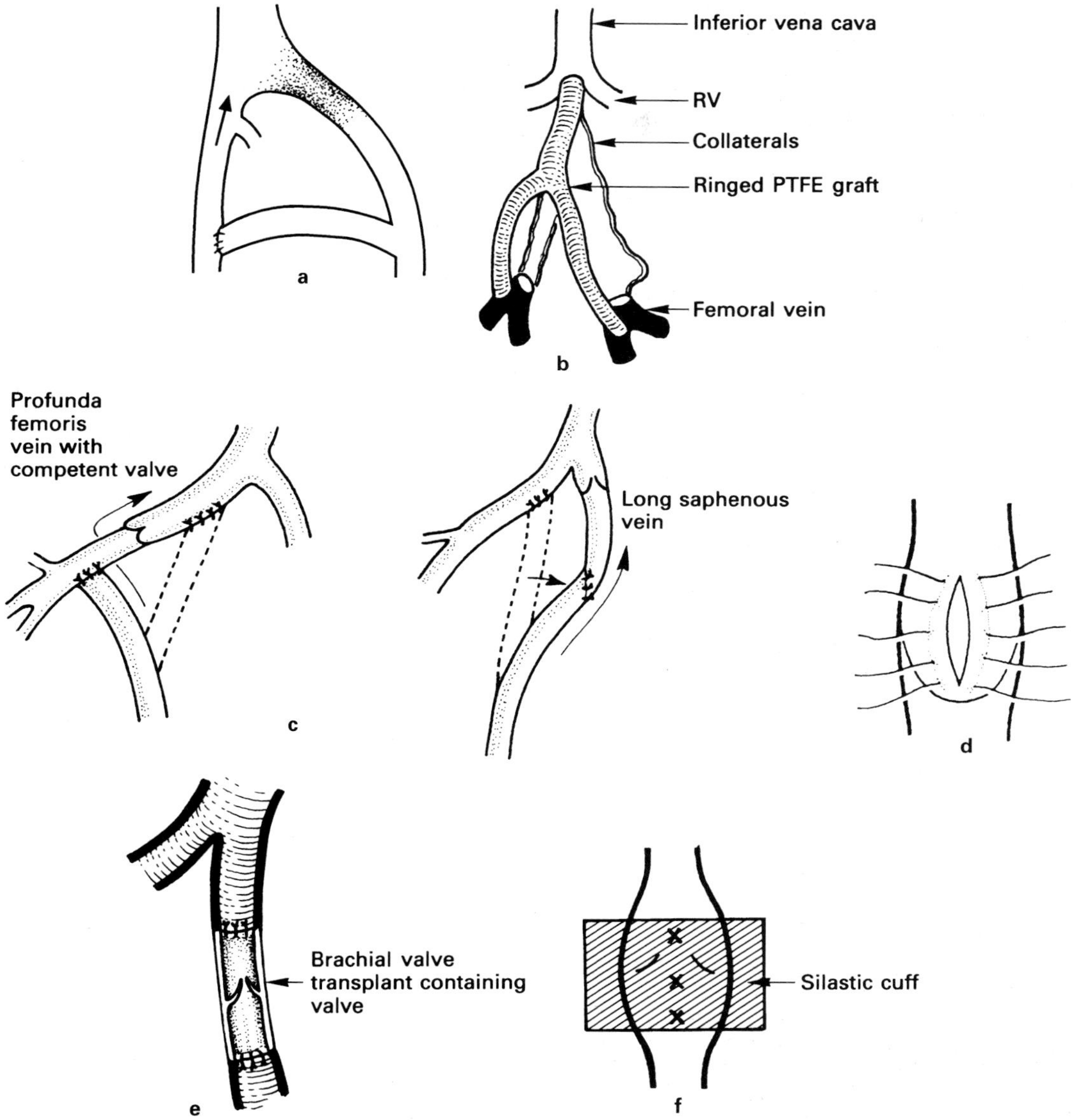

Fig. 11.23 Techniques that have been used to bypass obstructed deep veins or restore valular competence: (**a**) Palma; (**b**) Dale; (**c**) Kistner; (**d**) Jones; (**e**) Taheri; (**f**) Lane.

Although smoking has been shown to damage venous endothelium, it has been suggested that there is a lower incidence of deep vein thrombosis in smokers compared to non-smokers, although the mechanism by which cigarette smoking prevents thrombosis is not known. Prolonged sitting in air-raid shelters, or nowadays on international airline flights, is another factor; similarly immobility on the operating table may predispose to thrombosis.

Pathology

Aschoff[133] gave the first classic description of the pathogenesis of venous thrombosis. Initially platelets adhere to the endothelial surface and form a grey amorphous cluster. More platelets then adhere, with fibrin and red cells becoming deposited between the layers of platelets giving the laminated appearance known as the lines of Zahn (Fig. 11.24). The coralline (coral-like) thrombus so formed extends into the blood stream, becoming bent in the direction of flow. The flow past the thrombus decreases and eventually ceases with the rapid extension of red jelly-like propagated thrombus consisting of a fibrin and red cell meshwork extending up the vein as far as the next tributary.[134,135] The thrombus can continue to extend up the vein if the orifice of the tributary becomes occluded and may reach several feet in length. At this stage the thrombus that is loosely attached or lying free becomes easily detached increasing the risk of pulmonary embolism. Thrombus that becomes tightly adherent to the wall contracts and organizes, producing valve destruction and luminal occlusion,

REFERENCES

133. Aschoff L Beitr Pathol Anat 1912; 52: 207
134. Sevitt S J Clin Pathol 1974; 27: 517
135. Hadfield C J R Coll Surg Engl 1950; 6: 219

Table 11.2 Risk factors for deep vein thrombosis

Age
Sex
Season
Race
Occupation
Type of operation
Type of anaesthetic
Length of operation
Pregnancy and puerperium
General injury
Local injury
Immobilization
Bed rest
Malignancy
Previous venous thrombosis
Varicose veins
Obesity
Cardiac failure
Myocardial infarction
Arterial ischaemia
Contraceptive pill
Intravenous saline (haemodilution)
Haemostatic drugs
Other drugs
Vasculitis (Buerger's disease, Behçet's syndrome)
Congenital venous abnormalities: Klipper–Trenaunay syndrome

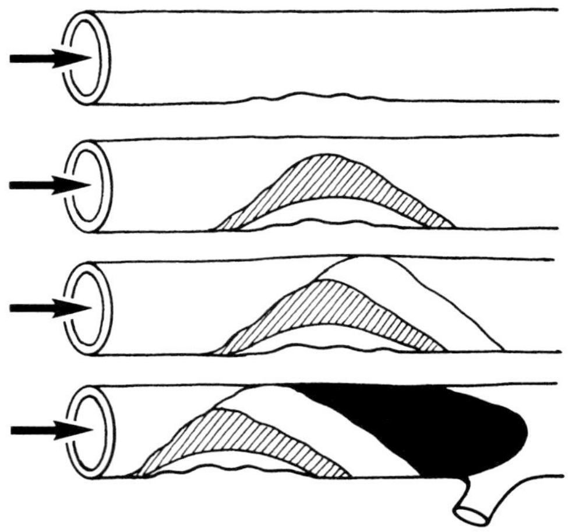

Fig. 11.24 Stages in the development of a venous thrombosis. **1.** The initial platelet cluster adheres to the vein wall as a grey amorphous thickening. **2.** Laminated coralline thrombus develops on the surface of the platelet cluster, with alternative layers of fibrin and red cells trapped between layers of fibrin and platelets (the lines of Zahn). **3.** As the thrombus grows across the flowing blood, it bends in the direction of the blood flow, making the lines of Zahn oblique. **4.** When the vein is totally occluded, non-adherent, jelly-like propagated thrombus spreads up the vessel as far as the next major tributary. This thrombus is dark red and consists only of fibrin and red cells.

responsible for the eventual development of the post-thrombotic limb. This process usually starts in the valve cusps of the soleal sinusoids (Fig. 11.25) although thrombosis may originate in the profunda femoris, common femoral, internal iliac and even the renal veins.

Clinical features

The symptoms of deep vein thrombosis include limb swelling, calf pain, tenderness, and a low-grade pyrexia. Even with extensive deep vein thrombosis, symptoms may not be experienced; a

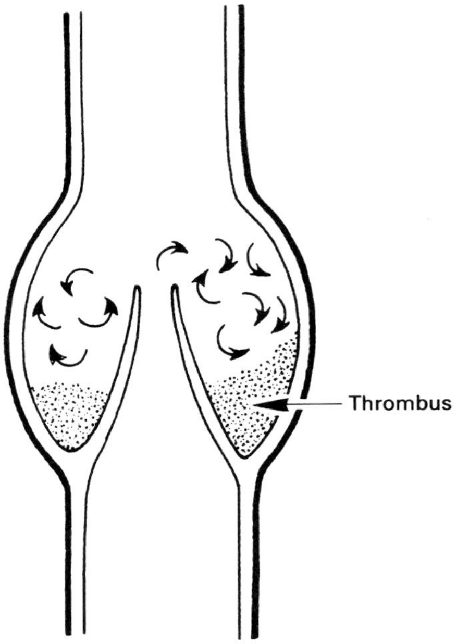

Fig. 11.25 Thrombus developing in a valve pocket.

pulmonary embolism or the subsequent development of a post-thrombotic limb may be the only indication of a previous venous thrombosis.[136] Occasionally patients with a severe ileofemoral thrombosis present with a very swollen white oedematous limb (phlegmasia alba dolens). More commonly a massive proximal thrombosis causes a blue leg (phlegmasia cerulea dolens) and this may eventually progress to true venous gangrene in a few patients (Fig. 11.26). Confirmation of swelling, tenderness over the deep veins, ankle oedema (especially if it is unilateral), and dilated superficial veins support the diagnosis. Homan's dorsiflexion test is inaccurate and should be abandoned. Clinical signs are often unreliable

REFERENCE

136. Jeffrey B C, Immelman E J, Banatar S R S Afr Med J 1957; 643

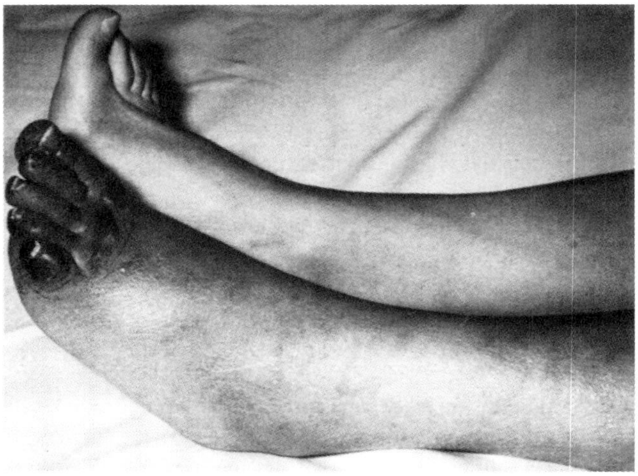

Fig. 11.26 Leg with venous gangrene of the toes. From Browse et al[183] with kind permission.

and special tests are essential to confirm the diagnosis. Only half of the patients with deep vein thrombosis present with clinical signs and 30–50% of patients with an indicative history and physical signs have normal deep veins on phlebography.[137] Ruptured Baker's cyst (Fig. 11.27) cellulitis, lymphoedema, torn calf muscles and calf haematomas can all mimic the signs of deep vein thrombosis. The full differential diagnosis is given in Table 11.3.

Investigations

All the tests that have been used to confirm the diagnosis of deep vein thrombosis have been compared with bipedal ascending contrast phlebography, which outlines the thrombus with a high degree of accuracy (Fig. 11.28). Venous imaging using B-mode ultrasound appears to be an alternative method of diagnosis,[138] but is less accurate than phlebography in the diagnosis of calf thrombosis. Nevertheless many are now advocating this as the investigation of first choice. Thrombus may be imaged or assumed if the vein cannot be compressed (Fig. 11.29). If this test is negative follow-up investigation should be undertaken, using phlebography in patients in whom there is a high suspicion of deep vein thrombosis or a repeat ultrasound in 2–3 days in those in whom there is a low suspicion. Isotope phlebography, although simple to perform, does not achieve the diagnostic accuracy of contrast phlebography.[139] The radioactive I^{125} fibrinogen uptake test was a valuable research tool but has now been withdrawn because of the risk of AIDS.[140]

Plethysmography, which detects a reduced venous capacitance and reduced venous outflow, may be used as a screening test,

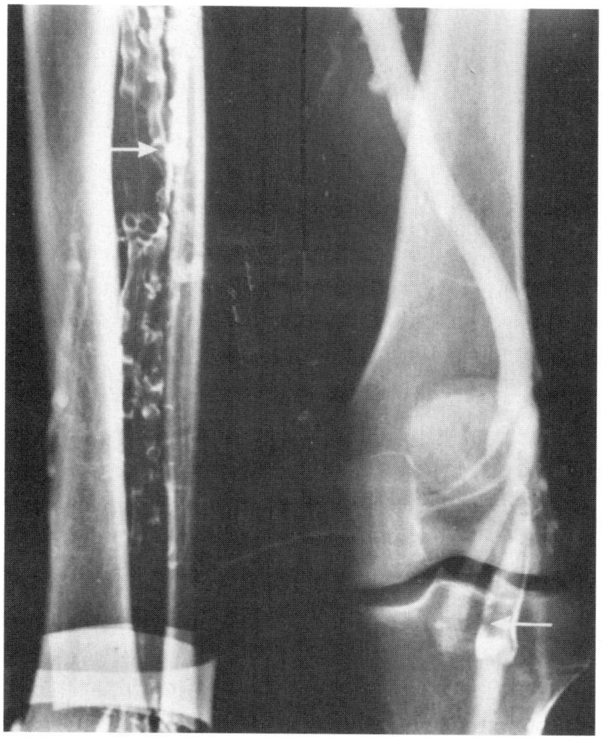

Fig. 11.28 Phlebogram showing deep vein thrombosis.

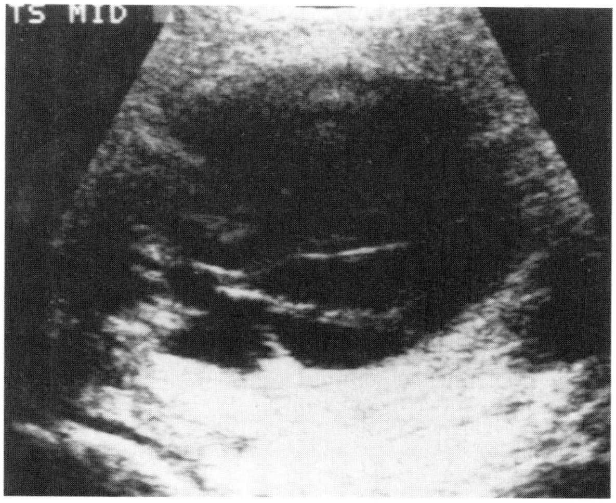

Fig. 11.27 An ultrasound of a ruptured Baker's cyst.

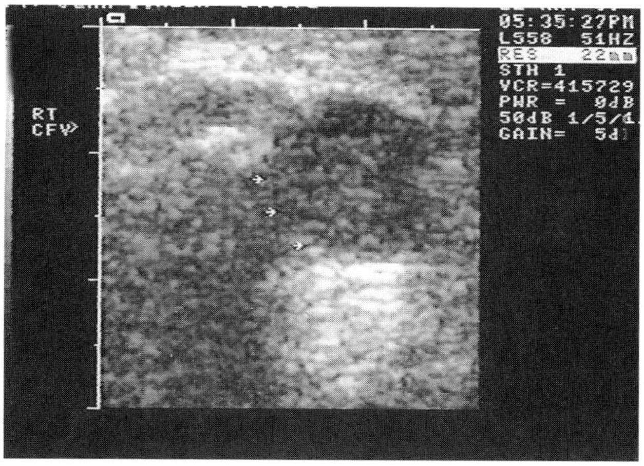

Fig. 11.29 Duplex scan showing thrombus.

Table 11.3 Differential diagnosis for deep vein thrombosis

Torn gastrocnemius muscle
Ruptured Baker's cyst
Calf haematoma
Lymphoedema with cellulitis
Acute arterial ischaemia
Extrinsic obstruction of veins and lymphatics in pelvis
Pathological fracture of femur
Superficial thrombophlebitis
Acute arthritis of the knee
Haemarthrosis of the knee
Torn meniscus
Achilles tendonitis
Oedema from congestive cardiac failure of the nephrotic syndrome
Rapidly growing sarcoma
Myositis ossificans
Münchhausen's syndrome

REFERENCES

137. Kakkar V V Arch Surg 1972; 104: 152
138. Sullivan E D, Peter D J, Cranley J J J Vasc Surg 1984; 1: 465
139. Hyman J H, O'Sullivan E, Thomas E Br J Surg 1973; 60: 52
140. Negus D, Pinto D J et al Br J Surg 1968; 55: 835

but its accuracy for non-occlusive calf thrombi is poor.[141] Thermography has also been used to screen for thrombosis, but its specificity is poor[142] and the equipment is expensive to purchase.

Prevention

The risk of death from pulmonary embolism has resulted in much attention being paid to deep vein thrombosis prophylaxis in the postoperative period. Patients can be classified into high risk (elderly, previous thrombosis, malignancy, extensive pelvic surgery), medium risk (most major operations) and low risk (young and minor surgery).[143] The methods employed fall conveniently into mechanical methods of prophylaxis and antithrombotic methods. Graduated compression stockings, intermittent pneumatic compression devices and electrical calf stimulation[144–147] have all been shown to reduce the incidence of venous thrombosis. Graduated compression stockings provide a simple and economical form of prophylaxis that is suitable for all low- to medium-risk patients. Intermittent pneumatic compression using either single or multichamber devices is also effective in reducing the incidence of deep vein thrombosis and is preferred by some. The use of pneumatic devices combined with graduated elastic compression stockings appears to be synergistic.[148] Electrical stimulation is now rarely used.

Full-scale anticoagulation is unpopular because of the risk of postoperative bleeding, although the use of warfarin has proved to be the most effective means of reducing the incidence of pulmonary embolism after hip fractures.[149,150] Subcutaneous heparin has been the most widely studied method of prophylaxis and has been shown to be effective in low doses (5000 u b.d.)[151] in reducing the incidence of both postoperative venous thrombosis and pulmonary embolism, albeit at the expense of an increased risk of bleeding. Combinations of heparin with graduated elastic compression stockings may prove more effective, although trials to date have proven inconclusive.[152] Ultra-low doses of intravenously administered heparin (1000 u b.d.) may reduce the risk of bleeding without losing prophylactic potency. Low molecular weight heparin fragments have also been shown to be effective in reducing the incidence of deep vein thrombosis, and they may be associated with a reduced incidence of bleeding complications. A lower dose given over a day seems to provide adequate prophylaxis even in patients having hip replacements, and the reduced frequency of administration and increased efficacy have now made this the most popular form of prophylaxis.[153–155]

Dextran 70 does not conclusively reduce the incidence of deep vein thrombosis, although it does appear to reduce the incidence of fatal pulmonary embolism.[156] Antiplatelet agents are of low but mild efficacy.[157] Combinations of prophylactic methods, including heparin, graduated compression stockings and intermittent pneumatic compression devices, have been shown to be synergistic.[158] However, even with 'ideal' prophylaxis, between 5 and 20% of all patients still develop a deep vein thrombosis and up to 0.2% still have a fatal pulmonary embolism.[158] Patients remain at risk even after they have been discharged home, and prophylactic measures should ideally be continued for several weeks.

Treatment of established deep vein thrombosis

Treatment cannot be based on a clinical diagnosis because this is so inaccurate, and the presence and extent of the thrombosis should be established by duplex scan or phlebography.[159]

Established thrombosis requires urgent anticoagulant therapy, and heparin is usually given via the intravenous route, although subcutaneous administration is also effective.[160,161] A single intravenous dose of 70 i.u./kg (about 5000 u for most adults) is recommended, followed by a constant infusion of about 20–30 i.u./kg per hour. The dosage is usually monitored by measuring the activated partial thromboplastin time although there is little evidence that this is accurate.[162] Alternatively, 10 000 i.u. heparin can be given subcutaneously every 12 hours. There may however be some resistance to heparin in severe thromboembolism which can usually be overcome by increasing the dose. In a minority, heparin resistance is marked, the result of an unusual immune response which results in thrombocytopenia, intravascular coagulation and bleeding.[163,164] These patients may require controlled defibrination with intravenous Arvin, or thrombolytic therapy. Low molecular weight heparin can be used in some of these patients without inducing this immune response. This can be monitored by daily estimation of platelet count.

Warfarin therapy may be begun after 24 or 48 hours. Several flexible dose schedules for warfarin therapy have been devised and if a 10 mg loading dose is given on the first day, followed by 5 mg on the second, third and fourth days, the majority of patients will fall within the therapeutic range of the international normalized ratio, as long as the sample has been collected less than 12 hours after stopping the heparin infusion.

REFERENCES

141. Barnes R W, Collicott P E et al Surgery 1972; 72: 971
142. Cooke E D, Pitcher M P Br J Surg 1974; 61: 971
143. Browse N L Ann Roy Coll Surg 1977; 59: 138
144. Scuff J H, Ibrihim S Z et al Br J Surg 1977; 64: 371
145. Allen A, Williams J T et al Br J Surg 1983; 70: 172
146. Nicolaides A N, Myles C, Hoare N Surgery 1983; 94: 21
147. Doran F S A, White H M Br J Surg 1967; 54: 686
148. Scurr R H, Coleridge Smith P D, Hasty J H Surgery 1987; 5: 816
149. Ockelfjord P A, Kesteven P J, Patterson J et al Br J Surg 1989; 56: 178
150. Eriksson B I, Zachrisson B E, Teger-Nilsson A C, Risberg B Br J Surg 1988; 7.5f: 1053
151. A multicentre controlled trial. Lancet 1974; ii: 118
152. Kakkar V V, Stamatakis J et al JAMA 1979; 241: 39
153. Lassen M R, Borris L C, Christiansen H M et al Semin Thromb Hemost 1991; 17(suppl 3): 284
154. Nurmohamed M T, Rosendaal F R, Büller H et al Lancet 1992; 340: 152
155. Leizorovicz A, Haugh M C, Chapuis F R, Samama M M, Boissel J P Br Med J 1992; 305: 913
156. Bergqvist D, Efsing H O, Hallböök T, Lindblad B Acta Chir Scand 1980; 146: 559
157. European Consensus Statement Int Angiol 1992; 11: 151
158. Willie-Jorgensen P, Fischer A et al Br J Surg 1985; 72: 574
159. Ramsay L E Br Med J 1983; 286: 698
160. Bentley P G, Kakkar V V et al Br Med J 1987; 294: 1189
161. Walker M G, Shaw J W et al Br Med J 1987; 294: 1189
162. Blaisdell W Cardiovasc Surg 1996; 4(6): 691
163. Kapsch D, Adelstone E et al Surgery 1979; 86: 148
164. Towne J B, Berhard V M et al Arch Surg 1979; 114: 372

The heparin infusion should be stopped at 9 p.m. on the last day and a sample for the international normalized ratio taken 12 hours later; this allows the warfarin dose to be adjusted when the result is reported in the afternoon. Patients receiving antibiotics or other drugs known to interfere with the vitamin K: warfarin balance require smaller loading and maintenance doses. Warfarin treatment is normally maintained for 3–6 months, and there is now clear evidence that early cessation leads to an increased risk of re-thrombosis.[165]

In some patients with coagulation abnormalities, such as antithrombin III deficiency or recurrent venous thrombosis, it may be necessary to give warfarin indefinitely. The dosage of warfarin is maintained by weekly or twice-weekly international normalized ratio estimations.

The fibrinolytic agents streptokinase, urokinase and tissue plasminogen activator may be used selectively if patients are shown to have an extensive fresh venous thrombosis. Given into a peripheral vein these agents have not been shown to be effective in reducing the incidence of post-thrombotic limb but the use of high doses delivered directly into the thrombus is currently being studied. The role of surgical thrombectomy has never been clearly established. In the acutely ischaemic limb with phlegmasia cerulae dolens as the result of an iliofemoral thrombus, surgical thrombectomy is indicated and may prevent limb loss.[166] After the femoral vein or veins have been exposed and snared, Fogarty catheters are passed in an antegrade and, if possible, in a retrograde direction to remove thrombus. Pulmonary embolism caused by catheter disruption is prevented by positive pressure ventilation. Further thrombus can be squeezed from the leg by compressing the calf with an Esmarch elastic bandage. An arteriovenous shunt made beyond the venotomy may help to prevent re-thrombosis[167] and full anticoagulation is required postoperatively. Thrombectomy has no place in the management of early distal venous thrombosis or in thrombus that is more than 5 days old. All thromboses are associated with intimal and valvular damage, and although thrombus can be removed, valves may still be permanently destroyed.[168,169] The risk of pulmonary embolism increases if extensive loose venous thrombosis is present and under these circumstances the place of venous interruption must be considered, especially if the patient has had a small herald embolus.[170] Ligation of major veins can lead to outflow obstruction and the eventual development of the post-thrombotic syndrome in a proportion of limbs. The insertion of transvenous filters to prevent venous emboli reaching the lung is now clearly preferable to distal vein ligation.

Direct methods of partially occluding the vena cava have now become obsolete unless the patient is undergoing surgery for another reason. The Mobin-Uddin filter was the first effective transvenous filter but the high incidence of thrombosis led to the development of the Greenfield–Kimway filter (Fig. 11.30a). There are now many other 'filters' which can be inserted percutaneously by radiologists (Fig. 18.30b). The Greenfield–Kimway filter is positioned into the vena cava via the internal jugular vein. This can be approached through a vertical or transverse incision placed over the sternomastoid muscle in the lower part of the neck but is now usually inserted percutaneously. The filter, which is shaped like a shuttlecock, is held closed within a special introducing catheter.

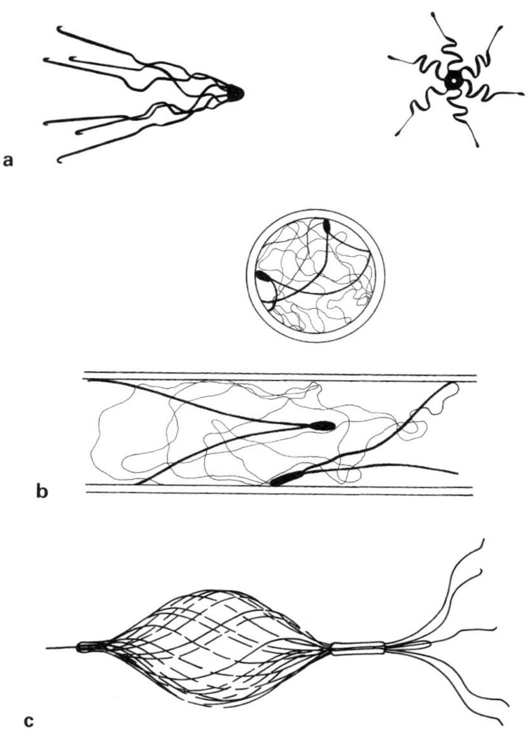

Fig. 11.30 Types of filter for interruption of inferior vena cava: (**a**) the Greenfield filter; (**b**) birds nest; (**c**) Günther.

This catheter is passed through the right atrium until the tip of the catheter comes to lie within the vena cava beneath the renal veins. Correct positioning of the filter is confirmed by contrast radiography before it is ejected. As the filter springs out, the little barbed feet hook into the vein wall and prevent it from becoming dislodged. The principal indication for inserting an inferior vena cava filter remains recurrent pulmonary embolism in patients who have received or are receiving full and adequate anticoagulation. Filters are also inserted into patients who cannot be given anticoagulants because of the risk of haemorrhage,[171,172] for example from a peptic ulcer.

Complications and recurrences

All patients who have had one deep vein thrombosis have an increased risk of developing another. Some patients develop recurrent spontaneous venous thromboses and these patients should be tested for activated protein C resistance, antithrombin III and

REFERENCES

165. Lagerstedt C I, Olsson C G et al Lancet 1985; ii: 518
166. Mahorner H, Castleberry J W, Coleman W C Ann Surg 1957; 146: 510
167. Eklof B, Linarsson E, Plate G In: Bergan J J, Yao J S T (eds) Surgery of the Veins. Grune & Stratton, Orlando 1985
168. Edwards A E, Edwards J E Surg Gynecol Obstet 1937; 65: 310
169. Plate G, Einarsson E et al Vasc Surg 1984; 1: 867
170. Browse N L, Lea Thomas M et al Br Med J 1969; 3: 382
171. Greenfield L J, Zocco J et al Ann Surg 1977; 185: 692
172. Scurr J H, Jarrett P, Wastell C Ann R Coll Surg 1983; 65: 233

protein C deficiencies, anticardiolipin antibodies and protein S deficiency (thrombophilia). These tests need to be performed when the patient is not on any form of anticoagulation which interferes with their accuracy.[173] Patients should also be screened for an occult neoplasm, and the fibrinolytic system should be assessed by measuring the euglobulin clot lysis time with and without venous compression.[174] Long-term anticoagulation is advisable in those patients who develop recurrent venous thrombosis or have a thrombophilia. Many patients with recurrent, apparently idiopathic thromboses are later found to have an occult malignancy.[175,176]

Relationship of deep vein thrombosis to pulmonary embolism

The majority of pulmonary emboli arise from venous thromboses developing within the lower limbs or pelvis. Most clinically significant pulmonary emboli arise from the femoral, iliac and pelvic veins. Venous thromboses in the calf veins seldom give rise to large pulmonary emboli until they propagate into the proximal veins.[177] There is good circumstantial evidence to suggest that reducing the incidence of deep vein thrombosis in the lower leg reduces the incidence of propagated thrombus in the proximal axial veins, and as a consequence the incidence of pulmonary embolism is reduced.[178]

Venous gangrene

The development of venous gangrene is a rare complication of massive iliofemoral thrombosis. The initial phase of phlegmasia alba dolens (white leg) usually precedes phlegmasia cerulae dolens (blue leg) but is often overlooked. The peripheral pulses are impalpable, and patients become toxic and ill as the signs of acute ischaemia develop. Venous gangrene may follow this stage if the condition remains untreated. Gangrene may be limited to the feet (Fig. 11.26) but can extend further up the limb. The symmetry of the gangrenous change in the toes distinguishes the condition from arterial ischaemia.

Pulmonary hypertension

Pulmonary hypertension develops after recurrent pulmonary emboli. It is the result of progressive obstruction of the pulmonary vasculature. The emboli are often extremely small and the onset of pulmonary hypertension is insidious. Pulmonary artery pressures are found to be high on right heart catheterization. Medical treatment is generally unsuccessful. Surgical interruption of the inferior vena cava to prevent further emboli has a place if further defects develop on lung scanning despite adequate anticoagulation. Lung transplantation is rarely indicated.

Paradoxical embolism

A patent foramen ovale, a ductus arteriosus or a ventricular septal defect allows a paradoxical embolism to occur. This is an embolus arising in the venous circulation which passes into the arterial circulation producing an arterial occlusion. This rare phenomenon should be suspected in any patient with a cardiac murmur who has a swollen leg and develops evidence of an acute arterial obstruction in the limbs or brain. Treatment involves not only removing the embolus, but also treating the venous thrombosis and subsequently closing the cardiac defect.

PULMONARY EMBOLISM

98% of pulmonary emboli originate from thrombi in the leg and pelvic veins. The symptoms of a pulmonary embolism include acute onset of pleuritic pain, dyspnoea, haemoptysis and sudden death. Many patients remain symptom-free and the diagnosis is only made on special tests or inferred from the subsequent development of pulmonary hypertension. The symptoms and signs of a deep vein thrombosis may predominate, but the presence of cyanosis, raised neck veins, a pleural rub and a fixed split second heart sound are all indicative of a pulmonary embolism.

The diagnosis of pulmonary embolism is supported by: oligaemia; wedge-shaped areas of consolidation and enlarged hilar shadows on chest radiograph; an S wave in lead 1, a Q wave in lead 3 and inverted T waves over the right chest on electrocardiogram (Fig. 11.31); and hypoxia combined with hypocarbia in the arterial blood. Ventila-tion perfusion scanning provides useful confirmation (Fig. 11.32), but pulmonary angiography (Fig. 11.33) remains the only absolute way of diagnosing embolism if the scan is equivocal. It is wrong to consider all emboli together as the size, significance and outcome of a pulmonary embolus are so variable. Miller[179] suggests they can be classified into one of four main groups:

1. Acute minor.
2. Acute massive.
3. Subacute massive.
4. Chronic (pulmonary hypertension).

In patients with a minor embolism, anticoagulation using heparin is appropriate providing the source of the embolism is confirmed and further embolism is prevented. Acute massive embolism is associated with significant pulmonary artery occlusion and marked outflow obstruction indicated by a significant rise in the pulmonary artery pressure. Emergency embolectomy can save the patient's life in these circumstances.[180,181] With smaller emboli anticoagulation or fibrinolytic treatment may be effective.

After all types of pulmonary embolism the following outcomes

REFERENCES

173. Browse N L, Burnand K G, Lea Thomas M Diseases of the Veins. Arnold, London 1988
174. Nilsson I M, Ljunger H et al Br Med J 1985; 290: 1453
175. Sproul E E Am J Cancer 1938; 34: 566
176. Lagattolla N R F, Burnand K G, Irvine A, Ferrar D Ann Roy Col Surg 1996; 78: 336
177. Gibbs N M Br J Surg 1957; 19: 15
178. Gaylan J E, Alpert J S Prog Cardiovasc Dis 1975; 17: 259
179. Miller G In: Browse N L, Burnand K G, Lea Thomas M (eds) Diseases of the Veins. Arnold, London 1988
180. Trendelenberg F Arch Klin Chir 1908; 86: 686
181. Clarke D B, Abrahams L D Lancet 1972; i: 767

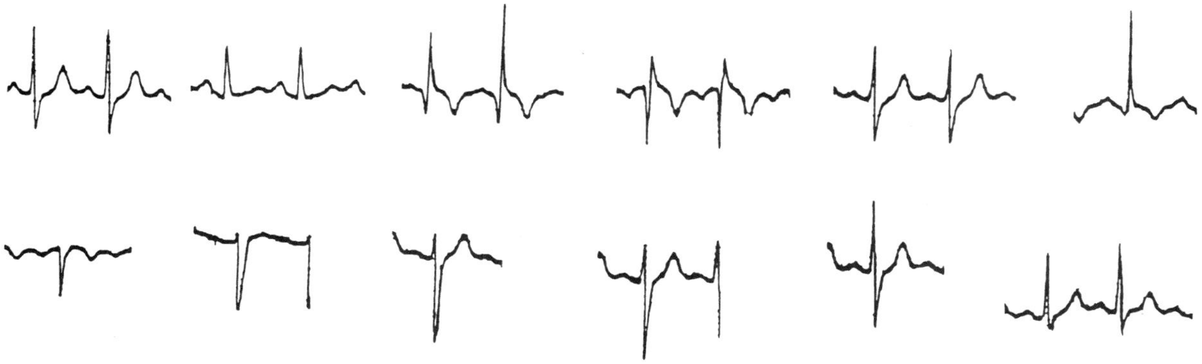

Fig. 11.31 An electrocardiogram showing the classical changes associated with a moderately severe pulmonary embolism.

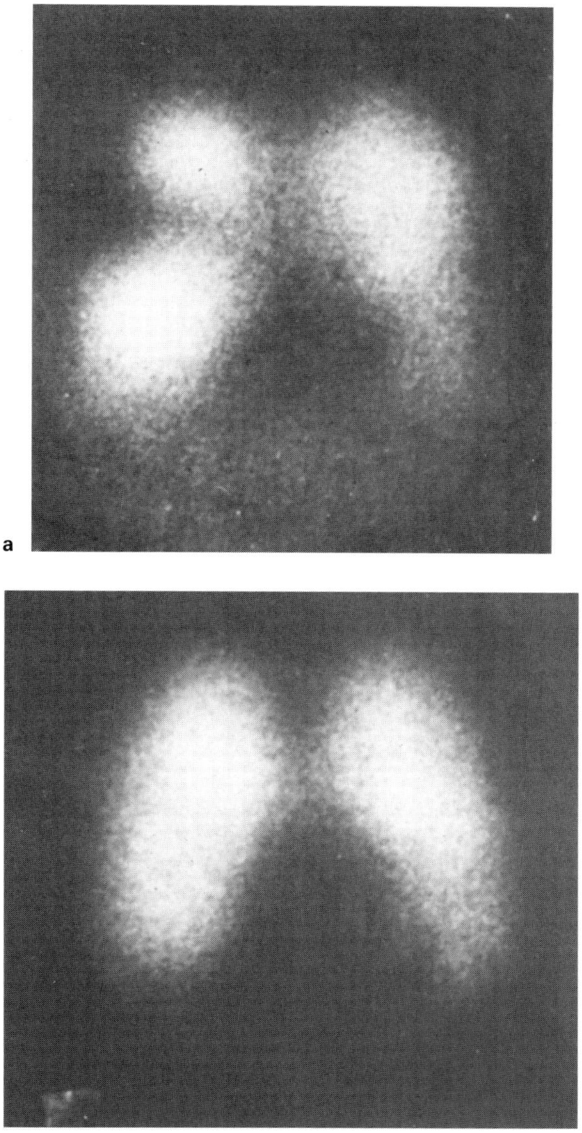

Fig. 11.32 A ventilation perfusion lung scan showing unmatched perfusion defects indicative of a pulmonary embolism.

have been found:[182,183] 10% of patients die within the first hour before the diagnosis can be confirmed or an emergency embolectomy

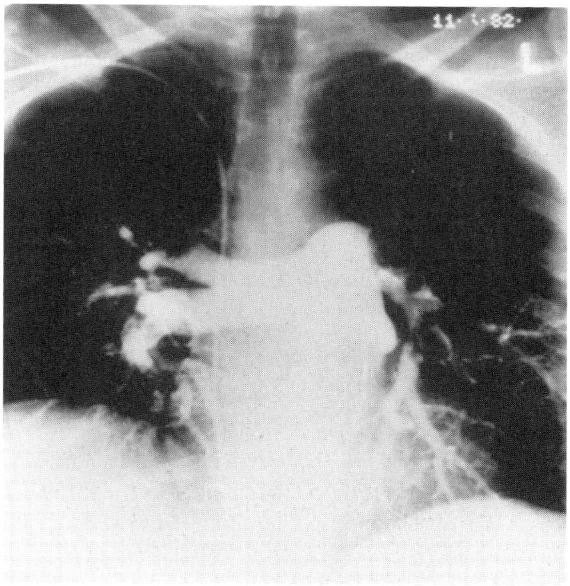

Fig. 11.33 A pulmonary angiogram showing multiple filling defects from repeated emboli.

performed; of the 90% or so who survive the initial insult the diagnosis is only confirmed in one third; when the diagnosis is made and appropriate treatment instituted the mortality is still 15%. Treatment is not instituted in patients in whom the diagnosis cannot be confirmed and in these patients the mortality is even greater than 50%.

Up to 70% of those patients presenting with the clinical features of a pulmonary embolism have normal pulmonary arteriograms. Clearly it is important to establish the diagnosis beyond doubt with pulmonary arteriography before starting treatment or attempting emergency embolectomy. Spiral CT angiography and magnetic resonance angiography may improve the diagnositic accuracy of standard contrast studies.

Once the patient has survived the initial pulmonary embolus, bipedal ascending phlebograms or duplex Doppler scans must be

REFERENCES

182. Gaylan J E, Alpert J S Prog Cardiovasc Dis 1975; 17: 259
183. Browse N L, Burnand K G, Lea Thomas M (eds) Diseases of the Veins. Arnold, London 1988

obtained to assess the presence and extent of any residual thrombus within the deep veins of the lower limbs although the detection rate of these studies is disappointing (about 20–30%). The further management of the patient depends upon these findings.

In some patients, despite adequate doses of heparin, further emboli occur.[184] Recurrent embolism in the presence of adequate anticoagulation is the best indication for interrupting the inferior vena cava.

SUPERFICIAL THROMBOPHLEBITIS

Thrombosis may affect the superficial veins. Varicose veins[185] and sclerotherapy are the most common predisposing causes of superficial thrombophlebitis. Trauma, chemical irritation and local sepsis may also play a part.[186] Patients present with a painful, hard, hot and reddened subcutaneous cord. Surgical treatment is now rarely indicated, unless the upper end of the long saphenous vein is involved when the vein should be ligated.

The majority of patients can be treated by analgesics and external elastic support. The condition is usually self-limiting, but recurrences should suggest the possibility of thrombophlebitis migrans, often associated with an underlying carcinoma.[187] Berquist & Jaroszewski[188] have shown that many patients with superficial thrombophlebitis have a coexistent deep vein thrombosis which may require treatment.

AXILLARY OR SUBCLAVIAN VEIN THROMBOSIS

This condition was originally described by Sir James Paget in 1875[189] and independently by Von Schrotter in 1884.[190] It accounts for 1–2% of all venous thromboses and may be idiopathic or secondary to a recognized cause.

Thrombosis is more common on the right, often developing after excessive or unusual exercise, and therefore has been nicknamed 'effort thrombosis'.[191] It often occurs in patients with cervical ribs or thoracic inlet obstruction and some have suggested that this is the cause of all axillary vein thromboses.[192] A number of studies have, however, shown that the aetiology is multifactorial.[193,194] Thrombosis may also occur following the insertion of catheters into the subclavian vein (central vein lines, Swan–Ganz catheters or venous access for chemotherapy).

Most patients are men between 35 and 45 years of age who present with discomfort and swelling in their dominant arm 24 h after an episode of excessive or unusual exercise. The hand and forearm feel cool and are swollen and blue. The finger movements are often diminished. There is usually pitting oedema on the dorsum of the hand and the subcutaneous veins are distended with enlarged collateral veins later becoming visible over the shoulder and chest. A tender cord can sometimes be felt along the course of the axillary vein. In the early stages, arterial ischaemia may be suspected, and external compression of the vein by a Pancoast tumour or secondary malignant lymph glands produces similar symptoms and signs.

A chest radiograph and a CT scan of the lungs may be helpful in excluding the above conditions but brachial phlebography is required to confirm the diagnosis and provide the necessary information for the proper management of the condition (Fig. 11.34a,b).[195] Duplex scanning is now an alternative but the therapeutic infusion of fibrinolytic drugs requires venous access.

Many patients present days or weeks after the onset of symptoms when active management has no part to play, but if patients are seen early and the diagnosis is confirmed, treatment by chemical thrombolysis (streptokinase or urokinase) or thrombectomy combined with decompression of the thoracic inlet may reduce late sequelae.[196,197] Angioplasty and stent placement are alternative treatment options. If incapacitating late symptoms of discomfort

REFERENCES

184. Barritt D W, Jordan S C Lancet 1960; i: 1309
185. Edwards E A Surg Gynecol Obstet 1938; 66: 236
186. Woodhouse C J R Ann R Coll Surg Engl 1980; 62: 364
187. Edwards E A New Engl J Med 1949; 240: 1031
188. Berquist D, Jaroszewski H Br Med J 1986; 292: 658
189. Paget J Clinical Lectures and Essays. Longman's Green, London 1875
190. Von Schrotter L In: Nothnagel C N H (ed) Handbuch der Pathologie und Therapie. Holder, Vienna 1884
191. Kleinsasser L J Arch Surg 1949; 59: 258
192. Adams J T, McEvoy R K, De Weese J A Arch Surg 1965; 91: 29
193. Tilney N L, Griffith H J G, Edwards E A Arch Surg 1970; 101: 792
194. Sundquist S B, Hedner U et al Br Med J 1981; 283: 265
195. Stevenson I M, Parry E W J Cardiovasc Surg 1975; 16: 580
196. Dunant J H Int Angiol 1984; 3: 157
197. Witte L C, Smith A C Arch Surg 1966; 93: 664

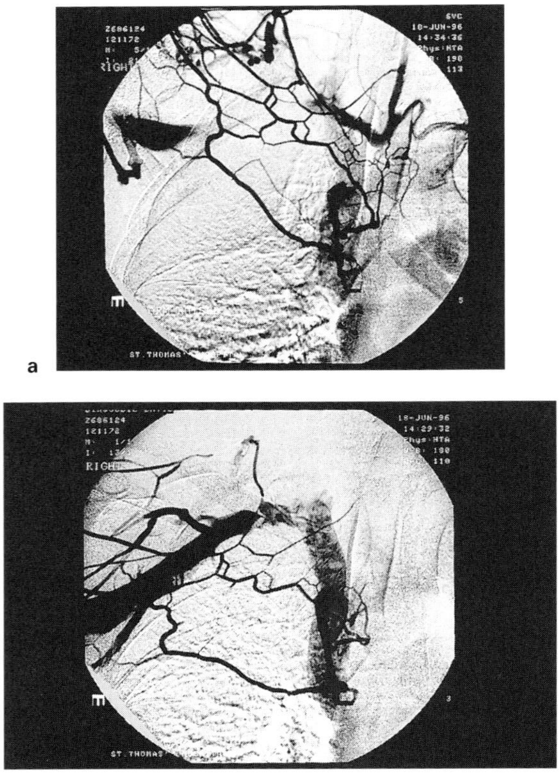

a

b

Fig. 11.34 Axillary phlebograms showing axillary vein thrombosis (a) pre lysis, (b) post lysis.

and oedema of the arm develop the occluded segment can be bypassed: the internal jugular vein appears to be the bypass of first choice.[197] Anticoagulants are usually given for 3 months to prevent propagation of thrombus or the faint possibility of pulmonary embolism. Most untreated patients develop good collateral pathways and after a few months become symptom-free.[192]

SUPERIOR VENA CAVAL THROMBOSIS

Thrombosis of the superior vena cava is usually an acute event and is often associated with a rapidly enlarging carcinoma of the bronchus, although it may also be caused by other neoplasms such as thymomas, lymphomas, and carcinoma of the thyroid.[198] A more chronic obstruction of the superior vena cava may develop in patients with a retrosternal goitre, in benign or slow-growing mediastinal tumours and in patients with constrictive pericarditis or mediastinal fibrosis. Acute thrombosis now most commonly follows intravenous cannulation of the internal jugular and subclavian veins for intravenous feeding, in which hyperosmolar solutions are usually infused.[199]

Patients present with swelling of the neck and face, accompanied by shortness of breath. Rare symptoms include tinnitus, epistaxis, a non-productive cough, and dysphagia. On examination the head and neck are suffused and cyanosed with obviously distended neck veins which do not collapse on elevation or with respiration.[198]

A chest radiograph often shows a bronchogenic or mediastinal tumour and CT scanning may be helpful in defining the extent of the neoplasm. Bilateral brachial vein injections of contrast determine the extent of the occlusion, but a tissue diagnosis should be obtained before treatment is begun.

Radiotherapy produces a rapid improvement in symptoms by shrinking bronchogenic and other rapidly growing neoplasms but this improvement is always temporary unless the patient dies of another cause before symptoms recur. Individual cases of caval bypass have been reported using vein or synthetic graft anastomosed to the right atrium.[200] Thrombolysis, angioplasty and stenting are now the treatment of choice, especially if the condition is a complication of intravenous feeding.

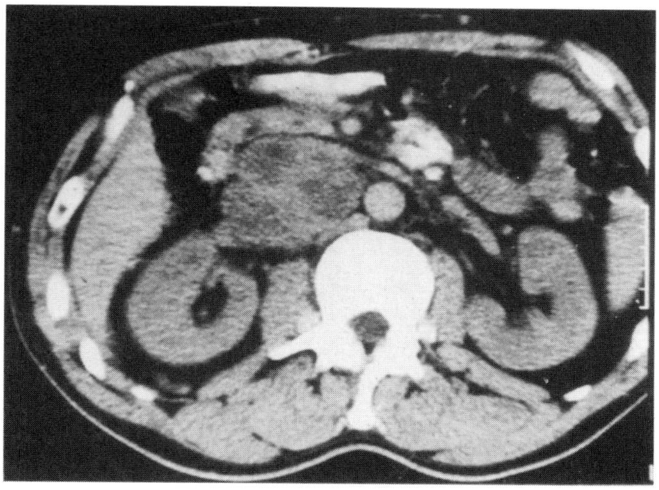

Fig. 11.35 A CT scan of the abdomen showing a leiomyosarcoma of the inferior vena cava.

VENOUS TUMOURS

Leiomyomas, which are usually low-grade leiomyosarcomas, are rare tumours arising in the vein wall; the inferior vena cava is the most common site of occurrence.[201] They present with symptoms and signs of venous obstruction and a mass may be palpable. Their extent can be determined by phlebography and CT scanning (Fig. 11.35). If possible the tumour should be resected and the vein bypassed or reconstructed.[200] These tumours often recur locally and the eventual prognosis is poor though the patients may live for many years.

REFERENCES

198. Browse N L, Burnand K G, Lea Thomas M (eds) Diseases of the Veins. Arnold, London 1988
199. Woodhouse C R J Ann R Coll Surg Engl 1980; 62: 364
200. Skinner D B, Saltzman E W, Scannell J C J Thorac Cardiovasc Surg 1976; 53: 549
201. Kieffer E, Berrod J L, Chomettor G In: Bergan J J, Yao J S T (eds) Surgery of the Veins. Grune & Stratton, Orlando 1995

12 Disease of the lymphatics

J. H. N. Wolfe   H. M. Hafez   K. G. Burnand

Lymphoedema is an accumulation of tissue fluid as the result of a fault in the lymphatic system; the term 'lymphoedema' should be confined to describing oedema in patients in whom a lymphatic abnormality has been confirmed. Lymphoedema principally affects the legs (80%), although the arms, genitalia and face can also become swollen. In the past many patients were diagnosed as having lymphoedema when the oedema was from another cause.

DIFFERENTIAL DIAGNOSIS

Other causes of tissue oedema must be considered before a diagnosis of lymphoedema is made (Table 12.1). The most common conditions do not usually represent a diagnostic problem.

Cardiac oedema should be apparent from examination of the central venous pressure, heart and lungs, while the oedema of chronic renal failure and hypoproteinaemia from malnutrition, malabsorption or hepatic cirrhosis should be diagnosed from the initial blood investigations.

Allergic disorders must also be considered, but they can usually be diagnosed from the history. Hereditary angioedema, from a deficiency in the complement system regulation, is inherited as an autosomal dominant. It presents with attacks of swelling of the face and extremities that subsequently resolve. The oedema is sometimes associated with erythema.

Idiopathic cyclic oedema, which commonly occurs in young females during their child-bearing years, can be mistaken for mild bilateral distal lymphoedema and this condition has been shown to be exacerbated by diuretics.[1] The cyclical nature of the swelling, which usually occurs in the week before their period, should also alert the clinician to this diagnosis. The lymphatics are entirely normal, and patients may be helped by remedies designed to help premenstrual syndrome.[2]

Table 12.1 Differential diagnosis of lymphoedema

Systemic disorders
Cardiac failure
Renal failure
Hepatic cirrhosis
Hypoproteinaemia
Allergic disorders
Hereditary angioedema
Idiopathic cyclic oedema
Venous disorders
Post-thrombotic syndrome
Iliac venous (obstructive) disease
Extrinsic pressure, e.g. by tumour, pregnancy, retroperitoneal fibrosis
Klippel–Trenaunay syndrome
Miscellaneous disorders
Arteriovenous malformations
Lipoedema/lipodystrophy
Disuse and factitious oedema
Gigantism

The most common cause of unilateral ankle oedema is long-standing venous disease. The diagnosis is usually indicated by the presence of abnormal cutaneous veins, an ankle flare or lipodermatosclerosis in the ankle skin. These changes may not, however, be present in limbs with iliac vein compression syndrome, or in patients with an inferior vena caval occlusion. If there is any doubt then a lower limb Duplex scan and a venogram should establish the diagnosis. Unless there is a failure of the lymphatic system venous occlusion cannot cause lymphoedema. Subclinical lymphoedema may occasionally become apparent as a result of venous thrombosis. Under these circumstances, poorly functioning lymphatics which were able to drain the interstitial space cannot cope with the extra fluid and protein forced out of the capillary bed. The interstitial proteins cannot then be cleared rapidly enough and clinical oedema starts to appear.

Klippel–Trenaunay syndrome, in which congenital varicose veins are associated with bony and soft tissue deformity, elongation of the limb, capillary naevi and often an abnormal deep venous system, may also cause limb oedema. Some patients with this syndrome have an associated primary abnormality of their lymphatics—55% in one report.[3]

Malignant disease may also cause unilateral oedema and as the lymphatic obstruction is frequently deep in the pelvis the clinical diagnosis is easily missed. Pelvic ultrasound or computed tomography scanning can usually detect enlarged pelvic lymph nodes with a reasonable degree of accuracy.

Disuse or hysterical oedema is produced by voluntary or involuntary immobility. This condition may develop in patients with long-standing paralysis from causes such as poliomyelitis (Fig. 12.1) but it may also occur in patients with psychological disturbances.

REFERENCES

1. MacGregor G A, Markandu N D, Roulston J E, Jones J C, de Wardener H E Lancet 1979; i: 397–400
2. Streeten D P H, Dalakos D G et al Clin Sci Mol Med 1973; 45: 347
3. Baskerville P A, Ackroyd J S et al Br J Surg 1985; 72: 232

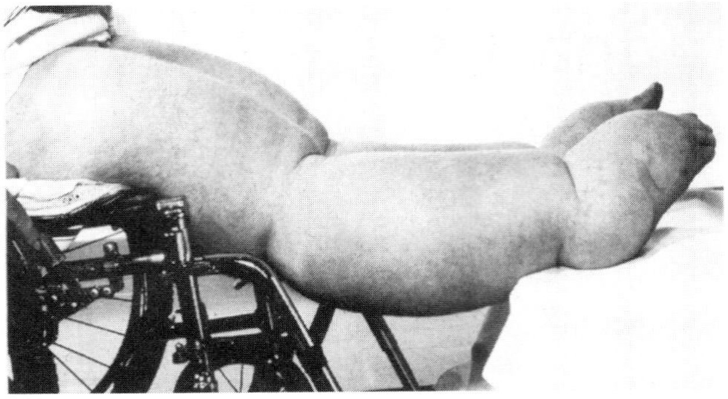

Fig. 12.1 Leg swelling due to poliomyelitis.

There remain a few obscure causes of leg swelling that must be differentiated from lymphoedema. In lipodystrophy or lipoedema there is excessive deposition of fat in the legs. Almost all patients with this condition are female and some have generalized gross obesity (Fig. 12.2). In others, the subcutaneous fat deposition is confined to the lower half of the body or the legs alone. Most patients complain of pain and admit that their ankles have always been 'heavy'. Their 'swollen' limbs do not pit and an isotope lymphogram is normal. The lymphogram shows a normal number of slightly wavy lymphatics. Erythrocyanosis frigida is a relatively common condition in young, often heavily built women, in whom the skin is cold to the touch and has reddish blue blotchy areas of discoloration owing to sluggish cutaneous circulation. The condition is almost always bilateral and the ankles are thickened, but the feet are not usually swollen. There is an overlap of this condition with lipodosis.

True gigantism of a limb is rare. It may be associated with varying degrees of hypertrophy of the subcutaneous tissue, but the skin texture, the blood supply and lymph drainage are all normal. Patients with multiple arteriovenous fistulae (the Parkes–Weber syndrome) also develop limb swelling and lengthening. The limb feels hot and bruits may be heard.

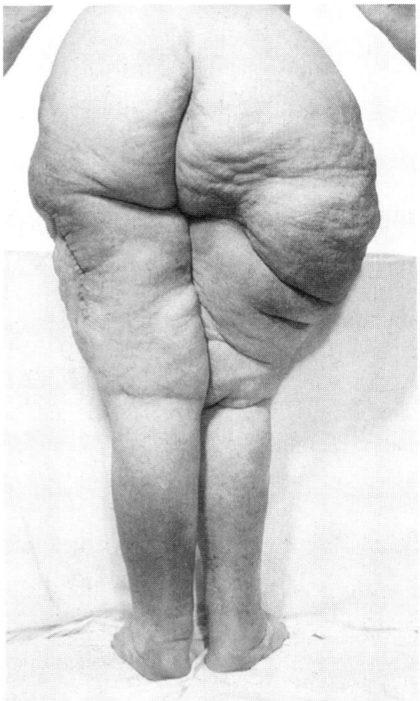

Fig. 12.2 Gross obesity should not be confused with lymphoedema.

PRIMARY LYMPHOEDEMA

The incidence of primary lymphoedema remains poorly documented. The frequency at birth of those who will develop primary lymphoedema is thought to be 1 : 6000 with a male to female ratio of 1 : 3.[4]

Once other causes of oedema have been excluded, the diagnosis of primary lymphoedema must be confirmed before the condition can be successfully managed. Several fundamental questions on the pathophysiology of the condition remain unanswered. The initial abnormality that leads to lymphatic failure is not known; nor is the reason for late-onset primary lymphoedema in what in the past has been thought to be a congenital disease. Furthermore, there is still disagreement on exactly how the lymphatic system develops. Despite this lack of knowledge, several aspects of the problem are now clearly understood.

SECONDARY LYMPHOEDEMA

Secondary lymphoedema in Europe and North America is usually the result of surgical excision and radiotherapy of local lymph nodes to treat malignant spread but, on a global scale, infection is of much greater importance.

Filariasis causes lymphoedema because the *Wuchereria bancrofti* worm enters the lymphatics and produces a fibrotic inflammatory reaction, particularly in the lymph nodes. Many textbooks incorrectly quote this as the major infective cause. This was disproved by Price[5] who carried out important studies in East Africa. He showed that elephantiasis was associated with areas where the soil was rich in silica. These silica particles, which became surrounded by dense fibrotic reaction, could be seen in the inguinal lymph nodes of the barefoot tribesmen. He also found that the problem seemed to run in families and surmised that recurrent chronic infections choked the lymphatic channels and nodes of individuals who were predisposed to the problem. Tuberculosis and other chronic infections can elicit the same effect.

The incidence of secondary lymphoedema following surgical excision of pelvic and inguinal lymph nodes varies considerably. The main determining factors are the primary pathology and whether adjuvant radiotherapy was given. Whereas the incidence of lymphoedema following iliac and inguinal lymphadenectomy for vulval and penile carcinoma is 15%,[6–10] that following inguinal

REFERENCES

4. Dale R F J Med Genet 1985; 22: 274–278
5. Price E W Trans R Soc Trop Med Hyg 1972; 66: 150
6. Petereit D G, Mehta M P, Buchler D A, Kinsella T J Int J Radiat Oncol Biol Phys 1993; 27: 963–967
7. Ornellas A A, Seixas A L, De Moraes J R J Urol 1991; 146 (2): 330–332
8. Lin J Y, Du Beshter B, Angel C, Dvoretsky P M Gynecol Oncol 1992; 47: 80–86

lymphadenectomy for cutaneous carcinoma can be as high as 55%.[11] Surgical interruption of inguinal lymphatics most commonly occurs following varicose vein surgery with a redo groin incision. The incidence of lymphoedema following this type of surgery is reported to be in the range of 0.5%.[12] Secondary lymphoedema of the upper arm usually follows an axillary clearance with or without adjuvant radiotherapy for breast cancer. The incidence varies between 2.7% and 7.6% depending on level of axillary clearance.[13,14] As the lymphatics have excellent regenerative properties, lymphoedema becomes more likely if the lymphatic extirpation is associated with infection or irradiation. The subsequent block of fibrous tissue cannot be transgressed by the new lymphatic pathways and lymphoedema ensues. In a number of patients an associated venous occlusion may increase the lymphatic load and tip the balance towards clinical oedema.

Rarely a patient will tie a tourniquet around the leg to produce lymphoedema artefacta. This may be recognized by a sharp cut-off to the swelling and a dent where the tourniquet is applied. The isotope lymphogram is normal. The merits of confronting the patient with the diagnosis are debated.

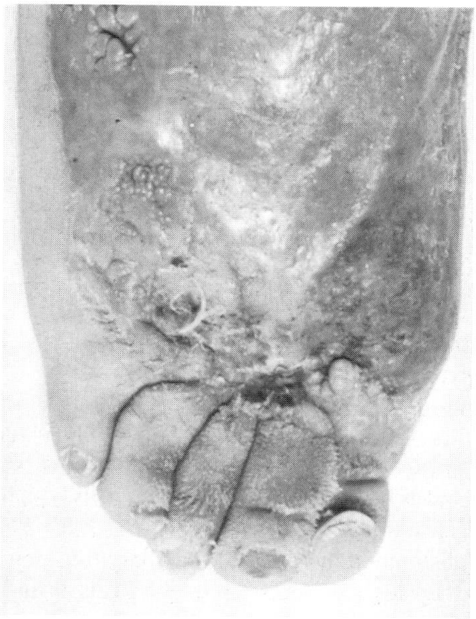

Fig. 12.3 Warty excrescences on toes. The typical skin changes associated with lymphoedema.

CLINICAL PRESENTATION

The majority of patients present with swelling of one or both lower limbs. At this stage the oedema usually pits readily; much later the chronic subcutaneous fibrosis leads to greater tissue resistance, which many textbooks have referred to as 'non-pitting'. This is incorrect as prolonged firm pressure will always produce indentation in even the most long-standing lymphoedematous limb. The patient may attribute the onset of the swelling to a minor infection, insect bite or a mild injury such as a twisted ankle. It is quite conceivable that such an episode did, indeed, produce the lymphatic overload that initiated the irreversible process of lymph accumulation in a patient with already inadequate or damaged lymphatics.

Warty skin excrescences start to develop on the toes, which 'square off' (Fig. 12.3) since the oedema is confined in shoes. The skin of the lower leg is thickened and pigmentation and ulceration are severe.

The inguinal nodes may be enlarged, particularly in patients with a proximal pelvic lymphatic obstruction. Small lymph vesicles or blisters may be visible and a cutaneous capillary naevus is suggestive of a megalymphatic problem. A few patients have chylous vesicles, chylometrorrhoea, chyluria, chylous ascites or chylothroax—all features of megalymphatics and the associated lymphatic fistulae. Some affected individuals have other associated congenital abnormalities which include yellow nails, distichiasis (two layers of eyelashes), cardiac anomalies and other rare conditions like Pierre Robin and Turner's syndrome.

MECHANICAL FUNCTION OF THE LYMPHATIC SYSTEM

The major mechanical function of the lymphatic system is to clear the interstitial space of large molecules and excess fluid. Starling's original hypothesis, which proposed that there was no protein transport across the capillary endothelium,[15] was modified by Pappenheimer & Soto-Riviera,[16] who demonstrated that the rate of capillary filtration is a function of hydrodynamic and colloid osmotic pressures and is directly proportional to their difference. Four factors govern this exchange: the capillary blood pressure (hydrostatic pressure); the oncotic (osmotic) pressure of plasma proteins in the blood; the interstitial pressure (hydrostatic pressure), and the oncotic (osmotic) pressure of proteins in the interstitial fluid. The terminal lymphatics are permeable, but the lymphatic collecting ducts do not allow transmural fluid transfer.

The protein content of blood and lymph are different and there is always relatively more albumin than globulin in lymph.[17] Between 50% and 80% of the intravascular protein is returned to the blood stream every day via the thoracic duct. Even when the lymph flow is reduced, some 40% of the intravascular plasma proteins passes through the thoracic duct in 24 hours.[18] This vast flux of protein can only occur in a fully functional lymphatic system.

LYMPH FLOW

Lymph flow depends mainly on the intrinsic contractility of the lymphatic vessels and extrinsic factors. This is a potent force in the

REFERENCES

9. Ravi R Jpn J Clin Oncol 1993; 23: 53–58
10. Cavanagh D, Fiorica J V et al Am J Obstet Gynecol 1990; 163: 1007–1015
11. James J H Scand J Plast Reconstr Surg 1982; 16: 167–171
12. Ouvry P A, Guenneguez H. 1993; Phlebol 46: 563–568
13. Siegel B M, Mayzel K A, Love S M Arch Surg 1990; 125: 1144–1147
14. Hoe A L, Iven D, Royle G I, Taylor I Br J Surg 1992; 79: 261–263
15. Starling E H J Physiol (Lond) 1896; 19: 312
16. Pappenheimer J R, Soto-Riviera A Am J Physiol 1948; 152: 471
17. Wooley G, Courtice F C Aust J Exp Biol Med Sci 1962; 40: 121

propulsion of lymph in the resting leg, but may be assisted during exercise by other extrinsic factors. These include muscular activity, thoracic and abdominal pressure changes, and even perhaps the pulsation of local blood vessels.[19]

Lymph flow is sluggish at rest and under these circumstances lymph nodes may produce a significant resistance to flow. The role of a lymph node is to act as a filter and this function causes a reduction in flow as the lymphatic drainage is interrupted at each lymph node.

THE UNKNOWN CAUSE OF PRIMARY LYMPHOEDEMA

The initial cause of lymphatic failure in primary lymphoedema remains an enigma, unlike secondary lymphoedema. Theoretically the condition can be caused by abnormalities in lymph formation or of lymph clearance.

Venous obstruction increases the capillary filtration by causing a persistent elevation in venous pressure. This in turn increases lymph formation. Despite the undoubted effect of venous disease on an inadequate lymphatic system, the hypothesis that lymphoedema develops secondary to venous disease is very unlikely.

There is general agreement that lymphoedema is caused by an abnormal clearance of lymph, which may occur at the level of the lymphatic capillary bed. The collecting vessels have been found to be abnormal on histological examination.[20] There is evidence of perilymphangitis and endolymphangitis proliferans, while other biopsies show lymphangiectasia (a dilated lymphangiole with atrophy of its wall). Almost all adults with primary lymphoedema have evidence of abnormal or occluded lymph vessels in their feet. Total aplasia of the lymph trunks is extremely rare except in congenital hereditary lymphoedema (Milroy's disease).[21] In a few patients there is a radiologically demonstrable abnormality of the thoracic duct that may interfere with lymph flow and these patients tend to have increased numbers of distal lymphatics[22] (see classification below). In 1948 Mowlem[23] suggested that abnormalities in the lymph node were the cause of primary lymphoedema, but this suggestion was not critically re-examined for many years. Extensive nodal fibrosis has been found in some patients with primary lymphoedema;[24] and it has been suggested that this may be the cause, rather than the result, of the condition (Fig. 12.4). The reason for this fibrosis remains obscure and particularly occurs in those with complete limb swelling.

Thirty per cent of patients with primary lymphoedema have a family history of swollen legs,[23] which suggests that a genetic defect may be an important factor, although true Milroy's disease (congenital familial lymphoedema) is a rare form of primary lymphoedema, accounting for only about 3% of cases. In the majority of patients the oedema does not develop until adolescence or later. At present a number of families with large numbers of affected individuals are being screened for candidate genes in the hope that one or more genes will be responsible. It is possible that a genetic abnormality may control either abnormalities in the structure of the lymphangiole or the lymph flowing through them, e.g. a defect in plasminogen activators. It appears to be dominantly inherited.

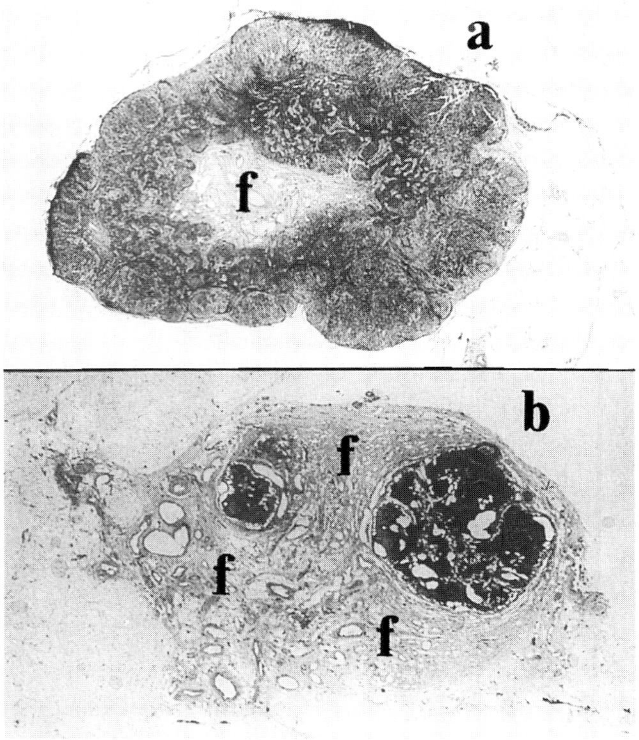

Fig. 12.4 (**a**) Normal lymph node with central fibrosis (f). (**b**) Fibrotic lymph node from patient with primary lymphoedema.

The fact that many girls develop lymphoedema around the age of puberty had led to conjecture that increased lymphatic return secondary to fluid retention caused by an increase in reproductive hormones may play a part in precipitating lymphoedema.

CLASSIFICATION OF PRIMARY LYMPHOEDEMA

The classification of lymphoedema into congenital, praecox and tarda does little to help differentiate between the different disease processes or aid management. Kinmonth developed a classification[25] based on lymphography but the terms used, such as aplasia, implied a congenital absence of lymphatics. Although these patients do not have lymphatics that can be cannulated for a lymphangiogram, there is histological evidence that damaged

REFERENCES

18. Yoffey J M, Courtice F C Lymphatics, Lymph and the Lymphomyeloid Complex. Academic Press, London 1970
19. Parsons R J, McMaster P D J Exp Med 1938; 68: 353
20. Casley-Smith J R In: Zweitach B W (ed) The Inflammatory Process. Academic Press, New York 1973
21. Pfleger L, Kaindl F et al In: Collette J M (ed) New Trends iii Basic Lymphology. Birkhauser Verlag, Basel 1967
22. Kinmonth J B Lymphatics, Surgery Lymphography and Diseases of the Chyle and Lymph System, 2nd edn. Edward Arnold, London 1982
23. Mowlem R Br J Plast Surg 1948; 1: 48
24. Wolfe J H N Ann R Coll Surg 1984; 66: 251–257
25. Kinmonth J B Clin Sci 1952; 11: 13

Table 12.2 Kinmonth classification of patients with lymphoedema

Hypoplasia or aplasia, distal	The lymph vessels are small and few (fewer than five vessels shown in the thigh) or obliterated
Hypoplasia, proximal	Lymph vessels and nodes are small and few in the groin and pelvis; vessels in the limbs distal to the site of hypoplasia are numerous and dilated, i.e. obstructed and distended
Hypoplasia, distal and proximal	A combination of the two previous conditions: vessels and nodes are small and few in limb and pelvis
Hyperplasia	Numerous lymphatics are seen in both limbs, with many large nodes in the groin and trunk, and a non-filling or distorted thoracic duct. Megalymphatics, many large, tortuous, varicose lymphatics in limbs and trunk, with diffuse scattered nodes often numerous, and almost always unilateral

lymphatics are present in the subcutaneous tissues. A variation of the original classification is shown in Table 12.2 Kinmonth. This classification essentially classifies all lymphoedema into obstructive or refluxing categories and then further subdivides based on the site of obstruction. The distal obstructive variety found in young females is usually mild and bilateral, fading out by knee level. The more proximal groin node obstruction affects either sex and causes whole leg swelling, often with foot sparing if the distal lymphatics are not affected. Although this is a lymphographic classification, the clinical presentation of the patient often identifies a particular subtype of the disease: a capillary naevus on the trunk associated with lymph vesicles suggests the presence of megalymphatics, and patients with this condition often have symptoms related to chylous fistulae in the abdominal or thoracic cavity. Patients with lymphoedema affecting the whole of one leg, including the thigh and buttock, are likely to have pelvic obstruction (this process affects men and women almost equally), whereas patients with mild ankle and foot oedema are much more likely to be women with distal obliteration of the lymphatics below the groins (Fig. 12.5). Browse & Stewart have also reclassified lymphoedema (Table 12.3).

Table 12.3 The Browse–Stewart classification of patients with lymphoedema

Secondary lymphoedema	All forms of lymphoedema caused by disease not originating in the lymph-conducting elements of the vessels and nodes
Primary lymphoedema	Lymphoedema caused by abnormalities or disease originating in the lymphatics or the lymph-conducting elements of the lymph nodes
CONGENITAL	
Congenital aplasia or *hypoplasia* of peripheral lymphatic	(lymphatic abnormality and/or oedema present at or appearing within 2 years of birth)
Congenital abnormalities of the abdominal or thoracic lymph trunks	
Congenital valvular incompetence	This is always associated with megalymphatics and often with chylous reflux
ACQUIRED	
Intraluminal or intramural lymphangio-obstructive oedema:	Distal: acquired obliteration of the distal limb lymphatics, of unknown cause Proximal: acquired obliteration of the lymphatics in the proximal part of the limb, usually associated with distal dilatation, of unknown cause Combined: acquired obliteration of all the lymphatics of the limb
Obstruction by the lymph nodes	Obliteration of the lymph-conducting pathways through the node by hilar fibrosis. This may cause the changes classified above as lymphangio-obstructive oedema. These two conditions often coexist, and acquired valvular incompetence may follow any form of obstruction

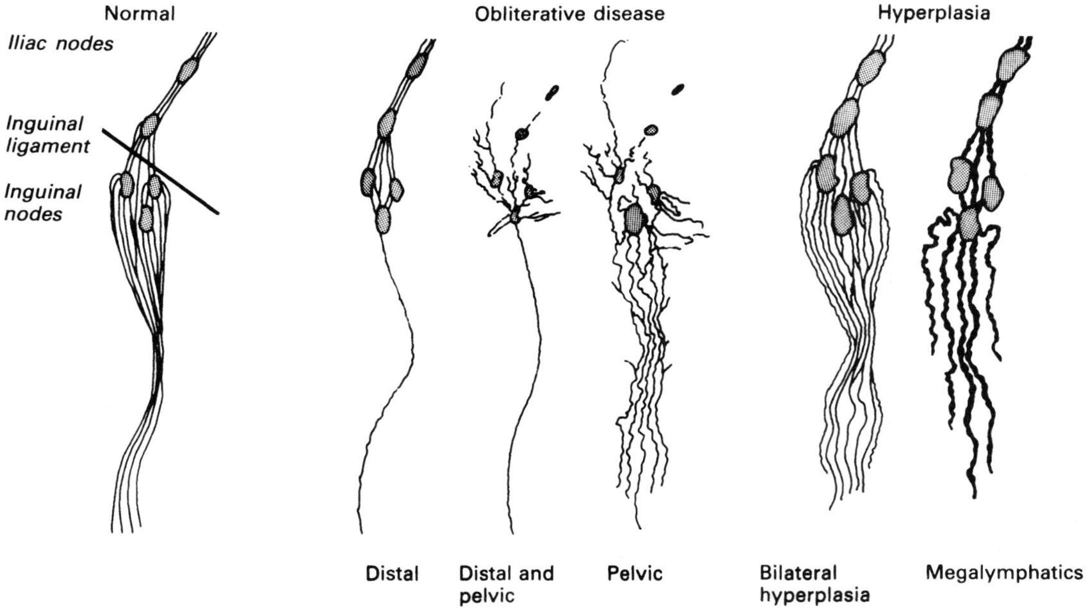

Fig. 12.5 Wolfe Classification of primary lymphoedema.[24]

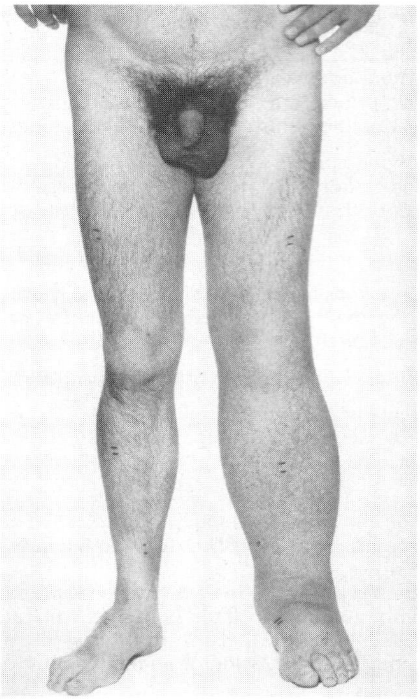

Fig. 12.6 Primary lymphoedema—the clinical diagnosis in this patient is evident, but lymphography may be useful for confirmation and in considering treatment.

DIAGNOSIS

An absence of venous stigmata makes the diagnosis of lymphoedema very likely if the appearances are typical (Fig. 12.6). Isotope lymphography should however always be performed to confirm the diagnosis and determine whether a proximal block is present and requires further assessment with a view to bypass surgery. Isotope lymphography is also the investigation of first choice if the diagnosis is in doubt. Rhenium and antimony sulphide microcolloids labelled with technetium^{99m} are taken up by the lymphatic system, when injected into a web space,[16] which pass up through the lymphatics to be concentrated in the inguinal nodes. The percentage of uptake can therefore be measured and, although normal values should be ascertained by each laboratory, an ilioinguinal colloid uptake of less than 0.3% at 30 minutes after the injection is probably diagnostic of lymphoedema.[26] An abnormally rapid clearance occurs in patients with venous oedema, resulting in early ilioinguinal lymph node uptake.

Other methods for interpreting lymphoscintigrams are the Kleinhans transport index where a score of >10 is considered diagnostic and time–activity curve analysis of different limb segments.[27] Lymphoscintigraphy is minimally invasive and moderately reliable in diagnosing lymphoedema but does not discern between the various subgroups of primary lymphoedema and between primary and secondary lymphoedema[28] (Fig. 12.7). Both false-positive and false-negative scans occur. False-positives scans are common when there is a proximal block associated with normal distal lymphatics or nodal uptake is normal and the region of interest continues to accumulate isotope. False-negatives occur when the isotope is incorrectly injected.

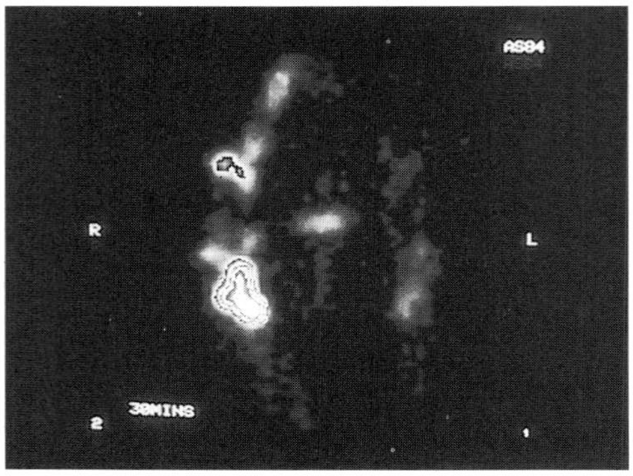

Fig. 12.7 A lymphoscintigram with technetium-labelled rhenium sulphur colloid. Inguinal lymph nodes are taking up isotope on the right but there is no uptake on the left, indicating poor distal lymphatic function.

Formal contrast lymphography using an oily contrast medium (Lipiodol) is now reserved for equivocal results from the isotope lymphography, especially if a proximal lymphatic block is suspected and bypass is being considered. It is also very valuable if reflux is suspected and the site and extent need to be carefully determined before treatment is undertaken. Patent blue green violet is injected between the web spaces before an incision through the skin on the dorsum of the foot defines a lymphatic and allows direct cannulation under an operating microscope. Immediate and delayed radiographs define the lymphatic anatomy with precision (Fig. 12.8).

TREATMENT

Ninety per cent of all patients with primary or secondary lymphoedema respond readily to active conservative treatment. Too often patients are given pessimistic, nihilistic advice and feel frustrated and impotent in the face of an incurable condition. Interstitial fluid can be compressed out of the subcutaneous tissues by the regular use of an intermittent pneumatic compression device (Flowtron, Lymphapress),[30] which is then maintained by adequate elastic stockings (40 mmHg compression or more). The adoption of these measures as part of a complex physical therapy regimen often produces good results.[31,32] Potential portals of entry of infection must be rigorously eradicated and cellulitis treated immediately with systemic antibiotics.

Many private clinics now specilize in a combination of regular massage and tight bandaging to bring the swelling under control. This is followed by application of tight correctly fitted elastic

REFERENCES

26. Stewart G, Gaunt J I et al Br J Surg 1985; 72: 906
27. Kleinhans E, Baumeister R G H, Hahn D, Siuda S, Bull U, Moser E Eur J Nucl Med 1985; 10 (7–8): 349–352
28. Cambria R A, Gloviczki P, Naessens J M, Wahner H W J Vasc Surg 1993; 18: 773–782
29. Golvete P J, Montgomery R A et al J Vasc Surg 1989; 10 (3): 306–312
30. Zelikovski A, Monoach M et al Lymphology 1980; 13: 68
31. Casley-Smith J R, Casley-Smith J R Australas J Dermatol 1992; 33: 69–74
32. Pecking A Bull Cancer Paris 1991; 78: 373–377

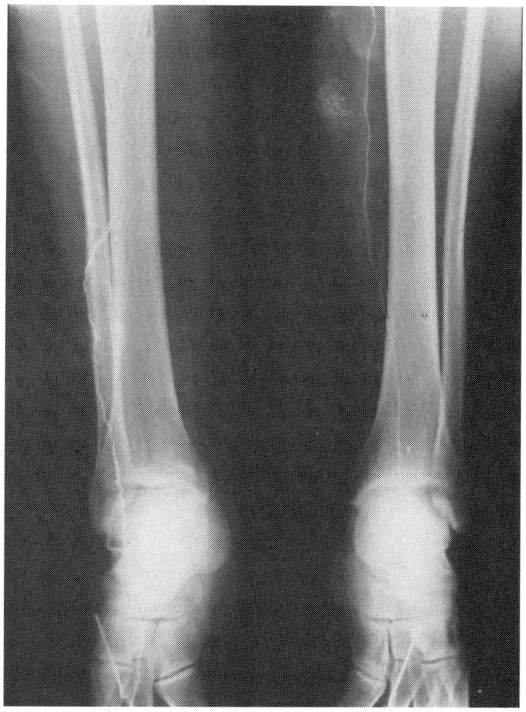

Fig. 12.8 A contrast lymphogram showing a single lymphatic passing up to the groin.

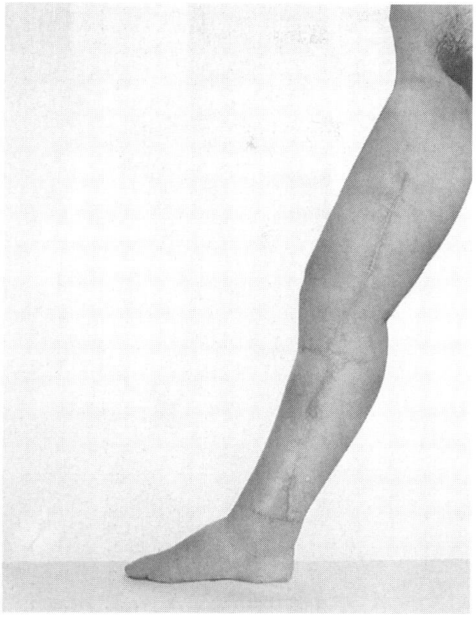

Fig. 12.9 The result of a Homans' reducing operation (the medial calf and thigh also required a reducing operation).

stockings. Patients should also be advised to lose weight and elevate the leg whenever possible. Exercise is not however contra-indicated.

Benzopyrones statistically reduce the size of lymphoedematous limbs but the reduction achieved is small.[33,34] They act through enhancing macrophage activity and the best results are usually achieved in combination with physiotherapy.[35] Reinfestation of these patients must be prevented if good results are to be maintained.[33]

Diuretics are inadvisable as fluid depletion throughout the body eventually results in only a marginal reduction in the size of the oedematous limb.

Surgery should only be considered for a few patients:

1. In 2 or 3% it is possible to improve lymphatic drainage with an operation designed to bypass the lymphatic occlusion.
2. In a limb that has become functionally impaired bulky tissue can be removed.
3. Patients with megalymphatics and lymphatic fistulae can be treated effectively by the judicious use of lymphatic ligation.[22]

Fortunately, the removal of excess bulk also appears to reduce the number of attacks of cellulitis. Cosmetic surgery for lymphoedema is fraught with pitfalls and adequate conservative treatment should suffice, particularly as the patient, having no experience of the results, is often overly optimistic about the possible improvement that will be achieved by the operation.

DE-BULKING OPERATIONS

The descriptions of many operations have filled the surgical literature over the past 80 years. Most of these have been attempts to improve the lymphatic drainage of the subcutaneous tissues while reducing the bulk of the leg. Kondoleon[36] hoped that by cutting windows in the deep fascia some lymph would drain into the deep compartment. Sistrunk[37] modified this operation with the same end in view.

Homans' operation[38] (first described by Auchincloss[39]) is moderately successful, but leaves large scars on the leg. Providing the skin is healthy, flaps are raised and a segment of subcutaneous tissue is removed. The anterior and posterior skin flaps are then sutured together to lie snugly on the deep fascia, once a gusset has been removed to avoid redundant skin. The first operation is usually performed on the medial side of the leg (Fig. 12.9) and sometimes a second operation is required on the lateral side. The circumference of the limb is usually reduced by about a third for each operation and the surgery can be repeated.

Thompson & Wee tried to combine tissue excision with an improvement in lymphatic drainage.[40] They hoped that by burying a dermal flap, lymph would pass through skin lymphatics into the deep fascial compartment. The results are no better than Homans' operation and the complications are greater. There is no sign of the buried dermal flap if the operation has to be revised. Pilonidal

REFERENCES

33. Casley-Smith J R, Wang C T, Casley-Smith J R, Cui Zi-hai. Br Med J 1993; 307: 1037–1041
34. Casley-Smith J R, Morgan R G, Piller N B N Engl J Med 1993; 329: 1158–1163
35. Casley-Smith J R, Casley-Smith J R, Cluzan R V Progress in Lymphology XIII. Elsevier, Amsterdam 1992 pp 537–538
36. Kondoleon E Munch Med Wochenschr 1912; 59: 525
37. Sistrunk W E JAMA 1918; 71: 800
38. Homans J N Engl J Med 1936; 215: 1099
39. Auchincloss H Puerto Rico J Pub Health Trop Med 1930; 6: 149
40. Thompson N, Wee J T K Chir Plast (Berl) 1980; 5: 147

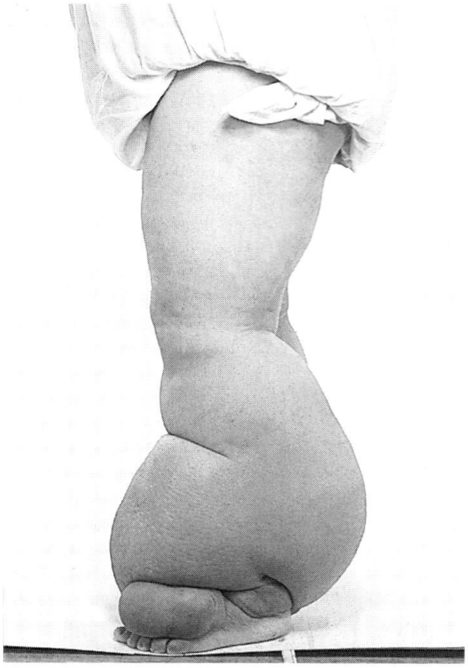

Fig. 12.10 Massive lymphoedema of the leg.

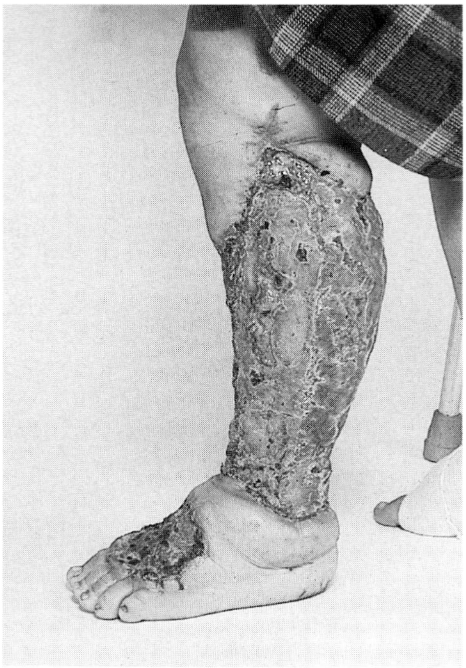

Fig. 12.11 A successful Charles reduction in the same patient.

sinuses in the buried flap provide additional complications and this procedure has now been abandoned.

A Charles procedure is indicated if the skin has become grossly thickened and involved in the lymphoedematous process.[41] It is also the best way of treating massive swelling (Fig. 12.10). All the skin and subcutaneous fat are excised between the ankle and knee before split-skin grafts are placed on the denuded deep fascia (Fig. 12.11). Care must be taken to shape flaps at the upper end to avoid a pantaloon effect and to keep the mature skin over both joints to ensure mobility.

Some patients who develop gross keratotic and warty excrescences after a Charles procedure protruding from a deeply fissured surface benefit by having these keratoses shaved down.

LYMPH DRAINAGE OPERATIONS

Many different procedures have been tried in an attempt to drain lymph from an affected leg but most have failed. The insertion of silk threads was introduced by Handley[42] in the hope that lymph would drain along them. This does not work and has been abandoned. Two operations that are moderately successful are the mesenteric bridge procedure and lymphovenous anastomosis.

Lymphovenous fistulae

Lymphonodal to venous anastomosis was originally attempted by Nielbowicz & Olszewski,[43] but the results were disappointing in patients with primary lymphoedema. Direct lymphovenous anastomosis may be more effective in patients with secondary lymphoedema than in patients with primary lymphoedema.[44] Nevertheless, there are several advocates of this painstaking technique in which lymphatics are dissected out with the operating microscope and anastomosed to nearby veins. Good results are claimed but they are masked by the concomitant use of improved conservative management and additional excisional procedures. In many countries initial enthusiasm has given way to total disillusionment.

Bridging operations

Many bridging operations have failed because lymphatic communication was not achieved. Omentum does not have sufficient lymphatics to be of value, but the introduction of the enteromesenteric bridge was a breakthrough in the management of primary lymphoedema caused by pelvic obstruction (Fig. 12.12). It is, however, only of value for a small number of patients. The rich submucosal lymphatics of the ileum are utilized by isolating and opening up a pedicle of small bowel. The bowel is opened along its anteromesenteric border and the mucosa is then stripped off to expose the rich lymphatic submucosal plexus which is brought into direct apposition with a bivalved lymph node or group of nodes in the iliac or inguinal region. As lymphatics have considerable powers of regeneration a 'low-resistance' connection soon develops between the lymph nodes of the lymphoedematous leg and the enteromesenteric pedicle. Providing the main lymphatic drainage

REFERENCES

41. Charles R H In: Latham A, English T C (eds) Elephantiasis Scrotii, A System of Treatment, vol 111. J & A Churchill, London 1912
42. Handley W S Lancet 1908; i: 783
43. Nielbowicz J, Olszewski W, Minerva Card Angio 1967; 15 (3): 254–256
44. O'Brien B McC Microvascular Reconstructive Surgery. Churchill Livingstone, Edinburgh 1977

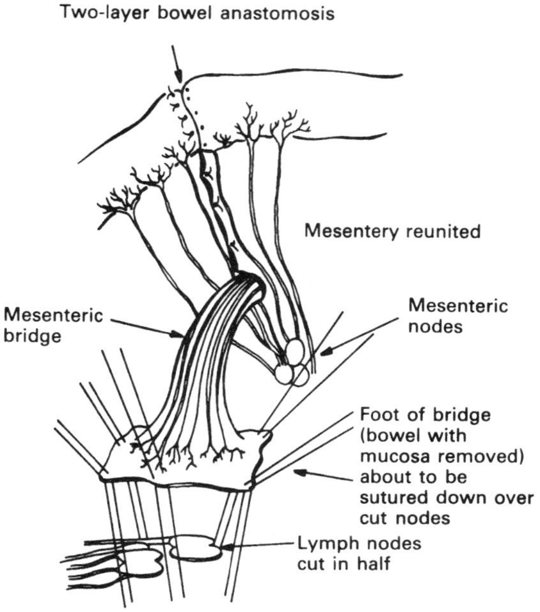

Fig. 12.12 A representation of the ileal mesenteric bridging operation (with thanks to Mr P A Hurst).

is patent at the level of the cisterna chyli, or more proximally in the thoracic duct, good results can be obtained in just over half the patients in whom it is attempted.[45,46] It is a relatively major operation and carries the potential risk of small bowel obstruction from strangulation around the mesenteric pedicle. Previous radiation is usually a contraindication and it is not effective when a long-standing proximal obstruction has caused distal lymphatic obliteration (Fig. 12.13).

SUMMARY OF SURGICAL OPERATIONS FOR LYMPHOEDEMA

There is no surgical procedure that returns a severely lymphoedematous limb to total normality. Patients should be referred to a specialist centre where appropriate investigations and careful assessment based on experience offer the optimum management.

The published results of the different procedures described above are summarized in Table 12.4. These results must be accepted with caution as none was subjected to independent scrutiny and most are only categorized into good, moderate and poor.

CHYLOUS REFLUX

Chylous reflux occurs when there is massive lymphatic ectasia with valvular incompetence. Leakage of chyle from vesicles, chyluria and chylous ascites are common. Lymphangiography with contrast may determine the site of leakage and allow ligation or excisional operations to be carried out. Chylous ascites may also be treated by peritoneovenous shunts but these often block and need to be replaced. Chylothorax is well-treated by pleurectomy.

PROGNOSIS

The clinical pattern of the disease appears to be determined early in its natural history. Although girth of an affected limb can increase,

REFERENCES

45. Kinmonth J B, Hurst P A E et al Br J Surg 1978; 65: 829
46. Hurst P A E, Stewart G et al Br J Surg 1985; 72: 272–274

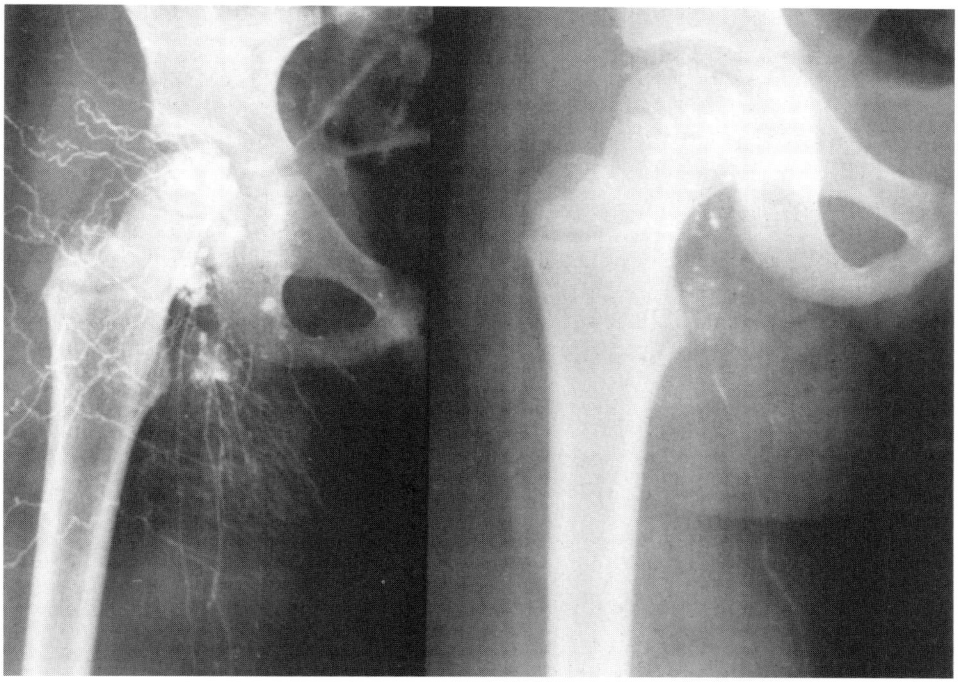

Fig. 12.13 The lymphogram on the left shows pelvic obliteration of lymphatics and collaterals but 9 months later (right) the distal pathways have also been obliterated.

Table 12.4 Results of surgical procedures for primary and secondary lymphoedema

Procedure	*No. of patients*	*Outcome*	*Reference*
Charles	34 with primary and filarial lymphoedema	Good functional results, 88% graft take	47,48
Modified Thompson's	74	Good 21.6%, moderate 60.8%, poor 17%	49
Lymphovenous anastomosis	91 with secondary lower limb lymphoedema	Good 72%, moderate 15%, poor 4%	50
Enteromesenteric bridge	8 primary lower limb	75% showed improvement	51
Microlymphatic anastomosis	79	Good results in 30%, fair results in 53%	52

it is unusual for the oedema to spread up the leg if only the lower leg has been involved for more than 5 years. Furthermore, if oedema develops in the opposite leg it is usually less severe. These observations have direct implications for management.

The majority of patients with primary lymphoedema have obliterated distal lymphatics (90%). This process predominantly affects the distal lymphatics of ovulating women and can be contained by a pneumatic compressin device and adequate compression stockings. The less common pelvic lymphatic obstruction may be amenable to lymph drainage procedures as the distal lymphatics often remain patent. As time passes these distal lymphatics obliterate so that the opportunity for successful surgery is lost[53] (Fig. 12.13).

Lymphoedema may also affect the eyelids and the genitalia, where excisional operations may be beneficial.

REFERENCES

47. Dellon A L, Hoopes J E Plast Reconstr Surg 1977; 60: 589–595
48. Dandapat M C, Mohapatro S K, Mohanty S S Br J Surg 1986; 73: 451–453
49. Thompson N, Wee J I K Chir Plastica (Berl) 1980; 5: 147–161
50. Huang G K, Hu-RQ, Liu Z Z, Shen Y L, Lan T D, Pan G P Plast Reconstr Surg 1985; 76: 671–685
51. Hurst P A E, Stewart G, Kinmonth J B, Browse N L, Br J Surg 1985; 72: 272–274
52. Kylov V, Milanov N, Abalmasov K Ann Chir Gynaecol 1982; 71: 77–79
53. Fyfe N C M, Wolfe J H N, Kinmonth J B Lymphology 1982; 15: 66–69

13 The face, mouth, tongue and jaws

M. McGurk K. Hussain

CRANIO-MAXILLOFACIAL DEFORMITY

Many acquired conditions, as well as congenital and developmental deformities of the craniofacial skeleton are now treated using the principles and techniques of craniofacial surgery (Table 13.1). The congenital and developmental conditions described below require a team of maxillofacial surgeons, neurosurgeons and plastic surgeons, psychologists, ophthalmologists and audiologists and geneticists to properly assess and treat the affected children.

Table 13.1 The scope of cranio-maxillofacial surgery

Congenital and developmental deformities	Craniosynostosis Craniofacial clefts Craniofacial cephaloceles Orthognathic deformities
Acquired conditions	Cranio-maxillofacial trauma Tumour access

CRANIOSYNOSTOSIS

This is a group of conditions in which the cranio-maxillofacial deformity is caused by premature fusion or synostosis of the cranial base synchondroses and/or the cranial sutures.[1] Cases are classified as simple, when only one or two sutures are affected, and complex when several sutures are involved.[2]

In Crouzon's syndrome fronto-orbital remodelling is required to relieve raised intracranial pressure by increasing the intracranial volume. Improvements can also be made in the frontal area providing bony and eyelid protection for the eyes and this can be combined with a midfacial advancement.

It is now becoming evident that better results are achieved if fronto-orbital remodelling can be delayed, provided that raised intracranial pressure is not present, until the child has reached the age of two years. The midfacial advancement usually requires a Le Fort III maxillary osteotomy, which ideally is undertaken after growth is completed at about 13 years of age, but can be performed earlier when indicated. Le Fort I or Le Fort II osteotomies may provide adequate correction with lesser degrees of maxillary deformity. Coexisting deformities of the mandible also require corrective surgery.[3–5]

CRANIOFACIAL CLEFTS

Craniofacial clefts can be simply defined as areas of partial or complete failure of development of one or more tissues and can be classified into true and pseudo-clefts. True facial clefts are the result of failure of the facial processes to fuse whereas pseudo-clefts arise from faulty differentiation of tissues after the fusion of the processes has occurred normally.

Clefts can be further classified according to the region affected: craniofacial, cranial or facial. Tessier proposed a classification relating the site of the cleft to the orbits.[6] This system has been widely adopted. The management of clefts of the lip and palate (facial cleft 2), hemifacial microsomia (facial clefts 6, 7) and Treacher Collins syndrome (facial clefts 6, 7, 8) is important.

Clefts of the lip and palate

A knowledge of the embryology of the head is essential for understanding the development and management of clefts of the lip and palate.

Embryology

The lip cleft deformity becomes established in the first 6–8 weeks of pregnancy and is usually considered to be caused by failure of fusion of the maxillary and median nasal processes[7] (Fig. 13.1). Another theory suggests that it may be caused by incomplete mesodermal ingrowth into these processes with subsequent breakdown of epithelium.[8]

The median nasal processes grow more rapidly than the lateral processes and approach each other in the midline. They fuse to give rise to the central part of the lip (the philtrum), the alveolus and the palate in front of the incisive foramen.

REFERENCES

1. Cohen M M Jr Birth Defects 1975; 11: 137
2. Cohen M M Jr (ed) Craniosynostosis, Diagnosis, Evaluation and Management. Raven, New York 1986
3. Marchac D, Renier D World J Surg 1989; 13: 358
4. Mulhbauer W, Anderl H et al World J Surg 1989; 13: 366
5. Marsh J L, Galic M, Vannier M W Clinic in Plastic Surg 1991; 18: 251
6. Tessier P J Maxillofac Surg 1976; 4: 69
7. Berkovitz B K B, Holland G R, Moxham B J Colour Altas and Textbook of Oral Anatomy. Wolfe Medical, London 1978
8. Veau V, Politzer J Ann d'Anat-Path 1936; 12: 275

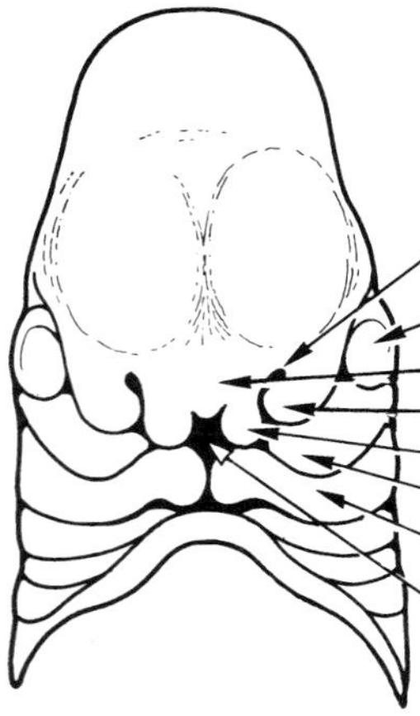

Fig. 13.1 Head of embryo at 6 weeks' gestation.

The extent of the deficiency in mesodermal migration determines the degree of clefting. This varies from a notch in the vermilion (an incomplete cleft) to a fissure extending through the lip to the nostril and involving the alveolus and anterior palate. The nostril is deformed and the columella is deflected to the opposite side.

In bilateral cleft lip, the central portion of the alveolus is covered anteriorly by the skin of the columella and philtrum and hangs from the tip of the nasal septum. Teeth which should develop at the site of the cleft are often deformed, unerupted or absent altogether.

Palatal cleft is the result of failure of fusion of the palatal shelves of the maxillary processes. These shelves are initially separated by the tongue, which descends by the eighth week of pregnancy, allowing the shelves to fuse (Fig. 13.2). This starts anteriorly and is followed by the development of centres of ossification which form the hard palate. Differentiation into the muscles of the soft palate occurs posteriorly from mesoderm which has migrated from the pharyngeal wall. The extent of the cleft may range from complete, extending bilaterally on either side of the premaxilla, to a simple bifid uvula. Submucosal clefts are probably the result of failure of mesodermal migration and consist of notching of the hard palate, bifid uvula and diastasis of the palatal muscles.

Aetiology

The aetiology of cleft lip is multifactorial, involving both genetic and intrauterine exogenous factors. The mode of inheritance is not clear but it is likely that it is polygenic.[9] Cleft palate alone is genetically and embryologically distinct, being inherited as a simple dominant with variable penetrance.[10] When unaffected parents have a child with a cleft lip, there is a 5% risk of a subsequent child having cleft lip and palate, rising to 9% if there are two affected siblings. If one parent and one child are affected, the risk is three times greater than normal.[11] Although heredity is the most important aetiological factor in typical cleft deformities, drugs such as thalidomide and cytotoxic agents have been incriminated in the formation of facial clefts.[12] Many cases are associated with anomalies or syndromes affecting other parts of the body, with a frequency varying from 10–50%.[13]

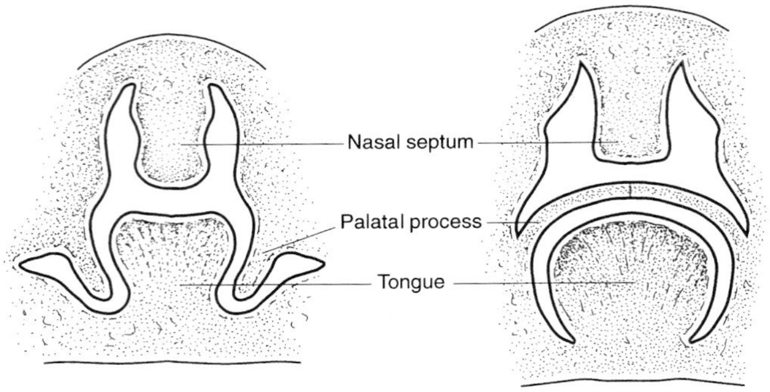

Fig. 13.2 Development of the palate at 7 weeks' gestation.

Clefts of the lip are amongst the most common birth defects, occurring in about 1 in 750 live births in the United Kingdom and affecting males more frequently than females.[14] However, clefts of the palate are rarer, occurring in about 1 in 2000 live births and affecting females more often than males.[15] In about half of the cases clefts of the lip and palate occur together.

Classification

Several methods of classification have evolved since that of Veau[16] and most are based on the system recommended by Kernahan & Stark.[17] Clefts of the lip and palate are classified in Table 13.2. Cleft lip may be incomplete or complete, with or without involvement of the alveolus. It may occur unilaterally (70% on the left side), bilaterally (25%) or, rarely, in the midline.

Clefts of the palate alone (32%) involve the soft palate and posterior third of the hard palate. They may be complete, incomplete or submucous.

Table 13.2 Classification of clefts of the lip and palate

Site of facial cleft	*Type*	*Severity*
Cleft lip	Unilateral Bilateral Median	Complete Incomplete
Cleft palate	Unilateral Bilateral Midline	Complete Submucous Incomplete (soft palate)

REFERENCES

9. Fogh-Andersen P Inheritence of Harelip and Cleft Palate. Nyt Nordisk Forlag, Arnold Busck, Copenhagen 1942
10. Roberts J A F Multifactorial inheritance and human disease. In: Steinberg A G, Bern A G (eds) Advances in Medical Genetics. Grune & Stratton, New York 1964
11. Fogh-Anderson P In: Edwards M, Watson A C H (eds) Advances in the Management of Cleft Palate. Churchill Livingstone, Edinburgh 1980 p 43
12. Poswillo D Oral Surg 1973; 35: 302
13. Gorlin R J, Pindborg J J, Cohen M M Syndromes of the Head and Neck, 2nd edn. McGraw-Hill, New York 1976 p 137
14. Drillien C M, Ingram T T S, Walkinson E M The Causes and Natural History of Cleft Lip and Palate. E & S Livingstone, Edinburgh 1966
15. Wilson M E A Brit J Plast Surg 1972; 25: 224
16. Veau V Division Palatine. Masson, Paris 1931
17. Kernahan D A, Stark R B Plast Reconstr Surg 1958; 22: 435

Clefts of the soft and hard palate involving the alveolus and associated with cleft lip (52%) may be unilateral or bilateral.[17] About 85% of bilateral cleft lips and 70% of unilateral cleft lips are associated with a cleft palate.[18]

Treatment

The fundamental principles in the management of craniofacial clefts are the functional and anatomical repair of both bony and soft tissues of clefts of the lip and palate to promote normal speech, hearing, growth and social integration.

Presurgical orthopaedics

Sometimes intraoral or extraoral appliances are employed to approximate the palatal cleft segments into a symmetrical arch form so as to facilitate cleft lip and palate repair.[19]

Cleft lip and palate repair

Most units undertake repair of the cleft lip at about 3 months of age, when the baby has grown a little to make surgery technically simpler, as well as safer. A gingivo-periosteoplasty can be undertaken at the same time if required. A soft palate repair is undertaken at about 6 months of age, and the hard palate is repaired at about 14–15 months of age (about 6–9 months after soft palate repair).[20]

Cleft lip repair

A detailed appreciation of the anatomy of the cleft lip deformity and identification of the normal landmarks are of vital importance in its repair (Figs 13.3 and 13.4).

The cleft lip deformity affects not only the skin but also the orbicularis muscle and the underlying maxilla which is hypoplastic and may have an alveolar cleft.

Although there are many techniques described for cleft lip repair, dating back to ancient times, probably the most commonly used today is the advancement-rotation method of Millard (1957)[21] (Fig. 13.5). This technique involves equalizing the heights of the lip on either side of the cleft by rotation of the medial edge of the cleft down to its normal position, and then advancing the lateral edge of the cleft across to meet the medial edge. In this way a symmetrical cupid's bow is created. The technique requires carefully made measurements in order to develop medial (M), lateral (L) and central (C) flaps. The medial flap is rotated down, thereby opening a gap into which the lateral flap is advanced. The central flap is used to lengthen the shortened columella.

In bilateral cleft lips, setting back the premaxilla causes retardation of forward maxillary growth; Millard's technique for closure of the bilateral cleft lip is therefore performed in two stages. Initially, the muscle layer is brought behind the prolabium and in front of the premaxilla. At the second stage the lip is freed from the septum, the columella is lengthened and the tip of the nose is raised.

A recent development in the surgery of primary cleft lip repair was the introduction by Delaire in 1975 of the concept of a functional repair.[22] The objective is to facilitate normal growth, thus avoiding the development of compensatory secondary deformities and the need for their later correction. Functional repair

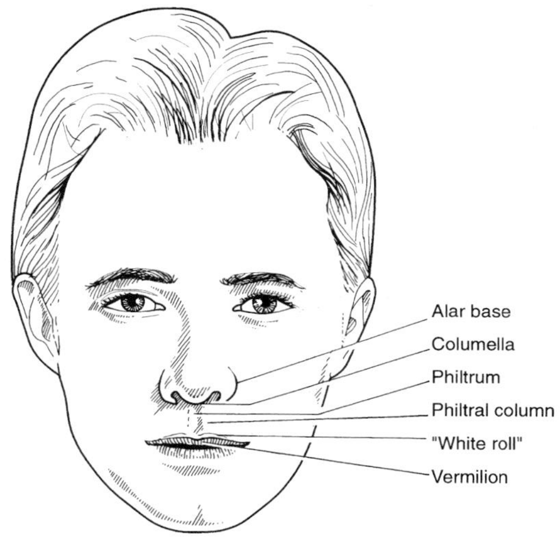

Fig. 13.3 Normal features of the nasolabial region.

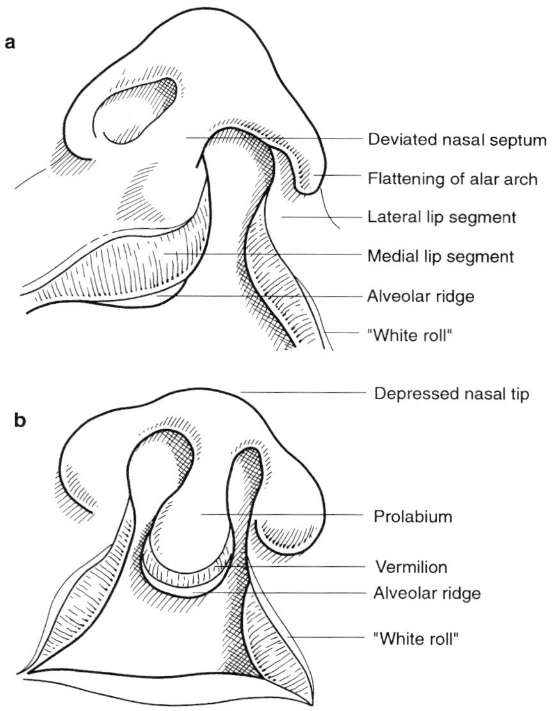

Fig. 13.4 Features of the nasolabial region of **(a)** unilateral and **(b)** bilateral cleft lip.

REFERENCES

18. Reidy J P Br J Plast Surg 1960; 12: 215
19. Jackson I T, Vandevord J E et al Brit J Plast Surg 1976; 29: 295
20. Markus A F, Smith W P, Delaire J Brit J Oral Maxillofac Surg 1993; 31: 281
21. Millard D R Cleft Craft. Little Brown, Boston 1976
22. Markus A F, Delaire J Brit J Oral Maxillofac Surg 1993; 31: 281

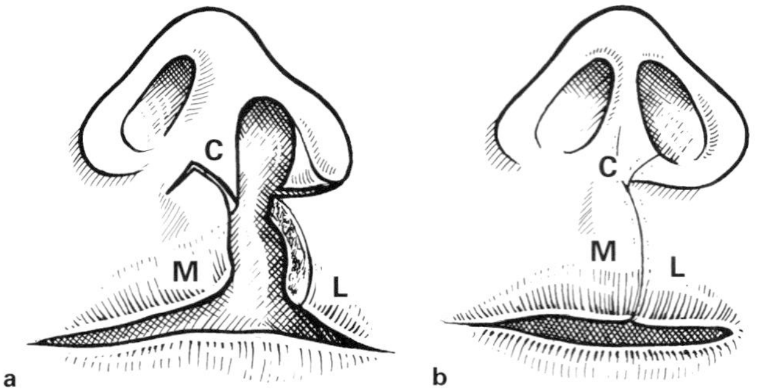

Fig. 13.5 (**a**) Inset of the flaps of rotation-advancement technique of cleft lip repair. (**b**) The completed unilateral cleft lip repair by the rotation-advancement method.

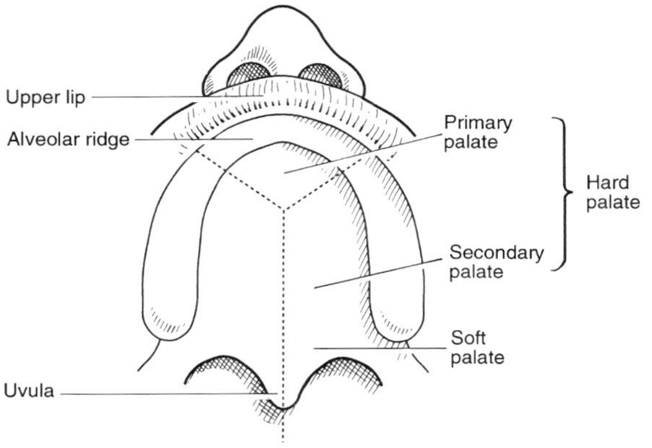

Fig. 13.6 The normal anatomy of the palate.

involves repositioning of displaced nasal skin on the lip back into the nostril, anatomical reconstruction of the nasolabial musculature, and correct positioning of distorted neighbouring soft tissues.

Cleft palate repair

As with cleft lip, a detailed appreciation of the anatomy of palatal cleft deformities is essential for their treatment (Figs 13.6 and 13.7). In addition to the clefting deformity the muscles of the soft palate are oriented anteroposteriorly rather than transversely, and inserted into the posterior edge of the hard palate and along the medial edge of the cleft. The correct repositioning of the soft palate muscles is essential to avoid nasal escape of air during speech.

The principles of cleft palate repair can be classified according to whether the hard and soft palate repair is undertaken at the same time or as a two-staged procedure.

There are a number of techniques available for repairing palatal clefts. In the one-stage procedure of Von Langenbeck,[23] long mucoperiosteal flaps are first raised in the hard palate by making medial incisions along the cleft margins and lateral incisions close to the gingival margins (Fig. 13.8). The latter are extended posteriorly onto the anterior pillar of the fauces and may be joined with medial incisions anteriorly (Veau flaps).[16] The muscles of the soft palate are then detached from their abnormal insertions and the flaps which have been raised on either side are transposed medially before closure is achieved in three layers—nasal mucosa, muscular, and oral mucosa.

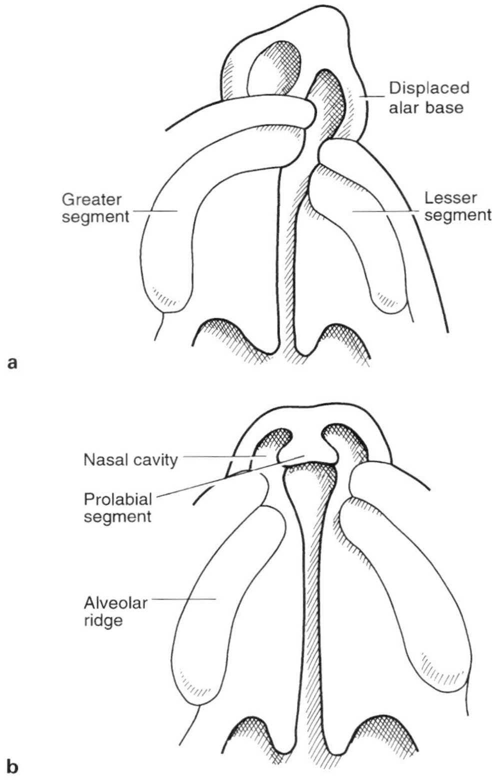

Fig. 13.7 (**a**) Anatomy of a unilateral cleft of the lip and palate. (**b**) Anatomy of a bilateral cleft of the lip and palate.

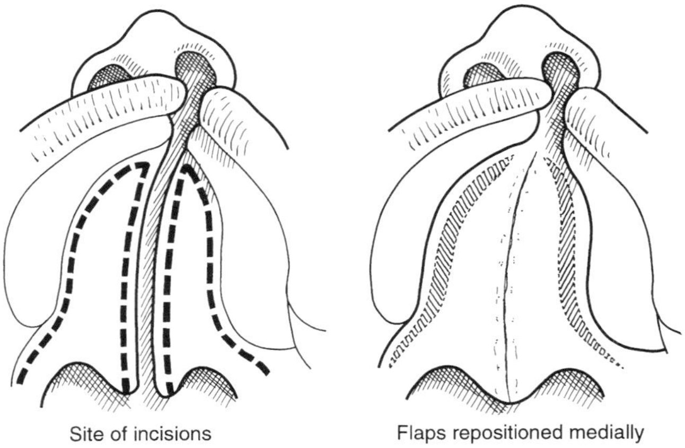

Fig. 13.8 The use of Veau flaps for repair of the cleft palate.

Based on careful investigations, Delaire has emphasized the importance of a precise anatomical and functional repair of clefts of the soft palate (functional palatoplasty).[20] The latter involves radical mobilization and repositioning of the muscles of the soft palate and closure of the nasal and oral mucosal layers.

REFERENCE

23. Von Langenbeck O B 1861. Cited by Watson A C H Advances in Management of Cleft Palate, Ch. 12. Churchill Livingstone, Edinburgh 1980

In the two-stage procedure, growth occurring after the initial repair of the soft palate brings the palatal segments closer together, reducing the width of the palatal defect. This makes the subsequent repair of the hard palate easier and more successful.

An alveolar cleft associated with a cleft lip should be closed at the same time as the lip is repaired, otherwise a troublesome oronasal fistula will result. The nasal floor may be closed in one layer by elevating the septal mucoperichondrium and suturing to the mucoperiosteum of the lateral wall of the nose. The second oral layer may be obtained from the labial mucosa, as described by Muir[24] and Burian.[25]

Speech

Normal speech can be expected in about three quarters of the children who have had cleft palates repaired. Correct phonation depends on the ability of the soft palate to complete a sphincter between the lateral and posterior walls of the oronasal pharynx; this can be objectively assessed using cinefluoroscopy and endoscopic examination, enabling selection of the most appropriate procedure for the correction of velopharyngeal incompetence should this persist following cleft palate repair.[26]

Hearing

Many children with cleft palates become deaf from recurrent middle ear infection. This may be the result of drainage problems along the eustachian canal associated with abnormalities of the tensor palati muscles.[27] Treatment of the ear infections must be prompt and effective, as loss of hearing has additional deleterious effects on the development of speech.

Secondary procedures

Throughout the formative years, an orthodontist must monitor the growth and development of the jaws. Teeth are often congenitally absent, deformed or displaced at the site of the cleft. Maintenance of oral hygiene and preservation of the secondary dentition are important measures that encourage oral rehabilitation.

Collapse of the dental arch may be corrected orthodontically at any time after the mixed dentition stage and the alveolar cleft bone-grafted; this enables displaced teeth to be aligned and produces a united maxilla. Any residual oronasal fistulae should be repaired at this stage.

In a proportion of cases the maxilla will fail to develop partly because of surgically induced inelastic scar tissue, leaving the patient with a flat or dish-face appearance. Osteotomies of the maxilla to advance the dental arch and nasal base can then be performed but should be designed to ensure that the velopharyngeal sphincter is not compromised.[28]

Later cosmetic adjustments may be required for the lip and any residual nasal deformity.

Hemifacial microsomia—facial clefts 6 and 7

Synonyms: first and second branchial arch syndrome, otomandibular dysostosis and craniofacial microsomia

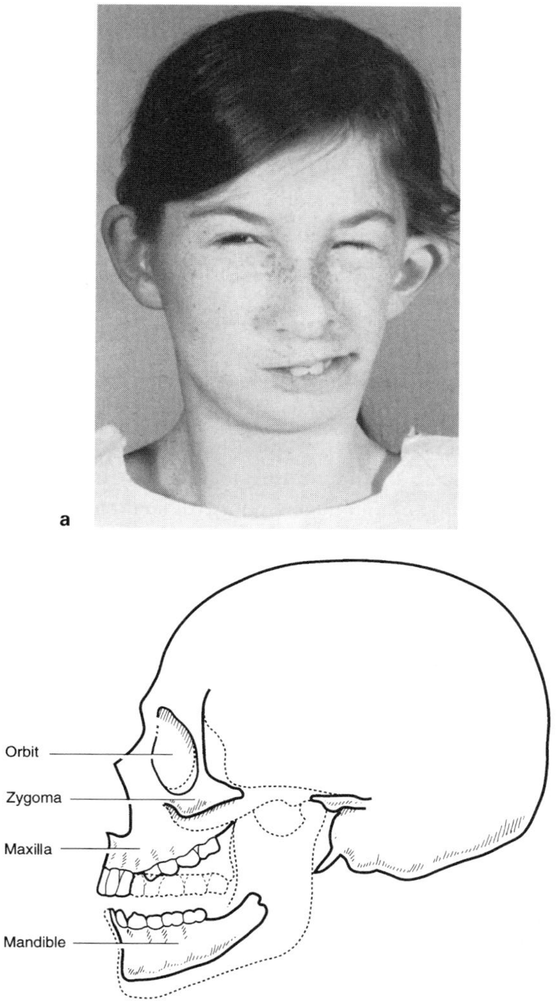

Fig. 13.9 The appearance of hemifacial microsomia. (a) With permission from Wolfe publications (Courtesy of Drs Henderson and Poswillo).

This defect was originally believed to be the result of bleeding from the stapedial arterial system during early embryonic development.[29]

The clinical features consist, to a varying degree, of inferior displacement of the lateral canthus, prominent and inferiorly displaced ear, midfacial flattening (zygomatic hypoplasia), deviation of chin, a hypoplastic mandible, upward tilting of the occlusal plane, nasal deviation, facial paresis, upper eyelid colobomas ('V'-shaped defects), and occasionally cleft lip and palate (Fig. 13.9).[30] When syndactyly, fusion of fingers and toes, is also present the condition is termed Goldenhar's syndrome. The

REFERENCES

24. Muir F K Br J Plast Surg 1966; 29: 30
25. Burian F The Plastic Surgery Atlas. Macmillan, New York 1978
26. Moore F T Br J Plast Surg 1960; 47: 424
27. Bluestone C Ann Otol Rhinol Laryngol 1971; 80: 1
28. Obwegeser H L, Lello G E, Farmand M In: Bell W H (ed) Surgical Correction of Dentofacial Deformities. W B Saunders, Philadelphia 1985 p 592
29. Poswillo D E Oral Surg 1973; 35: 302
30. Poole M D World J Surg 1989; 13: 396

deformity is essentially unilateral although in up to a third of cases the features may be bilateral.

The treatment varies according to the severity of the deformity. Some deformities, such as skin tags and macrostomia, are treated during early childhood whereas the treatment of the bony deformity is delayed until growth can be assessed. Some believe in delaying treatment of the mandibular hypoplasia until growth has ceased, when the deformity can be fully corrected in a single stage.

When there is a functional temporomandibular joint and only mild facial asymmetry, treatment is usually deferred until after the completion of growth. In moderately severe cases, hypoplasia is restricted to the condyle and coronoid processes but the temporomandibular joint is still present. These cases are treated between 12 and 16 years of age by performing an inverted 'L' osteotomy of the ramus of the mandible on the affected side. In severe cases there is hypoplasia of the entire mandible on the affected side including the ramus, condyle and temporomandibular joint. These cases are treated much earlier, between the ages of 6 and 10 years, using a costochondral graft to lengthen the mandible and provide a potential cartilaginous growth centre for the condyle.

The hypoplasia of soft tissues is an important aspect of the deformity and may require augmentation. This is now usually achieved by free tissue transfer.

Treacher Collins syndrome —facial clefts 6, 7 and 8

Also known as mandibulo-facial dysostosis, this is an autosomal dominant disorder. The syndrome produces a symmetrical deformity of varying severity (Fig. 13.10). The clinical features consist of antimongoloid palpebral fissures, a lower eyelid coloboma, absence of medial half of lower eyelashes, hypoplasia of external and middle ears, zygoma and mandible, a 'V'-shaped patch of hair extending onto the cheeks, a parrot-beak shaped nose, dental crowding, and an anterior open bite with class II malocclusion.[31]

Treatment of this condition requires correction of both the mid and lower facial deformities. The mid facial bony deformity is corrected by a split-rib or calvarial onlay and inlay bone grafts through a wide exposure provided by a bicoronal scalp flap. The bilateral mandibular hypoplasia is corrected by the same techniques already described above. Treatment of the soft tissue deformity involves a lateral canthopexy to correct the antimongoloid orientation of the palpebral fissure. The lower eyelids, which are particularly short of tissue, are lengthened by Z-plasties.

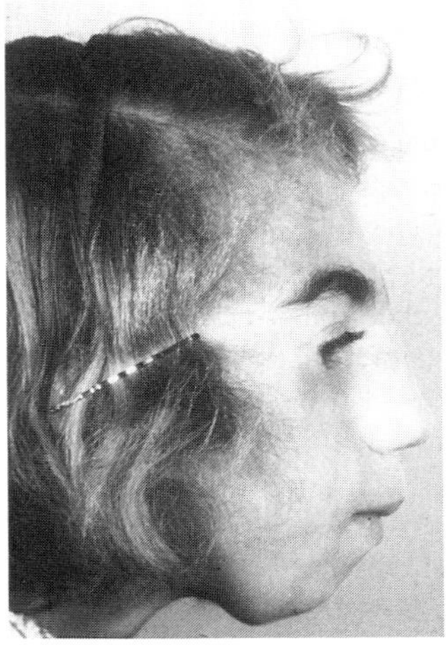

Fig. 13.10 The appearance of Treacher Collins syndrome. Courtesy of Professor D E Poswillo, Guy's Dental School.

CEPHALOCELES

Cephaloceles are herniations of the cranial contents through defects in the cranial bone. The herniated tissues consist of the meninges (meningocele) and may also include brain tissue (meningoencephalocele). They can either be primary and idiopathic or secondary to surgery or trauma.[32] Congenital cases may result from propulsion of the cranial contents between developing cranial plates or from a failure of fusion of the cranial plates.

These abnormalities are rare, occurring in about 1 in 10 000 live births, and are most frequently seen in South East Asia (Fig. 13.11).

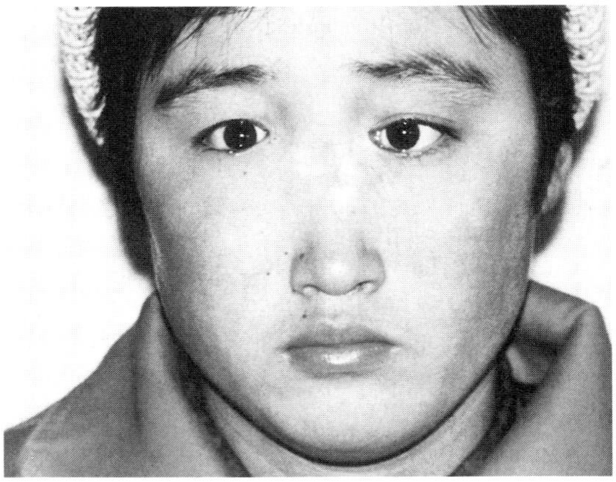

Fig. 13.11 The facial appearance associated with a fronto-ethmoidal encephalocele.

Naso-ethmoidal and nasofrontal encephaloceles may be associated with telecanthus, an increased distance between the medial canthi. Disturbance of visual acuity and ocular displacement are common and hydrocephalus, mental retardation and epilepsy may also occur. Hypertelorism, if present, can be corrected during the repair procedure.[33]

ORTHOGNATHIC DEFORMITIES

Orthognathic surgery involves repositioning parts of the facial skeleton to correct facial deformity. In addition to the improvement in the facial appearance there are functional improvements in the temporomandibular joints and dental occlusion.

REFERENCES

31. Argenta S C, Iacobucci J J World J Surg 1989; 13: 401
32. David D J World J Surg 1989; 13: 349
33. David D J, Shefield L, Simpson D, White J Br J Plast Surg 1984; 37: 271

Analysis of the deformity

Clinical evaluation

Clinical assessment is the most important aspect in the evaluation of facial deformity. Facial symmetry is the single most important feature of a pleasing facial appearance (Fig. 13.12).[34] Palpation from behind the patient allows assessment of retrusion of the supraorbital and infraorbital margins, the zygomatic prominences and paranasal areas.

The facial profile is particularly useful in the assessment of the deformity. The profile of the nose, lips and chin should take the shape of a cupid's bow. This is influenced by the relationship of the maxilla to the mandible and the inclination of their incisor teeth. The inclination of the teeth often compensates for the underlying skeletal deformity. Normally the upper incisor teeth are 1–2 mm in front of the lower ones. The teeth may, however, be proclined, retroclined or even reversed with the lower teeth occluding in front of the upper ones. Normally, only about 1–2 mm of the crowns of the upper incisor teeth show beneath the upper lip at rest, whereas about two thirds of the crowns are visible on smiling.

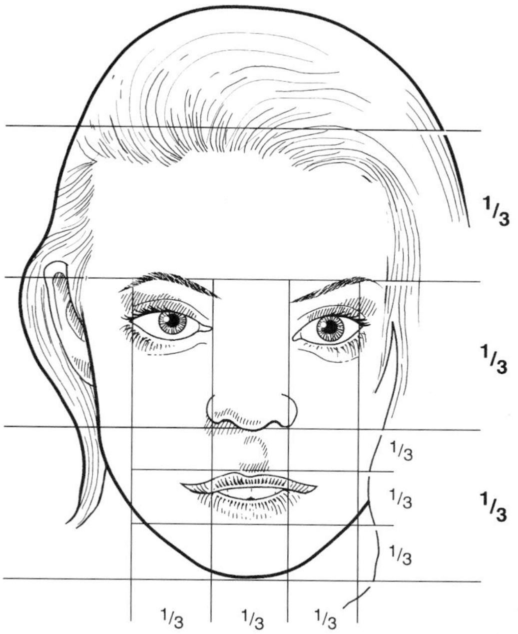

Fig. 13.12 Illustration of the ideal frontal facial proportions.

Radiological evaluation

By analysing standardized cephalometric radiographs from a large population, the average lengths, proportions and angles of various parts of the skull have been ascertained. These allow quantitative comparisons of measurements to be made between these 'norms' and individual cases in order to identify the areas of deformity and grade their severity.

Treatment planning

The objective of treatment is to achieve an optimal functional dental occlusion. Treatment usually begins with a prolonged course of orthodontics to align and correct the angulation of the teeth and to coordinate the dental arches into compatible shapes. Osteotomies are made in the maxilla and mandible to shift them appropriately to correct the facial deformity.

Maxillary osteotomies

The Le Fort I osteotomy is the most commonly performed maxillary procedure. It allows correction of both anteroposterior and vertical facial disproportions—namely, midfacial retrusion, as well as long or short faces (Figs 13.13 and 13.14). The Le Fort II and III maxillary osteotomies are mainly used to advance different areas of the mid-face. Segmental osteotomies of the maxilla allow the correction of more localized deformities.

Mandibular osteotomies

Osteotomies can be performed on the mandible at various sites. The ramus is the site most commonly chosen for both advancement and setback procedures, the sagittal split osteotomy being the most commonly used[35–37] (Figs 13.15 and 13.16). Other advancement procedures of the mandible include the vertical subsigmoid and inverted 'L' osteotomies, both of which require interpositional bone grafts.

Genioplasties

These procedures enable correction of deficient or excessive chin projection and lower anterior dental height discrepancies. An osteotomy is made in the anterior part of the mandible below the teeth and repositioned.

CRANIO-MAXILLOFACIAL TRAUMA

Cranio-maxillofacial-trauma is common, occurring in all age groups. Its aetiology can be classified into falls, impacts, assaults, road accidents, sports, occupational and 'others'. Most soft tissue injuries are the result of falls and impacts, with furnishings and fixtures, whereas fractures are commonly caused by assaults and road accidents.[38]

As cranio-maxillofacial trauma is often associated with other injuries a full assessment must be made of other systems. The advanced trauma life support (ATLS) is an excellent protocol for diagnosing and treating injuries.[39] Maxillofacial trauma may

REFERENCES

34. Epker B N, Fish L C Dentofacial deformities—integrated orthodontic and surgical correction, Vols 1 & 2. St Louis, Mosby 1986
35. Obwegeser H Oral Surg 1957; 10: 677, 787, 899
36. Dal Pont G J Oral Surg Anaesth and Hosp Dent Serv 1961; 19: 42
37. Hunsuck E E J Oral Surg 1968; 26: 249
38. Hussain K, Wijetunge D B, Grubnic S, Jackson I T J Trauma 1994; 1: 106
39. Advanced Trauma Life Support Student Manual. Committee on Trauma, American College of Surgeons, Chicago Illinois 1989

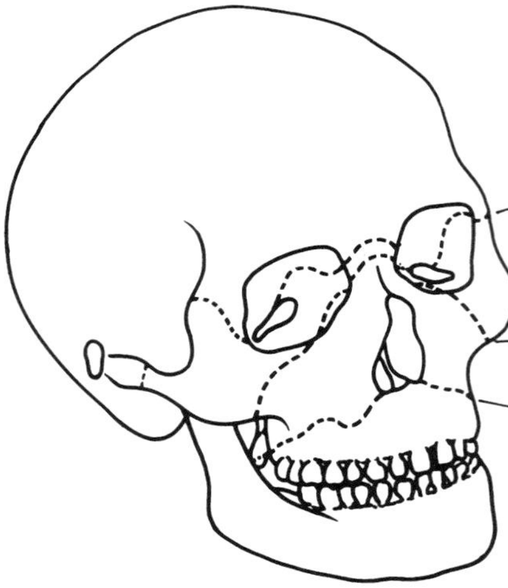

Fig. 13.13 The sites of the Le Fort maxillary osteotomies and fractures.

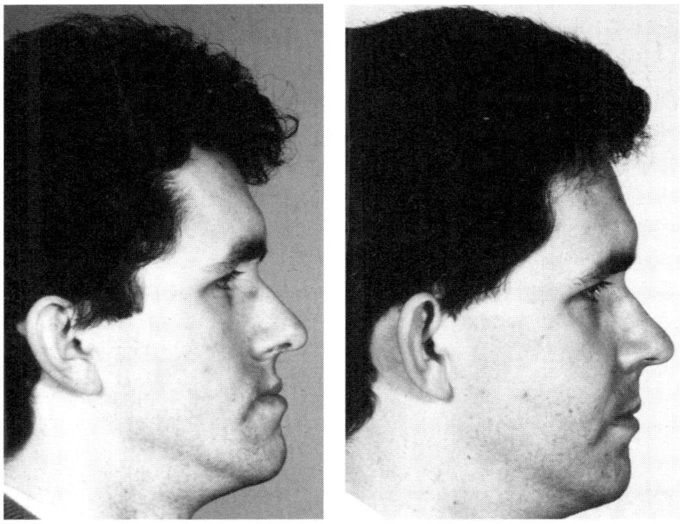

Fig. 13.14 A clinical case of maxillary hypoplasia before (**a**) and after (**b**) an advancement by Le Fort I maxillary osteotomy. Courtesy of Mr P D Robinson, Guy's Dental School.

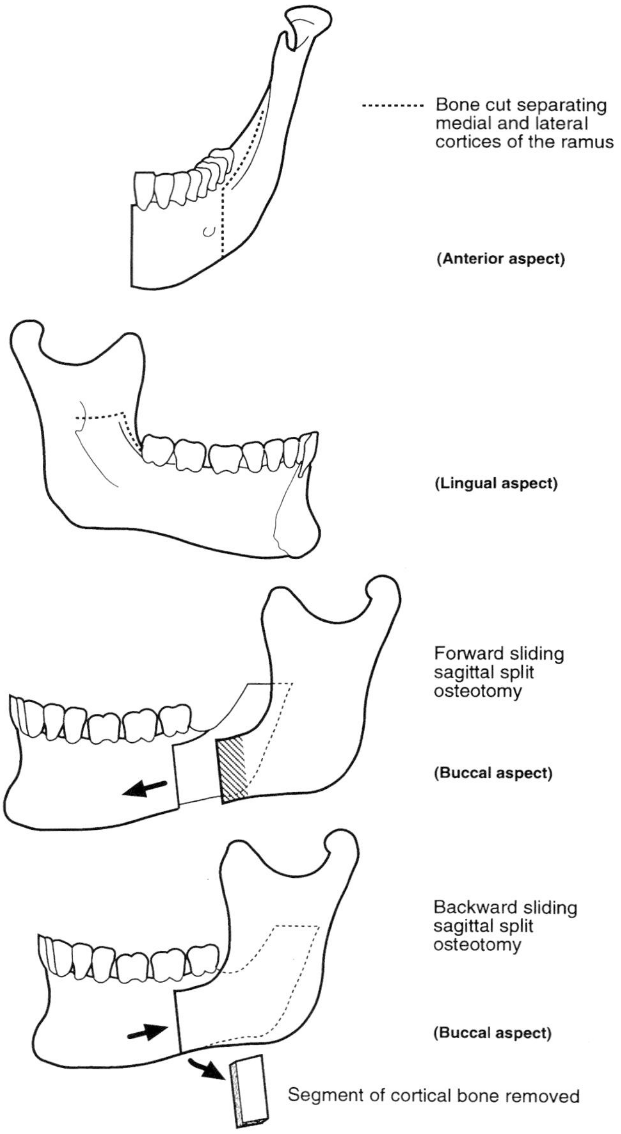

Fig. 13.15 The mandible, sagittal-split osteotomy.

compromise the airway and circulation, and cervical and head injuries also often occur.

Conscious patients with facial fractures are often able to guard their airway by sitting up and leaning forwards,[40] while those who are unconscious can not. Multiple dental fractures and fractured dental restorations are liable to be inhaled and obstruct the airway. They need to be removed with the aid of a good light and a suction catheter. With a posteriorly displaced Le Fort maxillary fracture, the soft palate may contact the pharyngeal walls and base of the tongue, obstructing the airway. This may be overcome by the insertion of an oropharyngeal or nasopharyngeal airway, an endotracheal tube or immediate manual disimpaction of the maxilla. Occasionally, midfacial fractures may be associated with torrential nasopharyngeal haemorrhage, preventing endotracheal intubation, and postnasal packing and/or cricothyrotomy may then be necessary as an emergency procedure.

The airway may also be compromised after some types of mandibular fracture. In bilateral parasymphyseal mandibular fractures, the central fragment is displaced posteriorly by the pull of the genioglossus muscles, allowing the tongue to fall back against the posterior pharyngeal wall and occlude the airway. Insertion of an oropharyngeal or nasopharyngeal airway relieves the obstruction. If these are not available a large suture is placed through the tongue and forward traction can then be applied.

Haemorrhage resulting from midfacial fractures is not normally prolonged but persistent haemorrhage is usually readily controlled by anterior and posterior nasal packing. If packing fails, carotid

REFERENCE

40. Rowe N L, Williams J L (eds) Maxillofacial Injuries. Churchill Livingstone, Edinburgh 1985

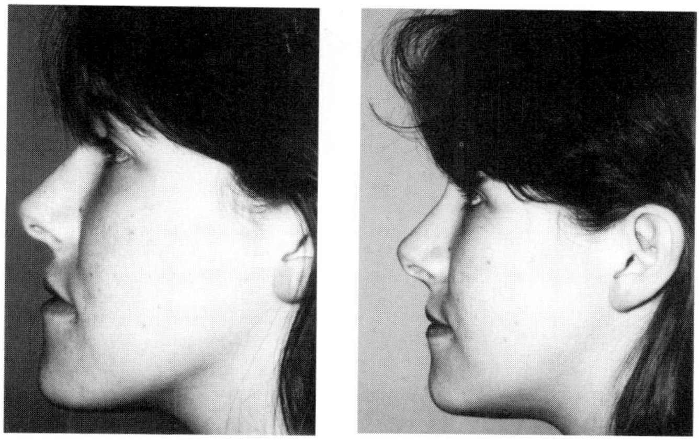

a b

Fig. 13.16 The lateral appearance of a case with mandibular prognathism before (**a**) and after (**b**) a sagittal-split backward sliding osteotomy. Courtesy of Mr P D Robinson, Guy's Dental School.

angiography may be indicated to identify bleeding vessels prior to ligation of, for example, the anterior ethmoidal or external carotid arteries. Therapeutic embolization is a possible alternative.

Cranio-maxillofacial examination begins with an inspection of the cranium: this may reveal the presence of haematomas and lacerations, suggesting an associated intracranial injury. Concomitant orbital injuries may also be present.

Orbital examination

It is important to undertake a basic ocular examination (visual acuity, pupillary size and reactivity, and depth of the anterior chamber) of the traumatized eye even when the lids are closed by swelling. Infraorbital nerve hypoaesthesia is usually associated with fractures of the infraorbital canal along the floor of the orbit; surgical emphysema is indicative of an orbital fracture involving one or more of the para-nasal air sinuses. It can also be caused by direct blunt injury of the nerve where the infraorbital nerve emerges from the infraorbital foramen. The presence of diplopia is also important.

Fractures of the orbital walls are inevitable with nasoethmoidal, zygomatic, and Le Fort complex fractures. However, an isolated 'blow-out' fracture of the orbital wall can result from direct impacts. Prolapse of periorbital fat and/or extra-ocular muscles through the defect may produce enophthalmos and restriction of ocular movement can result in diplopia.

Nasal and naso-ethmoidal examination

The naso-ethmoidal complex extends from the dorsum of the nose and the cribriform plate above to the palate below, and from the lateral nasal and medial orbital walls on one side to those on the other side.

The clinical features associated with nasal fractures are contusion, epistaxis, and nasal deformity. The nose may be displaced laterally or posteriorly. Powerful frontal blows displace the nasal structures posteriorly into the space between the medial orbital walls, producing naso-ethmoidal fractures. Additional signs of naso-ethmoidal fractures are a laceration over the root of the nose, telecanthus, an upturned nasal tip, a stretched columella, and CSF rhinorrhoea.

Zygomatic examination

Although zygomatic fractures may only involve part of the bone, for example its arch, parts of adjacent bones such as the frontal process of the maxilla, the zygomatic process of the temporal bone and the floor and lateral walls of the orbit are also often involved and fractures are, therefore, known as zygomatic complex fractures. The clinical signs associated with these fractures are tenderness and 'stepping' of the infraorbital margin and the zygomatico-frontal suture, midfacial flattening, and trismus in conjunction with those associated with orbital fractures.

Maxillary examination

Fractures of the maxilla are the result of considerable force and are often associated with craniocerebral injury. The maxilla offers a high resistance against forces directed upwards but relatively little resistance if the impact is horizontally directed. Fractures may occur at three levels—Le Fort I, II, and III—and may be unilateral or bilateral (Fig. 13.13). The palate may also be fractured in the midline.

The Le Fort I fracture passes from the lower end of the pyriform fossa backwards, across the maxilla above the roots of the teeth to the pterygo-maxillary fissure. The fracture also extends from the piriform fossa along the lateral walls of the nose and nasal septum at the same level. The Le Fort I segment therefore consists of the teeth, their supporting alveolar bone, and the hard palate.

The Le Fort II fracture is pyramidal in shape, passing from the dorsum of the nose backwards across the medial walls of the orbit (posterior to the nasolacrimal apparatus) to the inferior orbital margins, medial to the infraorbital foramina. It then continues across the maxilla, below the bodies of the zygomatic bones and above the roots of the maxillary teeth, to the pterygo-maxillary fissure.

Le Fort III. fractures are the most severe of all facial fractures and are the result of disjunction of the midfacial skeleton from the anterior cranial base. The fracture line passes from the dorsum of the nose and cribriform plate, along the medial walls of the orbit, to the inferior orbital fissures; it then continues up across the lateral walls of the orbits to the zygomatico-frontal sutures. The zygomatic arches are also fractured.

The clinical symptoms and signs vary according to the level of fracture. Dental malocclusion is associated with displaced fractures at any level. Le Fort II and III fractures cause the features of orbital wall and naso-ethmoidal fractures. The symptoms and signs of Le Fort III maxillary fractures are fairly characteristic and include panda/raccoon appearance (bilateral black eyes), gross midfacial swelling, bilateral epistaxis, cerebrospinal fluid rhinorrhoea, and dental malocclusion (Fig. 13.17). The face swells like a balloon because of the absence of a deep fascial layer the tissues

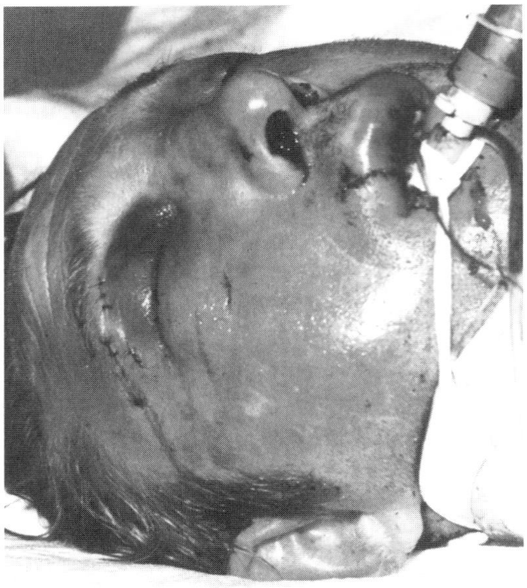

Fig. 13.17 The gross facial oedema associated with Le Fort II and III maxillary fractures.

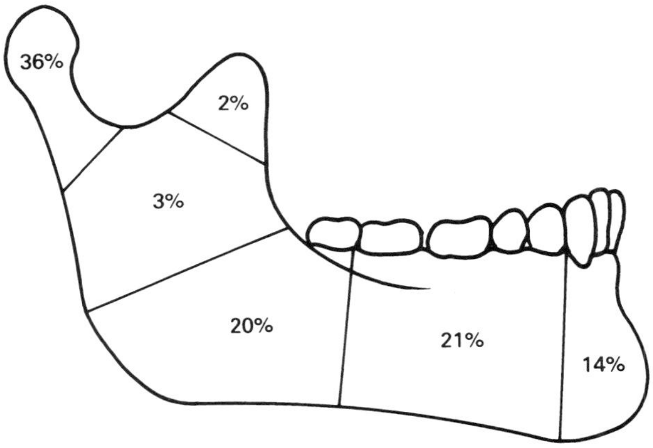

Fig. 13.18 The incidence of fractures occurring at various sites of the mandible.

offer little resistance to oedema formation. The clinical diagnosis of a Le Fort fracture is confirmed by mobility of the fractured segment.

Mandibular examination

The symptoms and signs of a fractured mandible include pain and swelling over the affected area as well as trismus and malocclusion. Displaced fractures of the body of the mandible may produce hypoaesthesia of the lower lip. The relative incidence of fractures of the mandible at various sites is shown in Figure 13.18.

Investigations

Radiology is necessary to diagnose facial fractures with certainty and assess their severity. 15° and 30° occipitomental plain radiographs are useful to diagnose maxillary, zygomatic, and orbital fractures (Fig. 13.19). They may show the classical 'hanging drop'

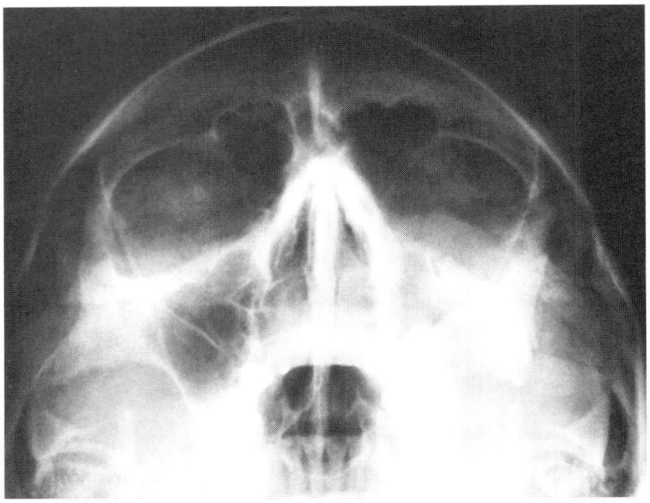

Fig. 13.19 A 15° occipitomental radiograph showing a zygomatic complex fracture.

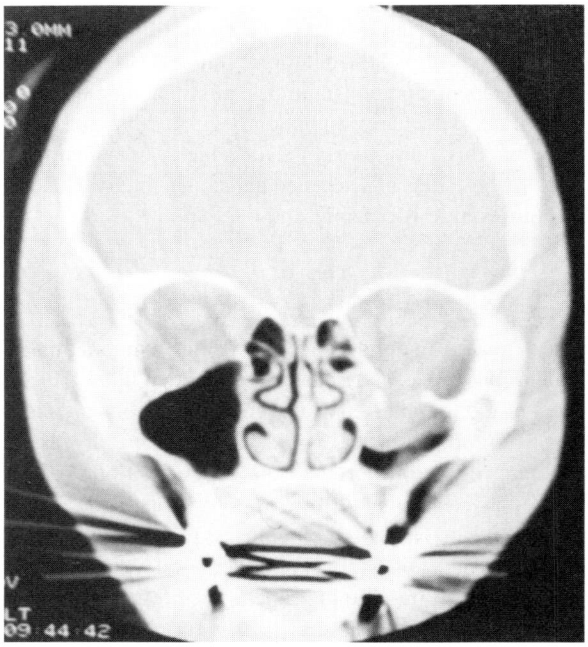

Fig. 13.20 An orbital coronal CT image showing an orbital blowout fracture with herniation of periorbital tissues into the maxillary sinus.

sign in the maxillary antrum which is indicative of an orbital floor injury. High-resolution cross-sectional CT and MR imaging is invaluable for demonstrating midfacial fractures and herniation of orbital soft tissues (Fig. 13.20). The range of eye movements is assessed by means of a Hess chart, which identifies restriction in ocular movement that could be the result of muscle entrapment or paralysis.

An orthopantomograph (OPG) and a postero-anterior mandibular radiograph show the vast majority of fractures of the mandible in two planes (Fig. 13.21). Transpharyngeal and transcranial views with the mouth open and closed allow a detailed assessment of intracapsular condylar fractures but are difficult to interpret. Mandibular fractures do not normally pose a diagnostic problem

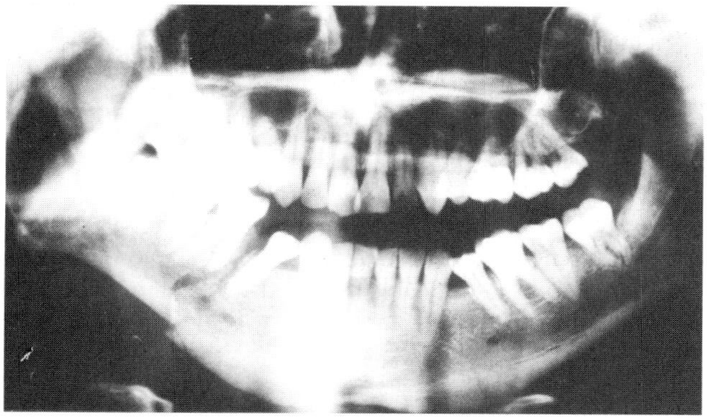

Fig. 13.21 An orthopantomograph view showing mandibular fractures.

but condylar fractures are easily overlooked. Preauricular tenderness, especially if accompanied by a laceration on the point of the chin, demands a careful radiological evaluation of the condyle.

Stabilization

The patient's condition should be stabilized before definitive treatment is undertaken. Fractures that are compound into the sinuses, mouth, or through the skin require antibiotic prophylaxis against the development of bony infections.

Orbital fractures

The objectives for the treatment of orbital fractures are the restoration of orbital wall continuity and volume. This involves replacing herniated periorbital soft tissue within the orbital cavity and reconstructing the defect with bone graft or an alloplastic material.

Nasal fractures

Nasal fractures are the most common type of craniofacial fracture (44%). Despite this, they are often inadequately treated with adverse affects on the facial appearance and nasal airway.[41] The 'open book' and laterally displaced types of nasal fracture are usually treated by closed reduction. Care should be taken to ensure that the septum is in its correct position to avoid the risk of late nasal deformity; nasal fractures must be carefully splinted postoperatively. Displaced naso-ethmoidals are treated by internal fixation and reconstruction of the orbital walls.

Zygomatic fractures

Non-displaced fractures do not require operative treatment. Simple displaced fractures are the result of low impact trauma and are usually adequately treated by one of a number of closed reduction techniques, the most common being that of Gillies' temporal reduction (Fig. 13.22). Grossly displaced and comminuted zygomatic complex fractures result from high impact trauma and require anatomical open reduction and internal fixation.

Residual midfacial flattening, neuropraxia of the infraorbital nerve and trismus are complications of poorly treated zygomatic complex fractures. Diplopia and enophthalmos may persist after the treatment of orbital fractures.

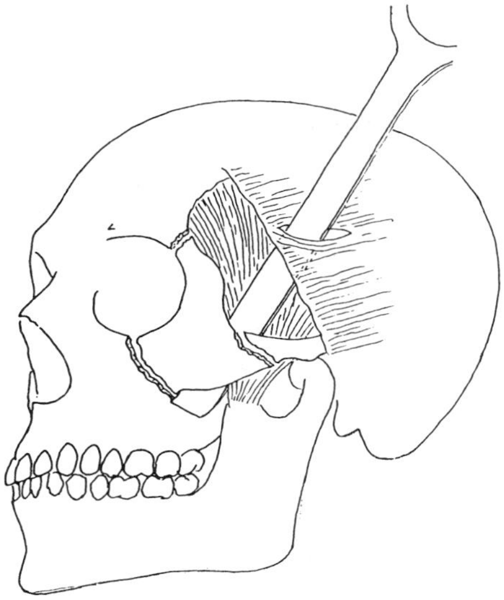

Fig. 13.22 The Gillies temporal approach for reduction of a zygomatic complex fracture.

Maxillary fractures

Undisplaced fractures are treated conservatively. Displaced fractures are now normally realigned by open reduction and internal fixation by using miniplates through a wide exposure of the fractures, although occasionally the traditional method of closed reduction and external fixation is still used. The mandible is used to align the maxilla using the dentition or dentures as a guide. If the mandible is fractured its continuity should be restored first. Once correct jaw alignment is achieved repositioning and immobilization of adjacent bone fragments is undertaken.

The complications of maxillary fractures include suboptimal restoration of the midfacial projection, altered dental occlusion, and infraorbital paraesthesia. Malunion is rare.

Mandibular fractures

The mandibular condyle is unusual in two ways; it acts as a growth centre and in children with condylar injuries some degree of mandibular growth retardation can develop in a quarter. This may produce secondary facial deformity. Fractures of the condyle heal spontaneously without immobilization of the jaw. This may be a disadvantage when the fracture is intracapsular, particularly in children below 10 years of age when the condyle may fuse with the temporal bone with disastrous consequences for facial growth. All condylar fractures should be mobilized early to forestall such an event.

Fractures of the condyle are usually extracapsular although a few involve the intracapsular portion of the joint. These fractures

REFERENCE

41. Stell P M Clin Otolaryngol 1980; 5: 362

are usually treated conservatively especially in children. If the dental occlusion is not affected, the jaw must be rested by giving a soft diet and providing appropriate analgesia. Immobilization by means of mandibulo-maxillary wire or, preferably, elastic fixation is required for a period of about 3 weeks if malocclusion is present. The management is similar even when the head of the condyle is dislocated medially from the glenoid fossa by traction from the lateral pterygoid muscle, although open reduction and internal fixation is becoming more popular in this situation and is definitely indicated when displacement dislocation is such that it interferes substantially with dental occlusion. It is also indicated when both condyles are fractured and displaced, leading to a reduction in height of the ramus and gagging of the mandible on the molar teeth particularly if the maxilla is also displaced and therefore, reliant on the mandible to establish the correct jaw alignment.

Mandibulo-maxillary fixation is achieved by eyelets and tie-wires, or arch bars and elastics (Fig. 13.23). The latter is preferred as it allows some mobility of the joint to continue during the period of 'immobilization', reducing the degree of postoperative joint stiffness and trismus. In edentulous patients, Gunning splints are used to reduce the condylar fractures and restore the correct occlusal relationship. These modified dentures are secured to their respective jaws by the use of circum-mandibular wires for the mandible and circumzygomatic, piriform fossa, or transpalatal wires for the maxilla. The two Gunning splints can then be wired to immobilize the fracture.

Angle and body fractures

These fractures are usually caused by a direct blow over the affected area or an indirect force transmitted from a blow over the contralateral parasymphyseal area of the mandible.

Undisplaced angular fractures, without mobility or dental malocclusion, are treated conservatively with rest, a soft diet and analgesia. If the fracture site is mobile or dental occlusion is affected, then reduction and immobilization of the fracture is indicated.

In the last two decades the management of facial fracture and mandibular fractures in particular has been revolutionized by the introduction of mini- and microplating systems that allow almost immediate restoration of function without a period of mandibulo-maxillary jaw fixation. The vast majority of fractures can now be adequately treated via an intraoral approach with minimal complications.

The presence of teeth is of great benefit as they enable the dental occlusion to be checked, allowing the correct relationship of the fracture fragments to be restored. Fractures of an atrophic edentulous mandible are traditionally managed by Gunning splints but more recently open reduction and internal fixation with bone plates has found favour, particularly in the presence of pulmonary disease. These pencil-thin mandibles are at particular risk of malunion.

Complications arising from the treatment of mandibular fractures are surprisingly uncommon and include infection, malocclusion, trismus, delayed union, nonunion, and growth reduction in children. The accurate reduction and fixation of fractures with miniplates is technically more demanding than traditional methods of mandibulo-maxillary wire fixation and can lead to a higher incidence of minor malocclusion.

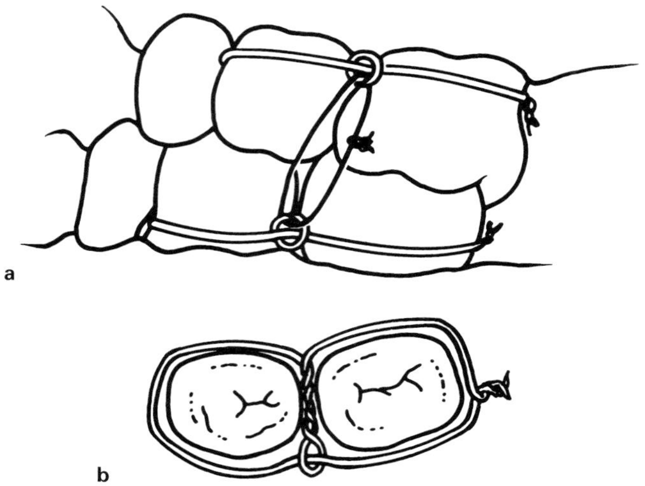

Fig. 13.23 Eyelet wiring.

Panfacial (multiple) fractures

The management of multiple facial fractures is the same as that of fractures of the individual bones. These are normally high-velocity injuries and consist of comminuted fractures of the orbital, naso-ethmoidal, zygomatic and maxillary complexes, as well as of the mandible; they are difficult to treat. With careful preservation of the multiple fractured bony fragments and their anatomical open reduction and internal fixation, excellent results can be achieved.

CRANIOFACIAL ACCESS SURGERY

It has in the past been both difficult and hazardous to gain surgical access to the skull base and upper cervical spine. This has, however, been overcome by carrying out osteotomies on the craniofacial skeleton to improve the surgical exposure.

The skull base can be divided into anterior, posterior, medial and lateral zones in relation to the carotid canals to help in understanding the surgical exposure of these areas.

Skull base tumours

Clinical features

The clinical presentation of skull base tumours varies according to the region affected and whether intracranial disease is present. The latter presents with the symptoms of raised intracranial pressure, such as headache and vomiting. Low-grade tumours can either enter or leave the cranium through its basal foramina and this gives rise to characteristic localizing signs (Table 13.3).

Investigations

The staging of tumours is important in determining whether or not they can be resected. Cross-sectional imaging with CT or MR has been a major advance in this respect as the full extent of the lesion and its relationship to adjacent structures can be established and

Table 13.3 Clinical features associated with skull base tumours

Area of skull base	*Structures affected*	*Clinical features*
Anterior segment	Orbit (through inferior orbital fissure)	Proptosis
	Temporal fossa	Swelling
	Parapharyngeal	Dyspnoea and dysphagia
Central segment	Middle ear	Pain and palsy
Posterior segment	Parapharyngeal space Parapharyngeal mass	May present as a deep lobe of parotid tumour

the treatment planned accordingly. Detailed evaluation of the local vascular anatomy and cross-flow across the circle of Willis is now possible with magnetic resonance angiography.

Treatments

Access to the skull base can involve subcranial (transoral or transfacial) or transcranial osteotomies. The approach chosen depends principally on the site of the pathology.

INFECTIONS OF THE MOUTH

Bacterial infection

Dental caries is the most common bacterial disease of the head and neck and results from acid demineralization of first enamel and then the dentine of the crowns of teeth; this process can be arrested in the early stages. The tooth decay results in destruction of the tooth and infection of the pulp which in turn leads to necrosis and death of the tooth. Infection may then extend along the root canal to the periapical tissues within the alveolar bone.

Dentoalveolar abscess

This may form as a result of an acute infection at the apex of a tooth and discharge pus into the mouth via a sinus on the alveolus or, more rarely, spread to cause a facial abscess. Involvement of submandibular lymph nodes, especially in children, may result in large swellings and abscess formation.

A periapical abscess requires drainage and elimination of the source of infection. A minor infection can be alleviated by a root canal therapy which may be performed in conjunction with open drainage of the abscess. Alternatively, tooth extraction provides drainage and removes the cause.

The infection from a periapical abscess penetrates the adjacent bony cortex and if left untreated tracks beneath the periosteum to discharge into the mouth. This is usually accompanied by significant pain relief. Most abscesses point into the oral cavity but in the posterior aspect of the mandible where the mylohyoid attachment becomes superficial and the apices of the teeth project below it, an infection can drain into the submandibular space. Infection beneath a wisdom tooth may spread into a variety of spaces and can present unexpectedly as a parapharyngeal or submasseteric abscess. The retromolar infections can be distinguished from a tonsillar quinsy because they invariably cause trismus.

Soft tissue infections

Soft tissue infection of dental origin may be acute or chronic. Acute infection may take the form of an abscess, which in most instances presents as a submandibular swelling or periorbital oedema if the maxillary teeth are involved. The majority of such infections can be easily controlled by drainage, antibiotics and removal of the source of the infection. Occasionally a virulent bacterium such as the β-haemolytic streptococcus can cause a spreading 'cellulitis' which in its severe form may result in Ludwig's angina (vide infra).

It is important with cervicofacial infections to exclude predisposing conditions such as diabetes mellitus and immunosuppression. Patients are unwell with systemic symptoms such as fever and malaise. Spreading infection can cause a compromised airway, preceded by an elevated tongue and difficulty in swallowing. The presence of trismus makes intraoral examination difficult but an orthopantomograph helps to identify carious teeth. The infection can spread to involve the sublingual space anteriorly, and the superficial pterygoid, deep temporal and parapharyngeal spaces posteriorly.

All patients except those with limited submandibular swellings are admitted to hospital and given intravenous antibiotic therapy and rehydrated if necessary. The abscess is then incised and drained. Intubation may be a real problem for the anaesthetist and the surgeon should remain at hand during induction in case the airway is lost and a tracheostomy is required. Hilton's method of blunt dissection is used to avoid damage to the mandibular branch of the facial nerve, and the fibrous septa in the abscess cavity are broken digitally.

Ludwig's angina

This condition causes bilateral infection of the submandibular, sublingual and submental spaces (Fig. 13.24). Most cases arise from dental sepsis, usually in a mandibular molar tooth, but other foci of infection in the mouth can also be responsible for this condition.

The infection may spread rapidly along the deep cervical and parapharyngeal fascial planes to produce supraglottic oedema and airway obstruction. Dyspnoea, dysphagia and dysphonia are sinister symptoms of impending airway obstruction. During the initial stages the patient is able to compensate for partial obstruction, however, patient exhaustion and complete airway obstruction can quickly supervene. This condition is a surgical emergency. The first priority in severe cases is to secure airway control by endotracheal intubation or tracheostomy. Intravenous antibiotics are commenced.

The submandibular, sublingual and submental spaces are decompressed, the cause removed (carious tooth), and the underlying infection treated with intravenous antibiotics.

Viral infections

Herpetic stomatitis

The primary infection usually occurs in childhood and may be accompanied by a severe systemic upset. While herpes type I virus is

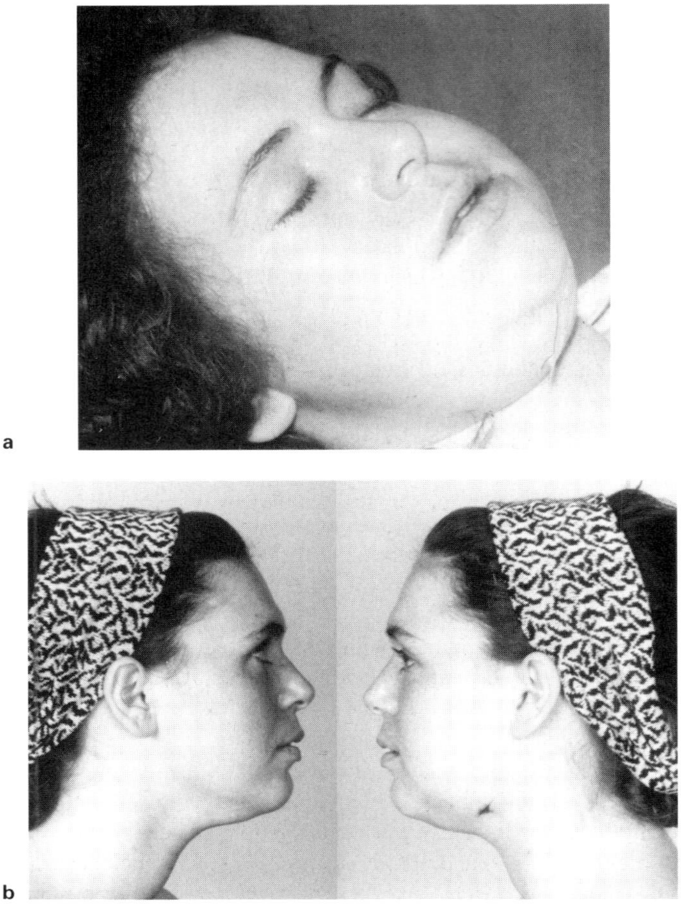

Fig. 13.24
A case of Ludwig's angina: (**a**) pre-treatment, (**b**) post-treatment.

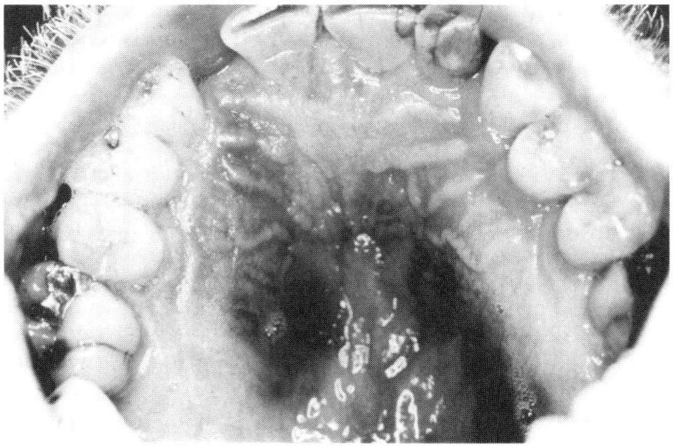

Fig. 13.25 Kaposi's sarcoma.

the common cause of infection, the type II virus, which is normally associated with genital disease, has become an increasing cause of herpetic stomatitis. The condition is characterized by multiple small painful ulcers, preceded by vesicles, affecting any part of the oral mucosa but mostly occupying the gingivae, hard palate and tongue. There is accompanying cervical lymphadenopathy. Recovery may take a week or more. Topically applied antiviral agents such as idoxuridine or acyclovir can be used in severe cases[42] but are not very effective once the infection is established.

Herpes labialis

About one third of the population who have had primary herpes are subject to recurrent herpetic lesions affecting the lips. The virus persists in latent form in the trigeminal ganglia and is reactivated by local or systemic factors such as fevers or overexposure of the lips to sunshine, cold or local trauma. The first sign is swelling of the lip and a crop of vesicles which burst and form the familiar cold sore. Treatment with acyclovir is effective if begun early[42] and is indicated in the immunocompromised.

Hand, foot and mouth disease (caused by strains of the Coxsackie A virus)

This is an acute but mild viral infection. It often produces minor epidemics in children and is characterized by painful oral ulceration with a rash on the hands and feet.[43] There is no specific treatment.

Herpes zoster of the trigeminal nerve (shingles)

This condition is more common in the elderly or the immunologically compromised patient and is accompanied by prodromal pain and a vesicular rash in the distribution of one or more divisions of the nerve.[44] The trigeminal nerve is affected in 15% of cases. Involvement of the ophthalmic division may lead to corneal ulceration (see Chapter 15). In a few cases the facial nerve is the focus of the viral infection, resulting in intense pain over the mastoid, followed by vesicles on both the soft palate and external auditory meatus in conjunction with a facial palsy (Ramsay Hunt syndrome). Herpes zoster responds to topical application of idoxuridine or acyclovir. Antibiotic creams are useful to prevent secondary infection of skin lesions and analgesics are usually necessary. Postherpetic neuralgia is an uncommon but troublesome complication in the elderly and responds poorly to treatment.

Human immunodeficiency virus

This virus can cause oral ulceration, Kaposi's sarcoma, candidiasis and hairy leucoplakia in the mouth; only Kaposi's sarcoma is pathognomonic of the virus (Fig. 13.25).[45]

Fungal infections

Candidiasis

The single-celled yeast organism *Candida albicans* is a commensal in man. Infection occurs in patients whose resistance is diminished

REFERENCES

42. Jaffe E C, Lehner T Br Dent J 1968; 125: 392
43. Cawson R A, McSwiggan D A Oral Surg 1969; 217: 451
44. Hudson C D, Vickers R A Oral Surg 1971; 31: 494
45. Lozada F, Silverman S et al Oral Surg 1983; 56: 491

or where local factors such as chronic trauma or maceration from dentures encourage establishment of the infection.

Acute infection (thrush). This is characterized by creamy white patches which can be rubbed off. They are produced by proliferation of the invaded epithelium. Acute infection complicates malnutrition, postoperative debility, antibiotic therapy and immunosuppressive treatment.[46] Antifungal agents such as nystatin or amphotericin B should be prescribed, and antibiotics should be withdrawn if possible.

Chronic infection. This is associated with ill fitting dentures where the underlying mucosa becomes red and oedematous. The infection is often associated with angular cheilitis, in which the epithelium at the angle of the mouth is broken down, inflamed and crusted.[47] Persistent white hyperplastic plaques, indistinguishable from leucoplakia, may also be found on the buccal mucosa, tongue and occasionally the palate. The diagnosis of chronic hyperplastic candidiasis can only be made with certainty by biopsy. Antifungal agents have variable success rates in the treatment of established chronic infection.[48] Dentures should be kept scrupulously clean and constructed to support the lips in order to eliminate the skin folds at the corners of the mouth. Thick white patches sometimes need to be removed by surgical excision.

Actinomycosis

Actinomycosis is a chronic suppurative infection of the cervicofacial region caused by *Actinomyces israelii* (see Chapter 4). It is characterized by widespread fibrosis and multiple skin sinuses. The matted colonies form into 'sulphur granules' and are discharged in the pus. Penicillin or tetracycline should be given for several weeks and will eventually produce complete resolution.[49] The condition is uncommon in the head and neck.

Fusospirochaetal infections

Acute ulcerative gingivitis (Vincent's gingivitis, trench mouth)

This is an acute ulcerative infection of the gingivae from synergistic infection by the spirochaete *Borrelia vincentii* and the spindle-shaped bacterium *Fusobacterium nucleatum*. Predisposing factors (apart from a neglected mouth) are stress, anxiety, smoking and upper respiratory tract infections. The term 'trench mouth' was coined in the First World War. The main symptoms are painful bleeding gums and marked halitosis. Treatment is with penicillin and improved oral hygiene. The condition is uncommon today.

Cancrum oris (noma, phagedaena)

This disease occurs mainly in tropical countries. It commences as an acute ulcerative gingivitis and progresses to necrosis of the soft tissues overlying the jaws. It affects debilitated children and seriously ill adults suffering from malnutrition. The ulceration and necrosis are progressive, affecting the lips, cheek and tongue and exposing large areas of alveolar bone. A fatal outcome from exhaustion and bronchopneumonia occurs in 90% of untreated cases.[50] Treatment is with penicillin and metronidazole combined with correction of the nutritional deficiency. Treatment must also be given for underlying diseases such as anaemia from hookworm infestation and malaria. The lesions heal by fibrosis, causing contractions, extra-articular ankylosis and severe disfigurement.

Tuberculosis and syphilis (see Chapter 4)

These conditions are relatively uncommon in the western population today, especially as a cause of oral ulceration. The primary tuberculosis complex is rare and presents as an indolent painless ulcer associated with marked regional lymphadenopathy. Primary syphilitic ulcers are also painless with a raised indurated edge. The regional lymph nodes are enlarged at this stage but serological tests are often negative. The second stage (6–8 weeks) is associated with a mild febrile illness, lymphadenopathy and the appearance of body rashes and flat, greyish oral ulcers, enlarging in a snail track manner. Tertiary syphilis presents several years later and classically affects the hard palate.[51]

ORAL ULCERATION

Persistent oral ulceration which cannot be identified with certainty as any of the following conditions must be regarded as neoplastic and biopsied to establish a diagnosis.

Traumatic ulceration

This is relatively common but seldom serious. The ulcers are in the buccal mucosa of the cheeks either at the level of dental occlusion or adjacent to a misaligned or sharp-edged tooth. Ulcers can arise on the lateral margins of the tongue where they may be mistaken for carcinoma, or on the buccal or lingual sulci in relation to ill fitting dentures. Removal of the source of irritation effects a cure within a few days, but if the ulcer persists it should be biopsied.

Aphthous ulceration

Aphthous ulceration is the most common disorder affecting the oral mucous membrane.[52] Three forms exist: minor, which occurs in crops of two or three ulcers which resolve within 10 days; major—large, deep and persistent ulcers which take a number of weeks to resolve leaving scars; and a herpetiform type which presents with multiple tiny ulcers. The minor form is most common. Suggested aetiological factors include infection, trauma, hormonal imbalance, immunological mechanisms and gastrointestinal disease.[53] Some patients may have low serum iron, folic acid or vitamin B_{12} levels.[54]

REFERENCES

46. Lehner T Dent Pract 1967; 17: 209
47. Holbrook W P, Rodgers G D Oral Surg 1980; 49: 122
48. Cawson R A Oral Surg Oral Med Oral Pathol 1966; 22: 53
49. Bramley P, Orton H S Br Dent J 1960; 109: 235
50. Emslie R D Dent Pract 1963; 13: 481
51. Meyer I, Shklar G Oral Surg 1967; 23: 45
52. Gayford J J, Haskell R Clinical Oral Medicine, 2nd edn. John Wright, Bristol 1979 p 1
53. Williams B D, Lehner T Br Med J 1977; 1: 1387

The condition begins in childhood, seems to affect patients with well cared for mouths and is rarely seen in the elderly edentulous patient. Minor aphthous ulcers vary in size, number and frequency and characteristically occur on the non-keratinized mucosa, lasting 3–7 days. They are round or oval, with a shallow grey/yellow sloughing base and surrounding erythema. There is no totally effective treatment but topical antiseptics and anaesthetics may be tried and some patients find relief from locally applied corticosteroid preparations.[55] Large ulcers may be several centimetres in diameter and persist for up to 3 months, resembling a carcinoma. When there is doubt, they should be biopsied.

Association with gastrointestinal disorders

Many of the disorders affecting the lower gastrointestinal tract also have oral manifestations. Patients with Crohn's disease have a characteristic cobblestone appearance of the oral mucosa and may suffer from mouth ulcers and granulomatous enlargement of the lips. Ulcerative colitis is associated with severe oral aphthous ulceration and coeliac disease with recurrent ulcers of the herpetiform variety.

Behçet's syndrome

This condition is a rare triple-symptom complex autoimmune disease characterized by oral ulceration (indistinguishable from aphthae), anterior uveitis and genital ulceration. Young males are mainly affected. Non-suppurative arthritis occurs in one third of cases. Treatment is symptomatic and systemic steroids are necessary in the acute condition.[56]

Agranulocytosis and neutropenia

The oral mucosa has a high rate of turnover, therefore any condition that interferes with cell proliferation can cause early symptoms or signs within the mouth. Oral ulceration may be the presenting feature of blood dyscrasias from cytotoxic drugs or bone marrow disease. The ulceration may progress to extensive necrotic lesions. Treatment should be directed at the underlying disease.[57]

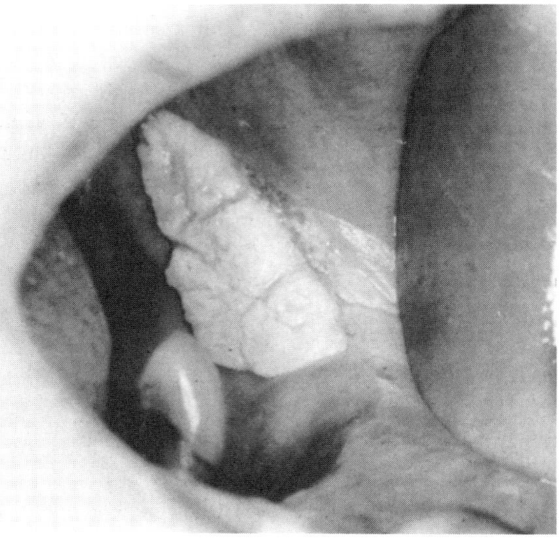

Fig. 13.26 Leucoplakia of the buccal mucosa.

Vesiculobullous lesions

Many dermatological conditions affect the oral mucosa. Vesiculobullous diseases often present with oral ulceration.

Epidermolysis bullosa is a rare inherited disorder. Intraepithelial bullae form in response to minor trauma.[58] A severe dystrophic form affecting the skin causes scarring and is sometimes fatal. There is no effective treatment.

Pemphigus is a progressive disease also characterized by intraepithelial bullae of the skin and mucous membranes. The epithelium may be rubbed off by light finger pressure—Nikolsky's sign.[59]

Benign mucous membrane pemphigoid in contrast consists of subepithelial bullae and results in scar formation. Immunosuppressive drugs may produce remission.

Erythema multiforme (Stevens–Johnson syndrome) is a rare but serious ulcerative condition of immune origin.[60] Drug allergy is known to produce it—especially sulphonamides and barbiturates—and certain infections such as mycoplasmal pneumonia, but often no cause can be found. Teenagers and young adults are predominantly affected. Oral ulceration can be diffuse with target lesions and extensive crusting of the lips at the mucocutaneous junction. Attacks may last up to 3–4 weeks and there may be associated conjunctivitis, tracheitis and dysphagia.[61] Corticosteroids, supportive treatment and antibiotics are given in severe cases.

WHITE PATCHES IN THE ORAL CAVITY

White patches commonly arise on the oral mucosa. It is estimated that they are present in 2% of the population; although the majority of cases are inconsequential approximately 2% have epithelial dysplasia. Leucoplakia is a term used to describe a white patch or plaque that cannot be characterized clinically or pathologically as any other condition (Fig. 13.26). This definition does not imply any specific histological changes.[62] White patches have three main histological features—abnormal keratinization, hyper- or hypoplasia of the epithelium and disordered maturation (dysplasia). Dysplasia is the only significant histological guide to the possibility of malignant change.

REFERENCES

54. Wray D, Ferguson M M et al Br Med J 1975; 2: 490
55. MacPhee I T, Sircus W, Farmer E D Br Med J 1968; 2: 147
56. Lehner T Gut 1977; 18: 491
57. Scully C, MacFadyen E, Campbell A Br J Oral Surg 1982; 20: 96
58. Winstock D Br J Dermatol 1962; 74: 431
59. Firkin B G, Whitworth J A (eds) Dictionary of Medical Eponyms. Parthenon, Lancs 1987 p 374
60. Ashby D W, Lazar T Lancet 1951; i: 1091
61. Lozada F, Silverman S Oral Surg 1987; 36: 628
62. Eveson J W Cancer Surv 2 1983; 3: 405

Frictional keratosis

This is caused by abrasion of the mucosa by irritants such as sharp teeth, ill fitting dentures, cheek-biting, etc. Removal of the cause effects a cure within a few days.

Smoker's keratosis

This is characteristically seen on the palate of heavy smokers. There is a pale white thickening of the mucosa and multiple small red swellings that mark the ducts of the minor mucous glands. It is not considered to be premalignant and disappears if the patient stops smoking. Reverse smoking, which is popular in some parts of the world, is definitely associated with an increased incidence of palatal cancer.[63]

Lichen planus

Lichen planus is the most common cause of persistent white patches in the mouth. The patches are often striated, forming a lace-like pattern, but can also be papular and confluent, especially on the tongue. They are often bilateral, affecting the cheek mucosa, and can be erosive and painful. Some patients may also have itchy skin papules on the flexor surfaces of their limbs. The condition is often associated with anxiety or stress. The oral lesions can be improved by removing any irritating factors or trauma and the erosive lesions should be treated with local application of corticosteroids.

Transient white patches

Other common causes of white patches are candida, infection and chemical burns, for example prolonged mucosal contact with aspirin. Small submucosal sebaceous glands (Fordyce spots) can also give the appearance of a white patch. Familial thickening of the mucosa occurs in white sponge naevus. Syphilitic leucoplakia is now only of historical interest.

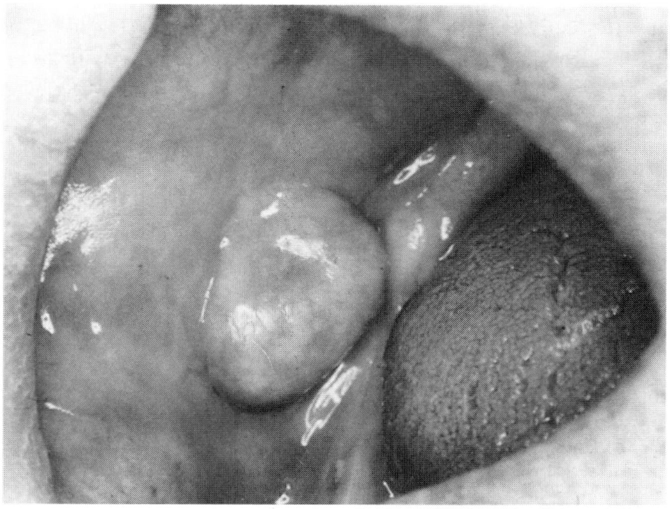

Fig. 13.27 A fibroepithelial polyp of the buccal mucosa.

GRANULOMATOUS SWELLINGS IN THE MOUTH

These are frequently the result of chronic inflammatory hyperplasia caused by recurrent minor injury or infection and are the most common localized swellings of the mouth. When they arise from the gingivae, the term 'epulis' (upon the gum) is used.

Pyogenic granuloma

These are caused by overproduction of granulation tissue in response to chronic infection or foreign bodies. They may be associated with chronic sinuses, infected tooth sockets, and gingival infection. Minimal provocation is required for their induction in pregnancy (pregnancy epulis).[64] They should be excised and any local cause should be treated.[65]

Fibroepithelial polyp

These swellings arise as the result of hyperplasia of the subepithelial tissue and are covered by stratified squamous epithelium.[66] They are caused by chronic irritation on the insides of the cheeks (occlusal trauma; Fig. 13.27) or at the periphery of ill fitting dentures. They are smooth pink swellings which are sessile or pedunculated and regress when the local irritant factor is removed. Occasionally an enlarged parotid papilla pouting from the cheek can be confused with a polyp. Phenytoin and cyclosporin A can stimulate an exuberant fibrous response to gingival inflammation producing gingival hyperplasia. This is managed with improved oral hygiene and gingival trimming.

Uncommon granulomatous conditions

Peripheral giant cell granuloma

These giant cell granulomas only arise anterior to the first molar teeth and are related to the process of deciduous tooth resorption. During removal the underlying bone should be curetted to prevent recurrence.[67]

Malignant granuloma

Two distinct conditions exist, Wegener's granuloma and midline lethal granuloma. They have a similar mode of presentation which normally consists of granulomatous inflammation in the nose and central maxilla. Wegener's granulomatosis is a vasculitis which also affects the kidneys and lungs[68] and is often fatal.[69] Midline lethal granuloma is a T-cell lymphoma, but the histological features may not be typical and in a third of cases the diagnosis is

REFERENCES

63. Roed-Peterson B, Banoczy J, Pindborg J Br J Cancer 1973; 28: 575
64. Angelopoulos A P J Oral Surg 1971; 29: 840
65. Bhaskar S N, Jacoway J R J Oral Surg 1966; 24: 391
66. Barker D S, Lucas R B Br J Oral Surg 1967; 5: 86
67. Killey H C, Kay L W J Int Coll Surg 1965; 44: 262
68. Fauci A S, Haynes B F, Katz P, Woff S M Ann Intern Med 1983; 98: 76
69. Butler D J, Thompson H Br J Oral Surg 1972; 9: 208

made on the clinical features alone. Treatment for the former disease includes steroids and cytotoxic drugs; the latter is treated with radiotherapy.

CYSTS OF THE MOUTH

Mucoceles

These probably occur from trauma to the ducts of minor salivary glands and are found particularly on the lip.[70] They are in reality mucus extravasation cysts as the histological appearances suggest that the duct has been torn allowing escape of mucus into the tissues.[71] They are superficial, bluish in colour and may fluctuate in size, reaching 1–2 cm in diameter (Fig. 13.28). They should be excised with an ellipse of overlying mucosa but the cyst wall is thin and fragile and unless care is taken they are easily ruptured at surgery. Recurrence is common. Mucoceles may also be treated by cryosurgery.[72]

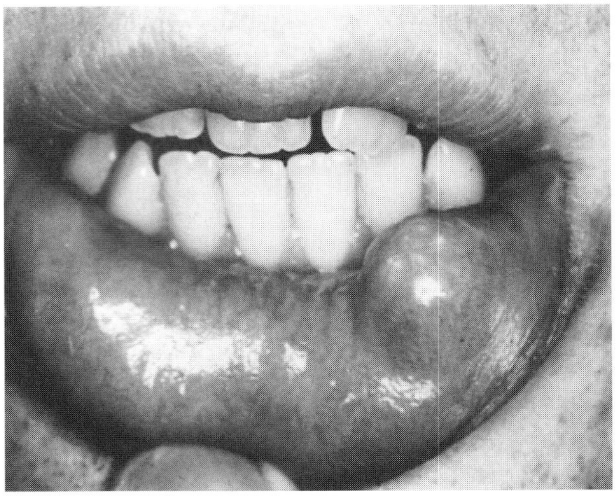

Fig. 13.28 A mucocele of the lip.

Ranula

This term ('like the belly of a frog') is used to describe a salivary extravasation cyst which develops in the floor of the mouth. It is larger than a mucocele because of the loose areola-filled spaces in the floor of the mouth into which it extends. It arises from the sublingual gland.[73] Ranulas develop on one side of the floor of the mouth and slowly enlarge to form a bluish dome-shaped fluctuant swelling beneath the sublingual mucosa (Fig. 13.29). They may extend between the muscle layers; if the mylohyoid diaphragm is penetrated they will present as a submental swelling or a plunging ranula. These cysts have very thin walls and are easily ruptured. If this occurs the cyst will recur unless the sublingual gland is removed.[74] Care must be taken not to damage the submandibular duct or the lingual nerve at the time of excision. Surgery is technically demanding and recurrence is common in inexperienced hands.

a

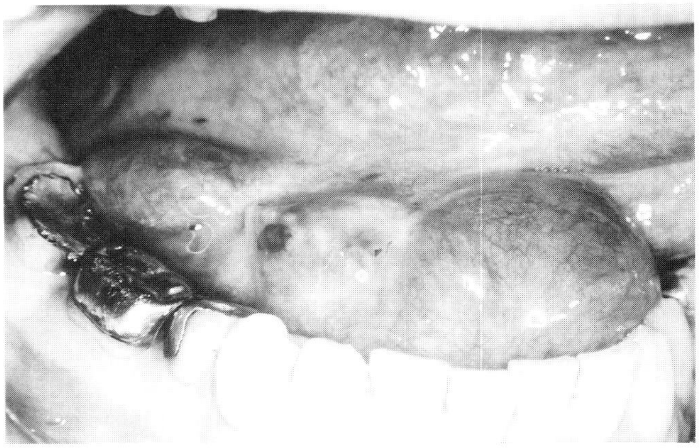

b

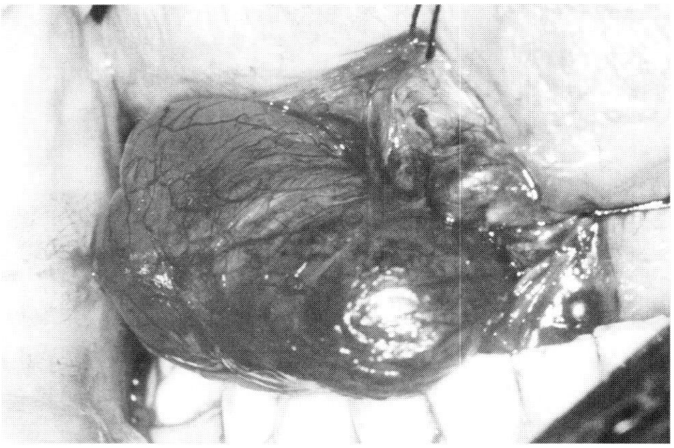

Fig. 13.29 Extravasation cyst in the floor of the mouth (ranula).

Other midline cysts

Sublingual dermoids are uncommon. They originate from embryonic branchial arches. They are thick walled, lined with squamous cell epithelium, and present as pink doughy swellings which may elevate the tongue. They may extend almost to the hyoid bone before the patient presents (Fig. 13.30). Large cysts or those which are adherent because of infection are more easily approached from the neck.[75]

Thyroglossal cysts rarely present in the mouth and occur more frequently in the hyoid area.

Lipomas, neuromas and other benign tumours may also present as a mass in the floor of the mouth and need to be correctly diagnosed.

BENIGN TUMOURS OF THE ORAL CAVITY

Squamous cell papilloma

These small tumours arise from the epithelium and occur mainly on the palate, fauces and gingivae in children and young adults.

REFERENCES

70. Cohen L Oral Surg 1965; 19: 365
71. Harrison J D Oral Surg 1975; 39: 268
72. Leopard P J Br J Oral Surg 1972; 13: 128
73. Roediger W E W, Lloyd P, Lawson H H Br J Surg 1973; 60: 720
74. Parekh D, Stewart M, Joseph C, Lawson H H Brit J Surg 1987; 74: 307
75. Seward G R Br J Oral Surg 1965; 3: 36

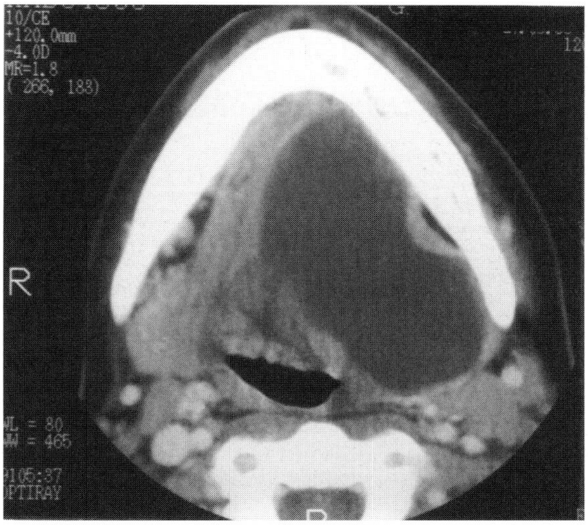

Fig. 13.30 CT scan demonstrating a large sublingual dermoid cyst.

They are of viral origin and their surface is covered in white finger-like processes or has a pink cauliflower-like appearance if the keratin is lost. They have no apparent malignant potential. Most are excised.

Lipomas

Intraoral lipomas are rare but may occur in the floor of the mouth or in the cheeks as slow-growing, soft lobulated fatty swellings.[76]

Haemangioma and lymphangioma

More than half of these angiomas occur in the head and neck and can present problems with respect to airway management, disturbed growth and haemorrhage.

Granular cell myoblastoma

This uncommon benign tumour usually occurs in the tongue and affects adults in middle age. The tumour presents as a small rounded swelling in or beneath the mucosa.[77] If the lesion is adequately excised, it does not recur.

Neural tumours

These are occasionally seen in the oral cavity as small painless nodules although a central neurilemmoma or schwannoma can develop in the mandible in the inferior dental nerve. Von Recklinghausen's neurofibromatosis (see Chapter 44) can involve the face and mouth, often extensively. The plexiform variety of neurofibroma infiltrates the facial tissues producing pendulous masses; it can involve the underlying bone, causing deformity and interfering with tooth eruption.[78] Surgery is undertaken for cosmetic and functional reasons (see Chapter 44).

MALIGNANT AND PREMALIGNANT TUMOURS OF THE ORAL CAVITY

Squamous cell carcinoma is the principal cancer of the upper alimentary tract. Much like its counterpart in the lung it is an aggressive tumour, and the untreated patient has a life expectancy of approximately 18 months from the time of diagnosis. Disease of the upper alimentary tract has an incidence of $12–15 \times 10^5$ per annum in the UK population but poses a much larger health problem in developing countries where it represents the third most common cancer.[79] In specialist centres 70–80% of patients with stage I or II tumours and half of those with stage III disease can be cured. In contrast only 25–30% with stage IV disease are curable.[80] This is a far cry from the situation at the beginning of this century when the condition was considered all but incurable.

One potential advantage of having a disease occur in the oral cavity is that the site is sensate as well as easy to examine. Thus, it might be assumed that early diagnosis of premalignant conditions should be the norm. However, half of the patients with oral cancer present with stage III or IV disease. Screening programmes are not considered to be cost-effective.

Premalignant conditions

Leucoplakia is a diagnosis established by exclusion of other known causes of oral white patches. Only a small proportion (2–4%) of leucoplakias progress to malignancy[81] and do so through a procession of identifiable stages, much like dysplasia of the cervix. Some areas become red and speckled—erythroplakias; half of these progress to cancer. Patches on the lateral border of the tongue or floor of the mouth also have a risk of malignant change. Factors which affect the risk of malignant change include increasing age, duration of the lesion, site, smoking/drinking habits and the degree of dysplasia.

Submucous fibrosis is peculiar to people of Asian descent[82] and is related to pan and betel nut chewing. The ingredients of pan (betel nut, slake lime and tobacco) cause a dense submucous fibrosis which caries a small risk of neoplastic change (4% over 15 years).

Lichen planus. This is an autoimmune disorder and presents usually as thin white striae within the buccal mucosa. At the extreme end of the disease spectrum is an atrophic and erosive

REFERENCES

76. Greer R O, Goldman H M Oral Surg 1974; 38: 43
77. Cawson R A, Eveson J W Oral Pathology and Diagnosis. Heinemann, London 1987 p 10.18
78. O'Driscoll P M Br J Oral Surg 1965; 3: 22
79. Johnson N W In: Johnson N W (ed) Risk Markers for Oral Diseases, vol 2, Oral Cancer. Cambridge University Press, Cambridge 1991 p 3
80. Franceshi D, Gupta R, Spiro R H, Shah J P Improved survival in the treatment of squamous carcinoma of the oral tongue. Am J Surg 1993; 166(4): 360–365
81. Harris M In: Johnson N W (ed) Risk Markers for Oral Diseases, vol 2 Oral Cancer. Cambridge University Press, Cambridge 1991 p 157
82. McGurk M, Craig G T Br J Oral Maxillofac Surg 1984; 22: 56

form of lichen planus and a small percentage of these can convert to squamous cell carcinoma (0.3%).

Sideropenic dysphagia. There is a significant association between cancer of the mouth and cervical oesophagus and sideropenic dysphagia (Paterson–Kelly syndrome).[83]

Aetiological factors in oral malignancy

A range of factors including syphilis, candidal infection, papilloma virus and repeated trauma are reported to induce oral cancer but definitive evidence is lacking. Epstein–Barr virus has an association with nasopharyngeal carcinoma[84] and women with iron deficiency anaemia and oesophageal stricture are at risk of hypopharyngeal cancer in Plummer–Vinson syndrome (see Chapter 20). The immune suppression that accompanies organ transplants is associated with skin rather than mucosal squamous cell carcinoma; similarly AIDS has not been associated with oral squamous cell cancer. Excessive exposure to sunlight is associated with lip cancer.[85]

The two overriding aetiological factors are excessive smoking and alcohol consumption. The effects are synergistic and the odds ratio over normal is as high as 15 for combined consumption and only 3–5 for single agent use.[86]

There is a hope that retinoids may help to stabilize the epithelium and protect against second cancers but the evidence of their efficacy is as yet unsubstantiated and a European study involving 3000 patients is waiting to report.

Clinical presentation

A delay of more than 3 months from the onset of symptoms to diagnosis occurs in about a third of cases. The patient is responsible for the delay in the majority of cases but the remainder relate to medical personnel (approx 20%).[87]

The median age at presentation is 61 years and men are more commonly affected than women. Tumours usually arise in the salivary gutters of the mouth (Fig. 13.31) and the four most common symptoms are ulcer, swelling, neck lump and pain. A history of pain radiating to the ear is an ominous symptom and demands careful evaluation.

Tumours normally metastasize to cervical lymph nodes, with systemic dissemination occurring in only 10% of cases if the primary cancer can be controlled. A palpable lymph node is present at presentation in 20% of cases and in a further 10% it is the only sign at diagnosis.[88] The latter mode of presentation can lead to mismanagement as open biopsy of the node may reduce survival by 30% by ensuring local dissipation of the tumour. The first step should be a careful evaluation of the upper alimentary tract, nasal passages and larynx which will normally reveal the primary tumour (see Chapter 20) but if this is unsuccessful a fine-needle aspiration biopsy (FNAC) of the neck lump is a preferred alternative procedure to open biopsy.

Approximately 5% of patients have a second synchronous tumour at presentation and a further 10% will develop a metachronous tumour within 6 months.[89] It is estimated that in the group of patients cured of their disease there is a 2% accumulative risk of developing a second primary cancer per year of life.

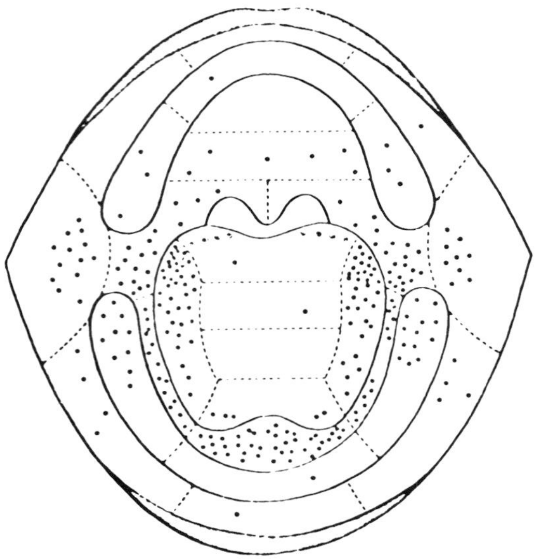

Fig. 13.31 Typical distribution of squamous cell carcinoma in the oral cavity.

Treatment

The criteria for staging have been formulated, amongst others, by the American Joint Committee on Cancer. T staging is governed both by size and involvement of local structures, therefore the criteria vary through the upper aerodigestive tract.[90] A simplified description is shown in Table 13.4.

In the past there has been a debate whether radiation or surgery is the more effective in treatment; this has now been resolved.[91] Unequivocal indications for surgery are failed radiotherapy, bone invasion and cervical metastasis. Small stage 1 and 2 tumours can be equally well treated by radiotherapy or surgery and the choice depends on the preference of the clinician. Small tumours in the anterior two thirds of the tongue can be treated by local implantation of radioactive needles (caesium wire[192] 5–7 days) under general anaesthesia[92] or can equally well be excised as the morbidity is low compared to a course of external beam radiotherapy. Large tumours, stage 3 and 4, or those with cervical metastasis respond best to surgery followed by adjuvant radiotherapy. The role of

REFERENCES

83. Larsson L G, Sandstrom A, Westling P Cancer Res 1975; 35: 3308
84. Yip T T C, Ngan R K C et al Cancer 1994, 74: 2414
85. Jorgensen K, Elbrand O, Anderson A P Acta Radiol Oncol Rad Phys Biol 1973; 12: 177
86. Binnie W H In: Johnson N W (ed) Risk Markers for Oral Diseases Vol 2, Oral Cancer. Cambridge University Press, Cambridge 1991 p 64
87. Kowalski L P, Franco E L et al Oral Oncol Eur J Cancer 1994; 30B: 267
88. Lefebvre J L, Coche-Dequeant B et al Am J Surg 1990; 160: 443
89. Pamosetti E, Luboinski B, Mamelle G, Richard J M Laryngoscope 1989; 99: 1267
90. American Joint Committee on Cancer Handbook for Staging of Cancer, 4th edn. J B Lippincott Company, Philadelphia 1992 p 27
91. Wennerberg J Acta Otolaryngol (Stoach) 1995; 115: 465
92. Fletcher G. Textbook of Radiotherapy, 2nd edn. Lea & Febiger, Philadelphia 1973 p 214

Table 13.4 Simplified staging criteria

Stage I:	T_1, N_0, M_0
Stage II:	T_2, N_0, M_0
Stage III:	T_3, N_0, M_0
	T_{1-3}, N_1, M_0
Stage IV:	T_4, N_0, M_0
	T_{1-4}, N_{1-3}, M_{0-1}

1. T_1 = 0–2 cm, T_2 = 2–4 cm, T_3 = 4–6 cm, T_4 > 6 cm)
   T staging is not strictly based on size but also takes account of invasion of anatomical structures and varies with position in the aerodigestive tract
2. N_0 No cervical node involvement
   N_1 Single ipsilateral node < 3 cm
   N_2 a. Single ipsilateral node > 3 and < 6 cm
   b. Multiple ipsilateral nodes < 6 cm
   c. Bilateral contralateral nodes < 6 cm
   N_3 node > 6 cm
3. M_0 No distant metastasis
   M_1 Distant metastasis

chemotherapy is limited with an estimated maximum improvement in survival of 0–6%.[93]

The single most important prognostic indicator of survival is cervical node metastasis, which halves survival.[94] The prognosis is also reduced if the capsule of the tumour has been breached, the chance of which increases with increasing size of the tumour and the number of metastatic lymph nodes. Adjuvant radiotherapy is advocated if more than two metastatic nodes are present in a specimen. The rationale for avoiding open node biopsy without continuing to perform a neck dissection is obvious.

Squamous cell carcinomas of the oral cavity, including the tongue, cheek and floor of mouth, are treated the same way irrespective of where they arise and it is artificial to consider them separately. The tumour is resected with at least 1 cm and preferably a 2 cm margin of normal tissue. Small tumours (<4 cm) can normally be resected through an oral approach but a careful preoperative evaluation is advised as these tumours are frequently larger than is at first appreciated. Repair is usually achieved by local flaps or direct closure when possible.

The key to the successful treatment of larger tumours is adequate access; if the neck has to be entered to gain access to the primary lesion a lymph node dissection should be carried out. Local infiltration of the mandible can be dealt with by marginal resection. If a hemimandibulectomy is required, the deformity that results is generally minor and it may be possible to repair the area with soft tissue rather than bone. Anterior mandibular defects are a different proposition but reconstruction is much improved now that microvascular osseocutaneous grafts are available.

Treatment of the neck

There are preferential routes of lymphatic drainage in the neck; oral tumours tend to metastasize to the upper cervical lymph nodes whereas tumours of the larynx and hypopharynx tend to involve the lower nodes.[95] This has led to the adoption of an array of neck procedures which entail less morbidity than the traditional radical neck dissection[96] but which are technically more demanding to perform. A modified radical dissection appears to be safe as long as there is limited nodal disease. Patients with large primary lesions and those with multiple cervical metastasis in lower lymph nodes should have the traditional radical procedure. With a combination of surgery and adjuvant radiotherapy, the control of neck metastasis is no longer a major problem as recurrence is only seen in 9–11% if the primary tumour has been eradicated.[97] Carcinoma of the tongue and oropharynx is also discussed in Chapters 13 and 20.

Minor salivary gland tumours of the oral cavity

Although the management of these tumours is similar to that of major salivary gland tumours, there are subtle differences.

General characteristics

Benign and malignant tumours arise from the submandibular and minor salivary glands with about the same frequency and together represent approximately 30% of salivary neoplasms. The rest originate in the parotid (see Chapter 14). It should be appreciated that because salivary gland cancers are often slow growing about 60% will present as an apparently benign lump.[98] The risk of encountering a malignant salivary gland tumour changes with the site of origin (Table 13.5), increasing from parotid to submandibular and being greatest in the minor salivary glands.

The histological classification of salivary gland cancers is unwieldy (see Chapter 14) and adds little to the surgical management which is simply governed by tumour stage (notably size of the lump) and clinical grade of tumour. Salivary gland cancers can be broadly divided into three prognostic groups. The histological subtypes that have a large proportion of high-grade lesions are malignant pleomorphic carcinoma, squamous cell carcinoma and anaplastic carcinoma. Low-grade tumours are mucoepidermoid carcinoma (although 20% of these are high grade) and acinic cell carcinoma. An intermediate group consists of adenoid cystic carcinoma and adenocarcinoma. The relative incidence of the different histological types is similar in the mouth and parotid but the submandibular gland has a higher proportion of adenoid cystic carcinomas (Table 13.6).[99] This fact has been used erroneously to explain the poor prognosis of tumours at the latter site. Wide local

Table 13.5 The proportion of benign and malignant salivary gland neoplasms by site

Parotid	*Submandibular*	*Minor salivary glands*
20% malignant	50% malignant	60% malignant
80% benign	50% benign	40% benign

REFERENCES

93. Munro A J Brit J Cancer 1995; 71: 83
94. Gamel J W, Jones A S Br J Cancer 1993; 67: 1071
95. Shah J P, Andersen P E Br J Oral Maxillofac Surg 1995; 33: 3
96. Shah J P Am J Surg 1990; 160: 405
97. Leemans C R, Tiwari R et al Laryngoscope 1990; 100 (11): 1194
98. Renehan A, Gleave E N et al Br J Surg 1996; 83: 1750

Table 13.6 Relative proportion of the 7 main histological cancers by site in a review of 670 minor, 585 submandibular and 2150 parotid cancers[99]

Tumour site	*Mucoepidermoid carcinoma*	*Adenoid cystic carcinoma*	*Adenocarcinoma*	*Malignant pleomorphic carcinoma*	*Acinic cell carcinoma*	*Squamous cell carcinoma*	*Anaplastic*
Minor salivary glands	41%	27%	19%	5%	3%	3%	2%
Parotid	31%	13%	14%	13%	12%	6%	10%
Submandibular gland	22%	41%	9%	12%	2%	7%	7%

Table 13.7 Distribution of benign and malignant minor salivary gland tumours by site in a review of 3079 reported cases[99]

Tumour	*Palate*	*Floor of mouth*	*Retromolar*	*Lip*	*Tongue*	*Cheek*
Benign	50%	12%	9%	54%	9%	41%
Malignant	50%	88%	91%	46%	91%	59%

excision of the submandibular triangle with some form of selective neck dissection ensures survival rates comparable to those achieved in the parotid and mouth.[100]

Clinical presentations

The majority of oral salivary gland neoplasms present as a smooth lobulated mass that may have a blue appearance. Benign tumours present at a median age of 48 years, about a decade earlier than malignant tumours. A delay in presentation of 2–3 years is a feature of these slow-growing tumours. Malignancy is suspected when an indurated lump is fixed to the overlying mucosa (Table 13.7).

Perineurial invasion is a feature of adenoid cystic carcinoma, as is pain, although this symptom is still uncommon (10–20% of cases) as is cervical lymph node metastasis.[99] The difference in management between major and minor salivary gland neoplasms is that, because the latter are superficial, they are amenable to open biopsy and the site can easily be included in the subsequent excision. The definitive diagnosis can therefore be established prior to surgery in the majority of instances. Where this is not possible fine-needle aspiration cytology will identify, in experienced hands, over 90% of malignant tumours.[101] Surgery is the treatment of choice for both benign and malignant salivary neoplasms.

Pleomorphic adenoma

Pleomorphic adenomas can be removed with a thin margin of normal tissue without fear.[102] As most will be at the junction of the hard and soft palate, the subperiosteal plane (the surgeon's friend) should be used for dissection whenever possible.

Carcinoma

Norman made the point that minor salivary gland cancers are minor in name only.[103] Small malignant lesions (T_1) can be treated adequately by wide local excision but with increasing size the management is similar to that for squamous cell carcinoma at this site, namely an in-continuity local and selective neck resection.

Several studies have demonstrated that both local control and improved survival are achieved with adjuvant radiotherapy and its application is advocated particularly in large or high-grade cancers. The prognosis for minor salivary gland cancers in the oral cavity is similar to that expected for major salivary gland cancer—75%, 62% and 56% at 5, 10 and 15 years respectively.[104]

Mucosal malignant melanoma

This tumour is uncommon in the face and oral cavity and represents only 1–2% of all malignant melanomas, consequently few institutions have a large experience in its treatment. Slightly more than half occur in the nose and paranasal sinuses, the remainder arise in the mouth and oropharynx. The mean age of presentation is in the fifth decade and most have an insidious onset. Symptoms involve nasal obstruction, discharge and bleeding if the primary tumour is in the nose or a mass if it is in the oral cavity. Delay in presentation is usual but the disease is often confined to the primary site. Cervical lymph node metastasis is uncommon at presentation.

Local resection has been the traditional approach to treatment, but it is difficult to ensure that the surgical margins are adequate because of diffuse submucosal lymphatic permeation. Local control is associated with prolonged survival if the focus of the disease is small and resectable.

The prognosis for this rare condition is, however, poor. The 5-year survival is 10–40%.[105] Local recurrence and distant metastasis is common. The use of super-radical surgery for a disease which in many cases is already incurable should therefore be tempered. Local disease may progress quite slowly in some patients and is held in check by simple debulking procedures. This cancer may also occasionally be responsive to radiation therapy[106] but immuno- and chemotherapy have no established place in its management.

REFERENCES

99. McGurk M, Williams R G, Calman F M B In: de Burgh Norman J E, McGurk M (eds) Color Atlas and Text of the Salivary Glands. Diseases, Disorders and Surgery. Mosby-Wolfe London 1995 p 181
100. Spiro R H, Armstrong J et al Arch Otolaryngol Head Neck Surg 1989; 115: 316
101. McGurk M, Hussain K. Role of fine needle aspiration cytology in the treatment of the discrete parotid lump. Ann R Coll Surg Engl 1997; 79: 198–202
102. McGurk M, Renehan A, Gleave E N, Hancock B D Brit J Surg 1996; 83: 1747
103. de Burgh Norman J E In: de Burgh Norman J E, McGurk M (eds) Colour Atlas and Textbook of the Salivary Glands. Diseases, Disorders and Surgery. Mosby-Wolfe London 1995 p 197
104. Spiro R H, Thater H T et al Am J Surg 1991; 162: 330
105. Stern S J, Guillamondegui O M Head Neck 1991; 13: 22

Sarcoma

Sarcoma of the head and neck is another relatively uncommon condition, constituting about 15% of all sarcomas but fewer than 1% of malignant tumours in the head and neck. Sarcomas are biologically diverse and the response to treatment can be affected by site, grade or age of the host, for example adult or child. The majority of tumours occur in adults, with a median age at presentation of 45 years, and most arise in soft tissue (80%) rather than bone (20%). The common presenting symptoms include a mass, pain, and skin involvement.

The natural history of this group of rare tumours is further confused by the fact that a wide range of histological types exist depending on the mesodermal site of origin. Prognosis is related principally to the grade and tumour size; histological type is of less influence except in the sense that some, such as rhabdomyosarcoma, have a greater proportion of high-grade tumours. The prognosis for patients with high-grade lesions is less than 40% at 5 and 10 years compared to approximately 80% for low-grade sarcomas.[107] The pattern of failure is usually local recurrence, normally within 2 years, with or without distant metastasis. Distant metastasis is a feature of high-grade tumours.

Wide surgical excision remains the mainstay of treatment. Dissemination is mainly by the haematogenous route so prophylactic neck dissections, except for access purposes, are not advocated. Multivariate analysis of prognostic factors has shown that local recurrence is largely a function of the adequacy of excision.[107] Microscopic extension of the tumour makes this difficult to achieve in half the cases but adjuvant radiotherapy has proved effective in reducing local recurrence.[108]

Lymphoreticular neoplasms

This group of tumours more commonly presents in the head and neck region as a cervical lymphadenopathy (see Chapter 17). Multiple myelomatosis may affect the jaws: deposits cause pain and swelling and even pathological fracture. The osteolytic lesions, which are also common in the skull bones, need to be distinguished from other causes of radiolucency. A raised sedimentation rate and Bence Jones proteinuria is often seen.

Burkitt's tumour

This is a tumour of lymphoid tissue occurring in children in tropical Africa and Brazil.[109] It is thought to be associated with the Epstein–Barr virus.[110] The jaws are initially affected with rapidly enlarging swellings destroying bone, often at several sites (Fig. 13.32). Deposits later appear in all the abdominal organs. Treatment is by cytotoxic drug regimens which may provide rapid remission but the overall mortality is high. Remission for more than 2 years is associated with a survival rate of 50%.[111]

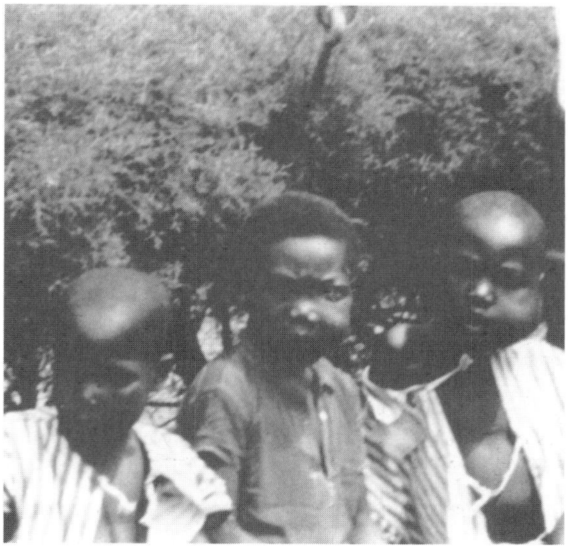

Fig. 13.32 Burkitt's lymphoma.

Lymphoma

Non-Hodgkin's lymphomas (see Chapter 34) can present in the oral cavity as isolated extralymphatic deposits but more commonly present as cervical lymphadenopathy or enlargement of Waldeyer's ring. Patients with Sjögren's syndrome can develop mucosa-associated lymphoid tissue (MALT) lymphomas which normally present as a discrete parotid mass.[112] The diagnosis of a 'benign lymph epithelial tumour' should be questioned: with time they invariably prove to be lymphomas.

Leukaemia

Oral manifestations of acute leukaemia are seen in half the patients with this disease and may be the primary lesion. Mucosal pallor, gingival bleeding or purpura are the first signs, followed by gingival swelling which may progress to ulceration. Necrotic ulcers and osteolytic lesions may also develop.[113]

Secondary neoplasms

Metastases occasionally occur in the mouth from primary tumours elsewhere in the body. Spread is via the bloodstream from sites such as the bronchus, breast, kidney, prostate and thyroid. The deposits develop as rapidly proliferating masses within the gingival tissues or they may present as osteolytic lesions in the jaws. Pain, anaesthesia or even pathological fracture can occur. The underlying disease should be treated if possible and the local lesion can be excised or irradiated.[94]

REFERENCES

106. Sause W T, Cooper J S et al Int J Rad Oncol Biol Phys 1991; 20: 429
107. Mandard A M, Petiot J F Cancer 1989; 63: 1437
108. Elias A D, Antman K H Sem Oncol 1989; 16: 305
109. Burkitt D J Dent Res 1966; 45: 554
110. Klein G N Engl J Med 1975; 293: 1353
111. Ziegler J L, MacGrath I T, Olweny C L M Lancet 1979; ii: 936
112. Isaacson P G In: de Burgh Norman J E, McGurk M (eds) Color Atlas and Text of the Salivary Glands. Diseases, Disorders and Surgery. Mosby-Wolfe London 1995 p 289
113. Pollock A Br Dent J 1977; 142: 369

THE TONGUE

Congenital abnormalities

Bifid tongue

This may occur as an isolated phenomenon or can be associated with chromosomal syndromes. It sometimes occurs in the Pierre Robin syndrome, may be associated with a medial cleft of the lower lip, and is a constant feature in the orofacial–digital syndrome.[114]

Fissured tongue

In this condition the dorsum of the tongue is crossed by irregular 3–4 mm deep fissures running longitudinally or diagonally. The mucosa is covered in normal papillae and the only significance of the condition is that some patients may complain of soreness from inflammation at the base of the fissures. Antifungal agents may then be beneficial.

Tongue tie (ankyloglossia)

This condition is the result of varying degrees of shortness of the lingual fraenum, which in the most extreme case attaches the tip of the tongue to the mucosa behind the lower incisor teeth. Children with tongue tie cannot protrude the tongue but treatment is only indicated if the tongue's contribution to controlling food and oral hygiene is compromised. Ankyloglossia rarely, if ever, affects speech.

Fraenectomy is carried out by excising the fraenum from its attachments, allowing the tip of the tongue to be pulled away from the floor of the mouth.[115] The resulting defect, which runs from behind the incisors between the submandibular duct orifices and along the ventral surface of the tongue, should be carefully sutured to prevent scarring.

Geographical tongue (erythema migrans linguae)

This common condition is characterized by smooth red patches which appear to migrate across the dorsum of the tongue like fairy rings. The scalloped edge is well defined by mild hyperkeratinization of the unaffected mucosa.[116] Histologically, there is thinning of the epithelium for which there is no explanation. The patient should be reassured that the appearance is of no significance and can be ignored.

Median rhomboid glossitis

This reddish diamond-shaped patch arises in the midline of the dorsum of the tongue anterior to the circumvallate papillae. It is only seen in adults and its cause is unknown though it was once thought to be the result of persistence of the tuberculum impar. Histologically, there is depapillation with acanthosis, irregular hyperplasia and chronic inflammatory infiltration. It is not premalignant. There are no symptoms and the patient should be reassured.[117]

Black hairy tongue

This is the result of overgrowth of the filiform papillae which form a thick, brownish-black hairy mat on the dorsum of the tongue.[118] The discoloration is from pigment-producing organisms or fungi. The cause is unknown although heavy smoking, sucking antiseptics and antibiotics have been blamed. The patient should be reassured that the condition is not dangerous and advised to scrape or brush the tongue to remove the overgrowth.

Glossitis

This is a term used to describe a red, smooth (depapillated) and sore tongue. It occurs in iron deficiency and pernicious anaemia and other vitamin B group deficiencies which are now rarely seen. It may also be caused by candida infection.[119]

Sore tongue

There are usually no abnormal appearances; once haematological abnormalities have been excluded, the cause is usually ascribed to psychogenic disorders.[120] In reality it is probably a degenerative disorder as it occurs principally in postmenopausal females and hormonal changes are known to induce mucosal atrophy.

Macroglossia

Enlargement of the tongue occurs in acromegaly and sometimes in multiple neurofibromatosis. The tongue may also be enlarged when it contains a vascular malformation such as a haemangioma, lymphangioma or more often a mixture of the two. The growth of these haematomas can have a secondary effect on the size of the mandible.[121] The tongue may also contain an angioma in patients with the Sturge–Weber syndrome.

Macroglossia can develop in a quarter or more of patients with primary amyloidosis.[122] Macroglossia also occurs in the mucolipidoses, especially Hurler's syndrome, in the mucopolysaccharidoses and in other genetic syndromes.[123] Hemihypertrophy of the face is associated with diffuse or unilateral macroglossia which may be associated with hypertrophy of the fungiform papillae. Macroglossia is a major component of the Beckwith–Wiedeman

REFERENCES

114. Gorlin R J, Pindborg J J, Cohen M M Syndromes of the Head and Neck, 2nd edn. McGraw Hill, New York 1976 pp 32, 91
115. Killey H C, Seward G R, Kay L W An Outline of Oral Surgery, Part 1. John Wright, Bristol 1975 p 65
116. Hume W J J Dent 1975; 3: 25
117. Baughman R A Oral Surg 1971; 31: 56
118. Neville B W, Damm D D, Allen C M, Bouquot J E In: Neville B W, Damm D D, Allen C M, Bouquot J E (eds) Oral and Maxillofacial Pathology. W B Saunders, Philadelphia 1995 p 12
119. Jensen H, Kjerulf K, Hjorting-Hansen E Acta Med Scand 1965; 178: 651
120. Lamey P-J, Lamb A B Br Med J 1988; 296: 1243
121. Gupta O P Arch Otolaryngol 1971; 93: 378
122. Keith D A Br J Oral Surg 1972; 10: 107
123. Neville B W, Damm D D, Allen C M, Bouquot J E In: Neville B W, Damm D D, Allen C M, Bouquot J E (eds) Oral and Maxillofacial Pathology. W B Saunders, Philadelphia 1995 p 8

syndrome.[124] The apparent enlargement of the tongue in the Pierre Robin syndrome and some muscle dystrophies is caused by glossoptosis.

The enlarged tongue may have its size reduced by wedge resection of the anterior two thirds to treat some of these conditions.[125]

INFECTION OF THE JAWS

The most common dental infection is dental caries and it may go on to produce dentoalveolar and soft tissue infection.

Acute osteomyelitis

This condition is still encountered but, in view of the large number of dental infections that arise from within the medullary bone, it has a surprisingly low incidence. The virulence of the organism and reduced host response from immunosuppression play a part in its development. It causes intense pain, fever and, if the mandible is involved, paraesthesia of the inferior dental nerve. After 5–10 days pus starts to discharge and the teeth loosen. Treatment is by a combination of antibiotic therapy and debridement as required.[126] Early disease may be aborted by intravenous penicillin or clindamycin until the systemic symptoms improve, when oral medication can commence. It is important to culture the organism whenever possible and determine antibacterial sensitivities as a number of patients will progress to a subacute or chronic form. Sequestration, decortication or even resection may be required to eradicate the infection if fistulae develop or the purulent discharge persists.

Infantile osteomyelitis is an uncommon but serious condition which carried a significant mortality before the introduction of antibiotics. The infection is disseminated through the bloodstream and targets highly vascularized bone, for example the maxilla or temporomandibular joints. The destruction and scarring that result can have a deleterious effect on growth. The condition usually presents in the first few weeks of life with local periorbital cellulitis and systemic malaise, fever and pyrexia. The organism is usually a staphylococcus and intravenous penicillin is the treatment of choice together with simple drainage where necessary.

Chronic osteomyelitis

The mandible may respond to chronic irritation by forming focal condensations of sclerotic bone in young adults.[127] The source of the irritation is usually a chronically infected tooth. Garré's sclerosing osteomyelitis is similarly a proliferative response to irritation in the periosteum of the jaw that leads to thickening of the membrane and cortical proliferation of bone.[128] The condition is primarily seen in children and young adults and reflects the underlying growth and proliferative potential of the tissues at that age.

Perhaps the most common cause of chronic osteomyelitis is radical radiation to the jaws. The mandible with its envelope of dense cortical bone is the most commonly involved bone. The effect of the radiation is two fold, endarteritis reduces the blood supply and many of the osteoblasts cannot proliferate and take part in repair. Chronic osteomyelitis often begins after tooth extraction. The risk can be minimized by scrupulous attention to dental health both during and after radiotherapy; if extractions are necessary a limited number of teeth (2–3) should be removed at any one time as atraumatically as possible. Prophylactic antibiotics should be prescribed. The mandible has two sources of nourishment, a central artery that fails with increasing age and the enveloping periosteum which becomes more important with time. Periosteal stripping of the bone should be avoided wherever possible.

Initially the condition is painless with dark ebony-like bone exposed in the floor of the mouth. Later it becomes painful as secondary infection develops. Long courses of tetracycline may improve the symptoms but the mucosal defect seldom heals. Hyperbaric oxygen increases the perfusion of the mandible by stimulating new vessel formation and is useful in containing early or focal disease but once osteomyelitis is established it is ineffective. Minor surgical debridement with primary mucosal closure may be successful in localized disease and is worth trying. In the advanced case new vascularized tissue is required to facilitate healing. This may best be achieved by surgical excision and reconstruction with a vascularized bone graft.

CYSTS OF THE JAWS

Cysts are a frequent occurrence in the jaws because epithelial remnants persist in the bone after tooth formation—odontogenic cysts (Table 13.8). Other cysts develop from epithelial residues at the lines of fusion of embryonic processes, so-called 'fissural cysts'.

For an understanding of the origin of the odontogenic cysts and also the rarer odontogenic tumours of the jaws a brief description of tooth development is necessary.[129]

At about the sixth week of fetal life, a band of proliferating oral epithelium called the dental lamina protrudes into the underlying mesoderm along the tooth-bearing region of each jaw. Small clumps of mesenchymal cells form in regions which correspond to those of the subsequent tooth germs and become surrounded by stalks of proliferating epithelium, thus establishing the toothbuds. The cap of epithelium, now known as the enamel organ, remains joined to the oral epithelium by a chord of cells, but like the dental lamina between the toothbuds, this eventually breaks down and disappears. Residual epithelium may remain as cell rests (Fig. 13.33).

The enamel organ now undergoes differentiation: cells on the inner aspect become cuboidal, there are central star-shaped cells, and somewhat flatter cells form the outer enamel epithelium. The condensation of mesenchymal cells known as the dental papilla is continuous with a layer of connective tissue surrounding the

REFERENCES

124. Gorlin R J, Pindborg J J Syndromes of the Head and Neck. McGraw Hill, New York 1976 p 42
125. Hendrick J W, Antonio S Surgery 1956; 39: 674
126. Adekeye E O, Cornash J Br J Oral Maxillofac Surg 1985; 23: 24
127. Eversole L R, Stone C E, Strub D Oral Surg Oral Med Oral Path 1984; 58: 456
128. Felsberg G J, Gore R L, Schweitzer M E Oral Surg Oral Med Oral Path 1990; 70: 117
129. Osborn J W, Tencate A R Advanced Dental Histology, 3rd edn. John Wright, Bristol 1977

Table 13.8 Classification of cysts of the jaws

Odontogenic cysts		*Non-odontogenic cysts*	
Inflammatory	*Developmental*	*Epitheliated*	*Non-epitheliated*
Apical	Dentigerous	Globulomaxillary	Aneurysmal
Lateral peridontal	Primordial	Median palatine	Solitary bone
Residual	Keratocyst	Nasopalatine	Stafne's bone cavity
	Calcifying odontogenic		

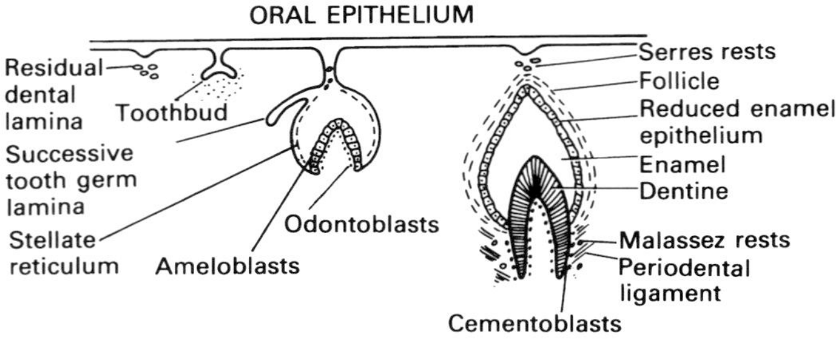

Fig. 13.33 A composite diagram illustrating the stage of tooth development and the origin of various cell remnants.

enamel organ called the dental follicle, and eventually this forms the periodontal membrane. The cells immediately adjacent to the enamel epithelium differentiate into a single layer of odontoblasts which form the dentine. Once this process begins, the cells of the enamel epithelium start laying down enamel and are then known as ameloblasts.

When the crown of the tooth has been formed, the rim of epithelium around its base proliferates downwards as the sheath of Hertwig, inducing cells to form the dentine of the root. The coronal part of the sheath breaks up and cementoblasts differentiate from the follicular tissue around the root and lay down cementum on the root surface, incorporating collagen fibres which make up the periodontal ligament. Residual epithelium remains in this membrane throughout life as the cell rests of Malassez.

Odontogenic cysts

Inflammatory cysts

Apical/residual cysts

Apical cysts occur most frequently (55%) and are the result of dental infection stimulating the epithelial remnants to coalesce. They are usually symptomless but may present with acute pain if they become secondarily infected.[130] Radiologically they appear as well defined unilocular radiolucencies (Fig. 13.34). Multilocular cysts or those that erode teeth suggest that a more aggressive pathological process is responsible. Small cysts (< 1 cm diameter) often resolve after root canal therapy or extraction of the tooth but occasionally may persist. Large cysts require enucleation and, if very large, may warrant marsupialization.

Lateral periodontal cyst

Lateral periodontal cysts are uncommon and have the same aetiology and pathogenesis as apical cysts. Their treatment is the same as apical cysts.

REFERENCE

130. Killey H C, Kay L W, Seward G R In: Killey H C, Kay L W, Seward G R (eds) Benign Cystic Lesions of the Jaws, their Diagnosis and Treatment. Churchill Livingstone, Edinburgh 1977 p 75

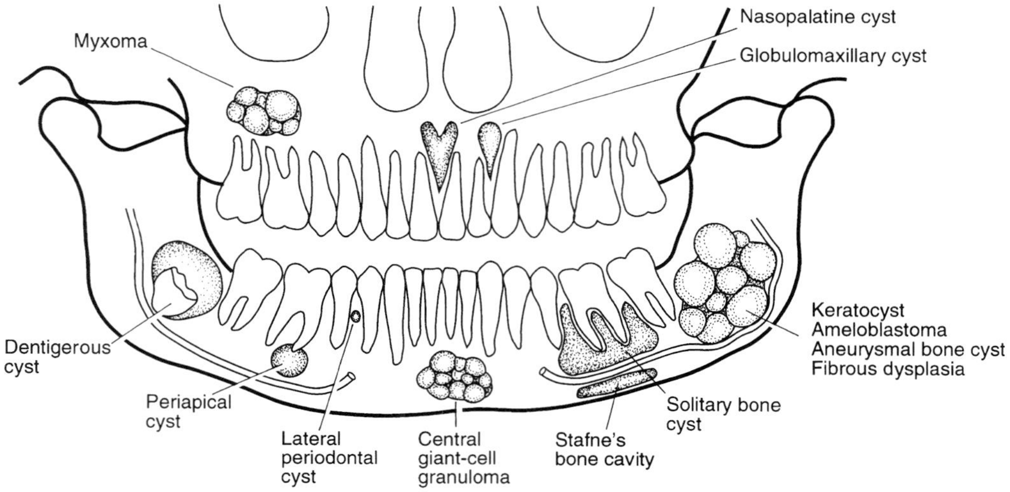

Fig. 13.34 Radiolucent lesions of the jaws and their sites of predilection.

Developmental cysts

Follicular or dentigerous cyst

Follicular or dentigerous cysts are relatively common and are the result of a cystic degeneration within the follicle around the crown of the tooth. They present as a slowly enlarging painless swelling and are seen as a unilocular radiolucency related to the crown of a tooth. They need to be differentiated from simple dilatation of a normal tooth follicle, which should not exceed 4 mm in width. They most commonly occur in the posterior part of the mandible.

Primordial keratocyst

Primordial keratocysts arise from degeneration of the dental stellate reticulum before the tooth forms and thus replace it. They are usually symptomless and present late as painless swellings of the jaw. The mandible is primarily involved either at its angle, the body or ramus. The cyst lining divides rapidly; this is presumably responsible for the large and multilocular nature of the cysts. They are capable of aggressive behaviour and must be correctly diagnosed preoperatively if recurrence is to be avoided. Diagnosis is possible because the aspirated cystic fluid is characterized by a soluble protein content of < 3.5 g/dl. Smaller unilocular cysts are treated by simple enucleation, but this technique is not effective for large multilocular lesions and a recurrence rate as high as 60% is reported.[131] Recurrence can be reduced by tanning with Carnoy's solution for 3 minutes immediately prior to removal.

Other odontogenic cysts

Calcifying epithelial odontogenic cysts are very rare. There are two types: one is a simple cyst, the other a neoplasm. They present as painless swelling of the anterior parts of the jaws and radiographs demonstrate calcification within the cyst. The simple cysts are treated by enucleation, the others usually by local marginal resection.

Epstein's pearls (Bohn's nodules)

These are gingival cysts, common in the newborn, which tend to rupture spontaneously or involute and are rarely seen after 3 months of age. They form small white nodules 2–3 mm in diameter and are found on the crest of the maxillary and mandibular ridges and in the midline of the palate.[132] They are thought to arise from epithelial remnants of the dental lamina which proliferate, keratinize and form small cysts. Those arising along the mid-palatal raphe develop from epithelial inclusions in the line of fusion of the palatal processes.[133] No treatment is required.

Non-odontogenic cysts (non-epithelial cysts)

The non-odontogenic cysts are classified according to the lining of the cyst wall. Fissural cysts are lined by epithelium, whereas aneurysmal and solitary bone cysts are only lined by connective tissue.

Aneurysmal bone cysts are rare. Their cause is unknown and they also affect the axial skeleton (usually the vertebrae and long bones of middle-aged adults). In the jaws the mandible is affected more frequently than the maxilla, and there is a predilection for the posterior regions of the jaws. Clinically they present as painful firm swellings with displacement of the associated teeth. Despite their name they are not pulsatile nor are they associated with a bruit. They may present radiologically as unilocular or multilocular radiolucencies (Fig. 13.34). They are treated by curettage and have a recurrence rate of about 25%.

Solitary bone cysts are idiopathic and tend to occur in a younger age group (10–20 years) than aneurysmal bone cysts. They are usually diagnosed as an incidental radiographic finding, but can present with swelling and pain. They have a similar distribution in the jaws to aneurysmal bone cysts and radiographically appear as scalloped radiolucencies above the level of the inferior dental canal (Fig. 13.34). They contain straw-coloured liquid and are treated by curettage.

Stafne's bone cavities are not cysts of the jaws but simply depressions on the lingual aspect of the mandible produced by the submandibular salivary gland. Radiographic images depict the depression as a well-circumscribed unilocular radiolucency below the level of the inferior dental canal (Fig. 13.34).

Non-odontogenic (epithelial fistula) cysts

All four fissural cysts occur infrequently and can be surgically enucleated.

Nasopalatine cysts are the most common type of fissural cyst, occurring in about 1% of the population. They develop from epithelium trapped between the median nasal and palatal processes and are located between or above the roots of the maxillary central incisor teeth (Fig. 13.34).

Globulomaxillary cysts develop from epithelium trapped between the median nasal and maxillary processes and therefore present as discrete radiolucencies between the maxillary lateral incisor and canine teeth (Fig. 13.34). They are usually an incidental radiographic finding but when infected are acutely painful.

Median palatal cysts develop from epithelium trapped between the palatal processes and usually present as non-painful swellings in the affected area.

Median mandibular cysts develop from epithelium entrapment between the mandibular processes.

OSTEODYSTROPHIES

The diseases of bone included under this heading are neither inflammatory nor neoplastic but are genetic, metabolic or of unknown cause.

REFERENCES

131. Killey H C, Kay L W, Seward G R In: Killey H C, Kay L W, Seward G R (eds) Benign Cystic Lesions of the Jaws, their Diagnosis and Treatment. Churchill Livingstone, Edinburgh 1977 p 62
132. Fromm A J Dent Child 1967; 34: 275
133. Shear M. Cysts of the Oral Regions, 2nd edn. John Wright, Bristol 1983 p 35

Genetic bone diseases

Osteogenesis imperfecta

This is a hereditary disorder in which the bones are poorly formed and fragile. The underlying defect is one of collagen synthesis—although cartilaginous growth is normal, cortical plates of compact bone are not formed.[134]

Cleidocranial dysostosis

This is a rare familial disorder in which anodontia and delayed eruption of teeth are accompanied by defective formation of the clavicles, delayed closure of fontanelles and maxillary hypoplasia.[135]

Metabolic bone diseases

Rickets

Disorders of calcium and phosphorus metabolism caused by deficiency of vitamin D, in rickets or chronic renal disease, result in defects in the development of bone but rarely of the teeth. Eruption of the teeth may be delayed and hypocalcification of dentine only occurs in severe cases.[136] A diagnosis is made on clinical and radiological examination and is confirmed by finding low serum levels of calcium and phosphorus with a raised alkaline phosphatase.

Hyperparathyroidism

The jaws are commonly affected by the giant cell 'tumours' (brown tumours) which occur in hyperparathyroidism.[137] This condition should always be considered, in the older female patient, when giant cell granuloma of the jaw is diagnosed histologically or if there is a recurrence after adequate excision. Granulomas can develop in either jaw causing radiolucent cyst-like swellings of the bone and loosening of the teeth. Successful treatment of the hyperparathyroidism causes the osteolytic lesions to regress.

Central giant cell granuloma

These are idiopathic lesions of the jaw bones which occur most commonly in young adults and females. They present clinically with swelling and tooth displacement. The anterior parts of the jaws and particularly the mandible are the most commonly affected sites. Radiologically these lesions have a unilocular appearance. The diagnosis is established by means of an incisional biopsy. A small proportion of these granulomas are also associated with secondary hyperparathyroidism, when they are known as 'brown tumours' or 'von Recklinghausen's disease of bone'. Thus patients with these 'tumours' should be investigated for the presence of hyperparathyroidism.

The treatment usually consists of enucleation, although a favourable response to calcitonin has also been described.[138] Those cases caused by hyperparathyroidism respond to treatment of the underlying condition.

Histologically the granulomas consist of focal collections of giant cells and they need to be distinguished from other intraosseous giant cell lesions such as osteoclastomas and aneurysmal bone cysts. They are now considered to be an exuberant proliferative process and not a neoplasm.

Scurvy

Deficiency of vitamin C (ascorbic acid) is normally the result of gross dietary deprivation. It may occur subclinically in elderly people whose diets do not include fresh fruit.[139] Various metabolic systems are affected causing defective formation of collagen and osteoid tissue.

Swollen oedematous and bleeding gums occur in patients with poor oral hygiene. There is a haemorrhagic tendency from increased capillary fragility. The Hess capillary fragility test produces capillary rupture, and areas of ecchymosis are common both intraorally and on the skin. Patients with these symptoms may have leukaemia.

Bone disease of unknown cause

Paget's disease (osteitis deformans) (see Chapter 42)

The aetiology of this condition is unknown. It affects patients past middle age and occurs in 3% of patients over 40 years. The incidence rises with age to 70% in men and 30% in women in their seventh decade.[140] The bones most frequently involved are the pelvis, femora, vertebrae and skull, when the jaws may also be affected.

There is a rapid, irregular and exaggerated resorption and replacement of bone, causing thickening, swelling and increased vascularity, often with severe intractable pain. Serum calcium and phosphorus levels are normal but the alkaline phosphatase level is raised.

When the skull is affected it slowly enlarges, as do the jaws—the maxilla more frequently than the mandible, necessitating frequent adjustments to dentures.[141] The teeth may become displaced and are affected by hypercementosis which fuses them to the bone, complicating extractions. In the osteolytic phase of the disease oral surgery can be complicated by severe haemorrhage and in sclerotic disease surgery may be followed by chronic osteomyelitis.

The main radiological changes are irregular patches of sclerosis and radiolucency (cotton-wool appearance), enlargement of the bone and hypercementosis of the roots of the teeth.[142] When the jaws alone are affected, general treatment to suppress bone metabolism is not required.

REFERENCES

134. Lewis N A et al Oral Surg 1958; 11: 289
135. Gorlin R J, Pindborg J J Syndromes of the Head and Neck. McGraw-Hill, New York 1976
136. Cawson R A Brit Dent J 1964; 117: 141
137. Silverman S Jr, Ware W H, Gillooly C Jr Oral Surg 1968; 26: 184
138. Harris M Br J Oral Maxillofac Surg 1993; 31: 89
139. Tillman H T Oral Surg 1961; 14: 877
140. Collins D H Lancet 1956; ii: 51
141. Smith B J, Eveson J W J Oral Pathol 1981; 10: 233

Fibrous dysplasia

Fibrous dysplasia may be monostotic or polyostotic: the latter can be further classified as Jaffe's disease and Albright's syndrome.[143]

Albright's syndrome has an insidious onset between 10 and 20 years of age with skeletal, cutaneous and endocrine manifestations. The skeletal involvement tends to be unilateral and affects the cranium (50%), mandible (30%) and long bones. Bone pain is the most common presenting symptom. Involvement of the facial bones can cause significant disfigurement. Café-au-lait spots are a feature and there are endocrine abnormalities of the pituitary, thyroid and parathyroid glands. Sexual precocity occurs in females.

Jaffe's variety of polyostotic dysplasia has a more restricted bony involvement than Albright's syndrome. Café-au-lait spots are also present but endocrine abnormalities do not occur.

In the monostotic variety single bones are affected: the skull base, zygoma or maxilla. It presents as a slow progressive facial deformity with displacement of teeth and visual disturbance from orbital wall and optic canal involvement.

A familial form of fibrous dysplasia called cherubism occurs—there is bilateral deformity. When the maxilla is affected there is subperiosteal deposition of bone on to the floor of the orbits, displacing the eyes upwards and exposing the sclerae, producing the appearance of a 'cherub'. The condition stabilizes at about 7 years of age when the deformity can be corrected.

TUMOURS OF THE JAWS

Primary tumours of bone can arise in the jaws, invade the jaws from adjacent structures or they may be the site of metastasis. Tumours can also arise from odontogenic tissue (Table 13.9). This tissue, which is responsible for the highly complex process of tooth formation, can be the origin of true neoplasms, malformations of dental tissues known as odontomes, or mixtures of both of these.

Both primary and odontogenic tumours are uncommon. The most common cause of a jaw tumour is local invasion from adjacent epithelium.

Odontogenic tumours

Ameloblastoma

The most common odontogenic tumour is the ameloblastoma with an annual incidence of 1 per 10^6 in the UK population, thus most of these odontogenic tumours are little more than curiosities. They are generally low grade.

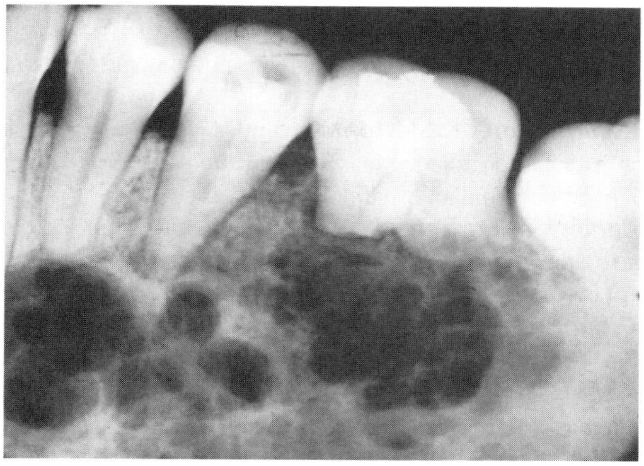

Fig. 13.35 The multilocular appearance of an ameloblastoma.

Ameloblastoma is so called because the cells have histological similarity to ameloblasts. It is virtually restricted to the jaws, and is locally invasive.[144] Various histological patterns are seen, some closely resembling the enamel organ. Cyst formation is common and occurs as microcysts in a predominantly solid tumour or as large unilocular cysts, often indistinguishable from non-neoplastic cysts.[145] Most tumours develop in middle age, predominantly in the mandible, and usually in the molar region or ascending ramus. They present as symptomless slow-growing swellings, sometimes attaining a large size if left untreated. Radiologically, there is a well defined radiolucent area which is characteristically multilocular with small daughter cysts on the periphery (Fig. 13.35). Variants range from a honeycomb appearance to a single well defined cyst. There may be resorption of dental roots and invasion of the soft tissues with ulceration into the mouth.

Table 13.9 Classification of primary odontogenic neoplasms of the jaw bones

Epithelial (ectodermal) origin
Ameloblastoma
Calcifying epithelial odontogenic tumour
Adenomatoid tumour
Ameloblastic odontoma
Ameloblastic fibroma
Ameloblastic fibro-odontoma
Ameloblastic fibrosarcoma
Connective tissue (mesodermal) origin
Cementoblastoma
Myxoma

Treatment

The ameloblastoma tends to penetrate medullary spaces and thus should be removed with a margin of up to 1 cm of cancellous bone.[146] The cortical plate is less readily invaded and a subperiosteal excision can be carried out with less chance of recurrence.

If the cortical plate has been penetrated, extraperiosteal excision is necessary, including an adequate amount of soft tissue. Some cases require a full-thickness excision of the affected part of the jaw and restoration with a bone graft.

Follow-up should be indefinite as recurrences may occur up to 20 years or more later.[147]

REFERENCES

142. Beeching B Interpreting Dental Radiographs. Update Books, London 1981 p 137
143. Neville B W, Damm D D, Allen C M, Bouquot J E In: Neville B W, Damm D D, Allen C M, Bouquot J E (eds) Oral and Maxillofacial Pathology. W B Saunders, Philadelphia 1995 p 460
144. Small I A, Waldron C A Oral Surg 1955; 8: 281
145. Robinson L, Martinez M G Cancer 1977; 40: 227
146. Kramer I R H Br J Oral Surg 1963; 1: 13
147. Gardner D G, Pecak A M J Cancer 1980; 46: 2514

Cementoma

These tumours are characterized by continuing proliferation of cementum.[148]

Benign cementoblastoma mainly develops in young adults as an irregular or rounded mass of cementum attached to the root of a mandibular molar or premolar tooth.

Cementifying fibroma is a mass of connective tissue which forms within the jaw, containing nodules of cementum-like material. It occurs in the molar region in middle-aged patients.

Gigantiform cementoma Several tumours may coalesce and grow until there is enlargement of the jaw. Radiographically, the lesions appear as lobulated radiopaque masses with a radiolucent border.

Myxoma

This tumour is only seen in the jaws and is regarded as being of odontogenic origin. It is a different entity from the myxomatous change that occurs in other tumours. The lesions consist of spindle-shaped cells, scantily distributed in a mucoid intercellular material showing a resemblance to dental mesenchyme. Young people are mainly affected and present with a slow-growing, painless swelling of the jaw.[149]

Radiologically, a finely trabeculated 'soap-bubble' radiolucency is seen expanding the bone. The lesion is infiltrative and recurrence after excision is common.

Odontomes

This term is now used for malformations of dental tissue of developmental origin. These 'tumours' are really hamartomas in that the enamel, dentine, pulp and cementum are found in relationship to one another and are thus composite in nature.

Compound composite odontome This malformation is caused by small portions of dental lamina forming separate and multiple tooth germs. The resulting simple tooth forms or denticles are surrounded by a fibrous capsule which may become cystic (Fig. 13.36). These odontomes cause painless swellings unless they become infected, when they should be removed.[150]

Complex composite odontome This tumour consists of a disordered arrangement of the dental tissues and produces a mass of enamel, dentine and cementum together with pulp and periodontal membrane in varying amounts. A hard painless swelling is usually seen in young people; radiologically it appears as an irregular, radiopaque mass.

Benign non-odontogenic tumours of the jaw

Fibroma

This rare tumour may arise in the bone or beneath the periosteum. Histologically, it consists of fibroblasts and bundles of collagen fibres in a whorled arrangement. Fibromas present as a slow-growing, round mass on the surface of the jaw or, if endosteal, will eventually expand the bone. They may invade the antrum and become quite large before symptoms occur.[151]

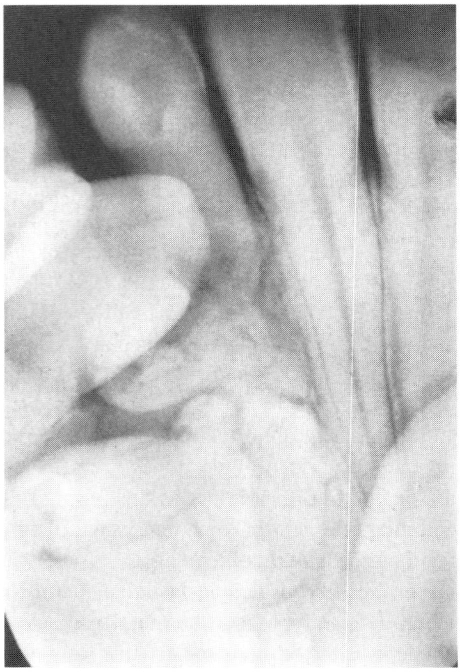

Fig. 13.36 Compound composite odontome.

Ossifying fibroma

This uncommon tumour usually arises in children's mandibles and presents as a slow-growing painless swelling. Radiologically, it appears as a well defined radiolucent area with speckled opacities throughout; these are small areas of calcification which are seen in the cellular fibrous tissue.[152] Local surgical excision is indicated.

Chondroma

Chondroma rarely occurs in the jaws. It consists of hyaline cartilage in which calcification may occur. The tumour presents as a rounded hard mass which may cause asymmetry of the mandible or a radiolucent expansion of either jaw.[153] Sarcomatous change may be seen in some, and wide excision is necessary.

Osteoma

Compact or cancellous osteomas are occasionally seen in either jaw but localized overgrowths known as exostoses are more common, especially in the maxilla.

Torus palatinus. This is an exostosis peculiar to the palate, and develops in early adult life as a smooth rounded symmetrical

REFERENCES

148. Pindborg J J, Kramer I R Histological Typing of Odontogenic Tumours. World Health Organization, Geneva 1971 p 31
149. Killey H C, Kay L W Br J Oral Surg 1964; 2: 124
150. Hitchin A D Br Dent J 1971; 130: 475
151. Wesley R K, Wysocki G P, Mintz S M Oral Surg 1975; 40: 235
152. Langdon J D, Rapidis A D, Patel M F Br J Oral Surg 1976; 14: 1
153. MacGregor A B Br Dent J 1952; 94: 39

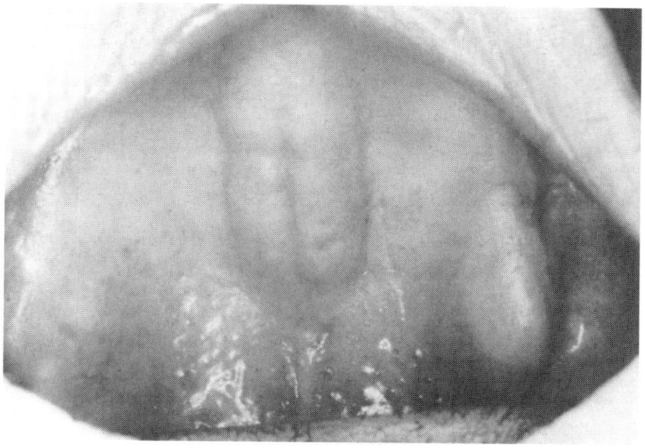

Fig. 13.37 Torus palatinus.

swelling in the midline of the hard palate (Fig. 13.37).[154] It need only be removed if it interferes with a denture.

Torus mandibularis. This is a similar exostosis found bilaterally on the lingual side of the mandible in the premolar region. It need not be removed.

Juvenile angiofibroma

This neoplasm occurs primarily in males and is characterized by aggressive local growth. It arises from the pterygo-palatine area and is particularly vascular. It extends as finger-like protrusions into local structures especially the nose, pterygo-maxillary fissure, maxillary antrum, ethmoid and sphenoidal sinus. Occasionally it extends through foramina in the skull base to enter the cranial cavity. It presents usually as a nasal mass accompanied by frightening epistaxis.

Almost all tumours occur in males between 10 and 20 years of age and they are known for spontaneous regression.[155] Its predominance in adolescent males suggests an endocrine origin, especially as anomalous sexual development is found in 20% of cases. Androgen therapy, however, is unpredictable in effect. Numerous ways have been found to manage these cases (cryotherapy, embolization, sclerotherapy, chemotherapy and endocrine therapy); the traditional method is surgery in conjunction with embolization.[156,157] Radiotherapy has been used in difficult cases, but surgery is preferred and is successful in 80–100%.

Malignant tumours of the jaw

Osteogenic sarcoma

This is a highly malignant tumour which rarely develops in the jaws. It usually affects young adults but may occur in the elderly after irradiation.[158] The tumour is necessarily osteoproliferative with osteoblasts, fibroblasts or cartilage cells seen on histological examination. The presence of osteoid is diagnostic.

The tumour forms a rapidly growing swelling which may be painful. Radiographs show resorption of normal bone with expansion and occasional radiopacities from bone formation throughout the tumour. Metastasis may already be present in the lungs at the time of diagnosis. Treatment is the same as that for soft tissue sarcomas (see Chapter 54).

Secondary neoplasms in the jaws

Metastatic deposits in the jaws usually arise from primary growths in the bronchus, breast, liver, thyroid or kidney. Deposits tend to occur at the lingula (mandibular foramen) or the mental foramen. The jaws are occasionally the site of the first apparent metastasis but a skeletal survey often shows widespread symptomless secondaries elsewhere.[159]

Common symptoms are pain and swelling of the gingival tissue overlying the bone. Anaesthesia of the lip is often present as the result of sensory nerve involvement at an early stage. Biopsy confirms the diagnosis. Treatment is palliative and symptoms may be relieved by local excision or by radiotherapy.[160]

Carcinoma of the maxilla

Carcinoma affecting the upper alveolus or palate is a consequence of oral cancer. Tumours at these sites present as a swelling or oral ulceration. The treatment is usually surgical excision of part or the whole of the maxilla depending on the site and the extent and type of tumour. A neck dissection is not normally indicated but otherwise the same principles apply as in other tumours of the mouth.

Squamous cell carcinoma of the maxillary antrum is a different entity. It is the most common malignant tumour of the maxilla (63%) and arises from the mucosal lining of the paranasal sinuses. Adenocarcinoma accounts for a further 16%, and various sarcomas, reticuloses and salivary gland tumours are occasionally seen.[161] Adenocarcinoma has a predilection for the ethmoid air cells; wood dust has been confirmed as one aetiological factor.[162]

Squamous cell carcinoma of the maxillary antrum has a high mortality (60%) because of the advanced stage of the disease at first diagnosis. Lymph node involvement is uncommon and is present in less than 10% of patients when they are first seen. It is an ominous sign and has been interpreted as a contraindication to aggressive curative surgery.[163,164]

This tumour arises in a hidden bony compartment of the maxilla and late presentation is the norm. Pain, swelling and nasal obstruction are the usual complaints although, to some extent, the character of the symptoms depends on the route of tumour invasion. If

REFERENCES

154. Kolas S, Walperin V et al Oral Surg 1953; 6: 1134
155. Cummings B J In: Harris D F N (ed) Dilemmas in Otolaryngology. Churchill Livingstone, Edinburgh 1988 p 223
156. Fitzpatrick P J, Briant T D, Berman J M Arch Otolaryngol 1980; 106: 234
157. Witt T R, Shah J P, Sternberg S S Am J Surg 1983; 146: 212
158. Garrington G E, Scofield H H et al Cancer 1967; 20: 377
159. Hatziotis J C, Constantinidou H, Papanayotou P H Oral Surg 1973; 36: 544
160. Henk J M, Langdon J D Malignant Tumours of the Oral Cavity. Edward Arnold, London 1985 p 211
161. Lewis J S, Castro E B J Laryngol Otol 1972; 86: 255
162. Hadfield E H Ann Coll Surg Engl 1970; 46: 301
163. Stell P M Proc Royal Soc Med 1975; 68 (2): 83
164. Harrison P F Laryng Otol 1976; 90(1): 69

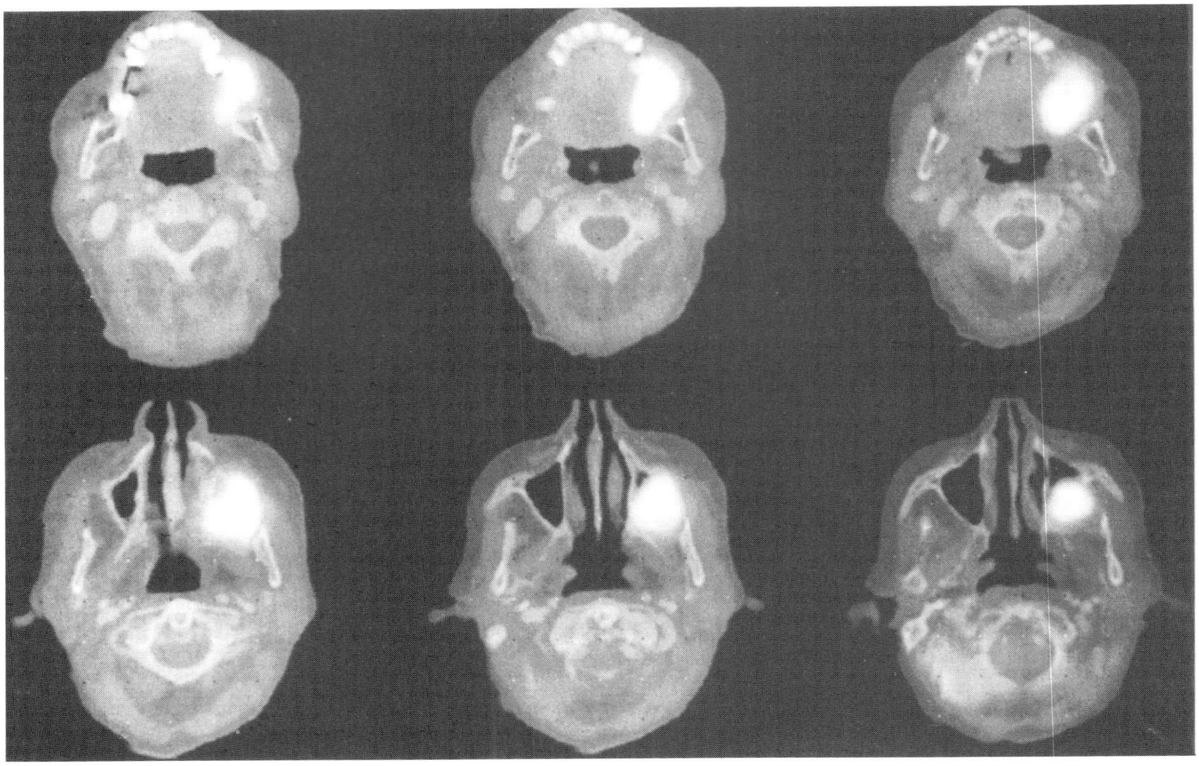

Fig. 13.38 Co-localized PET and CT images help to delineate a maxillary carcinoma.

there is invasion of the orbit superiorly, proptosis develops. Anterior invasion is associated with infraorbital nerve paraesthesia and medial invasion causes nasal obstruction. If the pterygoid plates and muscles become involved, with accompanying trismus, the disease is advanced and has a poor prognosis.

Radiological investigation, including computerized tomography, is essential for estimating the size and extent of the tumour. Recent advances that allow accurate superimposition of positron emission tomography images on CT or MRI scans have improved the clinician's appreciation of tumour extent (Fig. 13.38).[165] Biopsy may be carried out via a Caldwell–Luc approach but is best done via the intranasal route as the lateral wall of the nose will always be removed in the subsequent operation.

Treatment

The prognosis for this condition is relatively poor—6 out of 10 patients are incurable because of advanced disease. Surgery is disfiguring, especially when it involves maxillectomy with enucleation of the eye, although a dental obturator maintains good function. Traditionally there has been a reliance on radiotherapy as primary treatment with cure rates of only 10–15% for advanced disease. Surgical resection with adjuvant radiotherapy gives the best prospect of cure.[166] The Japanese have pioneered a combination of chemotherapy and radiotherapy, with surgery reserved as a de-bulking procedure.[167] This technique is similar to that being introduced for the larynx[168,169] but has not as yet received widespread acceptance for use in the maxilla.

Maxillectomy

This is a difficult operation to perform as there are no fascial planes to follow and the tumour frequently extends to the posterior maxillary wall and into the pterygoid area. A temporary tarsorrhaphy should be performed first. The Weber–Fergusson skin incision is most commonly employed (Fig. 13.39).[170] This begins in the midline of the upper lip and then, skirting the ala margin, runs upwards along the lateral border of the nose to the medial canthus. The incision is continued laterally about 5 mm below the lower lid to end over the zygoma. A cheek flap is then elevated in a supraperiosteal plane by incising the mucosa along the buccal sulcus. The alveolus and palate are split in the midline and the nasal process of the maxilla is divided by an oscillating saw or a fissure burr.

The orbital contents may be preserved if the orbital floor is not involved, in which case the antral wall in entered just below the orbital rim. One of the practical problems of this approach is that few eyes remain functional following postoperative radiotherapy.[171]

REFERENCES

165. Wong W L, Hussain K et al Am J Surg 1996; 172: 628
166. Ketcham A S, Van Buren J M Tumours of the paranasal sinuses: a therapeutic challenge. Am J Surg 1985; 150(94): 406
167. Sakai S, Hohki A, Fuchilate H, Tanaka Y Cancer 1983; 52: 1360
168. Lefebvre J-L, Chevalier D et al J Natnl Cancer Inst 1996; 88: 13
169. The Department of Veterans Affairs, Laryngeal Cancer Study Group N Engl J Med 1991; 324: 1685
170. Stell P M, Maran A G D Head and Neck Surgery, 2nd edn. Heinemann, London 1978 p 270

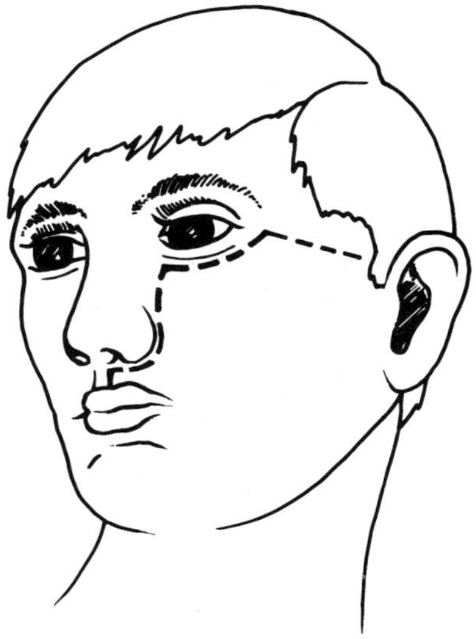

Fig. 13.39 The Weber–Fergusson approach for a maxillectomy.

The ethmoids are sectioned below the ethmoidal arteries if the eye is not to be preserved, and the bone cut continued inferiorly across the orbital floor to meet the inferior orbital fissure.

The malar process is divided or, if this bone is also to be removed, the zygomatic arch and frontal process of the maxilla must be separated by division of the fronto-zygomatic suture down through the lateral orbital wall to the inferior orbital fissure.

If the tumour has breached the posterior maxillary wall the ramus or coronoid process of the mandible can be resected to give free access to the infratemporal fossa and pterygoid plates. The latter are separated from their attachment to the base of the skull with an osteotome. The soft palate is now divided as dictated by the tumour extension before the maxilla is mobilized. Much of the final dissection in the nasopharynx has to be done blind.

After the antrum has been removed it is essential to support the cheek. Traditionally the raw surface of the cheek flap is skin-grafted to prevent scarring and the cavity packed using gutta percha attached to a previously constructed base plate or denture and held in place by wire.[172] If the zygoma and orbital rim have been removed, frontal wiring should be employed to retain the prosthesis.

The definitive obturator, usually soft-lined and of hollow box construction, may be fitted when healing has been completed and in most cases overcomes major disfigurement (Fig. 13.40). Primary reconstruction with microvascular flaps and dental implants is now an alternative. This helps to improve the stability of the eye prosthesis.

THE TEMPOROMANDIBULAR JOINT

The anatomy must be known in order to understand some of the disorders that affect this joint. It should be viewed as a tripartite structure comprising the bilateral articulation of the mandibular condyles with the glenoid fossa and the articular eminence of the temporal bone, and centrally the occlusion of the teeth. The joint capsule is relatively lax but is thickened laterally by the temporomandibular ligament which runs between the root of the zygoma and the neck of the condyle and prevents posterior displacement (Fig. 13.41). The meniscus, which is composed of fibrocartilage, fills the space between the condyle and the glenoid fossa and is firmly attached to the condyle medially and laterally where it blends with the capsule. Anteriorly, it gives rise to part of the insertion of the lateral pterygoid muscle. The thickened posterior edge consists of fibroelastic tissue which is loosely attached to the capsule and allows forward movement of meniscus and condyle. Centrally, there are two transverse thickenings or bands which form a protective cushion from compression forces during mastication.[173]

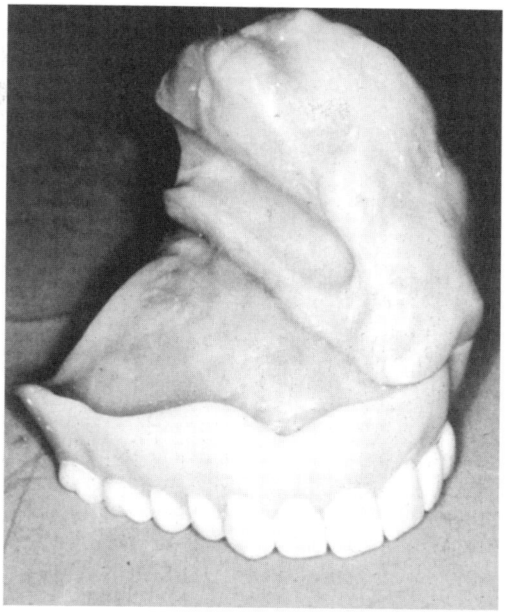

Fig. 13.40 A hollow box obturator attached to an upper denture.

The initial movement on opening the jaw is rotational between the condyle and meniscus, then the meniscus glides down the slope of the articular eminence. Maximal opening is again a rotational movement.[174]

Dislocation of the jaw

Dislocation of the mandible can be acute or chronic: the latter may be divided into recurrent or of long duration. The mandibular condyle can be displaced superiorly, posteriorly or anteriorly, the latter being the most common. In the presence of a fracture the condyle can also be displaced laterally or, more commonly,

REFERENCES

171. Stern S J, Goepfert H et al Otolaryngol Head and Neck Surg 1993; 109: 111
172. Harrison D F N In: Dudley H, Carter D (eds) Rob and Smith's Operative Surgery, Nose and Throat, 4th edn. Butterworths, London 1978 p 145
173. Rees L A Brit Dent J 1954; 96: 125
174. Rayne J In: Norman J, Bramley P A Textbook and Colour Atlas of Temporomandibular Joint Diseases, Disorders and Surgery. Wolfe Medical, London 1990 p 151

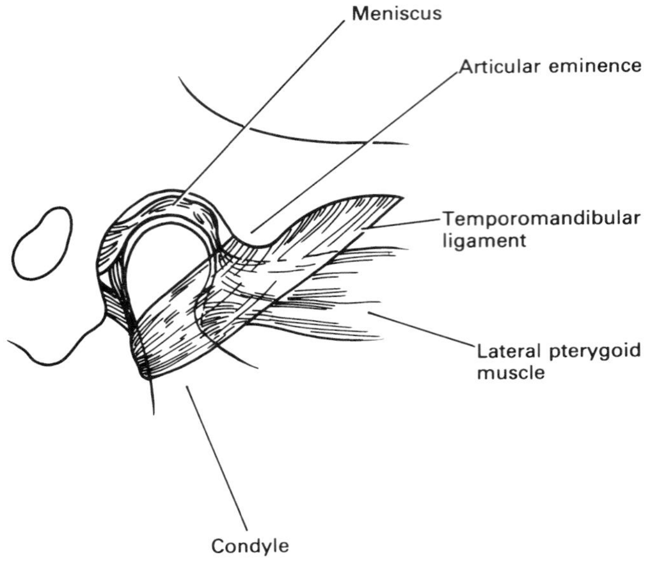

Fig. 13.41 Diagram of the temporomandibular joint showing the principal ligaments and meniscus.

medially as this is the direction of muscle pull. Acute dislocation is relatively common and may be the result of trauma or excessive mouth opening. It can also occur in patients with psychiatric disorders. In chronic disease, lax ligaments predispose to recurrent dislocation; longstanding dislocation is often overlooked, especially in a withdrawn psychiatric or geriatric patient.

Condylar dislocation normally occurs on one side and results in the chin deviating to the opposite side with an inability to close the mouth (Fig. 13.42). A pre-auricular depression and radiological evidence of an empty glenoid fossa confirm the diagnosis. The acute dislocation is painful and the masticatory muscles soon go into spasm. Simple reduction may prove impossible unless undertaken immediately; muscle relaxants and intravenous valium are otherwise required. Reduction is accomplished by applying downward pressure in the molar region with thumbs well protected by padding and at the same time elevating the chin point with the fingers.

Recurrent dislocation is a distressing condition in that each acute episode is accompanied by pain and requires reduction. The restraining capsule around the joint can be tightened with sclerosing agents or surgery. Alternatively the articulating eminence can be removed to allow the condyle to move freely over the surface or conversely augmented with bone grafts to block the passage of the condyle. All these surgical procedures induce a degree of local fibrosis which contributes to limitation in joint movement. A long-standing dislocation can be difficult to reduce and coronoidectomy may be required to release the powerful temporalis muscle. Under general anaesthesia traction may be applied by transcutaneous hooks placed at the sigmoid notch or wires attached at the angle of the mandible.

Trismus

Trismus is a functional inability to open the mouth and is a symptom rather than a disorder in its own right. The most frequent

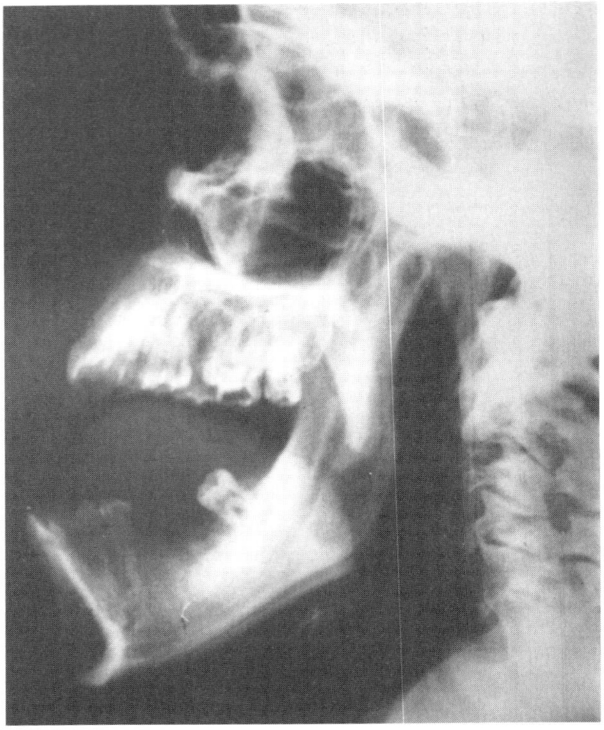

Fig. 13.42 A lateral skull radiograph showing bilateral dislocation of the temporomandibular joints.

cause is temporomandibular joint dysfunction and it may also follow an inferior dental nerve block due to trauma or haematoma in the medial pterygoid muscle. Direct invasion of muscles by a carcinoma is another unremitting cause of trismus. Disorders of the central nervous system in which trismus is an incidental feature include tetanus, motor neurone disease, dyskinesia produced by phenothiazine drugs, and hysteria. Symptoms regress with the treatment of the underlying condition.

Ankylosis

Permanent limitation of movement of the jaw may be caused by fibrous or bony ankylosis or mechanical obstruction of mandibular movement. There may be an associated deficiency in mandibular growth if it occurs in childhood but the child's general development remains normal. The majority of patients have surprisingly little difficulty in taking an adequate diet and the general nutrition is not impaired. Oral hygiene is, however, difficult to maintain and restorative dental work is not possible.

Ankylosis is a relatively uncommon condition in developed countries. The majority of cases follow injury or occasionally infection in children under 10 years of age. Ankylosis has been classified as intracapsular or extracapsular. Even in the intracapsular type a rudimentary joint space can often be identified and total fusion is rare. In extracapsular ankylosis the condyle and coronoid process may be discernible structures but they are enlarged and deformed or simply replaced by a broad block of bone. Discernable joint space may be present. In children bilateral ankylosis results in a 'bird face' with a tiny retruded mandible and compensatory growth of the alveolar bone around the teeth in an attempt to maintain dental occlusion. Unilateral ankylosis causes deviation of the mandible to the affected side, and on radiographic examination there is marked notching of the mandible indicating an overactive pterygo-masseteric muscle sling.

Management

In the child, the primary concern is to re-establish mandibular mobility and function. Facial aesthetics are of secondary concern as children maintain a potential for growth; reconstructive procedures are delayed until the patient is a teenager. In adults, once the ankylosis has been convincingly eradicated (recurrence is common) reconstruction of the mandible is undertaken. The details of the operative procedure have been described by Norman.[174] The operation can be demanding because of limitations in access. In long-standing ankylosis it is also necessary to remove both the coronoid processes to release the vice-like grip of the now fibrotic temporalis muscles. Once the segment of ankylosed bone is removed from around the condyle a strip of temporalis muscle is rotated inferiorly to line the glenoid area and an interpositional graft is used to replace the condylar segment to maintain the vertical height of the ramus and stop the pterygo-masseteric sling lifting the freed ramal segment back into contact with the skull base. A range of materials and techniques have been used but a free costochondral graft is the most reliable. The key to success is early mobilization of the joint if re-ankylosis is to be avoided. Forcing an increasing number of tongue spatulas between the incisor teeth is a simple and effective method of exercising the joint.

Temporomandibular joint dysfunction

This troublesome condition is characterized by one or more of the symptoms of pain, clicking and limited opening. A great deal has been written about this disorder but it is still ill understood.

The underlying aetiology is related to abnormalities of the tripartite joint structure. There is a strong psychological component in many patients and they exhibit an increased incidence of neuroticism, anxiety and depression. Apart from these cases, it is a self-limiting condition and the vast majority of patients spontaneously improve within a few months.[175] The underlying mechanism is probably related to over-loading of the joint due to bruxism or abnormal joint use. Treatment should be aimed at reducing these forces. Surgery is unpredictable in result and in the majority of cases it should be limited to arthroscopy and lavage unless identified pathology is present. Over-zealous treatment, bearing in mind the psychological components, can result in a cripple with intractable pain.

Arthritis of the temporomandibular joint

Rheumatoid arthritis

The temporomandibular joint is never involved alone: patients usually seek treatment for other affected joints. In adults, surgical intervention is rarely required but in Still's disease the childhood condyle may lose its growth potential leading to a bird face.

Osteoarthritis

Although the mandibular joint is not weight-bearing, degenerative changes are occasionally seen.[176] The condition is self-limiting.

Suppurative arthritis

Suppurative arthritis is rare as most infections are now promptly treated with antibiotics. The joint is swollen and painful with marked trismus, and destruction of bone may lead to ankylosis if untreated.

REFERENCES

175. Toller P A Scientific Foundation in Dentistry. Heinemann, London 1974 p 596
176. Ogus H Brit J Oral Surg 1979; 17: 17

14 Disease of the salivary glands

R. W. Ruckley

INTRODUCTION

A surgeon is most likely to encounter major salivary gland disease because of stones, inflammation, tumours or trauma. All but the latter are associated with swelling of the salivary gland — either a diffuse enlargement of the whole gland or a discrete swelling within it. A minor salivary gland may become enlarged because of tumour formation or blockage of its duct.

Swelling of the parotid gland has many causes. It is important to distinguish between swelling of the whole gland, and smaller swellings within the gland. The former usually signifies benign disease (Table 14.1) which is often inflammatory in nature. Discrete swellings within the parotid gland, by contrast, usually indicate benign neoplasia, and rarely replace the entire gland until very late on in the disease process. Intraparotid lesions such as facial nerve neuroma, aneurysms of the temporal artery and lymph node enlargement may occasionally confuse the diagnosis. Several extra parotid conditions such as subcutaneous lipoma, masseteric hypertrophy, winged mandible, or an abnormally large transverse process of the atlas or axis may occasionally be mistaken for parotid tumours. Parapharyngeal and infratemporal fossa tumours can also present as parotid swellings.

Submandibular gland disease usually presents as swelling of the whole gland, often with tenderness and pain. The most common cause is acute inflammation associated with a stone in the submandibular duct, but the submandibular triangle also contains lymph nodes which drain the oral cavity. Metastatic lymphadenopathy from an oropharyngeal cancer is one of the most common causes of a neck mass in the middle-aged patient and must not be missed. In comparison to the parotid gland, primary submandibular gland tumours are twice as likely to be malignant.

Table 14.1 Parotid gland swelling

Swellings of the whole parotid gland
Acute sialadenitis
Chronic recurrent sialadenitis (sialectasis)
Sialolithiasis
Sjögren's syndrome
Human immunodeficiency virus salivary gland disease
Sialosis (sialadenosis)
Sarcoidosis
Discrete swellings within the parotid gland
Tumours
Parotid lymph node enlargement
Facial nerve neuroma
Temporal artery aneurysms
Extraparotid swellings mimicking parotid gland enlargement
Lipoma
Dental infection
Hypertrophy of masseter muscle
Winged mandible
Transverse process of atlas/axis
Infratemporal fossa tumours
Parapharyngeal tumours

PAROTID GLAND TRAUMA

Penetrating injuries of the parotid gland will often lead to the development of a fistula with leakage of saliva through the wound. In minor injuries these fistulae seal spontaneously with little further trouble, while a salivary fistula developing after a deep penetrating injury involving the major duct system is likely to be persistent.[1] The majority of these injuries arise as a result of stab wounds, lacerations from broken glass, road traffic accidents or shrapnel from bomb blasts. Fistulae may also develop iatrogenically following parotidectomy or major head and neck resection, although this is uncommon, occurring in fewer than 1% of parotidectomies.[2]

Recent parotid injury

Parotid injuries often go undetected in the casualty department. All facial injuries in the parotid area should be explored carefully in the operating theatre under either local or general anaesthesia. Inadvertent damage to the facial nerve must be avoided and debridement should be conservative with meticulous haemostasis. The use of a peripheral nerve stimulator may help to identify the position of the facial nerve branches and the use of a loupe or operating microscope may at times be invaluable. The parotid duct should be cannulated using a lacrimal probe from inside the mouth. Major duct defects will be immediately obvious, but injection of saline or methylene blue through a lacrimal cannula may help to show up less obvious injuries to the duct. Sialography clearly

REFERENCES

1. Norman J E, McGurk M Colour Atlas and Text of the Salivary Glands, Diseases, Disorders and Surgery. Mosby-Wolfe, London 1995
2. Shaheen O H Problems in Head and Neck Surgery. Baillière Tindall, London 1994
3. Van Sickles J E, Alexander J M Oral Surg Oral Med Oral Pathol 1981; 52: 4

shows extravasation from a damaged duct if the diagnosis remains uncertain.

Parotid duct injuries can be classified[3] according to their location into three types:

1. Site A injury within the gland.
2. Site B injury to the duct overlying the masseter muscle.
3. Site C injury to the duct anterior to the masseter muscle.

Site A injuries should be treated by conservative debridement, careful approximation of the glandular tissue and repair of the capsule.[1]

Site B injuries are best managed by primary repair of the duct.[3,4] An appropriately sized sialogram catheter is used as a stent, and the duct ends approximated with 6/0 or 8/0 monofilament sutures. The catheter should be sutured to the buccal mucosa to prevent displacement and left in situ for 10 days. A broad-spectrum antibiotic is given during this period and the patient encouraged to use frequent mouth washes and regular secretgogues to stimulate salivary flow. Duct reconstruction is most difficult at the junction of the duct with the gland. If successful repair cannot be achieved then the proximal duct should be ligated, and the resultant gland atrophy accepted.[1] Risk of inadvertent damage to branches of the facial nerve must be kept in mind at all times. It is always safer to abandon attempts at repair rather than compound the injury by an iatrogenic facial nerve palsy.

Site C injuries of the duct should be managed by transecting the duct at the site of injury and reimplanting it into the mouth, avoiding undue tension and acute angulation of the duct.[4]

Long-standing parotid injury

Unrecognised parotid gland injury eventually presents with either a sialocoele or external salivary fistula.

Sialocoele

Saliva extravasates into the remaining parotid tissue to produce a parotid effusion when a major duct injury goes unnoticed for several days. This is frequently unrecognised and the gland swelling is usually attributed to post-traumatic oedema or haematoma formation. Once a parotid effusion is diagnosed then an urgent sialogram should be performed to identify the site of the duct injury. Duct injuries at sites B and C can be successfully repaired up to 72 hours following injury.[1] A parotid effusion eventually leads to the formation of a sialocoele if left untreated. This is recognized as a cystic swelling in the parotid region, usually occurring 1–2 weeks after injury. This pseudocyst is contained by a chronic inflammatory membrane and can be aspirated using a needle and syringe. The high amylase content in the saliva will readily distinguish it from a serous collection.[1]

External fistula

Leakage of saliva through the external skin wound usually occurs within 5–7 days of the injury, whether it is traumatic or surgical. By reducing salivary flow to a minimum these chronic fistulae can often be encouraged to heal spontaneously.[1] In glandular as opposed to duct injuries, the anticholinergic drug propantheline bromide, used to reduce salivary flow and repeated needle aspiration, may be all that is required. With a major duct injury, however, the patient needs to be kept off all oral fluids and food until the fistula has sealed. In persistent cases it may be necessary to create a permanent fistula into the mouth using the method described by Demetriades & Rabinowitz.[5] A small skin incision is made in the fluctuant area adjacent to the opening of the fistula and a small pair of artery forceps is passed through the incision, across the underlying cavity and out through the masseter muscle into the oral cavity. A fine Jacques catheter is then grasped in the forceps and pulled back into the cavity. It is secured to the buccal mucosa with sutures and the skin incision is closed. The patient is allowed to eat and the catheter is removed 2 days after it has stopped draining. Scar tissue may lead to stricture formation, high salivary back-pressure and eventual gland atrophy with long-standing parotid injuries.[5]

INFLAMMATORY DISORDERS

Acute suppurative sialadenitis

Although acute suppurative sialadenitis may involve either the parotid or the submandibular gland it tends to occur mainly in the former.[6] It arises as a result of salivary stasis, either from duct obstruction by a calculus or stenosis, or from decreased production of saliva. An ascending bacterial infection then occurs, leading to suppuration in the gland. The submandibular gland is thought to be more resistant to infection than the parotid gland because its saliva contains high molecular-weight glycoproteins with greater bacteriostatic activity. Predisposing factors include dehydration and poor oral hygiene. Although such conditions should now be rare in postoperative patients, they may still occur in the older patient with chronic debilitating disease, terminal malignant conditions and those receiving intensive chemotherapy.[1] These patients may be at risk not only as a result of the increase in oral flora associated with a dry mouth, but also because they may be taking medications which reduce salivary flow, or multiple antibiotic therapy which alters the balance of the oral flora. The situation may be further aggravated if the patient is not eating, because there is a loss of the stimulatory effect of mastication on the salivary glands and the cleansing action of the food itself. Hospital admission data for Trent, Yorkshire and Merseyside regions suggests an incidence of sialadenitis of 0.04 per 1000 population.[1]

Most cases of acute suppurative sialadenitis are caused by *Staphylococcus aureus*, although *Streptococcus pneumoniae*, *Escherichia coli* and *Haemophilus influenzae* are also commonly found.[7] Anaerobic organisms, including *Bacteroides*, may also be present, particularly if there is dental-related sepsis.[8]

REFERENCES

4. Stevenson J H Br J Plast Surg 1983; 36: 81–82
5. Demetriades D, Rabinowitz B Br J Surg 1987; 74: 309
6. Seifert G, Miehlke A, Haubrich J, Chilla R Diseases of the Salivary Glands. Thieme, Stuttgart 1986
7. Raad I, Sabbagh M F, Caranasos C J Rev Infect Dis 1990; 12: 591–601
8. Speirs C F, Mason D K Scott Med J 1972; 17: 62–66

Acute parotid sialadenitis

The commonest infection of the parotid glands is the result of the mumps virus and this is the most frequent cause of bilateral parotid swelling in children.[9] In teenagers viral parotitis is usually caused by an echovirus or coxsackievirus infection.[9] Acute suppurative parotitis is usually secondary to duct obstruction by a calculus, stenosis or epithelial debris; epithelial debris is probably the most common cause.[9]

Clinical features

The acute inflammatory response within the parotid gland leads to oedema of the gland parenchyma with obstruction of the intraglandular ducts. Initially this gives rise to discomfort or mild pain in the parotid area; however the pain becomes very severe when the patient attempts to eat. Secretomotor stimulation of the parotid gland increases the flow of saliva and in the presence of duct obstruction merely results in further swelling of the already tense gland. This causes severe pain often radiating to the jaw, ear and down into the neck. As the infection progresses the patient becomes pyrexial and often toxic. The pain and swelling of the gland may cause spasm of the adjacent masseter, temporalis and pterygoid muscles, giving rise to trismus. The reluctance to eat compounds exacerbates the already poor state of oral hygiene.

The patient is pyrexial and miserable, often with severe halitosis. There is diffuse tender enlargement of the whole parotid gland which is red and hot (Fig. 14.1). The orifice of Stensen's duct may also be swollen and inflamed. A stone may be palpable in the terminal portion of the parotid duct distal to the anterior border of the masseter muscle. Gentle massage of the gland may produce purulent secretions from the duct orifice. Such secretions must be sent for bacterial culture with a request for mycology as well. It is always prudent to obtain viral titres. Cervical lymphadenopathy is likely to be present in the upper deep cervical chain.

The differential diagnosis includes dental sepsis, unerupted molar teeth and arthritis of the temporomandibular joint. The facial nerve is resistant to infection and if facial weakness is present other parotid pathology must be excluded.

Investigations

A lymphocytosis indicates the presence of a viral infection, and a neutrophilia signifies bacterial sepsis. The C-reactive protein is high but falls rapidly once appropriate antibiotic therapy is commenced. Should it remain elevated in the presence of a very high erythrocyte sedimentation rate then a diagnosis of Sjögren's disease should be considered.

It should not be forgotten that tuberculosis may cause an acute parotitis. This is usually from infected lymph nodes within the parotid gland rather than direct involvement of the parotid parenchyma.[6] Fine-needle aspiration cytology of the gland, culture, tuberculin testing, chest radiography and sputum analysis for acid-fast bacilli will often help to confirm the diagnosis. Combination therapy is often effective but multi-drug resistant disease may occur in patients with human immunodeficiency virus infection.[1]

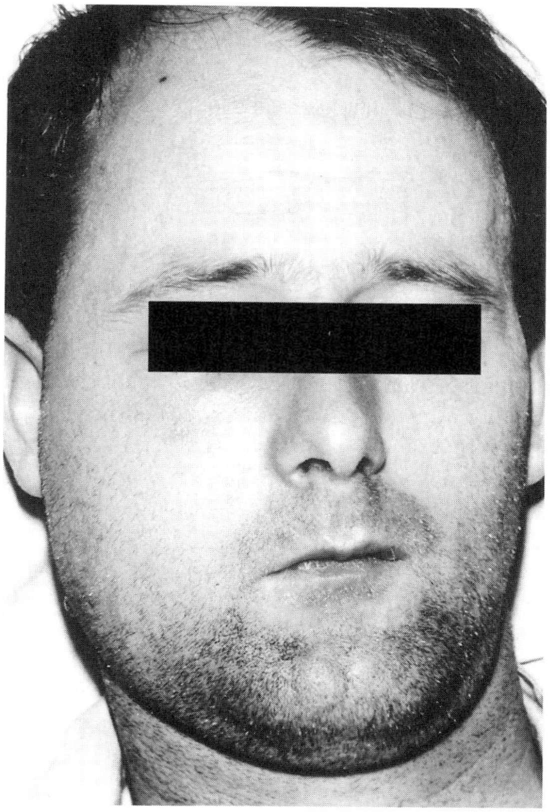

Fig. 14.1 Acute suppurative sialadenitis of the right parotid gland.

Radiology

The vast majority of parotid stones are radiolucent and plain X-rays are therefore an inappropriate investigation. Sialography should never be carried out in the acute phase of the illness. Once the infection has resolved, sialography should be performed under the cover of an antibiotic to establish the state of the duct system and identify the presence of calculi. The examination is often therapeutic in irrigating the duct system.

Fine-needle aspiration cytology

An experienced cytologist will be able to confirm the diagnosis of suppurative parotitis, although in the majority of cases clinical diagnosis alone will be sufficent.

Treatment

Medical treatment

The patient should be treated in hospital with intravenous antibiotics. A β-lactamase resistant anti-staphylococcal antibiotic should be started while awaiting the results of culture. Electrolyte imbalance is restored and the patient rehydrated with intravenous

REFERENCE

9. Kerr A G Scott-Brown's Otolaryngology. Butterworths, London 1987

fluids if necessary. Nutrition should be maintained with high-calorie fluids. Regular analgesia and mouth washes should be administered. Local heat applied to the parotid area is soothing and appreciated by the patient. Any anticholinergic medication should be discontinued.

Surgical treatment

Other than removing a parotid duct calculus, surgery is seldom required to treat acute parotitis. However, if conservative measures fail to produce an improvement in the patient's condition within 48–72 hours then an abscess may be forming. This is particularly likely if there is increasing pain, evidence of septicaemia or extension of infection into the periglandular tissues. An untreated abscess may rupture causing a fistula with the drainage of purulent secretions. An abscess may track via the pterygomaxillary fissure into the pterygopalatine fossa or via Santorini's fissure into the external auditory meatus.[6]

Computed tomography (CT), magnetic resonance imaging (MRI) or ultrasound may be used to confirm the diagnosis when a parotid abscess is suspected. MRI scanning with increased signal on T2-weighted images involving the parotid gland may demonstrate periparotid soft tissue oedema.[10] Because the parotid gland is enclosed between layers of the deep cervical fascia, abscess formation may occur with little evidence of fluctuation. Ultrasound-guided needle aspiration may well obviate the need for formal incision and drainage. If this fails, surgical drainage of a parotid abscess should be carried out under general anaesthesia avoiding the use of paralysing agents after induction so that facial nerve stimulation can be carried out perioperatively. A standard parotid cervicofacial incision is made and an anterior skin flap is raised. The parotid capsule is then incised in the direction of the facial nerve and the parenchyma gently disrupted with sinus forceps. These are opened in a line parallel with that of the facial nerve. A silastic corrugated drain is installed in the wound. It must be remembered that in children the mastoid process develops relatively late and therefore the facial nerve is in an exposed superficial position.

Acute submandibular sialadenitis

In the vast majority of patients acute infection of the submandibular gland is secondary to a calculus within Wharton's duct. Other less common causes are surgical scarring in the floor of the mouth or radiation stricture of the duct. Infection progresses with ascending bacterial sepsis. Acute inflammation within the gland causes obvious swelling of the whole gland, often filling the submandibular triangle. The gland is tender and the patient is usually pyrexial and in pain. The swelling and pain are made worse by attempts to eat with further distension of the gland from saliva which cannot drain away.

It may be possible to palpate a calculus within the line of Wharton's duct. Sometimes a stone may be visible at the duct orifice. There is often considerable mucosal oedema in the floor of the mouth and the duct orifice is inflamed and swollen. Gentle massage of the gland may produce purulent secretions (Fig. 14.2).

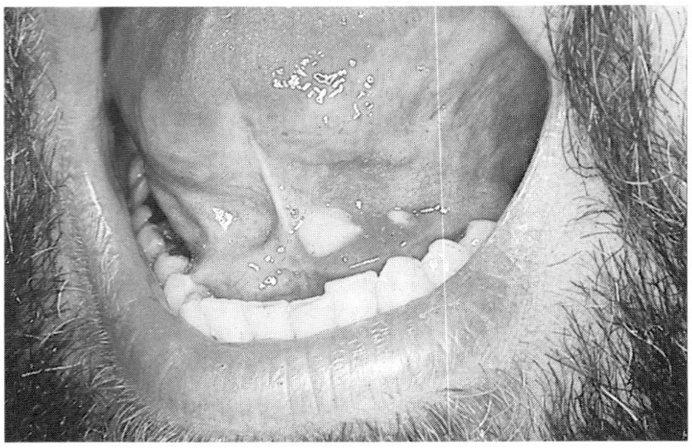

Fig. 14.2 Pus at opening of left Wharton's duct.

In a small number of cases submandibular gland infection may progress to abscess formation with erythema and oedema of the overlying skin and fluctuation of the submandibular swelling.

Investigations

Any pus obtained from the duct orifice must be sent for bacteriological and fungal culture. An elevated white count may be present with a predominant neutrophilia. Intraoral plain X-rays of the floor of the mouth often confirm the presence of one or more stones within the line of Wharton's duct. Submandibular sialography should not be attempted during acute infection.

Treatment

Treatment is centred on relieving the obstruction of Wharton's duct. Calculi within the terminal portion of the duct should be removed perorally.

The patient should be treated with a broad-spectrum antibiotic and given sialgogues such as apples, oranges or grapefruit to encourage drainage of the gland. Frequent mouth washes, adequate hydration and analgesics should be administered.

External incision and drainage are required if the submandibular gland infection has progressed to abscess formation. A small skin crease incision is made low down in the submandibular triangle at least 2 cm below the lower border of the mandible to avoid damaging the marginal mandibular branch of the facial nerve. The incision is deepened through the oedematous soft tissues towards the capsule of the gland at its inferior border until a collection of pus is released. A silastic corrugated drain is installed into the abscess cavity and left until drainage has ceased.

Once the acute infection has settled, submandibular sialography should be carried out under antibiotic cover. Parenchymal, hilar or proximal duct stones can only be treated by excising the submandibular gland. Proximal duct stones cannot be extracted satisfactorily through the floor of the mouth and attempts to do so run the risk of damaging the lingual nerve which is in close proximity to Wharton's duct in this location. Sialography may also

REFERENCE

10. Rice D H, Becker T S The Salivary Glands. Thieme, New York 1994

demonstrate a duct stenosis or sialectasis, which requires treatment to prevent or lessen the risk of recurrent infection.

A submandibular gland that has been the seat of chronic recurrent sepsis over many years is called a frozen gland.[1] It is shrunken and scarred by periglandular fibrosis and the patient becomes aware of a tender persistent hard swelling in the submandibular triangle. This type of gland has to be removed. This can be an exceedingly tedious operation because the normal tissue planes are completely obliterated by extensive fibrosis. The identification of the lingual nerve is particularly difficult and the operating microscope may come in useful.

Chronic recurrent sialadenitis

This is an incompletely understood condition of the parotid gland where there is recurrent unilateral or bilateral parotid swelling which may be associated with parotid pain. It can occur in children as well as adults and in some adults the disease originates in childhood. Chronic recurrent sialadenitis in adults is more common in women but in children, boys predominate. Some patients with chronic recurrent sialadenitis subsequently go on to develop Sjögren's syndrome.

The underlying pathological process is believed to be a reduced secretion of saliva with subsequent stagnation. There are currently two theories of initiation. The first is that one or more acute episodes of suppurative sialadenitis leads to ductal mucous metaplasia. The resulting increase in the mucus content of the saliva will contribute to the salivary stasis.[1,11,12] The second theory is that colonisation with opportunistic oral flora leads to chronic recurrent sialadenitis and subsequent mucous metaplasia of the duct epithelium. Mucus plugs block off the finer ducts and cause parotid swelling.[12]

As the condition advances, sialectasia, ductal ectasia and progressive acinar destruction develop and are accompanied by lymphocytic infiltration of the gland. The progressive disintegration of the acini eventually leads to the formation of cysts. The lymphocytic infiltrate appears to be a response to ductal and acinar damage with progressive replacement of secreting glandular elements by the infiltrate.[1,12]

Epithelial debris from the cysts intermittently sludges up and blocks off the ducts causing hypertrophy, stenosis and duct dilatation. This soft debris eventually enters the major duct system where it can cause intermittent duct obstruction. Either the whole gland or just part of it swells up at meal times when saliva production is increased depending on whether it is the main duct or a terminal branch that blocks. Eventually the sludge is forced out and the obstruction is overcome. This may occur after just hours or minutes, but sometimes the gland swelling may persist for days. In the latter situation there is more likely to be acinar damage and fibrosis from prolonged back-pressure effects.

Clinical features

The patient usually complains of mildly painful and tender parotid swelling, invariably made worse by food. The swelling may be in one or both parotids and each episode of swelling may last from a few minutes to several days. The intervals between attacks are variable, occurring every day, every week or even longer. Between times the gland may be completely normal. The acute exacerbations are associated with an unpleasant taste and occasional foetor oris. Massage of the gland may produce scant turbid secretions. Apart from the pain and swelling the patient remains well without any constitutional upset.

Investigations

A sialogram is the most useful investigation. This may be normal, or may demonstrate a duct stricture or occasionally a calculus. It usually shows evidence of sialectasis (Fig. 14.3). There may be dilatation of the main duct system, or alternating areas of dilatation and stricture, the so-called string of pearls appearance (see Fig. 14.3). The snowstorm appearance is when discrete beads of contrast are seen outside the duct system and this is often referred to as globular or saccular sialectasis. It occurs as the result of the contrast medium leaking from inflamed ducts into the gland

REFERENCES

11. Maynard J D Recurrent parotid enlargement. Br J Surg 1965; 52: 784–789
12. Maynard J D J R Soc Med 1979; 72: 591–598

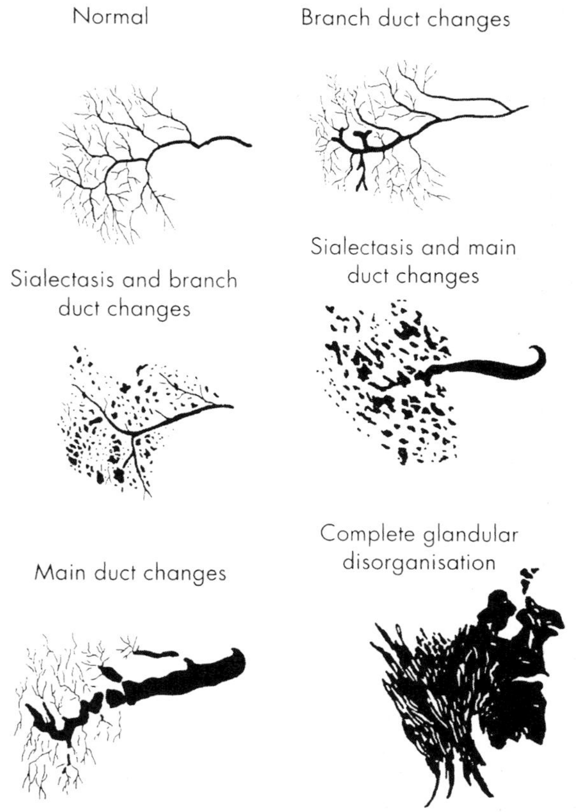

Fig. 14.3 Sialograms: the progressive changes seen in chronic recurrent sialadenitis. (Reprinted with kind permission of J E de B Norman and M McGurke from *Salivary Glands, Diseases, Disorders and Surgery* London: Mosby-Wolfe, 1995.)

parenchyma. The main duct may appear relatively healthy, with the abnormalities only occurring in the branch ducts. In severe cases there are abnormalities in the main ducts combined with multiple areas of cystic sialectasis produced by coalescence of the acini. In end-stage disease branch duct detail is lost completely and the contrast gives a streaky appearance, indicating glandular destruction and disorganisation (see Fig. 14.3).

Treatment

Any predisposing cause such as calculus or stricture, demonstrated by the sialogram, should be treated appropriately. The remainder should be treated conservatively. This includes the use of sialogogues (apples, oranges or grapefruit), massage and repeated courses of antibiotics.[1] Total obliteration of the gland by radiotherapy has been advocated in the past,[1] but the dosage necessary to achieve this could induce malignant change and has now been abandoned.

Tympanic neurectomy only produces a transient suppression of secretion, and is therefore of only short-term benefit.[9] Duct dilatation and duct ligation, while occupying the surgeon, have shown to be of infrequent benefit to the patient.[9]

Fortunately, in the childhood disease spontaneous improvement often occurs by puberty.[1] The only definitive treatment for this condition is total parotidectomy. There is no logic in performing a superficial parotidectomy for sialectasis; which after all, it involves the whole gland. Total parotidectomy in these cases is usually extremely difficult because of the extensive fibrosis and scarring. The risk of damage to the facial nerve is extremely high and therefore radical surgery should be reserved for the most severe cases.[1]

Sialolithiasis—salivary calculi

Sialolithiasis affects 12 per 1000 of the adult population.[13] Calculi can occur in both the submandibular and the parotid glands, although the majority, 80%, arise in the former.[6] In only 3% is more than one gland involved. In 75% of cases of symptomatic stone disease a single calculus will be present.[6] Sialolithiasis occurs most commonly in the 40–50 year age group; it is slightly more common in men. Over half the patients with chronic sialadenitis develop calculi, but many calculi are not associated with any other salivary gland disease.[6] Salivary calculi are unusual in children.

Predisposing factors for salivary calculi formation include reduced salivary flow rates, duct obstruction, changes in salivary pH and dehydration.[1,6] The central part of a typical stone is composed of organic material, mucoprotein or micro-organisms, whereas the outer part of the stone is composed of various forms of calcium phosphate with small quantities of carbonate, ammonium and magnesium.[1] Stone composition is independent of the gland in which it originated. Uric acid salivary calculi can occur in patients who have gout.[1,6]

It is thought that stones grow at the rate of 1 mm a year.[1] The submandibular gland is probably more susceptible to stone formation because its saliva has a higher pH, a higher mucus content and a greater concentration of calcium and phosphate.[1] Also in the upright posture, the submandibular duct has to ascend and curve round the posterior edge of the floor of the mouth so that saliva has to flow against gravity.[1] Salivary stones have been associated with diabetes mellitus in a quarter of cases, hypertension in 20% of cases, and chronic liver disease in 10% of cases.[14] Most calculi form in the large ducts of the salivary glands; those arising in the gland parenchyma have formed in the intraglandular branch ducts.

Clinical features

The signs and symptoms of salivary calculi will depend upon their location. A stone within the gland may cause no symptoms at all, whereas a stone within the duct system is likely to cause painful swelling of the gland dependent on the degree of duct obstruction caused. The usual history is of recurrent swelling and pain in the involved gland, usually precipitated by eating. After a meal is finished the gland frequently decreases in size and the pain and tenderness subside until the next meal. It may be possible to palpate a calculus in the terminal portion of the relevant duct by inserting a finger along the floor of the mouth. Bimanual palpation can also be used. Massage of the gland is likely to produce turbid secretion. Salivary calculi may be complicated by the development of acute suppurative sialadenitis, ulceration of the duct or stricture formation. Benign tumours can occasionally cause intermittent duct obstructions.

Investigation

Approximately 20% of calculi in the submandibular duct and nearly 66% of calculi in the parotid duct are radiolucent and not visible on the plain X-ray film.[10] Demonstration of submandibular duct calculi is best achieved by intraoral occlusal views, while oblique and puffed-cheek lateral views are frequently helpful in searching for the few parotid calculi which are radiopaque. Sialography can demonstrate intraductal calculi as filling defects and detects radiolucent calculi not seen on the initial plain film screening. Sialography also has the advantage of showing associated salivary gland disease. Intraglandular calculi can clearly be seen on CT scanning (Fig. 14.4).

Treatment

Submandibular calculi

Calculi in the terminal part of the submandibular duct can be removed through the floor of the mouth by an incision placed directly over the stone. A silk suture is placed around the duct behind the stone to prevent it moving back into the gland. After the stone is removed the opening in the duct is marsupialised with

REFERENCES

13. Rauch S, Gorlin R J Diseases of the salivary glands. C V Mosby, St Louis 1970
14. Laforgia P D, Favia G F, Chiaravalle N, Lacaita M G, Laforgia A Minerva Stomatol 1989; 38: 1329–1336

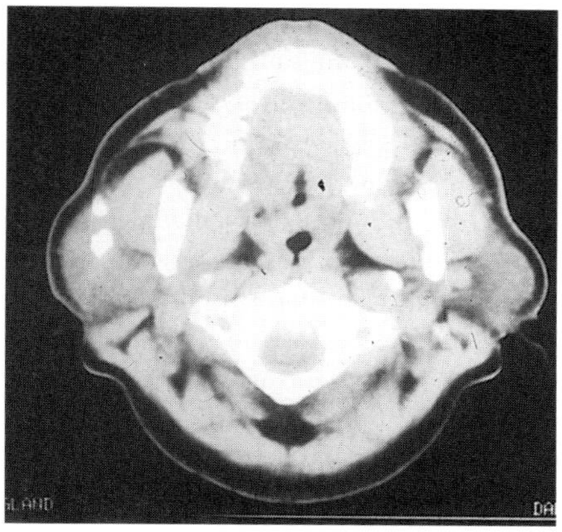

Fig. 14.4 Computed tomographic scan demonstrating two calculi in the right parotid gland.

approximation of the duct edges to the adjacent mucosa using fine absorbable sutures (Figs 14.5 and 14.6).

Stones in the proximal half of the duct, at the hilum of the gland or within the gland substance are best dealt with by excision of the submandibular gland including the proximal portion of the duct.

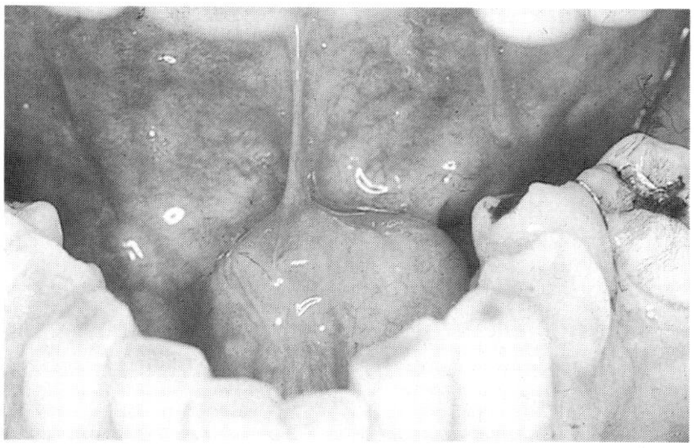

Fig. 14.5 Calculus in terminal part of left submandibular duct.

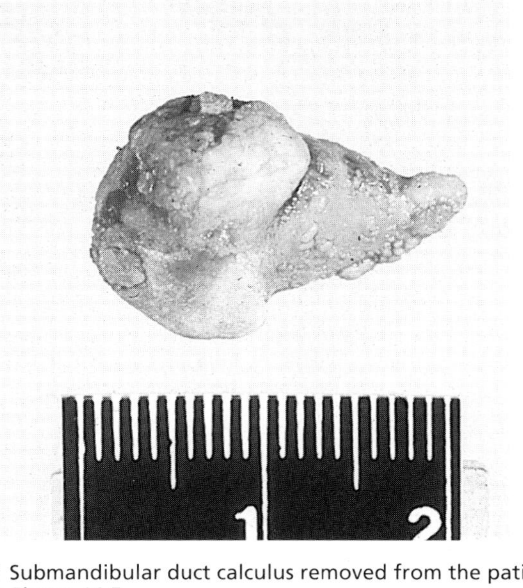

Fig. 14.6 Submandibular duct calculus removed from the patient shown in Figure 14.5.

Parotid calculi

Parotid calculi are often smaller than their submandibular counterparts. The stone may be extracted through a duct meatotomy in the mouth if it lies at or within 1 cm of the orifice of Stensen's duct. The mucosal edge of the incised duct is sutured to the adjacent buccal mucosa to prevent stricture formation as the duct heals. More proximal calculi are unlikely to be removed successfully through an intraoral approach without risking damage to adjacent local branches of the facial nerve. Calculi may be successfully extracted from the distal portion of Stenson's duct using a Fogarty embolectomy catheter.[15] The parotid gland should be formally explored if attempts to deliver a proximal duct stone fail. The stones are located and removed after the gland, duct and facial nerve have been dissected free. It is helpful to insert a lacrimal probe into Stenson's duct at the start of the procedure. During the subsequent dissection of the parotid gland, the presence of the probe helps to identify the origin of the main duct and acts as a useful reference point for locating intraglandular calculi when used in conjunction with the preoperative sialogram. In this way an awareness of the likely position of the stone within the gland substance often means that only those branches of the facial nerve going towards this area need be dissected out and the remainder of the gland does not have to be disturbed.

Extracorporeal shock-wave lithotripsy is a useful technique to treat renal stones. Specifically designed salivary lithotripters have now been used successfully to treat patients with both submandibular and parotid calculi.[16–18] In one recent study fragmentation of 19 parotid stones with complete duct clearance was achieved in 81% of cases. In 42 patients with submandibular stones, 84% became symptoms free after sialolithotripsy. Complete clearance of stone fragments from the duct was only achieved in 40% of cases; the remainder had retained duct fragments visible on ultrasonography.[16] This technique is still in its infancy, but these results are very encouraging and may improve the management of salivary calculi in the future.

SJÖGREN'S DISEASE

The salivary glands can be damaged by autoimmune disease and this can cause swelling of one or all of the salivary glands which may be either intermittent or constant.[19] Although the autoimmune inflammatory process predominantly involves the salivary glands, the lacrimal glands can also be affected and there is frequently an association with rheumatoid arthritis.[9] Autoimmune salivary gland disease is often loosely called Sjögren's disease. Sjögren's

REFERENCES

15. Ruckley R W 1997 in preparation.
16. Iro H, Schneider H T et al Lancet 1992; 339: 1333–1336
17. Kater W, Meyer W W, Wehrmann T, Hurst A, Buhne P, Schlick R J Endourol 1994; 8: 21–24
18. Brouns J A, Hendrikx A J M, Bierkens A F J Cranio-maxillofac Surg 1989; 17: 329–330
19. Maran A G J Laryngol Otol 1986; 100: 1299–1305

syndrome[20] is a distinct clinical diagnosis that may be made if two or three of the following triad are present:

1. Keratoconjunctivitis sicca (dry eyes).
2. Xerostomia (dry mouth).
3. Rheumatoid arthritis or other connective tissue disorders, such as disseminated lupus erythematosis, scleroderma, polymyositis or polyarteritis nodosa.

Primary Sjögren's syndrome (sicca syndrome) consists only of xerostomia and xerophthalmia with no connective tissue component.[6,19,21]

Secondary Sjögren's syndrome consists of xerostomia, xerophthalmia and a connective tissue disease which in nearly half of cases is rheumatoid arthritis. Benign lymphoepithelial lesion (myoepithelial sialadenitis) is a distinctive sialadenopathy of the parotid glands which may progress to lymphoma.

In Sjögren's syndrome there is a lymphocyte-mediated destruction of the exocrine glands causing xerostomia and keratoconjunctivitis sicca. Most cases (90%) occur in women and it is the second most common autoimmune disease after rheumatoid arthritis.[9] The average age of occurrence is 50 years. Almost 30% of patients with rheumatoid arthritis go on to develop Sjögren's disease.[9] The parotid gland is the most commonly involved major salivary gland but up to two-thirds of patients never have salivary gland enlargement.

Aetiology

The underlying cause of Sjögren's syndrome is thought to be B-cell hyper-reactivity with an associated loss of suppressor T cell activity and an alteration in the T-suppressor to helper cell relationship. It has been suggested that cytomegalovirus damages the salivary ducts and these damaged duct cells act as the antigen which cause B-lymphocyte proliferation.[6]

Histology

The characteristic histological features are lymphocyte and plasma cell infiltration, duct dilatation and fibrosis with acinar destruction.

Clinical features

Sjögren's syndrome runs a benign but progressive course. Patients complain of dry, burning oral discomfort and dry gritty eyes. One or both parotids enlarge more commonly in primary Sjögren's syndrome than in the secondary type. Patients with secondary Sjögren's also complain of joint pain and dysfunction if there is associated rheumatoid arthritis. Lacrimal dysfunction leads to thick mucoid tears. The ocular symptoms are progressive, leading eventually to filamentary keratopathy and corneal erosions.

The small amount of saliva that is produced from the diseased salivary glands is thicker than normal. Often the dry mouth is associated with *Candida* infection, stomatitis and glossitis, while the incidence of dental caries and periodontal disease is much higher.[6] In advanced xerostomia the tongue becomes glazed, red and fissured, and the lips are often adherent. The lipstick sign occurs in women, when lipstick adheres to the incisor teeth because of the lack of saliva. Chewing and swallowing dry food becomes more difficult.

Because Sjögren's syndrome is a disease involving multiple organs, there can be numerous associated symptoms resulting from interstitial pneumonitis, Raynaud's phenomena, achlorhydria, hepatosplenomegaly, primary biliary cirrhosis, pancreatitis, hyposthenuria and myositis. Raynaud's phenomena, renal involvement and lymphadenopathy tend to be more common in primary Sjögren's syndrome. Patients with Sjögren's syndrome are 40 times more likely to develop a lymphoma, which is usually a B-cell non-Hodgkin's type.[22]

Investigations

Routine blood tests confirm non-specific signs of inflammation, such as a raised C-reactive protein level, a raised erythrocyte sedimentation rate and increased plasma viscosity.

An immunoglobulin screen often reveals raised levels of all gamma-globulins but predominantly IgG. Anti-salivary duct antibodies are present in a quarter of patients with primary Sjögren's syndrome and 70% of patients with secondary Sjögren's syndrome.[6] They are also present in a quarter of the patients with rheumatoid arthritis who do not have Sjögren's syndrome.[21] Other autoantibodies may be present, such as antinuclear factor in approximately half, anti-gammaglobulin factors, parietal cell antibodies (27%), thyroglobulin antibody (18%) and thyroid microsomal antibody (21%).[10] In addition, elevated levels of antibody to secretory IgA have been reported.[10] Rheumatoid factor will be present in half the patients with secondary Sjögren's syndrome.[10] There are two antinuclear antibodies which are specific for Sjögren's syndrome. These are anti-SSA-Ro and anti-SSB-La. The former have been shown to be present in half the patients with secondary Sjögren's syndrome, while the latter occurs in three-quarters of patients with primary Sjögren's syndrome.[1]

Schirmer's test can be used to confirm xerophthalmia. A strip of filter paper is inserted into each fornix, and wetting of less than 5 mm in 5 minutes confirms hyposecretion of tears. Slit-lamp examination of the cornea may reveal filamentary keratitis after staining with Rose Bengal dye.

Histological confirmation of the disease can be obtained by examination of the minor salivary glands obtained from a lip biopsy. This can be carried out under local anaesthesia through a small incision on the inside of the lower lip. Depending upon the degree of periductal lymphocyte infiltration seen, the disease can be graded in severity from one to four.[9]

Parotid sialography may show multiple small punctate contrast collections throughout the gland early on in the disease, but as the

REFERENCES

20. Sjögren H Acta Ophthalmol 1933; 11: 1–151
21. Moutsopoulos H M, Chused T M et al Ann Intern Med 1980; 92: 212–226
22. Kassan S S, Thomas T L, et al Ann Intern Med 1978; 89: 888

disease progresses the contrast collections become larger and more globular.[10] These appearances are caused by extravasation of the contrast medium from the duct system, as the result of destruction of the duct wall. CT of the parotid glands may show multilocular cystic changes and calcification.[23] A tumour mass within the parotid gland will be seen if the disease is complicated by the development of a non-Hodgkin's lymphoma.

Treatment

At the present time there is no treatment which will halt the natural progression of this disease. The xerophthalmia may be helped by the use of artificial tears, but regular review by an ophthalmologist to monitor the state of the cornea is essential (see Chapter 15). The xerostomia may be helped by the use of artificial saliva. Patients should be advised to clean their teeth frequently, use topical fluoride treatment and be closely monitored by their dentist.

If there is severe parotid swelling and pain, this may be controlled with the use of systemic steroids.[9] The patient should be under the care of an appropriate physician for the management of associated collagen disease, or organ-specific autoimmune disease. Because of the increased risk of the development of lymphoma in these patients they should be reviewed regularly, ideally in a lymphoma follow-up clinic.

LYMPHOEPITHELIAL LESION

This predominantly occurs as an isolated lesion in the parotid gland and accounts for 1.5% of major salivary gland tumours.[24] The lesion usually begins as a soft painless swelling within the parotid gland and may be mistaken for a parotid tumour. It is more common in women between the ages of 50 and 70 years,[10] although it can occur at any age. Approximately half of the cases are associated with Sjögren's syndrome but in the remainder there is no xerostomia or autoimmune disease. The condition is sometimes referred to as myoepithelial sialadenitis.[24]

The gland is again infiltrated with lymphocytes, but this is combined with acinar atrophy and ductal epithelial proliferation, leading to the formation of the classical histological appearance of an epimyoepithelial island.[24] This consists mainly of duct cells embedded in a hyalinised stroma composed of basement membrane material infiltrated with lymphocytes. Although histologically very similar to Sjögren's disease, the lymphoepithelial lesion should be considered as a separate clinicopathological entity. The hyperplasia of salivary lymphoid tissue may be stimulated by an autoimmune process in Sjögren's disease but the cause of the lymphoepithelial lesion remains unknown.

While the course of the disease is usually benign, some lesions can progress and become aggressive developing into pseudolymphomas, lymphomas or carcinomas.[24] Lymphomas occur in 20% of lymphoepithelial lesions and are non-Hodgkin's B-cell in type.[24,25] The sudden development of hypogammaglobulinaemia or leukopaenia, a rapid increase in size or lymphadenopathy may herald the onset of lymphoma. When carcinomas develop they are usually anaplastic.[10] Many of the reported cases have been in Eskimos.[10]

HIV-ASSOCIATED SALIVARY GLAND DISEASE

Salivary gland disease may be associated with HIV infection and is referred to as HIV–salivary gland disease.[26] Clinically the salivary gland involvement is very similar to Sjögren's disease. Almost always it is the parotid glands that are involved and it usually causes painless enlargement. Both parotids are swollen in 80% of cases and it usually causes xerostomia. HIV–salivary gland disease is quite common, occurring in 20% of HIV-positive children with infected mothers.[1] There is usually diffuse enlargement of both parotid glands.

Pathology

The salivary glands contain cystic masses which histologically resemble "lymphoepithelial lesions". The epimyoepithelial islands may contain central cystic areas. Lymphoepithelial cysts may be quite large and are lined with non-keratinising squamous epithelium surrounded by lymphoid tissue containing germinal centres. It is not known whether the salivary gland lesion arises from intraparotid lymph nodes or from lymphocytic infiltrate within the parotid parenchyma.

The involved salivary glands show lymphocyte infiltration which is similar to that found in Sjögren's syndrome. The infiltrate is predominantly CD8-positive T-cells, whereas in Sjögren's disease CD4-positive T-cells predominate.[26] The T-cell status may be useful in the prognosis of HIV disease. CD4-positive T-cell counts of less than 200 cells/mm^3 in HIV patients who have lymphadenopathy is associated with a greater than 80% chance of progression to acquired immunodeficiency syndrome (AIDS) within 4 years; counts of 400 cells/mm^3 have only an 18% progression to AIDS within the same period.[27] The majority of patients with HIV–salivary gland disease have helper T-cell counts greater than 200 cells/mm^3 and it seems that salivary gland involvement in HIV-infected patients may have some prognostic benefit in adults.[27]

Immunological findings

Patients with HIV–salivary gland disease may have salivary autoantibodies, similar to those found in patients with Sjögren's syndrome. They do not however have anti-SSA-RO, anti-SSB-LA or antibody to DNA which are characteristic of Sjögren's syndrome.

Clinical features of HIV–salivary gland disease

Patients usually have enlargement of one or more of the major salivary glands. Parotid gland involvement usually accompanies the

REFERENCES

23. March D E, Rao V M, Zillenberg D Arch Otolaryngol Head Neck Surg 1981; 115: 105
24. McGee J O, Isaacson P G Oxford Text Book of Pathology. Oxford University Press, Oxford 1992
25. Falzon M, Isaacson P G Am J Surg Pathol 1991; 15: 59–65
26. Schiodt M Oral Surg Oral Med Oral Pathol 1992; 73: 164–167
27. Batsakis J D Tumours of the Head and Neck. Williams & Wilkins, Baltimore 1979

initial lymphadenopathy syndrome of early HIV infections. Accompanying xerostomia is variable. In one series parotid gland involvement occurred in 98% of cases of HIV–salivary gland disease, while submandibular gland enlargement occurred in only 2%.[26] Only one parotid gland was swollen in 40% while both were swollen in 60% of the cases in this study.

Diagnosis

The diagnosis of HIV–salivary gland disease should be considered in all patients with enlargement of the major salivary glands who have risk factors of HIV infection. HIV cannot be cultured from the saliva of patients with HIV–salivary gland disease despite positive cultures being obtained from the blood of these patients.[1] Fine-needle aspiration cytology may well be diagnostic and can often exclude Kaposi's sarcoma and lymphoma.[1] MRI scanning shows the characteristic multicentric cystic nature of the salivary gland disease.

Treatment

There is no specific treatment for HIV–salivary gland disease. Xerostomia should be managed with artificial saliva. As with Sjögren's disease, it is imperative that a high standard of dental hygiene is maintained with topical fluoride treatment and regular dental inspections. Superficial parotidectomy may be necessary where the diagnosis is in doubt, or in extreme cases for cosmetic reasons.[1]

SIALOSIS

Sialosis or sialadenosis is a term applied to recurrent swelling of the salivary glands which is not caused by neoplasia or inflammation.[6] Any of the major salivary glands can be involved but it mostly affects the parotid glands. Typically the swelling is painless, bilateral and gives the patient a hamster-like appearance. It is usually independent of eating. Men and women are affected equally, and it tends to occur after the fourth decade. An important distinguishing feature from other forms of parotidomegaly is the fact that in sialosis the gland, although enlarged, remains soft and is not indurated. Degenerative damage of the autonomic nervous system which innervates the glands is suggested to be the underlying cause of the condition.[6]

Sialosis can occur in association with endocrine disorders, metabolic disturbances and certain drugs.[6] It has been described in Cushing's disease, myxoedema, diabetes mellitus, diabetes insipidus, gout, gonadal dysfunction and during puberty and the menopause.[6] It is recognized in patients with nutritional disorders such as starvation and vitamin deficiency and also with anorexia nervosa and bulimia.[6,28,29] Dextropropoxyphene (Distalgesic), clonidine, guanethidine, psychotropic drugs and the oral contraceptive pill have all been reported as causing sialosis.[9]

Histologically, irrespective of the cause, sialosis is typified by swelling of the salivary acini. The swollen acinar cells may show a variable proportion of granular or vacuolated changes and the nuclei are generally displaced to the base of the cells.[6]

Endocrine sialosis is usually resistant to treatment and it is not unusual for the parotid gland enlargement to persist even in well-controlled diabetics. Drug-induced sialosis usually resolves after withdrawal of the drug but may persist in some cases.[6] In extreme cases where sialosis results in cosmetically unacceptable parotidomegaly, then superficial parotidectomy may be considered.

SARCOIDOSIS

Up to 6% of patients with sarcoidosis may develop salivary gland involvement, resulting in parotidomegaly.[6] A chest X-ray usually shows hilar enlargement and a Kveim test confirms the diagnosis. Uveoparotid fever (Boeck's sarcoidosis) or Heerfordt's syndrome is a rare cause of salivary gland swelling in which there is associated uveitis and pyrexia.[6]

SALIVARY GLAND TUMOURS

Salivary gland tumours account for 3% of all head and neck tumours. Of these, 80% occur in the parotid gland and 10% in the submandibular gland.[24] The remainder occur in the sublingual and minor salivary glands. The most common site for minor salivary gland tumours is in the oral cavity, with half occurring in the palate. Overall, benign tumours are more common than malignant tumours in the major salivary glands, with 80% of parotid tumours and 60% of submandibular gland tumours being benign.[24] In tumours of the minor salivary glands the situation is reversed and malignant tumours are more common. The only known risk factor for salivary gland tumours is exposure to radiation.[30]

A new classification of salivary gland tumours has been produced by the World Health Organisation[31] and is summarized in Table 14.2. The most common malignancies are mucoepidermoid and adenoid cystic carcinoma, followed by adenocarcinoma, malignant pleomorphic adenoma, acinic cell carcinoma and epidermoid carcinoma. Adenoid cystic carcinoma is the most common malignant tumour of the submandibular gland, whereas in the parotid gland mucoepidermoid carcinoma predominates.[32]

Histogenesis

The salivary gland unit comprises of acini of serous or mucous cells drained by an intercalated duct which connects to a striated duct which in turn empties into an excretory duct (Fig. 14.7). Myoepithelial cells are located around the acini and the intercalated duct. They contain contractile elements and are responsible for the propulsion of saliva into the duct system. Basal or reserve

REFERENCES

28. Levin P A, Falko J M et al J Intern Med 1980; 938: 827
29. Rauch S D, Herzog D B Am J Otolaryngol 1987; 8: 376–380
30. Rice D H, Batsakis J G, McClatchy K D Arch Otolaryngol 1976; 102: 699
31. Seifert G, Sobin L H Cancer 1992; 70: 379–385
32. Spiro R H Head Neck Surg 1986; 8: 177–184

Table 14.2 Simplified version of the World Health Organisation's histological classification of salivary gland tumours

Adenomas
Pleomorphic adenoma
Myoepithelioma
Warthin's tumour (adenolymphoma)
Oncocytoma
Basal cell adenoma
Carcinomas
Adenoid cystic carcinoma
Mucoepidermoid carcinoma
Acinic cell carcinoma
Adenocarcinoma
Squamous cell carcinoma
Carcinoma in pleomorphic adenoma
Malignant lymphomas
Secondary tumours
Unclassified tumours

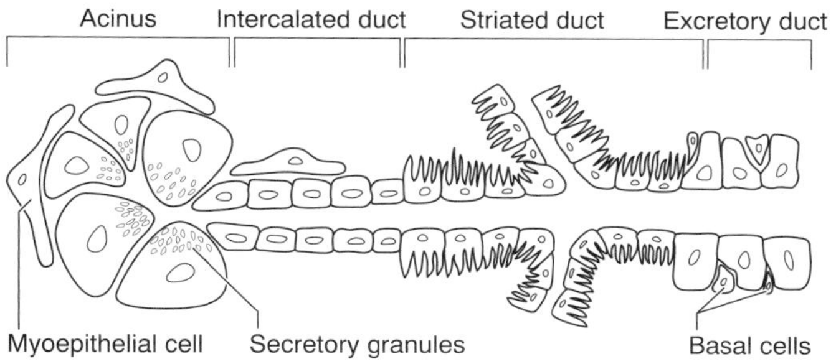

Fig. 14.7 The salivary gland unit.

cells of the excretory duct give rise to the columnar and squamous cells of the excretory duct while the reserve cells of the intercalated ducts give rise to the acinar cells, replacement intercalated duct cells, striated duct cells and the myoepithelial cells. It is now generally accepted that all salivary gland epithelial tumours arise either from the undifferentiated excretory cells or the intercalated duct reserve cells, and not by dedifferentiation of their mature counterparts.[27] Pleomorphic adenoma, Warthin's tumour, oncocytoma, acinous cell carcinoma, adenoid cystic carcinoma and oncocytic carcinoma arise from the reserve cells of the intercalated ducts and squamous cell carcinoma and mucoepidermoid carcinoma originate from the reserve cells of the excretory ducts. The myoepithelial cell is therefore responsible for the mesenchymal components of these tumours.

Benign salivary gland tumours

The most common benign tumour occurring in the parotid gland is the pleomorphic adenoma which accounts for 80% of all benign parotid tumours.[33] The remaining 20% comprise of Warthin's tumours, oxyphil adenomas (oncocytomata) and basal cell adenomas. Benign tumours of the submandibular gland and minor salivary glands are almost always pleomorphic adenomas. Benign tumours of the major salivary glands can occur in children but are very rare.

Pleomorphic adenoma

This is the commonest benign salivary gland tumour and is virtually the only benign neoplasm to occur in the submandibular, sublingual and minor salivary glands. It can occur at any location within the parotid gland. The most common site is in the tail, superficial to the upper part of the sternomastoid muscle in the retromandibular sulcus. When it arises in the deep lobe of the parotid gland it may present as a parapharyngeal mass.

Pathology

The tumour is made up of glandular and stromal elements which may be myxoid, chondroid or hyaline but are of epithelial origin. It does not have a true capsule but a pseudo-capsule resulting from fibrosis of the surrounding compressed salivary tissue. The surface of the tumour is irregular with multiple projections extending out into the normal surrounding gland. The tumour may contain areas of cystic degeneration or haemorrhage.

Clinical features

Pleomorphic adenomas present as a slow-growing painless mass in the parotid gland, or as a slow-growing enlargement of the submandibular gland. There is seldom any compromise of the facial nerve and patients may tolerate the swelling for many years before seeking medical advice. They must be differentiated from other benign and malignant salivary tumours and from other swellings such as lymph nodes, lipomata and sebaceous cysts.

Investigations

The clinical diagnosis of a pleomorphic adenoma can usually be confirmed histologically by means of fine-needle aspiration cytology. Unlike the Tru-cut needle biopsy technique, fine-needle aspiration cytology does not give rise to tumour implantation along the needle track.[34]

MRI will clarify doubts about any possible deep lobe involvement. Pleomorphic adenomas are demonstrated as a heterogeneous well-circumscribed mass of low signal on T1-weighted images, with increasing signal on T2-weighted sequences (Figs 14.8 and 14.9). In contrast, more aggressive tumours have low T1 and T2 characteristics and poorly defined margins.[35] There will be areas of high signal on both T1- and T2-weighted images if there has been recent haemorrhage within the tumour. At times it can be difficult to distinguish a deep lobe tumour from a primary parapharyngeal space mass. If MRI scanning demonstrates a fatty plane at all levels between the mass and the parotid gland, then this is suggestive of a tumour arising as a primary growth in the parapharyngeal space.

Treatment

Parotid pleomorphic adenomas should be removed by means of a superficial parotidectomy when the tumour is in the superficial

REFERENCES

33. Johns M E, Goldsmith M M Oncology 1989; 3: 47–56
34. Engzell U, Esposti P L et al Acta Radiol 1971; 10: 385–398
35. Som P M, Biller H F Radiology 1989; 173: 823–826

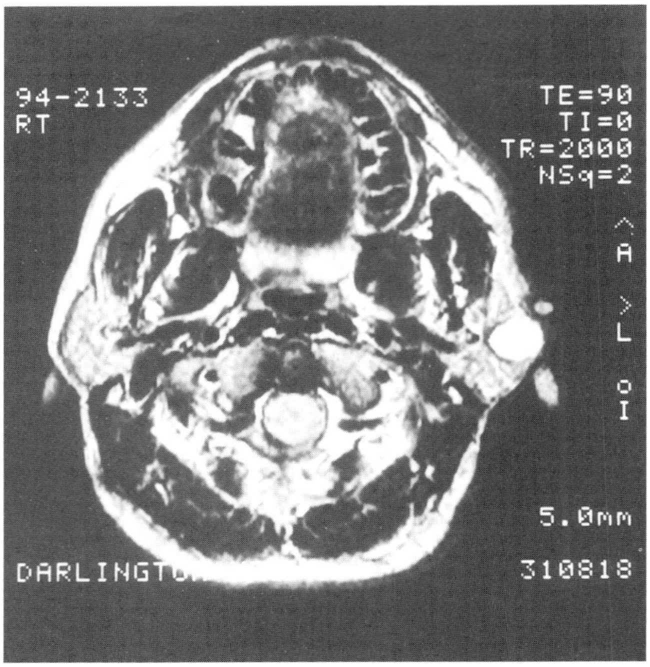

Fig. 14.8 MRI scan: transverse T2-weighted image showing left pleomorphic adenoma.

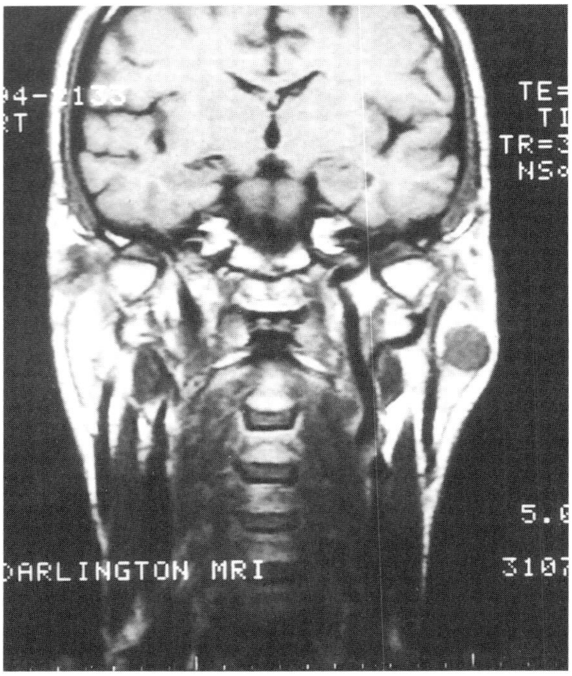

Fig. 14.9 MRI scan: coronal T1-weighted image showing left pleomorphic adenoma.

lobe of the gland or by total parotidectomy, with preservation of the facial nerve, in those tumours arising in the deep lobe or involving both lobes. There is no place for simple enucleation of a pleomorphic adenoma as this leads to unacceptably high rates of recurrence, estimated at 40% over a 25–30 year period.[9] In all operations the facial nerve trunk and its branches should be exposed at the beginning of the procedure before the tumour is removed with a surrounding cuff of normal healthy salivary tissue. In situations where branches of the facial nerve are adherent to the surface of the tumour then such a safe margin cannot be achieved. Under these circumstances the patient should be offered postoperative radiotherapy to minimize the chance of tumour recurrence.[36,37]

Pleomorphic adenomas arising in the submandibular gland should be treated by excision of the submandibular gland. Only in very long-standing tumours will the capsule of the gland be breached by tumour and therefore a safe margin of excision can usually be achieved.

Minor salivary gland pleomorphic adenomas should be excised with a wide healthy margin. Depending upon its site, reconstructive surgery may be required to close a fistula but this should not detract from the need for adequate excision.

Recurrent pleomorphic adenoma

Recurrence of a pleomorphic adenoma is usually considered to be because of inadequate excision at the time of the original surgery. This is perhaps a little harsh in that even the most careful surgeon will find it impossible to obtain total tumour clearance when branches of the facial nerve are adherent to the deep surface of the tumour.[1]

The diagnostic difficulty of distinguishing a pleomorphic adenoma recurrence from postoperative fibrosis in a patient with a discrete swelling in the parotid area can be overcome to some extent by an MRI scan. If used with the intravenous contrast agent gadolinium, an MRI scan will show only slight contrast uptake with postoperative fibrosis but with recurrent pleomorphic adenoma there is marked enhancement.

Recurrent pleomorphic adenomas do not develop as a single discrete tumour mass but as multiple tumour nodules anywhere within the site of the previous surgical exposure. Attempts to re-operate on such patients are fraught with danger.[38] In parotid tumours the multiplicity of the lesions together with the scarring from the original operation make identification of the facial nerve very difficult and hazardous. Under these circumstances it is most unlikely that complete tumour clearance will be achieved but it is very likely that the facial nerve will be damaged. It is therefore a much wiser option to treat these patients with radiotherapy.[38]

Long-standing pleomorphic adenomas may undergo malignant change. This is usually thought to occur when tumours have been present for 15–20 years or longer. The incidence is estimated at approximately 6% in such elderly tumours.[39] Sudden rapid growth in size and facial palsy are both suggestive of malignant change.

REFERENCES

36. Guillamondegui O M, Byers R M et al J Roentgenol Ther Nucl Med 1975; 123: 49–54
37. Tu G, Hu Y, Jiang P Arch Otolaryngol 1982; 108: 710–713
38. Maran A G, MacKenzie I J, Stanley R E Arch Otolaryngol 1984; 110: 167–171
39. Granick M S, Hanna D C. Management of Salivary Gland Lesions. Williams & Wilkins, Baltimore 1992

Warthin's tumour

This lesion accounts for 10% of all salivary gland tumours.[24] Warthin's tumour or adenolymphoma is the second most common benign tumour in the parotid gland. It can arise in the submandibular or minor salivary glands but is most unusual. Although approximately 10% are bilateral, they are usually not synchronous.[24] This tumour tends to occur predominantly in men mostly between the ages of 40 and 70 years. It has been reported in one series that 93.8% of patients with Warthin's tumour of the parotid gland were smokers[40] and it is postulated that tobacco consumption has an important role in its development.

Histologically the tumour is composed of a lymphoid stroma containing cysts and lymphoid follicles. The cysts are lined by a double layer of epithelium.

Clinically Warthin's tumour presents as a painless, well-defined soft mass, usually in the tail of the parotid gland. Because of the lymphoid component of the tumour it can become inflamed in association with upper respiratory tract infections. The patient may report that the tumour fluctuates in size and is intermittently painful. In severe cases a massive increase in size may be alarming, raising the possibility of a malignant tumour. Although malignant transformation within a Warthin's tumour can occur it is very rare.[39] The main differential diagnosis is from a pleomorphic adenoma which usually feels firmer. The other differential diagnoses of a pleomorphic adenoma must also be excluded.

Warthin's tumours should be excised with a margin of healthy salivary gland tissue to ensure complete removal just as with a pleomorphic adenoma. Should the tumour be ruptured during the course of its excision, then the surgeon will be alerted by the appearance of chocolate-coloured fluid oozing from the specimen.

Oncocytoma

Oncocytoma or oxyphil adenoma account for less than 1% of all salivary gland tumours.[24] They most commonly occur in the parotid gland and are unusual in other sites. This tumour tends to occur in elderly patients over the age of 55 years. It is twice as common in women and is very slow-growing. The tumour is composed entirely of oncocytes which are found in normal salivary gland tissue in the elderly. The oncocytes contain an abundance of mitochondria. It is probable that most oncocytic lesions are in fact hyperplastic and not neoplastic. The tumour tends to occur in the outer part of the parotid gland and the treat-ment is surgical excision as described for pleomorphic adenomas.

Basal cell adenoma

These tumours occur in the elderly, mostly in the parotid gland or the minor salivary glands. The male to female ratio is equal. Treatment is by excision with a margin of normal salivary gland tissue as described for pleomorphic adenomas.

Vascular and lymphatic swellings

Haemangiomata may be present in the parotid gland at birth or develop later in life. In the congenital type it is usual for the vascular malformation to undergo spontaneous involution within the first 5 years of life (see Chapter 10). Those occurring later on in life often require surgical excision. This is usually extremely difficult and, not surprisingly, associated with persistent and often considerable bleeding. Haemangiomata may also occur in the submandibular or sublingual glands, often presenting as a vascular mass in the floor of the mouth.

Lymphatic malformations, unlike their vascular counterpart, do not have a definable capsule and infiltrate widely across anatomical boundaries. They completely engulf blood vessels and nerves and deeply penetrate muscles and other adjacent soft tissues. The indeterminate margins of lymphangiomata make them exceedingly difficult to excise completely.

MALIGNANT TUMOURS OF THE SALIVARY GLANDS

Malignant tumours of the salivary glands are uncommon, occurring in 1–2 per 100 000 population per year.[1] They occur more frequently in women, predominantly in the fifth to seventh decades. Malignant tumours can occur in infants and children, but fortunately this is rare.[10] The frequency of malignant tumours occurring within the different salivary glands varies. Only 20% of parotid tumours are malignant, but this increases to 40% with submandibular tumours and 50% in the minor salivary glands.[1] Tumours arising in the sublingual gland are almost all malignant. Minor salivary gland tumours occur most frequently on the palate, followed by the upper lip and the buccal mucosa.

Although the cause of salivary gland malignancy is unknown, there does appear to be an increased incidence of the disease following exposure to radiation. It has been reported that the incidence of malignant salivary gland tumours in people surviving the Hiroshima atomic bomb explosion was 10 times greater than expected in a comparable population.[41] There was a latent period of 15–25 years after exposure before the development of these tumours. Similarly, patients irradiated for conditions of the tonsil or the nasopharynx have been shown to have a higher incidence of subsequent salivary gland malignancy.[42] In the USA dental radiology has also been linked to the development of salivary gland tumours.[10]

Pathology

Overall, the biological behaviour of salivary gland tumours varies according to their histopathological classification and whether the tumour is high-grade or low-grade.[32,43–45] Grading of the tumour is

REFERENCES

40. Ebbs S R, Webb A J Br J Surg 1986; 73: 627
41. Takeichi N, Hirose F, Yamamoto H, Ezaki H, Fujikura T Cancer 1983; 52: 377–385
42. Shorw-Freedman E, Abrahams C et al Cancer 1983; 51: 2159–2163
43. Afify S E, Maynard J D Ann R Coll Surg 1992; 74: 186–191
44. Hobsley M Ann R Coll Surg 1992; 74: 191
45. Ball A B S, Rajagopal G, Thomas J M Ann R Coll Surg 1990; 72: 247–249

based on the mitotic rate, cellular pleomorphism and stromal invasion. The high-grade tumours tend to be poorly differentiated adenocarcinomas, carcinomas ex-pleomorphic adenoma, undifferentiated carcinomas, squamous carcinomas, anaplastic carcinomas and some mucoepidermoid carcinomas. The more favourable low-grade tumours are acinic cell carcinomas and some of the mucoepidermoid carcinomas. A variable pattern of aggressiveness may be demonstrated by the adenoid cystic carcinoma which is usually classified by the pathologist as high, intermediate or low-grade.

Mucoepidermoid tumour

This is the most common malignant salivary gland tumour.[24] It predominantly occurs in the parotid gland and the minor salivary glands. There are lymph node metastases on presentation in 15% of cases, while a further 15% go on to develop metastases in the lungs, bones and brain.[9]

Histologically this tumour is composed of epidermoid cells and mucous cells; the latter secrete mucus into the stroma of the tumour and this explains its cystic nature. Tumours are graded high if 90% or more of their area is made up of tumour cells and less than 10% from cysts. The reverse applies for low-grade tumours.[9] Local recurrence is common in high-grade tumours, usually within 12 months of primary surgery.[9] The 10-year survival rate in patients with high-grade tumours is less than 40% compared to 80% in low-grade lesions. Although grading of this tumour can be helpful, the biological behaviour of the tumour, to a large extent, remains unpredictable.

Adenoid-cystic carcinoma

This is the most common malignant tumour to occur in the submandibular gland, sublingual gland and the minor salivary glands. It accounts for only 2% of parotid gland tumours.[9] It is a slow-growing tumour and may be present for many years before the patient comes to see a doctor. It has a tendency to spread by perineural infiltration and as a result nearly a third of patients will have some degree of facial paralysis at the time of presentation.[46] Distant metastases may appear several years after apparently successful removal of the primary tumour. The metastases tend to occur in the lung and bones, the former being more common. Lymph node involvement tends to occur by direct extension, but is uncommon. Local recurrence however tends to occur eventually in almost half of patients with this tumour.[47]

Four histological types of tumour are described—basaloid or solid, cribriform, cylindromatous and tubular.[27] The solid type has the worse prognosis; the others tend to be better differentiated. Perineural spread tends to occur both distally and proximally. Between 50 and 70% of patients survive 5 years but less than 30% are alive at 10 years.[39] Perineural spread of the tumour may result in intracranial extension and this is best detected by MRI scanning. A small proportion of patients with these tumours have facial pain early on in the course of the disease, in some cases before the tumour is palpable clinically, and therefore this diagnosis should always be considered in a patient with unexplained persistent facial pain.

Acinic cell carcinoma

This tumour occurs most frequently in the parotid gland. It is a slow-growing tumour which often metastasises after many years.[9] In a very small proportion of patients these tumours may be bilateral. It tends to occur more commonly in women and presents in the fourth and fifth decades. In common with other tumours it presents as a painless, slow-growing salivary gland swelling. Although various histological types have been described, there is little correlation with clinical behaviour, which is often very variable. Metastases tend to occur late by vascular dissemination to the lungs and bones.

Adenocarcinoma

This tumour occurs frequently in the parotid gland and the minor salivary glands, particularly in the nasal sinuses and the larynx. It is slightly more common in women. Facial palsy is evident on presentation in 5% of patients.[9] Invasion of the lymphatics and blood vessels are common and 20% of patients have nodal metastases when first seen. Histologically these tumours are found to have neoplastic duct or tubular formation. Lung metastases occur in 25% of cases and the 5-year survival rates range from 49 to 78%.[10]

Squamous cell carcinoma

This is an unusual salivary gland tumour which tends to occur in the elderly, usually in the seventh decade.[10] Men are more often affected and the parotid gland is the most frequent site. It grows rapidly and half of the patients have metastatic lymph node involvement at the time of presentation. It causes pain and facial paralysis, commonly associated with early skin fixation and ulceration (Fig. 14.10). Clinically it is important to establish that this tumour is not a metastasis from a distant primary tumour of the head and neck.

Malignant pleomorphic adenoma

This is a very rare tumour and three separate subtypes are described under this heading.[27] The majority arise in a pre-existing benign pleomorphic adenoma and are referred to as carcinoma ex-pleomorphic adenoma. The other two types are malignant from the outset. One is a carcinosarcoma and the other is a histologically benign pleomorphic adenoma which metastasises.

The risk of carcinomatous transformation in a benign pleomorphic adenoma increases with the age of the tumour.[10] It is the epithelial component which undergoes malignant transformation and the original benign tumour has often been present for 15 years or more.[1] It occurs most commonly in the parotid followed by the

REFERENCES

46. Ballantyne A J, McCartes A B, Ibinex M L Am J Surg 1963; 106: 651
47. Conley J Salivary Glands and the Facial Nerve. Thieme, New York 1974

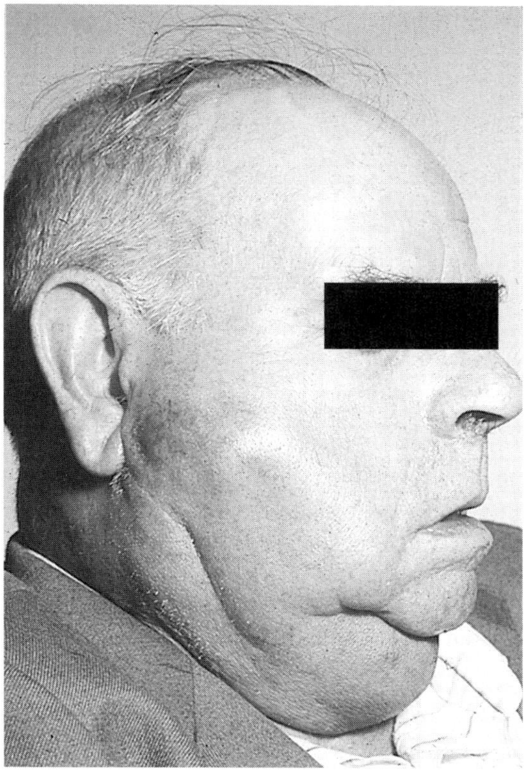

Fig. 14.10 Squamous cell carcinoma of the right parotid gland

submandibular gland and then the minor salivary glands of the palate, lip, paranasal sinuses and nasopharynx.[6] It is an aggressive tumour with a high incidence of metastases and carries a very bad prognosis. The 5-year survival rate varies from 50 to 75% but the 20-year survival rate approaches zero.[10]

Lymphoma

The majority of lymphomas occurring within the salivary glands arise in lymph nodes either within the gland substance or adjacent to it. The majority tend to be non-Hodgkin's lymphomas (see Chapter 34). Primary salivary gland lymphomas do occur but are uncommon, accounting for 10% of all salivary malignancies.[48] They run an indolent clinical course whereas lymphomas arising in intra-salivary gland lymph nodes usually present as rapidly enlarging swellings within the gland. Some arise in association with a benign lymphoepithelial lesion. Patients with Sjögren's syndrome have an increased risk of developing a primary salivary lymphoma (see Chapter 34).

Clinical features

Because two-thirds of malignant salivary gland tumours are of the intermediate or low-grade type, the majority of patients with salivary gland malignancies present with symptomless mass within a salivary gland. The history often extends back 2 or 3 years. Even with the high-grade tumours it is usually several months before the patient seeks advice. Associated pain is not a reliable indicator of malignancy, but when pain occurs in a histologically proven malignancy then the prognosis is worse.[49] The overall 5-year survival rate is only 33% whereas for those without pain it is 66%.

Presentation with facial nerve palsy is very suggestive of a malignant tumour. It is particularly likely to occur in high-grade tumours, especially adenoid cystic carcinomas which have a propensity towards perineural spread. It must always be remembered that facial nerve palsies can also occur in a small proportion of benign parotid lesions. There may well be displacement of the tonsil (if present) and/or the lateral oropharyngeal wall medially if a parotid malignancy involves the deep lobe. Tumours extending into the infratemporal fossa may present with trismus and in some cases referred pain via the trigeminal nerve.

A quarter of all patients with malignant parotid tumours have cervical lymphadenopathy at the time of presentation, and up to a third in those with submandibular lesions. Lymph node metastases are usually associated with high-grade tumours or extensive local spread.

Diagnosis and investigation

The only way to diagnose a salivary gland tumour accurately is to excise the whole tumour for histological examination. Whether the tumour is benign or malignant determines the extent of the surgery required to remove the lesion adequately. Preoperative cytological diagnosis by means of fine-needle aspiration cytology helps the surgeon to plan the appropriate surgery and prepare the patient for the possible radical nature of the operation proposed and the need for facial nerve excision.[1,45] Incision biopsy of a salivary gland tumour will inevitably lead to tumour seeding in the wound and is therefore to be condemned. Wide-bore needle biopsy with a Tru-cut runs the same risk. There are no reported cases of wound seeding following fine-needle aspiration cytology[34] and this is the safest way of attempting to obtain preoperative histological information of a salivary gland tumour. The success of the technique however depends upon the experience and enthusiasm of the histocytopathologist.

MRI scanning is now regarded as superior to CT scanning for evaluating salivary gland tumours.[50,51] There is no exposure to ionizing radiation, soft tissue discrimination is excellent and imaging can be carried out in multiple planes. The scan is not affected by dental metallic artefact. Malignant lesions often have diffuse irregular margins and usually obvious infiltration into surrounding soft tissues. Heterogeneous signal intensity is a common feature but is not a reliable sign of malignancy. The use of intravenous contrast agents such as gadolinium can enhance tumour delineation and show clinically unsuspected infiltration beyond the margins of the gland.[10,51] MRI scanning can also give an indication of the vascular nature of a lesion and is better than the CT scan in demonstrating cervical lymphadenopathy.[10,51]

REFERENCES

48. Auclair P L, Ellis G L, Gnepp D R Surgical Pathology of the Salivary Glands. W B Saunders, Philadelphia 1991
49. Eneroth C M, Hamburger C A Laryngoscope 1974; 84: 1732
50. Casselman J W, Mancuso A A Radiology 1987; 165: 183
51. Stark D, Bradley W Magnetic Resonance Imaging. Mosby, London 1992

MRI scanning of malignant parotid tumours gives valuable information concerning the involvement and relationship of adjacent structures. The external carotid artery, retromandibular vein and adjacent muscles such as the digastric and masseter are easily seen. In some cases the facial nerve may be identified. It can be invaluable in demonstrating tumour extension into the deep lobe or the parapharyngeal space and involvement of the skull base or mandible.

Treatment of malignant parotid salivary gland tumours

A primary malignant tumour of the parotid must be excised totally with a generous margin of healthy tissue to ensure its complete removal. In very small lesions confined to the superficial lobe of the parotid gland this may be achieved by means of a superficial parotidectomy. In larger tumours which penetrate between the branches of the facial nerve into the deep lobe, or in those tumours which are wholly within the deep lobe, the only safe way to ensure adequate excision is by means of a total parotidectomy. Tumours of the deep lobe of the parotid gland can be difficult to remove as this necessitates working between the intact branches of the facial nerve. Improved access may be achieved by mandibulotomy.

Where at all possible the facial nerve should be preserved. In parotid malignancy the only indication for sacrificing the facial nerve or its branches is if there is direct infiltration of the nerve by tumour, observed during the course of the resection. In this situation, having confirmed the tumour is malignant by frozen section histology, the nerve should be excised in continuity with the tumour. Frozen section histology of the remaining nerve stumps should confirm that the tumour does not extend to the margins of resection. It is worth attempting a nerve graft in this situation, even though the patient will have postoperative radiotherapy. Graft function does not seem to be affected by irradiation.[1]

Enlarged lymph nodes found at the time of surgery but not recognised preoperatively occur in less than 10% of patients with low-grade lesions, but are found in close to half the patients with high-grade tumours.[1,45] It is therefore logical for patients who are found to have nodal involvement at the time of surgery, confirmed by frozen section histology, to have their primary tumours removed in continuity with a radical block dissection of the neck.[1,45] Doubts remain as to whether it is beneficial to include a radical neck dissection in high-grade tumours where there is no obvious lymph node enlargement at operation.[52]

When there is tumour infiltration of the overlying skin or mandible, a radical excision of these structures is required in continuity with the growth. Again frozen section proof of clearance is helpful. Subsequent reconstruction can be achieved either by means of a chest flap or a free forearm flap.[1]

There is no doubt that low- and high-grade parotid tumours require different treatment. Studies have shown[43–45,53] that low-grade tumours can be managed by surgery alone and seldom require the facial nerve to be sacrificed. Prevention of overtreatment therefore requires the knowledge of tumour grade. When exploring a tumour known to be malignant by fine-needle aspiration cytology, or suspected to be so, then frozen section histology should be performed to establish the tumour grade.

Postoperative radiotherapy should be given to all patients with high-grade tumours and in all cases where there is doubt about the adequacy of surgical excision.[32,43] This is particularly likely to be the case where the tumour is found to be close to a branch of the facial nerve, but it is a fact that the nerve is not directly involved.

REFERENCES

52. Spiro I J, Wang C C, Montgomery W W Cancer 1993; 71: 2699–2705
53. Nnochiri C, Watkin G T, Hobsley M Br J Surg 1990; 77: 917–918

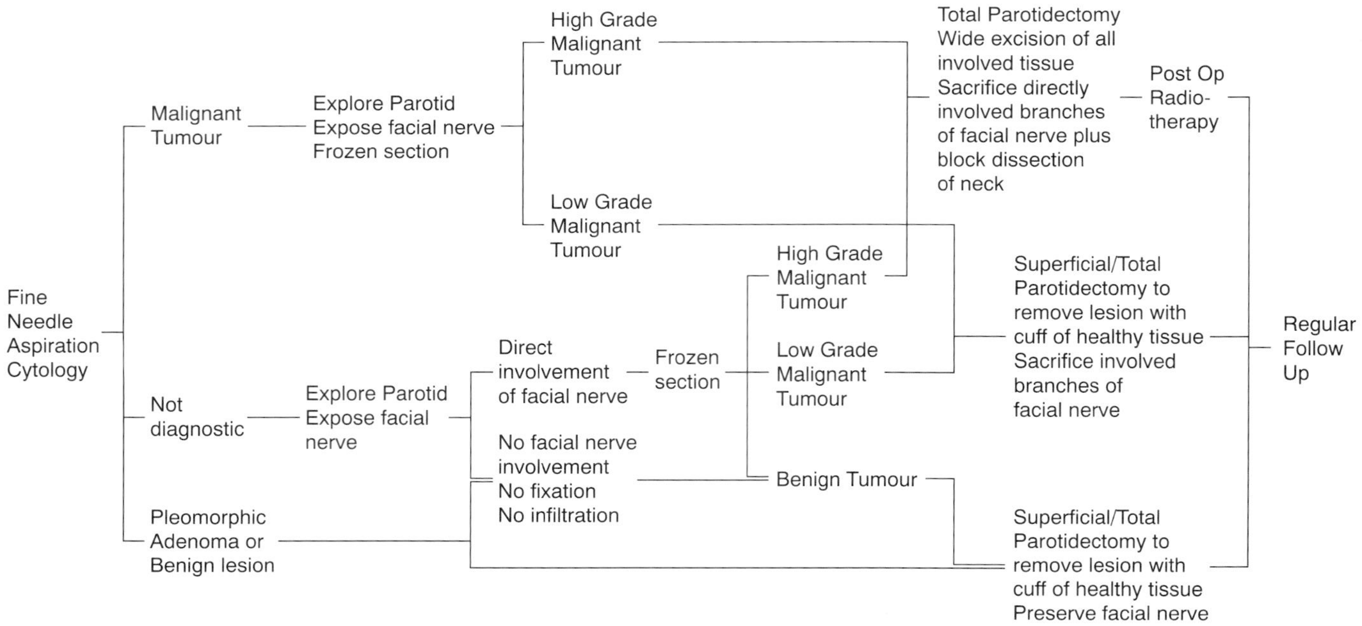

Fig. 14.11 Flow diagram of the treatment of parotid tumours.

Preserving the integrity of the nerve in this situation probably means that at best the margin around the tumour will be very narrow and it is prudent to treat the patient with postoperative radiotherapy. It is doubtful whether adjuvant postoperative radiotherapy is necessary in low-grade tumours and stage 1 and 2 tumours.[1] As yet, cytotoxic chemotherapy has a very small part to play in the management of malignant salivary gland tumours.[1]

Treatment of malignant submandibular gland tumours

With small tumours it may well be possible to remove the cancer by means of total submandibular gland excision with adequate margins confirmed by frozen section.[1] Larger tumours however require more radical surgery to ensure disease-free margins. This may require removal of the digastric muscle, a portion of the mylohyoid muscle and the adjacent floor of mouth.[1]

If there is direct tumour infiltration the lingual or hypoglossal nerves must be excised along with the specimen as far proximally and distally as possible in order to totally encompass the perineural spread. The nerve stumps should be confirmed to be free of tumour by frozen section histology. Resection of the mandible is required if the tumour is fixed to bone. Involvement of overlying skin by tumour infiltration requires wide excision in continuity with the growth. The resulting defect can usually be repaired by means of a myocutaneous pectoralis major flap or free forearm graft (see Chapter 8).

As with malignant parotid tumours, when there is adjacent cervical lymph node enlargement, frozen section histology should be carried out to confirm metastatic spread. Tumour excision should be carried out in continuity with a radical block dissection of the neck if the lymph nodes contain tumour deposits. High-grade tumours are best managed by always adding a radical block dissection of the neck to the resection of the submandibular gland.

The incision should be planned in such a way that it may be extended to permit a radical neck dissection and facilitate the use of flaps for reconstruction.

Adjuvant therapy

There is no doubt that adjuvant radiotherapy can improve local tumour control and should be given postoperatively to all patients with high-grade tumours and where there are any doubts about the adequacy of surgical margins.[32,43] In unresectable tumours hyperfractionation technique has been reported to give good results[54] but fast neutron therapy is even more effective and is considered by some to be the treatment of choice.[55] However, severe tissue necrosis can occur many years after the treatment, requiring extensive reconstructive surgery.

Prognosis

The treatment of salivary gland malignancy is complicated not only by the wide range of different tumours but also the variable behaviour of each type. Malignant salivary gland tumours have a poor prognosis when the tumour is of high grade, of advanced clinical stage, has a facial palsy or pain on presentation or if the patient's age is greater than 60 years. Epidermoid carcinomas, adenocarcinomas, malignant pleomorphic tumours and anaplastic carcinomas have the worst prognosis.[6] Adenoid cystic carcinomas run a long and protracted course and even though there may be

REFERENCES

54. Wang C C, Goodman M Int J Radiat Oncol Biol Phys 1991; 21: 569–576
55. Laramore G E Int J Radiat Oncol Biol Phys 1987; 13: 1421–1423

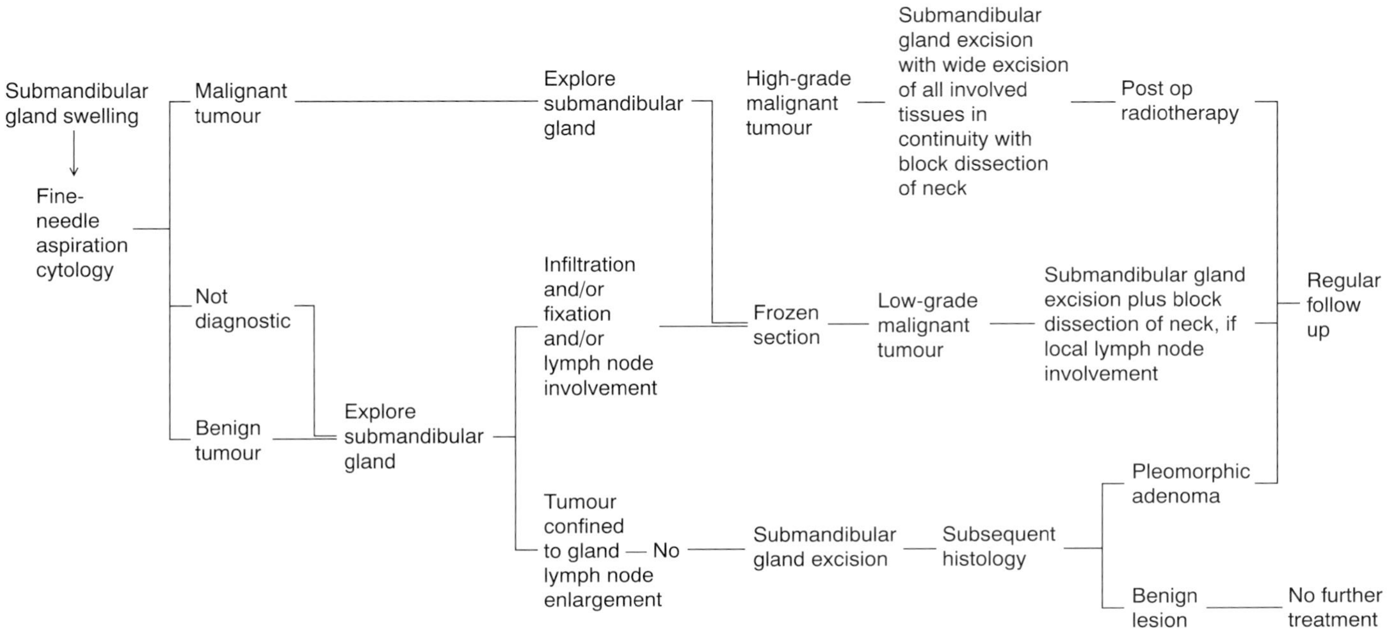

Fig. 14.12 Flow diagram of the treatment of submandibular gland tumours.

several disease-free years following initial surgery,[6] disseminated disease may occur after many years. Ten-year survival rates in parotid tumours have been reported at 90% in patients with low-grade tumours but only 25% in those with high-grade carcinomas.[32] Patients with tumours less than 3 cm in diameter and no lymphatic metastases had a 10-year survival rate of over 90% compared with the rate of 22% in patients with bigger tumours or lymph node metastases.[32] A greater proportion of high-grade tumours occur in the submandibular gland.[32] It is therefore not surprising that malignant tumours of this gland carry a much worse prognosis than those of the parotid gland.

Malignant salivary gland tumours in children

Half of all parotid tumours in children are malignant. More than half of these are mucoepidermoid carcinomas, followed by acinic cell carcinomas and adenoid-cystic carcinomas.[1,10] Childhood tumours tend to occur in teenagers. Surgical excision with adequate margins and facial nerve preservation is the treatment of choice. Postoperative radiotherapy should not be given routinely because of the potential for epiphyseal damage and latent tumour induction.[10]

Salivary gland surgery

For a detailed description of specific procedures the reader is referred to standard works on operative surgery.[56] The important principles of salivary gland surgery are as follows.

Informed consent

Obtaining a patient's informed consent for surgery involves giving information in a manner which the patient can readily understand.[57–59] Studies have shown that most of what is discussed with a patient prior to surgery is quickly forgotten. Information sheets specifically written for the proposed operation help to overcome this problem.[60]

The surgeon must provide patients having parotidectomy with details of the surgical risks. A full description of the danger of damage to the facial nerve and its consequences is imperative. The surgeon's explanation should distinguish between temporary and permanent facial weakness and should allude to the prolonged recovery period to be expected if a facial nerve graft has to be used. When the fine-needle aspiration cytology demonstrates malignant cells, a much more detailed explanation should be given on the consequences of radical surgery. Patients should also be made aware of the inevitable anaesthesia of the pinna and the skin of the cheek that occurs, with a warning that this may take 3–4 months to return to normal. Men should be warned to be careful when shaving during this time.

Patients undergoing submandibular gland excision should receive advice about the small risk of damage to the mandibular branch of the facial nerve and the resultant wry lip. The potential risks of damage to the lingual and hypoglossal nerves should also be discussed.

Parotidectomy

This can be partial, superficial or suprafacial, when that part of the parotid gland deep to the facial nerve is left undisturbed, or total, where the whole gland is excised. The procedure is *conservative* if the facial nerve is preserved intact or *radical* if the nerve is sacrificed.

The fundamental principle of operating on the parotid gland is the safe location and exposure of the facial nerve (Fig. 14.13). When towelling up it is important to leave the whole of the side of the face exposed so that any movement of the facial muscles during the operation can be observed. A sterile disposable peripheral nerve stimulator can be invaluable in helping to identify the nerve. The anaesthetist must be informed before the start of the operation that facial movements are going to be monitored so that paralysing agents can be avoided after induction. Nerve stimulation causes a twitch in the muscle group supplied by the nerve. It should be kept to a minimum using the lowest current setting. Repeated stimulation should be avoided as this may lead to damage of the nerve by myelin and axon degeneration.[61] Continuous facial nerve monitoring may also be employed throughout the operation to give the surgeon audible warning of any stimulation of the facial nerve or its branches. There are several ways the facial nerve may be located:

1. Expose the tragal cartilage down to its tip. The nerve trunk is located approximately 1 cm inferior and deep to this point surrounded by fat.
2. Expose the posterior belly of the digastric muscle and trace this to the tympanic plate. The facial nerve bisects the angle between these two structures.

REFERENCES

56. Dudley H, Carter D. Operative Surgery. Mosby Butterworths, London 1986
57. Edwards M H Br J Surg 1990; 77: 463–465
58. Gunning R The Technique of Clear Writing. McGraw-Hill, New York 1971
59. Edwards M H Medical Audit News 1991; 5: 69–70
60. Ruckley R W, Edwards M H ENT News 1996; 4: 67
61. Hughes G B, Chase S G, Dudley A W, Sismanis A In: Proceedings of the Fifth International Symposium on the Facial Nerve 1985 Masson, New York (Eds) M Portman; pp 381–384

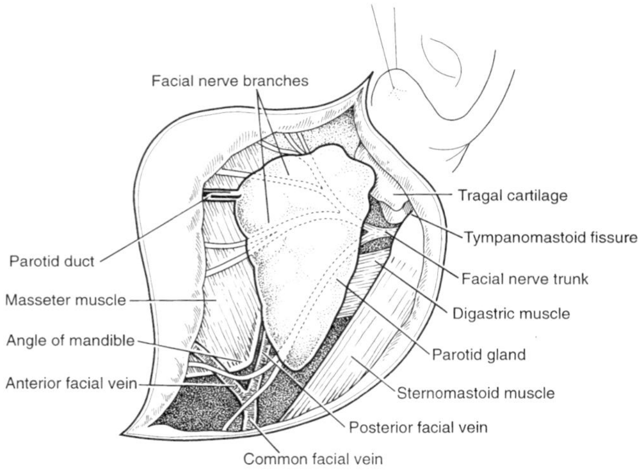

Fig. 14.13 Parotidectomy. Surgical anatomy.

3. The buccal branch may be identified at the anterior margin of the gland as it runs 1 cm below and parallel to the zygomatic arch to the angle of the mouth. Once this nerve has been found it can be traced backwards to the main trunk.
4. The posterior facial vein may be identified at the inferior margin of the parotid gland. If this is traced superiorly the mandibular branch of the facial nerve will be identified as it crosses over the vein. Again this can be traced backwards to the main trunk.

The first method is probably the best but with large tumours overlying the facial nerve trunk or when operating on a parotid for the second time, it may be advisable to work from the periphery back towards the trunk.

Having correctly identified the facial nerve it is then exposed. This is achieved by using fine artery forceps which are used to create a tunnel in the parotid tissue on top of the nerve. The artery forceps are carefully opened, thus producing a bridge of parotid tissue which can be safely divided with scissors or a small scalpel blade without damaging the underlying nerve. The cut edges of the bridge are held apart with artery forceps to allow another tunnel to be created. If there is any doubt that the bridge of salivary tissue contains a branch of the facial nerve, then it should be stimulated before it is cut. Only when the facial nerve trunk and its branches in the vicinity of the tumour have been carefully exposed is it then safe to divide the remaining parotid tissue and remove the specimen. During the dissection haemostasis should be meticulous. Bleeding points should be secured with carefully placed ligatures. In areas well away from the facial nerve and its branches bipolar diathermy may be used.

Even benign parotid tumours may extend into the deep lobe or may be located entirely within it. In either of these situations it is necessary to excise the deep lobe of the parotid gland. After a superficial parotidectomy has been performed the facial nerve branches are carefully separated from the underlying parotid tissue, carefully elevating the nerve as the dissection progresses using a sympathectomy hook. The external carotid artery is identified entering the deep lobe inferiorly. Once it is confirmed that this artery has branches and is therefore not the internal carotid artery, it is divided and suture ligated. Superiorly the superficial temporal and maxillary arteries are identified, divided and suture ligated. Any accompanying veins are also divided, and the deep lobe can then be carefully mobilized from the ascending ramus of the mandible in front, the temporal bone behind, and the lateral wall of the pharynx medially. It may be necessary to divide the stylomandibular ligament to improve access. Dislocating the mandible anteriorly increases the space between the mastoid process and the posterior border of the ascending ramus. In large tumours of the deep lobe it may be necessary to perform a mandibulotomy. Closed suction drainage of the wound is prudent.

Complications

Nerve injury

If any part of the facial nerve is transected during the operation, immediate end-to-end primary repair should be carried out. If it is not possible to approximate the ends then a nerve graft should be undertaken using a segment of the greater auricular nerve.[1]

Haematoma

Reactionary haemorrhage may occur within the first 2–3 hours after surgery. This is recognised by the rapid filling of the suction bottle, or by the appearance of a large haematoma. In either event the wound should be re-explored promptly and the bleeding point secured. There is an increased risk of wound infection following a re-exploration and therefore the patient should be started on appropriate antibiotics.

Temporary facial weakness

Unless there has been deliberate sacrifice of branches of the facial nerve during the excision of a malignant tumour, then most postoperative facial weakness is caused by a neuropraxia and is therefore transient. The surgeon can be reassured if the integrity of the facial nerve and its branches was confirmed by satisfactory stimulation at the end of the procedure. There is usually evidence of improving facial nerve function within 2–3 weeks of operation, but full function may take several months to recover.[1]

Frey's syndrome[62]

This syndrome consists of sweating over the anterior skin flap when the patient eats. There is associated pain in the auriculotemporal nerve distribution and facial flushing. It is caused by the reinnervation of divided sympathetic nerves to the facial skin, from the fibres of the secretomotor branch of the auriculotemporal nerve. When the patient eats, the salivary reflex causes the blood vessels to dilate and the sweat glands to secrete. The reported incidence after superficial parotidectomy varies widely between 5 and 59%.[63] It may be apparent within 18 months of operation, although in some cases the presentation may be many years after surgery. Severe symptoms may justify tympanotomy and division of Jacobson's nerve[64] on the promontory of the medial wall of the middle ear. This is successful in approximately half the cases and helpful in a further quarter.[64] Successful control of symptoms has also been achieved by local applications of aluminium chloride hexahydrate in an alcoholic solution using a roll-on applicator.[65]

Numbness of the ear

It is impossible to carry out a superficial parotidectomy without dividing the greater auricular nerve. This results in loss of sensation to the pinna. Recovery takes place slowly during the 12 months following surgery.

REFERENCES

62. Frey L Rev Neurol 1923; 40: 97–104
63. Johns M E, Shikhani A H Head Neck Surg 1986; 154–162
64. Hayes C L Laryngoscope 1978; 88: 1796
65. Black J M, Gunn A Ann R Coll Surg Eng 1990; 72: 49–52

Salivary fistula

Following a superficial parotidectomy there is a large surface area of exposed salivary gland tissue which continues to secrete saliva. In a surprisingly small amount of cases this may leak through the wound. The resulting fistula is a nuisance, but fortunately invariably dries up spontaneously within the first postoperative month.

Wound dimple

A parotidectomy, whether superficial or total, always leaves a depression behind the ascending ramus of the mandible. Although this is often quite pronounced immediately after the operation it tends to fill in to a certain degree over the following weeks. When the wound is fully healed a shallow dimple may persist.

Submandibular gland excision

The mandibular branch of the facial nerve, the hypoglossal and the lingual nerve (Fig. 14.14) are all at risk during excision of a submandibular gland.

The mandibular branch of the facial nerve can be protected by making the skin crease incision at least 4 cm below the lower border of the mandible and exposing the lower margin of the submandibular gland before raising the upper skin flap. The investing fascia propria is incised and, working in a subfascial plane, the upper flap is developed, exposing the entire lateral surface of the gland. This keeps the mandibular branch of the facial nerve safely within the flap and out of harm's way.

Mobilisation of the gland commences by identifying the facial artery and vein at the posterior margin of the gland and again superiorly one finger's breadth in front of the angle of the jaw. The vessels are divided and ligated at both sites. As the dissection proceeds the gland is retracted downwards and backwards to reveal the lingual nerve. This curves down towards the gland and is identified as a broad white ribbon. It is connected to the gland with a band of tissue containing many small blood vessels. This should be divided between fine artery forceps and ligated, taking care not to tent part of the nerve into the upper ligature. As soon as the sutures are cut the lingual nerve springs upwards out of view.

Anteriorly the submandibular duct should be exposed as far forwards as possible beneath the mylohyoid muscle. The duct is often accompanied by accessory glandular tissue which should be mobilized and removed along with the duct. Before dividing the duct as far forward as possible, the hypoglossal nerve should be sought and retracted out of the way. Once the duct has been divided and ligated the gland can be safely removed.

Prophylactic antibiotics should be employed when the submandibular gland has been removed for chronic sialadenosis.

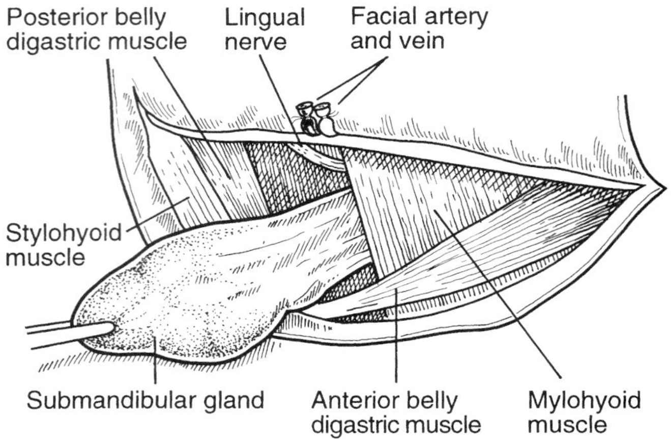

Fig. 14.14 Submandibular right gland excision. Surgical anatomy.

Complications

Nerve injury

The mandibular branch of the facial nerve is protected within the skin flap if it has been raised in the manner described. Overenthusiastic retraction of the upper flap can produce a temporary neuropraxia, resulting in a degree of wry lip.

Both the lingual and hypoglossal nerves may be damaged during the operation, particularly if there is poor haemostasis. Nerve injury may then occur from inaccurate application of artery forceps or injudicious use of diathermy. Lingual nerve damage results in ipsilateral anaesthesia and hemiplegia of the tongue. Injury to the hypoglossal nerve restricts the mobility of the tongue.

Haematoma

This is rare.

15 The eye and orbit

J. S. Shilling

The eyeball is a globe with an anterior cornea and posterior opaque sclera. The intraocular structures are contained within this closed system. The eyeball and its associated structures lie within the bony orbit. The optic nerve leaves the posterior aspect of the globe and passes through the optic foramen to join the posterior visual pathway which includes the optic chiasma, the optic tract, radiations and cortex. The anterior aspect of the globe is protected by the eyelids, and the inner surface of the eyelids and anterior surface of the eye are covered by the conjunctiva. The lacrimal gland and glands within the conjunctival sac lubricate the cornea. The movements of the eye are controlled by the extraocular muscles.

Common conditions affecting the eye and orbit are classified in Table 15.1.

Table 15.1 Classification of conditions affecting the eye and orbit

1. External eye disease: diseases of lids, conjunctiva, cornea, lacrimal apparatus	
2. Acute painful visual loss: uveitis, acute glaucoma.	
3. Painless visual loss:	
Acute	*Chronic*
Retinal artery occlusion	Cataract
Retinal vein occlusion	Glaucoma
Vitreous haemorrhage	Macular degeneration
Retinal detachment	
4. Trauma	
5. Extraocular muscle disorders	

EXTERNAL DISEASE

Eyelids

The eyelids and their normal movements are essential to protect the ocular environment. Lubrication of the cornea is carried out by blinking which distributes fluid over the surface of the eye. Exposure of the cornea or failure of the lubrication system results in rapid opacification of the cornea and blindness.

Poor lid closure is commonly the result of paralysis of the facial nerve. This may be congenital but is more usually an acquired problem (Bell's palsy). It often develops in middle age or later, and the patient may present with a red eye from corneal exposure. Treatment consists of lubricant drops, and antibiotic ointment can be added if any infection occurs. Lateral tarsorrhaphy is indicated if corneal exposure and ulceration develops. Recovery usually occurs over a few weeks but facial palsy may be permanent.

Loss of upper lid tissue causes corneal exposure and requires repair. Defects may be caused by facial injury or may result from the excision of tumours such as basal cell carcinoma from the eyelids. Repair is achieved either by skin-grafting or by the fashioning of flaps using tissue from the other lid or by rotating flaps from the cheek or the forehead.

Entropion and ectropion (Figs 15.1 and 15.2)

These malpositions of the eyelids are usually the result of defective lid support that occurs in the elderly, or they may occur because of conjunctival scarring (cicatricial type).

- *Entropion* causes discomfort because the lashes abrade the conjunctiva and cornea.
- *Ectropion* is unsightly and leads to an uncomfortable eye associated with chronic conjunctivitis and watering.

These conditions are treated by oculoplastic operations.[1] Entropion can be temporarily treated by strapping the lower lid to the cheek with tape.

Ptosis

Unilateral or bilateral drooping of the upper eyelid is unsightly and annoying. It may be either congenital[2] or acquired. Acquired ptosis can be the result of oculomotor nerve damage, muscle abnormalities such as dystrophia myotonica and myasthenia gravis, progressive external ophthalmoplegia and occasionally syphilis. Horner's syndrome may present with minor ptosis (Fig. 15.3). Surgical correction of ptosis can be achieved by a suspension technique using either fascia lata or artificial tissues, or by resection of part of the levator palpebrae muscle.[3]

Inflammation of the eyelids

Inflammation of the eyelids is a common clinical problem. Generalized inflammation called blepharitis may occur. This can be the result of staphylococcal and other bacterial infections or

REFERENCES

1. Collin J R O, Rathbone J E Arch Ophthalmol 1978; 96: 1058
2. Spaeth E B Am J Ophthalmol 1943; 26: 1326
3. Beard C Ptosis, 3rd edn. CV Mosby, St Louis 1981

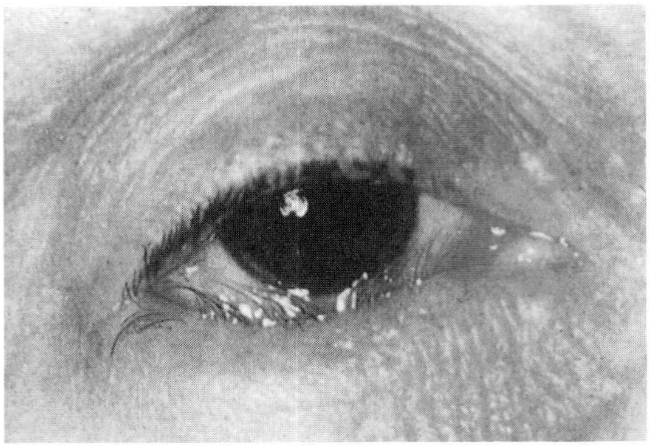

Fig. 15.1 Lower lid entropion.

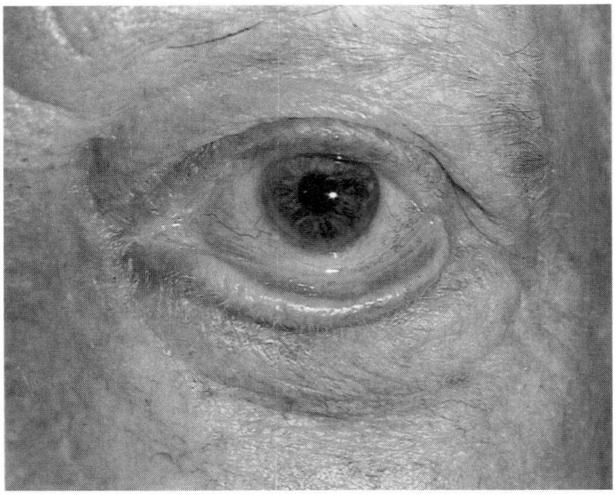

Fig. 15.2 Lower lid ectropion.

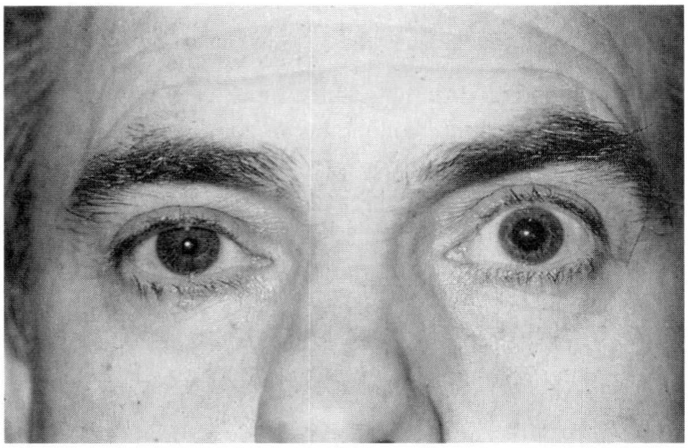

Fig. 15.3 Miosis due to Horner's syndrome.

may be part of seborrhoeic dermatitis.[4] It causes irritation and discharge from the eyelids, and can be associated with considerable scaling of the lids, particularly in the seborrhoeic variety. It is very difficult to cure this condition but regular eyelid hygiene which removes sebaceous material and discharge often provides symptomatic relief. Systemic doxycycline is prescribed for 3 months to patients with rosacea, and may also help others with this problem.[5]

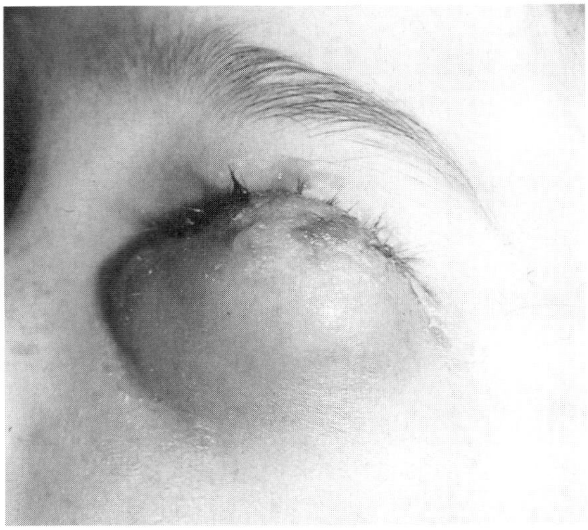

Fig. 15.4 A severe internal stye in a child.

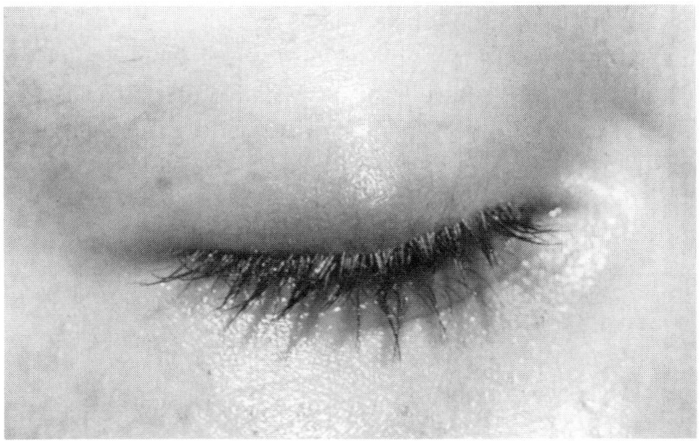

Fig. 15.5 An upper lid chalazion.

Stye (hordeolum) (Fig. 15.4)

An eyelash follicle (external stye) or meibomian gland (internal stye) may become infected. Styes are treated by heat, chloramphenicol drops and ointment. Removing the eyelash allows pus to escape from the offending follicle and encourages resolution.[6]

Internal styes are usually more persistent and may result in the formation of a meibomian cyst (chalazion; Fig. 15.5). This is a granuloma which causes a localized swelling within the tarsal plate. Chalazions may resolve spontaneously, but it is often necessary to incise and curette the granulomatous tissue under local anaesthetic in order to produce complete resolution.[6]

REFERENCES

4. McCulley J P, Dougherty J M, Deneau D G Ophthalmology 1982; 89: 1173
5. Mannis M J In: Duane's Ophthalmology, vol 4. Ch 5 Lippincott-Raven 1997
6. Ostler H B In: Duane's Ophthalmology, vol 4. Ch 22 Lippincott-Raven 1997

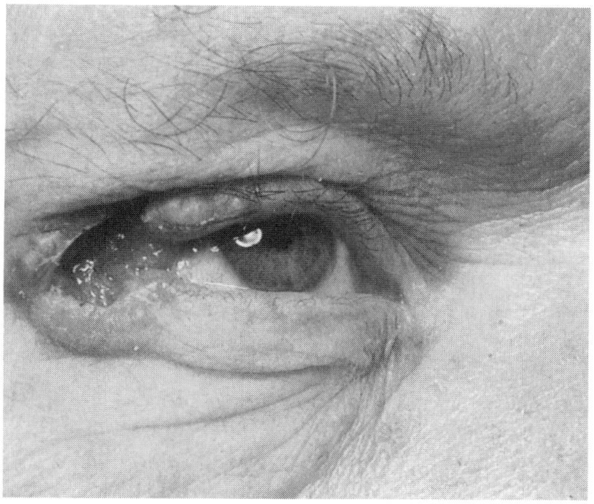

Fig. 15.6 An advanced basal cell carcinoma at the outer canthus.

Eyelid tumours

The most common tumour of the eyelid in adult life is a basal cell carcinoma which may occur in any part of either lid[7] (Fig. 15.6). It is important to diagnose and treat basal cell tumours early and adequately because invasion of the orbit may eventually necessitate exenteration. They are usually diagnosed on clinical appearance but they are often 'atypical' and biopsy evidence may be useful before definitive treatment is undertaken.[8,9] The choices are surgical excision or radiotherapy. The risks of irradiation are small if the eye is protected to avoid causing a cataract or retinal damage.

Squamous cell carcinomas of the eyelid are rare and are only seen in elderly patients. They grow rapidly and metastasize early. Treatment is again by surgical excision or radiotherapy.

The lacrimal gland

The lacrimal gland lies in the upper outer aspect of the orbit and secretes 'tears' into the conjunctival sac. The conjunctival cells also produce much of the lubrication fluid. The 'tears' circulate in the conjunctival sac and drain via the lacrimal canaliculi into the nasolacrimal sac and duct into the nose. Viral dacryoadenitis is the most common abnormality and causes a painful swelling of the lacrimal gland. Tumours of the lacrimal gland are important but rare. Lymphomas, pleomorphic adenomas and, occasionally, carcinomas occur and must be surgically excised or biopsied. The gland may be approached from in front but a lateral orbitotomy is necessary to remove some tumours completely.[10] This is particularly true for pleomorphic adenomas, which must be removed within their capsules to prevent orbital recurrence.[11]

The lacrimal drainage apparatus

Blockage of the lacrimal drainage system causes watering of the eye (epiphora). The blockage may occur in the first months of life if there is an incomplete formation of the nasolacrimal duct with a blockage at its lower end.[12] This abnormality usually resolves spontaneously but, if symptoms persist, the nasolacrimal duct can be probed under general anaesthesia to break down the obstruction.[13]

The lacrimal puncta may not be positioned correctly to ensure proper drainage. The lower punctum is not in contact with the globe in patients with ectropions. The position of a lacrimal punctum may be corrected by surgery.[14] The retropunctal conjunctiva can be cauterized causing it to scar and shrink and pull the lid into a normal position, or a triangle of conjunctiva and adjacent lid may be excised to produce the same result.[15]

The canaliculi may be obstructed by infection with herpes simplex virus or actinomycosis;[16] injury is another important cause of occlusion. The nasolacrimal sac or duct may also be blocked by chronic infection which predisposes to stone formation.[17] Dacryocystorhinostomy is an operation used to relieve blocked tear ducts. An incision is made through the skin of the nasofacial crease to expose the medial side of the lacrimal sac. The sac is opened and flaps are anastomosed to the nasal mucosa through a surgically created defect in the bones of the lacrimal fossa. The operation is very effective providing the lacrimal canaliculi are not involved; if they are involved, the success rate falls to around 60–70%.[18,19]

Acute dacryocystitis

Acute inflammation of the lacrimal sac causes pain, epiphora and swelling at the side of the nose. Treatment is by broad-spectrum systemic antibiotics and the infection usually resolves without requiring drainage. This condition often leads to blockage and a dacryocystorhinostomy is then necessary.

The conjunctiva

Conjunctivitis (Fig. 15.7) presents with a red sticky watery eye. It usually causes some discomfort but severe pain is not a feature and vision is not affected. Conjunctivitis is usually the result of bacterial or viral infection and can occasionally be caused by *Chlamydia*.[20] Streptococci and pneumococci are the most common

REFERENCES

7. Beard C Am J Ophthalmol 1981; 92: 1
8. Mohs F E Arch Ophthalmol 1986; 104: 901
9. Collin J R O Br J Ophthalmol 1976; 60: 806
10. Rose E R, Wright J E Br J Ophthalmol 1992; 76: 395
11. Font R L, Gamel J W, Jakobiec F A (eds) Ocular and Adnexal Tumours. Aesculopius, Birmingham AL 1978 p 787
12. Nelson L B, Calhoun J H, Menouke H Ophthalmology 1985; 92: 1187
13. Kushner B J Arch Ophthalmol 1982; 100: 557
14. Collin J R O A Manual of Systemic Eye Lid Surgery. Churchill Livingstone, Edinburgh 1982 p 31
15. Tse D T Am J Ophthalmol 1985; 100: 339
16. Ellis P P, Bausor S C, Fulmer J M Am J Ophthalmol 1960; 52: 36
17. Jones L T Am J Ophthalmol 1965; 60: 111
18. Hallum A V Trans Amer Ophthalmol Soc 1948: 46: 243
19. Welham R A N, Henderson P H Trans Ophthalmol Soc UK 1973; 93: 601
20. Jones B R, Al Hussani K, Dunlop E Revue de Trachoma 1965; 42: 27

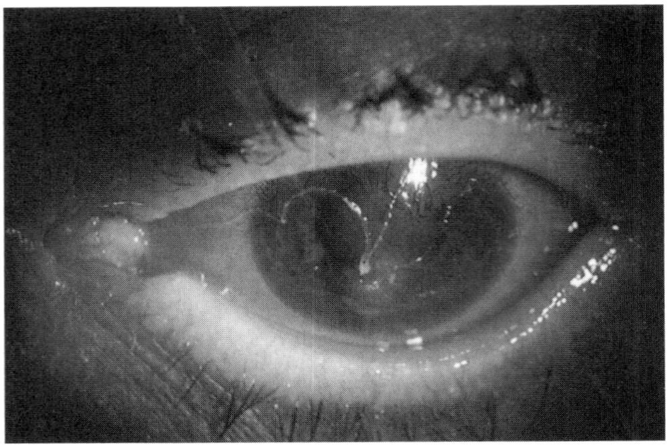

Fig. 15.7 An acute conjunctivitis.

bacterial pathogens, and the most common virus is an adenovirus.[21] Conjunctivitis may also be the result of allergens and toxins.[22] There is a diffuse reddening of the conjunctival sac with the greatest inflammation being furthest from the corneal margins. Follicular hypertrophy of the tarsal conjunctiva is usually associated with viral infection; papillary overgrowth is a feature of chlamydial infection and allergic conditions. The cornea is usually bright and clear, and intraocular examination is entirely normal. Conjunctivitis must be differentiated from more serious eye conditions such as uveitis or acute glaucoma.

Cultures from the conjunctival sac should be obtained; treatment is with antibiotic drops and ointment. The most commonly prescribed antibiotics are chloramphenicol, gentamicin and fucidin.[23] The safety of chloramphenicol has been questioned. Antiviral treatment is sometimes considered necessary and acyclovir may be given. Allergic conjunctivitis may respond to the removal of the offending allergen and desensitization may also be tried.[24] Disodium cromoglycate (Intal) and antihistamines are often administered.[25,26] Steroid drops are not used until herpes simplex virus infection has been excluded.

Dry eye syndrome

A reduction in tear secretion is a commonly underdiagnosed cause of chronic conjunctivitis. Patients present with uncomfortable eyes associated with some mild discharge, which may be associated with dryness of other mucous membranes (Sjögren's syndrome).[27] Therapy consists of lubricant eye drops, protection of the eyes by glasses and occlusion of the lacrimal puncta. Occasionally severe visual loss occurs as a result of corneal opacification and vascularization.

Other conjunctival conditions

The conjunctiva may occasionally be severely damaged by burns with alkalis or acids.[28] There is also a group of mucocutaneous syndromes in which conjunctival contracture and scarring develop resulting in loss of tear secretion and corneal opacification. The most common of these syndromes is ocular pemphigoid which may progress to cause bilateral blindness.[29]

Cornea

It is essential for good vision that the cornea is clear and has a smooth regular refractive surface. Any abnormality of this transparent window of the eye is likely to result in some reduction of vision. The two main problems are irregular astigmatism and opacification.

Astigmatism

A number of conditions cause irregularities of the corneal surface. A scar from healed injury, for example, causes irregular astigmatism and there are a number of conditions in which the corneal curvature is abnormal. The most important is keratoconus (conical cornea) which is usually a bilateral slowly progressive condition.[30] There is usually no underlying cause but it is sometimes associated with excessive eye-rubbing in allergic conditions and there is an increased incidence in patients with Down's syndrome.[31] Corneal irregularities are usually treated successfully by contact lenses but it is occasionally necessary to carry out a corneal graft operation.[32]

Corneal opacities

Corneal opacities have many causes. There are a group of corneal dystrophies in which opacities develop to a variable degree. The three best recognized are granular, macular and lattice dystrophy.[33] The most important is lattice dystrophy: this is inherited as an autosomal dominant and often requires corneal graft surgery to restore sight.[34] Injury to the cornea may also cause opacity, as may scarring following corneal infections.

Corneal infections

Viral infection

The most important infection in the United Kingdom is herpes simplex keratitis which presents initially with a superficial dendritic ulcer (Fig. 15.8); a disciform keratitis may develop later, resulting in a dense corneal opacity associated with intracorneal inflammation. Initial treatment is with acyclovir ointment; further therapy requires careful ophthalmic supervision.

REFERENCES

21. Jawetz E, Thygeson P et al Am J Ophthalmol 1957; 43: 579
22. Jones D B Ophthalmology 1981; 88: 714
23. Fraunfelder F J, Bagley G C Jr, Kelly D J Am J Ophthalmol 1982; 93: 356
24. Rocklin R E, Sheffer A L et al N Engl J Med 1980; 302: 1213
25. Easty D, Rice N S C, Jones B Trans Ophthalmol Soc UK 1971; 91: 491
26. Odenram H, Bjorgsten B, Klercher T et al Allergy 1989; 42: 432
27. Bloch J N J, Buchanan W W et al Medicine (Bait) 1965; 44: 187
28. Roper-Hall T Trans Ophthalmol Soc UK 1965; 85: 631
29. Mondino B J, Brown S I Ophthalmology 1981; 88: 95
30. Krachmer J H, Feder R S, Belin M W Surv Ophthalmol 1984; 28: 293
31. Zajacz M Klin Monatsbl Augenheilkd 1963; 143: 503
32. Paton D 1980 Transactions of the New Orleans Academy of Ophthalmology. CV Mosby, St Louis 1980 p 198
33. Duke Elder S System of Ophthalmology, vol III, Part 2. Henry Kimpton, London 1864 p 865
34. Lanier J D, Fine M, Togni B Arch Ophthalmol 1976; 94: 921

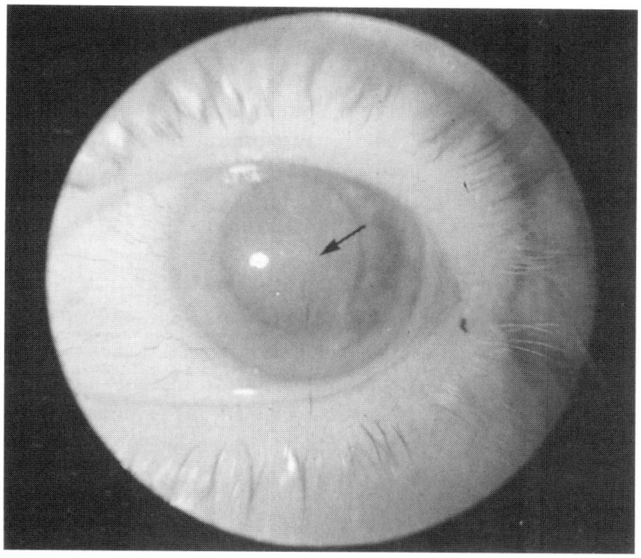

Fig. 15.8 An acute dendritic ulcer due to herpes simplex virus.

Bacterial and fungal infections

Staphylococcal and pneumococcal infections can also affect the cornea.[35,36] Gonococcus used to be a common cause of corneal opacification in the newborn but since the advent of effective antibiotics this is now rare.[37] *Candida albicans* and other fungal infections are particularly resistant to treatment.[38] Accurate bacteriological, viral or fungal diagnosis should be made as quickly as possible so that appropriate antimicrobial therapy can be started. Conjunctival swabbing may be adequate but it is often necessary to scrape the cornea or take a formal biopsy to obtain an accurate diagnosis. Antibiotics, antiviral and antifungal drugs are usually given in the form of drops, and systemic medication is usually unnecessary.[39]

PAINFUL VISUAL LOSS

Uveitis

The uveal tract consists of the iris, the ciliary body and the choroid. Iritis causes an acute, painful red eye with reduced vision. The inflammation is sterile: its causes include sarcoidosis, ankylosing spondylitis and other immunologically based disorders.[40] Cells can be seen in the anterior chamber of the eye with the slit lamp, and keratic precipitates (deposition of white cells) may be present on the posterior surface of the cornea (Fig. 15.9). The inflammation is sometimes severe enough to cause a hypopyon (a dense layer of cells deposited in the inferior part of the anterior chamber). The pupil is usually small as the result of ciliary spasm, and the intraocular pressure may be either depressed or elevated. Redness is mainly seen around the corneal margin (circumcorneal or ciliary injection). Multiple posterior synechiae (adhesions between the iris and lens) can develop and cataract formation is a late complication if the condition is not adequately and aggressively treated. Local steroids reduce the inflammation; mydriatic drops dilate the pupil and prevent the formation of adhesions.[40] Intraocular

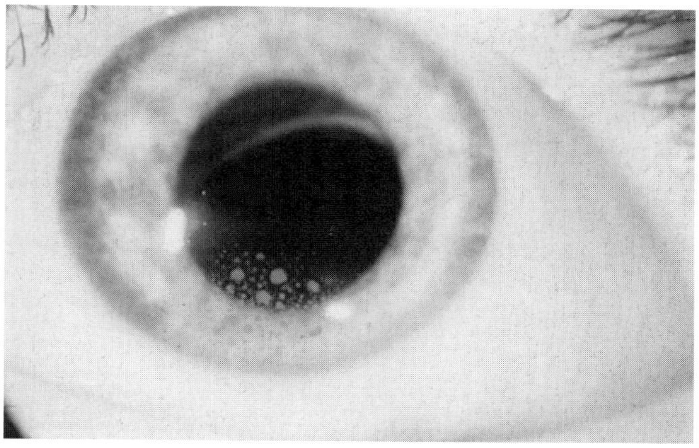

Fig. 15.9 An eye with anterior uveitis showing keratic precipitates, and a dilated pupil due to atropine treatment.

pressure should be lowered by acetazolamide tablets and β-blocker drops if it becomes elevated.[40] The acute attacks may now be treated very effectively but recurrent attacks may cause loss of vision and cataract formation.

Inflammation of the posterior part of the uveal tract (choroiditis) does not usually cause a painful red eye but presents instead with blurred vision as a result of the large numbers of inflammatory cells in the vitreous cavity, and sometimes an associated retinal vasculitis and macular or disc oedema.[41] The aetiology of choroiditis is similar to iritis but toxoplasmosis is a common additional pathogen.[42] Systemic prednisolone is used for some cases in a dose of 40–60 mg/24 h, with progressive reduction as the inflammation resolves. Antibiotics are also used. Other immunosuppressants are also tried if steroids fail.[43] The amount of visual loss is unpredictable, and may be significant and permanent if the condition becomes chronic or recurrent.[43]

Acute glaucoma

Acute closed-angle glaucoma causes a painful red eye (Fig. 15.10). This is dramatic in its onset with severe pain, marked debilitation and visual loss. It occurs in patients who are long-sighted (hypermetropic) with shallow anterior chambers. Pupillary dilatation leads to the iris blocking the passage of aqueous humour from the anterior chamber. The resultant severe corneal oedema is

REFERENCES

35. Jones D B Symposium on Medical and Surgical Disease of the Cornea. Transactions of the New Orleans Academy of Ophthalmology. CV Mosby, St Louis 1980 p 86
36. Jones D B Ophthalmology 1981; 88: 814
37. Ridgeway G L Trans Ophthalmol Soc UK 1986; 105: 41
38. Graybill J R Eur J Microbiol Infectious Dis 1989; 8: 402
39. Barza M, Baum J In: Duane T D, Jaeger E A (eds) Biomedical Foundations of Ophthalmology 1987, vol 2, Ch 16. Harper & Row, Philadelphia 1987
40. Smith R E, Nozik R A (eds) In: General Principles in Uveitis. Williams & Wilkins, Baltimore 1983 p 2
41. Sanders M D J Roy Soc Med 1979; 72: 908
42. Tabbara K F In: Tabbara K F, Hyndiuk (eds) Infections of the Eye. Little Brown, Boston 1986 p 635
43. O'Connor G R Bull N Y Acad Med 1972; 50: 192

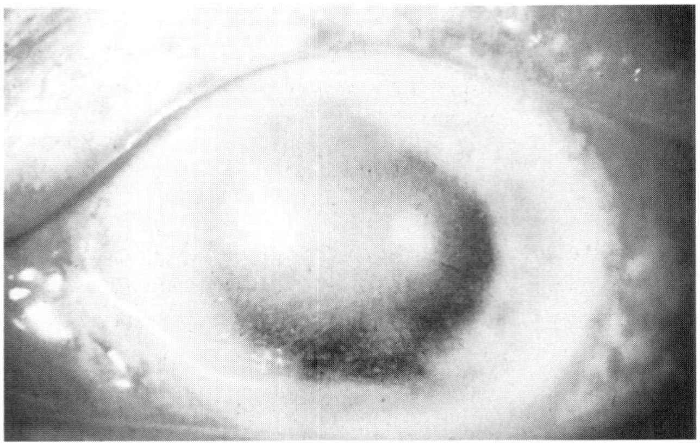

Fig. 15.10 An eye with acute closed-angle glaucoma.

responsible for the visual loss.[44] Patients are usually over the age of 40 years. It is essential that this condition is diagnosed and treated urgently by inducing a miosis of the pupil by pilocarpine drops. Acetazolamide should also be given systemically by intravenous injection to reduce the intraocular pressure as quickly as possible. Oral glycerol or intravenous mannitol is also sometimes necessary.[45] Therapy is highly successful so long as it is instituted early.

Recurrence is prevented by carrying out an iridectomy. This must be performed on both eyes because the condition is potentially bilateral. Surgical iridectomy was required in the past but now lasers can be used to avoid open operation. The window in the iris allows aqueous humour to drain from the posterior chamber whatever the degree of pupillary dilation.

The most common conditions responsible for a 'red' eye are conjunctivitis, acute anterior uveitis and acute glaucoma. Conjunctivitis is a painless condition, but the other two are extremely painful and therefore should not be confused.

PAINLESS LOSS OF VISION

The most common causes of blindness in the developed world are cataract, glaucoma, macular degeneration, diabetic retinopathy and a number of retinal and optic nerve diseases.

Cataract

A cataract is an opacity of the crystalline lens of the eye. There are a number of morphological types of cataract, which may be classified as either congenital or acquired.[46] Congenital cataracts are an important cause of blindness in infancy and childhood. Some are inherited, some are the result of intrauterine infection such as rubella, and some are associated with metabolic diseases such as galactosaemia. Others are associated with syndromes such as Down's syndrome. There are also a number of cases of congenital cataracts for which no cause is found.

The most common cause of cataract in adult life is old age. It is almost inevitable that some opacification of the lens develops with age. Patients with diabetes mellitus develop cataracts at an earlier age. There are a number of other diseases, such as dystrophia myotonica, which are associated with the development of cataracts.[47]

Secondary cataracts are caused by diseases within the eye, the most important being intraocular inflammation (see above). Iatrogenic cataracts may develop after prolonged steroid medication or may follow intraocular surgery. Eye injuries are another important cause of cataract: blunt trauma may cause cataracts after a variable time interval, while perforating trauma will inevitably cause cataract if the lens capsule is ruptured.

Symptoms of cataract

The most common symptom of cataract is progressive visual loss which may be either for distance or near vision. Other symptoms include glare (difficulty with bright lights), rapid changes in the refraction of the eye as the result of changes in the refractive power of the lens, and monocular diplopia. Haloes are also sometimes seen when the patient looks at bright lights; these haloes are monochromatic, in contrast to the multi-coloured haloes associated with acute glaucoma.

Treatment of cataract

Not all cataracts require surgical treatment. Localized cataracts may remain unchanged for many years, and a senile cataract may not require treatment if the vision is relatively unaffected. In children it is possible to remove the lens by simple aspiration.[48] In adult life the development of a central nucleus prevents this simple technique from being used. Cataracts may be removed from the adult eye by intra- or extracapsular extraction.[49] The lens is completely removed in the former while the opaque lens matter is removed with the retention of the posterior lens capsule in the extracapsular technique. Phakoemulsification, using ultrasound to break up the lens nucleus,[50] is increasingly popular and cutting instruments may be used to break up the lens[51] under special circumstances.

Vision must be corrected after the operation. For many years highly hypermetropic lenses (aphakic spectacles) were the only method of achieving useful vision and they can still be used today.[52] Contact lenses are a more recent and perfectly satisfactory method of correcting vision following cataract surgery[53] but intraocular lens implantation is now the most common method of

REFERENCES

44. Chandler P A, Grant W M Lecture on Glaucoma. Lea & Febiger, Philadelphia 1965
45. Campbell D G Perspect Ophthalmol 1980; 4: 123
46. Kanski J J Clinical Ophthalmology, 2nd edn. Butterworths, London 1989 p 234
47. Millar N R Walsh & Hoyts Clinical Neuro-ophthalmology, vol 2. Williams & Wilkins, Baltimore 1985 p 709
48. Stark W J, Taylor H R et al Ophthalmology 1979; 86: 1571
49. Cataract Surgery in the 1980s Ophthalmology 1988; 92(suppl): 54
50. Maloney W F Lincoln Grindle Textbook of Phacoemulsification. Lasenda 1988
51. Kanski J J, Crick M D P Trans Ophthalmol Soc UK 1977; 27: 52
52. Davies J K Proceedings of the Society for Photo-optical Instrumentation Engineers 1973; 39: 65
53. Oxford Cataract Treatment and Evaluation Team Eye 1990; 4: 138

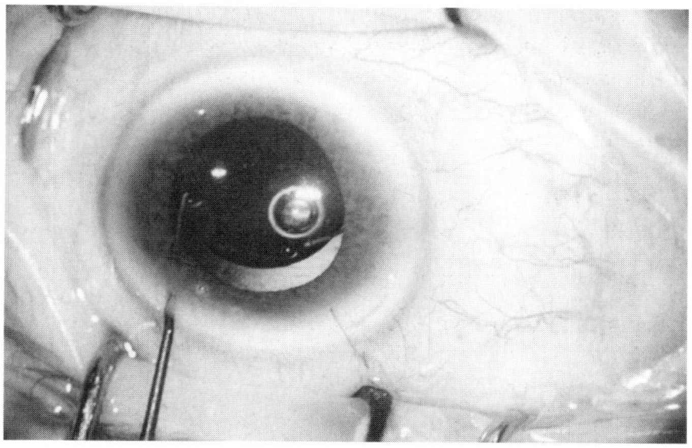

Fig. 15.11 An intraoperative photo showing insertion of a posterior chamber intraocular lens.

correcting aphakia in the developed world.[54] Lens implants may be inserted at a second operation but are now normally placed within the eye during the initial cataract operation. The lens may be placed in the anterior chamber, in the iris plane or behind the iris (the posterior chamber). The most popular operation performed at the present time is an extracapsular operation carried out either manually or by phakoemulsification with insertion of a posterior chamber intraocular lens (Fig. 15.11). There is an extremely high success rate from this operation and as many as 95% of patients may expect good vision following surgery. Opacification of the posterior lens capsule following surgery may occur some time after the initial operation, and this may require division (capsulotomy) to restore vision. This is usually performed using a YAG laser.[55]

The modern cataract operation can be performed under general or local anaesthetic and although some patients are admitted to hospital the operation may be performed equally satisfactorily as an out patient procedure.[56]

Complications of cataract surgery still occur despite modern techniques. Corneal oedema (aphakic bullous keratopathy) and glaucoma are rare. Retinal detachment remains an important complication and intraoperative expulsive haemorrhage is also rarely seen.[57] Postoperative infection is the most feared complication.

Glaucoma

The term 'glaucoma' is used to describe a number of eye conditions in which the vision is damaged by pathological elevation of the intraocular pressure. There are a number of causes of glaucoma. In infancy raised pressure results in enlargement of the eyeball because the coats of the eye are elastic.[58] The adult eye is unable to expand and therefore the type of damage sustained is different. A rapid elevation of pressure causes corneal oedema while less dramatic elevation causes damage to the optic nerve head with increased cupping of the optic disc, damage to the visual field and, finally, loss of visual acuity.

Elevation of intraocular pressure is the result of a disturbance in the production and drainage of the aqueous humour. Aqueous humour is formed by the ciliary body and circulates in the anterior chamber. It then drains through the trabecular meshwork into the canal of Schlemm before entering the veins on the surface of the eye. Increased aqueous secretion is a recognized but very uncommon cause of glaucoma, and the condition is usually caused by a reduction in drainage.

Congenital glaucoma

Congenital glaucoma, a rare condition of infancy, is the result of an incomplete cleft in the angle of the anterior chamber. A sheet of mesoderm persists across the drainage angle, preventing the fluid escaping. The intraocular pressure therefore rises and the infant eye enlarges, i.e. buphthalmos. Children with this condition almost invariably require an operation to divide the abnormal tissue (goniotomy) or drain the fluid externally (trabeculectomy).

Chronic glaucoma

The most common type of glaucoma, affecting 1–2% of the elderly population, is chronic open angle glaucoma in which there is a slow progressive deterioration in the function of the trabecular meshwork, resulting in a reduction of outflow and a slow increase in the intraocular pressure. This slow elevation of pressure causes damage to the optic nerve head, producing visual field loss seen first as an arcuate scotoma (loss of field in the distribution of the superior or inferior arcuate nerve fibres entering the optic nerve), followed by loss of the nasal visual field and progressive deterioration of the peripheral visual field. The central vision is maintained until late in the natural history, and it may be 5–10 years from the origin of the process before the vision is finally extinguished.[59–61] During this time the patient may remain symptomless.

The physical signs of chronic glaucoma are a raised intraocular pressure to a level of between 25 and 40 mmHg, increased cupping of the optic disc, i.e. an abnormally large cup in comparison with the neural rim, and visual field loss (Fig. 15.12). The eye is neither painful nor red and the condition is only diagnosed if doctors and opticians are constantly aware of the condition and carry out appropriate examination of all eyes.

Chronic glaucoma can be treated by drugs or surgery. β-blockers, pilocarpine, sympathomimetic and Trusopt drops, amongst others, reduce intraocular pressure.[62] Acetazolamide tablets are also sometimes used. The most common surgical procedure is a trabeculectomy which creates a fistula from the anterior chamber, draining the aqueous humour into the subconjunctival tissues.[63] Laser treatment to the drainage angle is also used in some patients.[64]

REFERENCES

54. Roper Hall M J Trans Ophthalmol Soc UK 1985; 105: 500
55. Terry A C, Stark W J et al Am J Ophthalmol 1983; 96: 716
56. Davies P D, Limacher E, Powell K Eye 1987; 1: 728
57. Speaker M G, Guerriero P N et al Ophthalmology 1990; 98(2): 202
58. Morin J D, Bryars J H Arch Ophthalmol 1980; 98: 1575
59. Drance S M Invest Ophthalmol 1969; 8: 84
60. Werner E B, Drance S M Arch Ophthalmol 1977; 18: 1173
61. Hart W M, Becker B Ophthalmology 1982; 89: 268
62. Watson P G, Grierson I Ophthalmology 1981; 88: 175
63. Cairns J E Am J Ophthalmol 1968; 5: 673
64. Reiss G, Wilensky J T, Higginbottam E J Surg Ophthalmol 1993; 35: 64

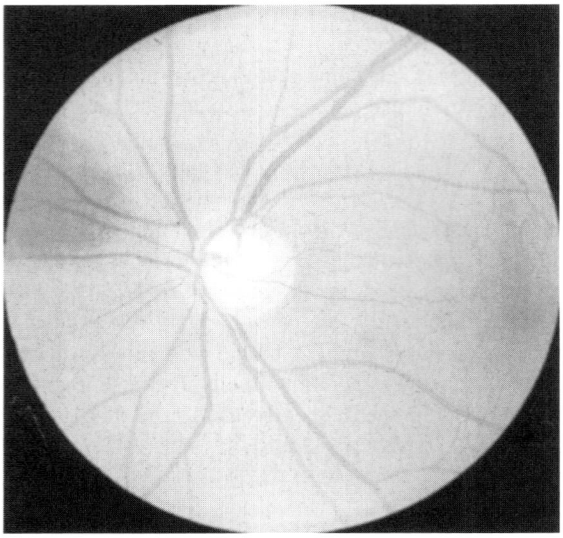

Fig. 15.12 A retinal photo showing a cupped optic disc due to chronic glaucoma. (It also shows a choroidal naevus.)

Progressive loss of visual field will not occur or may be slowed if the condition is diagnosed early and treatment instituted promptly, although damage already sustained will not be reversed.[65]

Other glaucomas

Other rarer causes of glaucoma include pseudoexfoliation,[66] pigmentary dispersion syndromes and intraocular inflammation.

Retinal diseases

Macular degeneration

Central visual loss in the elderly is often caused by degeneration of the macula (Fig. 15.13). It is important to inform these patients that it is only their central vision which is affected and that their peripheral vision will not deteriorate. Navigational vision is maintained, and an independent existence is possible.[67]

Macular degeneration is not a single disease entity but a group of conditions divided broadly into an atrophic type, in which there is slow degeneration of the retinal pigment epithelium and neuroretina, and disciform degeneration in which new subretinal vessels develop into a subretinal scar. A few patients with the latter type respond to laser treatment.[68]

Diabetic retinopathy

Diabetic retinopathy is an extremely common complication of diabetes mellitus. It is the most common cause for blind registration in the 30–60 year age group.[69]

Diabetic retinopathy is divided into a number of different types. Background retinopathy consists of haemorrhages, exudates and vascular changes in the absence of neovascularization. The macula is not affected. This type of retinopathy does not require treatment other than continued observation and good diabetic control.[70]

Diabetic maculopathy occurs when macular function is damaged by the diabetic process. This takes various forms. The most important subtype from the therapeutic point of view is focal exudative maculopathy in which exudate and oedema arising from localized areas of vascular abnormality encroach on the macula (Fig. 15.14). This condition may result in loss of macular function and responds well to argon laser photocoagulation.[71] Diffuse oedema and ischaemia of the macula respond less well to laser treatment.[72]

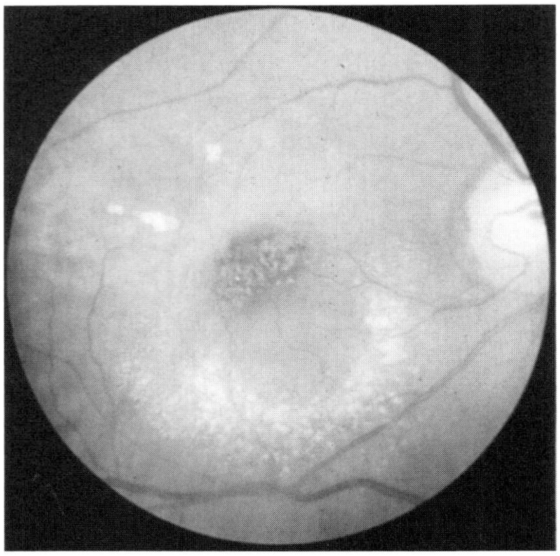

Fig. 15.13 The typical appearance of advanced macular degeneration.

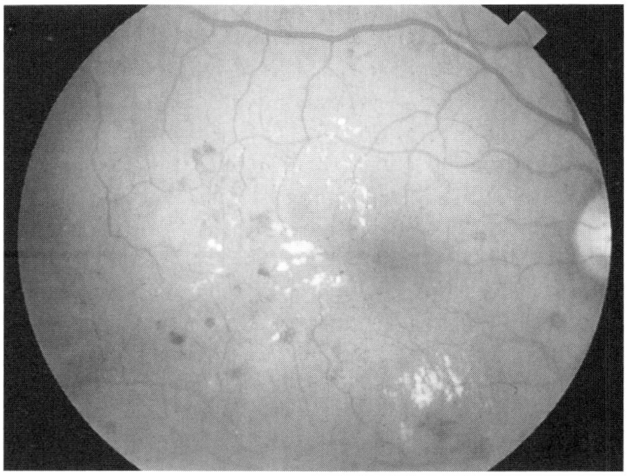

Fig. 15.14 A typical example of exudative diabetic maculopathy requiring laser treatment.

REFERENCES

65. Armaly M F Arch Ophthalmol 1969; 81: 25
66. Gradle H S, Sugar H S Am J Ophthalmol 1947; 30: 12
67. Ghafour I M, Allan D, Foulds W S Br J Ophthalmol 1983; 67: 209
68. Macular Photocoagulation Group Arch Ophthalmol 1982; 100: 912
69. Caird F L, Burditt A F, Draper G J Diabetes 1968; 17: 121
70. DCCT Research Group N Engl J Med 1993; 329: 977
71. ETDRS Group Arch Ophthalmol 1985; 103: 1796
72. Ticho U, Patz A Am J Ophthalmol 1973; 76: 880

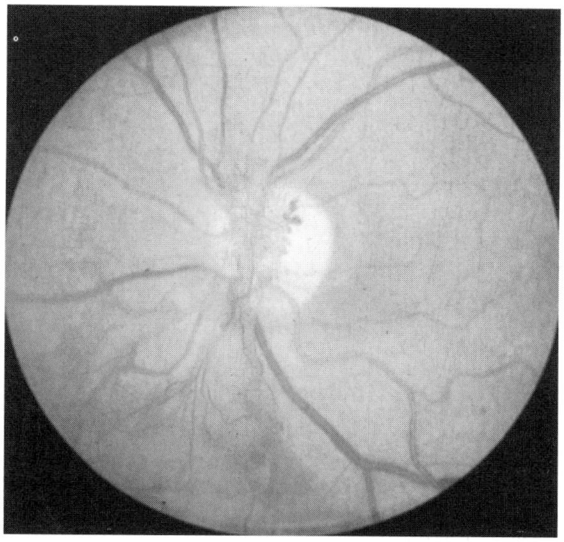

Fig. 15.15 Neovascularization arising from the optic disc in a patient with proliferative diabetic retinopathy.

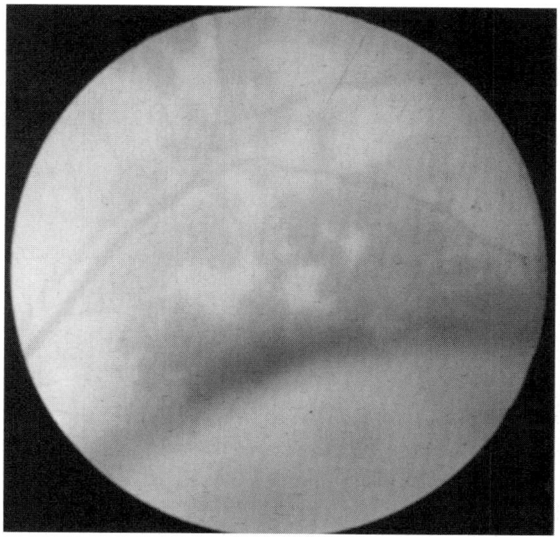

Fig. 15.16 An elevated malignant melanoma of the choroid causing retinal detachment.

The third form of retinopathy, which is the most severe and causes severe loss of vision if untreated, is proliferative diabetic retinopathy. Neovascularization grows from the optic disc (Fig. 15.15) or from areas of peripheral retina. The new vessels develop in response to retinal ischaemia and cause recurrent haemorrhages into the vitreous with the development of fibrovascular traction retinal detachment. These complications of proliferative retinopathy eventually lead to blindness. Proliferative retinopathy may be controlled by argon laser photocoagulation which is used to destroy areas of ischaemic retina. There is an 80% chance that the neovascularization will resolve with this form of therapy.[73]

Some patients are seen in whom either the treatment has been ineffective or who have presented too late for photocoagulation. It is possible to improve some of these patients by performing microvitreoretinal surgery to remove blood from the vitreous humour and to relieve areas of traction retinal detachment. Visualization in the eye is achieved by fibreoptic illumination and cutting instruments are inserted through small incisions to dissect and cut away the traction bands and the intraocular blood. The intraocular pressure is maintained during the operation by a continuous infusion into the vitreous cavity. The results of vitreous surgery are less satisfactory than argon laser photocoagulation applied at the correct time[74] (i.e. before complications have occurred).

Retinal detachment

Retinal detachment is the development of a separation between the neuroretina and underlying retinal pigment epithelium. This cleavage occurs in the embryological plane of invagination of the optic vesicle which forms the optic cup. Retinal detachment has three major causes:

Pathology beneath the retina such as inflammation or an intraocular tumour (for example, a malignant melanoma) can cause detachment (Fig. 15.16). The treatment depends upon the primary cause, for example it may be necessary to enucleate the eye for an intraocular malignant melanoma or give radiotherapy. The treatment of inflammatory detachments depends on the cause but often requires the use of steroids and immunosuppression.

Preretinal traction as the result of fibrous tissue developing on the vitreous side of the retina is another important cause of detachment. This may complicate diabetic retinopathy and may also follow other retinal vascular diseases,[75] or ocular injury. The retina is usually elevated in one area initially but may progress to total detachment. Treatment of this type of retinal detachment requires microvitreoretinal surgery, as described in diabetic retinopathy, to remove the sources of traction.

Tears or breaks in the retina are the most common cause of retinal detachment. They allow fluid to pass from the vitreous cavity into the subretinal space (Fig. 15.17). Breaks may be the result of peripheral retinal degeneration, sometimes occurring as a familial abnormality. They may also develop as a result of injury or following traction on the retina from a vitreous detachment. The latter is a normal occurrence during life and usually does not cause serious complications, but abnormal vitreoretinal adhesions are responsible for the retinal break. This condition is much more common in patients with severe myopia.

Retinal breaks may be symptomless, but flashes of light and floaters in the vision may occur and alert the physician to their onset. As the retina detaches the patient senses a shadow or curtain coming over the vision; if the macula becomes detached there is a severe loss of visual acuity.

Symptomatic retinal tears can be sealed by laser therapy or cryotherapy.[76] These techniques create a chorioretinal adhesion

REFERENCES

73. Diabetic Retinopathy Study Research Group Ophthalmology 1981; 88: 583
74. Diabetic Retinopathy Vitrectomy Group Arch Ophthalmol 1985; 103: 1644
75. Aaberg T M, Abrams G W Ophthalmology 1987; 94: 7755

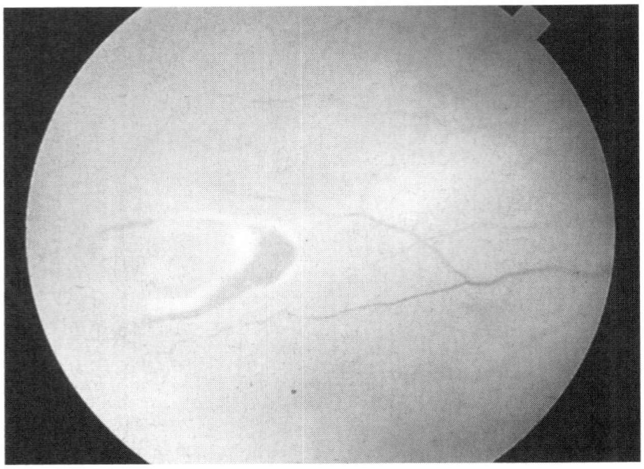

Fig. 15.17 Retinal detachment due to a U-shaped peripheral retinal tear.

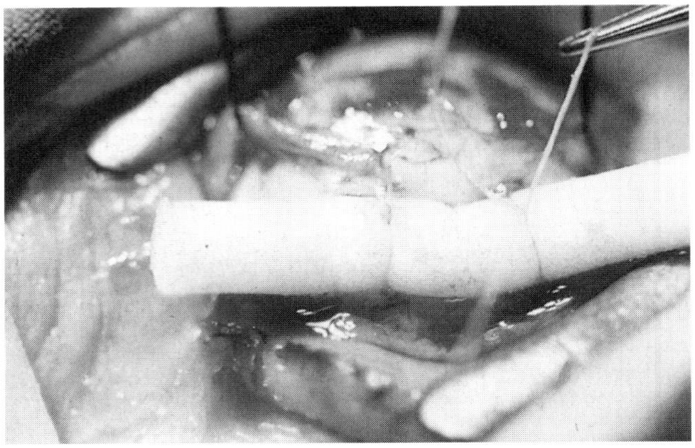

Fig. 15.18 Intraoperative photo showing the suturing of a Silastic sponge explant to indent the sclera against retinal breaks.

around the retinal tear to prevent it detaching. This is only possible while the retina remains flat. Once the retina has detached and the break is not in contact with the underlying pigment epithelium it is necessary to appose the break to the pigment epithelium. This usually involves indenting the sclera against the break using Silastic explants (Fig. 15.18). It is sometimes preferable to perform the operation from within the globe by injecting air and thus flattening the retina from inside. This latter technique is used particularly for superior bullous detachments in which the retinal break is difficult to localize from an external examination, thus making scleral indentation unpredictable. It is also used for complex cases.

The success rate of retinal surgery depends upon the extent of the detachment at the time of diagnosis. A flat retinal break can be successfully treated in 99% of cases with a good prospect of maintaining almost full vision.[77] Once the retina has detached the success rate of surgery falls to 85%, and restoration of good vision is rarely achieved if the macula has been detached prior to surgery. It is therefore very important that symptoms of retinal detachment are taken seriously and that the condition is diagnosed at an early stage by careful ophthalmoscopy through dilated pupils.

Retinal vascular disease

Occlusion of the retinal vasculature results in loss of part or all the vision in the affected eye. The most severe event is a central retinal artery occlusion which results in sudden complete loss of vision. The ophthalmoscope reveals closed arteries and a cherry-red spot at the macula (Fig. 15.19). This catastrophe is usually caused by an embolus which normally arises from the carotid artery and should stimulate a search for carotid vascular disease (see Chapter 10). Emboli may also arise from the heart or great vessels and a full cardiac examination is essential.[78] Cranial arteritis[79] is responsible for a few central retinal occlusions; if this diagnosis is suspected, the erythrocyte sedimentation rate and temporal artery biopsy should be urgently obtained.[80]

Treatment of central retinal artery occlusions is rarely successful but massage to reduce intraocular pressure and vasodilators occasionally reverse the condition.[81]

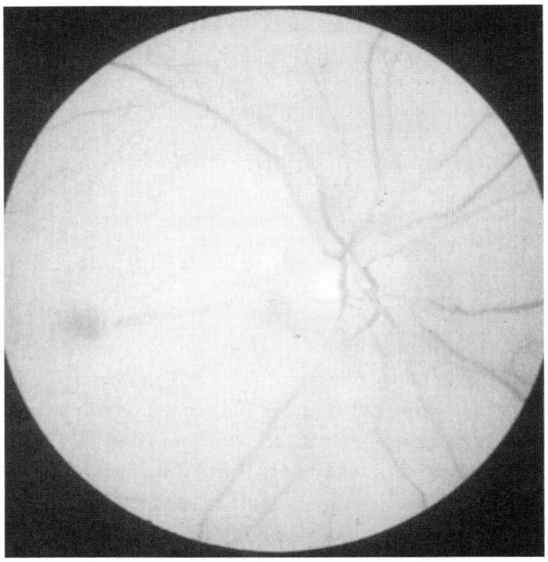

Fig. 15.19 An ischaemic retina with a cherry-red spot at the macula due to a central retinal artery occlusion.

Branch artery occlusions may cause a partial loss of vision. These are also usually embolic but are occasionally due to inflammation.[82]

Retinal vein occlusions

Occlusion of the central retinal vein causes blurring of the vision (Fig. 15.20). Some patients with this problem have glaucoma[83] and it is important that this condition is excluded. The most important

REFERENCES

76. Benson W E Retinal Detachment, 2nd edn. J B Lippincott, Philadelphia 1988 p193
77. Chignell A H, Shilling J S Br J Ophthalmol 1973; 57: 291
78. Arruga J, Sanders M D Ophthalmology 1982; 98: 1336
79. Wang F M, Henkind P Surv Ophthalmol 1979; 32: 264
80. Wagener H P, Hollenhorst R W Am J Ophthalmol 1958; 45: 617
81. Ffytche T J Trans Ophthalmol Soc UK 1974; 94: 468
82. Sanders M D Eye 1987; 1: 941
83. Frucht J, Shapiro A, Merin S Br J Ophthalmol 1984; 68: 26

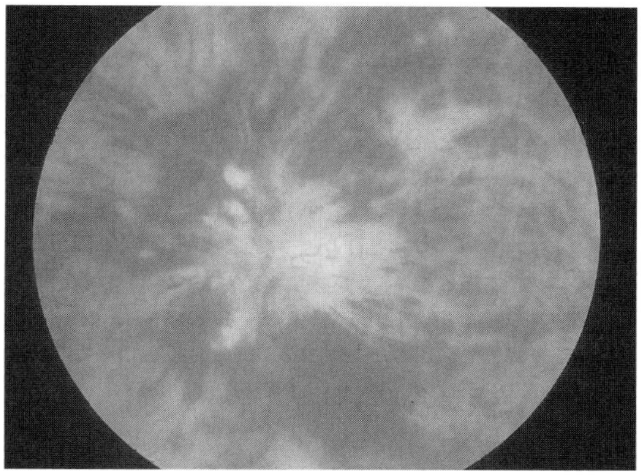

Fig. 15.20 An acute central retinal vein occlusion.

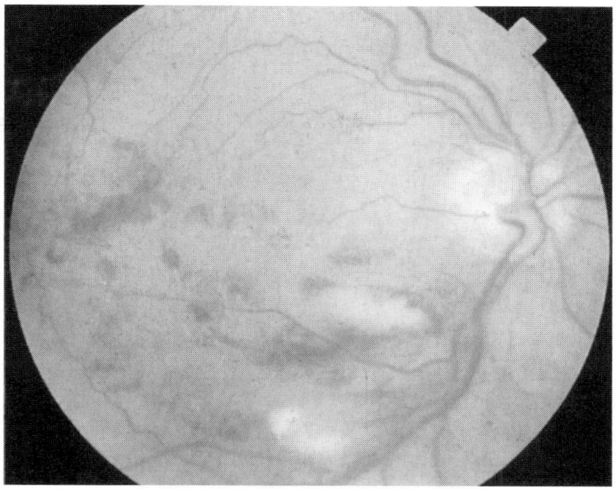

Fig. 15.21 A recent inferotemporal retinal branch vein occlusion.

complication of central vein occlusion is thrombotic glaucoma caused by new vessels occluding the drainage angle of the anterior chamber, resulting in a painful blind eye. This may be prevented by laser treatment, performed before new vessels develop.[84]

Branch retinal vein occlusions are common and cause a partial loss of vision (Fig. 15.21). They occur at arteriovenous junctions where the vein is compressed by an arteriosclerotic artery.[85] The initial loss of vision may improve spontaneously but sometimes macular oedema is persistent and in other patients the development of retinal neovascularization causes vitreous haemorrhage. Argon laser photocoagulation is sometimes helpful in preventing and treating these complications.[86] The systemic blood pressure is often raised, and should be lowered.

Retinal vasculitis

Inflammation of retinal vessels may result from a number of systemic diseases including sarcoidosis, Behçet's disease and syphilis. These patients may develop macular oedema or neovascularization.

Diseases of the optic nerve

Disease of the optic nerve results in variable loss of vision. Disease of the anterior part of the nerve initially causes disc oedema with subsequent optic atrophy. Posterior pathology causes optic atrophy. The most common conditions that affect the optic nerve are demyelinating, ischaemic and inflammatory diseases, optic nerve compression, and intrinsic optic nerve tumours.

Demyelinating disease

Acute optic neuritis or retrobulbar neuritis caused by demyelinating disease presents with acute visual loss with a dense central scotoma and is usually associated with pain on moving the eye. This visual loss is usually reversible over a few weeks; if recovery does not occur other causes of optic nerve disease must be excluded, particularly the presence of compression. Treatment with systemic steroids is used in some of these patients to shorten the period of visual loss.

Ischaemic optic neuropathy

Middle-aged, hypertensive atherosclerotic patients may develop arcuate scotomata or loss of central visual acuity. There is typically a reduction in colour sense and an afferent pupil. In the acute phase there is swelling of the optic disc, often localized to one half of the disc. A degree of optic atrophy subsequently develops. This condition starts unilaterally but over a period of years there is a high incidence of involvement of the second eye.[87]

There is no definitive treatment for this condition but steroid therapy is sometimes used to reduce swelling in the nerve during the acute episode. It is important that these patients are investigated for vascular disease, hypertension and diabetes.

Inflammatory disease

In the elderly patient severe ischaemic neuropathy can be caused by cranial arteritis. Patients with this condition usually have headaches associated with scalp tenderness, jaw claudication and general debility. The visual loss is initially unilateral but may rapidly progress to involve the second eye if treatment is not instituted.[88] It is therefore essential that these patients are investigated urgently. The erythrocyte sedimentation rate is usually very high and a temporal artery biopsy usually confirms the diagnosis.[89] High-dose steroid therapy is essential and should prevent progression of the disease especially in the second eye.[87] At least 60 mg prednisolone are given daily; double this dose is often necessary to prevent progression of the disease and involvement of the second eye. Treatment should be continued for some months and the high dose must be maintained until the erythrocyte sedimentation rate has returned to normal.

REFERENCES

84. Magargal L E, Brown G C et al Ophthalmology 1982; 89: 780
85. Clemett R S Br J Ophthalmol 1974; 58: 548
86. Branch Vein Occlusion Study Group Am J Ophthalmol 1984; 98: 271
87. Beri M, Klugman M R et al Ophthalmology 1987; 94: 1020

Other causes of inflammatory optic nerve disease include toxoplasmosis, sarcoidosis, tuberculosis and Behçet's disease.

Optic nerve compression and optic nerve tumours

There are a number of tumours which compress the optic nerve. These may be either extrinsic or intrinsic. The most common extrinsic cause of compression is a meningioma of the optic nerve sheath. Optic nerve gliomas are the most common intrinsic tumours and may arise in childhood.

It is important to remember that intracranial masses may compress the visual pathway; for example, a pituitary tumour may affect the optic chiasma and this possibility must always be considered in patients with unexplained visual loss. Visual field examination is essential in these patients and special investigations include magnetic resonance imaging, computerized tomography and electrodiagnostic tests (i.e. cortical visual evoked potentials and pattern electroretinograms).

EXTRAOCULAR MUSCLE DISORDERS

Squint

A squint is a condition in which the optic axes are misaligned. The angle of deviation may be constant in all positions of gaze (concomitant squint) or it may be variable (incomitant squint).

Concomitant squint

Concomitant squint usually presents in childhood. Refractive errors are a common cause of squint. A difference in the refractive power of the two eyes (anisometropia) may result in the failure of binocular function. Defects of the accommodation convergence mechanism are also an important cause, and eyes that are hypermetropic (long-sighted) may develop a squint because of excess accommodation which is necessary for clear vision.[90] Cataracts or corneal opacities which prevent the normal development of binocular function may also result in a squint of this type. Retinoblastoma is a rare but important cause of squint in childhood and it is essential that this condition is carefully excluded. Ophthalmoscopy is essential in all patients.

The management of a child with a squint requires refraction to exclude and treat refractive errors. Amblyopia is treated by occlusion of the normal eye to stimulate the vision in the affected eye, and orthoptic exercises are used to stimulate binocular function.[91] Muscle surgery is sometimes required to align the optic axes. The muscles are either shortened by resection or the position of the insertion is recessed to lessen its effect. Many squint operations are performed entirely for cosmetic reasons but in some cases restoration of binocular function may be obtained.[92]

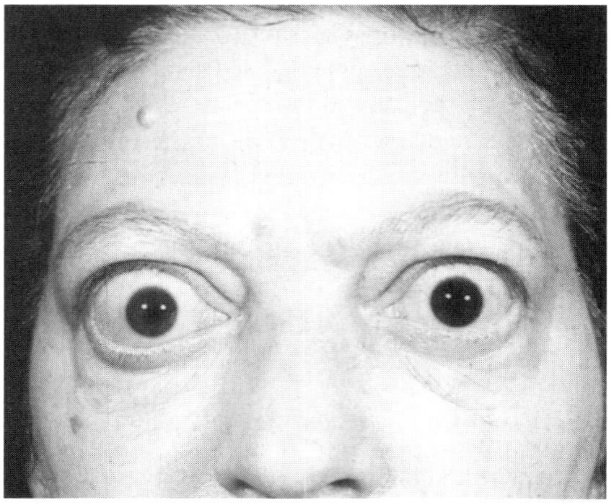

Fig. 15.22 Thyrotoxicosis with proptosis and lid retraction.

Paretic squint (Incomitant)

Paralysis of the extraocular muscles by nerve, muscular or mechanical lesions may result in a paretic squint. The eye movements are abnormal and the angle of squint is variable in different positions of gaze. The management of paretic squint depends on its aetiology, e.g. third, fourth or sixth nerve palsy, myasthenia, thyroid disease and trauma. Prisms are often helpful and surgery may be required to strengthen muscles or to weaken the opposing overaction of their antagonists. Surgical treatment is only advisable if the condition has been stable for a considerable length of time because results are otherwise unpredictable. The use of botulinum toxin injections to weaken muscles temporarily is increasingly used as an adjunct to surgery.

THE ORBIT

Proptosis

Proptosis is the most common presentation of orbital disease. Acute unilateral painful proptosis is usually the result of bacterial orbital cellulitis which often originates from paranasal sinus infection. This condition is common in childhood and requires urgent antibiotic therapy.[93] Orbital cellulitis can cause compression of the optic nerve, resulting in blindness if neglected, and surgical drainage is indicated if the visual acuity deteriorates or if an afferent pupillary defect develops during the course of the disease.

Thyroid eye disease is another important cause of proptosis. The proptosis is usually bilateral (Fig. 15.22) but can be unilateral. Thyroid exophthalmos may result in exposure of the cornea and may also cause compression of the optic nerve with loss of central vision. Defects of extraocular movement are common with thyroid disease because of involvement of the extraocular muscles. Involvement of the optic nerve requires urgent decompression of the orbit to prevent blindness. This may be achieved with systemic steroids but surgical decompression may be necessary. The most

REFERENCES

88. Sanders M D Trans Ophthalmol Soc UK 1971; 91: 369
89. Klein R G, Campbell R J, Hunter G G, Carney J A Mayo Clinic Proc 1986; 51: 504
90. Marshall Parks M M Arch Ophthalmol 1958; 59: 364
91. Von Noorden G U Investigative Ophthalmol & Vis Sci 1985; 26: 1704
92. Ing M R Trans Am Ophthalmol 1981; 79: 625

common operation performed is removal of the medial and inferior wall of the orbit through an anterior ethmoidal approach. Diplopia may respond to muscle surgery, with recession of the inferior rectus being the most common operation. The hyperthyroidism must also be treated appropriately (see Chapter 18).

Tumours within the orbit produce progressive proptosis. The most common are lymphomas and haemangiomas. Pseudotumours produced by inflammatory disease are an important differential diagnosis.

Acute bilateral proptosis is a serious but rare condition. It may be caused by cavernous sinus thrombosis, which is usually secondary to infection and often has an extremely poor prognosis resulting in death if appropriate therapy is not instituted urgently.[94] Caroticocavernous and dural fistulae are alternative causes of bilateral proptosis. These conditions are usually associated with audible bruits and are invariably preceded by a history of head injury. Cavernous sinus thrombosis requires urgent antibiotic therapy. Embolization of fistulae is sometimes indicated.

Pseudoproptosis

A large globe, often associated with high myopia, may cause a pseudoproptosis which must be differentiated from true proptosis.

ENOPHTHALMOS

Enophthalmos usually results from a defect in the bony walls of the orbit which allows tissue to extrude. A blow-out fracture of the floor of the orbit or the ethmoid wall is a common cause. This is the result of a blow on the eye in which the thin walls of the orbit rupture and the tissue escapes into the sinus cavities (Fig. 15.23). This may cause double vision in addition to enophthalmos and some patients need to have the walls of the orbit surgically reconstructed. Some patients, however, improve spontaneously and surgery is only required if diplopia persists after a period of 2–3 weeks or if there is significant enophthalmos. The usual surgical approach is through the eyelid. The orbital tissues are dissected from the fracture and the orbital wall is reconstructed using a plate of artificial material.

TRAUMA (Table 15.2)

Injuries to the eye and surrounding tissues may be the result of blunt trauma, perforating wounds, foreign bodies and burns.

Blunt trauma

Blunt trauma to the orbit may produce blow-out fractures, as described above. Subconjunctival haemorrhages are common and require no specific treatment. Haemorrhage into the anterior chamber (hyphaema) may result in raised intraocular pressure and blurred vision (Fig. 15.24). Hyphaemata usually settle with bed rest, and the raised intraocular pressure responds to medical therapy with acetazolamide tablets. Drainage of blood from the anterior chamber is rarely necessary and is often hazardous because visualization of intraocular structures is difficult during the procedure. Haemorrhage into the vitreous cavity results in severe loss of vision but usually improves spontaneously. The possibility of retinal damage must be considered when this occurs

a

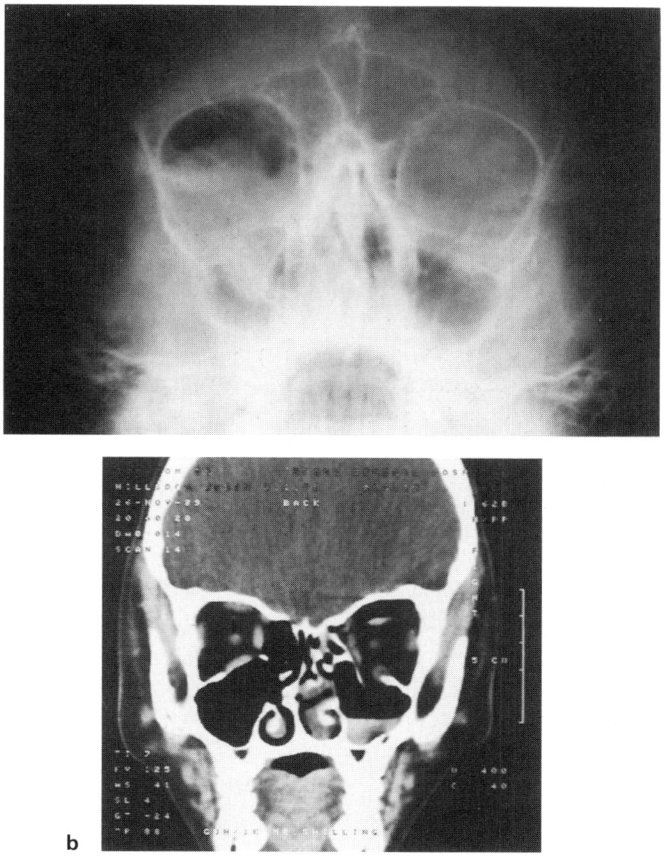

b

Fig. 15.23 (a) Radiograph showing a blow-out fracture of the orbital floor with the 'hanging drop' sign. **(b)** Computerized tomographic scan showing a blow-out fracture of the left orbital floor and the nasal wall of the orbit.

Table 15.2 Early management of eye injuries

1. Measure visual acuity in all cases.
2. Examine:
   - lids, conjunctiva, cornea (with torch)
   - extraocular movements
   - pupils
   - discs
   - slit-lamp examination by ophthalmologist when in doubt.
3. *Blunt injury* – look for extraocular and intraocular haemorrhage. Only urgent problem is high intraocular pressure.
   Sharp injury – look for lids, scleral and corneal perforation. Pad and arrange repair as soon as possible.
   Foreign body – look for foreign body. X-ray if in doubt.
   Chemical injury – wash out urgently with water.
   Burns – look for lagophthalmos. Needs urgent eye lid surgery.

REFERENCES

93. Gonnering R, Harris S J Infection of the Orbit. Little Brown, Boston 1986 p 517
94. Keltner J R, Satterfield D, Dublin A B, Lee B C P Ophthalmol 1987; 94: 1585

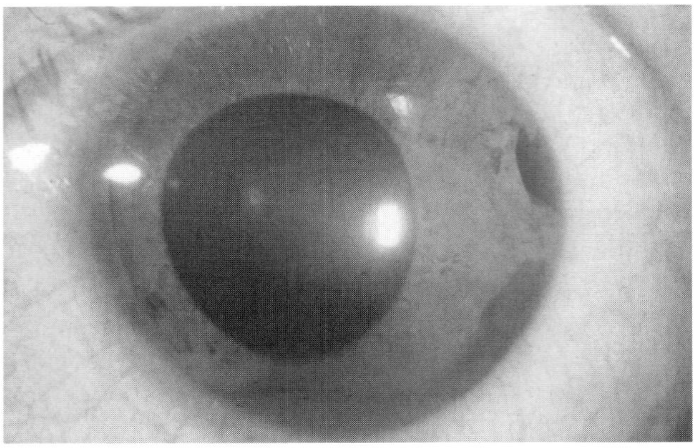

Fig. 15.24 Hyphaema due to blunt trauma. This photo shows iris damage with the haemorrhage arising from this area.

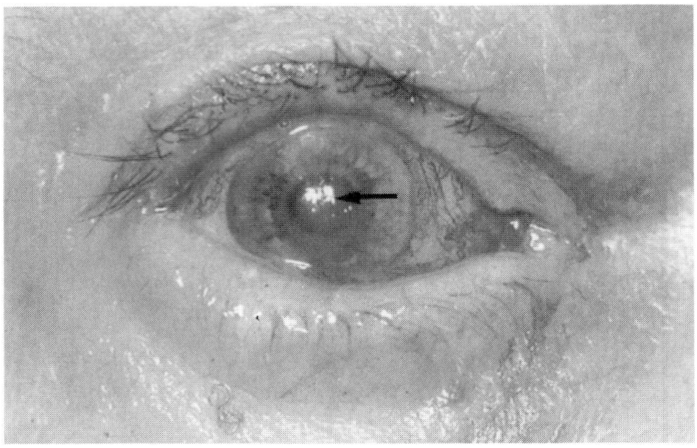

Fig. 15.25 A large epithelial defect stained with fluorescein.

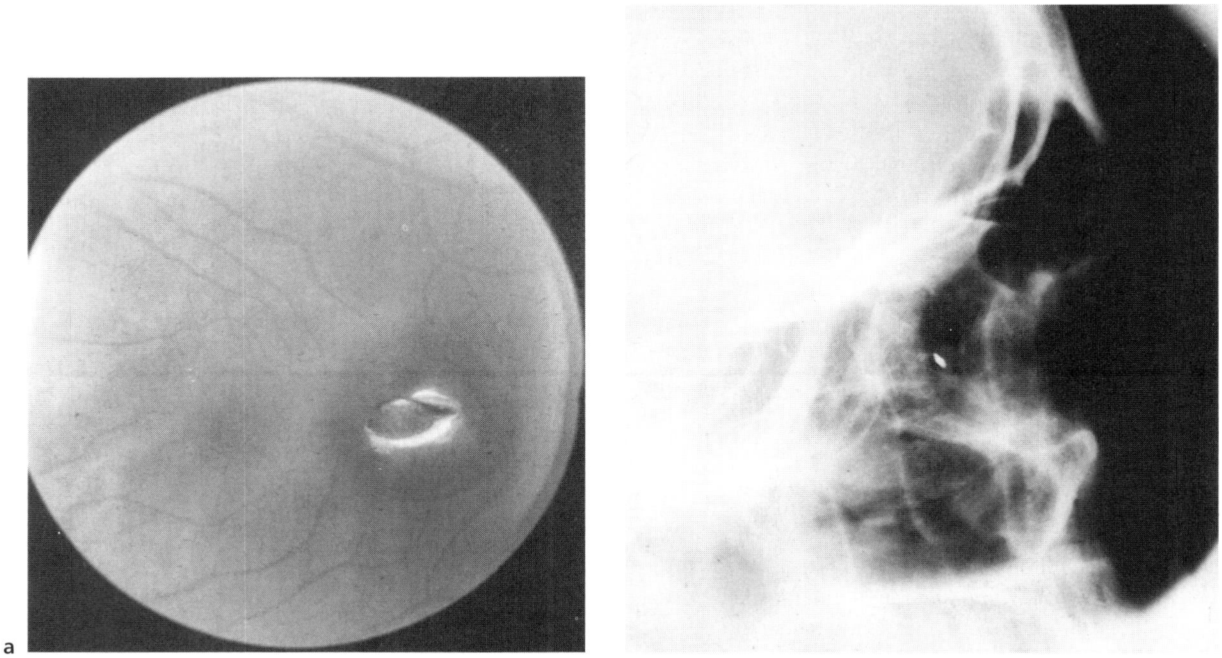

Fig. 15.26 (a) An iron foreign body lying on the surface of the retina. **(b)** A lateral radiograph showing an intraocular metallic foreign body.

and in particular the presence of retinal tears and detachment must be suspected and treated appropriately. Damage to the lens is common in blunt trauma. Cataract may develop or alternatively the lens may be displaced in position (subluxation or dislocation). All lens abnormalities may lead to severe loss of vision and surgery may be required to restore vision. Damage to the iris is common, often leading to pupillary abnormalities. Damage to the macula and optic nerve may result in severe permanent loss of vision.[95]

Corneal trauma

Corneal trauma is very common. Abrasions of the epithelium cause an exquisitely painful eye (Fig. 15.25). The diagnosis is made with a slit-lamp microscope after fluorescein drops have been instilled to stain the defect. Healing is hastened by closing the eye; antibiotic ointment, for example chloramphenicol, is given to prevent secondary infection. A mild mydriatic is often advocated. Corneal foreign bodies are best removed with a sharp needle, using slit-lamp magnification, following instillation of a local anaesthetic such as amethocaine. It is very important to assess the depth of corneal injury. This can only be achieved using a slit-lamp microscope. A full-thickness wound of the cornea requires surgical repair unless it is small and self-sealing. An intraocular foreign body must always be suspected in patients with corneal perforation, and radiography of the orbit is essential (Fig. 15.26).

REFERENCE

95. The Israeli Ocular Injuries Study Arch Ophthalmol 1988; 106: 776

Lacerations

Eyelid

It is important to classify eyelid lacerations correctly so that repair may be satisfactorily performed. Injuries not involving the lid margin can usually be sutured without cosmetic blemish. Lacerations transgressing the lid margin require careful apposition of the tarsal plate before the muscles and skin are sutured. The most important eyelid injuries are those involving the lacrimal canaliculi which, if not repaired accurately, may result in a watering eye. The best mode of repair is subject to debate but intubation of the canaliculi for a period of weeks may be necessary.[96]

Globe

It is important not to miss perforating wounds of the cornea or sclera. The diagnosis is usually obvious but it can be difficult and should be suspected if there is distortion of the pupil or hypotony of the globe (Fig. 15.27). Perforations require microsurgical repair[97,98] and late complications are common. The visual prognosis of perforating eye injuries is variable but with careful repair at least partial restoration of vision may be achieved. It is rare to remove an eye at the initial operation; an attempt should almost always be made to repair the injury even if the eye is severely damaged. The eye can be excised later if there is no vision or if severe inflammation occurs.

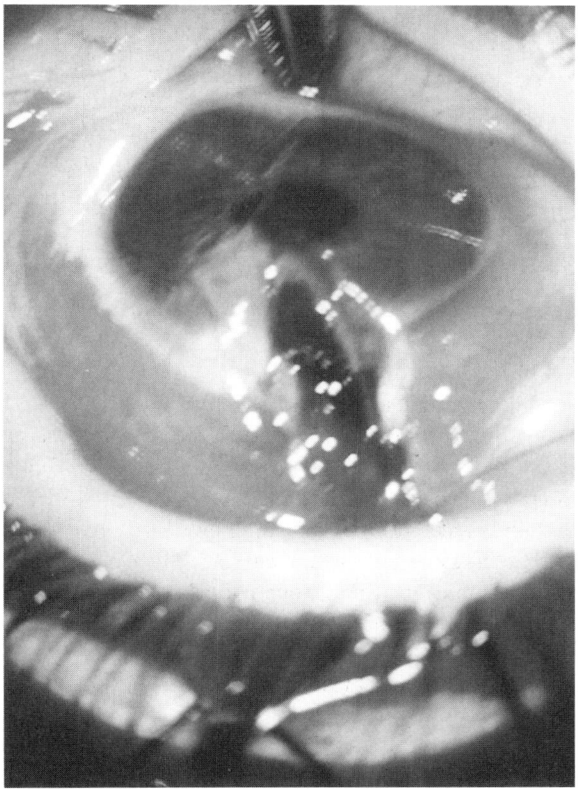

Fig. 15.27 An intraoperative photo showing a severe corneoscleral laceration.

The possibility of sympathetic ophthalmitis, a severe inflammation of both eyes following injury to one eye, must be remembered as a very important complication of perforating trauma, particularly if there is prolapse of uveal tissue. The incidence of this complication has lessened with improvements in surgical repair.[99]

Foreign bodies

Foreign bodies on the surface of the eye may be removed easily in the outpatient department using a sharp needle, local anaesthetic and a slit-lamp. Fragments which have entered the eye require careful management. The most important foreign body is an iron fragment because siderosis bulbi may lead to blindness if this remains undiagnosed.[100] Copper foreign bodies are also important as they cause severe inflammation of the eye if left in situ (chalcosis).[101] Vegetable matter may cause an inflammatory reaction while some foreign bodies, including glass, do not cause any problem over many years.[102]

The diagnosis of an intraocular foreign body must be suspected from the history. Radiopaque foreign bodies are diagnosed by plain radiograph. Ultrasound and computerized scans are useful.[103] Foreign bodies are removed, using microsurgical methods, if they are considered to pose a risk to vision (the famous magnet method for iron is now rarely used).

Burns

Burns may be either thermal or chemical. The latter damage the conjunctiva, cornea and intraocular structures.[104] Alkalis are the most important cause of chemical injury because rapid penetration of the globe occurs, causing severe damage (Fig. 15.28). The eye should be thoroughly irrigated as soon as possible. Later treatments are less effective by comparison. Antibiotics, steroids and vitamin C are helpful[105] but late complications may require corneal grafting or other surgical intervention. The success of surgery following severe chemical burns is very limited and patients presenting with these problems should be given a guarded prognosis.[105] Early adequate irrigation of the eye and rapid removal of any chemical matter remains the most important therapeutic manoeuvre.

Most thermal burns primarily affect the eyelids rather than the eye because the blink reflex protects the globe (Fig. 15.29). Blindness may result however because contraction of the burned

REFERENCES

96. Iliff W J In: Shingleton B J, Hersh P S, Kenyon K R (eds) Eye Trauma. CV Mosby, St Louis 1991 p 334
97. Eagling E M Br J Ophthalmol 1976; 60: 732
98. Eagling E M Trans Ophthalmol Soc UK 1975; 95: 335
99. Rao N A, Wong V G Trans Ophthalmol Soc UK 1981; 101: 357
100. Von Graefe V Graefes Arch Ophthalmol 1860; 6: 134
101. Rosenthal A R, Appleton B, Hopkins J L Am J Ophthalmol 1974; 78: 671
102. Ewart O, Lancet 1903; ii: 315
103. Lobes L A, Grand M G et al Ophthalmology 1991; 99: 26
104. Wright P Trans Ophthalmol Soc UK 1982; 102: 85
105. Pfister R R, Paterson C A Ophthalmology 1980; 87: 1050

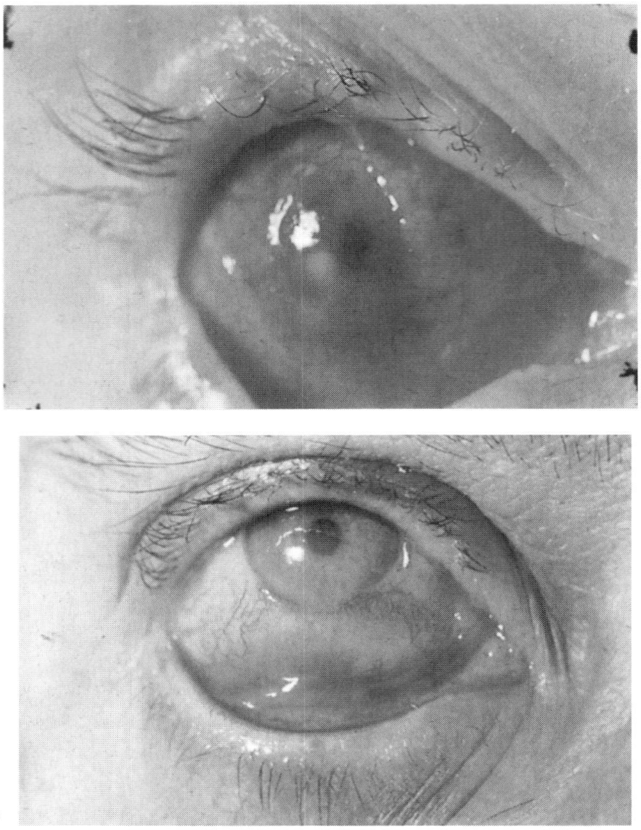

a

b

Fig. 15.28 **(a)** Acute conjunctival and corneal damage due to an alkali burn. The epithelial loss is stained with fluorescein. **(b)** Chronic severe conjunctival and corneal damage resulting from an alkali burn.

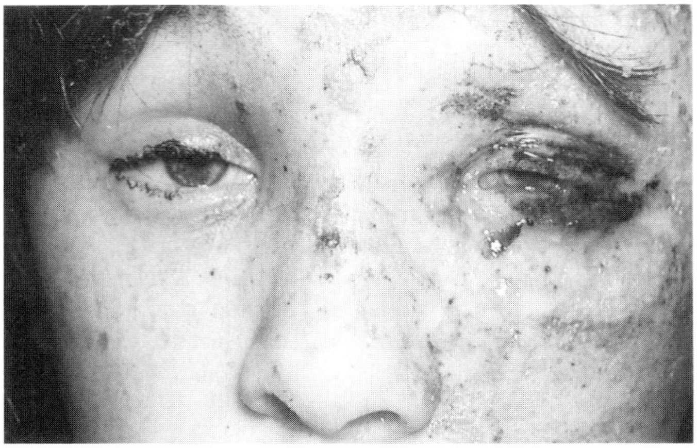

Fig. 15.29 Damage to eyelids due to thermal burn.

eyelids causes prolonged exposure of the eye and rapid opacification of the cornea. Eyelid burns should be treated by early application of skin grafts to replace any potentially damaged or contracting tissue.[106] Multiple grafts may be required.

REFERENCE

106. Fox S A Ophthalmic Plastic Surgery, 5th edn. Grune & Stratton, New York 1976

16 The skull and brain

Peter Bullock

INTRODUCTION

The recent advances in imaging and intraoperative monitoring have led to more accurate diagnosis and safer surgical management of intracranial pathology. Improvements in anaesthesia and intensive care have significantly improved the outcome of neurosurgery. Even so, the basic skills of taking a clear, intelligent clinical history and performing a detailed and thorough physical examination remain critically important to the successful management of the patient. The symptoms and signs of the most common conditions encountered in neurosurgery are now discussed with their relevant investigations, differential diagnosis and management.

CONGENITAL DISORDERS OF THE SKULL AND BRAIN

CRANIOSYNOSTOSIS

Craniosynostosis is characterized by the premature fusion of one or more of the cranial sutures, and has an overall incidence of 0.4 per 1000.[1] The most common form of craniosynostosis involves the sagittal suture and leads to an elongation of the skull termed scaphocephaly. The lambdoid and coronal sutures can also be independently involved and this produces flattening of the ipsilateral region termed plagiocephaly. In the majority of cases cranial synostosis is essentially a cosmetic problem but the premature closure of multiple cranial sutures may lead to raised intracranial pressure and visual failure.[2]

It is important to recognize any skull deformity early as timely surgical intervention in the first six months of life allows the rapidly growing brain to help bring about the skull correction with the minimum of operative intervention. After the age of one year more surgical refashioning is required. The surgical procedures undertaken range from excision of a single fused suture in sagittal synostosis, to complex staged craniofacial reconstructions undertaken by a multidisciplinary team for Crouzon's and Apert's syndromes.[3]

The condition can be classified into primary craniosynostosis, where there is a congenital abnormality of skull development, and secondary craniosynostosis with premature closure of all the sutures which results from primary failure of brain growth. This condition of secondary craniosynostosis is manifest as microcephaly in infants who have suffered severe perinatal hypoxic brain damage.

Moulding of the infant's skull is common and leads to flattening of the lambdoid region. This condition can mimic craniosynostosis but usually resolves spontaneously and does not require surgical intervention. Craniosynostosis can be excluded by demonstrating that the sutures are open on a CT scan.[4]

ENCEPHALOCELE

An encephalocele is a congenital midline defect with herniation of neural tissue into a meningeal sac. The majority occur in the occipital region and are recognized at birth. They occur once in every 5000 live births. The prognosis depends upon the size of the encephalocele and the amount of brain in the sac.[5] Those that occur anteriorly may present later in infancy with nasal obstruction and need to be distinguished from nasal polyps. The nasal encephalocele presents with characteristic physical signs when examined from the nose. The septal mucosa is continuous over the tumour; the swelling pulsates and is compressible, and its size increases with coughing or straining. The roof of the nose is often widened and there may be other craniofacial anomalies present, such as hypertelorism and cleft palate. Anterior encephaloceles require the attention of a multidisciplinary craniofacial team.

A midline dimple or dermal sinus in the occipital region may harbour an underlying abnormality and communicate with a dermoid cyst in the posterior fossa.[6] Patients with this condition may have recurrent episodes of bacterial or aseptic meningitis. A midline discharging cyst or sinus therefore requires detailed investigation with CT or MRI brain scan before excision from the scalp.[7]

HYDROCEPHALUS

Over the past 100 years there have been many innovative approaches to the treatment of hydrocephalus. Walter Dandy excised the choroid plexus from the lateral ventricles in order to reduce the formation of cerebrospinal fluid (CSF) in 1918.[8] This procedure only partially reduced the formation of cerebrospinal fluid, had a high morbidity and was soon discarded.

REFERENCES

1. Hunter A G W, Rudd N L Teratology, 1976; 14: 185
2. Reiner D, Saint-Rose C, Marchac D, Hirsch J J Neurosurg 1982; 57: 370
3. Hockley A D, Wake M J, Goldin H Br J Neurosurg 1988; 2: 307
4. McComb J G Neurosurg Clin North Am 1991; 2: 665
5. Mealey J Jr, Dzentis A J, Hockley A A J Neurosurg 1970; 32: 209
6. Schijman E, Monges J, Cragnaz R Child's Nerv Syst 1986; 2: 83
7. Floodmark O AJNR 1992; 13: 483
8. Dandy W E Ann Surg 1918; 68: 569

Dandy also developed the idea of internal diversion of the cerebrospinal fluid within the brain by third ventriculostomy.[9] With the improvement in fibreoptics this approach has recently become popular again.[10] A third ventriculostomy is an opening made with an endoscope through the floor of the third ventricle into the suprachiasmatic cistern. It is of particular value in patients with congenital aqueduct stenosis and avoids the need for a shunt.

Over the past two decades the ventriculo-peritoneal shunt has become the standard treatment for hydrocephalus but in the past the distal catheter has been placed in many other spaces including the pleural space, the gallbladder, the ureter, and the bladder itself.[11] The early shunt systems were valveless and the catheter was made from rubber or polyethylene. These early catheters often caused a foreign-body reaction and frequently became obstructed.[12] Real advances were not made until the rubber tubing was replaced by the Silastic catheter in 1954.[13] The ventriculo-atrial shunt remained popular for many years but, with the recognition of the rare but serious vascular and infective complications of pulmonary hypertension and shunt nephritis, it has been replaced by the ventriculo-peritoneal shunt.[14] This shunt has now become the system of choice, not just because it reduces the risk of serious complications but also for its ease of insertion and revision.

Advances in shunt design which control the flow of cerebrospinal fluid have further reduced the risk of complications from ventriculo-peritoneal shunts.[15] These advances include the facility to reprogramme the pressure setting by telemetry to give even finer control of fluid drainage.[16]

The annual incidence of new cases of congenital hydrocephalus as an isolated disorder is 1–2 per 1000 births.[17] The overall incidence is higher because hydrocephalus often occurs in association with other conditions.

Each day an adult produces over 400 ml of cerebrospinal fluid at a rate of 20 ml per hour. The majority is actively secreted from the choroid plexus within the lateral, third and fourth ventricles (Fig. 16.1). The remainder arises from fluid which directly passes across the ependymal lining throughout the central nervous system. The lateral ventricles communicate with the third ventricle via the foramina of Monro. The aqueduct of Sylvius transmits cerebrospinal fluid from the third down to the fourth ventricle. Cerebrospinal fluid then passes out of the fourth ventricle through the foramina of Magendie and Luschka to enter the subarachnoid space. The cerebrospinal fluid is reabsorbed mainly at the arachnoid villi which project into the sagittal venous sinuses.

Classification and pathology

Normally, the rate of ventricular cerebrospinal fluid production is balanced by its absorption from the subarachnoid space; when absorption is reduced or subarachnoid flow is obstructed, hydro-

REFERENCES

9. Dandy W E Bull Johns Hopkins Hosp 1922; 33: 189
10. Drake J M Neurosurg Clin North Am 1993; 4: 657
11. Matson D D J Neurosurg 1949; 6: 238
12. Davidson R I J Neurol Neurosurg Psychiatry 1976; 39: 640
13. Pudenz R H Surg Neurol 1981; 15: 15
14. Ames R H J Neurosurg 1967; 27: 525
15. Drake J M, Sainte-Rose C The Shunt Book. Blackwell Scientific, New York 1995; pp 75–108
16. Chapman P H, Griebel R et al In: Chapman P H (ed) Concepts in Paediatric Neurosurgery, vol 6. Karger, Basle 1995 pp 15–132
17. Lemire R J JAMA 1988; 259: 558

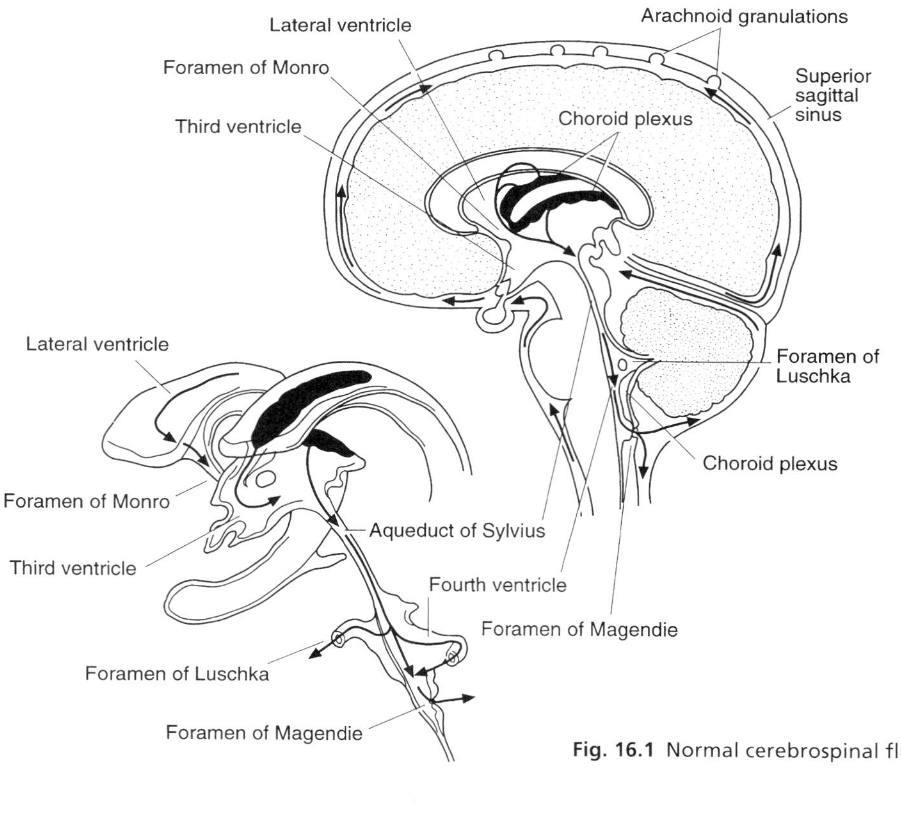

Fig. 16.1 Normal cerebrospinal fluid pathways.

cephalus results. This concept forms the basis of the usual classification of hydrocephalus into obstructive or communicating. Obstructive or non-communicating hydrocephalus results from an obstruction within the ventricular system such as aqueduct stenosis. When the absorption of cerebrospinal fluid is restricted at the arachnoid villi, it is termed a communicating hydrocephalus.

Hydrocephalus in infancy and early childhood is frequently found to be caused by congenital structural abnormalities of the brain. It can also result from intrauterine infection such as toxoplasmosis and cytomegalovirus and can be detected by ultrasound in utero.[18] In adults the most common cause is a tumour, resulting in an obstructive, non-communicating hydrocephalus.

Communicating hydrocephalus

Bacterial meningitis causes inflammation and scarring of the subarachnoid space and often the development of a transient communicating hydrocephalus. Haemorrhage into the subarachnoid space from trauma, the rupture of a cerebral aneurysm or a bleed from an arteriovenous malformation can cause a chemical meningitis and obstruction of arachnoid villi, which in a minority of patients results in a permanent hydrocephalus.

Obstructive, non-communicating hydrocephalus

In infancy and childhood congenital structural abnormalities of the hindbrain are frequently associated with hydrocephalus. 85% of children born with open spina bifida develop hydrocephalus.[19] The associated hindbrain anomaly (Chiari II malformation) fills the foramen magnum and prevents the cerebrospinal fluid leaving the fourth ventricle. The Dandy–Walker syndrome is a malformation where the outlet foramina of the fourth ventricle are absent, which leads to an expanded fourth ventricle and hydrocephalus. Congenital cerebral aqueduct stenosis may present at any age. The presence of long-standing raised intracranial pressure may be discovered by the 'copper beaten' appearance of the skull vault on a plain skull radiograph (Fig. 16.2). The most common cause of obstructive hydrocephalus in older children and adults is a tumour, either within the ventricular system or distorting it from outside (Fig. 16.3).[20]

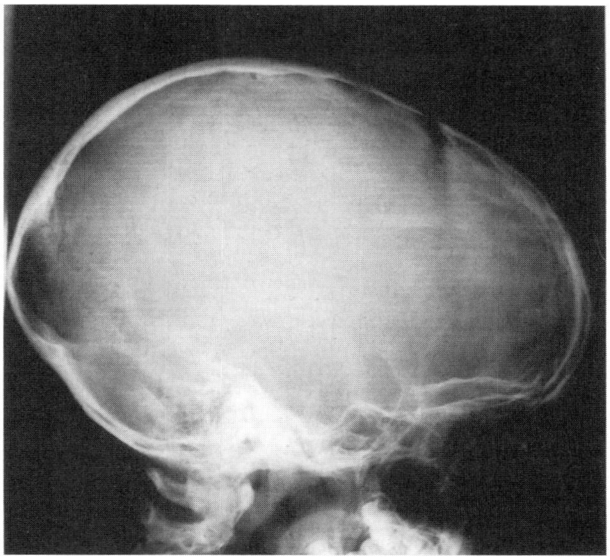

Fig. 16.2 Lateral skull radiograph showing 'copper beaten' appearance of the skull in raised intracranial pressure. Note the widened coronal suture and, in this case, relatively little erosion of the clinoid processes.

Clinical features

The clinical presentation of hydrocephalus depends upon the age of the patient and whether the cranial sutures and fontanelle are open. Infants present with accelerated head growth, widening of the sutures and a bulging fontanelle. Prominent scalp veins and sunsetting of the eyes are seen in more advanced cases. The downward deviation of the eyes may also be associated with unilateral or bilateral sixth nerve palsies. There is commonly a delay in development with motor skills being lost and head control being impaired. The tone in the lower limbs is disproportionately increased. The child can appear well in the early stages, but irritability, poor feeding and a high pitched cry develop in the later stages.[21]

Older children are more likely to present with headache, vomiting, lethargy and papilloedema, although other more subtle changes such as a deteriorating school performance can often be recognized. In adults an acute presentation with headache, vomiting and drowsiness is often precipitated by an underlying tumour which determines the speed and nature of the accompanying signs.

A chronic presentation is seen in the elderly; communicating hydrocephalus is characterized by a disorder of gait, failing intellect, poor memory, and urinary incontinence.[22]

Investigations

An ultrasound scan in infants, making use of the open anterior fontanelle, provides a rapid and accurate serial assessment of ventricular dilatation particularly in premature infants with intraventricular haemorrhage.[23] Skull radiographs can be of value in confirming suture separation in the younger child as well as the 'copper beaten' appearance in the older child with more chronic symptoms. CT or MRI scans complement the other investigations in the young but are the investigation of choice in the older child and adult. They provide a clear evaluation of ventricular size and the presence of any periventricular lucency (Fig. 16.4).[24] MRI is the investigation of choice in long-term follow-up because of the hazard of repeated irradiation with CT scans. MRI scan is able to give more detailed information on any underlying structural abnormalities and is more sensitive to changes in the transependymal movement of the cerebrospinal fluid, which reflects the increased CSF fluid pressure.

REFERENCES

18. Oi S, Matsumoto S et al Child's Nerv Syst 1990; 6: 338
19. Bamforth S J, Baird P A Am J Hum Genet 1989; 44: 225
20. Rappaport Z H, Zalit M N Acta Neurochir 1989; 96: 118
21. Kirkpatrick M, Engleman H, Minns R A Arch Dis Child 1989; 64: 124
22. Wood J H, Bartlett D et al Neurology 1974; 24: 517
23. Shinnar S, Gammon K et al J Paediatr 1985; 107: 31
24. Nadiach T P, Epstein F et al Radiology 1976; 119: 337

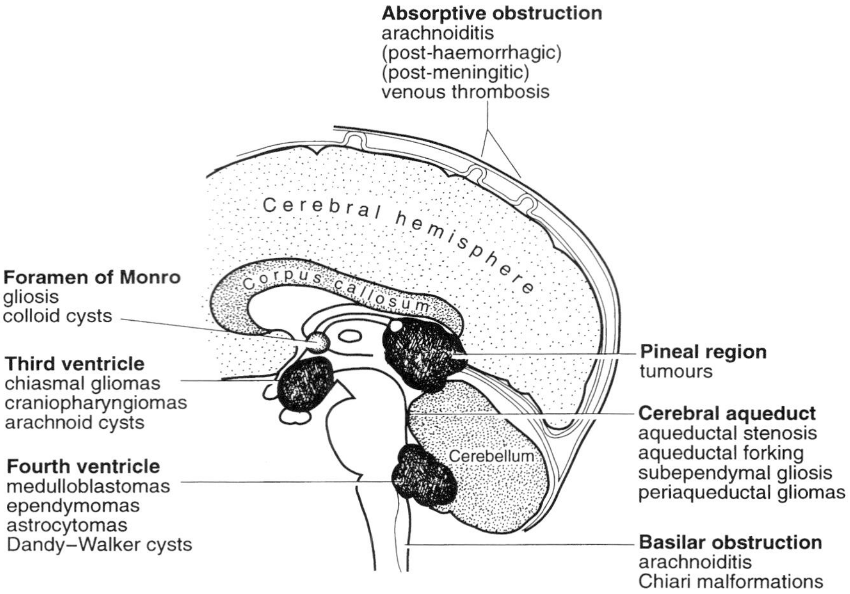

Fig. 16.3 Causes of hydrocephalus.

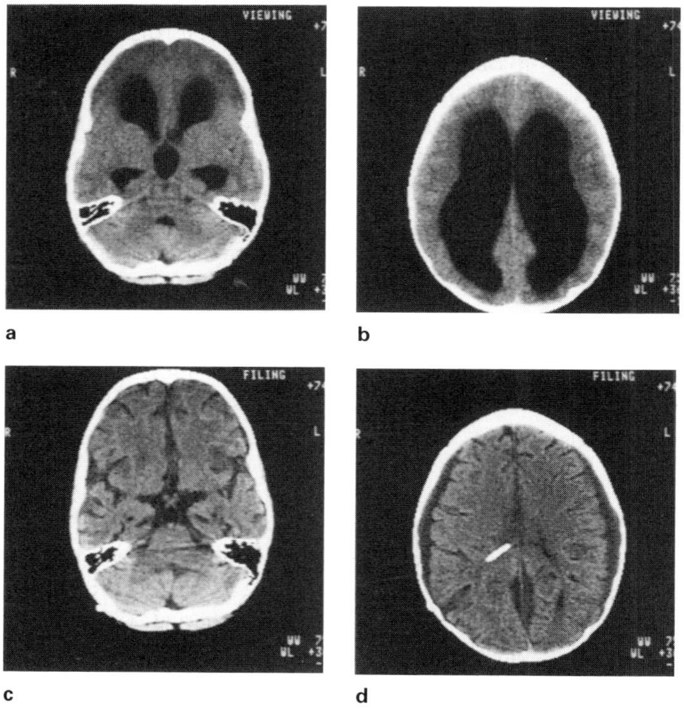

Fig. 16.4 **(a,b)** CT scans showing dilated ventricles in obstructive hydrocephalus caused by congenital cerebral aqueduct stenosis in an 8-year-old boy. Note dilated temporal horns and third ventricle and periventricular lucencies. **(c,d)** Same patient after ventrico-peritoneal shunting, demonstrating satisfactory increase in ventricular size but residual, small, bilateral subdural collections.

Management

Medical treatment

Surgery is the only effective treatment for hydrocephalus in adults but medical treatment can be of temporary benefit in post-haemorrhagic hydrocephalus of infancy.[25] Premature babies weighing less than 1.25 kg have a 50% incidence of intraventricular haemorrhage from the germinal matrix.[26] The cerebrospinal fluid is often bloody with a high protein and an early shunt may not be viable. In many cases the post-haemorrhagic hydrocephalus resolves with a combination of diuretics and repeated drainage of the cerebrospinal fluid by lumbar puncture or ventricular tapping.[27] The ventricular taps can be carried out with the help of a ventricular access device.

The diuretics acetazolamide and frusemide reduce cerebrospinal fluid production and can be continued for many months provided the ventricles do not continue to increase in size. Acetazolamide is used, 25 mg/kg per day, in divided doses by mouth. Acetazolamide is a carbonic anhydrase inhibitor and can cause acidosis. Supplements of tricitrate are required and the electrolytes must be regularly monitored.

Repeated ultrasound scans are undertaken and, if there is progressive enlargement of the ventricles and the cerebrospinal fluid has cleared, then a shunt is recommended for long-term control of the hydrocephalus and the diuretic therapy discontinued.

Surgical treatment of hydrocephalus

Hydrocephalus can be treated surgically by inserting a shunt or removing the obstructing lesion. A ventriculo-peritoneal shunt is now most frequently used. A burrhole is sited and a ventricular catheter passed into the frontal horn of the lateral ventricle. This is connected to a small reservoir and a one-way valve. The reservoir

REFERENCES

25. James H E, Bejar R et al Neurosurgery 1984; 14: 612
26. James H E, Boynton B R, Boynton C A Child's Nerv Syst 1987; 3: 110
27. Gurtner P, Bass T et al Child's Nerv Syst 1922; 8: 198

sits in the burrhole or immediately adjacent to it for ease of access. The distal Silastic tubing is tunnelled subcutaneously before its lower end is placed in the general peritoneal cavity (Fig. 16.5).

A ventriculo-atrial shunt can be of benefit in patients with previous abdominal complications and in premature infants who have suffered necrotizing enterocolitis.[28]

The pleural cavity provides an alternative site of drainage if the peritoneum is hostile. A ventriculo-pleural shunt is generally only considered in children over the age of 7 years; there is a significant risk of a major hydrothorax in younger children because the pleura is not able to absorb all of the cerebrospinal fluid.[29]

A lumbo-peritoneal shunt can be used as an alternative in adults with communicating hydrocephalus or in patients with benign intracranial pressure.[30] These shunts are not recommended in young children or infants because of the risk of precipitating cerebellar tonsillar herniation, which is known as an acquired Chiari I malformation.[31]

The pressure regulation and flow control of shunt valves

The majority of patients in the past had a medium pressure shunt inserted which was usually satisfactory. Many different systems of regulating CSF flow have now been developed. These specialized valves can reliably reduce the rate of complications such as overdrainage with the formation of subdural collections in patients with large heads and large ventricles.[32] The different types of valves currently available include both flow control and pressure control as well as variable pressure valves that can be reprogrammed externally by telemetry.[33]

Most systems incorporate a reservoir or chamber through which cerebrospinal fluid can be aspirated percutaneously. The chamber can also be palpated or pumped with a finger which allows the shunt function to be checked. These reservoirs can be palpated close to the burrhole. Burrholes are found in either the frontal or occipitoparietal regions, but the tip of the ventricular catheter is ideally positioned only in the frontal horn of the lateral ventricle to avoid blockage of cerebrospinal fluid drainage by the choroid plexus.

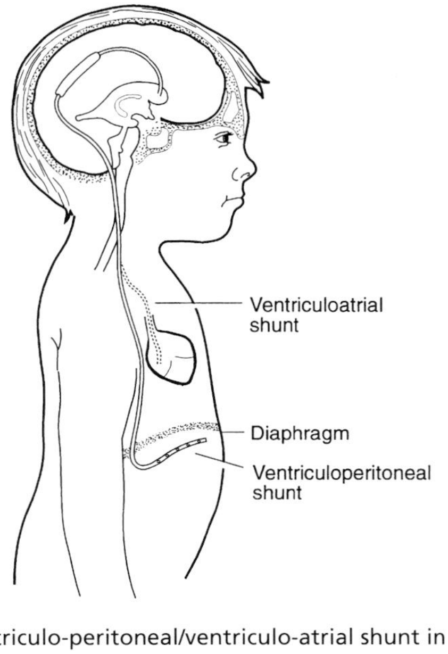

Fig. 16.5 Ventriculo-peritoneal/ventriculo-atrial shunt in situ.

Complications of ventriculo-peritoneal shunts

Mechanical. Disconnection, kinking or breakage of the tubing may occur at the site of the reservoir and the connectors. Migration of the tubing can also occur. A plain radiograph of the whole shunt system is often requested when there is some type of shunt dysfunction in order to determine if there is any disconnection or migration.

In the past, many children required lengthening of the distal catheter by the age of 6 years as it had ridden up to the chest wall and stopped working. This complication can be prevented by inserting a longer catheter, even in neonates, to allow for the future growth of the child.[34]

Obstruction. The management of a patient with a suspected blocked shunt can be considered a surgical emergency. The ventricular catheter is often blocked by the choroid plexus, which is why this catheter is ideally placed in the frontal horn in front of the choroid plexus.

The patient presents with the signs and symptoms of raised intracranial pressure. The patient's vision and even his or her life can be threatened if left untreated. The patient becomes increasingly drowsy and comatose. Decerebrate posturing may occur and be mistaken for seizures. The diagnosis can be made from the history and clinical findings and confirmed by CT scan. The reservoir can be palpated: it should empty and refill in 10–20 seconds.[35] A distal blockage is suspected if it is difficult to empty, while failure to refill suggests a proximal obstruction. The reservoir can be tapped by a fine butterfly needle under aseptic conditions to determine whether there is flow and to measure the pressure by connecting it to a manometer. It is not safe to undertake a lumbar puncture in any patient with a suspected blocked shunt because of the likelihood of precipitating downward herniation and coning of the hindbrain.

Infection of ventriculo-peritoneal shunts

Most shunt infections are thought to result from contamination at the time of the insertion. Elective shunt surgery is carried out at the beginning of the operating list to reduce the risk of on infection and prophylactic antibiotics can be given. Over half of the cases present within 2 weeks, and 70% of patients with shunt infections present within 2 months of insertion.[36]

Among the factors that increase the risk of shunt infection are age and the nutritional and immune status of the patient (neonates

REFERENCES

28. Perzotta S, Locatelli D, Bonfanti N Child's Nerv Syst 1987; 3: 114
29. Jones R F C, Currie B G, Kwok B C T Neurosurgery 1988; 23: 753
30. Aoki N Neurosurgery 1990; 26: 998
31. Chumas P D, Armstrong D C et al J Neurosurg 1993; 78: 568
32. Portnoy H D, Schulte R R et al J Neurosurg 1973; 38: 729
33. Cosman E R, Zervas N T et al Surg Neurol 1979; 11: 287
34. Piatt J H Jr, Carlson C V Paediatr Neurosurg 1993; 19: 233
35. Sainte-Rose C, Piatt J H et al Paed Neurosurg 1991; 17: 2
36. Yogev R Pediatr Infec Dis 1985; 4: 113

have the highest incidence of infection). Intercurrent infection is another important factor, and patients must be carefully assessed before shunt insertion to try to exclude other sources of infection.[37]

Patients frequently present with the symptoms and signs of shunt obstruction. The staphylococcus organism is most frequently responsible. The presentation may also be non-specific with a low grade fever, headache and irritability. Erythema and tenderness along the shunt tube may be elicited. Chronic bacterial colonization is a common cause of distal shunt obstruction.

Blood cultures should be taken if shunt infection is suspected. Cerebrospinal fluid aspirated from the shunt reservoir should be sent for microscopy and culture. All the shunt system must be removed and an external ventricular drain inserted. The old shunt system must also be sent to microbiology for culture. Both intravenous and intraventricular antibiotics are given for 7–10 days until the cerebrospinal fluid becomes clear, when a fresh shunt system can be inserted.[38]

Cranial complications of ventriculo-peritoneal shunts

Subdural haematoma. Subdural haematomas can often be anticipated: if this is the case a special shunt can be used to reduce the risk of this complication. Children with large heads and a thinned cortical mantle from chronic ventricular distension as well as the elderly are most at risk of developing subdural collections. In these groups of patients the cortical mantle folds in after the shunt has been inserted, causing tearing of the bridging veins. A flow-control or programmable valve allows a more gradual release of the cerebrospinal fluid and may avoid this problem.[39]

An established symptomatic subdural haematoma should be managed by drainage of the collections through burrholes and increasing the pressure level of the valve to allow the ventricles to re-expand.[40]

Slit ventricles. Chronic overdrainage of the ventricles can lead to the 'slit ventricle syndrome', where the lateral ventricles completely collapse. This results from the insertion of an inappropriately low pressure valve or the absence of an anti-siphon device. Many patients may have this appearence on CT scan while remaining symptomless but a small number experience symptoms of intermittent obstruction with headache and lethargy. The ventricular catheter intermittently blocks in these patients but no dilatation of the ventricles is seen because of their 'stiff walls'. Patients are treated by upgrading the pressure of the valve or inserting an anti-siphon device which allows a small degree of ventriculomegaly and prevents the walls of the ventricles collapsing around and intermittently occluding the ventricular catheter.[41]

Epilepsy. Onset of epilepsy is more related to the underlying pathology than the site of the ventricular catheter, but the risk of epilepsy related solely to the ventricular catheter has been estimated as 1% in the absence of revisions or infection.[42]

Abdominal complications of ventriculo-peritoneal shunts

Metastasis through the shunt. This risk can be theoretically reduced by a cell filter but in practice this often increases the chance of shunt blockage, and the possibility remains that the few documented cases of peritoneal seeding have been actually blood-borne.[43] Malignant brain tumours may occasionally spread via the catheter into the peritoneal cavity.

Erosion through the skin. The introduction of smaller shunt units and improved nutrition has reduced the incidence of local wound breakdown. It is still, however, important that infants with very large heads are not laid continuously on the same side as the shunt reservoir or tubing, as this can lead to disruption of the overlying skin.

Inguinal hernia and hydrocele. Inguinal hernia and hydrocele are frequently seen after the insertion of a new shunt in male infants because the increased peritoneal fluid distends a previously unsuspected patent processus vaginalis. These changes are often transient but can be alarming to the parents if they discover the tip of the shunt catheter in the scrotum. The hernias require repair and the shunt tubing is placed back into the general peritoneal cavity at the time of the repair.

Abdominal pseudocyst. Abdominal pseudocysts can present as masses, often associated with increasing local discomfort. Although the cerebrospinal fluid is often clear and water-like, careful microbiological studies can often demonstrate a low-grade colonization by *Staphylococcus albus*. The peritoneal end of the shunt is brought onto the surface and once the cerebrospinal fluid is sterile a new system is inserted.

Bowel obstruction. It is rare for shunts to cause intestinal obstruction in the absence of infection. The catheter tip can erode through the bowel and may even present per rectum.[44] Patients with these complications can be managed by bringing the end of the shunt onto the surface and treating the peritonitis with antibiotics. The shunt may be reinserted when the infection has disappeared. Perforation of the vagina and the bladder have also been reported.[45]

Management of a patient with a ventriculo-peritoneal shunt who is suspected of having appendicitis. If peritonitis is confirmed the shunt should be brought onto the surface until the infection has been treated; it can then be reinserted.

Complications of ventriculo-atrial shunts

Complications arising from ventriculo-atrial shunts can be more serious than those seen with ventriculo-peritoneal shunts. Cardiac tamponade, vascular thrombosis, pulmonary emboli and glomerulonephritis are specific complications of ventriculo-atrial shunts, which is why they are no longer the procedure of first choice.

REFERENCES

37. Ammirati M, Raimondi A Child's Nerv Syst 1987; 3: 106
38. Drake J M, Kulkarni A V Neurosurgical Quarterly, 1993; 3: 282
39. Aschoff A, Kremer P et al Child's Nerv Syst 1995; 11: 193
40. Samuelson S, Long D M, Chou S N J Neurosurg 1972; 37: 548
41. Keikens R, Mortier W et al Neuropaediatrics 1982; 13: 190
42. Dan N G, Wade M J J Neurosurg 1986; 65: 19
43. Berger M S, Baumeister B et al J Neurosurg 1991; 74: 872
44. Schulof L A, Worth R M, Kalsbeck J E Surg Neurol 1975; 3: 265
45. Mozingo J R, Cauthen J C Surg Neur 1974; 2: 195

Complications of ventriculo-pleural shunts

These shunts are considered when there is a contraindication to placing the distal catheter in the peritoneal cavity. A small pneumothorax is often seen after placement and should be followed in the postoperative period with regular chest radiographs.

The ventriculo-pleural shunt is not recommended in infancy or younger children because of the risk of poor absorption of the cerebrospinal fluid and the development of large pleural effusions.

Complications of lumbo-peritoneal shunts

These shunts have been regularly employed to overcome benign intracranial hypertension in adults and may also be of benefit in the treatment of a communicating hydrocephalus, but pressure regulation is difficult. They commonly give rise to low pressure headaches in the early postoperative period. Low pressure headaches are made worse by standing and usually respond to a further period of bed rest followed by gradual mobilization. These shunts are prone to migration and blockage and require frequent revision.[46]

A further potential complication has recently been recognized in children who develop progressive cerebellar tonsillar herniation—Chiari I malformation—and it has been recommended that these shunts are not employed in growing children.[47]

Prognosis

The prognosis for the individual patient depends upon several factors including the underlying disease process, the speed with which the original hydrocephalus was diagnosed and treated, and the frequency of complications. Excluding children with meningomyeloceles and tumours, the survival rate at 10 years is as high as 95%, with 70% having normal intelligence.[48] Patients with hydrocephalus associated with a myelomeningocele have a reduced survival rate which is related to the severity of the associated congenital abnormalities. It is sometimes difficult to decide whether to shunt symptomless patients with no evidence of physical or mental deterioration who are found to have a large head and distension of the ventricles on CT scanning. These patients have arrested their hydrocephalus spontaneously. A decision to shunt may be helped by serial CT scans, psychological testing and even intracranial pressure monitoring.

All patients and their families should be instructed about the signs and symptoms of shunt dysfunction and the need for regular follow-up. The patient is likely to need the shunt for life. The patient should be instructed not to pump the shunt, indeed many shunts now have solid reservoirs and cannot be pumped. Prophylactic antibiotics are recommended in patients with ventriculo-atrial shunts undergoing dental procedures or bladder catheterization.

HEAD INJURY

Introduction

One million patients attend accident and emergency departments every year with a head injury. The majority are cared for outside neurosurgical units but guidelines have been developed to make it easier to recognize those at risk of intracranial complications who need referral.[49] All patients with severe head injuries are referred for a neurosurgical opinion. The early recognition and treatment of these severe injuries has largely been learnt from military campaigns over the ages.[50] Ambroise Paré, the personal physician to four French kings, described the injury that Henry II suffered, 'after complaining of headache, he became drowsy and hemiplegic and then lapsed into coma, a post-mortem confirmed the diagnosis of subdural haematoma.'[51] In more recent times most severe head injuries have resulted from road traffic accidents, with alcohol often contributing. Sport, assault and accidents at home or at work account for the remainder.[52]

PATHOPHYSIOLOGY OF RAISED INTRACRANIAL PRESSURE

Normal compensatory mechanisms

The normal adult intracranial pressure measured at the level of the foramen of Monro in the supine position is 0–10 mmHg.[53] In the early stages of head injury there is a non-linear relationship between an expanding haematoma and the elevation of the intracranial pressure. First cerebrospinal fluid is displaced from the cranial to the spinal compartment[54] and then the venous vascular volume is reduced. During this early phase a haematoma may expand without any significant rise in the pressure (Fig. 16.6). Once this early compliance is lost the pressure will rapidly rise.[55]

REFERENCES

46. Johnston I, Besser M, Morgan M K J Neurosurg 1988; 69: 195
47. Chumas P D, Drake J M, del Bigio M Br J Neurosurg 1992; 6: 593
48. Storrs B B, McLone D G Concepts Pediatr Neurosurg 1988; 8: 51
49. Brookes M, MacMillan R et al J Epidemiol Community Health 1990; 44: 147
50. Gurdjian E S J Neurosurg 1974; 39: 157
51. Paré A In: Johnson T (trans) The Workes of that Famous Chirurgion Ambroise Parey. Richard Coates, London 1649
52. Jennett B, Frankowski R In Braakman R (ed) Handbook of Clinical Neurology Elsevier, Amsterdam 1990; 13: 57
53. Albeck M, Gjeris F et al J Neurosurg 1991; 74: 597
54. Lofgren J, Zwetnow N N Acta Neurol Scand 1973; 43: 575
55. Weinstein J D, Langfitt T W et al J Neurosurg 1968; 28: 513

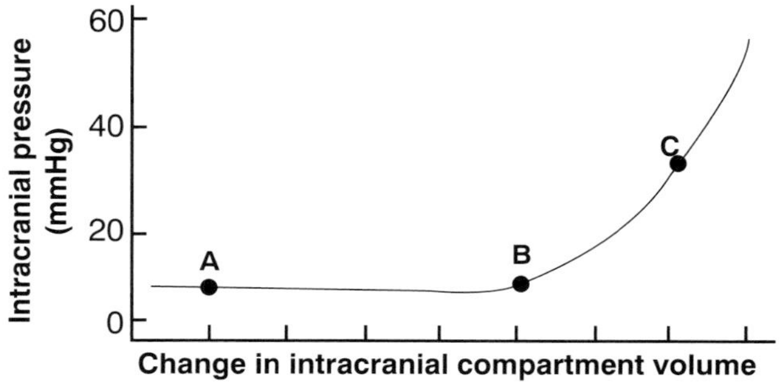

Fig. 16.6 Development of intracranial hypertension: the pressure–volume curve. **A.** The intracranial mass (e.g. haematoma) begins to expand but intracranial pressure (ICP) does not increase because of displacement of cerebrospinal fluid and venous blood. **B.** The intracranial pressure is still normal but 'compensatory' mechanisms are exhausted. **C.** Any further increase in volume of the intracranial mass causes a marked increase in intracranial pressure.

The magnitude of any pressure change depends upon the rate of expansion of the haematoma within the rigid skull. Thus an acute extradural haematoma due to a bleeding meningeal artery can cause loss of consciousness within hours. When intracranial pressure equals the mean systemic arterial pressure then cerebral perfusion ceases and brain death occurs.[56]

The focal damage from haematomas progressively leads to brain shift, herniation and ultimately brainstem compression. The most frequently recognized clinical syndrome from displacement of the brain is herniation of the medial temporal lobe through the tentorial hiatus because of a haematoma in the supratentorial compartment.[57] The parahippocampal gyrus and uncus on the medial aspect of the temporal lobe are displaced through the tentorial hiatus. This results in the classical triad of progressive deterioration of conscious level, dilation of the ipsilateral pupil due to third nerve compression and hemiparesis of the contralateral side due to compression of the cerebral peduncle. By the time the pupil dilates the patient is drowsy and passing into deeper coma. If the process continues the patient develops progressive signs of more severe brainstem compression, with irregular respiration and abnormal posturing. The agonal event is often accompanied by a rise in the blood pressure and a fall in the pulse rate – Cushing's reflex.[58] Once a patient shows signs of drowsiness, irreversible brainstem involvement may be imminent and urgent investigation and intervention are required.

The concept of the pressure – volume curve (Fig. 16.6) is a useful model to explain how, once the normal compensatory mechanisms are exhausted, even a small rise in brain swelling can result in a massive rise in intracranial pressure and a rapid deterioration in the patient's clinical condition (Fig. 16.6 — point C).

PATHOLOGY

Injury to the scalp

Cephalohaematoma (subpericranial haematoma). This is the most common form of scalp injury in young infants, possibly because of the greater vascularity of the pericranium in this age group. It may occur at birth when the amount of blood lost from the circulation into the haematoma may be significant.[59] The haematoma is rigidly demarcated by the attachment of the pericranium at suture lines, so that the swelling assumes the outline of the cranial bone it overlies. The scalp can remain tense and tender for several weeks as the haematoma is gradually absorbed. During this time the infant is often irritable but the haematoma should not be aspirated because of the risk of infection. The haemoglobin should be monitored as there is an occasional need for a transfusion.

Subaponeurotic haematoma. This haematoma arises in the space between the galea and the pericranium.[60] It can occur at any age following head injury. After a few days it takes the form of a large fluctuant swelling under the scalp. It often extends from the frontal region to the occiput and is associated with swelling of the eyelids. The patient is frequently restless and unwell in the early stages. This haematoma is not aspirated and gradually resolves over a number of weeks.

Scalp lacerations should be fully debrided before closure under local anaesthetic. Even simple scalp wounds are treated seriously and the possibility of an underlying skull fracture should be excluded. If there is any doubt a skull radiograph is requested. The wound is thoroughly debrided under local anaesthetic, and hair and other debris are removed. The scalp is ideally closed in two layers with absorbable sutures to the galea and then the skin is closed with non-absorbable sutures which control any bleeding.

Scalping. may result from hair being caught in moving machinery but is thankfully uncommon.[61] The detached scalp usually hangs by a narrow pedicle. Healing can still be successful, even with a narrow pedicle, provided there is no excessive tension of the suture line. A large scalp loss can be repaired by a formal rotation flap under a general anaesthetic or by being microsurgically reimplanted.

Injuries to the skull

Fractures of the skull vault may be linear, comminuted or depressed in form. They may be simple or compound (Fig. 16.7). Compound fractures of the vault carry the risk of intracranial infection. Fractures of the skull base are also compound as they can open into the pharynx, nose, ear or sinuses. They may be associated with cerebrospinal fluid rhinorrhoea or otorrhoea as well as cranial nerve palsies. Fractures of the anterior fossa are suggested by the presence of bilateral black eyes – 'panda sign', and fractures of the petrous bone by bruising over the mastoid process 'Battle's sign'.[62] The danger of these, and all compound fractures, is infection, meningitis and abscess formation. Patients with cerebrospinal fluid rhinorrhoea should be advised not to blow their nose as there is a risk of forcing air inside the head and causing a severe headache with the increased risk of infection.

The detection of skull fractures is important as they alert one to the risk of an intracranial haematoma. A linear fracture can be seen in 90% of patients with extradural haematomas, and in two thirds of patients with an intradural haematoma.[63] Patients who develop an intracranial haematoma in the absence of a fracture almost always show signs of impaired conscious level from the time of injury.[64]

Injuries to the brain

The pathological sequelae of injuries to the brain can be subdivided into those effects caused by the initial impact and those

REFERENCES

56. Braunstein P, Korein J et al Am J Roentgenol Radium Ther Nucl Med 1973; 118: 757
57. Byrnes D P Am Surg 1979; 45: 139
58. Cushing H Bull Johns Hopkins Hosp 1901; 12: 290
59. Argenta L C, Adson M H In: McLaurin R L et al (eds) Pediatric Neurosurgery. Surgery of the Developing Nervous System, 2nd edn. WB Saunders, Philadelphia 1989
60. Bruce D, Schut L, Sutton L N In: Wilkins R H, Rengachary S S (eds) Neurosurgery. McGraw-Hill, New York 1985; 1622–1623
61. Buncke H J, Rose E H, Brownstein M J, Chater N L Plast Reconstr Surg 1978; 61: 666
62. Harwood-Nash D C Am J Roengenol Rad Ther Nucl Med 1970; 110: 598
63. Mendelow A D, Teasdale G et al Br Med J 1983; 287: 1173
64. Galbraith S, Smith J Lancet 1976; I: 501

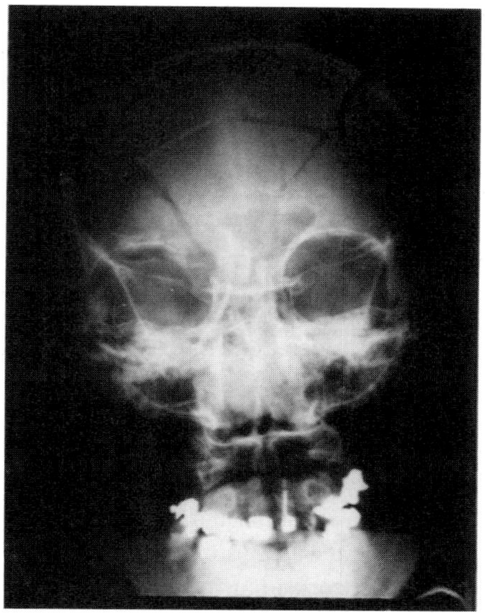

Fig. 16.7 Skull radiograph showing comminuted compound depressed frontal fracture. Fracture lines are usually straight and are darker than suture lines or vascular markings.

arising from secondary complications, both intra- and extracranial. The damage caused by the initial impact can be seen when a head strikes a surface such as a windscreen at high speed. The frontal and temporal regions of the brain impact on the inside of the skull leading to local contusions. A contre coup injury of the occipital pole can also be seen. Such a pure antero-posterior movement is exceptional[65] and there is more often major rotational force leading to widespread damage by shearing of the white matter tracts.[66] Thus acceleration and deceleration forces result in local cortical contusions at the site of impact as well as a more diffuse axonal injury. The significance of cortical contusions is that they can enlarge, coalesce and produce a significant mass effect termed a 'delayed traumatic intracerebral haematoma' (Fig. 16.8).[67]

Diffuse axonal injury is part of a spectrum; in its most severe form, patients are in deep coma from the time of the impact. At post mortem, patients with diffuse axonal injury (DAI) are found to have widespread axonal damage which can be seen on microscopy as axonal retraction balls and microglial clusters with tissue tears in the corpus callosum.[68] Open head injuries by contrast are generally caused by lower impact forces.[69] Thus patients with compound depressed skull fractures often report that they have not lost consciousness.

Patients with moderate and severe head injuries frequently suffer secondary brain damage from hypoxia and ischaemia.[70] Respiratory obstruction is one of the most common reasons for deterioration in patients with head injury.[71] All patients with severe head injuries require early intubation and ventilation to prevent hypoxia and hypercarbia. Almost 50% of patients with severe head injuries have additional injuries such as a ruptured viscus and 5% have an associated spinal injury.

Treatment is directed principally at preventing secondary brain damage by keeping the patient well oxygenated and normotensive and by early identification of intracranial haematoma. Fits also aggravate the primary damage and need to be rapidly controlled (Fig. 16.9). Over the past decade there has been considerable research into the cellular mechanisms that underlie brain injury.[72] The studies have largely focused on the biochemical changes related to acidosis, altered calcium haemostasis and the release of free radicals.[73] Acidosis develops rapidly in the cerebral tissue after injury because of the absence of oxygen delivery or blood flow to the damaged area. Anaerobic metabolism follows which leads to the production of lactate from pyruvate. Lactate continues to accumulate until the intracellular stores of glucose and glycogen

REFERENCES

65. Gennarelli T A, Thibault L E et al Ann Neurol 1982; 12: 564
66. Adams J H, Graham D I et al J Neurosurg Neurol Psychiatry 1991; 54: 481
67. Young H A, Gleave J R W et al Neurosurgery 1984; 14: 22
68. Strich S J Lancet 1961; 2: 443
69. Braakman R J Neurol Neurosurg Psychiatry 1971; 35: 995
70. Popp A J, Fortune J B Contemp Neurosurg 1988; 10: 1
71. Gildenberg P L, Makela M In: Dacey R G Jr, Winn H R et al (eds) Trauma of the Central Nervous System. Raven Press, New York 1985 p 79
72. Siesjo B K J Cereb Blood Flow Metab 1981; 1: 155
73. Wilberger J In: Current Techniques in Neurosurgery 2nd edn. Current Medicine, Philadelphia 1996 pp 159–167

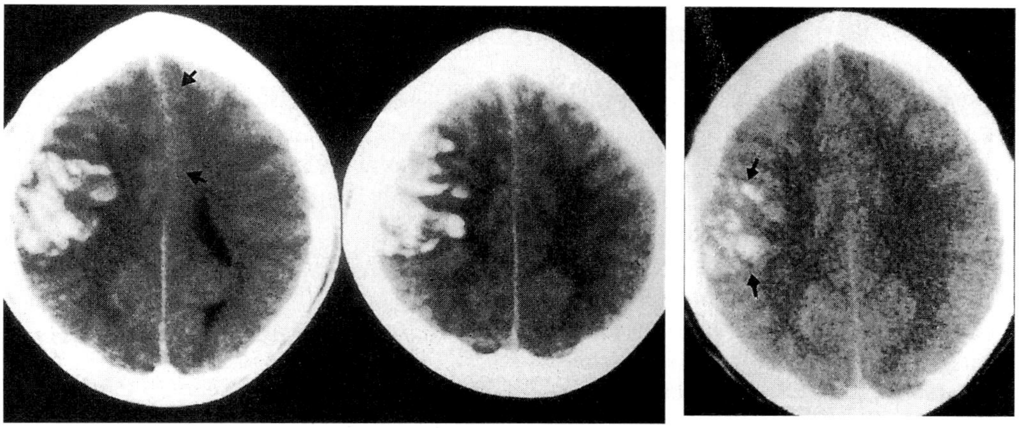

Fig. 16.8 Cerebral contusion.

Mechanisms of brain damage

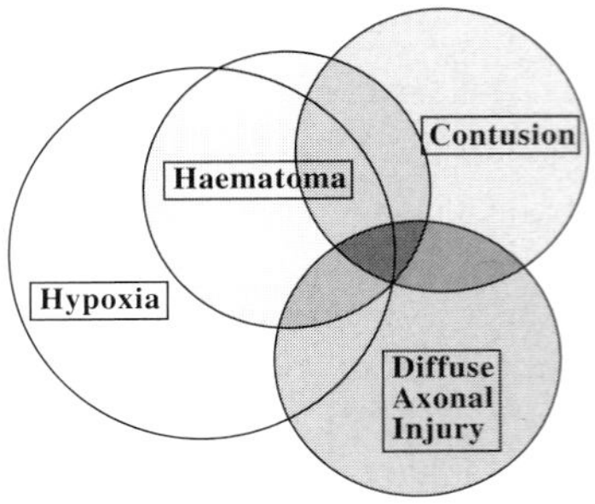

Fig. 16.9 Causes of brain damage after severe head injury.

are exhausted. These stores are depleted in minutes. The tissue acidosis is toxic to the surrounding uninjured neurons which in turn leads to further acidosis and spreading damage. Theoretically this secondary cellular damage may be limited by intervention at an early stage and although there are no specific agents available at the current time there are many clinical trials in progress. At present there is no single factor that accelerates recovery from head injury and the main goal is to maintain cerebral perfusion and prevent secondary injury.[74]

Assessment in the accident and emergency department of a patient with a normal conscious level following a head injury

- Establish a clear history and if necessary question any available witness, police or ambulance personnel.
- Fully examine the patient with a careful assessment of the head itself. Bruising and laceration of the scalp often accompany a skull fracture. An apparently innocent laceration can be the site of a penetrating injury.
- Undertake a detailed neurological examination in the conscious patient.
- Assess the post-traumatic amnesic period, which is a good guide to the severity of the injury.[75] Amnesia, even for a few moments, is evidence of diffuse brain damage. The post-traumatic amnesia is the interval from the time of impact to the stage when the patient has recovered full orientation.
- In each patient decide whether the patient has suffered a superficial head injury or a brain injury. Those patients who have been knocked unconscious for any period should undergo a skull radiograph.
- Keep good legible notes, entries being dated and timed as well as being clearly signed.

Head injuries are classified by their severity as well as by the mechanism of injury. Over 80% of all patients with head injuries seen in accident and emergency departments have suffered mild head injuries, with Glasgow coma scores between 13 and 15.[76] Those patients who are fully alert with a normal skull radiograph can be sent home with a head injury card. It is important that they are discharged to the care of a responsible adult who has written instructions to return if there is any deterioration in the patient's condition.

Table 16.1 Risk of haematoma

Conscious level	*Skull fracture*	*Adult*	*Child*
full	absent	1 in 8000	1 in 12000
impaired	absent	1 in 180	1 in 580
full	present	1 in 45	1 in 150
impaired	present	1 in 4	1 in 25

No patient should be discharged from the accident department unless fully alert and free of major headache. Follow-up in the department or with the general practitioner should be arranged.

Guidelines have been developed to select patients at risk of intracranial complications (Table 16.1) and the indications for skull radiographs are being replaced by the need for an early CT brain scan.[77] Patients with coma scores of 9–12 have a moderate risk of an intracranial haematoma and are all admitted for observation. Plain skull radiographs may still have an important role in the management of both minor and major head injuries in the accident and emergency department, particularly in hospitals where CT scanning is not available 24 hours a day. Identification of a skull fracture remains important because, despite the patient appearing well when first seen, it alerts one to the possibility of an intracranial haematoma. A skull radiograph may also reveal an unsuspected depressed skull fracture. Many of the patients with compound depressed fractures are fully alert when first seen, indeed they may never have lost consciousness and are well when first examined except for the scalp laceration.

Assessment of a patient with a depressed level of consciousness

The priorities for all clinicians involved in the early resuscitation of an injured patient are the same regardless of specialty (see Chapter 7). Rapid assessment and management take place along the lines recommended by the Advanced Trauma Life Support system, the airway and breathing being given the first priority.[78] Immobilization of the neck is important until a cervical spine injury has been excluded. After any bleeding is controlled and hypoxia corrected the nervous system is examined. The first neurological examination is diagnostic and the most comprehensive. The best level of motor response, eye opening and verbal response are elicited. Subsequent assessments are performed to monitor progress. The object is to assess the best Glasgow coma score and determine whether there is any focal damage as witnessed by a difference in motor response of the two sides and by recognizing changes in the pupils. There is no need for a very detailed neurological examination; the tendon reflexes and plantar responses are not usually helpful at this stage.

REFERENCES

74. Ward J D, Gadisseux P et al Prog Neurol Surg 1987; 12: 15
75. Lezak M D Cortex 1979; 15: 63
76. Levin H S, Eisenberg H M, Benton A L (eds) Mild Head Injury. Oxford University Press, Oxford 1989
77. Teasdale G, Murray G et al Br Med J 1990; 300: 363
78. Stein S C, Ross S E J Neurosurg 1992; 77: 562

Severe head injuries are defined as those with a Glasgow coma score of 8 or less and are frequently the result of high speed road traffic accidents.[79] The severity of the brain injury is judged by the conscious level. The Glasgow Coma Scale (Table 7.4) has been widely accepted as a practical method of assessing impaired consciousness after a head injury.[80] Loose terms such as 'semi-conscious' should be avoided. The best Glasgow coma score is elicited on each occasion, by painful stimulation if indicated. Hypotension in an adult with a head injury is almost always due to an extracranial injury. The more severe the head injury the more likely there is to be an associated systemic injury.[81] Chest injury and aspiration are common and lead to hypoxia. Hypotension and hypoxia are associated with a significantly worse outcome.[82] It is never safe to assume that a patient's impaired conscious level is due to alcohol or drugs. Strokes, epileptic fits and subarachnoid haemorrhage can also cause diagnostic difficulties and each may occur in association with a head injury.

Effective management of the airway, breathing and circulation is essential to prevent secondary brain damage. Patients with severe head injuries are intubated and ventilated after the early assessment as they are unable to protect their airway. They have frequently aspirated or suffered a chest injury. Continuous monitoring of the patient's circulation and oxygen saturation is essential during this early period when there may be transfer between hospital departments.[83] All patients with a depressed conscious level require a CT brain scan. Hypotension is almost always due to an extracranial injury in an adult, for example a ruptured spleen. Overall, one third of head injured patients in coma have a major injury elsewhere in the body.[84]

In patients who are not being ventilated the level of responsiveness and the pupillary responses are reviewed regularly. A patient with focal neurological signs and a deteriorating conscious level is likely to harbour an intracranial haematoma and requires urgent referral. Almost half of severe head injuries are complicated by significant intracranial haematoma.[85] A patient with impaired conscious level from the time of the accident and no lateralizing signs is likely to have a diffuse head injury without any significant intracranial haematoma. *The most important indicator of an intracranial haematoma and the need for urgent neurosurgical consultation is a decreasing conscious level.*

The more severe the head injury, the more likely there is to be an associated injury of the spine.[86] An associated spinal injury can be difficult to recognize: radiographs of the cervical spine as well as X-rays of the chest and pelvis are taken in all comatose patients. It is obviously important to think in terms of craniofacial–spinal injury in every patient; abrasions of the forehead should alert one to the possibility of a hyperextension injury of the neck. It is essential to be able to view all seven cervical vertebrae as well as T1, as C7/T1 injuries are not uncommon. The posterior aspects of the vertebral bodies should be aligned to form a smooth, concave curve. The spinous processes should be equally spaced. A normal vertebral alignment does not rule out the possibility of significant neurological damage, and it is important to inspect the prevertebral soft tissue line as swelling here may be the only clue to a significant neck injury. Flexion extension views should not be undertaken in a comatose patient. If there is any doubt about the appearance of the cervical spine a CT scan should be requested. Spinal cord injury without a bony abnormality is more frequent in children than in adults because of their increased mobility. As many as 50–60% of children with traumatic spinal cord injuries have no associated radiographic abnormalities.[87]

Trauma in children

Road traffic accidents are the most common cause of severe head injuries in childhood,[88] and head injury is overall the most common cause of death and disability in children of school age.[89] Children who suffer severe head injuries are less likely than adults to develop an intracranial haematoma but are more likely to suffer brain swelling.[90] Non-accidental injury should be excluded in any infant presenting with a severe head injury and without a history of road traffic accident.[91]

In infants a large scalp haematoma or intracranial haemorrhage can lead to hypovolaemia and collapse. A bulging fontanelle and widened sutures in an infant reflect a marked increase in the intracranial pressure. Cranial ultrasound and a haemoglobin estimation can provide a rapid assess-ment. Infants and toddlers suffer penetrating injury more frequently than older children. A careful history is important to prevent a small compound depressed fracture being overlooked in young children; the only visible sign may be an apparently innocent laceration as the object may have been removed by the time the child is seen in Casualty.

A modified Glasgow Coma Scale (Table 16.2) has been developed for the assessment of children of various ages and is particularly valuable in the under-5 age group.[92]

Transfer to a neurosurgical unit

Transfer to a neurosurgical centre is preceded by a telephone consultation and often an image link transfer. The condition of the patient should be fully stabilized before transfer. All patients with a Glasgow coma score of 8 or less, and those at risk of airway compromise require endotracheal intubation before transfer. Bladder catheterization is also valuable. The personnel accompanying the

REFERENCES

79. Jennett B, MacMillan R Br Med J 1981; 282: 191
80. Jennett B J Neurol Neurosurg Psychiatry 1976; 39: 647
81. Saul T G, Ducker T B J Neurosurg 1982; 56: 498
82. Frost E A M J Neurosurg 1979; 56: 699
83. Andrews P J D, Piper I R et al Lancet 1990; 355: 327
84. Miller J D Br J Surg 1990; 77: 241
85. Gentleman D, Teasdale G, Murray L Br Med J 1986; 292: 449
86. Huelke D F, O'Day J, Mendelsohn R A J Neurosurg 1981; 54: 316
87. Pang D, Wilberger J E Jr J Neurosurg 1982; 57: 114
88. Kraus J T, Mayer T A, Storrs B B, Hylton P D Am J Dis Child 1990; 144: 684
89. Luerssen T G Neurosurg Clin North Am 1991; 2: 399
90. Chan K H, Yue C P, Mann K S Child's Nerv Sys 1990; 6: 27
91. McClelland C Q, Rekate H, Kaufman B, Persse L Child's Brain 1980; 7: 225
92. Cheek W R, Marlin A E et al (eds) Paediatric Neurosurgery: Surgery of the Developing Nervous System, 3rd edn. WB Saunders, Philadelphia 1994 pp 274–275

Table 16.2 Glasgow Coma Scale score for adults and children

Function	*Adults*	*Infants and children*	*Score*
Eye opening	Spontaneous to command	Spontaneous	4
		To sound	3
	To pain	To pain	2
	None	None	1
Verbalization	Oriented	Appropriate for age Fixes and follows Social smile	5
	Disoriented	Cries but consolable	4
	Inappropriate	Persistently irritable	3
	Incomprehensible	Restless, lethargic	2
	None	None	1
Motor	Obeys commands	Spontaneous	6
	Localizes pain	Same	5
	Withdraws	Same	4
	Reflex flexion	Same	3
	Reflex extension	Same	2
	None	Same	1
Total score			15

patient must be familiar with the equipment and working environment of the transfer vehicle, and must be able to monitor the patient's condition accurately and perform any necessary procedures. It is also vital to ensure that all the documents and radiographs are sent with the patient.

Interhospital transfer of head injured patients is potentially an area of clinical risk. In a study of comatose patients transferred to neurosurgical units, Gentleman & Jennett found that 45% of patients had at least one untoward event or an inadequately treated extracranial injury. The most common problems were hypoxia and hypotension, and these were considered to have adversely affected the final outcome.[93]

Management of intracranial haematoma

Acute extradural haematoma

Prompt evacuation of acute extradural haematoma is associated with an excellent outcome as there is often associated primary brain injury.[94] It is therefore vital to diagnose the condition early. Frequently the initial injury is not severe, often a blow to the temporal region where the relatively thin skull overlies the meningeal artery. The patient may have been knocked down or briefly lost consciousness. Patients will quickly recover and then complain of increasing headache. Vomiting and drowsiness follow; the patient readily falls asleep and is difficult to rouse. There may be a boggy swelling in the temporal region due to bruising of the scalp. Lateralizing signs develop with an ipsilateral dilated pupil and a contralateral hemiparesis; finally there is coma with bilaterally fixed pupils, terminating in a respiratory arrest. The well known 'lucid interval' of an extradural haematoma is in fact the exception — the majority of patients progressively deteriorate from the time of the injury.[95] It is important not to wait until the patient is in coma before making the diagnosis. Clinicians must be mindful that there is a high risk of intracranial haematoma in any patient with a skull fracture and an impaired conscious level; a CT scan must be requested.[96] An urgent CT brain scan should be obtained in all patients whose level of consciousness deteriorates or who develop localizing signs.[97] The outcome is directly related to the patient's conscious level before surgery; for those with a coma score of 9 or above, the mortality is close to zero.[98] Extradural haematomas occurring in the posterior fossa are extremely rare but should be suspected in patients with occipital fractures.[99] In this group of patients there may be changes in the respiratory rate and cardiovascular system before there is a deterioration in the conscious level.

Surgical treatment of extradural haematoma

Only rarely are surgical procedures such as burrholes and craniectomy indicated in an emergency if a neurosurgeon is not on site. When rapid neurological deterioration occurs in a patient an exploratory operation must be undertaken immediately. Exploratory burrholes are indicated if a previously alert patient rapidly deteriorates into coma and develops a fixed and dilated pupil that is on the same side as the skull fracture. Such a procedure should only be undertaken after neurosurgical consultation or better still by a trained neurosurgeon.

The aim is to identify and evacuate the haematoma and reduce the intracranial pressure. A potent osmotic diuretic, 20% mannitol, is given in a dose of 0.5 g/kg body weight in adults as a single

REFERENCES

93. Gentleman D, Jennett W B Lancet 1990; 335: 330
94. Bricolo A P, Pasut L M Neurosurgery 1984; 14: 8
95. Rivas J J, Lobato R D et al Neurosurgery 1988; 23: 44
96. Kwan-Hon C, Mann K S et al. J Neurosurg 1990; 72: 189
97. Mendelow A D, Teasdale G et al Br Med J 1983; 287: 1173
98. Cordobes F, Lobato D et al J Neurosurg 1981; 54: 179
99. Roda J M, Giminiz D et al Surg Neurol 1983; 19: 419

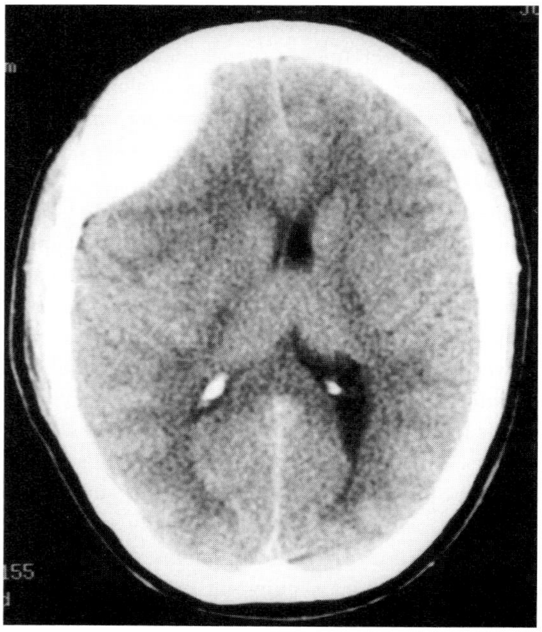

Fig. 16.10 CT scan appearance of an extradural haematoma—typically a biconvex high density mass lesion causing midline shift.

intravenous bolus over 15 minutes and the patient is catheterized 'to buy time' on the way to theatre or during transfer.

Burrholes are sited in the standard positions (Fig. 16.11) commencing on the side that the pupil dilated first, or on the side of the skull fracture if a CT scan is not available. Neurosurgeons use a variety of power tools to make burrholes and turn craniotomies. All surgeons who deal with trauma should be acquainted with the Hudson brace, to which is attached the perforating bit and subsequently the burr. Single burrholes are made through a straight scalp incision. The pericranium is reflected and the perforating bit employed to open just the inner table of the skull. When this is achieved the smooth rotation of the Hudson brace will become rough and erratic, an indication that it is now time to change to the burr, a conical or spherical drill bit used to enlarge the small hole made by the perforator.

In an emergency, once the burrholes are fashioned the extradural haematoma will often deliver itself through the burrhole. Under these circumstances the scalp incision is extended and a craniectomy performed by nibbling the surrounding bone, to get a better exposure of the bleeding vessel. In a neurosurgical unit a formal craniotomy would be turned. The clot is then evacuated and the bleeding meningeal artery coagulated. If no haematoma is found and the dura bulges outwards and is blue then a significant subdural haematoma may be present. Under such circumstances a small opening is made in the dura to release the haematoma.

Acute subdural haematoma

Acute subdural haematoma is seen more commonly than extradural haematoma and usually results from high speed injuries. It is associated with a more severe brain injury and often systemic injuries which lead to hypoxia and hypotension.[100] A clinical characteristic of this group of patients is that they are found unconscious at the site of the accident and deteriorate with focal signs. There is often major damage to the underlying hemisphere which is swollen, and its torn surface gives rise to the subdural haematoma which extends widely over the surface of the hemisphere (Fig. 16.12). The priorities are to evacuate the haematoma and then control the brain swelling.

The subdural haematoma is evacuated through a craniotomy or trephine. For a craniotomy, a scalp flap is first raised to expose the pericranium or temporalis muscle. Bleeding from the scalp edges is prevented by Raney clips or curved artery forceps applied to the galea. Burrholes are joined together by saw cuts using a Gigli saw passed from one hole to another using a curved guide. The bone flap cut in this way is generally left attached to its overlying muscle or pericranium which acts as a hinge along one margin of the craniotomy.

There are a few basic rules governing scalp incisions for craniotomies. Wherever possible, incisions should remain within the hair line (Fig. 16.13); the forehead should be avoided. Craniotomies in the frontotemporal region can be approached via a question-mark shaped scalp incision, beginning anterior to the tragus of the ear. Extensive lacerations or previous surgery may demand modification of these basic skull flaps. The width of the scalp flap should be at least a third of the height to ensure viability.

The timing of the operation is known to influence the outcome,

REFERENCE

100. Jones N R, Blumbergs P C, North J B Aust NZ J Surg 1986; 56: 907

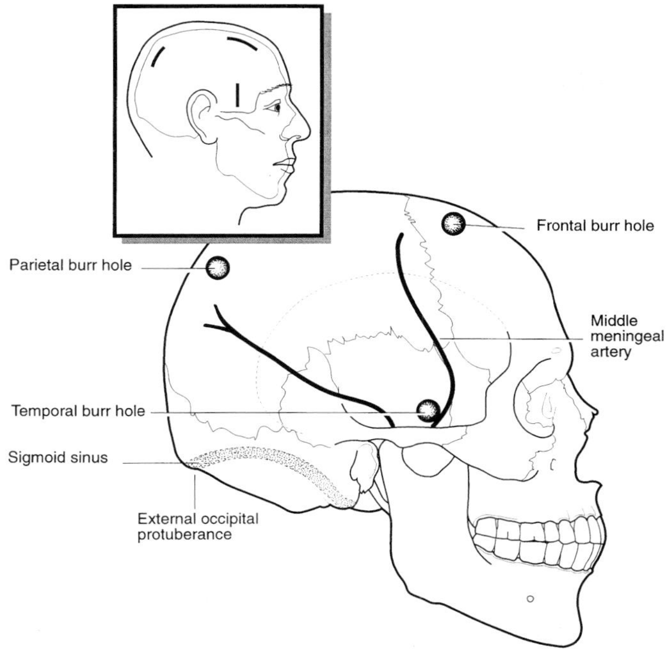

Fig. 16.11 Cranial landmarks, standard positions of exploratory burrholes.

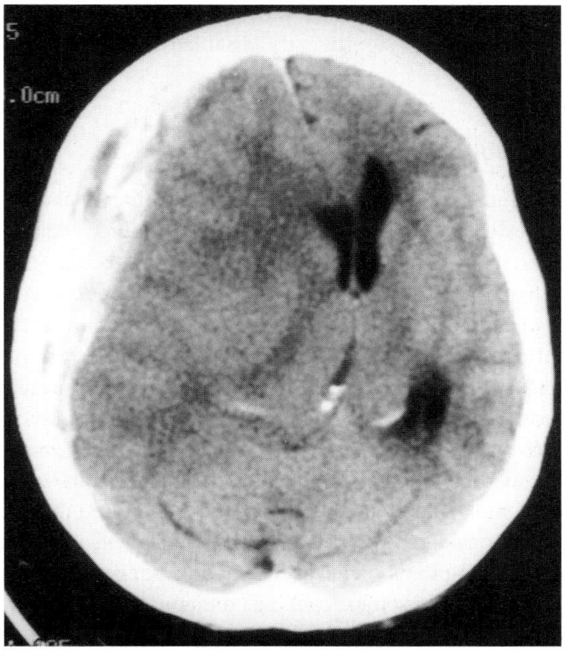

Fig. 16.12 CT scan appearance of a typical subdural haematoma which follows the surface of the brain.

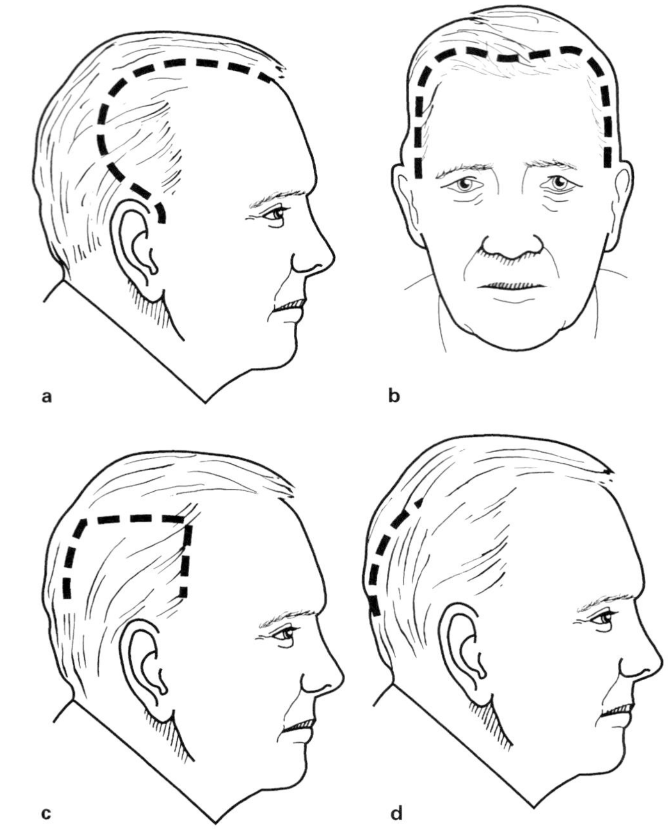

Fig. 16.13 Diagram of scalp incisions for craniotomies: (**a**) the 'question-mark' flap; (**b**) the bicoronal flap; (**c**) the square-sided flap; (**d**) a linear incision.

with early evacuation reducing morbidity and mortality.[101] The overall outcome is considerably worse than with an extradural haematoma. The mortality rate varies between 30% and 45%, the same number being significantly disabled and 20% making a moderate recovery.[102]

Chronic subdural haematoma

Chronic subdural haematomata in adults have their peak incidence in the elderly. They are collections of altered liquid blood that can be drained by burrholes. They are often triggered by minor trauma; the atrophied brain is mobile and as a result this puts the surface bridging veins at risk of stretching and rupturing from modest injury. Epileptics, alcoholics and patients on anticoagulants also have an increased incidence. Patients may not become symptomatic for many days or weeks after an otherwise minor head injury. The history of the head injury may not be forthcoming until after the subdural haematoma has been drained and the conscious level restored. The diagnosis of chronic subdural haematoma should be considered in the differential diagnosis of a stroke. Progressive symptoms of headache, failing intellect, hemiparesis and a fluctuating conscious level are common. The results of treatment of chronic subdural haematoma are generally good in spite of the advanced age of many of the patients, with up to 90% recovering their normal premorbid function (Fig. 16.14).[103]

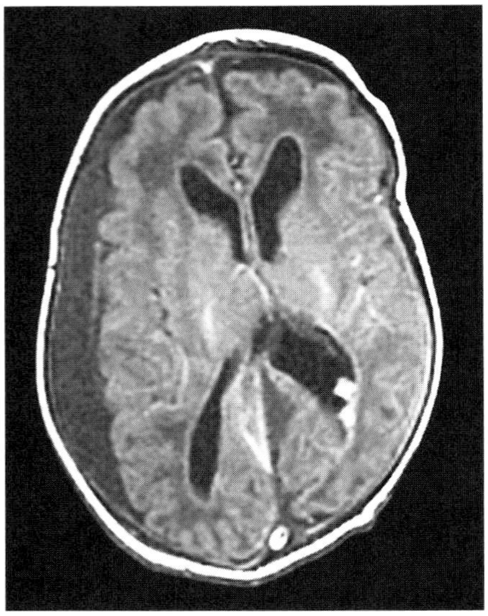

Fig. 16.14 CT scan showing chronic subdural haematoma.

Compound depressed fractures of the skull

Patients with depressed fractures (Fig. 16.15) have often been struck over the head. These injuries are usually associated with only focal brain damage and many patients never lose consciousness or do so only briefly.[104] The diagnosis may be overlooked in the accident department because scalp lacerations are so common. If in doubt the wound can be explored with a gloved finger, but often radiographs are needed to make the diagnosis. CT scan is essential to reveal an underlying brain contusion, intracerebral haematoma or air. When the inner table is displaced to a depth equivalent to the full thickness of the skull the dura is likely to have been torn. Treatment is aimed

REFERENCES

101. Wilberger J E, Harris M, Diamond D L J Neurosurg 1991; 212
102. Howard M A, Gross A S et al, J Neurosurg 1989; 71: 858
103. Robinson R G J Neurosurg 1984; 61: 263
104. Braakman R J Neurol Neurosurg Psychiatry 1971; 34: 106

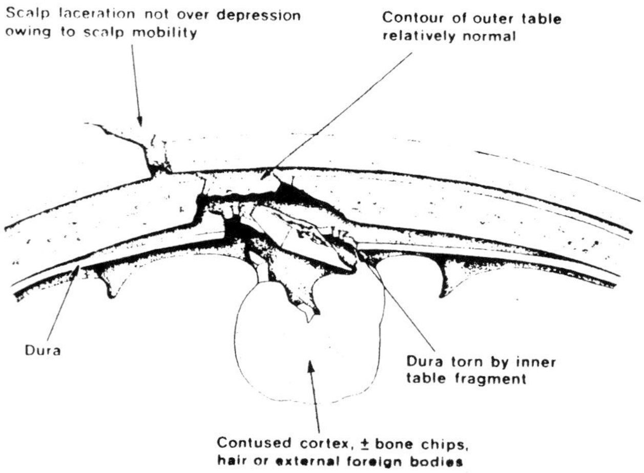

Fig. 16.15 Compound depressed fracture.

at the prevention of infection and therefore should be undertaken as soon as is convenient after the injury, and certainly no later than 24 hours. There is no evidence to suggest that elevation of the depressed bone fragments either improves neurological outcome or reduces the likelihood of post-traumatic epilepsy.[105]

Such wounds should be explored and debrided and the depressed bone fragments elevated to allow inspection of the dura. Elevation of depressed skull fractures usually requires a single burrhole in the intact skull alongside the area of the fracture. Curved elevators are then used to lift the depressed fragments after they have been mobilized. Depressed fractures overlying major venous sinuses should be approached with caution and not be explored except by experienced surgeons as there is a risk of major haemorrhage. If the dura is found to be intact it should not be opened unless there is evidence of a significant underlying haematoma. A torn dura should be opened further and the brain surface inspected and carefully debrided. The dura is closed with absorbable sutures and hitched up to the pericranium. A lattice of free bone fragments may be used to fill the defect if there is no gross contamination of the wound and the repair has been undertaken within 24 hours of injury. If in doubt, the bone fragments are not replaced. Patients who have not had the bone fragments replaced may require an acrylic or titanium cranioplasty at a later stage. Complex craniofacial injuries have traditionally been managed in several stages with early debridement of the wound and removal of loose bone fragments; the definitive reconstruction is delayed.[106] Over the past decade however, craniofacial teams have reported increasingly successful outcomes with an early single-stage repair in patients with complex craniofacial injuries and Glasgow coma scores of 10 or better on admission.[107,108] Prolonged anaesthesia and multiple operative procedures have not been found to cause any increased neurological morbidity in patients with a Glasgow coma score of 10 or better, and early surgical repair with primary bone grafting does not increase the risk of infection.[109,110] One advantage of the early repair is that technically there is easier dissection and mobilization of the bone fragments.[111,112] Early repair by an experienced team also achieves a better functional and cosmetic outcome in this group of patients, who are often young, and there are the additional savings from the reduced time spent in hospital. Clearly the success of this approach is dependent on all members of the multidisciplinary team being available at short notice and on a full radiological assessment having been completed. In all patients a team approach with involvement of the maxillofacial, ophthalmic and neurosurgical teams should be routine. Despite the enthusiasm for early craniofacial repair a more conservative approach is recommended for patients with more severe head injuries who have a significantly raised intracranial pressure (ICP) or a deteriorating conscious level where surgery is still limited to evacuating an intracranial haematoma and simple debridement of any open wounds.

Compound brain injuries from bullet wounds are increasing in the civilian population.[113] Fracture by bursting is seen in its most extreme form with high-velocity rifle injuries. The entry point of the bullet tends to be small but at its exit point it causes a large gaping wound caused by the high-pressure shockwave which immediately precedes the path of the bullet.[114] The pressure wave which follows in the wake of the bullet sucks hair and other debris into the track across the cranial cavity with resultant contamination and risk of infective complications if the casualty survives.[115] The management of such wounds is sadly not only restricted to military conflicts. The patient is resuscitated and the entrance and exit wounds identified. If a major dural sinus is found to be bleeding the patient is taken to theatre without delay, otherwise a CT brain scan is undertaken. A number of patients who survive the initial wounding are likely to succumb soon after admission. A patient in deep coma with fixed pupils and a through-and-through wound is very unlikely to survive. Those patients who survive the original injury and who receive early treatment undergo debridement of only the entry and exit wounds, in an attempt to preserve the maximum functioning brain tissue. Thus, in patients without any major intracranial haematoma or large indriven bone fragments, the entry wound is fully debrided and the superficial path irrigated, but metal fragments lying deep along the entry path and small bone chips lying deep that are not easily accessible are left. This again applies to a patient who is treated within a short time of the injury and where maximum dosage of appropriate antibiotics is available. There is a high incidence of epilepsy in patients with missile injuries and prophylactic anticonvulsants are routinely prescribed.[116]

Careful planning of the scalp incision is usually required to allow scalp closure without any tension, particularly if there is both an entrance and an exit wound. The most important guideline for the closure of both the dura and the scalp is that neither should ever be closed under tension. Attention is paid to ensuring a water-tight dural closure using a pericranial or fascia lata graft if necessary. It must be emphasized that patients presenting late and with established infection require a vigorous and wide resection/debridement of all necrotic brain, and removal of all retained bone and metal fragments, even those lying deep.

MANAGEMENT OF THE PATIENT WITH A SEVERE HEAD INJURY IN THE INTENSIVE CARE UNIT

Intracranial pressure monitoring

The current management of patients with severe head injuries but without intracranial haematomas includes sedation and controlled

REFERENCES

105. Jennett B, Miller J D, Braakman R J Neurosurg 1974; 41: 208
106. Lauritzen C, Lilja J, Valfors B Ann Plast Surg 1986; 17: 503
107. Jones N, Bullock P et al Interdisciplinary Approach to Craniofacial Injury. Oxford University Press, Oxford 1997
108. Pool M D, Briggs M Ann Roy Coll Surg Engl 1989; 71: 187
109. Theograraj S D Management of Facial Injuries following Craniofacial Trauma. WB Saunders, Philadelphia 1989
110. Gruss J S, Philips J H Clin Plast Surg 1989; 16: 93
111. Derdyn C, Persing J A et al Plast Reconstr Surg 1990; 86: 238
112. Benzil D L Neurosurgery 1992; 30: 166
113. Kaufman H H Neurosurgery 1993; 32: 962
114. Benzel E C, Day W T et al Neurosurgery 1991; 29: 67
115. Kaufman H H, Makela M E et al Neurosurgery 1986; 18: 689
116. Salazar A M, Jabbari B et al Neurology 1985; 35: 1406

hyperventilation to reduce brain swelling and prevent hypoxia or ischaemia. The neurological examination is restricted in ventilated patients apart from monitoring the pupillary responses, where changes are seen only after major rises in intracranial pressure. Intracranial pressure monitoring is therefore of value and provides a means of ensuring that there is effective cerebral perfusion, as well as detecting early rises in intracranial pressure due to brain swelling, or the formation of an intracranial haematoma (Fig. 16.16).

The maintenance of an adequate cerebral perfusion pressure is considered to be one of the fundamental aims in the management of patients with severe head injuries. It is calculated by subtracting the intracranial pressure from the mean arterial blood pressure. The optimum range is 60 mmHg–75 mmHg.

Steroids are very effective in controlling raised pressure in patients with brain tumours but are not effective in controlling brain swelling after head injuries.[117] Hyperventilation remains the primary method by which intracranial pressure is controlled. Under normal circumstances hypercapnia causes cerebral vasodilatation and cerebrospinal fluid is expelled from the intracranial compartment.[118] With severe head injuries the cerebrospinal fluid has already been maximally displaced and even mild hypercapnia causes a marked rise in intracranial pressure. Controlled hyperventilation aims to reduce the partial pressure of arterial carbon dioxide to between 3.5 and 4.0 kPa. Reducing the levels below this can result in excessive vasoconstriction and ischaemia in the normal areas of the brain. The patient's position in bed is important, and the simple manoeuvre of elevating the head and upper body to 30° will maximize cerebral venous return and lower the intracranial pressure. Intravenous mannitol given in regular small doses can be effective (0.2 g/kg) in the absence of a raised osmolality over many days. In a single larger dose (0.5 g/kg) it can reduce intracranial pressure rapidly when there is evidence of imminent cerebral herniation despite adequate hyperventilation.[119] Most centres have written protocols on the stepwise introduction of therapeutic measures to control a rising intracranial pressure (Fig. 16.17). Whilst the medical management of raised intracranial pressure forms an important part of the treatment of the head injured patient, it must be remembered that surgical evacuation of an intracranial haematoma provides the most effective means of controlling this life-threatening condition, and a repeat CT scan should be considered in ventilated patients with an unexplained rise in intracranial pressure to exclude a delayed haematoma.[120a]

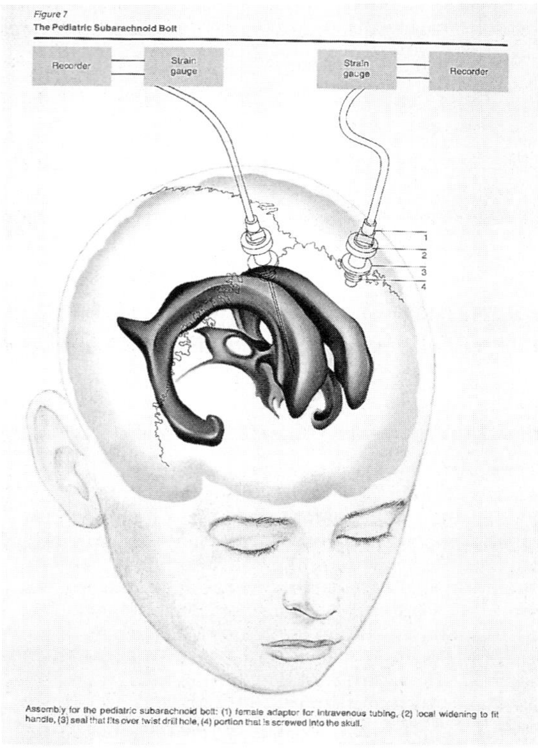

Fig. 16.16 Methods of monitoring intracranial pressure.

Complications of head injuries

Cerebrospinal fluid leak, pneumocephalus and meningitis with base of skull fracture

Patients who suffer fractures of the skull base with laceration of the overlying meninges may present with rhinorrhoea (CSF from the nose), or otorrhoea (CSF from the ear). The leak may occur immediately or within a few days, but in some patients it may not commence until several weeks or longer after the injury. In most cases of rhinorrhoea, the fracture is in the anterior cranial fossa and

REFERENCES

117. Gianotta S L, Weiss M H, Apuzzo M L J, Martin E Neurosurgery 1984; 15: 497
118. James H E, Langfitt T W et al Acta Neurochir 1977; 36: 189
119. Marshall L F, Smith R W et al J Neurosurg 1978; 48: 169
120. Antimicrobial prophylaxis in neurosurgery and after head injury. Lancet 1994; 344: 1547

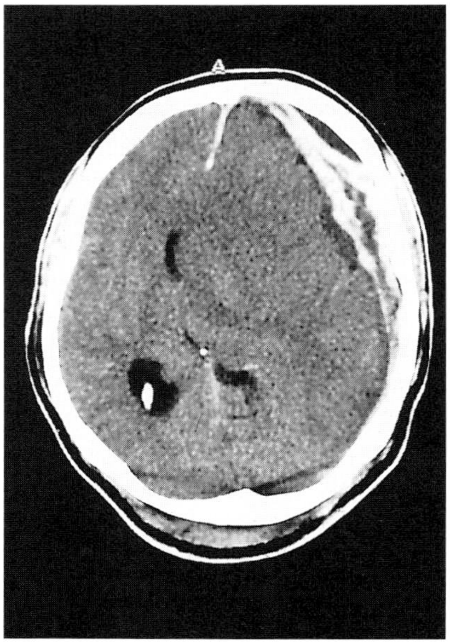

Fig. 16.17 A CT scan at this stage may reveal midline shift and ablation of the basal cisterns, providing radiological evidence of raised intracranial pressure.

crosses the cribriform plate or roof of the frontal sinus, so that it is often associated with anosmia due to olfactory nerve damage. Rarely, the fracture involves the middle ear, the tegmen tympani of the petrous temporal bone, and cerebrospinal fluid drains down the eustachian tube to the nose. In most basal fractures involving the middle and posterior cranial fossae the cerebrospinal fluid leak (otorrhoea) usually stops spontaneously within two weeks. A British working party in 1994 recommended against the routine use of prophylactic antibiotics whilst the CSF leak is present.[120]

The anatomical site and extent of the fractures is best delineated by a CT scan.

In patients with wide or comminuted fractures of the anterior fossa, there remains a small risk of meningitis or abscess formation even when the rhinorrhoea has stopped. The leak often stops because the brain plugs the dural defect, but there remains a potential portal of entry into the cranial cavity for microorganisms from the sinuses, *Streptococcus milleri* in particular, with a risk of meningitis.[121] If cerebrospinal fluid leakage persists, or there is a wide or comminuted fracture in a patient who has had a leak, exploration and dural repair are undertaken after the acute stage of the brain injury has passed. The dural defect is exposed via a frontal craniotomy and is repaired with an intradural patch of fascia lata or pericranium.

A variable amount of intracranial air is frequently seen on the CT scans of patients with fractures of the skull base. Rarely a patient with cerebrospinal fluid rhinorrhoea may blow his nose, resulting in severe headache and collapse due to a tension pneumatocele. If not recognized and treated, this can lead to significant morbidity from the acute rise in intracranial pressure. A single burrhole positioned to allow decompression of the air may be life-saving.

Post-traumatic epilepsy

Early seizures are those seen in the first week after injury; they occur more frequently in patients with contusions, acute subdural haematomas and penetrating injuries.[122] Fits need to be treated promptly because they cause cerebral hypoxia and venous congestion leading to a rise in intracranial pressure and aggravating the primary injury.[123] The risk of seizures is very low with an uncomplicated extradural haematoma. Children appear more prone to immediate or early seizures than adults, particularly under five years of age.[124] Early seizures increase the risk of late epilepsy.[125]

Although rapid control of the seizure is important, the use of drugs such as diazepam should in general be avoided as they can cause apnoea. The drug of first choice is phenytoin administered intravenously. After the loading dose, maintenance can usually be achieved by the oral route. Blood levels are checked to ensure that the level remains within the therapeutic range. In status epilepticus the risk of further damage from the epilepsy itself may justify the use of sedating drugs. Clonazepam is probably safer in this respect than diazepam, but both may depress respiration. Chlormethiazole given rapidly intravenously brings seizures under control. It may be given by continuous infusion until adequate blood levels of phenytoin are achieved. If, despite such measures the fits persist, the patient may require paralysing and ventilating with the addition of barbiturates. A cerebral function monitor (portable EEG machine) may help to establish if a ventilated patient is still fitting.

The overall risk of late epilepsy after head injury is about 5%.[122] The three most significant factors that increase the likelihood of late epilepsy after a head injury are: an early seizure, an intracranial haematoma or a depressed fracture.[122] When none of these factors is present the incidence is only 1%. Three quarters of patients developing late epilepsy suffer their first fit within 1 year after the injury. After a depressed fracture the overall risk of late epilepsy is 15% but this is increased by the presence of a dural tear, focal signs, post-traumatic amnesia over 24 hours, or early epilepsy.[126] The risk of late epilepsy is not influenced by whether the bone fragments are elevated or not.[127]

Prophylactic anticonvulsants remain controversial but are not given routinely in head injured patients because trials have not shown convincingly that they reduce either the incidence of early seizures or the prevention of late epilepsy.[128] Prophylaxis is, however, recommended in subgroups of patients with penetrating injuries or those patients who have suffered an infective complication where the risk of developing seizures is very high.

Carotico-cavernous sinus fistula

Carotid–cavernous fistulas are abnormal communications between the carotid artery and the cavernous sinus. A traumatic fistula may result from a fracture of the floor of the middle cranial fossa tearing the wall of the carotid artery at its entry to the cavernous sinus. Stab wounds and other penetrating injuries may also result in a direct fistula.[129] It is a high flow fistula and leads to considerable back pressure in the orbital draining vessels. This causes marked proptosis and hyperaemia, and eventually pulsatile proptosis with the patient complaining of the noise from the fistula. A bruit can be heard over the eye. The dangers of this fistula are loss of vision, ophthalmoplegia, and a small risk of death from a catastrophic intracranial or nasal haemorrhage.

Direct and indirect attempts at occlusion by surgery have now been superseded by endovascular techniques.[130] This involves a catheter being passed up to the site of the fistula at the point where the intracranial carotid artery traverses the cavernous sinus. It is important that cross flow from the contralateral carotid has been identified. A number of flow guided detachable balloons or coils are then released to close the fistula and maintain the patency of the parent vessel.

REFERENCES

120a. Harland S, Bullock P Surgery 1995; 13: 101
121. Eijemel M S M, Foy P M J Neurosurg 1990; 4: 479
122. Jennett B Epilepsy after Non-missile Head Injuries, 2nd edn. Heinemann Medical, London 1975
123. Delgado-Escueta A E, Wasterlain C, Treiman D M, Porter R J N Engl J Med 1982; 306: 1337
124. Jennett B Arch Neurol 1974; 30: 394
125. Jennett B Develop Med Child Neurol 1973; 15: 56
126. Jennett B, Miller J D, Braakman R J Neurosurg 1974; 41: 208
127. Steinbok P, Floodmark O et al J Neurosurg 1987; 66: 506
128. Temkin N R, Dikmen S S et al N Engl J Med 1990; 323: 497
129. Haddad F S, Haddad G, Taha J J Neurosurg 1991; 28: 1
130. Barrow D L, Spector R H et al J Neurosurg 1985; 62: 248

INFECTION OF THE BRAIN AND SKULL

BRAIN ABSCESS

In ancient times head injury was the main cause of intracranial sepsis, and the resulting brain fungus which appeared through the penetrating wound was dressed and allowed to discharge spontaneously.[131] Patients occasionally survived who had a well encapsulated cortical abscess which had undergone external drainage. The first successfully treated series of brain abscesses was described by a Scottish surgeon William MacEwan in 1893. Most of his patients had a chronic ear infection as the primary focus but many of his observations are relevant today. He considered that his success was the result of good cerebral localization and improved aseptic techniques. He emphasized that a high fever was unusual in patients with a brain abscess but was the rule in patients with meningitis and infective venous sinus thrombosis.[132]

In recent years the incidence of brain abscess has fallen to around 4 cases per million per year in the United Kingdom because of improved treatment of chronic ear disease and the widespread use of more potent antibiotics.[133] Also, the more radical surgical correction of congenital cyanotic heart disease has led to a reduced number of blood-borne infections.

Pathology

A brain abscess may be solitary or multiple and commonly arises from one of four different routes. By far the most common route is direct infection from the frontal sinus or from the middle ear. Mixed organisms are usually responsible – *Streptococcus milleri*, *Bacteroides* and Gram-negative enterobacteria.[134]

The next most frequent source is blood-borne infection from dental sepsis, chronic lung suppuration or bacterial endocarditis associated with congenital heart disease with streptococci predominating and giving rise to multiple abscesses.[135] Immunocompromised individuals are likely to harbour a different range of organisms such as fungi, candida, aspergillus, nocardia and other opportunistic organisms, listeria and toxoplasmosis.[136]

Direct implantation following a penetrating injury or after cranial surgery is the least common cause. Abscesses following head injury are often caused by skin commensals such as staphylococcus, streptococci, enterobacteria and clostridia. A small number of patients remain in whom the primary source of the infection is never identified and these abscesses are often called cryptogenic.

Clinical features

The clinical course is very variable, with the classical triad of pyrexia, headache and focal neurological signs being seen infrequently.[137] Pyrexia only occurs in about one half of the patients, and is usually low grade. Headache is more frequent, with the other signs of raised intracranial pressure ranging from drowsiness, lethargy and coma being seen to some degree in most patients.

Focal signs depend on the site of the abscess. A small visual field defect, a superior quadrantanopia, and a mild hemiparesis may be present in patients with a temporal lobe abscess. Nystagmus and ataxia localize an otogenic abscess to the cerebellum. Rarely a middle ear infection can spread up to the temporal lobe and back to the cerebellum at the same time.

Epilepsy develops in most patients with a supratentorial abscess at some time, either during treatment or follow-up, so this group of patients are prescribed prophylactic anticonvulsants early in their management.[138]

Investigations

The most valuable investigation is a CT scan of the brain with contrast enhancement. This reveals a fine ring enhancing cystic lesion with mass effect and surrounding oedema, although there is a spectrum of appearances from early inflammation to the mature ring enhancing capsule (Fig. 16.18). The typical ring enhancement seen with an abscess can be mimicked by other conditions, such as brain metastases, resolving haematoma and infarction.[139]

Blood cultures are rarely helpful and direct aspiration of the abscess provides a positive culture in the majority of cases. Lumbar puncture is to be avoided as it is unlikely to provide any useful information and will make the patient worse.

Management

Treatment is aimed at draining the abscess, introducing the highest dose of antibiotics systemically and at the same time reducing the risk of recurrence from the original focus of infection. Aspiration of the abscess is undertaken free-hand through a burrhole sited immediately over a superficial abscess or by image-guided stereotactic aspiration if the abscess is deep or multiple.[140] The frontal sinus or mastoid (whichever is the source of the infection) is drained at the same time. The abscess is aspirated daily; once it is dry, follow-up imaging is repeated to confirm satisfactory resolution. In a minority of cases there is no shrinkage of a tough thick-walled abscess cavity and it may then require craniotomy and excision.[141] Cerebellar abscesses are normally drained by a single open procedure (posterior fossa craniectomy).

Once a bacteriological diagnosis is confirmed the antibiotic regimen can be tailored and a 3-week course of high dose intravenous antibiotics is started. Topical instillation of the antibiotics is not usually required. Cefotaxime and metronidazole are frequently used in combination for infections arising from the frontal sinus to cover both aerobic and anaerobic organisms.

REFERENCES

131. Ingham H R, Sisson P R et al Pyogenic Neurosurgical Infections. Edward Arnold, London 1991
132. MacEwan W Pyogenic Infective Disease of the Brain and Spinal Cord. Meningitis, Abscess of Brain, Infective Sinus Thrombosis. James Maclehose, Glasgow 1893
133. Editorial Lancet, 1988; I: 219
134. Manpalam T J, Rosenblum M L Neurosurgery 1988; 23: 451
135. Garvey G J Neurosurg 1983; 59: 735
136. Levy R M, Pons V G, Rosenblum M L J Neurosurg 1984; 61: 9
137. Carey M E, Chou S N, French L A J Neurosurg 1972; 36: 1
138. Legg N F, Gupta P C, Scott D F Brain 1973; 96: 259
139. Britt R H, Enzmann D R J Neurosurg 1983; 59: 972
140. Dyste G N, Hitchon P W et al J Neurosurg 1988; 69: 188
141. Taylor J C Br J Neurosurg 1987; 1: 173

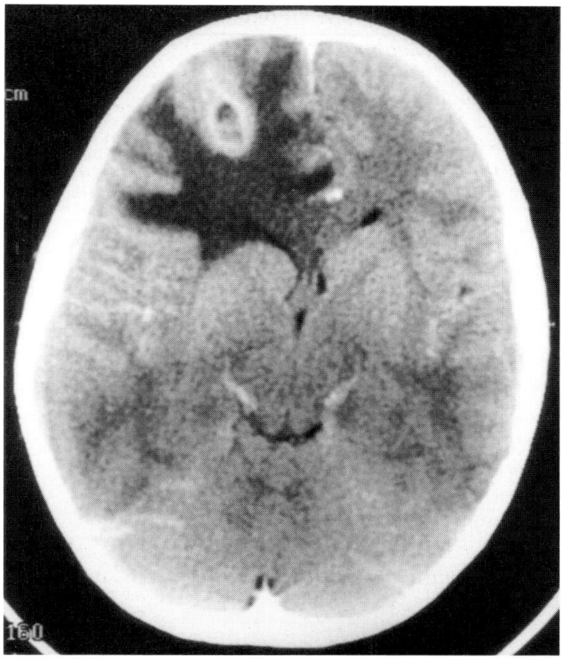

Fig. 16.18 CT appearances of an intracerebral (frontal) abscess, showing contrast enhancement in its wall, surrounding oedema, compression of the frontal horn and displacement of the falx cerebri.

Prolonged intravenous therapy is usually followed by a course of oral antibiotics. Once the organism responsible has been identified and the antibiotic sensitivity defined, steroids may be of value in patients with uncontrolled intracranial pressure.[142] This, however, remains controversial and steroids are not routinely prescribed.

Outcome

An improved outcome for patients with brain abscesses has followed the introduction of more accurate techniques for surgical localization and the availability of more potent antibiotics.[143] An individual's prognosis is closely related to the conscious level at the time of presentation. The outlook is best for the patient who is alert and orientated, and poorest for the patient in coma at the time of diagnosis. In the long term most patients treated for brain abscess develop epilepsy.[144]

SUBDURAL EMPYEMA

Infection between the surface of the brain and the dura is less common than intracranial abscess and has a worse prognosis.[145] It usually follows an infection of the mastoid, middle ear or frontal sinus, with the organisms reaching the subdural space through the skull along thrombosed emissary veins.[146] Multiple organisms are often present and include anaerobes such as *Strep. milleri* and *Bacteroides*, as well as aerobes, of which *Strep. pneumoniae* is the most common.

Clinical features

Symptoms and signs develop more rapidly than in patients with a cerebral abscess. Patients complain of severe progressive headache and tenderness over the infected sinus. They are often febrile and unwell and there are signs of meningeal irritation. The pus spreads rapidly and widely over the hemisphere and leads to thrombosis of the cortical veins. Infarction and swelling of the brain follows, manifested by a progressive hemiparesis, decreasing conscious level and fits. Epilepsy is almost invariable with both focal and generalized seizures which are often difficult to control. The diagnosis of a subdural empyema should be considered in any patient with meningeal irritation and focal signs.

Investigations

A CT or MRI brain scan should be obtained rather than a lumbar puncture which could make the patient worse due to 'coning' and brainstem compression. The CT scan may not be grossly abnormal in the early stages and an MRI scan may be more sensitive. In later stages the brain swelling becomes more obvious but the hallmark of subdural infection on an early CT scan is a narrow line of lucency running along the falx in the midline. MRI scan is diagnostic in the majority of cases, particularly for posterior fossa collections.[147]

Management

A generous craniotomy should be carried out; this may need to be reopened or extended if there is any suggestion of a re-collection of the pus. Pus and blood are sent for culture and sensitivity testing. High dose antibiotics are continued for a minimum of three weeks, usually via a central venous line. It is often valuable to obtain an early opinion from an otolaryngologist so that the frontal sinus or mastoid can be drained at the same time as the craniotomy is undertaken.[148] The mortality rate has fallen from 30% to 10%, with a corresponding increase in morbidity.[149]

MENINGITIS

Meningitis can rapidly follow the onset of a cerebrospinal fluid leak from a base of skull fracture. Once CSF rhinorrhoea or otorrhoea has been identified, prophylactic antibiotics and further investigations are recommended. In patients with recurrent bacterial meningitis it is important to exclude a dural fistula with intermittent cerebrospinal fluid leak or a congenital sinus.[150]

OSTEOMYELITIS OF THE SKULL

Infection of the skull can arise from chronic frontal sinusitis, an unrecognized or partially treated compound depressed skull

REFERENCES

142. Rosenblum M L, Manpalam T J, Pons V G Clin Neurosurg 1986; 33: 603
143. Rosenblum M L, Hoff J T et al J Neurosurg 1978; 49: 658
144. LeBeau J, Creissard P et al J Neurosurg 1973; 38: 198
145. Van Alphen H A M, Dreissen J J R J Neurol Neurosurg Psych 1976; 39: 481
146. Bannister G, Williams B, Smith S J Neurosurg 1981; 55: 82
147. Weisberg L Arch Neurol 1986; 43: 497
148. Beeden A G, Marsen C D et al J Neurol 1969; 9: 261
149. Shearman C P, Less P D, Taylor J C Br J Neurosurg 1987; 1: 179
150. Lewin W Br J Surg 1954; 42: 1

fracture, or more frequently as a complication of a craniotomy or cranioplasty.

Percival Pott described extradural pus with osteomyelitis of the skull bones secondary to frontal sinusitis in 1779; this has been regularly recalled by undergraduates ever since as 'Pott's puffy tumour', when the overlying scalp becomes inflamed and swollen.[151]

A skull radiograph confirms the chronic changes. Treatment consists of drainage of pus and excision of necrotic bone edges followed by a course of high dose antibiotics.

BRAIN TUMOURS

Cranial surgery was undertaken by general surgeons until the end of the nineteenth century. Early pioneers in neurosurgery in Britain and the United States included Sir Victor Horsley in London[152] and Harvey Cushing in Boston.[153] Cushing is considered the father of modern neurosurgery; his interest in pituitary tumours led to the clinical picture of excessive ACTH production from a pituitary adenoma being named after him – Cushing's disease.

The first successful operation for a brain tumour was accomplished by Sir Rickman Godlee, who was Lord Lister's nephew, in 1884. This was an important landmark for the neurologist and the surgeon because it reflected the increasing confidence in functional localization, and took place many years before any form of brain imaging was available. Sir Rickman Godlee's patient had presented with focal motor seizures and then developed a hemiparesis. Dr Bennett made the diagnosis and attended the operation in the company of Dr Hughlings Jackson and Dr David Ferrier, distinguished neurologists who had made important contributions in functional localization of brain pathology. Sir Godlee made a small cortical incision in the region of the motor strip and removed the tumour. The patient survived the operation only to die later from infection.[154]

Incidence

The average annual incidence of newly diagnosed primary brain tumours is 8 per 100 000,[155] although twice this number of secondary brain tumours are diagnosed in the same period. In adults, supratentorial malignant gliomas and meningiomas are the most common primary brain tumours and the incidence increases with age. Females have a slightly higher incidence of meningiomas and pituitary tumours than males. Infratentorial tumours are more common in children than in adults.[156]

Pathology

Table 16.3 shows how all primary brain tumours are classified. Primary intracranial tumours can be intrinsic, arising from the cells of the brain parenchyma (gliomas), or be extrinsic and arise from the meninges (meningiomas). Gliomas are unlike other primary tumours in the body because even when frankly malignant they do not usually metastasize. The common intracerebral tumours are discussed in detail after the clinical features and treatment, which are common to all tumours of the brain.

Table 16.3 Classification of brain tumours

I. Tumours of neuroepithelial origin
Astrocytoma
Oligodendroglioma
Ependymoma
Choroid plexus tumour
Pineal cell tumour
Neuronal tumours
Medulloblastoma
II. Tumours of nerve sheath cells
Schwannoma (acoustic neuroma)
Neurofibroma
III. Tumours of the meninges
Meningioma
IV. Primary lymphoma
V. Tumours of blood vessel origin
Haemangioblastoma
VI. Germ cell tumours
Germinoma
Choriocarcinoma
Teratoma
VII. Other tumour-like lesions
Craniopharyngioma
Dermoid cyst
Colloid cyst of the third ventricle
VIII. Tumours of the anterior pituitary gland
IX. Metastatic tumours

Familial brain tumours

In the following group of conditions, termed phakomatoses, there are cutaneous and ocular manifestations of an inherited disorder with an increased incidence of brain tumours. Patients are therefore regularly screened to identify lesions early, and families receive genetic counselling to advise them of the risks of future offspring being affected.[157]

Both type 1 and type 2 neurofibromatosis are dominantly inherited (see Chapter 9). The cutaneous manifestations of café-au-lait patches, multiple cutaneous neurofibromata, axillary freckling and Lisch nodules (hamartoma) of the iris are seen in type 1; there is a predisposition to optic nerve and brainstem gliomas as well as nerve sheath tumours. In type 2, which is genetically distinct from type 1, there is an increased incidence of bilateral acoustic neuromas, astrocytomas, meningiomas and spinal nerve root tumours, without the overt cutaneous manifestations seen in type 1 disease.[158]

Haemangioblastomas of the cerebellum are seen in families with von Hippel–Lindau disease, an inherited disorder predis-

REFERENCES

151. Bullitt E, Lehman R A W Surg Neurol 1979; 11: 163
152. Bennett A H, Godlee R J Lancet 1884; 2: 1090
153. Cushing H The Pituitary Body and Its Disorders. Clinical States Produced by Disorders of the Hypophysis Cerebri. J B Lipincott, Philadelphia 1912 pp 1–341
154. Gowers Sir W R, Horsley V Med-chir Trans 1888; 71: 379
155. Young L J, Ries L G et al Cancer 1986; 58: 598
156. Farwell J R, Dahnmann G J, Flannery J T Cancer 1977; 40: 3123
157. Martuza R L, Rouleau G In: Youmans J R (ed) Neurosurgical Surgery, 3rd edn, vol 2. W B Saunders, Philadelphia pp 1061–1080
158. Mulvihill J J, Parry D M et al Ann Int Med 1990; 113: 39

posing to retinal angiomas and spinal cord haemangioblastomas.[159] There is also a high risk of cancer in other organs, with renal cell carcinoma being a common cause of death.

In tuberose sclerosis, an autosomal dominant disorder, there is a predisposition to subependymal giant cell astrocytomas and tuberose hamartomas of the cerebral cortex in association with sebaceous adenomata of the face, mental retardation and epilepsy.[160]

Brain tumours in acquired immune deficiency syndrome (AIDS)

Primary lymphoma of the central nervous system has increased in incidence with the emergence of AIDS and the increasing use of immunosuppressant therapy.[161] Since the recognition of AIDS in the late 1980s there has been an overall increase of primary lymphoma from 2% to 5%. The prognosis is uniformly poor despite a good early response to adjuvant therapy.[162]

Symptoms and signs

The symptoms and signs produced by intracranial tumours fall into three broad categories: those of raised intracranial pressure, focal symptoms dependent on the location of the tumour, and epilepsy.

Headache, vomiting and drowsiness are the three cardinal symptoms of raised intracranial pressure and warrant urgent investigation. Headache typically occurs early in the morning and may wake the patient. It is commonly accompanied by vomiting which is often not preceded by nausea and may relieve the headache to some extent. The headache is not usually localized to the side of the tumour and is usually severe and progressive. Drowsiness occurs with more advanced neoplasms and is an ominous sign of impending deterioration. Alteration in the conscious level generally begins with lethargy and somnolence, often associated with subtle changes in personality and performance, and progresses to drowsiness and coma. A rising blood pressure with a slowing pulse is a very late sign of raised intracranial pressure and is a result of distortion and ischaemia of the brainstem (Cushing's reflex).

Failing vision is another late feature of raised intracranial pressure. Chronic papilloedema at first causes enlargement of the blind spot and restriction of the visual fields but may progress to episodes of obscuration of vision with transient blindness which, if not recognized, will progress to permanent blindness. Serial recording of the visual acuity and fields is essential in suspected space-occupying lesions and vital during follow-up.

Focal neurological deficits clearly depend on the location of the tumour. Tumours of the frontal region present with mental apathy, loss of volition, personality disturbance and occasionally with incontinence. Anosmia may result from a tumour of the olfactory groove and be the only localizing sign in a patient with a large subfrontal meningioma and dementia. Dysphasia results from tumours in the temporal region of the dominant hemisphere.

Hemiparesis and sensory disturbance are seen with tumours in the parietal lobe. Visual field defects, such as homonymous hemianopia, are seen with hemiplegia in association with deep intrinsic tumours of the thalamus, but the visual pathways are often of value in localizing lesions at other sites. Bitemporal hemianopia is the classical finding with a pituitary adenoma. In contrast, double vision is a poor localizing sign when caused by a sixth cranial nerve palsy because of its long intracranial course.

Tumours of the cerebellum present with poor coordination; if the tumour is in the midline the ataxia may only be evident when standing or walking, when truncal ataxia is present.

Epilepsy is a relatively uncommon presenting symptom of an intracranial tumour. Less than 10% of adults presenting with epilepsy after the age of 25 years prove to have an underlying neoplasm, and in children the proportion is even smaller.[163] Focal seizures where the character of the attacks alters with time are most typical, and are the presenting feature in approximately one third of patients with gliomas.

Investigations

Most patients undergo a CT scan to confirm the diagnosis of a cerebral tumour, but the MR scan is the investigation of choice as it often reveals that the tumour is more extensive than it appears on CT. The success of any surgery is dependent upon careful interpretation of the images in all planes. When a malignant posterior fossa tumour is suspected in a child the whole cranio-spinal axis is imaged preoperatively in order to stage the tumour, as there may be dissemination of the tumour throughout the subarachnoid space.[164] Angiography is not undertaken so commonly in the preoperative assessment of tumours because CT and MR scans give a clear picture of both vascularity and adjacent structures. MRI is of particular value in the preoperative assessment of patients with pituitary tumours to demonstrate any invasion of the cavernous sinus and to exclude an intrasellar aneurysm.

Although tumours often have a characteristic appearance on the CT and MRI scan, the pathological diagnosis cannot be made with certainty until a biopsy has been obtained and the histology confirmed

The principles of the treatment of brain tumours

The surgical management of brain tumours ranges from craniotomy and complete excision of superficial benign tumours such as meningiomas to the stereotactic biopsy of a deeply seated malignant tumour of the brainstem.[165] The advances in both imaging and intraoperative technology enable a very accurate biopsy to be taken of a tumour in any site with very low morbidity and mortality.[166]

REFERENCES

159. Seizinger B R Ann N Y Acad Sci 1991; 615: 332
160. Martuza R L In: Wilkins R H, Rengachary S S (eds) Neurosurgery. McGraw Hill, Toronto 1985 pp 511–22
161. Gail M H, Pluda J M et al Natl Cancer Inst 1991; 83: 695
162. Remick S C, Diamond C et al Medicine 1990; 69: 345
163. Page L K, Lombroso C T, Matson D D J Neurosurg 1969; 31: 253
164. Brody A S In: Cohen M E, Duffner P K (eds) Brain Tumours in Children. Neurol Clin 1991; 9: 273
165. Giunta F, Grasso G, Marini G, Zorzi F. Acta Neurochir 1989; 46: 86
166. Kelly P Neurosurgery 1989; 25: 185

In most cases a biopsy is recommended to establish the diagnosis, once a solitary space-occupying lesion has been demonstrated on the CT scan. Some patients with suspected malignant tumours are not however referred for biopsy, and the diagnosis, treatment and subsequent prognosis is based on the CT appearance alone. The diagnosis may then be incorrect and the management have to be revised in 5–10% of cases.[167]

The surgical management of malignant brain tumours includes tumour biopsy and debulking procedures in order to improve the quality and length of survival, and provides the best platform for adjunctive radiotherapy and chemotherapy.

Biopsies of cerebral tumours may be undertaken by free-hand burrhole biopsy or directed by an image guidance system.

Sophisticated planning of approaches to tumours is possible with three-dimensional reconstruction of both CT and MR images, which is particularly valuable for tumours around the base of the skull. Intraoperative localization by frameless stereotaxy or ultrasound is now routinely available, as is endoscopy for intraventricular tumours.[168]

Intraoperative monitoring of the facial and auditory cranial nerves ensures identification and preservation of function.[169] Electrocorticography and functional mapping can be of value in tumours which are adjacent to the motor strip[170] or the craniotomy can be undertaken under local anaesthetic for temporal lobe tumours to preserve speech function.[171]

Removal of deeply sited thalamic tumours by ultrasonic aspirators and lasers can be improved by overlapping the computer generated tumour image onto the view seen through the microscope to ensure that the full extent of the tumour has been reached.[172] Robotic surgery is also being developed.[173] Virtual reality is being explored for training purposes, allowing the neurosurgeon to rehearse different approaches to the same region and identify various anatomical structures en route.[174]

The overall outcome for patients with brain tumours undergoing surgery has been dramatically improved since the introduction of dexamethasone, which rapidly restores the patient to sensibility by its effect on both the tumour and the surrounding oedema.[175] The side-effects of high dose steroids are unfortunately significant: the patient rapidly becomes 'Cushingoid', gaining weight and developing diabetes mellitus if the medication is not reduced promptly (see Chapter 35).

Chemotherapy has a primary role in some rare brain tumours. Cisplatin and its derivatives are successful in the treatment of intracranial germ cell tumours,[176] but most common malignant brain tumours are relatively unresponsive to chemotherapy. The nitrosoureas are of benefit in a third of patients with malignant gliomas,[177] they are fat soluble and cross the blood–brain barrier without difficulty.

Radiotherapy plays an important role in the treatment of malignant brain tumours. It usually takes the form of external beam irradiation which can be delivered focally or to the whole brain. Radiosurgery, or a gamma knife, is the sophisticated delivery of a more finely focused beam.[178] The dose by any form of application is limited by the tolerance of the surrounding brain. Recurrent tumours may be treated with stereotactic focal irradiation or stereotactic implantation of a radiation source, brachytherapy, which delivers a continuous high dose locally.[179] The side-effects from radiation include early hair loss, and years later hypopituitarism and radiation necrosis which are irreversible. Radiation necrosis can be distinguished from recurrent tumour by a positron emission tomography scan.[180] An additional late risk is the development of a second malignancy.

COMMON INTRACRANIAL TUMOURS

The gliomas

Glial cells form the connective tissue or supporting framework of the brain, and most primary intrinsic neoplasms of the brain are known by the collective term 'glioma', because they are thought to arise from the astrocyte, oligodendrocyte or ependymal cell.

This is a widely diverse group of tumours: the low-grade pilocytic astrocytoma of childhood is often cured by surgery while at the other extreme is the glioblastoma multiforme of the elderly which rapidly leads to a fatal outcome despite aggressive surgery and adjuvant therapy. Histological assessment and grading of the gliomas is important for therapy and prognosis but can prove difficult when there is considerable heterogeneity within one tumour.[182]

The most common classification is that described by Kernohan[182] which is based on the degree of anaplasia, the frequency of mitotic figures, the cellularity of the tumour and any vascular proliferation as well as the presence of necrosis. Tumours are graded I–IV, with grade IV carrying the worst prognosis. There is inevitably an overlap of the boundaries between the grades and a biopsy from one area of the tumour may be unrepresentative of the entire tumour.

Grade I tumours are essentially cerebellar lesions that arise in children and young adults. These tumours are often cystic and can be cured by complete resection.[183] Only 10% of these cerebellar

REFERENCES

167. Coffey R J, Lunsford L D, Taylor F H Neurosurgery 1988; 22: 465
168. Apuzzo M L J, Chandrasoma P T et al Neurosurgery 1984; 15: 502
169. Ojemann R G, Levine R A, Montgomery W M, McGaffigan P J Neurosurg 1984; 61: 938
170. Bandettini P, Wong E et al Magn Reson Med 1992; 25: 390
171. Ojemann G, Dodrill C Adv Epileptol 1987; 16: 327
172. Kelly P J In: Apuzzo M L J (ed) Neurosurgery for the Third Millennium. American Association of Neurological Surgeons, Park Ridge Ill, 1992; pp 35–45
173. Apuzzo M L J, Chin L S, Chen T, Valencia P In: Apuzzo MLJ (ed) Neurosurgery for the Third Millennium. American Association of Neurological Surgeons Park Ridge Ill 1992; pp 11–33
174. Weinberg R In: Apuzzo MLJ (ed) Neurosurgery for the Third Millennium. American Association of Neurological Surgeons, Park Ridge Ill 1992 pp 47–64
175. Galicich J H, French L A Am Pract Dig Treat 1961; 12: 169
176. Kobayashi T, Yoshida J et al J Neurosurg 1989; 70: 676
177. Walker M D, Green S B et al N Engl J Med 1980; 303: 1323
178. Lunsford L D, Flickinger J, Coffey R J Arch Neurol 1990; 47: 169
179. Berstein M, Gutin P H Neurosurgery 1981; 9: 741
180. Rozenthal J M, Levine R L, Nickles R J, Dobkin J A Arch Neurol 1989; 46: 1302
181. Kim T S, Halliday A L et al J Neurosurg 1991; 74: 27
182. Kernohan J W, Mabon R F et al Proc Mayo Clin 1949; 20: 71
183. McCormack B M, Miller D C, Budzilovich G N Neurosurgery 1992; 31: 636

hemisphere tumours display infiltrative potential and recur following complete macroscopic excision. Pilocytic tumours that occur in the optic chiasma and hypothalamus are often more diffuse and associated with neurofibromatosis. Macroscopic surgical excision is not usually possible and adjuvant therapy using radiotherapy or chemotherapy is employed.[184]

Grade II astrocytomas are infiltrative lesions of the cerebral hemispheres and the pons and have a variable clinical course. In the hemisphere they may present with epilepsy and remain otherwise clinically silent for many years. Ultimately, widespread infiltration causes intellectual deterioration and motor deficits. The cytological grading may deteriorate and become frankly malignant. The management remains controversial, with early biopsy and radiotherapy being compared to a more conservative approach.[185]

Grade III, or anaplastic astrocytomas, and IV or glioblastoma multiforme present with a short history of raised intracranial pressure and focal signs which may include headache and a progressive hemiparesis.

The surgical management of grade III and IV astrocytomas is directed at making a histological diagnosis and reducing tumour bulk prior to radiotherapy.[186] Frequently a radical excision may not be possible and a stereotactic biopsy is undertaken. Despite radiotherapy and occasionally chemotherapy, over 90% of patients with grade IV tumours do not survive more than two years.[187,188] The prognosis for grade III tumours is only marginally better (Fig. 16.19).

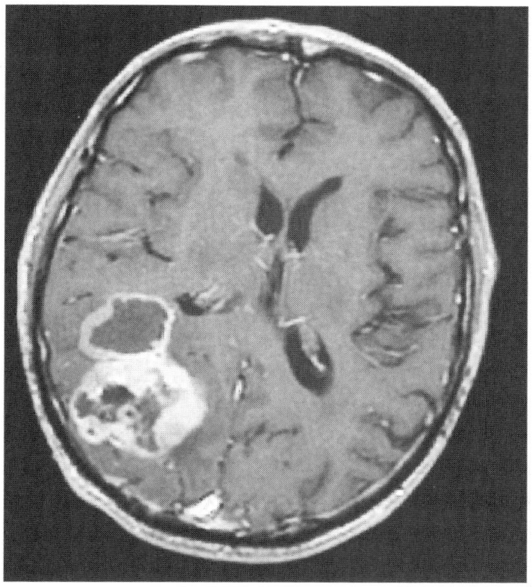

Fig. 16.19 Intrinsic malignant astrocytoma, right parieto-occipital region. Grade IV.

Oligodendroglioma

These tumours, comprising about 5% of all gliomas, almost always occur in the cerebral hemispheres.[189] The most characteristic presentation is similar to that of low-grade astrocytomas with a long history of epilepsy. Calcification is common and usually visible on skull radiographs or CT scan. Haemorrhage from these tumours is not uncommon and can cause a precipitous deterioration.[190] Patients may survive for a decade or more because of the slow growth rate of the tumour but, like the astrocytomas, most oligodendrogliomas eventually undergo anaplastic change and become frankly malignant. Biopsy, tumour debulking where possible, and radiotherapy are standard management. Despite its less ominous reputation, the mean postoperative survival is 4.3 years, and 80% of patients are dead within 5 years of diagnosis.[191,192]

Ependymoma

Ependymomas, which comprise about 6% of intracranial gliomas, occur most commonly in young patients.[193] They are found most frequently in the cavity of the fourth ventricle arising from the ependymal lining of the ventricles. Histologically they can be of mixed grade. The more malignant forms in the fourth ventricle and spinal cord may produce seeding within the subarachnoid space and full craniospinal irradiation is then required. Repeat resection and chemotherapy has been of benefit for recurrent tumour. The 5-year survival rate is 35–60%.[194]

Medulloblastoma

This is the most common glioma of childhood, occurring mainly in the first decade of life and arising in the roof of the fourth ventricle.[195] It is a malignant tumour which infiltrates widely into the cerebellum, the fourth ventricle and its floor, and frequently presents with obstructive hydrocephalus. Like the ependymoma, it too metastasizes through the subarachnoid space. With radical tumour removal via a posterior fossa craniectomy followed by craniospinal irradiation and chemotherapy long-term survival rates exceeding 70% have been reported at 5-year follow-up.[196,197] High dose irradiation, however, has been found to cause serious impairment in mental function of young children and many of the long-term survivors show a fall in intelligence quotient with multiple psychological and behavioural problems. Protocols for radiotherapy and chemotherapy have been revised in order to reduce these complications.[197]

REFERENCES

184. Weiss L, Sagerman R H et al Cancer 1987; 59: 1000
185. Cairncross J G, Laperriere N J Arch Neurol 1989; 46: 1238
186. Leibel S A, Sheline G E J Neurosurg 1987; 66: 1
187. Burger P C, Vogel F S et al Cancer 1985; 56: 1106
188. Kyritsis A P, Levin V A Adv Oncol 1992; 8: 9
189. Wilkinson I M S, Anderson J R, Holmes A E J Neurol Neurosurg Psych 1987; 50: 304
190. Ludwig C L, Smith M T, Godfrey A D, Armbrustmacher V W Ann Neurol 1986; 19: 15
191. Winger M J, Macdonald D R, Cairncross J G J Neurosurg 1989; 71: 493
192. Mork S J, Halvorsen T B, Lindegaard K F, Eide G E J Neuropath Exp Neurol 1986; 45: 65
193. Dohrmann G J, Farwell J R, Flannery J T J Neurosurg 1976; 45: 273
194. Undjian S, Marinov M Child's Nerv Syst 1990; 6: 131
195. Hoffman H, Hendricks E, Humphreys R Clin Neurosurg 1982; 30: 226
196. Packer R, Sutton L et al J Neurosurg 1988; 68: 383
197. Packer R, Sutton L et al J Neurosurg 1989; 70: 707

Meningioma

These tumours are discrete, well encapsulated and arise from the arachnoid layer outside the brain and therefore lend themselves to complete removal by surgery. They are slow growing and cause symptoms by gradual compression of the brain. They may, however, reach a considerable size before causing any symptoms because of the inherent deformability of the brain.

Meningiomas most commonly occur over the convexities or at the skull base, and are classified according to their anatomical site.[199] Women are affected twice as often as men, and the incidence increases with advancing years.

Meningiomas can generate local overgrowth in the overlying skull, resulting in a palpable lump on the skull. This exostosis can be mistaken for a simple osteoma but a skull radiograph reveals locally hypertrophied vascular markings, and a CT scan with contrast confirms the presence of a meningioma.[200]

Histologically these tumours display considerable plemorphism with occasional mitotic figures and even necrosis; recurrences can occur even after a wide excision of an apparently benign meningioma.

Parasagittal meningiomas often occur in front of the central sulcus and typically produce frontal or parietal lobe syndromes. They also tend to invade the sagittal sinus making complete excision difficult at times. The majority of these tumours are benign but infiltration of the brain implies that malignant transformation has occurred and makes tumour recurrence more likely. The recurrence rate for parasagittal tumours is up to 40% when invasion of the sagittal sinus has occurred. Symptomatic recurrence may be delayed for many years,[201] thus it is important that patients with partially excised meningiomas undergo long-term follow-up with serial imaging.

Cerebral metastases

The majority of cancers are widely disseminated by the time they involve the brain and spinal cord; the treatment is palliative.

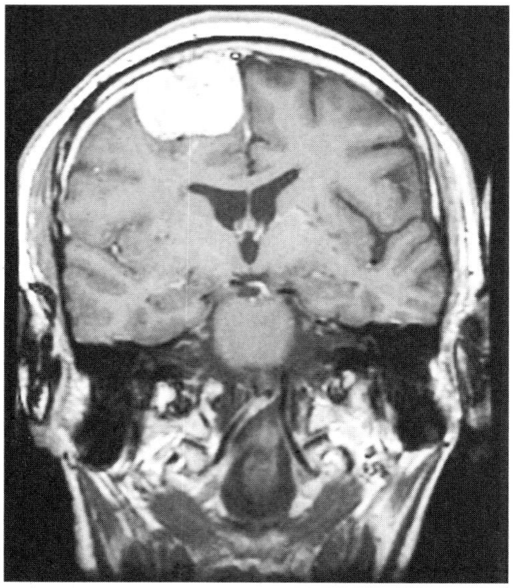

Fig. 16.20 Right parasagittal meningioma.

Cerebral metastases commonly arise from carcinoma of the bronchus and breast. Carcinomas of the colon and kidney and malignant melanoma are also frequent primary sources.

Even when only one lesion is visible on the CT brain scan, MR scanning with contrast often reveals multiple deposits.[202] A chest radiograph remains an essential investigation in patients with a suspected solitary brain metastasis and an unknown primary.

The surgical treatment is limited in its scope but excision of a solitary metastasis in symptomatic patients provides valuable palliation.[203] Treatment clearly involves not only the neurosurgical management but also further control of the primary source. The average survival for those undergoing complete removal of a solitary metastasis followed by whole-brain radiotherapy is approximately 12 months.[204]

Patients with multiple metastases are generally not offered any neurosurgical intervention once the diagnosis has been confirmed and other pathologies such as multiple cerebral abscesses have been excluded. External beam radiotherapy, dexamethasone and hormonal manipulation may produce useful symptom relief and palliation in women with cerebral secondaries from a breast carcinoma.

Pituitary tumours

Pituitary adenomas arise from the anterior lobe and are classified by their size and endocrine function. The most common pituitary tumours secrete prolactin, growth hormone or corticotrophin.[205] Non-secreting pituitary adenomas are less frequent and present with hypopituitarism or the local mass effect causing neurological signs.

Tumours larger than 2 cm in diameter expand the pituitary fossa and are called macroadenomas. They may extend into the suprasellar region causing optic chiasmal compression and visual failure.[206] It is therefore essential that any patient with a pituitary macroadenoma has the visual fields and acuity recorded. The cavernous sinus can be involved and local invasion is often heralded by facial pain, double vision and sensory changes from compression of the exiting cranial nerves. Downward growth into the sphenoid sinus also occurs and in advanced cases can lead to the tumour being mistaken for a nasal polyp. Giant tumours can distort the hypothalamus and obstruct the third ventricle leading to hydrocephalus.

REFERENCES

198. Levin V, Rodriguez L et al J Neurosurg 1988; 68: 383
199. Cushing H, Eisenhardt L Meningiomas: their Classification, Regional Behaviour, Life History and Surgical End Results. Charles C Thomas, Springfield, Illinois 1938
200. Latchaw R E, Hirsch W L In: Al-Mefty O (ed) Meningiomas. Raven Press. New York 1991; pp 195–207
201. Jaaskelainen J, Haltia M, Servo A Surg Neurol 1986; 25: 233
202. Coffey R J, Flickinger J C et al Int J Radiat Oncol Biol Phys 1991; 20: 1287
203. White K R, Fleming T R, Laws E R Mayo Clin Proc 1981; 56: 424
204. Patchell R A, Tibbs P A et al N Engl J Med 1990; 322: 494
205. Ezrin C, Kovacs K, Horvath E In: Bloodworth J M B Jr (ed) Endocrine Pathology, General and Surgical, 2nd edn. Williams & Wilkins, Baltimore Md 1982 pp 101–132
206. Wilson C B A decade of pituitary microsurgery: the Herbert Olivecrona lecture. J Neurosurg 1984; 61: 814

Prolactinomas are four times more common in women than men and usually present in young women in their second and third decades with a history of amenorrhoea and galactorrhoea.[207] The tumour is frequently less than 1 cm in diameter and is known as a microadenoma. It can be responsible for infertility. In men the clinical presentation is later in life, in the fourth and fifth decades, with a history of impotence or loss of libido, and the tumours are larger and more aggressive.

Acromegaly is an insidious process: patients have frequently bought larger footwear or had their rings increased in size over many years. It affects men and women equally and the diagnosis is usually made in middle age. In addition to the cosmetic effects, acromegaly causes hypertension, cardiomyopathy and diabetes mellitus, and untreated patients have a reduced life expectancy.[208] Gigantism results from a growth hormone secreting adenoma in childhood.[209]

The adrenocorticotrophic hormone (ACTH) secreting pituitary microadenoma which causes Cushing's disease is typically seen in women of middle age. The diagnosis can be difficult, particularly in distinguishing Cushing's disease of central origin from a more peripheral source. Adrenal tumours are a peripheral cause of steroid excess Cushing's syndrome, as is ectopic ACTH production from an oat-cell tumour of the lung[210,211] (see Chapter 35). The diagnosis should be suspected in any patient with hypertension, central obesity, easy bruising, violaceous abdominal and axillary striae and depression. Untreated, this group of patients have a 50% mortality in 5 years.

Large pituitary tumours may undergo sudden infarction or haemorrhage and present as an emergency with a suspected subarachnoid haemorrhage, termed pituitary apoplexy.[212] On examination multiple ocular nerve palsies are often found, and the CT scan is diagnostic. These patients require urgent surgery to decompress the optic chiasma.

The overall management of pituitary tumours is aimed at restoring normal endocrine function and reducing any mass effect of the pituitary adenoma. A combination of therapies is often required and thus patients are ideally managed by a multidisciplinary team including the neurosurgeon, endocrinologist and radiotherapist. Surgical excision is the preferred treatment for the majority of the patients with acromegaly, Cushing's disease and non-functioning pituitary adenoma.[213] Radiotherapy may be indicated for any residual or recurrent tumour demonstrated on follow-up imaging. Operations for pituitary microadenomas have a very low morbidity and mortality and often preserve normal pituitary function. Cushing himself popularized the trans-sphenoidal route in 1910.[214] The use of MR scanning (Fig. 16.21) provides essential preoperative detail of the anatomical relationships of the tumour. Even large macroadenomas with considerable suprasellar extension can be approached by the trans-sphenoidal route provided there is no restriction at the diaphragma sellae and the tumour is not found to be unusually fibrous.

Microprolactinomas can be treated medically with dopamine agonists such as bromocriptine and carbergoline, or by trans-sphenoidal surgery. Surgery is the first line of treatment in acromegaly, with octreotide being reserved for those patients whose growth hormone levels remain high following trans-sphenoidal surgery and radiotherapy.[215] Cushing's disease from a microadenoma is cured in up to 80% of cases by trans-sphenoidal surgery, but patients with larger tumours have a much poorer outcome even with radiotherapy.[216]

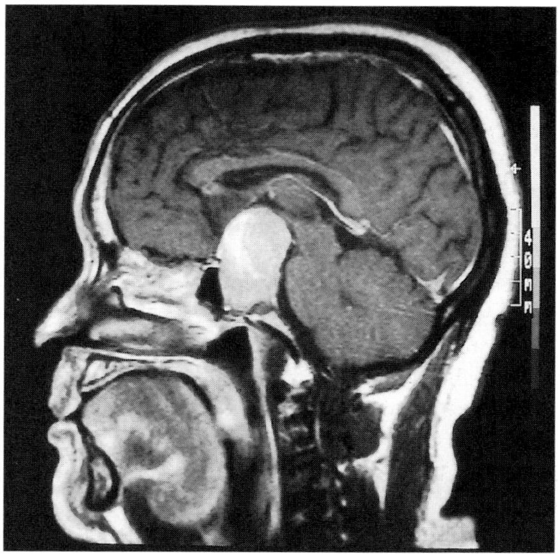

Fig. 16.21 MR scan of a pituitary macroadenoma.

Craniopharyngioma

These are cystic tumours arising in the suprasellar region, possibly from remnants of Rathke's pouch and therefore of congenital origin.[217] They are histologically benign but can be more aggressive in childhood. They present at any age from early childhood to old age, but have a peak incidence between 5 and 10 years and a second smaller peak between 50 and 60 years.[218] Overall, 40% occur in children younger than 16 years and 60% of all craniopharyngiomas are seen in patients older than 16 years. They cause pituitary and hypothalamic compression, visual failure and hydrocephalus as a result of invagination of the third ventricle (Fig. 16.22). There is little doubt that total excision is the treatment of choice but, because of their situation, complete excision may not

REFERENCES

207. Nabarro J D N Clin Endocrinol (Oxf) 1982; 17: 129
208. Laws E R Jr, Scheithauer B W et al J Neurosurg 1985; 63: 35
209. House W F, Brackman D E Otolaryngeal Head Neck Surg 1985; 93: 184
210. Oldfield E H, Doppmann J L et al N Engl J Med 1991; 325: 897
211. Salassa R M, Laws E R et al Trans Am Clin Climatol Assoc 1982; 94: 122
212. Cardoso E R, Peterson E W Neurosurg 1984; 14: 363
213. Hardy J Clin Neurosurg 1968; 16: 185
214. Jefferson A In: Fahlbusch R, Werder K V (eds) Treatment of Pituitary Adenoma. Thieme, Stuttgart 1978
215. Daughaday W H Am Intern Med 1990; 112: 159
216. Boggan J E, Tyrrel J B, Wilson C B J Neurosurg 1979; 50: 617
217. Adamson T E, Wiestler O D, Kleihues P, Yasagril M G J Neurosurg 1990; 73: 12
218. Camel P W In: Youmans J R (ed) Neurological Surgery, 3rd edn, vol 5. W B Saunders, Philadelphia pp 3233–3249

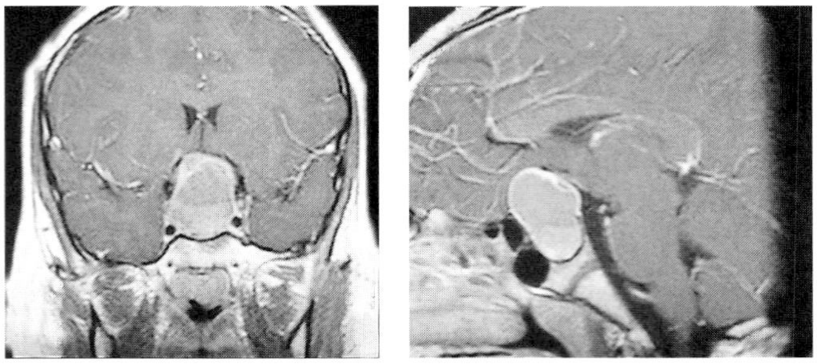

Fig. 16.22 Craniopharyngioma.

always be possible (Fig. 16.23).[219] As with pituitary adenomas, radiotherapy improves the long-term prognosis by delaying recurrence.[220]

Acoustic neuroma (schwannoma)

An acoustic neuroma should always be considered as a possible diagnosis in a patient presenting with unilateral deafness, which may be preceded or accompanied by tinnitus (see Chapter 20). There is often little to find in the early stages apart from the deafness, and frequently the diagnosis is not made until there is considerable distortion of the brainstem. The corneal reflex may be lost when the trigeminal nerve is elevated by the tumour but a seventh nerve palsy is a rare and late manifestation of the tumour. The importance of early diagnosis is considerable as the morbidity and mortality associated with surgery is directly related to the size of the tumour (Fig. 16.24).[221]

BRAIN TUMOURS IN CHILDREN

The worldwide incidence of brain tumour in childhood ranges from 2–5 new cases per 100 000.[222] In Britain there are approximately 350 new cases of brain tumour each year. Tumours of the posterior fossa are more common in children than in adults. 60% of all brain tumours in children arise in the posterior fossa compared to 20% in adults.[223] Tumours that involve the cranial nerves, such as acoustic neuromas, are rarely seen in childhood.

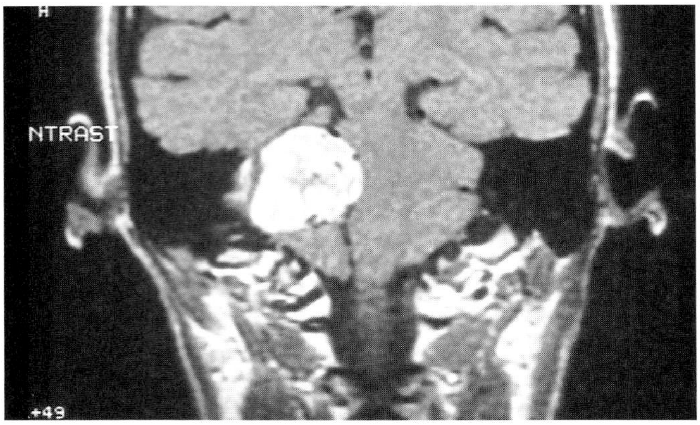

Fig. 16.24 A large acoustic neuroma.

Clinical features

Children with fourth ventricular and cerebellar tumours often have symptoms of raised intracranial pressure from obstructive hydrocephalus (Fig. 16.25) at the time of diagnosis.

REFERENCES

219. Raimondi A J, Rougerie J In: Concepts in Pediatric Neurosurgery. Karger, Basel pp 1–34
220. Manaka S, Teramoto A, Takatura K J Neurosurg 1985; 62: 648
221. Samii M In: Samii M, Draf W (eds) Surgery of the Skull Base. An Interdisciplinary Approach. Springer-Verlag, New York 1989 pp 377–395
222. Dahnman G J, Farwell J R Dis Nerv Syst 1976; 37: 396
223. Russell D, Rubenstein L Pathology of Tumours of the Nervous System, 5th edn. Williams & Wilkins, Baltimore 1989 251–279

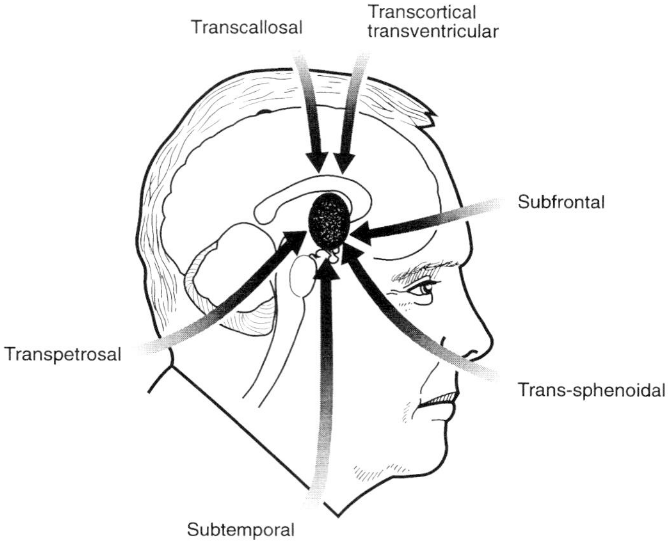

Fig. 16.23 Different approach options for the removal of craniopharyngiomas.

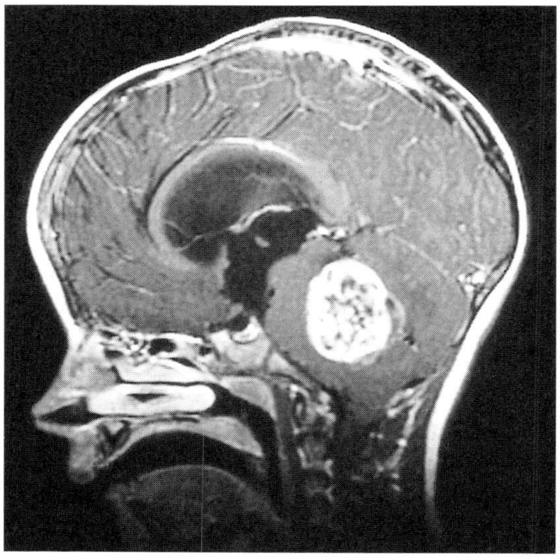

Fig. 16.25 Large posterior fossa tumour with hydrocephalus.

Headaches are the most frequent complaint and are commonly misdiagnosed as atypical migraine. Typically these headaches are generalized and associated with vomiting. They are often worse in the morning and can wake the child from sleep. The headaches may not always have the characteristic features of raised intracranial pressure, and in infants the manifestations are more likely to be of irritability and macrocephaly.

Disturbances of vision are the rule, nystagmus being a good localizing sign. Double vision can occur from a lateral rectus palsy which is a poor localizing sign, and results from the general rise in intracranial pressure. Head tilt is another characteristic manifestation of a posterior fossa tumour in childhood, often the result of compensation for the double vision. Papilloedema is a frequent finding with occasional loss of visual acuity to the point of blindness which may be transient, obscuration of vision, or permanent.

Children with brainstem tumours in contrast present with focal signs and do not complain of headache in the early stages. Hydrocephalus if it occurs at all, is late in the natural history. Disturbances of eye movements are common and occur early as a result of direct involvement of the nuclei and tracts in the brainstem. Nystagmus is often present. Unsteadiness and disturbances of gait are often regarded as the child being clumsy. Truncal ataxia is a feature of a 'vermian' midline cerebellar tumour such as a medulloblastoma or ependymoma. In these cases the child has satisfactory coordination when sitting, but is very unsteady when standing or walking. A laterally placed tumour such as a cerebellar astrocytoma gives rise to unilateral ataxia and nystagmus when sitting or standing.

Management

A third of children with brain tumours are unwell by the time the diagnosis is finally made; many are drowsy as a result of raised intracranial pressure and their vision may be threatened. Some are in a poor nutritional state because of persistent vomiting. In the majority of children steroids can be started, e.g. dexamethasone 1 mg/kg daily, with a gastroprotective drug such as ranitidine, and the child placed on the next available operating list for excision of the tumour. The hydrocephalus is treated by an external drain, which is inserted at the time of surgery and monitored for up to one week in the hope that the cerebrospinal fluid pathways will reopen and a permanent shunt will not be required. Less than half will require internalization of the drain. Shunting before the tumour is excised is not recommended, as the child may not require a long-term shunt and the patient is placed at risk from the attendant complications of shunting without the underlying problem having been treated.

Outcome

5-year survival has improved to 75% in children with medulloblastomas. This improved survival is not without some problems.[224] Children who have been successfully treated with chemotherapy and radiotherapy may suffer long-term disabling neuropsychological sequelae as a result of the therapy on the developing brain. There also remains a small risk of the development of a second tumour as a result of the treatment.

SKULL TUMOURS

A wide range of skin tumours can involve the scalp, but if the lesion is fixed to the skull a tumour arising from the skull itself must be suspected. The differential diagnosis of such a lump includes primary bone tumours as well as an exostosis from an intracranial meningioma. Definitive imaging with CT scan is indicated if there is any doubt before attempting excision under local anaesthetic.

Dermoid cysts can occur anywhere in the scalp but often cluster around the anterior fontanelle in infants. Posterior midline dermoids may be associated with a dermal sinus resulting from a midline fusion defect. This tract communicates through the skull with the subarachnoid space, and may cause repeated attacks of bacterial meningitis or abscess formation.

Epidermoid cysts also arise from embryonic dermal rests but consist of only epithelial cells whereas the dermoid has all elements including epithelial tissue and hair follicles. Epidermoid cysts can occur in the skull or the roof of the orbit. Both epidermoid and dermoid cysts slowly enlarge with time and can be readily distinguished from other lesions by CT scan. They are generally excised for cosmetic reasons alone but in the orbit may require surgery for progressive proptosis.

Rarely dermoid and epidermoid cysts can be found within the cranium, involving the brain directly from dermal cell rests without any cutaneous manifestation.

Primary benign tumours of the skull

Ivory osteomas of the skull vault are the most common benign tumour.[225] They produce a slow-growing sessile mass which, radiologically, may resemble the sclerotic reaction produced by a meningioma, so that a CT scan is indicated. Treatment is by excision for cosmetic reasons. Osteomas of the paranasal air sinuses may be associated with infective intracranial complications by eroding into the anterior cranial fossa and causing a cerebrospinal fluid leak and meningitis.[226]

Chondroma and chondrosarcoma

These tumours arise in cartilaginous elements in the skull base, particularly around the foramen lacerum, and thus tend to involve the parasellar region or cerebellopontine angle. Surgical treatment for skull base tumours has become very successful for tumours that were previously considered inoperable.

Chordomas arise from notochordal remnants and thus develop in the region of the sphenoid sinus, the clivus and around the foramen magnum, where they erode the skull base and produce multiple cranial nerve palsies. They tend to be slow-growing but are locally invasive; with the developments in skull base surgery they can be more radically excised.[227]

REFERENCES

224. Hirsch J, Renier D et al Acta Neurochir 1979; 48: 1
225. Abbott K H, Courville C B Bull Los Ang Neurol Soc 10: 19
226. Hallberg O E, Begley J W Arch Otolaryngol 1959; 41: 750
227. Sen C N, Sekhar L N, Schramm V L, Janecka I P Neurosurgery 1989; 25: 931

Primary malignant bone tumours of the skull[228]

Primary malignant tumours of the skull are very rare. Osteogenic sarcoma has an increased incidence in patients with Paget's disease of the skull and is then manifest as a rapidly enlarging vascular tumour. The usual radiological appearance of bone destruction associated with new bone formation and spicules of bone laid down at right angles to the surface may be obtained.

Secondary tumours of the skull

Multiple osteolytic lesions can arise from carcinoma of the lung, breast, kidney, thyroid, prostate and gastrointestinal tract tumours, as well as with myeloma. Other malignancies involving the skull include leukaemia and lymphomas.

INTRACRANIAL HAEMORRHAGE

INTRACRANIAL ANEURYSMS AND SUBARACHNOID HAEMORRHAGE

Rupture of an intracranial aneurysm is a cause of unexpected sudden death in adult life. It often occurs in a previously healthy individual in the most productive phase of life. In Britain, approximately one person in 10 000 will suffer a subarachnoid haemorrhage, of which nearly half will be fatal;[229] this is similar to the worldwide incidence of subarachnoid haemorrhage—estimated to be 12 in 100 000 people.[230]

Pathology

The causes of spontaneous subarachnoid haemorrhage (SAH) include aneurysms (85%), arteriovenous malformation (5%), vasculitis, coagulopathy and, rarely, tumour.[231]

Intracranial saccular or berry aneurysms occur most frequently at the points of bifurcation around the circle of Willis. It is considered that there are congenital defects in the arterial wall at the points of bifurcation which are further weakened by natural haemodynamic stresses as well as by degenerative changes produced by hypertension and atherosclerosis.[232]

90% of berry aneurysms are found in the internal carotid artery territory with the most common locations being the anterior communicating complex, the internal carotid/posterior communicating artery and the bifurcation of the middle cerebral artery.[233]

10% of aneurysms involve the posterior circulation in the vertebro-basilar territory. 20% of patients have multiple aneurysms. The anatomical distribution of cerebral aneurysms is shown diagrammatically in Figure 16.26. There is an association between berry aneurysms, polycystic kidneys, coarctation of the aorta and Marfan's syndrome. A small number of patients with aneurysms have a strong family history of the condition.[234]

Symptoms and signs

The clinical picture of subarachnoid haemorrhage is characteristic, with the sudden collapse of a middle-aged person with the worst headache of his or her life. Examination reveals an obtunded patient with neck stiffness. Fundoscopy may reveal subhyaloid haemorrhages. Lumbar puncture confirms the diagnosis with uniformly bloodstained cerebrospinal fluid and xanthochromia in the supernatant.

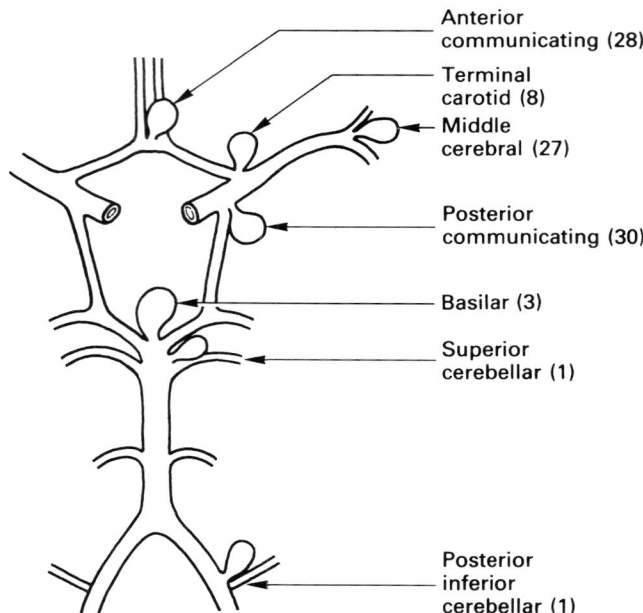

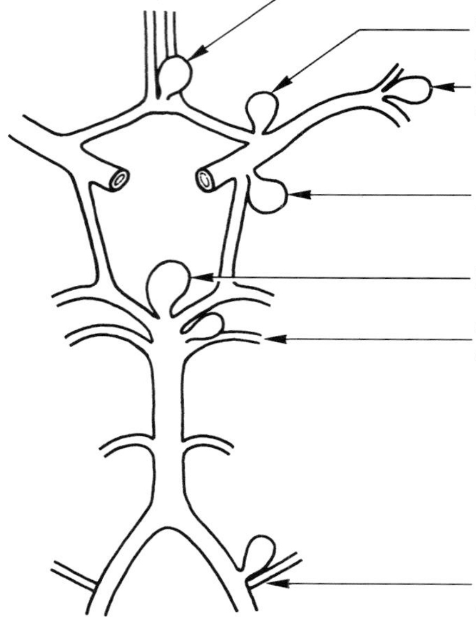

Fig. 16.26 Sites of aneurysms (figures denote percentage of total).

Berry aneurysm rupture is most likely to occur in middle age, reaching a peak in males in the fifth decade, and in females in the sixth decade. Many patients suffer warning headaches that are sudden and severe but are not diagnosed. Diagnosis at this time carries a good prognosis but unfortunately patients may be sent home from casualty because there may be few abnormal physical signs, only to suffer a fatal rebleed.[235] A painful third nerve palsy is the presenting sign of an expanding aneurysm of the posterior communicating or terminal basilar arteries and requires urgent treatment. The risk of epilepsy is highest with middle cerebral artery aneurysms (20% incidence in 5 years) because of the frequently associated intracerebral haematoma.[236]

Diagnosis

A non-enhanced CT brain scan is often diagnostic—blood can be detected in the subarachnoid space in the majority of cases within

REFERENCES

228. Dahlin D C, Unni K K Bone Tumours. Thomas Springfield 1986 pp 224–267
229. Linn F H H et al Stroke 1996; 27: 625
230. Haley E C Jr, Kassell N F, Torner J C Stroke 1992; 23: 205
231. Wirth F P Clin Neurosurg 1986; 33: 125
232. Sekher L N, Heros R Neurosurgery 1981; 8: 248
233. Weir B In: Weir B Aneurysms Affecting the Nervous System. Williams & Wilkins, Baltimore 1987
234. Bannerman R M, Ingall G B, Graf C J Neurol 1970; 20: 283
235. Verweij R D, Wijdicks E F M, van Gijn J Arch Neurol 1988; 45: 1019
236. Rose F L, Sarner M Br Med J 1965; 1: 18

48 hours of the ictus.[237] The site of the ruptured aneurysm can be predicted in many cases by the early CT scan, which is valuable as 20% of patients have multiple aneurysms.[238] CT scanning also reveals any degree of hydrocephalus and the extent of the haemorrhage, which is of value in predicting the risk of vasospasm. Patients with a thick blood clot in the basal cisterns have a higher risk of vasospasm and consequent development of a delayed cerebral ischaemic deficit (Fig. 16.27).[239]

Lumbar puncture is undertaken if the CT scan is normal or if there is any possibility of a bacterial meningitis; a xanthochromic supernatant is diagnostic of subarachnoid haemorrhage.[240] MR angiography and CT spiral imaging are improving but four-vessel cerebral angiography is still essential to provide detail prior to any surgical procedure. MR angiography is of more value in screening asymptomatic individuals at risk of developing berry aneurysms.

Principles of management

Patients who survive the initial subarachnoid haemorrhage are at risk of rebleeding and the development of a delayed ischaemic deficit as a result of vasospasm.[241] Surgery for ruptured aneurysms is prophylactic to prevent rebleeding and patients have a good outcome provided they are in optimum condition before surgery.[242] The patient's clinical condition on admission therefore determines the timing of surgery. Early surgery is recommended in patients who are in a good neurological condition. Those patients in a poor condition undergo surgery when their clinical condition has improved.[243] The importance of the patient's clinical condition in relation to management has led to the development of several classifications which also allow the response to novel therapies to be assessed.[244] The modified Hunt & Hess classification (Table 16.4) is the most widely accepted and is often combined with the Glasgow Coma Scale to monitor the patient's condition.

Patients in grades 1 and 2 are in the best condition and have the lowest risk of developing vasospasm. Patients in this group should

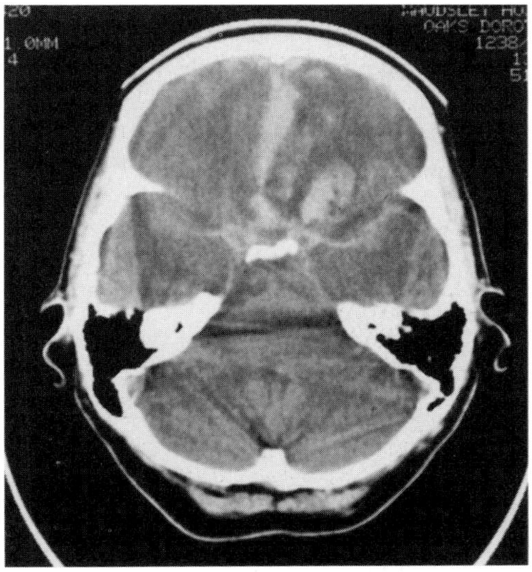

Fig. 16.27 CT scan in subarachnoid haemorrhage showing blood in the anterior interhemispheric fissure, suggesting an anterior communicating artery aneurysm.

Table 16.4 The Hunt & Hess classification of patients with subarachnoid haemorrhage

Grade 1	Symptomless, mild headache and minimal neck stiffness
Grade 2	Moderate or severe headache, meningism; no neurological deficit (except an oculomotor or lateral rectus palsy)
Grade 3	Drowsy or confused with mild focal deficits
Grade 4	Stupor with moderate or severe hemiparesis
Grade 5	Deep coma, moribund

undergo surgery on the next operating list and are very likely to have a good outcome.[245] All patients receive active measures to reduce the risk of an ischaemic deficit from vasospasm, including maintenance of normal perfusion and hydration as well as calcium channel blocking agents such as Nimodopine.[246] Patients who develop neurological deficits due to vasospasm are treated in the intensive care unit by hypervolaemia, haemodilution and elevation of the blood pressure if the aneurysm has been secured.[247]

Surgery

Surgical treatment by craniotomy and clipping of the aneurysm is the definitive treatment in the majority of patients.[248] Microsurgical technique with the application of an aneurysm clip is usually satisfactory but any residual sac may need to be reinforced with gauze. Some aneurysms are inaccessible, such as an internal carotid artery aneurysm within the cavernous sinus, so embolization is more appropriate for these cases. Very fine steerable catheters deliver coils into the sac to encourage spontaneous thrombosis. This endovascular technique has also been shown to be of benefit in basilar and other posterior circulation aneurysms.[249]

Outcome

More than half of all those who suffer a subarachnoid haemorhage from a ruptured aneurysm die or remain seriously disabled.[250] The operative mortality is between 5 and 10%, and a third of the patients who undergo successful clipping of the aneurysm return to their premorbid state.[251] 60% of those who undergo successful

REFERENCES

237. Lilliquist B, Lindqvist M Acta Radiol (Diagn) 1980; 21: 327
238. Takayasu M, Shintana A, Negoro M, Asai T Neurol Med Chir 1985; 25: 27
239. Mizoi K, Yoshimoto T et al Neurosurgery 1991; 28: 807
240. McMenemy W H Proc R Soc Med 1954; 47: 701
241. Grosset D G, Straiton J et al J Neurosurg 1993; 78: 183
242. Saveland H, Hillman J et al Acta Neurol Scand 1967; 43 (suppl 29): 1
243. Solomon R A, Onesti S T, Klebanoff L J Neurosurg 1991; 75: 56
244. Hunt W E, Hess R M J Neurosurg 1968; 28: 14
245. Sundt T M Jr, Kobayashi S, Fode N C, Whisnant J P Mayo Clin Proc 1985; 6: 230
246. Pickard J D, Murray G D et al Br Med J 1989; 298: 636
247. Kassell N F, Peerless S J et al Neurosurgery 1982; 11: 337
248. Yasargil M G, Fox J L Surg Neurol 1975; 3: 7
249. Guglielmi G, Vinuela F et al J Neurosurg 1992; 77: 515
250. Bailes J E, Spetzler R F et al J Neurosurg 1990; 72: 559
251. Saveland H, Hillman J et al J Neurosurg 1992; 76: 729

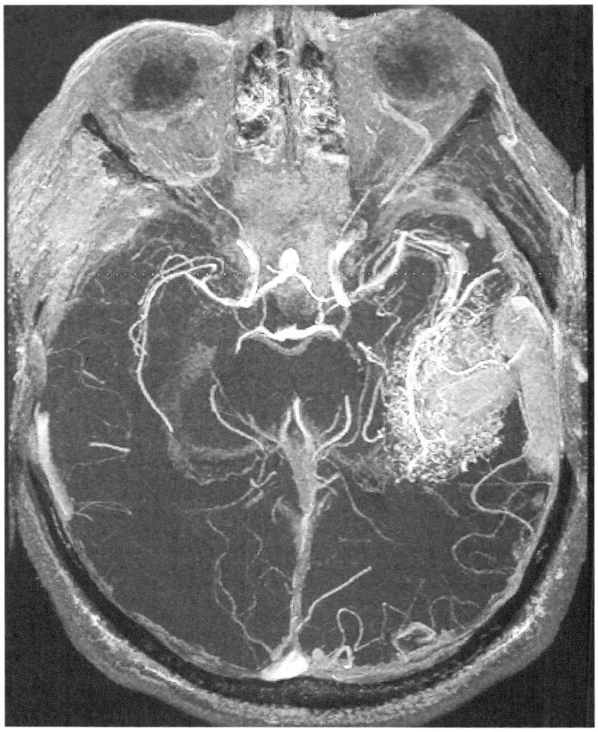

Fig. 16.28 MR Angiogram. Extensive left temporal arteriovenous malformation with aneurysm pointing forward in anterior communicating artery complex.

surgery describe a reduced quality of life because of difficulties with concentration, memory and the psychological sequelae.[252]

ARTERIOVENOUS MALFORMATIONS

Arteriovenous malformations in the brain can be discovered incidentally and do not all require active management. Those that have bled are likely to rebleed and need to be treated. Arteriovenous malformations that bleed differ from aneurysmal bleeds in that they do not precipitate the same degree of vasospasm despite extensive haemorrhage and there is not the high risk of early rebleeding.[253] Some arteriovenous malformations present with epilepsy and are too extensive for treatment (Fig. 16.28).[254]

Pathology

Arteriovenous malformations allow blood to pass directly from arteries into veins because of the failure of the embryonic capillary bed to develop; the veins become arterialized. They have been classified by their size, the number of feeding vessels, the location and whether the venous drainage is superficial or deep.[255] There are frequently other associated vascular abnormalities.[256] High flows generate an increased incidence of aneurysms on the arterial feeding vessels; on the venous side varices and stenoses are frequently seen.

Clinical presentation

An intracranial haemorrhage is the most common presentation, occurring in over half of patients with arteriovenous malformations.[257] The haemorrhage is usually intraparenchymal, but rupture into the ventricles or subarachnoid space is common. The majority of patients survive the ictus and unlike aneurysmal bleeds the risk of rebleeding or vasospasm is very small. Fits are the next most frequent presentation and these may be focal or generalized without signs of haemorrhage. Headaches are not infrequent and can be mistaken for migraine, they may be unilateral or generalized. Progressive neurological deficit developing over a long period can also result from ischaemia, due to a chronic 'steal syndrome'.[258]

Therapeutic options

Complete excision of a typical arteriovenous malformation that is running from the surface with an apex pointing deep into the cerebral hemisphere removes the risk of further bleeding, but the arteriovenous malformation may be more complex and require a combination of therapies.[259] Embolization and focused radiotherapy are the other techniques currently available and can be used individually or in combination with surgery.[260]

Selective catheterization of the feeding vessels and embolization with glue, coils or other particles can fully occlude the feeding vessels and obliterate the nidus. Radiosurgery, also called stereotactic radiotherapy, is another option for small deep malformations; this accomplishes a more gradual occlusion, with the risk of rebleeding remaining for up to a year or longer before the nidus disappears.[261]

TRIGEMINAL NEURALGIA

This condition has been recognized for over 200 years and was known as 'tic douloureux' because the electric-shock like pain causes a sudden contraction of the facial muscles.[262] It is a very severe and disabling pain which can lead to depression and suicide. It is most frequently seen in adults over 50 years of age. The unilateral facial pain occurs suddenly, lasting for a few seconds; as the condition worsens, the paroxysms become more frequent and the patient develops a more constant, aching background discomfort. The pain is often confined to one or two divisions of the trigeminal nerve. The second and third divisions of the nerve are most frequently affected.[263]

REFERENCES

252. Stenhouse L M, Knight R G et al Neurol Neurosurg Psych 1991; 54 (10): 904
253. Jane J A, Kassell N F et al J Neurosurg 1985; 62: 321
254. Spetzler R F, Martin N A et al J Neurosurg 1987; 67: 17
255. Hamilton M G, Spetzler R F Neurosurgery 1994; 34: 2
256. Brown R B Jr, Wiebers D O, Forbes G S J Neurosurg 1990; 73: 859
257. Drake C G Clin Neurosurg 1979; 26: 145
258. Crawford P M, West C R et al J Neurol Neurosurg Psychiatr 1986; 49: 1
259. Vinuela F, Dion J E et al J Neurosurg 1991; 75: 856
260. Lawton M T, Hamilton M G, Spetzler R F Neurosurgery 1995; 37: 29
261. Heros R C, Korouse K N Engl J Med 1990; 323: 127
262. Sweet W H N Engl J Med 1986; 315: 174
263. Penman J Postgrad Med 1950; 26: 627

The pain is characteristically 'shooting' or 'burning' in nature and may occur spontaneously or in response to touching trigger areas. Normal activities such as talking, shaving or chewing are impossible and the patients have difficulty eating and often lose weight.

A neurological examination is normal in trigeminal neuralgia, but patients with secondary trigeminal neuralgia from an underlying cerebellopontine angle tumour or multiple sclerosis may have evidence of other cranial nerve or brainstem involvement. Acoustic neuromas are by far the most common tumours occurring in the cerebellopontine region but metastases, epidermoid cysts and meningiomas are also found.[264]

The most widely accepted hypothesis on the pathogenesis of trigeminal neuralgia is that it results from vascular compression of the trigeminal sensory root at its entry into the brainstem.[265] Vascular loops from the superior cerebellar artery or adjacent vessels indent the nerve and cause irregular demyelination within the nerve root producing short-circuiting of the nerve impulse. A similar mechanism is implicated in hemifacial spasm and glossopharyngeal neuralgia.

An MR scan must be obtained in all cases to exclude a cerebellopontine angle lesion and to define any vessels adjacent to the origin of the nerve from the brainstem. The initial treatment is medical and carbamazepine (Tegretol) is the drug of choice. It is started at a low dose, 100 mg b.d., increasing to a level which controls the pain. Carbamazepine is usually highly effective and if it does not control the pain the diagnosis should be reviewed. Up to 1200–1800 mg in divided doses is usually the maximum tolerated daily dose. If side-effects such as nausea, unsteadiness and ataxia become intolerable at a dose which does not control pain, then surgery is considered. Carbamazepine can cause skin rashes and a rapidly fatal desquamation syndrome in allergic individuals.[266]

Surgical treatment

A surgical procedure is considered in patients unwilling or unable to tolerate carbamazepine. Many younger patients with trigeminal neuralgia benefit from a microvascular decompression of the trigeminal nerve. Loops of vessels compressing or traversing the trigeminal nerve are lifted away from the root entry zone and fine gauze interposed, leaving facial sensation undisturbed. This technique was originally described by Walter Dandy.[267] Jannetta has reported a contemporary series of patients with a pain-free period of 10 years in over 80%.[268] If no obvious vascular compression is found then the lateral third of the root is sectioned. The resulting reduction in facial sensation is usually well tolerated.[269]

Selective thermocoagulation of the retrogasserian portion of the nerve root by a percutaneous approach through the foramen ovale is a well tried technique and is particularly of benefit in older patients suffering from involvement of the second and third divisions of the trigeminal nerve.[270] There is a risk of ophthalmic complications when the first division of the trigeminal nerve is included in the lesion leading to corneal anaesthesia.[271]

The alternative approaches in the elderly who may not tolerate a general anaesthetic include peripheral destructive procedures with avulsion or cryosurgery but this gives a shorter respite, leaves numbness and can precipitate additional dysaesthetic pain after multiple procedures.[272,273]

REFERENCES

264. Bullitt E, Tew J M, Boyd J Neurosurg 1986; 64: 865
265. Janetta P J J Neurosurg 1967; 26: 159
266. Killian J M, Fromm G H Arch Neurol Chicago 1968; 19: 129
267. Dandy W E Johns Hopkins Med J 1925; 36: 105
268. Janetta P J Arch Neurol 1985; 42: 800
269. Sweet W H Clin Neurosurg 1985; 32: 294
270. Lunsford L D, Apfelbaum R I Clin Neurosurg 1985; 32: 319
271. Taha J M, Tew J M Neurosurgery 1996; 38: 865
272. Guidetti B, Fraioli B, Refice G M J Maxillofac Surg 1979; 7: 315
273. Sweet W H In: Wilkings R H, Rengachary S S (eds) Neurosurgery, 2nd edn. McGraw Hill, New York 1995

17 The neck

A. E. Young

The predominant clinical problem encountered in the neck by surgeons is a swelling. The assessment and diagnosis of such swellings is one of the classical exercises in clinical expertise. It requires not only a knowledge of the anatomy of the neck but also the skills of focused history taking and careful examination. These two alone will yield a diagnosis in the majority of cases.

A swelling in the neck may be of a type common elsewhere in the body such as a sebaceous cyst or lipoma; if the swelling is lymphadenopathy it may reflect systemic disease, but the majority of lumps that present in the neck are, or reflect, specific local disease (Fig. 17.1). The causes of such swellings are reviewed in this chapter, but the details of specific disease may be described in other chapters, particularly those dealing with the salivary glands (Chapter 14), the mouth and tongue (Chapter 13), the thyroid (Chapter 18), ear, nose and throat (Chapter 20), the arteries (Chapter 10) and lymphoma (Chapter 34).

For the sake of completeness and because they do not appear elsewhere in the book thyroglossal sinus and branchial fistulae are dealt with in this chapter.

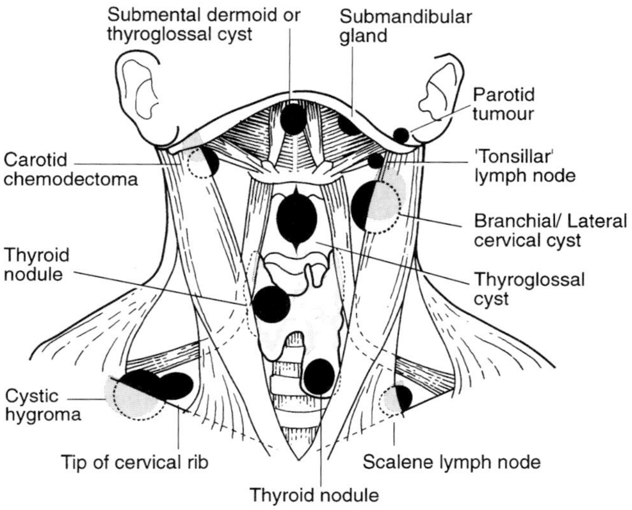

Fig. 17.1 Anatomical location of the most common swellings in the neck.

CAUSES OF A SWELLING IN THE NECK

The specific causes are summarized in Table 17.1.

Table 17.1 Causes of a swelling in the neck

Congenital abnormalities
Thyroglossal tract abnormalities
Branchial (lateral cervical) cysts
Cystic hygroma
Cervical rib
Tumours
Thyroid tumours (see Chapter 18)
Salivary gland tumours (see Chapter 14)
Sarcoma, lipoma, neuroma, fibroma, etc.
Chemodectoma
Lymph node enlargements
See Table 17.2
Benign enlargements of glands
Salivary gland (see Chapter 14)
Thyroid gland (see Chapter 18)
Diverticulae
Laryngocele (see Chapter 20)
Pharyngeal pouch (see Chapter 20)
Traumatic
Sternomastoid 'tumour'

Thyroglossal tract

The thyroglossal tract is the remnant which marks developmental descent of the thyroid gland. The thyroid appears as a midline diverticulum at the fourth week of development, and promptly descends ventrally to the pharynx between the developing second branchial arch (Fig. 17.2). The duct formed during descent becomes solid and then normally involutes. Various clinical results obtain if this process is not smooth:

1. Persistence of the origin of the tract may remain as a midline dimple at the junction of the filiform and valate papillae of the tongue—the foramen caecum.
2. The tract itself may persist whole as a thyroglossal duct or in part as a thyroglossal cyst.
3. Solid thyroid tissue may persist and develop at any stage along the tract, in particular as a lingual thyroid, as tissue in the wall of the patent duct or cyst or, most commonly, as a pyramidal lobe of a normal thyroid (see Lingual Thyroid, Chapter 18)

Thyroglossal cyst

Thyroglossal cysts may appear in association with patent or closed thyroglossal ducts. Some 40% present during the first decade of

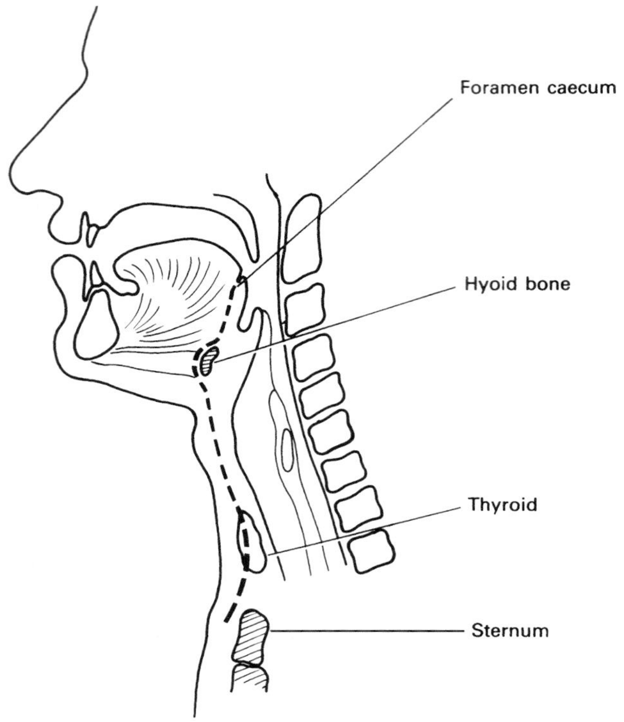

Fig. 17.2 The thyroglossal tract. Thyroglossal cysts are usually located between the hyoid and the pyramidal lobe but can occur anywhere from the foramen caecum to the sternum.

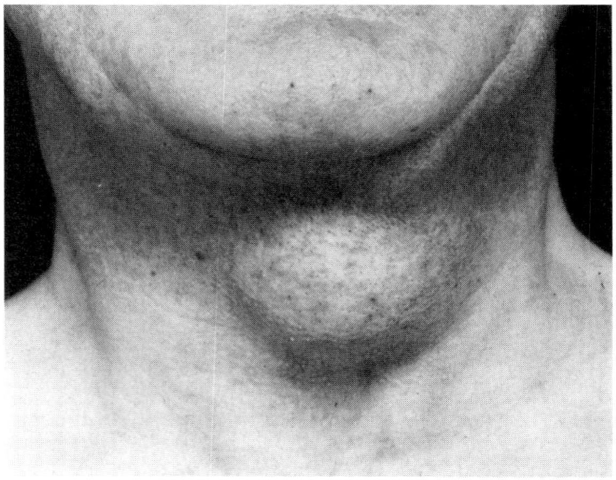

Fig. 17.3 A large thyroglossal cyst located just below the hyoid.

life, the remainder at any time; these cysts even appear in octogenarians. Only rarely is a thyroglossal cyst noted at birth. The incidence is approximately equal in males and females. Both variants are smooth, rounded, unattached to the strap muscles and typically in the midline, though a quarter may be a little to the right or the left (Fig. 17.3). Very occasionally a cyst is found as far out as the lateral tip of the hyoid. The cysts are usually just above or just below the hyoid, attached to a remnant of the thyroglossal tract. Thus, a cyst may rise on protrusion of the tongue and during deglutition. Elevation on protrusion of the tongue differentiates a thyroglossal cyst from a nodule in the thyroid isthmus or pyramidal lobe. Thyroglossal cysts rarely transilluminate.

Thyroglossal cysts are the most common midline neck tumour of infancy and may be confused with epidermoid cysts, dermoid cysts, enlarged lymph nodes, subhyoid bursae and pyramidal lobe thyroid nodules. The cysts are lined by stratified squamous epithelium or ciliated pseudostratified columnar epithelium. There may be thyroid or lymphoid tissue in the wall, and any of these elements may undergo malignant change. Indeed it has been asserted that the thyroid tissue is usually dysplastic and thus particularly at risk of malignant change. Malignancies are most commonly of thyroid papillary type[1] but there is no evidence that the disease is multicentric, and it is not necessary to excise the thyroid as well as the thyroglossal tumour.

Thyroglossal fistula (sinus)

A thyroglossal fistula is almost invariably an acquired lesion and is unlike congenital branchial fistulae. It originates following rupture or incision of a thyroglossal cyst. The external opening is usually directed cranially and overlaid by a crescent shaped fold of stretched skin. There is intermittent seropurulent discharge. It is difficult, either surgically or with dyes, to show any communication between the orifice and the foramen caecum of the tongue, and these fistulae are more appropriately classified as sinuses as they do not connect two epithelial surfaces. It is not known whether infection occurs in thyroglossal cysts by spread down a microscopically patent track from the tongue or by haematogenous spread.

Treatment of thyroglossal cyst and fistula

Where part or all of the thyroglossal duct is patent, the treatment of choice for both cyst and sinus is 'Sistrunk's operation'. A patent track may be injected with dye before the operation is begun. The cyst or sinus is then mobilized via a transverse incision made over it. The track is followed up between the infrahyoid muscles to the level of the hyoid bone. Its relationship to this bone is complex and the only sure way of ablating the track is to excise the central portion of the hyoid bone. The track is then followed upwards and backwards to the base of the tongue. Usually in this part of its course the track is incomplete and represented only by isolated fragments of epithelial tissue. A blind dissection must therefore be done in the midline between the geniohyoids and genioglossae. This suprahyoid part of the operation may be omitted where the cyst is infrahyoid and no proximal track can be demonstrated. It may be employed, however, with suprahyoid cysts and should ideally be taken to the foramen caecum. Failure to excise the central portion of the hyoid bone is associated with a high incidence of recurrence.[2] Excision of the hyoid is not attended by any disability, and is not associated with osteomyelitis when performed in the presence of sepsis.

REFERENCES

1. Saharin P C Br J Surg 1975; 62: 689–691
2. Pollock W F, Stevenson E O J Surg 1966; 112: 225–231

Branchial (lateral cervical) cyst

The second most common congenital swelling in the neck is the so-called branchial cyst. This name presupposes an origin from embryonic branchial cleft tissue remnants. This view is encouraged by the fact that when such cysts become infected they discharge through the skin and the sinus that may subsequently develop is at the anterior border of the sternomastoid muscle at a similar site to the external opening of a true branchial fistula (see below). Further evidence of a branchial cleft origin is supported by the very occasional tract that is discovered running from the deep surface of these lesions towards the pharynx. By contrast it has been noted that almost all branchial cysts have lymphoid tissue in their walls and may thus represent merely cystic degeneration in cervical lymphatic tissue. Linking these two disparate hypotheses is the notion that trapped embryological remnants or acquired additional epithelial tissue originating from the tonsil may stimulate this degeneration.[3] The cysts themselves are lined by heterotopic squamous epithelium. The debate is arcane and of little practical value except that it supports the view that these cysts should be defined as 'lateral cervical cysts' rather than 'branchial cysts', and that at operation 'what you see is what you get'; thus there is no requirement to dissect out a hypothetical deep tract leading to the pharynx.

Most lateral cervical cysts present in the third decade. There is no dominant side or predilection for either sex. Patients complain of an enlarging lump, usually presenting from behind the junction of the upper and middle thirds of the sternomastoid muscle, though it may present anywhere behind or just in front of the upper sternomastoid (Fig. 17.4). There may be pain and even frank infection, which is usually responsive to antibiotics. Established or recurrent infection can lead to the development of a brawny or fibrotic mass with fixity to surrounding structures. The diagnosis is primarily clinical, backed up if there is doubt by fine-needle aspiration biopsy which produces an opalescent fluid containing cholesterol crystals or frank pus.

Once diagnosed, the lateral cervical cyst should be treated by surgical excision. This should be preceded by a course of antibiotics if there is infection. The cyst which has never been infected can be readily excised through an oblique skin crease incision and a plane developed outside the cyst. The previously infected cyst will, however, be fixed wholly or in part to surrounding structures including the jugular vein and excision may be difficult. Care must be taken to excise the whole of the cyst; failure to do so risks recurrence or the development of a chronic, discharging sinus in the wound. There is no need to search for a tract leading to the pharynx from the deep surface.

Branchial fistulae and sinuses

The term 'branchial' is derived from the Greek word for a gill. At five weeks the human embryo exhibits four branchial clefts externally and five matched pharyngeal pouches internally.[4]

The first pair form the middle ear and eustachian tube. Anomalies of the first cleft may appear as a sinus posterior or anterior to the external ear and are rarely appreciated until they become infected, usually in a young adult (Fig. 17.5). These sinuses extend deeply and may be difficult to eradicate surgically. If the surgeon is tempted to operate on a recurrent sinus anterior to the meatus, it should be remembered that the deeply extending track will pass close to the facial nerve, which is therefore at risk.

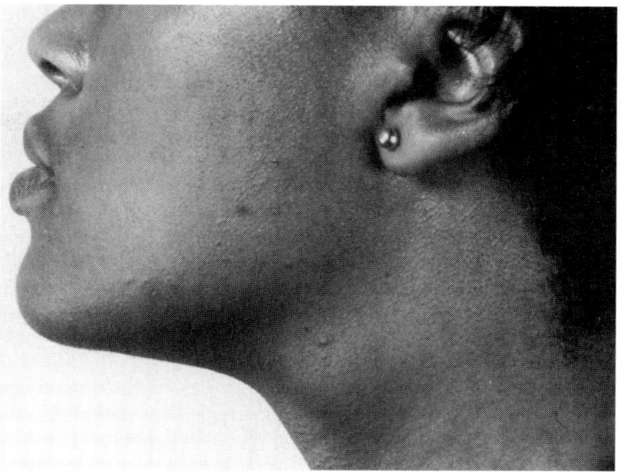

Fig. 17.4 A branchial cyst emerging anteriorly to the upper third of the sternomastoid.

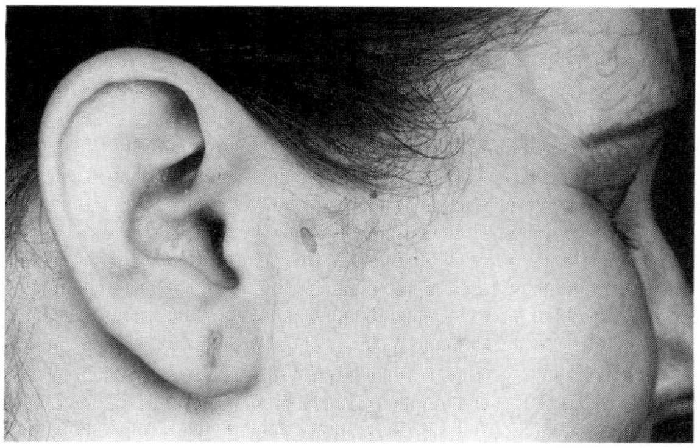

Fig. 17.5 A large, quiescent preauricular sinus.

Second cleft anomalies are uncommon. True fistulae may be bilateral; their anterior openings are in the line of the anterior border of the sternomastoid muscle. From this opening the fistula passes deeply between the stylohyoid muscles and the posterior belly of digastric, anterior to the hypoglossal nerve through the bifurcation of the internal and external carotid arteries and enters the pharynx in the tonsillar fossa.[5]

Cystic hygroma

This is an old but widely used term describing a congenital, cystic, lymphatic malformation at the root of the neck. Cystic hygromas probably represent a developmental anomaly during the coalescence of primitive lymph elements into the adult pattern. The malformation consists of thin-walled, single or multiple interconnecting

REFERENCES

3. Golledge J, Ellis H J Laryngol Otol 1994; 108: 653–659
4. Wendell Todd N Surg Clin North Am 1993; 73: 599–610
5. Parke W W, Settles H E Clin Anat 1991; 4: 285

or separate cysts which insinuate themselves widely into the tissues at the root of the neck. 50–65% are present at birth and if very large may even obstruct delivery. After delivery large cysts may obstruct respiration and swallowing.[6] Presentation is occasionally delayed until adulthood.

The diagnosis is usually made by clinical examination of these transilluminable thin-walled cysts, but a chest radiograph is important to map their caudal extents, and CT or MRI may be helpful if they are complex. The injection of sclerosant after aspiration may be effective treatment, but in general excision is necessary and this should preferably be performed as a one stage procedure. Partial excision may resolve symptoms.[7]

Cervical rib

About 1% of the population have a supernumerary rib arising from the lowest cervical vertebra. It is bilateral in 80%. The rib is an incomplete stub and its anterior portion can be felt as a fixed, hard swelling in the supraclavicular fossa where it may mimic metastatic disease. Cervical ribs themselves rarely cause symptoms, though occasionally symptoms of thoracic outlet syndrome may be produced due to disturbance of the adjacent brachial plexus or subclavian vessels. These do not pass over the rib, however, and other causes of thoracic outlet syndrome should be sought before the symptoms are attributed to cervical rib.

The rib is readily identified on simple radiography. Resection of cervical ribs is only indicated in the rare circumstances of their being confidently shown to be the cause of thoracic outlet syndrome. Both anterior and posterior routes have been described, but the standard approach is a supraclavicular collar incision with exposure of the upper and mid trunks of the brachial plexus before excision of the rib as far back as is necessary to relieve pressure on nerves or vessels[8] (see also Chapter 10).

TUMOURS IN THE NECK

Thyroid

Thyroid disease, whether solitary nodules or multinodular goitre, often presents as the finding of a nodule in the neck. A nodule located in the upper pole of the thyroid may be felt surprisingly high in the neck. Nevertheless, in all cases the thyroid nodule will move on swallowing; its relationship to the thyroid may be confirmed on ultrasound scanning and its nature initially investigated with a fine-needle aspiration biopsy (see Chapter 18).

Salivary gland

Salivary gland tumours and benign swellings are common causes of a swelling in the neck. The uninitiated will often mistake a tumour in the tail of the parotid as a cervical node (Fig. 17.6) but the history distinguishes benign whole gland swellings such as sialectasis and Sjögren's syndrome whilst fine-needle biopsy can diagnose tumours (see Chapter 14).

Chemodectoma (carotid body tumour)

Chemodectomas are tumours of the paraganglion cells of the cartoid body located at the bifurcation of the common carotid artery (see Chapter 10). These tumours are usually benign but locally invasive. Occasionally they are malignant and have potential to metastasize to local lymph nodes. They may be bilateral and

REFERENCES

6. Bill A H, Sumner D S Surg Gyn Obstet 1965; 120: 79–86
7. Kirschner P A Surgery 1966; 60: 1104–1107
8. Sharrard W J W In: Paediatric Orthopedics and Fractures. Blackwell, Oxford 1993 p 915

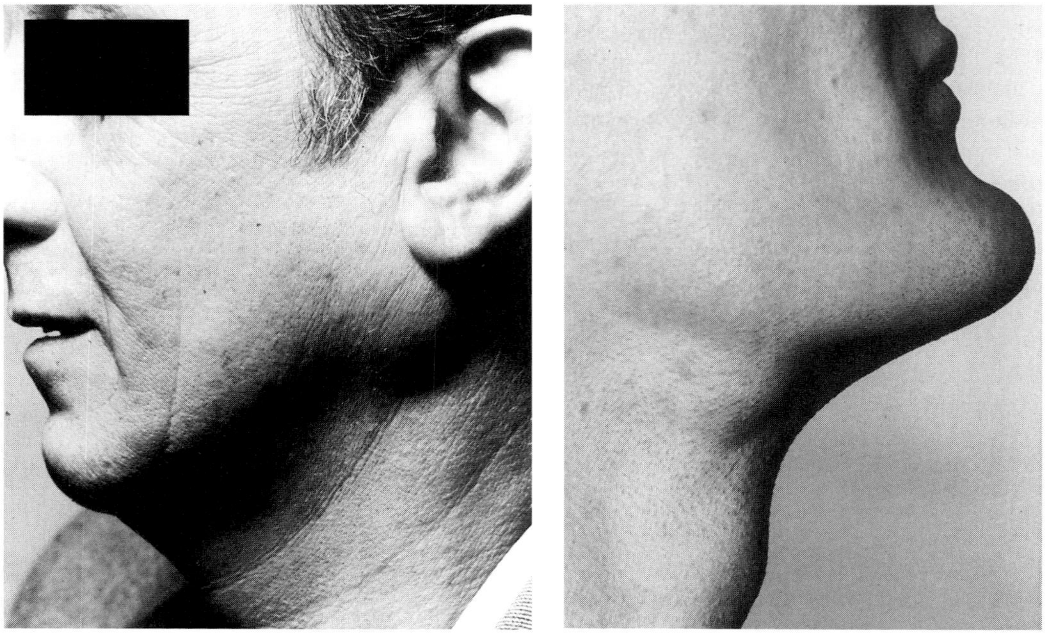

a b

Fig. 17.6 (**a**) A pleomorphic adenoma in the tail of the parotid. (**b**) Enlargement of a submandibular gland obstructed by a stone.

may also be familial.[9] Patients with chemodectomas may have other head and neck paraganglionic tumours, including vagal and glomus jugular tumours.

The tumour presents as a slow-growing, often painful pulsatile mass at the angle of the jaw; if untreated it spreads cranially to the base of the skull as well as forwards to become a more pronounced tumour in the neck. Investigation is initially by Doppler ultrasound to confirm the diagnosis and then by angiography. If there is doubt about the extent of the tumour a CT or MR scan may be helpful.

The preferred management is by surgery (see Chapter 10), but it should be remembered that there is only endothelium between the tumour and the lumina of the carotid artery. Surgery should only be undertaken when the necessary vascular surgical skills are available. If the tumour is large but resectable, surgery of these highly vascular tumours may be made more straightforward by preoperative embolization.[10,11] This is, however, a potentially dangerous addition to the management. Wax & Briant have described the use of the ultrasonic surgical dissector to facilitate removal of these tumours.[12]

Excellent results have been achieved with radiotherapy instead of surgery in patients who are unfit for surgery or who have large tumours. There are a number of reports of excellent long-term follow-ups without progression of disease in these patients.[13]

CERVICAL LYMPHADENOPATHY

Cervical lymph nodes may be enlarged by inflammatory changes or by primary or metastatic malignancy (see Table 17.2).

The most common cause of a swelling in the neck is cervical lymphadenopathy, and the causes are usually benign. Although only one node may be visible or palpable, other adjacent nodes are often enlarged. One third of the lymph nodes in the body are situated in the head and neck region[14] and an understanding of the possible causes of cervical lymphadenopathy requires a knowledge of their anatomy (Fig. 17.7). The habit of naming particular groups of cervical nodes might imply that there are anatomically discrete groups of such nodes. In fact, these names are largely a conventional way of subdividing an extensive interconnecting network of nodes and do not imply anatomical separateness. The surgeon must understand the pattern of lymph drainage in the head and neck if the correct investigations are to be undertaken in a patient with metastatic disease in lymph nodes (Figs. 17.8–10).

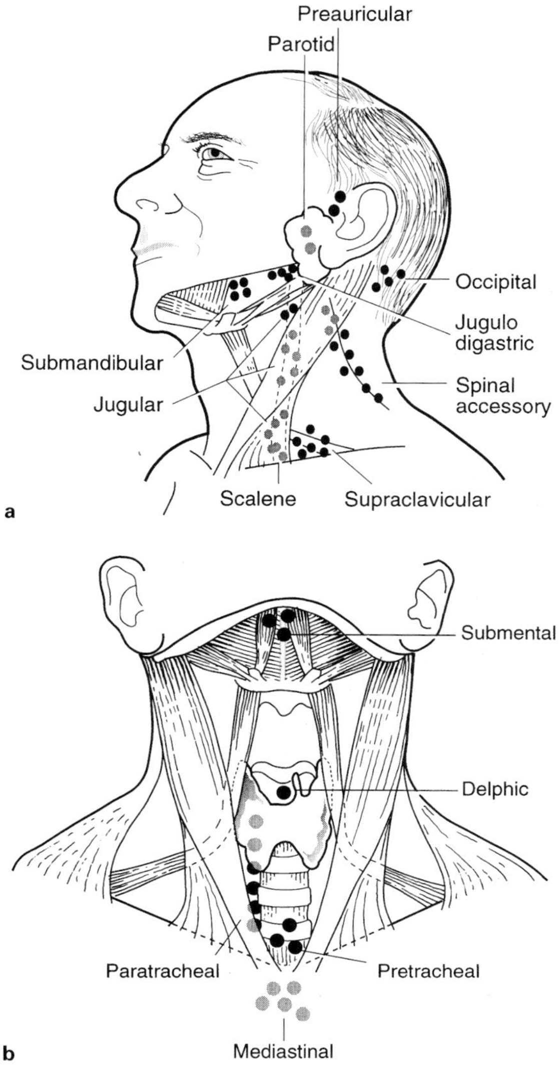

Fig. 17.7 Lateral view of the neck (**a**) and anterior view (**b**) to show typical grouping of lymph nodes.

Table 17.2 Causes of cervical lymphadenopathy

Primary malignancy
Lymphoma (Hodgkin's and non-Hodgkin's)
Leukaemia (especially chronic lymphatic leukaemia)
Metastatic malignancy
Skin—melanoma, squamous cell carcinoma
Nasopharynx—nose, sinuses, pharynx, larynx
Mouth—oral cavity, tongue, lips
Oesophagus
Thyroid
Infraclavicular—lung, bronchus, gastrointestinal tract, seminoma, breast, cervix
Occult primary
Lymphadenitis
Non-specific—sore throat, tonsillitis, idiopathic histiocytic necrotizing lymphadenitis, infected scalp
Specific—infectious mononucleosis, HIV/AIDS, toxoplasmosis, cat scratch fever
Granulomatous—tuberculosis, sarcoidosis, fungal
Other—Rosai–Dorfman disease, Castleman's disease, angioimmunoblastic lymphadenopathy

REFERENCES

9. Gardner G et al Am J Surg 1996; 172: 196–199
10. Fruhwith J et al Eur J Surg Oncol 1996; 22: 88–92
11. Guerrier B et al J de Chirurgie 199; 132: 287–294
12. Wax M K, Briant T D Otolaryngol Head and Neck Surg 1994; 114: 678
13. Schild S E et al Mayo Clin Proc 1992; 67: 537–540
14. Savoury L W, Gluckman J L In: Paparella M M et al (eds) Otolaryngology. W B Saunders, Philadelphia 1991 p 2565

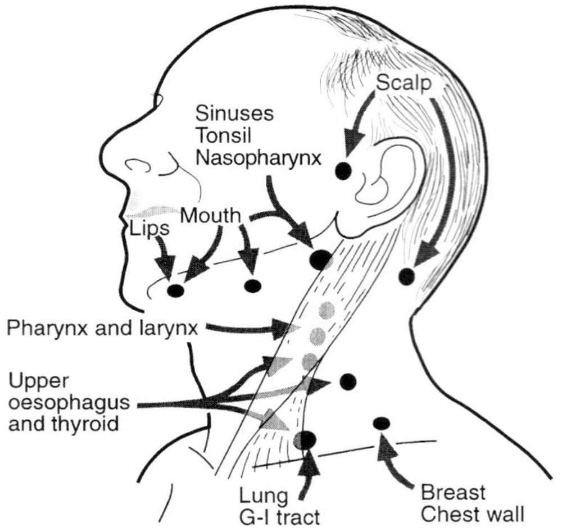

Fig. 17.8 Diagram to show typical lymph drainage pattern towards cervical lymph nodes. These patterns are not exclusive: there are extensive interconnections of lymphatic pathways in the neck.

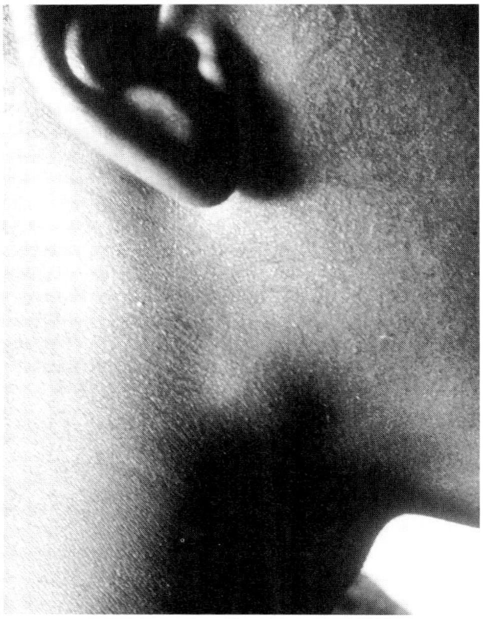

Fig. 17.9 A jugulo-digastric node enlarged by tonsillitis.

Identifying the cause of cervical lymphadenopathy

Careful clinical history taking and examination yield a diagnosis in the majority of cases. Particular note should be taken of ear, nose and throat symptoms, weight loss, fever, rashes or night sweats. Pain in lymph nodes after drinking alcohol is said to be a symptom of lymphoma but has been recorded in other non-malignant causes of lymphadenopathy. The social history should include enquiry about risk factors for HIV infection, about foreign travel and contact with animals. Examination should include the scalp, to exclude hidden melanoma, the tongue, lips and tonsils and the thyroid gland. A more general examination should seek evidence of distant malignant disease or hepatosplenomegaly.

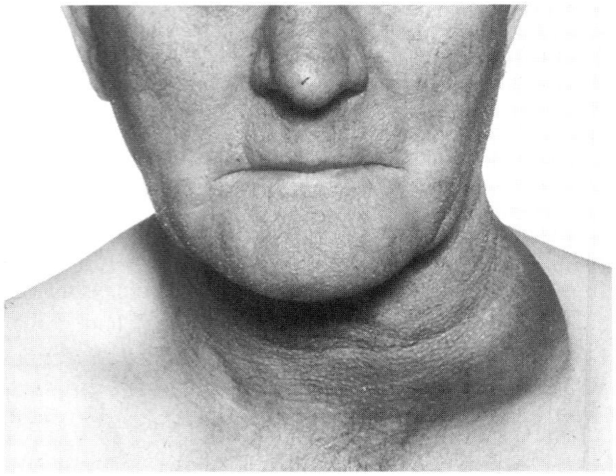

Fig. 17.10 A mass of indurated nodes in the root of the neck with reddening of the overlying skin. The differential diagnosis lies between inflammatory lymphadenitis, including TB, and metastatic nodes. In this patient the nodes were metastatic and the presenting feature of a carcinoma of the bronchus.

The first step in investigation is the taking of a fine-needle aspiration biopsy. A review by Donahue et al[15] showed that most studies of fine-needle biopsy show a false negative rate of around 1–10% and a false positive rate of 0–3%. If the samples are taken by an experienced clinician who can reduce the number of smears that are inadequate for diagnosis, and if the cytologist has appropriate experience, then in almost all patients useful information may be gleaned. An exact diagnosis is not always crucial. The questions particularly to be answered are:

- Is it malignant?
- If so, is it a squamous cell malignancy?
- Is it inflammatory?
- If so, is it tuberculous?

A diagnostic biopsy of a cervical lymph node should never be undertaken without a preliminary fine-needle biopsy. This is particularly important in cases of squamous malignancy and tuberculosis. An open lymph node excision biopsy in squamous malignancy may spoil the field for subsequent block dissection of the neck and, indeed, even reduce the potential of that operation to cure the patient.[16] If squamous metastatic disease is detected on fine-needle aspiration biopsy, there should be prompt referral to an ENT surgeon for a full assessment which will usually include panendoscopy. If this does not disclose a primary tumour, random biopsies from multiple sites are sometimes necessary, though it is very rare to discover the primary site from such blind biopsies. Chest radiographs and sputum cytology should also be obtained. The subsequent management of head and neck squamous cancers where the primary site is discovered is discussed in the relevant sections elsewhere. Sometimes, however, no primary site is discovered (see below, 'the occult primary').

REFERENCES

15. Donahue B J, Cruickshank J C, Bisop J W ENT Journal 1995; 74: 483–486
16. McGuirt W F, McCabe W F Laryngoscope 1978; 88: 594

If fine-needle biopsy of a node in the supraclavicular fossa discloses adenocarcinoma a search for a gastric, pancreatic or other abdominal malignancy is begun. Such marker nodes are usually found on the left and referred to as Virchow's nodes but they may also be found on the right. A previously treated breast cancer is also sometimes found to be the cause of isolated adenocarcinomatous metastatic nodes in the neck.

Mobile metastatic nodes of squamous malignancies are in general treated by block dissection of the nodes (see below) in conjunction with treatment of the primary tumour. Radiotherapy may be added. Where the cervical node or nodes are fixed at presentation, the prognosis is grave regardless of the site of the primary tumour. 5–10% of patients present with fixed nodes in the neck, and only 1% of these survive a year if untreated. When radical surgery and radiotherapy are feasible 15% survive to 5 years.[17] The most common group within the category of patients presenting with fixed nodes are those without a demonstrable primary tumour, a third of whom present in this way.

Cervical lymph node metastases from an occult primary

In a 12-year study reported in 1983 from the Sloan–Kettering Cancer Center,[18] it was noted that in 6% of all cases of head and neck malignancy no primary malignancy was apparent and in 60% of these cases the tumour was squamous. All were treated with radical neck dissection or with radiotherapy. Interestingly, half were alive 5 years later—a much better result than would have been predicted from identified primary squamous carcinomas in the neck. In only 15% was the site of the primary tumour ever discovered from its later appearance and detection at follow-up.

In the 1940s and 1950s, tumours where no primary was found were considered to be the result of malignancy arising in squamous inclusions in cervical lymph nodes, the so-called 'branchogenic carcinomas'. In the 1960s and 1970s this concept was largely abandoned,[19] but the issue remains unresolved. The proposed treatment policy for such patients is one of a basic search for a primary tumour, as outlined above, followed by radical neck dissection as failure to offer radical treatment is followed by a high incidence of uncontrolled local recurrence. Radiotherapy is advised if more than one lymph node is involved or if there is extracapsular spread.

Specific infections

Infectious mononucleosis (Epstein–Barr virus infection)

This viral infection, a consequence of infection with the Epstein–Barr herpes virus, begins as a prodromal systemic illness with fever, malaise, a headache and sometimes abdominal pain. The patient then typically develops pharyngitis or exudative tonsillitis and sometimes a rash, particularly if penicillin is prescribed. The lymphadenopathy which appears after the prodrome is predominantly cervical. Although the nodes may be substantially enlarged the enlargement is always of multiple nodes and the distribution is symmetrical. The great majority of patients are adolescents, teenagers or young adults, and the diagnosis is readily confirmed by the appearance of atypical mononuclear cells in the blood film associated with a positive 'monospot' or Paul–Bunnell serological test. The lymphadenopathy often persists for several months and is associated with hepatosplenomegaly in 10–20% of patients. There is almost never an indication to biopsy a node to establish the diagnosis. There are reports of emergency tonsillectomy being required for life-threatening upper airway obstruction occurring during the pharyngitic phase of this illness,[20] but this is an exceptionally rare event.

Toxoplasmosis

Toxoplasmosis is a consequence of infection with the parasite *Toxoplasma gondii*; it may occur congenitally as a consequence of infection in utero, or be acquired. Lymphadenopathy is only a feature of the acquired disease. The neck is the most common site of lymphadenopathy and usually only a few nodes are enlarged, hence the presentation of these patients to surgeons. The nodes are usually tender for the first 1–2 weeks after their appearance but after that are painless and may persist for many months; they never suppurate. There are usually few if any concomitant symptoms with the lymphadenopathy; sometimes there is slight fever and malaise. Fine-needle biopsy of the nodes shows non-specific changes. The blood may show slight leucopenia with some atypical lymphocytes but these are not diagnostic. Specific IgG antibodies appear two weeks after the onset of the illness but are a poor guide to diagnosis as there is a high prevalence in the normal population. Seropositivity rates are normally quoted for a population of fertile women: the rate is 72% in Paris and 21% in London, probably reflecting dietary differences. Toxoplasmosis is seen as an opportunistic infection in AIDS patients and in these patients specific antibody levels may be low. The node enlarged because of toxoplasmosis is thus difficult to diagnose with certainty. If the patient is well no specific treatment is required, but if the patient is unwell a 1–2 month course of Spiramycin is indicated.[21]

Cat scratch fever[22]

Lymphadenopathy is the most common presenting feature of cat scratch disease. The infecting bacillus, *Rochalimaea henselae*, enters through a scratch from a cat, usually a kitten, and causes the development of a local inflamed papule 3–10 days later, 1–7 weeks afterwards there is enlargement of the regional lymph nodes. These are initially painful, may suppurate and may persist for up to four months in association with vague systemic symptoms in 30% of

REFERENCES

17. Stell P M et al Cancer 1984; 53: 336–341
18. Spiro R H, DeRose G, Strong E W Am J Surg 1983; 146: 441–446
19. Batsakis J G Tumours of The Head and Neck, Williams & Wilkins, Baltimore 1979
20. Stevenson D S, Webster G, Stewart I A J Laryngol Otol 1992; 106: 989–991
21. Courvieur J, Thulliez P In: Oxford Textbook of Medicine, 3rd edn. Oxford University Press Oxford 1996 pp 865–869
22. Perkins B A In: Oxford Textbook of Medicine, 3rd edn. Oxford University Press, Oxford 1996 pp 745–746

patients. The diagnosis is made by aspiration of a node and the microscopic demonstration of the bacillus by Warthin–Starry silver stain. A skin test with prepared antigen is available but not widely used now. Usually no treatment is needed though large pus-filled nodes may need to be aspirated, and antimicrobial therapy is occasionally needed for systemic symptoms.[23]

Granulomatous lymphadenitis

Sarcoidosis

30% of patients with sarcoidosis have palpable cervical nodes, and in 75% of all patients with sarcoidosis scalene node biopsy discloses the diagnosis even when the nodes are impalpable. In white patients sarcoidosis only presents as a cervical lymphadenopathy in 3% as the disease is usually predominantly mediastinal; by contrast nodal disease is the presenting feature in 17% of Asians and 34% of blacks. The nodes are discrete, painless, rubbery and similar in feel to the nodes encountered in Hodgkin's disease. They do not suppurate. The diagnosis is by fine-needle or open biopsy backed up by a significant elevation of serum angiotensin I–12 converting enzyme or the Kveim–Siltzbach skin test.[24]

Tuberculosis in cervical lymph nodes

Tuberculosis may involve cervical nodes by lymphatic or haematogenous spread. Historically, the most common situation is for the organism to enter through the tonsillar bed as a consequence of drinking infected milk, and this pharyngeal point of entry leads to jugulodigastric node enlargement as part of the primary complex. More common in developed countries is the appearance of tuberculous lymphadenitis low in the neck secondary to pulmonary tuberculosis; in this instance infection is noted primarily in the supraclavicular nodes, the lower jugular or posterior triangle nodes. In these patients radiology of the chest may disclose a mediastinal lymphadenopathy. Although tuberculous lymphadenitis is now uncommon in western countries it is nevertheless seen in immigrants from other countries, especially the Indian subcontinent, where tuberculosis is still endemic and is also commonly encountered in the socially disadvantaged and malnourished and in immunocompromised patients, especially those with HIV/AIDS.

In developing countries tuberculosis remains extremely common and is the most common cause of cervical lymphadenopathy.[25]

Tuberculosis notifications in England and Wales show that there is a racial difference in the form of presentation of extrapulmonary tuberculosis. In whites, 37% present with cervical node involvement whereas the figure for those originating from the Indian subcontinent is 52%.

In spite of the relative infrequency of cervical tuberculosis in developed countries, it should always remain in the differential diagnosis of cervical lymphadenopathy because less than 50% will have any systemic symptoms and the enlarged or suppurating neck nodes may be the only marker of the disease.

In the early stages of tuberculous lymphadenitis the nodes enlarge but remain discrete. With progression of the disease the nodes caseate and coalesce; if the process proceeds slowly then there is gross surrounding fibrosis. Eventually marked, dense induration is noted mimicking malignancy. Progressive caseation leads to coalescence of caseous foci into a deep abscess with softening of the node mass. If the nodes are deep-seated the pus penetrates the deep fascia and forms a fluctuant cold abscess under the skin. This is the famous but rarely seen 'collar stud abscess'. Whenever tuberculous infection appears under the skin it causes a dusky cold induration of that skin and eventually discharges through the skin with the development of a chronic sinus. Secondary infection can now occur. Chronic tuberculosis in the skin produces the changes identified as 'scrofula'.

Management

Once tuberculosis has been suspected it is readily diagnosed by fine-needle aspiration biopsy cytology; this will show caseous changes and/or epitheloid cells in 85%,[26] but acid-fast bacilli will be seen in the cytological preparation in only 50%. Pus should therefore be aspirated for culture. Aspiration is not only crucial in providing material for determining antibiotic sensitivities but is also therapeutic when combined with drug therapy. Ultrasound or radiographic imaging is not useful in confirming a diagnosis of tuberculosis but may help to map abscesses and guide aspiration. A positive or suspicious fine-needle aspiration biopsy coupled with a strongly positive purified protein derivative/Heaf skin test is sufficient diagnosis to allow initiation of treatment without the need for open biopsy. It should, however, be remembered that the immunocompromised patient may have an anergic response to skin testing; these and other patients where the diagnosis is uncertain may still need diagnostic excision of a node for histology and culture.

The role of surgery in the treatment of tuberculous lymphadenitis is very limited; it should be avoided if possible because of the risk of development of chronic sinuses at the site of biopsy or drainage. It should be considered only if there is a persistent large mass or a sinus after a full course of medical treatment. Surgery should take the form of extirpation of the tuberculous mass as if it were a low-grade malignancy. The procedure is technically difficult, and surrounding structures are at considerable risk. If sinuses or ulcers have developed then surgery combined with medical therapy helps to obtain a cosmetically acceptable scar.[27]

Atypical mycobacterial infection

Several other mycobacteria can cause cervical lymphadenitis, mostly *M. avium* or *M. intracellulare*, and the infections occur almost exclusively in children and the immunocompromised, especially those who have had contact with birds. The patients tend to

REFERENCES

23. Margileth A M Pediatr Infect Dis J 1992; 11: 474
24. Studdy P R In: Oxford Textbook of Medicine, 3rd edn. Oxford University Press, Oxford 1996
25. Watters A K Br J Surg 1997; 84: 8–14
26. Dasgupta A et al J Indian Med Assoc 1994; 92: 44–46
27. Subramanyam M Br J Surg 1993; 80: 1547–1548

present with nodes higher in the neck than is found in tuberculous patients; the lymphadenopathy is more often unilateral and there is usually no concomitant systemic illness. This form of lymphadenitis often shows minimal response to drug therapy[28] and surgical treatment, ideally with node excision, should be undertaken.[29]

HIV/AIDS and cervical lymphadenopathy

Cervical lymphadenopathy is often encountered in patients with HIV infection and in those with AIDS. Persistent generalized lymphadenopathy is a feature of the pre-AIDS state. In these patients, as well as in patients with established AIDS, the clinical decision to be made is whether the appearance of enlarged cervical nodes is part of the lymphadenopathy associated with the disease itself, or whether it signals the appearance of an associated lymphoma, tuberculosis or other opportunistic infection in an immunocompromised patient. Fine-needle aspiration biopsy is indicated in an attempt to resolve this issue, especially if there is asymmetrical primarily cervical lymphadenopathy. The results of this will indicate the small number of patients in whom biopsy excision is justified. Widespread open excision biopsy of enlarged lymph nodes in these patients is rarely justified. In an analysis of studies of unselected biopsy for persistent, generalized lymphadenopathy in HIV positive patients, the management was only shown to be altered in 3% of patients as a consequence of the histological findings.[30]

Kikuchi–Fujimoto disease

Kikuchi–Fujimoto disease (necrotizing histiocytic lymphadenitis) is a disease of unknown aetiology predominantly affecting Japanese women between ages of 20 and 30. Usually it presents as posterior cervical lymphadenopathy. It may be associated with a flu-like prodrome and a relapsing course. Although C reactive protein levels and the ESR may be raised and the white count low, there is no means to confirm the diagnosis other than by seeing the complex but typical histological changes in an excision biopsy of the involved node.[31]

STERNOMASTOID TUMOUR

Sternomastoid tumours appear 1–2 weeks after birth, usually following a complicated or breech birth. The tumour is unilateral, usually occupies the lower half of the muscle and occupies both heads. At the outset it is in fact an interfascicular haematoma of the sternomastoid with associated muscle degeneration. It is at first tender and often associated with torticollis. If sternomastoid tumour is diagnosed early the optimal treatment is conservative with active stimulation and passive stretching; during this regime the tumour normally disappears over the first 4–6 months of life. Only those cases which are noted late and are unresponsive to conservative treatment require surgery.[32] If the condition is not treated a permanent wry neck deformity may begin to develop at about four years of age.

SURGERY OF CERVICAL LYMPH NODES

Lymph node biopsy

Excision of a cervical node for biopsy is necessary if fine-needle biopsy has failed to produce a diagnosis where it is clinically necessary to achieve one. It is also important if the proposed diagnosis is lymphoma, in which instance a whole node is required for detailed histology and marker studies. The most discrete, mobile, superficial yet clearly abnormal gland should be chosen for excision. Biopsy under local anaesthetic is feasible but general anaesthetic is often preferred as the surgery may prove more difficult than appears at first sight.

Damage to the spinal accessory nerve is a particular risk during biopsies in the posterior triangle. The nerve is intimately related to the posterior triangle nodes, is only 2 mm in diameter and is surprisingly superficial. Damage leads to pain in the shoulder and arm, paralysis of the trapezius muscle, winging of the scapula and frequently also to litigation. If the injury is recognized the patient should be promptly referred for neurolysis or nerve grafting.[33,34]

An inexperienced surgeon should not be allowed to undertake an unsupervised biopsy of posterior neck nodes without being apprised of the anatomical dangers.

Block dissection of the neck

The classical block dissection of the neck for clearance of the cervical lymph nodes has remained unchanged for most of this century and it remains the standard operation for extensive nodal disease from squamous carcinoma, malignant melanoma and patients with extensive medullary carcinoma of the thyroid. The classical procedure removes the sternomastoid muscle, the jugular vein and the accessory nerve (Fig. 17.11), leaving a considerable cosmetic and functional deficit. Therefore in many situations more limited operations are now undertaken; a stance reinforced by the widespread use of high-quality, effective adjuvant radiotherapy. Differentiated thyroid cancer has always been managed effectively with limited block dissection[35] and it is only in medullary or very advanced papillary/follicular tumours that radical procedures are undertaken (see Chapter 18). It has been proposed that, for node negative and early node positive oral and oropharyngeal carcinoma, a supraomohyoid dissection will suffice, and that for hypopharyngeal and pharyngeal tumours a lateral neck dissection is sufficient.[36]

REFERENCES

28. Bailey W C Chest 1983; 84: 625
29. Tunkel D E, Romaneschi K B Laryngoscope 1995; 105: 1024–1028
30. Godley M J Br J Surg 1986; 73: 170–171
31. Louis N, Hanley M, Davidson N M J Laryngol Otol 1994; 108: 1001–1004
32. Cheng J C, Au A W J Paediatr Orthop 1994; 14: 802–808
33. Williams W W et al Ann R Coll Surg Engl 1996; 78: 521–525
34. London J, London N J, Kay S P Ann R Coll Surg Engl 1996; 78: 146–50
35. Orsenigo E et al Eur J Surg Oncol 1997; 23: 286–288
36. Shah J P, Andersen P E Ann Surg Oncol 1994; 1: 521–532

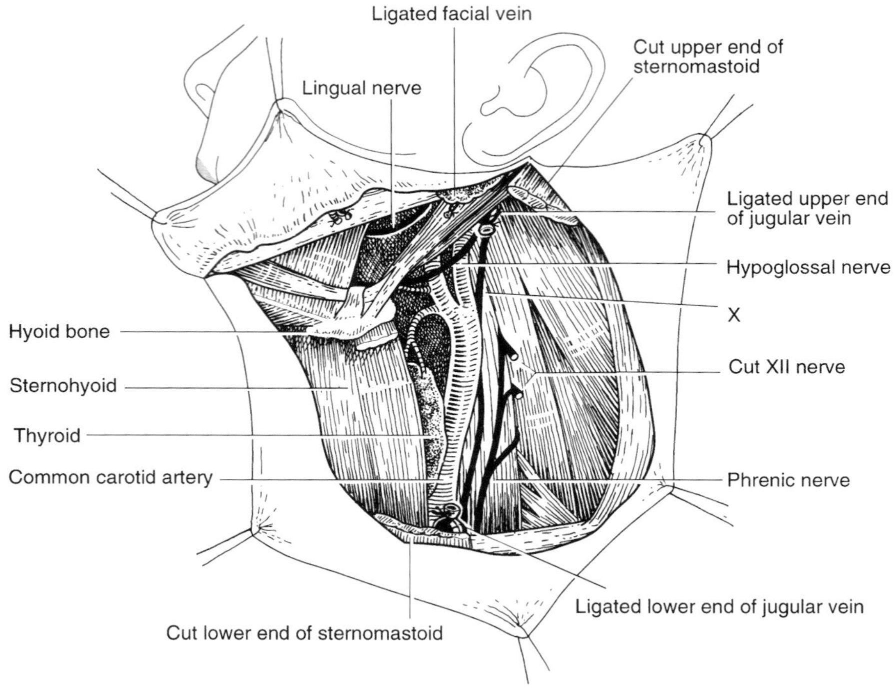

Fig. 17.11 Anatomical structures exposed at the end of a radical block dissection of the neck. Note the cut ends of the excised sternomastoid, accessory nerve and jugular vein.

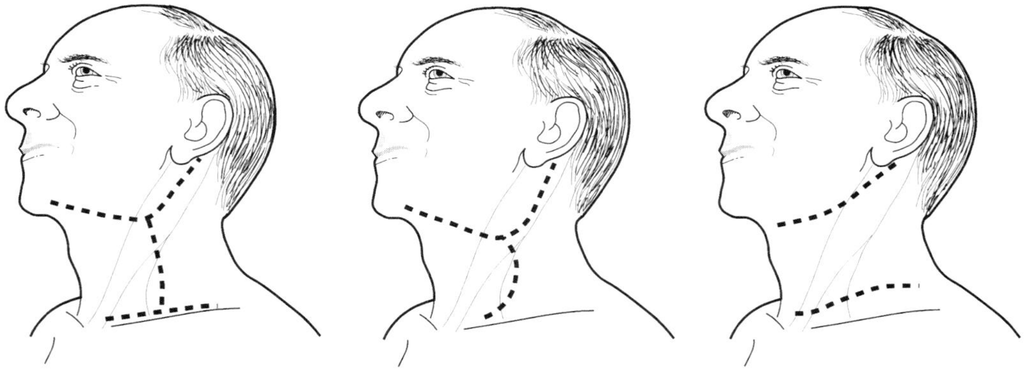

Fig. 17.12 Examples of incisions used for block dissection of the neck: (**a**) 'wine glass'; (**b**) Standard Y incision; (**c**) McFee.

Radical neck dissection

The purpose of the standard, full radical neck dissection is the clearance of all lymphatic tissue from the mandible above to the clavicle below and from the midline to the anterior border of the trapezius muscle laterally. Normally, only unilateral block dissection is undertaken but with the introduction of modified operations, particularly those sparing the jugular vein, bilateral dissections are sometimes feasible.

Many incisions are in use (Fig. 17.12). The McFee incision consists of two horizontal limbs, one below the mandible and the other above the clavicle, and is particularly used if the patient has been previously irradiated. The standard Y incision comprises a horizontal component which extends from the mastoid to the hyoid bone and then up to the point of the chin. The vertical component commences in the centre of the horizontal incision and descends vertically in a 'lazy S' shape to the clavicle.

Skin flaps are raised together with the platysma, taking care to protect the mandibular branch of the facial nerve under the upper skin flap. The lower limit of the dissection is extended and the distal end of the sternomastoid muscle is divided. Next the internal jugular vein is exposed and divided. The divided upper end of the vein, together with the lymphatic and connective tissues surrounding it, is lifted away from the common carotid artery and the vagus nerve. This block of mobilized tissues is now gently separated from the prevertebral fascia, sparing the phrenic nerve on the anterior surface of scalenus anterior. During the mobilization the transverse cervical artery and vein are divided and ligated. The anterior border of the trapezius is defined and the posterior triangle is cleared, dividing the accessory nerve centrally and distally to the mobilized block of lymphatic tissue. The dissection is continued upwards beside the common carotid artery to its bifurcation. The cranial end of sternomastoid is then separated from the mastoid process; the internal jugular vein is exposed, ligated and divided.

The dissection continues forwards, ligating the posterior facial vein and usually dividing the tail of the parotid gland. The hypoglossal nerve is traced forwards to the submandibular triangle and spared. The upper border of the submandibular gland is freed by dividing and ligating the facial vessels. The lingual nerve is identified and separated from the submandibular duct, which can then be divided. The gland is delivered after the facial artery has again been divided on its posterior border. If the tumour is situated in the anterior portion of the oral cavity the submental triangle should also be included in the dissection.

If the skin flaps are involved, irradiated or unhealthy, extra tissue may have to be brought in to close the wound of a block dissection of the neck. This can either be a free graft, skin flaps or free tissue transfer with microanastomosis (see Chapter 9).

18 The thyroid gland

A. E. Young

CONGENITAL ABNORMALITIES

Thyroglossal duct abnormalities (see Chapter 17)

Lingual thyroid

The lingual thyroid represents non-descent of all or part of the embryonic thyroid. It lies behind the foramen caecum at the back of the tongue, and may lie there symptomless or suffer from any of the diseases to which the thyroid is liable. In 75% of cases it constitutes the whole bulk of the thyroid; in the remainder it may be accompanied by thyroid tissue in the normal site or it may represent the lateral lobes and isthmus. The pyramidal lobe is found at a lower level in front of the trachea. The great majority of patients in whom lingual thyroid presents clinical problems are young women, where enlargement is due to the physiological hyperplasia of pregnancy or to the development of an adenoma.[1] The lesion is clinically apparent as a smooth, hypervascular reddish-brown mucosal-covered projection at the back of the tongue, often only clearly visible by use of laryngoscope. On rare occasions it may cause dysphagia, dysphonia or airways obstruction, and it may bleed. Malignant change in lingual thyroids has been reported.[2]

If a lingual thyroid is suspected, its presence may be confirmed and the extent or absence of other thyroid tissue explored by use of an iodine or technetium isotope scan.[3] If the patient is given atropine, confusing uptake by the salivary glands is minimized. A lingual thyroid which is stationary in size and does not produce symptoms is not interfered with. Hypertrophy may be limited by therapeutic doses of thyroxine, by antithyroid drugs or by radioiodine. Excision may be necessary, particularly if malignant disease has occurred. Removal is then undertaken by translingual pharyngotomy bisecting the tongue longitudinally to obtain access to the tumour. If a functionally normal lingual thyroid must be removed and there is no other thyroid tissue, then thin slices of the excised thyroid may be implanted in the strap muscles of the neck or in the rectus muscle, with a fair hope that it will function autonomously, alleviating the need for thyroxine replacement.[4]

Other ectopic thyroid tissue

Apart from a lingual site and in association with the thyroglossal tract thyroid tissue is only rarely found ectopically. The so-called lateral aberrant thyroid in lymph node areas deep to the sternomastoid muscle was once believed to arise as ectopic thyroid tissue derived from the ultimobranchial body. This concept is no longer valid.[5] Such lesions which have a papillary structure are invariably lymph node metastases from differentiated intrathyroid cancers. The primary may be so small as to escape all but the most vigilant pathologist. Nicastri et al[6] reported inclusions of small amounts of totally normal follicular thyroid tissue in lateral neck nodes removed in the course of block dissection for a different malignancy. This should, however, not detract from the general concept that such tissue is usually metastatic, and the presence of papillary tumour in cervical lymph nodes is an indication for ipsilateral hemithyroidectomy.

Thyroid tissue is sometimes identified as discrete nodules physically separate from the thyroid, but immediately adjacent to it. Such nodules may be mistaken for parathyroid glands. They are developmentally normal thyroid tissue and not metastases.

Thyroid tissue may also occur in the mediastinum as far distal as the pericardium, and within the wall of the trachea or oesophagus. A case has been reported of fatal asphyxia from hyperplasia of tracheal thyroid tissue during pregnancy.[7]

GOITRE

Goitre is a non-specific term indicating enlargement of the thyroid. Simple euthyroid (non-toxic) goitre is the commonest form of thyroid abnormality; it is described as endemic when it occurs frequently in a defined geographic area or sporadic when it occurs elsewhere. Simple goitres may be categorized on the basis of clinical findings as *diffuse* when the enlargement is even or *nodular* when more than one nodule is palpable within the gland.

Simple goitre is the result of hyperplasia of the thyroid to meet physiological demands for thyroxine. The hyperplasia occurs either because a normal gland must meet increased demands for thyroxine, as in puberty, pregnancy and lactation, or because the production of thyroxine is impaired. Inadequate levels of circulating thyroxine then increase thyroid-stimulating hormone production which in turn stimulates thyroid hypertrophy until an

REFERENCES

1. Montgomery M L West J Surg Gynecol Obstet 1935; 43: 661–669
2. Fah J, Moore R M Anat Surg 1963; 157: 212–222
3. Knight P J, Hamoudi A B, Vassy L E Surgery 1983; 93: 603–611
4. Swan H, Harper F, Christensen F P Surgery 1952; 32: 293
5. Wozencraft P, Foote F W, Frazell E L Cancer 1948; 1: 574
6. Nicastri A D, Foote F W, Frazell E L JAMA 1965; 194: 113
7. Cooper T V J Clin Pathol 1950; 3: 48

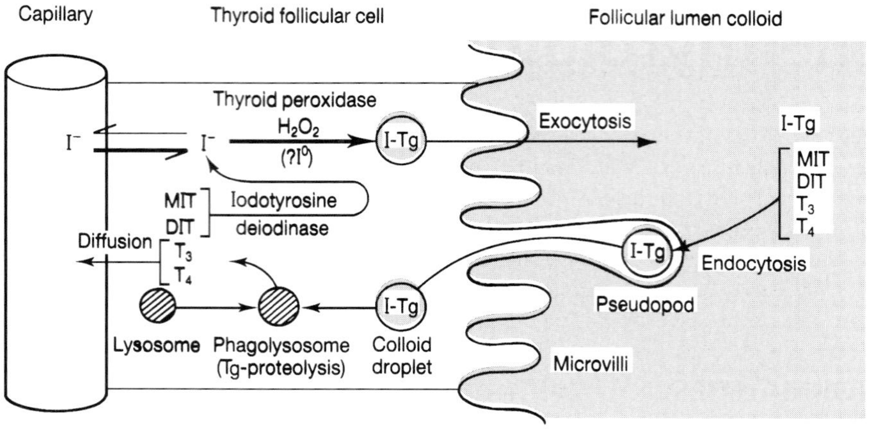

Fig. 18.1 Pathways of thyroid hormone synthesis. Tg = Thyroglobulin; MIT = monoiodotyrosine; DIT = di-iodotyrosine; T_3 = tri-iodothyronine; T_4 = tetraiodothyronine (thyroxine) From Clark.[8]

increased volume of gland becomes available to produce the necessary quantity of thyroid hormone. The pathways of thyroid hormone synthesis are shown in Figure 18.1.

The reasons for defective production of thyroid hormones are:

1. Iodine deficiency (i.e. less than 50 μg/day).
2. Ingestion of antithyroid substances as drugs or food.
3. Defective enzyme systems.
4. Radiation.
5. Thyroiditis.

The pathophysiological processes by which demand-led hyperplasia produces first a smooth (parenchymatous) goitre and then, if sustained, a nodular goitre are difficult to define and vary slightly depending on the exact cause. Thus with a severe inborn error of thyroid metabolism thyroid-stimulating hormone levels are very high and the infant gland becomes diffusely enlarged, the columnar epithelium is very tall and there are small follicles containing little or no colloid. More typically the underproduction of thyroxine is less severe and may be intermittent. In such cases a smooth diffuse enlargement first occurs as follicles become distended with excessive quantities of colloid (colloid goitre). As time passes some of these follicles rupture producing inflammatory changes or they outurn their blood supply producing infarction, haemorrhage, fibrosis, calcification and cyst formation. New follicles develop within an inelastic fibrous stroma. The overall effect of these changes is to produce a gland studded with nodules of varying size, maturity, activity and physical structure. The nodules may function autonomously of thyroid-stimulating hormone control.

Iodine-deficiency goitre

The earliest records of goitre occurring amongst the inhabitants of specific areas are Pliny's references to goitre in the Swiss Alps which contemporaries accurately ascribed to the drinking of water from melted snow which had of course a negligible iodine content.[9] The World Health Organization has identified 7% of the world population as suffering from clinically apparent goitre,[10] with prevalences ranging from almost zero in Japan, South Africa and the USA to 80% in parts of the Andes, Zaire and New Guinea. Although the role of inadequate dietary iodine in the majority of these cases is well-recognized and iodine has been introduced as a public health measure into salt, food or water, endemic goitre remains a common problem. Clinically it is revealed in its worst form as hypothyroidism in infants causing cretinism. The features of cretinism are mental and growth retardation, a thickened skin and tongue. Sometimes there is deaf mutism and spastic diplegia. In less severe forms the patient is euthyroid and has a progressively enlarging goitre, at first diffuse and then nodular.

Worldwide differences in the prevalence of iodine-deficiency goitre are not entirely attributable to iodine intake. Familial and racial traits of dyshormonogenesis and the intake of goitrogenic foods are also considered to play a role. The widespread use of dietary iodine has diminished but not eradicated endemic and sporadic multinodular goitre. Also impossible to explain on a dietary basis is the ninefold predominance of multinodular goitre in women. Whilst the extra demands of pregnancy and the cyclical demands of menstruation may be relevant, these are unlikely to be the only factors.

Goitrogens

These substances impair thyroxine synthesis by a variety of routes and the resultant increase in thyroid-stimulating hormone secretion causes the hypertrophy which is apparent as goitre. The substances may be grouped as follows:

1. Drugs: propylthiouracil and carbimazole interfere with organic binding of iodine, perchlorate and thiocyanate prevent its trapping; lithium prevents colloid droplet formation by cyclic adenosine monophosphate, while iodides, as in seaweed tablets or in amiodarone, inhibit thyroid peroxidase. Resorcinol,

REFERENCES

8. Clark O H Endocrine Surgery. C V Mosby, St Louis 1985
9. Medvei V C A History of Endocrinology. MTP Press, Lancaster 1982 pp 58, 59, 159
10. Kelly F C, Snedden W W Bull WHO 1958; 18: 5–173

sulphonamides, cobalt and aminoglutethimide also interfere with thyroxine synthesis.

2. Dietary agents have an ill-understood role. Excess intake of halogens such as chloride or fluoride displaces iodine; high levels of calcium in drinking water from limestone areas appear to influence the incidence of goitre where there is coexisting iodine deficiency. The mechanism is not understood. Pollution of drinking water by *Escherichia coli* is also implicated. *E. coli* has been found to produce the strongly goitrogenic substance thiopyramide nucleotide.[11] Cassava and soya beans contain goitrogens[12] but although substances derived from the members of the *Brassica* genus of vegetables can be shown to be goitrogenic in animals, there is no evidence of an effect in humans. Cigarette smoking increases serum thiocyanate concentrations and is thus theoretically a co-factor in goitrogenesis.

Radiation

Low doses of radiation (2–15 Gy), at one time used predominantly in the USA to treat a variety of benign head and neck diseases of childhood, have been implicated not only in the later development of cancer but also in a 20% incidence of nodular goitre 10–30 years later.[13] The nuclear accident in Chernobyl has been succeeded by a dramatic rise in the incidence of thyroid cancer in nearby parts of the Ukraine.

Thyroiditis (see below)

Dyshormonogenesis

The enzymes responsible for thyroxine synthesis may be partially or completely deficient. Such defects are familial. Enzymatic steps which may be affected are the transport of iodine, thyroid peroxidase, iodotyrosine coupling, iodotyrosine deiodinase and thyroglobulin synthesis.[14]

Severe defects tend to cretinism but less severely affected individuals develop an enlarging goitre, usually from childhood. This goitre may be smooth or nodular and the patient is usually euthyroid. Peroxidase deficiency may be associated with deafness as well as goitre.[15] This is known as Pendred's syndrome. It is neither necessary nor feasible in routine clinical practice accurately to identify the specific defect as treatment is the same for each variant, namely thyroxine replacement and thyroidectomy when indicated for the reasons outlined below.

Multinodular goitre

Clinical features

Almost all patients with epidemic or sporadic nodular goitre are euthyroid both clinically and biochemically. The patient presents for one or more of the following reasons:

1. Cosmetic.
2. Discomfort.
3. Tracheal compression.
4. Oesophageal compression.
5. Retrosternal extension.
6. Anxiety about malignancy.
7. Development of hyperthyroidism.
8. Hoarseness.

A goitre normally becomes visible when it is three times the normal size, i.e. it exceeds 50 g. Whether a goitre is cosmetically acceptable depends on the patient's personality and the culture in which he or she lives; in some cultures a goitre is a sign of beauty, while in others the appearance of a goitre is more likely to raise anxieties about cancer and obesity. When genuine discomfort is experienced, the goitre is either of acute onset caused by haemorrhage into a nodule or it is an episodic discomfort felt during neck movements or swallowing. Tracheal compression is insidious in its onset and may be made more severe by lateral deviation of the trachea by an asymmetrical goitre. A persisting minor cough is an early sign. Stridor develops late. Oesophageal compression is unusual unless there is retrosternal extension. Food may occasionally stick but if there is persistent dysphagia other causes should be sought before the cause is attributed to the goitre.

Many goitres enlarge harmlessly but impressively forwards from the neck. Some 10% will extend by preference into the chest. One in 10 of these has a low-set thyroid or a short neck which will confine the whole of the thyroid to the thorax. Such goitres are not aberrant anatomically and they maintain their connections with the cervical thyroid and its normal cervical vasculature.[16] Extension is generally into the anterior mediastinum but a posteriorly situated nodule may extend into the posterior mediastinum behind the oesophagus. Once in the confined space of the mediastinum, the possibilities of complications increase. Tracheal and oesophageal compression are common and the great veins may be obstructed (Fig. 18.2).

Many multinodular goitres may declare themselves because only one nodule is palpable, thus raising the possibility of a thyroid malignancy. Although careful examination, ultrasonography or isotope scanning will show the gland to be multinodular, this does not exclude the possibility cancer in a multinodular gland. Although the incidence of neoplasia in areas with endemic goitre is higher than in areas without, there is no clear-cut evidence that multinodular goitre itself carries a greater risk of neoplasm. Nevertheless a rapidly enlarging or dominant nodule in a multinodular goitre must never be ignored, particularly if there is associated lymphadenopathy or a recurrent laryngeal nerve palsy. If there is any doubt fine-needle aspiration biopsies should be performed.

Patients whose thyroids were exposed to low-dose radiation in childhood have a 30% incidence of malignancy in their goitres and nodules should be investigated early and a total thyroidectomy performed if cancer is discovered.

REFERENCES

11. Carbon J A, Hung L, Jones D Fed Proc 1965; 24: 486
12. McCarrison R M Chir Tr 1906; 89: 437
13. Greenspan F S JAMA 1976; 237: 2089–2091
14. Barsano C P, De Groot L J Clin Endocrinol Metab 1979; 8: 145–165
15. Fraser G R, Morgans M E, Troller W R Q J Med 1960; 53: 279–295
16. Lahey F H Surg Clin North Am 1945; 25: 609–618

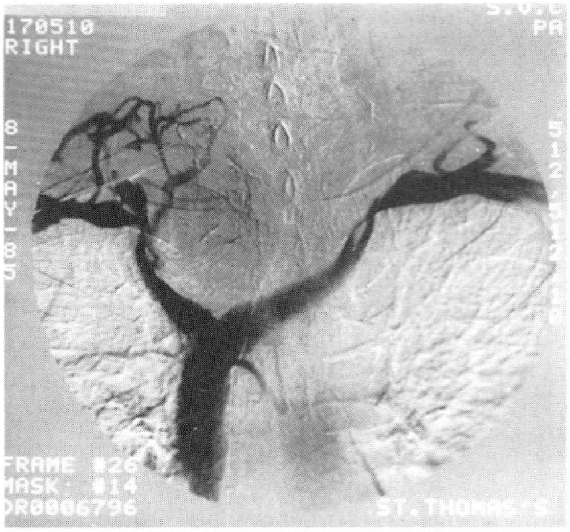

Fig. 18.2 Digital subtraction angiogram showing compression of the great veins by a retrosternal multinodular goitre.

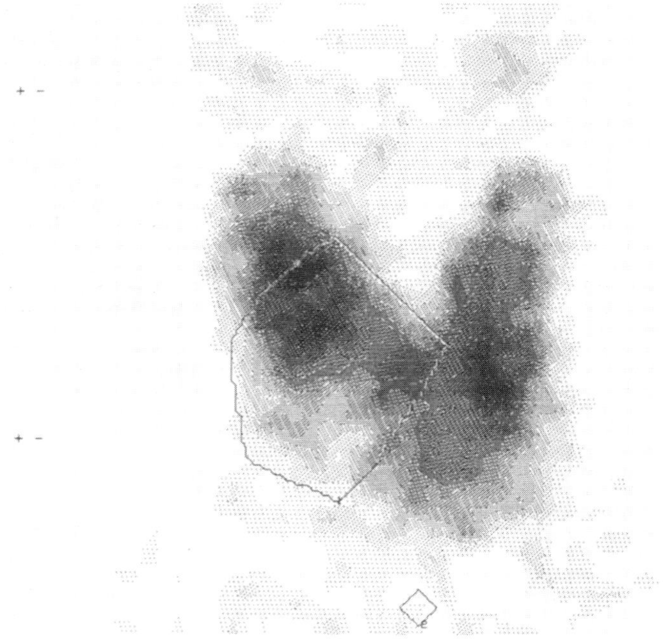

Fig. 18.3 Technetium scintiscan of the thyroid. The palpable nodules have been outlined. The fragmented pattern of isotope uptake reveals that this is a multinodular goitre.

Hyperthyroidism occurs in a small number of untreated nodular goitres due to the development of one or more autonomous hyperfunctioning nodules. The condition is known as Plummer's syndrome.[17] It is insidious in onset and rare under the age of 40. The resultant hyperthyroidism is usually mild and unassociated with exophthalmos, myopathy or the serological changes seen in Graves' disease.

Hoarseness

Voice changes may be produced by distortion of the larynx by the goitre or by recurrent laryngeal nerve palsy. This latter should be taken as a warning of the possibilities of thyroid neoplasia but it can occur simply by stretching of the recurrent laryngeal nerve by a benign nodule and is usually not reversed by operation.

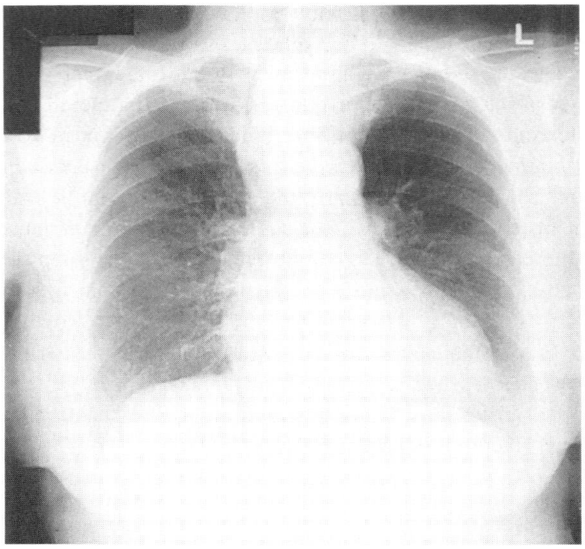

Fig. 18.4 Chest radiograph showing a retrosternal goitre. Note the trachea narrowed and displaced to the right.

Investigation

Tri-iodothyronine, tetraiodothyronine (thyroxine) and thyroid-stimulating hormone should be assessed in all patients. If there is any suspicion of thyroiditis, autoantibodies should be assayed. Ultrasonography will identify the dimensions of the goitre and the nodules and identify cysts suitable for aspiration. Alternatively a technetium scintiscan can be used for the demonstration of the diagnosis of multinodular goitre if only one nodule is palpable (Fig. 18.3). It will also identify hyperfunctioning nodules and cold nodules worthy of fine-needle biopsy. In retrosternal goitres radioiodine scans give better imaging. If there is anxiety about malignancy, a computer tomography scan may show that the gland capsule has been transgressed. Normal chest radiography is a reliable way of noting progression in a retrosternal goitre and may show benign calcification in it (Fig. 18.4). Dysphagia should always be investigated by contrast studies before it is confidently ascribed to pressure from the thyroid.

If tracheal compression is suspected it should be assessed by chest radiography with lateral and posteroanterior views of the cervical airway if it is not clearly seen on the chest radiograph.

Treatment

Medical

Endemic goitre may be partly prevented and treated by ensuring a daily iodine intake of 150–300 μg iodine. Older patients with developed multinodular goitre should not however be given iodine

REFERENCE

17. Plummer H S, Boothby W M J Iowa State Med Soc 1924; 14: 666

therapy as thyrotoxicosis may be induced (the Jod–Basedow effect). Goitrogens should be excluded from the diet.

Thyroxine has been widely used in the treatment of multinodular goitre because of the presumed role of a raised thyroid-stimulating hormone in its genesis. Some 70% of smooth dyshormogenic goitres in young people may regress with suppressive doses of thyroxine[18] but in the established nodular goitre a useful response is less common because the nodules are usually functionless or, if functional, are frequently autonomous. A trial is however often worthwhile if there are no pressing indications to proceed to surgery. The recommended dose for thyroxine in children is 3–4 μg/kg per day and in adults 2.5 μg/kg per day. Thus in adults the dose required to suppress thyroid-stimulating hormone is 0.1–0.3 mg per day. Regression when it occurs is predominantly of the non-nodular part of the gland and is only partial. It should be achieved within 3 months of starting therapy. Regression is unlikely to be achieved in more than 30–50% of patients.[19]

Where hyperfunctioning nodules have led to thyrotoxicosis the treatment is as for Graves' disease but in large glands surgery is preferable to radioiodine therapy.

Cystic nodules may be aspirated and the fluid should always be examined cytologically, remembering the limitations of cytology in this context. For example, fine-needle biopsy of large nodules which are cystic has a 30% chance of failing to detect a carcinoma if it is present.[20] True cysts may be destroyed by the instillation of tetracycline if they recur after simple aspiration.[21]

Surgery

The indications for surgery are:

1. Obstructive symptoms.
2. Continuing growth on adequate thyroxine therapy.
3. Retrosternal extension.
4. Suspicion of malignancy.
5. Cosmesis.
6. Thyrotoxicosis.

It is neither practical nor necessary to remove all multinodular goitres that have not regressed with thyroxine therapy. Neither is there any indication for surgery as a prophylaxis against malignant change[22] (with the sole exception of the irradiated thyroid). Discomfort and pressure symptoms are the usual indication. Any tracheal narrowing by a multinodular goitre may be regarded as an indication for surgery as sudden worsening may occur following haemorrhage into a degenerate nodule. If there is already stridor, surgery should be undertaken urgently. If all risk of recurrence is to be avoided total thyroidectomy should be performed for multinodular goitre but the risks of laryngeal nerve damage and hypoparathyroidism are however lessened if instead a generous bilateral subtotal thyroidectomy is performed removing all gross nodules in the remnant. Postoperatively the patient should be started on a replacement dose of thyroxine, though it may be wise to avoid this in the elderly patient if sufficient remnants have been left to allow normal thyroid function.

Surgery is indicated for true retrosternal goitre, i.e. goitres whose lower border do not rise out of the chest when the patient swallows with the neck extended. Surgery is indicated because these patients are particularly at risk of compressive symptoms, respond little to thyroxine therapy and because continued growth of the goitre may be difficult to assess. Furthermore the hazards of surgery increase proportionately with the size of the goitre. Even large retrosternal goitres can be safely extracted via the cervical incision as they derive their blood supply from normal thyroid vessels in the neck. However if the nodules are very large they may need to be removed piecemeal.[23,24] If there is definite malignant change with fixity of the goitre in the chest an upper midline sternotomy may be necessary.

TUMOURS OF THE THYROID GLAND

In all, 5% of the population have a clinically palpable thyroid nodule[25] and at autopsy 50% of adults are found to have a thyroid nodule[26] and 30% of all adults can be shown by ultrasound to harbour a nodule.[27] The incidence is substantially higher in areas of iodine deficiency and endemic goitre. By contrast however, the incidence of true thyroid cancer is low—around 4/100 000 per annum.[28] Therein lies the clinical problem. The palpable nodule is the end-point of many different pathological processes including hyperplasia, degeneration, inflammation, cysts and metastatic neoplasia, as well as benign and malignant thyroid tumours. Differentiation between these on the basis of simple clinical examination is difficult or impossible and referral to specialists therefore is appropriate and common. The death rate from thyroid cancer (6/million per year) is low but this reflects not just the relative indolence of some thyroid cancers but also the success of treatment. For this reason the proper assessment of thyroid nodules and the aggressive treatment of thyroid cancer is fully justified.

Thyroid tumours may be classified as shown in Table 18.1.

Benign thyroid tumours

Almost all of these are follicular adenomas. It is sometimes stated that benign papillary adenomas exist but this is unsound and all such lesions must be considered malignant. Follicular adenomas are a discrete pathological category not to be confused with the degenerative or regenerative nodules of a multinodular goitre. True follicular adenomas are discrete lesions with glandular or acinar patterns. They are encapsulated and usually 2–4 cm in diameter at

REFERENCES

18. Astwood E B, Cassidy C E, Amback G D JAMA 1960; 174: 459–464
19. Hennemann G J Clin Endocrinol Metab 1979; 8: 167–179
20. Meko J B, Norton J A Surgery 1995; 118: 996–1004
21. Goldfarb W B, Bigos S T, Nishigama R H Surgery 1987; 102: 1096
22. Sokal J E JAMA 1959; 170: 405–412
23. Katlic M R, Grillo H C, Chiv-an Wang Am J Surg 1985; 149: 283–287
24. Allo M D, Thompson N W Surgery 1983; 94: 969–977
25. Vander J B, Gaston E A, Dawber T R Ann Intern Med 1968; 69: 537–540
26. Hellwig C A Am J Clin Pathol 1935; 5: 103–111
27. Brander A, Viikinoski P et al Radiology 1991; 181: 683–687
28. Thompson N W, Kiskiyama R H, Harknen J K Curr Probl Surg 1978; 15: 1–67

Table 18.1 Classification of thyroid tumours

Benign
Follicular adenoma
Teratoma
Malignant
Differentiated carcinoma
Papillary
Mixed papillary–follicular
Follicular
Medullary
Undifferentiated (anaplastic)
Lymphoma
Miscellaneous
Squamous
Sarcoma
Teratoma
Plasmacytoma
Metastatic

presentation. The clinical difficulty with follicular adenomas is that they are solid on ultrasound, 'cold' on scintiscanning and cannot be confirmed as benign on fine-needle or even core biopsy. They are therefore indistinguishable from follicular carcinomas until they have been excised in toto and examined in detail by the histologist. They probably represent a continuum with malignant follicular cancers.

The follicular adenoma encompasses many categories such as embryonal, fetal, simple, colloid, macrofollicular and microfollicular adenomas. The embryonal adenomas are at one end of the spectrum, having rudimentary acini and no colloid, whereas the colloid adenomas at the other end are bulging with colloid. A difficult category to assess is the Hürthle cell adenoma (Askanazy cell tumour, oncocytoma, oxyphil tumour). In these there are featureless large granular cells of varying size distributed in poorly defined groups through a fibrous stroma. They may be particularly difficult to differentiate from malignant tumours and it is claimed that some will develop metastases. Nevertheless, in general these tumours may be regarded as benign and lobectomy is adequate treatment.[29]

Thyroid cysts

True cysts (i.e. those with a completely smooth wall) are very rare. The majority identified ultrasonographically are composite lesions representing colloid degeneration, necrosis or haemorrhage in benign or malignant tumours. Neither an ultrasound report of a 'thyroid cyst' nor the aspiration of clear fluid from a cystic lesion guarantees that it is harmless: only if the lesion is completely and permanently abolished by aspiration can it be considered benign (Fig. 18.5). Even acellular or benign cytology of the aspirate is no guarantee. One study has shown that 32% of 395 thyroid swellings were cystic and 46% of the cystic swellings were neoplastic, i.e. 14% overall were malignant (29% in men). A third of the malignant thyroid cysts had false-negative cytology.[30]

Toxic adenomas

Plummer was the first to differentiate toxic adenoma from Graves' disease. Toxic adenomas account for 5% of patients with thyrotoxicosis: 9 out of 10 cases are female. They can occur at any age. Some 54% present because of a nodule, 37% because of thyrotoxicosis;[31] 90–96% of such adenomas are benign.[32] The thyrotoxicosis may be of thyroxine or tri-iodothyronine type and is not normally associated with exophthalmos. Diagnosis is easily made with an iodine or technetium scintiscan which shows uptake of the isotope solely in the nodule; the remainder of the gland is not imaged. Such solitary 'hot' nodules may also be seen in euthyroid patients but most will probably progress in time to clinical toxicity.[31] ('Hot' nodules are also noted in multinodular goitre.) Solitary toxic adenomas are usually treated by lobectomy. Temporary thyroxine therapy is occasionally necessary after operation until the residual, suppressed lobe returns to normal function. Radioiodine treatment can be used instead of surgery but may not be effective and may allow a neoplasm to go undiagnosed. In addition it may result in postoperative hypothyroidism.

Malignant thyroid neoplasms

Aetiology of thyroid neoplasia

Thyroid neoplasia can occur in any part of the thyroid or in ectopic thyroid tissue. In the vast majority of cases no aetiological factor is evident. In laboratory animals, anything which causes excessive

REFERENCES

29. Bondeson L, Bondeson A G et al Am Surg 1981; 194: 677–680
30. Cusick E L, McIntosh C A et al Br J Surg 1988; 75: 984–987
31. Bransom C J, Talbot C H et al Br J Surg 1979; 66: 590–595
32. Johnson I D A Br J Surg 1975; 62: 765–768

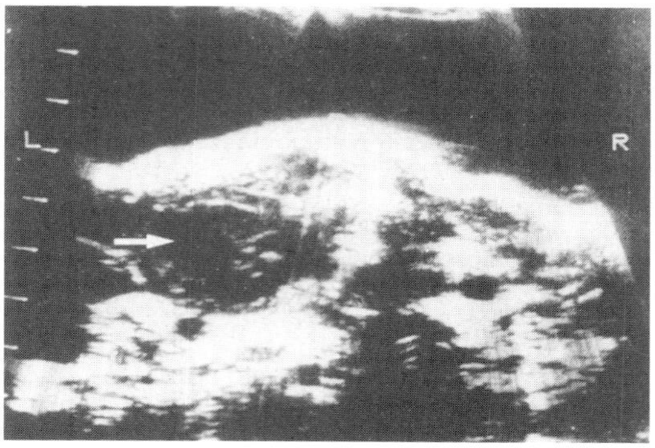

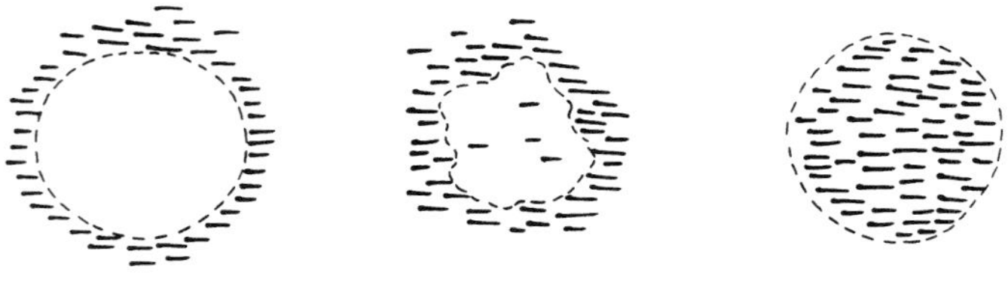

Fig. 18.5 Ultrasound appearance of a thyroid 'cyst' (arrowed). Such cysts are rarely the true cysts but more usually the fluid centre of an otherwise solid nodule, as in this ultrasound.

thyroid-stimulating hormone secretion can produce benign and malignant thyroid tumours.

Thyroid-stimulating hormone elevations occur with goitrogenic drugs and radiation. Human thyroid tumours carry active thyroid-stimulating hormone receptor sites but the growth of thyroid cells is normally also influenced by other growth factors. Their continued growth in neoplasia may be due to autocrine production of interstitial growth factors[33] and/or differences in the types or function of cellular thyroid-stimulating hormone receptors, possibly associated with gene changes. The sequence of genetic and hormonal events involved in the induction of differentiated thyroid malignancy is complex and incompletely understood.[34] Most differentiated thyroid cancers need thyroid-stimulating hormone for continued growth but undifferentiated and medullary cancers do not. The small doses of radiation once administered to the neck or thymus of children for the management of a range of minor childhood ailments is now known to be a potent carcinogen. This outcome was first noted by Duffy & Fitzgerald in 1950.[35] Faithfully recording it in the first edition of this book, Aird noted that 'it is hardly conceivable that a short course of low voltage X-rays could be carcinogenic'. It is, and when there is a history of such radiation therapy, the risk of malignancy in a palpable nodule may be as high as 50%.[36] The larger dose of radiation administered in the treatment of, for example, Hodgkin's disease may also lead to thyroid cancer after a latent period of 6–35 years.[37] The use of iodine 131 for the treatment of thyrotoxicosis has not been shown to lead to an increase in thyroid malignancy.

A family history of multiple endocrine neoplasia type II is a risk factor in medullary carcinoma of the thyroid. Papillary carcinoma may also be familial but only very rarely so.[38,39] Lymphocytic thyroiditis is associated with the development of thyroid lymphoma in a tiny minority of cases.

Assessment of thyroid nodules

Thyroid cancer cannot be excluded by the feel of a thyroid nodule. Hardness and fixity to surrounding structures are nevertheless suspicious and the presence of one or more palpable nodes in the deep cervical, supraclavicular or low posterior triangle groups makes cytological or histological assessment mandatory. The presence of a multinodular goitre does not exclude malignancy and the occurrence of a dominant nodule, especially with associated lymphadenopathy, is suspicious. Recurrent laryngeal nerve palsy or persisting pain and dysphagia may also be indicators of malignancy. Concomitant thyrotoxicosis makes malignancy less likely but does not exclude it.

More women suffer thyroid cancer than men but as men are less prone to develop thyroid nodules, the chance that a man's thyroid nodule will be malignant is substantially higher than a woman's. As a general rule, the younger a patient, the more likely that a nodule will be malignant, although rapidly growing nodules in the elderly are also particularly suspect.

Traditionally the investigation of a nodule relies on iodine 123 or technetium 99m scintiscanning, associated with ultrasonography. Isotopically 'cold' nodules which are solid or partly cystic are regarded as suspicious of malignancy and excision biopsy is advised (Fig. 18.6). One or other of these two tests is still useful in demonstrating whether an apparently solitary nodule is in fact part of a multinodular goitre, but fine-needle aspiration biopsy is becoming the definitive means of assessing the chance of malignancy in a thyroid nodule. Excision of the thyroid nodule can then be avoided if the fine-needle biopsy is unequivocally benign but many patients with solitary nodules will however have presented because of pressure symptoms or cosmetic anxieties and require excision regardless of the cause. Where such a nodule can be judged on straightforward clinical grounds as requiring excision, there is little to be gained from extensive investigation prior to operation.

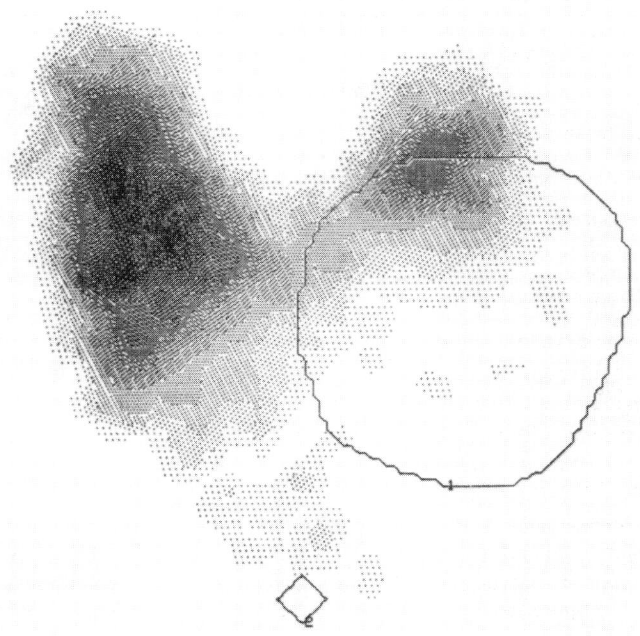

Fig. 18.6 Technetium scintiscan of the thyroid. The palpable nodule has been outlined. There is no uptake by the nodule which is therefore described as 'cold'.

Fine-needle biopsy

Although the technique dates back to 1900 fine-needle cytology of the thyroid was not generally practised until after the pioneering work of the Swedes in the 1960s.[40] There was transiently a vogue

REFERENCES

33. Duh Q Y, Clark O H Prog Surg 1988; 19: 205–222
34. Wynford-Thomas D In: Wheeler M H, Lazarus J H (eds) Diseases of the Thyroid. Chapman & Hall, London 1994
35. Duffy B J, Fitzgerald P J J Clin Endocrinol 1950; 10: 1296
36. Favus M J, Schnieder A B et al N Engl J Med 1976; 294: 1019–1025
37. Naunkeim K S, Kaplan E L Surgery of the Thyroid and Parathyroid Glands. Churchill Livingstone, Edinburgh 1983 pp 51–62
38. Ozaski O et al World J Surg 1988; 12: 565–571
39. Camiel M R et al N Engl J Med 1968; 278: 1056–1059
40. Lowhagen T, Granbery P O et al Surg Clin North Am 1979; 59: 3

for core biopsy of the thyroid[41] but fine-needle aspiration biopsy has now largely superseded it because it is more acceptable to the patient, requires no anaesthesia, has a low complication rate and in addition the processing of the sample is quicker, easier and cheaper. In the standard technique of fine-needle aspiration biopsy a 22-gauge needle attached to a syringe is passed through the lesion four to eight times in different directions without withdrawing the needle from the cutaneous entry site. Taking adequate specimens and making satisfactory slides is not difficult but requires experience.[42] Cytological assessment in experienced hands allows a confident diagnosis of benign colloid, involutional or cellular nodules, papillary, medullary and anaplastic carcinoma but cannot reliably differentiate between follicular adenoma and follicular carcinoma as the distinction between these lesions is based on the presence of vascular or capsular invasion.

Difficulties in interpretation are also encountered with aspirates from cystic lesions; when differentiating between hyperplastic nodules and follicular adenomas, and when differentiating between atypical lymphoid thyroiditis and Hürthle cell adenoma. Additionally there are sampling problems when biopsying multinodular goitres. Fine-needle aspiration biopsy of the thyroid requires the services of an experienced cytologist. Where a hospital has no previous experience in thyroid cytology, it should be implemented in stages; full clinical weight should only be given to the cytologist's opinion after considerable experience. Extensive reported experience of fine-needle aspiration biopsy in the literature shows a false-positive rate for malignancy of less than 2% and a false-negative rate of around 5%,[43] though in some situations such as large and partly cystic nodules the false-negative rates may be as high as 30% but for all diagnoses these rates are higher (Fig. 18.7). Although fine-needle aspiration biopsy is currently the most sensitive investigation of thyroid swellings it should be taken in conjunction with clinical assessment and if after

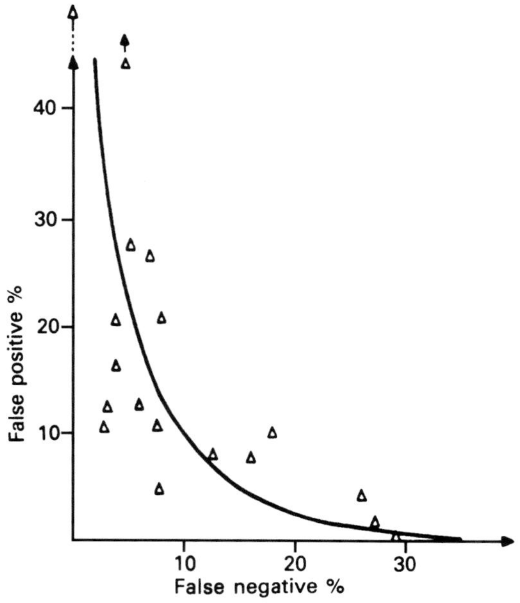

Fig 18.7 Relationship between false-negative and false-positive results with thyroid cytology reported by 18 different pathologists in the literature. From Kohler & Kohler.[44]

biopsy there remains any doubt about the benignity of the thyroid swelling it should be excised surgically. A management plan for thyroid nodules is shown in Figure 18.8.

Management of differentiated thyroid cancer

Differentiated thyroid cancer accounts for 80% of thyroid neoplasms and encompasses two major groups—papillary cancer and follicular cancer. The latter group falls into three categories:

1. Follicular tumours in which no invasion of capsule or blood vessels can be detected and which may be effectively considered benign.
2. Follicular tumours with papillary differentiation which are regarded as variants of papillary cancer and treated as such.
3. Invasive, purely follicular, carcinoma.

Papillary and follicular thyroid cancers are biologically different tumours. Papillary is multifocal, unencapsulated, invades lymphatics and spreads to lymph nodes. It is common in high-iodine intake areas. Follicular cancer, by contrast, is solitary, encapsulated, invades veins, spreads to bones and is common in low-iodine areas. The correction of iodine deficiencies in areas of endemic goitre results in a change in the ratio of papillary and follicular tumours encountered. Currently 70–80% of differentiated thyroid cancers are papillary and 20–30% follicular.

Papillary and mixed tumours

Differentiated thyroid carcinomas have a 4:1 predominance in women and tend to present in the young and middle-aged, although the elderly are not exempt. The tumours tend to be small at presentation (50% <2 cm in diameter) and to have a propensity for early lymph node metastasis and multicentricity. The incidence of multicentricity has varied between reports but is generally in the range of 30–50% with a similar incidence of tumour present in the contralateral lobe. The more extensive the search, the higher the incidence. This multicentricity is frequently cited as an indication for treatment of all papillary cancers by total thyroidectomy rather than by lobectomy.[45] Others have however noted that when papillary cancer is treated solely by lobectomy and lowering of thyroid-stimulating hormone levels by the administration of thyroxine, the incidence of recurrence in the opposite lobe is very low and the mortality rate just as low as with total thyroidectomy.[46,47]

REFERENCES

41. Wang C A, Vickery A L, Maloof F Surg Gynecol Obstet 1976; 143: 365–368
42. Abele J S, Miller T R Endocrine Surgery of the Thyroid and Parathyroid Glands. C V Mosby, St Louis 1985 pp 293–366
43. Gharib H Mayo Clin Proc 1994; 69: 44–49
44. Kohler F, Kohler H In: Romer H-D, Clark O H (eds) Thyroid Tumours. Karger, Basel 1988
45. Clark O H Am Surg 1982; 196: 361–370
46. Farrar W B, Cooperman H, James A G Am Surg 1980; 192: 701–704
47. Rossi R L, Cady B et al World J Surg 1986; 10: 612–622

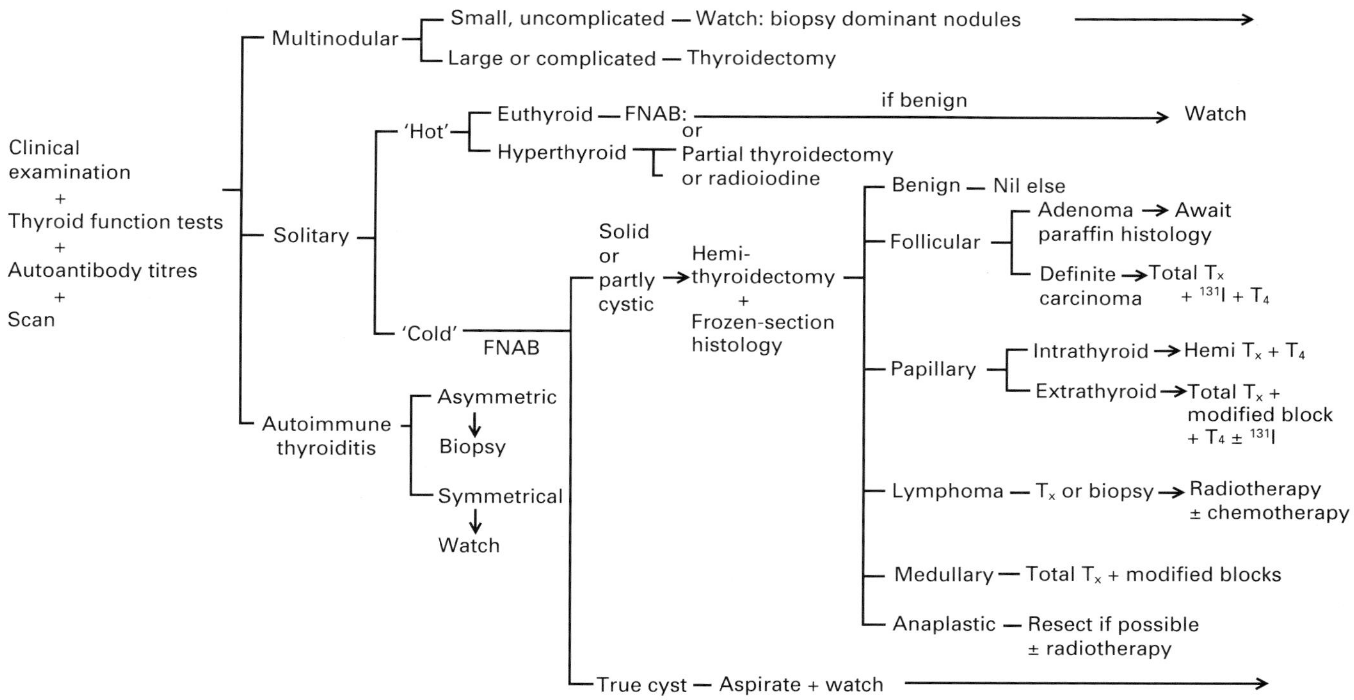

Fig. 18.8 Management plan for a thyroid nodule. T_x = Thyroidectomy; T_4 = suppressive thyroxine therapy; FNAB = fine-needle aspiration biopsy.

Further controversy surrounds the necessity for adjuvant lymph node dissection.[48] Noguchi et al[49] noted an 80% incidence of microscopic metastases in lymph nodes removed at prophylactic neck dissection for papillary cancer but not all studies show an effect of nodal status on survival.[50] Unfor-tunately no randomized studies exist which compare radical with conservative thyroid resection of papillary disease and the surgeon seeking advice is more likely to be confused than assisted by trying to find advice in the journals. The roots of this problem seem to lie in the composition of the groups of patients usually reviewed—usually all cases of differentiated thyroid cancer treated in one institution over the years. Analyses do however show that patients at high and low risk can be separated[51,52] and treatment tailored appropriately.

There is a need to identify some patients as suitable for conservative surgery because the complication rate of total thyroidectomy when generally applied is substantially higher than the 1–2% achieved by specialists. Foster,[53] for instance, analysing 24 108 thyroidectomies performed in the USA, identified an incidence of hypoparathyroidism of 8% after total thyroidectomy compared with 1.5% after subtotal thyroidectomy. Patients at low risk are those with a tumour less than 2 cm in diameter, which has not breached the capsule of the thyroid, where the regional nodes are not palpably involved, and where there is no evidence of distant metastases. Females under the age of 50 and males below 40 are also at lower risk. Studies of DNA content confirm the differences in behaviour of these tumours. Those with a diploid or tetraploid pattern have an indolent unaggressive course while those with an aneuploid pattern tend to behave aggressively.[54] In low-risk patients with a tumour confined to within a single lobe, treatment by unilateral total lobectomy is adequate if followed by lifelong thyroxine therapy at a dose sufficient to reduce thyroid-stimulating hormone to immeasurable or very low levels. The dose to achieve maximal thyroid-stimulating hormone suppression without toxicity usually lies between 200 and 300 μg/day thyroxine.

The use of thyroxine postoperatively significantly reduces recurrence and improves survival in papillary neoplasia.[55] Patients who do not fall into the favourable category (i.e. those with tumours larger than 2 cm, and/or those which have broached the thyroid capsule or who have nodal involvement) should be treated by total thyroidectomy. Papillary carcinoma in children behaves aggressively and should be treated by total thyroidectomy.[56] The fact that papillary carcinoma can be multifocal is not a sound reason for advocating total thyroidectomy for all patients. There is continuing vigorous debate on the value of different adjunctive therapies, not all of which can be shown to extend life expectancy, though they are effective at local control of disease. These adjunctive therapies include nodal excision, radioiodine, external irradiation and chemotherapy.

REFERENCES

48. Simon D, Goretzki P E et al World J Surg 1996; 20: 860–866
49. Noguchi S, Noguchi A, Marakami N Cancer 1970; 26: 1053
50. Hirabayaski R N, Lindsay S J Clin Endocrinol 1961; 21: 1596
51. Hay I D, Grant C S et al Surgery 1987; 1088
52. Mazzaferri E L, Young R L Am J Med 1981; 70: 511–518
53. Foster R S Surg Gynecol Obstet 1978; 146: 423
54. Backdahl M, Wallin G, Auer G Prog Surg 1988; 19: 40–53
55. Clark O H World J Surg 1981; 5: 39
56. Harrach H R, Williams E D Br J Cancer 1995; 72: 777–783

Follicular carcinoma

Where a clear histological diagnosis of invasive follicular carcinoma is made, the proper treatment is total thyroidectomy, as this allows subsequent treatment with radioiodine therapy. The absence of involved lymph nodes in follicular carcinoma does not exclude distant metastases, because vascular invasion is common. Where regional nodes are involved they should however be excised by modified block dissection. All patients must receive lifelong suppressive thyroxine therapy.

Where a follicular lesion has been removed at operation and the frozen section diagnosis is uncertain, it is best to complete the removal of the involved lobe and await paraffin section histology. If this confirms the follicular carcinoma, the residual lobe can be removed at a second operation or if small, ablated with radioiodine, though if the only indication of malignancy is minimal capsular invasion and the patient is less than 50, further therapy can be avoided.

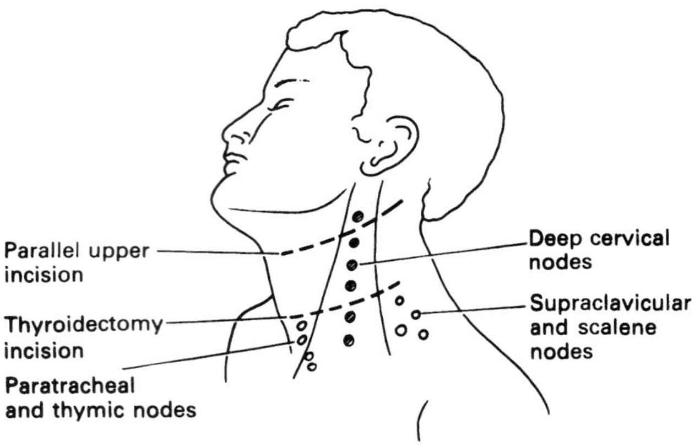

Fig. 18.9 Modified block dissection is carried out through an extended thyroidectomy incision supplemented, if necessary, by a higher parallel incision. All regional nodes in the neck can be removed through these incisions.

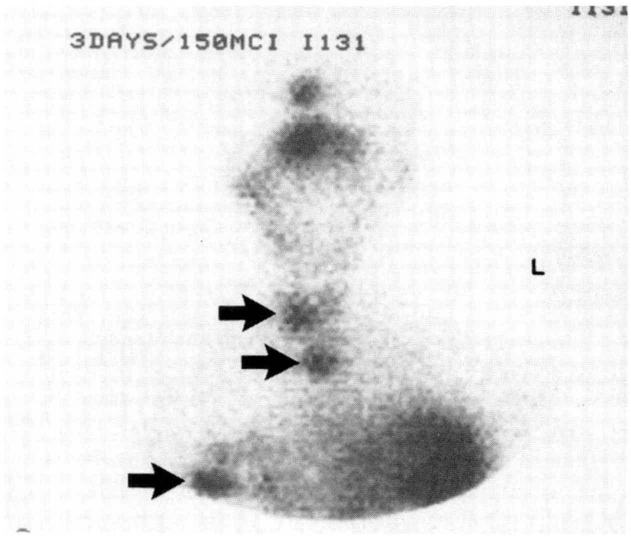

Fig. 18.10 Radioiodine scan showing metastatic follicular thyroid carcinoma in the neck and lungs (arrowed).

Adjunctive therapy for thyroid carcinoma

Prophylactic excision of the regional lymph nodes does not improve survival but clinically involved nodes should be removed. This can be done by individual excision 'berry-picking' or more confidently by modified block dissection. As metastatic cancer in lymph nodes rarely escapes from the confines of the nodes, traditional forms of radical block dissection sacrificing the jugular vein, the sternomastoid and nerves are almost never indicated and the appropriate operation of modified block dissection spares these structures. It can be performed through the extended thyroidectomy incision, sometimes supplemented by another higher parallel skin crease incision on the affected side (Fig. 18.9). The dissection need not be carried above the hyoid but needs to extend distally into the upper mediastinum, especially along the trachea-oesophageal groove.

Radioiodine therapy is indicated in follicular cancer and in papillary and mixed tumours where there is extracapsular disease and where the histology has demonstrated colloid formation by the tumour.

Radioiodine therapy

Following operation patients are rendered euthyroid with tri-iodothyronine 60–100 µg/day until recovery from operation is complete. The tri-iodothyronine is then discontinued 2 weeks before the planned time for radioiodine therapy. The resultant hypothyroidism stimulates maximal thyroid-stimulating hormone secretion, thus encouraging uptake of the isotope by residual functioning thyroid tissue. Initially a scanning dose of approximately 1 mCi of radioiodine is given. The whole body is imaged and assessments of iodine uptake made. If iodine uptake is imaged or demonstrated, a therapeutic dose is given (30–150 mCi). If multiple avid metastases are demonstrated a further higher dose up to 200 mCi is sometimes given. Where uptake has been demonstrated the process may be repeated at annual intervals to a total dose of 800–1000 mCi (Fig. 18.10). Thyroglobulin is only produced by functioning thyroid tissue and its presence in the serum after total thyroidectomy at levels in excess of 10 ng/ml suggests recurrent disease. It can be used as a guide for the need for further radioiodine therapy.[57,58] In patients with metastases there is a treatability rate of 60% and a response rate of 30% in papillary tumours and 50% in follicular lesions.[59] Although no randomized study exists, treatment with iodine 131 seems to confer survival advantages.[60,61]

External radiotherapy

In differentiated cancer, external radiotherapy is primarily of value where there is residual metastatic disease after radioiodine therapy,

REFERENCES

57. Ericson U B, Tegler L et al Acta Chir Scand 1984; 150: 367–375
58. Ashcroft M W, Van Herle A J Am J Med 1981; 71: 806
59. Leeper R D J Clin Endocrinol Metab 1973; 36: 1143
60. Varma V M, Bierwaltes W H, Nofal M M JAMA 1970; 23: 1437
61. Bierwaltes H W, Nishiyama R H et al J Nucl Med 1982; 12: 561

where there is no uptake of radioiodine by metastases which can be imaged by alternative means or where there is a large unresectable primary tumour. It is of course also of value in lymphomas and undifferentiated tumours.

Prognosis

The prognosis of differentiated thyroid cancer even when metastases are present at the time of discovery is excellent (Fig. 18.11). Prognosis is particularly favourable in patients between the age of 20 and 50. Although differentiated thyroid carcinoma is uncommon in children, the rates of recurrence are higher and prognosis less good than in the 20–50 age group.

Medullary thyroid cancer

Medullary thyroid cancer is cancer of the parafollicular cells, also called C cells. These are derived from ultimobranchial bodies. They produce calcitonin, a polypeptide which lowers blood calcium. Cancer of these cells was first clearly identified by Hazard et al in 1959.[63] Cancer of parafollicular cells accounts for 2–8% of all thyroid neoplasms and it occurs in several distinct clinical contexts:

1. Sporadic—90%.
2. Familial, in association with multiple endocrine neoplasia type II.
3. Familial, without other stigmata of multiple endocrine neoplasia.

Clinical features

Most sporadic cases present as thyroid masses or nodules and 25% of patients have palpable lymph node metastases at the time of presentation. Those with the disease as a manifestation of multiple endocrine neoplasia IIa may also have clinical signs of phaeochromocytoma and/or hyperparathyroidism. In multiple endocrine neoplasia IIb they will additionally display multiple mucosal neuromas, especially of the lips and tongue, together with a recognizable marfanoid habitus. Multiple endocrine neoplasia has an autosomal dominant inheritance and medullary thyroid cancer will be identified in known families by hormonal or genetic screening prior to its declaration as a thyroid tumour. Such screening should begin before puberty as medullary thyroid cancer can occur in patients of any age. In sporadic familial and in multiple endocrine neoplasia type IIa disease patients will show mutations on exons 11 and 10 of the RET proto-oncogene, whereas in multiple endocrine neoplasia type IIb exon 16 will be affected. Where present these mutations carry a 100% risk of developing medullary carcinoma and prophylactic thyroidectomy is indicated in childhood.[64]

In the sporadic diseases, patients are usually, however, over the age of 40. Medullary thyroid cancer produces not only calcitonin but also other substances including serotonin, prostaglandin, 5-hydroxyindoleacetic acid, carcinoembryonic antigen, histaminase, adrenocorticotrophic hormone and prolactin. These can be used to assess the presence, extent and recurrence of the disease. Usually however only calcitonin and carcinoembryonic acid are assayed.

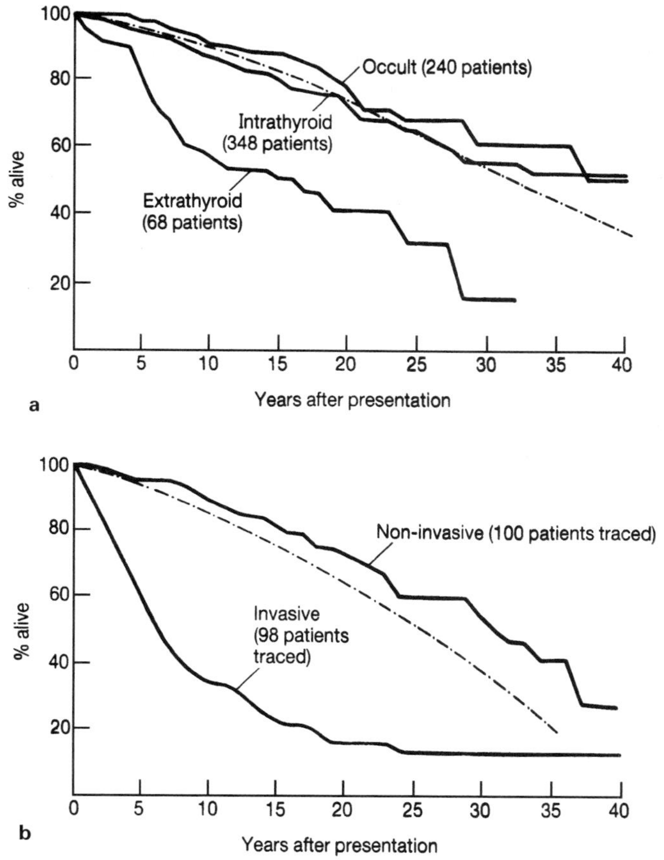

Fig. 18.11 Survival after treatment of **(a)** papillary and **(b)** follicular thyroid carcinoma. Broken line shows the survival of a normal population. From Woolner et al.[62]

High circulating levels of other substances may be responsible for the diarrhoea which is often associated with extensive medullary thyroid cancer.

Sporadic medullary thyroid cancer is usually solitary and unilateral, whereas hereditary forms are bilateral and multicentric. They may be preceded by C cell hyperplasia and predominantly occur in the middle to upper third of the gland where the C cells are most numerous.

There is no place for measuring calcitonin in all patients with thyroid nodules but if medullary thyroid cancer is suspected on fine-needle aspiration biopsy or from the clinical history or if there is bilateral upper polar calcification or the signs of phaeochromocytoma or hypercalcaemia, then calcitonin should be measured. If calcitonin is raised urinary vanillylmandelic acid and/or urinary catecholamines should be measured preoperatively to exclude a coexisting phaeochromocytoma. All relatives of patients discovered to have medullary thyroid cancer must have calcitonin levels assayed. If calcitonin is normal then the test is repeated using a

REFERENCES

62. Woolner L B et al In: Young S, Ingman I R (eds) ICRF Symposium on Thyroid Neoplasia. Academic Press, London 1968
63. Hazard J B, Hawk W A, Gile G J Clin Endocrinol 1959; 19: 152
64. Pacini F, Romeri C et al Surgery 1995; 118: 1031

provocative test with pentagastrin.[65] If a familial trait is identified then formal family tree analysis and reporting to the national multiple endocrine neoplasia database is appropriate.

Treatment

Medullary thyroid cancer is more aggressive than other forms of differentiated thyroid cancer; 50% of cases have involved nodes at operation even where the primary lesion is tiny. The mainstay of treatment is radical surgery. The addition of node dissection to thyroidectomy has been shown to improve the 10-year prognosis from 43 to 67%.[66]

The diagnosis of medullary thyroid cancer should if possible be established preoperatively by fine-needle aspiration biopsy. Total thyroidectomy should be performed as well as ipsilateral resection of all lymphatic tissue from the thyroid cartilage to the upper mediastinum, including the thymus and laterally to the outer border of the sternomastoid. If there is multicentric or familial disease, bilateral neck dissection should be performed. If the diagnosis was not made preoperatively or if the thyroidectomy is performed in a familial case with impalpable disease, later neck dissection is only indicated if calcitonin levels do not fall to normal or near normal levels postoperatively. Radical surgery is the key to cure. Radioiodine, external radiotherapy and chemotherapy have no role in the management of the primary disease.

After successful surgery patients must be followed by sequential calcitonin assays. Prognosis is shown in Figure 18.12. Although a raised postoperative calcitonin does not guarantee recurrent or persistent disease it strongly suggests it, particularly if the levels continue to rise. It should be noted that other causes for raised calcitonin include other malignancies, renal failure and pregnancy. After successful total thyroidectomy and node resection for medullary carcinoma the serum calcitonin should be immeasurably low. Many surgeons dealing with this condition are however familiar with the scenario of a low but stable calcitonin level which does not seem to be associated with progressing disease,[65] but others favour extensive investigation and aggressive reoperative strategies for such patients. Recurrent disease may be imaged with DMSA (i.e. ^{99m}Tc (111 dimercaptosuccinic acid) or octreotide isotope scans.

Metastatic medullary thyroid cancer may be troublesome because of local recurrent disease or diarrhoea. Debulking of metastases or therapy by external radiotherapy[68] or chemotherapy is occasionally feasible. Nutmeg therapy may relieve the diarrhoea.[69]

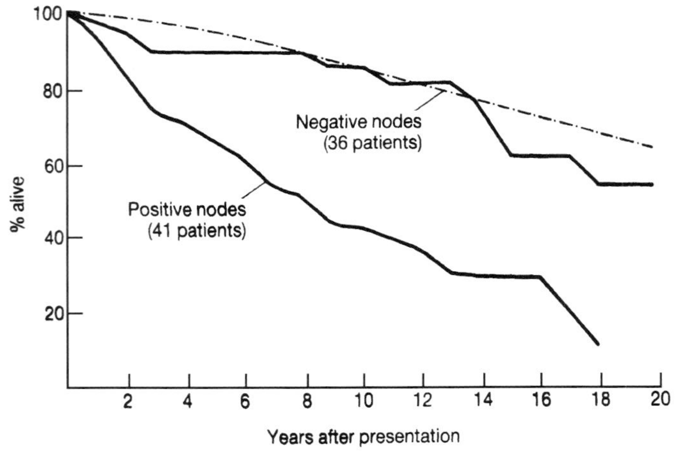

Fig. 18.12 Survival after treatment of medullary thyroid carcinoma. From Woolner et al.[62]

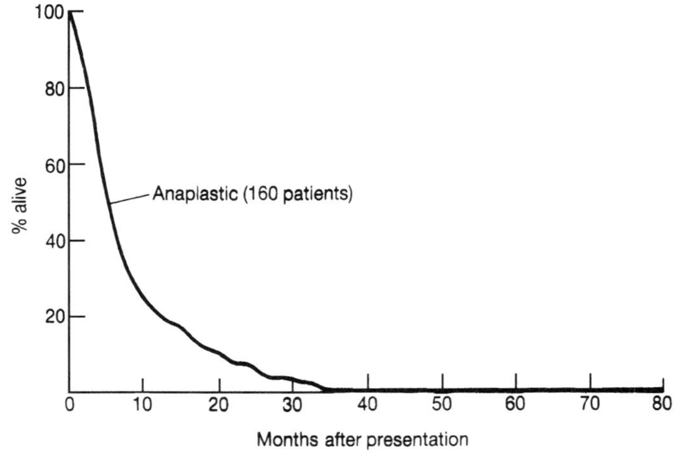

Fig. 18.13 Survival after presentation with anaplastic thyroid carcinoma. Note that the survival of these patients is recorded in months, not years, as in other graphs. From Woolner et al.[62]

Anaplastic thyroid cancer

Anaplastic malignancies of the thyroid—those which on histology show few or no differentiated structures—are the worst of all thyroid malignancies and one of the most aggressive of all human neoplasms. They are justly infamous for their unpleasant course. Death occurs within a year of diagnosis in 90% of patients (Fig. 18.13). They account for 3–30% of all thyroid neoplasms depending on the geographic area. They are commonest in areas of endemic goitre and women are more often affected than men. The tumour is almost entirely confined to elderly patients in whom it presents late, probably having begun as an unrecognized or ignored differentiated tumour of papillary or follicular type. Such tumours histologically coexist with anaplastic cancer in many cases.

At presentation the patient usually has a fixed mass in the centre of the neck surrounding the trachea and infiltrating local structures with great tenacity; even the carotid arteries and the lumen of the trachea are not excluded from invasion. Stridor from tracheal invasion, dysphagia from oesophageal involvement and recurrent nerve palsy and pain are all common.

REFERENCES

65. Wells S A Jr et al Ann Surg 1978; 188: 377–383
66. Ellhorn J Surgery 1993; 1078
67. Van Heerden J A, Hay I D In: Wheeler M H, Lazarus J H (eds) Diseases of the Thyroid. Chapman & Hall, London 1994 pp 400–401
68. Steinfeld A B Radiology 1977; 123: 745–746
69. Fawell W N, Thompson G N Engl J Med 1973; 289: 848–858

Management

Biopsy is the first essential with the object of differentiating between lymphoma and true anaplastic cancer. This distinction is not always possible on fine-needle aspiration biopsy and open or core biopsy may be necessary. The large cell anaplastic tumours readily diagnosed on fine-needle aspiration biopsy are certainly true anaplastic tumours. Diffuse small cell tumours are more difficult to classify and the survivors are found only in this group. Such patients may in fact be suffering from thyroid lymphoma.[70] As histopathological techniques improve an increasing proportion of anaplastic thyroid cancer becomes categorized as lymphoma. In the absence of a definite histopathological diagnosis the presence of multiple lymph nodes and a rapid response to radiotherapy allow a clinical diagnosis of lymphoma to be made. When undifferentiated and differentiated cancer are found to coexist the prognosis is no better than when the tumour is solely undifferentiated.

Curative surgery is almost never feasible; even Jereb et al who operated on 37 of 79 cases could only obtain macroscopic clearance in 5 patients and even with adjuvant radiotherapy only 1 of these patients survived for 10 years.[71] Traditionally debulking surgery is attempted when feasible but in fewer than half the patients the limited objective of freeing the trachea and oesophagus from encroachment is achievable.[72] Indeed the sole result may be to allow tumour to fungate through the wound. Super-radical surgery — even as extensive as pharyngolaryngectomy — has been advocated but is not generally accepted as useful.[73] Preoperative radiotherapy has not been found to shrink the tumour sufficiently to allow radical surgery. Some have advocated following surgery by radiotherapy and chemotherapy[74] but most older patients cannot tolerate this triple insult and such aggressive intent should be restricted to the rare younger patient presenting with this disease. For the majority of patients biopsy followed by attempted palliation with radiotherapy is all that is indicated.

Lymphoma of the thyroid

Lymphoma may involve the thyroid primarily or secondarily. Some 20% of those dying with disseminated lymphoma can be shown at autopsy to have thyroid involvement.[75] Primary lymphoma must be distinguished from small cell anaplastic cancer. There is sometimes a history of coexisting lymphocytic thyroiditis and histological changes of Hashimoto's thyroiditis are found in 36% of resected lymphomas of the thyroid, though only a tiny fraction of a per cent of patients with Hashimoto's progress to thyroid lymphoma. The lymphoma is usually of the B-cell type.[76] Treatment of the lymphoma confined to the thyroid may be by total thyroidectomy followed by irradiation of the neck and upper mediastinum. There is however no evidence that surgery improves the prognosis of patients presenting with extrathyroid disease and following a confident biopsy result these patients should be treated by radiotherapy. Recurrent or distant metastatic disease is treated by chemotherapy.[77]

The 5-year survival is 86% when the disease is confined at presentation to the thyroid, but only 38% where soft tissue or nodal involvement is present (Fig. 18.14). Prognosis is also critically

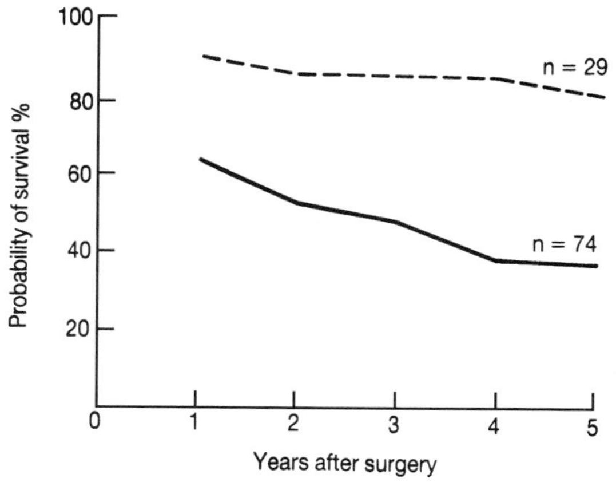

Fig. 18.14 Survival after presentation with primary thyroid lymphoma. Dashed line = intrathyroid; continuous line = extrathyroid. From Devine et al.[78]

related to the grade of the tumour: low and intermediate-grade tumours have a 5-year survival of around 80%, whereas for high-grade lesions it is less than 20%.[76] Age and sex have no influence on the prognosis. Solitary plasmacytoma of the thyroid with associated monoclonal gammopathy has been reported.[79]

Squamous carcinoma

This is very rare and should be distinguished from squamous metaplasia in papillary carcinoma. True squamous carcinoma arises in embryonal remnants and may coexist with adenocarcinoma. Squamous carcinoma of the thyroid is an extremely aggressive, essentially untreatable malignancy.[80]

Teratomas

These tumours contain tissue from all three germ layers. They are benign in children but usually malignant when encountered in adults, in which context they are very aggressive and prognosis is usually survival for less than 1 year.[81]

HYPERTHYROIDISM

Hyperthyroidism is the result of increased levels of thyroid hormone in the blood. The usual causes are diffuse toxic goitre

REFERENCES

70. Walt A J, Woolner L B, Black B M J Clin Endocrinol Metab 1957; 17: 45–60
71. Jereb B, Stjernsward J, Lowhagen T Cancer 1975; 35: 1293–1295
72. Nel C J C, Heerden J A et al Mayo Clin Proc 1985; 60: 51–58
73. Djalilian M, Beakro O H et al Am J Surg 1974; 128: 500–504
74. Rogers J D, Lindberg R H, Hill C S Cancer 1974; 34: 1328–1332
75. Meissner W A, Phillips M J Arch Pathol 1962; 74: 291–297
76. Aozasa A, Inique A et al Cancer 1986; 58: 100–104
77. Edmonds C J In: Wheeler M H, Lazarus J H (eds) Diseases of the Thyroid. Chapman & Hall, London 1994 pp 387–392
78. Devine R M, Edis A J, Banks P M World J Surg 1981; 5: 33–38
79. Beguin Y, Coniver J et al Surgery 1987; 101: 496–500
80. Harada T, Shimaoka K, Yakumaruk Ho K J Surg Oncol 1982; 19: 36–43
81. Kimler S C, Mulh W F Cancer 1978; 42: 311

Table 18.2 Causes of hyperthyroidism

Diffuse toxic goitre (Graves' disease)
Hyperfunctioning adenoma
Toxic multinodular goitre (Plummer's syndrome)
Overdose of thyroxine (iatrogenic or factitious)
Subacute or acute thyroiditis
Thyroid-stimulating hormone-secreting tumours (choriocarcinoma, hydatidiform mole, embryonal testicular cancer)
Functioning thyroid carcinoma
Overtreatment of nodular goitre with iodine (Jo–Basedow effect)
During ^{131}I therapy
Struma ovarii

(Graves' disease, von Basedow's disease) and hyperfunctioning adenomas or multinodular goitres (Plummer's disease). Other rarer causes are listed in Table 18.2.

Graves' disease

Aetiology

What we have now called Graves' disease was first clearly recognized by Caleb Hillier Parry in 1786.[9] More than 200 years later the details of its aetiology remain unclear. It is currently considered that Graves' disease is an autoimmune disorder in which polyclonal immunoglobulins activate thyroid-stimulating hormone receptors on the thyroid cell membrane. These thyroid-stimulating immunoglobulins are found in 90% of patients and are not the same as the long-acting thyroid-stimulating substance originally implicated.

The stimulus to thyroid-stimulating immunoglobulin production is unknown. Patients of human leukocyte antigen tissue type DW3 seem particularly at risk. Many patients relate the onset of their disease to a fright or stressful period in their lives.

The aetiology of the eye changes is more complex. Thyroid-stimulating immunoglobulin and other humoral immunoglobulins seem partly to be responsible for the exophthalmos but there may also be a cell-mediated immune process at work and binding of thyroglobulin to ocular muscles may be involved in the extraocular myositis. This complex topic is well-reviewed by Havard.[82]

Clinical features

Graves' disease is predominantly a disease of women, amongst whom the incidence is 20 per 1000—10 times greater than the incidence among men. The peak incidence is at 20–40 years but any age from birth to death may be affected. The onset is usually insidious, though in the young adult symptoms are usually florid at presentation with a visible goitre and abnormal eye signs. In the older patient neither of these pointers may be present and cardiovascular and neurological features then predominate.[83] In children the behavioural and growth abnormalities may be the only presenting features.

The clinical features of Graves' disease are listed in Table 18.3. Most are the result of excessive circulating thyroxine but exophthalmos, pretibial myxoedema and thyroid acropachy have a different causation. On examination of the patient the thyroid may be found to be uniformly enlarged, smooth and firm, though occasionally it is bossellated. It is rarely very large but is frequently hypervascular; a thrill may be palpable and a strong bruit audible.

Table 18.3 Clinical features of hyperthyroidism

General	Weight loss Increased appetite Fatigue Sweating Heat intolerance
Cardiovascular system	Palpitations Angina Sinus tachycardia or atrial fibrillation Cardiac failure Vasodilation Palpitations
Neuromuscular	Tremor Emotional lability, psychosis Proximal myopathy Myasthenia gravis Choreoathetosis
Gastrointestinal	Vomiting Diarrhoea Steatorrhoea
Skin	Increased pigmentation Thyroid acropachy Spider naevi Palmar erythema Pretibial myxoedema Onycholysis
Reproductive	Oligomenorrhoea Gynaecomastia Reduced libido
Eyes	See Table 18.4
Bones	Osteoporosis

A total of 75% of cases have associated eye disease but only 2–3% develop severe exophthalmos.[84] The typical appearances of exophthalmos are a combination of proptosis caused by increased retrobulbar orbital contents, lid retraction due to a direct effect of thyroxine on the muscles, conjunctival oedema and redness due to direct irritation by exposure of the conjunctive, and oedema of the eyelids. In severe cases there is ophthalmoplegia following paralysis of the voluntary eye muscles. This may cause squint. Finally optic nerve damage and loss of vision may occur. The severity of the eye disease has been categorized by Werner[85] (Table 18.4).

Diagnosis

Even when the diagnosis seems clinically obvious investigation must be undertaken; the anxious young woman with a non-toxic goitre can mimic Graves' disease closely. The measurement of thyroxine is central to the confirmation of the diagnosis but when assayed as total thyroxine may be misleading because:

REFERENCES

82. Havard C W H Br Med J 1979; 1: 1001–1004
83. Davis P J, Davis F B Medicine 1974; 153: 162–181
84. Hamilton R D, Vikinoski P et al Mayo Clin Proc 1967; 42: 812
85. Werner S C J Clin Endocrinol Metab 1977; 44: 203

Table 18.4 Classification of exophthalmos

Class	Mnemonic	Signs of exophthalmos
0	N	No signs or symptoms
1	O	Only signs (lid lag, stare, proptosis up to 22 mm or less than 3 mm between the eyes); no symptoms
2	S	Soft tissue changes (periorbital swelling, chemosis)
3	P	Proptosis 3 mm or more above upper limit of 18 for Japanese, 20 for whites, and 22 for blacks
4	E	Extraocular muscle involvement (limitations of motion at extreme of gaze and restricted gaze)
5	C	Corneal involvement
6	S	Sight loss (optic nerve involvement)

From Werner.[85]

1. Thyroid-binding globulin may have been increased by pregnancy or oestrogen therapy (low thyroxine).
2. Thyroid-binding globulin may have been decreased by liver disease, nephrotic syndrome or systemic lupus erythematosus (high thyroxine).
3. The hyperthyroidism may be due to surplus tri-iodothyronine (T_3 Toxicosis).

The commonest cause of a spuriously raised thyroxine is the taking of oral contraceptives. Because of these confusing factors it is better to measure free tri-iodothyronine and free thyroxine. The diagnosis should always be confirmed by a low thyroid-stimulating hormone level.

An isotopic thyroid scan will differentiate true Graves' disease from toxic nodular goitre or a hyperfunctioning adenoma (Fig. 18.15). A quantitative measure of the uptake of the isotope will also indicate the severity of the disease. Technetium or iodine 125 are the preferred agents. Other more sophisticated tests of thyroid function such as the thyrotrophin-releasing hormone test are available but not generally applicable in the assessment of straightforward Graves' disease. In some centres thyroid auto-antibodies are routinely assessed in all patients.

Treatment

If untreated, 25% of patients with Graves' disease will spontaneously recover but 25% will die and 50% will be left incapacitated to some degree. All patients with Graves' disease must therefore be treated. There are three forms of treatment: antithyroid drugs, radioiodine and surgery. No one form of treatment is optimal and the timing and choice of treatment must be carefully matched to the patient's disease, social circumstances and wishes. All treatment must therefore be preceded by full discussion of the benefits and complications of each form of treatment. A consensus statement for good practice in the management of hyperthyroidism has been produced by the Royal College of Physicians of London.[86]

Medical treatment

Medical treatment does not cure the underlying pathology; it merely ameliorates the symptoms either allowing time for natural remission to occur or for the patient to be prepared for surgery or radioiodine treatment. The primary agents are specific antithyroid drugs. β-Blockers may also be given to ameliorate the cardiac effects of excessive circulating thyroxine. The agents used for definitive treatment are the thionamides (propylthiouracil, methimazole, carbimazole) and potassium perchlorate. The thionamides inhibit thyroid peroxidase and are generally preferred to perchlorate which interferes with iodide transport. A dose of 5–100 mg propylthiouracil 6-hourly or 10–20 mg carbimazole 8-hourly can control thyrotoxicosis within 10–14 days; sometimes however it may take 2 months to achieve control and that control may be erratic. Divided doses are more effective than one daily dose. Some clinicians give thyroxine to ensure euthyroidism during treatment.

There is no agreement as to the optimal duration of the first course of treatment. Advice varies from 3 to 18 months. When the

REFERENCE

86. Vanderpump M P J , Ahlquist J A et al Br Med J 1996; 313: 539–544

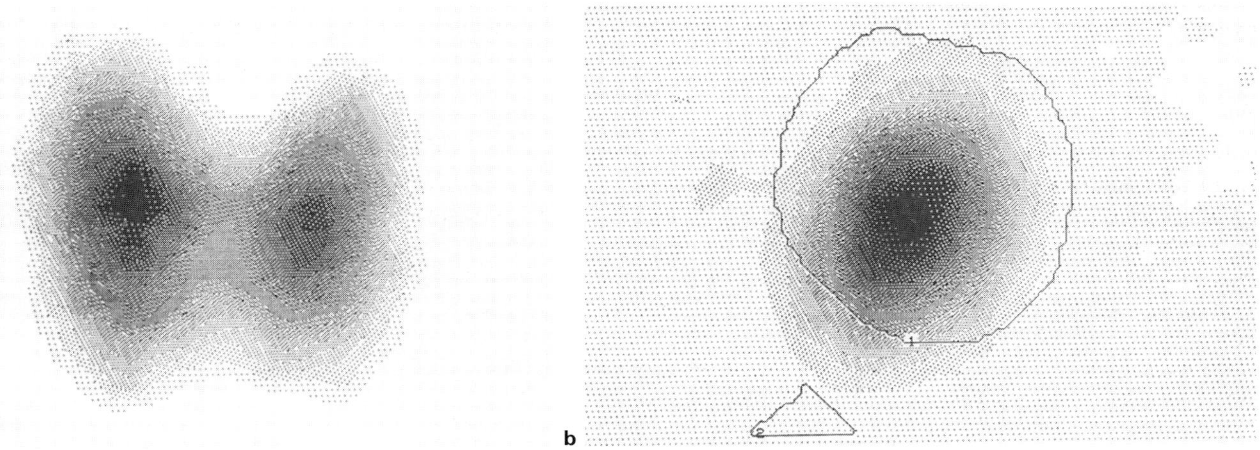

a b

Fig. 18.15 Technetium isotope scans: (a) Graves' disease. Uptake of the isotope was 5.3%; normal is 0.7–3% at 20 min. (b) Functioning thyroid adenoma. The triangle marks the sternal notch. Uptake was 5.16%. The right lobe is not imaged as it is suppressed by the hyperfunctioning left lobe.

drug has been discontinued at the end of that time about 20% of patients will stay in remission, though quoted figures for remission range from 15 to 80%. If recurrence occurs, it is usually within 6 months and a second course of antithyroid drugs is unlikely to be more effective than the first. A second course is however instigated for recurrence in preparation for definitive radioiodine or surgical treatment.

Remissions are most likely to occur where the goitre is small, the thyrotoxicosis mild and where there is a rapid response to the treatment by the shrinkage of the gland. Raised autoantibody levels are good predictors of remission; age is not.

Antithyroid drugs are not without side-effects; many patients find them unpleasant, as they produce dyspepsia and headaches; 3% will develop a sensitivity rash and about 0.4% develop the serious complication of agranulocytosis. A sore throat usually heralds this complication and patients must be warned to discontinue treatment and seek medical advice when this happens.

The choice between radioiodine and surgery is controversial and the decision often arbitrary, relying on preferences of the patient and the physician and the availability of a surgeon skilled in thyroid surgery. In essence though, radioiodine should be regarded as the treatment of choice for thyrotoxicosis and in elderly patients it may even be best first-line treatment before medical therapy. In many centres as few as 5% of thyrotoxic patients are treated surgically, with pregnancy and lactation the only absolute contraindications to radioiodine therapy.

Radioiodine

Radioiodine as ^{131}I is given as a single oral dose and exerts its action by direct radiation damage to the replicative mechanisms of the follicular cells. ^{125}I has not proved effective in this context because of its different radiation characteristics.[87] A dose of ^{131}I is chosen to match the estimated weight of the gland and its isotope uptake on scanning. This basic calculation is then modified by the physician's view on the acceptability of late hypothyroidism. The maximum dose allowable is 100 μCi/g of thyroid tissue, usually resulting in a total dose between 3 and 8 mCi. A response is generally achieved in 6–10 weeks and control of hyperthyroidism by drugs will be necessary in the interim. If no control is achieved at 4 months further radioiodine is given.

The benefits of radioiodine therapy are the ease of its administration, its cheapness and its short-term safety. The risks in theory include the possible induction of thyroid and other malignancies, especially leukaemia, and the induction of genetic abnormalities in future children. These risks appear to be very small. One study of 182 pregnant women given radioiodine showed two spontaneous abortions, two stillbirths and two significant congenital abnormalities. Six of the babies were however hypothyroid.[88] A study of 25 000 patients with Graves' disease treated between 1946 and 1968 showed that in the first year more thyroid neoplasms were found in the surgical group (incidental neoplasms were found in the resected specimen at a rate of 2 per 1000). The subsequent incidence of revealed thyroid cancer in a group treated with radioiodine was only 1 per 1000 but there was a high incidence of thyroid nodules in younger patients.[89]

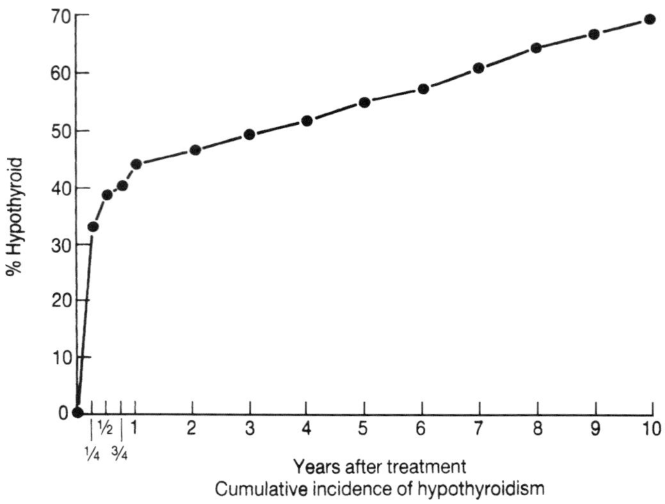

Fig. 18.16 Progressive incidence of hypothyroidism after ^{131}I treatment for thyrotoxicosis. First 6 months = 5.5%/month; second 6 months = 1.3%/month; after first year = 2.8%/year. From Nofal et al.[91]

Other risks include accelerated hyperthyroidism during treatment and late hyperparathyroidism.[90] The major problem however is the high incidence of late hypothyroidism and the unpredictability of its time of onset. The incidence of hypothyroidism varies with dose in the first 3 years and ranges from 10 to 40%. After 3 years there is a 3% per annum increment regardless of the initial dose (Fig. 18.16). Although widely applicable as definitive treatment, ^{131}I therapy is in some centres reserved for those over the age of 40 and for those who are unfit or unwilling to undergo surgery. It is the treatment of choice for those with thyrotoxicosis recurring after surgery.

Surgery

Surgery is appropriate therapy for the toxic patient who is pregnant or who wishes to become so within 4 years; for anyone under the age of 30; for those with large or nodular goitres and those who refuse radiation therapy. It is also preferable for those for whom follow-up or compliance with medical treatment is uncertain. The reasons for inclusion of this last group is the lower incidence of hypothyroidism in surgically treated patients and the fact that the great majority of postoperative hypothyroidism declares itself within 1 year of operation (Fig. 18.17).

Preparation for surgery

History recounts that surgery of the toxic thyroid was difficult and dangerous.[92] That it is not so now reflects not just improvements

REFERENCES

87. McDougall I R, Greig W R Ann Intern Med 1976; 85: 720–723
88. Stoffer S S, Hamburger J I J Nucl Med 1970; 17: 146–149
89. Dobyns B M, Sheline G E et al J Clin Endocrinol 1974; 38: 976–998
90. Tisell L E Surgery of the Thyroid and Parathyroid Glands. Churchill Livingstone, Edinburgh 1983

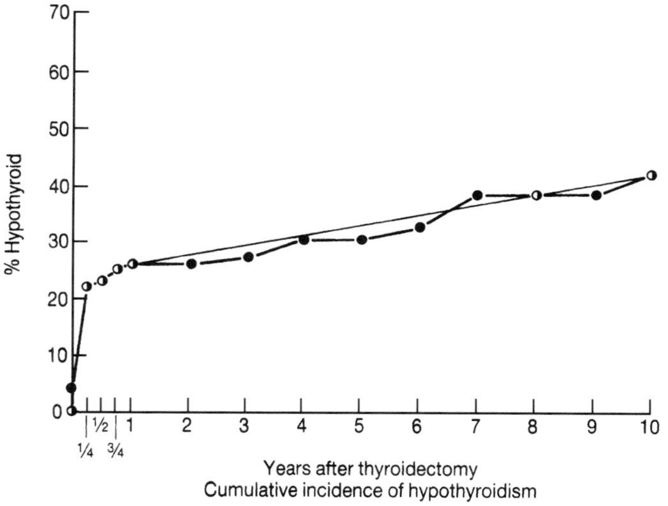

Fig. 18.17 Progressive incidence of hypothyroidism after thyroidectomy for thyrotoxicosis. First 6 months = 3.7%/month; second 6 months = 0.51%/month; after first year = 1.7%/year. From Nofal et al.[91]

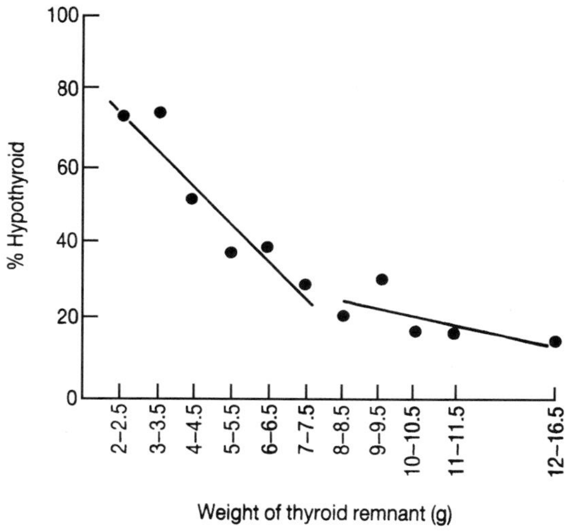

Fig. 18.18 Hypothyroidism in relation to size of thyroid remnant. From Michie.[96]

in surgical technique but also the habit of careful preparation of the patient.

The patient should be euthyroid when operated upon. Carbimazole or propylthiouracil are usually appropriate and control can be achieved within 2 weeks. The euthyroid status must be confirmed by laboratory testing prior to surgery. Preparation is generally improved by the addition of adrenergic β-blockade. Not only does this ameliorate the cardiac and psychological effects of thyrotoxicosis but it also specifically reduces peripheral conversion of thyroxine to tri-iodothyronine and reduces thyroid vascularity. Propanolol 5–40 mg 6-hourly has been used in the past but the long-acting agent nadolol may be preferred.[93] Iodine as potassium iodide or Lugol's iodine will reduce thyroid vascularity if given for 7–10 days preoperatively and alters the texture of the gland, making if firmer.[94] The use of β-blockade and iodine as sole preparation for surgery has been proposed but is not generally accepted as safe.[95] β-Blockade is potentially dangerous in patients with asthma, obstructive airways disease, cardiac failure and in pregnancy and in those on tricyclic and monoamine oxidase inhibitors or psychotropic drugs.

The addition of thyroxine to propylthiouracil during preparation for surgery will in theory reduce the associated rise in thyroid-stimulating hormone and diminish vascularity. It is however not normal practice to require this.

Operation

The operation usually performed is bilateral subtotal thyroidectomy. This satisfies the object of optimizing control of the thyrotoxicosis whilst minimizing complications. The risks of operation are the normal risks of thyroidectomy to which is added the risk of fulminating hyperthyroidism after operation if preoperative antithyroid and anti-adrenergic treatment has not been used. This treatment should be continued for 2 days following surgery as occasionally fulminating thyrotoxicosis may occur after the operation if medication has been discontinued on the day of surgery.

The weight of the thyroid remnants left to attain postoperative euthyroidism is difficult to judge both in theory and practically at the time of operation. It is however reasonable to aim to leave remnants that weigh between 4 and 10 g (Fig. 18.18).[97,98] Although claims have been made that avoiding ligation of the inferior thyroid artery will reduce the incidence of postoperative hypothyroidism,[99] this has not been confirmed by others.[100]

The technical difficulties of operating on the patient with Graves' disease should never be underestimated. Even in the fully controlled patient, the gland remains very vascular and difficult to handle, especially in the young patient. It is never an operation to be delegated to a novice or an inexperienced surgeon.

Results of surgery

Successful operation produces immediate control of thyrotoxicosis but does not guarantee long-term euthyroidism. The recurrence rate is about 5% at 5 years and recurrences continue especially in areas of high iodine intake. Kalk et al[101] noted that only 57% of recurrences in their series of 94 had occurred by 5 years. Early recurrence is associated with raised levels of thyroid-binding inhibitory immunoglobulin and antimicrosomal haemagglutination

REFERENCES

91. Nofal M M et al JAMA 1966; 197: 608
92. Mansberger A R Am Surg 1988; 207: 724–729
93. Peden N R, Browning M C K et al J Med 1985; 56: 579–591
94. Marigold J H, Morgan A K et al Br J Surg 1985; 72: 45–47
95. Feek C M et al N Engl J Med 1980; 302: 883–885
96. Michie W Br J Surg 1975; 62: 673
97. Michie W, Pegg C A S, Bewsher P D Br Med J 1972; 1: 13–17
98. Cusick E L, Krukowski Z H, Matheson N A Br J Surg 1988; 74: 780–783
99. Bradley E L, Leichty R D Surgery 1983; 94: 955–958
100. Corbett R C et al Surg Gynecol Obstet 1988; 166: 418–420
101. Kalk W J, Kantor S, Durback D Lancet 1978; i: 291–294

antibodies.[102] Recurrence can occur up to 50 years after apparently successful surgery.[103] Recurrence is treated with radioiodine because further surgery carries an unacceptable risk of damage to the recurrent laryngeal nerves or parathyroid glands.

Postoperative hypothyroidism develops in between 9%[104] and 49%[105] of patients. The incidence is higher with small remnants, pronounced lymphocytic infiltration of the gland, raised thyroid autoantibody titres and low iodine intake. It is not related to the patient's age or to the size of the original goitre. The reported incidence of hypothyroidism depends on its definition. Many patients will show a raised thyroid-stimulating hormone and a marginally low thyroxine in the first few months after surgery but many of these will remain clinically euthyroid and the thyroid function reverts to normal after 6–12 months.[97] Such patients need not take replacement thyroxine but need regular careful review. Definite clinical hypothyroidism requires lifelong replacement therapy with thyroxine. The dose will be between 100 and 200 μg and, once the proper dose is confirmed by thyroid-stimulating hormone and thyroxine testing, review is only necessary in pregnancy or if cardiac disease develops.[106] Although 90% of incidences of continuing postoperative hypothyroidism will declare themselves in the first year, there is a 1–2% addition to this total in each of the following years and follow-up should not therefore be discontinued after an apparently successful thyroidectomy as both recurrent hypothyroidism and hyperthyroidism can occur many years later.

Eyes

In the great majority of cases there will be regression or arrested progression of exophthalmos after successful management of the thyroid gland in Graves' disease. Progressive eye disease will however occur in 3–10%[107] and may require high-dose steroids, immunosuppression or even surgical orbital decompression.[81]

Thyrotoxicosis in childhood

Medical control of thyrotoxicosis in childhood may be difficult and more complicated than it is in the adult but should always be the first line of treatment. When control cannot be achieved or maintained the tendency in the past has been to prefer surgical treatment[108] but there is now enough long-term experience with radioiodine treatment to confirm that it is safe in this age group.[109,110]

Thyrotoxicosis in pregnancy

The prevalence of thyrotoxicosis in pregnancy is 0.05%.[111] The diagnosis is difficult as more than 50% of pregnant women have a goitre and the signs of pregnancy can mimic thyrotoxicosis. Serum thyroid-stimulating hormone, tri-iodothyronine and thyroxine are normally raised in pregnancy, though free tri-iodothyronine and thyroxine are not. If the diagnosis is made during pregnancy cautious treatment with the lowest effective dose of carbimazole, methimazole or propylthiouracil is indicated;[112] β-blockers and iodides are contraindicated and there is an absolute ban on investigation or treatment with radioiodine. The fetal loss may be as high as 14% and neonatal hypo- and hyperthyroidism can occur. As there is a real risk of abnormal pregnancy there is an argument for undertaking subtotal thyroidectomy in the second trimester.[113,114]

Toxic multinodular goitre

The preferred treatment for toxic multinodular goitre is thyroidectomy if the hyperthyroidism is serious or if the gland is large. Those with mild hyperthyroidism in small multinodular glands can be successfully treated with radioiodine. There is a high incidence of hypothyroidism after surgery—70% at 2 years in the Mayo Clinic series.[115]

HYPOTHYROIDISM

Hypothyroidism exists when there is inadequate thyroid hormone action on the peripheral tissues. This can occur by reduced production of hormone by the gland (primary hypothyroidism); failure of thyroid-stimulating hormone production (secondary hypothyroidism); failure of production of thyroid-stimulating hormone-releasing hormone (tertiary hypothyroidism) or resistance of the peripheral tissues to thyroxine. The causes of hypothyroidism are outlined in Table 18.5. The end-results of all these processes are the same and may be symptomatic (myxoedema) or asymptomatic.

Table 18.5 Causes of hypothyroidism

Primary hypothyroidism
Hashimoto's thyroiditis
Radioactive iodine therapy for Graves' disease
Thyroidectomy
Antithyroid drug therapy for Graves' disease
Excessive iodide intake
Subacute thyroiditis
Miscellaneous rare causes
Iodide deficiency
Goitrogens
Inborn errors of thyroid metabolism
Secondary hypothyroidism
Ablative therapy for pituitary adenoma
Chromophobe pituitary adenoma
Other causes of pituitary destruction
Tertiary hypothyroidism
Peripheral resistance to thyroxine

REFERENCES

102. Sugino K, Mimura T et al World J Surg 1995; 19: 648–652
103. Thompson J A, Wilson R, McKillop J H Br J Surg 1986; 73: 896
104. Caswell H T, Maier W P Surg Gynecol Obstet 1972; 134: 218–220
105. Michie W Br J Surg 1975; 62: 673–682
106. Toft A D N Engl Med J 1994; 331: 174–180
107. Kriss J P et al J Clin Endocrinol Metab 1970; 31: 315
108. Soreide J-A, van Heerden J A et al World J Surg 1996; 20: 794–800
109. Hamburger J I J Clin Endocrinol Metab 1985; 60: 1019
110. Safa A M, Schumacher P, Rodriguez-Antunez A N Engl J Med 1975; 292: 167–171
111. Drury M I J R Soc Med 1986; 79: 317–318
112. Herbst A L, Selenkow H A N Engl J Med 1965; 273: 627–637
113. Mujtaba Q, Burrow G N Obstet Gynaecol 1975; 46: 282–286
114. Bell G O, Hall J Med Clin North Am 1960; 44: 363–367
115. Mensen M D, Gharib H et al World J Surg 1986; 10: 673–680

Clinical symptoms

The hypothyroid infant (cretin) is somnolent, feeds poorly, fails to thrive and is constipated. The tongue is large, the face puffy, the abdomen is protruberant and umbilical hernias are common. Onset of hypothyroidism in childhood leads to growth failure and slowing of sexual, physical and intellectual development. In adults the onset of hypothyroidism is usually insidious and subtle and unnoticed by patient and relatives. There is weight gain, coldness, thickening and dryness of the skin, facial puffiness and pallor, dry brittle scanty hair and hoarseness. Sometimes there is anorexia, deafness, dyspnoea or palpitations. In almost all patients there is noticeable slowing of the intellect.

Once suspected, myxoedema is readily diagnosed if the thyroid-stimulating hormone is raised. Thyroid-stimulating hormone will however be low in secondary and tertiary myxoedema. Free thyroxine and tri-iodothyronine and serum are low in established myxoedema. Serum tri-iodothyronine may however initially be normal for, during progressive thyroid failure, thyroid-stimulating hormone increases tri-iodothyronine proportionally more than thyroxine to produce compensated hypothyroidism.

Treatment is ideally by synthetic thyroxine. It has a predictable biological activity, long half-life (1 week), is palatable and cheap. The normal dose is 2 μg/kg, i.e. 100–150 μg/day. In elderly patients and those with coronary atherosclerosis thyroxine therapy must be introduced with extreme care if angina is to be avoided. It is usual to start with one-tenth to one-fifth of the full replacement dose and increase gradually to the full dose over 2 months.[116]

Sick euthyroidism

Critically ill patients may show a decrease in tri-iodothyronine and thyroxine, and if this is not associated with a raised thyroid-stimulating hormone it is not true hypothyroidism. Treatment with thyroxine is contraindicated.

THYROIDECTOMY

For the comfort of both the patient and surgeon this is usually performed under full general anaesthesia with endotracheal intubation. Where the trachea is narrowed or distorted intubation may be difficult and failed intubation carries the risk of tracheal obstruction by oedema or submucosal bleeding. The site of such obstruction in the presence of a large goitre may make the salvage of such patients by tracheostomy impossible. Where extreme difficulty in intubation is expected it is sometimes advisable to use a simple face-mask or a laryngeal mask for the administration of the anaesthetic, though this approach carries risk and requires the assistance of an experienced anaesthetist. Where the patient is really unsuitable for general anaesthesia, regional anaesthesia is sometimes feasible.[117]

The operative technique of thyroidectomy is standard. A symmetrical skin crease incision always gives a better scar than an asymmetric one and a wide scar is no worse than a short one as the latter sometimes bowstrings between the sternomastoids. Division of the sternohyoid and sternothyroid muscles is a prudent step during exposure of the thyrotoxic or large goitre. It is easy and has no unsatisfactory functional or cosmetic sequelae.[118]

The commonest cause of difficulty when mobilizing the thyroid lobes is failure to identify and enter the false sheath of the thyroid gland. Once this is done mobilization of the lateral border of the gland is readily achieved and the parathyroid and recurrent laryngeal nerves more easily avoided.

The rule that the inferior thyroid artery should be ligated in continuity laterally where it emerges from under the carotid artery should always be followed in subtotal thyroidectomy. In total thyroidectomy however the branches are carefully ligated individually on the gland after identification of the parathyroids and the whole course of the recurrent laryngeal nerve. By doing this the blood supply to the parathyroid glands is more likely to be preserved.

In both total and subtotal thyroidectomy the superior thyroid artery and vein should be ligated separately and as close to the upper pole as possible to avoid damage to the external branch of the superior laryngeal nerve.

The key to avoiding nerve damage is recognition of the risk. The surgeon who is not constantly anxious about the possibility of damaging the recurrent laryngeal nerve should not be performing thyroid surgery. For details in relation to the recurrent and superior laryngeal nerve see below.

When operating for a solitary nodule the usual operation should be a near total or total lobectomy, though if the nodule is at the apex of a pole or in the isthmus a partial lobectomy is feasible. 'Shelling out' of a nodule is never acceptable. In primary toxic goitre the amount of thyroid tissue left should correspond in size to approximately one-third of a normal lobe (this should leave between 5 and 10 g and can be judged as approximately equivalent in size to the distal two-thirds of the surgeon's little finger). When the operation is done for toxic multinodular goitre a larger proportion of the gland should be left. When the operation is done for a simple goitre the proportion left should be slightly larger than the normal thyroid lobe. In total or subtotal thyroidectomy care must be taken to remove the whole of the pyramidal lobe as compensatory hypertrophy of any remnant leads to an unsightly centrally placed nodule in the neck.

It is normal and prudent after completion of thyroidectomy to insert small vacuum tube drains, though it has been claimed that this is not necessary.[119] Surgeons will always argue the merits and demerits of various forms of wound closure after thyroidectomy but almost all thyroid wounds will heal to produce an excellent scar regardless of the method used, so long as the platysma is closed and there is neat and careful apposition of the skin edges. Patients have traditionally been kept in hospital for 3–7 days after thyroid

REFERENCES

116. Rapoport B Endocrine Surgery of the Thyroid and Parathyroid Gland. C V Mosby, St Louis 1985 pp 144–171
117. Saxe A W, Brown E, Hamburger S W Surgery 1988; 103: 415–420
118. Jaffe V, Young A E, Ann R Coll Surg Engl 1993; 75: 118
119. Kristoffersson A, Sandzen B, Jarhult J Br J Surg 1986; 73: 121–122

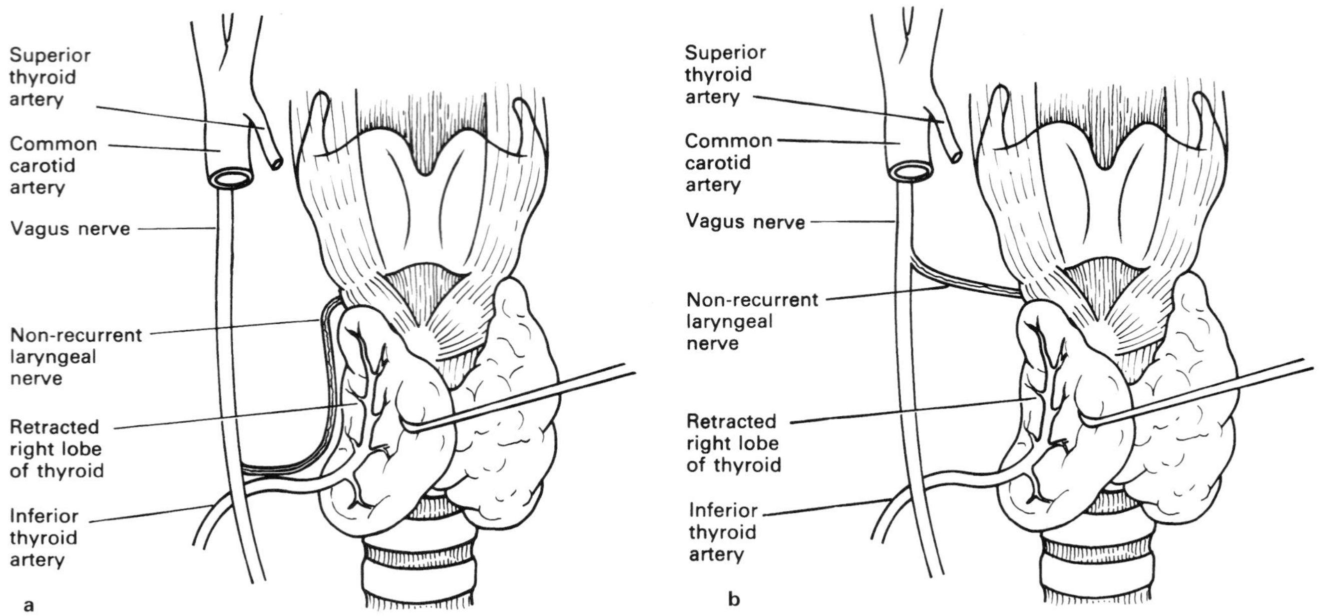

Fig. 18.19 Possible positions for a non-recurrent laryngeal nerve (**a**) with the inferior thyroid artery; (**b**) passing directly to the larynx.

surgery but current experience shows that with careful case selection and supervision some may be suitable for discharge after 24 hours.[120]

THE LARYNGEAL NERVES

The recurrent laryngeal nerve

The recurrent laryngeal nerve is motor to all the intrinsic laryngeal muscles except cricothyroid and is sensory to the subglottic area. It arises from the vagus nerve, on the right where it crosses the subclavian artery and on the left where it crosses the aorta. The nerves loop anteroposteriorly around these vessels ascending not exactly in the tracheo-oesophageal groove but in the loose fat just lateral to it, being at the lower pole of the thyroid 1–2 cm lateral to the trachea. The nerve bears a variable relationship to the inferior thyroid artery passing behind, in front of or between its terminal branches.[121] Some 40% bifurcate or rarely trifurcate into extra-laryngeal branches. This branching occurs within the last 4 cm before entering the larynx. The anterior branch is usually the larger and more important motor branch. Because it contains adductor and abductor fibres partial damage may be more injurious than total interruption as the cords may be left immobile in the fully adducted position rather than in the cadaveric partly adducted position.

In somewhat less than 1% of patients the right laryngeal nerve arises directly from the cervical vagus and runs transversely across the neck to reach the thyroid at any point from the superior to the inferior pole.[122] It is most at risk when it is adherent to the inferior thyroid artery and may thus be included in a ligature passed around that artery. Non-recurrence has been encountered on the left side but is exquisitely rare. Its occurrence on the right is thought to be due to failure of the fourth arch vessel to develop, the right subclavian arising dorsally from the aorta and sometimes passing posterior to the trachea and oesophagus (Fig. 18.19).

The superior laryngeal nerve

This nerve through its external motor branch supplies the cricothyroid muscle. Its internal branch transmits supraglottic sensory information. The external branch is at risk during any thyroid procedure which involves mobilization of the upper pole. The nerve is small and flattened and usually passes just medial to the superior thyroid artery lying on the inferior pharyngeal constrictor (Fig. 18.20). However in 20% it may be intimately involved with the superior thyroid artery, sometimes winding around it.[123] Many surgeons are heedless of the nerve since no obvious defect appears after damage to it. Careful studies show that damage causes a variable huskiness and weakness of the voice and a decrease in volume, range and pitch which may be of crucial importance to public speakers and to singers. Damage should therefore be avoided whenever possible. The superior branch enters the larynx 2 cm above the position of the normal upper pole but may none the less be damaged with enlarged lobes or by a high ligation. Damage can lead to a permanent post-deglutition cough with occasional choking.

The key to avoidance of recurrent laryngeal nerve injury is recognition of the risk. Arguments vary as to whether the nerve should be exposed. Certainly mobilization or the placing of slings around the recurrent nerve may itself produce a palsy of this delicate structure. This is however not an argument for allowing ignorance of the course of the nerve. Therefore its course should be

REFERENCES

120. Marohn M R, La Civita K A Surgery 1995; 118: 943–947
121. Nemiroff P M, Katz A D Am J Surg 1982; 144: 466–469
122. Stewart G R, Mountain J G, Colcock B P Br J Surg 1972; 59: 379–381
123. Moosman D A, De Weese M S Surg Gynecol Obstet 1968; 122: 1011–1016

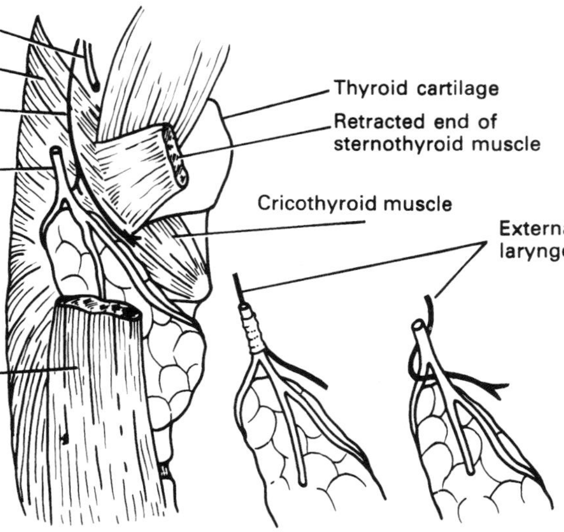

Fig. 18.20 Anatomy of the external branch of the superior laryngeal nerve with two common variants.

routinely identified early during thyroidectomy by palpation and by carefully teasing a window in the fat and connective tissue below and lateral to the junction of the inferior thyroid artery and thyroid gland. This is not the only place where the nerve is at risk but will allow the surgeon to begin to trace the whole of its course in the neck.

Complications of thyroidectomy

Haemorrhage

If haemorrhage occurs it does so within a few hours of operation and may quickly give rise to asphyxia, particularly if the trachea has been softened and flattened by the pressure of a large gland. The escaping blood collects in the pre-tracheal space and initially very little swelling may be obvious in the neck. The condition is recognized by deterioration in the patient's condition and by a crowing respiration not dissimilar to that of recurrent laryngeal paralysis. The danger is not so much in the haematoma itself as in the secondary laryngeal oedema that can occur even in the face of quite small amounts of blood in the neck. The prior insertion of drains is not a safeguard against the effects of haemorrhage. When haemorrhage or marked laryngeal oedema occurs the patient should be promptly re-intubated and the neck wound reopened. It is unusual to find a specific bleeding point and not all the haematoma can be evacuated as it tends to suffuse all the layers of the neck. After re-exploration the wound should loosely be resutured with generous drainage; because sepsis is common, prophylactic antibiotics should be given.

Wound complications

Sepsis

This is uncommon in thyroid surgery and prophylactic antibiotics are not normally indicated. When sepsis does develop it may be in the form of cellulitis or an infected haematoma. Both may present within days of surgery and discharge through the wound. When non-absorbable ligatures are used low-grade sepsis may occur round one or more of the sutures, leading to the development of a sinus in the wound weeks or months after operation. If the patient is fortunate the infected suture will discharge through the original wound. If not, re-exploration is indicated. A tender nodule felt through the skin may mark the involved area. The use of non-absorbable sutures is no longer necessary in thyroid surgery and synthetic absorbable materials should be used.

Oedema of the wound

Oedema of the wound flaps is common and may persist for weeks after operation, particularly in the upper flap.

Hypertrophic scarring

Although most thyroidectomy wounds will heal with almost invisible scars, some will become hypertrophic, especially in their centre. Local steroid application will sometimes be of benefit. In known keloid formers, an approach to the thyroid through bilateral submammary excisions has been proposed.[124]

Respiratory obstruction[125]

Respiratory obstruction after thyroidectomy may be due to oedema of the laryngeal mucosa, clot formation deep to the strap muscles, bilateral recurrent laryngeal nerve paralysis, mediastinal emphysema with extrapleural pneumothorax or collapse of a trachea whose cartilage has been made soft by long-standing compression by a goitre. This last is known as tracheomalacia; it is very rare.

REFERENCES

124. Aghaji M A C Br J Surg 1988; 75: 1034
125. Wade J S H Ann R Coll Surg Engl 1980; 62: 15–24

Whenever there is progressing airways obstruction after thyroidectomy as evidenced by stridor, prompt re-intubation is indicated. Unless a definite cause of the obstruction is known, subsequent extubation should be in the presence of an ear, nose and throat specialist equipped to assess the airway endoscopically.

Nerve damage

The recurrent and superior laryngeal nerves are at risk and in extensive thyroid surgery the vagus and the sympathetic trunks are also at risk.

Recurrent laryngeal nerve damage may be unilateral or bilateral and may be due to bruising, stretching, division, devascularization or ligation of the nerve. Paralysis may be incomplete with slight dyspnoea on exertion and little or no alteration in the voice; the cord lies at the midline. In complete laryngeal paralysis all the muscles of the larynx are paralysed except the cricothyroid and part of the arytenoideus; the cord lies in the cadaveric position midway between the normal resting position and the midline; the opposite cord can be adducted to meet the paralysed one but the difference in tension of the two cords gives a peculiar hoarse voice. In bilateral incomplete paralysis both cords lie in the midline and there is severe dyspnoea with stridor soon after operation. In bilateral complete paralysis the two cords occupy cadaveric positions. No abduction or adduction is possible; the voice is lost, but the dyspnoea is not so dramatic.

The vocal cords need not be inspected in all thyroidectomy patients prior to operation. A few will already have symptomatic or asymptomatic recurrent laryngeal nerve palsy, either idiopathically or secondary to the thyroid disease itself or as a consequence of previous thyroid surgery. It is reasonable to restrict preoperative laryngoscopy to those with a history of voice change or of previous thyroid surgery. If both cords function preoperatively and the surgery is unilateral then there is no virtue in having the anaesthetist inspect the vocal cords at the end of anaesthesia. If however both cords have been at risk very close attention must be paid to the patient in the immediate postoperative phase to confirm an adequate airway. It is not necessary for the anaesthetist to make a routine examination of the cords prior to the patient leaving the operating room as such assessments are both difficult and unreliable but all thyroidectomy patients must be very closely monitored in the recovery area and any doubts about the adequacy of the airway reported immediately to the anaesthetist and surgeon. If recurrent laryngeal nerve palsy is suspected at any time it should be documented by an ear, nose and throat surgeon. Most cases will recover spontaneously and re-operation is not indicated. Resuture of the nerves is not generally beneficial either early or late. It usually results in misdirected regeneration causing paradoxical cord movements,[126] though there have been claims that accurate resuture will improve phonation.[127]

The occurrence of recurrent laryngeal nerve palsy often leads to litigation, usually because the risks have not been explained before the operation or because the diagnosis has been delayed or concealed after the operation. If the patient has been properly warned and normal care taken then the presence of a recurrent laryngeal nerve palsy should not of itself be considered to be evidence of negligence. It will happen even with the most competent care in the most experienced hands, but its incidence in routine, non-malignant thyroid surgery should be no more than 1 or 2% of cases.

Hypocalcaemia

Calcium levels may fall after thyroidectomy for two reasons—metabolic and anatomical.

Metabolic

Some degrees of hypocalcaemia is almost invariably seen even in unilateral thyroidectomy but the fall is rarely to below 2.0 mmol/l and almost never symptomatic. The cause is not understood but the release of calcitonin during manipulation, the reversal of thyrotoxic osteodystrophy and a reduction of renal tubular reabsorption of calcium without a change in parathormone or calcitonin levels have been proposed.[128,129]

Anatomical

Deliberate or inadvertent excision of all parathyroid tissue en bloc with the thyroid during total thyroidectomy will lead to hypoparathyroidism and hypocalcaemia. Simple damage or devascularization during the operation may have similar effects. The risk of clinically significant hypocalcaemia is small and attempts have been made to obviate the risk by excluding lateral ligation of the inferior thyroid arteries from which, in theory, the parathyroids derive their blood supply. However routine use of this manoeuvre cannot be shown to obviate the problem and may lead to difficulties in haemostasis. The primary problem is not devascularization but local trauma. Careful identification and preservation of the parathyroids during thyroidectomy remains the most appropriate prophylaxis. Parathyroid glands removed inadvertently at the time of total thyroidectomy should be diced and inserted into pockets in the sternomastoid muscle where in due course they may revascularize and function.

Mildly symptomatic hypocalcaemia with circumoral dysaesthesia and digital paraesthesia need not normally be treated if the calcium is over 2.0 mmol/l. It will usually resolve within 2 days. If it does not or if the calcium continues to fall, treatment with oral calcium supplements or 10% calcium gluconate given slowly via a central vein may be necessary. If the hypocalcaemia persists, treatment with synthetic vitamin D and oral calcium will be necessary. Parathyroid function will usually eventually return with the growth of ectopic islands of parathyroid tissue or the revascularization of retained parathyroid tissue. This process may however take 3–6 months.

REFERENCES

126. Gordon J H, McCabe B F Laryngoscope 1968; 78: 236–239
127. Ezaki H, Ushio H et al World J Surg 1982; 6: 342–346
128. Percival R C, Hargreaves A W, Karis J A Acta Endocrinol (Copenh) 1985; 220–226
129. Michie W, Duncan T et al Lancet 1976; i: 508–514

Pneumothorax

Pneumothorax is uncommon except during extraction of retrosternal goitres.

Air embolism

This is also rare but may be produced if a large vein in the neck is opened when the patient is in the head-up position.

Thyroid crisis

This only occurs when the thyrotoxic patient is operated upon without adequate preliminary preparation. It occurs soon after operation and takes the form of fulminating thyrotoxicosis with hyperpyrexia, arrhythmias and cardiac failure. It is treated by large doses of carbimazole (60–120 mg) or propylthiouracil (600–1200 mg) followed by Lugol's iodine. The cardiac effects are blocked with propranolol; digoxin may also be necessary. Dexamethasone reduces the conversion of thyroxine to bi-iodothyronine peripherally and hyperpyrexia is treated by largactil and cooling. Extreme cases may require plasmapheresis or even exchange transfusion.

Recurrent hyperthyroidism

Recurrent hyperthyroidism may occur after thyroidectomy for thyrotoxicosis and is discussed under that heading.

Hypothyroidism

All patients treated by total thyroidectomy will develop hypothyroidism but only a small percentage of those treated by bilateral subtotal thyroidectomy will develop thyroid insufficiency unless the underlying disease is thyrotoxicosis, in which case the incidence is much higher and is discussed under that heading.

THYROIDITIS

Inflammatory changes in the thyroid are common and may or may not be associated with a change in the function of the gland. Their categorization is confused by ignorance of their aetiology but from a clinical point of view the traditional groupings of acute, subacute, Hashimoto's and Riedel's thyroiditis are adequate. However, as there are several definite clinical variants among patients previously categorized as Hashimoto's thyroiditis, the term 'autoimmune thyroiditis' is now more appropriate.

Acute suppurative thyroiditis

This condition—now rarely encountered—is a secondary rather than a primary disease. It results from the involvement of the thyroid by haematogenous or local spread of bacterial, fungal or parasitic infection from elsewhere in the body. Typically *Staphylococcus aureus*, haemolytic streptococci and *Streptococcus pneumoniae* are found but also reported are anaerobic organisms, *Escherichia coli* and salmonella, together with actinomycosis and ecchinococcus. The goitrous gland is more commonly involved than the normal one.

The clinical features are those of acute infection: pain in the thyroid radiating to the ear, occiput or jaw and worsened by movement or swallowing; fever, tachycardia, and local oedema that may involve the larynx, trachea or oesophagus. The diagnosis is clinical. Imaging and thyroid function tests are non-contributory. Identification of the organism may require needle aspiration and culture. Treatment is by the appropriate antibiotic but occasionally open drainage or thyroidectomy is indicated.[130]

Syphilis may involve the thyroid. In tertiary syphilis a solitary gumma or diffuse sclerosis may occur and mimic chronic thyroiditis or malignancy.

Subacute thyroiditis (de Quervain's)

This is a self-limiting inflammation of the gland, pathologically characterized by giant cells and granulomata. Although there is an association with the human leukocyte antigen B35 haplotype, the aetiology is probably primarily viral: mumps, measles, influenza, Epstein–Barr, coxsackie and adenoviruses have all been implicated. Thyroid symptoms are usually preceded by a sore throat and an upper respiratory tract infection. The gland then becomes tender and enlarged, usually bilaterally, though the enlargement may be unilateral. The gland may enlarge to two to three times its normal size. The patient is somewhat unwell, has a low-grade fever and sometimes an associated myalgia. In 50% of patients there may be transient signs of mild hyperthyroidism due to release of stored thyroxine by destruction of the thyroid parenchyma. Over ensuing weeks or months, the gland shrinks. Thyroid function tests return to normal but a quarter of patients become mildly hypothyroid.

Investigation shows a raised erythrocyte sedimentation rate, usually above 50 mmHr. The hyperthyroidism can be distinguished from Graves' disease by the low uptake of technetium or radioiodine on scintiscanning. Biopsy confirmation is not necessary. Usually no clinical treatment is indicated as the disease is self-limiting but non-steroidal anti-inflammatory drugs may ease the discomfort in the acute stage and steroid therapy is very occasionally necessary. Antithyroid drugs are of no value in the hyperthyroid stage but β-adrenergic blockade may produce symptomatic relief.[131]

Riedel's thyroiditis

Riedel in 1896[132] described 'a specific inflammation of mysterious nature producing a iron hard tumefaction of the thyroid'. The process is pathologically one of dense fibrosis of all or part of the gland and surrounding tissues. It is probably related to other idiopathic fibroses (retroperitoneal, mediastinal, retro-orbital and sclerosing cholangitis). The patients are middle-aged; clinically

REFERENCES

130. Levine S N Arch Intern Med 1983; 143: 1952–1956
131. Volpe R The Thyroid. Harpers & Row, Hagerstown 1978 pp 986–994
132. Riedel B M C L Verh Dtsch Ges Chir 1896; 25: 101–105

Table 18.6 Classification of autoimmune thyroiditis

Type	*Name*	*Haplotype*	*Aetiology*	*Autoimmune*
Acute suppurative	–	–	Infection	No
Subacute granulomatous	de Quervain's*	HLA Bw35	Viral and genetic predisposition	Possible in part
Subacute lymphocytic	'Silent' or 'painless' thyroiditis	HLA DR4	Thyroid stimulation in pregnancy or increased iodine intake	Probably
Chronic lymphocytic	Atrophic	HLA DR3	Surface expression of antigens activates T cells *and*	Definitely
	Goitrous (Hashimoto's†)	HLA DR5, B8, Dw3	organ-specific defect in suppressor T cells *leads to* autodestructive antibody production	Definitely
Chronic fibrous	Riedel's‡	–	Systemic fibrosis of unknown origin	Possible

*Fritz de Quervain (1868–1940) became reader to Kocher in Bern and succeeded him as Professor of Surgery. He described the thyroiditis which bears his name in 1902.
†Hakura Hashimoto (1881–1934), a Japanese surgeon, described thyroiditis in 1912, and in 1956 it was found to be autoimmune.
‡Bernhard Riedel (1846–1916), Professor of Surgery at Jena, described thyroiditis in 1896.
HLA = human leucocyte antigen.

the gland is non-tender, very hard and of normal or reduced size. Thyroid function tests and autoantibodies are normal and the diagnostic difficulty is in distinguishing the change from malignancy. Fine-needle aspiration biopsies produce an acellular specimen and although this is helpful it is not diagnostic. Steroids are of no proven value in treatment. Surgery may however be necessary to release the trachea or oesophagus.[133]

Autoimmune thyroiditis (Table 18.6)

Goitre associated with lymphocytic infiltration was first described by Hakura Hashimoto in 1912[134] but its aetiology remained a mystery until in the 1950s it was shown that thyroid extracts injected into animals could produce the disease and that autoantibodies could be demonstrated in the serum of the human patient. Autoimmune thyroiditis is a common disease, predominantly of females. It is histologically demonstrable in 20% of the population at autopsy and appears to be becoming more common. The terminology is confusing. Hashimoto used the term 'lymphomatous thyroiditis' but many thyroid diseases show lymphocytic infiltration and the term 'autoimmune thyroiditis' is to be preferred. These latter conditions have the common denominator of infiltration by lymphoid cells organized in clumps or germinal centres and associated with hyperplasia, fibrosis and increased oxyphil (Askanazy) cells. Although there is a clinical spectrum of autoimmune thyroiditis ranging from a goitrous form (Hashimoto's) to an atrophic form, there are serological differences between the groups. The human leukocyte antigen DR3 haplotype is common in atrophic thyroiditis, while the DR5/B8/DW3 is seen with goitrous thyroiditis. A third identifiable subgroup of autoimmune thyroiditis has been named 'silent' or 'painless thyroiditis' and is often associated with the human leukocyte antigen DR4 haplotype.[135]

All variants of autoimmune thyroiditis are characterized by presence of thyroid autoantibodies in the serum. Many autoantibodies have been identified and those in common clinical use are the anti-thyroglobulin and anti-microsomal antibodies. They are detected by a haemagglutination or radioimmunoassay method. These antibodies can be demonstrated in 15% of all middle-aged women and 8% of the normal population. Some 50% of the relatives of patients with clinical autoimmune thyroiditis will have raised autoantibodies; however in those without clinically demonstrable thyroid disease, the titre rarely exceeds 1/250.

The incidence of autoimmune thyroiditis is high in patients with Down's and Turner's syndromes and is sometimes associated with other autoimmune diseases such as pernicious anaemia, Sjögren's, rheumatoid arthritis, temporal arteritis, diabetes mellitus, Addison's disease and autoimmune liver disease.

The immunological mechanism is probably a defect in suppressor T cell function allowing helper T cells to be sensitized to thyroid antigens and thus stimulating B cells to produce the antithyroid antibodies. The pathological changes seen in the disease are a joint result of lymphocyte infiltration, antibody effect and increased stimulation of the gland by thyroid-stimulating hormone or growth-promoting substances released by the lymphocytes themselves.

Clinical patterns

Goitrous (true-Hashimoto's thyroiditis)

The gland is enlarged by infiltration with lymphocytes. The enlargement is usually moderate but sometimes gross. In texture the gland is rubbery and the goitre overall feels knobbly and sometimes asymmetric, mimicking multinodular goitre or malignancy or even solitary nodule. The enlargement is painless and the symptoms are due only to pressure. The patient is euthyroid or mildly hypothyroid. The diagnosis is primarily by autoantibody titre estimations. Antithyroglobulin is initially raised and later antimicrosomal titres rise and remain elevated. The presence of raised autoantibodies does not however exclude other thyroid pathology and the diagnosis can be confirmed by fine-needle aspiration biopsy. If the goitre is asymmetrical this is mandatory to exclude

REFERENCES

133. Woolner L B, McConabey W M, Beahrs O H J Clin Endocrinol Metab 1957; 17: 201
134. Hashimoto H Arch Klin Chir 1912; 97: 219–248
135. Belifiore A, Bottazzo G F Monogr Allergy (Basel) 1987; 21: 215–245

coexisting malignant disease. Thyroid scans shows a patchy uptake and are not diagnostic.

Treatment is primarily medical. Thyroxine is always given if the patient is hypothyroid. In the euthyroid patient, thyroxine treatment will decrease the size of the gland in 75% of patients. In many patients progression of the disease will however produce fibrosis and shrinkage of the gland even without treatment. There is no indication for the use of steroids. Surgery is only indicated where the goitre is large but unresponsive to thyroxine or where malignancy is suspected on clinical, histological or cytological grounds.[136]

Hashimoto's and neoplasia

Many reports based on retrospective studies of excised thyroid glands suggest an increased incidence of differentiated thyroid neoplasm in patients with Hashimoto's thyroiditis. This probably represents a sampling artefact. Nevertheless a prospective study of 829 patients with Hashimoto's followed for 8 years and compared with 829 controls with colloid goitre showed a sevenfold increase of malignant lymphoma in the Hashimoto patients.[137]

Atrophic thyroiditis

The end-point of autoimmune thyroiditis is often a fibrous atrophic hypofunctioning gland and this can occur without a preliminary goitrous phase. Clinical presentation is usually as hypothyroidism and autoimmune thyroiditis is the commonest cause of this. Overt myxoedema is readily recognized but milder degrees of hypothyroidism are easily missed.

Silent thyroiditis

This variant presents at any age. The female to male ratio is less than in other forms of autoimmune thyroiditis. Initially patients present with mild hyperthyroidism and this is never associated with infiltrative ophthalmopathy or pre-tibial myxoedema. The thyroid is moderately enlarged; tri-iodothyronine and thyroxine are initially raised. Radioiodine uptake is decreased. The hyperthyroid phase lasts for 2–12 months. After returning to the euthyroid state the patient may remain euthyroid or progress to hypothyroidism which is usually transient. The disease may recur episodically. This disease is distinguishable from de Quervain's by the absence of pain, by the presence of raised autoantibody titres and by the absence of giant cells on histological examination. Silent thyroiditis occurs in about 5% of post-partum women.[138]

REFERENCES

136. Thomas C G, Rotledge R G Am Surg 1981; 193: 769–776
137. Holm L E, Blomgrem H, Lowhagen T N Engl J Med 1985; 312: 601–604
138. Amino N, Mori H et al N Engl J Med 1982; 306: 849–852

19 Parathyroid glands

J. Farndon R. Mihai

Sandstrom described the macroscopic and microscopic appearance of the parathyroid glands over 100 years ago.[1] The first operations for hyperparathyroidism were carried out over 70 years ago by Mandl[2] and the physiology of the parathyroids was originally elaborated 50 years ago by Albright & Reifenstein.[3] In his inimitable style Albright said in 1948: 'In the final analysis very little is known about anything, and much that seems true today turns out to be partly true tomorrow, but as things go in medicine our knowledge of the interrelation one to another of all the sequelae which result from this action of the parathyroid hormone is probably clearer than that for any other hormone'.[3]

The physiology, embryology and anatomy that are relevant to clinical disorders of the parathyroid glands are described before parathyroid disease and its treatment are considered.

EMBRYOLOGY AND CLINICAL ANATOMY OF THE PARATHYROID GLANDS

Present knowledge on the development of the parathyroid glands comes largely from the work of Gilmour[4] and Boyd[5] in the Departments of Pathology and Anatomy of the London Hospital over 50 years ago. The two parathyroid glands develop from the endoderm of pharyngeal pouches III and IV with the probable incorporation of placodal ectoderm, which explains how parathyroid glands can be accommodated within the amine precursor uptake decarboxylation system (see below). Pouch III also gives rise to the corresponding half of the thymus gland and the caudal descent of this component carries the parathyroid with it until the time of its separation. Parathyroid III, therefore, comes to lie below parathyroid IV (Fig. 19.1).

During separation of the parathyroid 'buds' from the endoderm, microscopic fragmentation is observed and failure of this to occur might account for the accessory parathyroid glands which are sometimes uncovered. Retained fragments of parathyroid III within the thymus gland explain the rare clinical findings of ectopic parathyroid tissue within the thymus in the thoracic cavity.

Gilmour[6] demonstrated the variability of gland number in a consecutive series of 428 necropsies: 0.2% had only two glands, 6.1% had only three glands, 87% had four glands, 6% had five glands and 0.5% had six glands. He acknowledged that not all glands may have been found in every post-mortem. These figures should be borne in mind as the surgeon struggles to find four glands at each exploration. It is not clear whether the corpse is more or less tolerant and revealing than the anaesthetized patient!

The presence of detectable plasma levels of parathyroid hormone after total parathyroidectomy in patients with renal failure[7] also suggests that additional/ectopic parathyroid tissue might exist more frequently than had previously been considered.

A more recent autopsy study[8] suggested that a fourth gland was missing in only 3% of subjects and supernumerary glands were found in 13%, most often in the thymus. Symmetry can be expected in 80% of subjects. The commonest position for the superior gland is just above the intersection of the recurrent laryngeal nerve and the inferior thyroid artery and for the inferior gland more ventrally close to the lower pole of the thyroid, in the thymus or in the thyrothymic ligament. The 'lower' glands sometimes appear higher in the neck because of failure of descent during development. The relative frequency with which the glands are found in different sites is demonstrated in Figure 19.2.

In hyperparathyroidism the 'normal' anatomical relationships may be disrupted. Thompson et al[9] reviewed the anatomy of the glands in primary hyperparathyroidism in 273 subjects. The pathology of the glands also appeared to influence their distribution. A single adenoma was found in 80% of patients, four-gland hyperplasia in 15%, multiple adenomas in 2.5% and 'normal' glands in 2.5%. Only 2% of adenomas were entirely surrounded by thyroid tissue and these were all inferior glands. Most patients in whom a neck exploration fails eventually prove to have adenomas located in the upper mediastinum.

HYPERPARATHYROIDISM

Excess production of parathyroid hormone causes hypercalcaemia and this is called hyperparathyroidism. Most patients have a single adenoma, although up to 15% of patients have multiple gland hyperplasia. Carcinoma of the parathyroid is very rare (1%).

REFERENCES

1. Sandstrom I Upsala Lakarforenings Forth 1880; 15: 441
2. Mandl F Arch Klin Chir 1926; 143: 245
3. Albright F, Reifenstein E L The Parathyroid Glands and Metabolic Bone Disease. Williams & Wilkins, Baltimore 1948
4. Gilmour J R J Pathol Bacteriol 1937; 45: 507
5. Boyd J D Ann R Coll Surg Engl 1950; 7: 455
6. Gilmour J R J Pathol Bacteriol 1938; 46: 133
7. Nicholson M L, Feehally J Br J Surg 1995; 82: 1427
8. Akerström G, Malmaeus J, Bergstrom R Surgery 1984; 95: 14
9. Thompson N W, Eckhauser F E, Harness J Surgery 1982; 92: 814

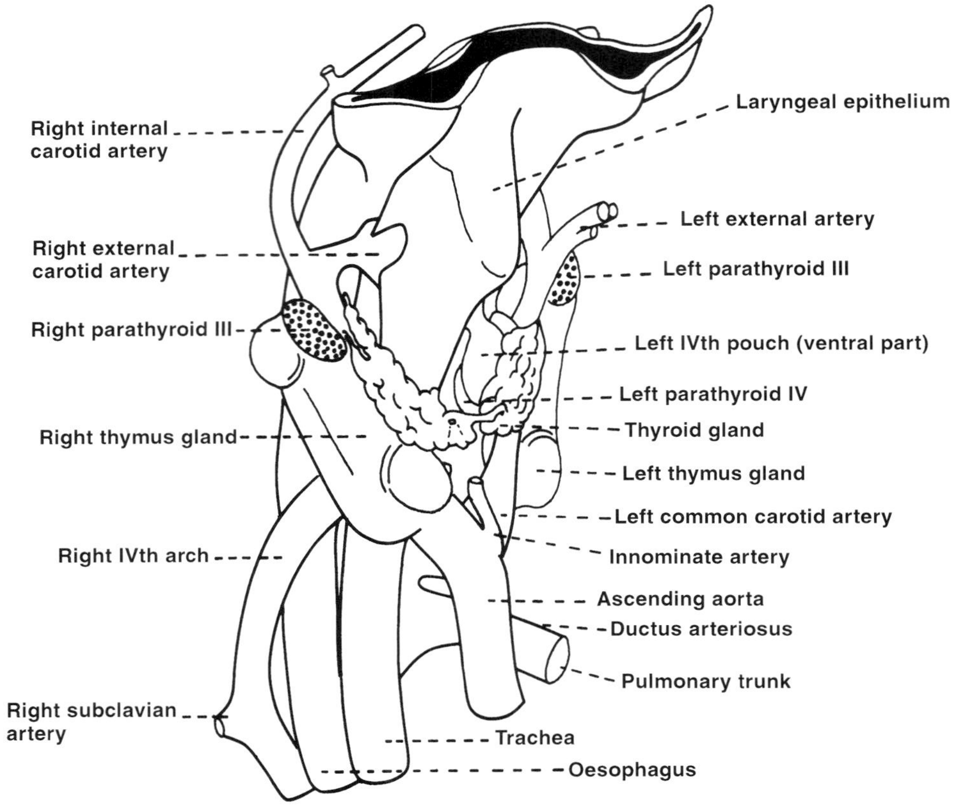

Fig. 19.1 The pharyngeal and laryngeal regions and associated pharyngeal derivatives of a human embryo of around 16.8 mm.

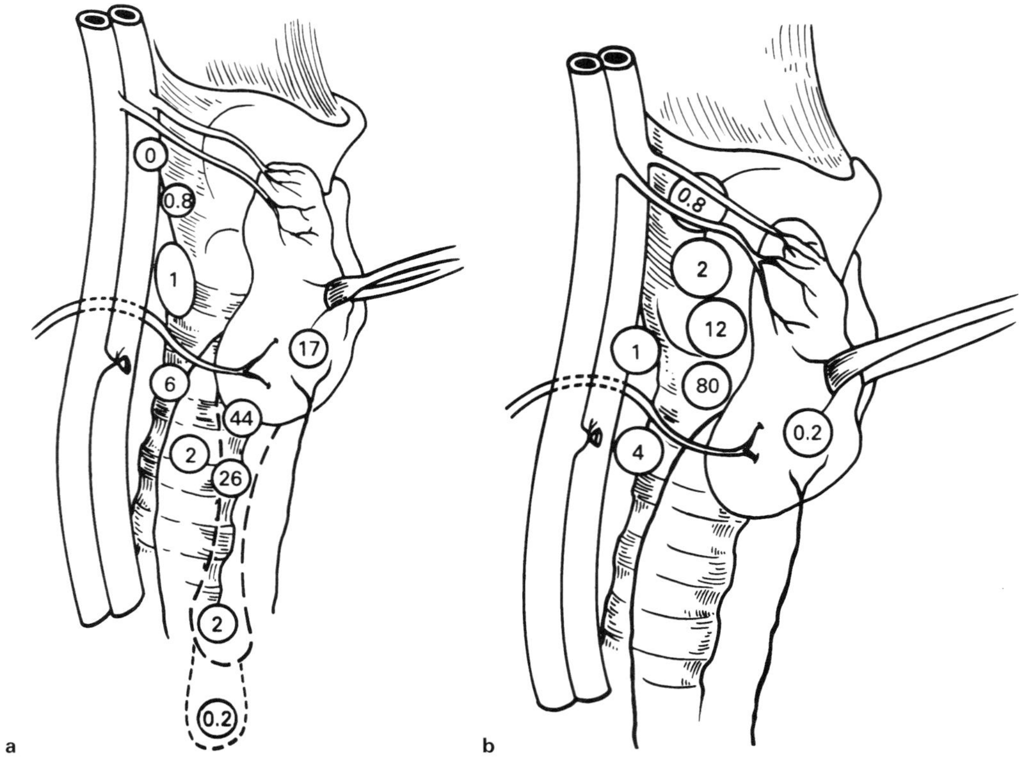

Fig. 19.2 Schematic diagram to show the relative frequency of location of (**a**) the lower parathyroid glands and (**b**) the upper parathyroid glands (modified from Akerström et al[8]).

Mineral metabolism and hyperparathyroidism

Calcium

Calcium is a vitally important cation concerned with cell membrane stability, nerve conduction, muscle contraction, enzyme and hormone activation, blood coagulation, bone mineral deposition and milk synthesis. All but 1% resides within the skeleton and plasma concentrations remain remarkably constant in health. Physiological changes occur about the mean level, e.g. a slight increase following food and a decrease of ionized calcium associated with alkalosis from whatever cause. The physiologically active calcium is in a free or ionized form within plasma and measurement of this fraction provides the most accurate marker of a calcium abnormality.[10] Some 40% of circulating calcium is bound to proteins: 80–90% to albumin and 10–15% to globulins, 10% is complexed to phosphate, lactate, bicarbonate etc. and half is ionized. Hypercalcaemia is almost a prerequisite for a diagnosis of hyperparathyroidism but normocalcaemic hyperparathyroidism can occur.[11]

Calcium-sensing receptor

A calcium-sensing receptor has recently been cloned from parathyroid cells.[12] Activation of this receptor induces a rise in intracellular calcium levels and enables the parathyroid cells to detect and respond to minute changes in the concentration of extracellular calcium. Inactivating mutations of this receptor cause two inherited autosomal dominant hypercalcaemic disorders: familial hypocalciuric hypercalcaemia and neonatal severe hyperparathyroidism.[13] Similar mutations have not been identified in parathyroid tumours[14] but calcium receptor expression appears to be substantially reduced in patients with parathyroid adenomas,[15] perhaps explaining the abnormal control of parathyroid hormone secretion by extracellular calcium. A member of the low-density lipoprotein receptor superfamily has recently been found to be another putative calcium sensor protein on parathyroid cells[16] and its expression is reduced in primary hyperparathyroidism.[17]

Parathyroid hormone

Parathyroid hormone is an 84-amino-acid peptide with a molecular weight of 9500 which has a short half-life of a few minutes in the circulation. It is rapidly cleaved into an amino-terminal fragment consisting of amino acids 1–34 and a carboxy-terminal fragment, which have half-lives of minutes and several hours respectively. Only the 1–34 amino-terminal fragment retains biological activity. Assays have been devised which measure the intact hormone, the amino-terminal carboxy-terminal and mid-portion fragments. Each hospital laboratory must derive its own normal concentrations of these hormones in health and disease. The amount of detectable parathyroid hormone need not be elevated in hyperparathyroidism but detectable amounts of parathyroid hormone in the face of hypercalcaemia are considered diagnostic of the condition. Most of the assays have in the past been radioimmunoassays but chemiluminescent immunoassays which have been recently developed give better specificity and sensitivity.[18]

Parathyroid hormone binds to specific receptors on the membrane of target cells and induces activation of several intracellular second messengers such as cyclic adenosine monophosphate, inositol triphosphate and calcium. Parathyroid hormone receptors are widely distributed in a variety of cells besides the traditional renal and bone targets, including fibroblasts, chondrocytes, vascular smooth muscle, fat cells and placental trophoblasts.[19]

Parathyroid hormone reacts with specific receptors on the proximal and distal renal tubular cells, leading to an increased excretion of phosphate, sodium, potassium and bicarbonate and a decreased excretion of magnesium and hydrogen ions. Although parathyroid hormone decreases the urinary excretion of calcium, in hyperparathyroidism this effect is rapidly overcome and hypercalcaemia-induced hypercalciuria occurs. Hyperchloraemia ensues secondarily. The intracellular signalling for these effects relies on intracellular cyclic adenosine monophosphate, which is secreted in the urine in increased amounts and can be used as a biochemical marker of hyperparathyroidism.

Parathyroid hormone stimulates bone reabsorption by the osteoclasts, resulting in an increase in the alkaline phosphatase and an increase in the urinary excretion of hydroxyproline. Elevated amounts of collagenase produce increased breakdown of bone matrix.

Several of these parathyroid hormone-induced changes are used to refine a possible diagnosis of hyperparathyroidism:

1. Hypophosphataemia.
2. Hyperchloraemia.
3. Increased chloride to phosphate ratio.
4. Hypercalciuria.
5. Increased serum alkaline phosphatase.
6. Increased urinary excretion of cyclic adenosine monophosphate.
7. Increased urinary excretion of hydroxyproline.

The different causes of hypercalcaemia and the variable parathyroid hormone secretory responses can make the differential diagnosis difficult. The urinary or nephrogenous cyclic adenosine monophosphate and the tubular reabsorption of phosphate are sometimes obtained to increase the sensitivity and specificity of the diagnosis. These measure the proportion of cyclic adenosine monophosphate produced by the action of parathyroid hormone on renal tubular cells alone, and the theoretical maximum of tubular reabsorptive capacity for phosphate related to the glomerular filtra-

REFERENCES

10. White T F, Farndon J R et al Clin Chim Acta 1986; 157: 199
11. Smith L H N Engl J Med 1979; 299: 270
12. Brown E M, Gamba G et al Nature 1993; 366: 575
13. Pollak M R, Brown E M, Chou Y H W Cell 1993; 75: 1297
14. Hosokawa Y, Pollak M R et al J Clin Endocrinol Metab 1995; 80: 3107
15. Kifor O, Moore F D et al J Clin Endocrinol Metab 1996; 81: 1598
16. Saito A, Pietromonaco S et al Proc Natl Acad Sci USA 1986; 91: 9725
17. Juhlin C, Klareskog L et al Endocrinology 1988; 122: 2999
18. Aston J P, Wheeler M H et al World J Surg 1988; 12: 454
19. Brown E M, Segre G V, Goldring S R Baillière's Clin Endocrinol Metab 1996; 123–161

tion rate. These tests of mineral metabolic effects have variable efficacy.[20] Disodium ethylenediaminotetra-acetic acid-induced hypocalcaemia produces increased intact and midportion parathyroid hormone secretion in those with hyperparathyroidism but not in those with hypercalcaemia from other causes.[21] This test may be of value when all the other investigations are equivocal.

Phosphate

Phosphate is contained mainly within the skeleton (85%), some as organic and some as inorganic pools of intracellular phosphates. Fifteen per cent of serum phosphate is bound to protein and the rest is ionized or complexed with cations. It is largely excreted by the kidneys and variations in plasma concentrations directly affect the concentration of serum calcium. Increased plasma levels of phosphates have a direct stimulatory effect on the parathyroid glands, and are the pathogenic mechanism responsible for secondary hyperparathyroidism in patients with renal failure.

Vitamin D

Vitamin D is in the form of two sterols: ergosterol in plants and dihydrocholesterol in the skin, which are converted upon exposure to ultraviolet light to vitamin D_2 and D_3 respectively. These forms are absorbed from the small intenstine by a process which requires the presence of bile salts. Vitamin D_3 becomes protein-bound in the portal venous blood and is 25-hydroxylated in the liver, before a second hydroxylation occurs in the kidney under parathyroid hormone control to produce 1,25-dihydroxycholecalciferol ($1,25(OH)_2D_3$)—a very potent form of vitamin D.

Active vitamin D_3 is an important regulator of parathyroid cell growth and inhibits parathyroid hormone gene transcription by binding to its receptor in specific regions of the parathyroid hormone gene promoter. It is assumed that impaired effects of vitamin D_3 may contribute to the enhanced secretion of parathyroid hormone and proliferation of the glands seen in secondary hyperparathyroidism. The vitamin D receptor genotype found in the majority of postmenopausal women with primary hyperparathyroidism is linked to decreased transcriptional activity and/or messenger RNA stability[22] and might account for reduced vitamin D receptor expression and the impeded regulatory actions of vitamin D in these patients.

Patients with hyperparathyroidism are more likely to develop vitamin D deficiency in countries with populations which have low circulating levels of 25-hydroxycholecalciferol and low exposure to sunlight.[23] In these countries preoperative treatment with vitamin D may reduce the subsequent bone hunger which follows parathyroidectomy.

Symptomatic hyperparathyroidism

The physiological disturbances associated with primary hyperparathyroidism account directly or indirectly for most of its symptoms. What is not understood or explicable is the protean way in which the disease presents. The same degree of biochemical disorder can be associated with renal disease, bone disease or a combination of the two with the same length of history. Relatively mild elevations in serum calcium produce severe systemic effects in some patients and no symptoms in others. There is also little doubt that the pattern of the disease is changing with time.

Bone disease

Bone disease in its florid form is called 'osteitis fibrosa cystica generalizata' and is now rarely seen. In 1947 Norris[24] found evidence of bone disease in 91% of those with a parathyroid adenoma. The earliest changes are seen on X-rays of the hands where subperiosteal erosions can be detected in the phalanges, especially on the radial aspect of the middle phalanges, and terminal tufts are also seen (Fig. 19.3). The skull demonstrates a

REFERENCES

20. Wells S A, Leight G S, Ross A J Primary Hyperparathyroidism in Current Problems in Surgery, vol XVII. Year Book Medical Publishers, Chicago 1980
21. Ljunghall S, Benson L et al World J Surg 1988; 12: 45
22. Carling T, Kindmark A et al Nature Medicine 1995; 1: 1309
23. Ingemansson S G, Hugosson C H, Woodhouse N J Y World J Surg 1988; 12: 517
24. Norris E H Arch Pathol 1947; 42: 261

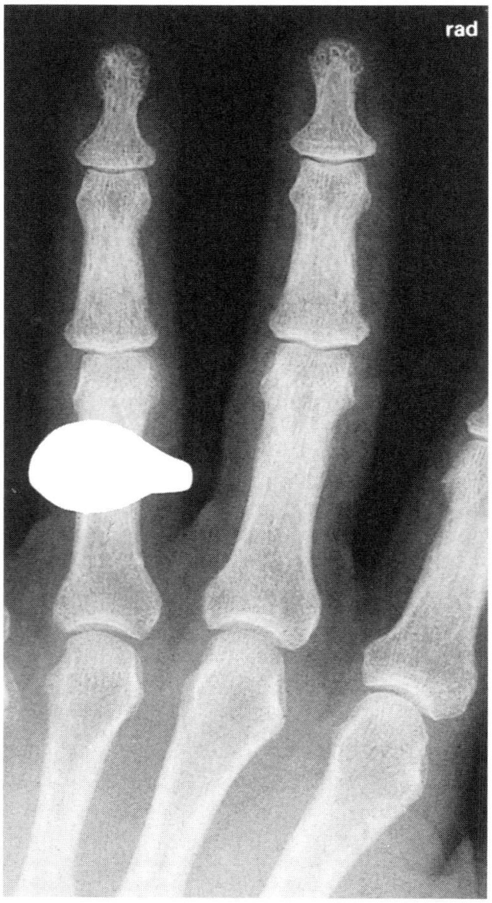

Fig. 19.3 Magnified view of the middle and ring fingers of a young man with hyperparathyroidism showing erosion of the terminal tufts of the distal phalanx and subperiosteal erosion—especially on the radial side (rad)—of the proximal phalanges.

mottled appearance with lucent cystic areas, called the 'pepperpot skull,' in its most florid form (Fig. 19.4) and any bone may demonstrate cystic lesions caused by osteroclastomas or brown tumours. These bone changes cause skeletal pain and may lead to pathological fractures. Subtle bone changes are rarely detected on skeletal surveys and there is little justification for obtaining a skeletal survey to aid diagnosis unless there are specific bone symptoms.

Dual-energy X-ray absoptiometry is now widely used to evaluate bone mass. There are region-specific differences in bone mass, with low values in areas with cortical bone such as the radius and normal or high values in the vertebrae and the iliac crest which are mostly composed of trabecular bone. In many patients there seems to be an initial rapid loss of bone mass followed by a period of stable disease with little progression by the time that the primary hyperparathyroidism is diagnosed.

Renal disease

Renal disease usually presents as a result of stone production or nephrocalcinosis with the patient complaining of polyuria, polydypsia, ureteric colic, renal pain, haematuria and symptoms of renal tract infection. In a Swedish study in 1986[16] renal calculi were the presenting symptom in approximately 65% of men but in only about 25% of women. The degree of hypercalcaemia was often not severe and a high proportion of patients had chief cell hyperplasia. Successful surgery is more difficult to achieve in these circumstances and some have postulated that this early presentation with a mild biochemical abnormality and hyperplastic glands might be the precursor of more severe adenomatous disease.[25,26]

Hypertension

Hypertension is present in many patients with hyperparathyroidism but there are no ready explanations for this. Only subtle differences in renal function have been found in those with hypertension compared with those without.[27] Recently a *parathyroid hypertensive factor* has been purified from the plasma of spontaneously hypertensive rats and its levels have been found to correlate with hypertension in patients with primary hyperparathyroidism. The levels of this factor fall after parathyroidectomy as the blood pressure returns to normal.[28]

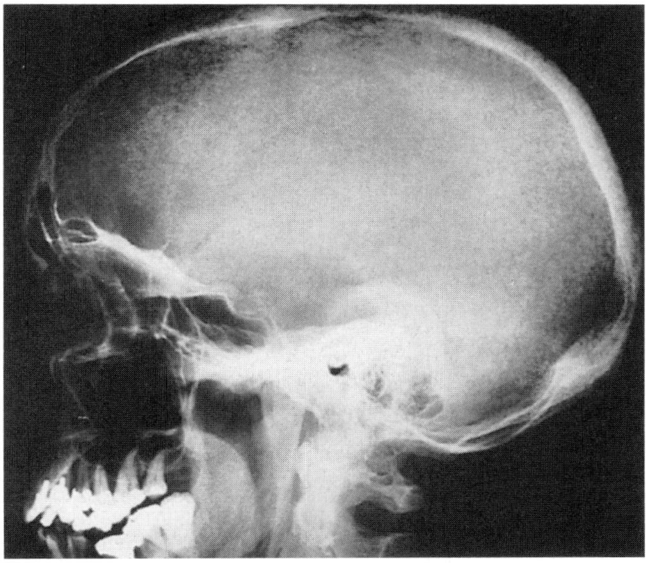

Fig. 19.4 Skull X-ray of the patient shown in Figure 19.3, demonstrating a classical 'pepperpot' skull.

Gastrointestinal symptoms

Gastrointestinal symptoms may be the result of peptic ulcer disease, constipation, acute pancreatitis or gallstones, all of which are variously linked to hyperparathyroidism with varying degrees of certainty. These are all common conditions and their association may be by pure chance, although in some situations the link appears to be clear-cut, e.g. peptic ulcer from hypergastrinaemia, where the excess gastrin is produced by a pancreatic tumour. This is associated with multiple parathyroid adenomas as part of the multiple endocrine neoplasia type I syndrome (see below).

Psychiatric and neuromuscular symptoms

Vague psychiatric and neuromuscular symptoms are recognized in 30% of patients presenting with hyperparathyroidism.[25] This form of presentation may be dismissed as coincidental. The advent of multichannel blood autoanalysers coupled with a low threshold on the physician's part to initiate investigation if a patient presents in this way results in 'patients' being uncovered or discovered! These symptoms can however be reversed by parathyroidectomy.[29] Their severity is not related to the degree of hypercalcaemia, and they may be dependent upon the turnover of central nervous system monoamines. A direct effect of parathyroid hormone on axon conduction times in different areas of nervous system has also been reported.

The incidence of asymptomatic hyperparathyroidism

It is difficult to put a precise figure on the incidence of hyperparathyroidism as this is likely to vary with the population studied and the means of diagnosis. The advent of multichannel biochemical analysers has influenced the prevalence of the disorder and encouraged the concept of asymptomatic or minimally symptomatic disease. Patients presenting to physicians with a specific complaint not normally associated with hyperparathyroidism or with non-specific complaints, such as malaise, depression or tiredness have a blood test arranged in the hope that it may cast light on the nature of the complaints. A serum calcium determination is

REFERENCES

25. Akerstrom G, Bergstrom R et al World J Surg 1986; 10: 696
26. Famebo L O, Sandersjoo G, Granberg P O World J Surg 1988; 12: 534
27. Salahudeen A K, Thomas T H et al Clin Sci 1989; 76: 289
28. Lewanczuk R Z, Benishin C G et al J Cardiovasc Pharmacol 1994; 23: S23
29. Jobom C, Hetta J et al World J Surg 1988; 12: 476

reported as part of the biochemical screen and this may be the first intimation of an abnormality. The pursuit of this abnormality may then demonstrate other features compatible with a diagnosis of primary hyperparathyroidism. Aird (p. 486) hinted at this aspect of the condition: 'the disease is commonest where physicians are most alert to the chance of its occurrence' and 'rarely, it is a general weakness or malaise'. In most current series it is exactly this form of the disease which dominates and it is presumed that awareness and improved diagnostic facilities have detected and treated almost all patients with severe bone disease.

This changing pattern of disease is exemplified by three different studies. Haff and his colleagues[30] in 1970 suspected this change and reported an incidence of hyperparathyroidism of 1 in 2000 of the population. Boonstra & Jackson[31] looking at a blood donor panel estimated the incidence to be 1 in 1000 and, more recently, in a hospital population the incidence was found to be as high as 1 in 680.[32] In the UK the incidence of hyperparathyroidism is estimated to be about 25 per 100 000 of the general population and it has been shown that the majority of these patients are symptomless.[33] In 1961 the incidence of symptomless disease was only 15%.[34] The definition of no symptoms can be very difficult: what might be attributable to old age in an 80-year-old would be unacceptable to most 40-year-olds. Symptoms can develop so insidiously over months or years that they are often ascribed by the patient to ageing. It is only after restoration of biochemical normality that patients are able to say that 'things were not quite right'. A short period in hospital associated with nursing and medical care and a cervical exploration, however, is no mean placebo!

The diagnosis of hyperparathyroidism

The simplest and cheapest of investigations can begin to make the diagnosis definitive. The serum phosphate and serum chloride are measured together as the chloride to phosphate ratio, the ionized calcium and plain radiographs of the chest, skull and hands are taken. Parathyroid hormone measurement might be considered the most important determination to clinch the diagnosis but care is required in its interpretation, especially if there is any evidence of renal failure. In this situation the carboxy-terminal, biologically inactive, parathyroid hormone fragments may accumulate and give a falsely reassuring weight to the diagnosis. Despite this, mid-region and carboxy-terminal assays still appear to be the best discriminator, while it is acknowledged that some overlap occurs in patients with other diagnoses, such as the hypercalcaemia of malignancy.[35]

The daily excretion of calcium in the urine is an invaluable assessment; excess calcium spillage can support the diagnosis of primary hyperparathyroidism but, more importantly, loss of less than 2 mmol of calcium per day must alert the clinician to the diagnosis of *familial hypercalcaemic hypocalciuria*. This latter condition may mimic primary hyperparathyroidism very closely, with normal levels of parathyroid hormone which are judged to be inappropriate in the face of hypercalcaemia. A repeat urinary calcium determination, an enquiry into the family history and measurement of the serum calcium in first-degree siblings, as it is inherited as an autosomal dominant disease, confirms the correct diagnosis and saves the patient an unnecessary exploration of the neck.

As has already been stated, the differential diagnosis can be difficult, and this has led to the recent development of a hypocalcaemic stimulation test in which an infusion of disodium ethylenediaminotetra-acetic acid or an intramuscular injection of salmon calcitonin induces hypocalcaemia in patients with hyperparathyroidism, malignancy or sarcoidosis. In patients with primary hyperparathyroidism ethylenediaminotetra-acetic acid always induces an increase in the mid-region intact hormone. Calcitonin also has the same effect in 80% of those with hyperparathyroidism. No such rise is demonstrated in patients with other causes of hypercalcaemia.[36]

Localization techniques

In earlier years arteriography and selective venous catheterization with sampling for parathyroid hormone levels (Fig. 19.5) were used to locate parathyroid adenomas and gave reasonable results. These techniques were costly and invasive and newer developments have allowed other procedures to be adopted. Almost 90%

REFERENCES

30. Haff R C, Black W C, Ballinger W F Ann Surg 1970; 171: 85
31. Boonstra C E, Jackson C E Am J Clin Pathol 1971; 55: 523
32. Harrop J S, Bailey J E, Woodhead J S J Clin Pathol 1982; 35: 395
33. Mundy G R, Cove D H et al Lancet 1980; i: 1317
34. Keynes M Br Med J 1961; i: 239
35. Lufkin E G, Kao P C, Heath H Am Intern Med 1987; 106: 559
36. Ljunghall S, Benson L et al World J Surg 1988; 12: 496

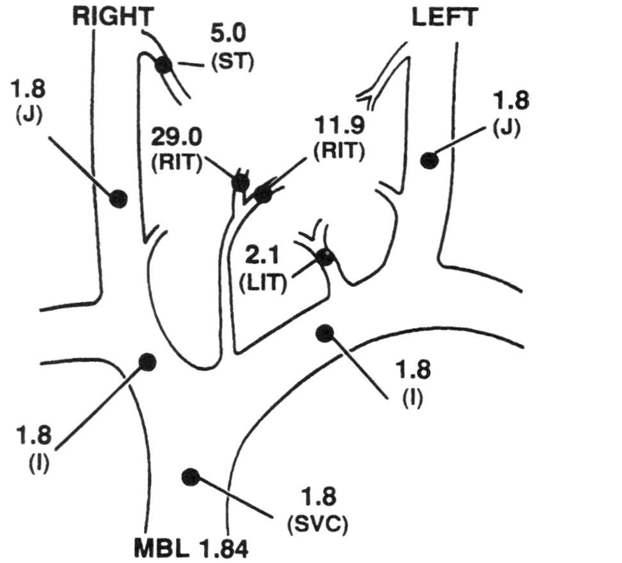

Fig. 19.5 Results of selective venous sampling for parathyroid hormone estimation in a patient with a parathyroid adenoma in the right lower position. The mean blood level of mainstream and vena caval samples represents a background reading of 1.84. The selective samples from the right inferior thyroid (RIT) vein demonstrate a marked gradient consistent with an adenoma in this position. ST = Superior thyroid vein; J = jugular vein; LIT = left inferior thyroid vein; I = innominate vein; SVC = superior vena cava; MBL = mean blood level.

of some series have been located by less invasive techniques and most surgeons agree that localization procedures are not justified before a first exploration of the neck.

Ultrasonography has an accuracy of 76%, a sensitivity of 82% and a positive predictive value of 81%. The accuracy can be further improved if the ultrasonographic findings are confirmed with fine-needle aspiration biopsy for cytology. The suspect lesion is biopsied and the cells are stained and examined or the aspirate is assayed for parathyroid hormone.[37] This approach is still experimental at present.

Although good results are reported for computed tomography (accuracy 76%, sensitivity 57% and positive predictive value 80%[38]), most feel that magnetic resonance imaging is even better.

Isotope scans using thallium-technetium or thallium-iodine isotopes have been used in the past with considerable success (Fig. 19.6) but recently scintigraphy using *technetium-sestamibi*[39] appears to be even more accurate and is now the initial investigation of choice. A combination of ^{99m}Tc-MIBI scanning with magnetic resonance imaging appears to be a very effective approach.

A preoperative infusion of methylene blue stains adenomas and hyperplastic glands a deep purple colour at surgery[40] and intraoperative high-resolution ultrasound has excellent sensitivity and positive predictive value.[41]

The differential diagnosis of hypercalcaemia

The list of causes of hypercalcaemia must be daunting for any student. Aird (p. 488) listed hyperparathyroidism, multiple myeloma, skeletal carcinomatosis, thyrotoxicosis, Paget's disease, sarcoidosis and skeletal metastasis from breast cancer. The following contemporary causes should be added: excess intake of vitamin D and/or calcium, Addison's disease, the use of thiazide diuretics, tuberculosis and familial hypocalciuric hypercalcaemia.

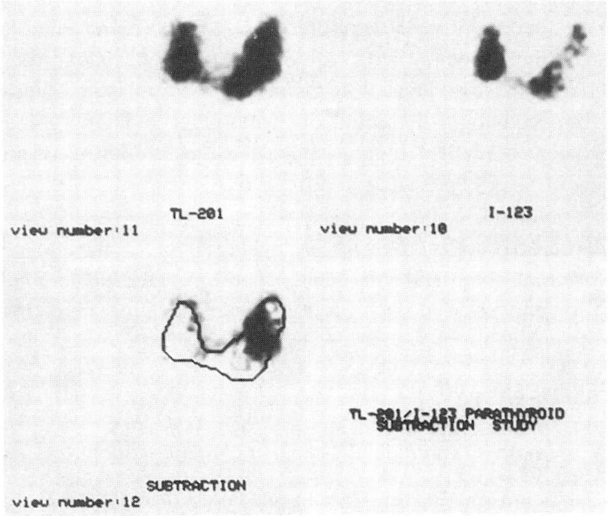

Fig. 19.6 A thallium/iodine subtraction scan. Top left: thallium image. Top right: iodine image; there is a suggestion of a filling defect consistent with poor uptake in a parathyroid nodule compressing the left lobe of the thyroid. Subtraction of the images (bottom left) reveals excess thallium uptake confined solely within a large parathyroid adenoma behind the left thyroid lobe.

This list and its application must however be kept in perspective. More than 80% of patients with persistent hypercalcaemia will have either hyperparathyroidism or malignancy and in general, the history and physical examination can often provide pointers to the correct diagnosis without recourse to too many complex or expensive investigations.[42] The history should highlight suspicious facts which might relate to the diagnosis. A careful drug history is needed to uncover the use of diuretics or antacids. A family history of hypercalcaemia or other endocrine tumours raises the possibility of multiple endocrine neoplasia syndrome or familial hypocalciuria. Weight loss and anorexia are obvious symptoms suggestive of malignancy.

It is hoped that sarcoidosis, thyrotoxicosis, tuberculosis and Addison's disease will have been excluded by careful clinical examination by referring physicians but surgical perspectives might uncover an occult neoplasm with skeletal metastases, e.g. from kidney or breast.

The inter-relationships between malignancy and hyperparathyroidism appear quite complex. A parathyroid hormone-like peptide derived from tumours has been described[43] which is similar to human parathyroid hormone through its first 13 amino acids. It was suggested that parathyroid-related peptide had paracrine and autocrine functions after it was identified in many adult and fetal tissues[44] and tumour cells. Although its coding genes and chemical structure differ from PTH, the two peptides act on similar or identical receptors.[19]

To complicate the issue further, primary hyperparathyroidism and breast cancer occur so frequently in the population that the two diseases can often be present in the same patient. Those with hyperparathyroidism, however, are usually distinguishable from those with hypercalcaemia of malignancy. Those with hyperparathyroidism have earlier-stage breast disease whereas 97% of those with hypercalcaemia of malignancy have advanced disease. Patients with primary hyperparathyroidism appear to survive better when compared with patients of similar stage of disease without parathyroid disease. This cannot be readily explained.[45]

Pathological basis of primary hyperparathyroidism

Adenomas

Chief cells, oxyphil cells and water-clear cells are present in differing proportions in parathyroid adenomas. An acinar pattern can be observed in some tumours. The presence of a rim of compressed normal tissue supports the diagnosis of an adenoma. Their weight ranges from 70 mg to 20 g.

REFERENCES

37. Karstrup S, Hegedus L et al Br Med J 1985; 290: 284
38. Grant C S, Van Heerdon J A et al World J Surg 1986; 10: 555
39. Mitchell B K, Kinder B K et al J Clin Endocrinol Metab 1995; 80: 7
40. Bambach C P, Reeve T S Aust N Z J Surg 1978; 48: 314
41. K-em K A, Shawker T H et al World J Surg 1987; 11: 579
42. Fisken R A, Heath D A et al Lancet 1981; i: 202
43. Broadus A E, Mangin M et al N Engl J Med 1988; 319: 556
44. Suva L J, Winslow G A et al Science 1987; 237: 893
45. Axelrod D M, Bockman R I et al Cancer 1987; 60: 1620

Double adenomas

Double adenomas are probably a distinct entity. Patients with persistent or recurrent hyperparathyroidism from missed or unrecognized double adenomas are older than patients with persistent or recurrent hyperparathyroidism caused by hyperplasia.[46] Nephrolithiasis is less common while muscle weakness, neuropsychiatric disorders, constipation, and weight loss are more severe.

Hyperplasia

Primary hyperplasia is not amenable to medical therapy. Its aetiology is not understood and surgical treatment is required for symptomatic disease. The first intimation of hyperplasia might be the uncovering of four-gland disease in a patient presenting in a conventional way. Intraoperative assessment is not always easy, even with the help of frozen sections and a skilled pathologist. Four-gland enlargement is unusual in the hyperplasia of sporadic primary hyperparathyroidism and as normal-sized glands frequently coexist with enlarged ones, the histological diagnosis may be difficult.

Primary hyperplasia of the chief cells and, more rarely, of the water-clear cells can occur alone or in association with certain familial endocrinopathies. It is usually inherited in an autosomal dominant fashion.

Carcinomas

Carcinomas of the parathyroids are extremely rare and represent less than 1% of cases.

Ectopic parathyroid hormone secretion

Ectopic parathyroid hormone secretion is extremely rare, quoted only in case reports of small cell lung cancer[47] and ovarian carcinoma, where DNA rearrangement and amplification in the regulatory region of one parathyroid hormone gene allele have been demonstrated.[48]

Neonatal hyperparathyroidism

Neonatal hyperparathyroidism is a genetically transmitted autosomal dominant disease characterized by life-threatening marked hypercalcaemia and intense parathyroid hyperplasia and hypercellularity. The disease is the result of a mutation in the calcium receptor gene which induces chief cell hyperplasia, leading to severe hypercalcaemia which is fatal if not recognized and treated early. Patients appear to be homozygotes for mutations of the calcium-sensing receptor which determines familial benign hypocalciuric hypercalcaemia in heterozygotes.[49] Near-total parathyroidectomy controls the disease.

TREATMENT OF PRIMARY HYPERPARATHYROIDISM

Once the diagnosis of primary hyperparathyroidism has been made, surgery may have to be undertaken urgently. An operation may not be seriously considered by either doctor or patient however if the biochemical disturbance is slight in an elderly patient with few or no symptoms.

A patient with a markedly elevated serum calcium can present as an emergency, with a hypercalcaemic crisis indicated by drowsiness, loss of consciousness, dehydration, severe weakness, vomiting and impaired renal function. Intensive medical treatment is required to prepare the patient for operation. Intravenous fluids correct dehydration and restore urine output, facilitating the renal excretion of calcium. *Diphosphonates* which prevent resorption have become one of the mainstays for lowering severe hypercalcaemia and pamidronate is equally effective. Calcitonin has the advantage of a very rapid onset of action, within minutes, and its main indication is in the first 24–48 hours of treatment of acute severe hypercalcaemia, when it can be used in conjunction with more potent but slower-acting therapies such as disphonates. Intravenous phosphate solution has only limited use because of the risk that it precipitates calcium salts.

The majority of patients can be managed electively. Surgeons have a responsibility to counsel patients about the accepted operative morbidity, for example, persistent hypercalcaemia because of a failure to recognize and/or remove all the abnormal ectopic glands, recurrent laryngeal nerve injury and persistent hypocalcaemia following damage or removal of normal parathyroid tissue.

Surgical strategy for neck exploration in primary hyperparathyroidism

Once the biochemical diagnosis has been confirmed there is no need to locate the diseased parathyroids precisely and neck exploration can be undertaken forthwith. Over 40 years ago Albright & Reifenstein[50] wrote: 'much mischief has been done by the "let's have a look" approach to the problem, "a good thyroid surgeon is not enough" and "there is no time like the first operation to uncover a small adenoma".' A comparison of ultrasonography and thallium radioisotope scanning showed no benefit in those with primary disease attending for first exploration.[51] It is more important to be aware of the frequency and usual location of ectopic adenomas. All the glands must be located as the search for a missing gland can then proceed logically based on anatomical and embryological knowledge. Excellent monographs exist describing the technical details of neck exploration and those by Gunn[52] and Wells et al[53] are recommended

A curved collar incision is made about 2 cm above the suprasternal notch and this is deepened through platysma before superior and inferior flaps are mobilized elevating the skin and

REFERENCES

46. Tezelman S, Shen W et al Surgery 1995; 118: 1115
47. Yoshimoto K, Yamasaki R, Sakai H J Clin Endocrinol Metab 1989; 68: 976
48. Nussbaum S R, Gaz R D, Arnold A N Engl J Med 1990; 323: 1324
49. Pearce S H S, Brown E M J Clin Endocrinol Metab 1996; 81: 1309
50. Albright F, Reifenstein E C The Parathyroid Glands and Metabolic Bone Disease. Williams & Wilkins, Baltimore 1948
51. Carlson G, Clayton B et al Br J Surg 1990; 77: 327
52. Gunn A Parathyroid Exploration. Wolfe, London 1988
53. Wells S A, Leight G S, Ross A J Primary Hyperparathyroidism. Year Book Medical Publishers, Chicago 1980

subcutaneous tissue to the level of the thyroid notch superiorly and the suprasternal notch inferiorly. The flaps are held open with a self-retaining retractor such as Joll's. Prior infiltration with local anaesthetic with adrenaline is unnecessary, though some prefer it.

The strap muscles are separated in the midline and separated from the underlying thyroid. They need never be cut. The surgical planes beneath platysma and the strap muscles are easily dissected by tissue separation with minimal sharp dissection. If this is not the case, the surgeon is in the wrong plane!

It may be necessary to divide the middle thyroid or the inferior thyroid veins but this should be avoided if at all possible. The middle thyroid veins are sometimes so short that they have to be divided to allow mobilization of the lateral thyroid lobes. Preservation of the veins may be important if the exploration is unsuccessful and selective venous sampling is subsequently required. Care must be taken as the thyroid is mobilized and the strap muscles are lifted from its surface. Thin-walled veins on the surface of the thyroid are easily damaged. Spilled blood stains the operative field and makes parathyroid detection more difficult.

One lateral thyroid lobe is then gently retracted toward the midline by the surgeon's finger while areolar tissue is swept away from those areas where the parathyroid glands are most likely to be found—just above the inferior thyroid artery and behind the lower thyroid pole. The carotid sheath is the lateral boundary of the dissection, the trachea and oesophagus the medial boundary and the prevertebral muscles and fascia lie posteriorly. The recurrent laryngeal nerve must be protected. Its feeding vessel is very small and usually easily seen lying on its anterior surface. Undue dissection or rough palpation near or directly on the recurrent nerve can cause an intraneural haematoma which may interfere with its function. The recurrent laryngeal nerve is sometimes situated very close to an abnormal parathyroid and must be carefully dissected free. Diathermy should not be used in the vicinity of the nerve. The parathyroid glands are often enclosed within a fat pad beneath some fascia and this has to be opened before the gland 'pops out'. This is especially true of the parathyroid glands within the thyrothymic ligament or thymus gland, when the capsule of these structures must be incised. The thymus often contains separate nodules which are usually small lymph nodes, that may be mistaken for normal parathyroid glands. They often contain carbon, however, and their cut surface is firmer and more granular than the smooth, tan, bulging surface of a parathyroid gland.

The vessels supplying the parathyroid glands can be seen coursing into their substance and care must be taken not to devascularize normal glands unwittingly. If a biopsy is taken, it should only be a sliver taken from the distal pole of the gland away from the feeding vessels. A silver clip placed across the distal third of a gland both marks the gland and allows a bloodless biopsy.

All four glands should be identified correctly before a policy of resection and biopsy is decided upon. If there appears to be one large adenoma and three apparently normal glands, then excision of the adenoma and biopsy of one of the normal glands should allow the pathologist to confirm the diagnosis. Too aggressive a biopsy policy leads to an unacceptably high incidence of hypoparathyroidism.[54]

A competent surgeon can successfully identify and remove abnormal tissue in 95% of patients by concentrating on the likely sites of the parathyroids.[55] The presence of four normal glands probably means that the patient does not have hyperparathyroidism as a fifth ectopic and abnormal gland is rare. Familial hypocalciuric hypercalcaemia is the commonest confounding diagnosis. The surgeon should not close the neck however without being as sure as possible that an abnormal gland is not still present. The exploration of the neck must be carried superiorly as far as possible and certainly above the upper thyroid pole, behind the pharynx and oesophagus. A full exploration and excision of the thymic upper poles should also be performed, opening the carotid sheath and exploring the lower thyroid poles. Intrathyroidal adenomas may be detected by intraoperative ultrasonography. A careful description of the whole exploration with a map should be kept, showing the location of all the parathyroid glands, with a notation on whether they were proven at biopsy or not. It is also helpful to indicate the presence of identifying landmarks, such as non-absorbable sutures or silver clips which might mark retained glands or biopsy sites.

Irrigation of the wound with saline removes any blood or clots and allows the identification of the smallest bleeding vessel. With full illumination tiny 'whiffs' or 'puffs' of blood can be easily seen.

Haemostasis can be totally secure, especially if care has been taken to tie or clip veins. Drains need not be placed.[56] Most surgeons reapproximate the strap muscles and platysma with an absorbable suture and close the skin with clips or staples. No dressing is required. Clips can be removed on the second postoperative day and if the serum calcium is normal the patient may be allowed home.

Unilateral exploration

The advantage and cost-effectiveness of preoperative localization and unilateral neck exploration in primary hyperparathyroidism are still controversial issues. Some propose that preoperative localization of a solitary parathyroid adenoma hopefully coupled with confirmation of excision of all hyperfunctional tissue by a quick parathyroid hormone assay, may allow unilateral neck exploration with a reduction in the operating time.[57,58] Others report unacceptably high surgical failure rates for unilateral neck exploration guided by preoperative localizing studies compared with a bilateral neck exploration by an experienced endocrine surgeon.[59]

Treatment of primary hyperplasia

Hyperplasia, with or without adenomas of the parathyroid glands, is always a possibility. The first indication of hyperplasia might be

REFERENCES

54. Kaplan E L, Bartlett S et al Surgery 1982; 92: 827
55. Thompson N W, Eckhauser F E, Harness J K Surgery 1982; 92: 814
56. Kristoffersson A, Sandzen B, Jarhult J Br J Surg 1986; 73: 121
57. Wei J P, Burke G J Am J Surg 1995; 170: 488
58. Irvin G L, Prudhomme D L et al Ann Surg 1994; 219: 574
59. Zmora O, Schachter P P et al Surgery 1995; 118: 932

the uncovering of four-gland disease on neck exploration. Intraoperative assessment is not always easy, even with the help of frozen sections and a skilled pathologist. The density of the gland might be a better marker of single or multiple gland disease than histology.[60]

Primary hyperplasia of the chief cells (and more rarely the water-clear cells) can occur alone or in association with certain familial endocrinopathies. It is usually inherited in an autosomal dominant fashion. Its aetiology is not known. When this parathyroid hyperplasia is associated with pancreatic islet cell and pituitary tumours it is called multiple endocrine neoplasia type I.[61] Occasionally adrenocortical, thyroid and carcinoid tumours are also associated. Ninety per cent of patients with multiple endocrine neoplasia type I syndrome have parathyroid hyperplasia with less pronounced hypercalcaemia presenting at an earlier age than its non-familial or sporadic counterpart.[62] The Zollinger–Ellison syndrome links hypergastrinaemia, from a non-beta islet cell tumour, with hyperparathyroidism in multiple endocrine neoplasia I, parietal cell hyperplasia, gastric acid hypersecretion and a fulminating peptic ulcer diathesis.[63] The association of medullary thyroid carcinoma, phaeochromocytoma and hyperparathyroidism constitutes the multiple endocrine neoplasia type II syndrome.[64] Some 20–60% of patients with this syndrome have parathyroid hyperplasia but the disease is usually mild and insignificant compared with the effects produced by the other endocrine tumours.

There is no value in screening for these familial syndromes by measurement of other hormonal products in a population of patients undergoing surgery for uncomplicated primary hyperparathyroidism, unless there is a positive family history or suggestive symptoms.[65]

In the multiple endocrine neoplasia I syndrome total parathyroidectomy and autotransplantation appear to give the best results.[66] Persistent or recurrent disease can be a problem with subtotal resections; it is encountered in 88% of those having 1–2½ glands resected and 33% of those with 3–3½ glands resected. Long-term follow-up studies have shown that autotransplantation is the best means of restoring optimum calcium levels in patients who have undergone total parathyroidectomy for primary hyperplasia of whatever cause.[67]

Management of asymptomatic hyperparathyroidism

Coe & Favus[68] were amongst the first to question whether mild, symptomless hyperparathyroidism required surgery. They felt that surgery should usually be offered because renal damage will develop in some untreated patients and because of the expense of intensive medical follow-up. Others have shown, however, that by 4 years there was no sign of deterioration in the blood pressure or plasma creatinine when age-matched unoperated controls were compared with patients who had undergone parathyroidectomy.[69] Clodronate sodium has been used as a form of medical treatment for hyperparathyroidism, particularly in those patients in whom suppression of bone disease is desirable before surgery or when surgery is contraindicated.[70]

The debate continues. Stevenson & Lynn[71] advocate parathyroidectomy for all patients with symptomless mild primary hyperparathyroidism because:

1. Subtle physical and psychological changes are only appreciated on restoration of biochemical normality.
2. There is a risk of developing renal failure in the long term.
3. There is a risk of bone loss—this is especially important in elderly females.
4. Hypercalcaemia may contribute to confusion in the elderly.
5. There is a risk of hypercalcaemic crisis in the elderly, especially if there is intercurrent illness producing dehydration.
6. The incidence and mortality from cardiovascular disease may be increased.

Heath[72] felt that the workload of adopting such a policy would be considerable—perhaps as many as 170 new patients from Birmingham over 70 years of age with symptomless hyperparathyroidism every year. He concluded: 'I would find it difficult on the present evidence to ask a fit, asymptomatic, elderly patient to undergo parathyroidectomy'. The jury remains out on this issue and a middle course would appear to be the most pragmatic.

Recurrent and persistent hyperparathyroidism

Persistent hyperparathyroidism is the commonest cause of postoperative hypercalcaemia, which is defined as continued hypercalcaemia in the immediate postoperative period or recurrence within 1 year of surgery. Recurrent hyperparathyroidism is defined by Muller[73] as hypercalcaemia recurring when the following criteria have been met:

1. Identification and biopsy proof of all four parathyroids at the initial operation.
2. Complete removal of all abnormal tissue.
3. A normocalcaemic phase of 1 year or longer.
4. Abnormal tissue uncovered at re-exploration at a site of previously normal gland.

True recurrent disease may account for 1% of recurrent hypercalcaemia.

REFERENCES

60. Welsh C L, Taylor G W World J Surg 1984; 8: 522
61. Wermer P Am J Med 1954; 16: 363
62. Lamers C B H, Froeling P G Am J Med 1979; 66: 442
63. Zollinger R M, Ellison E H Ann Surg 1955; 142: 709
64. Sipple J H Am J Med 1961; 31: 163
65. Farndon J R, Geraghty J M et al World J Surg 1987; 11: 252
66. Mahnaeus J, Benson L et al World J Surg 1986; 10: 668
67. Wells S A, Farndon J R et al Ann Surg 1980; 192: 451
68. Coe F L, Favus M J N Engl J Med 1980; 302: 224
69. Van't Hoff W, Ballardie F W, Bicknell E J Br Med J 1983; 287: 1605
70. Douglas D L, Kamis J A et al Br Med J 1983; 286: 587
71. Stevenson J C, Lynn J A Br Med J 1988; 296: 1017
72. Health D Br Med J 1988; 296: 1398
73. Muller H Br J Surg 1975; 62: 556

The diagnosis must be checked and confirmed if persistent disease is suspected. If hyperparathyroidism is present the next steps require careful thought. There is no virtue in attempting to localize the abnormal tissue if the patient's general condition would not withstand re-exploration and its associated morbidity. A conservative approach may be considered if the disease is symptomless, especially if it can be shown that kidneys, bones and eyes are not being damaged by the disease.

Most surgeons use localization procedures preoperatively if the diagnosis is confirmed and a decision is made to offer re-exploration. This is carried out after careful scrutiny of the previous operation notes, operative maps and histology reports as these often indicate the likely site of abnormality. If, for example, three glands had been identified and had normal biopsies but the left lower parathyroid had not been biopsied, radiologists would try to image this area to detect any intrathyroid masses or mediastinal adenomas.

An initial surgical failure is nearly always the result of an inadequate neck exploration. This may be the result of a joint error between the surgeon, endocrinologist and pathologist; for example, failure to recognize familial hyperparathyroidism or multiple endocrine neoplasia syndromes.[74] The lower pole of the thyroid often harbours a parathyroid adenoma if the lower glands were not found at the first exploration. Intraoperative ultrasonography may detect these tumours but often incision of the thyroid lobe or thyroid lobectomy is required.[75]

The mortality of re-exploration should be very low or non-existent but there is an increased morbidity—6% temporary recurrent laryngeal nerve neuropraxia, 4% permanent unilateral cord paralysis and 13% rendered hypoparathyroid.[38] The adenoma is usually in the neck and with these potential complications redo surgery should not be undertaken by the occasional surgeon.

PARATHYROID CARCINOMA

The incidence of parathyroid carcinoma remains very low and only accounts for about 1% of all patients with primary hyperparathyroidism. There is an equal male and female incidence and the mean age of onset is around the age of 50. There are no obvious clinical or biochemical markers which distinguish patients with carcinoma from those with an adenoma. Definitive histological studies do not always help because they lack precision. The presence of a rim of normal or atrophic parathyroid gland, the nuclear characteristics, the presence of fibrous bands, the stromal and intracytoplasmic fat content, the number of mitotic figures and the presence of vascular and capsular invasion have all been used to help distinguish carcinoma from hyperplasia and adenoma, but the accuracy of all these criteria is low. Unfortunately carcinoma is often only confirmed when the patient subsequently develops local recurrence or metastases.[76]

Chief cells predominate in carcinomas but oxyphil and transitional oxyphil cells may also be found. The architecture varies from a more solid to a trabecular pattern but there are no other great structural differences between an adenoma and a carcinoma.[77] An oxyphil cell carcinoma can only be recognized with certainty when metastases develop 5–8 years after the initial surgery. Electron microscopy then shows the typical cell type packed with numerous mitochondria.[78]

Flow cytometric analysis of the DNA content of parathyroid lesions does little to enhance the distinction between benign and malignant lesions. It has been suggested that tetraploid and near triploid aneuploid patterns in adenomas and some chief cell hyperplasias may be early markers of malignant potential.[79]

Unfortunately most parathyroid carcinomas continue to function and troublesome hypercalcaemia adds considerably to the patient's suffering. Occasionally carcinomas are non-secretory although they have similar light and electron microscopic features to functioning tumours and parathyroid hormone immunoreactivity is demonstrable on histology. Flow cytometric analysis of the DNA content of parathyroid glands does little to enhance the distinction between benign and malignant. In patients with clinical or pathological parathyroid cancers, flow cytometry may differentiate slow-growing tumours (diploid tumours) from aggressive ones (aneuploid).[80] Mitotic activity is also a prognostic risk factor but is again of limited diagnostic significance. In half of the carcinomas, the frequency of mitoses does not exceed values recorded in benign parathyroid lesions.[81]

Treatment

If the condition is recognized preoperatively, perhaps by suggestive appearances on a computed tomography scan or the presence of palpable lymph nodes, en bloc resections offer the best results in combination with central compartment dissection when there is evidence of regional node metastases.

The serum calcium and parathyroid hormone measurements are postoperative markers of tumour recurrence. Recurrence in the neck or lungs can often be treated by further surgery with en bloc radical dissections, mediastinal lymph node clearance and limited pulmonary resections.[82] This surgery is rarely curative but good palliation may be achieved if the hypercalcaemia is reduced. Radiotherapy is of little use. Mithramycin is a potent hypocalcaemic agent which is often effective for many months[83] and more recently symptomatic relief has been obtained by using disodium clodronate.[84] The outlook is variable and, as with many

REFERENCES

74. Clarke O H, Way L W, Hunt T K Ann Surg 1976; 184: 391
75. Wheeler M H, Williams E D, Wade J S H World J Surg 1987; 11: 110
76. Roth S In: Silverberg S G (ed) Principles and Practice of Surgical Pathology. John Wiley, New York 1983
77. Grimelius L, Akerstrom G, Johansson H The Parathyroids: Location and Histopathological Diagnosis. Institute of Pathology and Department of Surgery, University of Uppsala 1981
78. Obara T, Fujimoto Y et al Cancer 1985; 55: 1489
79. Bowlby L S, Debault L E, Abraham S R Am J Pathol 1987; 128: 338
80. August D A, Flynn S D et al Surgery 1993; 113: 290
81. Bondeson L, Sandelin K, Grimelius L Am J Surg Pathol 1993; 17: 820
82. Fujimoto Y, Obara T Surg Clin North Am 1987; 67: 343
83. Trigonis C, Cedermark B et al Clin Oncol 1984; 10: II
84. Jungst D Lancet 1984; ii: 1043

endocrine tumours, some patients survive for many years with known metastatic disease.[85]

HYPOPARATHYROIDISM

At the turn of this century Halsted[86] was only too well aware of the tetany which could accompany thyroid surgery. He wrote: 'The cause of tetany at the hands of well-versed operators is, I believe, less often removal of the parathyroids than interference with their circulation' and 'I fear to do an operation . . . which does not contemplate the leaving of a slice of the thyroid gland in the region of the ultimate distribution of the inferior thyroid artery'. These observations encouraged Halsted to study parathyroid transplantation and led to his 'law of deficiency' which caused him to believe erroneously that parathyroid allografts could survive. Aird (p. 490) was also well aware that tetany could follow parathyroid exploration—'a sure sign of success'! It is likely that his patients, however, had severe bone disease with 'an unnatural avidity of the bones for calcium'.

Hypoparathyroidism can arise idiopathically but this is extremely rare. It develops in young people and is usually associated with other endocrine disorders.[87] Surgery is the usual cause of the condition and it may often follow major extirpative surgery for cancer, for example after pharyngolaryngo-oesophagectomy.[88]

In a study of over 37 000 patients undergoing thyroid or parathyroid surgery an incidence of early tetany of 0.32% with an incidence of permanent tetany after more than 5 years of 0.16% was described.[89] Medical treatment at that time was not ideal and the authors examined the possibility of treating the condition by vascularized parathyroid fetal homografts—with little success. It has now been shown that total thyroidectomy as a treatment for non-medullary carcinoma of the thyroid does not give survival or recurrence-free benefit when compared with partial thyroidectomy (see Chapter 18). It is, however, associated with far greater morbidity, with 17% showing transient and 6% permanent hypocalcaemia whereas none was seen following partial thyroidectomy.[90]

An operative strategy which includes a more aggressive biopsy and resectional policy of parathyroid glands leads to a higher incidence of temporary hypocalcaemia without necessarily improving the overall success of the surgery.[91] It is difficult to be dogmatic or objective about an ideal biopsy policy and clearly the surgeon–pathologist team is trying to steer a course between curative surgery without temporary or permanent hypocalcaemia and the certainty that all the parathyroid glands have been seen and only normal glands have been left. It is essential to monitor calcium levels in the postoperative period and it is advisable to counsel patients that a normally temporary period of hypocalcaemia may follow parathyroid surgery. This may relieve anxiety over any symptoms of hypocalcaemia which might develop. The biochemical threshold at which symptoms appear is variable and unpredictable. Prior explanation also clarifies the apparent paradox of a requirement for calcium and vitamin D when the whole object of the exercise has been to lower an abnormally high calcium!

The requirement for an intravenous bolus or infusions of calcium is rare but is necessary for a few elderly patients with severe bone disease—'hungry bones'! When infusions are required, it is essential to monitor the serum calcium concentration to ensure adequate treatment and to prevent overdosage. It must be remembered that 10% calcium gluconate can cause severe phlebitis if undiluted and tissue damage if there is extravasation. It should therefore be diluted or delivered centrally. Mild hypocalcaemia need not prevent the patient being discharged but it is essential to arrange outpatient checks of the serum calcium in follow-up. It is surprising how quickly postoperative hypocalcaemia can reverse and the patient's devotion to replacement therapy may then result in hypercalcaemia of a greater magnitude than that found at initial presentation.

It is now easier to treat established permanent hypoparathyroidism and normocalcaemia can be maintained by balancing increased calcium absorption against its obligatory loss in the urine. Pharmacological doses of vitamin D or near physiological doses of the hydroxylated metabolites calcitrol or alphacalcidol are used. A combination of larger doses of oral calcium with a vitamin D preparation can often achieve stable, normal serum calcium concentrations and this form of replacement becomes an automatic medication, similar to thyroxine for myxoedema. Some oral calcium preparations are rich in potassium and must not be prescribed for patients with concomitant renal failure. In the elderly or in those with some renal impairment, measurement of the urinary calcium and creatinine concentrations allows an index to be generated which reflects the calcium load presented to the kidney (calcium excretion in mmol/l glomerular filtrate) and the renal tubular calcium reabsorption. This can be used to predict the likely calcium requirement and identify those patients at risk of developing hypercalcaemia.[92]

SECONDARY HYPERPARATHYROIDISM—MULTIGLANDULAR DISEASE AND PARATHYROID AUTOTRANSPLANTATION

Secondary parathyroid hyperplasia occurs in response to a stimulus which is usually biochemical. The commonest cause is the hyperphosphataemia, relative hypocalcaemia and disordered vitamin D metabolism associated with chronic renal failure. The duration of the renal failure and the length of dialysis contribute to the severity of the disease.

Secondary hyperparathyroidism can evolve into an autonomous condition which is not reversed even if renal function is restored to normal, for example, after renal transplantation. This is sometimes called tertiary hyperparathyroidism. A dominant adenoma or adenomas will be found within hyperplastic glands causing the hypercalcaemia.

REFERENCES

85. Van Heerden J A, Weiland L H et al Arch Surg 1979; 114: 475
86. Halsted W S Am J Med Sci 1907; 134: 1
87. Simpson H K L, Howden C W et al Br Med J 1993; 296: 1316
88. Buchanan G, West T E T et al Clin Oncol 1975; 1: 89
89. Watkins E, Bell G O et al JAMA 1962; 182: 140
90. Schroder D M, Chambers A, France C J Cancer 1986; 58: 2320
91. Kaplan E L, Bartlett S et al Surgery 1982; 92: 827
92. Newman G H, Wade M, Hoskins D J Br Med 1983; 287: 781

Secondary hyperparathyroidism with metastatic calcification leading to arterial disease and bone disease is one of the most important problems in patients with chronic renal failure. In spite of medical measures to control the serum calcium and phosphate levels and the use of a variety of vitamin D sterols, hyperparathyroidism responds transiently or not at all and parathyroidectomy is necessary. The criteria indicating the need for surgical intervention are however still not clearly defined.[93]

Two options are available: subtotal resection leaving behind at least one-half of a parathyroid gland in the neck or total parathyroidectomy with autotransplantation of fragments taken from the most normal gland into the forearm flexor muscles.

The majority of patients with secondary hyperparathyroidism benefit from parathyroidectomy with resolution or disappearance of non-visceral soft tissue calcification in 60% of patients.[94] Significant reductions in plasma parathyroid hormone concentrations occurred with concomitant falls in the serum calcium and phosphate. Improvements were also found in the subperiosteal erosions and the histological grade of osteitis fibrosa, but arterial calcification in the small vessels still developed or progressed in nearly 60% of patients. There is little evidence to support subtotal parathyroidectomy as a better treatment than total parathyroidectomy and autografting in secondary disease. There are significant advantages with the latter technique:

1. The parathyroid mass can be reduced effectively with immediate biochemical benefit.
2. Graft-dependent recurrent disease can occur but is readily treated by graft reduction under local anaesthetic, obviating the need for re-exploration of the neck with its attendant morbidity.
3. Graft function can be closely monitored by measuring parathyroid hormone directly in antecubital veins which drain directly from the graft site.[95]

Macroscopic nodules within hyperplastic glands behave more abnormally than diffuse hyperplastic areas when studied in vitro.[96] Autotransplants should therefore be taken from homogeneous parts of the parathyroid glands as this may reduce the incidence of graft-dependent recurrence.

Parathyroid autotransplantation

The parathyroid glands are remarkably resilient and can withstand relatively adverse conditions before resuming apparently normal function after transplantation.

When autotransplantation is undertaken all four parathyroid glands are removed from the neck. The most normal gland, which is usually the smallest, without nodule formation and showing diffuse hyperplasia on frozen section, is taken and sliced into slivers or chips 3 × 1 × 1 mm and placed in a bath of ice-cold saline. About 15 such fragments are placed, each in its own muscle pocket, in the forearm flexor mass, which is exposed through a longitudinal incision between 3 and 8 cm below the anticubital fossa. Each pocket is closed by reapproximating the fascia with a non-absorbable suture. This prevents graft extrusion and marks the site of implantation to aid re-exploration if necessary. Some fragments can be cryopreserved using the technique described by Wells & Christiansen.[97] Primary graft failure is extremely rare.

It cannot be predicted with certainty whether permanent hypocalcaemia will ensue after reoperation for persistent or recurrent hyperparathyroidism. When cryopreserved material is still available it may subsequently be used to restore normocalcaemia, sometimes as long as 18 months after surgery.[98] Cryopreserved parathyroid tissue is resilient and normally functions well after late implantation.[98]

White et al[99] have suggested that cryopreservation should be an essential part of reoperative parathyroid surgery, not only as a means of holding tissue in reserve, but also to enable definitive histology to be carried out to exclude a carcinoma. However the distinction between an adenoma and a parathyroid carcinoma cannot always easily be established on histology.

SUMMARY

Although major insights have been made into the management and pathophysiology of primary hyperparathyroidism, there are still many unsolved questions. The genetic alterations and molecular pathways involved in parathyroid gland physiology and pathology and the relationship between abnormal parathyroid cell growth and hormone secretion are not yet integrated into a simple model. The appropriate treatment for patients with mild or symptomless disease is still not agreed. There is continued controversy concerning the advantages of unilateral versus bilateral neck dissection in patients with positive imaging of one parathyroid adenoma. Following the identification of the plasma membrane calcium receptor, the development of pharmacological control of parathyroid hormone secretion by interfering with the function of this receptor is an exciting prospective.

REFERENCES

93. Drueke T, Zingraff J, Dubost C Advances in Nephrology. Year Book Medical Publishers, Chicago 1982
94. De Francisco A M, Ellis H A et al Q J Med 1985; 55: 289
95. Rothmunds M, Wagner P K Ann Surg 1983; 197: 7
96. Wallfelt C H, Larsson R et al World J Surg 1988; 12: 431
97. Wells S A, Christiansen C Surgery 1974; 75: 49
98. Brennan M F, Brown E M et al Ann Surg 1979; 189: 139
99. White J V, Logerfo P et al Lancet 1983; ii: 461

20 Ear, nose and throat

A. F. Fitzgerald O'Connor   Valerie J. Lund

THE EAR

Surgical anatomy

The ear may be divided into:

1. An external portion, comprising the pinna and external auditory meatus.
2. The middle ear cleft, composed of the middle ear, the eustachian tube and the mastoid air cells.
3. The inner ear or labyrinth, comprising the cochlea and vestibular labyrinth supplied by the VIII (vestibulo-cochlear or auditory) nerve (Fig. 20.1).

In the adult, the external ear canal is between 2 and 3 cm in length and is slightly curved. Thus, to view the tympanic membrane or eardrum which divides it from the middle ear, the canal must be straightened by gently retracting the pinna upwards and backwards. The tympanic membrane is divided into a small upper portion, the pars flaccida, so called because it lacks much fibrous support, and a lower portion, the pars tensa, which is responsive to sound and appears relatively transparent, exhibiting a light reflex on otoscopic examination due to its conical shape (Fig. 20.2). The malleus handle can be seen embedded in the drum and with the stapes and incus forms the ossicular chain. Sounds transmitted through the ossicular chain result in motion of the perilymphatic fluids that stimulate the hair cells of the cochlea.

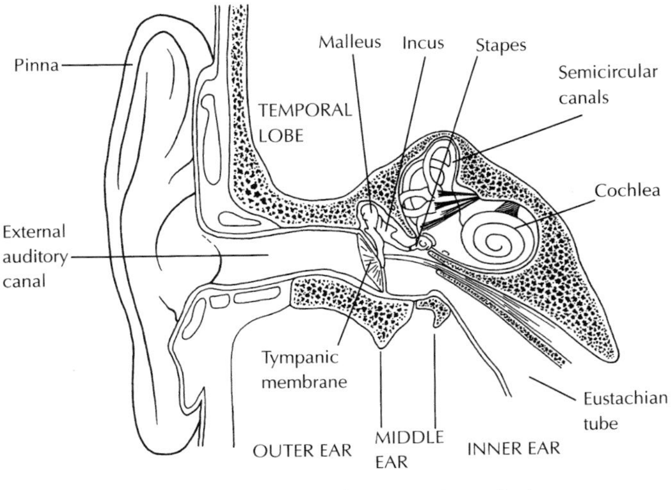

Fig. 20.1 Diagram showing coronal section through the ear.

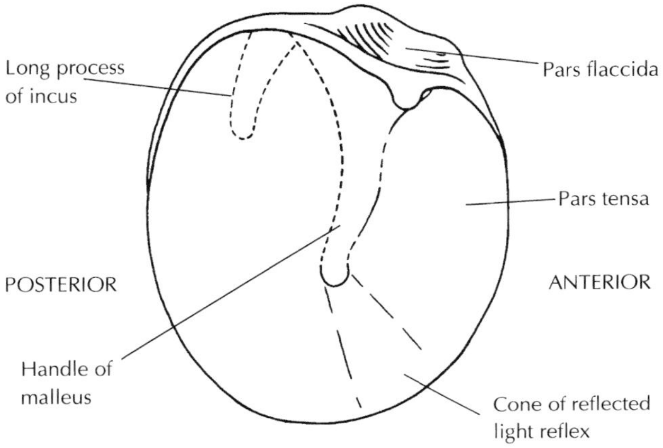

Fig. 20.2 Diagram showing right eardrum.

The middle ear lies in close proximity to important structures which may be involved by infection. The temporal lobe in the middle cranial fossa lies superiorly and is only separated from the middle ear by a thin bony plate, the tegmen tympani. Posteriorly the mastoid air cells are adjacent to the cerebellum in the posterior cranial fossa and lateral (sigmoid) sinus. Medially the lateral semicircular canal allows access to the inner ear and the facial nerve passes through the middle ear from the internal auditory meatus to the stylomastoid foramen. The eustachian tube connects the middle ear to the nasopharynx and is important to keep pressure equal between the two. It is relatively short and horizontal in infancy but during childhood becomes elongated with a more downward angulation.

The cochlea is a spiral structure of two and a half turns containing perilymph and endolymph partitioned by membranes. Sound vibrations are transmitted in the perilymph compartment vibrating the basilar membrane and thus stimulating the hair cells which generate neural impulses along the cochlear division of the VIII nerve. The organs of balance are contained in the bony labyrinth. Angular acceleration is detected by the three semicircular canals and linear acceleration by the saccule and utricle. The VIII (vestibulo-cochlear) nerve passes medially and runs into the internal auditory canal where it is joined by the facial nerve crossing the cerebello-pontine angle to the brainstem.

Clinical examination

The five main symptoms of ear disease are earache, deafness, discharge, tinnitus and vertigo. In a full otological examination,

examination of the external ear and eardrum may be performed with an otoscope, an aural speculum and a headlight or microscope, or with a rigid endoscope. The mobility of the drum may be assessed by observing it while the patient autoinflates the middle ear with a Valsalva manoeuvre or by gently insufflating the external canal with air. Tuning fork tests and free field speech testing may give a crude indication of hearing loss but a wide variety of audiometric and vestibular tests are available, the most common of which are a pure tone audiogram and impedance tympanometry. The audiogram can quantify a hearing loss and indicate whether it is sensorineural, due to lesions in the cochlea and VIII nerve, or conductive, due to lesions of the external auditory meatus to the oval window. Tympanometry is mainly used to demonstrate mobility of the drum and thus the presence of fluid in the middle ear. Other tests include speech audiometry, electric response audiometry, otoacoustic emissions, caloric testing and electronystagmography. Electroneuronography is used in the assessment of facial nerve function. Plain radiographs have been superseded by high-resolution CT scanning and MRI in the investigation of ear pathology.

Trauma and foreign bodies

The auricle may suffer lacerations, avulsion, thermal injury and blunt injury causing a haematoma (Fig. 20.3). The haematoma forms between the perichondrium and the pinna cartilage, depriving the cartilage of its blood supply and resulting in cosmetic deformity—a cauliflower ear. The haematoma should be drained under antibiotic cover through an incision at the anterolateral aspect of the concha; a supportive pressure dressing, contoured to the external ear, is then applied and removed daily for inspection.

The external meatus may also be injured; inserted foreign bodies require careful removal to avoid perforation of the eardrum.

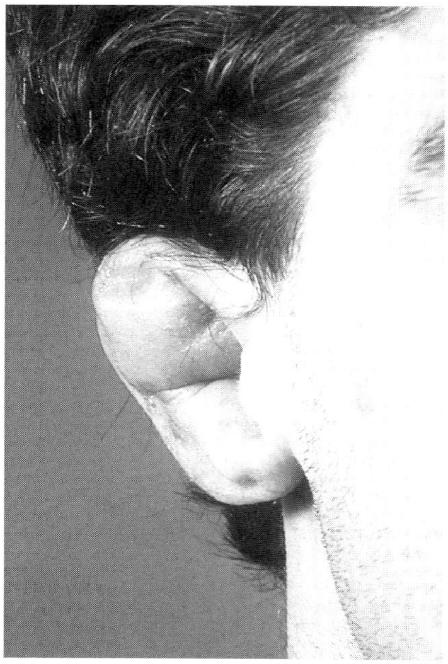

Fig. 20.3 Haematoma of right pinna.

In addition to penetrating injuries, the middle ear may be injured by severe barotrauma, e.g. bomb blasts, or overzealous ear syringing. Perforation of the eardrum, ossicular disruption, haemotympanum and/or a perilymph fistula may result and are characterized by varying degrees of hearing loss, tinnitus and vertigo.[1]

Wax may become impacted in the external canal, a condition often exacerbated by the patient trying to clean the ear with cotton-wool buds or other objects. The hearing loss is generally small unless there is complete obstruction. If the wax is hard, sodium bicarbonate drops may be used for a couple of weeks to soften it sufficiently to allow syringing. Alternatively the wax may be removed under direct vision using a headlight or microscope. Syringing is contraindicated immediately after injury to the ear or when there is a history of otorrhoea or tympanic perforation. Occasionally a mass of wax and desquamated epithelium can accumulate deep in the canal producing erosion of adjacent bone and eventually pain. This is termed keratosis obturans; its removal usually requires a general anaesthetic.

45% of skull base fractures extend to the temporal bone to involve the middle and inner ear, producing temporary or permanent hearing loss. These fractures may be longitudinal or transverse or a combination of the two (Fig. 20.4). Facial nerve paralysis is more often associated with transverse fractures (50% v 20%) as are vertigo and cerebrospinal fluid leaks.[2,3] Bruising over the mastoid bone (Battle's sign), blood in the external ear and a cerebrospinal fluid leak, either through a perforated drum or into the nose via the eustachian tube, strongly suggest a temporal fracture. Prophylactic antibiotics should be given while CT scanning is performed and audiological, vestibular and facial nerve function are assessed. The role of systemic steroids and surgical exploration is subject to debate.

Infection

Otitis externa

Non-specific inflammation of the external auditory canal usually represents a form of eczema or seborrhoeic dermatitis produced by irritants, e.g. perfume or hair spray, and may be exacerbated by a hot humid climate. A variety of organisms may be found, e.g. haemolytic streptococcus, *Staphylococcus aureus*, *Pseudomonas aeruginosa*, anaerobes and occasionally fungi such as aspergillus. The canal is swollen, weeping and full of debris. The inflammation may spread to the pinna and is often associated with discomfort and itching. Frequent suction cleaning of the canal using a microscope and packing with gauze or a wick soaked in a topical agent such as aluminium acetate solution are more effective than oral antibiotics. The patient is advised to keep irritants and water away from the ear.

A much more severe form, malignant otitis externa, can occur in diabetics; this can produce significant skull base destruction and

REFERENCES

1. Ballantyne J C Proc R Soc Med 1966; 59: 535
2. Aguilar E A, Yeakley J W, Ghorayer M, Hauser M, Cabrera J, Jahrsdoerfer R A Head Neck Surg 1987; 9: 162
3. Avrahami E, Chen Z, Solomon A Neuroradiology 1988; 30: 166

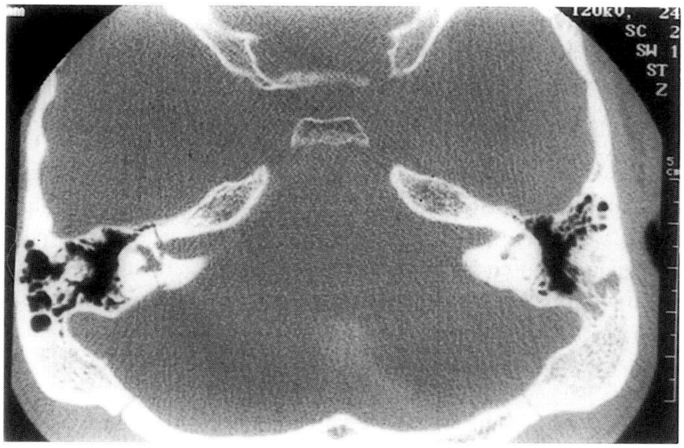

Fig. 20.4 Axial CT scan showing transverse fracture of left temporal bone. With kind permission of Dr P D Phelps.

cranial nerve palsies.[4] It often necessitates radical surgical debridement and high-dose parenteral antibiotics which cover pseudomonas and anaerobes, e.g. ciprofloxacin and metronidazole.

Localized infection of a hair follicle, usually with staphylococcus, produces a furuncle which causes severe pain. This condition is also more common in diabetics. It must be distinguished from acute mastoiditis (a complication of acute otitis media), impacted wax (keratosis obturans), viral infections such as herpes simplex or zoster, fungal infections (otomycosis) or bacterial infections associated with foreign bodies. It is usually more painful than diffuse eczematous otitis externa. An infiltrating squamous cell carcinoma, although very rare, should be considered, particularly in an individual with a history of chronic otitis media.

Other features which distinguish furunculosis from acute mastoiditis are summarized in Table 20.1. Hearing is impaired only when the canal is occluded. In addition to topical treatment combined with adequate analgesia and oral flucloxacillin, a furuncle may require drainage if it does not burst spontaneously.

Acute otitis media

Acute infection of the middle ear cleft is extremely common, especially in children. The patient complains of severe otalgia which may diminish when the drum perforates. Perforation is accompanied by some blood and purulent discharge. Hearing is reduced but in young children the clinical features are more diffuse with generalized malaise, pyrexia and gastrointestinal upset masking otologic features. In simple infections the pinna is normal and there is no swelling or tenderness of the mastoid though the drum is red and bulging if it is intact; following perforation there will be purulent secretion in the canal. In suppurative otitis media, respiratory pathogens such as *Streptococcus pneumoniae* and haemophilus are commonly found and respond to a broad-spectrum oral antibiotic such as amoxycillin or erythromycin. Some surgeons advocate myringotomy if perforation has not already occurred.

Chronic suppurative otitis media

Once the acute phase has settled, the perforation usually heals spontaneously; occasionally a more chronic infection develops. Chronic suppurative otitis media is generally divided into 'safe' and 'unsafe'. The latter is usually associated with cholesteatoma and represents a more destructive process. The exact cause of cholesteatoma is unknown but is related to a collection of keratinizing squamous epithelium in the middle ear, possibly in a retraction pocket in the tympanic membrane, which gradually erodes into the middle ear and adjacent structures.[5] Apart from some unpleasant smelling discharge and a degree of deafness the condition is often insidious until it produces severe vertigo, hearing loss or facial nerve paralysis. Cholesteatoma must be suspected if careful examination of the eardrum under the microscope reveals a perforation or pocket full of white debris in the attic or uppermost part of the drum. By contrast perforations in the pars tensa are usually 'safe'. The hearing loss is conductive though it may be less than expected because of conduction of sound through the cholesteatoma. Whilst 'safe' chronic suppurative otitis media may often be managed medically, cholesteatoma requires exploration of the middle ear and mastoid with regular follow-up.[6] Reconstruction of the ossicular chain may be undertaken at a later date.

Chronic serous otitis media

Following acute otitis media, a serous effusion or 'glue ear' may persist within the middle ear cavity, especially in younger children (Fig. 20.5). Myringotomy and grommet insertion is performed to improve hearing loss and its sequelae (Fig. 20.6). Predisposing factors thought to be important include eustachian dysfunction,

REFERENCES

4. Mendelson D S, Som P M, Mendelson M H Radiology 1983; 149: 745
5. Michaels L Ear, Nose and Throat Histopathology. Springer Verlag, Heidelberg 1987: 47–51
6. Wayoff M, Charachon R, Rouleau P, Lacher G, Deguine Ch Adv Otorhinolaryngol 1987; 36: 215

Table 20.1 Differentiation between furunculosis and acute mastoiditis

	Furunculosis	*Mastoiditis*
Postauricular tenderness	Diffuse	Maximal over mastoid antrum
Displacement of pinna	Forwards	Forwards and downwards
Enlarged lymph nodes	Present	Absent
Pressure on tragus, moving pinna	Pain	No pain
Mastoid radiographs	Mastoid air cells clear	Mastoid air cells cloudy
Examination of eardrum	If visible normal, usually hidden by swelling of canal	Before perforation, red and bulging

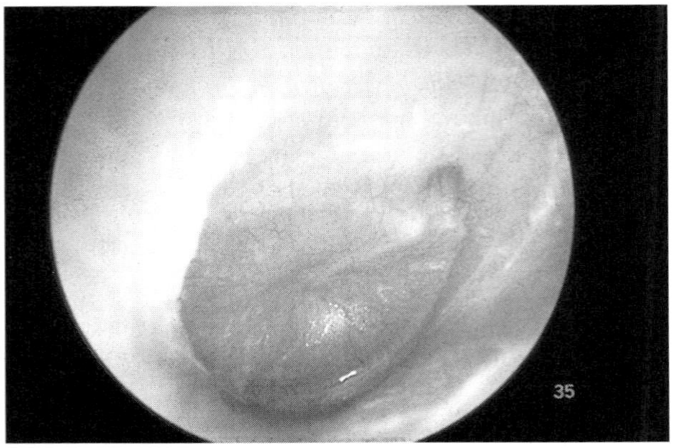

Fig. 20.5 Endoscopic photograph showing chronic serous otitis media of right ear. With kind permission of Prof A Wright.

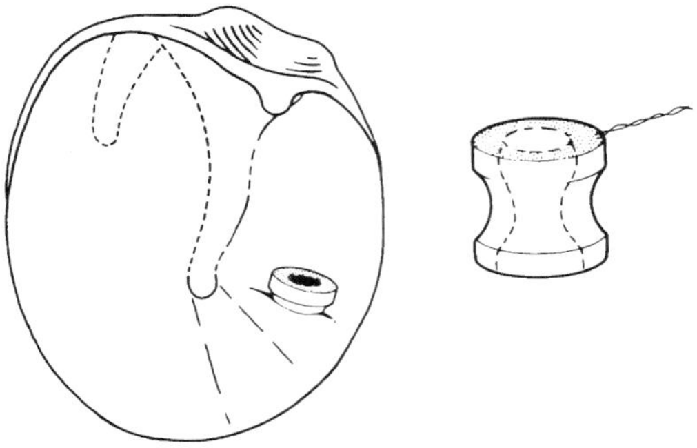

Fig. 20.6 Diagram showing position of myringotomy in anterior tympanic membrane and grommet in situ.

adenoidal hypertrophy and allergy which, if present, should be appropriately treated. A persistent unilateral middle ear effusion in an adult requires further investigation to exclude a nasopharyngeal tumour.

Complications of otitis media

In the acute phase, if there is any suggestion of mastoid tenderness or swelling or excessive malaise, headache or drowsiness, the local and intracranial complications of acute otitis media must be considered: middle ear infection is one of the commonest sources of a brain abscess, either in the temporal lobe or cerebellum[7] (Table 20.2). Spread may occur by direct extension through the intervening bone or tegmen tympani and/or by venous thrombophlebitis.

Acute mastoiditis is now relatively uncommon in the West. It affects children more often than adults and is due to extension of infection from the middle ear cleft into the pneumatized mastoid. From there it may spread to adjacent structures, notably the intracranial cavity. In addition to the clinical signs of the otitis, there is significant pain and swelling over the bone which displaces the pinna forwards and downwards (Fig. 20.7). The clinical presentation may be less obvious if the patient has partially responded to oral antibiotics, i.e. 'masked mastoiditis'. A plain radiograph will show opacification of the mastoid cells but a CT scan is preferable if readily available as it can demonstrate intracranial involvement. However, a normal CT scan does not exclude intracranial suppuration.

Acute mastoiditis responds to high-dose parenteral broad-spectrum antibiotics if treated promptly; if there is incomplete resolution or progression mastoid exploration is required. Other clinical symptoms and signs of intracranial extension may be apparent, in addition to headache and deep-seated otalgia, indicating the need for an early neurosurgical opinion and intervention combined with mastoid exploration. A lumbar puncture should not be performed in patients with raised intracranial pressure.

Sudden deafness

The majority of cases of sudden deafness are conductive, caused by occlusion of the external auditory meatus (wet wax or impacted wax on the drum) or due to middle ear effusion. Tuning fork tests highlight the conductive nature of the lesion. Sudden sensorineural deafness is most frequently idiopathic and probably related to a viral infection or vascular accident. Treatment with steroids and vasodilators is controversial. Care must be taken not to miss a retrocochlear lesion as 10% of acoustic nerve tumours present with a sudden hearing loss. After middle ear surgery the possibility of a perilymphatic fistula must be considered and an exploratory tympanotomy may be required to seal the leak.

Acute vertigo

Vertigo can be defined as the inappropriate sensation of motion. Acute vertiginous symptoms most commonly follow a viral infec-

REFERENCE

7. Gower D, McGuire W F Laryngoscope 1983; 93: 1028

Table 20.2 Intracranial complications of otitis media

Condition	*Clinical features*
Meningitis	Neck stiffness, photophobia, positive Kernig's sign
Lateral sinus thrombosis	Headache, rigors, spiking temperature, papilloedema, positive blood culture
Extradural abscess	Headache, early meningism
Temporal lobe abscess	
Initial	Chills, rigors, meningism, nausea, vomiting, headaches, psychological changes, tachycardia
Latent (may last for weeks)	Malaise, epileptiform attacks, neurologic signs, temperature and periodic slowing of the pulse
Manifest with raised intracranial pressure	Papilloedema, cranial neuropathies III–VII, nominal aphasia, central hearing disorders, acoustic hallucinations, visual disturbance, e.g. homonymous hemianopia, contralateral paralysis
Terminal	Increasing headache, vomiting, stupor, coma, bradycardia, Cheyne–Stokes respiration
Cerebellar abscess	Headache, ataxia, cerebellar signs, e.g. rhombergism, dysdiadochokinesia
Otitic intracranial hypertension	Headache, papilloedema, VI nerve palsy

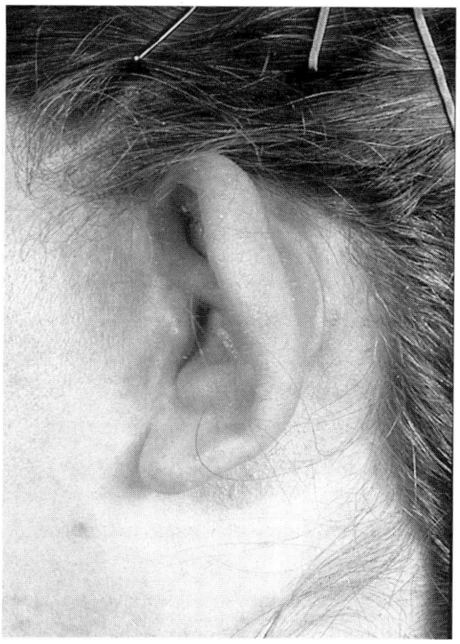

Fig. 20.7 Acute mastoiditis associated with acute otitis media pushing pinna forwards.

tion (acute labyrinthitis) when no hearing loss occurs. The vertigo is rotational and associated with nausea and vomiting. Other peripheral causes of vertigo include Menière's disease (associated fluctuant hearing loss, episodic tinnitus and a feeling of fullness in the affected ear), chronic suppurative otitis media and benign paroxysmal positional vertigo, a condition of undetermined aetiology where the vertigo is associated only with positional changes.

When the vertigo is not associated with vegetative symptoms a central lesion, e.g. tumour or multiple sclerosis, must be considered. An important aspect of the examination of the vertiginous patient is that of eye movements. Nystagmus is simply involuntary eye movements; in cases of peripheral vestibular disease it is characterized by a fast and a slow component. When the lesion is irritative the direction of the fast component is towards the affected ear. When the lesion becomes paralytic the fast component is directed away from the affected ear. Treatment is with labyrinthine sedatives, of which rectal prochlorperazine is the most useful.

Facial nerve paralysis

The VII cranial or facial nerve passes from the brainstem via the cerebello-pontine angle into the internal auditory meatus in the company of the auditory nerve. It has a complex path through the middle ear within a bony canal and mastoid cells to emerge in the neck through the stylomastoid foramen deep to the tip of the mastoid. It then divides into a number of branches within the parotid gland to supply the muscles of facial expression. A lower motor neurone paralysis may result from damage at any point in its course, conveniently divided into intracranial, intratemporal and extratemporal (Table 20.3). A careful history with ENT and neurological examination usually determines a likely cause. Displacement of the tonsil or lateral pharyngeal wall due to a mass in the deep lobe of the parotid should be sought. Appropriate audiometry, electroneuronography, CT and MRI should be requested.

Table 20.3 Causes of facial nerve paralysis

Intracranial	
Cerebrovascular accident	
Acoustic neuroma	
Meningitis (rarely)	
Intratemporal	
Acute and chronic otitis media	
Trauma:	surgical
	accidental, e.g. skull base fracture
Herpes zoster (Ramsay Hunt syndrome)	
Idiopathic (Bell's palsy)	
Tumours (rarely):	glomus, paraganglioma
	squamous cell carcinoma of external or middle ear
	metastases, e.g. breast
Extratemporal	
Parotid malignancy	
Trauma:	surgical
	accidental, e.g. facial lacerations

Bell's palsy is a diagnosis of exclusion when no other cause has been found. It has been assumed that this idiopathic lower motor neurone paralysis probably arises from a viral infection, though vascular and autoimmune factors have been suggested. In the majority (85%) of cases, recovery is complete and spontaneous so the relative value of steroids, vasodilators and surgical decompression is difficult to determine. A small number of patient are left with significant weakness. In common with all facial palsies, protection of the cornea is most important as the cornea may ulcerate without a blink reflex. Corneal protection is achieved by a lateral tarsorrhaphy, either temporary or permanent, combined with lubricants and artificial tears.

In addition to the treatment of an established cause for the facial palsy, e.g. parotidectomy for a malignant tumour or removal of an acoustic neuroma, the entire course of the facial nerve is accessible for repair where appropriate. This may include an 'end to end' repair or the interposition of a nerve graft.

Tumours

Fortunately, malignant tumours of the ear are very rare but several benign growths may have serious consequences because of their site of origin. An acoustic neuroma may arise from the auditory nerve within the internal auditory canal, which it expands causing unilateral hearing and tinnitus (Fig. 20.8). Other cranial nerve palsies, raised intracranial pressure and compression of the brainstem ultimately ensue. In von Recklinghausen's disease bilateral lesions may occur. A low threshold of suspicion should lead to early diagnosis and treatment with a commensurate reduction in operative morbidity and mortality. MRI is the most reliable diagnostic technique.[8]

Another benign lesion which is also best demonstrated by MRI is the glomus tumour arising from paraganglionic tissue (Fig. 20.9). This can be found in a number of sites in the head and neck including the middle ear (glomus tympanicum) and jugular bulb (glomus jugulare). It characteristically produces pulsatile

REFERENCES

8. Phelps P D, Lloyd G A S Diagnostic Imaging of the Ear, 2nd edn. Springer Verlag, London 1990: 175–192

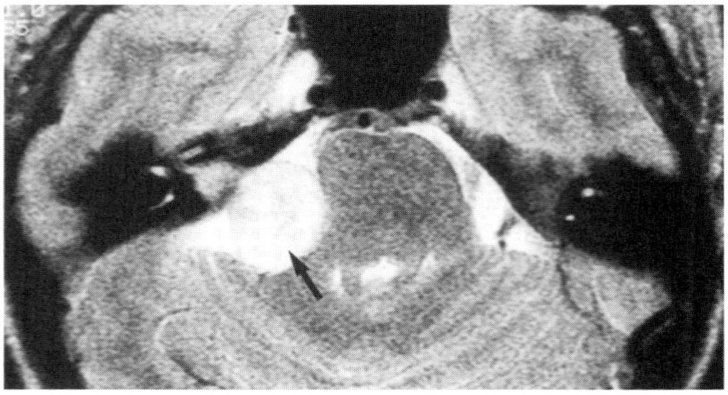

Fig. 20.8 Axial MRI scan (T_2-weighted sequence) showing left acoustic neuroma (arrowed). With kind permission of Dr P D Phelps.

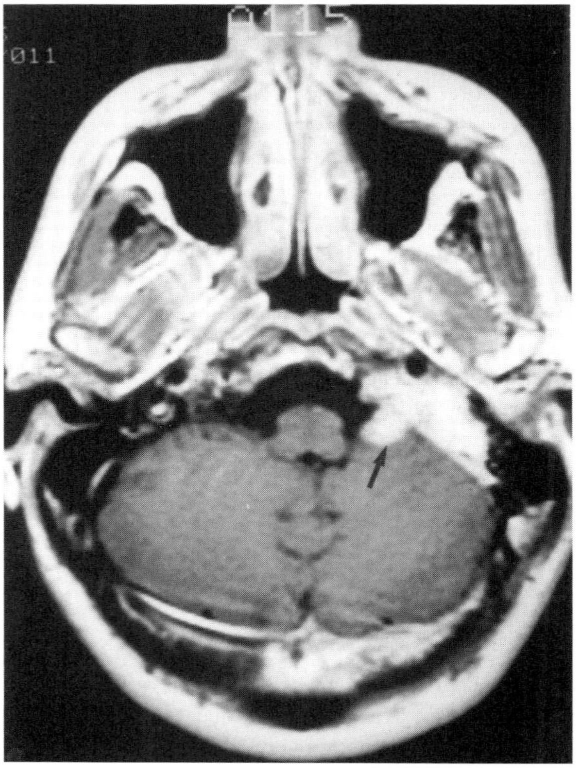

Fig. 20.9 Axial MRI scan (T_1-weighted sequence with gadolinium-DTPA) showing left glomus jugulare (arrowed). With kind permission of Dr P D Phelps.

tinnitus, hearing loss and ultimately cranial nerve palsies (VII, IX, X, XI, XII). The size of the lesion and age of the patient determine whether treatment is by surgery, radiotherapy or a combination of both.

THE NOSE

Surgical anatomy[9]

The nose consists of two nasal cavities beginning anteriorly at the nasal vestibule and ending at the posterior choana where the nasopharynx begins. The nasal cavities are divided by a nasal septum composed of an anterior cartilaginous portion consisting of a large quadrilateral cartilage with a small contribution from the upper and lower lateral alar cartilages, and a posterior bony part made up of the perpendicular plate of the ethmoid and vomer (Fig. 20.10). The lateral wall of the nose has three (or sometimes four) turbinates covering meatuses into which the sinuses drain. The anterior ethmoids, maxillary and frontal sinuses drain into the middle meatus (sometimes termed the 'ostiomeatal complex'), the posterior ethmoids into the superior meatus, and the sphenoid into the sphenoethmoidal recess above the posterior choana. The naso-lacrimal duct drains into the inferior meatus.

Most of the nasal mucosa is respiratory ciliated epithelium (Fig. 20.11), with a small area of skin in the vestibule, some areas of squamous metaplasia on the anterior ends of the turbinates and, superiorly, olfactory epithelium extending down from the nasal roof a variable distance on to the superior turbinate and nasal septum. The cilia waft mucus produced by seromucinous glands and goblet cells from the sinuses and nasal cavity via the nasopharynx, into the oropharynx whence it is swallowed. The sinuses drain by predetermined pathways into the nose through clefts which are vulnerable to obstruction leading to secondary bacterial infection. The close proximity of the sinuses to the orbit and anterior cranial cavity renders the latter structures at risk of involvement in severe acute infection and, less commonly, from the spread of sinonasal malignancy.

Investigation

The nose can be examined with a headlight and nasal speculum, a fibre-optic speculum and rigid or flexible endoscopes. Examination is assisted by the use of local anaesthetics and vasoconstrictors, e.g. cocaine, lignocaine and adrenaline. Plain sinus radiographs can be used to screen for rhinosinusitis but a CT scan is preferred for its optimal demonstration of the anatomy and pathology.[10] CT may be combined with MRI in the imaging of neoplasia.[11,12] Other investigations include tests for allergy, airway, mucociliary clearance and immune function.

Rhinosinusitis

Rhinosinusitis may be broadly defined as inflammation of the nose and sinuses characterized by one or more of the following symptoms: nasal congestion, rhinorrhoea, sneezing, itching and hyposmia. It may be classified as allergic and non-allergic (Table 20.4) but a number of other conditions must be considered in the differential diagnosis.

Infectious rhinosinusitis covers a range of acute and chronic infections—viral, bacterial and fungal (Table 20.5). Acute

REFERENCES

9. Maran A G D, Lund V J. Clinical Rhinology. Thieme, Stuttgart 1990: 5–22
10. Zinreich S J, Kennedy D W, Rosenbaum A E, Gayler B W, Kumar A J, Stammberger H J Radiol 1987; 163: 769
11. Lund V J, Howard D J, Lloyd G A S, Cheesman A D Head Neck Surg 1989; 11: 279
12. Lund V J, Lloyd G A S, Howard D J, Cheesman A D, Phelps P D Laryngoscope 1996; 106: 553

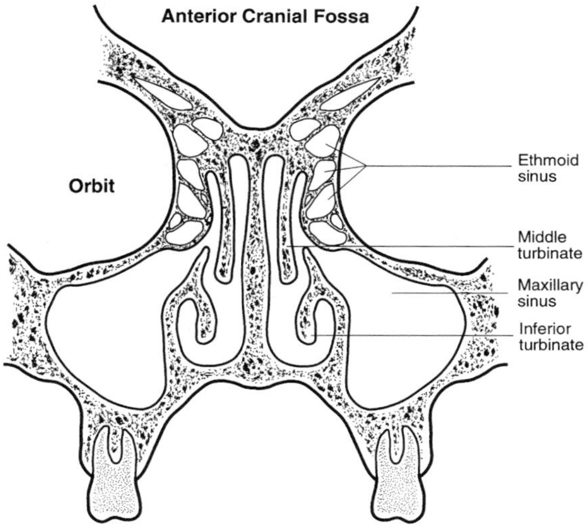

Fig. 20.10 Diagram showing coronal section through nasal cavity.

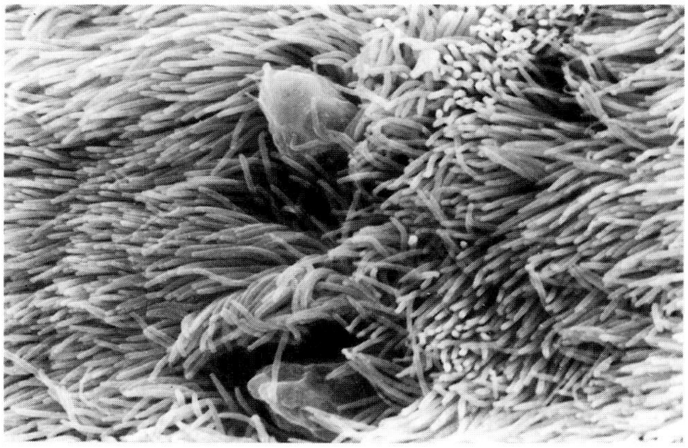

Fig. 20.11 Scanning electron micrograph (× 2300) showing ciliated columnar epithelium of nasal mucosa.

rhinosinusitis usually resolves spontaneously or with a short course of oral antibiotics but may be seen in hospital practice when a serious complication occurs. Involvement of the orbit and/or intracranial cavity constitutes a medical emergency (Table 20.6) (Fig. 20.12). In the orbit, vision may be lost and rarely recovers. The intracranial complications can be life-threatening, requiring neurosurgical intervention[13,14] (Figs 20.13 and 20.14). Complications are multiple in 30% of cases and the mortality from intracranial spread has not changed significantly in the last twenty years.[15]

In addition to the usual symptoms of nasal obstruction, purulent discharge, facial pain/headache and pyrexia there may be significant swelling around the eye, with additional proptosis, limitation of eye movement and visual loss depending upon the degree of orbital involvement. It is mandatory that the eye be adequately examined and kept under review irrespective of the associated discomfort. Symptoms of intracranial involvement such as headache, malaise and pyrexia may be obscured by those of the sinusitis but signs of meningism, raised intracranial pressure, focal neurological signs and drowsiness should alert the physician to this possibility.

Table 20.4 Classification of rhinosinusitis

1. *Allergic*
Seasonal
Perennial
2. *Non-allergic—infectious*
Acute
Chronic
3. *Non-allergic—non-infectious*
Idiopathic
Occupational
NARES
Hormonal
Drug-induced
Irritants
Food
Emotional
Atrophic
Differential diagnosis
Polyps
Mechanical factors
Deviated septum
Hypertrophic turbinates
Adenoidal hypertrophy
Anatomical variants in the ostiomeatal complex
Foreign bodies
Choanal atresia
Tumours
Benign
Malignant
Granulomas
Wegener's granulomatosis
Sarcoid
Infective—tuberculosis
leprosy
Malignant—midline destructive granuloma (T cell lymphoma)
Cerebrospinal rhinorrhoea

Table 20.5 Microbiology from rhinosinusitis (acute and chronic)

Viral
Rhinovirus
Influenza
Parainfluenza
Bacterial
Haemophilus influenzae
Streptococcus pneumoniae
Staphylococcus aureus
Streptococcus milleri
Streptococcus pyogenes
Pseudomonas aeruginosa
Klebsiella spp
Moraxella catarrhalis
Anaerobes
Fungal
Aspergillus
Dermatiacetes — Curvularia
— Bipolaris
— Alternaria
Mucormycosis, etc.

REFERENCES

13. Clayman G L, Adams G L, Paugh D R, Koopman C F Laryngoscope 1991; 101: 234
14. Chandler J R, Langenbrunner D J, Stevens E R Laryngoscope 1970; 80: 1414
15. Singh B, Van Dellen J, Ramjettan S, Maharaj T J Laryngol Otol 1995; 109: 945

Table 20.6 Complications of rhinosinusitis

Acute	
Local	
Orbital	Preseptal cellulitis
	Orbital cellulitis without abscess
	Orbital cellulitis with sub- or extraperiosteal abscess
	Orbital cellulitis with intraperiosteal abscess
	Cavernous sinus thrombosis
Intracranial	Abscess: extradural
	subdural
	intracerebral
	Meningitis
	Encephalitis
	Cavernous or sagittal sinus thrombosis
Bony	Osteitis/osteomyelitis (Pott's puffy tumour)
Dental	
Distant	
Toxic shock syndrome	
Chronic	
Mucocoele/pyocoele	
Associated diseases	
? Otitis media, adenotonsillitis, bronchiectasis	

High-dose broad-spectrum parenteral antibiotics covering likely aerobes and anaerobes should be commenced immediately and intranasal vasoconstrictor drops may be used. A plain sinus radiograph will demonstrate opacification of the sinuses and a CT scan will confirm the sinusitis and define the complications. Time should not be lost, however, if the orbit is involved and vision is clearly failing; under these circumstances, drainage of the sinuses should be undertaken forthwith.[16]

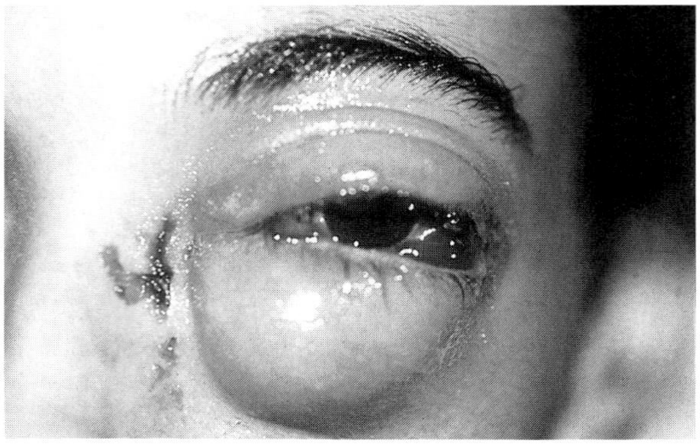
a

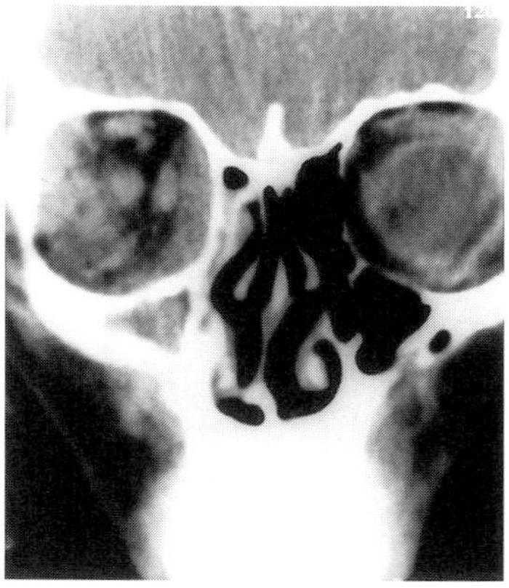
b

Fig. 20.12 (**a**) Acute orbital cellulitis with intraperiosteal abscess associated with acute pansinusitis. (**b**) Coronal CT scan of same patient.

Injury

The nose is frequently subject to injury, either as a circumscribed injury or as part of a more severe midfacial injury as in a road traffic accident. Fractures may be linear or severely comminuted 'smash' fractures involving frontal and lacrimal bones, the orbital rim and ethmoid, including the cribriform plate.[17] The latter may produce a leak of cerebrospinal fluid and/or loss of the sense of smell. A C-shaped fracture of the nasal septum frequently accompanies fractures of the nasal bones.[18] Radiographs of the nasal bones are frequently unhelpful but facial views may be required to exclude more extensive injury. Oedema of the overlying tissues usually obscures the deformity unless the patient is seen within 1–2 hours of the injury so the majority of patients are referred to an ENT surgeon for manipulation under anaesthesia. This should

REFERENCES

16. Lund V J In: Mackay I S, Bull T R (eds) Scott Brown's Otolaryngology—Rhinology. Butterworth-Heinemann 1997; 4: 1–11
17. Starkhammar H, Olofsson J Clin Otolaryngol 1982; 7: 405
18. Murray J A M, Maran A G D Injury 1986; 17: 338

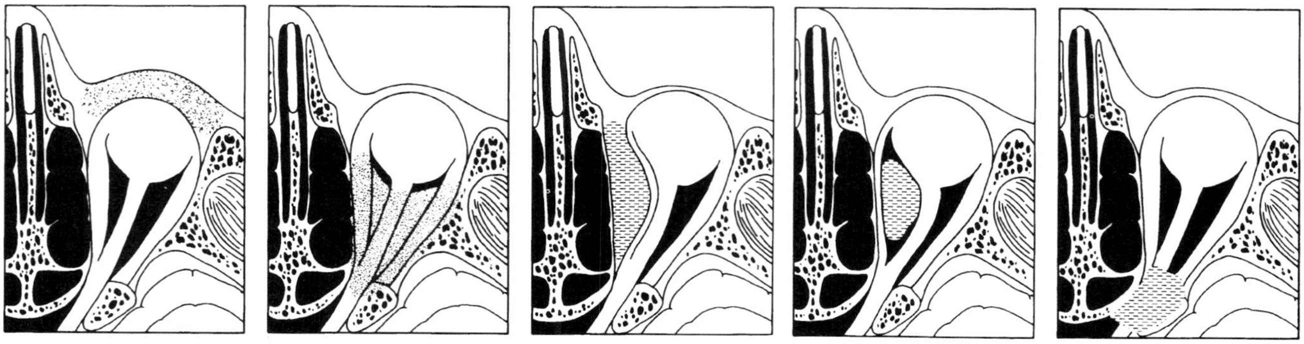
a b c d e

Fig. 20.13 Diagram showing spectrum of orbital complications associated with acute sinusitis: (**a**) preseptal inflammation; (**b**) orbital cellulitis; (**c**) orbital cellulitis with subperiosteal (extraperiosteal) abscess; (**d**) orbital cellulitis with intraperiosteal abscess; (**e**) cavernous sinus thrombosis. With permission of Butterworth–Heinemann, Scott-Brown's Otolaryngology 6th edition. Volume 4, Rhinology 1997.

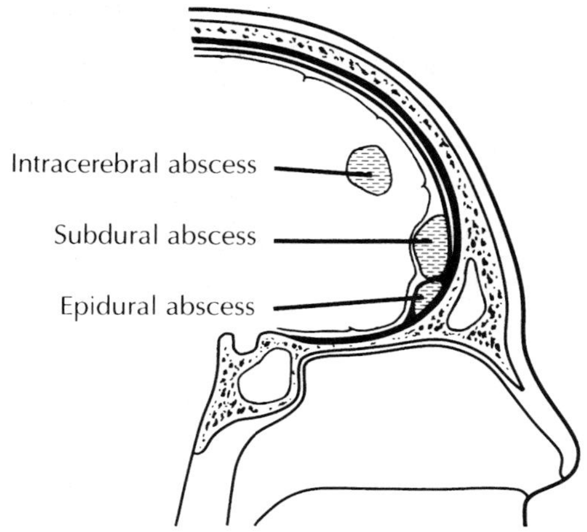

Fig. 20.14 Diagram showing spectrum of intracranial complications associated with acute sinusitis. With permission of Butterworth–Heinemann, Scott-Brown's Otolaryngology 6th edition. Volume 4, Rhinology 1997.

ideally be performed within 10 days of the injury. If a septal haematoma is suspected, however, this should be immediately drained under antibiotic cover to avoid necrosis of septal cartilage and cosmetic deformity.

Foreign bodies

The nose is a favourite site for insertion of a wide variety of foreign bodies. There is often a unilateral foul-smelling purulent discharge which, together with mucosal swelling, may obscure any view even with an endoscope; a radiograph will only help if the object is radiopaque. If the history is strong enough, the patient should be referred for an ENT opinion and examination under general anaesthetic.

Epistaxis

Nose bleeds can result from a wide range of local and systemic conditions, of which trauma is the most common (Table 20.7). The nose has an excellent blood supply and bleeding can occur from any area, though the most common is on the anterior nasal septum, from Little's area. Bleeding can range from occasional slight spotting to torrential life-threatening haemorrhage and the severity obviously dictates management. Many minor bleeds stop with simple pressure, with or without intranasal instillation of local anaesthetic/vasoconstrictor and cauterization of an obvious bleeding spot. More severe bleeds necessitate general resuscitation with intravenous fluid replacement, emergency cross-matching of blood, and appropriate haematological investigation (full blood count, haematocrit, clotting studies). If bleeding is too profuse to adequately examine the nose, a nasal pack should be inserted, preferably using 2 cm wide Vaseline gauze (Fig. 20.15). If layered carefully, 2 metres of gauze can be inserted in each nostril. If bleeding continues despite this, a postnasal pack may be required. In either case the patient must be admitted for observation and placed on antibiotics. Sedatives should not be given as they may further compromise respiration; anti-hypertensive agents are not required as an initially raised blood pressure will generally settle with bed rest. Occasionally packing under general anaesthesia and arterial ligation or embolization may be required.

Table 20.7 Causes of epistaxis

Local	
Idiopathic	
Trauma	Self-inflicted
	Facial fractures
	Iatrogenic—surgery
	Septal deviation
	Foreign bodies
	Septal perforation
Inflammatory	Atrophic rhinitis
Infectious	
Tumours	Benign, e.g. angiofibroma
	Malignant
General	
Atherosclerosis	
Bleeding dyscrasia	
a. Coagulation disorders	
Congenital	Haemophilia
	Christmas disease
	Von Willebrand's
Acquired	Renal and liver failure
	Massive transfusion
	Vitamin deficiency
	Anticoagulants
	Myelosuppressive drugs
b. Haemopoietic	Leukaemia
	Aplastic anaemia
	Lymphoma
	Widespread metastases
Hereditary haemorrhagic telangiectasia	
Endocrine	Vicarious menstruation
	Pregnancy

Nasal polyps

Nasal polyps are pedunculated masses composed of oedematous mucosa arising within the clefts of the lateral wall of the nose and

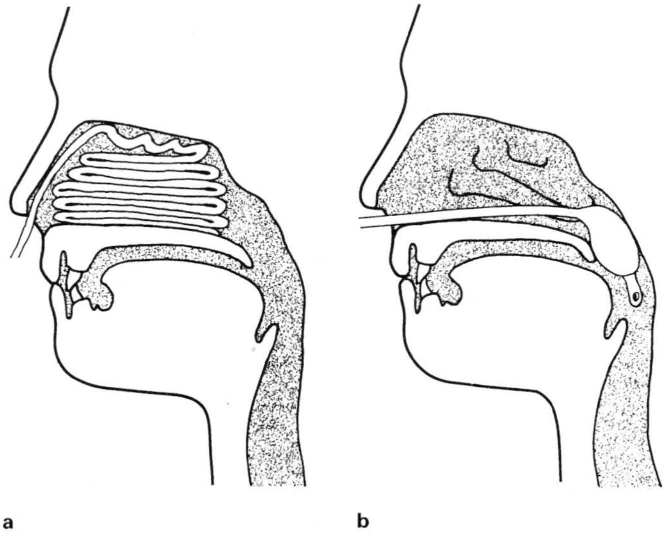

Fig. 20.15 (**a**) Diagram showing the placement of anterior nasal packing for epistaxis. (**b**) Diagram showing the placement of a Foley urinary catheter to control posterior nasal bleeding. After Skinner, Cambridge Textbook of Emergency Medicine. 1997

sinuses (Figs 20.16 and 20.17). They may occur in association with cystic fibrosis (25% in children,[19] 45% in adults[20]), asthma[21] and as part of aspirin idiosyncrasy[22] (acetylsalicylic acid sensitivity, sinusitis and asthma) but they most commonly occur alone. Infection, inflammation and imbalance of the arachidonic acid pathway have all been suggested as aetiological factors though allergy is not a cause. Complete cure is unusual but symptomatic relief can be achieved by a combination of steroids (intranasal and parenteral) and surgical removal.[23]

Chronic rhinosinusitis

Chronic rhinosinusitis is deemed to exist after symptoms have persisted for more than 12 weeks.[24] Allergy, mucociliary disturbance and immune deficiency may predispose certain individuals to the development of chronic infection. Patients may improve with intensive medication, e.g. long-term oral antibiotics and intranasal steroids, but surgery is frequently required. A more conservative approach has prevailed in recent years, complemented by the improved visualization afforded by CT scanning and the rigid endoscope; procedures such as the Caldwell–Luc operation are now rarely performed[25] (Fig. 20.18) The term 'functional endoscopic sinus surgery' has been applied to precise endoscopic surgery dictated by the pathology commencing in the middle meatus.[26]

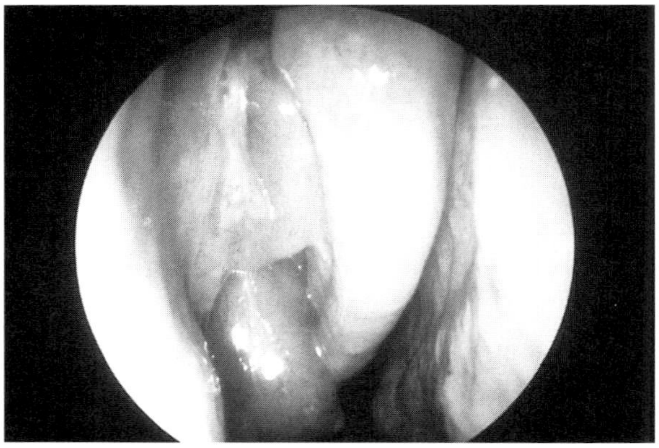

Fig. 20.16 Endoscopic view of nasal polyps in right middle meatus.

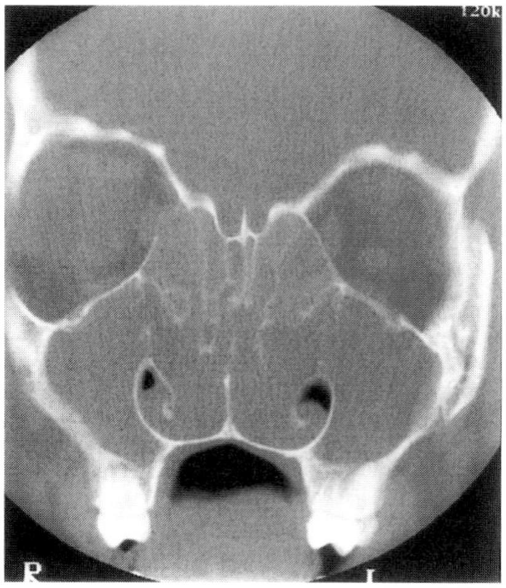

Fig. 20.17 Coronal CT scan showing extensive opacification of the nose and paranasal sinuses in nasal polyposis.

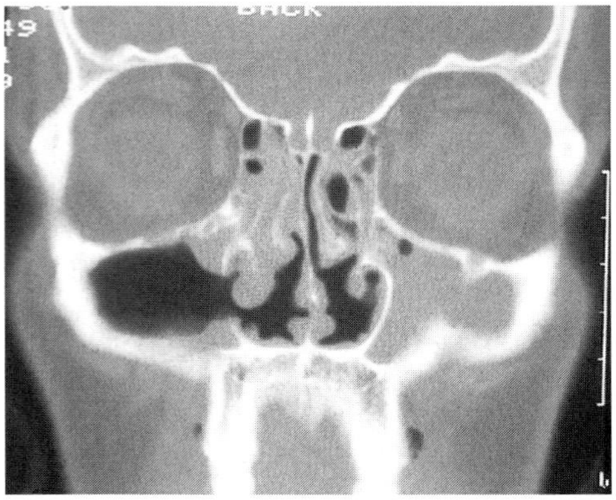

Fig. 20.18 Coronal CT scan showing chronic rhinosinusitis in a patient who has already undergone a right inferior meatal antrostomy.

Tumours

Sinonasal neoplasia is relatively rare but should be suspected when symptoms persist, particularly if they are unilateral. A comprehensive examination of the nose and sinuses must be undertaken. Similarly, serious systemic conditions such as Wegener's granulomatosis and sarcoidosis may first manifest themselves in the nose and sinuses.[27] Malignant sinonasal tumours comprise less than 3% of head and neck malignancy and are found in less than 1 in 100 000 of the population. Patients often present with advanced disease and oncological treatment is frequently compromised by the close proximity of the orbit and intracranial cavity (Fig. 20.19). Although squamous cell carcinoma is the commonest tumour encountered, this region offers the greatest histological diversity in the body. Men are more frequently affected than women, as in the rest of the aero-digestive tract, but the ratio is a less extreme 2:1. Smoking and alcohol have less impact in this location, whereas inhaled carcinogens in an occupational setting have a greater impact. Lengthy exposure to hardwood dust increases the relative risk of adenocarcinoma of the ethmoid to 70 times normal. Specialized histology and imaging (contrast-enhanced CT and

REFERENCES

19. Stern R C, Boat T F, Wood R E Am J Dis Child 1982; 136: 1067
20. DiSant'Agnese P A, David P B Am J Med 1979; 66: 121
21. Drake-Lee A B, Lowe D, Swanston A, Grace A J Laryngol Otol 1984; 98: 783
22. Spector S L, Wangaard C H, Farr R S J Allergy Clin Immunol 1979; 64: 500
23. Lund V J Br Med J 1995; 331: 1411
24. Kennedy D, Stammberger H, Lund V J Ann Otol Rhinol Laryngol 1995; (Suppl 167)
25. Stammberger H Otolaryngol Head Neck Surg 1986; 94: 143
26. Kennedy D W, Zinreich S J, Rosenbaum A E et al Archiv Oto-Rhino-Laryngol 1985; 111: 576
27. Lund V J, Howard D J In: Gershwin M E, Incaudo G A (eds) Diseases of the Sinuses. Humana, Totowa New Jersey 1996: 291–310

a

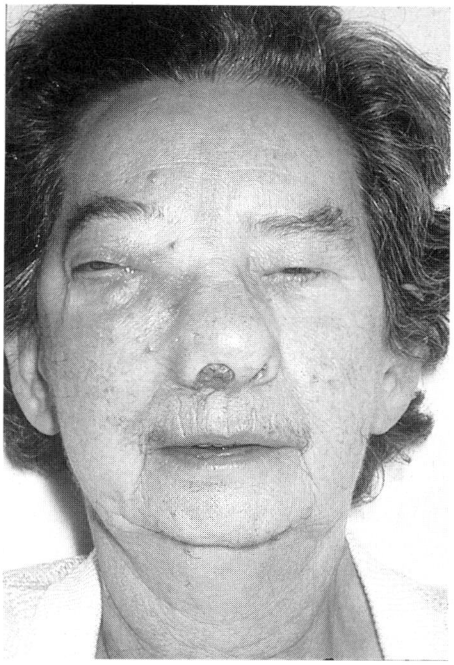

b

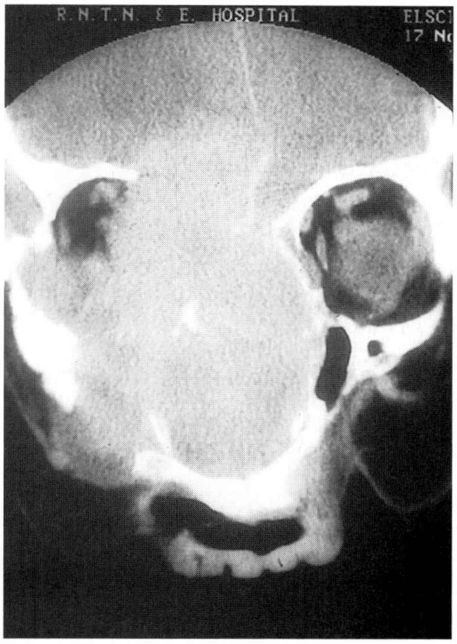

Fig. 20.19 **(a)** Patient with advanced poorly differentiated squamous cell carcinoma of the right antroethmoid and nasal cavity. **(b)** Coronal CT scan of above showing extensive intracranial extension.

MRI) are necessary to determine the diagnosis and extent. Depending upon histology, therapy consists of surgery and/or radiotherapy with occasional additional chemotherapy. A number of surgical approaches are available. For any tumour which has transgressed the anterior skull base, a craniofacial resection offers the best chance of cure. For lesions of the nasal cavity and maxillary sinus, a lateral rhinotomy, midfacial degloving approach and maxillectomies of varying extent may be chosen. An obturator can be inserted at the end of surgery to allow immediate resumption of speech and eating whilst prosthetic replacements of the orbit are available for cases where disease spread necessitates orbital clearance. Fixation of these prostheses can be enhanced by osseointegration techniques.

NASOPHARYNX

Surgical anatomy

The nasopharynx or postnasal space is situated with the posterior choana anteriorly and the soft palate inferiorly. Superiorly it is related to the skull base and posteriorly to the vertebral bodies. The cartilaginous pharyngeal eustachian tube enters the space superolaterally and forms the anterior border of the fossa of Rosenmüller. The adenoids are found on the posterior pharyngeal wall (Figs 20.20 and 20.21). Their lymphatic drainage is via the retropharyngeal nodes to both sides of the neck passing to the deep cervical nodes and posteriorly to the nodes in the posterior triangle.

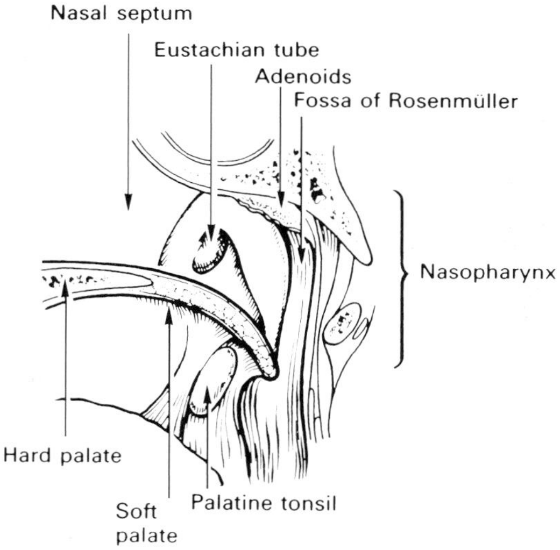

Fig. 20.20 The nasopharynx: sagittal section.

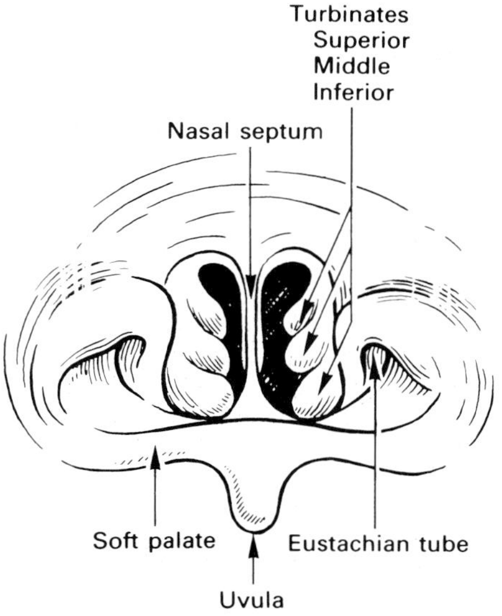

Fig. 20.21 The nasopharynx: view by posterior rhinoscopy.

The adenoids are collections of lymphoid tissue covered by squamous epithelium, present in childhood but tending to regress during adolescence (Fig. 20.22). Examination of the postnasal space can be achieved by retrograde mirror examination from the mouth or using either a flexible or rigid endoscope.

Adenoidectomy

Adenoidectomy is still one of the most frequently performed operations in paediatric practice. Indications for surgery include nasal blockage, especially when associated with a sleep apnoea syndrome, persistent nasopharyngeal infection and chronic otitis media with effusion (glue ear).[28,29]

Surgical excision is performed through the mouth under general anaesthesia using an oral tube. The adenoids are curetted from the posterior pharyngeal wall using an adenotome. Care is taken not to damage the eustachian tube opening laterally or the anterior arch of the atlas posteriorly. Haemostasis is obtained by means of a temporary postnasal pack. Primary haemorrhage is uncommon and usually follows inadequate removal of the adenoids, necessitating recuretting and repacking. Adenoidectomy is contraindicated in children with cleft palate abnormalities as a speech defect, rhinolalia aperta, may result.[30]

Nasopharyngeal carcinoma

Nasopharyngeal carcinoma generally accounts for only 4% of head and neck tumours but in China it accounts for 21% of all malignant neoplasms.[31] Many aetiological factors have been suggested—a genetic basis (Cantonese Chinese), the increased deposition of carcinogens in the fossa of Rosenmüller and the Epstein–Barr virus. Antibodies to the Epstein–Barr viral capsid antigen and the early antigen are found in advanced cases.[32]

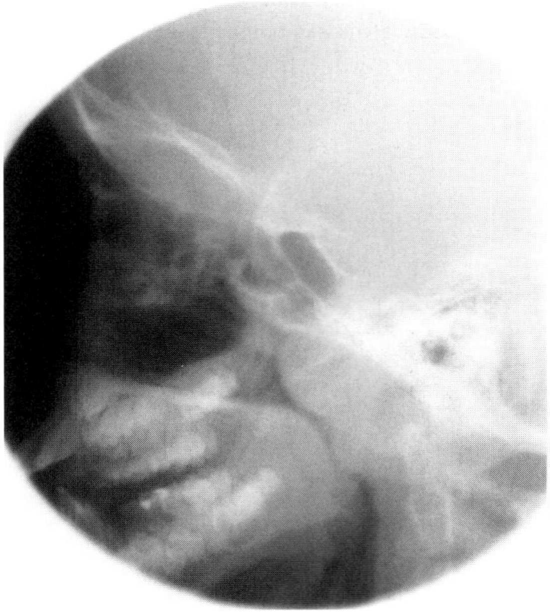

Fig. 20.22 Lateral plain radiograph showing adenoid mass in postnasal space. With kind permission of Dr P D Phelps.

Nasopharyngeal carcinoma most frequently presents in the fourth decade and is more common in men by a ratio of 4:1. The tumours are frequently poorly differentiated and when significant lymphoid infiltration has occurred the term 'lymphoepithelioma' has been used. However, this does not suggest any lymphoid neoplasia.

The most common presentations are nasal blockage with a sanguinous rhinorrhoea, sometimes frank epistaxis, a conductive hearing loss due to fluid in the middle ear and cervical lymph node enlargement. Pain, usually perceived in the ear as a referred otalgia, and cranial nerve neuropathies may occur.

The postnasal space must be carefully examined under general anaesthetic and even if no tumour is visible, blind biopsies must be taken in any adult with persistent unilateral fluid in the middle ear. A full examination of the cranial nerves must be made as 20% of patients will have at least one cranial nerve palsy. Plain radiography of the skull base may reveal lucent areas in the region of the foramen lacerum and the greater wing of sphenoid or hyperostosis in adjacent vertebrae. Computerized tomography and MRI scanning will optimally delineate the tumour and act as an aid for planning radiotherapy (Fig. 20.23).

The tumour may be biopsied through the nose while the nasopharynx is examined by a mirror inserted through the mouth aided by traction from a catheter which has been passed through the nose and delivered back through the mouth. Alternatively the area may be biopsied under direct vision using a rigid endoscope through the nose. In cases where no overt tumour is seen but the patient has cervical lymphadenopathy of unknown origin or persistent unilateral middle ear effusion, blind biopsies of the

REFERENCES

28. Bluestone C D, Cantekin E I, Berry Q C Laryngoscope 1975; 85: 113
29. Merck W HNO (Berlin) 1974; 22: 198
30. Goode R L, Ross J Arch Otolaryngol 1972; 96: 223
31. Buell P J Cancer 1965; 19: 459
32. Henle W J Natl Cancer Inst 1970; 44: 225

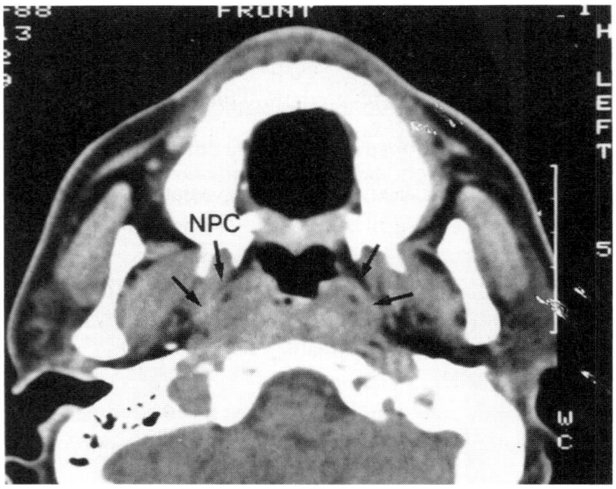

Fig. 20.23 Coronal CT scan showing a normal nasopharynx. Arrows indicate Fossae & Rosenmüller.

nasopharynx should be taken as up to 25% will be positive for tumour.[33]

Radiotherapy is the primary modality of treatment.[34] The field must include the cervical nodes even if they are clinically free of disease. Radiosensitizers may be used but chemotherapy has little place in treatment.[34] The 5-year survival rate for T1 tumours is in the region of 75%, falling to less than 15% in tumours that have spread laterally from the nasopharynx.[35] The presence of lymphatic metastases reduces these figures, although not greatly[36] (Table 20.8).

Other tumours may arise or present in the nasopharynx including neurilemmoma, chordoma, lymphoma, plasmacytoma and rhabdomyosarcoma. Juvenile angiofibroma, a hamartomatous lesion occurring exclusively in young males, arises in the region of the spheno-palatine foramen and extends from the nasal cavity into the nasopharynx where it presents as a unilateral polyp. Biopsies should never be undertaken as the angiofibroma is highly vascular in nature but a definitive diagnosis may be made with the pathognomonic features seen on CT scanning and MRI.[38] (See also Chapter 13).

Benign lymphoid hyperplasia may occur in HIV infection, and the nasopharynx is also the site of a number of congenital cysts and clefts (e.g. Thornwaldt's cyst).

THE TONGUE AND OROPHARYNX

Surgical anatomy

Although the tongue is anatomically part of the oral cavity, malignant tumours do not always respect these geographical divisions. It may be considered from an embryological perspective as divided into an anterior two thirds (anterior to the vallate papillae) and a posterior third. The interlacing muscle fibres of the tongue form an easy pathway for tumour spread with the median septum providing no barrier; the rich blood and lymphatic supply also facilitate embolic spread through the tongue substance and early dissemination to the cervical lymph nodes, which may be bilateral. The tip drains to submental nodes and the deep jugular chain. The sublingual part drains to the submandibular nodes and the rest of the anterior two thirds drains to the deep jugular chain from the level of the omohyoid to the posterior belly of digastric. Thus lesions on the lateral border of the tongue may only produce enlargement of the jugulo-omohyoid node.[36] The posterior third drains to the upper deep jugular nodes.

The oropharynx stretches from the soft palate to the pharyngoepiglottic fold. The pharyngeal wall lies posteriorly and the anterosuperior margin of the laryngeal vallecula forms the posterolateral boundary. Anterolaterally are the faucial pillars (anterior pillar: the palatoglossus muscle; posterior pillar: the palatopharyngeus muscle) which guard the palatine tonsils. Anteroinferiorly is the posterior third of the tongue bounded anteriorly by the sulcus terminalis and inferiorly by the lingual tonsil (Fig. 20.24). The lymphoid drainage of this region is often to both deep cervical chains with the tonsil specifically draining to the jugulodigastric node. The palatine tonsils tend to hypertrophy physiologically during childhood but in the adult are hardly visible because of the faucial pillars (Fig. 20.25).

Table 20.8 Three-year survival rates of nasopharyngeal carcinoma

Classification	*Affected area*	*3-year survival*
Stage I	Nasopharynx alone	93%
Stage II	Upper neck nodes	79%
Stage III	Lower neck nodes	60%
	Bone/cranial nerves	
Stage IV	Supraclavicular nodes	No data
Stage V	Distant metastasis	16%

From Neel[37]

The tonsils

Acute tonsillitis is characterized by a severe sore throat which usually produces difficulty in swallowing and may be associated

REFERENCES

33. Cowley J J JAMA 1971; 215: 456
34. Chew C T In: Kerr A G (ed) Scott Brown's Otolaryngology. Butterworth, London 1988
35. International Classification of Diseases for Oncology ICD-O 1977 In: Manual of the International Statistical Classification of Diseases, Injuries and Causes of Death, vol 1. World Health Organization, Geneva
36. Maran A G D, Gaze M, Wilson J A Stell and Maran's Head and Neck Surgery, 3rd edn. Butterworth-Heinemann, Oxford; 1993

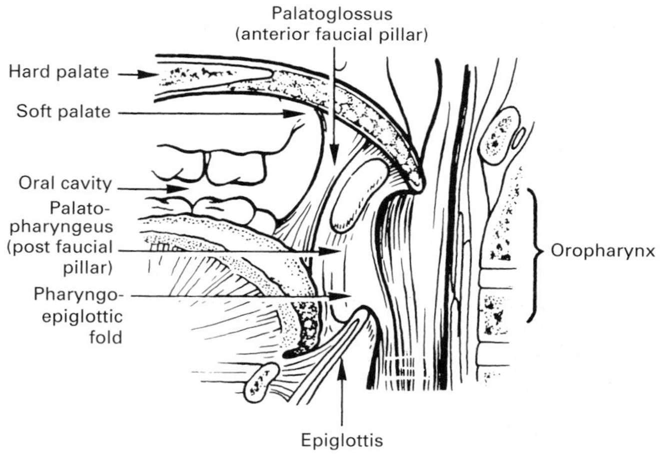

Fig. 20.24 The oropharynx: sagittal section.

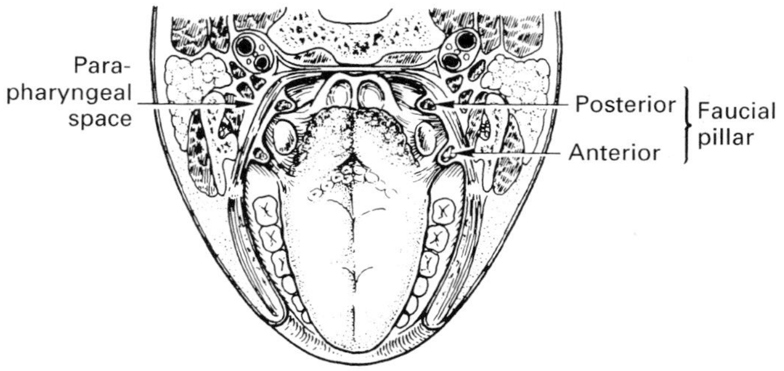

Fig. 20.25 The mouth and oropharynx: coronal section.

with pyrexia, general malaise and earache (Fig. 20.26). This last symptom is due to referred pain along the glossopharyngeal nerve running in the tonsillar bed to the tympanic plexus. A range of organisms are responsible for both acute and chronic tonsillitis (Table 20.9). Tonsillar enlargement, both unilateral and bilateral, may occur when neoplasia affects the lymphoid tissue, e.g. leukaemia and lymphoma. Diagnosis may be assisted by a throat swab, full blood count and differential and a Paul–Bunnell test. A broad-spectrum antibiotic should be given for acute bacterial tonsillitis, though amoxycillin should be avoided if glandular fever is suspected as this may result in the complication of a maculopapular rash.

Simple tonsillar hypertrophy is not necessarily pathological and its presence is not an indication for tonsillectomy. If however there is respiratory obstruction (sleep apnoea), recurrent attacks of acute follicular tonsillitis (more than four attacks per year) or more than one peritonsillar abscess, tonsillectomy is indicated.[39]

Tonsillectomy is usually performed under general anaesthesia using a nasotracheal tube and a Boyle–Davis gag in an adult. In the child an oral tube is used because of the likelihood of a coincidental adenoidal mass. A mucosal incision is made lateral to the edge of the anterior faucial pillar. The peritonsillar space is opened and, with the tonsil being retracted medially and inferiorly, it is dissected out of its fossa (Fig. 20.27). As the tonsil is continuous inferiorly with the base of the tongue, this area is snared off to reduce haemorrhage and so deliver the tonsil. Haemostasis may be achieved by diathermy or individual ties.

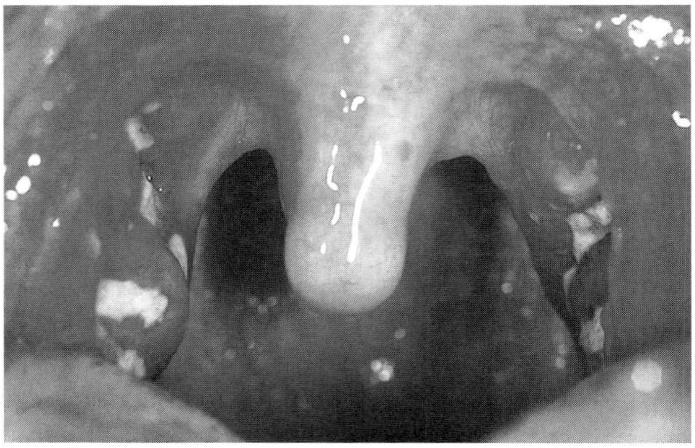

Fig. 20.26 Acute follicular tonsillitis.

Table 20.9 Acute tonsillitis

Viral	Rhinovirus Adenovirus Enterovirus Epstein–Barr/infectious mononucleosis HIV
Bacterial	β-haemolytic streptococcus *Staphylococci* spp *Pneumococci* spp *H. influenzae* *E. coli*
Rarely	*Corynebacterium diphtheriae* *Treponema pallidum* *Mycobacterium tuberculosis* Candida (in association with AIDS) Anaerobes (*Bacteroides fragilis*)

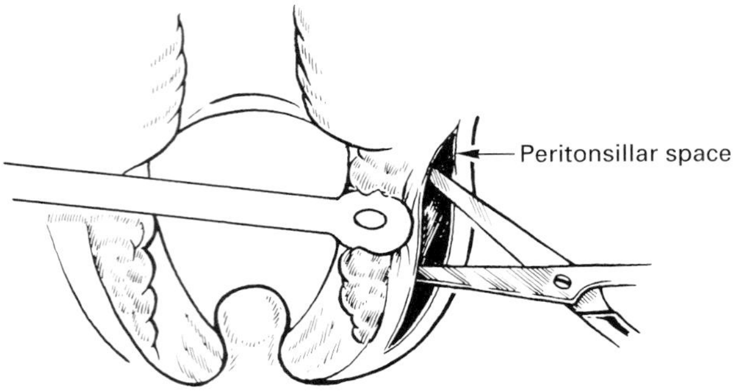

Fig. 20.27 Dissection of peritonsillar space.

Postoperative bleeding from the tonsillar bed may occur immediately after surgery (primary) or within the first 48 hours (reactionary). It may respond to a local adrenaline 1:10 000 pack

REFERENCES

37. Neel HB Otolaryngology: Head and Neck Surgery. Mosby, St Louis 1986
38. Lund V J, Lloyd G A S, Howard D J Rhinology 1989; 27: 179
39. Mawson S R, Adlington P, Evans M J Laryngol 1968; 82: 963

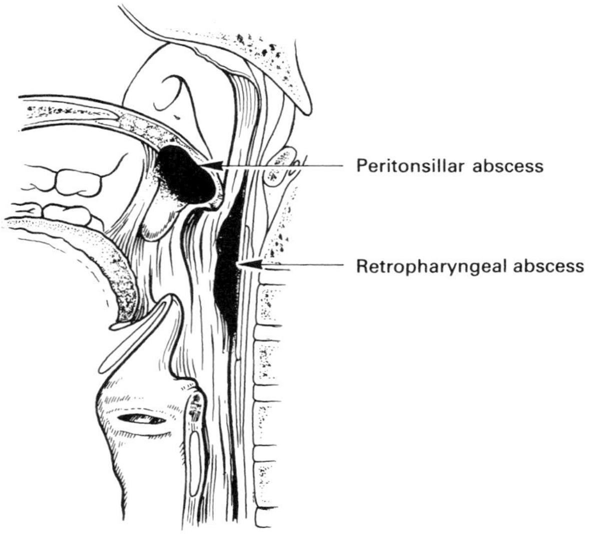

Fig. 20.28 The pharynx and larynx: midsagittal section.

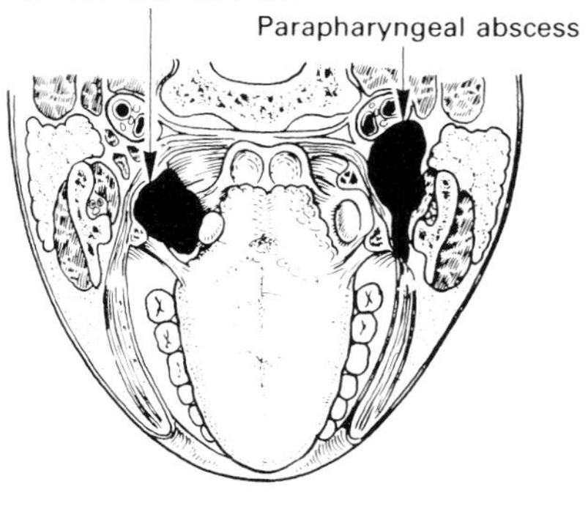

Fig. 20.29 Position of pharyngeal abscesses.

applied to the fossa but frequently re-exploration is necessary especially in a child. The induction of anaesthesia in such a situation is fraught with difficulty as the anaesthetist battles with a restless patient, a pharynx full of blood and a very poor view of the larynx.[40,41] Secondary haemorrhage occurs in approximately 1% of patients, usually between the 5th and 8th day postoperatively and usually due to infection.[42] Operative intervention is usually not indicated; simple supportive measures and parenteral antibiotic therapy suffice.

Foreign bodies

The most common foreign body found in the oropharynx is a fishbone which is usually found embedded in the palatine or lingual tonsil. Careful inspection after the application of good local anaesthesia often reveals the offending bone. Direct removal using Tilley's forceps is feasible for a bone stuck in the tonsil but the laryngeal mirror is usually required for those in the lingual tonsil/tongue base. Alternatively an anaesthetic laryngoscope may be employed with the patient lying flat and head extended. As fishbones are frequently not radiopaque, plain radiograph is of limited value.

Pharyngeal abscesses

The quinsy, or peritonsillar abscess, follows an acute tonsillar infection which results in pus collecting in the peritonsillar space. It presents with pain and excessive salivation and the speech is thick and muffled. Anatomically, the path of least resistance for the pus to track is superiorly and thus the abscess tends to point in the soft palate (Figs 20.28 and 20.29). Drainage is achieved under a local anaesthetic by lancing the abscess through the mouth using a guarded no. 11 blade. Trismus, due to inflammation of the medial pterygoid muscle, makes this approach difficult but can be overcome by local anaesthetic solution applied on cotton wool to the region of the spheno-palatine foramen on the lateral wall of the nose. The symptomatic relief of pain is nearly always instantaneous.

White concretions protruding from the tonsillar clefts, known as tonsilloliths, result from the collections of squamous epithelium in the crypts and are not associated with any symptoms or pathology.

The retropharyngeal nodes, which normally regress by the age of 7, may on occasion be associated with suppuration and abscess formation resulting in airway obstruction (Figs 20.28, 20.29). A lateral soft tissue radiograph of the neck clearly visualizes the size and extent of the abscess. Intubation is difficult and the child should be placed in the Trendelenburg position to reduce the risk of inhalation of pus. Treatment is again by simple drainage under general anaesthesia.

Parapharyngeal abscesses present in the lateral pharyngeal space which is bounded superiorly by the sphenoid and ends as the tip of an inverted cone at the level of the hyoid; laterally is the superficial layer of the deep fascia and medially the deep layer of the deep investing cervical fascia; posteriorly the carotid sheath and the cranial nerves IX–XII (Fig. 20.29). Pus in this space may have arisen in the peritonsillar space or may have followed pharyngeal trauma, either from a foreign body or during endoscopy. Drainage should be performed externally via an incision along the anterior border of the sternomastoid; the carotid sheath is retracted laterally. A corrugated or tube drain should be used without suction; parenteral antibiotics, providing cover for anaerobic organisms, should be administered.

Carcinoma of the tongue

The predominant tumour of the tongue is squamous cell carcinoma, most of which are well differentiated. This is a disease of middle-aged or elderly patients which is decreasing in frequency and was originally much more common in men (9:1) but in which there is now an almost equal sex incidence (1.5:1). Tobacco and, probably to a greater extent, alcohol are important aetiological factors but the decrease in syphilis, tobacco chewing and use of clay pipes and particularly improvements in oral hygiene are largely responsible for these changes.[43] Approximately 50% of tumours arise on the anterior two thirds of the tongue, of which 85% occur on the lateral border. Macroscopically the lesions may appear exophytic or ulcerative and infiltrative. However, the apparent size as judged by the mucosal lesion is deceptive and one should always assume that a further 2 cm of peripheral tissue may be infiltrated by disease. Palpation gives an indication of extent and this evaluation is best done under general anaesthetic when a deep biopsy can be taken. The lesion must obviously be differentiated from other pathology such as traumatic ulcers, infection (e.g. viral, syphilis, tuberculosis) and other mucosal diseases such as pemphigoid, pemphigus, erosive lichen planus and giant aphthous ulceration in Behçet's disease. Modern imaging with high-resolution CT and gadolinium-enhanced MRI can be very helpful but will not demonstrate micro-embolic spread.[44] The behaviour of the tumour generally becomes more aggressive the more posterior the lesion, with an increase in local and metastatic spread.[45] Thus at presentation the tonsil pillars, retromolar area, floor of mouth and pre-epiglottic space may be extensively infiltrated. Initially the lesion is not painful and may be ignored for some time by the patient until the tongue becomes fixed and extensive soft tissue involvement and associated necrosis and infection produce pain.

If a tongue lesion is detected at an early stage local excision (sometimes using a CO_2 laser)[46] or radiotherapy (interstitial or external beam)[47] may be appropriate; as already indicated, however, it is easy to underestimate the local extent of these

REFERENCES

40. Williams A J J Laryngol 1967; 81: 805
41. Davies D D Br J Anaesth 1964; 36: 244
42. Kristenson S, Tveteras K Clin Otolaryngol 1984; 9: 347
43. Johnston W D, Ballantyne A J Am J Surg 1977; 134: 444
44. Lenz M CT and MRI of Head and Neck Tumors. Thieme, Stuttgart 1993
45. Shah J P Am J Surg 1990; 160: 405
46. Panje W R, Scher N, Karnell M Arch Otolaryngol Head Neck Surg 1989; 115: 681
47. Mendenhall W M, Parsons J T, Stringer S P, Cassisi N J, Million R R Head Neck 1989; 11: 129

tumours and it has been strongly suggested that there be two operations—hemiglossectomy and total glossectomy—combined with some form of neck dissection even in the absence of palpable nodes, to provide a staging of the disease, followed by radiotherapy where any doubt still exists about the margins. These procedures may be performed without splitting the mandible and a range of myocutaneous and free flaps are available for reconstruction.[48] A small tumour of the tongue tip may be excised with a V-shaped wedge but special attention must be paid in these cases to possible bilateral cervical spread. Tumours which have extensively spread into the pre-epiglottic space and supraglottis may also require total laryngectomy.

Oropharyngeal neoplasia (see also Chapter 13)

80% of oropharyngeal neoplasms are epithelial tumours, 15% lymphomas, and 5% miscellaneous tumours including minor salivary gland tumours arising from the glandular epithelium in the oropharynx.[36] Of the squamous carcinomas, half present in the tonsil and half in the posterior third of the tongue, usually with ulceration. Referred otalgia via the glossopharyngeal nerve, dysphagia and a sore throat are common features in the history; some patients notice an ulcer on the tonsil and in 25% a node in the neck is the presenting feature. In an adult unilateral tonsillar enlargement which is not ulcerated must be considered a lymphoma until proven otherwise. Examination of the oropharynx must include mirror examination of the posterior third of the tongue and the lingual tonsil and a thorough manual palpation of this area. Tissue diagnosis is obtained by excision tonsillectomy or deep biopsy, for example of the tongue.

Management of a lymphoma is dependent on the histological and immunocytochemical features identified (see Chapter 34). It should be emphasized that such tumours are often associated with systemic disease and local surgery is only diagnostic. In squamous cell carcinoma, careful assessment of the staging must be performed under general anaesthesia. The use of printed diagrams may clarify the exact position of the tumour in relation to the local anatomical structures. This is particularly important when surgery is to be performed after radiotherapy, when removal of the entire primary tumour site is desirable. Radiography of the mandible is important as spread across the periosteum makes a radiotherapeutic cure significantly less likely.

The choice between primary radiotherapy and surgery is often difficult.[49] If there is no clinical lymph node involvement, radiotherapy is used as the primary treatment with salvage surgery held in reserve for any recurrent or residual tumour. When there is lymph node or bony involvement a combination of surgery and radiotherapy should be considered from the outset. Preoperative radiotherapy to the primary site, which includes a reduced dose to the lymph nodes (usually 4000 Gy), may be followed by radical surgery 4 weeks later.[50] Such surgery should include a radical neck dissection to remove palpable nodes and a suprahyoid block dissection in cases where the neck is clinically clear of metastases (Table 20.10). Composite en bloc resection of the primary tumour site allowing a 5–10 mm margin is achieved using a cutting diathermy and often results in partial glossectomy. If the lower jaw is then to be removed the muscle attachments are sectioned and a Gigli saw is used to divide the mandibular neck posteriorly and the body of the mandible at the level of the mental foramen.[52] Reconstruction following this radical procedure, often termed a 'commando operation', requires an internal lining for the pharynx which allows tongue mobility. Reconstruction can be by means of a pedicled forehead flap, a musculocutaneous flap based upon the pectoralis major, or a free flap taken from the forearm.[53] The advantages of the forearm flap are that it is obtained from outside the radiotherapy field, its size can be accurately designed and it is a very resilient viable flap.[54] The skin and subcutaneous tissue of the pronator aspect of the forearm, based on and including the radial artery and vein, is dissected free and re-anastomosed in the neck to a branch of the external carotid or as an end-to-side anastomosis to the external carotid itself. The venous anastomosis utilizes the most convenient available vein. If reconstruction of the mandible is needed then an en bloc resection of the inner plate of the radius can be taken and inserted along with the flap between the two ends of the mandible: as this is a vascularized autologous graft it offers the best chance of survival.[55] The effects of not reconstructing the mandible are predominantly cosmetic in that mastication is not unduly impaired but difficulty with speech is the predominant problem and the reconstruction should be designed to produce as mobile a tongue tip as possible.

Table 20.10 Five-year survival rates of tonsillar carcinoma

Classification	*Tumour size*	*Grade*	*5-year survival*
Stage I	Tumour < 2 cm	N^0M^0	93%
Stage II	Tumour > 2 cm	N^0M^0	57%
Stage III	Tumour > 4 cm	N^0M^0	27%
Stage IV	Tumour with deep invasion or fixed nodes or metastasis		17%

From Gleave[51]

Care must be taken not to misdiagnose deep parotid tumours presenting as a mass in the lateral oropharyngeal wall. A biopsy in such cases is contraindicated as it tends to seed the tumour into the pharynx.

Imaging of head and neck neoplasia

Routine radiography for diagnostic and management purposes has been superseded by advanced scanning techniques. CT and MRI

REFERENCES

48. Conley J, Sachs M E, Parke R B Otolaryngol Head Neck Surg 1992: 90: 58
49. Stell P M, Nash J R C In: Kerr A G (ed) Scott Brown's Otolaryngology. Butterworth, London 1988
50. Fleming P M Surg Clin North Am 1976; 56: 126
51. Gleave E W Operative Surgery: Head and Neck Part II. Butterworth, London 1981
52. McGregor I A In: McGregor I A, Howard D J (eds) Robin Smith's Operative Surgery—Head and Neck, Part 1. Butterworth-Heinemann, Oxford 1992
53. Panje W R Otolaryngol Clin 1984; 17: 401
54. McGregor I A, McGregor F M Cancer of the Face and Mouth. Churchill Livingstone, Edinburgh 1986
55. Ostrup L T, Frederickson J M Plast Reconst Surg 1975; 55: 563

scans alone or in tandem may give information on the gross extent of tumour; CT scanning provides an accurate assessment of bone erosion. However, when considering nodal disease, neither has a sensitivity better than that attained by palpation. Positron emission tomography offers greater diagnostic strength especially when co-registered with CT images. Preliminary studies suggest that digital positron emission tomography scanning has a significant role to play in post-therapy follow-up where early evidence of tumour recurrence may allow salvage with reduced morbidity and mortality.

Sleep apnoea and snoring

Recent interest in the sleep apnoea syndrome and snoring, caused by oropharyngeal obstruction secondary to large tonsils and a redundant soft palate, has led to the rather controversial use of surgical intervention by uvulopalatopharyngoplasty for these conditions.[56] In the case of sleep apnoea care must be taken to ensure that the patient is not suffering from centrally induced apnoea and that the apnoeic attacks are really significant. Patients are usually obese and may be polycythaemic due to Pickwickian syndrome. There is a body of opinion which believes that the upper respiratory tract obstruction is a result of laxity of the posterior and lateral pharyngeal lining rather than redundancy of the palate. This may explain why the results of surgery have not been as good as had been anticipated. Improvements in snoring are, however, achieved in over 90% of cases.[57] It is important that all other causes of upper respiratory tract obstruction, such as nasal pathology, have been excluded.

Uvulopalatopharyngoplasty consists of removal of the tonsils and a variable amount of the faucial pillars and soft palate including the uvula. Postoperative infection and bleeding are uncommon but rhinolalia aperta (nasal escape speech) and oropharyngeal reflux of fluids occur in most patients in the early postoperative period; fortunately most symptoms settle within 6 weeks.

THE HYPOPHARYNX

Surgical anatomy

Anteriorly the hypopharynx descends from the pharyngoepiglottic fold to the level of the cricopharyngeus and cricoid cartilage. It may be conveniently divided into three separate anatomical areas:

1. The posterior pharyngeal wall extends from the level of the pharyngoepiglottic fold as far as the oesophageal opening.
2. The piriform sinus or fossa lies below the pharyngoepiglottic fold and is bounded laterally by the mucosa covering the inner aspect of the thyroid cartilage and medially by the back of the aryepiglottic fold. Inferiorly it extends down to the oesophageal opening and posteriorly it opens into the hypopharynx proper. The pyriform fossa is often called the 'lateral food channel' because it is the normal route for food to pass between the posterior aspect of the tongue and the oesophagus (Fig. 20.30).
3. The postcricoid region extends from the level of the arytenoid cartilages above to the lower edge of the cricoid cartilage below.

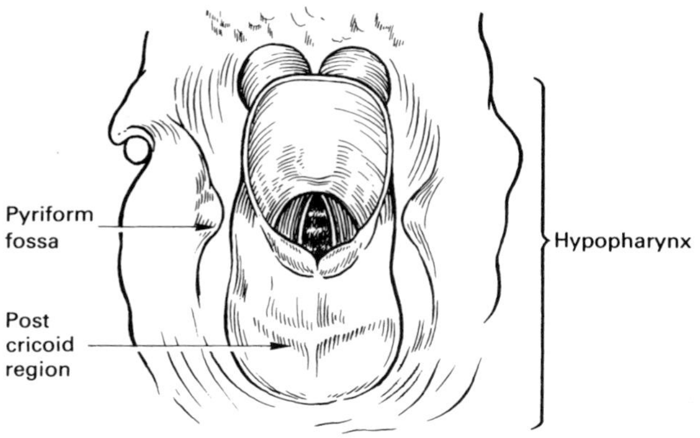

Fig. 20.30 Posterior aspect of the hypopharynx.

Clinical features

The primary symptom of any hypopharyngeal disorder is dysphagia, often associated with pain. The pain is classically referred to the ear, being conducted through the internal branch of the superior laryngeal nerve and the auricular branch of the vagus (Alderman's nerve). It is important to distinguish these symptoms which may indicate malignancy from globus sensation characterized by the 'feeling of a lump in the throat', often worse when swallowing saliva. Although there may be a functional element to globus it is now known to be associated with the reflux of gastric juice into the hypopharynx. A high proportion of cases have an associated hiatus hernia with substantial reflux, confirmed by endoscopic evidence of oesophagitis. In all disorders of swallowing indirect mirror examination of the larynx and pharynx and flexible endoscopy, followed if necessary by video fluoroscopy swallow and often direct endoscopy under general anaesthesia, are necessary. Lesions may be missed when an examination of the hypopharynx is made by a flexible endoscope because the redundant mucosa closes around the endoscope and restricts the view.

Management is by antacids with reduction of acid production (e.g. omeprazole), drugs which improve gastric motility (e.g. metoclopramide) and H_2-receptor antagonists.

Foreign bodies

Hypopharyngeal foreign bodies are usually found at or just above the cricopharyngeal sphincter. They impact on the sphincter and produce acute dysphagia, commonly complete, pain and sometimes voice change. The history of ingestion is usually clear. Plain lateral radiographs of the cervical spine demonstrate radiopaque foreign bodies anterior to the body of the C6 vertebra. An air shadow is often seen in the upper oesophagus which is normally closed. In cases where there has been penetration of the foreign body through the pharyngeal wall, surgical emphysema occurs with its characteristic radiological features. If there is any doubt

REFERENCES

56. Blair Simmonds F, Guilleminault C, Silvestri R Arch Otolarngol 1983; 109: 153, 503
57. Fujita S, Conway W A, Zoric R Laryngoscope 1985; 95: 70

about the diagnosis a barium swallow should be performed; this may be enhanced by asking the patient to swallow a small piece of cotton wool soaked in barium which will be caught on the tiniest bone spicule. The barium examination may also demonstrate extraluminal spread. In any of these circumstances, and even with negative findings but a good history, fairly urgent rigid endoscopy is performed. If the mucosa has been perforated either by the foreign body itself or during instrumentation, a nasogastric tube should be passed and the patient kept nil by mouth and given parenteral broad-spectrum antibiotics. One must be alert clinically to the development of a mediastinal abscess and also, in the older patient, to the possibility of a malignant stricture underlying the problem.

Pharyngeal palsies

Pharyngeal palsies cause poor coordination of the peristaltic wave travelling down the pharynx which is often associated with spasm of cricopharyngeus. This results in dysphagia, reflux and overspill of pharyngeal contents into the larynx, causing coughing and choking. Pharyngeal palsies are usually the result of brainstem damage and are often associated with a clinical pseudobulbar palsy.

The management of this condition is difficult especially if the hypoglossal nerve is affected because the food bolus cannot then be easily made to enter the pharynx. A cricopharyngeal myotomy may produce relief of symptoms when the bolus can be transferred to the pharynx but is not retained by the cricopharyngeus.

Cricopharyngeal myotomy

The pharynx is approached via an incision along the inferior half of the anterior border of the sternocleidomastoid. Care is taken to avoid the thyroid vessels. The cricoid ring is palpated and a rigid oesophagoscope is passed into the pharynx and positioned above the oesophageal opening. With the operating room lights lowered, the oesophagoscope light is visible through the pharyngeal mucosa and the fibres of the cricopharyngeus are clearly displayed. A wedge of muscle is excised from its lateral and posterior aspects without entering the pharynx. The wound is drained and closed in two layers. A nasogastric tube is not needed and the patient is encouraged to swallow soft food as soon as possible.[58] Laryngeal overspill, though relatively rare, can be a major problem as inhalational pneumonia may develop. This can be reduced by an epiglottopexy where the free edge of the epiglottis is scarified and sewn down on to the aryepiglottic fold;[59] surprisingly the airway or voice is hardly compromised by this technique.

Pharyngeal web

A pharyngeal web, which usually develops in the postcricoid area of middle-aged women, presents with dysphagia and with symptoms of an iron-deficiency anaemia (Paterson–Brown Kelly/Plummer–Vinson syndrome).[60] Care should be taken to examine the patient for koilonychia, angular cheilitis and glossitis along with splenomegaly. Following a barium swallow all patients with webs should have a rigid oesophagoscopy, both to rule out an associated neoplasm and as a treatment to break down the web and relieve dysphagia.[61] Close follow-up is required in all patients as the incidence of postcricoid carcinoma is significant.

Pharyngeal pouch

Pharyngeal pouches are most commonly seen in the elderly where they often have a long and symptom-free natural development. Patients eventually complain of dysphagia associated with regurgitation of undigested foods and consequent weight loss. Pulmonary overspill is a problem and on occasions hoarseness and chest infections may be the only presenting symptoms. A mass low down in the anterior triangle of the neck may be felt and deep palpation over this may produce a squelching sound, caused by free fluid in the pouch. Neoplasia has been reported in less than 1% of pouches.

The aetiology of pharyngeal pouches is not known but cineradiography and pressure studies suggest that there is neuromuscular incoordination resulting in high intraluminal pressure in the pharynx leading to herniation of the mucosa through its muscular coat. The spasm may be caused by acid reflux associated with a hiatus hernia in some patients. The weakest point is Killian's dehiscence between the thyropharyngeal and cricopharyngeal muscles that make up the inferior constrictor (Figs 20.31 and 20.32). Barium swallow examination is usually diagnostic and may be followed by rigid endoscopy if cancer is suspected. In very infirm patients endoscopic resection of the posterior party wall by diathermy is possible (Dohlman's procedure);[62] more recently an endoscopic stapling device has been used which reduces the incidence of a fistula and consequent mediastinitis. Many surgeons prefer a formal excision of the pouch.

Surgical excision

Preoperative preparation should include absence of solids for at least 24 hours prior to the operation. The anaesthetist should be

REFERENCES

58. Bowdler D A In: Kerr A G (ed) Scott Brown's Otolaryngology. Butterworth, London 1988
59. Brookes G B, McKelvie P Ann R Coll Surg Engl 1983; 65: 293
60. Patterson D R J Laryngol 1919; 24: 289
61. Richards S H J Laryngol 1970; 85: 141
62. Dohlman G, Mattson O Arch Otolaryngol 1960; 71: 744

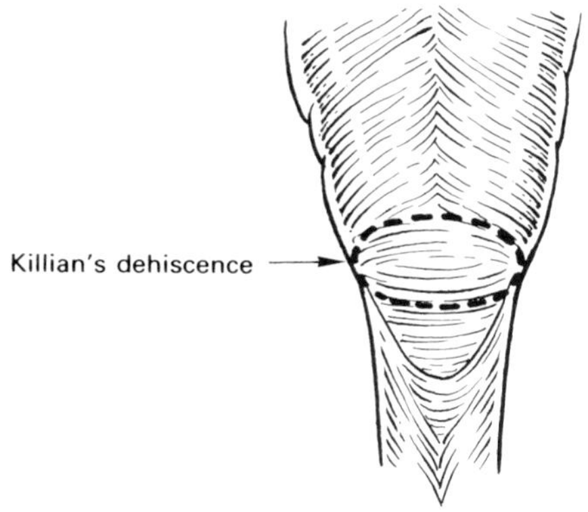

Fig. 20.31 Posterior view of pharyngo-oesophageal junction.

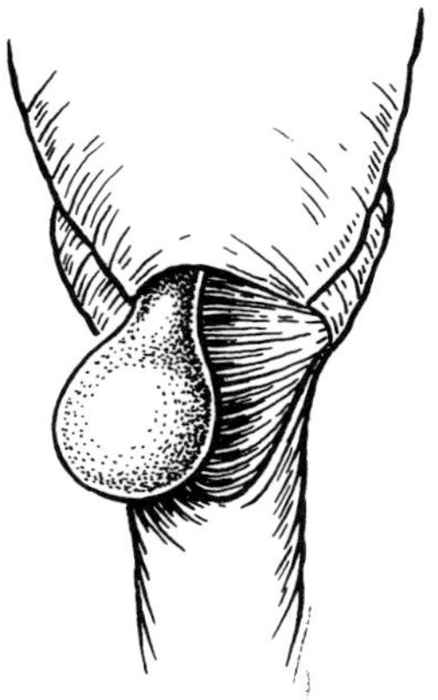

Fig. 20.32 Pharyngeal pouch.

warned of the possibility that the pouch could still contain saliva and foodstuff and that, following induction, the pouch contents may be inhaled, resulting in Mendelssohn's syndrome.[63] A nasogastric tube should first be passed into the oesophagus; this is often the most difficult part of the operation. The oesophageal lumen is often located with difficulty as the rigid oesophagoscope always tends to enter the pouch. The pouch is then packed with proflavine-impregnated gauze with a free end left trailing from the mouth to aid eventual removal and make the identification of the pouch much easier.

The approach is as for a cricopharyngeal myotomy. When the pouch has been dissected free the flavine gauze is removed by the anaesthetist, the neck of the pouch clamped by a small Payr's clamp and the pouch is excised. A continuous looped stitch placed over the clamp allows closure of the resulting pharyngeal defect without any spillage of pharyngeal contents. A second layer of interrupted absorbable sutures may be used to complete the repair.

Concomitant cricopharyngeal myotomy should be performed. The postoperative fistula rate should be low with nasogastric feeding for 5 days.

Diverticulectomy may be replaced by simple inversion and oversewing in high-risk patients.[64] Postoperative radiological studies suggest that after inversion the pouch atrophies very quickly and the patient's symptoms are soon relieved. However, this technique does not allow histopathological examination of the sac and there is a possibility that a diverticular carcinoma may be missed.

Hypopharyngeal neoplasia

The management of patients with tumours of the hypopharynx depends on accurate localization of the neoplasm. Plain radiographs of the neck, especially in the lateral position, can be helpful. A soft tissue shadow anterior to the vertebral bodies can usually be seen (Fig. 20.33). Gas may be seen beneath the tumour if the oesophagus is stented open. Barium studies are valuable in delineating the lower extent of a postcricoid tumour although care must be taken as barium can fail to delineate a tumour of the posterior pharyngeal wall as it courses laterally down the food channel of the pyriform fossa (Fig. 20.34). Panendoscopy must be performed with a careful examination being made of the oro- and hypopharynges, oesophagus, larynx, trachea and bronchi, along with an assessment of the vocal cord mobility. Deep biopsies are

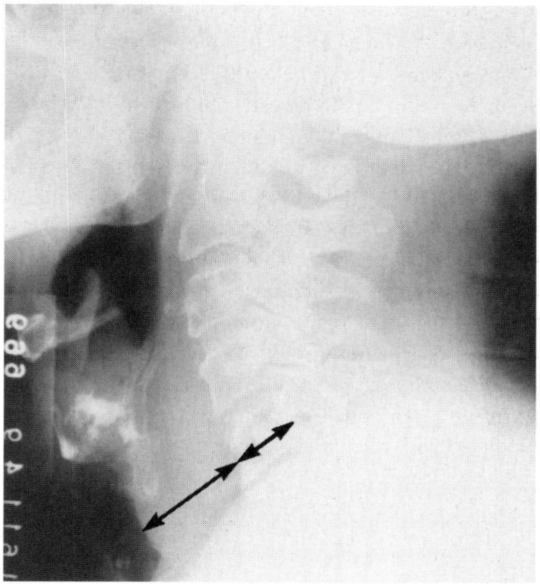

Fig. 20.33 Lateral radiograph showing the position of soft tissue shadow anterior to vertebral bodies due to hypopharyngeal tumour.

REFERENCES

63. Bannister W K, Satjilarroa J Anaesthesiology 1967; 23: 251
64. Bevan A D Surg Clin Chicago 1917; 1: 449

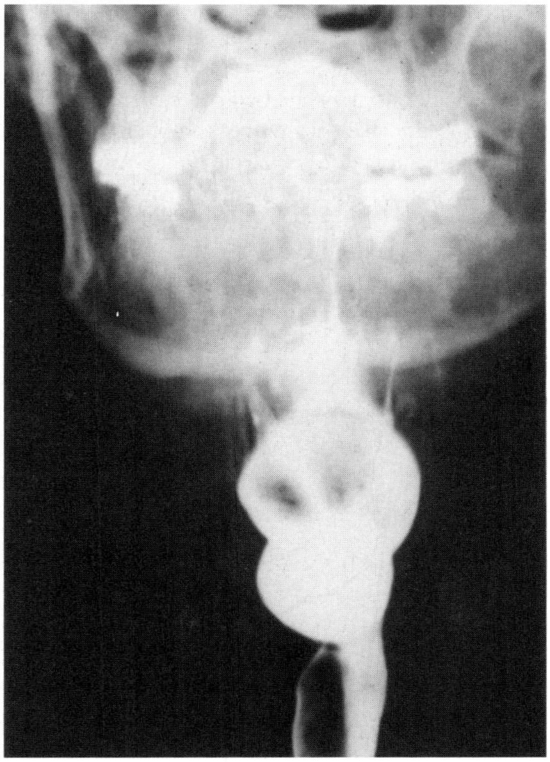

Fig. 20.34 Barium swallow showing filling defect.

taken of the tumour mass as it is often necrotic and a superficial biopsy can give spurious results. A biopsy of adjacent normal tissue allows an accurate estimate of the tumour size as it is quite common for such tumours to spread submucosally.[65] The presence of cervical lymphadenopathy and an assessment of any fixity may also influence the method of treatment. Patients with a hypopharyngeal tumour tend to lose weight and therefore preoperative nutritional support is often valuable (see Chapter 2).

It is important to recognize at the outset those patients whose tumours are incurable. In such cases surgical excision or radiotherapy provides little or no palliation, increases the morbidity of the condition and does not influence survival.[66] Though each case must be individually assessed, tumours that have spread outside the pharynx, those producing bilateral vocal cord paralysis and those associated with bilateral fixed nodes may be considered to be in this category (Fig. 20.35).[65]

Pyriform fossa neoplasms unfortunately expand silently in a relatively distensible area and are frequently associated with lymph node metastases at presentation; cure by radiotherapy is uncommon and surgery must be considered the primary treatment.[67]

When the tumour is confined to the lateral aspect of the pyriform fossa a partial pharyngectomy with conservation of the posterior pharyngeal wall and the contralateral pyriform fossa may allow a primary closure.[68] Postoperatively a surprisingly good swallow may be obtained through a relatively tight passage. If there is any doubt that a stenosis will result a vascularized graft should be used to close the defect. If only the posterior pharyngeal wall is involved excision and grafting may suffice. When the medial wall of the pyriform fossa is involved or there is a vocal cord palsy total laryngopharyngectomy must be performed.

In cases where lymph node metastases are present a contiguous block dissection is indicated. The value of a prophylactic block dissection in conditions associated with a high incidence of occult nodes is still questionable. In Europe[65] prophylactic neck dissection is not as frequently performed as in the USA.[67,69] The survival of patients who come to a total pharyngolaryngectomy is poor (see Fig. 20.35) and some regard the operation only as palliative; it is therefore particularly important that palliation should be good and the patient should be able to leave hospital in the shortest possible time. The choice of pharyngeal reconstruction must thus be the technique which carries the least operative morbidity. A gastric pull-up perhaps best satisfies this criterion (Fig. 20.36). The alternatives include: colon transplant, free jejunal graft, and skin flaps which may be either pedicled[70,71] or free[71] utilizing a microvascular anastomosis.[69,72]

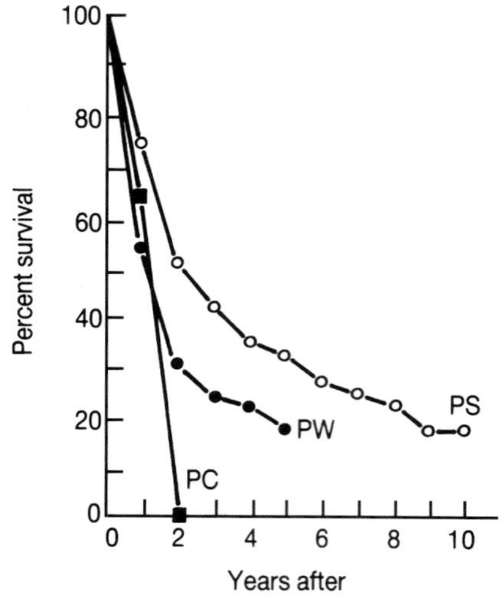

Fig. 20.35 10-year survival of hypopharyngeal cancer.

Pharyngolaryngectomy and stomach pull-up

There is no indication for primary tracheostomy unless there is coincidental airway obstruction. The patient is positioned supine with moderate extension of the cervical spine. A total laryngopharyngectomy can be performed through a single collar incision located just below the midpoint between the hyoid and the upper edge of the sternum.[72] The superior skin flap is raised deep to the platysma including the superficial layer of the deep investing fascia. The larynx is then mobilized by dissecting along the medial border of the sternocleidomastoid to display the carotid sheath which is retracted laterally. The omohyoid is divided and the superior middle and inferior thyroid vessels are ligated and divided. The strap muscles are then divided just above the sternum and at the lower border of the hyoid bone. The hyoid is then skeletonized by using cutting diathermy along its superior surface, thereby releasing the mylohyoid and the digastric sling. Dissection continues up to the greater cornua and the stylohyoid ligament is released from the lesser cornua of the hyoid. The cervical trachea is then mobilized by dissection in the plane between the oesophagus and the trachea; care is taken to ensure that the inferior thyroid artery has been located and well ligated. At this stage close cooperation between the surgeon and the anaesthetist is necessary. In order to keep the patient anaesthetized and oxygenated, quick transfer from the orotracheal tube to a cuffed tracheostomy tube is important. When the trachea has been fully mobilized it is transected obliquely so that it will lie at right angles when it is brought through the skin.

As soon as the trachea is open a cuffed tracheostomy tube is inserted and ventilation continues through this route. The free end of the trachea is loosely attached by catgut stay sutures to the circular skin incision above the sternal notch. This allows the trachea to be accurately aligned to the skin. Intermediate stitches appose the mucosa of the trachea and the skin edge circumferen-

REFERENCES

65. Stell P M, Swift A C In: Kerr A G (ed) Scott Brown's Otolaryngology. Butterworth, London 1988
66. Harrison D F N, Thompson A E Head Neck Surg 1986; 8: 418
67. Kirchner J A Ann Otol 1975; 84: 793
68. Ogura J H, Mallen R W Cancer of the Head and Neck. Appleton-Century-Crofts, St Louis 1967
69. Harrison D F N J Laryngol 1971; 84: 349
70. Wright D, Kenyon G In: Kerr A G (ed) Scott Brown's Otolaryngology, vol 5. Butterworth, London 1988
71. Langman J Medical Embryology, 4th edn. Williams & Wilkins, Baltimore 1985
72. Leonard J R, Maran A G Laryngoscope 1970; 80: 849

tially. An incision is then made into the pharynx above the hyoid, care being taken not to enter the pre-epiglottic space. As soon as the pharynx is open the epiglottis becomes visible and may be grasped. The opening in the pharynx is extended laterally, exposing the tumour and ensuring a clear margin of resection. When the mucosa on the posterior wall has been divided, the specimen may be reflected downwards off the anterior vertebral wall. The specimen is then only attached to the cervical oesophagus. This may be mobilized by a blunt finger dissection (Fig. 20.36).

The abdominal surgeon mobilizes the stomach, retaining the right gastric and right gastro-epiploic arteries. The short gastric and left gastric arteries are ligated and divided. Kocher's manoeuvre allows the duodenum to be mobilized medially and a pyloromyotomy is performed. The peritoneum over the oesophagus is divided and the opening in the right crus is defined. The vagi are divided and the mediastinum is entered by blunt dissection. The hiatus is enlarged and a hand is passed up into the mediastinum. The oesophagus is cored out by blunt dissection with the hand and fingers keeping close to its outer wall. The neck dissection and the mediastinal dissection are joined and gentle traction on the fully mobilized oesophagus brings the stomach up into the neck. The oesophago-gastric junction is divided and closed with staples or sutures and the fundus of the stomach is anastomosed end-to-end with the pharynx using interrupted Dexon or Vicryl (polyglycolic acid) sutures. The wounds are closed with suction drains and chest drains inserted.

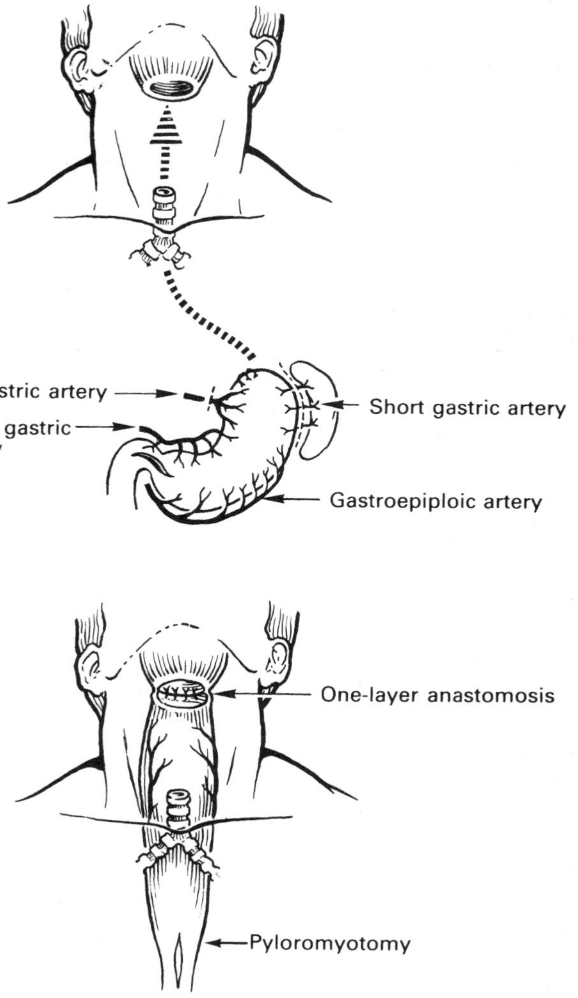

Fig. 20.36 Diagrams showing gastric pull-up procedure.

THE LARYNX

Surgical anatomy

The larynx, trachea and bronchi develop embryologically from the foregut in the form of an outpouching.[71] Functionally the larynx is primarily a protective sphincter for the lungs and only later phylogenetic development results in phonation. The larynx lies in the neck in front of the third to sixth cervical vertebrae. The laryngeal framework or skeleton consists of the hyoid bone, the thyroid, cricoid, epiglottic and arytenoid cartilages: all these may be seen on a lateral cervical spine radiograph. The larynx lies in the hypopharynx and inferiorly is in continuity with the trachea. It extends from the free edge of the epiglottis and aryepiglottic folds to the false vocal cords (ventricular folds), the laryngeal ventricle with the laryngeal saccule as its appendix anteriorly, the true vocal cords (vocal folds) and the area below the vocal cords and inferiorly to the cricoid cartilage (Fig. 20.37).

Surgically the larynx is divided into supraglottic, glottic and subglottic areas. The supraglottic area extends from the free margin of the epiglottis and aryepiglottic folds to a line drawn tangentially across the superior margin of the vocal cords. The glottis lies below this line but above the conus elasticus which runs from the inferior free edge of the cord to the cricoid. The subglottis lies below the conus elasticus and above the lower margin of the cricoid cartilage. These landmarks are important as the TNM classification of laryngeal cancer relates to them.[35] The vocal folds (two cords) consist of the thyroarytenoid muscle covered by loose connective tissue lined by stratified squamous epithelium. The rest of the larynx is lined by a respiratory epithelium with areas of squamous metaplasia. The amount of squamous metaplasia increases with age and smoking but is evident even in infancy.[73]

The extrinsic muscles of the larynx can broadly be divided into elevators of the larynx—namely the thyrohyoid, stylopharyngeus, palatopharyngeus, mylohyoid, geniohyoid and stylohyoid muscles—and depressors consisting of the sternohyoid, sternothyroid and omohyoid muscles. Such movement is important in deglutition as elevation and tilting of the larynx allows airway protection by apposing the epiglottis to the aryepiglottic folds, so encouraging the food bolus to pass into the lateral food channels.

The intrinsic muscles may be divided into abductors and adductors of the vocal cords. The posterior cricoarytenoid is the sole abductor of the vocal cord and arises from the posterior aspect of the cricoid lamina, being inserted into the back of the muscular process of the arytenoid. Abduction of the cord occurs by rotation of the body of the arytenoid combined with medial movement of

REFERENCES

73. Stell P M, Gregory I, Watts J Clin Otolaryngol 1980; 3: 13

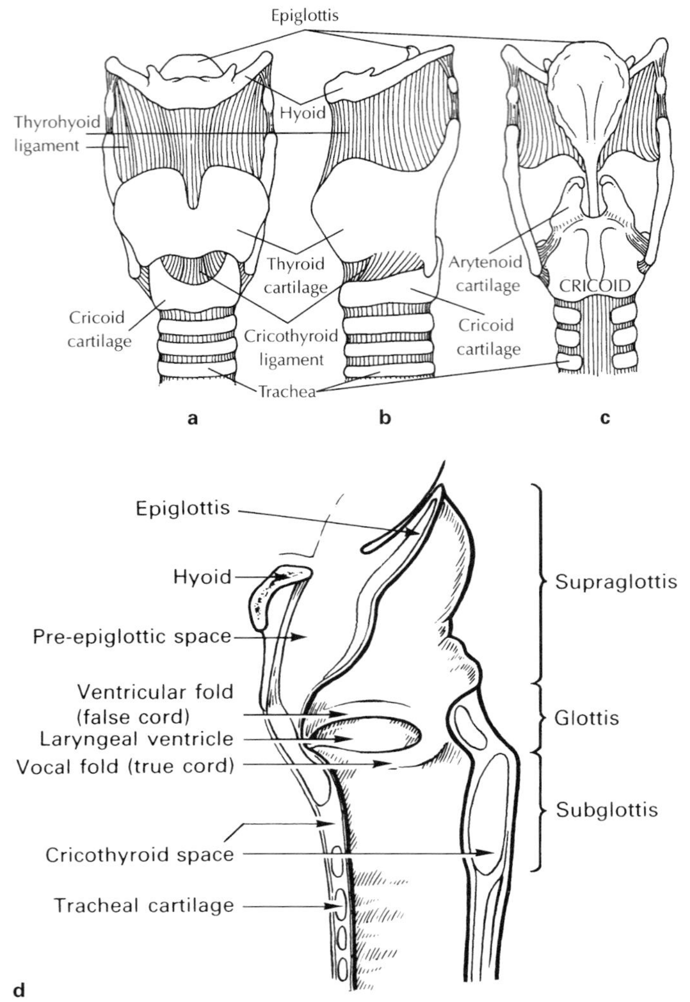

Fig. 20.37 Diagram showing the anatomy of the larynx: (**a**) anterior, (**b**) lateral and (**c**) posterior views. (**d**) Sagittal section.

the muscular process and lateral movement of the arytenoid in relation to the cricoid.

The adductors of the larynx are the lateral cricoarytenoid and the transverse and oblique arytenoids. These are supported by the tensors of the vocal cord, the thyroarytenoid (the vocalis) and the cricothyroid muscles. The aryepiglottis and thyroepiglotticus are the muscles which protect the vocal tract during deglutition.

The nerve supply to the larynx is contained in the vagus. The superior laryngeal nerve leaves the vagus just beneath the skull at the level of the inferior ganglion and descends posteriorly to the internal carotid artery, branching on the medial constrictor just below the level of the hyoid. The internal branch pierces the cricothyroid membrane above the superior laryngeal artery and provides sensory input to the larynx above the cords, in addition to having a parasympathetic secretor motor function. The smaller external branch continues down into the inferior constrictor entering the cricothyroid muscle and acting as its motor nerve. Contraction of the cricothyroid increases the distance between the vocal process of the arytenoid and the thyroid notch, thus increasing the tension of the vocal cord. The recurrent laryngeal nerve on the left leaves the vagus as it crosses the aorta, passing under the arch and the ligamentum arteriosum before ascending again in the groove between the oesophagus and trachea. On the right the nerve originates from the vagus as it crosses the subclavian artery, passing under the artery to ascend in the tracheo-oesophageal groove. At the lower border of the cricopharyngeus both nerves pass deeply with the laryngeal branches of the inferior thyroid artery to enter the larynx. The recurrent laryngeal nerve is the motor supply of all muscles of the larynx, with the exception of the cricothyroid.

In infancy the larynx is proportionally smaller than the adult larynx and thus small changes in its dimensions may lead to significant reduction in the airway.[74]

Clinical examination of the larynx and its function

Indirect and fibreoptic laryngoscopy

In order to achieve good visualization of the larynx and vocal cords in particular, practice is required (Fig. 20.38). The patient should be positioned on a seat with an upright back and the light source is angled on to a head mirror giving a clear, well focused bright light on the patient's mouth.[75] The tongue is then gently held by thumb and forefinger with the index finger balanced on the upper teeth. If the patient's gag reflex is too active local anaesthesia in the form of 1% Xylocaine spray may be used. Alternatively a flexible nasoendoscope may be passed through the nose into the nasopharynx. The examination should include an inspection of the entire larynx and adjacent pharynx. Vocal cord function during phonation is assessed with the patient phonating 'ah-ah'. This may more accurately be assessed using a stroboscope.

Direct laryngoscopy

This procedure is done under a general anaesthetic. It allows an excellent examination of the larynx but cannot assess laryngeal function with the exception of simple adduction and abduction. The patient is positioned on the operating table with the cervical vertebrae flexed and the atlanto-occipital joint extended—the so-called 'sniffing the morning air' position. Nasotracheal intubation is preferable as the tube then lies across the posterior commissure enabling maximum view of the larynx.

Microlaryngoscopy

An operating microscope is used to facilitate endoscopic surgery during direct laryngoscopy. This may be combined with a carbon dioxide laser system, though special ventilation techniques are required. Laser surgery most commonly utilizes a carbon dioxide laser system using an exposure time of 0.05 ms and a power of 15–20 watts.[76] When using the laser great care is taken to protect

REFERENCES

74. Batch A J B J Laryngol 1988; 99: 783
75. McCormick M S In: Kerr A G (ed) Scott Brown's Otolaryngology. Butterworth, London 1988
76. Carruth J A S J Laryngol 1985; 99: 573

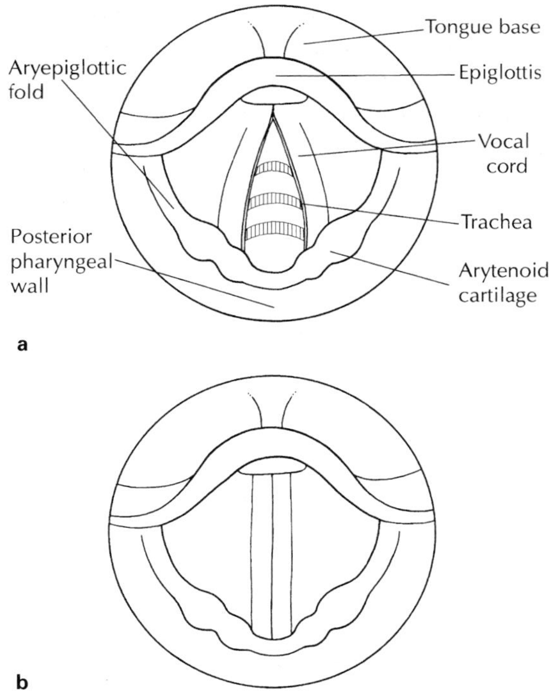

Fig. 20.38 Diagram showing a view of the larynx on indirect laryngoscopy in (**a**) abduction and (**b**) adduction.

the endotracheal tube as ignition of the combustible elements of the tube in a high oxygen environment is possible. The tube may be covered by silver paper (cooking foil) or alternatively it may be retracted into the pharynx and the patient oxygenated and anaesthetized by a diffusion process.[77] An alternative is to use the Venturi technique, in which the anaesthetic mixture is forced into the airway under high pressure through a small nozzle placed on the endoscope.[78] By using intermittent bursts of a gas–air mixture, anaesthesia and oxygenation can be maintained.

In addition to microlaryngoscopy, the mucosa can also be scrutinized with a large rigid endoscope which, with an angled view, is particularly helpful in examining the ventricle and subglottis.

Laryngeal disorders in childhood

Laryngomalacia

This not uncommon condition presents with inspiratory stridor (Table 20.11) usually without evidence of central cyanosis. The baby is worse in the supine position and the diagnosis is made by laryngoscopy. The epiglottis is characteristically omega-shaped and on inspiration is sucked backwards over the laryngeal aditus. When the laryngoscope is advanced beyond the epiglottis the arytenoids are seen to collapse inward on inspiration. Laryngomalacia reflects laryngeal immaturity although histological evidence suggests that the chondrocytes are defective.[79] Management rarely requires tracheostomy and parents can usually be reassured of the benign nature of the disorder. Any inflammatory disease of the larynx or trachea can however cause severe respiratory obstruction in these children. It should be remembered that airflow through the airway is proportional to the square of its radius.[80]

Table 20.11 Conditions producing stridor

Lumen	Impacted foreign body
Mural	
a. Congenital	Laryngeal web
	Laryngomalacia
	Subglottic stenosis
b. Acquired	
Inflammatory	Angioneurotic oedema
	Granulomas, e.g. Wegener's, sarcoid
Traumatic/iatrogenic	Post-tracheostomy
	Post-irradiation
Infective	Laryngotracheobronchitis
	Epiglottitis
Neoplasia	Laryngeal papillomas
	Malignancy
Extramural	
Traumatic/iatrogenic	Thyroidectomy
Neoplasia	Bronchus, oesophagus, thyroid lymphadenopathy
Neurological	Lower motor neurone disease

Laryngeal web

Congenital laryngeal webs present with stridor and dysphonia. They are most commonly sited at the anterior commissure but may also occur posteriorly. Management in the first instance is by laser excision which may need to be repeated several times.[81] A laryngotomy with insertion of a stent after the web has been excised offers the best chance of avoiding a recurrence, but is unfortunately associated with permanent voice problems. Care should be taken when excising a web with the laser as there is often a subglottic extension.

Laryngotracheobronchitis

In children this condition usually arises from a simple upper respiratory tract infection when inflammation spreads to the entire respiratory tract, producing tenacious mucus and mucosal oedema. The common causative organism is a haemolytic streptococcus. The clinical presentation is that of a common cold, usually in a child below the age of 8 years, progressing to a harsh cough, stridor and voice change. In the early stages the dyspnoeic child is inevitably agitated but later becomes 'calm' as hypercapnia and respiratory acidosis develop. Aggressive antibiotic therapy with penicillin and humidification of the inspired air are the initial treatment. Any evidence of deterioration calls for an alternative airway.[82] Tracheostomy is preferred to nasotracheal intubation, and frequent and thorough aspiration of the respiratory tract is of paramount importance.

REFERENCES

77. Vivori E Br J Anaesth 1980; 52: 638
78. Carruth J A S In: Kerr A G (ed) Scott Brown's Otolaryngology. Butterworth, London 1988
79. Hollinger P H, Brown W T Ann Otol Rhinol Laryngol 1967; 76: 744
80. Biller H F, Harvey J E, Bowe R C Ann Otol Rhinol Laryngol 1976; 79: 1048
81. Benjamin B Otolaryngology. Head and Neck Surgery. C V Mosby, St Louis 1986
82. Lockhart C H, Battaglia J D Pediatr Ann 1977; 6: 262

Epiglottitis

Acute inflammation of the supraglottic region leads to submucosal oedema producing a 'hot potato' quality to the voice and the sudden onset of stridor and dyspnoea, often with early cyanosis. The child, classically 5–7 years of age, presents with a short history of sore throat followed by stridor and dyspnoea which are worse on lying down. As a consequence the child sits in bed drooling and gasping for breath. Within hours he or she may be in extremis and an alternative airway is needed. The inflammation is caused by *Haemophilus influenzae* type B and responds readily to amoxycillin.[83] The choice of method to maintain the airway depends upon the facilities and the experience of the unit. Nasotracheal intubation is preferable but must be performed with great care and the facilities for tracheostomy should be available.[84] Preoperative investigation should be minimal as time is often precious in preventing sudden death and any attempt at examination may precipitate respiratory collapse. Maintenance of the airway may be combined with intravenous fluid replacement, appropriate broad-spectrum antibiotic and steroids.

Laryngeal clefts

Failure of the formation of the septum between the developing pharyngotracheal canal and the oesophagus results in an open communication between the larynx, the upper trachea and the oesophagus. Children with this defect present with continuous aspiration problems and a characteristic toneless cry. At microlaryngoscopy the intra-arytenoid area must be palpated carefully or the diagnosis will be easily missed.[85] Treatment is by direct suture through a lateral pharyngotomy incision although an endolaryngeal approach has been described.[86]

Subglottic stenosis

Both congenital and acquired subglottic stenoses are characterized by a thickened cricoid cartilage which becomes oval in shape (Fig. 20.39). The acquired variety may be an extension of an underlying congenital stenosis needing endotracheal intubation. The diagnosis is made at laryngoscopy and bronchoscopy. The smallest diameter neonatal bronchoscope (3.5 mm) should be passed through the subglottis without force: failure indicates a severe degree of stenosis. Dilation of the stenosis has little part to play and open laryngotracheoplasty is the treatment of choice.

Laryngeal papillomatosis

Laryngeal papillomata in childhood are associated with maternal vaginal papillomatosis; a papovavirus is implicated in the aetiology.[87] Medical management is by the use of the antiviral agent, interferon.[88] When the airway has been compromised surgical removal with the carbon dioxide laser is indicated.[89] If a laser is unavailable suction diathermy may be used instead.[90]

Acute laryngitis

Acute laryngitis is a complication of the common cold and is caused by an adenovirus or influenza virus. The condition is self-limiting and the symptoms consist of hoarseness and paroxysmal cough with sore throat. Resting the voice, abstinence from cigarettes and soluble aspirin gargles usually control the symptoms.

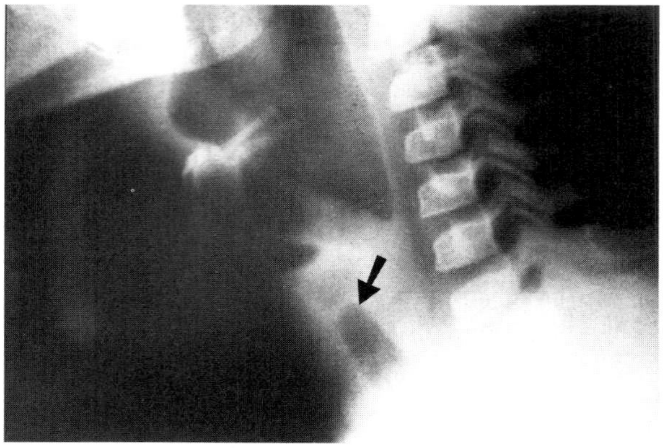

Fig. 20.39 Lateral radiograph of neck showing subglottic stenosis.

Chronic laryngitis

Hoarseness is usually of insidious onset and may be associated with a discrete attack of laryngitis. Sufferers are most frequently smokers and there is usually very little accompanying pain. Examination may reveal leucoplakia of the vocal cords, which on histological examination can display a spectrum of epithelial change from simple hyperplasia or keratosis, through keratosis with cellular atypia to carcinoma in situ.[91] The term 'leucoplakia' thus only indicates the naked-eye appearances of the larynx and not a histological diagnosis.

The most important form of treatment for chronic laryngitis is removal of the contributory factors such as tobacco, alcohol and purulent postnasal drip. However, because of its chronic nature the epithelial changes may become irreversible and the condition will only respond to stripping of the mucosa using a microlaryngoscopy technique.[92] If the presence of a carcinoma in situ is confirmed on subsequent histology, careful follow-up and review microlaryngoscopy 3 months later are necessary.[91]

Vocal polyps and nodules

As a result of poor or excessive voice usage, the vocal cords may develop nodules or become oedematous and develop polyps.

REFERENCES

83. Drake-Lee A B, Broughton S J, Grace A Br J Clin Pract 1984; 38: 218
84. Cantrell R W, Bell R A, Morioka W T Laryngoscope 1978; 88: 994
85. Glossop L P, Smith R J, Evans J N Int J Paed Otorhinolaryngol 1984; 7: 133
86. Evans J N Ann Otol Rhinol Laryngol 1985; 94: 627
87. Bettersby E F In: Kerr A G (ed) Scott Brown's Otolaryngology. Butterworth, London 1988
88. Lusk R P, McCabe B F, Mixon J H Ann Otol Rhinol Laryngol 1987; 96: 158
89. Birchall J P, Hattab M et al Ann R Coll Surg 1983; 65: 209
90. Hennessy T P J, Doyle-Kelly W, Brady M P Ann R Coll Surg 1984; 66: 343
91. Helquist H, Lundgren J, Oloffson J Clin Otolaryngol 1982; 7: 11

Nodules are seen more frequently in children and women, while polyps are more common in adult men. Smoking tends to accentuate any vocal cord trauma. Nodules are usually found at the anterior end of the cord about a third of the way from the anterior commissure (Figs 20.40 and 20.41). This position is governed by the actual length of the mobile cord which is the anterior two thirds of the visible cord length, whilst the posterior third is the vocal process of the arytenoid. Thus the point of maximum stress is at the midpoint of the mobile cord.

Such lesions can resolve in the acute phase if the voice is rested and re-educated[93] but the chances of spontaneous resolution decrease markedly when the lesions have undergone fibrous organization. Precise surgical removal is then required.

Vocal cord polyps can occur anywhere along the vocal cord but are frequently seen close to the anterior commissure. When well formed and pedunculated they do not resolve. Surgery for polyps and nodules may permanently damage or alter the patient's voice.[94] Although surgery can easily remove offending lesions care must be taken not to damage the adjacent cord and the underlying vocalis muscle. When the lesion is at the anterior commissure there is a danger that an anterior web may form after surgery.

Reinke's oedema

Generalized oedema of the vocal cord is probably the most common laryngeal response to noxious stimuli. The attachment of the vocal ligament along the medial edge of the cord and its extension on to the conus elasticus restricts the oedema to the upper aspect of the cord, thus giving it its characteristic appearance. Treatment is by surgical excision of the mucosal lining using the microlaryngoscope followed by complete voice rest and speech therapy.

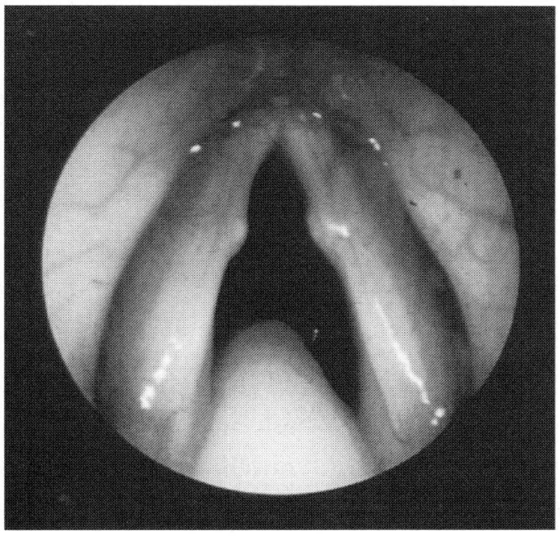

Fig. 20.40 Endoscopic view of vocal cord nodules.

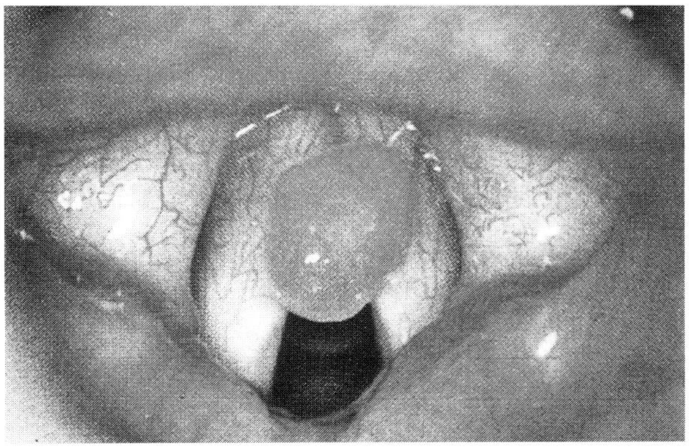

Fig. 20.41 Endoscopic view of benign laryngeal polyp.

Intubation granuloma

It is perhaps surprising, considering the number of intubations taking place, that vocal cord damage occurs so infrequently. A granuloma occurs at the posterior end of the vocal cord where the epithelium is firmly attached to the underlying arytenoid cartilage and probably results from pressure necrosis by the endotracheal tube during surgery rather than actual intubation trauma.[95] However recurrences are unfortunately common.

Laryngocele

When the laryngeal saccule is expanded with air it is termed a laryngocele. Any activity that increases intraglottic pressure, such as straining or blowing wind instruments, may cause laryngoceles. These may spread superiorly and present in the false cord (internal laryngocele) or may pass through the thyrohyoid membrane and present as a lump in the neck. Internal laryngoceles can be compressed through the false cords but external laryngoceles must be approached through the neck, with the dissection and excision taken as close to their origins as possible.[96]

Laryngeal paralysis

The position of the vocal cords following paralysis of either or both the superior or recurrent laryngeal nerves is contentious. The time-honoured 'Semon's law' is contradicted by contemporary physiological and pathological evidence.[97] Two positions of the vocal cords are recognized in the normal conscious patient: full adduction, the median position, occurring on phonation; and full abduction on inspiration (Fig. 20.42). The two well-recognized abnormal positions are the paramedian position and the intermediate or cadaveric position. However, it should be made clear that accurate assessments are often difficult as only a few millimetres separate all these positions and recovery of vocal cord function makes assessment even more difficult.

Superior laryngeal nerve palsy

Lesions of this nerve are often not recognized clinically unless the patient uses his or her voice professionally, particularly if he or she

REFERENCES

92. Kleinsasser O Microlaryngoscopy and Endolaryngeal Surgery. Saunders, Philadelphia 1976
93. Boone H The Voice and Voice Therapy, 3rd edn. Prentice Hall, New York 1981
94. Monday L A, Cornut G et al Ann Otol Rhinol Laryngol 1983; 92: 124
95. Benjamin B, Croxon G Ann Otol Rhinol Laryngol 1983; 92: 124
96. Stell P M, Maran A G D J Laryngol 1975; 89: 915
97. Wyke B D, Kirschner J A Scientific Foundations of Otolaryngology. Heinemann, London 1976

is a singer. A cricothyroid muscle palsy results in a loss of adduction and tension causing a slightly bowed cord and an asymmetrical larynx (Fig. 20.42b).[98] On phonation there is some air wastage but this is often not enough to cause the patient to seek medical advice. With time, compensation occurs and the voice may return in strength. As the superior laryngeal nerve is sensory to the supraglottis, problems with overspill and coughing may occur.

Recurrent laryngeal nerve palsy

A unilateral recurrent laryngeal nerve palsy rarely produces inspiratory problems, but as the cords tend to lie in the paramedian position the voice is often seriously compromised, being very breathy and hoarse, and the patient will be unable to count from 1 to 10 without taking a breath. As compensation occurs the contralateral vocal cord crosses the midline, probably due to activity of the intra-arytenoid muscle, and the voice disability is reduced (Fig. 20.42c).[99]

The aetiological factors known to cause recurrent laryngeal nerve palsy include injury, operative surgery (thyroidectomy, thoracic surgery), neoplasm (bronchial and thyroid carcinomas), neurological lesions, infections and inflammations: 40% of cases are idiopathic.[36]

The management of a cord palsy depends on defining the underlying pathology. A significant proportion of idiopathic palsies recover spontaneously and speech therapy may aid compensation by increasing glottic closure on phonation.[100] In palsies of malignant origin, e.g. carcinoma of the lung, or if at least 9 months have elapsed following surgical damage at thyroidectomy, measures should be taken to obtain glottic closure. Vocal cord injection by Teflon or collagen can be performed using microlaryngoscopy.[101] The injection is made into the cord just lateral to the vocalis muscle. More recently the use of a silastic shim has proved a popular alternative. This is placed through a window in the thyroid cartilage via a small external incision which allows accurate medialization of the cord.

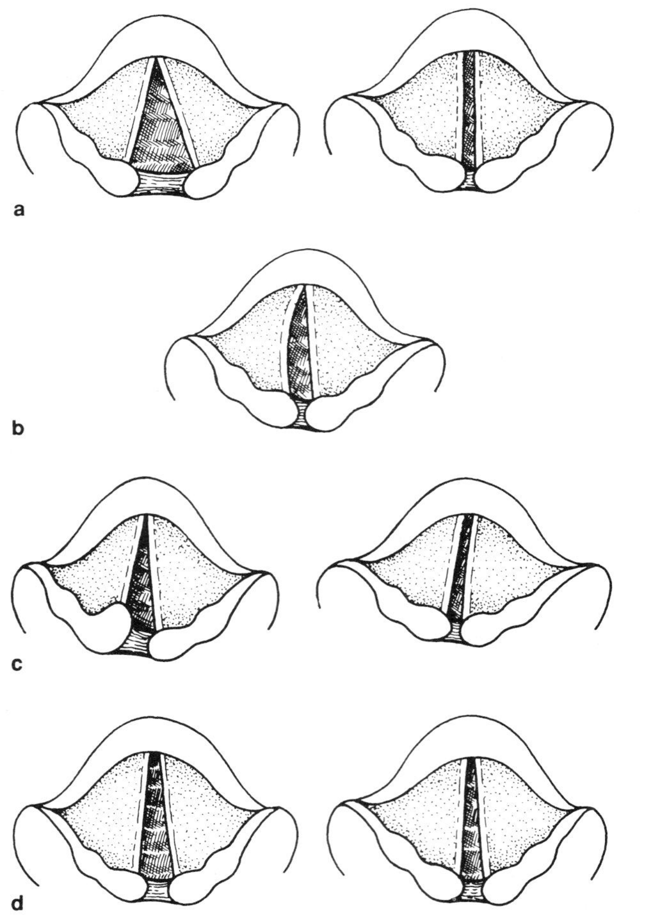

Fig. 20.42 (**a**) The normal larynx in abduction (left) and adduction (right). (**b**) Unilateral superior laryngeal nerve palsy in adduction. (**c**) Unilateral recurrent laryngeal nerve palsy: adduction in acute palsy (left) and after compensation (right). (**d**) Bilateral recurrent laryngeal nerve palsy in abduction (left) and adduction (right).

Bilateral recurrent nerve palsy

Damage to the recurrent laryngeal nerve during thyroidectomy is the most common cause of this problem. In the acute phase, often on awaking from the anaesthetic, the patient has a good voice but significant inspiratory stridor. A careful clinical assessment will indicate if an immediate tracheostomy is necessary (Fig. 20.42d). Paradoxically, on some occasions very little stridor is evident; the patient complains of dysphonia, which is only complicated by stridor when associated with an upper respiratory tract infection. Long-term management of the bilateral vocal cord palsy is based on the provision of an adequate airway with the best possible voice; obviously the larger the airway the poorer the voice. Decannulation can be achieved in 90% of cases. Laser arytenoidectomy is currently the most reliable treatment and results in a large glottic chink.

Laryngeal trauma

Blunt injuries

Fortunately the larynx is protected from most injuries by the anterior position of the mandible which on flexion of the head absorbs most traumatic forces. Thus mandibular fractures are significantly more common than laryngeal fractures. If the larynx is damaged by blunt injury the cartilage may be crushed against the cervical spine. Surprisingly symptoms may not develop immediately, stridor only appearing as laryngeal oedema accumulates. When the oesophagus or hypopharynx is damaged surgical emphysema results. Early formation of a tracheostomy is required if there is any question of airway obstruction. The anaesthetist should be warned that intubation may be difficult and tracheostomy, using local anaesthesia, may be necessary. Reconstruction of the larynx demands preserva-

REFERENCES

98. Howard D H, Lund V J Br Med Bull 1986; 42: 234
99. Dedo H, Urrea R D, Lawson L Ann Otol Rhinol Laryngol 1973; 82: 661
100. Howard D H In: Kerr A G (ed) Scott Brown's Otolaryngology. Butterworth, London 1988
101. Montgomery W W Ann Otol 1979; 88: 647

tion of as much laryngeal cartilage as possible and the fixation of the laryngeal skeleton around a solid stent kept in place by stainless steel sutures. Problems may arise from dislocation and rupture of the epiglottis or tearing of the anterior commissure which can be reconstructed by a keel repair.[102]

Sharp injuries

Stab injuries and self-inflicted knife wounds are frequently fatal but if they reach medical care they should be treated by protection of the airway while the haemorrhage is controlled. Induction of anaesthesia in such cases often results in venous relaxation overcoming post-traumatic spasm, causing a brisk haemorrhage and loss of the airway. A slick induction by a skilled anaesthetist avoids this problem.

Foreign body in the larynx

The glottis protects the airway by initiating a marked cough reflex but occasionally a foreign body still manages to become impacted in the larynx and this may prove fatal. Such a situation arises in the 'cafe coronary' or 'diner's death' syndrome.[103] The victim, who has been eating, suddenly collapses, perhaps clutching the throat, and quickly becomes cyanosed; as there is impaction no air can be expelled from the larynx so no cry is made. Treatment must be immediate. The victim is grasped from behind with the operator's fist placed just below the sternum and jerked with a strongly upward thrust with the intention that the air displaced from the lungs will pop the offending bolus from the larynx (Heimlich's manoeuvre).[104] An alternative, if time and facilities are available, is a cricothyroidotomy. Biros and penknives have been used to achieve this. A child may be held upside down while the lungs are forcibly compressed.

Tumours of the larynx

Malignant

The great majority of malignant laryngeal tumours are squamous carcinomas developing from the squamous epithelial lining of the vocal cord or from respiratory-type epithelium that has undergone squamous metaplastic change.

The incidence of laryngeal cancer in the UK is 4 in 100 000 of the population, which is considerably less than that found in Brazil and the USA (> 10:100 000 population) but more than Japan or Sweden (< 3:100 000).[105] It represents about 1% of all British malignancies. There is usually a long history of cigarette smoking often combined with alcohol abuse. Men (aged 60–70 years) are affected significantly more frequently than women, in a ratio of 6:1. Most laryngeal cancers develop on the vocal cords although in Sweden, Finland and Mediterranean countries a greater proportion arise in the supraglottis.[106] Hoarseness is the symptom most usually associated with laryngeal cancer: it is always continuous and often progressive. Stridor and dyspnoea are late features.

Examination by indirect laryngoscopy usually reveals the tumour clearly but a microlaryngoscopy should always be performed and biopsy taken. General anaesthesia in patients with laryngeal cancer may be hazardous and the anaesthetist should be forewarned to expect a difficult intubation. Intubation may be aided by railroading the naso- or orotracheal tube over a flexible fibreoptic endoscope. In some cases an initial tracheostomy must be performed but this procedure is not without its own problems as airway obstruction may occur when the patient is placed in the supine position and the tracheostomy must be placed below the tumour's inferior limit. The use of respiratory sedatives (benzodiazepines) should be avoided.

Inspection of the hypopharynx, upper oesophagus and trachea must be routine when the larynx is examined under anaesthesia. All biopsies should be taken using the microlaryngoscope to avoid missing tumours or causing unnecessary damage to the vocal cords. Tumours arising from the paraglottic space are often notoriously difficult to biopsy; the mucosa is intact and only deep biopsies will provide adequate material for histology. The mobility of the larynx should be carefully assessed as the patient is awakening from anaesthesia (Fig. 20.43).

Examination of the neck may identify the spread of the tumour in the form of a mass adjacent and fixed to the laryngeal skeleton or as lymph node metastases. Incisional biopsy of the cervical lymphadenopathy associated with clinical laryngeal neoplasia should be avoided although fine-needle aspiration is useful. General examination of the patient should include chest radiography and an assessment of liver function as the lifestyle of patients presenting with laryngeal cancer is often associated with chronic airway disease and cirrhotic liver disease. Distant metastases are uncommon although a second primary squamous carcinoma in the head and neck occurs in 10% of patients.[36]

Management of laryngeal cancer

The morbidity of laryngeal cancer reflects the local spread of the disease and so treatment, whether palliative or curative, can usually be confined to the larynx and adjacent neck (Fig. 20.44). Palliation is aimed at the relief of upper airway obstruction, dysphagia and pain. Radiotherapy given selectively may suppress local symptoms although with advanced disease the tumour bulk precludes anything but radical treatment. When airway obstruction is the major problem early tracheostomy is indicated as dyspnoea and stridor with associated hypoxia are extremely uncomfortable and very frightening.

Curative treatment usually involves radiotherapy, surgery or a combination of the two. Chemotherapy in the form of radiosensitizers may be used but there is no evidence to suggest that cytotoxic agents either increase survival or decrease morbidity.[107] The aim of a curative treatment must include the preservation of as

REFERENCES

102. McNaught R D Laryngoscope 1950; 60: 264
103. Adams G L, Boies L R Jr, Paparella M M (eds) Boies's Fundamentals of Otolaryngology. Saunders, Philadelphia 1978
104. Heimlich H J JAMA 1975; 234: 398
105. Robin P E, Olofsson J In: Kerr A G (ed) Scott Brown's Otolaryngology. Butterworth, London 1989
106. Newhouse M L, Gregory M M, Shannon H International Agency for Research on Cancer 1990

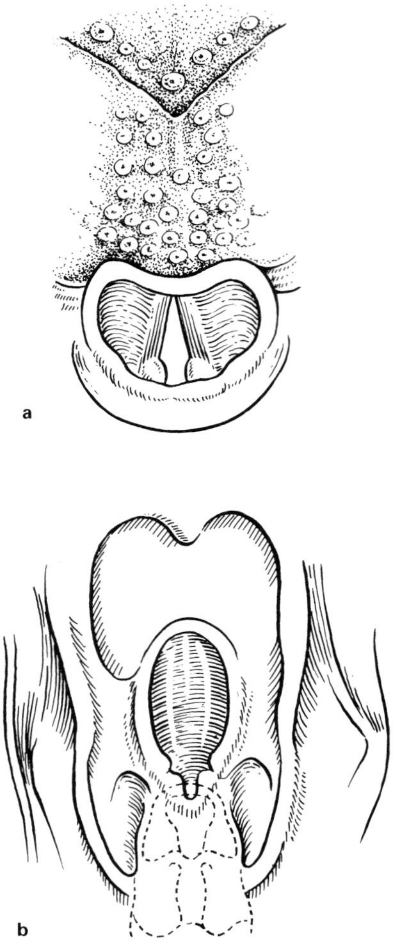

Fig. 20.43 Diagram showing (**a**) the larynx; (**b**) the hypopharynx.

much normal function as possible. With carcinomas of the larynx this precept is of paramount importance and this is why radiotherapy is the primary form of treatment in early lesions (T1 and T2). Primary surgery is indicated for carcinoma in situ where local excision in the form of vocal cord stripping may be effective. The CO_2 laser may also be used with good effect for this purpose and for the earliest T1 lesions which do not involve the anterior commissure. More extensive surgery should be selected for more extensive tumours (most T3 and T4 tumours), especially those associated with cervical lymphadenopathy, and for non-squamous carcinomas including adenocarcinomas, chemodectomas and chondrosarcomas where radiotherapy is less satisfactory or ineffective.

Emergency laryngectomy has been advocated for the patient with advanced malignant disease and stridor because of the danger of stomal recurrence following a primary tracheostomy.[108] However the logistics associated with this treatment, such as the need to obtain positive histological confirmation of the neoplasm and the absence of clear confirmatory evidence of increased stoma recurrence, have dissuaded most surgeons from this course of management.

Following radical radiotherapy, salvage surgery is indicated if the tumour is still present or if it recurs. Assessment of the larynx after radiotherapy is difficult and care should be taken in inter-

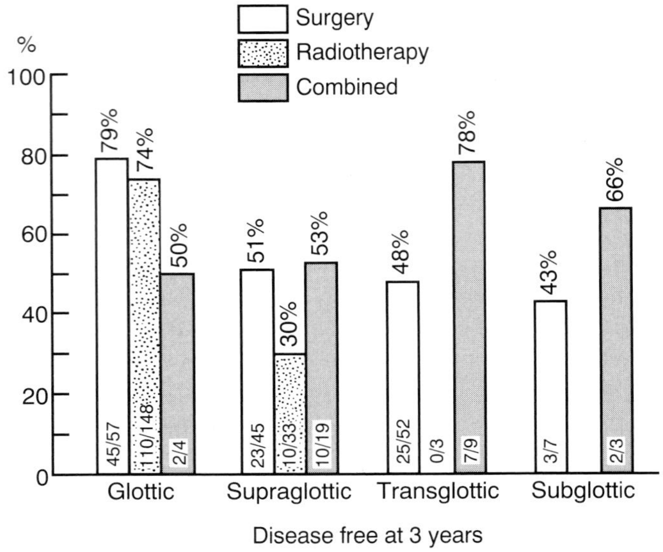

Fig. 20.44 3-year survival rates in laryngeal cancer.

preting biopsies in the first 3 months following a course of radiotherapy. Perichondritis after radiotherapy can produce symptoms which are very akin to those of recurrent tumour; if these symptoms do not respond to antibiotics and steroids, a laryngectomy is probably the treatment of choice.[107] Computerized tomographic scanning has been most useful in making this difficult decision. Although total laryngectomy is by far the most common definitive surgical operation for laryngeal cancer, a range of partial and subtotal laryngectomies are sometimes indicated.[109]

Total laryngectomy

A consequence of total laryngectomy is an end-tracheostome. When healed this does not normally require a tracheostomy tube but should be covered by a small gauze sponge which is kept permanently damp, to prevent entry of foreign material and to moisten air entering the lower respiratory tract.

Billroth performed the first laryngectomy for laryngeal cancer in 1873 although it was not until the early 20th century that the operative mortality fell to acceptable levels. In most cases primary tracheostomy is not required and anaesthesia is given through an orotracheal tube. The perioperative mortality is now in the region of 1%.

Incision. The operation is usually performed through a collar incision situated midway between the hyoid and the sternum with a separate circular incision for the tracheostomy. The Gluck–Sorenson incision[110] creates a U-shaped flap which includes the tracheostome and enables the surgeon to obtain good exposure

REFERENCES

107. Stell P M In: Harrison D F N (ed) Dilemmas in Otorhinolaryngology. Churchill Livingstone, Edinburgh 1988
108. Kiem W F, Shapiro M J, Rosin H D Arch Otolaryngol 1965; 81: 183
109. Robin P E, Olofsson J In: Kerr A G (ed) Scott Brown's Otolaryngology. Butterworth, London 1988

of the subglottis and paratracheal lymph nodes but may be associated with a postoperative stenosis of the tracheostome. Removal of the larynx is performed by the technique already described for laryngopharyngectomy. Closure of the pharynx must always be most carefully performed with a Connell inverted stitch; in the irradiated patient this should be continuous and should not contain a T junction.

Complications following laryngectomy. Pharyngocutaneous fistulae are not uncommon in the irradiated patient and usually occur in the second postoperative week. They often take a considerable time to heal and the patient should be fed by nasogastric tube until the fistula closes.[111] Re-operation should not be considered until after 6 weeks of conservative therapy which includes adequate nutrition, blood transfusion if the haemoglobin falls below 10 g/dl and antibiotic therapy including cover for anaerobic bacteria. Operative closure of the fistula involves the introduction of non-irradiated skin; this may be achieved by a free forearm flap which is constructed in order to cover the pharyngeal defect as well as the skin defect caused by the fistula.

Although simple closure using a deltopectoral or pectoralis flap may cover the skin defect this can lead to fibrosis of the pharynx and swallowing problems at a later date.

Voice rehabilitation. Following total laryngectomy approximately one third of patients are able to communicate with oesophageal speech. Phonation occurs when air swallowed into the oesophagus is allowed to pass across the cricopharyngeal sphincter producing a vibratory phonation which can then be articulated in the mouth. A mechanical phonation can be produced by means of a vibrator placed over the neck, under the mandible, once again with oral articulation. However this technique suffers from a loss of spontaneity and results in a monotonic Dalek-type voice. Recently several techniques have been used to improve the oesophageal voice by allowing the passage of air into the oesophagus by means of a valve placed in the posterior wall of the trachea. These valves are unidirectional and prevent aspiration.[112]

Partial laryngectomy

When any laryngeal function can be preserved without compromising the chance of cure, partial laryngectomy must be considered. As the cure rate associated with radiotherapy compares well with that of surgery, partial laryngeal surgery is predominantly used for radiation failures. Thus in cases of cordal recurrence cordectomy by vertical laryngofissure is indicated;[113] if more of the hemilarynx is involved a vertical hemilaryngectomy can be performed. Whenever such surgery is contemplated it is important to relate the operative excision to the position of the tumour before radiotherapy rather than the site of the recurrent tumour.

Supraglottic tumours may be managed by horizontal supraglottic laryngectomy. All partial surgery is performed with a tracheostomy in situ, and the postoperative management includes nasogastric feeding for the first 7 days. The tube is then removed and if there is no evidence of fistulation the patient is slowly encouraged to return to normal eating starting with soft solids. Some aspiration inevitably occurs and coughing tends to distress patients. However, normal swallowing is usually re-established within 3 days.

Tracheostomy

Tracheostomy may be an emergency or elective procedure. The commonest indications are respiratory and ventilation failure, usually associated with retained bronchial secretions and upper airway obstruction (Table 20.12). It is always important to remember the old surgical rule: 'do a tracheostomy when you think about it; don't wait until it becomes an emergency'.

Surgical technique. Tracheostomy is best performed under general anaesthesia in an operating theatre. The inexperienced surgeon should not be inveigled into performing the operation in an intensive care unit or ward except as a dire emergency; little advantage is gained and complications are more difficult to cope with. A horizontal skin incision is marked on the skin midway between the lower edge of the thyroid cartilage (cricoid ring) and the suprasternal notch. In the emergency situation a vertical midline incision may be used but the surgeon must take care not to veer laterally from the trachea (Fig. 20.45). At all times the surgeon should check the position of the trachea by manual palpation and thus avoid dissection into the paratracheal space. When the thyroid isthmus is recognized it should be divided between arterial clamps and ligated with transfixion sutures. On occasions it may be retracted upwards or downwards.

The cricoid ring is identified and retracted upwards by means of a cricoid hook. In children a vertical incision is made in the second and third tracheal rings; no cartilage is removed. In the adult a square window is excised between the second and fourth rings large enough to accept the tracheostomy tube—30–34 Fg in women, 32–38 Fg in men. At this stage the anaesthetist should be asked to remove the orotracheal tube slowly from the mouth and when its distal end moves past the tracheostomy the anaesthetist pauses while the tracheostomy tube, with its obturator inside, is inserted. Haemostasis is achieved and the tracheostomy tube is securely fastened by means of tapes around the neck tied with the head in flexion. As an additional precaution the flange of the tube may be sewn to the skin by a heavy suture which can be removed at the first change of tube. The skin incision should only be loosely sutured in order to avoid surgical emphysema.

Postoperative management. As the cough reflex is lost the patient is unable to clear secretions from the tracheobronchial tree, so frequent suction is necessary. There is usually no need to

REFERENCES

110. Sorensen P, Thompson A E Head Neck Surg 1986; 8: 418
111. Robin P E, Olofsson J In: Kerr A G (ed) Scott Brown's Otolaryngology. Butterworth, London 1988
112. Singer M I, Blom E D Ann Otol 1986; 89: 529

Table 20.12 Indications for tracheostomy

Emergency—acute upper airway obstruction	
	Foreign body
	Infection, inflammation
	Haemorrhage into upper airway
Elective—protection of the airway when laryngeal and cough reflexes are suppressed.	
	Coma
	Neurological disease
	Prolonged ventilation
	Bronchiolar toilet
	To decrease dead space

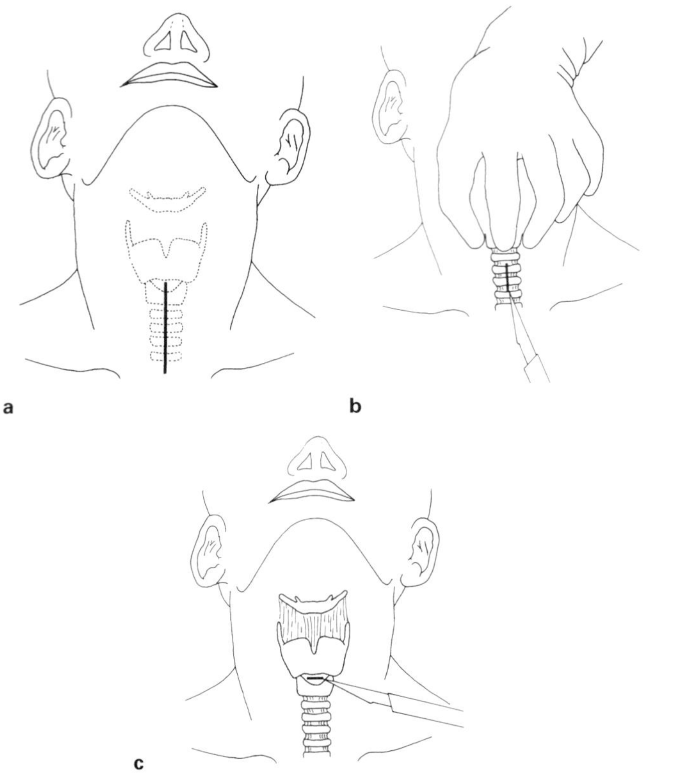

Fig. 20.45 (a) Drawing showing position of skin incision in relation to laryngeal landmarks for emergency tracheostomy. (b) Drawing showing position of vertical incision at the level of the second to fourth tracheal rings. (c) Drawing showing position of incision for a cricothyroidotomy (laryngotomy). After D J Howard, Emergency and elective airway procedures. In: MacGregor IA, Howard DJ (eds) Rob and Smith's Operative Surgery. Head and Neck Part 1. Butterworth 1992.

change the tracheostomy tube in the first 48 hours and indeed to change a tube during this period can be positively dangerous as the track has not organized, making replacement of the tube difficult. Crusting frequently occurs as cold dry air thickens the tracheobronchial secretions and therefore humidified air should be administered either by means of a commercial humidifier or by a regular droplet infusion into the tracheostomy tube. More serious complications can occur in the immediate postoperative period or some time later (Table 20.13).

Tracheostomy tubes

Non-metal. Silastic is the material most frequently used for tracheostomy tubes (Fig. 20.46a). These tubes may be cuffed or uncuffed, and low-pressure cuffs that produce less tracheal pressure are now available.[114] The obturator from the tracheostomy tube should be kept by the patient in case emergency re-intubation is necessary.

Metal tubes. Silver tubes are used for long-term tracheostomy patients (Fig. 20.46b). They have an outer and an inner tube which allows cleaning of the inner tube whilst maintaining the airway. The inner tube is designed to be slightly longer than the outer tube thus allowing secretions to be collected on removal of the tube. A third tube, which is placed inside the other two, is fitted with a small flap valve and allows phonation.

Table 20.13 Complications of tracheostomy

Early complications	*Late complications*
Haemorrhage	Difficult decannulation
Accidental extubation	Tracheo-cutaneous fistula
Tracheal and paratracheal trauma	Tracheo-oesophageal fistula
Tube lumen obstruction	Tracheo-innominate artery haemorrhage
Subcutaneous emphysema	Tracheal stenosis
Pneumothorax	
Infection	
Swallowing dysfunction	
Apnoea/death	

Laryngotomy/cricothyrotomy

Emergency entry to the airway in the absence of a previously positioned endotracheal tube is best achieved via the cricothyroid membrane.[82] The thyroid cartilage is steadied and slightly rotated upwards before a scalpel blade is used to make a vertical incision down to and through the cricothyroid membrane. A pair of artery forceps may be inserted to widen the aperture so that a small endotracheal tube may be inserted. Once the airway has been secured a formal endotracheal intubation or tracheostomy is performed.

Mini-tracheostomy

In cases where tracheobronchial toilet alone is needed the mini-tracheostomy is a useful technique.[83] A cricothyrotomy is performed and a small-gauge cannula is railroaded over a flexible introducer. Care should be taken to ensure that the cannula tip has not passed the carina.[115] This technique is not suitable for ventilation except in the very short term.[116]

REFERENCES

113. Ogura J H, Sessions D G, Spector G J Laryngoscope 1980; 85: 591
114. Sawada Y, Kozima Y, Fonkalsrud E W Surg Gynecol Obstet 1982; 154: 648
115. McGill J, Clinton J E, Ruiz E Ann Emerg Med 1982; 113: 61
116. Mathews H R, Hopkinson R B Br J Surg 1982; 71: 147

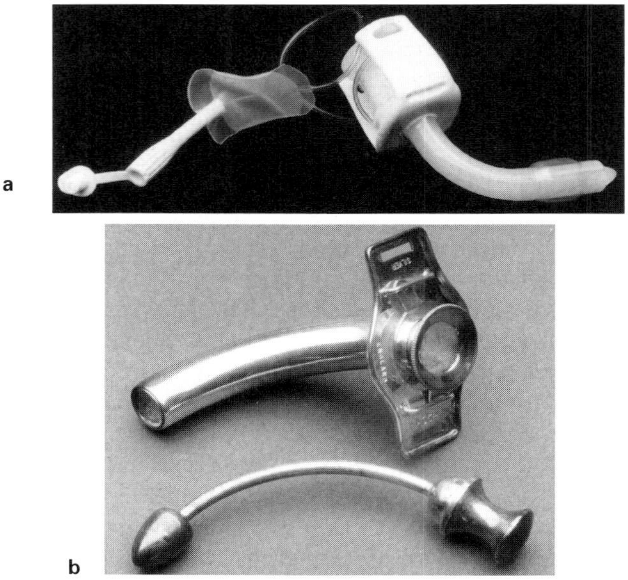

Fig. 20.46 Tracheostomy tubes: (a) cuffed portex tube; (b) silver Negus tube.

21 The oesophagus

J. Bancewicz W. J. Owen

CONGENITAL OESOPHAGEAL DISORDERS

Oesophageal atresia and tracheo-oesophageal fistula, which is often associated, are discussed in Chapter 41.

Dysphagia lusoria is caused by an anomalous subclavian artery or double aortic arch crossing the oesophaus. The aberrant artery can be divided with relief of symptoms.

INJURY

Oesophageal trauma is frequently lethal and therefore poses great problems in management. Damage to the oesophagus may arise in various ways, ranging from missile injuries and instrumental injury to damage by drugs or ingested corrosives.

Spontaneous rupture

Spontaneous rupture of the oesophagus has been reported many times since Boerhaave of Leiden first reported the case of Baron Wassenaar, Grand Admiral of the Dutch Fleet, a notorious glutton who had cultivated the Roman habit of autoemesis; exercising this habit after a meal he sustained a fatal perforation of the oesophagus just above the diaphragm.[1] Most cases still occur in similar, if less extreme, circumstances. The typical history is that severe pain in the chest or upper abdomen occurs suddenly after an episode of vomiting. This is followed rapidly by cardiovascular collapse as the result of a virulent chemical mediastinitis. When the pain is predominantly in the upper abdomen there is often some degree of abdominal rigidity as well, which may suggest gastroduodenal perforation. Otherwise the condition is most likely to be confused with myocardial infarction or dissecting aneurysm. The tear is usually on the left posterior aspect of the oesophagus just above the cardia. Occasional cases of intra-abdominal rupture have been recorded.

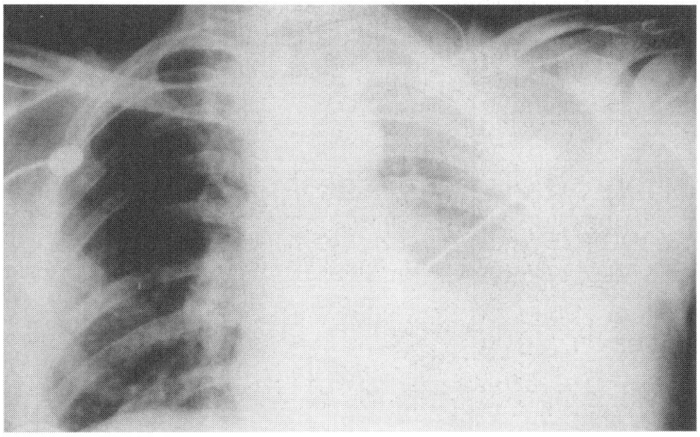

Fig. 21.1 Pleural effusion following oesophageal perforation.

In typical cases subcutaneous emphysema of the neck and upper chest appears, but this is not always marked and may be absent. Chest X-ray usually reveals mediastinal gas or a pleural effusion (Fig. 21.1), but a normal X-ray does not exclude rupture. A contrast swallow (Fig. 21.2) should always be done as soon as possible if the diagnosis is suspected as delay in making the diagnosis is the greatest single factor contributing to a poor prognosis.

Early diagnosis is the key to a successful outcome. Primary repair is the treatment of choice and should be carried out within a few hours of the rupture. Mortality can be as low as 10%,[2] but may be four or five times this level if the diagnosis is delayed.[3]

Penetrating injury

Penetrating injury is uncommon, even in war, as other intrathoracic organs present a much larger target. Bullets and knives are the usual implements, but chest drains may occasionally be responsible.[4] By far the largest experience in modern times is reported in the American literature.[5] Management is obviously affected by injuries to other organs. In the case of missile injuries, especially with high-velocity missiles, there may be a considerable amount of shock wave damage to surrounding tissues which is not apparent on gross inspection. In such circumstances generous resection may be the only option available. Continuity may be restored by oesophagogastric anastomosis. More complex reconstructions, for example by colonic interposition, should not be attempted in emergency cases.

Instrumental perforation

The less frequent use of the rigid oesophagoscope following the advent of flexible endoscopes has considerably increased the

REFERENCES

1. Boerhaave H 1724 Atroces, nec descripti primus. Morbi Historia. Secundem Artes Legis Conscripta. Lugdini Batavorum Boutesteniana: Medici
2. Triggiani E, Betsey R Thorax 1977; 32: 241
3. Sawyers J L et al Ann Thorax Surg 1975; 19: 233
4. Clifford P C Br J Surg 1980; 67: 451
5. Symbas P N et al Ann Surg 1980; 191: 703

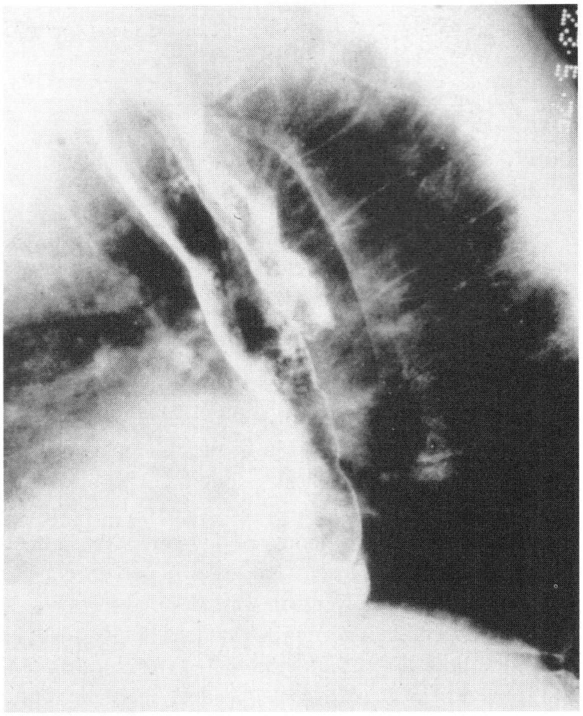

Fig. 21.2 Oesophageal perforation.

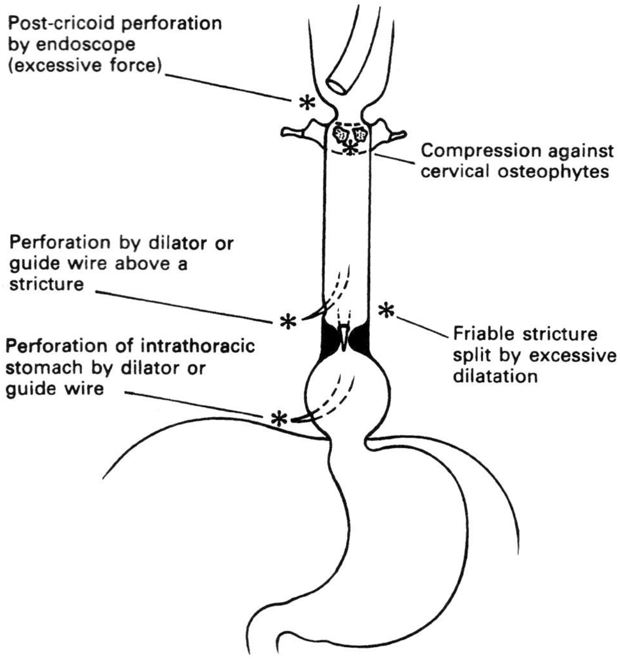

Fig. 21.3 Mechanisms responsible for instrumental perforation of the oesophagus.

safety of oesophageal instrumentation. A rigid oesophagoscope can be passed safely, but a great deal of skill is required. It can be virtually impossible in a kyphotic patient. Nevertheless, the rigid instrument is still occasionally required, for example, to remove an awkward foreign body.

An endoscope may perforate the oesophagus in its upper part, especially in a patient with prominent osteophytes in the cervical spine (Fig. 21.3). The thoracic or occasionally the abdominal oesophagus is more commonly injured during dilatation of strictures or pneumatic dilatation for achalasia.[6] Passage of dilators over a guidewire is normally safe, but only if the wire is correctly placed and its position does not change during instrumentation (Fig. 21.3).

Endo-oesophageal intubation for carcinoma may split a friable growth, but the leak is usually sealed, at least in part by the tube. It is now well-recognized that it is the dilatation that splits the tumour and that there is a significant risk in all tumour treatments, such as laser treatment that may involve prior dilatation.

Foreign body perforation

Foreign bodies of many sorts, including pins, dentures and other implements, can be retrieved safely from the oesophagus. However, perforation may occur during their removal and a foreign body that has been left in situ for several days may erode through the oesophageal wall.[7]

Pathological perforation

Pathological perforation of the oesophagus is unusual, but peptic ulcers and neoplasms may cause free perforation into the mediastinum or pleural cavity. Erosion into the aorta or even the ventricle may occur with rapidly fatal results.[8] Carcinomas, of course, more commonly cause tracheo-oesophageal fistulas which are discussed separately

Mediastinitis

Following oesophageal perforation the loose areolar tissues of the posterior mediastinum allow rapid spread of gastrointestinal contents. Mediastinitis is a very dangerous condition which produces marked systemic disturbance and cardiovascular collapse. Cardiac dysrhythmias are common.

The clinical signs of mediastinitis are those of severe systemic sepsis, but there is usually a more marked tachycardia than is expected from the patient's condition. Atrial fibrillation is the commonest dysrhythmia and may seriously interfere with cardiac output in an already compromised patient. There are few specific clinical signs, but a mediastinal 'crunch' may be heard on auscultation if gas is present around the pericardium. The crunching, which sounds like footsteps in soft snow, occurs in synchrony with the heart sounds.

Diagnosis of oesophageal perforation

Awareness of the possibility of oesophageal perforation is the most important aspect of diagnosis. Any upset or pain following

REFERENCES

6. Banks J G, Bancewicz J Br J Surg 1981; 68: 580
7. Wichern W A Am J Surg 1970; 119: 535
8. Ming S C In: Atlas of Tumor Pathology, Series 2, Fascicle 7. Armed Forces Institute of Pathology, Washington, DC 1973

oesophageal instrumentation should raise the suspicion of perforation. Severe chest or abdominal pain following an episode of vomiting is also suggestive of a spontaneous perforation.

Investigation has two purposes: first, to demonstrate the perforation, and second, to look for other oesophageal pathology which may influence treatment. A chest radiograph may show subcutaneous and mediastinal gas, a pleural effusion or a pneumothorax, depending on the site and size of the perforation. A contrast swallow is almost always required to provide firm proof of the diagnosis, to demonstrate the extent of the problem and to provide good anatomical definition of the injured oesophagus in order to determine the correct management. For this purpose barium is preferred to water-soluble contrast media which produce indifferent pictures. Contrary to popular belief barium is not harmful in such circumstances provided that it is used in moderation.[9] If a water-soluble contrast medium is used it should be one of the newer non-ionic agents which are not harmful to the respiratory tree when aspirated.

Occasionally careful endoscopy is required to give additional information.

Treatment

There is still controversy and even confusion about the best management of oesophageal perforation. Part of the reason is that no two patients are alike. An untreated perforation usually results in death unless it is very small or it drains into the pleural cavity and forms an empyema.[2] The factors that determine the outcome are the size and site of the perforation, the presence of mediastinitis and cardiovascular collapse, the general condition and previous health of the patient, the presence of other oesophageal pathology, and the interval between perforation and treatment. Delayed diagnosis is the most common reason for a poor outcome and failure to think of the possibility of oesophageal rupture is the main reason for diagnostic error. Paradoxically, the outlook is better in those who are not diagnosed for 48 hours or more.[6] This is presumably from selection of patients with the capacity for survival.

Recommended forms of management range from conservative treatment with intravenous fluids and antibiotics to total oesophagectomy. The range of options is given below.

1. Antibiotics, intravenous fluids, restriction of oral intake.
2. As above, plus pleural drainage using a percutaneous drain or thoracotomy.
3. Primary repair.
4. Exclusion of the oesophagus and drainage of the chest (Fig. 21.4).
5. Oesophageal resection with immediate or delayed reconstruction.
6. Chemical sclerosis.

Good results have been claimed for all of these methods,[2,10–13] but not all are applicable in every situation. Conservative treatment is appropriate for small perforations which are diagnosed promptly and which produce minimal pain and systemic disturbance. Occasionally oesophageal perforation is not diagnosed until several days after the event, when nothing more than drainage of

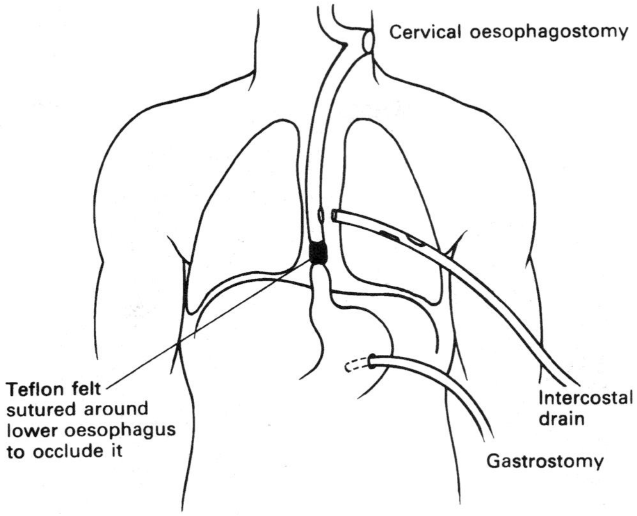

Fig. 21.4 Exclusion of the oesophagus for perforation.

an empyema is feasible, but this is rare. Chemical sclerosis[13] has been used to treat perforations that are diagnosed late and do not cause much systemic upset. Sodium hydroxide (20%) is applied to the edges of the perforation and then neutralized with 30% acetic acid in the hope that the defect will shrink more speedily.

In general the worse the systemic effects of the perforation, the greater the need for a surgical solution. Simple closure of the perforation is an effective form of management provided that this is done within 12 hours and, ideally, much sooner. When the diagnosis is delayed repair may be impossible because of the condition of the tissues and the problem of wound healing in the presence of sepsis. The defect in the mucosa is always longer than the defect in the muscle. The first stage is therefore to incise the muscle layer so that the edges of the mucosa can be clearly seen and sutured, preferably in layers. The repair may be strengthened by applying a flap of intercostal muscle, diaphragm,[14] or the adjacent fundus of the stomach.[15] Only normal oesophageal tissue should be closed. Resection should be considered if the perforation has occurred through or above a fibrous stricture.

Treatment by exclusion and drainage (Fig. 21.4) is appropriate for perforations that are diagnosed late and associated with heavy contamination.[12] Many other ingenious methods for excluding and draining the oesophagus have been reported using a variety of tubes.[16,17] The object is to drain the chest and divert salivary and gastric secretion away from the perforation. Subtotal oesophagectomy with construction of a cervical oesophagostomy and a

REFERENCES

9. Foley M J et al Radiology 1982; 144: 231
10. Cameron J L et al Ann Thorac Surg 1979; 27: 404
11. Lyons W S et al Ann Thorac Surg 1978; 26: 346
12. Urschel H C et al Ann Surg 1974; 179: 587
13. Gunning A J, Kingsworth A Br J Surg 1979; 66: 226
14. Westaby S Br J Surg 1980; 67: 801
15. Thal A P Ann Surg 1969; 168: 542
16. Hinder R A et al Br J Surg 1981; 68: 182
17. Barringer H, Meredith J Am Surg 1982; 48: 518

gastrostomy[2] is the ultimate treatment for the extreme situation. The obvious disadvantage is the need for subsequent reconstruction.

Mallory–Weiss syndrome

Mucosal tears at the cardia are quite common during prolonged or violent vomiting.[18] They present with haematemesis, usually of a modest degree. Endoscopy reveals a short longitudinal tear in the mucosa usually just distal to the cardia, or in the lower oesophagus just above the cardia. Some patients may develop chest pain, which raises the suspicion of complete rupture. Occasionally the bleeding may be so severe as to require surgical exploration and oversewing,[19] but this should be avoided if possible as it requires a laparotomy and the tear is usually small. Endoscopic diathermy or photocoagulation may be a useful manoeuvre for stopping severe bleeding.[20]

Removal of foreign bodies

Impacted foreign bodies, ranging from fishbone to false teeth, may present a considerable challenge to remove. There is no place for conservative management other than waiting for a few hours. Fishbones and coins are not usually difficult, but open safety pins and dentures may tax the skills of even the most experienced endoscopist. In general, the fibreoptic gastroscope is the best tool and an overtube is useful (Fig. 21.5). Most foreign bodies can be removed with simple grasping forceps, but dentures may need to be broken into small pieces with a cutter which can only be passed down a rigid endoscope. The classic problem is that of an open safety pin; the solution has been elegantly discussed by Chevalier Jackson.[21] When the point is downwards the pin may be held by forceps while the oesophagoscope (or overtube) is advanced over the pin. If the point faces upwards the pin can sometimes be pushed into the stomach and then drawn into the tube or endoscope. Alternatively, it may be turned in the oesophagus. This has to be done with a rigid endoscope and grasping forceps. In this manoeuvre the spring of the pin is grasped and moved to one side of the oesophagus. Continued lateral pressure is applied to widen the lumen and the instruments are carefully withdrawn.

Corrosive injury

Ingested corrosives are highly damaging to the upper gastrointestinal tract. The most commonly taken are caustic soda or sulphuric acid from car batteries in attempted suicide.[22] Bleach may be drunk by young children. All of these agents can cause extensive damage to the pharynx, larynx, oesophagus and stomach. Usually the pharynx is relatively spared because of the short contact time, but oedema of the laryngopharynx may produce respiratory difficulty.

The oesophagus takes the brunt of the injury, especially with caustic soda, and it may even perforate at a very early stage. More often there is severe mucosal and submucosal injury which later gives rise to strictures. The stomach is relatively protected because its contents dilute whatever has been swallowed. Gastric acid also neutralizes at least some of any ingested alkali. Despite this, injury

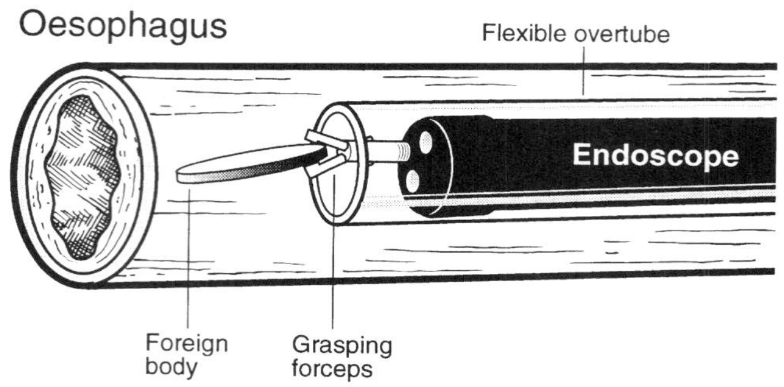

Fig. 21.5 Removal of foreign body from the oesophagus using an overtube and fibreoptic endoscope.

to the stomach may occur with perforation within a few hours or up to 3 weeks after the injury. Later on part or all of the stomach may contract if the injury has been severe.

The management of caustic injuries has been reviewed by Bremner.[23] Early endoscopy within a few hours of injury is the key. A fine fibreoptic gastroscope is passed by an experienced operator to inspect the whole of the oesophagus and stomach if possible. Complete endoscopy should not be attempted if there is a severe necrotizing lesion and air insufflation is kept to a minimum. Patients with minor injuries may be discharged early. Those with severe mucosal damage should be treated with steroids for 3 weeks and then have regular oesophageal dilatation. Early resection should be undertaken if full-thickness oesophageal necrosis is suspected.

Drug-induced injury

Medication may injure the oesophagus both by direct irritation and by its pharmacological effects. Many tablets and capsules lie in the oesophagus for long periods, especially if swallowed in the recumbent position without an adequate drink.[24] Release of irritant constituents in the oesophagus may then cause local damage, giving rise to pain, dysphagia and even stricture formation.[25]

Smooth muscle relaxants may induce gastro-oesophageal reflux and hence injure the oesophagus. They may also reduce the effectiveness of peristalsis and increase the risk of direct mucosal injury. For these reasons a full drug history must be taken from all patients with oesophageal symptoms, especially the elderly.

Radiation injury

Radiotherapy for carcinomas of the oesophagus, the lung or the breast may produce oesophageal damage. Usually the injury is

REFERENCES

18. Mallory G K, Weiss S Am J Med Sci 1929; 178: 506
19. Baue A E JAMA 1963; 184: 325
20. Sugawa C et al Am J Surg 1983; 145: 30
21. Jackson C Ann Otol Rhinol Laryngol 1924; 33: 1009
22. Paul A T S Surgery (Oxford) 1987; 49: 1156
23. Bremner C E In: Hennessy T P J, Cuschieri A (eds) Surgery of the Oesophagus. Baillière Tindall, London 1986
24. Channer K, Virjee J Br Med J 1982; 285: 1702
25. Heller S R et al Br Med J 1982; 285: 167

slight, but considerable dysphagia and odynophagia (painful swallowing) can occur. Inspection of the oesophagus usually reveals very little in the way of gross mucosal injury. Treatment is essentially supportive until the injury has subsided.

Radiation-induced strictures following treatment of oesophageal cancer may be troublesome.[26] They are often resistant to dilatation and may conceal a local recurrence.[27] They require resection if the patient's condition will permit, but this may be a technical challenge because of extensive radiation fibrosis.

Nasogastric intubation

Prolonged nasogastric intubation may occasionally cause an oesophageal stricture. Whether this happens in a normal oesophagus is open to debate.[28] Most of those developing a stricture have pre-existing oesophageal reflux and intubation simply aggravates matters. The upper oesophageal sphincter may also be rendered incompetent by intubation, increasing the risk of aspiration pneumonia.

DISORDERS OF THE PHARYNGO-OESOPHAGEAL JUNCTION

There are several conditions which may affect the pharyngo-oesophageal junction and cause dysphagia. Tumours and webs will not be mentioned here as they are discussed in Chapter 20. In practice, dysphagia arising from disorders of the upper oesophagus is often misdiagnosed and may be wrongly labelled as hysterical dysphagia. True psychogenic dysphagia is extremely rare and usually presents as obvious delusions about the act of swallowing.

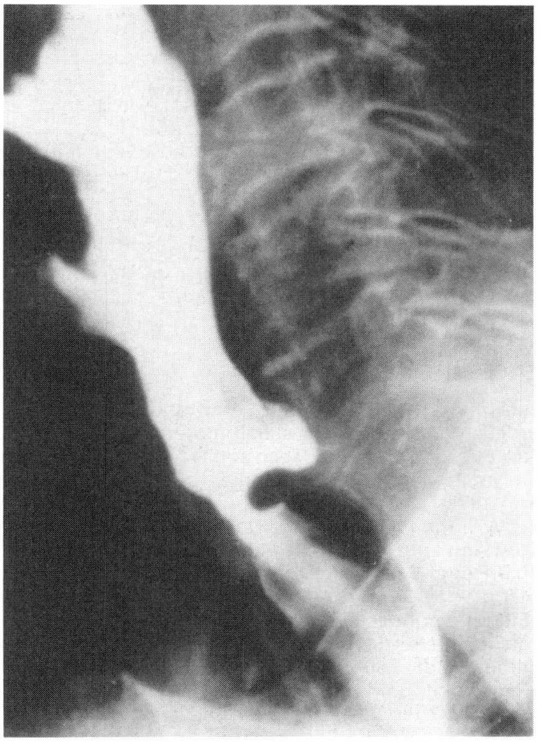

Fig. 21.6 Cricopharyngeal bar.

Functional disorders

Three types of problem may be encountered:

1. Diminished pharyngeal propulsion.
2. Relaxation difficulties.
3. Incoordination.

Diminished pharyngeal propulsion

This is essentially a neurological problem. Motor neurone disease and myasthenia gravis are the most common conditions which produce swallowing difficulty by reducing the power of pharyngeal propulsion.[29] Oculopharyngeal muscular dystrophy is an inherited condition which is mainly confined to French Canadians.[30]

Cerebrovascular accidents may also interfere with pharyngeal power if the 9th, 10th or 12th cranial nerves are affected, but there is also usually severe disturbance of coordination of the act of swallowing.[29]

Treatment is that of the underlying condition. Cricopharyngeal myotomy has a small part to play in palliative management.[31] Provided that some pharyngeal power is preserved, myotomy reduces the resistance of the upper sphincter and may improve swallowing.

Relaxation difficulties

These are uncommon and masquerade under a variety of unsatisfactory names such as cricopharyngeal bar and upper oesophageal achalasia.[31,33] Little is known of their nature, but this is now being remedied. Chronic inflammatory changes have been found in the cricopharyngeus muscle in a small number of patients.[34] This seems to produce stiffening of the muscle which cannot open up and allow food to pass. Cine or video barium studies are the most helpful form of investigation. The most common finding is a prominent indentation posteriorly at the level of the cricopharyngeus (Fig. 21.6). Endoscopy is essential to exclude a post cricoid carcinoma. Sometimes the resistance is so severe that it can actually be felt with an endoscope or a dilator.

Cricopharyngeal myotomy is usually very successful in the management of these conditions.[32–34]

Incoordination

Normally the upper oesophageal sphincter relaxes to receive the arriving pharyngeal contraction and allow food to enter the upper

REFERENCES

26. Hennessy T P J Br J Surg 1988; 75: 193
27. Xian Zhi Gu In: Huang G J, K'ai W Y (eds) Carcinoma of the Esophagus and Gastric Cardia. Springer Verlag, Berlin 1984
28. Ballfield W J, Hurwitz A L Arch Intern Med 1974; 134: 1083
29. Morrell R M In: Groher M E (ed) Dysphagia. Butterworth, London 1984
30. Duranceau A C et al Surg Clin North Am 1983; 63: 825
31. Duranceau A C et al Surg Clin North Am 1983; 63: 833
32. Blakeley W R et al Arch Surg 1968; 96: 745
33. Belsey R H J Thorac Cardiovasc Surg 1966; 52: 164
34. Cruse J P et al Histopathology 1979; 3: 223

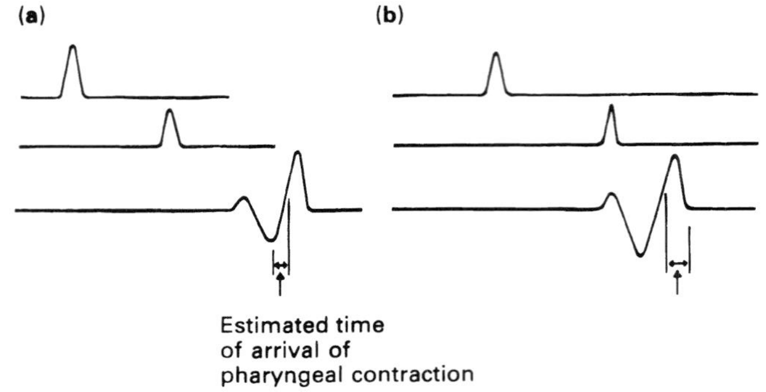

Fig. 21.7 Cricopharyngeal incoordination. (**a**) Coordinate response; (**b**) incoordinate response.

oesophagus. Dysphagia may occur if this response is disturbed (Fig. 21.7). Gross incoordination is common in patients with strokes and may occur in other neurological conditions.[29] Gastro-oesophageal reflux may also produce incoordination and high dysphagia is quite a common symptom in patients with reflux.[35] This dysphagia is not usually severe and the patient may not mention it unless prompted.

Treatment is again directed at the underlying condition, but cricopharyngeal myotomy may be required in severe cases. Caution should be exercised in patients with gross reflux as myotomy may leave the patient open to tracheal aspiration.[35]

Zenker's pharyngeal diverticulum[36]

A pharyngeal diverticulum is an outpouching of mucosa first observed by Ludlow in 1767. It protrudes from the back of the pharynx through Killian–Jamieson's dehiscence just above the cricopharyngeus muscle (Fig. 21.8). Large diverticula may extend into the mediastinum, reaching as low as the arch of the aorta. The reason why these diverticula occur has been the subject of speculation for many years. Most agree that it is likely to be the result of a chronic functional obstruction at the upper sphincter.[37] Establishing this as fact, however, has been impossible. Some report a high incidence of cricopharyngeal incoordination,[38] while others deny this.[39] The most convincing explanation is that there may be inflammatory degeneration in the cricopharyngeus muscle with a change in its elastic and contraction properties, similar to the relaxation anomalies mentioned above.[40] Diverticula may also be associated with severe symptoms even when they are small. Patients usually first find food sticking with attacks of hawking. Later food may be regurgitated and gas may escape, especially after neck pressure. Eventually progressive dysphagia, weight loss and aspiration pneumonia develop.

There are two classic problems in diagnosis. First, a diverticulum can be ruptured during injudicious endoscopy[41] and second, carcinomas may arise within the diverticulum itself, although this is really quite rare.[42] A barium swallow should be obtained before endoscopy if a pharyngeal diverticulum is suspected.

Treatment is by excision of the diverticulum and closure of the defect in two layers. This is preferably combined with a cricopharyngeal myotomy. Small diverticula may be left and treated by

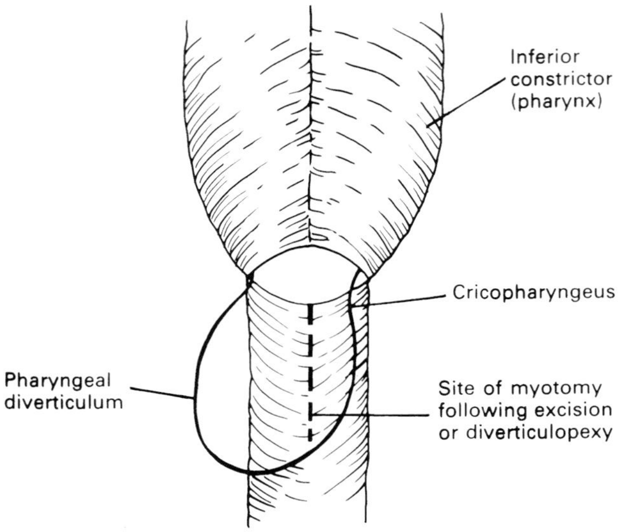

Fig. 21.8 Pharyngeal diverticulum: it presents posteriorly and (usually) to the left.

myotomy alone. Belsey[33] has suggested that large diverticula may be treated by myotomy and diverticulopexy so that the inverted pouch does not fill with food. An ingenious endoscopic method has been described by Dohlman & Mattsson[43] whereby the septum between the diverticulum and the oesophagus is divided by diathermy. The septum may also be divided safely with a laparoscopic linear cutter staple gun inserted via a short pharyngoscope,[44] but it is common to have slight residual dysphagia with this method.

GASTRO-OESOPHAGEAL REFLUX

The association between hiatus hernia, gastro-oesophageal reflux and symptoms was first described by Allison in 1951.[45] It is now known that hiatus hernia occurs in up to half the population over the age of 50, and that only one-third of those with a hiatus hernia suffer from reflux symptoms. Substantial gastro-oesophageal reflux also occurs in the absence of a hiatus hernia, and reflux can occur transiently in healthy symptomless individuals. This 'physiological' reflux occurs particularly in the upright posture

REFERENCES

35. Henderson R D The Esophagus: Reflux and Primary Motor Disorders. Williams & Wilkins, Baltimore 1980
36. Zenker F A, Ziemssen H In: Zeimssen H (ed) Handbuch des speciellen Pathologie und Therapie, vol 7 (suppl). F C Vogel, Leipzig 1877
37. Payne W S, King R M Surg Clin North Am 1983; 63: 815
38. Ellis F H Ann Surg 1969; 170: 340
39. Knuff T F et al Gastroenterology 1982; 82: 734
40. Lerut T et al In: Siewert J R, Holscher A H (eds) Diseases of the Esophagus. Springer-Verlag, Berlin 1988
41. Triggiani E, Belsey R Thorax 1977; 32: 241
42. Wychulis A R et al Surgery 1969; 66: 976
43. Dohlman G, Mattsson O Arch Otolaryngol 1960; 71: 744
44. Collard J M, Otte J B, Kestens P J Ann Thorac Surg 1993; 56: 573–576
45. Allison P R Surg Gynecol Obstet 1951; 92: 419

and the oesophagus can be exposed to acid for up to 2% of the time.[46] A survey of healthy hospital personnel revealed that 7% of those questioned complained of daily heartburn. Only a small proportion of subjects with gastro-oesophageal reflux seek medical attention and of those, as few as 5% eventually need surgical correction of reflux.[47]

Competence of the gastro-oesophageal junction is achieved by means of an effective lower oesophageal sphincter. This in turn is related to the pressure exerted by the sphincter, sphincter length, and in particular to that part of it which is situated below the diaphragm. The sphincter pressure varies throughout the day and is influenced by factors such as posture and eating. A sphincter less than 1 cm in length and one with an average pressure of less than 5 mmHg is likely to be incompetent.[46] Duodenogastric reflux, occurring especially after gastric resection, may promote reflux of alkaline duodenal contents into the oesophagus. Gastric outlet obstruction may raise intragastric pressure and encourage acid reflux into the oesophagus.

The effect of reflux is exacerbated if the clearing action of the oesophagus is defective. The best example of this is in scleroderma, where peristaltic activity of the lower oesophagus is reduced or abolished and reflux can be particularly troublesome.[48] Oesophageal motility can also be impaired by reflux, thereby setting up a vicious circle of acid reflux leading to defective clearing which in turn increases acid exposure.

Clinical features

Oesophaged reflux causes epigastric burning pain which is worse on lying flat or bending over. There are other presentations which may give rise to difficulty in diagnosis:

1. Anginal-type chest pain, where reflux is only suspected after cardiac investigations have failed to yield a diagnosis. Up to one-third of patients admitted to hospital with suspected cardiac pain have been found to have an oesophageal problem. About 40% of patients referred to a cardiologist with a diagnosis of angina and who are demonstrated to have normal coronary arteries are eventually found to have gastro-oesophageal reflux as a cause of their pain.[49] A group of patients has also been identified whose reflux is only related to exercise; diagnosis was made by pH monitoring while they exercised on a treadmill.[50]

2. Painful dysphagia occurring in the absence of a demonstrable stricture is usually intermittent and may be experienced particularly when swallowing hot drinks.

3. The reflux of food is often confused with vomiting. The clue is that reflux is effortless and provoked by bending or lying down, whereas vomiting involves a powerful contraction of the abdominal wall muscles.[51]

4. Globus refers to the sensation of a lump in the throat which usually does not interfere with swallowing. In the past this has been labelled as a hysterical symptom, but undoubtedly the majority of these patients suffer from gastro-oesophageal reflux with associated incoordination or over-activity of the cricopharyngeus. This can be seen radiologically as a prominent cricopharyngeal bar on a lateral barium swallow. This condition may progress to produce cricopharyngeal dysphagia, in some cases necessitating a cricopharyngeal myotomy.[52]

5. Pulmonary aspiration may result in nocturnal coughing, early morning hoarseness and a clinical picture akin to asthma. The association between respiratory symptoms and nocturnal acid reflux can be documented with pH monitoring.[53]

Diagnosis

No test is infallible but a carefully taken history is essential. Odynophagia is a good pointer towards reflux; this refers to the characteristic burning pain which patients experience immediately after ingestion of hot liquids or alcohol. The effects of posture on symptoms, the beneficial effects of antacids and the acidic taste of refluxed material in the mouth are also helpful indicators.

Barium swallow may confirm reflux and may also give additional useful information such as the presence of a pharyngeal pouch, stricture or coexisting hiatus hernia. Reflux cannot be demonstrated radiologically in 40% of patients who are proven to have reflux disease and therefore this cannot be regarded as a very sensitive investigation.[47] Mucosal changes resulting from reflux are visible at endoscopy and the earliest sign is the presence of small discrete erosions extending up from the squamocolumnar junction (Table 21.1). Later these erosions become confluent and involve the entire circumference of the oesophagus. Stricture or frank ulceration represents a more advanced stage of oesophagitis. Mucosal hyperaemia is not a reliable sign of reflux and it should be remembered that endoscopy may be normal in a third of patients with proven gastro-oesophageal reflux. Mucosal biopsies taken 5 cm above the gastro-oesophageal junction may show the characteristic hyperplasia of the basal zone and elongation of the papillae.[54] The presence of dilated capillaries associated with an

Table 21.1 Endoscopy

E0 = Normal
E1 = Erythema
Equivocal evidence of oesophageal reflux disease (GORD)
unequivocal evidence of GORD
E2 = (a) Erosions and/or patchy ulceration
(b) Confluent ulceration
E3 = Stricture or columnar-lined oesophagus

REFERENCES

46. DeMeester T R In: Watson A, Celestin L R (eds) Disorders of the Oesophagus. Advances and Controversy. Pitman 1984
47. Richter J E, Castell D O Ann Intern Med 1982; 97: 93
48. Cohen S J Clin Invest 1972; 51: 2663
49. Cook R A, Anggianasah A, Smeeton N C, Owen W J, Chambers J B Br Heart J 1994; 72: 231–236
50. Schofield P M et al Br Med J 1987; 294: 1459
51. Edwards D A W Clin Gastroenterol 1976; 5: 59
52. Henderson R D The Esophagus: Reflux and Primary Motor Disorders. Williams & Wilkins, Baltimore 1980
53. Pellegrini C A et al Surgery 1979; 86: 110
54. Ismail-Beigi F, Horton P F, Pope C E Gastroenterology 1970; 58: 163

increase in intraepithelial eosinophils is also taken as an indicator of reflux disease. A normal biopsy does not, however, rule out the disease as biopsies are normal in approximately 20% of those with reflux.

The Bernstein acid perfusion test has over the years proved useful in confirming the diagnosis of reflux in the absence of other evidence. Hydrochloric acid (0.1 mol/l) is perfused at the rate of 6 ml/min into the oesophagus through a tube whose tip is positioned 5 cm above the gastro-oesophageal junction. The response to acid is compared to saline which is used as a control solution. Acid perfusion reproduces the symptoms of oesophagitis in approximately 70% of those with reflux.

In 1969 Spencer[55] introduced pH monitoring of the oesophagus; the value of his technique in diagnosing reflux has now been confirmed[56,57] and it has become the accepted method of documenting reflux. The pH probe, which is either glass or antimony, is positioned 5 cm above the gastro-oesophageal junction and connected to a recorder. Patients are then told to resume daily activities but to avoid acidic drinks; they are asked to keep a diary of symptoms and events for the duration of the test. The results are expressed as the number and duration of reflux episodes over 24 hours; an abnormal result is indicated by a pH of less than 4 for more than 3% of the time when supine and 8.8% of the time when upright.[58] A scoring system has been evolved which incorporates supine and erect reflux, the total number of reflux episodes, the duration of the longest episode and the number of episodes lasting more than 5 minutes. A diagnostic sensitivity of 90% has been claimed.[59] pH monitoring is recommended when the clinical story indicates reflux and other investigations are normal, and also for those patients with atypical symptoms. It is particularly useful after antireflux surgery to check its effectiveness and to evaluate persistent symptoms.

Oesophageal manometry plays a relatively minor role in the routine evaluation of reflux, although of course it is the investigation of choice in the assessment of motility disturbances.

Complications

Oesophageal stricture

Strictures occur in approximately 10% of patients with gastro-oesophageal reflux and frequency increases with age. Benign strictures may be difficult to distinguish clinically from malignant strictures, although a short history of progressive or total dysphagia favours the latter. Endoscopy is essential and, if biopsy and brush cytology are carried out, a diagnostic accuracy rate of 95% can be achieved.[60] The inflammation may be mucosal or transmural and a particularly tight stricture may develop after prolonged nasogastric aspiration in association with reflux which may be resistant to dilatation therapy. Other causes which must be considered in a differential diagnosis of benign stricture include caustic strictures, following ingestion of certain tablets such as Slow-K, tetracycline or non-steroidal anti-inflammatory drugs; radiotherapy; fungal infections; tuberculosis; Crohn's disease and anastomotic strictures.

Most benign strictures are effectively treated by dilatation; 40% are satisfactorily treated by one dilatation; the remainder need an average of three dilatations in 3 years.[61] Some favour the use of Maloney mercury-filled dilators[62] which can be passed under simple sedation as a day-case. Other dilators in common use are the Eder Peustow and Celestin bougies which are introduced over a metal guidewire under X-ray control. Recently balloon dilators have been used which can be passed down the biopsy channel of an endoscope, allowing the stricture to be dilated under direct vision. A similar type of balloon dilator can be passed over a guidewire. Cransford & Cuschieri[63] advocate gradual dilatation to 45 FG or until pain or significant resistance is encountered. They feel that more aggressive dilatation is not beneficial as this increases the complication rate; the risk of rupture is about 0.5%. The rate of re-stricturing after dilatation can be reduced by the use of proton pump inhibitors such as omeprazole: the addition of cisapride as a prokinetic agent may provide further benefit thus reducing the need for further dilatation.[64]

Anti-reflux surgery should be considered in young patients and in those with a recurring stricture requiring increasingly frequent dilatation. The rare undilatable stricture with transmural inflammation may require resection and colonic interposition.[65] If oesophageal shortening is a problem then a Collis gastroplasty as an oesophageal lengthening procedure can be combined with a Nissen fundoplication, with good results.[66]

Barrett's oesophagus

In 1950 Barrett described the presence of a gastric-lined oesophagus, which is now recognized as a metaplastic response to reflux.[67] A Barrett's oesophagus can be recognized endoscopically when the lower oesophagus is covered with pink velvety gastric-type epithelium extending up from the gastro-oesophageal junction so that the squamocolumnar junction is at least 3 cm above the gastro-oesophageal junction. A study by Singh et al[68] compared patients with Barrett's oesophagus with patients with uncomplicated reflux and found a significant reduction in the lower oesophageal sphincter pressure and an increase in the acid exposure in the Barrett's group when compared to the uncomplicated

REFERENCES

55. Spencer J Br J Surg 1969; 56: 912
56. DeMeester T R et al J Thorac Cardiovasc Surg 1980; 79: 656
57. Branicki F J et al Gut 1982; 23: 992
58. Richter J E, Bradley L A, De Meester T R, Nu W C Dig Dis Sci 1992; 37: 849–856
59. Johnson L F, DeMeester T R In: DeMeester T R, Skinner D B (eds) Esophageal Disorders. Pathophysiology and Therapy. Raven Press, New York 1985
60. Witzell L et al Gut 1976; 17: 375
61. Watson A Br J Surg 1987; 74: 443
62. Sifris S E et al JAMA 1976; 235: 928
63. Cransford C A, Cuschieri A In: Hennessy T P J, Cuschieri A (eds) Surgery of the Oesophagus. Baillière Tindall, London 1986
64. Marks R D, Richter J E et al Gastroenterology 1994; 106: 907–915
65. Thompson A E In: Smith R L (ed) Operative Surgery. Butterworth, London 1983
66. Henderson R D, Marryatt G V Ann Thorac Surg 1985; 39: 74
67. Barrett N R Br J Surg 1950; 38: 175
68. Singh P, Taylor H, Colin-Jones D G Scand J Gastroenterol 1994; 29: 11–16

patients. Furthermore, they found that the length of the Barrett's oesophagus bore a direct correlation to the degree of acid exposure. Recent work using a bile probe (Bilitec 2000) claims increased bile reflux into the oesophagus in Barrett's patients as compared to patients with uncomplicated reflux.[69] Barrett's oesophagus is seen in about 10% of patients undergoing endoscopy for the assessment of reflux and carries with it a 30-fold increased risk of developing an adenocarcinoma of the oesophagus. This tumour may be multifocal and is often preceded by the development of high-grade dysplasia.[70] The discovery of dysplasia on biopsy is an indication for regular endoscopic surveillance. Few advocate prophylactic oesophagectomy,[71] most prefer to delay resection until invasive malignancy has been demonstrated on a biopsy.[72] Spechler et al have identified a group of patients who have what they term a short-segment Barrett's oesophagus and this is identified by the finding of columnar metaplasia within 3 cm of the squamocolumnar junction. The possible association between this finding and the development of adenocarcinoma has been raised.[73] The management of high-grade dysplasia is controversial; some advocate continued surveillance until an early adenocarcinoma is detected[74] while others recommend oesophagectomy because of the failure to differentiate high-grade dysplasia from adenocarcinoma. Certainly close liaison between the surgeons and pathologists is essential in such cases.[75]

Barrett's oesophagus may present as a benign stricture at the squamocolumnar junction and may be situated high in the oesophagus (Fig. 21.9). It may also be associated with deep penetrating ulcers involving the gastric-lined oesophagus which may bleed and, rarely, perforate. There are reports of regression of the columnar lined oesophagus after anti-reflux surgery but most would regard a Barrett's oesophagus as a late and irreversible change which does not regress after surgical or medical treatment.[76] Treatment is tailored to the attendant problems—dilatation for strictures, anti-reflux surgery if symptoms demand, surveillance for dysplasia and resection for carcinoma.

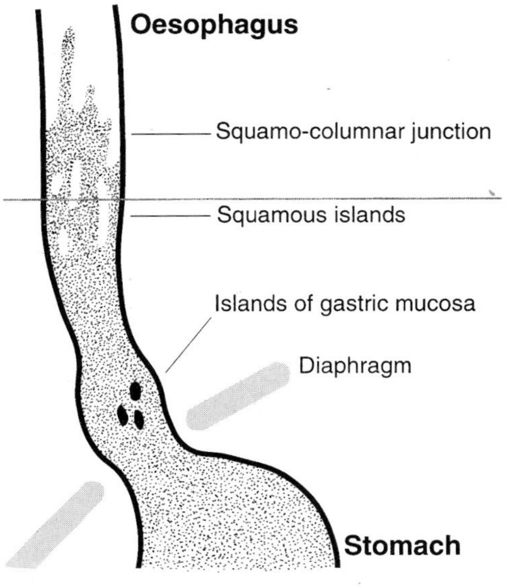

Fig. 21.9 Barrett's oesophagus showing replacement of the lower oesophagus with gastric-type mucosa (exceeding 3 cm) and also showing gastric mucosal islands amongst the squamous mucosa.

Haemorrhage

This is an uncommon complication of reflux, although severe haemorrhage can occur from a Barrett's ulcer or from an associated para-oesophageal hernia. Occasionally patients with oesophagitis are found to be anaemic but other more common causes of gastrointestinal bleeding should be excluded before ascribing the anaemia to the oesophagus.

TREATMENT OF UNCOMPLICATED GASTROINTESTINAL REFLUX

Medical

Some 90% of patients presenting to hospital with gastro-oesophageal reflux respond well to medical therapy. Many patients are overweight and volunteer that the onset of their symptoms coincided with their weight gain. Weight loss is often rewarding and simple measures such as elevation of the head of the bed significantly reduce nocturnal acid reflux.[77] Avoiding a large meal at night and limiting alcohol intake also often help. Antacids improve symptoms in 36% of patients[78] and can be conveniently given as an alginate antacid mixture which also acts as a mechanical barrier to reflux. Metaclopramide, which increases lower oesophageal sphincter pressure and promotes gastric emptying, relieves symptoms in half the patients. The mainstay of treatment is the anti-secretory drugs: H_2-blockers, cimetidine, ranitidine and fanotidine are effective in about half the patients in healing oesophagitis. Proton pump inhibitors (omeprazole 20 mg or 40 mg a day or lansoprazole 30 mg daily) have proved superior with symptom relief in up to 95%.[79] One study identified a group of patients who required up to 160 mg of omeprazole a day to stay in remission.[80] Long-term follow-up of such patients on high-dose proton pump inhibitors would be sensible in view of the unknown effect on gastric histology and the subsequent development of chronic gastritis.

REFERENCES

69. Vaezi M F, Lacamera R G, Richter J E Am J Physiol 1994; 267: G1050–G1057
70. Naef A P et al J Thorac Cardiovasc Surg 1975; 70: 826
71. Skinner D B et al Ann Surg 1983; 198: 554
72. Spechler S J, Goyal R J N Engl J Med 1986; 315: 362
73. Spechler S J, Zeroogian J M, Anatoniolo D A, Wang H H, Goyal R K Lancet 1994; 344: 1533–1536
74. Levine D S, Haggitt R C, Blount P L, Rabinovitch P S, Rusch V W, Reid B J Gastroenterology 1993; 105: 40–50
75. Peters J H, Clark G W B, Ireland A P, Chandrasom P, Smyrk T C, De-Meester T R J Thorac Cardiovasc Surg 1994; 108: 813–822
76. Bremner A P In: Watson A, Celestin L R (eds) Disorders of the Oesophagus. Advances and Controversies. Pitman, London 1984
77. Johnson L F, DeMeester T R Dig Dis Sci 1981; 8: 673
78. Vantrappen G, Jenssens J, Celestin L R In: Watson A, Celestin L R (eds) Disorders of the Oesophagus. Pitman, London 1984
79. Hallerback B, Une P et al Gastroenterology 1994; 107: 1305–1311
80. Klinkenberg Knol E C, Festen H P M et al Ann Intern Med 1994; 121: 161–167

Surgical

The early attempts at surgical correction of reflux concentrated on reducing the hiatus hernia and carrying out a crural repair,[81] but the most popular operation is now a Nissen fundoplication. It is not known exactly how this operation prevents reflux but it may improve the lower oesophageal sphincter tone and maintain the sphincter within the abdominal cavity.[82] This concept was reinforced when the lower oesophageal sphincter pressure was found to be increased by fundoplication, but more recently others have found that, while the lower oesophageal sphincter pressure increased in most of the group who achieved successful control of reflux, there was a sizeable group of patients in whom the pressure actually fell but who were still cured of reflux.[83] Furthermore no increase in the length of the abdominal oesophageal sphincter was found. It may well be that a relatively low sphincter pressure prevents reflux and this suggests that fundoplication acts partly as a flap valve. The wrap may also prevent distraction and weakening of the lower oesophageal sphincter when the intragastric pressure increases and threatens to produce reflux.[84]

The concept of the 'floppy' Nissen repair is important and has been well-described by Donahue et al.[82] The lower oesophagus is mobilized through a laparotomy incision. The greater curvature is then mobilized by division of the short gastric vessels so that the fundus of the stomach can be passed behind the oesophagus. The wrap-around is completed by suturing the mobilized fundus lying to the right of the oesophagus to the anterior surface of the stomach. The tightness of the wrap depends in part on the extent of gastric mobilization but also on the placement of sutures used to secure the wrap. The essential feature of the operation is a loose fundoplication using a fully mobilized fundus. This allows a short 2–3 cm wrap to be constructed around a 50 FG oesophageal bougie placed within the oesophagus. The looseness of the fundoplication is confirmed by the easy passage of a finger within the wrap. The lower suture picks up the oesophagogastric junction to prevent slippage, and a posterior crural repair is added to stop upward displacement of the fundoplication into the chest. This procedure has approximately a 90% chance of success;[85] the 'gas bloat syndrome' is reduced by keeping the wrap loose so that the patient maintains the ability to belch.[82] Postoperative dysphagia is nearly always mild and transient, only affecting approximately 10% of patients. Its occurrence is minimized by the use of the 50 FG bougie. Recurrent reflux is seen in about 5–10% and may be the result of anatomical disruption or slippage of the fundoplication.

The early results of laparoscopic Nissen fundoplication are also encouraging. The procedure is usually carried out through five ports and is in principle the same procedure as the open one. A loose short wrap is achieved with a crural repair when appropriate. The advantages are less postoperative wound pain and a shorter hospital stay of approximately 4 days[86] and a return to work within 2 weeks of surgery with a high patient satisfaction rate.[87] It is essential that this operation should be only carried out by trained surgeons in special centres well-versed with the pitfalls of laparoscopic oesophageal mobilization.[88] Some have pointed out the potential reasons for failure in this new approach and reiterate the need to adhere to the basic principles of the successful Nissen learnt from the open operation.

Another operative procedure is the Belsey mark IV anti-reflux procedure[89] is carried out through a transthoracic approach. The gastric fundus is mobilized and sutured on to the oesophagus in two layers in order to create a more acute angle at the oesophagogastric junction and also to provide a 270° wrap of the gastric fundus around the lower oesophagus. The repair is then sutured to the diaphragm (Fig. 21.10). The main advantage of this approach is in cases of short oesophagus where the transthoracic approach allows greater mobilization of the oesophagus with replacement of the wrap below the diaphragm. The disadvantages of this approach are the occasional post-thoracotomy neuralgia which may be troublesome and a higher rate of postoperative reflux when compared to a Nissen fundoplication.

The Hill repair[90] relies on fixation of the partly fundoplicated oesophagogastric junction to the median arcuate ligament of the diaphragm and may be combined with intraoperative manometry to gauge the magnitude of the lower oesophageal sphincter pressure.

Operations for recurrent gastro-oesophageal reflux

Reflux can occur when anti-reflux surgery has failed; it may also develop after vagotomy, and occasionally after cardiomyotomy for achalasia. Clearly further surgery after previous operations is attended by increased morbidity and mortality. If there is considerable scarring around the hiatus, making oesophageal dissection difficult, then the operation of antrectomy and Roux-en-Y duodenal diversion (Fig. 21.12) is a reasonable alternative. It is well-tolerated and has a success rate almost equal to that of fundoplication.[93] A vagotomy should be added to obviate the risk of stomal ulceration. If the previous operation failed because of oesophageal shortening then a Collis Nissen gastroplasty can be used to lengthen the oesophagus by constructing a neo-oesophagus from the stomach (Fig. 21.13). This is achieved by placing two light vascular clamps on to the stomach at the gastro-oesophageal junction so that they lie along the longitudinal axis of the stomach

REFERENCES

81. Allison P R Surg Gynecol Obstet 1951; 92: 419
82. Donahue P E et al Arch Surg 1985; 120: 663
83. Bancewicz J et al Br J Surg 1987; 74: 162
84. Jamieson G G Br J Surg 1987; 74: 155
85. DeMeester T R Ann Surg 1986; 204: 9–20
86. Jamieson G G, Watson D I, Britten-Jones R, Mitchell P C, Anvari M Ann Surg 1994; 2: 137–145
87. Hinder R A, Filipi C J, Wetscher G, Neary O, DeMeester T R, Perdikis G Ann Surg 1994; 4: 472–483
88. Collard J M, Romagnoli R, Kestens P J Dis Oesophagus 1996; 9: 56–62
89. Belsey R World J Surg 1977; 1: 475
90. Hill L D Ann Surg 1967; 166: 681
91. Gear M W L et al Br J Surg 1984; 71: 681
92. Bombeck C T In: Watson A, Celestin L R (eds) Disorders of the Oesophagus. Advances and Controversy. Pitman, London 1984
93. Payne W S In: Smith R A, Smith R E (eds) Surgery of the Oesophagus. The Coventry Conference. Butterworth 1977

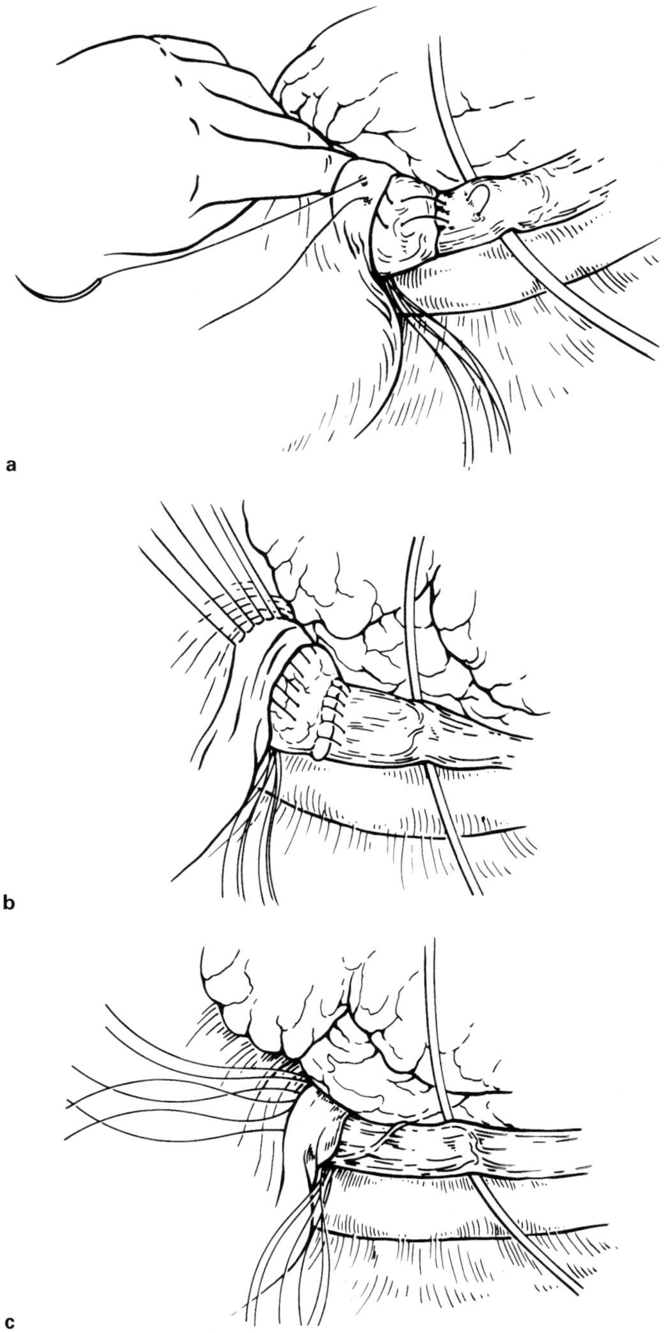

a

b

c

Fig. 21.10 Belsey transthoracic anti-reflux procedure which involves two layers of invagination sutures to produce a 270° wrap. **(a)** First layer of plication sutures. **(b)** Second layer of sutures placed between the diaphragm and the oesophagus. **(c)** Second layer tied.

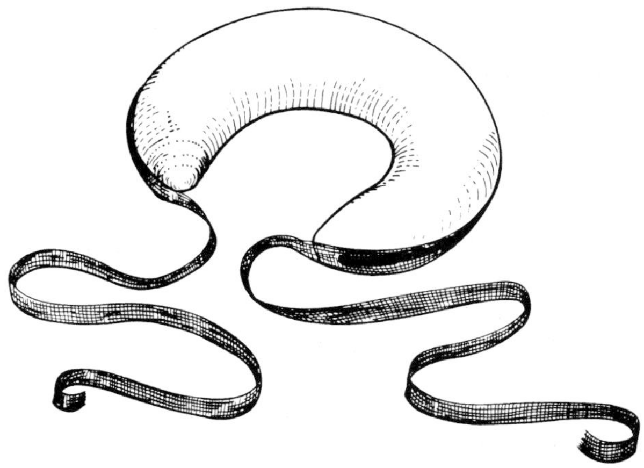

Fig. 21.11 Angelchik anti-reflux procedure involving minimal dissection to encircle the oesophagogastric junction and then placement of the prosthesis loosely around the junction where it is fixed by tying the attached tapes.

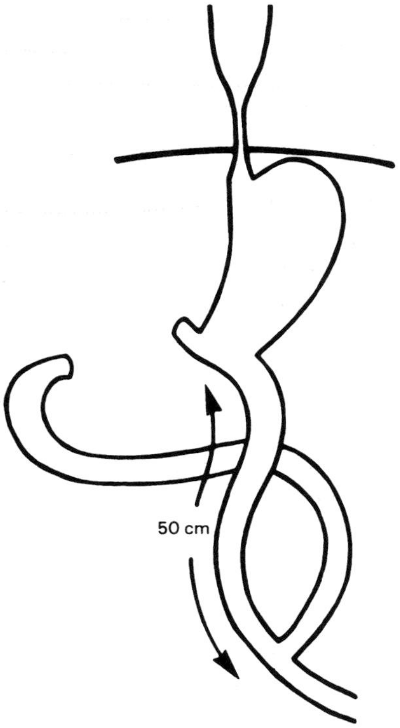

Fig. 21.12 Vagotomy and antrectomy-en-Roux. Truncal vagotomy combined with antrectomy and Roux-en-Y duodenal diversion of at least 50 cm.

and create a gastric tube. A size 60 FG oesophageal bougie is placed in the stomach before the clamps are applied to prevent narrowing of the gastro-oesophageal junction. The stomach is incised between the clamps and resutured creating a gastroplasty. The tube so formed allows a tension-free wrap to be carried out below the diaphragm. In this situation a 270° wrap has an unacceptably high failure rate and therefore a 360° Nissen-type wrap is preferred.[94] As a general rule, when a previous repair has been performed through the abdomen it is preferable to use a thoracic approach for the next procedure, while if the previous operation was a thoracic procedure then the subsequent repair is best carried out through a thoracoabdominal route.

REFERENCE

94. Orringer M B, Sloan H Ann Thorac Surg 1978; 25: 16

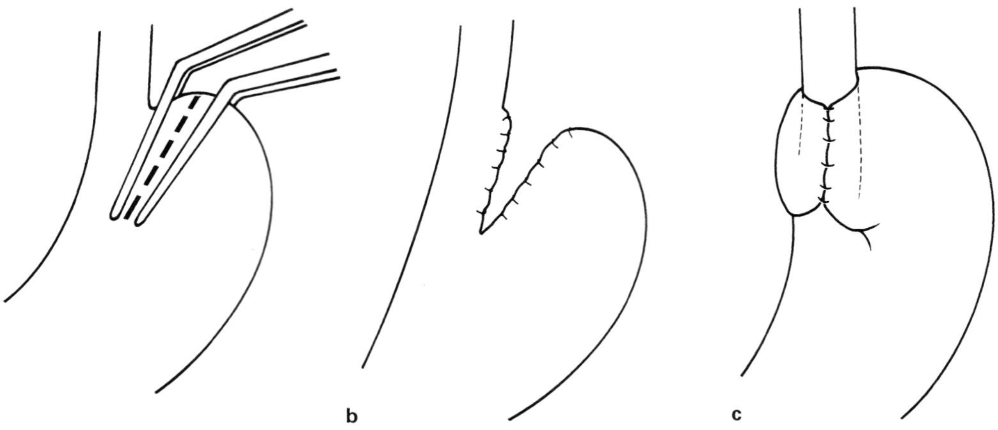

Fig. 21.13 Collis Nissen gastroplasty: a neo-oesophagus is formed by constructing a gastric tube. The redundant stomach is then used to produce Nissen completion wrap below the diaphragm.

The efficacy of a totally intrathoracic Nissen is occasionally mentioned. One report quotes a 33% incidence of gastric ulceration within the intrathoracic wrap;[95] this should mitigate against its use as a routine anti-reflux procedure. It also shows the importance of carrying out an adequate crural repair to lessen the chances of an abdominal Nissen repair migrating into the chest.

MOTOR DISORDERS OF THE OESOPHAGUS

The passage of a food bolus from the mouth to the stomach is initiated by pharyngeal contraction with simultaneous relaxation of the cricopharyngeus. This allows the bolus to enter the oesophagus. A coordinated peristaltic wave then sweeps the bolus down the body of the oesophagus to reach the lower oesophageal sphincter which then relaxes to allow the food to enter the stomach. Peristalsis is described as primary when it is initiated by swallowing and therefore follows a pharyngeal contraction, and secondary when it starts in the body of the oesophagus, usually in response to distension of the oesophagus by liquid or food bolus. Tertiary waves are non-propulsive synchronous contractions of the oesophageal body which are occasionally seen in health but when frequent they signify a motility disturbance. The term 'achalasia' was initially used by Hurst[96] to describe the absence of relaxation of the lower oesophageal sphincter and this is the most common primary disorder of motility. Osgood[97] described a condition which he called 'oesophagismus' and which is now known as 'diffuse oesophageal spasm'.

Oesophageal manometry

Manometry is used to study oesophageal motility and records pressure changes in the upper and lower oesophageal sphincter and in the body of the oesophagus. A manometry catheter is usually passed nasally with the pressure being measured at multiple points in the oesophagus and also in the upper stomach. Pressure is measured either by means of a low-compliance water infusion system[98] or with intra-oesophageal mini-transducers.

The lower oesophageal sphincter is assessed by gradual withdrawal of the catheter from the stomach into the oesophagus, measuring the rise in pressure in the sphincter zone from which its length can also be estimated. The ability of the sphincter to relax completely in response to a swallow is also noted. The catheter is then withdrawn further into the body of the oesophagus to record the motor activity, which may be peristaltic or non-peristaltic. Finally the upper oesophageal sphincter is studied, looking for co-ordinated relaxation of the cricopharyngeus in response to pharyngeal contraction. Oesophageal manometry is a particularly useful investigation in patients with obscure chest pain, unexplained dysphagia and suspected scleroderma.[99] Achalasia can be recognized by a failure of the lower oesophageal sphincter to relax, combined with absence of peristalsis in the body of the oesophagus. Scleroderma is characterized by diminished or absent peristalsis in the lower two-thirds of the oesophagus. Diffuse oesophageal spasm is identified by the presence of repetitive non-peristaltic multipeaked contractions of the body of the oesophagus. The picture can become blurred by variations in these classical patterns of motility, and very occasionally patients may change from one motility pattern to another over several years.

Scintigraphic measurement of oesophageal transit, studying the passage of an isotopically labelled bolus with technetium^{99m} from the pharynx into the stomach, can provide a useful test for abnormalities of oesophageal transit. There are many variations in the technique used to carry out this investigation but essentially the patient is studied by a gamma camera focused on a particular area of interest corresponding to the oesophagus and stomach. The time taken for 95% of the radioactivity to enter the stomach is measured. The bolus may be liquid, solid or semi-solid and the patient may be studied in the supine or erect position.[100] Some have found scintiscanning to be a sensitive screening test,[101] although

REFERENCES

95. Richardson J D et al Am J Surg 1982; 143: 29
96. Hurst A F Q J Med 1915; 8: 300
97. Osgood H Boston Med Surg J 1889; 120: 401–405
98. Arndorfer R C, Stef J J et al Gastroenterology 1977; 73: 23–27
99. Blackwell J, Castell D Br J Hosp Med 1984; 32: 267–271
100. Maddern G J et al Gastroenterology 1984; 87: 922–926
101. Blackwell J N, Castell D O In: Watson A, Celestin L R (eds) Disorders of the Oesophagus. Pitman, London 1984

manometry is still required to classify the abnormality. The test needs to be standardized before it can be fully accepted.

Achalasia

This condition affects 1 per 100 000 of the population and usually presents between the ages of 30 and 60 years.[101] Abnormalities have been found in the dorsal nucleus of the vagus, in the vagal trunks and there may be either a reduction or total absence of ganglia in Auerbach's plexus.[102] It has been suggested that the condition is caused by a neurotropic virus affecting the vagal nucleus and then travelling down the vagal trunk to the oesophageal ganglia but this theory remains unproven.[103] In the early phases, before oesophageal dilatation has occurred, the oesophageal body exhibits vigorous non-peristaltic simultaneous contractions—the so-called 'vigorous achalasia'. At this stage chest pain may be a prominent symptom, and may be confused with reflux pain or even anginal pain. Later on, as dilatation of the oesophagus occurs with retention of solids and liquids, dysphagia and regurgitation become prominent symptoms. Regurgitation of food is often delayed for some time after a meal and is often referred to by the patient as 'vomiting'. This may confuse the clinician into thinking of gastro-oesophageal reflux or even pyloric stenosis. Symptoms may be intermittent and exacerbated by stress, and the swallowing of both liquids and solids often presents equal difficulty to the patient.

Radiologically, achalasia is diagnosed by finding a dilated oesophagus with a tapering lower oesophageal segment, likened to a bird's beak, which fails to relax (Fig. 21.14). There is no gastric air bubble because the dilated oesophagus never completely empties and therefore swallowed air cannot pass into the stomach. In early cases of achalasia, before dilatation has occurred, the diagnosis may be missed by the radiologist. Examination of the patient in the prone position with barium may make it easier to show the characteristic aperistaltic oesophagus.

Manometrically, achalasia is characterized by the absence of peristaltic waves in the oesophagus with a high resting intra-oesophageal pressure. The normal pressure of the oesophageal body is below zero.[104] There is impaired relaxation of the lower oesophageal sphincter, which may have a high resting pressure. In health the lower oesophageal sphincter pressure relaxes to zero whereas in achalasia relaxation either does not occur or is incomplete.[105]

Pseudoachalasia can cause diagnostic difficulties and typically occurs in a patient over the age of 50 with a short history of dysphagia and with the radiological and manometric features of achalasia. This can be caused by a carcinoma of the lower oesophagus or of the cardia, by extrinsic compression produced for example by a pancreatic tumour or lymphoma.[106] Endoscopy may reveal a tumour but in some cases endoscopy, biopsy and brush cytology may still miss the diagnosis. The endoscope should 'pop' through the lower oesophageal sphincter in true achalasia and any resistance to its passage must put the diagnosis in doubt. A computed tomography scan or even surgical exploration may be the only means of establishing a diagnosis if genuine doubt remains.

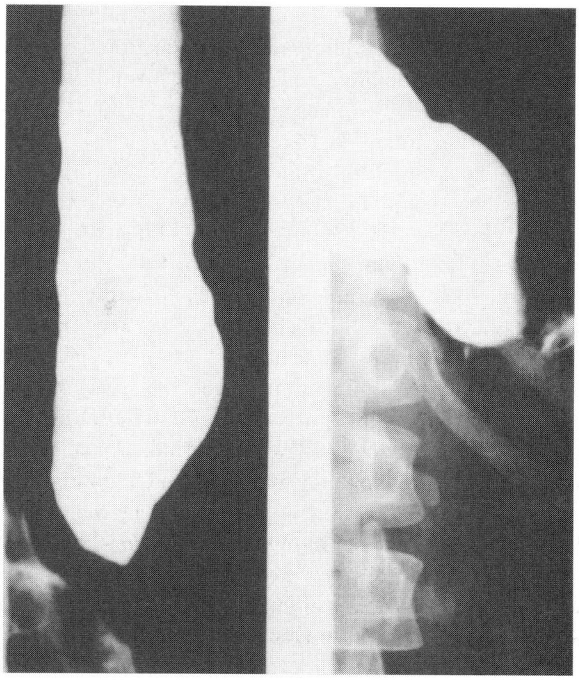

Fig. 21.14 Barium swallow in a patient with achalasia showing a dilated oesophagus with a constriction at the lower oesophageal sphincter.

Complications

Overspill from the dilated oesophagus into the bronchial tree may result in nocturnal lung aspiration and this may lead to bronchiectasis and lung abscess. Carcinoma complicates achalasia in 3% of cases and, when it occurs, is usually a squamous cell carcinoma developing in mid-oesophagus as a bulky tumour with a particularly bad prognosis.[107]

Treatment

This is designed to reduce the competence of the lower oesophageal sphincter without producing gastro-oesophageal reflux. The pneumatic oesophageal dilator, which is introduced over a guidewire under radiological control, represents a major advance in treatment.[108] The dilating balloon is carefully positioned in the lower oesophageal sphincter and inflated to a fixed pressure of 300 mmHg for 3 minutes. This is successful in relieving dysphagia in about 67% of patients, although repeated dilatations may be necessary. There is a low perforation rate of 3%.[109,110] Dilatation therapy is recommended in the first instance as it is relatively safe

REFERENCES

102. Trounce J R et al Q J Med 1957; 26: 433–443
103. Smith B Gut 1970; 11: 388–391
104. Castell D O Arch Intern Med 1976; 136: 571–579
105. Cohen S, Lipshutz W H Gastroenterology 1971; 61: 814–820
106. Vantrappen G et al Gastroenterology 1979; 76: 450–457
107. Lortal J J L et al Surgery 1969; 66: 969
108. Vantrappen G, Hellemans J Gastroenterology 1980; 79: 144–154
109. Tucker H J et al Ann Intern Med 1978; 89: 315–318
110. Fellows I W et al Gut 1983; 24: 1020–1023

and easy. Surgery is reserved for patients who still have symptoms after dilatation, and for children in whom dilatation seems ineffective. Post-dilatation rupture is usually managed conservatively and this is effective provided the oesophagus is empty before the dilatation and the condition is recognized early by means of a contrast examination after the dilatation. When balloon dilatation is compared to myotomy in a specialized centre the results were very similar except that the myotomized patients had a higher incidence of reflux.[111] It seems sensible therefore to recommend balloon dilatation as the primary treatment and to reserve myotomy for after failure of dilatation. There has been recent interest in laparoscopic and thoracoscopic myotomy but it is too early to assess the long-term efficacy of this method.

The standard operation for achalasia is Heller's cardiomyotomy which was first performed in 1913 as an anterior and posterior myotomy.[112] A single myotomy is now considered to be adequate and should be about 7 cm in length, extending no more than 1 cm on to the stomach; the oesophagogastric junction is recognized by the presence of small transverse extramucosal veins. The operation may be performed by the transabdominal or transthoracic route; the latter gives better exposure (Fig. 21.15). Controversy exists as to whether an anti-reflux procedure should be simultaneously performed to avoid postoperative gastro-oesophageal reflux, although if the operation is correctly performed with only minimal extension of the myotomy on to the stomach and minimal mobilization of the oesophagogastric junction, the incidence of reflux is less than 3%.[113] Vantrappen & Hellemans[108] reviewed a collected series of 1045 cases treated by myotomy and found the incidence of reflux to be 10%. If an anti-reflux operation is carried out it is important that any associated fundoplication should be short and loose to avoid postoperative dysphagia in view of the absence of peristalsis in the body of the oesophagus.

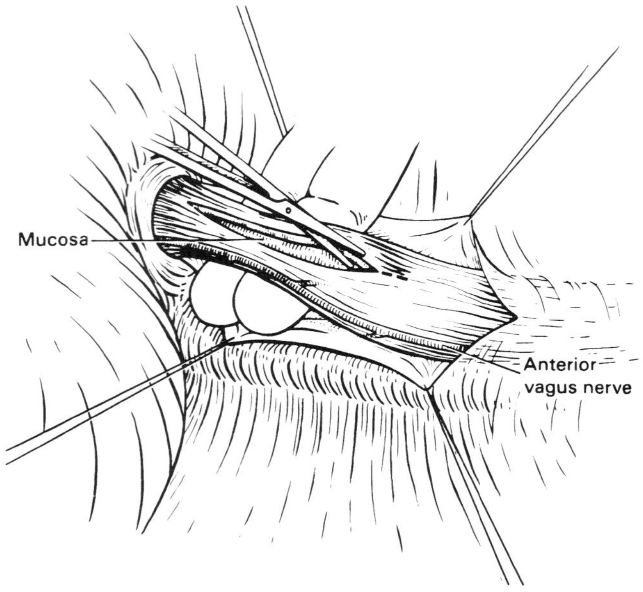

Fig. 21.15 Heller's cardiomyotomy.

Chagas disease

This interesting condition is found in rural South America and is a manifestation of chronic infection with the parasite *Trypanosoma cruzi*. The disease is most prevalent in certain parts of Brazil where about 25% of the population show evidence of infection.[114] As in achalasia, the intermuscular ganglion cells are destroyed and motility changes are evident when there is a 50% reduction in ganglion cell count; dilatation occurs when this figure rises to 90%.[115] The clinical features are identical to achalasia and treatment is along the same lines by balloon dilatation or cardiomyotomy. Very advanced cases may be complicated by extreme dilatation and tortuosity of the oesophagus so that resection may be necessary. Coincidental cardiomyopathy may give rise to sudden death from cardiac rupture. Chagas disease may also affect other parts of the gastrointestinal tract producing megacolon, megaduodenum and also possibly megaureter.[116]

Diffuse oesophageal spasm and related disorders

Interest in these conditions has increased since the use of coronary angiography for the investigation of presumed anginal chest pain. In the USA 30% of these patients were found to have a normal coronary angiogram and up to half this group were then found to have an oesophageal abnormality which was considered responsible for their symptoms.[117] Patients with diffuse oesophageal spasm present with episodic chest pain or dysphagia or both. Attacks may be severe and incapacitating, sometimes necessitating emergency hospital admission to exclude cardiac disease. The pain is usually felt retrosternally but may radiate to the jaws or the interscapular region, and the attacks may be associated with facial pallor and extreme sweating, mimicking myocardial infarction.

The intermittent nature of diffuse oesophageal spasm belies the difficulty there may be in making a diagnosis. Barium swallow is abnormal in less than half of the cases[118] (Fig. 21.16), and endoscopy is usually unremarkable. Oesophageal manometry characteristically shows a high proportion of high-amplitude simultaneous contractions of the body of the oesophagus which are of long duration and display multiple peaks (Fig. 21.16). Some peristalsis is maintained, thereby distinguishing it from achalasia. The 'nutcracker oesophagus' refers to the manometric finding of high-amplitude peristaltic contractions of long duration. This may be associated with chest pain and dysphagia.[119] In both diffuse

REFERENCES

111. Abid S, Champion G, Richter J E, McElvein R, Slaughter R L, Koehler R E Am J Gastroenterol 1994; 87: 979–985
112. Heller E Med Chir (JENA) 1913; 27: 141–145
113. Ellis F H et al J Cardiovasc Surg 1984; 88: 344
114. Earlam R J Am Dig Dis 1972; 17: 559–572
115. Koberle F Parasitology 1968; 63: 116
116. Bettarello A, Pinotti H W In: Bouchier I A D, Keighley M R B, Allen R N, Hodgson H J F (eds) Textbook of Gastroenterology. Baillière Tindall, London 1984
117. DeMeester T R et al Ann Surg 1982; 196: 488–498
118. Henderson R D The Oesophagus Reflux and Primary Motor Disorders. Williams & Wilkins, Baltimore 1980
119. Benjamin S B et al Gastroenterology 1979; 77: 478–483

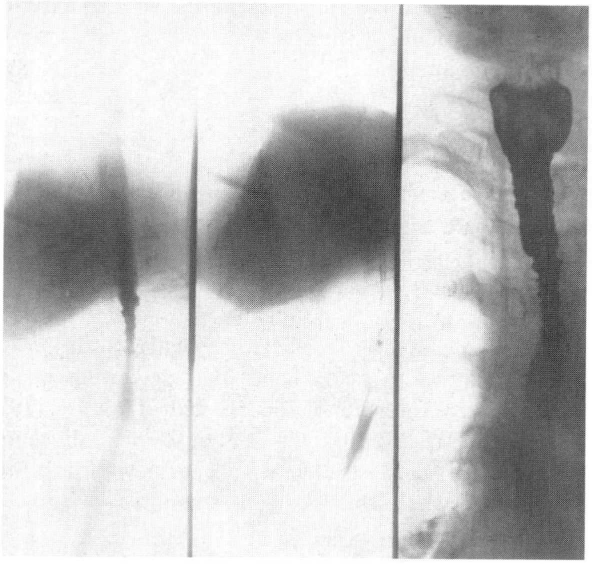

Fig. 21.16 Barium swallow in a patient with diffuse oesophageal spasm showing the area of intense muscle contraction mid-oesophagus.

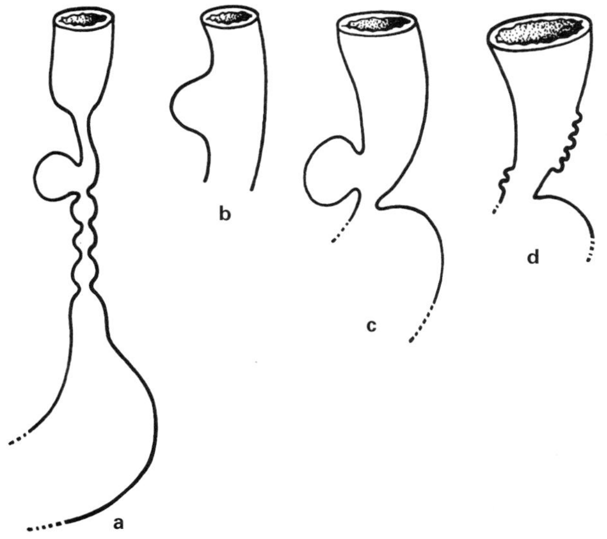

Fig. 21.17 Oesophageal diverticula: (**a**) pulsion; (**b**) traction; (**c**) congenital; (**d**) pseudodiverticula.

spasm and in the nutcracker oesophagus, relaxation of the lower oesophageal sphincter is normal.

Edrophonium can be used to precipitate the symptoms and the manometric abnormalities of both these conditions,[120] and has been shown to increase the diagnostic yield by 30%.[121]

The distinction between abnormalities of oesophageal motility can become blurred with the realization that achalasia may occasionally develop after many years of diffuse spasm. Gastro-oesophageal reflux may be the cause of diffuse spasm,[122] so ambulatory pH monitoring is necessary to clarify the precise cause of the manometric abnormality, and this clearly has important therapeutic implications. Occasionally during manometry a hypertensive lower oesophageal sphincter will be encountered which relaxes normally on swallowing but may nevertheless be associated with dysphagia.

The first line of treatment in a patient with diffuse oesophageal spasm is a thorough explanation of the cause of the pain and this in itself may occasionally suffice. If gastro-oesophageal reflux can be demonstrated on pH monitoring then a therapeutic trial with a proton pump inhibitor (omeprazole 40 mg or lansoprazole 30 mg daily) is indicated. Nifedipine, a calcium channel blocker, is effective in relieving symptoms in about half the patients,[123] but if symptoms persist and are sufficiently severe, balloon dilatation is helpful and this relieves symptoms in 70% of cases.[124] In a small group of well-selected patients with severe symptoms resistant to other therapy, long oesophageal myotomy may provide relief of symptoms but the results are not as good as achieved in patients with achalasia. The extent of the myotomy is controversial; Henderson[125] recommends a long myotomy of the whole thoracic oesophagus and combines this with an anti-reflux procedure.

Oesophageal diverticula

These have been classified into four types[126] (Fig. 21.17):

1. Pulsion diverticula, which are mucosal and usually caused by high intraluminal pressure associated with motor disorder of the oesophagus.
2. Traction diverticula, which are less common and historically associated with tuberculous mediastinal glands.
3. Congenital diverticula, which may be a type of oesophageal reduplication.
4. Pseudodiverticula, which usually represent oesophageal ulcers and are therefore devoid of an epithelial lining.

Mid oesophageal diverticula are usually of the pulsion variety, often symptomless and require no treatment. Rarely they may be complicated by fistula formation into the bronchial tree, into a major vessel or even by malignant change. Epiphrenic diverticula are often single and situated just above the diaphragm. They are usually of the pulsion variety and may be associated with achalasia, diffuse spasm or a hypertensive oesophageal sphincter. A large epiphrenic diverticulum may cause significant dysphagia, regurgitation or even nocturnal aspiration into the bronchial tree.[127] Bleeding, perforation and malignant change are rare complications.[128]

REFERENCES

120. London R et al Gastroenterology 1981; 81: 10–14
121. Linsell J C, Owen W J Br J Surg 1987; 74: 688–689
122. Bennett J R, Hendrix T R Gastroenterology 59: 273
123. Linsell J C, Owen W J, Anggiansah A In: Siewert J R (ed) Diseases of the Esophagus. Springer Verlag, Berlin 1987
124. Irving J D, Owen W J, Linsell J Gastrointest Radiol 1992; 17: 189
125. Henderson R Surg Clin North Am 1983; 63: 951–962
126. Hennessy T P J In: Cuschieri A, Hennessy T P J (eds) Surgery of the Oesophagus. Baillière Tindall, London 1986
127. Evander A, Little A G, Ferguson M K, Skinner D B World J Surg 1986; 10: 820
128. Duranceau A C In: Jamieson G G (ed) Surgery of the Oesophagus. Churchill Livingstone, Edinburgh 1988

Scleroderma

The oesophagus is involved in around 80% of cases of scleroderma and is also often affected in patients with the CREST syndrome[129] (calcinosis, Raynaud's, oesophagus, scleroderma and telangiectasis). The problems are related to the effects of gastro-oesophageal reflux combined with a relatively adynamic oesophagus so that eventually reflux strictures are formed, producing dysphagia. Manometrically, scleroderma is diagnosed by the presence of normal peristalsis in the upper part of the oesophagus and very-low-amplitude peristalsis or even feeble 'non-peristaltic' activity in the lower two-thirds.[130] The lower sphincter is hypotensive and this helps to distinguish the condition manometrically from achalasia. Lack of success with medical therapy may lead to a surgical referral, and if a fundoplication is considered, it should be a particularly lax type, for fear of causing postoperative dysphagia. Success rates of 86% have been claimed in this condition using the combination of a Collis gastroplasty with a Nissen fundoplication[131] and this combination is particularly useful in cases where the oesophagus is severely shortened as the result of long-standing reflux.[129,130]

Miscellaneous oesophageal conditions

Acquired immune deficiency syndrome and the oesophagus

Dysphagia and odynophagia may be presenting features of acquired immune deficiency syndrome as the patient is a potential host for *Candida albicans*, herpes simplex virus or cytomegalovirus.[132] The same infections can also be seen when the patient is immunosuppressed for other reasons, such as after transplantation or during chemotherapy. Barium swallow may show ulceration which can be confirmed by fibreoptic endoscopy, but routine diagnostic techniques of biopsy and brush cytology may fail to confirm the causative organisms, and in some cases the diagnosis will only be made at post-mortem.

Monilial oesophagitis

This condition is characteristically seen when an immunocompromised patient complains of painful dysphagia and is found to have oral thrush. Oesophagoscopy may reveal white specks of fungus on a friable hyperaemic oesophageal mucosa. The diagnosis may be confirmed by taking biopsies and brushings which should be placed directly into Sabouraud's medium.

Oesophageal moniliasis may complicate oesophageal cancer, reflux oesophagitis and achalasia but can also be seen in otherwise normal patients as a side-effect of antibiotic therapy. Complications include ulceration, fistula and bleeding, and treatment is with either nystatin lozenges or amphotericin elixir. Occasionally fibrous strictures need dilatation.

Other oesophageal infections

Rarely the oesophagus may be affected by other organisms producing oesophagitis, ulceration or fistulae. Syphilis is now only of historical importance but tuberculosis and actinomycosis, diphtheria, lactobacilli, streptococcus, histoplasmosis and blastomycosis are rare infectants.[133]

Crohn's disease

Crohn's of the oesophagus is rare and only a few cases have been described in the literature.[134] The diagnosis should be suspected if the patient with known Crohn's disease at another site develops an oesophageal stricture with ulceration and a cobblestone mucosa. These appearances must be differentiated from a reflux stricture and from a carcinoma by biopsy; some of the cases have been operated on in the mistaken belief that they were malignant strictures. There are reports of success with steroid therapy and one case report[135] describes the use of balloon dilatation of a tight cricopharyngeal stricture in a patient with small-bowel Crohn's disease whose swallowing was restored to normal after two dilatations.

OTHER NON-NEOPLASTIC CONDITIONS

Paraoesophageal hiatus hernia

Unlike a sliding hiatus hernia, the clinical significance of which is still debated, a paraoesophageal or rolling hiatus hernia is a severe mechanical disturbance which may cause serious complications. The pure paraoesophageal hernia is a pathological curiosity, confined to museum specimens and personal collections of interesting cases. The vast majority of rolling hernias are mixed hernias in which the cardia is displaced into the chest and a large portion of the stomach rolls up alongside the oesophagus (Fig. 21.18). As the hernia enlarges the stomach assumes an inverted position and the anatomical distortion of the cardia and the distal stomach is responsible for the symptoms.

The symptom pattern depends on the mechanical effects in the individual case. Distortion of the cardia produces dysphagia. Distortion of the distal stomach as it is drawn through the diaphragm may produce gastric outlet obstruction. Some patients have severe chest pain after eating. They are able to swallow, though with difficulty, but have difficulty belching and have poor gastric emptying. As a result the stomach may become markedly distended. This painful sequence is often eased if attempts to belch are successful. Occasionally the pain is so severe that the patient may be admitted as an emergency with a suspected myocardial infarction. Passage of a large-bore nasogastric tube gives instant relief. Gastric volvulus with strangulation and gangrene is a danger

REFERENCES

129. Hellemans J, Vantrappen G Diseases of the Esophagus. Springer-Verlag, Berlin 1974
130. Creamer B et al Gastroenterologia (Basel) 1956; 86: 763
131. Orringer M B et al Surgery 1981; 90: 624–630
132. Strohlein S et al Dysphagia 1986; 1: 84–87
133. Kramer P, Burakoff R Bockus Gastroenterology, 4th edn. Saunders, Philadelphia 1985
134. Cynn W S et al Am J Roentgenol 1975; 125: 359
135. Rowe P H et al Postgrad Med J 1987; 63: 1101

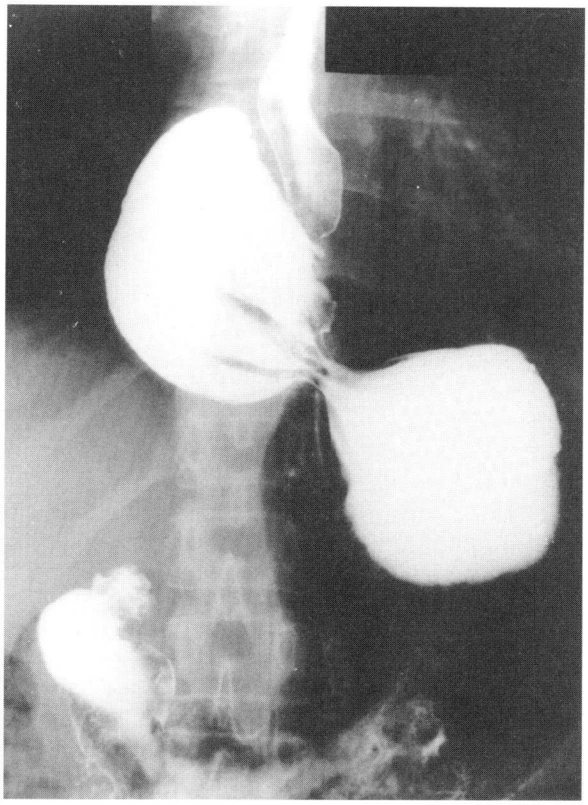

Fig. 21.18 Large mixed hiatus hernia.

in long-standing cases. Respiratory embarrassment may occur, but is uncommon even with very large hernias unless the patient has concomitant lung disease.

The only effective treatment is operative repair. Unfortunately many of the patients are elderly and the risks of operation must then be carefully weighed against the risks of leaving the hernia untreated. Repair may be done by the abdominal or thoracic route. Anatomical reduction is the main priority and may be maintained either by gastropexy as in the Hill operation,[136] by fixation to the anterior abdominal wall in the Boerema gastropexy or by a formal reflux-preventing operation such as a Nissen fundoplication. Despite opinions to the contrary,[136] reflux symptoms are common[137] and a formal anti-reflux procedure is entirely appropriate in many cases. It is now possible to do a very simple Boerema type of gastropexy by laparoscopy and this may be appropriate for the unfit or elderly.

Extrinsic problems at the cardia

After vagotomy

Dysphagia is an uncommon but well-recognized complication of vagotomy.[138] Usually it is transient and is presumably an effect of denervation and handling the oesophagus. Rarely, considerable fibrosis may develop in the tissues around the oesophagus at the hiatus. This can produce severe dysphagia. Oesophageal dilatation may be ineffective if this occurs, and operative release of the oesophagus is required.

After anti-reflux surgery

Any form of anti-reflux surgery may produce obstruction of the lower oesophagus. This may be an effect of the operation itself on the oesophagus, e.g. a Nissen wrap that is too tight or too long, or reaction to an Angelchik prosthesis, or it may be the result of overzealous tightening of the diaphragmatic hiatus. Whatever the cause the obstruction may be difficult to diagnose as there are other causes of persistent dysphagia following anti-reflux surgery. It may also be deceptively easy to pass tapered dilators through the obstruction, which is often elastic. The resistance to passage of large, at least 50 FG, olive dilators, such as the Eder–Puestow, gives a more accurate appreciation of the problem. As with post-vagotomy fibrosis, operative correction is usually required.

TUMOURS OF THE OESOPHAGUS

Benign tumours

Benign tumours of the oesophagus are exceedingly rare. Leiomyomas are the most frequent of these unusual lesions.[139] They are most common in the distal oesophagus and may become quite large before they cause dysphagia. They can be shelled out of the oesophageal wall at thoracotomy without breaching the mucosa.[140]

With the increasing use of endoscopy, small polyps are being found more frequently.[141] They may be squamous papillomas or true adenomas. Fibrovascular polyps have been reported, particularly in the upper oesophagus.[142] They can be large enough to cause symptoms and in about half of the cases the tumour may be regurgitated into the mouth or even outside the mouth![143] Lipomas,[144] chondromas,[145] granular cell tumours,[146] haemangiomas[147] and lymphangiomas[148] have all been described. Carcinoid tumours may occur, but they usually have malignant potential.[149] Nerve sheath tumours may arise from the vagi.

Malignant tumours

Sarcoma

Sarcoma of the oesophagus is excessively rare. Leiomyosarcoma[150] and rhabdomyosarcoma[151] have been reported. Other

REFERENCES

136. Hill L D, Tobias J A Arch Surg 1968; 96: 735
137. Walther B et al Am J Surg 1984; 147: 111
138. Spencer J D Br J Surg 1975; 62: 354
139. Seremetis M G et al Cancer 1976; 38: 2166
140. Storey C F, Adams W C Am J Surg 1956; 91: 3
141. Enterline H E, Thompson J Pathology of the Esophagus. Springer Verlag, Berlin 1984
142. Totten R S et al J Thorac Surg 1953; 25: 606
143. Jang G C, et al Radiology 1969; 92: 1196
144. Nora A F Am J Surg 1964; 108: 353
145. Stout A P, Lattes R In: Atlas of Tumor Pathology, Series 1, Fascicle 20. Armed Forces Institute of Pathology, Washington DC 1957
146. Hajdu S I In: Pathology of Soft Tissue Tumors. Lea & Febiger, Philadelphia 1979
147. Gentry R W et al Int Abstr Surg 1949; 88: 281
148. Armengol-Miro J R et al Endoscopy 1979; 3: 185

sarcomas are rarer still and in most instances are confined to single case reports.[141] Neurogenic sarcoma, osteogenic sarcoma and malignant granular cell tumours have been recorded. The oesophagus may be involved in T cell lymphomas, but this is usually secondary to involvement of adjacent mediastinal lymph nodes. There are only four convincing case reports of primary lymphoma of the oesophagus.[152]

A carcinosarcoma with adenomatous elements used to be described, but is now probably more accurately referred to as a polypoid carcinoma with dominant spindle cell elements.[153] It has a relatively good prognosis.

Carcinoma of the oesophagus

General

Carcinoma of the oesophagus is 1.5–3 times more common in men than in women.[141] Most of the patients are middle-aged or elderly and the condition is rare before the age of 40. Cancer is said to be most common at the points of physiological narrowing of the oesophagus—at its upper limit, at the arch of the aorta, at the level of transit of the left main bronchus, at the diaphragm and at the cardia—but many tumours are too long to permit precise determination of their site of origin.[141] Multiple cancers are as rare in the oesophagus as in the stomach, although submucosal secondary deposits, usually proximal to the primary, are not uncommon.[154] Approximately 55% of cases are in the upper and mid thoracic oesophagus, 34% in the lower and 8% in the cervical oesophagus. The remainder cannot be classified.[141]

Pathology and aetiology

Worldwide most carcinomas of the oesophagus are squamous cell tumours. Adenocarcinomas account for 0.8–8.0% of all carcinomas, depending on the local epidemiology.[151,155] Most are thought to arise as a result of Barrett's metaplasia.[156] Oat cell carcinoma, a small-cell undifferentiated carcinoma, is an unusual variant with a very poor prognosis.[157] Other epithelial tumours that have been described include adenoid cystic carcinoma,[158] mucoepidermoid carcinoma,[159] malignant melanoma[160] and the occasional carcinoid tumour.[147]

The incidence of squamous cell carcinoma of the oesophagus varies widely from one part of the world to another. There is a particularly high incidence in three areas—Northern China in the provinces of Henan, Hebi and Shanxi; the regions of Iran and Russia that border on the Caspian sea and in the black population of South Africa around Durban and in the Transkei.[141] In these areas the incidence is over 35 per 100 000 people, in contrast to 2–8 per 100 000 in most of Europe and the USA.[161] It is thought that diet is very important in the high-incidence areas. Four major factors have been identified: a diet high in nitrosamines; diets that include mouldy foods; foods raised on soils deficient in trace elements, especially molybdenum; and diets deficient in vitamins C and A, riboflavin, protein and caloric content.[141] Cigarette smoking and alcohol consumption are important factors in areas of the world that have a low or moderate risk.[161] Genetic factors may also play a part. A condition has been described in which oral leucoplakia and tylosis are associated with a high incidence of oesophageal cancer.[162] It is also suggested that oesophageal stagnation may increase the risk of carcinoma 22-fold in alkaline strictures, ninefold in oesophageal webs, sevenfold in achalasia and sixfold in peptic strictures.[163] Barrett's ulcer is also recognized as a premalignant condition. In many westernized countries the incidence of adenocarcinoma of the oesophagus and cardia has risen sharply in the last 20 years. As a result these are now relatively common lesions. The reason for the change is unknown, but obesity appears to be a risk factor.[164]

Table 21.2 Prognostic factors in squamous cell cancer of the oesophagus[152]

	Involvement	*5-year survival*
Size of tumour	<5 cm	20.9
	5–7.5 cm	20.4
	>7.5 cm	4.3
Depth of invasion	Muscle only	40.4
	Beyond	24.4
Lymph nodes	Not involved	43.3
	Involved	12.6

The poor prognosis of oesophageal cancer is proof of its ability to spread. Spread occurs directly through the wall of the oesophagus to adjacent organs, along the lymphatics in the submucosa or muscularis to form separate nodules, and to regional and distant lymph nodes; the pattern of spread depends on the primary site. Blood-borne distant metastases are also common, mainly to the liver and lungs. Pathological staging is a good predictor of prognosis.[154] The length of the tumour, depth of invasion, and presence of nodal metastases are the most important features (Table 21.2).

Clinical presentation

Dysphagia is the most common presenting symptom. It is relentlessly progressive unless the carcinoma is treated. Unfortunately this conceals the fact that symptoms may be very subtle at first. There may be minor retrosternal discomfort which the patient dismisses as 'wind' or which is treated as non-specific dyspepsia

REFERENCES

149. Rankin R et al Scot Med J 1980; 25: 245
150. Partyka E K et al Am J Gastroenterol 1981; 75: 132
151. Vartio T et al Virchows Arch (Pathol Anat) 1980; 386: 357
152. Stein H et al Dig Dis Sci 1981; 26: 457
153. Osamura R Y et al Am J Surg Pathol 1978; 2: 201
154. Huang G J, K'ai W Y Carcinoma of the Esophagus and Gastric Cardia. Springer Verlag, Berlin 1984
155. Bosch A et al Cancer 1979; 43: 1557
156. Cameron A J, Lomboy C T, Pera M, Carpenter H A Gastroenterology 1995; 109: 1541–1546
157. Briggs J C, Ibrahim H B N Histopathology 1983; 7: 261
158. Jacobsohn W Z et al Gastrointest Endosc 1980; 26: 102
159. Osamura R Y et al Am J Gastroenterol 1978; 69: 467
160. Sabanathan S, Eng J, Pradhan G N Am J Gastroenterol 1989; 84: 1475–1481
161. Fagelman K M et al J Ky Med Assoc 1979; 77: 637
162. Howel-Evans W et al Q J Med 1958; 27: 413
163. Joske R A, Benedict E B Gastroenterology 1959; 36: 749
164. Brown L M, Swanson C A et al J Natl Cancer Inst 1995; 87: 104–109

by a family doctor. Atypical chest pain from a secondary motility disorder is another early presentation which may cause difficulty. 'Pseudoachalasia' may occur with intermittent dysphagia and the radiological and manometric appearances of achalasia. The carcinoma in such cases is often a small tumour at the cardia which may be easily missed. Sometimes the initial presentation is with pulmonary symptoms, or frank pneumonia caused by overspill. More advanced cases may develop persistent cough during eating as the result of a tracheo-oesophageal fistula. Extensive tumours of the middle third of the oesophagus may cause a recurrent laryngeal nerve palsy. Anaemia or frank haematemesis is uncommon, but massive haematemesis from an aorto-oesophageal fistula may be a terminal event.

Physical signs are only seen in advanced cases and are those of malnutrition and disseminated cancer. Cervical lymphadenopathy may be detected, especially if there is a carcinoma of the cervical oesophagus.

Diagnosis

Barium swallow and endoscopy are the mainstays of diagnosis. Not every patient requires both investigations, but most do. Each has a slightly different purpose. Radiology is required to demonstrate the anatomy of the problem, and in operable lesions to assess the suitability of the stomach for reconstruction. Endoscopy yields material for histology or cytology and is a more accurate examination for small tumours and for those at the cardia. It should, however, be borne in mind that cancers may be missed by both types of investigation. Errors are most likely to occur at the entrance to the oesophagus and at the cardia. Fibreoptic endoscopes should be passed under direct vision as they may easily be pushed past a small tumour in the upper oesophagus. Sometimes the best views of the upper oesophagus will be obtained during withdrawal and it is a good practice to inspect the pharynx and vocal cords as the endoscope is removed.

Staging and general assessment

Once the diagnosis has been made it is essential to assess both the tumour and the patient to determine the best form of treatment. Unfortunately, many patients are only suitable for palliation because of advanced disease, advanced age or their poor general condition.

Liver metastases may be detected by ultrasound, computed tomography scanning, magnetic resonance imaging or laparoscopy, including laparoscopic ultrasound. Bronchoscopy is advisable before attempting resection of a tumour in the upper two-thirds of the oesophagus to exclude direct invasion or fistulation into the lung and bronchial tree. Laparoscopy is particularly useful for assessing adenocarcinomas of the distal oesophagus and cardia to assess transperitoneal spread. Computed tomographic and magnetic resonance imaging scanning are relatively inaccurate for assessing nodal spread.[165–167]

Endoscopic ultrasonography[165–167] provides the most accurate assessment of the primary lesion.[168] Assessment of the cardiovascular and respiratory systems is also an essential preliminary to radical treatment.

Preoperative preparation

Preliminary investigation excludes many patients as unsuitable for radical treatment, but many with potentially curable lesions are still in poor general condition and require some preoperative treatment. Fluid and electrolyte balance is easily corrected in most cases. Nutrition is more of a problem as there is simply not enough time for full nutritional resuscitation which may take several weeks. Nevertheless, some sort of nutritional support is often advisable (see Chapter 2). The simplest method of providing this is to withdraw all solid food and to start the patient on a high-protein liquid diet. It is surprising how much severe dysphagia improves once obstructing food material in the oesophagus has been cleared. Fine-bore nasogastric tubes and intravenous feeding have their occasional uses, but neither is a good solution for the severely obstructed oesophagus. Gentle oesophageal dilatation may help if a liquid diet cannot be tolerated. Ensuring that the patient can swallow is also good for the lungs as aspiration is an insidious and dangerous complication.

It is the respiratory system which requires the greatest attention as postoperative pulmonary problems are common. Most western patients with squamous cell cancers are smokers and even a short period of abstinence is a help. Good physiotherapy for the lungs and encouragement of exercise free of tubes and other medical encumbrances are also beneficial.

Treatment of malignant tumours

Curative treatment

Surgery

Surgical resection is the treatment of choice for adenocarcinomas of the oesophagus which are relatively radioresistant. Squamous cell cancers are more sensitive to radiation and the best form of management is therefore controversial. Unfortunately, no controlled trial has been done. The most quoted survival statistics following radiotherapy are those of Pearson.[169] He compared the results of surgery and radiotherapy in Edinburgh during the period 1948–1967. After 5 years only 11% of those treated surgically were alive, compared with 19% of those treated by radiotherapy. It must be stressed that this was not a controlled trial, but none the less the results achieved by radiotherapy were impressive at the time, mainly because the overall mortality was reduced by the absence of a postoperative mortality. No other radiotherapist has, however, been able to reproduce these results.

While the debate continues, the previously prohibitive operative mortality has been greatly reduced by improved methods of

REFERENCES

165. van Overhagen H, Lameris J S et al J Comput Assist Tomogr 1993; 17: 367–373
166. Sondenaa K, Skaane P, Nygaard K, Skjennald A Eur J Surg 1992; 158: 537–540
167. Takashima S, Takeuchi N et al Am J Roentgenol 1991; 156: 297–302
168. Botet J F, Lightdale C J, Zauber A G, Gerdes H, Urmacher C, Brennan M F Radiology 1991; 181: 419–425
169. Pearson J G Cancer 1977; 39: 882

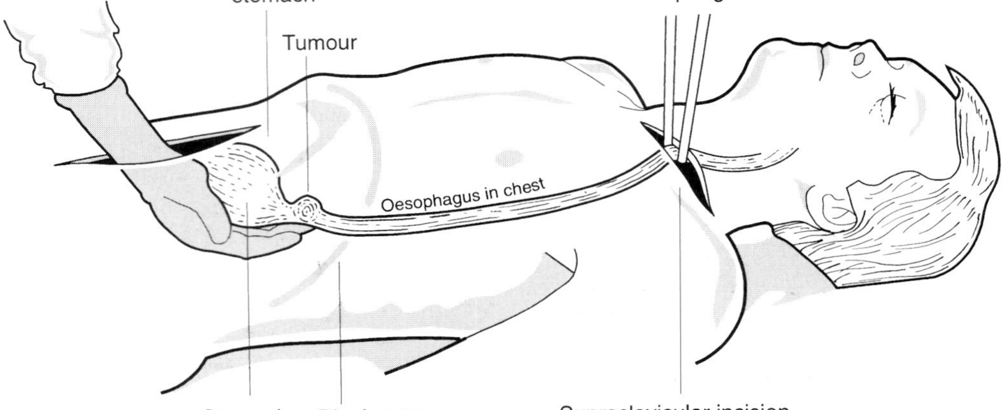

Fig. 21.19 Transhiatal dissection for oesophagectomy.

anaesthesia and perioperative care. For more than 10 years now most experienced surgeons have reported mortality rates of 10% or less for oesophageal resection at any level.[170,171] Unpractised surgeons still experience mortalities similar to those seen in the past.[172] In some countries such as China and Japan where oesophageal cancer is seen in younger and fitter patients, mortality rates of 5% or less have been reported. In 1980 Akiyama[173] reported 2 deaths in 279 resections (0.7%). This trend to safer surgery continues.

Many techniques have been described for resection of the oesophagus and its subsequent reconstruction. Safe resection usually involves thoracotomy, but some have returned to the older technique of resection of the oesophagus by blunt extraction popularized by Orringer.[174] This is appropriate for carcinomas in the lower oesophagus which can be mobilized by transhiatal dissection (Fig. 21.19). The normal oesophagus above the tumour is then removed by blunt dissection which is the well-established method of treating post-cricoid tumours.[175] Cancers in the mid-oesophagus may also be extracted, but there are occasional alarming unpublished reports of exsanguination from injury of the azygos vein which may be infiltrated by tumour.[176] Wong has reviewed the indications for transhiatal dissection.[176]

Tumours at the cardia may be removed via a left thoracotomy or a thoracoabdominal incision made through the sixth interspace. The distal oesophagus and the proximal stomach are resected. Adenocarcinomas at this site are discussed in Chapter 28.

A left thoracotomy gives poor access for adequate clearance and intrathoracic anastomosis if the cancer is above the cardia. In these circumstances a right thoracotomy through the fourth or fifth interspace is preferred.[177] The aortic arch is thus avoided and the only structure of note which runs across the oesophagus is the azygos vein which is easily divided. A midline or oblique laparotomy provides access to the abdomen for mobilization of the stomach and is usually done as the first stage of the operation. The next step is right thoracotomy and at least 6 cm of oesophagus should be resected proximal to the primary lesion. Because of the potential for submucosal spread it has been suggested that the entire intrathoracic oesophagus should be removed,[178] in which case a cervical incision is used to deliver the upper part of oesophagus. This approach also simplifies access for the anastomosis which need not be done deep in the chest. It is an attractive concept, but even if a cervical incision is used to mobilize the upper oesophagus a stump is left and the anastomosis may eventually lie in the upper thorax.

There is controversy about the role of extensive lymphadenectomy for oesophageal cancer. Five-year survival rates of 55% have been reported with three-field dissection in the neck, chest and abdomen[179] compared to 38.3% with conventional two-field dissection. Others feel that there is limited scope for such a major procedure.[180]

Minimally invasive surgical techniques have been used for oesophageal resection. Completely endoscopic procedures have been done, but are a lengthy tour de force at present. Thoracoscopic mobilization of the oesophagus is more practical, but has not yet reduced postoperative mortality.[181] An ingenious endoscope for performing transhiatal oesophagectomy under direct vision has been developed.[182]

It is fortunate that carcinomas of the upper thoracic or lower cervical oesophagus are rare as adequate removal is usually difficult. A small tumour may be amenable to removal by blunt dissection via a cervical incision, but full exposure is required if the cancer is adherent to the trachea. Injury to the trachea is a

REFERENCES

170. Dark J F et al Thorax 1981; 36: 891
171. Skinner D B Cancer 1982; 50: 2571
172. Matthews H R et al Br J Surg 1986; 73: 621
173. Akiyama H Curr Prob Surg 1980; 17: 55
174. Orringer M B Surg Clin North Am 1983; 63: 941
175. Ong G B, Lee T C Br J Surg 1960; 48: 193
176. Wong J Br J Surg 1986; 73: 89
177. Lewis I Br J Surg 1946; 34: 18
178. McKeown K C Br J Surg 1976; 63: 259
179. Akiyama H, Tsurumaru M, Udagawa H, Kajiyama Y Ann Surg 1994; 220: 364–372
180. Law S Y K, Fok M, Wong J Br J Surg 1996; 83: 107–111
181. Cuschieri A Endosc Surg Allied Technol 1994; 2: 21–25
182. Manncke K, Raestrup H, Walter D, Buess G, Becker H D Endosc Surg Allied Technol 1994; 2: 10–15

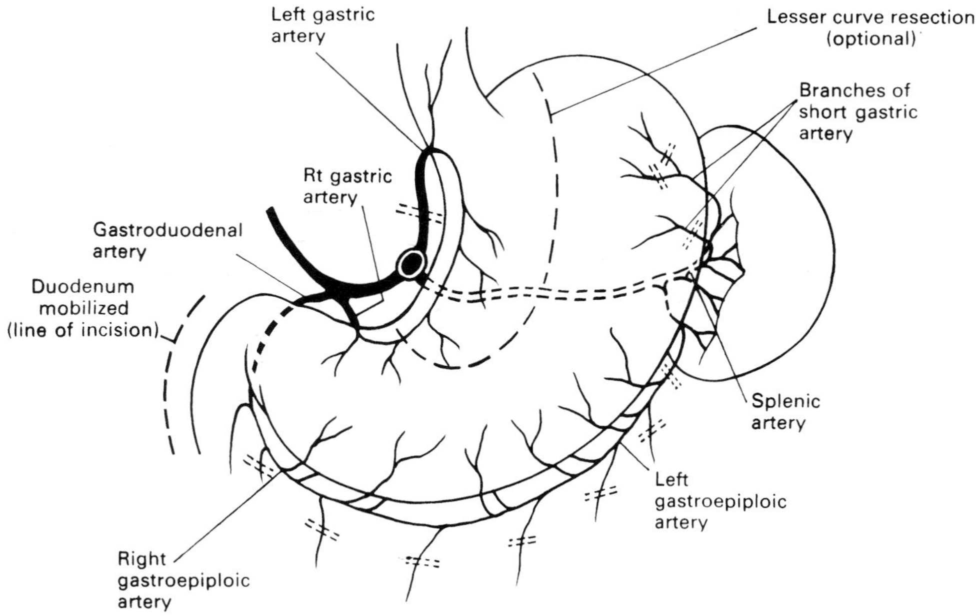

Fig. 21.20 Gastric mobilization for oesophageal reconstruction.

formidable complication which should not be risked. Exposure of the thoracic inlet may be through a 'trapdoor' incision with partial division and lateral reflection of the sternum and attached clavicle.

Oesophageal reconstruction

It is generally agreed that the stomach is the most suitable organ for reconstruction following resection of the oesophagus for cancer (see Chapter 20). With suitable mobilization it may be brought up to the neck (Fig. 21.20) unless a partial gastrectomy has been previously carried out. Troublesome postoperative reflux and stricture development are uncommon, but may be a problem after limited resections of the cardia. The anastomosis should therefore be as high in the oesophagus as possible or a generous gastric resection should be done.

More complex reconstructions using colon or jejunum are sometimes indicated, but pose a greater hazard for the debilitated patient.

Radiotherapy

Radiotherapy may be used for the treatment of a small primary squamous carcinoma as well as for the treatment of cancers which are not amenable to surgical resection.[169] There is a tendency to use suboptimal doses for palliative treatment to avoid the morbidity of radical treatment, but the benefit is usually disappointing and temporary.[183] Intubation or laser treatment is a simpler and better approach if palliation is all that is feasible.

There is as yet no evidence that routine pre- or postoperative radiotherapy improves the results of surgical resection. There have been few properly controlled studies of the value of preoperative radiotherapy. Launois et al[184] and Huseman[185] have both shown no benefit from this approach. Skinner et al[186] found that preoperative radiotherapy actually decreased survival at 6 and 12 months and abandoned its use. Reports of the possible benefit of adjuvant radiotherapy are mostly anecdotal and uncontrolled. An exception is a randomized study from China[187] which showed an increase in 5-year survival from 25.0 to 45.5% in patients under 65 years of age. The British Medical Research Council has performed a meta-analysis of all prospective randomized studies of preoperative radiotherapy that has shown identical survival curves in the two groups.[188] It is still possible that certain relatively favourable subgroups may benefit, but further study is required.

Chemotherapy

Cytotoxic chemotherapy is improving steadily and can now produce significant clinical benefits. Kelsen has pioneered the use of platinum-based regimens[189] that have been progressively improved and are now suitable for perioperative treatment.[190] Large prospective studies of pre- and postoperative chemotherapy are in progress in several countries. Chemotherapy has been shown to improve survival when given in conjunction with radiotherapy.[191]

REFERENCES

183. Earlam R, Cunha-Melo J R Br J Surg 1980; 67: 457
184. Launois B et al Surg Gynecol Obstet 1981; 153: 690
185. Huseman B In: Giuli R (ed) Cancer of the Esophagus in 1984. Maloine, Paris 1984
186. Skinner D B et al Ann Surg 1986; 204: 391
187. Huang G-J In: Giuli R (ed) Cancer of the Esophagus in 1984, Maloine, Paris 1984
188. MRC. Meta-analysis of the value of preoperative radiotherapy for oesophageal cancer. In press.
189. Coonley C J, Bains M, Hilaris B, Chapman R, Kelsen D P Cancer 1984; 54: 2351–2355
190. Kelsen D P, Minsky B, Smith M et al Preoperative therapy for esophageal cancer: a randomized comparison of chemotherapy versus radiation therapy. J Clin Oncol 1990; 8: 1352–1361

Palliative treatment

Intubation

Endoscopic intubation of malignant strictures is a simple form of management for those with incurable tumours. Several introduction systems[192,193] are available which rely on the initial insertion of a guidewire through the narrowed segment under direct vision using fibreoptic endoscopy and, ideally, X-ray control. A suitable tube mounted on its introducer is then passed over the guidewire (Fig. 21.21). Complications may still occur—mainly perforation of a friable growth—but the procedure is safe and effective in experienced hands.[194] Even if a split does occur it is usually small and partially sealed by the tube. Restriction of oral fluids for a few days and administration of antibiotics is usually sufficient treatment for these minor leaks.

A recent innovation is the expanding metal stent, of which there are several designs. These may be inserted at endoscopy or in the X-ray department. They are expensive, but provide excellent palliation with a very low complication rate and may well become the treatment of choice.[195]

Bypass or resection

It is possible to bypass an irresectable cancer or at least remove part of it. The Kirschner[196] operation has been used for this purpose. In this operation the oesophagus is divided in the neck and the abdomen. The stomach is brought up subcutaneously and anastomosed to the cervical oesophagus. The upper end of the excluded oesophagus is closed and the distal end is anastomosed to a loop of jejunum. Unfortunately, the postoperative mortality of this approach is 41.5%, which most would regard as prohibitive.[197]

It is quite true that better palliation of dysphagia may be achieved in those who survive palliative resection or bypass than by intubation. The benefit of a major procedure in patients with a limited life expectancy is questionable. Life may be so short that it is inappropriate to spend a large proportion of it in hospital or recovering from major surgery.

Laser phototherapy

Laser phototherapy for incurable lesions is capable of restoring swallowing to normal.[198] The laser probe is passed down the biopsy channel of a fibreoptic endoscope and vaporization is carried out under direct vision. A disadvantage of this approach is that it has to be done on several occasions, but eventually fibrosis seems to limit inwards growth of the tumour.[199] Laser therapy is now widely used, although the equipment is expensive. In general it is best for protruberant growths, while scirrhous cancers are still best treated by intubation. Similar results may be obtained with bipolar diathermy probes[200] or intratumoral injection of alcohol.[201]

Radiotherapy

External beam radiotherapy for palliation is superficially attractive, but is not without morbidity and the dose may need to be reduced to the tolerance of the patient. This limits its usefulness. Intraluminal radiotherapy, or brachytherapy, is a much more practical approach. A low-penetration radiation source with a suitable delivery system can treat a malignant stricture in 30 minutes or less. Results are comparable to other methods of intraluminal treatment.[202]

Malignant tracheo-oesophageal fistula

Fistulation of a cancer into the trachea or left main stem bronchus is a very distressing complication. Such tumours are incurable and are best treated by inserting an endo-oesophageal tube to seal the fistula and maintain swallowing.[192] Conventional rigid tubes, with or without a balloon cuff, or expanding stents may be used. Sometimes the oesophagus is not narrow enough to hold a tube. This problem may be overcome by wrapping a piece of Ivalon around the tube before insertion. This seems to give enough adhesion to grip the tube.[203] Bypass surgery has been advocated for this problem, but the disadvantages have already been outlined.

Complications of resection

Leaks

Leakage from an oesophageal anastomosis is a particularly lethal complication. The best management is not to get a leak in the first place! The low mortality rates following oesophageal resection quoted previously are largely from reducing anastomotic leakage by careful surgical technique. Meticulous and generous mobilization of the stomach with careful preservation of its blood supply is the best insurance against anastomotic problems. Even more care should be taken to ensure that the blood supply of the anastomosis is adequate if more complex methods of reconstruction are used. Prior angiography, careful inspection of arterial and venous anatomy and trial clamping of vessels before division are useful aids when long segments of colon are used.[204]

There is little point in attempting resuture of the anastomosis if leakage does occur. Except in the most fortunate circumstances this is doomed to failure. Small leaks may be managed conservatively with antibiotics, patience and nutritional support. Leakage of

REFERENCES

191. Herskovic A Martz K et al N Engl J Med 1992; 326: 1593–1598
192. Ogilvie A L et al Gut 1982; 23: 1060
193. Tytgat G N, den Hartog Jager F C Endoscopy 1977; 9: 211
194. Wilton A, Smith P M Eur J Gastroenterol Hepatol 1995; 7: 559–562
195. Rate A J, Nicholson D A, Brown T H, Kay C L, Bancewicz J Gut 1994; 35: 58
196. Kirschner M B Arch Klin Chir 1920; 114: 606
197. Wong J et al World J Surg 1981; 5: 547
198. Swain C P et al Br J Surg 1984; 71: 112
199. Krasner N et al Gut 1987; 28: 792
200. Jensen D M, Machicado G, Randall G, Tung L A, English-Zych S Gastroenterology 1988; 94: 1263–1270
201. Nwokolo C U, Payne-James J J, Silk D B, Misiewicz J J, Loft D E. Gut 1994; 35: 299–303
202. Low D E, Pagliero K M J Thorac Cardiovasc Surg 1992; 104: 173–178
203. Robertson C S, Atkinson M Lancet 1986; ii: 949
204. Shackelford R T In: Surgery of the Alimentary Tract, vol 1. Esophagus. Saunders, Philadelphia 1978

an anastomosis in the superficial part of the neck with a retrosternal reconstruction may produce a local fistula which heals spontaneously. Intrathoracic leakage is a much more serious problem. Large leaks producing cardiovascular collapse are likely to prove lethal and in a patient with a poor prognosis radical attempts at salvage may not be worthwhile. Exploration of the anastomosis may be worthwhile, if the patient is young or has benign disease, or a small cancer. If the leak is relatively small and the tissues are viable, carefully placed drains may control the contamination until healing occurs.[205] Otherwise further resection, with creation of an end cervical oesophagostomy and an appropriate abdominal stoma, is the only effective treatment.[206] Reconstruction is carried out some months later and should be delayed for as long as possible—ideally for 6–12 months.

Strictures

Anastomotic strictures are the result either of poor technique with the construction of a narrow stoma or postoperative reflux. The latter should be prevented by avoiding known pitfalls in reconstruction, such as a conservative excision of the cardia. Stapled anastomoses may stenose in a rather unpredictable way. Simple dilatation is effective if the stricture is not too fibrous. Mature strictures may require radial division with endoscopic diathermy.

REFERENCES

205. Wilson et al Am J Surg 1982; 144: 95
206. Triggiani E, Belsey R Thorax 1977; 32: 241

22 The chest wall, lungs, pleura and diaphragm

Peter Goldstraw

Much of the fascination of thoracic surgery lies in the broad spectrum of pathology which affects the thoracic contents. Its development has been spurred by successive 'epidemics': trauma and its complications during the First and Second World Wars, tuberculosis between the wars and into the 1940s and 50s, and latterly the rising tide of lung cancer. The legacy of rheumatic heart disease and the increasing incidence of coronary artery disease led to the development of cardiac surgical techniques (Ch. 23).

Whilst the physiological triumph of cardiopulmonary bypass still has considerable mystique, it is difficult for us now to appreciate how great a barrier the pleural space proved to the development of thoracic surgery. Before the importance of underwater drainage was appreciated, there was a high mortality associated with pleural intubation.[1] Early thoracic operations were undertaken with the patient breathing spontaneously, and were thus limited in duration and technical scale by the resultant pneumothorax. Subsequent progress has only been possible due to parallel developments in anaesthesia (see Ch. 5). The development of cuffed endotracheal tubes and mechanical ventilators permitted positive pressure ventilation and overcame the difficulties of the open pleura and resulting pneumothorax.

The spillage of infected material from the lung being operated upon into the dependent lung remained a problem. This was particularly important as most resections were originally carried out for bronchiectasis and other problems of pleuropulmonary sepsis. This difficulty was tackled in two ways. The first was to operate with the patient in the prone and slightly head-down position, so that all infected secretions drained into the trachea where they could be aspirated.[2] The second approach was to use endobronchial tubes which isolated each lung, preventing cross-spill[3] and allowing each to be ventilated independently. This latter approach has proven superior, as it allows the surgeon to operate with the patient in the lateral position which gives better access to the hilar structures and, by permitting the collapse of the ipsilateral lung, removes competition between surgeon and anaesthetist for space within the hemithorax. Any procedure using video-assisted thoracoscopic surgery (VATS) requires the ipsilateral lung to be collapsed to give access. Whilst some surgeons use compression by insufflating air under pressure, single-lung anaesthesia is more widely used. This 'minimally invasive surgery' parallels the development of laparoscopic surgery in the abdomen and requires considerable training. Many of its new applications are yet to be evaluated but it has already had a profound influence on many thoracic surgical procedures.

Selective endobronchial intubation is not, however, without its problems.[4] The tubes are positioned blindly and require considerable experience and expertise in placement. Despite such skill malposition can occur. The optimal position for such tubes is shown in Figure 22.1 along with some of the more common errors. Depending on the anatomy of the malposition, it may result in

REFERENCES

1. Graham E A, Bell R D Am J Med Sci 1918; 156: 839
2. Parry-Brown A I Thorax 1948; 3: 161
3. Bjork V O, Carlens E J Thorac Surg 1950; 20: 151
4. Goldstraw P In: Jackson J W, Cooper D K C (eds) Rob and Smith's Operative Surgery, Thoracic Surgery. Butterworths, London 1986 p 135

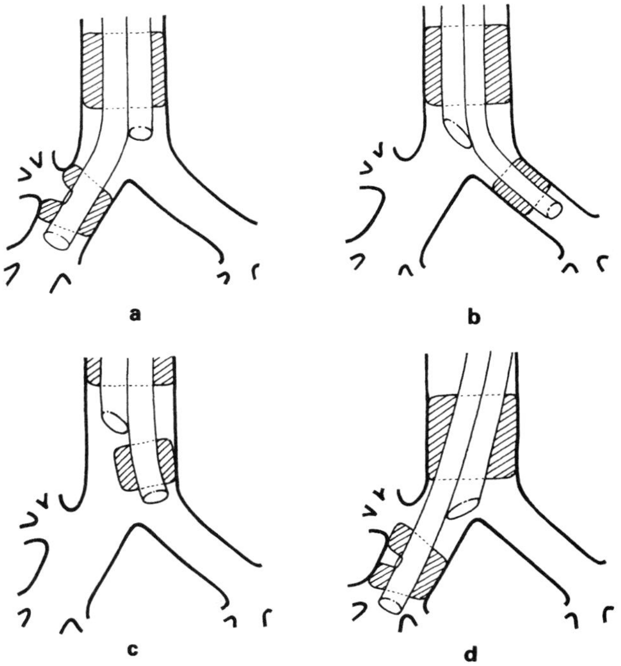

Fig. 22.1 The correct position for double-lumen tubes. **(a)** The right-sided tube used for left pneumonectomy; **(b)** the left-sided tube which because of its simpler design is used for all right-sided operations and any operation on the left where pneumonectomy is not anticipated. These tubes may go down the wrong side, may not be in far enough **(c)** and not protect the other lung from spillage, or may be down too far **(d)**, and fail to ventilate parts of that lung and even obstruct ventilation to the other lung.

unsuspected spill into the dependent lung or hyperinflation of the upper lung, with consequent difficulties for the surgeon.

Improved radiographic techniques have greatly aided the detection and diagnosis of thoracic disease. The quality of chest radiographs has improved considerably, greatly aiding preoperative evaluation and postoperative care. Within the last 10 years computerized tomography (CT) of the thorax has revolutionized thoracic radiology and has largely replaced the older techniques of conventional tomography and contrast radiology.

Improvements in intraoperative and postoperative monitoring, the emergence of intensive care as a specialty, increasing nursing expertise and the development of better physiotherapy techniques have allowed increasingly major thoracic operations to be undertaken safely in an ageing population.

THE CHEST WALL

The anatomy of the chest wall is a complex combination of skeletal, ligamentous and muscular structures supplied by neurovascular bundles. In addition to its role in respiration it also has an important protective function.

Chest trauma

Chest trauma is traditionally categorized as penetrating or blunt, depending on the mechanism of injury. Blast injury is responsible for a mixed variety of both blunt and penetrating trauma.

Penetrating trauma

Penetrating trauma is mechanically efficient, obtaining maximal injury by concentrating the maximum force on to a sharp point. Such a sharp implement or missile is often small enough to pass between the ribs, inflicting little damage to the chest wall, but injuring the underlying intrathoracic viscera.

Management of most penetrating injuries is not complex as injuries are commonly of low velocity. Such injuries may be accidental, such as impalement upon railings, or intentional with assault by knife or hand gun. The injury is limited to the track of the missile and management requires only a knowledge of the site and angle of entry, and an understanding of the underlying anatomical structures. In the majority of patients injury is confined to the lung with pneumothorax or haemothorax. In 95% of such cases the proper insertion of an intercostal drain will allow drainage of the collection and re-expansion of the lung.[5] Should the patient arrive in the accident and emergency department with a missile projecting from the chest, it should not be removed until a complete assessment has been undertaken, blood is available, and the patient is on the threshold of the operating theatre. Once removed, careful physiological and radiographic monitoring will dictate further management. Thoracotomy will only be necessary in a small minority, usually where major bleeding or air leak is not controlled by the insertion of a chest drain. Penetrating injuries over the precordium should be surgically explored if there is evidence of tamponade, with falling blood pressure and rising central venous pressure. Pericardial aspiration, by the subxiphoid approach, will confirm the diagnosis and temporarily relieve the situation whilst cardiothoracic advice is sought. If such cardiac injury requires surgical repair, a median sternotomy incision is best.[6] Penetrating injuries over the lower chest may result in damage to the abdominal viscera. Whilst a chest drain may deal adequately with the thoracic trauma, laparotomy may be necessary.

High-velocity injuries occur only with missiles travelling above the speed of sound. In these circumstances important secondary effects occur, with shock waves extending damage far beyond the track of the missile.[7] Such shock waves travel well through solid, water-filled viscera such as liver and spleen, but inflict relatively little damage on air-filled viscera such as lung. Such high-velocity missiles may pass directly through the chest, leaving little damage within the hemithorax, but causing extensive disruption and even infarction of organs within the abdomen and spinal canal, often several centimetres away from the track of the missile. High-velocity injury may be inflicted by high-powered hunting or military rifles, or shrapnel, and usually requires immediate surgical exploration to debride the wound, control bleeding and assess visceral damage.[8] Such injuries carry a high mortality.

Blunt injury

Blunt injury to the chest wall is mechanically inefficient as the force is spread over a wide area. As a result, the power of the human arm is incapable of causing major intrathoracic injury and mechanical assistance in the form of gravity or a vehicle is usually necessary to inflict serious injury. The incidence of blunt chest trauma is thus increasing in line with the rising number of road traffic accidents. The patterns of injury vary between pedestrians and other road users, and amongst vehicle occupants depending on the seat occupied.[9] Amongst those injuries which prove fatal, thoracic trauma is the commonest injury in vehicle occupants and second only to head injury amongst pedestrians. There is some evidence that the use of seatbelts is reducing the incidence and severity of thoracic trauma.[10]

The skeletal ring, composed of vertebral bodies, ribs and sternum, will when compressed distort to a variable degree, depending upon the suppleness of the ribcage, the energy applied and the area over which it is distributed. Such compression may contuse underlying structures such as the lung and heart, but once the bony resilience is overcome, the ribs or sternum fracture, and the force is then released upon deeper structures, causing more severe injuries.

Severe force applied over a broad area may fracture the bony ring at two points on its circumference producing a flail segment (Fig. 22.2). Such a segment may be lateral or anterior, depending

REFERENCES

5. Hood R M In: Sabiston D C, Spencer F C (eds) Gibbon's Surgery of the Chest. W B Saunders, Philadelphia 1983 p 291
6. Trinkle J K In: Trinkle J K, Grover F L (eds) Management of Thoracic Trauma Victims. J B Lippincott, Philadelphia 1980 p 67
7. Owen-Smith M High Velocity Missile Wounds. Arnold, London 1981
8. Gibbons J R P Eur J Cardiothorac Surg 1989; 3: 297
9. Fox J N, McLeod D A D Health Bull 1978; 36: 313
10. Galasko C S B, Edwards D H Injury 1975; 6: 320

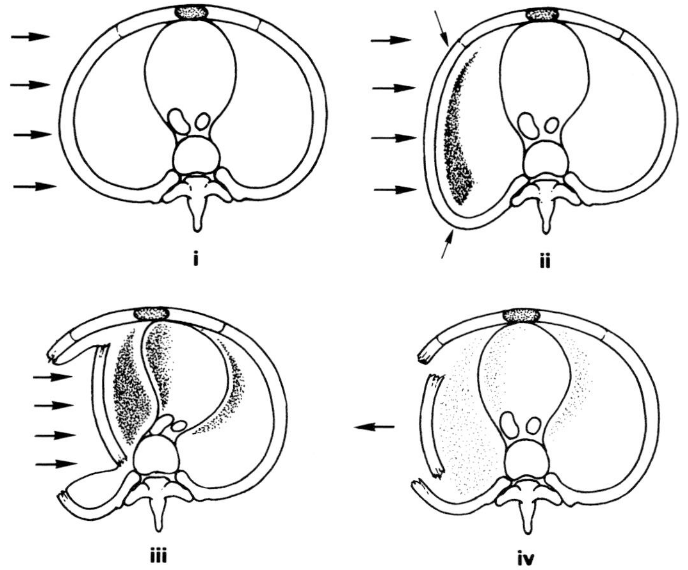

Fig. 22.2a The dynamics of lateral flail chest trauma. **(i)** Such injury requires major force to be applied over a large area of the chest wall. **(ii)** Initially the ribs flatten, restraining the force and limiting contusion to the lung immediately beneath. **(iii)** If the force is too great, the ribs fracture at the anterior and posterior angles, and the force drives the plate of chest wall medially, compressing and contusing the mediastinal structures and even the opposite lung. **(iv)** When the force is withdrawn, the flail segment recoils to lie within the arc of the chest wall. If intrapleural pressure becomes positive, as on coughing, or less negative, as with a pneumothorax, the flail segment will resume its anatomical position or even bulge outwards.

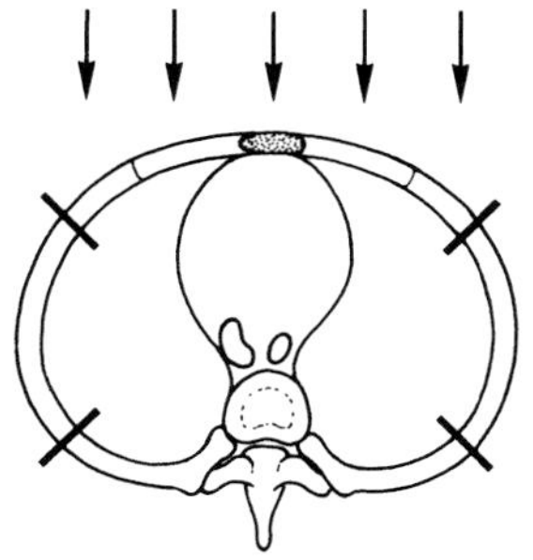

Fig. 22.2b Similarly, if considerable force is applied to the anterior chest wall, the ribs may fracture at the anterior and posterior angles, on one or both sides.

upon the mechanics of the injury.[11] If there is no pneumothorax or haemothorax, then the intrapleural pressure remains negative, and the flail segment lies within the usual arc of the ribs (Fig. 22.3), moving inwards as the intrapleural negative pressure increases during inspiration, and outwards during expiration.[12] If the intrapleural pressure becomes positive, as in coughing, then the flail segment bulges and becomes more obvious. Such paradoxical movement is an important physical sign, but has probably in the past received undue emphasis in the management of flail chest.[13]

Thoracotomy and mechanical fixation of the ribs enjoyed a vogue,[14] but are now not thought to be justified unless thoracotomy is necessary to control blood loss or massive air leak,[15] or to repair injury to other organs such as bronchial laceration[16] or diaphragmatic tears.[17] Similarly, ingenious methods of external fixation, using wires fixed to external traction beams, are also obsolete.[18] The significance of paradox lies in the severity of trauma necessary to produce a flail segment and the severe contusion such force can inflict on underlying structures.[19]

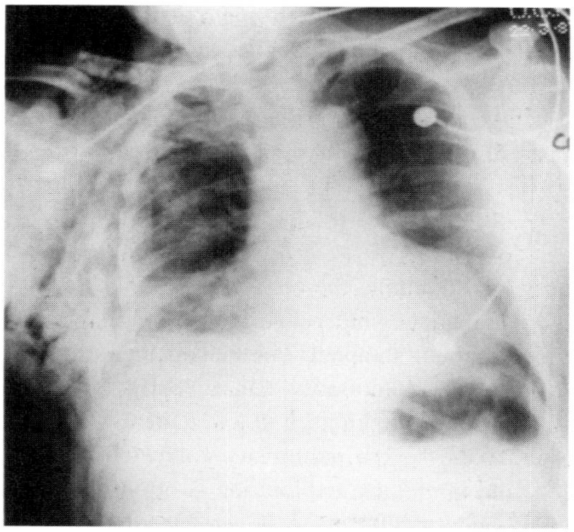

Fig. 22.3 The chest radiograph of a man hit by a car on the right side. There is a lateral flail segment lying just within the arc of the rest of the chest wall. There is contusion of the right lung, and surgical emphysema of the chest wall. Whilst the latter indicates air leak from the lung, the position of the flail segment confirms that there is no pneumothorax as intrapleural pressure is still negative.

As for all rib fractures, management should concentrate on minimizing further injury to the underlying lung. Paradoxical movement may appear for the first time up to a week following injury, and this is often ascribed to the loosening of rib fractures. It is, however, probable that such an occurrence reflects the increasingly negative intrapleural pressure and failing compliance when lung injury is complicated by oedema, further contusion or infection. Fractures of the first rib occurring with blunt trauma indicate severe force, as the rib is well protected by surrounding musculature and is short and stout. Such extreme injury may be associated with other severe intrathoracic injuries, such as transection of the aorta, or direct injury to the brachial plexus and subclavian vessels.[20]

REFERENCES

11. Mackay G M, Gloyns P F In: Williams H G, Smith R E (eds) Trauma of the Chest—The Coventry Conference. John Wright, Bristol 1977 p 63
12. Maloney J V, Schumtzer K J, Raschke E J Thorac Cardiovasc Surg 1961; 41: 291
13. Trinkle J K In: Trinkle J K, Grover F L (eds) Management of Thoracic Trauma Victims. J B Lippincott, Philadelphia 1980 p 39
14. Moore B P J Thorac Cardiovasc Surg 1975; 70: 619
15. Hurt R, Bates M (eds) Essentials of Thoracic Surgery. Butterworths, London 1986 p 145
16. Bates M In: Williams H G, Smith R E (eds) Trauma of the Chest—The Coventry Conference. John Wright, Bristol 1977 p 40
17. Harley H R S In: Williams H G, Smith R E (eds) Trauma of the Chest—The Coventry Conference. John Wright, Bristol 1977
18. Paris F In: Williams H G, Smith R E (eds) Trauma of the Chest—The Coventry Conference. John Wright, Bristol 1977 p 20
19. Trinkle J K et al Ann Thorac Surg 1973; 16: 568
20. Fisher R D, Rienhoff W F J Trauma 1966; 6: 579

Stress fractures of the first rib may result from well muscled young people carrying heavy loads on their shoulders.[21] Other ribs may fracture as a result of strenuous coughing. These fractures may cause little pain and are often seen when undertaking bone scans as part of the assessment of a malignancy.[22]

Blast injury

Blast injury may combine the blunt trauma of the explosion and resulting crush damage with penetrating damage caused by high-velocity fragments of shrapnel. The management of such injuries is thus complex and mortality consequently high. Whilst the insertion of intercostal drains will often deal with the haemo-pneumothorax, the severe pulmonary contusion will necessitate ventilation, and immediate exploration is often necessary to deal with the intra-abdominal damage. Severe bleeding follows damage to the spleen, kidneys or liver, and bowel ischaemia may result from mesenteric laceration. The later development of adult respiratory distress syndrome is common and requires appropriate management.

Chest wall tumours

Benign or malignant tumours may arise from any of the components of the chest wall,[23] but all are rare. Metastatic tumours and chest wall invasion from adjacent malignancies, especially the lung, are considerably more common.[24]

Benign tumours

Benign tumours of the chest wall should be excised. All rib tumours should be excised by wide extraperiosteal resection as malignancy can only be properly assessed by subsequent histological examination. Benign, non-neoplastic swellings of the ribs occur in fibrous dysplasia.[25] The expanded rib may be palpable and produce local pain and tenderness. The radiographic appearances are typical, with expansion of the rib and a foamy appearance. Although developmental, this abnormality usually presents in early adult life, but the development of new lesions is unusual after adolescence. If the patient is symptomatic, or if doubt persists as to the diagnosis, local excision is curative but may prove technically difficult if the first rib is affected.

Malignant tumours

Malignant primary tumours of the chest are radioresistant and wide resection should be undertaken. It may be necessary to resect the overlying skin with affected ribs, adjacent muscles and neurovascular bundles, the underlying parietal pleura and lung tissue, if invaded. If the resultant chest wall defect is large and unsupported by extrathoracic structures such as the scapula, a chest wall prosthesis should be inserted. The best prosthesis at present consists of two layers of polypropylene (Marlex®) mesh, filled and made rigid by methyl methacrylate cement.[26] This can be moulded to the contours of the thoracic wall before the cement hardens, and the mesh provides a suitable sewing ring around the margins of the prosthesis. Such a prosthesis will minimize resultant paradox and provide a satisfactory cosmetic result. Skin cover, if necessary, can be accomplished with a variety of rotation or myocutaneous flaps.[27]

Secondary deposits within the ribs are most commonly associated with primary tumours of the breast, bronchus, prostate, thyroid or kidney. Those from the kidney are particularly vascular and may well be associated with a bruit and be pulsatile. Multiple rib secondaries may be associated with myeloma or leukaemia. The radiographic signs are often unreliable and biopsy should be undertaken to establish diagnosis. Incision biopsy should be sited so that the scar can be excised should excision be shown to be desirable. Even if the tumour is pulsatile, a wide-bore needle biopsy may be safely performed if passed obliquely through the tumour so as to not penetrate the underlying pleura. Metastatic tumours of the chest wall, if symptomatic, are usually controlled by radiotherapy. However, excision may occasionally be justified if the primary lesion is controlled and the metastasis is solitary, or if symptomatic control is not achieved by radiotherapy.

Pectus deformity

Pectus deformities are believed to result from excessive growth of the costal cartilages, causing the sternum to be unusually prominent (pectus carinatum) or buckled inwards to produce an unsightly depression (pectus excavatum; Fig. 22.4). A mixed deformity may be produced, with a rolling convexity over one hemithorax, a deep sulcus over the other, and the sternum lying anteroposteriorly along its vertical axis. Such deformities may be evident at birth or become evident as the deformity increases during growth spurts. The cosmetic results may have social and psychological implications but, even if severe, it is rare for any physiological impairment to result from compression of the underlying heart or lungs.[28] The patient and parents should be reassured as to the cosmetic nature of the lesion, but many patients are disturbed by the appearance of the deformity, and despite reassurance will insist on surgical correction.

The implantation of prosthetic material to obscure the underlying deformity has disappointing long-term results. Surgical correction entails the excision of the abnormal cartilages from ribs 3 to 7 on each side.[29] With pectus carinatum deformity the sternum then falls back to occupy its more normal position. In an exca-

REFERENCES

21. Rademaker M, Redmond A D, Barber P V Thorax 1983; 38: 312
22. Hooper R G, Beechler G R, Johnston M C Am Rev Resp Dis 1978; 118: 279
23. Barrett N R Br J Surg 1955; 178: 113
24. LeRoux B T, Sharma D M In: Ravitch M M (ed) Current Problems in Surgery. Year Book, Chicago 1983 p 349
25. Pritchard J E Am J Med Sci 1956; 222: 313
26. Eschapasse H et al Ann Thorac Surg 1981; 32: 329
27. Al-Kattan K M, Breach N M, Goldstraw P Ann Thorac Surg 1995; 60: 1372
28. Morshuis W J, Folgering H T, Barentsz J O et al J Thorac Cardiovasc Surg 1994; 107: 1403
29. Ravitch M M In: Sabiston D C, Spencer F C (eds) Surgery of the Chest. W B Saunders, Philadelphia 1983 p 318

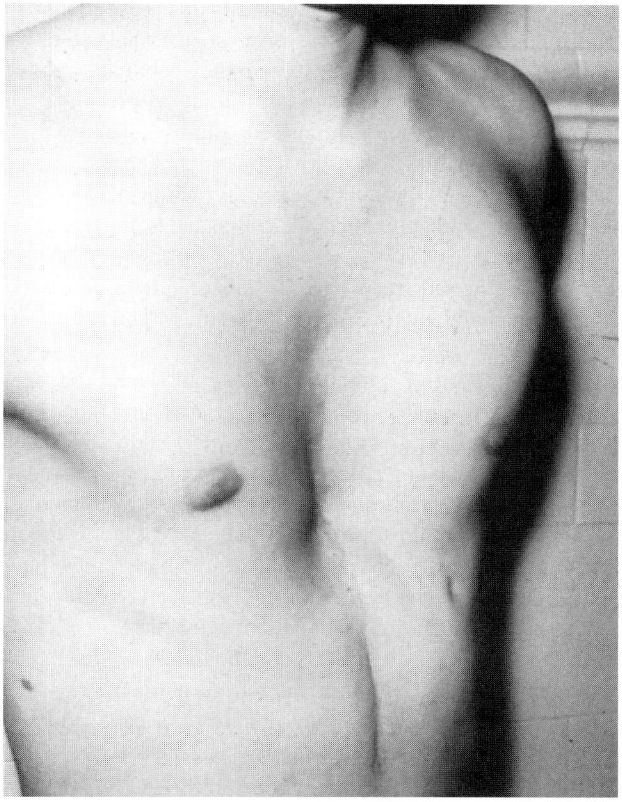

Fig. 22.4 Pectus excavatum deformity of the chest wall.

vatum deformity the sternum should be temporarily splinted with transverse plates of metal or rib. Once all the abnormal costal cartilages have been excised the sternum is usually found to be of satisfactory contour, but occasionally a transverse osteotomy or the shaving-off of undue prominences may be required. With further growth, the deformity may recur and surgical correction should be left as late as the patient will allow. Correction in infancy is not justified, but if evidence of psychological disturbance develops, correction may prove necessary at the time of school entry. Usually the patient presents at adolescence with the arrival of sexual awareness. A transverse submammary incision provides satisfactory access and a less unpleasant cosmetic result than the vertical incision previously utilized. This extensive surgery results in temporary chest wall instability and severe pain. Despite the evident risks, few patients are discouraged from seeking surgical correction.

Inflammatory conditions of the chest wall

Osteomyelitis of the ribcage is usually staphylococcal in origin.[30] Antibiotics are usually effective, but sequestra may form, requiring removal and drainage.

Chronic costochondritis (Tietze's disease)[31] is a painful inflammatory condition afflicting the costal cartilages, usually of the second, third or fourth ribs. The condition usually settles spontaneously, but may have a protracted course. Surgical excision should be avoided as an ugly scar results in this position, and the condition may reappear in the adjacent cartilages.

Tuberculous infections arising within an internal mammary lymph node may produce a fluctuant swelling on the chest wall adjacent to the sternum. Incision of the superficial abscess will result in a persistent sinus unless the dumb-bell extension through the chest wall is explored and the underlying lymph node excised. Tuberculosis may result in a cold abscess originating from the thoracic spine,[32] which may track around the intercostal bundles. The abscess may present as a fluctuant swelling at any point around the chest wall, most usually in the mid clavicular or mid axillary lines where perforating branches of the vessel penetrate the muscle bundles. If the tuberculous nature of these conditions is suspected, aspiration will establish the diagnosis, provide material for culture and may obviate the need for drainage. These abscesses may continue to enlarge on drug treatment, and if surgery proves necessary, it should be undertaken with appropriate drug cover.

Pyogenic empyema, if neglected by the patient or doctors, may present as a fluctuant subcutaneous swelling over an intercostal space (empyema necessitans).[33] Unless the underlying pathology is recognized, drainage of the superficial loculus will result in a persistent sinus.

THE LUNGS

Lung trauma

The lung may be damaged by penetration or blunt injury, but it must not be forgotten that blunt trauma may result in a penetrating wound of the underlying lung from rib fragments. If there is radiographic evidence of blood or air within the pleural space, an intercostal drain should be inserted. It is increasingly recognized that management of chest trauma depends on the management of the con-tused lung. It has been shown that the contused lung parenchyma is particularly susceptible to oedema from increased permeability of the alveolar capillary membrane.[34] Contusion and oedema may extend to adjacent lung tissue and pulmonary compliance may be further reduced by suprainfection.

Management depends on a number of key aspects, and the success or otherwise of treatment should be monitored with clinical evaluation supplemented by serial chest radiographs and arterial blood–gas estimations. These patients should be admitted to a well equipped unit, staffed by experienced nursing and medical staff, with facilities to undertake immediate ventilation should it prove necessary. The pathophysiology of chest trauma is of far greater significance than the anatomical extent of injury. Frail, elderly smokers with severe underlying lung disease may be precipitated into respiratory failure with a single rib fracture, whereas a healthy young adult may readily tolerate multiple rib fractures or a flail segment.

Intercostal drainage is only indicated if there is clear radiographic confirmation of a pneumothorax or haemothorax. The

REFERENCES

30. Jara F M, Yap A et al J Thorac Cardiovasc Surg 1979; 77: 147
31. Tietze A Berl Klin Wochenschr 1921; 58: 829
32. Teixera J Dis Chest 1968; 53: 19
33. LeRoux B T Br J Surg 1965; 52: 89
34. Trinkle J K et al Ann Thorac Surg 1973; 16: 568

insertion of a chest drain on clinical grounds alone may lead to further pulmonary contusion. If severe respiratory distress is evident, and the physical signs suggest a tension pneumothorax, with unmoving prominence of one hemithorax and mediastinal shift, then the insertion of a wide-bore intravenous cannula will relieve tension and permit time for proper radiographic evaluation. If respiratory distress is unrelieved then endotracheal intubation and ventilation are essential.

Pain control is of the utmost importance. Adequate analgesia should not be withheld for fear of causing respiratory depression or of obscuring neurological signs. Unrelieved pain is a potent cause of respiratory depression! Opiates should be given intravenously in small boluses (1–2 mg morphine or 5 mg pethidine) titrated against the patient's pain level. Intercostal blockade using local anaesthetic injections is appealing, but rarely practicable in a restless, distressed patient. Once the patient is stable and carefully monitored, an intravenous infusion of pethidine provides reliable and flexible analgesia. The drug is administered by syringe pump or metered-drop infusion, with 2 mg of pethidine per kg of patient body weight diluted in 100 ml of 5% dextrose given at 5–20 ml/h. The infusion may be temporarily increased when moving the patient for an X-ray, or undertaking physiotherapy. The baseline infusion should be titrated against the arterial partial pressure of carbon dioxide (pCO_2) and the clinical evaluation of pain control. A rising pCO_2 may indicate inadequate or excessive analgesia. Epidural analgesia may be valuable in the longer term, provided there is the anaesthetic expertise to insert the catheter and proper nursing supervision to maintain drug replenishment (see Ch. 5). Trauma victims may find it difficult to adopt a satisfactory position for the insertion of an epidural catheter.

Fluid overload will aggravate pulmonary oedema and increase the area of lung affected. Diuretics should be administered if large volumes of crystalloid have been given during resuscitation. If volume replacement is necessary to correct hypotension, careful monitoring of the central venous pressure is important and plasma expanders are to be preferred to crystalloids.

The contused lung is peculiarly susceptible to infection and in the days following injury careful monitoring of the temperature and white blood cell count should be performed. Any increasing radiographic density should be suspected to be infective in origin, and empirical broad-spectrum antibiotics initiated. Prophylactic antibiotics are of little benefit in patients whose lungs were normal prior to injury. Smokers, however, have changes within their bronchial tree predisposing to sputum retention, and in this group prophylactic antibiotics may be of benefit. Any fall in pulmonary compliance occurring after the first 24 h is usually the result of parenchymal infection and may be evident from an increasing respiratory rate, extending radiographic opacities, or changes in blood arterial gas concentrations with a rising pCO_2 and falling arterial partial pressure of oxygen (pO_2). Increasing the inspired oxygen concentration (FiO_2), humidified and applied through a facemask, may be necessary, but care should be taken in the chronic bronchitic patient who may be dependent upon hypoxia to maintain respiratory rate.[35] In such circumstances the inspired oxygen concentration should be slowly increased from 24% upwards, with careful monitoring of arterial gas concentration. Such patients have abnormal baseline levels and the titrating of FiO_2 against pO_2 and pCO_2 requires considerable experience. It is often difficult to provide adequate analgesia to enable smokers to expectorate the large volumes of sputum they habitually produce.

If analgesia and physiotherapy are failing to prevent sputum retention the insertion of a minitracheostomy tube is of great value.[36] This device may be inserted under local anaesthetic via a percutaneous incision through the cricothyroid membrane. This is widely used following pulmonary resection and is of great value in trauma victims.

Intravenous steroids reduce the alveolar capillary permeability only if administered within 30 min of the injury, and are therefore of little practical value.[37]

Intermittent positive pressure ventilation should be started immediately if respiratory distress is evident and not quickly reversible. In the majority of patients, however, a decision may be deferred whilst evaluation is undertaken. If, despite the best conservative management, respiratory distress progresses with increasing tachypnoea, rising pCO_2 or falling pO_2, then ventilation becomes essential. A previously unsuspected pneumothorax may rapidly expand immediately after ventilation has begun, and careful clinical and radiographic monitoring is important at this time.

Tracheostomy is now much less commonly used in the management of chest trauma. Careful monitoring of pulmonary contusion and the early treatment of infective complications have reduced the need for ventilation. Minitracheostomy, if inserted early, will deal with the mechanical problems of sputum clearance. Improved anaesthetic management of endotracheal tubes will now permit prolonged periods of ventilation without tracheostomy.[38] The use of nasotracheal tubes will allow intubation for 10–14 days[39] without laryngeal damage. Tracheostomy, however, still has some place, especially if assisted ventilation is anticipated for longer than this period, and is often valuable in assisting the weaning from ventilation in patients with chronic obstructive airways disease. Unless contraindicated by coagulopathy or anatomical considerations, tracheostomy is now performed percutaneously in the intensive care unit, usually by the intensivist.[40] The incidence of post-tracheostomy stricture is falling with better management of the tracheostomy and the use of tubes with low pressure/high volume cuffs, which are inflated to the recommended pressure. Stricture does still occur, however, and may later require tracheal resection.[41]

Adult respiratory distress syndrome

This may result from a variety of insults such as sepsis and burns, and commonly complicates trauma, especially to the chest. Adult

REFERENCES

35. Hutchinson D C W, Flenley D C, Donald K W Br Med J 1964; 2: 1159
36. Matthews H R, Hopkinson R B Br J Surg 1984; 71: 147
37. Frantz J L et al J Thorac Cardiovasc Surg 1974; 68: 842
38. Heffner J E Chest 1989; 96: 186
39. Marsh H M, Gillespie D J, Baumgartner A F Chest 1989; 96: 190
40. Toursarkissian B, Zweng T N, Kearney P A et al Ann Thorac Surg 1994; 57: 862
41. Grillo H C, Donahue D M, Mathisen D J et al J Thorac Cardiovasc Surg 1995; 109: 486

respiratory distress syndrome (ARDS) and the associated but less severe variant, acute lung injury (ALI) complicates 5% of lung resections,[42] and carries a high mortality. The risks of developing adult respiratory distress syndrome rise as the risk factors summate.[43,44] The final common pathway involves neutrophil activation, inflammatory mediators, and the release of free radicals[45] with increased alveolar capillary permeability. This results in the passage of large molecules into the alveolus and impaired gas exchange. The onset is usually insidious with increasing tachypnoea and hypoxia. The early radiographic signs are non-specific with diffuse alveolar shadows which may be thought to be caused by infection or fluid overload (Fig. 22.5). The diagnosis is usually made when the patient's condition continues to deteriorate despite empirical treatment of these reversible factors.

There is, as yet, no specific treatment and management consists of controlling additional risk factors whilst treating hypoxia. The inspired oxygen concentration, FiO_2, is increased as necessary and ventilation is invariably required. Care is needed to prevent fluid overload and to treat infective complications, especially in the lungs.

The prognosis is poor and is determined by the severity of the adult respiratory distress syndrome. In specialized units prolonged support by high-frequency, jet ventilation[46] or extracorporeal membrane oxygenation[47] may allow more time for recovery or act as a bridge to transplantation. Death results from severe hypoxia, hypercapnia, pulmonary hypertension and the secondary effects of these factors on renal, cardiac and hepatic function.

Inhaled foreign bodies

An immense variety of foreign bodies have found their way into the tracheobronchial tree. Young children are particularly at risk, being easily distracted whilst their mouths are full. In adults, inhalation most commonly occurs during anaesthesia, especially for dental treatment, or when consciousness is reduced by alcohol intoxication, head injury or epileptic seizure. Aspiration is classically accompanied by a paroxysm of coughing which may subside after several minutes. This symptom must never be lightly dismissed if foreign body aspiration is a possibility.[48] Radiopaque foreign bodies are easily seen on chest radiographs (Fig. 22.6) but are sometimes overlooked. Radiolucent foreign bodies, particularly those of organic material such as peanuts, are particularly dangerous. Chest radiographs may be normal, or show atelectasis. Obstructive emphysema may be evident on inspiratory and expiratory films (Fig. 22.7).

Whatever the radiographic appearance, if a history is suggestive of aspiration, then bronchoscopy is necessary to exclude a foreign body.[49] The anatomy of the carina ensures that the majority of inhaled objects fall into the right bronchial tree, but foreign bodies may impact at any point. Bronchoscopic removal of the foreign body should be carried out expeditiously by an experienced endoscopist who has to hand a range of instrument sizes and a variety of forceps, catheters and other devices. Metallic foreign bodies are well tolerated within the bronchial tree and removal has not proved

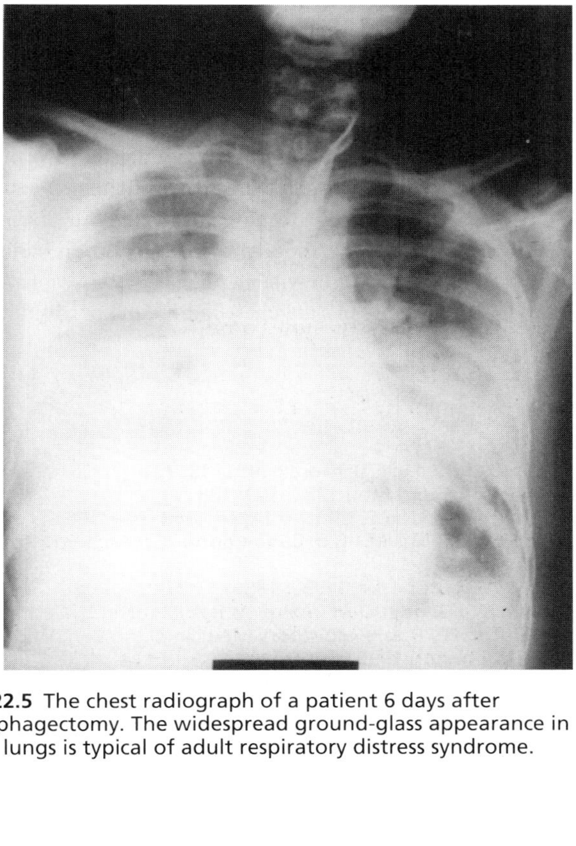

Fig. 22.5 The chest radiograph of a patient 6 days after oesophagectomy. The widespread ground-glass appearance in both lungs is typical of adult respiratory distress syndrome.

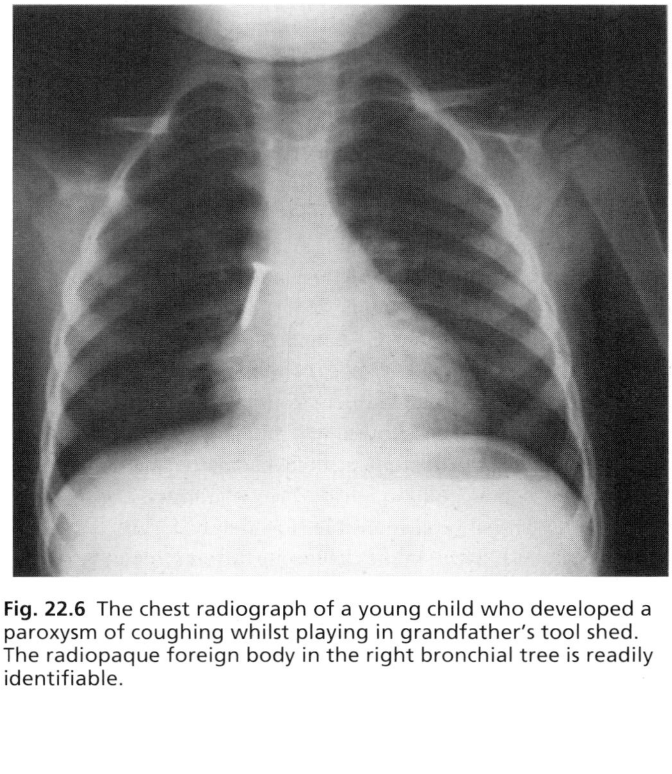

Fig. 22.6 The chest radiograph of a young child who developed a paroxysm of coughing whilst playing in grandfather's tool shed. The radiopaque foreign body in the right bronchial tree is readily identifiable.

REFERENCES

42. Hayes J P, Williams E A, Goldstraw P, Evans T W Thorax 1995; 50: 990
43. Fowler A A et al Ann Intern Med 1983; 98: 593
44. Cooper T J, Tinker J Hosp Update 1984; 10: 849
45. Hyers T M Semin Resp Med 1981; 2: 104
46. Carlon G C et al Crit Care Med 1983; 11: 83
47. Zapol W M et al JAMA 1979; 242: 2193
48. Goldstraw P, Venn G E Med Int 1986; 2: 1510
49. Aytac A et al J Thorac Cardiovasc Surg 1977; 74: 145

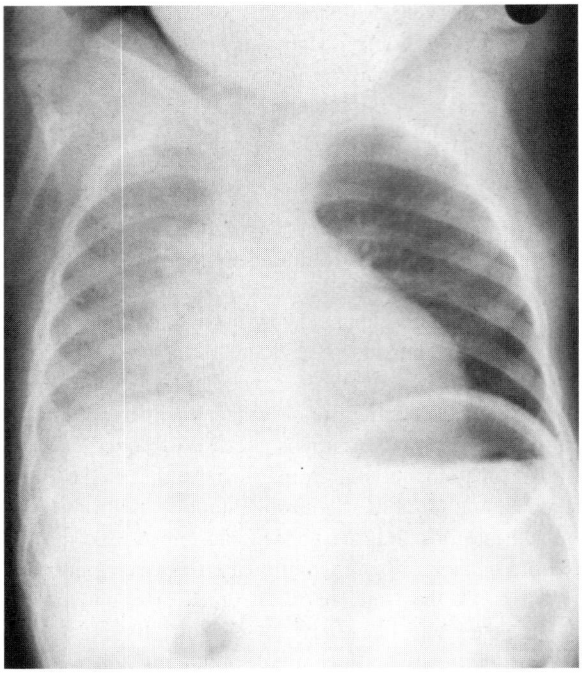

Fig. 22.7 Expiratory chest radiograph of a baby showing hyperlucency and air-trapping in the left lung due to a radiolucent foreign body.

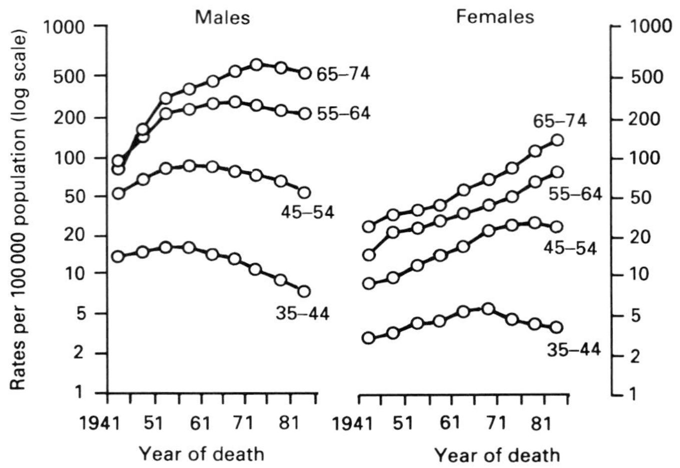

Fig. 22.8 Mortality for lung cancer amongst men and women in England and Wales over the last 40 years (by courtesy of the Cancer Research Campaign).

difficult, even after years in situ. Organic foreign bodies excite a ferocious inflammatory reaction, which is especially marked with the oily residue associated with peanuts.[50] Removal in such circumstances may prove difficult and bronchoscopic trauma may add to the difficulties. As the first attempts at removal have the greatest chance of success, referral to a specialist centre is recommended. If a foreign body is overlooked, then distal infection may lead to a lung abscess or bronchiectasis. Pulmonary resection is then necessary.

Carcinoma of the lung

There is now incontrovertible evidence that the most common forms of lung cancer are related to cigarette smoking.[51] Despite this, the impact of anti-smoking campaigns appears to have been slight. In men, lung cancer continues to be the most common malignant cause of death, although in the UK the incidence is no longer rising.[52] Amongst women, lung cancer continues to increase in incidence, although the steepness of the rise may be lessening[52] (Fig. 22.8). Already in the USA and Scotland lung cancer has displaced breast cancer as the most common cause of deaths from cancer amongst women.[53] Other environmental factors are clearly important. Early studies showed the high risk run by workers exposed to asbestos,[54] uranium, arsenic, haematite and other pollutants.[55] More subtle pollution from heavy industry and exhaust emissions is probably responsible for the differing incidence amongst smokers with similar habits in different countries, and between those living in towns and those in the rural areas. The evidence incriminating passive smoking is growing.[56] Recent years have seen considerable progress in understanding the sequential genetic changes associated with oncogenesis—chromosome deletion, oncogene expression and suppressor gene mutations which lead to loss of cell regulation.[57]

Screening programmes have attempted to improve the prognosis of lung cancer by detecting cases prior to the onset of symptoms using regular chest radiographs, sputum cytology and bronchoscopy. These expensive studies have resulted in few early cases being discovered, and improved survival in these patients may merely reflect the prolonged lead time before these tumours would have produced symptoms.[58] It must however be noted that the patients in the control arm of such studies were undergoing regular chest radiographs, and the study may be interpreted to show that intensive surveillance carries little advantage over such screening.

The symptoms of lung cancer are those of the primary tumour—cough, dyspnoea, pleuritic pain and haemoptysis; those of metastatic disease are bone pain, weight loss and neurological symptoms and those associated with a paraneoplastic syndrome such as inappropriate secretion of antidiuretic hormone or hypertrophic pulmonary osteoarthropathy.[59] In approximately 10% of patients coming to the surgeon, lung cancer has been discovered incidentally on routine chest radiographs taken for other conditions.

Central tumours may not be visible on chest radiographs. They may be too small to be seen on a chest radiograph or obscured by

REFERENCES

50. Fine A J, Abram L E Ann Allergy 1971; 29: 217
51. Doll R, Peto R Br Med J 1976; 2: 1525
52. Coggon D, Acheson E D Thorax 1983; 38: 721
53. Stolley P D N Engl J Med 1983; 309: 428
54. Selikoff I, Hammond E, Churg J JAMA 1968; 204: 106
55. Harris C C In: Straus M J (ed) Lung Cancer. Grune & Stratton, New York 1977 p 1
56. Wood A A Br Med J 1990; 300: 1650
57. Souhami R L, Geddes D M In: Brewis R A L, Corrin B, Geddes D M, Gibson G J (eds) Respiratory Medicine, 2nd edn. W B Saunders, London 1995, p 905
58. Spiro S G, Hansen H H In: Hoogstraten B, Addis B J et al (eds) Lung Tumours. Springer Verlag, Berlin 1988 p 9
59. Spiro S G, Rorth M In: Hoogstraten B, Addis B J et al (eds) Lung Tumours. Springer Verlag, Berlin 1988 p 59

the mediastinal outline or by the atelectasis and consolidation they produce (Fig. 22.9). Such tumours are within the reach of the bronchoscope, arising in the trachea or bronchi to segmental level.

Peripheral tumours may arise from the bronchial tree more distally, or from the lung parenchyma. Such tumours are visible on chest radiographs, being outlined by contrasting aerated lung tissue. Cavitation may be evident. The diagnosis is usually suspected radiographically and confirmed on sputum cytology. Bronchoscopy is a valuable staging investigation and will provide histology in 95% of central tumours.[60] Whilst most peripheral tumours are beyond the reach of the bronchoscope, this investigation may provide cytological diagnosis from brush or lavage specimens. Percutaneous fine-needle aspiration biopsy provides cytological diagnosis in 95% of peripheral lesions.[61] Management, however, should not be unduly influenced by the absence of cytological confirmation.

The World Health Organization describes four main histological categories of lung cancer:[62] small cell carcinoma, adenocarcinoma, squamous cell carcinoma and undifferentiated large cell carcinoma.

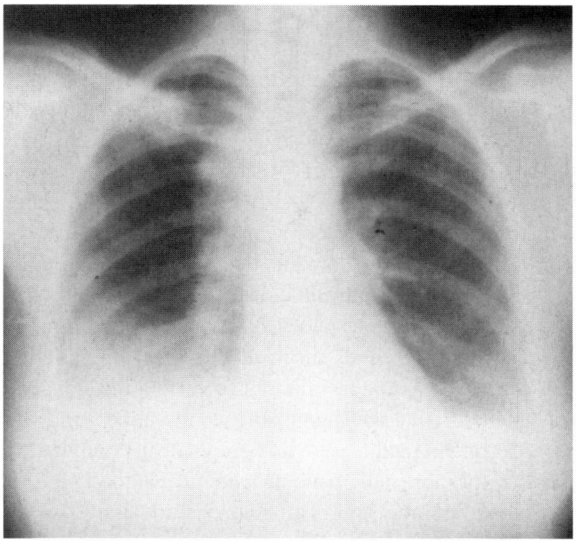

Fig. 22.10 A small peripheral tumour in the right upper lobe is associated with a pleural effusion and gross mediastinal node metastases. This appearance can occur with many tumours but is typical of small cell lung cancer.

Small cell lung cancer

Small cell lung cancer may exist in the classical oat cell form or as an intermediate cell type. These tumours are highly malignant and are usually disseminated at presentation. The chest X-ray frequently discloses mediastinal gland enlargement indicative of metastases (Fig. 22.10). Sophisticated investigations are rarely necessary to confirm the extensive nature of the malignancy. Less than 5% of such tumours are suitable for surgical management.[63]

For the majority of patients chemotherapy is the treatment of choice, but survival is usually measured in months.[64] Where the disease is limited to one hemithorax and the ipsilateral supraclavicular fossa (limited disease), survival may be improved from a mean of 9 to 18 months with chemotherapy. With more extensive disease, survival—even with treatment—has a mean of 9 months. Many chemotherapy protocols exist, the most common employing cyclophosphamide, Adriamycin and vincristine. For the otherwise fit, relatively young patient with limited disease, high-dose cyclophosphamide with bone marrow autotransplantation is being investigated.[65] Where a good response has occurred, mediastinal irradiation may be given to consolidate the chemotherapy, and prophylactic cranical irradiation may be given to patients achieving a complete response, with disappearance of all radiographic evidence of disease.[66] This additional treatment does not improve survival but may reduce the incidence of cerebral relapse with its disastrous social implications. Even with such combination treatment less than 10% of patients with limited disease will survive to 2 years, and survival beyond this is rare.[67]

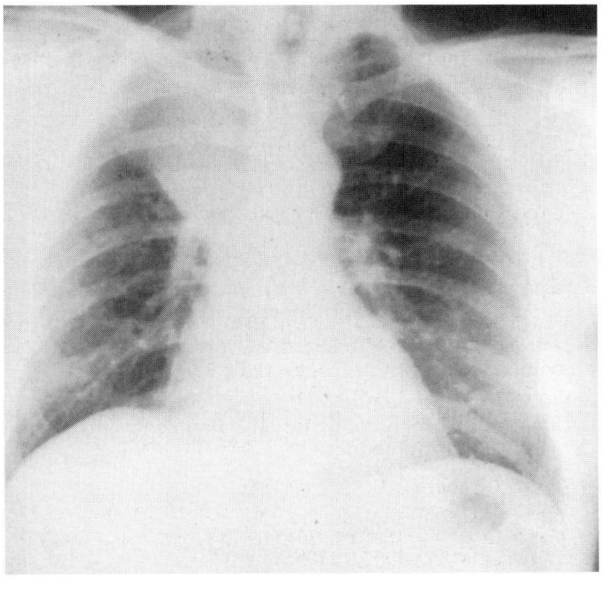

Fig. 22.9 A chest radiograph showing right upper lobe collapse and consolidation. The appearances suggest obstruction of the lobar bronchus, the most common cause being lung cancer.

Non-small cell lung cancer

Non-small cell lung cancer is the term used to group together the three other varieties of lung cancer: adenocarcinoma, squamous cell carcinoma and undifferentiated large cell carcinoma. Whilst there are differences in the natural history of each cell type, these

REFERENCES

60. Hansen H H, Spiro S G In: Hoogstraten B, Addis B J et al (eds) Lung Tumours. Springer Verlag, Berlin 1988 p 71
61. Oswald N C, Hinsen K F W et al Thorax 1971; 26: 623
62. World Health Organization Histological Typing of Lung Tumours. World Health Organization, Geneva 1981
63. Shah S S, Thompson J, Goldstraw P Ann Thorac Surg 1992; 54: 498
64. Bunn P A, Ihde D C In: Livingstone R B (ed) Lung Cancer. Martinus Nijhoff, The Hague 1981 p 169
65. Souhami R L et al Cancer Chemother Pharmacol 1982; 8: 31
66. Souhami R L et al Br Med J 1984; 288: 1642
67. Souhami R L, Law K Br J Cancer 1990; 61: 584

differences are of little importance in management. Surgical resection is possible in 10–15% of cases.[68] Much effort and resources are expended to identify this group since they are the only ones with prospects of cure. For the majority of patients, however, the disease is beyond surgery at presentation.

Preoperative assessment. Relatively simple assessment by clinical history, examination, chest radiographs and bronchoscopy shows that many patients are unfit for surgery. Radiotherapy is the most common choice for second line treatment if the tumour is inoperable. Whilst this may control the disease and relieve troublesome symptoms such as cough, dyspnoea, haemoptysis or bone pain, there is no evidence that it extends survival. Chemotherapy in non-small cell lung cancer is gaining in importance since a meta-analysis has shown a small survival advantage and such treatment may now be considered as an alternative to radiotherapy, or in combination with radiotherapy, for inoperable patients who have a good performance status.[69] There is some optimism that chemotherapy may prove effective as induction or neoadjuvant therapy to improve the results of surgery in non-small cell lung cancer, but the evidence is as yet experimental.[70] Inoperable patients should be assured that whilst cure is not possible, careful and sympathetic help will give them considerable symptomatic benefit.

Surgical treatment demands adequate patient fitness to tolerate an extensive pulmonary resection, and a tumour sufficiently localized to permit complete removal by pulmonary resection. Patient fitness is assessed clinically, taking note of the patient's age, coincidental medical disease and exercise tolerance. Lung function testing is by simple spirometry, measuring forced vital capacity (FVC) and forced expiratory volume in 1 s (FEV_1) and the ratio of FEV_1:FVC. The level of lung function necessary for pulmonary resection will depend upon the extent of the proposed resection and the function of the lung tissue to be removed. As a general guide, however, pneumonectomy is feasible if the FEV_1 exceeds 1.5 l and the FEV_1:FVC ratio is greater than 50%. Below these figures resection may still prove feasible, but the hazards of surgery increase. Where fitness for surgery is considered borderline, a period of inpatient preparation is often of help in controlling coincidental disease such as hypertension and angina, and optimizing lung function by physiotherapy and bronchodilators.

Staging. Pretreatment evaluation of any tumour entails the identification of prognostic determinants, usually expressed as tumour stage. Recent advances in molecular biology have identified chromosomal abnormalities and genetic markers[71–76] which have an adverse impact on survival. Most interest has focussed on the suppressor gene p53 and the *ras* group of oncogenes. It is now possible to detect the protein products of such genetic changes usuing immunohistochemistry. Such progress holds the promise that eventually there will be a battery of genetic markers from which prognosis may be inferred, but at present we are limited to anatomical descriptions of the tumour extent to express stage. The system most commonly employed is that of the American Joint Committee on Cancer Staging and End Results Reporting, subsequently revised.[77] An abbreviated version of this is shown in Table 22.1. Increasing numerical subscripts of the T stage indicate

REFERENCES

68. Thompson-Evans E W Thorax 1973; 28: 86
69. Stewart L A, Pignon J P, Parmar M K B et al Lung Cancer 1994; 11: 49
70. Rosell R, Gomez-Codina J, Camps C et al N Engl J Med 1994; 330: 153
71. Zimmerman P V, Hawson G A, Bint M H et al Lancet 1987; 2: 530
72. Kern J A, Schwartz D A, Nordberg J E et al Cancer Res 1990; 50: 5194
73. Slebos R J C, Kibbellalaar R, Dalesio O et al N Engl J Med 1990; 323: 561
74. Horio Y, Takahashi T, Koroishi T et al Cancer Res 1993; 51: 1
75. Bongiorno P F, Whyte R I, Lesser E J et al J Thorac Cardiovasc Surg 1994; 107: 590
76. Ogawa J, Sano A, Koide S, Shohtsu A, Kanagawa I J Thorac Cardiovasc Surg 1994; 108: 329
77. Mountain C F Cancer 1986; 89 (suppl): 225

Table 22.1 *The TNM staging classification for lung cancer*

Primary tumour (T)

T_x Tumour proven by the presence of malignant cells in bronchopulmonary secretions but not visualized roentgenographically or bronchoscopically, or any tumour that cannot be assessed as in a retreatment staging

T_0 No evidence of primary tumour

T_{IS} Carcinoma in situ

T_1 A tumour that is 3 cm or less in greatest dimension, surrounded by lung or visceral pleura, and without evidence of invasion proximal to a lobar bronchus at bronchoscopy*

T_2 A tumour more than 3 cm in greatest dimension, or a tumour of any size that either invades the visceral pleura or has associated atelectasis or obstructive pneumonitis extending to the hilar region. At bronchoscopy the proximal extent of demonstrable tumour must be within a lobar bronchus or at least 2 cm distal to the carina. Any associated atelectasis or obstructive pneumonitis must involve less than an entire lung

T_3 A tumour of any size with direct extension into the chest wall (including superior sulcus tumours), diaphragm, or the mediastinal pleura or pericardium without involving the heart, great vessels, trachea, oesophagus or vertebral body, or a tumour in the main bronchus within 2 cm of the carina without involving the carina

T_4 A tumour of any size with invasion of the mediastinum or involving heart, great vessels, trachea, oesophagus, vertebral body or carina or presence of malignant pleural effusion*†

Nodal involvement (N)

N_0 No demonstrable metastasis to regional lymph nodes

N_1 Metastasis to lymph nodes in the peribronchial or the ipsilateral hilar region, or both, including direct extension

N_2 Metastasis to ipsilateral mediastinal lymph nodes and subcarinal lymph nodes

N_3 Metastasis to contralateral mediastinal lymph nodes, contralateral hilar lymph nodes, ipsilateral or contralateral scalene or supraclavicular lymph nodes

Distant metastasis (M)

M_0 No (known) distant metastasis

M1 Distant metastasis present—specify site(s)

*The uncommon superficial tumour of any size with its invasive component limited to the bronchial wall which may extend proximal to the main bronchus is classified as T_1.
†Most pleural effusions associated with lung cancer are due to tumour. There are, however, some few patients in whom cytopathological examination of pleural fluid (on more than one specimen) is negative for tumour, the fluid is non-bloody and is not an exudate. In such cases where these elements and clinical judgement dictate that the effusion is not related to the tumour, the patients should be staged T_1, T_2 or T_3, excluding effusion as a staging element.

progressively more advanced tumours by size and bronchoscopic proximity or invasion of adjacent structures. Similarly advancing numerical subscripts in the N category denote more proximal nodal metastases within the thorax and supraclavicular fossa. Thus a 5 cm peripheral carcinoma without evidence of invasion to surrounding structures and with no nodal or distant metastases would be designated $T_2N_0M_0$; a tumour invading the chest wall with hilar node metastases but no distant spread, $T_3N_1M_0$; a central carcinoma extending to the carina on bronchoscopy, with paratracheal node metastases and bone secondaries, a $T_4N_2M_1$, and so on. Tumours with these TNM subsets may be grouped to give larger populations for study, as in Table 22.2.

The preoperative staging process may be considered to have intrathoracic and extrathoracic components. Although it may be easier to understand this evaluation if these components are discussed separately, in practice their assessment usually proceeds concurrently.

Extrathoracic staging entails a search for distant metastases. These may be evident clinically, with organ-specific features in the history or physical examination suggesting metastases in the liver, brain or skeleton. Bone secondaries may produce pain or local tenderness, brain secondaries, epileptiform convulsions, personality changes or confusional states, and liver secondaries may be obvious on abdominal examination. Careful palpation of the neck may reveal lymph node deposits. Unexplained weight loss—greater than 3 kg in 6 months—unexplained anaemia or abnormal liver function tests are useful indicators of metastases, but are not organ-specific. If this relatively simple evaluation reveals none of these organ-specific or non-specific features of metastases, more intensive evaluation is unnecessary. However, if any of these features is present, further evaluation should include isotopic bone scan, assessment of the liver by ultrasound or CT scanning, and evaluation of the brain using CT scanning. Bone scan abnormalities may be due to non-metastatic conditions such as degenerative conditions, and any hot spots should be further evaluated with skeletal X-rays. CT scanning of the brain, chest and abdomen is now essential prior to surgery and provides a single non-invasive assessment of the brain, liver, adrenals, retroperitoneal lymph nodes and contralateral lung.[78] Such a scan also provides valuable information in determining intrathoracic stage. Positron emission tomography (PET) scanning using ^{18}F-fluorodeoxyglucose is proving an interesting investigational tool to detect tumour deposits in the chest and elsewhere and can help characterize abnormalities discovered on CT.[79]

Intrathoracic staging seeks to identify the T and N determinants of the tumour. The T stage may be established for peripheral tumours by measuring the size of the tumour on chest radiographs (Fig. 22.11), whilst for central tumours bronchoscopy will demonstrate the proximal extent of the tumour. There may be clinical evidence of chest wall invasion or X-rays may disclose rib erosion. A pleural effusion on chest X-ray should be aspirated, and if it is bloody or contains malignant cells, this indicates the presence of pleural metastases, and the patient is inoperable.

Whilst N stage seeks to identify all nodal metastases, those within the lung or ipsilateral hilum (N_1) usually have no influence on the desirability of surgical treatment, only affecting the extent of pulmonary resection. In contrast, mediastinal gland involvement (N_2) is of critical importance since, if this is so extreme as to be determined preoperatively, there is little chance of surgical cure.[80] N_2 disease may be suggested clinically by dysphagia, recurrent laryngeal palsy or superior vena caval obstruction, or be evident on a chest radiograph. Significant mediastinal involvement may be present in up to one third of patients without these clinical or radi-

Table 22.2 Stage grouping of TNM subsets

	Stage grouping		
Occult carcinoma	T_x	N_0	M_0
Stage 0	T_{IS}	Carcinoma in situ	
Stage I	T_1	N_0	M_0
	T_2	N_0	M_0
Stage II	T_1	N_1	M_0
	T_2	N_1	M_0
Stage IIIa	T_3	N_0	M_0
	T_3	N_1	M_0
	T_{1-3}	N_2	M_0
Stage IIIb	Any T	N_3	M_0
Stage IIIb	T_4	Any N	M_0
Stage IV	Any T	Any N	M_1

REFERENCES

78. Grant D, Edwards D, Goldstraw P Thorax 1988; 43: 883
79. Lewis P, Griffin S, Marsden P et al Lancet 1994; 344: 1265
80. Gibbons J R P Br J Dis Chest 1972; 66: 162

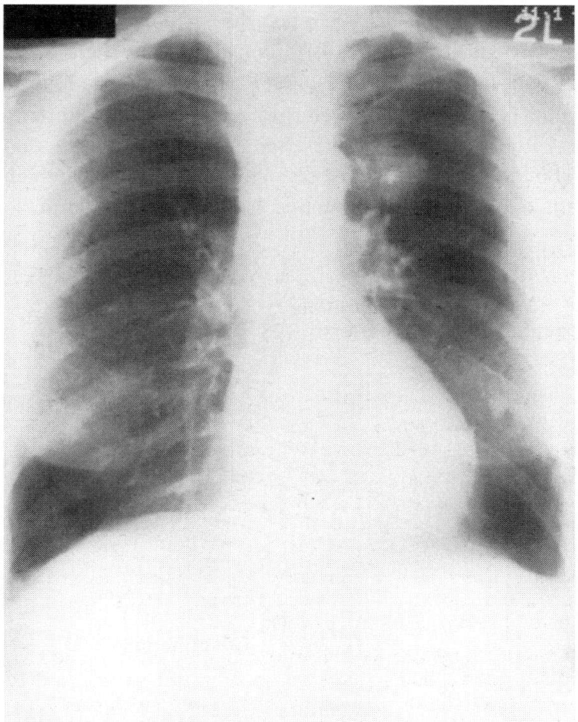

Fig. 22.11 A peripheral tumour in the left upper lobe surrounded by aerated lung tissue. Its size is readily measured to establish T stage.

ographic features, and should be excluded preoperatively by mediastinal exploration using the techniques of cervical mediastinoscopy and anterior mediastinotomy.[81]

Cervical mediastinoscopy is an endoscopic evaluation of the superior mediastinal lymph nodes, undertaken through a short transverse cervical incision midway between the thyroid cartilage and the suprasternal notch. Dissecting inferiorly into the mediastinum within the pretracheal fascia allows lymph nodes on both sides of the trachea and at the main carina to be inspected and biopsied (Fig. 22.12). This evaluation helps determine resectability, and the extent of nodal secondaries has a profound influence on the desirability of surgery.[82] The lymphatic pathways from tumours arising at various primary sites are shown in Figure 22.13. It will be appreciated that mediastinoscopy through the cervical approach allows an accurate evaluation of right upper lobe tumours and reasonable evaluation of tumours originating in either lower lobe. On occasions, however, lower lobe tumours may prove inoperable at thoracotomy due to direct invasion or metastases beyond the reach of the mediastinoscope. Tumours originating within the left upper lobe may become inoperable by invasion of the mediastinum around the aortic arch or by involvement of lymph nodes within the subaortic fossa. These factors cannot be assessed by cervical mediastinoscopy, but are amenable to left anterior mediastinotomy, a digital examination of these areas using a short incision through the second intercostal space, to the left of the sternal margin.

CT of the mediastinum has become a valuable adjunct to mediastinal exploration in the assessment of mediastinal invasion and glandular metastases.[83] CT scanning of the mediastinum, with contrast enhancement of the vascular structures, can detect lymph nodes larger than 5 or 6 mm in diameter (Fig. 22.14). As the size of lymph nodes increases, so does the incidence of metastatic deposits. Mediastinal nodes of 1 cm in size on a CT scan of a patient with lung cancer have a 30% chance of containing metastases, nodes of 1.5 cm diameter 40%, and 75% of lymph nodes above 2 cm will contain metastases.[84] However, there is no size limit above which nodes must be metastatic, nor below which they are certain to be benign. In practice, however, nodes too small to be demonstrated on CT scanning are unlikely to be metastatic and will not be detected by mediastinal exploration. If, therefore, a CT scan of the mediastinum is normal, mediastinal exploration may be omitted and the surgeon can proceed directly to a thoracotomy.[85] If CT scanning demonstrates enlarged glands or suggests invasion, these features should be checked by mediastinal exploration as false positives are common.

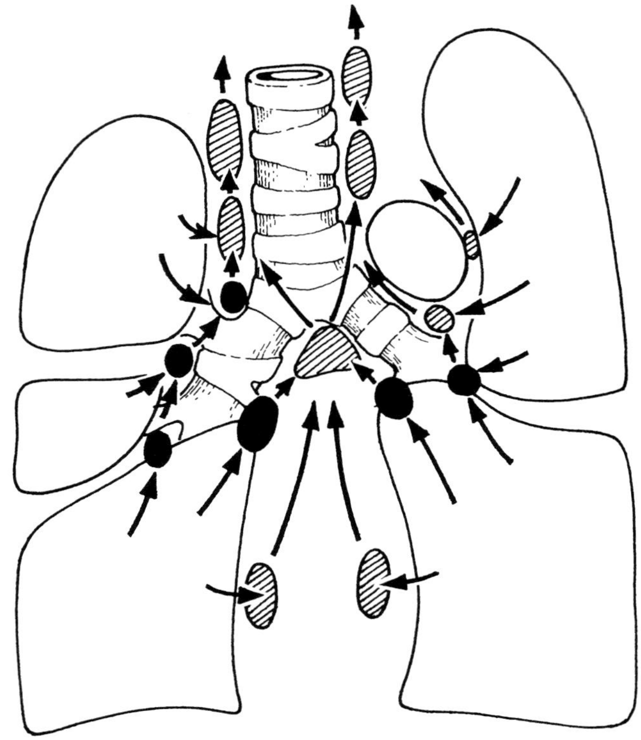

Fig. 22.13 The usual lymphatic pathways of tumour dissemination from different lobes of the lung. ● = hilar nodes, ◎ = mediastinal nodes.

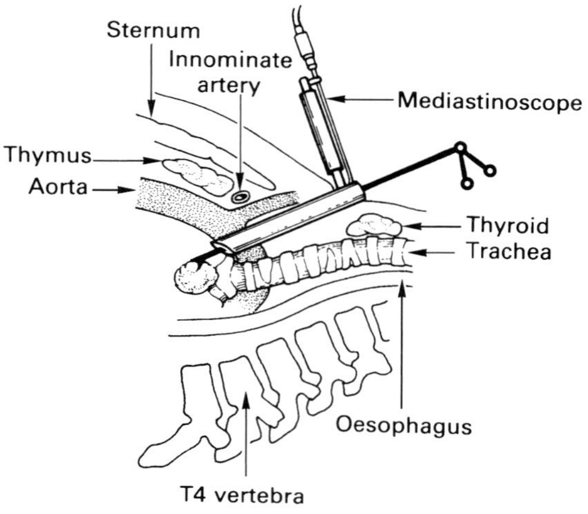

Fig. 22.12 A diagram to illustrate the passage of the mediastinoscope to the main carinal lymph nodes. Some of the structures at risk are readily apparent.

The value of video-assisted thoracoscopic surgery (VATS) in the staging of lung cancer is presently under investigation.[86] Mediastinal nodes which are enlarged on CT and lie beyond mediastinoscopy can be reached with such techniques, although involvement of these nodes may not have the same adverse impact on the prospects for surgical cure as metastatic nodes higher in the mediastinum, within reach of the mediastinoscope. The assessment of mediastinal invasion by video-assisted thoracoscopic surgery may not equate with irresectable disease.

No matter how careful the preoperative staging has been, it is now accepted that careful re-evaluation is essential at thoracotomy

REFERENCES

81. Goldstraw P Br J Dis Chest 1988; 82: 111
82. Pearson F G, Nelems J M et al J Thorac Cardiovasc Surg 1972; 64: 382
83. Goldstraw P In: Hansen H H (ed) Lung Cancer: Basic and Clinical Aspects. Martinus Nijhoff, Boston 1986 p 183
84. McKenna R J, Libshitz H I et al Chest 1985; 88: 206
85. Goldstraw P, Kurzer M, Edwards D Thorax 1983; 38: 10
86. Naruke T, Asamura H, Kondo H et al Ann Thorac Surg 1993; 56: 661

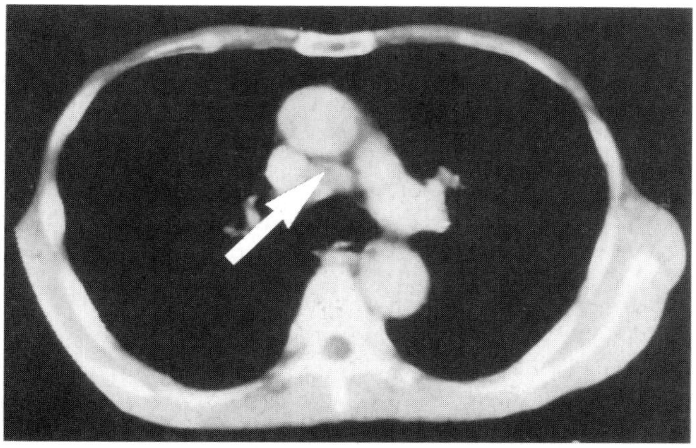

Fig. 22.14 A computerized tomography cut through the mediastinum. A large lymph node is arrowed lying in the pretracheal, retrocaval space.

before proceeding with pulmonary resection.[87] This entails assessment of T stage and a detailed dissection of all nodes, especially those in the mediastinum. Such steps are necessary to ensure that the prospects for cure are sufficient to merit resection and also to determine the minimum resection which will achieve complete removal of the tumour.

The steps utilized in intrathoracic staging are shown diagrammatically in Figure 22.15.[88]

Prognosis. The results of surgical excision are shown in Table 22.3.[89–96] Stage I and II tumours are ideal for surgical resection. The results achieved in these tumours greatly outweigh the risks of surgery and are far superior to the results possible with other forms of therapy. In addition, squamous tumours in category IIIa may be suitable, but the scale of surgery is more extensive and hence greater fitness of the patient is necessary if risks are to be kept low.

REFERENCES

87. Goldstraw P, Rocmans P, Ball D et al Lung Cancer 1994; 11: s1
88. Spiro S G, Goldstraw P Thorax 1984; 39: 401
89. Kirsh M M et al Ann Thorac Surg 1981; 21: 371
90. Shields T W et al J Thorac Cardiovasc Surg 1972; 64: 391
91. Wilkins E W et al J Thorac Cardiovasc Surg 1978; 76: 364
92. Immerman S C et al Ann Thorac Surg 1981; 32: 23
93. Williams D E et al J Thorac Cardiovasc Surg 1981; 82: 70
94. Naruke T et al J Thorac Cardiovasc Surg 1978; 76: 832
95. Piehler J M et al Ann Thorac Surg 1982; 34: 684
96. Pearson F G et al J Thorac Cardiovasc Surg 1982; 83: 1

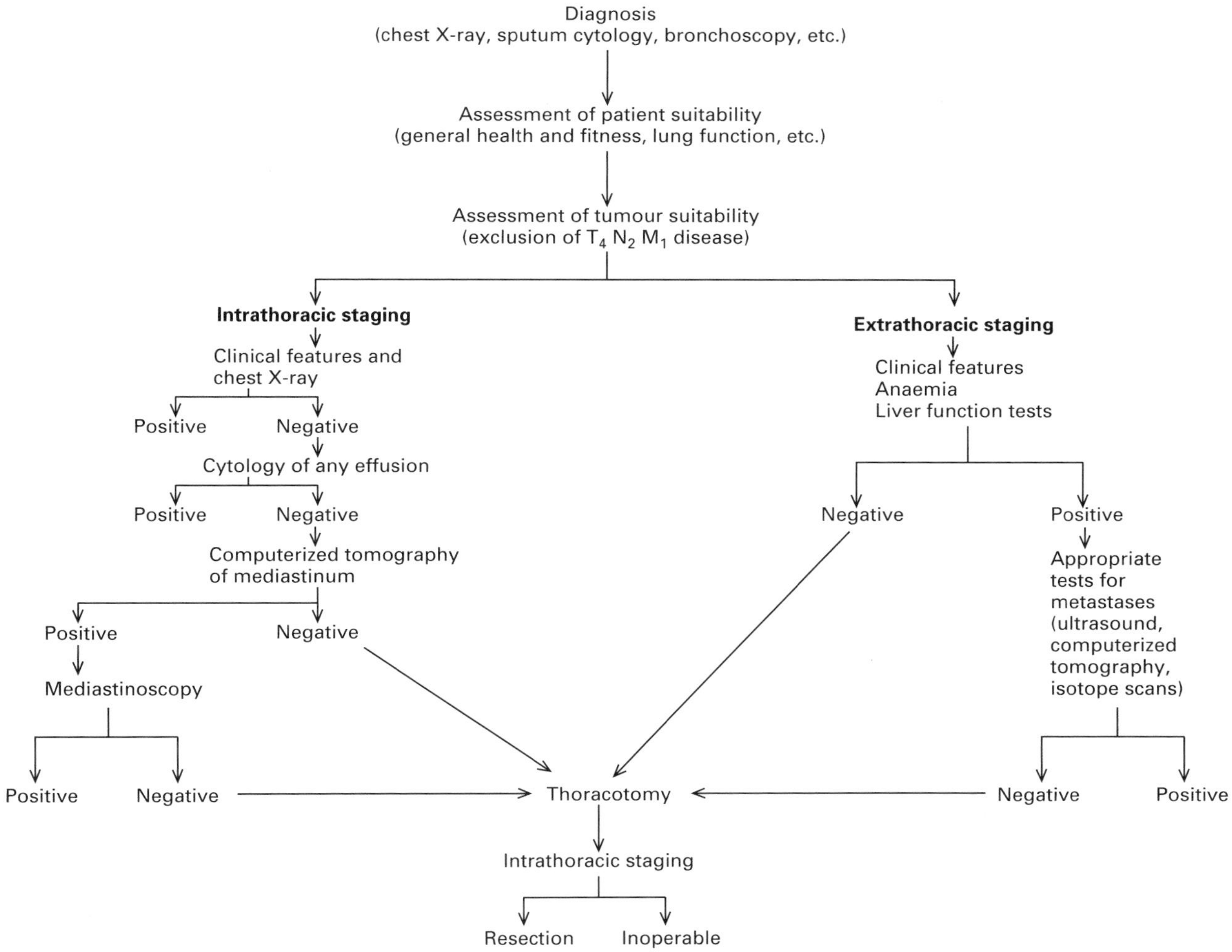

Fig. 22.15 A flow diagram to show the steps in preoperative evaluation of a patient with lung cancer.

Table 22.3 5-year survival rates following resection of non-small cell lung cancer

Category	*% Survival*
Complete resection:	
—any stage —any cell line	28–33[89,90]
Complete resection:	
—all squamous carcinoma	40[91]
Resections:	
Stage I or II squamous carcinoma	
—all stages	65[92]
—T_1N_0	80[93,94]
Stage IIIa	
—T_3N_0 (chest wall invasion)	50[95]
—T_1 or T_2N_2 (very limited mediastinal node involvement)	24[96]

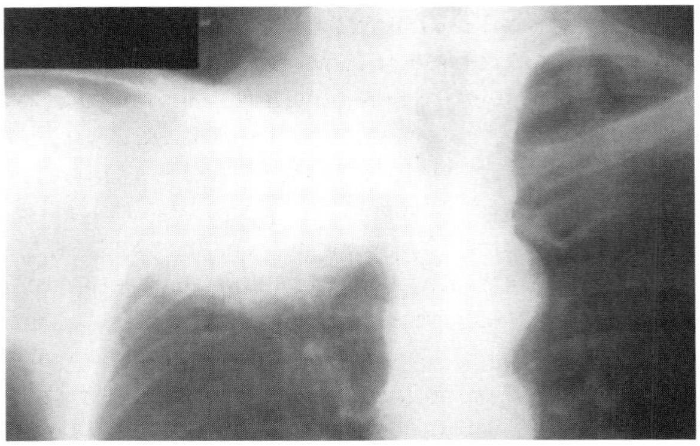

Fig. 22.16 A Pancoast tumour at the right apex. The erosion of the first and second ribs is seen.

Pancoast tumours

Pancoast tumours[97] present a difficult and peculiar problem. These tumours arise at the very apex of the lung, and present with pain from involvement of the first rib, the vertebral bodies, and the lower divisions of the brachial plexus. Horner's syndrome (ptosis, miosis, anhidrosis and enophthalmos) from invasion of the sympathetic chain, and invasion of the subclavian artery and vein may also occur (Fig. 22.16). Such extensive tumours would not normally be considered for surgical resection but palliation with radiotherapy is often short-lived and the intractable nature of the pain has caused a re-evaluation of the role of surgery. It has been suggested that in selected cases preoperative radiotherapy followed by extensive local resection may provide good palliation in the majority of patients, and long-term survival in one third of cases.[98] Dartevelle[99] has described an antero-cervical approach for tumours at the apex of the lung which provides superior access to the conventional thoracotomy approach, but it remains to be seen whether this allows cure rates to be improved.

Management of carcinoma of the lung

Thoracotomy is undertaken if preoperative evaluation suggests that the patient is fit enough to tolerate surgery and has a tumour sufficiently localized to be suitable for resection.

Thoracotomy is performed through a lateral incision, usually through the bed of the fifth or sixth rib. It is unnecessary to resect a rib. This incision permits a thorough evaluation of the ipsilateral lung and hilum and further evaluation of the mediastinum. Intraoperative assessment entails considerable dissection to obtain sufficient information to answer four questions.

Question 1: What is the diagnosis? The histological diagnosis may have been established preoperatively, but often surgery is recommended on the basis of a suspicious chest radiograph, sometimes supported by cytological evidence. In these circumstances biopsies should be taken at thoracotomy and submitted to frozen-section evaluation. This step is not always easy, since considerable inflammation may surround and obscure the true pathology. The surgeon must ensure that biopsies are representative, but efforts must be cautious so as not to damage hilar structures.

Question 2: Can the tumour, now proven to be present, be removed by pneumonectomy? The hilar structures are cleared of adventitia and the pleural reflection is incised. The surgeon should check that each hilar structure can be divided at a point which is free of macroscopic tumour. Occasionally it is necessary to open the pericardium to gain access to the intrapericardial portion of the pulmonary veins or pulmonary artery, but the pericardial incision should be sited so as not to damage the phrenic nerve at this stage.

Question 3: If pneumonectomy is possible, is it justified? Whilst evaluating resectability, mediastinal lymph nodes around the hilum will be encountered and should be removed for histological evaluation. In most cases this can be done macroscopically by slicing the nodes at the operating table, but if doubt exists, frozen-section analysis of these nodes is important. In approximately 25% of cases lymph node metastases within the mediastinal glands which have eluded preoperative evaluation are detected at thoracotomy.[100] In 85% of such cases complete resection is still possible and is justified as 5-year survival following resection in the presence of such minor mediastinal node involvement is 20%.[101] If nodal secondaries are more extensive, resection is unlikely to be curative and the surgeon may retreat without having inflicted permanent damage to lung parenchyma.

Question 4: If resection by pneumonectomy is possible and justified, is a lesser resection feasible? It is at this stage that the surgeon turns the attention to the pulmonary hilum to explore the possibility of lesser resections such as lobectomy or segmentectomy. It is important to proceed in this order since when undertaking lesser resections it is not unusual to find impalpable extension into the hilum necessitating pneumonectomy. With thorough preoperative assessment and diligent preoperative evaluation resection is justified in 95% of patients undergoing thoracotomy.[82,100]

REFERENCES

97. Pancoast H K JAMA 1932; 99: 1391
98. Paulson D L J Thorac Cardiovasc Surg 1975; 70: 1095
99. Macchiarini P, Dartevelle P G, Chapelier A et al Ann Thorac Surg 1993; 55: 611
100. Gaer J A R, Goldstraw P Eur J Cardiothorac Surg 1990; 4: 207
101. Goldstraw P, Mannam G C, Kaplan D K, Michail P J Thorac Cardiovasc Surg 1994; 107: 19

Historically it was believed that the best results for lung cancer treatment would come from pneumonectomy.[102] More conservative resections were initially developed and introduced for patients with poor lung function who were unable to tolerate pneumonectomy.[103] Each compromise has produced superior survival figures to pneumonectomy. It is now realized that for tumours to be suitable for lesser resections they must be localized and have other favourable staging characteristics, and that there is no survival advantage in undertaking resections greater than that required to remove the tumour and its involved lymph nodes. In 60% of patients resection can be accomplished by lobectomy or bilobectomy, in 35% pneumonectomy proves necessary, and in the other 5% resection is feasible by segmentectomy or bronchoplastic procedures.

A randomized trial has shown that local recurrence rates are higher for stage I tumours treated by local resection by segmentectomy or wedge excision when compared with lobectomy, and this had an adverse effect on survival.[104] Compared with lobectomy, local recurrence was twice as common after segmentectomy and four times as frequent after wedge excision. Lobectomy must now be considered the minimal resection for localized tumours, but segmentectomy may be justified for patients who are suitable for such surgery and have limited lung function. Wedge excision cannot be considered as an option for cure, and this has implications for those surgeons who are evaluating the role of video-assisted-thoracscopic surgery resection for lung cancer.[105] Lobectomy and pneumonectomy[106] have been undertaken using video-assisted thorascopic surgery but there is doubt as to whether intraoperative evaluation and nodal dissection is adequately performed using those techniques.

Segmentectomy[107] is the removal of one or more bronchopulmonary segments. There are 10 such segments in the right lung and nine in the left, and therefore segmentectomy entails minimal loss of lung tissue. Each bronchopulmonary segment has its own bronchus and arterial supply, and shares its venous drainage with adjacent segments through intersegmental veins.[108] The hilum is dissected to identify the segmental branch of the pulmonary artery and this is doubly ligated and divided. The segmental bronchus is clamped and divided and the segment becomes progressively atelectatic. If the anaesthetist then ventilates the remaining segments, the segment to be removed can be dissected from within the lung parenchyma, ligating and dividing its tributaries to the intersegmental veins. The raw surface left within the lobe will leak air for several days, requiring prolonged chest drainage.

Lobectomy[107] is the removal of one of the three lobes within the right lung, or one of the two lobes within the left lung. The fissures separating these lobes are somewhat variable in extent. If well developed, the visceral pleura envelops each adjacent lobe, allowing the removal of one lobe from its neighbours with minimal air leak. On the right, bilobectomy is possible, removing the middle lobe with either the upper or, more usually, the lower lobe. When undertaking lobectomy the segmental branches of the pulmonary artery are identified, ligated and divided. The draining vein is tied and the lobar bronchus is divided and sutured. Using the technique of differential inflation it is then possible to complete the dissection of the fissure.

Pneumonectomy[107] entails the removal of the whole lung. It is necessary to divide the main pulmonary artery to that lung, both pulmonary veins and the main bronchus. There is no evidence to suggest that division in any particular sequence has an advantage. The surgeon therefore chooses those structures which are easiest to isolate, as access then becomes progressively easier. Bronchial closure using mechanical staples is gaining in popularity but is of no proven superiority over manual suture techniques.

Bronchoplastic or sleeve resection[107] entails the resection of the stem bronchus with re-anastomosis of the distal bronchus, to salvage distal lung tissue. This operation is most commonly undertaken for tumours of the right upper lobe (Fig. 22.17). If proximal extension along the bronchus is the only contraindication to lobectomy, then a sleeve resection of the main bronchus may permit the re-anastomosis of the distal bronchus, conserving the middle and lower lobes. Pneumonectomy is to be preferred if lobectomy is

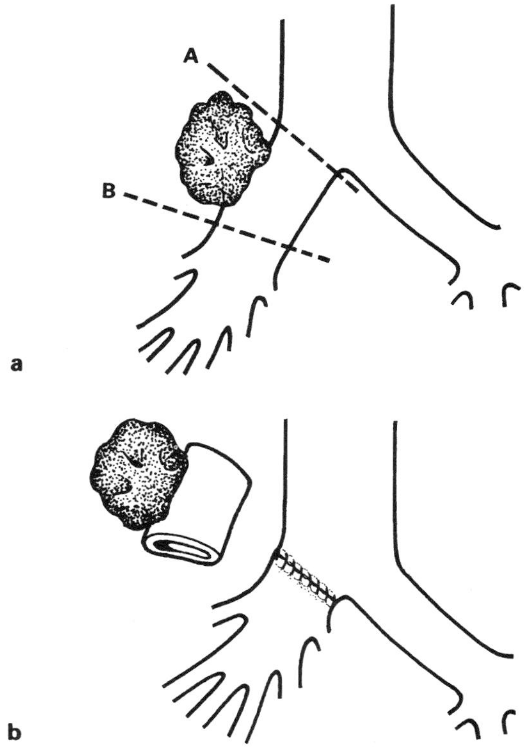

Fig. 22.17 Right upper lobectomy with sleeve resection. A tumour of the right upper lobe has extended to the descending bronchus, and this is the only feature preventing lobectomy. **(a)** The main bronchus is divided at A as for a pneumonectomy, the intermediate bronchus at B, and **(b)** their anastomosis thus preserves the lower and middle lobes.

REFERENCES

102. Ochsner A, Debakey M Surgery 1940; 8: 992
103. Belcher J R Lancet 1956; i: 349
104. Ginsberg R J, Rubenstein L V Ann Thorac Surg 1995; 60: 615
105. Ginsberg R J Ann Thorac Surg 1993; 56: 801
106. Giudicelli R, Thomas P, Lonjon T et al Eur J Cardiothorac Surg 1994; 8: 254
107. Paneth M, Goldstraw P, Hyams B Fundamental Techniques in Pulmonary and Oesophageal Surgery. Springer Verlag, London 1987

contraindicated by proximal extension of the primary tumour or involved lymph nodes on to the pulmonary artery. Sleeve resection may still prove feasible and is justified if N_1 disease is limited to the lobar or segmental nodes and even if there are small, involved nodes around the lobar bronchus.[109] Tumours of low-grade malignancy are often excised with a sleeve of bronchus, preserving all lung tissue, but for lung cancer sleeve resection is usually coupled with lobectomy.

The complications of pulmonary resection

The mortality of pulmonary resection varies not only with the skill of the hospital team but also with the selectivity of the surgeon. In-hospital mortality for lobectomy should, however, be between 3 and 4% and that for pneumonectomy between 5 and 8%.[110,111] As the majority of these operations are for smoking related disease, sputum difficulties are an ever-present threat. Sputum clearance requires intensive physiotherapy aided by optimal pain control. Several methods of analgesia have been validated and all have a place in selected patients. Epidural analgesia is probably superior[112] but carries the risk of urinary retention, especially in elderly men. Intravenous analgesia by infusion or by patient-controlled devices is a useful alternative, and intrapleural infusion is gaining popularity.[113] This measure is supplemented by intravenous pethidine infusion for the first 24–48 h and thereafter oral analgesia suffices. Minitracheostomy should be undertaken early if sputum problems develop.[36]

Pneumonia developing following pulmonary resection is a serious complication with a high mortality. It nearly always follows inadequate management of sputum problems. Broad-spectrum antibiotics are justified if the chest radiograph shows any evidence of parenchymal opacity or if fever develops with purulent sputum.

Supraventricular dysrhythmias, particularly atrial fibrillation, may occur following extensive resection in the elderly, usually 2–5 days after operation. There is controversy as to whether prophylactic digoxin decreases the incidence of supraventricular dysrhythmias,[114] but most surgeons continue to use digoxin selectively depending upon the patient's age, previous cardiac history and the extent of resection. Most also routinely administer low-dose heparin as prophylaxis against thromboembolic disease, although the evidence to support this practice is not conclusive.[115]

Wound infection occurs in up to 10% of patients undergoing pulmonary resection. The incidence is reduced by prophylactic antibiotics commenced at the induction of anaesthesia,[116] and continued for 48 hours which is more effective than shorter regimens.[117] Troublesome postoperative bleeding occurs in 1–2% of patients and is usually related to the scale of resection. It most commonly complicates pneumonectomy where there is an absence of lung tissue to tamponade small bleeding points.[118] Blood clot within the pneumonectomy space may expand as the result of an osmotic effect and may compromise the remaining lung. Re-exploration and evacuation of the clot should be undertaken as soon as this problem is appreciated. Following pneumonectomy, chest X-rays are taken daily to monitor the rising fluid level within the pneumonectomy space and to ensure the optimum position of the mediastinum. Ideally, following pneumonectomy the mediastinum should deviate towards the side of surgery, ensuring unimpeded expansion of the remaining lung. If fluid accumulates rapidly, the mediastinum may be pushed away from the side of operation and in these circumstances fluid and air must be aspirated to bring the mediastinum towards the side of operation. A chest drain is not routinely inserted following a pneumonectomy unless bleeding is anticipated. Following closure of the wound, air is aspirated from the space to bring the mediastinum over. During the succeeding weeks bloody fluid collects within the pneumonectomy space and air is progressively absorbed. Within 6 weeks this process is usually complete with full opacification of the hemithorax and loss of the fluid level (Fig. 22.18). Over the next few months there is fibroblastic proliferation within the pneumonectomy fluid which may proceed to complete fibrous obliteration of the space. Usually however fluid remains, often as a single large collection surrounded by a thick fibrous capsule. The pneumonectomy space contracts with progressive narrowing of the intercostal spaces, steady elevation of the hemidiaphragm and further mediastinal shift to the side of surgery. As long as fluid remains—usually the lifespan of the patient—it may be colonized by bacteraemic infection causing an empyema. Prophylactic antibiotics must be given to patients who have had a pneumonectomy if they are to have any other surgical procedure, including minor operations, endoscopy or dental treatment.

Following lesser resections, an alveolar air leak occurs from the raw lung surface and chest drains are necessary until the air leak has stopped. If the remaining lung tissue fails to fill the hemithorax, a persistent air leak and the consequent need for drains may lead to intrapleural sepsis requiring antibiotics and long-term drainage.

Empyema following pneumonectomy may present within a few weeks of surgery if related to intraoperative contamination or an unsuspected bronchopleural fistula. Empyema may present many years later with the development of a bronchopleural fistula or by haematogenous spread, often due to the bacteraemia occurring during dental treatment or cystoscopic examination.[118] An empyema may be of insidious onset without fever or leucocytosis. The patient steadily deteriorates and a recurrence of malignancy

REFERENCES

108. Boyden E A Segmental Anatomy of the Lung. McGraw Hill, New York 1955
109. Deslauriers J, Gaulin P, Beaulieu M et al J Thorac Cardiovasc Surg 1986; 92: 871
110. Ginsberg R J et al J Thorac Cardiovasc Surg 1978; 94: 673
111. The Society of Cardiothoracic Surgeons of Great Britain Annual Returns in Thoracic Surgery, 1985 (unpublished)
112. Brichon P Y, Pison C, Chaffanjon P et al Eur J Cardio-thorac Surg 1994; 8: 482
113. Bachmann-Mennenga B, Biscoping J, Kuhn DFM, et al Eur J Cardio-thorac Surg 1993; 7: 12
114. Ritchie A J, Danton M, Gibbons J R P Thorax 1992; 47: 41
115. Sutton G, Hosking S, Johnson C D Ann R Coll Surg Engl 1991; 73: 111
116. Ilves R, Cooper J D et al J Thorac Cardiovasc Surg 1981; 81: 813
117. Bernard A, Pillet M, Goudet P, Viard H J Thorac Cardiovasc Surg 1994; 107: 896
118. Kirsh M M et al Ann Thorac Surg 1975; 20: 215

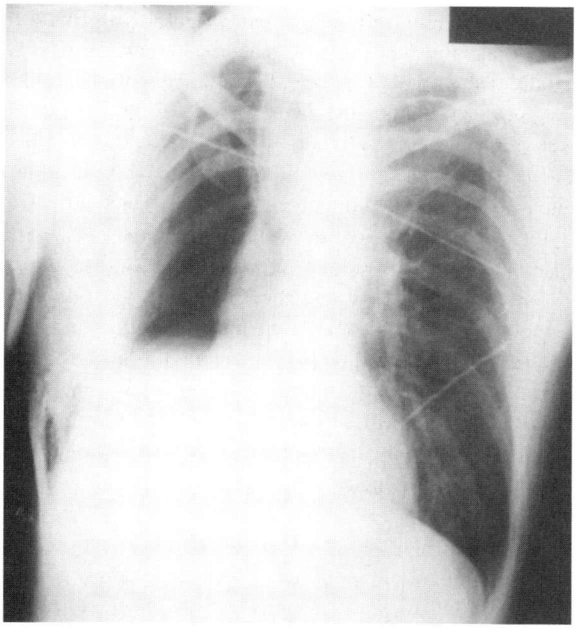

a

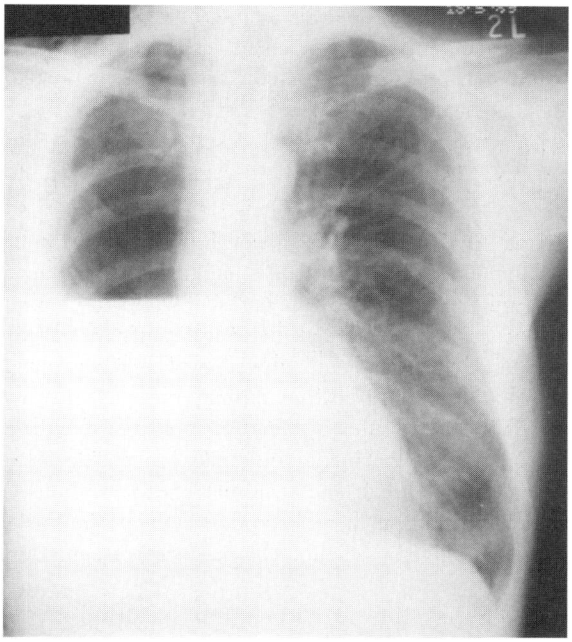

b

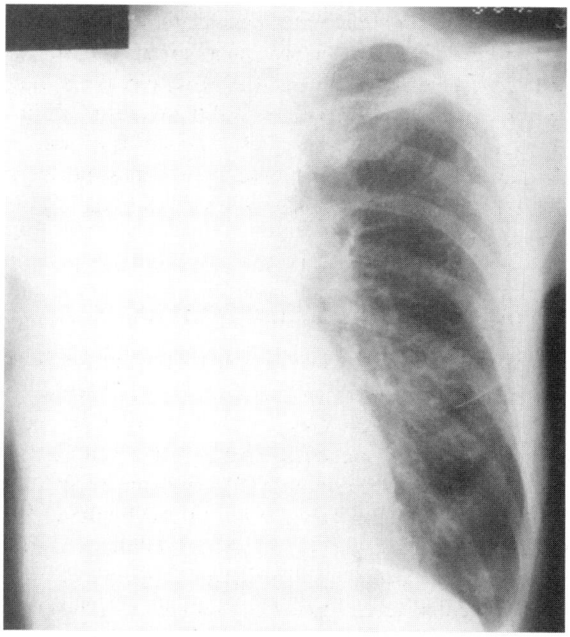

c

Fig. 22.18 A sequence of chest radiographs showing progress following pneumonectomy. **(a)** The immediate postoperative film shows the hemithorax containing only air and reduced in volume by mediastinal shift and elevation of the diaphragm. **(b)** Three days later, the pneumonectomy space now contains a fluid level as air is absorbed and an exudate accumulates. **(c)** By 4–6 weeks there is complete opacification of the space.

may be suspected. Aspiration of the pneumonectomy space should be undertaken in such circumstances to exclude an empyema. Cultures may prove negative in up to 30% of patients despite clear evidence of infection within the pneumonectomy space, and turbid fluid on aspiration is sufficient evidence to merit surgical drainage. Further treatment of the empyema will depend upon the presence of complicating fistulae, but once these have been closed, the pneumonectomy space can usually be irrigated, sterilized and then closed.[119] A one-stage treatment, closing the fistula and obliterating the empyema cavity using myoplastic and omental flaps is gaining popularity and has been shown to be safe.[120] *Staphylococcus aureus* is the organism most commonly encountered but other respiratory pathogens may be incriminated. A mixed growth of upper gut organisms strongly suggests an underlying oesophagopleural fistula.

Bronchopleural fistula is a serious but infrequent complication of pulmonary resection.[121] It is rare following lobectomy and in such circumstances it is usually associated with a persistent alveolar leak and empyema. A bronchopleural fistula developing soon after pneumonectomy is related to technical deficiencies in the closure of the bronchial stump. Thin bloody fluid from within the pneumonectomy space is expectorated in large volumes and may flood into the remaining lung, causing immediate death or severe pneumonitis. The immediate insertion of a chest drain to remove the remaining space fluid may be life-saving. If doubt exists as to the diagnosis a chest radiograph discloses increased translucency of the pneumonectomy space and a drop in the fluid level from its previously observed position. Immediate re-exploration and reclosure of the bronchial stump are necessary, but mortality remains approximately 50%. Small bronchopleural fistulae following pneumonectomy may be evidenced by the development of empyema or by the failure of the pneumonectomy space to become

REFERENCES

119. Goldstraw P Thorax 1979; 34: 740
120. Wong P S, Goldstraw P Eur J Cardio-thorac Surg 1994; 8: 345
121. Al-Kattan K M, Cattalani L, Goldstraw P Ann Thorac Surg 1994; 58: 1433

completely opaque on serial chest radiographs. Following drainage of the space most such fistulae close spontaneously, but re-operation may be occasionally necessary.

Other lung tumours

Carcinoid tumours have a variable, but usually low-grade, degree of malignancy.[122] Those demonstrating typical histological features are probably benign, and conservative resection is possible unless long-standing bronchial obstruction has led to distal bronchiectasis and lung damage. The patient usually presents with recurrent pneumonia or haemoptysis and the history is often very long. Carcinoid tumours arise from the Kulchitsky cells of the amine precursor uptake and decarboxylation (APUD) system within the bronchial mucosa, from which small cell carcinoma is also believed to arise.[123] They contain argyrophilic material on staining, and dense core granules may be visible on electron microscopy. Within the spectrum of tumours arising from the Kulchitsky cell, malignant carcinoid tumours occupy an intermediate position between the benign typical carcinoid and the highly malignant small cell carcinoma. Malignant carcinoid tumours exhibit atypical histological features. There may be cellular atypia and nuclear pleomorphism; local invasion may be evident; regional lymph node metastases are found in 25% of cases and distant metastases appear in 5%.[124] More extensive resections are necessary to deal with these tumours. Carcinoid syndrome is rare with tumours of bronchial origin and only occurs with extensive pulmonary or hepatic metastases.

All other primary lung tumours are rare.

Adenoid cystic carcinoma, previously termed cylindroma, usually affects the trachea or major bronchi.[124] Although highly malignant locally, it does not frequently metastasize and growth is often surprisingly slow. Long-term survival is common and patients often survive 3–5 years without radical treatment.[125] These tumours infiltrate extensively beyond the macroscopic margins of the tumour and frozen-section evaluation of resection margins is necessary to ensure complete clearance. Resection, if feasible, is the treatment of choice, but radiotherapy may be needed to control inoperable tumours. Valuable palliation can be achieved by the measures described later.

Mucoepidermoid carcinoma and carcinosarcoma are rare but highly malignant tumours.[126]

Chondroma of the lung is a benign, well circumscribed lesion and debate continues as to whether it should be considered hamartomatous or a mesenchymoma.[127] Local excision is possible and enucleation usually feasible.

The lungs are frequent sites for *metastatic tumours*. If the radiographic abnormalities are multiple and there is a history of previous malignancy, the diagnosis is not difficult. If there is a solitary lesion, it may be difficult to exclude a benign nodule or a primary carcinoma of the lung. The typical cannonball appearance on chest radiography is often seen with primary lung tumours and metastatic disease may assume a variety of radiographic appearances from finely nodular disease to an infiltrative, poorly defined opacity.

In selected cases surgical excision of pulmonary metastases may be feasible and worthwhile. A 5-year survival of 35–55% has been reported following the surgical excision of carcinomatous and sarcomatous deposits.[128,129] Selection for such surgery must be rigorous.[130] In addition to ensuring that the patient's fitness is sufficient for the scale of resection proposed, selection should ensure that: the primary tumour has been reliably controlled, usually by excision; extrathoracic metastases have been excluded using the most sensitive investigations appropriate; the extent of intrathoracic metastases has been documented by CT scans of the whole of both lungs. The disease-free interval and the number of metastases do not appear to influence the effectiveness of pulmonary resection.[131] Bilateral pulmonary metastases, if small and favourably sited, may be resected through a median sternotomy incision.[132] In other situations a staged approach via lateral thoracotomy incisions is to be preferred. The excision of each metastasis is performed by the most conservative resection feasible—usually removing only the deposit with a thin surrounding rim of normal lung. If metastases are large or impinge on hilar structures, segmentectomy or lobectomy may be necessary. Pneumonectomy is rarely justified for the removal of metastatic disease.

The results of lung resections are similar for most carcinomata and sarcomata but melanoma fares badly with nearly all patients relapsing within 1 year.[131] Even in melanoma there is some suggestion that pulmonary metastasectomy, combined with immunotherapy,[133] offers some hope of long-term survival. The role of adjuvant chemotherapy remains controversial except where effective agents exist, as for osteosarcoma and testicular teratoma[134] (see Chapters 54 and 40).

Tumours of the trachea and main bronchi

Obstruction to the trachea or major bronchi may result from primary tumours that are usually malignant, or by metastatic involvement. Whilst the latter may present with a discrete intraluminal metastasis, more commonly it results from extrinsic compression due to malignant involvement of adjacent glands.

Patients with tracheal obstruction may present with haemoptysis or stridor but the latter is often overlooked or may be misinterpreted as asthma. Obstruction of a main bronchus is associated with a unilateral wheeze and recurrent chest infections. If the obstruction is complete then absorption collapse and atelectasis result, but ball-valve obstruction can produce profound dyspnoea

REFERENCES

122. Lawson R M et al Thorax 1976; 31: 245
123. Bensch K G, Gordon G B, Miller L R Cancer 1965; 18: 592
124. Goldstraw P J Thorac Cardiovasc Surg 1976; 72: 309
125. Conlan A A et al J Thorac Cardiovasc Surg 1978; 76: 369
126. Turnbull A D et al Ann Thorac Surg 1972; 14: 452
127. Van den Bosch J M M et al Thorax 1987; 42: 790
128. McCormack P M, Martini N Ann Thorac Surg 1979; 28: 139
129. Mountain C F, McMurtrey M J, Hermes K E Ann Thorac Surg 1984; 38: 323
130. Goldstraw P In: Slevin M L (ed) Management of Metastases. Clinical Oncology. Baillière Tindall, London 1987 p 601
131. Venn G E, Sarin S, Goldstraw P Eur J Cardiothorac Surg 1989; 3: 105
132. Johnston M I R J Thorac Cardiovasc Surg 1983; 85: 516
133. Tafra L, Dale P S, Wanek L A, Ramming K P, Morton D L J Thorac Cardiovasc Surg 1995; 110: 119
134. Hendry W F, Goldstraw P, Peckham M J Br J Urol 1987; 59: 358

in the presence of normal radiographs unless air-trapping is sought on a chest radiograph taken in expiration.

Benign tumours of the trachea are most commonly carcinoid in type, but many other benign growths have been described, including mucous adenoma[135] and lipoma.[136] Benign tumours may be removed bronchoscopically if pedunculated, but there is commonly an intramural component necessitating resection.[137] Segmental resection of the trachea or sleeve resection of the main bronchus is frequently feasible without loss of lung tissue.

Metastatic deposits may rarely occur as endobronchial tumours within the tracheobronchial tree, usually from a primary in the colon, breast or kidney.[138]

All primary malignant tumours of the trachea are rare. They are usually squamous carcinomas or adenoid cystic carcinomas.[139] Once the condition has been considered, bronchoscopy is diagnostic. Chest physicians may be reluctant to undertake biopsy through a fibreoptic bronchoscope for fear of precipitating total obstruction or severe bleeding. Endoscopic resection provides relief of stridor and permits a more leisurely assessment of the tumour. Using the rigid bronchoscope, the tumour may be cored out or resected using large biopsy forceps.[140] A good lumen can usually be achieved using a diathermy loop.[141] Laser photoresection is more elegant, vastly more expensive and has not been shown to be any more effective.[142] Laser resection may be undertaken through the fibreoptic instrument but increasingly endoscopists are returning to the rigid instrument as it allows large fragments to be removed and bleeding to be controlled.

Tracheal resection may be undertaken for benign or malignant conditions. Resection of up to 50% of a child's trachea may be undertaken without difficulty, but with the inelastic trachea of adults, resection is more difficult and release techniques may have to be utilized.[143] The anatomical considerations of tracheal resection have been studied by Grillo and large series have been reported.[144,145] Resection of more than 50% of the trachea is not usually possible. Prosthetic replacement of the trachea has not been successful, but techniques of transplantation with revascularization are being developed in animal models.[146] For inoperable lesions radiotherapy may be of some value. For the majority of patients presenting with malignant obstruction of the trachea only palliative measures are possible. There is often an appreciable extramural component producing severe extrinsic compression. The intraluminal component of the tumour may be dealt with by repeated endoscopic resection using any of the techniques described above. If the tumour recurs following external irradiation, further external treatment may not be feasible because of the intolerance of the surrounding normal tissues. Endobronchial irradiation can be given using catheters inserted bronchoscopically, and provide valuable palliation.[147] When all else fails, the insertion of an internal hollow tracheal or tracheobronchial stent (Fig. 22.19) may prevent asphyxia and allow clearing of the obstructed secretions from the distal bronchial tree.[148] A wide range of stents have been developed to palliate airway obstruction due to malignant and benign strictures[149] (Fig. 22.20).

Lung infection

Postoperative atelectasis may progress to pneumonia if not effectively treated. It is a common problem after operations on

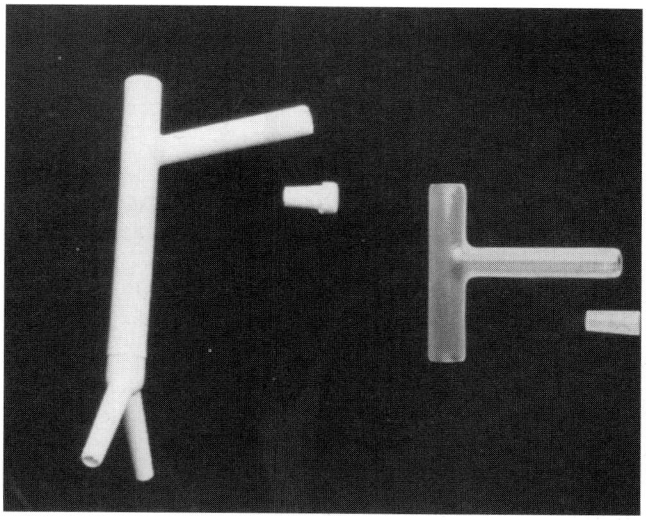

Fig. 22.19 Silicone rubber stents used to alleviate compression of the tracheobronchial tree.

smokers, particularly through upper abdominal or thoracic incisions.[150] Treatment by analgesia and physiotherapy has already been discussed, as has the value of a minitracheostomy tube.

Pulmonary tuberculosis was declining in Western countries until the last decade. Since that time the incidence has risen, mainly in association with AIDS. In Africa and Asia tuberculosis has never been controlled and is now epidemic.[151] Bacteriological insensitivity is rare in the UK, although it is on the increase in many countries. In the UK, 90% of patients are treated with the combination of rifampicin and isoniazid, usually with the addition of ethambutol or pyrazinamide.[152] Treatment is necessary for at least 6 months and may have to be modified if toxicity is encountered. There is concern as to the ocular toxicity of ethambutol but this drug is safe if the visual acuity is checked prior to treatment, and the patient is advised to discontinue the drug if vision becomes

REFERENCES

135. MacArthur C G C Br J Dis Chest 1977; 71: 93
136. Edwards C W, Matthews H R Thorax 1981; 36: 147
137. Halttunen P, Meurala H, Standertskjold-Nordenstam C G Thorax 1982; 37: 688
138. Shepherd M P Thorax 1982; 37: 362
139. Hetzel M R In: Brewis R A L, Gibson G J, Geddes D M (eds) Respiratory Medicine. Baillière Tindall, London 1990 p 823
140. Mathisen D S, Grillo H C Ann Thorac Surg 1989; 48: 469
141. Petrou M, Goldstraw P Eur J Cardiothorac Surg 1994; 8: 436
142. Toty L, Personne C, Colchen A, Vourch G Thorax 1981; 36: 175
143. Montgomery W W Arch Otolaryngol 1974; 99: 155
144. Mulliken J B, Grillo H C J Thorac Cardiovasc Surg 1968; 55: 418
145. Grillo H C Thorax 1973; 28: 667
146. Delaere P R, Liu Z Y, Hermans R, Sciot R, Feenstra L J Thorac Cardiovasc Surg 1995; 110: 728
147. Burt P A et al Thorax 1990; 45: 765
148. Montgomery W W Ann Otol Rhinol Laryngol 1968; 77: 534
149. Goldstraw P Endobronchial stents. In: Hetzel M (ed) Minimally Invasive Techniques in Thoracic Medicine and Surgery. Chapman & Hall, London 1994
150. Parfrey P S, Harte P J et al Br J Surg 1977; 64: 384
151. Benatar S R Thorax 1995; 50: 487
152. British Thoracic Association Lancet 1980; i: 1182

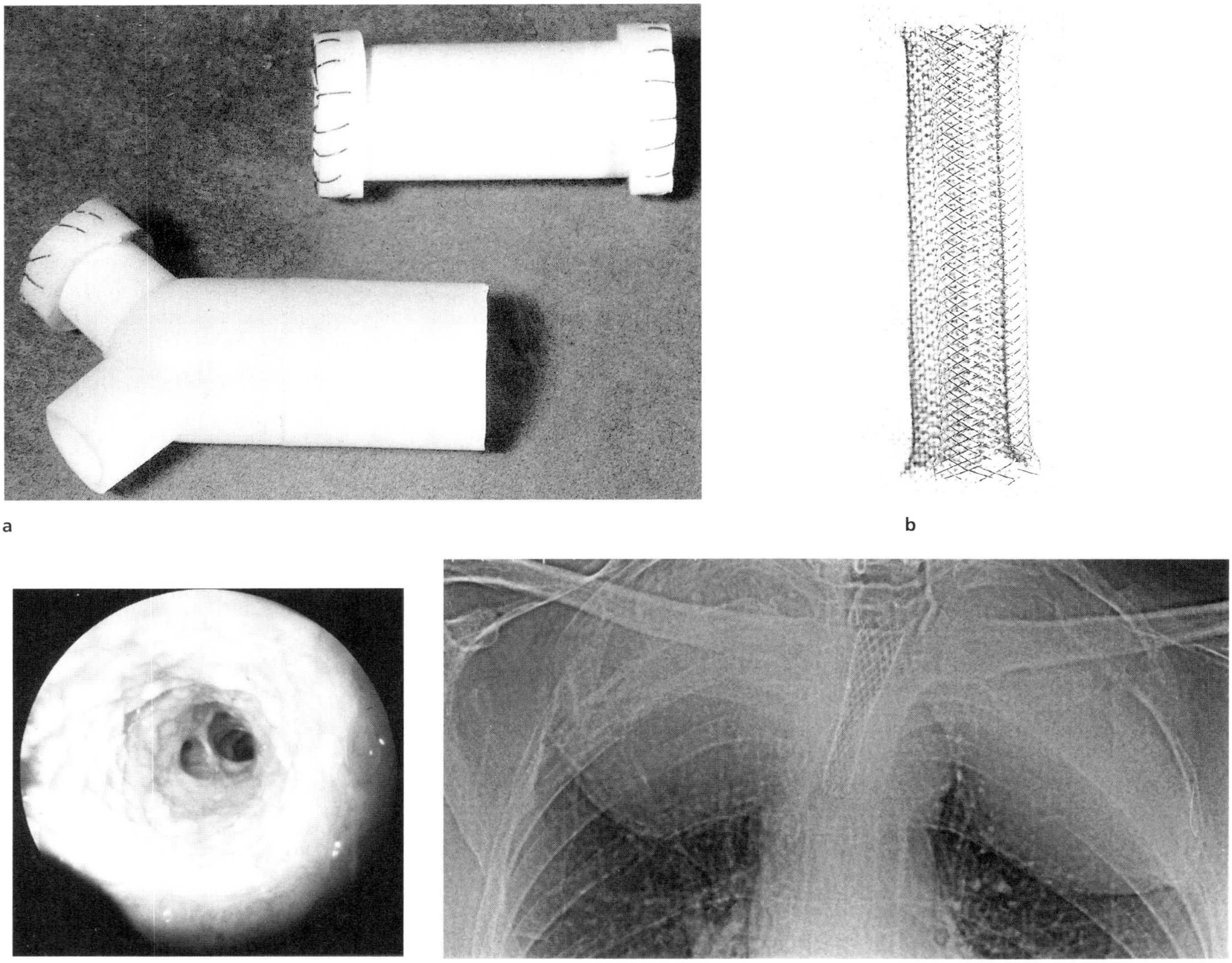

a b c d

Fig. 22.20 **(a)** Tailored straight and bifurcated silicone stents inserted bronchoscopically into the trachea and bronchi. **(b)** Wire stent inserted through the bronchoscope into the trachea or bronchi. Wall stent pattern. **(c)** Bronchoscopic appearances 3 years after insertion of a Wall stent for a benign stricture. The stent is almost completely epithelialized. **(d)** A chest radiograph showing a wire stent supporting the trachea.

blurred.[153] Cure is achieved in 98% of patients.[154] The older techniques of lung collapse therapy, utilizing artificial pneumothorax, phrenic crush, plombage and thoracoplasty, are now obsolete. Surgery still has a place in the management of tuberculosis, dealing with the increasing problem of multiple drug resistant organisms[155] and complications such as bronchiectasis or empyema. Cavities can be resected which persist after drug treatment and cause life-threatening haemoptysis or harbour bacteria, preventing cure by drugs.[156]

A *lung abscess* may follow any suppurative pneumonia, particularly if accompanied by bronchial obstruction.[157] Chest radiographs disclose cavitation with an air–fluid level (Fig. 22.21), but the appearances are variable and non-specific and are often indistinguishable from a cavitating peripheral carcinoma of the lung. Bronchoscopy is essential to exclude bronchial obstruction by benign or malignant conditions, and bronchial lavage may obtain useful bacteriological specimens. Conservative management is usually successful with physiotherapy and appropriate antibiotics.[158] Percutaneous catheter drainage of a lung abscess may speed recovery in the toxic, ill patient, and may thus avert the need

REFERENCES

153. Citron K M, Thomas G O Thorax 1986; 41: 737
154. McNicol M W In: Brewis R A L, Gibson G J, Geddes D M (eds) Respiratory Medicine. Baillière Tindall, London 1990 p 984
155. Treasure R L, Seaworth B J Ann Thorac Surg 1995; 59: 1405
156. Goldstraw P Surgery 1987; 1: 1071
157. Brock R C Lung Abscess. Blackwell Scientific, Oxford 1952
158. Moore-Gillon J, Eykyn S In: Brewis R A L, Gibson G J, Geddes D M (eds) Respiratory Medicine. Baillière Tindall, London 1990 p 974

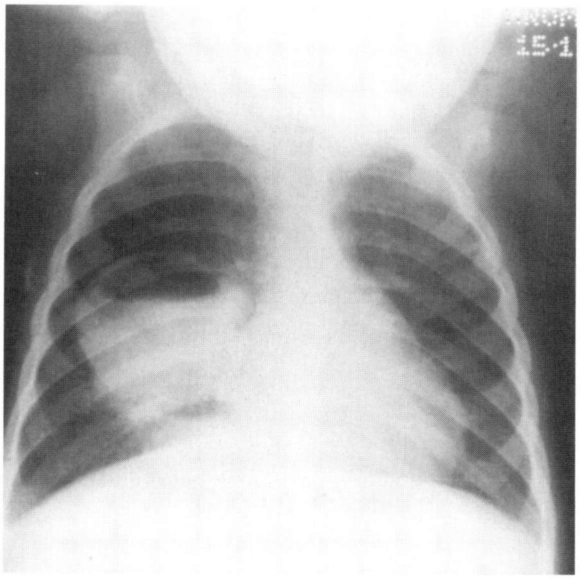

Fig. 22.21 The posteroanterior chest radiograph of a child with a lung abscess which had resulted from infection of a bronchogenic cyst.

for surgery.[159] Pulmonary resection is necessary if there is concern that the abscess is malignant, or if conservative therapy fails to relieve fever, cough and sputum production, or if the radiographic abnormality persists. Particular care should be taken during surgery in positioning the endobronchial tube to prevent the spillage of pus into the dependent lung. Alternatively an endobronchial blocker may be inserted into the lobar bronchus to prevent spillage into the opposite lung and ipsilateral lobe.

Bronchiectasis results from destruction of the normal bronchial architecture. The damage is usually initiated in childhood when severe infection may be exacerbated by bronchial obstruction.[160] The small airways of children lack firm cartilaginous support and are more susceptible to compression from adjacent reactive lymph nodes. With chronic infection there is progressive bronchial dilation and mucus gland hyperplasia. The process is then self-perpetuating, even if the bronchial obstruction is relieved.

Repeated infective exacerbations produce parenchymal lung damage and progressive loss of lung tissue. Tuberculosis remains an important aetiological factor in developing countries[161] but in developed countries has been superseded by the pyogenic sequelae of such common conditions as measles, whooping cough or a retained foreign body. Bronchiectasis may also result from systemic diseases such as cystic fibrosis or hypogammaglobulinaemia or from local defects in host defence, as in Kartagener's syndrome[162] in which there are defects in ciliary function. Bronchiectasis results in excessive and chronic sputum production with frequent infective exacerbations during which large volumes of purulent sputum may be expectorated, often associated with systemic illness and fever. Small children may fail to thrive. Bronchiectasis may be complicated by recurring pneumonia, but the classic complications of chronic infection, amyloid and brain abscess, are now rare.[163] Haemoptysis is usually minor, but may on occasions prove life-threatening.

Bronchiectasis is no longer as common as it was and the vast majority of patients can be managed medically.[164] If antibiotics and postural drainage do not control symptoms, surgery should be considered. Bronchography has been superseded by CT scanning in the evaluation of bronchiectasis (Fig. 22.22).

Pulmonary resection is only appropriate if the bronchiectasis is localized and usually unilateral. Resection is conservative, removing only the abnormal areas shown on bronchography, usually by segmentectomy or lobectomy or a combination of these procedures. Pneumonectomy or bilateral resection is justified only in the most severe circumstances. The prognosis of bronchiectasis, which used to be poor, has been dramatically improved with antibiotics, and the vast majority of patients now lead an active life.

Bullous emphysema

Emphysema may be focal or generalized. The localized variant may present in infancy, where it is often associated with congenital abnormalities of the lobar bronchus,[165] or later in life as a solitary air-filled cyst.[166] The homozygous chromosomal abnormality leading to α_1-antitrypsin deficiency produces severe generalized emphysema early in adult life,[167] and characteristically in this

REFERENCES

159. Yellin A, Yellin E O, Lieblerman Y Ann Thorac Surg 1985; 39: 266
160. Davidson M, Lee-Lander F B Br J Radiol 1938; 11: 65
161. LeRoux B T, Mohlala M L et al Current Problems in Surgery. Year Book Medical Publishers, Chicago 1986 p 97
162. Chang K H R, Niguidula F N, Ramos A J Thorac Cardiovasc Surg 1962; 43: 127
163. Cole P In: Brewis R A L, Gibson G J, Geddes D M (eds) Respiratory Medicine. Baillière Tindall, London 1990 p 726
164. Cook J C et al Thorax 1987; 42: 272
165. Lincoln J C R et al Ann Surg 1971; 173: 55
166. Soosay G, Baudouin S V et al Histopathology 1991; 20: 517
167. Tobin M J, Cook P J L, Hutchinson D C S Br J Dis Chest 1983; 77: 14

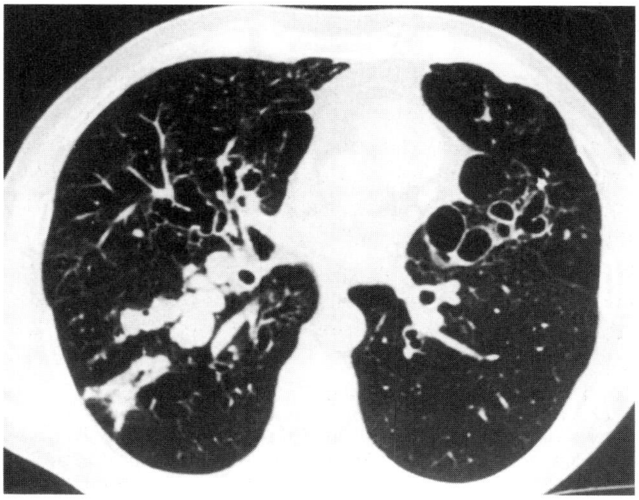

Fig. 22.22 A CT scan showing extensive, cystic bronchiectasis in the lingular segments of the left upper lobe and the right lower lobe.

condition the bullae are predominantly situated at the base of both lungs.

Generalized emphysema is far more commonly related to smoking. Radiographically the abnormality is predominantly within the upper zones of the lungs. The patient may present with progressive dyspnoea or there may be a sudden deterioration with the development of a pneumothorax. The radiological differentiation between a pneumothorax and severe emphysema is not always easy, particularly when interpreting chest X-rays in elderly smokers (Fig. 22.23). The inadvertent intubation of a bulla by an intercostal drain carries serious morbidity in an elderly patient with incipient respiratory failure. Many patients with progressive emphysema are content with their diminishing exercise capacity; most of those who are not cannot be helped surgically. Occasionally a patient is encountered who finds the dyspnoea unacceptable and who has, within the context of generalized lung disease, a localized and often expanding bulla. Occasionally such a dominant bulla may benefit from surgical treatment, especially if there is radiographic evidence suggesting compression of adjacent, less abnormal lung tissue. Lobectomy or resection of the bulla has been used but has now been superseded by operations which conserve lung parenchyma. Intracavitary drainage can be used if there is a dominant bulla, and this small operation can result in improvement in lung function.[168] Others have resected peripheral strips of emphysematous lung parenchyma to increase the radial forces maintaining airway patency during expiration and reducing chest wall and diaphragmatic distension. This operation of bilateral pneumectomy,[169] requires a median sternotomy which is a major undertaking in patients with poor lung function. Video-assisted thorascopic surgery techniques are being evaluated to undertake laser coagulation of bullae,[170] and pneumectomy procedures. Transplantation offers hope for the occasional patient who is unusually young, and single lung transplantation allows better use of the limited supply of donor organs.[171] The selection of patients best suited for this expanding field of surgery is still being evaluated.[172]

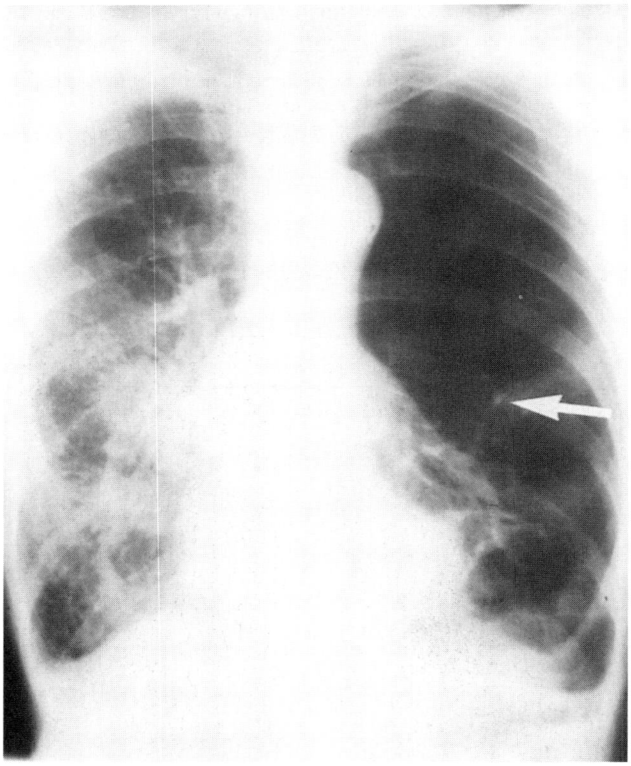

Fig. 22.23 The chest radiograph of an elderly patient with severe emphysema. A bulla in the left lung has completely filled the hemithorax, obscuring the less abnormal lung on that side and causing mediastinal shift to the right. The inexperienced might interpret these features as those of a pneumothorax. The absence of any lung margin and the strands of lung tissue (arrow) extending into the translucent area should alert the wary.

Hydatid disease

Hydatid disease is now rare in Europe but infestation occurs in areas of North Africa, Turkey and Cyprus. The worm responsible, *Echinococcus granulosus*, infects the gut of dog and other carnivores such as wolves, which act as the primary host. The ova, shed in the faeces of the primary host, are ingested by the intermediate host, principally sheep. The organism then erodes into the portal vessels and spreads to the liver where it develops into a cyst. If the organism passes through the hepatic capillary bed it will spread to the lungs, and if it traverses the pulmonary capillaries it may reach the brain, bones or other organs.[173] Man usually becomes an unwitting intermediate host from contact with dogs. Hydatid cysts are therefore more common in the liver, and when found in the lung are usually associated with liver involvement. Lung cysts may be bilateral and multiple. Lung cysts are characteristically ovoid, often notched by hilar structures (Fig. 22.24). Most cysts are symptomless, but if large may produce cough, chest pain or dyspnoea. If the cysts rupture spontaneously the patient expectorates clear, salty water, which may contain the 'grape skins' of the cyst membrane. There is usually some associated bronchospasm and anaphylaxis may be fatal. The cyst may die without rupture, shrinking away from the host lung tissue and allowing a crescent of air to enter the space. If the cyst collapses further, the dead cyst may be seen lying in the base of the lung cavity, producing the 'water lily' sign (Fig. 22.25). The cavity left in the lung may become infected, producing a complicated cyst—a lung abscess. Lung cysts should be treated surgically.[174] It is possible to enucleate the cyst, taking care not to rupture the thin cyst wall. There is usually a small bronchus at the base of the cavity. The anaesthetist may aid delivery of the cyst by gently inflating the lung. The bronchus is then sutured and the lung defect repaired. Should the cyst rupture

REFERENCES

168. Venn G E, Williams P R, Goldstraw P Thorax 1988; 43: 998
169. Cooper J D, Trulock E P, Triantafillou A N et al J Thorac Cardiovasc Surg 1995; 109: 106
170. Wakabayashi A Ann Thorac Surg 1995; 60: 936
171. Kaiser L R, Cooper J D, Trulock E P et al J Thorac Cardiovasc Surg 1991; 102: 333
172. Goldstraw P, Petrou M Chest Surg Clin N Amer 1995; 5: 777
173. Crofton J, Douglas A Respiratory Diseases. Blackwell Scientific, Oxford 1969
174. Qian Z Ann Thorac Surg 1988; 46: 342

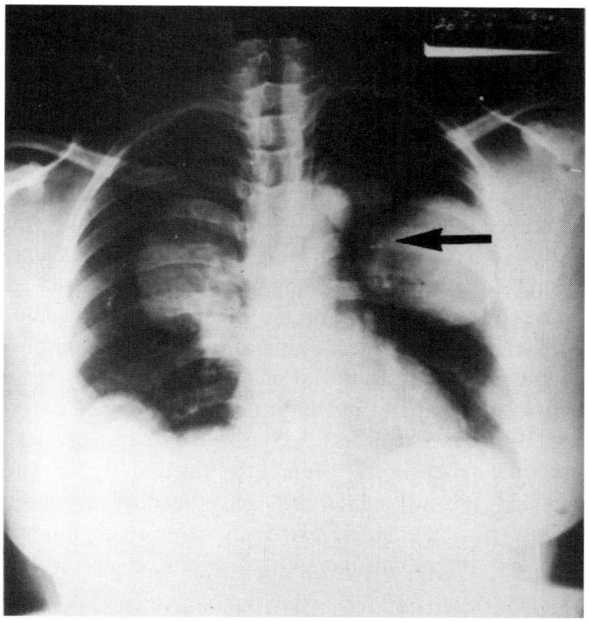

Fig. 22.24 Large, bilateral hydatid cysts, one clearly notched (arrow) by normal hilar vessels.

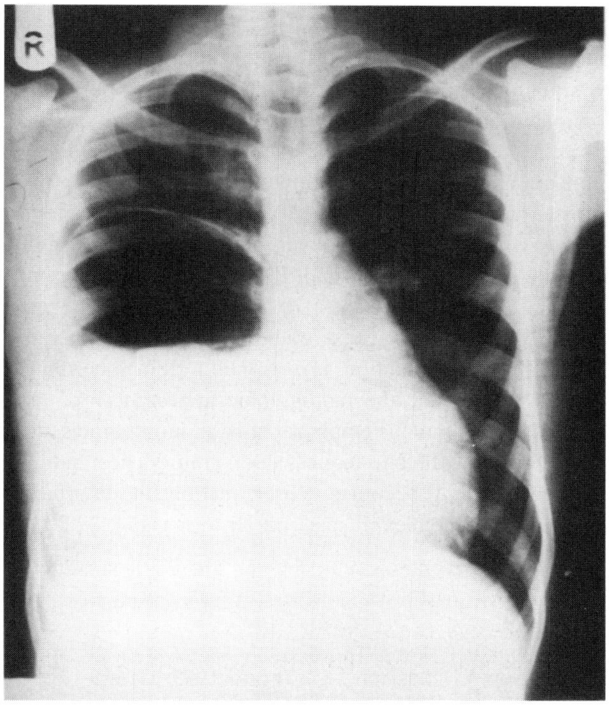

Fig. 22.25 An enormous hydatid cyst in the right lung. The cyst has ruptured and the patient expectorated 'grape skins'. The remaining cyst membrane can be seen at the base of the lung cavity, giving the 'water lily' appearance.

during removal, secondary cysts may be seeded around the pleural space. It is usual therefore to limit any possible spillage by placing swabs around the lung, and it may help to irrigate the soiled pleura with water or a solution of formalin. Antihelminthic drugs such as albendazole,[175] which are effective in patients with hepatic cysts may not help patients with lung cysts, as the dead organism may lead to a lung abscess which requires more extensive pulmonary resection. Such drugs are useful as an adjunct to surgery, combined with agents such as praziquantel which is active against the exposed scolices, or when operation is impractical.

Fungal infections of the lung

Fungal infection of the lung may occur with coccidioidomycosis, histoplasmosis, blastomycosis and aspergillosis.[173] All but the last are rare in the UK, although the others are endemic in areas of North and South America.

Aspergillosis is most commonly the result of infection by *Aspergillus fumigatus* whose spores are ubiquitous, but other species will be found occasionally. There are four clinical entities recognized:[173] allergic bronchopulmonary aspergillosis, aspergilloma, aspergillus colonizing areas of pulmonary infarction and systemic aspergillosis complicating immunosuppression.

Allergic bronchopulmonary aspergillosis results from bronchial hyperreactivity to the organism, with an asthma-like illness. There is wheeze and the chest radiograph shows transient pulmonary infiltrates caused by bronchial plugs. There is a florid reaction to skin prick testing with the organism, and serum precipitins may be found. The manifestations of the illness are suppressed by steroids.

A fungal ball, or aspergilloma, occurs when the organism colonizes a lung cavity, usually the result of chronic fibrosing lung diseases such as tuberculosis or sarcoidosis. The chest radiograph shows the ball outlined by air in the cavity (Fig. 22.26). CT scanning is more sensitive in showing this diagnostic feature[176]

REFERENCES

175. Leader Lancet 1984; i: 675
176. Roberts C M, Citron K M, Strickland B Radiology 1987; 165: 123

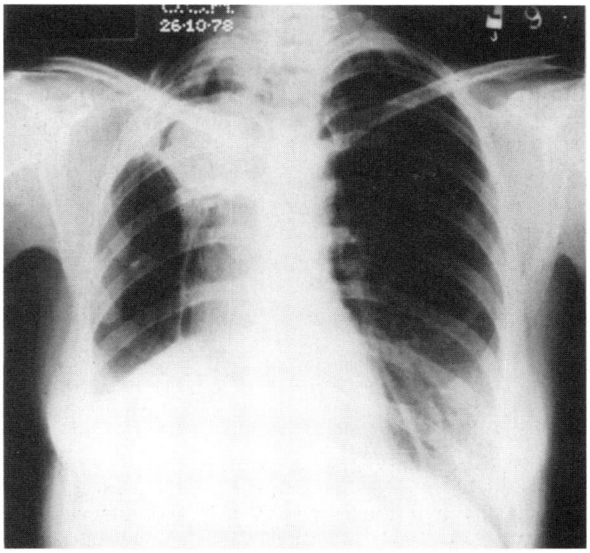

Fig. 22.26 A chest radiograph showing a fungal ball or aspergilloma in a contracted right upper lobe.

(Fig. 22.27). There is only shallow invasion of the cavity wall and little surrounding inflammation, but the appearance of fungal colonization is often accompanied by increasing haemoptysis and other symptoms, such as a low-grade fever with a distressing cough and purulent sputum. Skin prick tests are negative but serum precipitins are always found.

Pulmonary resection may be necessary if haemoptysis is life-threatening or other symptoms are troublesome. The associated lung disease makes surgery difficult, and a severe reduction in lung function is a common contraindication to resection.[177] Medical treatment with antifungal drugs, administered systemically or irrigated into the cavity by bronchoscopy or percutaneously, has been tried with little success.[178]

Bronchial artery embolization may stop haemoptysis temporarily,[179] and irradiation of the lung has also been used.[180] Fortunately, massive haemoptysis usually settles on conservative therapy, and only recurs in a minority of patients.[181] The prognosis is better for the fortunate minority whose lung function permits pulmonary resection.[177]

Aspergillus may colonize areas of pulmonary infarction, usually in patients who are immunosuppressed by chemotherapy, and life-threatening haemoptysis can result unless urgent surgery is undertaken.[182]

Lung and heart–lung transplantation

Over the last 30 years single-lung transplantation has been attempted sporadically to deal with end-stage lung disease, often caused by paraquat poisoning.[183] The results have been poor due to the difficulty of detecting rejection at an early stage and because of the infective problems caused by the immunosuppression. Recently progress has been made by the use of cyclosporin to control rejection, allowing reduced steroid dosage and a consequent reduction in infective problems. Heart–lung transplantation has been successful in patients with cystic fibrosis.[184] Single-lung transplantation is now being re-evaluated.[185]

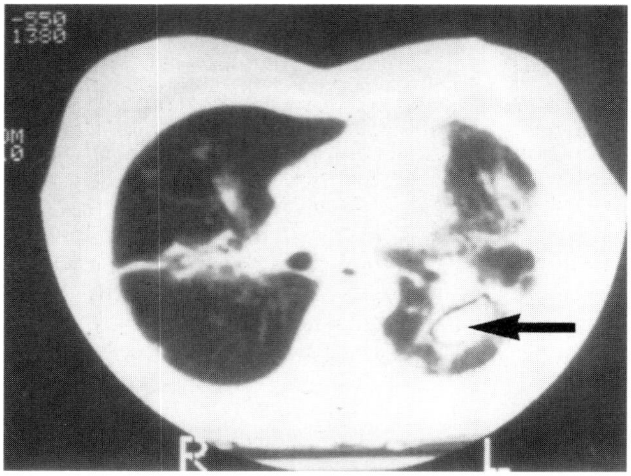

Fig. 22.27 The computerized tomographic scan of a patient with chronic and bilateral lung fibrosis, with clear evidence of a fungal ball in one of the cavities (arrow).

THE PLEURA

The pleura represents a single mesothelial membrane into which the lung is invaginated to produce parietal and visceral pleural surfaces. The pleural reflection runs around the hilum of the lung and extends downwards as the inferior pulmonary ligament.

There is an enormous fluid flux across the pleural space. The hydrostatic pressure gradient between the systemic and pulmonary capillaries causes fluid transudation from the parietal pleura into the pleural space and its absorption by the visceral pleura. Pleural lymphatics resorb 10–20% of the pleural fluid in addition to protein molecules and other large molecular weight substances.[186] In health there is only 10–15 ml of fluid in the pleural space, but this may increase rapidly and dramatically with any disturbance of the homeostatic mechanisms.

Abnormal collections within the pleural space produce compression of the underlying lung leading to dyspnoea. Unilateral effusions can, if extremely large, compromise both lungs because the mediastinum moves over to compress the other lung.

Intercostal drainage

Any pathological fluid accumulation within the pleural space may be aspirated through a wide-bore needle, often providing useful diagnostic samples. However, an intercostal tube is preferable in many situations since it has a larger lumen and also provides more continuous drainage so that changes of posture and spontaneous coughing lead to more complete evacuation of the pleural space. Complications are common following inappropriate or inexpert intercostal drainage.[187] The pleural space can only be safely intubated if its visceral and pleural layers are separated by an abnormal accumulation, be it of air or fluid. Except in the most unusual and pressing circumstances a chest drain should never be inserted unless a good-quality chest radiograph shows unequivocal evidence of such a collection. It is as well to remember that other conditions may mimic the radiographic appearances of a pneumothorax, such as bullous emphysema or an intrathoracic stomach (Fig. 22.28). It may help to request an expiratory chest radiograph. The underlying lung becomes denser, making the interface with the air trapped in the pleural space easier to see (Fig. 22.29).

REFERENCES

177. Jewkes J, Kay P H et al Thorax 1983; 38: 572
178. Henderson A H, Pearson J E G Thorax 1968; 23: 519
179. Remy J et al Diag Radiol 1977; 122: 33
180. Shneerson J M, Emerson P A, Phillips R M Thorax 1980; 35: 953
181. Rafferty P, Biggs B A et al Thorax 1983; 38: 579
182. Robinson L A, Reed E C, Galbraith T A et al J Thorac Cardiovasc Surg 1995; 109: 1182
183. Editorial Br Med J 1968; 3: 755
184. Whitehead B F, Rees P G, Sorensen K et al Eur J Cardio-thorac Surg 1995; 9: 1
185. Cooper J D, Patterson G A, Trulock E P J Thorac Cardiovasc Surg 1994; 107: 460
186. Millard F J C, Pepper J R In: Brewis R A L, Gibson G J, Geddes D M (eds) Respiratory Medicine. Baillière Tindall, London 1990 p 1407
187. Daly R C, Mucha P et al Ann Emerg Med 1985; 14: 865

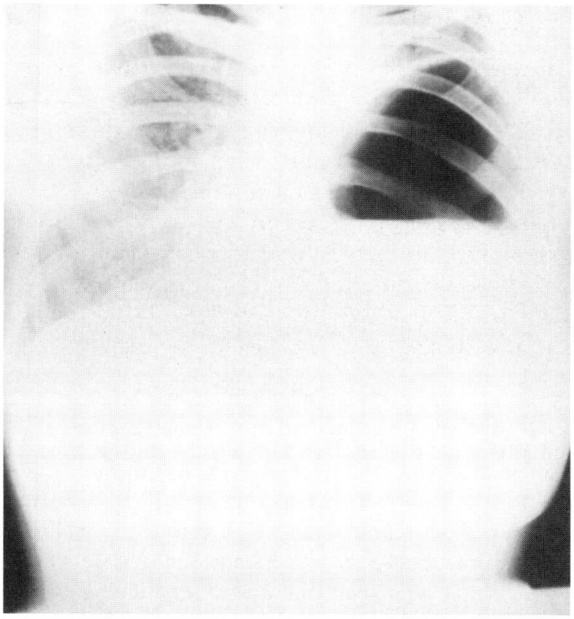

Fig. 22.28 The chest radiograph of a young patient with chest pain and dyspnoea. The air–fluid level was interpreted as a hydropneumothorax. However, the unusual upward displacement of the lung should have alerted the wary to other possibilities, such as a hernia.

In deciding the site of drain insertion it matters little whether air or fluid is being removed from the pleural space. During profound expiration the diaphragm may rise to the fifth interspace and chest drains should not be inserted below this level. Drains inserted anterior to the anterior axillary line will produce an ugly and visible scar and on the left may imperil the heart. Drains inserted posterior to the posterior axillary line are uncomfortable when the patient is sitting or lying. Chest drains should therefore be inserted into the line of the axilla, above the fifth interspace.[188] The size of chest drain used is limited by the width of the intercostal space. The largest tube which can be comfortably accommodated should be inserted at all times. A small chest drain is no less uncomfortable, also its small lumen produces greater resistance to drainage and it may kink more easily. In most situations a size 28 French gauge chest drain should be used in an adult.

The technique of insertion is important. Severe force is unnecessary, always painful, and may be dangerous. After thorough infiltration of local anaesthetic, a generous skin incision should be made and a track through the intercostal muscles created using a spreading action with strong scissors or an artery forcep. The track should be created to, if not through, the parietal pleura so that the chest drain and its introducer may be inserted without force. When it is correctly positioned, it may be held in place with a single suture which has both a pursestring and retention components (Fig. 22.30). The pleural drain should be connected to an underwater seal device which functions as a one-way valve (Fig. 22.31). The Heimlich valve[189] (Fig. 22.32) is undesirable as the leaflets adhere when wet. However, this device affords increased mobility which may be of crucial importance in the battlefield setting.

The rapid removal of large effusions may result in re-expansion

a

b

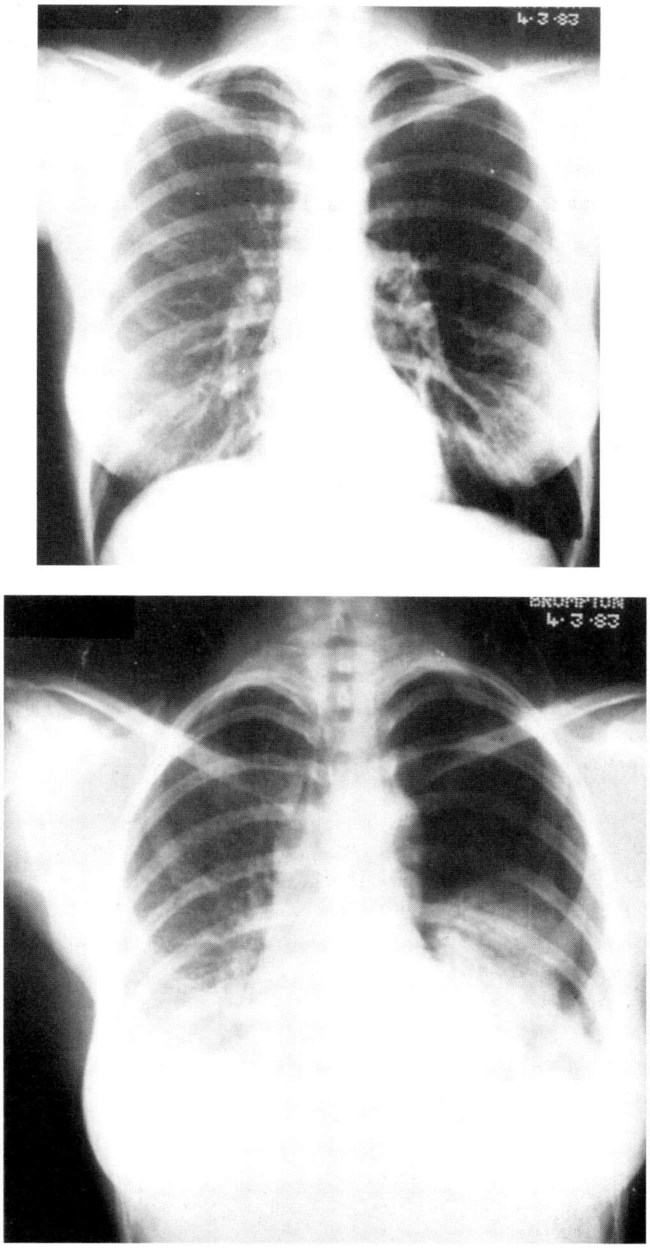

Fig. 22.29 **(a)** An orthodox and inspiratory chest radiograph taken on the suspicion of a left pneumothorax. A lung edge is visible but requires a strong light to be clearly seen. **(b)** An expiratory radiograph is unequivocal. The edge of the lung, now more dense, can be seen against the air trapped in the pleural space.

pulmonary oedema.[190] Although this is rare, it is prudent to remove large effusions slowly over the course of a few hours. Gentle suction may be desirable to drain the pleural space more effectively and to overcome the slight hydrostatic resistance of the

REFERENCES

189. Hemlich J H Dis Chest 1968; 53: 282
188. Goldstraw P In: Brewis R A L, Gibson G J, Geddes D M (eds) Respiratory Medicine. Bailliere Tindall, London 1990 p 349
190. Trapnell D H, Thuston J G B Lancet 1970; i: 1367

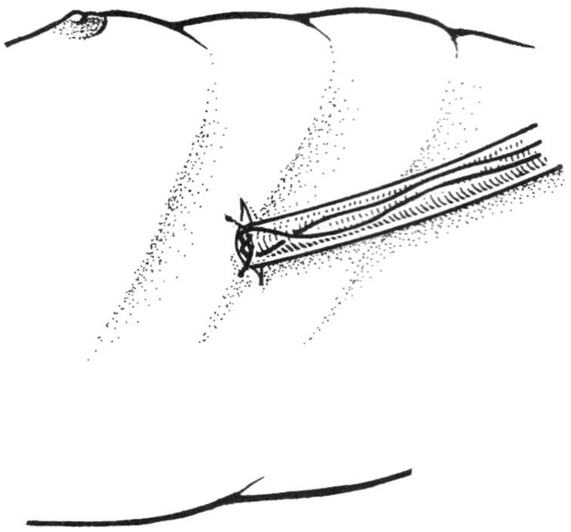

Fig. 22.30 A suitable suture to secure a chest drain. The pursestring prevents air entering the chest or fluid draining around the tube. It is drawn tight around the tube with a double throw which does not lock. The tails of the suture then surround and grip the tube 5 cm from the skin, preventing outward displacement of the drain. When the drain is removed the tails are cut near this knot and the pursestring suture closes the skin defect and is tied tight.

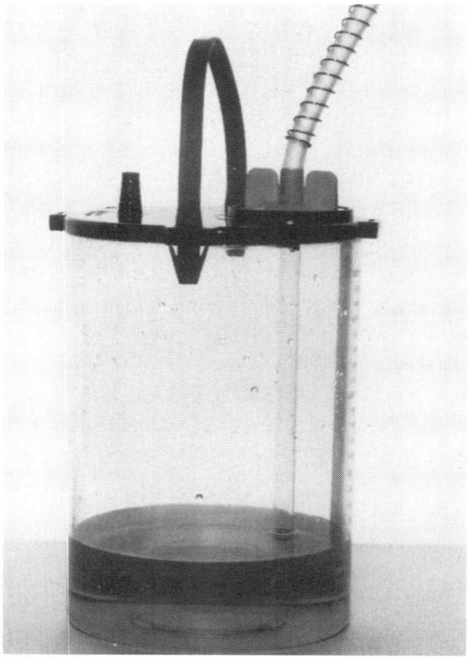

Fig. 22.31 An underwater drainage bottle used to provide one-way drainage of an intercostal tube. The long limb passing under the water is attached to the drain in the patient; the short limb above the level of the fluid in the bottle is left open or, if desired, may be connected to suction.

underwater seal. Suction at 2–5 kPa (15–40 cm of water) should be administered by a well regulated device capable of dealing with the high volumes of air which leak from a damaged lung. The Roberts suction pump does not fulfil these criteria and if wall suction is not available a high-volume suction device such as the Vernon-Thompson or Clements pump should be used.

It is self-evident that chest drains cannot function if obstructed,

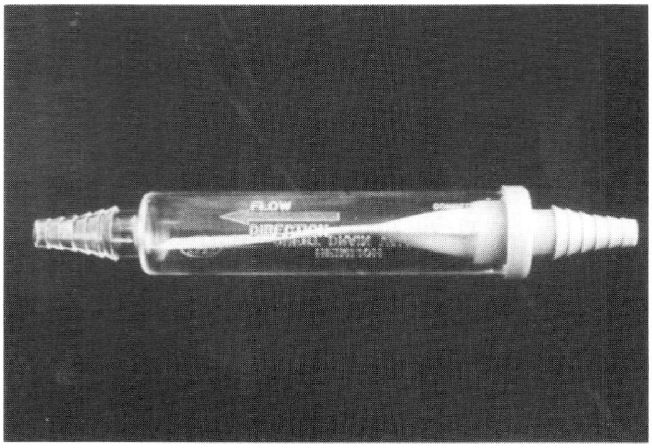

Fig. 22.32 The Heimlich valve used by some as a portable one-way valve on intercostal drains. Unfortunately the leaflets adhere together when wet and the valve becomes obstructive.

and they should never be clamped. It is perfectly possible to devise safe nursing practices to permit patients to move freely around the ward or hospital with their chest drain continuing to function. When transporting patients to and from the operating theatre or X-ray department the chest drain and its connecting tubing should be clearly visible on top of the bedclothes, passing down the middle of the bed or trolley to an underwater seat bottle securely retained in a basket fixed to the foot of the bed, but below bed level. All connections should be secure; the use of tape is unnecessary and may merely obscure disconnection. Daily chest radiographs should be taken to check that the chest drain is positioned satisfactorily and fulfilling the desired task. The removal of chest drains should be undertaken when they are no longer functioning, once there is full radiographic expansion of the lung, and air and fluid have ceased to drain. It is desirable to delay removal of the drain until respiratory fluctuation on the underwater seal is less than 2 or 3 cm. This indicates that the pleural space is obliterated by fibrinous adhesions, at least in the region of the chest drain. A pneumothorax will not develop, even if air enters the chest during removal of the drain. The retention knot should be cut and the chest drain removed smoothly but quickly whilst the patient holds a Valsalva manoeuvre. The pursestring suture is then tied. A further chest radiograph should then be taken immediately after removal.

Pneumothorax

Air may enter the pleural space through a chest wound or by damage to the oesophagus, trachea or main bronchus, but in most situations the leakage of air occurs from the lung itself. Air leak from the lung may be spontaneous or secondary to trauma. Such injury may result from blunt or penetrating chest trauma such as the insertion of a central venous line. Pneumothorax may occur during intermittent positive pressure ventilation or during severe asthmatic attacks.

A spontaneous pneumothorax may result from localized or generalized lung disease. Focal lung disease responsible for a pneumothorax includes an air-filled cyst, a solitary and presumably congenital bulla, but is very commonly associated with localized scarring and blebs beneath the visceral pleura. These blebs are usually localized to the apex of the lung but can on occasions be found elsewhere, such as on the apical segment of the lower lobe. The aetiology of this condition is unknown, but it is most common in tall, asthenic, otherwise fit young men.[191] Fanciful explanations have been suggested, including that the blebs result from trauma due to a sharp second rib.[192] Such focal lung abnormalities are found in Marfan's syndrome and it has been suggested that a forme fruste of this condition may be responsible for other sufferers.[193] There is a strong family history in many cases of spontaneous pneumothorax, but this may be related to stature. Spontaneous pneumothorax may complicate tuberculosis or be related to a carcinoma of the lung. Pneumothorax associated with generalized lung disease is most commonly secondary to severe bullous emphysema but also occurs with cystic fibrosis, sarcoidosis and other fibrosing lung conditions. The incidence of spontaneous pneumothorax thus has a bimodal age distribution. The first peak occurs in patients in their late teens and early twenties and is usually related to localized apical blebs. The second peak is found in the sixth and seventh decade, usually in elderly smokers with severe generalized emphysema.

Pneumothorax, whether spontaneous or secondary, may be complicated by intrapleural bleeding. Such a haemopneumothorax is a serious problem as the volume of blood lost is frequently underestimated. The bleeding may occur from trauma to the intercostal vessels, damage to the lung parenchyma, or by rupture of vascular adhesions across the pleural space.

The immediate management of a pneumothorax is largely uninfluenced by its aetiology. Shallow pneumothoraces may be treated conservatively as long as sequential chest radiographs show that a further air leak has not occurred and that resorption is proceeding. If the lung has collapsed more than 2 cm from the chest wall, more aggressive treatment is indicated. Whilst air may be removed by repeated aspiration, an intercostal drain will allow more continuous drainage and carries less risk of further trauma to the underlying lung. Surgery should be undertaken to control the air leak if it continues at a brisk level, and especially if there is a failure of expansion of the lung. Clearly it is prudent to proceed more swiftly to surgery in an otherwise fit young adult, and persist with intercostal drainage for a longer period of time in a frail old patient with severe generalized lung disease. Surgery should be considered, however, if the air leak persists beyond 1 week.

Recurrent spontaneous pneumothorax may prove troublesome and with each recurrence the risk of further incidence increases. In the healthy young adult the risk of a second pneumothorax following successful treatment of the first is 40%. Following first recurrence, this risk rises to 60%, and with second and subsequent recurrences may be as high as 80%.[194] It is usual to recommend surgical pleurodesis following the first or second recurrence. In the elderly patient more recurrences are permitted before undertaking pleurodesis and less satisfactory methods of pleurodesis may have to be used.

Conventional surgery for troublesome pneumothorax is through a limited lateral thoracotomy,[195,196] when the parietal pleura is abraded or excised (pleurectomy) and the air leak controlled. The results of such surgery are excellent with low morbidity and long-term protection against recurrence. However, video-assisted thoracoscopic surgery techniques are gaining in popularity[197]. These minimally invasive approaches result in better cosmesis, may reduce hospital stay and produce less pain in the short term. It remains to be seen whether the long-term results are as good, and early experience suggests this might not prove to be the case.

A tension pneumothorax is rare, but potentially lethal. It results from a ball-valve effect which allows air to enter the pleural space but not to leave. There is a progressive accumulation of air and an increasingly positive pressure develops in the pneumothorax. Tension most commonly results from the chest wound and is extremely rare following spontaneous pneumothorax. The presence of tension is evident clinically with respiratory distress, unmoving prominence of one hemithorax, mediastinal and tracheal shift towards the other hemithorax, and an absence of breath sounds on the side of the pneumothorax. It calls for immediate relief of the tension by the insertion of a large-bore drip catheter. When the tension is relieved radiographs should be taken prior to intercostal drainage. With any large pneumothorax the intrapleural pressure on the affected side becomes less negative than on the opposite side, resulting in mediastinal shift to the other side, but this does not indicate tension.

Catamenial pneumothorax occurs in young women recurrently within a few days of menstruation.[198] The aetiology of this fascinating condition is unknown. On rare occasions it may be associated with pleural endometriosis, or pleuroperitoneal defects may be noted at thoracotomy. In most such cases, however, the underlying condition is the apical pleural blebs so common in this age group, and the timing is presumably related to the changes in lung compliance with the fluid retention which precedes menstruation.

Surgical emphysema results from air tracking into subcutaneous tissues. It may be evident clinically from the typical crackling sensations on palpation and, if severe, may produce a strange 'helium' quality to phonation. Surgical emphysema may be evident on a chest radiograph and is sometimes restricted to the mediastinum. If gross, surgical emphysema may obscure the chest radiograph, making the detection of an underlying pneumothorax difficult (Fig. 22.33, 22.34). Severe surgical emphysema may track superiorly into the neck and face, making opening of the eyelids impossible (Fig. 22.34), or even track inferiorly into the scrotum. Although sometimes distressing, surgical emphysema requires no treatment. The patient should be strongly reassured and attention should focus on the underlying cause. Surgical emphysema following oesophagoscopy is of serious import as it indicates oesophageal rupture. If surgical emphysema is associated with a

REFERENCES

191. Withers J N, Fisback M E, Kiehl P V, Hannon J L Am J Surg 1964; 108: 772
192. Stephenson S F Thorax 1976; 31: 369
193. Wood J R, Bellamy D et al Thorax 1984; 39: 780
194. Gaensler E A Surg Gynecol Obstet 1956; 102: 293
195. Beardsley J M, Pahigian V M, Providence R I Surgery 1951; 30: 967
196. Martini N, Bains M S, Beattie E J Cancer 1975; 35: 734
197. Naunheim K S, Mack M J, Hazelrigg S R et al J Thorac Cardiovasc Surg 1995; 109: 1198
198. Grevy Ch, Anderen H J et al Thorac Cardiovasc Surg 1987; 35: 238

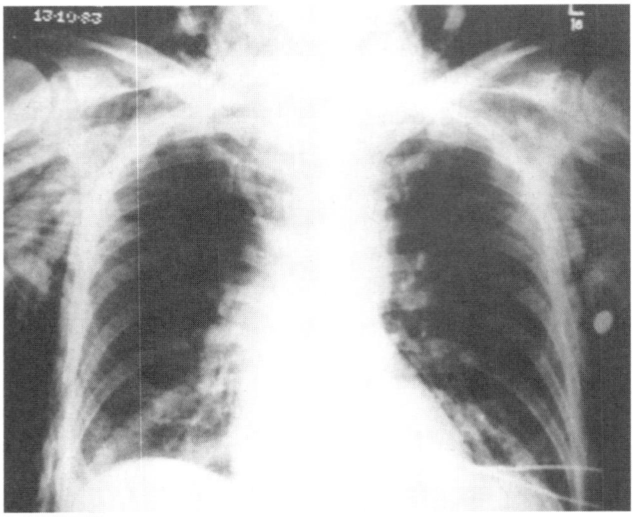

Fig. 22.33 A chest radiograph of a patient with gross surgical emphysema. Air can be seen in the soft tissues of the neck and chest wall. There was an underlying right pneumothorax but this was difficult to see.

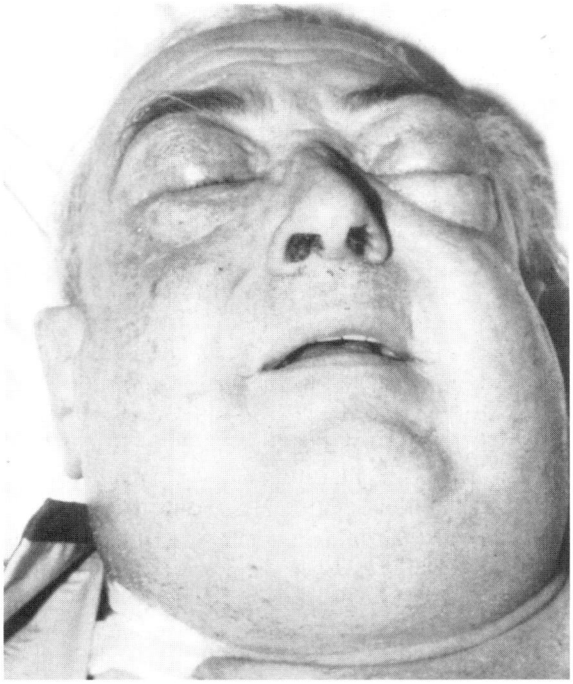

Fig. 22.34 Gross surgical emphysema causing swelling of the face and preventing the eyelids from opening.

pneumothorax, intercostal drainage should be undertaken. However, great caution must be taken in interpreting chest radiographs in this situation. If surgical emphysema results from chest trauma and lung injury is not apparent, damage to other hollow viscera should be sought by barium or gastrografin contrast swallow and bronchoscopic examinations. Localized surgical emphysema will occur around any penetrating chest wound and need not be associated with an underlying pneumothorax.

Malignant pleural effusion

Malignant pleural effusions are the ones most commonly referred to the thoracic surgeon. Malignant bronchial obstruction will lead to consolidation of the lung and may result in a benign effusion. Once these have been shown to be serous and cytologically negative they have little impact on the management of the underlying condition.[77] Malignant effusions, however, may result from visceral pleural invasion by a peripheral carcinoma of the lung or by metastatic involvement of the pleura by adenocarcinoma derived from the lung, breast or other sites. On occasions the primary may not be identified.

The diagnosis is usually made by aspiration cytology or needle biopsy of the pleura. Should these techniques fail, then surgical biopsy by open pleural biopsy through a limited thoracotomy or by video-assisted thorascopic surgery is indicated. Biopsy should not be taken from the visceral pleural surface as a troublesome air leak may result. If repeated pleural aspiration has led to fibrin deposition, open pleural biopsy is to be preferred, since thoracoscopy may in these circumstances be hazardous, or biopsy may fail to detect the underlying condition.[199] Metastatic involvement of the pleura precludes surgical cure and only palliative treatment is possible. Metastatic tumours from the breast may respond to hormonal manipulation (see Ch. 25). If malignant effusions are symptomatic and recurrent, pleurodesis should be undertaken. This is usually performed using video-assisted thorascopic surgical techniques, but occasionally fibrin or adhesions prevent good access and a limited thoracotomy is necessary. If the lung is prevented from expanding to fill the hemithorax then pleurodesis is ineffective and the insertion of a pleuro-peritoneal shunt is necessary. Successful palliation can be achieved by pleurodesis or shunting in over 90% of patients.[200] The patient may lead an active and enjoyable life once the pleural effusion has been controlled, until other manifestations of the malignancy occur, which may on occasions be as long as 2 or 3 years later. In contrast, repeated attempts at pleural aspiration may lead to empyema, a troublesome complication which seriously blights the patient's remaining life.

Haemothorax

Blood may collect in the pleural space as a result of trauma or following pneumothorax: 2–3 litres may accumulate without overt signs of loss. Treatment consists of volume replacement and intercostal drainage. Thoracotomy is indicated if blood loss continues or if significant clot remains within the pleural space. Pleural endometriosis is a rare cause of this condition.[201]

Chylothorax

Chylothorax is discovered on aspirating an effusion and discovering the typical milky fluid of chyle. It must be differentiated from

REFERENCE

199. Page R D et al Ann Thorac Surg 1989; 48: 66
200. Petrou M, Kaplan D, Goldstraw P Cancer 1995; 75: 801
201. Stern H, Toole A L, Merrin M Chest 1980; 78: 480

the chyliform appearance of a long-standing effusion or haemothorax. The latter is caused by large amounts of cholesterol in the fluid, but chylomicrons and triglycerides are only found in true chylous effusions. Chylothorax may result from trauma to the thoracic duct or from malignant obstruction to lymphatic return. Trauma to the thoracic duct may result from blunt or penetrating chest injury, or following thoracotomy to repair a patent ductus arteriosus or to undertake oesophageal resection. Malignant obstruction of the thoracic duct is common with lymphomas but has been reported when lymph nodes are replaced by carcinoma, most commonly of breast or lung origin.[202,203]

Chylothorax may be associated with congenital lymphatic defects and lymphatic reflux, usually associated with chylous ascites. Spontaneous chylothorax may occur, but is a diagnosis of exclusion. CT of the mediastinum is a sensitive test to detect enlarged lymph nodes which may be obscured by the mediastinal outline or by large effusions. With treatment of the underlying condition the chylothorax may resolve. If the effusion is unresponsive or large, intercostal drainage should be undertaken.

The continued loss of large volumes of chyle has profound nutritional and immunological consequences. Whilst the nutritional consequences may be minimized by the initiation of an elemental diet and the addition of medium-chain triglycerides, the immunological consequences of lymphocyte depletion will predispose to infection after 10–14 days.[204] If chylous leak continues beyond 1 week, surgical treatment should be undertaken. Chylothorax following thoracotomy is unlikely to settle on conservative management, and re-exploration is usually necessary within 3 or 4 days. If the site of the leak cannot be determined, mass ligation of the thoracic duct should be performed as it courses through the aortic hiatus. Mass ligation of the structures in this area may be undertaken by thoracotomy or laparotomy.[205] Recurrent chylothorax may be prevented by video-assisted thoracoscopic surgical control of the site of leak,[206] with or without pleurodesis. Pleuroperitoneal shunting is an attractive alternative in children.[207]

Pleurodesis

Pleurodesis is the obliteration of the pleural space and successfully prevents recurrence of pneumothorax, haemothorax, effusion or chylothorax. Pleural obliteration may occur spontaneously following a single episode of inflammation or be induced by the insertion of a chest drain. The older rubber tubes provoked a brisk inflammatory response, and may have been more effective in this respect than the inert plastic material used in modern chest drains.

A variety of sclerosants have been utilized to produce pleurodesis. These include blood, tetracycline, bleomycin and lyophilized *Corynebacterium parvum*.[208] The action of these agents is that of a chemical irritant and is independent of their other properties. These agents may be injected into the pleural space or instilled through a chest drain. The choice of agent will depend on the underlying condition, but the best agents—bleomycin and *Corynebacterium parvum*—will prevent recurrence in approximately 70% of patients with malignant pleural effusion.[209] Talcum powder insufflated into the pleural space is extremely effective, achieving pleurodesis in 90% of cases,[210] but the severe pain induced requires general anaesthesia. Talc is insufflated through the videothoracoscope at the time of pleural biopsy if lung expansion appears satisfactory. Surgical pleurodesis, at thoracotomy or using video-assisted thoracoscopic surgical techniques, may be achieved by abrading the pleura with a dry gauze,[195] or by pleurectomy, stripping the parietal pleura from the lateral chest wall and superior mediastinum.[196] These surgical methods are extremely effective and will prevent recurrence of a pneumothorax in all patients with localized lung disease. Where lung disease is generalized surgical treatment should be supplemented with talc insufflation.

Any technique of pleurodesis reduces chest wall excursion and the resultant restrictive ventilatory defect may reduce lung function temporarily. Young patients in particular must be encouraged to undertake vigorous exercise with adequate analgesia, and will then regain normal lung function within a few months of surgery.

Empyema

Pus within the pleural space—an empyema—may result from a number of medical or surgical conditions. A pre-existing effusion or haemothorax is often evident, and in other cases may be presumed to have been present. Bacteria migrate into this fluid from adjacent infective sources or reach it by haematogenous spread. The site of origin can sometimes be inferred by bacteriological analysis of the empyema fluid.[211] Empyema most commonly results from infection of the underlying lung by pneumonia or lung abscess, and lung pathogens such as *Streptococcus pneumoniae*, *Klebsiella pneumoniae* or staphylococci will be found in the pleural fluid. Less commonly, infection may extend through the diaphragm from an adjacent subphrenic abscess, and coliform organisms may be found in the empyema pus. If empyema complicates surgery or results from penetrating chest trauma, *Staphylococcus aureus* is the most common organism. Empyema from upper-gut organisms may originate in the mediastinum following perforation of the oesophagus. Overall the organisms most commonly responsible for empyema are the staphylococci but in as many as one quarter of cases no organism is found, presumably because of prior antibiotic treatment.

Bacterial contamination of a sympathetic effusion results in protein exudation and migration of white blood cells and fibroblasts. With time, the effusion becomes increasingly viscous, and

REFERENCES

202. MacFarlane J R, Holman C W Am Rev Resp Dis 1972; 105: 287
203. Bessone L N, Ferguson T B, Burford T M Ann Thorac Surg 1971; 12: 527
204. Selle J G, Snyder W H, Schreiber J T Ann Surg 1973; 177: 245
205. Ross J K Thorax 1961; 16: 12
206. Inderbitzi R G C, Krebs T, Stirnemann P, Althaus U J Thorac Cardiovasc Surg 1992; 104: 209
207. Murphy M C, Newman B M, Rodgers B M Ann Thorac Surg 1989; 48: 195
208. Fentiman I S Br J Hosp Med 1987; 37: 421
209. Austin E H, Flye M W Ann Thorac Surg 1979; 28: 190
210. Daniel T M, Tribble C G, Rodgers B M Ann Thorac Surg 1990; 50: 186
211. Bartlett P C et al Lancet 1974; i: 338

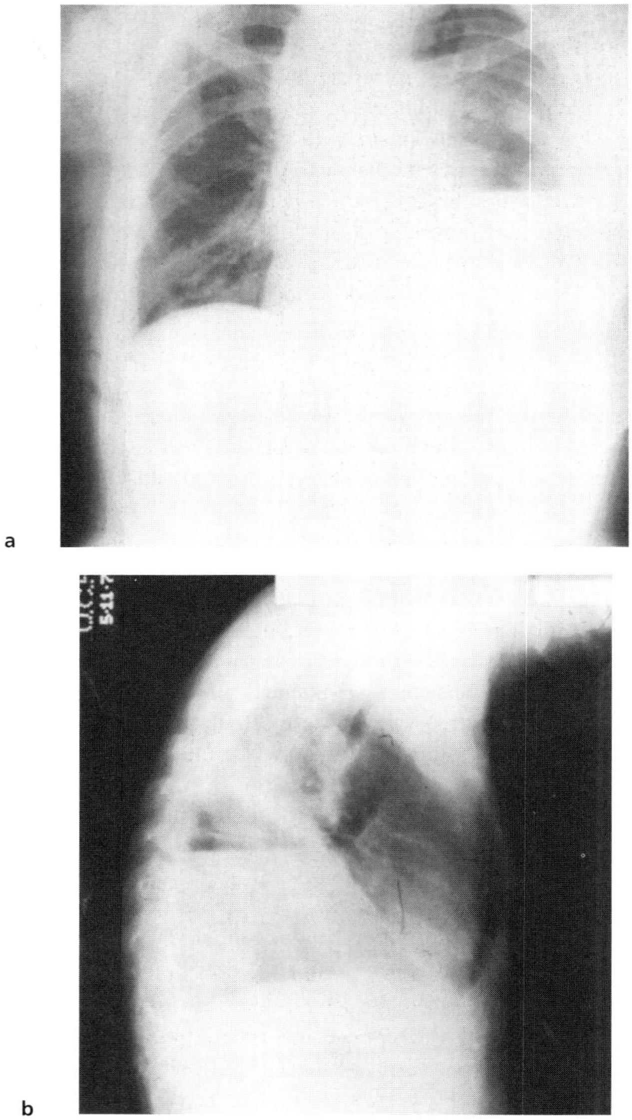

Fig. 22.35 The (a) posteroanterior and (b) lateral chest radiograph of a patient with a large left empyema. The abscess typically lies posteriorly at the lowest point of the pleural space. The fluid level indicates that, in this case, the abscess communicates with the lung through a bronchopleural fistula.

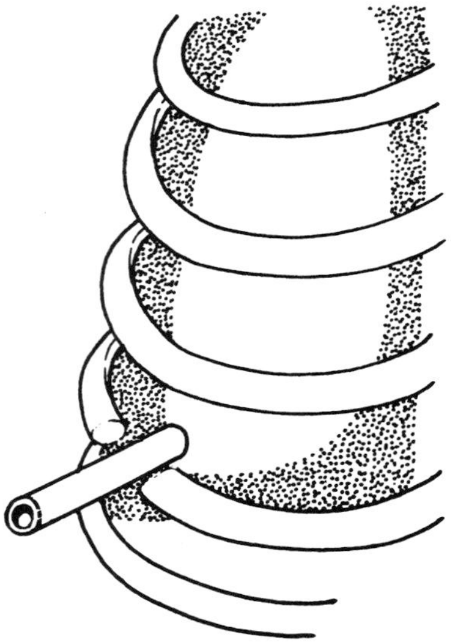

Fig. 22.36 A diagram to show an open drain inserted through a short rib resection into the base of a chronic empyema.

the viscosity of the pleural fluid is a good indication of the chronicity of the infection. The infective process becomes localized, as lamellae of fibrin and maturing fibrous tissue progressively form on the visceral and parietal pleura. Gravity and the configuration of the pleural space ensure that the majority of empyemata lie posteriorly adjacent to the diaphragm, at the most dependent area of the pleural space (Fig. 22.35). The fibrous cortex is continuous, but may be considered as having a visceral component, covering the pleura over the lung, and a parietal component, over the pleura of the mediastinum, diaphragm and lateral chest wall. The visceral cortex restricts movement of the lung and the parietal cortex causes progressive contraction and immobility of the overlying chest wall.

Management depends upon the chronicity of the empyema, as indicated by the viscosity of the pus, and the degree of illness of the patient. Early in the development of any empyema, watery pus is aspirated, providing evidence of an infected effusion. The appropriate antibiotic should be commenced and all the infected fluid removed. Whilst successes undoubtedly occur using repeated pleural aspiration, the insertion of a chest drain ensures continued and complete evacuation of all infected fluid. The reports of successful video-assisted thoracoscopic surgical treatment of empyema are probably in this situation, and amount to little more than debridement of fibrinous material.[212]

When the aspirated pus is thick and turbid, the empyema is already chronic and will be associated with a thick fibrous cortex. Antibiotics at this stage may reduce toxicity, but are unlikely to be curative. A chest drain should be inserted. Such a drain is not within the pleural space, but into the abscess cavity within the pleural space. The surrounding fibrous cortex prevents collapse of the underlying lung, and underwater seal is unnecessary. The tube may be left open, draining into a dressing or colostomy bag. Such an open drain may be required for some months and hence a large tube is inserted by removing a short segment of the underlying rib (Fig. 22.36). Preliminary injection of a dense radiopaque material into the empyema space defines its inferior margin (Fig. 22.37) and allows the rib resection to be optimally sited.

Following rib resection, long-term open drainage usually improves the patient's general condition. Serial chest radiographs will demonstrate progressive obliteration of the empyema cavity. Such long-term care can be managed with the patient at home, mobilizing and resuming normal activities. Pus will drain into a colostomy bag which the patient empties each day. The district nurse will supervise the changing of this bag every few days and the patient should be seen by the surgeon at 3- or 4-weekly

REFERENCE

212. Ferguson M K Ann Thorac Surg 1993; 56: 644

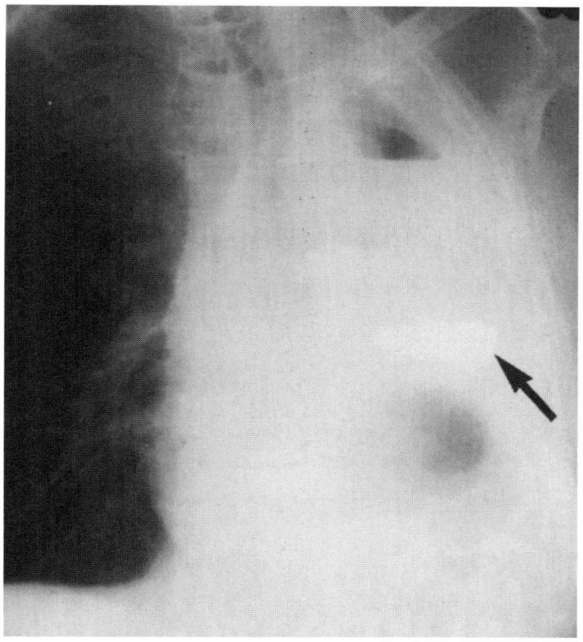

Fig. 22.37 The posteroanterior chest radiograph of a patient with a post-pneumonectomy empyema. To aid the siting of a drain, contrast has been injected into the empyema (arrowed) to provide an empyemagram, showing the most dependent limits of the empyema.

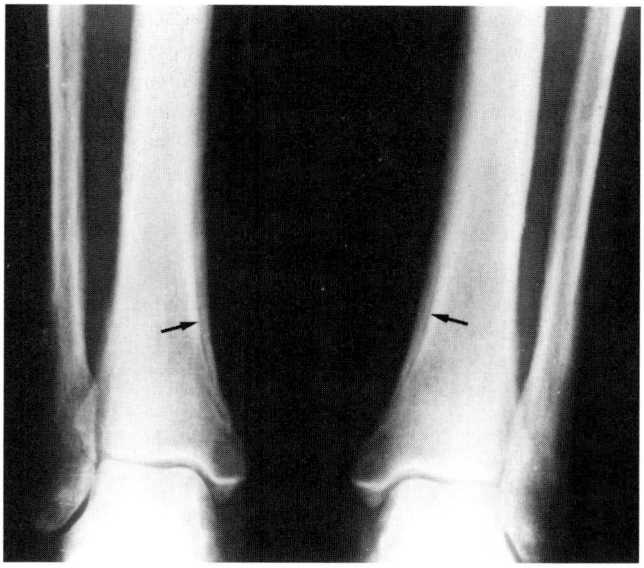

Fig. 22.38 Subperiosteal new bone formation of the tibia (arrowed) is evident on this radiograph of a patient with hypertrophic pulmonary osteoarthropathy.

intervals so that the open drain can be replaced and chest radiographs taken to monitor progress.

Once the cavity is too small to be seen on a chest radiograph, its further resolution should be checked periodically by inserting radiopaque dye through the drainage tube. When such a sinogram shows the cavity is completely obliterated, the tube is removed. Success usually takes many months, and in some circumstances a drain may be necessary indefinitely.

Thoracotomy will achieve a more rapid resolution and should be considered as a primary treatment in fit young adults or in older patients following a period of open drainage, if fitness permits and resolution is slow.[213] Surgical treatment entails decortication[214] to remove the fibrous cortex, allowing re-expansion of the underlying lung. If the lung is irretrievably damaged by pyogenic or tuberculous infection, usually evident on CT, concurrent pulmonary resection may be necessary. Access at thoracotomy may be difficult because of crowding of the ribs and the rigidity of the underlying cortex. The parietal cortex is stripped from within the chest wall by removing it with the parietal pleura. Excision of the abscess cavity is then completed by removing the visceral cortex from the lung, taking care not to damage the visceral pleura. If difficulties are encountered in removing the cortex over the diaphragm it may be left over this area. With full expansion of the underlying lung the pleural space is obliterated and infection eradicated. Any breach in the visceral pleura will result in a persistent air leak which may require intercostal drainage for 2 or 3 weeks.

Decortication is frequently confused with parietal pleurectomy. In the former, removal of the parietal pleura is a tactical expedient to facilitate excision of the parietal cortex, whereas in the latter its removal is to produce a pleurodesis.

If an empyema is neglected it may rupture into the bronchial tree, forming a bronchopleural fistula, or erode into the subcutaneous tissues, presenting as an empyema necessitans. Such chronic infection may result in amyloid disease or hypertrophic pulmonary osteoarthropathy or be complicated by systemic abscesses in the brain.

Pleural tumours

Benign tumours of the pleura are rare, the most common being a fibroma, otherwise known as a benign localized mesothelioma.[215] These tumours are sharply demarcated, usually pedunculated, and arise from the visceral pleura. They may be associated with hypertrophic pulmonary osteoarthropathy. This fascinating condition is associated with gross finger-clubbing and there is subperiosteal new bone formation, most commonly on the distal tibia and fibula (Fig. 22.38), proximal tibia and fibula, and distal radius and ulna. This condition may be associated with many other pulmonary conditions,[216] but the vast majority of such cases are associated with non-small cell carcinoma of the lung. Pleural fibromata may become extremely large and produce dyspnoea. This, and diagnostic difficulty, makes resection justified.

Primary pleural malignancy—mesothelioma—is associated with a known exposure to asbestos in 50% of sufferers. There is evidence that the incidence of this disease will continue to increase well into the next century because of the delay between exposure

REFERENCES

213. LeRoux B T, Mohlala M L et al Current Problems in Surgery. Year Book Medical Publishers, Chicago 1986 p 5
214. Sampson P C, Burford T H J Thorac Cardiovasc Surg 1947; 16: 127
215. Briselli M, Mark E J, Dickersin R Cancer 1981; 47: 2678
216. Goldstraw P, Walbaum P R Thorax 1976; 31: 205

and development of the disease.[217] Mesothelioma is locally malignant, with widespread but superficial invasion of the lung, diaphragm and chest wall (Fig. 22.390). Mediastinal node secondaries or peritoneal deposits are found at post mortem in 25% of patients.[218] The diagnosis is often difficult and frequently delayed. Patients may present with an effusion but more usually there is a long history of persistent chest pain and progressive pleural shadowing. Aspiration cytology is unreliable, but closed-needle biopsy may be diagnostic. Frequently open pleural biopsy is necessary to diagnose malignancy confidently and to determine the cell type.[219] Mesothelioma is only slowly progressive. The mean survival following diagnosis is around 2 years[220] and there are anecdotal reports of long-term survival without treatment.

Mesothelioma is resistant to chemotherapy, but radiotherapy may be effective in relieving pain from localized chest wall invasion, which may occur at sites of biopsy or through a thoracotomy incision. Prophylactic irradiation of biopsy sites has been shown to considerably reduce the frequency of such implants.[221] Surgical excision has been attempted, but success has been limited to the occasional fit patient who has an unusually localized tumour of the epithelial variant of mesothelioma.[222] Surgery is devastatingly extensive, usually requiring excision of the underlying lung and diaphragm. The high mortality of this operation and the long-term prognosis without treatment make attempts at resection unjustified in the vast majority of patients. Pain control is important. If analgesic drugs fail, neurosurgical intervention may help. If effusion is recurrent and troublesome, surgical palliation by pleurodesis or pleuro-peritoneal shunting is effective.[200] The unfortunate sufferers of this uniformly fatal disease are eligible for compensation but this is far greater if an unequivocal industrial link can be established.

Secondary carcinoma of the pleura may occur with mesothelial metastases from adenocarcinoma of the lung, breast or other sites. These patients present with recurrent pleural effusion which is usually unilateral. The condition is incurable, but the surgeon may help by establishing the diagnosis and preventing troublesome effusions by pleurodesis or pleuro-peritoneal shunting.[200]

a

b

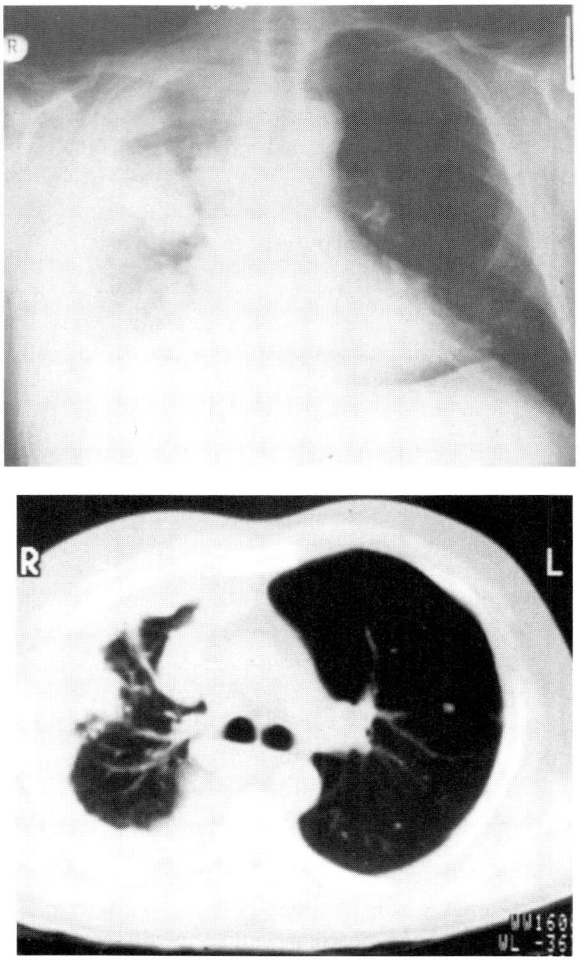

Fig. 22.39 (a) The chest radiograph of a patient with mesothelioma. There is irregular and nodular thickening of the pleura, extending into the fissures, and contraction of the hemithorax. **(b)** The computerized tomography scan shows these features more readily.

THE DIAPHRAGM

The diaphragm is an important muscle of respiration. Respiration requires a negative intrapleural pressure, and the diaphragm prevents the migration of abdominal viscera into the potential vacuum. Migration may occur through the normal foramina, such as the oesophageal hiatus, or through traumatic or congenital defects in the diaphragm (see Chapter 21).

Eventration

Eventration of the diaphragm is a symptomless anomaly, usually limited to the right hemidiaphragm and affecting the anteromedial quadrant.[223] In this area the diaphragm is thin and fibrous, and does not contract normally. It may be the result of a congenital defect but does not cause symptoms. Its main significance lies in its confusion with other more serious defects which have a similar radiological appearance.

Diaphragmatic paresis

When paralysed, the diaphragm is higher than usual on the chest radiograph and fails to contract when vigorous inhalation is studied by fluoroscopy. This paradoxical movement is more general than with eventration, and affects the whole of the hemidiaphragm. The phrenic nerve may be affected by neurological disease, such as poliomyelitis or shingles, or involved by intrathoracic malignancy,

REFERENCES

217. Peto J, Hodgson J T, Matthews F E, Jones J R Lancet 1995; 345: 535
218. Hillerdal G Br J Dis Chest 1983; 77: 321
219. Rudd R M In: Brewis R A L, Gibson G J, Geddes D M (eds) Respiratory Medicine. Baillière Tindall, London 1990 p 1254
220. Law M R, Hodson M E, Heard B Thorax 1982; 37: 810
221. Boutin C, Rey F, Viallat J Chest 1995; 108: 754
222. Sugarbaker D J, Mentzer S J, Strauss G Ann Thorac Surg 1992; 54: 941
223. Heitzman E R Clin Radiol 1990; 42: 15

such as lung cancer or a mediastinal tumour.[224] Phrenic paresis occasionally results from cardiac surgery, most commonly from damage during dissection of the left internal mammary artery for bypass grafting.[225] If all such causes are excluded, the paralysis may be attributed to a viral illness, and recovery usually occurs in a period of months.

Trauma to the diaphragm

Any severe compressive force applied to the lower thorax and upper abdomen may burst the diaphragm with immediate herniation of abdominal viscera through the stellate laceration in the central tendon (Fig. 22.40). This condition is often difficult to diagnose and a high level of awareness is necessary when treating patients with severe trauma.[226] Rupture occurs on the left in 90% of cases, and bilateral rupture has been reported.[227] On chest radiographs the superior margin of the herniated stomach may mimic a high hemidiaphragm, but identical radiological features are found with phrenic paralysis or congenital diaphragmatic eventration. The passage of a nasogastric tube or a limited barium examination may help visualize the position of the stomach, but cannot differentiate a diaphragmatic rupture from these other conditions.

If a diaphragmatic rupture is suspected, thoracotomy should be undertaken as soon as is allowed by the competing claims of other injuries. At thoracotomy the herniated viscera are inspected for damage, reduced, and the diaphragmatic tear sutured. Such tears are frequently stellate and may radiate to transect the phrenic nerve. Whilst plication of the diaphragm may reduce its paradoxical movement, it cannot restore normal contraction and some mechanical inefficiency is inevitable.[228]

The diaphragm may be perforated by penetrating trauma or impaled by sharp fragments of rib following blunt trauma. In such circumstances the force is applied predominantly from above the diaphragm, and there is usually no immediate herniation. It may be weeks or even years before the abdominal viscera exploit the diaphragmatic defect and herniate into the chest. A large hernia may result and the tight neck of the hernia predisposes to strangulation. Operative repair should always be undertaken.[229]

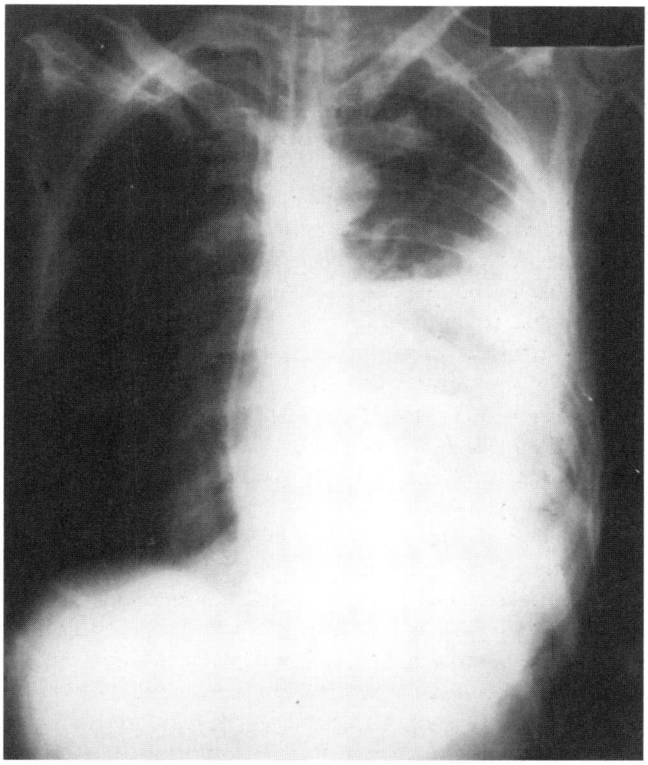

Fig. 22.40 The chest radiograph of a patient following major trauma in a road traffic accident. There is compression of the left lung and the left hemidiaphragm is obscured by pleural fluid and a complex shadow containing translucencies. Rupture of the left diaphragm must be suspected and thoracotomy was performed.

Congenital diaphragmatic hernia

Congenital diaphragmatic defects represent localized persistence of the pleuroperitoneal canal from a failure in septation. Such defects may be in the central tendon of one hemidiaphragm or peripherally and usually posteriorly, where the septum transversum fails to unite with the intercostal component of the diaphragm, resulting in a foramen of Bochdalek. Such defects may be evident at birth or cause respiratory distress in infancy. There is usually gross herniation of abdominal contents and hypoplasia of the ipsilateral lung, suggesting that herniation occurred in utero. Immediate repair should be undertaken once the general condition has been made optimal and respiratory acidosis temporarily corrected. Laparotomy provides adequate access. The prognosis depends on the severity of the associated pulmonary hypoplasia.

Herniation through the foramen of Morgagni usually presents in early adult life and may be found as a symptomless anterior mediastinal mass on routine chest radiographs. If very large, such hernias cause dyspnoea. The underlying defect in the diaphragm is presumably congenital. Reduction and repair may be undertaken via the chest or abdomen.

Tumours of the diaphragm

These are rare. All such tumours have similar radiological features. Rhabdomyosarcoma, fibrosarcoma and malignant fibrous histiocytoma have all been described,[230] and the diaphragm may be involved by more widespread pleural malignancy. The treatment of primary tumours is by wide excision of the diaphragm with prosthetic replacement using Marlex mesh. Adjuvant chemotherapy may be of value.

REFERENCES

224. Green M, LaRoche C M In: Brewis R A L, Gibson G J, Geddes D M (eds) Respiratory Medicine. Baillière Tindall, London 1990 p 1373
225. Estenne M, Yernault J C, De Smet J M, De Troyer A Thorax 1983; 40: 293
226. Arom K V In: Trinkle J K, Grover F L (eds) Management of Thoracic Trauma Victims. J B Lippincott, Philadelphia 1980 p 47
227. Lucido J L, Wall C H Arch Surg 1963; 86: 989
228. Graham D R et al Ann Thorac Surg 1990; 49: 248
229. Pearson S Arch Surg 1953; 66: 155
230. Venn G E, Gellister J et al J Thorac Cardiovasc Surg 1986; 91: 234

23 The heart and pericardium

Tom Treasure

OPERATING ON THE HEART

About 35 000 heart operations are performed each year in the United Kingdom. The majority are for coronary artery disease and, at a rate of about 400 per million of the population, this represents 65% of all heart surgery.[1–3] In the context of contemporary surgical methods, the heart is particularly amenable to the mechanistic approach that a surgeon can offer with restoration of blood supply and correction of mechanical and structural abnormalities.

It was the development of methods that enable the surgeon to interrupt the heart's function for long enough to perform the operation that permitted the enormous growth of cardiac surgery. The increasing complexity of conditions amenable to surgical correction, the extension of surgery into treatment of increasingly severe heart disease and the steady improvement in results have all depended upon refinement of cardiopulmonary bypass techniques. Operations for congenital abnormalities, valve disease and coronary atherosclerosis depend on the skilled application of the basic techniques for supporting the circulation, protecting the brain and preserving myocardial function, and these are therefore outlined first. It should be noted that there is renewed interest in operating on the heart while it continues to beat, avoiding the necessity to support the circulation.[4,5] Some coronary operations can be performed without cardiopulmonary bypass and the range of catheter and balloon techniques, although out of the hands of surgeons, is nevertheless part of the overall picture of treatment of heart disease by operative means.[6]

In 1925 Souttar wrote, on the subject of mitral stenosis: 'the problem is to a large extent mechanical, and as such should already be within the scope of surgery, were it not for the extraordinary nature of the conditions under which the problem must be attacked . . . and that apart from them the heart is as amenable to surgery as any other organ'.[7] In his day the only solution open to him was that 'in view of the extreme danger to the brain from even the shortest check to its blood supply . . . any manipulations which are carried out must therefore be executed in the full flow of the blood stream, and must not perceptibly interfere with the contractions of the heart'.[7]

Two strategies were developed and are now used, often in combination, to overcome this problem. First came the use of varying degrees of hypothermia to prolong the tolerance of the brain to ischaemia[8,9] and, secondly, the development of cardiopulmonary bypass—the biggest single advance in heart surgery.[10]

Hypothermia

The limit of the brain's tolerance to circulatory arrest is generally given as 3 minutes and while this is an accurate enough estimate, it is based upon collective experience rather than any precise knowledge of the tolerance of the different populations of neurones. It has also often been observed that children who have cooled rapidly by falling into icy water have survived long periods of cerebral ischaemia without evident brain damage. The protective effect of cooling is largely due to a reduction in oxygen requirement of the brain.[7] This knowledge was used to permit the earliest successful open heart surgery. Patients were anaesthetized with a vasodilating agent, cooled in a bath filled with ice and water until their core temperature approached 30°C and then the intracardiac part of the operation was performed during a few minutes of inflow occlusion and circulatory arrest.[9] This method was highly successful in the surgery of simple fossa ovalis atrial septal defects[11,12] but the time available was not long enough to permit more complex cardiac surgery to be performed, and allowed little time for thought. Any inaccuracy in the preoperative diagnosis or unexpected variation in the anatomy was disastrous.

Profound hypothermia was the logical extension of the method. It emerged empirically with uncertain time limits; sometimes an hour or more of circulatory arrest was used. More rigorous evaluation of clinical experience and laboratory experiments indicates that the technique allows up to about 40 minutes if the temperature is below 20°C.[13] It is now used in conjunction with cardiopulmonary bypass.

REFERENCES

1. UK Cardiac Surgery Registers for calendar years from 1979 to 1992 and for financial year 1993/4
2. Kumar P, Treasure T Coronary artery bypass graft trials Br J Hosp Med 1996 56(1): 33–36
3. Treasure T Br J Hosp Med 1990; 43: 459
4. Buffolo E, de Andrade J C S et al Ann Thorac Surg 1996; 61: 63
5. Westaby W Br Heart J 1995; 73: 203
6. Treasure T Recent Advances: Cardiac Surgery BMJ 1997; 314: 104–107
7. Souttar H S Br Med J 1925; 2: 603
8. Ross D N Guy's Hosp Rep 1954; 103: 97
9. Sellick B A Lancet 1957; i: 443
10. Gibbon J H Recent Advances in Cardiovascular Physiology and Surgery. University of Minnesota, Minneapolis 1953, p 107
11. Bedford D E, Holmes Sellors T et al Lancet 1957; i: 1255
12. Holmes Sellors T Ann R Coll Surg Engl 1970; 46: 1
13. Treasure T Ann R Coll Surg Engl 1984; 66: 235

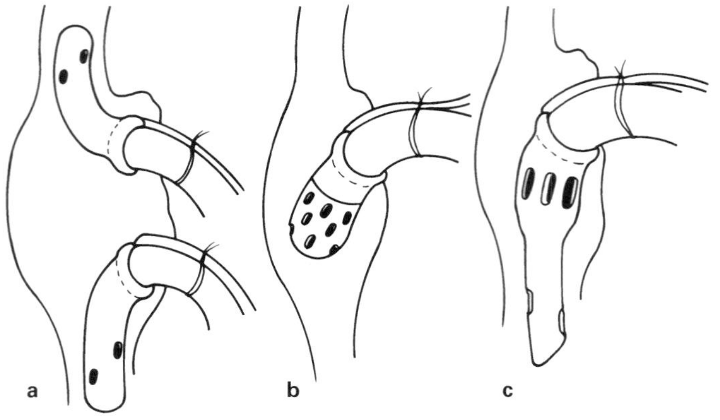

Fig. 23.1 (**a**) The venous return to the heart may be diverted by separate cannulation of the superior and inferior venae cavae which may be encircled with snares permitting operations to be performed within the right atrium. The coronary sinus venous return must then be collected separately. (**b**) A Ross basket in the right atrium permits total venous drainage and is the simplest technique for coronary artery surgery when the cardiac chambers are not opened. (**c**) A refinement with an extension into the inferior vena cava helps ensure that venous drainage is maintained as the heart is displaced to permit surgery to lateral or inferior coronary branches.

Cardiopulmonary bypass

Credit for the first pump oxygenator used clinically goes to Gibbon;[10] soon after, Kirklin[14] reported the first series of cases from the Mayo Clinic. Cardiopulmonary bypass is now routine. Blood is drained from the patient by a gravity siphon, either through a single cannula in the right atrium or separate cannulation of the superior and inferior venae cavae, depending on how much control of the right heart is required (Fig. 23.1). The blood runs through an oxygenator in which it is separated from a gas mixture by a system of membranes. The blood is then returned to the patient under pressure through a cannula which is usually positioned in the ascending aorta (Fig. 23.2). The flow is determined by an estimate of body surface area and is usually set at 2.4 litres/m^2. Reduction of temperature by 5–10°C is common practice but there are unresolved debates about the ideal pressure limits, the desirability of pulsed perfusion, and the optimum temperature.[15]

As judged by survival and relief of cardiac disease, results are excellent, but cardiopulmonary bypass is far from perfect. Deleterious effects on end-organs including the brain,[16,17] lungs, kidneys, liver, and on the total body inflammatory response occur with increasing severity with longer bypass time. There have been many studies showing changes in complement, neutrophil activation, free radical activity, and generation of cytokines.[18,19]

Myocardial protection

On cardiopulmonary bypass, the myocardium may be perfused normally through the coronary arteries as blood flows from the arterial cannula into the aortic root and the coronary ostia, but for many cardiac operations the perfusion of the heart muscle must be interrupted. In any operation where the left side of the heart is opened the aorta must be cross-clamped for periods of time to ensure that the heart does not eject air into the arterial circulation. When the aorta is to be opened, for example to replace the aortic valve, a cross-clamp must be applied between the perfusing cannula and the coronaries, rendering the myocardium ischaemic until the valve is replaced and the aorta closed again. A still, bloodless field is ideal if fine work is to be done (e.g. coronary artery surgery, neonatal surgery). Under all these circumstances the heart must be protected from the consequences of ischaemia. This may be kept to a minimum by direct cannulation of the coronary ostia during aortic valve surgery, or by intermittently releasing the clamp during mitral valve or coronary surgery.[20] Myocardial ischaemia seems to be well tolerated for up to about 15 minutes in a non-working heart, especially with the help of moderate cooling on bypass. More thorough cooling of the heart, especially by infusion of cold potassium solutions (about 20 mmol/l) into the

Components of a standard cardiopulmonary bypass circuit

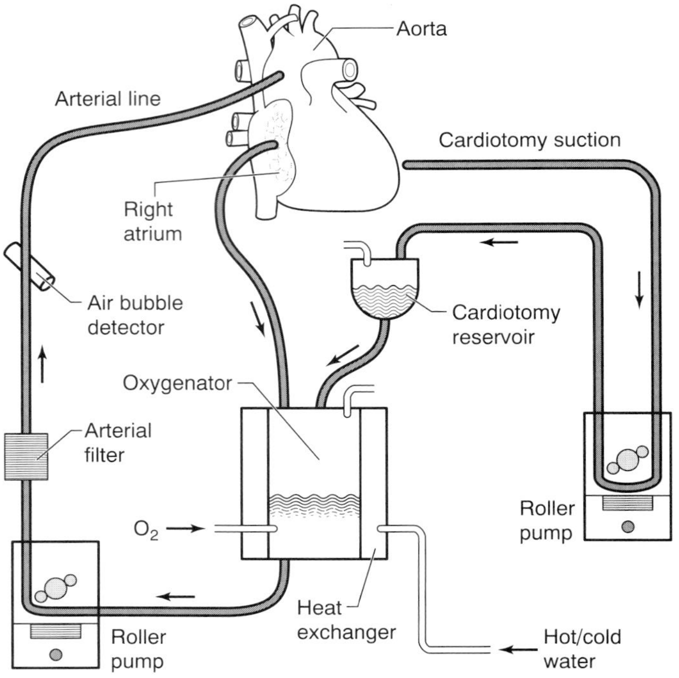

Fig. 23.2 The simplest and most commonly used system of venous drainage from the right atrium with arterial return to the ascending aorta thus bypassing the heart and lungs. The circuit includes a reservoir, oxygenator, a pump to deliver the blood and usually a filter of 40 μm pore size to remove gaseous microemboli.

REFERENCES

14. Kirklin J W, DuShane J W et al Proc Staff Meet Mayo Clin 1955; 30: 201
15. Perfusion 1989; 4(2): 83–161 (whole issue)
16. Smith P L C et al Lancet 1986; i: 823
17. Treasure T in: Yacoub M Y, Pepper J (eds) Annual of Cardiac Surgery, 7th edn. Current Science 1994 pp 161–169
18. Kirklin J K, Westaby S et al J Thorac Cardiovasc Surg 1983; 86: 845
19. Butler J, Rocker G M, Westaby S Ann Thorac Surg 1993; 55(2): 1033
20. Millner R, Treasure T Explaining Cardiac Surgery. BMJ, London 1995

aortic root or directly into the coronary orifices, greatly prolongs the protection and improves working conditions for the surgeon and the subsequent performance of the heart. The relative merits of these two techniques—intermittent ischaemic arrest and cold cardioplegic arrest—are debated[21] but the importance of preserving myocardial function cannot be over emphasized.

The use of cardioplegia, that is heart paralysis, has been a very important part of the changing and expanding practice of cardiac surgery. The essential components of the various techniques have depended on manipulation of chemical composition and temperature of the coronary perfusion. It is now usual to selectively perfuse the heart with oxygenated blood, but to modify it in one of a variety of ways, nearly all of which include raising its potassium content to between 15 and 20 mmol/l to arrest the heart in asystole. Cooling was central to most techniques but, with increasing experience, some surgeons have returned to more physiological temperatures.[22,23] The cardioplegia may also be given, or supplemented, by retrograde perfusion into the coronary sinus.

INVESTIGATION OF SURGICAL CARDIAC DISEASE

For the most part, the diagnosis and assessment of cardiac disease is in the hands of cardiologists, and the surgeon is asked to see the patient only when the diagnosis has been made. Under these circumstances it is easy for the surgeon to be seen merely as the technician, operating at the behest of the physician. While the relationship may degenerate to this level there is no reason why it should. Most units work cohesively, with a high level of shared responsibility and mutual reliance. The best cardiac surgeons are also very shrewd diagnosticians and know which of the symptoms, clinical signs and investigations really influence diagnosis and management, and which are best ignored, or at least kept in proportion.

Chest radiograph

The plain chest radiograph provides a two-dimensional image of the cardiac chambers and great vessels superimposed upon each other. The cardiac surgeon, familiar with the heart exposed in three dimensions, becomes very familiar with identifying the position and relative size of these chambers (Figs 23.3 and 23.4).

The electrocardiogram (ECG)

The surgeon has the ECG displayed during and after all operations, and recognizes unhesitatingly the repertoire of common heart rhythms, and the evidence of ischaemia, which may come and go during surgery on the heart. The oscilloscope screen is glimpsed as frequently and as familiarly as a car driver uses the rear-view mirror.

Of particular preoperative diagnostic importance in the investigation of coronary artery disease is the exercise (or stress) ECG which is usually performed (e.g. the Bruce protocol) while the patient walks on a moving platform which becomes steeper and faster in 3-minute stages. Symptoms, changes in pulse and blood pressure, and the development of ST and T wave changes are documented.

Echocardiography

Two forms of echocardiography are in routine use in cardiology. M-mode provides a single beam and identifies movement (hence M for motion) towards and away from the ultrasound source. It requires considerable skill to obtain and interpret the images and is largely dependent on the skill of the operator. Two-dimensional echocardiography, which is essentially the same as abdominal ultrasound familiar to all surgeons, provides a more readily interpretable image which can be stored and replayed. It has emerged as the most powerful tool in the investigation of congenital heart disease, permitting repeated non-invasive observation of anatomy and function of the heart in outpatients, at the bedside, in the operating theatre, and even in utero (see Fig. 23.25c). Transoesophageal echo (TOE) produces even better images, particularly of the mitral valve and the descending aorta.

Radionuclide investigation

In myocardial perfusion scintigraphy a gamma camera detects the distribution of intravenously injected thallium-201. This isotope behaves like potassium, entering cells, and its distribution is proportional to blood flow. In the diagnosis of myocardial infarction, technetium pyrophosphate is able to enter infarcted cells and bind to intracellular calcium. For left ventricular studies the technique of ECG 'gating' is employed. The red cells are labelled with technetium-99. At any given moment the scintillation counts over the heart cannot usefully be distinguished from the background. The counts from many cardiac cycles are therefore stored and divided into 16 subdivisions of the R–R interval 'gated' from the ECG. The cumulative counts provide a series of measurements of the volume of the heart in systole and diastole and from these measurements the ejection fraction can be calculated.

Cardiac catheterization

In spite of the growth of non-invasive methods such as echocardiography, Doppler imaging, and nuclear cardiology, cardiac catheterization remains important in many areas of diagnosis. Catheters are inserted into the arteries and veins by a Seldinger technique in the groin or by cutting down on the vessels in the antecubital fossa. All chambers and vessels can be reached. Pressures are measured, blood is withdrawn for oxygen saturation measurements, and radiopaque contrast media injected for cine angiography. Complete information can be obtained about narrowed or leaking valves, (Figs 23.5 and 23.6) abnormal shunts between the right and left heart can be demonstrated and the coronary arteries can be visualized.

REFERENCES

21. Anderson J R, Hossein-Nia M et al Ann Thorac Surg 1994; 58: 768
22. Treasure T, Edwards R (unsigned editorial) Lancet 1992; 339: 841
23. Warm Heart Investigators Lancet 1994; 343: 559

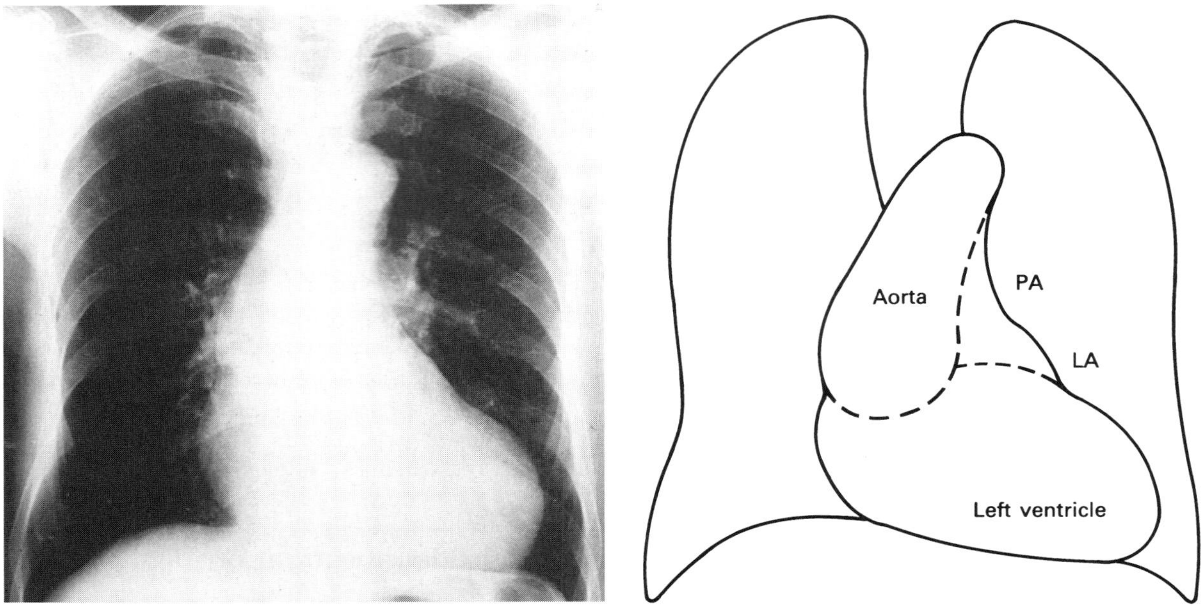

Fig. 23.3 Plain posteroanterior chest radiograph of a case of aortic stenosis. Note that the ascending aorta forms the mid-portion of the right heart border. The arch of the aorta is prominent on the left and in this case the concavity of the left border is striking because of the prominent left ventricle but normal-sized pulmonary artery (PA) and left atrium (LA).

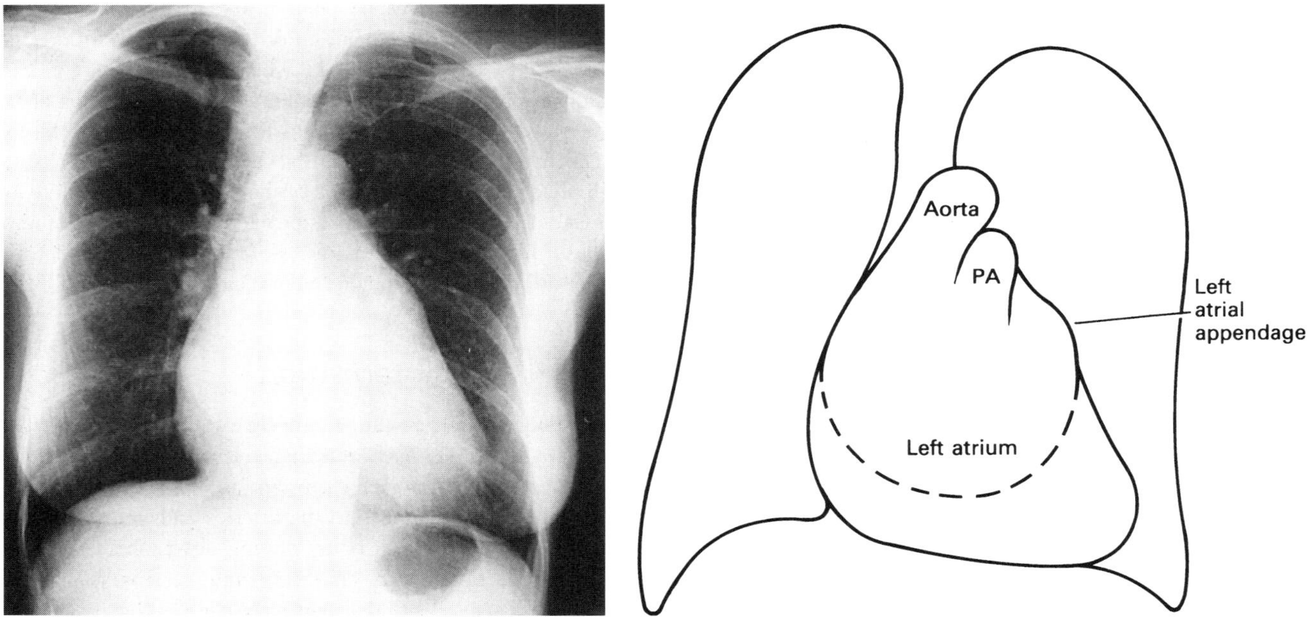

Fig. 23.4 Chest radiograph of a patient with mitral stenosis. The left border is filled out by the prominent pulmonary artery (PA) and left atrial appendage. The left atrial enlargement also creates a double shadow on the right.

CONGENITAL HEART DISEASE

The continuing advance in the surgical correction of many forms of congenital heart disease has realized Souttar's prediction.[7] The surgery is obvious enough in its more simple forms such as closure of a persistent ductus arteriosus or patching a septal defect. More complex procedures such as the Senning and Mustard[24,25] operations (both means of switching the venous inflow in transposition of the great vessels) are conceptually brilliant. The surgery requires an appreciation of disordered three-dimensional anatomy and allows little room for error. Congenital heart surgery, apart from simple procedures in older children or adults, is in most countries in the hands of a relatively small number of very expert surgeons working in specialized units.

REFERENCES

24. Senning A Surgery 1959; 45: 966
25. Mustard W T Surgery 1964; 55: 469

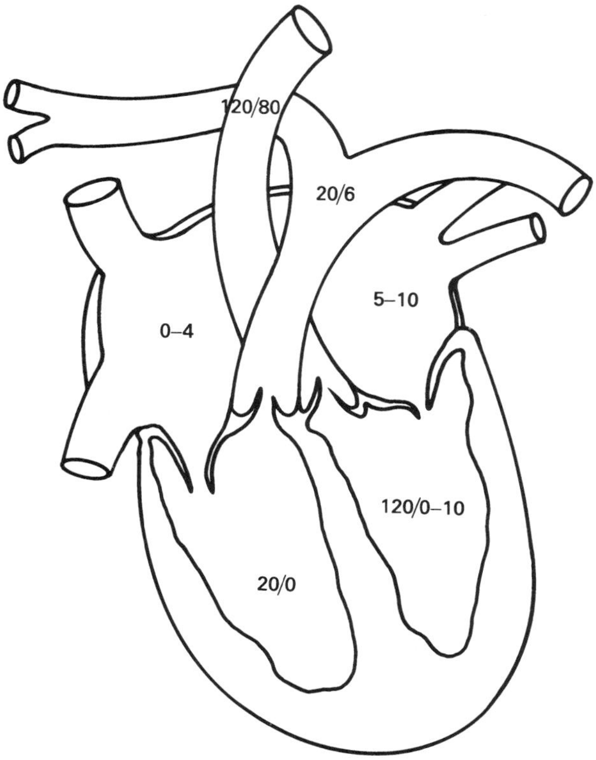

Fig. 23.5 Typical normal pressures in mmHg in the cardiac chambers and great vessels.

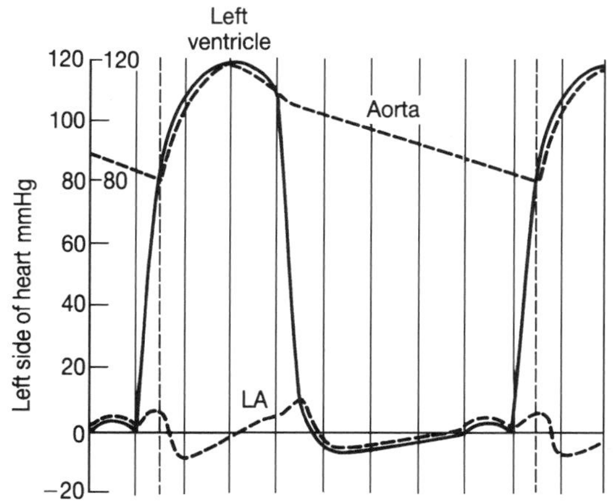

Fig. 23.6 The left-sided pressures against a time-base marked each 0.1 s. Note that the left ventricular pressure goes from just below left atrial pressure when the mitral valve is open to just above aortic pressure when the aortic valve is opened. As the lines cross a valve opens or closes. Knowledge of these pressure changes is fundamental to a logical appreciation of valve disease and its symptoms and signs.

Palliative operations for congenital heart disease

The earliest procedures were palliative. To understand them it must be appreciated that, from a functional point of view, many patients with congenital heart disease fall into two large groups: those who are cyanosed either because of inadequate pulmonary blood flow or a failure to direct the returning venous blood to the lungs; and those in whom pulmonary flow is excessive because of a shunt from the left side of the heart into the more compliant pulmonary circulation. When the abnormality in the heart is too complex to correct, or if there are reasons to want to improve the situation as a temporizing manoeuvre until the child is bigger, palliative procedures are used.

Systemic–pulmonary shunt operations

In cyanotic congenital heart disease the child's arterial blood may be desaturated because of a reduction in pulmonary blood flow. In Fallot's tetralogy, for example, there is a combination of restricted blood flow into the pulmonary artery (due to obstruction) and a communication between the ventricles. Desaturated blood flows into the systemic circulation. Because the predominant feature is cyanosis, the label 'blue baby' was almost diagnosis enough for this whole group of conditions before corrective heart surgery was possible. Very effective palliation became possible with the first description of a systemic to pulmonary artery shunt to bypass the obstructive pulmonary lesion and improve pulmonary blood flow.[26] The circulations are still mixed but the patient may derive great benefit from the improvement in systemic oxygenation.

The first technique described was the Blalock–Taussig shunt.[26] The right subclavian artery is mobilized, divided, swung down and anastomosed to the main right pulmonary artery (Fig. 23.7a). Alternatively, the ascending aorta used to be anastomosed directly to the right pulmonary artery (the Waterston shunt) or the descending aorta to the left pulmonary artery (Potts shunt). Finally, a length of vascular graft may be used to make the anastomosis, and this has gained popularity as better synthetic material for small calibre grafts has become available. The size of the anastomosis must be judged so that the patient is improved but flooding of the lungs is avoided.

Pulmonary artery banding

If there is a communication between the left and right sides of the heart (ventricular septal defect, for example) the more compliant pulmonary circulation permits a high left-to-right shunt and an increased pulmonary blood flow to the detriment of the lungs. The systemic blood flow is maintained and thus the total cardiac output is very much increased. If there is a common ventricle or multiple ventricular septal defects, closure in infancy is often too hazardous and then narrowing (or 'banding') the pulmonary artery to increase the resistance to pulmonary blood flow may provide useful palliation.

Closed cardiac operations

Operations for patent ductus arteriosus and coarctation were possible before the use of cardiopulmonary bypass and are grouped together to distinguish them from open or intracardiac operations.

REFERENCE

26. Blalock A, Taussig H B J Am Med Assoc 1945; 128: 189

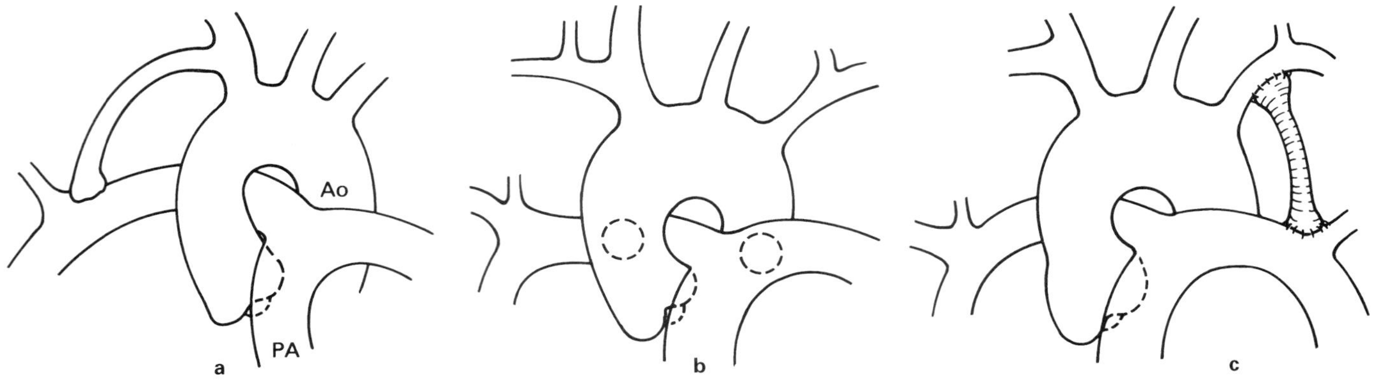

Fig. 23.7 Systemic to-pulmonary artery shunts for the palliation of cyanotic heart disease. (**a**) The Blalock–Taussig shunt in which the subclavian artery is divided just before the vertebral and internal mammary arteries branch off and is anastomosed end-to-side into the right main pulmonary artery (PA). Ao = aorta. (**b**) Direct side-to-side anastomoses used to be made between the ascending aorta and the right pulmonary artery (Waterston) or the descending aorta and the left pulmonary artery (Potts). Neither is now employed but may be seen in some adults who have had palliation in childhood. (**c**) Interposition of a tube graft is now used in some cases.

Persistent ductus arteriosus

In the fetal circulation the relatively poorly oxygenated blood from the superior vena cava passes via the right atrium and right ventricle into the pulmonary artery. From the main pulmonary artery the majority of blood bypasses the airless lungs and flows via the ductus arteriosus into the upper end of the descending aorta. These three vessels form a continuous conduit in the fetus (Fig. 23.8).

The ductus contains muscle in its wall and normally closes after birth, largely in response to a rise in oxygen tension as the lungs begin to function. Prostaglandins keep the duct patent and can be used therapeutically for this purpose in cases where, due to intracardiac abnormalities, the blood flow to the lungs is so poor that survival depends upon the presence of the ductal flow. In normal infants the duct closes within about 12 hours of birth and is obliterated within a few weeks.

Persistence of the ductus arteriosus is one of the most common forms of congenital heart disease, accounting for approximately 12% of congenital cardiac defects. As the pulmonary vascular resistance falls in the days and weeks after birth, blood flows increasingly from left to right and clinical manifestations depend on how large a shunt results. If the duct is large there is a free flow of blood at arterial pressure into the pulmonary circulation, the pulmonary vasculature is engorged and the left ventricle runs at high filling pressure and high output. On the other hand, a narrower ductus limits flow and the patient may be symptom free. The abnormally high blood flow may nevertheless result in pulmonary vascular disease in due course. The physical signs are a collapsing pulse and a continuous 'machinery murmur'. If the flow is small, resulting in a less than 2:1 pulmonary to systemic flow ratio, the patient may be symptomless throughout life and the only important risk is then of endocarditis (see later).

Gross[27] ligated a ductus arteriosus for the first time in 1938. A simple tie may suffice, or in infants a clip, but these may fail to obliterate the lumen and some advocate division and suturing in all cases. The ductus is fragile and it has a very large vessel at either end! The recurrent laryngeal nerve is very close. The operation is

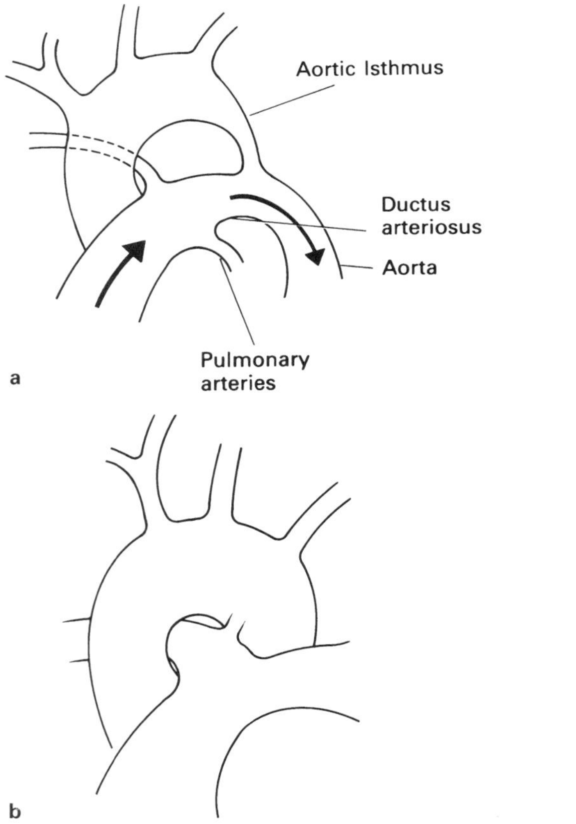

Fig. 23.8 (**a**) In the fetus the bulk of the desaturated blood passing through the right heart passes in the descending aorta and reaches the placenta via the umbilical artery. Failure of the ductus to close results in the condition of persistent ductus arteriosus. The blood flow reverses resulting in excessive pulmonary blood flow. (**b**) The ligamentum arteriosum remains as a fibrous band in the adult; the recurrent laryngeal nerve passes around it.

REFERENCE

27. Gross R E, Hubbard J P J Am Med Assoc 1993; 112: 729

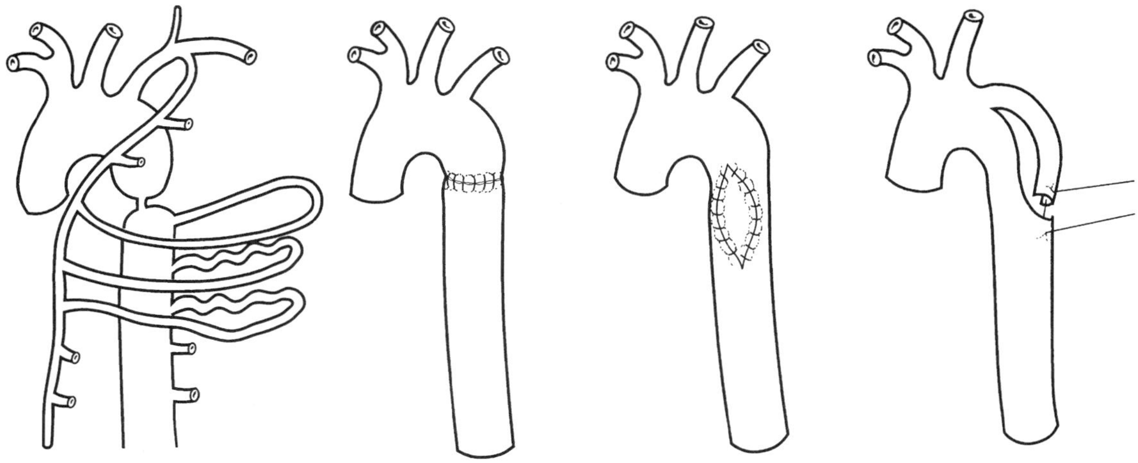

Fig. 23.9 **(a)** Coarctation is a narrowing of the aorta in the area just beyond the left subclavian artery which probably develops after birth due to abnormal ductus tissue. **(b)** Excision and end-to-end repair was the first and probably most common method of surgical management. **(c)** Widening the area with a gusset is a simpler alternative, particularly if the aorta is immobile or there is need for speed to avoid spinal cord ischaemia. **(d)** Mobilization of the left subclavian artery permits repair with normal arterial tissue and may allow for natural growth.

treated with considerable respect by cardiothoracic surgeons because disaster is always close and yet complete cure of the problem should be possible unless pulmonary vascular disease has supervened. Closure by a balloon, introduced from the femoral artery and passed retrogradely, is now a very successful way of closing the duct.

About 200 operations per annum are performed in the cardiothoracic units of the UK (a reduction by 60% compared with the figures quoted in the previous edition of this book).[1] The mortality is consistently about 1%. Operation for patent ductus arteriosus in the adult has become quite uncommon but it provides particular problems when there is calcification or aneurysm formation.[28]

Coarctation of the aorta

Almost invariably the site of coarctation is in the upper aorta opposite the ductus arteriosus. There may be a shelf-like narrowing with a pinhole orifice or a longer, tube-like narrowed segment, or a combination of these two. In severe cases there is considerable collateral development augmenting blood supply to the lower half of the body.

The problem may present as heart failure in infancy but in most cases there is then a major associated abnormality. Those patients surviving to childhood are symptom free, unless they have associated anomalies. The majority are hypertensive. The femoral pulses are delayed and attenuated and a systolic murmur can be heard over the coarctation. The collateral circulation is between the branches of the subclavian artery, notably the internal mammary arteries and scapular vessels which arise above the coarctation and feed the intercostal vessels from the third down. These have reversed flow into the descending aorta. They may be felt and heard clinically, and seen as rib notching on the chest radiograph. Quite a high proportion of patients—at least a quarter—have a congenitally abnormal aortic valve, usually bicuspid, and berry aneurysms in the intracranial vessels are a sometimes fatal association.

Symptoms due to left ventricular failure occur in time but by then the hypertension, which has a renal component, is irreversible. For this reason coarctation should be relieved before symptoms appear.

The techniques of repair are end-to-end anastomosis, patching, and use of the left subclavian artery as a flap (Fig. 23.9). The first operation for this condition was performed by Crafoord[29] in 1944. About 250 operations per year are performed in the UK[1] with a mortality of 1–2%.

Open cardiac operations for congenital defects

Atrial septal defect

There is a normal communication between the atria up to the time of birth; this is the foramen ovale which remains probe-patent in a proportion of hearts throughout life. It is valve-like and permits a flow of oxygenated blood from the placental vein passing via the hepatic vein to stream through to the left side of the heart. As the lungs expand and the left atrium fills, the valve is held closed and in most cases seals. Except where there are other abnormalities causing the right atrial pressure to exceed the left, blood does not pass through and a patent foramen ovale is rarely a problem although it can cause problems with right to left shunting in divers.

There are three patterns of atrial septal defect. The most common (about 80%) are defects in the fossa ovalis, also called ostium secundum defects. About 15% are ostium primum defects and are part of the spectrum of atrioventricular septal defects. High defects associated with minor anomalies of pulmonary venous drainage are called sinus venosus defects (Fig. 23.10).

....

REFERENCES

28. John S J Thorac Cardiovasc Surg 1981; 82: 314
29. Crafoord C J Thorac Surg 1945; 14: 347

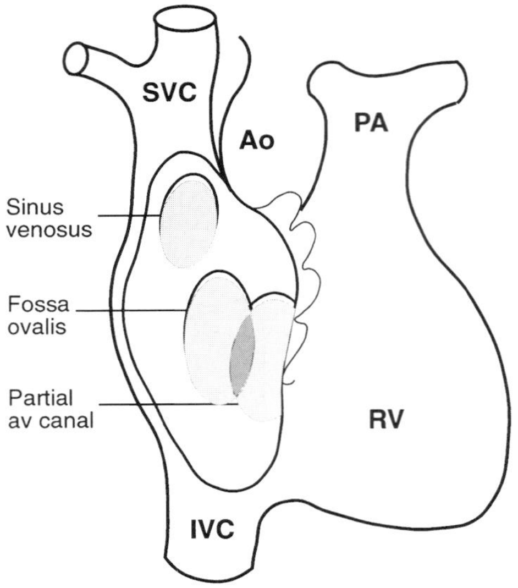

Fig. 23.10 Defects in the atrial septum. A defect of the fossa ovalis (also called an ostium secundum defect) is the most common form of atrial septal defect. A partial atrioventricular canal defect is also known as an ostium primum defect; both terms suggest the supposed embryological abnormality. It is part of a complex of atrioventricular septal defects. A sinus venosus defect may be associated with various anomalies of venous drainage into the atria.

The haemodynamic problem is that although the pressures in the atria are low and not very dissimilar, the thin-walled right ventricle is very compliant and permits a large left-to-right shunt. This is very well tolerated for many years even when the pulmonary to systemic flow ratio (QP : QS) is in excess of 3 : 1. Heart failure is rare but a tendency to 'chestiness' in childhood is typical. Gradually the heart size increases, the pulmonary artery pressure may rise and the heart rhythm may change to atrial fibrillation. On examination a systolic murmur can be heard as a result of the increased flow through the pulmonary valve. The lung fields are usually plethoric on radiographs. It is usual to advise operation if QP : QS, as estimated from the measurement of oxygen saturation in the right atrium, pulmonary artery and aorta, is greater than 2 : 1.

There was great enthusiasm for operating on this lesion in the early days of cardiac surgery, before cardiopulmonary bypass, and some ingenious methods were devised to satisfy Souttar's admonition that we should operate without halting the flow of blood or interfering with the heart beat.[7] These included suturing the free atrial wall on to the defect, placing a pursestring externally between the atria and suturing a well to the atrium and then operating by feel alone. The technique of moderate hypothermia was the most successful, and Holmes Sellors perfected the technique of using surface cooling to about 30°C to permit safe closure of fossa ovalis defects.[11,12] Cardiopulmonary bypass has replaced all these techniques. In the UK over 500 operations are performed each year—the majority in childhood—with a mortality of under 1%.[1] In fossa ovalis defects (ostium secundum) there is adequate tissue to permit direct suture. In other more complex types of atrial septal defect, where suturing would cause distortion of the entry of great veins or interfere with the functioning of the atrioventricular valves, a patch is used to close the defect.

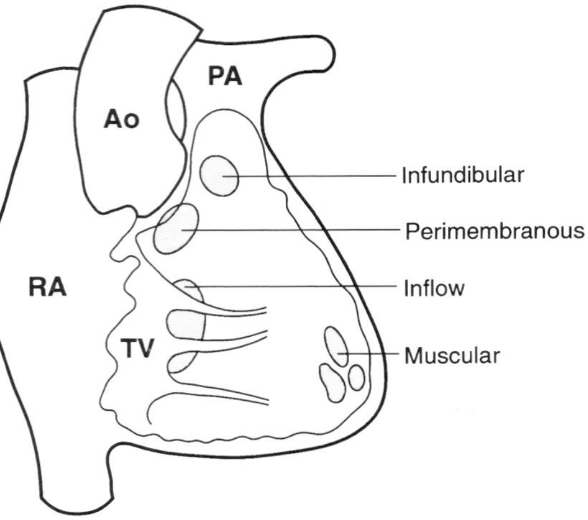

Fig. 23.11 Cut-away view of the heart from the right side to show the common sites of ventricular septal defects. Ao = aorta; TV = tricuspid valve; RA = right atrium; PA = pulmonary artery.

Ventricular septal defect

Defects in the ventricular septum vary widely in site and size. They may coexist with other lesions, for example pulmonary stenosis in Fallot's tetralogy or with atrial septal defect in complex atrioventricular defects, when the site is of diagnostic importance. In isolated ventricular septal defect the site affects the surgical approach and technical difficulty involved (Fig. 23.11). The size of the defect governs the haemodynamic consequences and therefore symptoms and is the major determinant of the eventual outcome for the patient.

In the presence of a ventricular septal defect there are two routes of exit for blood from the pressure-generating left ventricle; in addition to the normal route through the aortic valve, blood flows through the ventricular septal defect to the right ventricle. The volume of blood passing through the defect depends on both the size of the ventricular septal defect and the pressure generated in the right ventricle during systole, which in turn depends on the vascular resistance in the lungs. If the hole is as large as the aortic orifice, the pressure in the two ventricles will equalize, and flow is governed by the relative resistance of the pulmonary and systemic vasculature. In utero the pulmonary vascular resistance is relatively high in the airless lung and blood passes preferentially through the ductus arteriosus. This resistance takes some time to fall and initially there may be little left-to-right shunt and no murmur. Within a few days the pulmonary vascular resistance falls and then the ratio of pulmonary to systemic flow (QP : QS) may well be over 4 : 1 in a sick baby. Clinically, the baby is tachypnoeic and fails to thrive. The murmur is pansystolic. If the pulmonary vascular resistance rises again later, the shunt falls and eventually balances or reverses with the development of cyanosis. This is the phenomenon referred to as the Eisenmenger complex and by this stage the condition is inoperable.

The natural history of ventricular septal defect includes a high incidence of spontaneous closure. A substantial proportion of those detected in infants under 1 month of age eventually close spontaneously. The likelihood of closure diminishes as time passes and those still open by the time the child is of school age are very unlikely to close. Surgery is therefore only indicated in infancy if heart failure occurs. If the defects are multiple or the infant is very sick, pulmonary artery banding to protect the pulmonary vasculature until the child grows may be a wiser policy although the combined risks of the palliative operation and its subsequent revision are not inconsiderable.

In the UK about 100 babies under 1 year of age are operated on for this condition each year, and nearly twice as many older children, with mortality of under 1%.

Pulmonary stenosis

Pulmonary stenosis can exist as an isolated lesion at the valve itself or as part of a variety of more complicated conditions when the stenosis may amount to hypoplasia which may affect the whole of the right ventricular outflow tract.

Severe forms present in infancy. The baby is tachypnoeic and hypoxic. As the ductus closes, blood shunts from right to left at atrial level because of the obstruction to outflow from the right ventricle. Milder degrees are well tolerated and may present in childhood, when a murmur and a large heart are discovered. If the peak pressure in the right ventricle is under 75 mmHg and the gradient across the pulmonary valve is less than 50 mmHg the cardiac state may be stable, and there are no symptoms. There is a loud systolic murmur maximal to the left of the sternum. The heart shadow is large on the routine posteroanterior chest radiograph and, in particular with valvar stenosis, there is marked poststenotic dilatation of the pulmonary artery. The ECG provides evidence of right ventricular hypertrophy. The simplest indicator is that the normally small upward deflection, the R wave, in V1 is larger than the S wave.

Patients who develop symptoms or who have limited exercise tolerance should be offered surgery. The stenosis is relieved with conservation of the valve as far as possible.

Aortic stenosis

Congenital stenosis related to the aortic valve may be valvar, subvalvar or supravalvar. The severe forms, presenting in infancy and childhood, are treated rather unsatisfactorily by an operation designed to open the commissures and relieve obstruction while leaving some competence to the valve. Balloon valve dilatation has replaced surgery as the first treatment for most cases. It is also less than ideal but less invasive.

The mildest form of congenital abnormality is a bicuspid valve where two of the cusps, usually the right and left coronary cusps, have failed to separate. These valves usually function well but tend to calcify and present as aortic stenosis in the seventh decade. They are vulnerable to endocarditis. If this occurs they may present as severe aortic regurgitation at a much younger age. Aortic valve disease is most commonly encountered in adult life and is dealt with later.

Complex congenital heart disease

The isolated abnormalities of development already described are relatively easy to understand; the haemodynamic consequences are clear and the mechanics of correction are obvious. In complex lesions the whole development of the heart is abnormal and the description of the morphology itself is contentious. The work of Anderson[30] has done a great deal to clarify this subject and the system of sequential chamber analysis promulgated in his writing is widely (although not universally) accepted. In essence it recognizes that the terms 'right' and 'left', 'mitral' and 'tricuspid' cease to have clear meanings in the most complex cases and the system identifies structures by their morphology, irrespective of the actual 'side' of the chest, and by their 'connections'.

The exact mixture of symptoms and signs in an individual case is of limited use in making the final anatomical diagnosis. In most it merely serves to indicate that the heart is the cause of the infant's failure to thrive and denotes the relative severity of the physiological abnormality and the urgency with which it must be treated.

Fallot's tetralogy. This is perhaps the best known of the complex congenital heart conditions, largely because of its memorable eponym. Fallot correlated the clinical and anatomical abnormalities. He identified four components:

1. A ventricular septal defect.
2. The aorta over-rides it with the result that it receives desaturated right ventricular blood.
3. Obstruction to the right ventricular outflow.
4. Abnormal thickness of the right ventricular wall.

In an extreme form the aorta can arise from the right ventricle—a rare but well recognized condition called double-outlet right ventricle. Those with a special interest in cardiac morphology describe the anatomy of tetralogy in great detail. The severity and extent of the infundibular, valvar or pulmonary artery obstruction and the relationship between the ventricular septum and the aorta must be clearly understood if a surgical correction is to be achieved.

The most severe cases present in infancy, although the condition is associated with a classical clinical presentation at a slightly later age. It is noticed that the normally highly active toddler becomes blue and adopts a characteristic squatting posture after running around in the course of play. The degree of arterial desaturation becomes more severe with exercise and the child learns that squatting will relieve its hypoxia by abruptly raising the resistance to flow in the systemic circulation and thus forcing a little more blood to the lungs. The discovery of the systolic murmur generated by the pulmonary stenosis virtually confirms the diagnosis when this almost pathognomonic history is elicited from the mother.

About 300 operations are performed each year for this and related conditions and the overall mortality is about 5%.[1] An alternative is to perform palliative surgery, and this was the first use of the Blalock anastomosis.[26] The usual approach is to perform total correction when the anatomy is in any way favourable and the child is large enough. Otherwise a carefully planned shunt may be

REFERENCE

30. Shinebourne E A, McCartney F, Anderson R H Br Heart J 1976; 38: 327

performed to allow the child to grow as the risks then fall. The balance of risks and benefits of one- versus two-stage correction continues to be debated.

Transposition of the great arteries. In transposition the great vessels leaving the heart are reversed in position with the aorta arising from the right ventricle and the pulmonary artery from the left ventricle. This abnormality occurs once in 2000–3000 live births and accounts for around 5% of congenital heart disease. The pulmonary and systemic circulations are essentially parallel but if there is enough mixing across the atrial septum through the foramen ovale, and between the great vessels via the ductus arteriosus, the condition is compatible with survival for a time. The condition usually presents at birth with cyanosis which worsens as the ductus closes. Only 10% of cases survive to a year without intervention.

There are usually a number of associated abnormalities, of which pulmonary stenosis and ventricular septal defect are the most common. The presence of a ventricular septal defect permits mixing and pulmonary stenosis reduces the magnitude of pulmonary blood flow which would otherwise result in heart failure as the pulmonary vascular resistance falls. The diagnosis may be suspected in an infant cyanosed from birth and is confirmed and the anatomy defined by echocardiography. In a particularly interesting form there is also discordance of the atrioventricular connections, a condition called corrected transposition; in these cases the physiology is essentially normal.

The initial treatment in sick, cyanosed babies is aimed at increasing the amount of mixing of the circulations to permit survival. Rashkind balloon septostomy is a useful palliative measure.[31] A catheter is passed transvenously to the right atrium and then through the foramen ovale into the left atrium. A balloon at its tip is inflated and the catheter sharply jerked back to tear the septum.

The aim of surgery is to correct the anatomical abnormality. The obvious anatomical correction of resiting the great arteries is made difficult by the problem of connecting the child's tiny coronary arteries to the oxygenated systemic outflow. Also the left ventricle is unprepared to carry the systemic load unless it has remained hypertrophied due to associated pulmonary stenosis.

Truncus arteriosus. Failure of division of the truncus arteriosus into the aorta and pulmonary artery results in a single great vessel leaving the heart through a common valve before giving rise to systemic and pulmonary branches. This is a rare condition which usually presents with heart failure in infancy.

Atrioventricular septal defects. Abnormalities of development resulting in deficiency of tissue immediately above and below the atrioventricular junction result in a wide spectrum of cardiac abnormalities, which are particularly common in Down's syndrome. At the mildest end of the spectrum, an actual communication is only present between the atria—this is the condition already described under atrial septal defects as an 'ostium primum atrial septal defect' and was also known in the past as 'partial atrioventricular canal'. In the more severe form of atrioventricular defect, commonly known as 'complete atrioventricular canal', there are deficiencies of atrial and ventricular septation with abnormalities of both atrioventricular valves. These abnormalities are also grouped together as 'endocardial cushion defects', suggesting at least a nodding acquaintance with the embryological abnormality.

The presentation and clinical course of these cases are similarly diverse. The mild cases are similar in presentation to atrial septal defect although the course is less benign and the surgical correction is technically more exacting. Involvement of the ventricular septum results in a natural history more akin to ventricular septal defect, but with a much greater risk of developing severe pulmonary vascular disease. Associated atrioventricular valve regurgitation results in rapidly progressing congestive heart failure. The morphological description and the meticulous techniques involved in reconstructing the heart to create two valves and four chambers from a common atrioventricular canal are very complex.

Total anomalous pulmonary venous drainage. In this rare condition the pulmonary veins, carrying oxygenated blood, are not connected to the left atrium but instead drain into the right atrium. They most commonly (45%) drain above the heart through a vein reminiscent of a persistent left superior vena cava. In other cases they drain through the coronary sinus, or below the diaphragm into the portal system.

Presentation is with severe cyanosis from birth, without cardiac murmurs. Survival depends on the size of the atrial septal defect, which permits blood to reach the left atrium and thence the systemic circulation. A balloon septostomy therefore helps but early surgery is the treatment of choice. Surgical mortality is around 15%.

Left superior vena cava and coronary sinus anomalies. These are uncommon, relatively benign, but interesting abnormalities related to the formation of the coronary sinus. In the course of development there are paired superior venae cavae. Normally the left innominate vein enlarges and the left-sided superior vena cava regresses, leaving as a remnant the oblique vein of Marshall while its lower end becomes the coronary sinus, draining cardiac venous blood into the right atrium. Failure of this process may result in persistence of the left-sided superior vena cava, which may be no more than a coincidental finding. As an isolated anomaly it is excessively rare. More often it is associated with abnormalities of atrial septation and of coronary sinus development. These abnormalities can present as atrial septal defects or as abnormalities of systemic venous connections, associated with more complex cardiac conditions.

Abnormalities of lateralization. The term 'dextrocardia' means that the heart points towards or is largely on the right, rather than the left. The normal arrangement—with the right atrium inferior vena cava and the liver on the right—is called 'situs solitus'. The reverse is called 'situs inversus'. Situs ambiguus describes states in which there may be right- or left-sided 'mirror image' or isomerism. In right-sided isomerism there is no spleen. Asplenia is known to be associated with bizarre cardiac malformations with mirror-image atria, failure of septation and abnormal connections.

REFERENCE

31. Rashkind W J, Miller W W JAMA 1966; 1966: 991

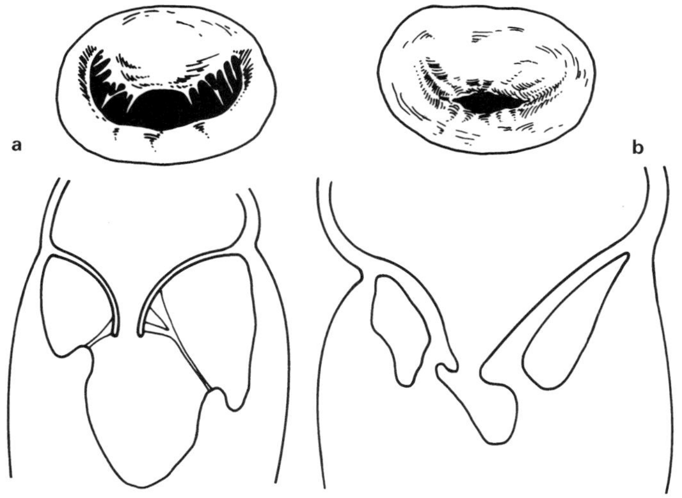

Fig. 23.12 (**a**) The normal mitral valve with a large anterior cusp and a crescent-shaped posterior cusp which can open to the full size of the atrioventricular orifice. (**b**) At its most severe the rheumatic valve has fused commissures, thickened immobile cusps, and short matted chordae. Of these, commissural fusion is the only component easily corrected by conservative valve surgery.

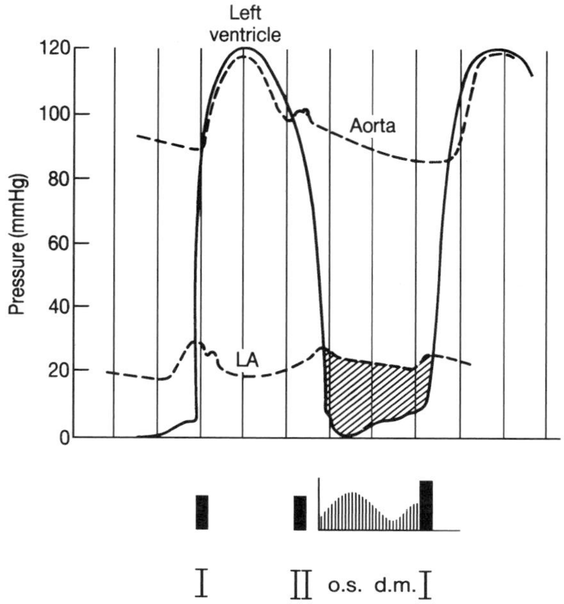

Fig. 23.13 The pressure diagram (Fig. 23.6) modified to show the effects of mitral stenosis. There is now a pressure difference between the left atrium (LA) and the left ventricle when the valve is opened. This creates a murmur in diastole due to turbulent flow and the valve opens with a snap as the tension is taken up and closes more noisily, making a loud S1.

SURGERY OF THE VALVES OF THE HEART

Mitral stenosis

Before cardiopulmonary bypass was available, mitral stenosis was consistently and safely relieved in large numbers of patients in the 1950s by valvotomy performed within the beating heart.[32,33] Virtually all cases of mitral stenosis—other than a few very rare congenital malformations—are the result of rheumatic fever. Women outnumber men by about 3:1. The condition follows throat infections with β-haemolytic streptococci whose antigens cross-react with those of various tissues of the body. The manifestations of acute rheumatic fever include involvement of several of the large joints in sequence, the basal ganglia causing Sydenham's chorea (St Vitus' dance) and, most importantly, the heart including valves, muscle, conducting system and pericardium. It is a disease associated with overcrowding and poor living conditions and has become uncommon in the more affluent nations.[34]

After the acute illness there are usually years of freedom from symptoms during which one or more valves becomes progressively thickened. The mitral valve is most commonly and most severely affected. The commissures become adherent, the cusps thickened and the chordae shortened (Fig. 23.12). Left ventricular filling is obstructed and the left atrial pressure rises, producing the symptoms of tiredness as the result of limited cardiac output and breathlessness as the atrial and therefore pulmonary capillary pressures reach the critical point where the drying effect of the intravascular oncotic pressure is exceeded. The alveoli become moist and oxygenation is impaired. The characteristic feature is that breathlessness becomes worse on lying flat due to alterations in the pressure and volume relationships of the pulmonary circulation. Symptoms may progress steadily or appear suddenly with pregnancy or the onset of atrial fibrillation. Patients may also present with systemic embolization, most commonly with stroke, but mitral stenosis must always be considered as a source of embolus to the leg or mesenteric arteries.

The natural history is of steady deterioration with 40% of patients dying within 10 years of presentation and only 20% surviving for 20 years, but sometimes deterioration is very slow. In older patients seen now, the history often includes a previous conservative mitral valve operation.

Clinical signs

At some stage atrial fibrillation supervenes but the heart may stay in sinus rhythm for years. The apex beat has a tapping quality due to the abrupt nature of the first sound; on auscultation there is a loud first sound, an 'opening snap' and a rumbling diastolic murmur. The explanation for these sounds and their interpretation is important in making surgical decisions. The diastolic murmur is the result of turbulence as the left ventricle fills through the stenosed valve. Its loudness is related to the severity of stenosis but also to the cardiac output so it may be very quiet even when stenosis is severe. The loud first sound and the opening snap are the result of the sudden tensing of the valve to and fro as the ventricular pressure abruptly changes in relationship to the left atrial pressure (Fig. 23.13). The louder the sounds, the more

REFERENCES

32. Treasure T, Hollman A Ann Roy Coll Surg 1995; 77: 145
33. Treasure T J Royal Soc Med 1996; 89(1): 19
34. Hall R J C, Treasure T In: Julian D G, Camm A J, Fox K M, Hall R J C, Poole-Wilson P A (eds) Diseases of the Heart, 2nd edn. Saunders, London 1996

mobile is the mitral valve. A mobile valve may be conserved but if the tissues are rigid from fibrosis or calcification the valve should be replaced.

Investigations

The chest radiograph shows a straight or bulging left border to the cardiac shadow where the enlarged pulmonary artery and left atrial appendage fill out the normal concavity below the aortic knuckle (Fig. 23.4). Other signs of left atrial enlargement are a double atrial shadow and widening of the subcarinal angle to more than 90 degrees. The ECG shows abnormal notched P waves (P mitrale) if atrial fibrillation has not supervened. There is evidence of right ventricular hypertrophy and a digitalis effect on S–T segment in advanced cases.

The diagnosis of pure mitral stenosis is made clinically and investigations are aimed at diagnosing and quantifying other factors such as left ventricular function, pulmonary hypertension, the presence and severity of concomitant aortic valve disease and the state of the coronary arteries. The usual indication for cardiac catheterization is to establish the state of the coronary arteries, particularly if the patient is male, above middle age or has had chest pain. Otherwise echocardiography provides excellent information about the state of the mitral valve.

Mitral stenosis, unless trivial, should be relieved because of the ever-present risk of arterial embolization and the progressive nature of the condition with often irreversible changes in pulmonary artery pressure and right heart function. The classical closed operation has lost favour in the developed world where commissurotomy is most often performed on cardiopulmonary bypass or in the catheter laboratory by balloon cathether, but closed mitral valvotomy remains an efficient and effective operation for those patients who have pure commissural fusion with a pliable valve as it spares the patient the deleterious effects of cardiopulmonary bypass.

Closed mitral valvotomy

The heart is approached through a left lateral or anterolateral thoracotomy in the fifth interspace. The pericardium is opened anterior to the phrenic nerve; with the right index finger inserted through the left atrial appendage and a specially designed dilator inserted through the apex of the left ventricle, the commissures are opened within the beating heart.

Even from this brief description it can be appreciated that the operation may become dramatic if haemorrhage, hypotension or rhythm disturbance occurs and yet, in practised hands, the mortality is around 1%. Sometimes the attempt results in severe mitral incompetence so facilities for cardiopulmonary bypass should be available. The surgeon must choose the patients well and retain control during the operation. The largest contemporary experience with this operation is now in the less developed countries: the report from the Christian Medical College, Vellore, India[35] describes the practice of closed mitral valvotomy in an environment where it provides an extremely effective and economic solution to a common problem.

Enthusiasm for percutaneous balloon techniques is growing amongst cardiologists; the cases most suitable for closed valvotomy are amenable to balloon dilatation for the same reasons.

Mitral regurgitation

Rheumatic heart disease may result in acute, severe mitral valve incompetence; more commonly a mild degree of regurgitation coexists with mitral stenosis. Occasionally attempts to relieve mitral stenosis, whether by open or closed operation, result in mitral regurgitation. The most common cause of pure mitral regurgitation is now floppy valve disease, where the leaflets become soft and spongy and the chordae elongated because of a basic biochemical abnormality of the valve collagen.[36] The papillary muscles may infarct as a result of ischaemic heart disease, resulting in varying degrees of regurgitation. If a papillary muscle ruptures after myocardial infarction this results in catastrophic regurgitation in an already sick patient. Infective endocarditis may involve the mitral valve, causing or exacerbating mitral regurgitation, and occurs particularly in floppy valve disease.

The haemodynamic consequence is that the larger proportion of the stroke volume, and therefore the ventricular work, is wasted in blood passing to and fro through the mitral valve. The lungs are subjected to high pressure, although in the early stages this is intermittent and the pressure falls to the ventricular diastolic pressure. Symptoms may therefore be mild while the heart compensates by increasing in size. Eventually breathlessness on exertion or attacks of pulmonary oedema occur. On examination the heart is abnormally large and active and there is a murmur lasting throughout systole, heard all over the chest but not radiating to the neck.

The chest radiograph typically shows generalized cardiac enlargement with all four chambers becoming involved due to volume load on the left side of the heart and eventually pressure load on the right side, as the pulmonary artery pressure rises. The ECG may have features of left atrial and left ventricular hypertrophy. Echocardiography is usually sufficient to make the diagnosis. Doppler imaging helps to quantify the severity of regurgitation. Cardiac catheterization is only needed to assess any associated coronary artery disease.

Surgical management

The decision to recommend operation may be very difficult.[37] Pulmonary oedema occurs in acute cases with gross regurgitation into a small atrium and surgery is essential. In chronic cases when mitral regurgitation is relatively mild or has progressed slowly, it is tolerated very well and surgery is hard to justify in a symptom free patient, especially as the results of mitral valve replacement are far from perfect and include a risk of thromboembolic problems, with possibly the added inconvenience and danger of anticoagulants.

REFERENCES

35. John S et al Circulation 1983; 68: 891
36. Barlow J B et al Am Heart J 1963; 66: 443
37. Wells F C, Shapiro L M Mitral Valve Disease. Butterworth Heinemann, Ch 20 p 187

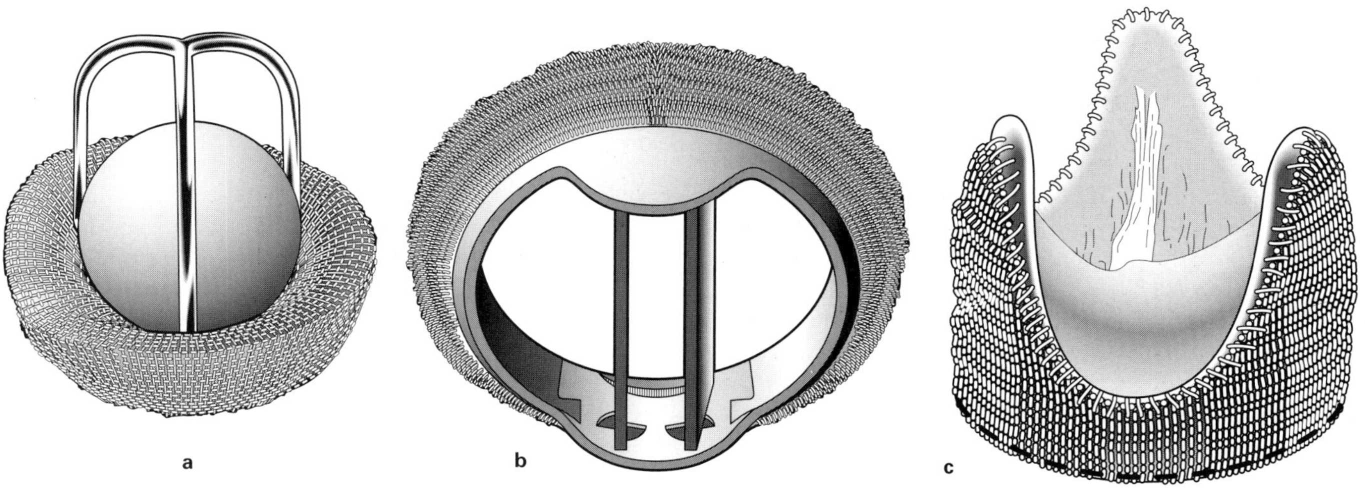

Fig. 23.14 (**a**) A 'ball in cage' aortic prosthetic heart valve (note the 3 struts). (**b**) A bi-leaflet mechanical valve. (**c**) A stentless porcine xenograft valve.

Once the heart begins to enlarge on serial chest radiographs taken at yearly intervals surgery is usually recommended to halt a progressive and then irreversible deterioration in the left ventricle.

The mitral valve is replaced in most patients with mitral regurgitation severe enough to justify surgery. The operative mortality (death within 30 days) has levelled off at 6–7% for all cases of mitral valve replacement.

There is an increasing trend back to conservative operations on the mitral valve, reflecting disillusionment with the performance of mitral prostheses. Procedures to refashion the cusp tissue, repair the chordae and reduce the annulus size permit the surgeon to restore function to the mitral valve.[38]

Mitral valve replacement

The usual approach is now through median sternotomy. Bypass is established, usually with separate cannulation of the superior and inferior venae cavae (Fig. 23.1). The left atrium is opened from the right side through an incision just behind and parallel to the interatrial septum. Access may be difficult and attention to details of exposure and operating conditions is important. Most of the skill lies in performing the operation quickly and accurately within the constraints of limited space and time.

The mitral valve is usually excised, although preservation of the posterior cusp with its chordae has been said to reduce the risk of posterior ventricular rupture—an uncommon and disastrous complication—and may also preserve left ventricular function. A variety of suture techniques are used: continuous and interrupted, with and without buttresses. A continuous technique has the advantage of speed and, when access is good, is surgically very satisfactory. Interrupted suturing techniques are easier in that individual stitches are inserted and spaced in the annulus and then in the sewing ring, as independent steps, making it more reliable in inexperienced hands or when access is difficult.

The choice of valve. The indications and techniques for mitral, aortic and tricuspid valve replacement differ considerably, but many aspects of cardiac valve prostheses can be considered in common. The first consideration is whether to use a valve made, as far as possible, of natural tissues or to opt for a mechanical valve of the best available materials. The first tissue valve used was the human cadaveric aortic valve (known as a 'homograft' in cardiac surgical literature)[39] and at a similar time a caged ball valve was tried.[40]

Engineers have continued to work on mechanical valve design and three basic patterns have evolved: caged ball, single disc and bi-leaflet.[41,42] The most widely used tissue valves to date have been made of a pig's aortic valve, glutaraldehyde-fixed and mounted on a frame. They are known generically as 'xenografts' or 'bioprostheses' and have the advantage over homografts of ready availability in a range of sizes with a high degree of quality control.

In essence, mechanical valves have a high risk of thromboembolic complications and patients receiving them must be rigorously controlled on anticoagulants for the rest of their lives. On the whole the valves are durable but there are sporadic examples of sudden mechanical failure.[43] In general, the tissue valves are safer but eventual failure seems inevitable. The median valve life is 12–14 years, leading to re-operation in many patients who live longer than that.[41,42] The haemodynamic characteristics, which include the pressure drop across the valve and the magnitude of any regurgitation, are satisfactory in all the currently available artificial valves (Fig. 23.14) but these valves share a serious and perpetual risk of endocarditis which affects about 2% per year.

The current trend for aortic valve replacement is once again towards a more natural valve, with a resurgence of free sewn homografts, stentless valves, and the Ross operation in which the patient's own healthy pulmonary valve is replaced with a homograft so that it can be used to replace a diseased aortic valve.[44]

REFERENCES

38. Carpentier J Thorac Cardiovasc Surg 1980; 79: 338
39. Ross D N Lancet 1962; ii: 487
40. Starr et al Circulation 1963; 27: 779
41. Treasure T Lancet 1990; 336: 1115
42. Treasure T Curr Opinion Cardiol 1995; 10: 144
43. Treasure T Br Heart J 1991; 66: 333
44. Treasure T Lancet 1994; 343: 1308

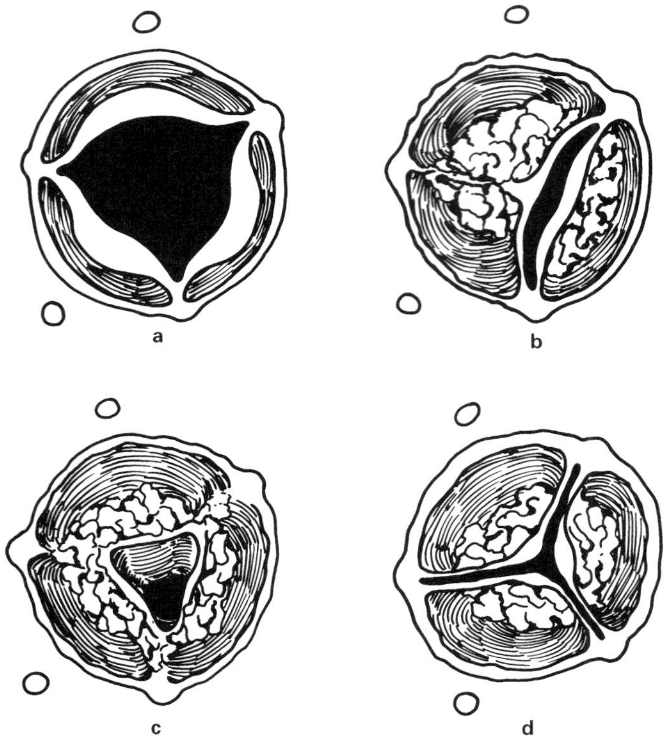

Fig. 23.15 Aortic valve. (a) Normal valve with three cusps opening symmetrically. The right coronary orifice is shown anteriorly and the left coronary posteriorly. (b) A congenitally abnormal valve with failure of development resulting in a bicuspid appearance which is likely to become calcified and stenotic in later life. (c) Rheumatic fever obliterates the commissures and leads to thickening and later calcification. (d) Some anatomically normal valves become calcified in old age.

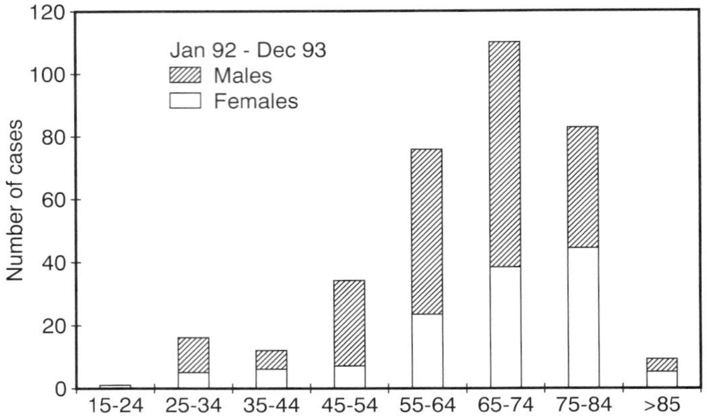

Fig. 23.16 Age and gender distribution of a series of our own patients undergoing aortic valve replacement at St. George's in 1992 and 1993.

Aortic valve disease

Aortic stenosis

Congenital abnormalities of the aortic valve are relatively common but only a minority are severe enough to present with aortic valve disease in infancy. Usually there is a variable degree of fusion between cusps; the right and left coronary sinuses most frequently share the common cusp and as long as this remains flexible there is no significant obstruction to flow. These abnormal valves tend to stiffen and calcify, and over half of the patients presenting for aortic valve replacement in middle and old age are found to have a congenitally malformed bicuspid valve. Rheumatic heart disease causes progressive commissural fusion and cusp rigidity which may be the only cardiac lesion or may coexist with mitral valve disease. The third form of aortic stenosis is generalized calcification of what appears to have been an anatomically normal valve.[45] This is more common over the age of 70 (Fig. 23.15).

The characteristic symptoms of aortic stenosis are: effort syncope, where the patient suddenly falls to the ground after exertion; angina pectoris (which may occur without any coronary disease); and breathlessness on exertion. Many cases are discovered because a systolic murmur is heard or an abnormality is detected on incidental investigation. The chest radiograph may be passed as normal because obvious cardiac enlargement is a relatively late feature. The heart does have a characteristic shape with prominence of the aorta and left ventricular apex, exaggerating the concavity on the left side which is lost in mitral valve disease. Calcification of the valve should be looked for on the lateral chest radiograph. The ECG has the characteristic changes of left ventricular hypertrophy, most easily recognized by increased voltage of the QRS complex in the chest leads (e.g. S in V1 plus R in V6 > 35 mm), with flattening and inversion of the lateral chest leads in more advanced cases. Echocardiography provides a measure of left ventricular hypertrophy and function and the degree of thickening and calcification of the valve. Cardiac catheterization is usually performed to measure the gradient across the valve, which remains an important determinant of the need for operation, and to visualize the coronary arteries.

Surgery for aortic stenosis. Aortic valve replacement is indicated in most cases of aortic stenosis causing symptoms, however well tolerated, because of the poor prognosis and the risk of sudden death. Even in the absence of symptoms a peak systolic gradient of greater than 60 mmHg represents a risk of sudden death and surgery is advised. This improves symptoms and prognosis and can be performed with a mortality of about 3%.[1] The peak incidence of aortic valve replacement in contemporary practice is around the age of 70 (Fig. 23.16) and more than 25% of our patients are over 75.

Aortic regurgitation

Incompetence of the aortic valve may be due to congenital (usually bicuspid) abnormality, endocarditis, rheumatic fever, syphilis, ankylosing spondylitis or Reiter's syndrome. Progress is insidious and patients may remain apparently well until the heart is enormously enlarged and the left ventricle is damaged beyond recovery. The natural history is very variable and some patients with a known regurgitant valve remain well without cardiac

REFERENCE

45. Davies M J, Treasure T, Parker D J Heart 1996; 75: 174

enlargement. Symptoms include breathlessness, and some patients have a sensation like angina, particularly on lying down.

The signs can be very dramatic. The long-standing increased pulse pressure results in massive arterial pulsation in the neck and the phenomenon of the collapsing, Corrigan or 'water hammer' pulse is well known to medical students. The heart is abnormally active but the diagnostic high-pitched decrescendo diastolic murmur is easily missed. It is sought carefully at the left sternal edge, immediately after the second sound. It can be heard more easily by asking the patient to breathe out while sitting forward.

The usually benign but unpredictable course makes timing of surgery difficult. The patient is followed until symptoms justify surgery or there is evidence of left ventricular deterioration, either with cardiac enlargement on the radiograph or deterioration of the ECG.[46]

Aortic valve replacement. The operation is performed through median sternotomy and a single venous cannula is sufficient. Cardioplegic arrest of the heart, which can be achieved or supplemented by direct coronary cannulation, has greatly improved the protection of the hypertrophied and vulnerable left ventricular muscle from ischaemic damage. Again, both interrupted and continuous suture techniques have their proponents. The risk is around 3% for all cases[1] but is very low in patients with well preserved left ventricular function. The addition of coronary artery grafting does not greatly complicate the operation and is safer than leaving unrelieved left ventricular ischaemia.

Tricuspid valve disease

Isolated tricuspid valve disease is rare.[47] The tricuspid valve may be involved with rheumatic fever along with the mitral valve or it may become incompetent as a secondary phenomenon due to high right-sided pressures as a result of left-sided valve disease. Endocarditis of the tricuspid valve is rarely seen apart from in drug addicts, in whom it is characteristic. Tricuspid incompetence occasionally presents with a large pulsating liver which is felt as a tender mass in the epigastrium.

The characteristic clinical signs are a raised jugular venous pressure with systolic waves and a pulsatile liver. The systolic murmur is not readily distinguishable from mitral regurgitation with which it may coexist.

The majority (about 85%) of tricuspid valve operations are performed at the same time as mitral valve surgery. These patients have a particularly high operative risk (20%) largely because of their preoperative state and the damage done to the pulmonary vasculature and the liver over many years of high pulmonary and systemic venous pressure.

Tricuspid valve surgery

Superior and inferior vena caval cannulation with encircling snares is essential so that the right atrium can be opened. The tricuspid valve is rarely abnormal and its triangular configuration makes replacement difficult. Competence can be restored by suturing the annulus to a suitably sized and shaped prosthesis.

Infective endocarditis

The term 'infective endocarditis' includes all infections seated on valvular and congenital abnormalities of the heart and great vessels and includes the very important group of prosthetic valve endocarditis. Endocarditis on previously normal valves is rare except in drug addicts. The rate of progress varies widely between acute fulminating cases and those that are so insidious as to defy detection for months, making the demarcation into acute and subacute unhelpful. Rickettsia or fungi, not just bacteria, may be the infecting agent, therefore the still familiar term 'SBE' (subacute bacterial endocarditis) is now obsolete.

Streptococci remain the most common organism although less predominantly. They are released into the bloodstream in the normal course of life, or in larger numbers with dental treatment. Gram-negative organisms may originate from large bowel abnormalities. Staphylococci of skin origin, including coagulase-negative staphylococci, are increasingly important and particularly difficult to treat. These organisms predominate in prosthetic valve endocarditis occurring within the first year after surgery when primary infection is suspected, and in drug addicts, related to recurrent dirty injections.

The symptoms are typically like influenza with aching muscles and alternating fever and shivering. All too often an ill considered course of antibiotics is given: this is in any case inappropriate for influenza and merely conceals the diagnosis. The combination of fever with any cardiac lesion on history, clinical examination or suspicion should lead to a working diagnosis of endocarditis. A series of blood cultures should be secured without delay.

The clinical signs include splenomegaly, splinter haemorrhages and, in long-standing cases, sometimes clubbing. Anaemia, a high erythrocyte sedimentation rate and leucocytosis are typical. Urgent and complete microbiological diagnosis is of paramount importance. Thereafter management should be carried out in consultation with a cardiologist and microbiologist. Surgery has a life-saving role in resistant cases and, particularly with prosthetic valve endocarditis, the surgeon should be involved early.

The cardiac condition, which often includes regurgitation of one or more valves, should be treated as appropriate. Indications for surgery include uncontrollable and life-endangering haemodynamic abnormalities that are amenable to surgical correction, for example valve replacement, closure of septal defects or ligation of a persistent ductus arteriosus. Surgery may be required if infection cannot be brought under control, which may be as a result of an intracardiac abscess.

Although absolute evidence will never be available, it seems likely that a short-term high-dose prophylactic antibiotics, given before predictable episodes of bacteraemia, may reduce the incidence of endocarditis in susceptible individuals. All patients with an abnormal heart should take antibiotics before even the most minor dental treatment (including scaling) and probably a number

REFERENCES

46. Treasure T Br J Hosp Med 1993; 49: 613
47. Treasure T (unsigned editorial) Lancet 1988; ii: 1061

of other events such as instrumental delivery of a baby, cystoscopy and other forms of instrumentation.

CORONARY ARTERY DISEASE

The advances in diagnosis and management of coronary artery disease have been formidable in the last 30 years. When Aird wrote on the subject in 1957 coronary angiography had not been performed and the surgery described, aimed at relieving angina, is now of only historical interest. It included creating pericardial adhesions with asbestos, a futile approach as these adhesions are bloodless. Cardio-omentopexy, in which the omentum was brought up through the diaphragm, and Vineberg's operation[48] where the internal mammary artery was tunnelled into the myocardium, may have had more hope of success but both depended on chance formation of a capillary network without direct access to the coronary system.

Since the late 1960s bypass grafting for coronary artery disease has become one of the most commonly performed operations. Favoloro[49] described the technique of saphenous vein bypass grafting from the Cleveland Clinic in 1967; in the 1980s over 10 000 operations per year were performed in the UK and over 200 000 in the USA. Operation rates range from 200 to nearly 1000 per million of the population in developed countries but after the enormous growth rate in the 1970s there are signs that both the epidemic of coronary artery disease and the numbers of operations performed are now levelling off. Medical management has also improved greatly with the availability of accurate methods of diagnosis and effective drugs.

Pathology

Deposition of atheroma in the coronary arteries is part of the spectrum of occlusive arterial disease. The diet and way of life in developed countries is of clear epidemiological importance with family history, lipid disorders, smoking, hypertension and diabetes being risk factors for the individual (see Chapter 10).

Presentation

The consequence of occlusive coronary artery disease is myocardial ischaemia: the mode of presentation depends on whether this is reversible, as is the case in patients who suffer recurrent episodes of angina pectoris, or irreversible resulting in myocardial infarction. Any combination of sequences of these clinical states may occur.

Angina pectoris is the key symptom; it may be very characteristic but diagnostic uncertainty is common. Its time scale and precipitating and relieving factors are of more diagnostic help than the exact site or subjective description of the attack. The sensation is most typically described as crushing or choking but some patients call it sharp or burning or describe a feeling of breathlessness; pain is often denied. Radiation, which is usually into the left arm, to the elbow or the wrist or into the jaw, is strongly in favour of the diagnosis, but not necessary for it; onset with exercise, relief by rest and exacerbation by wind, cold, or a recent large meal should be sought, with specific questioning if necessary.

Unfortunately the history may be inconclusive. There are many patients who are misdiagnosed as suffering from indigestion or from oesophageal or biliary pain; the cardiac condition is overlooked until the patient is admitted with acute infarction. The reverse is also true, and unexpected gallstones have been seen in the corner of a normal coronary angiogram! Clinical examination may be negative but hypertension and aortic valve disease should be specifically considered and excluded.

The other common and characteristic presentation of myocardial ischaemia is myocardial infarction. The symptoms accrue over several minutes (not suddenly) and persist for well over an hour with sustained intensity. The sensation may be similar or worse and more persistent than angina attacks which the patient has experienced or it may be the first ever experience of cardiac symptoms. It is accompanied by distress, pallor, sweating, nausea and sometimes vomiting. Although the clinical features of myocardial infarction are well known, the differential diagnosis is not always easy and the various causes of acute chest pain, including aortic dissection, pulmonary embolism, pneumothorax, and oesophageal pain must be considered in the differential diagnosis. Acute abdominal conditions also have to be considered, especially acute cholecystitis. The most valuable diagnostic test is a 12-lead ECG which virtually always shows evidence of ischaemia in the presence of evolving myocardial infarction. The immediate management should be active but is rarely surgical.

Surgical management of angina pectoris

Investigations

Clinical examination, chest radiograph and ECG are characteristically normal. Exercise ECG is important in confirming the diagnosis and assessing severity. Nuclear techniques can demonstrate perfusion abnormalities and document the state of the left ventricle reasonably well but coronary angiography is the important investigation that determines management.

Coronary angiography. This technique was developed and pioneered at the Cleveland Clinic. Preformed catheters are passed retrogradely into the aortic root from the femoral or right brachial artery. The ostia of the coronary arteries are selectively cannulated and injected with contrast medium and the angiogram recorded on cine film or CD ROM. At least two views, and often more, are taken of each of the coronary arteries to define the exact site and severity of any stenoses or occlusions.

Coronary anatomy

See Figure 23.17.

Medical management

The initial assessment is clinical. The best care of the patient with angina is holistic and should include removal of known and

REFERENCES

48. Vineberg Niloff Surg Gynecol Obstet 1950; 91: 551
49. Favoloro R G J Thorac Cardiovasc Surg 1969; 58: 178

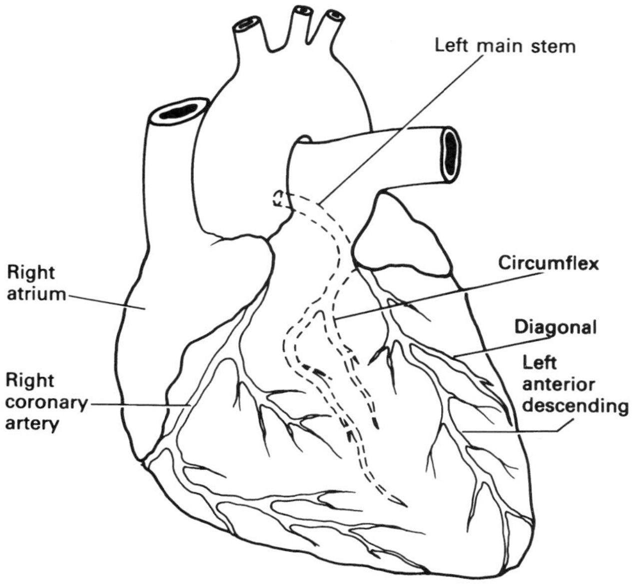

Fig. 23.17 In simple terms there are two coronary arteries arising from the aortic sinuses which, upon division of the left coronary artery into its anterior descending (anterior interventricular) and circumflex branches, comprise with the right coronary artery three functional systems supplying the heart approximately in thirds.

avoidable risk factors, judicious use of drugs, consideration of relief of obstruction with surgery or angioplasty, and sensible advice about changes in lifestyle. An adverse family history cannot be changed but a smoking habit can. Hypertension, diabetes and hypercholesterolaemia are factors which can be ameliorated to some extent.[50] Drug treatment of angina includes vasodilator drugs, β-blockers and calcium antagonists. The beneficial effects of vasodilators have been known for many years. The first described was amyl nitrate. Glyceryl trinitrate has been the mainstay for many years: it is used sublingually as tablets and spray and can also be given percutaneously and intravenously. A wide range of nitrates which can be given orally and in sustained-release preparations are now available. It is likely that the effect on coronary circulation itself is the least important and that venous dilatation, reducing the preload or wall stress during diastole, and arteriolar dilatation which reduces afterload (that is, the work done in systole) are more important in relieving angina. Full medical treatment may include all three agents—vasodilators, β-blockers and calcium antagonists.

If symptoms are readily brought under control with medical treatment and there are no particular features in the history to identify the patient as particularly at risk, no further action may be taken at this stage. Surgery is only indicated in symptomless patients if they have an anatomical pattern of disease known to be an independent hazard (for example left main stem stenosis) which could be neutralized by surgery. Angina which is uncontrolled by medical treatment should be considered for active intervention.

Selection of patients for surgery

Surgery produces the most dramatic and rewarding relief of severe disability in a high proportion of patients. The ideal case has tight proximal stenoses and large healthy distal vessels beyond, but surgeons long ago extended surgery to include almost any severity of coronary disease while still gaining symptomatic relief for the great majority. The question of whether surgery can extend life has been the subject of considerable debate. Three large multicentre prospective randomized trials have addressed this issue: the Veterans' Administration Cooperative Study,[51,52] the European Coronary Surgery Study Group[53] and the Coronary Artery Surgery Study.[54] The problem that underlies this debate is that there is little relationship between the symptom—angina—and the fatal consequence of coronary narrowing—myocardial infarction. Some patients live for years with daily angina but have an undamaged left ventricle while others suffer a massive infarction without warning and without subsequent angina.

Cardiologists and surgeons have used the information from these studies and other published series to formulate rational treatment policies.[55,56] We have now identified certain clinical and anatomical descriptors of good and bad prognostic groups. Patients with only one or two vessels involved, relatively distal lesions, unimpaired left ventricular function and stable angina have a very good chance—better than 90% probability—of being alive 5 years later and this has not been improved upon by operation. The margin of improvement which might be gained by surgery is in any case small because of the age and underlying pathology in these cases. In patients with a good natural history the decision depends on the severity of symptoms and limitation of the enjoyment of life, after medical measures have been tried. On the other hand, left main stem stenosis, proximal left anterior descending disease, three-vessel involvement, angina coming on at rest (unstable angina), and a left ventricle already damaged by infarction are all predictors of an increased likelihood of death; in these cases an operation significantly improves the probability of survival up to and beyond 5 years. In addition to these specific questions about probability of long-term survival with and without operation, the decision should take into account the various other risks which must be weighed up as the balance of risks and benefits is considered.

Coronary artery surgery

The operation is nearly always performed on cardiopulmonary bypass but, since none of the cardiac chambers need be opened, this can be set up in its simplest form (see Fig. 23.2). A single cannula is adequate for venous drainage, an arterial cannula is placed in the ascending aorta and no intracardiac vent is necessary, so the risks of air embolism are minimized. The coronary arteries are about 1.5–2.0 mm in diameter at the sites usually selected for grafting so a still bloodless heart is ideal. The use of cardioplegia

REFERENCES

50. ASPIRE Steering Group Heart 1996; 75: 334
51. Detre et al Lancet 1977; ii: 1243
52. Detre et al Circulation 1981; 63: 1329
53. European Coronary Surgery Study Group Lancet 1982; ii: 1173
54. Coronary Artery Surgery Study Principal Investigations N Engl J Med 1984; 310: 750
55. Kumar P, Treasure T Br J Hosp Med 1996; 56(1): 33
56. Hadorn D C, Holmes A C Br Med J 1997; 314: 135

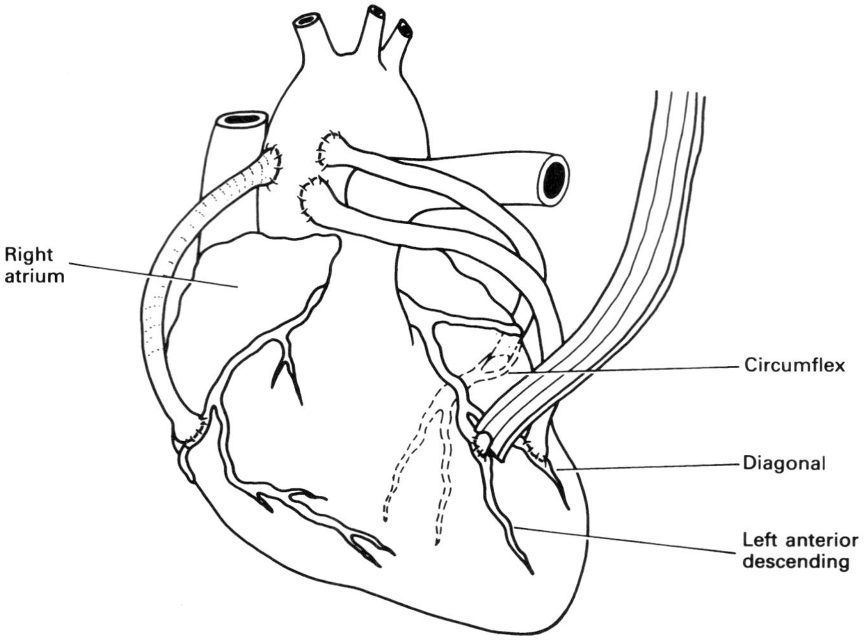

Fig. 23.18 A typical coronary operation with a left internal mammary artery anastomosed to the anterior descending coronary artery and aortocoronary vein grafts to three other branches.

or short periods (5–10 minutes) of ischaemia and ventricular fibrillation are equally well tolerated.

The use of the left internal mammary artery as the graft of first choice for the left anterior descending coronary artery has become widespread since 10-year follow-up results from the Cleveland Clinic[57,58] and other centres revealed that the long-term results were superior to saphenous vein grafts, not only in terms of graft patency but also infarct-free survival. Three or four coronary branches are usually bypassed (Figs 23.18 and 23.19) and various permutations of mammary and other arterial grafts (such as the free radical artery, or pedicled gastroepiploic artery) and vein grafts are used, often with two or more sequential anastomoses. Endarterectomy is avoided by most surgeons but may be the only means of access in a totally blocked system, most commonly the right coronary artery. The vessel is then grafted at this site but patency at 1 year is not as good as when a graft can be placed directly to a more normal segment of the vessel.

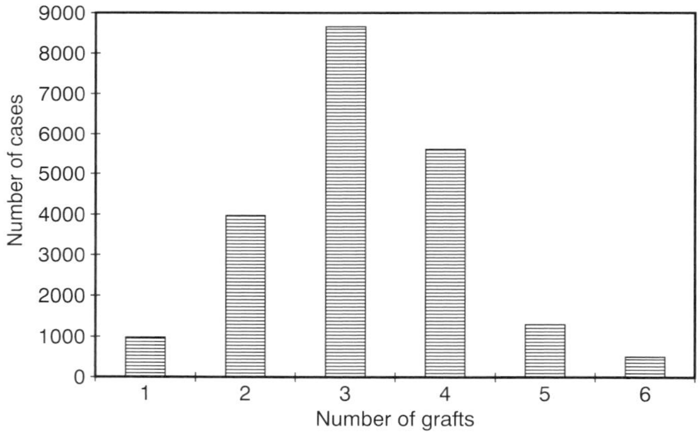

Fig. 23.19 Frequency distribution of numbers of vessels grafted in current coronary surgery practice from UK register[1] for 1993–1994.

Results of operation

The operative mortality (30-day or in-hospital) is 2–3% for national figures and large multicentre trials. The risk is increased with age over 70, female gender, increasing number of grafts (representing more extensive disease), poor left ventricular function, and coexistent disease. For elective male cases the true risk can be as low as under 1%. Morbidity includes a small risk of major stroke (about 1%), and a larger risk of transient focal neurological deficit, probably embolic in origin (2–4%). A high proportion of all patients who undergo cardiopulmonary bypass have transient neuropsychological impairment which is usually subclinical but can be detected with sensitive tests.[17,59] Significant wound infection complicates 2–3% of operations.[60,61]

The majority of patients have complete relief of angina but 10–15% have some residual symptoms and a small minority are no better. Failure to relieve angina is associated with failure to bypass all diseased vessels or early graft occlusion. Most patients leave hospital 8–10 days after surgery but convalescence can take several weeks.

The 1-year patency rate for vein grafts is about 80–90% with an attrition rate of 3–4% per year thereafter; a similar proportion of

REFERENCES

57. Treasure T (Unsigned editorial) Lancet 1985; 2: 1253
58. Loop et al N Engl J Med 1986; 314: 1
59. Smith P L C et al Lancet 1986; i: 823
60. Wilson A P R et al Eur J Cardiothorac Surg 1987; 1: 158
61. Luckraz H, Treasure T Curr Opinion Surg Inf 1996; 4: 1

patients develop recurrent angina, either due to graft occlusion or progression of disease in native vessels. There is evidence that treatment to reduce platelet adherence may improve graft patency:[62] this is now usually achieved with low-dose aspirin.

Surgery for the complications of myocardial infarction

By the time a patient presents with an evolving infarction, the area of myocardium beyond the blocked coronary is usually beyond surgical salvage. Immediate (within 3 h) thrombolysis minimizes myocardial damage. Surgery has only rarely a useful part to play. Various angioplasty techniques may be applicable in certain cases although, as with surgery, it is the time to get to this specialized form of treatment that will determine how generally applicable it is.

In the days that follow infarction about 3% of patients, typically in the group who are doing well, suddenly deteriorate due to rupture of the infarcted muscle. Rupture follows one of three characteristic patterns. Rupture of the free wall of the left ventricle results in sudden death with cardiac tamponade. Rupture of the ventricular septum results in left-to-right shunt, which if severe (resulting in a pulmonary to systemic flow ratio of over 2:1) is poorly tolerated. The third pattern is severe mitral regurgitation due to papillary muscle necrosis. The last two are amenable to surgical correction.

The diagnosis should be suspected in a patient who collapses suddenly with poor cardiac output and develops pulmonary oedema about 3–6 days after a myocardial infarction. Swan–Ganz pulmonary artery catheterization at the beside is the most valuable approach to the problem because a step-up in saturation will confirm a shunt while the pressure tracing from the pulmonary artery wedge may support the diagnosis of torrential mitral regurgitation. Few patients survive either of these complications without urgent surgery.

Surgical management of acute myocardial rupture

Investigation and resuscitation must be undertaken urgently and in parallel. At the same time plans to operate on the patient must be initiated. The information gained from Swan–Ganz catheterization is a valuable first step but most surgeons would prefer to have more information about the number and site of coronary obstructions, the state of the left ventricle and as much certainty as possible about the site and exact nature of the rupture. Modern two-dimensional echo techniques, particularly with the use of intracardiac Doppler flow studies, will provide much of the anatomical and haemodynamic information required but only formal cardiac catheterization will provide information about the coronary arteries. A quick, definitive operation may be the only hope of success so the surgeon must have as precise a diagnosis and operative plan as possible before embarking on surgery.

During cardiac catheterization, it is useful to place an intra-aortic balloon pump (see Fig. 23.24) to help support the circulation while the patient is being transferred to the operating theatre.

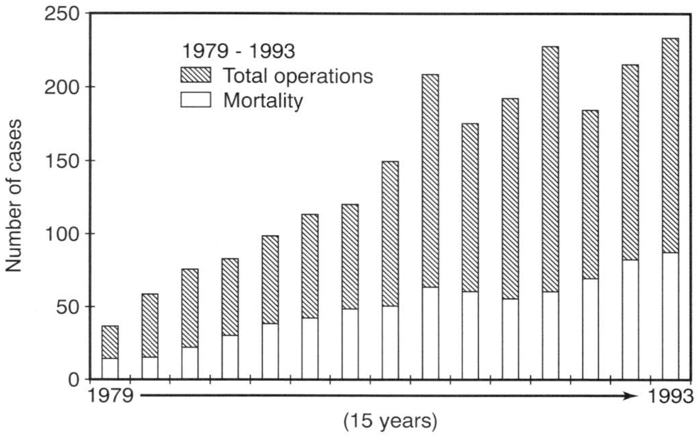

Fig. 23.20 Operations for ventricular septal rupture for 15 years from 1979 to 1993 showing a mortality of around 40% throughout.[1]

Mitral valve replacement under these circumstances is made a little more difficult by the small, as yet undilated, atrium and the delicate nature of the annulus in an essentially normal valve, but is otherwise a standard procedure (see above). The operation of repair of ventricular septal rupture is obvious in principle but can be very difficult in practice (Fig. 23.20). The necrotic tissues take sutures extremely badly and patches must be secured with Teflon felt buttresses so that they will not tear out, but this must be done without sacrificing functioning myocardium (Fig. 23.21).

Left ventricular aneurysm

In patients who survive a large full-thickness myocardial infarction the left ventricular scar may begin to stretch and become aneurysmal. This area contributes nothing to ejection and left ventricular work is wasted in the process. It may therefore be a reversible cause of heart failure. Left ventricular aneurysm may also be a source of embolism and of life-endangering ventricular arrhythmia.

Left ventricular aneurysm may present in any of these three ways but the history is quite non-specific. Clinical signs are described but are unhelpful. The ECG characteristically has Q waves in the anterior chest leads, absent R waves and an elevated ST segment. Echocardiography will detect left ventricular aneurysm but angiography is essential to define the coronary anatomy. The ideal case is a large anteroapical aneurysm occurring as a result of proximal left anterior descending coronary artery occlusion with good functioning muscle elsewhere. Inferior and lateral aneurysms are much less common. Paradoxical filling of the aneurysm during systole can be demonstrated angiographically or by nuclear techniques.

The patients must be carefully selected because not all will benefit from surgery and the risks are relatively high; mortality of around 10% is probably still a reasonable figure to quote (Fig. 23.22). Although the ideal case has single-vessel disease the

REFERENCE

62. Chesebro J H et al N Engl J Med 1984; 310: 209

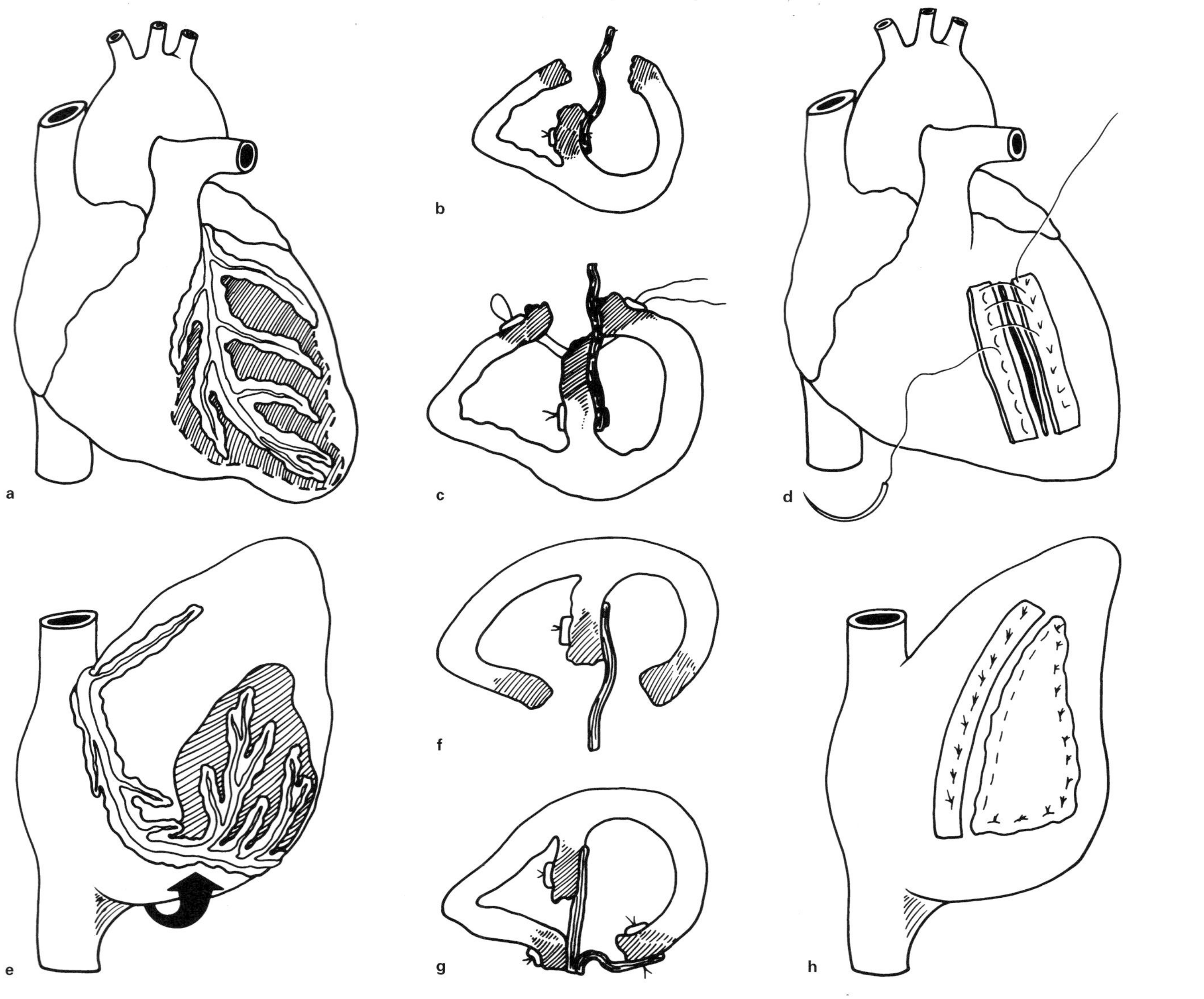

Fig. 23.21 Surgical repair of ventricular septal rupture following acute myocardial infarction. Shading shows the affected area. (**a**) Occlusion of the proximal left anterior descending coronary artery in a patient with little collateral supply results in extensive infarction of the anteroapical portion of the left ventricle and the septum. (**b**) An incision is made through the area of infarction and a patch sutured to the left side of the septum with exclusion or excision of infarcted tissue. (**c**) The patch is brought out through the ventricular incision. (**d**) The defect is closed with buttressed sutures. (**e**) Complete occlusion of the right coronary artery results in an inferior infarction. (**f,g**) Rupture of the posterior part of the septum is much more difficult to close but the principles are similar. (**h**) Closure of the left ventricle with a patch is required with inferior infarction. Infarction of right ventricle is usually associated and right ventricular function is a determinant of outcome in these cases.

majority of patients considered for surgery have disease in other vessels; where these have been grafted at the time of aneurysm resection the mortality is, if anything, less amongst those expected to be at more risk, which supports this policy.

Operation for resection of left ventricular aneurysm

The aneurysm is resected leaving a margin of tough scar tissue to take sutures. With careful attention to restoration of the left ventricular architecture this can be a very satisfactory operation but it requires some judgement (Fig. 23.23).

Intra-aortic balloon counterpulsation

The intra-aortic balloon pump is a valuable means of supporting the failing heart. The approximately cylindrical balloon is mounted on the end of a catheter through which it can be inflated and deflated abruptly with a low-viscosity gas such as helium. The balloon is inserted via the femoral artery and is sited in the descending aorta. The external pump is triggered from the patient's ECG so that it inflates during diastole and deflates again at the onset of systole (Fig. 23.24). It cannot therefore generate any cardiac output; however it displaces its own volume of blood and

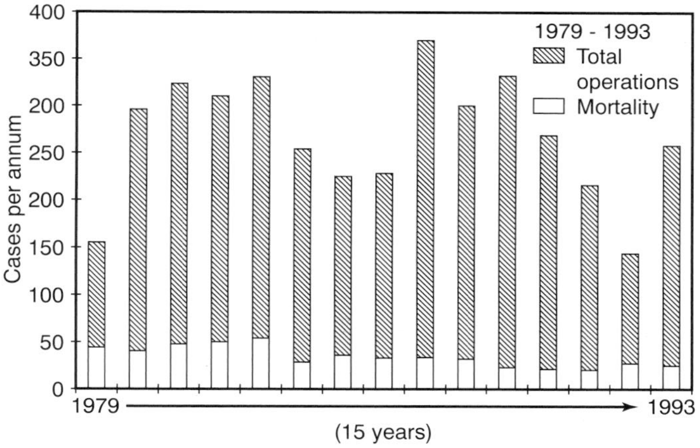

Fig. 23.22 Operations for left ventricular aneurysm. There is probably a decline in the frequency with which this operation is performed which, if viewed in comparison with other increases, is quite striking.[1]

enhances coronary blood flow as the myocardium relaxes in diastole; then, because it relaxes abruptly in systole, it permits ejection against a lowered peripheral vascular resistance.

It should only be used if there is a realistic prospect of the patient's condition improving or of being improved by surgery, as in the case of septal or papillary muscle rupture after myocardial infarction.

MYXOMA

Primary cardiac tumours are very uncommon and the only one that appears with sufficient frequency to merit discussion in a general clinical text is myxoma. This is a fascinating condition which can manifest itself in a variety of ways and can lead to great diagnostic confusion. Whenever it is considered, echocardiography should be performed and is diagnostic. About 50 cases per annum are operated upon in the UK.[1]

Pathology

In 80% of cases the myxoma is in the left atrium; in 15% it is in the right atrium and the remainder are ventricular or multiple. Myxomas vary in morphology but usually arise from the atrial septum on a short pedicle. Sometimes they are relatively solid and present late as they begin to obstruct the mitral valve. Others are friable, with sago pudding appearance and, in this form, are particularly likely to present with stroke or other embolic arterial occlusion. The old debate about whether these are true primary tumours or some form of organizing thrombus can now be forgotten. Their clinical behaviour and appearance at surgery are sufficiently characteristic for myxomas to be recognized as a discrete pathological entity. Their tendency to recur if incompletely removed and the occurrence of metastasis, albeit extremely rare, confirms that they are a form of tumour.

Clinical features

Myxoma can present in three quite distinct ways. As the tumour enlarges within the atrium it begins to obstruct blood flow and in

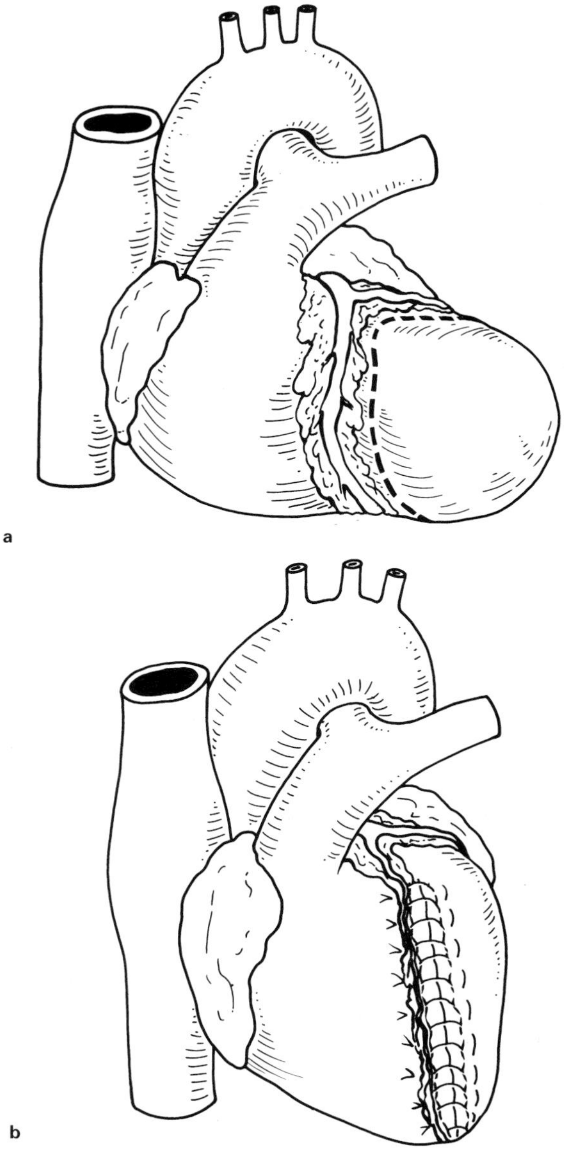

Fig. 23.23 (**a**) Left ventricular aneurysm due to stretching of a full-thickness scar in a survivor of myocardial infarction due to left anterior descending occlusion. (**b**) Resection and repair of the ventricular aneurysm.

the most common site, on the left side, mimics mitral stenosis. Breathlessness, orthopnoea and paroxysmal nocturnal dyspnoea may all occur. On examination the signs tend to support a diagnosis of mitral valve disease and although characteristic features such as variability of the murmur, postural changes and a 'tumour plop are described, it is a very astute clinician who even suspects the diagnosis. Aird's statement: 'Myxoma of the auricle has not been recognized during life' is no longer true but the diagnosis is still clinically elusive.

Embolism should always prompt a search for a cause: if the embolus is removed histological examination may make the diagnosis. Stroke is so common that it may not arouse suspicion. Finally, some cases present with rather non-specific systemic effects such as fever, high erythrocyte sedimentation rate and

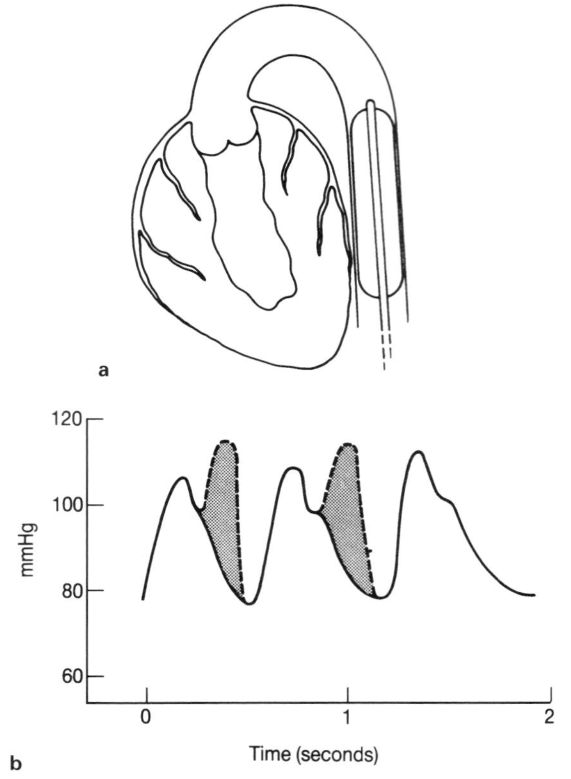

Fig. 23.24 (**a**) The balloon positioned in the descending aorta (see text). (**b**) The augmentation of the pressure trace (hatched area) due to balloon inflation during diastole, beginning at aortic valve closure.

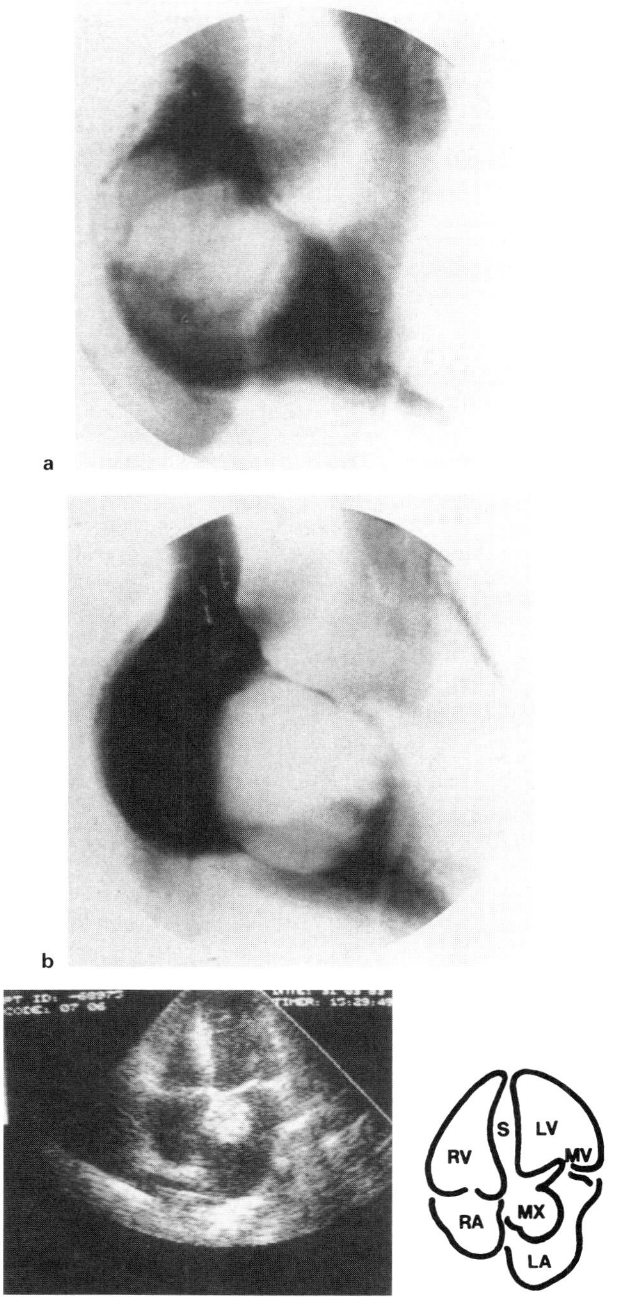

Fig. 23.25 Atrial myxoma. Digital subtraction angiogram of a myxoma seen as a white filling defect surrounded by contrast medium (black) which in this uncommon example is in the right atrium (**a**). With atrial systole it prolapses into the ventricle (**b**), seeming to fill the orifice completely. (**c**) Apical four chamber view of the heart with 2-dimensional echocardiography. The four chambers are labelled. RV, LV are right and left ventricles, and the septum (S) is easily seen between them. LA and RA are the two atria. The mitral valve (MV) is well seen and the myxoma (MX) is in the most common site, attached to the atrial septum.

plasma protein abnormalities and it may be a long time before the diagnosis is reached. Whichever way the patient presents, if the possibility of a cardiac cause is considered and an echocardiogram is performed the diagnosis is made with ease and certainty (Fig. 23.25).

Management

These tumours are removed as a matter of urgency because there is an ever-present risk of embolism or acute obstruction within the heart. Only about 50 operations per year are recorded for this condition in the UK Cardiac Surgical Register[1] and although it is a rare condition, it is likely that many more are missed. Operation should include complete removal of the attachment and careful exclusion of all fragments from the heart.

AORTIC DISSECTION

Dissection is the most common aortic emergency. If the ascending aorta is involved in the process the patient has little chance of surviving the acute event without surgical repair of the dissection. The real incidence of dissection is difficult to ascertain because these cases may be diagnosed as myocardial infarction and the true diagnosis may never be made, even though thoracic aortic dissection is 2–3 times more common than rupture of an abdominal aneurysm and occurs at a rate of 5–10 per million of the population per year. It presents as an emergency under various guises and may be seen on medical or surgical take.

The condition is rare below the age of 40 and most cases occur between 50 and 70 years of age. The sexes are about equally affected. Hypertension is the important aetiological factor. In

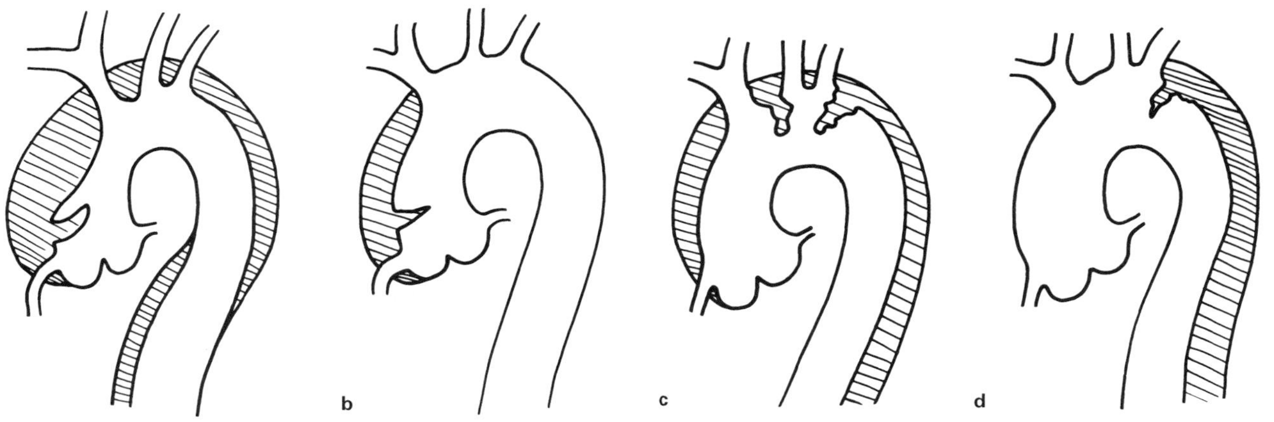

a b c d

Fig. 23.26 (**a**) The commonest pattern of aortic dissection with a tear in the ascending aorta and dissection extending retrogradely to the aortic valve and antegradely into the descending aorta (type I in DeBakey's classification). (**b**) Sometimes the dissection stops short of the arch (type II in DeBakey's classification). (**c**) Some cases with extensive dissection have a tear in the arch, or multiple tears. These do not fall easily into DeBakey's classification. (**d**) The second most common site for the tear is just beyond the left subclavian artery and then the tear may be confined to the descending aorta (type III DeBakey).
In a simpler classification all cases where the ascending aorta is involved in dissection (irrespective of the site of the tear) are called type A (i.e. **a**, **b** & **c**). These have a very high mortality without surgery. Dissection confined to the descending aorta, type B (**d**) may be managed conservatively in selected cases.

Marfan's syndrome[63] there is a propensity for aortic dissection due to a generalized abnormality in elastic tissue and it is one of the conditions which produces a histological appearance known rather imprecisely as 'cystic medial necrosis'. Aneurysmal dilatation of the proximal aorta is characteristic and may be seen without the other features. Both pregnancy and bicuspid aortic valve predispose to aortic dissection but considering the prevalence of these conditions the association is a weak one.

Pathology[64]

In aortic dissection the intima of the aorta suddenly gives way, producing a transverse or spiralling tear; blood enters the media, tracks longitudinally in the aortic wall, and splits it along a plane of cleavage in the outer part of the media. There is some evidence that the intramural haematoma is the first event and that the tear is secondary.[65] The intimal tear usually involves half to two thirds of the aortic circumference. The commonest sites are, in order of frequency:

1. 2–3 cm beyond the aortic valve—the majority, about 65%.
2. The uppermost part of the descending aorta just beyond the origin of the left subclavian—about a quarter occur here.
3. In the aortic arch itself—the remainder.

The longitudinal component, or 'dissection', which usually involves half to two thirds of the aortic circumference, may extend antegradely and retrogradely for a variable distance. Retrograde extension is usually right back to the aortic valve while antegrade dissection may extend along branches and beyond the aortic bifurcation with or without a re-entry tear. The dissection may obstruct the coronary arteries (particularly the right), the arch vessels, or impair the blood supply to the spinal cord, kidneys or gut producing appropriate clinical syndromes.

Aortic dissections are best classified according to their anatomical extent (Fig. 23.26). The diagnostic watershed depends on whether the ascending aorta is dissected. If it is, the dissection is of type A irrespective of the site of the tear, which is most commonly in the ascending aorta. If the dissecting process is confined to the descending aorta it is type B. This has tended to replace the time-honoured DeBakey classification (Fig. 23.26). Dissections are further classified as acute and chronic depending on the interval from occurrence to diagnosis, arbitrarily placed at 2 weeks.

The restraining adventitia may rupture at any time. In the case of type A dissections, rupture occurs within the pericardium and tamponade results. This is the cause of death in most cases. Any of the aortic branches may be occluded as a result of the dissection. In type A the right coronary artery is particularly vulnerable and the association of dissection with ECG changes of inferior myocardial infarction may add to diagnostic difficulty. Stroke may occur if the arch vessels are involved and paraplegia may result from interference to the arterial supply to the cord via the anterior spinal artery. Less commonly, acute renal failure or intestinal infarction may follow occlusion of visceral arteries, and iliac occlusion may produce ischaemia of the lower limbs.

Retrograde dissection to the aortic root results in aortic valve regurgitation. This is a very typical and almost diagnostic feature of type A dissection.

In type A dissection 40% of patients are dead within 24 hours and 80% in 2 weeks.

Presentation and diagnosis

The usual presentation is with chest pain of very sudden onset—tearing in quality and going through to the back. Collapse is

REFERENCES

63. Treasure T Br Heart J 1993; 69: 101
64. De Sanctis R W et al N Engl J Med 1987; 317: 1060
65. Davies M J, Treasure T, Richardson P D Heart 1996; 75: 434

common; the patient may lose consciousness and is often pale, clammy and pulseless. In those who survive to reach hospital, and in whom the diagnosis is suspected, a careful history should be taken of any transient neurological deficit, either cerebral or spinal.

Any information about the arterial pressure before the event should be carefully documented.

Examination

Documentation of the pulses is of particular importance because missing and varying pulses lend great weight to the diagnosis of dissection. Listen specifically for the soft, early diastolic murmur of aortic regurgitation, which is easily overlooked but may clinch the diagnosis. The findings on neurological examination should be recorded—an evolving stroke is a contraindication to surgery.

Investigation

Radiology

The majority present as emergencies to local general hospitals. The plain chest radiograph shows widening of the mediastinum and relative inward displacement of the crescent-shaped streak of calcification which marks the athermatous intima of the aorta in many cases. On reasonable suspicion of the diagnosis hypotensive management should be initiated. Nitroprusside by intravenous infusion should be given, titrated against the arterial pressure which is measured by an intra-arterial cannula. A β-blocker is added to reduce the force of contraction of the ventricle and thus the shear stress.

Steps should be made to transfer the patient for specialist assessment. This usually includes a cine aortogram although the diagnosis can be confirmed non-invasively by computerized tomography or with minimal interference by digital subtraction angiography, but insistence on performing these tests may delay definitive management.[66,67]

Echocardiography

This can be performed at the bedside in the Intensive Care Unit and, if positive, may give sufficient diagnostic information in an emergency.[68]

Surgery

The demonstration of dissection involving the ascending aorta (type A) is now generally accepted as sufficient indication to operate. Operation is contraindicated if there is an established or evolving stroke or if there is anuria because of established renal failure attributable to renal vascular involvement. Spinal involvement would deter most surgeons and of course extreme old age and the existence of intercurrent illness are arguments against operation.

While dissections confined to the descending aorta (type B) are managed conservatively from choice, life-endangering progression as indicated by continued pain or enlargement of the sac requires surgery.

Surgical treatment of type A dissections

Bypass is established with a femoral arterial cannula. The patient is cooled on bypass, initially to about 28°C but cooling to 18°C with circulatory arrest may be required if the arch is involved. Every effort is made to conserve the aortic valve. If there is dilatation of the aortic root itself, as occurs in Marfan's syndrome, it is then necessary to replace the aortic root and the valve and re-implant the coronaries (Fig. 23.27).

Results

The hospital mortality for medically managed type A dissections is over 90% while the UK Cardiac Surgical Register reports a mortality of about 25% for operated cases in recent years. There is little doubt that this group of patients stands the best chance of survival if the diagnosis is made promptly and they are referred for urgent surgery.[69,70]

TRAUMA TO THE HEART AND GREAT VESSELS[71,72]

The assessment of the multiply injured patient should take into account the pattern of the injury and all the systems that may be involved, whether primarily or as a result of blood loss, hypotension, hypoxia, or sepsis. Care of the patient cannot follow a leisurely sequence of assessment, investigation and treatment with each phase completed before the next is embarked upon, and the principles of acute trauma life support (ATLS) are now widely known and practised. As minutes, then hours and then days go by, the team has to reassess priorities and it is against this background that injury to a particular organ or system should be considered.

Blunt trauma

In something as apparently random as a motor accident the possible combinations of injuries may seem infinite and yet there are patterns that occur with sufficient frequency to be recognized. The three cardiothoracic injuries that may confront the trauma team are rupture of the aorta, myo-cardial contusion and rupture of cardiac valves.

Rupture of the aorta

In patients who have died after deceleration accidents such as aeroplane crash or a motor vehicle collision, rupture of the aorta is a

REFERENCES

66. Treasure T, Raphael M J Lancet 1991; 338: 490
67. Treasure T Br Heart J 1993; 70: 497
68. Treasure T, Brecker S J Heart Valve Dis 1996; 5: 623
69. Treasure T, Simpson I A In: Jackson G (ed) Difficult Concepts in Cardiology Martin Dunitz, p 183
70. Treasure T In: Russell R C G (ed) Recent Advances in Surgery 12. Churchill Livingstone, Edinburgh 1986
71. Sutherland G R, Calvin J E et al J Trauma 1981; 21: 1
72. Symbas P N In: Grillo H C, Eschapass H (eds) International Trends in General Thoracic Surgery, vol 2. W B Saunders, Philadelphia 1987

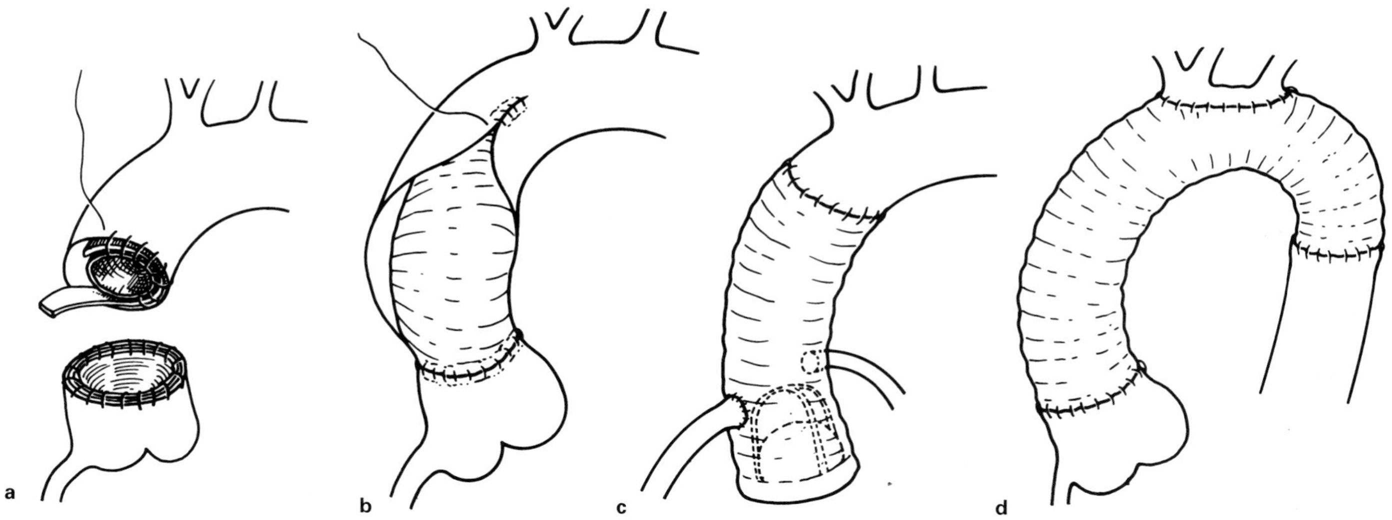

Fig. 23.27 Operations for aortic dissection. The operative approach ranges from transection and repair (**a**) through tube graft replacement (**b**), replacement of aortic root and aortic valve (**c**) to total aortic arch replacement (**d**) depending on the extent of the pathology and the judgement and skill of the surgeon.

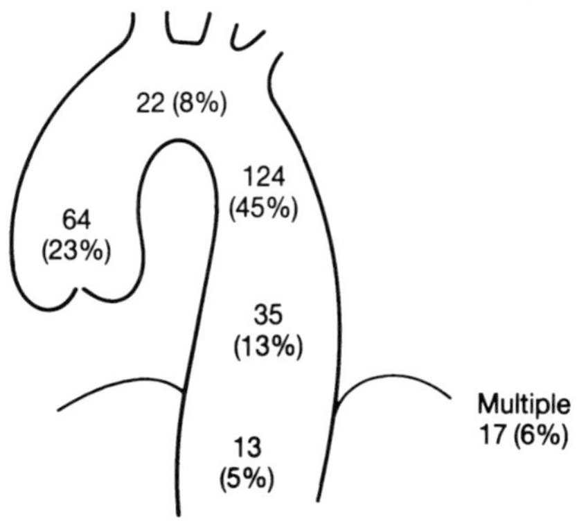

Fig. 23.28 Frequency with which various parts of the aorta are involved in traumatic rupture (data from Parmley).[73]

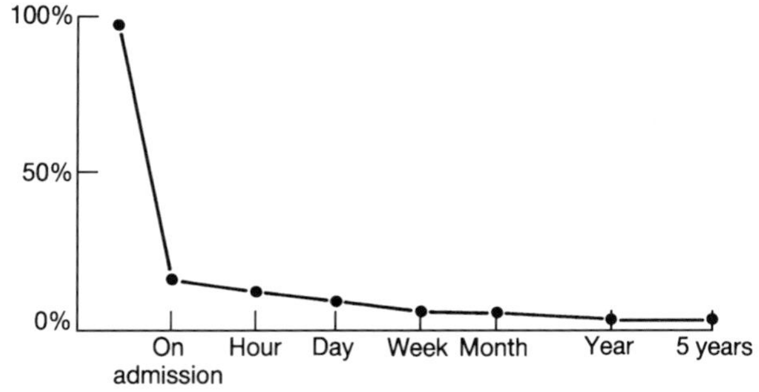

Fig. 23.29 Survival after traumatic aortic rupture (see text).

common finding.[73] In those who reach hospital alive, the most common site for the tear is in the uppermost part of the descending aorta, just beyond the left subclavian artery with the aortic adventitia and mediastinal pleura containing the rupture (Fig. 23.28). The likely explanation for the rather constant site of this lesion is that the heart with the ascending aorta and the arch swing forward as thé body is brought to an abrupt halt by the impact. The descending aorta with its pairs of intercostal branches is a more fixed structure, tethered to the vertebral column, and the tear occurs at the junction of the two.

The relevant features on examination are absent or weak femoral pulses or unequal blood pressure in the arms. A chest radiograph is usually taken supine under these circumstances and is of very little help in making the diagnosis since it always enlarges the mediastinal shadow compared with a posteroanterior view. Fluid in the left chest is also missed or underestimated. If at all possible, an upright chest radiograph taken under careful supervision greatly helps thoracic diagnosis. Imaging by aortography, digital subtraction angiography or computerized tomography scan will confirm the diagnosis in most cases but there may be false-negative results, especially with lack of experience in the investigation or its interpretation.

Once the suspicion has been raised, the problem may be an extremely difficult one. The condition is likely to prove fatal and requires emergency surgery, yet the process of investigation and transfer to a cardiothoracic unit has its own hazards for a patient under these circumstances.[74] An unnecessary journey for investigation may not be in the best interests of a multiply injured patient but attempts at local look-and-see surgery are unlikely to have a beneficial outcome. The best policy is to discuss the case with the cardiothoracic unit by telephone so as to plan the logistics of investigation and surgery in the light of the available facilities. It is of some comfort to realize that the patient who has survived the first few hours has a good chance of surviving long enough to get to expert help, having reached a flatter part of the survival curve (Fig. 23.29). Some patients contain the injury and survive for years, when a calcified false aneurysm is observed.

REFERENCES

73. Parmley L F Circulation 1958; 17: 1086
74. Unsworth-White M J, Treasure T, Buckenham T Ann Roy Coll Surg Engl 1994; 76: 381

Surgery is performed through a left thoracotomy. The mediastinum is featureless due to a spreading haematoma and the first manoeuvre is to attempt to cross-clamp the aorta, ideally between the left carotid and the left subclavian artery, without entering the haematoma. This may be very difficult. In the typical accident victim, direct suture may be possible.

Any additional procedures or unnecessary complexity may involve prolonged clamping, shunts or supportive bypass, and with the bleeding problems that are entailed, greatly reduce the chances of success.

Blunt cardiac injury

The heart may be compressed between the sternum and the vertebral column. Severe force may rupture the right ventricle, the septum or the atrioventricular valves. With complete rupture the patient is likely to die with tamponade before reaching hospital but there are three patterns which are worth recognizing.

Myocardial contusion

If the myocardium is contused but remains intact the consequences are similar to myocardial infarction. ECG changes are likely and may show classical Q waves or more usually generalized ST segment abnormality. Cardiac enzymes are elevated but their interpretation is difficult in the presence of other muscle injury. The course is similar to myocardial infarction and depends on the area of damage.

If the injury is full-thickness it may rupture at some later stage. Direct rupture into the pericardium is likely to be fatal but if the injury has become contained by pericardial adhesions, or rupture is delayed, a false aneurysm results which can be assessed and dealt with electively.

Ruptured valves

Rupture of the atrioventricular valves (tricuspid more often than mitral) is likely to occur at the time of the injury. The clinical signs are those of acute valvular regurgitation for any other reason but may well prove difficult to sort out in a multiply injured patient!

Sharp trauma[75]

The management of stab wounds to the heart is a technical challenge to the emergency surgeon since if the patient arrives alive with a stab wound it should be technically possible to repair the damage.

The history is of interest but is often unavailable, incomplete or deliberately misleading. The site of the wound is important because some thought as to the structures which might have been reached from that entry wound will influence the need for surgery and the incision. Clinical examination and repeated assessment of the state of the patient are vital. If the cardiac output is adequate to maintain consciousness and a palpable pulse, think carefully, because an ill judged manoeuvre may upset a delicate balance. If the patient is pulseless and apparently dead then there is nothing to be lost by performing a thoracotomy in the emergency department but this is very rarely successful.

There are two factors to be considered. Is the patient at risk from continuing haemorrhage? In this case, in addition to pallor, tachycardia, a weak pulse and arterial hypotension, the veins are empty. Or is there cardiac tamponade? In this case the neck veins are engorged and the volume of blood lost may be small. The clinical distinction between the two is usually dramatic—the aspiration of as little as 50 ml of blood from the pericardium in a case of acute tamponade may greatly improve cardiac filling, and thus cardiac output. The bleeding may be at low pressure if it is atrial and a temporarily stable equilibrium may be reached. Ventricular bleeding may stop for a while. In the marginal case where the cardiac output is good and there is debate about the need for emergency surgery it is wisest to allow a cardiothoracic surgeon to supervise if possible.

Surgical management

The first decision is whether or not to insert a drain. If there is haemopneumothorax an intercostal drain should be inserted and this may be essential if there is tension. It is best to insert the drain laterally. If there is major cardiac or vascular injury the drain will permit copious bleeding and if the situation was previously balanced because atrial, pulmonary or right ventricular haemorrhage was limited by a rise in intrathoracic pressure, it may now become out of control and require urgent surgery. Suction should not be used under these circumstances as it may lead to rapid exsanguination and there may even be circumstances when the drain should be clamped while the chest is opened rapidly to control haemorrhage. This is occasionally justifiable on the grounds that a brief period of tamponade, which is then relieved, may be preferable to exsanguination.

A cardiac surgeon would prefer a median sternotomy for speed and access but the equipment and expertise to make this incision are not always available. Those who have had even minimal exposure to cardiothoracic surgery will appreciate this incision, which can be made in an emergency using a Gigli saw. The more usual emergency incision is a left anterior thoracotomy through which reasonable access can be obtained and which can be made with the patient supine or, more easily, with the chest tilted with sandbags bringing the left side up. The fifth interspace is identified by counting the ribs down from the manubriosternal angle. The skin incision is in the line of the interspace, approximately equivalent to the submammary fold, and extends laterally in a gentle curve which passes 2–3 cm below the angle of the scapula. The anterior part of latissimus dorsi should be divided to give the generous access required under emergency conditions. The serratus anterior can be split along the length of its fibres. The periosteum is incised with diathermy along the upper border of the sixth rib and stripped off with a periosteal elevator as far back as can be reached. The ribs are spread with some form of geared or ratchet retractor, without

REFERENCE

75. Editorial Br Med J 1987; 294: 1630

which access is extremely difficult. The pericardium is incised longitudinally from the apex upwards, parallel and 2 cm anterior to the phrenic nerve.

The left ventricle with its thick walls can be controlled with 3/0 atraumatic sutures. A buttress may be necessary to achieve haemostasis in the thinner-walled right ventricle but it is wise to avoid foreign material and we prefer to employ pledgets of the readily available pericardium. The atria can be sutured directly, or controlled with a side-biting clamp to give more time. Haemorrhage from coronary arteries is a particular problem. Small branches, well away from the interventricular and atrioventricular grooves, can be oversewn if necessary but usually it is possible to control haemorrhage by taking delicate bites of epicardium on either side with 4/0 sutures and sealing the haemorrhage without occluding the artery.

The pericardium can be left open, but widely, so that the heart cannot be strangulated if it prolapses through. The pericardium and hemithorax should be drained; if there is any pulmonary injury, which might leak air, drainage should be with underwater seal. The ribs are approximated and the intercostal muscle and periosteum of the fifth space sutured to the intercostal muscle below the sixth rib. The closure is completed in layers.

CARDIAC TRANSPLANTATION

Under this heading we could discuss the possible therapies for an irretrievably damaged heart. These include heart transplantation, mechanical heart replacement, and dynamic cardiomyoplasty with latissimus dorsi. At the time of writing only heart transplantation is proven to be of any practical benefit.

Heart transplantation has become a standard and accepted surgical technique. Any discussion about indications and patient selection should begin with an awareness that it is strictly limited by an external factor—the availability of donor organs. The most common source of organs is relatively young patients (males < 55, females < 60) who have irrecoverable brain damage and are declared brain dead by strict criteria, and yet remain in reasonable physiological condition on a ventilator. They are most commonly victims of road accidents or intracranial haemorrhage.

Pre-existing cardiac disease, and malignant disease with the possible exception of primary brain tumours, must be excluded. Donors must have adequate cardiac performance as judged by adequate arterial pressure, at low filling pressure, and good urine flow. This must be without drug support. About 300 such hearts become available for transplantation in the UK each year. The donor heart must be within about four hours retrieval and journey time of the recipient hospital.

Potential recipients vastly outnumber the available donors. Here is an instance where 'selection' and the concept of 'rationing' are understood by doctors because donor availability is entirely subject to external factors.

Recipients are typically very symptomatic with end-stage left ventricular failure, most commonly due to ischaemia or dilated cardiomyopathy. Patients in terminal failure, in hospital, on support drugs or technologies, may be saved but are frequently excluded because they are often in, or on the verge of, multisystem failure, and the donor heart wastage in these cases is not justified when much better yield can be gained by offering the hearts to a chronically disabled, but relatively stable, outpatient pool. The latter group of patients has a median survival of about a year without transplantation.[76]

REFERENCE

76. Murday A J P, Madden B P Surgery 1996; 41(1): 18

24 The mediastinum

P. Goldstraw

The mediastinum is an area of great surgical interest, reflecting the wide variety of structures contained in this region and the broad spectrum of pathology encountered. This interest greatly exceeds the incidence with which these diseases are encountered, perhaps reflecting the value of this area as an examination topic. This chapter does not attempt to cover comprehensively all the diseases of the mediastinum but, with the exception of the oesophagus (see Chapter 21), does cover those subjects that are commonly encountered in general surgical practice.

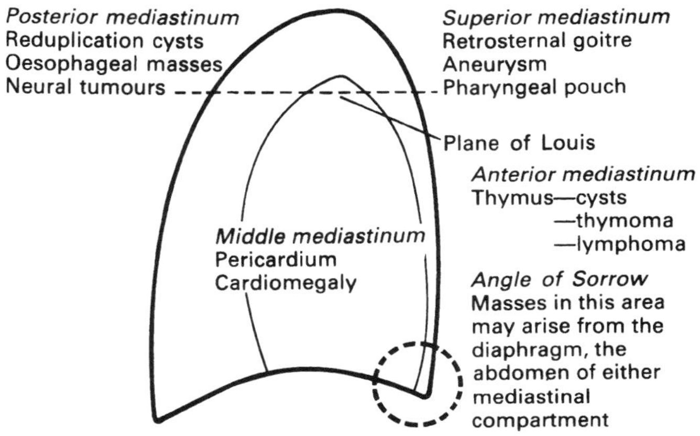

Fig. 24.1 Mediastinal compartments as seen on a lateral chest radiograph, and the commoner masses contained in each.

ANATOMY

The mediastinum includes all the structures located between the mediastinal pleura on each side, and extends from the diaphragm below to the thoracic inlet above, and the sternum in front to the vertebral bodies and paravertebral gutters behind. All these structures form a single confluent shadow on the chest radiograph. Special radiographic techniques may be used to visualize individual organs and the impact of computed tomography (CT) has been considerable. It is conventional to divide the mediastinum into superior, anterior, middle and posterior compartments based on anatomical landmarks identifiable on the lateral chest radiograph (Fig. 24.1). Such a classification remains useful as it allows the construction of a differential diagnosis.

The superior mediastinum is limited above by the thoracic inlet and below by the plane of Louis, passing transversely from the manubriosternal angle to the lower border of the fourth thoracic vertebra. It contains the arch of the aorta with its branches, the confluence of the innominate veins which form the superior vena cava, the trachea, proximal thoracic oesophagus, the thoracic duct, the thymus or its remnant, many lymph nodes and a number of nervous structures, namely the phrenic and vagus nerves on each side, the recurrent laryngeal branch of the left vagus nerve and the sympathetic chain.

The anterior mediastinum is bounded on the lateral radiograph by the posterior margin of the sternum in front, and the anterior surface of the pericardial outline behind. It contains a variable amount of fatty tissue in which there are many lymph nodes, and the thymus or its remnant.

The middle mediastinum contains the pericardium and intrapericardial structures—the heart, ascending aorta, main pulmonary artery and the phrenic nerves.

The posterior mediastinum is bounded in front by the posterior border of pericardium, and behind by the vertebral bodies and the paravertebral gutters. It contains the descending aorta with its branches, the oesophagus, thoracic duct, lymph glands and the vagus nerve and sympathetic chain on each side.

THE INVESTIGATION OF MEDIASTINAL PATHOLOGY

The chest radiograph is often the first indication of mediastinal disease. A lateral film allows of the pathology to be located in one of the four compartments and facilitates the construction of a differential diagnosis. Fleck calcification may be evident or a fluid level may be seen. A barium swallow examination is of value if the disease is adjacent to the oesophagus. It is particularly useful if dysphagia is a symptom, but is also useful when planning surgical exploration.

Conventional tomography has been largely superseded by CT. The wealth of additional information this provides has made CT a valuable investigation in mediastinal disease, often showing additional diagnostic features, and also allowing an assessment of adjacent structures. By localizing the abnormality, it is often possible to identify the organ of origin, and its relationship to adjacent structures. The vessels may be enhanced by intravenous injection of contrast material (Fig. 24.2), and this is particularly important before attempting surgical biopsy or resection. Lymphadenopathy, unsuspected on chest radiographs, may be seen on CT scanning, and these nodes may be amenable to biopsy, so facilitating diagnosis. When tumours are well-encapsulated, the margins on CT

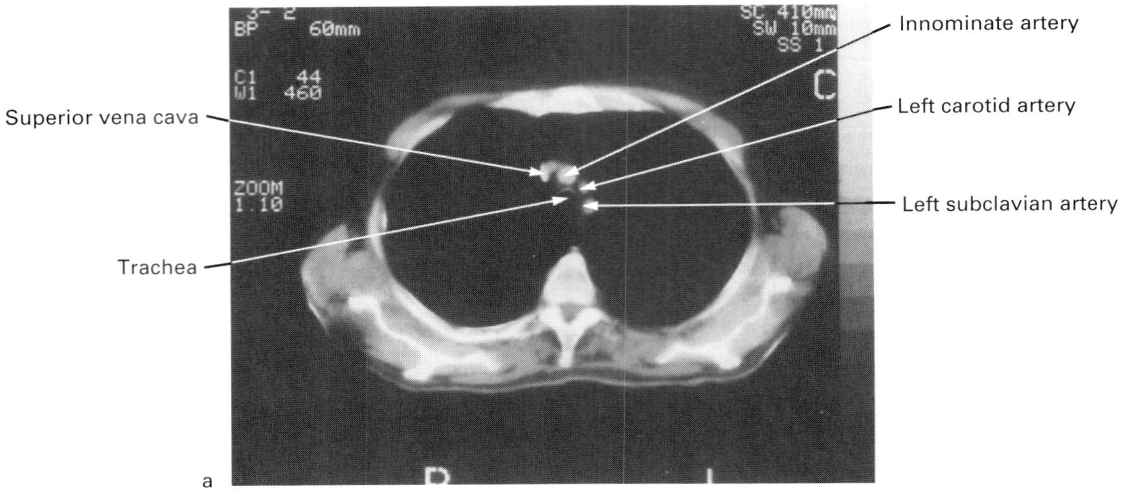

a

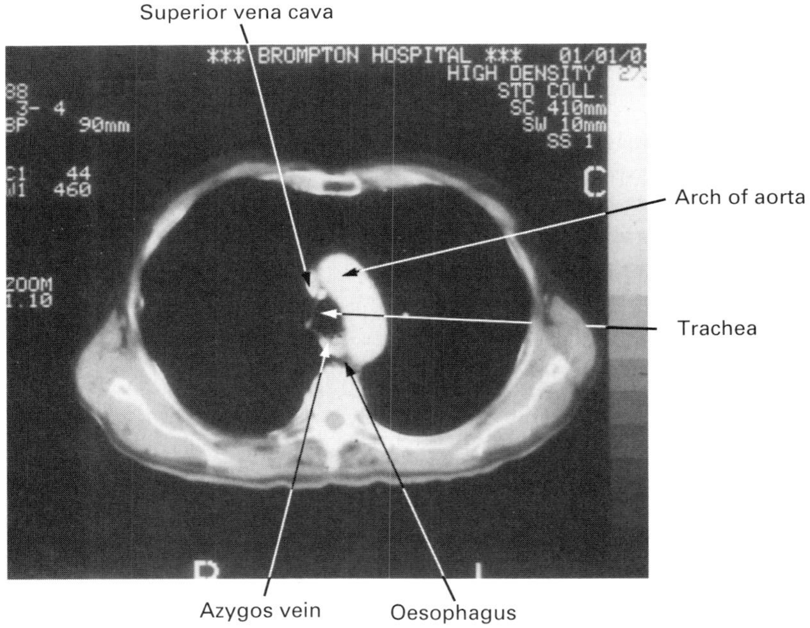

b

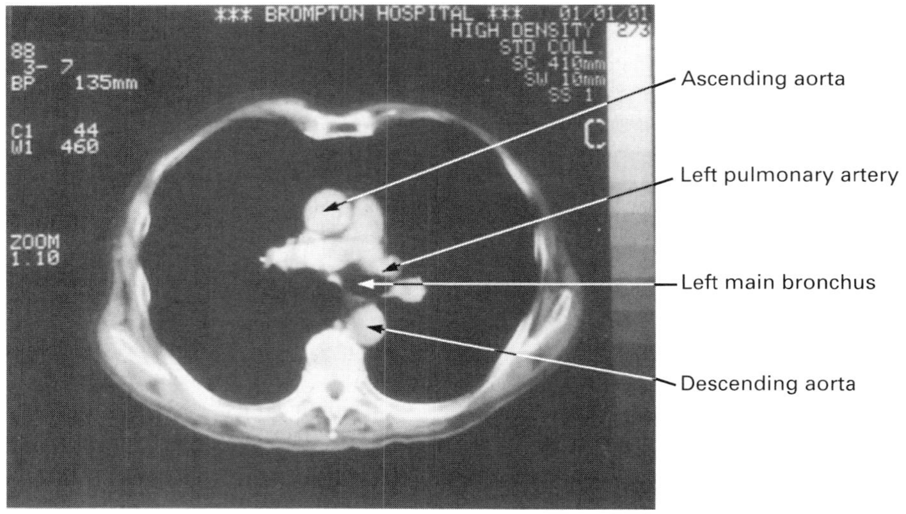

c

Fig. 24.2 CT cuts through the normal mediastinum with intravenous contrast to enhance the vessels (**a**) at the level of the head vessels; (**b**) at the level of the aortic arch; (**c**) at the plane of Louis.

may be highlighted by the preservation of the normal surrounding fatty tissue. The loss of this translucent line is suggestive of invasion.

Additional scanning techniques are occasionally of value. Radioiodine scans of the thyroid may confirm the thyroid origin of tumours in the superior mediastinum. Ultra-sound examination is developing into a valuable method of imaging, particularly when it is used by the transoesophageal route,[1] when the whole of the aorta can be imaged. Magnetic resonance imaging (MRI) has not as yet proved useful in the mediastinum as the present images seem inferior to those obtained by CT scanning.

Angiography and digital subtraction imaging techniques have now largely been superseded by enhanced CT scanning, but may be appropriate when investigating extremely vascular tumours or a suspected aneurysm. Endoscopy may be an important investigation in appropriate cases, and bronchoscopy or oesophagoscopy often shows evidence of extrinsic compression of these hollow viscera, and provides a diagnosis in primary tumours of the main airways and oesophagus.

The mediastinum is somewhat inaccessible, and if biopsy is to be performed safely and representative tissue reliably obtained, imaging must accurately locate the site for biopsy so that the optimum approach can be selected. Access may be gained from the front using an anterior mediastinotomy, through the thoracic inlet by cervical mediastinoscopy or by a lateral approach across the pleural cavity using video-assisted thoracoscopic surgery. Cervical mediastinoscopy[2] is an endoscopic examination of the superior mediastinum in the region of the trachea and main carina. Lymph nodes in this region are frequently involved by malignancy within the chest, and if these nodes are seen to be radiologically enlarged, a positive biopsy can be reliably and safety obtained by this route. Anterior mediastinotomy[2] is undertaken through a short transverse incision through the second or third intercostal space, to the left or right of the sternal margin. It provides reliable access to tumours within the anterior mediastinum.

Video-assisted thoracoscopy requires single-lung anaesthesia, using an endobronchial tube, so that the ipsilateral lung can be collapsed to allow access to the lateral aspect of one side of the mediastinum. The new technology of video-assisted thoracoscopic surgery and the development of specific instrumentation allow biopsy of previously inaccessible areas and, in suitable cases, provide sufficient access to excise some masses.[3]

Fine-needle aspiration biopsy can be used to obtain cytological material from masses within the mediastinum, and larger needles can be used to obtain small tissue samples if the mass is adjacent to the chest wall. For the differentiation of anterior mediastinal tumours, however, such tissue is often inadequate and open biopsy by anterior mediastinotomy is to be preferred. In practice aspiration biopsy is of limited value, as in other areas adjacent vascular structures may be at risk, and surgical excision is usually indicated for all tumours of the middle and posterior mediastinum.

When the imaging and clinical features raise the possibility of a germ-cell tumour, the measurement of serum tumour markers (see later) offers a unique opportunity to obtain a reliable diagnosis without undertaking biopsy.

MEDIASTINAL MASSES

Mediastinal masses are often symptomless, being discovered on routine chest radiographs or those taken for the investigation of other illnesses. Whilst only 5% of symptomless tumours are found to be malignant, 50% of those producing symptoms are malignant.[4] Pressure-related symptoms may be non-specific and are associated with malignant tumours and bulky benign tumours. Specific compressive symptoms may arise when tumours impinge on the trachea, superior vena cava or produce nerve compression with hoarseness, intercostal neuralgia or Horner's syndrome. Systemic symptoms of pruritus, pyrexia and alcohol-induced pain may be associated with lymphomas (see Chapter 34). Gynaecomastia may be present in males with germ-cell tumours (see Chapter 18).

The commonest mediastinal masses are grouped in Table 24.1

REFERENCES

1. Eerbel R, Borner N et al Br Heart J 1987; 58: 45
2. Goldstraw P Br J Dis Chest 1988; 82: 111
3. Coltharp W H, Arnold J H et al Ann Thorac Surg 1992; 53: 776
4. Sabiston D C, Oldham H N In: Sabiston D C, Spencer F C (eds) Surgery of the Chest. Saunders, Philadelphia 1983

Table 24.1 Masses found in each mediastinal compartment

Site	*Mass*
Superior compartment	
Thyroid	Goitre
Oesophagus	Pouch
	Reduplication cyst
Trachea	Bronchogenic cyst
Great vessels	Aneurysm
Anterior compartment	
Thymus	Hyperplasia
	Cysts
	Thymoma
	Lymphoma
	Germ-cell tumour
Thyroid	Goitre
Foramen of Morgagni	Hernia
Middle compartment	
Vascular	Aneurysm
	Anomalous vessels
Pericardium	Effusion
	Cysts
	Diverticula
Heart	Cardiomegaly
	Left ventricular aneurysm
Posterior compartment	
Neural	Tumours: benign or malignant, somatic, autonomic or of paraganglial origin
Oesophagus	Dilatation
	Benign or malignant tumours
	Gastroenteric cyst
Diaphragm	Paraoesophageal hernia
	Bochdalek hernia
Vascular	Descending aorta aneurysm
Masses common to all compartments	
Lymph nodes	Primary tumours
	Hodgkin's
	Non-Hodgkin's
	Secondary tumours
	Sarcoid
	Tuberculosis
Connective tissue	Tumours: benign or malignant, from fibrous tissue, vessels, fat or muscle
	Malignant fibrous histiocytoma

according to their compartment of origin. It should be remembered that large tumours can extend into adjacent compartments, widening the differential diagnosis, and that some tumours, especially those of lymph node origin, may arise in more than one compartment. Particular difficulty is encountered with masses arising at the anterior cardiophrenic angle, where the anterior and middle mediastinal compartments converge with the diaphragm. Masses in this area may arise from either compartment of the mediastinum, the diaphragm or from structures below the diaphragm.

Whilst the localization of a mass allows the construction of a differential diagnosis and may direct investigation, the final diagnosis must always be based on firm evidence, which in the vast majority of cases, requires histology obtained at biopsy or at excision. Undue reliance upon an assumed radiological diagnosis may be disastrous (Fig. 24.3). The superior mediastinum is another area where interpretation may prove difficult as masses in this area may have extended cephalad from other compartments within the mediastinum, or caudad from the root of the neck.

Retrosternal goitre

A goitre developing in the neck may extend inferiorly through the thoracic inlet, usually coming to lie anteriorly in the superior mediastinum (Fig. 24.4). Occasionally such masses are deflected posteriorly, passing behind the trachea and oesophagus. At exploration the thyroid is usually diffusely abnormal, but the cervical component may be impalpable. With careful examination whilst the patient swallows, the superior pole of the retrosternal mass is usually palpable. The classic rise of the thyroid gland on swallowing may be absent as the result of anatomical restriction. Rarely, there is an enlargement of ectopic thyroid tissue within the superior mediastinum. Symptoms arise from compression of the oesophagus, superior vena cava or trachea.

These tumours are extremely vascular and occasionally present with sudden onset of dysphagia or stridor when bleeding occurs into the goitre. Often however they are discovered as incidental findings on routine chest radiographs. Once considered, the diagnosis can only be conclusively proven at surgical exploration. Isotope scans of the thyroid are often unhelpful, as the intrathoracic extension is usually non-functioning. If the tumour does take up iodine, however, the diagnosis is assured. Computerized scans of the thoracic inlet show the characteristic heterogeneous density of a goitre, and often show calcification not visible on plain radiographs. Sequential CT slices demonstrate contiguity between the mediastinal mass and the lower pole of the thyroid gland. The patient should be advised to have the retrosternal mass excised, even if it is not causing symptoms, as doubt will persist as to the nature of the pathology, its possible malignancy and concern about the rare but serious complication of haemorrhage.

Exploration is undertaken through a cervical incision. Once the inferior thyroid vessels have been controlled, the retrosternal extension can be delivered through the thoracic inlet. The use of a suitably shaped spoon aids delivery and it is only occasionally necessary to enlarge the thoracic inlet by a limited median sternotomy. It is not usually essential to perform a subtotal thyroidectomy as it is only necessary to relieve mediastinal compression, and excision of the retrosternal component is adequate. Haematoma may collect in the large space left following resection and suction drainage for 2–3 days is desirable.

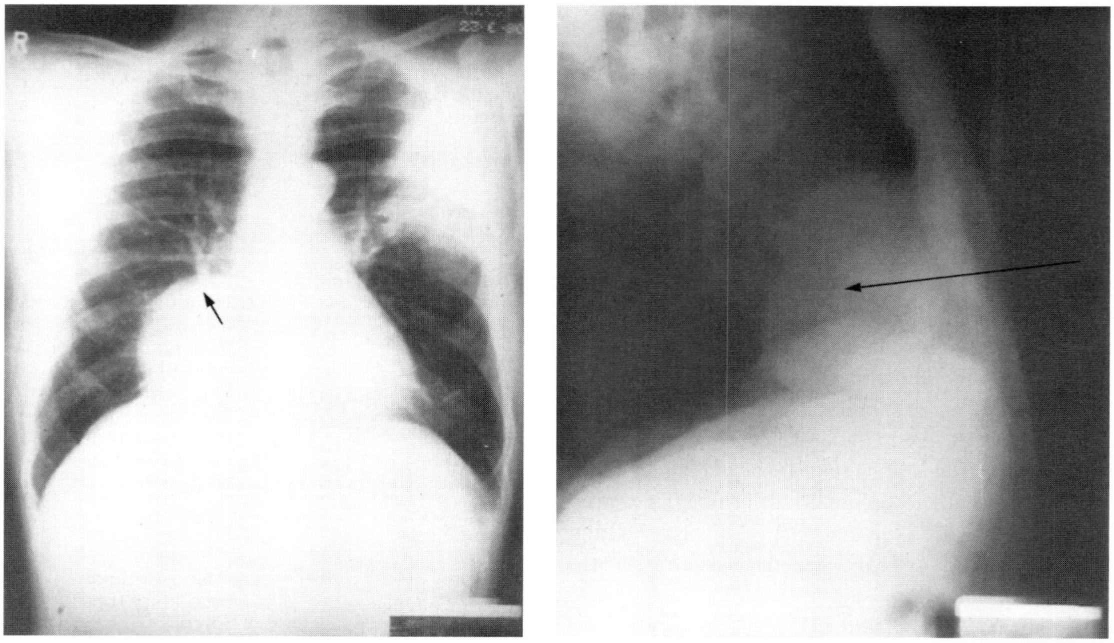

a b

Fig. 24.3 (**a**) The posteroanterior and (**b**) lateral chest radiographs of a patient presenting with left upper lobe pneumonia. The mediastinal mass (arrow) was noted, shown to be lying anteriorly and dismissed as a pleuropericardial cyst.

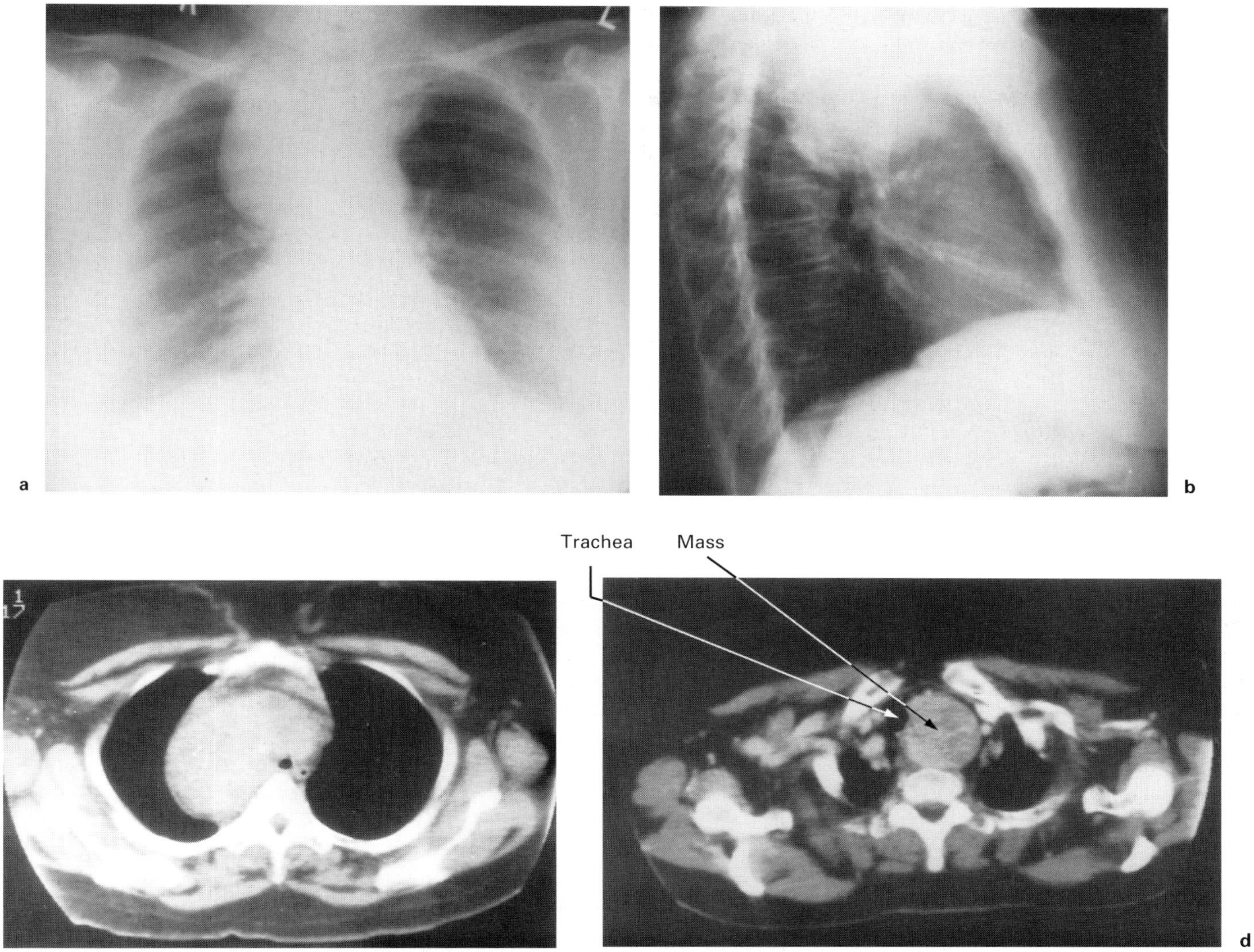

Fig. 24.4 (**a**) The posteroanterior and (**b**) lateral chest radiographs of a patient presenting with stridor and superior vena caval compression due to a large retrosternal goitre. The CT cuts show a mass in the right paratracheal area (**c**), producing severe tracheal compression at the thoracic inlet (**d**), and extending above the clavicles.

Thymic masses

The normal thymus has small, tubular, superior horns extending into the neck, and larger thoracic horns extending into the superior mediastinum and the upper portion of the anterior mediastinum. Whilst the gland progressively enlarges from birth until puberty, it is unusual to visualize the normal thymus on chest radiographs after the first 5 years of life. After puberty there is progressive replacement of the thymus by fatty tissue, but small islands of thymic tissue are detectable in the fatty gland even in advanced age. This thymic tissue may become hyperplastic in response to repeated immunological challenges. Such hyperplasia may be evident on chest radiographs in children recovering from chemotherapy and lesser degrees of thymic rebound may be detectable in adults using CT.[5] The normal size of the thymus gland in each age group has been determined by autopsy studies.[6]

Thymoma

Whilst tumours may develop from any of the components of the normal thymus gland, the term 'thymoma' should be reserved for neoplasms originating in the epithelial skeleton of this gland. On microscopy, lymphocytic elements may predominate and on occasions it may be difficult on microscopy to detect the true neoplastic, epithelial components.[7] When they are benign, thymomas are encapsulated forming a round, sharply demarcated opacity in the anterior mediastinum (Fig. 24.5a,b). Thymomas can

REFERENCES

5. Tait D M, Goldstraw P, Husband J Eur J Surg Oncol 1986; 12: 385
6. Kendall M D, Johnson H R M, Singh J J Anat 1980; 131: 483
7. Marchevsky A M, Kaneko M Surgical Pathology of the Mediastinum. Raven Press, New York 1984

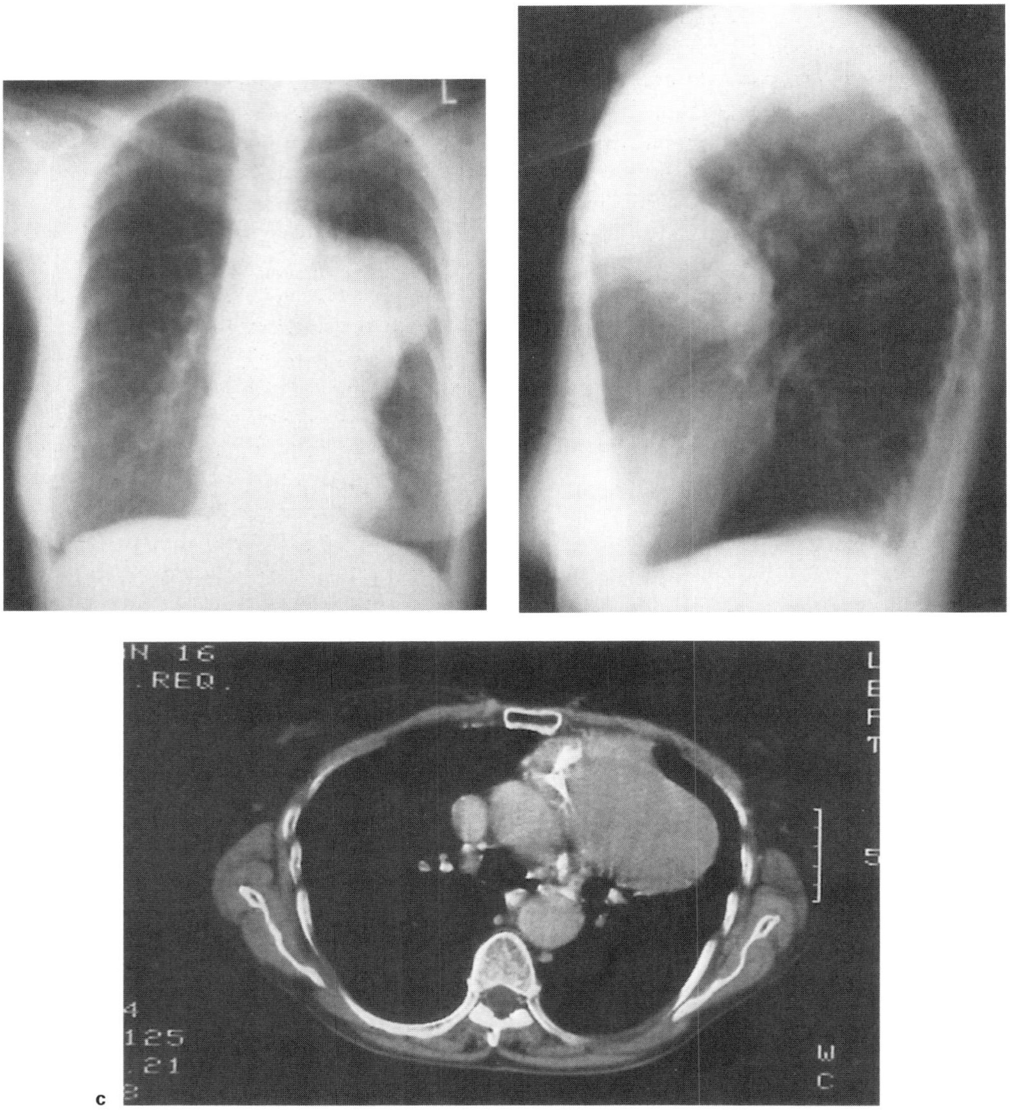

Fig. 24.5 (**a**) and (**b**) An anterior mediastinal mass subsequently found to be a benign thymoma. (**c**) The CT scan shows the mass to be well-demarcated and to contain calcification.

lie anywhere in the anterior compartment, and it is as well to remember the full anatomical extent of this compartment, occasionally a thymoma may lie low upon the diaphragm.[8] Calcification may be seen on the chest radiograph, flecked throughout the tumour, but is more commonly seen on a CT scan (Fig. 24.5c). There may be clinical or radiological evidence of malignancy with invasion of adjacent structures or pleural metastases, but the benign nature of a thymoma can only be finally established when the tumour has been completely excised, and its capsule examined microscopically.

Malignant thymoma is categorized as stage 1 if there is only microscopic invasion of the capsule; stage 2 if there is invasion into adjacent mediastinal fat or other structures such as lung and pericardium; or stage 3 if there are metastases.[9] Once the pleura has been invaded metastases may be widespread throughout the pleural space. Such nodules are detectable on chest radiographs, if gross, and smaller deposits may be seen on CT scanning. Metastases may be microscopic, and detected only on routine examination of macroscopically normal pleura. As local invasion progresses, adjacent mediastinal structures such as the superior vena cava, pericardium, lung and phrenic and vagus nerves may be invaded. Pleural metastases are present in a third to a half of such cases.[9] With such extensive tumours, regional lymph node metastases are common, but distant metastases remain rare. Such distant metastases have however been reported in the liver and in bony sites, principally the spinal column.

The association of a thymoma with myasthenia gravis is well established,[10] but there are other rare systemic manifestations, of

REFERENCES

8. Bradford R, McLelland J, Goldstraw P Postgard Med J 1984; 60: 611
9. Bergh N P, Gatinsky P et al Ann Thorac Surg 1978; 25: 91
10. Wilkins E W, Castleman B Ann Thorac Surg 1979; 28: 252

which the commonest is red cell aplasia.[11] Benign thymoma has also been associated with immune deficiency syndromes such as hypogammaglobulinaemia, and autoimmune disorders such as rheumatoid arthritis and systemic lupus erythematosus.[12]

CT scanning of the mediastinum allows clearer visualization of the relationships of the tumour and its margins. It may demonstrate invasion of adjacent structures such as the lung and it is more sensitive than chest radiographs in detecting pleural deposits. Needle biopsy is unreliable as the material obtained is insufficient to study the architecture of the tumour. Only incidental lymphoid elements may be obtained.[7] Open biopsy should be performed routinely to exclude other tumours such as lymphomas which can be treated without surgery.

Biopsies are easily undertaken through a short anterior mediastinotomy incision through the second intercostal space. The incision is sited immediately lateral to the sternum, over the side of the main radiographic abnormality. A deep incision biopsy can be taken. Whilst this demonstrates the thymomatous nature of these tumours it cannot be relied upon to diagnose the degree of malignancy. If the tumour appears encapsulated on CT scanning, total excision is recommended through a median sternotomy incision. The tumour is excised with the adjacent mediastinal fat and the whole of the thymus gland. Particular attention should be paid to any evidence of extracapsular spread, with invasion of mediastinal fat or adjacent structures such as the pericardium and pleura. Unless there is pleural invasion, the pleura need not be opened to inspect for pleural metastases.

When pathological examination shows none of the features of malignancy then the prognosis is excellent, although occasional recurrences have been reported,[13] presumably from tumour deposits developing in residual thymic tissue, or where capsular invasion has not been detected on microscopic examination. If there is only microscopic capsular invasion the prognosis remains excellent, and the role of adjuvant radiotherapy is unproven.[14] When there is preoperative evidence of malignancy on clinical or radiographic grounds, the situation is more difficult. These tumours are radio- and chemoresistant and surgical excision remains the only hope for cure.

Exploration via a median sternotomy provides satisfactory access to resect involved mediastinal structures such as the pericardium, innominate vein and superior vena cava. Many surgeons prefer a lateral thoracotomy incision if the tumour is predominantly invading laterally into the adjacent lung tissue, as it allows better access to the hilum if pulmonary resection proves necessary, and allows pleural deposits to be looked for and, if found, removed. The surgeon should be radical in an attempt to remove all macroscopic tumour. Small tumour deposits may be left to avoid sacrificing important structures such as the phrenic nerve or superior vena cava. These deposits should be tagged with metallic markers to facilitate postoperative radiotherapy.

Where surgical excision of a malignant thymoma has been apparently complete, many would argue in favour of a course of adjuvant radiotherapy to the mediastinum,[15] whilst others have not found this to be of value.[16] Unfortunately the unpredictable and usually slow progression of this tumour has made controlled studies impossible and no firm data exist as to its value.

Occasionally preoperative CT scanning shows that the bulk of the tumour is already outside the anterior mediastinal compartment, with bulky lymph node metastases. In this situation it is unlikely that surgical excision will remove an appreciable proportion of this tumour and radiotherapy may be the only treatment worth trying. Chemotherapy for thymoma is as yet experimental.[17] Local recurrence of tumour or the development of pleural masses can occur many years after the excision of a malignant thymoma. Repeated surgical excision remains the best hope of long-term disease control and death may be delayed for 10–17 years following the initial diagnosis.[16]

The role of the thymus gland in myasthenia gravis is now accepted, although its precise role in the pathogenesis remains obscure.[18] Remission of the myasthenia may be obtained by excising a normal or hyperplastic thymus. Remission may take several months following thymectomy and is more common in young female patients.[19] The prognosis is better in those patients with a short history prior to surgery, and in those in whom the gland is hyperplastic and where germinal centres are numerous.[20,21] Thymomas are found in 10–15% of patients with myasthenia gravis and approximately 30% of patients with thymoma have myasthenia gravis at presentation or on relapse.[13] Remission of the myasthenic symptoms is less likely if a thymoma is discovered but resection is justified to exclude malignancy.

Video-assisted thoracoscopic surgery techniques have been used to excise small benign thymomas and to resect the thymus in myasthenic patients. This is being explored with caution as complete excision of all thymic tissues must be assured.[22]

Lymphoma

Lymphoma of Hodgkin's and non-Hodgkin's type may occur in the thymus gland as an isolated deposit or as part of more generalized disease[23] (see Chapter 34). The clinical presentation and radiographic appearance precisely mimic a thymoma but 'B' symptoms may be present with weight loss, night sweats, fever and pruritis. Needle biopsy provides insufficient tissue to exclude other tumours and to subclassify the tumour precisely. Open biopsy via an anterior mediastinotomy approach should therefore be undertaken. Whilst there are historical reports of surgical cure following excision, treatment should now be undertaken by an oncologist.

REFERENCES

11. Korn D, Gelderman A et al N Engl J Med 1967; 276: 1333
12. Alarcon-Segovia D, Galbraith R F et al Lancet 1963; ii: 662
13. Maggi G, Giaccone G et al Cancer 1986; 58: 765
14. Tait D Cancer Topics 1986; 5: 117
15. Penn C R H, Hope-Stone H K Ann Intern Med 1972; 59: 533
16. Cohen D J, Ronnigen L D et al J Thorac Cardiovasc Surg 1984; 87: 301
17. Giaccone G, Musella R et al Cancer Treat Rep 1985; 69: 695
18. Mulder D W Mayo Clin Proc 1977; 52: 334
19. Eaton L M, Clagett O T Am J Med 1955; 19: 703
20. Rubin J W, Ellison R G et al J Thorac Cardiovasc Surg 1981; 82: 720
21. Monden Y, Nakahara K et al Ann Thorac Surg 1984; 38: 287
22. Sugarbaker D J Ann Thorac Surg 1993; 56: 653
23. Johnson D W, Hoppe R T, Cox R S Cancer 1983; 52: 8

Germ-cell tumours

These tumours most commonly occur in the testes or ovaries (see Chapter 40), but on rare occasions may be found in a variety of extragonadal midline sites, of which the anterior mediastinum is the most common. The pathogenicity of these tumours is debated but those of the mediastinum are believed to develop within the thymus gland.[24] Germ-cell tumours are subclassified into seminomatous type, or a variety of other subtypes grouped together as non-seminomatous, of which the most common is teratoma.

Teratomas may be benign and cystic (Fig. 24.6), or infiltrative and highly malignant. These tumours may contain ectodermal, mesodermal and endodermal elements. In the benign cystic teratoma the ectodermal elements may include sebaceous material, immature dental structures and hair follicles. The epithelial lining of the cyst is usually of keratinizing, stratified squamous type, often with bronchial or gastrointestinal types in some areas. This predominance of ectodermal structures has led to the term 'dermoid cyst' being applied to these benign teratomas. Other structures may be represented, including pancreas, thyroid, neural tissue, bone and cartilage. Benign teratomas have an equal distribution in men and women and may be found in all age groups.[25] The tumour may be an incidental finding on chest radiographs but in young children it usually presents with mediastinal compression. On occasions it may present with recurring pericardial or pleural effusions, usually attributed to a 'leaking dermoid'. However, at operation there is usually no evidence of any penetration of the capsule but there is considerable surrounding inflammation and the tumour may be extremely adherent to adjacent mediastinal structures and the lung.

On chest radiographs these cysts are often large and lobulated, with a smooth margin. Calcification is commonly seen in the cyst wall, but the diagnostic appearance of dental structures within the cyst is rarely seen. CT scanning may show the characteristic heterogeneous density of these tumours and may demonstrate additional calcification not seen on the chest radiograph (Fig. 24.6b). Biopsy via an anterior mediastinotomy incision may be unnecessary prior to resection if the appearances are typical. Excision is advisable as these cysts enlarge and may cause trouble later, by causing compression or recurrent effusions. Excision is usually performed through a median sternotomy incision, but if the tumour is markedly asymmetrical some surgeons prefer a lateral thoracotomy approach.

The extragonadal origin of malignant, primary mediastinal germ cell tumours is largely one of exclusion. An occult testicular primary should be sought by ultrasound. Seminomatous and non-seminomatous types both occur in the mediastinum. The latter is slightly commoner and occurs only in young men around the third decade. These tumours are highly malignant and often extremely large at presentation (Fig. 24.7). Symptoms usually arise from mediastinal compression with superior vena caval obstruction, cough or dyspnoea. Some 95% of non-seminomatous tumours are associated with grossly elevated serum levels of α-fetoprotein or human chorionic gonadotrophin.[26] Gynaecomastia may be a presenting symptom.

Biopsy via an anterior mediastinotomy incision should be undertaken unless tumour markers are diagnostically elevated. Seminomatous tumours are curable by chemotherapy or radiotherapy but the non-seminomatous variant is more difficult to treat. These are variously categorized as embryonal carcinomata, endodermal sinus or yolk sac tumours and choriocarcinomas. This subclassification has little influence on treatment. Initial therapy with combination chemotherapy using cisplatinum, bleomycin and vinca alkaloids results in tumour marker levels returning to normal

REFERENCES

24. Bergh N P, Gatinsky P et al Ann Thorac Surg 1978; 25: 107
25. LeRoux B T, Kallicharum M D, Shama D M Mediastinal Cysts and Tumors. Current Problems in Surgery. Year Book, Chicago 1984
26. Kuzur M E, Melody A et al Cancer 1982; 50: 766

a 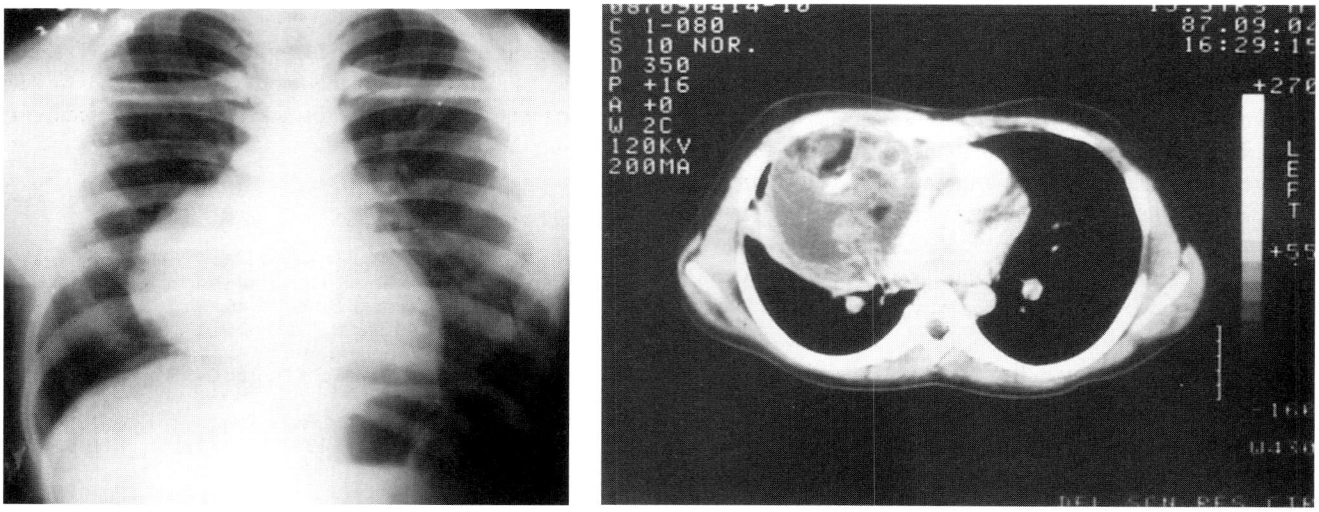 b

Fig. 24.6 **(a)** A chest radiograph of a young man with chest pain. The large anterior mediastinal mass, projecting to the right, was subsequently shown to be a benign cystic teratoma or dermoid. **(b)** A CT scan shows the heterogeneous density of the tumour and calcification.

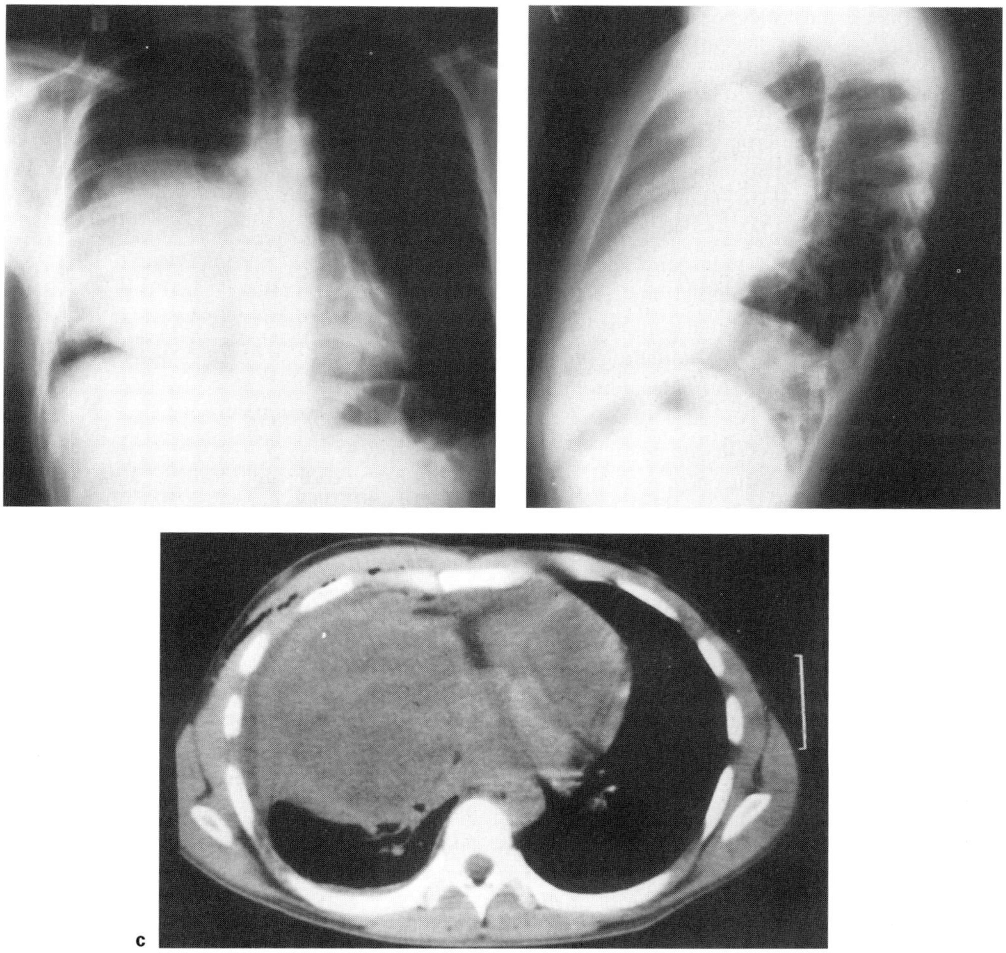

a b c

Fig. 24.7 (**a**) The posteroanterior and (**b**) lateral chest radiographs of a young man with chest pain. (**c**) The CT scan shows a large tumour with heterogeneous density, compressing the right lung and associated with a pleural effusion. The tumour mass is contiguous with the mediastinum. His tumour markers, human chorionic gonadotrophin and α-fetoprotein, were grossly elevated but his testes were normal. A biopsy was unnecessary to diagnose a primary mediastinal, malignant, non-seminomatous germ cell tumour. The patient was treated with chemotherapy. After normalization of the tumour markers, the residual tumour mass was excised successfully.

in three-quarters of patients.[27] Bulky residual disease should then be excised.

The prognosis after completion of this combined treatment is excellent.[28] Excision is however extremely difficult and often requires wide excision of the mediastinum with adjacent involved structures. For those patients in whom response to chemotherapy is less satisfactory there is no hope of cure and surgical excision is inappropriate.

Other thymic tumours

The thymus gland may on rare occasions be the site of other malignancies such as carcinoid tumour, small cell carcinoma or metastatic deposits.[7]

Thymic cysts

Cysts of the thymus gland are congenital in origin and are most commonly seen in small children. They are usually symptomless but may cause symptoms in young children, and if large, may present in adults with features of mediastinal or pulmonary compression. CT scanning discloses the characteristic low density of the cyst contents but excision is recommended as cystic change may be present in thymic tumours.

Oesophageal masses

Oesophageal carcinoma is dealt with elsewhere (Chapter 21). Occasionally oesophageal tumours are bulky enough to project from the mediastinal outline, causing an opacity in the superior or posterior mediastinum. The oesophagus, obstructed by a carcinoma, rarely dilates sufficiently to be visible on plain radiographs of the mediastinum. Dilation can, however, become gross in

REFERENCES

27. Horwich A, Peckham M J Proceedings of the Second Germ Cell Tumour Conference. Pergamon Press, Oxford 1985
28. Kay P H, Wells F C, Goldstraw P Ann Thorac Surg 1987; 44: 578

benign conditions,[29] such as the classical megaoesophagus associated with achalasia. Such gross dilation causes the oesophagus to project to the right of the mediastinal outline, widening the mediastinal shadow and with a characteristic curvilinear opacity extending above the clavicle on the anteroposterior chest radiograph. The oesophageal nature of the opacity may be disclosed by the presence of a fluid level or the typical speckled appearance of air trapped within solid food residue. Should the oesophageal contents be evacuated, spontaneously or at endoscopy, the thickened wall of the oesophagus may be seen running parallel to the right heart border, separated from the mediastinal contour by the air-filled viscus (Fig. 24.8). A barium swallow examination proves the oesophageal nature of the opacity but provides unreliable evidence as to the cause of the obstruction.

The paraoesophageal or rolling type of hernia is frequently visible on plain chest radiographs as a translucency, usually associated with a fluid level, superimposed upon the cardiac outline. A lateral chest radiograph shows the posterior position of this air-filled viscus (Fig. 24.9). A barium examination gives some insight into the anatomy of this abnormality, with axial rotation of the stomach, and the greater curve forming the superior margin of the hernia (Fig. 24.9). Chest radiographs are usually diagnostic but a barium examination provides useful additional information regarding the position of the cardia, and may show a coexistent stricture or shortening of the oesophagus.

Pharyngeal pouch

A pharyngeal pouch, whilst arising within the neck, may extend inferiorly, and present as an opacity within the superior mediastinum with a characteristic fluid level. The presence of a fluid level in a well patient, without evidence of sepsis, strongly suggest an oesophageal condition.

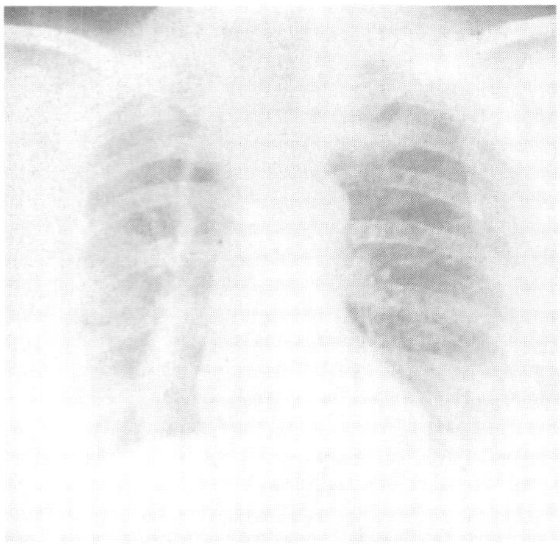

Fig. 24.8 The chest radiograph of a patient with achalasia of the oesophagus. Following endoscopy the oesophagus is empty and its thick right wall is seen as a curvilinear shadow, parallel to the right border of the mediastinum.

Benign smooth muscle tumours of the oesophagus—leiomyomas

These may present with dysphagia which is usually mild and does not progress. More commonly however such tumours are discovered incidentally as a mediastinal mass on a routine chest radiograph (Fig. 24.10). There is a characteristic smooth indentation on the barium swallow. Leiomyomas can become large, but malignant change is rare. These tumours can be enucleated from within the wall of the oesophagus, leaving the mucosal tube intact.[30] It is

REFERENCE

29. Venn G E, DaCosta P, Goldstraw P Thorax 1985; 40: 684

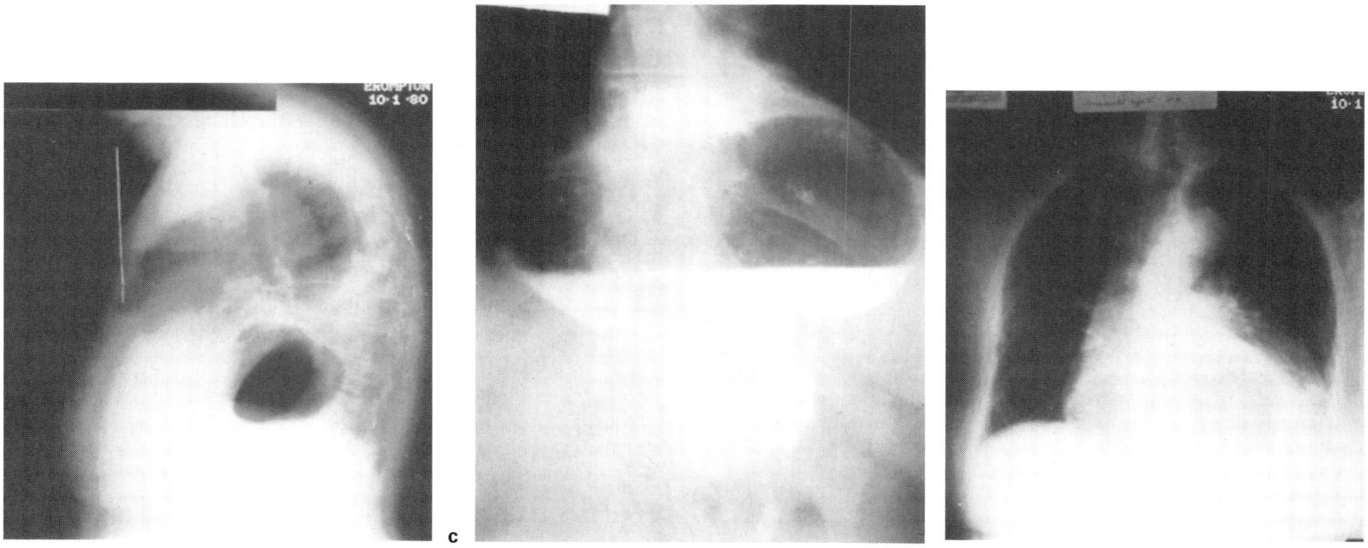

b c a

Fig. 24.9 (**a**) The posteroanterior and (**b**) lateral chest radiographs of a patient with a rolling or paraoesophageal hernia. A gas-filled opacity is seen to lie behind the heart. This is characteristic, but a barium examination (**c**) confirms the anatomy, and shows the volvulus of the stomach. The superior margin of the hernia is the greater curve of the stomach.

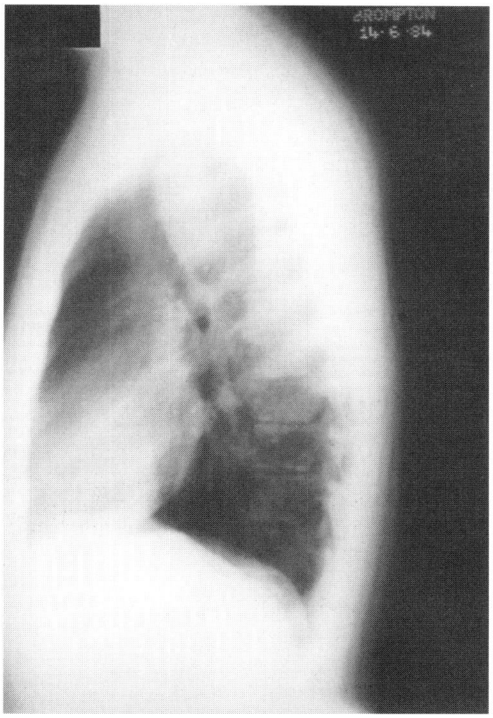

a

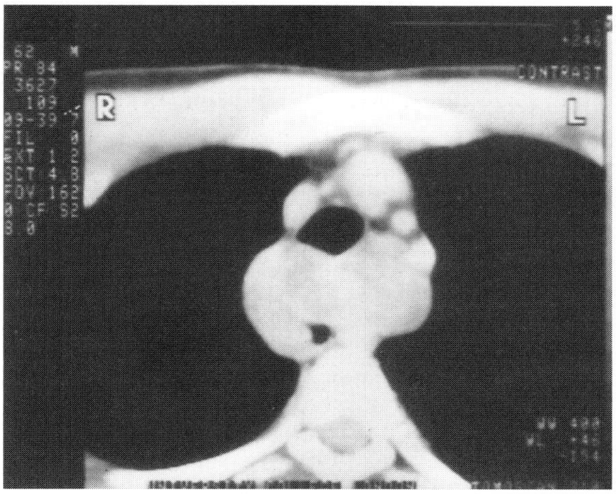

b

Fig. 24.10 (**a**) A lateral chest film of a leiomyoma showing the mass to lie posteriorly, displacing the trachea. (**b**) The CT scan shows the mass encircling the oesophagus.

unwise to attempt biopsy at endoscopy, as the plane of dissection is disturbed and a fistula may follow resection. Leiomyoma occurring in the lower oesophagus can be approached through a left thoracotomy incision, but elsewhere within the intrathoracic oesophagus a right thoracotomy approach provides better access.

Developmental cysts

Developmental cysts arise from the primitive foregut and may be associated with any of the structures derived from this embryological structure. Such cysts lying along the course of the oesophagus are usually labelled as gastroenteric cysts or oesophageal reduplication cysts.[31] They may have a variety of mucosal linings with oesophageal, small intestinal or gastric features, and the wall typically has the double muscular layer associated with the gastrointestinal tract.

Cysts elsewhere in the mediastinum may be associated with the trachea or bronchial tree and are usually termed bronchogenic.[32] They characteristically have cartilaginous elements within their wall and the mucosal lining may be ciliated or squamous. All such developmental cysts may be considered together as foregut reduplication cysts as often they lack any features to permit more precise histological classification. Reduplication cysts should be excised as there is usually doubt as to the diagnosis and they can become symptomatic, producing dysphagia, cough or stridor. Excision is performed through a lateral thoracotomy incision, but here also the application of video-assisted thoracoscopic surgery technology is being explored.[33]

Pleuropericardial cysts

Thin-walled mesothelial cysts may develop from pericardial or pleural origins. They are typically low-pressure cysts containing crystal-clear 'spring water' fluid. They are commonest at the pericardiophrenic angle, and may enlarge into the middle or anterior mediastinal compartments. They have a characteristic low density on CT scanning and if the diagnosis is confirmed by aspiration of clear fluid which is cytologically negative, they may be left intact. Frequently, however, excision is recommended because of diagnostic doubt. They may become very large and lead to the development of symptoms—usually cough or dyspnoea.

Vascular masses

Post stenotic or aneurysmal dilatation of the great vessels may be large enough to show on plain chest radiographs. Aneurysms developing from the ascending aorta will enlarge to the right and anteriorly and may mimic other anterior mediastinal tumours. Aneurysms of the aortic arch distort the superior mediastinal contour, whilst those of the descending aorta produce a mass within the posterior mediastinal compartment (Fig. 24.11). It is important to consider these unusual abnormalities within the differential diagnosis since biopsy is ill advised! CT scanning is usually diagnostic (Fig. 24.12) and transoesophageal echocardiography is also very accurate, but if doubt persists, aortography should be undertaken. Aneurysms developing in the region of the ligamentum arteriosum may

REFERENCES

30. Hennessy T P J In: Hennesy T P J, Cushieri A (eds) Surgery of the Oesophagus. Baillière Tindall, London 1986
31. Silverman N A, Sabiston D C Curr Probl Cancer 1977; 2: 1
32. Abel M R Arch Pathol 1956; 61: 360
33. Lewis R J, Caccavale R J, Sisler G E Ann Thorac Surg 1992; 53: 318

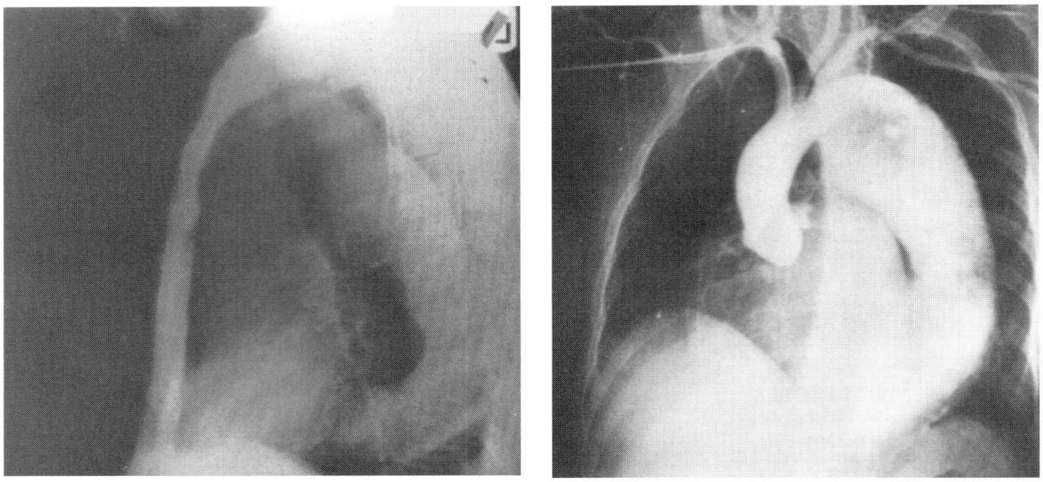

a b

Fig. 24.11 (a) A lateral chest radiograph showing a mass projecting from the left border of the mediastinum; the mass is seen to lie posteriorly, and has the appearance of a tortuous and aneurysmal descending aorta. (b) The aortogram confirms the diagnosis.

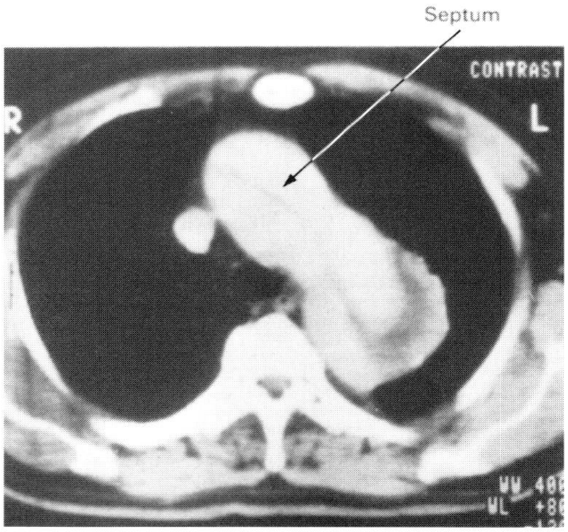

Fig. 24.12 CT scan showing a grossly aneurysmal aorta. The septum (arrow) indicates its origin as a dissection, and separates the true and false lumens.

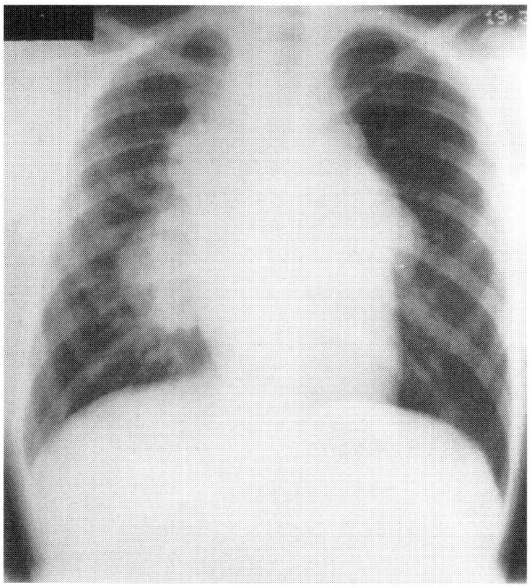

Fig. 24.13 The chest radiograph of a boy with Hodgkin's disease. The lobulated appearance, extending to right and left of the mediastinum, is typical of lymph node masses.

produce traction on the left recurrent laryngeal nerve causing hoarseness, and raising fears of a malignant tumour. The surgery of these aneurysms is difficult[34] and associated with a high mortality and morbidity. The decision whether to operate is therefore frequently difficult but surgery should be undertaken if there is radiographic evidence of progressive enlargement (see Chapter 24).

Lymph node masses

Lymph nodes are ubiquitous within the mediastinum. The differential diagnosis may be extremely difficult if a single lymph node is enlarged. Usually however several lymph nodes are enlarged, giving a characteristic lobulated appearance on the chest radiograph (Fig. 24.13). Lymph nodes involved by chronic inflammatory conditions or malignancy may be sufficiently enlarged to be visible on plain chest radiographs.

The differential diagnosis includes chronic inflammatory conditions such as tuberculosis or sarcoidosis; primary malignancies such as Hodgkin's or non-Hodgkin's types of lymphoma, and involvement by secondary malignancies principally from a primary site within the lung or breast. A CT scan of the mediastinum with contrast enhancement of the vessels is of considerable practical advantage in identifying the most convenient route for biopsy (Fig. 24.14). Lymph node masses lying in either the paratracheal chain or at the carina are accessible by cervical mediastinoscopy, those within the anterior mediastinum can be reached by anterior mediastinotomy, and elsewhere video-assisted thoracoscopic surgery may be appropriate. Mediastinal lymph nodes draining intrathoracic malignancy may show granulomatous or

REFERENCE

34. Bahnson H T In: Sabiston D C, Spencer F C W (eds) Surgery of the Chest. Saunders, Philadelphia 1983

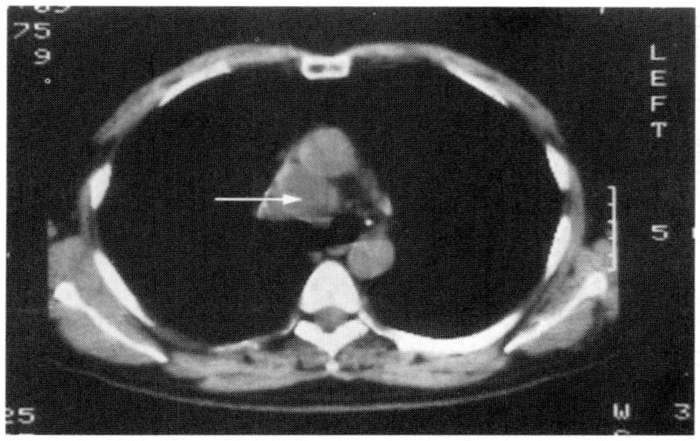

Fig. 24.14 A CT scan, without contrast, showing a large lymph node (arrow) in the retrocaval, pretracheal area, within reach of the mediastinoscope.

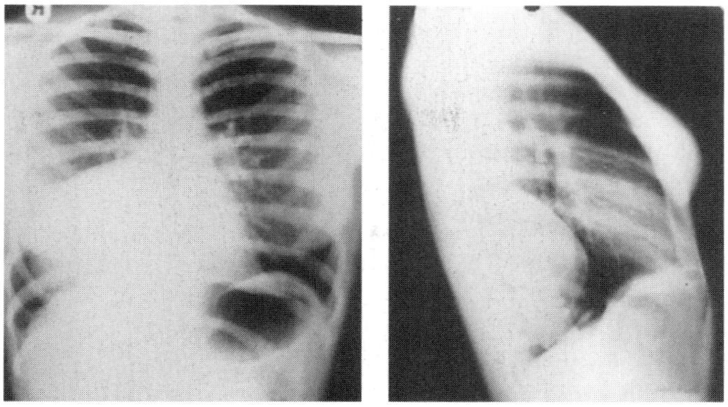

Fig. 24.15 A large tumour in the posterior mediastinum. After excision it was shown to be a benign neurilemmoma.

sarcoid change. This presents a common pitfall in the biopsy of such abnormalities, and the surgeon should biopsy several lymph node groups within the mediastinum to be sure of determining the underlying diagnosis.

Neural tumours

Neural tumours account for the great majority of posterior mediastinal tumours. They are the most common of all mediastinal masses in children, and second only in incidence to thymomas in adults.[4,25] These tumours may arise from peripheral nerves, autonomic nervous tissue or paraganglionic tissue. There are benign and malignant variants of each tumour type (Table 24.2), but the benign varieties are considerably more common.

Neurilemmoma is the most common of all neural tumours of the mediastinum[35] (Fig. 24.15). In common with neurofibroma, they are usually symptomless and an incidental finding on a routine chest radiograph in an adult. These tumours cannot be differentiated clinically or radiographically, and often histological differentiation is difficult. Both usually originate from an intercostal nerve. They may, on rare occasions, extend through the intervertebral foramen, forming a dumb-bell, intraspinal extension.[36] This possibility should be considered in all cases as it has a profound influence on surgery. A CT scan is not always conclusive and MRI may give a clearer view of the intraspinal structures. If an intraspinal extension is suspected, the assistance of a neurosurgeon allows all the tumour to be resected at a single operation. These tumours may become large and produce symptoms of nerve compression, with intercostal neuralgia, hoarseness or Horner's syndrome. They may produce dyspnoea if very large. These tumours may be plexiform, involving several intercostal nerves and the sympathetic chain. Excision requires the division of these nerves. Thoracotomy is desirable for large nerve tumours and for any that prove malignant, but video-assisted thoracoscopic surgery can be used for small tumours.[37]

Table 24.2 Neural tumours—benign and malignant variations

Tissue of origin	*Benign tumour*	*Malignant variant*
Somatic nerve—commonly intercostal nerve, but occasionally the vagus or phrenic nerves	Neurilemmoma (schwannoma)	Malignant schwannoma Neurofibrosarcoma Neurofibroma
Autonomic nerve—commonly the sympathetic chain	Ganglioneuroma	Neuroblastoma Ganglioneuroblastoma
Paraganglionic tissues	Chemodectoma Phaeochromocytoma	Malignant paraganglioma

Multiple neurofibromata, arising from intercostal, vagus and phrenic nerves, may be associated with subcutaneous tumours and the café au lait spots typical of von Recklinghausen's disease. In this condition it is impossible to excise all the nodules but, as malignancy may develop in up to one-quarter of such tumours, any nodules seen to enlarge should be excised.

Ganglioneuroma may occur in adults, but they are the most common neural tumour in children (Fig. 24.16). They may arise as a neuroblastoma, maturing spontaneously or under the influence of chemotherapy. Neural tumours in childhood may be associated with skeletal abnormalities such as hemi-vertebrae or scoliosis (Fig. 24.17). Such tumours may arise from the sympathetic chain, often at the apex in the region of the stellate ganglion.

Malignant tumour of nerve sheath origin

This is a general term incorporating those tumours previously termed malignant schwannoma and neurofibrosarcoma. Such a term acknowledges the difficulty of differentiating these tumours.[7] Total excision may provide local control, but local relapse is common and distant metastases occur.

Biopsy is unnecessary as all neural tumours should be excised. Excision is the only reliable way to exclude malignancy and the excision of benign tumours is justified to prevent the later development of symptoms.

Diaphragmatic herniae

Hiatus hernia is dealt with in Chapter 21, and paraoesophageal hernia has been discussed above. Congenital herniae develop

REFERENCES

35. Davidson K G, Walbaum P R, McCormack R J M Thorax 1978; 33: 359
36. Grillo H C, Ojemann R J et al Ann Thorac Surg 1983; 36: 402
37. Riquet M, Mouroux J et al Ann Thorac Surg 1995; 60: 943

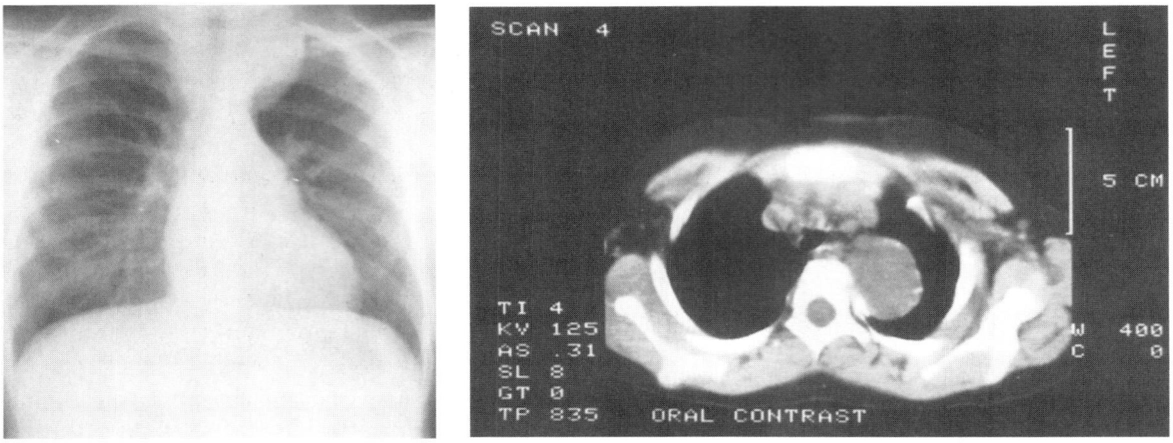

a b

Fig. 24.16 (**a**) A mass in the superior mediastinum of a young boy. (**b**) The CT scan shows the mass to lie posteriorly and to contain calcification. Histology was of a ganglioneuroma.

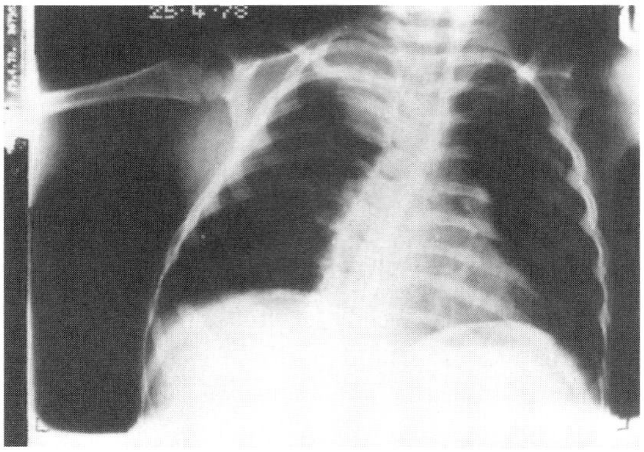

Fig. 24.17 An apical ganglioneuroma in a young child associated with scoliosis and vertebral anomalies such as hemi-vertebrae.

through persistent pleuroperitoneal communications. These may occur anteriorly, through the foramen of Morgagni, or posteriorly through the foramen of Bochdalek. On chest radiographs these form large lobulated masses, with gas translucencies when bowel is included in the hernia. A Morgagni hernia expands into the anterior mediastinal compartment and pushes posteriorly into the middle mediastinum (Fig. 24.18), whilst a Bochdalek hernia lies in the posterior compartment. The diagnosis is usually established by CT scanning. A barium examination with follow-through films may demonstrate the viscera contained within such herniae. All diaphragmatic herniae should be repaired surgically as they may assume a large size and are at risk from incarceration, strangulation or perforation.

Rarely tumours may arise from the fibrous or muscular components of the diaphragm.

Soft tissue tumours

Mesenchymal tumours of the mediastinum may develop from lymphoid tissue, blood vessels, fat, muscles or skeletal tissues, and may be located in any of the mediastinal compartments. Increasingly such spindle cell malignancies, lacking any diagnostic features, are termed 'malignant fibrous histiocytomas' (see Chapter 54). They may occur anywhere within the mediastinum

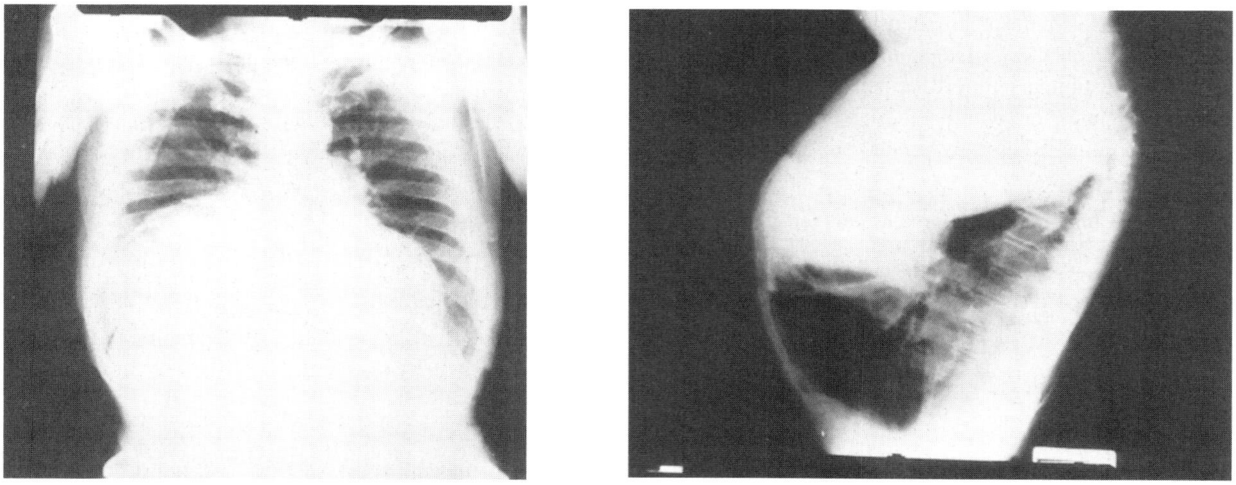

a b

Fig. 24.18 (**a**) Posteroanterior and (**b**) lateral chest radiographs showing a large mass in the anterior mediastinum, extending into the right chest. The air densities in the viscera within it show it to be a Morgagni hernia. This diagnostic clue may only be evident on a CT scan.

and assume large proportions. The treatment of these highly malignant tumours is difficult but total excision is desirable.[38] Lipomata may become large and are most common within the posterior mediastinum. They may undergo sarcomatous change. Surgical excision may be difficult but is recommended. The CT scan appearances are typical with a mass of low density from fat tissue (Fig. 24.19). A barium swallow is useful when planning surgery to disclose the course of the oesophagus through these large lobulated tumours.

ACUTE MEDIASTINITIS AND MEDIASTINAL ABSCESS

Mediastinitis and abscess formation may follow penetrating trauma, spontaneous and instrumental perforation of any mediastinal viscus, most commonly the oesophagus,[39] but nowadays most commonly results as a complication of surgery, especially after cardiac operations.[4] Oesophageal obstruction favours the development of such infection and perforation of an obstructed oesophagus leads to a rapid and severe mediastinitis. The chest radiograph may show widening of the mediastinum, and a fluid level may be visible in the posterior mediastinum adjacent to the oesophagus. There is usually a sympathetic pleural effusion on one or both sides (Fig. 24.20). The surgical management depends on the aetiology and the associated pathology. Thoracotomy, drainage of the mediastinum and broad-spectrum antibiotics are important components of treatment.[40] If mediastinitis is neglected, or if the initial trauma is severe, the infection may spread to either pleural space, with colonization of the sympathetic effusion and empyema formation. Infection may extend superiorly into the neck, displacing the trachea anteriorly and leading to life-threatening laryngeal obstruction.

REFERENCES

38. Venn G E, Gellister J et al J Thorac Cardiovasc Surg 1986; 91: 234
39. Crofton J, Douglas A In: Crofton J, Douglas A (eds) Respiratory Diseases. Blackwell Scientific Publications, Oxford 1969
40. Marty-Ane C H, Alauzen M et al J Thorac Cardiovasc Surg 1994; 107: 55

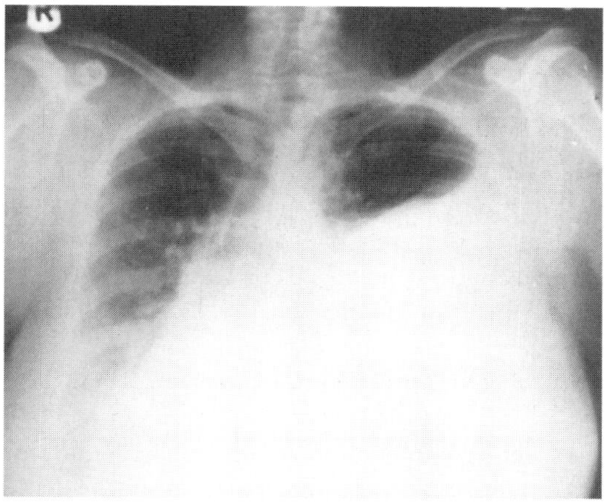
a

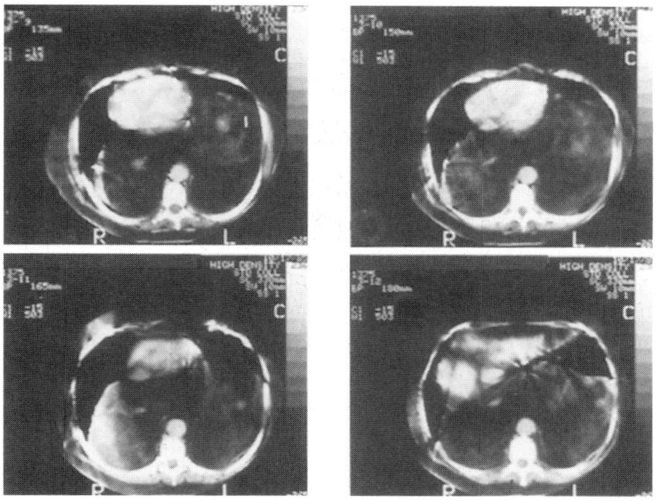
b

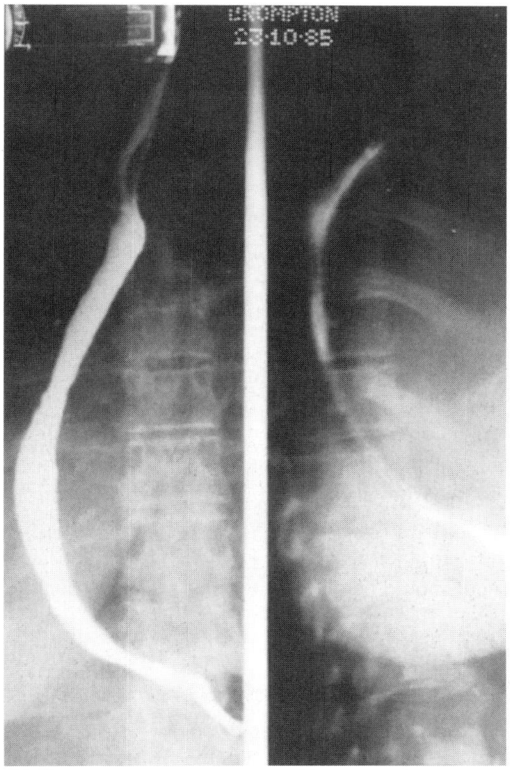
c

Fig. 24.19 (**a**) A large mass filling the left hemithorax and displacing the mediastinum to the right. (**b**) The CT scan shows the mass to be in the posterior mediastinum, and to be of fat density (–40 Houndsfield units). (**c**) In the planning of its excision, a barium swallow was of value in showing the abnormal position of the oesophagus. Histology showed a liposarcoma.

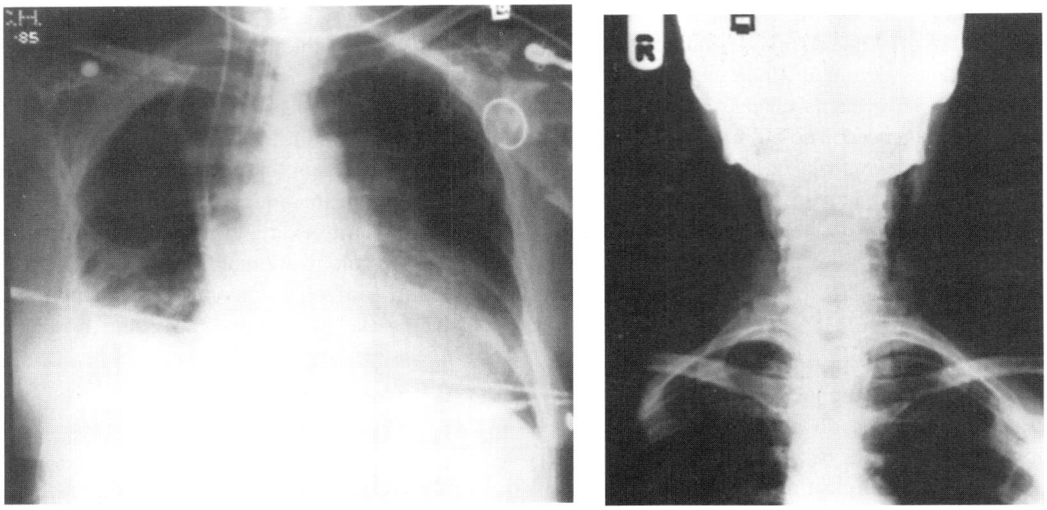

a b

Fig. 24.20 (**a**) The chest radiograph of a patient with oesophageal carcinoma, admitted severely ill 7 days after laser endoscopy. There is gross mediastinal widening and a right-sided effusion. (**b**) In another patient, an oesophageal tear after endoscopy was evidenced by surgical emphysema in the neck, seen on a chest radiograph.

CHRONIC MEDIASTINITIS AND MEDIASTINAL FIBROSIS

The aetiology of mediastinal fibrosis is obscure but it may be associated with retroperitoneal fibrosis.[41] The patient is usually an otherwise fit young adult who presents with superior vena cava compression. Fibrosis may narrow the trachea or oesophagus. The diagnosis is usually one of exclusion. The chest radiograph may show widening of the superior mediastinum but CT scanning does not demonstrate any space-occupying lesion such as lymphadenopathy. Biopsy by cervical mediastinoscopy is hazardous and the pathology is non-specific. Exploration by lateral thoracotomy may be necessary to establish a firm diagnosis, but this can usually be inferred from the clinical and radiological findings.

There is no effective treatment, but as with most causes of superior vena caval obstruction, symptoms lessen with time with development of collaterals. Patients with distressing and persisting obstruction of the superior vena cava may benefit by venous bypass or venous stenting.

MEDIASTINAL EMPHYSEMA

Mediastinal emphysema may be present as an isolated radiological finding or as part of more generalized, and clinically evident, surgical emphysema (Fig. 24.21). It occurs most commonly with pneumothorax of any aetiology. Whilst mediastinal emphysema does not require treatment, it is a valuable radiological sign and its occurrence without a pneumothorax should suggest an injury to one of the hollow viscera within the chest. Following blunt trauma it may indicate tracheal or bronchial transection and bronchoscopy is necessary. Following vomiting or endoscopy oesophageal injury is likely, and contrast radiology should be undertaken to exclude an oesophageal leak.

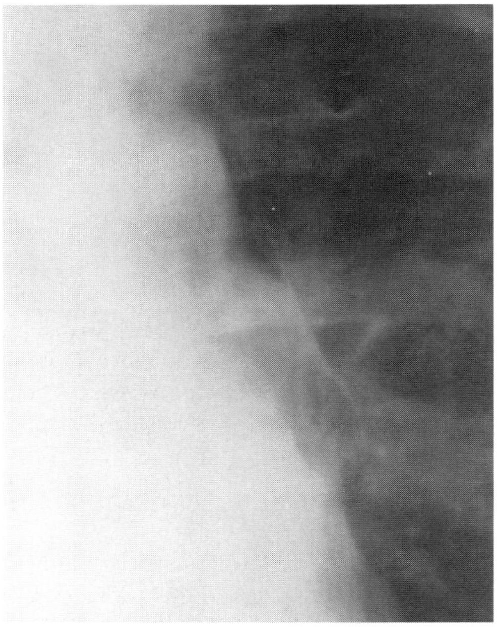

Fig. 24.21 A chest radiograph showing a pneumopericardium in a patient with mediastinal emphysema.

Spontaneous mediastinal emphysema may occur during violent coughing, or may be associated with asthma or whooping cough.[4] It can occasionally be precipitated by a strong Valsalva manoeuvre, by vigorous attempts at a resuscitation or by positive pressure ventilation when high airway pressures are necessary.[4] Treatment should be directed to the underlying condition.

REFERENCES

41. Editorial Br Med J 1962; 2: 720

25 The breast

J. M. Dixon R. E. Mansel

BENIGN CONDITIONS

INTRODUCTION

Benign conditions of the breast are important because they are more common than breast cancer and so account for the majority of attendances to hospital. Many are frequently difficult to differentiate from breast cancer and some benign conditions are incorrectly diagnosed and inappropriately treated. Patients with benign conditions present with a lump, breast pain, nipple retraction or discharge or are referred with a clinical or radiological abnormality found at screening.

Benign conditions have been separated into aberrations of normal development and involution and true breast disease.[1] Tables 25.1 and 25.2 provide a framework for the classification and understanding of benign breast disease.

History

The most important pointer to the diagnosis in women presenting to a breast clinic with a palpable breast lump is the patient's age (Fig. 25.1). Although cancer classically presents as a lump, others can present as nipple discharge, nipple retraction, change in contour and, rarely, breast pain.

Investigation

All patients over the age of 35 presenting with a breast complaint should have single oblique mammography. Before this age the breasts are usually too dense to show any abnormality, but mammography may be of value in patients with a palpably suspicious breast mass. The addition of craniocaudal views at mammography doubles the dose of radiation but significantly increases its sensitivity. Two-view mammography with oblique and craniocaudal views should normally be restricted to the age group at greatest risk of breast cancer, that is, all women attending a breast clinic over the age of 50 years.

Ultrasound examination can be a useful investigation in patients who are under 35 years of age or in those who have dense breasts on mammography. It is also of great value in measuring the exact size of any abnormality and demonstrating whether a clinical or mammographic lesion is cystic; it is also valuable in helping to determine whether a palpable mass is benign or malignant.

Fine-needle aspiration cytology

Neither clinical examination nor mammography can detect breast cancers with complete certainty.[2] For this reason all patients presenting with a solid breast lump should have either fine-needle aspiration cytology or a biopsy. The indications for fine-needle aspiration cytology are a solid mass which is suspicious of cancer, or as an alternative to biopsy in those patients whose lump appears clinically and mammographically to be benign.

Fine-needle aspiration is performed with a 10 ml syringe and a 21G needle. An aspiration gun is not required, although some find it useful. The needle is advanced into the suspicious lesion and suction applied as the needle is moved in different directions within the mass. Before the needle is withdrawn, the suction is released. The aspirated material is then spread on to slides, half of which should be air-dried and the other half fixed in alcohol.[3]

Benign diseases are more difficult to aspirate cells from than breast cancers. An acellular aspirate needs to be interpreted within the context of the physical findings and in the presence of benign impression on clinical examination and lucent mammograms may provide sufficient information to assess the need for biopsy.[4]

CONGENITAL ANOMALIES OF THE BREAST

Absence and asymmetry of a breast

Because the terms 'amastia' (absence of a breast) and 'amazia' (absence of a breast with the nipple present) are seldom used correctly, amastia has been replaced by the term 'absence of a breast' and amazia by 'hypoplasia of a breast'[5] (Fig. 25.2). Ninety per cent of patients with true unilateral absence of a breast have either absence or hypoplasia of the pectoral muscles,[6] although 90% of patients with pectoral muscle defects have normal breasts.[7] Some patients who have abnormalities of the pectoral muscles and

REFERENCES

1. Hughes L E, Mansel R E, Webster D J T Lancet 1987; ii: 1316–1319
2. Dixon J M, Anderson T J, Lamb J, Nixon S J, Forrest A P M Br J Surg 1984; 71: 593–596
3. Dixon J M, Lamb J, Anderson T J Lancet 1983; ii: 564
4. Dixon J M, Mansel R E Br Med J 1994; 309: 722–726
5. Berakha G J In: Gallager H S, Leis H P, Snyderman R K, Urban J (eds) The Breast. Mosby, St Louis 1978 pp 442–451
6. Trier W C Plast Reconstr Surg 1965; 36: 430
7. Pers M, Scand J. Scand J Plast Reconstr Surg 1968; 2: 125

Table 25.1 Classification of common benign conditions: aberrations of normal development and involution

Stage	*Normal process*	*Aberration*	*Clinical presentation*	*Pathology*
Development	Lobule formation	Fibroadenoma—small or large	Discrete lump	Fibroadenoma
	Stromal development	Juvenile (virginal) 'hypertrophy'	Large breasts	Excess stroma
Hormonal activity	Cyclical changes	Exaggerated cyclical changes	Cyclical mastalgia; nodularity—generalized or discrete	No pathological abnormality
Involution	Lobular involution (including microcysts, apocrine changes, fibrosis, adenosis)	Macrocysts	Discrete lumps Breast pain	Benign cysts
		Excess fibrosis	Lump, pain X-ray abnormality	Sclerosing adenosis Radial scar
Duct ectasia	Ductal involution and dilatation with age	Duct ectasia	Nipple discharge Nipple retraction Lump; no inflammation	Duct ectasia

Table 25.2 Classification of common benign conditions: benign breast disease

Abnormality	*Clinical presentation*	*Pathology*
Lactating breast abscess	Tender inflamed lump	Breast abscess
Periductal inflammation	Lump + inflammation Non-lactating breast abscess Mammillary fistula Breast pain	Periductal mastitis
Florid epithelial hyperplasia + atypia	Chance finding Mass Nipple discharge X-ray abnormality	Epithelial hyperplasia + atypia Complex sclerosing lesion
Fat necrosis	Lump Skin retraction X-ray abnormality	Fat necrosis
Duct papilloma	Nipple discharge (blood-stained)	Papilloma

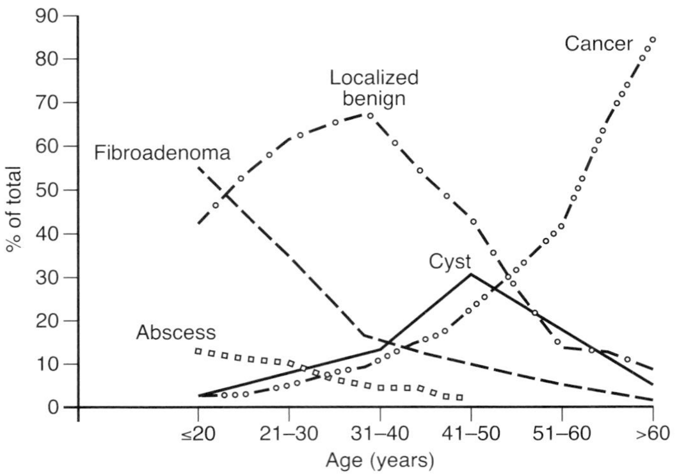

Fig. 25.1 Cause of breast lumps in women of different ages.

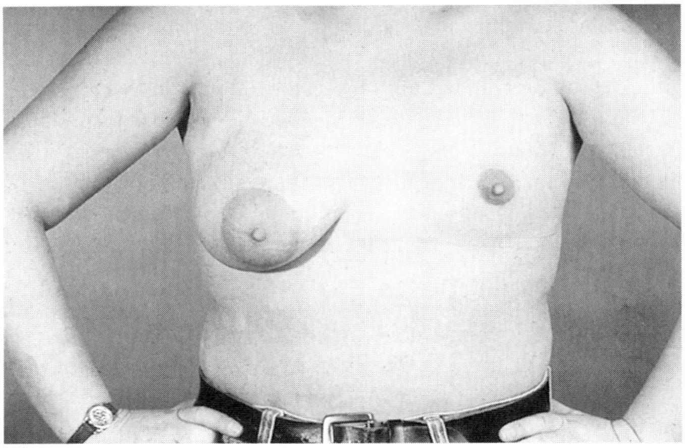

Fig. 25.2 Hypoplasia of the left breast.

absence of or hypoplasia of the breast have a characteristic deformity of the upper limb and this cluster of anomalies is known as Poland syndrome. This is thought to be an erroneous eponym, because Poland in his 1841 description did not recognize the association between chest wall deformities and a hand deformity, which is characteristic of this syndrome. The typical hand abnormality is synbrachydactly with hypoplasia of the middle phalanges and skin webbing.[5]

Some degree of breast asymmetry is normal rather than the exception, the left breast being usually the larger of the two. Apart from developmental anomalies, tumours, surgery, radiation therapy and injury can all result in breast asymmetry. Abnormalities of the chest wall such as pectus excavatum and deformities of the thoracic spine can make symmetrical breasts appear asymmetrical.

True breast asymmetry can be treated by enlarging the smaller breast, reducing or elevating the larger breast, or combining the two procedures.[5]

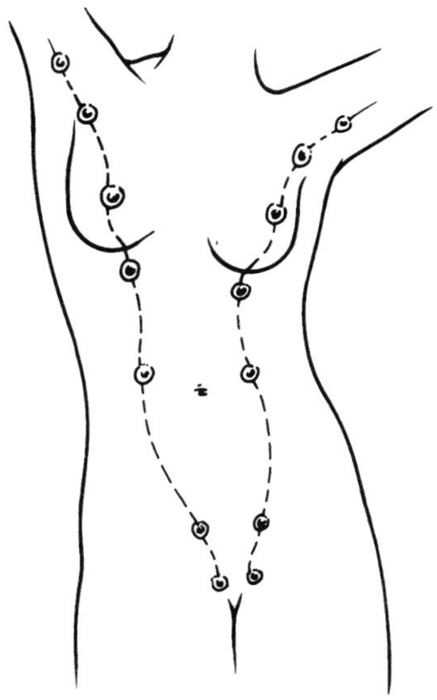

Fig. 25.3 The milk line.

Absence of a nipple

This was previously known as 'athelia' and is exceedingly rare. Absent nipples can be reconstructed by free grafts taken from the other areola or from the upper inner thigh or vulva.[5]

Extra (supernumerary or accessory) breasts or accessory nipples

These are the result of persistence of extramammary portions of the breast ridge. In the sixth week of embryonal development an ectodermal ridge, called the milk line, develops and extends from the axilla to the groin on both sides (Fig. 25.3). Segments then coalesce into nests and in humans all but one normally disappear. One or more of the other nests persist in 1–5% of people[8] as a supernumerary or accessory nipple (Fig. 25.4). Occasionally a supernumerary breast or breasts develop. This condition was previously known as polymazia. Supernumerary breasts are usually found in the axilla (Fig. 25.5) whereas accessory nipples are most common in the milk line, below the normally sited breasts and above the umbilicus. Accessory breasts have been reported at other sites, including the groin, labia majora, inner side of thigh and buttock. They need not be bilateral and, if they are bilateral, they need not be symmetrical. The extra breast may be a small nodule of mammary tissue beneath a supernumerary nipple or fully developed and capable of lactation. Accessory nipples rarely require treatment. Accessory breast tissue is of no benefit but it should only be excised if it is unsightly or uncomfortable.

After the breast has developed, it undergoes changes with the menstrual cycle. Pregnancy causes a doubling of breast weight at term which then involutes after pregnancy. In nulliparous women, breast involution begins some time after the age of 30. During involution the breast stroma is replaced by fat so that the breast becomes less radiodense, softer and ptotic. Changes in the glandular tissue during involution include fibrosis, formation of small cysts (microcysts) and an increase in the number of glandular elements (adenosis). The life cycle of the breast consists of three main periods: development (and early reproductive life), mature reproductive life and involution. Most benign breast conditions occur during one specific period and are so common that they are best considered as aberrations rather than disease.

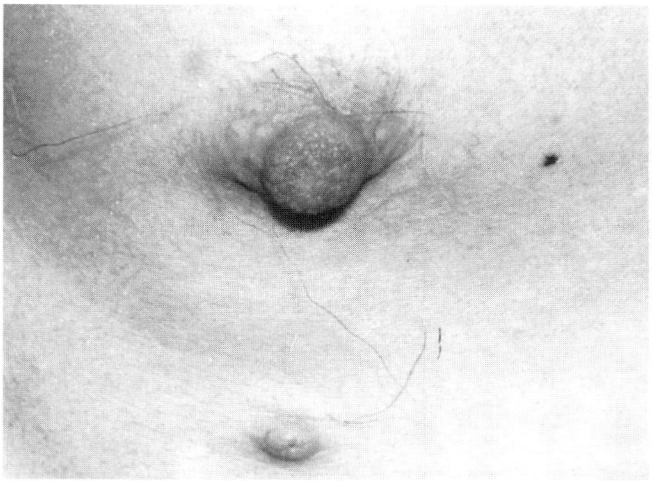

Fig. 25.4 Extra supernumerary or accessory nipple.

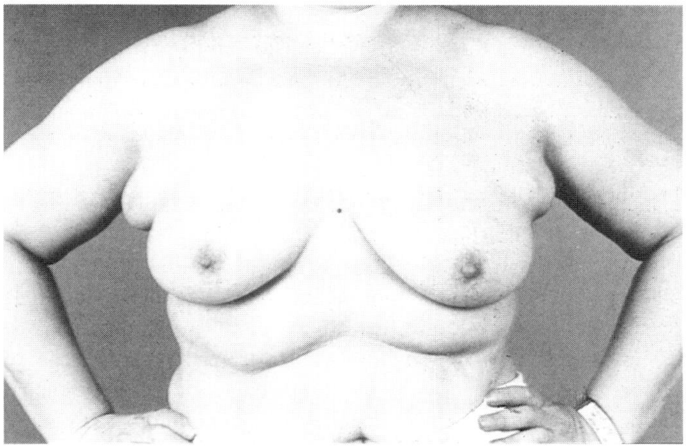

Fig. 25.5 Bilateral accessory breasts.

DISORDERS OF DEVELOPMENT

Abnormal breast enlargement

Female

Continued enlargement of the breast bud in the first week or two of life occurs in about 60% of normal newborn babies[9] and the gland may reach several centimetres before regressing. Enlargement may be unequal and is frequently associated with secretion of a colostrum-like substance known as 'witch's milk'. Involution

REFERENCES

8. Gerschickter C F. Disease of Breast. Lippincott, Philadelphia 1943
9. August G P, Chandra R, Hung W J J Pediatr 1972; 80: 259

usually occurs over several weeks but enlargement may persist for several months in breast-fed babies.

Prepubertal breast enlargement in girls is a common occurrence in the absence of other signs of sexual maturation.[8] Only if this is associated with other signs of sexual development is there an indication for investigation. In these patients hormone-secreting ovarian and adrenal tumours must be excluded by assays of hormones in blood and urine and by imaging techniques.

Uncontrolled overgrowth of breast tissue occurs occasionally in adolescent girls[5,9,10] whose development begins normally at puberty, but after a few months to a year the breasts grow rapidly. Histological examination of the breast usually shows overgrowth of periductal connective tissue associated with proliferation and increased branching of ducts, but no lobule formation. The appearance is similar to gynaecomastia in the male and is no more than an exaggeration of the structure of normally developing breast tissue. These changes are usually bilateral, but may be limited to one breast or part of one breast.

This overgrowth is often referred to as virginal or juvenile 'hypertrophy' and the condition is considered to be an aberration, rather than a true disease. Endocrine abnormalities have not been detected in these girls. Cosmetic surgery is by reduction mammoplasty in carefully selected patients. Patients with large breasts frequently complain of pain in the shoulder, neck and back or under the bra straps. They may also suffer irritation where the breasts rub against the abdominal wall.

There are a variety of methods for performing a reduction mammoplasty but most rely on maintaining the nipple and areola on a pedicle and re-siting this after excision of skin and breast tissue.[11] Excision of a horizontal wedge from the inferior part of the breast is combined with a vertical wedge with the base facing the horizontal excision and the apex corresponding to the summit of the new breast. The scars left by this procedure leave an inverted-T incision. Figure 25.6 shows the preoperative marking using an inferior dermal flap technique; the areola-carrying glandular flap is based in the inframammary fold.

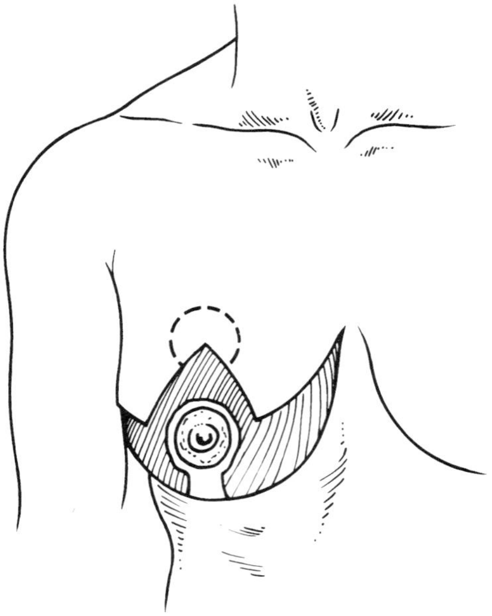

Fig. 25.6 Markings for a reduction mammoplasty.

Hormonal manipulation using danazol in the rapid phase of breast enlargement has been reported to be of benefit,[1] but as long-term studies of the effects of this treatment are not available, it cannot be confidently recommended.

Fibroadenoma

Fibroadenomas are classified in most texts as benign tumours. It is now felt that they too are aberrations of development, rather than true neoplasms.[1] The reason for this is that each fibroadenoma develops from a single lobule and not from a single cell—the prerequisite of a neoplasm. Hyperplastic lobules which are histologically identical to clinical fibroadenomas are also commonly present in normal breasts but are usually impalpable.[12] Fibroadenomas also show hormonal dependence which is similar to normal lobules. They lactate during pregnancy and involute in the perimenopausal period. This hormonal response is greater than that associated with any other benign neoplasm.

There are four separate clinical entities which do not have specifically different histological patterns. The four entities are 'common' fibroadenoma, giant fibroadenoma, juvenile fibroadenoma and phyllodes tumours. There is no universally accepted definition of what constitutes a giant fibroadenoma but most consider that it should measure at least 5 cm in diameter.[13] Giant fibroadenomas may be more common in certain African countries.[13,14] Juvenile fibroadenomas occur in adolescent girls and sometimes undergo rapid growth. They are often large and tend to be more cellular than ordinary fibroadenomas (Fig. 25.7). These three entities are treated in an identical way. Phyllodes tumours are distinct pathological entities but cannot always be differentiated clinically from fibroadenomas.

As they are disorders of development so-called 'common' fibroadenomas present most frequently immediately after the period of breast growth, that is, in the 15–25-year age group. These fibroadenomas are also common causes of a discrete breast lump in older women. In the third decade they account for 15% of all discrete palpable breast tissues and 20% of all benign breast masses. They are more common in this decade than cysts (Fig. 25.1). On examination they are usually well-circumscribed, firm, smooth, mobile lumps and may be multiple or bilateral. They are said to occur more frequently in Afro-Caribbean populations.[15]

It is important to recognize that a clinical diagnosis of fibroadenoma may be incorrect in up to 50% of cases. Although a small

REFERENCES

10. Seashore J H In: Gallager H S, Leis H P, Snyderman R K, Urban J (eds) The Breast. Mosby, St Louis 1978 pp 502–507
11. Strömbeck J O In: Strömbeck J O, Rosato F E (eds) Surgery of the Breast. Thieme, Stuttgart 1986 p 277
12. Parks A G Ann R Coll Surg Eng 1959; 25: 235–251
13. Fechner R E. In: Page D L, Anderson T J (eds) Diagnostic Histopathology of the Breast. Churchill Livingstone, Edinburgh 1987 p 72
14. Azzopardi J G. Problems in Breast Pathology. Saunders, London 1981
15. Dixon J M Br Med Bull 1991; 47: 258–271

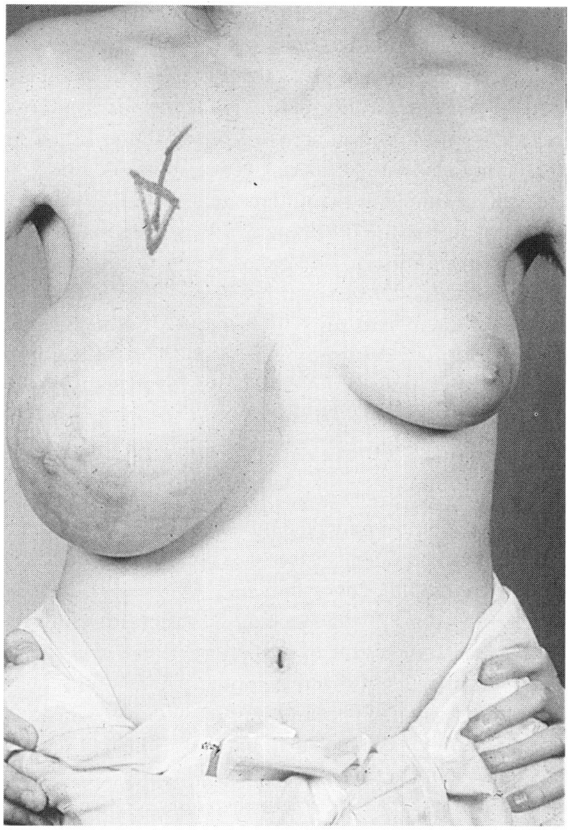

Fig. 25.7 Giant (juvenile) fibroadenoma of the right breast.

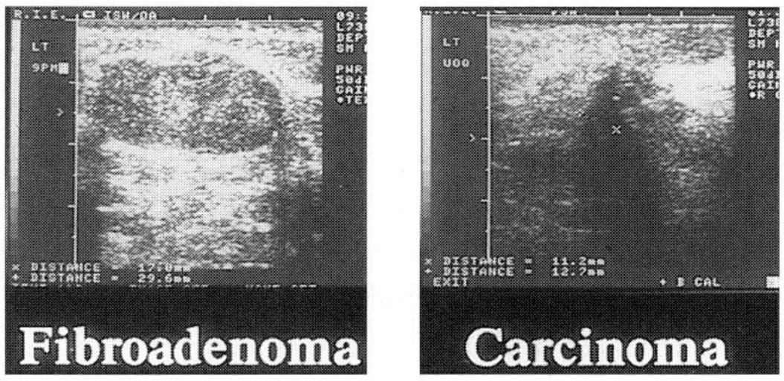

Fig. 25.8 Ultrasound scan of a fibroadenoma and a breast cancer. The scan of the fibroadenoma shows clear edges with an easily visible posterior wall. In contrast, the edges of the cancer are indistinct and there is a posterior acoustic shadow.

number of fibroadenomas increase in size the majority do not and over a third get smaller and disappear within 2 years.[16] Because of the inaccuracy of clinical diagnosis, management should not be based on this alone and all patients should have a fine-needle aspirate or an excision biopsy. Breast ultrasonography is useful in all ages and fibroadenomas have a characteristic appearance with easily visualized margins which allows the size of the lesion to be measured accurately (Fig. 25.8). If the fine-needle aspirate and ultrasound confirm a fibroadenoma, then the patient can be reassured and given the option of observation or removal. Observation is with a single follow-up ultrasound to ensure the mass has not increased in size or developed features indicating that the initial diagnosis was incorrect.

Clinical fibroadenomas over 4 cm in diameter should be excised. Giant or large juvenile fibroadenomas are best removed through an incision in the inframammary crease. Unfortunately, removal of very large fibroadenomas can result in breast distortion and subsequent revisional surgery is often required. Excision of smaller fibroadenomas can easily be performed under local anaesthesia. As with all procedures for benign disease, the incision should follow skin crease lines and, if possible, the mass should be excised through a circumareolar incision tunnelling to the lesion in the plane between the fat of the breast and the subcutaneous tissue. The fibroadenoma can be shelled out if there has been a preoperative diagnosis by fine-needle aspiration cytology; otherwise excision should include a small portion of surrounding normal breast tissue. The distinction between peri- and intracanalicular fibroadenoma is no longer considered important.

On mammography a fibroadenoma is seen as a well-rounded opacity. As up to 5% of such opacities are carcinomas, deferral of further investigation on the basis of mammography is unwise. During involution some fibroadenomas disappear and others calcify: when they do calcify a definitive mammographic diagnosis is possible.

Carcinoma arising in a fibroadenoma is rare, with an incidence of approximately 1 per 1000.[14] The carcinoma is usually of a lobular type and frequently not invasive.[17] The prognosis of carcinoma limited exclusively or almost exclusively to a fibroadenoma is excellent.[14,17]

DISORDERS OF CYCLICAL CHANGE

Mastalgia and nodularity

Premenstrual nodularity and breast discomfort occur so commonly that they are considered to be normal. When the pain is severe, this condition is classified as cyclical mastalgia.[18] Painful nodularity has been called ‘fibroadenosis’, which is an unfortunate term as there is no correlation between mastalgia, nodularity and the histological appearances of fibrosis and adenosis. The term ‘fibroadenosis’ is therefore inappropriate and should be abandoned. The cause of cyclical mastalgia is unknown, but there is some evidence that women with this condition may have an underlying abnormality which can be demonstrated by an excessive prolactin release from the pituitary gland following stimulation of the hypothalamic–pituitary axis.[19] It is known that the symptoms are not psychologically based.[20] A less common but nevertheless significant problem is non-cyclical mastalgia.[18] Differentiation between the two types of mastalgia is best achieved by the use of a pain chart (Fig. 25.9).

REFERENCES

16. Dixon J M, Dobie V, Lamb J, Walsh J S, Chetty U Br J Surg 1996; 83: 264–265
17. Oyyello L, Gump F E Surg Gynecol Obstet 1985; 116: 99–101
18. Preece P E, Hughes L E, Mansel R E, Bolton P M, Gravelle I H Lancet 1976; ii: 670–673
19. Kumar S, Mansel R E et al Cancer 1984; 53: 1311–1315
20. Preece P E, Mansel R E, Hughes L E Br Med J 1978; i: 29–30

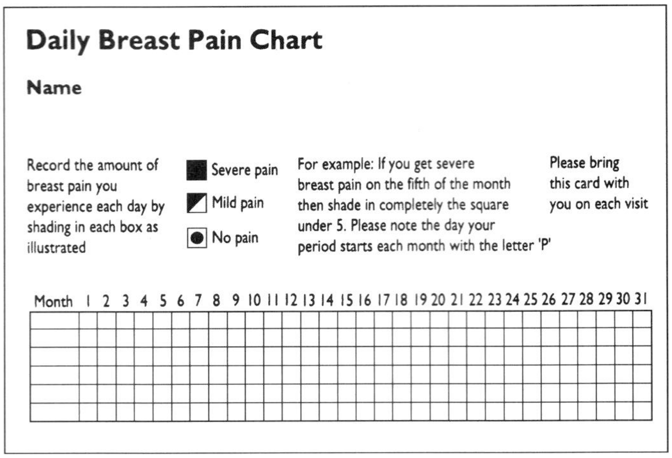

Daily breast pain chart.

Fig. 25.9 Breast pain chart.

Cyclical mastalgia

Most cyclical breast pain is of minor or moderate degree and the only real indication for treatment is pain which interferes with everyday activities.[21] Patients with cyclical breast pain are by definition premenopausal and the average age is 34. Because certain benign conditions and, very rarely, breast cancer can present with pain, it is important to exclude these by full clinical examination and mammography in women over 35 years of age. Localized areas of abnormality require further assessment by ultrasound and fine-needle aspiration cytology. It is important then to give some reassurance that cancer is not responsible for their symptoms and patients should also be given an explanation of the hormonal basis of the pain. This is the only treatment that is necessary in 85% of women with cyclical mastalgia. Some women gain relief from simple measures such as wearing a soft support bra 24 hours a day. Antibiotics, vitamin B_6, progestogens and diuretics are not effective in the treatment of breast pain.[21] There are three drugs with a product licence for the treatment of cyclical mastalgia and these include evening primrose oil (prescribed as Efamast), danazol and bromocriptine. Their effectiveness gauged from a number of studies into the treatment of mastalgia is shown in Table 25.3.

Evening primrose oil, whose active ingredient is gamolenic acid (each 500 mg capsule of evening primrose oil contains 40 mg of gamolenic acid), is used as the initial treatment in a dose of 6–8 capsules per day because it has only minor side-effects. A trial of this treatment should last at least 4 months and the effects of treatment should be monitored with pain charts.[21]

The full course of treatment with Efamast should last 6 months. Danazol in a dose of 100 mg per day should be used for patients with very severe pain or patients who fail to respond to evening primrose oil.[21,22] Tamoxifen and luteinizing hormone-releasing hormone factor analogues are both effective[23] in cyclical breast pain but do not yet have a product licence for this condition. Surgical excision of painful areas of breast tissue in the absence of palpable nodules or so-called 'trigger spots' is almost always unsuccessful in relieving symptoms and should be discouraged. Very occasionally, if the breast pain is so severe that it is making the patient's life a misery, and it has failed to respond to all the treatments discussed above, or it has relapsed following previous successful treatment and fails to respond to other agents, then following appropriate counselling, a unilateral or bilateral mastectomy is effective, if drastic. An alternative is subcutaneous mastectomy with prosthetic replacement.

Table 25.3 Response of cyclical and non-cyclical mastalgia to drug treatment

	Useful response to treatment		
	Cyclical mastalgia (%)	*Non-cyclical mastalgia (%)*	*Side-effects (%)*
Danazol	79	40	30
Gamolenic acid	58	38	4
Bromocriptine	54	33	35

Nodularity

Nodularity in the breast may be either diffuse or focal. Focal nodularity is the most common cause of a breast lump and is seen in women of all ages (Fig. 25.1). Patients with focal nodularity often report that the breast lump fluctuates in size in relation to the menstrual cycle and careful examination reveals that the lump is usually tender and is not discrete. Some patients present with an acute episode of localized breast swelling and overlying erythema. This usually settles spontaneously and is presumably due to either a change in plasma hormones or a change in the breast reactivity to normal circulating levels of hormones. This is difficult to distinguish from an episode of breast infection and if there is doubt that infection is present then antibiotics should be administered. Breast cancer must be excluded in patients with localized asymmetric areas of nodularity. Fine-needle aspiration cytology usually allows exclusion of malignancy without resort to open biopsy and is the investigation of choice in these patients.[24] Mammography in women over the age of 35 or ultrasound in younger women should also be obtained. Excision or core biopsy is indicated if the nodular area is reported as benign on fine-needle aspiration but there is clinical, mammographic or ultrasonographic suspicion of malignancy.

Non-cyclical mastalgia

Localized pain in the chest wall, referred pain and diffuse true breast pain must be differentiated. Up to 60% of patients with a persistent localized painful area in the chest wall can be effectively treated by infiltration with local anaesthetic and steroid injection (2 ml of 1% lignocaine and 1 ml containing 40 mg of methylprednisolone).[21] Injection of local anaesthetic confirms the diagnosis is correct if it cures the pain. Costochondritis (Tietze's syndrome) is often alleviated by oral non-steroidal anti-inflammatory agents.

REFERENCES

21. Mansel R E Br Med J 1995; 309: 866–868
22. Gateley C A, Miers M, Skone J F, Mansel R E In: Mansel R E (ed) Recent Developments in the Study of Benign Breast Disease. Parthenon, Carnforth, Lancs 1991 pp 17–21
23. Hamed H, Chaudary M A, Caleffi M, Fentiman I S Ann R Coll Surg Engl 1990; 72: 221–224
24. Cooper A P Diseases of the Breast. Part 1. Longmans, London 1829

Full clinical examination and, if appropriate, mammography, should be performed in patients with true non-cyclical breast pain. In the majority no cause for the pain is found and these patients may gain relief from wearing a well-supporting bra 24 hours a day. Initial systemic treatment should be with a non-steroidal anti-inflammatory agent. If this fails, some women respond to the drugs used for cyclical mastalgia (Table 25.3).[21] The cause of the pain remains obscure.

DISORDERS OF INVOLUTION

Involutional changes in the breast are usually obvious by the age of 35. The changes include disappearance of both lobular epithelium and specialized lobular connective tissue with replacement by the fibrous tissue found in the interlobular region. Aberrations from this normal process include cyst formation, sclerosis, epithelial hyperplasia and a failure of all breast tissue to involute at the same rate.[1]

Breast cyst formation

Astley Cooper was the first to distinguish cysts from breast malignancy in 1829.[24] The term 'cystic breast disease' is now restricted to a clearly defined group of women with a palpable cyst. Cystic disease of the breast affects 7% of women in the western world and cysts constitute 15% of all discrete masses in the breast. Cysts occur most frequently in women between the ages of 38 and 53 (Fig. 25.1). Cysts are distended and involuted lobules and are seen most frequently in perimenopausal women. These women do not appear to have different hormonal profiles from symptomless age-matched women and the mode of cyst formation is unknown.[25] Patients who have cystic disease in the perimenopausal period and who take hormone replacement therapy continue to develop cysts until they stop this treatment. Most present as a smooth discrete breast lump which can be painful and are sometimes visible. Although they are usually fluctuant, non-fluctuant, so-called 'tension cysts' also occur and can mimic a carcinoma.

Mammography should be performed in patients over the age of 35 with a suspected cyst prior to aspiration, as 1% of patients will have a visible carcinoma on their mammogram (Fig. 25.10). Cysts appear smooth and circumscribed; they have characteristic halos on mammography. They can, however, be incorrectly interpreted as malignant or suspicious lesions on mammography and are more reliably diagnosed by ultrasonography. A needle aspiration (with a 21-gauge needle) should be performed if a breast cyst is suspected to confirm or refute the diagnosis. Once a cyst has been confirmed, it should be aspirated completely. Fluid aspirated from cysts varies in colour from pale yellow, through dark-green, to brown. Only evenly blood-stained cyst fluid should be submitted for cytological examination.

Carcinomas presenting as breast cysts are rare and these should be separated from carcinomas adjacent to cysts, which are slightly more common. Following cyst aspiration, a patient should be re-examined and if there is a residual mass, this should be assessed by imaging and fine-needle aspiration cytology. All patients should be reviewed 4–6 weeks after the initial cyst aspiration and re-examined.

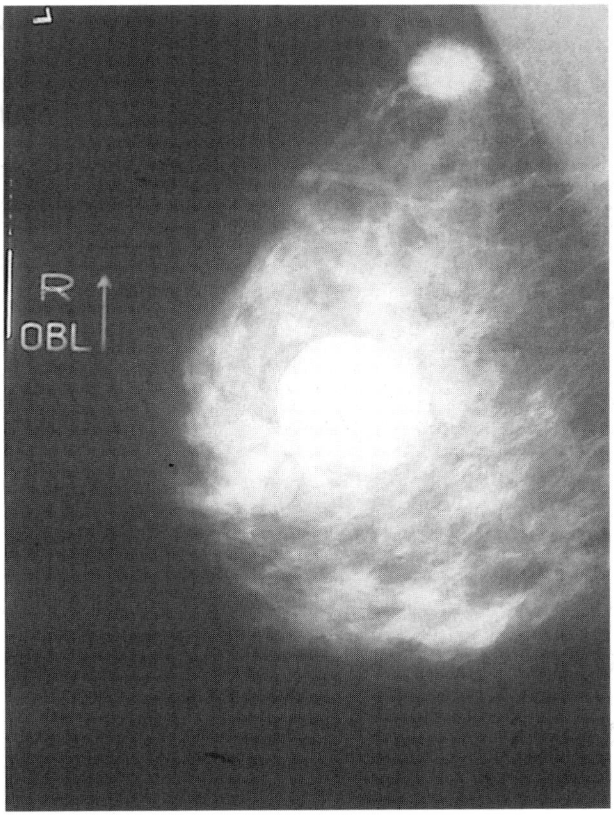

Fig. 25.10 Mammogram showing a cyst in the central part of a breast and a carcinoma in the upper part of the breast.

Indications that cancer might be present are an evenly blood-stained cyst aspirate, a suspicious persistent residual mass or refilling on more than two occasions of a cyst.[25] Approximately half of all women with cysts only develop a single palpable cyst, a third form between two and five cysts and the remainder develop more than five cysts.[26] Two per cent of patients with breast cysts develop over 25 cysts and 1% will form more than 100 cysts. In these latter groups, cyst formation can be arrested by treatment with danazol.[25] In patients with multiple cysts ultrasound is useful in confirming that all palpable lesions are cystic.

There appears to be an increased risk of breast cancer in women with palpable breast cysts but the magnitude of this risk is likely to be less than four times that of the general population and so it is not clinically significant.[25] The difficulty is in diagnosing the malignancy correctly in a breast containing multiple cysts.

Sclerosis

Sclerosing adenosis, radial scars and complex sclerosing lesions are all terms that are now used to describe the pathological changes that were previously called sclerosing papillomatosis or duct adenoma. These are all examples of sclerosis occurring in the

REFERENCES

25. Dixon J M Curr Pract Surg 1995; 7: 118–122
26. Haagensen C D, Bodian C, Haagensen D E. Breast Carcinoma Risk and Detection. Saunders, London 1981 p 55

period of breast involution.[27] These breast abnormalities cause diagnostic problems to the surgeon, radiologist and pathologist. Patients with these conditions may present with a breast lump, breast pain or they may be picked up when a mammographic abnormality is found on screening. Clinically and radiologically these conditions can simulate cancer and excisional biopsy is often required to make a definitive diagnosis. Sclerosing adenosis and radial scars are both associated with distortion of breast lobules and ducts without any evidence of epithelial hyperplasia and can be regarded as aberrations of involution.[1] Complex sclerosing lesions are less common and are more frequently associated with significant degrees of epithelial hyperplasia.

Epithelial hyperplasia

An increase in the number of layers of epithelial cells lining the terminal duct lobular unit is known as epithelial hyperplasia. Previously this change was called epitheliosis or papillomatosis, but these terms can now be regarded as obsolete. The degree of hyperplasia can be graded as mild, moderate or florid.[28] If the hyperplastic cells also show evidence of cellular atypia, the condition is called 'atypical hyperplasia'. Some degree of epithelial hyperplasia is common in the premenopausal period and may regress later.[12] Moderate or florid epithelial hyperplasia is associated with a slightly increased—although again not clinically significant—risk of subsequent breast cancer and is of little clinical importance.[29]

The hyperplastic cells may be classified as ductal if they are large, differ in size and shape and have angular hyperchromatic nuclei, or lobular if they are uniformly round or oval, with regular round or oval nuclei.[30] This classification is based on histological features and not the site where the cells originate as both types of cell arise from the epithelium of the terminal duct lobular unit. The original view that ductal hyperplasia arises in the breast ducts and lobular hyperplasia arises in the lobules is almost certainly incorrect.[30,31] The importance of identifying atypical ductal and atypical lobular hyperplasia lies in their association with subsequent malignancy. There is a 4–5 times increased risk of women with these changes developing breast cancer when compared with the general population and there is an association between atypical hyperplasia and a family history of breast carcinoma. Women with atypical ductal hyperplasia who have a first-degree relative (mother, daughter or sister) with breast cancer have an absolute risk of 20–30% of developing breast cancer over the next 15–20 years (Fig. 25.11).[29] When they develop breast cancer they do so in the breast from which the biopsy was taken, unlike patients with atypical lobular hyperplasia who develop breast cancer with an equal frequency in either breast.

Patients with atypical hyperplasia may present with a breast lump, nipple discharge or a mammographic abnormality. There are no particular clinical signs which allow separation of these patients from those with prominent nodular breast tissue or lesser degrees of hyperplasia. Fine-needle aspiration cytology is usually reported as showing features which are suspicious of malignancy.[2] On mammography, atypical hyperplasia can cause areas where the architecture is distorted by a complex sclerosing lesion or it can be

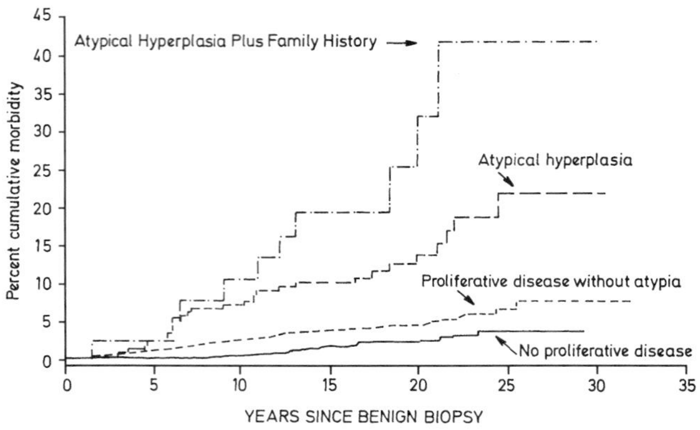

Fig. 25.11 Actual risk of breast cancer in patients with atypical hyperplasia with or without a family history.

associated with microcalcification and may only be diagnosed after a localization biopsy.[32] The majority of patients with epithelial hyperplasia are however symptomless.[1,31] Because of the increased risk of subsequent breast cancer, patients with this condition are usually recommended to have regular annual mammography. There is unfortunately no evidence that this type of breast screening in these high-risk individuals reduces mortality. Studies are underway to assess the value of tamoxifen in reducing the risk of cancer in these patients but the results from these studies will not be available for at least 10 years. Women with atypical hyperplasia and a family history of breast cancer or women with atypical hyperplasia who are found to carry a mutation in the BRCA1 or BRCA2 gene by DNA analysis may be offered mastectomy. Operations in these patients should be performed by experienced surgeons who must ensure that all the breast tissue is removed and should then normally proceed to immediate breast reconstruction.

Mastectomy for high-risk women

The goal of mastectomy in high-risk women is to reduce the chance that breast cancer develops by removing all breast tissue. In addition to removing risk, it is hoped that this procedure will reduce anxiety levels when compared with surveillance alone. Breast cancer has been reported after prophylactic mastectomy and significant amounts of breast tissue in the subareolar and peripheral breast regions have been reported after this procedure. The patient must be made aware that there is some risk of developing breast cancer even after surgery. Any procedure should

REFERENCES

27. Page D L, Anderson T J, Diagnostic Histopathology of the Breast. Churchill Livingstone, Edinburgh 1987
28. Dupont W D, Page D L N Engl J Med 1985; 312: 146–151
29. Page D L Breast 1992; 1: 3–7
30. Page D L, Dupont W D, Rogers L W, Rados M S Cancer 1985; 55: 2698–2708
31. Wellings S R, Jenson H M, Marcum R J J Natl Cancer Inst 1975; 55: 231–273
32. Kinne D W, Dershaw D D, Rosen P P In: Harris J R, Hallman S, Henderson I C, Kinne D W (eds): Breast Diseases. Lippincott, Philadelphia 1991 pp 113–117

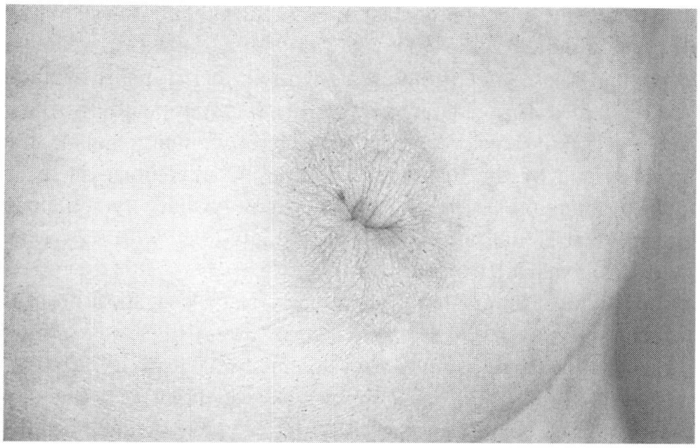

Fig. 25.12 Slit-like retraction of the nipple characteristic of duct ectasia.

attempt to remove all breast tissue. There remains debate whether subcutaneous mastectomy is an adequate procedure for prophylaxis. Reconstruction after these prophylactic procedures can be achieved using implants or myocutaneous flaps.

Duct ectasia

Duct dilatation or duct ectasia without marked periductal inflammation occurs as a consequence of normal involution[1] and accounts for the frequency with which it has been reported in various studies.[33] Symptomatic duct ectasia is best considered an aberration of normal breast involution (Table 25.1). Duct dilatation was thought to occur as a consequence of destruction of the supporting elastic lamina of breast ducts by preceding periductal mastitis. The periductal mastitis and duct ectasia complex has usually been considered to be a single entity[34–36] but as the two conditions affect different age groups and produce different symptoms, and they are best considered separately.[34,37]

Duct ectasia principally affects older women and presents with a symmetrical slit-like retraction of the nipple (Fig. 25.12) or nipple discharge. This discharge can be from single or multiple ducts and no specific treatment is required unless the discharge is troublesome, when a microdochectomy or an operation to excise all the ducts should be performed. Dilated ducts and surrounding fibrosis can cause a palpable mass which may resemble a carcinoma and in these instances cytology is useful in establishing a diagnosis.

The majority of patients with this condition have normal mammograms,[34] although some radiographs may show thickening of the ducts behind the nipple and coarse calcification.

Residual breast tissue

The breast tissue may involute at different rates in some women. This causes clinical and mammographic asymmetry which can sometimes be difficult to differentiate from breast cancer. Fine-needle aspiration cytology and repeat mammography after an interval of 3–6 months are the best methods of establishing the diagnosis.

Table 25.4 Causes of gynaecomastia

Physiological		
Neonatal—high maternal oestrogen +? high hCG		
Pubertal—? oestrogen/androgen imbalance		
Old age—? LH/FSH imbalance		
Hypogonadism		
Gonadotrophin deficiency—pituitary disorders		
Reduced androgen production, e.g. Leydig cell insufficiency		
Androgen resistance		
Neoplasms		
hCG-producing—seminomas, teratomas, choriocarcinomas		
Oestrogen-producing—Leydig, Sertoli and granulosa theca cell tumours, adrenal tumours		
Oestrogen precursor-producing—adrenal tumours		
Gonadotrophin-producing—bronchogenic carcinoma, hepatomas, renal cell and gastric carcinomas, lymphomas		
Systemic disease		
Hepatic disease		
Testicular suppression		
Increased precursor availability		
Increased SHBG		
Renal failure on dialysis		
Increased testosterone		
Increased LH		
Increased oestrogen		
Starving and refeeding, e.g. anorexia nervosa		
Hypothalamopituitary axis disturbance		
Hyperthyroidism		
Increased SHBG		
Increased testosterone, increased oestrogen		
Drug-induced		
Hormones and inhibitors		
oestrogens	spironolactone	digitalis
androgens	cimetidine	
hCG	ketoconazole	
Neurotransmitter agonists—affect prolactin secretion		
methyldopa	tricyclic agents	
phenothiazines	metoclopramide	
Cytotoxic chemotherapeutic agents—impair Leydig cell function		
busulphan	nitrosoureas	
vincristine		

hCG = Human chorionic gonadotrophin; LH = luteinizing hormone; FSH = follicle-stimulating hormone; SHBG = sex hormone-binding globulin.

Gynaecomastia

Any enlargement of breast tissue in males of any age is known as gynaecomastia. It is an entirely benign condition and is usually reversible. The amount of enlargement varies and the size and shape in extreme cases may be similar to that of a female breast. In approximately a quarter it is bilateral.[38] The histological changes are identical to those of virginal hypertrophy.

Gynaecomastia occurs in three different age groups. The neonatal form is identical to that found in female infants.

REFERENCES

33. Frantz V K, Pickering J W, Melcher G M, Auchinloss H Cancer 1951; 47: 62–83
34. Dixon J M World J Surg 1989; 13: 715–720
35. Sandison A T, Walker J C Br J Surg 1962; 50: 57–64
36. Thomas W G, Williamson R C N, Davis G D, Webb A J Br J Surg 1982; 69: 423–425
37. Dixon J M, RaviSekar O, Chetty U, Anderson T J Br J Surg 1996 83: 820–822
38. Crichlow R W In: Gallager H S, Leis H P, Snyderman R K, Urban J A (eds) The Breast. Mosby, St Louis 1978 pp 508–523

Gynaecomastia also occurs commonly at puberty and in old age. Pubertal gynaecomastia occurs in 30–70% of boys if carefully sought. Persisting pubertal gynaecomastia accounts for a quarter of all cases seen in adults. The aetiology, which must have a hormonal basis, is not completely understood, although it is probably the result of an oestrogen-androgen imbalance. It does not usually require treatment as 80% of cases resolve spontaneously within 2 years.[38] Tamoxifen (20 mg daily) and danazol (300 mg daily) have been found to be effective treatments for gynaecomastia, producing complete resolution in approximately half of all patients treated.[39] Subcutaneous mastectomy, which should be performed through a circumareolar incision, is occasionally required for persistent embarrassing enlargement resistant to drug treatment. Unless it is performed for Klinefelter's syndrome where a total mastectomy should be performed, a small disc of breast tissue should be left attached to the undersurface of the areola and some fat should be left on the skin flaps to ensure that the end-result is not an unsightly depression.

Senescent 'hypertrophy' accounts for a quarter of all adult males with gynaecomastia and occurs in the fifth and sixth decades of life. In the majority it does not appear to be associated with any endocrine abnormality, although there may be an underlying hormone imbalance between luteinizing hormone and follicle-stimulating hormone. Specific causes of gynaecomastia need to be excluded in all patients.[39] These include hypogonadism (15% of cases), neoplasm (3%), systemic disease (12%) and drugs (20%) (Table 25.4).

Gynaecomastia is usually soft or rubbery to palpation and involves the whole gland. It is often bilateral. Unilateral, eccentric, tender, hard or ulcerating lesions indicate a male breast cancer. Where there is doubt, mammography is useful and fine-needle aspiration cytology should confirm malignancy.

INFECTIVE AND INFLAMMATORY LESIONS

Mastitis neonatorum

The continued enlargement of the breast bud in the first week or two of life has been described earlier. Occasionally the breast may become infected, usually with *Staphylococcus aureus* and an abscess can then develop (mastitis neonatorum). The child may be severely ill. In the early stages antibiotics (flucloxacillin) may suppress the infection, but prompt incision, placed as far peripherally in the breast as possible to avoid damage to the breast bud, is required if fluctuation develops.

Lactating breast abscess

Puerperal mastitis and lactating breast abscess are now less common in developed countries but are still a frequent problem in many parts of the world. Lactating breast abscesses are caused by *Staphylococcus aureus* but can also be caused by *S. epidermidis* and streptococci. Infection is usually related to abrasions or cracks of the nipple and it is probable that increased numbers of bacteria are present on the skin of these areas. Organisms which enter the breast multiply in areas that are draining poorly which contain stagnant milk. Infection is most often seen in the first month after delivery, although some women develop infection during weaning. Lactating breast infection presents with erythema, pain, swelling and tenderness. In the later stages a fluctuant mass with overlying shiny, red skin develops.[40] The tight fascial compartments of the breast bound by the ligaments of Astley Cooper however often make fluctuation an unreliable late sign. Axillary lymph node enlargement is unusual. Patients are usually toxic with a pyrexia, tachycardia and a leucocytosis.

Antibiotics administered at an early stage can abort abscess formation. As over 50% of staphylococci are resistant to penicillin, flucloxacillin or, in patients with a penicillin sensitivity, erythromycin should be given. In the past most patients with a lactating breast abscess have been treated by incision and drainage of the abscess under a general anaesthetic.[41] Patients whose condition does not improve rapidly on antibiotic therapy and those with clear evidence of abscess formation can now be treated by applying local anaesthetic cream to the skin overlying the point of maximum tenderness and leaving this in place for 1 hour.[40] A 19-gauge needle is inserted in those patients where the overlying skin is normal and if pus is obtained, it is aspirated, while the patients continue on oral antibiotic therapy; aspiration is then repeated every 2–3 days until pus is no longer obtained.[40] The mean number of aspirations is between three and four per patient. There are some patients whose abscess cavities fill up with milk. Providing this is not purulent then this does not require to be aspirated. Antibiotics can usually be discontinued within 10 days of initial aspiration. If pus is not aspirated, a sample of cells is removed from the abnormal area and sent for cytology.

If the skin overlying the abscess is thinned, a small incision is made with a 15 blade through the skin and the pus drained: drainage does not need to be dependent. If the skin overlying the abscess is necrotic, then this can be excised without the application of local anaesthetic cream. Following incision and drainage or excision of necrotic skin, the cavity of the abscess is irrigated daily with saline. This conservative approach of aspiration and antibiotics or mini-incision and drainage is usually effective in lactating abscesses and only rarely is more extensive drainage of the cavity under general anaesthetic necessary. Even in these patients dependent drains are unnecessary.

It has been common practice in women with lactating breast infection either to discontinue breast-feeding completely or to breast-feed from the normal breast and to express and discard milk from the affected breast. Patients find this extremely painful and it is much more comfortable and more effective mild drainage is achieved by continuing to breast-feed from both breasts.[40] The infant is not harmed by the bacteria and certain antibiotics, including flucloxacillin, co-amoxiclav and erythromycin, within the milk. Antibiotics which are contraindicated during lactation include tetracycline and ciprofloxacin as they enter the milk and can affect the child. It is advisable to transfer to bottle-feeding and

REFERENCES

39. Dixon J M, Mansel R E Br Med J 1994; 309: 797–800
40. Dixon J M Br Med J 1994; 309: 946–949
41. Preece P E Surgery (Medicine Group, Lond) 1983; 1: 28–33

in some instances to suppress lactation with hormones if the mother finds breast-feeding too painful.

Non-lactating breast abscesses

Non-lactating infections can be divided into those occurring centrally within the breast in the periareolar region which are usually associated with periductal mastitis and those affecting the peripheral breast tissue.

Periareolar infections

Periareolar infection is most commonly seen in young women with a mean age of 32 years. Periductal mastitis is usually the cause. If the inflammatory tissue is biopsied it shows inflammation around undilated subareolar breast ducts. This condition has been confused with and mistakenly called duct ectasia; duct ectasia is a separate condition affecting an older age group.[37,39] Current evidence suggests that smoking is an important aetiological factor in periductal mastitis but not in duct ectasia: about 90% of women who get periductal mastitis or its complications smoke cigarettes compared with 38% of the same age group in the general population.[37] Substances absorbed orally from cigarette smoke may either directly or indirectly damage the wall of the breast ducts.[42] Damaged tissues then become infected by *Staphylococcus aureus* or more often anaerobic organisms, including *Bacteroides* and anaerobic streptococci.

The clinical syndrome of periductal mastitis is characterised by periareolar inflammation, a non-lactating breast abscess and a mammary duct fistula[40] (Fig. 25.13). Patients may also present with breast pain. Nipple discharge from one or both breasts is present in 15–20% of women. Nipple retraction occurs early at the site of the diseased duct in periductal mastitis and is present in up to three-quarters of patients who present with periareolar inflammation. Early in the disease, the retraction is slight and can be missed. Marked retraction or inversion occurs after recurrent episodes of infection.

Co-amoxiclav or a combination of erythromycin and metronidazole[40] is used to treat periareolar inflammation in the first instance even if there is an associated mass. Care should be taken to exclude an underlying neoplasm if the mass or inflammation does not resolve after an appropriate course of antibiotics. Non-lactating breast abscesses should be managed by aspiration or by incision and drainage. Periareolar abscesses secondary to periductal mastitis are now more common in the UK than puerperal abscesses.[34] Up to a third of patients develop a mammary duct fistula after drainage of a non-lactating periareolar abscess. Recurrent episodes of periareolar sepsis should be treated by excision of the diseased duct by an experienced breast surgeon[34,40] while the patient continues to take antibiotics.

Mammary duct fistula

A mammary duct fistula is a communication between the skin, usually in the periareolar region, and a breast duct (Fig. 25.14). It is believed that almost all mammary duct fistulae develop as a complication of periductal mastitis.[34,43] One in three events precedes the development of a fistula: a periareolar inflammatory mass discharging spontaneously, a periareolar mass is biopsied; or a non-lactating breast abscess is incised and drained.

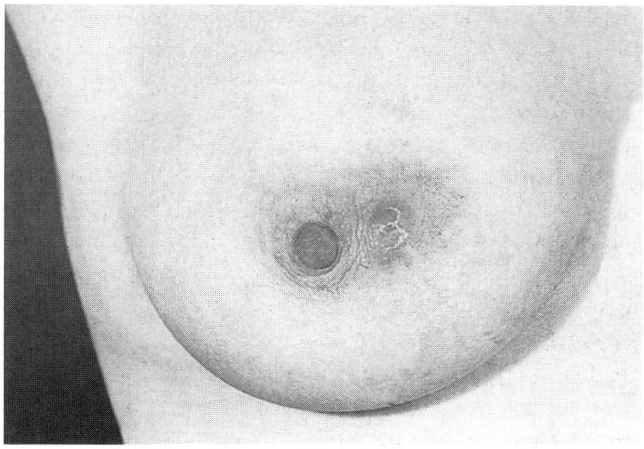

Fig. 25.13 Periareolar inflammation and abscess characteristic of periductal mastitis.

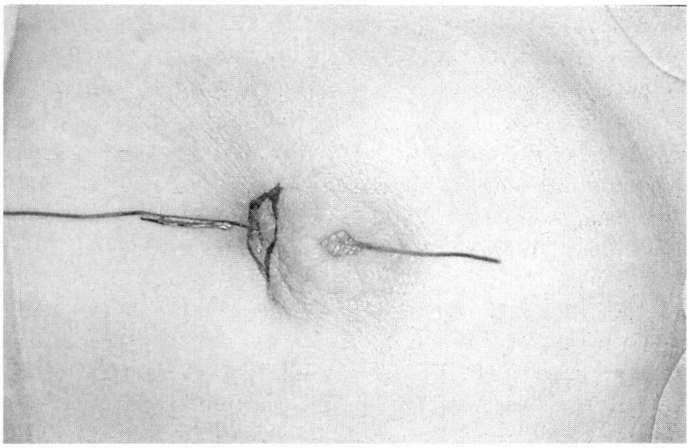

Fig. 25.14 Patient with a mammary duct fistula with a probe demonstrating the fistula.

The underlying pathology is either periductal mastitis or, rarely, granulomatous mastitis[43] and older theories that mammary duct fistulae result from duct obstruction or congenitally lined squamous tracts are incorrect. Women developing mammary duct fistulae have a median age of 35 years. Retraction of the nipple at the site of the involved duct is present in almost all patients. Occasionally there can be more than one opening at the areolar margin from a single diseased duct.

There is no optimal method for surgically treating mammary duct fistula at present. If the fistula is laid open or the fistula tract is excised, healing occurs by secondary intention, which leaves an ugly scar across the areola and nipple. The most efficacious method of treatment appears to be to excise the fistula with its

REFERENCES

42. Bundred N J Breast 1993; 2: 1–2
43. Dixon J M, Thompson A M Br J Surg 1991; 78: 1185–1186

associated duct through a circumareolar incision incorporating the external opening of the fistula. The wound is then closed primarily while the patient continues to take co-amoxiclav or a combination of erythromycin and metronidazole.[40,43] The excision should incorporate a portion of nipple skin to ensure complete removal of the diseased duct. The nipple should be everted to prevent recurrence.[44] Total duct excision is required in patients in whom the nipple cannot be everted after excision of the fistula and involved duct and in patients undergoing surgery for recurrent mammary duct fistula.[43]

Peripheral non-lactating breast abscesses

Peripheral breast abscesses are less common than periareolar abscess associated with periductal mastitis. This type of infection may be associated with other diseases such as diabetes, rheumatoid arthritis and with steroid treatment or trauma.[40] The majority, however, develop in the absence of any predisposing factor and a suspicion of underlying malignancy must always be entertained. Pilonidal abscesses affecting the skin of the breast in sheep shearers and barbers have been reported.[40]

Staphylococcus aureus is usually responsible but some abscesses do contain anaerobic organisms. These abscesses are more common in premenopausal than in postmenopausal women and the patient characteristically presents with a tender lump which is associated with inflammatory changes in the overlying skin and occasionally with oedema of the whole breast, seen as peau d'orange.

A needle should be inserted to confirm the diagnosis. Treatment with co-amoxiclav or a combination of erythromycin and metronidazole will often abort abscess formation if pus is not aspirated but infection is still suspected. Treatment is as already outlined if pus is aspirated.

Primary infection of the skin of the breast

Primary infection of the breast skin can present as cellulitis or an abscess. It most commonly affects the skin of the lower half of the breast.[40] These infections may often recur in women who are overweight, have large breasts or who have poor personal hygiene. Cellulitis of the skin is seen more commonly after surgery or radiotherapy (Fig. 25.15). *Staphylococcus aureus* is the usual infecting organism. Cellulitis in the male breast is uncommon but is seen in the neonatal and pubertal periods. Treatment is the same as for cellulitis at other sites with antibiotics and drainage, or aspiration if an abscess is present. Women with recurrent skin infection should be advised about weight reduction and keeping the area as clean and dry as possible. This includes careful washing of the area up to twice a day with Hibiscrub or Betadine solutions, avoiding skin creams and talcum powder and wearing either a cotton bra or cotton vest worn inside the bra.

Sebaceous cysts are common in breast skin and may become infected. Modified sebaceous glands are also present on the areolar as Montgomery's glands below the tubercules and these likewise can become infected. Some recurrent infections in the inframammary fold are the result of hidradenitis suppurativa (Fig. 25.16). In this condition the infection should be initially controlled by a combination of antibiotics and drainage of any pus. The same organisms are found in hidradenitis as in periareolar infection. Conservative excision of the infected skin is effective in stopping further infection in about half the patients. The remainder continue to have episodes of infection despite surgery.[44]

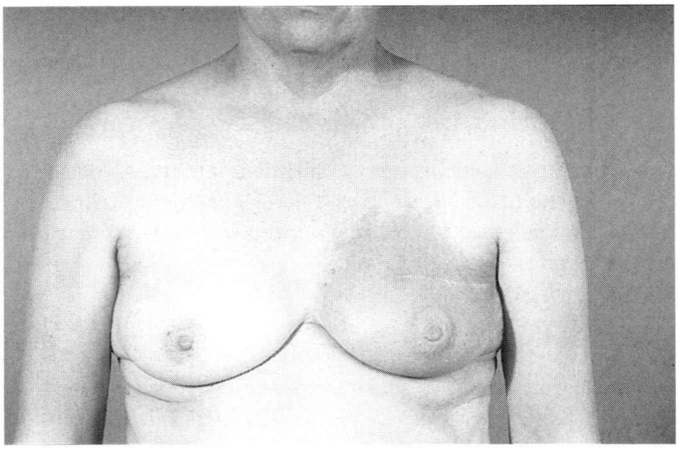

Fig. 25.15 Cellulitis of the left breast following previous surgery and radiotherapy for breast cancer.

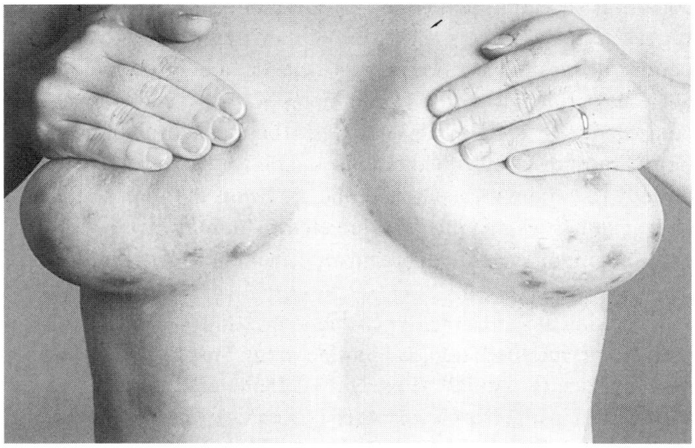

Fig. 25.16 Infection of the skin of the lower half of the breast in a patient with hidradenitis suppurativa.

Granulomatous lobular mastitis

This form of mastitis is classified separately from periductal mastitis,[45] although it is likely to be a variant of this condition. Surgical intervention is often complicated by wound infection and a mammary duct fistula and there is a strong tendency for this condition to persist or recur despite surgery.[40] Operation is best avoided and, if granulomatous mastitis is diagnosed on fine-needle

REFERENCES

44. Hughes L E, Mansel R E, Webster D J T Benign Disorders and Diseases of the Breast: Concepts and Clinical Management. Baillière Tindall, London 1989
45. Kassler E, Wolloch Y Am J Clin Pathol 1992; 58: 642–644

aspiration cytology, surgery should be restricted to dealing with the complications, such as abscess formation or mammary duct fistula.[46]

Fat necrosis

Traumatic fat necrosis most often occurs in older women,[47] although in at least half of the patients there is no history of trauma. Extensive fat necrosis is sometimes seen as a consequence of seat belt damage following a road traffic accident (Fig. 25.17). It is of interest that the breast in its exposed position is subjected to almost daily trauma, yet fat necrosis is an uncommon condition, though it often occurs in other parts of the body which are less frequently injured.

In the early stage a focus of haemorrhage can usually be seen. Later the fat undergoes liquefaction necrosis and the surrounding area is densely infiltrated by liquid-filled macrophages and polymorphonuclear leucocytes. Foreign-body giant cells are a frequent histological finding. The focus eventually becomes converted to a dense fibrous scar, which may contain microcalcification. Fat necrosis has to be distinguished from breast cancer, because the focus of fibrosis often becomes attached to the overlying skin, resulting in skin dimpling or retraction. Focal calcification and scarring may also resemble a carcinoma on mammography. Aspiration cytology or excision biopsy is sometimes required to confirm the diagnosis of fat necrosis and exclude a breast carcinoma.

Tuberculosis

Tuberculosis of the breast was first described by Astley Cooper.[24] Infection usually reaches the breast by lymphatic spread from axillary, mediastinal or cervical nodes or it can pass directly from an infected rib, costochondral junction or the pleura.[48] Haematogenous spread from a primary focus in the lung is very uncommon. In 3% of patients both breasts are affected; the axillary nodes are involved in 60% and these may caseate.[48,49] Tuberculosis of the breast predominantly affects women in the latter part of the child-bearing period and because it is now rare, the diagnosis is difficult to make from the clinical history and examination. A clue to diagnosis is a history of costal, sternal or axillary tuberculosis: the presence of a sinus in the breast or axilla which is present in half the patients also strongly suggests the possibility of tuberculosis. In the early stages it causes an ill-defined mobile swelling, but later caseation occurs and an abscess or sinus develops. As the disease progresses and fibrosis becomes the predominant feature, a firmer mass often becomes palpable; this can mimic breast cancer by producing skin-tethering and nipple inversion and a biopsy may be required to establish the correct diagnosis. It is important to appreciate that a great many conditions can produce microscopic changes which are indistinguishable from tuberculosis, including sarcoidosis, mycotic infections (cryptococcosis, histoplasmosis, blastomycosis), metazoal infections (hydatid, cysticerosis), periductal mastitis/duct ectasia, Wegener's granulomatosis and granulomatous mastitis.[49] It is also important to recognise that tuberculosis and breast cancer can coexist.[47–49] Treatment is with appropriate antituberculous chemotherapy, based if possible on the results of laboratory sensitivity testing (see Chapter 4).

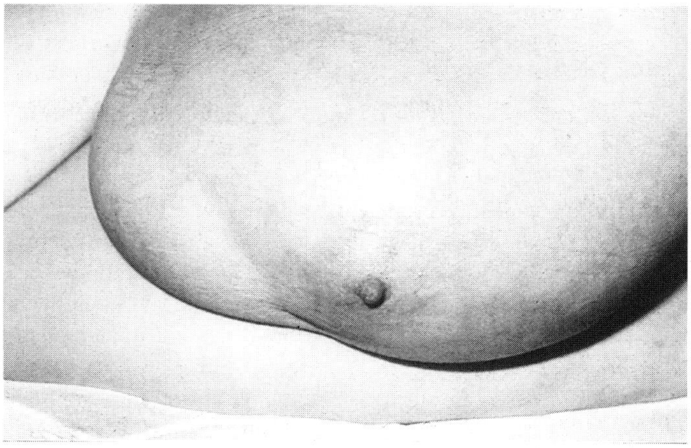

Fig. 25.17 Consequence of extensive fat necrosis following a seat belt injury in a road traffic accident.

Syphilis

This is now exceedingly rare. A primary chancre usually develops on the nipple or areola from kissing or from nursing an infected child. In the initial stages, single or multiple painless ulcers develop, and organisms can be seen in the serum of the ulcer on dark-ground microscopy. Axillary lymphadenopathy is also present in the majority of patients with chancres. Gummata occasionally affect the breast in tertiary syphilis. Serology is only positive in the secondary or tertiary stages. Treatment is with appropriate antibiotics (see Chapter 4).

Actinomycosis

Primary actinomycosis of the breast occurs rarely[50] and secondary spread from pulmonary actinomycosis is also exceedingly uncommon. The disease involves the pleura, ribs and pectoral muscle and extends through them to the breast. Penicillin is the treatment of choice (see Chapter 4).

Herpes

Herpetic ulceration of the nipple has been reported[51] but is rare.

Molluscum contagiosum

This can affect the areola and presents as wart-like lesions.

REFERENCES

46. Dixon J M, Chetty U Br J Surg 1995; 82: 1143
47. Lee B J, Edair F E Ann Surg 1920; 37: 189–191
48. Apps M C P, Harrison N K, Blauth C I A Br Med J 1984; 288: 1874–1875
49. Symmers W S In: Payling Wright G (ed) Systemic Pathology, vol 1. Longman Green, London 1966 p 953–955
50. Lloyd-Davies J A Br J Surg 1951; 38: 378–381
51. Oertel Y C Fine Needle Aspiration of the Breast. Boston, Butterworths 1987 p 74

BENIGN NEOPLASMS

Duct papilloma

These lesions can be single or multiple. They are very common and it has been suggested they may be more of an aberration of development rather than a true benign tumour as they show minimal, if any, malignant potential.[1] Some believe patients with the 'multiple papilloma syndrome' are at increased risk of subsequent breast cancer,[26] but this remains disputed.[28] Papillomas are usually small and only cause symptoms when they arise in major breast ducts. The most frequent symptom is a blood-stained nipple discharge.

Mammography may show a dilated duct behind the papilloma or a small round opacity in the retroareolar region, although there is usually no visible abnormality. The treatment is to excise the involved duct (microdochectomy). A number of methods are available to identify the involved duct at operation. Usually the duct is so dilated that it can be visually identified during dissection, but some prefer to place a lacrimal probe in the discharging duct. A circumareolar incision is made over the site of the dilated duct. Care is taken during the dissection to preserve the other ducts on the undersurface of the nipple. The diseased duct is excised with a portion of tissue out to the limit of the probe or beyond the extent of the duct dilatation, which is usually 2 cm or less. A total duct excision should be performed when it is clear at operation that the patient has multiple sites of discharge. It is only necessary to excise 1–2 cm of the major subareolar ducts for this operation to be effective. Excision of all ducts has been reported to be associated with loss of nipple sensation in up to 20% of patients.[40] One reason for loss of sensation may be the incision described for this operation, which encompasses 50% of the circumareolar margin. It can be performed through a much smaller incision which damages fewer nerves and probably limits the loss of nipple sensation.

Lipoma

These soft, lobulated, radiolucent masses are common in the breast. Interest lies in the confusion with a 'pseudolipoma', which is a soft mass which can be felt around a small breast cancer caused by indrawing of fat by a spiculated carcinoma. For this reason all patients over 35 thought on clinical examination to have a lipoma should have mammography and fine-needle aspiration cytology.

Granular cell myoblastoma

These lesions can mimic breast cancer, but are rare. They present as firm homogeneous masses. Their histogenesis is unclear but they are composed of uniform cells with abundant periodic acid–Schiff-positive cytoplasm and large vesicular nuclei.

Other benign tumours, including leiomyoma, chondroma, chondrolipoma, myxoma, ganglioneuroma and osteoma, have been described in the breast but are rare. Benign skin adnexal tumours are also occasionally seen over the skin of the breast.

NIPPLE DISCHARGE

Up to two-thirds of all normal non-lactating women produce fluid from the nipple if a small negative pressure is applied to the major breast ducts.[52] The fluid varies in colour from clear through yellow to dark green and is never blood-stained. It may arise from single or multiple ducts. The other causes of nipple discharge include:

1. *Duct papilloma*—the discharge is usually from a single duct and often frankly blood-stained.
2. *Duct ectasia*—the discharge is usually 'cheesy' and is positive to blood on Haemo-Stix testing in 60%. It is rarely frankly blood-stained and often comes from more than one duct.
3. *Periductal mastitis*—this can be watery or purulent and usually contains bacteria on culture.
4. *Epithelial hyperplasia*—the discharge may be blood-stained and is usually from a single duct.
5. *Galactorrhoea*—this is the confirmed frank discharge of breast milk and the prolactin levels must be checked. It may be associated with a pituitary adenoma which secretes prolactin.
6. *Breast cancer*—there is usually a discharge from a single duct, which may be watery or serous with microscopic red cells present. Frequently it is blood-stained and associated with a palpable mass. It is a rare cause of nipple discharge.

Investigation includes Haemo-Stix testing, clinical examination and mammography. Ductography has no role in routine investigation and cytology of the discharge is only of value in the investigation of patients who present with an isolated blood-stained nipple discharge.

Surgical excision of the involved duct should be performed if the investigations suggest there is a suspicion of an underlying malignancy (e.g. if the discharge is obviously blood-stained) or it is troublesome or persists over a period of months.[4] Further discharge from other ducts is common when a microdochectomy has been performed for periductal mastitis or duct ectasia and total duct excision is the recommended treatment for these conditions. A total duct excision should also be performed in patients who have troublesome discharge from multiple ducts.[4] The great majority of nipple discharges are totally innocent and require neither treatment nor investigation.

In troublesome multiduct discharge a total duct excision should be performed.

NIPPLE RETRACTION

This may be either congenital or acquired. The cause of congenital nipple retraction is not known, but the inversion often corrects itself during pregnancy. It is only of clinical importance because it may frustrate attempts at breast-feeding and may be confused with acquired retraction. Plastic surgical procedures have been devised to correct this problem.

Acquired causes of nipple retraction include periductal mastitis, duct ectasia, tuberculosis, previous biopsy and malignancy. In the

REFERENCE

52. Wynder E L, Hill P Lancet 1977; ii: 840–842

absence of suspicious clinical, mammographic or cytological features, no treatment is required.[4]

PROBLEMS OCCURRING DURING PREGNANCY AND LACTATION

The majority of patients who present with breast lumps in pregnancy have the same conditions as those found in non-pregnant women. Rare breast masses include localised breast infarcts from overgrowth of a pre-existing fibroadenoma or a spontaneous infarct. The likelihood of diagnosis of cancer is similar to that in the non-pregnant population. Nipple discharge with blood present, either visibly or cytologically, during pregnancy or lactation is common and unless it persists or becomes troublesome does not require any specific investigation. There are specific lesions which occur and these include galactocoele. This is a cystic lesion containing breast milk which may become inspissated. It is thought to occur in women who stop breast-feeding suddenly.[4] Treatment is by aspiration, which both confirms the diagnosis and usually cures the condition.

MISCELLANEOUS LESIONS

Fibromatosis

This poorly understood condition originally presents as a breast mass. It is caused by a benign proliferation of myofibroblasts and behaves in a similar manner to other extra-abdominal fibromatosis (desmoid tumours), in that it frequently recurs after excision.[53] The treatment is still by wide local excision.

Nodular fasciitis

This usually develops in the pectoral fascia beneath the breast and presents as a deep-seated breast lump. It occurs as a result of fibroblastic proliferation and, like fibromatosis, it is treated by wide local excision.

Lymphocytic lobulitis

The pathogenesis of this condition is unknown. It is associated with other autoimmune conditions and presents with a mass that can resemble breast cancer. It is different from granulomatous lobular mastitis and is characterised by lymphocytic infiltration around the breast lobules, with lymphocytic vasculitis and epithelioid fibroblasts in the stroma.[54]

Diabetic mastopathy

Patients with diabetes can develop dense, keloid-like areas of fibrosis within the breast which both clinically and mammographically can be mistaken for breast cancer. The diagnosis is often only established by open biopsy. This condition is not well-understood.[55]

Sarcoidosis

Involvement of the breast by sarcoidosis is rare but, when present, may again simulate a neoplasm. Sarcoidosis should be distinguished from granulomatous lobular mastitis and a diagnosis of sarcoidosis should only be made after other causes of granulomatous infection, such as microbacterial, fungal and parasitic infections or reactions to foreign materials, have been excluded. Histologically the breast tissue contains typical non-caseating granulomas with varying numbers of giant cells. It can present either with a mass in the breast or as enlarged intramammary or axillary lymph nodes.

Amyloid

Amyloid deposits have been reported in the breast.[56]

Haematoma

This may follow injury, especially from car seatbelts, and can occur spontaneously in patients on anticoagulant therapy. A supporting bra should be worn and aspiration may occasionally be helpful. A breast haematoma may progress to fat necrosis. Occasionally breast carcinoma may present as a seemingly spontaneous haematoma. Surgical drainage of such lesions should therefore always include the taking of a biopsy.

Hamartoma

Hamartomas are uncommon breast lesions. They are also known as fibroadenolipomas. Mammographically these lesions consist of fibroglandular tissue admixed with fat and surrounded by a capsule of connective tissue. The halo of connective tissue surrounding the lesion differentiates these from fibroadenomas and they have a classic mammographic appearance.

Intramammary lymph nodes

These are common and are often misdiagnosed as fibroadenomas or small carcinomas. Fine-needle aspiration cytology establishes the correct diagnosis. Enlargement of lymph nodes may be secondary to local pathology or may be the result of systemic disorders such as infectious mononucleosis, toxoplasmosis, skin conditions such as psoriasis or lymphoreticular malignancy.

Paraffin and silicone granulomas

The desire for larger breasts has led women to seek augmentation. This was originally accomplished by injecting liquid paraffin into the submammary space. Later a silicone compound was used. Unfortunately both substances can migrate into the breast and cause a low-grade inflammatory reaction, characterised

REFERENCES

53. Rosen Y, Papasozomenos S, Gardner B Cancer 1978; 41: 1409–1413
54. Schnitt S J, Connolly J L In: Harris J R, Lippman N, Morrow M, Hellman S (eds) Diseases of the Breast. Lippincott-Raven, Philadelphia 1996 p 39
55. Sideman J D, Schnapper L A, Philips L E Hum Pathol 1994; 25: 819–824
56. Fernandez B B, Hernandez F J Arch Pathol 1973; 95: 102–105

histologically by the presence of granulomata and foreign-body giant cells. Clinically this can cause a lump, which may mimic breast cancer. The preferred method of augmentation is now the placement of silicone gel enclosed in a Silastic envelope in the submammary space, although this still often results in capsule formation.

Lactational change

Lactational change is occasionally seen in the breasts of non-pregnant women and may be focal or diffuse. The patient may present with a focal breast lump. This occurs as a result of abnormally high levels of prolactin, from either a prolactin-secreting tumour of the pituitary or, more commonly, from stimulation of the pituitary by drugs, particularly psychotropic drugs.[57]

Blocked Montgomery's tubercle

Montgomery's tubercles are blind-ending ducts in the areola. Secretions from the lining cells may become inspissated and present as a periareolar lump which can be locally excised.

Mondor's disease of the breast

Superficial thrombophlebitis of the veins over the breast is known as Mondor's disease.[58,59] In the early stages the vein is very tender, but with time it becomes a string-like band and may be associated with skin dimpling. There is no specific treatment. There was a report of a patient with breast carcinoma presenting initially with Mondor's disease, but this was considered to be coincidental.[59]

Arteritis

Patients with generalized vasculitis can get vasculitic changes in the breast which cause breast lumps.[60] These lesions are usually part of a much more widespread vasculitis and many can only be diagnosed by biopsy.

Aneurysm

Aneurysmal dilatation of a vessel within the breast has been described and presented as a discrete mass, with an audible bruit on auscultation.[61]

Sebaceous cyst

These cysts quite frequently affect the skin of the breast.

Eczema of the nipple

This may be a local problem, or it can be part of generalized eczema. The problem lies in differentiating eczema from Paget's disease, and frequently a biopsy is necessary to establish the correct diagnosis. A clue is that eczema almost always involves the areola first, whereas Paget's disease always starts on the nipple. The eczema may be caused by a local sensitivity and removal of the sensitising agent results in rapid resolution. Topical steroids are often effective if no sensitising agent can be identified.

Skin dimpling

This can result from involution of breast tissue. It may follow previous surgery or can occur as a consequence of fat necrosis, sclerosing adenosis, radial scars and fibromatosis. Breast cancer must always be excluded.

Nipple adenoma

This presents as an abnormal ulcerated area on the nipple. Histologically there is benign epithelial hyperplasia of the major ducts behind the nipple. The biopsy may be cellular and have cytological atypia, but despite these appearances the lesion is benign and cured by wide excision.[27]

Factitial disease

Artefactual or factitious breast disease is created by the patient, often through complicated or repetitive actions. Such patients may undergo many investigations and operations before the nature of the disease is recognised. The diagnosis is difficult to establish but should be considered when a clinical situation does not conform to common appearances or pathological processes.[44]

Jogger's nipple

The nipple is occasionally the site of trauma and the condition of jogger's nipple is well-recognized.[62] The changes are presumably the result of constant friction between an unprotected warm or moist nipple on ill-fitted clothing. It is sometimes severe enough to produce bleeding. A cyclist's nipple is a similar condition which appears to be a cold injury causing pain lasting for several days.[63] A tassel dancer's nipple has also been described.[64]

MALIGNANT DISEASE

CARCINOMA

Carcinoma of the female breast is the most common female cancer and affects some 1 in 12 adult women during their lifetime. In 1984 there were 24 471 new cases of breast cancer in the UK and in 1986 a total of 15 245 women died of the disease. These figures make the disease the leading cause of death in women between the ages of 40 and 50 years.

REFERENCES

57. Mason R C, Miller W R, Hawkins R A, Brown M S, Forrest A P M Breast Cancer Res Treat 1983; 3: 331–338
58. Oldfield M C Lancet 1962; i: 994–996
59. Veronesi P, Zurrida S Breast 1995; 4: 170–171
60. Stephenson T J, Underwood J L E Br J Surg 1986; 73: 105
61. Dehn T C B, Lee E C G Br Med J 1986; 292: 1240
62. Levit F N Engl J Med 1977: 297: 1197–1198
63. Powell B North Am Med Assoc 1982; 249: 2457–2458
64. Collins R E C Br Med J 1981; 283: 1660

Aetiology

The aetiology is not known but genetic, endocrine and dietary factors are implicated in its genesis. The development of the disease is probably multifactorial with no predominant cause. The disease is commoner in females who are nulliparous and live in developed countries. Conversely, multiparous women who had their first pregnancy to term at an early age and who live in underdeveloped countries have a low incidence of the disease. The protective effect of multiparity is almost certainly related to the fact that fecund women tend to have their first child young. The protective effect of breast-feeding is also related to a young age at first birth.

The mechanism by which endocrine events alter the susceptibility of breast tissue to malignant change is unclear, but Korenman[65] has suggested that overexposure to oestrogens unopposed by progesterone—a circumstance which happens in nulliparous women—may be implicated. This oestrogen window hypothesis is consistent with the higher incidence of breast cancer in women who have an early menarche and late menopause. Similarly, an artificial early menopause induced by ovarian irradiation or oophorectomy has been shown to be a protective factor. Hyperoestrogenism has also been thought to explain the observation that obese women have a higher incidence of breast cancer, as it is known that aromatization of androgens to oestrogens occurs in peripheral fat. Direct measurement of oestrogens in the blood has however failed to show any differences between women with cancer and control subjects. Indeed, no consistent endocrine abnormality has been recorded in women with breast cancer compared with age-matched controls.

Genetic and environmental factors

In the mouse transmission of breast cancer from one generation to another has been demonstrated but this was found to be caused by transmission of the Bittner virus in the mother's milk. No such mechanism has been shown for human breast cancer. Breast cancer in women is generally a sporadic disease; clusters of cases within families are not common but do occur in around 5% of patients.[66] A family history of premenopausal breast cancer in a mother or sister certainly carries an increased risk of breast cancer, but the risk increase is only some two- to fourfold,[67] demonstrating that mendelian inheritance is not usual. Up to 20% of breast cancer patients have a first-degree relative with breast cancer. The percentage of affected first-degree relatives is even higher if the patient has bilateral premenopausal breast cancer. Recently two major breast cancer genes have been identified (BRCA1 and BRCA2) and these have been shown to be definitely associated with inherited breast cancer in several large affected families.[68,69] BRCA1 is located on chromosome 11 and is associated with both breast and ovarian cancer development, while BRCA2 is on chromosome 17 and is associated solely with breast cancer. The clinical usefulness of these two new breast cancer genes is currently being explored, but because they are large and complex genes with a large number of mutations already identified, it is likely that routine testing will only be relevant to a small number of women with an identified family history of breast cancer.

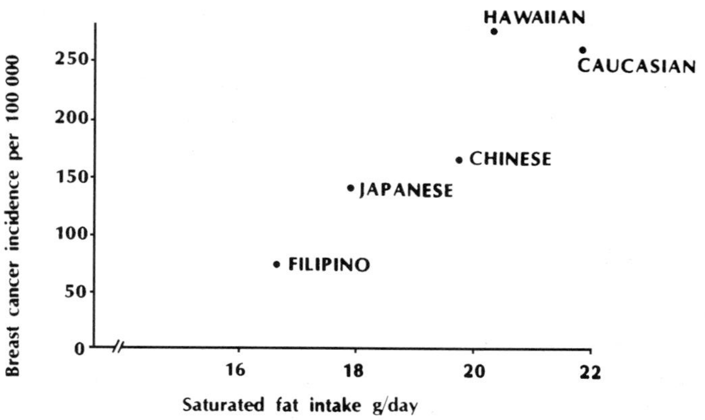

Fig. 25.18 Graph showing the close correlation between saturated fat intake per caput and breast cancer incidence per 100 000 women in defined racial populations.

It is likely that environmental factors are more powerful than genetic factors, and this is supported by the observation that second-generation Japanese women in Hawaii who eat American-style diets tend to increase their breast cancer incidence.[70] The role of hormones and genes is probably a permissive one, in conjunction with an unidentified environmental carcinogen or carcinogens. There is a great deal of current interest in the role of dietary saturated fats in breast cancer as there is a close correlation of fat intake nationally with breast cancer incidence (Fig. 25.18). Recently the National Cancer Institute of the USA has recommended that women should reduce their intake of saturated fat to lower their risk of breast cancer.

Previous benign breast disease

Many older reports suggested an increased incidence of breast cancer in women who had been diagnosed as having benign breast disease, but the varying and confused terminology and the use of retrospective analyses made these reports unreliable. More recent reports by several American pathologists relating the component parts of benign breast histology to future cancer risk have clarified the situation. Dupont & Page[71] have shown that only hyperplasia with atypia is associated with increased risk, especially if a family history of breast cancer is also present. Most of the lesions formerly included in the non-specific umbrella terms of fibroadenosis or fibrocystic disease have not been shown to have any increased risk of subsequent breast cancer.[72] This confused area

REFERENCES

65. Korenman S G Lancet 1980; i: 700–701
66. Lynch H T, Albano W A et al Cancer 1984; 53: 612–622
67. Brinton L A, Hoover R, Fraumeni J F Jr Br J Cancer 1983; 47: 757–762
68. Miki Y, Swenson J, Shattick-Eiders D et al Science 1994; 266: 66–71
69. Wooster R, Bignall G, Swift S et al Nature 1995; 378: 789–792
70. Brinton L A, Hoover R, Fraumeni J F Jr J Natl Cancer Inst 1982; 69: 817–822
71. Dupont W D, Page D L N Engl J Med 1985; 312: 146–151
72. Page D L, Vander Zwagg R et al J Natl Cancer Inst 1978; 61: 1055–1063

Table 25.5 Association of benign breast conditions

No increased risk	
Adenosis—sclerosing or florid	Hyperplasia (mild)
Apocrine metaplasia	Mastitis
Duct ectasia	Periductal mastitis
Fibroadenoma (simple)	Squamous metaplasia
	Fibrosis
Slightly increased risk (1.5–2 times)	
Hyperplasia—moderate or florid, solid or papillary	
Papilloma with a fibrovascular core	
Cysts (relative risk)	
Moderately increased risk (5 times)	
Atypical hyperplasia (ductal or lobular)	

was the subject of a recent consensus conference organized by the American College of Pathologists and has resulted in a much simplier classification of cancer risk (Table 25.5). Only lobular or ductal hyperplasia with atypia are thought to be histological markers of increased cancer risk but as these histological entities occur in just 4% of breast biopsies they are not useful as population markers, as only 15% of women have ever had a breast biopsy.

Exogenous hormones

The most important exogenous hormones are the oestrogens and progestogens contained in the modern oral contraceptive pills which are taken by millions of women from their early teens to their fourth decade. Although the doses of hormones are smaller in current oral contraceptives, the potential effects are still causing much controversy. Despite several large case-control studies, no clear effect has been noted on breast cancer incidence, unlike benign breast disease where a large reduction in incidence has been documented.[73] Although some studies have suggested a higher risk of breast cancer in early pill users,[74] the overall situation seems to suggest no great effect on breast cancer incidence in users of the modern combined oral contraceptive.

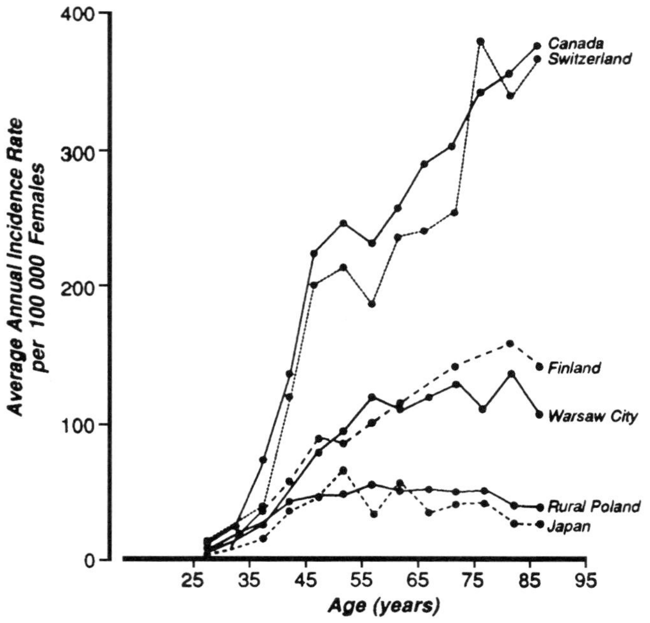

Fig. 25.19 The annual incidence of breast cancer by age in different countries. Note the high incidence in Europe and Canada compared with Japan, and the continuing rise with age in the high-incidence countries. Redrawn from Haagensen.[76]

The chairman of the Committee on Safety of Medicines in the UK has reviewed current evidence on the relationship between oral contraceptive use and breast cancer and concluded that no change in current policy is needed,[75] as modern oral contraceptives have lower oestrogen levels than those generally reported in the studies that demonstrated an increase in breast cancer after oral contraceptive use. Some studies[74] suggest an increased relative risk of breast cancer in young women who started the contraceptive pill early, but the national incidence figures show no corresponding increase in young women. The question of a link between oral contraceptives and breast cancer remains speculative.

Clinical features

Cancer of the breast is seen most commonly in females from their fourth decade of life but, as the age–incidence graph shows, the incidence of the disease continues to increase indefinitely (Fig. 25.19).

Presentation

The commonest presenting feature is a painless dominant lump in the breast; change in shape, pain and skin ulceration are less common presenting features. Often the patient has known about the lump for some considerable time but has not consulted her general practitioner because of fear. This reticence of some patients to consult a doctor at an early stage may be because of their fear of the diagnosis or the mutilating effects of ablative surgery which may be used in the treatment of the disease.

The lump is usually hard and irregular in outline and fixed to adjacent breast tissue, skin or muscle. In early cases there may be no skin changes and the diagnosis rests on the discovery of a lump. In more advanced cases secondary nodal masses or skin ulceration may occur (Fig. 25.20). The clinical examination must be conducted in a good light with the patient stripped to the waist in order to detect early signs of skin tethering. These are best demonstrated by elevating the arms (Fig. 25.21). Slight fixity to the skin may only be seen by moving the lump within the breast while watching the overlying skin for dimples. Asking the patient to contract her pectoral muscles and to lean forward are other good ways of demonstrating skin fixity. Deep fixity is demonstrated by fixation of the underlying pectoral or serratus muscles and assessment of the mobility of the mass in two planes. Occasionally pseudofixity can be produced by benign lesions such as cysts, especially those close to the major ducts, and inflammatory conditions such as plasma cell mastitis or abscess. Previous breast

REFERENCES

73. Vessey M P, Baron J et al Br J Cancer 1983; 47: 455–462
74. Editorial Lancet 1989; i: 973
75. Oral Contraceptives and Carcinoma of the Breast. Committee on Safety of Medicine, Current Problems no. 26. CSM, London 1989

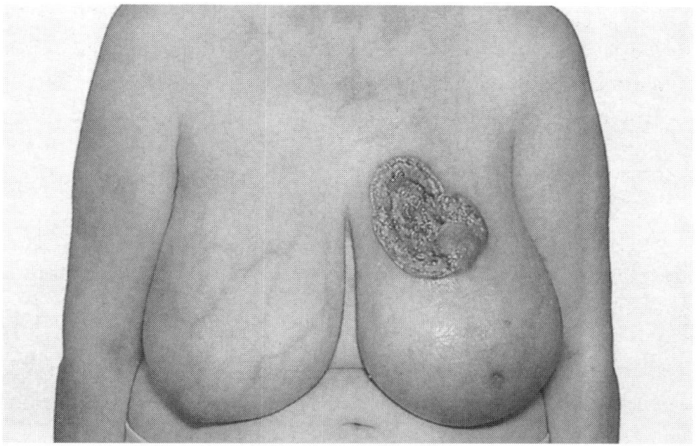

Fig. 25.20 Advanced cancer of the left breast showing ulceration of the skin and elevation and retraction of the nipple. The cancer shows the typical rolled edge of a malignant ulcer.

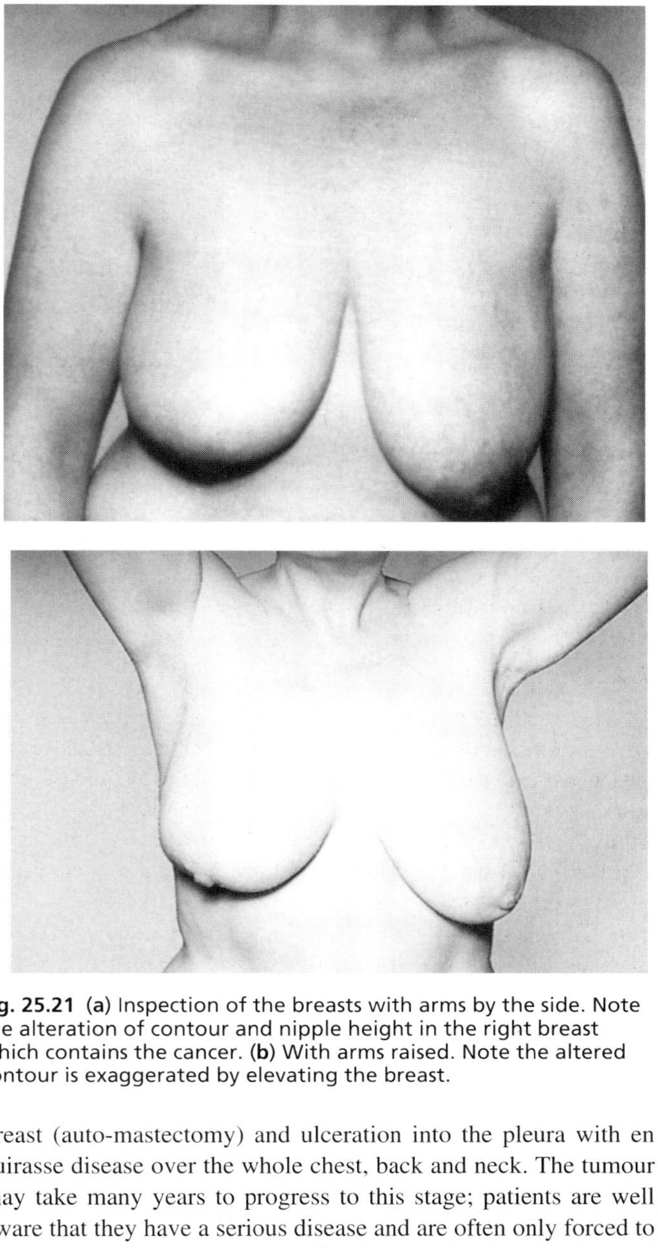

a

b

Fig. 25.21 **(a)** Inspection of the breasts with arms by the side. Note the alteration of contour and nipple height in the right breast which contains the cancer. **(b)** With arms raised. Note the altered contour is exaggerated by elevating the breast.

biopsy may also produce tethering as a result of the scar tissue, especially if the breast was sutured too close to the breast defect produced by tissue removal.

As cancers frequently arise close to the major ducts, their presence is often revealed by retraction of the nipple. Nipple retraction of slight degree is best appreciated by raising the arms and looking for differences in nipple height in the vertical and horizontal planes. More severe degrees of retraction are obvious on simple inspection (Fig. 25.22); however, the time course of the retraction should be sought in the history as retraction over many years is more likely to be from duct ectasia and congenital retraction is also common.

A more subtle change in the nipple is the intraepidermal infiltration of the nipple skin by large clear cancer cells giving rise to the condition of Paget's disease. The early signs can be difficult to perceive as they include slight reddening of the skin with mild excoriation not dissimilar to eczema, but eventually erosion takes place (Fig. 25.23). Ultimately the whole nipple may be destroyed and the process may extend into the areolar skin (Fig. 25.24). It is important to appreciate that Paget's is always associated with carcinoma but there may not be a palpable mass or a radiological cancer in many cases of Paget's disease.

Further local advance of the disease gives rise to the signs of oedema, satellite nodules and eventually infiltration of the skin of the chest, back and neck, known as cancer en cuirasse, as it has been likened to the steel breastplate worn in a suit of armour. Localised oedema can best be seen in the areolar or dependent skin of the lower half of the breast and when marked shows the pitted appearance of an orange skin or peau d'orange (Fig. 25.25). In fact, skin oedema is readily seen on mammograms and can be detected in a large proportion of cancers. Mammographic skin thickening has been shown to be a prognostic indicator for breast cancer.[77]

Continued local growth of breast cancer eventually results in ulceration, usually over the primary tumour mass and infiltration of the surrounding skin with satellite nodules which may be some distance from the original primary growth (Fig. 25.26). Areas of secondary ulceration may arise from the axillary or supraclavicular nodes. The final stage of local disease results in destruction of the breast (auto-mastectomy) and ulceration into the pleura with en cuirasse disease over the whole chest, back and neck. The tumour may take many years to progress to this stage; patients are well aware that they have a serious disease and are often only forced to seek medical help when the offensive smell of their ulcerated cancer attracts attention. Infiltration of the brachial plexus or axillary nerves can make the end-stage of the disease very painful.

Pain in the breast is a fairly uncommon primary presentation of a small breast cancer. Preece et al[78] noted mastalgia as a presenting complaint in about 10% of operable breast cancer. Pain may be a more prominent feature in advanced breast cancer, especially in cases where breast cancer has metastasised to bone or liver.

Other presentations associated with metastatic disease are weight loss, debility, ascites or jaundice with liver secondaries and central

REFERENCES

76. Haagensen C D (ed) Diseases of the Breast. W B Saunders, London 1986
77. Shukla H S, Gravelle I H et al Br Med J 1984; 288: 1338–1341
78. Preece P E, Baum M et al Br Med J 1982; 284: 1299–1300

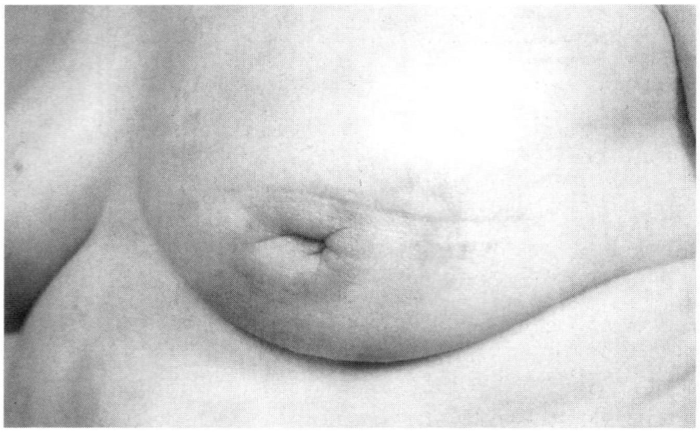

Fig. 25.22 Gross nipple retraction caused by breast cancer with the characteristic retraction of the whole nipple. The bruising is from a recent needle biopsy.

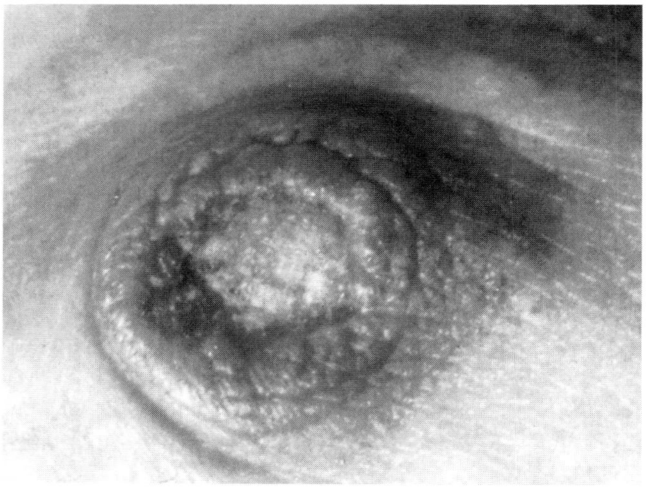

Fig. 25.23 Paget's disease of the nipple. Note the loss of normal skin markings due to erosion of the nipple skin, giving a well-defined crater.

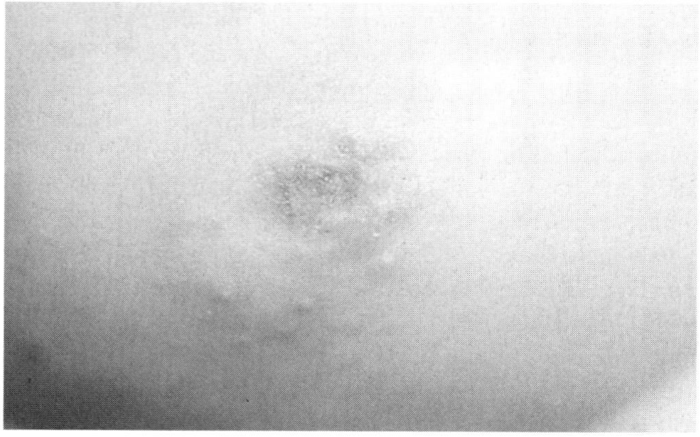

Fig. 25.24 Advanced Paget's disease of the nipple showing loss of the nipple and extension of the disease into the areolar skin.

nervous symptoms with brain metastases. Rarely hypercalcaemia as the result of massive osteolysis and leucoerythroblastic anaemia from marrow infiltration is seen. Patients with bony secondaries may present with pathological fractures, especially of long bones and ribs.

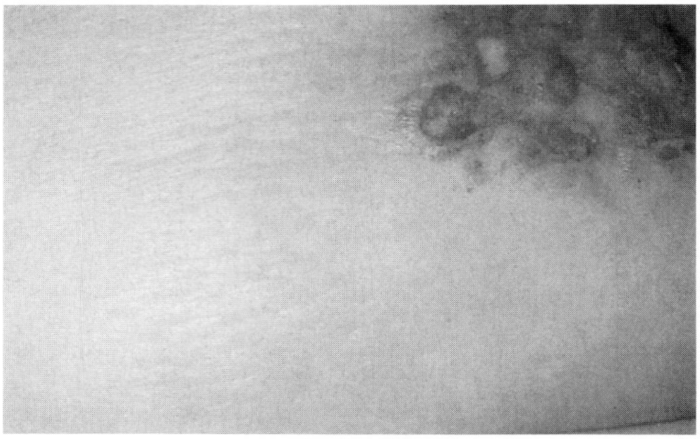

Fig. 25.25 Peau d' orange adjacent to an extensive ulcerating breast cancer.

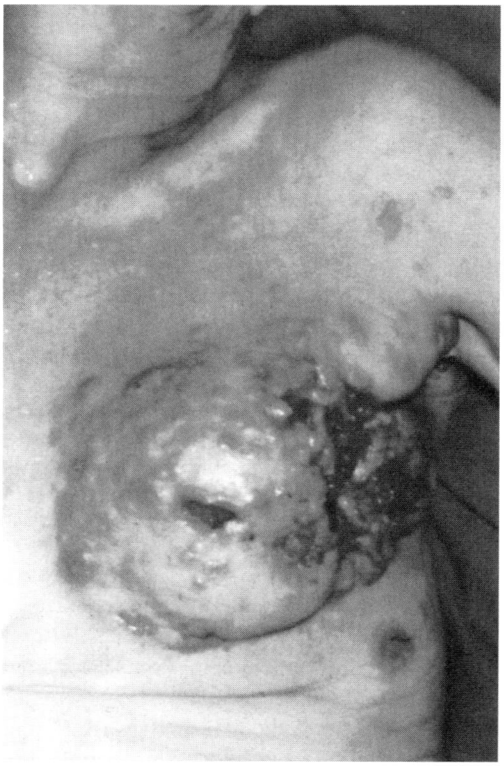

Fig. 25.26 A grossly neglected advanced breast cancer showing total involvement of the breast by tumour with widespread skin nodules at some distance from the breast.

Occasionally a bloody nipple discharge is produced by an underlying ductal carcinoma but this is more commonly associated with duct ectasia or intraduct papilloma. In practice both sero-sanguinous and watery discharges may be seen in association with breast cancer but in the series of 2437 cancers seen by Leis et al[79] only 3.4% presented with nipple discharge.

REFERENCE

79. Leis H P Jr, Greene F L et al South Med J 1988; 81: 22

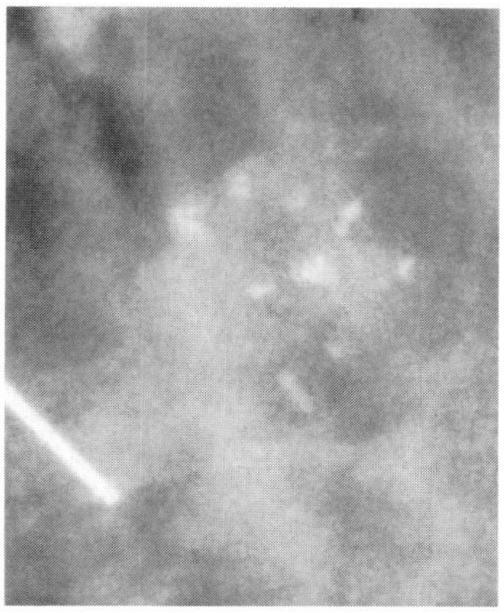

Fig. 25.27 Magnification view of a mammogram showing microcalcification caused by ductal carcinoma-in-situ. The wire marker inserted to localize the calcifications is also seen.

A new and increasingly important presentation is the discovery of a subclinical cancer on routine screening of the breast by mammography. This presentation is now seen much more frequently as a result of the introduction of population screening for the 50–64-year group in the UK following the implementation of the Forrest report.[80] Some 20% of the cancers detected by this method are non-invasive (Fig. 25.27) and the invasive lesions tend to be smaller with less node involvement than in symptomatic cases and are presumed to be biologically early lesions.[81] There is good evidence that screening by mammography reduces mortality from breast cancer in women over 50 in European and US studies.

Staging

Breast cancer can be staged in a variety of ways but the three major clinical systems are the Union Internationale Contre le Cancer (UICC), Manchester and Columbia classifications which are essentially similar. All three systems describe the clinical staging of the disease by reference to the primary tumour, regional nodal areas and systemic disease, but the more universal and comprehensive UICC system is to be preferred. The UICC system is summarised in Table 25.6 and describes the size of the primary tumour from T0 (subclinical) to T4 (any size with fixity or ulceration). Local signs of advanced disease such as fixity, ulceration or peau d'orange are denoted by the suffixes a–c in the T4 category. Node involvement, determined clinically, is denoted by the N0–N3 codes which describe the extent of regional node involvement for ipsilateral axillary and internal mammary nodes. Metastatic disease is either absent (M0) or present (M1).

The approximate equivalent terms of the three main staging systems are shown in Table 25.7. The clinical staging systems are accurate for definition of tumour size but estimation of nodal involvement by palpation is inaccurate as studies show that palpable nodes are frequently not invaded by tumour on microscopic examination and vice versa. In the fourth revision of the TNM classification[82] a separate pathological classification has been added.

Table 25.6 The UICC TNM classification (4th revision 1987)[82]

Primary tumour = T		*Nodes = N*	
TX	Not assessable	NX	Not assessable
T0	No primary tumour	N0	No node metastasis
TIS	Carcinoma-in-situ/Paget's disease	N1	Ipsilateral* axillary (mobile)
		N2	Ipsilateral* axillary (fixed)
T1	2 cm or less	N3	Ipsilateral* internal mammary nodes
T1a	< 0.5 cm		
T1b	0.6–1 cm		
T1c	1.1–2 cm		
T2	> 2 cm but < 5 cm		
T3	> 5 cm		
T4	Any size with chest wall or skin extension		
T4a	Chest wall		
T4b	Oedema/ulceration/nodules		
T4c	Both 4a and 4b		
T4d	Inflammatory cancer		
Distant metastases = M			
MX	Not assessable		
M0	No distant metastases		
M1	Distant metastases present		

*Any other lymph node metastases are coded M1.

Table 25.7 Breast cancer staging systems*

TNM	*Manchester*	*Columbia*
T0–T1 N0–N1a	Stage I	Stage A
N1b T2	Stage II	Stage B
T3–T4 N2–N3	Stage III	Stage C
M1	Stage IV	Stage D

*These are approximate equivalents as all three sections are different in points of detail.

Pathology

The classification of breast cancer used to be based on tumours arising from the lobule and those arising from the duct but it has increasingly become clear that it is impossible to say which cells give rise to most tumours. The 1982 revision of the World Health Organisation classification[83] simply divides the tumours into those arising from epithelial cells and those arising from connective tissues (Table 25.8). This classification is based on histological appearance alone and thus recognises the difficulty in determining the cell of origin of each individual tumour. The malignant tumours of epithelial origin are divided into the non-invasive lobular or ductal in-situ carcinomas, and the invasive tumours which have many subgroups. By far the commonest type of all is the invasive ductal carcinoma of no special type, which in most symptomatic series forms around 80–90% of all carcinomas of the breast.

The non-invasive tumours are becoming increasingly important as modern screening methods are detecting more of these types.

REFERENCES

80. Forrest Report: Breast Cancer Screening. DHSS/HMSO, London 1986
81. Walls J, Boggis et al Br J Surg 1993; 80: 436–438
82. International Union against Cancer TNM Classification of Malignant Tumours, 4th edn. Springer-Verlag, London 1987
83. Azzopardi J G, Chepick O F et al Am J Clin Pathol 1982; 806–816

Table 25.8 The pathology of primary breast cancer (World Health Organisation classification)

Epithelial tumours	
Non-invasive	
Intraductal carcinoma (DCIS)	
Lobular carcinoma-in-situ (LCIS)	
Invasive	
Invasive ductal carcinoma (not otherwise specified; NOS)	80–90%
Invasive ductal with predominant DCIS component	
Invasive lobular	1–2%
Mucinous carcinoma	5%
Medullary carcinoma	1–5%
Papillary carcinoma	rare
Tubular carcinoma	2%
Adenoid cystic carcinoma	rare
Secretory carcinoma	
Apocrine carcinoma	1%
Carcinoma with metaplasia	rare
Paget's disease	2%
Mixed connective tissue and epithelial	
Miscellaneous, e.g. skin or soft tissue	
Unclassified tumours	

Based on World Health Organisation classification.[83]
Percentages indicate proportions of all carcinomas.

Lobular carcinoma-in-situ is uncommon, being seen in some 1% of biopsies, and usually occurs as an incidental finding. Haagensen et al[84] thought it to be so benign in behaviour that they call it lobular neoplasia, but long-term follow-up of lobular carcinoma-in-situ treated by simple excision shows that invasive cancer subsequently occurs in up to 40% of women in either breast.[85]

Ductal carcinoma-in-situ in isolation forms only 3–5% of pathological series of breast cancers but is much more common in association with invasive ductal cancers. Series of screen-detected cancers however show a much higher incidence of ductal carcinoma-in-situ—up to 30% in some series. This is because it is readily detected as fine microcalcification on mammography. In this condition the cells are packed into the ducts in varying architectural patterns but do not show invasion outside the wall of the duct. There are several different types of ductal carcinoma-in-situ, such as comedo, cribriform, solid, papillary and clinging, depending on the pattern within the tumour. Mixtures of these subtypes may be seen but the tumour is classified by the predominant pattern. The comedo type is more likely to be associated with multicentric disease and is thought to have a worse prognosis than the cribriform type. More recent developments are based on cytonuclear grade and the presence or absence of necrosis. The recently described van Nuys classification has been shown to correlate well with prognosis in locally excised ductal carcinoma-in-situ.[86]

The significance of ductal carcinoma-in-situ is that it is a premalignant condition; some 30% of women who have been followed after incomplete local excision of this entity have gone on to develop ipsilateral invasive carcinoma.[87,88] The risk of metastasis (1%) in pure ductal carcinoma-in-situ is very low. The rare intracystic type also comes into the in-situ part of this classification. When ductal carcinoma-in-situ is seen around an invasive cancer the morphology of the invasive cancer determines the classification.

Invasive ductal cancers form the majority of breast cancer, especially the category of 'not otherwise specified'. This term simply recognises the fact that most invasive ductal cancers are undifferentiated and cannot be easily classified in terms of morphology. The specified types of invasive ductal cancer are listed in Table 25.8, but invasive lobular medullary, mucinous and tubular are the commonest variants, although Haagensen et al[84] maintain that apocrine cancer is commoner than usually stated in the literature. These special subtypes form only 10% of all breast cancer. The differentiation between these subtypes is a microscopic one and the only significance of the invasive subtypes is that they tend to be better differentiated and hence have a better prognosis than the 'not otherwise specified' type.

Paget's disease of the nipple is a special category of invasive epithelial cancer where histologically the nipple skin is infiltrated by large pale cells and eventually nipple erosion occurs (Fig. 25.23). This condition is invariably associated with an underlying invasive or intraductal carcinoma. When Paget's disease is associated with an invasive cancer at a separate site in the breast then it is classified as an invasive cancer.

In the mixed connective and epithelial section of the classification, the most common tumour is the phyllodes tumour (formerly known as cystosarcoma phyllodes). This is a circumscribed neoplasm with a leaf-like structure with varying degrees of cellularity. The assessment of the behaviour of this tumour is difficult but lesions with a high mitotic rate, cellular atypia and infiltrative margins tend to be locally recurrent after simple excision.

Pathological prognostic factors

Cancerous invasion of the regional nodes demonstrated on histology (positive nodes) is an excellent predictor of subsequent prognosis, as shown in Figure 25.28. Fisher et al[90] in their analyses of 505 patients with known nodal involvement enrolled in the National Surgical Adjuvant Breast and Bowel Project, showed that an increasing number of positive nodes correlated very well with worsening prognosis. Patients with greater than five positive nodes have a 5-year survival rate of less than 20%. Histological examination of the regional nodes is the only reliable method of determining lymph node invasion. Nodes can be obtained by a sampling operation which removes the lower axillary nodes or by an axillary clearance which gives the whole population of nodes. It has been shown that at least four nodes must be examined to achieve acceptable accuracy of axillary staging (Danish Co-Operative Breast Group).[91] Vascular invasion seen in the primary tumour and multicentric tumour within the breast are also accurate pathological markers of poor prognosis.

Tumour grade is also a good predictor of subsequent prognosis and is based on cytological and structural patterns in the primary

REFERENCES

84. Haagensen C D, Lane N et al Cancer 1978; 42: 737
85. Van Dongen J A, Fentiman I S et al Lancet 1989; ii: 25–27
86. Van Nuys
87. Rosen P P, Brown D W, Kinne D W Cancer 1980; 46: 919–925
88. Page D L, Dupont W D et al Cancer 1982; 49: 751–758
89. Donegan W L, Spratt J S (eds) Cancer of the Breast, 3rd edn. Brace Harcourt, London 1988 p 351
90. Fisher B, Bauer M et al Cancer 1983; 52: 1551–1557
91. Danish Co-Op Group

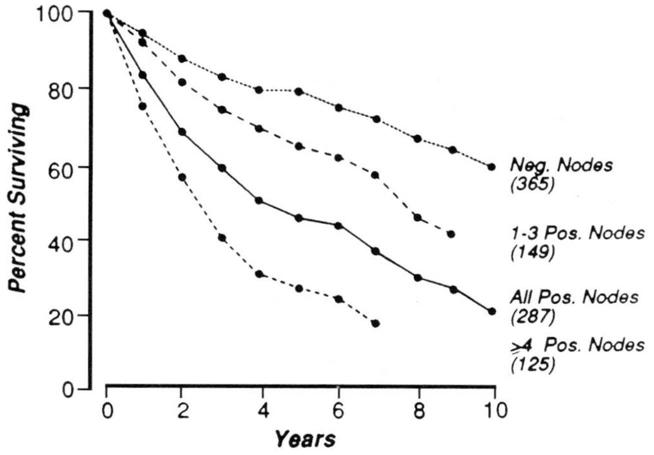

Fig. 25.28 Life table survival curve showing the effect of increasing numbers of pathologically involved axillary nodes on survival. Nodal status is the most powerful prognostic factor. Numbers in parentheses indicate patient numbers; Neg. = negative; Pos. = positive. Redrawn from Donegan & Spratt.[89]

breast cancer. Most systems are based on the Bloom & Richardson classification[92] which allocates three grades from 1 (well differentiated) to 3 (poorly differentiated). This system is based on the amount of tubule formation, pleomorphism and mitotic activity. The well-differentiated histological types of breast cancer such as tubular and lobular carcinomas have a good long-term prognosis[93] but tend to be uncommon, as noted above. Some subtypes such as the medullary tumour would score grade 3 on the Bloom & Richardson scale but are known to have a good prognosis. As observer variation is a problem in tumour grading, more objective methods such as measurement of DNA ploidy by flow cytometry are currently being evaluated.

Biochemical prognostic factors

Several biochemical markers of prognosis have been proposed but few have been demonstrated to be of clinical value. Oestrogen/androgen excretion indices[94] have now been shown to be of no value but the content of oestrogen receptor protein in the primary tumour has been found to be useful for predicting response to endocrine therapy and for survival.[95,96] Progesterone receptor, which is itself regulated by oestrogen receptor, was reported to be of even greater prognostic value[97] but its place as an independent prognostic marker is currently in dispute.[98]

Attempts have been made to incorporate the several different prognostic factors into a single index, devised by multifactorial analyses of the individual weighting of each prognostic factor to the whole.[99] In these analyses the most important prognostic factors are positive nodes, tumour grade and the size of the primary tumour.

Diagnosis

A history of the presenting complaint and the relevant reproductive and family histories should be taken, although the vast majority of patients will simply complain of a lump. Clinical examination consists of careful palpation with the flat of the hand examining all four quadrants, the nipple areolar area and the axillary tail in turn. The regional nodes should then be palpated. In cases of suspected cancer the lungs and liver should also be assessed. In women over 35 years mammography should be performed both as a diagnostic test on the breast showing the symptoms and as a check on the symptomless breast. All dominant lumps should be aspirated and, if the mass is a cyst and the fluid is blood-stained, the aspirate should be sent off for cytology. If a residual lump remains, a fine-needle aspiration of the solid element should be taken for cytological assessment.

Accurate diagnosis requires pathological examination of the tumour, as clinical diagnosis is unreliable even in the presence of signs normally associated with cancer, such as skin fixity, as these can be seen in benign conditions such as duct ectasia and plasma cell mastitis. A preoperative diagnosis can be accomplished in most cases by either fine-needle aspiration with cytological examination of the aspirate[100] or needle biopsy using a Tru-cut or similar needle with histological examination of the resulting core. The method used depends on the experience of the surgeon and the pathologist. Both methods can give false-positive results, although this occurs infrequently, and the sampling error increases in tumours smaller than 2 cm in diameter. Most clinics are now using image-guided aspiration with ultrasound to increase the accuracy of the diagnosis of small tumours. Before embarking on mastectomy for a breast mass, the surgeon should obtain definite and unequivocal evidence of cancer in order to prevent the disaster of breast removal for a benign condition.

Fine-needle aspiration cytology is easy and quick to perform: the skill of the operator will determine the quality of cytological smears produced, especially the rate of acellular smears. The technique only requires a 21-guage needle with a syringe (Fig. 25.29); the needle tip is passed backwards and forwards through the palpable lump, which is steadied with the fingers of the other hand while suction is maintained on the barrel of the syringe. The handling of the syringe is made easier by a specialized syringe holder which allows good control and suction to be applied simultaneously. After passing through the lump a number of times—some would say at least 10 times—the suction is released and the needle withdrawn. The contents of the needle are then blown on to a glass slide and fixed or air-dried, depending on the local cytologist's preference.

Dominant lumps larger than 2 cm in diameter can be biopsied by a wide-bore cutting needle such as the Tru-cut needle which has

REFERENCES

92. Bloom H J G, Richardson W W Br J Cancer 1957; 11: 359–377
93. Dixon J M, Page D L et al Br J Surg 1985; 72: 445–448
94. Moore J W, Thomas B S, Wang D Y Cancer Res Surv 1986; 5: 537–559
95. Clark G M, McGuire W L Breast Cancer Res Treat 1983; 3(suppl): 69
96. Howell A, Barnes D M et al Lancet 1984; i: 588–591
97. Clark G M, McGuire W L et al N Engl J Med 1983; 309: 1343–1347
98. Howat J M T, Harris M et al Br J Cancer 1985; 51: 263–270
99. Todd J H, Dowle C et al Br J Cancer 1987; 56: 489–492
100. Dixon J M, Anderson T J et al Br J Surg 1984; 71: 593–596

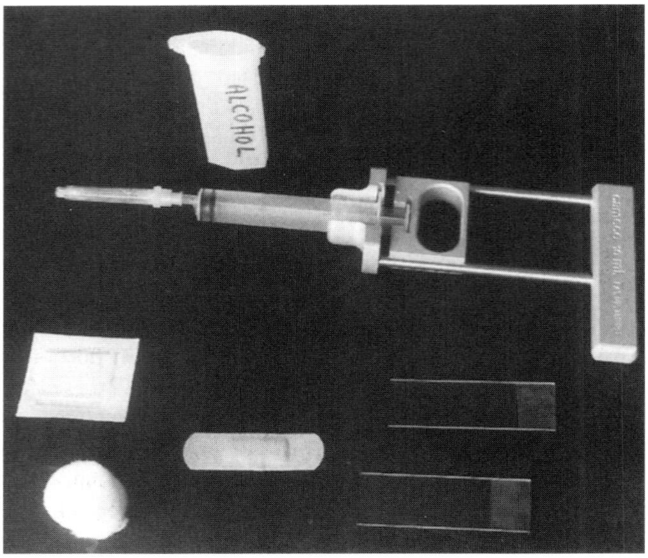

Fig. 25.29 Items needed for fine-needle aspiration cytology of the breast. The syringe holder allows manipulation of the syringe by one hand while the other holds the breast lump.

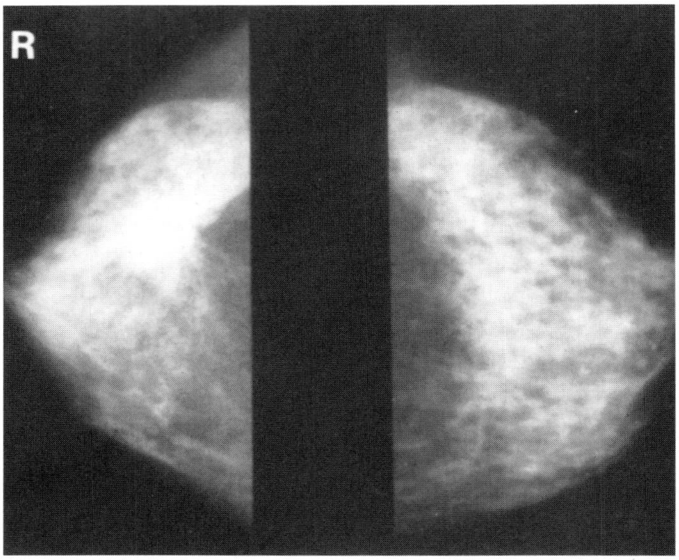

Fig. 25.30 Craniocaudad mammographic views of both breasts showing a mass lesion with irregular margins and tentacles in the outer half of the right breast, typical of carcinoma of the breast.

the advantage of producing a core of tissue which can be paraffin-embedded and read as a normal histological specimen. When a modern spring-loaded wide-bore needle device is used with local anaesthetic in the skin, a series of high-quality cores can be obtained rapidly and almost painlessly. A further advantage of wide-bore needle biopsies is that a large amount of prognostic information can be obtained on the needle biopsy specimen, including the histological grade, receptor levels and DNA analyses.[101]

Mammography is an accurate diagnostic method in breast cancer with rates of 80–95% depending on the experience of the radiologist.[102] It is less accurate in the younger denser breast and in deep-seated or axillary tail tumours. The mammographic signs of malignancy are a mass lesion with irregular edges, called spiculation, or long tentacles called tentaculation and fine scattered microcalcification. Distortion of the normal parenchymal markings may also be seen and thickening is often evident in the skin over the quadrant harbouring the cancer. Some cancers may appear as discrete rounded masses with smooth edges and mimic fibroadenomas. A clear example of a mammographic cancer is shown in Figure 25.30 but it should be remembered that approximately 10–15% of palpable cancers are invisible on mammography.

Ultrasound examination of poorly defined masses on mammography may also be useful to show underlying cystic disease and this imaging technique is now being used routinely in most specialist clinics.

The validity of mammography as a screening technique is currently being examined in population screening of women aged 50–64 years in the UK. The accuracy of diagnosis can be increased to over 95% by a combination of clinical examination, mammography and fine-needle aspiration cytology[103] and this triple technique should be routinely used in the diagnosis of all symptomatic breast masses. A further advantage of preoperative cytological diagnosis is that oestrogen and progesterone receptor levels in fine-needle aspirates can be measured using immunohistochemistry in order to obtain prognostic information before the definitive treatment is selected.[104]

Special techniques for screen-detected cancers

The small cancers detected on mammography in symptomless women are often impalpable and require localisation before biopsy. These cancers show up as small mass lesions or as clustered microcalcifications. New methods of stereotactic fine-needle aspiration are being evaluated for diagnosis of these tumours and these techniques are becoming routine in screening clinics. Prior to conventional open biopsy, there are two principal techniques of localisation which are performed by the radiologist in order to guide the surgeon to the impalpable lesion: the double-dye and the hooked-wire technique. In the double-dye technique a mixture of radiological contrast and Patent Blue dye is injected as close to the mammographic abnormality as possible and further mammograms are taken to show the relationship of the mixture to the radiological abnormality. The surgeon then seeks the blue colouration in the breast tissue after incising the skin and calculates from the mammogram where the abnormal area lies in relation to the dye.

In the hooked-wire or needle technique, which has now become the preferred method (Fig. 25.31), a needle is similarly placed in or as close to the abnormality as possible and a hooked wire is pushed down the needle and engaged in the breast tissue. The wire is left in the breast and acts as a guide to the surgeon to the location of the radiological abnormality.

REFERENCES

101. Baildam A D, Turnbull L et al Br J Surg 1989; 76: 553–558
102. Locker A P, Manhire A R et al Lancet 1989; i: 887–889
103. Smallwood J, Khong Y Ann R Col Surg 1984; 66: 267–269
104. Weintraub J, Weintraub D et al Cancer 1987; 60: 1163–1172

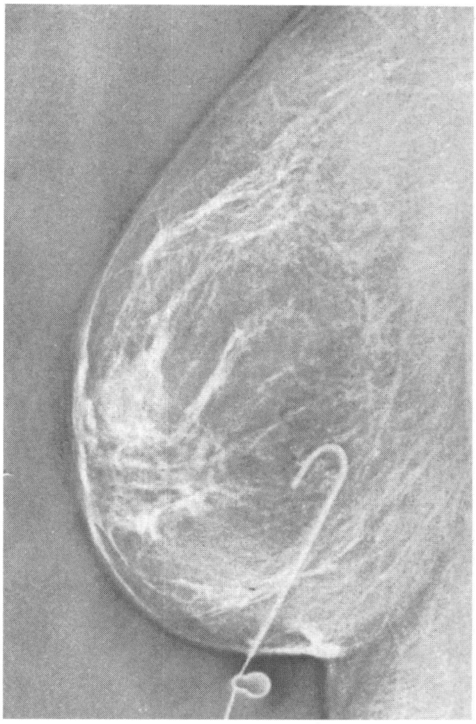

Fig. 25.31 Mammogram with a hooked needle in situ before biopsy. The mammographic abnormality is a small cluster of calcifications shown within the head of the hooked needle.

Both methods work well in experienced hands but it is essential to send the excised tissue for immediate radiography of the specimen to confirm that the abnormal area has been excised. A further rule is that localisation biopsies are always subjected to paraffin histology and not frozen section, as the differentiation between ductal carcinoma-in-situ and hyperplasia is difficult and depends on optimal cytological detail. Additionally the margins of the surgical specimen require histological assessment. This can be made difficult if a sample has been taken for frozen section.

Other investigations

Patients with palpable cancers should have a routine chest X-ray and liver function tests performed to exclude pulmonary and hepatic metastases. Routine bone scans are not usually employed in T1 and T2 tumours as the detection rates are very low. In large tumours a bone scan and ultrasound scan of the liver are helpful, especially if operative treatment of the primary disease is contemplated. The need for other specialised investigations such as computed tomography scans is determined by symptoms suggestive of metastatic disease. Areas of acute bone pain in the long bones should be radiographed to pick up pathological fractures and lytic or sclerotic deposits.

Differential diagnosis

As breast cancer can occur from the age of 16 years upwards, it may be confused with any of the benign diseases that give rise to a lump or skin changes. The main differential diagnoses are given in

Table 25.9 Differential diagnosis of breast cancer

20–30 years	Fibroadenoma
30–60 years	Cystic disease ANDI* Intraduct papilloma
Any age	Duct ectasia Plasma cell mastitis Fat necrosis
Radiological	Sclerosing adenosis Microcystic disease ANDI Radial scars Fibroadenoma

ANDI = Aberrations of normal development and involution.

Table 25.9 but most confusion occurs in women in the 30–50-year group where cysts and breast nodularity are often misdiagnosed as carcinoma. Cysts can be confused when they are multilocular with extensive fibrosis around them or when they produce skin tethering by distorting the breast architecture. Circumscribed carcinomas in younger women are often mistaken for fibroadenomas. The best mimic of breast cancer is, however, the inflammatory phase of duct ectasia which produces induration, redness and nipple retraction and can be indistinguishable clinically from an inflammatory breast cancer. Indeed, this condition has led to mastectomies being performed in the past on the grounds that the evidence for clinical cancer was so strong that biopsy was unnecessary. This underlines the point that biopsy by cytology or histology is essential before mastectomy is undertaken.

Radiologically the most confusing problem is the microcalcification seen in common conditions such as cystic disease or sclerosing adenosis. It can be impossible to differentiate between intraduct cancer and some of these benign conditions, although the number and size of the particles of calcium can be helpful as numerous small sharp spicules suggest cancer. Most series however only show a 30–40% accuracy for cancer when localisation biopsy of an area of microcalcification is performed.[105] The stellate appearance of complex sclerosing lesions is also difficult to distinguish from small scirrhous cancers.

Treatment

The treatment of breast cancer depends on the stage of the disease at presentation and has three specific aims:

1. The control of local disease.
2. The control of systemic disease.
3. The maintenance of cosmesis if possible.

Historical note

The early concept of breast cancer was that it spread from the breast via lymphatics to regional nodes and thence systemically. Treatment was directed at removal of the breast and regional nodes in the Halsted mastectomy. The continuing mortality from breast

REFERENCE

105. Aitken R J, MacDonald H L et al Br J Surg 1990; 70: 673

cancer after radical local therapy brought the realisation that early spread by the blood stream was a more common means of dissemination, and the micrometastases responsible are probably present at the time of diagnosis in most patients with symptomatic breast cancer. The fact that the axillary nodes are involved in some 40–60% of operable breast cancers was realised to be a prognostic marker of systemic metastases rather than a filter mechanism trapping cancer cells escaping from the breast. Micrometastases may arise from very small invasive cancers, although they are unusual in cancers smaller than 5 mm in diameter. The rate of growth of micrometastases can be quite slow, taking many years to appear as secondary disease. Indeed, data from long-term studies suggest that distant disease may appear up to 40 years after removal of the primary tumour by mastectomy[106] and it could be argued that only some 20% of breast cancer patients are truly cured of their disease. These considerations and observations have become embodied in the current philosophy that the outlook for most patients with breast cancer is predetermined by the biological fact of early metastatic spread by the blood stream and local therapy is therefore likely to affect only the control of the primary disease and systemic adjuvant therapy is needed to control micrometastases. Local therapy can be curative when the cancer is truly confined to the breast but it is not possible to say whether the disease is totally confined when the patient presents.

Current treatment—operable disease

Most women diagnosed as having breast cancer bring with them to the consultation many preconceptions—and often misconceptions—about the options for managing the disease. A frank discussion between the surgeon and patient, assisted by a breast counsellor or specialist nurse, must therefore always precede the defining of an agreed treatment plan.

For operable carcinoma, usually defined as T1–3, N0–1 and M0 by the UICC staging, or stages 1, 2 and some 3 by the Manchester staging, the treatment has changed from the historical emphasis on mastectomy to breast conservation techniques which excise the tumour and preserve the breast form.[107] A survey conducted in 1986[108] showed that mastectomy was the most favoured treatment among British surgeons but the trend has more recently moved towards conservation of the breast.[109] Formerly, Halsted radical mastectomy was predominant, especially in the USA, but the modified radical mastectomy (Patey) then became more popular. This in turn was supplanted by simple mastectomy with radiotherapy to the axilla to cover disease in the axillary nodes.

A large study carried out by the National Surgical Adjuvant Breast and Bowel Project in the USA comparing radical mastectomy with total mastectomy with or without radiation found no differences in overall survival or local recurrence between the groups at 10 years. In this study 50 Gy was given to the axilla in clinically node-negative patients and a further boost of 10 Gy to the node-positive patients.

In general, local recurrence rates of around 8% in node-positive patients and 4% in node-negative patients at 5 years are obtainable by surgical treatment with mastectomy and axillary clearance or simple mastectomy with adjuvant radiotherapy.[110,111] Surgical

Table 25.10 Histological node involvement in stage I and stage II breast cancer

Series	*Number of cases*	*Positive nodes (%)*	
		Stage I	*Stage II*
Haagensen[76]	1036	31	72
Veronesi[113]	701 (Stage I only)	25	–
Fisher B–04[114]	641		54
Fisher B–06[110]	1843		37
Forest[112]	199		40

clearance of the axillary nodes, as in a Patey mastectomy, has the advantage of accurate staging of lymph node metastases for prognostic purposes, but node sampling or excising the level I and II nodes has been reported to be as accurate.[112] In stage I and II cancers involved nodes are very common when assessed histologically, as shown in Table 25.10, even when nodes are not clinically palpable, as in the Milan trial.[113] Most series show that if the axilla is cleared and examined pathologically about 27% will have involved nodes in stage I cases and 40–50% in stage II cases. A large Danish study showed that the extent of the nodal dissection was inversely correlated with the risk of local recurrence.[115]

More recently there has been a marked move towards breast conservation on the grounds that better cosmesis can be obtained with an equivalent mortality. The concept of breast conservation is not new and has been championed over the last 50 years or so by Keynes[116] in the UK, Crile[117] in the USA, Calle et al[118] in Paris and Spitalier et al[119] in Marseilles. These groups have tended to treat selected patients with small, good-prognosis tumours and so their conclusion that conservation is safe could not be applied to breast cancers in general.

Controlled studies have however been carried out in the last decade by Veronesi et al[113] in Milan and Fisher et al[111] in the USA. Veronesi and colleagues compared conventional Halsted mastectomy with quadrantectomy, surgical axillary clearance and radiotherapy to the breast (QUART) and reported no survival differences between the two groups, although there was a higher rate of local recurrence within the QUART group, which they attributed to second primary tumours rather than recurrences. This trial was run from 1973 to 1980 and involved 701 patients, all with T1 tumours and without palpable axillary nodes. At 8 years the

REFERENCES

106. Brinkley D, Haybittle J L Lancet 1984; i: 118
107. Lippman M E Cancer 1987; 60: 2050–2053
108. Greenberg E R, Stevens M Br Med J 1986; 292: 1487–1491
109. Morris J, Royle G T, Taylor I J Soc Med 1989; 82: 12–14
110. Fisher B, Redmond C et al N Engl J Med 1985; 312: 674–681
111. Fisher B, Bauer M et al N Engl J Med 1985; 312: 665–673
112. Steele R J C, Forrest A P M et al Br J Surg 1985; 72: 368–369
113. Veronesi U, Zucali R, Vecchio M D World J Surg 1985; 9: 676–681
114. Fisher B, Wolmark N et al Surg Gynecol Obstet 1981; 152: 765–772
115. Graversen H P, Blichert-Toft M et al Eur J Surg Oncol 1988; 14: 407–412
116. Keynes G Br Med J 1937; 2: 643–647
117. Crile G Ann Surg 1975; 181: 26–30
118. Calle R, Pilleron J P et al Cancer 1978, 42: 2045–2053
119. Spitalier J M, Gambarelli J et al World J Surg 1986; 10: 1014–1020

disease-free survival was 77% in the Halsted mastectomy group, and 80% in the QUART group. A dose of 50 Gy (5000 rad) was given to the breast with a local boost using high-energy photons of 10 Gy to the tumour bed.

The American trial run by Fisher (B-06) compared lumpectomy with axillary irradiation against total mastectomy with axillary dissection in 1843 women.[110] In the segmental mastectomy patients the margins of excision were examined to ensure that they were clear of microscopic tumour. A total mastectomy was carried out if the margins were found to contain tumour and this occurred in some 10% of the patients. In the segmental mastectomy and irradiation group, a minimum of 50 Gy was given over 5 weeks with no boost to the scar. The results of this trial showed that segmental mastectomy alone did not control local recurrence in the ipsilateral breast as 30% of patients suffered from this problem. When radiation to the breast was added to segmental mastectomy the local recurrence rate fell to around 10% at 5 years. No survival differences were however shown between the lumpectomy plus radiotherapy and mastectomy groups.

Several studies have now shown no differences in mortality between mastectomy and breast conservation but local recurrence is often slightly higher in the conserved breast. In stage I disease local recurrence after conservation tends to occur at the rate of 1% per year with a higher rate for stage II tumours. Factors which predispose to local recurrence are large central tumours, poor histological differentiation, vascular invasion and widespread intraduct cancer around the invasive component.[120–122] Although the Milan trial and the National Surgical Adjuvant Breast and Bowel Project trial showed good results for conservation, it should be remembered that the tumour excision was radical in the conservation arms in both trials, as quadrantectomy was performed in the Milan trial and clear pathological margins were confirmed in the National Surgical Adjuvant Breast and Bowel Project trial, and axillary clearance was used in both. Further, some 10% of the lumpectomy group in the National Surgical Adjuvant Breast and Bowel Project trial failed to obtain clear pathological margins despite an intention to do so, and these patients underwent mastectomy. These results highlight the need to confirm tumour excision margins pathologically if a policy of breast conservation is adopted. A further Milan trial compared quadrantectomy and radiation (QUART) with tumorectomy and radiation (TART) and showed that the narrower excision margins resulted in a higher local recurrence, although survival was unaffected.[123]

The results of a more general acceptance of lumpectomy and radiotherapy will almost certainly be worse than the published results as larger tumours may be treated inappropriately and the margins are not always checked histologically for clearance. Recently Veronesi has acknowledged that the current practice in Milan is to perform rather less than a quadrantectomy in conservation cases. This highlights the problem that the extent of excision is hard to define and may vary considerably from surgeon to surgeon.[124] The guiding principle of all conservation surgery should be the excision of the whole tumour and any surrounding ductal carcinoma-in-situ with confident histological confirmation that the excision margins are free of disease.

A further problem is that the anticipated psychological benefits of conservation therapy have not clearly emerged in practice, as research has shown no differences in psychological debility between mastectomy and conservation patients given a choice of therapy.[125] The expected improvement in psychiatric morbidity in the patients with conserved breasts may be replaced by an increased anxiety regarding recurrence in the conserved breast; the end-result appears to be similar short-term morbidity in both conservation and mastectomy groups. The recent trend is certainly towards greater use of conservation techniques although, as mentioned, local recurrence will be higher and careful follow-up of these patients is important. Detection of a recurrence in an irradiated breast can be difficult as the post-radiation fibrosis makes both palpation and mammography difficult to interpret. Magnetic resonance imaging (MRI) has proved to be useful if detecting recurrence in an irradiated breast. The detailed long-term follow-up may be one of the factors producing anxiety in the patient with a conserved breast. The main value of long-term follow-up is surveillance of the contralateral breast by mammography.

When local recurrence does occur it is usually treated by mastectomy or, occasionally, re-excision. These salvage mastectomies can be technically difficult and may need a myocutaneous flap to give sound healing in previously irradiated tissues. It is reported that the outlook after salvage mastectomy for local recurrence secondary to conservation is as good as the initial conservation group but so far follow-up is short and series are small. Kurtz et al[126] reported 118 salvage operations for local recurrences in the breast after conservation treatment of stage I and II cancers. They performed mastectomy in 56% and further wide excision in the others. After a median follow-up of 7 years they reported an actuarial survival of 72% at 5 years and 58% at 10 years. Further local recurrence occurred in 17% of the patients.

Operative surgery for breast cancer

There are basically three general procedures:

1. Excision of the tumour for diagnosis or treatment.
2. Mastectomy in some form with or without axillary dissection.
3. Reconstructive procedures.

Excision of tumour

When performed as a diagnostic open biopsy this should be done through a circumareolar incision or a circumferential incision placed in such a way that the scar can be re-excised if a mastectomy is found to be necessary at a later date. Transverse incisions

REFERENCES

120. Locker A P, Ellis I O et al Br J Surg 1989; 76: 890–894
121. Harris J R, Connolly J L et al Ann Surg 1985; 201: 164–169
122. Bulman A, Lindley R P et al Ann R Coll Surg Engl 1988; 70: 289–292
123. Quart v Tart
124. Benson E A, Thorogood J Eur J Surg Oncol 1986; 12: 267–271
125. Fallowfield L J, Baum M, Maguire G P Br Med J 1986; 293: 1331–1334
126. Kurtz J M, Amalric R et al Ann Surg 1988; 207: 347–351

can be used in the medial half of the breast. Radial and vertical incisions should be avoided as these heal poorly, especially in the upper half of the breast.

When performed as part of conservation treatment in a proven cancer the tumour should be excised with a margin of surrounding 'normal' breast tissue which should be at least 2 cm wide of the palpable tumour. Excision of a whole quadrant, as advocated by the Milan group, gives a wide clearance but the cosmesis is less good. Microscopic clearance should ideally be obtained and optimal management includes the verification of this by biopsies of the cavity walls. The specimen should be orientated for the pathologist and the margins should be inked to allow proper histological evaluation. Some surgeons believe that closure of the cavity in the breast is not necessary unless a quadrantectomy has been performed. Suturing may cause distortion of the breast. Good haemostasis is essential as haematoma is the major complication of this technique, but should occur in less than 5% of cases. If an axillary dissection is to be performed it should be done simultaneously through the same incision for upper outer quadrant cancers or via a separate incision in the axilla for tumours located in other parts of the breast.

Mastectomy procedures

These operations are performed for tumours that are unsuitable for conservation, for widespread ductal carcinoma-in-situ, as a salvage procedure for recurrent or locally advanced cancers and when the patient prefers this treatment for an operable breast carcinoma after discussion with the clinician.

The terminology can be confused but excision of the breast alone should be called total rather than simple mastectomy; removal of the breast with or without pectoralis minor and the axillary contents is termed a modified radical or Patey mastectomy, and excision of the breast, both pectoral muscles and axillary contents a radical mastectomy or Halsted mastectomy. The extended radical, which also removes the internal mammary nodes, has fallen into disrepute. When only the breast tissue is removed, leaving the nipple and areola, this is called a subcutaneous mastectomy, although many variations on this operation are performed. As noted above, the recent trend has been towards total mastectomy with radiation of the axilla as the most common therapy but the Patey mastectomy both treats and stages the axilla at the same time, thus obviating the need for local radiotherapy.

Operative technique

Total mastectomy is performed with the patient's arm on a sideboard, but only the chest and axilla are prepared. In the Patey-type operation it is helpful to be able to move the arm into flexion and abduction and this is best done by preparing the arm and wrapping it in sterile towels at the start of the operation. Alternatively an arm-board mounted on a universal joint, which allows movement in any plane, can be used.

In all forms of mastectomy except the subcutaneous skin flaps are raised; the nipple and areola are removed with the breast. A transverse elliptical incision is made and the flaps are reflected to the midline, to the clavicle superiorly, to the anterior border of latissimus dorsi posteriorly and to the rectus sheath inferiorly. The subcutaneous vessels are retained within the flaps to ensure flap survival. The flaps should be thin distally but thicker towards the chest wall. In both total and modified radical operations the breast is removed from the pectoral fascia and the internal thoracic perforating vessels coming through the second to fourth anterior intercostal space are ligated.

In a total mastectomy the axillary tail is dissected from the axillary fat and the lower nodes may be taken as a sampling procedure. Some surgeons only remove palpable nodes for sampling but it is worthwhile determining whether the nodes are pathologically negative, as this may be crucial to determining a need for postoperative adjuvant therapy. At this stage the total mastectomy operation is complete; haemostasis is secured and the flaps are closed with suction drainage. A skin graft may be needed if the flaps are tight but this is rarely necessary. In the total mastectomy no muscles or nerves are sacrificed.

In a Patey mastectomy the axilla is dissected free of all nodes; the boundaries of the dissection are the axillary vein superiorly, the latissimus dorsi laterally, the subscapularis muscle posteriorly and the chest wall medially. The axillary vein is displayed by dissection of the tough anterior layer of the clavipectoral fascia which invests the axillary fat. The nodes are swept downwards from the axillary vein and the level III or apical nodes (Fig. 25.32) are dissected free from the apex of the axilla. During this phase of the dissection it is important to ligate and divide only the branches going to the axillary vein and to avoid damaging the vein. Access to the apex of the axilla is improved by flexing the arm at the shoulder joint to relax the pectoralis major muscle. The axillary fat and nodal mass is mobilised and then swept downwards and the pectoralis minor is divided at its origin from the ribs and taken with the specimen. The medial pectoral nerve running to the pectoralis major muscle is carefully preserved on the underside of that muscle. Some operators merely retract the pectoralis minor and do not excise it, especially if only level I and II nodes are to be

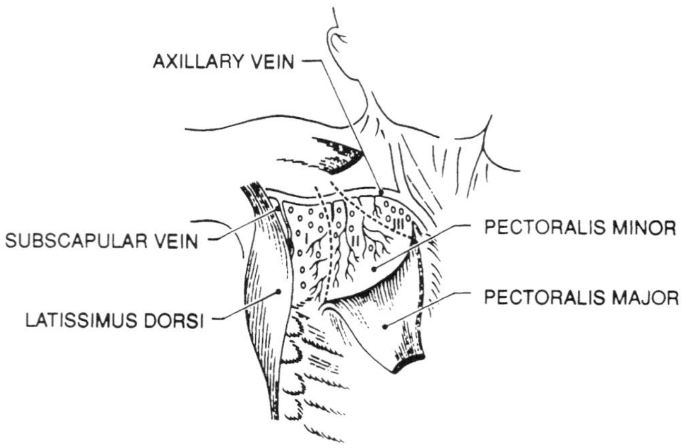

Fig. 25.32 Nodal areas in the axilla. Area I lies lateral to the lower border of pectoralis minor muscle; area II lies beneath that muscle and area III (the apex) lies medial to the upper border of pectoralis minor. In practice most axillary sampling takes a portion of area I, and full axillary clearance with division of pectoralis minor should clear all three areas and yield upwards of 20 nodes in the specimen.

removed. During the clearing of the mid-axilla the intercostobrachial nerve is divided as it emerges from the chest wall just posterior to the origin of the pectoralis minor muscle. Some surgeons now try to preserve this nerve. The thoracodorsal and long thoracic nerves are preserved if at all possible but occasionally the thoracodorsal nerve needs to be excised if surrounded by involved nodes. At the end of the procedure the wound is drained by two suction drains and the skin flaps are closed. The drains are left in for 3–5 days or until the volume of daily drainage falls to 50 ml. Recent studies have shown that patients may be safely sent home with the drain in situ, reducing the hospital stay.[127] Postoperative complications are uncommon but seromas often occur in the axilla and can be treated by simple aspiration. When the intercostobrachial nerve has been divided the patient should be warned that she will have an anaesthetised patch of skin in the axilla and upper medial part of the arm.

Subcutaneous mastectomy is performed via a submammary, axillary or circumareolar incision and is usually indicated for prophylaxis of breast cancer in women at high risk of the disease. This includes women with a strong family history or those with atypical proliferative disease or ductal carcinoma-in-situ. These operations are not easy to perform and the cosmetic results may be poor. A further problem is that not all the breast is removed and instances of late breast cancer have been recorded. After excision of the breast tissue the breast shape is reformed by a gel-filled implant. This operation is best performed in consultation with a plastic surgeon or breast surgeon with interest in reconstruction. All breast tissue removed should be carefully examined for occult carcinoma. This operation has also been used to treat small invasive cancers.

Breast reconstruction

Some 10–20% of women undergoing mastectomy will experience lifelong distress from the damage to the perceived body image that may follow mastectomy. It is not always easy to predict which women will be affected. The option of breast reconstruction must therefore be discussed with all patients. Not all women will wish to undergo reconstruction, particularly if the complications, the need for an implant and the possibility of a second operation are explained. If chosen, these operations may be performed at the same time as the mastectomy or at a later date. The aim is to produce a mound on the chest wall which resembles the lost breast: the patient should not be given the impression that a normal breast can be reproduced.

The techniques vary from simple placement of an implant under the skin flaps to the more complicated insertion of a myocutaneous flap into the mastectomy defect (Table 25.11). The techniques employing an implant alone are simpler but probably produce less satisfactory cosmetic results. As in subcutaneous mastectomy the implant should be placed subpectorally (i.e. under pectoralis muscles) to reduce the incidence of capsular contraction. A simple implant can only be used when plenty of skin is available after completion of the mastectomy. The main problem however with a subpectoral implant is that it lies above the level of the natural inframammary fold, giving a high breast. Enlarging the muscular pocket inferiorly by dissecting underneath the serratus anterior can help this problem.

Table 25.11 Breast reconstruction operations

Subcutaneous prosthesis
Submuscular implant
Tissue expander
Rectus abdominis myocutaneous flap ± implant
Latissimus dorsi myocutaneous flap + implant

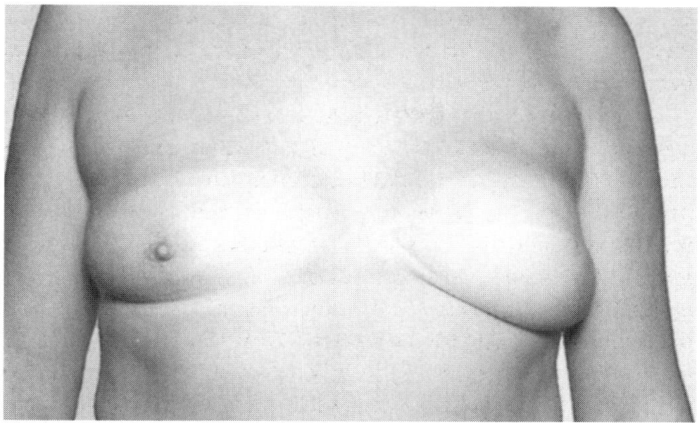

Fig. 25.33 Breast reconstruction using a latissimus dorsi myocutaneous flap with a silicone gel implant. This procedure was done as an immediate reconstruction at the same time as the mastectomy. Note the symmetry and the recreated inframammary fold, highlighted by the patient's suntan.

Tissue expanders offer a slightly more complicated approach[128] as at least two operations are needed to place and remove the implant and to complete the reconstruction. In order to make the new inframammary fold at the correct level, a submuscular pocket is created beneath both the pectoral and serratus anterior muscles. The expander is then filled slowly in outpatients over the next 3–6 months until an over-expansion of some 100–200 ml over the desired breast size is achieved. A permanent implant is then exchanged for the tissue expander at a second operation. Although appearing to be a simple operation, numerous complications have been reported[129] and the technique is still being developed. It does offer the patient a reconstruction without an additional donor scar on the back or abdomen. This technique is becoming more popular and tissue expanders have now been developed for permanent implantation (Becker type), which makes the second stage much simpler as the filling port can be removed without disturbing the implant.

Myocutaneous flaps can produce good cosmetic results and are especially useful where skin and muscle are short after an extensive mastectomy or where the skin flaps have been irradiated (Fig. 25.33). These complicated techniques involve longer operating times and greater blood loss and are best done as a team approach between cancer surgeon and plastic surgeon. They can however be

REFERENCES

127. Early Drain
128. Argenta L C, Marks M W, Grabb W C Ann Plast Surg 1983; 11: 188–195
129. Dickson M G, Sharpe D T Br J Plast Surg 1987; 40: 629–635

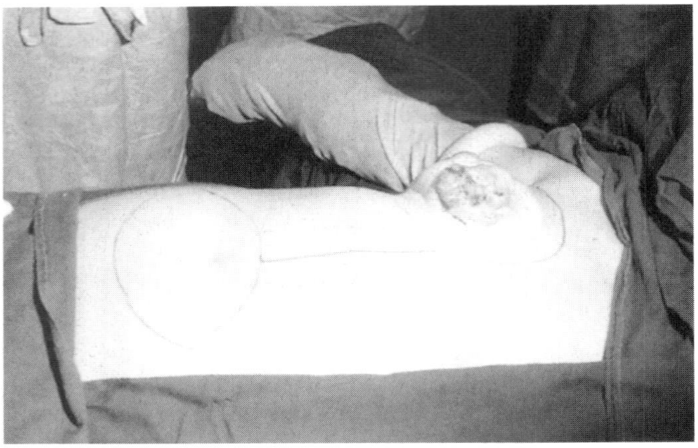

Fig. 25.34 Operative photograph of a patient with locally advanced breast cancer about to undergo a radical mastectomy with closure using a rectus abdominis myocutaneous flap. The outline of the flap and rectus muscle have been drawn on the abdomen at the start of the operation.

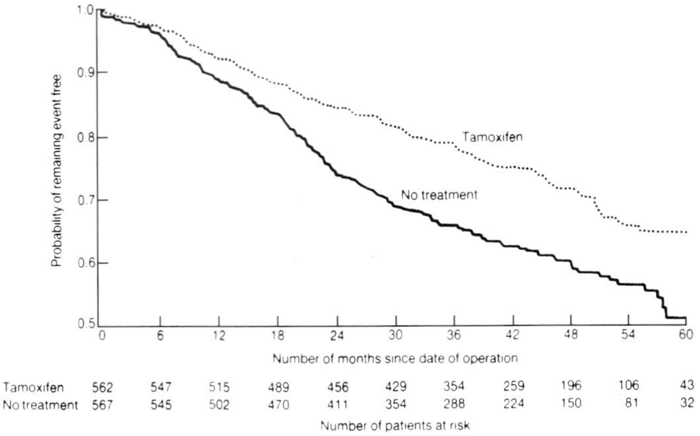

Fig. 25.35 Life table of the Nolvadex Adjuvant Trial Organization trial showing significantly higher event-free levels (event = recurrence or death) in the tamoxifen-treated patients.[134]

performed satisfactorily by general surgeons with appropriate experience[130] and are particularly useful for salvage surgery for recurrence in the conserved breast and for locally advanced disease[131] (Fig. 25.34). The choice between a latissimus dorsi reconstruction or a rectus flap depends on patient preference and the amount of abdominal fat present. Extensive abdominal scarring precludes the use of a rectus flap as the blood supply to the muscle may have been damaged by the previous surgery.

Adjuvant therapy

The use of adjuvant therapy in operable breast cancer is based on the hypothesis that early treatment by either chemotherapy or hormone therapy destroys the micrometastases which are present but undetectable at the time of surgery on the primary cancer. The results of randomized trials of adjuvant therapy support this concept in part and this is one area in the therapy of breast cancer which has seen significant advances, although the absolute gains in terms of reduction in mortality are not great. The important studies of chemotherapy were first run in the Milan Cancer Institute by Bonadonna et al[132] and in the USA by Fisher et al[133] who used the combination of cyclophosphamide, methotrexate and fluorouracil (CMF) in both pre- and postmenopausal patients. The drugs were given for 12 months after surgery in patients with positive axillary nodes.

Both trials showed a definite advantage for the treated patients over control patients in both disease-free interval and subsequent mortality. This advantage was greatest in premenopausal patients with one to three metastatic nodes in the axilla. However, the toxicity of the therapy was a problem: some 30% of patients experienced significant side-effects. It is now clear that 6 months of adjuvant therapy with CMF is as good as 1 year, and so this should be the treatment of choice.

Later studies of antioestrogen therapy using tamoxifen for 2 years have also confirmed an advantage over control patients, especially in postmenopausal patients with positive nodes.[134–136] The large Nolvadex Adjuvant Trial Organization study of 1285 patients in the UK[134] showed an increased survival in the tamoxifen-treated group with very low toxicity (Fig. 25.35). This trial treated both pre- and postmenopausal patients with tamoxifen 10 mg twice daily for 2 years and was compared against controls who were given no adjuvant treatment. The results suggested that the benefit of Nolvadex was also found in the oestrogen receptor-negative patients, although only about half the patients had their receptors assayed. These findings were surprising as tamoxifen was thought to act via the oestrogen receptor pathway, but other studies have now reported similar results in both oestrogen receptor-positive and -negative patients.[137] A trial in Scotland of 1312 patients on tamoxifen 20 mg/day for 5 years showed a highly significant delay in relapse in the treatment group which was independent of nodal or menopausal status.[138] Again the beneficial effect was seen in all the oestrogen receptor categories, although the greatest benefit was demonstrated in patients with oestrogen receptor levels of greater than 100 fmol/mg protein.

The overall 10-year results of adjuvant therapy were recently summarised by Peto in a meta-analysis of 40 trials of tamoxifen in 30 000 women and 46 trials of adjuvant chemotherapy in 26 000 women.[137] He found that tamoxifen reduced the odds of death by 17% and this effect was mainly seen in older women. Chemotherapy gave a reduction of 16% in the odds of death, but this effect was mainly in younger premenopausal women. Adjuvant chemotherapy with multiple drug combinations offered better results than single-agent regimens. A further recent overview of ovarian ablation by the same group reported on 2102

REFERENCES

130. Mansel R E, Horgan K et al Br J Surg 1986; 73: 813–816
131. Flook D, Webster D J T et al Br J Surg 1989; 76: 512–514
132. Bonadonna G, Brussamolino E et al N Engl J Med 1976; 294: 405–410
133. Fisher B, Carbone P et al N Engl J Med 1975; 292: 117–122
134. NATO trial Lancet 1985; i: 836–840
135. Report Lancet 1987; ii: 171–175
136. Ribeiro G, Swindell R Eur J Cancer Clin Oncol 1985; 21: 897–900
137. Peto R Lancet 339; 1–15, 72–85
138. Scottish Tam Trial

premenopausal women and showed a 6% improvement in survival at 15 years for the ovarian ablation group.[139]

This suggests that mortality can be reduced modestly by adjuvant chemotherapy in young women and by adjuvant tamoxifen in older women. These treatments should be the standard for patients with positive nodes. Patients with negative nodes have been regarded as having such a good prognosis that adjuvant therapy is unnecessary, but a trial of node-negative, oestrogen receptor-positive patients has shown a significant prolongation of disease-free survival in patients treated with tamoxifen 20 mg/day for 5 years.[140] It is currently considered that because of the small but real risk of induced uterine malignancy, tamoxifen should not be taken for longer than 5 years.

Current treatment—inoperable and advanced disease

Patients who present with locally advanced or metastatic disease are deemed incurable because local treatment, whether surgical or radiotherapeutic, cannot save the patient. When a patient is likely to die within a few months as a result of her breast cancer, then mastectomy should not be performed as this procedure does not help the patient, and often increases her distress. Mastectomy may however be a useful manoeuvre when used together with radiotherapy or chemotherapy to obtain local control of the cancer. Signs of inoperability are skin oedema and peau d'orange, skin ulceration, chest fixity and satellite nodules. The patient may have had a history of a primary breast mass for many years without any overt signs of distant spread.

When the disease is locally advanced it is useful to ascertain the oestrogen receptor status to see if the disease is likely to run a slow or rapid course. Where the primary tumour is deemed inoperable or where the patient presents with metastases then radiotherapy is often the treatment of choice for the local problem as it is cosmetically superior to surgery and can be given as an outpatient. More recently, courses of chemotherapy have been given prior to local treatment in an attempt to reduce the size of the tumour so that the radiation is more effective or conservative surgery can be used as a treatment instead of mastectomy. This combined therapy, sometimes referred to as neoadjuvant treatment, is still being evaluated and although increased responses defined in terms of tumour shrinkage are being obtained, there appears to be no survival advantage when compared with radiotherapy alone. Where the tumour is found to be oestrogen receptor-positive or the biopsy is of a slowly growing tumour, endocrine therapy is often worthwhile as the first-line therapy, keeping radiotherapy in reserve for later progression. Endocrine therapy, usually with tamoxifen 20–40 mg/day, has an initial complete and partial response rate of 30–40% compared with chemotherapy rates of 50–60%, although endocrine therapy is less toxic. Assessment of response is usually defined by shrinkage of measurable disease and the UICC criteria[141] are generally employed. These classify responses as complete, partial, no change and progression: to conform with these definitions response should be maintained for at least 6 months. Even if the primary tumour becomes impalpable as a consequence of neoadjuvant chemotherapy, there may still be surviving malignancies and surgery or radiotherapy is still required.

Metastatic disease

Similar principles apply to women presenting with stage IV disease. Treatment is directed at the relief of symptoms as cure is not possible and the less toxic endocrine therapies are used if the tumour is slow-growing and is oestrogen receptor-positive. When the oestrogen receptor status is unknown, then response will be most likely in a patient who is postmenopausal with slow-growing disease confined to the bones or soft tissues. Tamoxifen is almost universally used as the first-line hormone therapy as it has a very low toxicity. In premenopausal women either surgical oophorectomy or ovarian radiation can be used to ablate ovarian function. Studies are underway to assess the efficacy of luteinizing hormone-releasing hormone agonists in premenopausal women. Endocrine responses are more likely in patients with bony and soft tissue disease and tend to be longer-lasting than chemotherapy responses.

On relapse a second-line hormone such as a progestogen or aminoglutethimide can be used to obtain a further response as a good first endocrine response predicts a better chance of a second response. As aminoglutethimide is associated with adrenal suppression it has been replaced with second-generation aromatase inhibitors such as anastozole or letrozole which have lower side-effects. Ablative endocrine procedures such as adrenalectomy and hypophysectomy have now been supplanted by the wide range of 'medical' hormonal therapies that are available and should no longer be used. Combination cytotoxic chemotherapy is usually used as the first-line therapy if the disease involves viscera or is likely to be rapidly life-threatening. Combinations of cytoxic drugs are used, as few single agents apart from Adriamycin have much activity in breast cancer.

Localised painful bony metastases are best treated by palliative radiotherapy and analgesics. Brain metastases are treated by radiotherapy and high-dose steroids. Metastatic disease may produce many different disease states, such as leucoerythroblastic anaemia when the bone marrow is infiltrated, or hypercalcaemia when massive osteolysis occurs; these require specific therapy. Involvement of the spinal canal may produce paresis which will require urgent spinal canal decompression by laminectomy (see Chapter 46). Fixation of pathological fractures of the long bones by intramedullary nails may also be needed.

The place of surgery in advanced disease is limited to salvage mastectomy for local control of residual disease after failure of radiotherapy or chemotherapy. These salvage operations are often massive, requiring excision of chest wall as well as the breast and pectoral muscles as the disease has often infiltrated widely in the breast and chest wall. The resulting defect can be filled by a myocutaneous flap (see Fig. 25.34) or omental graft.[142] These large excisions are intended to be palliative and aim to produce local

REFERENCES

139. Early Breast Cancer Trialists Collaborative Group. Lancet 1996; 348: 1189–1196
140. Fisher B, Costantino P H et al N Engl J Med 1989; 320: 479–484
141. Hayward J L, Hewson J C Cancer 1977; 39: 1289–1294
142. Williams R J L, Fryatt I J C et al Br J Surg 1989; 76: 559–563

control until the patient dies of distant recurrence. The outlook for most patients with stage IV disease is very poor—only 10% survive 5 years.

When it is clear that the disease is advancing despite treatment, it should be recognised that the doctor's duty is to palliate distressing symptoms. Pain should be managed by adequate and frequent doses of oral opiates which may reach doses of many hundreds of milligrams in 24 hours (see Chapter 5); locally painful areas can often be usefully palliated by radiation given in single treatment sessions. Constipation induced by the opiates can be treated by regular laxatives. Pleural effusions are treated by tapping and instillation of bleomycin or talc into the pleural space. Ascites should be tapped and if chronic can be managed by a peritoneovenous shunt (see Chapter 27).

When it is clear that death will soon occur then frank but sympathetic discussion with the patient and her relatives is beneficial. These patients need a lot of counselling and many different agencies may need to be involved. Home care is the ideal situation but when available a hospice is a better environment for a dying patient than an acute surgical ward. The growing hospice movement is better versed in the specific physical and emotional problems of patients dying of advanced malignancy.

MALE BREAST CANCER

Male breast cancer is 100 times less common than the female variety and represents only 0.7% of all cancers in males. The peak age incidence is 5–10 years older than that in females. The aetiology, like that of female breast cancer, is unknown but there is an increased incidence in patients with Klinefelter's syndrome. Gynaecomastia is seen in some 30% of males and is not a risk factor for breast cancer.

The presenting features are identical to those in females: a discovered and palpable lump, skin or nipple retraction and occasionally nipple discharge are the main symptoms. The only difference between the sexes is that the male tumour infiltrates skin and nipple at an early stage because of the smaller breast volume and the closer proximity of the chest skin (Fig. 25.36). All the common histological varieties of breast cancer are seen in the male, with the exception of lobular carcinoma, as no lobular development occurs in the male breast. The differential diagnosis is gynaecomastia.

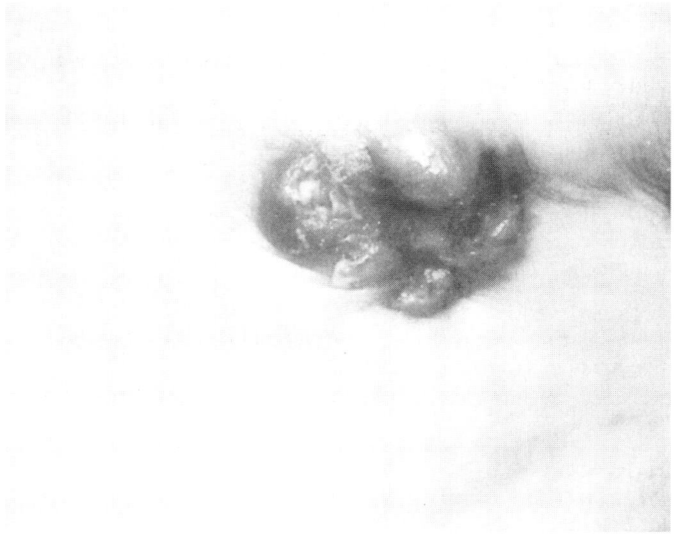

Fig. 25.36 Male breast cancer showing ulceration of the skin and infiltration of the nipple. These changes tend to occur early in breast cancer in the male as the skin is very close to the gland tissue. Courtesy of Dr G Riberio.

The prognosis of male breast cancer is now thought to be identical to that of the female type when compared stage for stage but, as noted, the male tends to present with skin infiltration more often than the female and therefore is seen at a later stage. The preferred treatment in males is mastectomy which must usually be radical because of early infiltration of the pectoral muscles. Although the hormonal milieu is different in males, breast cancer still appears to respond well to hormonal therapy when it is oestrogen receptor-positive. As in the female, castration has been reported to produce a good remission in advanced male breast cancer.[143]

NON-EPITHELIAL TUMOURS OF THE BREAST (SARCOMA)

There are several types of non-epithelial tumour, although all are rare in comparison to ductal carcinomas. The sarcomas form the largest group and are divided into fibrosarcomas, leiomyosarcomas, rhabdomyosarcomas and angiosarcomas, depending on the predominant cell type. The angiosarcoma is the commonest subtype, although in 1989 a review of the world literature only yielded 87 cases.[144] The tumour presents as a lump, or diffuse infiltration of the skin, and skin discoloration is seen in 30% of cases. There is considerable variation in the size of the primary tumour, with a range from 2 to 11 cm and macroscopically the tumour may appear spongy with multiple blood-filled spaces. Donnell et al[145] divided the tumour into three groups based on histology, with 12 out of 13 group I patients alive at 5-year follow-up, compared with 4 out of 18 group III patients. The other sarcomas form less than 1% of malignant tumours and are thus very rare in the breast (Fig. 25.37).

Fibrosarcoma presents as a poorly defined mass in the breast and microscopic examination shows the typical spindle cells with multiple mitotic figures. Simple mastectomy is indicated for local control and node dissection is not indicated as the distant spread is usually via the blood stream to the liver. The prognosis is poor and chemotherapy is usually ineffective. One long-term survivor of metachronous bilateral breast tumours has been reported with disease-free survival up to 13 years after the first tumour.[146]

Occasionally the breast is the site of other primary tumours, with the lymphomas or leukaemia being the most common group.

REFERENCES

143. Meyskens F L, Tormey D C, Neifeld J P Cancer Treat Rev 1976; 3: 83–93
144. Chen K T K, Kiregaard D D, Bocian J J Cancer 1989; 46: 368–371
145. Donnell R M, Rosen P P et al Am J Surg Pathol 1981; 5: 629–642
146. Bundred N J, O'Reilly K, Smart J G Eur J Surg Oncol 1989; 15: 263–264

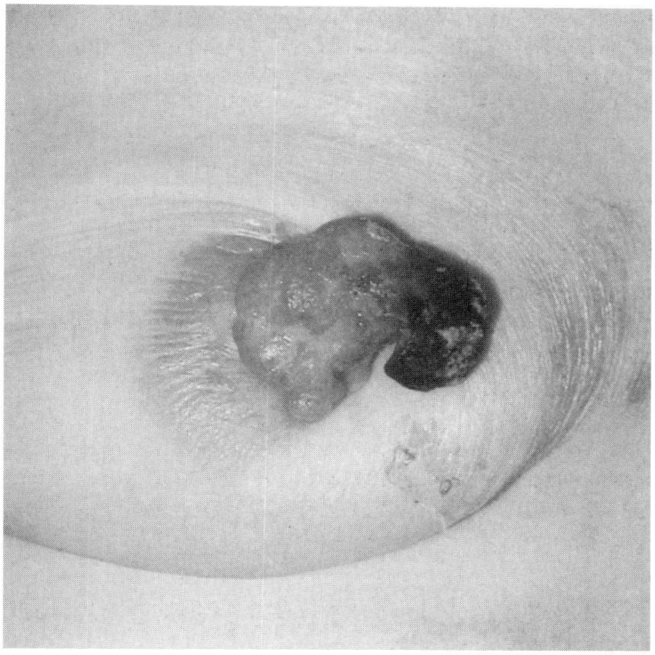

Fig. 25.37 Spindle cell sarcoma of the breast presenting as a rapidly growing ulcerating mass destroying the nipple. Note the necrotic tip of this fast-growing tumour which showed many mitotic figures on microscopy.

The skin over the breast may be affected by any skin primary cancer and occasionally secondary deposits from adenocarcinomas at other sites are seen in the breast.

BREAST SCREENING

The Health Insurance Plan study, set up in New York as a randomized study of breast screening, was the first to demonstrate a survival advantage for women whose carcinoma was detected by mammography.[147] These findings have now been validated in European studies in the Netherlands and Sweden where screening was performed by mammography alone. The first Dutch study[148] reported 30 000 women over 35 years old screened by a single-view mammogram every 2 years, and demonstrated a halving of the mortality rate from breast cancer in the screened group. Another non-randomised case-control Dutch study screened 14 000 women by mammography and clinical examination and showed a significant reduction in mortality.[149] A major randomised study from Sweden studied 134 000 women in a mammographic screening programme and recorded a high attendance rate and a 40% reduction in mortality from breast cancer in women aged 50–74 years screened by a single-view mammogram.[150] As a result of these and other studies the British government has instituted a population-based screening programme for women aged 50–64 by a single-view mammogram.[80] This programme is now in place, although some believe that this form of screening may not be as useful as the early studies suggested[151] and the first report of the British experience failed to show a significant reduction in mortality.[152]

The latest review of the quality of the National Screening programme showed that most targets were being met by all the screening clinics (see Table 34.60 in NHSBSP Review 1996). The take-up rate for most units was well above the target of 70% of the population. This performance is encouraging, but it is too early yet to see if there is a reduction in breast cancer mortality because of the screening programme.

Another possible approach is to prevent breast cancer by endocrine or other agents taken by high-risk women prior to the onset of breast cancer, but these studies are currently only research projects.[153,154] There is an international breast intervention study (IBIS) currently studying prevention of breast cancer by tamoxifen in women at high risk of breast cancer measured by family history, but results will not be available for some years.

REFERENCES

147. Shapiro S, Venet W et al J Natl Cancer Inst 1982; 69: 349–355
148. Verbeek A L M, Holland R et al Lancet 1984; i: 1222–1224
149. Collette H J A, Rombach J J et al Lancet 1984; i: 1224–1226
150. Swedish Trial
151. Skrabanek P Lancet 1985; ii: 316–319
152. UK Trial of Early Detection of Breast Cancer Group Lancet 1988; ii: 411–416
153. Powles T J, Wang D Y, Bulbrook R D Lancet 1986; i: 83–86
154. Pike M C, Ross R K et al Br J Cancer 1986; 60: 142–148

26 The abdominal wall and hernias

H. B. Devlin A. N. Kingsnorth

ABDOMINAL INCISIONS

In 1946 Sir Heneage Ogilvie[1] defined a good incision as one which affords access, extensibility and the greatest possible safety to the abdominal wall, the structures it encloses and the patient. Additional features include speed of access, ease of closure, security from early dehiscence, avoidance of long-term wound failure or herniation and the cosmetic appearance. Cultural differences also influence a surgeon's choice of incision: the Anglo-Saxons show a preference for vertical incisions and the Latins, especially the French, are enthusiasts for transverse abdominal access.[2]

Longitudinal vertical median, paramedian or transrectus incisions provide speed of access, extensibility to the pubis and xiphoid (with easy extension by median sternotomy to the chest). Median incisions through the linea alba are relatively bloodless and allow surgery in all four abdominal quadrants. The gastrointestinal tract is developed from a midline primitive gut and can be mobilized on its mesentery to the midline. Laterally based structures—the renal tract, for instance—are less accessible through a midline abdominal incision; oblique flank incisions are needed to approach these and other retroperitoneal structures. Lateral oblique and transverse incisions through the red muscle bellies of the abdominal wall and horizontal incisions across the rectus muscle are less desirable than longitudinal incisions in the aponeurosis. Division of red muscle involves more blood loss and less secure closure (red muscle does not hold sutures well). All lateral incisions can damage intercostal motor nerves to the abdominal wall.

When a median incision is utilized a vertical skin cut is employed; the umbilicus is grasped in a stout tissue forceps and held to one side while the incision is made through the skin at the base of the cicatrix and vertically through the umbilicus.[3] Subcutaneous haemostasis is achieved with either diathermy coagulation or absorbable ligatures. The linea alba is incised along with the peritoneum which directly underlies it. The fat, subcutaneous tissue and epimysium should not be dissected away from the aponeurosis: this devitalizes the margins of the aponeurotic wound and can lead to later wound failure. Similarly, division of the aponeurosis by diathermy scalpel causes more tissue damage and ischaemia than is necessary. Damage to the aponeurosis by diathermy, excessive retraction and sepsis is the herald of dehiscence.

Paramedian incisions are very popular in the UK. The traditional paramedian with vertical incisions through the anterior and posterior rectus sheaths not more than 1.5 cm from the midline, with the rectus muscle retracted laterally, has little advantage compared with the midline incision and the disadvantage that it takes longer to make. On the other hand, the lateral paramedian incision where the rectus sheath is divided over the lateral rectus muscle about 3.5 cm from the midline to form wide flaps of anterior and posterior rectus sheath for closure confers significant benefits for postoperative wound stability.[4]

The most frequently used transverse incision in adults is the Pfannenstiel suprapubic incision. This affords excellent access to the female reproductive organs for caesarean section, and for bladder and prostate operations. It is also invaluable in extraperitoneal approaches to groin hernia repairs in adults and for hernia repair and orchidopexy in infancy. The Pfannenstiel incision, if carefully constructed and repaired, is most cosmetic. The skin is incised in a downwardly convex arch in the suprapubic skin crease 2 cm above the pubis. The scar should lie within the pubic hair. The upper flap is raised and the rectus sheath incised transversely about 1 cm or more cephalic to the skin incision. This is an important technical detail; it is essential to avoid making the skin and rectus sheath incisions in the same plane if the best cosmesis is to be obtained. Only the rectus sheath should be opened; extending the aponeurotic incision laterally into the external oblique may be complicated by the subsequent development of a Spigelian or direct inguinal hernia. The rectus muscles are separated in the midline and access can be made to the lower peritoneal cavity and pelvis. Closure is in layers. Haemostasis may be troublesome and suction drainage may avoid haematomas.

Transverse abdominal incisions are of particular advantage in neonates and children.[5] At an early age the subdiaphragmatic and pelvic recesses do not exist and a girdle-shaped transverse incision gives excellent access to the entire abdominal cavity in small children. In adults these incisions have the disadvantages already mentioned.

Oblique incisions, including the Kocher subcostal, the Leclerc rooftop incision, the McBurney gridiron, the Rutherford Morrison lower oblique and the thoracoabdominal upper oblique, all fulfil

REFERENCES

1. Ogilvie H Proc R Soc Med 1946; 39: 234
2. Chevrel J P (ed) Chirurgie des parois de l'abdomen. Springer Verlag, Berlin 1985
3. Paes T R F et al Br J Surg 1987; 74: 822
4. Guillou P J et al Br J Surg 1980; 67: 395
5. Jones P F, Towns F M Br J Surg 1983; 70: 719

distinct advantages of local access without providing the complete access and extensibility afforded by the vertical incisions (Fig. 26.1).

Kocher's incision is made 2.5 cm below the costal margin, to avoid the eighth intercostal nerve.[6] Medially the incision extends to the midline and laterally to the tip of the ninth costal cartilage. The incision is continued obliquely through the anterior rectus sheath which is divided for the same length as the wound. Laterally, the external oblique muscle is split in the direction of its fibres. Kocher did not extend the incision more laterally and he only divided one (the ninth) neurovascular bundle.[6] This incision has been criticized because many surgeons extend it laterally, dividing more neurovascular bundles. Surgeons have also used absorbable material to close the incision and placed drains through its lateral extremity. These neurovascular insults, inadequate suturing and drains have earned the subcostal incision an undeservedly bad reputation for dehiscence and herniation. Kocher's incision gives good access for cholecystectomy on the right or splenectomy on the left. It is incapable of caudal extension, which limits its usefulness in biliary or pancreatic surgery. When it is closed with non-absorbable monofilament sutures it is a good incision.

The double Kocher, Leclerc or rooftop incision affords easy access to the liver and spleen. For intrahepatic surgery it is invaluable.[2] It may also be employed for radical pancreatic and gastric surgery and for bilateral adrenalectomy.

The McBurney incision,[7] preferably with a skin-crease horizontal skin cut, is a time-honoured approach to the appendix. McBurney described the incision as 'an inch or so medial to the anterior superior iliac spine at right angles to a line drawn from the anterior superior iliac spine to the umbilicus'. In modern practice the incision is made at the junction of the outer third and medial two-thirds of a line from the anterior superior iliac spine to the umbilicus; it is safe and heals with a good cosmetic scar providing wound infection is avoided. The lower incision, called a Lanz incision, is more transverse and medial than the classical McBurney incision and provides better cosmesis at the expense of poorer access to a high retrocaecal appendix. Herniation should not be a complication of a McBurney incision. The lower Lanz incision risks damage to the iliohypogastric and ilioinguinal nerves with subsequent atrophy of the posterior inguinal wall and an increased risk of subsequent herniation.[8]

The gridiron incision can be extended cephalad and laterally as a Rutherford Morrison incision,[9] obliquely splitting the external oblique to afford a good route to the caecum, appendix and right colon. A similar incision on the left allows access to the left colon but not to the rectum.

The right or left thoracoabdominal incision is the time-honoured road to the lower thorax and upper abdomen. Any vertical or oblique upper abdominal incision can be extended into the chest by division of the costal margin and then by a radial incision through the diaphragm to the oesophagus or great vessels. This incision is used in liver and biliary surgery on the right and for oesophageal, gastric and aortic surgery on the left.[10]

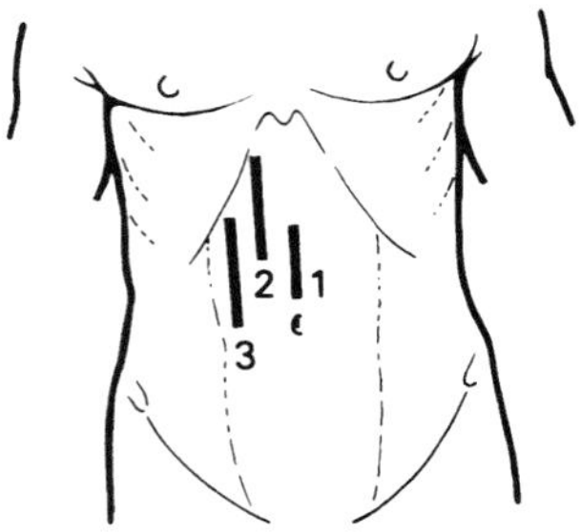

Fig. 26.1a Vertical incisions. **1** Median; **2** paramedian; **3** lateral paramedian.

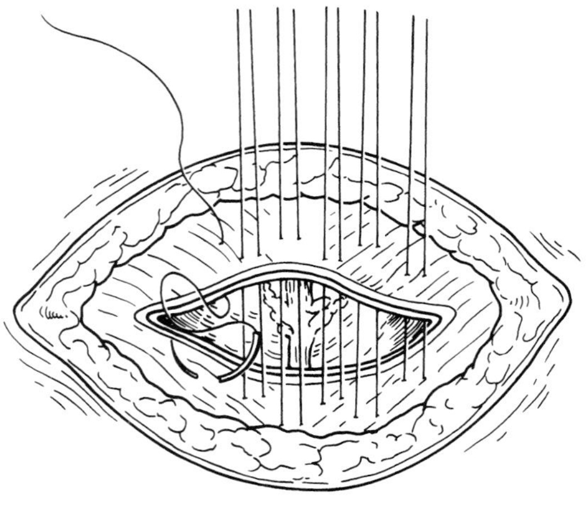

Fig. 26.1b Oblique incisions. **1** Kocher; **1 and 2** Leclerc rooftop; 3 McBurney gridiron; **4** thoracoabdominal.

Pulmonary considerations

Whether the choice of incision for upper abdominal surgery should be influenced by constraints of pulmonary pathophysiology is an unresolved debate. The upper abdominal wall is an important ventilatory muscle; its impairment might be expected to reduce pulmonary function and increase postoperative pulmonary complications. Observations made on young and middle-aged male patients in the late 1960s demonstrated a fall of 25% in the functional reserve capacity with hypoxaemia after abdominal surgery through an epigastric incision.[11] A postoperative fall in vital capacity was confirmed by other studies:[12] with a supraumbilical midline incision the vital capacity falls by 70%; with an infraumbilical midline incision it falls by 60%, while a major transverse incision gives a reduction of only 50%.[12] Pneumoperitoneum may also cause pulmonary collapse.[13] Others have found no difference in postoperative ventilatory function between midline and transverse incisions in patients undergoing upper abdominal surgery.[14] A well-conducted randomized study failed to demonstrate any

REFERENCES

6. Kocher T Chirurgische Operationslehre. Verlag von Gustav Fischer, Jena 1907
7. McBurney C Ann Surg 1894; 20: 38
8. Arnbjornsson E Am J Surg 1982; 143: 367
9. Morrison R Br Med J 1906; 2: 1005
10. Schwartz A, Quenu J Paris Med 1919; 9: 162
11. Alexander H et al Clin Sci 1972; 3: 137
12. Edouard A et al Cahiers Anesth 1979; 27: 25
13. Bevan P G Br Med J 1861; 2: 609
14. Williams C D, Breowitz J B Am J Surg 1975; 130: 725

difference in pulmonary complications whether a vertical or transverse incision is used.[15]

The choice of incision should therefore be made for anatomical rather than pulmonary criteria.

The contaminated wound

Particular problems can occur when an incision is made into a grossly infected or contaminated abdominal cavity. Some principles warrant reiteration.

A peritoneal drain should never be placed through an incised wound. Infection, dehiscence and herniation follow. If the wound itself needs draining a suction drain shall be placed through a nearby stab incision. The skin should not be closed if the wound needs draining because it is microbiologically contaminated. The wound should also be left open if the abdomen is heavily infected or contaminated. The omentum can be spread over the viscera and a patch of inert mesh may be sutured to the wound edges to hold the viscera in place with a non-stick antiseptic dressing laid in the wound.[16]

ABDOMINAL WOUND CLOSURE

Aponeurotic wound healing and sutures

There is slow healing in aponeurosis after division. This process[17] is conveniently considered in three stages. First is the lag or inflammatory phase, during which blood vessels are plugged, the wound is enmeshed in fibrin and an inflammatory response occurs. During this phase the only strength the wound possesses is derived from the sutures. This phase lasts up to 4 days in human aponeurosis. Next is the proliferative or fibroblastic phase, during which macrophages and fibroblasts migrate into the wound and primitive collagen is laid down. This phase continues for up to 21 days, during which the wound rapidly gains strength. After this there is a long remodelling or maturation phase of collagen realignment. At 50 days the aponeurosis has regained half of its initial strength. Thereafter the process is slow; after 1 year the aponeurosis achieves 80% of its initial tensile strength.[18] These rates of healing are modified by co-morbidity, sutures and foreign bodies in the wound.[19,20]

Malnutrition,[21] vitamin C deficiency,[22] smoking,[23] increasing age,[24] immunosuppression and numerous other factors delay aponeurotic healing.[24] Sepsis delays wound healing.[25] Clearly some of these conditions can be modified therapeutically. Genetic anomalies of collagen synthesis, Marfan and Ehlers–Danlos syndromes and prune belly syndrome are important examples of collagen malsynthesis.[26] Of equal importance in determining the rate and quality of wound healing is the suture technique and material used. The choice of suture is critical. The older biological sutures made of human and animal tendon and catgut are later digested by macrophages. They excite a powerful inflammatory response. This response delays the onset of collagen repair.

The strong inflammatory response to animal collagen rapidly weakens sutures made from it and causes knots to slip. After 2 or 3 days plain catgut provides no strength at all to the healing aponeurotic wound. Chromic catgut is little better, losing half of its strength in 14 days.[27] This time span is not congruent with the time cycle of aponeurotic wound healing. Silk and linen are biological suture materials that keep their strength for longer periods but they, too, excite strong inflammatory responses in human aponeuroses. Biological-based fibres also have other disadvantages; they are difficult to sterilize; once infected they remain so until removed from the tissues, and they are difficult to manufacture in a standardized manner.[28] For all these reasons they are no longer recommended for abdominal incision repair. There has been a revolution in sutures. The choice of suture is critical to rapid and sound wound healing.[29] Sutures today are a far cry from Aird's statement in 1957: 'the material used for sutures is probably not very important'.[30]

Suture choice

Modern sutures are the products of polymer chemistry. They are manufactured by extrusion of the polymer and may be used in surgery in either braided or monofilament forms. Their durability in the body and their rates of absorption are dictated by their chemistry. They all excite little, if any, biological response. The choice of suture should be related to the expected rate of healing of the tissue being sutured. As aponeurotic incisions are slow to heal they need support for 4–6 months. Therefore slowly absorbable, polydioxanone (PDS), polyglactin (Vicryl) or polyglycolic acid (Dexon) or non-absorbable polyesters (Mersilene, Ethibond), polyamides (nylon) or polypropylene (Prolene) fulfil these requirements.[31]

There can be problems even with inert modern non-absorbable sutures. Persistent infection and sinus formation can develop if braided non-absorbable sutures become infected. Non-absorbable monofilaments are difficult to knot and can saw through tissue, causing herniation months or years later.[32] Persistent sinuses can also complicate wounds sutured with monofilament materials.

Monofilament stainless steel wire has similar properties to polymers and, indeed, before the new polymers were readily avail-

REFERENCES

15. Greenall M J, Evans M, Pollock A V Br J Surg 1980; 67: 188
16. Mughal M M, Bancewicz J, Irving M H Br J Surg 1986; 73: 253
17. Douglas D M Br J Surg 1952; 40: 79
18. Van Winkle W Surg Gynecol Obstet 1969; 129: 819
19. Douglas D M et al Br J Surg 1969; 56: 219
20. Van Winkle W et al Surg Gynecol Obstet 1975; 104: 7
21. Kraybill W G Am J Surg 1944; 66: 220–225
22. Levene C I et al Virchow's Arch Part B 1977; 23: 325
23. Schilling J A Ann Surg 1985; 201: 268
24. Hobsley M J R Soc Med 1982; 75: 870
25. Bucknall T E, Ellis H Surgery 1981; 89: 672
26. McKusick V A Heritable Disorders of Connective Tissue. Mosby, St Louis 1974
27. Lawrie P et al Br J Surg 1959; 46: 638
28. Stotter A T et al In: Russell R C G (ed) Recent Advances in Surgery, vol 12. Churchill Livingstone, London 1986
29. Artandi C Surg Gynecol Obstet 1980; 150: 235
30. Aird I Companion in Surgical Studies, 2nd edn. Livingstone, Edinburgh 1957
31. Van Winkle W, Hastings J C Surg Gynecol Obstet 1972; 135: 115
32. Krukowski Z H, Matheson N A Br J Surg 1987; 74: 824

able was the suture material of choice for the elective repair of abdominal hernias. Monofilament stainless steel is difficult to use and prone to fracture during insertion. Stainless steel wire is no longer recommended.

Laparotomy closure

The peritoneum adds little, if any, strength to abdominal closure and some question the necessity to close it.[33] Most surgeons do, however, suture it for aesthetic reasons and to facilitate closure of the overlying rectus aponeurosis. Because the peritoneum is unimportant as a source of strength to the healing abdominal wound it is closed with an absorbable polymer.

The aponeurosis must be closed with a non-absorbable monofilament nylon or polypropylene or a very slowly absorbable synthetic polydioxanone or polyglactin suture. The least amount of foreign body should be left in the wound, hence the thinnest practicable suture should be used.

Apart from the choice of suture material the geometry of the suture technique is important for wound stability. Big bites of aponeurosis with sutures placed at least 1 cm from the wound margin are essential. The sutures should be close together so that the length of suture is at least four times greater than the length of wound if continuous suturing is employed. This is Jenkins rule,[34] which reduces the incidence of dehiscence. Mass closure, in which the suture is passed through all the layers of the abdomen with each bite, is recommended for midline and medial paramedian incisions.[35] Lateral paramedian incisions should be closed in layers.

With adequate pre- and postoperative care of the patient, avoidance or correction of the recognized risk factors, careful technique and correct choice of suture material, early wound dehiscence should be very rare.[36] It does however still occur, generally some 5–10 days after surgery. Dehiscence is heralded by a serosanguineous discharge. The patient may notice 'something giving way'; inevitably, within 24 hours omentum or intestine is seen bulging subcutaneously and between the skin sutures. The emergent gut is usually covered with warm towels and the wound is resutured with through-and-through all-layers sutures.[30] Whether this is always appropriate is not known. Reduction of the gut and repair with polypropylene mesh sutured to the margins of the aponeurosis is easily achieved, less traumatic and probably better for the ill patient in the intensive therapy unit.[37]

DISEASES OF THE UMBILICUS (Table 26.1)

Umbilical tumours

Squamous carcinoma is a rare primary cancer of the umbilicus caused by irritation from retained sebaceous material and other debris. It is treated by complete excision of the umbilicus and the surrounding skin, together with the whole thickness of the periumbilical wall. Metastases to the inguinal nodes can develop. Secondary deposits may occur by direct extension of malignant disease along the ligamentum teres from the liver or from malignant glands in the porta hepatis. Primary tumours of the breast, colon, ovary or other[38] intra-abdominal malignancies can spread in this manner. A primary adenocarcinoma of urachal elements at the umbilicus has been described.[39] Endometrioma of the umbilicus resembles a tumour. It enlarges and bleeds at the time of the menses.[40]

Table 26.1 Classification of umbilical defects

Congenital defects, omphalocoele, hernia of the cord and gastroschisis (see Chapter 00)
Hernias
Childhood
Adult
Tumours
Primary
i. Benign—skin papilloma, lipoma, etc.
ii. Malignant—squamous carcinoma
Secondary—breast, ovarian, colon carcinoma and other tumours
False tumours—endometriosis
Fistulas
Urinary tract
Gastrointestinal tract
Suppuration
Primary
Secondary

Suppuration in children

Omphalitis in newborn children may give rise to septicaemia with distant pyogenic inflammation, or to thrombophlebitis of the portal vein with fatal liver suppuration and jaundice. Tetanus neonatorum can complicate neonatal omphalitis. Most umbilical infections of the infant are however purely local and heal quickly with adequate hygiene. They are usually associated with an umbilical polyp if they persist. This is really an overgrowth of granulation tissue which should be dealt with by ligature or application of a caustic stick.

Superficial remnants of the omphalomesenteric duct may be in the form of local gut mucosa remaining at the umbilicus or cysts deep to the umbilicus. These and similar urachal remnants can lead to local suppuration in children. It is important to screen the intestine and urinary tract for other defects which frequently coexist if there is an umbilical anomaly. Treatment is by local excision.

Umbilical fistula

These are abnormal communications between the umbilicus and the urinary or gastrointestinal tract or the embryonic structures related to them. Urinary tract fistulas can result from a persistent patent urachus; this is uncommon. Cysts of urachal remnants do,

REFERENCES

33. Ellis H, Heddle R Br J Surg 1977; 64: 633
34. Jenkins T P N Br J Surg 1976; 63: 873
35. Pollock A V, Greenall M J, Evans M Proc R Soc Med 1979; 72: 889
36. Kirk R M Proc R Soc Med 1973; 66: 1092
37. Voyles C R et al Ann Surg 1981; 94: 219
38. Quenu J, Longuet J P Rev Chir 1896; 16: 97
39. Blumenthal N J South Afr Med J 1980; 58: 457
40. Steck R, Helwig H JAMA 1950; 191: 167

however, occur and present as suppurative masses just below the umbilicus. The drainage of such a cyst may lead to a urinary fistula and this is a real risk if the patient has bladder neck outflow obstruc-tion. A urinary fistula can complicate a long-healed umbilical wound in an elderly man who develops prostatic hypertrophy.

Umbilical sepsis in the adult

Umbilical sepsis also occurs in adults, most commonly in obese women. It arises from local collections of sebum, body hair or cosmetics, sometimes as the result of stenosis of the umbilical orifice. A pilonidal sinus is rare at the umbilicus and is more frequent in hirsute males than in females.[41] The clinical features are those of local infection. The suppuration may spread inwards to involve the peritoneal cavity. The umbilicus is the thinnest part of the abdominal wall and any intraperitoneal suppurative process may present as an abscess at the umbilicus. Chronic intrahepatic and subphrenic suppuration can extend to the umbilicus along the ligamentum teres. Before any surgery is undertaken, developmental abnormalities and abdominal tuberculosis should be excluded, as also should neoplastic disease of the stomach, gallbladder, colon and pelvic organs.

The treatment of an umbilical infection is, on general grounds, that if suppuration occurs, drainage should be established. Deep fungal infections are treated with topical antifungal ointment. Omphalectomy is necessary if recurrent infections are associated with severe umbilical scarring.

TUMOURS OF THE ABDOMINAL WALL

Musculoaponeurotic fibromatosis—desmoid tumour

Fibromatosis is the generic term for a group of related conditions—Dupuytren's palmar contracture (see Chapter 44), Ledderhose's plantar contracture, Peyronie's disease, fibromatosis coli or congenital torticollis and desmoid tumours. They have five common characteristics: proliferation of well-differentiated fibroblasts; an infiltrative pattern of growth; variable but usually abundant collagen between the fibroblasts; no cytological features of malignancy and an aggressive clinical behaviour with frequent local recurrence. The tumour has no capacity to produce distant metastases.[42]

A desmoid tumour classically arises in the intermuscular fibrous septa of the lower rectus in parous women of child-bearing age. It may also occur in young people and even in children. Despite its classical description in most series, the tumour is as common in men as in women! The tumour is not encapsulated: it slowly infiltrates the rectus muscle and, in the late stages, the peritoneum, the subcutaneous tissues and even the pubic bones. The limits of the rectus sheath at first impose upon the tumour its vertically elongated shape. Desmoid tumours are associated with intestinal tumours, Gardner's syndrome, which consists of colonic polyps and multiple osteomata and familial polyposis coli.[43]

The treatment is by wide excision. The whole breadth of the lower rectus is removed with part of its sheath and, if necessary, with portions of the adjacent lateral abdominal muscles, parietal peritoneum and skin. The resultant defect in the abdominal wall is closed with a prosthesis. A computed tomography scan is useful to outline the tumour prior to surgery. Adequate local excision is never followed by local recurrence.[44]

Haematoma of the rectus sheath

This may result from spontaneous rupture of an epigastric artery or disinsertion of abdominal wall muscles.[45]

Haemorrhage within the rectus sheath may arise in five separate ways:

1. An epigastric vessel may be injured by direct violence, usually when the rectus muscle is tightly contracted in expectation of a blow and with or without demonstrable damage to that muscle. Seat-belt injuries are a common example of this type of injury.
2. A deep epigastric vessel may be torn, perhaps with a few fibres of rectus muscle, in young men at the beginning of a sports season. A similar episode may occur during tetanic spasms.
3. Bleeding may occur within the rectus sheath, not only in typhoid fever, in which Zenker's degeneration especially affects the rectus abdominis, but also in other infectious fevers and debilitating disorders such as typhus, tuberculosis, influenza and ulcerative colitis.
4. Spontaneous haematoma may develop in the rectus sheath of patients with haemophilia, scurvy and leukaemia, and in those on anticoagulants.
5. Haematomas may also arise, apparently spontaneously, from such minor strains as coughing or sneezing, or without obvious trauma or disease.

Disinsertion of the abdominal wall muscles is recorded with high-velocity trauma when either the ribs or the pelvis are fractured. A concomitant diaphragmatic injury and diaphragmatic hernia can develop if the lower ribs are damaged. In pelvic fractures the rectus abdominis of the contralateral side can be pulled off its attachment, leading to an inguinal hernia.[46]

Injury and abdominal wall loss

Abdominal wall injuries are treated by debridement followed by primary or delayed closure. There is no longer any necessity to achieve abdominal closure at all costs. If the wound can be debrided and closed this is ideal but, if not, replacement of an area of abdominal wall by either polypropylene or polytetrafluoroethylene mesh which can be covered by saline dressings should be

REFERENCES

41. Sroujiell A S, Dawoud A Br J Surg 1989; 76: 687
42. Rosai J Ackerman's Surgical Pathology. Mosby, St Louis 1981
43. Parks T G Ann R Coll Surg Engl 1990; 72: 181
44. Posner M C et al Arch Surg 1989; 124: 191–196
45. Siddiqui M N et al J R Soc Med 1992; 85: 420–421
46. Ryan E A Surg Gynecol Obstet 1971; 133: 440

carried out. The wound should be left to granulate. If the wound is already infected and associated with intra-abdominal sepsis, so that the peritoneal contents are fixed, this is called laparostomy. A silicone rubber dressing speeds this process. Any residual defect is repaired secondarily.

The intestines should, if possible, be covered by omentum and the mesh placed over this. Ideally, the mesh should overlap the margins of the defect for at least 3 cm and be sutured to the parietes carefully with many sutures, to ensure adherence. Granulations develop through the mesh and short-term cover can be obtained using split skin. When a hernia develops later there is no need to remove the mesh; an ellipse is withdrawn and the mesh is tightened to reduce the hernia size. Myocutaneous sartorius and latissimus dorsi flaps are also useful for replacing abdominal wall defects.[47]

GROIN HERNIAS

Epidemiology and aetiology of inguinal hernias

Indirect inguinal hernias occur in 4% of male infants born in the UK. These hernias are more frequent in low-birth-weight and premature male infants.[48] Inguinal hernias develop most frequently in the first 3 months of life; thereafter their occurrence falls off with age. Hernias are rare after 3 years of age. These infantile hernias all represent an intrauterine or periparturition failure of the processus vaginalis to close. They are congenital. At all ages inguinal hernias are more frequent on the right side (5 : 4) than the left; in the male this may be related to the later descent of the right testis and later closure of the right processus vaginalis.[49]

Indirect inguinal hernias also occur in female infants, but they are much less frequent than in males. In females they may be an isolated congenital anomaly. In phenotypical females, the testicular feminization syndrome or the complete androgen insensitivity syndrome may first be suspected when a unilateral or bilateral inguinal hernia appears.[50] A female child with inguinal hernias should always have chromosome studies performed to exclude testicular feminization syndrome. Some 60% of inguinal hernias in babies and children first present with incarceration. In young children incarceration very rarely proceeds to strangulation and 95% of incarcerations resolve spontaneously with sedation and traction in the Solomon position[51] (Fig. 26.2).

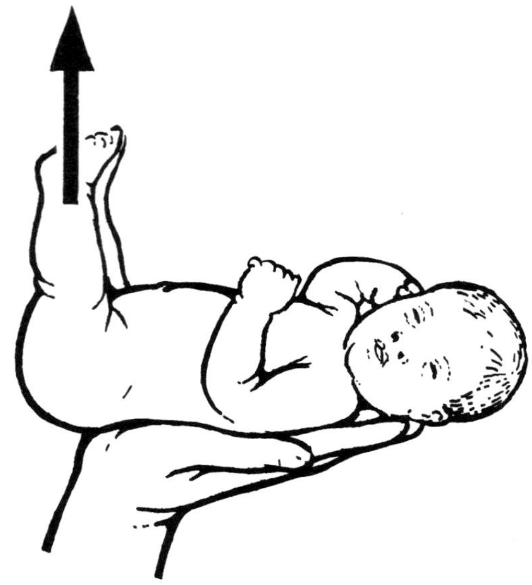

Fig. 26.2 Gallows traction for infant groin hernia incarceration —named 'Solomon' after the supposed role of King Solomon (I Kings 3:25).

In the adult, inguinal hernias are 10 times more frequent in males than females. Of inguinal hernias in male adults, 60% are indirect, 35% direct and 5% are a combination of direct and indirect, saddlebag or pantaloon hernias.[52] Indirect hernias are more frequent in younger men while the direct type are more frequent in older men. In women, indirect inguinal hernias are as common as femoral hernias.[53] Direct inguinal hernias are exceptionally rare in woman.[54] Both direct and indirect inguinal and femoral hernias are more frequent on the right than the left side at all ages: the ratio of right to left is 5 : 4.[49]

Indirect inguinal hernias are congenital; a patent processus opens under the stress of extrauterine intra-abdominal pressure—the saccular theory of Russell.[55] The co-determinants of an open processus vaginalis are prematurity, twins, low birth weight and race—Africans have a much higher incidence than Europeans;[56] indeed, on the island of Pemba off the East African coast, 30% of adult males have indirect inguinal hernias.[57] The African pelvis is more oblique and has a lower arch than the European pelvis; this lowness of the pubis is associated with a narrower origin of the internal oblique muscle from the lateral inguinal ligament. The narrow origin of the internal oblique muscle fails to protect the deep ring, and consequently indirect herniation is encouraged[58] (Fig. 26.3).

Another variant of abdominal wall anatomy is causally related to the development of direct inguinal herniation. The internal oblique and the transversus aponeurosis insertion into the superior aspect of the pubis where it forms the conjoint tendon normally extends laterally beyond the pubic tubercle and for 1–2 cm along the pectineal line where it is continuous with the iliopectineal ligament of Astley Cooper. In 10% of adult white subjects this lateral extension is lacking; these subjects are particularly liable to direct herniation.[59]

REFERENCES

47. Neidhardt J P H et al In: Chevrel J D (ed) Chirurgie des parois de l'abdomen. Springer Verlag, Berlin 1985
48. Rowe M I et al J Paediatr Surg 1969; 4: 102–107
49. Devlin H B Management of Abdominal Hernias. Butterworths, London 1988
50. Berkovitz G D et al Clin Endocrinol Metab 1983; 12: 155
51. Palmer B V Ann R Coll Surg Engl 1978; 60: 121
52. Qvist G Br J Surg 1977; 64: 442
53. Devlin H B In: Russell R C G (ed) Recent Advances in Surgery, vol II. Churchill Livingstone, Edinburgh 1982
54. Glassow F Br J Surg 1973; 60: 342
55. Russell R H Lancet 1906; iii: 1197
56. Badoe E A Afr J Med Sci 1973; 4: 51
57. Yordanov Y S, Stoyanov S K East Afr Med J 1969; 46: 867
58. Zinanovic S East Afr Med J 1968; 45: 41
59. Isaac R E Br J Surg 1961; 49: 204

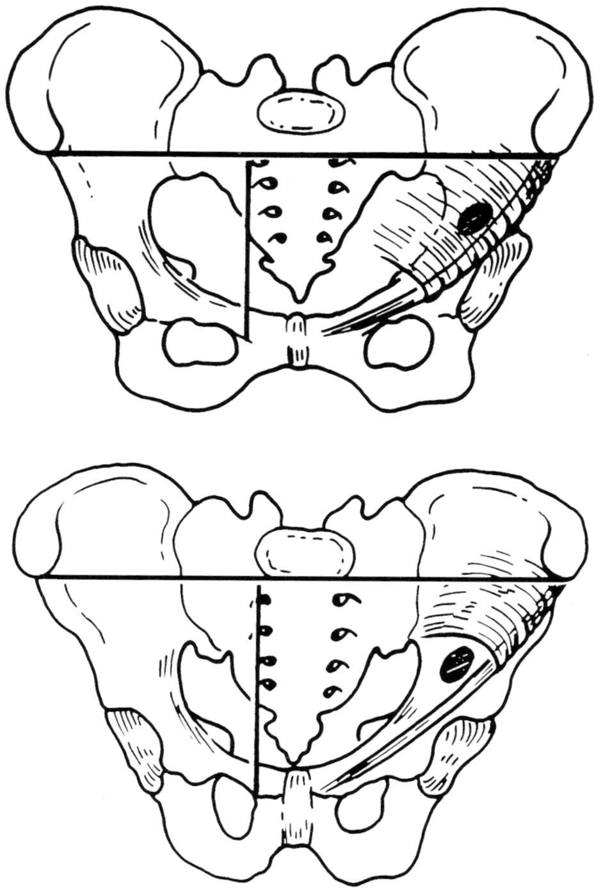

a

b

Fig. 26.3 The European pelvis (a) is wider than the African pelvis (b), which has a deeper pubic arch. Consequently the origin of the internal oblique muscle in the African provides a less competent closure of the deep inguinal ring. This predisposes to indirect inguinal herniation in the African.

Direct herniation is associated with smoking and with aortic aneurysm. Smoking is said to result in metastatic emphysema of collagen tissue,[60] although the concept of high levels of circulating elastase has not been confirmed. The link with aneurysm is confined to the saccular type; patients with occlusive disease or coronary artery disease do not share the same risk, implying a selective fibre degeneration.[61,62] A collagen defect has been demonstrated in these patients.[63] This is characterized by disorganized collagen fibrils in the aponeurosis, a raised leucocyte count, raised α_1-antitrypsin in the serum and delayed and deficient aponeurotic healing. Fibroblasts from inguinal hernia patients secrete increased quantities of II-procollagen which results in incomplete fibril assembly.[64] A genetic element has been suggested in Eskimos because of a high frequency of the human leucocyte antigen B27 allele which is associated with an increased prevalence of diseases associated with instability of mesenchymal tissues.[65]

Indirect hernias and hydrocoeles may occur as a complication of intraperitoneal fluid accumulation from any cause, including cardiac failure, cirrhotic or carcinomatous ascites and continuous ambulatory peritoneal dialysis. The mechanism of herniation is the opening up of a pre-existing processus vaginalis.[66]

TYPES AND DEFINITIONS OF GROIN HERNIAS

Indirect (oblique) inguinal hernia

An indirect inguinal sac is the remains of part or the whole of the processus vaginalis, a protrusion of peritoneum which accompanies the testis in its descent from the abdomen. The sac is congenital, even though the hernia may often not appear until late in adult life. It is considered congenital for the following reasons. Its anatomical relations are the same as those of the processus vaginalis and an empty sac in this position is often found at other operations when there is no actual hernia. Simple removal of the sac in childhood is curative and infantile hernias are occasionally associated with other anomalies such as an imperfectly descended testis.

The sac starts at the deep inguinal ring and may extend down the inguinal canal through the external ring and sometimes reaches the scrotum or labium majus. It is said to be incomplete or a bubonocoele if the sac is limited to the inguinal canal, and may be described as an inguinoscrotal or inguinolabial hernia if complete. If there is a complete vaginal sac, the testis will be lying free in the fundus of it. An interstitial hernia between the layers of the abdominal wall is found in 60% of boys with ectopic testicles.[67]

Direct inguinal hernia

In a direct inguinal hernia the sac lies behind the cord and the inferior epigastric artery lies lateral to the neck. The hernia passes directly forwards through the defect in the posterior wall of the inguinal canal formed by the fascia transversalis.

The hernia only rarely goes down along the cord to the scrotum; it is usually visible or palpable on coughing or standing and disappears during recumbency. Direct hernias are almost unknown in women.[51]

Femoral hernia

A femoral hernia comes through the femoral canal below and lateral to the inguinal ligament. The sac initially lies within the femoral sheath, then emerges through the fossa ovalis and bends upwards over the inguinal ligament where it may closely resemble a bubonocoele. The neck of a femoral hernia always lies below the inner end of the inguinal ligament, lateral to the pubic tubercle. A bubonocoele is above the inguinal ligament and may be medial to the pubic tubercle. An inguinal hernia is reduced by pressure laterally and backwards: a femoral hernia, if it is reducible at all, must be reduced downwards in the first instance, then backwards and upwards.

REFERENCES

60. Cannon D J, Read R C Ann Surg 1981; 194: 270–276
61. Lehnert B, Wadouh F Ann Vasc Surg 1992; 6: 134–137
62. Hall K A et al Am J Surg 1995; 170: 572–576
63. Cannon D J et al Arch Surg 1984; 119: 387
64. Friedman D W et al Ann Surg 1993; 218: 754–760
65. Harvald B Clin Genet 1989; 36: 364–367
66. Nelson H et al Surg Gynecol Obstet 1983; 157: 541
67. Spangen L, Andersson R, Ohlsson L Am Surg 1988; 54: 574

Clinical features of groin hernias

Pain and swelling are the cardinal symptoms of a groin hernia. The pain may be a dull dragging sensation which leads the patient to feel the groin and find the swelling. None the less, severe pain in the groin has a special clinical significance. Pain is complained of: at the first appearance of the hernia; if the hernia becomes strangulated; and sometimes in small, sometimes impalpable inguinal hernias in women.[63] The swelling of a groin hernia is usually intermittent at first. It is most frequently present in the evening, or after walking or on exertion.

The patient should first be examined relaxed and lying on the couch. Even if an inguinal hernia is not actually present at the time of examination, enlargement of the cord at the superficial inguinal ring may be felt by careful palpation as it emerges from the abdomen. Invagination of the canal with the examining finger thrust up the scrotal wall is uncomfortable and only gives useful information in very large hernias—when the diagnosis is obvious anyway. When the hernia is not obvious, a cough may send the abdominal contents down into the sac, and cough impulse may be felt by a finger placed over the external ring.

The patient should also always be examined standing up. In men, the position and size of the testicles must be checked when standing and in both sexes an inguinal or femoral hernia may only be apparent when the patient stands up and coughs. A second hernia of which the patient is unaware may be detected on standing.

Hypertrophy of the cord is another useful sign in infants and adults. The cord is gripped, and its constituents allowed to slip one by one through the examining fingers. Thickening of the cord contents may be detected on the side of the hernia — this is known as the 'rolled-silk' sign.

Differential diagnosis of groin hernias

A hernia needs to be differentiated from other groin lumps. This depends on demonstrating the clinical features of a hernia, which is a lump of varying size with an expansible cough impulse. However not all hernias are reducible and not all lumps that are reducible, such as varicocoeles, are hernias.

The anatomy of the hernia should be very carefully ascertained. While it is usually possible to distinguish inguinal from femoral hernias, there are many inaccuracies in preoperative diagnosis.[68] Some 10% of femoral hernias are misdiagnosed as inguinal.[69] It may not always be possible to differentiate between direct and indirect herniation. Although careful examination usually allows the hernia to be classified into one or other diagnostic categories, research has shown that this differential diagnosis is prone to error, even in experienced hands.[70] The accuracy of diagnosis of direct hernia is little better than 50%, whilst indirect hernia can be correctly diagnosed in 90% of patients.[71]

Other conditions which must be distinguished from hernias in the groin include the following:

1. Hydrocoeles of the cord or of the canal of Nuck. These may appear and disappear. They are usually oval, smooth, transilluminable and can be manipulated in the long axis of the cord. When they are pulled the testicle moves too, because it is attached to the cord. The testicle does not move when a hernia is reduced.
2. An ectopic testicle can easily be mistaken for an inguinal hernia if the patient is inadequately or cursorily examined. The scrotum and its contents must always be examined with the patient lying relaxed on the couch and standing erect.
3. A lipoma of the spermatic cord is soft and lobulated and does not vary with coughing.
4. Swellings of inguinal lymph nodes are generally multiple and extend laterally as well as lying medial to the femoral vessels.
5. A lipoma of the fat in the femoral canal can be differentiated from a femoral hernia only at operation; enlargement of this pad of fat often precedes the development of a femoral hernia and is sometimes said to be responsible for the hernia.
6. A saphenous varix presents as a cystic swelling which is easily emptied by pressure and disappears when the patient lies down. It usually has a bluish appearance and demonstrable thrill on coughing. A percussion impulse can be felt when dilated veins at the saphenofemoral junction are percussed.
7. A psoas abscess may transmit a cough impulse but is usually lateral to the femoral vessels. The patient will have symptoms and signs related to the primary pathology in the spine or retroperitoneum.
8. An iliofemoral aneurysm has an expansile pulsation (see Chapter 10).

Clinical examination remains the mainstay of diagnosis for inguinal and femoral hernias, but clinical differentiation between these groin lumps is notoriously unreliable. Much greater accuracy can be obtained by ultrasound scanning and this is recommended whenever there is doubt. Persistent intermittent groin pain in obese women is difficult to diagnose; in these cases, ultrasound may demonstrate an impalpable hernia.[67]

IMAGING AND THE ABDOMINAL WALL

Modern imaging has enabled more precise diagnosis of abdominal wall hernias, tumours, fistulas and infections. Standard X-rays (plain films) show alterations of tissue density in abdominal wall tumours, subcutaneous gas in gas-forming infections, gas shadows within gut in hernias, dilated intestine and fluid levels in obstructed hernias. Contrast films outline sinuses and fistulas at the umbilicus. A small bowel enema may demonstrate a Meckel's diverticulum. A barium enema may demonstrate the caecum or sigmoid colon in groin hernias and transverse colon in an umbilical hernia.

An intravenous urogram in a small child may show 'bladder ears' sliding into indirect inguinal hernias.[72] This investigation may also show a 'bladder hernia' within a direct inguinal hernia of

REFERENCES

68. Hardy J C, Costin J R J Am Osteopath Assoc 1969; 68: 696
69. Glassow F Ann Surg 1966; 163: 227
70. Ralphs D N L et al Br Med J 1980; 1: 1039
71. Cameron A E P Br J Surg 1994; 81: 250
72. Allen R P, Condon V R Radiology 1961; 77: 979

an adult, especially in males with bladder outflow obstruction. It may also show a sliding bladder in the femoral sacs of women. The ureter is rarely seen in the wall of a large femoral hernia.

Herniography is performed by injecting water-soluble contrast into the peritoneal cavity to outline a hernia sac.[73] It is a sensitive investigation capable of demonstrating hernia in the groin, even when physical examination has revealed nothing.[74] Hernias are often found in patients with obscure groin pain when investigated with herniography and subsequent surgical treatment relieves the discomfort. The use of this investigation in patients with symptoms after an inguinal hernia repair is particularly helpful (Fig. 26.4) because a normal herniogram provides important evidence that the hernia has not recurred, eliminating the need for re-exploration.[75] It is also occasionally useful in diagnosing hernias in infants.[76]

Ultrasound is very useful in diagnosing tumours and other disorders of the abdominal wall, especially in examining the groin for femoral or inguinal hernias (separating solid groin lumps from hernia sacs containing gut) and, most particularly, for diagnosing small incisional and spigelian hernias. Tumours and haematomas of the rectus sheath and muscles can also be readily diagnosed by this simple technique[77] (see Chapter 30).

Computed tomographic scanning is useful in assessing all tumours of the abdominal wall, but its resolution is inadequate to diagnose small hernias.

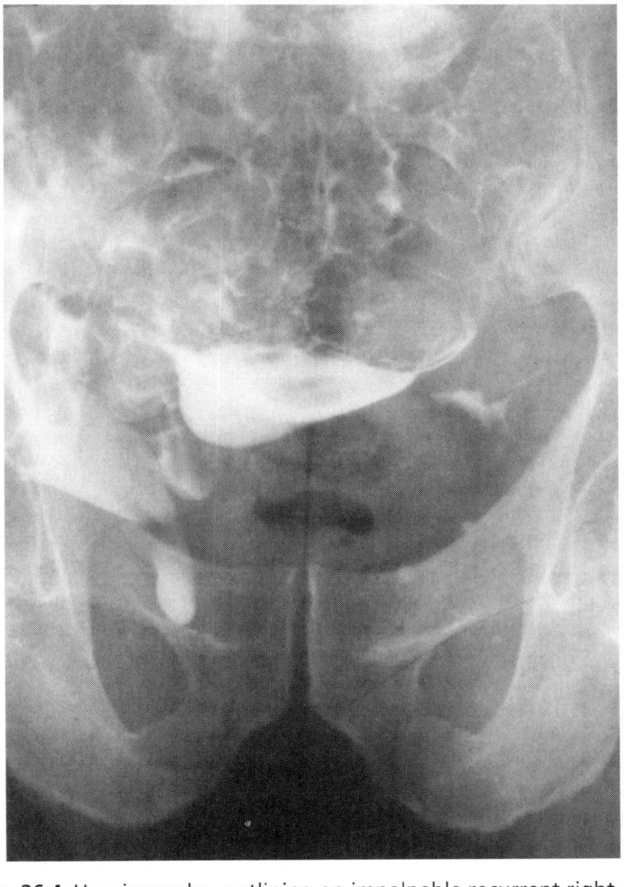

Fig. 26.4 Herniography, outlining an impalpable recurrent right inguinal hernia.

THE COMPLICATIONS OF HERNIAS

Incarceration, irreducibility, obstruction and strangulation

The constricting agent is the neck of the peritoneal sac which is often fibrosed and rigid where it traverses the parietal defect. In indirect inguinal hernias this defect is in the fascia transversalis at the deep ring; in direct inguinal hernias the defect is again in the fascia transversalis, this time more medially in the inguinal canal. The external ring may occasionally be the site of constriction in large inguinoscrotal hernias. In babies and small male children who have not yet developed an oblique inguinal canal the constricting agent is the rigid aponeurotic margin of the superficial inguinal ring.

In a femoral hernia the constriction is caused by fibrosis of the peritoneum in the neck of the sac at the femoral ring where it abuts on the inguinal ligament anteriorly, the lacunar ligament medially and the pectineal ligament posteriorly. The femoral vein, situated laterally, is rarely compressed and obstructed by a strangulated femoral hernia, suggesting that the constriction is in the wall of the sac rather than by the adjacent structures. The saphenous vein may however occasionally be occluded by a strangulated femoral hernia. In umbilical hernias the rigid aponeurotic margins which surround the neck of the peritoneal sac constrict the sac and its contents.

Strangulated small bowel is more frequently found in right groin hernias than left-sided ones (in a ratio of 2 : 1). This phenomenon is related to the anatomy of the small intestine rather than to the anatomy of hernial orifices (Fig. 26.5a).

The clinical features of strangulation are those of intestinal strangulation (see Chapter 29) with pain and tenderness localized over the irreducible hernia. Subcutaneous ecchymosis is often seen over strangulated hernias, especially in femoral or obturator hernias in emaciated elderly females.

Taxis — reduction en masse

Reduction by taxis can be attempted in all irreducible hernias. The risks are considerable as it may cause rupture of the bowel at the neck of the sac or return devitalized bowel to the abdomen. It may also result in reduction en masse of the hernia sac and strangulated contents out of sight through the abdominal ring or between the muscle layers of the abdominal wall. This can also be produced by the patient him- or herself (auto-reduction en masse), and the hernia may have been reduced for some days before the signs of strangulation arise (Fig. 26.5b,c).

The bowel may occasionally develop a stricture following the relief of strangulation by taxis—the intestinal stenosis of Garre. A

REFERENCES

73. Gullmo A World J Surg 1989; 13: 560–568
74. Smedberg S G G et al Am J Surg 1985; 149: 378–382
75. Hamlin J A, Kahn A M West J Med 1995; 162: 28–31
76. Hall C et al Br J Surg 1990; 77: 902
77. Deitch E A, Engel J M Surg Gynecol Obstet 1980; 151: 484

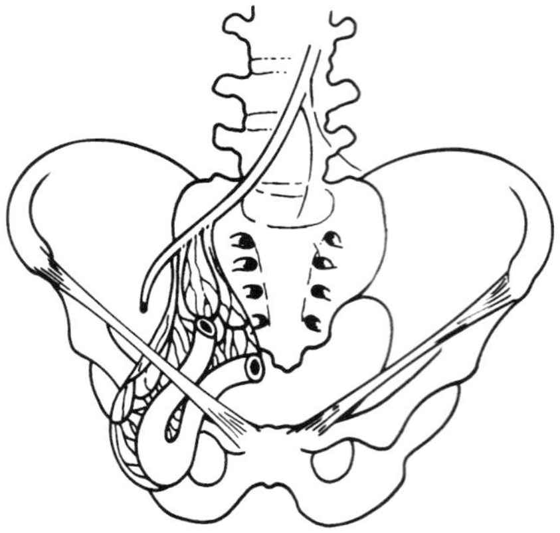

Fig. 26.5a Strangulated hernias containing small bowel are more frequent on the right than the left. This is determined by the anatomy of the mesentery.

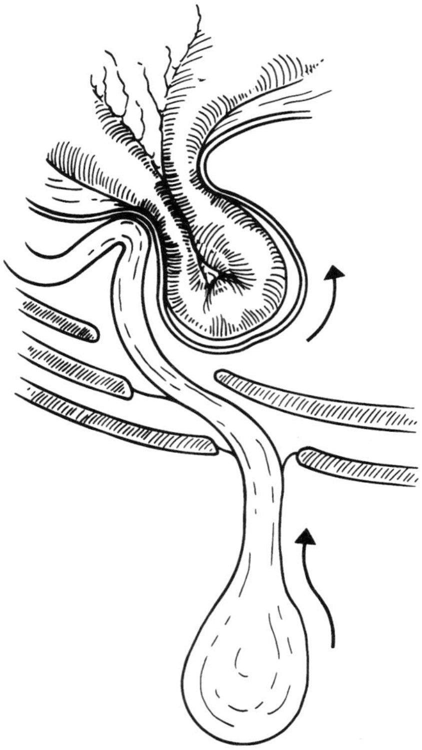

Fig. 26.5b Reduction en masse. Forcible reduction may rupture the parietal attachments of the sac, allowing the contents to be reduced, but with the constricting neck still intact and strangulating the bowel. The bowel is still strangulated in the sac pushed deep to the parietes, the cord is fore-shortened and the testicle drawn up. Traction on the testicle gives a pain and a tender mass is felt in the abdomen (Smiddy's sign).

double stricture can arise at the two sites of constriction of the afferent and efferent bowel within the hernia sac. This is caused by a reduction of devitalized gut into the peritoneal cavity. The patient develops diarrhoea and melaena, then progressive obstruction a few days after the hernia has been reduced.[78]

Operation is therefore almost always necessary when strangulation is suspected. The approach used should allow full inspection of the bowel proximal and distal to the obstruction, and of all the bowel reduced from the hernia sac. The bowel is observed and its colour, sheen and peristalsis assessed. If the bowel is red or blue, suffused with blood, oedematous and infarcted (Latin *infarcire*—to stuff), it is wrapped in warm saline soaks for 5 minutes and then reviewed again. It should be resected if the vitality does not return. Non-vital gut should not be returned to the peritoneal cavity as it may cause a postoperative stricture or even bowel mixture and peritonitis. If there is colonic infarction an anastomosis should not be performed; in these circumstances exteriorization of gut ends as stomas is a much safer option.

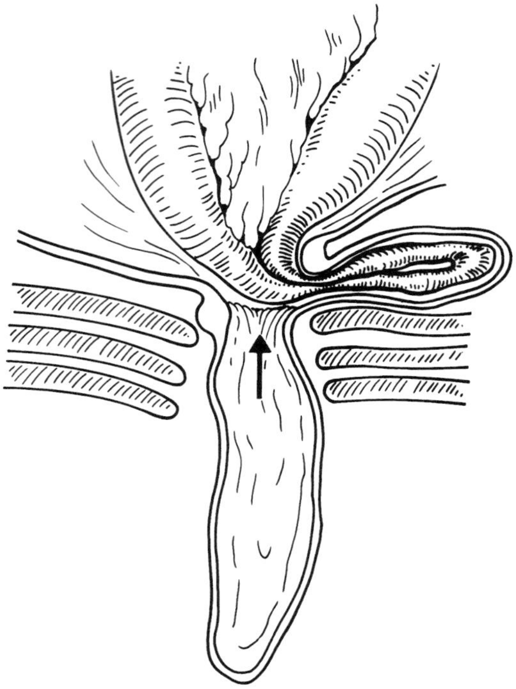

Fig. 26.5c Reduction en masse. Moynihan reported reduction en masse in a bilocular sac, the contents being moved from the external to the interstitial sac.

Maydl's hernia, afferent loop strangulation, Richter's and Littre's hernia

Maydl's hernia is a complication of large hernial sacs, especially right scrotal hernias in Africans, when a W loop of small gut lies in the sac. The intervening loop is strangulated within the main abdominal cavity by the constriction of the neck of the sac.[79] Afferent loop strangulation, again often seen in Africans, occurs when the gut of the afferent loop entering the hernial sac becomes entwined about the afferent and efferent loops leading to and from the sac.[80] Richter's hernia is present when part of the bowel, the antimesenteric margin, is strangulated in the sac. The intestinal obstruction is incomplete but the hernia is tender and irreducible and toxaemia occurs as gangrene develops in the strangulated portion of gut. This complication can develop in all tender and irre-

REFERENCES

78. Vowles K D J Br J Surg 1959; 47: 189
79. Bayley A C Br J Surg 1970; 57: 687
80. Philip P J Br J Surg 1967; 54: 96

ducible hernias, making exploration essential. Richter's hernia most often occurs in femoral, obturator and small incisional hernias (Fig. 26.6).

Littre's hernia is an oddity and rarity;[81] a hernia sac containing a strangulated Meckel's diverticulum. Littre's hernia can resolve spontaneously with gangrene, suppuration and formation of a local fistula. An inflamed Meckel's or appendix within the hernial sac can give similar signs.[82]

Spontaneous rupture of hernia sac

Spontaneous rupture of an incisional hernia sac and its overlying integument is well-recognized; the most frequent antecedent is a caesarean section. This is a surprisingly benign occurrence; peritonitis is rare and most patients survive reduction and repair. Presumably adhesions and oedema at the neck of the sac protect the main peritoneal cavity from immediate contamination, although urgent laparotomy is recommended.[83] Blunt trauma to the abdomen or when an inguinal hernia is 'down', or over-enthusiastic attempts at taxis can lead to rupture of the gut at the neck of the sac.[30]

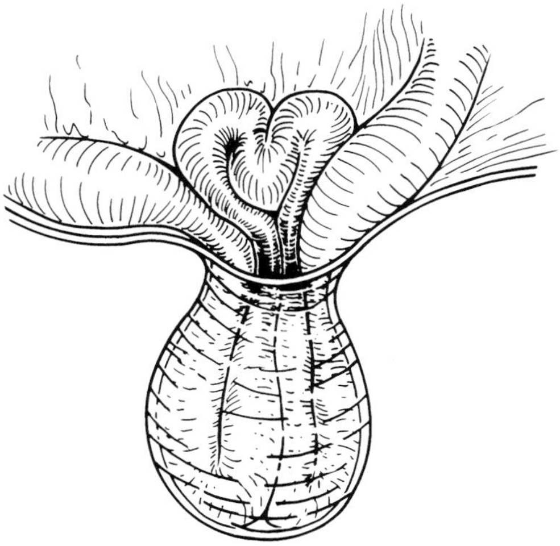

Fig 26.6a Maydl's or W-loop hernia strangulation.

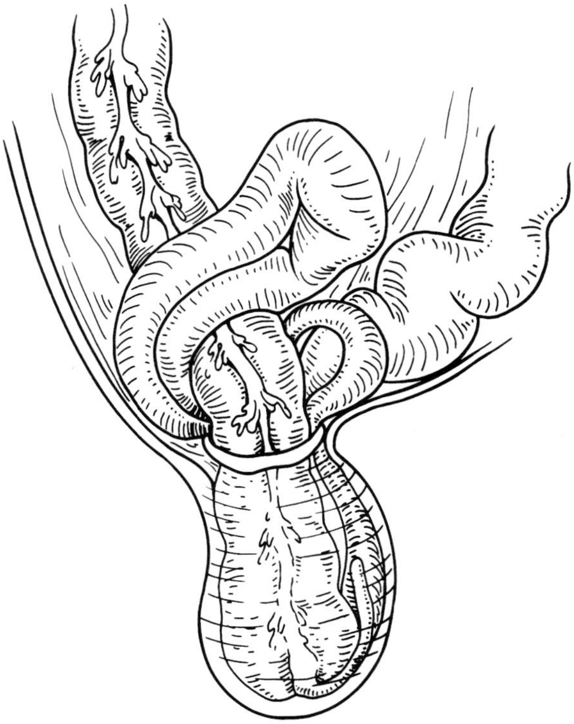

Fig. 26.6b Afferent loop strangulation.

REFERENCES

81. Treves F Medico-Chirurgical Transactions. London 1887; 52: 149–167
82. Cronin K, Ellis H Br J Surg 1959; 46: 364–367
83. von Helwig H Schweiz Med Woch 1958; 27: 662

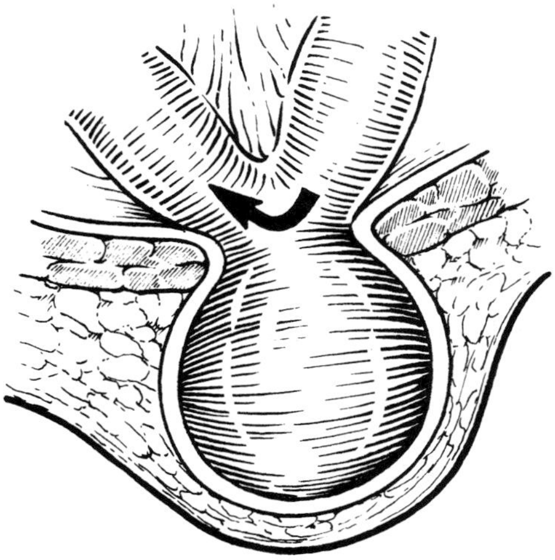

Fig. 26.6c Richter's hernia or partial enterocoele.

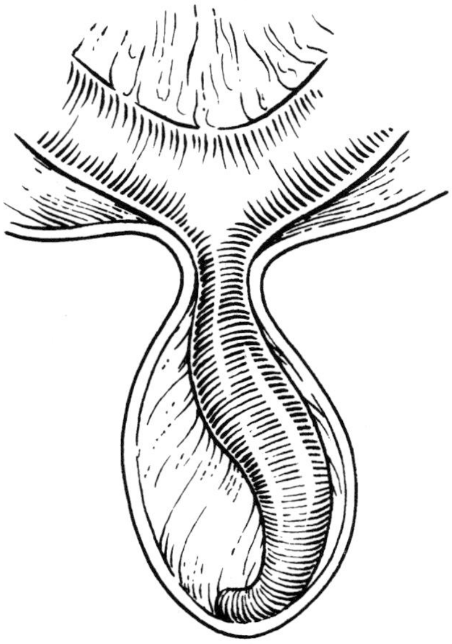

Fig. 26.6d Littre hernia—strangulation of a Meckel's diverticulum.

Involvement in peritoneal disease processes

Hernial sacs can become involved with many intra-abdominal disease processes. In infancy repeated incarcerations of the gut in the growing hernial sac can lead to local peritoneal hyperplasia, sometimes referred to as mesothelial hyperplasia. This is an exuberant reactive phenomenon and must be distinguished from true peritoneal mesothelioma (see Chapter 27).[42]

Any abdominal carcinoma can involve a hernia sac by transcoelomic seeding or direct invasion from a permanently incarcerated organ: colon, stomach and ovarian cancers can present in hernial sacs. When unexpected ascites and thickening of a hernia sac are found at operation, cytological examination of the ascitic fluid and histological examination of the sac should be performed. Routine histology of all hernial sacs to detect occult malignancy has been advocated but a critical review of the detection rate shows this strategy is not cost-effective—3×10^6 normal specimens have to be examined to find one occult carcinoma.[84]

A mini-laparotomy through the sac wall gives additional information if malignancy is found in a hernia sac. It is probably best to proceed with the hernia repair, taking care not to implant malignant tissue in the repaired wound. The patient should have a laparotomy as soon as possible if resection is considered feasible. To perform major cancer surgery at the time of the original hernioplasty operation on an unprepared and inadequately assessed patient is not advisable.

Intra-abdominal mesothelioma (see Chapter 27) can spread into a hernia sac. This malignant condition must be distinguished from the reactive mesothelial hyperplasia encountered in infancy.[85] Endometriosis sometimes occurs in hernia sacs of menstruating women. It is most frequently found in incisional hernias after gynaecological operations or caesarean delivery.[49] Peritonitis, from whatever cause, can lead to a pus-filled hernia sac.[86] Appendicitis has been described in inguinal, femoral and umbilical hernias.[87] A blood-filled hernial sac can develop in patients with leaking aneurysms or ruptured ovarian cysts.

Sliding hernia—hernie en glissade

'Sliding hernia' is the term applied to a hernia whose sac wall is composed in part of its circumference by a viscus such as the caecum or colon which does not have a complete investment of peritoneum. The bowel forms part of the hernia, but lies outside the cavity of the sac. Sliding hernias are common at the extremes of life; in children sliding hernias of the bladder are frequent in the medial wall of indirect sacs in boys, and sliding hernias can contain the ovary and tubes in girls. Large and long-standing sliding hernias occur in elderly subjects. Sometimes a huge part of the sigmoid or caecum may be extruded, with a small sac related to only the upper part of the hernia (Fig. 26.7).

At operation any patulous redundant sac is removed and the hernial contents are mobilized before being reduced back into the abdominal cavity. In any hernia containing colon great care must be taken to avoid opening bowel in mistake for sac. Reduction of the visceral contents and sac behind the repaired fascia transversalis is all that is necessary.[88]

Herniation of female internal reproductive organs—pregnancy

The ovary and tubes are commonly found in inguinal hernias in small girls. They must be carefully preserved and returned to the

REFERENCES

84. Kasson M A et al Surg Gynecol Obstet 1986; 163: 518
85. Brenner J et al J Surg Oncol 1981; 18: 159
86. Cronin K, Ellis H Br J Surg 1959; 46: 364
87. Thomas W E G et al Ann R Coll Surg Engl 1982; 64: 121
88. Ponka J L Am J Surg 1966; 112: 52

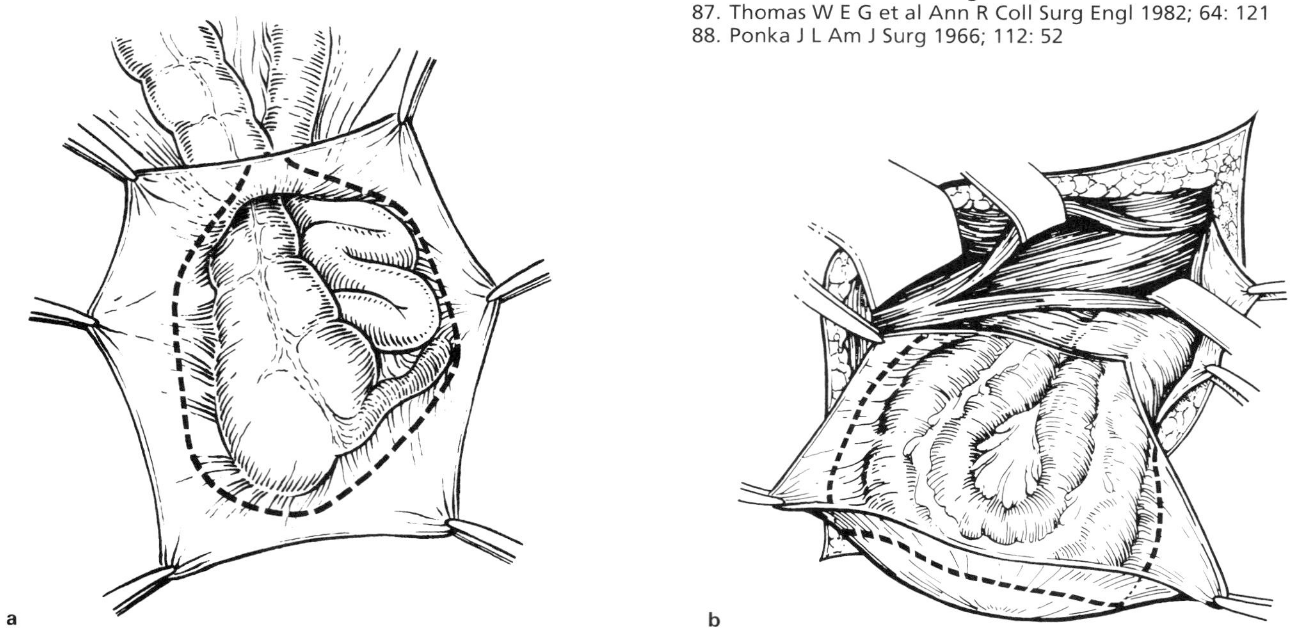

Fig. 26.7 A sliding hernia usually contains the large bowel as a component of the wall of an inguinal hernia. (**a**) The caecum is on the right; (**b**) the sigmoid colon is on the left.

abdomen. In older women sliding hernias of the ovary and tubes are not infrequent in femoral, inguinal and obturator hernias. In 1757 Sir Percival Pott described a woman with bilateral inguinal hernias containing the ovaries.[89] Pott performed a bilateral herniotomy and removed both ovaries; he observed that the woman ceased her menstrual flow and developed the breast and body changes of old age. The uterus is a rare finding in a hernial sac but none the less pregnancy in incarcerated umbilical and inguinal hernias is well-recorded in the literature.[90]

Testicular complications

Infarction or ischaemia of the testicle may occur in infants with an incarcerated inguinal hernia. The testicular vessels are compromised at the superficial inguinal ring. At operation the testicle is discoloured, blue and swollen. The testicular vessels should be carefully dissected off the sac, the testicle preserved and left in the scrotum. Postoperatively the testicle feels hard, but many of these testicles recover, or at least maintain endocrine function, and are hormonally and cosmetically useful in later life. The incidence of postoperative testicular ischaemia is reduced if the testicle is not dislocated from its scrotal bed at operation (see below).[91] Spontaneous testicular infarction occurs as a complication of giant indirect inguinal hernias in adult Africans, the testicular vessels being occluded at the deep inguinal ring.[92]

Transient ischaemic orchitis is a well-recorded complication of a groin hernia repair in adults.[93] The condition is slow in onset after operation. Oedema and swelling of the testicle is the first change to be noted followed by shortening and tenderness of the cord, local pain and a low-grade fever. The pathophysiology is thrombosis of the pampiniform plexus, usually with incomplete venous infarction, progressing to partial testicular atrophy. Frank testicular gangrene is very rare. The condition is more frequent after repair of recurrent inguinal hernias. Ischaemic orchitis complicates 0.3% of primary inguinal hernia repairs.[94] The incidence of the condition is reduced if the dissection of the cord is not extended medial to and below the pubic tubercle and if the testicle is not disturbed in the scrotum.[95] Avoidance of dissection of the cord medial to the pubic tubercle preserves the superficial pudendal-to-cord anastomosis. This cord-to-pudendal anastomosis and the testicular blood supply itself are sometimes precarious in patients who have had a previous vasectomy; in these cases every care must be taken if the testicular blood supply is to be maintained (and subsequent litigation avoided).

An indirect inguinal hernial sac which extends medial to the pubic tubercle or into the scrotum should never be dissected out because this dissection will damage the cord vessels and is followed by a higher incidence of testicular ischaemia. The large indirect sac should be transected at its neck, the parietal peritoneum closed and the distal sac left open and undisturbed in the cord.

The management of ischaemic orchitis is expectant. Most testicles recover with a scrotal support. Antibiotics are not indicated—it is a vascular, not an infective condition.

Postoperative hydrocoele is a rare complication of inguinal hernia repair. Hydrocoele is more likely if much of the fat and as a result the lymphatic is dissected out of the cord. Halsted in 1889[96] abandoned skeletonization of the cord to avoid this hazard. Today the incidence of post hernial hydrocoele is less than 0.5%. Virtually all these hydrocoeles resolve spontaneously; if they cause discomfort they should be aspirated once. Operation is rarely required.[97]

PRINCIPLES OF HERNIA MANAGEMENT

There are three principles which govern hernia management:

1. The patient must be resuscitated.
2. The hernia must be reduced.
3. The defect must be repaired.

Resuscitation and the management of any co-morbidity are crucial in hernia management and this is especially true in neonates and the elderly.[98] The mortality for elective groin hernia repair is almost zero at all ages, but in strangulated hernia repair the mortality increases with age: at 60 years it is 3%, at 70 years it is 6%, at 80 years it is 12%.[46]

This mortality is related almost entirely to haemodynamic, respiratory and renal disease. Time spent resuscitating the patient lowers this mortality. To quote Moynihan: 'We have made surgery safe for the patient; we must now make the patient safe for surgery'.[99]

Reduction and repair of individual hernias are described in the separate sections.

PROSTHESES

Many abdominal hernias occur through parietal defects that are too large to close by simple coaptation of the tissues. To close these defects prostheses must be used and over the years many materials have been tried. A distillation of this experience indicates that a successful prosthesis must be chemically and biologically inert; easily sterilizable, flexible and not prone to physical change or hardening in the body. Prostheses must be strong enough to last until the patient's death.

Modern polymer chemistry has produced many of the present prostheses. Monofilament knitted polypropylene (Marlex® mesh) is a popular and proven prosthesis.[100] There are four major problems associated with biomaterials:[101] rejection, infection, fixation

REFERENCES

89. Pott P Treatise on Ruptures. Hitch and Hawes, London 1757
90. Watson L F Hernia. Kimpton, London 1938
91. Puri P et al J Paediatr Surg 1984; 19: 44
92. Magogunje O A et al Trans R Soc Trop Med 1980; 74: 749
93. Wantz G E Surg Gynecol Obstet 1982; 154: 570
94. Wantz G E Surg Clin North Am 1984; 64: 287–298
95. Fong Y, Wantz G E Surg Gynecol Obstet 1992; 174: 399–402
96. Halsted W S Bull Johns Hopkins Hosp 1889; 1: 12
97. Obney N J Can Med Assoc 1957; 77: 463
98. Buck N, Devlin H B, Lunn J N Report of a Confidential Enquiry into Perioperative Deaths. Nuffield Provincial Hospitals Trust and King's Fund, London 1987
99. Moynihan B G A Harvein oration. Lancet 1926; 2: 789
100. Lamb J P et al Surgery 1983; 93: 643
101. Amid P K et al Postgrad Gen Surg 1992; 4: 150–155

and host tissue incorporation. Polypropylene mesh shows rapid, complete fixation without wrinkling with good fibroblast penetration and collagen ingrowth. A minimum mesh pore size of at least 10 μm allows the polymorphs to enter and seek out any bacteria. The repair of many thousands of groin and incisional hernias with no ensuing problems of infection or rejection and with low recurrence rates is evidence for the efficacy of Marlex® mesh.[102,103] Other monofilament meshes such as Prolene® are available[104] and French surgeons have favoured the multifilament material Dacron® in the preperitoneal approach to recurrent groin hernia.[105] Removal of monofilament biomaterials from infected wounds is generally not necessary, antibiotic treatment being effective in eradicating bacteria.[106] The treatment of infection in multifilamentous material is more problematic.

Expanded polytetrafluoroethylene (ePTFE) is useful in incisional hernia repair, particularly where there is a risk of the prosthesis coming into contact with bowel.[107] The risk of development of adhesions to ePTFE leading to intestinal obstruction is small.[108] Inlay ePTFE has been used to repair primary, complex and recurrent inguinal hernia, but has been largely abandoned in laparoscopic repair.[109,110]

The prostheses should be fixed in position with sutures of a compatible suture material. It is important to allow the prosthesis to overlap the edges of the defect to permit fibroblast invasion to bond the prosthesis to the aponeurosis. A minimum overlap of 2–3 cm is advisable and the mesh should be quilted to the adjacent tissue. The quilting sutures are not essential if the mesh is put into the extraperitoneal layer between the intact peritoneum and the parietes.

INGUINAL HERNIA IN BABIES AND CHILDREN

Ten per cent of children with inguinal hernias present as emergencies with incarceration, which has its highest incidence in the first 3 months of life. Although incarceration is common, strangulation is rare.[111] In infants prompt elective surgery for inguinal hernia is essential, whatever the age of the child. The probability of incarceration is 1 in 4 for all inguinal hernias in male children before the age of 1.

Until the inguinal canal develops its obliquity at the age of 11–12 years, simple herniotomy is sufficient to repair the common indirect inguinal hernia. The operation should be carefully performed to avoid testicular vessel damage and to give a good cosmetic scar.[112] A skin-crease incision is made 1 cm cephalad to the external inguinal ring. The cord is defined as it emerges from the inguinal canal, and the fibres of the cremaster are gently opened to display the blue peritoneal sac on the anterosuperior aspect of the cord. The sac is separated from the cord structures and, if the sac is complete, extending into the scrotum and containing the testicle, it is divided across and the distal sac is left in situ without dislocating the testis from the scrotum. The sac is dissected proximally and its neck with the parietal peritoneum is identified. Any contents are returned to the peritoneal cavity; this is especially important in the female when the fallopian tube and ovary can be a sliding component of the hernia sac wall. The sac is tranfixed and ligated at its junction to the peritoneal cavity and any redundant sac excised before the wound is closed.

The testicle should not be dislocated from the scrotum during the operation as this causes a higher incidence of testicular ischaemia. The surgeon must check that the testicle is in its proper place in the scrotum at the completion of the operation, to avoid iatrogenic ectopic testicles.

INGUINAL HERNIA IN ADULTS

It is important to recognize, as Bassini did over 100 years ago,[113] that inguinal hernia, both indirect and direct, is the result of failure in the transversalis fascia of the abdominal wall.[114] Repairing or reinforcing this layer should cure inguinal hernias.[115] Bassini himself always divided and repaired the transversalis fascia[116]—a fact overlooked by many British surgeons.

Reinforcement of the inguinal canal by darning between the conjoint tendon and the inguinal ligament is an old concept. Darns with kangaroo tendon,[117] human fascia lata,[118] floss silk[119] and wire[120] have all been tried and found wanting. Darning with monofilament nylon was popularized by Moloney of Oxford immediately after the 1939–1945 war.[121] Moloney himself reported impressive results; in his initial series of 400 cases he had no recurrences at 2-year follow-up. Moloney was meticulous in his technique; he always dissected and sutured the fascia transversalis at the deep ring before he darned the direct area. This attention to the fascia transversalis may have accounted for his excellent results. Others have omitted this fascia transversalis repair and obtained poor results. The most recent report of a darn technique reported a cumulative recurrence rate greater than 10% at 62 months.[122]

Three open techniques to repair the transversalis fascia are recommended: the Shouldice operation,[123] the McVay–Cooper ligament operation[124] and the Lichtenstein hernioplasty.[125] The French extraperitoneal open mesh operation for recurrent hernia is also reported to give good results.[126]

REFERENCES

102. Molloy R G et al Br J Surg 1991; 78: 242–244
103. Shulman A G et al Am Surg 1992; 58: 255–257
104. Capozzi J A et al Surg Gynecol Obstet 1988; 167: 124–128
105. Stoppa R E et al Surg Clin North Am 1984; 64: 269–285
106. Gilbert A I, Felton L L Surg Gynecol Obstet 1993; 177: 126–130
107. Hamer-Hodges D W, Scott N B J R Coll Surg Edinb 1985; 30: 65
108. Deysine M Am J Surg 1992; 163: 422–424
109. Kennedy C M, Matyas J A Am J Surg 1994; 168: 304–306
110. Pailler J L et al Postgrad Gen Surg 1992; 4: 168–170
111. Nussbaum A Munch Med Wochenschr 1913; 60: 1434
112. Harvey M H et al Br J Surg 1985; 72: 485
113. Bassini E Arch Klin Chir 1890; 40: 429
114. Read R C Surgery 1980; 88: 682
115. Berliner S et al Am J Surg 1978; 135: 666
116. Catterina A Bassini's Operation. Lewis, London 1934
117. Marcy H O Trans 7th Int Med Congress. London 1881; 2: 446
118. McArthur L L JAMA 1901; 37: 1162
119. Maingot R Br Med J 1941; 1: 777
120. McGavin L Br Med J 1909; 2: 357
121. Moloney G E, Gill W G, Barclay R C Lancet 1948; ii: 45
122. Lifschutz H, Juler G L Arch Surg 1986; 121: 717
123. Glassow F Ann R Coll Surg Engl 1976; 58: 133
124. McVay C B, Chapp J D Ann Surg 1958; 148: 499
125. Lichtenstein I L Am J Surg 1987; 153: 553–559
126. Stoppa R et al Chirurgie 1982; 108: 570

Shouldice operation

In the Shouldice operation (Fig. 26.8) an oblique groin incision is made 2 cm cephalad and parallel to the inguinal ligament. The external oblique aponeurosis is opened in the line of the incision. The cremaster muscle is removed from the cord to give good access to the deep ring. The margins of the deep ring are dissected from the cord and the fascia transversalis is opened medially down to the pubic tubercle. The fascia transversalis is cleared of extraperitoneal fat to expose the deep surface of the conjoint tendon. This tendon is seen as a 'white line' through the fascia transversalis. The fascia transversalis is also cleared of extraperitoneal fat as it plunges into the thigh, posterior to the inguinal ligament, to become the anterior layer of the femoral sheath.

If an indirect sac is present it is excised and the neck is sutured where it is continuous with the parietal peritoneum. A direct sac does not usually need excision, but the transversalis fascia is opened, the sac is inverted and the peritoneum is kept deep to the fascia transversalis when it is repaired.

The lower lateral fascia transversalis flap is then sutured to the undersurface of the upper medial flap along the 'white line' of the transversalis flap. The upper flap of fascia transversalis is overlapped and sutured to the anterior surface of the lower lateral flap of fascia transversalis. This reconstructs and tightens the fascia transversalis in the posterior wall of the inguinal canal. The suturing is taken laterally to make a new deep ring flush with the emergent cord. The fascia transversalis repair is then reinforced by suturing the aponeurotic conjoint tendon to its anterior surface and the lowermost aponeurosis of the external oblique adjacent to the inguinal ligament medially. The cord is replaced. The external oblique aponeurosis is closed anterior to the cord. All the suturing is now done with continuous monofilament non-absorbable sutures.

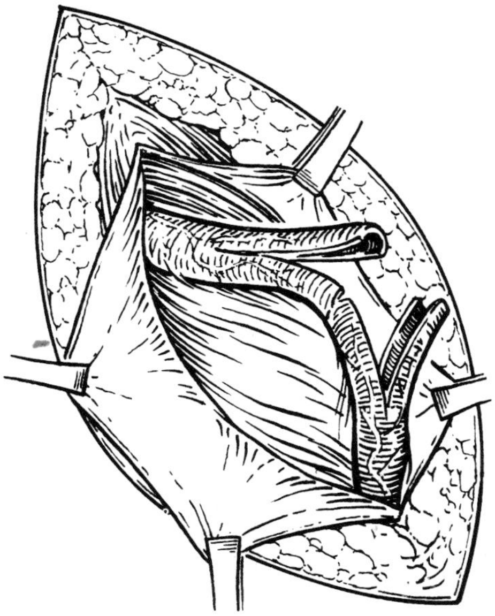

Fig. 26.8a The Shouldice repair for inguinal hernia. **(a)** After a conventional skin incision the external oblique muscle is split in the length of the canal to give access to the cord and fascia transversalis. The cremaster is removed from the cord. This enables an indirect sac to be identified and the deep ring dissected.

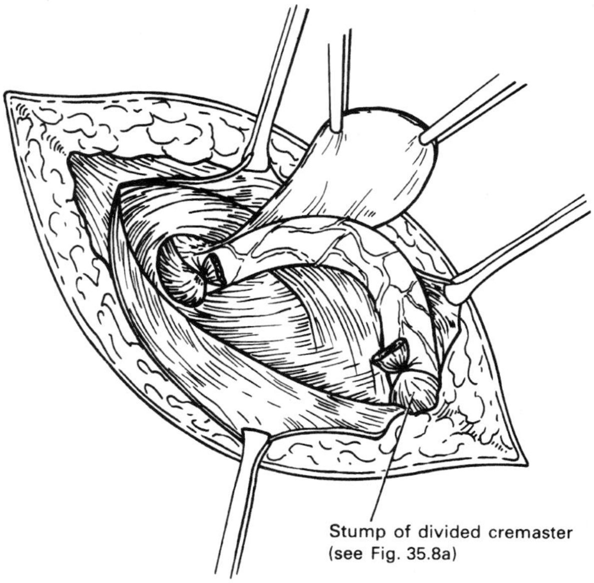

Fig. 26.8b The indirect sac on the anterosuperior aspect of the cord is cleared.

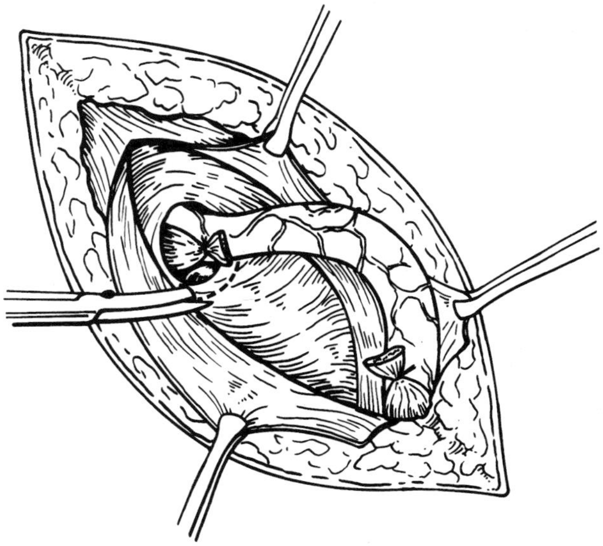

Fig. 26.8c The deep ring is defined about the cord. Any small crescent of peritoneum is noted. The deep ring is dissected clear of the emergent cord.

McVay–Cooper repair

In the McVay–Cooper ligament repair the deep ring in the fascia transversalis is repaired tightly around the cord and then the transversalis lamina is reinforced by suturing the aponeurotic conjoint tendon from medial to lateral to the iliopectineal or Cooper's ligament.[127] This invariably puts the aponeurosis under strain and is not conducive to healing, so a rectus muscle slide (Wöfler, Bloodgood, Reinhart or Tanner) is needed to ease the tension.[128] To

REFERENCES

127. Rutledge R H Surgery 1988; 103: 1
128. Tanner N C Br J Surg 1942; 29: 285

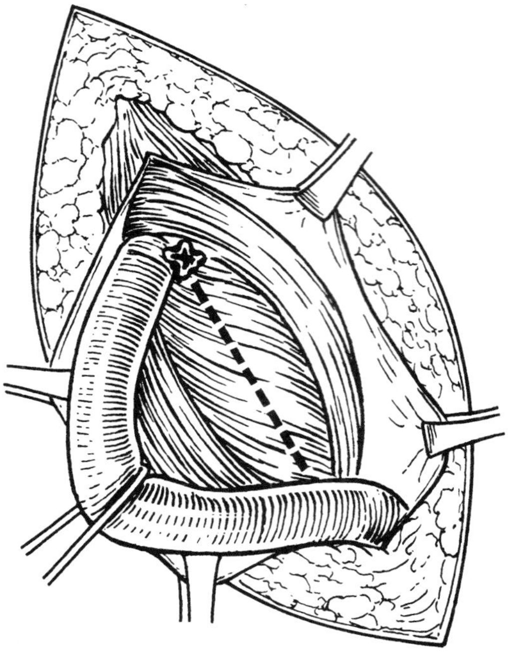

Fig. 26.8d The fascia transversalis is dissected and opened throughout the posterior wall of the canal.

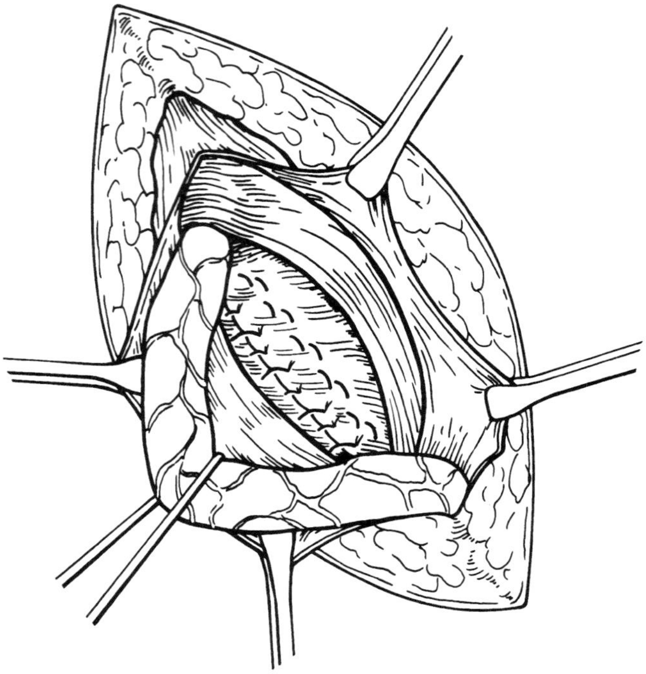

Fig. 26.8f The repair is completed by bringing the upper medial flap of fascia transversalis down to double-breast the layer and suturing to the anterior surface of the lower flap just proximal to where the lower fascia transversalis goes deep to the inguinal ligament and becomes the anterior femoral sheath.

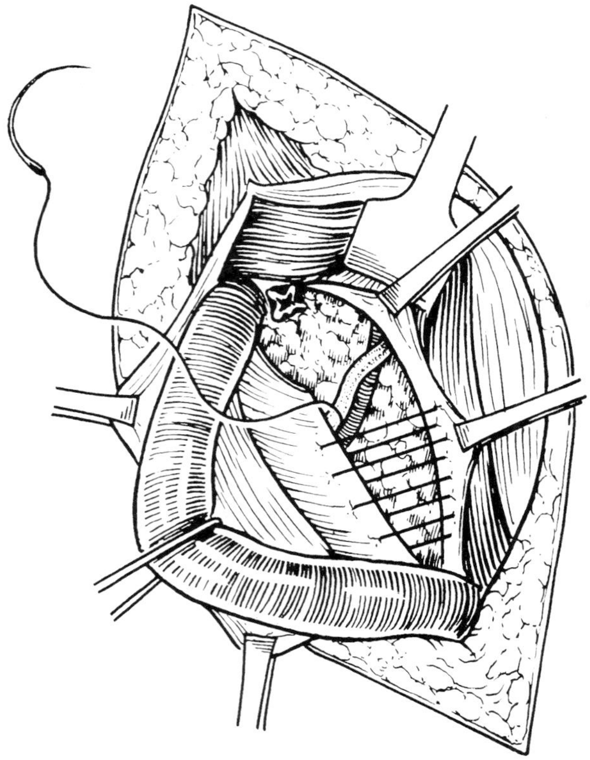

Fig. 26.8e The repair is made by suturing the cut margin of the lower lateral flap of fascia transversalis to the undersurface of the upper medial flap along the 'white line' of the conjoint tendon or arch.

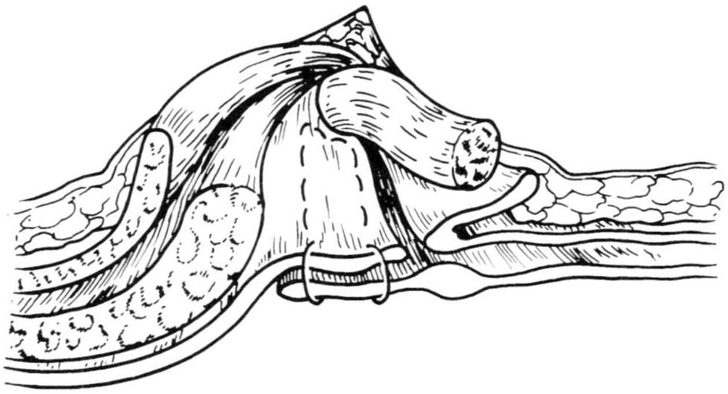

Fig. 26.8g This double-breasting allows a snug closure of the fascia transversalis up to the medial side of the cord to form a new competent deep ring.

make the slide the external oblique in front of the lowermost rectus sheath is retracted as far medially as possible. Then a vertical incision is made in the deep lamina of the anterior rectus sheath to expose the underlying rectus muscle. This incision should be 1 cm from the midline and 5–7 cm long (Fig. 26.9).

Lichtenstein mesh repair

In the Lichtenstein mesh hernioplasty the approach to the inguinal canal and herniotomy is identical to the Shouldice operation, but the fascia transveralis is left undisturbed. Excision of the cremaster

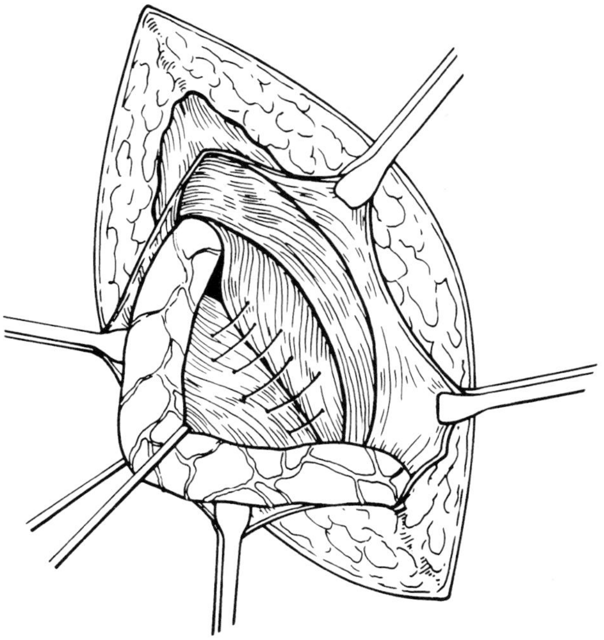

Fig. 26.8h The medial repair is reinforced by attaching the white aponeurotic anterior surface of the internal oblique to the external oblique medially.

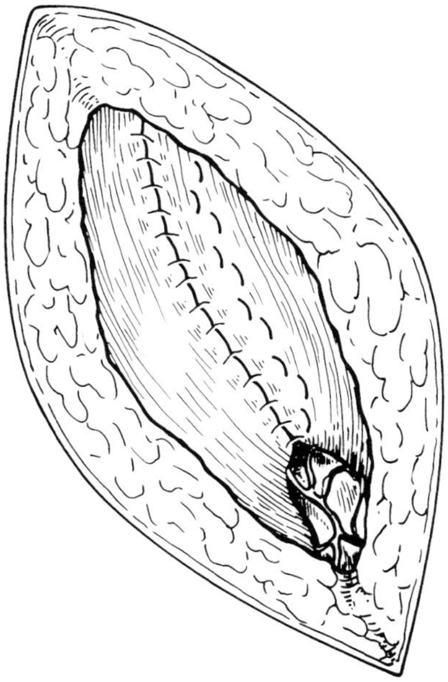

Fig. 26.8i The cord is replaced and the external oblique closed anteriorly to it with an overlap. Non-absorbable monofilament sutures are used throughout.

is unnecessary; fenestration to inspect the cord contents and search for an indirect sac is adequate. A bulging direct sac may be inverted by a running suture to flatten the posterior wall without tension. A pre-cut rectangle of mesh (Fig. 26.10a) is now tailored to the individual patient's requirements by trimming it appropriately to fit between the inguinal ligament and reflected external oblique (Fig. 26.10b). The mesh is now placed to lie side-to-side with the inguinal ligament with the medial corner overlapping the pubic tubercle by 1–2 cm. It should lie over the internal oblique/conjoint tendon with wide overlapping.

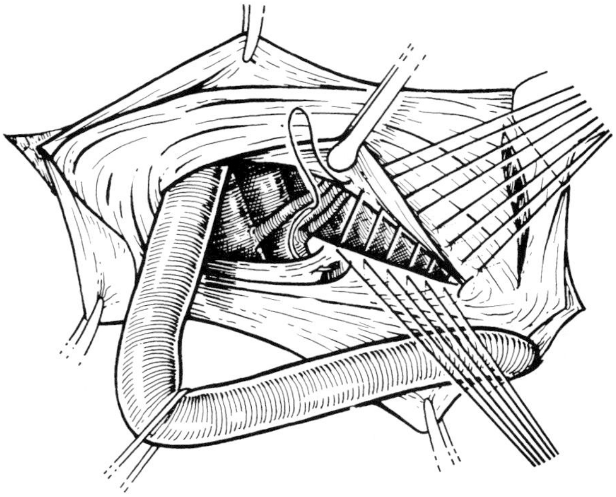

Fig. 26.9 The McVay–Cooper ligament operation. The fascia transversalis is repaired to adjust and tighten the deep ring by suturing the divided fascia transversalis and the conjoint tendon, the triple layer of Bassini, to the pectineal ligament medially and the fascia transversalis laterally as far as the emergent cord. A relaxing incision in the deep lamina (internal oblique) of the anterior rectus sheath will allow the medial structures to be slid down to facilitate the medial repair. The triple layer is sutured laterally to the inferior fascia transversalis so that the femoral cone is also closed.

The mesh must be sutured in position in order to prevent it shifting and developing gaps between the mesh and the underlying aponeurosis.[129] A running monofilament suture should fix the mesh to the aponeurosis and the reflected edge of the inguinal ligament from 2 cm beyond (medial) the pubic tubercle and a point just lateral to the internal ring. The mesh is slit horizontally from its lateral margin to accommodate the cord. The 'fish-tails' so produced are brought around the cord (Fig. 26.10c). Two or three interrupted sutures are placed between the upper edge of the mesh and the underlying aponeurosis and a suture is used to close the internal ring which secures the lower edge of the upper and lower flap to the inguinal ligament (Fig. 26.10d). The tails are then trimmed and tucked laterally beneath the external oblique aponeurosis. This hernioplasty is rapidly gaining in popularity.[130,131]

The French extraperitoneal mesh repair

The extraperitoneal space is opened through a midline or lateral Pfannenstiel incision. The groin is approached from behind the muscles of the abdominal wall; any peritoneal sacs are eased out of the parietal defects and then excised. A large sheet of prosthetic mesh is placed between the peritoneum and parietes to reinforce the fascia transversalis (Fig. 26.11).[126]

REFERENCES

129. Lichtenstein I L et al Am J Surg 1989; 157: 188–193
130. Davies N et al Br J Surg 1994; 81: 1478–1479
131. Kark A E et al Ann R Coll Surg Engl 1995; 77: 299–304

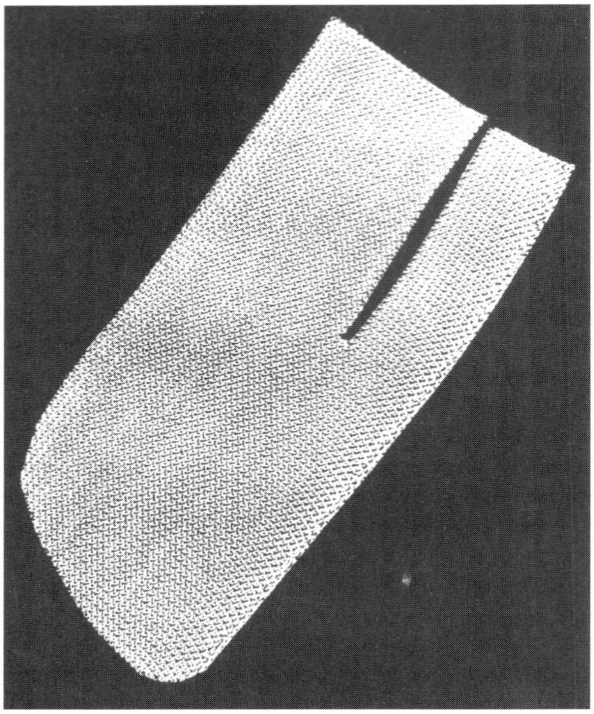

Fig. 26.10a Mesh prior to suturing.

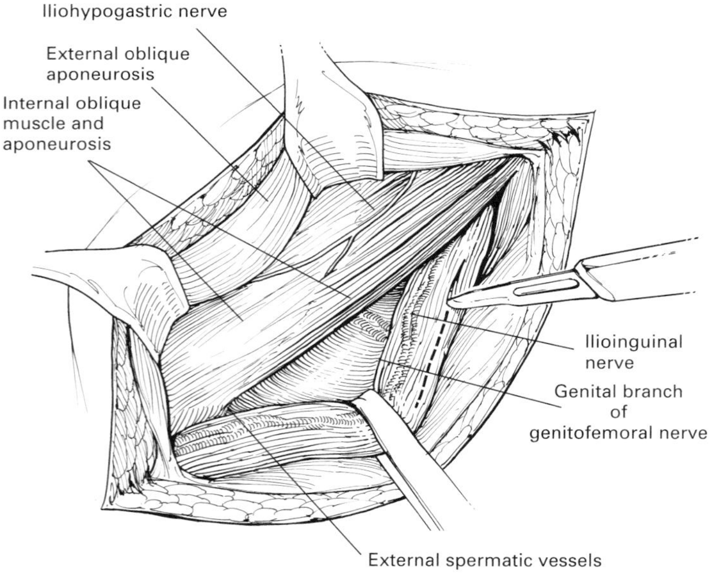

Fig. 26.10b The spermatic cord, together with its cremasteric covering, external spermatic vessels and genital nerve, is raised and the cremasteric fibres are cut transversely or longitudinally at the level of the internal ring.

Overview

The above techniques all have the following principles in common:

1. All the possible hernia sites are carefully inspected at each operation, avoiding the possibility of a missed hernia.
2. The transversalis fascia is repaired.

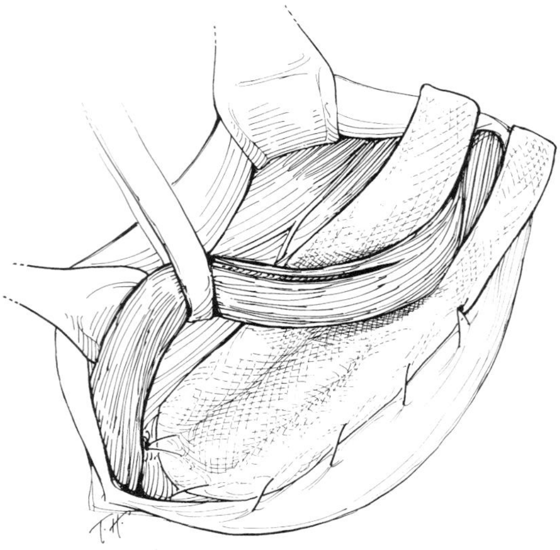

Fig. 26.10c The spermatic cord is placed in between the two tails of the mesh.

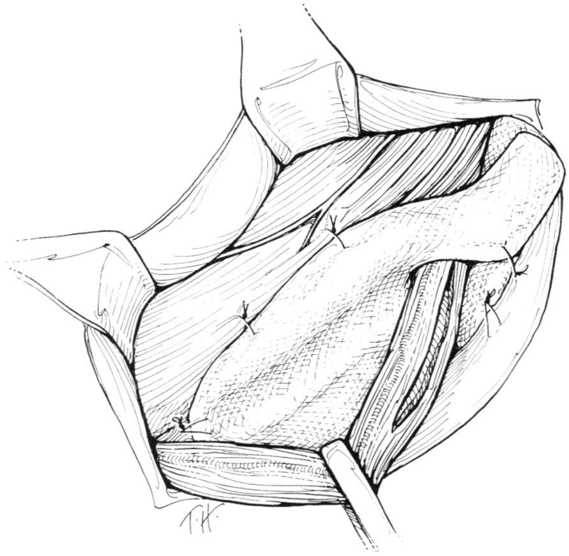

Fig. 26.10d The lower edges of the two tails are sutured to the shelving margin for creation of a new internal ring made of mesh.

3. Non-absorbable sutures or prostheses are used for the repair as aponeurotic healing is slow.
4. Only aponeurotic tissue is sutured or used for fixation of prosthesis as red muscle possesses no intrinsic strength.

The recurrence rate for all groin hernias should be less than 2% at 5 years, if one of these techniques is used and all of these principles are applied. Sepsis and tissue necrosis must be avoided by careful technique[96] and damage to the vas and testicular vessels is also essential.

LAPAROSCOPIC REPAIR

Laparoscopic hernia repair is feasible technically and is efficacious in the short term. In 1994 an expert panel of the European

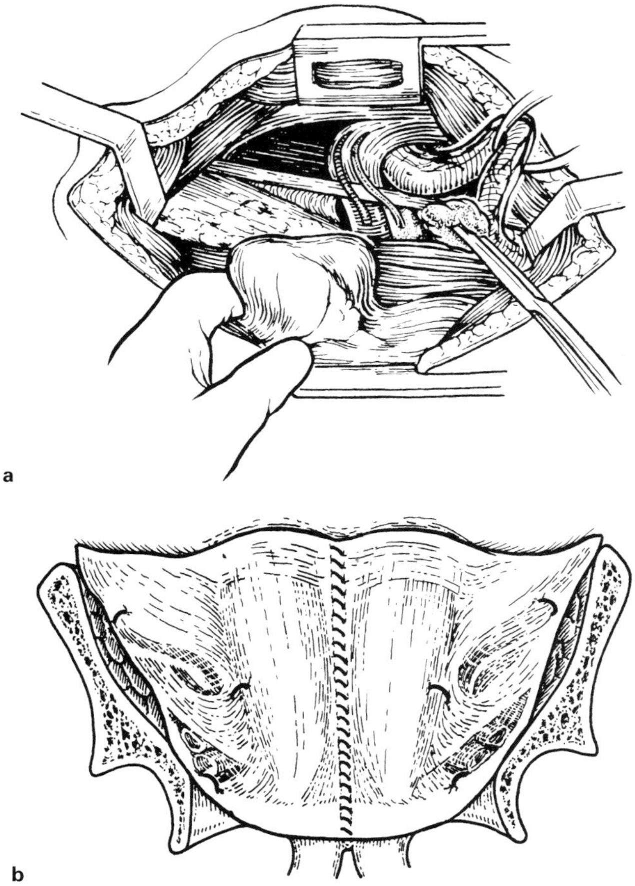

a

b

Fig. 26.11 The French extraperitoneal prosthetic groin repair operation. **(a)** The extraperitoneal space is opened, femoral or inguinal hernia sacs are identified and then 'milked' out of the parietes and excised. **(b)** A large sheet of mesh is placed in the extraperitoneal space to repair the defects. The mesh is held in position by a few sutures and abdominal pressure, like ham in a sandwich. It should completely cover the anterior pelvic peritoneum and close each of the potential hernia defects—direct and indirect, inguinal and femoral.

Association of Endoscopic Surgeons (EAES) stated: 'we recommend that endoscopic hernia repair should only be performed after appropriate training and with some sort of quality control'.[132] The results of properly conducted multicentre randomized trials are not yet available. The EAES also stated that laparoscopic repair had not yet reached the effectiveness stage where it could be recommended for general practice. Detailed analysis of cost-effectiveness and cost–benefits are lacking and safety aspects have not been sufficiently evaluated. Many laparoscopic surgeons are reluctant to abandon the transabdominal approaches with the attendant risks to intra-abdominal viscera in favour of the totally extraperitoneal approach favoured by a new wave of laparoscopic enthusiasts.[133] Hernias may be repaired by a transabdominal approach with the sac being either amputated or invaginated. A mesh is then placed in the preperitoneal space (as in the French method) and the peritoneum closed. The alternative is a totally extraperitoneal approach to the same layer using extraperitoneal balloon dissection. Again the sac is invaginated or amputated and closed. A mesh is placed between the peritoneum and the abdominal wall.

FEMORAL HERNIA

Femoral hernia is two-and-a-half times more common in females than in males in the UK, although in females indirect inguinal hernia is as common as femoral hernia.[134] The incidence of femoral hernias varies around the world; femoral hernias are very rare in native Africans.[135] It is postulated that chronic foot infections lead to repeated inflammation of groin lymph nodes and the consequent fibrosis of the femoral canal prevents herniation.[136]

The femoral sac is an acquired downward extension of peritoneum through the femoral canal which is normally occupied by extraperitoneal fat and Cloquet's lymph node. The sac has inguinal ligament in front of it, the lacunar ligament medial to it, the femoral vein lateral and the pectineal ligament and pectineus muscle behind as it passes through the femoral ring. The anterior layer of the femoral sheath, lying in front of the sac, is a downward continuation of the transversalis fascia; the posterior wall is a downward continuation of the fascia iliaca. Thus the femoral sheath is a funnel-shaped extension of the fascia transversalis into the thigh (Fig. 26.12).[137]

The hernial sac is considered to be acquired because a preformed sac has never been found at autopsy on a newborn infant. The hernia commonly arises late in life; it is most frequently seen in multiparous females. Weight loss predisposes to femoral herniation in both sexes. Ten per cent of femoral hernias follow a previous operation for an inguinal hernia; this is especially true of adult males.

Femoral hernia is more common in females than in males because the inguinal ligament makes a wider angle with the pubis in the female and an increase in fat of the femoral canal occurs in obese middle-aged females and stretches the femoral sheath. When the obesity disappears in old age a femoral hernia develops. Pregnancy increases the intra-abdominal pressure and may stretch the fascia transversalis and predispose to femoral herniation.

When a femoral hernia enters the thigh, it lies below the fossa ovalis and enlarges forwards, stretching the cribriform fascia over its fundus. The upper edge of the fossa ovalis has a strong, tight and sharp edge and the hernia twists over this edge before extending upwards and medially in the superficial fascia, over the inguinal ligament, into the angle between the superficial external pudendal and superficial epigastric veins. As a femoral hernia enlarges through the cribriform fascia it may obstruct the saphenous vein which becomes dilated.

A femoral hernia is rarely large, and in an obese patient may be difficult to find. It is not usually reducible and frequently patients have no cough impulse. It usually contains omentum and rarely contains bowel. Richter's hernia is more common here than at any other site, and more common in the right femoral canal than in the left.

REFERENCES

132. Neubauer E et al Surg Endosc 1995; 9: 550–563
133. Fitzgibbons R J et al Ann Surg 1995; 221: 3–13
134. Glassow F Ann J Surg 1971; 121: 637–641
135. Cole G J Trans R Soc Trop Med Hygiene 1964; 58: 441–447
136. Wosornu L Trop Doctor 1974; 4: 59
137. McVay C B Surg Clin North Am 1971; 51: 1251

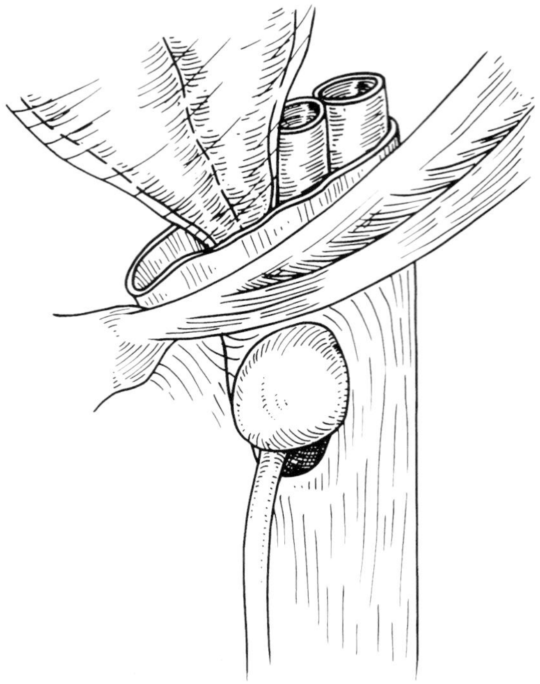

Fig. 26.12a Femoral hernia. (a) A femoral hernia exploits the medial femoral sheath to enter the thigh and emerge through the saphenous opening.

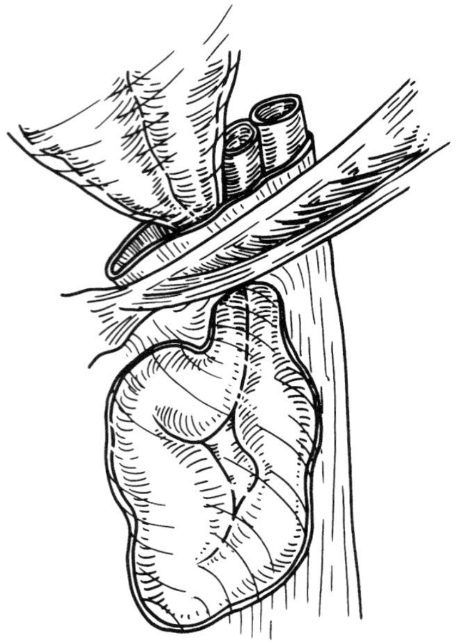

Fig. 26.12b The sac descends along the femoral sheath to the saphenous opening where it enters the superficial tissues of the thigh.

Certain rare varieties of femoral hernia are recognized. They are listed in order of frequency:

1. A prevascular hernia (Narath's hernia) protrudes in a long narrow sac in front of the femoral artery. It is the prolongation of the transversalis fascia which constitutes its sheath.[138] Its relation to the inferior epigastric artery is variable. The sac lies lateral to the saphenous opening and shows no tendency to protrude forwards or to ride up over the inguinal ligament. A hernia of this type may complicate congenital dislocation of the hip, or follow surgery on the innominate bones or the external iliac vessels. A similar hernia can complicate any groin wound when the inguinal ligament has been divided.[139]

2. An external femoral hernia (Hesselbach)[140] enters the thigh lateral to the deep epigastric vessels and the femoral vessels. It is usually associated with an indirect inguinal hernia.

3. A transpectineal femoral hernia (Laugier)[141] enters the thigh through a defect in the pectineal part of the inguinal ligament or through the lacunar ligament.

4. Deep femoral hernia (Callisen or Cloquet):[142] the sac descends deep to the femoral vessels and spreads out fanwise under the deep fascia. It cannot protrude through the saphenous opening.

5. A multilocular deep femoral hernia (Cooper)[143] enters the thigh deep to the investing deep fascia. Loculi spread out and can be mistaken for an obturator hernia.

6. An extremely rare variant of a femoral hernia associated with maldescent of the testicle had been described once in the literature. In this case the testicle descended behind the inguinal ligament, causing a femoral hernia with the testicle as a sliding component of its wall.[144]

Differential diagnosis

A femoral hernia must be differentiated from:

1. An inguinal hernia which lies above the inguinal ligament. Difficulties may arise when the fundus of a femoral hernia turns upwards and lies in front of the inguinal ligament. The neck of the sac can usually be felt below and lateral to the pubic tubercle.

2. A saphena varix often has a bluish tinge, is very soft, is associated with a dilated long saphenous vein and disappears on lying down. It frequently has a palpable thrill on coughing and a tap impulse (see Chapter 10).

3. An enlarged lymph node may be impossible to diagnose with certainty unless other enlarged nodes are present. Ultrasound or fine-needle aspiration cytology may be useful.

4. A psoas bursa is usually associated with an osteoarthritic hip and disappears on hip flexion. Ultrasound and aspiration confirm the diagnosis.

5. A psoas abscess is normally fluctuant and there may be cross-fluctuation above the inguinal ligament with an iliac abscess. There are signs in the back and radiographs of the spine, computed tomographic scanning and ultrasound confirm the diagnosis.

6. A lipoma may be impossible to differentiate from a femoral hernia.

REFERENCES

138. Narath A Arch Klin Chir 1899; 59: 396
139. Keynes G Br J Surg 1932; 20: 55
140. Hesselbach F K Neueste Anatomisch-Pathologische. Baumgartner, Wurzburg 1814
141. Laugier S Arch Gen Med Paris 1833; 2: 27
142. Callisen H Herniaerarioram Hanniae 1777; 2: 321
143. Cooper A The Anatomy of Hernia. Cox, London 1804
144. Stirk D I Br J Surg 1955; 43: 331

7. A femoral aneurysm has an expansile pulsation.

8. A sarcoma usually enlarges rapidly but slow-growing leiomysarcomas of the femoral vessels can be difficult to differentiate.

9. An ectopic testis is suspected if the testis is not present in the scrotum. Ultrasound should confirm the diagnosis.

10. An obturator hernia feels deeper and more lateral but can be mistaken for a femoral hernia in a very thin thigh.

The treatment of femoral hernia

Operation should always be recommended. Elective operation is advised as soon as possible, as femoral hernias have a real risk of strangulation and elective operations on relatively fit elderly patients have a lower morbidity than emergency operation. Emergency operation for obstruction or strangulation should be preceded by the most careful resuscitation[145] (see Chapter 5).

A femoral hernia is caused by a defect of the fascia transversalis and overlying parietes which allows a peritoneal protrusion to occur. Repair is by removing the peritoneal sac, repairing the fascia transversalis and reinforcing the aponeurosis. Three approaches to femoral hernia repair are described:

1. The abdominal, suprapubic, retroperitoneal, preperitoneal or extraperitoneal (eponyms: Cheatle, Henry, McEvedy[146]).
2. The inguinal or high (eponyms: Annandale, Lothiessen or Moschowitz[147]).
3. The crural or low (eponyms: Bassini or Lockwood[148]).

The extraperitoneal approach utilizes a midline vertical or a Pfannenstiel incision to undertake bilateral repairs. A transverse incision and oblique muscle split can be used for unilateral operations. The extraperitoneal space is opened by blunt dissection; the sac is found and evacuated from the parietes. The peritoneum can be opened to inspect or resect contents (Fig. 26.13).

The inguinal approach opens the inguinal canal and then divides the posterior fascia transversalis wall of the canal to gain access to the femoral canal from above (Fig. 26.14).

The crural approach uses an oblique incision in the groin about 1 cm below and parallel to the medial two-thirds of the inguinal ligament. The femoral sac is found in the subcutaneous tissue; the sac is then cleared, isolated and opened (Fig. 26.15). It is then transfixed or closed and excised.

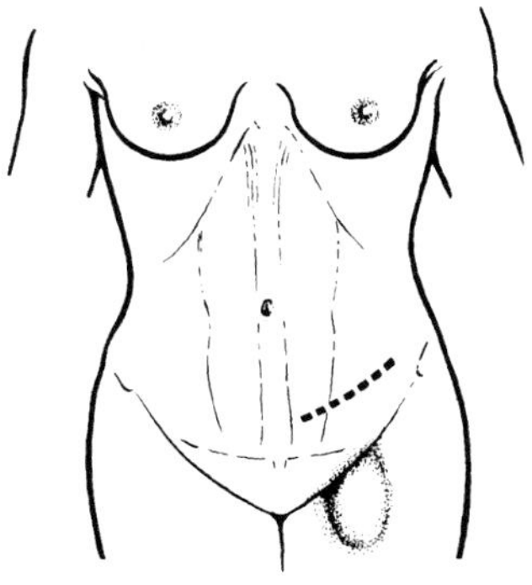

Fig. 26.13a Extraperitoneal approach to femoral hernia. (a) The approach to the unilateral hernia.

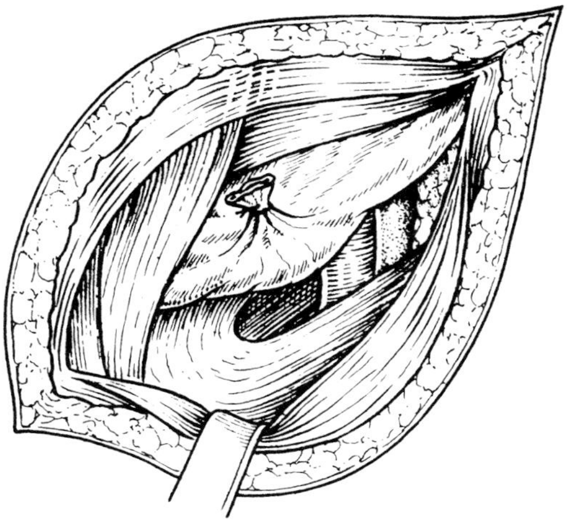

Fig. 26.13b The sac is reduced and excised.

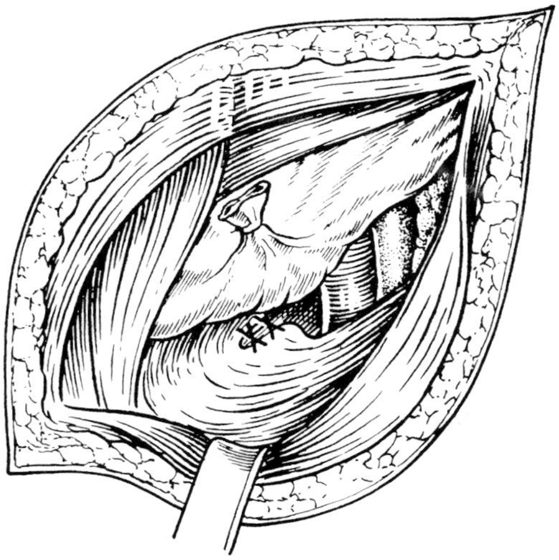

Fig. 26.13c The repair is effected by suturing the medial inguinal ligament to the pectineal ligament.

The extraperitoneal approach is the most useful approach for a strangulated hernia. The inguinal approach enables inguinal and femoral hernias to be repaired simultaneously but the posterior wall of the inguinal canal must be repaired to avoid an inguinal hernia developing. The crural operation is easy to do and is best reserved for elective situations. A standard paramedian incision should be made to deal with the devitalized bowel or omentum if it is used on an emergency case.

The parietal repair is achieved by suturing the medial inguinal ligament to the Cooper's pectineal ligament with a non-absorbable monofilament polymer. Care should be taken not to compress or damage the femoral vein which lies immediately laterally.

REFERENCES

145. Nicholson S, Keane T E, Devlin H B Br J Surg 1990; 77: 307
146. McEvedy P G Ann R Coll Surg Engl 1950; 7: 484
147. Moschowitz A V NY State J Med 1907; 7: 396–400
148. Lockwood C B Lancet 1893; ii: 1297

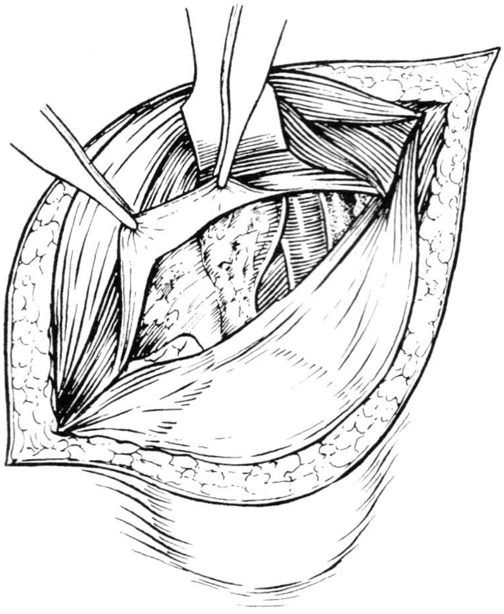

Fig. 26.14 The inguinal approach to femoral hernia.

Iliofemoral vein thrombosis and fatal pulmonary embolism have occurred after femoral hernia repair when the vein has been compressed.[149]

This repair can be reinforced by placing extraperitoneal mesh or by suturing the lower aponeurotic fibres of the conjoint tendon to the pectineal line. A flap of pectineal fascia can also be turned up and sutured over the defect.

The high extraperitoneal approach is ideal when the hernia is strangulated and the low crural operation is the simplest for the elective case. The overall recurrence rate for femoral hernia operations by either of these routes is 15%; this doubles to 30% if the inguinal approach is made.[150] However, when the inguinal

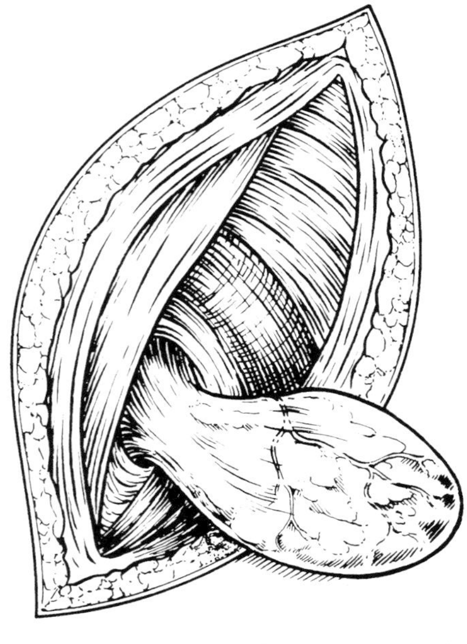

Fig. 26.15a The crural approach to femoral hernia. **(a)** Exposing the sac.

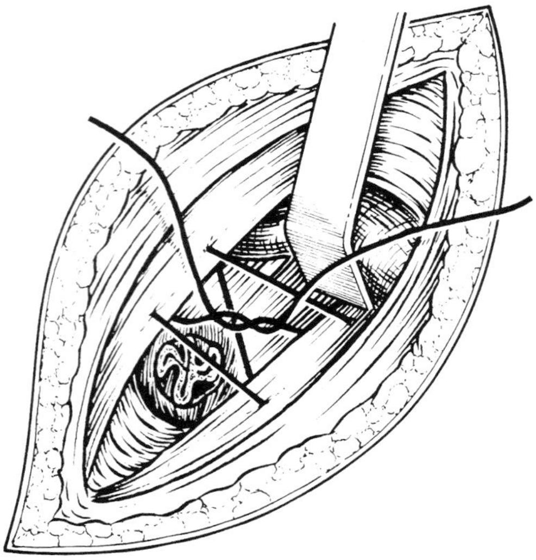

Fig. 26.15b After excision of the sac, the femoral cone is closed by suturing the medial inguinal ligament to the pectineal ligament. Care must be taken to avoid femoral vein compression or damage.

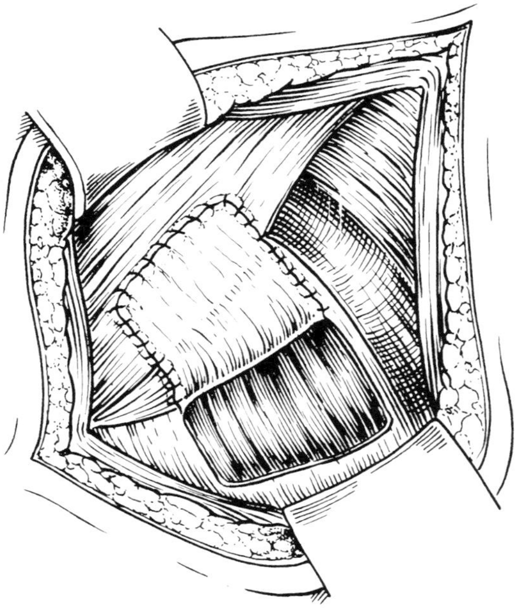

Fig. 26.15c The initial repair is reinforced with a pectineal fascia flap.

approach is used electively and combined with a Shouldice repair of the inguinal canal, an impressively low recurrence rate of under 2% has been recorded.[145,151]

The principles which govern the management of strangulated femoral hernia are the same as those employed in strangulated inguinal hernia. The constricting agent is usually the thickened neck of the sac where it abuts the femoral ring. The neck is then

REFERENCES

149. Brown R E et al Surgery 1980; 87: 230
150. Wheeler M H Proc R Soc Med 1975; 68: 177
151. Glassow F Ann Surg 1966; 163: 227

divided but division of the edge of the lacunar ligament is not required. Rarely, the strangulating agent of a large hernia is the edge of the fossa ovalis. A formal laparotomy should always be carried out if there is any doubt about the viability of the sac contents.

THE RECURRENT GROIN HERNIA

All series of groin hernia repairs have reported recurrences. Nowadays using one of the four modern transversalis repairs described above, scrupulous technique and non-irritant synthetic polymer sutures, recurrence rates at 5 years should be less than 2%.[152] After surgery 30% of recurrences are present at 2 years, 60% at 5 years and 90% at 10 years. When inguinal hernias recur 55% of the recurrences are indirect and these tend to be early recurrences, 45% of recurrences are direct and usually occur late and 5% are femoral hernias.[153] Recurrence is related to the experience of the surgeon, technical failure at the original operation, sepsis, haematoma, inept tight suturing and missed hernia. Missed hernia is the worst sin and every possible hernia site must always be inspected. To repair the direct bulge and miss the small crescentic indirect sac is a poor advertisement for a surgeon's skill!

Repair of recurrent groin hernia requires an experienced surgeon. If it is a first-time recurrence an anterior approach, careful dissection of each anatomic layer and local reoperation will suffice. If it is a second recurrence or if there has been previous sepsis, to go through the old scar is foolish and runs the risk of cord damage. To reoperate through the virgin extraperitoneal plane and insert mesh is simple and gives a very satisfactory result.[126]

UMBILICAL HERNIA IN INFANTS AND CHILDREN

Minor degrees of umbilical herniation are present in many neonates but the majority of these hernias resolve spontaneously. The incidence of umbilical hernias in the newborn which subsequently require surgery is about 3 per 1000 live births in the UK. The incidence of umbilical herniation is higher in black than white children.[154]

The hernia forms a small protrusion at the umbilicus; it is more prominent when the child cries. The hernia consists of a peritoneal sac penetrating through the linea alba umbilical cicatrix to lie in the subcutaneous tissues. It characteristically has a narrow rigid neck as it passes through the aponeurosis.

All childhood umbilical hernias undergo spontaneous reduction in size as the child grows and few, if any, persist after puberty. Some can incarcerate but only a minority require operation. It is important to preserve the umbilicus in children for cosmetic reasons. The Mayo 'vest-over-pants' operation is an effective method of repair. A subumbilical curved incision is used and the operation is performed as described below for adults.

ADULT UMBILICAL HERNIA

Adult umbilical hernia occurs with equal frequency in both sexes. It is uncommon before the age of 40 except as a complication of cirrhotic or malignant ascites. The hernia is not congenital but is the consequence of increased intraabdominal pressure on the umbilical cicatrix which may be associated with multiple pregnancy, malignancy, ascites, continuous ambulatory peritoneal dialysis or obesity. The hernia is always progressive and sometimes reaches a huge size. It usually contains omentum and sometimes transverse colon, small intestine and even stomach. The skin, superficial fascia, rectus sheath, transversalis fascia and sac stretch over the hernia and fuse into a parchment-like membrane through which peristalsis may be observed. Redness, excoriation, frank ulceration and even gangrene may occur in the overlying skin. Infection may spread and lead to a spontaneous faecal fistula. The neck of the sac is often surprisingly narrow and very fibrous in comparison with the volume of the contents. The contents usually adhere to each other and to the coverings, especially at the fundus. Adherent omentum divides the sac into complex multilocular cavities, and as a consequence umbilical hernias are usually irreducible.

Clinical features

Abdominal pain from incarceration and subacute obstruction are frequent. Strangulation by the rigid fibrous neck of the sac is a common complication. Backache as the result of mesenteric tension and the lordosis caused by the hernia may also occur.

Treatment

In older patients cardiovascular, pulmonary and renal disease are common. Obesity and diabetes are other co-morbidities which combine to increase the risk of operation. This should be attempted nevertheless, as the chance of strangulation is quite high and operation for strangulated umbilical hernia has a high mortality. Before elective operation weight reduction is beneficial if the hernia is strangulated. Resuscitation is essential.

Elective operation is also often hazardous because the return to the abdomen of bulky omentum, mesentery and bowel may raise the intra-abdominal pressure enormously. This may interfere with blood flow through the abdominal veins and impede the diaphragmatic movements so that both circulation and respiration are embarrassed. A pneumoperitoneum induced preoperatively can be used to enlarge the peritoneal cavity and make reduction of the contents easier.[155]

Mayo's repair is the operation of choice.[156] The stretched integument over the hernial protrusion is incised as a horizontal ellipse which is deepened to reach the rectus sheath and to expose the neck of the sac. This incision is enlarged laterally if necessary to give a long transverse exposure. The sac is opened near its neck where adhesions are least likely to be present. Protruding bowel is

REFERENCES

152. Glassow F Ann R Coll Surg Engl 1984; 66: 382
153. Glassow F Br Med J 1970; 1: 215
154. James T J R Soc Med 1982; 75: 537
155. Caldironi M W et al Br J Surg 1990; 77: 306
156. Mayo W J Ann Surg 1901; 31: 276

returned to the peritoneal cavity and omentum is excised to lessen the volume of contents to be reduced. The whole sac is removed together with the adherent overlying skin. The lower edge of the rectus is now sutured behind the upper flap, which is similarly carried down in front so that the two flaps overlap (Fig. 26.16). Interrupted mattress absorbable monofilament polymer sutures are used.

EPIGASTRIC HERNIA

Epigastric hernia may occur in children or in adults. It is caused by a protrusion of extraperitoneal fat through one of the fissures which are commonly found between the fibres of the linea alba. The protruding fat may draw peritoneum after it as a small hernia sac. Reflex digestive disturbance and epigastric pain may occur and can be out of all proportion to the size of the hernia, sometimes simulating a duodenal ulcer. Care should be taken to determine before operation that the patient's symptoms are caused by the hernia and not by coexistent intra-abdominal disease, which was present in a third of the patients in some series.[157] Excision of the sac and repair of linea alba cure the hernia.

INCISIONAL HERNIA

Incisional hernia is a diffuse extrusion of peritoneum and abdominal contents through a weak scar after an operation or accidental wound. They represent a partial abdominal dehiscence where the deep layers separate but the skin remains intact. Incisional hernias were one of the first long-term complications of abdominal surgery to be reported in the 19th century: Gerdy repaired an incisional hernia in 1836 and Maydl another in 1886.[158]

Patients with an incisional hernia complain of a lump which gradually increases in size and which may disappear on lying down. Episodic subacute intestinal obstruction, incarceration, strangulation and skin excoriation, particularly in the sulcus below the lump can occur, but spontaneous rupture of the hernia is rarely seen. Spontaneous rupture is a particular complication of caesarean and gynaecological wounds.[159] Strangulation and spontaneous rupture are complications that require urgent operation.

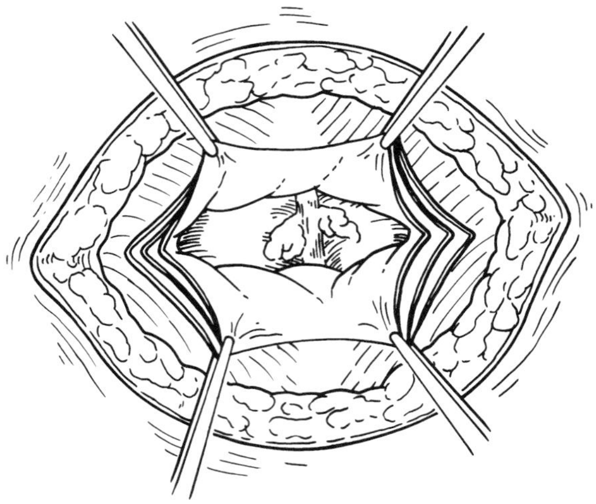

Fig. 26.16a Umbilical hernia: Mayo operation. (**a**) Mayo's vest-over-pants' operation for umbilical hernia.

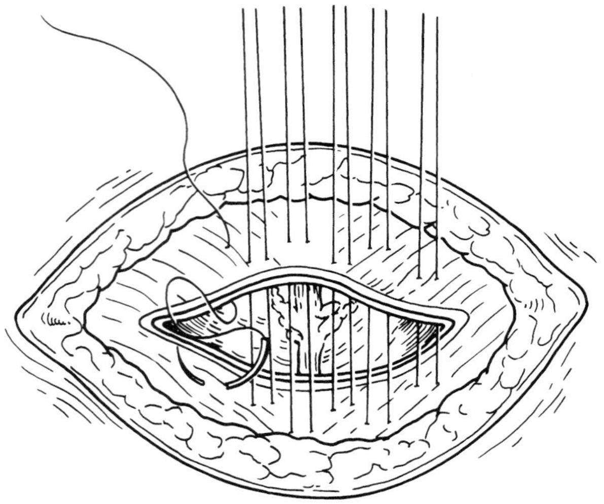

Fig. 26.16b The sutures are placed.

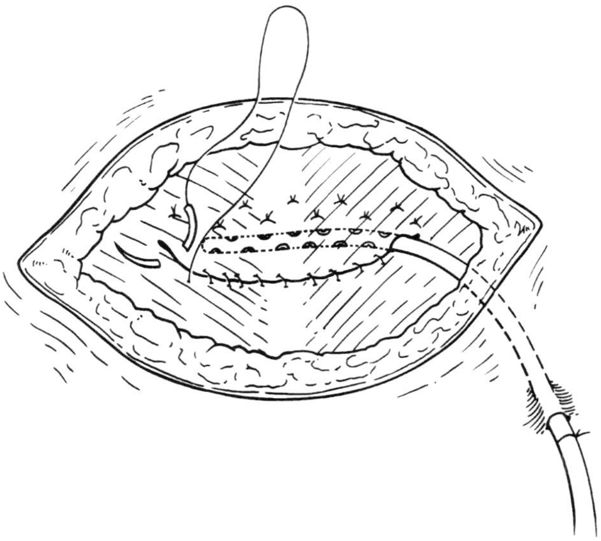

Fig. 26.16c The sutures are tied and the top layer of the repair is completed. When doing a Mayo repair it is always sensible to drain the dead space between the peritoneum and the aponeurosis with a suction drain.

Persistent discomfort in an abdominal wound can be caused by a small extraperitoneal fatty hernia through the wound or through the suture holes alongside it. Ultrasound or herniography can detect these small incisional hernias which are often impalpable, especially in the obese.[160]

It is difficult to quote an accurate incidence of incisional hernias because unless they cause significant symptoms they are not referred to hospital for treatment. Patients followed up after

REFERENCES

157. Pemberton J de J, Curry F S Minn Med 1936; 19: 109
158. Lason A H Hernia. Blakiston, Philadelphia 1941
159. Senapati A Br J Surg 1982; 69: 313
160. Krukowski Z H, Matheson N A Br J Surg 1987; 74: 824–825

abdominal surgery have shown that incisional hernia complicates 6% of abdominal wounds at 5 years and 12% at 10 years.[161,162] The continued increase in incidence of these hernias years after surgery is unexplained, but suggests failure or attrition of the collagen in healed wounds. Incisional hernias have an almost equal incidence in both sexes (males 55%, females 45%).

Risk factors associated with the development of incisional hernias can be put down to technical failure by the surgeon and tissue failure of the patient.

Technical factors include:

1. Postoperative haematoma, necrosis and sepsis.
2. Inept closure—using absorbable sutures on aponeuroses, too small bites and knots may come undone.
3. Placing drains or stomas through wounds.
4. Inappropriate or badly made incisions.

Tissue factors include:

1. Age.
2. Immunosuppression, diabetes, jaundice and renal failure.
3. Obesity.
4. Malignant disease.
5. Gross abdominal distension from obstruction or ascites.

Midline lower abdominal incisions are most at risk for incisional herniation. Other incisions commonly followed by incisional hernias are upper midline, lateral muscle-splitting (McBurney), subcostal/Kocher's, parastomal and transverse.[53] There is no satisfactory controlled study of the incidence of incisional hernias in competently closed incisions and it is therefore difficult to make specific criticisms of different incisions.

Incisional hernias should be surgically repaired after the patient has had cardiopulmonary disease corrected, with as much weight loss as possible, and had local skin sepsis treated. The induction of a preoperative pneumoperitoneum is a useful aid to surgery[155] if the hernia is large and the peritoneal cavity contracted. This enlarges the main peritoneal cavity and stretches the hernia sac and the adhesions within facilitating dissection. A plastic cannula with a micropore filter is used to inject increasing volumes of air into the peritoneum in the 4 weeks prior to operation; it is usual to start with increments of 500 ml and increase every few days until the abdomen and hernia are blown up as tight as a drum.

The two techniques of surgical repair most commonly used are layer-to-layer anatomical repair, if there is no tissue loss or mesh graft insertion across the defect. A mesh is essential if there is loss of aponeurotic tissue (Fig. 26.17).

The best results are obtained by experienced surgeons who are interested in incisional hernia repair. Recurrence rates with suture or layer techniques vary from 1.6 to 46%, while those reported with prosthetic mesh replacement are much lower (10%),[163] and this appears to be the best technique.[164] The mesh must have an adequate overlap over normal tissue if it is to be successful.

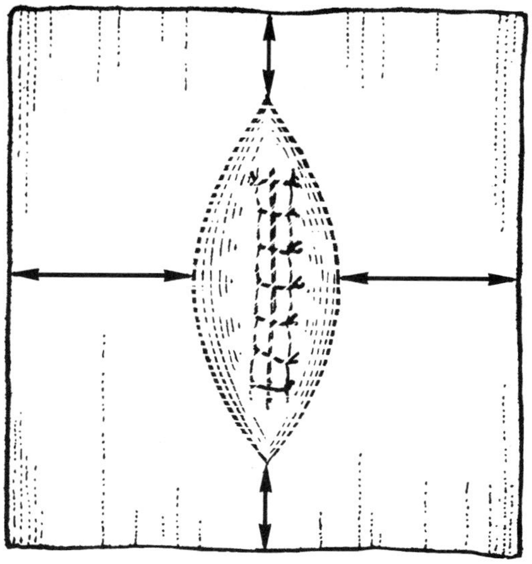

Fig. 26.17a Mesh repair of incisional hernia. (**a**) The mesh is cut and positioned: it must overlap the margins of the defect by 2 cm.

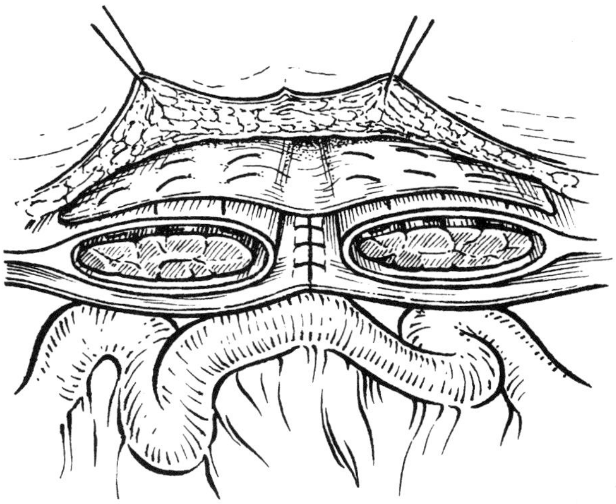

Fig. 26.17b Multiple suture lines to attach the mesh to the adjacent virgin aponeurosis securely.

OBTURATOR HERNIA

Obturator hernia was first described by Arnaud de Ronsil in 1724 but the Royal Academy of Sciences in Paris refused to accept his findings. Laparotomy was first performed for the condition by Hilton in 1848.[165] A preoperative diagnosis was rarely made until recent years and the operative mortality is still more than 30%.[49]

Obturator hernia is six times more common in women than in men, three times more common after than before the age of 50 and nearly twice as common on the right side as on the left. The hernia is more frequent in oriental people than caucasians or blacks. An obturator hernia has been described in a child of 12 but nearly half the patients are aged over 60 years.[166] It particularly affects elderly women who have had a recent rapid weight loss.

REFERENCES

161. Ellis H et al Br J Surg 1983; 70: 290
162. Mudge M, Hughes L E Br J Surg 1985; 72: 70
163. Usher F C Am J Surg 1979; 138: 740
164. George C D, Ellis H Ann R Coll Surg Engl 1986; 68: 185
165. Wakeley C P G Br J Surg 1939; 26: 515–525
166. Kwong K H, Ong G B Br J Surg 1966; 53: 23

The peritoneum protrudes through the obturator canal, which is a 3 cm long fibro-osseous channel between the obturator groove of the lower surface of the pubic ramus and the upper border of the obturator membrane. The obturator nerve lies on the anteromedial side of this channel and the artery lies posterolateral. Emerging from the obturator canal, the hernia comes into contact with the deep surface of pectineus muscle. It then protrudes forwards between the pectineus and abductor longus muscles to enter the femoral triangle. It may be mistaken for a femoral hernia in the upper thigh.

The sac usually contains small intestine, rarely caecum, pelvic colon, ovary and fallopian tube. A Richter's hernia is not unusual. The hernia does not usually attract attention until intestinal strangulation occurs and even then the cause of the strangulation may not be obvious until after the abdomen has been opened. A strangulated obturator hernia may have the Howship–Romberg sign: pain is referred along the geniculate branch of the obturator nerve to the inner aspect of the knee. The signs of intestinal obstruction accompanied by pain and tenderness on the inner side of the femoral vessels should raise the suspicion of strangulated obturator hernia, even if a swelling is not palpable in the thigh. The hernia may be felt as a palpable mass on vaginal examination. The diagnosis of obturator hernia is rarely made until it strangulates.

Because the diagnosis is seldom made until laparotomy, it is fortunate that the abdominal route is the most satisfactory approach to this hernia. Only when the foramen is viewed from within the pelvis can the tight obturator canal be opened up without the risk of damaging the obturator vessels and nerve, which are easily visible. Once the contents have been released it is usually unnecessary to repair the obturator canal, though if the defect is considerable it can be closed by an extraperitoneal mesh plug.

SEMILUNAR LINE (SPIGELIAN) HERNIA

The semilunar line was described by Adrian van der Spieghel (1578–1625); and herniation through this line was first described by Klinkosch in 1764.[167] Sir Astley Cooper collected 23 cases of spigelian hernia, of which 19 were below the umbilicus, and proposed the theory that herniation occurred through stretched neurovascular openings which occur in the line.[168] This theory was accepted until Zimmerman and his associates demonstrated 'banding' of the internal oblique muscle in 1942.[169] As the internal oblique muscle enters the semilunar line it forms bands that contribute alternately to the anterior or posterior rectus sheaths. There are slit-like defects between these bands and peritoneal protrusions exploit these defects to produce hernias. Usually the hernial sac is deflected by the overlying external oblique muscle as it emerges, forcing it to lie interparietally. The hernia is usually deflected laterally so that it forms a mass near the iliac crest. Rarely it enters the rectus sheath where in the acute phase it can be confused with a ruptured rectus muscle or inferior epigastric haematoma. Most hernias occur below the umbilicus adjacent to the line of Douglas where the anatomy of the posterior rectus sheath changes.

Spigelian hernias are more frequent in women than men, in a ratio of 1.5 : 1. They represent fewer than 1% of abdominal wall hernias. The clinical features include a lump which aches more and more as the day goes on and disappears when the patient lies down in bed. The pain in the lump is exacerbated by raising the arm on the ipsilateral side above the head. The hernia may contain small and large bowel or omentum. It may strangulate and if this occurs the rigid aponeurotic margins of the hernia cause early tissue pressure necrosis. The diagnosis can be confidently made by ultrasound scanning.[170]

Spigelian hernias are repaired by excising the peritoneal sac and closing the aponeurotic defect. This is best achieved by a modified Mayo-type 'vest-over-pants' operation using non-absorbable polymer sutures.

LUMBAR HERNIA

Lumbar hernias may follow renal operations, surgical drainage of lumbar abscesses or paralysis of the lateral lumbar muscles by poliomyelitis or spina bifida. It may also appear spontaneously through one of two anatomically weak points in the lumbar region. The first is the lumbar triangle of Petit, which is bounded by the crest of the ilium, the posterior edge of obliquus externus and the anterior edge of latissimus dorsi. The neck of such a hernia is nearly always wide and its contents, either the omentum or the right or left colon, are usually easily reducible. A prosthesis can be used to carry out an extraperitoneal repair. The second is through the superior quadrilateral lumbar space. It is bounded by the 12th rib, the lower border of the serratus posterior inferior, the anterior border of erector spinae and the internal oblique. Hernias through this space, along the 12th intercostal neurovascular bundle, are as common as through Petit's triangle.

GLUTEAL AND SCIATIC HERNIA

Gluteal hernias protrude through the greater sciatic notch and a sciatic hernia passes through the lesser sciatic notch. Both gluteal and sciatic hernias are very rare and, like obturator hernias, are usually discovered in the course of a laparotomy performed for the relief of an obstruction of unknown cause. Rarely, a palpable swelling or tenderness in the buttock or pain referred along the sciatic nerve may suggest the diagnosis.

PELVIC HERNIA

A false pelvic hernia is the protrusion of peritoneum with a cystocoele, rectocoele or prolapse of the rectum. This is a variety of sliding hernia and the viscus which is either at the bladder or the rectum forms one side of the sac. A true pelvic or vaginal hernia which is a hernia of the pouch of Douglas may occur

REFERENCES

167. Klinkosch J J Programma quo Divisionem Herniorum. Beman, Rotterdam 1764
168. Cooper A Hernia. Longman, London 1807
169. Zimmerman L M, Anson B J et al Surg Gynecol Obstet 1944; 78: 535
170. Spangen L Acta Chir Scand 1976; 462: 1

spontaneously in the multiparous woman or, more commonly, as a result of trauma at childbirth. The hernia protrudes into the posterior vaginal wall and vulva. The swelling may be differentiated from a rectocoele by synchronous vaginal and rectal examination. The patient or her partner may complain of peristalsis or gurgling gas in the hernia.

A postoperative pelvic hernia can develop after vaginal hysterectomy or, more commonly, after abdominoperineal resection of the rectum. A lateral pelvic hernia is a protrusion of peritoneum and its abdominal contents through a persistent hiatus of Schwalbe which is a gap in the line of origin of the levator ani from the fascia of the obturator internus. Such a hernia may appear in the ischiorectal fossa or the labium major, when they are called ischiorectal or pudendal hernias.

INTERNAL HERNIA

Internal hernias have lost their glamour and surgical interest. Treitz,[171] Waldeyer,[172] Treves[173] and Moynihan[174] each wrote monographs about them but with the advent of safer surgery, fluid replacement and modern imaging, few surgeons would think them worth reporting.

Internal hernias attract attention either as a cause of recurrent, severe episodes of vomiting or because of acute small bowel obstruction which rapidly progresses to strangulation. When the patient is complaining of recurrent small bowel obstruction, investigation by small bowel contrast enema can allow a preoperative diagnosis to be made. With acute strangulation the diagnosis is confirmed by plain abdominal X-rays and confirmed at laparotomy.

A brief description of difficult internal hernia is given below:

1. Into the lesser sac:
   (a) Through the epiploic foramen.
   (b) Through a congenital defect in the transverse mesocolon.
   (c) Postoperatively, alongside the loops of a posterior gastroenterostomy or retrocolic gastrectomy. Strangulation of the afferent loop in these hernias can be confused with acute pancreatitis.
2. Paraduodenal—these are often associated with anomalies of midgut rotation:
   (a) Left paraduodenal hernia—the mouth of the sac is to the right and the sac extends to the left of the duodenum. The inferior mesenteric vein and the ascending branch of the left colic artery lie in the anterior peritoneal fold that forms the neck of this hernial sac.[173]
   (b) Inferior duodenal hernia of Treitz—this sac extends downwards behind the transverse peritoneal fold which runs from the fourth part of the duodenum to the inferior mesenteric vein.[171]
   (c) The mesentericoparietal hernia of Waldeyer[172] enters the sac from the left behind the mesentery and extends to the right. It lies immediately inferior to the third part of the duodenum. The superior mesenteric artery (which crosses the third part of the duodenum) lies in the anterior free margin of the neck of the sac.
   (d) Retroduodenal hernias pass from right to left behind the ascending fourth part of the duodenum.
3. Hernias through mesenteric defects. These defects occur in the distal ileum and are frequently multiple. They cause intestinal obstruction in neonates, but can occur at any age. Laparotomy and closure of the defect is an effective treatment.
4. Paracaecal hernias occur in the various folds about the appendix and caecum. The best remembered is the bloodless fold of Treves which extends from the ileum to the appendix.[173]
5. Intersigmoid hernias occur into the potential sac which extends upwards and laterally between the two limbs of the sigmoid colon. They are very rare and may be associated with gut malrotation.
6. Supravesical hernias are associated with weight loss which allows a hernia sac to develop anterior to the bladder in the rectovesical space. These hernias are more frequent in males than females. They occur in the triangular space bounded by the medial umbilical ligament forced by the obliterated urachus, the lateral umbilical ligament forced by the obliterated umbilical artery and the reflection of the peritoneum on to the fundus of the bladder below. They present with obstruction when a loop of small bowel becomes imprisoned in the sac. The development of a supravesical hernia is sometimes associated with symptoms of reduced bladder capacity.
7. Hernia through the broad ligament is very rare. It usually occurs in elderly women who have undergone a previous gynaecological operation with preservation of the tubes and ovaries.

The management of internal hernia

Large-necked peritoneal sacs are rarely compromised by the strangulation of their contents but small-necked sacs frequently have critical strictures in their margins and these cannot be divided. If the hernia is strangulated and irreducible the distended bowel should have its contents withdrawn by needle aspiration prior to reduction.

Closure of the defect prevents recurrence. These rare hernias and their treatment are well-reviewed.[175,176,177]

REFERENCES

171. Treitz W Hernia Retroperitonealis. Credner, Prague 1857
172. Waldeyer H W, von Waldeyer-Hartz Hernia Retroperitonealis. Jungfer, Breslau 1868
173. Treves F The Anatomy of the Intestinal Canal. Lewis, London 1885
174. Moynihan B G A Retroperitoneal Hernia. Baillière Tindall, London 1906
175. Chevrel J P (ed) Surgery of the Abdominal Wall. (English translation.) Springer Verlag, Berlin 1987
176. Devlin H B Management of Abdominal Hernias. Butterworths, London 1988
177. Schumpelick V Hernien. Enke Verlag, Stuttgart 1987

27 The peritoneum, the mesentery, the greater omentum and the acute abdomen

S. Paterson-Brown

The peritoneal cavity provides the internal environment for the abdominal viscera, and has received somewhat scant attention since James Douglas in 1730[1] first suggested that its role was to act as a lubricating lining for these organs. The pathophysiology of the peritoneum, mesentery and omentum is now being studied in much greater detail.

PERITONEUM

Embryology and structure

Both the visceral and perietal peritoneal membrane lining the intestines and abdominal cavity are formed of a layer of mesothelial cells. These are flattened and polyhedral in appearance, being only one layer thick. Electron microscopic studies have shown that these cells have microvilli and cilia on their intraperitoneal border,[2] which increases the surface area and helps to circulate intraperitoneal fluid in an upwards direction towards the diaphragm. Peritoneal cells contain many vesicles which are involved in fluid transport and have lacunae with valves at the entrance of the lymphatics.[3]

The blood peritoneal barrier behaves like a capillary wall with both large (25 nm) and small (5 nm) pores.[4] About 80 cm^2 or 0.4% of the mesothelial surface is available for diffusion. During peritonitis the number of large pores increases, augmenting the transport of macromolecules including immunoglobulin G and immunoglobulin M from the blood into the peritoneal cavity, while there is no alteration in the number of small pores and solute transport remains constant.

Apart from the openings of the fallopian tubes, the peritoneal cavity is a completely closed sac unless there is a failure of full development of the anterior abdominal wall. The peritoneal cavity is divided into greater and lesser sacs which communicate through the foramen of Winslow (Fig. 27.1). The peritoneum may be subdivided into a visceral component lining the intra-abdominal organs and a parietal component lining the wall of the abdominal cavity (Fig. 27.2). Both parts of the peritoneum receive visceral innervation but the parietal peritoneum also has somatic sensation. Thus pain arising from intra-abdominal pathology which involves the parietal peritoneum leads to pain which is experienced in the abdominal wall.[5] It is also responsible for the pain which is experienced when a needle or trocar is inserted into the peritoneal cavity. Primitive reflexes caused by peritoneal stimulation can produce bradycardia and ileus.

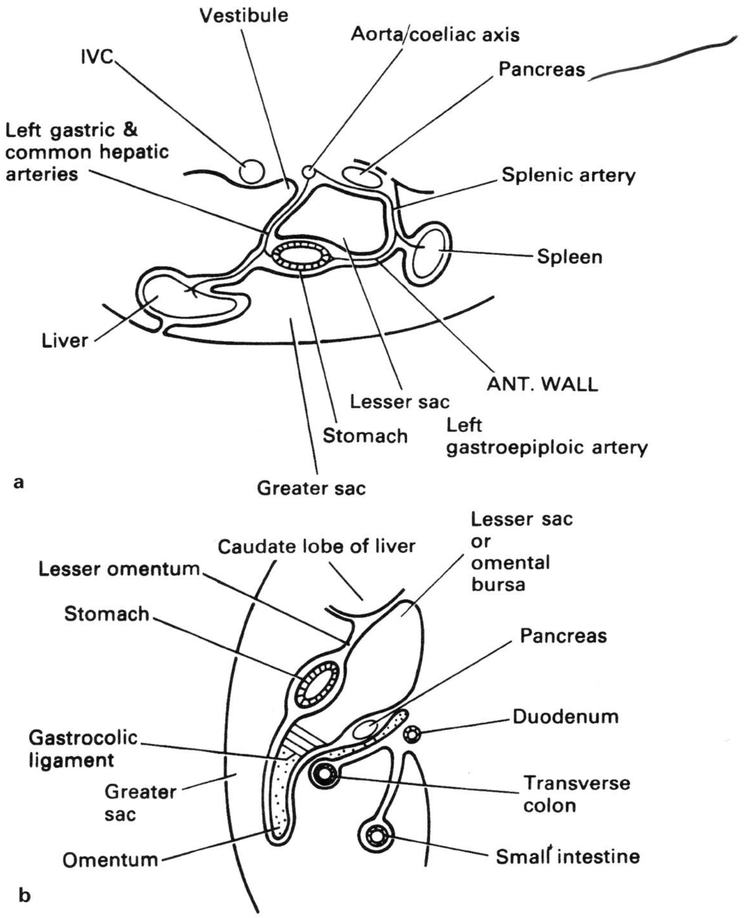

Fig. 27.1 (**a**) Transverse section through peritoneal cavity. (**b**) Longitudinal section. The greater and lesser sacs are shown.

REFERENCES

1. Douglas J A Description of the Peritoneum. Warwick Lane, London 1730
2. Andrews P M, Porter K R Anat Rec 1973; 177: 409
3. Granger H J, Laine G A et al In: Stanb N C, Taylor A E (eds) Edema. Raven Press, New York, 1984 pp 189–228
4. Nolph K D J Lat Clin Med 1979; 94: 519
5. Capps J A, Coleman G H An Experimental and Clinical Study of Pain in the Pleura, Pericardium and Peritoneum. Macmillan, New York 1932

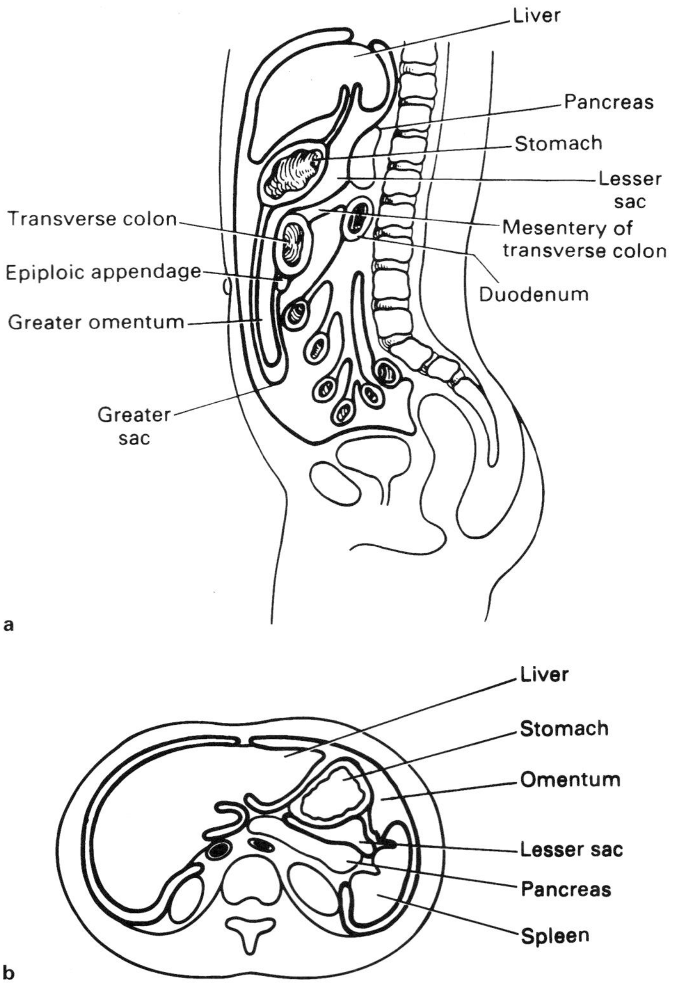

Fig. 27.2 (**a**) Coronal section of the peritoneal cavity showing peritoneum lining the abdominal cavity (somatic) and surrounding the organs (visceral). (**b**) Transverse section of the abdominal cavity.

Function

The peritoneal membrane provides lubrication for the loops of intestine by secreting a slightly viscous fluid. Under normal conditions the amount of peritoneal fluid that is produced is minimal and just enough to lubricate the abdominal contents. The mesothelial cells with their abundance of rough endoplasmic reticulum and prominent Golgi apparatus are also able to secrete lytic enzymes, an angiogenic factor, prostaglandins, interferon, lymphokinase and oxidative free radicals,[6] some of which probably discourage infection.

The peritoneal surface area is almost 2 m^2, which is larger than that of all the glomeruli. The large fluid and electrolyte movements which this allows can be utilized to provide access for insulin, bactericidal and cytostatic drugs, and provides a semi-permeable membrane for dialysis of patients with renal failure.

The fluid and particulate matter which enters the vesicles and lacunae of the mesothelial cells passes along the lymphatics towards the diaphragm. This forms an interface with the pleural cavity which probably accounts for the pleural effusions found in association with some ovarian tumours—a phenomenon described as Meigs syndrome.[7]

CONGENITAL ABNORMALITIES

During foetal development the exteriorized intestine elongates and undergoes rotation,[8] before being accommodated within the developing abdominal cavity. Changes also occur in its vascular supply which lead to the formation of a number of common but inconstant peritoneal folds.[9] As the third part of the duodenum becomes fixed to the posterior abdominal wall the ligament of Treitz is formed.[10]

Occasionally paraduodenal fossae are formed by folds of peritoneum in association with the ligament of Treitz (Fig. 27.3a). A loop of jejunum can herniate into one of these fossae causing intestinal obstruction.[10] The bloodless fold of Treves[11] can develop during fixation of the caecum and may make the appendix difficult to find at operation (Fig. 27.3b). The fold of Treves is too small to strangulate or obstruct bowel, but the peritoneal folds associated with branches of the superior mesenteric artery can cause clinical problems. When rotation of the caecum is incomplete, Ladd's band (fold of peritoneum) comes into relationship with the duodenum on the posterior wall of the abdominal cavity and can cause small bowel obstruction (see Chapter 29). Laparotomy and division of Ladd's band, with rotation of the caecum to the left, are required to prevent further problems.

PERITONITIS

Although micro-organisms are the commonest cause of peritonitis, bacteria, enzymes and chemicals all cause a similar inflammatory response. Peritonitis may be generalized or localized. Anatomical partitions can in the case of lesser sac abscesses prevent dissemination. Post-mortem and radiological studies have demonstrated that the peritoneal cavity is effectively divided into four compartments. The two infracolic compartments situated below the transverse mesocolon and above the pelvic brim are divided into left and right by the longitudinal barrier formed by the lumbar spine, abdominal aorta, inferior vena cava and small bowel mesentery. The pelvic cavity is situated below the pelvic brim, psoas muscles and iliac vessels. The supracolic compartment is situated below the diaphragm and above the transverse mesocolon.[12] Infected material from the supracolic compartment is directed down over the surface of the omentum, along the paracolic gutters into the pelvic basin where it can collect without embarrassing the diaphragm. Fluid escaping from a perforated duodenal ulcer passes down over the colon to the right paracolic gutter before entering the pelvis or passing up into the right subphrenic space. Fluid collecting within

REFERENCES

6. Steinhauer H B, Gunter B, Schollmeyer J J Clin Invest 1985; 15: 1
7. Meigs J V, Cass J W Am J Obstet Gynecol 1937; 33: 249
8. Haymond H E, Dragstedt L R Surg Gynecol Obstet 1931; 53: 16
9. Kiewswetter W B, Smith J W Arch Surg 1958; 77: 483
10. Treitz W, Prag F A Hernia Retroperitonealis. Ein Beitrag zur Geschichle Inner Hernien. Crednar 1957
11. Treves F. Cassell, London 1884 (Jacksonian Prize Essay)
12. Mitchell G A Q Br J Surg 1941; 28: 291

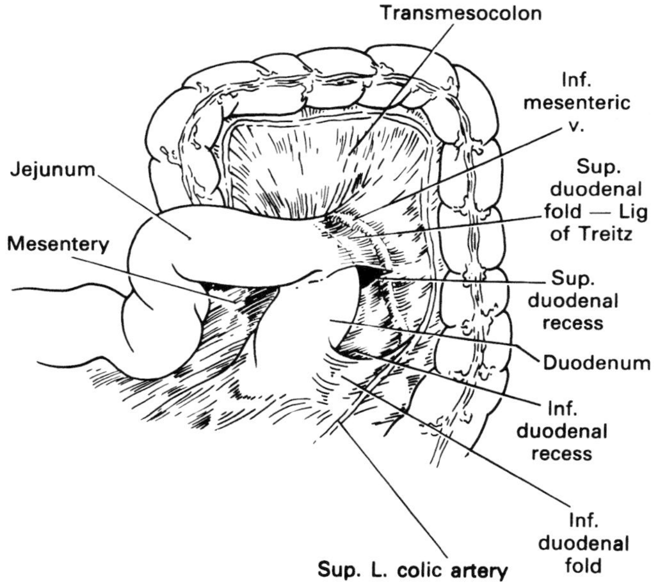

Fig. 27.3a The paraduodenal fossae and the ligament of Treitz.

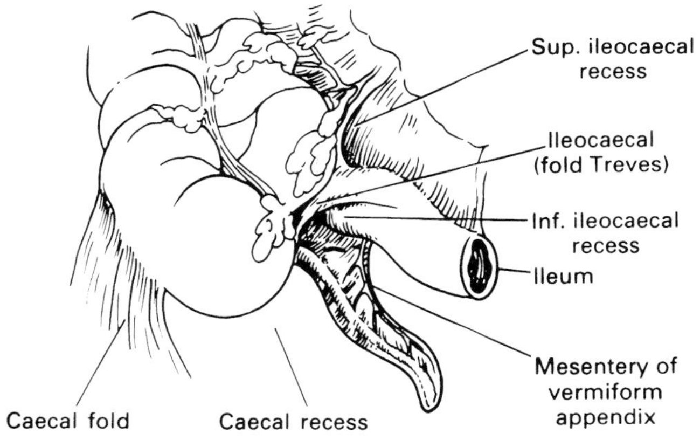

Fig. 27.3b The paracaecal fossae and the fold of Treves.

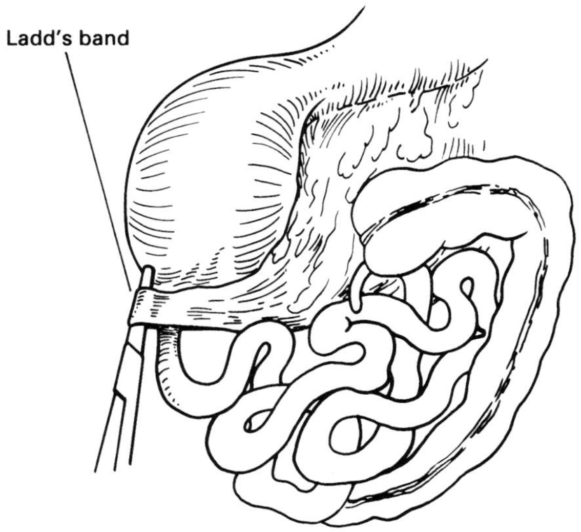

Fig. 27.3c Malrotation of the bowel associated with a Ladd's band.

the pelvic cavity is often contained within this space and fluid collections within the pelvic cavity are often prevented from entering the upper abdomen for some time.

The greater omentum, which constantly alters its position within the peritoneal cavity as a result of intestinal peristalsis and abdominal muscular contractions, adheres to and surrounds any inflamed viscus with which it comes into contact. Fibrinous peritoneal exudate glues the bowel and omentum to the inflammatory focus, walling it off and preventing a generalized peritonitis. The spread of infection around the peritoneal cavity is further reduced when toxic exudate inhibits intestinal peristalsis.

Infection may reach the peritoneum directly from an abdominal wound, from a suppurative process in one of the intraperitoneal viscera, after an operation on an infected viscus, through the blood stream, through lymphatic spread from the pleura, or directly via the open ends of the fallopian tubes. It is an important diagnostic exercise to determine whether peritonitis is primary or secondary to pathology of an intra-abdominal viscus in order to determine the correct treatment. For the surgeon, the most important decision will be whether to select non-operative treatment with intravenous fluids and antibiotics or to operate.

Gram-positive organisms, Gram-negative bacilli, mixed synergistic infections and anaerobic organisms can all be pathogenic in the peritoneal cavity. Acute suppurative peritonitis is most commonly the result of perforation of the appendix or the large bowel from infection or ischaemia. Sigmoid diverticular perforations are usually more localized than caecal perforations which are often secondary to a distal obstruction and are followed by a rapid escape of liquid faeces which has a high bacterial content into the general peritoneal cavity.

Perforations of the stomach and duodenum do not lead to such a profuse bacterial contamination and to a lesser extent the same is true of small bowel perforations because of the low bacterial counts in the small bowel content. Nevertheless a significant chemical peritonitis follows the escape of gastric juice or small bowel fluid into the peritoneal cavity.

Peritonitis without perforation occurs in relation to any acute inflammatory process and in women the differential diagnosis must always include pelvic inflammatory disease. The organisms most commonly isolated in peritonitis are listed in Table 27.1. Inflammation of the peritoneum results in an increase in its blood supply and local oedema. Transudation of fluid into the peritoneal cavity is followed by the accumulation of a protein-rich fibrinous exudate containing leucocytes and antibodies which escapes through the large pores which increase in number as a result of

Table 27.1 Organisms responsible for peritonitis

Organisms	%
Aerobes	
Escherichia coli	100
Proteus	24
Klebsiella	24
Pseudomonas	24
Streptococci	33
Anaerobes	
Bacteroides fragilis	90
Clostridia	52

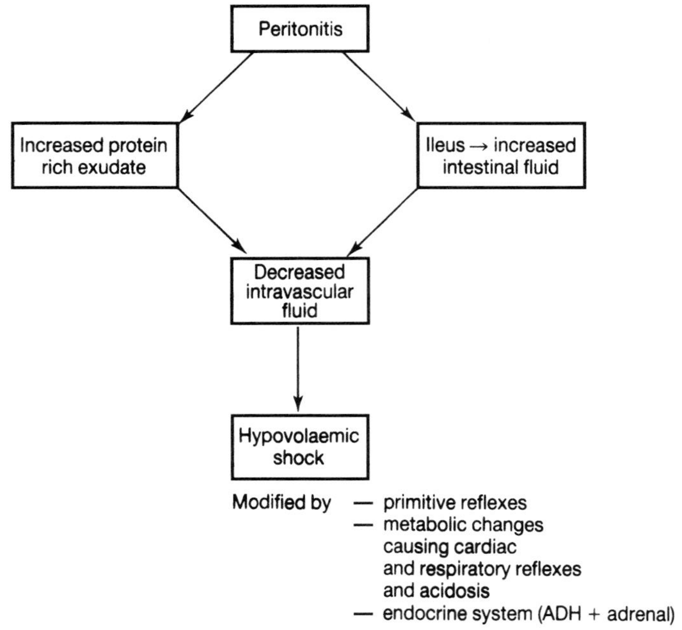

Fig. 27.4 The metabolic and fluid changes caused by severe prolonged and generalized peritonitis. ADH = Antidiuretic hormone.

inflammation.[13] The clinical consequences of peritonitis will vary depending on a number of factors which include its pathogenesis, whether it is localized or generalized, the duration of the symptoms and the age of the patient. If the infection is mild or slow in developing, localization by omentum and adhesions is likely to occur with the formation of an intraperitoneal abscess. When the infection is severe or fulminating it floods the peritoneal cavity, localization fails and profuse peritonitis develops. The peritoneal fluid becomes turbid and later frankly purulent.

Peritonitis causes fluid shifts and metabolic changes, especially if it is generalized and prolonged. These changes are summarized in Figure 27.4. The general response is modified by a number of secondary reactions. The heart and respiratory rate increase initially as a result of volumetric, intestinal, diaphragmatic and pain reflexes. Subsequently cardiac output and respiration are influenced by metabolic changes brought about by acidosis and increased secretion of aldosterone, antidiuretic hormone and catecholamines.[14] Mobilization of hepatic glycogen and catabolism of protein form part of the metabolic response which is now recognized to be much more complex.

Clinical features

Clinically the symptoms and signs of peritonitis have been well-recognized for many centuries and the characteristic facies of a sick dehydrated patient with peritonitis were originally described by Hippocrates.[15] The most common symptom is pain which may be either localized or diffuse and is usually constant and of a sharp pricking character. A visceral perforation causes a severe pain of sudden onset which is usually first appreciated in the area of the perforation[16]—upper epigastric in the case of a duodenal ulcer and the left iliac fossa following perforation of a colonic diverticulum. Shoulder-tip pain is present if the diaphragmatic peritoneum is inflamed. The pain may later become more generalized as the infection spreads. Intermittent colicky abdominal pain may precede established peritonitis in appendicitis or strangulating obstruction. The pain often follows a period of malaise and is accompanied by anorexia, nausea and vomiting. There is usually associated constipation unless a pelvic abscess develops, which can cause diarrhoea.

The patient lies relatively motionless and supine with shallow respiratory excursions. The abdomen becomes increasingly rigid and board-like as peritonitis develops. The knees are sometimes flexed and drawn up, reducing tension in the abdominal wall and relieving pain. The face is drawn, pale and anxious. The eyes are sunken. This reflects the extent of any accompanying hypovolaemia which can be confirmed by finding a tachycardia and a thready peripheral pulse.

Palpation of the abdomen increases the pain and should be undertaken gently when assessing abdominal guarding and rigidity which are initially voluntary and subsequently become involuntary reflexes. The site of maximum tenderness is usually related to the site of the pathology. The increasing ileus is confirmed by auscultation of the bowel sounds which diminish and finally disappear. In diffuse peritonitis the whole abdominal wall is rigid, wooden and no longer moves on respiration. The rigidity gradually resolves if localization occurs and a mass or abscess may become palpable through the slackening abdominal wall. If the peritonitis remains diffuse, distension and dehydration continue and end in circulatory failure, coma and death.

The demonstration of gas under the diaphragm on an erect chest or lateral decubitus abdominal radiograph confirms the diagnosis of a perforated viscus. A serum amylase concentration below 1000 iu/l excludes acute pancreatitis as the cause of peritonitis (see Chapter 33). Peritoneal tap and lavage can be useful in doubtful cases to differentiate peritonitis from other conditions, as can ultrasonography, computed tomography (CT) scanning and laparoscopy, all of which will be discussed later in more detail.

Pneumonia is sometimes accompanied by peritonism and can be misdiagnosed, especially in children, as peritonitis. Other conditions which must be considered in the differential diagnosis include ureteric calculi, gastroenteritis, hepatitis and urinary tract infections. Acute intermittent porphyria, the lightning pains of syphilis, diabetes mellitus and the coxsackie virus can also give a similar picture, although they are far less common (p. 755).

Treatment

Surgical treatment

Once the diagnosis has been established, antibiotics that are effective against anaerobes and aerobes should be started immediately.

REFERENCES

13. Verger C, Luger A et al Kidney Int 1983; 23: 823
14. Clowes G H A, Farrington G H, Zuschneid W Ann Surg 1970; 171: 663
15. Hippocrates 'On Surgery' 400 BC. The Genuine Works of Hippocrates. F Adams, Sydenham Society, London 1849
16. Doran F S A Br J Surg 1961; 49: 376

As a general rule most patients suspected of having suppurative peritonitis should be prepared for laparotomy. Intravenous fluid replacement with both crystalloids and colloids with urinary catheterization and monitoring of the urinary output are required if there are signs of hypovolaemia or shock. Nasogastric aspiration reduces abdominal distension and prevents repeated vomiting with the risk of aspiration. Oxygen and vasoactive drugs may be required to support the respiration and circulation in severe cases. Strong opiate analgesics should be given as soon as a working diagnosis has been clearly established. It has often been argued that early administration of opiate analgesia to patients with acute abdominal pain should be withheld as it may interfere with the clinical signs. This has now been shown to be untrue[17] and early relief of the patient's pain is an essential part of good surgical practice. The patient should not be taken to theatre until dehydration and fluid and electrolyte imbalance have been corrected.

Laparotomy is normally undertaken through an upper or lower midline incision depending on the suspected site of the pathology. Transverse incisions are popular with some surgeons but access to the opposite end of the peritoneal cavity can be difficult if the incision is incorrectly sited or the patient is very obese. The first objective is to establish the cause of the peritonitis and then to remove the inflamed or ischaemic organ or to close the perforated viscus. Specific procedures are discussed in the section on the acute abdomen (p. 721). Removal of infected material by peritoneal lavage is thought to reduce mortality.[18,19] The chief benefit of this measure probably results from physically washing out large numbers of bacteria, but irrigation with agents such as tetracycline which also have an antibacterial effect is now common practice.

The value of draining the peritoneal cavity is more controversial.[20,21] It is probably unnecessary in patients with generalized peritonitis, if a satisfactory closure of the perforation can be achieved, but may be of value in more localized forms of peritonitis such as a pericolic abscess. Non-suction tube drains have theoretical and practical advantages over both suction drains and the old-fashioned corrugated drains. Suction drains tend to become attached to adjacent viscera and bowel can be damaged by being sucked into the drainage holes.[22] Mass closure of the abdomen[23] is undertaken using either interrupted or continuous monofilament sutures. There is no evidence that the use of deep tension sutures provides additional advantages to interupted mass closure.

Normally peritoneal healing and re-peritonealization of denuded areas of abdominal wall is rapid, being completed within a few days.[24] Much work has been carried out over the last 20 years on the mechanism of adhesion formation and it appears to be related to a reduction in tissue plasminogen activator activity in the peritoneal mesothelial cells which follows drying, trauma, ischaemia and inflammation.[25,26] This reduction in tissue plasminogen activator activity may be caused by the presence of a specific inhibitory substance which is produced by the peritoneal cells following inflammation.[27] Adhesions are also produced by lavage fluid and experimental studies in rats have demonstrated that lavage with high concentrations of tetracyline (10 mg/ml) produces ultrastructural damage to the peritoneum with loss of serosal microvilli.[28] Tetracycline lavage at concentrations of 1 mg/ml which is the usual concentration used in clinical practice and with normal saline still produced more adhesions than no lavage following 'clean' surgery. This advantage was lost if bacterial contamination was introduced.[28]

Non-operative treatment

There are many occasions for managing patients with peritonitis without operation, depending on the underlying diagnosis. In some circumstances, such as on board ship or when medical help is limited or poorly equipped, non-operative treatment becomes the only option. Every effort should be made to assist the peritoneum to localize infection in a safe location, preferably below the pelvic basin. Food is withheld and nutrition is maintained parenterally if possible. Opioid analgesics are liberally prescribed. A nasogastric or Miller–Abbott tube is passed to provide continuous gastric or intestinal drainage and the patient is nursed sitting up with the head of the bed elevated on blocks (the Fowler's position).[29] A broad-spectrum antibiotic or a combination of antibiotics (a cephalosporin or an aminoglycoside with metronidazole) is administered intravenously. As the patient's condition improves and the temperature settles, food is re-introduced, the nasogastric tube is withdrawn and the patient is allowed out of bed. If the temperature fluctuates widely an abscess must be suspected and once localized may require drainage.

Prognosis

The mortality of peritonitis depends on the underlying cause and increases with the bacterial count, the delay in treatment and the age of the patient. The mortality of peritonitis caused by appendicitis is 10% above the age of 80, but in peritonitis secondary to large bowel perforation the mortality is 20% below the age of 40 and rises to 80% in those over 80 years of age.[30] The overall mortality for perforated peptic ulcer is 26%, but for those over 70 years rises to 34%.[31] When acute suppurative peritonitis is suspected treatment should be regarded as an emergency before local changes progress to renal failure with secondary cardiovascular collapse and respiratory failure.[32]

REFERENCES

17. Attard A R, Corlett M J et al Br Med J 1992; 305: 554
18. Hudspeth A S Arch Surg 1976; 110: 1233
19. Stewart D J, Matheson N A Br J Surg 1975; 65: 54
20. Broome A R, Hanson L C, Tyger J F Acta Chir Scand 1983; 149: 53
21. O'Connor T W, Hugh T B Aust NZ J Surg 1979; 41: 253
22. Seely M F, Hyde W A, Irving M H Br J Surg 1979; 66: 657
23. Jenkins T P N Br J Surg 1976; 63: 873
24. Ellis H, Harrison W, Hugh T B Br J Surg 1965; 52: 471
25. Raftery A T Br J Surg 1981; 80: 107
26. Thompson J N, Paterson-Brown S et al Br J Surg 1989; 76: 382
27. Wawell S A, Vipond M N et al Br J Surg 1993; 80: 107
28. Phillips R K S, Dudley H A F Br J Surg 1984; 71: 537
29. Fowler G R Med Rec NY 1900; 57: 617
30. Bothen J, Boulanger M et al Arch Surg 1983; 118: 285
31. Irvin T T Br J Surg 1989; 76: 215
32. Renvall S Acta Chir Scand 1976; 142: 407

Table 27.2 Types of peritonitis

Primary
Spontaneous
Secondary
Acute suppurative
Granulomatous
Aseptic (chemical)
Miscellaneous
Interventional
Drugs
Carcinomatosis
Foreign bodies

Varieties of peritonitis

Peritonitis may be classified according to its pathogenesis (Table 27.2).

Primary peritonitis

Primary bacterial peritonitis which occurs without any obvious source for the infection being demonstrated is much more common in those with some intercurrent disease, such as children who have undergone a splenectomy or who have a nephrotic syndrome[33] and adults with cirrhosis.[34] In true spontaneous peritonitis only one organism is found in the cultures of the peritoneal fluid. Pneumococci used to be the most commonly isolated organisms but *Escherichia coli* and *Klebsiella* are now more frequently cultured.[35] In cases where bacteria cannot be identified, raised viral titres are sometimes found. The route of entry of organisms into the peritoneal cavity cannot usually be determined but transmural spread as well as blood stream spread have both been postulated. Primary peritonitis is more common in young girls than young boys and as a consequence it has been suggested that the female genital tract may be a portal of entry.[36] Aird reported that the pneumococcus could be isolated from the vaginas of many young girls in Edinburgh. Pneumococcal peritonitis, however, appears to be declining in incidence and an intraperitoneal foreign body must always be excluded in cases of primary peritonitis.

Clinical features

All grades of severity occur. In the milder forms there is a low-grade peritonitis associated with a gelatinous exudate, while in the fulminant variety there is a rapidly spreading purulent peritonitis with pneumococcal septicaemia, collapse and often extreme cyanosis. Patients present with abdominal pain, pyrexia and vomiting. At a later stage abdominal rigidity and distension develop. Labial herpes may be present.

The differential diagnosis from conditions such as appendicitis is often only made at the time of laparotomy[37] when a predisposing cause is excluded and peritoneal ascitic fluid is cultured. Laparoscopy and/or peritoneal tap and culture can be considered if the condition is suspected clinically. However, caution must be exercised in accepting the diagnosis of spontaneous peritonitis, for the dangers of missing unusual pathology such as a pneumococcal abscess are far greater than the dangers of an unnecessary laparotomy. Unless a primary pathology is found, drainage of the peritoneal cavity is unnecessary and treatment is by an appropriate antibiotic such as benzylpenicillin combined with the non-operative measures outlined above.

Aseptic chemical peritonitis

The most common form of aseptic peritonitis occurs after perforation of a duodenal ulcer when the gastric contents and bile enter the peritoneal cavity. Secondary overgrowth with intestinal flora occurs if the peritoneal contamination persists for some hours without treatment. Bile escaping from a ruptured gallbladder (see Chapter 32) and pancreatic enzymes collecting in patients with acute pancreatitis can also cause chemical peritonitis. Bile peritonitis usually requires drainage. It can also occur when a T-tube becomes dislodged or an accessory hepatic duct is inadvertently divided at the time of cholecystectomy. Blunt abdominal trauma can release blood, pancreatic enzymes, bowel and urine into the peritoneal cavity following rupture of the relevant organs. Blood within the peritoneal cavity can cause pain and peritonism.

Meconium peritonitis can occur in neonates following intestinal rupture any time after the third month of intrauterine life. The term should not be used unless meconium, calcified meconium, mucus droplets or lanugo hairs are demonstrated in the peritoneal cavity. Initially the peritonitis is sterile but infection may develop later. Usually the bowel perforation causing the condition has closed before birth, but it occasionally persists. In half the cases of meconium ileus, atresia, volvulus or hernia is responsible. In viable infants there are signs of intestinal obstruction, distension and pneumoperitoneum. The meconium may have become calcified and is visible on plain radiographs of the abdomen. Treatment entails relief of obstruction and closure of any perforations that are present.

Interventional peritonitis

Following abdominal surgery, bowel and gastric contents, blood and urine may all escape and cause aseptic peritonitis which later becomes infected with bacteria. Invasive diagnostic procedures such as percutaneous transhepatic cholangiography and barium enema causing perforation of a diverticulum can give rise to a similar clinical picture. Diagnostic endoscopy may perforate the oesophagogastric junction, the caecum, sigmoid colon and bladder leading to peritonitis. An increasing number of patients are now treated by continuous ambulatory peritoneal dialysis for chronic renal failure and this is known to predispose to peritonitis despite careful tunnelling and positioning of the catheters[38] and the use of an aseptic technique when changing bags.

REFERENCES

33. Rubin H M, Balu E B, Michael R H Paediatrics 1975; 56: 508
34. Correira J P, Conn H O Med Clin North Am 1975; 59: 963
35. Bartlett J G, Miao P V W, Gorbach S L J Infect Dis 1977; 135 (suppl 80)
36. Fraser & McCartney quoted by Aird I Companion in Surgical Studies. Livingstone, Edinburgh 1958
37. Curry N, McCallum R W, Gath P H Am J Dig Dis 1974; 19: 685
38. Bengmark S The Peritoneum and Peritoneal Access. Wright, Bristol 1987

Drugs

Clinical symptoms similar to acute peritonitis have been described during treatment with isoniazid. A chronic form of plastic peritonitis with the formation of matted loops of bowel and greatly thickened visceral peritoneum (sclerosing peritonitis) resulted from the chronic usage of the β-blocking drug practolol which has now been withdrawn.[39,40] Treatment consisted of careful division of the thickened fibrotic cocoon from around the bowel. Intraperitoneal chemotherapy for malignant disease may also cause a peritoneal reaction.[41]

Foreign bodies

Talc, which is a magnesium silicate powder, and starch may stimulate foreign-body granulomata if they are inadvertently introduced into the peritoneal cavity on surgical gloves.[42,43] The associated inflammation encourages adhesion formation. Mechanical washing of surgical gloves before they are inserted into the peritoneal cavity is of some help but not completely effective.[44] Modern operating gloves are now starch- and talc-free and this condition should be effectively extinct. Starch peritonitis presents with abdominal pain, distension and pyrexia. Ascites is present with matted omentum and bowel causing abdominal masses. Appropriate signs can be detected on clinical examination or on imaging with abdominal ultrasound. The diagnosis is confirmed on a wound or peritoneal biopsy when birefringent granules are seen. Malignant and tuberculous peritonitis have to be considered in the differential diagnosis. Treatment is largely supportive and expectant but systemic steroids may prove beneficial in some cases.[45]

Special forms of peritonitis

The signs of peritonitis may be masked in patients on steroids, in immunosuppressed patients (those with acquired immunodeficiency syndrome or on immunosuppressive drugs), in young children and in the very old and infirm.

Complications

These include adhesive obstruction (p. 735) and intraperitoneal abscesses (see below).

INTRAPERITONEAL ABSCESSES

An intraperitoneal abscess is formed when peritonitis remains localized or when generalized peritonitis fails to resolve completely. Localization can occur as a result of developmental folds, adhesions between local intestinal loops or when the omentum prevents the spread of infection. Occasionally a bacteraemia may cause a retroperitoneal infection which leads to a localized peritoneal reaction and abscess formation. Abscesses usually develop close to the original source of infection. Localized abscesses in the peritoneum are most often found in the subphrenic region or in the pelvis. *Escherichia coli* and *Bacteroides* are the commonest organisms to be isolated from these collections of pus (see Chapter 4).

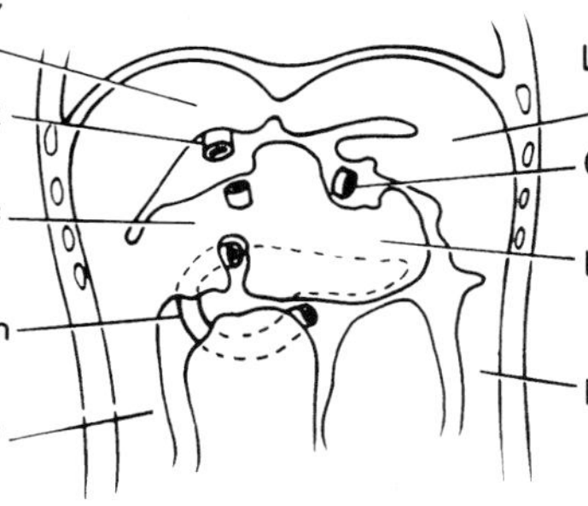

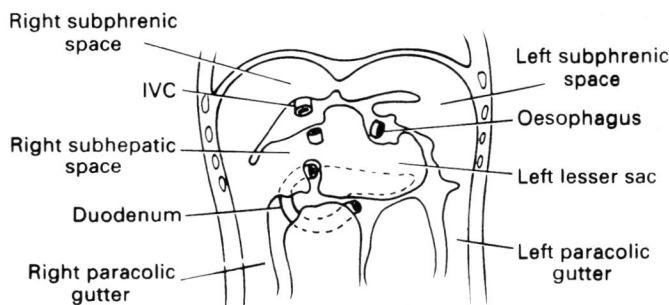

Fig. 27.5 The subphrenic spaces beneath the diaphragm. IVC = inferior vena cava.

Subphrenic abscesses

There are seven anatomical spaces and potential spaces in relation to the abdominal surface of the diaphragm where pus can collect: three on each side and one placed centrally (Fig. 27.5). In practice pus is usually bounded by inflammatory adhesions rather than the ligaments of the liver but a broad anatomical classification is helpful when considering approaches to drainage.

The right anterior intraperitoneal space (right subphrenic space)

This lies in front of the liver and right coronary ligament, below the diaphragm and behind the abdominal wall. Its left boundary is the falciform ligament; inferiorly it communicates over the liver edge with the general peritoneal cavity. This space is commonly infected from the gallbladder or from a perforation of the stomach or duodenum. An abscess in this space tends to point towards the right costal margin.

The right posterior intraperitoneal space (the right subhepatic space)

This is the hepatorenal pouch of Rutherford–Morison. It lies behind and below the right lobe of the liver, in front of the peritoneum covering the diaphragm and the kidney. It is bounded above by the posterior leaf of the paracolic gutter. Infection commonly reaches this space from the appendix, the gallbladder, the right colon, the duodenum or the right perinephric tissues. An abscess in this space points towards the loin.

The right extraperitoneal subphrenic space

This is a potential space between the bare area of the liver and the diaphragm. In front and behind are the two layers of the coronary

REFERENCES

39. Brown P, Baddeley H et al Lancet 1974; 11: 1477
40. Eltringham W K, Espiner C W D et al Br J Surg 1977; 64: 229
41. Sugarbaker P H, Gianola F J, Speyer J C Surgery 1985; 98: 414
42. Antapol W Arch Pathol 1933; 76: 326
43. McAdams G B Surgery 1956; 39: 329
44. Kent S J S, Burnand K G, Owen D Ann R Coll Surg Engl 1975; 57: 212
45. Bates B Ann Inter Med 1965; 62: 335

ligament, which fuse in the right corner. On the left the space is bounded by the inferior vena cava. This space is usually infected by a perinephric infection arising from the right kidney. Abscesses in this space tend to track forwards in front of the vena cava to a point in the epigastrium between the layers of the falciform ligament. An abscess in this space is unusual.

The left anterior intraperitoneal subphrenic space (left subhepatic space)

This is similar to its fellow of the opposite side. Anteriorly is the abdominal wall, superiorly the diaphragm, posteriorly is the left triangular ligament and inferiorly the left lobe of the liver. The falciform ligament lies to the right and the spleen to the left. The space communicates over the liver edge with the anterior peritoneal compartment in front of the omental curtain. This space is infected by an anterior gastric perforation, or from infection associated with the left colon, pancreas or spleen. An abscess in this space points below the left costal margin.

The left posterior intraperitoneal space (left subhepatic space)

This is the lesser sac situated between the stomach and lesser omentum anteriorly and the under-surface of the left lobe of the liver superiorly, the peritoneum and the transverse mesocolon and transverse colon inferiorly. The lienorenal ligament and the gastrosplenic ligament form the left boundary and it communicates with the greater sac behind the porta hepatis through the foramen of Winslow on the right. It is usually infected from the pancreas or following gastric surgery. Abscesses in the lesser sac tend to point anteriorly through the lesser omentum or greater omentum below the greater curvature of the stomach.

The right and left extraperitoneal spaces

These are unimportant and their names are applied to the areolar tissue around the upper poles of the kidney. An abscess in these spaces is usually classified as a perinephric abscess.

Microbiology

Subphrenic abscesses are almost always pyogenic, although tuberculous abscesses have been reported[46] complicating tuberculosis of the gallbladder, liver, spleen, kidney and lung.

The clinical picture depends upon the site and size of the abscess. The presentation and signs are frequently obscure, when it is described by the surgical aphorism: 'pus somewhere, pus nowhere, pus under the diaphragm'. A subphrenic abscess is suspected when a patient develops a swinging fever associated with marked toxaemia after an intra-abdominal infection or operation. A fever and abdominal pain with tenderness which persist and defy diagnosis should suggest the possibility of a subphrenic abscess, especially if there is a raised sedimentation rate and accompanying leucocytosis. Pain may be entirely absent or may be referred to the chest wall, loin, upper abdomen, back or shoulder. Pain may be produced or exacerbated by pressing the rib margins together. Hiccup is common and may be distressing. Tenderness can usually be elicited at one of the points of Vegni:[47]

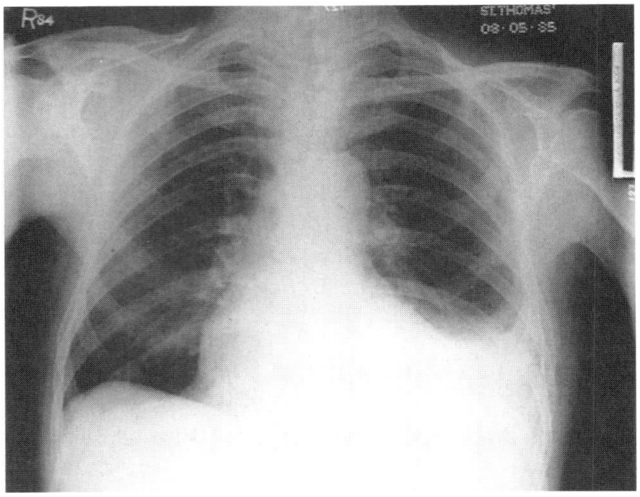

Fig. 27.6 Chest X-ray showing a small pleural effusion above a subphrenic abscess.

1. The anterior phrenic point at the tip of the 10th rib.
2. The posterior phrenic point where the edge of the erector spinae crosses the 11th intercostal space.
3. The superior phrenic point which is situated over the phrenic nerve between the two heads of sternomastoid.

The liver is usually depressed and its edge is palpable. The signs of a pleural effusion may be present and occasionally hyper-resonance indicates the presence of gas in the subphrenic space, as a result of a perforation or an anaerobic infection. Rarely a palpable swelling is present in the upper abdomen or lower chest. The extent of the apparent liver dullness is often decreased.

A leucocytosis is invariably present and chest X-ray may show a small pleural effusion or even an empyema (Fig. 27.6). Air may be seen in the subphrenic space and occasionally an air–fluid level is seen. Other diagnoses which should be considered include liver abscess, empyema, lung abscess, pelvic abscess, deep vein thrombosis and septic pulmonary embolism, portal pyaemia and pneumonia.

Subphrenic abscess have in the past been diagnosed by finding reduced movement on screening of the diaphragms, but now most are well-demonstrated by ultrasound or CT (Figs 27.7 and 27.8). Radiolabelled leucocytes, using indium, are concentrated in abscess cavities and this is an alternative means of locating a collection of pus.

Treatment

Once a subphrenic abscess has been diagnosed a decision has to be made between conservative management with antibiotic therapy

REFERENCES

46. Piquand G Rev Chir 1909; 40: 336
47. Vegni cited in Aird I Companion in Surgical Studies. Livingstone, Edinburgh 1958

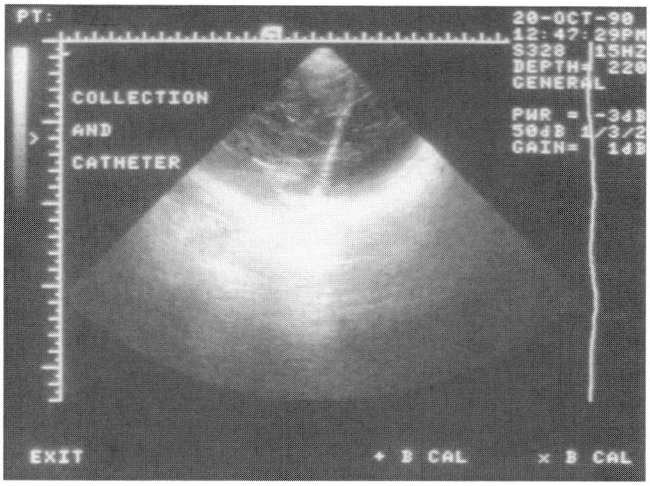

Fig. 27.7 Ultrasound scan demonstrating a collection of pus in the subhepatic space (Rutherford–Morrison's pouch). A catheter can be seen within the abscess.

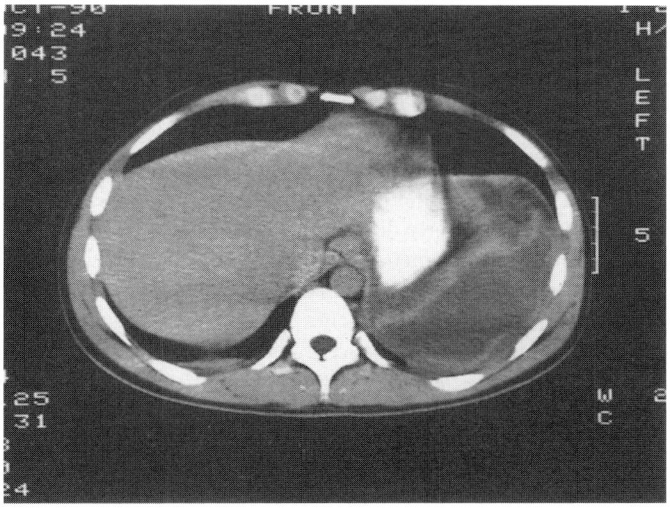

Fig. 27.8 CT scan of a subphrenic abscess.

and drainage. Many abscesses can now be treated by ultrasound or CT-guided placement of a drainage tube inserted under local anaesthesia.[48] This drain can be left in place or the pus can be aspirated and antibiotics instilled into the cavity. The aspiration may be repeated on several occasions, provided the clinical picture is improving but deterioration should indicate the need for open surgical drainage.

Surgical drainage

The presence of a swelling or the position of an abscess on CT scanning or ultrasound may indicate the best approach for drainage. An anterior approach may be used for a right subphrenic abscess (Fig. 27.9). However, both right and left subphrenic abscesses are often best approached from behind through the bed of the 12th rib (Fig. 27.10). Care must be taken to avoid opening the pleura and producing an empyema. The pleura should be pushed gently upwards and a finger can then be inserted below the diaphragm and above the kidney to explore the subphrenic space (see Fig. 27.9b). An area of induration may be entered with a resultant satisfying gush of pus. If this technique fails to locate the abscess, a long wide-bore needle attached to a syringe can be used to explore the subphrenic space. It is important to stay in the extraserosal plane if possible. Once the abscess cavity is entered it must be widely explored, opened and drained to avoid loculi developing. A large tube drain is then inserted. Regular and repeated sinograms down the drainage tube indicate that the cavity

a

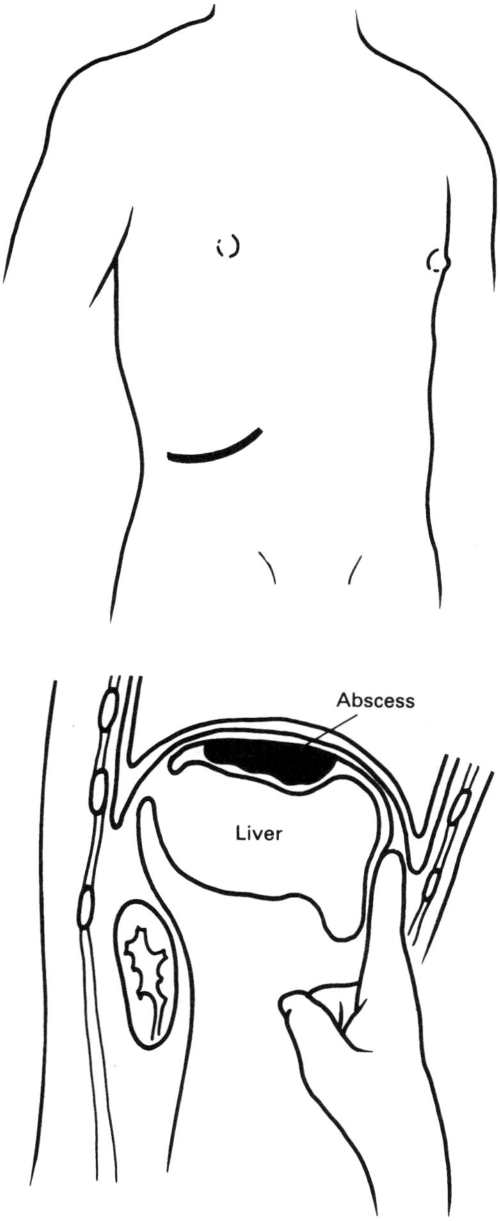

b

Fig. 27.9a,b The incision and extraperitoneal approach to drain a subphrenic abscess; usually best approached by an anterior subcostal route.

REFERENCES

48. Russell R C G J R Soc Med 1987; 80: 471

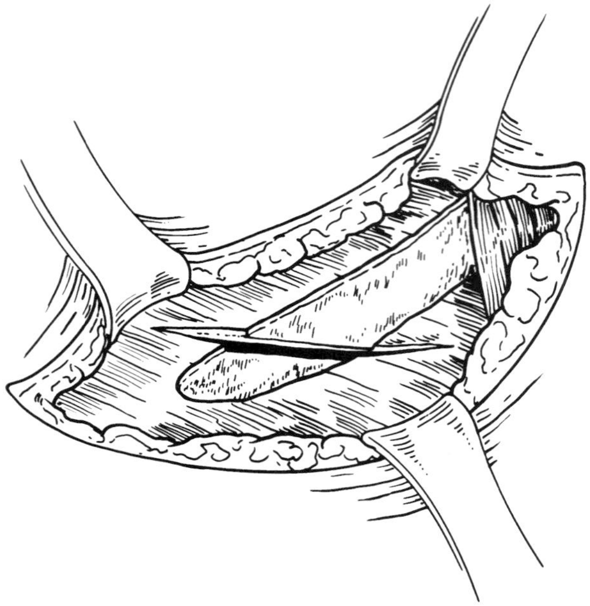

Fig. 27.10 The posterior approach used to drain a subphrenic abscess, through the bed of the 12th rib.

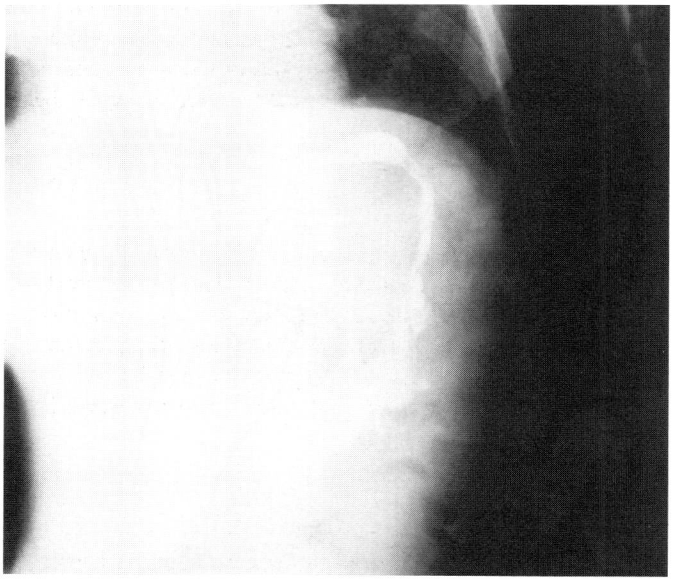

Fig. 27.11 Sinogram outlining a subphrenic abscess cavity in the left subphrenic space after a splenectomy.

has shrunk and this should be confirmed before the tubes are removed (Fig. 27.11).

Pelvic abscess

Many of the features of a pelvic abscess are similar to those of a subphrenic abscess from which it must be differentiated. A pelvic abscess is the commonest variety of intraperitoneal abscess. An inflamed appendix, pelvic inflammatory disease and acute diverticulitis can all cause local pelvic peritonitis and eventually lead to pelvic abscess formation. Pus can also track down into the pelvis from a perforated peptic ulcer.

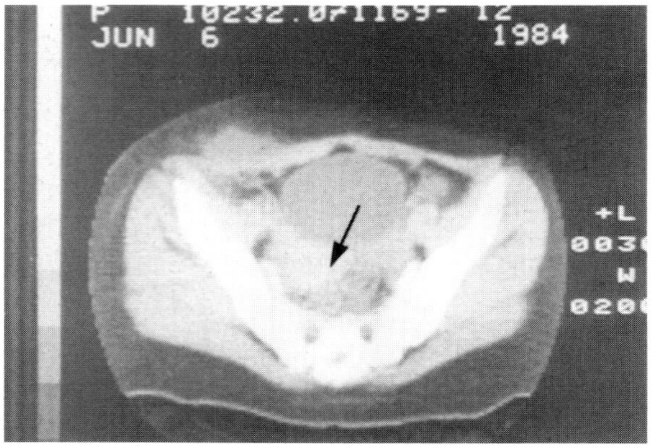

Fig. 27.12 CT scan showing a pelvic abscess developing after acute appendicitis.

The condition must be suspected in any patient, known to have had one of the predisposing conditions or pelvic surgery, who develops a swinging pyrexia some days after the initial event. Pelvic abscesses often cause few symptoms but a frequent call to stool and the excessive passage of mucus on defecation indicate that the abscess is beginning to point into the rectum. Occasionally urinary frequency occurs. A palpable boggy mass felt on digital examination of the rectum confirms the diagnosis, but this may not be present in the early stages when rectal examination may only elicit pain. Ultrasound and CT scanning provide a more accurate means of making an early diagnosis (Fig. 27.12). There is usually a marked accompanying leucocytosis.

Many pelvic abscesses drain spontaneously into the rectum, requiring no additional treatment. This can be encouraged by gentle finger pressure at the site of maximal swelling. If spontaneous drainage does not occur, the abscess should be formally drained under general anaesthesia with the patient in the lithotomy position. A proctoscope or operating sigmoidoscope is inserted into the rectum. If the abscess is clearly seen to be pointing, a pair of sinus forceps can be gently pushed into its centre, but if uncertainty exists a large-bore aspirating needle and syringe can be used to locate the pus. Good drainage must be obtained. All loculi should be broken down with a finger. Occasionally pelvic abscesses can drain through the vagina but rectal drainge is always preferable.

ABDOMINAL TUBERCULOSIS

Intestinal tuberculosis

This is discussed in Chapter 29.

Tuberculous mesenteric adenitis

This was and still is in some parts of the world a common disease of childhood. It usually follows the entry of bovine bacillus via a Peyer's patch or a solitary lymph follicle. The pathology is similar to tuberculosis of the cervical glands. It is normally discovered incidentally as a calcified symptomless lymph node or on routine abdominal X-ray (Fig. 27.13). Enlarged tuberculous nodes are

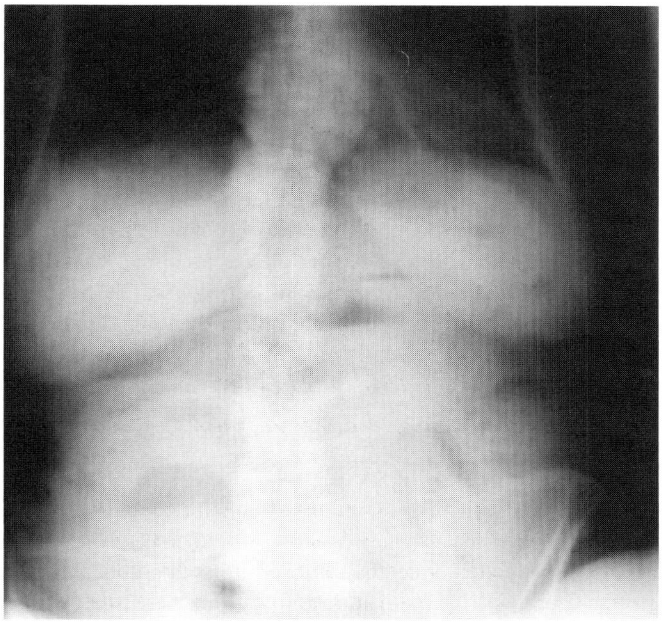

Fig. 27.13 Calcified tuberculous lymph node.

hardly ever palpable. The bowel occasionally becomes adherent to a tuberculous gland which can then cause intestinal obstruction. Tuberculous mesenteric glands can caseate and rupture causing tuberculous peritonitis.

Tuberculous peritonitis

This can develop from miliary tuberculosis, from direct spread from the bowel or the fallopian tubes, or from rupture of a tuberculous mesenteric lymph node. Blood stream spread to the peritoneum from a focus outside the abdominal cavity such as the lung, a bone or joint, or the urinary tract is unusual. Women are affected twice as commonly as men, perhaps because the female genital tract is an important portal of infection. Although the disease has declined in western countries since the early part of this century, it is still common in India and the Far East,[49] and population migration has increased the incidence in many western countries.[50]

Four forms of the disease have been described—ascitic, adhesive, acute and caseous—but these are often not clearly defined and more than one type of response may be present in the same patient.

The ascitic variety

This is characterized by liberal peritoneal exudate and numerous tubercles. It has an insidious course with vague abdominal symptoms, vomiting, constipation or diarrhoea, weight loss, evening temperature, malaise, night sweats, abdominal distension and congested abdominal veins. Occasionally the ascites fills a hernial sac causing persistent protrusion. Shifting dullness or a fluid thrill can usually be detected and a doughy abdominal mass represents the matted greater omentum studded with tubercles. Localized encysted collections can occur and may be mistaken for a mesenteric cyst or an abdominal tumour.

Ascitic tuberculosis has to be distinguished from other types of ascites and if a laparotomy is performed, fat necrosis, starch peritonitis and widespread carcinomatosis are usually considered in the differential diagnosis. A strongly positive Mantoux test supports the diagnosis. Ultrasound and CT scans confirm the presence of ascites and may show irregular soft tissue masses within the peritoneal fluid. If the ascites is tapped for diagnostic purposes, a pale yellow fluid is obtained with a high specific gravity. Tubercle bacilli are rarely demonstrated even after centrifugation, but may be confirmed by culture after 6 weeks. Because of the delay in making a bacteriological diagnosis and starting treatment, laparoscopy and biopsy are usually necessary to establish the diagnosis.[51] Ziehl–Neelsen staining of bacilli in the biopsy specimens and typical histological findings usually confirm the diagnosis. Laparoscopy should be performed with care, preferably using the 'open' technique (see Chapter 32) as adhesions may make insertion of the Veress needle dangerous, with risk of bowel perforation.

Adhesive variety

Bowel loops are matted together at first by tubercles and later by fibrous bands. This type usually presents with subacute intestinal obstruction, though acute obstruction can develop. If surgery is required careful separation of small bowel loops by division of adhesions is preferable, with intestinal resection or bypass being kept in reserve for inoperable disease.

Acute form

This presents as a purulent peritonitis with abdominal pain and distension. It may be suspected if there is a history of tuberculosis, or if ascites is detected, although a presumptive diagnosis of carcinomatosis is often made in western countries. At operation the adhesions should be divided and the tubercles biopsied.

Carcinomatosis, fat necrosis and starch peritonitis are again the important differential diagnoses.

Caseous form

This is a rare variety of abdominal tuberculosis which presents with large collections of caseous pus within the abdominal cavity. Cold abscesses may develop within the abdomen and these often point towards the umbilicus, or burst into the lumen of the bowel with the development of intestinal fistulae. Previous abscesses may require surgical drainage and the fistulae require operative closure.

Clinical features

In summary, chronic debility, abdominal pain, fever, night sweats, abdominal distension, weight loss and anorexia are all common

REFERENCES

49. Bhansali S K, Desai A N Ind J Surg 1968; 30: 218
50. Wells A D, Northover J, Howard E R J R Soc Med 1986; 79: 149
51. Udwadia T E Ind J Surg 1978; 40: 91

complaints while the presence of ascites, a doughy abdomen and irregular abdominal masses are the most common clinical findings.[52,53]

Treatment

Beside the operative measures outlined above all patients are placed on antituberculous combination chemotherapy for 9–12 months which usually consists of rifampicin, ethambutol and isoniazid (see Chapter 4). This often causes complete cessation of the symptoms, although surgery may occasionally be required to divide fibrous adhesions.[50,51]

GRANULOMATOUS PERITONITIS

Yeast, amoebae, fungi and parasites are rare causes of non-specific granulomatous peritonitis.

TUMOURS OF THE PERITONEUM

Solid primary tumours of the peritoneum are rare. The most common tumours are secondary carcinomas, usually derived from transcoelomic dissemination from another abdominal tumour or occasionally by blood or lymphatic spread from an extra-abdominal primary site. Peritoneal metastases may take the form of discrete nodules, plaque-like masses, diffuse malignant adhesions, flat subperitoneal deposits, cystic masses (usually ovarian) and pedunculated tumours. Bizarre deposits with tufts of hair are associated with secondary teratomas. Ascites is often present.

The differential diagnosis of peritoneal metastases may be extremely difficult. Other conditions that can give similar appearances include tuberculosis, encapsulated foreign bodies, talc granulomata, chronic sepsis, fat necrosis, infestation by parasites (schistosomiasis, cysticercosis, hydatids), polyarteritis nodosa, gas cysts, splenosis, actinomycosis, leprosy, infection with *Pasteurella* and *Brucella*. Carcinomatosis of the peritoneal cavity usually presents with pain, weight loss and abdominal swelling.

The diagnosis is by biopsy, although if ascites is present a cytological diagnosis is possible. The biopsy may be obtained at laparotomy or at laparoscopy (see below).

Treatment is usually supportive with measures designed to relieve pain, vomiting, constipation and abdominal distension. Occasionally intraperitoneal chemotherapy can cause a useful regression.

The best recognized primary tumour of the peritoneum is the mesothelioma or the endothelioma which occurs in benign and malignant forms and is similar to the well-recognized pleural tumour (Chapter 22). The malignant variety usually responds to radiotherapy but recurrence is invariable.

Pseudomyxoma peritonei

After rupture of a pseudomucinous cystadenoma of the ovary or, more rarely, of a mucocoele of the appendix, mucus-secreting cells are liberated into the peritoneal cavity where they become implanted on the peritoneal surface. The abdominal cavity becomes filled with tumour masses and fluid. Biopsy of the tumours shows a fibrinous network with mucin or pseudomucin in its spaces: the masses may be enclosed in a veil of epithelium, or may project from the serous surfaces of the viscera into the peritoneal cavity. In places, scattered islands of columnar cells are found.

The symptoms are those of progressive abdominal distension and weight loss. If pseudomyxomatosis is found at operation, an effort should be made to clear out all the abnormal tissue. The causative appendix or ovary should of course be removed. Unfortunately, recurrence is common and further laparotomies and peritoneal toilet may be required. It is a condition that is better avoided than treated.

ASCITES

This is the name given to an increased amount of fluid collecting within the peritoneal cavity. Ascites can either be the result of increased production or decreased absorption of peritoneal fluid. It is often a protein-rich exudate resulting from increased capillary and mesothelial permeability following peritonitis or carcinomatous infiltration and irritation, or it may be a transudate in patients with cardiac failure, constrictive pericarditis, tricuspid incompetence or Budd–Chiari syndrome. These all cause an increase in the hydrostatic pressure. When ascites occurs in cirrhosis of the liver the mechanism is complex, but raised portal venous pressure, hyperaldosteronism and reduced oncotic pressure from osmotic low albumin levels all play a part. Rupture of hepatic lymphatics may also contribute to fluid formation. Patients with hypoproteinaemia also develop ascites, as do patients with abnormal lymphatic drainage (chylous ascites).

Clinical features

Abdominal distension, nausea, constipation and weight loss are the main symptoms. Patients often notice that their clothes no longer fit, or that they have to let out their belts. The physical signs are of shifting dullness when the fluid collection is small and a percussion thrill when it is tense. Ascites (fluid) must be differentiated from the other five fs—fetus, faeces, flatus, fat and fibroids—which can also cause abdominal enlargement. A large ovarian cyst is the main differential diagnosis but tuberculous peritonitis must also be considered.

Investigations

The patient must be investigated in order to confirm the diagnosis and if possible determine the cause. Urea and electrolytes and liver function tests may confirm the nephrotic syndrome, liver failure or hypoproteinaemia. Plain X-rays of the abdomen usually show a ground-glass appearance with a paucity of gas shadows. Abdominal ultrasound and CT scanning confirm the presence of

REFERENCES

52. Dineed P, Homan W P, Grafe W R Ann Surg 1976; 184: 717
53. Addison N V Ann R Coll Surg Engl 1983; 65: 105

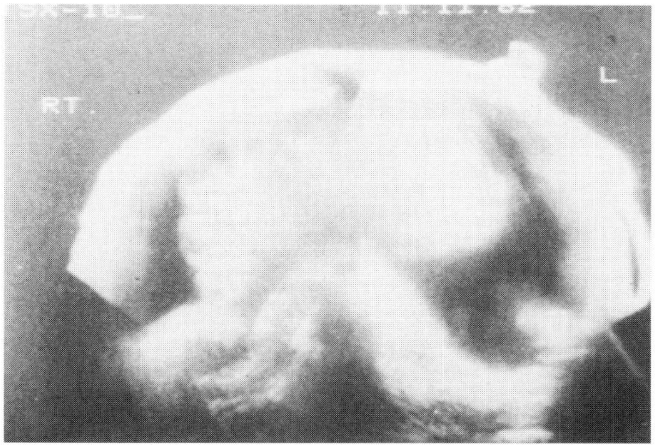

Fig. 27.14 Ultrasound scan demonstrating free fluid in the peritoneal cavity (ascites).

intraperitoneal fluid (Fig. 27.14). The fluid should be tapped and sent for chemical analysis, microbiological microscopy and culture and cytology to look for malignant cells. The patient should be re-examined for signs of cardiac disease, hypoproteinaemia, lymphatic disorders, chronic liver disease and tuberculosis. A milky tap suggests chylous ascites and requires lymphography to determine the presence of megalymphatics and if possible to define the site of leakage.

The finding of malignant cells may occasionally encourage the search for the primary tumour as carcinoma of the ovary has a good long-term prognosis following surgery and chemotherapy.[54] Liver biopsy and laparoscopy may be required to exclude chronic liver disease, tuberculosis and Meigs syndrome (ascites associated with a benign ovarian fibroma).[7] Occasionally laparotomy functions as the final court of appeal if all other causes have been excluded, but under these circumstances it rarely provides the answer.

Treatment

When a cause can be found this should be treated (e.g. heart failure, hypoproteinaemia, tuberculosis, ovarian malignancy). Cirrhotic ascites usually responds to diuretics and a combination of a thiazide diuretic with an aldosterone antagonist such as spironolactone is usually effective. Dietary sodium restriction may also be helpful. Repeated paracentesis became unpopular on the grounds that it induced hypoproteinaemia, although recently its value has again been championed.[55] The ascites is tapped through a peritoneal dialysis catheter and great care is taken with sterility to avoid introducing infection which can be rapidly fatal in patients with cirrhosis.

Insertion of a peritoneovenous shunt between the abdominal cavity and the internal jugular vein has been used to treat patients with a severe refractory ascites. This type of shunting is rarely successful in patients with a heavy proteinaceous exudate as the one-way valve mechanism used to prevent venous reflux within the shunt rapidly blocks up, even if the open end of the tubing remains patent. Two types of shunt are commercially available—the Le Veen[56] and the Denver[57] shunts. They are tunnelled subcutaneously from the peritoneal cavity to the internal jugular vein. They are made of Silastic and contain a non-return valve to prevent blood reflux and allow manual compression in an effort to overcome blockage. Large quantities of ascites must be present and being continuously formed for the shunt to remain patent. Dangers include fluid overload, cardiac failure, disseminated intravascular coagulation and blood stream spread of malignancy.[58]

Chylous ascites may be reduced by ligation of lymphatic fistulae, by resection of abnormal small bowel (leaking lymph from its surface) and by forming a lymphovenous anastomosis to bypass an obstructed thoracic duct.[59,60]

Malignant ascites may improve with intraperitoneal or systemic chemotherapy.

HAEMOPERITONEUM

Blood within the peritoneal cavity may occur from the following causes:

1. Traumatic injury to abdominal organs, vessels, omentum, mesentery or a trivial injury to a diseased organ (e.g. a malarial spleen or a vascular malformation of the liver).
2. Ruptured ectopic pregnancy.
3. Ruptured ovarian cyst, torted uterine fibroid, torted ovarian cyst or tumour.
4. Rupture of splenic or hepatic artery aneurysm.
5. Ruptured aortic or iliac aneurysm.
6. Rupture of atherosclerotic mesenteric artery.
7. Torted omentum.
8. Acute pancreatitis.
9. Perforated bleeding peptic ulcer or carcinoma of the stomach.
10. Haemorrhage from an intra-abdominal tumour, especially a hepatic adenoma or hepatocellular carcinoma.
11. Haemorrhagic disorders such as thrombocytopenia or over anticoagulation.
12. Primary amyloid.

The signs and symptoms of haemoperitoneum depend on the underlying cause, but include severe abdominal pain, abdominal distension and hypovolaemic shock. The diagnosis is confirmed by a peritoneal tap, peritoneal lavage or laparotomy. Treatment is that of the underlying condition. Urgent laparotomy after appropriate resuscitation is usually essential, although there is an increasing tendency to manage some cases of traumatic haemoperitoneum conservatively if the patient remains stable.

LAPAROSCOPY/PERITONEOSCOPY

This was first performed in 1902 by Kelling[61] on the dog using a cystoscope. In 1937 Ruddock[62] went on to develop an end-vision

REFERENCES

54. Raju K S, McKinna J A et al Am J Obstet Gynecol 1982; 144: 650
55. Editorial Lancet 1988; ii: 475
56. Le Veen H H, Wapnick S et al Ann Surg 1976; 184: 574
57. Lund R H, NewKirk J B Contemp Surg 1979; 14: 31
58. Lund R H, Mortz M W Arch Surg 1982; 117: 924
59. Kinmonth J B The Lymphatics. Edward Arnold, London 1972 p 243
60. Suhrland L G, Weisberger A S Arch Intern Med 1965; 116: 431

endoscope which was introduced by a stab incision through the rectus sheath after first producing an artificial penumoperitoneum. Since then gynaecologists were quick to see the advantages of laparoscopy for diagnosis of both acute and chronic pelvic disease in addition to tubal sterilization. Surgeons were however more reluctant to do so, despite numerous reports in the surgical literature demonstrating its value in the diagnosis of liver disease, ascites of unknown origin, tuberculous peritonitis, gall-bladder disease and other intra-abdominal masses and unexplained pain.[51,63,64]

Following the demonstration by Mouret in 1987 that laparoscopic cholecystectomy was possible,[65] combined with the recent improvement in instrumentation and video-technology, general surgeons have finally recognized the value of diagnostic and therapeutic laparoscopy, both of which have now become firmly established in the surgical armamentarium.

PERITONEAL LOOSE BODIES

Most peritoneal loose bodies arise by torsion and separation of epiploic appendices, but larger ones may originate from tubal abortions. Loose bodies should be distinguished from foreign bodies such as fish or meat bones that have perforated the intestine. All peritoneal loose bodies have a central crystalline core of calcium phosphate with a laminated fibrinoid capsule derived from peritoneal exudate. Loose bodies are usually symptomless. Most of them gravitate to the pelvis and there has been at least one case of acute retention from impaction of a large loose body in the retrovesical pouch.[66]

THE MESENTERY

Embryology

Like the omentum the mesentery develops from splanchnic mesoderm.[67] The dorsal mesentery of the gastrointestinal tract undergoes a great change during development, as the intestine elongates outside the embryo and subsequently rotates before returning to the peritoneal cavity. In the course of this process there is an anticlockwise rotation of the small bowel around the superior mesenteric artery. The mesentery fixes the intestines to the posterior wall of the abdominal cavity and allows the vascular and lymphatic vessels access to the bowel. The mesentery also contains lymph nodes, visceral nerve fibres and fat. The cells covering the mesentery are identical to those that lie in the peritoneal cavity, which have already been described. The mesentery of the small bowel arises from the posterior abdominal wall, passing obliquely from the duodenojejunal flexure to the ileocaecal junction (see Fig. 27.15). Although the root of the mesentery is only about 15 cm in length it fans out to be attached to the entire length of the small bowel. The ascending colon is usually without a mesentery but the transverse colon has a long mesocolon fused with the greater omentum (Fig. 27.1b). The descending and sigmoid colons also have mesenteries of variable lengths.

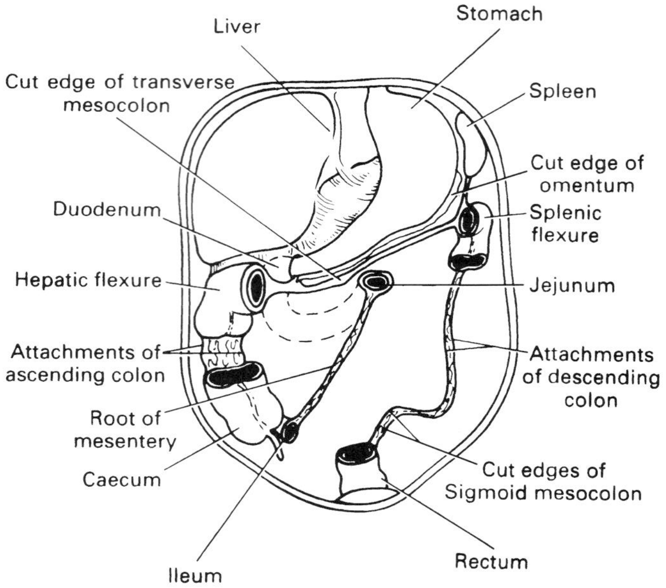

Fig. 27.15 The mesenteric attachments to the posterior abdominal wall.

Physiology and anatomy

The mesentery acts as another site of absorption from within the peritoneal cavity, having a cell structure and intracellular pore size similar to that of the peritoneum. It also acts as the vascular pedicle for the intestine and allows lymphatic transport to and from the mucosa. The splanchnic bed, contained in the bowel and mesentery, receives up to 30% of the cardiac output and large vascular alterations and fluid movements occur during stress and digestion. The superior mesenteric artery passes from behind the neck of the pancreas and in front of the third portion of the duodenum before entering the mesentery (Fig. 27.16). The small bowel is richly supplied with vascular arcades, but the terminal branches of the colonic vessels are less frequent and arise from a marginal artery close to the wall of the colon. The preservation of this marginal artery is therefore of great importance in the blood supply of the colon during resection and anastomosis. The inferior mesenteric artery which supplies the splenic flexure of the transverse colon, the descending colon, sigmoid colon and proximal part of the rectum arises from the lower aorta and is not uncommonly compromised by severe atherosclerotic disease. Both the superior and inferior mesenteric veins drain into the portal venous system. The haemorrhoidal veins which drain into the inferior mesenteric vein form a communication between the portal and systemic venous systems (Fig. 27.16). The importance of this communication

REFERENCES

61. Kelling G Munch Med Wochenschr 1902; 49: 21
62. Ruddock J C Surg Gynecol Obstet 1937; 65: 623
63. Gaisford W D Am J Surg 1975; 130: 671
64. Cuschieri A Br J Hosp Med 1980; 24: 254
65. Cuschieri A, Dubois F et al 1991; 161: 385
66. Shepherd J T Br J Surg 1951; 39: 185
67. Hamilton W J, Mossman H W Human Embryology. Macmillan, London 1976

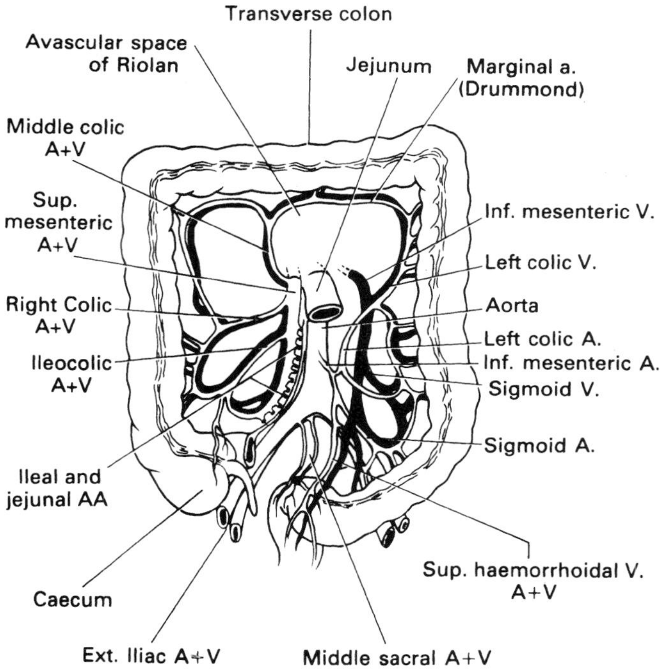

Fig. 27.16 The arterial supply and venous drainage of the small and large intestines.

is recognized when abscesses around the perineum and rectum are complicated by development of portal pyaemia.

The lymphatic vessels of the mesentery accompany the arteries and veins. After ingestion of food they are prominently outlined by chylomicrons from fat digestion and after a fatty meal can be easily observed at operation. They drain lymph to the proximal nodes within the mesentery and thence to the pre-aortic nodes and cisterna chyli before joining the thoracic duct which passes to the left subclavian vein in the neck. Mesenteric lymph nodes are frequently enlarged and may cause symptoms which have to be differentiated from acute appendicitis, especially in children.[68] Mesenteric adenitis may be the result of both viral and bacterial infection. The mesenteric lymph nodes are a common site for tuberculous infection and are often involved in the secondary spread of malignant disease within the peritoneal cavity.

CONGENITAL ABNORMALITIES

Malrotation of the bowel

On re-entering the peritoneal cavity the intestine may fail to rotate and the mesentery may not adhere to the posterior peritoneal wall.[69,70] Abnormal peritoneal folds are common. Intraperitoneal hernias can occur as a result of these anatomical variations. Herniation may take place through congenital defects in the mesentery of both the large and small intestine. Mesenteric defects may also follow injury or surgery. The window through which the bowel herniates may be associated with a vascular pedicle and care must be taken to avoid damaging blood vessels at the time of surgery to release the herniated bowel. Herniation through the foramen of Winslow has been reported, and bowel may be caught in a congenital fold around the duodenum (paraduodenal herniation) or in a fossa in the sigmoid mesocolon.[71,72] Such patients present with unexplained small bowel obstruction (p. 735).

VASCULAR DISEASE

Diseases of the mesenteric arteries and veins are described in Chapters 10 and 29. Arteriovenous fistulae are occasionally seen in the mesentery as a result of a penetrating injury or, rarely, following surgery.[73] They are treated by ligation and excision, repair being rarely feasible.

CYSTS

Mesenteric cysts[74,75] are uncommon in adults and even rarer in children. Most are loculated, indicating their origin from several abnormal lymphatic vessels. The walls of the cyst are formed from endothelial cells but may contain fibrous tissue and smooth muscle. The first such cyst was described by Benevieni, the Florentine anatomist in 1507.[76] Cysts vary in size and may grow to over 20 cm in diameter. They can resemble a reduplication of the bowel and their contents may be clear or chylous.

Acquired cysts of the mesentery also occur. These may follow trauma and rupture of lymphatic vessels, or contain enzyme-rich secretions following rupture of the pancreas. Occasionally cysts arise from degeneration of a tumour or as a result of certain infections such as tuberculosis and infestation such as hydatid disease (see Chapter 31). Dermoid cysts can also occur in the mesentery.

Many mesenteric cysts are symptomless until the swelling is noticed by the patient. Some cause abdominal pain which may be colicky in nature while as many as one-third cause intestinal obstruction or volvulus. Some rupture, some become infected and some present with anaemia following repeated haemorrhage into the cyst. If the cysts are palpable the attachment of the mesentery ensures that they are mobile in a transverse direction but restrained from moving vertically. They can now be diagnosed with reasonable certainty by ultrasonography or CT (Fig. 27.17) and, although needle aspiration under imaging control may be useful for diagnostic purposes, surgical excision is the definitive form of treatment,[77] with or without resection of the adjacent segment of intestine. If the anatomical position of the cyst makes surgical excision hazardous, marsupialization can be performed, leaving the open cyst to drain into the peritoneal cavity.

REFERENCES

68. Foster A K Arch Surg 1939; 38: 131
69. Kanagasuntheram R J Anat 1957; 91: 188
70. Aird I Br Med J 1945; 2: 680
71. Hansmann G H, Marton S A Arch Surg 1939; 39: 333
72. Fiddian R V Br J Surg 1961; 49: 186
73. Sumner R G, Kistler P C et al Circulation 1963; 27: 934
74. Moynihan B Ann Surg 1897; 26: 1
75. Kurzweig F T, Daron P B et al Am J Surg 1974; 40: 462
76. Benevieni cited by Warfield J O Ann Surg 1932; 96: 329
77. Carpreso P Arch Surg 1974; 108: 242

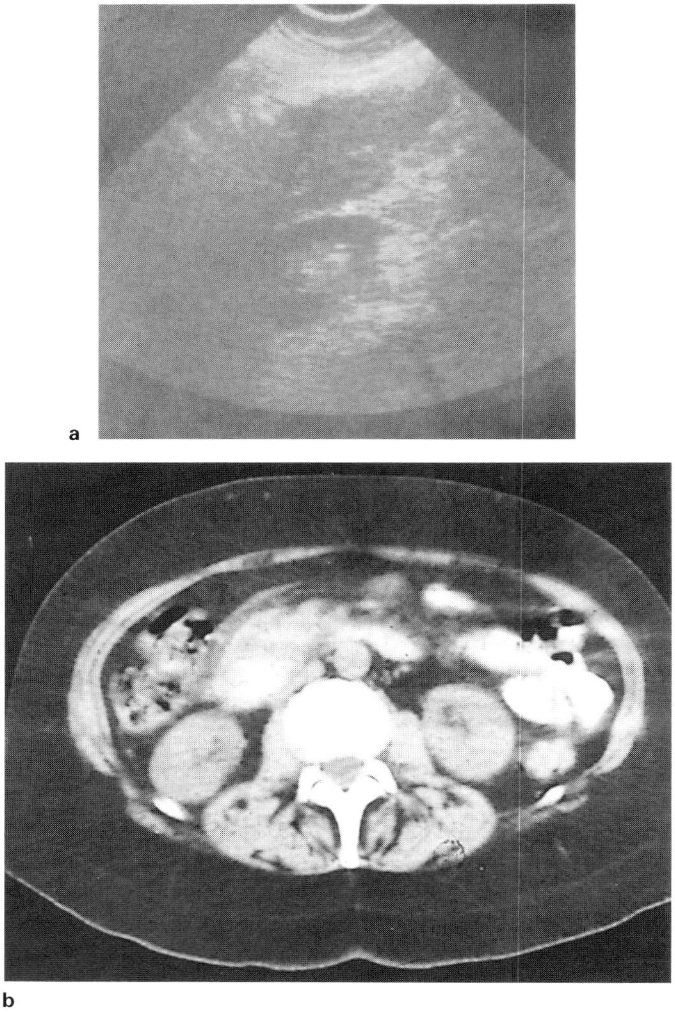

Fig. 27.17 A mesenteric cyst shown by (a) ultrasound and (b) CT scanning.

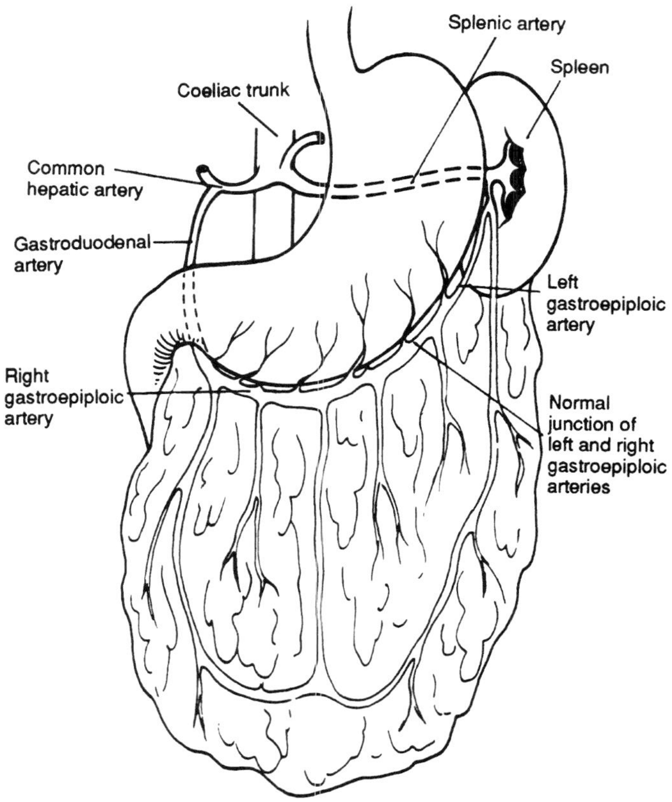

Fig. 27.18 The left and right gastroepiploic arteries supplying the omentum and greater curvature of the stomach.

TUMOURS

Solid primary tumours of the mesentery[78] are rare. They are most commonly sarcomas, desmoid tumours or neurofibromas. In addition, the mesentery may contain deposits of lymphoma and other metastases from intra-abdominal and distant primary carcinomas. Rare benign tumours of the mesentery include lipomas, fibromas and haemangiomas (hamartomas).

THE OMENTUM

The omentum is a fold of visceral peritoneum which is related to the stomach and transverse colon composed of a thin double layer of mesothelium, containing a large amount of fat and a rich vascular network. The surface area of the omentum is as much as 1500 cm^2.

The lesser omentum lies between the lesser curve of the stomach and the undersurface of the liver. The greater omentum forms the walls of the lesser sac and becomes fused into an apron of tissue which hangs from the transverse colon. The gastrocolic omentum lies between the greater curvature of the stomach and transverse colon. The gastrocolic ligament stretches from the fundus of the stomach to the lower surface of the diaphragm. The spleen, which is developed from the same embryonic mesoblastic tissue, lies between the gastrosplenic omentum and the lienorenal ligament.

Anatomy

The omentum contains many aggregates of lymphoid tissue measuring between 0.5 and 3 mm in diameter, in addition to the trabecular framework of vessels and adipose tissue. These lymphatic deposits were initially described as milky spots and are in effect individual lymphoreticular organs. These aggregates become involved in the immunological responses in the peritoneal cavity. In addition to macrophages they contain T and B lymphocytes and mast cells and they can increase in size dramatically with intraperitoneal infection.[79]

The arterial supply of the omentum is from the right and left gastroepiploic arteries (Fig. 27.18) which are derived from the coeliac axis and pass along the greater curvature of the stomach.

REFERENCES

78. Weinberger H A, Ahmed M S Surgery 1977; 82: 754
79. Beelen R H J, Fluitsma D M, Hoefsmit E C M J Reticuloendothial Soc 1980; 28: 601

The gastric branches are more numerous than the epiploic branches. The right gastroepiploic artery is larger and longer than the left. The right gastroepiploic artery is about 2.8 mm in diameters at its origin while the left gastroepiploic is usually half this diameter. Both arteries diminish in size and usually anastomose about two-thirds of the way along the greater curvature from the duodenum. In about one-third of specimens the only communication is by peripheral anastomoses.

The venous drainage runs in conjunction with the arterial supply. The right gastroepiploic vein joins the superior mesenteric vein and the left gastroepiploic vein drains into the splenic vein. These veins provide a ready access to the portal venous system.

There is an extensive network of lymphatic vessels within the omentum; these arise as bulbous pouches in the milky spots. The lymphatics of the omentum drain into the subpyloric, splenic and coeliac nodes and eventually lymph passes on to the thoracic duct.

Nerve fibres have been described in connection with the omental vessels, but there is a lack of sensory perception and the nerves probably only subserve vascular reflexes.

Physiology

In addition to its plasticity, the omentum adheres to injured and inflamed surfaces.[80] It is also very useful in achieving haemostasis and neo-vascularization and provides a large surface area for fluid movement and the absorption of molecular substances from the peritoneal cavity. The omentum does not have the capacity for active movement although passive movement readily occurs.[81] The overall function of the omentum is encapsulated in the phrase 'the abdominal policeman', used originally by Rutherford–Morison.[82]

Clinical features of omental disease

It is usually difficult, if not impossible, to differentiate between primary omental pathology and omental disease originating from other intra-abdominal organs. Patients who have primary omental pathology present with the signs and symptoms of intra-abdominal inflammation, acute vascular occlusion or space-occupying lesions.

Inflammation of the omentum may develop as the result of any of the acute intra-abdominal infections, such as acute cholecystitis, diverticulitis and appendicitis. Adhesions may then form which can cause acute or subacute obstruction. Tuberculous peritonitis can cause diffuse omental adhesions. Vascular occlusions can occur in the omentum as a result of torsion, adhesions, trauma, atherosclerosis and embolism. They usually cause non-specific abdominal pain and local tenderness.

Primary, solid or cystic lesions in the omentum are rare but may occur at any age. The usually cause abdominal distension and pain. Haemorrhage into a cyst or solid tumour may present as a rapidly increasing abdominal mass.

Investigation of omental disease

Plain abdominal radiographs may show a soft tissue mass or cystic lesion within the abdominal cavity and if this is seen to be lying anteriorly on the lateral film an omental lesion should be suspected. Ultrasonography and CT are now the main methods of diagnosis. Occasionally laparoscopy is undertaken to confirm an omental lesion and establish the pathology by biopsy. Laparotomy is required for treatment of omental injuries, inflammatory disease associated with other organs, omental torsion, tumours and cysts.

INJURIES OF THE OMENTUM

Blunt abdominal trauma may lead to omental disruption and haemorrhage. An omental defect may result, through which a loop of bowel may herniate and later obstruct. The omentum may also be injured at operation and by penetrating abdominal injuries such as stab wounds. The defects caused by these injuries are also potential sites for future herniation.

HERNIATION OF OMENTUM

Either small bowel or omentum may herniate into the paraduodenal fossa. Other rare sites of omental herniation include the foramen of Winslow, the transverse mesocolon, the supravesical fossa and the diaphragm. Omentum may also enter any external hernia, and it is often found within a partial dehiscence of the abdominal wall. A penetrating injury can cause prolapse of the omentum through the abdominal wall, and omentum may herniate through the site of a surgical drain. It is now a common finding inside a poorly closed laparoscopy port site.

The symptoms depend on the site of the hernia. Treatment is often required to reduce the omentum and repair the defect to prevent future problems.

ADHESIONS

Trauma, ischaemia, inflammation and foreign bodies can cause peritoneal adhesions which often involve the omentum. The symptoms and signs depend upon the site and extent of the adhesion formation. Adhesions may be silent or they may cause obstruction (p. 735).

INFLAMMATION

The inflammation in generalized peritonitis also involves the omentum. Occasionally the inflammatory process is localized to the omentum and may arise spontaneously, postoperatively or following injury.[82] The classical distinction between omentitis plastica simplex, adhesiva and purulenta is not now used as it has little if any clinical relevance. Spontaneous inflammation of the omentum occurs with bacterial infection and may follow intraperitoneal infection in another viscus. Parasites and tuberculosis can also cause omentitis, and postoperative and post-traumatic omentitis follows the introduction of foreign material.

REFERENCES

80. Myllainie H Acta Chir Scand 1967; 377 (suppl): 1
81. Walker F C Ann R Coll Surg Engl 1963; 33: 282
82. Crofoot D D Am J Surg 1980; 139: 262

Laparotomy may be required to exclude another interperitoneal disease if the symptoms and signs are of sufficient severity. Resection of part of the omentum may be necessary if the inflammation is sufficiently severe to produce areas of infarction.

TORSION OF THE OMENTUM

Primary torsion of the omentum is a rare condition that has most often been recorded in men of between 30 and 50 years who are of obese build. It was first described by Eitel.[83,84]

Secondary torsion is much more common, accounting for more than half of the reported cases. Adhesions of the omentum to the parietal peritoneum, to any old focus of infection or to a hernia may lead to torsion.

Clinical features and treatment

Sudden severe abdominal pain, nausea and vomiting are usually abdominal present. The twisted omentum may be felt as a mobile mass or it may be obscured by abdominal rigidity. Sometimes a string of several masses may be felt which are several twists of omentum. Free fluid is usually present in the peritoneal cavity. Most cases come to operation with a mistaken diagnosis of acute appendicitis. At operation the strangulated omentum should be resected.

TUMOURS

Fibromas, lipomas, haemangiomas and lymphangiomas are benign tumours that have been found to arise in the omentum. Primary malignant tumours account for less than 3% of all malignancy arising in the omentum. Fibrous histiocytoma, malignant haemangiopericytoma, malignant mesothelioma and a number of sarcomas including liposarcoma, leiomyosarcoma and rhabdomyosarcoma have all been described.[85,86] The majority of malignant tumours of the omentum are secondary deposits. These have been described from almost every site but deposits from the ovary, stomach and colon are particularly common and secondaries from malignant melanomas are also well-recognised.

Although both primary and secondary tumour deposits in the omentum are often discovered by chance at the time of laparotomy, if sufficiently large or numerous, symptoms and signs may arise. These include pain, abdominal distension, intestinal obstruction and ascites. On occasions, large space-occupying tumours cause pressure symptoms on neighbouring organs.

Surgery is often confined to a diagnostic biopsy at the time of laparotomy. Resection of large deposits causing pressure symptoms or obstruction can give symptomatic relief. The omentum is usually excised at the time of radical surgery for gastric and ovarian carcinomata as a debulking manoeuvre, even if it is not involved with tumour.[87] The plane of dissection for omental resection begins at the fusion between the omentum and transverse mesocolon. It should be divided from its attachment to the greater curvature of the stomach in ovarian cancer and it is removed en bloc with the stomach for gastric cancer (see Chapter 28). The resection of the omentum with deposits of ovarian carcinoma is important as a means of reducing tumour bulk before chemotherapy.[88,89]

RARE TISSUE DEPOSITS

Abnormal fat deposited in the omentum has been described in Christian–Weber disease.[90] Splenic rupture may lead to splenosis (see Chapter 34). Endometriosis of the omentum has also been described.[91] Limited resection of the omentum is undertaken in these conditions for diagnosis but radical omentectomy may be required if symptoms persist.

CYSTS

Lymphatic cysts and lymphangiomas may arise as developmental abnormalities. Diagnostic laparotomy and resection is required if these cysts become large enough to produce symptoms. In addition rare dermoid and urogenital cysts resulting from tissue displacement have been described.[92–94] Care must always be taken at the time of surgery to remove omental cysts intact as some may be the result of hydatid disease, which disseminates throughout the peritoneal cavity on rupture (see Chapter 31).

RECONSTRUCTIVE SURGERY

In recent years the omentum has increasingly been used for reconstructive surgery. Initially it was used within the peritoneal cavity to repair defects in the intestinal wall at various sites. These have included the duodenum and colon.[95] Much attention has recently been focused on the value of omentum for closing pelvic fistulae, including those of rectum, vagina and bladder.[95] Because of the ability of the omentum to be mobilized on either the left or right gastroepiploic pedicle it can also be transposed to distant sites outside the peritoneal cavity. It has been used in reconstructive procedures on the chest wall,[96,97] the buttock, groin and leg[95] and it has also been transposed to the arm for a limited period to revascularize devitalized tissue. Free omental grafts have also been undertaken for head and neck reconstructive surgery using a microvascular anastomosis.[98]

REFERENCES

83. Eitel G G Med Rec N Y 1899; 55: 715
84. Tolenaar P L, Bast T J Br J Surg 1987; 74: 1182
85. Pack G T, Taborh E J Int Abstr Surg 1945; 99: 209
86. Braasch J W, Mon A B Surg Clin North Am 1967; 47: 663
87. Desmond A M Proc R Soc Med 1976; 69: 867
88. Griffiths E T, Grogan R M, Hall T C Cancer 1972; 29: 1
89. Bereic J S, Hacker N F et al Obstet Gynecol 1983; 58: 192
90. Soerell K H, Hensley G T Gastroenterology 1966; 51: 529
91. Venter P F South Afr Med J 1980; 57: 895
92. Handfield-Jones R M Br J Surg 1924; 12: 119
93. Nichols H M Ann Surg 1947; 126: 340
94. Howarth V S Br J Surg 1950; 37: 329
95. Libermann-Meffert D, White H The Greater Omentum, Anatomy Physiology Pathology with a Historical Survey. Springer Verlag, New York 1983
96. White H A Colour Atlas of Omental Transposition for Advanced Breast Carcinoma. Wolfe, London 1987
97. Williams R J L, Fryatt I J C et al Br J Surg 1989; 76: 559
98. Brown R, Nahai F, Silverton J Br J Plast Surg 1978; 13: 58

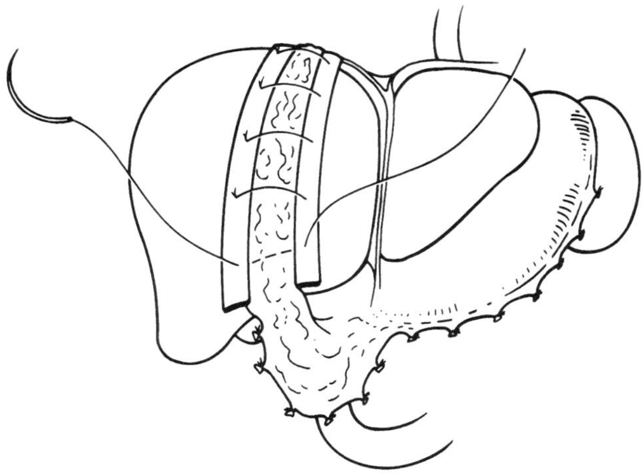

Fig. 27.19a Omentum used to plug a damaged liver.

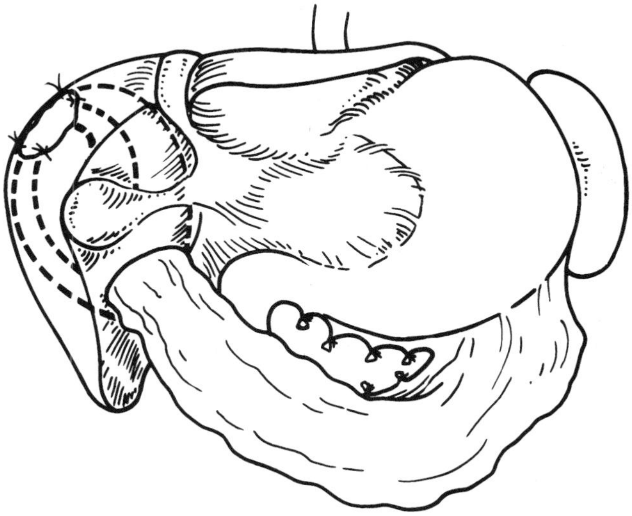

Fig. 27.19b Omentum used to fill the cavity left by the excision of a hydatid cyst.

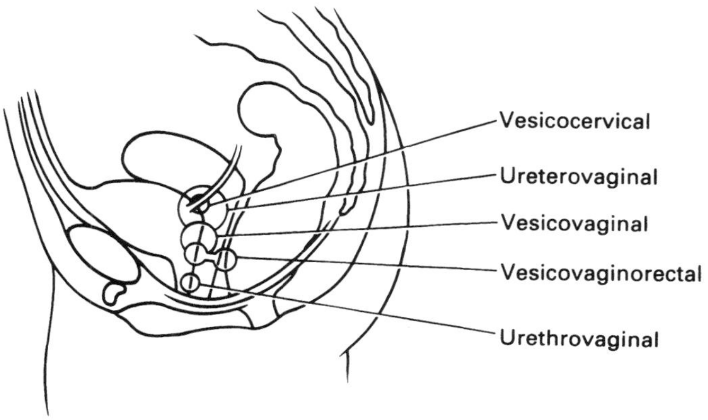

Fig. 27.19c Use of omentum to close fistulae between the pelvic organs of a woman.

Figure 27.19 shows some of the sites where omentum is used in reconstructive surgery. The benefit of the omentum in these reconstructions is largely as a result of its excellent blood supply.

MISCELLANEOUS INTRA-ABDOMINAL USES

Occasionally the omentum is of value to tamponade hepatic trauma (Fig. 27.19a) and to obliterate the dead space in the liver after excision of cysts and tumours see Chapter 31. (Fig. 27.19b).[99] It may also be used to fill the presacral space after anterior resection or pelvic exenteration.[100] It is thought to be of value in protecting anastomoses with a poor blood supply and in those threatened by previous or subsequent radiotherapy.[101]

When foreign material such as a vascular prosthesis is inserted within the abdomen, omentum may be used to separate organs from the prosthesis, as for example at the duodenal flexure where an aortic graft enteric fistula may develop if the prosthesis is allowed to adhere to the duodenal wall (see Chapter 10.)[102]

The omentum has also been used in patients with retroperitoneal fibrosis to wrap the ureters after they have been successfully lysed to help prevent further fibrosis from developing.

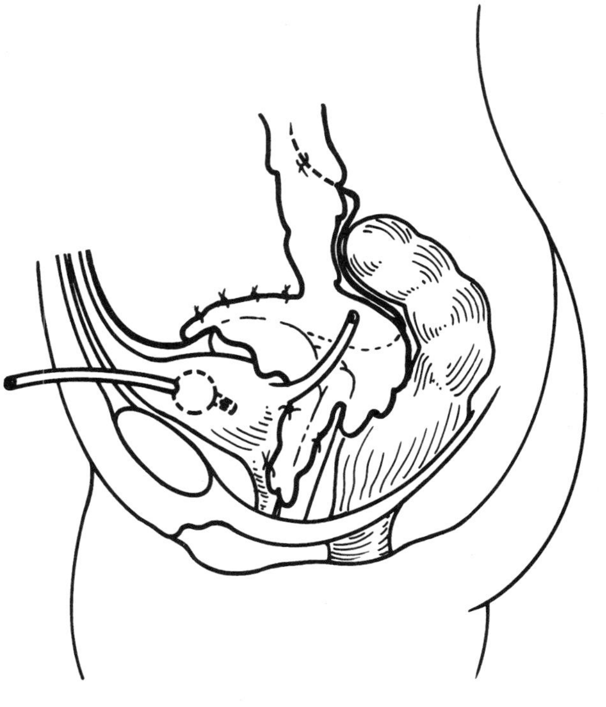

Fig. 27.19d Omentum transposed between bladder and vagina to close a vesicovaginal fistula.

REFERENCES

99. Fabian T C, Stone H H South Med J 1980; 73: 1487
100. Poston G J, Smith S R G, Baker W N W Ann R Coll Surg Engl 1991; 73: 229
101. Greenburg B M, Low D, Rosato E F Surg Gynecol Obstet 1985; 161: 487
102. Bunt T J, Doer Hoff C R, Haynes J L Surg Gynecol Obstet 1984; 158: 591

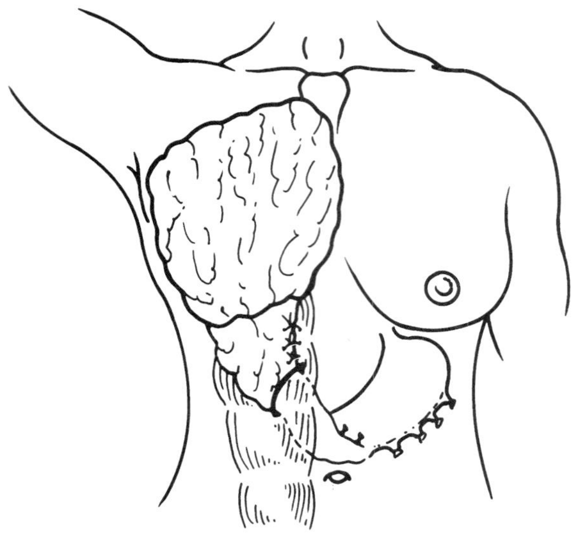

Fig. 27.19e Omentum used to close a thoracic wall defect. This is especially useful after post-irradiation necrosis when the blood supply has been damaged.

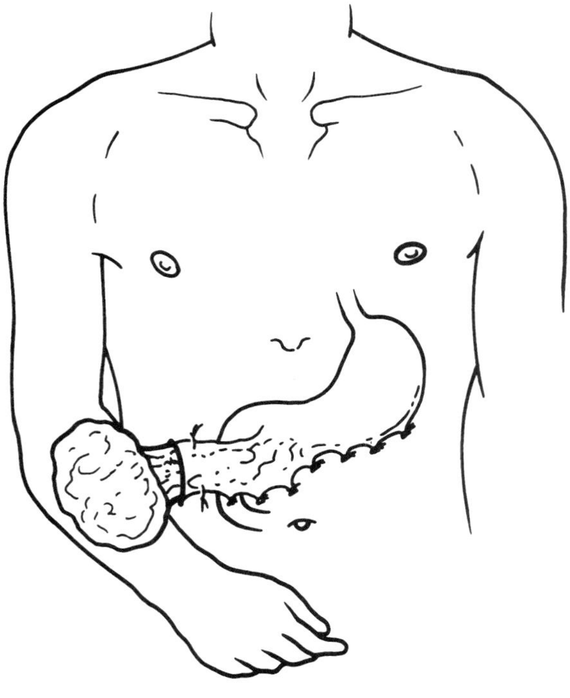

Fig. 27.19f Omentum can also be pedicled to the forearm.

TRANSPOSITION TO THE EXTREMITIES AND CRANIUM

Attempts to reduce lymphoedema of the extremities by establishing lymph drainage through transposed omentum have proved of little value (see Chapter 12) and likewise transposition of omentum to the cranium to improve the blood supply of patients with carotid occlusions[103] has not found widespread application.

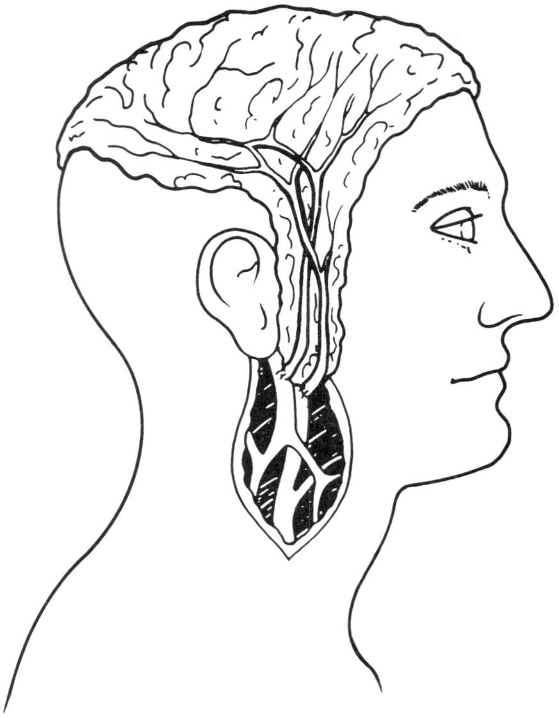

Fig. 27.19g Free graft of omentum to the superficial temporal vessels to cover a scalp defect before applying split-skin grafts.

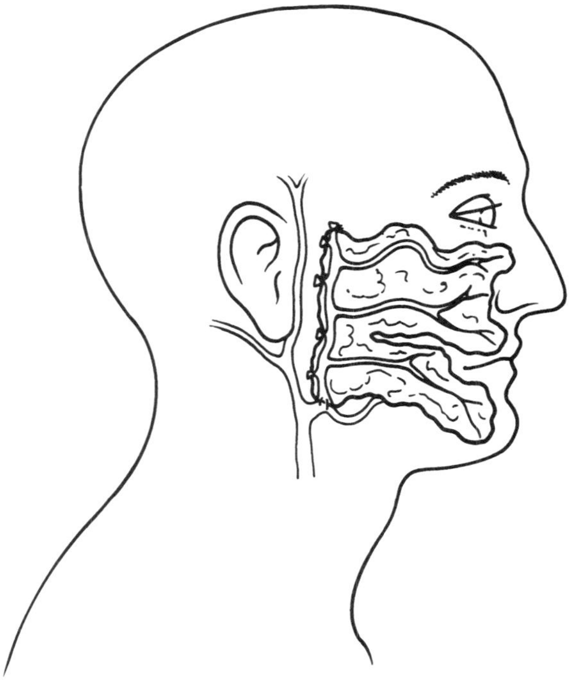

Fig. 27.19h Another free graft of omentum to the external carotid artery to provide bulk replacement of hemifacial atrophy.

REFERENCE

103. Goldsmith H S, Chen W S, Dickett S W Arch Surg 1973; 106: 965

RETROPERITONEAL TUMOURS

These are listed below:

1. Neuroblastomas in the adrenal gland or lumbar sympathetic chain are common tumours in children.
2. Ganglioneuromas or phaeochromocytomas of the adrenal or lumbar sympathetic chain (see Chapter 35).
3. Sarcomas, usually of a small round-celled type, histiocytic, myxomatous or lipomatous (see Chapter 52).
4. Lymphoma in the lumbar glands (see Chapter 34).
5. Vascular malformations, usually of a cavernous type. These often originate in the pelvis and may cause bleeding from the rectum, bladder or vagina and may be part of the Klippel–Trenaunay syndrome or consist of congenital arteriovenous fistulae.
6. Lipoma. This is the commonest retroperitoneal tumour and accounts for as many as 60% of all retroperitoneal masses in some series. Most tumours contain mixed elements of fibrous tissue, myxomatous tissue and sometimes fibrosarcomatous tissue. The majority start in the perirenal fat; the largest may extend from the diaphragm to the pelvis. Patients often present between 40 and 50 years of age and females outnumber males.
7. Teratoma may occur in the retroperitoneal tissues of both women and men. They may arise from totipotential blastomeric cells misplaced along the cavity of the primitive coelom, or from aberrant germ cells. Like teratomas elsewhere they may develop malignancy in one of their component elements. They usually present as palpable tumours with pressure effects such as gross oedema of the lower limb. A teratoma is probably responsible for the retroperitoneal chorion epithelioma. Retroperitoneal seminomas or teratomas can develop in undescended testes (see Chapter 40) and may be encountered in hermaphrodites.
8. Adrenogenital urinary tumours. These are solid tumours resembling renal or ovarian tissue. Others are neuroblastomas or adrenocortical tumours (see Chapter 35).
9. Renal and pancreatic tumours (see Chapters 36 and 33) are strictly speaking retroperitoneal but are usually classified individually.

Most retroperitoneal tumours are diagnosed on CT scan, and can be confirmed by biopsy. Arteriography may give an indication of resectability.

The surgical approach to retroperitoneal tumours is always difficult. Large retroperitoneal tumours are best approached through a midline abdominal incision or a left-sided thoracoabdominal incision. The right colon and duodenum are mobilized medially if they lie on the right side, or the left colon, spleen, body and tail of pancreas and the splenic vessels are reflected to the left if the tumour lies on the left side. The prognosis is poor except in the case of cystic tumours. The only retroperitoneal tumours which can be removed with a confident hope of cure are ganglioneuromas, neurofibromata and lipomas. Unfortunately the lipoma is frequently a liposarcoma and the teratoma usually contains malignant elements.

Retroperitoneal germ cell tumours can be preoperatively diagnosed if circulating tumour markers are detected (B human chorionic gonadotrophin and α-fetoprotein). They are initially treated with aggressive chemotherapy, and if the markers return to normal and the tumour shrinks or disappears on CT scan, surgical resection of residual tissue is attempted to prevent the possibility of recurrence from surviving cell nests in an otherwise 'dead' tumour.

RETROPERITONEAL CYSTS

1. Nephrogenic cysts of wolffian origin usually occur in adult women. They are often large, may be unilocular or multilocular and are usually situated laterally. The wall is formed of fibrous tissue with a lining of high cylindrical epithelium.
2. Epidermoid cysts of wolffian duct.
3. Dermoid cysts.
4. Renal cysts (see Chapter 36).
5. Pancreatic cysts (see Chapter 33).

Treatment

These cysts may be ignored, aspirated or resected.

THE ACUTE ABDOMEN

Many of the conditions responsible for acute abdominal pain are described in detail elsewhere in this book, but the acute abdomen is such a common and important entity that it merits a separate section reviewing all the causes of acute abdominal pain and providing a coherent approach to their management. For the purposes of multicentre studies, initially to examine the role of computer-aided diagnosis in the acute abdomen, the definition of acute abdominal pain is considered as abdominal pain of less than 1 week's duration requiring emergency admission to hospital.[104]

Hippocrates in 477 BC[105] recognized the importance of peritonitis and the acute abdomen and was the first to use the term 'ileus' to describe intestinal obstruction. The condition of intestinal volvulus was later recognized by Celsus,[106] but many centuries passed before strangulated hernia and acute appendicitis were appreciated as life-threatening abdominal emergencies.[107–109]

PATHOLOGICAL PROCESSES CAUSING THE ACUTE ABDOMEN

Inflammation and infection

These conditions are usually characterized by a febrile illness with localized signs of peritonitis. The origin of the inflammation can

REFERENCES

104. de Dombal F T, Leaper D J et al Br Med J 1972; 2: 9
105. Adams E F The Genuine Works of Hippocrates. Sydenham Press, London 1949
106. Celsus A Of Medicine in eight books. Translated by Greive J. Wilson Durham, London 1956
107. Cope Z A History of the Acute Abdomen. Oxford University Press, New York 1965
108. Heister J Chirurgie 1970
109. Fitz R H J Med Sci 1986; 184: 321

frequently be determined from the history and onset of the pain and by the site of maximum tenderness. Common intra-abdominal inflammatory conditions include acute appendicitis, acute cholecystitis, acute diverticulitis, acute pancreatitis, acute salpingitis (pelvic inflammatory disease) and mesenteric adenitis. Other less common inflammatory conditions which can cause abdominal pain are Crohn's disease, Meckel's diverticulitis, pyelonephritis and cystitis. Very occasionally *Yersinia* infection of the small bowel can also present with an acute abdomen.

Perforation

Perforation of an abdominal viscus usually results in the sudden onset of severe abdominal pain. Identification of which viscus has perforated may be determined from a history of previous abdominal pain. In the early stages, the site of maximum tenderness may also indicate the organ which has perforated. However, the usual end-point of generalized peritonitis is a rigid board-like abdomen when selective tenderness can no longer be elicited. The cause of the perforation must then await the findings at laparotomy. The most common causes of perforation excluding acute appendicitis are peptic ulceration—either of the stomach or duodenum—and diverticular disease. Perforated diverticular disease is usually the result of generalized diverticulitis, although rarely a solitary diverticulum in the ascending colon can perforate. Other less common causes of a perforated viscus include: carcinoma of the colon; Crohn's disease; ulcerative colitis; lymphoma; foreign bodies; acute cholecystitis; perforation of the oesophagus (Boerhaave's syndrome) and perforation of a segment of strangulated bowel. Occasionally the caecum may perforate in severe cases of large bowel obstruction. This may be either mechanical or associated with a pseudo-obstruction. Perforation of any intra-abdominal viscus may also result from trauma.

Obstruction

Obstruction of any hollow viscus within the abdominal cavity usually causes acute abdominal pain. Obstruction of of all viscera except the gallbladder tends to produce colicky pain while obstruction of the gallbladder (biliary colic) usually presents with a more continuous type of pain, often punctuated by acute exacerbations. Renal or ureteric colic is also a background pain with frequent excruciating exacerbations that make the patient sweat and roll around. Unless a complication such as strangulation or perforation has occurred, there will not in most instances be signs of peritonitis. The identity of the obstructed viscus can sometimes be determined from the history of the pain.

Infarction

There are a number of processes that can cause an abdominal viscus to infarct. These include torsion of the viscus, occlusion of its arterial inflow by thrombosis or embolus, venous thrombosis and haematological disorders which lead to arterial occlusion. The vascular supply of the small bowel may be occluded by an adhesion or a hernial orifice causing a strangulating obstruction which ultimately leads to infarction and perforation. An acute aortic dissection can occlude the origins of the mesenteric vessels as the false lumen extends. Organs that may undergo infarction include ovaries, usually from torsion of associated cysts, appendices epiploicae, the omentum, the testes or testicular appendices and segments of intestine. Infarction of the spleen occurs in a number of haematological disorders, especially sickle cell disease, and the kidney may occasionally infarct as a result of atherosclerotic disease. Uterine fibroids that twist or outgrow their blood supply may also infarct. In severe cases of acute pancreatitis infarction and necrosis of the pancreas can occur.

Haemorrhage

Blood within the peritoneal cavity produces the symptoms and signs of an acute abdomen. This may initially be localized to the site of the bleed, but rapidly becomes more generalized. The history and the original site of abdominal pain again should give some indication as to the source of the haemorrhage. In addition to abdominal trauma, conditions causing intraperitoneal bleeding include ruptured abdominal aortic aneurysms, aneurysms of mesenteric vessels including the splenic, coeliac and hepatic arteries, ruptured ovarian cysts, ruptured ectopic pregnancies, retrograde menstruation, endometriosis, spontaneous rupture of liver tumours or a pathologically abnormal spleen.

Medical causes of the acute abdomen

There are a number of medical conditions that give rise to the symptoms and signs of an acute abdomen.[110] In many instances these can be differentiated from surgical conditions by a careful history and examination but occasionally they are responsible for an unnecessary laparotomy. These important conditions are discussed in detail at the end of this chapter.

CLINICAL FEATURES

The site, onset, character and duration of the abdominal pain provide important pointers to the diagnosis. For example, a pain felt in the right hypochondrium, of gradual onset, continuous in nature, perhaps with acute exacerbations, should indicate the likelihood of gallbladder disease. Radiation of the pain, progression or alteration of its site or character, factors that aggravate the pain or relieve it, and any associated symptoms are also helpful in refining the diagnosis. The site of the abdominal pain is usually related to one of nine areas (Fig. 27.20). These regions are demarcated by the mid clavicular lines in the vertical axis and by the transpyloric and transtubercular lines in the horizontal axis. Figure 27.20 also indicates some of the common organs and pathological processes that cause pain experienced in these regions. This figure is not meant to be comprehensive or to indicate that the pain arising from these viscera is exclusively felt in these sites.

REFERENCE

110. Harvard C W H B J Hosp Med 1972; 443

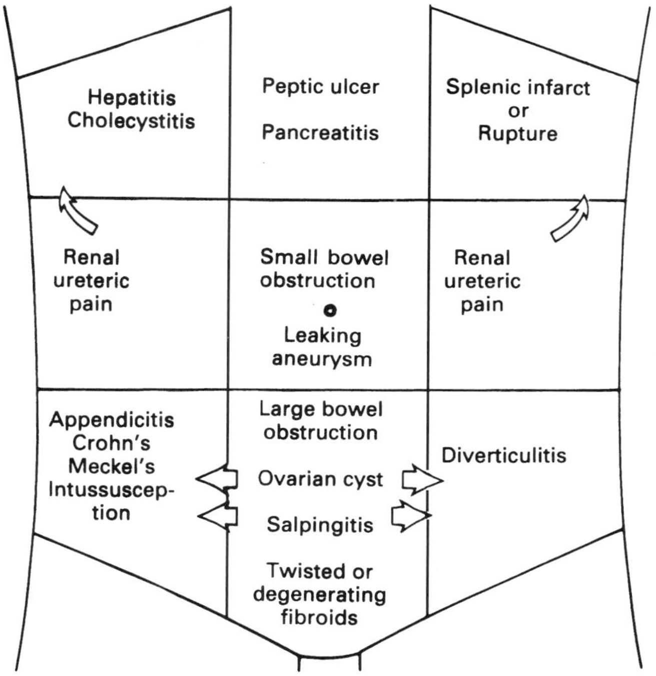

Fig. 27.20 The nine regions of the abdomen and some of the commoner conditions responsible for pain in these areas.

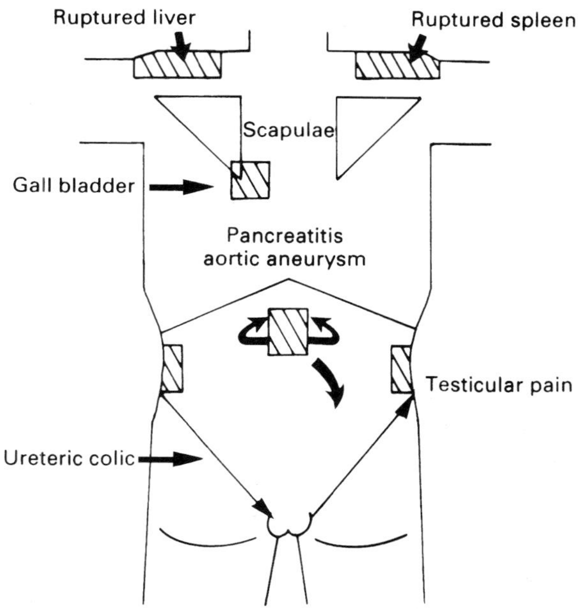

Fig. 27.21 Some of the well-recognized sites of radiation of pain derived from intra-abdominal viscera.

The onset of abdominal pain may be either sudden or gradual. Pain from underlying inflammatory conditions tends to be insidious in development. A sudden onset can be caused by perforation, infarction or haemorrhage. Patients with a sudden onset of pain usually remember exactly what they were doing when the pain occurred.

The character of the pain may be colicky, or continuous with either a background ache or acute exacerbations. A pain made worse by moving and coughing suggests 'peritonism'—in other words underlying peritoneal inflammation—whereas pain which makes the patient roll around or double up is typical of 'colic'. True colic is a griping pain which gradually reaches a crescendo before dying away, often completely.[111] It is usually severe and causes the patient to writhe around, often accompanied by sweating and vomiting and an inability to lie still. This description is true of intestinal and renal colic but biliary colic is a misnomer as patients tend to complain of a continuous pain with exacerbations of severe pain.[112] Strangulation should be suspected when an intestinal colic alters to become a continuous pain.

There are many other descriptions of abdominal pains and adjectives such as stabbing, gripping, wrenching, boring, or crushing are used by individual patients but are of little help in coming to a diagnosis.

The severity of any abdominal pain is difficult to judge and is often more dependent on the personality of the individual with the pain rather than the pathological process responsible. Pains of very short (a few minutes) or very long duration (several years) are often difficult to assess. In contrast specific areas of radiation are characteristic of certain causes of abdominal pain and help to confirm a tentative diagnosis. Some of the classic sites of radiation are shown in Figure 27.21.

The progression and movement of the pain may also be valuable in diagnosis, as shown by the obvious example of acute appendicitis when a central intermittent pain moves to the right iliac fossa and becomes constant.

Factors that aggravate or relieve pain are also important in making a diagnosis and information on the influence of movement, injury, position, food, antacids, vomiting, bowel action and micturition on the pain must always be sought. A history of previous trauma, however minor, may be important. At the same time it is important to ask about associated symptoms such as vomiting, diarrhoea, dysuria or a missed period that preceded or followed the onset of the pain as these may again provide important diagnostic clues.

It is impossible to list every direct question that could or should be asked to elucidate possible disorders of the gastrointestinal, genitourinary, cardiorespiratory and reproductive systems. Some of these questions will become apparent from reading the remainder of this chapter while others will only be learnt by the practical experience of talking to many patients with acute abdominal pain.

The history should conclude with details of past illnesses or operations, the family and social history, details of alcohol intake and any regular medication, especially corticosteroids, anticoagulants and monoamine oxidase inhibitors, in addition to any known allergies. A general systems enquiry should also be made. Identification of the 'best questions' to ask is obviously important and in his studies on acute abdominal pain de Dombal revealed not only how important enquiry as to aggravating factors to the pain was, but that this simple question was omitted in half the patients being questioned in a single hospital.[113]

REFERENCES

111. Stokes M A, Moriarty K T, Catchpole B N Lancet 1988; i: 211
112. French E B, Robb W A T Br Med J 1963; ii: 135
113. de Dombal F T J R Coll Phys 1979; 13: 203

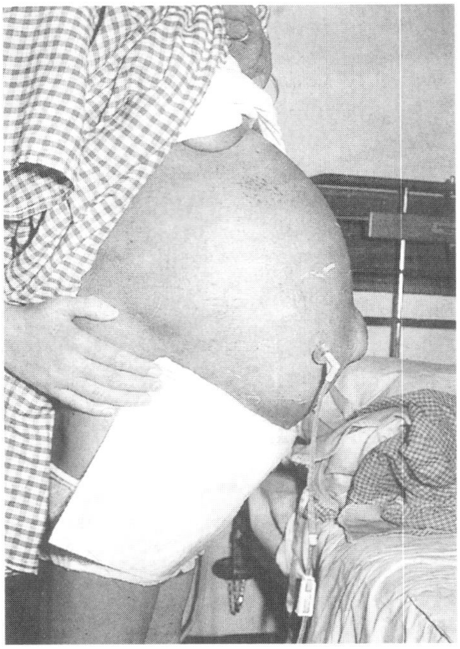

Fig. 27.22a A swollen abdomen caused by massive ascites which is being drained.

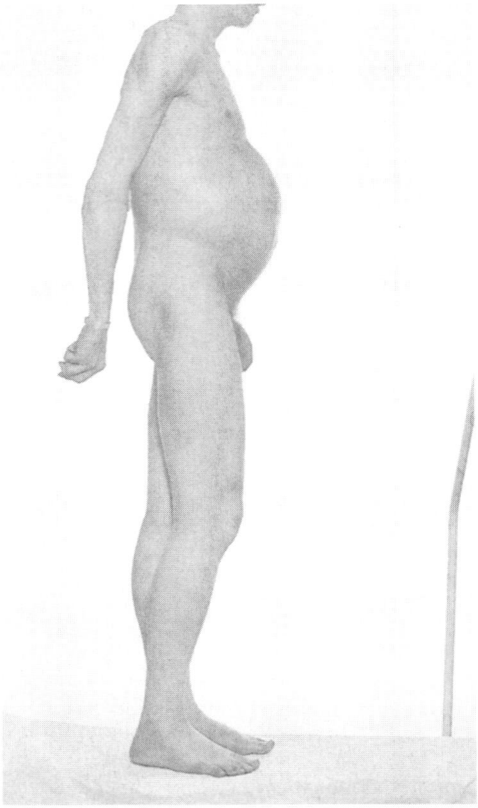

Fig. 27.22b A distended abdomen caused by a large retroperitoneal sarcoma.

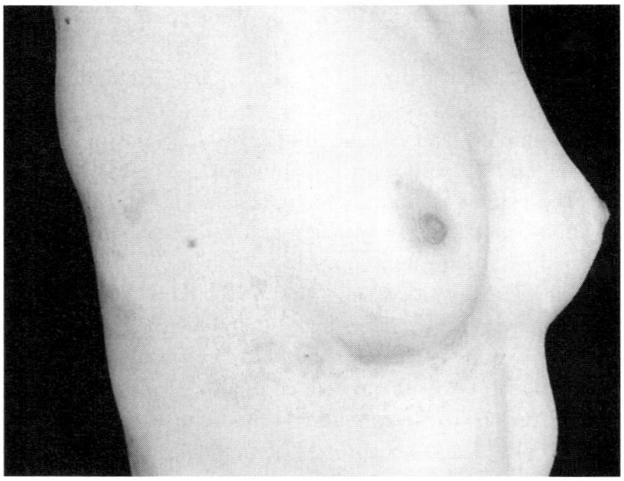

Fig. 27.23 A circular skin eruption caused by herpes zoster.

The patient should then be carefully examined. Anaemia, pallor, cyanosis, jaundice, lymphadenopathy, dehydration, foetor and pyrexia are some of the important physical findings that may be found by a thorough general examination. A rapid pulse and low blood pressure may indicate signs of shock. A rapid or irregular pulse may also be relevant.

The chest should be examined next, looking especially for signs of pneumonia, pleurisy and chronic obstructive airways disease. Examination of the cardiovascular system may uncover evidence of cardiac failure, hypotension, hypertension or valvular disorders. For the abdominal examination, the patient should be suitably undressed and lying flat in warm surroundings. The patient must be inspected from the nipples to the mid-thigh region. This ensures that genital abnormalities and groin lesions are not overlooked, and that the type of respiration is assessed. Abdominal swellings caused by enlargements of the liver, spleen, kidneys and bladder or tumours of the bowel or ovary and other intra-abdominal or retroperitoneal structures may be visible on careful inspection. The expansile pulsation of an abdominal aneurysm may also be seen. All abdominal scars must be noted and tested for an incisional hernia. Distension, which is usually caused by ascites, intestinal obstruction or a large intra-abdominal tumour, is usually readily apparent (Fig. 27.22). Skin eruptions caused by herpes zoster (Fig. 27.23), distended veins as a result of portal hypertension or occlusion of the inferior vena cava (Fig. 27.24), hernial swellings (Fig. 27.25) and visible peristalsis (Fig. 27.26) are other physical signs that may be detected by a careful inspection.

Palpation should be carried out in a systematic manner beginning with a gentle, superficial examination of the whole abdomen in an anticlockwise direction, progressing from the left iliac fossa to the right iliac fossa (assuming the examiner is right-handed). This precedes a more thorough detailed and deeper palpation once it has been determined that this will not cause undue pain or distress. It is important to establish the site or sites of a maximum tenderness which can be determined by repeated gentle pressure at different points on the anterior abdominal wall. At the same time the presence of abdominal wall rigidity and involuntary guarding should be assessed. Deeper palpation allows hepatomegaly, splenomegaly and renal enlargement, if present, to be confirmed, providing guarding and rigidity do not interfere. Tumours and other intra-abdominal masses such as a distended gallbladder, an

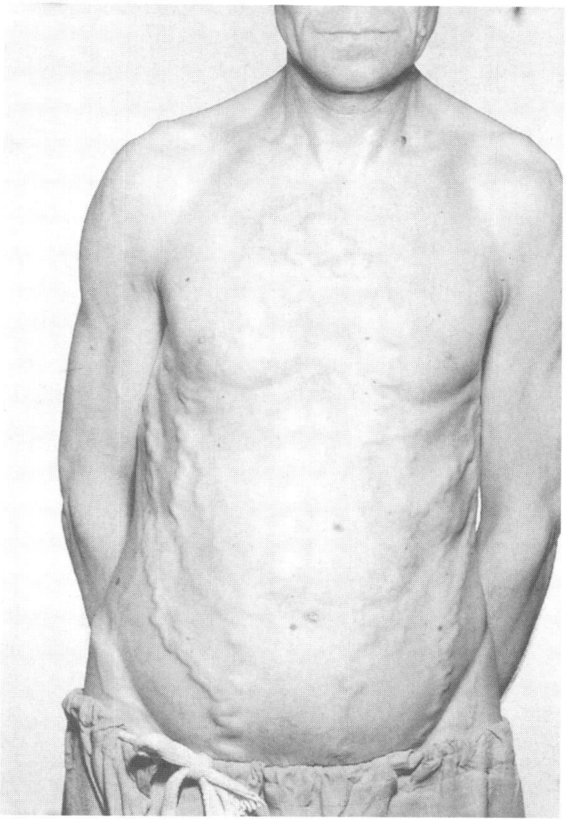

Fig. 27.24 Distended veins on the anterior abdominal wall acting as collaterals for an occluded inferior vena cava.

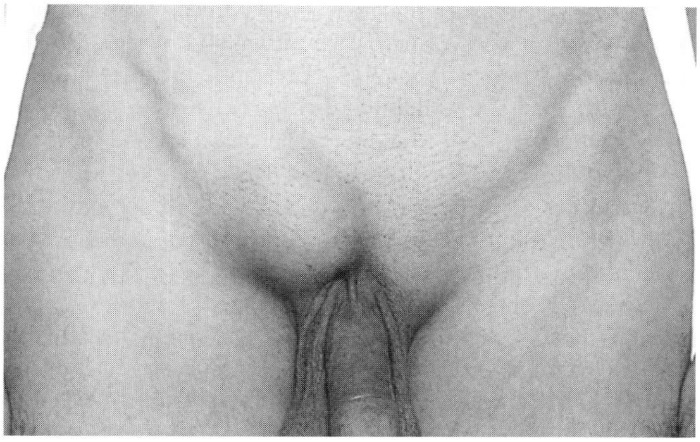

Fig. 27.25 An inguinal hernia containing strangulated bowel.

aortic aneurysm or a pancreatic phlegmon may also be identified on careful palpation. The hernial orifices must be specifically examined, as must the male genitalia, looking especially for tenderness and masses within the scrotum.

The presence of rebound tenderness indicates underlying peritoneal inflammation and is best examined by using percussion, although pain on coughing is also indicative of rebound tenderness.[114] Percussion is also useful to detect liver dullness, splenomegaly and an enlarged bladder.

Auscultation is used to assess the characteristic bowel sounds produced by an obstructed intestine, and the total absence of bowel

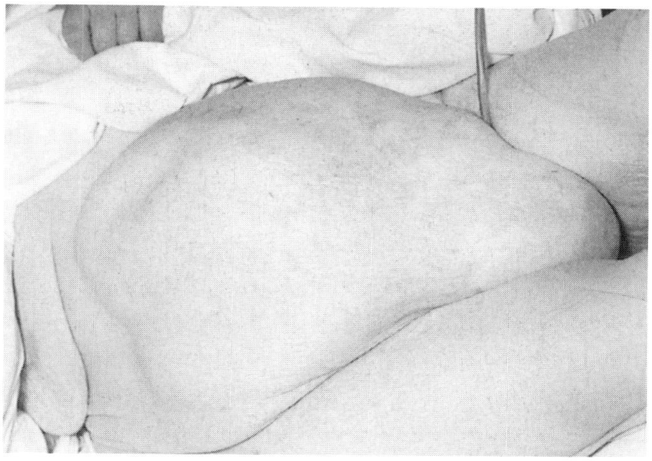

Fig. 27.26 A patient with visible peristalsis caused by small bowel obstruction.

sounds found in patients with a severe generalized peritonitis or paralytic ileus. Abdominal bruits may also be detected but are of dubious diagnostic value. The abdominal examination should include rectal and vaginal examinations and the urine should be tested by dipsticks and microscopy.

Specific signs such as those of Cullen,[115] Grey Turner,[116] Rovsing,[117] Murphy,[118] Boas[119] and Cope[120] may be sought, and specific tests such as the psoas stretch test, the obdurator internus stretch test, straight leg raising and hyperaesthesia in Sherren's[121] triangle may be performed when indicated. These specific signs and tests are described under the individual conditions which they help to diagnose.

FURTHER MANAGEMENT

On completion of the clinical examination a working or differential diagnosis should be made. Additional specific investigations may then be ordered to confirm the presumptive diagnosis or help to reduce the number of differential diagnoses. In many instances additional blood tests, X-rays or other methods of investigation will be considered unnecessary, and the patient can be managed on the basis of the history and clinical examination alone. Patients with acute abdominal pain may be reassured and discharged, admitted for observation and repeated re-examination, investigated further, or treated for a confidently diagnosed condition.

In those patients thought to have intra-abdominal pathology in whom a definite diagnosis cannot be made, a full blood count including a white cell count, serum amylase, abdominal and chest

REFERENCES

114. Bennett D H, Tambeur L J M T, Campbell W B Br Med J 1994; 308: 1336
115. Cullen Am J Obstet Gynecol 1918; 78: 457
116. Grey Turner G Br J Surg 1920; 7: 394
117. Rovsing G Z Chir 1907, 34: 1257
118. Murphy J B Surgical Clinics of J B Murphy 1912; 1: 459
119. Boas I Dtsch Med Wochenschr 1893; 19: 940
120. Cope Z Br Med J 1970; 3: 147
121. Sherren Br Med J 1925; 1: 727

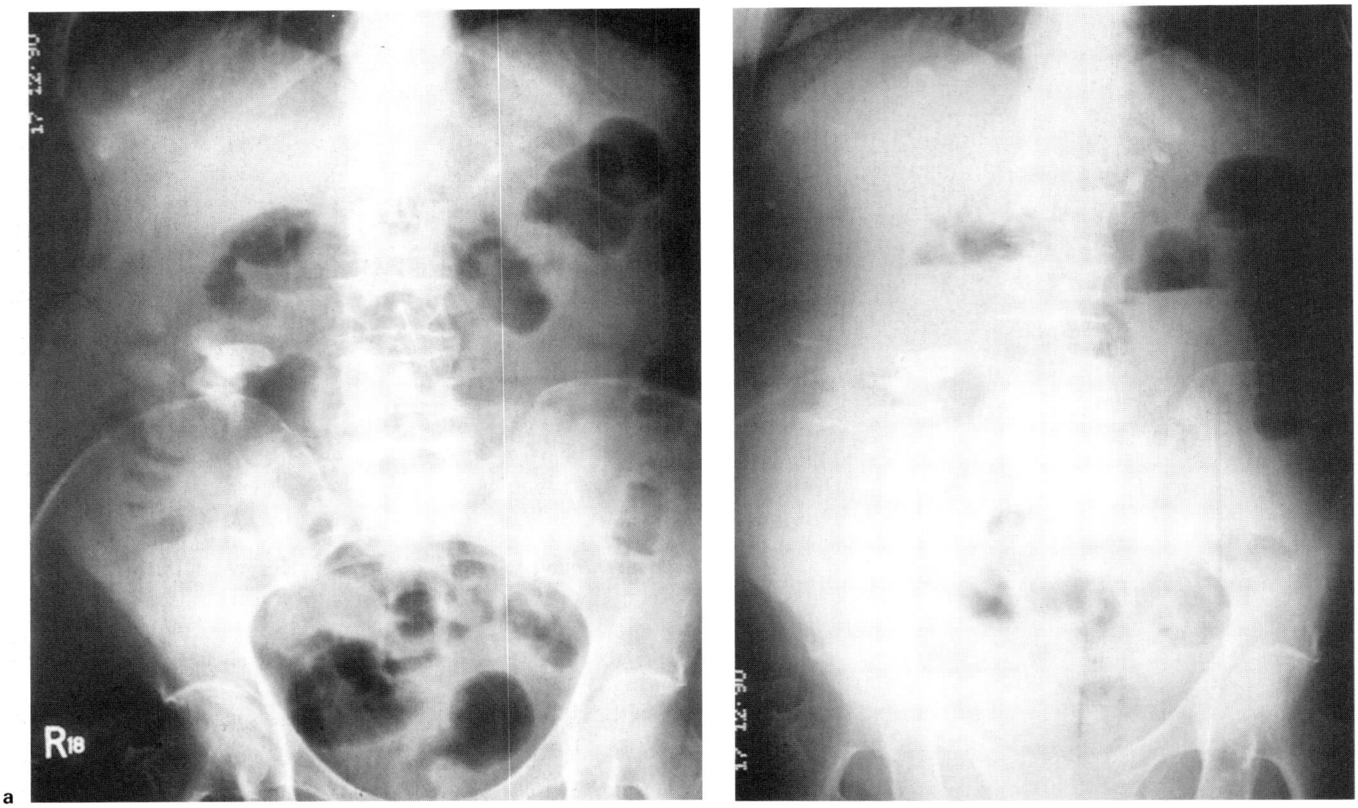

Fig. 27.27 (a) A plain abdominal radiograph taken in the supine position showing some dilated small bowel loops; (b) erect film taken at the same time showing multiple small bowel fluid levels.

radiographs are often helpful initial investigations. There has been considerable debate over the value of all these investigations. An amylase level in excess of 1000 iu/l is indicative of acute pancreatitis, but lesser values can be the result of any number of underlying diseases including perforated peptic ulcers, obstruction and mesenteric infarction. The initial white cell count, like the first temperature reading,[122] is often of little value, but sequential measurements are much more helpful as a trend can be observed.[123] The value of plain abdominal X-rays in the overall assessment of the acute abdomen has come under some considerable scrutiny over the last two decades. Conflicting evidence exists regarding the role of the plain abdominal radiograph,[124,125] but there is little doubt it is overused and in most cases of acute abdominal pain a supine film will suffice, the erect abdominal film rarely adding any further information.[126] There is no doubt that with experience the plain abdominal X-ray can be extremely helpful to the surgeon when certain conditions are considered—obstruction, ureteric colic, trauma, ischaemia and gallbladder disease[127]—and its use in these circumstances is to be encouraged. Occasionally fluid levels on the erect abdominal film, in the presence of a relatively normal supine radiograph, help to raise the suspicion of intestinal obstruction (Fig. 27.27), and for this reason is probably most use in uncertain cases rather than the more obvious ones. Free gas from a perforated intra-abdominal viscus is best seen on the erect chest X-ray (Fig. 27.28) or the lateral decubitus abdominal view.[126,128,129]

The desirability of other investigations obviously depends to some extent on the initial working diagnosis or the differential diagnosis reached on completion of the clinical examination. It also depends to some extent on the availability of the diagnostic equipment and laboratory facilities. Urea and electrolyte measurement is essential if dehydration or renal failure is suspected and liver function tests are required for all hepatobiliary and pancreatic conditions. Hepatitis A and B antigens may also be tested for, and the Paul–Bunnell test may be used if glandular fever is considered. The serum calcium, methaemalbumin, fibrinogen and C-reactive protein may all be helpful in diagnosing and assessing the severity of acute pancreatitis. Blood should be sent for a sickle test if the patient is black[130] and the urinary porphyrins can be measured if acute porphyria is considered.[131] A pregnancy test is helpful if a tubal pregnancy is suspected and antibody titres may be sent for amoebic and viral disease.

Better images of the intra-abdominal viscera can now be obtained with ultrasound, CT and magnetic resonance imaging. These investigations are of considerable value in the investigation

REFERENCES

122. Howie C R, Gunn A A J R Coll Surg Edinb 1984; 29: 249
123. Thompson M M, Underwood M J et al Br J Surg 1992; 79: 822
124. Lee P W R Br J Surg 1976; 63: 763
125. Stower M J, Amar S S et al Soc Med 1985; 78: 630
126. Field S, Guy P J et al Br Med J 1985; 290: 1934
127. Eisenberg R L, Heineken P et al Ann Intern Med 1982; 97: 257
128. Delacey G J, Wignall B K et al Clin Radiol 1980; 31: 453
129. Miller R E, Nelson S W Am J Roentgenol 1971; 112: 574
130. Tomlinson W J Am J Med Sci 1945; 209: 722
131. Stein J A, Tuschudy D P Medicine 1970; 49: 1

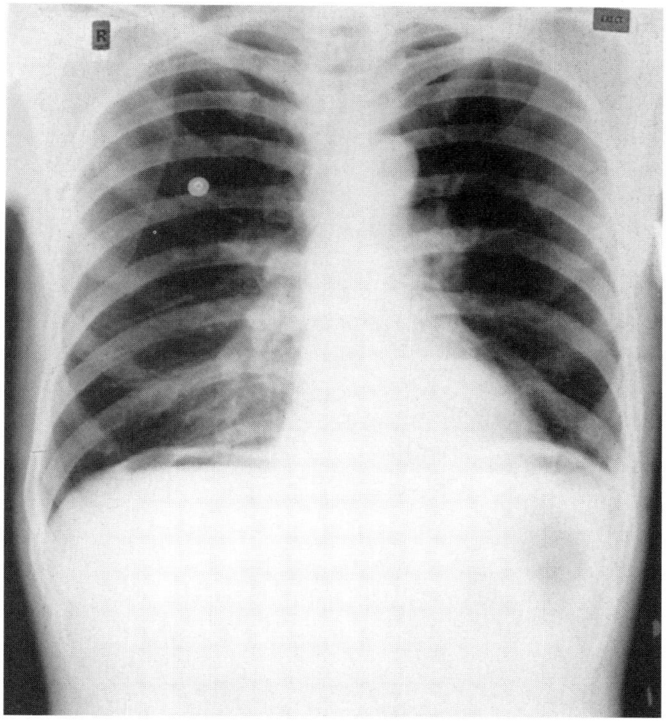

Fig. 27.28 An erect chest X-ray showing air under the diaphragm.

of some intra-abdominal conditions.[132,133] Contrast studies may also be helpful in patients suspected of having a gastric volvulus (Fig. 27.29), pyloric obstruction or Crohn's disease (Fig. 27.30) or when a perforated peptic ulcer is suspected but no free gas is seen on the erect chest radiograph.[134] A contrast enema is essential in the assessment of large bowel obstruction to differentiate between pseudo-obstruction and a mechanical cause.[135,136] Intravenous pyelography or ultrasound confirms renal obstruction from calculi (Fig. 27.31) and may be helpful in elucidating other causes of renal pain. Upper gastrointestinal endoscopy is useful in making an early diagnosis of a peptic ulcer, but is contraindicated if a sealed perforation might have occurred. Urgent colonoscopy can be used therapeutically to decompress acute colonic pseudo-obstruction and is occasionally used to assess colonic bleeding. Needless to say, before embarking on any investigation of the large bowel, rigid sigmoidoscopy must be performed to exclude local causes within the anorectum.

Laparoscopy was originally regarded as the province of the gynaecologist but it is now regarded by many as a useful tool in diagnosing patients with an acute abdomen of unknown cause.[137,138] Laparoscopy is particularly useful in young women when gynaecological causes, such as ovarian cyst rupture, ectopic pregnancy and salpingitis, often mimic acute appendicitis.[139] Its use is associated with a reduction in unnecessary appendicectomies[140,141] and it can also confirm the diagnosis in other causes of peritonitis. Retroperitoneal structures are not suitable for laparoscopic examination because of their position.

Peritoneal lavage is now widely accepted as one of the first-line investigations in patients suspected of intra-abdominal haemorrhage as the result of trauma, particularly in the unconscious

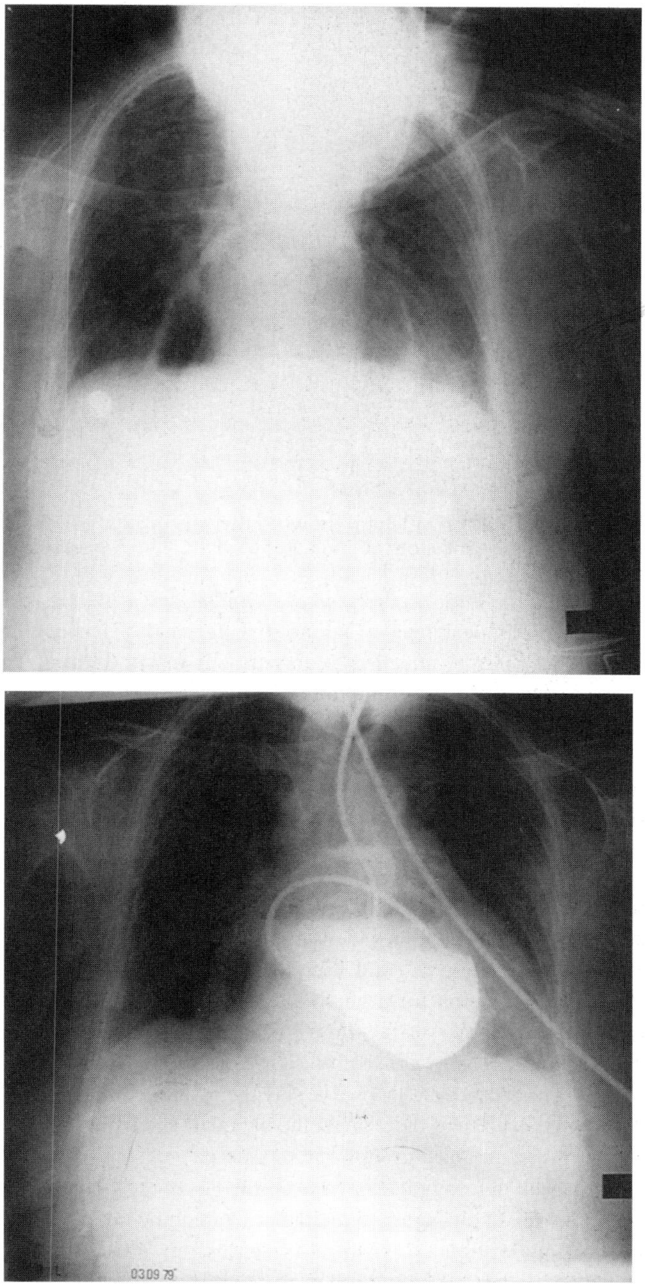

a

b

Fig. 27.29 (**a**) A chest radiograph and (**b**) a gastrografin swallow showing a gastric volvulus. The gastrografin (put down a nasogastric tube) enters a blind-ending pouch.

REFERENCES

132. Warys B T, Barr H et al Br J Surg 1987; 74: 611
133. Federle M P, Crass A et al Arch Surg 1986; 117: 645
134. Wellwood J M, Wilson A N, Hopkinson B R Br J Surg 1971; 58: 245
135. Stewart J, Finan P J et al Br J Surg 1984; 71: 799
136. Koruth N M, Koruth A, Matheson N A J R Coll Surg Edinb 1985; 30: 258
137. Paterson-Brown S, Ekersley J R et al Br J Surg 1986; 73: 1022
138. Leape L L, Ramentofsky M L Ann Surg 1980; 91: 410
139. Paterson-Brown S, Eckersley J R T, Dudley H A F J R Coll Surg Edinb 1988; 33: 13
140. Paterson-Brown S, Thompson J N et al Br Med J 1988; 296: 1363
141. Clarke P J, Hands L J et al Ann R Coll Surg Engl 1986; 68: 68

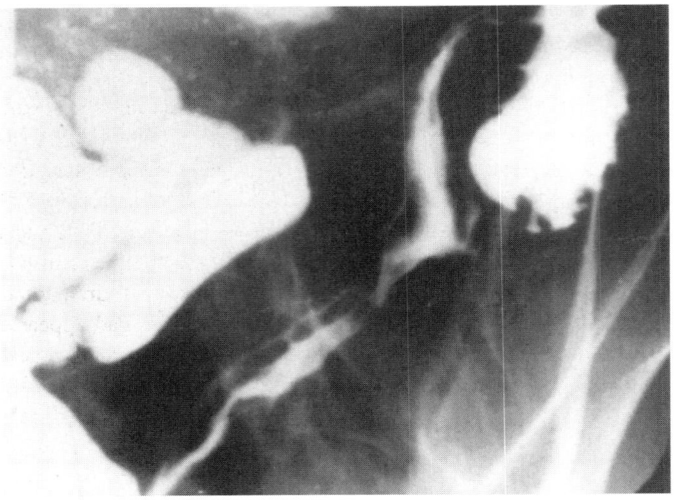

Fig. 27.30 A small bowel meal showing the 'string sign' in the terminal ileum, typical of the long stenosis of Crohn's disease.

patient with multiple injuries where clinical assessment is difficult.[142,143] Peritoneal lavage has now replaced the four-quadrant tap—when a needle attached to a syringe is inserted through the abdominal wall in each of the four quadrants and aspirated—in the assessment of abdominal trauma (see Chapter 7) and has more recently been used to assess acute abdominal pain.[144]

Peritoneal lavage is performed by inserting a dialysis catheter into the peritoneal cavity under direct vision, using a small incision below the umbilicus. One litre of normal saline is infused and the patient's position altered to ensure 'mixing'. The effluent is then removed and analysed for red and white cell concentration, amylase levels and the presence of intestinal contents, confirming perforation. A return of frank blood on insertion of the catheter is usually an indication for urgent laparotomy. Otherwise a red cell concentration above 100 000/mm^3 or a white cell concentration above 500/mm^3 are considered indications for laparotomy.[145] Injuries which produce a 'positive' lavage result do not necessarily require surgery[146] and there are some data that laparoscopy may be useful in the equivocal group.[147–149]

Peritoneal cytology has been examined over the last few years as a relatively non-invasive method of obtaining intraperitoneal information without resorting to laparoscopy. This was first described by the late Richard Stewart,[150] and subsequently verified by other groups.[151–153] A small (14-gauge) venous cannula is inserted into the peritoneal cavity halfway between the umbilicus and the symphysis pubis after infiltration with local anaesthesia. An umbilical catheter (size 3.5 Ch) is then passed down the cannula and aspirated. The resultant aspirate is deposited on a glass slide, stained and the percentage of polymorphonuclear cells in one high-powered field determined by light microscopy. A percentage greater than 50% is indicative of significant inflammation. Although extremely useful in differentiating those patients without an intra-abdominal inflammatory process, peritoneal cytology on its own cannot indicate the need for surgery as some inflammatory conditions such as pelvic inflammatory disease which do not require surgery cannot be differentiated from those such as acute appendicitis where operation is required.

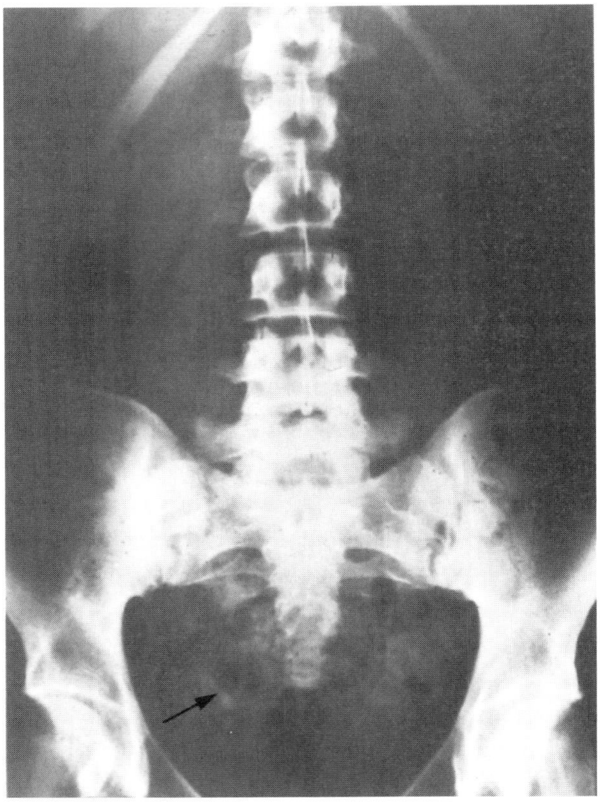

Fig. 27.31 (a) A plain radiograph showing a radiopaque calculus lying in the lower end of the right ureter.

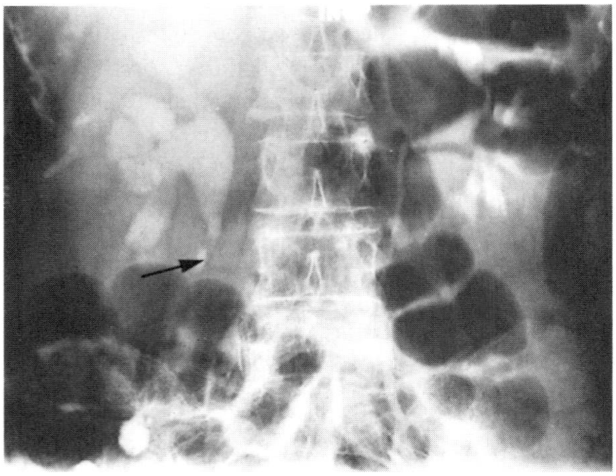

Fig. 27.31 (b) An intravenous urogram showing a calculus obstructing the pelviureteric junction. The right kidney is obstructed and hydronephrotic.

REFERENCES

142. Myers R A, Agrawalnn M, Crowley R A Surg Gynecol Obstet 1981; 153: 739
143. Root H O, Hauser C W et al Surgery 1965; 57: 633
144. Hoffmann J Acta Chir Scand 1987; 153: 561
145. Alyono D, Perry J F J Trauma 1981; 21: 345
146. Sorenson V, Vincent G et al J Trauma 1983; 23: 666
147. Sherwood R, Berci G et al Arch Surg 1980; 115: 672
148. Berci G, Dunkelman D et al Am J Surg 1983; 146: 261
149. Cushieri A, Hennessy T P J et al Ann R Coll Surg 1988; 70: 153
150. Stewart R J, Gupta R K et al Lancet 1986; ii: 1414

Arteriography, whether selective, flood, conventional or digital, is rarely helpful,[154] and isotopic scanning is also of little practical value at an early stage in the assessment of the acute abdomen. Repeated reassessment is an important part of the decision-making process[155] and initial uncertainty may often be resolved one way or another by a few hours of observation. Occasionally laparoscopy and even laparotomy still have to be undertaken where the risk of failing to treat a potentially curable condition outweighs the danger of an unnecessary operation.

The laparotomy incision is made in an appropriate site to allow extension and for all the intra-abdominal viscera to be inspected. This usually requires a midline incision at the level of the umbilicus.

Computer-aided diagnosis has been used by a number of hospitals for some time to improve diagnostic accuracy in the acute abdomen.[104,156] Multicentre studies have confirmed that diagnostic accuracy increases by 20% in association with computers[157] but it would appear that much of the improvement results from the use of structured proformas which are used to record the clinical details rather than the direct use of the computer.[158,159]

SPECIFIC CAUSES OF THE ACUTE ABDOMEN

ACUTE APPENDICITIS

History

Certain Coptic jars containing bowel are inscribed with references to the 'worm of the bowel', and the Hermetic Books of Thoth and the Books of the Dead contain statements which probably refer to the appendix. The appendix is crudely represented attached to the bowel in Greek votive jars from Cos and Gnidos, but Aristotle and Galen were ignorant of it, as their anatomical studies were confined to the lower mammalian orders. Aretaeus of Cappadocia[160] in AD 30 described the case of a patient who recovered from either an appendiceal or a perinephric abscess after simple drainage of the abdominal wall, Berengar Da Carpi[161] gave the first full account of the condition and Farnelius[162] described ileus following an appendix perforation. None of these authors recognized that the inflammation began in the appendix, neither did any anatomist, from Vésalius[163] who described the organ, to Verhegen[164] who named it, without knowing anything of the pathological process which afflicted it.

Creése[165] makes it clear that the first appendicectomy was performed in 1736 by Claudius Amyand, Fellow of the Royal Society, Surgeon to St George's Hospital and Sergeant Surgeon to King George II. Amyand removed the appendix, a pin which it contained, and the surrounding omentum from a scrotal hernia, complicated by faecal fistula, in a boy of 12 years. In 1753 Heister[166] described the post-mortem appearances of a gangrenous perforated appendix. Mestivier[167] opened an abscess in the right iliac fossa in a patient; autopsy subsequently showed this patient had a pin in the appendix. While the autopsy confirmed a relationship between the abscess and a gangrenous caecum, there was no mention of any continuity between the abcess and the appendix.

In 1819 Parkinson[168] recognized that 'appendicitis' was a frequent and important cause of death. Melier[169] gave a classical description of appendicitis and stated it was often responsible for pain in the right lower abdomen and might be curable by appendicectomy. He later retracted these revolutionary ideas when his senior colleague Dupuytren sneered at them. A clear description of acute appendicitis was also given by Bright & Addison.[170] Numerous German authors in the succeeding decade accurately described the symptoms of appendix abscess, ascribing its cause to 'perityphlitis'. In 1848 Hancock[171] recognized and drained an appendix abscess before fluctuation and crepitation had appeared and Parker,[172] in the USA, described the three stages of appendicitis gangrene, perforating ulcer and abscess. Symonds[173] in 1885 removed a calculus from a retrocaecal appendix which had been diagnosed by palpation, via a posterior retroperitoneal route. Fitz[174] coined the term 'appendicitis' and advised early operation. Mikulicz (cited by Kronlein[175]) in 1884 also suggested treatment by appendicectomy, and in the following year Kronlein[175] operated for appendicitis and removed a perforated appendix; unfortunately the patient died. A second case, 2 days later, also presented with peritonitis: this time Kronlein did not remove the appendix, but washed out the peritoneal cavity and the patient recovered. In 1887 Morton[176] first successfully removed the appendix with the intention of curing appendicitis. In 1902 Sir Fredrick Treves did much to popularize the condition by removing the appendix of the Prince of Wales (see Chapter 1).

REFERENCES

151. Vipond M N, Paterson-Brown S et al Br J Surg 1990; 77: 86
152. Baigrie R J, Saidan Z et al Br J Surg 1991; 78: 167
153. Caldwell M T P, Watson R G K Br J Surg 1994; 81: 276
154. Bewes P C Br J Hosp Med 1983; 402
155. Jones P F Br J Surg 1990; 77: 365
156. Gunn A A J R Coll Surg Edinb 1976; 21: 170
157. Adams I D, Chan M et al Br Med J 1986; 293: 800
158. Lawrence P C, Clifford P C, Taylor I F Ann R Coll Surg Engl 1987; 69: 233
159. Paterson-Brown S, Vipond M N et al Br J Surg 1989; 76: 1011
160. Aretaeus the Cappadocian. The extant works of Aretaeus the Cappodocian. F Adams (ed & trans) Sydenham Society, London 1856
161. Berengar Da Carpi Commentaria cum amplissimis additionibus super anato mica. Mundini una cum textu ejusdem in pristinum et verum rutorem vedacto. Bononiae Impression H. de Benedictus 1521
162. Farnelius J Universa Medicina. Wechelus, Frankfort 1581 p 295
163. Vesalius A De fabricio corporis humani librorum epitome. Basileae ex off J. Oporini 1543
164. Verhogen Corporis humani anatomia 1699
165. Creese P G Surg Gynecol Obstet 1953; 97: 643–652
166. Heister L Institutions, Chirurgie (1770). Reeves J, London 1755
167. Mestivier J Med Chir Pharmacol 1759; 10: 441
168. Parkinson, Med Chir Trans 1812; 3: 57
169. Melier J Gen Med Chir Pharmacol 1827; 100: 317
170. Bright H, Addison T Elements of the Practice of Medicine 1839; 1: 498
171. Hancock H Lancet 1848; 2: 380
172. Parker W Med Rec N Y 1867; 2: 25
173. Symonds C J Trans Clin Soc Lond 1885; 18: 285
174. Fitz R H Am J Med Sci 1886; 92: 32
175. Kronlein R Arch Klin Chir 1886; 33: 507
176. Morton T G Trans Coll Phys Surg Phil 1887; 12: 1

Incidence

In the 100 years since the first successful removal of the appendix for acute appendicitis, appendicectomy has become the commonest emergency surgical operation. It has been estimated that more than 80 000 people are admitted to hospital annually in the UK with a diagnosis of acute appendicitis[177] and Ashley[178] estimated that up to 12% of any western population will suffer an episode of acute appendicitis during their lifetime. Extrapolating from Irvin's figures,[179] this may be an overestimation of the current incidence, which looks like being between 10 000 and 20 000 per year in the UK.

The increase in appendicitis in the UK and Europe is thought to have begun abruptly between 1890 and 1895.[180–183] Death rates from the condition rose from 1901 until 1911, then remained steady and only began to fall in the late 1930s.[184] It has been suggested that the incidence rose more steeply than the mortality as the case fatality fell sharply during the first decade of this century.[185] It is also possible that the apparent rise in prevalence may have been exaggerated by a wider recognition of the condition.[186] Between 1920 and 1935 the case fatality declined,[187,188] and it has been suggested that this was the result of earlier admission to hospital and the widespread application of appendicectomy.

There appears to have been a true decline in the prevalence of appendicitis in England and Wales over recent years. Annual discharge rates for acute appendicitis fell progressively from 27 per 10 000 in 1959 to 13 per 10 000 in 1980.[189] A detailed review of appendicectomies in 1965–1978 also showed a steady decline which was not caused by a reduction in the rate of removal of normal appendices.[190] A similar decline in acute appendicitis has also been recorded in the USA and in other countries.[191–193]

Aetiology

The underlying cause of this common condition remains uncertain. A number of theories have been proposed; these include abnormalities in the diet, genetic factors and a variety of infectious agents. The latter may be related to poor domestic hygiene.

Diet

In the early part of this century when appendicitis was increasing in incidence, it was suggested that a lack of fibre in the diet might cause acute appendicitis.[180,194] The increase in appendicitis occurred during the time that imported flour, which had a low cellulose content, was being used more widely. It was also observed that the upper classes, who were the major users of white flour, had a higher incidence of acute appendicitis. Acute appendicitis is an uncommon disease in developing countries where the population consumes a high-fibre diet, but there is an increasing incidence of appendicitis when the diet changes to a low-fibre western-type diet. Burkitt suggested that the high-fibre diet produced bulkier stools which had a faster transit time through the intestine.[195–197] It is thought that a slower transit time associated with a low-fibre diet leads to an alteration in the bacterial flora which may also contribute to a higher incidence of appendicitis.

More recently the validity of the dietary fibre theory has been challenged. Epidemiological evidence shows that appendicitis in western Europe[184,190,198,199] and the USA[185,193] has been declining steadily for the past 30–40 years, although the dietary fibre intake[199,200] has not altered, and studies performed in South Africa have shown that urban blacks continue to have a very low incidence of acute appendicitis in spite of diets that are lower in fibre than those of the urban white population.[201] A positive correlation has been found between potato consumption and appendicitis, whereas a high intake of fruit and vegetables other than potato is associated with a lower incidence of the condition.[184] It appears that the influence of diet in the aetiology of acute appendicitis is not understood and the role of fibre is less convincing than was originally thought.[202]

Genetic factors

A number of authors have demonstrated a familial tendency in acute appendicitis.[203–206] The reason for this is not known, although it has been suggested that shared dietary habits,[190] genetic resistance

REFERENCES

177. Lee E C G In: Weatherall D J, Ledingham J G G, Warrel D A (eds) Oxford Textbook of Medicine. Oxford University Press, Oxford 1987 pp 12.178–12.181
178. Ashley D J Gut 1967; 8: 533–538
179. Irvin T T Br J Surg 1989; 76: 1121
180. Rendle Short A Br J Surg 1920; 8: 171–189
181. Murray R W Lancet 1914; ii: 227–230
182. Spencer A M Br Med J 1938; i: 227–230
183. Aschoff L Appendicitis, its Aetiology and Pathology. Translated by Pether G C. Constable, London 1932
184. Barker D J P Br Med J 1985; 290: 1125–1127
185. Editorial Lancet 1910; ii: 1835
186. Fitz R H Am J Med Sci 1886; 184: 321–345
187. Young M, Russell W T Appendicitis, a Statistical Study. Medical Research Council Special Report series no 233. HMSO, London 1939
188. Boyce F F Acute Appendicitis and its Complications. Oxford University Press, New York 1949
189. Report on the Hospital In-patient Enquiry. HMSO, London 1957 and following years
190. Raguveer-Saran M K, Keddie N C Br J Surg 1980; 67: 681
191. Mortality Statistics from General Practice, Studies on Medical and Population Subjects, nos 14 and 26. HMSO, London 1958, 1975
192. Castleton K B, Puestow C B, Sauer D Arch Surg 1959; 78: 794–801
193. Palumbo L T Am J Surg 1959; 98: 702–703
194. Williams O T Br Med J 1910; ii: 2016–2021
195. Burkitt D P Br J Surg 1971; 58: 695–699
196. Burkitt D P, Walker A R P, Painter N S Lancet 1972; ii: 1408–1412
197. Walker A R P, Walker B F et al Postgrad Med J 1973; 49: 243–249
198. Noer T Acta Chir Scand 1975; 141: 431–432
199. Arnbjornsson E, Asp N-G, Westin S I Acta Chir Scand 1982; 148: 461–464
200. Robertson J Nature 1972; 238: 290–292
201. Segal L, Walker A R P Nutr Cancer 1986; 8: 185–191
202. Heaton K W Br Med J 1987; 294: 1632–1633
203. Baker E G S Heredity 1937; 28: 187–191
204. Andersson N, Griffith H et al Br Med J 1979; ii: 697–698
205. Arnbjornsson E Curr Surg 1982; 39: 18–20
206. Brender J D, Marcuse E K et al Am Dis Child 1985; 139: 338–340

to bacterial flora[203] or inheritance of fibrous band anomalies related to the appendix[207] may be the cause.

Infection

The relationship between viral infections and acute appendicitis has been based on the findings of raised viral antibody titres,[208] the association between appendicitis and coincidental viral illness,[209] the clustering of appendicitis during particular seasons[210] and the presence of lymphoid tissue within the mucosa and submucosa of the appendix.[211] Lymphoid hyperplasia is not, however, always present in appendices resected for acute appendicitis[212] and not all patients have raised viral antibody titres during acute appendicitis.[213]

It has been shown that the incidence of appendicitis closely relates to the percentage of homes without fixed baths and hot water systems, suggesting that the lack of these facilities is associated with domestic overcrowding and a greater risk of respiratory and enteric infection.[214] Continued improvements in hygiene may reduce the exposure to infection and as a consequence reduce the risk of appendicitis.[215]

Pathology

For whatever reasons the wall of the appendix becomes inflamed and oedematous, and pus eventually fills the lumen.[183,216] This oedema and inflammation causes venous congestion which may impair the arterial inflow leading to thrombosis and gangrene. Organisms from the lumen of the appendix then enter the devitalized wall causing it to liquefy and perforate. If this occurs early, before surrounding adhesions have formed, generalized peritonitis develops, but if the inflammatory process is more gradual, small bowel and omentum adhere to the appendix and localize the sepsis.

It has been thought for many years that occlusion of the appendix is a very significant event in the development of appendicitis.[217,218] Faecoliths, hyperplasia of the lymphoid tissue, foreign bodies, congenital or inflammatory strictures of the appendix, carcinoid tumours or rare congenital bands may cause obstruction and subsequent appendicitis. The incidence of obstruction by faecoliths and the extent of the lymphoid hyperplasia vary considerably in studies where the cause of appendicular obstruction has been sought.[212,219]

Infection is thought to be initiated by luminal bacteria; the organisms enter the submucosa by way of an ulcer or through a devitalized portion of the appendix.[216] Haematogenous spread of bacteria—particularly streptococci—may also occur.[209]

Clinical features

The onset of acute appendicitis is associated with vague abdominal pain, sometimes colicky in nature, which is situated in the centre of the abdomen at the level of the umbilicus. There may be associated nausea and vomiting and in most cases anorexia is present. The temperature is usually only mildly elevated. The pain usually shifts to the right iliac fossa after a variable time, which may be only a few hours or as long as 24 hours. The central abdominal pain may

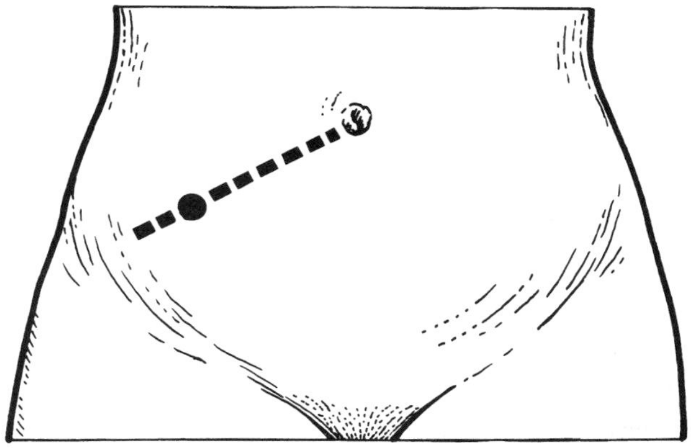

Fig. 27.32 McBurney's point.

persist or may be completely superseded by the pain in the right iliac fossa. This shift in pain occurs when the inflammation has spread to the serosal coat of the appendix and local peritonitis is present. The pain is usually sharp and localized and is aggravated by movement, walking or coughing. In many cases the initial central abdominal pain is not experienced and pain is first noticed in the right iliac fossa. Examination usually confirms a low-grade fever (up to 38°C) and a dry tongue with associated foetor.

Tenderness and guarding are frequently found on abdominal examination in the early stages, before the pain has localized to the right iliac fossa. After the pain has moved to the right iliac fossa the patient is usually able to localize the point of maximum tenderness with one finger. The site of this tenderness has classically been described as McBurney's point (one-third of the way between the anterior superior iliac spine and the umbilicus;[220] Fig. 27.32). Associated with the tenderness is muscular rigidity and percussion tenderness in the same area. Palpation in the left iliac fossa may produce pain at the site of tenderness in the right iliac fossa (crossed tenderness or Rovsing's sign). Rectal and vaginal examinations are frequently normal, although localized tenderness may be present if the inflamed organ lies below the pelvic brim. One study demonstrated that if rebound tenderness is present on abdominal examination, rectal examination does not provide any further diagnostic information.[221] In women a pelvic examination may provide helpful additional information of a possible gynaecological cause for the pain.

REFERENCES

207. Downs T M Ann Surg 1942; 115: 21–24
208. Tobe T Lancet 1965; i: 1343–1346
209. Galloway W H Br Med J 1953; ii: 1412–1414
210. Martin D L, Gustafson T L Am J Surg 1985; 150: 554–557
211. Bohrod M G Am J Clin Pathol 1946; 16: 752–760
212. Chang A R Aust NZ J Surg 1981; 51: 169–178
213. Morrison J D Br J Surg 1981; 68: 284–286
214. Barker D J P, Morris J Br Med J 1988; 296: 953–955
215. Larner A J Br J Hosp Med 1988; 540–542
216. Pieper R, Kager L et al Acta Chir Scand 1982; 148: 39–44
217. Wangensteen O H, Bowers W F Arch Surg 1937; 34: 496–526
218. Wangensteen O N, Dennis C Ann Surg 1939; 110: 629–647
219. Arnbjornsson E, Bengmark S Am J Surg 1984; 147: 390–392
220. McBurney C N Y Med J 1890; 52: 329
221. Dixon J M, Elton R A, Rainey J B, MacLeod D A D Br Med J 1991; 302: 386–388

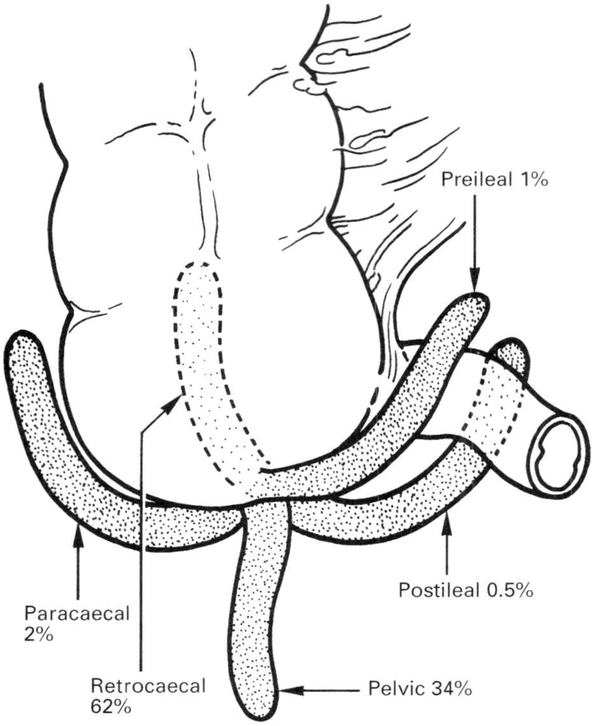

Fig. 27.33 The positions where the appendix lies.

The symptoms and signs of acute appendicitis are influenced by the position of the appendix (Fig. 27.33). It has always been accepted that the appendix is most often situated in the retrocaecal position[222] and usually lies free in the retrocaecal fossa. This was however produced from cadaveric dissections and more recent data from diagnostic laparoscopy have demonstrated that in vivo the appendix lies towards the pelvis in up to 50% of patients.[223] In some instances however it may be bound by a fold of peritoneum to the caecum or it may lie retroperitoneally between the caecum and the psoas muscle. Where the appendix is bound down in the retrocaecal fossa the symptoms of abdominal pain are often poorly localized and the muscular guarding may not be detected at McBurney's point; the signs are more marked further laterally towards the flank. When the appendix lies in close proximity to the psoas muscle, the patient tends to lie on the back with the hip flexed; passive extension or hyperextension of the hip increases the abdominal pain (psoas stretch sign). This is thought to occur as a result of muscle spasm caused by the appendix being in contact with the psoas. In this position the appendix may also be in contact with the ureter and a few red and white blood cells or protein may appear in the urine.

The symptoms of vomiting and diarrhoea may be more prominent if the appendix lies over the pelvic brim than in other forms of appendicitis and there may be very few signs, particularly in the early phase. In this position rectal examination more frequently reveals tenderness and swelling on the right side. The psoas stretch sign may be positive and on some occasions where the appendix lies in relation to the obturator internus, passive internal rotation of the hip may aggravate the pain (obturator stretch sign).

The pre- and post ileal positions are less common positions for the appendix. In the preileal or anterior position the signs of appendicitis may be very obvious as the appendix lies close to the anterior abdominal wall. The retro- or postileal position is possibly the most difficult of all positions for making an accurate diagnosis. The appendix lies behind the ileum and its mesentery, with its tip directed towards the spleen. The symptoms may be very vague with poorly localized abdominal pain and early vomiting. The abdominal signs may be non-specific with tenderness located high in the abdomen.

An inflamed appendix can also be situated in the right upper quadrant of the abdomen and may mimic acute cholecystitis or a perforated ulcer. This position is the result of non-descent of caecum—an anomaly of intestinal developmental rotation, which leaves the appendix closely related to the liver. With a very long appendix, the inflamed tip can be some distance from McBurney's point and give rise to tenderness in other sites. In very rare instances transposition of the viscera causes the caecum to lie on the left side and may produce signs in the left iliac fossa.

The clinical features of acute appendicitis may also be influenced by the patient's age and other conditions such as pregnancy. Acute appendicitis is an uncommon condition in neonates and children under the age of 3 years and in the past this has resulted in diagnostic delays and an associated increase in morbidity and mortality.[224,225] Better awareness has now rectified this state of affairs,[226] and the majority of deaths from appendicitis are now in the elderly, again often due to diagnostic problems. Very young children are unable to describe the pain clearly and vomiting may be the only presenting symptom. Diarrhoea is common, and when it occurs can lead to a misdiagnosis of gastroenteritis. In this age group it is important to consider the possibility of acute appendicitis even though it is much less common than in older age groups. Old age also modifies the symptoms of acute appendicitis. The initial pain is often less intense or entirely absent and the first symptoms may only occur with the onset of local peritonitis or perforation. Vomiting can precede the pain, and tenderness is often absent.

Acute appendicitis in pregnancy produces special problems. The later in pregnancy that appendicitis occurs, the more serious the disease is for both the mother and the foetus. In the first 7 months of pregnancy, appendicitis appears to have the same frequency as in women of child-bearing age who are not pregnant, although in the last 2 months of gestation it seems to be less frequent.[227] In a small series Horowitz et al reported one maternal death and the loss of three foetuses in 10 patients with acute appendicitis.[228] There are considerable difficulties in diagnosis

REFERENCES

222. Wakeley C P G J Anat 1933; 67: 277–283
223. Paterson-Brown S, Olufunwa S A, Galazka N, Simmons S C J R Coll Surg Edinb 1986; 31: 106–107
224. Williams H Br Med J 1947; 2: 730–732
225. Brown J J M J Coll Surg Edinb 1956; 1: 268–284
226. Hunter I C, Paterson J G, Davidson A I J R Coll Surg Edinb 1986; 31: 161–163
227. Johnson B Med J Aust 1944; 2: 379–383
228. Horowitz M D, Gomex G A et al Arch Surg 1985; 120: 1362–1367

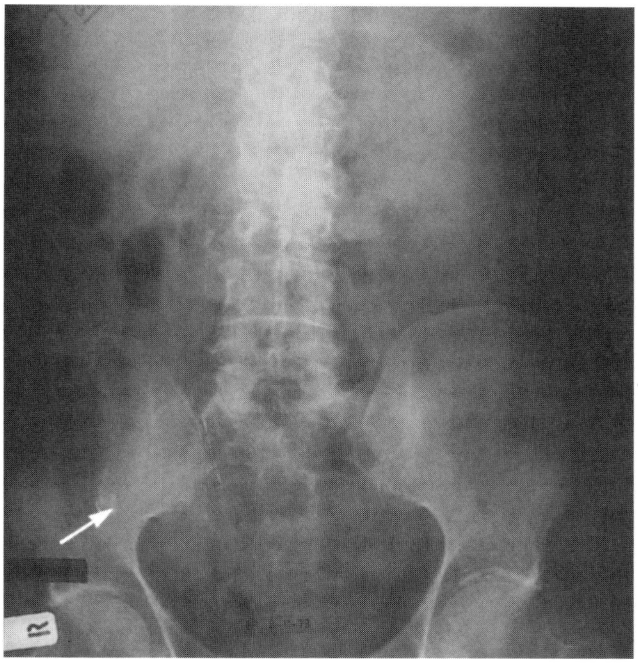

Fig. 27.34 (a) A plain radiograph showing an opacity in the right iliac fossa. This was an appendicular faecolith.

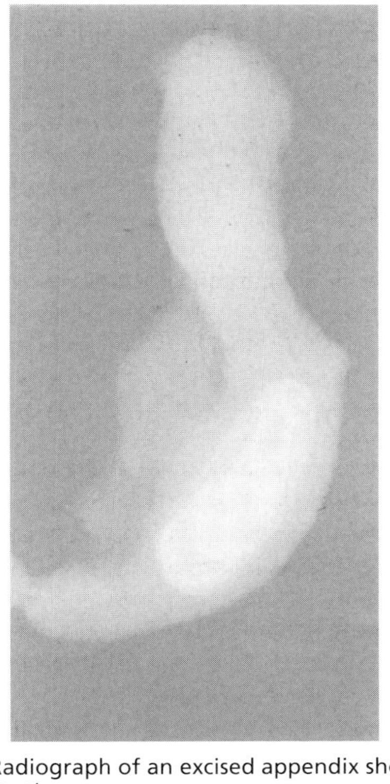

Fig. 27.34 (b) Radiograph of an excised appendix showing a faecolith near its tip.

because the initial symptoms are often confused with the onset of labour. Anorexia and constipation are inconsistent symptoms but nausea and vomiting tend to be more frequent. Because of the upward displacement of the appendix in advancing pregnancy, tenderness found anywhere in the right side of the abdomen can be caused by acute appendicitis. Guarding and rebound may not be present as the gravid uterus separates the inflamed appendix from the anterior parietal peritoneum. Six of Horowitz's 10 patients had perforated by the time of operation.

Laboratory investigations

Approximately 90% of patients with acute appendicitis have a moderate leucocytosis of about 15 000 cells/μl and 75% have a neutrophilia.[229] It must, however, be remembered that the white cell count is normal in 10% of cases. Urinalysis and microscopy are usually normal, but in patients with pelvic or retrocaecal appendicitis there may be red blood cells or leucocytes present in the urine.

X-ray investigations and imaging

Plain abdominal radiographs are generally unhelpful in diagnosing acute appendicitis.[229] Their main value is to exclude other causes of abdominal pain such as bowel obstruction, perforation or ureteric colic. It has been suggested that appendicitis can be excluded by the demonstration of a patent appendix that fills on barium enema.[230] Occasionally a faecolith is seen within the appendix (Fig. 27.34).

Other methods of diagnosing for acute appendicitis

Laparoscopy has been advocated to help differentiate acute appendicitis from gynaecological causes of the acute abdomen and it has been shown that if this investigation is performed in all women with suspected appendicitis, the incidence of unnecessary appendicectomy can be reduced.[140]

Ultrasound scanning is also useful in excluding other pelvic conditions such as ovarian cysts or a pyosalpinx and tubal pregnancy. It may also demonstrate a swollen inflamed appendix,[231,232] and a number of studies have shown a high sensitivity and specificity in diagnosing acute appendicitis.[233–236] However, other studies have failed to produce such good results[237,238] and ultrasound should probably be reserved for those patients in whom the diagnosis is uncertain, particularly young women. The diagnosis of acute appendicitis on ultrasonography is based on finding a non-compressible aperistaltic tubular structure with a dilated lumen and a thickened wall.

REFERENCES

229. Benry J, Malt R Ann Surg 1984; 200: 567
230. Abu Yousef M M, Blecher J J, Maher J W AJR 1987; 149: 53
231. Puyaert J, Rutgers P et al N Engl J Med 1987; 317: 666
232. Pearson R H Br Med J 1988; 297: 309–310
233. Puyaert B C M Radiology 1986; 158: 355–360
234. Jeffrey R B, Laing F C, Lewis F R Radiology 1987; 163: 11–14
235. Abu-Youseff M M, Bleicher J J, Maher J W Am J Radiol 1987; 149: 53–58
236. Karstnip S, Torppederson S, Roikjaer A Br J Radiol 1986; 59: 985–986
237. Puyaert J, Rutgers P et al N Engl J Med 1987; 317: 666–669
238. Takada T, Yasuda H et al Int Surg 1986; 71: 9–13

Both peritoneal cytology[153,239] and peritoneal lavage[240] have been used to detect polymorphonuclear cells within the peritoneal cavity, thereby confirming underlying inflammation. These techniques are valuable when negative, but if positive do not distinguish between acute appendicitis which requires surgery and pelvic inflammatory disease which does not. Laparoscopy can be used as the final arbiter before embarking on a laparotomy. As discussed earlier it is usually the young female in whom this diagnostic dilemma arises.

Differential diagnosis of acute appendicitis

Several conditions may be misdiagnosed as acute appendicitis.

Gastroenteritis

Vague gastrointestinal upsets are the most common disorders that are confused with appendicitis, and often a specific diagnosis is never established. Occasionally positive cultures can be obtained from the stools. Abdominal tenderness is usually less well-localized than in acute appendicitis.

Mesenteric adenitis in children and young adults poses a particular problem (see p. 756).

Disorders of the female pelvis (see p. 750)

An incorrect diagnosis of acute appendicitis is most commonly made in women of child-bearing age. The conditions that cause confusion include ruptured ovarian follicle, pelvic inflammatory disease, ruptured ectopic pregnancy and torsion of an ovarian cyst.

Ruptured ovarian follicle (mittelschmerz)

This diagnosis is suggested if the pain occurs in the middle of the menstrual cycle (at the time of ovulation). The pain is initially severe before gradually subsiding over the course of several days. There is usually some tenderness in the right lower quadrant but there are rarely any gastrointestinal symptoms and the patient does not look unwell.

Pelvic inflammatory disease (acute salpingitis)

In this condition the lower abdominal pain is associated with a high fever and tenderness which is usually most marked in the suprapubic region and in both iliac fossae. A vaginal discharge is often present, although this may be absent in the early stages. On pelvic examination a discharge may be observed coming from the cervix and bacteria can be cultured from a swab. Cervical manipulation usually exacerbates the pain.

Ruptured ectopic pregnancy

In this condition there is classically a history of a missed or abnormal period which precedes a sudden pain in the lower abdomen. This pain may be referred to the shoulder tip. On examination altered blood may be seen coming from the vagina. The patient may be pale and hypotensive, although in the early stages

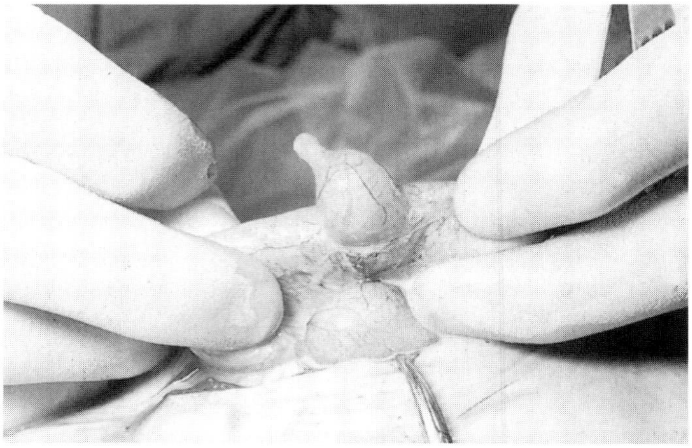

Fig. 27.35 A Meckel's diverticulum.

these signs are often not present. Tenderness is present across the lower abdomen with signs of guarding and rebound tenderness. There may be some periumbilical bruising (Cullen's sign). There is usually pain on movement of the cervix but vaginal examination should be performed with caution. The diagnosis is supported by a positive pregnancy test and evidence of an abnormality within the fallopian tube on ultrasound or at laparoscopy.

Torsion of an ovarian cyst

Torsion of an ovarian cyst can cause marked pain and a low-grade fever. There are few gastrointestinal symptoms, although the patient will often vomit with the pain. Tenderness is present in the lower abdomen, but usually confined to one iliac fossa. A mass may be felt arising from the pelvis if the cyst is large, otherwise there may be no evidence of any mass on palpation. The cyst can sometimes be palpated on pelvic examination, but can almost always be confirmed by abdominal ultrasound. The torsion involves the ovary and once the diagnosis has been made surgery is required.

Iliocaecal disorders

There are a number of disorders of the iliocaecal region which can mimic acute appendicitis.

Meckel's diverticulitis

This diagnosis is rarely made before operation for presumed acute appendicitis. The only differentiating features which occasionally arouse suspicion are a more medial point of maximal tenderness and possibly some evidence of mechanical small bowel obstruction. The small bowel must be inspected for a possible Meckel's diverticulum if the appendix is found to be normal when appendicitis is suspected (Fig. 27.35).

REFERENCES

239. Baigrie R J, Scott-Coombes D et al Br J Clin Pathol 1992; 46: 173–176
240. Hoffman J, Rasmussen O O Br J Surg 1989; 76: 774–779

Regional ileitis (Crohn's disease)

Acute forms of regional ileitis can be mistaken for acute appendicitis. The presence of a vague, tender mass in the right lower quadrant or symptoms of diarrhoea may suggest Crohn's disease. This condition is discussed in detail in Chapter 29. The appendix should be removed with careful repair of the caecum if Crohn's disease is discovered during an operation for presumed acute appendicitis. Although there is a risk of postoperative fistulation, this is small and removes potential diagnostic uncertainty during subsequent episodes of acute abdominal pain. *Yersinia* infection may cause a condition which appears on microscopic examination to be identical with Crohn's (see p. 731).

Carcinoma of the caecum

Occasionally this may cause acute appendicitis. It may also present with acute right iliac fossa pain if the caecum ruptures proximal to a carcinoma in the colon or a local perforation leads to a paracolic abscess (see Chapter30).

Foreign body perforation

When this occurs in the caecum or distal small bowel it can mimic acute appendicitis. The diagnosis is not usually made until laparotomy.

Genitourinary disorders

Several genitourinary disorders produce symptoms similar to those of acute appendicitis.

Ureteric calculus

This is usually differentiated from acute appendicitis because the pain of renal colic is quite different to the pain of acute appendicitis. It is much more severe, gets worse in waves and radiates from the loin to the groin. Nausea and vomiting occur with both conditions, and pelvic or retrocaecal appendicitis can be associated with haematuria and white cells in the urine. Haematuria is usually more marked with ureteric colic and although there may be right iliac fossa tenderness in ureteric colic, this is generally less marked than that found with acute appendicitis, and is usually associated with loin tenderness. Plain abdominal X-rays show a radiopacity in the line of the renal pelvis or ureter in 90% and the presence of obstruction can be determined by an intravenous urogram (Fig. 27.31).

Pyelonephritis

The presentation of this condition is usually with loin pain and urinary frequency associated with a high fever and chills which are uncommon in acute appendicitis. There is normally some renal tenderness and sometimes the tenderness is maximal in the right iliac fossa. Under these circumstances the differentiation from retrocaecal or pelvic appendicitis is difficult, especially as white and red cells may be found in the urine of patients with retrocaecal appendicitis. Organisms identified on a Gram stain of the urine will usually help to make the diagnosis and if a pyonephrosis is present ultrasound will be diagnostic. It is particularly difficult to differentiate between acute pyelonephritis and appendicitis in pregnancy.

Other less common conditions mimicking acute appendicitis

Cholecystitis, perforated ulcer and a number of medical conditions such as herpes zoster and acute porphyria (see p. 759) may be misdiagnosed as appendicitis.

Rupture of the inferior epigastric artery, causing a haematoma in the rectus abdominis muscle (see p. 754), particularly during a fit of coughing or unaccustomed exercise, may occasionally be mistaken for acute appendicitis. Other symptoms of acute appendicitis, such as anorexia and the typical colicky pain moving to the right iliac fossa, are absent.

Treatment of acute appendicitis

The treatment of acute appendicitis is appendicectomy in almost all cases in order to avoid the potentially serious complications associated with perforation and generalized intra-abdominal sepsis. Occasionally, early acute appendicitis may resolve spontaneously or be encouraged to do so with antibiotics and this has raised the possibility of avoiding operations in some patients.[241] Non-surgical treatment of acute appendicitis is only advocated in those situations where surgical treatment is not available or is contraindicated by the patient's poor general condition. Conservative treatment is also used in patients who have an appendix mass without signs of general peritonitis. Some of these patients do go on to develop an abscess that requires drainage, but in most the acute episode resolves. In the elderly it is essential to perform a barium enema or colonoscopy to exclude an underlying caecal carcinoma before considering an interval appendicectomy, which is usually carried out 6–8 weeks later to prevent further attacks.[242] Some young patients do not get further attacks and therefore in the younger age group a more pragmatic view can be taken regarding the need for interval appendicectomy.

If an appendix mass is managed conservatively it is essential to obtain an ultrasound scan to exclude an underlying abscess which requires drainage. Although it is common to use antibiotics, there is no clear evidence that they are either beneficial or harmful.[243,244] Persistent pyrexia, tachycardia, increasing abdominal pain, signs of generalized peritonitis, an increase in the size of the mass or a failure to reduce in size after 4–5 days indicate that an abscess is developing and requires drainage.[245] Cellulitis or fluctuation developing within the abdominal wall are late signs and indicate that drainage should have been carried out earlier.

REFERENCES

241. Neutra R In: Bunker J P, Barnes B A, Mosteller F (eds) Costs, Risks, Benefits of Surgery. Oxford University Press, New York, 1977; pp 277–307
242. Keddie N Br J Hosp Med 1975; 175
243. Paull D L, Bloom G P Arch Surg 1982; 117: 1017
244. Hoffman J et al Am J Surg 1984; 148: 379
245. Paull D L, Bloom G P Arch Surg 1982; 117: 1017–1019

Preoperative management

Patients who are dehydrated require several hours of rehydration with intravenous fluids. In most cases of uncomplicated appendicitis rehydration is not necessary and appendicectomy can be carried out once the diagnosis has been made.

Use of antibiotics

There have been many studies on the use of antibiotics to reduce postoperative wound sepsis after appendicectomy. Legions of different topical and parenteral agents have been investigated. In a review of the literature on the prevention of wound infection after appendicectomy, Krukowski[246] concluded that prophylactic antibiotics reduce the frequency of wound sepsis even in low-risk patients and that a single pre- or perioperative dose is normally sufficient for this purpose. The use of peroperative antibiotic lavage is also associated with a reduction in wound infection in both low- and high-risk patients.[247–249] In patients with gangrenous and perforated appendicitis most surgeons would advocate antibiotic lavage (with 1 g tetracycline in 1000 ml normal saline) in addition to antibiotics, which should be continued for at least 48 hours, if not 5 days. The antibiotic chosen should have a broad spectrum to cover both aerobes and anaerobes.

The appendix is normally approached through the Lanz or gridiron McBurney incision. The Lanz incision is nearly horizontal and is sited low in the right iliac fossa almost in the pubic hair, while the gridiron is made through McBurney's point at right angles to a line joining the anterior superior iliac spine to the umbilicus (Fig. 27.32). A right paramedian or lower midline incision is indicated in the elderly when there is diagnostic uncertainty or when a carcinoma of the caecum is suspected.

After the horizontal incision, the oblique muscles of the anterior abdominal wall are split in the line of their fibres and retracted until the peritoneum is exposed. Once the peritoneum has been opened the caecum is located and gently eased on to the surface using a finger, or atraumatic Babcock's or Denis Brown's forceps. As the caecum is turned forwards the appendix is usually exposed lying in the retrocaecal fossa and this too is delivered on to the surface with the aid of gentle pressure exerted by a finger passed up and hooked behind the inflamed organ.

Babcock's forceps can be applied to the base of the appendix once this has been reached to prevent the caecum and appendix slipping back inside the abdomen. The abdominal wound should be extended if it is difficult to deliver the appendix and the muscles may have to be divided. In these circumstances the appendix is often in a high retrocaecal or extraperitoneal position and it may be necessary to mobilize the caecum along its lateral border by dividing the peritoneal reflection. Once the caecum has been delivered on to the surface, the appendix is held up to enable the mesentery to be divided between artery forceps. The appendicular vessels are then ligated. The base of the appendix is crushed, ligated and inverted using a pursestring or Z suture, or simply ligated (Fig. 27.36). It is important accurately to identify the base of the appendix, which lies at the junction of the taeniae coli, in order that a length of appendix is not left behind to cause further trouble. The wound is then closed.

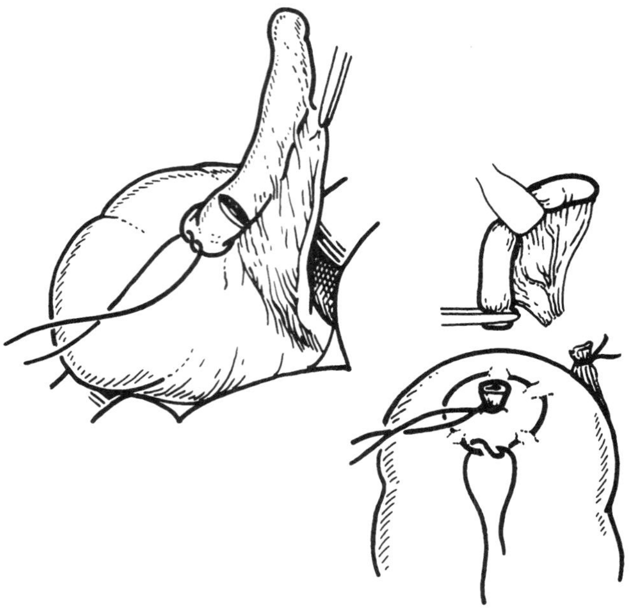

Fig. 27.36 Operative techniques for dealing with the appendix stump.

Several papers have questioned the need for invagination of the appendix stump, after showing that there is no significant difference in either the postoperative infection rate or the length of postoperative stay, whether the stump is invaginated or not.[250,251] Laparoscopic appendicectomy is now being advocated and large series of patients have been reported.[252,253] Randomized controlled trials have not demonstrated any advantage in this technique which takes longer and is more expensive than conventional surgery.[254,255] It has been suggested that return to work may be quicker after the laparoscopic approach.[256]

Postoperative management

In most instances bowel function resumes rapidly and the patient can start a normal diet on the first postoperative day. Hospital stay is variable but the majority of patients can be discharged within 4 days.[257]

REFERENCES

246. Krukowski Z H, Irwon S T et al Br J Surg 1988; 75: 1023–1033
247. Eklund A-E, Tunevall T G World J Surg 1987; 11: 263–266
248. Gottrup F Acta Chir Scand 1980; 146: 133–136
249. Krukowski Z H, Matheson N A Br J Surg 1988; 75: 857–861
250. Engstrom L, Fenyo G Br J Surg 1985; 73: 971–972
251. Watter D A K, Walker M A, Abernethy B C Ann R Coll Surg Engl 1984; 66: 90–91
252. Pier A, Gotz F, Bacher C Surg Laparosc Endosc 1991; 1: 8–13
253. Valla J, Limonne B et al Surg Laparosc Endosc 1991; 1: 166–172
254. Tate J J T, Chung S C S, Lau W T, Li A K C Lancet 1993; 342: 633–637
255. Martin L C, Puente I et al Ann Surg 1995; 222: 256–262
256. Kum C K, Ngoi S S, Goh P M Y, Tekhant Y, Isaac J R Br J Surg 1993; 80: 1599–1600
257. Baigrie R J, Dehn T C B, Fowler S M, Dunn D C Br J Surg 1995; 82: 933

Complications of acute appendicitis

The complications of acute appendicitis can be divided into preoperative, early and late postoperative complications. They include those that occur with any operative procedure and those that are specific for appendicitis (Table 27.3). In a recent survey of 8651 appendicectomies performed in England and Wales in 1992[257] the mortality rate was 0.24% and the morbidity 8%.

The complications of perforation, generalized peritonitis and appendiceal abscess are considered in detail. Other complications include septicaemia, portal pyaemia, haemorrhage, paracaecal, pelvic and subphrenic abscesses, intestinal obstruction, faecal fistula and urinary retention. These are discussed elsewhere.

Perforation

Gangrenous appendicitis and perforation follow a significantly longer period of pain than in patient with uncomplicated appendicitis.[258] The consequences of perforation are generalized peritonitis and the formation of an intra-abdominal abscess. In young women there is an increased risk of infertility following perforated appendicitis.[259,260]

Generalized peritonitis

Perforation of the appendix leads to a generalized perito-nitis if the appendix has not been walled off by surround-ing omentum and loops of bowel. The abdominal pain becomes more diffuse with tenderness and guarding over the whole abdomen. The patient has a high fever and appears very unwell, becoming dehydrated and hypotensive. At a later stage the abdomen becomes distended as a result of a paralytic ileus. Under these circumstances operation is better performed through a midline or right paramedian incision to enable general peritoneal lavage to be performed and to ensure that there is no other cause of the peritonitis.

Appendix abscess

An appendix abscess complicates a localized perforation of the appendix or gangrenous appendicitis when pus is prevented from entering the remainder of the peritoneal cavity as the result of adherent omentum and loops of small bowel. In the early stages an appendix mass is usually present. Many surgeons prefer to take a conservative approach to an appendix mass, providing there is no evidence of generalized peritonitis or advancing local sepsis. Some, however, prefer to operate early in the knowledge that appendicectomy is usually possible and this combined with the use of antibiotics prevents further sepsis. In the pre-antibiotic era McPherson & Kinmonth[261] believed that patients presenting with a palpable mass had an inflammatory phlegmon rather than an abscess. They were able to treat 67% of 129 patients without surgery, with only one death. Other subsequent studies produced similar results.[262–264] Drainage must however be performed if there is evidence that sepsis is continuing and one study demonstrated that 31 out of 35 patients with an appendix mass had well-defined abscesses at laparotomy.[243]

Table 27.3 Complications of appendicitis and appendicectomy

Preoperative
Perforation of the appendix
Generalized peritonitis
Appendiceal abscess
Early postoperative
Residual abscess
Paracaecal
Pelvic
Subphrenic
Faecal fistula
Postoperative obstruction
Paralytic ileus
Mechanical obstruction from adhesions
Caecocolic intussusception (appendix stump becoming intussuscepted into the colon)
Retention of urine
Chest complications
Bronchial pneumonia
Atelectasis
Empyema
Thromboembolism
Parotitis
Partal pyaemia and thrombosis
Ileocaecal actinomycosis
Persistent sinus
Late postoperative
Ventral hernia
Inguinal hernia
Adhesions causing bowel obstruction

The need for interval appendicectomy after successful conservative management or incision and drainage of an appendiceal abscess is also disputed. One study showed that one-third of 71 appendices showed no evidence of active inflammation at the time of interval appendicectomy.[265] Others have however reported that there was microscopic evidence of inflammation in the wall of 67%,[266] although only 4 of 16 patients had recurrent symptoms. Other studies have recorded attacks of acute appendicitis in about 5% of patients within 9 months (42 patients),[245] approximately 8% at 5 years (13 patients)[265] and in none out of 7 patients at 2.4 years.[264] The value of routine interval appendicectomy therefore still remains unproven.

Miscellaneous conditions of the appendix

Grumbling appendix (chronic appendicitis)

It is doubtful if the condition of chronic appendicitis exists, although appendicectomy is still performed for recurrent attacks of

REFERENCES

258. Moss J G, Barrie J L, Gunn A A J R Coll Surg Edinb 1985; 30: 290–293
259. Mueller B A, Daling J R et al N Engl J Med 1986; 315: 1506–1507
260. Mueller B A, Daling J R et al N Engl J Med 1987; 316: 1662
261. McPherson A G, Kinmonth J B Br J Surg 1945; 32: 365–370
262. Thomas D R Surgery 1973; 73: 677–680
263. Foran B, Berne T V, Rosoff L Arch Surg 1978; 113: 1144–1145
264. Mosegaard A, Nielsen O S Acta Chir Scand 1979; 145: 109–111
265. Barnes B A, Behringer G E, Wheelock F C et al JAMA 1962; 180: 122–126
266. Befeler D Arch Surg 1964; 89: 666–668

pain located in the right iliac fossa. Recurrent attacks of lower abdominal and right iliac fossa pain in childhood and adolescence is a common problem that is sometimes labelled 'grumbling appendix'. Such chronic abdominal pain in childhood rarely has an identifiable cause.[267] Clearly those patients who are in fact having attacks of acute recurrent appendicitis need to be differentiated from those who are not.[268]

An essential feature of recurrent appendicitis is a clear history that the recurrent abdominal pain followed an attack of acute appendicitis. It is therefore vital to establish the nature of the first attack of pain. Recurrent pains are frequently associated with anorexia, general malaise and tenderness over the appendix. When this type of story is obtained the appendix is often found to be inflammed or to show clear evidence of previous inflammation when it is removed.[269,270]

Some children with chronic recurrent right iliac fossa pain have psychological difficulties and the over-anxious parent is of real relevance. Others appear to be experiencing genuine attacks of pain which may be related to the irritable bowel syndrome, although this tends to be a problem of later life. Some children are found to have appendices containing *Enterobius vermicularis* and the role of these helminths as a cause of abdominal pain is ill-understood. Affected individuals should receive a course of piperazine. Constipation is the most common cause of abdominal pain in children.

Recurrent right iliac fossa pain in adolescent and adult life can be caused by Crohn's disease, pelvic sepsis, small bowel obstruction by bands or adhesions, irritable bowel syndrome, mittelschmerz (mid-cycle pain from a ruptured ovarian follicle), constipation, urinary tract infections and many other conditions which are extremely rare. Sensible investigations after a detailed history and examination will often elucidate a cause, but eventually laparotomy, laparoscopy or appendicectomy may be required. This will occasionally reveal an appendicular carcinoid tumour or clear evidence of prior inflammation.

Crohn's disease of the appendix

Crohn's disease presenting as an acute illness mimicking acute appendicitis has been reported to occur in as many as 10% of patients with Crohn's disease and the correct diagnosis is often not made until operation. Crohn's disease limited entirely to the appendix is, however, an uncommon condition,[271] as distinct from appendiceal involvement in Crohn's disease of the ileocaecal region which may be present in up to half of the cases.[272,273] Controversy exists over whether or not to perform an appendicectomy when ileocaecal Crohn's disease is encountered unexpectedly. Appendicectomy has been reported to be a safe procedure with a low incidence of postoperative fistula,[271] and removes subsequent diagnostic dilemmas when the patient represents with recurrent right iliac fossa pain. Local resection of the involved terminal ileum and caecum may, however, be a safer procedure if there is a broad-based appendix with inflammatory involvement in the caecum. This may also act as the definitive treatment for the Crohn's disease as approximately 50% of patients treated in this way do not develop recurrence. It has even been suggested that 90% of patients with acute regional enteritis do not progress to the chronic form.[274,275]

MECKEL'S DIVERTICULUM

This ilial diverticulum derives its name from Johann Friedrich Meckel the younger[276,277] who described its pathological and embryological features. It is a true diverticulum containing all the layers of the intestinal wall and is the commonest congenital anomaly of the small bowel. It is a remnant of the omphalomesenteric or vitelline duct and is normally found arising from the antimesenteric border of the ileum approximately 50 cm proximal to the ileocaecal valve (although this varies considerably). It may contain ectopic tissue, most frequently gastric or pancreatic mucosa. The incidence in the general population has been variously recorded at 0.6–2.3% in autopsy series, and a figure of 2% is the most widely accepted.[278]

A Meckel's diverticulum may cause abdominal pain in a number of ways. In the adult, the commonest complication is intestinal obstruction. This may result from volvulus or kinking of loop of small bowel round a congenital band running from the tip of the diverticulum to the umbilicus, the abdominal wall or the mesentery. Obstruction may also be caused by intussusception with the diverticulum as the apex of the intussusceptum. The next most common complication is inflammation of the Meckel's diverticulum. This can produce abdominal pain that is clinically indistinguishable from acute appendicitis; the diagnosis is rarely made until operation. The incidence of perforation in the presence of acute inflammation of a Meckel's diverticulum is reported to be as high as 50%. In children the most commonly encountered complications are intestinal obstruction and rectal bleeding.[279,280]

The diverticulum can usually be treated by simple excision, but in some cases ileal resection is necessary. A broad-based diverticulum may be difficult to excise without narrowing the lumen. Figure 27.37 shows two methods that are commonly used[281] to avoid this problem.

There is no consensus on the correct management of the incidentally discovered Meckel's diverticulum; some surgeons favour

REFERENCES

267. Apley J The Child with Abdominal Pains, 2nd edn. Blackwell Scientific, Oxford 1975
268. Anonymous Br Med J 1979; 294
269. Grossmann E B Surg Gynecol Obstet 1978; 146: 596–598
270. Savrin R A, Clausen K et al Am J Surg 1979; 137: 355
271. McCue J, Coppen M J et al Ann R Coll Surg Engl 1988; 70: 298–299
272. Warren S, Sommers S C Am J Pathol 1948; 24: 475–501
273. Larsen E, Axelsson C, Johansen A Acta Pathol Microbiol Immunol Scand (suppl), 1970; 212: 161–165
274. Kirsner J B, Shorter R G N Engl J Med 1982; 306: 775–785
275. Kirsner J B, Shorter R G N Engl J Med 1982; 306: 837–848
276. Meckel J F Arch Physiol 1809; 9: 421–453
277. Meckel J F Handbuch der pathologischen Anatomie, vol 1. Leipzig Reclam, CH 1812
278. Harkins H N Ann Surg 1933; 98: 1070–1095
279. Wansbrough M B, Thomson S, Leckey R G J Surg 1957; 1: 15–21
280. Meguid M, Canty T, Eraklis A J Surg Gynecol Obstet 1974; 139: 541–544

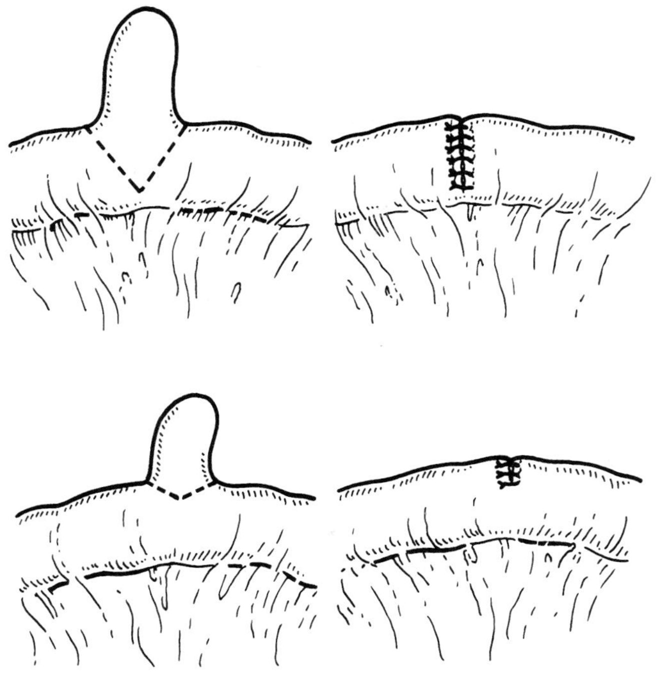

Fig. 27.37 Operative techniques for dealing with a Meckel's diverticulum.

surgical excision[282–284] while others advocate a less aggressive approach.[285,286] In coming to a decision it is necessary to weigh up the relative risks of developing a complication compared to the risk of surgical excision. Most complications occur in children[286] and the lifetime risk of a complication from Meckel's diverticulum is thought to be around 4%,[285] although after the age of 16 years the likelihood of developing complications reduces significantly towards zero in old age.[286]

The risk of developing complications from a Meckel's diverticulum is associated with the presence of ectopic mucosa, a length exceeding 4 cm and a base width less than 2 cm.[286] These factors may be used to select which Meckel's diverticula to resect and which to leave alone.

ACUTE CHOLECYSTITIS

The diagnosis and management of this condition are described in detail in Chapter 32. It is important to make a firm diagnosis of the condition, which is indicated by a history of severe central or right-sided abdominal pain and vomiting and signs of local peritonitis in the right upper quadrant. Patients are usually pyrexial and may be jaundiced. Zachary Cope, Murphy's and Boas's signs may be present. Ultrasound usually confirms the presence of a thick-walled gall bladder containing stones, but if this investigation is equivocal, and or normal despite the signs and symptoms of acute cholecystitis, an oral cholecystogram or HIDA scan may be obtained to confirm that the gallbladder is not functioning. Differential diagnoses to be considered include perforated or penetrating peptic ulcer, acute and even chronic pancreatitis, viral hepatitis, acute appendicitis, haemorrhage from a hepatic adenoma, Curtis–Fitz-Hugh syndrome, lower lobe pneumonia and myocardial infarction.

Intravenous fluids and antibiotics are administered and once the diagnosis has been made most patients are now managed by early cholecystectomy. This is increasingly by the laparascopic technique. The major complications include empyema and mucocoele, ischaemic perforation, ascending cholangitis, acute pancreatitis and septicaemia.

ACUTE PANCREATITIS

This condition is also considered in detail in Chapter 33. It is suspected when patients present with severe upper abdominal pain radiating to the back and shock, although many have less severe symtoms. The presentation may then be with a colicky or continuous upper abdominal pain, vomiting and distension. Many patients are thought to have cholecystitis and the pancreatitis is only diagnosed on finding a raised serum amylase, which remains the best diagnostic test.[287] Perforated peptic ulcer, perforated gall-bladder, mesenteric ischaemia, small bowel volvulus, ruptured aortic aneurysm and myocardial infarction must be carefully excluded. Finding a low serum calcium supports the diagnosis and other enzyme levels may also be assayed.[287]

There are now a number of prognostic indices which have been evaluated and found to be of value in assessing the severity of the attack. Patients with evidence of circulatory, respiratory and renal failure do poorly and detection of pancreatic necrosis and subsequent need for pancreatic necrosectomy can be aided by repeated contrast enhanced CT scanning and serial measurements of the C-reactive protein. Patients should be aggressively resuscitated with intravenous fluids, cardiorespiratory and renal support if necessary. Calcium may be required to prevent tetany.

Laparotomy is occasionally carried out inadvertently when the diagnosis is uncertain, usually when ischaemic bowel is being considered. Endoscopic retrograde cholangiography can be performed early in patients with gallstones and pancreatitis when papillotomy and removal of a stone in the common bile duct can be of value. These issues are discussed in more detail in Chapter 32.

CROHN'S DISEASE

This rarely presents as an acute abdomen, but may on occasions be mistaken for acute appendicitis or an appendix abscess. There is usually a history of some previous colicky abdominal pains and bowel upset. Crohn's disease usually presents with symptoms of chronic subacute obstruction but may occasionally present with an acute small bowel obstruction. Very occasionally it causes a free

REFERENCES

281. Williams R S Br J Surg 1981; 68: 477–480
282. Mackey W C, Dineen P Surg Gynecol Obstet 1983; 156: 56–64
283. Michas C A, Cohen S E, Wolfman E F Am J Surg 1975; 129: 682–685
284. Diamond T, Russell C F J Br J Surg 1985; 72: 480–482
285. Soltero M J, Bill A H Am J Surg 1976; 132: 168–173
286. Leijonmarck C-E, Bonman-Sandelin K et al Br J Surg 1986; 73: 146–149
287. Clavien P A, Burgan S, Moossa A R Br J Surg 1989; 76: 1234–1243

perforation and presents with severe peritonitis. The treatment of the condition is discussed in detail elsewhere (see Chapters 29 and 30), but essentially consists of resecting widening or defunctioning involved segments of bowel.

DIVERTICULITIS

Diverticulitis, pericolic abscess and perforations are the most frequent complications of colonic diverticular disease (see Chapter 30) and increase in frequency with age.[288] They are more frequent when the diverticular disease involves the whole colon. Inflammation can arise in solitary diverticulum of the caecum or the ascending colon. It is then difficult to differentiate from acute appendicitis and the diagnosis may not be made preoperatively.[289]

Diverticulitis is thought to arise when an inspissated faecolith obstructs the neck of a diverticulum. The resultant stagnation of the intraluminal contents is thought to encourage bacterial proliferation. The localized diverticulitis that develops may resolve by discharge of the contents of the sac into the colonic lumen. If this does not occur, inflammation may spread to the pericolic tissues and in particular into the pericolic fat. The ensuing oedema may then obstruct a number of other diverticula, resulting in a greater length of bowel becoming involved in the inflammatory process. It has also been suggested that the initiating event in diverticulitis is a localized perforation of a diverticulum followed by inflammatory reaction in the pericolic fat.[288]

Clinical findings

Inflammation associated with diverticulitis may be localized, or may result in abscess formation, fistula formation, or free perforation with peritonitis. The symptoms associated with diverticulitis have been described as left-sided appendicitis.[290] The pain may initially be crampy and intermittent in the central lower abdomen before becoming continuous and localizing in the left iliac fossa. Sometimes the pain begins and remains in the left iliac fossa. Other symptoms such as anorexia and nausea may be present, but vomiting is relatively uncommon in the early stages. An alteration in bowel habit is frequent with either diarrhoea or constipation predominating. There may also be symptoms of increased urinary frequency and dysuria. A low-grade fever is usually present and on abdominal examination localized tenderness can usually be elicited in the left iliac fossa which is often associated with guarding and rebound tenderness. An ileus may arise later, causing abdominal distension, and there are signs of generalized peritonitis if free perforation occurs. A palpable mass may be present in the left iliac fossa or on rectal examination, making distinction from carcinoma of the colon difficult.

In some cases a previous barium enema may have confirmed the presence of diverticular disease (Fig. 27.38) but in most instances there is no such evidence available. It is then preferable to defer the barium enema until the episode of acute diverticulitis has settled in order to avoid the risk of perforating the bowel during insufflation. Recent evidence suggests that the early use of water-soluble contrast enemas appears to help detect the presence of perforation and may influence subsequent management.[291] CT scanning may also be used to detect any associated periodic or pelvic abscesses.[292]

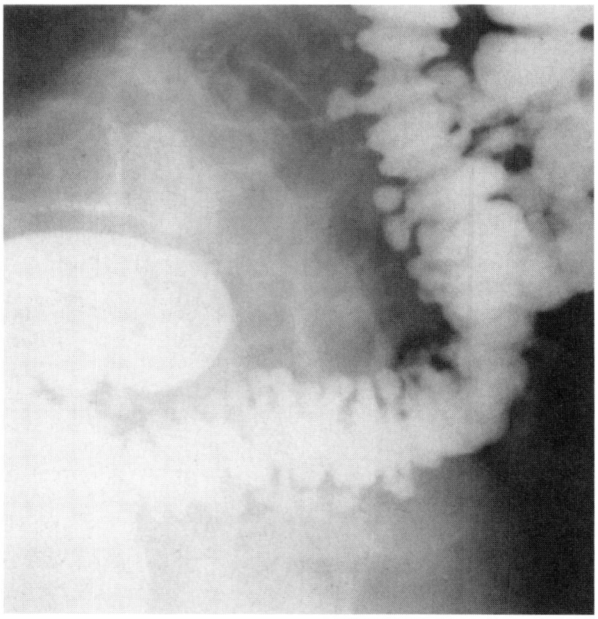

Fig. 27.38 Barium enema showing severe diverticular disease of the sigmoid colon.

Treatment

The initial treatment is usually conservative: patients are given a course of intravenous antibiotics and restricted to a low-residue diet.[293] In most instances this results in gradual resolution of symptoms and signs within 2–3 days. If the pain and signs persist, surgical resection of the affected (usually sigmoid) colon may be necessary, but this is rare in uncomplicated cases (see Chapter 30). Once the acute episode has resolved, a high-fibre diet is recommended in order to keep the stools soft and bulky in an attempt to limit the frequency of further episodes of diverticulitis.

Complications

The major complications associated with acute diverticu-litis are large bowel obstruction, perforation and fistula formation. Colonic obstruction may result from the oedema and inflammation of acute diverticulitis. After resolution of the acute episode subsequent obstruction is usually the result of fibrosis and stenosis. The management of diverticular obstruction is discussed later in this chapter.

REFERENCES

288. Berman L G, Burdick D et al Surg Gynecol Obstet 1968; 127: 481
289. Painter N S Br Med J 1968; 3: 475
290. Bolt D E Ann R Coll Surg Engl 1973; 53:
291. Kourtesis G J, Williams R A, Wilson S E Aust N Z J Surg 1988; 58: 801–804
292. Shrier D, Skucas J, Weiss S Am J Gastrol 1991; 86: 1466–1471
293. Parks T G, Connell A M Br J Surg 1970; 57: 775

When free perforation occurs, it causes the signs and symptoms of generalized peritonitis. This is often the result of a pericolic abscess perforating into the peritoneal cavity rather than a free perforation of the bowel wall causing frank faecal peritonitis, although the latter is not uncommon.

Fistula formation occurs in only a small proportion of patients with diverticulitis and may involve any adjacent organ (Fig. 27.39). Management of colonic fistulae is discussed in Chapter 30.

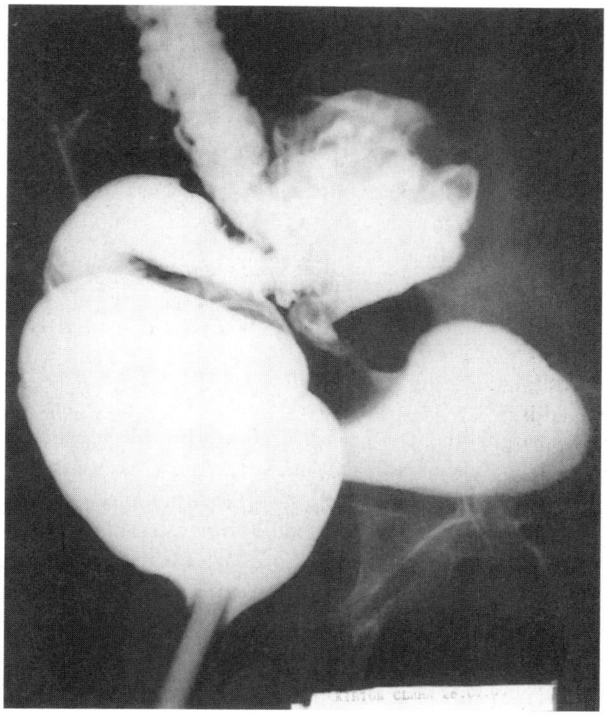

Fig. 27.39 Colovesical fistula from diverticular disease.

Treatment of perforated or obstructed diverticular disease

The options for treating perforated or obstructed diverticular disease include:

1. Excision of the affected segment of colon with a primary anastomosis covered by a transverse colostomy. When the anastomosis has healed, the colostomy can be closed.[294]
2. Hartmann's procedure, consisting of resection of the diseased colon with formation of an end colostomy and closure of the rectal stump, or resection with an end colostomy and mucous fistula. The end colostomy is made in the left iliac fossa.[295]
3. Some surgeons are now prepared to perform resection and primary anastomosis without fashioning a defunctioning stoma when sepsis is minimal. Although an on-table lavage to wash out the proximal bowel is advisable, it is not always essential.

There is now little place for simple closure of the perforation with drainage and defunctioning colostomy, which is associated with a higher morbidity and mortality[296] (see Chapter 30).

PERFORATION OF THE GASTROINESTINAL TRACT

Perforation of the oesophagus, stomach, duodenum, small bowel or colon causes sudden onset of acute abdominal pain. Perforations of the stomach or duodenum are usually the result of a peptic ulcer, though sometimes an ulcerated carcinoma of the stomach may perforate. In the small bowel, perforation may be associated with trauma, foreign bodies,[297] bowel wall infiltration by Crohn's disease,[298] leukaemia or lymphoma and peptic ulceration developing within a patch of ectopic gastric mucosa.[299] A Meckel's diverticulum may perforate, as occasionally may ulceration of the terminal ileum caused by chronic ingestion of potassium chloride tablets.[300] In the colon the commonest cause of perforation is diverticular disease, and less commonly, carcinoma. Typhoid can cause perforations in both the large and small bowel in countries where the disease is endemic,[301,302] as can amoebic and tuberculous infections of the bowel.[303] Radiation damage, Crohn's disease and ischaemia are rarer causes of colonic perforation. Oesophageal perforation may be spontaneous, when it is known as Boerhaave's syndrome, or it may follow surgery or instrumentation.[304]

All perforations cause severe abdominal pain which may commence in the upper or lower abdomen but later becomes generalized. The organ that has perforated may be indicated by the initial site of the pain. Upper abdominal pain is more likely to be the result of a duodenal or gastric perforation whereas lower abdominal pain is indicative of a perforation of the colon. In many cases, however, this differentiation cannot be made.

On examination the patient is febrile, the abdomen is rigid and bowel sounds cannot be heard. Shoulder-tip pain is caused by irritation of the diaphragm. Liver dullness is reduced if air lies between the liver and the abdominal wall. Symptoms and signs are often minimal in elderly sick patients.

An erect chest X-ray is the first-choice investigation to show free intra-abdominal air (Fig. 27.28),[305] but this may not be seen in as many as half the patients.[134] In these circumstances a decubitus abdominal film in the left lateral position can be helpful or alternatively a water-soluble contrast meal can be carried out.[134,306]

The management of perforated peptic ulcers is described in Chapter 28 and perforations of the small and large bowel in Chapters 29 and 30.

REFERENCES

294. Krukowski Z H, Matheson N A Br J Surg 1984; 12: 921
295. Roxburgh R A, Dawson J L, Yeo R Br Med J 1968; 3: 465
296. Botsford T W, Zollinger R M, Hicks R Am J Surg 1971; 121: 70
297. Leader Br Med J 1976; 2: 737
298. Steinberg D, Cooke W T, Alexander Williams J Gut 1973; 14: 865
299. Johns T N P, Wheeler J R, Johns F S Ann Surg 1959; 150: 241
300. Davies D R, Brightmore T Br J Surg 1970; 57: 134
301. Bitar R, Tarpley J Rev Infect Dis 1985; 7: 257
302. Egeelston F C, Verghese M, Handa A K Br J Surg 1978; 65: 748
303. Prakash A, Sharma L K, Pandit P N Br J Surg 1974; 61: 162
304. Trriggiani E, Belsey R Thorax 1977; 32: 241
305. Miller R E, Nelson S W AJR 1971; 112: 574–585
306. Fraser G M, Fraser I D Clin Radiol 1974; 25: 397–402

FOREIGN BODY PERFORATION OF THE INTESTINES

A variety of ingested foreign bodies can produce abdominal pain as the result of perforation at any site in the alimentary tract. These include fish and their bones, pins, needles, toothpicks, broken glass, razor blades, metal fragments and a host of other solid objects.[307] In most instances these foreign bodies pass through the alimentary tract without problems; radiopaque objects are monitored by serial X-ray. Complications can arise, particularly from sharp objects which may perforate the bowel causing peritonitis, or more commonly a localized abscess.

The main symptom is abdominal pain which may start as the colic of bowel obstruction before developing the features of a localized peritonitis. The clinical findings include fever, tenderness and sometimes a palpable mass. Diagnosis is often difficult because of the non-specific nature of the symptoms and signs: a mistaken diagnosis of acute appendicitis is often made. Free gas may be seen beneath the diaphragam. Once the signs of peritonitis are present laparotomy is required to remove the offending object and repair the site of perforation.

PERFORATIONS OF OTHER ORGANS

The appendix, gallbladder and bladder (see Chapters 32 and 39) may also rupture but do not release gas into the peritoneal cavity.

INTESTINAL OBSTRUCTION

Intestinal obstruction is a common and dangerous surgical emergency which, improperly managed, is associated with a high mortality rate. If it is recognized and treated early, the results are usually good.

Small bowel and large bowel obstruction are fundamentally different in both their aetiology and management and will therefore be considered separately. Although differentiation between the two merges in distal small bowel and proximal large bowel obstruction, in general small bowel obstruction presents with colicky abdominal pain and vomiting, whereas in large bowel obstruction distension and absolute constipation tend to be more common.

SMALL BOWEL OBSTRUCTION

Obstruction of the small bowel may be subdivided into mechanical and paralytic. In mechanical obstruction there is a physical occlusion of the bowel lumen preventing the intestinal contents from passing along the intestine. The obstruction may be either partial or complete. Mechanical obstructions can be further subdivided into simple obstruction in which there is obstruction to the passage of intestinal contents alone, and strangulation obstruction, where there is impairment of the blood supply to the obstructed segment of bowel.

In paralytic obstruction the contents are unable to progress because the smooth muscle within the intestinal wall is unable to provide the necessary propulsive force. This is synonymous with neurogenic or functional obstruction of the bowel. It should be emphasized that the distinction between a mechanical and a functional obstruction is not always clear-cut, and the two may coexist in the early postoperative period following a laparotomy. It is, however, important to attempt to make the distinction as the management differs considerably.

Mechanical obstruction

Aetiology

Obstructions of the small bowel comprise approximately 80–85% of all intestinal obstructions.[308] The relative frequency of different causes of small bowel obstruction has changed considerably through the 20th century.[308–310] Earlier in this century strangulated external hernias were responsible for a high proportion of cases, but widespread elective hernia repair has made this complication relatively less common. In contrast, the increasing frequency of abdominal surgery has made adhesions an increasingly important cause of small bowel obstruction. For instance, out of a total of almost 7000 cases of intestinal obstruction of both the small and large bowel between 1925 and 1930, almost half were the result of strangulated hernias, and fewer than 10% were caused by adhesions.[311] In the second half of this century, reports show that adhesions now predominate over strangulated hernia as a cause of small bowel obstruction.[312] Indeed, some reports of small bowel obstruction have found that adhesions account for more than 80% of the cases.[313]

Demographic factors also play a major role, and indeed marked geographic variations in causation can be demonstrated. Even today in less developed communities, strangulated hernias remain the most common cause whilst obstructions caused by adhesions are almost invariably a consequence of pelvic sepsis rather than surgery.[314]

Mechanical obstruction of the small bowell has many different causes. These are usually placed into three categories—luminal, intrinsic, that is, caused by disease in the bowel wall itself, or extrinsic, that is from pressure from without. Some of the causes of small bowel obstruction are listed here:

1. *Luminal*—foreign bodies, faecoliths, gallstones, bezoars, parasites, polypoidal tumours.
2. *Intrinsic*—atresia, inflammatory strictures (tuberculosis, Crohn's disease), tumours.
3. *Extrinsic*—adhesions, hernias, volvulus, intussusception, bands, inflammatory or neoplastic masses.

REFERENCES

307. Editorial Br Med J 1976; 673
308. Ellis H Br Med J 1981; 283: 1202–1204
309. Bevan P G Ann R Coll Surg 1984; 66: 164–169
310. McEntee G, Pender D et al Br J Surg 1984; 74: 976–980
311. Vick R M Br Med J 1933; 2: 546–548
312. Bevan P G Br Med J 1968; 1: 687–690
313. Bizer L S, Liebling R W et al Surgery 1980; 89: 407–413
314. Chiedozi L C, Aboh I O, Piserchia N E Am J Surg 1980; 139: 389–393

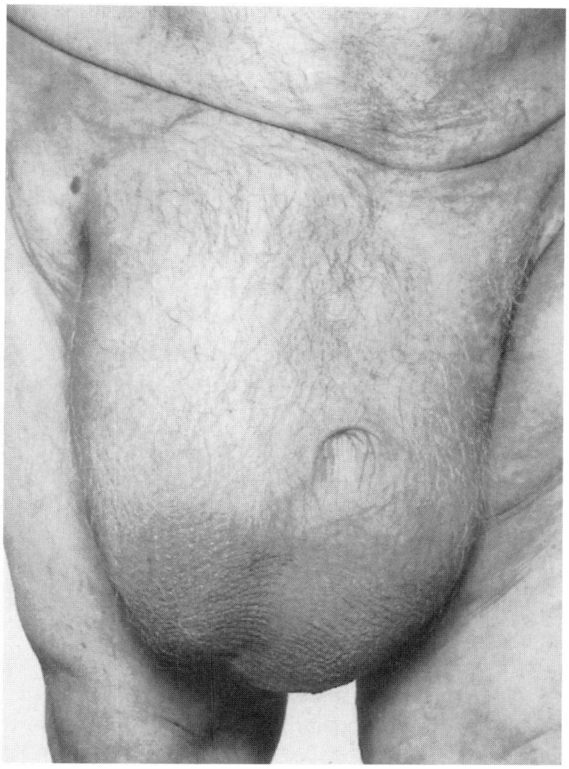

Fig. 27.40 A large incarcerated inguinal hernia causing obstruction.

Table 27.4 Cause of small bowel obstruction

Cause	*Approximate incidence*
Adhesion	60–80%
Strangulated hernia	10–15%
Neoplasm	5–10%
Others	<5%

Table 27.4 shows, however, that adhesions, hernias and intra-abdominal neoplasms account for 95% of all cases of small bowel obstruction and that all the other conditions are relatively rare.

The more important causes of small bowel obstruction are briefly considered below.

Adhesions

These form after most laparotomies. Their cause has been the subject of much speculation. Animal experiments[315] have suggested that they develop in areas of ischaemia. Many adhesions cause no symptoms and they have often been present for many years before becoming a source of symptoms. Those that form after lower abdominal procedures such as appendicectomy or gynaecological operations are most likely to cause trouble.

Irritant materials or particles, such as talcum powder or starch on surgical gloves, can induce a granulomatous reaction and have been shown to cause adhesions.[316] Peritonitis from any cause, whether localized or generalized, can also result in troublesome adhesion formation. There is some recent evidence that a local decrease in the tissue fibrinolytic activity of the bowel wall may encourage adhesion formation,[26] and the incidence of postoperative adhesions may be reduced by instilling tissue plasminogen activator into the peritoneal cavity.[317]

Congenital bands and adhesions are often found in association with malrotation of the bowel, or arising from a Meckel's diverticulum, but are an uncommon cause of obstruction.

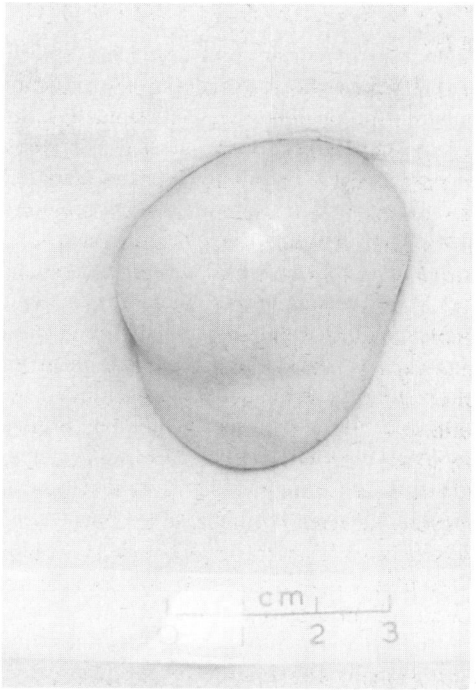

Fig. 27.41 A loop of bowel strangulated within a paraumbilical hernia.

Hernias

Incarceration of an external hernia (inguinal, femoral epigastric, paraumbilical or one of the rarer varieties) is the second most common cause of small bowel obstruction (Figs 27.40 and 27.41; see Chapter 26). This is now less of a problem than it was earlier this century but nevertheless occurs frequently enough to warrant a careful examination of the hernial orifices in all cases of small bowel obstruction. The hernia may have been present for many years or in some instances the patient may be unaware of the defect. This underlines the importance of a thorough groin examination, which may be difficult if the patient is obese. A small femoral or obturator hernia is easily missed (see Chapter 26).

Internal hernias through anatomical defects, such as the foramen of Winslow or the paraduodenal fossae, are rare but must always be considered, and very occasionally the small bowel may be caught in an omental or mesenteric defect.[318,319]

REFERENCES

315. Ellis H Br J Surg 1962; 219: 11–16
316. Jagelman D G, Ellis H Br J Surg 1973; 60: 111–114
317. Dunn R C et al Prog Clin Biol Res 1990; 358: 113
318. Natt P C H Postgrad Med J 1983; 59: 790
319. Fiddian R V Br J Surg 1961; 49: 168

Neoplasms

Extrinsic tumour involvement from secondary spread is much more likely to be responsible for small bowel obstruction than is a primary tumour of the small bowel (see Chapter 29). Small bowel obstruction from metastatic disease arises when loops of small bowel become trapped within a malignant mass. Carcinomas of the ovary, colon, stomach and pancreas are the most common cause of this type of small bowel obstruction.[320]

Primary tumours of the small intestine can cause bowel obstruction either by occluding the lumen or by acting as a nidus for an intussusception. Benign tumours tend not to cause obstructive symptoms unless they intussuscept. Malignant tumours, of which adenocarcinomas, lymphomas and carcinoid tumours are the most common,[321] usually present with a long history of recurrent colicky pain, but they rarely cause an acute obstruction. Obstructing caecal carcinomas arising near the ileocaecal junction may simulate a small bowel obstruction (see Chapter 30).

Foreign bodies and bezoars

Luminal obstruction may arise as a result of the ingestion of foreign bodies, usually by children or psychiatrically disturbed patients. Bezoars usually form in the stomach and may migrate into the small intestine before impacting in the terminal ileum where they can cause an obstruction. They are comprised of human hair (trichobezoar) or undigested vegetable matter or fibre. Obstruction by foreign bodies or bezoars is particularly likely to occur when the bowel is narrowed as a result of previous gastrointestinal surgery.[322] Small bowel obstruction from bezoars arising in intestinal diverticula has also been described.[323]

Other causes

Small bowel obstructions caused by intussusception, volvulus and meconium ileus are discussed separately (see p. 748). Crohn's disease and intestinal atresia are discussed elsewhere (see Chapter 30 and 41).

Pathophysiology

The small intestine may be considered to have two functional components:[312] a proximal part which has a predominantly secretory role, and a distal segment for absorption. Table 27.5 shows the average volume of alimentary juice secreted in 24 hours by a normal 70 kg man. One-fifth of the total body fluid is secreted and reabsorbed through the intestine each day and any interference with this process rapidly causes fluid sequestration in the bowel with effective fluid depletion (see Chapter 2).

Table 27.5 Approximate amounts of alimentary secretions occurring within 24 hours in a 70 kg man

Secretion	*Litre*
Saliva	1.0
Gastric juice	3.0
Bile	1.0
Pancreatic juice	1.0
Intestinal secretions	2.0
Total	8.0

Simple obstruction

The bowel distal to the point of obstruction is emptied by absorption or evacuation of its fluid and gas content and it shrinks as it is no longer kept distended. Peristalsis in this collapsed segment ultimately ceases. This is well-illustrated at laparotomy when the bowel distal to an obstruction is found to be empty, collapsed and quiescent. In contrast, the bowel proximal to the obstruction distends with gas and fluid, which is persistently augmented by the continuous secretion of biliary, pancreatic and gastrointestinal juices.

In the early stages the major source for the intestinal gas is swallowed air which is responsible for approximately 70% of the gas in the distended bowel.[324] The major component of atmospheric air is nitrogen which, unlike oxygen, is poorly absorbed. With time, the amount of oxygen within the bowel steadily falls, and this is associated with a concomitant rise in carbon dioxide. Gas arising from bacterial fermentation becomes increasingly important if the obstruction is not relieved. This process is responsible for the production of other gases such as hydrogen sulphide, ammonia and a variety of other amines.[325] These gases lower the partial pressure of nitrogen within the lumen and, in so doing, establish a gradient for the further diffusion of nitrogen from the congested vessels in the mucosa into the lumen. This provides a third and important source of luminal gas.

Large quantities of isotonic fluid pass into the bowel lumen and, because this fluid is not reabsorbed, it is lost from the extracellular compartment. This loss is augmented by the continual addition of biliary, pancreatic and gastrointestinal juices into the obstructed segment. The colour and nature of the fluid within the lumen of the bowel proximal to the obstruction slowly change. Although initially the fluid contains recognizable food, this is soon replaced by turbid biliary fluid and gradually the colour of the intestinal juice darkens. Eventually, the intestinal contents become brown or even black as a result of the leakage of blood into the intestine and the continued fermentation and digestion by proliferating microorganisms. This is responsible for the faeculant odour of obstructed small bowel content.

Under normal circumstances, a bidirectional flux of salt and water exists but this is disrupted in the presence of an obstruction.[326] The movement of salt and water from the blood to the lumen increases, whilst movement from the lumen to the blood either remains static or decreases. Thus, not only is absorption

REFERENCES

320. Osteen R T, Buyton S et al Surgery 1980; 67: 611
321. Southam T A Ann R Coll Engl 1974; 55: 129–133
322. Moriel E, Anjalon A et al Gastroenterology 1988; 84: 752–755
323. Billings P J, Farrington G H Br J Surg 1987; 74: 1186
324. Wangensteen O H Intestinal Obstruction, 2nd Edition. Thomas, Springfield, Illinois 1947
325. McIver M A 1934 Acute Intestinal Obstruction. Hoeber, New York
326. Shields R Br J Surg 1965; 52: 774–779

halted but fluid moves in the opposite direction, resulting in further losses of water, sodium and potassium from the extracellular space[326] (see Chapter 2).

In response to the loss of salt and water, a number of compensatory changes are set in motion. Salt and water excretion in the urine is reduced, in order to maintain plasma volume. This results in oliguria. Fluid moves from the interstitial space into the intravascular space in an endeavour to preserve plasma volume. The blood pressure is maintained for some time by these changes, although the clinical features of dehydration become apparent at a relatively early stage.

As well as the loss of sodium ions, potassium loss is usually considerable. This eventually causes a large deficit in the total body potassium, but because of shifts in potassium between the extravascular and intravascular compartments, hypokalaemia develops late. Acid–base control also becomes disrupted as bicarbonate ions are retained to compensate for the loss of chloride ions. Vomiting accentuates fluid and electrolyte deficits and causes further problems with acid–base homeostasis. Profound hypovolaemia is an important cause of death in untreated small bowel obstruction.

It is essential to understand these fluid and electrolyte changes in order to achieve optimal resuscitation. As the bowel becomes progressively more distended with gas and fluid, the intraluminal pressure rises and may reach a peak of 75 cm of water during a peristaltic wave. When the sustained intraluminal pressure reaches 10 cm of water, which is common during an obstructive episode in humans, venous drainage from the bowel wall becomes impaired. This in turn causes congestion and oedema of the mucosa, contributing to further intraluminal fluid losses and additional losses from the serosal surface of the bowel into the peritoneal cavity. Peristalsis becomes more vigorous in an endeavour to overcome the resistance imposed by the obstruction and audible peristaltic rushes are heard early in the course of an obstruction. Eventually, however, the smooth muscle becomes fatigued, especially when the bowel has become greatly distended and there is associated hypokalaemia, at which time bowel sounds are no longer heard.

Unobstructed small bowel has low bacterial counts, but microorganisms proliferate rapidly in the stagnant fluid of an obstructed bowel. Indeed this overgrowth of anaerobic bacteria is partially responsible for the faeculant nature of the vomitus and nasogastric aspirate. It has never been shown that the absorption of bacterial toxins from the distended loops of bowel is in any way responsible for the disordered physiology of uncomplicated obstruction, though this unquestionably becomes important once strangulation has occurred.

Strangulation obstruction

Strangulation occurs when there is an impairment of the blood supply to and from the bowel wall. It is the most feared complication in any mechanical obstruction but it is especially common in a closed-loop obstruction (see below). The effects of strangulation are rapidly fatal if left untreated.

If a segment of bowel becomes caught in a rigid and unyielding space, the venous outflow becomes impaired and causes capillary engorgement. This greatly increases the tension within the bowel wall which eventually compromises the arterial inflow to the involved segment of bowel, resulting in arterial occlusion. This in turn causes a haemorrhagic infarct of the bowel wall which is responsible for bleeding into the lumen of the bowel, which may be considerable at times. Bacteria pass through the damaged wall into the peritoneal cavity causing peritonitis. Eventually frank perforation occurs with signs of generalized toxaemia.

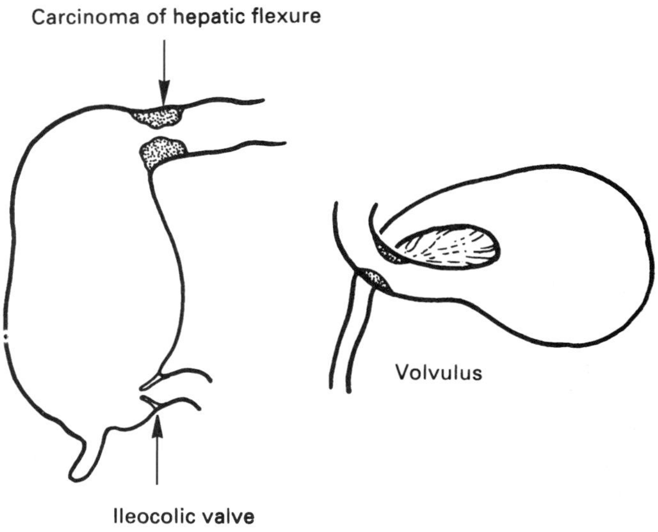

Fig. 27.42 Closed-loop obstruction.

Closed-loop obstruction

A closed-loop obstruction is a form of mechanical obstruction in which a segment of bowel is isolated by closure of both its ends (Fig. 27.42). This may occur as a result of a loop of small bowel becoming trapped in a hernia or twisting about an unyielding band, causing a volvulus. The rapidity of the onset of symptoms and signs depends on the length of the involved segment and the number of organisms present within the lumen. For example, if the intestinal contents are heavily colonized or the length of the affected loop is short, tension rises rapidly and devitalization and rupture swiftly follow.

Clinical features

There are certain clinical features which are common to all patients with mechanical small bowel obstruction and others which vary depending on the cause and nature of the obstruction. Certain signs and symptoms are likely to predominate depending upon the level of the obstruction.

The cardinal features of both large and small bowel obstruction are colicky abdominal pain, vomiting, absolute constipation and abdominal distension.

History

Abdominal pain is usually the first symptom that the patient notices. Two types of pain should be recognized and distinguished.

One is a colicky central pain which is difficult to localize, because it is a visceral pain. This pain tends to occur in waves several minutes apart, rising to a crescendo before subsiding. Between these episodes the patient is usually painfree. The length of the painfree interval gives an indication of the level of obstruction; it is a few minutes in high small bowel obstructions and up to 30 minutes or more in obstruction of the terminal ileum or large bowel. The other type of pain which may occur is a persisting pain, sharper in nature and easier to localize in the area of the distended loop of bowel. It may be associated with localized tenderness on palpation and occurs when the serous coat of the bowel becomes inflamed. When this type of pain develops it should be regarded as a warning of impending strangulation.

Whilst vomiting is usually a feature of bowel obstruction, its contribution to the clinical picture varies according to the level of obstruction. For example, in a high small bowel obstruction it is an early dominant feature, whereas in a low obstruction vomiting may occur much later and it is rarely a major symptom of large bowel obstruction.

It is quite common for the patient to have normal bowel movements in the initial period of obstruction and these may persist for some time if the obstruction is near the duodenojejunal flexure. Eventually, however, if the obstruction is complete and especially if it is low or in the large bowel, absolute constipation, that is the passage of neither flatus nor fluid, ensues. Paradoxically patients with a chronic low-grade obstruction may develop diarrhoea because the proximal bowel is over-stimulated in an effort to overcome the blockage. This results in the persistent passage of fluid faeces through the stenosed segment.

Examination

This must first be directed at establishing the general condition of the patient. At presentation, the patient may show signs of dehydration with a dry furred tongue, sunken dull eyes, a characteristic foetor and decreased tissue turgor—all of which reflect loss of extracellular fluid (see Chapter 2). In cases of simple obstruction the peripheral circulation is maintained until a late stage, when tachycardia, hypotension and cold, clammy extremities indicate the onset of hypovolaemic shock.

The degree of abdominal distension varies according to the level of obstruction. It is minimal in a high small bowel obstruction and becomes more prominent the lower the level of the obstruction. Abdominal distension tends to be mainly central in obstruction of the distal small bowel as the dilated loops lie one above the other in a ladder pattern. This is in contrast to colonic obstruction where distension is mainly in the flanks or in the upper abdomen. Visible peristalsis may be present (see Fig. 27.26) but this is not a reliable sign. Peristalsis may be seen in thin patients in the absence of obstruction.

Tenderness on palpation is not a feature of uncomplicated intestinal obstruction and its presence should alert the examiner to the possibility of impending strangulation. The presence of any abdominal masses suggests a neoplastic or inflammatory process. The hernial orifices, especially in the groins and periumbilical region, should be carefully examined as an unsuspected strangulated hernia is an important cause of small bowel obstruction. The abdomen tends to be especially tympanitic as a result of the over-distended gas-filled loops of bowel. Obstructive bowel sounds are invariably present at some stage but may disappear if the obstruction remains unrelieved or if strangulation develops.

Rectal examination confirms that faeces are present. The characteristic ballooning of the rectum below a large bowel obstruction may also be appreciated. A rectal tumour may be detected and extrarectal masses within the pelvis may also be palpable. A 'frozen' malignant pelvis often causes a shelf of tumour to project into the rectum—the so-called rectal shelf of Blumer.[327]

Investigations

Erect and supine plain abdominal X-rays usually confirm the presence of intestinal obstruction (Fig. 27.43). Gas-distended loops of small intestine with multiple fluid levels are suggestive of mechanical obstruction, although similar appearances can occur with severe peritonitis, mesenteric infarction and paralytic ileus.[328] The level of obstruction can usually be estimated from the supine film. Gaseous distension of the caecum indicates large rather than small bowel obstruction (Fig. 27.44). In a proximal small bowel obstruction the changes may be minimal at an early stage but eventually gaseous distension is seen in the upper left side of the abdomen. In obstructions of the mid small bowel, the valvulae conniventes of the jejunum are evident on plain radiography (the ladder pattern) with distended loops of small bowel tending to take on a horizontal lie. As a rule, the lower the level of the obstruction, the greater the number of distended loops which eventually involve the whole abdomen moving from the upper left side down to the bottom right. The distended ileum often appears cylindrical and free of valvulae conniventes. It is important to remember that the radiographic signs of obstruction are usually minimal or absent in the early stages and many never appear in some cases where the bowel is filled with fluid rather than gas. This is particularly seen in closed-loop obstructions.

There are other features apart from the distribution of bowel gas that may be seen on the abdominal radiographs which may help to make a diagnosis. For example, the presence of an opaque gallstone in the right iliac fossa associated with gas in the bilary tree is diagnostic of a gallstone ileus (see Fig. 27.51). Later radiopaque intraluminal foreign bodies may also be easily recognized.

There has been a trend for radiologists to dispense with the erect abdominal film, relying instead on the degree of gaseous distension seen on the supine film,[126] but subtle differences may be missed and the presence of multiple fluid levels on the erect abdominal radiographs should alert even the most exhausted and inexperienced surgeon in the middle of the night to the presence of serious intra-abdominal pathology.

Patients with a chronic long-standing history of obstructive symptoms should be investigated by a small bowel meal or, better

REFERENCES

327. Blumer G Albany Med Ann 1909; 30: 361
328. Bough M I, Gear M W L 1971 The Plain X-ray in the Diagnosis of the Acute Abdomen. Blackwell, London 1971

a

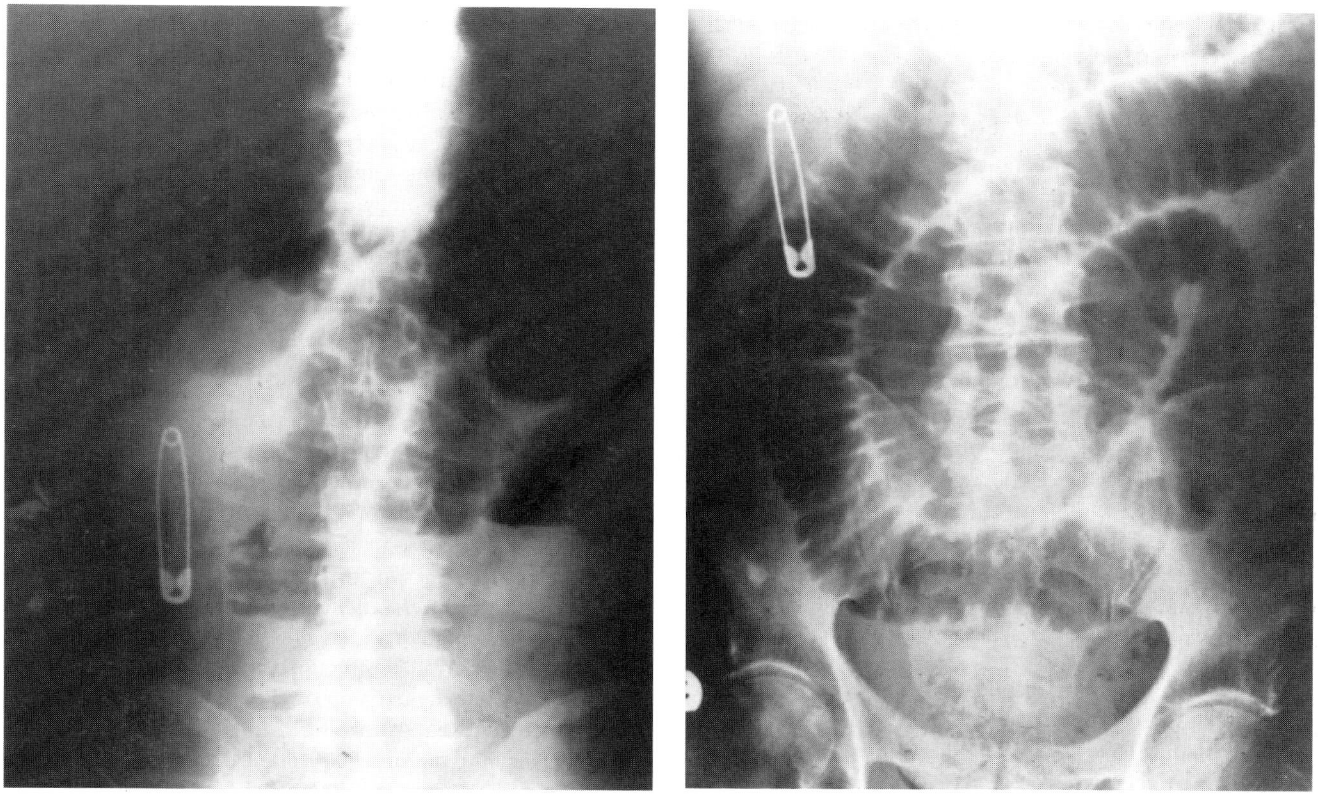

b

Fig. 27.43 (**a**) Erect and (**b**) supine abdominal X-rays showing distended gas-filled loops of bowel with a ladder pattern and multiple fluid levels.

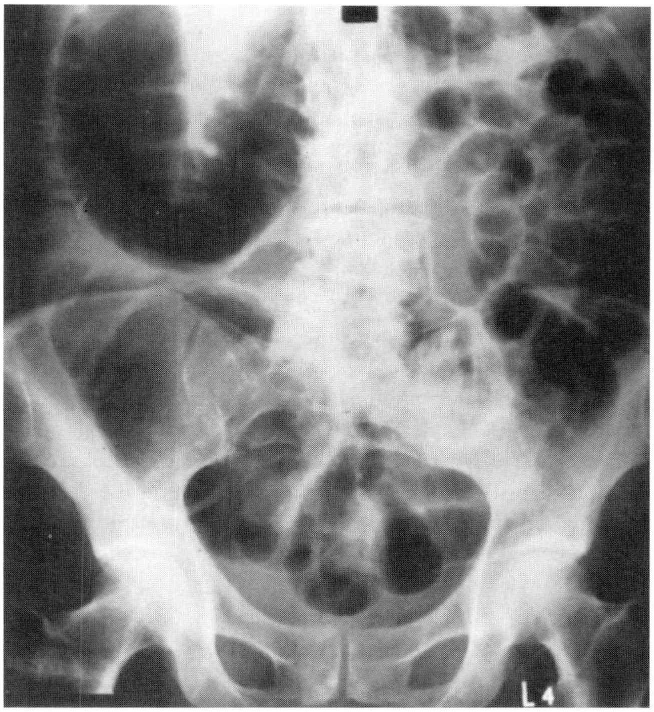

Fig. 27.44 Distension of the caecum in a case of large bowel obstruction.

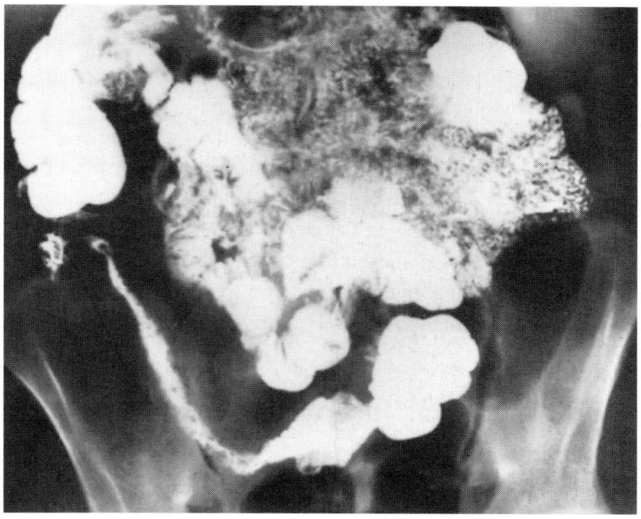

Fig. 27.45 A small bowel meal with Cantor's string sign and a swollen cobblestone mucosa indicating Crohn's disease.

still, a small bowel enema (Fig. 27.45), especially if these are associated with diarrhoea and a diagnosis of Crohn's disease is suspected. These contrast studies are often indicated in patients when the cause of the small bowel obstruction is not apparent, and may for instance reveal a rare primary tumour of the small bowel.

Distinction between simple obstruction and strangulation obstruction

The diagnosis of strangulation is important as it requires urgent surgery. Whilst there are certain clinical features which are suggestive of strangulation, the distinction from simple obstruction is often difficult. Indeed, one report has suggested that as little as 15% of strangulated obstructions are correctly diagnosed at the time of presentation.[329] A similar incidence of pain, vomiting, distension, tachycardia, pyrexia and abdominal tenderness was found in patients with strangulation and those with simple obstruction, though the finding of a mass on abdominal examination is more suggestive of strangulation.[330] It has been suggested that once a diagnosis of a small bowel obstruction has been made, even if there is nothing to suggest strangulation, the best treatment should still be urgent surgery.[308]

An attempt should nevertheless be made to make the distinction between simple and strangulated obstruction. A colicky pain that becomes a continuous or a parietal pain at a localized site is suggestive of strangulation. Evidence of localized tenderness, rebound tenderness and guarding make the diagnosis of strangulation even more likely. The presence of a tender mass which hardens on peristalsis is almost diagnostic. Surgery is long overdue by the time that toxaemia has developed.

Numerous studies have shown that the white cell count on its own is not a particularly helpful predictor of strangulation in patients who present with a mechanical obstruction. For instance, a white cell count in excess of 11 000 mm^3 was observed in 24 of 53 cases of simple obstruction, compared to 31 of 50 cases of strangulation obstruction.[331] However, if one or more of the four classic features of potential strangulation—continuous pain with peritonism, tachycardia, leucocytosis and a fever—are present, then the possibility of strangulation cannot be ignored and laparatomy is indicated.[332]

Plain radiographs showing widening of the spaces between adjacent loops of bowel are a late sign in strangulated obstruction and may also be seen in simple obstruction. Thumb-printing and loss of the mucosal pattern indicate ischaemic damage, whilst gas in the bowel wall and in the mesenteric and portal veins are late and sinister signs of putrefraction. Free intraperitoneal gas of course indicates perforation and is an unequivocal sign of strangulation.

Diagnosis and differential diagnosis

There are four steps that need to be undertaken in the diagnosis of a small bowel obstruction. These are:

1. Deciding whether or not obstruction exists.
2. Differentiating between a mechanical and a neurogenic obstruction.
3. Determining the level of obstruction.
4. Diagnosing the nature of the obstructing lesion.

The presence of all four cardinal signs of intestinal obstruction (colic, vomiting, absolute constipation and distension) usually indicates that a bowel obstruction has occurred. There are however numerous exceptions to this classical presentation. For instance, in low obstructions vomiting may occur late, while distension may be slight in high obstructions, and patients may often evacuate their bowels for some time after the onset of pain. Thus the absence of one or more cardinal features does not in any way preclude the diagnosis of a mechanical obstruction.

It is also important to distinguish obstruction from other acute intra-abdominal pathology. Inflammatory conditions of intraperitoneal organs and perforations of hollow viscera are usually associated with signs of peritonism at an early stage, although ultimately if left untreated peritonitis and ileus develop. This may make differentiation from strangulation obstruction very difficult. Patients with uraemia may also present with vomiting, distension and colicky abdominal pain.

The distinction between a mechanical and a neurogenic obstruction is sometimes also difficult to call. In paralytic ileus, abdominal colic and bowel sounds are usually absent and although the 'ileus' usually occurs in response to a recognizable cause, this is not always the case, as in the early postoperative phase following a laparotomy.

The clinical features vary according to the level of obstruction. Profuse early vomiting, which seldom becomes faeculant, is the dominant symptom in obstruction of the proximal small bowel, while distension is rarely apparent and plain abdominal radiographs often reveal surprisingly little. Although obstructions involving the third or fourth parts of the duodenum are uncommon, they may be associated with high fluid losses—up to 8 l/day—because the upper intestinal secretions are prevented from reaching the segment of bowel responsible for absorption. This type of problem is especially seen in children with duodenal atresia and in patients with advanced carcinoma of the pancreas or upper small bowel.

Colicky periumbilical pain is often the presenting symptom if the obstruction involves the mid small bowel, and vomiting follows after an interval which varies depending on the level of obstruction. Fluid losses occur but not to the same extent as those associated with proximal obstructions. Plain abdominal radiographs show multiple fluid levels and a ladder pattern.

Small bowel obstructions always need to be differentiated from large bowel obstruction, which is described in detail on p. 744. Having diagnosed the presence of small bowel obstruction it is important to ascertain the cause. It may be possible to predict this before operation in many cases but sometimes the exact cause is only discovered at laparotomy. The range of diagnoses can be narrowed down considerably on the basis of the clinical context under which the obstruction has occurred. Certain causes are more common at particular stages of life and the pattern of presentation often gives a clue to the aetiology. Obstructions at birth or in the neonatal period are caused by intestinal atresia, meconium ileus,

REFERENCES

329. Zollinger R M, Kinsey D L Ann Surg 1964; 30: 1–5
330. Shatila A H, Chamberlain B E, Webb W R Am J Surg 1976; 132: 299–303
331. Wolfson P J, Bauer J J et al Arch Surg 1985; 120: 1001–1006
332. Stewardson R H, Bombeck C T, Nyhus L M Ann Surg 1978; 187: 189–193

malrotation or volvulus neonatorum, whilst those presenting in infancy are most likely to be caused by an ileocaecal intussusception or hernia. In early adult life postoperative adhesions are now the most common cause (suggested by the presence of a laparotomy scar), whilst in the elderly, obstructions from strangulated hernia and malignancy must always be considered. When the patient appears to have obstruction and hypovolaemic shock, a diagnosis of mesenteric ischaemia should be suspected, especially if the patient is fibrillating or is known to have atherosclerotic disease in other vessels.

Mechanical small bowel obstruction may also be classified into acute, subacute, chronic and intermittent. Obstructions may be considered to be acute if they develop quickly and progress rapidly to become complete and irreversible. In subacute obstruction the symptoms are milder and the obstruction is often incomplete with some gas or fluid faeces passing distal to the obstruction. Low-grade inflammatory conditions of the small bowel, such as Crohn's disease, produce a chronic obstruction with mild symptoms experienced over many weeks. Paradoxically these patients often complain of intermittent bouts of diarrhoea because of the persistent passage of fluid faeces through the stenosed segment. Intermittent obstruction refers to recurrent acute short-lived bouts of obstruction, almost invariably caused by intraperitoneal adhesions, although this sort of presentation may be the harbinger of widespread malignancy in the elderly.

Treatment

General management

There are four main measures that are deployed in the management of intestinal obstruction—analgesia, nasogastric aspiration, intravenous fluid and electrolyte administration and operative correction. The successful management of patients with bowel obstruction depends on the prompt commencement, efficient conduct and adequate continuation of the first three of these measures and then choosing the correct moment to operate.

Nasogastric suction is begun immediately if a diagnosis of simple obstruction can be confidently made, and the patient's fluid and electrolyte requirements are estimated and replaced. The cornerstone of effective management is close monitoring, regular assessment and re-assessment. This requires the institution of accurate fluid balance charts, close monitoring of vital signs and repeated physical examination and radiological examination when required. A conservative regimen can in theory be continued indefinitely providing strangulation does not supervene, water and salt losses are replenished, the pain settles and the patient is showing clinical and radiological evidence of improvement. In addition to the effects of starvation, there is, however, a danger that strangulation will be overlooked and for this reason some have advocated early laparotomy in all cases.[308] In patients with a complete obstruction of the small intestine operation is usually indicated, especially if, after a period of close observation, the clinical picture is deteriorating.

As it has been demonstrated that as many as half the patients with adhesive small bowel obstruction settle with conservative management,[310] it is reasonable to try this treatment initially in all patients without overt signs of strangulation. Likewise it is usually instituted in the immediate postoperative period, in patients with a history of recurrent bouts of obstruction which have previously settled with conservative measures, and in patients with inflammatory bowel disease. It is unusual for small bowel obstruction to resolve without an operation if it has not done so within the first 24–48 hours of conservative management.

Where there is a history of radiation therapy or there have been numerous previous operations for obstruction, the risks of an operation must be weighed against the potential benefits. The decision on when to operate in these difficult cases demands mature judgement and careful monitoring. Avoiding an operation may sometimes be in the patient's best interests.

Patients dying with extensive intra-abdominal malignancy present a special problem and it is often better not to operate. These patients can usually be treated by analgesia and be made comfortable without nasogastric suction or intravenous infusion. It is important to make the distinction between patients who have had an intra-abdominal malignancy who present with small bowel obstruction, those who have known small bowel obstruction from malignancy and those who are obviously dying from advanced malignancy with associated small bowel obstruction. In the former two conditions surgery may well be beneficial and in one study 17 of 53 patients with small bowel obstruction who had had previous abdominal malignancy were found at laparotomy to have a benign cause for the obstruction.[333]

Nasogastric suction

Gastroduodenal suction following insertion of a nasogastric tube should be commenced immediately the diagnosis is made. This is of benefit as it relieves vomiting, avoids aspiration and reduces the contribution of further swallowed air to the abdominal distension. It also alleviates massive gastric dilation, making operations much easier and reducing the likelihood of vomiting and inhalation during induction of anaesthesia (see Chapter 5).

Ryles single-lumen tubes are less efficient than Salem double-lumen tubes with an air vent. This modification stops the mucosa from being sucked into the side holes, so preventing satisfactory aspiration. Continuous siphoned suction into a dependent reservoir should be supplemented by intermittent aspiration by a bladder syringe carried out at quarter- or half-hourly intervals in the early stages. This regimen may be relaxed if the aspirate reduces.

Some surgeons routinely pass a long intestinal tube. In one report it was shown that up to two-thirds of patients with adhesive small bowel obstruction could be managed by this means alone.[315] Intubation of the small bowel can be exceedingly difficult and is usually unnecessary. It may result in substantial fluid and electrolyte losses which are difficult to correct and this may even delay operative intervention.

REFERENCE

333. Walsh H P J, Schofield P F Br J Surg 1984; 71: 933–934

Fluid and electrolyte replacement

Intravenous cannulation is instituted immediately and intravenous fluids are continued until adequate amounts of fluid can be tolerated by mouth. The requirements for fluid and electrolytic replacement vary considerably depending on the level and duration of the obstruction. Isotonic saline replaces the salt and water losses and potassium must be added to correct a low serum level.

The precise volume and type of fluid and electrolyte replacement vary in each individual, with the amount being calculated from an estimate of the initial deficit, to which is added an amount equivalent to the continuing daily losses over and above the average daily requirements (see Chapter 2). All losses should be replaced in order to re-establish an optimal urine output. Fluid balance charts used in conjunction with the clinical evaluation of the patient's hydration provide the necessary guide to monitor treatment and calculate continuing requirements. A central venous pressure line and even a Swan–Ganz catheter may be of value if there is coexisting renal or cardiac disease.

Operative intervention

Ideally the operation should be timed to coincide with the period when the patient has been adequately resuscitated and the function of the vital organs has been restored. Obviously on occasions this is not possible as the toxic effects of strangulation make early operation necessary. Prophylactic antibiotics must be administered if there is a possibility of strangulation or the need for bowel resection.

The incision should be selected to afford direct access to the expected site of obstruction. For patients who have an incarcerated inguinal or femoral hernia, an appropriate groin incision is required (see Chapter 26). When the cause of the obstruction is not known, an abdominal incision which provides satisfactory access to the whole abdomen is essential. The choice of the incision may be influenced by previous abdominal scars but in general a vertical midline incision is recommended. Once the abdomen is opened, the surgeon passes a hand around the abdomen to try to determine the site and cause of the obstruction. The caecum should be felt first and, if collapsed, the lowest loop of ileum is withdrawn and collapsed bowel is followed upwards loop by loop until the obstruction is reached. When the caecum is distended, the pelvic, descending, transverse and ascending colons are palpated to determine the site of obstruction.

The precise operative procedure varies according to the cause of the obstruction. Adhesions or bands need to be carefully divided, because the morbidity and mortality are increased considerably if bowel is inadvertently opened. Obstructing tumours should ideally be resected but occasionally if this is not possible a bypass procedure is an acceptable alternative. Obstructing foreign bodies or gallstones can usually be milked back up the bowel and removed with ease through a transverse proximally placed enterotomy made in healthy bowel.

The surgeon must decide whether or not a strangulated loop of bowel is viable once the obstruction has been relieved. This assessment is not always easy. It may be helpful to wrap the loop of affected bowel in a warm saline-soaked pack and leave it undisturbed for several minutes. The pack is then removed and the bowel once again inspected for colour, mesenteric pulsation and peristalsis.[334] The bowel is considered viable when the sheen remains on the serosal surface, when the colour returns, when the affected segment transmits peristalsis and when there is demonstrable pulsation in the mesenteric vessels. Conversely the bowel is felt to be not viable if its sheen is lost, it has become purple, dark green or black in colour, it emits a detectable odour, it fails to conduct peristalsis or if the vessels in the mesentery have become thrombosed.

Another method which may occasionally be helpful in determining whether or not a loop of bowel is viable involves the injection of 1000 mg of fluorescein into a peripheral vein over a few minutes. The bowel is then inspected under an ultraviolet light.[335,336] A viable bowel with an adequate blood supply fluoresces, while a dead bowel does not. Special attention must be paid to any constriction rings where the bowel has often been tightly compressed. An overtly gangrenous segment of bowel obviously needs to be resected and if any doubt exists, it is best to err on the side of resection.

When the obstruction has been relieved a number of massively dilated loops of small bowel may make abdominal closure extremely difficult. It is often advisable to decompress these loops before closure is attempted. There are several methods by which this may be accomplished.[337] The best and safest procedure is to milk the small bowel contents back into the stomach where they can be aspirated via a large-bore nasogastric tube—the Monks–Moynihan procedure. Alternatively the gastrointestinal contents may be aspirated through a long gastrointestinal tube threaded down from above. Introduction of a suction catheter via a well-placed enterotomy surrounded by a pursestring suture affords rapid decompression but at the expense of possible contamination and a subsequent suture line, which usually has to be closed through distended and oedematous bowel.

Lysis of adhesions may be ill-advised when removal of the obstruction is impossible or hazardous, or in patients with severe radiation damage or carcinomatosis causing a frozen abdomen or pelvis. Anastomosis of a distended proximal loop of bowel to a collapsed distal loop of bowel may afford the safest option.

Prognosis

Despite improvements in fluid and electrolyte replacement, the conduct of general anaesthesia and postoperative intensive care, the mortality of acute uncomplicated small bowel obstruction may still be as high as 10%.[334] The mortality of strangulated obstruction is much greater.

REFERENCES

334. Ellis H Intestinal Obstruction. Appleton-Century Crofts, New York 1981
335. Buckley G B, Zuiderma C D et al Ann Surg 1981; 193: 628
336. Mann A, Fazio V W, Lucas F V Surg Gynecol Obstet 1982; 154: 53
337. Singleton A O, Montalbo P Ann Surg 1986; 167: 909

Recurrent small bowel obstruction

One group of patients that may pose particular difficulties with management are those that develop recurrent bouts of small bowel obstruction from adhesions. Where possible, surgery should be avoided in these patients as the capacity to reform adhesions is augmented by each new laparotomy.

Attempts to return the small bowel to the peritoneal cavity in a regular orderly fashion in the hope that new adhesions will fix the bowel and prevent recurrence is almost always unsuccessful. In order to fix the bowel while new adhesions develop, a method of complete small intestinal intubation by means of a Baker tube has been described.[338] This involves the introduction of a long tube via a gastrotomy which remains in place for 5–10 days following laparotomy, during which time it acts as an intraluminal stent. Plication of loops of the small intestine, as described by Noble[339] to prevent recurrent adhesive obstruction, has been shown to be of little benefit.[340]

Neurogenic obstruction (paralytic ileus)

Neurogenic obstruction or paralytic ileus occurs when intestinal peristalsis ceases, resulting in a functional obstruction of the bowel. As a consequence the bowel dilates and the patient develops features of intestinal obstruction.[341]

Aetiology

After laparotomy there is almost invariably a period of paralytic ileus. The stomach remains inactive for varying periods, though peristaltic activity in the small intestine often resumes within a few hours.[342] The return of bowel sounds following an operation is therefore often a poor indicator of the return of bowel motility.

The resumption of peristalsis is occasionally abnormally prolonged and when this occurs after a laparotomy the patient is said to have a paralytic ileus. Intraperitoneal sepsis, major abdominal trauma, retroperitoneal haemorrhage, fractures involving the spine and poor renal function are all factors that are recognized to predispose to a paralytic ileus.[343]

Pathogenesis

Sympathetic overactivity is thought to cause the paralytic ileus. The evidence for this is based largely on experimental work where it has been shown that paralytic ileus following manipulation of the bowel or peritonitis can be prevented by a total abdominal sympathectomy.[344] The small bowel undergoes massive distension along its length and at the same time salt and water are lost from the extracellular compartment as absorption of fluid from the lumen is impaired.

Clinical features

There is usually a recent history of an operation or another of the recognized precipitating causes. On the second or third postoperative day effortless vomiting occurs which is associated with abdominal distension. The patient does not complain of intestinal colic. There is silence on auscultation of the abdomen and neither flatus nor faeces are passed.

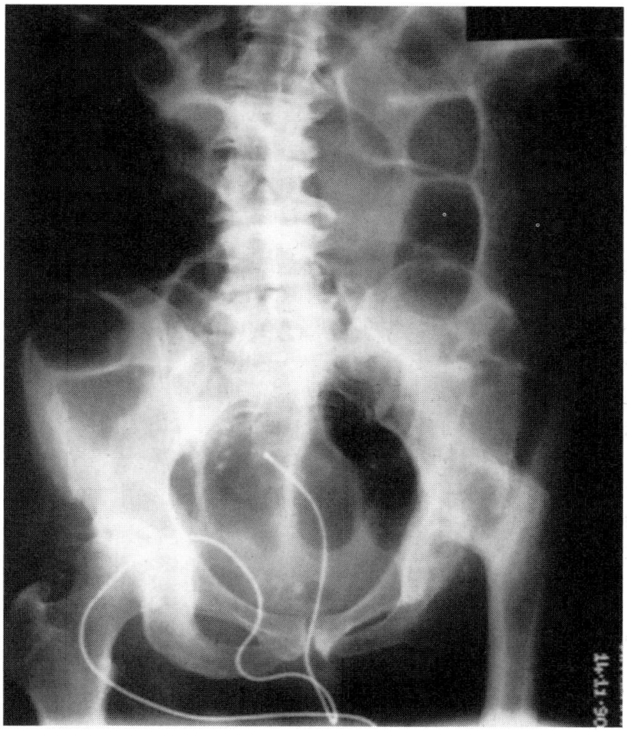

Fig. 27.46 A plain X-ray of a patient with pseudo-obstruction. There is generalized dilation of small and large bowel. A rectal thermometer indicates the patient is being monitored in the intensive care unit.

A plain abdominal X-ray confirms gas-distended loops of small intestine containing multiple fluid levels (Fig. 27.46). The colon is also often distended and contains multiple fluid levels, although it may be empty and collapsed.

Differential diagnosis

It is important to differentiate a paralytic ileus from a mechanical obstruction which tends to occur later in the postoperative phase and is usually associated with colicky abdominal pain and obstructive bowel sounds. Prograde contrast studies can be useful in the differentiation, not only of paralytic ileus from mechanical obstruction,[345] but also in recognizing mechanical obstruction which might settle from that which may not.[346] A postoperative

REFERENCES

338. Munro A, Jones P F Br J Surg 1978; 65: 123–127
339. Noble T B Am J Surg 1937; 35: 41–44
340. Bevan P G Br J Hosp Med 1982; 1: 258
341. Ogilvie W H Br Med J 1948; 2: 761–763
342. Catchpole B N Surgery 1969; 66: 811–820
343. Sykeb P A, Scholfield P F Br J Surg 1974; 61: 594
344. Nealy J, Catchpole B N Br J Surg 1971; 58: 21–28
345. Matheson N A, Dudley H A F Lancet 1963; i: 914–917
346. Riveron F A, Obeid F N, Horst H M, Sorensen V J, Bivins B A Surgery 1989; 106: 496–501

paralytic ileus must also be differentiated from a patient who has generalized peritonitis from a dehisced anastomosis causing a secondary ileus. This differential may be difficult to make and must always be considered in a patient developing an ileus 7–10 days after a bowel anastomosis.

Prophylaxis

Postoperative ileus can be limited by adhering to some simple rules of technique. Unnecessary exposure and handling of the intestine should be avoided. The practice of removing the small bowel from the peritoneal cavity and suspending it on its mesentery makes the bowel oedematous and congested, prolonging the duration of any postoperative ileus.

Treatment

Nasogastric suction and intravenous fluid replacement are required once a paralytic ileus has become established. The volume of replacement is based on the patient's needs, though particular attention should be paid to the serum potassium level which often tends to be low. Failure to correct this may perpetuate the condition.

Pharmacological agents have been used to try and counteract the sympathetic overstimulation that is thought to be responsible for the 'ileus'.[347] Good results have been obtained by blocking the sympathetic-derived inhibition with α-sympathetic blockers such as guanethidine, and then producing direct stimulation of the smooth muscle with parasympathomimetic agents. This nevertheless needs to be performed with caution, as it is contraindicated in the presence of a mechanical obstruction, which may be difficult to exclude. The drugs that are administered are known to possess significant cardiovascular side-effects. Cisapride is a more recent drug that has been shown to stimulate peristalsis in the postoperative period.[348]

LARGE BOWEL OBSTRUCTION

Mechanical obstruction

Aetiology

In western societies the most common cause of a mechanical large bowel obstruction is an adenocarcinoma of the colon. Indeed, this cause of colonic obstruction so far exceeds other causes that it should always be excluded before other conditions are even considered. Chronic diverticulitis and sigmoid volvulus are the other main causes of large bowel obstruction (Table 27.6). There are a host of rarer conditions which can cause large bowel obstruction and these include colonic intussusception, radiation and inflammatory strictures, external hernia and ischaemic strictures. It is exceedingly rare for adhesions to cause colonic obstruction.

In parts of Eastern Europe, Central Africa and Asia, volvulus of the sigmoid colon is the most common cause of colonic obstruction.[349] Conversely carcinoma of the colon is much less common in these countries and diverticulitis as a cause of colonic obstruction is virtually unknown.

Table 27.6 Causes of colonic obstruction in adults

Causes	*Approximate incidence*
Carcinoma of the colon	65%
Diverticulitis	10%
Volvulus	5%
Miscellaneous (including pesudo-obstruction)	20%

Pathophysiology

The pathophysiology of large bowel obstruction is influenced by the competency of the ileocaecal valve. In 10–20% of patients with large bowel obstruction it becomes incompetent,[350] colonic pressure being relieved by reflux of the colonic contents into the ileum. This results in distension of both the colon and the small intestine. When the ileocaecal valve remains competent and the colon is not decompressed, a closed loop is formed between the valve and the obstructing point (see Fig. 27.42). This in turn results in progressive colonic distension as the ileum continues to empty gas and fluid into the obstructed segment. Under these circumstances, intraluminal pressures may reach very high levels, impairing the circulation to the bowel wall, resulting in gangrene and perforation.

Although the sigmoid colon is the most common site of colon cancer, a large review of malignant bowel obstruction found that tumours of the splenic flexure were in fact more likely to obstruct the colon.[351]

Perforation of the colon occurs if a closed-loop obstruction is left unrelieved. As the wall of the right colon is thinner than that of the left and its luminal calibre is greater, this is the most common site of perforation. When the intraluminal pressure rises, distension and wall tension are maximal in the distended caecum, in accordance with the Laplace's law. Once a caecal diameter of 15 cm has been reached the threat of ischaemic necrosis and perforation is so great that surgery must not be delayed.[352]

Clinical features

Colonic obstruction often develops insidiously, in contrast to the presentation of small bowel obstruction. The colicky abdominal pain associated with colonic obstruction is usually not as severe as that of small bowel obstruction. The visceral pain is usually situated in the hypogastric region of the lower abdomen. The onset of sharp continuous severe pain is indicative of ischaemia or imminent perforation and is therefore an important symptom.

Faeculent vomiting, if it occurs, is also a very late symptom. It is only seen when the ileocaecal valve is incompetent and the features of a small bowel obstruction are added to those of colonic obstruction. Constipation is a consistent feature of complete

REFERENCES

347. Douglas D M, Mann F C Br Med J 1941; 1: 227–231
348. Verlinden M, Michiels G et al Br J Surg 1987; 74: 614
349. Rennie J A J R Soc Med 1979; 72: 654
350. Phillips S F, Quieley E M M, Kumar D Gut 1988; 29: 390
351. Phillips R K S, Hittinger R et al Br J Surg 1985; 72: 396–302
352. Addison N V J R Soc Med 1983; 76: 252

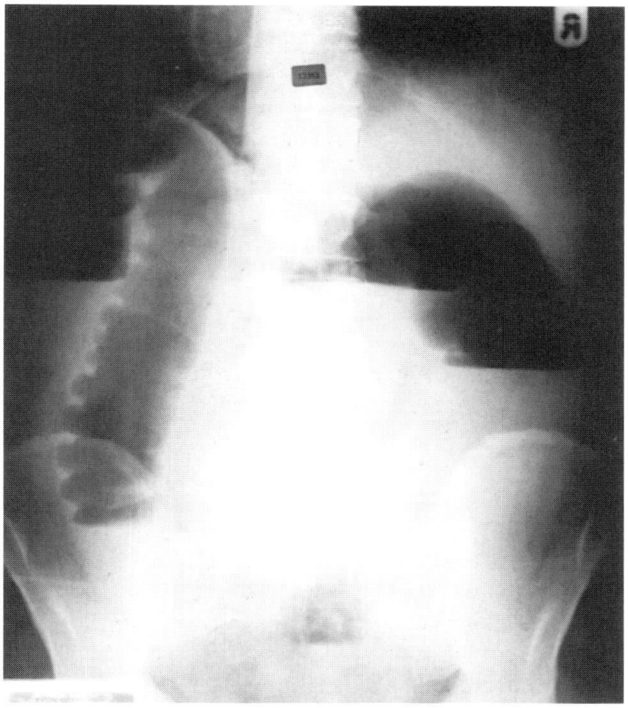

Fig. 27.47 Haustral markings in a case of large bowel obstruction.

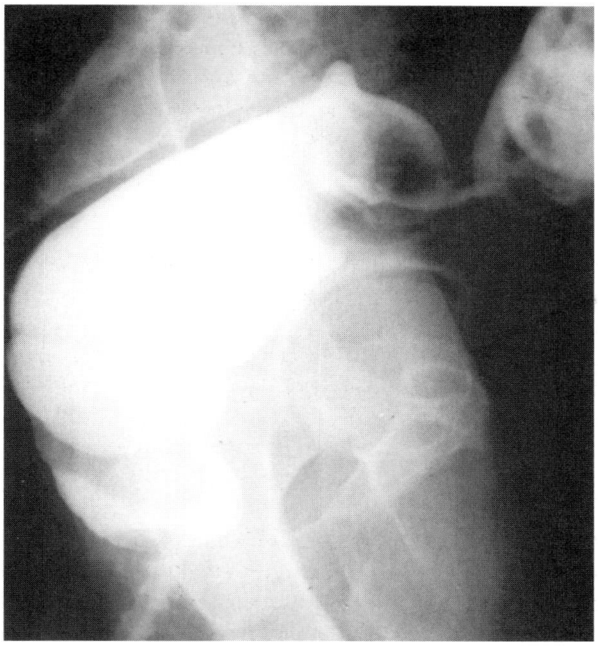

Fig. 27.48 Tumour causing large bowel obstruction.

colonic obstruction, although the rectum may be emptied in the early stages.

Abdominal distension tends to dominate the clinical picture. This is maximal in the flanks, although this is often difficult to appreciate. The abdomen rapidly becomes tympanitic, and amphoteric bowel sounds associated with rushes and gurgles may be heard.

Evidence of localized or generalized peritonitis indicates that gangrene or rupture of the bowel is imminent or has more than likely occurred. Particular attention must be paid to tenderness in the right iliac fossa as the caecum is the most likely part of the colon to rupture, and it often becomes tender when the mucosa is still intact but the serosa has started to split.

Sigmoidoscopic and rectal examinations are essential in all cases of colonic obstruction as the obstructing lesion may be palpated as seen.

Investigations

Radiological examination

Plain abdominal X-rays are often diagnostic. Typically the distended colon creates a 'picture-frame' outline of the abdominal cavity. The colon can be distinguished from the small bowel by its haustral markings which do not traverse the entire diameter of the lumen (Fig. 27.47). The specific findings associated with volvulus are discussed on p. 749. The bowel below the level of the obstruction is collapsed and the rectum does not contain gas. Occasionally only the small bowel is distended if there is an obstructing tumour of the caecum and ascending colon with an incompetent ileocaecal valve.

Any patient in whom colonic obstruction is suspected on clinical and radiological grounds must undergo a barium or water-soluble contrast enema to distinguish between a mechanical cause and pseudo-obstruction.[135,136] A contrast study is also able to identify the site and may be able to diagnose the nature of the pathology (Figs 27.48–27.50). The use of water-soluble contrast medium is favoured by some because if a perforation has occurred, barium is more irritant to the peritoneum. Also in an emergency setting the only important information required is whether or not there is a complete obstruction. Others dispute this and feel that barium gives better definition, even in an unprepared bowel. Further investigations like colonoscopy can always be undertaken at a later date if required once complete obstruction has been ruled out.

Diagnosis and differential diagnosis

There are two important alternative diagnoses that need to be considered. First colonic obstruction needs to be distinguished from a small bowel obstruction. This distinction may be difficult, as obstructing lesions of the right colon may produce radiological changes that are identical to those seen in low small bowel obstruction. The presentation of a small bowel obstruction in an elderly patient in whom there has been no prior history of surgery should always alert the clinician to the possibility of malignancy in the right colon.

Second, as mentioned above, a mechanical colonic obstruction needs to be differentiated from pseudo-obstruction, a condition in which massive colonic distension occurs in the absence of a physical obstruction. This condition often occurs in bed-ridden patients with serious intercurrent illnesses. Although the plain abdominal X-ray often reveals colonic distension, a contrast enema disproves any evidence of a mechanical obstruction.

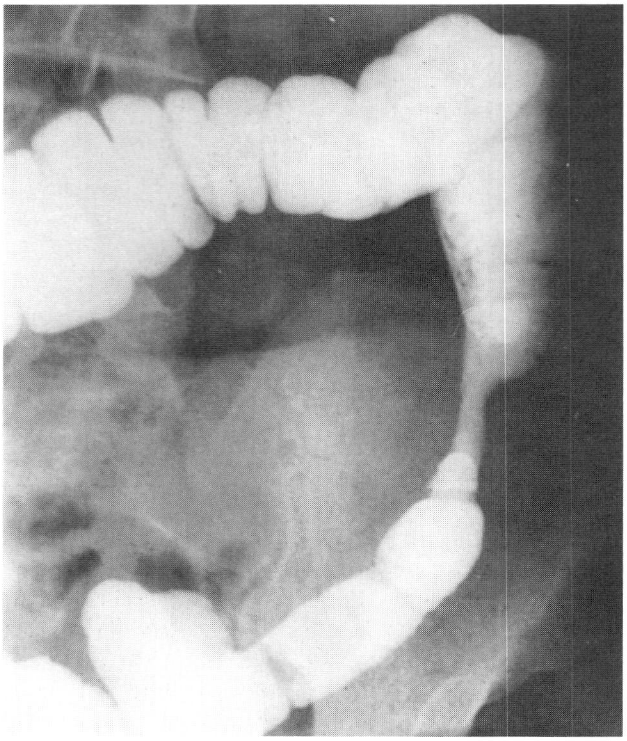

Fig. 27.49 An ischaemic stricture of the large bowel.

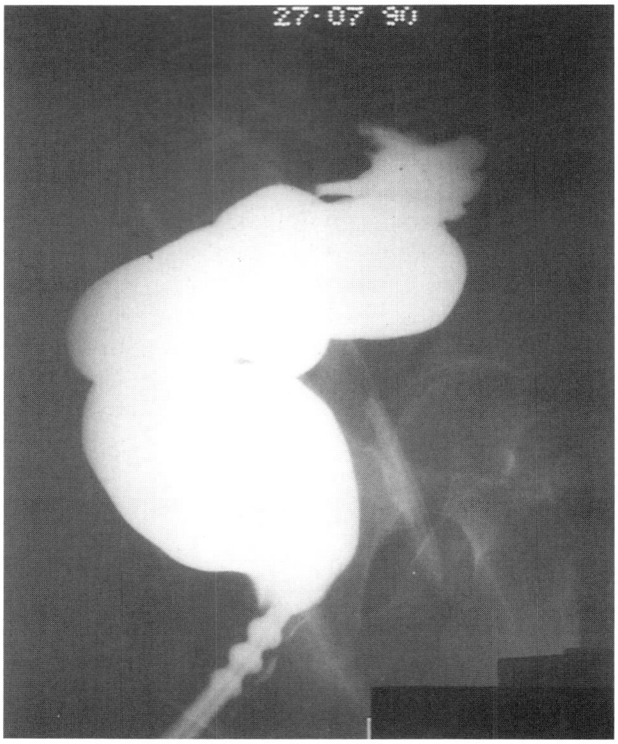

Fig. 27.50 Diverticular disease causing large bowel obstruction.

Treatment

The first aim in the management of colonic obstruction is to decompress the obstructed segment in order to prevent perforation. In mechanical obstruction this almost always requires an operation. The second aim is to remove the obstructing lesion and restore the continuity of the large bowel if possible.

Right-sided lesions

For tumours or other obstructing lesions of the right colon a one-stage right hemicolectomy with an ileotransverse anastomosis usually achieves both objectives as long as the patient is fit enough to withstand the procedure and the obstructing lesion is resectable. The obstruction can still be relieved by bypassing the obstruction with an ileotransverse anastomosis, even if it is not possible to resect the tumour in advanced cases. In the presence of perforation and gross contamination an anastomosis is not advisable. The obstructing lesion should then, if possible, be resected and the proximal bowel brought on to the surface as an end ileostomy. The continuity of the bowel can then be restored at a future date when the patient has fully recovered.

Left-sided lesions

The management of obstructing lesions of the left colon is more controversial. There are three main approaches:

1. The three-stage approach, where a defunctioning colostomy is performed, followed by resection and anastomosis and finally closure of colostomy.[353]
2. Resection of the tumour with a temporary end colostomy.[354] A second operation is then required a few months later for colorectal re-anastomosis.
3. Resection with primary anastomosis—this is becoming increasing popular.

A staged approach does allow time for meticulous preparation of the bowel so that definitive resection of the obstructing lesion and primary anastomosis can be performed under optimal conditions. Bowel decompression by transverse colostomy can be performed by inexperienced surgeons in the middle of the night and is less hazardous for the ill patient as major colonic resection of an obstructed bowel requires considerable expertise. The resection and closure of the colostomy can then be performed at leisure.

Proponents of a one-stage approach argue that the combined overall mortality rate of a staged approach is in fact greater than that of a single procedure.[355] This challenges the view that resection and primary anastomosis in the presence of an obstructed and unprepared bowel are associated with increased risk of anastomotic dehiscence. This argument is supported by evidence that faecal loading in an ill-prepared bowel does not appear to increase the risk of anastomotic dehiscence.[356] In the sick patient with a grossly distended and oedematous bowel the surgeon must take no

REFERENCES

353. Goligher J C, Smiddy F G Br J Surg 1957; 45: 270–274
354. Huddy S P J, Shorthouse A J, Marks C G Ann R Coll Surg 1988; 70: 40–43
355. Mealy K, Salman A, Arthur G Br J Surg 1988; 75: 1216–1219
356. Irving A D, Scrimgeour D Br J Surg 1987; 74: 580–581

risks. Intraoperative colonic lavage allows the anastomosis to be performed under the best possible conditions and has now become widely adopted.[357] Only in carefully selected patients is it advisable to perform a left-sided colonic anastomosis in ill-prepared bowel.

A number of surgeons have suggested that left-sided obstruction should be treated by a subtotal colectomy with ileorectal anastomosis.[358] This avoids many of the problems described above and can even be performed in the elderly with acceptable functional results, although the number of bowel actions is usually increased to three or more per day for the rest of their lives.[359] Because of the risks of postoperative diarrhoea, this procedure should probably be reserved for tumours in the transverse and descending colon only.

Thus the choice of operative management in patients with obstruction of the left colon is not straightforward. There are advantages and disadvantages of each approach and each case of left-sided colonic obstruction requires careful assessment and a management tailored to the specific circumstances of each patient.

Prognosis

The mortality of colonic obstruction is still about 30%[360] and this increases significantly if the caecum has perforated. The prognosis is worse in elderly patients, especially if they are in poor general health.

Pseudo-obstruction

This is a term applied to a condition which presents as colonic obstruction, but in which a mechanical cause cannot be found.[361] In 1948 Ogilvie suggested a cause for this functional problem, when he described it in 2 patients with malignant retroperitoneal infiltration of their coeliac plexus.[341] In some parts of the world it is still just called Ogilvie's syndrome.

Aetiology

A long list of conditions have been reported to be possible causes of pseudo-obstruction, though a substantial number of cases occur spontaneously and are classified as idiopathic.[362] Recognized causes are given in Table 27.7.

Table 27.7 Causes of pseudo-obstruction[363]

Idiopathic
Systemic disease
Cardiac disease
Renal disease and uraemia
Hypovolaemia
Hypoxia
Liver disease
Acute stress (e.g. burns)
Lead poisoning
Electrolyte abnormalities
Puerperium
Myxoedema
Drugs
Local disease
Retroperitoneal injuries and tumours
Pelvic injuries and surgery
Intra-abdominal sepsis
Infiltration of intrinsic plexus of bowel wall (e.g. amyloidosis, scleroderma, radiation and strongyloidiasis)

Pathophysiology

In the presence of such a diversity of causes the clinical picture of pseudo-obstruction may often simply be a manifestation of multiple adverse stimuli. The mechanism by which these disorders cause atonia of the large bowel appears to be linked with an imbalance in the parasympathetic and sympathetic innervation resulting in sympathetic reflex inhibition of colonic motility.[363]

Clinical features

The patient is often elderly and frequently bed-ridden. The abdomen gradually distends and bowel actions cease, though bowel sounds may still be heard and may even sound obstructive. The abdomen is tympanitic but is not tender and the clinical picture strongly resembles that of a mechanical colonic obstruction, usually without pain.[364]

Abdominal radiographs do not differentiate the condition from a mechanical obstruction, although they usually show that the colon is distended with gas with few or no fluid levels. Cut-off points may be noted and these may be seen to progress distally on serial X-rays. Gas is often present in the rectum.

Once it has been considered, the diagnosis can often be made in the context of its clinical setting. There is usually ample time to exclude a mechanical obstruction by a water-soluble enema[135,136] or by colonoscopy.[365]

Management

The management in most instances is expectant as pseudo-obstruction is usually a self-limiting condition. Any associated metabolic disorder needs to be corrected, once the diagnosis has been confirmed. This entails correction of fluid and electrolyte abnormalities, adequate oxygenation and nutritional support. It is not necessary to pass a nasogastric tube and cautious oral fluid may be continued.

In the early phases decompression is often successfully accomplished by passage of a sigmoidoscope and flatus tube. Colonoscopic decompression has also been described as a means of not only investigating but also treating this condition.[365]

REFERENCES

357. Dudley H A, Radcliffe A G, McGrechan D Br J Surg 1980; 67: 80–81
358. Deutsch A A, Zelikowski A et al Dis Colon Rectum 1983; 26: 227
359. Klatt G R, Martin W H, Cillespie J T Am J Surg 1981; 141: 577–578
360. Phillips R K S, Hittinger R et al Br J Surg 1985; 72: 296
361. Dudley H A, Sinclair I S et al J R Coll Surg Edinb 1958; 3: 206–217
362. Bullock P R, Thomas W E G Ann R Coll Surg 1984; 66: 327–330
363. Paterson-Brown S, Dudley H A F In: Williamson R C N, Cooper M J (eds) Emergency Abdominal Surgery. Churchill Livingstone, Edinburgh 1990 pp. 182–190
364. Dudley H A, Paterson-Brown S Br Med J 1986; 292: 1157–1158
365. Kukora J S, Dent L Arch Surg 1977; 112: 512–517

Caecal tenderness should be examined for at regular intervals as it is still possible for even a functionally obstructed colon to dilate to the point of caecal rupture.[364] A laparotomy may still be required to decompress a grossly distended caecum, especially if there is right iliac fossa tenderness and adequate decompression cannot be achieved by a flatus tube or by colonoscopy. The procedure of choice is caecal exteriorization and decompression, even when the caecum has become gangrenous or a pinhole perforation has occurred.[364] Occasionally resection may be required in advanced cases. Tube caecostomy is dangerous and is not recommended.[366]

Special causes of intestinal obstruction

There are several causes of bowel obstruction where the clinical features and management are so different from the general principles outlined above that they warrant separate discussion.

Meconium ileus

Meconium ileus, first described by Landsteiner in 1905,[367] is a condition in which the distal small bowel or colon becomes obstructed in the neonatal period as a result of inspissated intestinal contents. This condition occurs in children with the inherited metabolic disorder of cystic fibrosis or mucoviscidosis. Disordered intestinal secretion, including a lack of pancreatic juice, results in the formation of obstructing firm putty-like sticky meconium.

The clinical features and management in childhood are described in Chapter 41. A similar condition, known as 'meconium ileus equivalent', is now seen in teenagers and young adults who have survived childhood with cystic fibrosis. The lack of digestive enzymes reaching the intestine combined with reduced mucus secretion results in indigestible cellulose plugs obstructing the terminal ileum and causing bolus obstruction. These may have to be removed at open operation by milking them on into the large bowel or by extracting them through one or more transverse enterotomies.

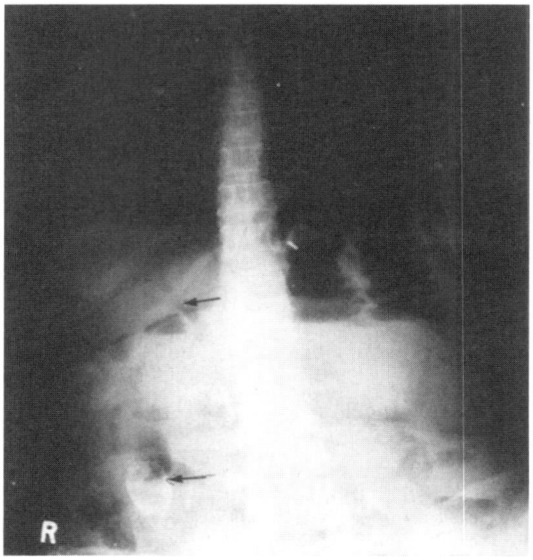

Fig. 27.51 Gallstone ileus.

Malrotation

Maltrotation of the intestine is an important cause of intestinal obstruction in infancy. Its pathophysiology, clinical features and management are discussed in Chapter 41.

Gallstone ileus

Gallstones are responsible for fewer than 1% of all cases of small bowel obstruction.[368] About 90% of gallstones entering the intestine lodge in the terminal ileum, though impaction at other sites, including the jejunum, duodenum, colon and rectum, has been described. The stone originates in the gallbladder and passes into the intestine through a biliary–enteric fistula, usually between the gallbladder and duodenum.

Clinical features

The patients are almost invariably elderly. They may have a history of chronic cholecystitis, but this is often not the case. Patients usually present with symptoms of acute intestinal obstruction which are sometimes preceded by recurrent attacks of subacute obstruction.

Investigations

The radiological appearances are those of an intestinal obstruction, and in addition a gallstone may be visible in an unusual location. A fistula is usually present if the bile ducts or gallbladder are outlined by gas (Fig. 27.51) and the diagnosis of gallstone ileus can then be made preoperatively. Gas in the biliary tree may follow a biliary–intestinal bypass or sphincterotomy and is rarely the result of gas-forming organisms multiplying within the biliary tract.

Treatment

An operation is required to relieve the bowel obstruction. The stone should be milked upwards into the healthy bowel to avoid opening the bowel at the point where the stone has impacted as this area heals poorly. The cholecystoenteric fistula is always encased in scar tissue and it is best left alone. The risk of further stones impacting is low and the potential dangers of unpicking the cholecystoenteric fistula and causing peritonitis from a duodenal or binary leak is considerable. Stones that have already passed into the proximal bowel should be sought and removed at the same time. Cholecystectomy is not required.

Intussusception

An intussusception occurs when a segment of bowel (the intussusceptum) invaginates into its adjoining lower segment (the intussuscipiens). Intussusception may be caused by the presence of a nidus

REFERENCES

366. Gierson E D, Storm F R et al Br J Surg 1975; 62: 383–386
367. Landsteiner K Z Allg Pathol Anat 1905; 16: 903
368. Hertz J Int Coll Surg 1950; 13: 644

in the bowel wall, such as a polyp or a Meckel's diverticulum, but often no abnormality is present.

Ileocaecal intussusception

This form of idiopathic intussusception classically occurs in healthy infants aged between 3 months and 2 years.[369] It is thought that the development of this type of infantile intussusception may be related either to an exaggerated protrusion of the ileocaecal valve into the caecum or a disproportionate amount of submucous lymphoid tissue in the Peyer's patches of the ileum which may be grasped and passed on as the apex of an intussusception.[370]

Although intussusception also occurs in children over the age of 2 years, the likelihood of a pathological cause for the intussusception becomes far more likely[355,371] (see Fig. 27.42).

The clinical features and management are described in Chapter 41.

Adult volvulus

A volvulus occurs when a segment of bowel twists through 360°. This often compromises the circulation of the affected segment of bowel and always causes a closed-loop obstruction.

Sigmoid volvulus

Volvulus of the sigmoid colon is responsible for approximately 4% of all cases of intestinal obstruction in western Europe and the USA but it is the major cause of colonic obstruction in parts of Eastern Europe, Africa and Asia.[372] The greatest incidence is in the sixth and seventh decades.

Predisposing factors

Essential prerequisites are a redundant sigmoid colon and a short mesenteric attachment which serve as the focal point about which the volvulus rotates. Most patients have a long history of disordered bowel habit with chronic constipation and laxative abuse. It commonly develops in psychiatric and senile patients, especially if they eat a diet that contains excessive quantities of fibre.[373] This may explain the high incidence of the condition in Uganda and Russia.[372]

Pathology

The bowel twists in an anticlockwise direction and the circulation is not impaired until one-and-a-half twists have occurred. At this point the associated closed-loop obstruction also interferes with the blood supply of the bowel wall, leading to gangrene, perforation and rapidly fatal peritonitis if left untreated.

Clinical features

An accurate history may not be forthcoming as patients are frequently senile or psychiatrically disturbed. There is usually a prior history of many years of constipation. The onset of the volvulus is accompanied by abdominal pain, nausea and vomiting. This is followed by absolute constipation, at times with distressing tenesmus if the twist produces traction on the rectum.

The abdomen soon becomes very distended and tympanitic as the loop of sigmoid colon fills with gas. A one-way valve seems to exists which allows faeces and air to continue to enter the volvulus but prevents their onward egress. Tachycardia, toxaemia and signs of peritonitis are indications of developing gangrene.

Radiological findings

The radiological features of a sigmoid volvulus are often diagnostic (Fig. 27.52). On plain radiographs a grossly distended loop of large bowel is seen arising from the pelvis and forming an omega loop or double cotyledon with its convexity lying away from the site of obstruction. A bird's beak narrowing of the air-filled colon points towards the site of obstruction.

Barium enema is usually not necessary to confirm the diagnosis but in doubtful cases it may be helpful (Fig. 27.52b). Characteristic features indicate narrowing at the site of the torsion spiral mucosal folds and the ace-of-spades deformity.[374] This investigation is contraindicated if gangrene is suspected.

Treatment

This should be prompt in order to prevent ischaemia of the bowel wall. A preoperative attempt should be made to untwist the colon. A sigmoidoscope is passed up to the obstruction and gently manipulated past the twist. This often results in a satisfying gush of wind which is usually followed by a large quantity of fluid faeces. Instantly the abdominal distension disappears and the patient feels greatly relieved. A flatus tube can be left in situ for 12–24 hours to prevent an immediate recurrence. This technique obviates the need for an urgent operation, but further assessment by a barium enema determines the necessity for planned surgery to excise a grossly redundant sigmoid colon.

Urgent surgery is required when the volvulus cannot be untwisted. At operation the volvulus is reduced by rotating the bowel in a clockwise direction. Sigmoid resection is necessary to prevent repeated recurrences or if the bowel is gangrenous. A primary anastomosis, Hartmann's or Mickulitz procedure can then be carried out, the choice depending on the state of the bowel and the condition of the patient.

Volvulus of the caecum

This condition is less common than volvulus of the sigmoid colon. It occurs when the caecum and ascending colon have not adhered to the posterior abdominal wall and are freely mobile on a lax

REFERENCES

369. Bond M R, Roberts J B M Br J Surg 1964; 57: 818
370. Strang R Br J Surg 1921; 9: 46
371. Reijnen J A M, Jooston H M, Festen C Br J Surg 1987; 74: 692
372. Shepherd J J Br J Surg 1969; 56: 353
373. Hall-Crages E C B Br Med J 1960; 1: 1015
374. Sackier J M, Wood C B Surgery 1989; 1: 1578

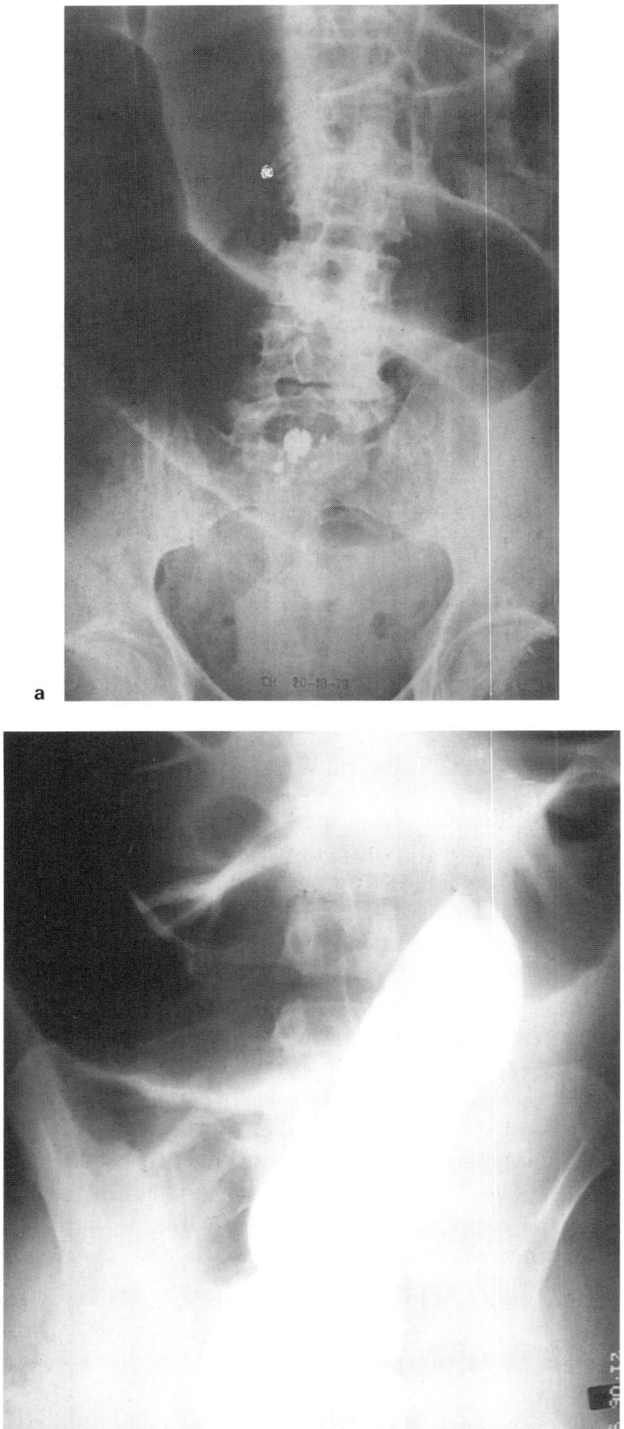

a

b

Fig. 27.52 (**a**) Plain X-ray of abdomen and (**b**) barium enema of a sigmoid volvulus.

mesocolon. It accounts for fewer than 1% of all cases of intestinal obstruction and about 30% of colonic volvuli.[375]

Caecal volvulus presents with the signs and symptoms of a low small bowel obstruction. Patients often describe previous similar minor attacks which resolve spontaneously. The caecum is visible as a distended, palpable and tympanitic swelling, lying centrally and rather to the left of the abdomen, while the right iliac fossa is relatively empty. Plain abdominal radiographs show a grossly distended gas-filled loop of bowel containing a large fluid level in the central abdomen, and an empty left colon (Fig. 27.53).

The caecum may perforate within a few hours unless it is decompressed. At operation the volvulus is untwisted and the safest method of preventing recurrent episodes is to perform a right hemicolectomy, although this opinion is the subject of controversy.[375–377] Caecopexy and caecostomy have also been advocated, although recurrence rates of 20% have been reported.[378]

Volvulus of the transverse colon can also occur but is incredibly rare.

GYNAECOLOGICAL DISORDERS

Several gynaecological disorders present as an acute abdomen. These include ruptured ectopic pregnancy, endometriosis, torsion or rupture of an ovarian cyst, ruptured ovarian follicle and pelvic inflammatory disease.

Ectopic pregnancy

Ectopic pregnancy occurs in fewer than 1% of pregnancies.[379] There is an increased incidence in patients with documented evidence of previous salpingitis, in those who use intrauterine contraceptive devices and in those who have had previous ectopic pregnancies. Ectopic pregnancies usually occur in the fallopian tube but they may also develop in the ovary, cervix and even occasionaly in the peritoneal cavity.

A tubal ectopic pregnancy is thought to be caused by defective transport of the fertilized ovum through the fallopian tube. This may be the result of scarring and irregularity from previous infection or tubal surgery, or it may be the result of a congenitally abnormal tube. The fertilized ovum lodging within the tube causes vascular engorgement and invasion of the wall leading to weakening and rupture. The symptoms and signs of shock develop if the bleeding is rapid, but there may be no haemodynamic disturbance if the blood loss is slow.

Clinical findings

The early symptoms and signs of a ruptured ectopic pregnancy are often misleading and variable, and the diagnosis can be easily overlooked. The typical history is of one or even two missed menstrual periods with other signs indicative of pregnancy. These include breast tenderness, morning sickness and urinary frequency. In some instances there is minor spotting at the time of the missed period, and the onset of symptoms may be associated with vaginal bleeding. Abdominal pain is at first crampy in nature, but

REFERENCES

375. O'Mara C S, Wilson T H et al Ann Surg 1979; 189: 725
376. Howard R G, Catto J Arch Surg 1980; 115: 273
377. Neil D H, Reasbeck P G et al Ann R Coll Surg Engl 1987; 69: 283
378. Weiss B D Postgrad Med J 1982; 72: 189
379. Wyper J F B Br Med J 1962; 1: 273

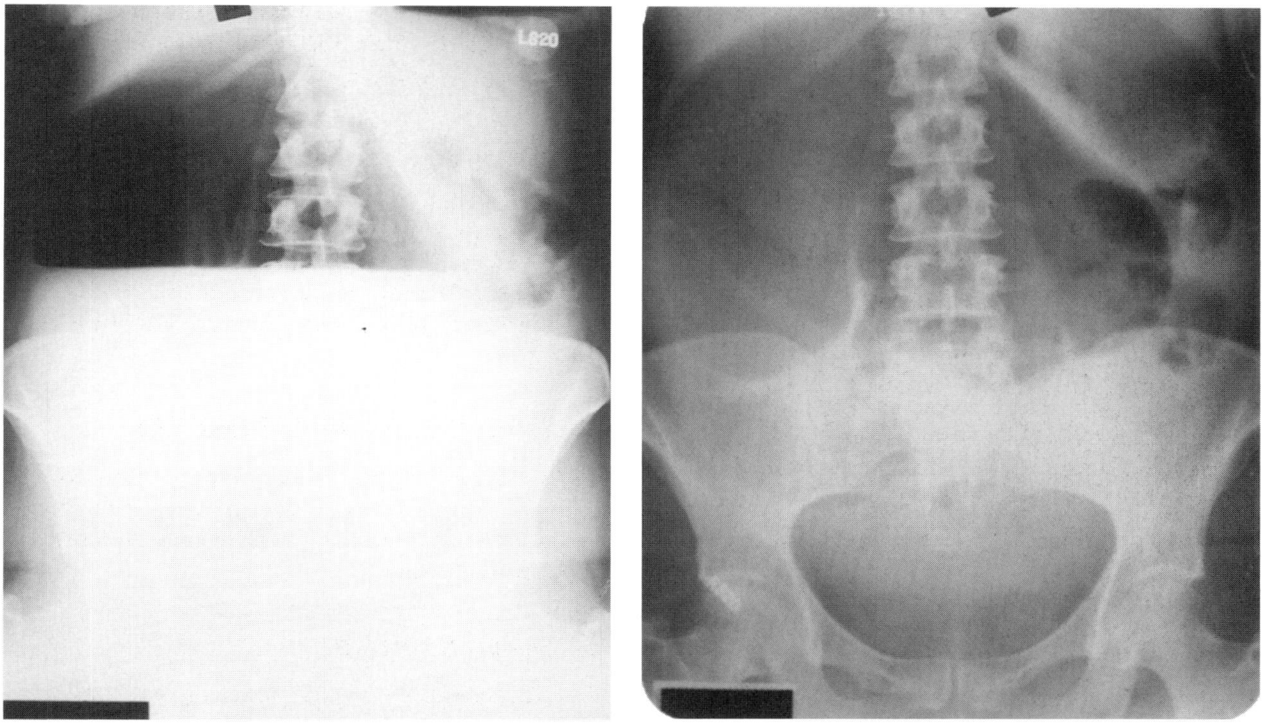

a b

Fig. 27.53 (a) Erect and (b) supine films of a caecal volvulus.

subsequently becomes more continuous and generalized throughout the lower abdomen. Shoulder-tip pain caused by the diaphragm being irritated by blood may be a prominent feature in some patients. Syncope may occur as a result of hypotension from major blood loss.

On examination the patient looks pale and other signs of hypovolaemic shock may be present, such as tachycardia and hypotension. There is abdominal tenderness, guarding and rebound tenderness which may be localized to the lower abdomen or may be generalized. Frequently altered blood is coming from the cervix, and movement of the cervix usually produces considerable abdominal discomfort. In some instances a mass may be felt in one of the adnexae and the uterus is frequently bulky and soft. Clumsy vaginal examination, excessive cervical manipulation or over-vigorous deep palpation all carry the risk of inducing further severe haemorrhage.[380] A full pelvic examination is essential, but if the clinical suspicion is high, this is best left to a gynaecologist. The haemoglobin and haematocrit are often low except in the early stages or in patients with a slow bleed when the haemoglobin may not have fallen. The diagnosis is strongly supported by a positive pregnancy test.

In many cases the clinical presentation does not fit this classical picture, and often there may not be a clear history of menstrual irregularity or symptoms suggestive of pregnancy. Initially the abdominal pain may be rather vague and mild in nature, and the abdominal signs may be insignificant. When the haemorrhage is slow there may be no evidence of shock. When the bleeding is gradual and continued, the only guide to the diagnosis is a falling haemoglobin and haematocrit. In difficult cases pelvic or vaginal ultrasound is extremely helpful,[381] but the most useful diagnostic test is laparoscopy which helps to differentiate tubal pregnancy from other conditions such as pelvic inflammatory disease, ovarian cyst rupture or torsion, endometriosis and appendicitis.[382]

Treatment

Prompt surgical intervention is imperative, once the diagnosis has been made and the patient has been properly resuscitated. In some cases it is possible to preserve the fallopian tube, particularly in unruptured tubal pregnancies, but a unilateral salpingectomy or salpingo-oophorectomy may be essential to save life. Tubal conservation should be attempted if at all possible to try to preserve future fertility.[383]

Endometriosis

This is a condition where functioning endometrial tissue is found as deposits outside the uterine cavity. The most commonly affected sites include the ovaries, the uterine tubes, the peritoneum, the uterosacral ligaments, the serosal surface of the uterus, the sigmoid colon and the small intestine. Endometrial tissue has occasionally been found in other sites, including the umbilicus, in abdominal scars, in the breasts and in the pleural cavity.[384,385]

REFERENCES

380. Lucas C, Hassim A M Br Med J 1970; 1: 200
381. Stiller R J, Deregt R H, Blair E Am J Obstet Gynecol 1989; 161: 930
382. Silva P D Obstet Gynecol Surg 1988; 72: 944
383. Seigler A M, Wang C F, Westcoffe C Obstet Gynecol Surg 1981; 36: 599

Symptoms

This condition characteristically develops during the third and fourth decades of life. Initially it may cause dysmenorrhoea with pain starting in the week before the period. In some cases there is a vague continuous lower abdominal pain throughout the menstrual cycle which is exaggerated during menstruation. In others it presents with low back pain and painful defecation. This is the result of endometrial deposits in the pelvic peritoneum and in the rectovaginal septum. Bladder involvement can cause dysuria and haematuria at the time of menstruation. Endometriosis in the sigmoid colon or rectum may produce signs of partial intestinal obstruction, which is particularly prominent during the menstrual periods.

Occasionally, large ovarian endometrial cysts may rupture and present with an acute onset of severe lower abdominal pain which is associated with low-grade fever and signs of lower abdominal tenderness, guarding and rebound. There is usually some tenderness on vaginal examination and occasionally endometrial deposits can be palpated on rectal examination. Rarely large cystic masses may be felt in the pelvis. The diagnosis is confirmed on laparoscopic examination when deposits of endometriosis can be seen on the serosal surface of the pelvis.[386]

Treatment

No immediate treatment is indicated if the diagnosis is made at laparotomy. A number of hormones have been tried in the treatment of this condition, including progesterone, medroxyprogesterone and norethisterone. Approximately 80% of patients with endometriosis have benefited from these agents.[387,388] Danazol, a synthetic androgen, has been found to be particularly effective in endometriosis. This is prescribed for 6–9 months and results in cessation of the symptoms in the majority of patients.[389]

Complicated endometrial cysts require elective surgical excision or laser ablation.[390] More radical treatments include bilateral salpingo-oophorectomy, or hysterectomy with ovarian preservation in young women who do not wish to become pregnant.

Torsion or ruptured ovarian cysts

Cysts of the ovary may be functional cysts of the follicles or corpus luteum or they may be proliferative cysts (dermoid cysts, serous or mucinous cyst adenomas or even cyst-adenocarcinomas; Fig. 27.54). Ovarian cysts can cause acute abdominal pain when they rupture, twist or infarct. Torsion may involve both the ovary and the fallopian tube.

Symptoms and signs

A ruptured or torted ovarian cyst produces severe lower abdominal pain of acute onset. There may be a low-grade fever and evidence of guarding and rebound in the lower abdomen. This can be localized to one side of the abdomen and may be difficult to differentiate from acute appendicitis when it occurs on the right side. A cyst can sometimes be palpated on pelvic examination or more easily on bimanual examination under anaesthesia.

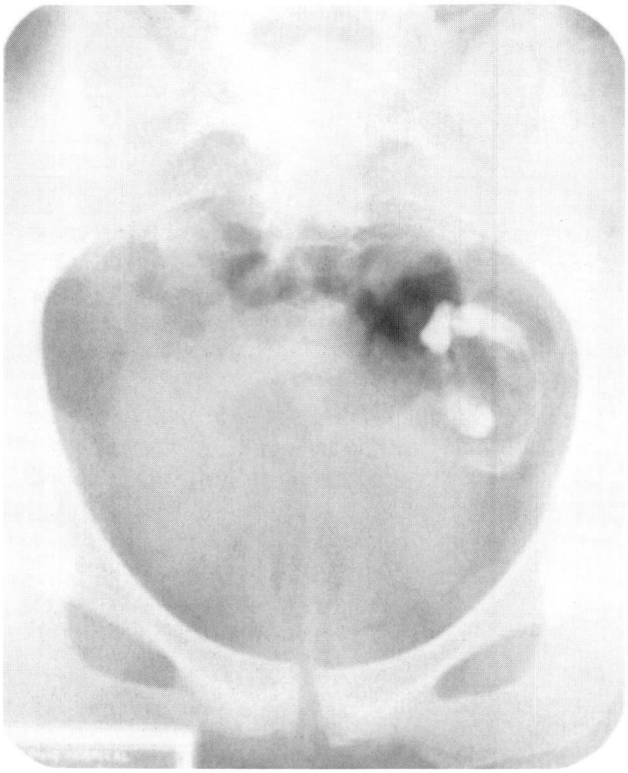

Fig. 27.54 An ovarian dermoid cyst.

The presence of an ovarian cyst can be confirmed by ultrasonography or laparoscopy.[391] Treatment depends on the size of the cyst; if large, the cyst and ovary should be excised. Laparasopic aspiration may be an alternative method of treating certain types of cyst.

Ruptured ovarian follicle (mittelschmerz)

Extensive bleeding from a graafian follicle at the time of ovulation can produce severe lower abdominal pain with signs of tenderness and guarding, and a low-grade fever. Mittelschmerz can be difficult to differentiate from acute appendicitis if a cyst in the right ovary ruptures. The diagnosis is suggested if pain develops acutely in the middle of the menstrual cycle. On careful questioning a similar mid-cycle pain may have occurred before. Patients are rarely pyrexial and the pain usually settles in a few hours. The diagnosis can be confirmed by laparoscopy, but in a small number

REFERENCES

384. Venter P F S Afr Med J 1980; 57: 895
385. Scott R B, Rinde R W Ann Surg 1950; 131: 697
386. Chamberlain G, Brown J C Gynaecological Laparoscopy: The Report of the Working Party of the Confidential Enquiry into Gynaecological Laparoscopy. Royal College of Obstetricians and Gynecologists, London 1978
387. Hammond C B, Haney A F Fertil Steril 1978; 30: 495
388. Anonymous Br Med J 1980; 281: 889
389. Noble A D, Letchworth A T Postgrad Med J 1979; 55: 37
390. Davis E D Obstet Gynecol 1986; 68: 442
391. Sema K, Mettler L Am J Obstet Gynecol 1980; 70: 948

of cases the diagnosis is not made until operation is mistakenly performed for appendicitis.

Pelvic inflammatory disease

Pelvic inflammatory disease develops in approximately 15% of patients in whom *Neisseria gonorrhoeae* has been cultured from the cervical swabs.[392] Once a gonococcal infection has produced damage to the fallopian tubes, further attacks of non-gonococcal infection may occur. The micro-organisms responsible include coliforms, aerobes, a number of anaerobes and *Chlamydia trachomatis*.[393] There is an increased incidence of pelvic inflammatory disease if an intrauterine contraceptive device is present.

The condition presents with acute lower abdominal pain and a high fever. The pain is usually severe and is accompanied by signs of tenderness in the lower abdomen. The tenderness is usually present in both iliac fossae but unilateral infections can occur. On vaginal examination a discharge may be seen coming from the cervix, and movement of the cervix causes exquisite tenderness.[394]

The diagnosis is usually suspected from the clinical features, the presence of a discharge from the cervix and a high fever which is not matched by the severity of the abdominal signs. The white cell count is usually markedly elevated. Laparoscopy can be used to confirm the diagnosis and exclude other causes of lower abdominal pain. Treatment is by antibiotics and bed rest. If an intrauterine contraceptive device is present, it should be removed.

In the more advanced stages of pelvic inflammatory disease, a tubo-ovarian abscess may develop and if this goes on to perforate, the patient complains of severe abdominal pain and has evidence of generalized peritonitis. This is usually treated by salpingo-oophorectomy and intravenous antibiotics.[395]

POSTOPERATIVE ACUTE ABDOMEN

After major abdominal surgery, complications are prone to occur and can cause an acute abdomen. The clinical features are often atypical and physical signs can be very difficult to elicit because of the masking effect of the abdominal surgery. The surgical team must always be aware of the possibility of this problem. The most common complication is small bowel obstruction with entrapment of a segment of the small bowel either in the abdominal wound or in some part of the abdomen.

Acute pancreatitis may occur after cholecystectomy, gastrectomy and splenectomy. Postoperative perforation of a viscus or leakage from a bowel anastomosis produces severe abdominal pain with signs of peritonitis. Postoperative intraperitoneal haemorrhage may occur when a ligature on a major vessel slips, or when an artery that has been in spasm later reopens. Mesenteric thrombosis is especially difficult to diagnose in the postoperative period and bowel ischaemia is often well-advanced by the time it is recognised.

Biliary peritonitis results in severe abdominal pain which is caused by the presence of free bile in the peritoneal cavity. This may be the result of damage to the common bile duct at the time of cholecystectomy, bile leakage from the liver bed or slipping of the ligature on the cystic duct. It may also occur following removal of a T-tube if a tract has not developed (see Chapter 32).

Postoperative cholecystitis can result from existing gallstones. Acalculous ischaemic cholecystitis also occurs in patients who are severely ill from another cause.[397] This condition is thought to result from an occlusion of the cystic artery in patients with severe splanchnic vasoconstriction or a primary bacterial infection. Treatment is by cholecystectomy (see Chapter 32).

ABDOMINAL WALL PAIN

Pain arising in the abdominal wall rather than the abdominal cavity may occasionally be mistaken for an acute abdomen.

Neurovascular bundle entrapment

Patients with this condition frequently present with recurrent pain in the abdomen for which no definite cause can be found.[396,397] The features which suggest that the pain is arising from the abdominal wall are the presence of one or two trigger points which can be accurately localized using one finger.[398,399] These usually lie just medial to the linea semilunaris of the rectus sheath.[400] Tensing the abdominal wall muscle results in persistence and, on some occasions, accentuation of the abdominal pain, whereas disappearance of the pain during straining is thought to indicate visceral disease.[398,401] The commonest sites for this pain are in the right iliac fossa and the right hypochondrium. Abdominal scars, felt to be the main source of pain in one series,[401] were thought not to be important in another series, where the site of pain was described as being at least 3 cm from any scar.[400] Injection of local anaesthetic[400,401] is often both diagnostic and curative. The beneficial effect of the local anaesthetic is often considerably longer than its expected duration of action.[401] In some instances a single injection cures the pain, and in others the pain is completely relieved by repeated treatment. Many other methods of treatment have been reported, each with some success. These include injecting a combination of local anaesthetic and steroids,[402] aqueous phenol,[396] the use of radiofrequency sound waves and surgical decompression of the affected area.

Clearly in making this diagnosis one needs to be convinced that there is no underlying visceral pathology. The response rates to one injection of local anaesthetic have been reported to be between 55 and 100%.[396,400,401]

REFERENCES

392. Meheus A Z Am J Obstet Gynecol 1980; 138: 1064
393. Paavonon J, Valtonen V V et al Lancet 1981; 293
394. Hare M J Br Med J 1986; 293: 1255
395. Horgan P G, Campbell A L, Gray C C, Gillespie G Br J Surg 1989; 76: 1296
396. Mehta M, Ranger I Anaesthesia 1971; 26: 330
397. Applegate W V Surgery 1972; 711: 118
398. Thompson H, Francis D M Lancet 1977; 1: 1053
399. Gray D W K, Seabrook G et al Ann R Coll Surg Engl 1988; 70: 233–234
400. Hall P N, Lee A B P Br J Surg 1988; 75: 917
401. Gallegos N C, Hobsley M J R Soc Med 1989; 82: 343
402. Tung A S, Tenicela R, Gioranetti J JAMA 1978; 240: 738

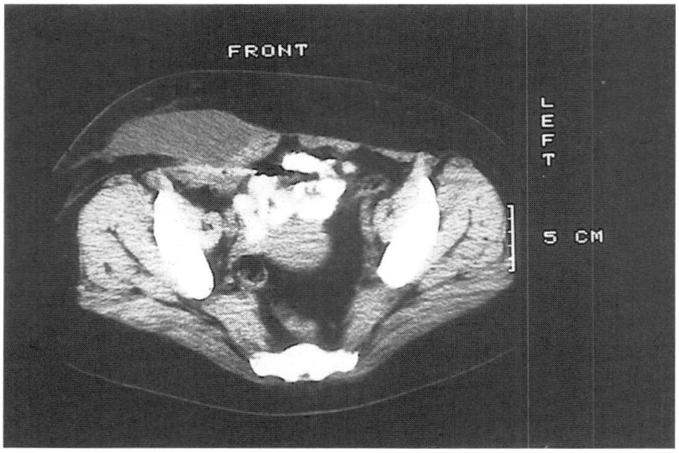

Fig. 27.55 An ultrasound scan of a rectus sheath haematoma.

Rectus sheath haematoma

This is an uncommon condition that may arise spontaneously, after minor trauma or after bouts of coughing or sneezing.[403–405] The underlying abnormality is thought to be poor elasticity of the arteries which results in a failure of the vessel to accommodate sudden, marked variations in length as the rectus muscle undergoes contraction and relaxation. When a rectus sheath haematoma occurs spontaneously it may be associated with an underlying disorder of coagulation, degenerative vascular disease, infectious diseases or haematological conditions such as leukaemia.[403–405]

It presents with an acute onset of abdominal pain and there may be associated symptoms of nausea and vomiting which suggest an intra-abdominal abnormality. Examination frequently reveals exquisite tenderness in the lower abdomen and a sensation of fullness or a mass in the abdominal wall which can still be felt when the muscles are tensed. The pain is accentuated by tensing the abdominal muscles during palpation. Later bruising and discoloration of the skin over the haematoma may develop. In cases where this is not evident, and a mass is not clearly palpable, a diagnosis of the acute abdomen may mistakenly be made. An ultrasound or CT scan may confirm the presence of a haematoma if the condition is suspected (Fig. 27.55).

The condition is usually treated conservatively with the pain settling in 2–3 days, although the mass may take several weeks to resolve. In some instances with severe abdominal pain, evacuation of the haematoma and control of the bleeding point may be considered.

The surgical causes of the acute abdomen are summarized in Table 27.8.

Table 27.8 Surgical causes of the acute abdomen

Inflammation and infection
Acute appendicitis
Acute cholecystitis
Acute diverticulitis
Acute pancreatitis
Salpingitis
Septic abortion
Mesenteric adenitis
Primary peritonitis
Crohn's disease
Meckel's diverticulitis
Pyelonephritis and cystitis
Yersinia infection
Perforation
Gastric ulcer
Duodenal ulcer
Diverticular disease
Carcinoma of the colon
Crohn's disease
Ulcerative colitis
Lymphoma
Foreign body perforation
Acute cholecystitis with perforation
Acute appendicitis with perforation
Perforation of the oesophagus (Boerhaave's syndrome)
Perforation of a segment of strangulated bowel
Perforation of the urinary bladder
Obstruction
Renal colic
Biliary colic
Small bowel
Congenital bands/atresia
Meconium ileus
Malrotation of the gut
Adhesions from previous surgery
Hernia
Intussusception
Gallstone
Tumours
Crohn's
Large bowel
Tumour
Volvulus
Inflammatory stricture
Infarction
Torsion of a viscus
Arterial thrombosis or embolus
Venous thrombosis
Dissecting aortic aneurysm
Haemorrhage
Ruptured abdominal aortic aneurysm
Aneurysms of mesenteric vessels
Dissecting aneurysm of the aorta
Ruptured ovarian cyst
Ruptured ectopic pregnancy
Ovulatory bleed
Endometriosis
Spontaneous rupture of liver tumour
Rectus sheath haematoma
Abdominal trauma

'MEDICAL' CAUSES OF THE ACUTE ABDOMEN

There are many conditions that involve the abdominal, retroperitoneal and intrathoracic organs and mimic the acute abdomen (Table 27.9). The common medical conditions that are mistaken for the acute abdomen but which do not require surgical treatment are discussed below.

REFERENCES

403. Fotergill W E Br Med J 1926; 1: 941
404. Brodel M Bull Johns Hopkins Hosp 1937; 61: 295
405. Cullen T S Bull Johns Hopkins Hosp 1937; 61: 317

Table 27.9 Non-surgical causes of the acute abdomen

Intra-abdominal
Disease of the liver
Liver tumours
Hepatic abscesses
Primary peritonitis
Bacterial peritonitis
Tuberculosis
Candida
Glove lubricants
Infective conditions
Acute viral gastroenteritis
Acute food-poisoning
Typhoid fever
Mesenteric adenitis
Yersinia
Curtis–Fitz–Hugh syndrome
Abdominal wall pain
Rectus sheath haematoma
Neurovascular enlargement
Retroperitoneal causes
Pyelonephritis
Acute hydronephrosis
Intrathoracic causes
Myocardial infarction
Pericarditis
Spontaneous pneumothorax
Pleurisy
Coxsackie B virus
Spontaneous perforation of the oesophagus
Strangulation of a diaphragmatic hernia
Dissection of the aorta
Metabolic disorders
Diabetes
Addison's disease
Uraemia
Porphyria
Haemochromatosis
Hypercalcaemia
Heavy metal poisoning
Neurological causes of the acute abdomen
Spinal disorders
Tabes dorsalis
Haematological disorders
Sickle cell anaemia
Haemolytic anaemia
Henoch–Schönlein purpura
Leukaemia
Lymphomas
Polycythaemia
Anticoagulant therapy
Immunological disorders
Polyarteritis nodosa
Systemic lupus erythematosus
Infections
Infectious mononucleosis
Herpes zoster

Intra-abdominal causes

Disease of the liver

Any condition that produces stretching of the liver capsule causes acute abdominal pain and signs of tenderness in the right upper hyperchondrium. Acute viral hepatitis often presents in this way, but is differentiated from acute cholecystitis by finding raised viral antibody titres and altered liver function tests. Congestive cardiac failure causes a similar pain from passive congestion of the liver, especially if there is tricuspid incompetence when the liver may be pulsatile. This is suspected when the patient has an elevated jugular venous pressure, peripheral oedema, chest crepitations or gallop cardiac rhythm and of course a systolic ejection murmur.

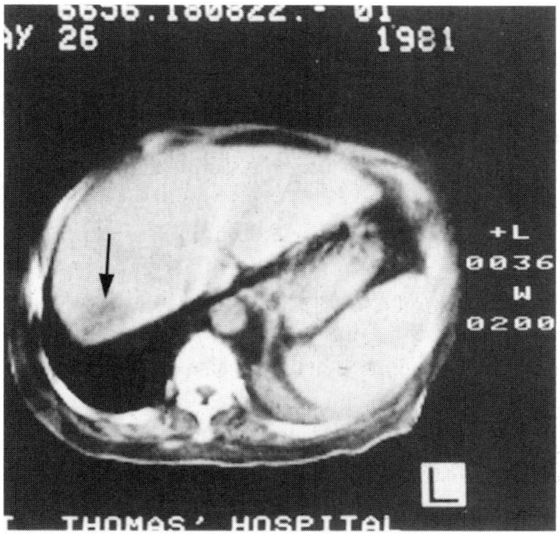

Fig. 27.56 A CT scan showing a liver abscess.

Primary or metastatic liver tumours may also present with abdominal pain, although these could probably be considered as surgical causes of acute abdominal pain as they occasionally require operations. The pain is caused by sudden enlargement of the liver as a result of rapid tumour growth or by secondary haemorrhage into a necrotic tumour. Free bleeding may also occur into the abdominal cavity. Liver neoplasms can be confirmed by imaging with ultrasound, CT or magnetic resonance.

Both pyogenic and amoebic hepatic abscesses (see Chapter 31) may present with abdominal pain, hepatic enlargement and tenderness.[406] The pain is usually in the right upper quadrant but may also be experienced over the right lower chest where there may be swelling and pitting oedema of the subcutaneous tissues. The pain may be referred to the shoulder if the abscess is in contact with the diaphragm. The upper abdominal signs are generally not as marked as the signs of systemic sepsis. Radiographs reveal an elevated or immobile diaphragm on the right side, the cardiophrenic angle is often obliterated and if there are gas-producing organisms within the abscess an air–fluid level may be seen within the cavity. Imaging of the liver usually demonstrates the presence of an abscess (Fig. 27.56). An amoebic abscess may be confirmed by a specific complement fixation test or the demonstration of amoebae within stools. The final diagnosis is invariably confirmed by aspiration of 'anchovy' pus from the abscess cavity (see Chapter 31).

REFERENCE

406. Rubin R H, Schwartz M N, Malt R Am Med J 1974; 57: 601

Primary peritonitis

Primary bacterial peritonitis is an uncommon condition in which there is no obvious abdominal source of infection (pp. 000–000). Pneumococci were formerly thought to be the most frequent infecting organism, but coliforms have now been shown to account for over half of the cases.[407–409] The condition has an insidious onset, and symptoms include abdominal pain and distension, vomiting, lethargy, fever and diarrhoea. This condition is seldom as severe as an acute suppurative peritonitis, and is often confirmed by peritoneal aspiration and culture of a specific organism. The major difficulty in making this diagnosis is to differentiate it from a secondary peritonitis which requires laparotomy. Abdominal exploration is often essential to exclude a primary source of infection.

Tuberculous and fungal peritonitis

Tuberculosis is now an uncommon cause of peritonitis. It is associated with granuloma formation and extensive adhesions[410,411] and there may be evidence of other tuberculosis infection elsewhere. Patients present with a dull abdominal pain, ascites and abdominal tenderness but most cases do not have signs of peritonitis. *Candida* and other yeasts may also produce peritonitis in immunosuppressed patients.[412]

Starch peritonitis

Contamination of the peritoneal cavity by starch or other glove lubricants such as talc, mineral oil, corn and rice starch or by cellulose fibres from drapes or packs used during operative procedures may cause abdominal pain with signs of peritonitis.[413] This generally occurs several weeks after an abdominal operation and may be associated with an abdominal mass. The peritonitis usually eventually resolves spontaneously and does not require laparotomy. Resolution may be hastened by the administration of oral steroids.[414]

Infective conditions

Acute viral gastroenteritis

This is a common condition in childhood when it is self-limiting. The abdominal symptoms are occasionally severe and may mimic the acute abdomen. It is characterized by watery diarrhoea, nausea and vomiting associated with crampy abdominal pain.[415] Tenderness in the abdomen is usually ill-localized.

Acute food-poisoning

This usually produces a similar picture to viral gastroenteritis. In some instances the abdominal pain is quite intense and may even be associated with tenderness and rebound. Diarrhoea is common and the causative organism or its toxin can often isolated from the stool. Differentiation from other abdominal emergencies may be difficult in some cases. Many cases of viral gastroenteritis or suspected food-poisoning are now being found to have *Campylobacter* in their stools, and giardiasis may also have to be excluded.

Typhoid fever

This may produce symptoms and signs which are similar to those of acute appendicitis.[416] The onset is generally less acute with several days of symptoms. Associated findings include Koplik's spots, a macropapular rash, leucopenia and at times a marked bradycardia. Patients appear extremely unwell, out of all proportion to their abdominal signs. The diagnosis is confirmed by culture of salmonella from the stools or blood. Perforation of the distal ileum occurs in a small proportion of cases and requires surgical treatment.[417,418]

Mesenteric adenitis

This is an enlargement of the mesenteric lymph nodes caused by adenovirus infection which particularly affects young children, and can at times be difficult to differentiate from acute appendicitis (pp. 721–730).[419] There is usually a history of an upper respiratory infection, which may either still be present or may have subsided. The upper respiratory tract infection is often associated with fever, pharyngitis and cervical lymphadenitis. The abdominal pain is usually more diffuse than in patients with appendicitis, and tenderness is rarely isolated to the right iliac fossa. The site of maximal tenderness may be altered by re-examining patients on their side. Guarding may be present but rebound tenderness is almost never elicited. A relative lymphocytosis may be present but cannot be relied upon to confirm the diagnosis. In most instances careful observation of the patient and repeated re-examination differentiate mesenteric adenitis from acute appendicitis.

Yersinia

Infection with *Yersinia* has been associated with acute appendicitis, mesenteric adenitis, acute terminal ileitis and non-specific abdominal pain.[420] *Yersinia enterocolitica* has been isolated from patients with gastroenteritis and right iliac fossa pain, while

REFERENCES

407. Cann H O, Fessel J M Medical 1971; 50: 161
408. Curry N, McCallum R W, Guth P H Am J Dig Dis 1974; 19: 685
409. Fowler R Aust Paediatr J 1971; 7: 73
410. Cromartie R S III Surg Gynecol Obstet 1977; 144: 876
411. Singh M M, Bhargava A N, Jain K P N Engl J Med 1969; 281: 1091
412. Solomkin J S, Flohr A B, Quie P G, Simons R L Surgery 1980; 88: 524
413. Warshaw A L Surgery 1973; 73: 681
414. Bates B Ann Intern Med 1965; 62: 335
415. Crist N R, Bell E J, Aasaad F Progress in Medical Virology. Karger, Basel, 1978
416. Woodward T E, Smadel J E Ann Intern Med 1964; 60: 144
417. Sitram V, Fenn A S, Moses B V, Kanduri P Ann R Coll Surg Engl 1990; 72: 347
418. Akgun Y, Bac B, Aban N, Tacyildiz I Br J Surg 1995; 82: 1512–1515
419. Jones P F Br Med J 1969; 1: 284
420. Attwood S E A, Mealy K et al Lancet 1987; i: 529–533

Y. pseudotuberculosis has been isolated from patients with non-specific abdominal pain. *Yersinia* infection can be confirmed by a rising titre of antibodies to *Y. enterocolitica* and *Y. pseudotuberculosis*. Using sequential samples, *Yersinia* was found to be present in 31% of cases of acute appendicitis, 12% of cases of non-specific abdominal pain and in 2 out of 6 cases with mesenteric adenitis.[421] Despite this study it is not known how often *Yersinia* causes these conditions.

Yersinia has also been found in patients with acute terminal ileitis[422] which may be discovered at the time of appendicectomy and can mimic Crohn's disease of the ileum. This type of ileitis does not go on to produce the recurrent problems associated with Crohn's disease.

Fitz-Hugh–Curtis syndrome[423,424]

This syndrome was initially thought to be caused by gonococcal salpingitis, but is now more commonly associated with *Chlamydia trachomatis*[425,426] infection. The pelvic infection tracks up either left or right paracolic gutters to produce perisplenitis or perihepatitis. As such these patients may present with both lower and upper abdominal pain,[427] which often mimics acute biliary disease.[428,429] The presentation is usually with severe right upper quadrant abdominal pain which may be associated with anorexia, nausea and a low-grade fever. The predominant tenderness is in the right upper quadrant. The presence of a pelvic infection must be sought and high vaginal and cervical swabs sent for culture. The disease is confirmed by the presence of elevated serum levels of specific antibodies. Treatment is by a course of doxycycline. The diagnosis may also be made at laparoscopy or even laparotomy when adhesions can be demonstrated around the capsule of the liver. The Fitz-Hugh–Curtis syndrome may also result in diffuse peritonitis and chronic ascites.[430]

Retroperitoneal renal causes of abdominal pain

Pyelonephritis and other conditions affecting the kidney such as hydronephrosis and renal colic can, at times, present as an acute abdomen.

Renal colic may at times mimic bowel obstruction, especially if there is an associated paralytic ileus (see Chapter 36). The differentiation between these two conditions relies very much on the history of the pain: renal colic tends to present with loin pain which radiates to the groin. The patient cannot lie still and often rolls around the bed or the floor during the colicky attacks. By contrast, intestinal obstruction produces a central colicky pain, causing the patient to double up, bringing the knees up to their chin.

Pyelonephritis

This can also be mistaken for acute appendicitis. Acute pyelonephritis develops fairly rapidly over a few hours and is normally associated with a high fever and rigors. There may also be symptoms of nausea and vomiting. Increased urinary frequency and dysuria usually occur before the onset of the fever, but occasionally they never develop. The pain is experienced in the loin, and may radiate to the groin. In some instances the presenting pain appears to be located in the iliac fossa. There is usually marked tenderness in one or both loins, and there is tenderness of varying severity in the iliac fossae. Bacteria and white cells are nearly always present in the urine.

Acute hydronephrosis

This may present with a pain in the upper abdomen referred from the kidney, and may be difficult to differentiate from other conditions such as biliary colic. There is usually pain in the loin and tenderness can generally be demonstrated on bimanual palpation. Ultrasound imaging demonstrates the dilated renal pelvis.

Intrathoracic causes of abdominal pain

A number of conditions affecting the thoracic organs may cause abdominal pain. Pain from a myocardial infarction may be localized to the epigastrium and may be associated with nausea and vomiting. This type of cardiac pain is usually of rapid onset and is a persistent, severe, crushing pain which may radiate to the neck and left arm. Shortness of breath and sweating may also be present. The abdominal muscles may be rigid, but the patient rarely complains of pain during palpation. General examination frequently reveals tachycardia or arrhythmia, sweating and hypotension with poor peripheral perfusion. Fever and a high white cell count are not normally present in the early stages. The diagnosis is confirmed by characteristic electrocardiographic changes and by finding a subsequent elevation of the cardiac enzymes over the next 48 hours. Myocardial infarction must be considered in all patients presenting with severe abdominal pain and shock, and is one of the differential diagnoses that must be considered in patients suspected of having acute pancreatitis, a perforated peptic ulcer, a ruptured aortic aneurysm, mesenteric infarction or a small bowel volvulus.

Pericarditis may also cause abdominal pain, particularly when the inflammation affects the diaphragmatic pericardium. This produces severe epigastric pain which has the peculiar feature of being relieved by sitting and accentuated by taking up other positions. A friction rub is usually present and should be listened for, both over the lung bases and in the precordium. The diagnosis of pericarditis can usually be made on an electrocardiogram where

REFERENCES

421. Wever, Finlayson N B, Mark J B D N Engl J Med 1970; 283: 172–174
422. Gurry J F Br Med J 1974; ii: 264–266
423. Curtis H JAMA 1930; 98: 1221
424. Fitz-Hugh T Jr JAMA 1934; 102: 2044
425. Muller-Schopp J W, Wang S P et al Br Med J 1978; 1: 1002
426. Wolner-Hanssen P Br J Obstet Gynaecol 1986; 93: 619–624
427. Gatt D, Heafield T, Jantet G Ann R Coll Surg Engl 1986; 68: 271–274
428. Wood J J, Bolton J P et al Br J Surg 1982; 69: 251–253
429. Shanahan D, Lord P H, Grogono J, Wastell C Ann R Coll Surg Engl 1988; 70: 44–46
430. Marbet U A, Stalder G A V et al Br Med J 1986; 293: 5–6

the widespread elevation of the ST segment differentiates the condition from myocardial infarction. Viral pericarditis, which is the most common form, has no additional symptoms or signs, but in other types of pericarditis, such as those associated with uraemia, tuberculosis, rheumatic fever and bacterial infection, additional features may be present which suggest the diagnosis.

A spontaneous pneumothorax can occasionally cause abdominal pain as the result of diaphragmatic irritation. Examination of the chest and a chest radiograph should confirm the diagnosis. Pain can also be referred to the abdomen from pleurisy, especially when this affects the diaphragmatic pleura. Abdominal pain is more frequent when there is an associated pneumonia or pulmonary infarct from a pulmonary embolus. There may be limited chest movement on the affected side, cough and haemoptysis, shortness of breath, signs of consolidation of the lung, a friction rub and some tightening of the abdominal muscles. Chest radiographs, blood-gas and sputum analysis, electrocardiography and lung scanning may be required to confirm the diagnosis.

Coxsackie B virus infection (Bornholm disease) or epidemic pleurodynia can present with severe pain in the chest or the abdomen. Other symptoms include shortness of breath, pain on respiration, headache and sore throat. The abdominal pain which is experienced in the upper abdomen and lower thorax is usually aggravated by movement and respiration. Patients are usually pyrexial but the white cell count is rarely elevated. The diagnosis is suggested by finding superficial hyperaesthesia over the upper abdomen and by the lack of signs on abdominal examination. An elevation of viral antibodies on repeat testing confirms the diagnosis after several weeks.

Spontaneous perforation of the oesophagus (Boerhaave's syndrome) is a condition in which the oesophagus ruptures and its contents enter the mediastinum and one of the two hemithoraces, usually the left[431] (see Chapter 2). This occurs more commonly in males and frequently follows an episode of excessive food or alcohol intake associated with violent vomiting or retching. Severe pain rapidly develops in the epigastrium and lower chest, and is aggravated by swallowing and breathing. On examination the patient is febrile, tachypnoeic and may even be cyanotic. Subcutaneous emphysema may be present and a friction rub may be heard over the left chest. In the early stages the rupture is confined to the mediastinum which appears widened on a chest radiograph (Fig. 27.57). A pleural effusion may be present in the left chest and there may also be evidence of mediastinal gas. The diagnosis is confirmed by a water-soluble contrast swallow or by aspirating stomach contents from the pleural cavity: this has a low pH or a high amylase content. Oesophageal perforation without associated perforation of the pleura can be managed non-operatively, but when the pleura has been breached the patient needs a thoracotomy, pleural lavage and oesophageal repair with pleural drainage and antibiotics (see Chapter 21).[432,433]

A *strangulated diaphragmatic hernia* is extremely rare and other conditions that produce acute mediastinitis can also produce similar symptoms and signs. It requires urgent surgery, especially if it is associated with a gastric volvulus (see Chapter 28).

Aortic dissection can also produce abdominal or chest pain which is similar to that of a myocardial infarction. The original site of the pain is usually in the back between the shoulder blades, but this may spread down into the abdomen even if the blood supply of the intestine is not compromised. The signs of mesenteric ischaemia indicate the need for urgent surgery. The anatomy of the dissection is shown by CT scanning, transoesophageal ultrasound or arteriography (see Chapter 23).

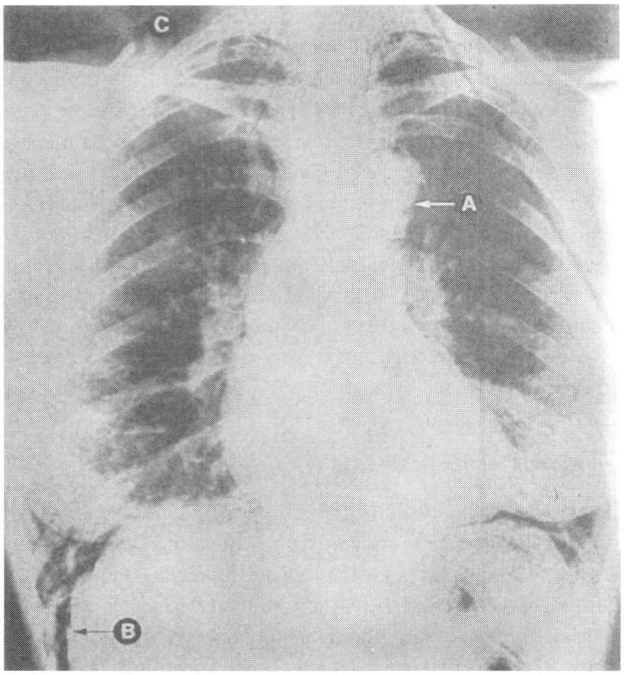

Fig. 27.57 A spontaneous rupture of the oesophagus. A chest X-ray showing (A) air in the mediastinum, (B) air under the diaphragm and (C) subcutaneous emphysema.

Metabolic disorders

A number of metabolic disorders can produce abdominal pain which is only occasionally severe enough to be mistaken for a surgical emergency.

Diabetes

Diabetic ketoacidosis can cause severe abdominal pain and tenderness. Nausea and vomiting are frequently present and the abdomen is diffusely tender on palpation without evidence of guarding or rebound tenderness. Diabetic ketoacidosis is usually differentiated from other causes of the acute abdomen by the knowledge that the patient has diabetes, although some patients present for the first time with diabetic ketoacidosis.[434] They may however give a prior history of polyuria, polydipsia, lassitude, anorexia and weight loss

REFERENCES

431. Boerhaave H, Lugd Bat Boutesteniana 1724 Trans Bull Med Lib Assoc 1955; 93: 28
432. Tilanus H W, Bossuyt P, Schattenkerk M E, Obertop H Br J Surg 1991; 78: 582–585
433. Jones W G, Ginsberg R J Ann Thorac Surg 1992; 53: 534–543
434. Beardwood J T JAMA 1935; 105: 1168

an careful questioning. The general appearance of the patient is characteristic with laboured breathing from air hunger and a ketoacidotic foetor from acetone on the breath. There is usually evidence of dehydration with hypotension, a thready pulse and oliguria. The diagnosis is made by testing the urine and the blood for glucose and ketones. It is important to be certain that an acute abdomen is not being overlooked in a patient with diabetic ketoacidosis, and that an acute abdomen has not precipitated the ketoacidotic episode. The abdominal signs of diabetic ketoacidosis resolve once the diabetes is brought under control and fluids have been replaced.

Addison's disease

Chronic deficiency of the adrenal cortex may at times be characterized by gastrointestinal symptoms which include anorexia, lethargy, weight loss, nausea, vomiting, diarrhoea and ill-defined abdominal pain (see Chapter 35). In an Addisonian crisis the abdominal symptoms may become intensified. The patient is usually severely dehydrated and hypotensive. A diagnosis of Addison's disease is suggested by the presence of pigmentation, which is a diffuse brown tan or bronze darkening of both exposed and unexposed areas of skin, and severe hypotension which is out of keeping with the rest of the clinical picture. The diagnosis is confirmed by finding a low plasma cortisol level and the failure of the cortisol to rise in response to stimulation (see Chapter 35).

Uraemia

Patients with chronic renal failure may develop anorexia, nausea, vomiting and bleeding from small ulcers in the gastrointestinal tract. Abdominal pain tends to be associated with severe vomiting and diarrhoea, or with the complications of pericarditis and acute pancreatitis. The pain is not usually severe but on occasions can be more marked and may be mistaken for an acute abdomen. The clinical picture of a dehydrated patient who is pale, with a yellowish skin and foetor, raises the clinical suspicion of chronic renal failure. The diagnosis is confirmed by finding an elevated blood urea and creatinine.

Porphyria (acute intermittent porphyria)

Porphyrins are iron-free pigments, produced during haemoglobin metabolism.[435] In the porphyrias there is a disorder of pyrrole metabolism resulting in the formation of large amounts of free porphyrins. Acute intermittent porphyria, which is the most common type, is transmitted as a Mendelian dominant and affects young and middle-aged adults. It is characterized by periodic attacks of intense abdominal pain which may be associated with nausea and vomiting, constipation, neuromuscular disorders and abnormal psychological behaviour. Colicky abdominal pain is the presenting complaint in many cases, but fever is rare and the abdominal signs are ill-defined. Patients with porphyria may have been erroneously treated in the past for acute appendicitis, cholelithiasis, renal colic or acute pancreatitis. Recurrent abdominal crises can occur for many years before a diagnosis is made.

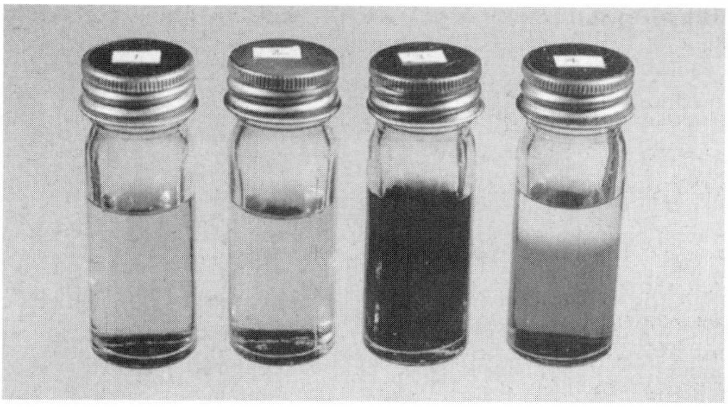

Fig. 27.58 Urine from patient with porphyria. The urine goes dark on standing.

The neurological damage usually causes vague neurotic complaints but occasionally patients may become comatose, confused or frankly psychotic. They may also develop peripheral neuropathy, neuritic pain in the extremities, paraplegia, quadriplegia and bulbar paralysis. The diagnosis is confirmed by finding porphobilinogen in the urine. The freshly voided urine is frequently normal in colour but on standing in sunlight turns to a burgundy or port-wine colour (Fig. 27.58). During a remission the porphobilinogen reaction of heating the urine with the addition of acid is usually positive, but a negative test does not entirely exclude the presence of porphyria.

Haemochromatosis

This is a disease of iron metabolism which results in an elevation of the plasma iron and saturation of the iron-binding protein transferrin, leading to iron being deposited in parenchymal cells in the form of ferritin and haemosiderin.[436] Increased amounts of iron are found in almost all body tissues, especially the liver and pancreas, and to a lesser extent in the heart, kidney, spleen and skin. Symptoms of haemochromatosis are related to skin pigmentation, diabetes, liver impairment and cardiac disease. Abdominal pain occurs in a number of these patients, and is only rarely severe enough to simulate an acute surgical emergency. The diagnosis is indicated by the presence of high serum iron and iron-binding protein levels and the definitive diagnosis is made on histological examination of a liver biopsy.

Hypercalcaemia

Hypercalcaemia may be associated with symptoms of muscular weakness, anorexia, nausea, constipation and abdominal pain (see Chapter 9). The site of the abdominal pain is variable and there are very few associated signs. Although it used to be thought that hypercalcaemia could cause acute pancreatitis, it is debatable whether this is in fact true.[437]

REFERENCES

435. Stein J A, Tuschudy D P Medicine 1970; 44: 1
436. Livingstone D J Scot Med J 1960; 5: 164
437. Shearer M G, Imrie C W Br J Surg 1986; 73: 282

Heavy metal poisoning

Lead poisoning is the commonest form of heavy metal poisoning to cause abdominal pain.[438] Arsenic and mercuric poisoning can cause similar symptoms. Lead is an accumulative poison that is slowly excreted from the body, and acute lead poisoning is virtually non-existent. Lead poisoning is caused by ingestion of lead-containing materials such as paint and water, or from the inhalation of fumes released by burning lead-containing substances such as solder or batteries. In the early stages the symptoms, which include vague muscular pains, lassitude and weakness, often pass unnoticed. Symptoms usually develop suddenly after chronic exposure. They include generalized abdominal colic, constipation and rigidity of the abdominal wall musculature. The colic is thought to be produced by tonic contractions of the small intestine. The attacks of colic may be exacerbated by intercurrent infections or alcoholic binges and are often not relieved by narcotic injections. There are usually no signs of infection or inflammation and abdominal examination is often unremarkable. Other complications include encephalopathy, peripheral neuritis and anaemia. The diagnosis is suspected when a blue line is seen in the gum around the margins of the teeth and confirmed by finding a raised lead level in the blood. The pain can be relieved by the intravenous injection of calcium salts. The exposure to lead should be reduced and penicillamine should be administered.[439]

NEUROLOGICAL CAUSES OF THE ACUTE ABDOMEN

Spinal disorders

Any disorder of the spine resulting in compression or irritation of a nerve root can produce abdominal pain[440–442] (see Chapter 46). Osteoarthritis, osteoporosis, disc degeneration, inflammatory conditions, neoplastic conditions and osteomalacia can all cause root compression. The onset of the pain may be gradual or acute when caused by prolapse of an intervertebral disc. The pain is usually positional and aggravated by movement or by coughing. It may be eased by adopting specific postures, especially lying down. The pain may be experienced on one or other side and is commonly associated with hyperaesthesia over the relevant dermatome. Abdominal palpation rarely increases the pain and examination of the back usually reveals the source of the pain, which is often associated with a limitation of straight leg raising. The diagnosis is confirmed by radiographs of the lumbar spine, isotopic bone scanning, myelography, radiculography, CT scanning or magnetic resonance imaging.

Tabes dorsalis

Approximately 10% of tabetic patients develop severe episodes of abdominal pain associated with nausea and vomiting.[443] These episodes, known as gastric crises, can last for several days and lead to dehydration. They usually settle spontaneously, and recur at regular intervals. Other signs of tabes dorsalis such as ataxia, Charcot's joints and an alteration in the pupils—Argyll Robertson pupil, meiosis, a poor reaction to light and a poor response to atropine—may indicate the diagnosis. This is confirmed by serological testing for syphilis, although in the later stages of tabes dorsalis the serology may be negative. This is a rare cause of abdominal pain today.

HAEMATOLOGICAL DISORDERS

A number of haematological disorders can produce abdominal pain. These include haemolysis, Henoch–Schönlein purpura, sickle cell disease, leukaemia, lymphoma, polycythaemia and disorders of coagulation.

Sickle cell anaemia

Sickle cell anaemia is a chronic hereditary haemolytic disease caused by the haemoglobin S gene. Haemolysed red corpuscles become trapped in small vessels, causing deoxygenation and a reduced pH, which in turn favours further sickling and increases blood viscosity. This leads to reduced tissue perfusion and in the long term may cause infarction and shrinkage of the spleen (see Chapter 34) aseptic necrosis of bone, haematuria, pulmonary infarction, disorders in the central nervous system, chronic leg ulcers and cholelithiasis. Affected patients often complain of episodic weakness, joint pains and chest pains. Between crises they usually adjust to the chronic haemolytic anaemia and require no specific treatment. Many patients with sickle cell anaemia are poorly developed, often with defective secondary sex characteristics.

During sickle cell crises there are sudden episodes of severe abdominal pain which are usually experienced in the epigastrium and associated with nausea and vomiting.[444] Patients may have a fever and an elevated white cell count with signs of tenderness and guarding in the epigastrium. The acute crises are managed by maintaining hydration and electrolyte balance and correcting any metabolic acidosis that occurs. The inspired oxygen should be kept at a high level.

Haemolytic anaemia

The onset of any type of haemolytic anaemia can result in an acute illness characterized by severe rigors, fever, malaise, headache, back pain and limb pain. Some patients also develop severe abdominal pain and marked muscular rigidity, simulating an acute abdomen. Severe haemolysis also causes hypotensive shock and anuria. Jaundice tends to develop rapidly and other symptoms of anaemia may also be present. A haemolytic anaemia is usually normocytic but may be macrocytic during phases of rapid blood regeneration when many immature cells are present. A raised reticulocyte count is usually present.

REFERENCES

438. Dagg J H, Goldberg A et al Q J Med 1965; 34: 163
439. Catsch A, Harmuth-Hoene A E Pharmac Ther 1976; Al: 118
440. Fernstorm U Acta Chir Scan 1957; 113: 436
441. Ashby E C Ann R Coll Surg Engl 1977; 59: 242
442. Carnett J B Surg Gynecol Obstet 1962; 42: 625
443. Harvard C W Br J Hosp Med 1972; 21: 443
444. Tomlinson W J Am J Med Sci 1945; 209: 722

Henoch–Schönlein purpura

This form of vascular purpura is characterized by serosanguinous effusions into the subcutaneous, submucous and subserous tissues. These are the result of perivascular inflammation. The pathogenesis of this disorder is obscure, although there is some evidence to suggest that it has an allergic basis.[445] It is more common in children and young adults. The haemorrhagic lesions in the skin vary considerably. They are usually located on the extremities and may be associated with allergic manifestations such as erythema and urticaria. The joint effusions cause swelling and pain. Severe abdominal pain is produced by haemorrhagic effusions developing within the subserosal layer of intestinal wall and these localized haematomas can lead to intussusception. Constitutional symptoms such as fever and malaise are present in most cases. The diagnosis is usually suspected because of the presence of skin lesions. If these are absent, the bouts of abdominal pain which may be accompanied by fever, leucocytosis and possibly melaena can be difficult to distinguish from other causes of the acute abdomen. Neutrophilia or eosinophilia may be present but the blood film, differential and coagulation tests are often normal. The diagnosis is made on histological examination of a biopsy taken from a skin lesion or occasionally by the characteristic appearances at laparotomy.

Leukaemia

Leukaemia can occasionally present with abdominal pain as a result of leukaemic infiltration of the spleen or liver. This can rarely lead to splenic infarction or even rupture. Leukaemic infiltration can also occur in the intestine, but in most instances this does not cause abdominal pain, although the involved bowel may very occasionally perforate during vigorous chemotherapy. Leukaemia is usually diagnosed on the peripheral blood film or on bone marrow examination.

Lymphomas

Abdominal pain can similarly be caused by lymphomas as a result of infiltration in the liver and spleen, but more commonly arises from disease in the retroperitoneal lymph nodes or involvement of the gastrointestinal tract. There is often evidence of recent weight loss and there may be signs of anaemia. A palpable abdominal mass may be present and there may be signs of small bowel obstruction. The diagnosis may be surmised if there are other constitutional symptoms or evidence of marked lymphadenopathy elsewhere. Radiological imaging may be required to demonstrate enlargement of the mesenteric or retroperitoneal lymph nodes when the disease is confined to the abdomen. Biopsy is usually required to obtain a histological diagnosis. The association of lymphomas with acquired immunodeficiency syndrome (AIDS) has increased the incidence of primary disease of the small bowel which may perforate or obstruct the affected segment.

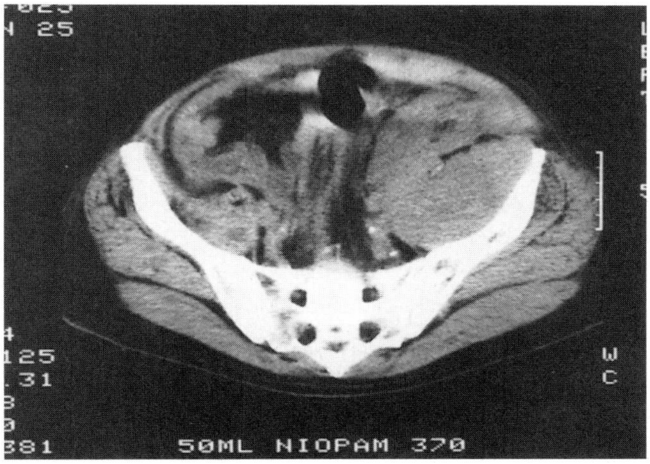

Fig. 27.59 A CT scan showing a large retroperitoneal haematoma.

Polycythaemia

Polycythaemia can give rise to abdominal pain by causing a thrombosis of the mesenteric vessels. Peptic ulceration is also more common in patients with polycythaemia. The condition is suspected from the patient's dusty-red hue which is most obviously seen in the lips, cheeks and nose. The diagnosis is confirmed by measuring the haemoglobin, haematocrit, red cell count and red cell mass.

Anticoagulant therapy

Poorly controlled anticoagulation can cause retroperitoneal bleeding which may present with abdominal pain. There is usually some abdominal tenderness on palpation and occasionally a mass may be felt. The diagnosis should be suspected when it is known that the patient is on anticoagulants, especially if the prothrombin ratio is elevated and the haemoglobin has dropped. CT scanning confirms the presence of a retroperitoneal blood clot (Fig. 27.59). The condition should usually be treated conservatively by reversal of the anticoagulation and if necessary blood transfusion, while waiting for the haematoma to resolve. Surgical drainage is rarely required.

IMMUNOLOGICAL DISORDERS

Polyarteritis nodosa

This is a rare condition in which there is necrotizing inflammation of the blood vessels of uncertain aetiology. The vasculitis can affect arteries, arterioles and also sometimes adjacent veins in any part of the body. Abdominal symptoms occur in 60–70% of the patients. Ulceration, haemorrhage, perforation and intestinal infarction can develop.[443] Many patients require laparotomy for these complications but the diagnosis may already be suspected if there are lesions in the skin or evidence of renal or cardiac involvement. Histological examination of the bowel, muscle or kidney usually enables the diagnosis to be made with certainty.

REFERENCE

445. Silber D L Pediatr Clin North Am 1972; 19: 1061

Systemic lupus erythematosus

This is an immunological disorder of unknown cause which predominantly affects women. Abdominal pain can occur when the vasculitis involves the visceral vessels and some patients progress to severe mesenteric ischaemia and infarction.

INFECTIONS

Infectious mononucleosis

Infectious mononucleosis or glandular fever is an acute infection most commonly seen in adolescents and young adults caused by the Epstein–Barr virus.[446] The characteristic clinical picture is one of fever, pharyngitis and lymphadenopathy. Splenomegaly occurs in approximately half the patients and is very occasionally complicated by spontaneous splenic rupture. Patients with hepatomegaly or splenomegaly can also experience abdominal pain, which arises from stretching of the sensitive capsules of these organs. The presence of a tender enlarged spleen or liver is confirmed by abdominal examination, and the diagnosis is made by a Paul–Bunnell test. On occasions this may take some time to become positive and may therefore have to be repeated.

Herpes zoster (shingles)

The virus responsible for this condition primarily affects the nerves of the skin. The thoracic intercostal nerves are involved in approximately half the cases, the cervical nerves in 20% and lumbar and sacral nerves in 15%.[443] The clinical presentation is usually with fever and pain over the affected dermatomes. A characteristic skin eruption develops over the involved dermatomes either at the same time as the onset of the pain or up to 4–5 days later. The pain may be very severe, sharp and burning or dull in nature. The skin usually becomes erythematous at first but then develops red papules that progress to vesicular, pustular and crusting eruptions over the next 2 weeks. The rash usually involves one or two dermatomes on one side of the body. In very rare instances the pain is experienced but the rash never develops. Before the skin eruptions appear, the severe abdominal pain and hyperaesthesia on palpation may be mistaken for an acute abdomen, although careful re-examination rarely demonstrates guarding or rebound tenderness.

Tetanus

The presence of pain, muscular stiffness and rigidity involving the abdominal musculature may mimic the acute abdomen (see Chapter 4). The clinical manifestations of tetanus follow an injury which occurred from 2 to 56 days before the onset of symptoms, although they usually develop within 14 days of injury. Non-specific symptoms such as restlessness, irritability and headache are the first to occur and the commonest presenting complaints are stiffness in the jaw, the abdomen and the back which is accompanied by difficulty in swallowing. There may be a low-grade fever, tachycardia, profuse sweating, brisk tendon reflexes and sustained clonus. Tetanus can usually be differentiated from other causes of intra-abdominal pathology by the presence of symptoms in other muscle groups.

DRUG-INDUCED ABDOMINAL PAIN

Quinine, chlorpromazine and primaquine may produce abdominal pain in the absence of other symptoms[447] and this may be mistaken for an acute abdomen. Oral contraceptives predispose to mesenteric venous thrombosis which can also cause abdominal pain (see Chapter 29). Corticosteroids can produce referred pain in the abdomen as a result of osteoporosis and crush fractures of the vertebral bodies.

MÜNCHAUSEN'S SYNDROME

There is a small group of patients with a strange psychological abnormality which leads them to feign symptoms and signs of the acute abdomen in order to fulfil a desire to expose themselves to surgery.[448–451] Many are itinerant drug abusers who crave attention and delight in baffling their medical attendants. The condition should be suspected if the level of pain appears out of keeping with the signs, if there are many abdominal scars or if there is a history of 'failed' operations, unhealed wounds or fistulae all occurring at another hospital. It is vital to obtain a clear history from the other hospitals visited by the Münchausen's patient as some do the rounds of many institutions before being found out. Psychiatrists appear to be of little help in managing this condition.

NON-SPECIFIC ABDOMINAL PAIN

This diagnosis is frequently used in the assessment of the acute abdomen when no cause for the patient's pain can be found. Many studies have looked into the possible causes in detail which have all been described under these 'medical' causes of the acute abdomen. It would appear that the incidence of this diagnosis varies between 30 and 45%[452] and therefore constitutes the single most common diagnosis which makes up the 'acute abdomen'. There is little doubt that a careful history, combined with a thorough examination and the appropriate investigations, including laparoscopy, can demonstrate a definitive diagnosis in many of these patients. It must be recognized that this is a diagnosis of exclusion, and when these patients are followed up important diagnoses may subsequently come to light, particularly in the elderly. De Dombal's work from computer-aided diagnosis revealed that 10% of patients over the age of 50 years who were discharged from hospital with a diagnosis of non-specific abdominal pain were later found to have an intra-abdominal cancer.[453] Half of these patients had primary tumours of the large bowel.

REFERENCES

446. Carter R I, Penman H G Infectious Mononucleosis. Blackwell, Oxford 1969
447. Oaton A Br Med J 1976; 2: 1179
448. Pearson K D, Buchingnal J S et al AJR 1972; 116: 256
449. Steligmann E, Singer H A Am J Med Sci 1936; 192: 67
450. Witherbee H R, Oearce M L Ann Intern Med 1958; 49: 876
451. Looff L J Med 1917; 294: 965
452. Gray D W R, Collin J Br J Surg 1987; 74: 239–242
453. de Dombal F T, Matharu S S et al Br J Surg 1980; 67: 413–416

28 Stomach and duodenum

R. C. Mason J. Fielding

INTRODUCTION

Surgery of the stomach and duodenum is currently undergoing changes as fundamental as those seen with the introduction of gastrectomy by Billroth and vagotomy by Dragstedt. Elective surgery for peptic ulceration has all but disappeared with the advent of histamine 2 (H_2)-receptor antagonists and proton pump blockers. The recognition of the important role of *Helicobacter pylori* in the aetiology of peptic ulceration further reduces the need for elective surgery. Surgery is now largely reserved for the acute management of complications of peptic ulceration, especially bleeding which is uncontrolled by interventional endoscopy. In the field of cancer, surgery still has a major role, although the extent of radical resection is currently being questioned, as is the role of adjuvant therapy.

CONGENITAL ABNORMALITIES

Congenital abnormalities of the stomach and duodenum, apart from pyloric stenosis, are rare and include duplication, atresia, diverticula, the presence of ectopic mucosa and megaduodenum or superior mesenteric artery entrapment syndrome.

In children with duplication, a cystic swelling is found adjacent to the stomach which can communicate with the gastric lumen. It can easily be removed.

Complete atresia presents with high intestinal obstruction at birth. This requires urgent surgical correction and bypass.

Diverticula of the duodenum are more common than in the stomach. They develop at the insertion of the ampulla of Vater in 60%, making cannulation of the bile and pancreatic ducts extremely difficult at endoscopic retrograde cholangiopancreatography (Fig. 28.1). They rarely cause symptoms and should be left alone.[1] Surgical excision can be hazardous, especially if the diverticulum lies within the head of the pancreas.

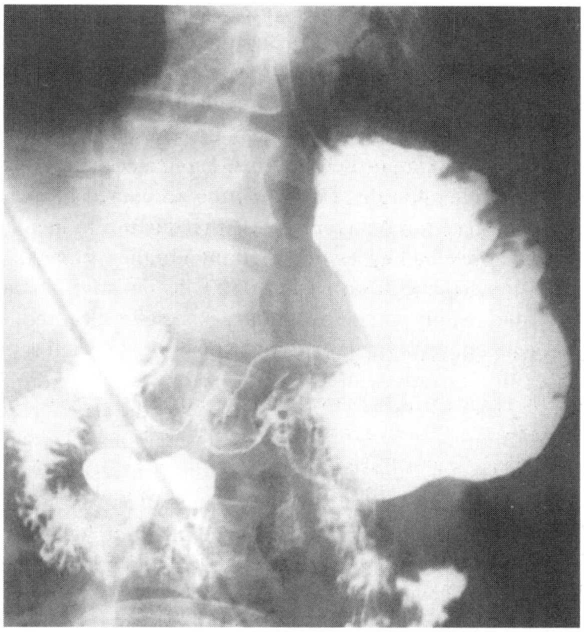

Fig. 28.1 A duodenal diverticulum.

Ectopic pancreatic tissue within the stomach wall rarely produces symptoms, although it can become inflamed and ulcerate. It may be confused with gastric cancer. Ectopic pancreas within the duodenum may encircle the second part of the duodenum as an annular pancreas (see Chapter 33), and is due to abnormal rotation of the ventral bud of the pancreas. Patients present with recurrent vomiting, obstruction and, in 20% of cases, peptic ulceration.[2] These symptoms are exacerbated by pancreatitis within the ring of tissue. Upper gastrointestinal endoscopy usually reveals no obvious cause, but the diagnosis can be made by barium meal which demonstrates a smooth constant constriction of the duodenum. For treatment, see Chapter 33.

Megaduodenum as the result of compression of the third part of the duodenum by the superior mesenteric vessels is another rare cause of high intestinal obstruction where the diagnosis is made by barium meal.[3] Treatment is as for annular pancreas.

The differential diagnosis for both these rare conditions is malignant duodenal obstruction from a primary duodenal carcinoma, pancreatic carcinoma, especially arising in the uncinate process, and renal cell carcinoma.

Congenital pyloric stenosis (see Chapter 41) usually presents in the third and fourth week of life as copious projectile vomiting and a failure to thrive. It rarely presents after 3 months.

The diagnosis is made by feeling a pyloric tumour as the baby feeds or by ultrasound examination, which can be successful in up to 90% of cases.

REFERENCES

1. Afridi S et al Am J Gastroenterol 1991; 86: 935
2. Thomford N et al Ann Surg 1972; 176: 159
3. Mansell P et al Gut 1991; 32: 334

Treatment is by Ramstedt's pyloromyotomy, but only after full resuscitation and correction of fluid and electrolyte imbalance. Feeding is recommenced within 12 hours of operation.[4]

Rarely, hypertrophic pyloric stenosis can present in adult life with vomiting and the finding of a smooth narrowed pyloric canal and no ulcer. The condition is relieved by performing a pyloroplasty[5] with either a vagotomy or acid suppression by H_2-receptor antagonists to prevent peptic ulceration.

PEPTIC ULCERATION

The true incidence of gastric and duodenal ulceration is impossible to acertain as the majority of acute ulcers never reach medical attention, resolving rapidly or being treated with non-prescription medications. Evidence from autopsies[6] suggests that approximately 20% of men and 10% of women have suffered from peptic ulcers at some time in their life. The number of patients presenting to hospital with complicated and uncomplicated peptic ulcers is steadily declining and this fall cannot be accounted for solely by access to H_2-receptor antagonists.[7] This reduction in incidence is not however matched by a similar fall in mortality. In 1990, peptic ulcers still accounted for nearly 4500 deaths in England and Wales[8,9] due mainly to complications, especially bleeding. Peptic ulcers occur more frequently in men than women and mortality increases significantly with age.[10]

Many factors have been associated with the development of peptic ulceration,[11–14] including socioeconomic class, stress, smoking, alcohol, duodenogastric reflux, ingestion of non-steroidal anti-inflammatory agents and steroids, burns—Curling's ulcer, neurotrauma—Cushing's ulcer and infection with *H. pylori*. The original observation that 'no acid equals no peptic ulcer' still holds true and all ulcers originate as the result of an imbalance between the production of luminal acid and pepsin and the ability of the mucosa to resist damage and repair itself. In duodenal ulceration, the imbalance tends to favour excess or inappropriate acid secretion, especially at night, and in gastric ulceration impaired mucosal defences are probably the major factor.[15]

Before discussing the aetiology and treatment of peptic ulceration it is important to understand the basic physiology of the gastric and duodenal mucosa. The factors controlling acid secretion and mucosal defences are summarized in Figures 28.2 and 28.3.

Acid secretion is stimulated by the vagus and gastrin by a direct action on the parietal cell or via their action on the intermediate enterochromaffin-like cell. Acid secretion is inhibited by the vagus and by the somatostatin cell under the influence of cholecystokinin.[16]

Mucosal defences fall into three categories: extramucosal, mucosal and microvascular. The extramucosal factors include the mucus cap and secreted bicarbonate.[17] It is now thought that the mucus does not form a sheet in normal conditions but forms ropes which coalesce when the mucosa is damaged to protect the repair processes outlined later.[18] Mucosal factors include the increased resistance to acid of the luminal surface of the epithelial cells, mucosal integrity and the presence of tight junctions between cells.[19] These are influenced by luminal growth factors which include mucosal integrity peptides (e.g. transforming growth factor-α) which maintains epithelial integrity, luminal surveillance peptides (e.g. epidermal growth factor) which acts via a receptor on the basal surface of epithelial cells and when damage occurs stimulates proliferation, and rapid response peptides (e.g. the trefoil peptides) which stimulate cell migration.[20] The most impor-

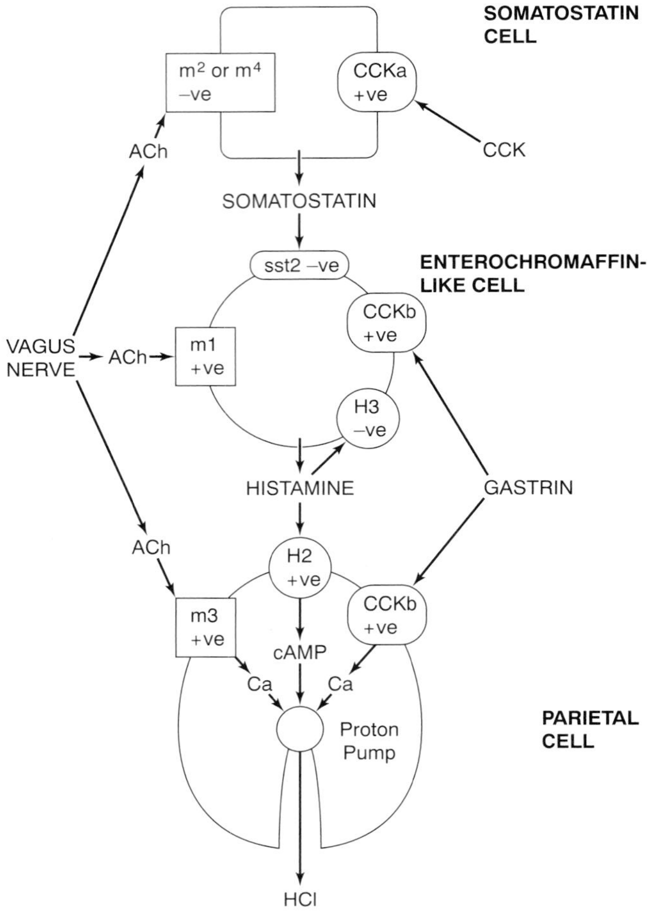

Fig. 28.2 Control of acid secretion by the stomach.

REFERENCES

4. Scherer C R, Grosfeld J L In: Surgery of the Oesophagus, Stomach and Small Intestine (Eds) Wastell, Nyhus, Donahue, 5th edn. Little, Brown New York 1995 p 164
5. Hiebert B, Farris A Am Surg 1966; 32: 712
6. Watkinson G Gut 1960; 1: 14
7. Kurata J et al Gastroenterology 1982; 83: 1008
8. Office of Population Censuses and Surveys Mortality Statistics 1990 HMSO London
9. Taylor T V Br Med J 1985; 291: 653
10. Beardon P H G et al Q J Med 1989; 71: 497
11. Langman M J S In: Diseases of the Gut and Pancreas Blackwell London (Eds) Misiewicz Pounder, 1994 p 249
12. Friedman G D et al N Engl J Med 1974; 290: 469
13. Griffin M R et al Ann Intern Med 1991; 114: 735
14. Rauws E A J, Tytgat G N J Lancet 1990; 335: 1233
15. Feldman M, Richardson C T Gastroenterology 1988; 90: 540
16. Hersey S J, Sachs G Physiol Rev 1995; 75: 155
17. Rees W D W, Turnberg L A Clin Sci 1982; 62: 343
18. Morris G P et al Virchows Arch Part B 1984; 46: 239
19. Sanders M J et al Nature 1985; 313: 52
20. Wright N A et al Nature 1990; 343: 82

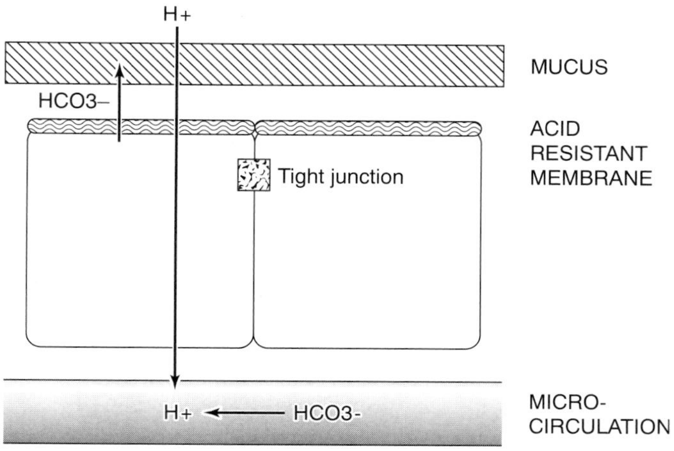

Fig. 28.3 Mechanism of the mucosal defence to luminal acid.

tant factor governing mucosal resistance is probably the microcirculation.[21] This is responsible for the alkaline tide which neutralizes acid and transports away toxic substances. Prostaglandins, neuropeptides and nitric oxide are important in maintaining this microcirculation and factors which interfere with them increase ulcer risk.[22]

Damage to the mucosa above the basement membrane repairs by a process of restitution in which cells migrate from the germinal zone to cover the defect.[23] This process does not require mitosis and can occur in 3–4 hours but is dependent on prostaglandins and an intact microcirculation. Deeper injury, breaching the basement membrane, produces an inflammatory response and healing is then by secondary intention which involves mitosis and in which epidermal growth factor has a role. This produces scar tissue and takes 4–5 days.[22]

Pathology

Peptic ulcers are characterized by an acute inflammatory response surrounding the ulcer with slough in the ulcer base.

Distribution

Gastric ulcers classically present at the incisura on the lesser curve at the junction of the body and antral mucosa. They can be divided into:

1. Type I—whose classical site is at the incisura.
2. Type II—which are associated with a duodenal ulcer.
3. Type III—which are prepyloric ulcers.

The latter two behave like duodenal ulcers.

Duodenal ulcers normally develop in the duodenal bulb. Ulcers occurring in the second part of the duodenum and beyond should raise the suspicion of Zollinger–Ellison syndrome (see Chapter 33). Peptic ulcers in the distal small bowel result from ectopic mucosa in a Meckel's diverticulum (see Chapter 29).

Presentation and diagnosis

Patients with peptic ulcer classically present with dyspepsia. Few patients with gastric ulcer however present with the classical picture of pain coming on while eating which is relieved by vomiting, nor do all patients with duodenal ulcer complain of hunger pain relieved by food, which may wake them in the early hours of the morning. Such dyspeptic symptoms exhibit periodicity and are more common in spring and autumn. Although some patients with peptic ulcer have symptoms which have little association with eating, on close questioning the majority of patients will have some association between their pain and food. When this link is lost and constant background pain and weight loss are present, gastric cancer must be excluded. The fact that early gastric cancer can cause symptoms similar to benign ulceration strengthens the argument for investigation of all new patients with dyspepsia prior to commencing treatment, especially if they are over 40 years of age.

Other and not infrequent presentations include waterbrash, epigastric tenderness and the complications of benign peptic ulceration. These complications include haemorrhage, which may be either overt as haematemesis and melaena or occult blood loss presenting with iron-deficiency anaemia. Patients may also present with an acute abdomen as the result of perforation, or gastric outlet obstruction causing vomiting or heartburn. The change of a benign gastric ulcer into a malignant one is now thought to be extremely rare. Such malignant ulcers were probably malignant all along.

Differential diagnosis

Almost any condition in the chest and upper abdomen can mimic the symptoms of peptic ulceration, including myocardial infarction, pulmonary embolus and lower lobe pneumonia. Common conditions include gallstones, pancreatitis, gastric cancer, gastro-oesophageal reflux, non-ulcer/non-gallstone dyspepsia, irritable bowel syndrome and mesenteric ischaemia.

Diagnosis

The clinical diagnosis of peptic ulcer is confirmed by endoscopy (Fig. 28.4). Barium meal examination has all but disappeared due mainly to the ability to undertake biopsy via the endoscope and is now only undertaken if endoscopy is contraindicated (Fig. 28.5). Multiple biopsies must be taken in all cases of gastric ulcer to ensure that a cancer is not missed. This is especially important in cases of gastric ulcer at sites other than the incisura. Whether all ulcers should be biopsied for *H. pylori* is debatable and will be discussed later. There is now no role for acid-secretory studies in the diagnosis of peptic ulcers other than in suspected cases of Zollinger–Ellison syndrome (see later).

Treatment

All uncomplicated peptic ulcers should receive medical treatment: the need for surgery in uncomplicated disease has all but disap-

REFERENCES

21. O'Brien P In: Splanchnic Ischaemia and Multiple Organ Failure Edward Arnold, 1990 p 145
22. Whittle B J R In: The Stomach (Eds) Gustavson, Kumar, Graham. Churchill Livingstone Edinburgh 1992; 81
23. Silen W, Ito S Annu Rev Physiol 1985; 47: 217

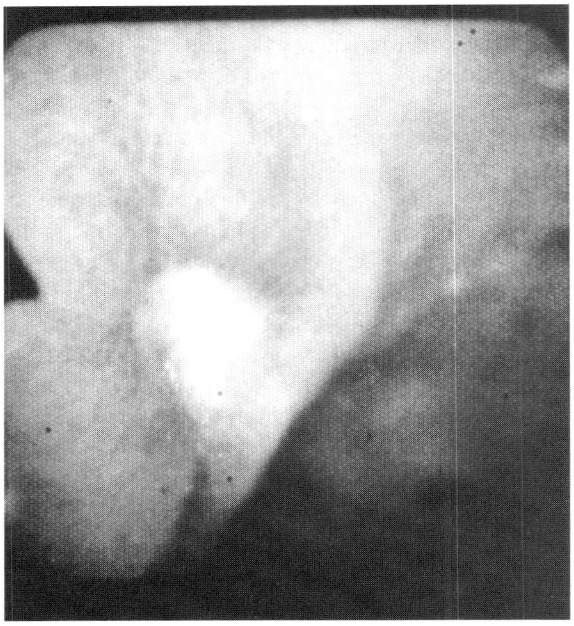

Fig. 28.4 Endoscopic view of a benign gastric ulcer situated at the incisura.

peared. Patients must be advised to stop smoking and if possible to avoid the use of non-steroidal anti-inflammatory drugs as failure to do so will increase the incidence of relapse.[24,25]

The drugs in common use are outlined in Table 28.1. The mainstay for first-line treatment is still the H_2-receptor antagonists.[26] It is now well-established that a once-daily treatment regimen given at night is as effective as multiple doses.[27] The use of proton pump inhibitors should be reserved for ulcers which are resistant to H_2-receptor antagonists or have produced complications such as bleeding. Although a combination of H_2-receptor antagonists and proton pump inhibitors will heal the vast majority of peptic ulcers, there is a small group of patients whose ulcers will not heal primarily and others that recur when treatment is stopped. For these, two avenues of treatment are indicated: maintenance therapy with H_2-receptor antagonists to prevent recurrence or eradication of *H. pylori* with combination therapy which may well heal resistant ulcers and prevent recurrence.[28,29]

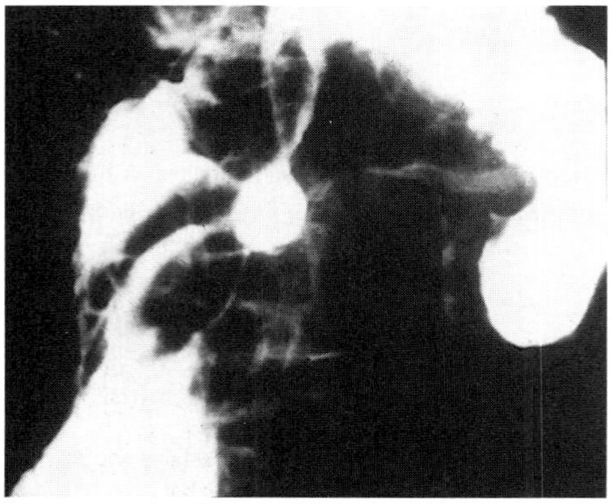

Fig. 28.5a Large gastric ulcer at the incisura.

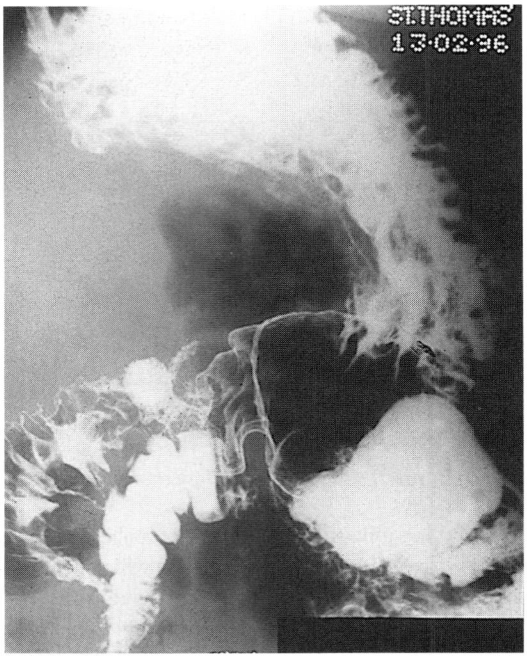

Fig. 28.5b A large duodenal ulcer in the first part of the duodenum.

HELICOBACTER PYLORI

The presence of spiral organisms in the gastric mucosa was first recognized over 50 years ago but the significance of this infection was only appreciated in the early 1980s.[30] It is an organism which has a worldwide distribution and its prevalence increases with age, with approximately half of the population over 60 years showing evidence of infection.[31] It is thought to produce problems as a result of its direct cytotoxic effect on gastric mucosal epithelial cells which produces an acute inflammatory response. It is also thought to produce hypergastrinaemia and hyperchlorhydria by interference in the somatostatin suppression of gastrin secretion.[32] The association between infection with *H. pylori* and acute gastritis is strong and antral infection can be demonstrated in over 90% of patients with duodenal ulcers and 66% of patients with gastric ulcers. The means of diagnosis are shown in Table 28.2. Eradication will increase the incidence of healing of the ulcer substantially and reduce the risk of recurrence.[33] The current first-line therapy for eradication of *H. pylori* is 7 days of omeprazole 20 mg b.d, amoxycillin 500 mg t.d.s. and metronidazole 400 mg t.d.s. (*British National Formulary*). The success for eradication is

REFERENCES

24. Taha A S et al Gut 1994; 35: 891
25. Sontag S et al N Engl J Med 1984; 311: 689
26. Pounder R C Baillières Clin Gastroenterol 1988; 2: 593
27. Chiverton S G, Hunt R H Baillières Clin Gastroenterol 1988; 2: 655
28. Jensen D M et al N Engl J Med 1994; 330: 382
29. Hentschel E et al N Engl J Med 1993; 328: 308
30. Marshall B J, Warren J R Lancet 1984; ii: 1311
31. Colin Jones D Dis Gut Pancreas (Eds) Misiewicz, Pounder, Venables Blackwell, London 1994; 261
32. Moss S, Callum J Gut 1992; 33: 289
33. Sung J J Y et al Am J Gastroenterol 1994; 89: 199

Table 28.1 Drugs in common use for the treatment of peptic ulcers

		Dose	*Acid suppression (%)*	*Healing rate (%)*
H_2-Receptor antagonists				
Ranitidine	8/52	150 mg b.d.	70	93
Cimetidine	8/52	400 mg b.d.	65	90
Proton pump inhibitors				
Omeprazole	4/52	40 mg	99	98
Mucosal protection				
Sucralfate	4/52	2 g b.d.		80
Denol	4/52	240 mg b.d.		80
Prostaglandin analogues				
Misoprostol	4/52	400 mg b.d.		50

Table 28.2 Tests for *Helicobacter pylori*

	Sensitivity (%)	*Specificity (%)*
Serology	90	90
13C Urea breath test	95	99
Histology	90	95
Urease test	90	99

in excess of 90% and should be confirmed by repeat breath testing.[34] This test is based on the capacity of *H. pylori* to hydrolyse urea labelled with the carbon isotope 13C to carbon dioxide, which is expelled in the breath.

Surgery for non-complicated peptic ulcer

With the advent of modern medical therapy for peptic ulcer the need for surgery has all but disappeared in modern surgical practice unless complications ensue. Indications for surgery include chronic unhealed ulcers, gastric ulcers which fail to heal after two courses of treatment where doubt occurs regarding the possibility of cancer, and peptic ulcers which present at an early age and require continuous full-dose medical treatment to prevent recurrence.[35]

Over the century many operations have been devised for the treatment of peptic ulcer (Table 28.3). Although these appear to have significant differences in mortality, in experienced hands little difference exists.[36,37]

In the case of gastric ulcer one operation has stood the test of time: the Billroth I partial gastrectomy (Fig. 28.6) in which the susceptible mucosa is resected and the stomach re-anastomosed to the duodenum. In cases of high lesser-curve gastric ulcer, a sleeve of lesser curve of stomach encompassing the ulcer is excised (Fig. 28.7). Billroth I partial gastrectomy has a lower recurrence rate than truncal vagotomy and drainage in treating gastric ulcer.[38,39]

Table 28.3 Operations for peptic ulcer

	Mortality (%)	*Recurrence rate (%)*
Bilroth I gastrectomy (GU)	1	1
Gastrojejunostomy (DU)	<1	40
Truncal/selective vagotomy and drainage (DU)	<1	8–10
Highly selective vagotomy (DU)	<1	10–20
Bilroth II gastrectomy (DU)	2	2 (stomal ulcer)
Truncal vagotomy and antrectomy (DU)	2	0.5

GU = Gastric ulcer; DU = duodenal ulcer

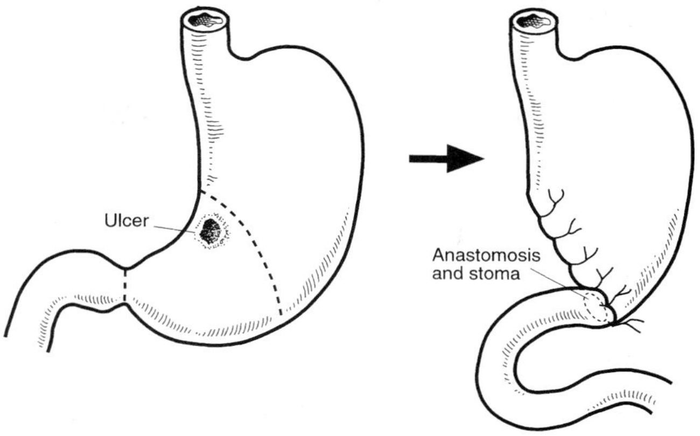

Fig. 28.6 A Billroth 1 gastrectomy.

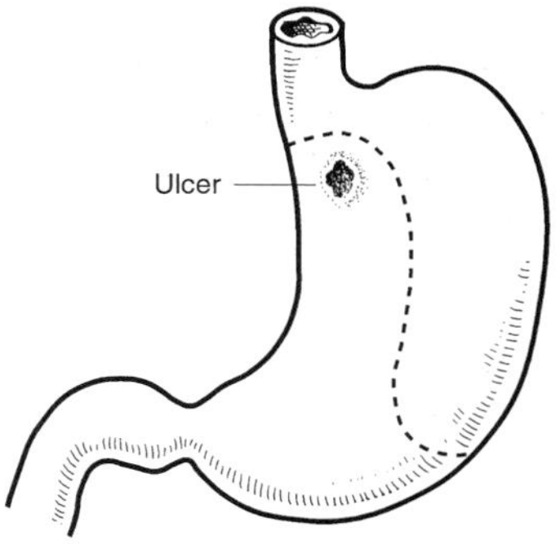

Fig. 28.7 Modification of the Billroth I gastrectomy for a high lesser-curve gastric ulcer.

The picture is more complicated with regard to duodenal ulcer. The aim of all the operations shown in Figure 28.8 is to reduce acid secretion either by reduction in the acid-secreting gastric mucosa (Billroth II partial gastrectomy), by resection of the gastrin-secreting antrum (antrectomy) or by denervation of the parietal cells (vagotomy).

The operation with the highest success rate for prevention of recurrence is truncal vagotomy and antrectomy with reconstruction by duodenogastrostomy (Billroth I) or gastrojejunostomy (Billroth II) or by a Roux-en-Y anastomosis (Fig. 28.9). This reduces acid secretion by 95% as compared to 70% for antrectomy alone and 65% for truncal vagotomy.[40,41] It is not however without significant morbidity and mortality and is usually reserved for recurrent peptic ulceration, bleeding and type 2 and 3 gastric ulcers.

In truncal and selective vagotomy, the total stomach (and gastrointestinal tract as far as the transverse colon in the case of truncal but not selective vagotomy) is denervated and they need to

REFERENCES

34. Hosking S W Lancet 1994; 343: 508
35. Taylor T V Br J Surg 1989; 76: 427
36. Golligher J C et al Br Med J 1968; 2: 781
37. Postlethwaite R W Surg Gynecol Obstet 1973; 137: 387
38. Thomas W E G et al Ann Surg 1982; 195: 189
39. Duthie H L, Kwong N K Br J Surg 1956; 44: 206
40. Kay A W J R Coll Surg Edinb 1962; 7: 275
41. Herrington J L et al Arch Surg 1977; 106: 469

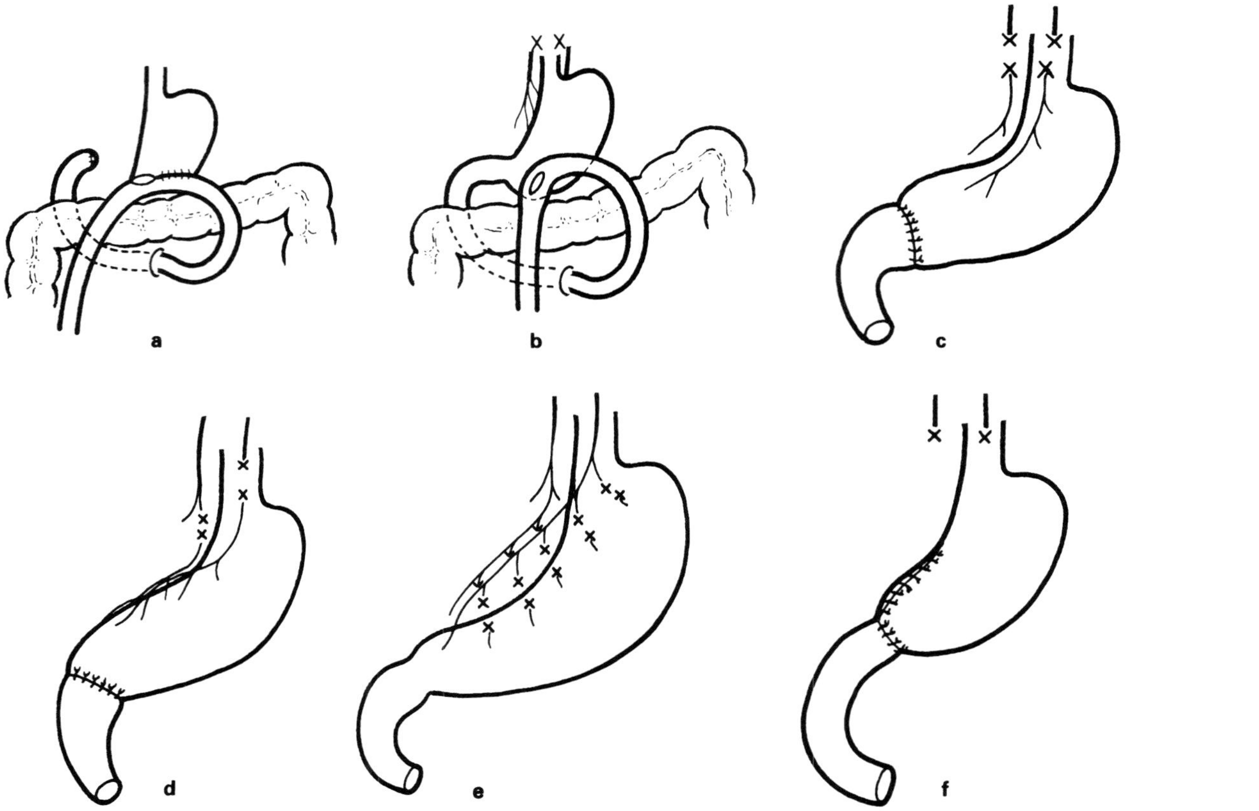

Fig. 28.8 Operations for duodenal ulcer: (**a**) Billroth II gastrectomy; (**b**) truncal vagotomy and gastrojejunostomy; (**c**) truncal vagotomy and pyloroplasty; (**d**) selective vagotomy and pyloroplasty; (**e**) highly selective vagotomy; (**f**) truncal vagotomy and antrectomy.

be combined with a drainage procedure such as Heineke–Mikulitz pyloroplasty or gastrojejunostomy to prevent gastric stasis which occurs in one-third of cases.[42] The gastrojejunostomy is best situated on the posterior gastric wall, via a window in the transverse mesocolon to which the anastomosis is sutured to prevent prolapse.

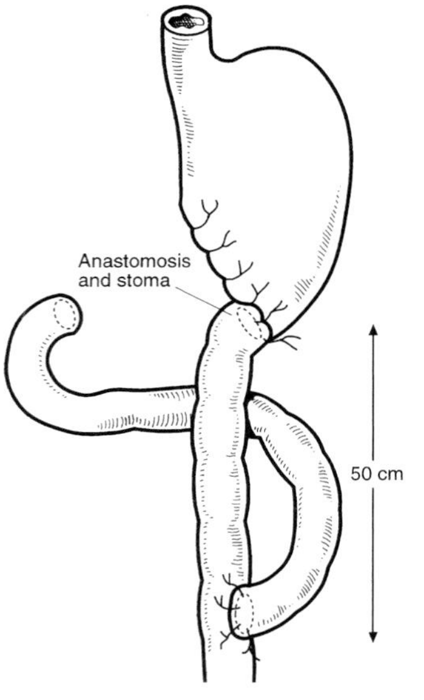

Fig. 28.9 Roux-en-Y reconstruction following partial gastrectomy.

The main indication for forming a gastrojejunostomy rather than pyloroplasty is when there is pyloric scarring.[43,44]

Billroth II partial gastrectomy is more frequently used for ulcers that develop complications but can be used as primary treatment of gastric ulcers if the ulcer is high on the lesser curve and insufficient stomach remains to fashion a gastroduodenal anastomosis.[45] Controversy exists especially over the size of the anastomosis and whether it is anti- or isoperistaltic. These factors do not affect the results of surgery.[46]

The most popular procedure for surgically treating uncomplicated duodenal ulcer is highly selective vagotomy in which denervation of the gastric body and fundus is achieved, preserving innervation to the rest of the gastrointestinal tract, especially the gastric antrum which is important for gastric emptying. This operation provides the best balance between ulcer healing and minimal complications.[47,48]

REFERENCES

42. Dragstedt L R, Schaffer P W Surg St Louis 1945; 17: 742
43. Goligher J C et al Br Med J 1972; 1: 7
44. Johnson A G Surgery of the Oesophagus, Stomach and Small Intestine (Eds) Wastell, Nyhus, Donahue , 5th edn. Little, Brown New York 1995; p 484
45. Fisher A B World J Surg 1984; 8: 293
46. Van Prohaska J et al Arch Surg 1954; 68: 491
47. Golligher J C Br J Surg 1974; 61: 337
48. Johnston D Br Med J 1975; 1: 716

There are several variants to the conventional highly selective vagotomy, the commonest being anterior seromyotomy and posterior truncal vagotomy. This combination is based on the observation that gastric emptying is the responsibility of the anterior vagal trunk. Its main attraction lies in the fact that it is easier to perform laparoscopically than conventional highly selective vagotomy.[49,50]

The relatively high recurrent ulcer rate following highly selective vagotomy has been blamed on failure fully to denervate the body and fundus of the stomach.[51,52] Various tests were designed to assess the completeness of vagotomy: the most popular was the Grassi test, which requires a pH electrode to be inserted via a small gastrostomy.[53] Most surgeons do not do this, preferring to adopt the maxim of being radical at the top end, clearing at least 5 cm of oesophagus and dividing the nerve of Grassi and being conservative at the lower end—the crow's foot. The lack of frequency with which such surgery is now undertaken strongly suggests that highly selective vagotomy should not be performed by an 'occasional' surgeon, for whom the recurrence rate will be unacceptably high.

Complications

Complications of peptic ulcers include ulcer recurrence, haemorrhage, perforation, obstruction, malignant change in a benign ulcer and fistulation into an adjacent viscus.

Recurrence

As mentioned in the earlier section on medical management, it is now possible to heal practically all peptic ulcers with a combination of H_2-receptor antagonists, proton pump inhibitors and combination treatment for the eradication of *H. pylori*.[54] It is also recognized that after completion of a course of treatment recurrence will occur in up to 80% of patients within 1–2 years.[55] This can be reduced to 10% if maintenance treatment is given with low-dose nocturnal H_2-receptor antagonists. The relapse rate is also reduced by removing the factors responsible for peptic ulceration, namely bad eating, smoking, ingestion of non-steroidal anti-inflammatory drugs (or combining them with prostaglandin analogues) and eradication of *H. pylori*.[33]

Recurrence of peptic ulcers after surgery is also a recognized problem and varies with the different procedures. After highly selective vagotomy the recurrence rate may be as high as 20% 10 years or more after surgery.[56] Recurrent ulcers even after surgery frequently respond well to medical treatment with H_2-receptor antagonists and rarely require further surgery. In the rare situation where the ulcer does not respond and if complications ensue, patients who have undergone previous highly selective vagotomy or truncal vagotomy and drainage are best converted to truncal vagotomy and antrectomy or, if adhesions prevent access to the oesophagus, a high Billroth II-type partial gastrectomy is an alternative, although it carries a higher mortality.

When recurrent ulcers occur after surgery and/or full-dose medical treatment, two possibilities must be considered: the retention of a small area of antrum after gastrectomy (Fig. 28.10) and Zollinger–Ellison syndrome. In the former this isolated pouch of antrum not exposed to acid will continue to excrete gastrin because of the loss of negative feedback on the G cells from luminal acid.

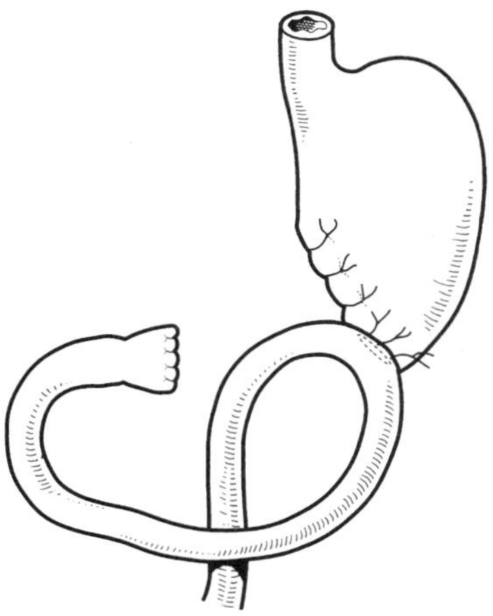

Fig. 28.10 Retention of a small antral pouch following Billroth II gastrectomy.

Zollinger–Ellison syndrome (see Chapter 33)

This condition is characterized by high levels of circulating gastrin and is the result of a gastrin-secreting tumour of the islet cells of the pancreas or, rarely, of the duodenum or gastric antrum. It often presents as intractable duodenal ulceration with a high incidence of bleeding and perforation. It is also associated with multiple endocrine adenopathy type 1 with an associated adenoma of the parathyroids in approximately 25% and hyperplasia of the adrenal and thyroid in 10%. The fasting gastrin level in the blood is in excess of 100 pg/ml. This on its own is not sufficient to make the diagnosis as any condition producing hypochlorhydria may produce elevated levels of gastrin (Table 28.4). The diagnosis is confirmed by acid secretion tests which show high levels of resting acid secretion (>15 mEq/h) which do not increase with administration of pentagastrin. Differentiation between a G cell tumour and G cell hyperplasia, in which high gastrin is associated with high acid secretion, can be made by the use of a secretin test in which a rise

Table 28.4 Conditions resulting in increased levels of serum gastrin

Pernicious anaemia
Atrophic gastritis
Medical treatment of peptic ulcers by acid suppression
Previous surgery for peptic ulcers
Excluded gastric antrum
G Cell hyperplasia

REFERENCES

49. Taylor T V et al Lancet 1982; 2: 846
50. Taylor T V et al Br J Surg 1985; 72: 620
51. Meisner S et al Ann Surg 1994; 220: 164
52. Jordan P, Thornby J Ann Surg 1994; 220: 283
53. Grassi G Surg Gynecol Obstet 1975; 140: 259
54. Fallahzadeh H Am Surg 1993; 59: 20
55. Penston J, Wormsley K Scand J Gastroenterol 1989; 24: 1145
56. Meisner S et al Ann Surg 1994; 220: 164

in serum gastrin (> 200 pg/ml) in response to a bolus of secretin (2 iu/kg body weight) is diagnostic of gastrinoma.[57]

It may be difficult to localize the gastrinoma as they are frequently invisible on computed tomographic scanning of the pancreas. In addition, selective venous sampling has little to offer. The best method of localization is probably intraoperative or endoluminal ultrasound or somatostatin receptor scintigraphy.[58]

Treatment is directed towards resection of the pancreatic tumour if it can be localized, as the majority of such tumours are malignant.[59] If the tumour cannot be found, blind pancreatectomy is not advised. Treatment is then directed at the target organ—the stomach—and acid secretion is suppressed by full-dose treatment with proton pump inhibitors. The need for total gastrectomy has largely passed.[60]

Haemorrhage from peptic ulcers

This complication is now the major cause of death from peptic ulceration.[35] It must be noted that bleeding can be overt—haematemesis and melaena—or occult, presenting with iron-deficient anaemia. It is vital to investigate the large bowel even if a cause is found in the stomach or duodenum as dual pathology may be present and cancer is a common finding.[61]

Acute and chronic peptic ulcers and erosions account for over 80% of all cases of upper gastrointestinal haemorrhage (Table 28.5). The other causes include gastric malignancy, angiodysplasia of the stomach, the Deulafoy syndrome, oesophageal varices, Mallory–Weiss tears, reflux oesophagitis, haemobilia, aortoduodenal fistulae and medical conditions resulting in thrombocytopenia and coagulopathies.[62] Factors from the history and examination (signs of liver failure—jaundice, ascites, history of peptic ulceration, ingestion of non-steroidal anti-inflammatory drugs, steroids and anticoagulants, presence of blood or melaena per rectum) may point to a diagnosis but it should be remembered that patients with known cirrhosis and varices are as likely to be bleeding from an ulcer as from varices.[63]

Management of upper gastrointestinal haemorrhage

The management is the same for all patients. The degree of shock should be assessed and the patient resuscitated (Fig. 28.11). This is achieved by placing a large intravenous cannula into the antecubital fossa and giving 1 litre of normal saline. At the same time blood samples are obtained for cross-match, full blood count (to exclude long-standing anaemia), urea and electrolytes and liver function tests, including prothrombin time. If the blood pressure does not respond to this fluid replacement, plasma expanders such as Gelofusine or Hespan are given and blood of the patient's own group or fully cross-matched is quickly substituted. In unstable patients more invasive monitoring is required and a central venous pressure line and urinary catheter are inserted. A nasogastric tube is passed to empty the stomach and check for evidence of fresh blood.

Table 28.5 Causes of upper gastrointestinal bleeding

Peptic ulcers and erosions	80%
Oesophageal varices	8%
Oesophagitis	5%
Gastro-oesophageal cancer	5%
Angiodysplasia	2%

Investigation

Upper gastrointestinal endoscopy is the most important investigation in these patients. Various stigmata seen on endoscopy can predict for the risk of further haemorrhage. These are an actively bleeding vessel, clot adherent to the ulcer base and the 'visible vessel'.[64,65]

Debate exists as to when endoscopy should be performed—either immediately or within 24 hours.

Endoscopy should be obtained without delay if the patient is actively bleeding, requires continued transfusion of intravenous fluid in excess of 350 ml/h to maintain a satisfactory blood pressure or has a high likelihood of oesophageal varices. Because of

REFERENCES

57. McGuigan J E, Wolfe M M Gastroenterology 1980; 79: 1324
58. de Kerviler E et al Eur J Nucl Med 1994; 21: 1191
59. Fraker D et al Ann Surg 1994; 220: 320
60. Metz D C et al In: Recent Advances in Research and Management. Karger 1995 p 240
61. Cook I J et al Br Med J 1986; 292: 1380
62. Holman R A E et al Gut 1990; 31: 504
63. Waldram R et al Br Med J 1974; 4: 94
64. Foster D N et al Br Med J 1978; 1: 1173
65. Storey D W et al N Engl J Med 1981; 305: 915

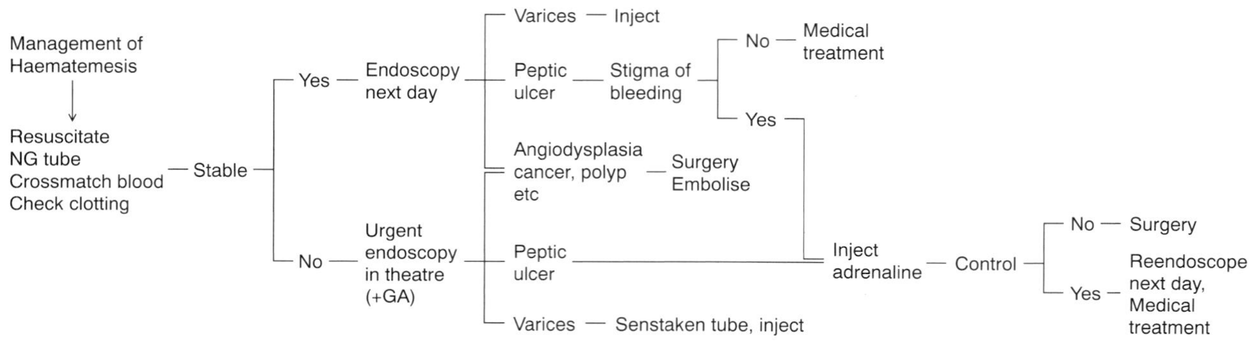

Fig. 28.11 Management plan for a patient with a haematemesis.

the risk of inhalation of blood and gastric fluids this should be performed in theatre with adequate suction and resuscitation equipment available or preferably under a crash general anaesthesia and endotracheal intubation.[66]

In 90% of patients, however, bleeding stops and the patient responds to simple resuscitation. In this situation it is safe to wait a least 6 hours for the stomach to empty and endoscope the patient under sedation on an elective endoscopy list.

In a small percentage of cases of persistent gastrointestinal haemorrhage, no source of bleeding is found on endoscopy. In this situation, rigid sigmoidoscopy must be performed and, if blood is seen coming from above, the patient is further investigated by radioisotope scanning with chromium-labelled red cells and, if positive, with selective mesenteric angiography[67,68] (Fig. 28.12). In young adults, when a Meckel's diverticulum with ectopic gastric mucosa is suspected, a technetium scan is indicated (see Chapter 29).

Treatment of bleeding from peptic ulcers

Medical

In spite of advances in medical treatment with the advent of H_2-receptor antagonists, no evidence exists that these drugs prevent rebleeding of peptic ulcers.[69] Despite this most patients receive 50 mg ranitidine intravenously on admission. No data exist on the intravenous use of proton pump inhibitors in this situation. Although no role exists in the acute phase, all patients should be commenced on a full course of medical treatment (preferably with proton pump inhibitors) and in high-risk patients, such as the elderly and those on ulcerogenic drugs, maintenance treatment for life should be considered.

Endoscopic

There are now several techniques by which the endoscopist can arrest haemorrhage from peptic ulcers and prevent rebleeding.[70] These include the use of a heater probe, laser to the ulcer and injection of sclerosants and adrenaline to the ulcer base. There are series showing significant improvements in outcome with all these techniques. The simplest and one that should be available in any endoscopy unit is to inject 1 in 1000 adrenaline (up to 10 ml) in and around the ulcer using an oesophageal varices injection needle. This technique is especially useful in treating Deulafoy syndrome—localized angiodysplasia where a single vessel appears through apparently normal mucosa.

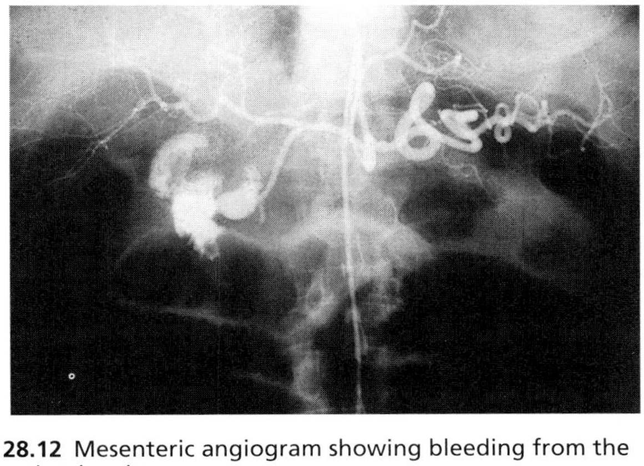

Fig. 28.12 Mesenteric angiogram showing bleeding from the gastroduodenal artery.

Radiological

In rare cases where the source of bleeding can only be identified on angiography, selective embolization may be possible, although care must be taken not to produce ischaemic bowel.[71]

Surgery

The decision about whom to operate on can only be taken by experienced surgeons. The absolute indication for surgery is persistent uncontrolled haemorrhage. Other indications include rebleeding and the presence of a large chronic ulcer with stigmata, which indicate a high probability of rebleeding, especially in patients over 50 years of age. If conditions permit, surgery in this latter group should be undertaken on the first available elective list.

The operation of choice for bleeding duodenal ulcers is to open the duodenum and under-run the ulcer with a long-lasting but absorbable suture such as 20 polyglycolate. This must be combined with an acid-reducing procedure such as truncal vagotomy with either a gastrojejunostomy if the duodenum is scarred or pyloroplasty if it is not. Advocates of a Billroth II partial gastrectomy can point to a slight reduction in rebleeding but expose the patient to an increase in mortality.[72]

The operation of choice for bleeding gastric ulcers is a Billroth I partial gastrectomy but if the patient's condition is too poor, exclusion of the ulcer with large polydioxone sulphate sutures can be life-saving.

Perforated peptic ulcers

The incidence of this complication is approximately 0.5% per year (0.8% males, 0.3% females), which compares to 2.8% per year for bleeding.[73] The patient usually presents with peritonitis, but there are a significant number of silent perforations found on erect chest X-rays, usually in old women taking non-steroidal anti-inflammatory drugs. These should be treated medically. The diagnosis of a perforated peptic ulcer is confirmed by an erect chest X-ray which demonstrates free gas under the diaphragm (Fig. 28.13). At least 10% of patients with a perforated duodenal ulcer do not have any free gas because fluid only escapes through the perforation. Patients usually also have a small increase in serum amylase (<100

REFERENCES

66. Whorewell P J et al Digestion 1981; 21: 18
67. Alavi A, Rung E J Am J Roentgenol 1981; 137: 741
68. Allison D J et al Lancet 1982; ii: 30
69. Haglund U Scand J Gastroenterol Suppl 1987; 137: 39
70. Steele R J C Br J Surg 1989; 76: 219
71. Eckstein M R et al Radiology 1984; 152: 643
72. Schiller K F R. Br Med J 1970; 2: 7
73. Pulvertaft C N Postgrad Med J 1968; 44: 597

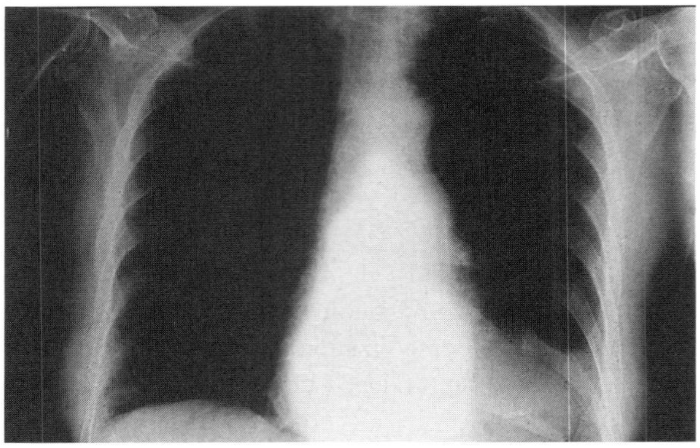

Fig. 28.13 Erect chest X-ray showing free gas under the right hemidiaphragm.

units per ml). The differential diagnosis is from acute cholecystitis, acute pancreatitis, perforated appendix and diverticulitis.

Treatment

The treatment is surgical, except in cases of silent perforations, as described above. The decision to operate is taken on clinical grounds—an acute abdomen, preferably supported by the finding of free gas under the diaphragm. The patient must be fully resuscitated before operation with intravenous fluids, a nasogastric tube, adequate analgesia and intravenous antibiotics (metronidazole 500 mg and cefuroxime 750 mg). The operation of choice for a perforated duodenal ulcer is patching with greater omentum loosely tied over the hole. This must be associated with full peritoneal lavage. Whether this should be combined with a definitive procedure is controversial. The majority of perforations are acute and not preceded by a previous ulcer history. These should be treated by simple oversew and medical treatment with intravenous ranitidine followed by long-term oral omeprazole 40 mg/day. Patching may be accompanied by truncal vagotomy and gastroenterostomy if a large chronic ulcer is present and the patient's condition is suitable.[74,75]

The use of the laparoscope to treat perforated duodenal is now being advocated. It is certainly feasable to close the defect with intracorporeal suturing but the extent of the lavage remains to be determined.

Perforated gastric ulcers should be treated by resection by either a Billroth I or Billroth II gastrectomy if the patient's condition permits. The ulcer can be excised if the patient is unfit, the defect closed and the patient treated with intravenous ranitidine followed by oral omeprazole 40 mg/day. In all such cases the ulcer should be biopsied to exclude cancer.

Complications of perforated peptic ulcer include intra-abdominal abscess formation, especially subphrenic abscess, prolonged ileus and associated haemorrhage.

Gastric outflow obstruction (pyloric stenosis)

Cases of gastric outflow obstruction from peptic ulceration present with weight loss and projectile vomiting. A pyloric stenosis may be caused by a duodenal ulcer adjacent to the pyloric canal or by a prepyloric ulcer of the gastric antrum. Patients with long-standing pyloric stenosis have a hypokalaemic metabolic alkalosis. This must be corrected with intravenous normal saline and added potassium. Once the hypokalaemia is corrected, the metabolic alkalosis corrects itself. A nasogastric tube is passed to empty the stomach, which may contain over 1 litre of gastric contents. Although lesser degrees of pyloric stenosis may resolve by medical treatment with proton pump inhibitors and balloon dilatation of the pylorus, the primary treatment is surgical. The operation of choice is a pyloroplasty or gastrojejunostomy if stricturing is marked. The addition of a truncal vagotomy is controversial. It will prevent stomal ulceration but may prolong ileus. If a vagotomy is not undertaken, the patient will require acid suppression by medical means for life. If the obstruction is of long standing, prolonged postoperative nasogastric decompression may be needed together with peripheral vein intravenous nutrition.[76,77]

Obstruction of the body of the stomach with large saddle gastric ulcers is a rarity and is treated by gastric resection.

Malignant change

Duodenal ulcers never turn malignant. Whether gastric ulcers do remains a matter of debate. If they do, the risk is probably less than 1%, although gastric ulcers initially diagnosed as benign may later turn out to be malignant as a result of the initial biopsy being taken from the wrong place.[78]

Fistulation

This is a rare complication of peptic ulcers. Gastric ulcers can fistulate into pancreas and transverse colon and duodenal ulcers into the gallbladder. They should be treated surgically as appropriate.

Post-gastrectomy syndromes

These now include complications of vagotomy, gastric resection and those resulting from the excision or bypassing of the pylorus. The presence of these complications together with the incidence of recurrent ulceration can be quantified using a Visick grade, which is a subjective scoring system based on patients' symptoms (Table 28.6).[79] The incidence of these complications is hard to quantify but they tend to occur more frequently in patients who have undergone gastric resection than in those who have had truncal vagotomy and drainage (Table 28.7). They fall into the following groups:

1. Deficiencies—malnutrition, anaemia (iron and vitamin B_{12}) and calcium deficiency.
2. Dumping—early and late.

REFERENCES

74. Griffin G E, Organ C H Ann Surg 1976; 183: 382
75. Irvin T T Br J Surg 1989; 76: 215
76. Lund O C et al World J Surg 1985; 9: 165
77. White C M et al Gut 1978; 19: 783
78. Mountford R A Gut 1980; 21: 9
79. Visick A H Ann R Coll Surg Engl 1948; 3: 266

Table 28.6 Visick grading

Grade	
Grade I	*No symptoms*
Grade II	Mild symptoms relieved by care
Grade IIIs	Mild symptoms not relieved by care but satisfactory
Grade IIIu	Mild symptoms not relieved by care and unsatisfactory
Grade IV	Not improved

'By care' is now meant medical treatment.
Grade IIIu and IV are considered treatment failures.

Table 28.7 Complications of surgery for peptic ulcer

	Truncal vagotomy and drainage (%)	*Billroth II gastrectomy (%)*
Diarrhoea	7	16
Dumping	11	14
Bile vomiting	5	10
Anaemia	27	38

3. Diarrhoea.
4. Disordered motility—delayed gastric emptying, afferent loop syndrome and increased risk of gallstones.
5. Duodenogastric reflux.
6. Gastric stump carcinoma.
7. Increased incidence of infection.

Deficiencies

Most patients who undergo any type of partial gastrectomy will fail to regain their preoperative weight.[80] This is the result of a small stomach and early satiety, together with rapid gastric emptying and intestinal transit. This usually improves with time and sensible patients alter their eating habit, taking frequent small meals and eating dry food separately from liquids. The need for surgical correction is rare. Any surgery should be delayed for at least 1 year and only be undertaken after full assessment by barium and gastric-emptying studies. An enteroenterostomy performed below the gastrojejunal anastomosis can help if there is a long afferent loop and failure of the food to mix with duodenal juices. Patients with a high Billroth II gastrectomy and tiny gastric remnant preventing any sizeable intake of food may be converted to a total gastrectomy with improvement.[81] Patients with malnutrition following a total gastrectomy and with a Roux-en-Y reconstruction may be improved by interposing a jejunal pouch between the oesophagus and duodenum[82,83] (Fig. 28.14).

Hypochlorhydria interferes with the absorption of iron and calcium. This can easily be corrected by dietary supplementation. Deficiency of vitamin B_{12} invariably develops after a total gastrectomy but can occur in patients who have undergone partial resection. This is corrected by 3-monthly injections of 1 mg hydroxocobalamin. This should be started before patients who have had a total gastrectomy are discharged.

Dumping

This is a disabling complication of gastric surgery which affects approximately a fifth of all patients after gastrectomy and a tenth of all patients following a pyloroplasty.[36,43] There are two main patterns of dumping—early and late.

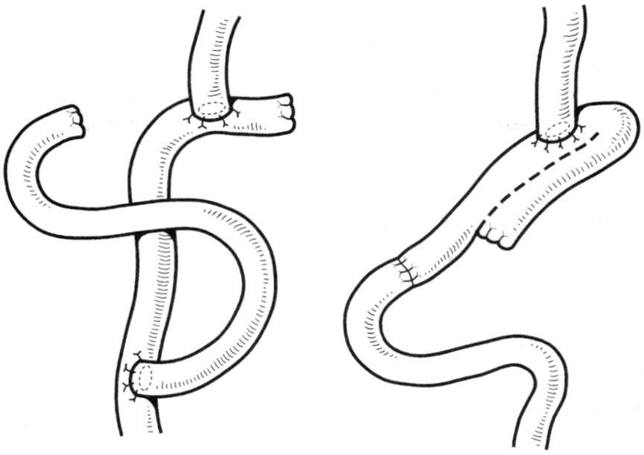

Fig. 28.14 Reconstruction following a total gastrectomy and Roux-en-Y by means of a jejunal pouch between the oesophagus and duodenum.

Early

This occurs approximately 30 minutes after eating, and is the result of the rapid gastric emptying of a hyperosmolar meal into the small intestine shortly after or during eating. This results in fluid leaking from the splanchnic circulation into the intestinal lumen, producing third-space loss and hypovolaemia, together with the release of vasoactive peptides. This causes weakness, faintness, dizziness, sweating, palpitations and a sensation of abdominal distension. Late symptoms include cramps and diarrhoea.

This can be confirmed by using a dumping provocation test which involves serial measurements of the haematocrit in patients given a provocation meal.[84] This usually improves with time, modification of the diet and lying down. There is no role for revisional surgery.[85]

Late

This results from an inappropriate hyperinsulinaemia after the glucose load has passed and comes on 1–2 hours after food and is the result of hypoglycaemia. This is much less common than early dumping and can be controlled by taking sugar. The symptoms are similar, with weakness, faintness, palpitations and hunger predominating.

Diarrhoea

Mild diarrhoea is a frequent problem after any form of gastric surgery and is usually self-limiting. Severe explosive diarrhoea associated with marked urgency occurs in approximately 20% of patients and may be the result of early gastric emptying or a small intestine which has lost the controlling influence of the vagus

REFERENCES

80. Tytgat G N J et al Hepatogastroenterology 1988; 35: 271
81. Eckhauser F H et al Ann Surg 1988; 208: 345
82. Cuscheri A Br J Surg 1982; 69: 386
83. Miholic J et al Ann Surg 1989; 210: 165
84. Linehan I P et al Br J Surg 1986; 73: 810
85. Sagar G R et al Br Med J 1981; 282: 507

nerve.[80,86] Investigation is by barium meal and follow-through. It may respond to medical management with bulking agents, intestinal sedatives or cholestyramine to bind bile salts. It is worth excluding steatorrhoea, milk allergy and giardiasis. Surgery in the form of reversed loops of jejunum or a reversed ileal patch in order to slow small bowel transit have been advocated but the results are disappointing[87] (Fig. 28.15). The risk of developing diarrhoea is substantially increased if a truncal vagotomy is performed in a patient who has previously undergone a cholecystectomy.[88]

Disordered motility

Delayed emptying

Many patients following partial gastrectomy or a vagotomy experience delayed gastric emptying in the immediate postoperative period.[80] This is a frequent problem following truncal vagotomy, antrectomy and Roux-en-Y anastomosis. This is probably related to the loss of the duodenal pacemaker and does not appear to be associated with the size of gastrojejunal anastomosis or, in the case of Billroth II gastrectomy, the type and direction of the gastrojejunal anastomosis. It is also a problem in patients with pre-existing pyloric stenosis who are treated by truncal vagotomy and gastrojejunostomy. Investigation by barium studies can be misleading as there appears to be a total obstruction at the anastomosis. The investigation of choice is gentle endoscopy at least 1 week after surgery. If there is no physical obstruction encountered at endoscopy, the treatment is to wait and feed the patient parenterally or to insert a long jejunal tube to enable enteral feeding. It can take up to 1 month for the stomach to empty satisfactorily for liquids and even longer for solids. The temptation to re-operate and refashion the anastomosis should be resisted. In this situation prokinetic drugs, of which cisapride 10 mg q.d.s. is an example, can be tried.[89]

Afferent loop syndrome

This results from kinking or too long an afferent loop following Polya gastrectomy. The obstruction of the flow of duodenal juices produces sudden epigastric pain which may be followed by massive bilious vomiting. It should be suspected if a smooth central abdominal mass (the obstructed loop) is felt and may be visible on plain abdominal X-ray. It may be associated with a raised serum amylase and difficulty entering the afferent loop on endoscopy. Differential diagnoses include acute pancreatitis and high small bowel obstruction.

It is corrected by fashioning an enteroenterostomy between efferent and afferent loops (Fig. 28.16).

Increased incidence of gallstones

This complication appears to result from decreased gallbladder motility following truncal vagotomy. It appears that up to 20% of patients develop this complication 5 years after surgery.[80]

Duodenogastric reflux

Any operation in which the pylorus is bypassed, excised or rendered incompetent can produce duodenogastric reflux. In the majority of cases, this produces no symptoms, but almost always produces some gastritis at the site of reflux.[80] Rarely, this gastritis goes on to erosions and bleeds, producing an iron-deficiency anaemia. In a small percentage of cases, reflux of duodenal contents produces pain in the post-prandial period and alkaline gastro-oesophageal reflux. Diagnosis is by exclusion of other causes of pain, such as recurrent ulcer, and can be confirmed by a provocation test.[90] This involves the passage of a nasogastric tube into the jejunum. Cholecystokin is given intravenously and the duodenal juice collected. The tube is withdrawn under screening into the stomach and acid, duodenal juice and normal saline are infused in rotation without the patient's knowledge. Revisional surgery can be contemplated if the patient's symptoms are repro-

REFERENCES

86. Condon J R et al Br J Surg 1975; 62: 309
87. Cuscheri A Br J Surg 1986; 73: 981
88. Taylor T V et al Lancet 1978; i: 295
89. Johnson A G Scand J Gastroenterol Suppl 1989; 165: 36
90. Meshkinpour H et al Gastroenterology 1980; 79: 1283

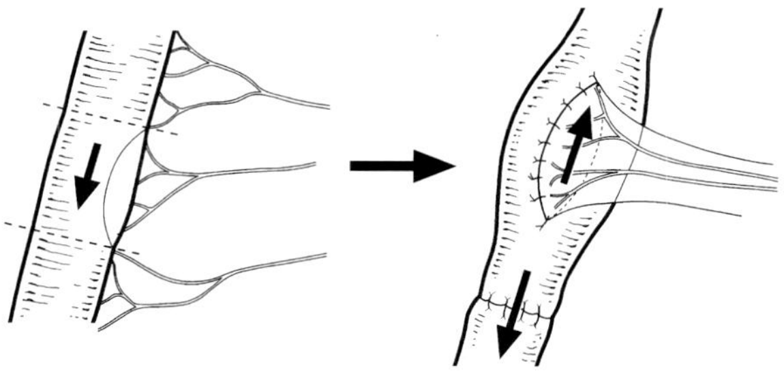

Fig. 28.15 Reversed ileal patch.

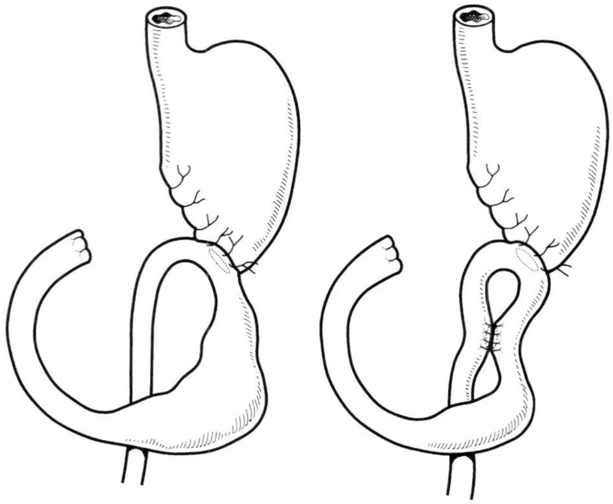

Fig. 28.16 Afferent loop syndrome—the afferent and efferent loops are anastomosed side-to-side below the gastrojejunostomy.

duced only by infusion of duodenal juice. This should only be carried out if medical treatment with cytoprotective drugs such as sucralfate 1 g four times a day or cholestyramine 4 g four times a day to bind bile salts have been tried and have failed.[91]

The pyloroplasty can be reversed or a gastrojejunostomy taken down in patients who have undergone truncal vagotomy and drainage. This should only be carried out after 1 year has elapsed from the time of surgery when the stomach has regained a normal emptying pattern. In patients who have had gastric resection, revisional surgery usually requires conversion to a Roux-en-Y anastomosis with a 50 cm Roux loop to prevent retrograde passage of duodenal contents.[92] This must be combined with a truncal vagotomy or lifetime acid suppression with omeprazelo to prevent stomal ulceration.

Gastric stump carcinoma

A serious consequence of duodenogastric reflux is an increased incidence of gastric cancer. These cancers occur at the gastrojejunal anastomosis at least 20 years after surgery. The exact cause is unknown but is possibly the result of chronic irritation of the gastric mucosa by duodenal contents.[93] It is now also recognized that following truncal vagotomy there is an increased risk of large bowel cancer, possibly because of excess bile salts reaching the colon.[94]

Increased incidence of infection

There is an association between an increased incidence of pulmonary tuberculosis and gastric mycosis and previous partial gastrectomy. This extremely rare complication is probably the result of loss of gastric acid which will kill the bacterium and fungus.[95]

INFLAMMATION OF THE STOMACH

Acute gastritis can follow any insult on the gastric mucosa by such things as drugs, spicy foods and acute infection with *H. pylori*. This will usually heal when the irritant is removed.

In patients on the intensive care unit, gastrointestinal haemorrhage can occur from acute gastritis which can progress to superficial widespread gastric erosions. This is the result of mucosal ischaemia failing to sweep away the hydrogen ions which have penetrated the epithelial cells. Prevention of this complication is achieved by maintaining a high intraluminal pH by intravenous ranitidine and coating the mucosa with sucralfate or neutralizing the gastric pH with antacids via a nasogastric tube. A total gastrectomy may be required if the bleeding becomes torrential, although the mortality of this is in excess of 80%.[96,97]

In contrast, chronic gastritis is characterized by a mucosal infiltration with lymphocytes and plasma cells. It is usually persistent and progressive to atrophic gastritis. In most cases this is associated with infection with *H. pylori*. If this progresses to intestinal metaplasia (type 3), in which differentiation is lost and which can be regarded as a form of dysplasia, an increased risk of gastric cancer appears.[98,99]

The link between the immune system and chronic gastritis has been established in those patients with pernicious anaemia in whom anti-intrinsic factor and antiparietal cell antibodies can be demonstrated. These patients have a fourfold increase in gastric cancer and should have regular surveillance by gastroscopy.[100]

Other forms of gastritis include granulomatous gastritis from Crohn's disease involving the stomach and hyperplastic gastritis in Ménétrier's disease.

In Crohn's disease of the stomach *there is* inflammation and ulceration may mimic extensive cancer. Biopsy is usually diagnostic if granulomata are seen and treatment is with high-dose steroids and H_2-receptor antagonists.

Ménétrier's disease is characterized by giant enlargement of the gastric rugal folds of the body and fundus of the stomach. The mucosa leaks large volumes of protein and there are reduced levels of acid secretion because of the loss of parietal cells. Patients present with atypical dyspepsia and hypoproteinaemia and, less commonly, iron-deficient anaemia as the result of blood loss. There is no increased risk of cancer and patients are treated symptomatically. Surgery in the form of total gastrectomy is reserved for the few patients with severe hypoproteinaemia.[101]

GASTRIC VOLVULUS

This condition is frequently symptomless and is a chance finding on a barium meal examination. When symptoms occur they are usually of sudden onset of vomiting and severe epigastric or retrosternal pain. It is invariably associated with a paraoesophageal hiatus hernia, especially if of the organoaxial type (Fig. 28.17). Treatment is surgical and involves repair of the diaphragmatic defect and fixing the greater curve of the stomach to the anterior abdominal wall by means of sutures or by performing a high greater-curve gastrostomy and posterior gastrojejunostomy.[102]

ACUTE GASTRIC DILATATION

This usually presents as a complication of upper abdominal surgery, especially splenectomy. The patient complains of shoulder-tip pain and hiccups. If not recognized, the patient can

REFERENCES

91. Meshkinpour H et al Gastroenterology 1977; 73: 441
92. Wickremesinghe P C et al Gastroenterology 1983; 84: 354
93. Clarke C G et al Br J Surg 1985; 72: 591
94. Mullan F J et al Br J Surg 1990; 77: 1085
95. Konok G et al Surg Gynecol Obstet 1980; 150: 337
96. Zuckerman G et al Am J Med 1984; 76: 361
97. Menguy R et al Arch Surg 1969; 99: 198
98. Ihamaki T et al Scand J Gastroenterol 1978; 13: 771
99. Jass J R, Filipe M I Gastric Carcinoma. Churchill Livingstone Edinburgh 1986 p 274
100. Tytgat G N J Diseases of the Gut and Pancreas (Eds) Misiewicz, Pounder, Venables, 2nd edn. Blackwell London 1994 p 221
101. Cooper B T et al Butterworths Intern Med Rev: Foregut (Eds) Baron, Moody London 1981; 141
102. Otterson M F, Condon R E Surgery of the Esophagus, Stomach and Small Intestine (Eds) Wastell, Nyhus, Donahue, 5th edn. Little, Brown New York 1995 p 697

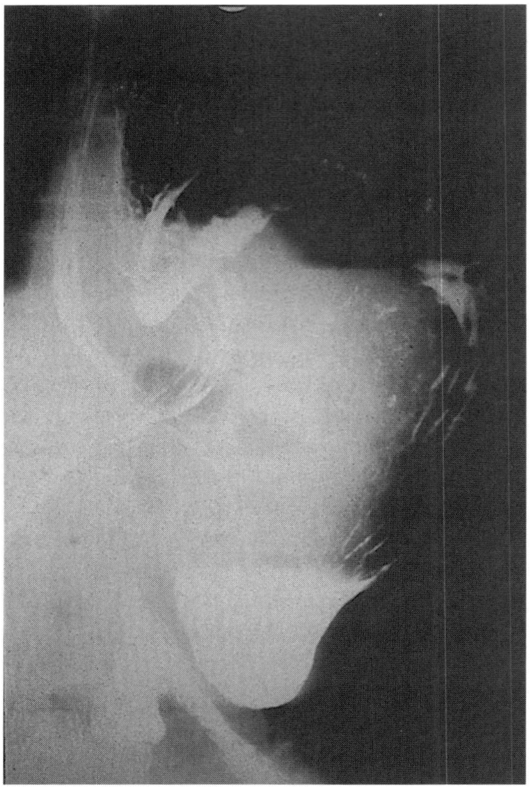

Fig. 28.17 Gastric volvulus with associated paraoesophageal hernia.

rapidly become shocked and may die from massive aspiration of vomit. Treatment is by passage of a wide-bore nasogastric tube. This condition can occur in patients suffering from anorexia nervosa and other psychiatric conditions such as depression, especially when they are prescribed large doses of psychotropic drugs.

GASTRIC BEZOARS

These can be composed of hair (trichobezoars) or vegetable matter (phytobezoars), which can be precipitated by gastric stasis post-vagotomy. Attempts can be made to break them up endoscopically or with pancreatic enzymes. If large, however, they will need removal by open surgery.

TRAUMA TO THE STOMACH AND DUODENUM

These organs are at risk from both sharp and blunt injury. In both cases the risk of injury to both stomach and duodenum is increased if the stomach is full at the time of injury. In all cases of gastric and duodenal trauma, care must be taken to exclude injury to other organs.

Sharp injury may be caused by either a stab wound or iatrogenically when a left-sided chest drain is inserted too low. Perforation of the stomach and duodenum by diagnostic and therapeutic endoscopy is virtually never seen, in contrast to oesophageal perforation. The patient will present with peritonitis and have free gas under the diaphragm on erect chest X-ray. In the case of a misplaced chest drain, the presence of gastric juice in the drain and the position of the drain on check X-ray—curved under the diaphragm—alerts one to the problem. Urgent laparotomy and primary repair are the correct treatment with gastric drainage either via a nasogastric tube or via a gastrostomy placed in the site of perforation.

Blunt injury to both is usually the result of deceleration injuries in road traffic accidents.[103,104] In the case of gastric trauma, the injury may be full-thickness with perforation or a contusion presenting with gastric bleeding, which may result in delayed rupture. Repair is dictated by the degree of injury and may require resection.

Duodenal blunt injuries classically involve the third part which is crushed by the seat belt against the spine. As the injury is contained retroperitoneally, diagnosis may be delayed. Such trauma to the duodenum is invariably associated with injuries to the pancreas. If suspected and if the patient is stable, contrast-enhanced computed tomographic scan is an important diagnostic tool. If such injury is found it must be repaired surgically and the stomach drained via a gastrostomy and the patient fed via a feeding jejunostomy inserted at operation.

GASTRIC SURGERY FOR MORBID OBESITY

Morbid obesity is defined as a body weight which is 100% greater than the ideal weight. Before contemplating surgery, endocrine disorders and hypothalamic lesions which cause obesity must be excluded. The need to reduce weight is based on the major increase in mortality associated with morbid obesity. There is a 14-fold increase if the patient is 100% above ideal weight.

The success of diet and psychological modification of eating habits are disappointing in this group. Early surgical procedures to help weight loss are either disappointing (jaw wiring) or have an unacceptable morbidity and mortality (jejunoileal bypass). Current surgical approaches centre on the stomach and are based on suppressing appetite by producing early fullness using a vertical banded gastroplasty (Fig. 28.18), or by a combination of reduced gastric capacity with malabsorption produced by a Roux-en-Y gastric bypass and biliopancreatic bypass (Fig. 28.19).

The importance of full medical and psychological preparation cannot be overstated and, in the postoperative period, patients need careful monitoring as they are at high risk of respiratory and thromboembolic complications. Patients often end up with a degree of malabsorption, and haemoglobin, iron, Vitamin B_{12} and calcium should be regularly monitored. Gastroplasty leads to a weight reduction to within 50% of the ideal weight in 23% of cases, compared to 55% for gastric bypass.[105,106]

REFERENCES

103. Courcy P et al Am Surg 1984; 50: 424
104. Hawkin M, Mullen J J Trauma 1974; 14: 290
105. Brolin R E Curr Pract Surg 1993; XIII: 8
106. Brolin R et al Ann Surg 1994; 220: 782

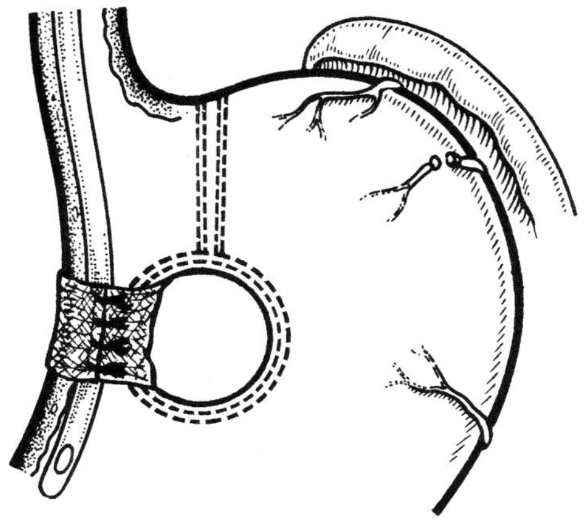

Fig. 28.18 Vertical banded gastroplasty.

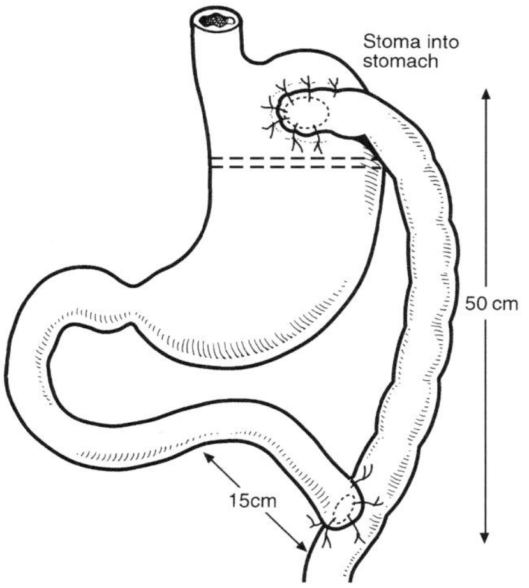

Fig. 28.19 Roux-en-Y gastric bypass and pancreaticobiliary bypass.

NEOPLASMS

Benign and malignant neoplasms originate from any of the elements that make up the stomach or duodenum. The most common neoplasm is adenocarcinoma of the stomach. As there is a relationship between benign and malignant neoplasms, it is appropriate first to consider adenocarcinoma of the stomach.

ADENOCARCINOMA OF THE STOMACH

Incidence and epidemiology

Gastric cancer is common, though there are international variations in incidence. Japan has the highest age-adjusted death rate, followed by Chile, Austria and Finland. In addition to international variations, the incidence can vary within a country. In the UK, the annual mortality rate is 23.4 per 100 000.[107] However, in Wales the incidence is higher (33.5 per 100 000 for men and 22.3 per 100 000 for women). In many parts of the world the incidence of gastric cancer has decreased. In the USA the annual stomach cancer mortality decreased from 28.8 to 13 per 100 000 between 1930 and 1955.[108] The highest incidence occurs in the 55–65-year age group and it is twice as common in males as females.

These variations in incidence implicate either genetic or environmental factors. A study of Japanese migrants to Hawaii demonstrates that the incidence of gastric cancer amongst first-generation Japanese is similar to that in Japan but the incidence in second-generation Japanese is significantly lower, although still higher than that seen in North American whites.[109] This alteration may be the result of environmental factors, but as the incidence is not that of the local population it leaves open the question of genetic influences. Insured patients with a family history of gastric cancer have a mortality about a third greater than other insured persons, and the risk of stomach cancer is four times greater than among the relatives of non-cancer patients.[110] Gastric cancer is more common in patients with blood group A in the UK but in Japan is associated with blood group B.[111,112] The existence of a relationship with social class is well-established, with the incidence being highest in social classes 3–5.[113]

Aetiology

The role of diet is unclear in the genesis of gastric cancer. In the USA the intake of beef, milk, citrus fruit and green vegetables has increased, whilst that of potatoes has decreased. In Japan striking changes in the incidence of gastric cancer have been associated with changes in diet, with a 28-fold increase of consumption of milk products and a significant inverse relationship between the increase in fatty food and vitamin A and the intake of yellow and green vegetables.[114]

There is also a link with ingestion of nitrate and a role for nitrate-reducing organisms in the hypochlorhydric stomach associated with increased risk of gastric cancer. The Correa hypothesis links the ingestion of nitrate reduced by bacteria to nitrite which combines with dietary amines to form nitrosamines—potent carcinogens. Vitamin C, found in fresh fruit and vegetables, inhibits the bacterial reduction of nitrate as well as being an antioxidant.[115]

There is now increasing evidence to link the presence of infection with *H. pylori* and increased incidence of stomach cancer, possibly via its role in producing inflammation and chronic gastritis.[116]

Pathology

Precancerous conditions and lesions

Polyps

Polyps arise in the gastric mucosa and are either hyperplastic or adenomatous. Hyperplastic polyps are covered with well-differen-

REFERENCES

107. Mortality Statistics Series DH2 no. 7. OPCS HMSO, London 1980
108. Haenszel W T J Natl Cancer Inst 1958; 21: 213
109. Haenszel W, Karibaru M J Natl Cancer Inst 1968; 40: 43
110. Lehtola J Scand J Gastroenterol 1978; 13 (Suppl 50)
111. Aird I et al Br Med J 1953; 1: 799
112. Hirayama T Early Gastric Cancer. University of Tokyo Press, Tokyo 1971
113. Stukons M, Doll R Int J Cancer 1969; 4: 248
114. Advances in Bioscience, vol 32. Pergamon Press London 1981
115. Correa P et al Lancet 1975; 2: 58
116. Correa P Cancer Res 1992; 52: 6735

tiated glands and the incidence of malignant change is rare. In adenomas the epithelium may be dysplastic and malignant change occurs in 18–75% of these. If the polyp is greater than 2 cm the incidence of malignant change is increased.[117]

Gastric ulcer

It is now felt that the incidence of malignant change in a benign gastric ulcer is extremely rare, and probably represents an error in diagnosis, with the endoscopic biopsy of the ulcer missing the cancer. In a large Japanese series the incidence of gastric cancer was 7.2% amongst 1286 patients with gastric ulcer, with only 2% of 2180 gastric ulcers detected on screening being malignant.[118]

Chronic gastritis

This is frequently found in association with gastric cancer. A total of 94% of superficial cancers are found in areas of gastritis, and carcinomas have been found in 10% of patients with chronic gastritis and intestinal metaplasia.[119] Chronic gastritis can be classified as autoimmune, hypersecretory and environmental, which is associated with infection with *H. pylori*.

Autoimmune gastritis is the gastritis of pernicious anaemia. The inflammatory process involves the body and fundus diffusely, leaving the antrum intact. This type of gastritis increases in prevalence and severity with age and is found more frequently in men than in women. Intestinal metaplasia commonly accompanies autoimmune gastritis and, as it is subject to dysplastic transformation (type 3), there is a high risk of malignancy.[99] Characteristically, when cancers develop they do so in the body of the stomach.

Hypersecretory gastritis is found in association with an ulcer. Histologically there is distortion of the glandular epithelium but no significant intestinal metaplasia or association with malignant change.

Environmental chronic gastritis is prevalent in some parts of the world. Its geographical distribution matches areas where there is a high risk of the intestinal type of gastric cancer. The changes in the gastric mucosa occur early in life, developing by the age of 25 years.[120] For populations with a low incidence of gastric cancer, chronic gastritis is found in less than 20%. This rises to 70% in areas of high incidence. This form of gastritis has a characteristic distribution: it is multifocal and involves the antrum and body of the stomach.[121] The earliest changes appear on the lesser curve below the incisura. Histologically, the milder areas of inflammation show the characteristic changes of acute gastritis with a dense inflammatory exudate below the lamina propria. As it progresses, atrophy of the mucosa develops, with a progressive loss of gastric glands. Regeneration produces an intestinal-type mucosa which undergoes dysplasia—intestinal metaplasia type 3.[99] This progresses to intestinal-type cancer.

The diffuse type of adenocarcinoma is not accompanied by gastritis. Differentiation of gastric carcinoma into intestinal and diffuse types is helpful when related to gastritis and geographical variations. The lack of gastritis in the diffuse lesions makes the relationship unclear. It may be that dysplasia is the important feature, as this can occur in foveolar epithelium as well as intestinal metaplasia, and it may be the important premalignant mucosal change.[122]

Macroscopic features

Until the last decade, the most common site for gastric cancer was the antrum, mirroring the distribution of chronic gastritis described above. It has become apparent in recent years that the distribution is changing, with a significant increase of cardia tumours.[123] The incidence has increased over 10-fold and is the fastest increasing cancer in the gastrointestinal tract. Histologically this is intestinal in type and the reason for this is not clear. Macroscopically, gastric cancer can be polypoid, ulcerative, stenotic or diffuse—linitis plastica.

Microscopic features

Gastric cancer can be classified on the basis of its histological appearance into well, moderately or poorly differentiated types. The most valuable classification is that described by Lauren into intestinal and diffuse types:[124] the former are composed of malignant glands and the latter of small groups or single cells. When such cells contain significant intracellular mucus, displacing the nucleus to one side, they are called signet-ring cancers. The prognosis of intestinal-type cancers is better than the diffuse type.[125]

THE SPREAD OF CANCER IN THE STOMACH

In 1932, Carnett & Howell[126] described the mechanisms of dissemination of gastric cancer as direct extension into adjacent organs, lymphatic embolization, lymphatic permeation, blood stream embolization and transplantation. Gastric cancer may spread luminally into the duodenum and oesophagus. It is not true that the pylorus is the invariable limit of distal spread. Duodenal involvement occurs in 24–30% of all gastric cancers.[127]

Lymph node metastases are common. The distribution of the nodes is shown in Table 28.8 and Figure 28.20. They have been simplified into two groups: N1, or within 3 cm of the primary growth: all others are classified as N2. Para-aortic nodes are classified as distant metastases.

Clinical features

Symptoms

All patients with gastric cancer develop symptoms, yet the diagnosis is often only made when the disease is advanced. The first symptoms are those of dyspepsia, epigastric pain, vomiting,

REFERENCES

117. Ming E C Gastrointest Radiol 1976; 1: 121
118. Yamagatu S, Hisamichi S World J Surg 1979; 3: 671
119. Freisen G et al Surgery 1962; 51: 300
120. Correa P Frontiers of Gastrointestinal Research. The Stomach. Karger 1980
121. Anatoli D A, Goldman H Cancer 1982; 50: 775
122. Morson B C et al J Clin Pathol 1968; 33: 711
123. Pera M et al Gastroenterology 1993; 104: 510
124. Lauren P Acta Pathol Microbiol Scand 1965; 64: 31
125. Ming S C Gastric Carcinoma. Churchill Livingstone Edinburgh 1986 p 197
126. Carnett J B, Howell J C Surg Clin North Am 1932; 12: 1351
127. Zinniger M, Collin W Ann Surg 1949; 130: 557

Table 28.8 Lymph node groups in gastric cancer

Site of primary lesion	*N1 nodes**	*N2 nodes*
Upper third	Left cardiac (1) Right cardiac (2) Lesser curve (3) Greater curve (4)	Supra- and infrapyloric (5, 6) Left gastric (7) Common hepatic (8) Splenic artery (9) Splenic hilum (10) Coeliac axis (11)
Middle third	Right gastric (12) Lesser curve (3) Greater curve (4) Supra- and infra pyloric (5, 6)	Splenic artery (9) Splenic hilum (10) Left cardiac (1) Left gastric (7) Common hepatic (8) Coeliac axis (11)
Lower third	Lesser curve (3) Greater curve (4) Supra- and infra pyloric (5, 6)	Right cardiac (2) Left gastric (7) Common hepatic (8) Coeliac axis (11)

*N1 nodes are within 3 cm of the primary; nodes in any of these groups more than 3 cm away become N2 nodes. Numbers in parentheses represent the node groups shown in Figure 28.20.

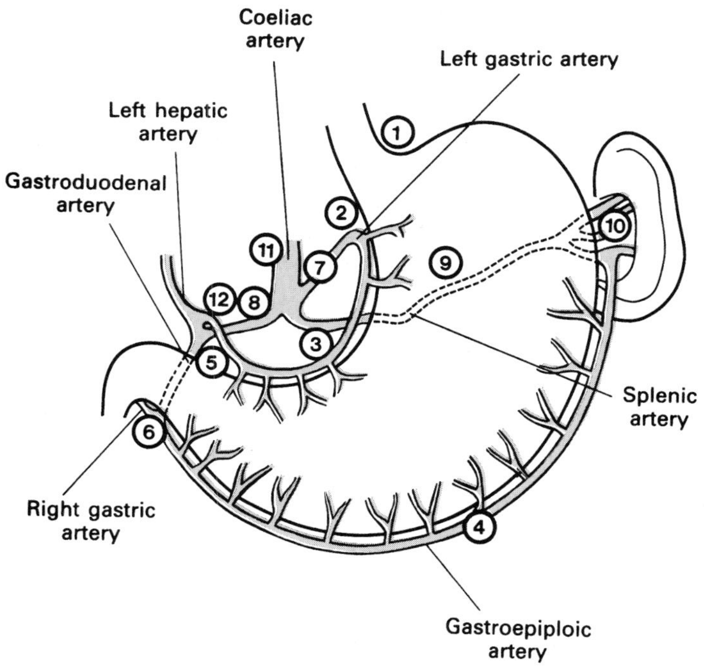

Fig. 28.20 N1 and N2 groups of gastric lymph nodes.

dysphagia and bleeding.[128] These are often impossible to differentiate on clinical grounds from benign peptic ulceration and the temptation to treat patients medically without confirmation of the diagnosis should be resisted as these symptoms in early gastric cancer may disappear with acid-reducing treatment. Only later in the disease do the constitutional effects of anorexia, malaise, weight loss and anaemia occur, with the recurrence of epigastric pain, which has lost its association with food.

Physical signs

The diagnosis should be made before any physical signs are apparent. The presence of a mass indicates spread to the omentum, and a palpable liver, ascites and jaundice implies extensive secondary spread either to the liver or portal nodes. The presence of a Virkov's node, which can be confirmed on fine-needle aspiration cytology, is diagnostic of advanced disease.

Differential diagnosis

This includes benign conditions, such as peptic ulcer gastritis and Crohn's disease of the stomach, and malignant conditions, such as oesophageal and pancreatic cancer, together with gastric lymphoma and leiomyosarcoma. The generalized presentation of gastric cancer—anorexia, anaemia and aesthenia—can be mimicked by cancer of the bronchus and right colon, together with pernicious anaemia, hypercalcaemia and uraemia.

Diagnosis

The diagnosis is invariably made by endoscopy with multiple biopsy of all suspicious lesions. Barium meal should be undertaken if endoscopy is apparently normal but the element of suspicion high. It is possible to miss linitis plastica on endoscopy as the tumour spreads in the submucosa and shallow biopsies may not be diagnostic. An inability to inflate the stomach should arouse suspicions and barium meal is diagnostic, although it cannot differentiate between linitis plastica and lymphoma (Fig. 28.21). The combined accuracy of endoscopy and barium studies is 98%.[129]

Screening

The Japanese have extensive experience of mass screening with indirect radiology followed by endoscopy. This significantly increases the incidence of stage 1 disease, reducing the death rate by 25%.[130]

Treatment

Ian Aird in the first edition of this book stated that: 'the only treatment which offers any prospect of cure is gastrectomy': nothing new has evolved to challenge this approach. Surgery for gastric cancer should accommodate the following factors:

1. The stage of disease at time of presentation.
2. The pattern of spread of disease.
3. The pattern of failure after resection.
4. The influence of resection on postoperative mortality and long-term survival.

Stage of disease at presentation

Of the current imaging techniques, computed tomographic scanning and endoluminal ultrasound offer the best means of staging

REFERENCES

128. Swynnerton B F, Truelove S C Br Med J 1952; 1: 287
129. Nagao F, Takahishi M D World J Surg 1979; 3: 693
130. Hirayama T Textbook of Gastroenterology (Eds) Bouchier, Allan, Hodgson, Keighley. Baillière Tindall London 1984

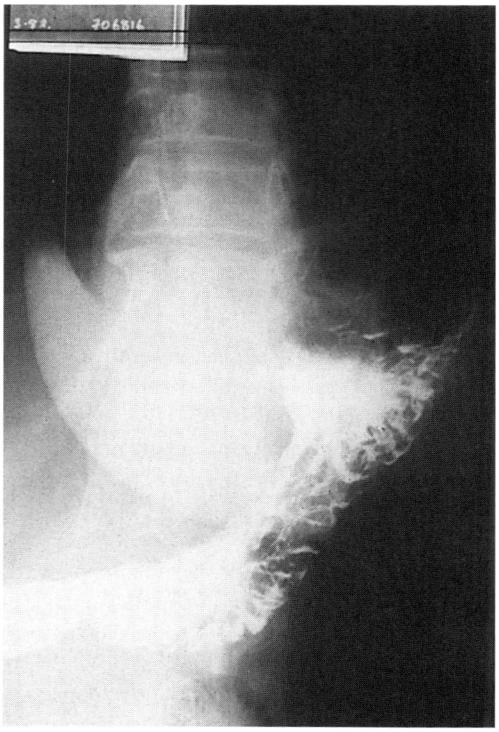

Fig. 28.21 A barium meal demonstrating linitis plastica with poor gastric distension.

the disease preoperatively; the two techniques complement each other.[131,132] Computed tomographic scans can detect liver metastasis, significant thickening of the gastric wall (Fig. 28.22) and lymph nodes over 1 cm in size. The degree of invasion of the gastric wall can best be assessed by endoluminal ultrasound, which will also detect lymph nodes adjacent to the gastric wall, particularly left gastric nodes. Laparoscopy may be of value in detecting small liver metastases and peritoneal deposits.[133] Laparotomy will often however provide the only means of assessing the disease.

Patterns of spread

Patients who demonstrate features of dissemination or blood stream embolization such as those with liver or lung secondaries are only suitable for palliation. Curative resection is only applicable in patients with tumours confined to the stomach and the N1 and N2 nodes.

Patterns of failure after resection

This has important implications for curative surgery. Recurrence occurs in the gastric remnant in 10–50% of cases—an argument for total gastrectomy.[134] The reported 5-year survival rate following a total gastrectomy as a routine operation for gastric cancer is not however significantly better than that for subtotal resections. Gundosa & Sosin found that 53% of reoperated cases had recurrent disease either in the gastric remnant or in the gastric bed.[135]

The value of lymphadenectomy is controversial: recent European trials have shown little benefit between a D2 resection which removes all N2 nodes and D1 resection, in which N1 nodes

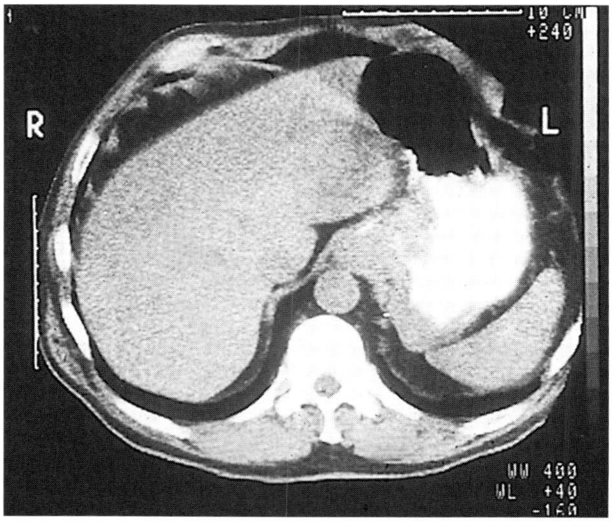

Fig. 28.22 A computed tomographic scan of the stomach demonstrating a carcinoma of the lesser curve with significant thickening of the gastric wall.

and some N2 nodes are removed.[136] The increased mortality associated with a D2 resection is largely related to the resection of distal pancreas which is performed as part of the radical operation and not the splenectomy. Current practice is to undertake resection of N2 nodes preserving pancreas and, if feasible, the spleen. In the Japanese literature a significant survival benefit is demonstrable for D2 over D1 and D0 resection, with operative mortality as low as 5% for such radical surgery.[137]

Radical surgery

This operation should remove the part of stomach containing the tumour with at least 5 cm clearance (excluding the duodenum) and all N1 and N2 nodes (Figs 28.23 and 28.24). Current practice however is to not remove pancreas but to strip the lymph nodes from the splenic artery and preserve the spleen unless the tumour is in the proximal stomach. The greater omentum is removed in all cases along with the left gastric, coeliac and common hepatic nodes.[138]

In distal cancers with at least 5 cm (preferably 10 cm) proximal clearance, the proximal stomach can be preserved. This may be reconstructed as either a Billroth I or II gastrectomy, although in the vast majority of cases the extent of resection necessitates a Billroth II reconstruction. This has the added advantage of removing the stomach and anastomosis from the gastric bed. An

REFERENCES

131. Mason R C et al Lancet 1987; 1: 108
132. Rankin S, Mason R Clin Radiol 1992; 46: 373
133. Shandall A, Johnson C Br J Surg 1985; 72: 449
134. Pichlmayr R, Meyer H J Advances in Biosciences, vol 32. Pergamon Press London 1981
135. Gundosa L C, Sosin H Int J Rad Oncol Biol Phys 1982; 8: 1
136. Cuschieri A et al Lancet 1996; 347: 995
137. Kajitani T, Miwa K WHO-CC Monograph 2. WHO, Tokyo 1979
138. Craven J L In: Cancer of the Stomach (Eds) Preece, Cuschieri, Wellwood. Grune & Stratton 1986, p 165

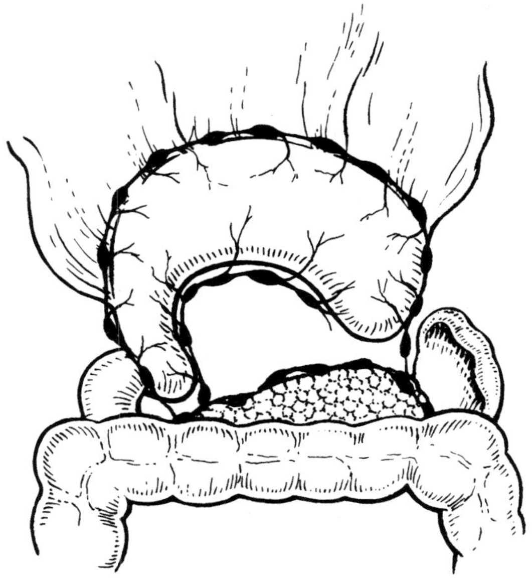

Fig. 28.23 Mobilization of stomach for a D2 gastrectomy showing lymph nodes to be removed.

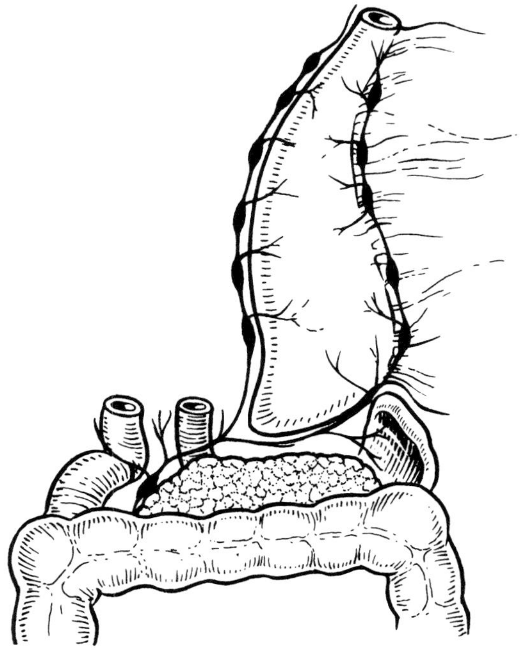

Fig. 28.24 Completed lymphadenectomy for a D2 gastrectomy.

alternative is to reconstruct with a Roux-en-Y anastomosis which prevents bile reflux (Fig. 28.25). This must be combined with truncal vagotomy or lifelong proton pump inhibitors to prevent stomal ulceration.

Following total gastrectomy (performed for body and proximal cancer) the classical method of reconstruction consists of anastomosing a 50 cm Roux-en-Y loop to the oesophagus. Because total gastrectomy is associated with higher morbidity than partial resection, largely as the result of dietary problems, deficiencies and dumping, modifications to the standard Roux loop have been

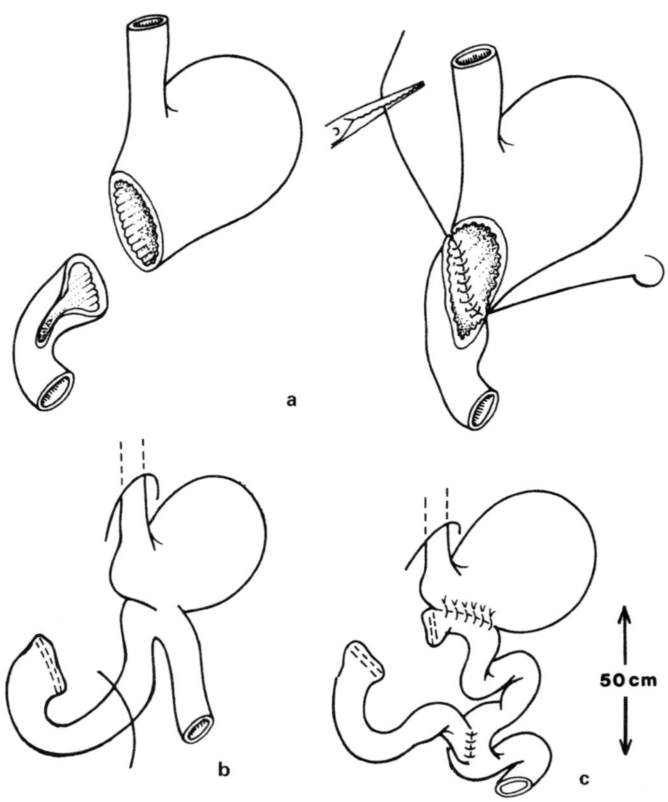

Fig. 28.25 Methods of reconstruction after a partial gastrectomy. (**a**) Billroth I; (**b**) Billroth II; (**c**) Roux-en-Y.

proposed. These are demonstrated in Figure 28.26. A standard 50 cm Roux loop constructed without kinking and a short proximal jejunal limb offer the best means of reconstruction if the patient takes vitamin and mineral supplements and eats little and often.

Palliative treatment

In the presence of advanced disease, treatment should be directed to the simplest means of alleviating the patient's symptoms and this should be tailored to the individual. The symptoms most commonly requiring palliation are obstruction, haemorrhage and pain. These can be treated by resection, bypass, exclusion, intubation with plastic or self-expanding metal stents and laser recanalization (Figs 28.27 and 28.28). In distal tumours, resection bypass and exclusion are the best options. In proximal tumours, the results of surgery are poor and intubation and/or laser ablation offer good palliation with minimum morbidity and mortality.[139,140]

Other therapeutic possibilities

Until recently, the results of cytotoxic chemotherapy for gastric cancer both as primary treatment and as adjuvant therapy have

REFERENCES

139. Watkinson A F et al Semin Intervent Radiol 1996; 13: 17
140. Mason R C et al Br J Surg 1991; 78: 1346

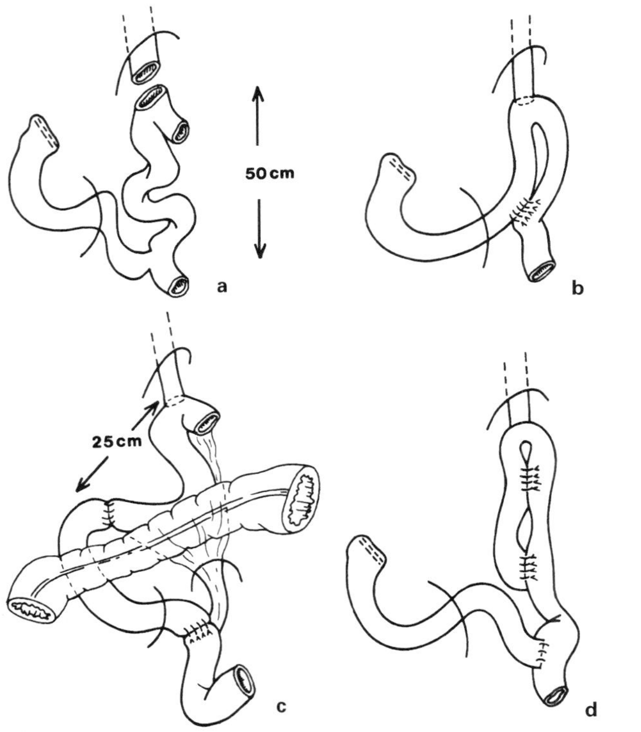

Fig. 28.26 Methods of reconstruction after a total gastrectomy. (**a**) Roux-en-Y; (**b**) Omega gastrojejunostomy; (**c**) Henley jejunal interposition; (**d**) Lydidakis modification of Roux-en-Y.

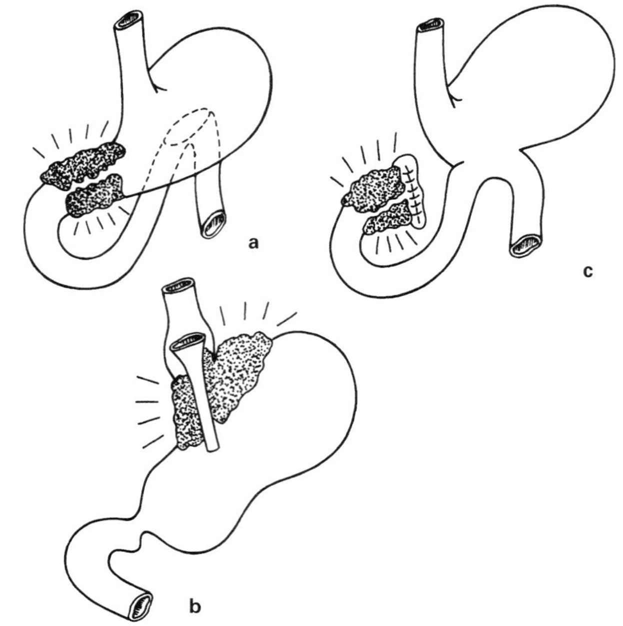

Fig. 28.27 Palliative procedures. (**a**) Gastroenterostomy; (**b**) intubation with plastic tube; (**c**) exclusion.

been disappointing.[141,142] The use of regimens based on cisplatin and the continuous infusion of 5-fluorouracil administered via a Hickman catheter and minipump have demonstrated a 60% response rate in advanced disease[143] and are currently under evaluation in the MRC Adjuvant Gastric Infusional Chemotherapy Trial (MAGIC) trial as neoadjuvant treatment in operable disease.

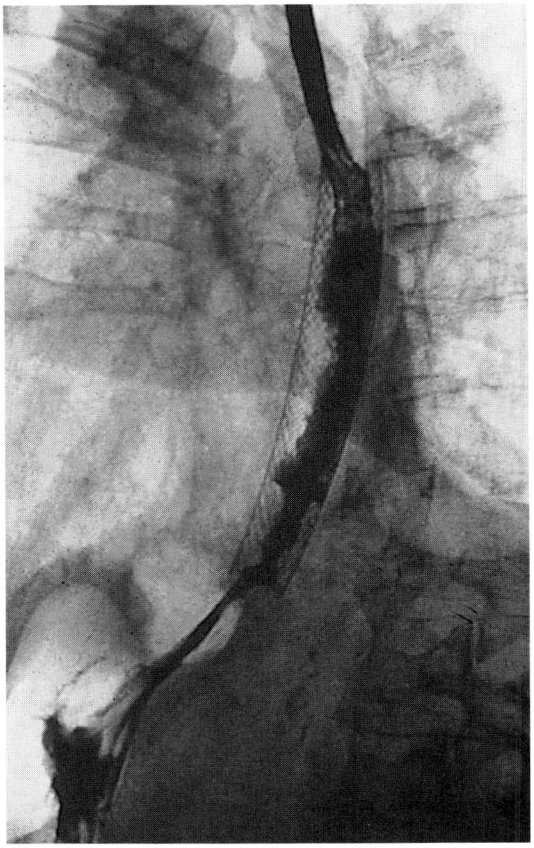

Fig. 28.28 Self-expanding metal stent at the oesophagogastric junction.

No evidence exists that external beam radiotherapy in gastric cancer is beneficial, but it can be useful in reducing bleeding in patients with advanced disease.

Results of treatment

There are many series demonstrating different survival rates. Series from Europe and North America show curative resection rates of 25–40% with 5-year survival figures of between 10 and 15%.[144,145] This contrasts with Japan, where the curative resection rate is over 50% and 5-year survival figures are between 20 and 30%.[146] The most important determinant of survival is the clinicopathological stage of the disease. The Tumour Node Metastasis staging system (Table 28.9) has been modified to allow identification of the group of patients having palliative resections (stage

REFERENCES

141. Hockey M S S, Fielding J W L Gastric Cancer in Randomised Trials in Cancer. Raven Press, 1986 p 221
142. Fielding J W L et al World J Surg 1983; 7: 390
143. Highley M S et al Br J Surg 1994; 81: 763
144. Inberg M V et al Arch Surg 1975; 110: 703
145. Scott A W et al Surgery 1985; 97: 55
146. Kajitani T et al Gann Monog Cancer Res 1979; 22: 77

Table 28.9 Staging system for gastric cancer

Stage	*Clinical*	*Pathology*
I	Radical resection (T1, N0, M0)	Mucosa +, submucosa +/–, muscularis propria –, serosa –, node – (T1, N0, M0)
II	Radical resection (T2–4, N0, M0)	Muscularis propria +, serosa +/–, node – (T2–4, N0, M0)
III	Radical resection (TX–4, N1–3,M0)	Muscularis propria +/–, serosa +/–, node+ (TX–4, N1–3, M0)
IVA	Palliative resection (TX–4, NX–3, M0–1)	Residual disease (TX–4, N0–3, M0–1)
IVB	No resection (TX–4, NX–3, M0–1)	Positive histology (T4,N0–3, M0–1)

IVA) as compared to those who have no resection (stage IVB).[147] This system accommodates the important clinicopathological features of gastric cancer:

1. Resectability.
2. Depth of penetration of the primary lesion.
3. The presence or absence of lymph node involvement and distant metastases.

The strength of this system is confirmed in the retrospective study from tumours in the Birmingham Cancer Registry (Fig. 28.29). When international comparisons are made between like-stage disease, similar results are then seen, although the Japanese do report a survival rate for stage 1 disease of 100%. It is likely that the apparent difference in overall results of treatment across the world are related to the variable distribution of stage. In Japan the incidence of stage 1 disease is as high as 30%.[148]

OTHER EPITHELIAL AND NON-EPITHELIAL TUMOURS

Squamous cell carcinoma and carcinoid tumours of the stomach are exceedingly rare—0.04–0.07% of all gastric cancers, and about four times more common in men than women. Presentation is similar to adenocarcinoma.[149] Similarly, argentiffinomas are not common and the diagnosis is frequently established at post-mortem. They occur with equal frequency in both sexes and present in a similar way to adenocarcinoma, though they may have a long preoperative history.

Radiologically, carcinoids appear as polypoid neoplasms. If it is a small tumour with no evidence of metastasis it should be locally excised. Where the neoplasm is over 2 cm in diameter or where there is evidence of metastasis, operation appropriate to the stage should be performed. The prognosis is good: among the 15 reported cases followed for more than 5 years there are 12 survivors. Amongst the 90 reported cases 6 had malignant carcinoid syndrome, producing high levels of 5-hydroxytryptophan and histamine.[150]

Lymphoma

The stomach is the most common extranodal site of non-Hodgkin's lymphoma but it is still uncommon, accounting for 1.2% of gastric malignancies. The mean age is 60 years, with a male to female

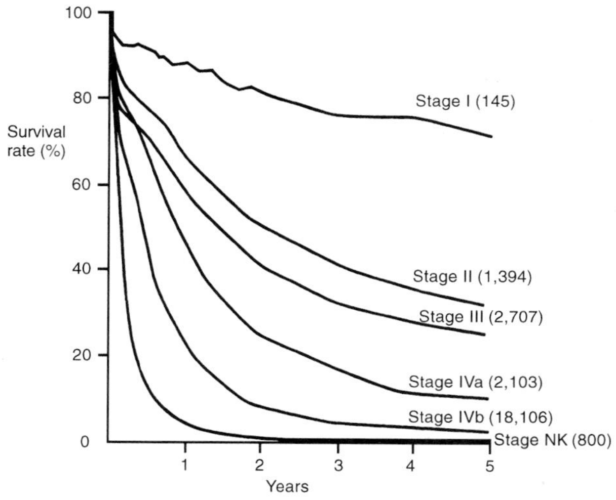

Fig. 28.29 The relationship of 5-year survival rate by stage in the West Midlands.

ratio of 1.3:1. The presenting symptoms are similar to adenocarcinoma, although a mass is found in 20%. Two-thirds of lesions are resectable and overall 5-year survival is 24%. Significant prognostic factors are tumour node metastasis staging and tumour size; survival can be doubled by the addition of radiotherapy to resection.[151] The role of chemotherapy regimens used for non-Hodgkin's lymphoma elsewhere remain to be confirmed.

Leiomyoma/leiomyosarcoma

These comprise 1–3% of all gastric tumours. The differentiation between leiomyoma and leiomyosarcoma is made on the number of mitotic figures seen in high-power microscopic fields. If there are none, the tumour is benign, whereas over 10 mitotic figures indicates a high likelihood of metastasis. They are most commonly situated on the anterior and posterior gastric walls. Macroscopically they are bulky and vascular, with multiple areas of ulceration. Microscopically they originate from smooth muscle. Direct spread is rare and lymph node metastasis does not occur. At laparotomy macroscopic dissemination is found in 10–45% of patients. The incidence is the same between the sexes. The most frequent presenting symptom is bleeding: 75% having either haematemesis or melaena. There may also be epigastric symptoms and an abdominal mass is found in up to 60% of cases. The diagnosis is established by a combination of endoscopy and radiology. Surgery is curative and consists of wide local excision without

REFERENCES

147. Fielding J W L et al Br J Surg 1984; 71: 677
148. Nishi M In: Cancer of the Stomach. Grune & Stratton (Eds) Preece, Cuschieri, Wellwood 1985 p 107
149. Eaton H Br J Surg 1972; 59: 382
150. Rogers L, Murphy R Am J Surg Pathol 1979; 3: 195
151. Hockey M S et al Br J Surg 1987; 74: 43
152. Skandalakis L J et al Surgery of the Oesophagus, Stomach and Small Intestine, 5th edn. Little, Brown 1995 p 607
153. Levison D A, Shepherd N A In: Cancer of the Stomach. Grune & Stratton (Eds) Preece, Cuschieri, Wellwood 1985 p 47

lymphadenectomy. The prognosis is quite good, with a 5-year survival rate ranging between 37 and 54%.[152,153] There is no benefit in palliative adjuvant chemo- or radiotherapy.

Other rare tumours of the stomach

These include schwannomas, chorioepitheliomas and carcinosarcomas. The diagnosis is usually made only after resection of a gastric mass. They should not be confused with benign hamartomas of the stomach associated with Peutz–Jeghers syndrome.[154]

DUODENAL NEOPLASMS

Benign duodenal tumours

These are found in 1% of endoscopies. Most are located in the first part of the duodenum with the risk of malignancy increasing the more distal they are found. Gastrointestinal haemorrhage is the most frequent presentation. Adenomas are the most common but villous adenomas do occur. Other rare tumours include Brunner gland adenomas, leiomyomas, lipomas and carcinoid tumours.[154]

Malignant duodenal lesions

Duodenal cancers are rare, accounting for only 0.3% of gastrointestinal malignancies. A third of small bowel neoplasms are however situated in the duodenum.

Adenocarcinomas are the most frequent tumours, but lymphomas and carcinoids also occur. The presentation depends on the site. In the periampullary region the patient presents with jaundice, whereas elsewhere they present with obstructive symptoms. In 25% of cases a mass may be felt.[154]

The most effective treatment is pancreaticoduodenectomy. If there is local invasion or distant metastasis, surgical or radiological bypass is indicated. Overall 5-year survival is 25%.

REFERENCE

154. Otterson M F, Condon R E In: Surgery of the Oesophagus, Stomach and Small Intestine, 5th edn. Little, Brown 1995 p 691

29 The small intestine

M. H. Jourdan

The small intestine is the segment of the gastrointestinal tract between the pylorus and the ileocaecal valve. The duodenum will only be considered as it relates to the small intestine in general and this chapter concentrates upon the small intestine which extends from the duodenojejunal flexure at the ligament of Treitz to the ileocaecal valve. In adult life this part of the small bowel, measured unstretched along the mesenteric border, is approximately 300 cm long, although precise measurement is meaningless. For convenience it is divided into the upper two-fifths, referred to as the jejunum in view of the fact that it was noted to be empty at post-mortem and at laparotomy, and the lower three-fifths, the ileum. In reality, it is impossible to determine an exact cut-off point between jejunum and ileum and there is a slow gradation in the middle third of the small intestine from the jejunum, with its thick highly vascular mucosa and tall multiple villi, to the ileum with its thinner mucosa and smaller villus height. The vascular arcades of the jejunum are numerous while those of the ileum are fewer.

The newborn infant has a sterile gastrointestinal tract, but within a few weeks bacterial colonization has occurred, especially in the terminal ileum and colon. The jejunal contents are normally bacteria-free, except for transient colonization with enterococci and lactobacilli. The ileal contents however contain coliforms and *Bacteroides* at concentrations of 10^5–10^8 organisms per ml of contents. These bacteria seem to be important in digestion; they live in symbiosis with the host, breaking down molecules such as taurocholic and glycocholic acid and gastrin, and liberating folate into the luminal contents; this is then absorbed to the host's advantage. In certain abnormal situations the bacteria in the small bowel may proliferate to levels found in the colon, where they produce malabsorption. The 'blind loop syndrome', in which bacterial overgrowth occurs in a blind-ending segment of bowel, may result from a number of causes, including the construction of surgical anastomoses and occasionally from congenital conditions such as multiple small bowel diverticulosis (Fig. 29.1).

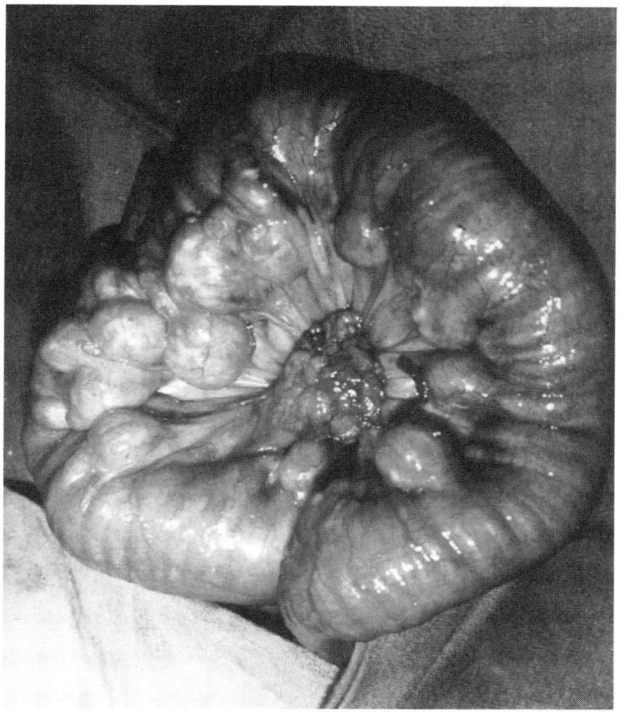

Fig. 29.1 Jejunal diverticulosis.

THE FUNCTIONS OF THE SMALL INTESTINE

1. The small intestine provides the site and means of digestion and absorption of all foodstuffs. In addition to the incomplete hydrolysis of carbohydrates and proteins, which occurs in the intestinal lumen, the brush border of the enterocytes contains enzymes such as peptidases and disaccharidases which complete the conversion of proteins and carbohydrates to amino acids and monosaccharides respectively. The absorption of fat is more complicated; the majority of absorbed triglycerides are converted to chylomicrons and absorbed into the lymphatic system of the small intestine. Small chain and medium chain triglycerides, if given as additional supplements, may be either hydrolysed to glycerol and fatty acids or absorbed directly into the portal venous system[1] (see Chapter 2).

Vitamin B_{12}, in association with intrinsic factor, is mainly absorbed in the final 50–100 cm of ileum, as also are the bile salts. Resection or disease of this part of the small intestine eventually results in vitamin B_{12} deficiency. Interference with the entero-hepatic circulation of bile salts may result in the formation of gall-stones and fat malabsorption. In the adult human, glucose, amino acids, water and electrolytes required for homeostasis can be satisfactorily absorbed by as little as 30–120 cm of jejunum, although

REFERENCE

1. Krause M V, Mahon L K In: Food, Nutrition and Diet Therapy. W B Saunders, Eastbourne 1979

with adaptation this function can occur in the ileum when extensive jejunal resection has been necessary.[2]

2. In the wall of the small intestine there are amine precursor uptake decarboxylase cells and these produce a variety of peptide hormones including gastric inhibitory peptide, vasoactive intestinal peptide, motilin and enteroglucagon, which appear to regulate locally the absorptive and motor functions of the bowel.[3]

3. The small intestine is richly endowed with cells of the immune system, including T and B lymphocytes and plasma cells. Immunoglobulin γ A is normally produced in large quantities and reduced production results in intestinal infection by such organisms as *Giardia lamblia*, with consequent malabsorption and diarrhoea. Coeliac disease, Crohn's disease and atrophic gastritis are all associated with immune deficiency.

EMBRYOLOGY OF THE SMALL INTESTINE

The small bowel is derived from part of the mid-gut with its supplying artery, the superior mesenteric artery. Its venous drainage from the superior mesenteric vein passes into the portal venous system. The lymphatic drainage follows the course of the arteries. Hence lymph drains from the small intestine through a series of mesenteric lymph nodes to the para-aortic nodes and from there to the cysterna chyli and thoracic duct. At 8 weeks of gestation the apex of the small bowel connects to the yolk sac via the vitellointestinal duct. As the intra-abdominal organs enlarge, the developing intestine is excluded from the forming abdominal cavity and comes to lie in the extraembryonic coelom as part of the umbilicus. The proximal limb of this intestinal loop, which forms the jejunum and most of the ileum, elongates considerably but at the 12th week of gestation this tube begins to pass back into the abdominal cavity and as it does so, rotates in an anticlockwise direction as viewed from in front. In this way the loop of the duodenum is formed; this becomes fixed retroperitoneally, and the more distal part of the mid-gut, which extends from the ascending colon to the splenic flexure, comes to lie anterior to the duodenum. The final position of the caecum at the time of birth is usually in the right hypochondrium.

This process may not proceed entirely smoothly and in consequence a number of congenital anomalies may occur which can present with surgical problems either early in life, or in some instances later.

DEVELOPMENTAL ANOMALIES

A wide variety of anomalies may present to the paediatric surgeon, e.g. exomphalos, volvulus neonatorum and other abnormalities of rotation,[4] enteric atresia, enterogenous cysts and duplication of the intestine (see Chapter 41). In some instances symptoms associated with congenital anomalies may not appear until adult life.

Ladd's bands

In 1932, Ladd[5] described duodenal obstruction as a result of the persistence of fibrous bands between the root of the small bowel mesentery and the liver, crossing and obstructing the second part of the duodenum. In this situation, which is found in 0.2% of barium studies of the gastrointestinal tract,[6] the rotation of the intestine was incomplete; the colon lay on the left of the abdomen while the small bowel was on the right. Although duodenal obstruction with bile-stained vomit usually occurs in children, it may present occasionally in adulthood.

Treatment is achieved by dividing the bands and the narrow peritoneum at the base of the small bowel mesentery, leaving the small intestine on the right and the colon on the left side of the abdomen. This results in a much longer base to the mesentery of the small intestine, making volvulus less likely.[7]

Diverticula of the small intestine

These were first described by Astley Cooper in 1807.[8] They are generally multiple and project between layers of mesentery (Fig. 29.1). The origin of these diverticula is uncertain. They may arise developmentally during canalization of the original intestinal cord, but they are found much more commonly in the jejunum, whereas enterogenous cysts, which are most definitely developmental abnormalities, are seen more frequently in the caecum and ascending colon. Diverticula may be associated with dyspepsia,[9] perforation, haemorrhage, inflammation and obstruction.[10]

The majority of patients with diverticula of the small intestine are symptom-free, but in addition to the complications mentioned above, blind-loop syndrome, associated with bacterial overgrowth in the diverticula and malabsorption of fats and vitamins, is occasionally seen.[11]

Anomalies of the vitellointestinal ducts

The vitellointestinal duct is the channel which passes from the middle of the mid-gut through the umbilicus to the yolk sac, in company with the vitelline artery, which is an extension of the superior mesenteric artery. There is persistence of the duct to some degree in 10 males and 2 females per 1000 population. This congenital antimesenteric diverticulum of the ileum was first illustrated by Ruysch in 1701;[12] the main effects of persistence of vitellointestinal duct remnants were grouped together by Meckel in 1809,[13] and the work was completed by Allen in 1882.[14]

REFERENCES

2. Williamson R C N et al Gastroenterology 1978; 74: 16
3. Solcia E, Polak J M et al In: Bloom S R (ed) Gut Hormones. Churchill Livingstone, Edinburgh 1978
4. Dott N M Br J Surg 1923; 11: 251
5. Ladd W E N Engl J Med 1932; 206: 277
6. Kantor J L Radiology 1934; 23: 651
7. Bill A H, Grauman D J Pediatr Surg 1966; 1: 127
8. Cooper A Anatomy and Surgical Treatment of Crural and Umbilical Hernia. Walters, London 1807
9. Hughes-Jones W E A Br J Surg 1934–1935; 22: 134
10. Milnes-Walker R Br J Surg 1944–1945; 33: 457
11. Donald J W Ann Surg 1979; 190: 183
12. Ruysch F Thesaurus Anatomicus. J Walters, Amsterdam 1701
13. Meckel J F Arch Physiol 1809; 9: 439
14. Allen J J Anat 1882; 17: 59

Meckel's diverticulum

This diverticulum lies on the antimesenteric border of the ileum about 50 cm proximal to the ileocaecal valve. It is caused by persistent patency of the intestinal end of the vitellointestinal duct, and although its presence is usually symptomless it can manifest itself in a number of ways. It is present in about 2% of the population (Fig. 29.2).

Inflammation

The opening of a Meckel's diverticulum is usually wide, but if it is narrow, material may accumulate in the diverticulum, giving rise to inflammation and features which are indistinguishable from acute appendicitis (see Chapter 27). An inflamed Meckel's diverticulum is always sought in an operation for acute appendicitis if the appendix is healthy. Treatment involves excision of the diverticulum with transverse closure of the ileum, or if this would narrow the lumen of the bowel a short length of ileum may need to be resected.

When a Meckel's diverticulum is discovered incidentally at laparotomy, its presence should be noted but no attempt should be made to remove it unless the neck is obviously narrow or the diverticulum is obviously diseased.

Intussusception

A Meckel's diverticulum may become inverted and then act as a focus for intussusception with the development of low small bowel obstruction. Treatment is by reduction and a short ileal resection, conserving as much bowel as possible.

Peptic ulceration

About 16% of Meckel's diverticula contain ectopic gastric mucosa capable of secreting hydrochloric acid.[15] This fact can be demonstrated using a pertechnetate technetium^{99m} scan (Fig. 29.2). The secretion of acid may so damage the surrounding mucosa that ulceration with perforation or haemorrhage may occur, often at the base of the diverticulum and sometimes in the ileum itself. Such ulcers are eight times more common in males than in females, and the average age of onset of symptoms is 10 years, though adult cases occasionally occur. In adults, post-prandial pain is the most common symptom, while in children the presentation is usually with melaena or the passage of obvious blood per rectum.[16] It must always be remembered however that the presence of a Meckel's diverticulum does not necessarily imply that it is responsible for the symptoms, and another cause such as intussusception or neoplasm may be the source of the problem.

Vitellointestinal band

Such a band uniting the umbilicus to the antimesenteric border of the ileum or to the mesentery represents the fibrous remnant of the vitellointestinal duct or the vitelline vessels. It may act as a focus around which a loop of bowel may twist, resulting in intestinal obstruction.

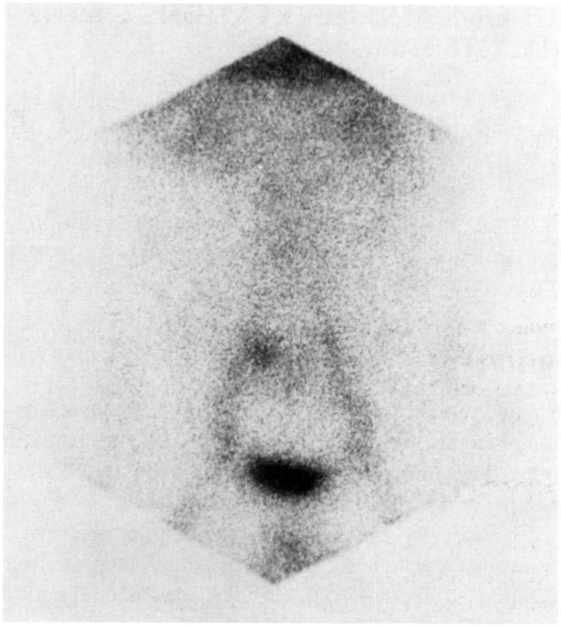

Fig. 29.2 Meckel's diverticulum demonstrated by a pertechnetate technetium^{99m} scan.

Perforation

A Meckel's diverticulum may perforate as a result of impaction of a foreign body, such as a fishbone within it, or as a result of the development of a peptic ulcer.

Tumours of the Meckel's diverticulum

These are rare, but the least rare is the carcinoid tumour. This usually presents as small bowel obstruction caused by cicatrization of the tumour, or occasionally, if liver metastases occur, the carcinoid syndrome may develop (see below).

When necessary the resection of a Meckel's diverticulum can be performed laparoscopically using an Endo GIA-type stapler. This is one of the few circumstances in current practice where laparoscopic surgery is applicable to the small intestine.

Hirschsprung's disease (see Chapter 41)

Congenital aganglionosis of the intestine occurs to some extent in 1 in 4500 live births.[17] Although it is familial, the inheritance pattern is not simple. The underlying pathological process is a failure of distal migration of ganglion cells in the submucous and myenteric plexuses of the intestine.

It is unusual for this to involve the small intestine, but there have been reports of the whole intestinal tract being affected.[18] Small intestinal involvement almost always results in small bowel obstruction in infancy.

REFERENCES

15. Soltero M J, Bill A H Am J Surg 1976; 132: 168
16. Rutherford R B, Akers D R Surgery 1966; 59: 618
17. Orr J D, Scobie W G Br Med J 1983; 287: 1671

INFECTIONS AND INFESTATIONS OF THE SMALL INTESTINE

A host of micro-organisms may find a temporary home in the small intestine, and some of these may cause conditions requiring surgery. The majority of infections, such as staphylococcal enteritis, cholera, *Giardia lamblia*, tapeworms, etc. produce diarrhoea, malabsorption, anaemia and pain as well as systemic illness but certain organisms can cause intestinal obstruction, haemorrhage and even perforation of the bowel.

Typhoid fever

This disease is endemic in most tropical countries and is caused by ingestion of the salmonella organisms. The most severe symptoms are produced by *Salmonella typhi*. In England and Wales about 200 cases occur each year.[19]

The organism may survive in the gallbladder or urinary tract, having invaded through the small intestinal mucosa following multiplication in the bile-rich area of the second part of the duodenum.[20] The organisms may be taken up in any part of the body, but usually enter the Peyer's patches, particularly in the ileum but also in the jejunum. Here ulceration develops, with possible subsequent haemorrhage or perforation, which occurs in the third week of the disease,[21] although if simple healing occurs, as in the majority of patients, there is little fibrous tissue formation. Consequently stricturing with obstruction is not a problem. Patients with sickle cell disease fare badly if they catch typhoid fever.[22] Surgical intervention with ileal resection is necessary for perforation or severe haemorrhage.

When perforation occurs, a fit patient shows all the signs of peritonitis, but the seriously ill patient may show little in the way of abdominal tenderness or guarding. An additional source of confusion is provided by the rupture of the inferior epigastric artery which sometimes occurs with typhoid fever and gives a similar rigidity in the right iliac fossa[23] (see Chapter 27). At operation the bowel is very friable and should be handled gently. The possibility of multiple perforations must be considered. Whether the perforation is oversewn or resection is performed depends upon the conditions found at laparotomy,[24,25] but in any event the patient should be given intravenously chloramphenicol 4 g/day for 2 weeks (adult dose).

Tuberculosis

In western countries tuberculosis of the terminal ileum from uptake of mycobacteria into Peyer's patches with subsequent ulceration and stricture formation is rare and Crohn's disease is a much more common cause of small bowel obstruction. With increasing migration and the influx of Asians into the UK, there are now reports of tuberculous enteritis being seen with increasing frequency in some parts of the UK where such communities settle.[26]

In tropical countries, such as India and Sri Lanka, Crohn's disease is virtually never seen and ileocaecal tuberculosis is relatively common. The condition may present with abscess formation and intestinal obstruction; occasionally perforation and surgical intervention may be necessary for drainage of pus, relief of obstruction or resection of the involved bowel. If a reasonably secure diagnosis of ileocaecal tuberculosis can be made before complications develop, a course of anti-tuberculous therapy may prevent the complications and make surgical intervention unnecessary. When surgery is necessary it should always be combined with anti-tuberculous chemotherapy, which may need to be continued for 1–2 years.

Actinomycosis

This chronic inflammatory condition is fortunately rare, and is because of intrusion by a Gram-positive anaerobic bacterial organism, *Actinomyces israelii*. In 70% of cases the condition starts in the cervicofacial area, usually following dental trauma,[27] but in 20% of cases the organism enters in the ileocaecal region, often following a perforation of the appendix.[28] Here it produces a chronic inflammatory response with dense fibrosis and multiloculate abscesses which may eventually discharge through multiple sinuses in the right iliac fossa. The pus characteristically contains the sulphur granules, which are dense, matted filaments of organisms with surrounding radially disposed club-shaped growths. The latter do not appear in artifical culture. The organisms travel in the portal vein to the liver if septicaemia occurs from the ileocaecal region where multiple abscess formation may result in the characteristic honeycomb appearance. Surgery may be necessary for the drainage of abscesses, but the organism is sensitive to a wide variety of antibiotics including penicillin and lincomycin.[29]

Syphilis

Varieties of tertiary syphilis such as tabes dorsalis may produce abdominal pain, tenderness and guarding leading to an unnecessary laparotomy (see Chapter 27). This situation is now rare in western countries, and even rarer are the gummata which may occur in the small intestine leading to ulceration, perforation or stricture formation. Secondary syphilis may occasionally produce diarrhoea due to ulceration involving the small bowel mucosa.

REFERENCES

18. Nixon H In: Goligher J (ed) Surgery of the Anus, Rectum and Colon. Baillière Tindall, London 1984
19. Public Health Laboratory Service Br Med J 1983; 287: 1205
20. Cook G C In: Misiewicz J J, Pounder R E, Venables C W (eds) Diseases of the Gut and Pancreas. Blackwell Scientific, Oxford 1987
21. Bitar R, Tarpley J Rev Infect Dis 1985; 7: 257
22. Cook G C Tropical Gastroenterology. Oxford University Press, Oxford 1980
23. Aird I In: Companion in Surgical Studies. Livingstone, Edinburgh 1958
24. Bitar R, Tarpley J Rev Infect Dis 1985; 7: 257
25. Butler T et al Rev Infect Dis 1995; 7: 244
26. Addison N V Ann R Coll Surg Engl 1983; 65: 105
27. Beradi R S Surg Gynecol Obstet 1979; 149: 257
28. Cope Z Actinomycosis. Oxford University Press, London 1938
29. Putnam H C, Dockerty M B et al Surgery 1950; 28: 781

Yersiniosis

These organisms used to be known as *Pasteurella*, and the *pestis* species causing the plague is the most notorious. Two other varieties of *Yersinia* may cause gastrointestinal illnesses—*Y. pseudotuberculosis* and *Y. enterocolitica*. These organisms are anaerobic Gram-negative rods from an animal reservoir, which probably secondarily infect humans through food, milk and contact with animal excreta.[30] *Y. pseudotuberculosis* mainly infects children, producing mesenteric adenitis, a condition clinically indistinguishable from acute appendicitis. The organism, when present, can be cultured from most body fluids, and produces in the lymph nodes epithelioid giant cell granulomas with areas of central necrosis surrounded by polymorphonuclear leucocyte infiltration. The microscopic appearances are distinguishable from those of Crohn's disease and tuberculosis.

Y. enterocolitica produces more widespread manifestations. Apart from mesenteric lymph node involvement, there may be an acute pyrexial gastroenteritis, diarrhoea and abdominal colic. The features may suggest acute appendicitis and at laparotomy an acute ileitis with bright-red inflammation of the terminal ileum may be found. The appendix may look normal and acute Crohn's disease is the main differential.[31] There is always a dilemma whether to remove the appendix or not. The theoretical risk of causing a fistula would seem to have been exaggerated, and if the caecum looks healthy, removal of the appendix with culture of the peritoneal fluid would appear to be appropriate initial management.[32]

Yersinia is sensitive to a wide range of antibiotics including chloramphenicol, co-trimoxazole and tetracycline and one of these should be used. Extraintestinal manifestations such as erythema nodosum and arthritis may also occur. In less acute cases, *Yersinia* infection might be suggested by the nodularity and aphthoid ulceration seen on barium follow-through examination in the terminal ileum.[33] The diagnosis can be confirmed by a rise in serum antibody titre to *Yersinia.*[34]

Other infestations

Ascaris lumbricoides infection may occasionally result in a matted collection of intertwined worms in the small bowel which produce obstructive symptoms. In subacute obstruction or where vague abdominal symptoms occur, investigation by small bowel enema may reveal barium in the intestine of the worms (Fig. 29.3). Worms may also migrate into the biliary tree producing cholangitis or pancreatitis.[35]

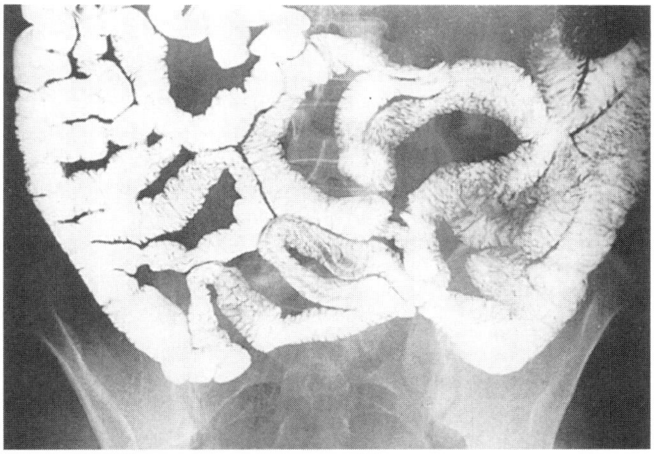

Fig. 29.3 *Ascaris* worms seen in the small intestine.

The hookworms (*Ancylostoma duodenale* or *Necator americanus*) probably infect 600 million of the world's population and can produce a chronic iron-deficiency anaemia. Although uncommon in western Europe, it may be appropriate to consider this organism in the differential diagnosis of some patients with iron-deficiency anaemia as the result of blood loss.

Strongyloides, *Trichuris* (whipworm) and tapeworm infestations when severe may produce abdominal discomfort, anaemia and even obstructive symptoms.

PNEUMATOSIS INTESTINALIS

Gas cysts of the intestines are rare and usually symptomless pathological curiosities which were first described by Bang[36] in 1876. The cysts are tiny collections of gas enclosed within a wall of connective tissue supporting an inner layer of endothelium. Sometimes within this wall there is a chronic inflammatory infiltration of lymphocytes and of foreign body giant cells. The gas contained within the cysts is unlike air; it has a hydrogen content of up to 20%, and is totally different from the lethal gas formed by micro-organisms which enter the intestinal wall in necrotizing enterocolitis or intestinal infarction.

The condition used to be considered three times more common in males than in females,[37] but more recent reports suggest an approximately equal sex frequency.[38] Although it used to be relatively common,[39] small bowel disease is now rare and colonic pneumatosis is more commonly seen. It is probable that the reduction in incidence of associated illness of severe peptic ulcer and pyloric stenosis may account for the reduction in incidence of small bowel disease.

Colonic pneumatosis is seen in patients with obstructive airways disease, pseudomembranous colitis, diverticular disease, jejunoileal bypass for obesity, sigmoid volvulus and occasionally following colonoscopy. The air cysts can be submucosal or subserosal and occasionally there is rupture into the peritoneal cavity with gas appearing under the diaphragm.

The mechanism of formation of the air cysts is not understood, but the high hydrogen content, continuous gas production and occurrence of this condition in the bypassed small intestine

REFERENCES

30. Misiewicz J J et al (eds) Diseases of the Gut and Pancreas. Blackwell Scientific, Oxford 1987
31. Savage A, Dunlop D Br Med J 1976; ii: 916
32. Schwartz S L, Ellis H (eds) Maingot's Abdominal Operation, 8th edn. Appleton-Century-Crofts, Norwalk, Connecticut 1985
33. Vantrappen G et al Gastroenterology 1977; 72: 220
34. Paff J R et al Am J Clin Pathol 1976; 66: 101
35. Pfeffermann R et al Arch Surg 1972; 105: 118
36. Bang J Nord Med Ark 1876; 8: 18
37. Nitch C A R Br J Surg 1923 1924; 11: 714
38. Yale C E, Balish E Dis Colon Rectum 1976; 19: 107
39. Koss L G Arch Pathol 1952; 53: 523

following jejunoileal bypass suggest that bacteria are responsible.[40] No causative organism has been cultured from the cysts however. There is also an epidemic form of pneumatosis intestinalis in pigs, and two specimens of this are present in the Hunterian Museum at the Royal College of Surgeons of England. The condition may be symptomless, but may present as diarrhoea, intermittent rectal bleeding, excessive passage of mucus and flatus or intestinal obstruction. Malabsorption may also occur.

In the colonic pneumatosis the cysts may be recognized at sigmoidoscopy, but in small bowel disease the gas shadows may be recognized in the bowel wall on plain radiography or as filling defects in the small bowel enema. The main differential diagnosis clinically and on barium studies of the small bowel is between lymphoma, carcinoma and Crohn's disease.

Treatment

This essentially consists of treating the underlying causative condition, but when the cysts themselves are causing symptoms the first line of treatment is to administer oxygen at a high flow rate, providing an oxygen concentration of 70% via a face-mask or nasal catheter for up to 5 days.[41,42]

Other treatments tried include antibiotic therapy with ampicillin and metronidazole, and treatment with an elemental diet—both have had variable success. Surgery is only necessary where a complication such as haemorrhage or volvulus supervenes. In any event recurrence of the intestinal air cysts is common.

CROHN'S DISEASE

In 1932 Crohn et al[43] published a report describing the clinical situation in 14 young adults with chronic inflammatory bowel disease of the ileum which was not tuberculosis and not neoplastic. In some of these patients multiple fistulae had developed and in some small intestinal obstruction associated with fibrotic strictures had occurred. This condition had almost certainly been described before by Dalziel in 1913,[44] and in 1806 a paper—later published in 1813—was delivered at the Royal College of Physicians by Combe & Saunders,[45] entitled 'A singular case of stricture and thickening of the ileum', in which the lower part of the ileum as far as the colon was contracted 'for the space of three feet to the size of a turkey's quill'. There were also colonic lesions. Moynihan[46] in 1907 described a benign stricturing of the colon resembling malignant disease which in retrospect was probably colonic Crohn's disease. The name 'Crohn's disease' has, however, become established in the literature and over the years many thousands of cases have been documented.[47]

Crohn's disease can affect any part of the gastrointestinal tract from the lips to the anus. It is apparently increasing in frequency in western societies but is very uncommon in the underdeveloped world. It has a considerable morbidity, some mortality and its cause is unknown. Treatment is therefore symptomatic.

The highest prevalence reported is from Scandinavia ($75/10^5$ population[48]). The incidence is increasing markedly in the UK and at the moment is $6.1/10^5$ population per year in Blackpool.[49] In western Europe and North America the incidence is greater in the Jewish population, with a tendency towards female preponderance.[50] The peak incidence of diagnosis is between 15 and 35 years of age. There is an interesting anomaly in the incidence figures from Cardiff[51] between 1971 and 1980 in those patients diagnosed over 65 years of age. At this time of life when the absolute numbers of patients is reducing, the incidence remains unchanged. Does this imply that Crohn's disease provides some protection in elderly people against death from other causes?

Aetiology

The cause of Crohn's disease is still not known. About 10% of patients have a first-degree relative affected by the disease, and there is a 30-fold increase in sibling incidence compared with the general population.[52] Although patients with Crohn's disease have no consistent human leucocyte antigen typing pattern, individuals with ankylosing spondylitis and human leucocyte antigen B27 have a ninefold increased prevalence of Crohn's disease compared with a control population.[53] There is some evidence that patients with Crohn's disease have an increased intake of refined carbohydrates[54] but as these were retrospective studies in patients who already had the disease it is difficult to know whether the high intake was simply a dietary response to the effects of the disease.

Patients with Crohn's disease are more likely to be smokers, and there may also be some association with oral contraceptive intake.[55]

Attempts to isolate an infective agent in Crohn's disease have so far been inconclusive, although some studies have suggested that a transmissible agent may exist. Because of the pathological similarity to tuberculosis, the mycobacteria have been studied in some detail, particularly *Mycobacterium kansasii*, but no good evidence that these agents are responsible has yet been advanced.[56] Many other possible aetiological factors have been suggested, including ingestion of toothpaste and cornflakes, and a possible autoimmune component has been suggested. No good evidence confirms any of these theories however. Recently two centres have promulgated the importance of measles exposure or a para-tuberculosis infection as the cause of Crohn's disease. Further work is required to support or refute these hypotheses.

REFERENCES

40. Van der Linden W, Hoflin F Eur Surg Res 1978; 10: 225
41. Forgacs P et al Lancet 1973; i: 579
42. Holt S et al Gut 1979; 20: 493
43. Crohn B B et al J Am Med Assoc 1932; 99: 1323
44. Dalziel T K Br Med J 1913; 2: 1068
45. Combe C, Saunders W Med Trans Coll Phys 1813; 4: 16
46. Moynihan B G A Edinburgh Med J 1907; 21: 228
47. Armitage G, Wilson M Br J Surg 1950–1951; 38: 182
48. Hellers G K G Acta Chir Scand 1979; Suppl 490
49. Lee F L, Costello F T Gut 1985; 26: 274
50. Acheson E Gut 1960; 1: 291
51. Mayberry J et al Gut 1979; 20: 602
52. Weterman I T, Pena A S Gastroenterology 1984; 86: 449
53. McBride J A et al Br Med J 1963; 2: 483
54. Thornton J R et al Br Med J 1979; 2: 762
55. Lesko S M et al Gastroenterology 1985; 89: 1046
56. Thayer W R et al Dig Dis Sci 1984; 29: 1080

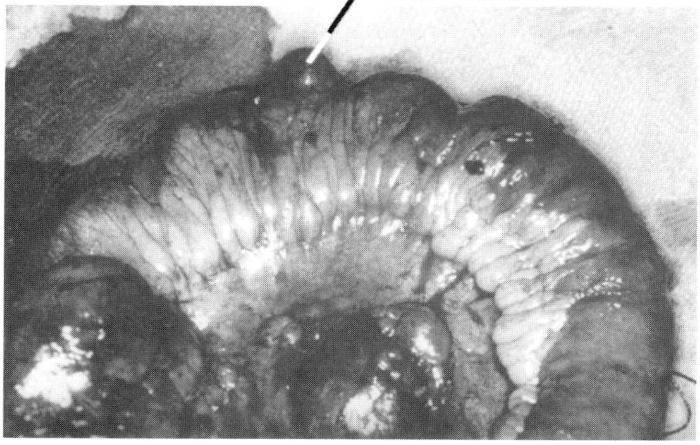

Fig. 29.4 Crohn's disease of the ileum, showing the march of fat from the mesentery on to the serosal surface of the bowel. In this case a Meckel's diverticulum is present and involved in the disease process.

Histopathology

It is possible that the primary lesion is a chronic inflammatory change in a submucosal lymphoid follicle leading to an overlying ulceration with the formation of aphthous-type ulcers. The inflammatory process spreads transmurally when it may lead to the formation of deep fissuring ulcers. When these fissures reach the serosal surface the bowel may become stuck to an adjacent organ and result in fistula formation. Thickening of the bowel wall with narrowing of the lumen may eventually result in obstruction. The lymphatic vessels in the bowel wall and mesentery become dilated and large fleshy lymph nodes develop. The whole process is often discontinuous, with 'skip' areas of involved bowel separated by normal segments. The non-caseating giant cell granuloma is the diagnostic histological feature found in the bowel wall, but it only occurs in 60% of the pathological specimens and presumably reflects some aspect of the immunological response to the disease by the patient. These granulomas are often subserosal in position, and may be found in rectal biopsies taken from patients with small bowel disease who have no macroscopic evidence of Crohn's disease in the rectum. Paneth cell hyperplasia may also be found in response to the chronic inflammatory process. The ileum and ascending colon region are affected in two-thirds of patients; the colon alone is involved macroscopically in 20% (Fig. 29.4).

Clinical presentation

The onset of the disease may be acute or insidious depending upon its site and severity. Abdominal pain is the most common symptom, with diarrhoea, loss of appetite and weight, intermittent fever, nausea, vomiting and lassitude frequently associated. Fistula formation is present in about 15% of patients and nutritional disturbances with anaemia (iron, folate or vitamin B_{12} deficiency), hypoalbuminaemia and weight loss are common. These nutritional disturbances may result from anorexia, but are often compounded by the presence of chronic sepsis or malabsorption from involvement of large sections of the small intestine.[57] Anal fissure and fistula formation does occur with ileal Crohn's disease but isolated anorectal involvement is less common than when the disease is present in the large bowel. Apart from the chronic blood loss from the ulceration of the bowel, massive haemorrhage may rarely occur from small bowel disease.

Systemic manifestations of the disease include finger clubbing, large joint arthritis, erythema nodosum, iritis, pyoderma gangrenosum, episcleritis, uveitis and conjunctivitis, sclerosing cholangitis and bile duct carcinoma, although liver problems are much more commonly found in ulcerative colitis. Crohn's disease affecting the gallbladder has been described and pathological evidence of Crohn's disease may be found in skin ulcers either directly related to enterocutaneous fistulae or at some remote site such as the scrotum. This may be regarded as metastatic Crohn's disease. Venous thrombosis and arterial occlusion may occur more commonly in patients with Crohn's disease than expected, particularly at the time of surgery.[58]

Renal stones are more commonly found in patients with Crohn's disease than in the general population.[59] Uric acid stones are found particularly in patients who have had an ileostomy, and calcium triple phosphate stones develop in patients on steroid medication, as the result of calcium mobilization from the bones. Patients with steatorrhoea have an increased colonic oxalate reabsorption and this may also increase the risk of stone formation.[60] In addition to enterovesical and enteroureteric fistulae, hydronephrosis may develop particularly in the right side in association with ileocaecal Crohn's disease.

The nutritional consequences of Crohn's disease may either be very severe or very mild depending upon the extent and the severity of the disease. The state of nutrition may also wax and wane with the disease activity, and may act as a useful guide to the extent of the inflammatory process. Anaemia, vitamin deficiencies, electrolyte imbalance, trace element deficiencies and hypoproteinaemia may all occur in association with weight loss.

Diagnosis

The diagnosis is often delayed for some time as the initial symptoms are often nebulous and non-specific. Confirmation of the diagnosis depends upon finding characteristic histological changes in a biopsy taken from an affected area. A small bowel biopsy can be taken at upper gastrointestinal endoscopy, by the use of a Crosby capsule, at full colonoscopy from the terminal ileum or at laparotomy. A small bowel enema may demonstrate the characteristic small bowel changes of Crohn's disease (Fig. 29.5), which include areas of luminal narrowing with an irregular thick bowel wall. There may be multiple skip lesions and areas of dilatation associated with obstruction. Deep fissuring ulcers or even fistulae

REFERENCES

57. Dyer N H, Dawson A M Br J Surg 1973; 60: 134
58. Misiewicz J J, Pounder R E, Venables C W (eds) Diseases of the Gut and Pancreas. Blackwell Scientific, Oxford 1987
59. Gelzavd E A et al Am J Dig Dis 1968; 13: 1927
60. Chadwick V S et al N Engl J Med 1973; 289: 172

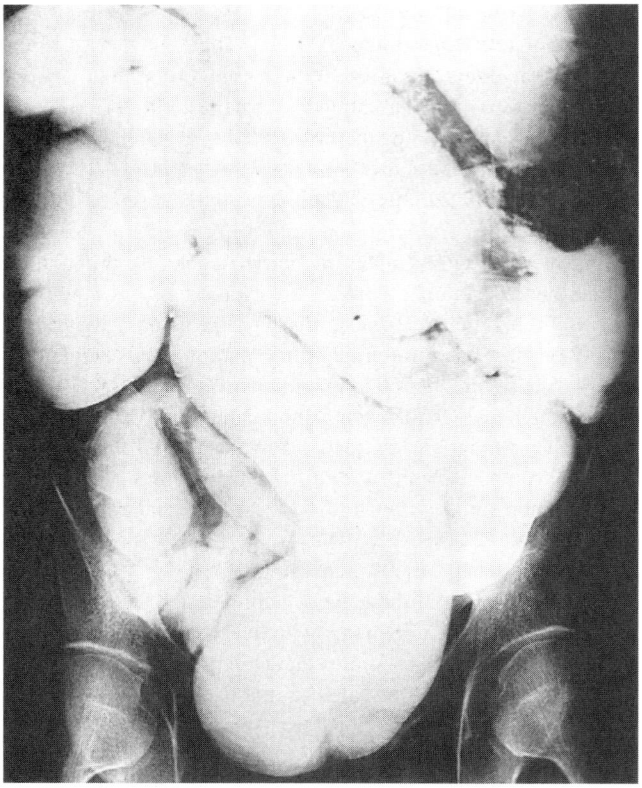

Fig. 29.5 Barium follow-through in a patient with chronic small bowel obstruction associated with Crohn's disease affecting the terminal ileum. In this patient, aged 24 years, a fistula had developed between the ileum and the caecum; the ileum was also the site of an adenocarcinoma.

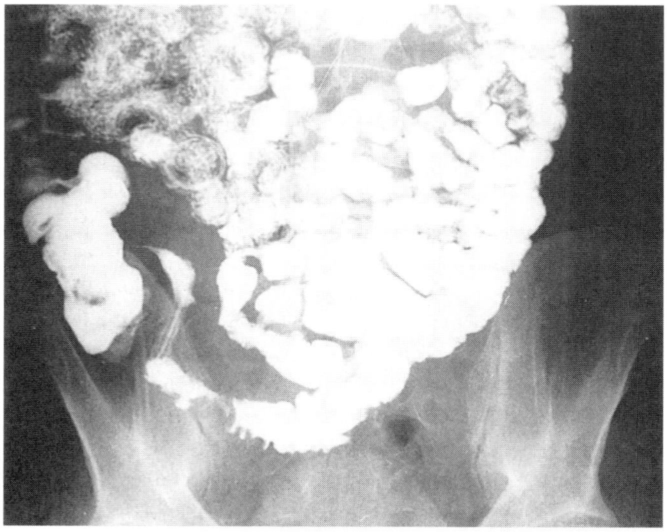

Fig. 29.6 Barium follow-through showing Crohn's disease of the terminal ileum.

may be demonstrated and if the terminal ileum is involved the characteristic string sign of Kantor[61] may be present (Figs 29.6 and 29.7). Between the areas of ulceration the mucosa may be thick and oedematous, giving rise to a 'cobblestone' appearance.

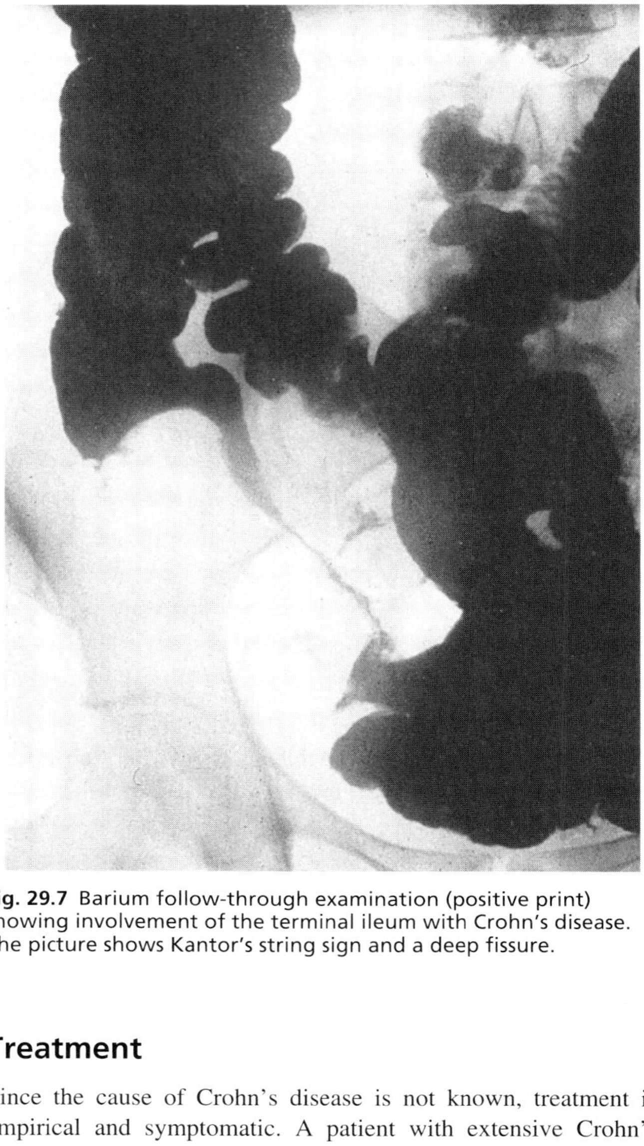

Fig. 29.7 Barium follow-through examination (positive print) showing involvement of the terminal ileum with Crohn's disease. The picture shows Kantor's string sign and a deep fissure.

Treatment

Since the cause of Crohn's disease is not known, treatment is empirical and symptomatic. A patient with extensive Crohn's disease but minimal symptoms requires minimal treatment. In view of the fact that Crohn's disease activity tends to wax and wane, and that there is a high frequency of recurrence of the disease after surgery, surgical intervention should be reserved for specific problems and should not be regarded as curative. There appears to be a tendency in some hospitals to regard surgical intervention as an admission of failure by the physician. The patient may experience a better quality of life with early removal of a small stenosing lesion from the terminal ileum rather than smouldering on with steroids and immunosuppressive therapy, even if the disease recurs. The best results are obtained when interested physicians and surgeons cooperate in a patient's management.

REFERENCE

61. Kantor J L JAMA 1934; 103: 2016

Medical treatment

Most patients with Crohn's disease receive a variable period of medical treatment. This is tailored to the extent and severity of the disease and includes a number of different treatments:

1. Nutritional: dietary alteration to provide palatable mix; replacement of nutritional deficiencies; enteral feeding; intravenous feeding[62] (see Chapter 2).
2. Drugs: steroids—most commonly prednisolone; immunosuppression—azathioprine, cyclosporin; sulphasalazine; metronidazole.
3. Mental and physical support facilities.
4. Antibiotics: for infective complications of Crohn's disease.
5. Anti-diarrhoea agents: codeine phosphate; loperamide; diphenoxylate atropine (Lomotil).

In the National Cooperative study,[63] prednisolone and azathioprine were found to be better than placebo in reducing the activity of Crohn's disease in the small bowel over a 17-week period. There is no evidence that corticosteroids maintain remission,[64] although most clinicians still use them in low doses for this purpose, as experience suggests that abrupt withdrawal of the steroids results in relapse.[65] Sulphasalazine, although useful for damping down colonic Crohn's disease, has not been shown to help small bowel disease.[66] Azothioprine (2 mg/kg body weight per day) when added to a corticosteroid regimen has been found to improve the patient's condition,[67] but is not effective when used alone. The role of cyclosporin in Crohn's disease has not been properly evaluated, but a few dramatic improvements in severely ill patients with Crohn's disease have been noted.[68]

Indications for surgery

As Crohn's disease cannot be cured in the accepted sense of the word, surgery is reserved for patients with specific problems:

1. Intestinal obstruction.
2. Abscess formation.
3. Fistula formation.
4. Failure of medical treatment for limited disease.
5. Need to raise an ileostomy to defunction diseased bowel.
6. Nutritional failure.
7. Small bowel perforation (rare).
8. Acute severe haemorrhage (rare).
9. Uncertainty of diagnosis.

Occasionally a patient may be admitted with acute small bowel obstruction from Crohn's disease, but usually the obstruction is chronic and insidious, with surgery being planned as an elective procedure. Occasionally a patient is operated upon with an 'acute abdomen', usually mimicking acute appendicitis, and Crohn's disease is found. Excisional surgery may or may not be appropriate on these occasions. Certainly excisional surgery should not normally be undertaken for acute ileitis, as the majority of these patients later prove to have an acute *Yersinia* infection (see above).

When there is an absolute indication for surgical intervention the decision to operate is easily made, and the procedure must be tailored to cope with the extent of the disease. In general the least surgical procedure that can solve the problem should be selected, and there is now no place for massive resection of the small bowel in an attempt to clear all disease. Indeed in the acute situation with active disease it can be very difficult to determine just how much small bowel is involved, and a judicious defunctioning split ileostomy may allow inflamed bowel to settle and limit the subsequent resection.

Acute small bowel perforation or haemorrhage are rare complications occurring in less than 2% of hospital admissions for Crohn's disease, but both must be treated by small bowel resection of the appropriate segment.[69] The patient with persistent or recurrent pain with or without obstruction who fails to respond to medical treatment is a candidate for excisional surgery if the disease is limited. This is particularly true where ileal disease is shown to be causing right ureteric obstruction.

Intra-abdominal abscesses should be surgically drained, although in certain situations ultrasound-guided percutaneous drainage of an abscess provides satisfactory resolution, at least in the short term. On many occasions however the abscesses are multiloculate and in these circumstances surgical drainage is more appropriate.

When a fistula forms surgery is often but not always necessary. A patient with an internal fistula between loops of small bowel causing minimal symptoms may be managed perfectly satisfactorily without surgery for many years. However where symptoms are troublesome and unremitting, surgical intervention is indicated. The dangers of urinary tract infection arising from an enterovesical fistula may justify surgery even if the bowel symptoms are minimal.

In recent years it has been recognized that nutritional failure may be an indication for surgery in patients with Crohn's disease that can be resected or bypassed. On occasions simply the construction of a split ileostomy defunctioning distal small bowel disease is enough to improve the state of nutrition. In one such patient an ileostomy disappeared into a valley of fat, and the restricting belt which the patient was forced to wear to hold the bag in place caused pressure necrosis of the skin.

All surgeons who deal with Crohn's disease have been gratified on occasions by the marked improvement in the nutritional status and general well-being of a patient following resection of disease, even when previous intravenous feeding has been ineffective. In children in whom the Crohn's disease has resulted in a failure to thrive, resection of the disease before the epiphyses fuse often allows the growth spurt to occur.

REFERENCES

62. Levi A J Gut 1985; 26: 985
63. Summers R W et al Gastroenterology 1979; 77: 847
64. Smith R C et al Gut 1978; 19: 606
65. Leading article Lancet 1983; ii: 831
66. Malchow H et al Gastroenterology 1984; 86: 249
67. O'Donoghue D P et al Lancet 1978; ii: 955
68. Allison M C, Pounder R E Lancet 1984; i: 1242
69. Greenstein A J et al Am J Gastroenterol 1985; 80: 682

Surgical options

Where surgery is necessary, it should be as limited as possible, and tailored to meet the particular needs of the patient. It used to be fashionable to examine the margins of bowel resection by frozen section until no evidence of Crohn's inflammatory pathology was found.[70] This has been shown to be an incorrect concept and resection only needs to remove the macroscopically obvious disease.[71,72]

As Emanoel Lee stated,[73] surgery should be regarded as 'an incident in a lifetime of disease, rather than an attempt at cure'. At operation diseased bowel should if at all possible be resected rather than bypassed, as recurrence occurs earlier after bypass surgery.[74] Sometimes a bypass at the first operation may allow sufficient resolution of the inflamed bowel for resection to be possible at a subsequent procedure 6–12 months later.

In recent years the concept of stricturoplasty has been introduced for the management of short strictures with chronic disease of the small bowel. The operation involves dividing the stricture longitudinally and suturing it horizontally with a continuous suture of long-lasting synthetic absorbable materials such as polyglactin polyglycolin acid (Vicryl) or Dexon.[75] Balloon dilatation of multiple strictures may also be undertaken at operation.[76] It is well-recognized that surgery of any sort may be complicated by the development of an enterocutaneous fistula. When this occurs, conservative management is usually successful.

It can be very difficult to distinguish operative mortality from mortality of the disease itself. The operative mortality is probably about 3%[77] and there is a twofold increase in the overall mortality compared with the general population at all ages.[78] Following any resection for small bowel Crohn's disease, whether a first or subsequent resection, recurrence requiring further surgery occurs in 40% at 10 years and 50% at 15 years—figures considerably higher than those for Crohn's colitis.[79] (see Chapter 30).

Carcinoma in Crohn's disease

Adenocarcinoma may develop in a small intestine which has been affected by chronic long-standing Crohn's disease. In two-thirds of cases the ileum is involved, although the complication appears to be rare.[80] The prognosis is poor—over 70% of patients die within 8 months of the diagnosis, despite surgery. The reason for this probably relates to a delay in diagnosis, as the symptoms may initially be ascribed to the Crohn's disease. But in addition these tumours do tend to be diffuse and infiltrating, arising in areas of epithelial dysplasia. There is no evidence that there is an increase or decrease in non-intestinal malignant tumours in patients with Crohn's disease.

OTHER INFLAMMATORY CONDITIONS AFFECTING THE SMALL BOWEL

Backwash ileitis

In patients with severe ulcerative colitis with total involvement of colon the terminal ileum may occasionally be the seat of an acute or chronic non-specific inflammatory change. It is important to recognize this possibility when surgery is undertaken for ulcerative colitis, and not to confuse the condition with Crohn's disease. The ileum can be preserved, and the inflammation will resolve once the diseased colon has been removed.

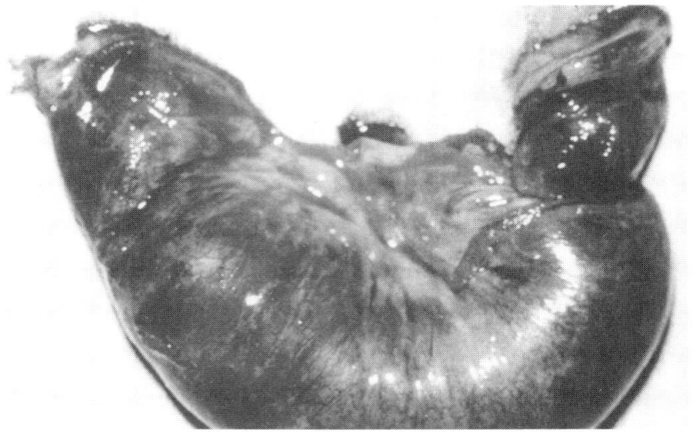

Fig. 29.8 Intussusception of the ileum in a patient with Henoch–Schönlein purpura.

Sarcoidosis

Involvement of the small intestine by sarcoid is very rare, but if the lymph nodes of the mesentery are involved a protein-losing enteropathy can result.[81]

Henoch-Schönlein purpura

Involvement of the small intestine by Henoch-Schönlein purpura occasionally occurs, usually in children, and may present as an acute abdomen either with the signs of peritonitis or by the development of intussusception at the site of a haemorrhage, resulting in small bowel obstruction (see Chapter 27). Laparotomy may be performed inadvertently, in which case it is important to recognize the condition, as reduction or resection of an intussusception may be necessary (Fig. 29.8).

Systemic sclerosis

Any of the connective tissue disorders may affect the small intestine, but the best documented is scleroderma, producing systemic sclerosis. Where the gastrointestinal tract is affected, about half the cases show involvement of the duodenum where the smooth

REFERENCES

70. Kyle J Br J Surg 1972; 59: 821
71. Lee E C G Gut 1984; 25: 219
72. Cooper J C, Williams N S Ann R Coll Surg Engl 1986; 68: 23
73. Lee E C G Gut 1984; 25: 219
74. Homan W P, Dineen P Ann Surg 1978; 187: 530
75. Alexander Williams J Int J Colorect Dis 1986; 1: 54
76. Alexander Williams J et al Ann R Coll Surg Engl 1986; 68: 95
77. Brooke B N et al Crohn's Disease. Macmillan, London 1977
78. Higgens C S, Allan R N Gut 1980; 21: 933
79. deDomball F J et al Gut 1971; 12: 519
80. Hawker P C et al Gut 1982; 23: 188
81. Popovic O S et al Gastroenterology 1980; 78: 119

muscle is replaced by fibrous tissue.[82] Involvement of the small intestine results in bacterial overgrowth, malabsorption and malnutrition, abdominal pain, bloating and eventually functional obstruction, often erroneously referred to as 'pseudo-obstruction'. The surgeon may have difficulty distinguishing mechanical obstruction from a single specific lesion from this form of functional obstruction, and occasionally an inappropriate laparotomy may be performed.

TRAUMA TO THE SMALL INTESTINE

Open wounds

Until recently it has been taught that wounds of the abdomen which are presumed to be penetrating should always be explored by laparotomy, since the consequences of adopting a policy of careful observation can prove fatal. This view has been challenged in recent years by reports suggesting that careful observation of the patient combined with intravenous fluids and antibiotics might result in a better selection of patients requiring laparotomy.[83] These reports have come from hospitals dealing with so many cases of abdominal injury that the workload might overwhelm the capacity to provide care, and it may be that in hospitals where fewer abdominal injuries are seen a policy of laparotomy for all patients with likely penetrating wounds of the abdomen is still more appropriate. The rising incidence of stab injuries in many parts of the UK[84] may result in a change in policy in the future.

When the small intestine is examined during an operation for a penetrating wound of the abdomen it may be found to be contused, perforated or transected. The mesentery may be damaged with the bowel or it may be damaged alone. The viability of the bowel will depend on to what extent the mesenteric vessels, and particularly the vessels of the peripheral arcade, have been divided or thrombosed.[85]

When examined soon after the injury the contused or perforated bowel is usually in tight spasm and the mucosa is everted through perforations that may be present. Later the bowel dilates and the edges of the tear, which gape more widely, may become swollen with oedema. Perforation of the bowel is followed by suppurative peritonitis (see Chapter 27). Contused bowel may recover completely, may perforate later with peritonitis, or heal with stricture formation.

Small perforations may be closed with two layers of sutures, such as inner 2/0 chromic catgut and outer 3/0 polyglycolic acid inserted so that the line of closure is transverse. Large perforations and multiple perforations placed close together usually require resection, with reconstitution by end-to-end anastomosis. Small contusions may be simply infolded by seromuscular sutures while large contusions or injuries causing division of the mesenteric vessels near the bowel usually require a length of intestine to be resected.

Occasionally the intestine is perforated from within, for example by a fishbone (Fig. 29.9), and the patient presents with a seropurulent peritonitis. Toothpicks, bristles, meatbones, nails, wood splinters and other sharp objects have all been described as perforating agents.

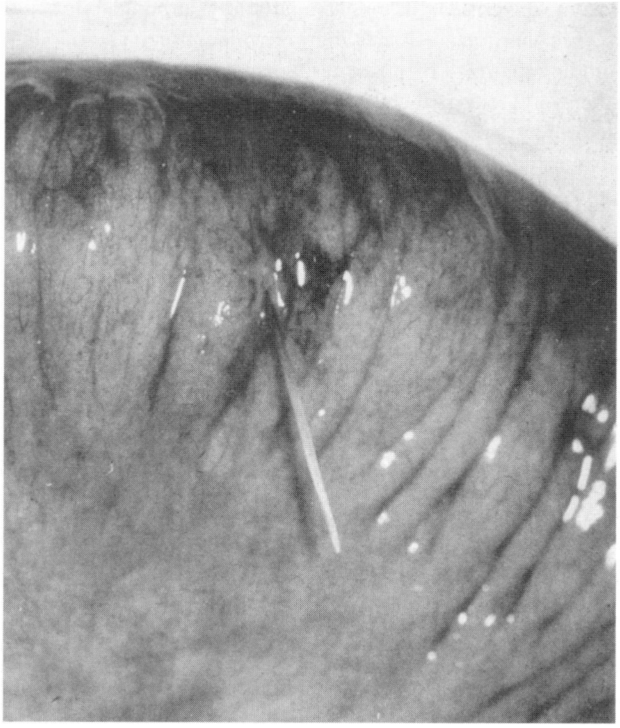

Fig. 29.9 A fishbone penetrating the small bowel and presenting in a patient as peritonitis.

Blunt trauma

The small intestine may be contused or divided by violence applied to the abdomen, without penetration (see Chapter 27). Small intestine partially fixed by adhesions is particularly prone to this type of injury. The normal non-adherent bowel is only injured by sudden trauma to the abdominal wall which catches the patient unprepared with the abdominal muscles uncontracted, allowing the bowel to be squeezed between the traumatizing agent and the vertebral column.

The upper jejunum and lower ileum suffer most commonly, as these are the segments that are prevented from escaping by their relatively fixed attachments to duodenum and caecum. The part of the small intestine where blunt trauma may produce its most dangerous effects is the duodenum, as injury here is often associated with pancreatic injury (see Chapter 33). This may not be immediately obvious, and serious retroperitoneal sepsis may have developed before the diagnosis is made. Morton & Jordan[86] reported 131 patients with duodenal injury; in 14 the injury was caused by blunt trauma. The liver was coincidentally damaged in 38% of cases, the pancreas in 28% and the inferior vena cava in 17%.

REFERENCES

82. Bluestone R et al Gut 1969; 10: 185
83. Oreskovich M R, Caricco C J Ann Surg 1983; 198: 411
84. Mariadson J G, Parsa M H et al Ann Surg 1988; 207: 335
85. Murless B C Br J Surg 1942–1943; 30
86. Morton J R, Jordan G L J Trauma 1968; 8: 127

Diagnosis is often difficult at laparotomy, although bile staining of the retroperitoneal tissues may provide a clue. The duodenum should be mobilized by a Kocher's manoeuvre and division of the ligament of Treitz if there is doubt about a duodenal injury. The surgeon may, however, be between Charybdis and Scylla, as the presence of a large retroperitoneal haematoma may be caused by an injury of the vena cava, and mobilization of the duodenum may release tamponade and result in torrential venous haemorrhage. Two options are open if this situa-tion seems likely. A catheter may be introduced into the duodenum through a gastrotomy and water-soluble radiopaque medium introduced. On-table radiographs are then taken, and a duodenal perforation sought. When the duodenum appears to be intact and the retroperitoneal haematoma is not expanding it is probably wiser not to mobilize the duodenum and simply to institute gastric aspiration. If the duodenum is seen to be ruptured then mobilization is necessary, and preparations must be made for dealing with a potential injury to the inferior vena cava (see Chapter 11). Pancreatic drainage may also be necessary, although Whipple's procedure is reserved for the most severe destructive injuries to the duodenopancreatic axis (see Chapter 33).

Mortality rates as high as 50% have been reported for duodenal injuries; the highest figures are found after blunt trauma. In the majority of patients with duodenal injury, debridement and simple suture with drainage are effective, although a serosal patch may be used[87] or a duodenal defunctioning procedure may be undertaken.[88]

Aird[89] commented on the association between blunt trauma, intestinal perforation and the presence of an inguinal hernia, particularly in men. When a hernia sac is present the increased intra-abdominal pressure at the time of injury causes a segment of intestine to balloon into the sac, causing it to rupture. The neck of the intestine immobilized in a hernia may occasionally be the site and cause of the rupture.

TUMOURS OF THE SMALL INTESTINE

Primary tumours of the small intestine are exceedingly rare, although secondary invasion either directly or by tumour deposits seeded into the peritoneal cavity is relatively common. Primary small bowel tumours are found in about 0.5% of autopsies,[90] although most of these tumours have not caused any symptoms in life. The surface area of the small intestinal mucosa is about 85% of the total surface area of the gastrointestinal tract, but nevertheless it contributes less than 2% of alimentary malignancies.[91] Malignancy is 100 times more common in the oesophagus, stomach and colorectum.

Tumour types (Table 29.1)

Benign tumours are more common than malignant tumours, but in some cases the tumour is of an intermediate variety; it appears to be benign initially but later develops malignant features.

Table 29.1 Types of tumour which may be found in the small intestine

Primary malignant tumours	*Intermediate tumours*	*Benign tumours*	*Hamartomas*
Adenocarcinoma	Leiomyoma/ leiomyosarcoma	Submucous lipoma	Peutz–Jeghers syndrome
Lymphoma	Carcinoid	Adenoma	Vascular malformations
Sarcomas	Gastrinoma Villous adenoma	Fibroma Neurofibroma	Ectopic pancreas

Adenomas

Histologically these benign tumours may appear tubular, tubulo-villous or villous in appearance. In the colon, villous adenomas, which carry a considerable risk of malignant change, make up about 10% of the total polyps while in the small intestine this figure is closer to 40%.[92] Adenomas are most commonly found in the second part of the duodenum, and seem on occasions to be part of the familial adenomatous polyposis syndrome (see Chapter 30).[93–95] In one report from the Cleveland Clinic[96] 22% of a series of patients with villous tumours of the duodenum had polyposis coli; the duodenal tumour was diagnosed at a mean of 17 years after colectomy.

Other small bowel tumours have also been found in familial adenomatous polyposis, for example in the ileum after colectomy.[97] The risk of malignancy in these adenomas seems to be very small.[98]

Polyps may present with intussusception (see Chapter 27), bowel obstruction or bleeding, and once confirmed on barium meal, small bowel meal examination or upper gastrointestinal endoscopy, can be removed either endoscopically or, if they are inaccessible, at laparotomy.

Carcinoid tumours (chromaffinoma: argentaffinoma)

The term 'carcinoid' was introduced by Obendorfer[99] in 1907 to describe a tumour of the small intestine with a capacity for metastasis, but which was slow-growing and had a good prognosis. The tumour was identified histologically by the staining of granules within its cells using silver preparations, and subsequently the carcinoid tumour has been identified as an example of an APUDoma, i.e. a tumour of the APUD cells (amine precursor uptake decarboxylation—which describes their biochemical properties).

The most common site for a carcinoid tumour is the appendix, and here it constitutes 85% of appendicular neoplasms. About

REFERENCES

87. Kobold E E, Thol A P Surg Gynecol Obstet 1963; 118: 340
88. Corley R O et al Ann Surg 1975; 181: 92
89. Aird I Br J Surg 1936–1937; 24: 529
90. Darling R C, Welch C E N Engl J Med 1959; 260: 397
91. Williamson R C N et al Ann Surg 1983; 197: 172
92. Perzin K H, Bridge M P Cancer 1981; 48: 799
93. Hoffman D C, Goligher J C Br J Surg 1971; 58: 126
94. Yao T et al Gastroenterology 1977; 73: 1086
95. Jarvinen H et al Gut 1983; 24: 333
96. Galandiuk S et al Ann Surg 1988; 207: 234
97. Hamilton S R et al Gastroenterology 1979; 77: 1252
98. Ross J E, Mara J E Arch Surg 1974; 108: 736
99. Obendorfer S Frankf Z Pathol 1907; 1: 426

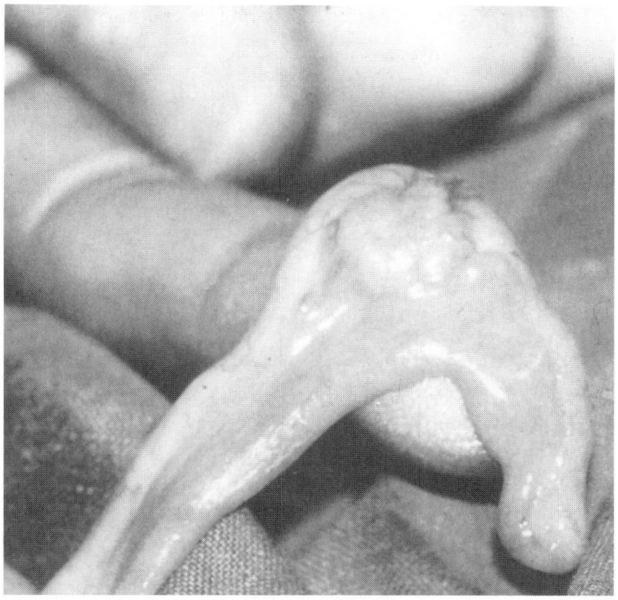

Fig. 29.10 A carcinoid tumour of the appendix.

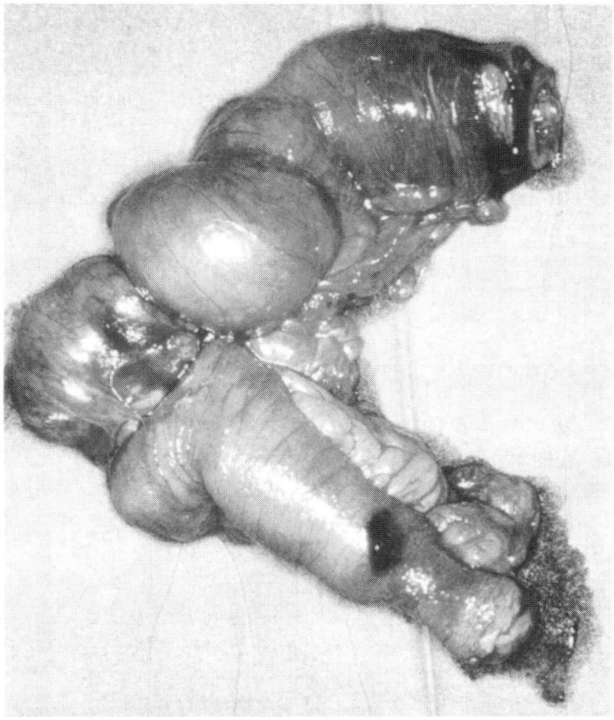

Fig. 29.11 A carcinoid tumour of the ileum producing small bowel obstruction.

0.5% of removed appendices are found incidently to contain a carcinoid tumour, which forms a submucosal yellow mass, usually nearer the tip of the appendix rather than the base (Fig. 29.10). The vast majority show no evidence of spread or metastasis, but if the muscle is involved and if lymph node spread has occurred then a right hemicolectomy is necessary.

Carcinoid tumours involving the small intestine should however be regarded as malignant. They are most commonly found in the ileum; 73% of malignant carcinoids are found at this site[100] (Figs 29.11 and 29.12). Some 7% occur in the bronchi (see Chapter 22) and 4% in the jejunum.

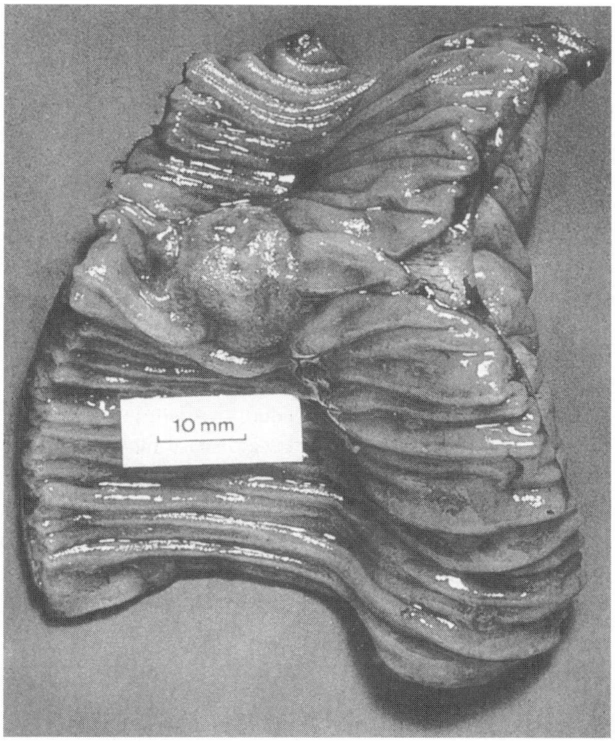

Fig. 29.12 A resected specimen of ileum opened to show a carcinoid tumour.

Small bowel carcinoid tumours usually present with intestinal obstruction: in 40% of cases metastases are found at laparotomy.[101] The tumours can be recognized by the intense cicatrization which they produce, and when the bowel is opened they appear as raised, yellow submucosal tumours sometimes with a central area of mucosal ulceration. They have to be differentiated from submucous lipomas, but look different.

About 4% of patients with small bowel carcinoid tumours develop the carcinoid syndrome, which is a combination of flushing, intestinal hypermotility and bronchospasm. The development of this syndrome depends on the tumour-secreting kinins such as 5-hydroxytryptamine, bradykinin and histamine, and on the tumour being of such sufficient bulk in liver metastases to secrete these kinins into the systemic circulation. The kinins are normally totally inactivated by the liver. The carcinoid syndrome may very rarely develop when a kinin-secreting tumour metastasizes on to the abdominal parietes, when again secretion of the kinins may occur directly into the systemic circulation.

Carcinoid tumours of the left colon and rectum do not seem to secrete kinins, and hence are not associated with the carcinoid syndrome even when liver metastasis has occurred.[102] An

REFERENCES

100. Norheim, I et al Ann Surg 1987; 206: 115
101. Bowers C R, Cheek J H Arch Surg 1952; 64: 92
102. Moertel G C et al Cancer 1968; 14: 901

association has been reported between duodenal carcinoid tumours and neurofibromatosis.[103] These duodenal carcinoids contain somatostatin, and macroscopically have psammoma bodies and a glandular growth pattern, so they can easily be confused with a duodenal adenocarcinoma. The precise mechanism of the association is unknown.

Carcinoid syndrome

The flushing found in this syndrome may be a transient erythema with facial telangiectasia and suffused conjuctiva. Bronchospasm occurs during episodes of kinin release, and intestinal hypermotility appears as watery diarrhoea and borborygmi, often associated with hypokalaemia. Right-sided cardiac lesions such as pulmonary stenosis and tricuspic valve disease may be associated with fibrosis, and since tryptophan is required for 5-hydroxytryptamine synthesis, patients may develop a nutritional deficiency of the amino acid. Tryptophan is also required for the synthesis of the vitamin niacin (nicotinic acid) as well as for protein, and its deficiency may result in pellagra and hypoproteinaemia.

Treatment

There seems little doubt that debulking of as much tumour as possible will relieve the unpleasant symptoms of the carcinoid syndrome. To some extent this may be possible surgically and should be preceded by appropriate antiserotonin therapy, such as methysergide maleate 2 mg t.d.s. Liver metastases can be reduced by a combination of hepatic chemotherapy infusion, with agents such as cyclophosphamide, Adriamycin and 5-fluorodeoxyuridine in combination and systemic chemotherapy, but at best only palliation is obtained.[104,105] Other drugs such as parachlorophenylalanine, phenoxybenzamine, chlorpromazine, cyproheptadine, α-methyldopa and corticosteroids may be valuable in reducing unpleasant side-effects such as diarrhoea and flushing.

Previous experience with two patients has shown that radiotherapy to the liver can abolish the carcinoid syndrome, at least for a time.

Prognosis

Malignant carcinoid tumour of the small bowel has a 25% 6-year survival rate, with 15% still alive at 10 years.[106]

Gastrinoma

This tumour is also one of the APUD series, and is found with a frequency of 2–3 cases per million of the population per year in western societies.[107] It has been suggested that up to 1% of all patients with duodenal ulcer disease may harbour a gastrinoma. Most gastrinomas are found in the pancreas (see Chapter 33), but a few occur in the duodenum when they may produce the Zollinger–Ellison syndrome.[108] Even small tumours, less than 5 mm in diameter, can produce the full syndrome and it is therefore not surprising that the primary tumour is often not found. The majority of duodenal gastrinomas are probably malignant.[109] It used to be the practice that if the primary tumour could not be located total gastrectomy was undertaken. The recent use of omeprazole, a potent inhibitor of the proton pump in the parietal cell, has however been found virtually to eliminate acid secretion and thus control symptoms.[110]

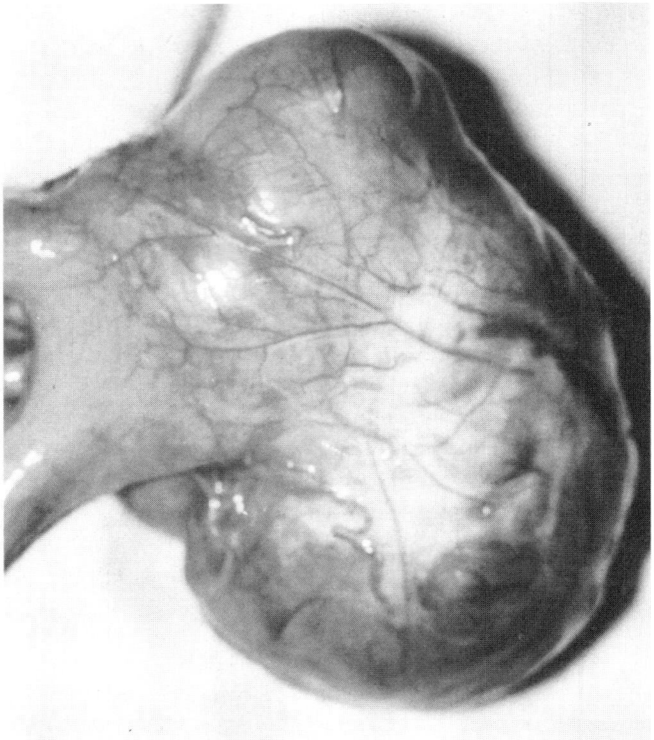

Fig. 29.13 An exenteric leiomyoma of the terminal ileum.

Leiomyoma/leiomyosarcoma

A leiomyoma is a neoplasm of the smooth muscle, but histologically it can be very difficult to state that this tumour is entirely benign and probably there is a gradation of invasiveness. Tumours with extensive nuclear pleomorphism and a high mitotic index may run a relatively benign course.

Leiomyomata usually occur singly and may be found with equal frequency in any part of the small intestine. As they grow they tend to ulcerate the overlying mucosa and often present with massive intestinal bleeding. They may cause obstruction or act as a focus for intussusception if they enlarge into the lumen of the bowel. If they grow by stretching the serosa (exenteric; Fig. 29.13), they may become very large before producing symptoms; an

REFERENCES

103. Griffiths D F R et al Q J Med 1987; 64: 769
104. Melia W M et al Br J Cancer 1982; 46: 331
105. Harris A L Cancer Chemother Pharmacol 1981; 5: 133
106. Davis Z et al Surg Gynecol Obstet 1973; 137: 637
107. Buchanan K D Br J Hosp Med 1980; 24: 190
108. Zollinger R M, Ellison E H Ann Surg 1955; 142: 709
109. Stable B E, Passaro E Am J Surg 1985; 149: 144
110. Lamers C et al N Engl J Med 1984; 310: 758

exenteric leiomyoma impacted in the pelvis may even produce colonic obstruction.[111] Central necrosis may occur if the tumour is a leiomyosarcoma, with the formation of either an abscess or a fistula into an adjacent loop of intestine. Treatment is by small bowel resection as these tumours are resistant to radiotherapy and chemotherapy. The 5-year survival rate for leiomyosarcomas is about 30%.

Lymphoma

Primary lymphomas of the intestine tend to present in the seventh decade and occur randomly throughout the small intestine. They are sometimes multiple. They usually produce an annular, constricting and ulcerating mass leading to obstruction and anaemia. They may complicate coeliac disease and diffuse nodular lymphoid hyperplasia. Both Hodgkin's and non-Hodgkin's lymphomas can occur, but they are mainly classified as diffuse or nodular lymphomas of the non-Hodgkin's variety. Some 30% of lymphomas present with perforation causing peritonitis and 40% are palpable as an abdominal mass, which may need to be differentiated from Crohn's disease or an intussusception.

Small bowel resection should be undertaken where possible, though palliative bypass may be all that is possible. Despite the fact that these tumours are sensitive to radiotherapy and chemotherapy, the overall 5-year survival rate has been reported to be less than 20%.[112]

The development of a lymphoma should be suspected if any patient with coeliac disease suddenly deteriorates despite adherence to a gluten-free diet. Investigations at an early stage may be unrewarding and a diagnostic laparotomy may be more appropriate.[113] These tumours are usually malignant histiocytomas and the outlook is extremely poor.

Mediterranean lymphoma, or α chain disease, is a special variety of intestinal lymphoma usually affecting the jejunum. It is of unknown aetiology,[114] although chronic intestinal infections may be a predisposing factor. It is found particularly in the Middle East in countries bordering the eastern Mediterranean and its development is often preceded by non-lymphomatous immunoproliferative small intestinal disease, involving the immunoglobulin γ A secretory system of plasma cells.[115] Severe malabsorption, finger clubbing and abnormal α heavy chain components of the immunoglobulins are usually found in blood and urine. Later, small intestinal obstruction and occasionally perforation from deep fissuring ulcers may develop. When possible, small bowel resection is the mainstay of treatment.

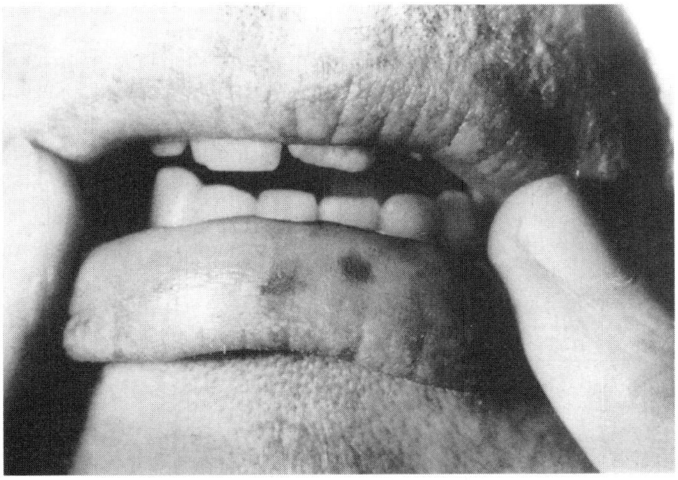

Fig. 29.14 Circumoral pigmentation of the Peutz–Jeghers syndrome.

Other sarcomas

Fibrosarcoma, liposarcoma and angiosarcoma are extremely rare in the small intestine,[116] although Kaposi's sarcoma, associated with the acquired immune deficiency syndrome, has been described in the small intestine and may in the future increase in frequency.[117]

Peutz–Jeghers hamartomas

The Peutz–Jeghers syndrome is a rare inherited autosomal dominant condition in which circumoral mucocutaneous pigmentation (Fig. 29.14) is associated with hamartomatous polyps in the small intestine, and hamartomas of the stomach and colon have also occasionally been described.[118,119] The blue-to-brown flecks of pigmentation may be found on the lips (especially the lower lip), the buccal mucosa, the hard and soft palate and the skin of the fingers and toes. The polyps are not adenomas but show the features of hamartomas, with a fibrous and smooth muscular core covered by well-developed normal small intestinal epithelium,[120] and may vary in size from a few millimetres to 5 cm (Fig. 29.15). The polyps are usually multiple and present in childhood. As the patient grows they may ulcerate, producing bleeding and anaemia, or may act as a focus for intussusception causing small bowel obstruction. Malignant change has also been described,[121] but is probably rare and occurs in 2–3% of patients. Surgery is necessary when the hamartomas produce symptoms, and sometimes multiple enterotomies with local excision or larger resections are required. This can be avoided if all the polyps are removed endoscopically through a single enterotomy at the time of laparotomy.

Adenocarcinoma

The most common site of occurrence for adenocarcinomas of the small bowel is the duodenum, and 80% of malignancies arising in the duodenum are carcinomas. Some 60% present with epigastric

REFERENCES

111. Cookson C C Lancet 1947; ii: 280
112. Awrich A E et al Surg Obstet Gynecol 1980; 151: 9
113. Cooper B T et al Medicine 1980; 59: 249
114. Al Saleem T I Lancet 1978; ii: 709
115. Lewin K J et al Cancer (NY) 1976; 38: 2511
116. Slavin G In: Booth C C, Neale G (eds) Disorders of the Small Intestine. Blackwell Scientific, Oxford 1986
117. Friedman S L et al Gastroenterology 1985; 89: 102
118. Peutz J L A Ned Maandschr Geneesk 1921; 10: 134
119. Jeghers H N Engl J Med 1944; 231: 88
120. Morson B C Dis Colon Rectum 1962; 5: 337
121. Cochet B et al Gut 1979; 20: 169

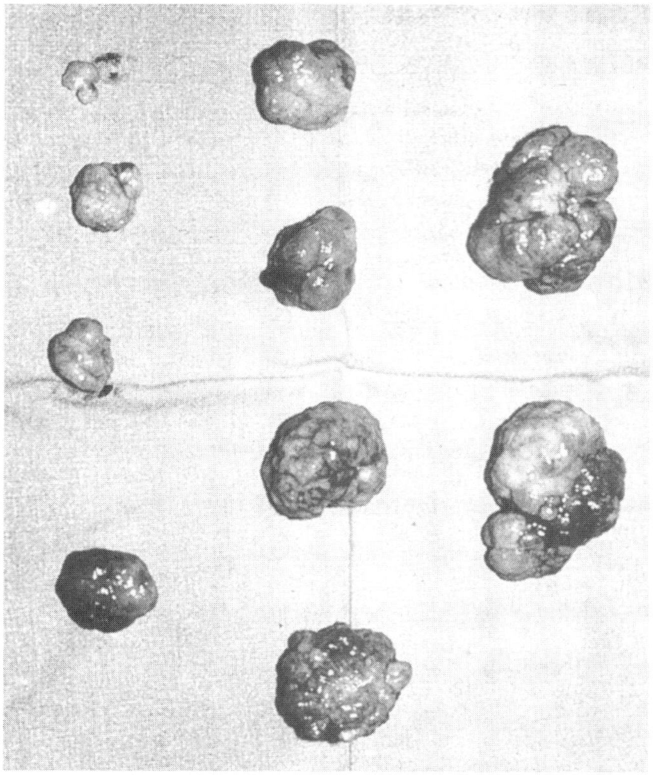

Fig. 29.15 Multiple hamartomas removed endoscopically from the small intestine through a single enterostomy made at the time of laparotomy.

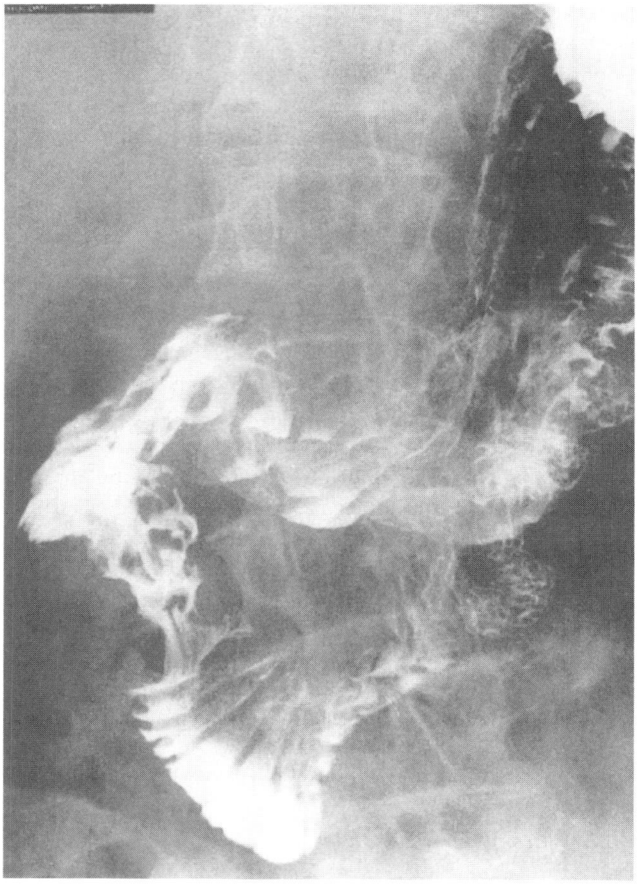

Fig. 29.16 Barium meal showing a carcinoma in the second part of the duodenum.

pain, usually associated with vomiting, weight loss and anaemia. When sited near the ampulla of Vater an adenocarcinoma may present with obstructive jaundice; 20–30% of patients have this feature (see Chapter 32).[122] A primary adenocarcinoma of the duodenum may be confused with an ampullary tumour, an infiltrating bile duct carcinoma or even an advanced carcinoma of the pancreatic head. Invasion by an external tumour may also be suspected. Apart from the history, the diagnosis depends on barium contrast studies (Fig. 29.16), endoscopy and biopsy. Ultrasound and computed tomography scanning may also delineate the tumour. There are usually no specific physical signs unless secondary spread has occurred. Surgery offers the only hope of cure. Local resection may occasionally be appropriate, but usually more radical surgery such as a pancreatoduodenectomy (Whipple's procedure) is necessary (see Chapter 33).[123]

Even if the tumour is not resectable palliative surgery, which may consist of gastrojejunostomy and either cholecystojejunostomy or choledochojejunostomy, may alleviate vomiting and clear the jaundice (see Chapter 32). Pain relief may be achieved by an alcohol block of the coeliac plexus. In the rare event of malignant change being found in the apex of an adenoma local excision using a diathermy snare down a fibreoptic duodenoscope is simple and effective. Where the polyp is sessile it will almost certainly not be possible to make this distinction until pancreatoduodenectomy has been performed. The 5-year survival rate is less than 20%.[124]

In the jejunoileal region the majority of adenocarcinomas occur in the first 50 cm of the bowel, and in this part of the small intestine equal numbers of carcinomata and other malignant tumours such as sarcomas and lymphomas are found.[125]

Jejunal carcinomas (Fig. 29.17) tend to be circumferential and ulcerating tumours, often producing chronic small bowel obstruction with bleeding and anaemia. Diarrhoea, weight loss and a palpable mass may be present and ileal tumours may perforate, although this is unusual. Probably most carcinomas of the ileum develop in pre-existing Crohn's disease, while in Meckel's diverticulum all types of small bowel tumour may be found.[126]

The diagnosis of jejunoileal carcinoma is often only confirmed at laparotomy although the history, physical findings and barium follow-through studies may be highly suggestive of the diagnosis. Surgical resection with end-to-end anastomosis offers the only hope of cure, but side-to-side entero-entero anastomosis may provide palliation for obstruction. The overall 5-year survival rate is less than 30%, but is about 50% if lymph node metastasis has not already occurred.[127]

REFERENCES

122. Lillemare K et al Surg Gynecol Obstet 1980; 150: 822
123. Whipple A O Ann Surg 1935; 102: 763
124. Lowenfels A B Lancet 1973; i: 24–26
125. Arthaud J B et al Am Gastroenterol 1979; 72: 638
126. Weinstein E C et al Int Abstr Surg 1963; 116: 103
127. Bridge M F, Perzin K H Cancer 1975; 36: 1876

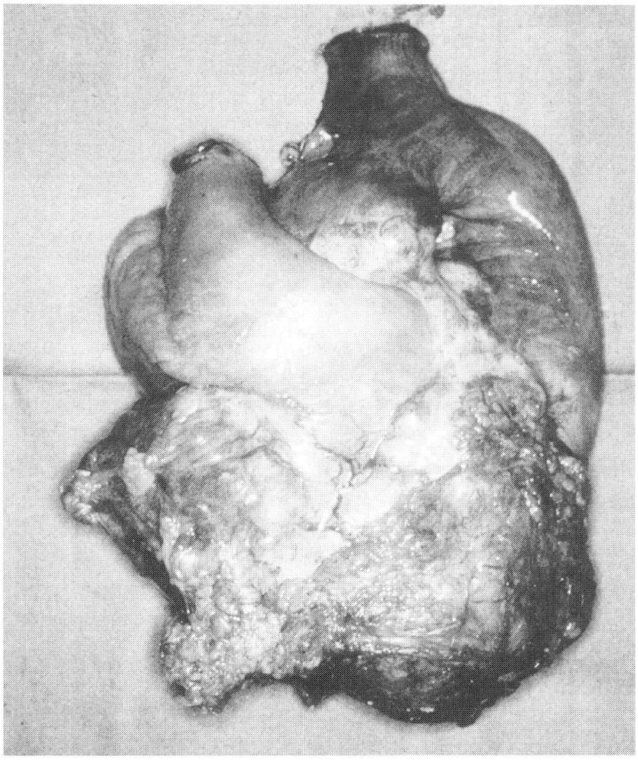

Fig. 29.17 A large adenocarcinoma of the jejunum presenting in an 80-year-old man with anaemia.

Occasionally extremely rare malignant tumours may be found in the small intestine, as for example the malignant fibrous histiocytoma of the ileum, which presents with perforation and peritonitis.[128]

Secondary deposits

The small intestine may become involved by a number of secondary cancers, but of interest is the report by Das Gupta & Brasfield,[129] suggesting that half the patients dying of malignant melanoma show intestinal metastases at autopsy.

ENDOMETRIOSIS

Endometriosis is a common condition and is believed to affect between 8 and 15% of menstruating women.[130,131] It has been estimated that foci of endometriosis occur in the intestines of about 4% of women,[132] but symptoms are thankfully rare.

These deposits usually occur on the large bowel, particularly the sigmoid colon, but occasionally the ileum is involved and here endometrosis may cause intestinal obstruction.[133–135] Menstrual bleeding from the intestine as the result of endometriosis is extremely rare as the endometriosis, invades from the serosal surface and only rarely ulcerates through to the mucosa. Treatment of the obstructive deposit is surgical, but in order to abort the endometriosis, danazol 200 mg twice dally or norethisterone 1 mg twice daily may be prescribed as long-term prophylaxis. Once the ovaries have stopped functioning or been removed, endometriosis regresses. Pregnancy has a similar beneficial effect.

SMALL INTESTINAL INFARCTION

Pathology

Infarction of the small intestine may be caused by an acute reduction in the arterial input as the result of a mechanical occlusion, embolus, thrombosis or poor cardiac output; blockage of the venous drainage by mechanical occlusion or thrombosis; or by a combination of both factors. Arterial insufficiency may also be caused by severe hypovolaemic and cardiogenic or septicaemic shock. The mucosa, which has the highest rate of cell turnover and metabolism, suffers most and if the ischaemic episode is transient, mucosal necrosis alone may occur with subsequent healing, sometimes with stricture formation. Otherwise the full thickness of the bowel is damaged and secondary bacterial invasion may produce gas within the bowel wall and eventually within the portal vein and liver.

When the superior mesenteric artery is occluded (see Chapter 10) there is a short-lived pallor of the bowel associated with muscular spasm; however, this was only observed in 7 of 359 cases in one series.[136] The capillaries and venules then dilate and the contained blood becomes anoxic, imparting a dusky blue appearance to the bowel. Oedema follows and then the small vessels become disrupted causing haemorrhage into the lumen and bowel wall. The increased peristalsis and spasm present at the outset give way to atony and paralysis and eventually gangrene. The vessels beyond the embolus or thrombosis become filled with propagated thrombus.

Small intestinal ischaemia and infarction

Infarction of the small bowel may be a localized or generalized process. When a loop of small intestine is strangulated in a hernial sac or twisted about an adhesive band, localised ischaemia and infarction may occur. In a Richter's hernia see (Chapter 26) the damage may be to only part of the circumference of the bowel (Fig. 29.18) but this situation is most dangerous as obstruction may be a late phenomenon and only occurs when perforation is impending. Patients with intestinal ischaemia often have a background of continuous pain, overlaid by episodes of colic, and may demonstrate little in the way of physical signs despite severe abdominal pain until peritonitis and perforation occur. Patients are usually pyrexial, dehydrated from vomiting, with low urine outputs, and high polymorphonucleocyte counts, often in excess of 25 000 cells per mm^3.

REFERENCES

128. Raju G C et al J R Soc Med 1987; 80: 385
129. Das Gupta T K, Brasfield R D Arch Surg 1964; 88: 969
130. Hawthorne H R et al Am J Obstet Gynecol 1951; 62: 681
131. Venter P F, S. AFr. Med J 1980; 57: 895
132. Ecker J A et al Am J Gastroenterol 1964; 41: 405
133. Kinder C H Br J Surg 1953–1954; 41: 550
134. Golditch I M Obstet Gynecol 1965; 26: 780
135. Bose A, Davson J Br J Surg 1969; 56: 109
136. Trotter W Embolism and Thrombosis of Mesenteric Vessels. Walters, London 1914

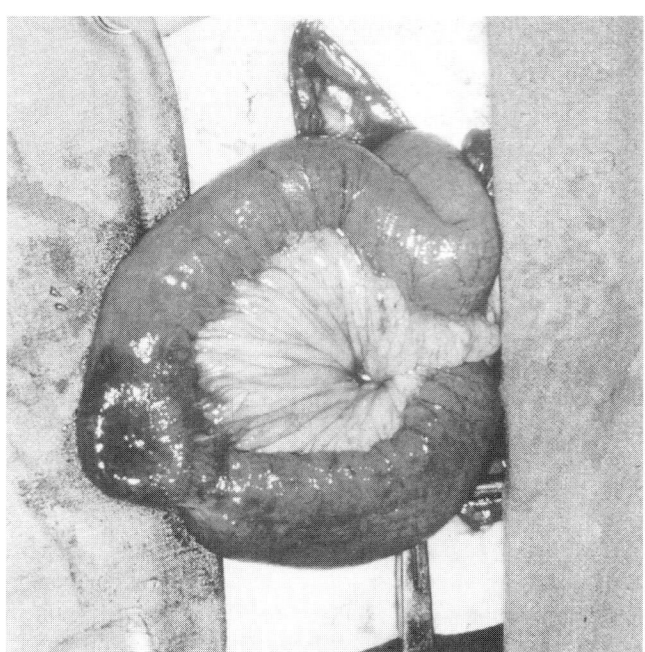

Fig. 29.18 Ileum caught in a femoral hernia—a Richter's hernia.

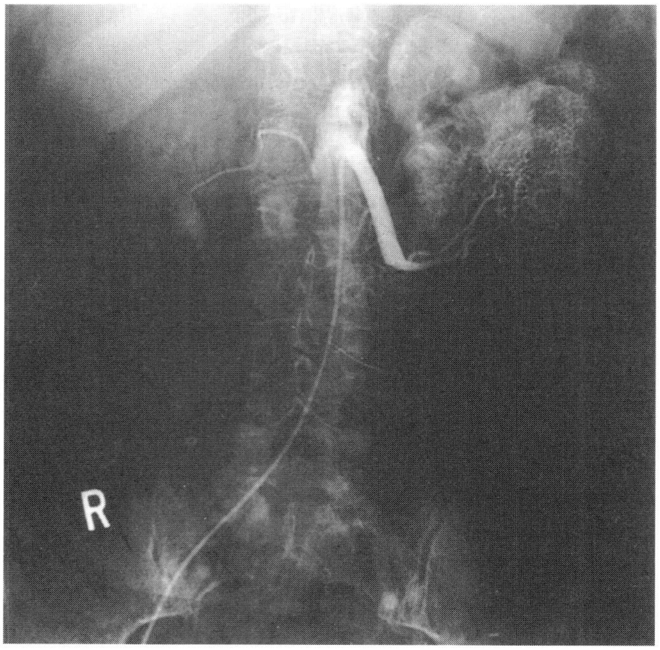

Fig. 29.19 Selective superior mesenteric arteriogram showing an embolus lodged just beyond the first jejunal branch of the artery. This 74-year-old woman was suffering from atrial fibrillation.

Mesenteric vascular occlusion

Mesenteric vascular occlusion was first described by Tiedmann in 1843.[137] Elliott[138] performed the first successful resection in 1894, but Klein[139] could only find records of 24 successful resections in 1921.

Mesenteric venous thrombosis

This condition accounts for fewer than 10% of all cases of intestinal ischaemia and may be the result of a variety of causes including trauma, increased blood coagulability (e.g. post-splenectomy), portal vein thrombosis, dehydration, ascending infection from, for example, an inflamed retroileal appendix, compression by neoplasms or bands, intestinal volvulus and the use of vasoconstrictor drugs such as vasopressin.[140] The onset of symptoms is often insidious with a low-grade fever, epigastric or periumbilical cramping pains, vomiting and diarrhoea, followed by abdominal distension and peritonism. This contrasts with the acute onset of symptoms associated with mesenteric arterial occlusion. The diagnosis may be suspected from the history, and is suggested by features of small bowel obstruction and thickening of the bowel wall on plain abdominal X-ray. The diagnosis can be confirmed by selective arteriography.

Treatment is by resection of infarcted bowel, venous thrombectomy and the creation of an intestinal stoma and mucus fistula. Primary anastomosis should not be attempted. In order to prevent extension or recurrence of the venous thrombosis long-term postoperative anti-coagulation is necessary. Some cases resolve spontaneously.

Mesenteric arterial embolus

Mesenteric embolism accounts for 25–30% of patients with intestinal ischaemia.[140] In all, 90–95% of emboli arise from the heart in patients with atrial fibrillation. Emboli may sometimes pass into branches of the superior mesenteric artery resulting in localized areas of infarction, but usually an embolus impacts just beyond the middle colic branch of the artery, hence sparing the upper jejunum and transverse colon[140] (Fig. 29.19). The majority of mesenteric emboli arise from the heart: from the left auricle in patients with atrial fibrillation, from a mural thrombus following a myocardial infarct or from vegetations or platelet thrombi on the mitral valve; they can also arise from a septic thrombus in a pulmonary vein, or from a plaque of atheroma in the aorta. Any illness resulting in vomiting and dehydration in elderly patients may so reduce the blood flow to the intestine that, coupled with some degree of atheromatous narrowing, a low-flow state may result in localized or extensive bowel ischaemia and necrosis. The condition is now a well-recognized complication of cardiac surgery. Where the main stem of the superior mesenteric artery is blocked with an embolus, the resulting catastrophe involves infarction of the intestine from a point about 15 cm beyond the duodenojejunal flexure, to the splenic flexure of the colon providing that the coeliac axis is functioning.

REFERENCES

137. Tiedmann T Vereng. u Schliessung d Pulsa. Krankheiten. Leipzig 1843
138. Elliott J W Ann Surg 1895; 21: 9
139. Klein T Surg Obstet Gynecol 1921; 33: 385
140. Marston A (ed) In: Vascular Disease of the Gut. Arnold, London 1986

The surgical options must be balanced against the quality of life that may be expected if the operation succeeds. In a younger patient the option of extensive resection followed by total parenteral nutrition, which may be continued at home, can be considered, but in elderly patients closure of the abdomen and effective pain control by the judicious use of opiates is likely to be more appropriate. Otherwise arterial embolectomy and revascularization procedures may be considered if the bowel is potentially viable (see below).

Mesenteric artery thrombosis (Fig 19.20)

Thrombosis of the superior mesenteric artery superimposed on atherosclerosis accounts for 10–15% of cases of acute intestinal ischaemia. The thrombosis usually occurs at the origin of the superior mesenteric artery and in consequence infarction is usually extensive from just beyond the ligament of Treitz to the splenic flexure. When a potentially reversible situation is found at laparotomy a bypass graft of autologous saphenous vein can be inserted between the aorta and the superior mesenteric artery; this is often technically very difficult in an obese patient. Alternatively a side-to-side anastomosis of the common iliac artery to the ileocolic artery produces retrograde revascularization.[140] Any frankly dead or dubiously viable bowel must be resected before revascularization is attempted as toxic washout of metabolites is often fatal if necrotic bowel is revascularized.

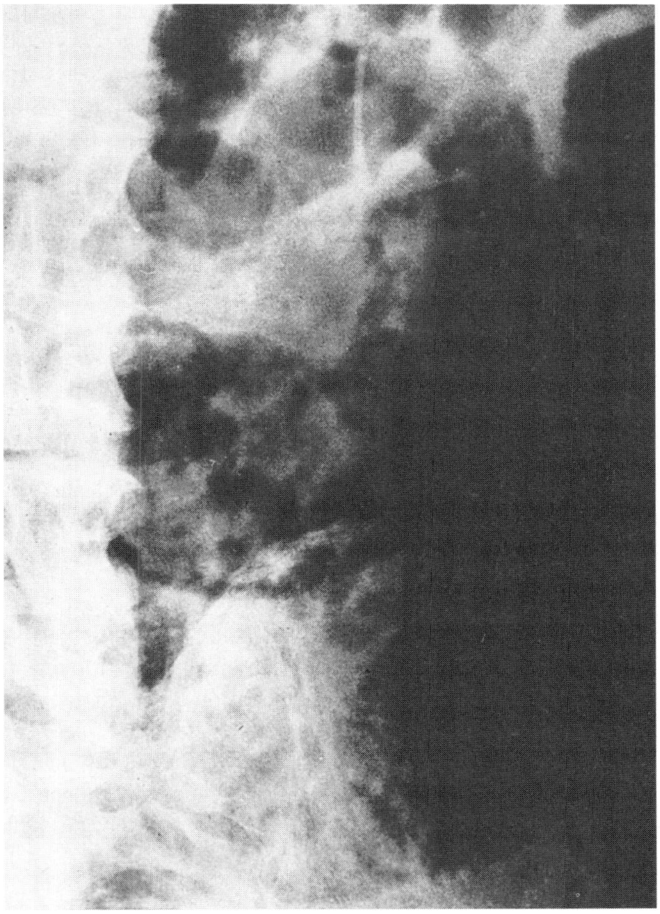

Fig. 29.20 Plain abdominal X-ray showing gas in the wall of the small bowel in a 75-year-old diabetic man with small bowel infarction due to thrombosis of the superior mesenteric artery.

Occlusion suggesting thrombosis may occasionally be produced by extension of an aortic dissecting aneurysm into the root of the superior mesenteric artery (see Chapter 10).

The mortality from acute intestinal ischaemia is between 70 and 100% and does not appear to have changed significantly over the last 50 years.[140] The peak age incidence for death occurs at 70 years for men and 85 years for women, and there is often a delay in diagnosis in view of the rather imprecise nature of the symptoms and signs. In middle-aged or elderly patients, particularly if they are known to have cardiac disease, who develop sudden prostating abdominal colic with rapid collapse, pallor and a fall in systolic blood pressure and subsequently the signs of acute obstruction should be suspected of having a mesenteric arterial blockage. Sometimes blood is passed per rectum, but this is relatively rare. There is often hyperamylasaemia, which may raise the suspicion of acute pancreatitis (see Chapter 33). There was a suggestion that the release of phosphate from the damaged bowel, producing hyperphosphataemia, might prove a useful guide to diagnosis,[141] but this has not proved to be accurate. The differential diagnosis of severe abdominal pain and shock includes a leaking abdominal aneurysm, small bowel volvulus, perforated peptic ulcer and acute pancreatitis.

Laparotomy should be performed early on suspicion of intestinal ischaemia, particularly in a patient with atrial fibrillation. Dead, flaccid, dusky blue or black small bowel with loss of serosal sheen should be resected if this is considered appropriate for the patient (see above). In general it is safer to bring out the jejunum as an end jejunostomy and the colon as a mucus fistula where subtotal small bowel resection is undertaken. When the infarction is more localized, direct anastomosis is appropriate. The state of the remaining bowel can immediately be assessed by looking at the stomas if anastomosis is not attempted. After direct anastomosis a deliberate policy of second-look laparotomy at 24 hours should be planned.[142]

Where the blood supply of the bowel is found to be compromised with lack of pulsation in the mesentric vessels, but the intestine is still viable at laparotomy, the superior mesenteric artery should be carefully mobilized after division of the ligament of Treitz below the transverse mesocolon (Fig. 29.21). The vessel is controlled, an arteriotomy made and Fogarty embolectomy is performed. This may also be carried out through a transected distal arcade at the time of bowel resection.

SMALL INTESTINAL RESECTION

Technique

The wide variation of techniques available for small bowel resection are described elsewhere,[142] but the general principles are

REFERENCES

141. Jamieson W G et al Br J Surg 1982; 69 (suppl S): 52–53
142. Schwartz S L, Ellis H Appleton-Century-Crofts Maingot's Abdominal Operations, 8th edn. Norwalk, Connecticut 1985

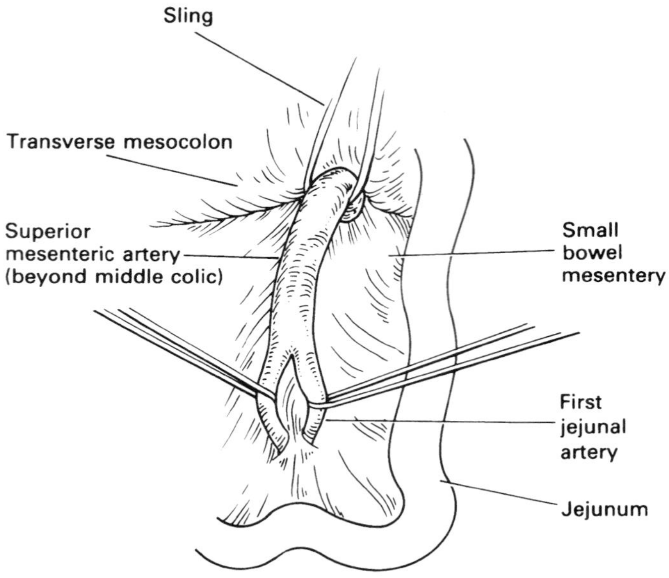

Fig. 29.21 The superior mesenteric artery.

accepted. The segment of small bowel to be removed is resected with a wedge of mesentery. The vessels in this mesentery should be individually ligated to leave the best possible blood supply to the ends of the bowel requiring anastomosis. The bowel ends should be seen to bleed after removal of any clamps and if there is any doubt about the blood supply, for example in radiation-damaged small intestine, it is better to avoid applying clamps. If the viability of the bowel is in doubt, it is wiser to bring the two ends of the small intestine out on to the abdominal wall rather than anastomosing them. The intestine should be handled gently, and the anastomosis made between the open ends of the intestine; spillage is often prevented by application of non-crushing clamps. The cut ends are often made slightly obliquely, with the anti-mesenteric side being shorter. Anastomosis may be made with either continuous or interrupted sutures in one or two layers using absorbable or non-absorbable materials, inverting or everting, including the mucosa, or sparing the mucosa by submucosal sutures. The results are probably closely related to the care with which the surgery is done, but the anastomosis should end up watertight with good blood supply, a satisfactory lumen and under no tension. In order to prevent herniation of bowel, the mesenteric defect is closed with a continuous suture. The speed of the anastomosis is thought to be increased by the use of staple guns, although this is debatable, and in this situation as opposed to oesophageal and rectal anastomosis there is a definite cost benefit for the hand-sewn technique.

The metabolic sequelae

The small intestine is 4 m long and perfectly adequate nutrition can be maintained after half has been resected. Long-term survival has been recorded in an adult with 15–45 cm of jejunum remaining along with the duodenum and colon, although the patient maintained a low weight. Special enteral feeding may be required and in a small number of patients suffering from the short bowel syndrome long-term intravenous feeding, which can be managed at home, is sometimes possible.[143] Malabsorption of vitamin B_{12} and bile salts, with consequent anaemia, malabsorption of fats and fat-soluble vitamins, and diarrhoea may occur after resection of 50–80 cm of ileum; steatorrhoea is a feature after 90 cm of resection. Following loss of small bowel the remainder undergoes adaptation with an increase in villous height and in the number of enterocytes.[144]

BLEEDING FROM THE SMALL INTESTINE

The majority of patients with either acute or chronic blood loss into the gastrointestinal tract are either bleeding from the upper gastrointestinal tract, including the oesophagus, stomach and duodenum, or from the colorectum. If, after investigation of such a patient, no source of the blood loss is found at any of these sites, then a source of bleeding within the small bowel must be sought.

Acute haemorrhage

Patients with acute bleeding into the small bowel may present with melaena or even the passage of frank blood per rectum. There may be intestinal colic and, depending upon the site of blood loss, features of shock may be present, including faintness, peripheral vasoconstriction with sympathetic sweating, tachycardia, hypotension and oliguria. The patient in this situation needs to be stabilized by resuscitation and, having excluded as far as possible bleeding from the upper or lower gastrointestinal tract, the nature of small bowel bleeding needs to be established. The possible causes of acute bleeding from the small intestine in adults are listed below:

1. Meckel's diverticulum.
2. Intussusception.
3. Angiodysplasia.
4. Peutz–Jeghers syndrome.
5. Leiomyoma/leiomyosarcoma.
6. Lymphoma.
7. Zollinger–Ellison syndrome.
8. Crohn's disease.
9. Non-specific ulceration (cytomegalovirus/fungus).
10. Haemangiomata (Rendu–Osler–Weber syndrome).
11. Aortoenteric fistula.

Following resucitation, an urgent labelled red cell or sulphur colloid scan may be carried out if the patient is continuing to bleed.[145] Technetium^{99m}-labelled sulphur colloid is given intravenously before the abdomen is scanned. Following rapid clearance from the blood by the liver, the technetium^{99m} marker accumulates at any site of active bleeding into the bowel lumen and this point can be identified on the scan. Alternatively red cells

REFERENCES

143. Weser E Gastroenterology 1976; 71: 146
144. Dowling R H N Engl J Med 1973; 288: 520
145. Alavi A et al Radiology 1977; 124: 753

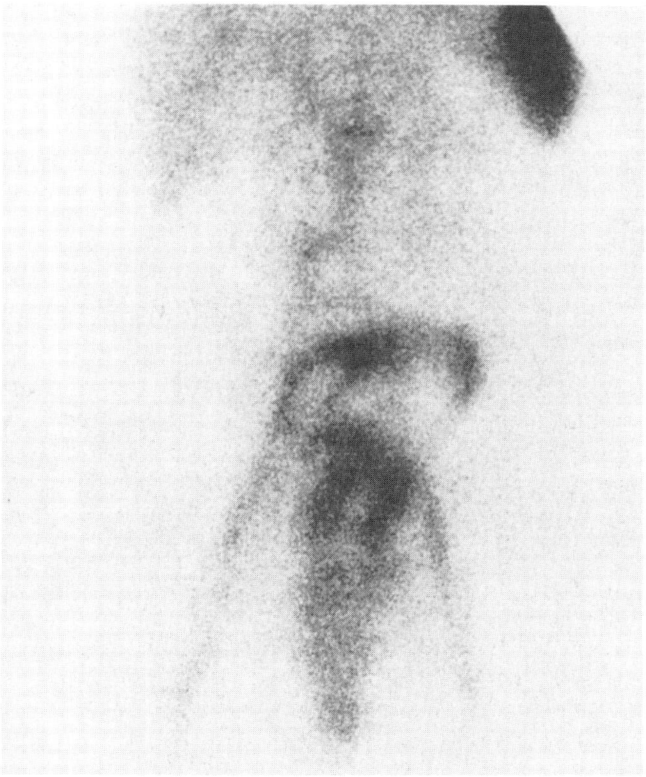

Fig. 29.22 A technetium^{99m} pertechnate red cell scan showing extravasation into the bowel which subsequently proved to be the terminal ileum. This was the result of non-specific ulceration in a patient with chronic renal failure on dialysis.

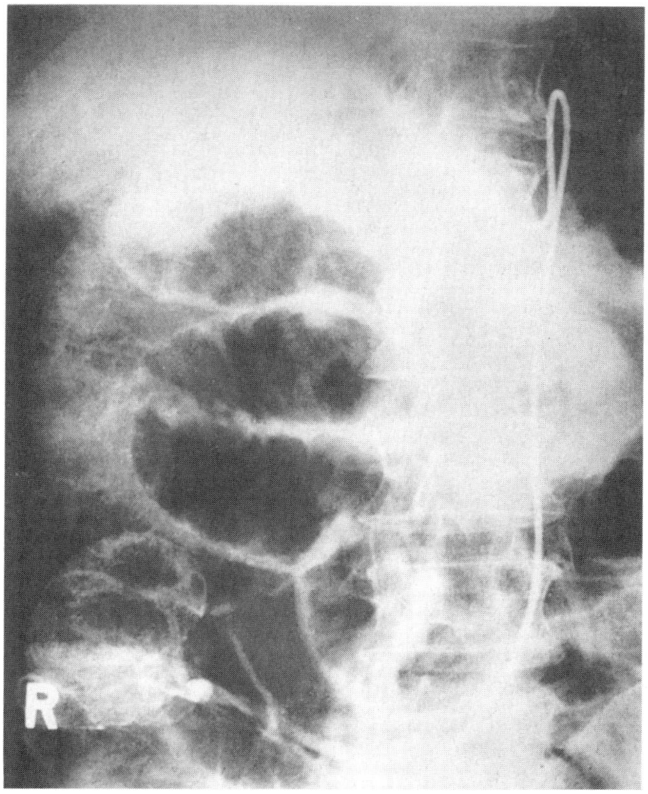

Fig. 29.23 Selective superior mesenteric arteriogram showing the circulation in a leiomyoma of the terminal ileum.

removed from the venous system are labelled with technetium^{99m} and re-injected when the radiomarker accumulates at the site of bleeding (Fig. 29.22). Where the facility for radionucleotide scanning exists it is often obtained before arteriography, which is only carried out if the scan is positive.

Selective arteriography may be performed to provide more precise identification of the site of small bowel bleeding, and the superior mesenteric artery is the vessel to be selectively catheterized. Bleeding from a duodenal source may best be outlined through a coeliac arteriogram, whereas left-sided large bowel haemorrhage is best identified through an inferior mesenteric arteriogram. An obvious tumour may be found (Figs 29.23 and 29.24) or a site of bleeding may be demonstrated by the accumulation of radiographic contrast material in the bowel, without revealing the exact cause (Fig. 29.25). In order to help the surgeon identify the bleeding site at laparotomy, the radiologist may be able to advance the arterial catheter into the feeding peripheral vessel so that at the time of operation methylene blue may be injected via the catheter to identify the segment of bowel involved prior to resection.[146] Occasionally multiple sites of bleeding are shown, as for example in the ulceration sometimes found in patients with immunosuppression when cytomegalovirus or a fungus, such as *Aspergillus fumigatus*, may produce many intestinal ulcers either synchronously or metachronously.[147]

Fibreoptic enteroscopy provides another method of determining the site of small bowel bleeding at operation.[148] A colonoscope

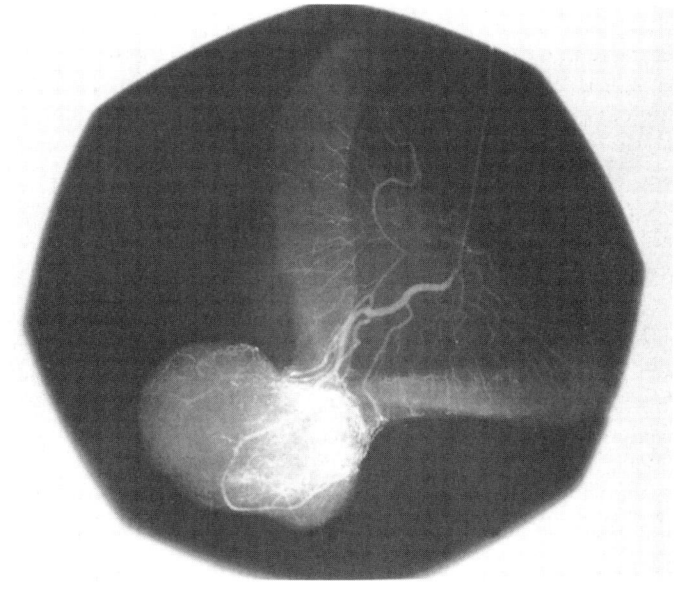

Fig. 29.24 Arteriogram performed on a resected portion of terminal ileum containing a leiomyoma.

REFERENCES

146. Lau W Y et al Br J Surg 1988; 75: 249
147. Kinder R B, Jourdan M H J R Soc Med 1985; 78: 338
148. Lau W Y et al Br J Surg 1986; 73: 217

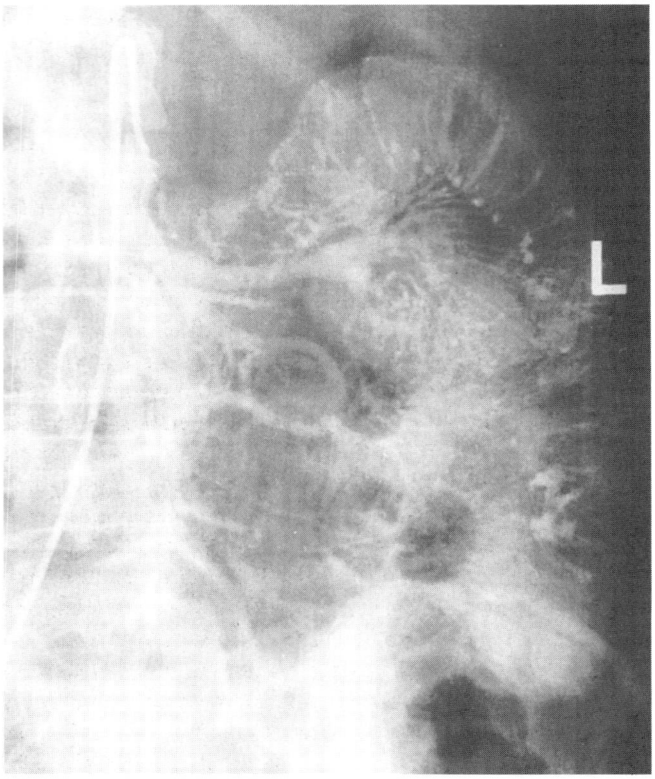

Fig. 29.25 Selective superior mesenteric arteriogram showing leakage of contrast into the upper jejunum. This proved to be the site of an area of ulceration associated with angiodysplasia.

may be fed into the small bowel through the stomach by a surgeon and endoscopist working in concert. The endoscope may be directly inserted into the small bowel by enterostomy.

Angiodysplasia

This is a vascular malformation associated with ageing in which tortuous venous channels open up in the submucosa of the bowel and may ulcerate through the mucosa, producing haemorrhage. Bleeding is often torrential as the vessels are fed from a submucosal arteriole.[149] Angiodysplasia is most commonly found in the elderly, and occurs most frequently in the right colon, though it may also be found in the jejunum and ileum (Fig. 29.26). It is only in recent years since the advent of selective splanchnic arteriography that its importance as a source of gastrointestinal bleeding has been recognized.

There does appear to be an increase in the frequency of angiodysplasia in patients with aortic valve disease and chronic airways disease, although the reason for this is not clear.[150] It has been suggested that the vascular anomalies occur as a result of degeneration of the mucosa associated with capillary and venular dilatation. Gradually an arteriovenous malformation develops.[151]

Although the colonic malformations tend to present in patients over the age of 50 years, the average age of presentation for patients with small bowel angiodysplasia is 30–35 years.[152] The diagnosis is usually made by arteriograph, but extravasation of contrast into the bowel lumen only occurs if the bleeding is greater

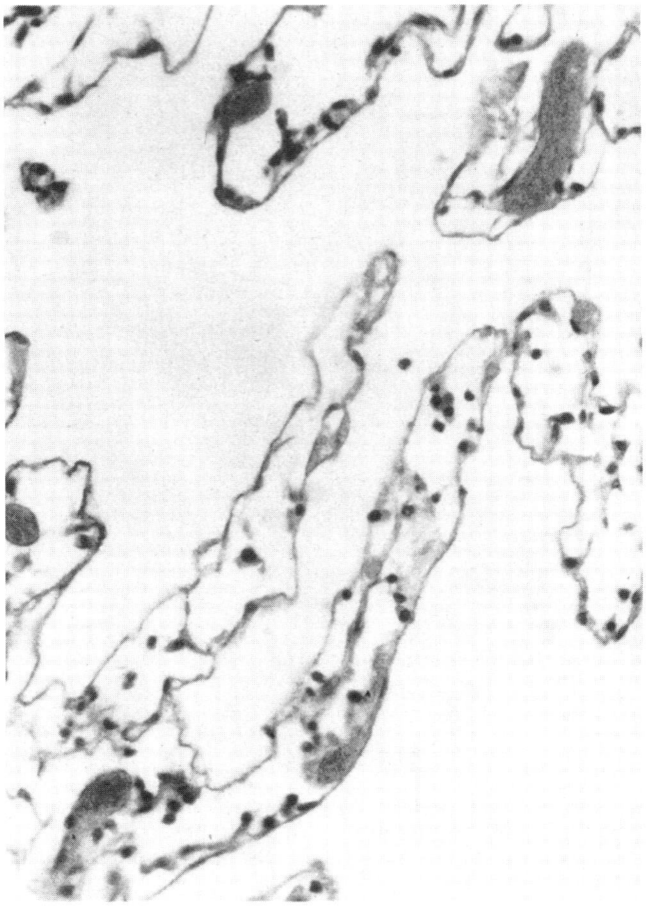

Fig. 29.26 An area of angiodysplasia in the villi of the jejunum. The specimen was injected into its feeding artery with a barium sulphate gel.

than 2 ml/min, and if it is occurring at the time of the angiogram. It must also be remembered that the demonstration of angiodysplasia does not necessarily mean that this is the source of the bleeding, but if the overall evidence leads to that conclusion, treatment of small bowel malformations is usually by resection. The radiologist can help the surgeon identify the segment of bowel involved at the time of laparotomy by leaving a catheter in place in the feeding vessel.[148] Angiodysplasia will only be demonstrated in the resected specimen if the barium sulphate gel is injected into the vessels of the specimen immediately after its removal from the body.[153]

Vascular anomalies

Occasionally intestinal haemangiomas are a cause of chronic small recurrent intestinal haemorrhages, particularly in childhood and adolescence. These vascular malformations are usually submucosal

REFERENCES

149. Marx F W et al Am J Surg 1977; 134: 125
150. Galloway S J et al Radiology 1974; 113: 11
151. Boley S J et al Gastroenterology 1977; 72: 650
152. Meyer C T et al Medicine 1981; 60: 36
153. Boley S J et al Am J Surg 1979; 137: 57

until ulceration occurs, and occasionally are part of a generalized haemangiomatous condition such as the Rendu–Osler–Weber syndrome.[154,155] In this syndrome, also called hereditary haemorrhagic telangiectasia, haemangiomas around the lips, in the buccal cavity, nasopharynx and gastrointestinal tract occur. It is inherited as a Mendelian dominant condition. Bleeding is usually seen in the nasopharynx, but in middle age, gastrointestinal bleeding may occur, although fortunately surgical intervention is only rarely necessary.

Cavernous haemangiomas, such as 'blue-rubber' bleb naevi, may also ulcerate and bleed.[156,157] Jejunal diverticular occur in the Ehlers–Danlos syndrome, and ulcers with bleeding may develop within the duodenum.[158] Occasionally disseminated neurofibromatosis may produce bleeding, as well as small bowel obstruction and perforation.[159]

Widespread Kaposi's sarcoma,[160] a malignant haemangioma, is being increasingly found in the western homosexual population. Gastrointestinal bleeding is a recognized cause of death in this condition.[161]

Ileostomy varices

As the numbers of patients in the developed world who have an ileostomy have increased, the number of complications has also increased. One such complication is the development of varices in the submucosa of the ileum associated with portal hypertension.[162] The classic situation is in the patient with ulcerative colitis who has had a total pan-proctocolectomy but who developed liver disease as a complication of the colitis (Fig. 29.27) (see Chapter 31). The varices may bleed at the point of maximum trauma from the faecal stream or from the appliance, i.e. at the mucocutaneous junction or at the point of passage of the ileum through the abdominal wall. Conservative or local treatment with injection sclerotherapy with 5% ethanolamine is usually effective, but on occasions refashioning of the ileostomy at a new site may be necessary. In general, ileostomy varices are easier to deal with than their oesophageal counterparts, and they may even prevent the development of oesophageal varices. Ileal varices may also develop in an ileal conduit fashioned in a patient who also has portal hypertension.[163]

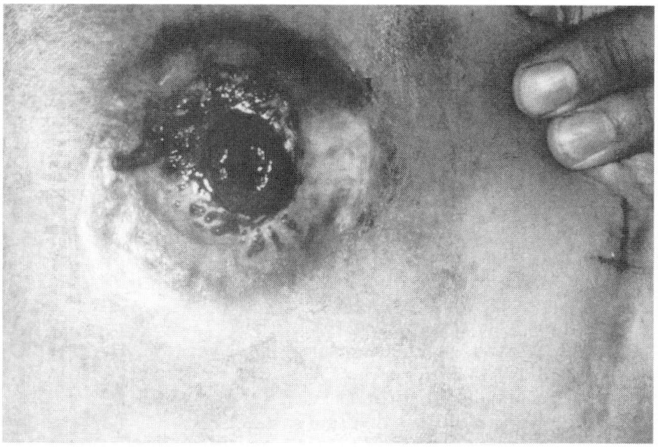

Fig. 29.27 Varices developing around an ileostomy in a 50-year-old man who developed portal cirrhosis and portal hypertension 15 years after pan-proctocolectomy for ulcerative colitis.

Aortoenteric fistula

Most fistulae developing between the aorta and small intestine do so as a result of a Dacron graft insertion on to the aorta, either because of an aortic aneurysm or as part of aortoiliac–femoral bypass (see Chapter 10). The pulsation of the graft may rub against and damage the duodeno–jejunal flexure, although any part of the small bowel may be involved. The inflammatory response so induced causes the bowel either to stick to the graft or to form a seroma between the bowel and graft. Gradually the mucosa of the bowel may ulcerate, infection spreads into the graft and eventually a pinhole connection is made into the aortograft anastomosis or into the graft itself. Alternatively a perigraft infection may burst into the bowel lumen and infection may then cause anastomotic dehiscence. Episodes of haemorrhage into the small bowel occur with increasing frequency over a period of several days, months or occasionally years. The diagnosis is often delayed and an episode of exsanguinating haemorrhage may cause the patient's death.

Investigation is difficult as the connection between the aorta and the bowel is often small and arteriography may fail to demonstrate any abnormality unless bleeding is torrential. Upper gastrointestinal endoscopy performed when the patient is bleeding may demonstrate the presence of blood in the duodenum and the graft sutures may occasionally be seen, but identification of the site of bleeding may not be possible. Computed tomography scan may show a soft tissue mass between the graft and the duodenum. Diagnosis is often made on suspicion and only confirmed at laparotomy.

Primary aortoenteric fistulae are uncommon, but may occur in association with periaortic arteritis or from an aneurysm of the right renal artery.

Treatment

Secondary aortoenteric fistulae should be treated by excision of the graft, closure of the aortic stump and revascularization of the lower limbs by a procedure such as axillobifemoral bypass, coupled with closure of the small bowel fistula.[164] A more conservative approach has also been advocated, replacing the aortic graft with omental interposition between the aorta and bowel[165] or simple repair of the fistula without graft replacement but with omental interposition

REFERENCES

154. Osier W Johns Hopkins Hosp Bull 1907; 18: 401
155. Bandier M Gastroenterology 1960; 38: 641
156. Berlyne G M, Berlyne N Lancet 1960; ii: 1275
157. Fretzin D P, Potter B Arch Intern Med 1965; 116: 924
158. Beighton P, Horan F Br J Surg 1969; 56: 255
159. Manley K A, Skyring A P Arch Intern Med 1961; 107: 182
160. Kaposi M Arch Dermatol Syph 1872; 4: 265
161. Friedman-Kien A E et al Ann Intern Med 1982; 96: 693
162. Ricci R L et al Gastroenterology 1980; 78: 1053
163. Eckhauser F E et al Ann Surg 1980; 192: 620
164. O'Hara P J et al J Vasc Surg 1986; 3: 725
165. Thomas W E G, Baird R N Br J Surg 1986; 73: 875

between the aortic graft and bowel.[166] These more conservative treatments are usually less satisfactory but may be of value in certain circumstances.

For the primary aortoenteric fistula it would seem reasonable to deal with the underlying aortic aneurysm, but even here, particularly in the sick patient, separation of bowel and aorta, local repair and omental interposition seem to work on occasions.

Chronic bleeding from the small intestine

Patients bleeding steadily from the small intestine are likely to present with symptoms of chronic anaemia. Gastrointestinal bleeding is often occult, but faecal testing for blood is usually positive. Initially attention is focused on the stomach and duodenum to exclude a chronic ulcer or gastric neoplasm, and on the right colon looking for a neoplasm, but once these have been excluded, chronic blood loss from the small intestine must be investigated. The possible causes are indicated.

1. Hookworm infestation.
2. Meckel's diverticulum.
3. Angiodysplasia.
4. Carcinoma of the ampulla of Vater.
5. Adenocarcinoma of the small bowel.
6. Other small bowel neoplasms.
7. Crohn's disease.
8. Coagulation defects, e.g. von Willebrand's disease, hereditary thrombasthenia, uraemia.
9. Rendu–Osler–Weber disease.
10. Ehlers–Danlos syndrome.
11. Peutz–Jeghers syndrome.
12. Haemangiomas.
13. Cavernous haemangiomas, e.g. blue rubber bleb naevi.
14. Polycythaemia rubra vera.
15. Systemic sclerosis.

Investigations, including upper gastrointestinal endoscopy to inspect the duodenum, colonoscopy with visualization of the terminal ileum, enteroclysis or small bowel enema, technetium^{99m} pertechnetate scan to detect a Meckel's diverticulum and arteriography, should be performed. Arteriography will delineate the problem in about 45% of patients where a small bowel source of bleeding has been confidently predicted.[167]

In some patients the diagnosis is not clearly determined by these investigations and a diagnostic laparotomy has to be performed, with facilities for on-table endoscopy of the small intestine which can be performed through one or two enterotomies. The theatre lights are dimmed and the small intestine may be inspected both internally and by observation of the light transmitted through the bowel wall, which may occasionally reveal abnormal shadows or vasculature. A single abnormality or several lesions close together may be resected to include the actively bleeding site, but where the problem involves a diffuse small bowel disorder, long-term management may be difficult and restricted to dealing with crises as and when they occur.

NEUROMUSCULAR DISORDERS IN THE SMALL INTESTINE

The term 'pseudo-obstruction' is a bad one, but has gained recognition by common usage to imply a failure of forward propulsion of intestinal contents in the absence of a mechanical cause. The obstruction that this produces however is very real. Acute colonic pseudo-obstruction is common, occurring in elderly patients with chronic obstructive airways disease, cardiac disease or pneumonia, but involvement of the small bowel is less oftenly seen.

Acute postoperative paralytic ileus is much less frequently found in surgical wards than was the case 20 years ago. The attention to fluid and electrolyte and particularly potassium balance,[168] and the enormous improvements in anaesthesia, with all its attendant advantages, have combined to reduce this frustrating complication which is believed to be caused by an overactivity of the sympathetic nervous system. The combination of a ganglion-blocking agent, guanethidine, with a parasympatheticomimetic drug, bethanicol,[169] was used to stimulate peristalsis in patients with a paralytic ileus, but has now been discontinued because of impleasant side-effects. Following operation, the small intestine usually regains normal motility within 24 hours,[170] while the stomach and colon may take several days to recover.[171]

Chronic alterations of small bowel motility can be divided into two types—idiopathic and secondary. Idiopathic pseudo-obstruction of the small bowel is rare, but a report suggests that when it occurs it may be related to elevated levels of prostaglandin E.[172]

Secondary pseudo-obstruction is the result of retroperitoneal damage from inflammation, bleeding, trauma (iatrogenic or otherwise) or infiltrating neoplasms. Ogilvie[173] described this situation producing pseudo-obstruction in the colon. Systemic disease such as amyloidosis, myxoedema and systemic sclerosis may produce the same effect on the small bowel from involvement of the intestine, as may jejunal diverticulosis and coeliac disease.

The diagnosis is often difficult as an element of mechanical obstruction may also be present. Surgery should be avoided if at all possible, but may become necessary if a mechanical obstruction cannot be excluded or a grossly distended bowel needs defunctioning or deflating.

RADIATION ENTERITIS

The small bowel may be damaged by the effects of abdominal radiation and this is now seen with increasing frequency. The most common cause is when a combination of intracavity and external beam radiation has been used to treat carcinoma of the cervix and

REFERENCES

166. Walker W E et al Ann Surg 1987; 205: 727
167. Sheedy P F et al Am J Roentgenol Rad Ther Nucl Med 1975; 123: 338
168. Ebrill D, Naftalin L Lancet 1953; ii: 411
169. Neely J, Catchpole B Br J Surg 1971; 58: 21
170. Ross B et al Gut 1963; 4: 77
171. Wilson J P Gut 1975; 16: 689
172. Luderer J R et al N Engl J Med 1976; 295: 1179
173. Ogilvie H Br Med J 1948; ii: 671

uterus,[174] although radiation damage following treatment of carcinoma of the prostate[175] and testicular tumours[176] is well-recognized. Despite precautions being taken to shield the rectum, there is inevitably some scatter which may affect the bladder or the contents of the pouch of Douglas, and it is in this latter site, particularly if it is bound by adhesions, that the small bowel may be damaged. If the rectum or sigmoid colon is involved a radiation proctitis or colitis ensues, sometimes with ulceration and bleeding and sometimes with fibrosis and stricture formation at a later stage (see Chapter 30).[177] In the narrower small bowel, fibrosis follows irradiation-induced vasculitis, with the development of strictures and small bowel obstruction. When the endarteritis induced by the radiation is sufficiently severe, then ischaemia, necrosis and perforation may occur, and it is interesting to observe at operation how the omentum appears not to be involved in any attempt to wall off the inflamed area (Fig. 29.28).

Radiation strictures in the small bowel are difficult to manage. As far as possible conservative measures should be employed, but resection of the involved bowel may become necessary. Every attempt must then be made to ensure that the two ends have the best possible blood supply. Clamps should not be used; all feeding vessels up to the cut edge should be preserved; the resection margins should be clear of obvious radiation damage and the cut ends should be seen to bleed. The anastomosis should be made with either a non-absorbable material such as Ethibond or Prolene, or a long-lasting material such as Vicryl, but even when performed in a meticulous manner, there is still a risk that it will break down with the development of a fistula or peritonitis.

There is a considerable mortality for this procedure, which in some reports is as high as 50%[178] and for this reason many surgeons prefer to undertake the safer side-to-side anastomosis above and below the stricture, without resecting any bowel.[178]

Resection is obviously essential however when perforation, gangrene or haemorrhage are presenting features, and often in this situation it is wiser to fashion a double-barrelled stoma.

When one or more fibrotic strictures develop as a result of radiation, stricturoplasty may be appropriate; the stricture is divided longitudinally and sutured with a non-absorbable material horizontally.

JEJUNAL–ILEAL BYPASS PROCEDURES FOR MORBID OBESITY

Kremen et al[179] in 1954 first proposed the exclusion of the majority of the small bowel from the foodstream as a treatment for morbid obesity, but it was Payne & De Wind[180] who in 1969 described optimal results in terms of weight loss using 35 cm of jejunum anastomosed end-to-side to the ileum 10 cm from the ileocaecal valve. The divided upper end of the jejunum was closed over and sutured to the small bowel mesentery in an attempt to prevent intussusception, a complication which has subsequently been reported[181] (Fig. 29.29). Thereafter different surgeons have varied the lengths of jejunum and ileum used in the bypass procedure in an attempt to overcome the side-effects, creating an end-to-end jejuno–ileal anastomosis and implanting the lower cut end of the jejunum into the ascending colon (Fig. 29.30).

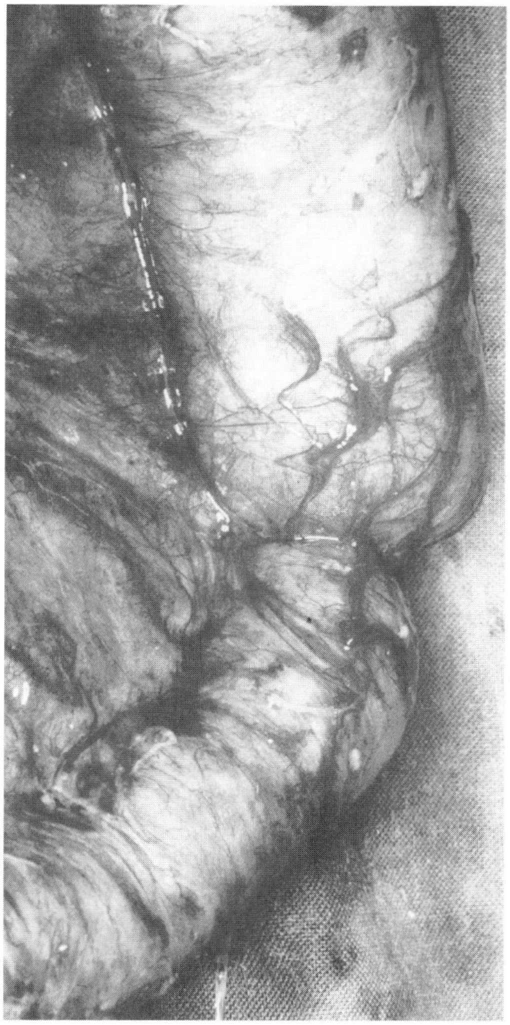

Fig. 29.28 A radiation stricture of the ileum.

In general, fewer side-effects have been associated with the preservation of a greater length of ileum, although Baddeley[181] found only a marginally greater weight loss when 10 cm of jejunum was anastomosed to 35 cm of ileum as opposed to 35 cm of jejunum to 10 cm of ileum.

When results from all the 'bariatric' centres undertaking this operation are reviewed the operative mortality is about 4%, with a further mortality of around 6% occurring later largely as a result of liver failure. Expeditious reversal of the bypass before this complication sets in may reduce the late mortality. Multiple complications have been reported after bypass surgery, including liver

REFERENCES

174. DeCosse J J et al Ann Surg 1969; 170: 369
175. Duggan F J et al Br J Urol 1975; 47: 441
176. Roswit B et al Am J Roentgenol 1972; 114: 460
177. Jackson B T Proc R Soc Med 1976; 69: 683
178. Swan R W et al Surg Gynecol Obstet 1976; 142: 325
179. Kremen A J et al Ann Surg 1954; 140: 439
180. Payne J H, DeWind L T Am Surg 1969; 118: 141
181. Baddeley R M Br J Surg 1979; 66: 525

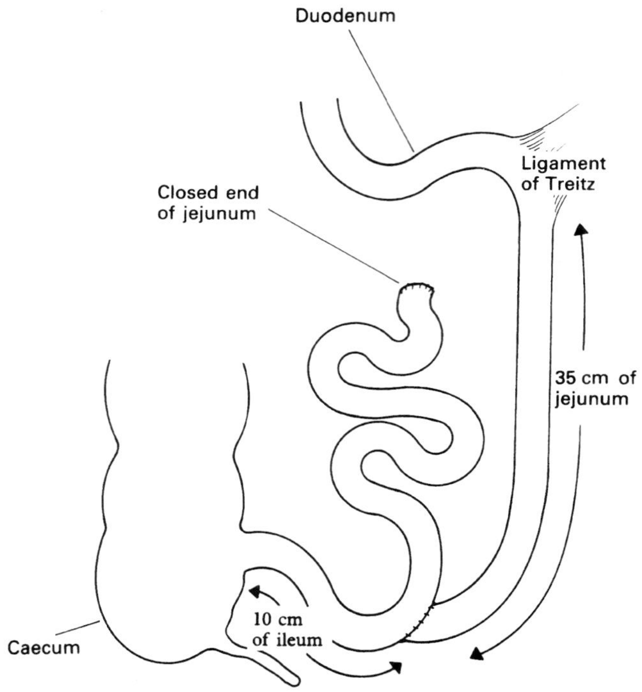

Fig. 29.29 Jejuno–ileal bypass: 35 cm jejunum: 10 cm ileum.

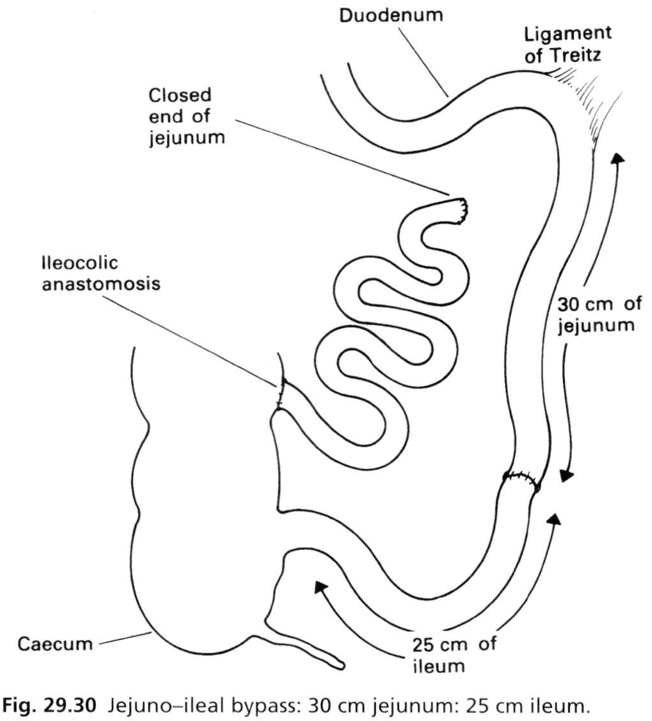

Fig. 29.30 Jejuno–ileal bypass: 30 cm jejunum: 25 cm ileum.

dysfunction, metabolic bone disease, polyarthralgia, polymyalgia, renal calculi and kidney failure.[182] These complications are largely the result of disturbances in the enterohepatic circulation and colonization of the small bowel with bacteria, and in 9% of patients a micronodular cirrhosis develops. Up to 35% have osteomalacia by 5 years after the procedure, and all these problems pose such a

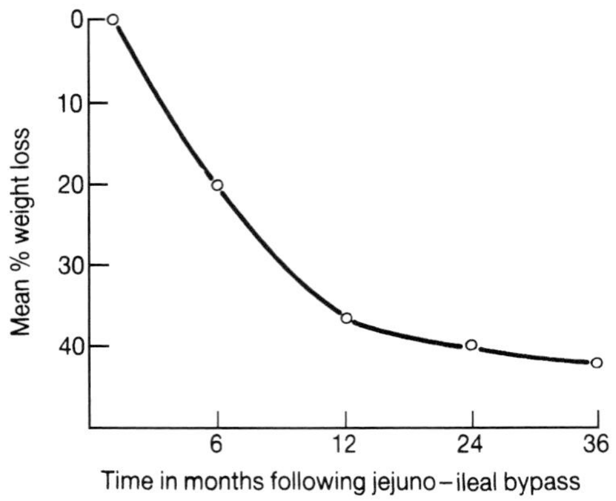

Fig. 29.31 Weight loss following jejuno–ileal bypass.

heavy and expensive clinical load on any centres undertaking the operation that the popularity of jejunal–ileal bypass has waned despite its undoubted ability to produce substantial weight loss (Fig. 29.31).

There are still occasional encouraging reports for jejuno–ileal bypass[183] and for selected patients it probably still has a place, but for the moment emphasis is passing to the technically more difficult but metabolically more satisfactory gastric bypass or banding procedures first introduced by Mason & Ito[184] in 1967 in the surgical management of gross morbid obesity.

In the UK the biggest single experience on jejuno–ileal bypass has been achieved at St George's Hospital in London, and this group has now published its last paper on this subject. However, the decline and fall of this operation were reported by Griffen et al as early as 1983.[185] Many patients are however still attending obesity clinics who need a lifetime of follow-up to monitor any metabolic complications that may develop.

SMALL BOWEL TRANSPLANTATION

In theory transplantation of the small bowel seems to offer an alternative to chronic intravenous feeding in patients with short bowel syndrome following massive intestinal resection. Experimental evidence in animal models has however highlighted the major rejection problems associated with a large amount of lymphoid tissue in the intestinal wall.[186] In addition graft-versus-host reaction is an important complication and immunosuppressive regimens, including cyclosporin, do not appear to prevent this at the moment. There have been a number of attempts at small bowel transplantation in human patients, sometimes in combination with other organs, but the results are not yet sufficiently beneficial. Future success will probably have to await better methods of coping with rejection.[187]

REFERENCES

182. Baddeley R M World J Surg 1985; 9: 842
183. Hope L, Engebretson L F Acta Chir Scand 1985; 151: 625
184. Mason E E, Ito C Surg Clin North Am 1967; 47: 1345
185. Griffen W O Jr et al Surg Gynecol Obstet 1983; 157: 301
186. Madara J L, Kirkman R L J Clin Invest 1984; 75: 502
187. Pritchard T J, Kirkman R L World J Surg 1985; 9: 860

SMALL BOWEL FISTULAE

Small bowel fistulae may develop internally to other loops of small bowel or other intra-abdominal organs, or may open on to the abdominal wall. They may be congenital or acquired.

A congenital small bowel fistula is caused by an incomplete closure of the vitellointestinal duct associated with a distal intestinal obstruction, such as an imperforate anus (see Chapter 41). It is very rare and occurs once in every 15 000 births. It usually presents in childhood, but may not become obvious until adult life when a distal obstruction such as a colonic carcinoma causes small bowel contents to spill out at the umbilicus.

Acquired fistula may be caused in a number of ways including trauma, sometimes iatrogenic following laparoscopy, after small bowel resection or appendicectomy, tuberculosis, actinomycosis, Crohn's disease (Fig. 29.32), malignant disease and small bowel diverticular inflammatory disease. A jejunostomy or ileostomy may be intentionally created by the surgeon. Small bowel fistulae tend to heal spontaneously unless there is distal obstruction or when inflammation proceeds unabated. Surgery is necessary on occasions, but the nutritional state of the patient can be managed during the healing process by the use of total parenteral nutrition[188] (see Chapter 2).

The output from a small intestinal fistula can impose a very significant burden on the fluid and electrolyte balance of the body. In some cases many litres of fluid may be lost, and intravenous replacement with appropriate electrolyte solutions is required (see Chapter 2). The enzyme content of the fistula fluid may produce severe digestive excoriation of the surrounding skin, and much skill and ingenuity may be required to protect the integument. Stomahesive, corya paste and aluminium paste may all be helpful in providing protection. Where an ileostomy or jejunostomy is created surgically, the construction of the everted stoma producing a spout ileostomy as described by Brooke[189] has proved one of the most significant advances in this field.

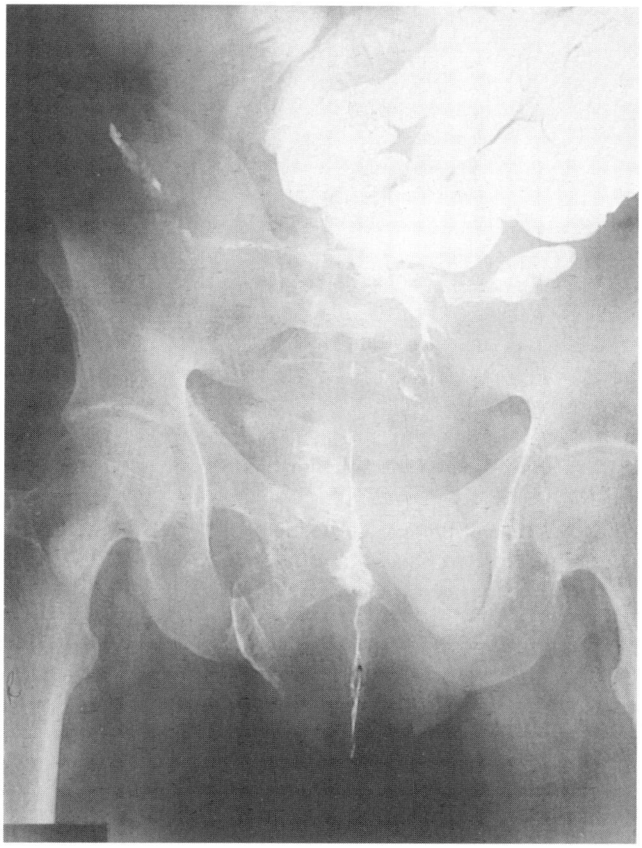

Fig. 29.32 Multiple small bowel fistulae demonstrated at small bowel enema in a patient with Crohn's disease.

CHRONIC CONDITIONS AFFECTING THE APPENDIX

Congenital anomalies of the appendix

Congenital absence of the appendix has been reported.[190] Such a diagnosis is permissible if the taenia coli are followed to a point of junction in the caecum at which there is not even a tiny vestige of an appendix, and if the patient has not been subjected to a previous abdominal operation.

Double appendix has been recorded.[191]

Congenital diverticula of the appendix differ from the acquired variety in that they are intramuscular, having a lining of smooth muscle in their walls.

Intussusception and torsion of the appendix have both been recorded.

Chronic appendicitis

This loose term is used to cover a multitude of conditions in which chronic intermittent right iliac fossa pain is subsequently found to be associated with some pathology of the appendix, and if the appendix is removed the pain disappears. The condition is clinically indistinguishable from a multitude of other causes of right iliac fossa pain including the irritable bowel syndrome, chronic salpingitis and ileoinguinal nerve entrapment.

Mucocoele of the appendix (Fig. 29.33)

Sometimes obstruction occurs at the mouth of the appendix without producing acute appendicitis. Mucus may accumulate in the appendiceal lumen, and the slow distension results in a thickening of the wall of the appendix. In such a way a mucocoele is created. Muscular contraction of the appendix may occur producing a diverticulum but also resulting in colicky pain—so-called appendicular colic.[192] A mucocoele of the appendix needs to be distinguished from the rare papilliferous cystadenoma or cystadenocarcinoma which can arise from the appendix, producing a mucoid tumour which, if it ruptures, may result in

REFERENCES

188. Williams J A, Irving M In: Intestinal Fistulas. Wright, Bristol 1982
189. Brooke B N Lancet 1952; ii: 102
190. Robinson J O Br J Surg 1952; 39: 344
191. Cave I J Anat 1936; 70: 283
192. Wilson R R Br J Surg 1950; 38: 65

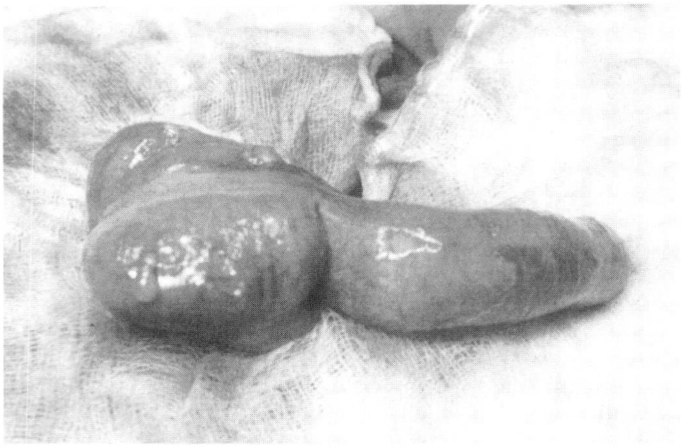

Fig. 29.33 Mucocoele of the appendix.

pseudomyxoma peritonei. Calcification and even heterotopic bone have rarely been described in appendix mucocoeles,[193] and intussusception into the caecum has also been recorded.[194]

Chronic inflammation of the appendix without obstruction, followed by subsequent fibrosis, seems to occur and such an appendix may be found incidentally during laparotomy for some other problem. Often no specific symptoms can be elicited on subsequent enquiry. The appendix may also become blocked by foreign bodies such as lead pellets (Fig. 29.34), fruit seeds, pins and *Ascaris* worms. The patient illustrated in Figure 29.34 had a history of recurrent colicky lower abdominal pains, and appendicectomy was associated with relief of symptoms—a true example of appendicular colic?

TUMOURS OF THE APPENDIX

Carcinoid tumour

(argentaffinoma: chromaffinoma; see Fig. 29.10)

The first tumour of the appendix, its nature still unknown, was described by von Pommer Esche;[195] the first undoubted primary adenocarcinoma by Beger.[196] The peculiarities of the carcinoid tumours were not appreciated, however, until the work of Obendorfer,[99] who introduced the term 'carcinoid'. The incidence of carcinoid is about 0.5%.[197]

Tumour of the appendix is most frequently found in the third decade, and appears to be commoner in women than in men. In 70% of cases the tumour lies near the tip of the appendix[198] and in only 2% of cases is there any evidence of metastasis to regional lymph nodes. Usually these tumours are discovered incidentally at laparotomy and there is always some difficulty in deciding the best course of action. On those rare occasions where obvious metastases have occurred, right hemicolectomy is indicated. The general opinion for the remaining cases is that tumours less than 1 cm in diameter should be removed by simple appendicectomy, but that the larger tumours require a limited right hemicolectomy to remove the draining lymph nodes.

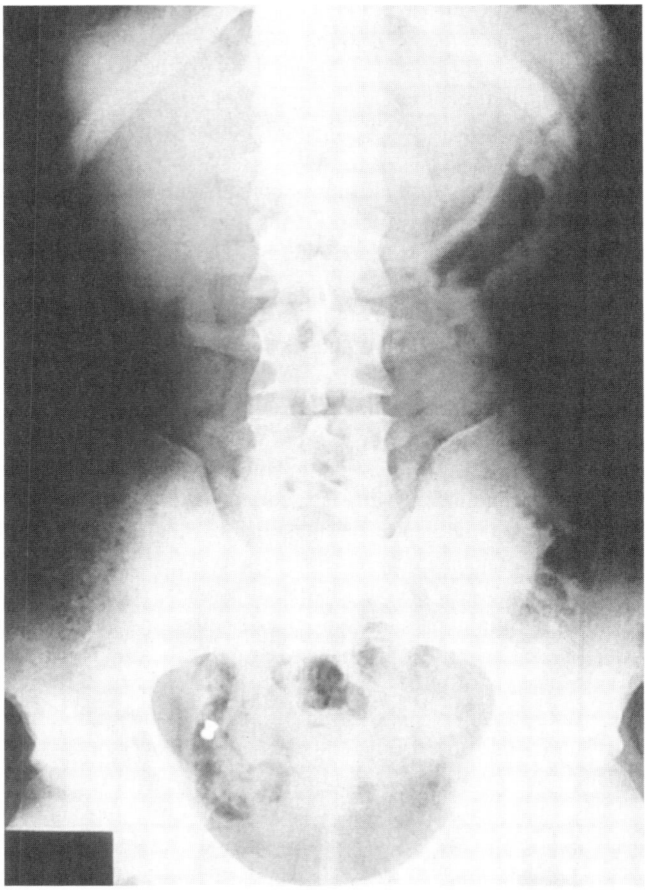

Fig. 29.34 Plain abdominal radiograph in a young man with intermittent colicky abdominal pain. The airgun pellet is seen to be in the appendix. Appendicectomy relieved his symptoms. A case of true appendicular colic?

Adenocarcinoma of the appendix[199]

This is the second most common tumour of the appendix and 10% of patients have widespread dissemination by the time of operation. Following right hemicolectomy the 4-year survival rate is 60%.

Lymphoma may affect the appendix, in which case the regional lymph nodes are usually involved[200] and benign tumours such as fibroma, myxoma, angioma, adenomatous polyp, myoma, myofibroma and neurofibroma have also been recorded. Endometriosis may also involve the appendix.

REFERENCES

193. Juvara U Borcesou Br Med J Surg 1948; i: 931
194. Ward McQuaid J N Br J Surg 1949; 37: 109
195. von Pommer Esche W Med Zeid 1837; 6: 133
196. Beger A Berlin Klin Wochenschr 1882; 19: 616
197. Glasser E M, Bhagavan B S Arch Pathol Lab Med 1980; 104: 272
198. McCartey A, McGrath C Ann Surg 1914; 59: 675
199. Wolff M, Ahmed N Cancer 1976; 37: 2493
200. Gallaway S, Owens B Br Med J 1949; ii: 1387

30 The colon, rectum and anus

N. J. Mortensen R. J. Nicholls J. M. A. Northover N. S. Williams

The colon is no longer regarded as pathologically distinct from the rectum as a result of new developments in diagnosis, pathological understanding, medical and surgical treatments. Many diseases affecting the colon and rectum are the same or analogous. Fibreoptic endoscopy introduced in the late 1960s has enabled precise diagnosis and surveillance of the large bowel, and snare polypectomy has greatly diminished the need for surgical operations for polyps. The air contrast barium enema has increased the sensitivity of contrast radiology fourfold and the developments of ultrasound, computerized tomography and magnetic resonance have also revolutionized diagnosis.

There is now a vast amount of epidemiological data on large bowel cancer and population screening may eventually reduce the mortality of this condition. The strategy of screening depends on an appreciation of the adenoma–carcinoma sequence, a greater understanding of risk factors and the natural history of colorectal cancer. Avoidance of colostomy through sphincter-preserving operations is another major advance. New anastomotic techniques have been established and properly assessed by prospective study. In cancer, risk factors for treatment failure are largely known, particularly with regard to local recurrence. Adjuvant treatments, including radiotherapy and chemotherapy, have formed a large new field of clinical research.

In inflammatory bowel disease, Crohn's colitis has been defined as an entity and the existence of anal disease in this condition established. The natural history, liability to recurrence and indications for surgery have been more fully appreciated. Bypass procedures have been replaced by resections which have become steadily more limited. Clinical trials have rationalized the medical management of colitis. Surgery for ulcerative colitis can now avoid ileostomy in most cases. The indications for surgery and the choice of operation in both emergency and elective cases have been defined.

Anal disease is an integral part of colorectal surgery and important developments in the treatment of haemorrhoids, fissure, carcinoma and sexually transmitted diseases have taken place. The management of anorectal sepsis has been simplified by the employment of an effective classification. Pelvic floor disorders have become of major importance in colorectal practice in the last 20 years. Increased knowledge of disordered function through physiological, radiological and pathological investigation has led to improvements in treatment. Anal ultrasound has transformed the investigation of incontinence and obstetric injuries. An improving understanding of the pharmacology of the anorectum will lead to new medical therapies for common anal conditions.

FISSURE IN ANO

Fissure in ano is a common condition and accounts for about 15% of referrals to a rectal clinic. The fissure is a longitudinal tear in the anoderm of the lower third of the anal canal, extending from the dentate line to the anal margin. It is almost always situated in the midline. In males about 90% are posterior and 10% anterior. In females anterior fissures are more common, comprising 20% of cases, and fissures appearing after childbirth are often associated with a low pressure sphincter. Rarely an anterior and posterior fissure coexist (in about 5% of cases). The condition is most common in young adults and the sex ratio is approximately equal. Fissures occasionally occur in infants and children but are rare in the elderly.[1]

The aetiology is unknown. There is no evidence to support the pecten band theory, where it was thought that constipation with the passage of a hard stool caused the anoderm to tear.[2] The pecten band is in fact a condensation of fibrous tissue occurring as a consequence of chronic inflammation rather than being the cause of the fissure. Only 20% of patients give a history of constipation, which may in any event have been the result of the fissure rather than the cause. Anal canal tone is increased but this may also be the result of reactive spasm rather than the cause of the fissure. Indeed sometimes a fissure complicates a bout of diarrhoea. Fissure is the most common anal abnormality in Crohn's disease and ulcerative colitis.[3] It often occurs in pregnancy and there is an association with chronic intersphincteric abscess in about 5% of cases.[4] This suggests that the fissure may be the result of anal crypt infection, especially given the midline distribution of both fissure and the internal openings of anal fistulae. A further suggestion is that a fissure arises from ischaemia as a result of impaired mucosal blood flow.

The fissure probably starts as a simple linear ulcer. Chronic inflammation then leads to undermining of the edges and the base deepens to expose the fibres of the internal sphincter.[5] A papilla may form at its upper limit level with the dentate line, and a skin tag or 'sentinel pile' develops at its distal end. The sphincter becomes hypertonic, probably in response to the pain produced by the fissure.

REFERENCES

1. Bennett R C, Goligher J C Br Med J 1962; 2: 1500
2. Miles W E Surg Gynecol Obstet 1919; 29: 497
3. Lockhart Mummery H E Br J Surg 1985; 72 (suppl): 595–596
4. Parks A G, Thomson J P S Br Med J 1983; ii: 537
5. Eisenhammer S S Afr Med J 1953; 27: 266

Clinical features

90% of patients have pain on defecation: typically it comes on just after defecation and lasts for 1–2 hours. The fear of defecation may lead to constipation. Bleeding frequently occurs and is usually seen on the toilet paper on wiping. Other symptoms include pruritus (50%), a watery discharge (20%) and constipation (20%).[6] An obstetric history in females is essential. A previous sphincter injury during childbirth with an additional 'injury' from treatment of a fissure may result in incontinence.

The diagnosis is made on inspection by gently parting the anal margin (Fig. 30.1). In 20% of cases a simple split is seen but in the remainder features indicating chronicity are found. Chronicity is recognized by the presence of any of the following: skin tag or papilla, undermining of the edges of the fissure or visible sphincter fibres in its base. Digital examination is contraindicated at this stage as it is painful and unhelpful, but it is usually possible to pass a paediatric sigmoidoscope to exclude proctitis without causing undue pain. A full anorectal examination is however essential and is most conveniently carried out during treatment of the fissure itself with the patient under general anaesthesia when the fissure is extremely painful.

The differential diagnosis is of other causes of severe anal pain, including a thrombosed perineal varix, an anorectal abscess, an anal carcinoma, leukaemic ulceration and sexually transmitted diseases such as warts, herpes simplex, and a syphilitic chancre. Conditions associated with fissure include inflammatory bowel disease, especially Crohn's disease and anorectal tuberculosis. A syphilitic ulcer may closely resemble an anal fissure but is relatively painless: an atypical site away from the midline and an obvious exudate should arouse suspicion. Serological tests should be requested when syphilis is considered and in cases with an associated proctitis rectal biopsy, stool microbiology and contrast radiology should be carried out.

Treatment

A chronic anal fissure should be treated conservatively at first unless the patient has intense anal pain and spasm. The recent introduction of topical glyceryl trinitrate 0.2% used three times daily may heal half the anal fissures and control anal pain. The two operative procedures that are currently used are lateral sphincterotomy and anal dilatation. Both carry a small risk of incontinence, and for this reason a careful history of obstetric sphincter injury should be sought in female patients. Anal dilatation was first used to treat fissures during the last century by Recamier.[7] It produces healing in 80–90% of cases. The stretch should be limited to four fingers as minor disturbances of continence have been reported in up to a third of cases where a more forcible dilatation is carried out.[8] Lateral sphincterotomy involves division of the distal internal sphincter up to the dentate line lateral to the anal orifice and therefore away from the fissure itself. Any papilla or tag is removed at the same time but the fissure is not disturbed. The sphincter division can be carried out by open exposure through a circumferential incision, or through a stab incision using a tenotomy knife.[9] The operation is best performed under general anaesthesia and healing occurs in 2–3 weeks in 95% of cases.[10] Posterior sphincterotomy is no longer favoured as disturbances of continence occur in up to a quarter of cases.[1]

Fig 30.1 Chronic anal fissure seen on displaying distal anal canal. The fissure has a thickened margin and granulating base.

Conservative treatment

Half the simple acute fissures without features of chronicity heal spontaneously.[6] A 2–3 week trial of conservative treatment should be considered when pain is not severe. Most fissures in pregnancy and childhood can be managed in this way. A laxative to loosen the stool and a local anaesthetic ointment are prescribed; 0.2% glyceryl trinitrate ointment has been shown to heal half the fissures.[11] There is no evidence that an anal dilator increases the prospect of healing. Surgery is indicated[12] if the fissure persists.

Fissure complicating crohn's disease

Fissure is the most common anal lesion in Crohn's disease. The site and symptoms are identical to an ordinary fissure in ano but there is a greater likelihood of another problem such as anorectal sepsis being simultaneously present. Treatment should be conservative. The majority (70%) heal spontaneously with or without resection of any simultaneously affected intestine. Sphincterotomy risks sepsis and should be avoided.[13,14]

ANORECTAL SEPSIS

Infection in the anorectal region can lead to abscess or fistula formation. Acute anorectal abscess is one of the most common

REFERENCES

6. Lock M R, Thomson J P S Br J Surg 1977; 64: 355–358
7. Recamier N Gaz d'Hop 1829; 1: 220
8. Watts J M, Bennett R C, Goligher J C Br Med J 1984; 11: 342–343
9. Notaras M J Br J Surg 1971; 58: 96
10. Hoffman D C, Goligher J C Br Med J 1970; 111: 673–675
11. Lund J N, Scholefield J H Dis Colon Rectum 1997; 40: 468–470
12. MacDonald P, Driscoll A, Nicholls R J Br J Surg 1983; 70: 25–26
13. Buchmann P, Keighley M R B et al Am J Surg 1980; 14: 642
14. Sweeney J L, Ritchie J K, Nicholls R J Br J Surg 1988; 75: 56–57

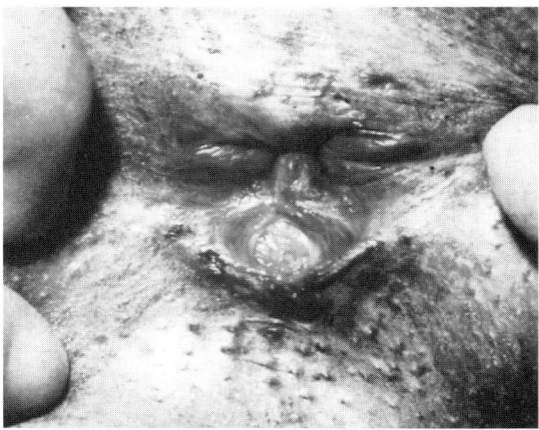

surgical emergencies. Drainage or spontaneous rupture results in resolution of the acute inflammation. Recurrence is common and about 80% of recurrences are associated with the formation of a fistula in ano.[15]

Aetiology

It was proposed more than 60 years ago by Gordon-Watson & Dodd[16] that many cases of anorectal sepsis originated from infection of an anal crypt gland, originally described by Chiari in 1878.[17] Subsequent research by Eisenhammer[18] and Parks[19] has shown the presence of cryptoglandular tissue within the track of many cases of fistula in ano. Others[20] have been unable to find such a strong relationship between the site of acute anorectal abscess and the anal gland bodies but, whatever the truth of the matter, the anal gland theory enables a simple classification to be devised which is essential for treatment.[21]

The reasons why patients develop cryptoglandular infection are not known. It is possible that there is a cultural factor, perhaps associated with diet.[22] In 19th-century Europe fistula in ano was a common affliction (Dickens was operated on by Salmon for the condition[23]) but it is less so now. This may in part be the result of a fall in the incidence of tuberculosis which can produce an anal fistula. Anorectal sepsis is also associated with other diseases including Crohn's disease, ulcerative colitis and hidradenitis suppurativa. It is important to exclude Crohn's disease in today's practice. Up to 70% of patients with rectal Crohn's disease have an anal fistula.[24,25] Rarely a fistula may result from a presacral dermoid cyst draining through the pelvic floor. In some cases, a perianal abscess is not the result of cryptoglandular infection but is caused by a simple furuncle arising from perianal skin. Grace et al[26] have shown that bacteriological culture of pus from abscesses can distinguish between these two origins. With the former, bacteria tend to be enteric in type, whereas with the latter the organisms identified are more likely to be skin pathogens.

Pathogenesis

The 10–12 anal glands are simple glands with a duct draining into the crypts of Morgagni. The gland bodies lie at varying depths from the submucosa to the tissue space between the internal and external sphincters. Anorectal sepsis, according to the cryptoglandular theory, starts with infection of a gland body lying within the intersphincteric space causing an intersphincteric abscess. It is already in anatomical communication with the crypt via the gland duct. As the abscess expands, pus may track longitudinally in various directions to present as a perianal, ischiorectal or supralevator abscess as shown in Figure 30.2. Tracking can also occur circumferentially leading to a 'horseshoe' extension which can spread into the intersphincteric space, the ischiorectal fossa or the supralevator space, the ischiorectal fossa being the commonest site.

A fistula in ano has the following anatomical features: an internal opening, which is usually single, and an external opening (which may be multiple) connected by the primary track. Upward extensions of pus within the intersphincteric space to the supralevator space or within the ischiorectal fossa are referred to as secondary tracks.

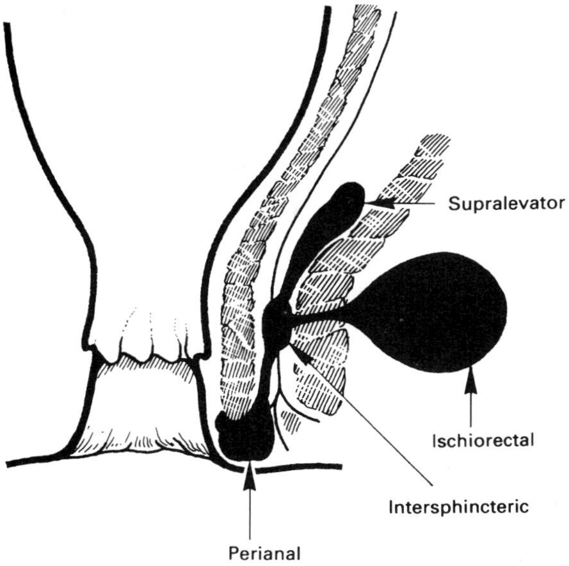

Fig 30.2 Pathogenesis of anorectal abscesses. Pus may track to various sites after initial formation of an intersphincteric abscess.

Classification

Anorectal abscesses or fistulae can be classified according to the relation of the primary track to the external sphincter and puborectalis muscle.[21] About 60% of cases are intersphincteric in type. Here the pus tracks within the intersphincteric space to appear at the anal verge as a perianal abscess and drainage results in an intersphincteric fistula. Occasionally an intersphincteric abscess becomes walled off by fibrosis and, while still communicating with the crypt, it does not track to the exterior. It may remain dormant for long periods but acute exacerbations causing anal pain may occur. It forms the distinct clinical entity of chronic intersphincteric abscess.[27]

In about 35% of cases, pus from the focal intersphincteric abscess penetrates the external sphincter to enter the ischiorectal fossa.[28] It then points to the perineal skin some distance away from the anal orifice. This is an ischiorectal abscess which on drainage

REFERENCES

15. Chabrot C M, Prasad M L, Abcarian H Dis Colon Rectum 1983; 26: 105
16. Gordon-Watson C, Dodd H Br J Surg 1935; 22: 303
17. Chiari H Med J Wien 1878; 419
18. Eisenhammer S Surg Gynecol Obstet 1956; 103: 501
19. Parks A G Br Med J 1961; 1: 463
20. Goligher J C, Ellis M, Pissides A Br J Surg 1967; 54: 977
21. Parks A G, Gordon P H, Hardcastle J D Br J Surg 1976; 63: 1–12
22. Grace R H Ann R Coll Surg Engl suppl 1990
23. Granshaw L In: St Mark's Hospital, London—a Social History of a Specialist Hospital. King's Fund Publishing, London 1985
24. Lockhart Mummery H E Br J Surg 1985; 72 (suppl 595)
25. Hellers T, Bergstrand O et al Gut 1980; 21: 525–527
26. Grace R H, Harper I A, Thompson R G Br J Surg 1982; 69: 401–403
27. Parks A G, Thompson J P S Br Med J 1983; ii: 537
28. Marks C G, Ritchie J K Br J Surg 1977; 64: 84–91

results in a trans-sphincteric fistula. Rarely (in 5% of cases or less) the pus from the intersphincteric focus extends upwards to the supralevator space and then enters the ischiorectal fossa by penetrating the levator ani muscle. This too produces an ischiorectal abscess but, owing to its relationship to the puborectalis, the corresponding fistula is suprasphincteric in type (Fig. 30.3).[21] Even more rarely, there may be a direct communication between the rectum and the perineum lateral to the puborectalis which is classified as an extrasphincteric fistula. This is not of cryptoglandular origin and may be caused by trauma, rectal disease including carcinoma or inflammation, e.g. Crohn's disease, gynaecological diseases and fistulas from the colon or small bowel.[29]

Clinical features

Anorectal abscess

Pain occurs in the anal region, worsening gradually over a few days. It is often very severe and aggravated by defecation. The patient may have a fever and there may be inguinal lymphadenopathy. Swelling and redness of the perianal skin with tenderness are usual but sometimes no external features are noted. When an abscess is suspected, digital examination of the rectum should not be performed until a general anaesthetic is given, when a full assessment can be made and appropriate drainage carried out. It is also essential to sigmoidoscope the patient to exclude proctitis, which is suggestive of Crohn's disease.

Chronic intersphincteric abscess

This condition causes episodic attacks of anal pain without evident discharge, usually resolving spontaneously after a few days. There is an absence of perianal swelling and redness and the diagnosis is made on digital examination of the rectum. As with the internal openings of fistula in ano (see below), about two thirds of chronic intersphincteric abscesses lie in the midline posteriorly. The abscess is identified on bidigital palpation and measures about 1 cm in diameter. It is usually tender and an internal opening into the crypt may be found.[27]

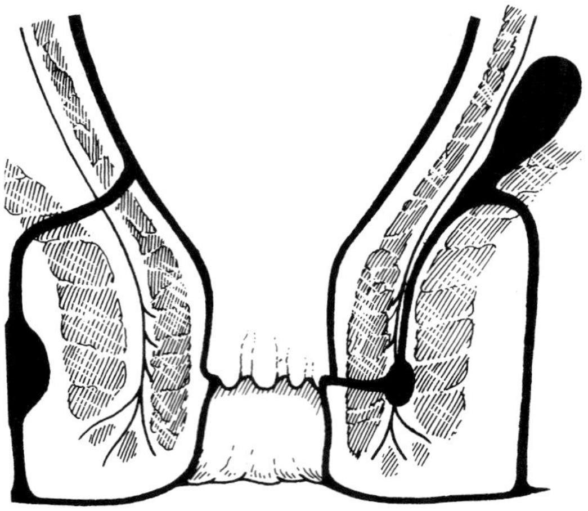

Fig 30.3 Extrasphincteric and suprasphincteric fistulae—the least common types and the most difficult to treat.

Fistula in ano

Fistula in ano is characterized by a discharge of pus from the external opening. This may be intermittent and associated with exacerbations of acute abscess formation causing pain which resolves when pus discharges from the external opening. Digital examination provides the key to correct treatment. The important physical sign is induration caused by an inflammatory infiltration around the tracks and associated abscesses. The examination sets out to identify the site of the primary track and the presence of any secondary tracks. The primary track is identified by finding the internal opening. This is usually felt as an area of induration at the level of the anal crypts. In two thirds of patients the internal opening lies in the midline posteriorly. In the remainder the internal opening lies in the anterior quadrant. Lateral openings are very rare in fistulae not associated with Crohn's disease. Goodsall's rule (Fig. 30.4).[30] generally applies. This states that if the external opening of a fistula lies behind a line drawn transversely across the anus the track should curve in a horseshoe-like manner towards the internal opening in the midline posteriorly. The track tends to pass radially in a straight line towards the internal opening if the external opening is in front of the transverse anal line. The presence of any secondary tracks is identified by feeling for supralevator induration. The finger is passed into the rectum and the levator ani palpated just above the anorectal junction. It is important to look for this physical sign on both sides of the rectum.

Treatment

Abscess

An anorectal abscess should be drained under anaesthesia. General anaesthesia is preferable as this allows a better examination of the anorectal region. This can be carried out as a day-case procedure. A sigmoidoscopy is performed and the anal canal is examined with

REFERENCES

29. Goligher J C In: Surgery of the Anus, Rectum and Colon, 5th edn. Baillière Tindall, London 1984
30. Goodsall D H In: Goodsall D H, Miles W E (eds) Diseases of the Anus and Rectum. Longmans, London 1900

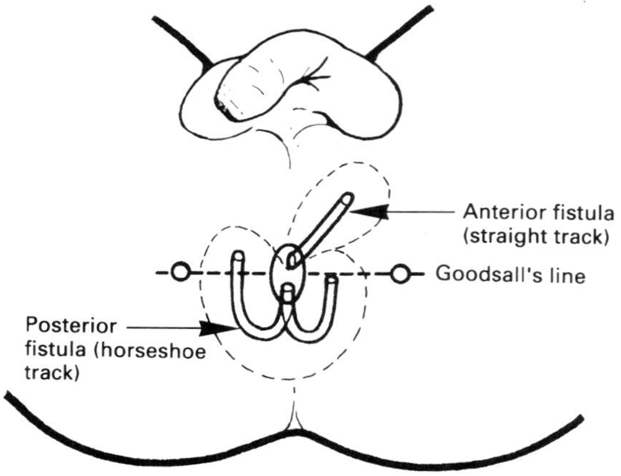

Fig 30.4 Goodsall's rule.

a proctoscope or speculum. Sometimes pus can be seen coming from an internal opening, but no great attempt should be made to find the internal opening if it is not immediately obvious. The abscess is drained by an incision over the point of maximal fluctuation which is usually in the perineum. The finger is gently inserted into the cavity and loculi broken down to release pus which is sent for culture. A small disc of skin should be removed at the point of incision to prevent early closure of the wound. The cavity is then kept open by a short drain which may be removed after 24 or 48 hours depending on the quantity of drainage. Antibiotics should only be given to patients who are at high risk of infection, e.g. those with diabetes mellitus, leucopenia or immunological incompetence.

Although recommended by some surgeons[31] it may be inadvisable to lay open an apparent fistula at this stage as the anatomy of the anal sphincter may not be easily identified. A routine examination under anaesthetic after 10 days has been advocated to look for an associated fistula when the pus culture has shown the presence of an enteric organism. This increases the likelihood of a fistula being present.[26] Growth of a cutaneous organism is strong evidence that the original abscess was furuncular in type and likely therefore to heal with simple drainage. Drainage with primary suture under antibiotic cover has been practised.[32] but the method has not been generally accepted. Nevertheless the results are quite impressive with primary healing rates of around 80%.[33]

Chronic intersphincteric abscess

In cases where an internal opening is evident, it is possible to pass a probe into the abscess, which can then be laid open. Alternatively the intersphincteric plane can be explored, starting at the inferior border of the sphincter, and the abscess dissected out. The internal sphincter should be divided up to the level of the crypt.

Fistula

The principle of surgical management is to lay open the primary track and to drain any secondary tracks. It is essential to assess patients preoperatively when they can voluntarily contract their sphincters. This allows the surgeon to determine the level of the internal opening in relation to the puborectalis muscle. Faecal continence is maintained provided the puborectalis and upper part of the external sphincter are preserved. With an adequate preoperative assessment, the surgeon knows at operation whether simple laying open will achieve this or not. The vast majority of anal fistulae are intersphincteric or trans-sphincteric in type, when the primary track enters at the level of the anal crypts and therefore well below the upper part of the sphincter. The track can then be safely laid open.[28]

With the patient in the lithotomy or jack-knife position, the primary track is probed from either the external or internal opening and the tissue between the probe and the perineal skin is divided. Any abscess cavity associated with the track is curetted. The probe is then passed into secondary tracks which are curetted and widened to allow good drainage and easy dressing postoperatively. Curettings from the track are sent for histological examination for Crohn's disease. The wound is trimmed to facilitate healing from above downwards and to make dressings easy to apply. Postoperatively the dressings are changed at about 24 hours and the wound is then dressed twice daily after baths for a few days until healing occurs. A subsequent examination under anaesthesia may be necessary if healing is not proceeding satisfactorily.

Suprasphincteric fistulae are rare but with these and with high trans-sphincteric fistulae, immediate laying open is contraindicated. Under these circumstances muscle in the upper sphincter should be preserved and a length of suture material, a seton (Latin; *seta* = bristle), is passed through the fistula track from the external to internal opening. Management of the seton can then proceed along two possible lines. Either it can be tied tightly with the aim of producing a slow division of the muscle over a period of weeks,[34,35] or alternatively the seton can be left loose to act as a drain while secondary tracks heal. At the end pf several weeks or months, the primary track may heal on removal of the seton, although this appears to occur in only about 40% of cases.[36] The primary track can be laid open with the expectation that the surrounding fibrosis will prevent retraction of the anal sphincter if healing does not occur. An alternative method of managing high fistulae is to drain the primary track externally while repairing the internal opening using an anorectal advancement flap.[37,38]

Continence after fistula surgery is related to the amount of functioning sphincter that has been preserved.[39,40] Only in cases with a high fistula of the type described above are disturbances of faecal continence likely although some difficulty in controlling the passage of flatus is often experienced. Minor leakage rates of 10–20% have been reported[28] and about 5% of patients with just a bar of puborectalis remaining have a significant degree of faecal leakage. These cases are rare, however, when compared with the total numbers of patients treated. Occasionally a sphincter repair may be necessary, but this should only be undertaken after all the sepsis has settled.

PRURITUS ANI

Irritation is very common in the anal region and can be extremely difficult to treat. Pruritus ani is a symptom, not a disease, and there are several causes. It is a disorder of the skin of the lower anal canal and the perianal region. It can be a primary condition caused by general dermatoses involving the perianal area or by local perianal conditions. It can be secondary to moisture, faecal soiling or the application of allergenic creams or ointments. Certain general medical diseases can also produce anal itching.

REFERENCES

31. Abcarian H Int J Colorectal Dis 1987; 2: 51
32. Ellis M In: Carling E R, Ross J P (eds) British Surgical Practice. Butterworth, London 1959 p 379
33. Wilson D H Br J Surg 1964; 51: 828
34. Arnous J, Parnaud E, Denis J Rev Practicien 1972; 22: 11
35. Parnaud E Int J Colorectal Dis 1987; 2: 56
36. Thompson J P S, Ross A H Int J Colorectal Dis 1989; 4: 247
37. Girona J Int J Colorectal Dis 1987; 2: 53
38. Aguilhar P S, Plaseucia G et al Dis Colon Rectum 1985; 28: 496–498
39. Belleveau P, Thomson J P S, Parks A G Dis Colon Rectum 1983; 26: 152–154
40. Sainio P Acta Chirurg Scand 1985; 151: 695–700

Aetiology

The causes of pruritus ani are listed in Table 30.1. Generalized dermatoses account for about 5% of cases and local perianal conditions for a further 30–40%. Pruritus is often associated with haemorrhoids.[41] Contact dermatitis, most often caused by the application of local anaesthetic, accounts for about 5% of cases. Occasionally fungal infection of the perineal skin may be the cause.[42] The most common single cause, however, is anal moisture and faecal soiling. The perianal area is normally colonized by skin flora but faecal organisms can be cultured in a high proportion of patients with pruritus. Faecal bacteria produce highly irritant metabolites, e.g. neuramidases, and this combined with moisture through sweat or mucus leads to maceration and excoriation of the skin. The resulting irritation leads to scratching, causing further damage to the skin and initiating a vicious circle. Any condition which causes an anal discharge can therefore cause pruritus.

Eyers & Thomson[43] identified a group of patients in whom an abnormality of the internal sphincter seems to be present. In these patients, internal sphincter relaxation occurs at a lower threshold of rectal distension and remains more profound than in normal subjects. A similar finding was reported by Allan et al,[44] who also showed that the saline infusion test was more likely to be abnormal in patients with pruritus than in age and sex-matched controls. This ready sphincter relaxation may result in subclinical leakage of irritant faecal material. More often, however, poor anal hygiene is the result of inadequate cleaning after defecation. This may be difficult in hairy people or where there are skin tags or prolapsing haemorrhoids. patients with diarrhoea often have anal soreness, presumably caused by frequent exposure of the perianal skin to liquid faeces. Infestation with threadworm is a common cause of pruritus, especially in children.

Table 30.1 Causes of pruritus ani

Primary	
Generalized dermatoses	Eczema Psoriasis Lichen planus Allergic eruptions
Perianal disease	
— Local lesion	Fissure Carcinoma Crohn's disease
— Infection	Fungal Yeast Worms Sexually transmitted diseases (condylomata acuminata, chancre, herpes)
— Contact dermatitis	Local anaesthetics Antibiotic ointment
Secondary	
Skin damage due to moisture and irritants	
— Sweat	Poor anal hygiene
— Mucus	Prolapse (rectal, haemorrhoids) Mucus overproduction (adenoma, carcinoma, solitary ulcer)
— Pus	Fistula in ano
— Faeces	Diarrhoea Incontinence Poor anal hygiene
General medical diseases	Diabetes mellitus Myeloproliferative disorders Obstructive jaundice Lymphoma
Idiopathic	

Diagnosis

The history should aim to determine the existence of any allergy, the use of allergenic cream or ointment, anogenital contact and symptoms suggesting any of the conditions listed in Table 30.1. The general examination with appropriate investigations aims to exclude dermatoses and general medical diseases. On anorectal examination any moisture and soiling of the perianal region, maceration or excoriation of the skin, or the presence of perianal lesions and prolapse should be looked for. A lax orifice may indicate a weak sphincter and possible rectal prolapse. Full rectal examination will identify cases of fistula, haemorrhoids, mucus-producing rectal lesions and sphincter incompetence. An anal skin scraping should be sent for microbiological examination to exclude fungal infection. Worm infestation can be diagnosed by examination of the stool or of a swab from the perianal skin for ova. Often no underlying explanation for pruritus is found.[45]

Management

Management involves general measures and specific treatment of any underlying cause. General measures include advice to avoid scratching or rough wiping after defecation. The anal region should be kept clean and dry, and preparations such as zinc starch dusting powder can be helpful. Local anaesthetic preparations and soap should be avoided. The anus should be carefully washed after defecation and gently dried. Most cases will respond to this approach. Operations on the perianal skin or local injections have not been found to be effective.

PILONIDAL SINUS

The term 'pilonidal sinus', first introduced by Hodges in 1880,[46] may be applied to any subcutaneous sinus which contains hair. The sinus may be epithelial or lined partly by epithelium and partly by granulation tissue. There is usually associated chronic inflammation with acute episodes of abscess formation. It is most commonly found in the natal cleft but other sites have been described. These include the webs of barbers' fingers, the umbilicus, the axilla, the scar in the perineal wound after rectal excision, and within pits in the anal canal. The condition is common and affects young adults with males predominating in a ratio of about 4:1.[47] It is rare in children, adolescents and in patients over the age of 40.[48]

REFERENCES

41. Murie J A, Sim A G W, MacKenzie I Br J Surg 1981; 68: 247–249
42. Alexander S Clin Gastroenterol 1975; 4: 651–657
43. Eyers A A, Thomson J P S Br Med J 1979; 11: 1549–1551
44. Allan A, Ambrose N S et al Br J Surg 1987; 74: 576–579
45. Friend W G Dis Colon Rectum 1977; 20: 40–42
46. Hodges R M Boston Med Surg J 1880; 103: 485
47. Buie L A, Curtiss R K Surg Clin North Am 1952; 9: 44
48. Allen Mersh T G Br J Surg 1990; 77: 123

A pilonidal sinus developing between the buttocks consists of one or more primary openings which communicate via the primary track with a subcutaneous cavity (Fig. 30.5). The primary track lies in the natal cleft and at its origin is lined by cutaneous epithelium. This soon peters out and the cavity itself is lined by chronic inflammatory granulation tissue, often containing foreign body giant cells. The cavity may ramify in various directions to open on to the surface via one or more secondary tracks. Secondary openings are usually found on either side of the midline. Hairs are almost always found in the primary track. Some are detached and lying loose but others may still be rooted in hair follicles in the surrounding skin. There are no hair follicles in the primary track itself.

Pathogenesis

There is argument as to whether the disease is congenital or acquired. A congenital origin was accepted for many years. The various theories that were advanced all had a common feature: namely the presence of an epithelialized structural abnormality in the natal cleft.[49,50] This could either be a pit or a subcutaneous inclusion sacrococcygeal cyst. Where a pit is present, it has been postulated[51] that hairs within it prevent the free escape of sebum, leading to infection and extension of the sinus. Only a little epithelium is however found in pilonidal sinus, and the observation that recurrence may occur after excision is also against the congenital theory.

Patey[52] produced evidence to support an acquired cause. He suggested that the sinus starts by penetration of the skin by hairs. Most patients, but not all, are hirsute with considerable hair growth in the natal cleft region. Penetration may occur by the point of a hair still rooted in the surrounding skin which is propelled by movement of the buttocks[53] and its own growth.[54] More usually, however, hairs found in the sinus are detached and are lying with their tips projecting from the opening. Some are too long to have originated from the buttock area and may well be detached capital hairs. This is consistent with the observation that a loose hair when rolled between the finger and the palm of the hand will tend to move in the direction of its root, because of the shape of the minute scales on the hair which project from the axis of the shaft at an acute angle towards the tip.

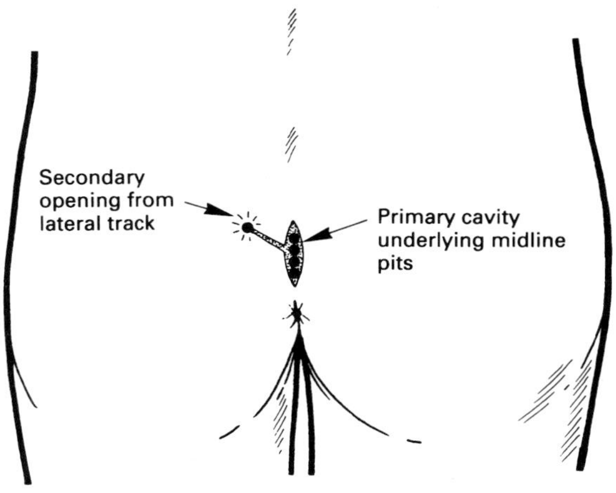

Fig 30.5 Pilonidal sinus—primary openings and secondary track.

Subsequent infection leads to abscess formation within the subcutaneous tissue. This may drain via the primary point of entry of the hairs or it may track laterally to form a secondary opening.

Clinical presentation

The disease presents as an acute abscess or as a chronic discharging sinus. The abscess produces pain and swelling in the natal cleft region, sometimes associated with inguinal lymphadenopathy. Occasionally it settles spontaneously but more often bursts to form a chronic sinus. A chronic pilonidal sinus is characterized by relapses and remissions of pain and discharge of pus. The diagnosis is clinched by finding one or more pits within the natal cleft, usually accompanied by an area of induration, where the chronic granulation tissue forms around the hairs. The differential diagnosis includes anal fistula, particularly if there is a posterior opening, hidradenitis suppurativa, a simple furuncle or an infected sebaceous cyst.

Treatment

An acute abscess should be drained and the inflammation allowed to settle. Occasionally healing occurs but more usually it will be necessary to treat the residual pilonidal sinus. Treatment of the sinus depends on the severity of symptoms and its size. A small sinus giving no trouble should probably be managed conservatively by keeping the area clean, dry and free of hairs and by shaving or using depilatory cream. In most cases, however, an operation is necessary. There are two surgical approaches: first, wide excision of the area to include all infected tracks and, secondly, simple laying open of tracks and deroofing of any abscess cavity.

With wide local excision the entire sinus is removed down to the sacral fascia. The resulting wound can then be left open to heal by secondary intention or a primary closure may be carried out. Healing of an open wound takes several weeks and attention to careful dressing and regular shaving is necessary. If the wound is closed by primary suture, care must be taken to avoid any dead space—techniques which employ skin flaps may be helpful. Healing by secondary intention following wide excision takes an average of 79 days, which is reduced to a mean of 27 days if the wound edges are sutured to the sacral fascia (marsupialization).[48] Failure and recurrence rates of these two techniques at 1 or more years following surgery are 13% and 4% respectively. Recurrence is most likely within the first 3 years of treatment.[55]

Wide excision with primary closure in the midline has a recurrence rate at 1 year of 15%. Recurrence is lower if primary closure is carried out asymmetrically away from the midline[56] or if closure

REFERENCES

49. Haworth J C, Zachary R B Lancet 1955; ii: 10
50. Chamberlain J W, Vawter G F J Paediatr Surg 1974; 32: 1247
51. Brihaye J, Gerard A, Kiekeus R Surg Neurol 1978; 10: 93
52. Patey D H Br J Surg 1969; 56: 463
53. Brearley R Br J Surg 1955; 42: 62
54. Millar D M Proc R Soc Med 1970; 63: 19
55. Notaras M J Br J Surg 1970; 57: 886–890
56. Karydakis G E Lancet 1973; ii: 1414

is effected by the use of skin flaps,[57] with reported average rates of less than 5% and less than 10% respectively.[48] Healing times are usually less than 2 weeks.

All tracks must be probed and identified if the sinus is to be treated by simple laying open. Granulation tissue and hairs are cleared away. The wound edges are trimmed to facilitate dressing. Healing occurs by secondary intention in an average time of 6 weeks but recurrence and failure rates range from 1 to 43% (average 13%).[48] In a simple variant of this procedure the external openings are enlarged under local anaesthetic and the tracks cleaned using curettage and brushing. With careful nursing healing occurs in most cases with a recurrence or failure rate of 3%.[58] Others have reported a failure rate of up to 10% for this treatment.[59] Injection of the track with pure liquid phenol can produce satisfactory results with failure or recurrence occurring in 0–35% of patients.[60,61]

HAEMORRHOIDS

Haemorrhoids (Greek; *haima*-blood; *rhoos* = flowing), or piles (Latin; *pila* = a ball), are an extremely common condition in all western countries. It is highly likely that aspects of western culture, particularly the refined diet, low in fibre, play a part in their aetiology. The Valsalva effect resulting from excessive straining at stool engorges the anal cushions and the shearing force of hard stools disrupts these cushions to cause piles. There may be a congenital deficiency of the supporting tissues in some patients, and the progestogenic effect on smooth muscle and the stretching of parturition explain the presence of haemorrhoids in women.

Pathological anatomy

The normal anal canal contains three cushions of vascular tissue underlying the mucosa of its upper third, consisting of vascular spaces in a fibrous stroma.[62] When internal piles develop, this tissue hypertrophies and may with time tend to be extruded downwards as the attachments to the underlying internal sphincter weaken; ultimately this results in prolapse through the anus.[63] As so-called 'internal piles' enlarge, their base extends below the dentate line, producing intero-external piles.

In addition to internal piles there is normally a continuous ring of external haemorrhoidal plexus beneath the skin of the distal anal canal. When this enlarges it may develop areas of thrombosis, sometimes known as perianal haematoma, but more correctly called thrombosed perianal varices.[64]

Symptoms

Many members of the normal population have symptomless enlargement of the internal haemorrhoidal plexus and if this is noticed on routine examination the temptation to treat must be firmly resisted. The symptom most likely to encourage the patient to see a doctor is bleeding. This is usually painless, fresh and confined to a smear on the toilet paper on wiping, though it is sometimes more spectacular. Rarely bleeding may be sufficient to produce the symptoms of anaemia. A tendency to mucous discharge may be noticed, perhaps leading to the complaint of pruritus. Prolapse may occur on defecation, which may require digital replacement; sometimes the piles may resist replacement or may tend to prolapse on exercise as well as during defecation. Prolapse can cause interference with venous drainage, which can lead on to strangulation and acute thrombosis. This presents with marked pain and swelling, and may occasionally progress to gangrene. This condition must be differentiated from thrombosed external piles (perianal varices).

It is very important to remember that there is a considerable symptom overlap between piles and other more serious anorectal conditions, in particular neoplastic diseases. Proper physical examination of the anorectum is therefore essential in a patient presenting with any of the above symptoms.

Physical examination

Physical examination must include a general and abdominal examination. When the anus is inspected it may look normal, though there are often skin tags around the margin. Piles may be seen to be prolapsed at rest or on the command to strain (Fig. 30.6); when prolapsed they usually conform to the triple pattern (3, 7 and 11 o'clock) and include tissue from above and below the dentate line to become continuous with the external haemorrhoidal plexus. Prolapsed piles are usually dark red or purple and, if subject to frequent prolapse and trauma, may be covered by variable pale areas of squamous metaplasia. Prolapsed piles must be differentiated from prolapse of the rectum, which is paler, has concentric mucosal rings and can be felt to contain bowel muscle on bidigital palpation.

Proctoscopy in a patient with non-prolapsing piles demonstrates a normal pale pink rectal mucosa, which gives way to darker haemorrhoidal tissue in the 3, 7 and 11 o'clock positions (the patient being in the lithotomy position) as the instrument is drawn down into the upper anal canal. On further withdrawal the piles may flop into the lumen of the scope. As the tip passes through the lower canal it is necessary to check whether the piles extend downwards, deep to the skin at and below the dentate line. The distal canal must also be checked for a concomitant anal fissure.

Treatment

There has long been a tendency to overtreat piles. Until the last half-century surgery formed the mainstay of treatment in the UK and in many countries this is still the case. Traditionally piles have been classified into four stages or degrees as follows: first degree,

REFERENCES

57. McDermott F T Aust NZ J Surg 1967; 37: 64
58. Lord P H, Millar D M Br J Surg 1965; 52: 298–300
59. Kobel T, Marti M C Coloproctology 1988; 10: 102
60. Stansby G, Greatorex R Br J Surg 1989; 76: 729
61. Stephens F O, Sloane D R Surg Gynecol Obstet 1969; 129: 786
62. Thompson W H F Br J Surg 1975; 62: 542–552
63. Haas P A, Fox T A, Hass G P Dis Colon Rectum 1984; 27: 442–450
64. Thompson W H F Lancet 1982; ii: 467–468

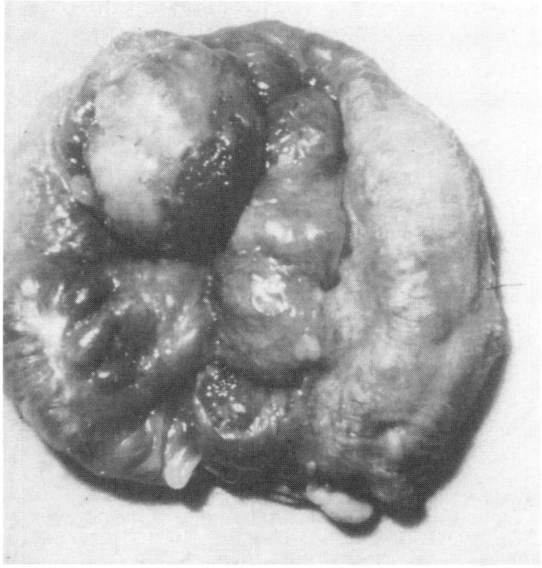

Fig 30.6 Prolapsed piles. Three primary 'internal' piles are seen with a circumferential ring of external plexus.

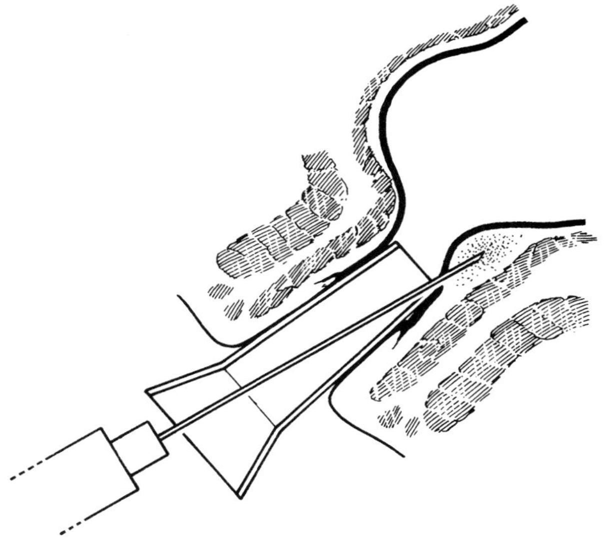

Fig 30.7 Injection sclerotherapy. The sclerosant should be injected at the level of the anorectal ring.

bleeding without prolapse; second degree, prolapse reducing spontaneously; third degree, prolapse requiring manual replacement; fourth degree, prolapse permanently present. This staging system does not however offer a convenient division upon which to base treatment. In broad terms the following guidelines to treatment[65] hold true today:

1. No symptoms—no treatment.
2. Small, non-prolapsing, symptomatic piles—bulking agents or injection sclerotherapy.
3. Prolapsing piles arising above the dentate line—elastic banding.
4. Prolapsing piles straddling the dentate line too large to band or having a large symptomatic external component—haemorrhoidectomy.

Bulking agents

Many patients with minor piles respond to this simple measure.[66] Failure to keep to the regimen in the longer term is likely to lead to relapse.

Injection sclerotherapy

Sclerotherapy has been employed in various forms for a very long time; in the late 1800s in the USA the method was practised by 'travelling pile doctors'—quacks—but soon became established amongst conventional practitioners.[67,68] Carbolic acid was widely used until the 1930s, when phenol became the standard sclerosant.

With the patient comfortably placed in the left lateral position the proctoscope is passed into the lower rectum. The instrument is withdrawn until the upper edge of the pile tissue is visible. The sclerosant (usually 5% phenol in arachis or almond oil) is injected using a 10 ml haemorrhoid syringe; 3 ml is injected just above the piles at the 3, 7 and 11 o'clock positions (Fig. 30.7). The needle is inserted firmly into the submucosal layer; if the tip is correctly placed a bleb appears, covered in semi-transparent mucosa containing visible blood vessels, as the injection proceeds. If, however, the injection is made below the mucosa, more pressure is required on the plunger and a white, featureless area appears on the mucosa. The procedure, though perhaps uncomfortable, should be painless when correctly performed. The patient should be seen again 6 weeks later to check the result; further injection is required only if symptoms persist although it is not unusual to see residual but symptomless persistent piles. The most serious potential complication is injection of sclerosant into the prostate or seminal vesicles which can lead to urinary symptoms and abscess formation.

Rubber band ligation

This procedure was described by Barron[69] and probably has a longer-lasting effect than sclerotherapy. It is to be preferred if the piles are large enough to allow application of bands.[70] The proctoscope should be positioned so that the dentate line can just be seen; the pile to be banded is grasped with forceps and the bander is slid over the pile so that the band can be released (Fig. 30.8). It is important to place the band above the dentate line to avoid severe pain. All three piles can be treated in turn but it is sometimes technically difficult to see the third pile sufficiently well after the first two bands have been placed; in this situation the third pile is best treated by sclerosant injection. The patient should be seen again in

REFERENCES

65. Nicholls R J, Glass R In: Coloproctology. Diagnosis and Outpatient Management. Springer-Verlag, Berlin 1985 p 84
66. Senapati A, Nicholls R J Int J Colorect Dis 1988; 3: 124–126
67. Swinford Edwards F Br Med J 1888; 2: 815–816
68. Anderson G Practitioner 1924; 113: 399–409
69. Barron J Am J Surg 1963; 105: 563–570
70. Sim A J W, Murie J A, Mackenzie I Surg Gynecol Obstet 1983; 157: 534–536

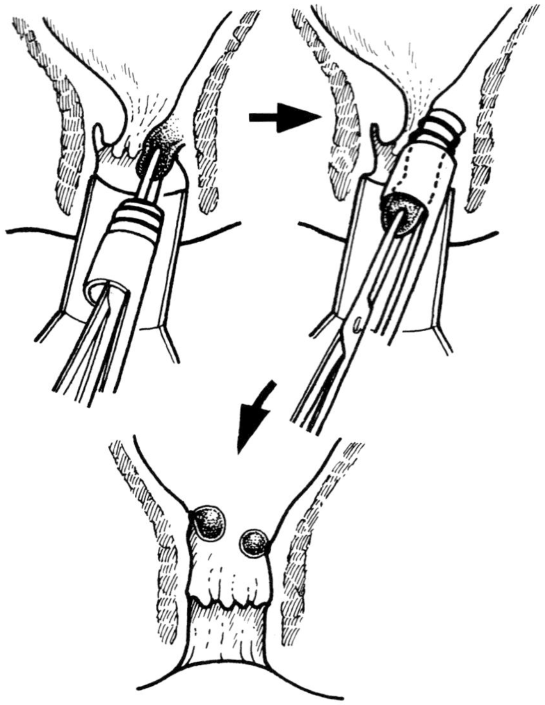

Fig 30.8 Rubber band ligation. Care must be taken to avoid including sensitive skin (below the dentate line) in a band.

6 weeks to check the result. Banding is not without complications—secondary haemorrhage may occasionally require admission, transfusion and re-operation. A few cases of fatal portal pyaemia have been reported.

Other outpatient techniques

Other methods include the application of a cryoprobe[71] or infrared irradiation.[72,73] These techniques have no obvious advantages over the methods mentioned above.

Surgery

This is now reserved for those patients with piles that are too large to band or which straddle the dentate line, making band application impossible because of the pain that would ensue. Only around 5% of piles need to be treated by operation. Of the many methods available the one most widely applied in the UK is the open, or Milligan–Morgan, haemorrhoidectomy (Fig. 30.9).[74] This method involves the dissection, transfixion and excision of the three main piles, preserving the intervening skin and leaving the wounds open. Closed haemorrhoidectomy involves closure of the defects in the lining of the canal after pile excision. This procedure is widely practised in the USA.[75] Submucosal haemorrhoidectomy, in which the mucosa and skin are opened over each pile, followed by excision of pile tissue and closure of the defects, is the most conservative of the excisional procedures[76] but has no demonstrable advantages to offset the added difficulty of the operation.[77]

Some would still advocate the use of manual dilatation of the anus as a primary elective operation for piles: four fingers are carefully inserted into the anus for 4 min.[78] It has the advantage of simplicity, though it probably carries an increased risk of subsequent incontinence for faeces or flatus and for this reason this technique has lost favour.

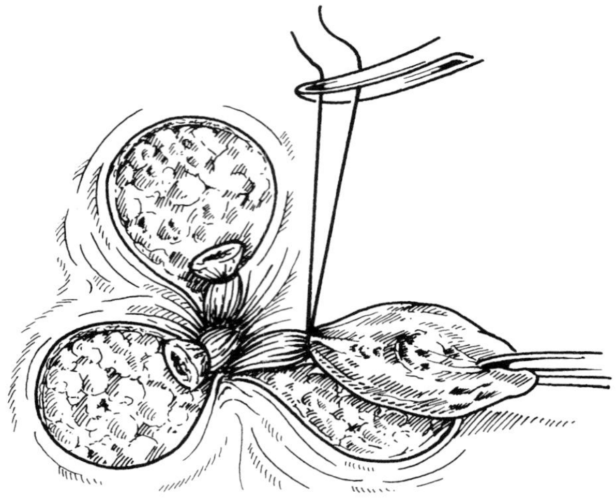

Fig 30.9 Open (Milligan—Morgan) haemorrhoidectomy.

Results

Many trials comparing treatments have been reported. The results depend on the duration of follow-up and on the stage of the disease at the time of treatment (Table 30.2). There is a tendency for recurrent symptoms to develop after all outpatient treatments. When patients are assessed at 1 year, in general rubber band ligation performs better than injection sclerotherapy.[87]

Treatment of strangulated piles

This acute emergency (Fig. 30.10) can be treated either conservatively or by immediate haemorrhoidectomy. The latter has the advantage that the patient is rapidly relieved of symptoms and the

REFERENCES

71. Oh C Dis Colon Rectum 1981; 24: 613
72. Leicester R J, Nicholls R J, Mann C V Dis Colon Rectum 1981; 24: 602
73. Ambrose N S, Morris D et al Dis Colon Rectum 1985; 28: 238–240
74. Milligan E T C, Naunton Morgan C et al Lancet 1937; ii: 1119–1124
75. Ferguson J A, Heaton J R Dis Colon Rectum 1959; 2: 176–179
76. Parks A G Br J Surg 1956; 43: 337–351
77. Watts J M, Bennett R C et al Br J Surg 1964; 51: 8
78. Lord P H Proc R Soc Med 1968; 61: 935–936
79. Keighley M R B, Williams J A et al Br Med J 1979; ii: 967
80. Cheng F C Y, Shum D W P, Ong G B Aust NZ J Surg 1981; 51: 458
81. Greca F, Hares M M et al Br J Surg 1981; 68: 250
82. Murie J A, Sim A J W, Mackenzie I Br J Surg 1982; 69: 536
83. O'Callaghan J D, Matheson T S, Hall R Br J Surg 1982; 69: 157
84. Hancock B Ann R Coll Surg Engl 1982; 64: 397
85. Templeton J L, Spence R A J et al Br Med J 1983; i: 1387
86. Ambrose N S, Hares M M et al Br Med J 1983; i: 1389
87. McRae M, McLeod R S Dis Colon Rectum 1995; 38: 687–694

Table 30.2 Haemorrhoids: results of clinical trials

	Follow-up (months)	*Symptom*	*No. of symptomless patients/no. of patients followed*						
			Injection	*RBL*	*MDA*	*IR*	*C*	*LS*	*H*
Keighley et al (1979)[79]	12	Not specified		16/35	11/37		4/36	6/34	
Cheng et al (1981)[80]	12	Bleeding	14/21	15/20	19/22				18/19
		Prolapse	4/9	10/10	5/8				11/11
Greca et al (1981)[81]	12	Not specified	13/33	15/28					
Murie et al (1982)[82]	42	Bleeding		27/38					32/38
		Prolapse		17/25					27/29
O'Callaghan et al (1982)[83]	48	Not specified					65/89		64/88
Hancock (1982)[84]*	60	1st, 2nd degree			19/22				
		3rd degree			12/26				
Leicester et al (1981)[72]	12	Bleeding	17/35			20/38			
		Prolapse		12/34		17/43			
Templeton et al (1983)[85]	3–12	Not specified		33/62		34/60			
Ambrose et al (1983)[86]	12	1st degree		6/17		8/22			
		2nd degree		20/62		26/68			

RBL = Rubber band ligation; MDA = maximal dilatation of the anus; IR = infrared coagulation; C = cryotherapy; LS = lateral sphincterotomy; H = haemorrhoidectomy.
*Non-controlled trial.

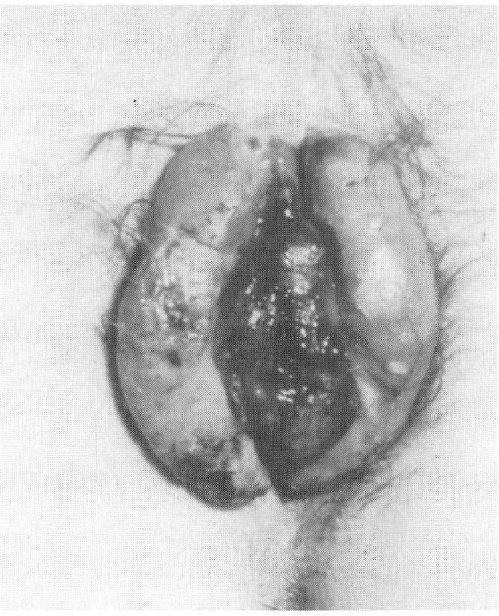

Fig 30.10 Prolapsed strangulated piles.

piles are permanently dealt with. The alternative entails bed rest, analgesia and local applications. The piles reduce over the ensuing few days if the procedure is successful; the patient requires a later haemorrhoidectomy to prevent recurrence.

Thrombosed perianal varix (perianal haematoma)

This condition is caused by a thrombosis in a sub-anodermal venous saccule and probably occurs as a result of sudden tearing of the anal margins by diarrhoea or constipation.[88]

It presents acutely with severe anal pain, difficulty with defecation and a perianal lump. It develops over 24–48 hours and the pain gradually subsides over the subsequent 3–5 days. On examination there is a blue, smooth, firm, tender lump at the anal margin. The lump settles over a period of 1–3 weeks, often leaving a small nodule. It is usually around 1 cm in diameter and hemispherical, though sometimes it is ovoid, occupying one lateral half of the anal circumference (Fig. 30.11).

The condition is self-limiting: if it has been present for several days, and the pain seems to be improving, it is best treated conservatively, with bed rest, cold compresses or topical local anaesthesia. It is best treated surgically, however, if it is acutely painful. Surgery can be performed under either local or general anaesthesia. The affected area can be incised, and the blood clot expressed or excised, thus avoiding the formation of a skin tag when the haematoma resolves. The condition has a tendency to recur in another part of the external venous plexus.

SEXUALLY TRANSMITTED DISEASES

Although sexually transmitted diseases involving the anorectum affect both sexes, it is in male homosexuals that the clinical problem is most apparent. Marked promiscuity and the use of anal

REFERENCE

88. Thompson W H F Lancet 1982; ii: 467

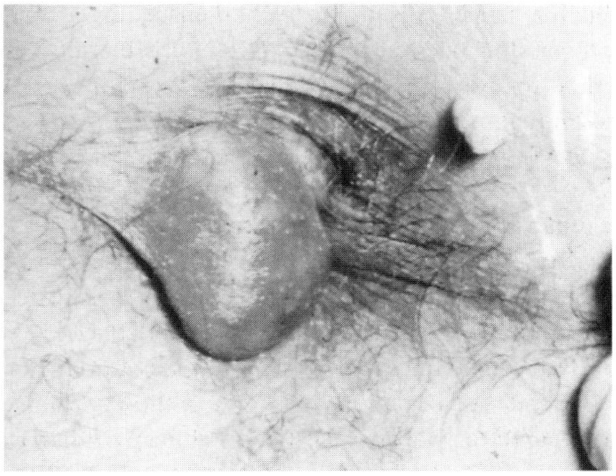

Fig 30.11 Thrombosed perianal varix.

sexual practices has led to the widespread development of several important conditions; many affected individuals carry more than one infection. Some of the more prevalent types, which have clinical features that overlap with conditions normally seen in surgical clinics, are discussed below.

Anorectal gonorrhoea

This infection may be symptomless; it is very common amongst homosexual males.[89] The symptoms are usually mild, but include constipation, tenesmus and mucopurulent discharge. Sigmoidoscopy reveals mildly erythematous areas, perhaps with small ulcers and mucopus. Diagnosis is made by Gram stain of a rectal swab. Treatment is by single doses of intramuscular procaine penicillin and oral probenecid[90] or an alternative antibiotic depending on the sensitivity of the organisms.

Anorectal herpes simplex

This is another common condition in the homosexual population. It presents with pain, often severe constipation, discharge and perianal ulceration. Typical vesicles and ulcers, are seen perianally and in the rectum. The diagnosis can be confirmed by finding the virus on electron microscopy. Oral or topical acyclovir shortens the clinical course of what is anyway a naturally remitting infection.[91]

Chlamydia trachomatis proctitis

This comes in two forms, those with positive lymphogranuloma venereum serology and those which are lymphogranuloma venereum negative.[92] The condition produces anorectal pain, tenesmus and discharge. Examination of the rectum reveals a friable rectal mucosa with discrete ulcers. In advanced cases fistulae and rectal strictures can suggest a diagnosis of cancer or Crohn's disease.[93] Diagnosis is by culture and lymphogranuloma venereum serology. Tetracycline is the treatment of choice.

Anorectal syphilis

This presents with a painless anal ulcer, the primary chancre, which can be mistaken for a fissure or a traumatic lesion. Untreated, the chancre disappears to be replaced by a condyloma latum, proctitis or mucosal polyps. Serology is the most dependable method for confirming the diagnosis. Penicillin remains the mainstay of treatment.

Anal warts (condylomata acuminata)

These are caused by human papilloma virus types 6 and 11.[94] Around 70% of those affected admit to anal sexual practices. The typical warty lesions may be confined to the perianal skin, but also may involve the anal canal (Fig. 30.12). Numbers vary from one or two, to hundreds of separate warts giving the appearance of a continuous carpet of wart tissue. Small numbers of discrete perianal warts can be treated with topical podophyllin. More widespread warts are best treated by scissor excision following subcutan-eous infiltration with saline containing dilute adrenaline (1:300 000).[95]

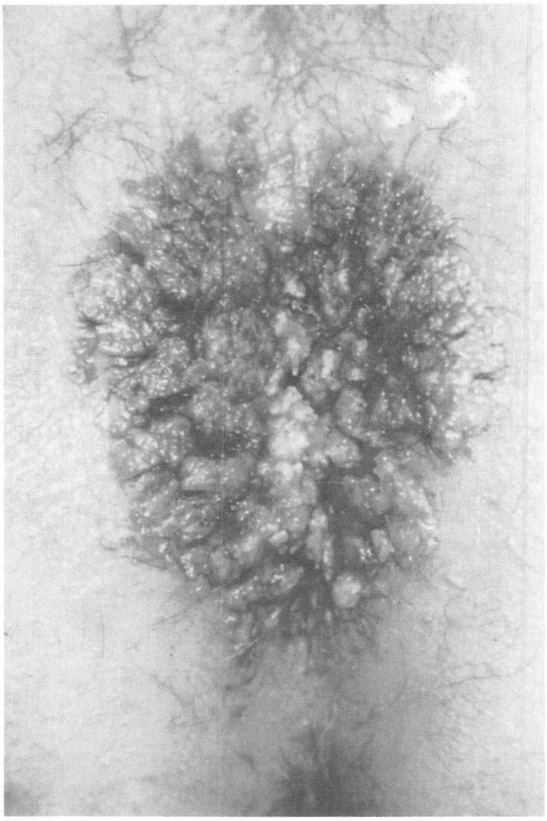

Fig 30.12 Condylomata acuminata.

Acquired immune deficiency syndrome

This condition has several anorectal manifestations. The patient may have a fissure or perianal sepsis indistinguishable from the standard conditions. Alternatively more florid lesions such as severe ulceration, rectal lymphoma[96] or Kaposi's sarcoma[97,98] can occur.

The advance of the human immune deficiency virus epidemic makes it necessary for the surgeon to suspect carriage of this virus in certain high-risk groups.[99,100] Those with anal warts or those who

REFERENCES

89. Quinn T C Med Clin North Am 1986; 70: 611–633
90. Centers for Disease Control. Sexually transmitted diseases; treatment guidelines. MMWR 1982; 31: 355
91. Rompalo A M, Mertz G J et al Clin Res 1985; 33: 58A
92. Quinn T C, Goodell S E et al N Engl J Med 1981; 305: 195–200
93. Levine J S, Smith P D, Brugge W E Gastroenterology 1980; 79: 563
94. Krzyzek R A, Watts S C et al J Virol 1980; 36: 236
95. Thomson J P S, Grace R J Proc R Soc Med 1978; 71: 180–185
96. Burkes R L, Meyer P R et al Arch Intern Med 1986; 146: 913–915
97. Kaposi M Arch Dermatol Syphilol 1872; 4: 265
98. Stern J O, Deiterich D et al Gastroenterology 1982; 82: 1189
99. Cone L A, Woodard D R et al Dis Colon Rectum 1986; 29: 60–64
100. Wexner S D, Smithy W B et al Dis Colon Rectum 1986; 29: 719–723

admit to active homosexual activity should be asked for their permission to be screened for human immune deficiency virus carriage prior to inpatient treatment. Meticulous attention to techniques of cleanliness, both during examination and in cleaning instruments in general surgical practice, is important to help prevent transmission of human immune deficiency virus.[101]

CONGENITAL DISEASES

Hirschsprung's disease

Hirschsprung's disease is a distinct disease in the rather ill defined area of chronic constipation. First described by Hirschsprung in 1888,[102] it is characterized pathologically by an absence of the ganglia in Auerbach's plexus and an increase in unmedullated innervation to the bowel wall muscle.[103,104] Although there is usually a well demarcated segment of abnormal bowel in the rectum, very occasionally the affected segment is ultrashort, being confined to the anal canal. In some cases it is much longer, extending proximally into the colon.[105] The aganglionic segment creates a functional obstruction leading to distension of the proximal bowel which is itself functionally normal.

Although the condition usually presents at birth, the diagnosis may not become apparent until the child is older. Rarely the patient does not present until adulthood.[106] The incidence is 1 in 5000 births, and males are affected about four times more than females.[107] There is an association with other congenital anomalies including Down's syndrome.[108,109] The affected neonate usually fails to pass meconium in the first 24 h. This can be associated with abdominal distension, feeding difficulties and vomiting. Rectal examination may reveal a mucous plug, dislodgement of which leads to a dramatic decompression. Recurrent episodes of this type will ensue if not diagnosed at this stage. The older child fails to thrive; this is associated with a chronically distended abdomen and refractory constipation.[110] Unlike other forms of chronic constipation, faecal soiling does not occur but the child may suffer recurrent episodes of acute enterocolitis[111] (see Chapter 41).

The diagnosis is made by a combination of barium enema examination, anorectal manometry and rectal biopsy. Barium studies show the typical megacolon above a narrow, aganglionic segment (Fig. 30.13). Manometry demonstrates the absence of the rectosphincteric inhibition reflex on rectal distension,[112] while biopsy, preferably by the simple suction method, confirms the absence of submucosal ganglia and proliferation of cholinergic nerve fibres.[113]

Hirschsprung's disease must be differentiated from other conditions causing constipation. In the neonate, meconium ileus associated with cystic fibrosis and infective gastroenteritis can produce similar features to Hirschsprung's disease. In the older child chronic constipation without aganglionosis is the most important alternative diagnosis. This may be associated with a large bowel of normal calibre or with a megarectum.

In most cases diagnosed in infancy and childhood a preparatory colostomy allows the child to be made fit and ensures that the dilated colon returns to normal calibre, making anastomosis easier. Three main curative procedures are available: Swenson's,[114] Duhamel's,[115] and Soave's[116] operations (Fig. 30.14) (see Chapter 41). Their aim is to resect the aganglionic segment and to construct an anastomosis between normal proximal bowel and the anal canal. Swenson's procedure was the first curative operation described for this condition. The rectum is excised and a coloanal anastomosis performed outside the anus, after the anal canal has been everted. The anastomosis then retracts spontaneously inside the anus. In Duhamel's operation the normal colon is brought

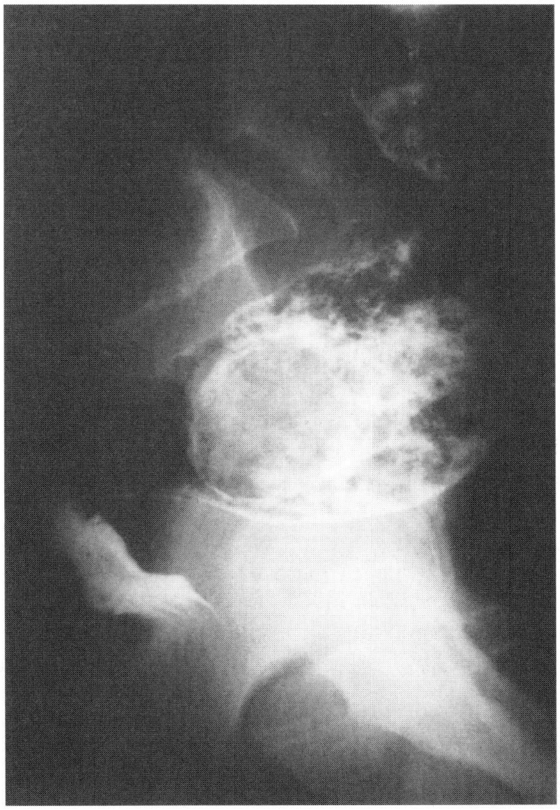

Fig 30.13 Barium enema showing Hirschsprung's disease in an adult. This lateral view of the rectum demonstrates the hold-up of barium and faecal residue above the aganglionic segment in the distal rectum.

REFERENCES

101. Symposium Int J Colorectal Dis 1990; 5: 61
102. Hirschsprung H Jahresbericht Kinderheilk 1888; 27: 1
103. Dalla Valle A Pediatria Napoli 1924; 32: 569
104. Bodian M, Stephens F D, Ward B L H Lancet 1949; i: 6
105. Nixon H H In: Goligher J (ed) Surgery of the Anus, Rectum and Colon, 5th edn. Baillière Tindall, London 1984 p 305
106. Todd I P Br J Surg 1977; 64: 311
107. Kleinhaus S, Boley S J et al J Pediatr Surg 1979; 14: 588
108. Passarge E N Engl J Med 1967; 276: 138
109. Swenson O, Bill A H Surgery 1948; 24: 212
110. Wyllie G G Lancet 1957; i: 847–850
111. Fraser G C, Berry C J Pediatr Surg 1967; 2: 205–211
112. Lawson J O N, Nixon H H J Pediatr Surg 1964; 2: 544
113. Noblett H R J Pediatr Surg 1969; 4: 406–409
114. Swenson O Ann Surg 1964; 160: 540–550
115. Duhamel B Presse Med 1956; 64: 2249
116. Soave F Arch Dis Child 1964; 39: 116–124
117. Todd I P Br J Surg 1977; 64: 311

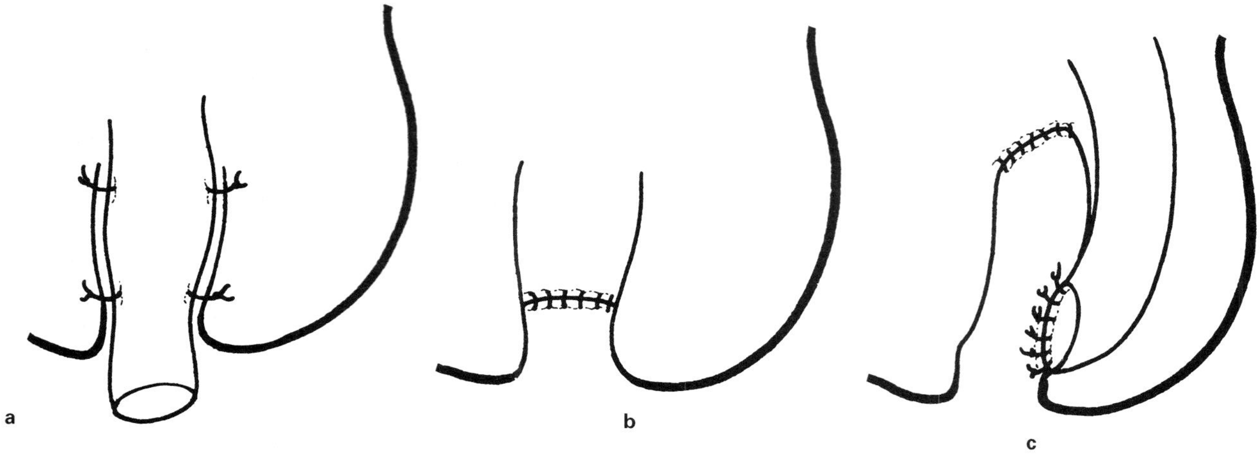

Fig 30.14 Principal operations in Hirschsprung's disease. (**a**) Soave; (**b**) Swenson; (**c**) Duhamel.

down behind the divided and closed rectum and an extended anastomosis is made between it and the back of the upper anal canal and the rectal stump. Soave's procedure consists of a rectal mucosectomy followed by a pull-through and anastomosis of the normal colon to the upper anal canal. Complications include disturbances of micturition (3.6%), enuresis (11%), anastomotic leakage (2%), and mild anal stenosis (5–14%). Some 85% have satisfactory longer term results.

Adults who are found on investigation to have Hirschsprung's disease usually have a history going back to early childhood. Investigation and treatment are broadly the same. Duhamel's operation is probably the best procedure for treating adults with this condition.[117]

Congenital anal anomalies

Anal anomalies occur in around 1:5000 births. They can be divided into two broad categories—low and high—depending on whether the abnormality extends below the pelvic floor.[118] In girls most anomalies are of the low variety while in boys there are rather more high anomalies (see Chapter 41).[119]

Low anomalies

The anus may be abnormally sited (ectopic anus) or may not be visible (covered anus). An ectopic anus in females is often found just inside or behind the vulva (Fig. 30.15). The external sphincter, which may be partially or completely formed, lies in its normal anatomical position. The majority of children can be treated by a cutback procedure, in which a pair of scissors is used to divide the skin behind the anus.[120] Regular dilatation leads to a satisfactory cosmetic and functional result. Sometimes, however, a definitive repair is needed, entailing mobilization of the distal few centimetres of bowel and re-routing it through the external sphincter (Fig. 30.16). The covered anus is usually simply treated by location of the sphincter and division of the overlying skin, followed by dilatation until healing is complete (see Chapter 41).

Low anomalies are relatively easily treated, producing good anatomical and functional results.

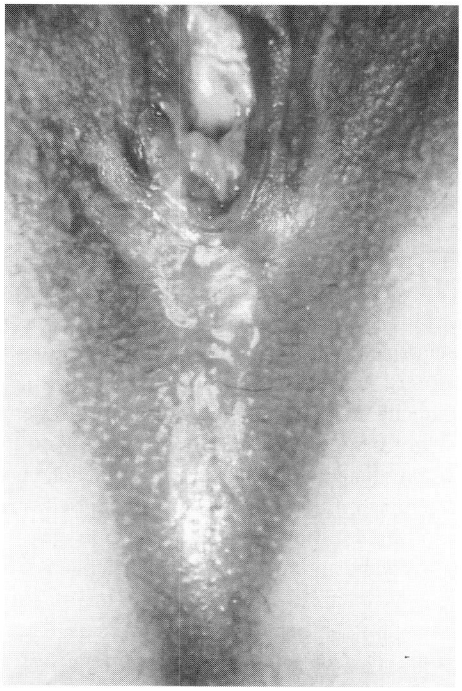

Fig 30.15 Vestibular anus. In this anomaly the anus is situated in the posterior part of the distal vagina.

High anomalies

In this group the rectum extends to the pelvic floor but there is absence of the anal mechanism, except perhaps for part of the external sphincter, below this level. The most common of these

REFERENCES

118. Stephens F D, Smith E D Anorectal Malformations in Children. Year Book Medical Publishers, Chicago 1971 p 133
119. Nixon H H In: Goligher J (ed) Surgery of the Anus, Rectum and Colon, 5th edn. Baillière Tindall, London 1984 p 285
120. Pena A Pediatric Surgery, 2nd edn. W B Saunders, Philadelphia1993 pp 372–392

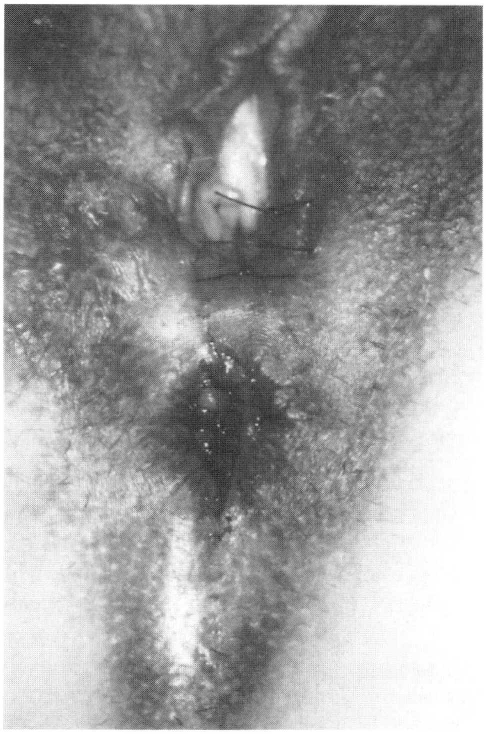

Fig 30.16 Vestibular anus. Appearance after anal transposition.

abnormalities is anorectal agenesis, sometimes with a recto-urethral fistula in the male and a high rectovaginal fistula in the female (Fig. 30.17). Instead of a fistula there may be a fibrous imperforate cord connecting the two systems. More bizarre abnormalities are thankfully rare. The perineum is blind in these cases and the passage of meconium from the vagina or in the urine of male infants confirms the abnormal connection. Inversion of the baby, followed by lateral radiography, should show the gas-filled blind extremity of the bowel in relation to the pelvic skeleton.

Repair of a high anomally is a complicated procedure. The principles of the classical pull-through technique include a sacral approach to open the space above puborectalis, followed by an abdominal approach to mobilize the mucosal tube from within the rectum. The fistula is not divided completely so as to preserve the surrounding nerve plexuses. An opening is made in the back of the rectal muscle tube to allow delivery of the mucosal tube through the anus. A perineal approach is then made to create a new anus and the mucosal tube is delivered from above and sutured to the anal skin. In many cases with a high anomaly, this procedure has resulted in poor function owing to failure to bring the mucosal tube through the correct point in the pelvic floor musculature. Pena & de Vries[121] have described a more anatomical reconstruction involving a sagittal incision to display the pelvic floor muscles on each side. The blind end of the intestine is mobilized and brought down to the perineum through the carefully identified sphincteric muscles which are then repaired accurately around it. The use of posterior sagittal anorectoplasty in older children after failed pull-through procedures has, however, been disappointing.[122]

INJURIES OF THE COLON, RECTUM AND ANUS

Abdominal trauma may damage the large bowel or its blood supply. This may be the result of penetrating or non-penetrating injuries, and is usually associated with damage to other abdominal organs. Iatrogenic injury from colonoscopic and radiological examinations can also occur.

REFERENCES

121. Pena A, de Vries P A J Pediatr Surg 1982; 17: 796
122. Brain A J L, Kiely E M Br J Surg 1989; 76: 57

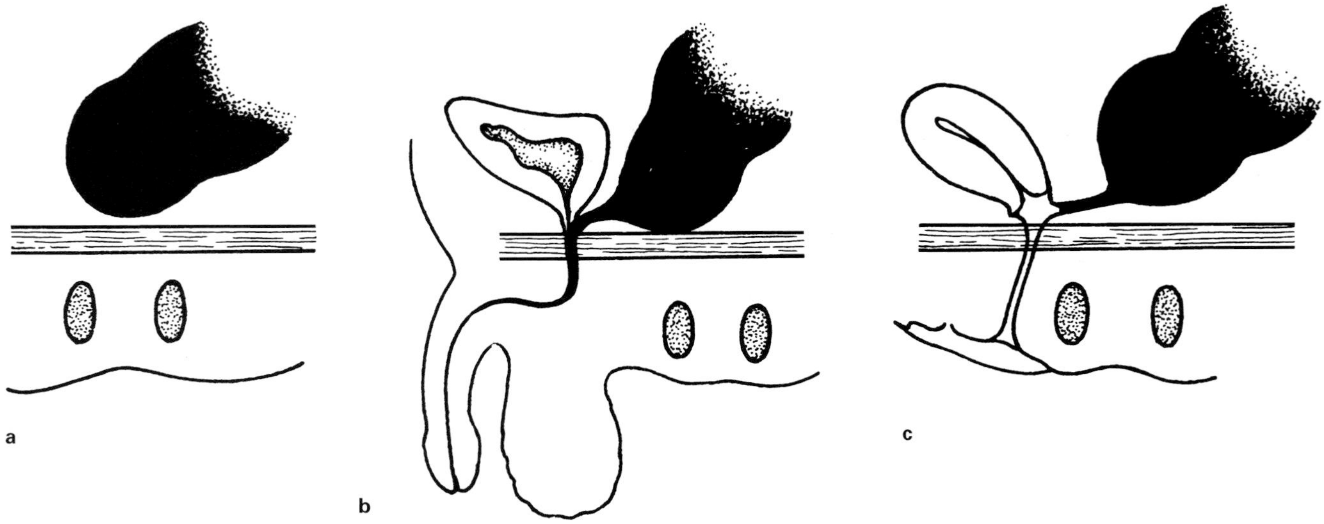

Fig 30.17 The three main varieties of 'high' anorectal anomaly. Anorectal agenesis (a) without fistula; (b) with recto-urethral fistula; (c) with rectovaginal fistula.

Colonic injuries

Road traffic accidents are the most common cause of blunt abdominal trauma,[123] but a fall or blow on the abdomen at work or during sport is also a well recognized source of injury. The colon is usually torn near a point of fixation, being crushed against the vertebral column, or burst by a rise in the intra-abdominal pressure. The severity of injury can vary from a tear of the serosa and muscle to a complete perforation with faecal peritonitis. Damage to the blood supply may cause serious haemorrhage or ischaemic necrosis of colonic wall. Seatbelt injuries, which usually damage the caecum and splenic flexure, can cause discrete perforations of the antimesenteric border or a complete transection of the colon (see Chapter 7).[124]

The outcome and severity of a penetrating wound usually depends on the nature of the injury. Whilst stab and gunshot wounds are the most common causes, bomb-blast injuries may not only result in blunt trauma but can also drive fragments of shrapnel, clothing and masonry into the abdominal cavity. High-velocity bullets entering through a small wound can cause massive cavitating injuries of the colon and surrounding tissues before passing out through a larger exit wound. Low-velocity bullets, shotgun pellets and shrapnel may by contrast lodge in the abdomen.

Pneumatic injuries are rare but highly dangerous. They usually result from practical joking in which compressed air is passed up the victim's anus. The sudden increase in pressure results in rupture of the intraperitoneal rectum with free abdominal gas and severe pain and shock.

Management

After initial resuscitation a rapid overall assessment must be made. Where the patient is fit enough, plain abdominal X-rays in two planes may reveal free gas and displaced bowel loops from a haematoma or a foreign body.

Physical signs usually determine the management of a patient with blunt trauma, and repeated reassessment is essential. Peritoneal lavage is less useful in diagnosing peritonitis than haemorrhage and may be misleading where there is retroperitoneal injury.[125] It may however be very valuable in an unconscious patient (see Chapter 7).

Although selected cases of abdominal stab injury can be managed conservatively,[126] gunshot wounds should always be explored. At laparotomy, the full extent of an injury must be carefully assessed through a long midline incision. It may be necessary to mobilize the colonic flexures to exclude retroperitoneal injury. Basic surgical principles apply, including stopping haemorrhage, minimizing contamination, excising any damaged or non-viable tissue, draining and irrigating contaminated areas, and closing skin wounds by delayed primary closure. In gunshot injuries the number of holes should be counted, applying the 'rule of two'. If an uneven number of holes is found there is probably a missed exit wound, unless there has been a tangential injury. Broad-spectrum antibiotics, usually metronidazole and a cephalosporin, are given by the intravenous route and the patient should have an injection of tetanus toxoid unless already immunized.

Every injury is different, and it is difficult to propose didactic and specific surgical treatment. There is a range of surgical options depending on the state of the patient and the expertise of the surgeon, as summarized below:

1. Primary suture of the damaged colon.
2. Primary suture of the colon with proximal decompression by colostomy.
3. Exteriorization of the perforation in the colon.
4. Colonic resection with a colostomy and mucous fistula.
5. Colonic resection with a colostomy and closure of the rectal stump.
6. Colonic resection with a primary anastomosis.
7. Colonic resection with an anastomosis and proximal decompression.

In general, right-sided colonic injuries can be managed more safely by primary suture, or resection and immediate anastomosis than those on the left side. Primary colonic closure is reasonable if there is a discrete injury of less than 4 h duration, with minimal peritoneal soiling, no major blood loss and few associated injuries. It is absolutely contraindicated when there is frank peritonitis, extensive contamination, blunt trauma, a high-velocity bullet wound, shattering of multiple bowel loops from an explosion or shotgun injury, severe mesenteric injury or associated damage of multiple organs, especially the pancreas and duodenum. Under the circumstances exteriorization or resection is preferable.[127,128]

Wounds of the transverse colon are best treated by exteriorization, converting the perforated area into a defunctioning colostomy. In injuries of the descending colon primary suture or primary resection should be protected by a proximal stoma, closing it subsequently when the colonic and any associated injuries are soundly healed. In carefully selected cases where there is a clean fresh localized wound with little contamination, primary suture is permissible but it should be the exception rather than the rule.[127] An anastomosis is best deferred if there has been extensive damage, and the proximal bowel end should be brought out as a colostomy, with closure of the distal stump or formation of a mucous fistula. The sigmoid colon is often mobile enough to be managed by exteriorization when the injury is at the apex of the loop, but wounds near the peritoneal reflection require resection.

The mortality and morbidity from colonic injuries are generally high, especially when there is associated haemorrhagic shock, gross peritoneal contamination, multiple visceral injuries or an undue delay in diagnosis. The mortality is also related to the number of associated injuries. In one series from Belfast there was a 17% mortality and the causes were usually multifunctional (see Chapter 7).[127]

REFERENCES

123. Towne J B, Coe J D Am J Surg 1971; 122: 693
124. Falcone R E, Carey L C Surg Clin North Am 1988; 68: 1307
125. Soderstrom C A, DuPriest R W, Cowley R A Surg Gynecol Obstet 1980; 151: 513–518
126. Feliciano D Trauma, Appleton & Lange, Norwalk, USA
127. Parks T G Br J Surg 1981; 68: 725

Injuries of the rectum and anal canal

The rectum and anal canal can be injured in a variety of ways. These are summarized in Table 30.3.

Clinical features

The site of injury is more accessible than in the colon, and a careful examination of the pelvis, perineum and anal margin is important. The rectum and anal canal should be carefully palpated, bearing in mind that small rectal lacerations can easily be missed. In gunshot wounds rectal injury should be suspected if the path of the projectile is anywhere near the rectum, if there is a blood in the lumen, or if there is an associated sacral fracture. It is important to exclude damage to adjacent organs, especially the bladder and urethra.

Sigmoidoscopy can be very helpful, but only a minimal amount of air should be insufflated. Impalement injuries are usually more serious than they at first appear, and where a patient presents with a stake or foreign body in situ it should only be removed in the operating theatre under a general anaesthetic with the abdomen open.[124] On removal there may be brisk haemorrhage and the direction of the track can be more easily seen through the laparotomy incision.

Management

A proximal colostomy is advisable if the injury is above the peritoneal reflection, especially where there is a large ragged defect in the colon. Debridement and repair are still best achieved from the abdomen for wounds below the peritoneal reflection. The pelvis can be adequately drained through an abdominal approach, and a colostomy raised, usually in the left iliac fossa. The rectum below the colostomy must be vigorously cleaned of faeces to prevent continuing contamination of the perirectal tissues.

When the anal sphincters are damaged, as much sphincter as possible should be preserved, and a primary or delayed primary repair carried out only if this is feasible. Unless the injury is minor, a colostomy is necessary and the rectum must be thoroughly washed out.[129] As with the colon, the morbidity and mortality from rectal injury depend upon the presence of other injuries.[130]

Table 30.3 Causes of rectal injuries

Swallowed foreign bodies	Chicken or fishbone, nail, needle
Objects inserted per anum	Enema/decompression tube Sigmoidoscope Thermometer Sexual objects
Impalement	
Gunshot	
Bomb blast	
Pelvic fractures	
Surgical complications	Gynaecological Urological Anorectal
Obstetric trauma	

Foreign bodies in the rectum

Most foreign bodies have been inserted per anum and sometimes can be difficult to remove. Extraction is best achieved under general anaesthetic, and the use of obstetric forceps, retractors and snares may be necessary. A catheter passed alongside larger objects high in the rectum will allow enough air to be inserted into the proximal bowel to facilitate removal.[131]

Occasionally the foreign body will have to be pushed upwards and removed through a colotomy.

VASCULAR MALFORMATIONS

Vascular malformations are a rare cause of colonic bleeding and may be very difficult to identify by conventional investigations. Aneurysms and malformations of the major colonic blood vessels are excessively rare. In clinical practice two distinct types of malformation are recognized.

Angiodysplasia

Angiodysplasia has been increasingly identified since the introduction of colonoscopy. Most of these lesions are of unknown aetiology, but they may occasionally occur in association with cutaneous and oral vascular malformations as in hereditary telangiectasia (Osler–Weber–Rendu disease). Histologically there is debate as to whether angiodysplasia is degenerative, hamartomatous or neoplastic.[132]

There is also an association with aortic valve stenosis but the relationship between these conditions remains obscure.

Clinical features

Rectal bleeding is the most common presenting symptom. On occasions this is torrential, but more often a series of repeated small bleeds or persistent occult bleeding results in anaemia. Angiodysplasia can occur anywhere in the colon but is most common in the right colon of elderly patients.[133] The physical signs of aortic valvular disease may be detected. Barium enema radiology is of no use in diagnosis and may make subsequent identification of the bleeding site more difficult.

At colonoscopy in a well prepared bowel the angiomatous lesions can usually be seen as multiple mucosal abnormalities up to 1 cm in diameter, resembling spider naevi (Fig. 30.18). When there is a major haemorrhage colonoscopy may be impracticable but selective mesenteric arteriography will then often demonstrate the characteristic blush of a malformation (Fig. 30.19).[134] Extravasation of contrast into the colonic lumen is only seen if the

REFERENCES

128. Kirkpatrick J R, Rajpal S G Am J Surg 1975; 129: 187
129. Haas P A, Fox T A Dis Colon Rectum 1979; 22: 17
130. Fallon W F Dis Col Rectum 1992; 35: 1094–1102
131. Eftaiha M, Hambrick E, Abcarian H Dis Col Rectum 1977; 112: 691
132. Price A B Int J Colorect Dis 1986; 1: 121
133. Boley S J, Di Biase A et al Am J Surg 1979; 137: 57
134. Sheedy P F, Fulton R E, Atwell D T Am J Roentgenol 1975; 123: 338

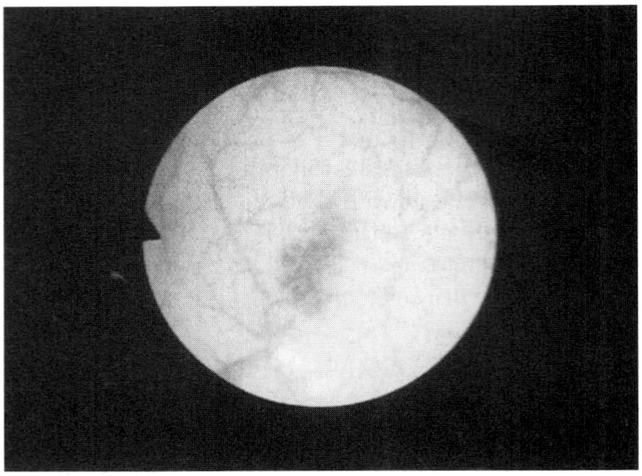

Fig 30.18 Angiodysplasia. A group of abnormal small vessels in the colonic mucosa is clearly seen via a colonoscope.

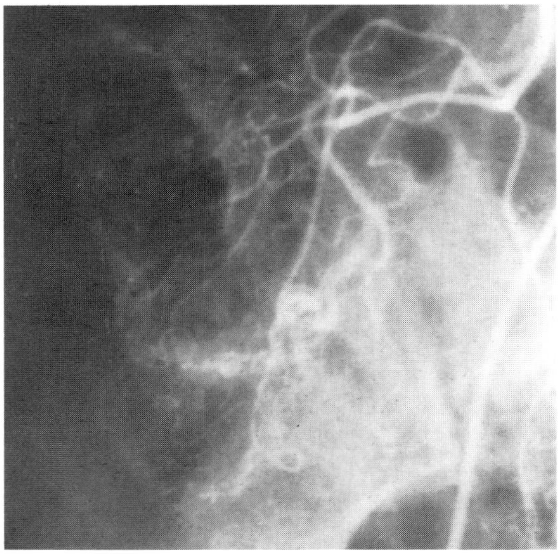

Fig 30.19 Angiodysplasia. A group of abnormal small vessels in the blush seen in the abnormal vessels in the caecum.

angiodysplasia is actively bleeding at the time of the investigation. Radiolabelled scintigraphy may also be useful in localizing the site of bleeding but it can not diagnose the pathological cause.[135]

Management

Small numbers of angiodysplastic malformations can be treated through the colonoscope by coagulation with hot biopsy forceps.[136] Extensive areas of angiodysplasia often require resection, usually by a right hemicolectomy. Intraoperative colonoscopy with transillumination of the colonic wall can be helpful in determining the extent of resection.[137] Torrential haemorrhage may require a total colectomy and ileo-rectal anastomosis if the bleeding site cannot be clearly identified preoperatively.

Other malformations

These are usually cavernous or giant haemangiomata, and involve the whole thickness of the colonic wall. The most common site is the rectum, but they may extend proximally to involve the colon. The angioma can usually be seen on endoscopy as a prominent red area, or as a collection of dilated tortuous submucosal vessels with a bluish tinge. Phleboliths may be seen on a plain X-ray, and MR scanning using a stir sequence demonstrates the full extent of a malformation (see Chapter 10).

Smaller lesions may be managed by electrocoagulation. Injection sclerotherapy with phenol may give temporary control. A large rectal cavernous haemangioma that is diffuse and symptomatic can be successfully treated surgically.[138] The rectum is excised to a few centimetres above the pelvic floor and the mucosa of the remaining angiomatous tissue above the dentate line is removed endoanally following infiltration with 1 in 300 000 adrenaline in saline. An endoanal and coloanal anastomosis using uninvolved proximal colon completes the procedure. The laser photocoagulator has been used with some success.

Patients with Klippel–Trenaunay syndrome may also develop pelvic venous abnormalities which can cause troublesome bleeding (see Chapter 11).

ISCHAEMIC DISEASE OF THE LARGE BOWEL

With an increasingly elderly population, ischaemic bowel disease has become more frequent. Two distinct clinical syndromes can be recognized in the colon: colonic gangrene and ischaemic colitis (see Chapters 10 and 30).[139,140]

Anatomy

Three visceral branches of the aorta supply the gastrointestinal tract. The proximal colon to mid transverse colon is supplied by the superior mesenteric artery, and the distal half by the inferior mesenteric artery, but this can be a variable watershed. As there are no vascular arcades, much depends on the marginal artery which may be absent or poorly developed at the splenic flexure.

Causes

Arterial thrombus/embolus

Arterial thrombus can develop on an atheromatous plaque of the inferior mesenteric artery at its origin. Although complete occlusion of the vessel at the aorta is quite common, it is normally compensated for by collaterals. The compensatory mechanisms may suddenly fail during low-flow states such as left heart failure or after total occlusion of an already critically narrowed vessel. The outcome can vary from an ischaemic colitis to colonic gangrene. Ligation of the inferior mesenteric artery at its origin

REFERENCES

135. Colacchio T A, Forde K A et al Am J Surg 1982; 143: 607
136. Danesh B J Z, Spiliadis C et al Int J Colorectal Dis 1987; 2: 218
137. Campbell W B, Rhodes M, Kettlewell M G Ann R Coll Surg 1985; 67: 290
138. Jeffrey P J, Hawley P R, Parks A G Br J Surg 1976; 63: 678
139. Abel M E, Russell T R Dis Colon Rectum 1983; 26: 113
140. Marston A Intestinal Ischaemia. Edward Arnold, London 1977

during aneurysm repair or colonic surgery occasionally results in left colonic ischaemia.

Small vessel disease

Vasculitides such as polyarteritis, Buerger's disease and systemic lupus erythematosus, together with microemboli from atheromatous disease and diabetes, can give rise to colonic ischaemia.

Low-flow states

In patients with severe heart failure or those with severe septic or hypovolaemic shock the colonic blood supply fails, allowing metabolically active bacteria, especially pathogenic strains of clostridia, to invade the colonic wall and induce necrosis, toxaemia and shock.[140]

Intestinal obstruction

Blood flow in the colonic wall is not only influenced by its blood supply, but also by intraluminal pressure and the radial tension and diameter of the colon. Sometimes typical ischaemic changes are seen proximal to an obstructing carcinoma of the colon.

Venous occlusion

The inferior mesenteric vein may be ligated without any obvious effect, but extensive venous thrombosis causes a haemorrhagic infarction closely resembling an arterial injury. It may be impossible in some cases to distinguish between venous and arterial infarction.

Idiopathic infarction

A number of cases appear to occur without any obvious precipitating cause.

Pathology

Whatever the cause, colonic ischaemia follows a characteristic evolution. After severe prolonged ischaemia there is progressive destruction of the bowel wall ending in full-thickness necrosis, sloughing and rupture. In contrast, a transient episode causes a limited degree of congestion and inflammation which usually resolves completely. An intermediate degree of ischaemia does not usually threaten the integrity of the bowel wall but does cause critical ischaemia of mucosa and muscle. Here the inflammatory response is followed by mucosal ulceration, haemorrhage and fibrosis extending into the muscle coat. The end-result may be a stricture which can be confused with an annular carcinoma or a segment of Crohn's disease (Fig. 30.20).

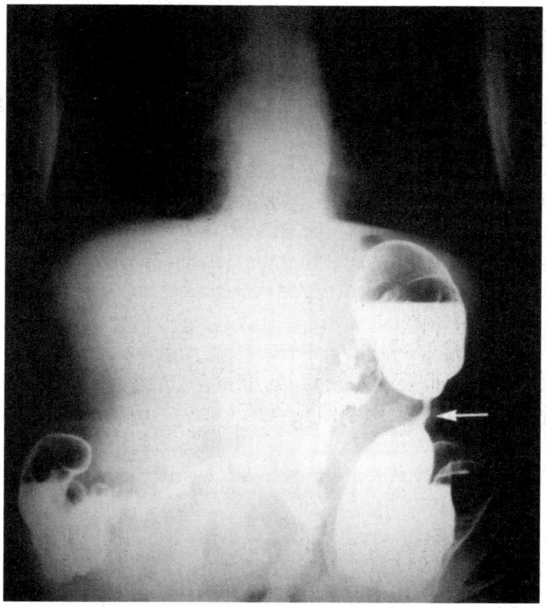

Fig 30.20 Ischaemic stricture. This barium enema shows the smooth stricture, typically situated near the splenic flexure.

Clinical features

Colonic gangrene

A middle-aged or elderly patient, often with a history of cardiovascular disease treated with digitalis and diuretics, presents with a sudden illness. Symptoms usually consist of severe generalized abdominal pain which is at first colicky and later becomes constant with associated vomiting and sometimes diarrhoea. Rectal bleeding is unusual. The patient's condition rapidly deteriorates with abdominal distension, restlessness and a rising respiratory rate as peripheral circulatory collapse ensues.

On examination the patient is pale, sweaty and dyspnoeic with a tachycardia and hypotension, and appears gravely ill. In the abdomen there are signs of generalized peritonitis and on rectal examination dark blood may be observed on the glove. This picture may be indistinguishable from mesenteric embolism, severe pancreatitis, ruptured abdominal aneurysm, perforation or strangulation obstruction, and the diagnosis is only made with certainty at laparotomy. The plain radiograph may be normal at first, but later shows progressive colonic dilatation resembling a volvulus or toxic megacolon. There is an early and often marked leucocytosis, a rise in the packed cell volume and a metabolic acidosis. Serum enzymes including the amylase and transaminases may be elevated. Barium enema and arteriography are of no value.

Management

The first step is resuscitation with crystalloid and colloid to restore the circulating blood volume while monitoring the central venous pressure. A nasogastric tube should be passed, oxygen administered, and a urinary catheter inserted to measure urine output. The patient is prepared for an emergency exploration of the abdomen and intravenous broad-spectrum antibiotics are started.

Treatment

On opening the abdomen, the presence of a length of necrotic colon and sometimes small bowel (see Chapter 29) is immediately apparent. The affected colon may have a deep red, purple, black or green blotchy appearance extending for a variable distance between sigmoid and caecum. The rectum is usually spared. A characteristic odour pervades the operating room. After excluding any other intra-abdominal pathology, the colon is gently examined and the mesenteric vessels inspected and palpated. The affected colon must be mobilized with great care and no attempt should be made to preserve the greater omentum. Thin necrotic colon is easily perforated and gross peritoneal contamination must be avoided if at all possible. The vessels are divided and the colon resected widely, making sure that the cut ends are viable. The proximal bowel is brought out as a colostomy and the distal colon brought out as a mucous fistula. There is absolutely no place for a primary anastomosis in the management of this condition.[140]

Colonic gangrene is an abdominal catastrophe with a high mortality. Timely resuscitation, safe surgery and the correction of cardiovascular and metabolic disturbances in the intensive care unit postoperatively can produce a successful outcome.[140]

Ischaemic colitis

The typical patient is middle-aged or elderly with a history of cardiovascular disease but no previous intestinal symptoms. There is usually an acute onset of pain in the left iliac fossa spreading across the abdomen up to the epigastrium. Diarrhoea often develops and the stool is characteristically dark, containing blood clots.

On examination there is tenderness in the left iliac fossa and dark blood on rectal examination, but often little in the way of systemic disturbance. The differential diagnosis includes complicated diverticular disease, carcinoma of the large bowel, sigmoid perforation, acute inflammatory bowel disease, left-sided renal colic, leaking abdominal aneurysm and acute infective gastroenteritis.

The affected colon is usually beyond the reach of the rigid sigmoidoscope. Colonoscopy is much more helpful and can be used to take biopsies for histology in mild cases. The colon has a heaped-up oedematous bluish purple mucosa, sometimes with ulceration and contact bleeding. The white cell count is usually raised. A plain abdominal radiograph may show an area of dilated colon with characteristic 'thumbprinting' or signs of small bowel obstruction. Arteriography may occasionally be helpful, but the most useful investigation is a barium enema. Here the changes are well demarcated and centred around the splenic flexure. The involved segment is of variable length and is usually narrowed; the mucosa is irregular and sometimes shows rounded filling defects caused by the oedematous mucosa called thumbprinting (Chapter 10). Later in the course of the disease stricturing is an important feature.

In elderly patients a transient episode of ischaemic colitis may be misdiagnosed as gastroenteritis or diverticular disease. In other patients it has to be distinguished from any other abdominal catastrophe, but a barium enema usually provides the answer.

Management

Once the diagnosis is established, the management is conservative with careful monitoring by repeated examination and the administration of intravenous fluids and antibiotics. The condition usually resolves, though it may progress to gangrene or to a late stricture. Surgery is only rarely required and usually the affected colon has to be resected. Provided care is taken over the blood supply the anastomosis usually heals uneventfully.

IRRADIATION BOWEL DISEASE

Irradiation for uterine or bladder cancer can result in proctitis, ulceration and stricture formation in the rectum, or a fistula into the vagina or bladder. The full effects may take years to develop.[141] Radiation proctitis can give troublesome bloody diarrhoea, and a diverting colostomy may be necessary. Provided the sphincter has not been damaged and recurrent tumour has been excluded, an omental interposition and rectal resection with coloanal anastomosis bringing down non-irradiated left colon may be successful. Where there is local destruction of the sphincter an abdominoperineal excision is required.[142]

INFLAMMATORY BOWEL DISEASE

When a patient presents with diarrhoea two broad groups of diseases must be considered. These include infective and non-infective inflammatory bowel disease. Although it is inappropriate in a surgical textbook to describe specific infectious diseases in detail, it is important to bear them in mind when considering the management of patients with severe diarrhoea so that inappropriate surgery can be avoided. Conversely, although altered bowel function with blood in the stool in an African or Arab patient is likely to be caused by bacillary or amoebic dysentery or schistosomiasis, other diseases such as ulcerative colitis must be considered. With the rise in foreign travel by western patients to tropical countries, infectious diseases must always be excluded in a business traveller or holiday maker.[143]

Amoebic dysentery

The disease is caused by the protozoan *Entamoeba histolytica* which, when ingested as a cyst, invades the large intestinal tissues; colonies in the colonic wall lead to ulceration, occasionally with brisk bleeding. Intestinal amoebiasis usually presents with fluctuating bleeding diarrhoea. Without treatment it may progress to chronic dysentery, amoebic appendicitis, or an amoeboma. Rectal amoebic ulceration can be mistaken for a carcinoma. Sigmoidoscopy often reveals ulceration which may be pinpoint or very large. In its more active form the amoebic ulcer may be very large and diamond-shaped, single or multiple, and with a raised ragged margin, undermined edges and a slough in the wall from which amoebae can be obtained.[144] More chronic lesions take the form of craters or pits with smooth edges and shallow bases.

REFERENCES

141. Allen-Mersh T G, Wilson E J, Hopestone H F, Man C V Surg Gynecol Obstet 1987; 164: 521–524
142. Cooke S A R, Wellsted M D World J Surg 1986; 10: 220
143. Cook G C Tropical Gastroenterology. Oxford University Press, Oxford 1980
144. Mandal B K, Scholfield P F Br Med J 1992; 305: 638–664

Occasionally an amoeboma is present, appearing as a localized oedematous swelling which may be mistaken for a carcinoma.

Fresh stool specimens must be rapidly examined for protozoa. Treatment with metronidazole (400 mg) is highly effective but must be supplemented with a contact amoebicide such as diloxanide furoate (0.5 g). Surgery is rarely necessary but it may be required for the complications of pericolic abscess, stricture, haemorrhage or perforation, or for amoeboma.[145]

Bacillary dysentery (shigellosis)

This is often an epidemic disease and a contact history can usually be obtained. The Shigella organisms rapidly multiply in the colon; in severe cases endotoxins can cause a coagulopathy or haemolytic anaemia.[146] Inflammation of the colon leads to necrosis of epithelium and desquamation with formation of a membrane and discrete ulcers. The diagnosis is usually made by stool culture. Most cases will settle with conservative and supportive measures, and treatment with the antibiotics ampicillin or tetracycline is usually reserved for resistant cases.

Schistosomiasis

The infective agent is a trematode worm of the genus *Schistosoma* and includes the species *Schistosoma mansoni, intercalatum* and *japonicum*. The lifecycle involves an intermediate host, the freshwater snail. The cercariae develop in the snail and are then released into fresh water where they infect humans by penetrating the skin, usually of the feet. They then enter the portal system to develop into adult worms. After sexual reproduction, the female lays ova that are released into the bowel lumen or into the general circulation to reach the lung, brain, spinal cord and urinary tract. Ova excreted in the faeces develop into larvae which, provided they find their way to fresh water, then infect the intermediate host encouraging continual infection cycles.

Repeated stool specimens have to be examined for parasites. Sigmoidoscopy may demonstrate ulceration and a rectal biopsy is often diagnostic. Barium enema shows an immobile irregular colon. Treatment of schistosomiasis has been simplified with the introduction of a very effective drug, praziquantel.[148]

Other specific colonic infections

Campylobacter and *Yersinia enterocolitica* infections predominantly involve the small intestine but may occasionally cause colitis with a characteristically infective clinical picture.[148]

Pseudomembranous colitis[149] is a severe form of antibiotic-induced diarrhoea caused by opportunistic infections by *Clostridium difficile*, the toxin of which can be measured in stool. It may follow the use of clindamycin, lincomycin and occasionally ampicillin or tetracycline.[150] The clinical picture varies from a simple diarrhoea to a severe colitis with epithelial necrosis characterized by a white membrane which can be seen on sigmoidoscopy (Fig. 30.21). Rectal biopsy shows the characteristic histology of a pseudomembrane. Treatment is with vancomycin or metronidazole; occasionally colectomy is required for severe necrotizing disease.[151]

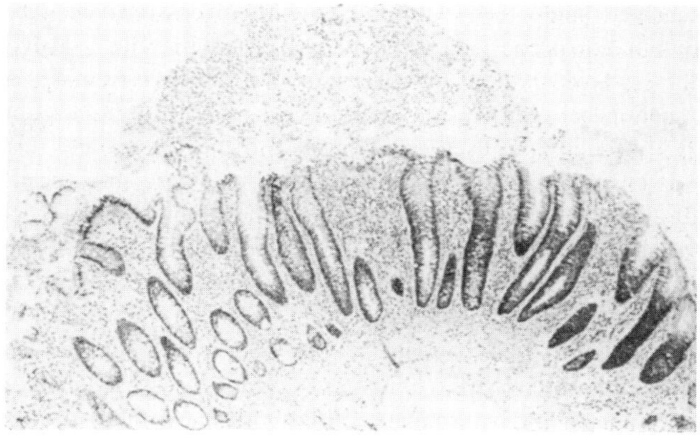

Fig 30.21 Pseudomembranous colitis. Histological section to show epithelial necrosis and pseudomembrane.

ULCERATIVE COLITIS

Ulcerative colitis most commonly occurs between the ages of 15 and 40 years. Its prevalence of 40 per 100 000 is static.[152] Genetic factors, immune mechanisms, environmental and dietary causes have all been considered but the aetiology is still not known.[153] About 15% of patients with an onset before 21 years of age have immediate family members with the disease, but careful studies have failed to confirm anything other than polygenic inheritance.[154] Although human leucocyte antigen B27 has been linked with ankylosing spondylitis no blood group antigens have been matched with inflammatory bowel disease. Ankylosing spondylitis is probably an associated disorder, though it has been considered to be a complication of the colonic disease.[155] Its incidence in ulcerative colitis is much higher than in the general population. No definite causative organism has been identified, but immune responses or autoimmune disorders in response to bacteria have been suggested. Dietary antigens, especially milk products, have been implicated but no direct causal relationship has been established.[156]

Pathology

Ulcerative colitis is a mucosal disorder which almost invariably involves the rectum and then spreads more proximally. It may relapse and remit, during which time its distribution can become

REFERENCES

145. Knight R J Antimicrob Chemother 1980; 6: 577
146. Keasch G J Clin Gastroenterol 1979; 8: 645
147. Editorial Lancet 1980; i: 635
148. Jewkes J, Larson H E et al Gut 1981; 22: 388
149. Editorial Br Med J 1979; 2: 349
150. Larson H E, Honour P et al Lancet 1978; ii: 1063
151. Keighley M R B, Burdon D W et al Br Med J 1978; 2: 1667
152. Langman M J S, Burnham W R In: Allan R N, Keighley M R B et al (eds) Inflammatory Bowel Diseases. Churchill Livingstone, Edinburgh 1983
153. Kirsner J B, Shorter R G N Engl J Med 1982; 306: 775, 837
154. Farmer R G, Michener W H, Mortimer E A Clin Gastroenterol 1980; 9: 271
155. Macrae I, Wright V Ann Rheum Dis 1973; 32: 16
156. Wright R, Truelove S C Br Med J 1965; 2: 142

extensive, and then decrease with successful treatment. Inflammation is confined to the mucosa except in acute and severe colitis, where fissures and transmural changes can make the distinction between severe Crohn's colitis and ulcerative colitis very difficult. The disease is confined to the rectum and distal sigmoid in 60% of cases, extension to the splenic flexure is seen in a further 25% and in the remaining 15% inflammation extends beyond the splenic flexure. This last group is said to have total or near total colitis and is at greater risk of developing severe acute colitis, possibly with toxic dilatation.[157] The cancer risk is also much greater in these patients.[158] Cases in which it is not possible to differentiate ulcerative colitis from Crohn's disease by histology are designated as indeterminate colitis.[159] It appears that indeterminate colitis behaves more like ulcerative colitis than Crohn's disease.[160]

Histologically there is a diffuse infiltration of acute and chronic inflammatory cells which are limited to the mucosa, together with numerous crypt abscesses, distortion of the glandular pattern and goblet cell depletion. In long-standing colitis epithelial dysplasia may occur; when this is severe, carcinoma is frequently found at other sites in the colon.[161] Surgery should be considered if severe dysplasia is found on rectal or colonic biopsies.

Clinical features

Bloody diarrhoea in an otherwise fit patient is the most common presentation. Patients with a limited proctitis may be constipated but they still complain of the passage of blood and mucus. In severe cases there may be almost constant diarrhoea with cramping abdominal pain, and urgency to defecate may be accompanied by episodes of incontinence. In severe disease systemic symptoms include anorexia and weight loss. Malnutrition, anaemia, water and electrolyte loss and toxicity also occur in severe disease. The recognized extraintestinal associations are listed in Table 30.4. They can be divided into those occurring transiently, related to activity of disease, and those which persist irrespective of activity.

On general examination there may be nothing of note. Rectal examination usually reveals blood and mucus on the glove and the mucosa may feel velvety. Sigmoidoscopy shows a diffuse proctitis with contract bleeding, ulceration and granularity. It is important to recognize patients with severe acute colitis. Local symptoms are severe with a frequency of often more than 10 stools/24 h, blood with each stool and an urgent desire to defecate. Systemic symptoms are usually present. These may be evident as wasting, pallor, tachycardia and pyrexia. Abdominal signs of tenderness or distension are very indicative of severe disease. Patients with severe acute colitis may progress to acute toxic dilatation of the colon, ultimately leading to perforation.

The differential diagnosis includes Crohn's colitis, ischaemic colitis, diverticular disease, carcinoma, irritable bowel syndrome, pseudomembranous colitis, Shigella and amoebic colitis.

Investigation

Investigation aims first to make the diagnosis and secondly to assess the severity of the disease. Sigmoidoscopy enables a biopsy to be taken but it also permits an assessment of the proximal anatomical extent of the disease in cases with inflammation limited to the rectum. The diagnosis is made by histological examination of the biopsy. Even in mild chronic cases there may be difficulty in differentiating ulcerative colitis from Crohn's disease. The anatomical extent is related to severity of the disease. A barium enema (Fig. 30.22) demonstrates the extent of macroscopic disease. Colonoscopy can be helpful as a primary investigation and is also invaluable for assessing strictures, doubtful radiology and taking biopsies from multiple sites around the colon. Neither investigation should be employed in patients with severe acute colitis as there is an increased risk of bowel perforation. Blood samples are taken for haemoglobin and markers of inflammation such as the erythrocyte sedimentation rate, orosomucoids, C-reactive proteins and albumin. All these investigations may show elevated levels compared to normal.

Table 30.4 Extraintestinal manifestations of inflammatory bowel disease

Related to disease activity	
Skin	Pyoderma gangrenosum, erythema nodosum
Mucous membranes	Aphthous ulcers of mouth and vagina
Eyes	Iritis
Joints	Activity-related arthritis of large joints
Unrelated to disease activity	
Joints	Sacroiliitis, ankylosing spondylitis
Liver	Chronic active hepatitis, cirrhosis
Biliary tree	Sclerosing cholangitis, bile duct carcinoma
Renal	Amyloidosis in Crohn's disease
Integument	Fingernail clubbing

Medical management

The severity of the colitis can be judged on the basis of its anatomical extent and the severity of both local and general symptoms. Medical management has several aims, which include reducing inflammation, controlling symptoms, water and electrolyte correction and nutritional replacement (see Chapter 2).

Anti-inflammatory

Steroids are used to induce a remission, and salicylic acid derivatives have been shown to maintain an established remission.[162,163] Topical steroid applications given as suppositories or enemas are used for rectal disease.[164] For more extensive disease, confined to the rectum or left colon, oral steroids should be given (e.g. prednisolone).

Sulphasalazine (Salazopyrin) is a combination of sulphapyridine and 5-aminosalicylic acid. It is poorly absorbed in the

REFERENCES

157. Edwards F C, Truelove S C Gut 1963; 4: 299
158. de Dombal F, Watts J et al Br Med J 1966; i: 1442
159. Price A B J Clin Pathol 1978; 31: 567
160. Wells A, McMillan I et al Br J Surg 1991; 78: 179–181
161. Morson B C, Dawson I M P et al Gastrointestinal Pathology, 3rd edn. Blackwell Scientific Publications, Oxford 1990
162. Dissanayake A S, Truelove S C Gut 1973; 14: 923
163. Misiewicz J J, Lennard Jones J E et al Lancet 1965; i: 185
164. Truelove S C Br Med J 1960; i: 464

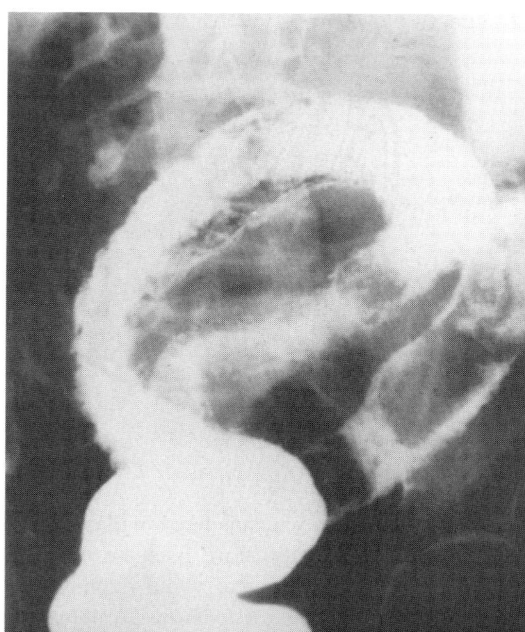

Fig 30.22 Barium enema appearance in severe ulcerative colitis. Undermining of mucosa by ulceration produces epithelial pseudopolyps.

small intestine and split by bacterial action in the colon to liberate the active 5-aminosalicylic acid moiety. It reduces inflammation and prevents relapse. The sulphapyridine fraction is responsible for most of the side-effects[165] which include dyspepsia, skin rashes and azoospermia. Patients who cannot tolerate the drug can be given an enteric-coated preparation or one of the recently developed preparations that contain 5-aminosalicylate alone (e.g. mesalazine). Maintenance treatment should be continued for at least 1 year.

In severe acute ulcerative colitis intravenous prednisolone (60 mg daily) is used in divided doses[166] and three quarters of the patients respond and avoid surgery.[167] In less severe cases prednisolone is given by mouth, starting with 40–60 mg/day. Recent trials of cyclosporin (2 mg/kg) in acute colitis show that half respond, but further results are awaited. Long-term high-dose steroids cause side-effects, so these regimens are only used to induce a remission. Topical applications and steroid enemas are poorly absorbed and are used to treat limited disease or proctitis.[168]

The new non-absorbable oral steroid budesonide and azathioprine can be used in patient's who are steroid intolerant. There is no evidence that antibacterial drugs are of any value in ulcerative colitis and they may induce the development of enteric pathogens.[169]

Symptomatic control

Antidiarrhoeal agents, including codeine phosphate, diphenoxylate and loperamide, can be used to reduce the number of bowel actions. They are relatively non-toxic and can be given in maximal dosage.

Nutrition

Patients who are acutely ill with associated malnutrition require nutritional supplements (see Chapter 2). Whether these are given by the enteral or parenteral route depends on the severity of disease. Iron supplements may also be necessary if patients are anaemic.

Surgical treatment

The indications for surgery are only rarely absolute; the ideal solution is joint management between an aggressive physician and a conservative surgeon (Fig. 30.23).[170] Clearly surgery is essential if the patient develops a dangerous acute complication such as perfo-

REFERENCES

165. Azad Kahn A K, Howes D C et al Gut 1980; 21: 232
166. Meyers S, Janowitz H D Gastroenterology 1985; 89: 1189
167. Truelove S C, Willerby C P et al Lancet 1978; ii: 1086
168. Truelove S C Br Med J 1958; 2: 1072
169. Chapman R W, Selby W, Jewell D P Gut 1986; 27: 1210
170. Jewell D P Int J Colorect Dis 1988; 3: 186

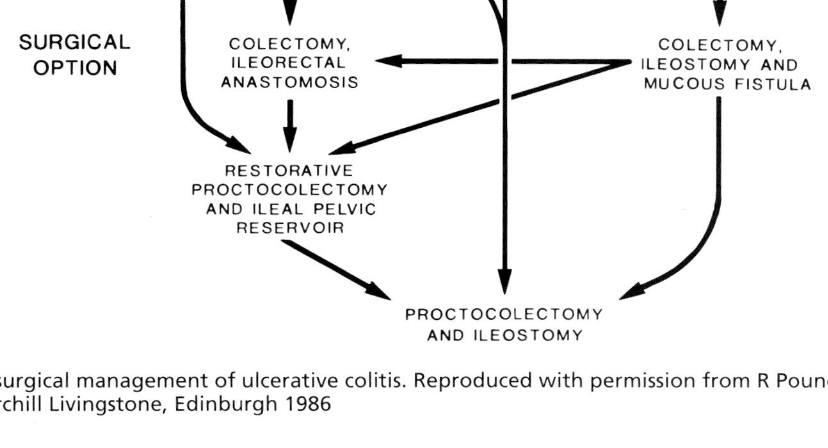

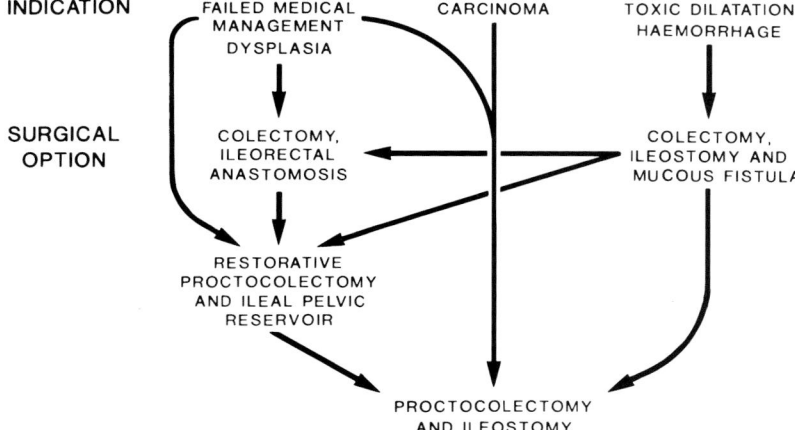

Fig 30.23 Algorithm for surgical management of ulcerative colitis. Reproduced with permission from R Pounder (ed) Recent Advances in Gastroenterology 6. Churchill Livingstone, Edinburgh 1986

ration, severe haemorrhage or toxic dilatation. When a severe attack fails to respond to high-dose parenteral steroid therapy, surgery should be considered after 4 or 5 days and especially under the following circumstances: more than 8 bloody stools per day; tachycardia of more than 100 beats/min; a fever above 38.5°C; dilatation of the transverse colon greater than 5 cm, and a falling serum albumin.[167]

Some patients have repeated attacks which respond promptly to steroids but which rapidly relapse or require continuing doses of steroid for control. Chronic disability or ill health can be an indication for surgery, as can growth retardation in children.[171] There is a risk of cancer developing in patients who have long-standing total colitis. The degree of risk is controversial[172] but it appears to be negligible up to 10 years from diagnosis. Thereafter there is a cumulative incidence of about 1% per annum so that about 10% of a cohort of patients diagnosed 20 years previously will have developed cancer.[173] Surgery is necessary when a cancer is found or if severe dysplasia is reported in colonoscopic biopsies on more than one occasion during surveillance.

Proctocolectomy with ileostomy

The patient is catheterized and placed in the modified lithotomy—Trendelenburg position. The chosen ileostomy site is trephined. Starting at the right colon the ileocolic junction is divided and the colon mobilized. The omentum is removed with the transverse colon if it is adherent.

The rectum is mobilized either in the perimuscular 'close rectal' plane or very carefully in the mesorectal plane, and the dissection taken to the pelvic floor. The anal canal is removed from below in the intersphincteric plane, and the pelvis and perineum closed. A Brooke spouted ileostomy[174] is brought out at the stoma site.

Complications of the procedure include problems with the ileostomy, such as retraction, prolapse, parastomal fistula and rarely necrosis. Intestinal obstruction from adhesions may also occur. Failure of primary healing of the perineal wound may lead to perineal sinus formation and perineal hernia.

Kock continent ileostomy

With modern appliances and the care offered by the stomatherapist, most patients with a Brooke ileostomy manage very satisfactorily. It does, however, function continuously and an appliance must be worn all the time. In the 1960s Kock[175] developed an operation which produced a continent ileostomy (Fig. 30.24), enabling the ileostomy bag to be dispensed with in successful cases. There are fewer indications now for this procedure than 10–20 years ago, because of the development of restorative proctocolectomy with ileoanal anastomosis. It still however, has a place for patients who have had a proctocolectomy with excision of the anal canal and who are keen to improve their quality of life. It is especially suitable for patients with an unsatisfactory Brooke ileostomy who are having difficulty in keeping an appliance in place.

After a conventional proctocolectomy a reservoir is constructed from 30 cm of terminal ileum leaving a length of 15 cm distally. This distal ileum is then invaginated into the reservoir to create a

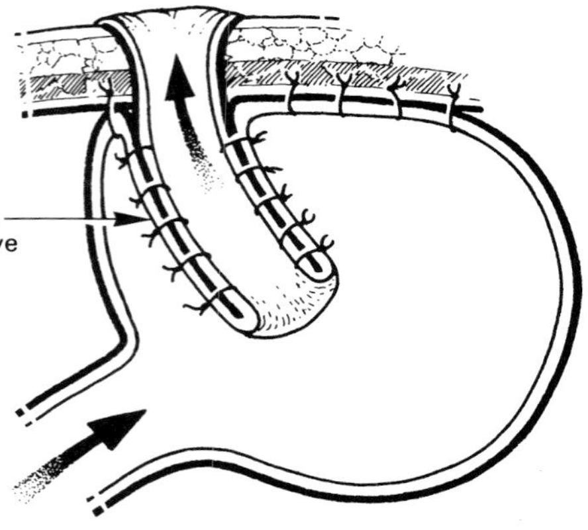

Fig 30.24 The Kock continent ileostomy.

nipple valve about 5 cm long which is fixed in place by four rows of staples placed longitudinally. Care must be taken to avoid damaging the small bowel mesentery while stapling the nipple. The reservoir is fixed to the anterior abdominal wall by interrupted sutures and the 5 cm length of terminal ileum projecting from it is brought through the anterior abdominal wall and sutured flush with the skin to form a stoma in the lower part of the right iliac fossa.[176] Postoperatively an indwelling catheter is left in the reservoir for 5 or 6 weeks, after which the patient is taught to evacuate by self-catheterization. In a successful case the stoma will remain continent and evacuation by catheterization is necessary about 4–5 times every 24 h.

The major complication of this procedure is slippage of the nipple valve leading to incontinence of the stoma. Re-operation with fixation is necessary to rectify this problem. The re-operation rate depends upon the experience of the surgeon and also on the method of fixation. Stapling (see above) is more effective than many of the techniques used previously. In an analysis of 314 patients Kock et al[176] have achieved a re-operation rate for valve slippage of 7%. Others have reported rates of 20–40%.[177,178] Pouchitis (non-specific inflammation) can occur in 30%.

Colectomy and ileorectal anastomosis

This offers an ileostomy-saving proctocolectomy in some patients. It has however become less popular since the advent of restorative proctocolectomy using an ileoanal reservoir.[179] A successful result depends upon there being only mild disease in the rectum. It is

REFERENCES

171. Berger M, Gribetz D, Korelitz B Paediatrics 1975; 55: 459
172. Dickinson R J, Dickson M C, Axon A T R Lancet 1980; i: 620
173. Lennard Jones J E, Morson B et al Gastroenterology 1977; 73: 1280
174. Brooke B N Lancet 1952; ii: 102
175. Kock N G Ann Surg 1971; 173: 545
176. Kock N G, Myrvold H E et al Acta Chir Scand 1981; 147: 67–72
177. Goligher J C In: Surgery of the Anus, Rectum and Colon, 5th edn. Baillière Tindall, London 1984 p 919
178. Palmu A, Sivala A Br J Surg 1978; 65: 645
179. Symposium 1986 Dozois R R et al Int J Colorectal Dis 1: 2

especially important to bear in mind that the use of rectal steroids may give a favourable but false impression of the degree of inflammation.[167] It is particularly good for younger patients, allowing them to mature through adolescence without a stoma. Persisting disease in the rectum is responsible for a high relapse rate, with failure, defined by conversion to a permanent ileostomy, being reported in 10–70% of cases.[180–182] Malignant change in the retained rectum occurs in 5–15% although this risk may have been overemphasized.[154,180,183] Areas of neoplasia may be difficult to identify in the presence of liquid stool, so the attending surgeon has a clear responsibility for long-term follow-up by sigmoidoscopy and biopsy at 6-monthly intervals.

Procedure. The operation consists of a colectomy as for a proctocolectomy. The rectum is transected at the sacral promontory and the terminal ileum anastomosed to it with adsorbable sutures.

The major complication is anastomotic leakage,[180] which requires a laparotomy and defunctioning ileostomy.

Colectomy with ileorectal anastomosis is a compromise operation in which the diseased rectum is left behind in order to avoid a permanent stoma. Patients are therefore susceptible to the effects of persisting disease in the rectum. Continued inflammation or the onset of malignant transformation may lead to failure. Published failure rates range from around 10%[181] to up to 40%.[180,182,184,185]

Restorative proctocolectomy

In this procedure all the diseased tissue is removed but the patient avoids a permanent stoma. It was first introduced in 1976 and the long-term effects are therefore still not known.[186] As it is a highly attractive alternative to a permanent ileostomy it is rapidly becoming the procedure of choice in the surgical treatment of ulcerative colitis.[179] Well motivated patients under the age of 60 years, aware of the possible complications and problems and not having Crohn's disease, are suitable candidates.[187]

Procedure. The colon is resected if it has not already been removed, but the rectum remains in place. The rectum is removed by a close dissection along its wall, keeping well clear of pelvic nerves. The rectum is transected at the pelvic floor, leaving a cuff of mucosa of no more than 2–3 cm above the dentate line (Fig. 30.25). The anal mucosa is removed in four strips from the level of the dentate line upwards after adrenaline has been infiltrated. Not everyone agrees that mucosectomy is necessary, and many surgeons preserve the entire anal canal fashioning a double stapled ileoanal anastomosis. The ileum is transected just proximal to the ileocaecal valve, usually after division of the ileocaecal artery.

Various designs of reservoir have been described (Fig. 30.26).[186,188,189] The site of the proposed ileoanal anastomosis is chosen at the apex of the first two loops of small bowel. It is tested to ensure that its length is suitable, either by offering the ileum to the anal canal before creating the reservoir or by seeing how far beyond the symphysis pubis it reaches. The anastomosis must not be made under any tension: if there is insufficient length, vessels in the mesentery must be judiciously divided. For a four-loop reservoir 10–15 cm lengths of the terminal ileum are laid out.

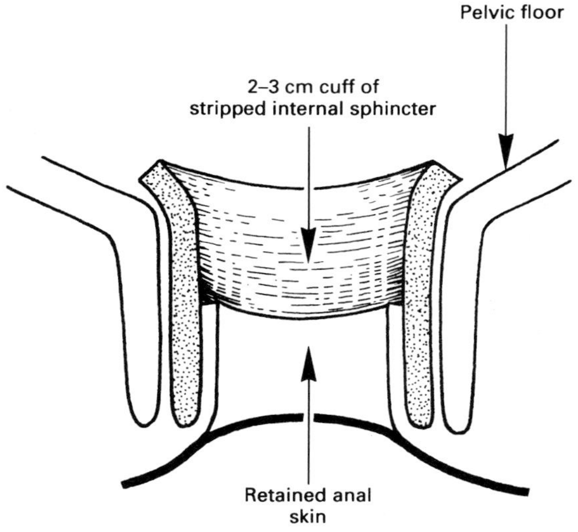

Fig 30.25 Anal remnant ready for ileal pouch—anal anastomosis in restorative proctocolectomy.

They are opened with cutting diathermy along their contiguous borders and adjacent loops are sewn together. The final anterior suture line is completed leaving a defect for the anastomosis. The reservoir can also be made using staples. A two-loop construction can be simply performed using a 90 mm linear stapling instrument. The three-loop reservoir has a length of distal ileum projecting from it. This should be as short as possible (1–2 cm) to avoid evacuation difficulties. The four-loop reservoir aims to give adequate volume without the presence of a distal ileal segment (Fig. 30.26). The pouch is then brought down into the pelvis. A perineal operator places a retractor into the anal canal. Stay sutures on the pouch are delivered through the anus to bring the mouth of the reservoir down to the dentate line without tension. Interrupted absorbable sutures are placed endoanally to complete the ileoanal anastomosis.

The exact level of the ileoanal anastomosis is controversial. Preserving the sensitive anal mucosa 1 or 2 cm above the dentate line may improve continence. A loop ileostomy is raised as near to the pouch as possible and placed in the right iliac fossa. This can be closed after 8–10 weeks provided the ileoanal anastomosis and pouch have healed uneventfully. The final result is shown in Figure 30.27. Radiological examination of the reservoir should be undertaken to check for leaks before the ileostomy is closed.

Complications. The most common complication is pelvic sepsis—usually the result of dehiscence of the ileoanal anasto-

REFERENCES

180. Jones P F, Munroe A, Ewen S W B Br J Surg 1977; 64: 615
181. Aylett S O Br Med J 1966; i: 1001
182. Hawley P R Br J Surg 1985; 72 (suppl): S75
183. Baker W N W, Glass R E et al Br J Surg 1978; 65: 862
184. Grundfest S F, Fazio V W Ann Surg 1981; 193: 9
185. Gruner O P N, Flatmark A et al Scand J Gastroenterol 1975; 10: 641
186. Parks A G, Nicholls R J Br Med J 1978; ii: 85
187. Mortensen N J Gut 1988; 29: 561
188. Utsunomiya J, Iwama T et al Dis Colon Rectum 1980; 23: 459
189. Fonkalsrud E W Surg Gynecol Obstet 1980; 150: 1

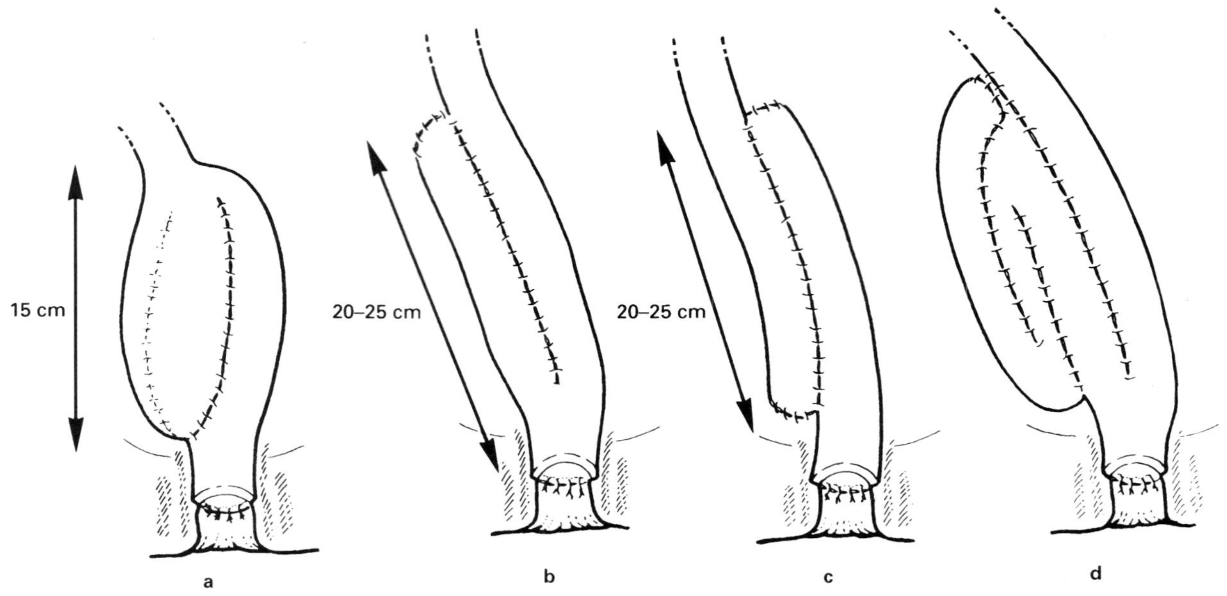

Fig 30.26 Various designs for ileal reservoir in restorative proctocolectomy. (**a**) S pouch; (**b**) J pouch; (**c**) H pouch; (**d**) W pouch.

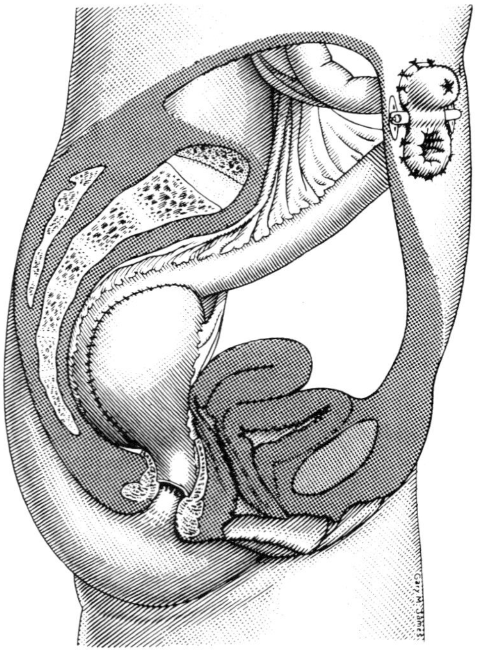

Fig 30.27 Ileal reservoir in situ in the pelvis. The loop ileostomy is closed at about 8 weeks after the pouch operation. Reproduced with permission from R Pounder (ed) Recent Advances in Gastroenterology 6. Churchill Livingstone, Edinburgh 1986.

mosis. It is reported to occur in 8–25% of published cases. The incidence decreases with experience, but sepsis in the pelvis can be troublesome. It does not always drain freely, and the resulting fibrosis and scarring may mar the eventual clinical result. A stricture develops in 10% of patients, but usually responds to simple dilatation. Adhesive obstruction is the other major problem; it can usually be managed conservatively, but a further laparotomy may be necessary in up to 15% of patients. The loop ileostomy may lead to dehydration and salt loss, and there is a small complication rate following closure. Nonetheless, over three quarters of patients do not have any complications from pouch formation.[187]

Postoperative function. When the ileostomy is closed patients have a normal desire to evacuate faeces and in three quarters this can be deferred without urgency. Fortunately patients who have had a pouch formed do not seem to make or pass much flatus. Whilst there is a range of frequency of defecation, a mean of 3–6 actions per 24 hours can be expected. Frank incontinence is unusual but around 10% have minor leakage of mucus, especially at night. Outright failure occurs in around 5% of patients for reasons of pelvic sepsis, undiagnosed. Crohn's disease or unacceptable stool frequency.[187]

No serious nutritional problems have emerged but the long-term consequences of the pouch are not known. In 10% of colitic patients a syndrome of acute pouch inflammation, excessive stool frequency and malaise has been recognized and is called 'pouchitis'.[190] Bacterial overgrowth is heavier in a pouch than in a conventional ileostomy, but there is no clear relationship between the microbiology, incomplete emptying and function.[187,191] 'Pouchitis' usually responds to treatment with metronidazole, ciprofloxacin, steroids or pouch drainage.

Acute severe colitis and toxic megacolon

Patients with fulminating colitis should be jointly managed by a physician and surgeon and reviewed on a daily basis. A sigmoidoscopy, biopsy and stool cultures are essential, but colonoscopy

REFERENCES

190. Handelsman J C, Fishbein R H et al Surgery 1983; 93: 247
191. Madden M V, Farthing M J G, Nicholls R J Gut 1990; 31: 247

and barium enema examination are proscribed. Daily plain abdominal films are taken to assess the degree of dilatation of the colon; any increase in diameter greater than 6 cm indicates the development of toxic megacolon.

The indications for emergency surgery include acute severe colitis that has not responded to intensive medical treatment, toxic megacolon, massive bleeding and perforation. Under close joint management, perforation has become rare with cases being referred for surgery before its development. A perforated colon has a high mortality. Massive bleeding is uncommon. When it occurs, the site is often located in the rectum.

When surgery is necessary a subtotal colectomy with an ileostomy and mucous fistula is the preferred option. It is effective in restoring the health of the patient with the minimum of surgical trauma. It spares a sick patient the morbidity of a pelvic dissection. As the rectum and anal sphincter are left undisturbed, future restorative surgery is possible. The surgical specimen may allow the histopathologist to make a firm diagnosis but in severely diseased bowel the distinction between ulcerative colitis and Crohn's disease may be difficult. In about 10% of cases the pathologist will report that the colitis is indeterminate in type.[159] The operative mortality of this procedure is less than 5%.

CROHN'S DISEASE

Crohn's disease can involve any part of the gastrointestinal tract from mouth to anus, and cannot be cured either medically or surgically. The most frequent site of involvement is the terminal ileum (see Chapter 29). Over 60% of patients have both small and large bowel disease, and 20% have large bowel disease only.[192] Because the distribution is so variable it is difficult to be specific about the management.

Aetiology

The presence of granulomata suggested a mycobacterial origin, but attempts to prove that *M. paratuberculosis* is the causative organism have not been successful. Many other infectious agents (viruses, cell wall deficient pseudomonads) have been proposed and a popular theory is a measles virus induced vasculitis. Intriguingly, smoking appears to accelerate recurrence after resection. Whatever the initiating factor, immunological mechanisms play a part in the eventual pathogenesis of the disease. The familial incidence of Crohn's disease is around 10–15%.

Histopathology

The disease is a chronic discontinuous granulomatous condition with transmural aggregates of inflammatory cells and deep penetrating fissures and ulceration. In the colon it differs from ulcerative colitis, which is confined to the mucosa except in very severe cases.[193] In Crohn's disease the bowel wall is thickened and pipe-like with strictures and fistulae into adjacent small bowel, colon or other organs such as the bladder. There are large fleshy lymph nodes in the mesentery and the mucosa is oedematous with linear ulceration, giving a cobblestone appearance (Fig. 30.28). Areas of

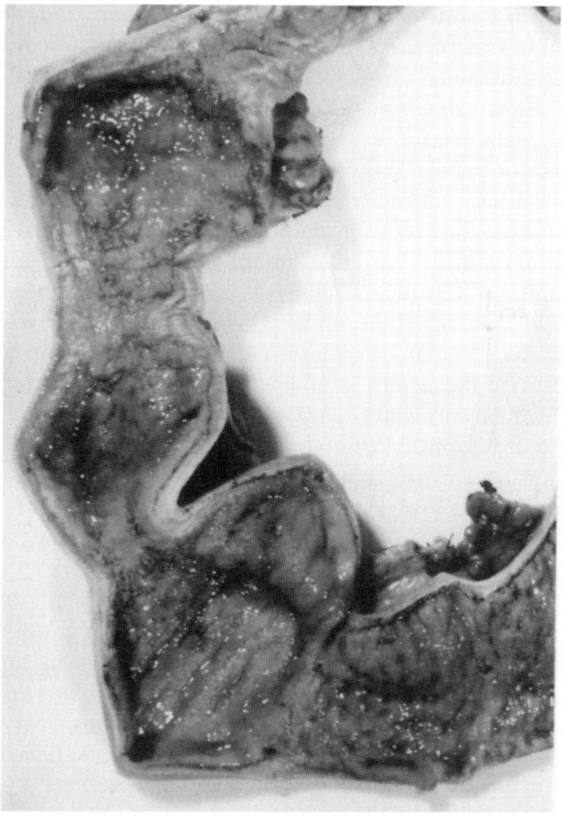

Fig 30.28 Crohn's disease. 'Skip' lesions are separated by normal segments. Diseased areas are characterized by cobblestoning and linear ulcers.

normal mucosa separate involved segments (skip lesions) but diffuse disease does occur in the colon. In less severely affected areas aphthoid ulcers are the earliest lesions and start as ulcerating lymphoid follicles.

Curiously, in small bowel disease (see Chapter 29) recurrences invariably occur on the ileal side of an ileocolic anastomosis.[161] In the colon the important distinguishing microscopic feature is the presence of granulomata, but these are only found in 60% of cases. Rectal biopsy is more helpful in diagnosing ulcerative colitis than Crohn's disease, where there may be a normal rectum and sampling errors may fail to find any abnormality.[194] Colonoscopic biopsies from multiple sites and the endoscopic distribution of disease are of more help in making the diagnosis of Crohn's disease.

Clinical features

In the small bowel, stricture formation leads to chronic intestinal obstruction. Local perforation may also occur and this can present either as abscess formation within the abdomen or fistulation either

REFERENCES

192. Allan R N In: Bouchier I A D, Allan R N et al (eds) Textbook of Gastroenterology. Baillière Tindall, London 1983 p 941
193. Lockhart-Mummery H E, Morson B C Gut 1960; 1: 87
194. Surawicz C M, Meisel J L et al Gastroenterology 1981; 80: 60

to the exterior or to other organs. Small bowel disease is discussed in detail in Chapter 29. Colorectal Crohn's disease presents with diarrhoea, bleeding, obstruction or perianal disease. In the large bowel both stricture formation and fistulation can also occur. The disease often causes extensive mucosal inflammation which presents as a colitis. This can be very similar to ulcerative colitis but the clinical and endoscopic differences shown in Table 30.5 allow a distinction to be made between the two diseases in the majority of cases. The most useful clinical features are the segmental involvement of Crohn's disease and the presence of anal disease. Rectal sparing is also very indicative of Crohn's disease. Anal disease is common in cases with large bowel involvement, particularly if the rectum is inflamed. An anal lesion is present in 50–70% of patients with large bowel Crohn's disease.[195] The most common anal problems are fissure and anorectal sepsis.[196,197] but ulceration, oedematous skin tags, stenosis (usually at the anorectal junction) and rectovaginal fistula can also occur. Patients with large bowel Crohn's disease may present with acute colitis which can occasionally progress to a toxic dilatation.[198]

As with ulcerative colitis, patients with chronic Crohn's disease may develop extra-alimentary manifestations which are listed in Table 30.5. Oral aphthous ulceration, erythema nodosum and fingernail clubbing are particularly indicative of Crohn's disease. In cases with rectal involvement, sigmoidoscopy may show aphthous ulceration or more deep ulceration when inflammation is severe. In these cases inflammatory polyps may be seen.

Investigation

A barium enema examination may show areas of discontinuous disease and stricture formation. Mucosal changes indicating aphthous ulceration, deep ulceration with fissure formation and fistulation may also be seen (Fig. 30.29). Colonoscopy provides a view of the proximal mucosa and may detect terminal ileal disease if the ileocaecal valve can be passed. It also enables multiple biopsies to be taken. Blood tests, including the erythrocyte sedimentation rate, C-reactive protein and orosomucoids, give an indication of disease activity. In cases with poor nutrition the serum albumin level is low. The presence of small bowel Crohn's disease should be confirmed or excluded by a small bowel meal examination (see Chapter 29).

Medical management

When considering medical management two clinical pictures should be distinguished. A flare-up of disease activity giving rise to mucosal ulceration and oedema is likely to respond to medical treatment, which must include steroids and occasionally azathioprine. In patients with strictures causing obstruction, or in those with fistulae or abscesses, medical treatment is unlikely to give long-lasting relief and surgery is invariably necessary. There is no evidence that long-term treatment with steroids or sulphasalazine reduces the chances of surgery becoming necessary.[199]

Patients with extensive intestinal involvement or sepsis may be severely nutritionally depleted. The serum albumin and the amount of weight loss are a rough guide to the degree of nutritional failure.

Table 30.5 Clinical differences between Crohn's disease and ulcerative colitis

	Crohn's disease	*Ulcerative colitis*
Symptoms		
Bleeding	Sometimes	Very common
Abdominal pain	Common	Sometimes
Urgent defecation	Sometimes	Very common
Abdomen		
Abdominal mass	Sometimes	Rare
Spontaneous fistulae	Sometimes	Never
Anal region		
Fissure	Common	Occurs
Ulceration	Common	Rare
Infection	Common and often complicated	Occurs
Lesions preceding bowel symptoms	Sometimes	Never
Endoscopy		
Rectal involvement	50%	> 95%
Appearance	Oedema, ulcers, normal patches	Uniform, continuous, granular, friable
Prognosis		
Medicine	Inadequate in 80%	80% successful
Surgery	Often recurrence	'Cure' possible
Cancer risk	Slight	Definite

Intravenous nutrition or, in some suitable cases, enteric feeding may be necessary.

Surgical management

Surgery is indicated for the complications of Crohn's disease, including obstruction, fistula, bleeding, abscess and intractable diarrhoea. As the disease cannot be cured, minimal surgery aims to restore bowel function and excise the active inflammation without removing any more bowel than is necessary.

Terminal ileal and ileocolic disease

This is the most common form of Crohn's disease and presents with either obstructive symptoms or abscess. Surgical treatment is usually necessary and a resection with anastomosis, preserving as much right colon as possible, minimize postoperative bowel frequency (see Chapter 29).[200] Resection may be followed by long or apparently permanent relief of symptoms. Recurrence requiring further resection is unfortunately common. The recurrence rate is cumulative with re-operation over a 5–10-year period being necessary in 40–60% of cases.[201–203] In patients with multiple strictures

REFERENCES

195. Hellers G, Bergstrand O et al Gut 1980; 21: 525–556
196. Lockhart Mummery H E Br J Surg 1985; 72 (suppl): S95
197. Buchanan P, Keighley M R B, Allan R N Am J Surg 1980; 140: 642
198. Buzzard A J, Baker W N W et al Gut 1974; 15: 416
199. Summers R W, Switz D M et al Gastroenterology 1978; 77: 847
200. Lee E C G Gut 1984; 25: 217
201. Hellers G Acta Chir Scand 1979; 490 (suppl): 1
202. Lock R M, Farmer R G et al N Engl J Med 1981; 304: 13
203. Higgens C S, Allan R N Gut 1980; 21: 933

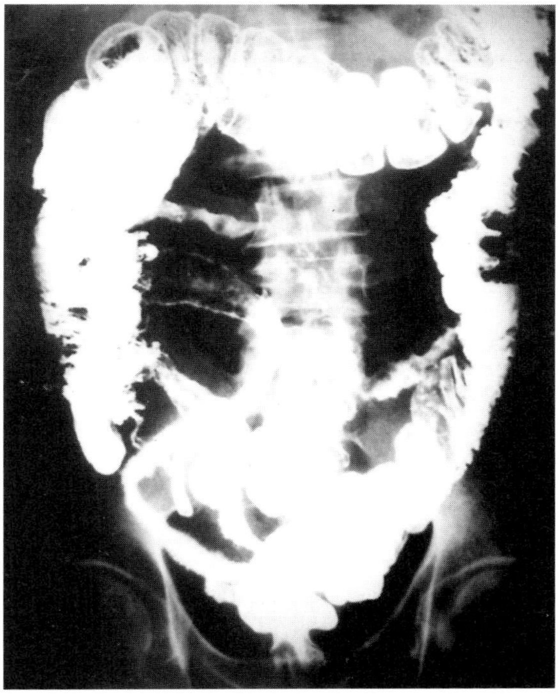

Fig 30.29 Crohn's disease. Barium enema with reflux into small bowel shows extensive narrowing of the distal ileum, with deep ulceration, wall thickening and cobblestoning.

in whom resection might lead to the possibility of short bowel syndrome, stricture plasty (Fig. 30.30) offers relief of obstruction without the need for resection. In this procedure the affected segments are left in situ and the stricture opened along the long axis of the gut and sewn transversely to widen the lumen. Some of these sites then heal and complications are remarkably low. There is as yet no effective adjuvant drug treatment which reduces the long-term recurrence rate.[199]

Colonic disease

The medical management of colonic Crohn's disease is similar to that for ulcerative colitis. Surgical treatment is different, however, in a number of respects. In patients with diffuse or multiple-site colonic disease, defunctioning the bowel may allow the disease to resolve and about one quarter can subsequently have their gut continuity restored.[204] There is evidence, however, that after this procedure long-term recurrence rates are high and any improvement is short-lived. Either a split ileostomy or loop ileostomy can be used. The latter has the advantage that closure does not require laparotomy, but the disadvantage that unless it is constructed properly, overspill occurs and defunction is incomplete. Segmental resection in patients with localized strictures or discrete areas of involvement may be successful.[205]

Where there is rectal sparing and a normal anus an ileorectal anastomosis saves the patient an ileostomy, but there is a recurrence rate at 5–10 years of 30%, and more than half require further

REFERENCES

204. Harper P H, Truelove S C et al Gut 1983; 24: 106
205. Allan A, Andrews H et al World J Surg 1989; 13: 611–614
206. Flint G, Strauss R et al Gut 1977; 18: 23

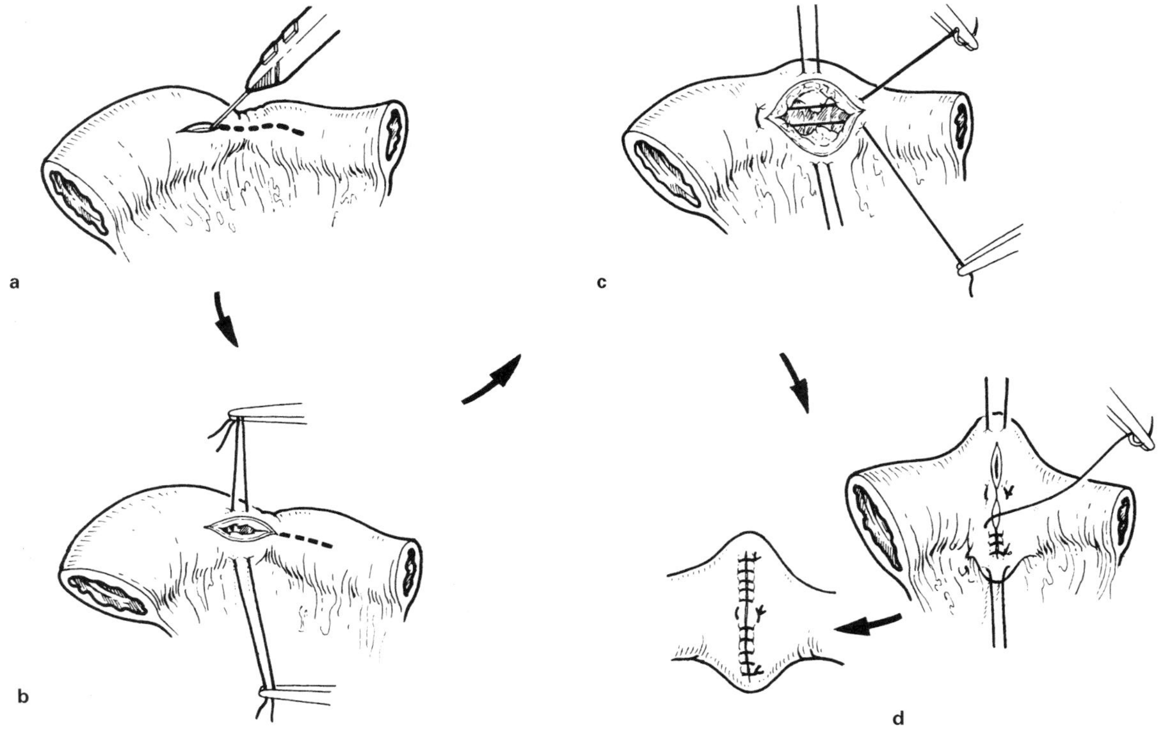

Fig 30.30 Stages in ileal stricture plasty for Crohn's disease.

resection or conversion to a proctocolectomy.[206–208] Using actuarial determined estimates of cumulative recurrence, Lockhart Mummery & Ritchie[209] reported a recurrence rate of 56% at 10 years after colectomy with ileorectal anastomosis, and a similar figure of 50% at 16 years was reported by Buchmann et al.[210]

In patients with widespread colonic disease a proctocolectomy and ileostomy may be indicated and the surgical technique is similar to that for ulcerative colitis.[211] The mortality for elective proctocolectomy is very low and the principal complication is a perineal sinus or delayed healing of the perineal wound. This is more likely to occur where there is pre-existing perianal sepsis or a fistula in ano. Recurrence of Crohn's disease in the ileum after a proctocolectomy is less common than after colectomy with an ileorectal anastomosis: recurrence rates of 10–30% have been reported.[208,209]

Anorectal disease

Over half the patients with large bowel Crohn's disease have an anal lesion, and the prevalence is greater in those with rectal involvement. An anal fissure is the most common problem although it may be symptomless. Fissures may heal with medical management or become chronic, when they can become the site of fistula formation.[212,213] Sometimes the pain is so severe that faecal division is necessary. Occasionally where there are other forms of perianal disease excision of the rectum is necessary. Anal surgery for the fissure should be avoided if possible.

A fistula in ano may develop either directly as a result of Crohn's disease or secondary to its effects upon the anal gland anatomy.[145] Fistulae are sometimes multiple and complex but can still be healed with conventional conservative surgery and a fistula is rarely the main indication for rectal excision.[214,215] Great care must be taken over division of the sphincter muscle in high fistulae, and conservative surgery with drainage of abscess cavities and insertion of a seton is more appropriate. Sometimes treatment with metronidazole will control recurrent episodes of sepsis in otherwise symptomless fistulae. In patients with a supralevator abscess there is less chance of successful conservative treatment and a defunctioning colostomy or proctectomy may eventually be necessary.[195,204] Very rarely a long-standing Crohn's fistula in ano may undergo malignant change.[216]

Rectovaginal fistula

Incontinence as a consequence of a rectovaginal fistula is often severe and the condition is difficult to manage. Patients without symptoms need no treatment although a low fistulae can be laid open.[217] Excision of the fistula may be successful provided there is no severe rectal disease. With the patient in the prone jack-knife position, the fistula is cored out, closed in layers and a rectal advancement flap brought down over the fistula site (Fig. 30.31). Intractable cases and those who develop incontinence require proctectomy.

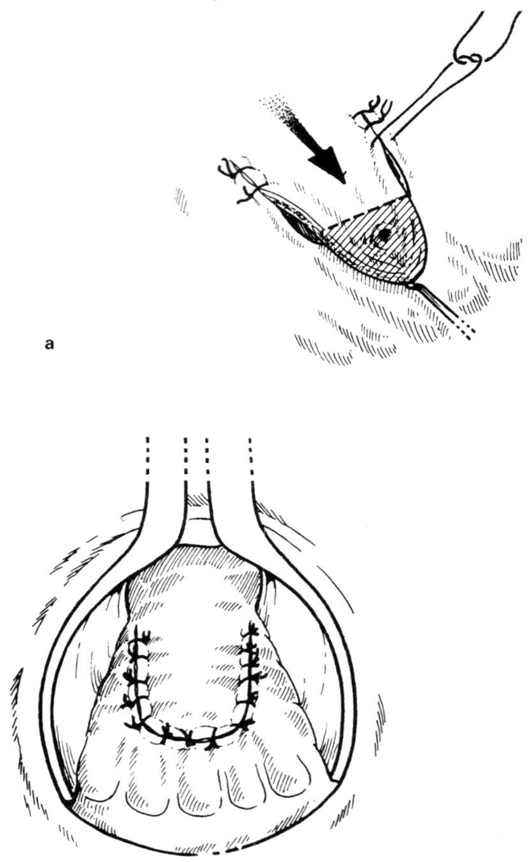

a

b

Fig 30.31 Advancement flap repair for rectovaginal fistula.

Perineal wound

Poor primary healing of the perineal wound after proctectomy is common.[218] It is sometimes related to the presence of pre-existing anal disease at the time of proctectomy.[219] The management of this problem can be difficult. Steroids may be tried but rarely work, and repeated examination under anaesthesia, curettage and dressings is the usual treatment. In patients with a long-standing perineal sinus a muscle flap may be effective in achieving healing.

Haemorrhoids

Great care should be taken when treating haemorrhoids in patients with Crohn's disease, and haemorrhoidectomy should be avoided

REFERENCES

207. Goligher J C Surg Gynecol Obstet 1979; 148: 1
208. Allan R N, Steinberg D M et al Gastroenterology 1977; 73: 72
209. Lockhart Mummery H E, Ritchie J K In: Allen R N, Keighley M R B et al (eds) Inflammatory Bowel Diseases. Churchill Livingstone, Edinburgh 1993 p 462
210. Buchmann P, Waterman I T et al Br J Surg 1981; 68: 7
211. Scammell B E, Andrews H et al Br J Surg 1987; 74: 671
212. Buchmann P, Allan R N et al Am J Surg 1980; 140: 462
213. Sweeney J L, Ritchie J K, Nicholls R J Br J Surg 1988 Jan; 75(1) 56–57
214. Marks C G, Ritchie J K, Lockhart Mummery H E Br J Surg 1981; 68: 525
215. Williams J A In: Lee E C G (ed) Surgery of Inflammatory Bowel Disorders. Churchill Livingstone, Edinburgh 1987 p 182
216. Jeffrey P J, Ritchie J K, Parks A G Lancet 1977; i: 1084
217. Francois Y, Descos L, Vignal J Int J Colorectal Dis 1990; 5: 12
218. Baudot P, Keighley M R B, Alexander-Williams J Br J Surg 1980; 67: 257
219. Scammell B E, Keighley M R B Br J Surg 1986; 73: 150

as it may lead to anorectal sepsis, sometimes requiring rectal excision.[216] Many patients' symptoms settle spontaneously or with local steroid applications.

DIVERTICULAR DISEASE

Diverticula of the colon were first reported by Voigtel in 1804[220] and were described in detail by Cruveilhier in 1849.[221] At least in its mildest form, diverticular disease is one of the most common afflictions of western people. It has been estimated that around a third of all British adults over the age of 60 years have abnormalities of the colonic wall which can be ascribed to this condition.[222] There have been great efforts over the past few decades to confirm the link between a low fibre intake and diverticular disease;[223] almost all the evidence is epidemiological. It has not been possible to produce an animal model of the condition, nor to perform long-term prospective dietary manipulation trials in human volunteers. There seems little doubt, however, that the causal connection is valid.

Pathophysiology

Hypertrophy of the circular muscle is the earliest abnormality (Fig. 30.32), perhaps the result of long-standing constipation resulting from low fibre intake. Diverticula develop as mucosal extrusions at weak points in the bowel wall, presumably as a result of raised intraluminal pressure produced by the uncoordinated action of hypertrophied muscle.[224,225] Most diverticula develop where blood vessels penetrate the colonic muscle at the edges of the anti-mesenteric taeniae (Fig. 30.33).[226] By far the most common site for diverticula is the sigmoid colon, though any part of the colon can be involved. In some oriental countries, where diverticular disease is becoming more prevalent, the right colon is the site of predilection.[227] The rectum never develops diverticula.

When diverticula are present but uninflamed (so-called 'diverticulosis') the individual is usually unaware of the condition. At most there may be episodic lower abdominal pain (painful diverticular disease; Fig. 30.34).[224] Diverticula are narrow-necked mucosal pouches (wayside inns of ill repute) and likely to collect inspissated faeces within them. This may cause ulceration within the diverticula, leading to pericolonic inflammation, perforation or bleeding from the associated penetrating artery. The inflammatory

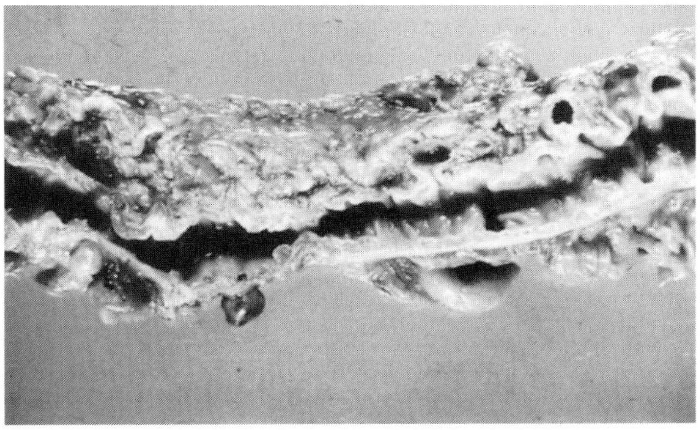

Fig 30.32 Diverticular disease. Marked thickening of the muscle layer and resultant diverticula formation.

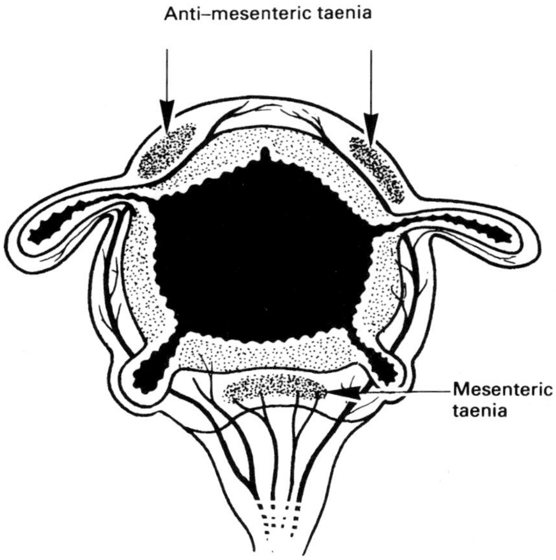

Fig 30.33 Diverticular disease. Transverse section of sigmoid colon to show sites of predilection for diverticula formation.

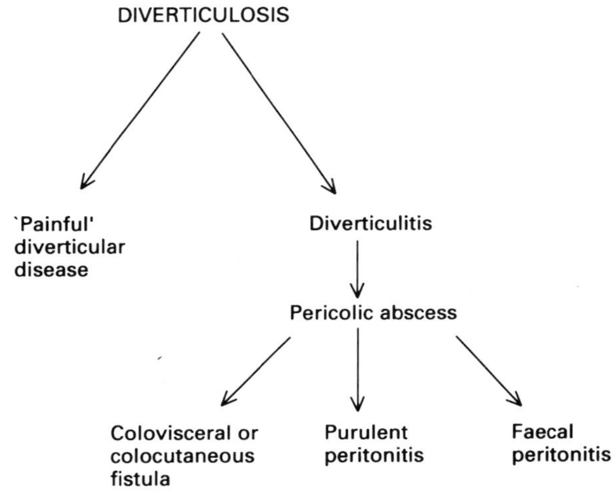

Fig 30.34 Diverticular disease. Alternative pathways in natural history.

changes can produce a chronic painful condition, an acute exacerbation of disease (acute diverticulitis), or a pericolic abscess (which may rupture into the general peritoneal cavity or into a neighbouring viscus to produce a fistula).

Clinical presentation

Diverticular disease can present in a wide variety of ways. Patients may present electively, via the outpatient department, or as an emergency.

REFERENCES

220. Voigtel F G Handbuch der Pathologischen Anatomie. Band 2. Halle, 1804
221. Cruveilhier J Traite d'Anatomie Descriptive. Paris, 1849
222. Parks T G Proc R Soc Med 1968; 61: 932
223. Painter N S, Burkitt D P Br Med J 1971; 2: 450–454
224. Arfwiddson S Acta Chir Scand (suppl) 1964; 342

Elective presentations

Painful diverticular disease

This is the most common and least serious clinical presentation, though some would dispute even its existence.[228] The patient usually complains of episodic lower abdominal pain, which may be associated with a change of bowel habit and a feeling of abdominal bloating. The symptoms are akin to those of the irritable bowel syndrome. Physical examination is usually unremarkable, but barium enema shows the presence of diverticula and the concentric indentations of muscle hypertrophy (Fig. 30.35). Fibreoptic endoscopy should be performed to exclude a carcinoma if there is any doubt about the radiological appearances.[229] Treatment, which is aimed at relieving symptoms and preventing progression of the disease, consists of a high-fibre diet and a trial of mebeverine or liquorice extract.[230]

Fistulae

The most common type is the colovesical fistula, followed by colovaginal, colocutaneous and coloenteric.[231]

Colovesical fistula. This condition is more common in males, presumably because the uterus intervening between the two organs has a protective effect in females. There may be a history suggestive of previous diverticulitis. The patient usually complains of recurrent cystitis, pneumaturia or the presence of solid (i.e. faecal) matter in the urine. Rarely the patient may pass urine per rectum. A lower abdominal inflammatory mass may be palpable. The differential diagnosis includes Crohn's disease, carcinoma of the colon, bladder and uterus, radiation damage, tuberculosis, actinomycosis and trauma. The most useful investigation is cystoscopy.[232] Contrast radiological investigations may not demonstrate the communication, although contrast or plain radiographs may show gas in the bladder or the upper urinary tract (Fig. 30.36). Fibreoptic endoscopy of the bladder and rectum with biopsy is worthwhile before a laparotomy is carried out.

Sigmoid colectomy with a primary bowel anastomosis and repair of the bladder is the procedure of choice when the bowel has been adequately prepared.[233] A defunctioning stoma may be indicated if there is severe local sepsis. The repair sites in the intestine and the bladder should be separated by interposing a pedicle of omentum between them. A urinary catheter should be left in situ for at least 10 days postoperatively.

Other fistulae. Colovaginal and colocutaneous fistulae from diverticular disease present with faecal discharge from the vagina or skin of the lower abdomen respectively.[234] Colo-ileal fistula presents with frequent loose excoriating stools, as small bowel contents pass directly into the rectum. Primary colonic resection and anastomosis is the treatment of choice for all these fistulae.

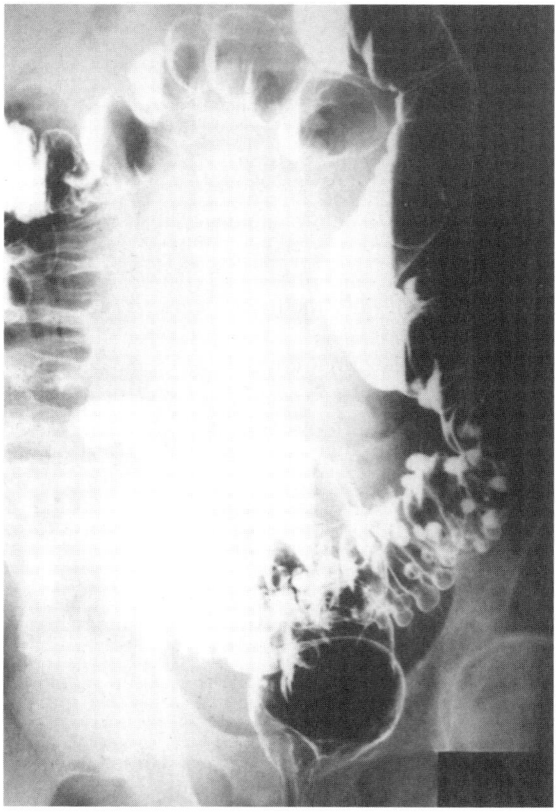

Fig 30.35 Diverticular disease. Barium enema showing concentric muscle hypertrophy and diverticula formation.

REFERENCES

225. Painter N S Ann R Coll Surg Engl 1964; 34: 98–114
226. Slack W W Br J Surg 1962; 50: 185–190
227. Sugihara K, Muto T et al Dis Colon Rectum 1984; 27: 531–537
228. Thompson W G Am J Gastroenterol 1986; 81: 613–614
229. Boulos P B, Karamanolis D G et al Lancet 1984; i: 95–96
230. Brod Ribb A J M Lancet 1977; i: 664
231. Small W P, Smith A N Clin Gastroenterol 1975; 4: 171
232. Mileski W J, Joehl R J et al Am J Surg 1987; 153: 75–79
233. Rao P N, Knox R et al Br J Surg 1987; 74: 362–363
234. Fazio V W, Church J M et al Dis Colon Rectum 1987; 30: 89–94

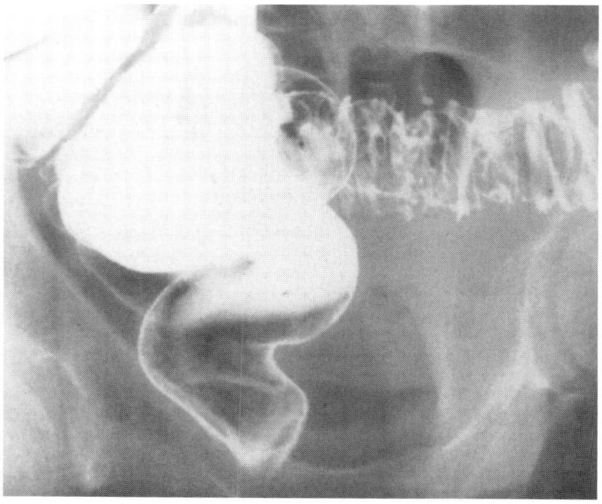

Fig 30.36 Diverticular disease. Barium enema incidentally revealing gas in the bladder, indicating a colovesical fistula.

Emergency presentations

Acute diverticulitis. The patient complains of severe lower abdominal pain, which is often accompanied by the frequent passage of loose stools. There are usually associated constitutional symptoms which may include sweating, nausea and vomiting. The temperature and pulse are invariably raised, and there is marked tenderness and guarding in the left lower quadrant where a mass may be palpable. Plain abdominal radiographs may show a non-specific increase in bowel gas in the lower abdomen (see Chapter 29).

Treatment should be conservative in the absence of signs of generalized peritoneal irritation. Oral intake should be withheld and fluids given intravenously. Broad-spectrum antibiotics (metronidazole and a cephalosporin) and analgesia are administered. Only if the patient's condition deteriorates—particularly if signs of spreading peritonitis develop—is surgical intervention indicated. Failure to improve suggests the development of a pericolic abscess, which may be further suspected if there is a persistent leucocytosis and a swinging pyrexia. Ultrasound or CT may show the pericolic fluid collection.

Pericolic abscess. Drainage is required if this complication develops. Percutaneous catheter drainage, guided by computerized tomography or ultrasound, should be used as the first-line treatment.[235] Faeces may 'drain' as well as pus. Usually the acute episode resolves satisfactorily but elective resection to prevent recurrent complications is a sensible precaution if the patient is sufficiently fit. Portal pyaemia and liver abscesses are now rare complications of pericolic abscess, presumably because of the newer and more efficient antibiotics that are invariably prescribed.

Generalized peritonitis. This may be caused by rupture of a pericolic abscess or by direct perforation of a diverticulum, in which case faeces spread freely throughout the peritoneal cavity and the prospects for survival are much reduced.[236] The patient often presents in septicaemic shock. The usual signs of generalized peritonitis are likely to be present, though these can be muted in the elderly. Plain radiographs often show free intraperitoneal gas (see Chapter 27).

After initial resuscitation with intravenous fluids and the administration of broad-spectrum antibiotics, the patient is taken urgently to theatre.[236] After general peritoneal toilet the affected segment of bowel is resected. If the proximal bowel is loaded with faeces, this should be cleared by on-table lavage. It is usually prudent to avoid primary anastomosis in the presence of gross faecal contamination. Bringing out a mucous fistula or oversewing of the rectal stump with a left iliac fossa colostomy (Hartmann's operation) is recommended.[237] Re-anastomosis can be performed when the patient has made a satisfactory recovery. A primary anastomosis may be performed, provided a temporary proximal colostomy is fashioned under favourable conditions. It has been clearly shown that leaving the affected segment in situ, and performing no more than a proximal colostomy, is associated with a worse prognosis.[238]

Intestinal obstruction. This can develop as a result of steadily advancing chronic diverticulitis with the development of pericolic fibrosis, but it may also be caused by the adhesion of a loop of small bowel to an acutely inflamed diverticular segment. Either way, this is best treated by operation with resection and either Hartmann's procedure or a protected primary anastomosis. Obstruction is not common in diverticular disease and its presence should make the clinician suspect a hidden carcinoma (see Chapter 29).[239]

Haemorrhage. For many years it was held that diverticular disease was a relatively common cause of large quantities of fresh rectal haemorrhage. More recently, investigation during such episodes has suggested that vascular malformations (angiodysplasia) are a more common cause.[240] Acute bleeding episodes are usually self-limiting, and best treated conservatively. When bleeding does not stop and surgery is required, a total colectomy with ileostomy and preservation of the rectal stump is the procedure of choice if the source cannot be identified by angiography.

BENIGN TUMOURS OF THE COLON AND RECTUM

POLYPS

A polyp is an abnormal elevation from an epithelial surface. It may be pedunculated, possessing a head and a stalk, or sessile. A sessile polyp may be flat or villous. Polyps may be acquired or inherited, symptomatic or symptomless; they may be single, occur in clusters or occupy virtually all of the large bowel mucosa. When the latter occurs, the term 'polyposis syndrome' is applied. There are numerous histological types of polyp which are best divided into neoplastic and non-neoplastic.

Neoplastic polyps

Adenoma

An adenoma is a benign neoplasm of the large bowel glandular epithelium and is the most common neoplastic polyp. Adenomas are the most important form of polyp from the clinical and pathological points of view, as they are believed to be the precursor of colorectal cancer. In the past there has been a good deal of confusion with regard to the nomenclature of adenomas, but the World Health Organization[241] agreed on a classification based on microscopic appearances which has now been adopted worldwide. In this, adeno-mas are split into three categories: tubular, villous or tubulovillous.

REFERENCES

235. Neff C C, van Sonnenberg E et al Radiology 1987; 163: 15–18
236. Killingback M Surg Clin North Am 1983; 63: 97
237. Krukowski Z H, Koruth N M, Matheson N A Br J Surg 1985; 72: 684–686
238. Dawson J L, Hanon I, Roxburgh R A Br J Surg 1965; 52: 354–357
239. Hughes L E Clin Gastroenterol 1975; 4: 147
240. Goligher J Surgery of the Anus, Rectum and Colon, 5th edn. Baillière Tindall, London 1984
241. Morson B C, Sobin L H International Histological Classification of Tumours, no 15. Histological Typing of Intestinal Tumours. WHO, Geneva 1976

Pathology

A tubular adenoma may involve no more than a single crypt or it may be several centimetres in diameter, though most are less than 2 cm. It may be pedunculated or sessile, and is usually darker in colour than the surrounding mucosa owing to its vascularity. Microscopically, it consists of closely packed epithelial tubules, separated by normal lamina propria, which grow and branch horizontally to the muscularis mucosae. The tubules may branch in a regular or irregular pattern. In a pedunculated adenoma, the pedicle consists of normal mucosa and submucosa.

A villous adenoma is often large and sessile with a shaggy surface made up of numerous fronds. It may be flat or protrude into the bowel lumen, and may extend over a considerable area of the bowel wall, hence the term 'carpet-like'. Microscopically, it consists of a core of connective tissue bearing numerous delicate frond-like branches or villi. The epithelial cells which cover the villi grow vertically towards the bowel lumen. Between the villi, the mucosa rests directly on the muscularis mucosae with no intervening connective tissue.

The tubulovillous adenoma is an intermediate form containing features of both morphological types.

Dysplasia and malignant transformation

The epithelial cells may show an increase in mitotic figures; they may form several layers and their nuclei may become pleomorphic, with loss of polarity. The term 'dysplasia' is applied to these changes. Any invasion of these abnormal epithelial cells through the muscularis mucosae to enter the submucosa constitutes malignant transformation. Dysplasia may be classified as mild, moderate or severe.[242–244] Severe dysplasia is termed 'carcinoma in situ' by some histopathologists, but the distinction between this term and true malignant change must be stressed. Carcinoma in situ in an adenoma which is still confined to the mucosa is not a cancer.

Approximately 60% of adenomas show mild dysplasia, about 30% exhibit moderate dysplasia, and the remaining 10% show severe dysplasia. It is generally believed that there is a gradual transformation through the various grades of dysplasia to frank malignancy—the so-called adenoma—carcinoma sequence.[245]

Another histological variant of which the pathologist must be aware is the presence of benign adenomatous epithelium deep to the muscularis mucosae. Gland-like structures are present in the submucosa of what is considered to be pseudocarcinomatous invasion.[246] These usually show the same degree of dysplasia as the surface epithelium of the polyp. The features of true malignancy are not present.

Incidence and anatomical distribution

The true incidence of adenomatous polyps is difficult to determine. Radiological studies in symptomatic patients reveal an incidence of 3–12%,[247,248] but obviously in such studies histological confirmation is lacking. In addition, these studies give no indication of the incidence within the total population, as only symptomatic patients were investigated. Autopsy studies ought to be more accurate. These, however, show a tremendous variation in incidence, from 6 to 69%.[249–252] A prospective autopsy study in a population with a high incidence of colorectal cancer shows prevalence rates of adenomas of around 35% in men and about 30% in women.[253] Colonoscopic and autopsy studies demonstrate that approximately two thirds of all colorectal adenomas occur beyond the splenic flexure.[254,255] This distribution is less pronounced when more than one polyp is present or the patients are elderly. Villous adenomas are more common in the rectum.

Age and sex incidence

Adenomas may occur at any age, but they increase in frequency with advancing age. Males seem to be more commonly affected than females. The average age at presentation is 55–60 years.[253,255,256]

Adenoma–carcinoma sequence

The evidence that there is a link between adenoma and colorectal cancer is most persuasive, yet it is still circumstantial. Virtually all pathologists believe that adenomas can develop into carcinomas but whether all carcinomas start life as an adenoma remains debatable. Adenomas and carcinomas have a similar topographical distribution.[257–259] Interestingly, with the trend in the incidence of carcinoma away from the left side of the colon towards the right side,[260] there has been a concomitant shift in the distribution of adenomas. The incidence of adenomas associated with carcinoma is higher than might be expected. In patients presenting with two synchronous carcinomas, Heald & Bussey[261] found that three quarters had associated adenomas. Similarly, patients with polyps in association with a carcinoma of the colon are twice as likely to develop a subsequent carcinoma after operation, compared with patients who have no polyps at the time of surgery.[262]

Epidemiological data also support the adenoma–carcinoma sequence, in that both conditions are more prevalent in a western-

REFERENCES

242. Potet F, Soullard J Gut 1971; 12: 468
243. Ekelund G, Lindstrom C Gut 1974; 15: 654
244. Kozuka S Dis Colon Rectum 1975; 18: 483
245. Morson B C The Pathogenesis of Colorectal Cancer. W B Saunders, Philadelphia 1978 pp 33–42
246. Muto T, Bussey H J R, Morson B C J Clin Pathol 1973; 26: 25
247. Wilson G S, Dale E H, Brines O A Am J Surg 1955; 9: 834
248. Miller C J, Day E, L'Esperance E S NY State J Med 1950; 50: 2023
249. Stewart M J Lancet 1931; ii: 565, 617, 669–674
250. Susman W J Pathol Bact 1932; 35: 29
251. Lawrence J C Am J Surg 1936; 31: 499
252. Atwater J S, Barwen J A Gastroenterology 1945; 4: 395
253. Williams A R, Balasoorya B A W, Day D W Gut 1982; 23: 835–842
254. Shinya H, Wolff W I Ann Surg 1979; 190: 679–683
255. Gillespie P E, Chambers T J et al Gut 1979; 20: 240–245
256. Minopoulos G L, McIntyre R L E et al Br J Surg 1983; 70: 51–53
257. Ekelund G Acta Pathol Microbiol Scand 1963; 59: 165–170
258. Helwig E B Dis Colon Rectum 1959; 2: 5–17
259. Berge T, Ekelund G et al Acta Chir Scand 1973; 4 (suppl): 38
260. Snyder D N, Heston J F et al Am J Dig Dis 1977; 22: 791–797
261. Heald R J, Bussey H J R Dis Colon Rectum 1975; 18: 6–10
262. Bussey H J R, Wallace M H, Morson B C Proc R Soc Med 1967; 60: 208

ized society in which a low-fibre, high-meat diet is typical. Experimental carcinogens, such as azoxymethane, which are capable of producing colorectal cancers, also induce adenoma formation. Careful histological studies of carcinomas frequently show elements of benign adenomas within the tumour. Similarly, there is an incidence of 3–4% of carcinomas in apparently benign adenomas.[263] Finally, there is the condition of familial adenomatous polyposis in which all patients eventually develop carcinomatous change within their polyps if left untreated.

The above outlines the circumstantial evidence for the adenoma–carcinoma sequence, but does not provide definite proof that all carcinomas develop from adenomas. It follows, however, that if the theory is correct, routine colonoscopic removal of adenomas should reduce the incidence of carcinoma within a population. With this in mind, the data from Gilbertsen[264] are interesting. In his study, 18 000 subjects underwent regular sigmoidoscopic surveillance over a 25-year period. All detected polyps were removed. This population was predicted to develop 75–80 rectal carcinomas during the period of follow-up. In fact, only 11 carcinomas developed, and each of these was an early growth.

The malignant adenoma

Malignant change within an adenoma is diagnosed when there is invasion by malignant cells deep to the muscularis mucosae. The incidence in colonoscopically removed polyps is between 4 and 5% (Table 30.6) and this incidence increases with increasing polyp size. Villous adenomas are far more likely to develop malignant change than the other histological types of polyp. The incidence of malignancy in large series of villous adenomas removed surgically varies between 4 and 55% (Table 30.7).

The incidence of spread to lymph nodes from a malignant polyp is difficult to determine because not all surgeons perform colonic resection for cancerous polyps. The general consensus, however, is that 10% of malignant polyps which can be colonoscopically removed have lymph node metastases. Certain pathological characteristics (e.g. a sessile lesion, poor differentiation and lymphatic invasion) help to identify those polyps with nodal spread. A quarter of villous adenomas showing malignant change which have been removed surgically have lymph node involvement.[271] These data have important implications when it comes to determining their correct management.

Clinical features

Adenomatous polyps are often symptomless and may be detected on routine screening after a positive occult blood test. When they cause symptoms the clinical features vary to some extent according to their size, number, site and the degree of villous component. Rectal bleeding may occur, and its hue will depend on the distance of the polyp from the anus. The larger rectal polyps may cause a change in bowel habit, with diarrhoea and the passage of mucus being prominent. Occasionally, a rectal polyp may prolapse through the anus on straining. Rarely, abdominal colic may be the result of a colo-colic intussusception of a polyp.

Table 30.6 Incidence of malignancy in colonoscopically removed adenomas

	Number of patients	*Percentage with malignant invasion*
Minopoulos et al (1983)[256]	180	4.4
Gillespie et al (1979)[255]	1047	4.7
Shinya & Wolff (1979)[254]	5786	4.9
Colacchio et al (1981)[265]	729	5.3
Coutsoftides et al (1978)[266]	416	4.3
Nivatvongs & Goldberg (1978)[263]	580	4.0

Table 30.7 Incidence of malignant change in villous adenomas

	Number of cases of villous adenoma examined	*Incidence of invasive carcinoma (%)*
Southwood (1962)[267]	180	12
Wheat & Ackerman (1958)[268]	50	16
Grinell & Lane (1958)[269]	216	32
Enterline et al (1962)[270]	81	55
Hanley et al (1971)[271]	217	11
McCabe et al (1971)[272]	169	28
Quan & Castro (1971)[273]	215	24
Orringer & Eggleston (1971)[274]	65	42
Nivatvongs et al (1973)[275]	72	4
Welch & Welch (1976)[276]	258	29
Chiu & Spencer (1978)[277]	331	29
Jahadi & Baldwin (1975)[278]	264	18

Large villous adenomas of the rectum frequently present with tenesmus or the passage of copious mucus, often tinged pink by blood. Incontinence is not infrequent. The fluid and electrolyte loss may be so great that the patient may develop severe metabolic disturbance and this may even lead to shock.[279–281] Thus the patient may complain of lethargy, weakness and oliguria and demonstrate acidotic breathing, mental confusion and hypotension.

Diagnosis

Villous tumours of the rectum may be palpated on digital rectal examination, but can be difficult to feel because of their soft

REFERENCES

263. Nivatvongs S, Goldberg S M Dis Colon Rectum 1978; 21: 8–11
264. Gilbertsen V Cancer 1974; 34: 931–939
265. Colacchio T A, Forde K A, Scantlebury V P Ann Surg 1981; 194: 704–707
266. Coutsoftides T, Sivak M V et al Ann Surg 1978; 188: 638–641
267. Southwood W F M Ann R Coll Surg Eng 1962; 30: 23
268. Wheat M W, Ackerman L V Ann Surg 1958; 147: 476
269. Grinell R S, Lane N Int Abstr Surg 1958; 106: 519–538
270. Enterline H T, Evans G W et al JAMA 1962; 179: 322–330
271. Hanley P H, Hines M D, Ray J E Ann Surg 1971; 37: 190
272. McCabe S C, McSherry B C K et al Am J Surg 1973; 126: 336
273. Quan S H, Castro E B Dis Colon Rectum 1971; 14: 267
274. Orringer M B, Eggleston J C Surgery 1972; 62: 378
275. Nivatvongs S, Balcos E G et al Dis Colon Rectum 1973; 16: 508
276. Welch J P, Welch C E Am J Surg 1976; 131: 185–191
277. Chiu Y S, Spencer R J Dis Colon Rectum 1978; 22: 493–495
278. Jahadi M R, Baldwin A Am J Surg 1975; 130: 729–732
279. McKittrick L S, Wheelock F C J Carcinoma of the Colon. Charles C Thomas, Springfield 1954 pp 61–63
280. Pheils M T Dis Colon Rectum 1979; 22: 406–407
281. Shnika T K, Friedman M H W et al Surg Gynecol Obstet 1961; 112: 609–612

consistency. Occasionally a pedunculated adenomatous polyp may be palpable. Digital examination may detect areas of hardness within the polyp suggesting the possibility of focal malignant invasion. Sigmoidoscopy using the rigid or flexible instrument can detect polyps up to 25 or 60 cm from the anal verge respectively. Polyp detection is three times as great with the flexible instrument.[282]

After a polyp has been detected by endoscopy the rest of the bowel should be examined, either by barium enema or colonscopy. Clearly, local factors influence the choice of investigation. Most now believe that if a polyp is suspected, colonoscopy is the better method of investigation as it is more sensitive and allows the polyp to be removed at the same time.[283]

Management

Once a polyp has been detected, it should be removed so that its histological type can be determined. Clearly, however, common sense should prevail. It would be quite wrong doggedly to pursue the removal of a 2 mm colonic polyp in a frail 85-year-old woman. Most rectal adenomas can be removed via the rigid or flexible sigmoidoscope using a diathermy snare. Larger sessile, usually villous, rectal adenomas are best removed surgically via the transanal route (see below). Alternatively, if a villous lesion is situated on the anterior rectal wall some surgeons prefer the trans-sphincteric approach of York Mason,[284] where the external and internal anal sphincters are completely divided in the vertical axis, and the rectal lumen is laid open like a book.

Transanal excision of a rectal villous adenoma.[285] This can be performed with the patient in either the lithotomy or jack-knife position. A Parks' self-retaining anal retractor is inserted. The submucosal plane beneath and around the tumour is infiltrated with 1 in 300 000 adrenaline solution. To aid repair of the defect at the end of the excision, it is helpful to place sutures in the rectal mucosa around the tumour just lateral to the proposed line of incision (Fig. 30.37). By a combination of sharp dissection and diathermy, the whole of the tumour can be excised from the underlying rectal muscle. The excised specimen should be pinned out on to a cork board before formalin fixation to facilitate the histopathological examination.

Transanal endoscopic microsurgery (TEM) is a new intraluminal technique for the full-thickness excision of villous lesions in the mid and upper rectum, where the Parks' procedure becomes increasingly difficult. A 40 mm diameter rectoscope is placed in the anal canal, the rectum insufflated with CO_2, and through gas-sealed ports long-handled instruments are manipulated to carry out the procedure and repair the defect. A stereoscopic optic provides clear views of the operation site.[286] Although experience with this new technique is limited it does seem to be safe and effective for small selected groups of patients who might otherwise have to undergo classical anterior resection.

A more extensive villous adenoma of the rectum may require removal by the abdomino-transanal coloanal pull-through technique.[287] In this operation, the lower part of the papilloma is excised from the rectal muscle via the transanal route, as described above. The upper part of the rectum and sigmoid colon containing the abdominal extension of the tumour are then resected via the abdominal route. Continuity is achieved by drawing the proximal colon down through the denuded rectal muscular cuff and anastomosing it to the anal mucosa via the transanal route. The operation is similar to that performed for certain very low carcinomas, and the details are described elsewhere. Alternatively a proctectomy and end-to-end coloanal anastomosis can be performed.

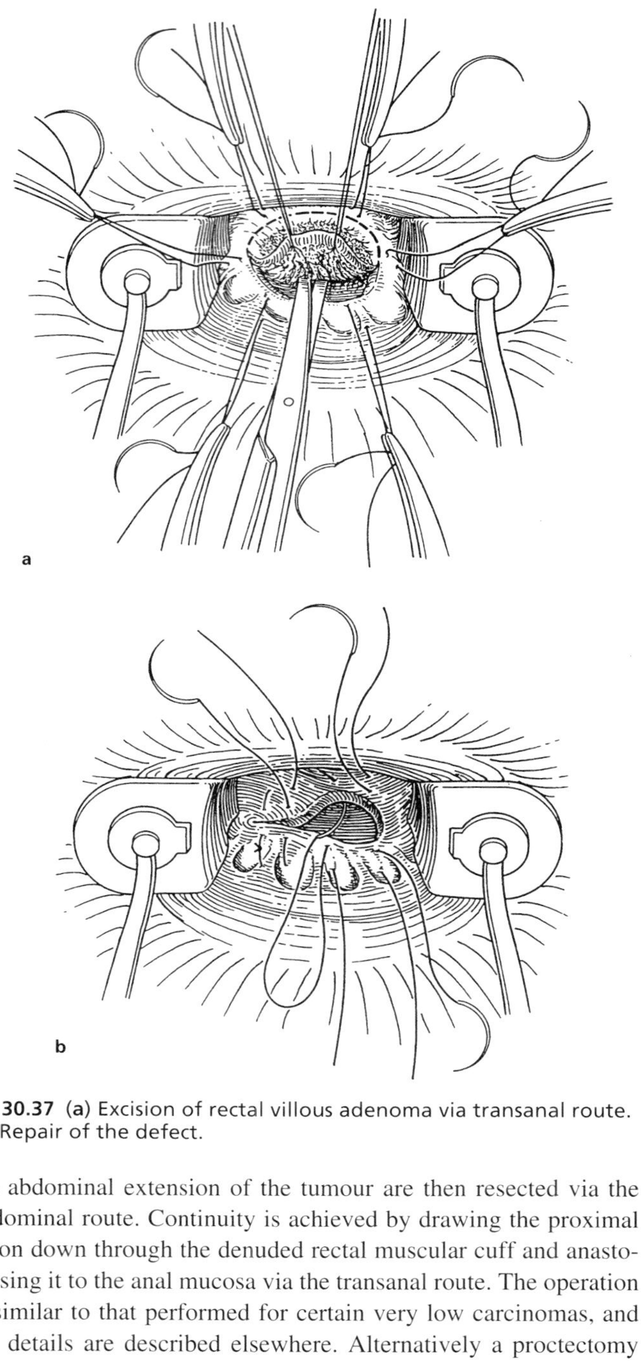

Fig 30.37 **(a)** Excision of rectal villous adenoma via transanal route. **(b)** Repair of the defect.

An alternative to surgical excision of a villous adenoma of the rectum is diathermy fulguration. This technique should however,

REFERENCES

282. McCallum R W, Meyer C T et al Am J Gastroenterol 1984; 79: 433–437
283. Durdey P, Weston P, Williams N J Lancet 1987; ii: 549
284. Mason A Y Progr Surg 1974; 13: 66–97
285. Parks A G, Stuart A E Br J Surg 1973; 60: 688–695
286. Mayer J, Mortensen N J McC Br J Surg 1995; 82: 435–437
287. Parks A G Proc R Soc Med 1972; 65: 975–976
288. Jahadi M R, Baldwin A Am J Surg 1975; 130: 729–732

only be regarded as a second-line treatment, as it is unlikely that the whole tumour can be destroyed. In addition, because the tumour is not removed in a form which allows adequate pathological assessment, it is not possible to be certain whether it has undergone malignant transformation. Nevertheless, the technique can be used as a palliative procedure in a patient who is unfit for a major procedure. The recurrence rate after transanal excision or diathermy has been reported to vary between 7 and 27%.[288–290]

Colonic adenomas. The treatment of colonic polyps has been revolutionized in the last 20 years by the introduction of the colonoscope. Surgical excision should never be undertaken without first attempting colonoscopic polypectomy, as some polyps that look sessile or malignant on barium enema prove to have small stalks on endoscopy. The indications for laparotomy and colotomy are nowadays very few. Colonic resection is necessary when a polyp is too large to be removed endoscopically. When it is still thought that the polyp needs removing and the colonoscopist has failed to remove a polyp for technical reasons, many now prefer the technique of operative colonoscopic removal in preference to resection. In this procedure, the colonoscope is passed at laparotomy, and with the help of the surgeon the polyp is removed. This manoeuvre allows polypectomy to be performed without opening the bowel.

Polyps with stalks can usually be removed by colonoscopic diathermy snare. Every attempt must then be made to retrieve the whole polyp in order that an adequate histological examination can be made. Large whole sessile polyps can rarely be removed satisfactorily, and a piecemeal resection is usually required. Even if this technique is necessary, it is still important to retrieve as much of the polyp as possible. For very small polyps which look entirely innocent, the 'hot biopsy' technique[291] may be used. In this, an electric current is applied to the biopsy forceps which coagulates the base of the polyp, while that part of the polyp grasped by the jaws of the forceps is preserved for histological examination.

Complications of polypectomy. These include bleeding, bowel perforation and occasionally gas explosion. The latter complication should no longer occur now that bowel preparation with mannitol has been abandoned. The incidence of haemorrhage requiring transfusion is approximately 2%.[292–294] Perforation occurs in 0.2–0.7% of polypectomies.[295,296] The overall mortality rate from perforation and haemorrhage from the technique is about 0.05%.

Follow-up after polypectomy for adenomas. There are no firm data upon which to base a follow-up policy. A full appraisal of the literature that is available on regrowth of adenomas[297] supports the following policy. All patients should be seen annually apart from those who are very old and infirm. At each visit, if patients remain symptom free, a flexible sigmoidoscopy should be performed as an outpatient procedure. Provided this examination does not show a problem, a full colonoscopy should be carried out every third year. If symptoms develop or a flexible sigmoidoscopy shows a polyp, a colonoscopy should be performed irrespective of whether this investigation was scheduled. Exceptions are patients who have had several adenomas removed, or whose adenoma, although benign, was greater than 2 cm in diameter, and those who have had a malignant adenoma removed. These patients should be endoscoped annually. This policy is purely empirical and awaits further evaluation.

Operative removal

Although laparotomy is rarely indicated for a colonic adenoma, there are certain specific indications:

1. When the adenoma is too large or sessile for colonoscopic removal. Endoscopists vary as to how large an adenoma should be before they recommend surgery. Most feel that 3 cm is usually the upper limit for a sessile lesion.
2. When the adenoma is inaccessible to the endoscopist, and is causing symptoms.
3. When the polyp has only partially been removed, but histological examination shows it to be malignant.

Several operative manoeuvres are available. These include operative colonoscopic polypectomy, colotomy and polypectomy, or colonic resection.

Management of a malignant adenoma removed via the colonoscope

The selection of this approach depends to some extent on the endoscopist's and surgeon's view concerning the incidence of lymphatic involvement from a malignant polyp. At one end of the spectrum there are those who believe that if a malignant polyp has been removed, all patients must be submitted to colonic resection, irrespective of whether biopsy of the base shows evidence of malignant invasion. There are others[298–300] who adopt a conservative approach. They feel that, provided the base that remains does not contain malignant cells on biopsy, the patient should be merely followed up by regular colonoscopic review. There is also a middle view represented by those who base their policy on histological criteria. Cooper[301] advocates that adenomas with a long stalk may be treated by polypectomy alone, except in cases of poorly differentiated carcinoma and where there is lymphatic invasion or carcinoma at the resection margin. Adenomas with a short stalk containing cancer limited to the head of the polyp may be treated similarly to long-stalked adenomas, but sessile adenomas should be surgically resected.

A sensible policy is to carry out a colonic resection on all patients with residual carcinoma after polypectomy, provided of course they are fit enough for operation. Sessile adenomas with

REFERENCES

289. Thomson J P S Dis Colon Rectum 1977; 20: 467–472
290. Adair H, Everett W J R Coll Surg Edin 1983; 28: 318–323
291. Williams C B Endoscopy 1973; 5: 215
292. Berci G, Panick J F et al Gastroenterology 1974; 67: 584–585
293. Frumorgen P, Demling L Endoscopy 1979; 11: 146–150
294. Williams C B, Tan G Gut 1979; 20: A903
295. Roseman D M Gastrointest Endosc 1973; 20: 36
296. Rogers B H G, Silvis E et al Gastrointest Endosc 1975; 23: 73–75
297. Williams C B Curr Opin Gastroenterol 1989; 5: 43
298. Morson B, Whiteway J et al Gut 1984; 25: 437–444
299. Christie J Am J Gastroenterol 1984; 79: 543–547
300. DeCosse J Gut 1984; 25: 433–436
301. Cooper H Am J Surg Pathol 1983; 7: 613–623

invasive malignancy but without residual disease should be treated in an identical manner. Short- or long-stalked adenomas with the same characteristics can however be treated by colonoscopic polypectomy alone, provided that patients are followed by frequent endoscopic review. The use of histological appearances is unreliable as a prognostic indicator because of the large inter- and intra-observer variation amongst pathologists.

Other benign neoplastic polyps

Compared with adenomas, other benign neoplastic tumours of the colon are rare.

Benign lymphoma

This is the most common non-epithelial benign tumour. It occurs in the large intestine and is usually seen in the rectum as a single reddish purple or grey rounded polyp varying in diameter from several millimetres to 3–4 cm. The cells form a follicular pattern with a well defined germinal centre, which differs from its malignant counterpart where the cells are arranged in a haphazard fashion and no germinal cell is present.[302] The differentiation between benign and malignant is difficult, but if the pathologist is sure of the diagnosis, the benign lesion can be treated by simple local excision.

Lipoma

A lipoma is the second most common non-epithelial benign tumour, but it is still rare, with an incidence of 0.2–0.3% in autopsy studies.[303] It is more commonly present in the caecum and right colon.[304] Most lipomas are situated in the submucosal layer, but some lie subserosally. They vary in size from a few millimetres to 6 cm or more. They are never reported to turn malignant, and in 20% of patients several lipomas may be present. They usually present with symptoms that are indistinguishable from an adenocarcinoma. Sometimes they may form the head of an intussusception but they often cause no symptoms, being discovered at autopsy or laparotomy for another condition. A barium enema shows a narrow line of barium surrounding a smooth lobulated filling defect, and colonoscopy shows a pedunculated lobulated spherical tumour projecting into the lumen, with an intact overlying mucosa. Ulceration of the mucosa normally takes place, and the lipoma then looks like a carcinoma.

Lipomas can sometimes be removed by a diathermy snare if they present as a polypoid tumour. A larger lipoma usually requires some form of resection, as it is not usually possible to make the diagnosis with confidence before operation.

Leiomyoma

Smooth muscle tumours of the large intestine are very rare. Stout[305] reported only 30 leiomyomas in a review of 200 benign tumours of the large bowel. Histological differentiation between benign and malignant is very difficult. The clinical features are identical to those of other benign tumours.

Fibroma

This rare colonic tumour is usually hard, mobile and pedunculated. It arises from the submucous layer and is covered by intact epithelium. It may contain muscle or glandular tissue, and often undergoes myxomatous or hyaline change. Histologically, it consists of whorls of spindle cells.

Haemangioma

This may be capillary or cavernous in type, and may arise in the colon or rectum. These lesions need to be differentiated from angiodysplasia. They occasionally cause profuse rectal bleeding and may then have to be treated by excision or embolization.

Non-neoplastic polyps

Metaplastic or hyperplastic polyps

These are the most common type of polyp found in the rectum, but they occur throughout the large bowel. Only 10% of small polyps in the colon however prove to be metaplastic. They are usually small in size, 2–5 mm in diameter, plaque-like and the same colour as normal mucous membrane. They are often seen at sigmoidoscopy in the elderly, but can occur at all ages. These polyps are usually flat-topped and rarely pedunculated. Histologically, they are made up of elongated tubules which often show cystic dilatation; the lining epithelium appears serrated because of patchy flattening of its cells, and the goblet cells are reduced in number. There is no evidence to suggest that they may develop dysplastic or neoplastic change.[306] These polyps are usually symptomless, only being discovered on routine sigmoidoscopy. Although the vast majority are tiny and insignificant, larger metaplastic polyps are occasionally found in the colon, and these may give rise to symptoms.

Hamartomatous polyps

A hamartoma is a tumour-like malformation in which the normal tissues of a particular part of the body are arranged haphazardly, usually with an excess of one or more of its components.[307] There are two types of colorectal polyp which are classified as hamartomas: the juvenile polyp and the Peutz–Jeghers polyp. The latter is uncommon in the colon, but does sometimes occur as part of the Peutz–Jeghers syndrome, considered later in this section and in Chapter 29.

REFERENCES

302. Price A B In: Morson B C (ed) The Pathogenesis of Colorectal Cancer. W B Saunders, Philadelphia 1978 pp 33–42
303. Haller D, Roberts T W Surgery 1964; 55: 773–781
304. Pemberton J, McCormack C J Am J Surg 1937; 37: 205–218
305. Stout A P Surg Clin North Am 1955; 1283
306. Grand Quist S, Gabriellson B, Sundelin P Endoscopy 1979; 11: 36–42
307. Albrecht E Verch Disch Path Ges 1904; 7: 153

Juvenile polyp

As the name suggests, this type of polyp occurs in infants and children, although occasionally adults are affected. It has characteristic appearances, being 1–2 cm in diameter, with a smooth surface. It has a slender stalk covered with normal colonic epithelium which, as it extends over the head of the polyp, becomes granulation tissue. The head consists of dilated cystic spaces filled with mucus, the spaces being lined by columnar mucus-secreting epithelial cells. In between these spaces, there is a large amount of connective tissue containing numerous eosinophils. These polyps are usually found in the rectum, and may sometimes present by prolapsing through the anus. Torsion or intussusception may also occur. Such polyps should be treated either by transanal excision or colonoscopic polypectomy, and the rest of the colon must be checked, as in 30% of patients the polyps are multiple.[308]

Inflammatory polyps

These polyps may be scattered throughout the colon. They consist of worm-like or thread-like (filiform) tags of essentially normal mucosa and are found in any patient suffering from ulcerative colitis or Crohn's disease.

Polyposis syndromes

There are several forms of polyposis syndrome—all are rare. They are best classified according to their histological types (Table 30.8).

Familial adenomatous polyposis

This is a dominantly inherited condition, the gene for which has been shown to be located on the short arm of chromosome 5.[310] Characterized by myriad colorectal adenomata, together with widespread extracolonic stigmata, it affects around 1 in 10 000 live-born and is responsible for the development of approximately 1% of all colorectal cancers.

Table 30.8 Classification of polyposis syndromes

Neoplastic	Familial adenomatous polyposis Turcot's syndrome Lymphosarcomatous (lymphomatous) polyposis Leukaemic polyposis
Inflammatory	Ulcerative colitis Crohn's disease Other inflammatory polyposis: amoebiasis, schistosomiasis, eosinophilic, granulomatous polyposis, diffuse histoplasmosis
Hamartomatous	Juvenile polyposis Peutz–Jeghers syndrome Neurofibromatous polyposis Lipomatous polyposis Cronkhite–Canada syndrome Cowden's disease
Unclassified	Metaplastic polyps Pneumatosis cystoides intestinalis

Modified from Morson (1962)[309]

Pathology

The key feature is the development, usually during the teenage years, of hundreds or thousands of adenomas on the mucosa of the colon and rectum. Left untreated, progression to malignancy is inevitable within about 20 years. Hamartomatous polyps in the stomach, adenomas in the duodenum, osteomata of the jaw, dental cysts, epidermoid cysts, retinal pigmentation and desmoid tumours in the abdomen or, rarely, elsewhere are other features of this condition. Duodenal adenomas may progress to malignancy. Desmoid tumours may develop after any type of abdominal trauma, for example bowel surgery or pregnancy. Desmoid tumours may cause no symptoms, or they may expand or invade locally, causing intestinal or ureteric obstruction, ulceration through the abdominal wall, bleeding from the bowel or severe abdominal pain. The term 'Gardner's syndrome' has been attached to patients with polyposis coli harbouring extracolonic lesions, but it has become apparent that most, if not all, individuals affected by familial adenomatous polyposis exhibit some of these features, so the eponym has been dropped.

Clinical features

This condition is increasingly diagnosed before symptoms develop by screening the children of affected individuals. When it is not identified in this manner, symptoms are likely to occur in the late teens or twenties. The passage of loose stools and blood or mucus per rectum is the usual early complaint. The associated features rarely produce symptoms.

Diagnosis

In the children of known patients, it is usual to examine the rectum by rigid sigmoidoscopy in the mid teens, when adenomata are likely to have appeared in those who will develop the condition. Annual repeat examination is necessary if the rectum appears normal. The diagnosis is confirmed by histological examination of suspect lesions. New mutations are responsible for cases with no family history. In this event, the diagnosis is likely to follow the onset of symptoms, perhaps even after cancer has developed. The diagnosis is then made on the basis of the large number of adenomata present. Conventionally, familial adenomatous polyposis is assumed in the presence of a hundred or more adenomata. The finding of other stigmata, including skin cysts and jaw abnormalities, adds strength to the diagnosis. Gene markers are being used increasingly in the diagnosis of the condition at a prephenotypic stage, perhaps even before birth.

Management

Treatment of the multiple polyps in the large bowel sometimes has two aims. In all cases there is the aim of diminishing the cancer

REFERENCES

308. Mazier P, Mackeigan J M et al Surg Gynecol Obstet 1982; 154: 829–832
309. Morson B C Dis Colon Rectum 1962; 5: 337–344
310. Bodmer W F, Bailey C J, Bussey H S R Nature 1987; 328: 614–616

risk, while in those who have already developed cancer, the tumour itself has also to be appropriately treated. Prophylactic surgery involves either removal of the whole colon alone, with ileorectal anastomosis, or total removal of the large bowel and replacement of the rectum with a small bowel reservoir, the so-called restorative proctocolectomy. Provided that postoperative surveillance is adequate, the former procedure is generally to be favoured, as it is a smaller operation with a more predictable outcome. Rectal adenomas regress partially or completely after surgery, and only large polyps of greater than 5 mm need be removed when seen at regular follow-up. Restorative proctocolectomy is to be favoured on grounds of cancer prevention when the rectum is badly affected, or if regular follow-up is for any reason likely to be difficult to implement. This procedure can be used at a later date in patients in whom a retained rectum appears to be passing out of conservative control.

The duodenum should also be examined on a regular basis in order to try to identify and remove large or severely dysplastic adenomas.[311,312] The most appropriate pattern of follow-up is still being assessed by prospective studies.

MALIGNANT TUMOURS OF THE COLON AND RECTUM

Approximately 19 000 patients die from colorectal carcinoma each year in the UK, and this neoplasm is now second only to lung cancer as a cause of death from malignant disease. The situation is similar in the USA, where in 1981 there were 54 000 deaths from the disease compared with 105 000 from cancer of the lung.[313] While progress has been made in understanding the aetiology of the disease, in improving early diagnosis and in the development of new surgical techniques for resection, the mortality from colorectal cancer has remained static for the last 50 years.

98% of malignant tumours of the colon and rectum are adenocarcinomas. Carcinoids and squamous cell carcinomas are other rarer tumours of colonic epithelial origin. Tumours of mesenchymal origin, sarcomas and malignant melanoma are relatively rare.

Geographical distribution (Table 30.9)

The highest incidence of colorectal cancer is seen in Western Europe and North America, whereas intermediate rates prevail in Eastern Europe.[314] The lowest rates are seen in Asia, Africa and South America. The incidence of rectal cancer varies less in different parts of the world than colon cancer. The disease is more common in urban areas than in rural areas.[315]

Aetiology

The precise causes of colorectal carcinoma are unknown, but both genetic and environmental factors seem to be involved. At present, it is believed that the latter are more important. Support for this thesis comes from the fact that migrants who move from an area of low incidence to one of high incidence become just as prone to develop cancer of the colon as the indigenous population of the high-risk area.[315]

Table 30.9 Incidence of colorectal cancer in different countries*

	Colonic	Rectal	Colorectal
Nigeria	1.3	1.2	2.5
India	4.6	4.4	9.0
Osaka (Japan)	6.3	6.9	13.2
East Germany	13.6	12.0	25.6
Vas (Hungary)	9.1	11.0	20.1
Connecticut (USA)	30.1	18.2	48.3
Detroit (USA)			
White	26.2	16.0	42.2
Black	24.5	13.8	38.3
Birmingham (UK)	16.5	16.1	32.6
Oxford (UK)	15.7	15.4	31.1
Ayrshire (UK)	16.6	14.0	30.0
Denmark	16.2	16.7	32.9
Finland	7.9	7.7	15.6
New Zealand			
Maori	7.4	4.6	12.0
Non-Maori	23.0	15.4	38.4
Hawaii			
Japanese	22.4	16.3	38.7
Caucasian	23.9	13.5	37.4
Hawaian	14.1	9.4	23.5

*Per 100 000 age-adjusted to world population.
Adapted from Waterhouse et al.[314]

Environmental factors

Dietary and digestive factors

Lack of fibre

From epidemiological studies, it appears that populations that consume a high-fibre diet are protected from cancer of the large intestine. Burkitt[316] believes that this is because high fibre intake speeds transit and reduces the exposure of the gut mucosa to potential carcinogens. There is much circumstantial evidence to support this theory, but little scientific proof.

Increased fat

There is some evidence suggesting that a western diet, rich in animal fat, is an important risk factor. The concept is that fat favours the development of a bacterial flora containing organisms which are capable of degrading bile salts to carcinogens.

Bile acids

Apart from the action of bacteria on bile acids converting them into carcinogens, evidence suggests they also have a direct toxic effect on colonic mucosa, which is capable of promoting the neoplastic

REFERENCES

311. Jones J R, Nance F C Am Surg 1977; 185: 565
312. Jagelman D G, De Cosse J J, Bussey H J R Lancet 1988; i: 1149–1150
313. Silverberg E Cancer Statistics 1981. New York American Cancer Society, New York 1981
314. Waterhouse J A H, Muir C S et al (eds) Cancer Incidence in 5 Continents, vol III. International Agency for Research in Cancer, Lyons 1976
315. Blot W J, Fraumeni J F et al J Natl Cancer Inst 1976; 57: 1225
316. Burkitt D Cancer 1971; 28: 3–13

process. Bile acids can promote colorectal cancer in animals.[317] Human epidemiological studies have found higher concentrations of bile acids in the faeces of high-risk populations.[318–320]

Previous cholecystectomy

Much has been written to suggest that previous cholecystectomy increases the risk of colorectal cancer, particularly carcinomas of the right colon.[321–323] Although such studies are of considerable interest, the case as yet remains unproven. Cholecystectomy does increase the production and turnover of degraded bile salts.

Inflammatory bowel disease

The risk of colorectal cancer developing in patients with long-standing ulcerative colitis is well appreciated and has already been discussed. The relationship between cancer and Crohn's colitis, however, is far more tenuous. Although diverticular disease and carcinoma frequently coexist, there is no evidence to link the two disorders.[324] Evidence from China suggests that there may be a link between schistosomiasis and colorectal cancer.[325,326]

Ureterosigmoidostomy

Although this technique is now rarely performed for urinary diversion, patients who have undergone the procedure seem to be at considerable risk of developing a carcinoma of the sigmoid.[327,328] Presumably, certain constituents of the urine are carcinogenic to colonic mucosa (see Chapter 37).

Irradiation

Patients who have received pelvic irradiation seem to be at higher risk of developing rectosigmoid carcinoma compared with the normal population.[329]

Genetic factors

Although environmental factors seem to be of most significance in colorectal carcinogenesis, there is evidence to suggest that genetic factors are more important than previously realized. The most obvious genetic link is with familial adenomatous polyposis where the abnormality is on chromosome 5.[309] There are two other dominantly inherited syndromes: the so-called cancer family syndrome, characterized by the development of multiple primary carcinomas of large bowel, breast, ovary and endometrium, and the site-specific colon cancer syndrome, in which only large bowel tumours develop.[330] The frequency of colorectal cancer developing in first-degree relatives of patients with large bowel carcinoma is significantly higher than expected.[331–334]

Pathology

Approximately half of large bowel tumours are situated in the rectum. Of those developing in the colon, approximately half occur in the sigmoid and a quarter occur in the caecum and ascending colon. The remaining quarter are distributed in order of frequency as follows: transverse colon, splenic flexure, descending colon and hepatic flexure.[335–337] The number of neoplasms arising in the right colon is steadily increasing.[338]

Synchronous tumours are those which are present at the time of presentation in addition to the primary carcinoma. Approximately 3% of patients have synchronous carcinomas. About three quarters of patients with a primary carcinoma, who are not suffering from ulcerative colitis or adenomatous polyposis, have associated benign adenomas.

Macroscopic appearances

Bowel cancers may be polypoid or ulcerating, and may spread around the circumference as a scirrhous, obstructing annular lesion.

Microscopic features and histological grading

Both Dukes[339] and Grinnell[340] introduced grading systems in which tumours were graded I–IV according to the degree of dedifferentiation of the cells, grade I being well differentiated and grade IV anaplastic. Grade IV also includes all colloid tumours. 10% of tumours are colloid, producing excessive mucus within the tumour. Approximately 60% of tumours are moderately differentiated (average grade) and the remaining 40% are divided up equally between well differentiated (low grade) and poorly differentiated (high grade or anaplastic). The histological grade is said to correlate with survival; however, interobserver variation between pathologists makes such conclusions difficult to interpret.[341]

REFERENCES

317. Hill M J In: De Cosse J, Sherlock P (eds) Gastrointestinal Cancer. Martinus Nijhoff, The Hague 1981 pp 187–226
318. Crowther J S, Drasar B J et al Br J Cancer 1976; 34: 191–196
319. Hill M J Cancer 1975; 36: 2387–2400
320. Hill M J Gut 1983; 24: 871–875
321. Linos D A, O'Fallon W M et al Lancet 1981; ii: 379–381
322. Turunen M J, Kivilaakso E O Ann Surg 1981; 194: 639–641
323. Vernick L J, Kuller L H Am J Epidemiol 1982; 116: 86–101
324. Stewart M Lancet 1931; ii: 669–674
325. Cheng M, Chuang C et al Cancer 1980; 46: 1661
326. Cheng M, Chuang C et al Lancet 1981; ii: 971–973
327. Thompson P, Hill J et al Br J Surg 1979; 66: 65
328. Harford F, Fazio V et al Dis Colon Rectum 1984; 27: 321–324
329. Sandler R, Sandier D Gastroenterology 1983; 84: 51–57
330. Lynch H T, Harris R E et al Cancer 1977; 40: 1849–1854
331. Lovett E Br J Surg 1976; 63: 13–18
332. Burdette W J In: Burdette W J (ed) Carcinoma of the Colon and Antecedent Epithelium. C C Thomas, Springfield 1970
333. Woolf C M Am J Human 1958; 10: 42
334. Macklin M T Am J Human Gen 1996; 10: 42
335. Fraser J Br J Surg 1938; 25: 647–648
336. Judd E S 5th Med J Nashville 1924; 17: 75–80
337. Smiddy F G, Goligher J C Br Med J 1957; i: 793–798
338. Welch C E, Hedberg S E In: Dunphy J E, Ebert P A (eds) Polypoid Lesions of the Gastrointestinal Tract, 2nd edn. Saunders, Philadelphia 1979
339. Dukes C E Proc R Soc Med 1937; 30: 371–376
340. Grinnell R S Ann Surg 1939; 109: 500
341. Thomas G D H, Dixon M F et al J Clin Pathol 1983; 36: 385–391

The DNA content of colorectal cancer cells seems to be a better indicator of prognosis than its histological grade. Flow cytometry can be used to divide up tumours into those that primarily consist of diploid cells and those that consist of aneuploid cells. Patients with aneuploid carcinomas have a significantly worse prognosis than those with diploid tumours.[342] As flow cytometry is a quantitative technique, observer variation is eliminated.

Spread

Direct spread

Direct lateral spread is far more common than spread in the longitudinal axis. Distal intramural spread is particularly pertinent to rectal cancer when the length of resection may determine whether the patient retains or loses the anal sphincter. Most studies suggest that distal intramural microscopic spread is rare, but when it is present it usually extends for less than 1 cm.[343] In those cases where it exceeds this distance, the tumour is advanced, and the patient is highly likely to die from widespread metastases without developing local recurrence.[343–345] As a result of these findings, the traditional 5 cm margin of clearance distal to a rectal cancer can be reduced to 2 cm if necessary, thus enabling more sphincter-saving operations to be accomplished.

Lymphatic spread

Spread from carcinoma of the rectum was originally considered to occur in three directions, upwards along the superior rectal and inferior mesenteric vessels, laterally along the middle rectal vessels in the lateral ligaments to the internal iliac nodes, and downwards through the sphincter muscles into the ischiorectal fossa and perianal skin, and finally to the inguinal nodes.[346] For these reasons, Miles[346] advocated abdominoperineal excision for all rectal carcinomas. Subsequent research, however, has demonstrated that although upward spread is usual, downward spread is rare, only occurring if the proximal route of drainage is obstructed.[347] Lateral lymphatic spread is unusual in tumours of the intraperitoneal rectum, being more common in extraperitoneal growths. These findings have important implications now that surgeons are performing more sphincter-saving procedures.

Blood-borne spread

This is usually first to the liver via the portal vein. In the past, liver metastases were considered to develop late in patients with colorectal cancer, but more recent data have shown that up to 30% of patients have occult liver metastases at the time of presentation.[348] Pulmonary metastases occur in about 5% of cases[349] and the adrenal glands, kidneys and bones are involved in about 10% of cases. Neoplastic cells have been found in the circulation at the time of surgery, but their viability is uncertain. It has not been proven that manipulation of the tumour at operation increases the risk of metastases. It may be that, although malignant cells are released into the circulation, they often do not survive.[349]

Transperitoneal spread

Spread by this route occurs in approximately 1 in 10 patients after resection. Spread to the ovaries may also occur by this route, resulting in Krukenberg tumours.

Spread by implantation

Several reports have suggested that this method of spread is possible, although uncommon. Thus, implantation metastases have been described in anal fistulae, haemorrhoidectomy wounds, abdominal incisions and around colostomies. Suture line recurrences may also be explained on the basis of implantation. There is considerable debate about the viability of cells released into the lumen of the bowel during surgery.[350] They may be an important mechanism of spread in patients having laparoscopic colonic resections, where port site recurrence is now well recognized, and may limit the feasibility of this type of surgery in cancers of the colon and rectum.[351]

Staging

Pathological stage

The standard method of staging patients with colorectal cancers is based on the pathological characteristics of the resected specimen. Dukes' system, originally described for rectal tumours only, is the accepted classification in the United Kingdom[352,353] and is as follows:

Stage A

The tumour is confined to the bowel wall with no involvement of lymph nodes.

Stage B

The tumour extends through the wall of the bowel without spread to lymph nodes.

Stage C

Lymph node metastases. When the highest lymph node is involved, the tumour is at Dukes' stage C2; otherwise the tumour is said to be at Dukes' stage C1 although this was not part of the original classification.

REFERENCES

342. Quirke P, Durdey P et al Lancet 1986; ii: 996–998
343. Quer E A, Dahlin D C, Mayo C W Surg Gynecol Obstet 1953; 96: 24–30
344. Black W A, Waugh J M Surg Gynecol Obstet 1948; 87: 457–464
345. Grinnell R S Surg Gynecol Obstet 1954; 99: 421–430
346. Miles W E Br Med J 1910; 2: 941–942
347. Williams N S, Dixon M F, Johnston D Br J Surg 1983; 70: 150–154
348. Finlay I G, Meek D R et al Br Med J 1982; 284: 803–805
349. Cole W H, Packard D, Southwick H W JAMA 1954; 155: 1549–1554
350. Umpleby H C et al Dis Colon Rectum 1984; 27: 803–809
351. Berends F J, Kazemier G et al Lancet 1994; 344: 58
352. Dukes C E Br J Surg 1930; 17: 643–648
353. Dukes C E J Pathol Bacteriol 1940; 50: 527

Since Dukes originally described his system, it has been customary also to include stage D for those patients with distant metastases. There are many other pathological staging systems, of which the most commonly used include the Astler–Coller[354] and the TNM classifications. Others have advocated staging systems which take operative and other clinical data into account. It remains to be seen whether these add power to the prognostic prediction.

Clinical stage

Patients can be classified into three broad prognostic groups following surgery.

Incurable because of the presence of distant metastases

Whenever possible, this should be supported by histological confirmation. Biopsy is however not necessary when metastases are clearly shown on imaging, e.g. lung or liver metastases detected on chest X-ray or CT scanning.

Incurable because of the presence of residual local disease

Included in this category are patients in whom the operative specimen contains tumour at any margin of the excision. The only group in which histological confirmation of residual local disease is not required is when the specimen has been perforated, either spontaneously or operatively.

Curative operations

Curative operations are defined as those procedures in which all demonstrable tumour has been removed, as judged by preoperative imaging assessment and postoperative histological examination of the specimen. When there is any doubt, the patient should be classified as having an operation (specified) which is indeterminate for cure.

Clinical features

Patients usually present in the sixth to eighth decade, although the disease may occur at any age. Approximately 250 patients below 35 years of age present each year with a colorectal cancer in the UK, and a small proportion are children. Colon cancer occurs with equal frequency in men and women, but rectal cancer is more prevalent in men.[355] In its early stages an uncomplicated carcinoma of the colon is usually symptomless. Symptoms include a change in bowel habit, bleeding per anum which is often dark in colour, the passage of mucus, and abdominal discomfort or distension. Occasionally, a mass may be felt by the patient. Anorexia and weight loss are rarely early features but may occur if the tumour becomes disseminated.

The site of the carcinoma often dictates the symptoms. Carcinoma of the right colon is soft and friable and bleeds easily. Thus the patient may present with symptoms of anaemia from occult bleeding which is mixed within the stool and invisible by the time it reaches the rectum. Sometimes the patient complains of abdominal pain and a mass may be palpable in the right iliac fossa.

Tumours in the left colon are more likely to constrict and cause obstruction, particularly so because the intraluminal contents are more solid on the left. Constipation, therefore, is a frequent initial symptom and is often accompanied by abdominal colic. Overt bleeding and the passage of mucus per anum are more common with tumours on the left side.

Carcinoma of the rectum often produces a classic symptom complex. Bleeding is common and resembles that coming from haemorrhoids in being bright red although often it is darker. A change in the bowel habit is frequent, with patients often suffering from explosive episodes of diarrhoea punctuated by periods of relative constipation. Tenesmus, the painful and repeated call to stool is usually a late feature and indicates an advanced tumour. These symptoms are often present in the morning and improve as the day wears on. The patient may also present with symptoms referable to the organ or organs invaded if local spread has occurred. Thus posterior invasion into the sacral plexus may cause back pain and sciatica, and extension downwards into the anal canal may produce anal pain, reminiscent of a fissure in ano. Invasion of the ureters, bladder or prostate may produce urinary tract symptoms, and extension of a rectal tumour into the vagina may form a rectovaginal fistula.

Differential diagnosis

The differential diagnosis includes diverticular disease, irritable bowel syndrome, amoebic and chlamydial proctitis, Crohn's disease, ulcerative colitis, ischaemia, solitary rectal ulcer, radiation enteritis and other tumours, including polyps, lymphoma, melanoma, etc.

Diagnosis

A combination of history, clinical examination, sigmoidoscopy, and either barium enema or colonoscopy, or both, will invariably determine the diagnosis. 70% of rectal tumours are situated within 12 cm of the anal verge, as measured on sigmoidoscopy, and are palpable on digital examination. Even if a tumour is discovered on rectal examination or sigmoidoscopy, the rest of the large bowel should be examined, preferably by colonoscopy, to rule out synchronous cancers and adenomas. There is some debate as to whether a colonoscopy or a barium enema should be the initial investigation if rectal examination and sigmoidoscopy are normal. Colonoscopy is more accurate in detecting neoplasms and more comfortable for the patient[356] and as a consequence many feel that this procedure should be the first investigation. A satisfactory compromise would be the use of flexible sigmoidoscopy and

REFERENCES

354. Astler V, Coller F Ann Surg 1954; 139: 846–851
355. Offices of Population Censuses and Surveys Cancer Statistics: Registration 1976. HMSO, London 1981
356. Durdey P, Weston P, Williams N J Lancet 1987; ii: 549

double-contrast barium enema. Once a tumour has been identified, it should be biopsied to confirm the diagnosis.

Screening

Despite advances in surgical technique there has been no improvement in the long-term survival of patients with colorectal cancer over the last 30 years. The earlier detection of colorectal carcinoma by screening populations might be expected to improve this situation. Screening can be divided into selective screening of high-risk groups and general screening of individuals of average risk. The high-risk group includes patients with a long history of ulcerative colitis, a past history of an adenoma or a colon cancer, female genital cancer and perhaps those with a strong family history.[357–361] This group should have a regular barium enema and/or colonoscopy every 3 years.

It is not yet known whether the cost of screening the general population justifies the benefit for the few positive cases identified. Using faecal occult blood testing, a carcinoma is detected in about 1–2 cases per 1000 screened, with a false-positive rate of approximately 2%. Several studies have shown that carcinomas can be detected at an earlier pathological stage by this method of screening.[362–365] It is not yet known whether the survival of the population screened will be improved. A trial of once-only flexible sigmoidoscopy in screening 55–64-year-old people without symptoms is in progress.

Complications

Obstruction

Carcinomas of the left colon are more likely to cause obstruction than those of the right, as they are often of the constricting variety. Occasionally a tumour may cause obstruction by acting as an apex for either an intussusception or volvulus. Patients with large bowel obstruction present with colicky central lower abdominal pain, distension and absolute constipation (see Chapter 27).

Perforation

Perforation may occur either through the carcinoma itself or more commonly at a site proximal to it. The latter occurs late, and the most common area to perforate is the caecum as a result of a closed loop obstruction. The perforation may cause either generalized faecal peritonitis or a localized abscess. The latter may mimic a diverticular abscess on the left side or an appendix abscess on the right.[366] Despite improvements in circulatory management and antibiotic therapy, the mortality from faecal peritonitis is still high. A perforated carcinoma is unlikely to be curable.

Fistula formation

A colorectal carcinoma may adhere to and eventually penetrate any abdominal or pelvic viscus. Although it is a rare occurrence, the organ most commonly involved is the bladder, and the carcinoma usually resides in the sigmoid colon. The resulting vesicocolic fistula may produce pneumaturia, faecuria and frequent urinary tract infections. The diagnosis is often difficult, and the differentiation from diverticular disease as a cause of the fistula may be impossible until the pathologist has examined the excised specimen.

Rectal cancer may invade the vagina and produce a rectovaginal fistula. A fistula may also develop between a tumour in the transverse colon and the stomach or duodenum, when the patient may present with faecal vomiting. Rarely, an external spontaneous fistula may develop but this is more commonly associated with Crohn's disease.

Rarer complications

Although a tumour frequently causes minor bleeding, massive haemorrhage can occur. Occasionally a large caecal carcinoma obstructs the base of the appendix and causes acute appendicitis (see Chapter 27). A carcinoma may cause a colo-colic intussusception. Half of all such intussusceptions in adults are caused by a carcinoma.[367]

Treatment

General principles

Surgical resection is the standard treatment for colorectal cancer although further improvements in survival rates are likely to come from adjuvant therapy. The aim of a curative excision is to eradicate the disease and also remove the regional lymphovascular drainage. Excision of the tumour should be attempted whenever possible, even if it is considered that an operation is only palliative, as it may prevent intestinal obstruction developing and avoid distressing symptoms.

Preoperative preparation

Patients must be carefully assessed before operation to determine their fitness for surgery and the extent of the spread of their disease. When there is any doubt about a patient's fitness, he or she must be seen by the anaesthetist. Conditions such as diabetes and chronic obstructive airways disease must be appropriately treated.

REFERENCES

357. Anderson D E, Ramsdahl M M In: Mulvihill J J, Miller R W, Fraumeni J F Jr (eds) Progress in Cancer Research and Therapy: Genetics of Human Cancer 1977, vol 3. Raven Press, New York 1977
358. Devroede G In: Winawer S J, Sherlock P, Shottenfeld D (eds) Colorectal Cancer: Epidemiology and Screening. Progress in Cancer Research 1980. Raven Press, New York 1980
359. Kushin S Z, Lipkin M, Winawer S J Am J Gastroenterol 1979; 72: 448–453
360. Lynch H T, Lynch J, Lynch P In: Mulvihill J J, Miller R M, Fraumeni J F Jr (eds) Progress in Cancer Research and Therapy. Genetics of Human Cancer, vol 3. Raven Press, New York 1977 p 235
361. Winawer S J, Sherlock P et al Gastroenterology 1976; 70: 783–788

In deciding which operation is applicable it is important to try to determine if metastases are present by imaging techniques as examination at operation is not sufficiently sensitive to find, for instance, deposits deep within the liver. An elderly patient with liver metastases and a relatively small rectal tumour may best be served by a local procedure rather than a major resection.

Similarly, it is good policy to determine the extent of local spread. A large rectal tumour with extensive local invasion may best be managed by a course of preoperative radiotherapy which will help to reduce the bulk of the tumour and often convert an inoperable growth to an operable lesion, although it may not necessarily improve the chances of survival.[368] Liver metastases are best shown by computerized tomography scan, but if this is not available, ultrasound is an acceptable alternative. Computerized tomography can also be used to assess local spread, but a cheaper and potentially more accurate technique is endoluminal ultrasonography.

Bowel preparation

The chief source of sepsis is the endogenous bacteria within the bowel lumen. Mechanical clearance is desirable as it reduces the possibility of contamination at operation. This can be achieved by purgatives, enemas and dietary restriction. The patient takes only liquids by mouth for 3 days preoperatively. Purgatives such as castor oil or magnesium sulphate have largely been replaced by sodium picosulphate (Picolax).[369] Two sachets in the 24 hours before operation achieve a satisfactory preparation in about 80% of cases. Using this preparation the need for a washout or enema is avoided. Whole-gut irrigation is now less popular than it was 10 years ago: it requires more nursing time and can cause water overload, particularly in the elderly or those suffering from heart disease. In patients who have obstructive symptoms, on-table bowel irrigation is safer and more effective, as a purgative may cause massive bowel dilation above the tumour, increasing the risk of caecal rupture.[370]

The other main advance has been the use of prophylactic antibiotics to reduce septic complications. Systemic antibiotic cover has dramatically reduced the incidence of postoperative wound infection. A high serum level of antibiotics which are bactericidal to both aerobic and anaerobic organisms must be achieved throughout the early postoperative period. A combination of metronidazole and a cephalosporin is now most popular. The administration of either one dose on induction of anaesthesia or three doses perioperatively reduces the risks of drug resistance and side-effects, while providing satisfactory prophylaxis (see Chapter 4).[371,372]

Counselling

It is important to inform the patient and relatives of the intended procedure, particularly if a colostomy is a possibility. Patients who have had an unexpectedly formed colostomy often complain afterwards that they were not given enough information before the operation.[373] A stoma therapist or experienced senior nurse must be available to indicate the ideal site for the stoma, explain precisely how it will function and provide advice and reassurance.

Surgical techniques for elective cases

The colon

The type of operation depends on the site of the tumour. As the lymphatic drainage accompanies the main blood vessels, the length of bowel resected depends on the extent of the lymphatic clearance that is required. Gastrointestinal continuity is restored by either colo-colic or ileo-colic anastomosis, depending on the type of resection which has been performed. Intraoperative irrigation, originally described by Muir,[374] is a useful method that allows a primary anastomosis to be performed if preoperative mechanical preparation has not been successful.[375] A large bowel anastomosis can be made in one or two layers. For the former, non-absorbable material, e.g. silk or nylon, or long-lasting absorbable material, e.g. polyglycolic acid, polyglactin, PDS or maxon, is used as interrupted sutures. The sutures are placed either through all layers of the colonic wall or extramucosally, taking serosa, muscularis propria and submucosa.[376] If a two-layer anastomosis is to be constructed, it is normal policy to use an absorbable suture for the full-thickness inner layer, and a non-absorbable suture on the outer seromuscular layer. Both layers may be continuous or interrupted, but the inner layer is usually inserted as a continuous suture while the outer layer is constructed using interrupted seromuscular or Lembert sutures.

The anastomosis is normally constructed with both ends of bowel open, spillage being avoided by placing non-crushing clamps approximately 5 cm from the end of the bowel. Irrigation of the open bowel with a cancerocidal agent, for example 1% cetrimide or povidone iodine, may be beneficial. Any loose viable malignant cells which might have been shed into the bowel lumen are killed: it is hoped that this reduces the risk of local implantation recurrences. The open technique allows sutures to be inserted more accurately than the closed aseptic techniques formerly recommended.[377,378]

A colonic anastomosis is usually constructed either end-to-end or end-to-side, depending on its location. Occasionally a side-to-

REFERENCES

362. Winawer S J In: de Cosse J J (ed) Large Bowel Cancer. Churchill Livingstone, Edinburgh 1981
363. Hardcastle J D, Farrands P A et al Lancet 1983; ii: 1–4
364. Siba S Hepatogastroenterology 1983; 30: 27–29
365. Gilbertsen V A, Church T R, Grewe F J J Chron Dis 1980; 33: 107–114
366. Patterson H A Ann Surg 1956; 143: 670–675
367. Sanders G B, Hazen W H, Kinnaird P W Ann Surg 1958; 147: 796–801
368. Gerard A, Berrod J et al Rec Res Cancer Res 1985; 110: 130–133
369. Johnston D Br J Surg 1987; 74: 553–554
370. Dudley H, Phillips R In: Fielding L P, Welch J (eds) Intestinal Obstruction. Churchill Livingstone, London 1984
371. Herter F P Surg Clin North Am 1972; 52: 859–870
372. Keighley M R B Br J Surg 1977; 64: 315–321
373. Devlin H, Plant J et al Br Med J 1971; 3: 413–418
374. Muir E G Proc R Soc Med 1980; 61: 401
375. McDermott F, Hughes E S R et al Surg Gynecol Obstet 1982; 154: 833–837
376. Matheson N A, Irvine A D Br J Surg 1975; 62: 239
377. Seton Pringle Br J Surg 1924; 12: 238
378. Schoemaker Surg Gynecol Obstet 1921; 33: 591

side anastomosis is performed. The end-to-side anastomosis is used most frequently when there is a gross disparity in size between the two bowel ends, which may be the case with an ileocolic or ileorectal anastomosis. Lesser degrees of disparity between the colonic ends may be compensated for by dividing the segment of colon with the smaller lumen in an oblique manner from mesenteric to antimesenteric borders or by making a Cheatle slit in the antimesenteric border of the piece of bowel with the smaller lumen.

Turnbull et al[379] advocated ligation of the major blood vessels before mobilization of the tumour in the belief that metastatic spread can occur as the result of mechanical disturbance of the tumour. In addition direct handling of the tumour was avoided: the so-called 'no-touch technique'. Using this early ligation technique, he reported a 58% 5-year survival rate for tumours of Dukes' stage C, which was much higher than that achieved by other surgeons working in the same department. He did not however compare this technique with his own control group having a 'late' ligation after mobilization. In a randomized controlled trial of early versus late ligation, no difference in survival was found.[380] Despite this, many surgeons still prefer to divide the vessels at an early stage in the operation.

Right hemicolectomy. This is used for growths of the caecum, ascending colon, hepatic flexure and the right half of the transverse colon. The right colon is supplied by branches of the superior mesenteric artery. Resection requires ligation of the appropriate colic branches as close as possible to their origins (Fig. 30.38).

The operation is performed through a right paramedian, a transverse or a midline incision. The intra-abdominal organs are examined and the liver is carefully palpated bimanually for metastases. The operability of the growth is assessed. If the tumour appears to be involving other organs, this does not preclude resection. As much of any adherent tissue or organs as possible should be excised en bloc with the tumour. Adhesions are often inflammatory and not neoplastic, and thus the prognosis may be better than anticipated.

The greater omentum is separated from the right side of the transverse colon and the peritoneum of the posterior abdominal wall is incised lateral to the ascending colon along the line of peritoneal reflection, which Moynihan[381] called the 'white line of physiological fusion'. This incision is carried round the hepatic flexure into the transverse mesocolon and down around the caecum and below the attachment of the mesentery of the terminal ileum. The right colon is then elevated from the posterior abdominal wall with its vessels and regional lymph glands, taking care to preserve the duodenum, the right ureter, the gonadal vessels and the genitofemoral nerve (Fig. 30.39).

Dissection is continued medially as far as the origins of the ileocolic and right colic vessels and the right edge of the superior mesenteric vein, and these are divided and ligated approximately 1–1.5 cm from their points of origin. The right colic vessels are absent in 18% of patients and abnormal in source and distribution

REFERENCES

379. Turnbull R B Jr, Kyle K et al Ann Surg 1967; 166: 420–425
380. Wiggers T, Jeekel J, Arendj S W et al Br J Surg 1988; 75: 409–412
381. Moynihan B G A Abdominal Operations, 4th edn. Saunders, Philadelphia 1926

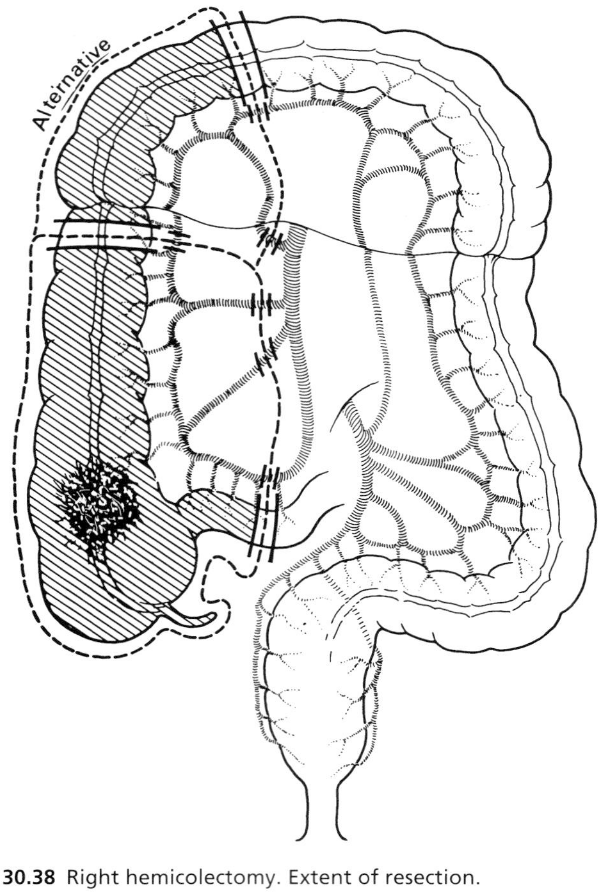

Fig 30.38 Right hemicolectomy. Extent of resection.

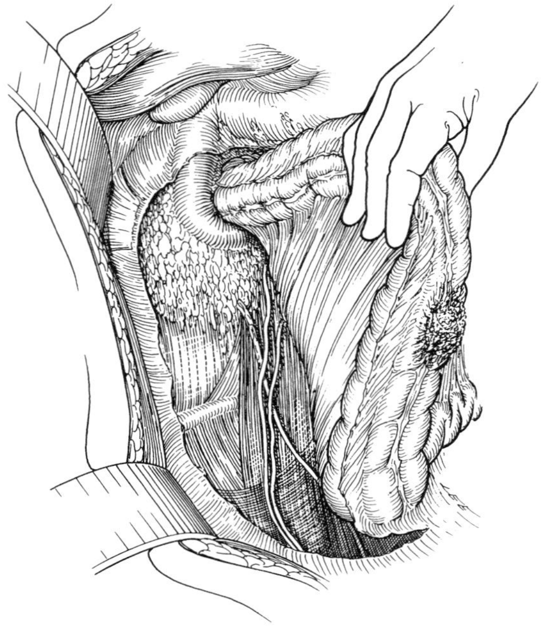

Fig 30.39 Right hemicolectomy. Mobilization reveals the duodenum, right ureter and gonadal vessels.

in a further 40%.[382] The mesentery is divided on each side from the proximally ligated vessels to the antimesenteric border of the bowel, and the ileum and colon are then divided between clamps (Fig. 30.40). Intestinal continuity is restored by an ileo-colic anastomosis.

Left hemicolectomy. This operation is used to treat cancers of the splenic flexure, descending and sigmoid colon. Radical resection involves ligation of the appropriate colic branches of the inferior mesenteric artery. Some surgeons believe that an even more radical excision is required for all tumours of the left colon in which the inferior mesenteric artery is divided at its origin. The whole of the left colon is excised and an anastomosis is constructed between the distal transverse colon and the upper rectum. This technique, known as extended left hemicolectomy, has not been shown to be any more successful than the segmental resections that are depicted in Figures 30.41 and 30.42. Furthermore a retrospective analysis has shown no significant difference in survival rates between the two techniques when applied to sigmoid colon carcinomas.[383]

Dissection begins with mobilization of the sigmoid colon. As with right hemicolectomy, the peritoneum lateral to the bowel is incised and the plane between the retroperitoneal structures and the sigmoid mesocolon is entered. The dissection is continued upwards, mobilizing the descending colon to the splenic flexure. Care must be taken during mobilization of the splenic flexure to avoid damage to the splenic capsule. During this dissection the gonadal vessels, the left ureter and the renal capsule are identified. The appropriate vessels are then divided and ligated close to their

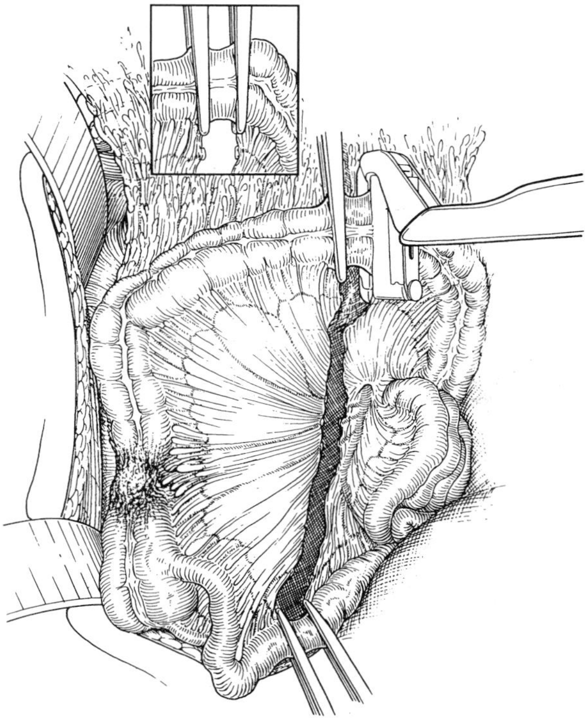

Fig 30.40 Right hemicolectomy. The transverse colon and terminal ileum are transected and the mesentery divided. Continuity is re-established by anastomosing ileum to transverse colon.

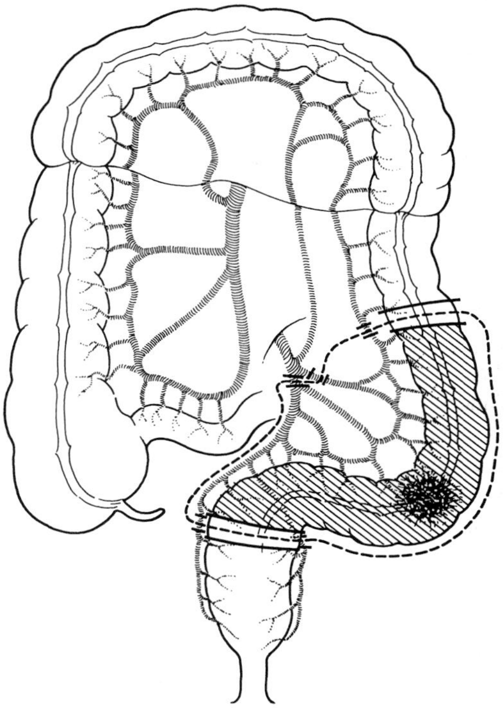

Fig 30.41 Sigmoid colectomy.

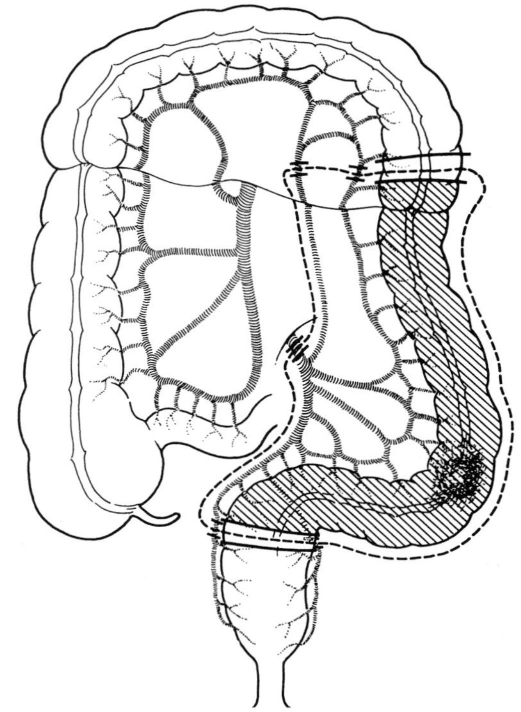

Fig 30.42 Standard left hemicolectomy. An extended left hemicolectomy would involve extension of the resection proximal to the splenic flexure.

REFERENCES

382. Stewart J A, Rankin F W Arch Surg 1933; 26: 843
383. Bonfanti G, Rozetti F et al Br J Surg 1982; 69: 305–307

origin, and a colo-colic or colorectal anastomosis is constructed using an end-to-end technique.

Transverse colectomy. A tumour situated in the middle of the transverse colon is removed by transverse colectomy. The middle colic artery is divided close to its origin. The splenic and hepatic flexures are mobilized and resected with the specimen and the anastomosis is made between the ascending colon and the descending colon. An extended right hemicolectomy can be used as an alternative means of resection with the terminal ileum being anastomosed end-to-end to the mobilized splenic flexure or descending colon.

The rectum

The first excision of the rectum for cancer seems to have been performed by Lisfranc in Paris in 1826,[384] but the first success was recorded by Czerny of Heidelburg in 1879.[385] Modern operations for the radical treatment of rectal cancer are derived from the pioneering work of Miles,[386] who first advocated the combined operation of abdominoperineal excision of the rectum. This entails removal of the rectum, lower sigmoid colon, anal canal and perianal skin. The regional lymphovascular pedicle and the levator ani muscle laterally to the pelvic wall are removed en bloc with the bowel (Fig. 30.43). Only in this way, according to Miles, could the zones of upward, lateral and downward spread of tumour be included in the removal. The operation was modified to be performed by two operators simultaneously, and the synchronized combined abdominoperineal excision of the rectum became the standard operation for the treatment of all rectal cancers for several decades.[387]

In the 1930s the pathological principles on which total rectal excision was founded were reassessed.[388] These pathological studies showed that Miles had not been entirely correct. Whilst upward and lateral spread were important, downward spread beyond 1 cm rarely occurred. This finding allowed Wangensteen and Dixon[389] to develop the operation of anterior resection, whereby a carcinoma of the upper third of the rectum could be resected and the proximal colon anastomosed to the rectal stump via the abdomen. It was still believed, however, that it was imperative to remove the tumour with a distal margin of at least 5 cm of normal rectum, the so-called '5 cm rule'.[390] This, coupled with the technical difficulties of performing a manual anastomosis deep in the pelvis, together with the belief that the receptors necessary for continence were situated in the rectal wall, inhibited surgeons from performing sphincter-saving operations for carcinoma of the lower two thirds of the rectum.

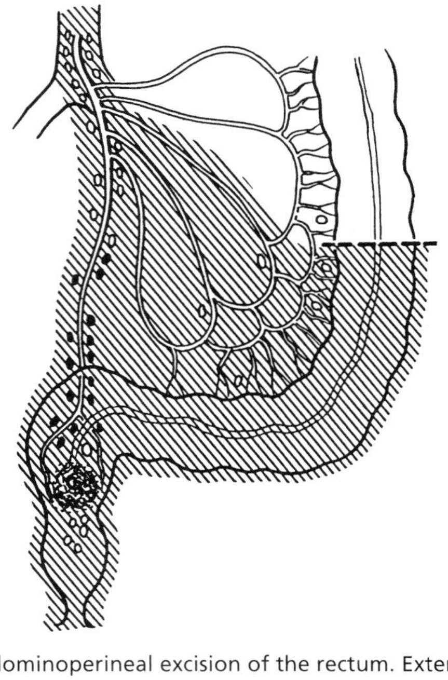

Fig 30.43 Abdominoperineal excision of the rectum. Extent of excision.

Within the last 40 years, however, the climate of opinion has changed. Pathological studies[391–393] have shown that distal intramural spread rarely exceeds 1 cm and that it is therefore safe to reduce the margin of distal clearance from 5 to 2 cm. In addition, it is now known that continence can still be achieved even if the whole rectum is excised and the colon is anastomosed to the anal canal.[394] New techniques have been developed which make simpler an anastomosis deep in the pelvis. In particular, the introduction of the stapling gun has revolutionized the surgery of this disease. Thus, prior to 1980, three quarters of middle third rectal cancers were treated by total rectal excision and a quarter by anterior resection. Since that time, the percentages for each procedure have been reversed and three quarters are now treated by anterior resection.

More conservative techniques are also used to treat rectal cancers—local excision,[395] diathermy fulguration,[396] radiation[397] and, more recently, laser destruction/vaporization may be used to treat selected tumours, usually in patients who are too frail to undergo a major resection. Local treatment can be applied successfully to a small group of otherwise fit patients with a lower third carcinoma that is confined to the rectal wall and not of anaplastic histological grade.

The choice between abdominoperineal excision of the rectum and sphincter-saving resections. It is generally agreed that carcinomas of the upper third of the rectum (more than 12 cm from the anal verge) should be treated by anterior resection. Most surgeons agree that tumours where the lower edge is 5 cm or less from the

REFERENCES

384. Lisfranc J Rev Med Franc Etrang 1826; 2: 380
385. Czerny P 1893 Quoted by Rankin F W, Bargen J A, Buie L A The Colon, Rectum and Anus. Saunders, Philadelphia 1932
386. Miles W E Br Med J 1910; ii: 941–942
387. Lloyd-Davies O V Lancet 1939; ii: 74
388. Westhues M Grundlagen der Chirurgie des Rektumkazin ans Leipzig. George Thieme Verlag, Stuttgart 1934
389. Dixon C Am J Surg 1939; 46: 12–17
390. Goligher J C, Dukes C E, Bussey H J R Br J Surg 1951; 39: 199–211
391. Quer E A, Dahlin D C, Mayo C W Surg Gynecol Obstet 1953; 96: 24–30
392. Williams N, Dixon M et al Br J Surg 1983; 70: 150–154
393. Penfold J B Aust NZ J Surg 1974; 44: 354–356
394. Lane R H S, Parks A G Br J Surg 1977; 64: 596–599
395. Mason A Y Aust NZ J Surg 1976; 46: 322
396. Madden J L, Kandalaft S Am J Surg 1971; 122: 347
397. Papillon J Proc R Soc Med 1973; 66: 1179

anal verge should be removed by an abdominoperineal excision. The treatment of cancers between these two levels is, however, controversial. The new sphincter-saving techniques result in a better quality of life than can be achieved after abdominoperineal excision.[398] Apart from numerous psychological problems related to the colostomy, patients who have undergone an abdominoperineal excision have a higher incidence of bladder and sexual disturbances.[398–400] As less tissue is excised during a sphincter-saving resection than during an abdominoperineal excision the fear is that recurrence and survival rates will be compromised. There is the theoretical risk that insufficient microscopic distal spread will be removed during sphincter-saving resection and anastomotic recurrence will consequently occur if the margin of distal clearance is reduced to less than the recommended distance of 5 cm. There is also the risk that the degree of lateral clearance will be reduced. In practice, neither of these fears has been justified. Studies which have carefully matched patients have found no significant difference in recurrence or survival rates for similar tumours treated by either type of operation.[375,401,402] The incidence of local recurrence is not influenced by the margin of distal clearance[403] and the degree of lateral clearance seems to be comparable.

It thus appears that, provided a distal clearance of 2 cm can be achieved, all low rectal cancers should if possible be treated by some form of resection and anastomosis. Of course, such an approach is not possible for some patients with extensive local spread, but in fact such cases are uncommon.

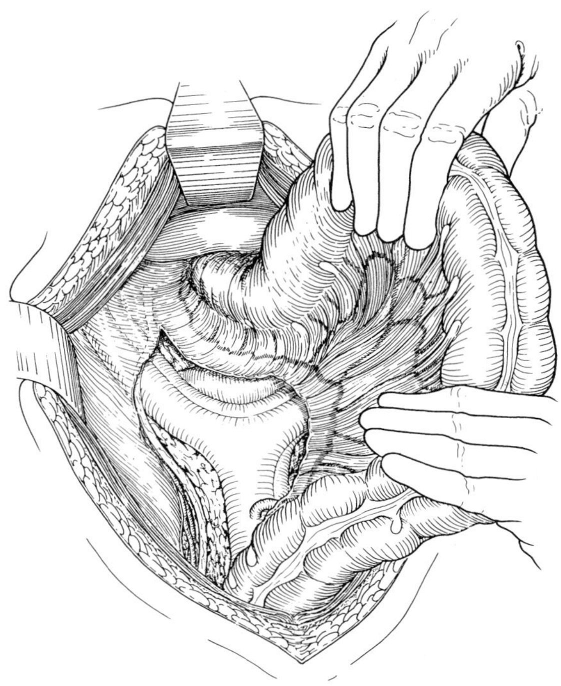

Fig 30.44 Anterior resection. Mobilization of sigmoid colon and upper part of the rectum by division of peritoneal attachments along the lateral border.

Sphincter-saving resections

Anterior resection with manual anastomosis. The patient is placed in the modified Trendelenburg position or the Lloyd Davies position with 20–30° of Trendelenburg tip and a urinary catheter is passed. The abdomen is opened and the liver and peritoneal cavity assessed for the presence of metastases. The mobility of the growth is assessed: provided the tumour is operable, and most are, the operation proceeds.

The sigmoid colon is mobilized along its lateral border by dividing any adhesions which bind it to the posterior peritoneum. The peritoneal incision is extended upwards and downwards to expose the gonadal vessels and the left ureter where it lies on the bifurcation of the common iliac artery. These structures are carefully preserved (Fig. 30.44).

The peritoneum on the right side of the sigmoid mesocolon and upper mesorectum is now divided and the right ureter is identified and preserved. The inferior mesenteric artery is defined close to its origin from the aorta, before being ligated and divided, taking care not to damage the central root of the presacral nerves. The inferior mesenteric vein is identified and divided separately.

The sigmoid mesocolon is divided obliquely from the point of ligation of the inferior mesenteric vessels to the site of proposed transection of the left colon. During division of the mesocolon, the following vessels are serially divided: the ascending left colic artery running to the splenic flexure, the left colic artery and the marginal artery between the left colic and first sigmoid vessels. After division of the mesocolon, the colon is divided. It is important at this point to ensure that the blood supply of the colon is adequate and that the descending colon has been sufficiently mobilized to reach into the pelvis, so that the subsequent anastomosis will be adequately performed and without tension. For very low anastomoses, it is necessary to mobilize the whole of the left colon, together with the splenic flexure and the distal transverse colon.

Attention now turns to the pelvic dissection, the extent of which depends on the height of the tumour. For an upper third growth it is usually not necessary to divide the lateral ligaments completely. The peritoneal incisions are continued down on each side of the rectum to the level of the seminal vesicles. The bowel is then held anteriorly and the rectosigmoid mesentery containing the divided vascular pedicle is stripped down from the front of the lower aorta, the right common iliac vein and the fifth lumbar vertebra to the promontory of the sacrum. The bilateral branches of the presacral nerve are identified and safeguarded. The retrorectal space is now entered between the mesorectum and the presacral fascia and this dissection is continued down to about 3 or 4 cm below the lower border of the growth (Fig. 30.45). Heald[404] has emphasized the importance of a full mesorectal clearance, claiming a low local recurrence rate because of this manoeuvre.

The anterior plane of dissection between the posterior wall of

REFERENCES

398. Williams N S, Johnston D Br J Surg 1983; 70: 460–462
399. Fowler J, Bremner D et al Br J Urol 1978; 50: 95–98
400. Williams N, Price R et al Br J Surg 1980; 67: 203–208
401. Nicholls R J, Ritchie J K et al Br J Surg 1979; 66: 625–627
402. Williams N, Johnston D Br J Surg 1984; 71: 278–282
403. Pollett W G, Nicholls R J Ann Surg 1983; 198: 159–163
404. Heald R J, Husband E M, Ryall R D H Br J Surg 1982; 69: 613

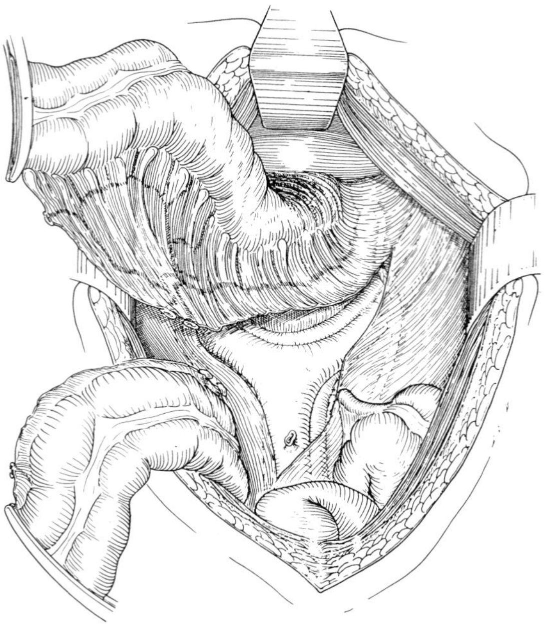

Fig 30.45 Anterior resection. The inferior mesenteric vessels have been divided and ligated, and the sigmoid mesentery and sigmoid colon have been transected.

the bladder or vagina and the anterior wall of the rectum is developed by scissor dissection (Fig. 30.46). The extent of anterior dissection depends on the height of the tumour, but in growths of the lower half of the rectum the dissection continues to the apex of the prostate or lower vagina. The lateral ligaments are divided

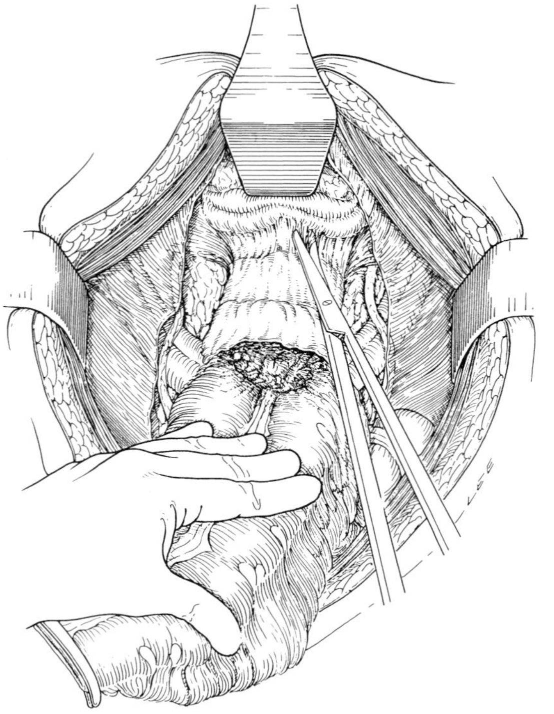

Fig 30.46 Anterior resection. The anterior dissection.

(Fig. 30.47) and a right-angled clamp is then applied transversely across the lower rectum at least 2 cm below the tumour (Fig. 30.48). The lower rectum is irrigated through the anus with a cancericidal solution such as 1% cetrimide or povidone iodine and transected below the clamp. A one- or two-layer anastomosis is then constructed between the descending colon and the rectal stump (Fig. 30.49). At the conclusion of the anastomosis, consideration is given to the need for a covering stoma. This decision depends on a number of factors, including the adequacy of bowel preparation, the difficulty experienced by the surgeon in performing the anastomosis and the experience of the operator. If a stoma is considered necessary, either a loop ileostomy or transverse colostomy is suitable, although the former is preferable.[405]

Anterior resection with stapled anastomosis. Mobilization of the rectum is exactly as for anterior resection with hand-

REFERENCE

405. Williams N S, Durdey P, Johnston D Br J Surg 1985; 72: 595–598

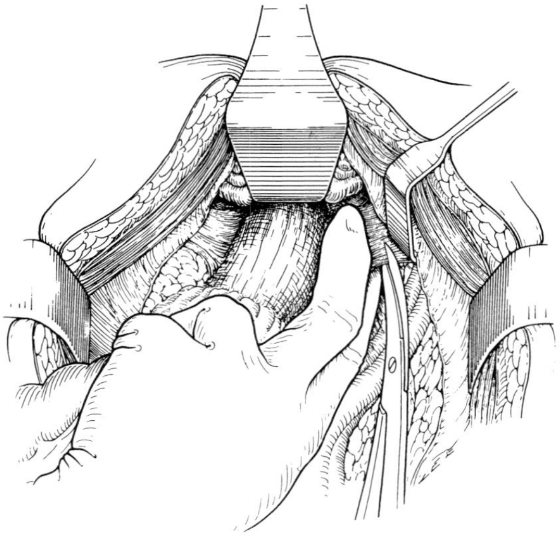

Fig 30.47 Anterior resection. Division of lateral ligaments.

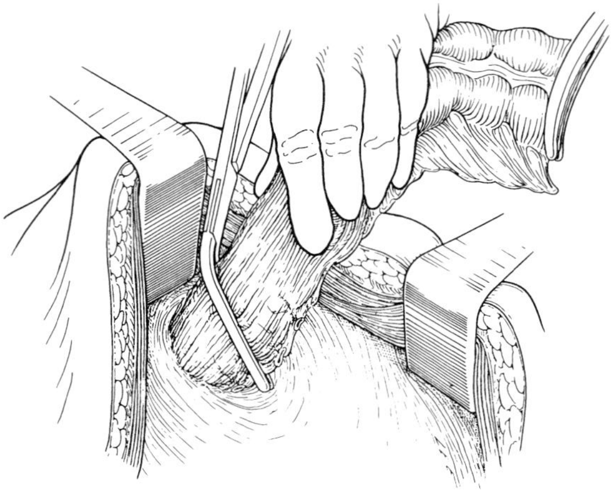

Fig 30.48 Anterior resection. Cross-clamping at least 2 cm distal to tumour prior to cancericidal washout and division of rectum.

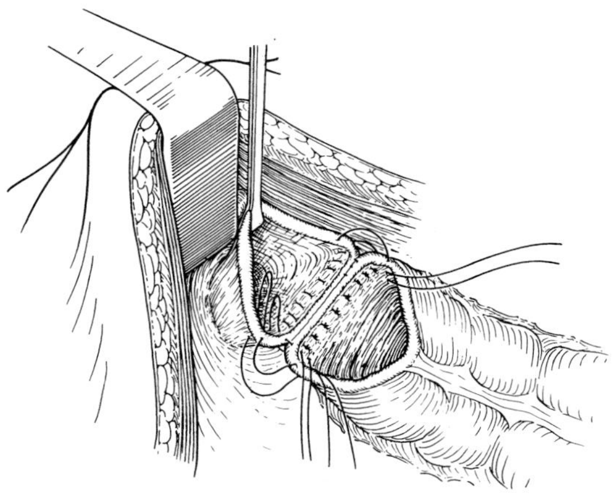

Fig 30.49 Anterior resection. One-layered manual anastomosis.

sutured anastomosis. The right-angled clamp is cut off with a long-handled knife, leaving the rectal stump open. A pursestring suture of nylon or prolene (gauge 0) is then inserted into the top of the rectal stump, and another is inserted into the open end of the distal descending colon which is to be used for the anastomosis. The appropriate-sized stapler is inserted through the anal canal so that its head emerges through the open rectal stump. The instrument is then opened to separate the head maximally from the anvil and the head is inserted into the open end of the colon. Both pursestring sutures are tied so that rectum and colon are firmly applied to the shaft of the gun. The instrument is closed to approximate the head and anvil and the gun is fired. In so doing, the circular knife cuts through the tissue contained outside each pursestring suture and simultaneously fires a double circular row of staples through both the rectal and colonic walls. The instrument is opened slightly and carefully removed. The two rings of tissue, 'donuts', are extracted from the head and anvil and inspected for completeness. If they are incomplete, it is necessary to place some reinforcing sutures across the anastomosis and to consider a temporary stoma.

An alternative stapling technique has been described. After irrigation of the rectum, a transverse stapler is applied below the clamp to close the rectal stump. The shaft of the circular stapling gun without its head is thrust through the top of the closed stump and the head is replaced on to the shaft (Fig. 30.50). The anastomosis then proceeds as already described. This technique eliminates the need for a pursestring suture on the rectal stump. It simplifies the operation considerably, for after excision of very low tumours insertion of the rectal pursestring suture may be very difficult. The leak rate after this technique, however, appears to be greater than with the conventional stapling procedure.

Other sphincter-saving resections. These include the abdominotrans-sphincteric operation, the abdominotrans-sacral technique and the abdominoperanal procedure described by Parks.[406] With the advent of the stapling gun, these techniques are employed less frequently but they are useful in cases where stapling is not feasible. The abdominal phase of the Parks procedure is the same as for anterior resection, except that the dissection is taken down to the pelvic floor. The rectum is transected at this level, and the operative specimen removed. After mobilization of

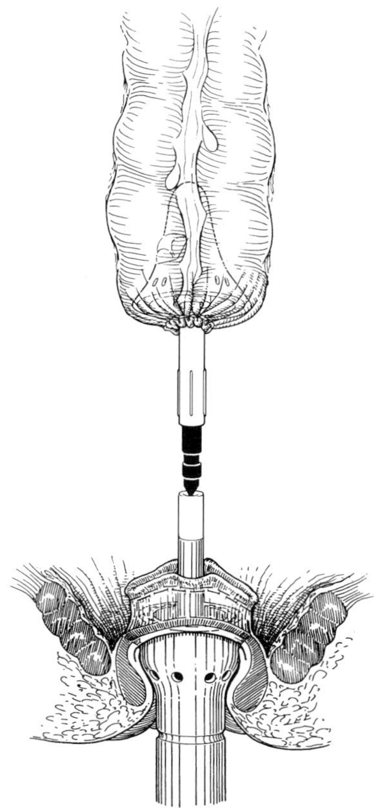

Fig 30.50 Low anterior resection using Premium CEEA stapling gun.

the splenic flexure, the colon is brought down through the anal canal and an anastomosis is made between the colon and anal canal via an endoanal approach (Fig. 30.51). This is covered by a loop ileostomy or proximal transverse colostomy.

Abdominoperineal excision. The abdominal part of the operation is exactly the same as for an anterior resection, except that the sigmoid colon is divided and its proximal end brought out as an end colostomy in the left iliac fossa. It is good practice to make the colostomy trephine before opening the abdomen. The site should be marked preoperatively after the patient has tried wearing an appliance to determine its optimal position. The trephine should be made through the rectus sheath without division of any fibres of the rectus abdominis muscle. While the rectum is being mobilized, the perineal phase is begun.

The anus is closed at the start of the procedure by a strong pursestring suture. An elliptical incision is made around the anus, beginning midway between the anus and the bulb of the urethra anteriorly, and extending posteriorly to the tip of the coccyx. The incision is deepened posteriorly through the fat until the coccyx is reached. The tip of the coccyx may be disarticulated and excised, although most surgeons prefer to leave it intact and divide the anococcygeal raphe just anterior to it (Fig. 30.52). By this manoeuvre access is gained to the pelvis. The fascia of Waldeyer,

REFERENCE

406. Parks A G Proc R Soc Med 1972; 65: 975–976

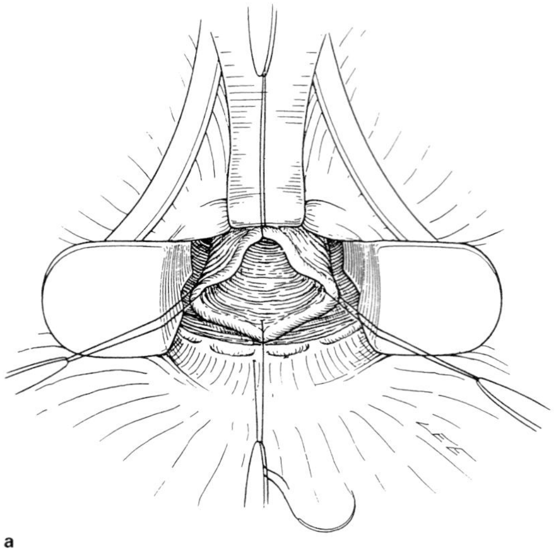

a

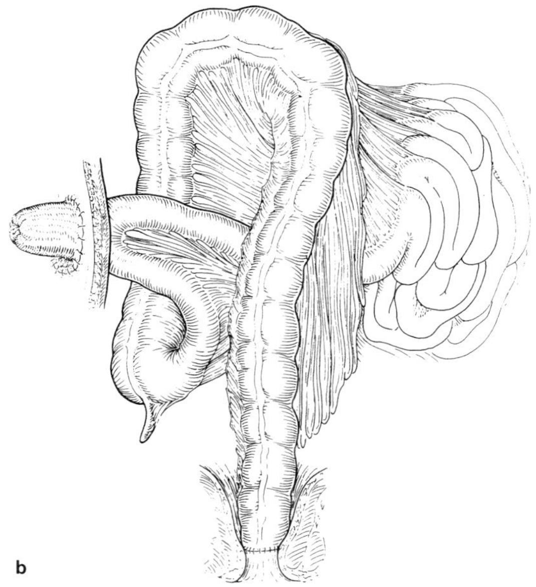

b

Fig 30.51 Abdominotransanal coloanal anastomosis. **(a)** The rectum has been excised and the mucosa of the upper part of the anal canal has been removed. The colon is brought down through the denuded anal canal, and is anastomosed transanally to the dentate line. **(b)** On completion of the procedure a covering ileostomy is fashioned to protect the healing anastomosis.

which separates the rectum from the pelvic nerves and sacral plexus and forms a fascial floor to the pelvis above the levatores ani, is divided in a horseshoe fashion from side to side in front of the coccyx. This avoids damage to the presacral veins.

Attention is now turned to the anterior dissection. In the male the transverse perineal muscles are identified and displaced anteriorly. Maintaining this line, the rectoprostatic plane is entered (Fig. 30.53). A finger is then inserted to develop the plane by blunt dissection to meet the abdominal operator's finger placed in the rectoprostatic septum above. Scissors are then inserted from below and the remaining tissue between the two operators is penetrated. The puborectalis muscle on each side is divided and, following

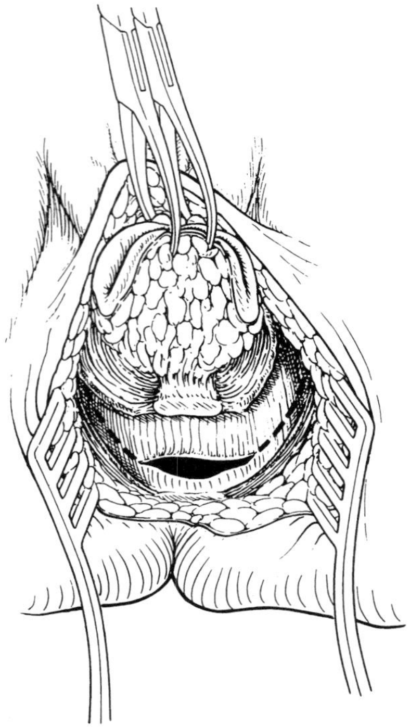

Fig 30.52 Abdominoperineal excision of the rectum. Posterior perineal dissection.

division of the lateral ligaments containing the middle rectal vessels, the specimen is freed and delivered through the perineal wound. The perineal wound is then closed.

The perineal dissection in the female is similar in its posterior and lateral parts. Anteriorly the posterior vaginal wall is taken along with the specimen. A longitudinal incision is made in the vagina on each side and the pelvis entered. A transverse incision is then made, freeing the specimen. Bleeding from the vaginal venous plexus is controlled by a running whip suture.

Perforation of the rectum confers palliative status on the operation because of the increased risk of local recurrence. The perineal dissection is therefore a matter of great responsibility. The proximal divided end of the sigmoid colon is brought out through the colostomy trephine incision. The space between the colon and the lateral abdominal wall (the lateral space) is then closed. This avoids internal herniation and gives support to the stoma itself. The extraperitoneal colostomy is little used today.

The pelvic peritoneum may then be sutured, although there is debate as to whether this manoeuvre is necessary. The abdominal wound is then closed. The colostomy is fashioned using interrupted absorbable mucocutaneous sutures.

Additional procedures

A hysterectomy should be combined with the rectal excision if the growth extends into the uterus, the two organs being removed en bloc. A portion of the ureter must be excised if it is involved by tumour. Reconstruction by uretero-ureterostomy may be necessary or it may be feasible to reimplant the ureter into the bladder with or without a Boari flap (see Chapter 36). Alternatively, provided the

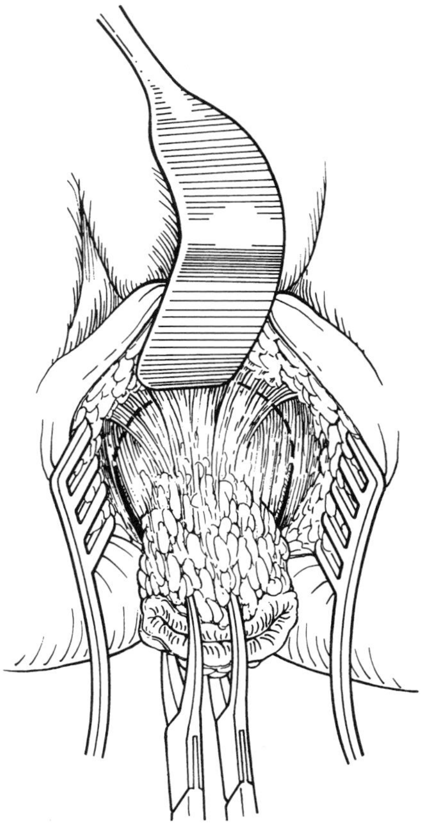

Fig 30.53 Abdominoperineal excision of the rectum. Anterolateral perineal dissection.

kidney on the opposite side is known to function normally, a nephrectomy may be simpler. It is rarely worthwhile to perform a total cystectomy and pelvic exenteration.

Hartmann's procedure. Occasionally, in patients with a rectal carcinoma, it is not feasible to perform either an abdominoperineal or a sphincter-saving resection. For instance, it is unwise to construct an anastomosis in the presence of pus. Similarly, it is unwise and probably unkind to perform either an abdominoperineal or sphincter-saving resection in the presence of extensive local spread when it is clear that recurrence is inevitable and life expectancy is likely to be considerably reduced. In these circumstances, excision of the tumour with closure of the rectal stump and construction of an end-colostomy may be the operation of choice. One of the simplest ways to perform Hartmann's procedure is to use a transverse stapling instrument to close the top of the rectal stump.

Postoperative care after rectal resection

The postoperative care is similar to that following any major abdominal procedure. Hydration is maintained by intravenous fluids until a normal oral intake has been re-established. Two further doses of the prophylactic antibiotic regimen are given, usually 6 and 12 hours after operation. The patient should receive adequate systemic analgesia which may be administered as epidural opiates (see Chapter 5). The urethral catheter is kept in situ for several days until the patient is relatively mobile. It is not unusual, however, for the establishment of normal micturition to be delayed after rectal excision. In most cases this problem rights itself after further bladder drainage, with or without the administration of bladder stimulants (see Chapter 37). If normal micturition is not achieved by these measures, the patient must be investigated for a denervated bladder or a mechanical obstruction to flow (see Chapter 37).

It is normal practice to cover the colostomy initially with an ileostomy drainable bag, because the effluent at first tends to be liquid rather than solid. As the days pass, the faeces thicken and the patient and stomatherapist can then decide on the best appliance. The patient must be encouraged at the earliest stage to take an interest in the stoma and under supervision be taught how to change the appliance.

There are two methods of long-term colostomy management. In the first the patient wears an appliance all the time and disposes of it when the stoma acts. Usually this occurs about twice a day after bowel function has re-established itself postoperatively. The second method avoids the need to wear an appliance by daily irrigation of the colon. Appliance manufacturers have devised irrigation sets which include a cone to fit the colostomy, a reservoir and tubing and adhesive pouches with a long sleeve. At a set time each day, the patient irrigates the bowel with about 1 litre of tap water which discharges spontaneously over the next 30 min or so, clearing faecal material at the same time. It is then possible to cover the stoma with a simple dressing until the next irrigation 24 hours later. It may, however, be advisable to put an appliance on at night.

Complications

Intestinal obstruction

Small bowel obstruction may occur from herniation of small intestine lateral to the colostomy loop, if the lateral space has not been closed, or through the pelvic peritoneal wound closure. Small intestine may also become adherent to the pelvic peritoneal closure. After sphincter-saving resections a small dehiscence in the anastomosis may become plugged by a loop of small bowel which may then become obstructed. The large bowel may become temporarily obstructed either as the result of oedema of the colostomy or from a bolus of faeces. The former settles in time; the latter may need suppositories or a gentle enema. It is unwise to treat this problem until at least 7 days have elapsed.

Urinary complications

Acute retention may be the result of denervation of the bladder or prostatic obstruction (see Chapter 37 and 38) Direct injury to the ureters may lead to hydronephrosis, pyonephrosis or urinary fistula. The bladder may be opened during the anterior dissection and the urethra may be injured in the perineal phase of abdominoperineal excision, leading to fistula or stricture at a later date.

Sexual dysfunction

Damage to pelvic nerves may also result in impotence or failure of ejaculation. The former is caused by injury to the nervi erigentes, the latter by damage to the presacral nerves. Impotence is more common after abdominoperineal excision (around 50%) than after anterior resection (20–50%).[407] In females, fibrosis around the vagina may result in dyspareunia.

Perineal wound

Primary, reactionary or secondary haemorrhage may occur. Infection is probably the most frequent complication: if drainage is not satisfactory, an abscess may form in the deep recesses of the cavity. Pressure necrosis of the wound edges may develop if the patient is not turned frequently. A perineal sinus may form if the wound fails to heal completely, and at a later date a perineal hernia may develop.

'Phantom' rectum

This is a condition akin to phantom limb (see Chapter 10) which may develop after amputation. About half of the patients feel that the rectum is still present and this produces a distressing sensation.[408]

Colostomy complications

The stoma may bleed, prolapse, retract or stenose if it has not been correctly made. The skin around the colostomy may become excoriated or a fistula may develop between the stoma and the skin. A paracolostomy hernia may also develop, though this complication was more frequent when the colostomy was brought out lateral to the rectus sheath, with a incidence of around 25% at 5 years.

Anastomotic dehiscence

This is the most dangerous complication and may present in a number of ways. Generalized peritonitis will develop if there is a perforation into the peritoneal cavity, while a pelvic abscess will develop if the leak remains localized. The abscess may subsequently perforate into the peritoneal cavity and once again peritonitis will result. Alternatively, the abscess may drain spontaneously through the defect in the anastomosis back into the intestinal lumen, resulting in the passage of pus per anum. The abscess may also track to the skin and discharge through either the main wound or drain track. The discharge of pus is then almost always followed by a discharge of faeces, indicating an established fistula. Most fistulae close spontaneously provided there is no distal obstruction.

Anastomotic dehiscence is related to two main factors: the level of the anastomosis, and the surgeon. After high anterior resection the leak rate is around 5%. This rises significantly where the anastomosis is constructed below the peritoneal reflection. After low anterior resection anastomotic leakage has been reported to range from 5% to more than 25% of cases.[409–411] These rates refer to a clinical dehiscence; radiological examination of the anastomosis using a water-soluble contrast medium reveals some degree of leakage in a much higher proportion.[412] In a multivariate analysis of factors relating to anastomotic dehiscence, other than the level, the only significant factor was the surgeon.[413] This strongly implies that good technique is vital. Randomized trials of stapled versus hand-sutured anastomosis have not shown any significant difference in the leak rate.[409,413]

Anastomotic stricture formation which is not related to local recurrence is usually caused by fibrosis. This seems to be more common after stapled anastomosis, being reported in 5–10% of cases.[414,415]

Haemorrhage is rare, occurring in about 1% of cases. It can be reactionary or secondary, and is either the result of inadequate haemostasis at the suture line or disruption of the anastomosis.

Increased bowel frequency and incontinence are more likely the lower the colorectal anastomosis. After coloanal anastomosis, the mean bowel frequency is around 3–4 times per 24 hours but some patients go considerably more often. Continence is normal in around 70%, with some soiling (usually minor) in the remainder.[416] Function tends to improve with time up to almost 1 year from operation. The addition of a colonic reservoir to coloanal reconstruction appears to improve bowel function significantly.[417,418]

Results of surgery for colorectal cancer

Carcinoma of the colon

Over the last 40 years, the proportion of colonic cancers amenable to resection has increased and the operative mortality has been reduced: respective rates are now 70–80% and 5–10%.[419] The overall crude 5-year survival for patients treated by surgery in most hospitals ranges between 50 and 70%.[420–423] The overall 5-year survival rate is much lower, 20–25% in the UK.[424,425] If all patients with the disease are included, however, irrespective of whether they have an operation, the survival rate is worse. Many of these patients are old and about 20–30% have disseminated cancers at presentation. This figure for disseminated cancer rises to around 50% in patients presenting with intestinal obstruction.

Various factors influence survival after surgery, the most important being the stage of the tumour. Thus the age-corrected 5-

REFERENCES

407. Williams N, Johnston D Br J Surg 1983; 70: 460–462
408. Druss R G, O'Connor J F, Stern L Q Arch Gen Psychiatry 1969; 20: 419–426
409. Beart R W, Kelly K A Am J Surg 1981; 141: 143–147
410. Weakley F L Dis Colon Rectum 1981; 24: 231–246
411. Blamey S L, Lee P W R Br J Surg 1982; 69: 19–22
412. Goligher J C, Simpkins K C, Lintott D J Br J Surg 1977; 64: 609
413. McGinn F P, Gartell P C et al Br J Surg 1985; 72: 603–605
414. Smith L E Dis Colon Rectum 1981; 24: 236–242
415. Waxman B P Br J Surg 1983; 70: 64–67
416. Parks A, Percy J Br J Surg 1982; 69: 301–304
417. Lazorthes F, Faget P et al Br J Surg 1986; 73: 136–138
418. Parc R, Tiret E et al Br J Surg 1986; 73: 139–141
419. Turunen M J Ann Chir Gynaecol 1983; 72: 317–323
420. Gilbertsen V A Surgery St Louis 1959; 46: 1027
421. Grinnel R S Surg Gynecol Obstet 1953; 96: 31–36
422. Hughes E S R Aust NZ J Surg 1966; 35: 183–188
423. Rankin F, Osen P Surg Gynecol Obstet 1953; 56: 366–371
424. Slaney G In: Modern Trends Surgery, 3rd edn. Butterworths, London 1971
425. Walker R M Annual Report of South Western Regional Cancer Bureau. UTF House, King Square, Bristol BS2 8HY, 1971

year survival rate for Dukes' C tumours is 30–40%, whereas that for Dukes' A and B tumours is 70–80%.[421] Younger patients appear to have a worse prognosis than older patients, and the shorter the history the worse the outlook.[424,426] The development of complications, particularly perforation or obstruction, also, adversely affects survival.[427–429]

Carcinoma of the rectum

The results of surgery for carcinoma of the rectum are similar to those for carcinoma of the colon. In specialized units or hospitals, the resectability rate may be as high as 95%, with an operative mortality of less than 5%.[430] Overall 5-year survival rates in these units are approximately 50%, but the rate falls to about 25% when the results of district general hospitals are included.[424] The most obvious reason for this difference is the higher proportion of advanced and emergency cases treated in the non-specialized hospitals. Survival rates are influenced by the Dukes' stage (see Table 30.10), and fixed or partially fixed tumours have a worse prognosis than mobile lesions.[431,432] The lower the tumour is in the rectum, the worse the outlook,[433,434] and the histological grade also influences survival.

Local recurrence

Local recurrence can occur after both anterior resection and abdominoperineal excision of the rectum. There are three major causes: inadequate clearance at the original operation, implantation of viable cancer cells[435] at the anastomotic site or a metachronous tumour arising in an unstable epithelium. In around one third of resection specimens, tumour is present at the lateral margins; positive margins are associated with a very high incidence of recurrence. Heald[404] showed that microscopic islands of tumour occur within the mesorectum beyond the tumour and that if these are removed as part of a total mesorectal excision, recurrence rates are less than 5%. Lateral pelvic nodal involvement is unusual but may account for a small number of recurrences.[436,437] These nodes are not normally removed in the standard operations for rectal cancer and are therefore almost certainly responsible for some cases of pelvic recurrence. Pelvic lymphadenectomy in addition to rectal removal has been claimed to improve survival. These results are in contrast however to experience with lymphadenectomy in other tumours.[437]

Most of the factors shown to influence survival also influence recurrence. Thus, Dukes' stage and the height of the lesion from the anal sphincter are important factors. On the other hand, the type of operation (i.e. abdominoperineal excision or anterior resection) performed for similar tumours in similar patients does not influence the incidence of recurrence. 80% of all local recurrences develop within the first 2 years after surgery.[438] The average incidence of local recurrence seems to be about 10%. There is however considerable variation from centre to centre and surgeon to surgeon. The variation between consultant surgeons recorded in the St Mary's Hospital Large Bowel Cancer Project was between 5% and 20%.[439]

Patients with local recurrence often complain of persistent pelvic pain, which may radiate down the legs if the sacral nerve roots are involved. Urinary symptoms develop if the bladder or urethra is invaded. A swelling or some induration may be visible or palpable in the perineum if there is a local recurrence after abdominoperineal resection. Alternatively an abscess or a discharging sinus may develop. Bilateral leg oedema may arise from invasion and obstruction of the lymphatics and veins.

Local recurrence after anterior resection may again cause a change in bowel habit or the passage of blood per rectum. As the pelvis is more accessible to examination after restorative resection than after abdominoperineal excision, it might be expected that the detected local recurrence rate would be higher. This in fact is not the case. Sigmoidoscopic biopsy of friable tissue at the anastomosis may confirm recurrence but it often develops extrarectally and may be detected as induration on digital examination or by computerized tomography. The best method of treating recurrence is by further surgical excision but this is often not possible because of the advanced stage of the tumour. Patients may develop an increase in serum carcinoembryonic antigen concentration before they develop clinical recurrence, and at present a controlled trial is being conducted to determine if monitoring for this tumour marker is worthwhile.[440] Radiotherapy and cytotherapy are merely palliative. Endoscopic resection and Nd Yag lasers have been used to create a lumen through a recurrence which has developed at the anastomosis after sphincter-saving resections.[441,442]

Table 30.10 Corrected 5-year survival for rectal cancer according to modified Dukes' classification

Dukes' stage	%
A	91.9
B	71.3
C1	40.0
C2	26.5
D	16.4

Local techniques for rectal cancer

Patients who are unfit for major surgery may receive useful palliation by electrocoagulation,[443] contact irradiation,[444] local excision

REFERENCES

426. Copeland E, Miller L et al Am J Surg 1969; 116: 875
427. Gerber A, Thompson R et al Surg Gynecol Obstet 1962; 123: 593–598
428. Irvin T T, Greaney M G Br J Surg 1977; 64: 741–746
429. Dudley H A F, Phillips R K In: Fielding L P, Welch J (eds) Intestinal Obstruction. Churchill Livingstone, London 1987
430. Lockhart-Mummery H E, Ritchie J K, Hawley P R Br J Surg 1976; 63: 673–679
431. Habib N A, Peck M A et al Br J Surg 1983; 70: 423–424
432. Wood C, Gillis L et al Br J Surg 1981; 68: 326–328
433. Gilchrist R K, David V C Am Surg 1947; 126: 421–426
434. Stearns M, Binkley G Surg Gynecol Obstet 1953; 96: 368–372
435. Umpleby H C, Fermore B et al Br J Surg 1983; 70: 680
436. Sauer L, Bacon H E Surg Gynecol Obstet 1952; 94: 229
437. Deddish M R, Stearns M W Ann Surg 1961; 154: 961–966
438. Morson B C, Vaughan E G, Bussey H J R Br Med J 1963; 2: 13
439. Phillips R K S, Hittinger R et al Br J Surg 1984; 71: 12–16
440. Northover J M A, Slack W W Dis Colon Rectum 1984; 27: 576
441. Wirsching R World J Surg 1987; 11: 499–503
442. Kettlewell M G W Curr Opin Gastroenterol 1988; 4: 19–25
443. Strauss A, Strauss S et al JAMA 1935; 104: 1480
444. Papillon J Proc R Soc Med 1973; 66: 1179

and Nd Yag laser therapy. These techniques can also be applied as the primary treatment for low-grade carcinomas which are confined to the bowel wall. These tumours only account for around 5% of all rectal cancers and can be identified and assessed by a combination of digital examination, biopsy and rectal endoluminal ultrasound.[445,446] 5-year survival rates of over 90% have been reported in these low-grade tumours.

Histopathological examination must confirm that the tumour is confined to the rectal wall. A curative resection should be undertaken if there is evidence of local spread beyond the bowel wall.

Adjuvant therapy. Much attention has been focussed on radiotherapy and chemotherapy because there has been no significant improvement in survival rates after surgery alone in the last 30 years.

Adjuvant radiotherapy is chiefly used in patients with rectal cancer as the rectum can be treated without damaging the small bowel. It may be given either pre- or postoperatively. Reports of trials using low-dose preoperative radiotherapy have been conflicting.[447–449] A recent Swedish trial of preoperative radiotherapy has shown much lower recurrence rates.[450] Preoperative radiotherapy may convert a growth deemed inoperable on clinical examination into an operable one[449] although long-term survival is poor. Postoperative radiotherapy has the advantage that it can be reserved for poor risk cancers. The few controlled trials have again produced conflicting results.[451,452]

Only 5-fluorouracil has been extensively investigated in randomized controlled trials and has been found to be disappointing. Combinations of 5-fluorouracil and methyl semustine and mitomycin have produced some benefit.[453] 5-fluorouracil combined with levamisole has been reported to improve survival of patients with Dukes' C tumours.[454] Further studies are necessary to confirm this benefit. Adjuvant chemotherapy may also be administered intra- and postoperatively by perfusing the liver with 5-fluorouracil through the umbilical veins although this technique is still of doubtful value.[455]

RARE MALIGNANT TUMOURS

Carcinoid

Carcinoid is a rare and usually malignant tumour of the large bowel derived from the Kulchitsky cells of the crypts of Lieberkuhn. Large bowel carcinoid tumours do not secrete 5-hydroxytryptamine, even when spread to the liver has occurred.[456,457]

The tumour usually arises as a polyp of yellowish hue, which often becomes ulcerated. Colonic carcinoids are more frequently malignant than rectal carcinoids.[458,459] The clinical presentation and treatment are the same as adenocarcinoma, but the prognosis is usually better.[460] Somatostatin analogues can successfully treat diarrhoea caused by metastatic carcinoid.

Primary malignant lymphoma

This tumour is also rare, accounting for only 0.1% of all malignant tumours of the large bowel. Malignant lymphomas occur more commonly in the caecum than in the left colon or rectum. The tumour may develop in patients with long-standing ulcerative colitis.

The degree of malignancy depends on the cell type and extent of spread at the time of diagnosis. Both Hodgkin's and non-Hodgkin's lymphomas can occur (see Chapter 34). Their clinical presentation is similar to adenocarcinomas. Radiotherapy and chemotherapy play an important adjuvant role to surgical excision, particularly when there is lymph node involvement. The large bowel may be secondarily infiltrated by lymphomas arising at other sites within the abdomen.

Leiomyosarcoma

These neoplasms which originate from the muscularis propria project either into the bowel lumen or on to its external surface. They are usually large, rubbery, lobulated tumours and half ulcerate through the overlying mucosa. Microscopically, they are often difficult to differentiate from their benign counterparts. Many pathologists believe that all tumours arising from the muscle coat should be labelled as smooth muscle tumours, and they should only be subsequently labelled as malignant or benign when their behaviour is known (see Chapter 54). The symptoms are similar to other tumours, but massive rectal haemorrhage is characteristic. Treatment is by surgical resection. Postoperative radiotherapy may prevent recurrence.

Other malignant tumours

Fibrosarcoma, haemangiopericytoma, plasmacytoma, endothelioma and malignant lymphomatous polyposis are very rare tumours of the large bowel.[459–464] Very occasionally a malignant melanoma or squamous cell carcinoma may arise in the colorectum, but these are much more common in the anal canal.

REFERENCES

445. Nicholls R J, York Mason A et al Br J Surg 1982; 69: 404–409
446. Hildebrandt U, Feifel G Dis Colon Rectum 1985; 28: 42–46
447. Stearn M, Deddish M et al Surg Gynecol Obstet 1974; 138: 584–586
448. Roswit B, Higgins G et al Cancer 1975; 35: 1597–1602
449. Gerard A, Berrod J L et al Cancer 1985; 55: 2373–2379
450. Frykholm G J, Glimelius B, Pahlman L Dis Colon Rectum 1993; 35: 564–572
451. Balslev I, Pedersen M et al Cancer 1986; 58: 22–28
452. GITSG N Engl J Med 1986; 315: 1294–1295
453. Wolmark N, Fisher B et al J Natl Cancer Inst 1988; 80: 30–36
454. Moertel C, Fleming T et al N Engl J Med 1990; 322: 352–358
455. Taylor I, Machind D et al Br J Surg 1985; 72: 359–363
456. Goligher J C Surgery of the Anus, Rectum and Colon, 4th edn. Baillière Tindall, London 1984
457. Peskin G W, Orloff M J Surg Gynecol Obstet 1959; 109: 673–678
458. Gabriel W B, Morson B C Proc R Soc Med 1956; 49: 472–477
459. Stout A P In: Turell R (ed) Diseases of the Colon and Anorectum, vol 1. W B Saunders, Philadelphia 1959
460. Orloff M J Cancer 1971; 28: 175–180
461. Morgan C N Proc R Soc Med 1932; 25: 1020–1025
462. Norbury L E C Proc R Soc Med 1952; 25: 1021–1026
463. Orda R, Bawbik J B et al Dis Colon Rectum 1976; 19: 626–631
464. Pack G T, Miller T R, Trinidad S S Dis Colon Rectum 1963; 6: 1–6

ANAL TUMOURS

Anal tumours are rare. Epidermoid squamous cancers, which are the most common type, only occur in only 300 new cases annually in the UK.[465]

BENIGN ANAL TUMOURS

Leiomyomas, lipomas and other mesodermal tumours can arise in the anal region.[466] The diagnosis should be confirmed by biopsy and treatment is by local excision.

MALIGNANT ANAL TUMOURS

Epidermoid tumours

This term refers to tumours variously known as squamous, basaloid, cloacogenic and transitional cell carcinomas. Neoplasms at the anal verge are more common in men, while tumours in the anal canal more frequently affect women. Evidence suggests that anal tumours occur more frequently in male homosexuals and are related to anal sexual practices.[467] Human papilloma virus has been shown to be associated with anal cancer in some cases.

These tumours present with bleeding, anal pain and discharge; sometimes a lump may be noticed by the patient. The tumour may look like a typical skin cancer, appearing as a raised ulcer or as an irregular plaque. It may have invaded the anal sphincters, or have spread upwards to involve the rectum. The inguinal nodes should be palpated for evidence of spread, although distant metastases are uncommon.

Operative excision is the standard treatment.[468,469] Tumours at the anorectal margin have been treated mainly by local excision, with around 50–60% of patients surviving for 5 years. Anal canal neoplasms, on the other hand, have usually been treated by radical anorectal excision, with about the same 5-year cure rates. In the past 20 years there has been mounting evidence that primary treatment by radiation alone with chemotherapy gives cure rates that are as good while avoiding a colostomy in most cases.[470]

Leucoplakia

Leucoplakia is a premalignant condition of the anorectum which is similar to the oral disorder (see Chapter 13). The firm white plaques may be circumscribed or confluent around the anus. Local excision often fails to prevent further disease and careful surveillance is required to detect invasive malignancy.

Malignant melanoma

This anal tumour is extremely rare. It presents as a pigmented lump, with bleeding and fluid discharge. The results of surgery are usually so poor that many feel palliative local excision is to be preferred to radical excision.

Lymphoma

This can arise in the anal region, usually as part of a generalized disease. More recently, in common with other rare tumours, it has been described as a complication of AIDS.[471]

Kaposi's sarcoma

This is now recognized as another complication of AIDS[472] and can cause rectal bleeding. Kaposi's sarcoma appears dark red and slightly raised; histology shows the typical haemangiomatous changes.

FUNCTIONAL DISORDERS OF THE LARGE BOWEL AND PELVIC FLOOR

There are a number of conditions in which symptoms arise from some failure of rectal function. Certain forms of constipation and diarrhoea in which no obstructive or inflammatory cause can be found are included. Abnormalities in intestinal transit or rectal capacitance are demonstrable in these patients. Abnormalities of the pelvic floor can cause incontinence, difficulty in evacuation, perineal discomfort and pain.

Conditions encompassed by the term 'functional disorders' are common and the physiological mechanisms that are responsible are largely unknown. Hirschsprung's disease, idiopathic slow transit constipation (Arbuthnot Lane's disease) and idiopathic megabowel have been recognized for many years; others such as the irritable bowel syndrome have only recently been defined.[473]

Pelvic floor disorders such as rectal prolapse and solitary rectal ulcer have been recognized for years, but the association between pudendal neuropathy and obstructed defecation has only recently been appreciated. This is really a syndrome and may occur in many functional disorders, which often appear to be inter-related.

These functional disorders are common and often cause great distress to patients. Investigations are now available which have enabled the nature of the disturbance to be identified in some cases. Many of these techniques are still however classified as research rather than clinical practice.

REFERENCES

465. OPCS 1983 HMSO London
466. Morson B C, Dawson I M P Gastrointestinal Pathology. Blackwell, Oxford 1990 p 754
467. Daling J R, Weiss N S et al N Engl J Med 1987; 317: 973–977
468. Greenall M J, Quan S H Q, DeCosse J J Br J Surg 1985; 72: S97–S103
469. Pinna Pintor M, Nicholls R J, Northover J M A Br J Surg 1989; 76: 806
470. Nigro N D Dis Colon Rectum 1984; 27: 736–766
471. Burkes R L, Meyer P R et al Arch Intern Med 1986; 146: 913
472. Stern J O, Deilerich D et al Gastroenterology 1982; 82: 118
473. Chaudhary N A, Truelove S C Q J Med 1962; 31: 307–322

Techniques of investigation

Colorectum

Intestinal transit can be estimated by following the passage of a known number of ingested radiopaque markers by plain radiographs. Delay is diagnosed when more than 80% of the markers are still present in the bowel after 5 days.[474] More frequent films taken during this period may localize the site of delayed transit in the colon.[475] Scintigraphy following insertion of a radionuclide marker in the caecum has also been used to study transit.[476]

Defecography may give useful information on a variety of functional abnormalities.[477] Spot films and videos are taken of the rectum during defecation after instillation of barium. The rate of emptying, the presence of internal prolapse, pelvic floor descent and spasm, and the size of the anorectal angle can be estimated by this method (Fig. 30.54). The changes seen on straining may however be difficult to interpret as some occur in normal subjects.[478] Dynamic defecography has been integrated with simultaneous pressure and electromyographic recordings of the anorectum.[479] The place of this technique in clinical practice has not yet been defined.

Rectal capacitance may be reduced in some patients with faecal urgency and can be estimated by distension of a balloon inserted per anum. In normal subjects the threshold of rectal sensation occurs at 20–60 ml of distension and the maximal tolerable volume ranges from 200 to 400 ml.

Pelvic floor

The pelvic floor musculature is both somatic and visceral. The somatic skeletal muscle includes the levator ani, the puborectalis and the external anal sphincter. These muscles are innervated by branches of the sacral plexus from segments S2 to S4. The levator muscles support the abdominal contents while the puborectalis is responsible for maintaining the anorectal angle at about 90°. The external sphincter contributes to anal canal closure. The internal sphincter, which is the splanchnic component, lies concentrically within the external sphincter and is continuous above with the circular smooth muscle of the rectum. The somatic component is in a constant state of tonic contraction maintained by muscle sphincter reflex activity.[480] Tone can be increased by voluntary contraction and sudden rises in intra-abdominal pressure, and is inhibited during defecation.[481,482] The internal sphincter is in a state of maximal contraction at rest and relaxes during defecation. Rectal distension produces a reflex relaxation of the internal sphincter. This is known as the rectosphincteric reflex,[483] which is mediated by nervous plexuses within the bowel wall.[484]

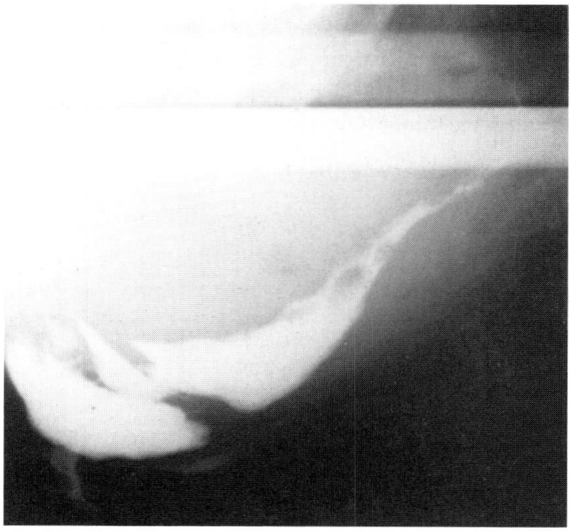

Fig 30.54 Defecating proctogram. Lateral view; the coccyx can be seen to the right, highlighting the gross perineal descent during straining.

Manometry

The pressure in the anal canal can be measured by a balloon probe, an open-tip tube or a directly inserted pressure transducer connected to a suitable recording device.[485] The resting pressure in normal individuals lies between 50 and 100 cm of water, 80% of which is derived from internal sphincter activity.[486] On voluntary contraction the anal pressure increases by 60–120 cm water, entirely caused by external sphincter activity. The resting anal pressure is low where the sphincters are weak. A low voluntary contraction pressure indicates a weak external sphincter.

The rectosphincteric reflex is elicited by inflation of a balloon (100–200 mm diameter) in the rectum while simultaneously measuring anal canal pressure. On rectal distension a sudden fall in anal pressure occurs followed by a slow spontaneous rise towards the basal level over a few seconds. This reflex is absent in Hirschsprung's disease.[487]

Other tests

The electromyographic activity of the somatic pelvic floor can be recorded using needle electrodes placed through the perianal skin. This technique is mainly used to assess if there is any neuromuscular denervation of the pelvic floor skeletal muscle by estimating the fibre density.[488] It may also be useful in locating residual func-

REFERENCES

474. Hinton J M, Lennard-Jones J E, Young A C Gut 1969; 10: 842–847
475. Kuijpers J H C, Bleijenberg G, de Morree H Int J Colorectal Dis 1986; 1: 44–48
476. Kamm M A, Thompson D G et al Gut 1987; 28: A1365
477. Mahieu P, Pringot J, Bodart P Gastrointest Radiol 1984; 9: 253–261
478. Shorvon P J, McHugh S et al Gut 1987; 28: A1361–1362
479. Womack N R, Williams N S et al Dis Colon Rectum 1987; 30: 319
480. Floyd W F, Walls E W J Physiol Lond 1953; 122: 599–609
481. Parks A G, Porter N H, Melzack J Dis Colon Rectum 1962; 5: 407–414
482. Porter N H Ann R Coll Surg Engl 1962; 31: 379–404
483. Gowers W R Proc R Soc (Lond) 1877; 26: 77–84
484. Lubowski D Z, Nicholls R J et al Br J Surg 1987; 74: 668–670
485. Miller R, Bartolo D C C et al Br J Surg 1988; 75: 40–43
486. Bennett R C, Duthie H L Br J Surg 1964; 51: 335–357
487. Lawson J O N, Nixon H H J Paediat Surg 1967; 2: 544
488. Stalberg E, Thiele B J Neurol Neurosurg Psychiatry 1979; 38: 874–880

tioning muscle in congenital anomalies or injuries of the pelvic floor. Estimation of the latency of conduction of the pudendal nerve[489] and of the spinal cord and cauda equina[490] also gives information on denervation. Incontinent patients have a reduced sensory awareness to electrical and thermal stimulation of the anal canal.[491,492] An objective test of continence has been described in which a constant-rate saline infusion is given into the rectum and the volume at which leakage occurs is measured.[493]

CHRONIC CONSTIPATION

Constipation is a symptom which surgeons tend to treat with levity; although Arbuthnot Lane[494] described the use of radical surgery to alleviate its more extreme forms, today most would regard this as over-zealous. Yet undoubtedly there are patients with severe intractable constipation who deserve the attention of the surgeon. Some are found on investigation to be suffering from Hirschsprung's disease; others, while having no evidence of aganglionosis, have a megacolon demonstrated on radiological investigation. The remainder, with normal macroanatomy and ample ganglia, are the group most likely to be labelled as having a psychosomatic or frankly psychiatric abnormality, yet this is a group in which surgery may sometimes have a role. The label 'idiopathic slow-transit constipation' has been used if all defined causes of constipation have been excluded and the symptoms continue despite an adequate high-fibre diet.[495] This may be confirmed using a 'shapes study'; the patient is asked to swallow 20 radiopaque markers and is then radiographed on the fifth day. Passage of less than 80% of the markers by this time is considered abnormal. Typically the patient is a young adult female with a variable past history. Some can trace their symptoms back to childhood, while others remember that symptoms started at puberty or following a hysterectomy. Bowel evacuation without strong laxatives is often very infrequent, perhaps once every several weeks. In addition the patient may complain of abdominal discomfort and bloating. Physiological investigations may demonstrate a pathological inability to pass a balloon inflated in the rectum[496] or there may be a paradoxical contraction of puborectalis detected by electromyography during straining.[497] These findings suggest an abnormality in the defecatory mechanism, though attempts to alleviate this by division of puborectalis have been generally unsuccessful.[498,499]

Initially treatment should consist of the regular use of osmotic laxatives such as magnesium sulphate. Patients whose lives continue to be made miserable by their symptoms should be offered a total colectomy and ileorectal anastomosis. This results in a significant improvement of constipation in 60–70% but in the remainder diarrhoea may occur and the abdominal pain and bloating are not relieved.[500] Lesser procedures, such as sigmoid colectomy in those with a 'redundant' sigmoid colon, or subtotal colectomy and caecorectal anastomosis, have generally failed to provide any benefit. Anorectal myectomy has also produced uncertain long-term results.[501] A better understanding of the pathophysiology of these problems should lead to better treatment.

RECTAL PROLAPSE

Rectal prolapse may be either complete or partial. In complete prolapse all layers of the rectum descend through the anal canal, whereas in partial prolapse only the rectal mucosa protrudes. Rectal prolapse is usually associated with haemorrhoids.

Complete rectal prolapse

There is an increased incidence in infancy, declining to a low level after 1 year, which is maintained throughout adult life until the age of 75. During these years the sex ratio is apparently equal but in old age, when the condition is much more common, females are affected 20 times more often than males.[502]

The two factors that appear to favour the development of rectal prolapse are increased rectal and colonic mobility and weakness of the pelvic floor musculature. A deep rectovaginal or rectovesical pouch, extensive peritoneal covering of the lateral aspect of the rectum and even the presence of a rectal mesentery may be seen at laparotomy.[503] The rectosigmoid and sigmoid colon are usually redundant. Patients with neurological diseases affecting the pelvic floor muscles sometimes develop prolapse and in many other patients it is possible to show evidence of neuropathic changes in the neuromuscular axis of the puborectalis and external and sphincter by testing motor unit fibre density and pudendal nerve conduction latency.[504] Progressive neuropathic pelvic floor weakness is a normal process occurring after the age of 65 but may also result from obstetric injury and possibly from chronic straining.[505]

Straining in itself may be an independent aetiological factor.[506,507] Often patients with prolapse give a history of long-standing chronic constipation. Some, particularly in the younger age group, are mentally defective or have personality disorders[508] and are prone to episodes of faecal impaction, perhaps exacerbated

REFERENCES

489. Kiff E S, Swash M Br J Surg 1984; 71: 614–616
490. Merton P A, Hill D K et al Lancet 1982; ii: 597–600
491. Roe A M, Bartolo D C C, Mortensen J N McC Br J Surg 1986; 73: 310–312
492. Miller R, Bartolo D C C et al Br J Surg 1987; 74: 511–515
493. Read N W, Harford W V et al Gastroenterology 1979; 76: 747–756
494. Lane W A The Operative Treatment of Chronic Constipation. Nisbet, London 1909
495. Hinton J M, Lennard-Jones J E, Young A C Gut 1969; 10: 842–847
496. Barnes P R H, Lennard-Jones J E Gut 1985; 26: 1049–1052
497. Preston D M Br J Surg 1985; 72: S8–S10
498. Barnes P R H, Hawley P R et al Br J Surg 1985; 72: 475–477
499. Kamm M A, Hawley P R, Lennard-Jones J E Br J Surg 1988; 75: 661–663
500. Kamm M A Int J Colorectal Dis 1987; 4: 229
501. Yoshioka K, Keighley M R B Br J Surg 1987; 74: 373–376
502. Kupfer C A, Goligher J C Br J Surg 1970; 57: 34
503. Moschcowitz A V Surg Gynecol Obstet 1912; 15: 7
504. Neill M E, Parks A G, Swash M Br J Surg 1981; 68: 531–536
505. Snooks S J, Swash M et al Lancet 1984; ii: 546–555
506. Porter N H Ann R Coll Surg Engl 1962; 31: 379–404
507. Parks A G, Swash M, Urich H Gut 1977; 18: 656–665
508. Altemeier W A, Cuthbertson W R et al Ann Surg 1971; 173: 993–1006

by the constipating effects of antidepressants. There is an association between rectal prolapse and the solitary ulcer syndrome in which difficulty in defecation and straining are major aetiological factors.[509] In infants excessive straining is often encouraged by parents. Prolapse can occur from sliding of the anterior rectal wall[503] or by intussusception of the upper rectum. Cine contrast proctography has shown that both mechanisms are probably involved.[510] The apex of the prolapse may become ulcerated and mucus production from the irritated mucosa is increased. Histological changes are identical with those seen in the solitary ulcer syndrome. Usually the prolapse reduces spontaneously but it can very occasionally become incarcerated, when strangulation and gangrene may develop.

Clinical features

In infants, the prolapse is usually noticed by the parent and may be accompanied by the passage of blood and mucus. The child may be wasted, but in most cases is normally developed. Prolapse in infants can be distinguished on digital examination from intussusception, in which the finger enters the rectum lateral to the intussuscipiens. Adults complain of the presence of the prolapsing mass itself, the passage of blood and mucus, and faecal incontinence (Fig. 30.55). The prolapse may descend only during defecation and reduce spontaneously afterwards but in more severe cases it occurs on standing or walking and sometimes it is permanently present. About half the patients have some degree of faecal incontinence, this is more common in the older patient.[511–513] Any history of previous obstetric or spinal trauma should be sought and a careful history of bowel function obtained.

The mental state of the patient should be noted and signs of neurological disease and perineal trauma must be carefully excluded. The diagnosis is made on inspection. Often it is necessary to ask the patient to strain down to demonstrate the prolapse. This may only be possible when the patient stands. Rarely the prolapse may become irreducible and strangulated.[514] Signs of pelvic floor weakness are usually present and include abnormal perineal descent on straining, poor voluntary contraction of the levators, puborectalis and external sphincter, and a poor anorectal angle, all of which are evident on digital examination. A patulous anus, seen on gently parting the anal verge, indicates a defective internal sphincter. Sigmoidoscopy is essential in all patients to exclude a coexisting carcinoma.

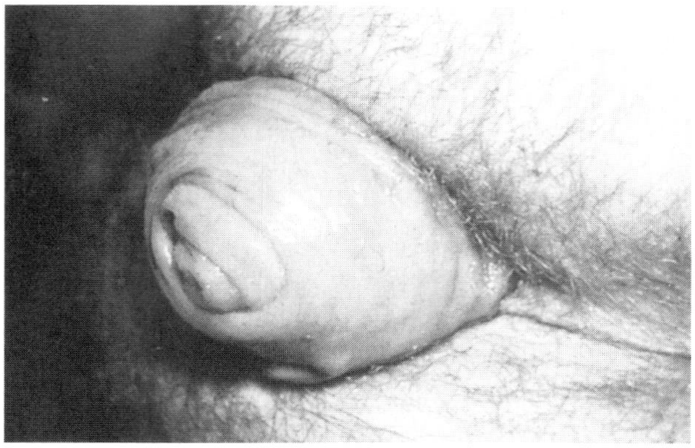

Fig 30.55 Full-thickness rectal prolapse.

Rectal prolapse can be simulated by other anorectal disorders including haemorrhoids, mucosal prolapse and low rectal polyps. Reddening of the rectal mucosa seen on sigmoidoscopy may be caused by inflammatory bowel disease and a biopsy should then be taken.

Treatment

Infants can almost always be treated successfully by correct bowel training. The parent should pot the child regularly for short periods and a mild laxative may be prescribed to avoid straining. The prolapse should be digitally replaced when it occurs. In a few children where this management fails, submucous injection of a sclerosant such as phenol in arachis oil may be effective. In principle, however, treatment should be conservative.

In adults rectal prolapse should be treated surgically. The numerous operations which have been described can be classified according to their aims. These are simple excision of the protruding bowel, improvement of the anal sphincter mechanism or fixation of the rectum. Rectosigmoidectomy is the best example of the first.[515] The prolapse is delivered and excised via a perineal approach. The bowel is anastomosed outside the anus, before being reduced. Delorme's procedure is similar but only the mucosa of the prolapse is resected. The operation is well tolerated even by the frailest patient, although the recurrence rate is high (60%) and as a consequence of this the operation has fallen from favour. Combined rectosigmoidectomy with a pelvic floor repair has a much lower recurrence rate,[508,516] suggesting that this operation should be re-evaluated. Repair of the pelvic floor sphincter mechanism alone or insertion of a Thiersch wire to encircle the anus has high recurrence rates (20–40%). The latter procedure can also cause difficulty in evacuation and the wire may become infected. For these reasons it has largely been discarded.

The treatment of choice at present for a fit patient is an abdominal rectopexy. This operation is well tolerated in the elderly and involves mobilization of the rectum followed by fixation. Many methods of fixation have been described. Some use an implant of foreign material, for example polyvinyl alcohol (Ivalon), polypropylene (Marlex) or polyfluorine (Teflon) to provoke fibrosis around the rectum. Fixation can be lateral,[517] posterior[518]

REFERENCES

509. Kennedy D K, Hughes E S R, Masterton J P Surg Gynecol Obstet 1977; 144: 718–720
510. Broden B, Snellman B Dis Colon Rectum 1968; 11: 330–347
511. Morgan C N, Porter N H, Klugman D J Br J Surg 1972; 59: 841
512. Holmstrom B, Ahlberg J et al Acta Chir Scand 1978; 482 (suppl): 51
513. Keighley M R B, Fielding J W L, Alexander-Williams J Br J Surg 1983; 70: 229–232
514. Neve C R Br J Surg 1953; 41: 221
515. Gabriel W B The Principles and Practice of Rectal Surgery, 4th edn. H K Lewis, London 1948
516. Watts J D, Rothenberger D A et al Dis Colon Rectum 1985; 28: 96–102
517. Loygue J, Huguier M et al Br J Surg 1971; 58: 847
518. Wells C Proc R Soc Med 1959; 82: 602–603

(Fig. 30.56) or anterior.[519] Infection of the implant is rare (< 5%) but it is a serious complication and antibiotic cover is obligatory. Recurrence rates of around 5% have been reported.

For posterior rectopexy, a midline incision is made and the abdominal contents inspected taking care to exclude a carcinoma. The redundant sigmoid colon is mobilized and, following division of the peritoneum on each side of the rectum, the plane between rectum and presacral fascia is entered with identification of the presacral nerves. Dissection is continued down to beyond the top of the coccyx and the lateral ligaments are divided. A sheet of polypropylene mesh measuring 12 × 6 cm is sutured in the midline to the pelvic floor anterior to the coccyx and the sacral periosteum just below the promontory. The tension is adjusted so that it forms a bowstring-like sheet across the sacral curvature. The lateral edges are then wrapped around the rectum which is pulled cephalad under moderate tension. Sutures are placed between the implant and the rectum on each side leaving about a quarter of the circumference of the rectum free anteriorly. The peritoneum is closed over the implant and the abdomen is closed. Laparoscopic methods of rectopexy are being developed but the long-term results of this approach are not yet known.

An alternative abdominal procedure involving a similar mobilization and fixation of the rectum followed by resection of the sigmoid has been described.[520] The results have been excellent with a recurrence rate of less than 5%. It has been claimed that this procedure avoids constipation,[521] which is said to occur in some cases of abdominal rectopexy.[522] Fixation of the rectum using a perineal approach to insert an implant[523] or plicate the protruding prolapse[524] is well tolerated by patients too frail for an abdominal procedure. Postoperative constipation must be avoided in all cases by suitable laxative administration. Continence is improved in 50–75% of patients following an abdominal rectopexy.[525,526]

Partial (mucosal) prolapse

Mucosal prolapse of the lower rectum may be overt, when it emerges from the anus, or it may be occult, when it is only detectable by proctoscopy. As a result the condition is often associated with prolapsing haemorrhoids and also with abnormal perineal descent and uterine prolapse in females. Only rarely is mucosal prolapse a precursor of complete rectal prolapse.[527] In many patients mucosal prolapse is one feature of the descending perineum syndrome which shares the clinical features described below.[528]

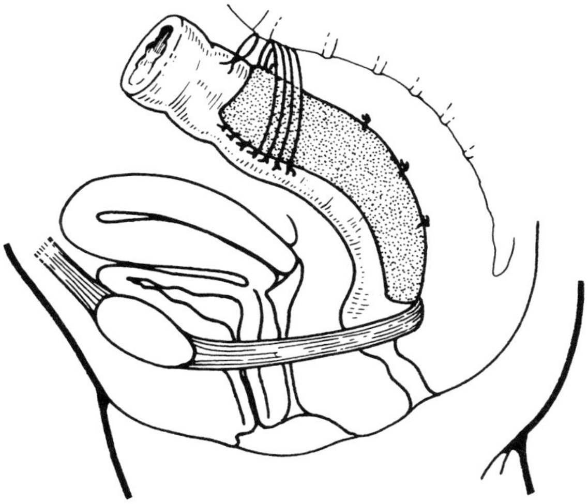

Fig 30.56 Wells' operation, or Ivalon rectopexy.

Clinical features

The symptoms are the same as those caused by haemorrhoids and include bleeding, a protruding swelling, pruritus ani, anal discomfort and mucus leakage. The discomfort is often described as a heaviness in the perineum akin to a feeling of incomplete evacuation. A similar sensation occurs in patients with the solitary ulcer syndrome. It is not known whether this symptom is caused by the mucosal prolapse itself or by the associated perineal descent. Some patients admit to straining at stool and there may be an evacuation disorder in these cases. The prolapse may be seen on direct inspection of the perineum but is more likely to be evident on proctoscopy. There is a tendency to overdiagnose the condition as the lower rectal mucosa is often somewhat redundant and can be persuaded to descend into the proctoscope when the patient is asked to strain. The prolapsing mucosa may be reddened and is occasionally ulcerated. Sometimes there is obvious mucus secretion from the surface. Anal sphincter weakness and perineal descent are present in many cases, as are haemorrhoids.

Treatment

The treatment involves correction of associated constipation by laxatives or suppositories. The nature of the condition should be explained to the patient who should be advised against straining. Injection or rubber band ligation of the prolapse may improve the symptoms of bleeding and mucus discharge. Symptoms appear to be episodic in most cases but a small group of patients (about 10%) develop a progressive deterioration with persisting discomfort, increasing perineal descent and sphincter weakness. A few of these may be alleviated by an extended haemorrhoidectomy. Management should, whenever possible, remain conservative.

REFERENCES

519. Ripstein C B Dis Colon Rectum 1975; 18: 458–460
520. Frykman H M, Goldberg S M Surg Gynecol Obstet 1969; 129: 1225–1230
521. Watts J D, Rothenberger D A et al Dis Colon Rectum 1985; 28: 96–102
522. Mann C V, Hoffman C Br J Surg 1988; 75: 34–37
523. Wyatt A P Br J Surg 1981; 68: 717–719
524. Delorme R Bull Soc Chirurg Paris 1900; 26: 459
525. Keighley M R B, Fielding J W L, Alexander Williams J Br J Surg 1983; 70: 229–232
526. Watts J D, Rothenberger D A, Goldberg S M In: Henry M M, Swash M (eds) Coloproctology and the Pelvic Floor. Butterworths, London 1985 pp 326–328
527. Allen-Mersh T G, Henry M M, Nicholls R J Br J Surg 1987; 74: 679
528. Parks A G, Porter N H, Hardcastle J D Proc R Soc Med 1966; 59: 477–482

SOLITARY ULCER SYNDROME

Although described in the 19th century by Cruveilhier,[529] the solitary ulcer syndrome was first defined clearly by Madigan & Morson in 1969.[530] At about the same time, Ihre[531] reported a series of patients with internal procidentia of the rectum. There is now reason to believe that these two accounts may be describing the same disorder. The condition is rare in general surgical practice. The incidence is estimated to be 1/100 000 population per year on the basis of 51 cases presenting over a 10-year period in Northern Ireland.[532] The condition most commonly affects young adults, although the age range extends from childhood to old age. The peak incidence in the third to fourth decades of life corresponds with the first peak in the incidence of rectal prolapse, the second of which occurs in old age.

There is clinical, radiological and histological evidence to link the solitary ulcer syndrome with rectal prolapse. Both complete and mucosal rectal prolapse have been reported to occur in 16–60% of patients with a solitary ulcer,[530,532,533] proctographic studies have demonstrated a rectal intussusception to be a common finding (between 70% and 58%) in patients with a solitary ulcer syndrome.[534,535] A study of 9 patients[536] investigated by proctography integrated with simultaneous measurements of pelvic floor electromyography and intrarectal pressure demonstrated proctographic abnormalities in 8 of the patients. These included anterior rectal wall prolapse in 2, intra-anal and extra-anal intussusception in 3 and complete rectal prolapse in 3. In another study[537] cine radiography was carried out in 1397 patients with symptoms of obstructive defecation, inadequate emptying, incontinence and/or bleeding 292 of these had a rectal intussusception and 211 a rectal prolapse. 190 patients with rectal intussusception were reviewed in detail, of whom 57% had obstructive symptoms, 43% pelvic pain and 27% bleeding. It seems likely that many of these patients had solitary ulcer syndrome.

The aetiology of the condition, however, is still unknown. There is undoubtedly a disorder of defecation which leads to a vicious circle of straining, producing internal prolapse and further difficulty in defecation, leading on to further straining. Many of these patients have been shown to have a paradoxical contraction of the puborectalis on straining.[538] The aetiology of this is not known. In a more recent study, a paradoxical contraction was present in 60% of patients studied,[539] but half the patients studied had evidence of partial denervation of the external sphincter. The inference was that prolonged straining over many years had led to secondary weakness of the pelvic floor. Histological abnormalities found in the solitary ulcer syndrome include obliteration of the lamina propria by fibroblasts and muscle fibres from the muscularis mucosae, reactive hyperplasia and mucin depletion within the tubules. These are identical to the changes seen in complete rectal prolapse.[538]

Almost all patients complain of bleeding (> 90%) and the passage of mucus (70–90%). Some also have pain (20%) and many report episodes of incontinence (57%). One of the most notable symptoms, however, is that of difficulty with evacuation, which on detailed questioning may have preceded the other symptoms. Although only about 40–50% of patients in Madigan & Morson's[530] original series had an abnormal bowel habit, it seems that there is a history of straining at stool with a feeling of incomplete evacuation in the majority of patients. Although patients' bowels may be open daily, it is not uncommon to find this to be the result of many visits to the lavatory with long periods spent there on each occasion. A persistent desire to defecate is common. Abdominal symptoms of the irritable bowel syndrome can also be present,

The term solitary ulcer is inaccurate as the pathological abnormalities may be multiple[530,532] and ulceration is not always present. Redness and oedema of the mucosa varying in length from a few millimetres to several centimetres are present in all cases, and may be the only physical sign in about 20%. In over half, however, frank ulceration occurs and in a further 20% the mucosa is elevated to give a polypoid appearance which is easily mistaken for a carcinoma. The majority (more than 60%) of ulcers lie anteriorly at 7–10 cm from the anal verge, often on the fold of a valve of Houston.

Conservative treatment includes the prescription of laxatives and advice to avoid straining. Explanation and suppositories are supplied. In a review of 34 patients treated between 1974 and 1984 at one hospital, no fewer than 10 different treatments had been used. Local treatment by rubber band ligation, cryosurgery and local excision gave poor results. 5 patients treated by defunctioning colostomy and 5 by anterior resection failed to improve. 13 patients were treated by a postanal repair, of whom 4 seemed to be improved. A posterior rectopexy improved 3 out of 10. Both patients who underwent total rectal excision were cured.[540] These poor results suggest that a combination of anterior and posterior rectopexy to prevent presumed intussusception of the most common site of ulceration might be the best option. About two thirds of patients were helped by this procedure[541] but constipation occurred postoperatively in about 10% of cases. The results were similar to those obtained by Johansson et al[537] using a similar operation.

FAECAL INCONTINENCE

Anal incontinence is defined as the involuntary loss of control of flatus or faeces. It can be subdivided into three orders of severity—incontinence to flatus only, to fluid faeces, and to solid faeces. Continence depends on the competence of the anal sphincter mechism. This serves two main functions: first the maintenance of the anorectal angle at rest by the forward pull of the puborectalis, and secondly closure of the anal canal by the combined action of

REFERENCES

529. Cruveilhier J In: Anatomie Pathologique du Corps Humain. Vol 2, Maladies du Rectum. J B Baillière, Paris 1870
530. Madigan M R, Morson B C Gut 1969; 10: 871–881
531. Ihre T Scand J Gastroenterol 1972; 7: 643–646
532. Martin C J, Parks T G, Biggart J D Br J Surg 1981; 68: 744–757
533. Schweiger M, Alexander-Williams J Lancet 1977; i: 70–71
534. Mahieu P H G Int J Colorectal Dis 1986; 1: 85–90
535. Kuijpers H C, Schreve R H, Hoedemakers H Dis Colon Rectum 1986; 29: 126–129
536. Womack N R, Williams N S et al Dis Colon Rectum 1987; 30: 319–323
537. Johansson C, Ihre T, Ahlback S Dis Colon Rectum 1985; 28: 920–924

31 The liver and portal circulation

I. S. Benjamin S. Papagrigoriadis

ANATOMY

Understanding of the surgery of the liver and portal circulation must be based on a thorough knowledge of the detailed anatomy of the liver, its blood supply and venous drainage. This account will inevitably overlap with the details of biliary anatomy covered in a previous chapter.

The obvious surface markings of the liver which divide it into the anatomical right and left lobes conceal a system of liver segments divided vertically by the scissuras occupied by the right, middle and left hepatic veins. Within each of the four resulting sectors of liver there is a segmental arrangement defined by the portal and arterial blood supply. This system of eight liver segments has now been universally adopted following its definition by the French surgical anatomist Couinaud,[1] and is illustrated in Figure 31.1. This is important because each liver segment is for practical purposes structurally independent, and resection of major parts of the liver is possible provided that whole segments with their associated blood supply, biliary apparatus and venous drainage can be left intact. These are sufficient to support life during the process of regeneration. Although the size of the liver segments is variable there is little variation in their arrangement. This is not true of the biliary tree, particularly around the region of the confluence of the main segmental hepatic ducts, and knowledge of these variations is important during major liver and biliary surgery.

There are important variations in the arrangement of hepatic venous drainage, which must be taken into account when planning liver resection. The right hepatic vein may be a single large trunk or may consist of two or more smaller vessels. In particular the possibility of a prominent inferior right hepatic vein draining directly into the vena cava via a very short trunk from the back of segment VI is important. It is often possible to isolate a sufficient length of right hepatic vein outside the liver to allow separate control of this vessel during resection of the right lobe of the liver. The junction between the left and middle hepatic veins, and the inferior vena cava is not constant and must be carefully defined during resections involving the left lobe of the liver. The caudate lobe (segment I) drains directly into the vena cava through a variable number of short veins, and this is important in the Budd–Chiari syndrome (see below). There are numerous anomalies of the extrahepatic portal venous system which result from variations in embryonic development. These range from a pre-duodenal portal vein which is often associated with malrotation of the bowel, situs inversus and polysplenia, through duplication of the portal vein, to abnormal direct communications with the great vessels in the mediastinum. A pre-duodenal portal vein is found in 4% of infants with biliary atresia.[2]

LIVER PHYSIOLOGY

The liver has a wide variety of functions and liver disease not surprisingly has many manifestations. The functions of the liver include metabolism of carbohydrates, lipids, protein and vitamins, production of bile, detoxification of numerous blood-borne substances, both exogenous and endogenous, and immune function via the fixed reticuloendothelial system of Kupffer cells. Furthermore the control of liver blood flow is complex and is significantly affected by parenchymal liver disease and liver tumours. It is not surprising therefore that there is no one test of 'liver function' and the term 'liver function tests' ('LFTs') covers a wide variety of investigations used for different purposes. The most commonly performed tests include serum bilirubin, which is a measure of conjugation and excretion of bile pigment; alkaline phosphatase, an enzyme associated with cholestasis; and the transaminases alanine aminotransferase (ALT) and aspartate aminotransferase (AST), which are elevated by hepatocellular necrosis. γ-Glutamyl transpeptidase (γ-glutamyl transferase, GGT) provides a sensitive measure of enzyme induction including that associated with alcohol abuse. Albumin is a measure of hepatocellular protein synthesis, as is the prothrombin time. This range of tests gives a broad picture of underlying liver pathology, though a spectrum of results is rarely specific for a single pathological activity.[3] They are nonetheless important and are considered in more detail below.

Bilirubin

Unconjugated bilirubin is the main breakdown product of the haem moiety of haemoglobin and is derived mostly from effete

REFERENCES

1. Couinaud Le foie. Etudes anatomiques et chirurgicales. Masson, Paris 1957
2. Howard E R In: Howard E R (ed) Surgery of Liver Disease in Children. Oxford: Butterworth-Heinneman, Oxford 1991
3. Preisig R, Tygstrup N, Price C In: Millward S-GH, Wright I R, Arthur M P J (eds) Wright's Liver and Biliary Disease, 3rd edn. Saunders, London 1992

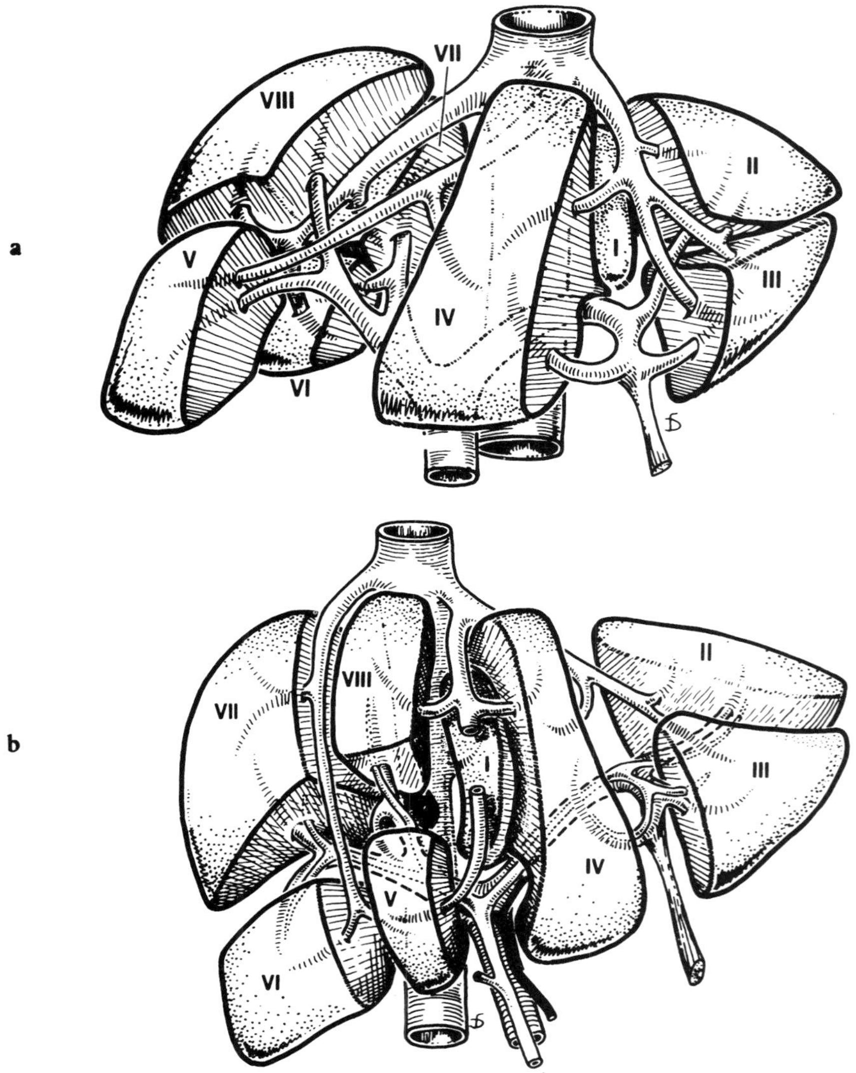

Fig. 31.1 Functional division of the liver and liver segments according to Couinaud's nomenclature: (a) as seen in the patient (b) in the ex vivo position. From Blumgart L H (ed) *Surgery of the Liver and Biliary Tract*. Churchill Livingstone, reproduced by permission of the publishers.

erythrocytes. Unconjugated bilirubin is insoluble in water and is transported bound to albumin in the plasma. Unconjugated bilirubin is transported across the hepatocyte membrane by a carrier protein, where it is bound to glutathione transferases, enters the endoplasmic reticulum and is conjugated to bilirubin monoglucuronide and bilirubin diglucuronide. These water-soluble conjugated moieties are then excreted by another carrier into the biliary canalicular lumen. Routine bilirubin measurement estimates total bilirubin, but in some circumstances it is useful to measure conjugated and unconjugated bilirubin separately.[4] *Unconjugated* hyperbilirubinaemia is caused by overproduction of bilirubin usually as a result of haemolytic disease such as congenital spherocytosis. It may also be caused by decreased hepatocyte uptake during sepsis and some drug reactions or decreased conjugation caused by some drug reactions, jaundice of prematurity, cirrhosis, hepatitis and Gilbert's syndrome. An increase of *conjugated* bilirubin may be the result of decreased secretion which can be caused by drug reactions, cirrhosis, hepatitis, cholestasis of pregnancy or Dubin–Johnson syndrome but more often is the result of biliary obstruction. The conjugated and unconjugated fractions of bilirubin are sometimes referred to as 'direct' and 'indirect', respectively, referring to former use of the van den Bergh reaction. Excess conjugated bilirubin in the urine results from extra- or intrahepatic biliary obstruction, and produces the dark urine of

REFERENCE

4. Zimmerman H, Richen J In: Blumgart L H (ed) Surgery of the Liver and Biliary Tract, 2nd edn: Churchill Livingstone, Edinburgh 1994

obstructive jaundice. In contrast, excessive urobilinogen in the urine implies increased load or failure of extraction. Jaundice becomes clinically apparent when the plasma bilirubin reaches 50 μmol/l, which is two to three times the upper limit of normal.

Alkaline phosphatase

Alkaline phosphatase is an enzyme which is present in liver, bone, intestine, placenta, kidney and white blood cells. Isoenzyme estimation differentiates alkaline phosphatase of hepatic and skeletal origin, although this is rarely performed. Simultaneous elevation of other liver-specific enzymes such as 5′-nucleotidase or GGT is indicative of a liver disorder. An increase in the serum alkaline phosphatase in hepatobiliary disease occurs because of stimulation of synthesis at the canalicular membrane, possibly by increased bile acids associated with biliary obstruction or stasis. It is a very sensitive marker of biliary obstruction, even when this is intermittent or incomplete, but it is also elevated in patients with space-occupying lesions in the liver.

γ-Glutamyl transpeptidase

This enzyme is also found in a number of other organs, but not in bone, increasing the diagnostic specificity of an elevated alkaline phosphatase. GGT activity is induced by a variety of drugs, including ethanol, and it may be significantly elevated even after a single episode of over-indulgence. In combination with a raised transaminase and increased erythrocyte volume (MCV), it is a sensitive though non-specific indicator of chronic alcohol abuse. *5′-Nucleotidase* is less commonly used these days, but is more specific than alkaline phosphatase in detecting liver disease.

Transaminases

The alanine and aspartate aminotransferases are intracellular enzymes. Aspartate aminotransferase is also found in other tissues, including the heart, skeletal muscle and kidney, while alanine aminotransferase is relatively specific for the liver. Both are significantly elevated in the presence of hepatocyte necrosis, though there is no direct relationship with the degree of functional liver impairment. Very high values are found in acute hepatitis and high levels in the absence of raised alkaline phosphatase suggest a hepatocellular rather than an obstructive cause for jaundice. The use of this phenomenon in differentiating 'surgical' from 'medical' jaundice becomes less reliable as the duration of the jaundice increases, when a mixed enzyme picture is frequently found.

Albumin

This protein is synthesized exclusively by hepatocytes and is therefore an indicator of their function. It is more useful in defining chronic malfunction as it has a half-life in the serum of 20 days.

Clotting factors

The liver is the major synthetic site for all coagulation proteins except von Willebrand's factor. The synthesis of factors II, VII, VIII and X is dependent on normal liver function and on adequate vitamin K levels. As vitamin K is fat soluble, deficiency develops in the presence of biliary obstruction with fat malabsorption. In vitamin K deficiency, a number of protein precursors known as PIVKA (protein induced by vitamin K absence or antagonists) can be detected in the plasma and these are sometimes used as specific markers for this deficiency. The prothrombin time must always be checked before invasive procedures are undertaken in patients with suspected liver disease. Parenteral administration of vitamin K usually corrects deficiencies caused by biliary obstruction, but is not effective in patients with prolonged or severe hepatocellular disease.[5]

Dynamic tests of liver function

All of the above tests are static indicators of individual components of liver function but more sensitive informa-tion may be obtained by quantitative or semi-quantitative dynamic tests.

Clearance tests

Antipyrine and aminopyrine are related minor analgesics and antipyretics, and their metabolism and clearance are associated with function of cytochrome P450, which may be profoundly affected by both biliary obstruction and hepatocellular disease. Aminopyrine metabolism is assessed by a breath test after administering [^{14}C]aminopyrine.[6] Antipyrine clearance is measured by its activity in plasma or saliva following intravenous administration, but requires high-pressure liquid chromatography for its measurement. This test may be a predictor of outcome in patients with obstructive jaundice.[7]

Caffeine clearance

This is also dependent on cytochrome P450, but it differs somewhat from the metabolism of aminopyrine/antipyrine. It has not been widely used, but has been shown to detect complications following liver transplantation.[8]

Lignocaine clearance (MEGX) test

Lignocaine clearance is flow dependent, but its breakdown to its main metabolite monoethylglycinexylide (MEGX) is dependent on hepatocellular function. It has been used to predict the outcome of liver transplantation when performed on liver donors, and may be a good short-term prognostic indicator in patients with cirrhosis awaiting transplantation.[9]

REFERENCES

5. Harrison P M, O'Grady J G, Keays R T, Alexander G J, Williams R Br Med J 1990; 301: 964–966
6. Gill R A, Goodman M W, Golfus G R, Onstad G R, Bubrick M P Ann Surg 1993; 198: 701–704
7. McPherson G A D, Benjamin I S, Boobis A R, Blumgart L H Am J Surg 1985; 149: 140–143
8. Nagel R, Dirix L, Hayllar K, Preisig R, Tredger J, Williams R J Hepatol 1990; 10: 144–148

Galactose clearance

This is a measure of metabolic capacity of the liver, although used in low doses it is flow dependent and may simply be a measure of liver blood flow.[10] The *maximum rate of urea synthesis* (MRUS) has been used by some for identi-fying patients at risk of encephalopathy following shunt surgery.[11] *Arterial ammonia* levels are sometimes measured in patients with suspected liver failure and portal systemic encephalopathy.[12]

Dye clearance tests

Sulphobromophthalein and indocyanine green are organic anionic dyes extracted by the hepatocytes. Sulphobromophthalein is rarely used because it can cause severe anaphylactic reactions, but indocyanine green is not metabolized and is rapidly cleared by the normal liver with very little extrahepatic extraction. It can be measured in various ways, including half-life, 15-minute retention, or more complex dynamic measurements, and has been used to predict complications after hepatic resection and rejection after liver transplantation.[13]

Other tests used in liver disease

Reliable markers for hepatitis A, B and C are now available and are important in patients with suspected liver disease. Antimitochondrial, antinuclear and anti-smooth muscle antibodies are used to investigate suspected primary biliary cirrhosis and autoimmune chronic active hepatitis. Iron, iron-binding capacity and serum ferritin are used in the diagnosis of haemochromatosis. Caeruloplasmin and urinary copper are used to diagnose Wilson's disease, and α_1-antitrypsin is also measured when deficiency of this enzyme is suspected.

Scoring systems in liver disease

Specific scoring systems have been used to predict the progression of certain conditions such as primary biliary cirrhosis and sclerosing cholangitis, and to predict when transplantation will be required. Probably the most commonly used scoring system for liver disease in general is the Child's grading system, modified by Pugh[14] (see Table 31.1). Originally designed to predict mortality and encephalopathy following portal-systemic shunting it has been extended to evaluate 'liver function'. Child's original system included a non-specific assessment of the nutritional status of the patient, but this has been replaced in Pugh's modification by measuring the prothrombin time. It must be said that this system has stood the test of time and remains the most commonly used general grading system for liver disease.

Table 31.1 Classification of liver reserve in cirrhotic patients (modified Child's grading)

	Grade A	*Grade B*	*Grade C*
Serum bilirubin (μmol/l)	<34	34–51	>51
In primary biliary cirrhosis	<69	69–170	>170
Plasma albumin (g/l)	>35	28–35	>28
Ascites	None	Mild	Moderate
Encephalopathy	None	Minimal	Advanced
Prothrombin time (prolongation compared with control)	<4 s	4–6 s	>6 s

REGENERATION OF THE LIVER

The liver has a unique capacity for restoration of normal mass and function after resection or partial destruction. The process is extremely reliable after resection of normal liver, and the timescale is more rapid than was previously thought. Early experimental observations of Higgins and Anderson in the laboratory rat[15] showed that after removal of two-thirds of the liver normal mass was restored within two weeks. Comparable studies in man have been difficult to obtain but scanning suggests that normal liver size is restored within three months of a hepatectomy.[16] The mechanisms which control regeneration are complex and subtle, and although circulating factors have been identified which promote liver cell growth during regeneration, the triggers which control these factors are still not clear.[17,18] 'Hepatotrophic' factors carried in portal venous blood were once thought to be responsible for the process, but are now recognized as being permissive agents rather than primary initiators. Insulin and glucagon from the pancreas are important because liver atrophy occurs when the liver is not perfused by portal blood and while regeneration still occurs, the final size is less than that of the normal liver.[19]

Regeneration is a process of cellular hyperplasia, and the liver architecture becomes abnormal, with double rather than single cell plates lining the hepatic sinusoids being. Apart from this, there may be little histological evidence that regenerative hyperplasia has occurred. The physical direction of liver growth is determined by the anatomy of the resection and the position of the liver remnant in relation to surrounding structures. The left lobe of the liver may regenerate laterally to cradle and almost surround the spleen (Fig. 31.20c). Removal of the liver substance is not a necessary stimulus to regenerative hyperplasia. Interruption of the portal blood supply to segments of the liver, segmental biliary obstruction, or combinations of both cause atrophy and fibrosis in those

REFERENCES

9. Oellerich M, Burdelski M, Lautz H U, Binder L, Pichlmayr R Hepatology 1991; 14: 1029–1034
10. Schirmer W J, Townsend M C, Schirmer J M, Hampton W W, Fry D E J Surg Res 1986; 41: 543–556
11. Kardel T, Ramsoe K, Norby Rasmussen S Scand J Gastroenterol 1975; 10: 29–32
12. Capocaccia L, Ferenci P, Fisher J E, Opolon P Gastroenterol Int 1989; 2: 131–140
13. Hemming A W, Scudamore C H, Shackleton C R, Pudek M, Erb S R Am J Surg 1992; 163: 515–518
14. Pugh R N H, Murray-Lyon I M, Dawson J L, Pietroni M C, Williams R Br J Surg 1973; 60: 646–649
15. Higgins G M, Anderson R M Arch Pathol 1931; 12: 186–202
16. Blumgart L H, Leach K G, Karran S J Gut 1971; 12: 922–928
17. Selden C, Johnstone R, Darby H et al Biochem Biophys Res Commun 1986; 139: 361–366
18. Selden C, Hodgson H J F J Hepatol 1989; 9: 167–176
19. Bucher N L R, Patel U, Cohen S In: Ciba Foundation Symposium No. 55: Hepatotrophic Factors. Elsevier, New York 1978

segments, and regenerative hyperplasia in the remaining liver.[20] This may lead to gross distortion of the liver anatomy, and in the case of right-sided atrophy and left-sided hyperplasia the liver may rotate about its axis, producing distortion of the bile ducts and portal vein in the porta hepatis, causing a significant hazard during operations in this area.

The process of regenerative hyperplasia is impaired in patients with liver disease, especially cirrhosis though it is still present. Major liver resection in cirrhotic patients therefore is hazardous as the liver remnant may be insufficient to support vital functions because of the retarded regenerative response.

THE CLINICAL SPECTRUM OF SURGICAL LIVER DISEASE

Liver disease has a wide spectrum of presentations. Jaundice is one of the most important and it must be determined whether this is caused by hepatocellular dysfunction or obstruction. The finding of hepatomegaly is also a common presentation, and imaging studies have revolutionised the evaluation of patients found to have a large liver. It is important to determine whether hepatomegaly is part of a generalized process or caused by a discrete liver mass. The stigmata of hepatocellular disease should be carefully sought, as these are clear indicators of severe liver dysfunction. They include palmar erythema, spider naevi, finger clubbing and leukonychia, gynaecomastia, spontaneous bruising, and scratch-marks from pruritus. These features should be taken in conjunction with a careful history, including a past exposure to hepatitis, contact with jaundiced patients, intravenous drug use, tattooing, and other high-risk behaviour. A drug history is important because there are a number of drugs associated with hepatocellular dysfunction. A detailed history of alcohol intake is also important.

IMAGING TECHNIQUES

Plain radiology

An enlarged soft tissue liver shadow may confirm hepatomegaly. Some gallstones are radio-opaque (10–15%), and gas within the biliary tree is associated with an abnormal communication between the biliary tract and the gut. This may be a pathological communication such as a cholecystoduodenal fistula, or as a result of previous biliary surgery, such as hepaticojejunostomy or choledochoduodenostomy. Associated features such as pancreatic calcification may also be seen (see Ch. 33).

Imaging techniques

Ultrasound

This is now the initial imaging investigation for imaging hepatobiliary disease, particularly in patients with jaundice. It has the advantage of being quick and non-invasive. It can also accurately guide invasive procedures such as drainage of collections and biopsies. Intrahepatic duct dilatation is indicative of biliary obstruction and ultrasound imaging of the biliary tree and pancreas establishes the level and cause of obstruction in more than 90% of cases.[21] This is as good as computed tomographic (CT) scanning. It is important to remember, however, that up to 10% of patients with biliary tract obstruction may not have duct dilatation, up to 16% in one series.[22] This is especially true of patients with parenchymal liver disease or long-standing obstruction. Ultrasound is much less reliable when large amounts of bowel gas are present. Portable equipment has brought ultrasound scanning into the operating theatre and the wards, and ultrasound may in future become the surgeon's stethoscope. The advent of miniature probes which can be used laparoscopically is beginning to have a significant impact on the staging and evaluation of liver and pancreatic disease, especially in evaluating the resectability of tumours.

Isotope scanning

Imaging using technetium 99m sulphur colloid imaging, taken up by the reticuloendothelial cells in the liver, has diminished in popularity since the availability of ultrasound and CT scanning. Iminodiacetic acid scans (HIDA, DISIDA, PIPIDA) are still used to evaluate biliary function (see Ch. 32). These compounds are handled in a similar way to bilirubin, and provide quantitative imaging of the biliary tract and liver function. The blood pool, liver, central bile ducts and the gut can have areas of interest selected, and dynamic measurements of uptake and excretion provide reproducible estimates of liver blood flow, hepatocyte extraction, excretory capacity and hold-up within the biliary system. Examples of these measures are shown in Figure 31.2. These scans are of particular value in diagnosing the causes of postoperative jaundice, and in evaluating the success of biliary drainage procedures.[23] They are rarely of use in the presence of deep jaundice.

Computed tomographic scanning

Routine CT scanning has little advantage over ultrasound in evaluating the biliary tree, though there are exceptions to this rule. The precise imaging obtained from CT scanning is extremely helpful in evaluating liver masses. Ultrasound and CT must be seen as complementary investigations, and the use of both procedures will, on occasion, increase the diagnostic yield. The simultaneous administration of intravenous contrast medium not only opacifies the hepatic parenchyma, but also allows the intrahepatic blood vessels to be differentiated from dilated bile ducts and from abnormal liver masses. This is illustrated in Figure 31.3. CT arterioportography (CTAP) is an extension of this principle. A catheter is introduced into the superior mesenteric artery via the femoral artery using the Seldinger technique and an angiogram of the liver

REFERENCES

20. Hadjis N S, Blenkharn J I, Hatzis G, Guzail M, Benjamin I S Surgery 1991; 109: 671–676
21. Gibson R N, Yeung E, Thompson J N et al Radiology 1986; 160: 43–47
22. Beinart C, Efremedis S, Cohen B, Mitty H A JAMA 1981; 245: 353–356
23. Zeman R K, Lee C, Stahl R S, Cahow C E, Viscomi G N, Neumann R D, Gold J A, Burrel M I Radiology 1982; 145: 109–115

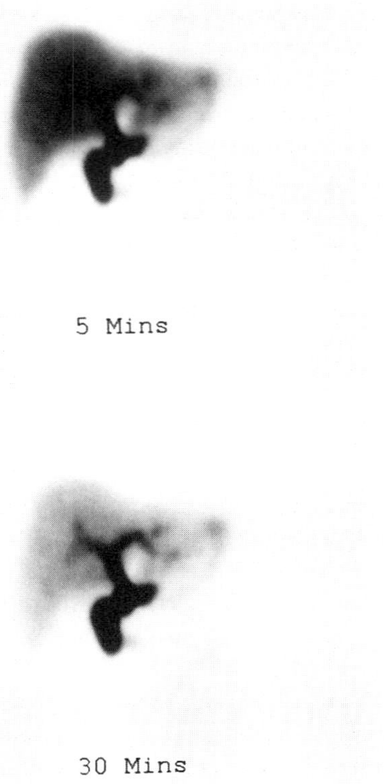

a

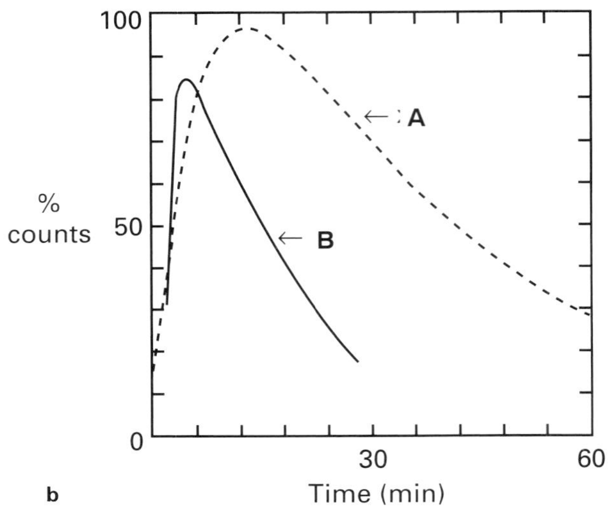

b

Fig. 31.2 HIDA scans in a patient who has a hepaticojejunostomy for a benign biliary stricture. (**a**) The scans show uptake of contrast by the liver and excretion into the central hepatic ducts and then into the Roux loop. (**b**) The derived curves demonstrate the different phases of uptake and excretion, and from these curves parameters can be calculated which give a quantitative estimate of hepatocyte biliary excretory function. A = 'raw' curve of liver uptake and excretion; B = calculated curve.

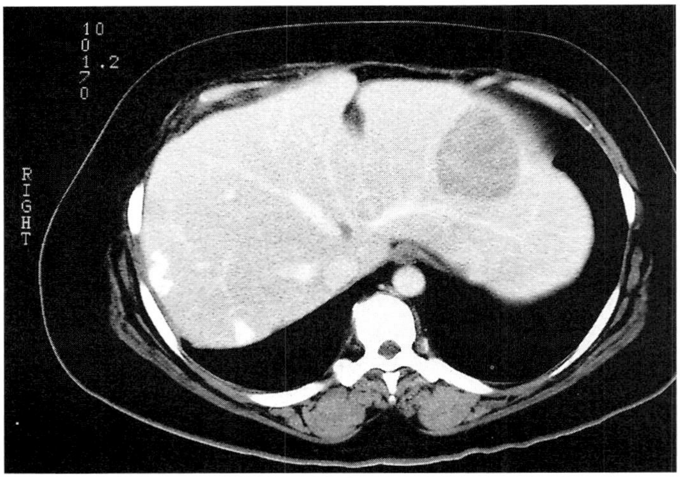

Fig. 31.3 A CT scan of the liver after intravenous contrast. The three main hepatic veins show up clearly, while the space-occupying lesion in segment II caused by a liver cell adenoma is displayed as a negative image on a bright background of liver parenchyma.

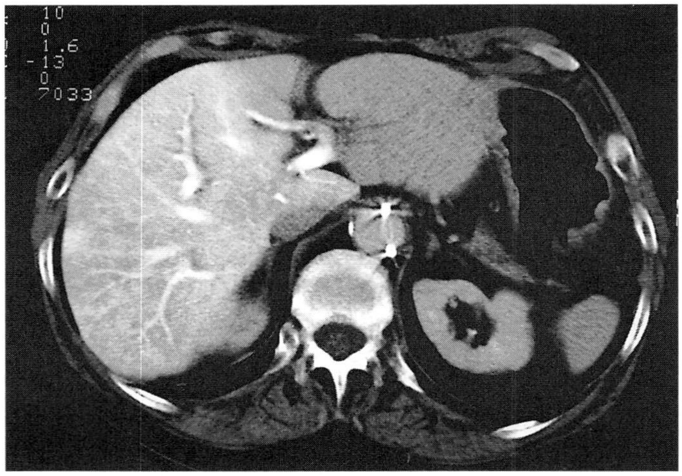

Fig. 31.4 A CT arterioportogram shows the excellent definition of the intrahepatic portal veins. The main left portal vein is truncated in the umbilical fissure, giving a branch to segment IV, but no portal filling of segment III because a metastatic tumour deposit blocks the vein at that point.

circulation can be obtained. The patient is moved to the CT scanner with the catheter in situ and a precisely timed sequence of bolus injection of contrast and acquisition of CT scanning images is carried out. This gives precise images of the intrahepatic circulation, including the hepatic veins, and also produces maximum contrast between avascular liver masses such as secondary deposits and the opacified hepatic parenchyma (Fig. 31.4). Many people now regard this as the best method for detecting small liver metastases.[24]

The lipiodol CT also provides useful additional information. When introduced into the hepatic arterial circulation lipiodol, an iodized oil suspension, is rapidly taken up by Kupffer cells which

REFERENCE

24. Soyer P, Levesque M, Elias D, Zeitoun G, Rosch A Am J Roentgenol 1992; 159: 741–744

are scattered throughout the normal liver. It is virtually cleared within 7–10 days. Liver tumours, and hepatocellular carcinomas in particular, lack Kupffer cells and the abnormal vascularity of these tumours traps the oily particles which show up very brightly on a subsequent CT scan after the rest of the liver has cleared. This is a particularly valuable method for detecting small primary hepatocellular carcinomas, particularly in a cirrhotic liver in which the presence of multiple nodules may mask a tumour (Fig. 31.5).[25]

Magnetic resonance imaging

Magnetic resonance imaging (MRI) provides images which are similar to those obtained by CT scanning but, because the scans rely on a different physical principle the information may be additional or complementary. While image acquisition with rapid 'spiral' CT scanners has become extremely fast, the length of time required to obtain an MRI image with present equipment is a major drawback, and scans often contain significant movement artefacts from breathing and cardiac pulsation. Numerous different 'sequences' are used in MRI scanning, but their place in liver disease has not yet been established. The availability of improved contrast media for use with MRI scanning has improved the resolution yet further.[26] Coronal and even three-dimensional reconstructions can be performed which can give valuable information for the surgeon in evaluating the position and resectability of liver tumours (Fig. 31.6) although these techniques can also be applied to CT scanning.

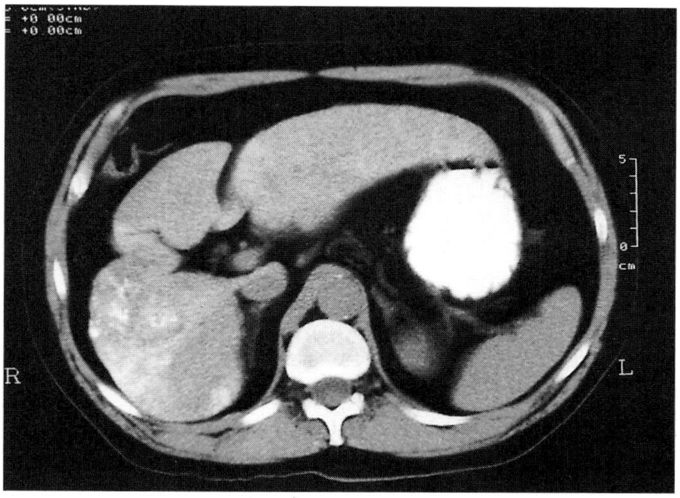

Fig. 31.5 A lipiodol angiogram in a patient with hepatocellular carcinoma in a cirrhotic liver. The lipiodol is retained in the area of the tumour after it has cleared from the rest of the liver.

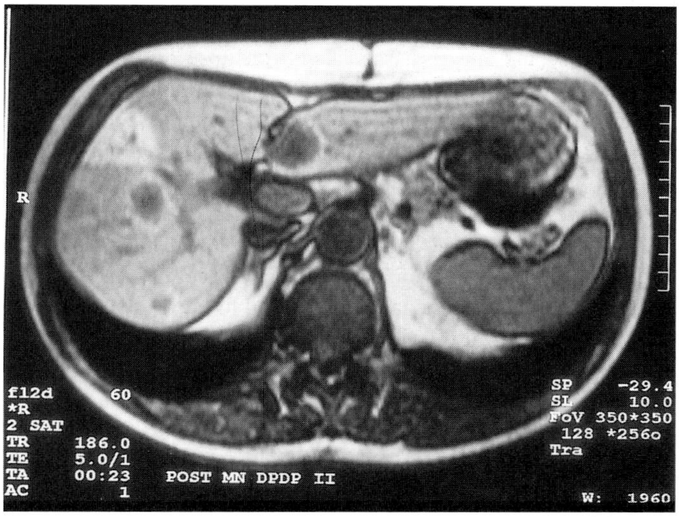

Fig. 31.6 A magnetic resonance scan with MnDPDP contrast medium which clearly shows the intrahepatic vessels (dark) and several secondary deposits with peripheral uptake of contrast.

Positron emission tomography (PET scanning)

This has not been used extensively to evaluate liver disease until now but it may have a place in examining the metabolic activity of the liver cells, which may relate to the viability of tumours which are being treated.

Biliary imaging

This is covered in greater detail in Chapter 32, but imaging of the biliary system is often of great importance in evaluating liver problems. Endoscopic retrograde pancreatography (Fig. 31.7) and percutaneous transhepatic cholangiography (Fig. 31.8) may both be used to see biliary strictures or tumours. They will not be considered further in this chapter.

Hepatic angiography

Hepatic angiography is usually performed using the Seldinger technique. It provides valuable information on the anatomical arrangement of blood vessels of the liver when resection is planned. This is particularly useful as anomalies of the arterial supply are frequent. The commonest of these is a right hepatic artery arising from the superior mesenteric artery, and a replaced left hepatic artery (Fig. 31.9) arising from the left gastric artery or directly from the coeliac axis is not infrequent. It is no longer considered essential to use hepatic angiography to obtain this anatomical information and most use it selectively for detection of small vascular tumours or as part of arterioportography.

Delineation of the portal venous system is of value in patients with portal hypertension (see below). Excellent images can be obtained by injection of contrast into the superior mesenteric artery with the use of modern digital equipment and delayed films outline the superior mesenteric and portal veins (Fig. 31.10). This form of 'indirect splenoportography' has largely replaced the use of the alternative direct methods of splenoportography via a needle/catheter placed in the splenic pulp, and retrograde portography obtained via a transhepatic needle. These latter procedures did, however, have the advantage of allowing pressure measurements

REFERENCES

25. Dawson P, Adam A, Banks L Eur J Radiol 1993; 16: 201–206
26. Power C, Ros P R, Stoupis C, Johnson W K, Segel K H Radiographics 1994; 14: 459–482

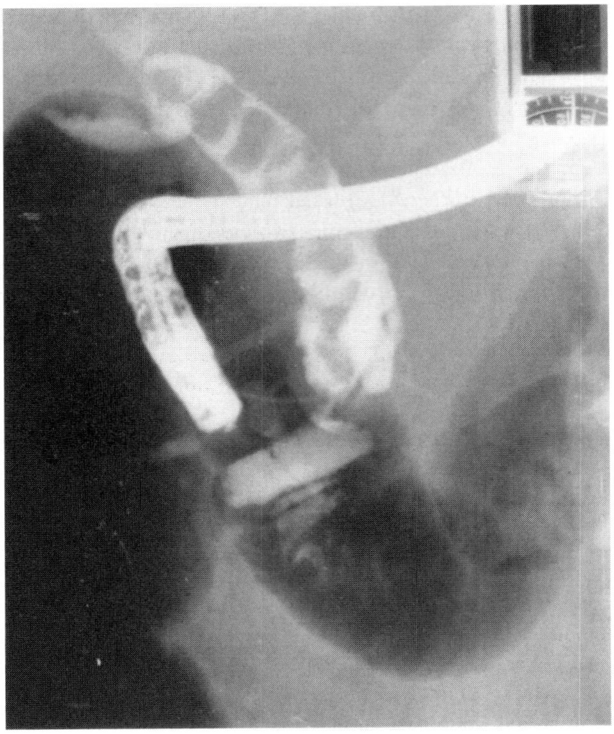

Fig. 31.7 Endoscopic retrograde cholangiopancreatogram showing multiple stones in the common bile duct.

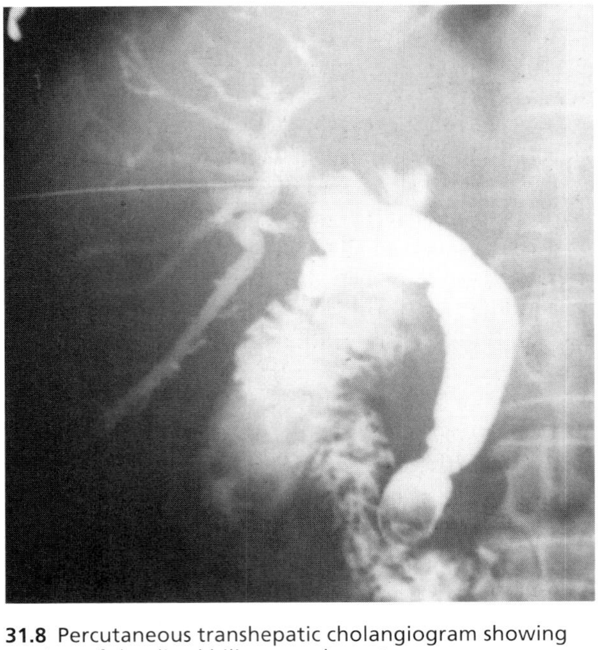

Fig. 31.8 Percutaneous transhepatic cholangiogram showing obstruction of the distal biliary tree by a stone.

to be taken which may be of useful in the diagnosis and treatment of portal hypertension.

Arterial embolization

Selective embolic occlusion of the arterial supply to part of the liver has a number of therapeutic indications. Arterioportal or

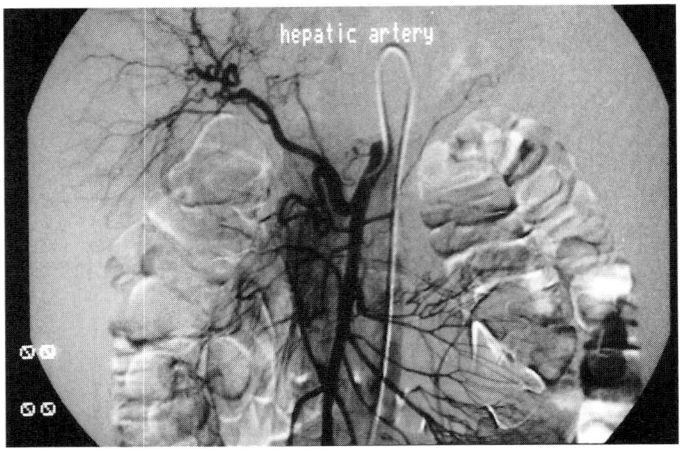

Fig. 31.9 A right hepatic artery arising from the superior mesenteric artery, which completely replaces the 'normal' blood supply to the right liver.

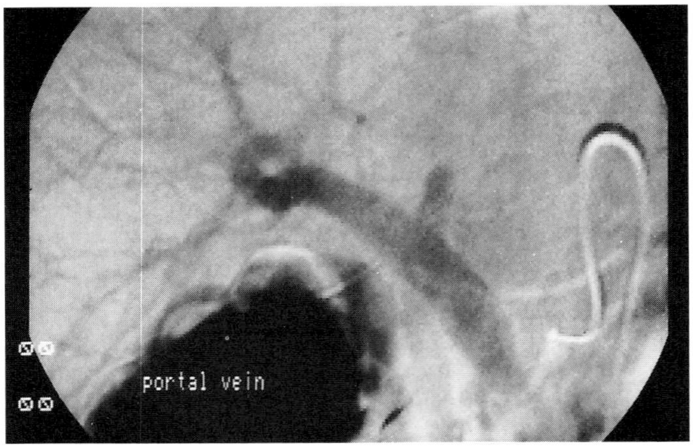

Fig. 31.10 An indirect portogram obtained by injection into the superior mesenteric artery shows clear outlining of the superior mesenteric and portal veins, including their hepatic branches. Digital imaging is necessary to obtain this degree of definition.

arteriovenous communications may develop after liver trauma and these may sometimes be associated with false aneurysms of an intrahepatic artery. This may occasionally occur after liver biopsy. Selective catheterization by the Seldinger technique allows occlusion of these aneurysms or arteriovenous malformations using a variety of materials including metal coils, human dura, gelfoam and other substances (see Ch. 10). Interruption of the hepatic artery may promote shrinkage of the tumour and cellular necrosis since many benign and malignant tumours of the liver have a rich arterial blood supply. The hepatic artery used to be ligated surgically outside the liver but revascularization through collaterals rapidly followed this procedure, even when the arterial supply to the liver was totally abolished by the division of all ligamentous attachments. Arterial embolization has therefore replaced surgical ligation in appropriate cases. This approach directly occludes small vessels which feed the tumour, and the interruption of the blood supply is more complete. It can also be repeated several times if necessary because access to the main arterial system remains intact. The combination of embolization with cytotoxic agents or radio-isotopes is discussed later in the section on liver tumours. Occasionally embolization may be carried out as a preliminary manoeuvre for very large tumours to reduce their volume and vascularity prior to resection. Portal venous embolization via a transhepatic approach has also been used to produce atrophy of a tumour-bearing segment of liver and hyperplasia of the contralateral liver in the hope of rendering major liver resection safer by producing a larger liver remnant.

ASSESSMENT OF A MASS IN THE LIVER

This is such a common problem that it merits separate consideration. Rapid recourse to percutaneous biopsy of a liver mass without careful diagnostic evaluation and planning of possible treatment is often inappropriate, and biopsy can often be avoided altogether. The importance of a careful history and examination has already been emphasized. Particular attention should be paid to signs of hepatocellular insufficiency and lymphadenopathy. A history of previous surgery or of malignant disease elsewhere is also very important. The characteristics of the liver mass should be determined by clinical examination, and it is useful to listen for a bruit which may be present in some cases of haemangioma or malignant liver tumours. A machinery murmur may be heard over an arteriovenous malformation. It must be remembered also that not every tumour apparently arising from the liver is necessarily a liver tumour. Particular pitfalls arise with large tumours of the right adrenal gland and kidney, but rare tumours such as those of the peritoneum (see Ch. 27) or leiomyomas/leiomyosarcomas of the inferior vena cava (see Ch. 11) may masquerade as liver tumours (Fig. 31.11).[27] Liver function tests, serum tumour markers including α-fetoprotein which is specific for hepatocellular carcinoma (+ testicular teratoma), carcinoembryonic antigen which is a ubiquitous tumour marker for cancers of gastrointestinal origin and CA19-9 should all be obtained. When appropriate fasting samples for measurement of gastrointestinal hormones and urinary 5-hydroxyindoleacetic acid (5-HIAA) for carcinoid tumours can

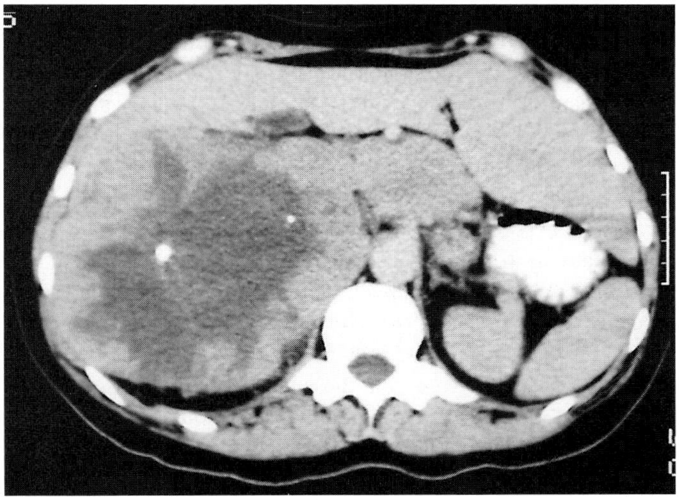

Fig. 31.11 A large adrenal tumour which presented as a suspected liver mass. Such masses may be difficult to distinguish even on scanning and angiography.

be measured. Patients with primary liver tumours of the fibrolamellar variant do not express α-fetoprotein, but the presence of neurotensin and elevated vitamin B12 binding capacity in the serum are relatively specific for this type of tumour.

Imaging

Radiological imaging is the cornerstone of diagnosis for focal liver lesions. Various algorithmic approaches have been described, virtually all of them starting with an ultrasound scan. The first questions to determine are whether the lesion is single or multiple and whether it is solid or cystic. Cystic lesions of the liver are considered later in this chapter. Solid lesions which are multiple and unlikely to be treated by liver resection may reasonably be biopsied under ultrasound guidance provided there are no other contraindications. Early biopsy of a lesion which is solitary, or likely to be considered for resection, does carry some drawbacks. Not only is there a risk of bleeding from vascular tumours, but there are numerous case reports of dissemination of tumour into the peritoneal cavity and indeed along the needle track following percutaneous needle biopsy.[28] Fine-needle aspiration cytology is undoubtedly safer, but is also harder to interpret, and has a higher false-negative rate for diagnosing tumours.[29] The solitary or resectable liver 'tumour' is therefore probably better evaluated by CT and when appropriate MRI scanning. CT arterioportography has already been described, and many now feel that this is the best method for detecting other small deposits, down to a few millimetres in size. Each of the benign and malignant tumour types has characteristic though not diagnostic appearances on ultrasound and CT scanning, and the diagnosis may be even clearer if dynamic contrast CT scanning is used. It should be possible to distinguish haemangiomas from most other tumours by this means (Fig. 31.12), though some vascular tumours may not be easily distinguished from haemangiomas. It is important not to forget that chest radiographs and whole-body CT scans of the chest may avoid unnecessary investigation by demonstrating that the patient has diffuse metastatic disease from a primary source, known or unknown, which renders further investigation with a view to surgery futile.

LIVER INJURIES

The liver is a large and vascular organ, and although protected by the thoracic cage it is a frequent site of injury following both blunt and penetrating trauma (see Ch. 27). Liver injuries are present in around a third of patients who undergo laparotomy for abdominal trauma.[30] In the UK the majority of liver injuries arise from road

REFERENCES

27. Collier N A, Allison D J, Vermess M, Blumgart L H Aust NZ J Surg 1984; 54(2): 113–118
28. Quaghebeur G, Thompson J N, Blumgart L H, Benjamin I S J R Coll Surg Edinb 1991; 36: 127
29. Ferrucci J T, Wittenberg J, Mueller P R et al AJR 1980; 134: 323–330
30. Feliciano D V, Jordan G L, Bitondo C G, Mattox K L, Burch J M, Cruse D A Ann Surg 1986; 204: 438–443

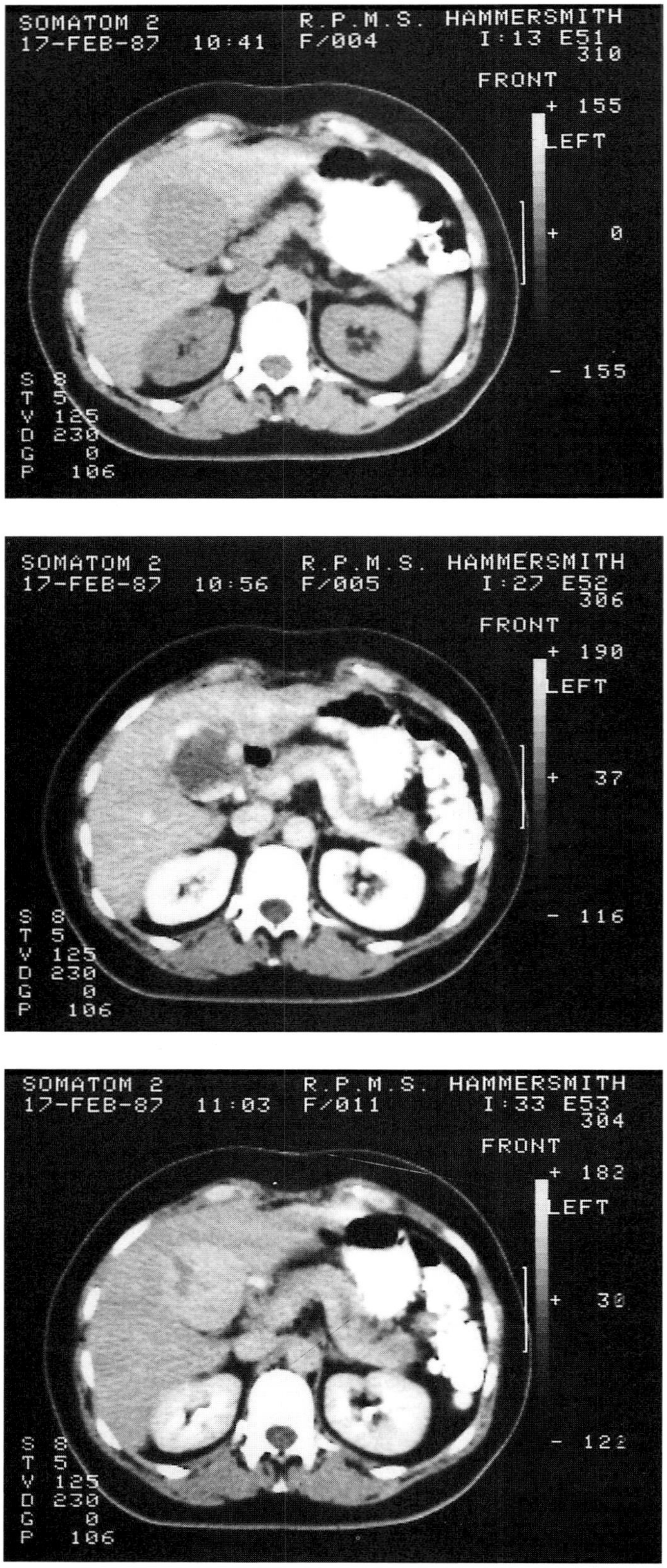

a b c

Fig. 31.12 Dynamic CT scanning through a haemangioma of the liver, in which successive films before and 15 and 22 minutes after intravenous contrast injection show gradual infilling of the lesion from the periphery to the centre, with incomplete opacification due to central fibrosis.

traffic accidents, while in North America the majority are caused by gunshot and stab wounds. It is important to maintain a high index of suspicion in patients injured in a road traffic accident.

Diagnosis and assessment

Severe liver injury is not difficult to diagnose in patients presenting with hypovolaemic shock, spreading peritonism and right shoulder tip pain. The diagnosis may, however, not be so simple in patients with other injuries or in unconscious patients. The general principles of evaluating the multiply injured patient and of resuscitation are discussed in Chapter 7. Specific manoeuvres aimed at diagnosing intra-abdominal haemorrhage and liver trauma include diagnostic peritoneal lavage and, increasingly, abdominal ultrasound and CT scanning. Ultrasound is quick and easy and can be used even in an urgent situation while other diagnostic tests and resuscitation efforts continue. Ultrasound can easily demonstrate free fluid (blood) in the peritoneal cavity and also shows up major hepatic parenchymal disruption. It may also demonstrate disruption of the splenic pulp (see Ch. 34). It is more dependent on the 'operator' than CT scanning, but CT scans are restricted to patients in a more stable condition: their use at a later stage in the patient with liver trauma is discussed below. Laparoscopy has been used in some centres to assess liver damage, but probably offers little advantage over diagnostic peritoneal lavage. Having briefly discussed these issues, it should not be forgotten that the patient who clearly has advancing intra-abdominal signs or hypovolaemic shock is likely to require a laparotomy and most tests are superfluous under these cicumstances.

Classification

A number of systems exist for classifying liver injuries. The one used by the American Association for Surgery of Trauma is shown in Table 31.2. The important variants are the different degrees of haematoma or of laceration. There is no doubt that, apart from associated injuries outside the liver, the mortality rate depends upon the extent of the injury, the number of segments involved, and in particular any associated damage to the inferior vena cava or major hepatic veins. Blunt injuries invariably produce more severe damage and have a higher mortality, stage for stage, than penetrating injuries.

Management

Stable patients in whom it appears that the bleeding has stopped are often best treated conservatively, even in the face of radiological evidence of significant hepatic trauma. When this approach is adopted it must be pursued in a centre with appropriate facilities, including intensive care, on the understanding that operating theatres are immediately available. Observation may be required for many days with repeated ultrasound or CT scanning. This policy was originally proposed for managing liver injuries in children, but has been increasingly adopted in adults.[31]

When surgery is required, the operative approach to the abdomen is often determined by the general condition of the

Table 31.2 American Association of Surgery for Trauma: Liver surgery scale

Grade	*Injury description*	
I	Haematoma	Subcapsular, non-expanding, <10% surface area
	Laceration	Capsular tear, non-bleeding with <1 cm deep parenchymal disruption
II	Haematoma	Subcapsular, non-expanding, <10–50%; intraparenchymal non-expanding, <2 cm diameter
	Laceration	<3 cm parenchymal depth, <10 cm length
III	Haematoma	Subcapsular, >50% of surface area or expanding; ruptured subcapsular haematoma with active bleeding; intraparenchymal haematoma > 2 cm
	Laceration	>3 cm parenchymal depth
IV	Haematoma	Ruptured central haematoma
	Laceration	Parenchymal destruction > 75% of hepatic lobe
V	Laceration	Parenchymal destruction involving 25–75% of hepatic lobe
	Vascular	Juxtahepatic venous injuries (retrohepatic cava/major hepatic veins)
VI	Vascular	Hepatic avulsion

Pachter H L, Spencer F C, Hofstetter S R, Liang H G, Coppa G F. Significant trends in the treatment of hepatic trauma: experience with 411 injuries. Am Surg 1992; 215: 492–499.

patient and the presence of other injuries. The injured liver is often approached via a long midline incision, through which a full exploration if necessary of the abdominal viscera and retroperitoneum can be carried out. Better access can be gained to the liver after such an incision, by extending horizontally through the right rectus muscle below the costal margin well out to the flank, when the whole of the liver can usually be satisfactorily mobilized.

A systematic approach must then be adopted.[32] The first priority is to detect the source of haemodynamic instability, and to control any obvious bleeding. Inspection of the right liver dome, the most frequent site of damage in blunt trauma, may require division of the right coronary ligament. A *Pringle manoeuvre*, which is compression of the contents of the free edge of the lesser omentum between finger and thumb or by a vascular or soft bowel clamp, may help to control bleeding while this is carried out. It is essential to exclude other intra-abdominal injuries at the same time. Injuries which are fairly minor or have stopped bleeding by the time of laparotomy should normally be left alone. Lacerations on the edge of liver which bleed persistently can be controlled by suturing, but measures have to be taken to prevent the stitches from cutting through the soft liver parenchyma. This can be achieved by suturing through and over buffers of fibrin (Biethium, Ethicon) or over pledgets of haemostatic material.[33] This technique should only be applied to peripheral lacerations, and no attempt should be made to suture the edges of deep or central liver lacerations. Suturing of this type of liver damage does not always stop bleeding and an expanding haematoma can then develop within the liver. A deeper wound should be explored digitally and individual bleeding points can be sutured, but this may be difficult particularly in inaccessible parts of the liver, and may indeed not be necessary.

Perihepatic packing has revolutionised the management of liver injuries of all grades. The cavity of the liver injury should not be packed itself, as this often causes more bleeding when the packs are removed. The liver should be mobilized as much as necessary to allow anterior, posterior, lateral and inferior packs to be placed.[34] This may require division of the right coronary ligament, but this manoeuvre should not take very long. The packs should be placed between the liver and diaphragm and beneath the liver in such a way as to afford satisfactory hepatic tamponade, and the abdomen should not be closed until control has been obtained. The abdomen is then closed without drainage and the packs are removed at a second laparotomy after 48–72 hours. CT scanning with contrast and occasionally hepatic arteriography can be performed before the packs are removed if there is concern about major intrahepatic damage. Major disruption of the intrahepatic arteries or arterioportal or arteriovenous fistula formation, can then be selectively embolized before the patient is returned to theatre for removal of the packs.

This policy of packing and re-laparotomy controls the great majority of liver injuries, even quite major injuries to the intrahepatic veins. On occasion, however, bleeding continues and is so severe that packing fails. These constitute the most serious liver injuries, and while techniques for placement of intracaval shunts, the use of partial and complete liver bypass and even cardiopulmonary bypass have been described, the survivors of such techniques are few. Vascular isolation of the liver can be obtained by placing a clamp or sling on the inferior vena cava below the liver, performing a Pringle manoeuvre, and either clamping the cava immediately above the liver or splitting the tendinous part of the diaphragm down to the inferior vena cava and clamping inside the mediastinum below or within the right atrium. This may provide sufficient access to the ruptured hepatic veins or vena cava and allow suturing, but if there is severe liver disruption then resectional debridement of separated fragments of liver and devitalised tissue substance is often required. This can be combined with packing of the dead space for later removal. The liver withstands normothermic ischaemia for more than 1 hour during these manoeuvres. Cooling techniques have also been described but are rarely used.

By application of these various techniques the number of patients requiring emergency liver resection following trauma has diminished considerably. The policy of exploration, early perihepatic packing before too much haemorrhage has taken place and coagulopathy becomes a problem, and transfer to a specialist centre has revolutionised the management of liver injuries.[32]

LIVER ABSCESS

These are classified according to the nature of the infecting organism and a useful working classification is shown in Table 31.3. In the

REFERENCES

31. Hiatt R H, Dale Harrier H, Koenig V, Ransom J Arch Surg 1990; 125: 101–103
32. Gryf-Lowczowski J V D, Benjamin IS Curr Prac Surg 1994; 6: 78–85
33. Wood C B, Capperauld I, Blumgart L H Ann R Coll Surg Engl 1976; 58: 401–404
34. Calne R Y, McMaster P, Pentlow B D Br J Surg 1979; 66: 338–339

Table 31.3 Aetiology of liver abscess

Pyogenic
Biliary tract origin
'Ascending' cholangitis
Stent occlusion
Primary sclerosing cholangitis
Portal origin
Appendicitis
Diverticular disease
Inflammatory bowel disease
Umbilical sepsis
Traumatic
Iatrogenic (e.g. biliary surgery, liver biopsy, post-embolization)
Penetrating injuries
Blunt liver trauma
Neoplastic
Degeneration
Post-embolization
Infected cysts
Simple
Choledochal
Parasitic
Contiguous spread
Gallbladder
Gastrointestinal perforation
Metastatic from systemic sepsis (especially in immunocompromised hosts)
'Cryptogenic'
Specific bacterial infections
Tuberculosis
Fungal
Parasitic
Amoebic
Hydatid
Clonorchis sinensis
Ascaris lumbricoides

past most pyogenic abscesses were the result of sepsis within the gut, often appendicitis or diverticulitis, and the decreasing frequency of severe untreated appendicitis over the years has led to a shift in the age spectrum of liver abscess to a proponderance in the fifth decade. Complicated diverticular disease is now a much more common portal source of origin (see Ch. 30). Umbilical sepsis remains common in poorer countries where the umbilical cords of infants may be dressed with infected materials. Immune compromise must be considered whenever an unexplained liver abscess develops, and in particular the possibility of acquired immune deficiency syndrome should be ruled out. Pyogenic liver abscesses of gastrointestinal tract origin are often multiple. The number of pyogenic abscesses for which no origin can be found has diminished, but they still account for up to 15% of cases.[35]

The biliary tract is now responsible for almost one-third of all pyogenic liver abscesses, which are usually associated with cholangitis and biliary obstruction. This has overtaken other gastrointestinal sources as the major site of origin of pyogenic liver abscess and direct spread from empyema of the gallbladder or severe acute cholecystitis can be included in this category. The late results of injury, including iatrogenic trauma such as liver biopsy and therapeutic embolization, are of increasing importance.

Abscesses caused by specific infections such as amoebiasis, fungi, tuberculosis and parasites which become secondarily infected are much commoner outside Western countries. For the majority of the world's population, a liver abscess is considered to be amoebic until proven otherwise and blind antimicrobial therapy

Table 31.4 Pathogenic aerobic organisms in 38 cases of liver abscess

Organism	*n*
Escherichia coli	16
Klebsiella pneumoniae	6
Streptococcus sp.	6
Enterococcus	4
Proteus sp.	4
Enterobacteriaceae	3
Other Gram-negative rods (*Pseudomonas aeruginosa* 1)	3
Staphylococcus aureus	1

Data from Barnes et al.[37]

is often prescribed in poorer countries. Hydatid cysts may also become secondarily infected with pyogenic organisms.[36]

Microbiology

Table 31.4 shows the pathogenic aerobic organisms found in a series of liver abscesses reported in 1987.[37] Most were enteric organisms. Anaerobic species have been more commonly identified recently, the commonest being bacteroides fragilis, with a significant incidence of *Streptococcus milleri* (see Ch. 4).

Clinical features

The classic presentation is with fever, sweating, anorexia, malaise, vomiting, weight loss and pain in the upper abdomen. The classical swinging fever actually occurs in only about one-quarter of cases.[38] About a quarter of patients also become jaundiced and this is an adverse prognostic sign in patients with multiple liver abscesses.

Physical examination may confirm hepatomegaly and tenderness in the right upper quadrant. Often, however, the features are very non-specific and pyogenic liver abscess should always be considered in the differential diagnosis of a patient presenting with pyrexia of unknown origin.

Investigation

Most patients have a marked leukocytosis and a raised sedimentation rate. They often have a raised alkaline phosphatase and the serum albumin may plummet to very low levels quite rapidly. A low albumin is associated with a high mortality. Plain abdominal radiographs may show hepatomegaly or even a gas/fluid level below the diaphragm or within the liver. Gas within the biliary tree indicates a communication between the biliary and the gastrointestinal tracts, but gas within portal radicles is a serious sign. A raised hemidiaphragm and associated pleural effusion is common with large liver abscesses. The diagnosis is usually made by upper abdominal ultrasound and is often confirmed by CT scanning. A

REFERENCES

35. Garrison R N, Polk H C In: Blumgart L H (ed) Surgery of the Liver and Biliary Tract. Churchill Livingstone, Edinburgh 1994
36. Blenkharn J I, Benjamin I S, Blumgart L H J Infect 1987; 15: 169–171
37. Barnes P F, DeCock K M, Reynolds T N, Ralls P W Medicine 1987; 66: 472–483
38. Ahmed L, el-Rooby A, Kassem M I, Salama Z A, Strickland G T Rev Infect Dis 1990; 12: 330–337

search for the source of sepsis is important, although this may have to await later investigation. The exception is in patients with liver abscesses associated with biliary tract obstruction, in which relief of the obstruction either operatively or by interventional endoscopy or radiology is an essential step in promoting resolution of the abscess.

Treatment

Antibiotics are always indicated, and although a blind selection of antibiotics to cover a broad spectrum of aerobic and anaerobic organism should be started, pus should be obtained as quickly as possible, in order to target antibiotic therapy. Blood cultures can be helpful but early needle aspiration of the abscess for aerobic and anaerobic culture is generally indicated. This should be done using ultrasound guidance, ideally at the time that the original diagnosis is made. The question of providing external drainage is considered in more detail below.

Antibiotics should be started intravenously and, if aminoglycosides are prescribed, careful attention must be paid to plasma levels and surveillance of renal function, especially in patients who are both septic and jaundiced (see Ch. 29). Sometimes prolonged antibiotic administration may cause resolution without the need to drain the abscess. This is especially true in patients with multiple miliary intrahepatic abscesses in whom focal drainage is not possible.

Abscess drainage

While open drainage was formerly the standard treatment for liver abscesses this has been overtaken in recent years by percutaneous drainage techniques which appear to be equally effective and somewhat safer in the majority of cases. Various non-randomized comparisons have been made between radiological and surgical drainage, but conclusions have to be rather tentative because the issue does not readily lend itself to controlled trials. A retrospective survey at the Mayo Clinic between 1977 and 1984[39] suggested that percutaneous closed drainage has some disadvantages, but with modern interventional radiological techniques wide-bore catheter drainage can be obtained even in the case of multilocular cavities containing thick material. Failure to respond to the initial insertion of a catheter should not be regarded as a total failure as it may be reinserted. The catheter may be used to break down internal loculi and this combined with repeated irrigation and aspiration may still be successful. Even quite large cavities may be treated in this manner and a laparotomy thus avoided. A transabdominal approach is preferable if surgical drainage becomes necessary. The site of the abscess in the liver is identified, using intraoperative ultrasound if necessary, and the rest of the abdomen packed away to avoid contamination. The abscess is approached at its most superficial point, and the contents are first aspirated with a wide-bore trocar and cannula. After this either a large drain can be inserted and irrigated, or if the roof of the abscess is sufficiently thin this can be excised to allow thorough removal and debridement of the abscess contents. Any bleeding from the edges of the excision is controlled with a series of simple sutures. Wide-bore closed tube drainage of the cavity is probably as good as any other method, though irrigating sump drains may be useful for large cavities. A flap of omentum may be laid into the cavity to help reduce the dead space and the tube or tubes are retained in situ until they cease to drain. The cavity should be evaluated by regular ultrasound or sinograms until it is seen to be closing down around the tube, at which point the drain can be removed.

Outcome

Before the 1970s liver abscesses had mortality rates of 80–90%. Now the mortality should be less than 10%, remembering that patients with biliary sepsis must have free biliary drainage. In some cases this may simply involve changing a blocked stent, but in others formal biliary drainage procedures may be necessary.

CYSTIC LIVER LESIONS

Cystic lesions of the liver are commonly encountered in surgical practice, though the majority are symptomless and discovered by chance. The increased use of ultrasound for the investigation of upper abdominal symptoms has led to the detection of many small simple liver cysts, which rarely pose a major diagnostic dilemma. Cysts occasionally cause symptoms or raise difficulties in differential diagnosis. Liver cysts can be classified as shown in Table 31.5.

Congenital simple cysts are intrahepatic cysts lined with a low cuboidal epithelium presumably derived from the biliary system, although they do not have any anatomical communication with the intrahepatic bile ducts. The pathogenesis of these cysts is obscure. These are the most commonly encountered liver cysts and they range from a few millimetres in diameter to more than 20 cm. While most are symptomless, those who do develop symptoms generally experience progressive dull pain as the result of gradual expansion of the cyst, with abdominal distension and post-prandial fullness. Spontaneous rupture is exceptional, as is spontaneous haemorrhage, but haemorrhage following trauma may cause a sudden increase in the cyst size with associated pain.

Table 31.5 Liver cysts

Congenital cysts
Simple cysts
Polycystic liver disease
Traumatic cysts
Parasitic cysts
Hydatid
Biliary cysts
Choledochal cysts (type IVA)
Caroli's disease
Neoplastic cysts
Cystadenoma
Cystadenocarcinoma

REFERENCE

39. Bertel C K, Van Heerden J A, Sheedy P F Arch Surg 1986; 121: 554–558

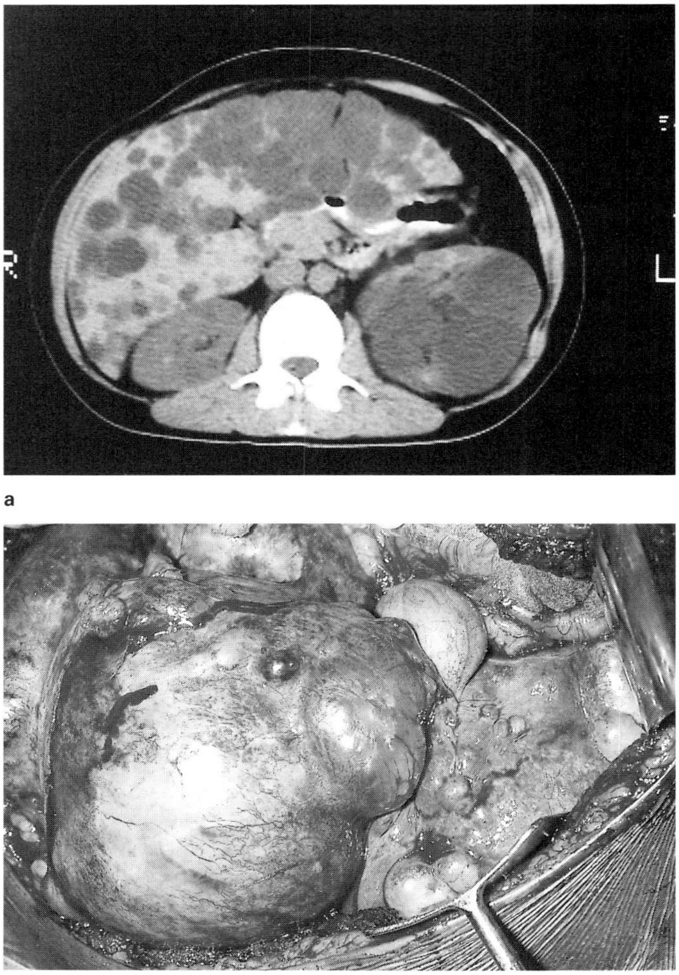

a

b

Fig. 31.13 (a) Polycystic liver and kidney disease, showing huge numbers of cysts throughout most segments of the liver, with some normal liver preserved in the inferior part of the right lobe. (b) Operative view of polycystic liver.

Polycystic liver disease is a genetic disorder, the majority of patients falling into the group with autosomal dominant polycystic kidney disease. There is an enormous spectrum in the site, size and number of cysts but the majority of patients present in early to mid-adult life with gradual onset of progressive abdominal distension (Fig. 31.13). Liver function is usually well preserved, but massive polycystic disease may be complicated by compression of the hilar bile ducts with obstructive jaundice and several cases of Budd–Chiari syndrome in association with polycystic liver disease have also been reported.[40] The prognosis in patients with polycystic liver and kidney disease is usually determined by the progression of the renal disease to end-stage renal failure rather than by the polycystic liver. Nevertheless gradual progression of the liver disease may produce symptoms which require therapy.

Traumatic cysts follow the formation of intrahepatic or subcapsular haematomas and are in fact pseudocysts. Most resolve spontaneously, but some may persist and require operative treatment. This should include assessment of any biliary communication and an attempt to close this.

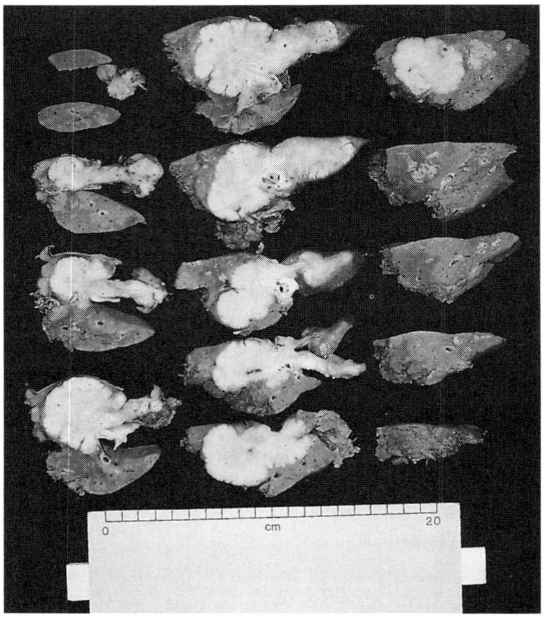

Fig. 31.14 A cystadenocarcinoma of the left liver, presenting with an upper abdominal mass. This patient was treated by resection, subsequently had a re-resection for recurrent tumour, and when the tumour recurred for the second time she was treated by liver transplantation. She remains alive and well six years after her transplant.

Neoplastic cysts, though uncommon, are important because they must be distinguished from simple cysts or polycystic liver disease. *Cystadenoma* and *cystadenocarcinoma* are not distinct entities, and malignant characteristics may only be evident in a few localized areas of the tumour in patients with an otherwise benign cystic tumour of the liver. Careful histological examination is therefore important after excision of these lesions. The majority present in women with non-specific upper abdominal symptoms. Histologically they are multiloculated cysts lined with cuboidal or columnar mucus-producing epithelium, and the carcinomatous elements often have a papillary appearance. Following incomplete resection of the malignant variant, local recurrence is possible and re-resection or even transplantation has been reported in a number of cases (Fig. 31.14). The Mayo Clinic reports a five-year survival rate of 25% for patients with resected cystadenocarcinoma.[41]

Investigations

There are no specific investigations for cystic liver disease apart from imaging studies. CT scans give the best anatomical information, and there is an enormous variation in the distribution, size and number of the cysts. Tumour markers may help to identify malignant cases, or secondary tumours in areas of polycystic liver.

REFERENCES

40. Uddin W, Ramage J K, Portmann B, Wilson P, Benjamin I S, Tan K C, Williams R Gut 1995; 36: 142–145
41. Que F G, Gores G J, Welch T J, Nagorney D M In: Pitt H A, Carr-Locke D L, Ferrucci J T (eds) Hepatobiliary and Pancreatic Disease: The Team Approach to Management. Little, Brown, London 1995

Management

Symptomless cysts should be left alone. Percutaneous aspiration is invariably followed by refilling, usually within a few weeks or months. Percutaneous aspiration followed by instillation of sclerosing agents is effective and well tolerated, but is also frequently followed by recurrence if the cysts are large. The most common sclerosing agent is absolute alcohol, of which 5–25 ml is instilled into the cyst and the patient moved around to wash the alcohol around the entire cyst lining. The fluid is reaspirated after 30 minutes. This may provide very good symptomatic relief, which may be permanent with smaller cysts, but recurrence within 12–24 months is the rule for the majority.

Surgical treatment may be easy for the very large cyst, in which wide deroofing ('fenestration') of the superficial surface can be undertaken. The walls of adjacent cysts can also be broken down and excised from within. There have been recent reports of this procedure being successfully carried out laparoscopically. This treatment is most successful for medium to large cysts, but it is virtually impossible for areas of liver with multiple grossly packed small cysts. A combination of partial liver resection and fenestration may be valuable in some cases. Resection is often possible because large areas of liver may be spared, presumably having regenerated in response to the growth of the cysts in the remainder of the liver. Twenty-nine of 31 patients treated by combined resection and fenestration at the Mayo Clinic had satisfactory results at follow-up between three months and eight years.[41] Reoperation is generally very difficult because of substantial adhesions if multiple fenestrations had been peformed.

Caroli's disease is considered elsewhere in this chapter.

HYDATID DISEASE

Hydatid disease or *echinococcosis* is a zoonosis which involves humans as the accidental intermediate host. Dogs and also occasionally wolves and foxes are the definitive hosts and sheep are the intermediate host. The cause is four species of *Taenia echinococci*: *Echinococcus granulosus*, *E. multilocularis*, *E. oligarthrus* and *E. vogeli*, of which the first is the commonest. It is very common in Mediterranean countries, the Middle and Far East, Africa, Australia and South America, but immigration, refugees and travel have contributed to its spread so it is common enough to be seen by most general surgeons.[42] In other Western countries it is found in sheep-farming areas.

The liver is the commonest site of infection but a third of affected patients have other organs involved, most commonly the lungs and the brain but also the kidneys, spleen and bones.

Biology of the parasite

Echinococcus granulosus, the commonest species, infects domestic and wild dogs but also wolves and foxes as definitive hosts, depending on the part of the world. The mature parasite lives in the ileum of the dog. It consists of a head (the *scolex*), which is attached to the intestinal mucosa by multiple hooklets, a neck and three to five segments, the last of which (the *proglottis*) is the largest and contains male and female gonads and thousands of eggs. At some stage in the life of the parasite the proglottis becomes detached and is excreted in the dog's faeces. The eggs and the proglottides can survive for weeks colonizing the dog's perineal area and are transferred by its tongue to other parts of its skin. Humans become infected by direct contact with dogs and ingestion of the eggs or indirectly from contaminated vegetables and water. Sheep, the intermediate host, ingest the ova through pasture. The eggs develop into embryos which are called *oncospheres*. Dogs are recontaminated through eating the viscera of sheep. When humans ingest the eggs, the oncospheres are released in the duodenum and attach to the duodenal mucosa by their hooklets and eventually enter the blood vessels. They can be carried by the portal and systemic circulation anywhere in the body, but the majority of them colonize the liver.

Formation of the hydatid cyst

The oncospheres lose their hooklets as soon as they arrive at the liver and within 12 hours form a microscopic follicle. An inflammatory response occurs with the local accumulation of mononuclear cells but, if the parasites overcome this they grow to cysts visible with the naked eye within three weeks. By five months the *pericyst* has been formed, which is a fibrous capsule produced by the liver. Although this is generally avascular it may contain occasional blood vessels and fine bile ducts. The fully developed cyst consists of the *ectocyst* or laminated membrane, whose role is to protect the cyst from pressure by the pericyst, host proteins and bacteria, and the *endocyst* or germinal membrane, which produces the scolices, capsules and daughter cysts as well as the fluid. The ectocyst is non-nucleated.

Clinical features

Hyatid infection is often contracted during childhood although it has been demonstrated that adults may develop it more rapidly. The cysts may remain latent for years, even decades, and during latency there are no symptoms or signs. Symptoms are caused in two ways: either by local compression of structures by the growing cyst or by complications such as rupture or suppuration. The vast majority of patients present with right upper quadrant pain (60–85%). Dyspepsia and vomiting may occur (19–29%). Approximately 10% of patients report an episode of fever or jaundice or have weight loss.

When spontaneous rupture of a cyst occurs it may cause anaphylactic shock, and if the rupture occurs into the biliary tree (5–10%) symptoms include biliary colic, cholangitis with intermittent jaundice and the presence of debris from the germinal membranes in the faeces. Rupture through the diaphragm into the lungs creates a bronchobiliary fistula which may present with bile-stained sputum, fever and thoracobilia. Rupture into the

REFERENCE

42. Matossian R M, Rickard M D, Smyth J D Bull World Health Org 1977; 55: 499–507

duodenum, small bowel and colon has also been reported. Spontaneous rupture of a large cyst into the peritoneum results in *secondary echinococcosis*, characterized by multiple intraperitoneal cysts, ascites and even intestinal obstruction. Clinical signs in the absence of complications are non-specific and are usually confined to hepatomegaly: this may be the result of compensatory hyperplasia of the healthy lobe of the liver.

Diagnosis

Immunological

Over 10 immunological serological tests have been proposed and used in the diagnosis of hydatid disease but none has satisfactory sensitivity and specificity to become established as the single diagnostic investigation. Intradermal tests such as the Casoni test have been abandoned and the current practice is to use initially either enzyme-linked immunosorbent assay (ELISA) or the indirect haemagglutination (IHA) test followed by the electrophoresis (IEP) test for confirmation of patients with a positive first test.[43] Immunological tests are not helpful for screening in endemic areas or in postoperative follow-up.

Imaging

Plain abdominal X-ray may show elevation of the right hemidiaphragm in a minority (~20%) of patients. Calcified cysts can also be demonstrated. A calcified cyst is not necessarily inactive so the presence of calcification alone should not affect the decision for intervention.

Nuclear scanning is no longer performed for hydatid disease, having been replaced by ultrasonography and CT scanning.

Utrasonography demonstrates the cysts as well-defined lesions containing fluid lined by daughter cysts. When the cyst is very young it may resemble a simple cyst of the liver and when it has been infected it can be misdiagnosed as an abscess or a tumour. Occasionally cysts can be filled with 'sludge' and have a semi-solid appearance or resemble an egg shell if they are calcified.[44]

CT scanning is the best way of imaging hydatid cysts[45] as it is clearly able to demonstrate the daughter cysts and any intraperitoneal spread. It also provides clear anatomical information on the relations of the cyst, which facilitates the subsequent operative planning (Fig. 31.15a).

MRI also provides excellent imaging of echinococcal cysts but is not superior to CT scanning. As it is more expensive and as the disease is endemic in the Third World, there is no place for its routine use in the diagnosis of hydatid disease.

Angiography and endoscopic retrograde cholangiopancreatography (ERCP) may be used in the investigation when the diagnosis is in doubt. ERCP and sphincterotomy may be of specific value in patients who present with intrabiliary rupture and intermittent biliary obstruction.

Biopsy or *percutaneous aspiration*, though reported, is to be avoided because of the risks of dissemination and of causing anaphylactic shock.

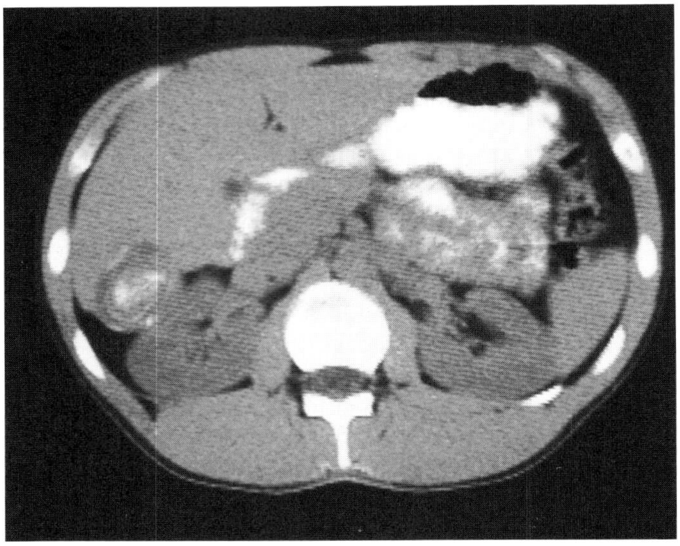

a

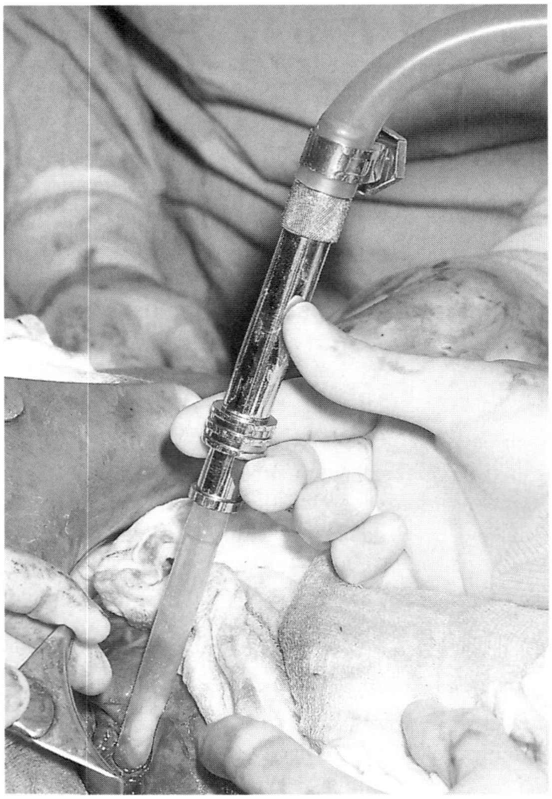

b

Fig. 31.15 (**a**) CT of a patient with hydatid disease. (**b**) Aspiration of the contents of a larger hydatid cyst with a large-bore sucker: a daughter cyst membrane can be seen entering the sucker.

REFERENCES

43. Kertesz V, Roberts P W, Sharp P Med J Aust 1979; 2: 678–680
44. Milicevic M In: Blumgart L H (ed) Surgery of the Liver and Biliary Tract, Vol 79. Churchill Livingstone, Edinburgh 1994
45. Choji K, Fujita N, Chen M et al Clin Radiol 1992; 46(2): 97–103

Treatment

Surgery

Although surgery is the only proven curative treatment for echinococcosis, there are occasionally cases where it may not be the best therapy for the patient. This is particularly true for elderly patients, who are at greater risk of developing postoperative complications. Little has claimed that patients over 60 have only calcified cysts[46] but Milicevic[44] presented a series which does not support this. Surgical treatment should be withheld if there is a single small cyst (< 4 cm) which is deeply seated, because cysts of that size rarely cause symptoms or complications and they require extensive surgery for their removal. Moreover, if they are left to grow under regular observation they almost always extend to the periphery of the liver capsule, making the surgical approach easier.

Cystopericystectomy is performed for peripherally located cysts mainly of the left lateral segment. This involves complete excision of the cyst with the pericyst. Although this treatment is theoretically ideal, it is performed in less than 15% of cases because removal of large cysts is associated with high morbidity.

Partial cystectomy (endocystectomy) with capitonage is the commonest[47] (70–80%) operation and has few recurrences and a low complication rate.

Partial cystectomy with capitonage plus omentoplasty is used to fill large residual cavities.

Liver resection is rarely (< 6%) required, and is usually performed for cysts of the left lobe. Liver resection should not be performed for large medial cysts because they are often in contact with the inferior vena cava and the hepatic veins. It is often only performed when the pathology is in doubt.

Marsupialisation (1%) is external drainage of the cyst which indicates the presence of infection and is associated with a very slow convalescence.

Roux-en-Y cystojejunostomy has been proposed and ERCP may be required if there are residual cystobiliary fistulae.

For all procedures the surgical approach to the liver is through a subcostal incision. The whole abdomen should be explored and all adhesions should be divided. The liver must be fully mobilized as for a liver resection and packs should be placed around it to prevent spillage. The cysts are decompressed with a large trocar and emptied before excision is attempted. The use of a large-bore gynaecological curettage apparatus facilitates aspiration of membranes and daughter cysts and reduces the risk of spillage (Fig. 31.15b). After aspiration deroofing of the cyst allows the removal of residual daughter cysts. Bile-stained fluid implies that there is a communication of the cyst with the biliary tree which will form a fistula if not interrupted. The endocysts are excised and then the cavities are washed with a protoscolicidal agent. Numerous such agents have been used in the past and these include formalin, hydrogen peroxide, Povidone iodine and hypertonic saline. The problem is that if these agents enter the biliary tree through an overlooked communicating duct they cause sclerosing cholangitis.[48] Hypertonic saline (20%) is the safest fluid but because even this can cause strictures it is advisable to dilute it to 3%, although its scolicidal action becomes weaker. Whatever the agent, mechanical cleansing of the cyst is the most important factor. Multiple drains are left in the subhepatic and subphrenic spaces, and occasionally have to stay for many weeks.

Results

Approximately a third of patients develop complications, the commonest of which is biliary fistula formation. Abscess formation is more rare. Recurrence varies in different reports from 0.9% to 22% and this may reflect the heterogeneity of material or lack of long-term follow-up as recurrence may occur several years later. Regular postoperative ultrasound or CT scanning has been suggested for follow-up.

Medical treatment

Medical treatment alone cannot control hydatid disease and it should be used only in elderly high-risk patients with small cysts or as adjuvant therapy in disseminated disease. Original encouraging reports on *mebendazole*,[49,50] were questioned later,[51] and mebendazole may cause significant toxicity. Hepatitis, glomerulonephritis and neutropenia have all been reported to occur. *Albendazole* and *flubendazole*,[52] especially in combination, have been found to give better results. Although these drugs can be detected in the cysts after several weeks of preoperative treatment,[50] it is not yet clear if their administration before and after operation can reduce the incidence of recurrence.

LIVER TUMOURS

Classification

Liver tumours may be primary or secondary, and secondary tumours may originate from a wide variety of extrahepatic primary growths. A classification of primary liver tumours is shown in Table 31.6.

Benign tumours of the liver

Miles Little and his colleagues drew attention to the problem of solid lesions found in the liver on imaging for unrelated symptoms. The majority of these proved to be benign and Little classified these under the label 'dystychomas', from the Greek, meaning that the lesion has been found by 'ill chance'.[53] Examination of the relative frequency of pathologies in this group showed that 73% of

REFERENCES

46. Little J M Med J Aust 1996; I: 903–908
47. Golematis B C, Peveretos P J Mt Sinai J Med 1995; 62(1): 71–76
48. Castellano G, Moreno-sanchez D, Gutierrez J et al Hepatogastroenterology 1994; 41(5): 458–470
49. Kayser H J S Afr Med J 1980; 58: 560–563
50. Morris D L, Gould S E Br Med J Clin Res 1982; 285: 175
51. Rudwan M A, Mousa A M, Muhtaseb S A Int Surg 1986; 71: 22–26
52. Gil-Grande L A, Rodriguez-Caabeiro F, Prieto J G et al Lancet 1993; 342: 1269–1272
53. Little J M In: Terblanche J (ed) Hepatobiliary Malignancy. Edward Arnold, London 1994

Table 31.6 Liver tumours

Benign	
Liver cell adenoma	
Bile duct adenoma	
Focal nodular hyperplasia	
Cystadenoma	
Mesenchymal hamartoma	
Haemangioma	
Haemangio-endothelioma	
Other rarities	
	Fibroma
	Lipoma
	Leiomyoma
	Teratoma
	Adenomatous hyperplasia
	Partial nodular transformation
	Inflammatory pseudotumour
Malignant	
Hepatocellular carcinoma	
Hepatoblastoma	
Cholangiocellular carcinoma	
Angiosarcoma	
Embryonal sarcoma	
Embryonal rhabdomyosarcoma	
Rarer primary tumours	
	Malignant lymphoma
	Malignant teratoma
	Yolk sac tumour
	Carcinoid and other endocrine tumours
	Malignant fibrohistiocystoma
	Fibrous sarcoma
	Leiomyosarcoma

tumours were not neoplastic and only 27% were true tumours; 10% were benign and 17% malignant (11% secondary and 6% primary hepatic cell carcinomas). Of the 73% non-neoplastic and the 10% benign tumours the breakdown was as follows: 52% were haemangiomas, 11% had focal nodular hyperplasia, 8% had liver cell adenoma and 8% had fatty infiltration. Three per cent of apparent liver 'growths' proved to be extrahepatic, such as chronic abscess cavities or adrenal tumours. These 'dystychomas' give rise to a great deal of anxiety, and engender much, often unnecessary, investigation. The general approaches have already been discussed in the section on diagnosis of the liver mass, and usually, particularly in young patients, the diagnosis of a benign disorder becomes clear at an early stage. It is, however, necessary for the clinician to be as certain as possible that he has excluded a malignant tumour, and in cases of doubt to keep the patient under regular surveillance by scanning and, when appropriate, the use of tumour markers. Sadly, no one test, even in some cases biopsy, can absolutely exclude malignancy. Dystychoma indeed!

The remainder of this section will deal with the more important tumours categorized here and discuss their pathology, clinical features and management.

Benign tumours

Haemangioma

This is the commonest mesodermal tumour of the liver and has an autopsy prevalence of about 7%. They are usually single and vary in size from 1 cm upwards. 'Giant' haemangiomas have been defined as those greater than 4 cm in size. They are hamartomatous in nature, consisting of a collection of well-defined large vascular channels with a soft spongy consistency, often containing areas of organized thrombosis and sometimes dystrophic calcification. The ultrasound appearances are characteristic though not diagnostic, and are most reliable for the smaller haemangiomas. Red blood cells labelled with technetium 99m have a high specificity and sensitivity. CT scans taken at intervals after an intravenous bolus of contrast material show the characteristic changes of peripheral enhancement progressing slowly to almost complete infilling of the tumour (Fig. 31.12). They have no propensity to malignant change, and a variable tendency to grow with time. Spontaneous rupture is at the very least exceedingly rare, and in some surgeons' opinions never occurs. Certainly rupture can be induced by trauma, including biopsy, which should be avoided for this reason. Several series have followed up haemangiomas over a number of years and a very small minority grow with time.[54] Nonetheless there is a small group of patients who do develop symptoms, usually associated with growth and stretching of the liver. Some may reach an enormous size. For these patients arterial embolization may have some effect on symptoms but may produce very little regression in size, presumably because of the fixed stroma. A minority of cases therefore come to resection, which may be by enucleation or formal anatomical resection. This group of patients benefit considerably from surgical treatment.[55]

Liver cell adenoma (LCA)

This tumour has an enormous preponderance in women, and has seen an increase in incidence in the last 30 years, thought to be the result of the use of oestrogen-containing oral contraceptive preparations. It is a true adenoma, usually found on scanning or at laparotomy, but more than occasionally presenting with abdominal pain resulting from an increase in size, intralesional haemorrhage or intraperitoneal rupture. An increase in size and rupture have both been reported to be associated with use of the oral contraceptive pill and also with pregnancy.[56] There are no specific features on ultrasound, CT scanning or arteriography, and adenomas vary in their vascularity. Histologically they consist of sheets of well-differentiated liver cells and usually bile ducts are not seen.

The malignant potential of these adenomata is controversial. Certainly elements of hepatic cell carcinomas can be found in some patients with oral contraceptive-associated adenomas, but the adenoma/carcinoma sequence is by no means clear.

Coexistent adenoma, hepatic cell carcinoma and peliosis hepatis, an associated spongy vascular change in the liver architecture, has been seen in a young bodybuilder who had been using anabolic steroids. He presented with intraperitoneal rupture and fatal haemorrhage.[57] Many adenomas regress on withdrawal of oestrogens.

REFERENCES

54. Pietrabissa A, Giulianotti P, Campatelli A et al Br J Surg 1996; 83: 915–918
55. Leading article Lancet 1988; ii: 882–884
56. Tsang V, Halliday A W, Collier N A, Benjamin I S, Blumgart L H Dig Surg 1989; 6: 86–87
57. Creagh T M, Rubin A, Evans D J J Clin Pathol 1988; 41: 441–443

Treatment is also controversial, but the consensus is that small adenomas of under 3 cm in size can be observed with annual ultrasound measurement. Larger adenomas, tumours which are growing or are symptomatic, and those in which there is a doubt about diagnosis should be resected with an adequate margin of clearance.[58] Biopsy is often not diagnostic and is inadvisable.

Focal nodular hyperplasia (FNH)

This curious condition has some similarities to the adenomas described above, though the evidence for a hormonal cause is less clear. The typical macroscopic appearance is of an irregular firm mass in the liver with prominent fibrous septa radiating from a central stellate scar which produces characteristic appearances on ultrasound and CT scanning. There is a frequent association with coexistent haemangiomas in the liver and some with vascular malformations elsewhere in the body. As with liver cell adenomas the relationship with liver cancer is controversial, but the comments on vigilance and life-long surveillance for patients apply to both conditions. The criteria for resection are similar.

Cystadenoma

This has been discussed under the section on liver cysts.

Other rare benign tumours

Of the many reported variants, the mesenchymal hamartoma and partial nodular transformation merit particular mention. Mesenchymal hamartomas often present during the first two years of life and may cause considerable diagnostic difficulty because of their rapid enlargement in size. Many are therefore surgically resected. Partial nodular transformation, a localized form of adenomatous hyperplasia of the hepatocytes, produces large and small nodules containing sheets of regenerating hepatocytes and fibrous bands. When concentrated around the porta hepatis it may cause portal venous obstruction and extrahepatic portal hypertension.

Malignant tumours

Hepatocellular carcinoma (HCC)

This is one of the most common malignancies in the world, largely because of its association with hepatitis virus infections. Although it is rare in Western Europe and the USA areas of high incidence coincide with areas of endemic hepatitis. While hepatitis B and C virus infections are the best-documented risk factors, any form of cirrhosis, including alcohol and haemochromatosis, increases the risk of hepatocellular carcinoma. Other factors implicated in its aetiology are contamination of crops by aflatoxin in some parts of the world, and this may be synergistic with the hepatitis virus in inducing mutation of the tumour suppressor gene *p53*.[59]

Most cases are diagnosed late and indeed in the West the average survival from the time of diagnosis is less than one year. Upper abdominal discomfort and distension associated with weight loss and sometimes low-grade fever are the common presenting features. Since the advent of liver transplantation, many small hepatocellular carcinomas are found incidentally after the removal of cirrhotic livers. A substantial minority of these tumours invade the biliary tract, causing obstructive jaundice by a tongue of tumour which grows down the bile ducts to obstruct the confluence, or by embolization of tumour fragments. The main portal veins may be similarly infiltrated.

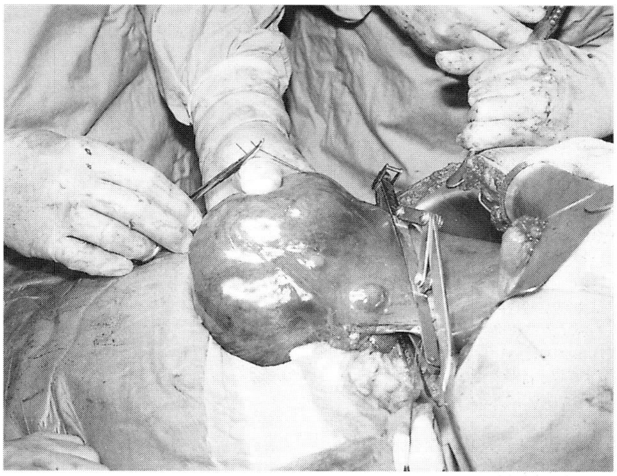

Fig. 31.16 A hepatocellular carcinoma arising in a pedunculated manner from the inferior segments of the right liver. Resection with a good clearance margin was easy in this case without loss of normal liver substance.

A number of different morphological variants have been described, which fall into three broad patterns: massive, consisting of a single large mass with our without small satellite nodules; nodular, in which multiple discrete nodules are present throughout the liver; and diffuse, where multiple minute indistinct nodules are found throughout the liver.[60] Others have described the tumours according to their behaviour, distinguishing between infiltrative and expansive tumours, which remain discrete, pushing the surrounding liver tissue aside.[61] Occasional rather striking variants are seen in which the tumour adopts a pedunculated appearance, often hanging down from the undersurface of the right or left lobe of the liver (Fig. 31.16). An important variant is the fibrolamellar hepatoma, a distinct histological type with large polygonal eosinophilic cells and a fibrous stroma. This usually occurs in younger patients without any underlying liver disease or known risk factors, behaves in a 'pushing' rather than infiltrative manner, and it may grow to a rather large size before presentation (Fig. 31.17). The mean age at presentation is younger, and unlike other variants of hepatic cell carcinomas, there is no male preponderance.

Eighty per cent of patients with hepatic cell carcinomas express the tumour marker α-fetoprotein in the plasma. Patients with

REFERENCES

58. Leese T, Farges O, Bismuth H Ann Surg 1988; 208: 558–564
59. Hsu I C, Metcalf R A, Sun T, Welsh J A, Wang N J, Harris C C Nature 1991; 350: 427–428
60. Eggel H. Beitr Z Pathol Anat Allg Pathol 1901; 30: 506–604
61. Nakashima T, Kojiro M Hepatocellular Carcinoma: An Atlas of its Pathology. Springer-Verlag, Tokyo 1987

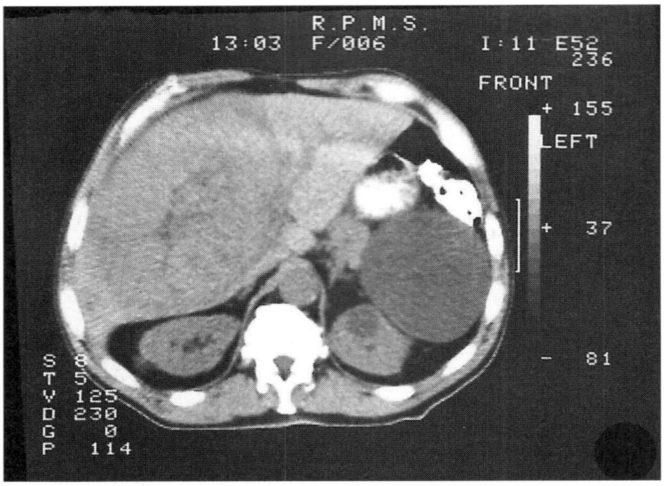

a

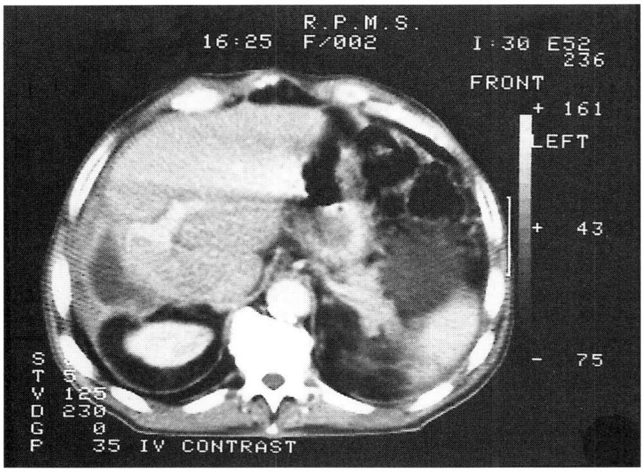

b

Fig. 31.17 CT scans of a patient with a large fibrolamellar hepatoma replacing much of the right liver. Extended right hepatectomy was performed and the second scan shows the regenerated liver three months later.

fibrolamellar hepatomas do not express α-fetoprotein, but the tumour has a high content of neurotensin, which can be detected in the plasma.[62] Vitamin B12 binding capacity is also increased in the majority of patients with fibrolamellar tumours.

The diagnosis of both types of tumour depends on the use of tumour markers and of imaging techniques. Biopsies are frequently obtained, though they do carry the distinct hazard of tumour implantation, which may be important if curative resection is being considered.[28]

Management options are often limited by the late presentation and the coexistence of liver disease, which may preclude major liver resection. Resection of solitary tumours in non-cirrhotic patients produce five-year survivals between 20% and 40%, and possibly 50% for the fibrolamellar variant.[63] The risk of resection in cirrhotic patients may be estimated by Child's grading, though some groups have attempted to use quantitative estimation of the functional residual capacity of the liver following resection, using techniques such as indocyanine green clearance (see above). Patients with irresectable primary tumours who are potential candidates for transplantation are now considered much more readily than in former times (see Ch. 8). Transplantation is at present probably the best choice for the patient with a less than 5 cm hepatic cell carcinoma in a cirrhotic liver, particularly if there is evidence of progressive liver disease which might merit transplantation at a future date.[64]

Non-operative treatment options include the percutaneous injection of ethanol, chemoembolization using lipiodol bound to a chemotherapeutic agent such as epirubicin, or lipiodol bound to iodine[131], though controlled trials have not produced impressive results.[65] Systemic chemotherapy with drugs such as epirubicin is of little or no value. There is some evidence that tamoxifen may be useful as oestrogen receptors are expressed by some tumours.[66] For patients with fibrolamellar hepatoma, resection should be attempted whenever possible and transplantation is also an option.

Cholangiocellular carcinoma

Related to but distinct from the hilar cholangiocarcinoma (the Klatskin tumour) this intrahepatic tumour is very variable in its appearance and presentation. It is often very scirrhous and infiltrates the liver widely. There is an association with Caroli's disease, ulcerative colitis and primary sclerosing cholangitis, and in the Far East with infestation with the liver fluke *Clonorchis sinensis*. Prior exposure to Thorotrast, a radiological contrast agent used in the 1930s and 1940s, was formerly a risk factor for several forms of primary liver tumour, including cholangiocarcinoma, angiosarcoma and hepatic cell carcinomas.[67]

Most patients present with an advanced tumour and survival is rarely longer than nine months from the time of diagnosis. Because of the late and insidious presentation, most tumours are irresectable. Previously regarded as resistant to chemotherapy, combination therapy, for example with 5-fluorouracil, folinic acid and cisplatin, has produced some useful responses.[68]

Angiosarcoma

As well as Thorotrast, this tumour is related to a number of industrial chemicals. Arsenicals used as insecticides in vineyards and vinyl chloride monomer in plastics factories are strongly associated with the development of this tumour. The presentation is entirely non-specific and the diagnosis is usually only made on biopsy or following resection. It is a highly malignant tumour and even after resection and chemotherapy the majority of patients survive for only a few months to one or two years.[69,70]

REFERENCES

62. Collier N A, Weinbren K, Bloom S R, Lee Y C, Hodgson H J F, Blumgart L H Lancet 1984; i: 538–540
63. Rosen C B, Nagorney D M In: Terblanche J (ed) Hepatobiliary Malignancy. Edward Arnold, London 1994
64. Ismail T, Angrisani L, Gunson B K et al Br J Surg 1990; 77: 985
65. Madden M V, Krige J E J, Bailey S et al Gut 1993; 34: 1598–1600
66. Boix L, Bruix J, Castella A et al J Hepatol 1993; 17: 187–191
67. Popper H, Thomas L B, Telle N C et al Am J Pathol 1978; 92: 349–376
68. Cunningham D Personal communication

Liver metastases

These are the commonest tumours in the liver and can arise from almost any primary metastasizing tumour. Tumours of the gastrointestinal tract are overwhelmingly the most common primary site, but breast and lung tumours may also metastasize to the liver. Metastases from cancer of the colon and rectum occupy a particularly important place in liver surgery because of their frequency (see Ch. 30). Of the 30 000 or so new cases of cancer of the colon and rectum each year in the UK about half have liver metastases at some time, and the majority of these are present at the time of diagnosis of the primary tumour.[71] There is a curious disjunction between the tendency for colorectal tumours to spread to the lymph nodes and their ability to metastasize to the liver via the portal venous system. Although tumour cells arrive within the liver via the portal system they quickly develop an arterial blood supply, and if they survive they grow at a variable rate in discrete spherical masses, varying from one to dozens. Many lodge near the surface of the liver, and when their growth reaches the liver capsule they take on a characteristic umbilicated appearance on the surface, because of central loss of blood supply. The capsular surface of the tumour is often adherent to adjacent peritoneal surfaces, including the diaphragm, but this is usually caused by inflammatory adhesions and adventitious blood supply, and is very rarely the result of direct tumour invasion.

A wealth of historical data indicates that the majority of patients with liver metastases die within two to three years of presentation, and practically all are dead within five years.[72] A similar wealth of experience from centres involved in liver resection shows a remarkable consensus in the five-year survival figures following resection of colorectal metastases.[73] Tumour clearance, including freedom from extrahepatic disease, is the most important determinant of survival after resection, though the Dukes' stage, degree of differentiation and number of tumour deposits, particularly if greater than four, influence survival. The size of the tumour may have an effect on the morbidity of the procedure, but has surprisingly little impact on survival. Allowing for all of these different factors the overall five-year survival for patients selected for resection of colorectal liver metastases averages around 35% in the majority of papers. Careful patient selection is, however, essential.

For patients with irresectable tumours, and arguably for those who have undergone resection, there is now good evidence that combination chemotherapy produces a useful response in around a quarter,[74] though survival improvement may be only a few months.

Other treatments have been introduced for irresectable lesions. Thermal ablation of the tumour either by heat delivered through laser fibres[75] or by cold applied using a liquid nitrogen cooled probe at operation[76] have both been tried. There is no doubt about the potential of these treatments to cause major tumour necrosis, though the overall effects on survival are not yet demonstrated. Some of these techniques may extend the application of liver resection, as resection of large tumours on one side of the liver and thermal ablation of tumours on the other side followed by combination chemotherapy may give the best chance of improved survival, if not cure, for some patients who would otherwise have been regarded as untreatable.

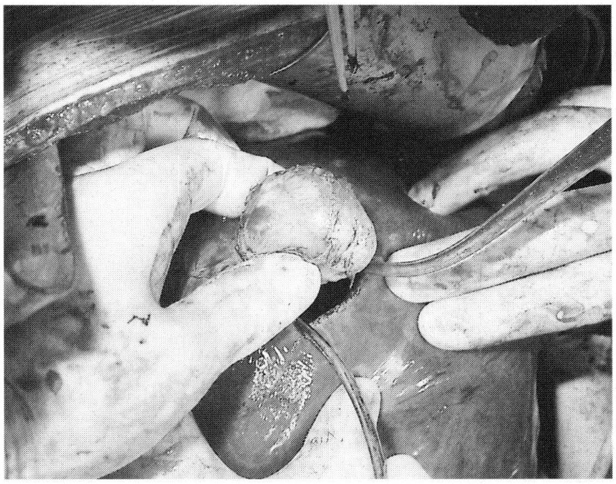

Fig. 31.18 Secondary deposits of carcinoid tumour in the liver in a patient suffering from severe carcinoid syndrome. Multiple metastasectomies were performed, which resulted in resolution of the syndrome, even though much disease was left behind.

Metastases from other sources are much less commonly treated by resection. An important though somewhat rare exception is that of patients with primary neuroendocrine tumours which have been removed and who have liver metastases. The criteria for resectability have been extended in these patients, because these are often slowly growing tumours which exert their effects mostly through associated endocrine syndromes. Perhaps the best example is that of the carcinoid syndrome (see Ch. 29), and unlike colorectal metastases, multiple metastasectomies performed by 'shelling out' tumours from the liver may produce both relief of symptoms and prolonged survival (Fig. 31.18).[77] This philosophy has been extended and liver transplantation is now a feasible option for patients with secondary neuroendocrine tumours of the liver.

Locoregional chemotherapy

Dissatisfaction with the results of systemic chemotherapy, and in particular with high rates of systemic toxicity, led to the use of intra-arterial infusion for liver metastases. Various techniques have been used for this, but most commonly a catheter is introduced through the gastroduodenal artery at laparotomy to allow direct infusion of cytotoxic agents into the hepatic circulation. This procedure may be complicated by the existence of multiple hepatic

REFERENCES

69. Forbes A, Portmann B, Johnson P, Williams R Gut 1987; 28: 668–674
70. Sundaresan M, Kelly S B, Benjamin I S, Akosa A B J Clin Pathol 1990; 43: 1036–1039
71. McArdle C S, Hole D, Hansell D et al Br J Surg 1990; 77: 280–282
72. Scheele J, Stangl R, Altendorf A Br J Surg 1990; 77: 1241–1246
73. Hughes K Surgery 1988; 103: 278–288
74. De Gramont A, Krulik M, Cady J et al Eur J Clin Oncol 1988; 24: 1499–1503
75. Masters A, Steger A C, Brown S G Br J Surg 1991; 78: 518–523
76. Ravikumar T S, Steele G Jr, Kane R et al Cancer Res 1991; 51: 6323–6327
77. Benjamin I S In: Terblanche J (ed) Hepatobiliary Malignancy. Edward Arnold, London 1994

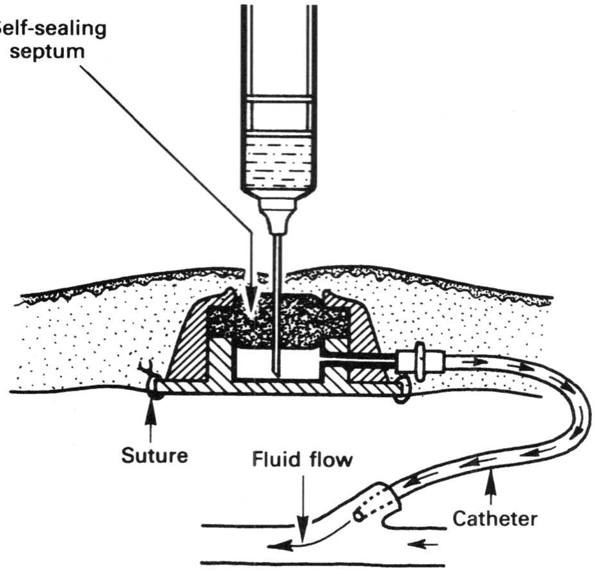

Fig. 31.19 Diagrammatic cross-section of a subcutaneous infusion port for intra-arterial chemotherapy.

arterial vessels such as the anomalous right hepatic artery from the superior mesenteric as described previously and special techniques may be required to overcome this.[78] The catheters may be led to a subcutaneous port into which intermittent infusions can be given (Fig. 31.19), or attached to a permanent pump for long-term constant-rate infusion. An implantable pump (Infusaid) has been used in the UK in what is now a very extensive trial, the final results of which are still awaited. Some studies have shown that while responses may be demonstrated in the liver tumours using these infusional techniques, they are almost invariably accompanied by progression of disease outside the liver. Work is in progress to develop a pharmacodynamic approach which will allow both adequate locoregional therapy and good conventional systemic therapy by the same route.[79] It has to be said that, although response rates seem to be improved, the evidence from controlled trials for survival advantages of intrahepatic therapy over continuous systemic intravenous infusion is not overwhelming.[80]

Liver resection

Anatomical liver resection now follows the segmental anatomy of Couinaud as described at the opening of this chapter. The common resections are right hepatectomy (segments V–VIII), left lateral segmentectomy (segments II and III, also called left lobectomy), left hepatectomy (segments II–IV, with or without segment I) and extended right hepatectomy (segments IV–VIII, with or without segment I, sometimes called trisegmentectomy, especially in the USA). The overriding principle is to stay within the anatomical plane while achieving optimal tumour clearance, and to leave intact inflow and outflow structures to the remaining segments. Recent improvements in technique have allowed removal of multiple segments from different parts of the liver, and resections such as central hepatectomy and extended left hepatectomies.[81] These are technically challenging and should be restricted to specialist centres.

The basic technique includes mobilization of the liver and control of the inflow vessels, either outside or just within the liver substance. Some surgeons routinely ligate the relevant hepatic veins outside the liver, and others approach them within the liver substance. Division of the liver itself may be carried out in a number of ways, but the most popular technique is the use of the cavitron ultrasonic surgical aspirator (CUSA).[82] This is a device held in the hand and controlled from a console. It's tip vibrates at ultrasonic frequency and shatters the hepatocytes leaving the vessels and biliary radicles intact so that they can be accurately and deliberately ligated or sutured. The use of this instrument leaves a relatively clean, smooth liver surface with little bleeding at the end of the resection, and any residual oozing from the surface can be controlled with diathermy, an argon beam coagulator, or the application of a fibrin tissue sealant.[83] It is usually possible to avoid occluding the vascular inflow to the liver remnant, except perhaps for a very short period, and this results in less postoperative liver dysfunction. Intra-operative blood losses have also been reduced with the development of modern surgical techniques, and many surgeons routinely perform major liver resection without blood transfusion.

Postoperatively a reduced liver cell mass is required to support all of the complex liver functions until the process of regeneration has restored the liver function to normal. The first few days require careful vigilance, with particular care being taken to avoid hypoglycaemia, coagulopathies and hypoalbuminaemia. Following large liver resections a transient period of jaundice is the rule, and this must be distinguished from jaundice caused by a technical complication such as damage to or kinking of the bile duct. This is one of the few settings in which separate measurement of conjugated or unconjugated bilirubin may be of value. HIDA scans may also help, and if there is serious doubt then ERCP may be necessary. The majority of patients now suffer few immediate complications following routine liver resection, and most are discharged in about one week.

Liver regeneration proceeds rapidly in the normal liver, though it is less reliable in the presence of cirrhosis. Normal liver size is generally restored in six to eight weeks, and conventional liver function tests have returned to normal well before that time (Fig. 31.20). The alkaline phosphatase may remain elevated for some time and is probably associated with remodelling of the intrahepatic canalicular membranes.

The mortality of elective liver resections should now be only 2–5%. Long-term survival depends upon the underlying pathology.

REFERENCES

78. Goldberg J A, Leiberman D P, McArdle C S Surg Gynecol Obstet 1989; 169: 71–72
79. Kerr D J, Lederman J A, McArdle C S et al J Clin Oncol 1995; 13(12): 2968–2972
80. Kemeny N E, Sigurdson E R In: Blumgart L H (ed) Surgery of the Liver and Biliary Tract, 2nd edn, Vol 2. Churchill Livingstone, Edinburgh 1994
81. Scheele J, Stangl R In: Blumgart L H (ed) Surgery of the Liver and Biliary Tract, 2nd edn, Vol 2. Churchill Livingstone, Edinburgh 1994
82. Hodgson W J, Del-Guercio L R Surgery 1984; 95: 230–234
83. Kram H B, Reuben B I, Fleming A W Trauma 1988; 28: 1195–1201

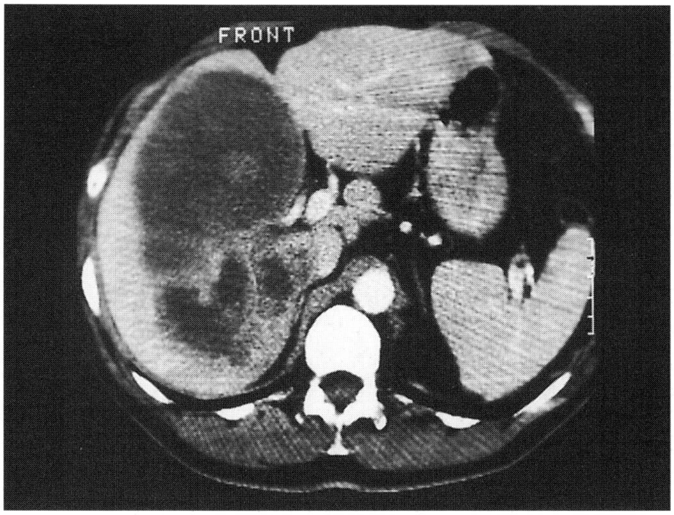

a

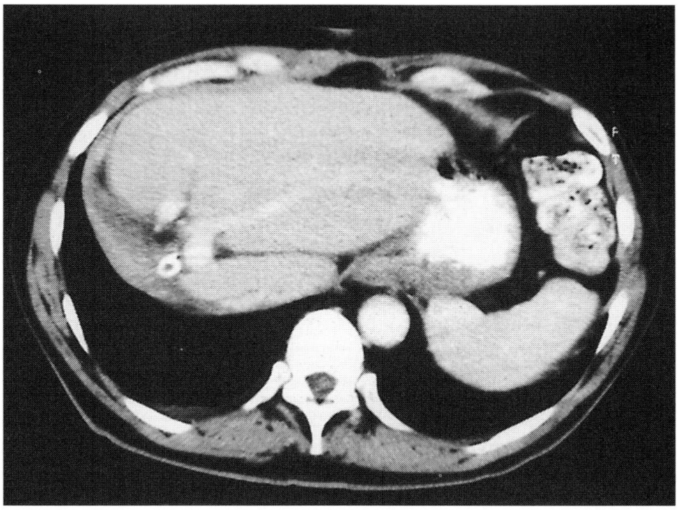

b

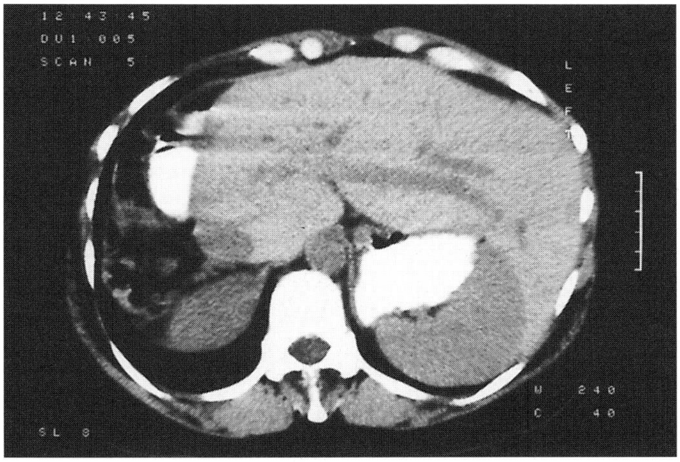

c

Fig. 31.20 (**a**) CT of a 70-year-old man with a large metastatic colorectal tumour replacing most of the right lobe of the liver. (**b**) Two months after extended right hepatectomy (segments IV–VIII) the remaining liver has undergone enormous hyperplasia. (**c**) In another case (six years after right hepatectomy) the liver has regenerated to the left and partially lies lateral to the spleen.

PORTAL HYPERTENSION

Portal hypertension is defined as an increase in portal vein pressure of more than 10 mmHg (normal values 5–10 mmHg). Portal blood flow through the liver may be greatly reduced or even reversed. The portal pressure can be measured directly at operation or indirectly through a needle introduced into the spleen as the splenic pulp pressure or via catheterization of the hepatic veins and measurement of the wedged hepatic venous pressure gradient (HVPG). This last method is of no value in the case of pre-sinusoidal venous block (see below).

Aetiology and pathophysiology

Portal hypertension has many causes and defining the cause is very important before planning treatment. In the Western world the leading cause is cirrhosis of the liver but worldwide schistosomiasis is responsible for the majority of cases. There are generally two mechanisms creating portal hypertension (Table 31.7): (a) increased resistance to portal flow; or (b) increased blood volume and flow in the portal vein. Portal hypertension caused by increased resistance to flow is classified into pre-hepatic, hepatic and post-hepatic. Portal hypertension created by increased blood flow is divided into that caused either by arteriovenous fistula or increased splenic flow.[84]

Table 31.7 Causes of portal hypertension

- Pre-sinusoidal
  - Extrahepatic
    - Portal vein thrombosis
    - Splenic vein thrombosis
    - Increased splenic blood flow
  - Intrahepatic
    - Schistosomiasis
    - Sarcoidosis
    - Indian childhood cirrhosis
- Sinusoidal
  - Cirrhosis
- Post-sinusoidal
  - Budd–Chiari syndrome
  - Congestive heart failure
  - Veno-occlusive disease

There is a subtle and complex interrelationship between hepatic arterial and portal venous blood flow. Reduction or interruption of portal venous inflow results in prompt dilatation of the hepatic artery, which can compensate for up to 45% of the total portal venous flow. This so-called 'buffer effect' has been much investigated, and seems to be mediated by adenosine and perhaps also by ATP. Both adenosine and ATP are important endothelial-derived vasodilators, found in the liver circulation as well as elsewhere. Their action differs in that adenosine acts on purinoceptors on the smooth muscle to cause vasodilatation while ATP acts on the

REFERENCE

84. MacMathuna P, Vlavianos P, Westaby D et al Dig Dis 1992; 10(Suppl 1): 3

endothelium, causing vasodilatation by the release of nitric oxide. This buffer effect may have a role in the preservation of liver blood flow and function after surgical creation of a portacaval shunt, and one report has demonstrated a lower incidence of hepatic encephalopathy and mortality in patients whose hepatic arterial blood flow increased by more than 100 ml/min after shunting.[85] Most cases of portal hypertension are caused by increased resistance at some point in the portal circulation. There is, however, evidence that hormonal factors cause a hyperdynamic circulation and splanchnic hyperaemia. Glucagon is believed to contribute to this effect and a chronic increase of nitric oxide levels is associated with hyperdynamic circulation in cirrhosis and portal hypertension.[86]

Intrahepatic portal hypertension can be caused by increased resistance at three levels:

1. *Presinusoidal*, of which schistosomiasis is the leading cause worldwide. The ova of the parasite colonize and obstruct the portal venules. Many of these patients also have hepatitis B and concomitant cirrhosis.
2. *Sinusoidal*: the main example is alcoholic cirrhosis where collagen accumulates in the space of Disse. In the early stages swelling of the cells by intracellular fat deposition also reduces sinusoidal flow. Alcoholic cirrhosis may also create post-sinusoidal portal hypertension because of pressure on the small hepatic veins from the regenerating nodules.
3. *Post-sinusoidal*, which is rare and is mainly the result of Budd–Chiari syndrome and congestive heart failure.

Pre-hepatic and post-hepatic portal hypertension are discussed separately.

All forms of portal hypertension induce circulatory changes of major significance. Numerous collaterals are created between the portal and systemic venous systems, both intrahepatically and extrahepatically, so that portosystemic shunting occurs at many sites. The most significant collateral circulation is that through the coronary and short gastric veins towards the azygos vein. This results in the creation of *oesophagogastric varices*, which are the major source of haemorrhage (Fig. 31.21) and mortality for these patients. Varices can develop in any other part of the gastrointestinal tract, which is generally congested. Other common bleeding sites are the stomach and rectum, where congestive gastropathy and anorectal varices respectively develop. Congestion of the splenic vein leads to splenomegaly. The epigastric and abdominal wall vessels are also enlarged through recanalization of the umbilical vein, and multiple retroperitoneal collaterals are created which do not bleed spontaneously but in case of surgery make even a simple operation difficult.

Cirrhosis

Cirrhosis is a diffuse condition of the liver parenchyma characterized by fibrosis and the conversion of the normal liver architecture into structurally abnormal regenerative nodules. It is the end stage of chronic liver disease which causes hepatocellular necrosis. It was first described in the fourth century BC by Hippocrates and the name is attributed to Laennec, derived from the Greek word 'kirrhos' which means of yellow colour. It is the fifth leading cause

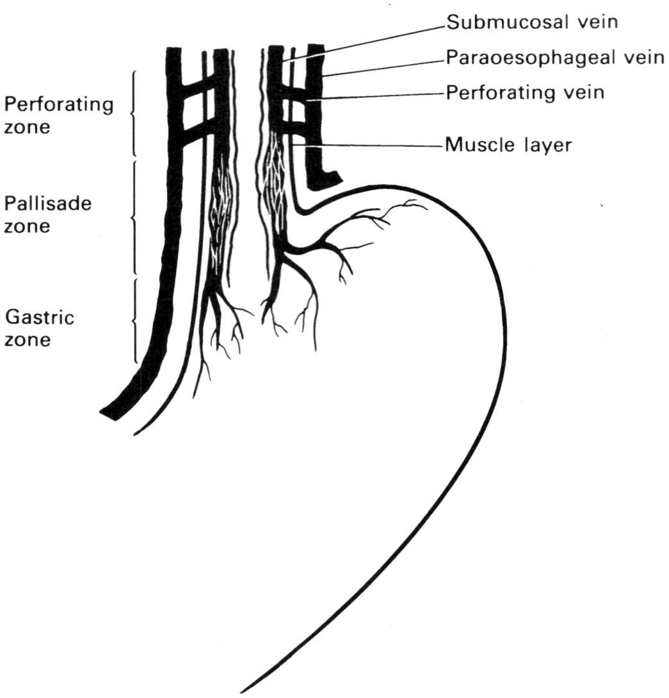

Fig. 31.21 The venous anatomy of the lower oesophagus.

of death in the USA between the ages of 35 and 55. Cirrhosis can be classified morphologically, as macronodular or micronodular, or on an aetiological basis. The latter classification is more useful to the surgeon.

Aetiology of cirrhosis (Table 31.8)

This shows marked geographical variation. In the Third World the majority of cases are of viral aetiology. In the UK, where the per capita consumption of alcohol is 6.2 litres of absolute alcohol per year, the incidence of cirrhosis is 5.7 per 100 000. In France alcohol consumption is 16.4 litres and the incidence of cirrhosis is 10 times higher (57.2 per 100 000).[87]

Alcoholic cirrhosis is micronodular and occurs only in 20% of heavy drinkers. The deleterious effects of alcohol are mediated by the metabolite acetaldehyde, which induces a cascade of adverse events, including glutathione depletion, decreased DNA repair, enzyme inactivation and promotion of free radical toxicity. This is followed by deposition of alcoholic hyalin and an inflammatory response. Women are more vulnerable.

Post-hepatitic cirrhosis (hepatitis B, hepatitis C, hepatitis D) is common in Asia and Africa but also in the Western world in certain high-risk groups namely drug abusers, homosexuals and health care workers.

REFERENCES

85. Burchell A R, Morens A H, Panke W F et al Ann Surg 1976; 184: 289–302
86. Cahill P A, Sitzmann J V Hepatol 1995; 23: 355–356
87. Sherlock S Diseases of the Liver and Biliary System. Blackwell Scientific Publications, Oxford 1989

Table 31.8 Aetiological classification of cirrhosis

Acquired	
	Alcoholic
	Post-hepatitic (hepatitis B, C, D)
	Biliary cirrhosis
	Primary biliary cirrhosis
	Secondary biliary cirrhosis
	Autoimmune
	Autoimmune chronic active hepatitis
	Sarcoidosis
	Drug-induced cirrhosis
	Indian childhood cirrhosis
	Post-intestinal bypass
	'Cryptogenic'
Congenital	
	Haemochromatosis
	Wilson's disease
	α_1-Antitrypsin deficiency
	Galactosinosis
	Type IV glycogen storage disease
	Tyrosinosis
	Fructose intolerance

Primary biliary cirrhosis accounts for 15% of cases in the UK, affecting women nine times more often than men, and is one of the commonest indications for liver transplantation. It is an autoimmune disease progressing to cirrhosis within four years in 80% of the patients and it is characterized by the circulation of antimitochondrial antibodies selectively directed against the enzyme pyruvate dehydrogenase, which is present in the biliary epithelium. The bilirubin level is the best prognostic factor (17 months mean survival when it exceeds 170 μmol/l) and patients are transplanted when the level exceeds 100 μmol/l.

Secondary biliary cirrhosis follows chronic obstruction of the extrahepatic biliary tree, often from choledocholithiasis or to iatrogenic common bile duct injury during cholecystectomy. It is associated with recurrent cholangitis which causes inflammation and scarring of the bile ducts and proliferation of the small bile ductules. *Biliary atresia* in infants, if untreated, leads to secondary biliary cirrhosis. Secondary biliary cirrhosis is obviously of particular concern to the surgeon as it is amenable to surgical prevention and treatment in the early stages by creation of biliary–enteric anastomoses. Early stages of biliary fibrosis may be reversible following good biliary decompression, but it is doubtful whether the changes of fully developed formed cirrhosis can be reversed.

Cirrhosis of autoimmune origin includes *autoimmune chronic active hepatitis* and *sarcoidosis* cirrhosis.

Drugs can induce cirrhosis, two common examples being methyldopa and methotrexate.

Patients who undergo multiple transfusions (e.g. thalassaemias) may develop cirrhosis from *secondary haemochromatosis*.

Patients who underwent *intestinal bypass* (jejunoileal or jejunocolic) for treatment of morbid obesity often developed fatty change in the liver which frequently progressed to cirrhosis. The cause is thought to be the resulting disturbance of the enterohepatic circulation and metabolism of bile salts.

Indian childhood cirrhosis is of unknown cause and affects children younger than three years old in India, Asia and the Middle East, with a grim prognosis.

Congenital causes of cirrhosis include a large group of conditions such as *primary haemochromatosis, Wilson's disease, a_1-antitrypsin deficiency, tyrosinosis, type IV glycogen storage disease, galactosaemia* and *fructose intolerance*.

When no cause can be identified, cirrhosis is called *cryptogenic*. In the past this group included almost a third of the total number of cases. Many cases formerly thought to be 'cryptogenic' cirrhosis are now thought to be caused by hepatitis C.

Diagnosis and assessment of the cirrhotic patient

As always the *history and physical examination* are essential. Usually the only complaints are non-specific: fatigue, weakness and weight loss. Occasionally severe gastrointestinal bleeding from oesophageal varices is the first manifestation of cirrhosis. A history should be sought of alcohol abuse, episodes of jaundice or cholangitis, operations on the biliary tract, hepatitis or a family history of liver disease. Physical examination may provide support for the diagnosis of chronic liver disease. Palmar erythema, leukonychia, Dupuytren's contracture, spider naevi, gynaecomastia and testicular atrophy raise suspicions which are confirmed by finding jaundice or ascites, the palpation of a hard liver, or an enlarged spleen and finding dilated periumbilical veins. In advanced cases the presence of mental confusion or hepatic coma indicates a poor prognosis.

Laboratory tests are very useful in establishing the diagnosis. Liver function tests are usually abnormal although it is not uncommon for them to be normal in patients with latent cirrhosis. Bilirubin values are raised according to the degree of liver damage and the presence of remaining parenchyma. Elevation of transaminases to more than three times normal is a marker of continuing hepato-cellular necrosis. A marked increase in the alkaline phosphatase and γGT denote intra- or extrahepatic cholestasis, though isolated elevation of γGT may reflect recurrent alcohol use.

Hypoalbuminaemia indicates chronic liver disease as well as malnourishment. The prothrombin time is usually prolonged because of decreased synthesis of coagulation factors. Non-specific changes include anaemia from malnutrition, bleeding, and haemolysis, leukopenia and thrombocytopenia from the hypersplenism (see Ch. 34). In advanced disease hyponatraemia, hypokalaemia and metabolic alkalosis are consequences of ascites, hyperaldosteronism and vomiting. The hepatitis markers are positive when the cirrhosis is post-viral.

Ultrasonography and *CT scanning* are the initial means of radiological assessment and usually show a heterogeneous liver parenchyma with increased reflectivity, intrahepatic or extrahepatic biliary tree dilatation, splenomegaly and possibly ascites. A duplex scan of the hepatic vessels can confirm portal hypertension. Investigation may proceed with aortoportography, ERCP or percutaneous transhepatic cholangiography according to the underlying disease.

Liver biopsy is the definitive method of establishing the diagnosis and can be obtained by direct percutaneous needle biopsy, by using a transjugular catheter, or at laparoscopy or laparotomy. It should be performed with caution when coagulation is impaired or marked ascites is present, as major bleeding and haemobilia are serious complications.

Assessment of hepatic functional reserve

Assessment of the hepatic functional reserve is necessary to balance the risks and benefits of either palliative or definitive treatment. In some centres dynamic tests of hepatocellular function are performed: these include the aminopyrine breath test, the galactose elimination capacity and the hepatic clearance of amino acids. The most useful assessment is still the Child–Pugh classification (see above). The operative mortality for Child's A patients is less than 5% while for Child's class C it is over 25%.

Ascites

Increased sinusoidal pressure and hepatic insufficiency result in the creation of ascites. Its pathophysiology is complex and not entirely clear but there is agreement that three factors contribute: (a) increased formation of lymph by both the liver and the intestine; (b) hyperaldosteronism with sodium and water retention; and (c) hypoalbuminaemia. Ascites rarely requires surgical intervention as medical treatment is effective in more than 90% of cases. Medical treatment consists mainly of a low-salt diet and diuretics, spironolactone (100–400 mg per day) being the first-line drug. The aim is to lose 500 g of weight per day. Clinical response together with 24-hour urinary sodium determination are the criteria for the use of stronger diuretics. Strong diuretics are needed if the 24-hour urinary sodium is less than 5 mEq. Frusemide and ethacrynic acid are always given in combination with spironolactone. No diuretics are necessary if the 24-hour urinary sodium is more than 25 mEq. A low-sodium diet is given but total sodium or water restriction is no longer considered necessary. Paracentesis was abandoned for some time but it has been recently reintroduced and may be valuable in the management of ascites in some patients. Albumin is often administered when a paracentesis is performed, otherwise serious circulatory and electrolyte disturbances may occur.

Five to ten per cent of patients with ascites are resistant to medical treatment ('refractory ascites') and these patients may need a LeVeen peritoneal–jugular shunt, which uses a subcutaneous silastic catheter to drain the ascitic fluid from the peritoneal cavity into the jugular vein. A modification incorporating a small subcutaneous pump which can be compressed externally is called the Denver shunt. Postoperatively an abdominal binder is applied. Complications include disseminated intravascular coagulation, septicaemia from infected ascites and obstruction of the catheter (~10%). A portacaval shunt is effective in controlling ascites but it is indicated only if it is intended also to treat concomitant bleeding varices. An exception is in the Budd–Chiari syndrome (see below).

Hepatic encephalopathy

Hepatic encephalopathy occurs in patients with advanced hepatic failure and in approximately 20% of patients who undergo a portacaval shunt. It is a metabolic neuropathy ranging from minor mental changes to lethargy and coma. Many factors play a role: the decompensated liver cannot sufficiently inactivate the *toxins* produced by the action of intestinal bacteria on protein and these toxins cross the blood–brain barrier, which also seems to be intrinsically defective. Neurotransmitters produced in the gastrointestinal tract also cross the blood–brain barrier, and particularly *GABA* as well as the *'false' neurotransmitters* octopamine, phenylethanolamine and aromatic amino acids have been implicated. In liver failure *ammonia* is not sufficiently converted to glutamine and accumulates in the blood and cerebrospinal fluid. Although it has been shown experimentally that ammonia produces symptoms similar to those of hepatic encephalopathy, its exact role in the syndrome remains to be resolved. Even in the absence of a surgically created shunt there are always multiple sites of intrahepatic and extrahepatic *shunting* in the circulation. Patients with hepatic failure may also be elderly, debilitated, with fluid and electrolyte disturbances from ascites, excessive diuretic therapy or suffering from infections, and all these factors add to the development of encephalopathy. Treatment aims at eliminating the bacterial load of the gut, restricting the dietary protein intake and correcting any coexisting metabolic and electrolytic abnormalities. Enemas, laxatives and oral neomycin are used to cleanse the bowel.[88] A high carbohydrate and vegetable protein diet together with lactulose, which also inhibits bacterial enzymes and reduces the amount of produced ammonia, are used for long term treatment.

Acute liver failure, with encephalopathy occurring within eight weeks from the onset of symptoms, has replaced the term fulminant hepatic failure, as many of these patients now survive today. This can be subdivided into three groups: hyperacute liver failure (encephalopathy within seven days of the onset of jaundice) which carries a better prognosis, acute (8–28 days) and subacute (5–12 weeks), in decreasing order of prognosis.[89] Death occurs as a result of cerebral oedema and sepsis, usually combined with multiorgan failure. Treatment should be attempted only in specialized units, with early ventilation, dialysis, intracranial pressure monitoring and with prophylactic antibiotics and antifungal agents. Prostaglandins and *N*-acetyl cysteine are currently being tested as possible cytoprotective agents. A major area of research is the '*bioartificial liver*',[90] a support system which consists of a sophisticated pump which directs the blood through fibre filters and cultured hepatocytes which are derived from human hepatoblastoma cells or pig hepatocytes. The bioartificial liver has produced some promising results and it may prove invaluable for temporary support of patients with acute liver failure until the organ regenerates or a graft is available for transplantation. The selective use of urgent liver transplantation has transformed the results in acute liver failure (see Ch. 8).

Hepatorenal syndrome

Although renal impairment accompanying liver disease had been recognized since the 19th century the term was used for the first time in 1956 by Hecker and Sherlock. The criteria for diagnosis have been revised repeatedly in 1978 and 1988 and new criteria

REFERENCES

88. Salmeron J M, Tito L, Rimola A et al J Hepatol 1992; 14: 280–285
89. O'Grady J G, Schalm S W, Williams R Lancet 1993; 342: 273–275
90. McNair A N B, Tibbs C J, Williams R Br Med J 1995; 311: 1351–1355

have been again proposed in 1996.[91] It occurs in patients with advanced hepatic failure and portal hypertension, and is characterized by impaired renal function and marked abnormalities in the arterial circulation and activity of the endogenous vasoactive systems. In the past, hypovolaemia and sepsis were considered to be precipitating factors but this is currently questioned. Recent evidence indicates that endothelial factors play a role in the creation of hepatorenal syndrome as well as in the general circulatory disturbances of cirrhosis.[92] For the diagnosis to be accepted, there must have been no previous renal disease or use of nephrotoxic agents. The urine volume is usually very low, less than 800 or even 500 ml/24 h, the urinary sodium is very low (< 10 mEq/24 h) and the urine output does not respond to administration of fluids. Kidney histology is normal, and if the patient has a liver transplant, renal function recovers. In other cases renal function deteriorates rapidly.

Oesophageal varices: acute bleeding

(Table 31.9)

Approximately one-third of cirrhotic patients die from variceal haemorrhage. The risk of haemorrhage is greater in those with severe hepatic decompensation (50% for Child's class C patients). Of those who bleed, half will die during that episode and a third of the survivors will bleed again within six weeks. The aim of treatment is to control the bleeding with as little invasion as possible as these patients are at very high risk for surgery. The general resuscitation principles for treating any acute haemorrhage apply. *Octreotide* is a somatostatin analogue that has a vasoconstrictive effect on the splanchnic circulation and as it has few side effects is tending to replace *vasopressin* and its analogues, which were previously used. *Emergency oesophagogastroscopy* establishes the diagnosis and also allows the best methods of first-line treatment to be carried out. The varices are treated either by *sclerotherapy*—injection of sclerosant such as ethanolamine oleate into and/or around the varices—or by *rubber band ligation* which has been recently reported to be the more effective of the two.[93] A repeat endoscopy is performed within 48 hours as the rebleeding rate within the same hospital admission is 25%. When endoscopy is not available and pharmacological therapy ineffective, *balloon tamponade* is applied. The Sengstaken–Blakemore tube (two balloons, three lumina) or the Minnesota variation (two balloons, four lumina) are used (Fig. 31.22). The first balloon is inflated in the gastric fundus, and the second in the oesophagus. The third

Table 31.9 Oesophageal varices: management of acute bleeding

Resuscitation
Urgent endoscopy
Rubber band ligation
Sclerotherapy
Balloon tamponade
Medical treatment
Octreotide
Vasopressin
Transjugular intrahepatic portosystemic shunt (TIPS)
Surgery
Oesophageal transection
Urgent portosystemic shunt

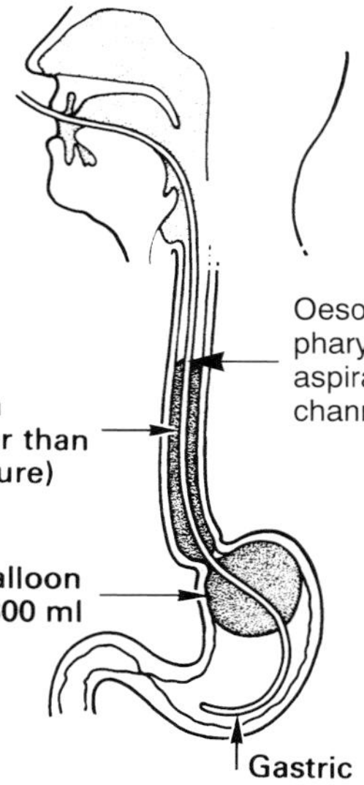

Fig. 31.22 A Minnesota modified Sengstaken–Blakemore tube.

lumen is used to aspirate the contents of the stomach and the fourth to aspirate oesophageal contents. It is important to make sure that adequate traction is applied to compress the fundal varices and to achieve the correct pressure (around 40 mmHg) in the oesophageal balloon using a manometer. Balloon tamponade is not free of complications, the main ones being the aspiration of pharyngeal secretions and oesophageal ulceration from pressure necrosis. When the bleeding stops (75% of patients) the tube is usually left in situ for 24 hours with the oesophageal balloon deflated. The early rebleeding rate is twice that of endoscopic treatment (50%) so this method should only be used when endoscopy is not available or occasionally when it is ineffective.

Transjugular intrahepatic portosystemic shunt (*TIPS*) is a way of creating a shunt through a catheter inserted into the liver via the jugular vein under radiological guidance. The catheter is forced into an intrahepatic branch of the portal vein and a metal stent is placed to maintain the communication. This technique is used when repeated sclerotherapy fails to control variceal bleeding, but it is not definitive as most stents thrombose within a year. Complications include intraperitoneal bleeding (mortality 1%), recurrent variceal bleeding (10–20%), encephalopathy (10–20%) and aggravation of the hepatic failure (25–35%). Randomized trials are needed to determine its real place but at the moment it is a useful 'bridge' towards liver transplantation for a certain group of patients.[94]

Surgery is the last solution if the previous methods fail to control variceal bleeding. An *emergency portacaval shunt* (end-to-side portacaval or H-mesocaval) is effective in stopping the

REFERENCES

91. Hecker R, Sherlock S, Lancet 1956; ii: 1121
92. Arroyo V, Gines P, Gerbes A L et al Hepatology 1996; 23(1): 164–176
93. Schrier R W, Aroyo V, Bernardi M et al Hepatology 1988; 8: 1151–1157

bleeding. A distal splenorenal shunt (see below) is not appropriate for emergency surgery. The survival depends on the preoperative status of the patient and the mortality approaches 50% in Child's class C patients, mostly as a result of postoperative encephalopathy. *Oesophageal transection* using a circular stapling device is an effective emergency procedure which has largely displaced the older manual methods of high, wide gastrotomy and oversewing of bleeding varices, but is still not a definitive treatment because varices usually recur a few months later.

Oesophageal varices: elective treatment

(Table 31.10)

The overall risk of bleeding in patients with oesophageal varices is 30% for those who have not bled before and 70% for those who have bled once before. Following control of a first bleed, it is therefore important to treat varices actively to prevent this major complication. Patients at high risk are Child's class C, or those whose varices are large, or show cherry-red spots or 'varices on varices'. Sclerotherapy should be repeated as frequently as necessary until the varices have been eradicated, when it is used as the only means of treatment. *Prophylactic endoscopic sclerotherapy*, however, has not been proven so far to reduce the risk of bleeding.

Pharmacological treatment is more promising. *Propranolol* has been shown to reduce the incidence of the first episode of bleeding by 40% and also reduces the mortality during the first bleed. It also reduces the frequency of rebleeding but it has not been shown to decrease mortality.[95] *Octreotide* is effective in preventing rebleeding, as are combinations of *vasopressin, glypressin* and *nitroglycerin* in the short term. Patients who do not reduce their portal pressure with propranolol may do so when *isosorbide mononitrate* is added.

Surgery has three strategies: liver transplantation, portosystemic shunts and devascularization procedures.

Liver transplantation is the definitive treatment with good results and low mortality.[96] The choice depends on the overall evaluation of the patient and the underlying disease as well as possible contraindications such as continuing alcoholism. A TIPS may be used for temporary control of bleeding if transplantation is planned.

Portosystemic shunts (Fig. 31.24) are divided into:

1. *Total shunts*, which decompress the entire portal system: end-to-side portacaval, side-to-side portacaval, mesocaval with use of a graft between the inferior vena cava and the superior mesenteric vein, or splenorenal.

Table 31.10 Oesophageal varices: elective treatment

Pharmacological treatment
Propranolol
Octreotide
Vasopressin/glypressin
Nitroglycerin
Isosorbide mononitrate
Endoscopic sclerotherapy
Transjugular intrahepatic portosystemic shunt (TIPS)
Surgery
Portosystemic shunts
Devascularization (Sugiura procedure)
Liver transplantation

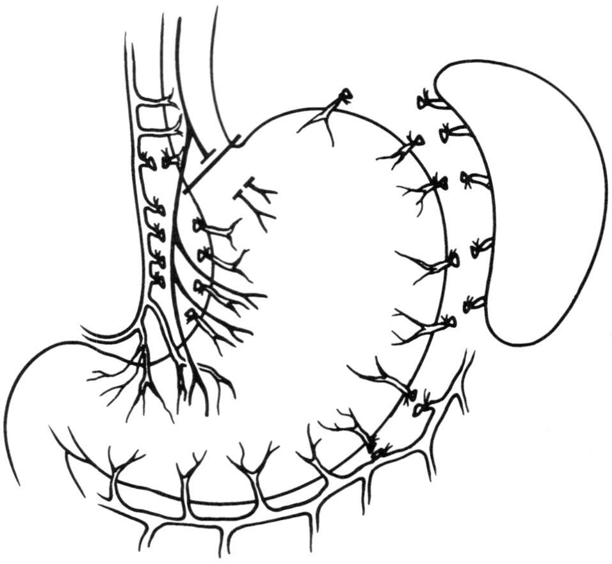

Fig. 31.23 Devascularization/transection operation.

2. *Selective shunts*, which decompress only the vulnerable oesophagogastric compartment, and aim to preserve hepatic portal perfusion. This shunt, the distal splenorenal or Warren shunt, creates an anastomosis between the distal end of the splenic vein and the renal vein, and is combined with ligation of the coronary vein. It is a technically demanding shunt, unsuitable for emergency treatment, and it does not improve ascites.

All shunts are equally effective in reducing rebleeding to 10% of cases. They all have a considerable mortality (~20% in Child's class C patients) and the same long-term survival, but they differ in the early postoperative encephalopathy rate, which is almost half in selective compared to total shunts (15% vs 25%). Shunts have not been shown to give any survival benefit over endoscopic sclerotherapy, and are now generally reserved as a second-line treatment when the latter treatment fails repeatedly, or for decompression of varices in ectopic sites.

The most popular *devascularization procedure* is the *Sugiura procedure*[97] (Fig. 31.23). This is performed in two stages: (a) thoracotomy with devascularization, transection and re-anastomosis of the oesophagus; and (b) six weeks later laparotomy, devascularization of the upper two-thirds of the stomach, vagotomy, pyloroplasty and splenectomy. Original excellent results with this operation reported in Japan were not confirmed in American studies, but the procedure is still widely used, for example, in the Middle East, where there is a high prevalence of schistosomiasis,

REFERENCES

94. Gimson A E S, Ramage J H, Panos M Z et al Lancet 1993; 342: 391–394
95. Laberge J M, Somberg K A, Lake J R, Gordon R L et al Gastroenterology 1995; 108: 1143–1151
96. Conn H O, Grace N D, Bosch J et al Hepatology 1991; 13: 902–912
97. Iwatsuki S, Starzl T E, Todo S et al Surgery 1988; 104: 697

as this responds poorly to portal diversion because of a high incidence of encephalopathy.

Pre-hepatic portal venous obstruction

Idiopathic portal vein thrombosis is rare in adults but is the commonest cause of portal hypertension in children. In adults it is caused by trauma, tumours, chronic pancreatitis, abdominal sepsis and hypercoagulable states. In children omphalitis, neonatal septicaemia or umbilical vein catheterization may be responsible, but it usually remains unnoticed until several years later when children present with either variceal bleeding or splenomegaly and pancytopenia. Liver function tests are normal and diagnosis is made by mesenteric angiography. Treatment is initially by sclerotherapy and at the age of 8–10 a portosystemic shunt may be performed[98] (Fig. 31.24). Splenectomy is contraindicated.

Splenic vein thrombosis is rare and may be caused by chronic pancreatitis, pseudocysts, trauma or tumours. The blood flow is diverted through the short gastric veins and the left gastric vein to the liver, and sometimes only gastric varices may be present–so-called 'left-sided portal hypertension'. Splenectomy is curative.

Budd–Chiari syndrome

This is a rare syndrome caused by various disorders that produce obstruction of hepatic venous outflow. Spontaneous thrombosis of the hepatic veins occurs with the use of oral contraceptives, in the presence of polycythaemia vera and a range of other pro-coagulant disorders. Tumours compressing the vena cava, as well as idiopathic membranous stenosis of the inferior vena cava, cause thrombosis of the hepatic veins. Intrahepatic veno-occlusive disease may also be caused by some toxic alkaloids found in herbal preparations. The clinical presentation consists of marked ascites and nonspecific gastrointestinal symptoms such as nausea and bloating.

••••••••••••

REFERENCE

98. Sugiura M, Futugawa S World J Surg 1984; 8: 673

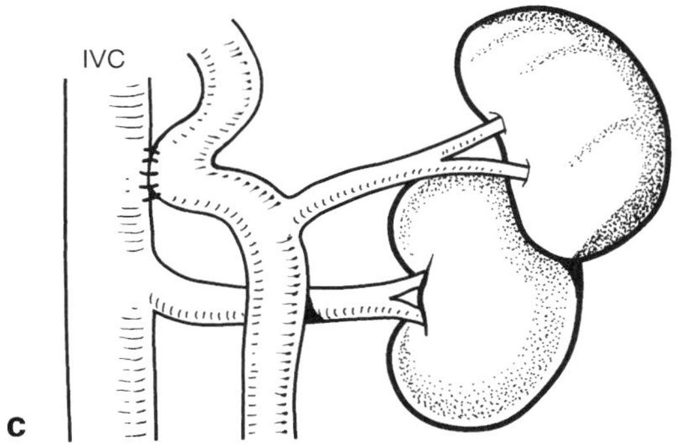

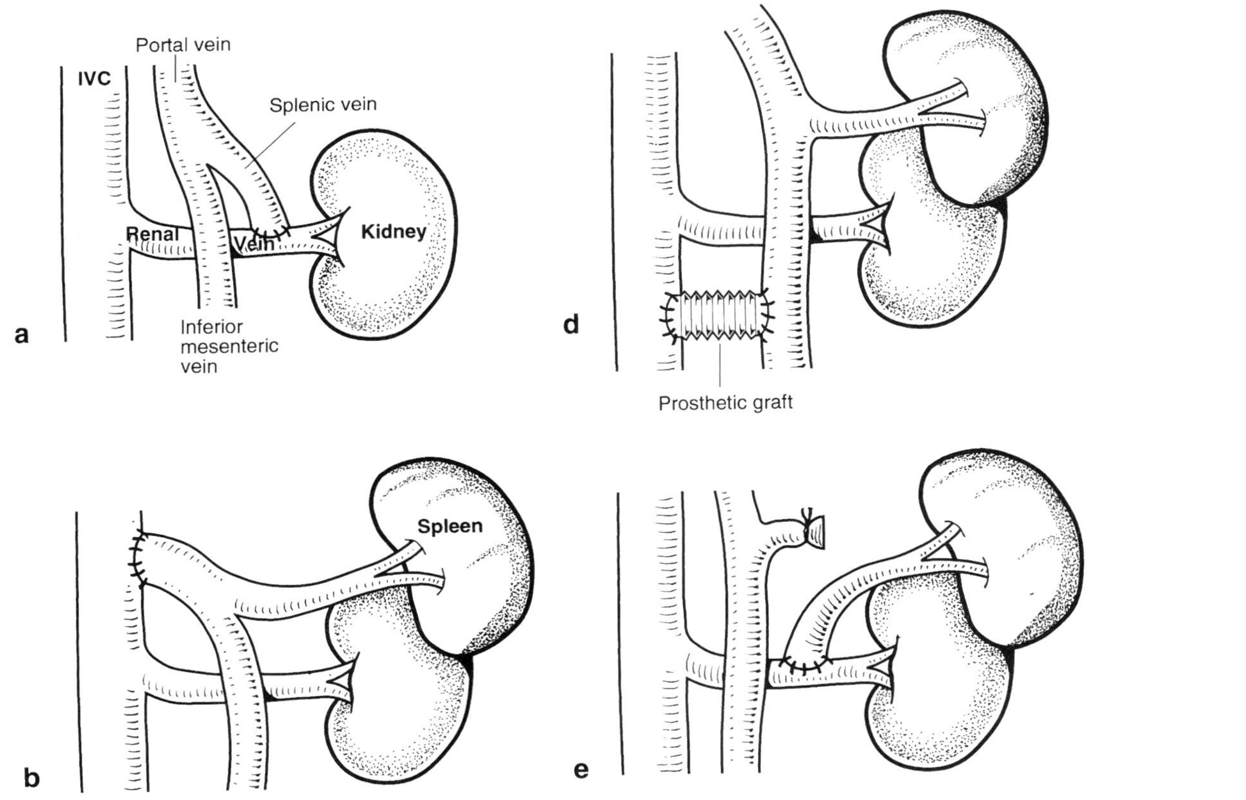

Fig. 31.24 Main types of portosystemic shunts: (**a**) standard splenorenal; (**b**) end-to-side portacaval; (**c**) side-to-side portacaval; (**d**) mesocaval H graft; (**e**) distal splenorenal.

The nerves to the extrahepatic bile ducts are derived from segments 7–9 of the thoracic sympathetic chain and from the parasympathetic vagi. Afferent nerves which include pain fibres from the biliary tract run in sympathetic nerves and pass through the coeliac plexus and the greater splanchnic nerves to reach the thoracic spinal cord via the white rami communicantes and dorsal ganglia. The preganglionic efferent nerves from the spinal cord relay with cell bodies in the coeliac plexus and the post-ganglionic fibres run with the hepatic artery to supply the biliary tract. A small contribution of pain afferents may travel within the right phrenic nerve and peritoneum below the right diaphragm.[3] These fibres may account for the radiation of gallbladder pain to the right shoulder tip during attacks of gallstone colic. Vagal fibres supply the hilum of the liver and the bile ducts. Although vagal stimulation results in gallbladder contraction and relaxation of the sphincter of Oddi, the effects are overshadowed by the action of gastrointestinal hormones such as cholecystokinin.

ANOMALIES OF ANATOMY

Gallbladder

The gallbladder is rarely absent or rudimentary,[4] but when this occurs it may be associated with other congenital anomalies such as tracheo-oesophageal fistula or imperforate anus. Left-sided or intrahepatic gallbladders must not be overlooked. Double and triple gallbladders have also been reported. Maingot[5] for example described 136 cases of double gallbladder, although some of these were small and rudimentary arising from the common bile duct along the free edge of the lesser sac. Discovery of duplications at operation, usually by operative cholangiography, should be followed by removal of both gallbladders. If only one organ is removed a second operation may be necessary later.[6]

The gallbladder may be abnormal in structure, for example the body may be divided completely or partially by a septum. Complete division may result in two separate cavities fused at their necks to form a single cystic duct or they may drain by two separate ducts.

Most of the commonly observed abnormalities of gallbladder structure are associated with gallstones. For example, the so-called Hartmann's pouch[7] is an enlargement of the neck, parallel with the cystic duct, which is associated with cholelithiasis.

Constriction of the body may be congenital but again is more usually associated with stones. Oral cholecystography may occasionally show a partial separation of the fundus from the body known as a Phrygian cap[8] which is caused by a thickening of the gallbladder wall. It is of little significance and gallbladder function is usually normal.

The anatomical position of the gallbladder may vary. It may be completely buried within the liver parenchyma (intrahepatic) or found on the undersurface of the left hepatic lobe, particularly in association with situs inversus. Complete investment of the gallbladder with peritoneum can predispose to torsion around its associated mesentery,[9] particularly when this is restricted to the neck of the organ so that the body and fundus remain free. Torsion of the gallbladder can occur at any age but is most common after 60 years. An acute onset of severe pain with enlargement of the gallbladder in a thin elderly patient is diagnostic. Gangrene and perforation commonly follow, and cholecystectomy is the treatment.

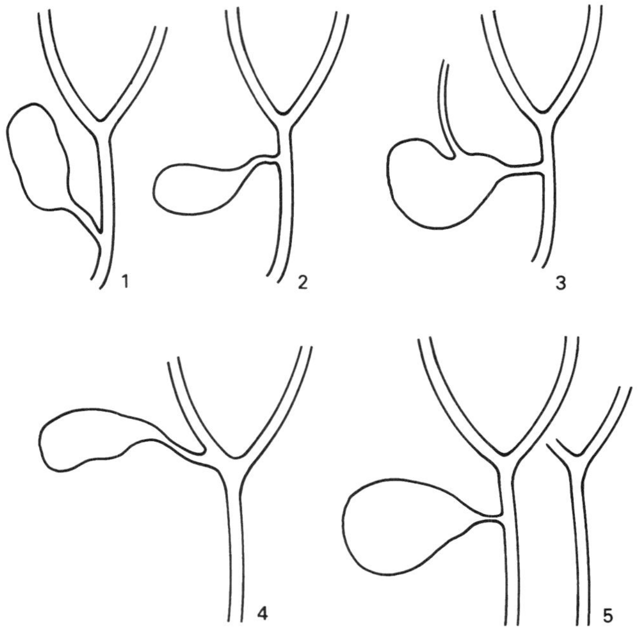

Fig. 32.1 Variations in normal anatomy. **1** Long cystic duct; **2** short cystic duct joining bifurcation; **3** accessory hepatic duct joining either gallbladder or cystic duct; **4** cystic duct joining right hepatic duct; **5** double common bile duct.

Bile ducts

Major variations in bile duct anatomy are not uncommon[10] (Fig. 32.1), and their frequency has been analysed recently in a review of 513 operative cholangiograms.[11] The most important, and potentially dangerous, variations involve different types of right subsegmental ducts and their drainage into the biliary tract via, or close to, the cystic duct.

A few examples of the commoner variations include:

1. A long cystic duct, running parallel to the common hepatic duct, with a low insertion into the common bile duct (20%).

2. A high insertion of the cystic duct into the region of the common bile duct bifurcation (3.1%).

3. An accessory hepatic duct, defined as a separate channel, draining a segment of the right lobe of the liver into the common

REFERENCES

3. Burnett W, Cairns F W, Bacsich P Ann Surg 1964; 123: 8
4. Ferris D O, Glazer I M Arch Surg 1965; 91: 359
5. Maingot R Abdominal Operations, 7th edn. Appleton-Century-Crofts, New York 1980
6. Harlaftis N, Gray S W, Skandalakis J E Surg Gynecol Obstet 1977; 145: 928
7. Wood D Am J Surg 1979; 138: 746
8. Joseph A E A, Grundy A In: Wilkins R A, Nunnerley H B (eds) Imaging of the Liver, Spleen and Pancreas. Blackwell Scientific Publications, Oxford 1990, p 309
9. Ashby B S Br J Surg 1965; 52: 182
10. Benson E A, Page R E Br J Surg 1976; 63: 853
11. Kullman E, Borch E et al Br J Surg 1996; 83: 171

hepatic duct, cystic duct or gallbladder. The incidence is probably 1–4%[12] and it may be the only drainage from the relevant segment. An injury can easily occur to these ducts during cholecystectomy and may result in partial or total occlusion of a portion of the biliary tract as there is a lack of interductal communications within the liver.

4. The cystic duct entering the right hepatic duct. This is an uncommon variation (0.2%), but this increases the risk of transection or ligation of the right duct during surgery.

5. The right and left hepatic ducts may joint the common hepatic duct in a variable manner, and occasionally this junction may be truly intrahepatic. The right duct occasionally fuses with the cystic duct.

Intraoperative cholangiography is used for the recognition of these anomalies. Accessory ducts may be tied off if small, but larger ducts should be preserved and implanted into a Roux loop if necessary. Bile peritonitis or fistula may be a consequence of the unrecognized division of such a duct. Anomalous ducts are particularly at risk during laparoscopic cholecystectomy as operative cholangiography is frequently omitted during the procedure.[13]

Anomalies of the common bile duct itself are very rare but ectopic drainage of accessory ducts into the stomach has been described on five occasions,[14] including an original report by Vesalius in 1543. The anomaly has been associated with symptomatic biliary gastritis.

Hepatic and cystic arteries

Variations of arterial supply are found in more than half the patients undergoing cholecystectomy.[15] The normal arrangement describes the hepatic artery as arising from the coeliac axis and giving off gastroduodenal and right gastric vessels. The common hepatic artery ascends anterior to the portal vein and medial to the common bile duct, dividing into right and left hepatic arteries behind the bifurcation of the bile duct in 80% of cases.

Major anomalies of vessel origin are particularly important during hepatectomy and pancreatectomy. The left hepatic artery arises from the left gastric, splenic or superior mesenteric in 3–6% of the population and may be especially at risk during gastrectomy. The right hepatic artery arises from the superior mesenteric artery in 10–20% and an accessory right hepatic artery arising from the superior mesenteric is found in 5% of patients.

The right hepatic artery is particularly at risk during cholecystectomy if it takes a tortuous course close to the cystic duct and neck of the gallbladder (known as the 'caterpillar hump'); the cystic artery may be very short in this variation.

The cystic artery not uncommonly runs in front of the common bile duct which increases its risk of damage during cystic artery dissection and ligation.

PHYSIOLOGY OF THE BILIARY TRACT

Bile is transported from the liver to the duodenum through the biliary tract. Some 50–60% of bile enters the gallbladder in the fasting state[16] where it is concentrated and modified in composition. Normal bile secretion pressures range from 12 to 15 cm of water. The ampullary sphincter provides a resistance to bile flow between meals, although the flow never ceases completely.

Bile secretion is inhibited when the bile duct pressure reaches 20 cm of water.[17] Cholesterol and phospholipid secretion is reduced rather more severely than bile salts by this rise in pressure but a high ductal pressure does lead to accumulation of bile salts within the liver and other body tissues.[18]

The resting pressure of the gallbladder varies between 0 and 16 cm of water but rises to 30 cm of water during a contraction. The pressures measured within the common bile duct vary according to the contractile and resorptive activity of the gallbladder as well as the resistance to flow afforded by the sphincter of Oddi.

The gallbladder capacity is approximately 40 ml and its function includes the absorption of water and electrolytes from hepatic bile. Both gallbladder contraction and relaxation of the sphincter of Oddi are under hormonal control; the most important hormone is cholecystokinin.

Gallbladder contractility

Cholecystokinin is released during absorption of fat and essential amino acids from the duodenum and small bowel mucosa.[15] It has a direct action on the gallbladder muscle and is the major stimulus for contraction.[19] Of the other hormones, secretin decreases contractility and motilin alters motility between meals. Motility is also affected by gastrin and the prostaglandins.

Hormones therefore play a major role in the control of gallbladder activity, and abnormalities in cholecystokinin release patterns and gallbladder response have been described.[20]

Hormone production from the gastrointestinal tract is inhibited by bile salts and this mechanism may allow the gallbladder to fill between meals.

In contrast to the hormonal effects on the biliary tract, neurological control is more difficult to measure. Reciprocal reflex activity between the gallbladder and duodenum has been demonstrated in dogs during vagal stimulation, but vagal effects are complicated by gastrointestinal secretion and hormone release. No direct vagal influence has been found on either the sphincter of Oddi[21] or on gallbladder contractility.[22] Vagotomy does not appear to affect gallbladder emptying in response to either cholecystokinin or a fatty meal.

REFERENCES

12. Knight M, Smith R, Sherlock S (eds) In: Surgery of the Gall Bladder and Bile Ducts. Butterworth, London 1981
13. Moosa A R, Easter D W et al Ann Surg 1992; 215: 203
14. Sieber W K, Wiener E S, Chang J J Pediatr Surg 1980; 15: 817
15. Bouchier I A D In: Smith R, Sherlock S (eds) Surgery of the Gall Bladder and Bile Ducts. Butterworths, London 1981, p 67
16. Watts McK, Dunphy J E Surg Gynecol Obstet 1966; 122: 1207
17. Strasberg S M, Dorne B C et al Gastroenterology 1971; 61: 357
18. Strasberg S M, Redinger R N et al Lab Clin Med 1982; 99: 342
19. Vagne M, Grossman M I Am J Physiol 1968; 215: 881
20. Thompson J C, Fried G M et al Ann Surg 1982; 195: 670
21. Pitt H A, Doty J E et al J Surg Res 1982; 32: 598
22. Sandblom P, Poegtlin W L, Ivy A C Am J Physiol 1935; 113: 175

Gallbladder resorption

The columnar epithelium of the gallbladder is composed of three types of cells—epithelial cells on a basement membrane, slender 'pencil' cells within the body of the gallbladder and basal cells.[23] The mucous membrane is thrown into folds when the gallbladder empties.

Active absorption of sodium, chloride and bicarbonate ions is followed by the passive absorption of water.[24] Lipid-soluble substances pass across the epithelium easily and there is slow absorption of conjugated bile salts. The absorption of unconjugated bile salts appears to be speeded up by mucosal damage and therefore deconjugation by bacterial activity within the gallbladder may result in a significant loss of bile salts, reduced cholesterol solubility and possibly gallstone formation.

Sphincter of Oddi

Details of the sphincteric structure at the lower end of the bile duct were described in several species by Oddi[25] in 1887. Anatomical studies in humans[26] clearly showed that the sphincteric muscle was separate from the muscle layers of the duodenal wall. Waves of relaxation and contraction with a rate of approximately 10 cycles per minute occur across the sphincter so that bile is actively expressed into the duodenum. The common bile duct, in contrast, contains only sparse numbers of muscle fibres and no significant motor activity has been demonstrated.

Cholecystokinin causes gallbladder contraction and reciprocal relaxation of the sphincter of Oddi. Glucagon also relaxes the sphincter but gastrin raises sphincter pressure and there are therefore marked changes in biliary tract function between fasting and feeding.

Vagal stimulation tends to reduce sphincter tone whilst vagotomy increases it[21] but the changes are insignificant compared with the hormonal mechanisms.

In summary, bile is stored and concentrated in the gallbladder, but passes through the common bile duct in a passive manner.

Common bile duct emptying is controlled by gallbladder activity and contractions in the sphincter of Oddi. Substantial common bile duct dilatation does not occur after cholecystectomy unless there is either mechanical or functional obstruction in the distal duct.

INVESTIGATION OF THE GALLBLADDER AND BILE DUCTS

The imaging techniques now available allow an accurate assessment to be made of the biliary tract in both the jaundiced and non-jaundiced patient.

Plain abdominal radiograph

Approximately 10% of gallstones are radiopaque and very occasionally the bile ducts are outlined by a high concentration of calcium in the bile. Enlargement of the gallbladder may be recognized as a soft tissue mass above the hepatic flexure of the colon. Air within the bile ducts may be associated with a spontaneous biliary–intestinal fistula or with gas-forming organisms in inflammatory disease, particularly severe cholangitis. Previous surgical procedures, for example sphincterotomy or choledochoduodenostomy, will also allow the free passage of air into the bile ducts.

Oral cholecystogram[27]

Oral contrast agents such as Telepaque (iopanoic acid) or Biloptin (sodium iopodate) are administered the night before the examination after a preliminary control radiograph. The contrast is absorbed from the gut, bound to albumin in the portal blood, extracted by the hepatocytes and secreted in bile. Visualization is obtained following concentration in the gallbladder and is optimal 10 hours after ingestion of the agent.

Jaundice, with a bilirubin level greater than 35 μmol/l, and recent inflammatory disease prevent successful opacification. Other reasons for failure of the test include a failure of absorption of the contrast in patients with pyloric stenosis or paralytic ileus, and liver disease. The gallbladder is presumed to be abnormal if there is no opacification after a double dose of contrast.[28]

Oral cholecystography has now been largely replaced by ultrasonography as the initial test of gallbladder disease and is reserved for equivocal cases, for example when the ultrasound scan is negative but the clinical history is very suggestive of gallstones.

Intravenous cholangiogram

Intravenous contrast agents such as Biligram (meglumine ioglycarnate) are excreted by hepatocytes in a large enough concentration to opacify the bile ducts, although gallbladder opacification is usually not very good. Tomography is employed to increase the bile duct definition. In many centres the investigation has been replaced by endoscopic retrograde cholangiography as the false-negative rate for stones in the common bile duct is approximately 15%.[29] Minor toxic reactions may occur from the iodine content and there may be severe, possibly fatal, reactions in patients with Waldenström's macroglobulinaemia. It is suggested that protein electrophoresis should be performed in all patients who are to undergo intravenous cholangiography.

Percutaneous transhepatic cholangiography
(Fig. 32.2)

The risk of bile leakage from needle puncture of the liver has been reduced by the development of thin, long needles, but bacteraemia and occasionally septic shock are well-known complications of the technique, particularly in patients with strictures or stones.

REFERENCES

23. Evett R D, Higgins J A, Brown A L Gastroenterology 1964; 47: 49
24. Diamond I M, Tormey I McD Nature 1966; 210: 817
25. Oddi R Arch Ital Biol 1887; 8: 317
26. Boyden E A Surg Gynecol Obstet 1957; 104: 641
27. Graham E A, Cole W H, Copher G H JAMA 1924; 82: 1777
28. Mujahed Z, Evans J A, Whalen J P Radiology 1974; 112: 1
29. Goodman M W Gastroenterology 1980; 79: 642

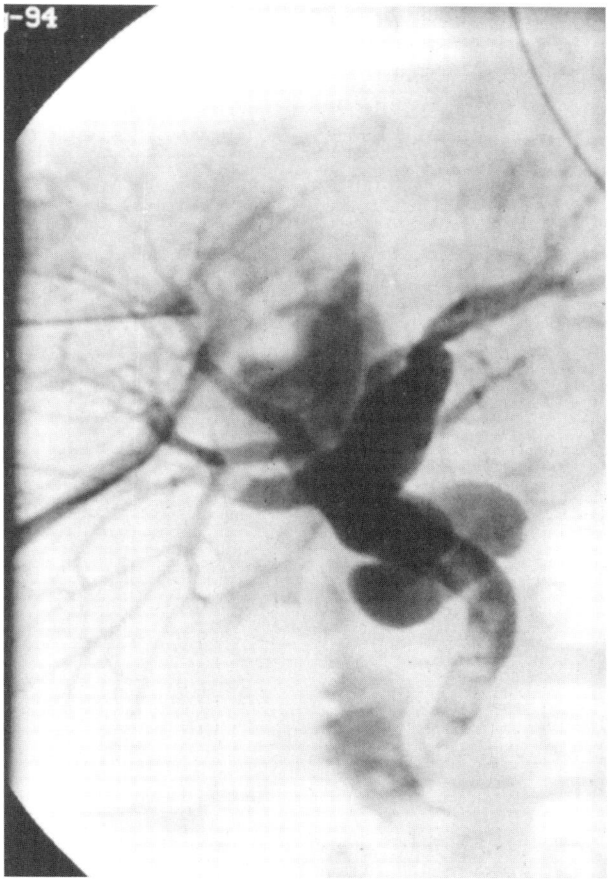

Fig. 32.2 Percutaneous transhepatic cholangiogram performed in a 2-month-old jaundiced infant. The cholangiogram shows that there is inspissated bile in the common bile duct.

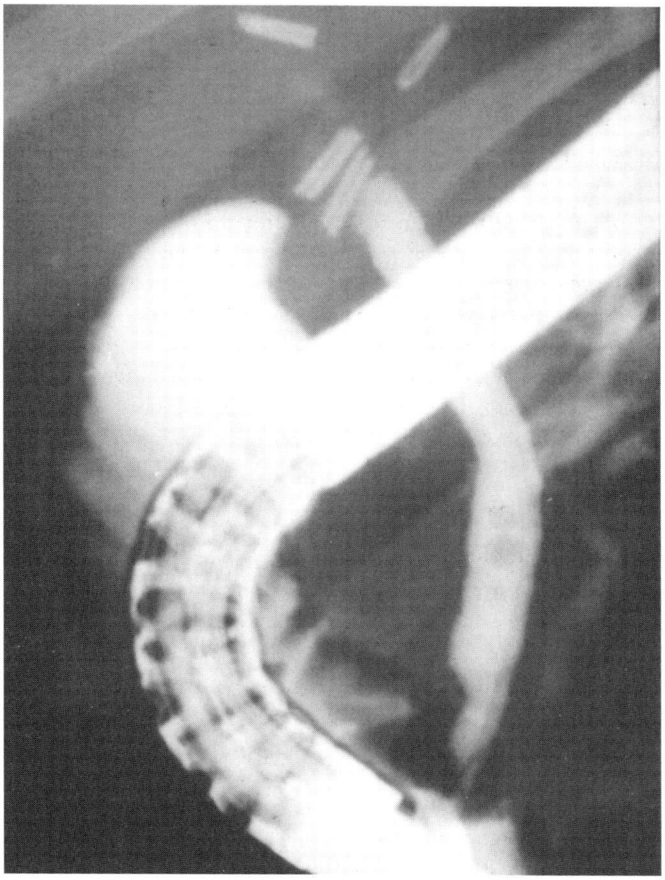

Fig. 32.3 This patient became jaundiced after laparoscopic cholecystectomy. The endoscopic retrograde cholangio-pancreatography shows that clips have been placed across the common bile duct, which has been mistaken for the cystic duct.

Antibiotic prophylaxis and coagulation studies are essential in these patients before the investigation is performed. Nearly 95% of dilated ducts can be demonstrated by percutaneous transhepatic cholangiography and more than half of all non-dilated ducts can also be entered.[30] The needle is passed through the seventh or eighth intercostal space into the right hepatic lobe and water-soluble contrast is injected as the needle is withdrawn. Hepatic or portal veins and lymphatics are commonly observed but contrast clears quickly. Contrast within bile ducts persists for a longer period. The technique is particularly useful for stones, strictures and tumours.

Endoscopic retrograde cholangiopancreatography (Fig. 32.3)

The ampulla of Vater is visualized with a side-viewing endoscope which allows cannulation of the common bile duct or pancreatic duct. Cannulation may fail for anatomical reasons, such as the previous construction of a Polya gastrectomy or if the ampulla is strictured.[31] The technique is very useful in the jaundiced patient, particularly if there are associated coagulation problems. Biopsy of the ampulla may be performed if tumour is suspected. Cholangitis and pancreatitis are uncommon complications.

Ultrasonography

Ultrasound is used increasingly as a screening test for gallstones and is an extremely sensitive method of detecting bile duct dilatation. It is very specific for stones of more than 4 mm diameter[32] and is invaluable in patients who are pregnant[33] or iodine-sensitive.

The examination is performed with the patient fasting: the biliary tract is therefore distended with bile. Stones are visualized as echogenic foci with acoustic shadowing; movement of the patient changes their position. Limitations of the technique include poor definition of stones in the common bile duct and small stones within the gallbladder, particularly those in the gallbladder neck. Calcium bilirubinate may be reported as 'sludge' on ultrasound but in the absence of stones is probably of no surgical significance.

REFERENCES

30. Howard E R, Nunnerley H B J R Soc Med 1979; 72: 495
31. Lintott D J In: Wilkins R A, Nunnerley H B (eds) Imaging of the Liver, Spleen and Pancreas. Blackwell Scientific Publications, Oxford, 1990 p 278
32. De Graaff C S, Dembner A G, Taylor K J W Arch Surg 1978; 113: 877
33. Machi J, Sigel B, McGrath E C Surg Gynecol Obstet 1985; 160: 119

Stones, gallbladder wall thickening and distension are highly suspicious of acute cholecystitis.[34]

Radionuclide scans (Fig. 32.4)

^{99}Tc-labelled derivatives of iminodiacetic acid administered intravenously give very good γ-camera images of the bile ducts after 15 minutes. The technique is useful for the diagnosis of acute cholecystitis, obstruction in the common bile duct, and bile duct anomalies in childhood (see below). The passage of radionuclide into the bowel can also be used to measure the patency of biliary–enteric anastomoses postoperatively.

The use of iminodiacetic acid scanning in acute cholecystitis secondary to cystic duct occlusion has proved diagnostic in 97% of patients with physical signs of gallbladder inflammation[35] when the test fails to demonstrate the obstructed gallbladder.

INVESTIGATION OF JAUNDICE

Type of jaundice

In the commonly used classification, jaundice is divided into prehepatic, hepatic and post-hepatic types.

Prehepatic

In this group of disorders the liver is presented with an excessive load of bilirubin which is unconjugated and therefore absent from the urine. The faecal and urinary urobilinogen levels are increased. Increased haemolysis is the usual reason and is seen in spherocytosis, thalassaemia and sickle cell disease. Rarer causes include Gilbert's syndrome[36] in which there is a defect in bilirubin transport to liver cells and the Crigler–Najjar syndrome[37] caused by a conjugation defect inherited as an autosomal recessive (type I) or dominant (type II) disorder.

Hepatic

Hepatocellular damage, for example from viral or alcoholic hepatitis, may result in a conjugated hyperbilirubinaemia. Conjugated bilirubin is water-soluble and therefore excreted in the urine. Cholestatic disorders caused, for example, by toxic drugs (e.g. phenothiazines), primary biliary cirrhosis and pregnancy present in a similar manner.

Post-hepatic

Bile duct obstruction causes a conjugated hyperbilirubinaemia with bile in the urine and pale stools. Commoner causes include pancreatic, bile duct and ampullary malignancies, calculi and strictures. Less frequently sclerosing cholangitis, chronic pancreatitis, choledochal cysts and metastatic lymphadenopathy present in a similar manner. Parasitic infestation of the biliary tract is unusual in the UK but over 600 million people throughout the world are infested with the worm *Ascaris lumbricoides* which can migrate into the common bile duct and the intrahepatic ducts. The worms may live in this site for approximately 1 month before they die and after death their fragmented bodies may become covered with a precipitate of calcium bilirubinate to form biliary tract calculi.

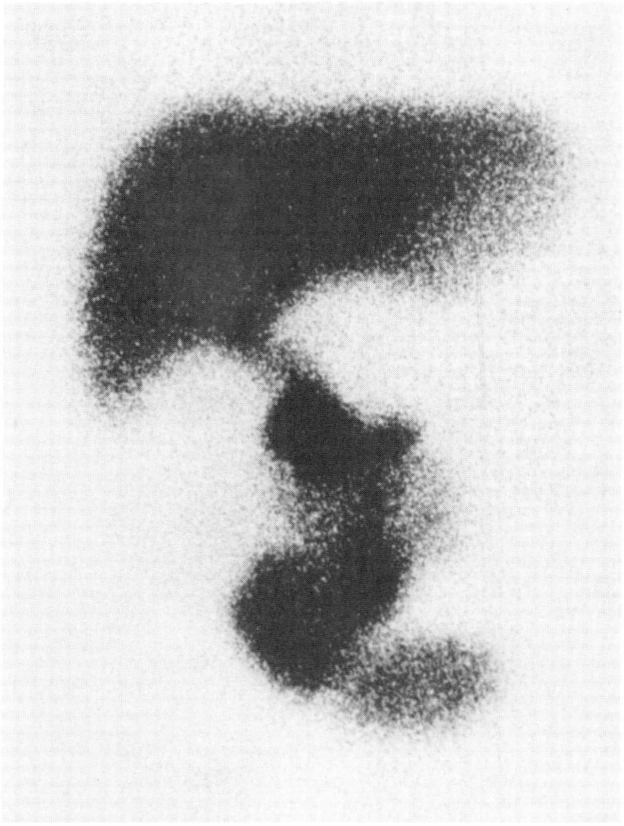

Fig. 32.4 A radionuclide scan performed after Roux loop reconstruction of the biliary tract in a 6-month-old infant with biliary atresia. There is excellent biliary excretion into the bowel.

The liver fluke, *Clonorchis sinensis*, which is prevalent in South-east Asia, is another example of a parasite which may colonize the bile ducts and cause complications with stone formation. *Clonorchis* infestation is also associated with an increased incidence of cholangiocarcinoma.[38]

The diagnosis and management of the jaundiced patient are very dependent on the clinical history and examination. Recent travel, or drug addiction, for example, may suggest hepatitis and the patient may present with tiredness, joint pains and anorexia.

Chronic alcohol abuse may be documented in a patient presenting with cirrhosis. Severe episodic right hypochondrial pain with fever and jaundice suggests gallbladder disease, whereas constant epigastric pain and weight loss are more indicative of malignant disease.

Pruritus is an important feature of both hepatic and post-hepatic cholestasis. Itching which is related to bile salt deposition within the skin is most severe on the extremities and worse in warm

REFERENCES

34. Rails P W, Colletti P M et al Radiology 1985; 155: 767
35. Suarez C A, Block F et al Ann Surg 1980; 191: 391
36. Foulk W T, Butt H R et al Medicine 1959; 38: 25
37. Crigler J F, Najjar V A Pediatrics 1952; 10: 169
38. Hou P C Cancer 1958; 2: 168

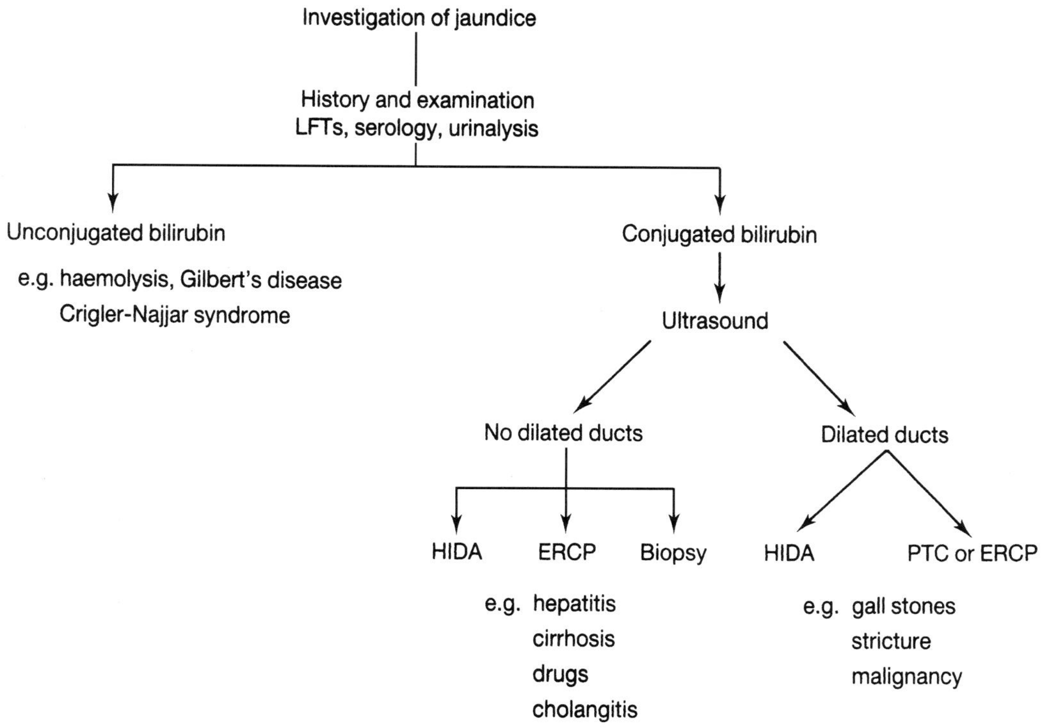

Fig. 32.5 Investigation of jaundice. LFT = Liver function test; HIDA = 2,6-dimethyl phenylcarbamoylmethyl-imindodiacetic acid; ERCP = endoscopic retrograde cholangiopancreatography; PTC = percutaneous transhepatic cholangiography.

weather. Hypoprothrombinaemia from either hepatocellular damage or malabsorption of vitamin K can present with severe bruising. Haemolytic disorders may be diagnosed from a family history of jaundice. Bilirubin is deposited within the elastic tissue of the sclerae, face and upper limbs and usually becomes obvious when the serum level is above 40 μmol/l. General examination may reveal the stigmata of chronic liver disease, such as spider naevi (angiomata), palmar erythema, finger clubbing, leuconychia, gynaecomastia and ascites. Splenomegaly and prominent abdominal wall veins suggest portal hypertension and cirrhosis. Features of specific types of liver disease include xanthomata in biliary cirrhosis and Kayser–Fleischer rings in Wilson's disease.[39]

Enlargement of the liver is recognized by palpation of the lower margin and percussion over the right lower ribs. The character of the liver edge may be diagnostic; for example, the irregular hard edge of malignant disease.

When jaundice is caused by a stone in the common bile duct dilatation of the gallbladder is rare, but when the duct is obstructed in some other way (e.g. carcinoma of pancreas) dilatation is common (Courvoisier's sign).[40] Clearly the obstruction in the latter case must be below the confluence of the cystic and common hepatic ducts.

Sequence of investigations in jaundice

Urinary, biochemical and serological tests are usually followed by an ultrasound scan which will reveal any ductal dilatation, gallstones or intrahepatic lesions. The cause of ductal dilatation may be shown and surgical treatment can proceed. Liver biopsy should be obtained if ductal dilatation is not present, providing the coagulation tests are satisfactory.

Further definition of the biliary tract can be obtained with either percutaneous transhepatic cholangiography or endoscopic retrograde cholangiography (Fig. 32.5). Biochemical tests of jaundice are often disappointing as sole diagnostic criteria. The hepatic alkaline phosphatase is produced in the epithelium of cholangioles and increased production occurs in liver disease. Levels may therefore rise in association with focal liver lesions (e.g. neoplasms) which are obstructing only a segment of the biliary tree. Levels may also rise in cholangitis.[41]

5′-Nucleotidase and leucine aminopeptidase are also produced by cholangioles and are elevated in cholestasis. γ-Glutamyl transferase is raised in all types of liver disease but most markedly in biliary tract obstruction. High levels are also seen with liver metastases.

Serum albumin and globulin rise in cirrhosis and globulin reaches particularly high levels in biliary cirrhosis. There is no change in these proteins with bile duct obstruction unless cirrhosis is also present.

Hepatocellular injury allows a leakage of cell contents into the circulation, which include the enzymes aspartate aminotransferase

REFERENCES

39. Nazer H, Ede R J et al Gut 1986; 27: 1377
40. Taylor I, Wright R In: Blumgart L H (ed) Surgery of the Liver and Biliary Tract, 2nd edn. Churchill Livingstone, Edinburgh 1994, p 184
41. Price C P, Sammons H G J Clin Pathol 1976; 29: 976

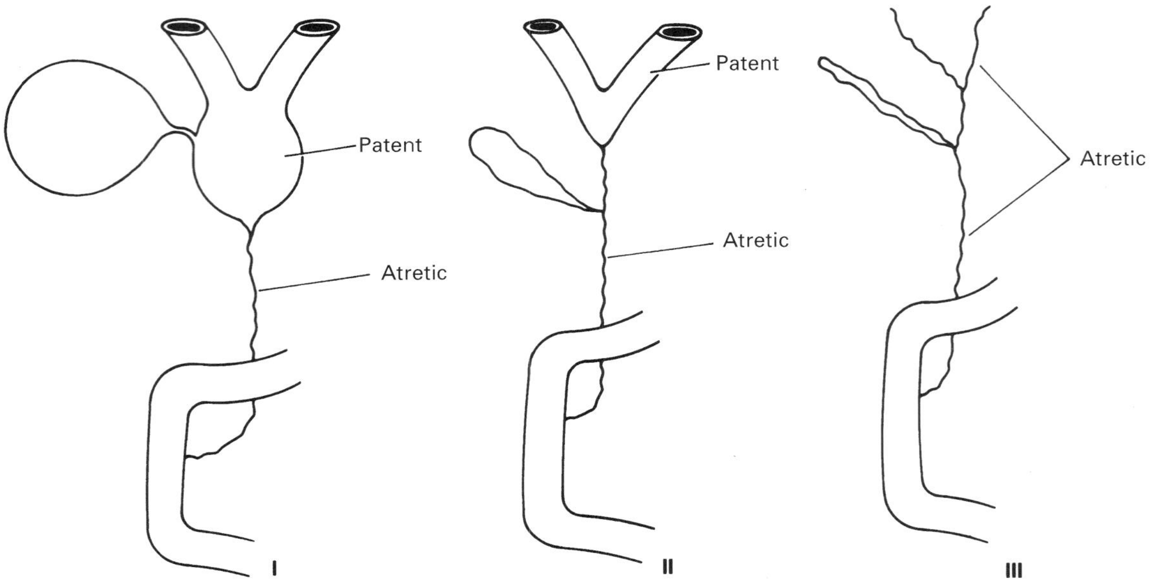

Fig. 32.6 Classification of biliary atresia. **I** Patent common hepatic duct; **II** patent hepatic ducts; **III** atresia of all extrahepatic ducts.

and alanine aminotransferase. The levels are highest in acute liver damage but are also raised in chronic liver disease and biliary tract obstruction.

Urobilinogen is completely absent from the urine if the bile duct is totally obstructed, but levels are high in prehepatic jaundice.

DISORDERS OF THE BILIARY TRACT IN CHILDHOOD

Conjugated hyperbilirubinaemia in infancy may be caused by structural changes within the biliary tract associated with extrahepatic biliary atresia or choledochal cysts. The presentation and biochemical abnormalities of these conditions may be difficult to distinguish from infective and metabolic causes of jaundice in infancy.

Rarer surgical conditions of the bile ducts in children include inspissated bile syndrome, spontaneous perforation of the bile ducts, gallstones and tumours.

Extrahepatic biliary atresia

This is the commonest cause of childhood biliary tract obstruction. The incidence is approximately 1 per 14 000 live births and the sexes are equally affected.[42] The extrahepatic bile ducts are progressively destroyed by an inflammatory process which starts around the time of birth. Intrahepatic changes also occur and eventually result in biliary cirrhosis and portal hypertension. The untreated child dies before 3 years of age of liver failure or haemorrhage.

The aetiology is unknown, although a viral infection has been proposed[43] and studies of the pancreaticobiliary junction in 8 infants with atresia revealed a long common channel at the ampulla in all cases.[43]

This inflammatory destruction of the bile ducts has been classified into three main types[44] (Fig. 32.6):

1. Type I atresia restricted to the common bile duct.
2. Type II atresia of the common hepatic duct.
3. Type III atresia of right and left hepatic ducts.

Associated anomalies are present in approximately 20% of cases and include cardiac lesions, polysplenia, situs inversus, absent vena cava and preduodenal portal vein.[42]

Histology of the obliterated (atretic) bile ducts shows fibrosis and variable numbers of inflammatory cells. Small segments of partially obliterated hepatic ducts can sometimes be identified, but are usually replaced by 'ductules' lined by either cuboidal or columnar epithelium. Intrahepatic changes include portal fibrosis, bile duct proliferation, and giant cell change in the hepatocytes. Hepatic fibrosis increases with age.[43]

Investigations include screening tests for infective and metabolic causes of jaundice. The stools are white from lack of pigment. Liver biopsy and radionuclide excretion scans are essential and some centres aspirate duodenal juice for bile analysis. Endoscopic retrograde cholangiopancreatography examination was reported in 26 of 30 cases of biliary atresia and occlusion of the bile duct was demonstrated in all the patients.[45]

Patent segments of proximal bile ducts are found in less than 10% of cases (type I lesions). A conventional biliary–enteric

REFERENCES

42. Howard E R In: Howard E R (ed) Surgery of Liver Disease in Children. Butterworth-Heinemann, London 1991 p 39
43. Morecki R, Glasser J H, Horwitz M S In: Daum F (ed) Extrahepatic Biliary Atresia. Marcel Dekker, New York 1983
44. Hays D M, Kimura K Curr Probl Surg 1981; 18: 546
45. Takahashi H, Kuriyama Y et al In: Ohi R (ed) Biliary Atresia. Professional Postgraduate Services, USA 1987 p 110

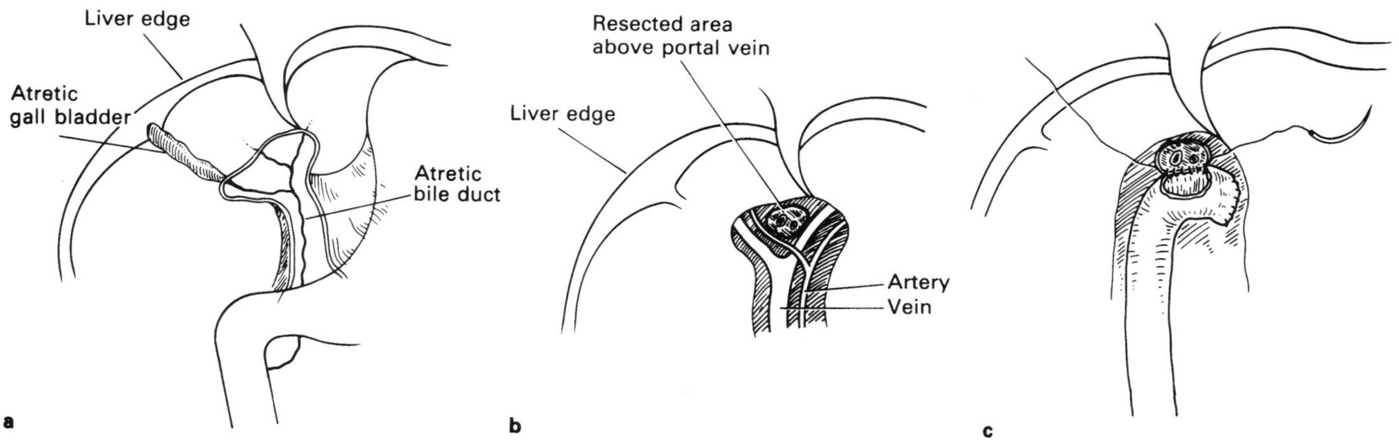

Fig. 32.7 Stages in the operation of portoenterostomy. **a** Atresic ducts exposed by dissection; **b** residual ductal tissue excised completely above the level of the portal vein; **c** anastomosis of Roux-en-Y loop of jejunum to edges of excised tissue.

anastomosis may be possible in this group and an analysis of 64 such cases showed satisfactory postoperative bile flow in 75%.[46] Progressive liver disease, however, results in a more disappointing long-term survival which varies between 25 and 50% at 5 years.

Type II and type III lesions, in which the atretic process affects more proximal portions of the extrahepatic bile ducts, are not amenable to conventional surgery. The affected tissue at the porta hepatic however frequently contains ductular structures which can communicate with intrahepatic bile ducts. These communications were first demonstrated by Kasai[47] and the operation of portoenterostomy was developed from his observations. Portoenterostomy consists of a radical excision of all bile duct tissue up to the liver capsule. A Roux-en-Y loop of jejunum is anastomosed to the exposed area of liver capsule above the bifurcation of the portal vein (Fig. 32.7). The chances of achieving effective bile drainage after portoenterostomy are maximal when the operation is performed before the age of 8 weeks, and approximately 90% of the children whose bilirubin falls to within the normal range can be expected to survive for 10 years or more.[48] Early referral for surgery is therefore critical.[49]

There is now an increasing number of adolescents and adults with successfully treated biliary atresia and Laurent et al (1990) reported 40 patients who had survived for more than 10 years.[50]

Postoperative complications of portoenterostomy include bacterial cholangitis which complicates the postoperative course in approximately 40% of cases.[42] Repeated attacks of infection cause increasing hepatic fibrosis. Portal hypertension also affects approximately 50% of long-term survivors with variceal bleeding in 20–30%.[51] Reduced bile flow may be associated with poor growth and deficiency of fat-soluble vitamins such as vitamin D.

Liver transplantation may be considered when portoenterostomy fails to relieve jaundice[52] and most transplants are required within the first 2 years of life when it becomes clear that bile drainage has not been achieved. Transplantation may be indicated in older cases of atresia for progressive liver failure or severe portal hypertension secondary to biliary cirrhosis.

Liver transplantation is not regarded as the primary treatment for biliary atresia in the UK but is considered to be complementary to the portoenterostomy operation.

Choledochal cysts

The triad of jaundice, pain and a mass in the right hypochondrium is often quoted as the classic presentation of congenital cysts of the biliary tree, although an early review of 740 cases[53] concluded that the triad was present in only 38%. In a more recent review of 72 children with cysts only 6% presented with the classic triad.[54] Jaundice was a feature in 69%, a mass in 3% and pain alone in 18%. Thirty of 31 patients investigated for recurrent abdominal pain were shown to have raised serum or biliary amylase levels. More than 80% of cysts occur in females and the condition appears to be more common in Japan.

The aetiology can be explained by a congenital weakness of the bile ducts associated with a functional obstruction at the lower end. Anomalous junctions of the biliary–pancreatic junction are frequently observed and long common channels result in high levels of biliary amylase in 70–80% of cases. Common pancreaticobiliary channels may be associated with repeated attacks of pancreatitis (Fig. 32.8).

Cysts of the common bile duct are divided anatomically into type 1, cystic or fusiform; type 2, diverticulum of the duct; type 3, choledochocoele of the intraduodenal portion, and type 4, cases with both intra- and extrahepatic cysts[55] (Fig. 32.9).

A survey of 1433 patients[56] showed that 51% of cases were type 1 cystic, 11% were type 1 fusiform and 28% were type 4. A diverticulum of the common bile duct is extremely rare. Investigations include ultrasonography, which is very specific for choledochal

REFERENCES

46. Ohi R In: Ohi R (ed) Biliary Atresia. Professional Postgraduate Services, Tokyo, Japan 1987 p 125
47. Kasai M: cited in Howard E R Br J Surg 1983; 70: 193
48. Ohi R, Hanamatsu M et al World J Surg 1985; 9: 285
49. Mieli-Vergani G, Howard E R et al Lancet 1989; 1: 421
50. Laurent J, Gauthier F et al Gastroenterology 1990; 99: 1793
51. Stringer M, Howard E R, Mowat A P J Pediatr Surg 1989; 24: 438
52. Beath S, Pearmain G et al J Pediatr Surg 1993; 28: 1044
53. Flanigan D P Ann Surg 1975; 182: 635
54. Stringer M D, Dhawan A et al Arch Dis Childhood 1995; 73: 528
55. Alonso-Lej F, Rever W B, Pessagno D J Int Abst Surg 1959; 108: 1
56. Yamaguchi M Am J Surg 1980; 140: 653

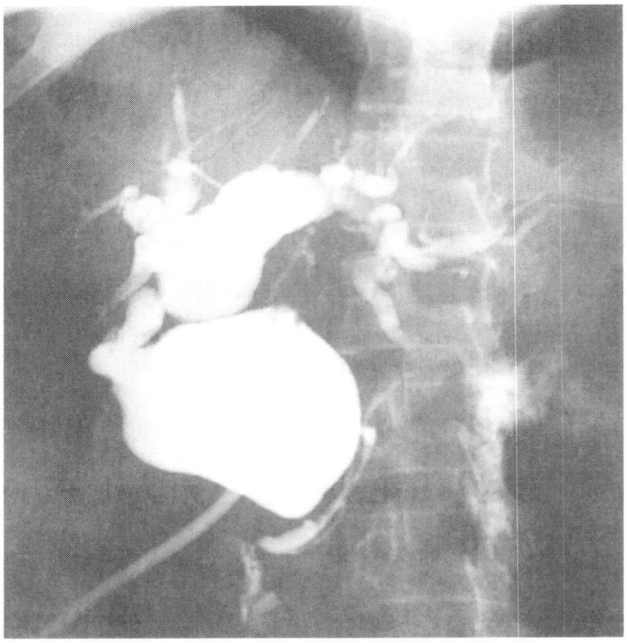

Fig. 32.8 Operative cholangiogram of cystic dilatation of the extrahepatic bile ducts in an adult female. The terminal portion of the narrow pancreatic duct forms a common channel with the bile duct.

cysts, endoscopic retrograde cholangiopancreatography and radionuclide scanning. Complications of the cysts include pancreatitis, spontaneous rupture, liver abscess, cirrhosis and portal hypertension. Carcinoma of the biliary tract is a well-recognized complication[57] and carries a poor prognosis, probably because of the difficulty of early diagnosis. It is, however, a very rare complication in children who have undergone surgical excision and is mostly confined to cysts detected in adult patients.

Radical excision of the cysts is the treatment of choice, with reconstruction of the biliary tract with a Roux-en-Y loop of jejunum. Lesser procedures such as internal drainage are complicated by recurrent cholangitis and anastomotic stenosis in approximately 40% of cases[58] and should be avoided.

Inspissated bile syndrome

Obstructive jaundice in early infancy is occasionally associated with inspissated bile within the common bile duct. It is sometimes secondary to haemolysis caused by blood group incompatibility.

REFERENCES

57. Kagawa Y, Kashihara S, Kuramoto S Gastroenterology 1978; 74: 1286
58. Trout H H, Longmire W P Am J Surg 1981; 121: 68

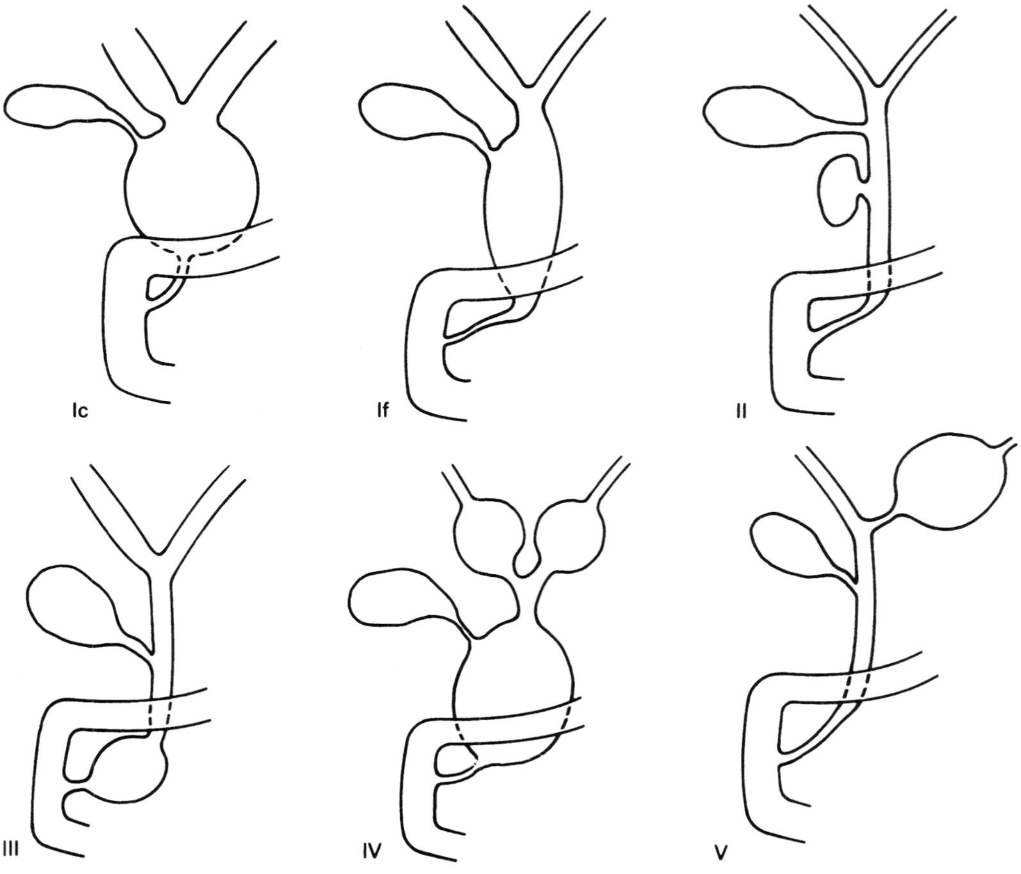

Fig. 32.9 Classification of types of choledochal cyst. **Ic** Extrahepatic cystic dilatation; **If** fusiform dilatation; **II** lateral diverticulum; **III** choledochocoele; **IV** combined intra- and extrahepatic cysts; **V** intrahepatic dilatation only.

Dilatation of proximal bile ducts and gallbladder is observed at laparotomy. The inspissated material is removed through a choledochotomy but occasionally an ampullary sphincterotomy is necessary.[59]

Spontaneous perforation of the common bile duct

This rare condition should be suspected when an infant of a few weeks of age develops fluctuating jaundice, acholic stools and dark urine. Less specific signs include weight loss, irritability and occasional vomiting. Examination shows biliary ascites which may cause a dark staining of the umbilicus or scrotum. More than 50 cases have been reported.[60,61] Investigations show raised serum bilirubin levels of between 100 and 120 μmol/l and normal liver enzymes. Radionuclide scans highlight the intraperitoneal bile and provide images of the peritoneal cavity. This confirms the diagnosis.

The perforation occurs at the junction of the cystic and common bile ducts. The cause is unknown but the condition may be associated with inspissated bile at the lower end of the common bile duct.[61]

Laparotomy is essential. Operative cholangiography confirms the site of perforation which is drained. The addition of a cholecystenterostomy has been suggested but in many cases the perforation has healed satisfactorily with drainage alone.[61]

Gallbladder disease in childhood

Acute gallbladder distension (hydrops of the gallbladder), unrelated to gallstones or inflammation, is a well-recognized condition in early childhood. The mean age of presentation of 29 cases was 5.1 years.[62] The condition often follows respiratory tract infections and may be related to cystic node enlargement. Abdominal pain, vomiting, tenderness and a mass in the right hypochondrium are typical signs. Ultrasonography confirms the diagnosis. Tube cholecystostomy is the treatment of choice and postoperative recovery is usually uncomplicated. Acalculous cholecystitis in children may follow burns and trauma and may also be seen as a postoperative complication of abdominal surgery. A review of 74 cases showed an age range of 1 month to 15 years[63] and revealed that the condition was frequently misdiagnosed as appendicitis. Cholecystostomy is the treatment of choice in these children.

Haemolytic anaemias and congenital anomalies may predispose to gallstone formation in children. Cholesterol stones also occur occasionally when the presenting symptoms and complications are similar to those of adults.[64]

Tumours in childhood

Benign inflammatory tumours have been described in the extrahepatic bile ducts.[65] The aetiology is unknown, but the tumours have a yellow-brown surface and are composed of fibroblasts, collagen and a mixture of inflammatory cells. The bile ducts show loss of epithelium and dense fibrous tissue in their walls. Excision is curative.

Rhabdomyosarcoma is the commonest malignant tumour of the bile ducts in children. It is extremely rare and only 32 cases have been reported.[66] Treatment consists of radical excision combined with cytotoxic therapy. It has been suggested that these lesions arise from multipotent splanchnic mesenchyme which is capable of differentiating into rhabdomyoblasts.[67]

GALLSTONES

Incidence and aetiology

The commonest gallstones are composed of a mixture of cholesterol (70–75%), bilirubin and calcium (as carbonate, phosphate and bilirubinate). They are smooth or faceted, light brown in colour, laminated and usually contain a dark nucleus. Pure cholesterol stones or solitaires are uncommon. Pure pigment stones, associated particularly with haemolytic disorders, are multiple, small, black and amorphous, soft and crystalline.

The precipitation of stones from bile occurs almost always in the gallbladder and 70–80% of stones are radiolucent. It has been estimated that approximately 35% of women and 15% of men in the UK will form gallstones during their lifetime, whilst in the USA there are approximately 20 million people with stones. American studies report 500 000 cholecystectomies per year and 10 000 deaths per year related to gallstone problems.[68]

Gallbladder disease previously occurred most commonly at about 40 years of age but the incidence now appears to be rising in younger age groups.

Pathogenesis

Normal bile contains soluble mixed micelles of cholesterol, lecithin and bile salts. Changes in the relative concentrations of these components may result in supersaturation and precipitation of cholesterol. The water content is important as the solubility of cholesterol is lowered in dilute bile.[69] Supersaturation also results from alterations in the enterohepatic recycling of bile salts which can alter the synthesis and secretion of bile lipids.[70] An example is the reported reduction of lecithin in the bile of patients with gallstones.

REFERENCES

59. Lilly J R J Pediatr Surg 1980; 15: 577
60. Howard E R, Johnston D I, Mowat A P Arch Dis Childhood 1976; 51: 883
61. Davenport M, Howard E R In: Howard E R (ed) Surgery of Liver Disease in Children. Butterworth-Heinemann, London 1991 p 91
62. Chamberlain J W, Hight D W Surgery 1970; 68: 899
63. Ternberg J L, Keating J P Arch Surg 1975; 110: 543
64. Kirtley J A, Holcomb G W Am J Surg 1966; 111: 39
65. Stamatakis J D, Howard E R, Williams R Br J Surg 1979; 66: 257
66. Mihara S, Matsumoto H et al Cancer 1982; 49: 812
67. Heaton N D, Howard E R In: Howard E R (ed) Surgery of Liver Disease in Children. Butterworth-Heinemann, London 1991 p 107
68. Sali A In: Schwartz S I, Ellis H (eds) Maingot's Abdominal Operations, 8th edn. Appleton-Century-Crofts, Norwalk, Connecticut 1985
69. Carey M C, Small D M Am J Med 1970; 49: 590
70. La Morte W W, Matolo N M et al Surg Clin North Am 1981; 16: 765

The bile acid content may be affected by a variety of factors, which include:

1. Impaired synthesis and secretion of bile acids by the liver.
2. Changes in gallbladder function, e.g. defective emptying in the last trimester of pregnancy.[71]
3. The influence of infection, diet and drugs.

In summary, supersaturated bile may be associated with high concentrations of cholesterol, increased water content and low levels of bile acids and phospholipids. The saturated bile may lead to the formation of microcrystals which can then provide the basis for subsequent stone growth. Crystal growth can radiate from nuclei of bacteria, shed cells and foreign bodies (e.g. sutures) but may also start from a core of bile pigment.

Local conditions within the gallbladder have also been implicated in gallstone formation. For example, the concentration of gallbladder bile is associated with a fall in pH, which can alter the solubility of bilirubin and calcium bilirubinate leading to precipitation and gallstone formation.[68]

Knowledge of the pathogenesis of gallstones helps to explain some epidemiological observations. For example, the risk of gallstones in vegetarians is half that of meat-eaters.[72] Morbidly obese patients have a high incidence and half develop gallstones within 3 years of surgery for obesity. Hypertriglyceridaemia, ingestion of the oestrogen-rich contraceptive pill and chronic liver disease are associated with supersaturated bile.[73] Crohn's disease and ileal resection, which may result in bile salt malabsorption and reduction in bile acids, are associated with an increased rate of cholelithiasis.[74] Clofibrate (Atromid-S) therapy for hyperlipidaemia promotes the excretion of cholesterol into bile and increased bile lithogenicity.[75]

Racial variations in the incidence of gallstones have often been observed. For example, the condition is more frequent in the white than the black population of the USA. The incidence is low in the nomadic tribes of East Africa, but is increasing in Japan as the consumption of fat and protein rises.[76] A study of the familial incidence in 100 patients showed that 72% of close relatives also had gallstones[62] and it was suggested that diet might be the important factor.

Pigment stones

Haemolytic anaemias, infection (both bacterial and parasitic) and cirrhosis predispose to stones composed mainly of bilirubinate. Pigment stones are more common in oriental countries,[76] accounting for up to 40% of cases. Infection of the biliary tract with *Escherichia coli* is an important causal factor through the production of the enzyme B-glucuronidase, which hydrolyses soluble conjugated bilirubin to form free bilirubin which then precipitates as the calcium salt.[77] Intrahepatic stones are usually pigment stones.

Summary of factors in gallstone formation

Metabolic factors, infection and biliary stagnation are all important but the solubility of cholesterol is crucial. Gallbladder function and motility have a role but their influence is not well-defined. Western countries have a higher incidence of cholesterol stones, while oriental countries favour pigment stones. Risk factors include increasing age, female sex, parity, diet, obesity, hypertriglyceridaemia, chronic liver disease, ileal dysfunction, clofibrate and oestrogen-rich contraceptive medication, haemolytic disorders and biliary tract infection.

Symptoms and signs of gallstones

Gallstones may cause intermittent obstruction of the gallbladder outlet, thereby causing gallbladder colic. They are also associated with inflammatory disease of the gallbladder wall and carcinoma of the gallbladder. Many stones, however, remain symptomless and may be chance findings during investigations for unrelated conditions. Autopsy reports from the UK have shown that only 10% of gallstones have been treated with surgery,[78] whilst prospective studies from North America concluded that 18% of men followed for 24 years developed symptoms from previously silent stones.[79] These studies have cast doubt on the value of prophylactic cholecystectomy, advocated in the past, and certainly the benefits of surgery for silent stones should always be weighed against the possible morbidity and mortality of operation.

Gallbladder dyspepsia

Non-specific symptoms of epigastric discomfort, flatulence and intermittent nausea exacerbated by fatty foods have been ascribed to gallbladder disease but also occur with hiatus hernia, peptic ulcer and duodenogastric reflux. These symptoms are believed to be caused by a functional disorder of the pylorus which fails to contract in response to a duodenal contraction.[80] Duodenogastric reflux, exacerbated by a fatty meal, is a direct consequence of the disorder which may occur with or without associated gallstones. Treatment by cholecystectomy is contentious. For example, cholecystectomy in 90 patients with gallstones and dyspepsia produced relief from symptoms in 46% and improvement in 24%; 30% were no better.[80] On the other hand, flatulent dyspepsia was not helped in patients who were symptomless before surgery. It has been suggested that dyspeptic symptoms associated with negative or equivocal ultrasonography can be assessed by provoking gallbladder contractions with cholecystokinin, for example by admin-

REFERENCES

71. Rains A J H In: Smith R, Sherlock S (eds) Surgery of the Gall Bladder and Bile Ducts. Butterworths, London 1981
72. Pixley F, Wilson D et al Br Med J 1985; 291: 11
73. Carey M C, Small D M J Clin Invest 1978; 61: 1988
74. Heaton K W, Read A E Br Med J 1969; 3: 494
75. Read A E In: Millward-Sadler G H, Wright R, Arthur M J P (eds) Wright's Liver and Biliary Disease, 3rd edn. WB Saunders, London 1992 p 1252
76. Brett M, Barker D J P Int J Epidemiol 1976; 5: 335
77. Maki T Ann Surg 1966; 164: 90
78. Godfery P J, Bates T et al Gut 1984; 25: 1029
79. Gracie W A, Ransohoff D F N Engl J Med 1982; 307: 798
80. Johnson A G Ann R Coll Surg 1975; 56: 69

istering an infusion of 0.02 mg/kg in saline over 5 minutes. The effects of cholecystokinin can also be assessed in association with oral cholecystography.[81] Gallbladder symptoms were assessed in 26 patients with normal cholecystograms who were given cholecystokinin. Ten showed no response but 16 either developed symptoms or showed less than 50% gallbladder emptying within 15 minutes of the cholecystokinin infusion. All 16 underwent cholecystectomy and no stones were found. Histology however showed chronic cholecystitis in all cases and 13 patients were relieved of their symptoms.

Biliary colic

Painful contractions of the gallbladder are referred to the epigastrium and right hypochondrium. The pain typically shows a gradual increase in severity, lasts for 1–2 hours and may radiate to the back or tip of the right scapula. Vomiting may accompany the pain which is caused by the movement of the gallstone into Hartmann's pouch or the cystic duct. The pain resolves if the stone falls back or passes on into the common bile duct. Impaction of the stone may cause inflammation of the gallbladder (chemical cholecystitis) or a mucocoele. Occasionally an impacted stone in the cystic duct can cause obstructive jaundice, known as the Mirizzi syndrome.[82,83] The impacted stone, with the associated inflammation, can cause jaundice when either the cystic duct is separated from the common hepatic duct by a thin mucosal-lined septum or when the cystic duct is very short, so that the swelling associated with the stone impedes the flow of bile through the common bile duct. Long-standing impaction may cause cholangitis.

Acute cholecystitis

Acute inflammation of the gallbladder is usually preceded by one or more attacks of biliary colic. It is the result of stones, concentrated bile and secondary infection and half the patients have positive bile cultures, especially with *Escherichia coli*.[84,85] Occasionally there is secondary infection with a gas-forming organism (e.g. *Clostridium welchii*) and gas may be identified within the gallbladder wall on a plain radiograph.

Severe pain in the right hypochondrium is made worse with movement. Signs include pyrexia, tachycardia and local peritonitis with guarding and tenderness.

The diagnosis is clear in many cases, but may be confused with perforated peptic ulcer, acute pancreatitis, pleurisy, cardiac pain, Curtis–Fitz-Hugh syndrome and occasionally with the pain caused by some liver secondaries.

A plain radiograph may reveal gallstones but unfortunately only 10–20% of calculi are radiopaque. The white count is usually raised and liver function tests may be mildly disturbed. Ultrasonography and radionuclide scanning are confirmatory.

Gas in the gallbladder wall (emphysematous cholecystitis) is a serious but rare complication. It is more common in diabetics who form 20% of all cases, and males predominate. The condition may lead rapidly to bacteraemia and hypovolaemic shock.

TREATMENT OF ACUTE CHOLECYSTITIS

Emphysematous cholecystitis

Anaerobic infection, particularly with clostridia and anaerobic streptococci, is recognized by gas within the gallbladder wall. Gallstones are not always present. The infection tends to progress rapidly and a high proportion of cases go on to perforation. The infection may be blood-borne with biliary colonization.

Treatment must include resuscitation with intravenous fluids and broad-spectrum antibiotics before cholecystectomy or cholecystostomy is performed. The choice of operation depends on the patient's general fitness.

Acute calculous cholecystitis

The common type of cholecystitis will usually resolve with bed rest, intravenous fluids and antibiotics. Gangrenous changes are rare in the gallbladder and previously it was common practice for cholecystectomy to be delayed for 2–3 months after an episode of inflammation. Urgent surgery is however necessary for persistence or worsening of the inflammatory process, demonstrated by a rising pulse rate, a swinging pyrexia and signs of spreading peritonitis.

An alternative strategy for managing acute cholecystitis involves early operation for all patients who are otherwise fit.[86,87] The proponents of early operations claim that the operation is no more difficult than elective cholecystectomy and that oedema often makes dissection easier. Patients spend less time in hospital[88] and a Swedish survey[89] reported that delayed elective cholecystectomy was 65% more expensive than early operation.

It must be emphasized that if a policy of early operation is considered:

1. Operative cholangiography must be available for all cases.
2. Accurate diagnosis is essential and may depend on radionuclide scanning if the ultrasound is equivocal.
3. Adequate resuscitation must precede operation.
4. If acute inflammatory change makes dissection difficult, then cholecystostomy with removal of stones is the procedure of choice.

In experienced hands the results of gallbladder surgery have been good. For example, in a series of 815 patients operated on in a district hospital the mortality rate was 0.7%.[90] Wound infections occurred in 10% and there were retained stones in 11%. The 6 deaths were all in patients with biliary peritonitis. Four of these

REFERENCES

81. Griffen W O O, Bivins B A et al Ann Surg 1980; 191: 636
82. Mirizzi P L J Int Chir 1948; 8: 731
83. Starting J R, Matallona R H Surgery 1980; 88: 737
84. Kune G A, Schutz E Med J Aust 1974; 1: 255
85. Keighley M R B Ann R Coll Surg 1977; 59: 328
86. Jarvinen H J, Hastbacka J Ann Surg 1980; 191: 501
87. Paterson-Brown S, Chan S T Br J Hosp Med 1987; 37: 546
88. Fowkes F G R, Gunn A A Br J Surg 1980; 67: 613
89. Alinder G, Herlin P et al World J Surg 1985; 9: 329
90. Crumplin M K H, Jenkinson L R et al Br J Surg 1985; 72: 428

were over 75 years of age and 4 underwent exploration of the common bile duct.

Deaths from cholecystectomy mostly occur in patients over 60 years of age and are associated with diabetes, cardiovascular disease and pulmonary complications.

Stones in the common bile duct or coexistent acute pancreatitis increase the risk of surgery but generally the mortality rate for cholecystectomy is less than 1%.[90]

Mucocoele of the gallbladder

A typical attack of biliary colic may be followed by aching in the right hypochondrium secondary to the development of a mucocoele. Examination reveals a large, tense gallbladder caused by the impaction of a stone in the neck. Bile pigment is absorbed but mucus secretion continues. The gallbladder may become enormous and cholecystectomy is then the treatment of choice.

Empyema

Infection of gallbladder contents after stone impaction can result in a pus-filled gallbladder and symptoms of persisting inflammation. The patient is toxic with a high swinging temperature and a high white cell count. Omental adherence, thickening and inflammation of the gallbladder result in a large tender mass. Intravenous fluids, antibiotics and surgery are the treatment of choice.

Perforation

The gallbladder perforates occasionally, usually in an elderly patient. The presentation may be one of generalized peritonitis of unknown cause. Urgent surgery is essential. Mortality rates as high as 50% have been reported.[91] Ischaemia and infection can lead to patchy gangrene which may be walled off by the omentum, duodenum and small bowel or this may progress to a pericholecystic abscess. These patients are very toxic and again surgery is essential.

Chronic calculous cholecystitis

Varying degrees of inflammation are found in gallbladders removed for stones which are thought to be the cause of the symptoms. Calculi may be symptomatic or symptomless. In advanced cases the gallbladders become thickened and contracted with fibrosis and loss of function. Treatment is by cholecystectomy.

Acalculous cholecystitis

Acute cholecystitis without gallstones has been reported as a complication of severe sepsis, burns, hyperalimentation, multiple injuries, recent childbirth and after unrelated surgery. The condition may be complicated by perforation of the gallbladder. Some patients have had gallbladder symptoms before the acute illness.[92] The aetiology of the inflammatory changes is unknown, although a blood-borne infection has been suggested. An inflammatory response by the gallbladder to a high concentration of bile salts has also been postulated, particularly in patients who are ill from burns, diabetes or other systemic conditions.

Adenomyomatosis

A thickening of the gallbladder wall which may contain intramural (Aschoff–Rokitansky) sinuses may be demonstrated with oral cholecystography as a partial occlusion of the gallbladder lumen. The changes are also known as cholecystitis glandularis proliferans and may be associated with stones. In the absence of stones the relationship of symptoms to the adenomyomatosis is difficult to assess, but cholecystectomy is often recommended.[93]

Cholesterolosis of the gallbladder

Inflammatory changes may cause a bright-red coloration of the mucosa. Cholesterol deposits show up as white flecks and the overall appearance has been given the name 'strawberry gallbladder'. Macrophages filled with lipid accumulate in the submucosa and can form cholesterol polyps which may be mistaken on ultrasound for small stones.[94]

Cholecystenteric fistula

Small bowel obstruction from impaction of a gallstone in the distal ileum is the most common presentation of fistulae between the gallbladder and duodenum. Elderly women over 70 years of age are most commonly affected. Gallstone ileus accounts for 20% of older patients with small bowel obstruction who do not have a history of a hernia or previous abdominal surgery.[95] Plain radiographs may show the triad of small bowel obstruction, a gallstone in the gut and gas in the biliary tree.

Treatment should include the following:

1. Removal of the gallstone by enterotomy proximal to site of impaction or crushing of the stone without an enterotomy.
2. A search for other gallstones in the gut.
3. Cholecystectomy at a later date if the patient is fit and if symptoms referable to the gallbladder occur. (In unfit elderly patients further surgery is probably best avoided.)

A cholecystenteric fistula follows adherence of an inflamed gallbladder to the stomach, duodenum or colon with subsequent pressure necrosis. Fistula formation may therefore follow an episode of acute cholecystitis, and it is diagnosed most commonly during an elective cholecystectomy.

REFERENCES

91. Cuschieri A In: Blumgart L (ed) Surgery of the Liver and Biliary Tract. Churchill Livingstone, Edinburgh 1988 p 535
92. Felice P R, Trowbridge P E, Ferrara J J Am J Surg 1985; 149: 466
93. Raghavendra B N, Subtramanyam B R et al Radiology 1983 146: 747
94. Zeman R K, Burrell M I Gallbladder and Bile Duct Imaging: A Clinical Radiological Approach. Churchill Livingstone, New York 1987
95. Clavien P A, Richon J et al Br J Surg 1990; 77: 737

Cholecystenteric fistula formation is a rare complication of diverticulitis, carcinoma of the hepatic flexure, or carcinoma of the gallbladder.

A cholecystocolic fistula may present with diarrhoea, caused by the discharge of bile into the colon. The diagnosis may be confirmed by:

1. A plain X-ray showing air in the biliary tree.
2. Barium studies demonstrating reflux of contrast into gallbladder.
3. A percutaneous transhepatic cholangiogram or endoscopic retrograde cholangiopancreatogram which may demonstrate the fistula very clearly.

Carcinoma of the gallbladder

Malignant change in the gallbladder is the fifth commonest cause of carcinoma in the gastrointestinal tract. The male to female ratio is 1:4.[96] The majority of cases are associated with gallstones and malignant change is found in approximately 0.9% of cholecystectomies.[97] The 5-year survival is only 1–3%.[96]

There is an association between carcinoma of the gallbladder and ulcerative colitis, usually without gallstones, and 9 cases have been reported.[98] Some 90% of these malignancies are adenocarcinomas and the remainder are squamous cell lesions.

Lymphatic spread is common and nodal enlargement may cause obstructive jaundice. Venous and local spread to the liver occurs early but spread to the adjacent bowel is uncommon.[96] Clinical signs are often indistinguishable from cholecystitis, although weight loss and jaundice are suggestive of a carcinoma.

The investigation is similar to that for calculous disease and cholangiocarcinoma of the bile ducts, with which it may be mistaken. If hepatic involvement by tumour is recognized on ultrasonography then endoscopic retrograde cholangiopancreatography and selective hepatic angiography should be considered in preparation for hepatic resection, which may be either a segmental resection or a formal right hepatectomy (see Chapter 31). The results of treatment remain poor: 90% of patients die within 1 year and less than 5% survive at 5 years.[99]

Medical treatment of gallstones

Approximately 20% of gallstones may be judged suitable for dissolution therapy by feeding the patient chenodeoxycholic acid or ursodeoxycholic acid. The bile acids dissolve gallstones by reducing cholesterol saturation in bile. Biliary cholesterol production is reduced. The criteria for the use of bile acids include a functioning gallbladder, radiolucent stones that are less than 2 cm in diameter (pigment stones are often radiopaque), and patients who are unfit for surgery.[100]

Retained stones in the common bile duct may be treated with bile acids if endoscopic sphincterotomy is contraindicated. Dissolution therapy demands patient compliance, and is not effective for pigment or mixed stones or when the cystic duct is obstructed. Chenodeoxycholic acid treatment in 916 patients over 2 years produced effective dissolution in only 19%.[101] Patients need repeated gallbladder examination to monitor gallstone size and the side-effects of treatment include diarrhoea (in 50%). Recurrence after cessation of treatment is common, half recurring in 3–60 months.[102]

Shock-wave treatment (lithotripsy)

The indications for lithotripsy are similar to those listed for bile acid dissolution. Patients with complications of gallbladder disease (e.g. cholecystitis or bile duct obstruction) are excluded and the gallbladder must be functioning. Stones must be radiolucent cholesterol calculi and number not more than three. Patients are pretreated with chenodeoxycholic acid and ursodeoxycholic acid for 1 week. Animal experiments have shown successful gallstone disintegration,[103] and in a recent series of patients 9 gallbladder and 5 common bile duct stones were treated successfully. However sphincterotomy was sometimes necessary for removal of stone fragments and biliary pain and mild pancreatitis occurred in most of the cases. In a further series[104] 101 patients have now been reported. If fragmentation fails at the first attempt a further treatment is given approximately 72 hours later.

Cholecystectomy

The indications for the surgical treatment of gallbladder disease have already been discussed above. It should be re-emphasized that in the elderly, particularly in those with severe medical conditions such as heart failure, surgery should be restricted to those with severe complications of emphysema, perforation, etc.

Mortality rates are increased by more than 10% in patients with cirrhosis and portal hypertension[105] and symptomless stones should not be treated in patients with these disorders.

The operative technique of open cholecystectomy

Patients should always be placed on a radiolucent table or an X-ray cassette-holder, and a laparotomy performed through a 10–15 cm subcostal (Kocher), a transverse or a right paramedian incision. The use of a small, 5–7 cm, transverse incision is known as a mini-cholecystectomy.[106] The cholecystectomy is started by defining the

REFERENCES

96. Khawaja H, Howard E R In: Allen-Mersh T G (ed) Surgical Oncology (Bailey & Love companion series). Chapman & Hall, London 1996 p 177
97. Brossart P A, Patterson A H, Zintel H A Am J Surg 1962; 103: 366
98. Ritchie J K, Allan R N et al Q J Med 1974; 43: 263
99. Adson M A Surg Clin North Am 1973; 53: 1203
100. Sali A, Iser J H Aust NZ J Surg 1978; 48: 484
101. Schoenfield L J, Lachin J M Ann Intern Med 1981; 95: 257
102. Dowling R H, Ruppin D C Br Med J 1982; 285: 132
103. Brendel W, Enders G Lancet 1983; i: 1054
104. Sackman M, Delius M et al Gastroenterology 1987; 92: 1608
105. Aranha G V, Sontag S J Am J Surg 1982; 143: 307
106. Downs S H, Black N A et al Ann R Coll Surg (Eng) 1996; 78 (part 2): 241

cystic duct. The cystic artery and common bile duct are identified and the ductal anatomy is confirmed with an operative cholangiogram. The exposure may be improved by aspirating a tense gallbladder or by manipulating stones out of Hartmann's pouch. Exposure is also improved by allowing air to enter between the liver and the diaphragm and by drawing Hartmann's pouch towards the operator with sponge-holding forceps.

The anatomical variations described earlier should be sought at the beginning of the dissection around the cystic duct; the position of the right hepatic artery, which may lie adjacent to the cystic duct, should be checked carefully. (Note that there are two cystic arteries in approximately 10% of cases.)[107]

After division of the cystic artery between ligatures the cystic duct is cannulated (e.g. with a small catheter possessing a bulbous end, such as a 6 FG ureteric catheter). Preliminary passage of a probe makes catheter insertion easier. Contrast medium (e.g. 45% Hypaque) is injected in volumes of 1, 2 and 3 ml and the three radiographs are inspected for:

1. Free flow of contrast to duodenum.
2. Calibre of bile ducts.
3. Filling defects.
4. Filling of the whole of the biliary tree.

If all of these points are satisfactory the catheter is removed and the cystic duct ligated, and the gallbladder removed. Occasionally catheterization of the cystic duct is not possible but cholangiography can if necessary be performed via needle puncture of the common bile duct. In one series this technique was used without complications in 500 examinations.[108] Most surgeons now prefer screening with digitalized equipment using a C-arm and an image intensifier. Prospective trials have shown that wound drainage is unnecessary after uncomplicated cholecystectomy. No significant differences were detected in the incidence of complications, wound infections or the length of hospital stay in 300 patients in whom the drain was omitted.[109]

Retrograde cholecystectomy

This technique is particularly useful when inflammatory change around the neck of the gallbladder makes the initial dissection of Calot's triangle hazardous.[110] A plane is developed between the gallbladder and liver capsule at the fundus. Preliminary aspiration of the gallbladder may ease the dissection. The cystic artery is identified and divided as the neck of the gallbladder is reached. Operative cholangiography is performed through the cystic duct as previously described.

Cholecystostomy

This is a useful method of treatment for acute gallbladder disease and in the gravely ill may be carried out under local anaesthetic. It is particularly useful when the anatomy is obscured by severe inflammatory disease, but the indications may vary with the experience of the surgeon. The procedure may be followed by cholecystectomy at a later date if the patient improves sufficiently. In one study, 39 of 53 patients who underwent cholecystostomy developed recurrent stones within 15 years,[111] and carcinoma has been reported some years after cholecystostomy.

The gallbladder should be aspirated before an incision is made in the fundus. Infected bile and stones are removed but stones impacted in the cystic duct can usually only be removed at subsequent cholecystectomy. The gallbladder is closed around a Foley catheter which allows irrigation. Percutaneous cholecystostomy with local anaesthetic and ultrasound control has been used occasionally.

Complications of cholecystectomy

General

Wound infection

This complication is seen in 15–20% of all operations on the gallbladder.[112] Factors which predispose to wound infection include age (over 70 years), emergency surgery, empyema, stones in the common bile duct and cholangitis. Positive bile cultures are obtained in 50–80% of patients in these groups,[112] and include *Escherichia coli*, *Klebsiella*, enterococci and *Proteus* spp. Administration of broad-spectrum antibiotics 1 hour before and 24 hours after surgery is essential in high-risk groups.[112] For example, the wound infection rate fell from 15 to 7% when 1 g of cephamandole was given 1 hour before surgery.[113]

Bleeding

Jaundiced patients are more at risk and vitamin K is given to correct an abnormal prothrombin time.

Bile duct injury

Excessive traction on the gallbladder may deform the common bile duct which may then be included in a cystic duct ligature. The bile duct is less likely to be mistaken for the cystic duct if cholangiography is performed routinely during surgery, although in one series of 65 cases of bile duct trauma, half had already been damaged before cholangiograms were performed.[114] More than 50% of injuries followed a 'fundus-first' technique of cholecystectomy.

Haemorrhage during cholecystectomy should be controlled by the Pringle manoeuvre (occlusion of the structures in the lesser omentum) before the application of clips or sutures to the bleeding

REFERENCES

107. Smadja C, Blumgart L H In: Blumgart L H (ed) Surgery of the Liver and Biliary Tract, 2nd edn. Churchill Livingstone, Edinburgh 1994 p 11
108. Turunen M T, Jarvinen J H et al Acta Chir Scand 1984; 150: 561
109. Cathcart R S, Gregorie H B Am Surg 1984; 50: 482
110. Baer H U, Blumgart L H In: Schwartz S I, Ellis H (eds) Maingot's Abdominal Operations, 9th edn. Appleton Lange, Norwalk 1989 p 1480
111. Norby S, Schonebeck J Acta Chir Scand 1970; 136: 711
112. Pollock A V In: Taylor I (ed) Progress in Surgery. Churchill Livingstone, Edinburgh 1985
113. Kune G A, Hunt R F et al Aust NZ J Surg 1985; 55: 19
114. Andren-Sandberg A, Alinder G, Bengmark S Ann Surg 1985; 201: 328

points. The blind application of forceps during haemorrhage may well damage the bile duct.

Damage to the common bile duct should be suspected if jaundice occurs after an uncomplicated cholecystectomy and early investigation with endoscopic retrograde cholangiopancreatography is essential. The differential diagnosis is mainly from a retained stone within the duct.

Excessive bile drainage

Excessive bile coming from a drain may follow major duct damage or unrecognized division of an accessory bile duct. Loosening of a cystic duct ligature may also be responsible. Persistence beyond 4 or 5 days should be investigated with endoscopic retrograde cholangiopancreatography and fistulogram. Bile peritonitis may be a sign of major duct damage and is also an occasional complication after T-tube removal from the common bile duct when a tract has not been walled off.

Laparoscopic cholecystectomy

Laparoscopic removal of the gallbladder was developed between 1988 and 1989 in an attempt to reduce the morbidity and cost of surgery.[115] The principles of the technique are similar to those of the open method of cholecystectomy. Good exposure of the abdominal cavity via the telescope is essential and this may be compromised by, for example, extensive adhesions from previous surgery. The cystic duct and the cystic artery must be clearly identified and the cystic duct must not be divided until it has been seen to widen into the neck of the gallbladder. Cholangiography may be performed through a 4 F or 5 F ureteric catheter placed through a small incision in the cystic duct made with fine scissors.

Briefly, the procedure of laparoscopic cholecystectomy is based on a four-trocar technique.[115] A 10 mm trocar may be inserted just below the umbilicus after the peritoneal cavity has been inflated with carbon dioxide through a Veress needle to a pressure of approximately 15 mmHg. This pneumoperitoneum provides a pressure against which the trocars can be pushed through the abdominal wall. It also provides a safe distance between the abdominal wall and underlying viscera and improves visibility within the peritoneal cavity. Many surgeons, however, prefer to insert the first trocar, through which the telescope is inserted into the peritoneal cavity, by dividing the rectus sheath and peritoneum under direct vision and inserting a blunt Hassan trocar through the opening. This reduces the complications of visceral vascular damage which are associated with the blind insertion of the Veress needle technique.

Two 5 mm trocars are inserted at suitable sites in the right hypochondrium and a further 10 mm operating trocar is placed in the midline 3–4 cm below the xiphoid process. Grasping forceps are inserted through the 5 mm trocars and are used to control the position of the gallbladder during dissection. The gallbladder is grasped and retracted above and over the liver. Retraction on Hartmann's pouch allows safe dissection of the cystic duct and artery as in the open operation. The artery and duct are divided between clips and the gallbladder removed with the aid of diathermy. The gallbladder is removed through one of the 10 mm trocars and the wounds are carefully repaired.

In a recent review a comparison has been made of the published results of laparoscopic cholecystectomy and open cholecystectomy.[106] This review concluded that there was no difference in clinical outcome up to 1 year after surgery and no statistical difference in mortality and complications. There was, however, some evidence that bile duct injuries were more common in the laparoscopic procedure (see below). As might be expected, there was clear evidence that postoperative pain was less after laparoscopic cholecystectomy but there was no evidence of any difference in patients' levels of physical activity 3 months after surgery.

Reported complications after laparoscopic cholecystectomy include wound complications of infection and of incisional hernia through the port sites. Bowel injury from trocar insertion or electrocautery, haemorrhage, ventilatory compromise from the pneumoperitoneum, thromboembolic problems and biliary tract damage have also been reported. Biliary tract damage has occurred because of errors in identification of the common hepatic or common bile duct which have been mistaken for the cystic duct. Perforation of the biliary tract has also followed injudicious use of the electrocautery. Despite all of these problems, most hospitals in the world have now taken up the laparoscopic operation and many surgeons are also removing bile duct calculi using the laparoscope. Some laparoscopic cholecystectomies are very difficult and all units should accept that conversion to open operation is wise in some circumstances.

COMMON BILE DUCT STONES

Both cholesterol and black pigment stones form in the gallbladder and can migrate into the bile duct, especially if the cystic duct is short and wide. By contrast, brown pigment stones are formed from non-polymerized unconjugated bilirubin, are common in Orientals and frequently form de novo in the bile duct and are associated with bacterial infection.[116] Predisposing causes of western-type bile duct stones include non-absorbable sutures at the time of cholecystectomy, stricture of the bile ducts after cholecystectomy and previous bile duct exploration for stones.[116] The prevalence of bile duct stones gradually increases with age, being present in 31% of patients undergoing cholecystectomy in the age group 61–70 and 52% in those aged between 71 and 90 years, giving an overall incidence, irrespective of age, of between 7 and 20%.[116–118]

Although bile duct stones may present with acute cholangitis or acute pancreatitis, silent stones have been reported with an incidence of between 1 and 12% at the time of cholecystectomy and may remain asymptomatic for some years or may pass spontaneously.[119–121]

REFERENCES

115. Olsen D O Am J Surg 1991; 161: 339
116. Perisat J, Huibrectse K et al Br J Surg 1994; 81: 799
117. Herman R E Am J Surg 1989; 158: 171
118. Heaton K W, Braddon et al Gut (Eds) Mountford, Hughes, Emmett 1991; 32: 316
119. Way L W, Admirand W H, Dunphy J G Ann Surg 1972; 176: 347

Acute cholangitis

Acute cholangitis, which usually presents as a combination of fever, rigors and jaundice (Charcot's triad), is a serious and potentially lethal condition. It is caused by complete or partial biliary obstruction in combination with ascending infection of the biliary tree. It in turn may lead to septicaemia and multiple hepatic abscesses. It is important to be aware that serious infection may not always present with the full Charcot's triad and so attention to the clinical state of the patient, the use of serial blood cultures and early parenteral administration of antibiotics are important in order to prevent serious complications developing. Acute suppurative cholangitis is a rare subgroup[122] in which pus is under tension within the biliary tree, causing a profound illness with Gram-negative septicaemia. It requires high-dose antibiotics and urgent decompression of the bile ducts. This may be achieved by passing a small plastic catheter via an endoscope through the ampulla of Vater above the site of the obstruction.

Acute pancreatitis

Acute pancreatitis is caused by gallstones in 13–19% of patients.[120] Small gallstones are particularly liable to cause this complication and there is now evidence that an attack is due to the impaction or passage of a stone through the ampulla of Vater—the data have been obtained from routine examination of faeces or from endoscopic appearances.[123] Diagnosis is based on an elevated serum amylase, the ultrasonic demonstration of gallbladder stones and the absence of alcohol ingestion.

The accepted management plan for the majority of patients with pancreatitis of biliary origin is early endoscopic retrograde cholangiography, with or without endoscopic sphincterotomy and laparoscopic cholecystectomy on the next available list (preferably within 7 days; see Chapter 33).

Detection of stones

Ultrasound is the initial examination of choice and is accurate in detecting dilatation of the bile duct. The upper limit of normal for the common bile duct is taken as 8 mm on ultrasound[124] and stones are rare in ducts of 6 mm or less.[125]

The ability to detect stones is limited because of the relative lack of bile surrounding the stones in the bile duct as compared to the gallbladder. The presence of surrounding structures also reduces the sensitivity of ultrasound.[126] False-negatives are common but false-positives relatively rare. Intravenous cholangiography may detect stones in patients who are anicteric or only mildly jaundiced with an elevation of the alkaline phosphatase. The use of meglumine iotroxate (Biliscopin) has increased the use of this investigation because it causes fewer allergic reactions.[126] Endoscopic retrograde cholangiography has a 95% success rate with excellent visualization of the bile duct, a very low mortality of 0.2% and a 3% risk of complications.[127] Identification of bile duct stones allows careful assessment of the size and number of stones. It also provides useful information on the anatomy of the bile ducts including whether any strictures are present. Intraoperative pre-exploratory cholangiography was used both as a routine procedure and on a selective basis in the era of open cholecystectomy but, with the advent of laparoscopic cholecystectomy and the increased precision of ultrasound, the majority of biliary surgeons would now favour the selective approach based on the identification of those patients at risk of having bile duct stones.[116,128–130] Patients judged to have a high chance of having bile duct stones include those with a past history of jaundice or acute pancreatitis where the amylase has been elevated to four times normal, or those with abnormal liver function tests, particularly those with a raised alkaline phosphatase. A common bile duct that has a diameter of 8 mm or more and the possibility of stones in the bile duct on ultra-sound are strong indications for selective peroperative cholangiography.

Where the number of stones in the gallbladder is greater than 10, the size is small and the cystic duct relatively wide, the chance of the stones passing into the bile duct is increased.[131]

Intraoperative ultrasound[132] has a limited application at the present time because of operator difficulties but improvements in technology in the future may make it a useful intraoperative investigation for confirming or excluding common bile duct stones.

Management depends upon the level of index of suspicion for the presence of bile duct stones. Clinicians now have a choice. Some may favour preoperative endoscopic retrograde cholangiography and endoscopic sphincterotomy on a selective basis, following which the patient should have a laparoscopic cholecystectomy. Others may prefer to carry out a laparoscopic cholecystectomy with intraoperative cholangiography.[116,128–130] If this shows common bile duct stones, patients can have postoperative endoscopic retrograde cholangiography with endoscopic sphincterotomy. The third alternative, if stones are demonstrated, is to explore the bile duct laparoscopically or convert to an open operation and supraduodenal exploration of the bile duct. Routine endoscopic retrograde cholangiography before every laparoscopic cholecystectomy is not recommended because of expense and because the number of bile duct stones identified is relatively small. Routine peroperative cholangiography has been debated but is also considered unnecessary due to the low yield, the relatively

REFERENCES

120. Stubbs R S, McCloy R F, Blumgart L H Clin Gastroenterol 1983; 1: 179
121. Perisat J, Huibregtse K et al Br J Surg 1994; 81: 799
122. Neoptolemos J P, Bouchier I A D In: Bouchier I A D, Allan R N, Hodgson N S F, Keighley M R B (eds) Gastroenterology: Clinical Science and Practice. WB Saunders, London 1993 p 1732
123. Mayer A D, McMahon M J et al Ann R Coll Surg (Engl) 1984; 66: 179
124. Neoptolemos J P, Carr-Locke D L Hepatogastroenterol 1991; 38: 243
125. Faris I, Thompson J P S et al Br J Surg 1975; 62: 966
126. Ansell G Invest Radiol 1970; 5: 374
127. Dawson P In: Dolery C T (ed) Therapeutic Drugs Churchill. Livingstone, Edinburgh 1991 p 161
128. Thompson M H Br J Surg 1996; 83: 724
129. Rieger R World J Surg 1994; 18: 900
130. Tronsden G World J Surg 1995; 19: 852
131. Corfield A P, Cooper M S, Williams R C N Gut 1985; 26: 724
132. Jakimowicz J J, Rutten H, Jurgens P J World J Surg 1987; 11: 628

high incidence of false filling defects and the prolonged operation time.[116,133]

Patients with a low index suspicion are those who have never been jaundiced or had pancreatitis. They have normal or transiently abnormal liver enzymes and a normal common bile duct size on ultrasound. The natural history of these symptomless bile duct stones is that some will pass and others will enlarge and become symptomatic.

Routine peroperative cholangiography has not been shown to reduce the incidence of bile duct damage in this group and therefore a selective policy, based on the finding of an elevated alkaline phosphatase, a doubtful ultrasound result, multiple stones in the gallbladder and a relatively wide cystic duct would appear to be appropriate indications for carrying out the technique.

Management of stones

The management of a definite bile duct stone depends on the diameter of the bile duct.[116] If the bile duct is less than 8 mm, the surgeon can attempt a laparoscopic removal at the time of laparoscopic cholecystectomy. The cystic duct approach is favoured provided that the cystic duct is short and wide, the stones are small and situated distal to the insertion of the cystic duct,[116] and the surgeon has the appropriate instruments and training. The incision in the cystic duct is dilated and a balloon catheter inserted. The stone is often pushed through the papilla but may be withdrawn through the cystic duct. The alternative is to hope that the stones pass spontaneously or to consider a postoperative endoscopic retrograde cholangiography if, or when, stones cause symptoms. In the younger patients it is probably better simply to dilate the papilla rather than carry out an endoscopic sphincterotomy. The final alternative is to use anti-spasmodics with or without oral ursodeoxycholic acid.

Where the bile duct is greater than 8 mm in diameter and the stones are relatively large, they are unlikely to pass spontaneously.[116] In this situation it may be better to carry out an endoscopic retrograde cholangiography and endoscopic sphincterotomy in the postoperative period or to explore the bile duct laparoscopically using the transcystic approach. With the larger bile duct, a direct laparoscopic choledochotomy and exploration can be attempted[116] or a decision may be made to convert to an open exploration as transcystic manipulation is inadvisable when the duct stones are very large.[116]

Peroperative endoscopic sphincterotomy has been attempted but is difficult and appears to be associated with a relatively high incidence of acute pancreatitis.

OPEN SURGERY OF BILE DUCT STONES

The standard approach to the common bile duct is the supraduodenal route: the duct is opened vertically between fine stay sutures.[134] Stones are removed with Desjardin forceps and a Fogarty balloon catheter but the use of blind probing of the papilla with Bakes dilators should be avoided as it can lead to the creation of false passages which can cause fistulae into the duodenum or sinus tracts into the pancreas or retroduodenum. Moreover it does not prevent calculi from being overlooked or facilitate the passage of residual calculi.

Complete clearance of stones from the ducts can be checked by choledochoscopy, although some still prefer postoperative cholangiography. Sometimes these two investigations are complementary for, although residual calculi can be accurately located and removed under direct choledochoscopic vision, the patency of the choledochoduodenal junction can only be confirmed with certainty on radiology. Passage of the choledochoscope through the normal narrow sphincteric region may cause damage.[135] Post-exploratory cholangiography may increase the incidence of re-exploration as air bubbles, which can be mistaken for stones, are difficult to eradicate. Opinions differ as to whether the duct should be closed primarily but most surgeons still prefer T-tube drainage after open duct exploration.[135] The presence of a T-tube allows further cholangiography, and if stones are found it provides access for their removal.[135] Specific complications related to the T-tube include kinking, dislodgement and infection.[136] The T-tube should not be removed before the 10th postoperative day in order to allow a tract to develop and thus prevent bile leakage into the peritoneal cavity when the tube is gently withdrawn.

Drainage procedures in patients with common duct stones

Transduodenal sphincteroplasty and external choledochoduodenostomy

When a stone is impacted in the sphincteric region the transduodenal route is preferred.[137] When multiple stones and biliary mud are present or when the bile duct is being re-explored for recurrent or residual calculi in patients in whom endoscopic sphincterotomy and stone extraction have failed, the transduodenal route is again favoured. It should not, however, be used in patients who have had recent pancreatitis.[135,138,139] The duodenum and head of the pancreas are fully mobilized, and the papilla carefully identified, aided if necessary by the passage of a ureteric catheter via the cystic duct (Fig. 32.10a). The papillary region is exposed through a vertical duodenotomy and gentle traction draws the papilla into view (Fig. 32.10b). A grooved director is then inserted into the common bile duct and kept in the same axis as the bile duct to avoid entering the pancreatic duct (Fig. 32.10c). The insertion of a line of stay sutures on either side of the papilla provides accurate control of the sphincterotomy which is enlarged to a size sufficient to permit easy stone extraction. The surgeon must identify the orifice of the pancreatic duct before the stay sutures are tied (Fig. 32.10d). The duodenotomy is carefully closed in its original axis.

REFERENCES

133. Tate J J T, Lau W Y, Li A K C Br J Surg 1994; 81: 720
134. Dudley H A F (ed) Alimentary Tract and Abdominal Wall, 4th edn, vol 11. Butterworths, London 1983
135. Johnson A G, Hosking S W Br J Surg 1987; 74: 555
136. Lygidakis N J Surg Gynecol Obstet 1986; 163: 153
137. Peel A L G et al Ann R Coll Surg (Engl) 1975; 56: 124
138. Allen B, Shapiro H, Way L W Am J Surg 1981; 142: 91
139. Lygidakis N J Surg Gynecol Obstet 1982; 155: 679

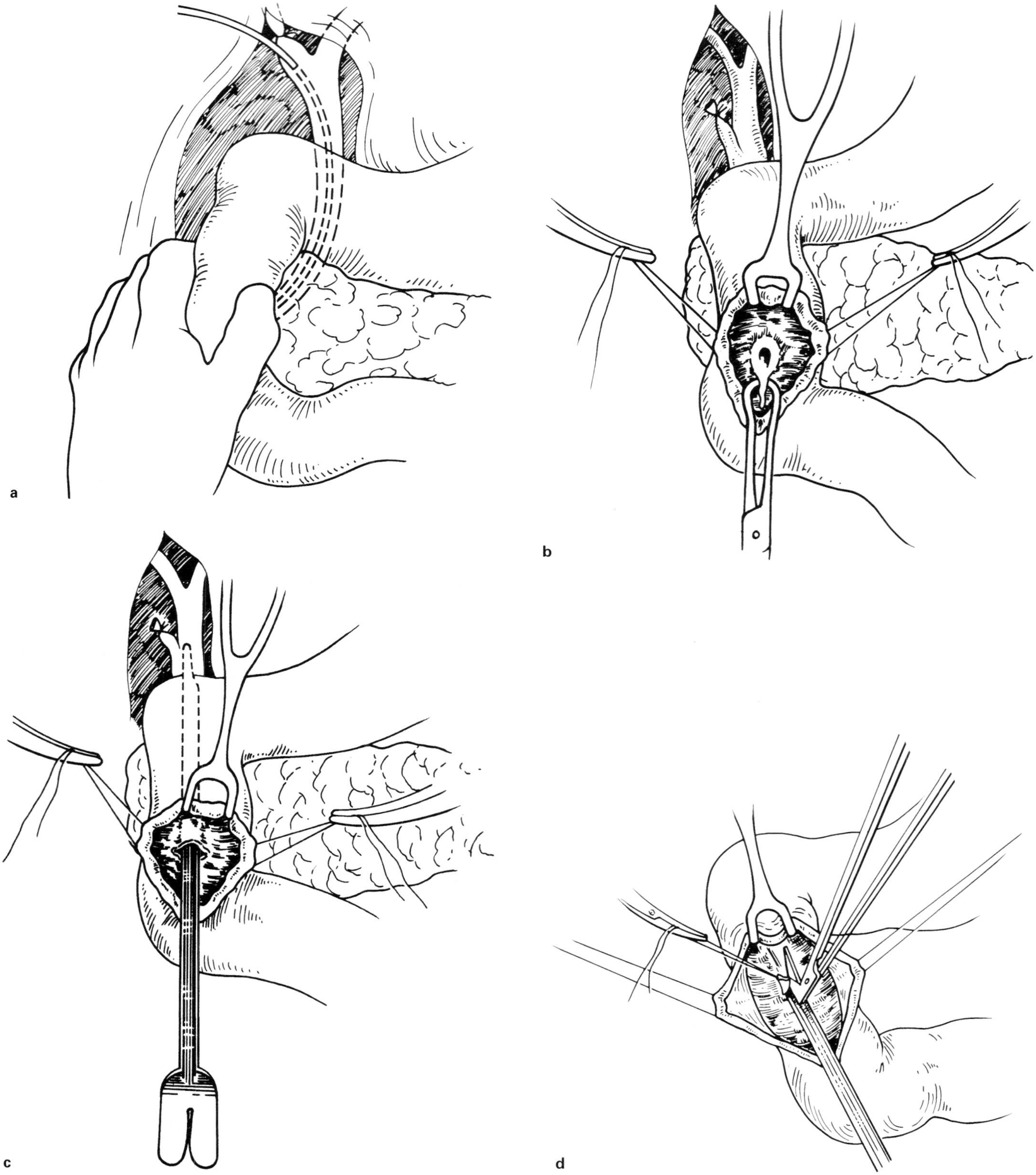

a b c d

Fig. 32.10 Operative technique for transduodenal exploration of the bile duct. **a** Mobilization and palpation of the papilla. **b** Exposure of the papilla with Babcock's forceps applied to the longitudinal fold, drawing the papilla into the duodenotomy. **c** The grooved director passed through the papillary orifice into the common bile duct. **d** The sphincterotomy and division of sphincter between stay sutures. Reprinted[134] with permission.

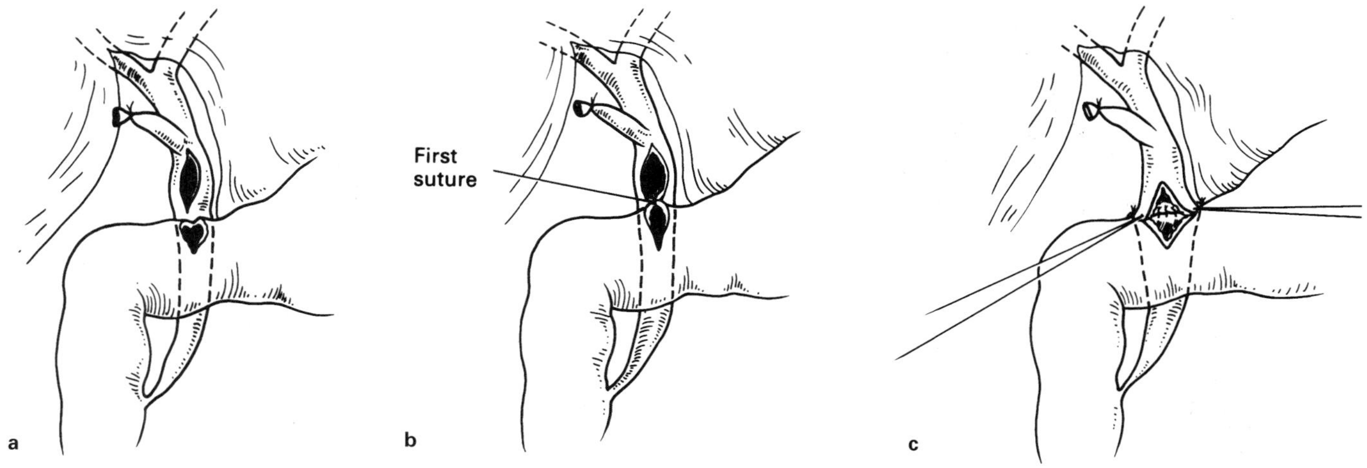

Fig. 32.11 External choledochoduodenostomy. **a** The creation of a stoma in the duodenum and a stoma in the supraduodenal part of the common bile duct. **b** The first suture in position tied on the mucosal side. **c** The posterior layer of sutures in situ and the start of the insertion of the anterior layer sutures. Reprinted[134] with permission.

Choledochoduodenostomy

A side-to-side anastomosis between the bile duct and the duodenum is used in patients with large bile ducts which are greater than 2 cm in diameter. This procedure is indicated particularly if the patient is elderly, the choledochoduodenal junction is narrow or if there has been difficulty in establishing complete clearance of calculi from the bile ducts.[139,140] For satisfactory long-term results the stoma should be more than 2.5 cm diameter and this is facilitated by full duodenal mobilization to ensure that the anastomosis is carried out without tension (Fig. 32.11). (Roux-en-Y hepatico- or choledochojejunostomy is reserved for patients with calculi above a bile duct stricture, and is discussed later.)

POSTOPERATIVE COMPLICATIONS

Infection

The use of prophylactic antibiotics has reduced the incidence of intra-abdominal and wound infection after surgery on the common bile duct.[141] Elderly patients with common bile duct stones causing cholangitis or pancreatitis are especially at risk. Either a single large dose of a broad-spectrum antibiotic such as cefuroxime is given at induction of anaesthesia or three doses at induction and at 8 and 16 hours postoperatively to all patients undergoing surgery for duct stones. Organisms most frequently cultured from the bile are *Escherichia coli* (15–50%), *Klebsiella spp* (10–20%), *Streptococcus faecalis* (10–15%) and, occasionally, *Proteus* species, clostridia and *Bacteroides*. A more prolonged course of antibiotics should be considered for patients with severe cholangitis or multiple small intrahepatic abscesses.

Localized subhepatic collections after common duct exploration may be suspected in a patient who develops a postoperative pyrexia. This is often associated with nausea, from delayed gastric emptying, and increasingly abnormal liver function tests. Treatment is by percutaneous aspiration or drainage under ultrasound control.

It is sensible to obtain an endoscopic retrograde cholangiogran to assess any bile duct damage and to discern the size of any leak. A nasobiliary tube may aid recovery in patients with large leaks.

Acute pancreatitis

This is a serious complication of bile duct exploration and is one of the major dangers of the transduodenal route, especially when both supra- and transduodenal approaches are combined. The danger can be minimized by avoiding blunt instrumentation of the lower bile duct, and ensuring that the pancreatic duct orifice is identified during sphincteric surgery. Serum amylase levels are elevated postoperatively in up to 30% of patients undergoing transduodenal sphincterotomy and in 10–15% of patients undergoing supraduodenal choledochotomy.[137]

Haemorrhage

Minor bleeds may occur after any exploration of a bile duct affected by severe cholangitis, and haemorrhage most frequently complicates transduodenal sphincterotomy (2–4%).[137] Surgical re-exploration is required on rare occasions only.

Fistulae

Fistulae usually result from blind instrumentation of the distal common bile duct, but they may complicate a duodenotomy or a choledochoduodenostomy. They rarely require active surgical treatment.

REFERENCES

140. Parilla P, Ramirez P et al Br J Surg 1991; 78: 470
141. Keighley M R B, Flinn R, Alexander-Williams J Br J Surg 1976; 63: 528

Stenosis

Stenosis of the distal common bile duct may develop as the result of choledocholithiasis. A stenosis can also be produced by excessive dilatation of the ampulla and may follow endoscopic sphincterotomy of a small bile duct. Stenosis may also occur at the site of insertion of a T-tube or as a result of accidental damage (see below). A sphincteroplasty may stenose but if the initial cut is adequate this is rare (less than 2%).[137,139] Late post-operative stenosis of the sphincter region may be associated with cholangitis and recurrent calculi and can be treated by endoscopic sphincterotomy.[135,142]

Sump syndrome

This occurs after choledochoduodenostomy and is caused by stones and debris collecting in the distal common bile duct between the anastomosis and the papilla.[140] It may cause epigastric discomfort, recurrent cholangitis and pancreatitis. It can usually be successfully managed by endoscopic sphincterotomy, although occasionally the anatomosis may have to be revised.[143]

ALTERNATIVES TO SURGERY FOR BILE DUCT STONES

Endoscopic stone removal

Endoscopic sphincterotomy can be carried out safely with a mortality of less than 1%, and a morbidity of less than 10%.[135,144] Stones may be allowed to pass spontaneously, or they may be extracted using Dormia baskets or balloon catheters. The insertion of a stent to provide good drainage and bypass large stones after sphincterotomy may be valuable, especially in the elderly.[145] A nasobiliary tube may also be inserted to irrigate the bile duct, initially with antibiotics and subsequently to perfuse it with mono-octanoin to dissolve the stones and to encourage them to pass. Complications of endoscopic sphincterotomy include haemorrhage, acute pancreatitis, and duodenal bile leakage into the retro-duodenal tissues as a result of the cut extending beyond the duodenal wall.[135,144] These complications are, however, relatively infrequent and usually resolve with conservative treatment. Massive haemorrhage may occasionally require surgical exploration and open sphincteroplasty.

The endoscopic approach to common bile duct calculi is particularly appropriate for elderly frail patients, those who are severely ill with acute suppurative cholangitis requiring emergency decompression, patients with acute pancreatitis, and patients with significant medical illness creating a higher than normal surgical risk.[135,144] Studies comparing surgical and endoscopic treatment of bile duct stones showed the latter to be associated with a lower mortality and morbidity.[146,147] In a prospective study of patients undergoing cholecystectomy who were also known to have common bile duct stones, preoperative endoscopic sphincterotomy resulted in slightly worse results than those achieved by cholecystectomy and surgical exploration of the bile duct.[148]

There is conflicting evidence as to the necessity for cholecystectomy after endoscopic duct clearance of calculi. Some feel that it should not be routine as only 5–10% subsequently require removal of the gallbladder,[149,150] but Classen[151] reported that half the patients whose gallbladders were left in situ developed complications from the residual gallbladder. Selective cholecystectomy is therefore generally recommended for all patients when the risk of surgery is acceptable.

Cystic duct obstruction demonstrated by a failure of the gallbladder to opacify is a clear indication for interval cholecystectomy. The gallbladder will often become small and fibrotic after the bile duct has been cleared, making laparoscopic cholecystectomy difficult.

Adjuncts to endoscopic retrograde cholangiography and endoscopic sphincterotomy

Gallstone dissolution may be considered for retained stones. Mono-octanion can be re-infused continuously via a nasobiliary tube for 7–14 days with complete dissolution of a quarter of the stones and partial dissolution in a further quarter, which enables stones to pass through the sphincterotomy.[152,153] Methyl tert-butyl ether may be infused twice daily for 4–13 days but is associated with problems.[152,154] Extracorporeal shock-wave lithotripsy is another option which is described in detail below.

INTRAHEPATIC DUCT STONES

Intrahepatic duct stones are frequent in Japan, China, Taiwan, Korea, the Philippines, Malaysia, Singapore and Indonesia, but rare in the west.[153,155] These calculi are composed of calcium bilirubinate rather than cholesterol, and are found in dilated intrahepatic ducts above a stricture, which is often situated at the liver hilum and frequently involving the left hepatic duct. The gallbladder does not contain calculi in half of the cases. Recurrent cholangitis leads to progressive fibrotic change in the liver parenchyma. Histology of the bile ducts shows an inflammatory infiltrate, fibrosis, granuloma formation and proliferation of ductal epithelium.[155] Bacteria are found in all cases and include *Escherichia coli*, *Bacteroides* spp. and *Clostridium perfringens*. Bile stagnation and duct dilatation behind the strictures are significant factors in the genesis of intrahepatic stones. Parasitic infestation by *Clonorchis sinensis*

REFERENCES

142. Lambert M E, Martin D F, Tweedle D E F Br J Surg 1988; 75: 896
143. Johnson A G, Rains A J H et al Br J Surg 1972; 59: 277
144. Rosseland A Q, Osnes M World J Surg 1989; 13: 178
145. Dalton H Q, Chapman R W L Gut 1995; 36: 485
146. Safrany L Lancet 1978; 2: 983
147. Thompson M H Br J Surg 1986; 73: 779
148. Neoptolemos J P, Carr-Locke D L, Fossard D P Br Med J 1987; 294: 470
149. Cotton P B Gut 1984; 25: 587
150. Martin D F, Tweedle D E F Br J Surg 1987; 74: 209
151. Classen M Clin Gastroenterol 1986; 15: 457
152. Neoptolemos J P, Hoffman A F, Moossa A R Br J Surg 1986; 73: 515
153. Palmer K R, Hoffman A F Gut 1986; 27: 196
154. Murray W R, Lafer L A G, Fullerton C M Gut 1988; 29: 143
155. Choi T K Br J Surg 1989; 76: 213

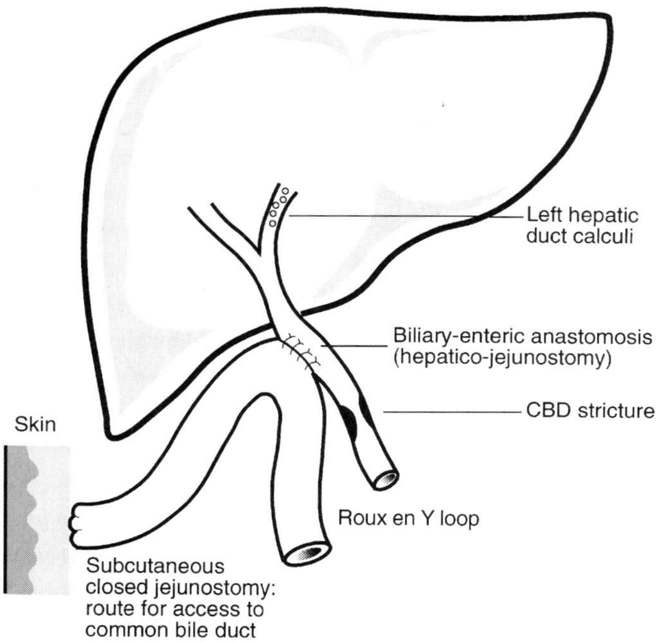

Fig. 32.12 Bile duct decompression. CBD = Common bile duct.

and *Ascaris lumbricoides* may also contribute to intrahepatic lithiasis by acting as a nidus for stone formation but may be incidental rather than causative.[156]

Calculi should be removed as completely as possible in order to eliminate bile stasis and a drainage procedure should be carried out to provide free egress for residual calculi. Sphincteroplasty, or a bilioenteric anastomosis, is required, although for simple cases without a strictured common duct, exploration and T-tube drainage may suffice. When residual or recurrent hepatic duct stones exist, often associated with a proximal stricture, they are best treated by a choledochojejunostomy combined with a subcutaneous closed jejunostomy (access loop) (Fig. 32.12). This will allow future percutaneous extraction of stones under sedation using either flexicholodochoscopes under ultrasound or radiological guidance. Extracorporeal or locally applied lithotripsy may be particularly helpful in this situation.[157] Occasionally it is necessary to perform a hepaticojejunostomy above a stricture or even a hepatic resection when stones are confined to one liver lobe. In a series of 56 patients complete stone removal was achieved in half of cases with good results in 70.8%.[158]

OVERLOOKED STONES

Common bile duct stones are left behind in between 3–15% of patients after common bile exploration. These patients may subsequently develop severe cholangitis or acute pancreatitis and revisional surgery is associated with a relatively high mortality (1.8–14.3%) and morbidity (12.3–45%).[120,159] Residual stones or new stone formation may be expected in 2.9–33% in those with previous stones in the ducts.[160] Avoidance of overlooked stones is based on the identification of risk factors which include elderly patients with multiple common bile duct stones, large bile ducts with poor drainage, stones within the hepatic ducts, strictures and cholangitis associated with haemobilia.[135] The incidence of retained stones may be reduced by the combination of pre-exploratory cholangiography and meticulous post-exploratory choledochoscopy or cholangiography which may reveal unsuspected stones in 14–30% of ducts.[135] In order to reduce the likelihood of retained stones, biliary–enteric drainage procedures should be considered for the elderly patient with multiple stones and widely dilated ducts. These procedures also have a place in patients with primary choledocholithiasis, or when stones are knowingly left behind (e.g. in the intrahepatic duct radicals).[135,139]

MANAGEMENT OF OVERLOOKED STONES

Overlooked stones may be detected on the postoperative T-tube cholangiogram. Small stones may pass in 10–25% of cases,[135] but with a T-tube in situ the bile ducts may be flushed with saline or irrigated with a gallstone dissolution agent. Simple flushing of the ducts with saline under manometric control, facilitated by pharmacological relaxation of the sphincteric region with Buscopan or glucagon,[152] may succeed in removing stones in 20–50% of cases. Various other irrigating agents have been used but some have been discontinued because of toxicity, such as ether and chloroform. Sodium cholate and mono-octanoin methyl-tertbutyl-ether both solubilize cholesterol and are preferable.[152–154] Calcium bilirubinate fragments may be dissolved by a bile solvent and ethylenediaminetetraacetic acid solution has been used.[154] Endoscopic sphincterotomy may be a useful adjunct at the time of flushing.[161,162]

Instrumentation of the T-tube tract was first described by Mondet[163] in 1962 and has been adapted by Mazzariello[164] who used pliable forceps and by Burhenne[165] who used a steerable catheter. These authors reported a success rate which approached 90%, but most achieve success in around 70%.[166] A T-tube tract larger than 14 French gauge is essential and the tract itself needs to be mature; this requires the T-tube to remain in situ for 6 or more weeks. Under fluoroscopic control a steerable catheter, through which a Dormia basket may be threaded, is used to capture the stone and extract it. Several attempts are often required.

Endoscopic sphincterotomy and extraction of stones is the preferred technique for stone retrieval and the overall success rate is between 85 and 95%.[167] Unfortunately, the technique is not always possible after Polya gastrectomy.[168] The mortality of

REFERENCES

156. Nakayama F, Koga A World J Surg 1984; 8: 9
157. Sauerbach T, Holl J et al Endoscopy 1988; 20: 305
158. Koga A, Miyazaki K et al World J Surg 1984; 8: 36
159. Classen M, Leuschner U, Schreiber H W Gastroenterology 1983; 1: 203
160. O'Doherty D P, Neoptolemos J P, Carr-Locke D L Br J Surg 1986; 73: 454
161. Motson R W Br J Surg 1981; 68: 203
162. Kurtz W, Classen M Gastroenterology 1984; 3: 91
163. Mondet A Bol Soc Gr (Buenos Aires) 1962; 46: 278
164. Mazzariello R Surgery 1973; 73: 299
165. Burhenne H J Am J Roentgenol 1973; 117: 388
166. Mason R R Clin Gastroenterology 1985; 14: 403
167. Koch H, Rosch W et al Gastroenterology 1977; 73: 1393
168. Osnes M, Rosseland A R, Aabakken L Gut 1986; 27: 1193

retained stones ranges from 0 to 1.4%[169–171] and early complications of cholangitis, pancreatitis and bleeding occur in 5–10% of cases.[170] Late stenosis develops in 4% and further stones in 10%.[169] Stone fragmentation by mechanical lithotripsy with a wire cage,[145] electrohydraulic lithotripsy[172] and laser lithotripsy[173] may be useful adjuvants.

Extracorporeal shock-wave lithotripsy[145] has also been used. It is safe and effective in 80% of cases but expensive. Recent improvements include ultrasound guidance and a water pad and sedation which avoid the necessity for anaesthesia.[145] Coexistent bile salt therapy is essential.

MANAGEMENT OF RESIDUAL STONES IN THE ELDERLY

Surgical exploration in the elderly carries a very high risk when there are large residual stones which cannot be removed by endoscopic sphincterotomy. In this group the insertion of pigtail or straight stents has been shown to be effective.[145] The stents appear to work by splinting the stones, preventing impaction and permitting flow through the bile duct so that, when the stent itself becomes blocked, the patients often remain symptomless. This is a different situation from stent insertion in malignancies of the bile duct. An additional sphincterotomy may be helpful.[174]

SYMPTOMS AFTER CHOLECYSTECTOMY

Symptoms often remain after cholecystectomy and common duct exploration and constitute the post-cholecystectomy syndrome. When jaundice develops an abnormality of the biliary tract is usually found, but investigation of less specific pain and discomfort is often unrewarding.[175] Physiological studies of the papillary region have proved disappointing. Irritable bowel syndrome may be responsible for similar symptoms in some of the patients.

ACUTE EXTRAHEPATIC BILE DUCT INJURY

Iatrogenic (accidental) injury

Cholecystectomy is the most frequent cause of bile duct injury. This may be related to abnormal anatomy, severe pathology or to surgical inexperience.[176] In open cholecystectomy, the importance of operative cholangiography has been emphasized by some authors. In one series[177] operative cholangiography was not done in 71% of patients who subsequently developed a bile duct stricture. In another series, however, injury had occurred before intraoperative radiographs were available for inspection in half of the cases.[176]

The overall incidence of bile duct damage is 0–0.5%, or 1 in every 200–300 cases.[176,177]

Bile duct injury may be suspected after cholecystectomy in patients who develop jaundice, rigors and subhepatic collections or a persistent bile leak following removal of a drain. Occasionally bile ascites may present as abdominal distension. Late presentation is commonly with pain, jaundice and fever from cholangitis developing proximal to a stricture. Serious complications such as hepatic lobar abscess, hepatic atrophy or biliary cirrhosis and portal hypertension may also develop but are thankfully rare.

Laparoscopic injury to bile ducts

Reports on the early experience of laparoscopic cholecystectomy indicated a higher incidence of bile duct injury (1–2.8%), but more recent publications show an incidence of 0.3–0.5% or 1 in every 100–200 patients.[178–186] Risk factors have been identified and include inexperience on the part of the laparoscopic surgeon, inadequate training, a difficult dissection in Calot's triangle, failure to recognize the correct anatomy and operations performed on patients who have had recent acute cholecystitis or acute pancreatitis.[179,180,183–185] Particular difficulties with laparoscopic cholecystectomy necessitating conversion to open operation may be anticipated in elderly males of short stature and in patients of both sexes where the gallbladder is seen to be contracted and thick-walled on ultrasound examination. At laparoscopic cholecystectomy, injuries usually occur because the operator mistakes the common bile duct for the cystic duct, with the result that the bile duct is clipped and ligated (Fig. 32.13a and b).

Sometimes part of the common hepatic duct is resected, the proximal common hepatic duct being divided just below the confluence.[179,183,185] The right or the left hepatic duct may not be recognized and may be left open and draining bile. Tenting up an undilated common bile duct during the dissection and display of Calot's triangle is dangerous and can result in the wall of the common bile duct being included in the cystic duct clip (Fig. 32.13c).[186] This may narrow the common bile duct and cause ischaemia and a subsequent stricture.[179,183,185]

The right hepatic duct may be mistaken for the cystic duct and as a consequence it may be clipped and divided (Fig. 32.13d).[117,119] Injury may also be caused by unipolar diathermy or the use of laser with subsequent fibrous stricture formation leading to recurrent jaundice and cholangitis.[180,183,185] Diathermy, laser or scissors may

REFERENCES

169. Rosseland A R, Osnes M World J Surg 1989; 13: 178
170. Lambert M E, Martin D F, Theobald D E F Br J Surg 1988; 75: 896
171. Neoptolemos J P, Davidson B R et al Br J Surg 1987; 74: 916
172. Ell C H, Kerzel W et al Gut 1989; 30: 680
173. Ell C H, Lox G et al Gut 1988; 29: 746
174. Dalton H R, Chapman R W G Gut 1995; 36: 485
175. Cairns S R, Dias L et al Gut 1989; 30: 535
176. Andren-Sandberg A, Alinder G, Bengmark S Ann Surg 1985; 201: 328
177. Blumgart L H, Kelley C J, Benjamin I S Br J Surg 1984; 71: 836
178. Dunn D, Fowler S et al Ann R Coll Surg (Engl) 1994; 76: 269
179. Fullarton G M, Bell G Gut 1994; 35: 1121
180. Metzler P, Camal E M Int Surg 1995; 80: 328
181. Go P M N Y H, Dirksen C C Int Surg 1995; 80: 304
182. Hobbs K E F Gut 1995; 36: 161
183. MacMahon A J, Fullarton G et al Br J Surg 1995; 82: 307
184. Windsor J A, Vaux D E Br J Surg 1994; 81: 1208
185. Scholl F P G, Go P M N, Gouma D J Br J Surg 1994; 81: 1786
186. Richardson M C, Bell G, Fullarton G M Br J Surg 1996; 83: 1356

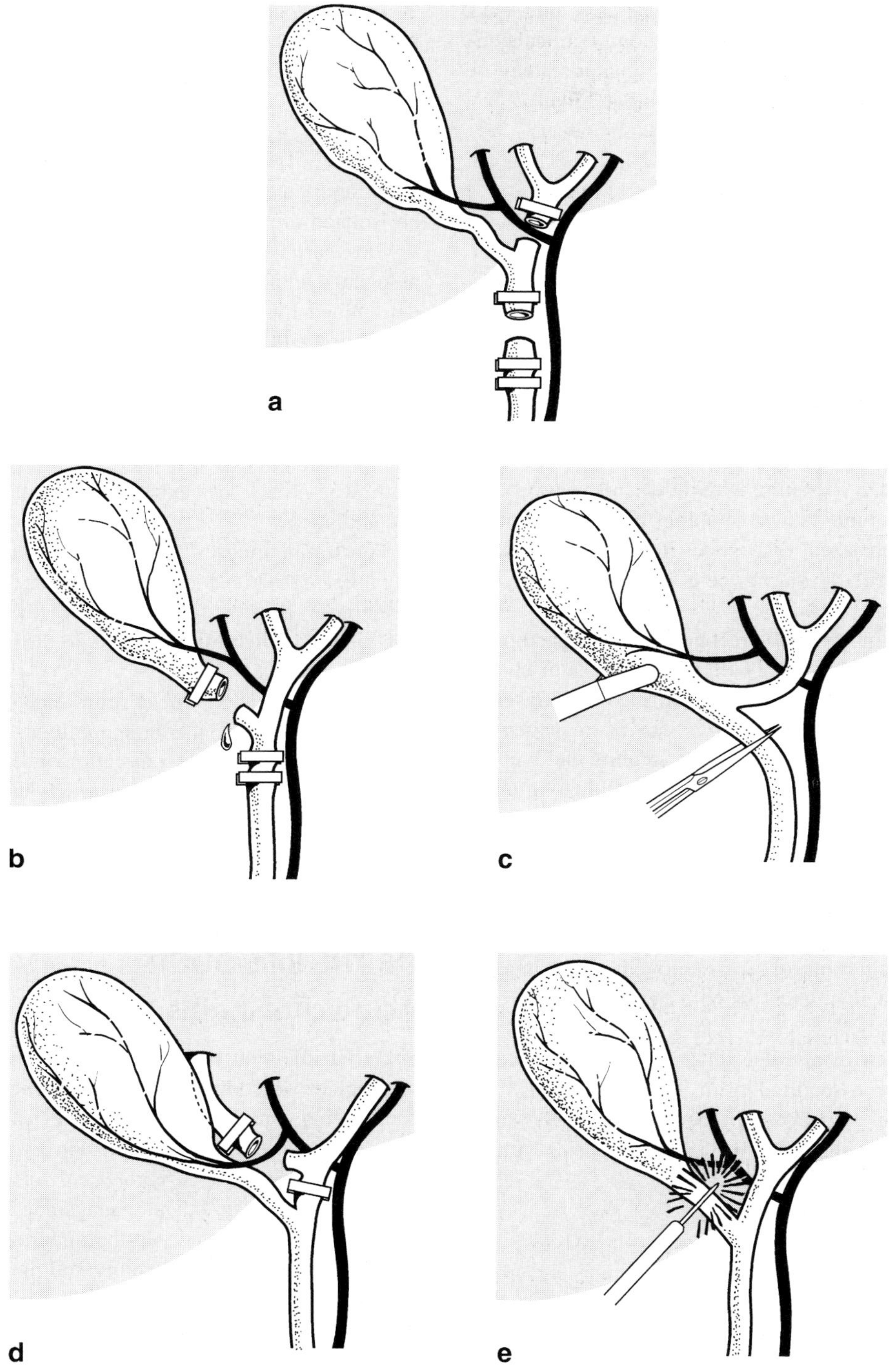

Fig. 32.13 **a** Classical injury (7 of 37 cases): misidentification of the common bile duct for the cystic duct with resultant clipping and division of the common duct and resection of a segment of common hepatic duct. Underlying right hepatic arterial injury associated. **b** Variant classical injury (3 cases): incorrect identification of common bile duct for proximal cystic duct with clipping. Upper cystic duct identified correctly, clipped and divided, leading to a bile leak. **c** Tenting injury (17 cases): lateral traction of gallbladder causes tenting of common duct with loss of angle of interception with cystic duct. Dissection low on cystic duct leads to inadvertent laceration (or clip involvement) of the common duct at this junction. **d** Confluence injury (5 cases): misidentification of right hepatic duct for cystic duct. Clipping and division around the confluence results in a high, severe injury. **e** Diathermy injury (5 cases): injudicious use of diathermy in Calot's triangle with resultant bile leak (necrosis) or late stricture. From *Br J Surg* 1996; 83: 1356–1360, with permission.

directly injure the bile duct and result in postoperative bile leaks (Fig. 32.13e) with subhepatic abscess formation. Percutaneous drainage of such a collection using ultrasound guidance may be followed by the development of a persistent biliary fistula.[180,183] Biliary peritonitis may also occur from an injured bile duct.[183]

Laparoscopic bile duct injuries have been classified into the following grades:[180,183]

I Minor, including erroneous incision into the bile duct.
II Clipping of the bile ducts.
III a. Complete transection with no tissue loss.
b. Complete transection with tissue loss.
IV Defect in the common hepatic duct, right hepatic duct or left hepatic duct.

Laparoscopic bile duct injury can be reduced by formal training and supervision of surgeons.[180,183,185] Conversion to an open operation rather than persisting with a difficult laparoscopic dissection may also be important in avoiding bile duct damage. It cannot be overemphasized that good intraoperative views must be obtained, particularly during the display of structures in Calot's triangle.

Although bile duct injury may be recognized in the postoperative period, more than half are only discovered after discharge from hospital.[184] The diagnosis is usually confirmed by ultrasound and scintigraphy. Fortunately many cases can be managed by endoscopic retrograde cholangiography with stenting and balloon dilatation (types I and II).[180,185] It is sometimes possible to intubate type III but types IIIa, IIIb and IV should be transferred to specialized centres for repair.[187] Early diagnosis has been shown to reduce morbidity and increase the effectiveness of repair and the chance of successful conservative treatment.[180,183] When the diagnosis is delayed or where a segment of bile duct is missing, the first essential is to establish drainage, control sepsis, allow the inflammation to settle and then repair this defect using a hepaticojejunostomy Roux-en-Y anastomosis.[183,187]

The outcome of repair of bile duct injuries after laparoscopic cholecystectomy has been reported from The Netherlands.[185,188] Three deaths occurred in 49 patients. Immediate end-to-end anastomosis was possible where there had been early diagnosis without gross tissue loss.

Open injury to bile ducts

Most injuries to the bile ducts at the time of open cholecystectomy can be avoided by a clear demonstration of the anatomy, a knowledge of anatomical variation and the use of operative cholangiography.[177] Adequate incision and exposure, good technique and a sufficient number of assistants are essential.[189]

Primary repair of the bile duct can be undertaken at the time of surgery when a major segment has not been contused or resected. End-to-end repair over a T-tube should then be considered. This is often difficult because of the thin wall and narrow lumen of a normal bile duct. A hepaticojejunostomy is required with more extensive injuries. In a series of 55 patients, primary repair produced good results in only 22% after end-to-end anastomosis but in 54% after biliary–enteric anastomosis.[176]

Bile duct repairs should be referred to surgeons in hepaticobiliary units experienced in this type of work and long-term follow-up is essential.[187]

Non-surgical trauma

Blunt injury to the biliary tree from road traffic accidents is rarely an isolated injury, and frequently involves other intra-abdominal viscera, particularly the liver, pancreas and duodenum. It is often associated with head and thoracic injuries. The prognosis is usually determined by the extent and severity of the associated injury. Injury to the portal vein and hepatic artery is infrequent.[180,187] The presence of retroperitoneal bile or the infiltration of periportal structures with blood and bile strongly suggests injury to the duodenum or bile duct. Delayed diagnosis is quite common and abdominal tap and lavage may be helpful. ^{99}Tc-iminodiacetic acid scans may be extremely useful in demonstrating bile accumulation.

Penetrating injuries by gunshots or stab wounds may occasionally involve the bile ducts. Most patients require immediate laparotomy but in a few (5%) laceration of the bile ducts leads to slow bile leakage which may give rise to difficulty in diagnosis and to delayed surgery.

Primary repair by direct suture and T-tube drainage may be possible when the contusion is minimal, such as a tangential tear, but more often complete transection or severe contusion requires a choledocho- or hepaticojejunostomy with a Roux-en-Y anastomosis. Coexistent hepatic injury significantly increases mortality and morbidity.[190]

INFLAMMATORY CONDITIONS OF THE BILE DUCTS

Acute cholangitis

Bacterial infection leads to acute cholangitis in the presence of incomplete or complete biliary obstruction, the most frequent cause being calculi. Micro-organisms can be recovered from the bile in nearly all cases and include *Escherichia coli*, *Klebsiella* spp., *Staphylococcus*, *Streptococcus*, clostridia, and, very rarely, *Bacteroides fragilis*.[191] The management of calculous disease has already been considered, but the importance of antibiotics should be stressed in reducing mortality and morbidity from septicaemia and intrahepatic abscesses. A 5-day course of broad-spectrum antibiotics such as a ureidopenicillin or a cephalosporin is preferred for the treatment of established cholangitis and allows urgent investigation to be undertaken prior to early elective surgery.

REFERENCES

187. Rossi R L, Schirmer W J et al Arch Surg 1992; 127: 596
188. Scholl F P G, Go P M N, Gouma D J World J Surg 1995; 19: 1997
189. Johnston G W Br J Surg 1986; 73: 245
190. Kitihama A, Alliott L F et al Ann Surg 1982; 196: 536
191. Keighley M R B In: Blumgart L H (ed) The Biliary Tract. Churchill Livingstone, Edinburgh 1982

Acute suppurative cholangitis is an uncommon but very serious infection of the biliary tree demanding emergency decompression. The condition is characterized by pain, jaundice and a high swinging pyrexia, with rigors, shock and central nervous system depression and has a 100% mortality if left untreated. Emergency endoscopic decompression has now replaced surgery as the treatment of choice. Often disimpaction of the stone during cannulation allows pus to drain and full endoscopic sphincterotomy with stone extraction may be deferred until the patient's condition improves.[192] Recurrent episodes of cholangitis after biliary surgery are usually the result of residual or recurrent calculi which can be caused by stenosis of the biliary outlet. This may also occur after biliary drainage procedures in the absence of stenosis,[193] stoma patency being judged by the free influx and efflux of barium. Achlorhydria, duodenal diverticula and foreign bodies are considered to be important predisposing factors.

Cholangitis may occur when there is slow emptying of dilated intrahepatic ducts and when bacterial colonization of the ducts is heavy. The dilatation is likely to diminish in the absence of distal obstruction over a period of many months with clinical reduction in the frequency of attacks. Recurrent pyogenic cholangitis or oriental cholangitis is related to intrahepatic duct stones and in some instances this is associated with parasitic infestation.

Parasitic infestation and involvement of the bile ducts

Round worm

Ascaris lumbricoides is endemic in many parts of the world where poor socioeconomic conditions and bad sanitation exist. Adult worms live in the human intestine (see Chapter 29) and when infestation is heavy one or two may enter the papilla and pass into the bile ducts; up to 60 or more worms may be found.[194] They cause biliary pain, partial obstruction and cholangitis with complications such as liver abscesses, perforation and stricture of the bile duct.

Children are most frequently affected. The diagnosis is based on the identification of worms in the biliary tree on ultrasound, intravenous cholangiography, barium meal or at endoscopic retrograde cholangiopancreatography.

Patients are initially treated with antibiotics and parenteral fluids to control infection and to correct dehydration and then with parenteral anti-spasmodics to relax the sphincter and allow egress of the live worms from the biliary tree. Anti-helminthics are also given. Persistent intraductal worms can be removed either endoscopically or surgically. Surgery may also be required for persistent worms in the gallbladder and for biliary stricture.[194] Liver abscesses can be drained percutaneously under ultrasound guidance.

Hydatid disease

The biliary tree may be involved when a hydatid cyst either compresses or ruptures into a biliary radical causing severe cholangitis (see Chapter 31). Compression by a hydatid cyst usually requires surgical drainage of the cyst; care must be taken to avoid spillage of the cyst contents and to oversew any open bile duct radicals. When rupture into the biliary tree has occurred, hydatid debris may be removed by endoscopic sphincterotomy and either extraction with a Dormia basket or flushing through a cannula.[195] The scolicidal agents, formalin and hypertonic saline, can unfortunately cause biliary strictures.[195]

Clonorchis sinensis

In South-east Asia infestation of the biliary tree by the liver fluke, which is ingested in contaminated fish, is frequent.[38] The worms live in the intrahepatic bile ducts and predispose to cholangitis, periductal fibrosis and stone formation. They are also associated with an increased incidence of bile duct cancer.[38] There is no satisfactory treatment of the parasite and management is directed towards the complications.[38]

Primary sclerosing cholangitis

This is a chronic fibrosing inflammatory condition of the biliary tree which affects both intrahepatic and extrahepatic ducts and may involve the gallbladder and pancreas. It is of unknown origin[196,197] and must be distinguished from secondary sclerosing cholangitis associated with choledocholithiasis, previous biliary surgery or cholangiocarcinoma. It is associated with inflammatory bowel disease, usually ulcerative colitis, in 50–70% of cases and these patients may be at greater risk of developing bile duct carcinoma.[196,197]

The patient, who is commonly between 20 and 50 years of age, presents with a progressive cholestatic disorder with right upper quadrant discomfort, jaundice, pruritus and fever. Investigation reveals a considerable elevation of the alkaline phosphatase and on cholangiography stricturing and beading of the bile ducts are seen (Fig. 32.14). Immunological studies show elevated immunoglobulin M, anti-smooth muscle antibodies but no rise in the anti-mitochondrial antibodies which differentiates the condition from primary biliary cirrhosis.

In 80% of the patients both the intra- and extrahepatic ducts are involved, but in 20% only extrahepatic involvement is present. Hepatic changes include periductal and portal fibrosis, bile ductular proliferation, with a reduction in the number of normal bile ducts, piecemeal necrosis and copper accumulation.[197] The average survival is only 5–7 years.[197]

Treatment aims to relieve episodes of cholangitis, pruritus, jaundice and discomfort. Antibiotics, vitamin K, cholestyramine, steroids and azathioprine do not usually help and colectomy does not alter the prognosis.[197] Surgical drainage by sphincteroplasty, biliary–enteric anastomosis and T-tube insertion has been used but is of dubious benefit.[198] Percutaneous transhepatic biliary stenting

REFERENCES

192. Ikeda S, Tanaka M et al World J Surg 1981; 5: 587
193. Goldman L D, Steer M L, Silen W Am J Surg 1983; 145: 450
194. Lloyd D A, White J A M In: Blumgart L H (ed) The Biliary Tract. Churchill Livingstone, Edinburgh 1982
195. Khodadadi D J, Kurgan A, Schmidt B Int Surg 1981; 66: 361
196. Lefkowitch J H Arch Intern Med 1982; 142: 1157
197. Chapman R W G, Arborgh B A M et al Gut 1980; 21: 870

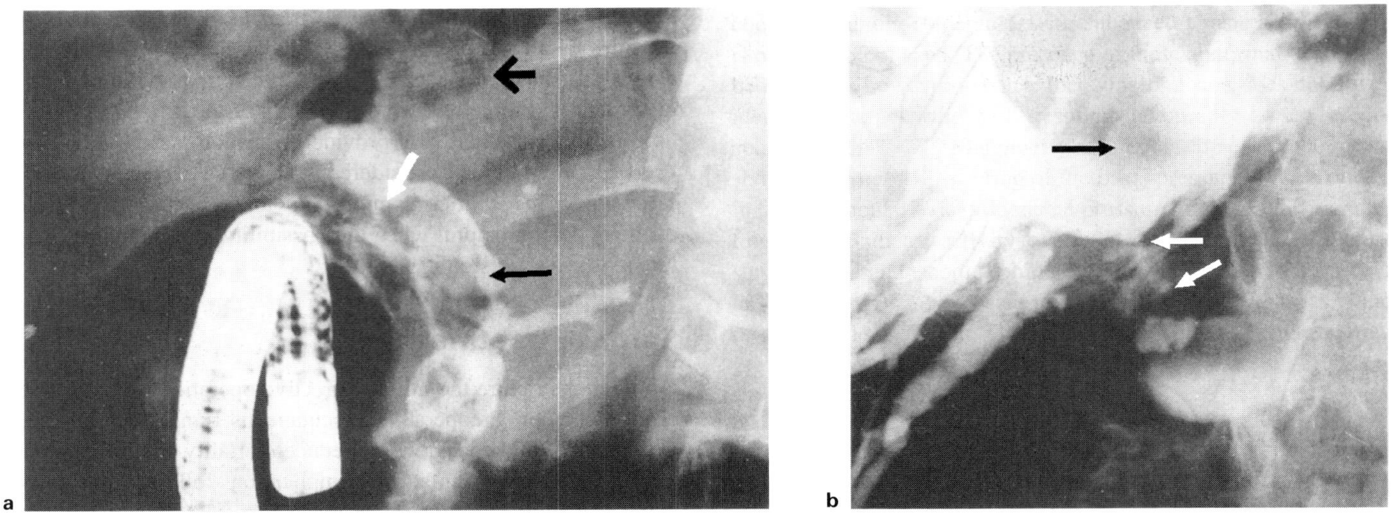

Fig. 32.16 A 43-year-old female patient with recurrent cholangitis. She had a previous history of cholecystectomy and choledochoduodenostomy for recurrent stone formation. Investigations revealed high bile duct stricture, probably secondary to cholecystectomy. **a** Endoscopic retrograde cholangiography. The thin black arrow shows stones within the distal common bile duct (sump). The open arrow shows the choledochoduodenostomy and the thick black arrow shows gas in the left hepatic duct. **b** Percutaneous transhepatic cholangiography demonstrates the high bile duct stricture (shown between the two open arrows) and calculi in the proximal biliary tree (black arrow).

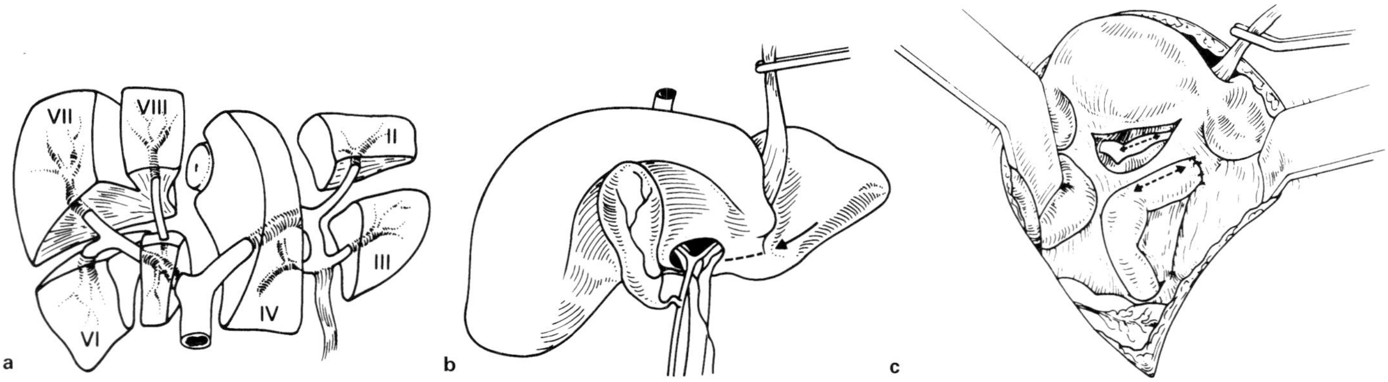

Fig. 32.17 **a** Segmental structure of liver demonstrating that the left portal triad is always extrahepatic beneath the quadrate lobe. **b** The bridge of liver tissue that needs to be divided in order to expose the depth of the umbilical fissure. **c** Exposure of the left hepatic duct and confluence by incision of the peritoneal reflexion at the base of the quadrate lobe, thus lowering the left hepatic duct in preparation for anastomosis to the Roux-en-Y jejunal loop. Dotted lines indicate lines of incision in left hepatic duct and jejunum. Reprinted[209] with permission.

Choledochoscopy is helpful in ensuring complete removal of all the calculi. Having gained access to healthy biliary mucosa, a biliary–enteric anastomosis can be constructed above the stricture. Care must be taken to ensure that there is adequate drainage of the right hepatic duct. Two hepaticoenteric anastomoses must be created if only a small bridge of mucosa is present at the con fluence or if the right or left hepatic ducts are separated.[205] Alternatives to this approach include prolonged stenting, often with a changeable transanastomotic stent, e.g. insertion of a U-tube.[213] Balloon dilatation of the stricture may be achieved percutaneously utilizing a similar technique to percutaneous transhepatic drainage.[209,214] The latter may be followed by stenting or repeated dilatation. Repeated endoscopic balloon dilatation is an alternative[210,215] which may be followed by stenting or repeated dilatation but recurrent episodes of cholangitis may require stenting[218] or surgical repair. The creation of a choledochojejuno-cutaneous fistula for ready access to prevent repeat dilatation has been particularly helpful where recurrent stone formation is anticipated.[216,217] Balloon dilatation is particularly helpful in elderly frail patients who are at high risk for surgery, especially if they have developed cirrhosis or portal hypertension.

REFERENCES

213. Hepp J World J Surg 1985; 9: 507
214. Praderi R Ann Surg 1974; 179: 937
215. Rao K J M, Blake H, Theodossi A Gut 1990; 31: 565
216. Hutson D G, Russell E et al Ann Surg 1984; 199: 637
217. Schweizer W P, Matthews J B et al Br J Surg 1991; 78: 559
218. Smits M E, Rauws A S et al Br J Surg 1996; 83: 764

cannot reliably differentiate a benign from a malignant bile duct stricture, particularly in the region of the hilum. Percutaneous fine-needle aspiration cytology is associated with a very low mortality and morbidity[206,228] but biopsy is probably better at achieving a definitive diagnosis, although it is unclear whether cells may be disseminated during this procedure.[206] Exfoliative cytology in the bile is highly specific[206,228] but a negative result is of less value. Endobiliary brush cytology produces a better cellular sample than exfoliative bile cytology[229] and is a valuable method of diagnosis. Endobiliary biopsy and endobiliary fine-needle aspiration cytology, in which a biopsy forceps is introduced into the biliary tree without a sphincterotomy in the former, and in which a needle is introduced into the biliary tree either percutaneously or endoscopically in the latter, both have useful potential.[206,229,230]

Surgical resection is usually only attempted for patients under 70 years of age. The site and spread of the cholangiocarcinoma must be determined by the techniques described above before surgery is undertaken. Proximal long strictures, vascular encasement, lymph node metastases, liver secondaries and multiple lesions within the biliary tree are contraindications to attempted surgical resection. Computed tomography angiography is of considerable value in assessing the presence of liver metastases, which can be confirmed by fine-needle biopsy and the relationship of the tumour to blood vessels. It is important to outline the biliary tree both proximal and distal to the obstruction and to fill both the right and left hepatic duct systems (Fig. 32.19). Incomplete mixing of contrast media with bile can occur and late films should be taken in the erect position to demonstrate the true level of the stricture.[231]

There is debate concerning the value of preoperative percutaneous transhepatic biliary drainage in relieving the biliary obstruction.[208] Although the bilirubin level falls, it is often accompanied by a fall in the albumin and it is likely that bacterial contamination of the biliary tree occurs within a short period of time. This may result in an unexpectedly high incidence of septic complications following surgery.[228]

Treatment

Potentially curable cholangiocarcinomas

High bile duct 'hilar' tumours should only be considered for resection by a surgeon who is experienced in the technique since a major liver resection is frequently required.[232,233] Reported resection rates range from 5 to 21%,[233] 47%[227] and 59%,[232] probably reflecting the differing referral patterns to specialized units. Operative mortality ranges from 10 to 25%, although in carefully selected cases this may be as low as 7.4%.[228] Average survival is in the order of 12–18 months with occasional patients surviving 5 or more years.[228] The survival time after resection, although longer is not statistically better than after surgical or intubation bypass. This must be weighed against the higher operative mortality when considering the management options. Carcinoma of the distal bile duct has a higher resectability rate (60–70%), a lower mortality (8%) and longer survival (28% at 5 years)[227] and laparotomy is usually worthwhile if there is no evidence of metastatic spread.

Palliative treatment

Unfortunately the majority of patients (80–90%) come into this category. The aim is to relieve symptoms of jaundice, cholangitis and itch.

Surgical measures

1. Hepaticojejunostomy, Roux-en-Y, the 'French connection', using the round ligament approach to the left hepatic duct or segment 3 duct with a mucosa-to-mucosa anastomosis may be feasible. Although this is a major operation and is not suitable for the frail or elderly, it does provide good palliation, relieving jaundice and preventing further attacks of cholangitis.[234]
2. Intraoperative insertion of an internal or an interoexternal stent (U tube) that can be changed are alternatives and may be combined with radiotherapy, producing some long-term survivors.[235] There is, however, considerable morbidity, particularly from septic complications.

Non-surgical measures

Endoscopic stenting has superseded percutaneous placement and is often achievable in over 90% of cases of malignant bile duct obstruction.[236,237] Causes of failure include the presence of a very tight stricture, a duodenal diverticulum, duodenal infiltration by malignancy and previous gastric surgery.[236] Percutaneous biliary stenting is far superior to external drainage in that it avoids electrolyte disturbance and reduces the risk of sepsis. The patient does not have to live with soreness resulting from a long-term indwelling tube coming through the skin and the inconvenience of carrying and emptying bile bags. Migration into the duodenum and occlusion with biliary sludge are less frequent problems with larger stents in the range of 10–16 French gauge. The expanding metal stent (Wall stent; Schneider UK) gives a satisfactory average patency period of 6–18 months and will be increasingly used.[237] It is important to remember that this type of stent is not removable and should not be inserted if surgery is being considered. If tumour overgrowth or biliary sludging causes stent occlusion, it can be treated either by reboring or insertion of an inner smaller flexible stent.[228,238]

Negotiation of the stricture may prove impossible at the first attempt if there is a widely dilated proximal bile duct. A period of

REFERENCES

228. Hadjis N S, Blenkarn J et al Surgery 1990; 107: 597
229. Kurzawinski T, Deery A et al Gut 1992; 33: 1675
230. Davidson B R Gut 1993; 34: 725
231. Williamson B W A, Blumgart L H, McKellar N J Am J Surg 1980; 139: 210
232. Launois B, Campion J P et al Ann Surg 1979; 190: 151
233. Beasley R M, Haqhis N et al Ann Surg 1984; 99: 623
234. Guthrie C M, Haddock G et al Br J Surg 1993; 80: 1434
235. Terblanche J Ann Surg 1979; 11: 249
236. Ede R S, Williams J J Br J Surg 1989; 76: 867
237. Kuvshinoff B W, Armstrong J G et al Br J Surg 1995; 82: 1522
238. Pogany A G, Kerlan R K, Ring E J Clin Gastroenterol 1985; 14: 387

decompression with an external catheter for several days permits the bile duct to contract down and makes subsequent passage of the stent much easier. Perforation is avoided by gentle technique and asepsis reduces the risk of cholangitis or septicaemia if external drainage is used. The subsequent choleresis demands careful management if electrolyte imbalance is to be prevented.[239] Complications are more frequent with proximal tumours but jaundice can be relieved in 75–100% of all ductal lesions, with a 30-day mortality of about 20% for proximal lesions and an overall survival of 6–13 months.[240]

Iridium 192 wire placed through the tumour at the time of operative tube drainage or through a percutaneous transhepatic catheter has also been found to be effective. Nearly half the patients so treated survived for more than 12 months.[241,242]

Ampullary carcinoma (see Chapter 33)

The majority of patients present with painless jaundice and, although some have an associated iron-deficiency anaemia, the clinical finding of a silver stool is a rarity. Ultrasonography shows dilatation of the intra- and extrahepatic bile ducts and an echogenic area at the ampulla may be detected. It is important to define the tumour with another test as calculi, lymph nodes and pancreatic nodules can be mistaken on ultrasound for an ampullary carcinoma. Endoscopic retrograde cholangiography with biopsy confirms the diagnosis in over 80%.[242] Endoscopic sphincterotomy may allow resolution of the jaundice and, indeed, in elderly frail patients it may be the only therapeutic measure that is necessary.

In fit younger patients a pancreaticoduodenectomy (see Chapter 33) should be considered or, if this is felt to entail an unduly high risk, a local excision of the tumour can be worthwhile. The ampullary region is approached transduodenally and after excision of the tumour the dilated bile and pancreatic ducts are reimplanted into the duodenum by direct mucosa-to-mucosa suture of the ductal and the duodenal walls. This procedure carries a low mortality and morbidity but has the disadvantage that the carcinoma may not be completely excised.

Guidelines for the management of patients with a primary malignancy of the biliary tract

Palliative non-operative measures should be selected for frail patients with concurrent disease and in those with metastases, since palliative operative surgery carries a high mortality and morbidity in this group. Surgical bypass avoids the recurrent longer-term septic complications of endoprostheses and external drainage and should be considered for the younger fitter patient with a localized but irresectable primary tumour.[243]

Most ampullary and periampullary tumours should be treated surgically by radical or local resections but when surgery is inappropriate endoscopic sphincterotomy is preferred to stenting. Mid common bile duct tumours can be treated by surgical bypass or intubation as resection is rarely feasible. Proximal tumours at the confluence should be considered for surgical bypass when irresectable, because of the high incidence of complications associated with stents. Insertion of iridium wire is an alternative method of treating hilar and mid bile duct tumours.

REFERENCES

239. Tytgat G N J, Huibregtse K et al Clin Gastroenterol 1986; 15: 249
240. Earnshaw J J, Teasdale C et al Ann R Coll Surg 1992; 74: 388
241. Fletcher M S, Brinkley D et al Br J Surg 1983; 70: 733
242. Venu R P, Geenen J E Clin Gastroenterol 1986; 15: 439
243. Gillen P, Peel A L G Br J Surg 1986; 73: 631

33 The pancreas

R. C. G. Russell

The pancreas originates from two separate embryonic anlagen: a ventral and a dorsal primordium. On or about the 24th day of gestation the hepatic diverticulum begins to bud from the duodenal portion of the primitive digestive tube to start to form the liver. Some 2 days later (26th day of gestation) a similar diverticulum becomes the dorsal anlage of the pancreas. The smaller ventral pancreatic anlage buds from the hepatic diverticulum on about the 32nd day of gestation.[1] The common bile duct, together with the ventral pancreatic anlage, then rotates into a dorsal position behind the primitive superior mesenteric vessels, bringing the dorsal and ventral portions of the pancreas together by the 37th day of gestation. The draining ducts fuse and the right dorsal leaf of the mesentery fuses with the posterior abdominal wall fixing the pancreas in its retroperitoneal position. By the 42nd day, the position and development of the pancreas are largely complete. The ventral anlage now constitutes the uncinate process and most of the pancreatic head. Its duct, the duct of Wirsung, fuses with the duct of the dorsal anlage and drains into the duodenum together with the common bile duct. The dorsal anlage constitutes the body and tail of the pancreas and the cranial part of its head. The distal part of its duct joins that draining the ventral anlage while its proximal portion, the duct of Santorini, drains via the minor papilla (Fig. 33.1).

CONGENITAL ANOMALIES

Total aplasia of the pancreas is rare and leads to death from growth retardation. Partial aplasia, usually of the dorsal pancreas (the body and tail) is equally rare and is usually described by the endoscopist as a 'congenital short pancreas'; it may be associated with an increased incidence of acute pancreatitis.

Ectopic (accessory or heterotopic) pancreas

Pancreatic tissue may occur in ectopic sites in the gastrointestinal tract and even elsewhere, either because of separation of some cells of the pancreatic anlage from the primary pancreatic mass early in embryonic life or because of 'pancreatic' differentiation of multipotent cells. The most common location for nodules of aberrant pancreas is in the wall of the stomach, duodenum or jejunum (Fig. 33.2). Approximately 75% of the nodules are found in the submucosa with the remainder either in the muscular layer or subserosa. The incidence of heterotopia is difficult to define, but when a search of the duodenum was made in 410 autopsies, pancreatic cells were found in 13.7%.[2] Although most nodules or ectopic pancreatic tissue contain acini, ducts and islets, any one of these may be missing. Many nodules of ectopic pancreatic tissue are symptomless; symptomatic cases are usually located in the stomach or duodenum and present with epigastric pain or haemorrhage. Heterotopic nodules may cause obstruction of the bile or

REFERENCES

1. O'Rahilly R Anatomy Embryol 1978; 153: 123
2. Feldman M, Weinberg T JAMA 1952; 148: 893

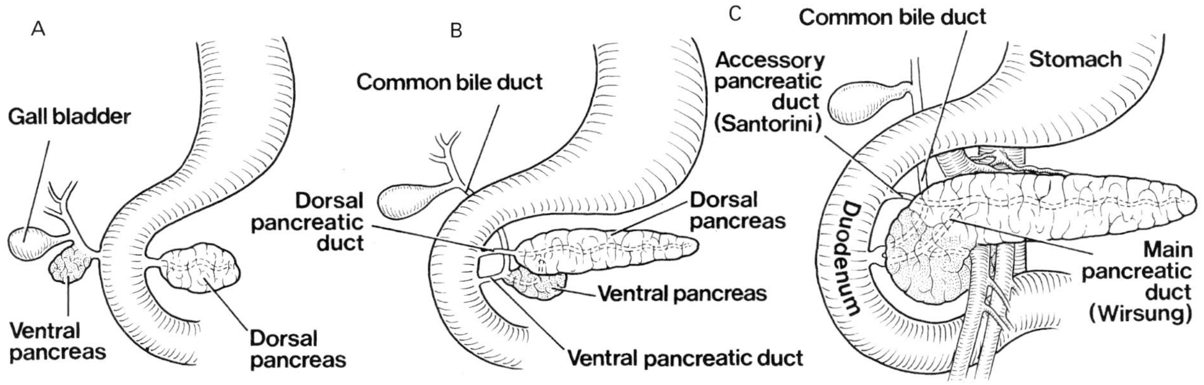

Fig. 33.1 The development of the pancreas. **(A)** Endodermal buds from the dorsal and ventral border of the foregut form between the 24th and 26th day. **(B)** The ventral bud rotates behind the foregut to form the pancreas at the 37th day. **(C)** The duct systems fuse by the 42nd day.

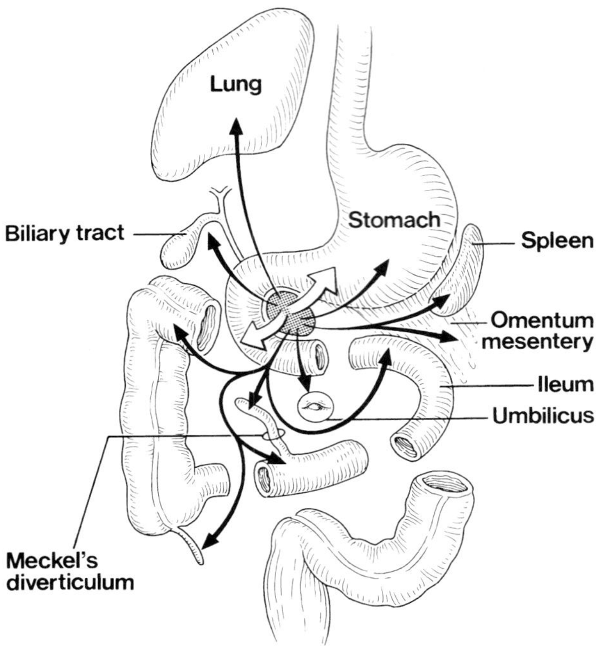

Fig. 33.2 Potential sites of heterotopic pancreatic tissue.

pancreatic ducts and can lead to intussusception.[3] These islands of pancreatic tissue may be diagnosed by gastroscopy or radiology. They appear smooth and rounded with umbilication and even a small duct. Treatment is by local excision. Rarely, they present as a carcinoma or islet cell adenoma; treatment is by excision.

Annular pancreas

The malformation of annular pancreas was first described by Tiedmann in 1818[4] and given its aptly descriptive name in 1862 by Ecker.[5] In the course of an anatomy demonstration he found a strip of pancreatic tissue overlying the second portion of the duodenum, which on closer examination was found to be a ring of pancreas surrounding the duodenum. It is now known that during rotation of the duodenum, pancreatic tissue from the ventral anlage may be carried with the second portion of the duodenum, subsequently fusing its free end above the head of the pancreas, thus creating an annular deformity. The aetiopathogenesis of annular pancreas is unknown. It may be a component of a more generalized disorder of embryogenesis when associated with trisomy 21, tracheo-oesophageal fistula or cardiorenal abnormalities, or may occur alone or with local duodenal abnormality. Recent evidence suggests that it is totally derived from the ventral pancreatic anlage and that the symptoms in the adult occur as a result of pancreatitis brought on by obstruction.[6] Its incidence is not known, but has been calculated at about 1 in 20 000. The presentation tends to be bimodal with peaks in the neonatal period and in the fourth and fifth decades, with equal numbers reported in adults and children.[7] It is responsible for 15% of all neonates presenting with duodenal obstruction. The pregnancy may have been associated with polyhydramnios. The obstruction is generally classified as intrinsic as pancreatic tissue is often intimately related to the wall of the duodenum. Other congenital abnormalities occur in about 80% of neonates and 20% of adults.

Vomiting is the principal symptom and bile may or may not be absent from the vomitus. Jaundice has been reported. The distended stomach and peristaltic waves are visible in the epigastrium. The plain film of the abdomen shows a distended stomach and may show a double-bubble sign. The obstruction is usually incomplete and the contrast studies show a sharp cut-off in the duodenum. An absolute differentiation between annular pancreas and duodenal atresia or stenosis is not possible before operation, and is of no consequence as operation must be undertaken urgently.

Adult presentation may be with duodenal stenosis, peptic ulceration, chronic pancreatitis or as an incidental finding. The most common adult symptom is upper abdominal pain. Diagnosis is made by ultrasound, computed tomographic (CT) scanning and endoscopic retrograde cannulation of the ducts.

At operation the annular pancreas is quite readily recognized as pancreatic tissue surrounding the duodenum. Division of pancreatic tissue should be avoided because leakage of pancreatic juices will occur and its intramural position may prevent opening up of the stenosis. The preferred operation is a duodenoduodenostomy or if this is difficult a duodenojejunostomy, which is best performed by the retrocolic route. In the adult these procedures are suitable for the inflamed pancreas with stenotic symptoms, but in the presence of pancreatitis a Whipple procedure is appropriate. Gastroenterostomy inadequately decompresses the duodenum, and carries the risk of an anastomotic ulcer.

Variations in pancreatic ducts[1]

In approximately 60% of subjects, the main pancreatic duct, which drains the tail and body of the pancreas, turns downwards and posteriorly into the head of the pancreas where it opens into the duodenum at the major papilla. The smaller accessory duct of Santorini runs as a continuation of the line of the main duct to drain into the duodenum some 2 cm proximal and anteriorly at the minor papilla. The pancreatic duct varies from 175 to 275 mm in length; the diameter in the tail varies from 1 to 2 mm, in the body from 2 to 3 mm and in the head from 3 to 4 mm. The duct is adequately filled by 2–3 ml of contrast (Fig. 33.3).

Pancreas divisum

The normal pancreas is formed by fusion of the dorsal and ventral pancreatic buds. Failure of fusion occurs in around 5–7% of individuals. At endoscopic retrograde cannulation of the pancreatic duct, a ventral remnant alone is shown while injection of contrast along the accessory duct opacifies the main ductal system of the pancreas (Figs 33.4 and 33.5).

REFERENCES

3. Lai E C S, Tomkins R K Am J Surg 1986; 151: 697–700
4. Tiedmann F Dtsch Arch Physiol 1818; 4: 403
5. Ecker A Z Art Med 1862; 14: 354
6. Dowsett J F, Rode J, Russell R C G Gut 1989; 30: 130–135
7. Lloyd-Jones W, Mountain J C, Warren K W Ann Surg 1972; 176: 163–170

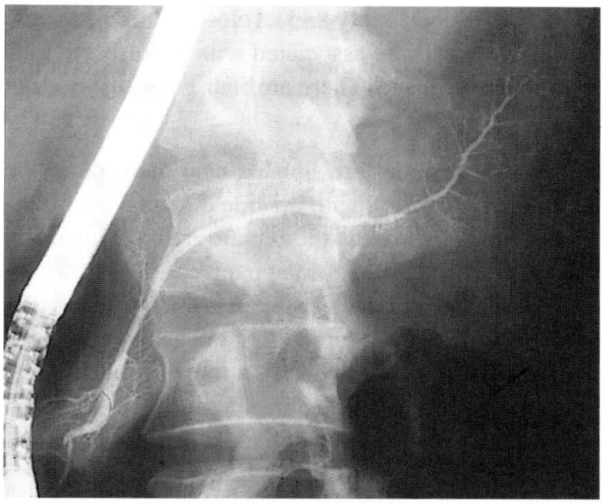

Fig. 33.3 A normal pancreatogram.

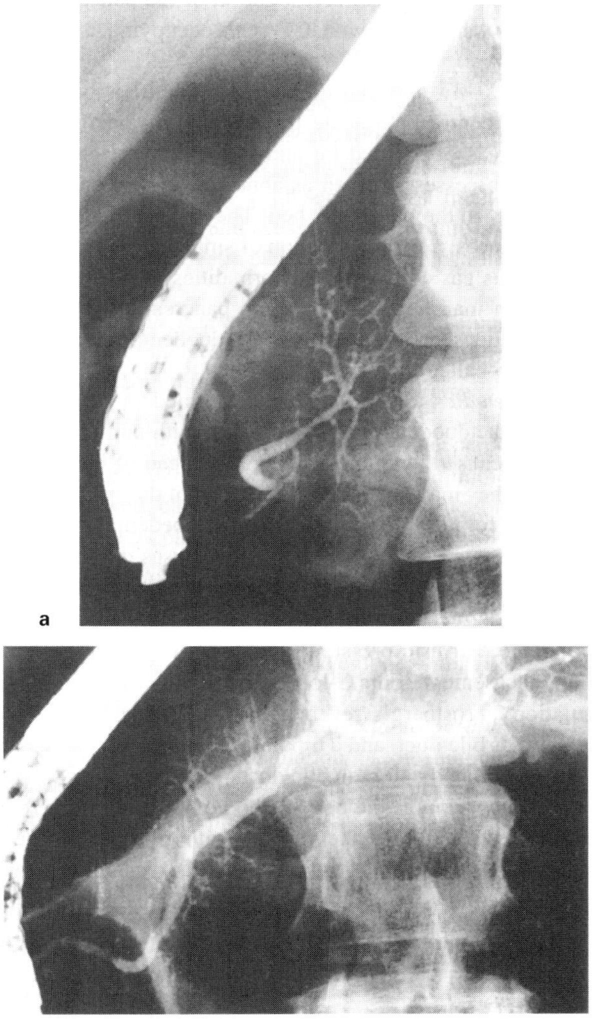

a

b

Fig. 33.4 (**a**) In pancreas divisum, injection of the main papilla fills the duct system of the ventral pancreas alone, with no communication to the dorsal duct. The ventral pancreas is normal. (**b**) Same patient as Fig. 33.4**a**. Injection of the accessory papilla fills the dorsal duct with no communication to the ventral duct. There are changes associated with chronic pancreatitis.

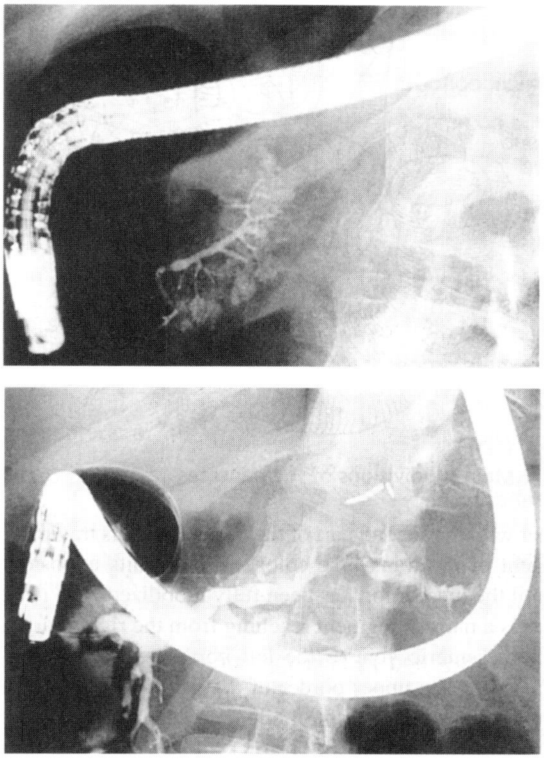

a

b

Fig. 33.5 (**a**) Pancreas divisum: a normal ventral pancreatogram with overfilling of the duct system to try and demonstrate a communication with the ventral pancreas—no communication was present. (**b**) Same patient as in Fig. 33.5**a**: dorsal pancreatogram showing a dilated pancreatic duct. An accessory sphincteroplasty was performed.

It is debatable whether this anatomical variant can be a cause of chronic pancreatitis and abdominal pain.[8] In the vast majority of people with this anomaly, no malfunction occurs, but in others there is definite evidence of obstruction at the accessory papilla. Sphincteroplasty of this sphincter usually improves symptoms and is the procedure of first choice in managing symptomatic patients with pancreas divisum.[9] It is preferable to confine this operation to those patients with recurrent acute attacks of pancreatitis, and to avoid this procedure in those with chronic pain, who should be treated on merit.[10]

SURGICAL ANATOMY

The pancreas is divided into the head (including the uncinate process), neck, body and tail (Fig. 33.6). The head is flattened 1–2 cm thick and firmly fixed on the right to the second and third parts of the duodenum. To the left it merges into the neck along an arbitrary line marked by the gastroduodenal artery above and the superior mesenteric and portal veins behind. Its anterior surface is covered by the pylorus above and the transverse colon below.

REFERENCES

8. Cotton P B Gastroenterology 1985; 89: 1431–1435
9. Staritz M, Meyer Z U M, Buschenfelde K-M Pancreas 1988; 3: 248–253
10. Keith R G, Shapero T F, Saibil F G, Moore T L Surgery 1989; 106: 660–607

compression against the handlebars of a bicycle or a lap-type seat belt can transect the pancreas. Pancreatic injury can be subdivided according to severity into:

1. *Minor*, in which there is contusion, abrasion or laceration to any portion of the gland not involving the main ducts.
2. *Intermediate*, in which there is distal laceration, transection or duct disruption.
3. *Major*, in which there is laceration of the head of the pancreas or a pancreaticoduodenal injury.

For *penetrating wounds* of the abdomen the criteria for performing laparotomy are discussed in Chapter 27. If a peritoneal lavage is performed, absence of blood or of a raised amylase level in the perfusate indicates that pancreatic injury is unlikely and observation is safe. Early diagnosis of a blunt pancreatic injury continues to be a surgical enigma. The retroperitoneal location of these injuries dampens the classic symptoms and signs of intra-abdominal mischief, thus causing delay in recognition. This delay is the single most important factor causing increased morbidity and mortality, particularly if the delay exceeds 24 hours. The most common physical findings in patients with retroperitoneal duodenal rupture or pancreatic injury are minimal abdominal pain and tenderness, which are present immediately after injury. These signs usually decrease over the next 1 or 2 hours only to worsen again within 6 hours. Absence of shock on admission does not preclude retroperitoneal injury. Those patients with a delayed presentation frequently do not have associated intraperitoneal injury.

Laboratory tests

No specific laboratory tests will lead to an early diagnosis of blunt pancreatic or duodenal injury. The serum amylase may or may not be elevated. A repeat amylase level is sometimes helpful after blunt abdominal trauma. The rise in serum amylase does not relate to the severity of trauma. Plain abdominal X-ray may be helpful, especially if there is an associated duodenal injury. Specific findings which may be seen are air bubbles distributed along the right psoas margin, the upper pole of the right kidney or along the lower mediastinum. Non-specific findings include obliteration of the psoas shadow and scoliosis. Gastrografin swallow, with the patient lying on the right side, may demonstrate the passage of contrast material into the retroperitoneal space. Late signs include a ground-glass appearance in the mid-abdomen as a result of the lesser sac being filled with fluid. The decision to operate depends upon repeated clinical observation with evidence of deterioration in the patient's general condition despite adequate conservative management. This will be influenced by signs of pancreatic disruption or damage on good-quality CT scans.

Operative treatment

Following appropriate resuscitation and induction of general anaesthesia, a midline laparotomy incision is made. All patients with possible pancreatic or duodenal injury require a full exploration of the lesser sac. Criteria for lesser sac exploration include:

1. Air bubbles in the retroperitoneal tissues.
2. Bile staining anywhere in the peritoneal cavity.
3. Haematoma along the border of the duodenum, the base of the mesentery or adjacent to the greater curve of the stomach.
4. Penetration or near penetration of the upper abdomen by a missile or knife.

Mobilization of the tail and body of the pancreas or mobilization of the head of the pancreas is not indicated unless there is evidence of intermediate or major pancreatic injury.

Minor and intermediate pancreatic injury such as contusion, haematoma or lacerations which do not involve the main pancreatic duct are best treated by haemostasis with drainage. It is unnecessary to suture the pancreatic capsule. Major pancreatic injury of the body or tail is best treated by distal pancreatectomy with splenectomy. Injuries to the head of the pancreas, especially if they are associated with a duodenal injury, are best treated by a pancreaticoduodenectomy; however, unless the operator is experienced and other injuries are minor, valuable holding time can be achieved by simple drainage, with patching of the duodenum by the laying of a serosal graft on the damaged surface from an adjacent loop of small intestine.

Occasionally, pancreatic injuries present at a later stage with a pancreatic fistula, pancreatic abscess, pseudocyst or bleeding. Ultrasound, computed axial tomography and endoscopic cannulation of the pancreatic duct in combination with contrast studies (Fig. 33.8) clearly define the extent of the problem and enable the correct treatment to be selected. Pancreatic resection is usually the most suitable treatment if these studies show that the duct has been transected or damaged.[19]

The postoperative management is exacting with great attention being paid to prevent respiratory problems, fluid balance disturbance and renal injury. These patients invariably require nutritional support. Once rehabilitated, the prognosis is excellent, with few sequelae. The nature of the wounding agent influences the extent of pancreatic injury, shotgun injuries being the most lethal (60%) and stab wounds the least (9%). Blunt injuries have a 20% mortality. The cause of death is usually sepsis, late haemorrhage and pancreatic necrosis secondary to acute pancreatitis.

INFLAMMATION OF THE PANCREAS

Classification

Some of the confusion surrounding pancreatitis has arisen on account of the inability to define and diagnose the condition adequately. Much thought has been given to this problem, and three broad groups of definitions have been found useful in describing the disorder: they are dependent on clinical presentation, pathological findings and associated complications.

The current definitions have been built on the experience gained with the original Marseilles classification presented by

REFERENCE

19. Carr N D, Cairns S J, Lees W R, Russell R C G Br J Surg 1989; 76: 1244–1246

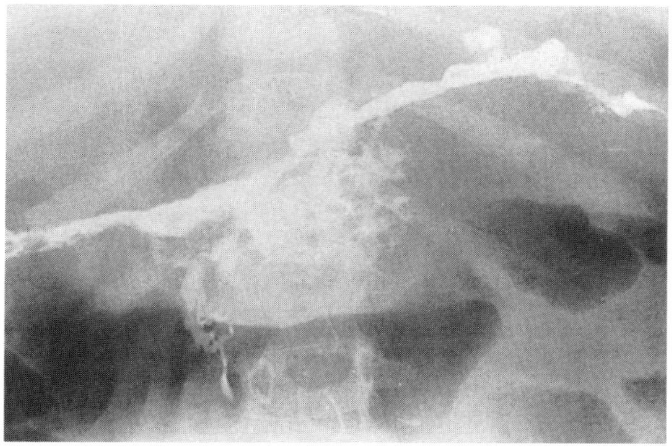

Fig. 33.8 Trauma: a 6-year-old boy was involved in a road traffic accident—he had two laparotomies with drainage of fluid without improvement. A fistulogram outlined the duct in the body and tail of the pancreas, but there was no communication with the duct in the head of the pancreas. He was cured by a distal pancreatectomy.

Sarles and colleagues in 1963. This was revised by the Cambridge workshop on pancreatitis,[20] and in 1984 a further Marseilles workshop.[21] The most recent classification emanated from a workshop held in Atlanta, Georgia in 1992[22] and it is these definitions which are now accepted.

ACUTE PANCREATITIS

Acute pancreatitis is defined as an acute inflammatory process of the pancreas, with variable involvement of other regional tissues or remote organs. The clinical manifestations are those of an illness with a rapid onset accompanied by upper abdominal pain and associated with variable clinical findings ranging from mild abdominal tenderness to rebound tenderness. An acute attack is accompanied by vomiting, fever, tachycardia, leucocytosis and an elevated pancreatic enzyme level in the blood or urine.

The pathological findings range from microscopic interstitial oedema and fat necrosis of the pancreatic parenchyma to macroscopic areas of pancreatic and peripancreatic necrosis and haemorrhage. The pathological changes represent a continuing process with interstitial oedema and minimal histological evidence of necrosis at the minor end of the scale to confluent macroscopic necrosis at the other extreme.[23]

The diagnosis is essentially a clinical diagnosis. Initial episodes of acute pancreatitis in patients who progress to chronic pancreatitis are defined as acute pancreatitis until the diagnosis of chronic pancreatitis has been clearly established. Severe acute pancreatitis is associated with organ failure or local complications such as necrosis, abscess formation or pseudocyst. Mild acute pancreatitis is defined as acute pancreatitis with minimal organ dysfunction and an uneventful recovery. Acute pancreatitis presents as an acute abdomen (see Chapter 27) and must be differentiated from other causes of severe abdominal pain and shock such as perforated peptic ulcer, acute gangrenous cholecystitis, mesenteric ischaemia, small bowel volvulus, and ruptured abdominal aneurysm.

Chronic pancreatitis is defined as a continuing inflammatory disease characterized by irreversible morphological change and typically causing pain and/or permanent loss of function. A distinct morphological form of chronic pancreatitis is obstructive chronic pancreatitis which is characterized by dilatation of the ductal system proximal to the occlusion of a major duct, diffuse atrophy of acinar parenchyma and uniform diffuse fibrosis.[21]

Complications

These are common to both acute and chronic pancreatitis. They may be systemic or local and may develop at any stage of the disease (Table 33.1). Systemic complications are derangements of the function of organs or systems (Table 33.2) and it is these derangements which frequently determine the outcome of severe disease. Local complications are defined as follows:

1. *Pancreatic phlegmon:* A non-suppurative inflammatory mass involving pancreatic and peripancreatic structures.
2. *Peripancreatic oedema:* Swelling of the peripancreatic tissues without necrosis or infection.
3. *Pancreatic effusion:* An encapsulated collection of fluid arising as a consequence of acute pancreatitis, typically in the pleural cavity.
4. *Pancreatic ascites:* Chronic generalized peritoneal enzyme-rich effusion usually associated with pancreatic duct disruption.
5. *Pseudocyst:* A pseudocyst is a collection of pancreatic juice enclosed by a wall of fibrous or granulation tissue which arises as a consequence of an episode of acute pancreatitis, pancreatic trauma or chronic pancreatitis.

REFERENCES

20. Sarner M, Cotton P B Gut 1984; 25: 756–759.
21. Singer M V, Gyr K, Sarles H Gastroenterology 1985; 89: 683–685
22. Bradley E L Arch Surg 1993; 128: 586–590
23. Bittner R, Block S, Büchler M, Beger H G Dig Dis Sci 1987; 32: 1082–1087

Table 33.1 Complications of pancreatitis

Systemic	*Local*
Cardiovascular	Phlegmon
Pulmonary	Oedema
Renal	Effusion
Haematological	Ascites
Metabolic	Infected effusion
Neurological	Pseudocyst
Gastrointestinal	Pancreatic abscess
	Necrosis

Table 33.2 Criteria for defining systems failure in acute pancreatitis

Systemic	*Local*
Cardiac	Hypotension, tachycardia >130 beats/min arrhythmias; electrocardiogram changes
Pulmonary	PO_2 <60 mmHg Adult respiratory distress syndrome
Renal	Urine output <40 ml/hour Rising blood urea and creatinine
Metabolic	Low calcium, magnesium, albumin
Haematological	Falling haematocrit; disseminated intravascular coagulation
Neurological	Irritability, confusion, localizing signs
Gastrointestinal	Severe ileus with fluid sequestration

6. *Pancreatic abscess:* A circumscribed intra-abdominal collection of pus usually in proximity to the pancreas, containing little or no pancreatic necrosis, which arises as a consequence of acute pancreatitis or pancreatic trauma.

7. *Pancreatic necrosis*: A diffuse or focal area of non-viable pancreatic parenchyma which is typically associated with peripancreatic fat necrosis.

8. *Pseudoaneurysm*: Bleeding from a major peripancreatic vessel confined as a clot by the surrounding tissues and often associated with infection. Recurrent bleeding is common, often culminating in fatal haemorrhage.[24]

Epidemiology

The incidence of acute pancreatitis has increased several-fold between the 1960s and the 1990s.[25] In the early 1970s an incidence of 21 per million population was recorded; by the mid 1980s the incidence had risen to 142 per million. The Scottish epidemiological data showed that between the 1960s and the 1980s there was an increase in admissions for both men from 69 to 750 per million population and women from 112 to 484 per million population.[26] The reason for these increases may be related to an increase in alcohol abuse or an improved ability to diagnose the disease.

Aetiology

Gallstones are the most common cause of acute pancreatitis, accounting for approximately 45–60% of cases.[27] Alcohol is the second most common cause, accounting for 35% of cases.[28,29] After gallstones and alcoholism, miscellaneous causes account for approximately 10% of cases and 10% of cases occur without a cause being found (Table 33.3).

The importance of the aetiology of pancreatitis is that a search should always be made for its aetiology, particularly after a mild attack. It is well-known that if the cause is not removed further and more severe, even fatal, attacks of the pancreatitis can occur. Thus, it behoves those looking after patients with acute pancreatitis to ascertain and eliminate any possible cause.

REFERENCES

24. Glazer G In: Glazer G, Ranson J H C (eds) Acute Pancreatitis. Baillière Tindall, London 1988 pp 37–50
25. Steinberg W, Tener S N Engl J Med 1994; 330: 1198–1210
26. Wilson C, Imrie C W Br J Surg 1990; 77: 731–734
27. Fan S T, Lai E C S, Mok F P T, Lo C-M, Zheng S S, Wong J N Engl J Med 1993; 328: 228–232
28. Steinberg W, Tenner S N Engl J Med 1994; 330: 1198–1210
29. Singh M, Simsek H Gastroenterology 1990; 98: 1051–1062

Table 33.3 Causes of acute pancreatitis

Obstruction	*Metabolic*
Choledocholithiasis	Hypertriglyceridaemia
Ampullary or pancreatic tumours	Hypercalcaemia
Worms or foreign bodies obstructing the papilla	*Inherited conditions*
Divisum with accessory duct obstruction	*Infection*
Choledochocoele	Parasitic
Periampullary duodenal diverticula	*Ascaris*
Hypertensive sphincter of Oddi	*Clinorchis*
Toxins	Viral
Ethyl alcohol	Mumps
Methyl alcohol	Rubella
Scorpion venom	hepatitis
Organophosphorous insecticides	Cocksackie B
Drugs	Echovirus
Azathioprine and mercaptopurine	Human immunodeficiency virus
Valproic acid	Bacterial
Oestrogens	*Mycoplasma*
Tetracycline	*Campylobacter jejuni*
Metronidazole	*Mycobacterium tuberculosis*
Nitrofurantoin	*Vascular abnormalities*
Pentamidine	Ischaemia
Frusemide	Hypoperfusion, e.g. after cardiac surgery
Sulphonamides	Atherosclerotic emboli
Methyldopa	Vasculitis
Cimetidine, ranitidine	*Miscellaneous conditions*
Erythromycin	Penetrating peptic ulcer
Salicylates	Crohn's disease
Trauma	Reye's syndrome
Accidental	Hypothermia
Blunt trauma to the abdomen	
Iatrogenic	
Postoperative trauma	
Endoscopic retrograde cholangiopancreatography	
Endoscopic sphincterotomy	
Manometry of the sphincter of Oddi	

Pathophysiology

The pathogenesis of acute pancreatitis remains poorly understood. A number of factors can apparently initiate this process, including obstruction or over-distension of the pancreatic duct, exposure to ethanol and other toxins, hypertriglyceridaemia, hypercalcaemia, an increase in the permeability of the pancreatic duct and hyperstimulation of the gland.[28] How these diverse factors initiate a disturbance of cellular metabolism with activation of zymogens has not been elucidated. Experimental models of acute pancreatitis show coalescence of zymogen granules with lysosome vacuoles allowing for possible premature activation of zymogen by hydrolases.[30] Ischaemia of the organ appears to transform mild oedematous pancreatitis into a severe haemorrhagic or necrotizing form of the disease.[31] Once triggered, the acinar cell follows an unpredictable cascade of events that can lead to mild localized interstitial inflammation or to severe necrosis with spread into peripancreatic spaces and the release of toxic factors into the systemic circulation or peritoneal space, leading to multi-organ failure. The intra-acinar activation of trypsin from trypsinogen is believed to be one of the initiating events.[32] Small amounts of intracellular trypsin are thought to be inactivated by endogenously secreted pancreatic trypsin inhibitor. Larger amounts of liberated trypsin, however, overwhelm the defence mechanisms of the pancreas and the system as a whole (circulating α_2-macroglobulin and α_1-antitrypsin) and activate other enzymes. The activation of phospholipase A_2 releases an enzyme with potent cytolytic properties that is thought to cause acute pulmonary injury by degrading surfactant.[33] The activation of elastase leads to the digestion of the elastic components of pancreatic blood vessels, thus contributing to intrapancreatic haemorrhage.[28] The release of trypsin activates complement and kinin, possibly playing a part in developing disseminated intravascular coagulation, shock and renal failure. Kallikrein is activated by circulating trypsin, leading to the release of bradykinin and kallidin which may be instrumental in causing vascular instability. Liberation of lipase in the peripancreatic region leads to fat necrosis. Recent evidence suggests that mediators produced and released by activated inflammatory cells may contribute to the recognized complications of pancreatitis, namely multi-organ failure, necrosis and sepsis. Neutrophil activation is a significant event in human pancreatitis, which induces injury directly by the production of elastase and superoxide ions which cause endothelial damage.

Platelet-activating factor, which can be raised ninefold, is important in the genesis of pancreatitis. It is known to encourage adhesion of granulocytes and is released from neutrophils when activated by tumour necrosis factor. A platelet-activating factor receptor antagonist has been developed, and trials to assess its therapeutic potential are in progress.[34]

The necrotic pancreas becomes secondarily infected in 40–60% of those affected, usually with Gram-negative bacteria translocated from the alimentary tract.[35,36] Infected necrotic tissue differs from a pancreatic abscess. The former is a diffuse infection of acutely inflamed necrotic pancreas and peripancreatic areas that occurs within the first 1–2 weeks of the illness and is associated with an increased mortality.[37] An abscess is a well-defined collection of pus occurring several weeks into the illness, after the acute inflammation has subsided. It is associated with a lower mortality rate.

Many years of alcohol abuse are required before acute alcoholic pancreatitis develops. As pancreatitis only develops in approximately 5% of alcoholics,[38] other unexplained factors must clearly predispose patients to this disorder. The precise pathogenesis of gallstone-induced pancreatitis also continues to be debated.[39] Opie's proposal at the turn of the century that a gallstone obstructing the ampulla of Vater would cause reflux of bile into the pancreatic duct is not universally accepted. Nevertheless, there is now no doubt that gallstone transit through the biliary tree into the lumen of the gut is associated with pancreatitis and once the gallbladder has been removed it is rare for further attacks to occur.[40]

Diagnosis

The diagnosis of acute pancreatitis and its differentiation from other abdominal diseases depend on both careful clinical assessment and the use of supportive laboratory and radiographic techniques. An elevation of the serum amylase is the cornerstone of diagnosis. Serum lipase is said to be more sensitive and specific but is a more difficult assay to perform.[41] Neither serial measurements of amylase nor amylase clearance in relationship to creatinine clearance add important diagnostic information. The exception is that a very low amylase–creatinine ratio is indicative of macroamylasaemia.[42]

Imaging techniques are now routinely used to confirm the diagnosis and to provide clues to its cause. Ultrasonography remains the most sensitive method of evaluating the biliary tract in acute pancreatitis. It has a sensitivity of 67% in the urgent diagnosis of acute pancreatitis and a specificity of 100%. The presence of overlying bowel gas limits its usefulness. Repeated sonograms may be required to demonstrate gallstones.

Contrast-enhanced CT is the imaging method of choice in delineating the pancreas as well as in determining the severity and

REFERENCES

30. Lerch M M, Saluja A K, Dawra R, Saluja M, Steer M L Gastroenterology 199; 104: 1768–1769
31. Klar E, Messmer K, Warshaw A L, Herfarth C Br J Surg 1990; 77: 1205–1210
32. Figarella C, Amourie M, Guy-Crotte O In: Beger H G, Büchler M (eds) Acute Pancreatitis: Research and Clinical Management. Springer-Verlag, Berlin, Germany 1987 pp 53–60
33. Büchler M, Malfertheiner P, Schädlich H, Nevalainen T J, Friess H, Beger H G Gastroenterology 1989; 87: 1521–1526
34. Skaife P, Kingsnorth A N Postgrad Med J 1996; 72: 277–283
35. Beger H G, Bittner R, Block S, Büchler M Gastroenterology 1986; 91: 433–438
36. Gerzof S G, Banks P A et al Gastroenterology 1987; 93: 1315–1320
37. Bittner R, Block S, Büchler M, Beger H G Dig Dis Sci 1987; 32: 1082–1087
38. Gullo L, Priori P, Labo G In: Banks P A, Porro G B (eds) Acute Pancreatitis: Advances in Pathogenesis, Diagnosis and Treatment. Masson Italia Editori, Milan, Italy, 1984 pp 87–89
39. Singh M, Simsek H Gastroenterology 1990; 98: 1051–1062
40. Moody F G, Senninger N, Runkel N Gastroenterology 1993; 104: 927–931
41. Gumaste V, Dave P, Sereny G Am J Med 1992; 92: 239–242
42. Pezzilli R, Billi P, Miglioli M, Guillo L Dig Dis Sci 1993; 38: 1265–1269

many of the complications of pancreatitis (Figs 33.9 and 33.10). CT scanning may indicate a normal pancreas in 15–30% of patients with mild disease. Pancreatitis that is moderately severe to severe, however, is nearly always accompanied by an abnormal CT scan of the pancreas. Dynamic CT pancreatography in which large doses of intravenous contrast are given rapidly and thin tomographic cuts of the pancreas are obtained is now used to identify pancreatic perfusion defects whose presence is correlated with pancreatic necrosis. The positive predictive value of dynamic CT scanning in diagnosing acute pancreatitis is 92%. Nearly all patients with clinically severe disease have necrosis.[43]

ERCP plays a part in the diagnosis of patients in whom no definite cause of acute pancreatitis is found after the initial history-taking and imaging studies (Fig. 33.11). ERCP and manometry of the sphincter of Oddi can provide useful information about the cause of pancreatitis and it also has an important role in the diagnosis and subsequent treatment of a stone in the bile duct.[44]

Plain radiology is relatively unimportant in the diagnosis of acute pancreatitis. Chest and abdominal films reveal some abnormality in 25–50% of cases; usually it is a small pleural effusion. Erect films help to eliminate a perforated ulcer by failing to demonstrate gas under the diaphragm. Radiological diagnosis is based on either the demonstration of a duodenal or gastric deformity accompanying the inflammatory process or a change in intestinal motility. In plain films a sentinel loop of distended small gut may be present or the hepatic flexure of the colon may be distended (colon 'cut-off' sign). The stomach may be pushed anteriorly by the enlarged pancreas. Barium studies may also show enlargement of the duodenal loop and reduced duodenal motility.

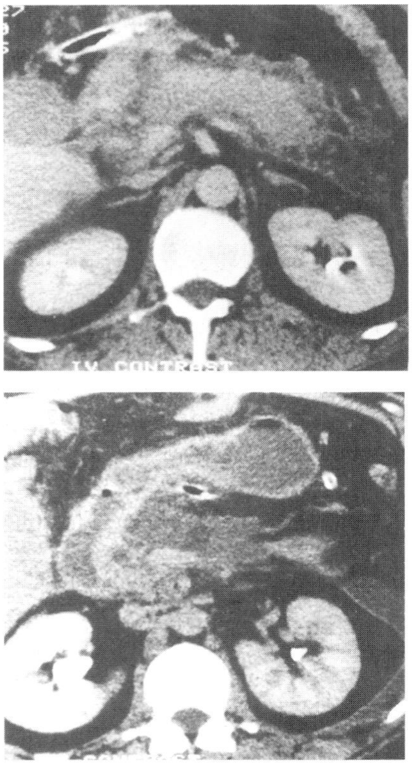

a

b

Fig. 33.9 (**a**) Acute pancreatitis: CT scan day 6. The body of the pancreas is oedematous and enlarged with surrounding collections of the fluid. A drainage tube lies in the lesser sac above the pancreas. Spontaneous resolution occurred. (**b**) Acute pancreatitis: CT scan day 6. Oedematous head of pancreas with thickened duodenal wall.

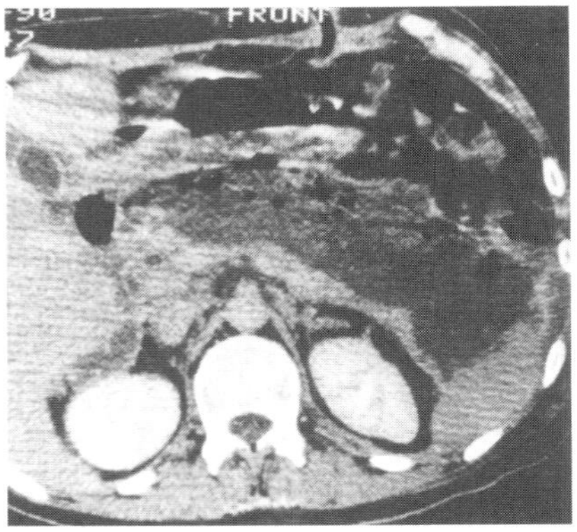

Fig. 33.10 Acute pancreatitis: CT scan day 40. Failure to resolve due to presence of a pancreatic abscess with gas formation. Slow resolution occurred after debridement.

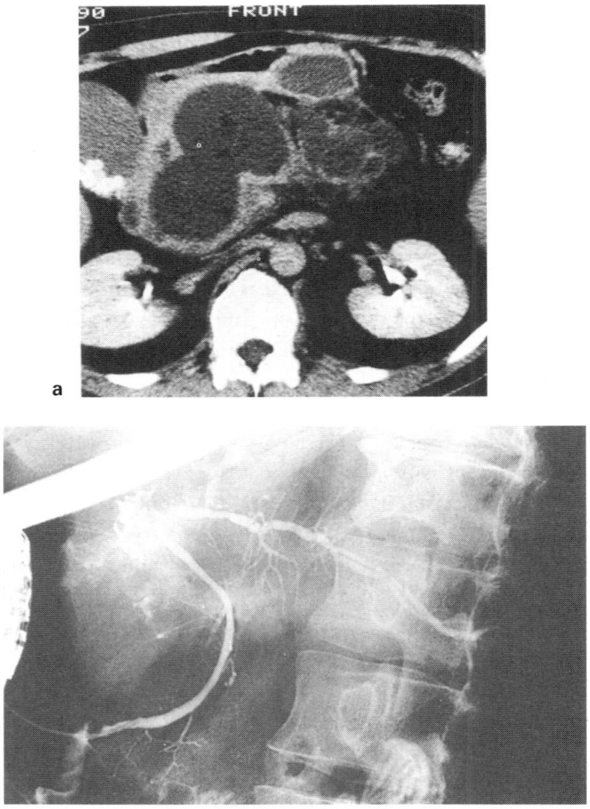

a

b

Fig. 33.11 (**a**) Recurrent acute pancreatitis: CT scan after third attack. The large pseudocyst occurred in the head of the pancreas due to duct disruption shown in the pancreatogram (**b**). Note the gallstones on the CT scan. Despite the apparent gland destruction, the duct is largely intact. Treatment by cholecystectomy and cyst-gastrostomy was appropriate.

REFERENCES

43. Nuutinen P, Kivisaari L, Schröder T Pancreas 1988; 3: 53–60
44. Neoptolemos J P, Carr-Locke D L, London N J, Bailey I A, James D, Fossard D P Lancet 1988; 11: 979–982

Prognostic indicators

Commonly used combinations of clinical and laboratory data that can indicate the severity of pancreatitis within the first 48 hours after admission have been developed by Ranson[45] and by clinicians from Glasgow[46] (Table 33.4). Patients with fewer than three of the risk factors present have a very low mortality. As the number of risk factors increases, there is a corresponding increase in the morbidity and mortality. For instance, those with one or two risk factors according to the Ranson criteria have a mortality rate of less than 1%; those with three to four risk factors, a 15% mortality and those with six to seven risk factors, a 100% mortality rate. The acute physiology and chronic health evaluation (APACHE II) illness grading system is another list of clinical and laboratory variables that can be used to predict the severity of pancreatitis. Its advantages over the other two systems is that it can be employed not just within the first 48 hours after admission but throughout the patient's illness.[47,48]

Individual laboratory tests also appear to be useful as indicators of severe disease within the first few days after admission. C-reactive protein,[49] trypsinogen activation peptides and leucocyte elastase are promising. For instance, a C-reactive protein above 140 mg/l in the first 48 hours is associated with a severe attack. A peritoneal tap can also be used to determine the severity of the disease in patients with acute pancreatitis.[50] Very dark fluid (the colour of prune juice) is characteristic of severe necrotizing pancreatitis. A peritoneal tap is occasionally helpful in differentiating an acute 'surgical' abdomen from pancreatitis. Fluid obtained from a patient with a perforated viscus may contain bacteria and be foul-smelling, unlike the sterile non-odorous fluid obtained from a patient with acute pancreatitis.

Table 33.4 Adverse prognostic factors in severe acute pancreatitis

RANSON'S CRITERIA
Pancreatitis not due to gallstones
On admission
Age > 55 years
White cell count >16 000/mm³
Glucose > 200 mg/dl
Lactic dehydrogenase > 350 U/l
Aspartate aminotransferase > 250 U/l
Within 48 hours of admission
Decrease in haematocrit > 10 points
Increase in blood urea nitrogen > 5 mg/dl
Calcium < 8 mg/dl
Partial pressure of oxygen < 60 mmHg
Base deficit > 4 mmol/l
Fluid deficit > 6 litres
Gallstone-induced pancreatitis
On admission
Age > 70 years
White cell count > 18 000/mm³
Glucose > 220 mg/dl
Lactic dehydrogenase > 400 U/l
Aspartate aminotransferase > 250 U/l
Within 48 hours of admission
Decrease in haematocrit > 10 points
Increase in blood urea nitrogen > 2 mg/dl
Calcium < 8 mg/dl
Base deficit > 5 mmol/l
Fluid deficit > 6 litres
MODIFIED GLASGOW CRITERIA
Within 48 hours of admission
Age > 55 years
White cell count > 15 000/mm³
Glucose > 180 mg/dl
Blood urea nitrogen > 45 mg/dl
Albumin < 3.3 g/dl
Calcium < 8 mg/dl
Partial pressure of oxygen < 60 mmHg

Natural history and complications

Between 10 and 25% of all attacks of acute pancreatitis are severe, leading to complications. The mortality rate overall approaches 9%. Autopsy studies show that 60% of deaths from acute pancreatitis occur within the first week and that pulmonary failure was the most common cause of death. Forty per cent of deaths occur after the first week and in this group sepsis is the commonest cause of death. Obesity remains a major risk factor for severe acute pancreatitis.[51] During the first week in hospital, severe acute pancreatitis is complicated by some degree of multisystem organ failure, most commonly involving the cardiovascular, pulmonary and renal systems. Cardiovascular collapse from bleeding, exudation of plasma into the retroperitoneum or myocardial infarction often occurs. Respiratory complications can be mild as manifested by mild hypoxaemia, atelectasis or pleural effusions, or severe as manifested by pneumonia and the adult respiratory distress syndrome. Renal failure, most commonly resulting from hypotension and acute tubular necrosis, occurs within the first week (Tables 33.1 and 33.2).

Sterile and infected pancreatic and peripancreatic necrotic tissue can also be seen in severe disease during the first 2 weeks of the illness. Infected necrotic tissue cannot be differentiated easily from sterile necrotic tissue by any particular physical signs.[52] This can only be determined by percutaneous aspiration of the pancreatic necrotic tissue under CT guidance. This is not recommended as it can introduce infection into a sterile necrosis along the needle track.

The late complications occur after the second week of the illness and include the formation of pseudocysts and abscesses. Pseudocysts complicate 1–8% of cases of acute pancreatitis and abscesses 1–4%. Other unusual complications include gastrointestinal haemorrhage from stress ulceration, gastric varices resulting from splenic vein thrombosis or rupture of pancreatic pseudoaneurysms and pancreatic encephalopathy (confusion, delu-

REFERENCES

45. Ranson J H C In: Glazer G, Ranson J H C (eds) Acute Pancreatitis. Baillière Tindall London 1988 pp 303–330
46. Blamey S L, Imrie C W, O'Niell J, Gilmour W H, Carter D C Gut 1984; 25: 1340–1346
47. Larvin M, McMahon M J Lancet 1989; 2: 201–205
48. Wilson C, Heath D I, Imrie C W Br J Surg 1990; 77: 1260–1264
49. Wilson C, Heads A, Shenkin A, Imrie C W Br J Surg 1989; 76: 177–181
50. McMahon M J, Pickford I R, Playforth M J Acta Chir Scand 1980; 146: 171–175
51. Funnell I C, Bornman P C, Weakley S P, Terblanche J, Marks I N Br J Surg 1993; 80: 484–486
52. Beger H G, Bittner R, Block S, Büchler M Gastroenterology 1986; 91: 433–438

sions and coma); Purtscher's angiopathic retinopathy (discrete flame-shaped haemorrhages with cotton-wool spots) leading to sudden blindness;[53] obstruction, necrosis or fistulation of the adjacent (usually left-sided) colon from pancreatic inflammation; and splenic rupture or haematoma formation caused by the spread of peripancreatic inflammation and hydronephrosis and hydroureter of the right kidney.[54]

Treatment

The treatment of acute pancreatitis is supportive. Patients with mild disease are treated by eliminating oral intake, instituting intravenous hydration and providing frequent parenteral analgesics. Controlled trials have shown that nasogastric tubes do not increase pain relief or shorten hospital stays. Nasogastric suction is appropriate in patients with ileus or severe vomiting to provide symptomatic relief.

Factors which may have precipitated the attack such as drugs or alcohol should be removed or stopped. Surgical or endoscopic extraction of gallstones retained in the common bile duct is a point of debate. Several studies have shown that removal of gallstones on an emergency basis by endoscopic sphincterotomy in patients with severe acute gallstone-induced pancreatitis lowers the morbidity and mortality.[20,44] It is accepted that if the initial ultrasound scan shows dilatation of the common bile duct and deranged liver function tests then an immediate endoscopic sphincterotomy is indicated and can be dramatically effective. Similarly, removal of obstructing ascarides accelerates the resolution of symptoms in those with parasitic pancreatitis.[55]

Severe acute pancreatitis requires intensive management of cardiovascular, pulmonary, renal and septic complications. Antibiotics have recently been shown to reduce morbidity and mortality. Imipenem is said to be the most effective antibiotic.[56,57] Specific therapies such as the use of antiproteinases, the use of peritoneal lavage and immediate surgery have not improved survival.[58] Therapies designed to put the pancreas to rest by inhibiting pancreatic secretion such as those involving nasogastric suction, cimetidine, atropine, calcitonin, glucagon and somatostatin have also not been shown to change the course of the disease.[25] The mainstay of treatment remains active supportive care and avoidance of infection.

The role of surgery is controversial. Early surgery increases mortality[59] but the role of pancreatic debridement in patients whose general condition is deteriorating is strongly advocated by its proponents. Removal of necrotic tissue with closed drainage,[60] removal of necrotic tissue with lavage of the lesser sac[61] and removal of necrotic tissue with open packing and planned re-exploration have all been tried.[62] No controlled study comparing early surgical treatment with medical treatment has shown distinct benefit.[63] The value of interventional radiology complicates the issue. The consensus view is that if the patient is deteriorating within the first 2 weeks of the acute attack then removal of the necrotic material with drainage or lavage is appropriate. For those patients who survive the first 2 weeks radiological techniques with CT-guided drainage appear superior to repeated operative intervention.

The following points require specific management during the early phase of disease:

1. *Pain*. Patients must receive appropriate analgesics in an appropriate dose based on body weight.
2. *Vomiting*. If repeated retching and vomiting occur, nasogastric aspiration is important to prevent aspiration pneumonia.
3. *Shock*. Pancreatitis should be considered as a burn: the more severe the pancreatitis, the greater the fluid loss. As there is no easy method of determining the severity of the 'burn', careful monitoring of central venous pressure, blood pressure, urine output, haematocrit and electrolytes must be undertaken. Replacement therapy with large volumes of fluid, electrolytes, plasma and blood are required.
4. *Renal failure*. Oliguria must be avoided by rapid restoration of circulating volume. If renal failure occurs, peritoneal dialysis has been shown to be safe and effective.
5. *Respiratory failure*. Treatment is with oxygen at high flows with recourse to endotracheal intubation and positive pressure ventilation if the blood gas analyses remain unsatisfactory. All patients with severe pancreatitis should have regular monitoring of arterial oxygen, carbon dioxide and pH.
6. *Metabolic*. Hypocalcaemia is a manifestation of the low albumin level and should be managed by the replacement of albumin. Should tetany develop, 20 ml 10% calcium gluconate is given intravenously. Hypomagnesaemia is treated with 25% magnesium sulphate by intramuscular injection.
7. *Diabetes*. Hyperglycaemia occurs during the acute phase and should be managed with an intravenous insulin infusion.

Management of complications

Complications and infection should be anticipated if the patient deteriorates. Diagnosis is by repeat CT scanning of the pancreas.

Pancreatic sepsis

The term 'sepsis' is preferable to abscess as the infection can be local, that is within the pancreas, in the surrounding peripancreatic tissues as an abscess, or distant, tracking along fistulous tracks in the retroperitoneum to distant parts. On the basis of ultrasound and

REFERENCES

53. Semlacher E A, Chan-Yan C Am J Gastroenterol 1993; 88: 756–759
54. Valderrama R, Pérez-Mateo M et al Digestion 1992; 51: 65–70
55. Khuroo M S, Zargar S A et al Br J Surg 1992; 79: 1335–1338
56. Pederzoli P, Bassi C, Vesentini S, Campedelli A Surg Gynecol Obstet 1993; 76: 480–483
57. Sainio V, Kemppainen E et al Lancet 1995; 346: 663–667
58. Mayer A D, McMahon M J et al N Engl J Med 1985; 312: 399–404
59. Teerenhovi O, Nordbach I, Isolauri J Br J Surg 1988; 75: 793–794
60. Warshaw A L, Jin G Ann Surg 1985; 202: 408–417
61. Beger H G, Buchler M, Bittner R, Oettinger W, Block S, Nevalainen T World J Surg 1988; 12: 255–261
62. Bradley E L III Ann Surg 1987; 206: 408–417
63. Schröder T, Sainio V, Kivisaari L, Puolakkainen P, Kivilaakso E, Lempinen M Ann Surg 1991; 214: 663–666

CT findings, the nature of the abscess is determined. Percutaneous drainage is the optimal therapy if it contains pus and is liquid. This drainage should be performed under antibiotic cover and continued until the cavity has resolved. Resolution can only be followed by repeated CT scanning. It is rare for such septic collections to require surgical drainage (Fig. 33.12). Resolution is to be anticipated but if the sepsis becomes uncontrolled the mortality can be as high as 20%.

Pseudocyst

This is a collection of fluid often starting as a peripancreatic collection and developing a wall of granulation tissue. These cysts can be drained percutaneously[64] but if symptomless are preferably left alone. Smaller cysts invariably resolve while larger cysts form a thick wall which can be drained percutaneously or transgastrically using an endoscopic approach.[65] Occasionally the larger cysts need to be managed by cyst-gastrostomy or cyst-jejunostomy.

Haemorrhage with or without haemetemesis

This complication is frequently the harbinger of doom in acute pancreatitis. It invariably indicates the disruption of a major blood vessel leading to pseudoaneurysm formation with rupture into the peritoneal cavity or the intestinal lumen. A stress ulcer is occasionally the cause. Frequently there is a warning bleed.[66] Such bleeds should be taken seriously and the cause elucidated by gastroscopy to exclude ulceration and angiography to exclude aneurysmal change. Vigorous treatment by antacids is required for the ulcer and an attempt may be made to embolize the aneurysm with steel coils or other foreign material. Surgical treatment of pseudoaneurysm is rarely effective because of the recurrence of infection and further aneurysm formation.

Duodenal obstruction

This complication is frequent in the acute stage of pancreatitis but rarely persists once the inflammation has resolved. Prolonged parenteral nutrition may be required until resolution, and is preferable to gastroenterostomy.

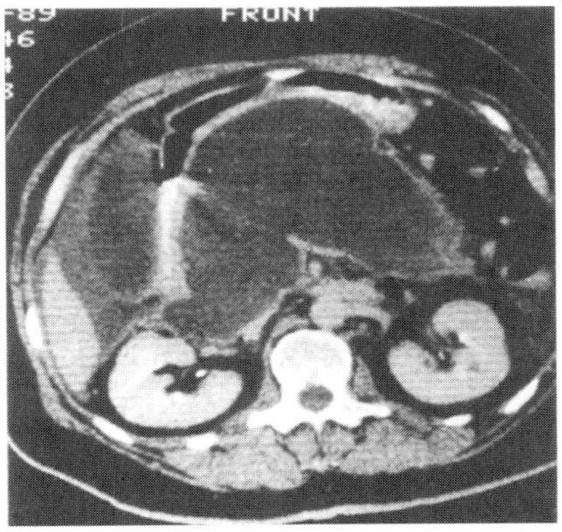

Fig. 33.12 Acute pancreatitis with an infected pseudocyst: CT scan day 30. Failure to resolve following conservative treatment due to a large infected pseudocyst. Open debridement of the body and tail of the pancreas was successful.

Colonic necrosis

This condition frequently occurs after surgical intervention when the middle colic or left colic artery is damaged during drainage or debridement of the pancreatic collection. Frequently spontaneous fistulation occurs of the necrotic pancreas into the colon and is often associated with resolution of the pancreatitis. It is extremely uncommon for primary necrosis of the colon to occur. It is treated by formation of a proximal colostomy or ileostomy.

Jaundice

Jaundice, especially if associated with a fever, requires urgent investigation at any stage of the illness. If it develops within 48 hours of presentation, a stone blocking the ampulla of Vater should be suspected and confirmed by ultrasound scanning. Immediate endoscopy should be performed if the common bile duct is dilated. Percutaneous drainage or endoscopic stenting should be undertaken if obstructive jaundice occurs as a complication of prolonged pancreatitis. Extrahepatic biliary obstruction in the presence of infection is associated with a poor prognosis and should be avoided.

Prognosis

There is good evidence that those patients who survive an attack of acute pancreatitis, even if this is very severe causing a prolonged illness, return to a normal state of health and have a reasonable life expectancy. The problems of diabetes and enzyme deficiency may also require correction. Above all, any factor or factors thought to be responsible for the attack must be removed. Cessation of all alcohol is the only therapy which will ensure freedom from further attacks in those patients for whom alcohol is thought to be the key component.

CHRONIC PANCREATITIS

Chronic pancreatitis is a chronic inflammatory disease in which there is irreversible progressive destruction of pancreatic tissue. Its clinical course is characterized by a dynamic progressive fibrosis of the pancreas. In the early stages of its evolution, it is frequently complicated by attacks of acute pancreatitis that are responsible for the recurrent pain which may be the only clinical symptom. An interval of years (on average 5 years) between the onset of symptoms and the manifestation of permanent pancreatic dysfunction and/or calcification is typical. Exocrine tissue is destroyed first and later endocrine tissue is also damaged.

Aetiology and epidemiology

The cause of the pancreatic inflammation plays an important role in the long-term progression of the disease and epidemiological

REFERENCES

64. Sacks D, Robinson M L AJR 1988; 151: 303–306
65. Sahel J, Bastid C, Sarles H Gastroenterol Clin Biol 1988; 12: 431–433
66. Shankar S, Russell R C G Br J Surg 1989; 76: 863–866

data reveal distinct differences between different forms of pancreatitis. Acute biliary pancreatitis virtually never progresses to chronic pancreatitis, in contrast with acute alcoholic pancreatitis which proceeds to chronic pancreatitis in the majority of patients. Chronic pancreatitis caused by alcohol has a much higher rate of progression of pancreatic dysfunction, causes more pain and is more often calcified than non-alcoholic pancreatitis. The parallel development of calcification and exocrine insufficiency is also more evident in alcoholic pancreatitis, whereas in non-alcoholic pancreatitis calcification precedes exocrine insufficiency in nearly half the patients. In gallstone pancreatitis and in other causes of acute pancreatitis stricture of the pancreatic duct may persist after the acute episode. This can consequently give rise to chronic pancreatitis[67] but this form of disease is not progressive and the proximal portion of the pancreas usually remains normal. Most authorities consider this a separate subgroup of chronic pancreatitis on account of the confined nature of the disease. Frequently the term 'chronic obstructive (non-progressive) pancreatitis' is used to describe this condition.

Few studies are available which document the frequency of chronic pancreatitis. In a prospective Danish study the incidence was 8.2 new cases per 1 million inhabitants per year and the prevalence was 27.4 cases per million population.[68] The average incidence collected from retrospective studies in Europe and North America is about 3–10 per million population. The incidence is increasing in that the number of patients discharged from hospital has risen fourfold in men and twofold in women when the periods 1960–64 and 1980–1984 are compared. Recent data from England and Wales show a correlation between alcohol consumption per head of population and the number of hospital discharges with chronic pancreatitis 6 years later.[69]

In the majority of patients, chronic pancreatitis is caused by nutritional factors. Chronic alcohol consumption, often in connection with a diet rich in fat and protein, is a common aetiological factor in industrialized countries. In areas with endemic protein deficiency, a diet lacking in various macro- or micronutrients may be associated with chronic pancreatitis in childhood. Other forms of chronic pancreatitis are caused by or associated with metabolic disorder (notably hypercalcaemia and hyperlipidaemia), ductal obstruction or ill-defined hereditary factors; in many patients a specific causal factor is not identified. Pancreatic insufficiency occurs in a substantial number of patients with cystic fibrosis; however the pancreatic findings in this disease should not be classified as chronic pancreatitis.

History and clinical examination

Pain is the outstanding symptom in the majority of patients with chronic pancreatitis. The site of the pain depends to some extent on the main focus of the disease and may be in the epigastrium or the right or left subcostal region. It frequently radiates through to the back either centrally or to one side. In some patients the back pain predominates while in others the pain is more diffuse; occasionally the pain radiates to the shoulder, more commonly on the left side. Certain positions may relieve the pain. Nausea is common during attacks of pain and vomiting may occur, although it rarely relieves the pain. The pain is a dull gnawing ache. Frequently there are no clear precipitating factors; rarely food may precipitate the pain, particularly meals with a high fat content. Alcohol rarely precipitates the pain but may do so, particularly after a binge drinking session. During an attack the pain is aggravated by eating food.

There is great variation in the pattern and periodicity of the pain of chronic pancreatitis. The attacks may be intermittent, lasting for hours or days, while some patients consider there is always a background pain present. Loss of sleep, time off work and the number of admissions to hospital are pointers to severity. The severity of the pain can frequently be assessed by the quantity of analgesics required. The type of analgesic should be documented. The amount of time that the patient loses from work should also be assessed.

The patient not infrequently presents to the surgeon with the complications of chronic pancreatitis. Weight loss can be dramatic and may be associated with swelling of the abdomen which can be caused by pseudocysts or ascites. Even a fistula can be the presenting feature of chronic pancreatitis, often as a complication of previous treatments. Jaundice occurs in 5–10% of patients, and haemorrhage, particularly into a pseudocyst or into the ducts, will be the presenting feature in 2–3% of patients. Offensive, pale and frothy stools indicative of steatorrhoea frequently bring the patient to the physician; approximately 10% of patients present in this way. Diabetes eventually develops in all patients with alcoholic chronic pancreatitis.

A careful evaluation of the whole patient must be made. Malnutrition and weight loss may be present. The complications of diabetes or drug addiction can be in evidence. The dishevelled appearance of the alcoholic or the drug abuser indicates the social disorder that this disease is associated with or can cause. Burn marks (erythema ab igne) on the abdomen or back may indicate the repeated use of heat pads or hot water bottles in an attempt to relieve the pain. Patients may be jaundiced as a result of common bile duct obstruction. A visible or palpable mass may be present in the upper abdomen, indicating that a large chronic pseudocyst may be present. Occasionally the signs of portal hypertension secondary to a thrombosis of the portal vein can be seen. Careful differentiation from cirrhosis is required.

Investigation

No single test is sufficiently sensitive or specific to establish the diagnosis of chronic pancreatitis with certainty so that a combination of tests is required.[70] Ultrasonography is likely to be the first test used to evaluate the outline of the pancreas, its size, contour and texture. Ultrasonography may also reveal calcification, duct dilatation, cysts, pseudocysts and abscesses and diseases affecting neighbouring organs such as the liver, biliary tree and spleen. Contrast-enhanced helical CT of the pancreas refines the informa-

REFERENCES

67. Sarles H Dig Dis Sci 1986; 31: 91–107
68. Copenhagen Pancreatitis Study Scand J Gastroenterol 1981; 16: 305–312
69. Johnson C D, Hosking S Gut 1991; 32: 1401–1405
70. Boyd E S, Walmsley K G Int J Pancreatol 1987; 2: 211–222

tion gained by ultrasound. Pre-contrast scans should be carefully examined for calcification. In the contrast-enhanced scans the outline of the pancreas should be carefully scrutinized, the presence of any abnormal swellings associated with the pancreas should be noted and the size of the pancreatic duct should be measured. The presence of duct obstruction, fistula formation, cyst formation, an abscess or pseudoaneurysm may also be demonstrated. Occasionally, a previously undiagnosed pancreatic tumour may be found. Endoscopic retrograde pancreatography complements the CT scan (Fig 33.13 and 33.14). It is possible to see whether the papilla is normal, whether pancreas divisum is present and whether there are stenoses within the duct system. The combined use of these investigations rarely leaves doubt about the diagnosis, although pancreatic carcinoma is difficult to exclude. Pancreatic exocrine function tests are rarely of value. A history of steatorrhoea is a better index of function than the complexity of a carefully performed pancreatic function test. Diabetes mellitus is best diagnosed by a series of random blood glucose estimations and monitoring of the glycosylated haemoglobin level.

Management

Assessment and management of patients with chronic pancreatitis are both difficult and time-consuming; they demand considerable skill and experience. Less than half the patients seen with chronic pancreatitis require surgical treatment. A multidisciplinary approach is required, with care often extending over many years. The main features of management are to confirm the diagnosis, to establish the cause and if possible eradicate it. The severity of the disease and the morphological changes should be assessed and any accompanying disease should be rectified (e.g. hyperparathyroidism, hyperlipidaemia). The occasional associated case of pancreatic cancer must be diagnosed. Pain is the major problem. It is essential to define the cause of this pain. It often occurs with acute exacerbations of inflammation but may also occur over the long term with exacerbations and remissions. The cause of the pain is unknown. The hypothesis that it is the result of nerve entrapment or increased pressure in the ducts remains open to question; however, some patients have pain associated with specific obstructive phenomena such as strictures or stones while others have pain from cysts, fistulae, infection or aneurysms.

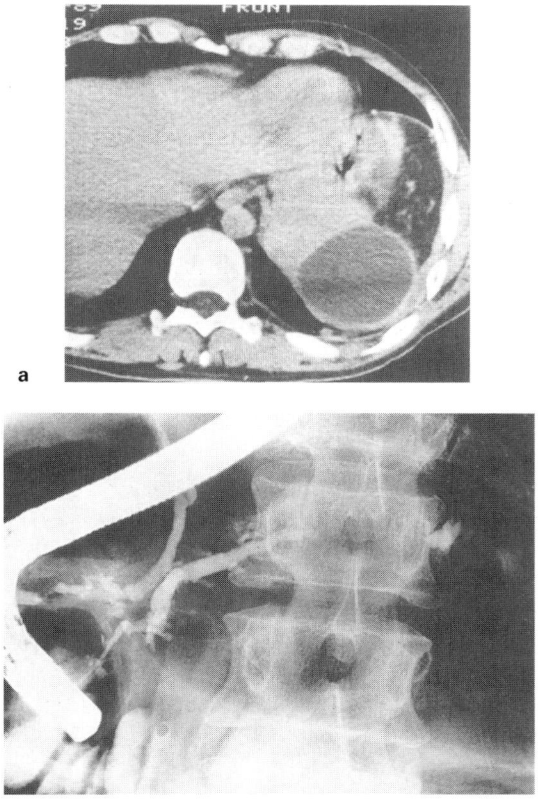

Fig. 33.13 (**a**) Chronic pancreatitis—CT scan: chronic cyst in the tail of the pancreas. (**b**) Chronic pancreatitis—pancreatogram: the duct in the body and tail was disrupted by the disease process, which prevented the ductal drainage of the cyst. A distal pancreatectomy resolved the persitent pain.

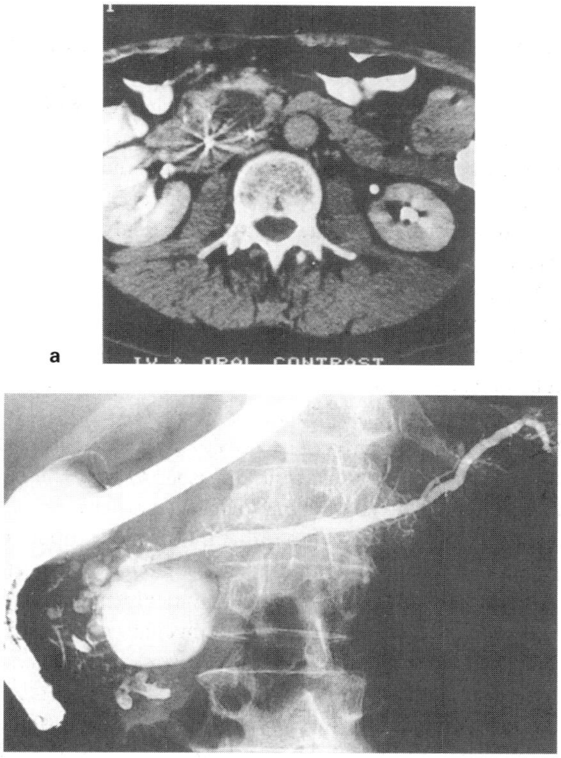

Fig. 33.14 Intrapancreatic cyst in the head of the pancreas in a patient with long-standing pancreatic pain. (**a**) CT scan showing calcification in the head of the pancreas and a cyst. (**b**) Filling of the cyst from an abnormal pancreatic duct. A pancreatoduodenectomy was effective treatment.

Acute exacerbations of chronic inflammation are easier to treat than the chronic pain. The cause for the acute exacerbation can be determined and eliminated. Otherwise a period of rest in hospital with intravenous fluids, cessation of oral intake and appropriate analgesics is invariably effective. In the great majority of cases symptoms are brought under control by this conservative approach. The question of surgical intervention frequently relates to the periodicity of these acute exacerbations and whether there is an appropriate abnormality which can be surgically corrected. With chronic pain the problems are different and more difficult. It is occasionally appropriate to admit a patient for a period of intestinal rest and withdrawal from analgesic consumption. On this regimen most patients who are not addicted to the analgesic can be withdrawn from medication and re-established on milder analgesics. Psychiatric appraisal is rarely of value and the use of coeliac plexus blocks or other temporary nerve-blocking techniques rarely helps in the long term. According to Amman et al,[71] the pain will gradually disappear with time without surgical intervention as endocrine and exocrine atrophy occur. Most surgeons find this does not happen in those severely afflicted, although it may well occur in patients with milder disease who are not referred to the surgeon. In patients with manageable pain, continued supervision and support are required and provided there is no underlying surgical disorder, many will manage satisfactorily over a number of years.

It is essential to remove the cause of the pancreatitis (Table 33.3) and so abstinence from alcohol is essential. Dietary considerations are rarely of value, although many have suggested avoiding high fat and high protein. It is said that this reduces stimulation of the pancreas by cholecystokinin. Indeed, some have suggested the use of pancreatic enzyme supplements in order to reduce the requirement for pancreatic secretion but this has no proven basis.

In the management of these patients, it is essential to treat their steatorrhoea with adequate doses of enzyme supplementation; it is also essential to treat their diabetes and it is important to maintain body weight as a low body weight appears to predispose to severe pain. Any complication such as biliary obstruction, vomiting as a consequence of duodenal stasis or haemorrhage from either an ulcer or a complication of pancreatitis should also be treated.

Indications for surgery

Chronic pancreatitis is not a surgical disease. The management belongs primarily to the gastroenterologist. Those patients who fail to respond to conservative management and whose debility interferes with life merit consideration for surgery. Those patients who have severe pain from a defined cause, those patients who are developing narcotic addiction despite good conservative management and those patients with weight loss which is not responding to treatment deserve operation. Those with complications will require relief by surgery if appropriate. It is improbable that an operation can slow down the progress of the underlying disease and this is not a reason for operating. Specific indications for operation include:

1. *Biliary stenosis*: Stenosis of the common bile duct is not as rare in chronic pancreatitis as was once thought. It occurs in approximately 20% of patients with severe disease.[72] A choledochoduodenostomy is appropriate if the stenosis occurs without pain, while if there is severe pain associated with disease in the head of the gland then a pancreatoduodenectomy or Berger procedure is appropriate.

2. *Duodenal stenosis:* Some degree of duodenal obstruction is common but it is extremely rare to find this is the sole problem.[73] A simple gastrojejunostomy is effective if it is associated with minimal pancreatic disease but the incidence of peptic ulceration is high and permanent H_2-receptor antagonists are required.

3. *Colonic stricture:* This is rare and usually settles with conservative management.[74] It is rare for the stricture to require treatment on its own but with severe disease in the body and tail of the pancreas, particularly with cyst or abscess formation, colonic resection may be indicated in combination with a distal pancreatectomy.

4. *Pancreatic duct stenosis or obstruction:* If this is considered to be the cause of the pain then drainage can be undertaken in the form of a pancreatojejunostomy, while if the duct is not sufficiently dilated (> 8 mm) or of sufficient length (> 8 cm) then resection of the head or the tail of the pancreas is indicated (Figs 33.15 and 33.16).

5. *Pancreatic pseudocysts:* These can be drained by a simple cyst-gastrostomy, occasionally a cyst-jejunostomy or even cyst-duodenostomy.

6. *Pancreatic ascites or pleural effusions:* There is invariably a fistula and once this is removed by surgery resolution occurs.[75] Appropriate drainage is the most usual answer to this problem.

7. *Haemorrhage:* Changes in the peripancreatic arteries are rarely seen, but if they are associated with a pseudoaneurysm, erosion will lead to massive haemorrhage and urgent intervention is required. If angiography and embolization fail the appropriate resection is required.

8. *Suspicion of pancreatic cancer:* There are occasions when pancreatic cancer cannot be excluded by all the techniques presently available, including biopsy. In these instances a resection is appropriate, even though the disease may be mild and the outcome benign. A full explanation must be given to the patient in order that he or she understands both the complications of the operation and the outcome related to the possibility of a cancer not being found.

REFERENCES

71. Amman R W, Akovbiantz A, Largiader F, Schueler G Gastroenterology 1984; 86: 820–828
72. Littenberg G, Afroudakis A, Kaplowitz N Medicine 1979; 58: 385–412
73. Prinz R A, Aranha C V, Greenlee H B Arch Surg 1985; 120: 361–366
74. Bradley E L III In: Bradley E L III (ed) Complications of Pancreatitis. Medical and Surgical Management. W B Saunders, Philadelphia

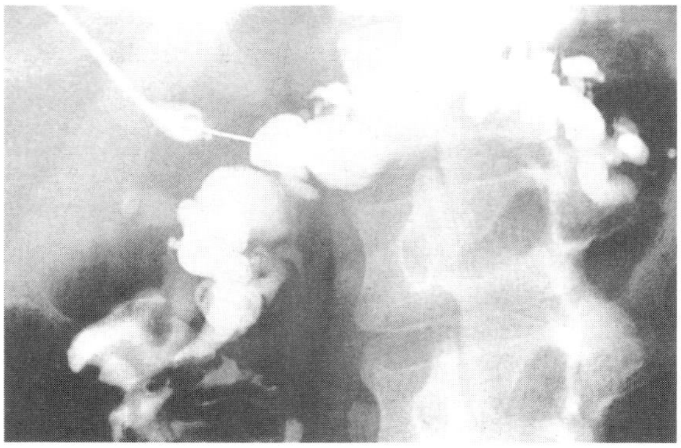

Fig. 33.15 Chronic pancreatitis: a percutaneous pancreatogram in a 24-year-old woman with dilating pancreatic disease of long standing. A pancreatojejunostomy was curative.

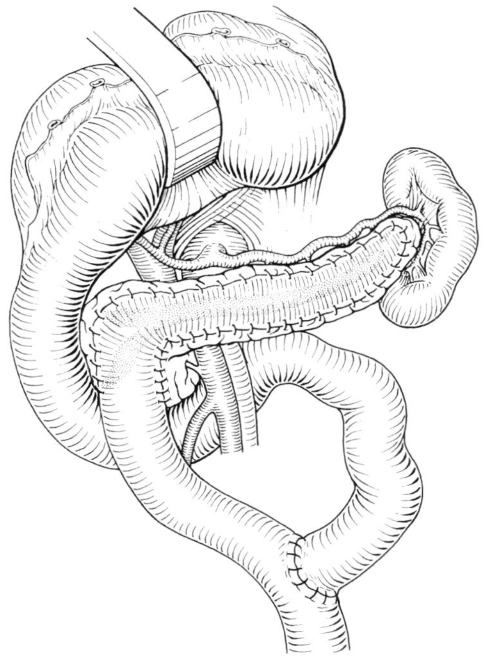

Fig. 33.16 A pancreatojejunostomy: the duct is laid open and covered with a Roux loop of jejunum.

Surgical options in chronic pancreatitis

The decision to operate must be made with care and after discussion with the other clinicians and the patient.[76] It is important in defining strategy to preserve as much functioning pancreatic parenchyma as possible. Indirect operations such as vagotomy, gastric resections, cholecystectomy and indeed even operations on the nerves to the pancreas are invariably unsatisfactory and do not alter the course of the disease.[77,78] Direct operations on the pancreas are divided into drainage and resection procedures. Drainage is indicated for pseudocysts, biliary obstruction and for pancreatic ducts dilated to a diameter of more than 8 mm. Currently the optimal drainage procedure is a long parenchyma-sparing side-to-side pancreatojejunostomy. The theoretical advantages of simple drainage notwithstanding, whenever mechanical obstruction involves several structures, for example the duodenum, bile duct or pancreatic duct, multiple drainage procedures seem less effective than resection. Resection procedures are indicated for localized complications, for painful small duct disease and whenever a carcinoma is suspected and cannot be excluded. As a rule chronic pancreatitis involves the entire gland. Frequently however, the 'pacemaker' is situated in the head of the pancreas, causing pain and stenoses of some or all the structures meeting there. Isolated pancreatitis of the tail of the gland is rare. Subtotal resections from the left have fallen into disrepute since poor long-term pain relief is coupled with a high incidence of diabetes. The standard Whipple pancreatoduodenectomy is the preferred resection procedure for most cases of painful complicated pancreatitis. Various pyloric and duodenal-preserving procedures provide equally good results but so far none of these procedures provide better results than the standard Whipple procedure. Total pancreatectomy is indicated in rare cases of end-stage disease when all else has failed.[79] There is no single ideal operation for the various problems of chronic pancreatitis; it is more important to select an appropriate method of management for each particular patient. The correct procedure must be adopted for the appropriate patient.

Long-term results of surgical treatment depend more on the type of patient operated upon and his or her ability to stop drinking alcohol.[80] It is usual to achieve an 80% response provided appropriate care has been taken in selection. Those that fail to respond to conservative surgery should rarely have a total pancreatectomy as the results of this procedure are no better than a 50% salvage rate.

TUMOURS OF THE PANCREAS

The first conclusive descriptions of human pancreatic tumours date back to Bigsby (1835) and Mondier (1836). Up to the first decades of this century neoplasms of the pancreas were uncommon. In Europe, pancreatic cancer is at present the seventh commonest form of cancer in men after tumours of the stomach, colon, rectum, lung, prostate and bladder. In the USA, pancreatic neoplasms take fourth place as a cause of cancer mortality in men and fifth place in women. Human pancreatic tumours are commonly classified according to the World Health Organization classification[81] or alternatively the detailed classification of Cubilla and Fitzgerald (Table 33.5).[82] The recent UICC classification of tumour stage strictly distinguishes between malignant tumours of the exocrine pancreas, the ampulla of Vater and the distal bile duct. This strict separation of ampullary and pancreatic carcinomas causes problems in cases where carcinoma infiltrates the ampulla as well as the head of the pancreas (Table 33.6).

The important clinical finding is that there are benign tumours of the pancreas as well as malignant neoplasms. Tumours in the ampulla can be simple adenomas and papillomas with a long life history. Similarly, tumours of the pancreas such as cystadenomas, tumours of the islets of Langerhans and a variety of miscellaneous neoplasms can complicate assessment of masses in the pancreas and necessitate a careful lesson that radical and dangerous surgery should not be undertaken when a more conservative approach is appropriate and safer.

Endocrine tumours of the pancreas

The islets of Langerhans are part of Feyrter's 'diffuse endocrine epithelial organ', which he described as a widely scattered system

REFERENCES

75. Fielding G, McLatchie G P Br J Surg 1989; 76: 1126–1128
76. Moosa A R Br J Surg 1987; 74: 661–667
77. Leung J W, Bowen-Wright M, Aveling W, Shorvon P J, Cotton P B Br J Surg 1983; 70: 730–732
78. Bengtsson M, Lofstrom J B Acta Chir Scand 1990; 156: 285–291
79. Linehan I P, Lambert M A, Brown D C, Kurtz A B, Cotton P B, Russell R C G Gut 1988; 29: 358–365
80. Mannell A, Adson M A, McIlrath D C, Ilstrup D M Br J Surg 1988, 75: 467–472
81. Gibson J B, Sobin L H Histological Typing of Tumours of the Liver, Biliary Tract and Pancreas. WHO International Classification of Tumours, vol 20. World Health Organization, Geneva 1978
82. Cubilla A L, Fitzgerald P F In: Atlas of Tumour Pathology, second series. American Forces Institute of Pathology, Washington DC 1984

Table 33.5 Classification of exocrine primary pancreatic neoplasia

Benign	Malignant
Epithelial origin	
Duct/ductile/centroductal (acinar) cell	Duct/ductule cell origin
Polyp	Duct cell carcinoma
Papilloma, papillomatosis, villous papilloma	Giant cell carcinoma (including osteoclastoid)
Adenoma	Adenosquamous carcinoma (including spindle cell type)
Solid	Microadenocarcinoma (solid microglandular)
Duct (ductule)	Mucinous ('colloid') carcinoma
Centroductular (centroacinar)	Mucinous–carcinoid carcinoma
Cystadenoma	Oat cell carcinoma
Serous	
Simple	
Papillary	Papillary cystic tumour
Mucinous	Mucinous ('colloid') carcinoma
Simple	
Papillary	
Carcinoid	Carcinoid
Oncocytoma	Oncocytic carcinoma/carcinoid
Ciliated cell	Ciliated cell carcinoma?
Acinar cell	Acinar cell
Adenoma	Acinar cell carcinoma
Cystadenoma	Acinar cell cystadenocarcinoma
Mixed epithelial cells	Mixed cell
Duct/islet; duct/acinar	Duct/islet; duct/islet/acinar
Duct/acinar/islet;	Acinar/islet; carcinoid/islet
Acinar/islet; carcinoid/islet	
Connective tissue origin	
Fibroma	Fibrosarcoma
Leiomyoma	Leiomyosarcoma
Neurilemmoma	Malignant neurilemmoma
Fibrous histiocytoma	Malignant fibrous histiocytoma
Vascular	
Lymphangioma	
Haemangioma	
Miscellaneous	Osteogenic/lipo/rhabdomyosarcoma
Mixed epithelial–connective tissue origin	
Fibroadenoma	
Uncertain histiogenesis/other	
	Pancreatoblastoma (simple and mixed types)
	Unclassified (large, small or clear cell type)

From Cubilla & Fitzgerald[82] with permission.

Table 33.6 Suggested TNM classification of pancreatic cancer

Tumour	
(add 'i' if local organs infiltrated)	
TX	not assessable
T_1	< 2 cm maximum diameter
T_2	2–3 cm maximum diameter
T_3	3–5 cm maximum diameter
T_4	> 5 cm maximum diameter
Nodes	
NX	Not assessable
N_0	No nodal involvement
N_1	Anterior and/or posterior pancreaticoduodenal groups
N_2	Above + superior and/or inferior head nodes
N_3	Above + superior and/or inferior body nodes
N_4	Above + other node groups
Metastases	
MX	Not assessable
M_0	No distant metastases
M_1	Distant metastases

of clear cells. These cells are distributed throughout the body and produce the polypeptide hormones. Their maximal aggregation is in the intestine, and its embryological derivatives the pancreas and liver. The term APUD, by which these cells are now known, is an acronym for their principal characteristics (amine precursor uptake and decarboxylation). Tumours of these cells are now characterized by the hormones they produce, and at least 12 such tumours have been clearly documented in the pancreas (Fig. 33.17). They are frequently grouped under the generic term 'apudomas' because they exhibit essentially similar morphological appearances and behavioural characteristics. These tumours are easily recognized as endocrine tumours, because of their closely packed polyhedral cells with a greater or lesser number of glandular lumina progressing to distinct acini. Their cytoplasm is eosinophilic. In appearance apudomas are thus usually benign but may demonstrate malignant characteristics by invading surrounding tissues and metastasizing. They all tend to grow slowly and patients survive for many years with metastases in the lymph nodes and liver.

In the pancreas, the apudomas so far described produce an excess of insulin from the β cell, glucagon from the α cell, vasoactive peptide (Verner–Morrison syndrome) from the Δ cell, and gastrin from the Δ cell. All these tumours may also secrete pancreatic polypeptide, which is produced by apud cells lying between the acinar cells of the exocrine parenchyma.

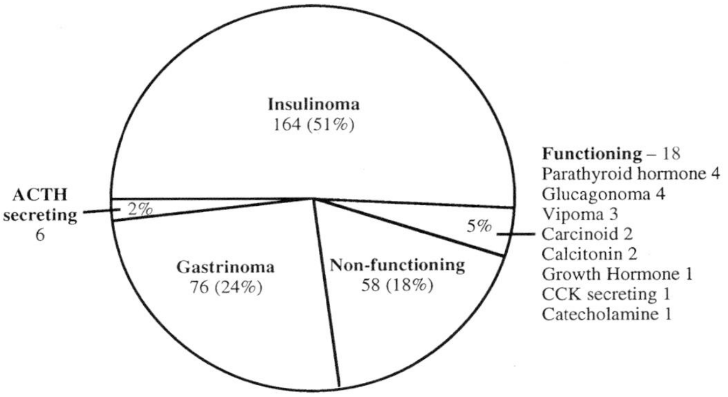

Fig. 33.17 Distribution of islet cell tumours in 322 patients treated at the Mayo Clinic 1960–1986. ACTH = Adrenocarticotrophic hormone; CCK = cholecystokinin. From Van Heerden & Thompson (1993).

Insulinoma

History

In 1924 Seale Harris reported three cases of hypoglycaemia which he suggested might be caused by hypoinsulinism. In 1927 a laparotomy was performed at the Mayo Clinic on a hypoglycaemic physician; a malignant tumour of the pancreas was found, with metastases of high insulin content in lymph nodes and liver. Roscoe Graham of Toronto published the first report of successful removal of an islet cell tumour of the pancreas, with consequent relief of hypoglycaemia in 1929. Since these early beginnings the condition has become established, but it is rare, with an incidence of 1 per million per annum in the general population.

Clinical features

A diagnosis of insulinoma is made, almost without exception, as a consequence of investigations initiated to elucidate the cause and nature of symptoms which appear to come from the central nervous system. Episodes of odd behaviour and disturbances of consciousness are the commonest complaints, but almost any neurological or psychiatric syndrome may be simulated. During neuroglycopenic episodes, conversation and movements are restricted, and behaviour patterns resembling mild to severe alcoholic intoxication develop. Characteristically, the patient feels well between attacks. A temporal relationship to meals is seldom noted. Chronic neuroglycopenia presents with insidious changes in personality, defective memory and mental deterioration. Very rarely an insulinoma may present with peripheral neuropathy and/or a progressive muscular atrophy.

Women are slightly more susceptible (55%) to insulinoma. The average age of diagnosis in 828 cases of insulinoma was 42; however, no age is exempt.

Pathology

Most insulinomas occur as solitary benign neoplasms 5–50 mm in size. Discrete tumours like the islets of Langerhans, they are evenly distributed throughout the pancreas. In 10% of cases there are two or more discrete tumours. In about 4% there is diffuse adenomatosis involving many, but not all of the pancreatic islets. A small but poorly defined proportion of all insulinomas represent the pancreatic element of the multiple endocrine adenopathy syndrome type I. In such cases the tumours are commonly multiple and may secrete more than one pancreatic hormone. Generalized hyperplasia of all islets has also been incriminated as a cause of spontaneous fasting hypoglycaemia. Conclusive proof has not been produced that this ever happens in adults. Between 5 and 10% of all insulin-producing tumours have already metastasized to the liver or elsewhere at the time of initial diagnosis. The amount of connective tissue in tumours varies greatly and possibly accounts for the differences in the appearances observed at operation, from a plum-coloured tumour to an almost pure white nodule. Ductular elements are sometimes recognizable between the endocrine cells, and amyloid is often discernible as in other peptide-secreting tumours. Rarely the tumour cells contain round colloid bodies, but mitoses are only occasionally seen except in metastasizing tumours. The diagnosis of an insulinoma can be confirmed by immunohistochemical techniques.

Diagnosis

The original diagnosis rested on the triad of Whipple:

1. A patient with symptoms of hypoglycaemia must develop the symptoms within 48 hours of total deprivation of caloric intake.
2. While the patient is having symptoms the blood sugar must be less than 2.5 mmol/l.
3. The symptoms must abate with the administration of glucose.

However, more sophisticated methods are now available to confirm the diagnosis and exclude other causes of hypoglycaemia.

Blood glucose. Demonstration that hypoglycaemia—defined as blood glucose concentration of less than 2.2 mmol/l—exists and is the cause of the patient's symptoms, is the first step in diagnosis. The period of fasting necessary to provoke hypoglycaemia in patients with insulinoma varies widely, but 90% of proven cases have hypoglycaemia on one or more occasions after a 15-hour overnight fast providing that three tests are performed.

Plasma insulin. Continued and *inappropriate* insulin secretion is characteristic of insulinomas during fasting, and is demonstrated by the occurrence of normal or raised plasma insulin and C-peptide levels in the presence of hypoglycaemia. Failure to demonstrate inappropriate insulin and C-peptide levels on at least one out of three overnight fasts should be taken as strong but not conclusive evidence that the diagnosis is not correct.

Glucagon test. By injecting 1 mg of glucagon intravenously and measuring the plasma insulin and blood glucose response the inappropriate secretion of insulin can be demonstrated in 80% of patients with an insulinoma.

There is no absolute test for an insulinoma, but the diagnosis should be treated with caution by the surgeon until the inappropriate secretion of insulin and C-peptide has been demonstrated either in the simple fasting state or in response to glucagon.

Once the diagnosis has been confirmed the site of the insulinoma must be determined. Ultrasound and CT scanning are the first-line investigations and should identify well over 90% of the tumours. Endoscopic ultrasound improves the yield of positive results so that it is now rare to require selective arteriography of coeliac and superior mesenteric arteries.[83]

Surgical treatment

Because of the malignant potential of these tumours, all insulinomas once diagnosed should initially be treated surgically rather than medically. The pancreas is exposed by division of the omental attachments to the transverse colon and flexures. Intraoperative ultrasound is used to define or confirm the position of the tumour.[84] The front of the pancreas is then inspected and palpated. If a tumour is found, it is enucleated and submitted for immediate histological confirmation before proceeding. If not, the head of the pancreas is mobilized and the posterior surface examined. Next the spleen and tail of pancreas are mobilized and the body and tail of the pancreas palpated between finger and thumb. If these manoeuvres fail to demonstrate the insulinoma, the tail of the pancreas is resected and submitted to immediate frozen section histological examination to exclude islet cell hyperplasia. A resection is preferable to an enucleation for tumours buried in the head of the gland in order to prevent fistula formation, which is the main cause of the high mortality for this procedure—3% following the first operation and 10% for subsequent procedures.

Postoperatively, transient hyperglycaemia which may require insulin therapy is common but lasts only 2–3 weeks. Persistent hypoglycaemia is the result of residual tumour.

Medical management

This is reserved for patients in whom the tumour has metastasized, or if it cannot be found at operation, or if it recurs following operation. Diazoxide is the drug of choice, inhibiting insulin release by the β cell. Complications encountered with this drug include hypotension, oedema, hirsuitism and granulocytopenia. Although plasma insulin levels can be lowered to concentrations where they do not cause symptoms and many patients may become symptom-free with diazoxide, the tumour will continue to grow and metastasize, because the drug has no tumoricidal activity. For this reason streptozotocin, although more difficult to use and more toxic, will by its semi-selective action on the β cell attain a biochemical response in 64% and objective regression of tumour in 50%. A synthetic somatostatin analogue, SMS 201–995 (Sandostatin), given by twice-daily injections also controls the symptoms.[85]

Nesidioblastosis

Hypertrophy of the islet cells is one of the rare causes of infantile hypoglycaemia, giving rise to inappropriate insulin levels. Many affected babies can be managed conservatively, but a few come to surgery. The appropriate procedure is a 95% duodenal-preserving pancreatectomy.[86]

Gastrinoma

History

Clinicians have for many years recognized that there was a relationship between an insulinoma, which did not produce hypoglycaemia, and duodenal ulcer, although no specific cause and effect could be proved. In 1955 Zollinger and Ellison reported 2 cases in which removal of the acid-secreting surface by total gastrectomy was required because of persistence of marked gastric hypersecretion and a fulminating ulcer diathesis. Non β islet cell tumours were found in both patients, and it was suggested that these tumours were producing a potent gastric secretagogue. Within 5 years Gregory and colleagues proved that the ulcerogenic tumours were producing a potent gastric secretagogue. They identified it as 'gastrin-like', so explaining gastric hypersecretion and the intractable ulceration. In an attempt to gain insight into this disease, a registry was established by Ellison & Wilson and there are now over 1000 patients in this registry, which provides a statistical basis for the knowledge of this tumour. The incidence is about 1 patient per 2 million population per annum which is half as frequent as an insulinoma.

Clinical features

Ninety per cent of patients with gastrinomas develop peptic ulcers. The ulcer may present in one of four ways:

1. A standard duodenal ulcer.
2. Peptic ulcers outside the stomach or duodenal bulb.
3. Multiple ulcers.
4. A peptic ulcer with a fulminating course.

In the first group the history may be long; 28% of all patients with a gastrinoma had a history which exceded 5 years, and only 21% had a history of less than 1 year. The symptoms usually respond poorly to the usual medical management, and diarrhoea was frequently associated with the ulcer. An ulcer outside the stomach and duodenum is observed in a quarter of all patients; a jejunal ulcer in the absence of previous surgery is pathognomonic of a gastrinoma. Multiple ulcers are present in 10–20% of patients, while the ulcer which is resistant to various surgical procedures is the hallmark of the condition; a patient who has anastomotic problems following the primary procedure for an ulcer should always be investigated to exclude a gastrinoma.

Diarrhoea is present in 30% of patients; 13% of all patients develop diarrhoea as the first symptom and 5% have diarrhoea as the sole complaint. Gastrointestinal bleeding is seen in a third of patients and perforation in 14%. Some patients have periods of remission, but most have a persistent and progressive course.

REFERENCES

83. Rossi P, Allison D J et al Radiol Clin North Am 1984; 27: 129–162
84. Norton J A, Cromack D T, Shawker T N Ann Surg 1988; 207: 160–168
85. Comi R J, Maton P N, Go V L W Ann Intern Med 1989; 110: 35–50
86. Gough M H Br J Surg 1984; 71: 75–78

Men are more susceptible (63%) to gastrinoma. The onset of symptoms is most common in the fourth decade, but the age range is from 9 to 90 years.

Pathology

Unlike insulinoma, a solitary tumour in the pancreas without metastases is unusual. Seventy-five per cent of patients have a pancreatic tumour to the right of the portal vein, often in the duodenal wall, 10% have only distant metastases and the remaining 5% have islet cell hyperplasia. Only 17% of all cases have a single localized tumour in the pancreas. The tumour size is variable; a duodenal tumour may be only 5 mm in diameter while metastatic deposits can be 10 cm in diameter. At least 30% are associated with other endocrine tumours (multiple endocrine adenopathy type I), 25% of gastrinomas being associated with hyperparathyroidism. Anterior pituitary, adrenal, thyroid and ovarian tumours are less frequent.

Sixty per cent of gastrinomas are malignant at the time of diagnosis, but only 19% of deaths from a gastrinoma are from tumour progression. Half of those patients who have had a total gastrectomy where there is evidence of metastatic disease will be dead by 5 years.

Gastrin has been shown by histochemical, immunofluorescent and direct assay to be present in very large quantities within the tumour. Ultrastructural studies show the tumour cells contain round secretory granules, resembling those seen in the antral gastrin G cell. The tumour cells are notably uniform with eosinophilic cytoplasm and nuclei. Mitotic figures are rarely seen. Light microscopy alone is unable to identify a gastrinoma.

Diagnosis

Because the presentation is often as an uncomplicated peptic ulcer, the first stage in diagnosis is to be aware of a gastrinoma in an aggressive or unusual ulcer (see Chapter 26). The first step in diagnosis is to perform a pentagastrin secretion study. If the basal acid output is greater than 60% of the maximal acid output, or if the 1 hour basal output is greater than 15 mmol (5 mmol if a partial gastrectomy has been performed) and there is minimal stimulation with pentagastrin, a serum gastrin estimation should be performed. A minimum of three fasting gastrin levels should be performed because of the fluctuation in the daily gastrin levels. A level twice the normal range raises the possibility of a gastrinoma. A level greater than 10 times the normal value in the presence of acid hypersecretion and a suggestive history confirms the diagnosis. Inhibitory and stimulation tests are required in the doubtful case. Following a meal, the gastrin level increases in patients with a duodenal ulcer, but remains stable if a gastrinoma is present. A 100% increase in the level of gastrin is found after a calcium infusion of 4 mg/kg per h over a 4-hour period if a gastrinoma is present. The provocation test infusing secretin at the rate of 1 unit per kilogram body weight over a 5-minute period is most helpful if doubt still remains. Secretin normally inhibits gastrin release, but in a patient with a gastrinoma there is an increase in the level of gastrin, and in the basal acid output.

There are unfortunately other patients who have an aggressive ulcer, increased acid secretion and a moderately raised gastrin level. There are two important causes: the first is hyperparathyroidism in which the calcium level is raised—a known stimulant of gastrin release—and the second is an antral gastrin cell hyperplasia. There are two possibilities if the calcium level is raised; either the raised level of gastrin is entirely the result of the raised calcium or the patient has multiple endocrine adenomatosis. The clinical decision on which condition to treat first is arbitrary, but experience has shown that it is safer to treat the hyperparathyroidism first, and observe the gastrin response to this procedure.

Antral gastrin cell hyperplasia must be considered if the calcium level is normal. In this condition there is a marked gastrin secretion in response to food, a variable response to calcium and inhibition of gastrin release by secretin. Confirmation of the diagnosis is obtained by endoscopic biopsy of the antrum when excessive numbers of g cells are demonstrated in the antral mucosa on immunofluorescent staining of histological sections. The return of the gastrin levels to below normal following vagotomy and antrectomy confirms the diagnosis.

Having established the diagnosis of a gastrinoma the same localization procedure as for an insulinoma should be undertaken.

Treatment

Thirty-five per cent of patients with this condition present as an emergency with perforation (18%) or haemorrhage (17%) from a peptic ulcer, while the remainder are diagnosed by a suggestive history or clinical course. Because of the fulminant course of many cases, surgical treatment was in the past often undertaken without adequate investigation. This should not now occur because histamine H_2-antagonist and proton pump inhibitors can control the excess acid secretion, so allowing adequate investigation with healing of the ulcer. Thus, even with a perforation (such as a jejunal perforation) simple closure can be undertaken with comparative safety.

The rationale behind this conservative approach is the high mortality associated with emergency surgical treatment of gastrinoma of around 20%. An H_2-receptor antagonist not only enables the ulcer to be healed and the diagnosis to be confirmed, but also allows the patient's nutritional state to be improved, by parenteral hyperalimentation if necessary.

A decision has to be made to determine whether operative intervention is appropriate once the clinical condition of the patient is stable and the symptoms are well-controlled by an H_2-receptor antagonist. If a single tumour is identified by scanning, it should be removed and the gastrin levels followed. A vagotomy and antrectomy should be performed as this makes future medical management easier if no tumour is found or if the surgeon fails to confirm the presence of an identified tumour. A total gastrectomy is reserved for the patient who has poor symptom control by medical therapy, is not compliant or who requests this operation after careful explanation.[87]

REFERENCE

87. Maton P N, Frucht H, Vinater R, Wank S A, Gardner J D, Jensen R T Gastroenterology 1988; 94: 294–299

In patients with metastatic deposits who are failing to thrive, combination chemotherapy using 5-fluorouracil with streptozotocin may be provide useful palliation.

Glucagonoma

The first report of a tumour arising from the α cells of the pancreas was in 1966. The patient presented with a bullous 'eczematoid' rash and had evidence of mild maturity-onset diabetes mellitus. At laparotomy a pancreatic islet cell carcinoma was found with hepatic metastases. Immunoassay of the tumour extract and serum showed high levels of glucagon. In 1974, 9 patients with a glucagonoma were described. All these patients had a skin rash which was present for more than a year, and in some cases for as long as 10 years. The rash begins as an erythematous area which tends to blister and crust; healing occurs within 2–3 weeks, but new lesions often develop elsewhere. Glossitis, diabetes and wasting are also present. Plasma glucagon levels are raised. Surgical treatment follows a similar pattern to that of an insulinoma.[88]

Vipoma

In 1957 Priest & Alexander called attention to the association of islet cell tumours with diarrhoea. The following year Verner and Morrison reported the association of watery diarrhoea and an islet tumour. Later it was noted that these patients had achlorhydria and hypokalaemia, hence the name watery diarrhoea hypokalaemia and basal achlorhydria syndrome. In 1973 it was shown that this syndrome was caused by the excessive secretion of vasoactive intestinal peptide. Extracts of this pancreatic tumour contained large quantities of vasoactive intestinal peptide, and plasma vasoactive intestinal peptide levels were raised. It has subsequently been shown that following resection of these tumours the vasoactive intestinal peptide levels return to normal, and the patient's symptoms improve, with bowel habit returning to normal. Sandostatin relieves diarrhoea at once.[85]

Tumours have been described in association with most of the apud series. Their surgical management rests on the principles outlined above.

Malignant tumours

Cystadenocarcinoma

The cystadenoma and its malignant counterpart the cystadenocarcinoma are rare tumours: 90% develop in middle-aged women. The tumour may arise in any portion of the gland, and is slow-growing, usually attaining a large size before it is detected. Patients usually present with an abdominal mass unless the mass causes pressure symptoms on an adjacent organ, for example jaundice, by pressure on the bile duct.

The tumours consist of multiple cysts on pathological examination, although there is a papillary form which is more solid. These tumours, if left untreated, undergo malignant change. The diagnosis is made at laparotomy, and resection should be undertaken if it is technically feasible. Emphasis has recently been laid on the difficulty of differentiating these tumours from a chronic pseudocyst; if the history does not suggest pancreatitis then the 'tumour' should be explored.[89] Extensive surgery with high mortality is unacceptable in the management of these patients, as the tumours are very slow-growing and prolonged survival is usual even without treatment.

Carcinoma of the pancreas

Carcinoma of the pancreas was first described by Mondine, who reported 2 patients in 1836, but the first full description relating autopsy findings with the signs and symptoms of the disease was in 1888. The classic sign of a palpable distended gallbladder, now often overemphasized, was described by Courvoisier in 1890. Pain as the predominant symptom was not recognized until 1908. Surgical treatment for malignant lesions of the pancreas was reported in 1884 when Billroth performed what was probably the first pancreatectomy. Intermittent reports of pancreatic operations appeared over the ensuing years. The first cases of en bloc resections of carcinoma of the ampulla of Vater were performed between 1912 and 1922 by Herschel, Kausch and Tenai. The modern era of pancreatic surgery began in 1935 when Whipple, Parsons and Mullins reported that they had succeeded in resecting a large part of the duodenum, the lower end of the bile duct and approximately 50% of the head of the pancreas. The first successful total pancreatectomy, which was performed for hyperinsulinism, was carried out by Priestly in 1944.[90]

Aetiology

The incidence of pancreatic cancer in cigarette smokers is twice that of non-smokers.[91] The mechanism is unknown but the carcinogen must be potent since as little as 10 cigarettes per day increases the risk. Those countries whose dietary fat intake is high have a higher incidence of pancreatic cancer, and the westernization of the Japanese diet is said to account for the fourfold increase in pancreatic cancer since 1950.[92] A possible mechanism for this increase has been the finding that nitrosamines, a potent pancreatic carcinogen in some animals, are formed during cooking from the nitrates used as a meat preservative.[93–96] The incidence of carcinoma of the pancreas in patients with diabetes appears to be about twice that in the general population, but this is debatable.[97,98] The

REFERENCES

88. Bloom S R, Polar J M Am J Med 1987; 32: 25–36
89. Warshaw A L, Rutledge P L Ann Surg 1988; 205: 393–398
90. Praderi R C In: Carter D C, Trede M (eds) Surgery of the Pancreas. Churchill Livingstone, London 1993 pp 3–15
91. Kahn H A The Dorn Study of Smoking and Mortality among US Veterans: Report on 8½ Years of Observation. NCI monograph 1966; 19: 127–204
92. Raymond L, Infante F, Tuyns A J, Voirol M, Lowenfels A B Alimentation et cancer du pancreas. Gastroenterol Clin Biol 1987; 11: 488–492
93. Druckrey H, Ivankovic S et al Z Krebsforch 1968; 71: 167–182
94. Reddy J R, Rao M S Cancer Res 1975; 35: 2269–2277
95. Pour P, Runge R G et al Cancer 1981; 47: 1573–1587
96. Longnecker D S Arch Pathol Lab Med 1983; 107: 54–58
97. Everhart J, Wright D JAMA 1995; 273: 1605–1609
98. Gullo L, Pezzilli R, Morselli-Labate A M, Italian Pancreatic Cancer Study Group N Engl J Med 1994; 331: 81–84

development of diabetes de novo or the development of instability in a previously controlled diabetic at the time of the appearance of carcinoma of the pancreas is well-known. There is also evidence that chronic pancreatitis predisposes to carcinoma of the pancreas.[99] The risk is similar to the risk posed by ulcerative colitis for carcinoma of the colon. Carcinoma of the pancreas can be readily induced in experimental animals by the implantation of carcinogens nitrofen, azinphos methyl, directly into the pancreas while a few carcinogens such as 2,2′-dihydroxy-di-N-propylnitrosamine, cause cancer of the pancreas after systemic administration.[100] No carcinogens acting on the human pancreas have yet been identified, but carcinoma of the pancreas is more common in workers in the chemical industry.[101]

Pathology

The tumour develops in the head of the pancreas in 85% of cases, and appears as a poorly demarcated, greyish white, scirrhous nodular growth in glandular substance. The cut surface may show scattered red or brown areas of necrosis or haemorrhage. Locules of turbid grey or brown liquid may be present. Because of the obstructive effects of the tumour, the duct of Wirsung is frequently dilated, and the body and tail of the pancreas is indurated.

The cancer spreads into and along both the bile duct and the duct of Wirsung. There may be direct extension into the duodenum and into the lymph nodes in the vicinity. The portal vein is frequently compressed and directly invaded. Nerve sheaths are infiltrated and distant spread is initially to the liver.

The most common histological type is the ductal adenocarcinoma with varying degrees of differentiation within the same tumour. Other tumours include squamous carcinomas, mucinous carcinomas and ciliated adenocarcinomas. Acinar carcinomas are rare tumours with a specific histological appearance consisting of groups of polygonal cells (Tables 33.5 and 33.6). Carcinoma of the head of the pancreas should be distinguished from carcinomas of the intrapancreatic portion of the common bile duct, the ampulla of Vater and the duodenal mucosa. Although exhibiting symptoms similar to tumours of the head of the pancreas, the three latter tumours are frequently resectable and have a more favourable prognosis.

Clinical features

The symptoms produced depend to some extent on the site of the tumour, although pain, jaundice and loss of weight are major symptoms in most patients whatever the anatomical site of the carcinoma. Pain is the presenting symptom in 50–80% of patients and occurs at some time in the course of the disease in between 75 and 90% of patients. The pain is variable in location and severity, but most frequently occurs as a dull aching or boring pain in the epigastrium; it is steadily progressive and often increased in severity at night. It may be aggravated by eating and by recumbency, but relieved by sitting forward. There is no doubt that the pain of carcinoma of the body and tail of the pancreas results in epigastric pain which radiates to the left upper quadrant, while neoplasms in the head of the pancreas radiate to the right upper quadrant. This bears out experimental studies in which direct stimulation of the pancreas, by means of very fine electrodes inserted into the head, body and tail of the pancreas, was performed during the postoperative period in a series of patients subjected to elective biliary tract surgery. It was found that the pain resulting from stimulation of the head of the pancreas was distributed over the right epigastrium, that from stimulation of the body to the mid-epigastrium, and that from stimulation of the tail to the lower epigastrium on the left and at times even to the left lower quadrant. Simultaneous stimulation of all three areas produced band-like pain across the epigastrium with radiation to the back. Pancreatic pain rarely occurs alone, and is usually associated with a general abdominal pain or discomfort.

Jaundice is the first symptom in 10–30% of patients, and by the time the patient is seen by the doctor is present in 30–60%. It occurs at some time in the course of the disease in up to 90% of patients. The jaundice is often accompanied by pain and is usually progressive, but spontaneous fluctuations in the degree of icterus early in the course of the disease have been reported in 10%. The jaundice is usually accompanied by pruritus, which can be very troublesome.

Loss of weight is probably the commonest symptom of carcinoma of the pancreas and usually precedes other symptoms, affecting 70–90% of patients by the time of diagnosis. The weight loss is rapid and progressive, being independent of the site of the tumour. The extent of the tumour is not related to the weight loss, and should not be used as an index of respectability. Despite the frequency of weight loss, anorexia and steatorrhoea are rare symptoms. Other symptoms which occur but are of limited diagnostic help are epigastric bloating and flatulence (31%), weakness or fatigue, or both (31%), diarrhoea (25%), vomiting (23%) and constipation (11%).[102]

The commonest physical findings are of obstructive jaundice, a palpably enlarged liver and abdominal tenderness. A palpable gallbladder is found in 12–37%, while thrombophlebitis occurs in less than 10% of patients. Physical signs of metastatic spread are common (70%) when the patient first seeks medical advice, particularly when the patient has carcinoma of the body and tail of the pancreas.

Investigations

The diagnosis of pancreatic cancer has been made easier by modern imaging. Ultrasound can identify over 90% of pancreatic tumours and give a correct anatomical description of the cause of jaundice. A contrast-enhanced helical CT scan of the pancreas usually defines the tumour and its operability (Fig. 33.18). Endoscopy identifies the presence or absence of duodenal involve-

REFERENCES

99. Lowenfels A B, Maisonneuve P et al N Engl J Med 1993; 328: 1433–1437
100. Pour P, Mohr U et al Cancer 1975; 36: 379–389
101. Garabrani D H, Held J et al J Natl Cancer Inst 1992; 84: 764–771
102. Gambill E E S Med J 1970; 63: 1119–1122

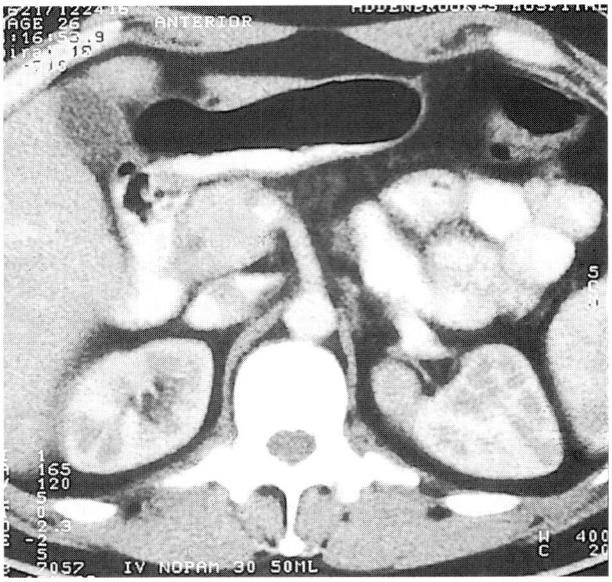

Fig. 33.18 Contrast-enhanced helical CT scan showing a carcinoma of the head of the pancreas which proved inoperable on account of portal vein involvement.

ment and confirms whether or not the tumour is ampullary in origin. The exact site of obstruction can be determined by an endoscopic retrograde pancreatogram and cholangiogram (Fig. 33.19). A cholangiogram may be obtained by the percutaneous approach if these endoscopic facilities are not available. Neither of these techniques are advocated unless immediate decompression is planned, as the incidence of infection is significant even with prophylactic antibiotics.

Antigens to human pancreatic cancer have been extensively tested to determine if there is a marker which would enable its early diagnosis which might increase its resectability. To date none of the antigens are tumour-specific.[103]

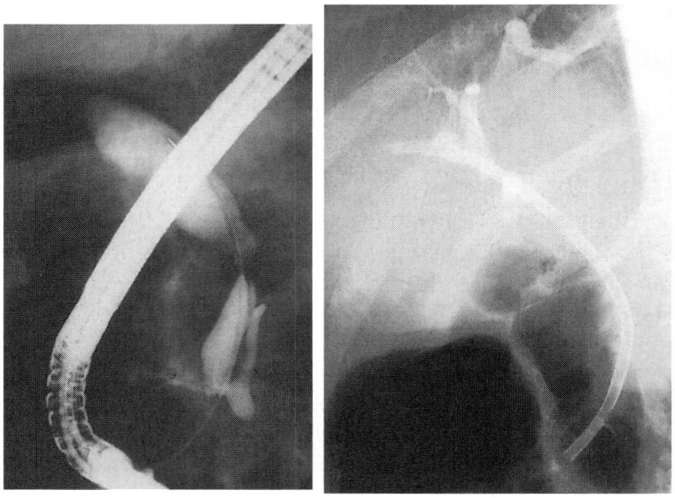

a **b**

Fig. 33.19 (**a**) An endoscopic retrograde cholangiopancreatogram showing obstruction by tumour of both the pancreatic and bile duct. A guidewire is placed through the stricture in preparation for the passage of a stent through it (Fig. 33.19**b**).

The diagnosis can now be confirmed by a percutaneous biopsy under imaging control to obtain a 1 mm tissue core suitable for histological assessment.[104]

Management

The only hope of cure in pancreatic cancer remains surgical resection, but the chance of cure is probably less than 1%.[105] Half the patients who present with cancer of the pancreas are over 75 years, and relatively unfit for major surgery. Consequently, palliative treatment is the appropriate therapy for most of these patients. For those who are fit for curative resection, a careful analysis of the tumour is undertaken by use of ultrasound, endoscopic ultrasound, CT scanning and endoscopy. A curative resection should be attempted if the tumour is small (< 2 cm), is not involving the major vessels, has not metastasized and has a favourable histological appearance, provided no untoward findings are revealed at laparotomy. For the very old or unfit patient endoscopic stenting relieves jaundice, while for the patient with duodenal obstruction, a laparotomy and surgical bypass is necessary. The remainder of the patients are equally well-served by surgical bypass or endoscopic stenting. It is essential by endoscopy to detect the tumour arising from the ampulla of Vater, for these tumours have a very much better prognosis and are more likely to be resectable than the standard pancreatic adenocarcinoma.[106]

The curable patient

Most patients are jaundiced and should have an endoscopic stent inserted to relieve the jaundice and allow the liver function to return towards normal. At the end of 6 weeks, their tumour should be reassessed and if still operable, they should be presented for surgery in good nutritional balance with near normal liver function and normal albumin, a normal blood count with normal clotting screen and an adequate fluid balance.

Only by rigorous attention to detail and careful selection of patients can the mortality be reduced from around 25%, which is the overall mortality for cumulative results, to the 5% level.[107]

Radical excision of the head of the pancreas—pancreaticoduodenectomy—Whipple's operation

The development of this operation is largely the result of Whipple's efforts, who in 1935 described a two-stage procedure.[108] At the first stage, a gastroenterostomy and cholecyst-gastrostomy were performed, followed later by excision of the duodenum and

REFERENCES

103. Metzgar R S, Asch H L Pancreas 1988; 3: 352
104. Jennings P E, Donald J J, Coral A, Rode J, Lees W R Lancet 1989; 1: 1369–1371
105. Gudjonsson B Cancer 1987; 60: 2284–2303
106. Warshaw A L, Swanson R S Ann Surg 1988; 208: 541–553
107. Lillemoe K D Ann Surg 1995; 221: 133–148
108. Whipple A O, Parsons W B, Mullins C R Ann Surg 1935; 102: 763–779

head of the pancreas, with closure of the pancreatic stump; this proved a successful management for ampullary growths. Brunchwig recorded the first successful removal of a cancer of the head of the pancreas, anastomosing gallbladder to jejunum, and isolating a jejunal loop and employing it for a jejunojejunostomy. The ligated lower end of the common duct, even though bypassed by cholecystenterostomy, proved liable to blow-out and Whipple suggested reconstitution of biliary drainage by end-to-side anastomosis of common bile duct to jejunum and Orr independently drained the common duct into the jejunum, even though cholecystostomy had previously been performed. In 1941 Whipple reported a one-stage procedure. Hunt suggested end-to-end burial of the stump of the pancreas into the open end of the jejunum, end-to-side choledochoenterostomy, and gastroenterostomy performed distal to the biliary and pancreatic anastomoses, with closure of the pylorus. Orr reported a modification of the one-stage procedure which included closure of the stomach and duodenal stump, gastroenterostomy and implantation of both pancreas and common duct into a loop of jejunum distal to the gastroenterostomy and isolated by lateral anastomosis.

Child brought up the divided end of the duodenum for anastomosis to the pancreas end-to-end and to the common bile duct side-to-end before uniting the stomach end-to-side to the distal jejunum in front of the colon. Most surgeons have come to accept the gastrojejunostomy as the last anastomosis in the sequence because it avoids reflux of chyme into the biliary and pancreatic ducts, and allows the gastrojejunostomy to be bathed in alkaline juice. Whether the pancreatic anastomosis or the choledochojejunostomy is made first appears to be a matter of preference, and the method of pancreaticojejunostomy is still open to debate (Figs 33.20 and 33.21).

The principles laid down in the second edition of this text still apply:

1. Ligation of the common bile duct, even after the establishment of the cholecystenterostomy, is liable to be followed by fistula.

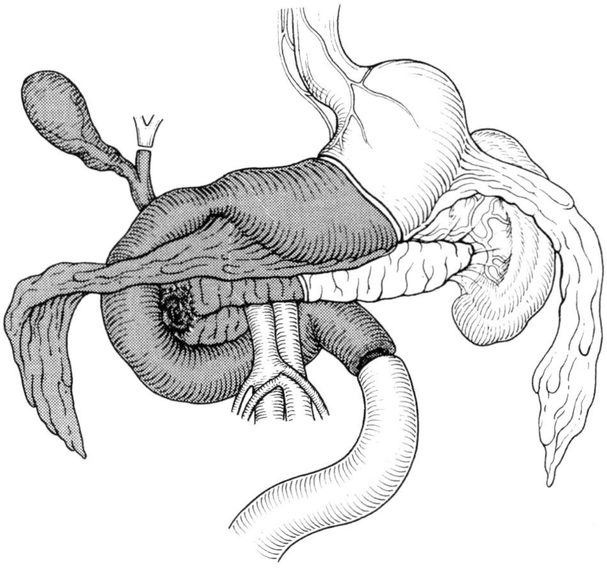

Fig. 33.20 The extent of resection in a standard Whipple procedure.

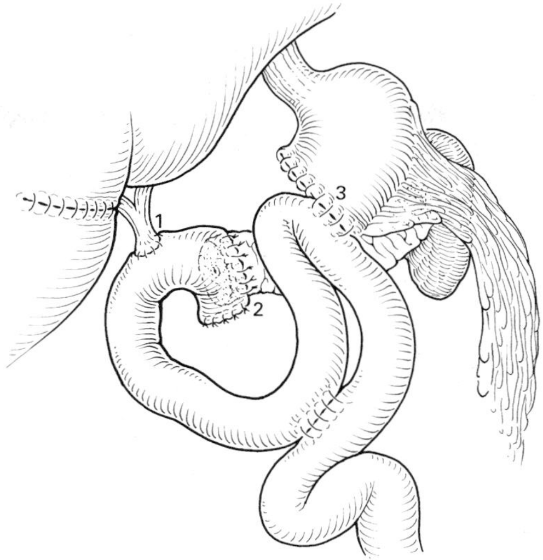

Fig. 33.21 The usual reconstruction following a Whipple resection: **1** choledochojejunostomy; **2** pancreatojejunostomy; **3** gastrojejunostomy.

2. Closure of the pancreatic stump is more liable to be followed by pancreatic fistula than is implantation of the pancreas into the jejunum.
3. Ascending infection of the biliary system can always occur after anastomosis between bile channels and jejunum; it is particularly likely to occur if both gallbladder and common duct are separately joined to jejunum and least likely to occur if the common duct alone is to be drained into the gastrointestinal canal and a cholecystectomy performed; ascending biliary infection is not prevented by lateral anastomosis of the limbs of the jejunal loop into which the common duct drains.

Technique of pancreaticoduodenectomy

The usual approach is by a long transverse incision. When the abdomen is opened a complete examination of the abdominal and pelvic cavities is carried out. Close attention should be paid to the liver, the caudal surface of the mesocolon and the ligament of Treitz. Any tissues showing fixation, puckering or implantation in these areas should be sent for frozen section examination. Any attempt at resection should be abandoned if tumour is found in these biopsies. The lesser sac is then opened by division of the gastrocolic omentum so that the head, neck and body of the pancreas are visible. If the tumour is still deemed operable, the duodenum is mobilized by division of the peritoneum on its lateral border extending the peritoneal incision up to the common bile duct and down to the hepatic flexure, which is then mobilized downwards and medially to expose the fourth part of the duodenum. The head of the pancreas within the duodenum can then be lifted off the vena cava and the aorta. Provided the uncinate process is not fixed to the superior mesenteric artery, the tumour is considered resectable.

The middle colic vein is defined, and traced down to the superior mesenteric vein. The right gastroepiploic vein and artery are followed down to the anterior surface of the pancreas where they are ligated and divided to give a better exposure of the anterior surface of the head of the pancreas. The superior mesenteric vein is traced upwards and greater exposure achieved by division of the inferior pancreatoduodenal artery. The portal vein is dissected from the pancreas and a tape is then passed around the neck of the gland. The common bile duct is next dissected and encircled with a tape. The stomach is divided just proximal to the pylorus. The ligament of Treitz is incised to the right of the superior mesenteric vessels so that the proximal jejunum can be delivered behind the colon into the supracolic compartment. The jejunum is divided, and the jejunal arteries between the inferior border of the pancreas and the line of resection are divided. The neck of the pancreas is then divided and the portal vein exposed. The common bile duct is next divided so that the pancreas is now suspended by the uncinate process and the vessels of the posterior arterial arcade. Lifting the duodenum in anterosuperior direction, the vessels between the head of the pancreas and the portal vein and superior mesenteric artery are divided. These vessels are easily torn, and transfixion ligation is an easier technique than simple ligation. The specimen is finally freed by dividing the pancreaticoduodenal arteries so joining the dissection already performed by the division of the bile duct.

At the start of the reconstruction, the end of the jejunum is oversewn and invaginated. The pancreatic duct is then identified, and intubated with a catheter which has been passed through the jejunal loop. A pancreaticojejunostomy is constructed over the catheter, and the cut surface of the pancreas sutured to the jejunal serosa. The bile duct is anastomosed end-to-side to the jejunum. Finally a gastrojejunostomy is performed.

It is fashionable to preserve the pylorus, and over half the procedures for cancer do so, but the disadvantage of delayed postoperative gastric emptying is not outweighed by the supposed benefit of improved gastric function in the long term. It is preferable to perform the procedure that is technically safest for that particular patient (Fig. 33.22).

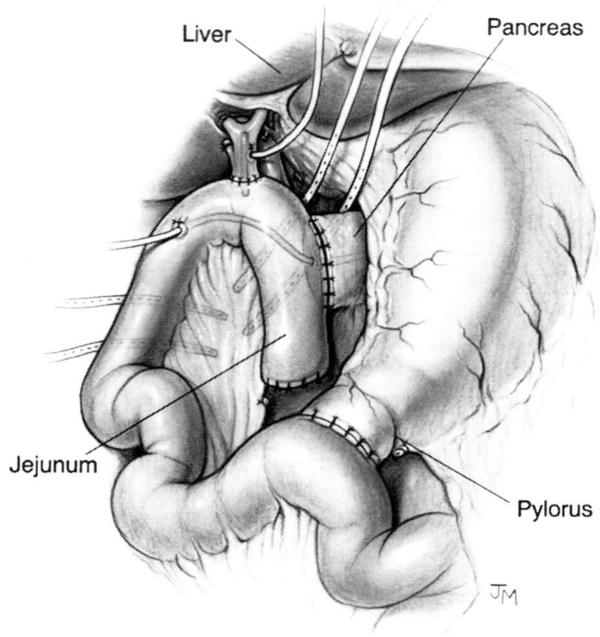

Fig. 33.22 A pylorus-preserving pancreatoduodenectomy.

Distal pancreatectomy

After full evaluation of the abdominal cavity to exclude distant spread the lesser sac is opened by dividing the attachment of the omentum to the colon so that the pancreas, from hilum of the spleen to the duodenum, can be examined. The spleen is mobilized and the plane between the pancreas and the posterior abdominal wall is entered if the tumour can be removed by a distal pancreatectomy. By this means the spleen and tail of pancreas can be delivered into the wound. The omentum is then separated from the splenic flexure and the splenic hilum, and mobilized completely by dividing the left gastroepiploic artery and the short gastric arteries. The splenic artery is then divided near the coeliac axis while the splenic vein is divided flush with the inferior mesenteric vein which is closed by suture. The pancreas is divided on the anterior surface of the portal vein. The duct is closed by ligature and the stump oversewn (Fig. 33.23).

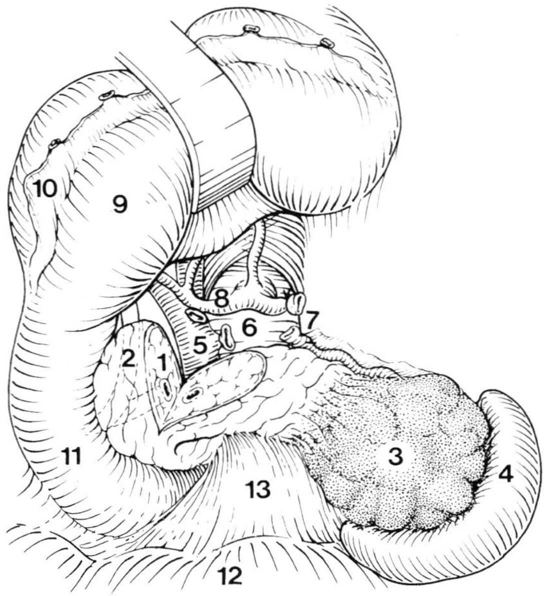

Fig. 33.23 A distal pancreatectomy at the stage when the spleen and tumour have been completely mobilized. The neck of the pancreas in the process of division. **1** Pancreatic neck and duct; **2** common bile duct; **3** tumour; **4** spleen; **5** portal vein; **6** stump of the splenic vein; **7** stump of the splenic artery; **8** hepatic artery; **9** stomach; **10** divided omentum; **11** duodenum; **12** transverse colon; **13** mesocolon.

Total pancreatectomy

The suggestion that total pancreatectomy may be indicated for malignant pancreatic disease is supported by the observation that the full extent of the tumour cannot be determined by inspection alone. Removal of the whole pancreas enables a more thorough cancer operation to be performed with the avoidance of a pancreatic anastomosis, which is a significant cause of morbidity. This operation has however not proved popular because the mortality is higher (10%), and there is no evidence of prolongation of survival.[109] Even the operation of regional pancreatectomy in which the pancreatic segment of the portal vein is excised with an en bloc total pancreatectomy and regional lymph node dissection has failed to show an improved survival and has thus been abandoned by most surgeons.[110]

Palliative procedures

The principal requirement, when the tumour has been deemed inoperable, is a simple procedure to prevent or relieve jaundice and duodenal obstruction. Decompression of the biliary tree is best accomplished by a choledochoduodenostomy. This procedure should be performed by excising a disc of bile duct at least 1 cm in diameter and a similar-sized disc of duodenum. An anastomosis between the two is easily performed using interrupted absorbable sutures. Only if there is evidence of tumour encroachment on the duodenum is a gastrojejunostomy performed. By selecting patients with evidence of duodenal obstruction and performing a gastrojejunostomy, the incidence of delayed obstruction can be reduced to less than 10%.

Postoperative care

The cardiorespiratory systems must be carefully monitored during the initial postoperative period, and ideally patients undergoing extensive pancreatic resections should be nursed in a high-dependence area until all observations are stable. Fluid balance must be maintained with care for the first 12 hours postoperatively. Colloid may be necessary because of the extensive retroperitoneal dissection. Sodium should be avoided because the urinary sodium loss is minimal in the first 48 hours; urinary electrolyte measurements are invaluable to aid initial fluid balance (see Chapter 2). Even after a partial resection of the pancreas, hyperglycaemia is common; insulin should be given if ketones appear in the urine or the blood sugar rises above 10 mmol/l. After the initial postoperative recovery period, parenteral nutrition should be started. Oral fluids are begun when gastrointestinal function returns, and the patient kept in hospital until their condition is stable.

Complications

The specific complications of this operation usually involve problems of the pancreatic anastomosis with the jejunum. Disruption of this anastomosis leads to fistula formation, abscess and haemorrhage. The biliary anastomosis leaks less commonly, although ascending infection may still be a problem. Patients after a major resection for pancreatic cancer are remarkably prone to the general complications of surgery and this accounts for the high morbidity associated with this procedure.[111,112]

Prognosis

Most studies have shown a mean survival after diagnosis of less than 6 months, with only 10% surviving 1 year without treatment. Even if the carcinoma is localized to the pancreas at the time of diagnosis, only 40% survived 6 months, 20% 1 year and less than 2% survived for 5 years. In patients with distant metastases 15% survived 6 months, 5% 1 year and all were dead within 2½ years.

Survival is increased by surgical excision; however, the increase in life expectancy must be weighed against the very substantial operative mortality. The results of 17 studies showed a mean operative mortality of 21% from 496 operations with a 5-year survival rate of 4%. It is probable that unless the operative mortality is 5% or less there is minimum benefit to the patient in performing a pancreaticoduodenectomy as compared to a palliative procedure.[113] In specialist centres the mortality has been reduced to 5% or less with a 5-year survival rate of 15–20%.

The specimen histology is a major determinant of prognosis after curative resection. A non-functioning islet tumour of the pancreas should have a 50% 5-year survival, while that of a true ampullary tumour has a 40% 5-year survival. On the other hand acinar carcinomas will have a median survival of only 18 months after resection, with all but 1% of patients being dead by 5 years.

Despite optimism, there is no evidence that radiotherapy or chemotherapy significantly prolongs survival or enhances the quality of life. Nevertheless, the newer regimen using continuous infusion with 5-fluorouracil with or without radiotherapy may enhance survival and the quality of life in 15–25% patients.[114]

There is much that can be done for patients with pancreatic cancer to ease their symptoms. Frequently their major problems are those of diarrhoea and polyuria. By careful control of their endocrine and exocrine requirements, further symptomatic relief can be achieved. If their pain cannot be controlled by simple analgesics, a coeliac plexus block is an extremely effective treatment and should be used early in the course of the disease.

REFERENCES

109. Van Heerden J A, McIlrath D C, Ilstrup D M, Welland L H World J Surg 1988; 12: 658–660
110. Satake K, Nishiwaki H et al. Surg Gynecol Obstet 1992; 175: 259–265
111. Connolly M M, Dawson P J, Michelassi F, Moosa A R, Lowenstein F Ann Surg 1987; 206: 366–373
112. Trede M, Schwall G Ann Surg 1988; 207: 39–47
113. Crist D W, Sitzman J V, Cameron J L Ann Surg 1988; 207: 39–47
114. Warshaw A L, Del Castillo F N Engl J Med 1992; 326: 455–465

34 The spleen and lymphoma

A. E. Young A. R. Timothy

The spleen

A. E. Young

Only in the second half of the 20th century has the function of the spleen been clarified. To the ancients it was the 'organ of mystery' and considered probably to be dispensable. This belief underpinned the surgical approach to the spleen which until the 1970s encompassed only one operation for splenic disease—splenectomy. Increasing knowledge of the untoward effects of splenectomy has led to conservatism in the management of splenic trauma. A greater knowledge of the pathology of the diseases which may require splenectomy for their management has led to a more careful selection of patients for elective splenectomy (Table 34.1).

SPLENIC FUNCTIONS[1]

The spleen is the second largest reticuloendothelial organ in the body and whilst it shares functions with other parts of that system many of its functions are unique. Its activities may be summarized as follows:

1. Immune function: the spleen captures and processes foreign antigen and is a major site of specific IgM production. The non-specific opsonins, tuftsin and properdin, are also synthesized in the spleen.
2. Filter function: macrophages in the splenic reticulum capture cellular and non-cellular material from the blood and plasma and this material includes bacteria, especially pneumococci.
3. Culling: the spleen recognises and removes old, deformed or defective platelets and red cells.
4. Pitting: this is the process of removing particulate inclusions from red cells and returning the repaired cell to the circulation. Inclusion bodies include denatured haemoglobin and parasites such as malaria.
5. Iron reutilization: phagocytic reticular cells remove iron from ingested degraded haemoglobin during red cell culling and return the iron to the plasma.
6. Pooling: up to 30% of platelets are normally pooled in the spleen by a process of reversible adhesion.
7. Reservoir function: in animals, especially the dog, up to a third of the blood volume may be sequestered in the spleen during sleep and returned to the circulation on waking. This does not occur in humans. The rapidly enlarging pathological spleen of blackwater malarial crises and sickle cell crises may however trap sufficient red cells to produce systemic shock.
8. Haematopoiesis: the human spleen is a haematopoietic organ only up to the fifth intrauterine month. Thereafter the only cells which are normally produced are some lymphocytes and plasma cells from the germinal centres. Haematopoiesis may however recommence in certain disease states.

Table 34.1 Medical indications for splenectomy

Regularly
Autoimmune thrombocytopenia
Autoimmune haemolysis
Hereditary spherocytosis (elliptocytosis)
Portal hypertension
Splenic vein thrombosis
Gaucher's disease
Occasionally
Thrombotic thrombocytopenia
Myelofibrosis
Thalassaemia major
Sickle cell disease
Thrombotic thrombocytopenia
Hodgkin's disease
Hairy cell leukaemia

CONGENITAL ABNORMALITIES

Asplenia

Asplenia is very rare and is normally associated with situs inversus and cardiac anomalies[2] there may also be biliary atresia.[3] In certain disease states, typically sickle cell disease, repeated silent infarctions of splenic tissue can lead to autosplenectomy and this may be mistakenly identified as asplenia.

Wandering spleen

Laxity of the peritoneal attachments of the spleen occasionally occurs in children and in thin nulliparous women and may allow ptosis of the spleen into the left iliac fossa or even the pelvis. Such spleens are at risk of either chronic or acute volvulus. The treatment of wandering spleen is ideally splenopexy, but splenectomy is needed if volvulus has occurred.[4,5]

REFERENCES

1. Crosby W H In: Williams W W et al (eds) Haematology. McGraw-Hill, New York 1983 pp 89–97
2. Puschar W G J, Manion W C Am J Clin Pathol 1956; 26: 429
3. Dyke M P, Martin R P, Berry P J Arch Dis Child 1991; 66: 636
4. Dawson J H McL, Roberts N G Aust N Z J Surg 1994; 64: 441
5. Peitgen K, Scweden K Eur J Surg 1995; 161: 49

Table 34.2 Location of accessory spleens in 335 patients

Location	*Number*	%
Splenic hilum—tail of pancreas	288	86
Greater omentum	53	16
Gastrosplenic ligament	21	6
Splenocolic ligament	10	3
Along the splenic artery	5	1
Other	38	11

From Baesl[6]

Accessory spleens

Accessory spleens occur in up to 20% of the population and may be multiple. They are rarely larger than 2 cm in diameter. They usually occur near the splenic hilum and along the splenic vessels (Table 34.2). They have also been identified in the retroperitoneum and the inguinal canal.[6] Faulty development of the spleen may lead to its appearing as multiple small spleens rather than as a single organ.

RUPTURE OF THE SPLEEN

Rupture of the spleen is usually a closed injury caused by direct external violence. It particularly occurs when the left lower ribs are struck, typically by the steering wheel of a car or the handlebars of a bicycle. Quite minor falls from bicycles, swings and trees can readily lead to rupture of the spleen in childhood as the ribs are more flexible and the spleen proportionately larger and less well protected. At all ages splenic enlargement from malaria, vascular malformations, haematological malignancies and infectious mononucleosis predisposes to easy rupture with minimal trauma, as also do perisplenic adhesions.[7]

Aird records that rupture may be occasioned by the physiological strains of coitus, pregnancy, labour and defecation, though this is exceptional. One of the most common reasons for splenic rupture remains incidental damage to the spleen during abdominal surgery, especially for gastric disease.[8]

Clinical features

The clinical effects of rupture of the spleen are those common to ruptures of all solid abdominal viscera, together with certain manifestations peculiar to the spleen. The main signs are those of internal haemorrhage, but often the haemorrhage is of a peculiar kind and the symptoms are characteristically biphasic. Initial trauma usually gives rise not to free intraperitoneal haemorrhage but to intracapsular rupture with the formation of a splenic haematoma. The haematoma remains restricted in extent while the blood pressure is low from initial shock. Sometimes, however, when the blood pressure rises the haematoma increases in size and may then rupture into the general peritoneal cavity.

A similar period of transient improvement may occur if a small rent in the spleen is first closed by adherent omentum or blood clot or if the spleen ruptures first into the extraperitoneal tissues at its hilum or between the layers of the gastrosplenic ligament. In classical cases the initial injury is followed by pain in the left side, often referred to the left shoulder (Kehr's sign). The patient may present with signs of progressive internal haemorrhage, but there may be only a slight fall in systolic pressure and a period of recovery may then follow, continuing for some hours or even a day or two. There may then be sudden collapse with left-sided or generalized abdominal pain and a severe and progressive fall in blood pressure. The physical signs are those of intraperitoneal haemorrhage; sometimes the spleen may be palpable, if enlarged by a splenic haematoma. Occasionally extraperitoneal bleeding in addition to the peritoneal bleeding gives rise to a phenomenon referred to as Ballance's sign. Haemorrhage into the extraperitoneal tissues causes a fixed dullness in the left flank whilst bleeding into the peritoneal cavity gives shifting dullness which is better appreciated in the right flank. If a rib has been fractured a plain radiograph may demonstrate it. Other non-specific radiological signs have been described and include increased density in the upper left quadrant of the abdomen, elevation of the left side of the diaphragm, displacement of the stomach or splenic flexure, dilatation of the stomach with serrations in the greater curve and fluid levels between loops of intestine.

Management

The diagnosis of ruptured spleen may be clinically obvious and signs of continued bleeding may render laparotomy essential after preoperative resuscitation. In all gunshot wounds and most knife wounds involving the spleen laparotomy is required to exclude other injuries. For closed injuries there has been a trend to conservatism since the 1960s. The mainspring of this has been the recognition of the serious potential late consequences of splenectomy, particularly in children, 2% of whom were found to have died of late fulminant infection after splenectomy for trauma. Non-operative management is sometimes feasible for splenic injuries, and splenic repair is often applicable when laparotomy is indicated. The management of splenic injuries has become more complex and difficult and requires more skill.[9]

If the patient is haemodynamically stable, and if other injuries can be excluded, investigation of the possibility of splenic injury should be undertaken using peritoneal lavage. If this demonstrates frank blood, further examination by technetium 99 m isotope scanning, ultrasound or computerized tomography (CT) is undertaken. Of these, CT is the most specific (Fig. 34.1) but all have a positive diagnostic accuracy in excess of 90%. A non-operative policy can cautiously be undertaken if there is continuing absence of evidence of progressive blood loss, i.e. no more than 4 units of transfusion in 48 hours in adults[10] or 40 ml/g in the first 24 hours in children[6] and in the absence of signs of other intra-abdominal injuries. If surgery is thus avoided the patient must be carefully observed in hospital for at least 6 days. Non-operative management carries the theoretical risk of delayed rupture and this has been reported as occurring

REFERENCES

6. Baesl T J, Filler R M Surg Clin North Am 1985; 65: 1269
7. Bauer T W, Haskins G E, Armitage J O Cancer 1981; 48: 2729
8. Danforth D D, Thorbjamarson B Ann Surg 1976; 183: 124
9. Wilson R H, Moorehead R J Injury 1992; 23: 5
10. Zucker K, Browns K et al Arch Surg 1984; 119: 400

a

b

c

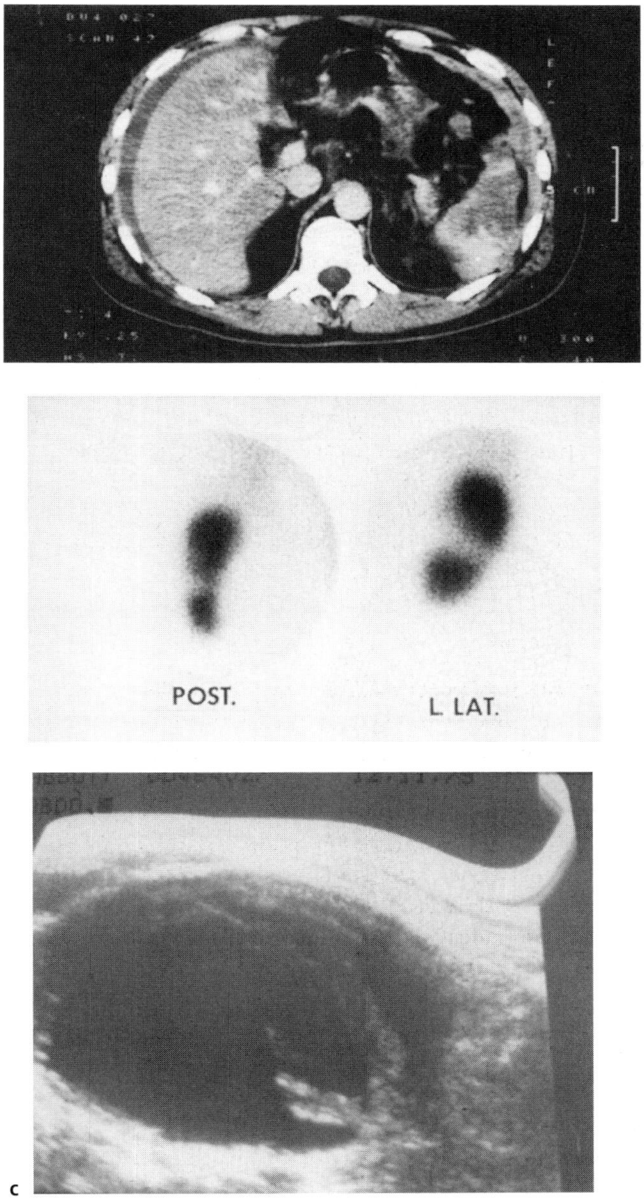

Fig. 34.1 Ruptured spleen: (**a**) CT scan; (**b**) isotope scan; (**c**) ultrasound scan.

as late as 2 weeks after injury.[11] It is, however, currently considered that delayed rupture more often represents delayed diagnosis of rupture rather than late rupture of an intrasplenic haematoma and experience has shown that when non-operative management is possible bleeding will normally have stopped within 12 hours of the injury.

Successful non-operative management in children has now been widely reported and in some series as many as 60–70% of children were managed non-operatively,[6] though in other series the figure has been less than 10%.[12] In general it is children who are more easily managed non-operatively than adults. Where continued bleeding or other injuries requires laparotomy, efforts should always be made to preserve the spleen. This has not been the policy in the past. In the first edition of this book Aird reflected the then current attitude, observing: 'Rupture of the spleen of course requires splenectomy'. Yet ever since the first successful partial splenectomy for trauma in 1734 efforts at conservation have been made, though it is only the recognition of overwhelming post-splenectomy infection that has changed the general attitude. John Gibbon in 1908 perhaps came close to the crux of the problem when he observed that 'if the spleen were not so easily removed fewer splenectomies for rupture would be reported'.[13]

Conservative surgery for splenic injury is now widely practised and experience shows that at the time of laparotomy there is a 30–50% chance of salvaging enough splenic tissue to be of value. The feasibility and techniques of splenic salvage are related to the severity of the injury and the skill and experience of the operator (Fig. 34.2). During surgery the spleen must be fully mobilized and inspected. Small tears may be managed by pressure and local application of haemostatic agents such as microfibrillary collagen. Fractures can be sutured with catgut on large blunt liver needles; the stitches may be buttressed on the capsular surface if necessary. The branches of the splenic artery are end arteries and so partial splenectomy is sometimes achievable after branch ligation; 84% of spleens are supplied by 2 major branches of the splenic artery and the remaining 16% by 3.[14] Avascular planes separate the territories of these arteries and ligation of the major branch assists in partial resection using that plane. The TA stapler has been found helpful in partial splenectomy.[15] Multiple fractures may sometimes be treated by an overall omental wrap or by firmly enclosing the whole spleen in an absorbable polyglactin mesh bag. Failure to achieve satisfactory haemostasis is an indication for splenectomy. Only very rarely is splenorrhaphy followed by a need for late re-operation for bleeding.[16]

Where splenectomy is necessary for trauma, attempts have been made to retain splenic function by implanting splenic fragments into the omentum.[17] Although there is ample evidence that such implants do function it is doubted that they provide a sufficient functional mass to prevent overwhelming post-splenectomy infection.[18]

Spontaneous splenic rupture

Truly spontaneous rupture of the spleen probably does not occur. The enlarged or engorged spleen can however rupture with minimal trauma and cases are particularly reported in patients with malaria or infectious mononucleosis. Splenic vascular malformations may also present as an apparent spontaneous rupture. Spontaneous rupture is treated as any other form of splenic rupture and conservative management may be appropriate.[19]

REFERENCES

11. Kluger Y, Paul D et al J Trauma 1994; 36: 568
12. Buyukunal C, Danismend N, Yeker D Br J Surg 1987; 74: 350
13. Gibbon J H Ann Surg 1908; 48: 152
14. Skandalakis P N, Colborn G L et al Surg Clin North Am 1993; 73: 747
15. Uranus S et al Am J Surg 1994; 168: 49
16. Stauch G O Am J Surg 1979; 137: 478
17. Kusminsky R E, Chang H H et al Surg Gynaecol Obst 1982; 155: 407
18. Moore G E, Stevens R, Moore E E, Aragon G E Am J Surg 1983; 146: 413
19. Schuler J G, Filtzer H Arch Surg 1995; 130: 662

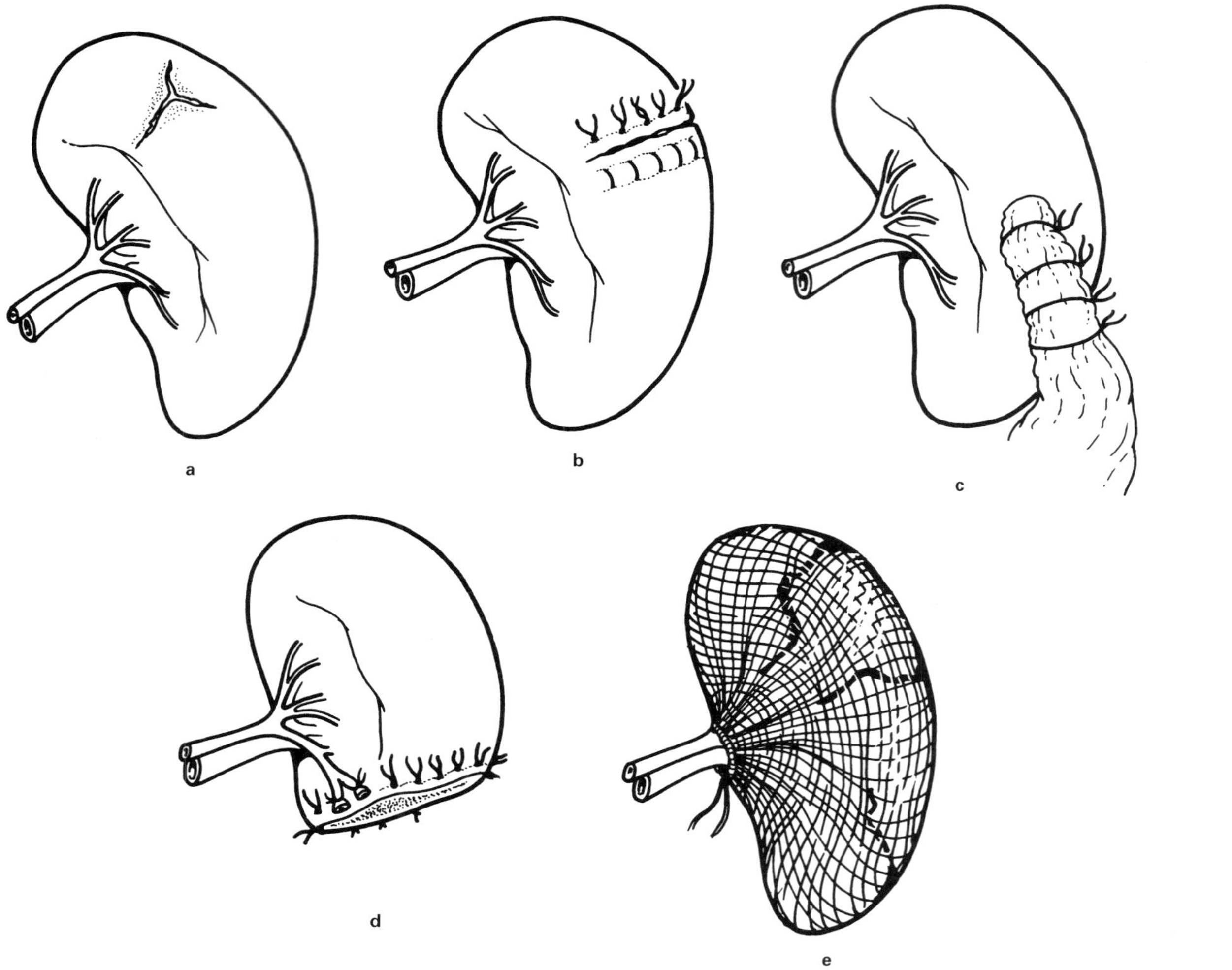

Fig. 34.2 Techniques of splenic conservation. (**a**) Capsular tear treated with thrombogenic agent; (**b**) rent in spleen closed with deep mattress sutures buttressed if necessary; (**c**) ragged tear packed with omentum; (**d**) traumatized pole amputated; (**e**) fragmented spleen packed together in an absorbable mesh bag.

Overwhelming post-splenectomy infection (OPSI)

One of the crucial functions of the spleen is the destruction of encapsulated micro-organisms in the circulating blood, especially *Streptococcus pneumoniae*, *Neisseria meningitidis* and *Haemophilus influenzae*. After splenectomy this ability is impaired and infection with one of these organisms can lead to a syndrome of overwhelming sepsis which carries a 50–90% risk of death. Typically there is a 2–3-day prodrome of a flu-like illness which then progresses to a high fever, malaise, vomiting and headache. Coma quickly develops and death usually follows within 24 hours. The organisms, usually *Streptococcus pneumoniae*, can be grown from the blood in huge quantities (more than 106/ml). Other investigations show acidosis, hypoglycaemia and disseminated intravascular coagulation. Post-mortem examination shows adrenal haemorrhage.

Splenectomy interferes with other host defences against sepsis, and splenectomized patients are generally more prone to infection than the normal population. However, other forms of sepsis, especially ordinary postoperative sepsis, should not be confused with overwhelming post-splenectomy infection which is a distinct clinical syndrome. Its true incidence is unclear[20] but for children who have been splenectomized for trauma it is probably around 1–2% whilst for adults it is 0.5% or less. Patients undergoing splenectomy for haematological reasons or malignancy have the highest incidence, the highest reported being after splenectomy for thalassaemia (10–14%).[21] Total splenectomy is unavoidable where the indications for operation are haematological; it is only in trauma patients that conservative splenic surgery is a realistic option for excluding the risk of overwhelming post-splenectomy infection. The incidence is sufficiently high in children to justify strenuous efforts at splenic conservation. However, the very low incidence in adults must be offset against the possible risk of attempts at splenic conservation.

REFERENCES

20. Dicataido A, Puleo S et al Br J Surg 1987; 74: 343
21. Posey D L, Marks C Am J Surg 1983; 145: 318

Table 34.3 Key guidelines for splenectomized patients. From Working Party of the British Committee for Standards in Haematology.[22]

- All splenectomized patients and those with functional hyposplenism should receive pneumococcal immunization (*A, B*).
- Documentation, communication, and re-immunization require attention (*A, B*).
- Patients not previously immunized should receive *Haemophilus influenzae* type b vaccine (*A, B*).
- Meningococcal immunization is not routinely recommended (*B*).
- Influenza immunization may be beneficial (*B*).
- Lifelong prophylactic antibiotics are recommended (oral phenoxymethylpenicillin or an alternative) (*A, B*).
- Asplenic patients are at risk of severe malaria (*A*).
- Animal and tick bites may be dangerous (*A*).
- Patients should be given a leaflet and a card to alert health professionals to their risk of overwhelming infection (*A, B*).
- Patients developing infection despite measures must be given a systemic antibiotic and urgently admitted to hospital (*A, B*).

A = Based on published evidence. *B* = Expert opinion.
N.B. There are no randomised controlled trials or case controlled studies on this issue.

Prophylaxis against post-splenectomy infection should be implemented in all patients who undergo total splenectomy. Long-term penicillins or erythromycin are of proven value in children, as the maximal incidence of overwhelming post-splenectomy infection occurs within 2 years of surgery. There is however a lifelong risk and prophylaxis with polyvalent vaccines against pneumococcus is also required. Additionally vaccination against *Haemophilus influenzae* is indicated in the non-immune, but meningococcal vaccination is not currently advised (see Table 34.3).[22] Vaccinations should ideally be given two weeks preoperatively and are not appropriate before the age of 2. The value of pneumococcal vaccines in adults is still debated; nevertheless, their value in autosplenectomized patients with sickle cell disease is proven. The long-term benefit in trauma patients remains to be assessed.

The doses of antibiotic used in prophylaxis and in treatment of post-splenectomy infection are summarized in Table 34.4.

SPLENOMEGALY

Palpable spleens are not always abnormal, and abnormal spleens are not always palpable. Of normal students, 3% have a palpable spleen;[23] by contrast the abnormal spleen of thrombocytopenic purpura is rarely enlarged. In general, however, the diseased spleen is larger than normal (200 g), even if it is impalpable. Size may be assessed by ultrasound or CT scanning or more quantitatively by radioisotope scanning. Very large spleens (i.e. more than 2000 g) extending into the lower half of the abdomen account for less than 20% of patients undergoing elective splenectomy in western practice (Table 34.5). Quite pronounced splenomegaly can develop with only minimal symptoms. Sudden enlargement will however produce aching upper abdominal pain whilst established splenomegaly may be felt as a dragging, dull pain in the left upper quadrant. Some very large spleens are completely symptomless. Giant splenomegaly can compress the stomach, producing significant

REFERENCES

22. Working Party of the British Committee for Standards in Haematology Br Med J 1996; 312: 430
23. McIntyre O R, Ebauch F G Ann Intern Med 1967; 66: 301

Table 34.4 Dosing regimens for antibiotic prophylaxis and treatment. From Working Party of the British Committee for Standards in Haematology.[22]

Antibiotic	*Oral prophylaxis*	*Treatment for suspected infection*†
Penicillin		
Adult	250–500 mg 12-hourly‡§	1.2 g 4–6-hourly*
Child aged 5–14 years	250 mg 12-hourly§	200–300 mg/kg per day in six divided doses (maximum 6 g)*
Child under 5 years¶	125 mg 12-hourly§	200–300 mg/kg per day in six divided doses (maximum 6 g)*
Erythromycin (base)		
Adult + child over 8 years	250–500 mg daily	0.5–1.0 g 6-hourly by mouth or intravenously
Child aged 2–8 years	250 mg daily	250 mg 6-hourly by mouth 12.5 mg/kg/day intravenously by infusion in four divided doses
Child under 2 years	125 mg daily	12.5 mg/kg/day by mouth or intravenously by infusion in four divided doses
Amoxycillin/co-amoxiclav (doses according to amoxycillin content)		
Adult	250–500 mg daily	0.5–1.0 g 8-hourly by mouth or intravenously
Child aged 5–14 years	125 mg daily	250 mg 8-hourly by mouth 90 mg/kg/day intravenously in three divided doses
Child aged 1–5 years	10 mg/kg/day	125 mg 8-hourly by mouth 90 mg/kg/day intravenously in three divided doses
Child under 1 year	10 mg/kg/day	62.5 mg 8-hourly by mouth 90 mg/kg/day intravenously in three divided doses
Cefotaxime		
Adult	Not suitable	2 g 8-hourly intravenously
Child under 14 years	Not suitable	100 mg/kg/day intravenously in three divided doses (maximum 12 g)
Ceftriaxone		
Adult	Not suitable	1–2 g once daily intravenously
Child under 14 years	Not suitable	80 mg/kg/day intravenously in a single dose (maximum 4 g)
Chloramphenicol (only patients allergic to penicillins and cephalosporins)		
All patients	Not suitable	Expert advice

†Established infection may require much higher doses given in hospital; ‡If compliance is a problem 500 mg once daily is acceptable; §Phenoxymethylpenicillin (oral); *Benzylpenicillin (intravenous); ¶Seek expert advice for neonatal doses

Table 34.5 Causes of truly massive splenomegaly*

Chronic
Chronic granulocytic leukaemia
Myeloid metaplasia
Polycythaemia vera (end-stage)
Primary thrombocythaemia (uncommon)
Malignant reticuloendotheliosis
Malignant lymphoma
Hairy cell leukaemia
Hodgkin's disease (rare)
Gaucher's disease
Cooley's anaemia
Sickle cell anaemia (rare)
Kala-azar
Malaria in combination with, for example, cirrhosis
Sarcoid (rare)
Felty's syndrome (rare)
Acute
Malaria: splenic crisis with blackwater fever
Sickle cell anaemia splenic crisis

*The spleen extends into one or both lower quadrants of the abdomen or weighs >2000 g

Table 34.6 A classification of causes of splenomegaly

Infections
Acute, subacute, chronic
Inflammatory diseases
Rheumatoid arthritis, sarcoid, lupus, amyloid
Neoplasms
Leukaemia, lymphoma, polycythaemia vera, myelofibrosis
Primary tumours, metastases, cysts
Haemolytic diseases
Hereditary, acquired: acute, chronic
Deficiency diseases
Severe iron deficiency anaemia, pernicious anaemia
Storage diseases
Gaucher, Niemann–Pick
Splenic vein hypertension
Cirrhosis, splenic and portal vein thrombosis and stenosis
Idiopathic
With or without hypersplenism

anorexia and early satiety. Severe pain is usually only the product of partial or total splenic infarction; if the diaphragmatic surface of the spleen is involved, referred shoulder-tip pain may be experienced.

Mild splenomegaly is a common association with many diseases but only those causes of substantial splenomegaly are identified here. It is useful to classify splenomegaly on the basis of its causative mechanism (Table 34.6).

Not all causes of splenomegaly will require splenectomy as part of their treatment. Elective splenectomy is indicated:

1. To treat haematological disease in the form of hypersplenism.
2. To diagnose an obscure splenomegaly.
3. To treat splenic cysts, tumours and abscesses.
4. For the relief of discomfort due to the volume of the spleen.
5. Occasionally to stage and sometimes to diagnose lymphoma, especially Hodgkin's disease.
6. As a consequence of surgery to adjacent organs, e.g. resection of a splenic artery aneurysm, distal pancreatectomy, radical gastrectomy.

HYPERSPLENISM

Splenectomy as part of the treatment of haematological disease is usually undertaken to reverse hypersplenism. Hypersplenism is a rather indefinite term classically implying the combination of:

1. Splenomegaly.
2. Any combination of anaemia, leucopenia or thrombocytopenia.
3. Compensatory bone marrow hyperplasia.
4. Improvement after splenectomy.[24]

A more pragmatic definition of hypersplenism is: 'the spleen has become more harmful than beneficial[25] or 'when a person is haematologically better off without a spleen, he had hypersplenism'.[26] Such pragmatic definitions contain an element of retrospection in the diagnosis and there in lies the problem for the haematologist and surgeon debating whether to embark upon splenectomy. The causes of hypersplenism vary and reflect the different functions of the spleen. Experience shows that for some causes of hypersplenism, splenectomy can be confidently anticipated to improve—though rarely to cure—the effects of the underlying disease. In others the benefit is much less predictable. The severity of hypersplenism tends to be proportional to the size of the spleen.

IMMUNE THROMBOCYTOPENIC PURPURA (IDIOPATHIC THROMBOCYTOPENIC PURPURA) (ITP)

ITP is a syndrome in which the dominant feature is a persistently low platelet count. In the great majority it is an immune or autoimmune disease. Although historically it is identified as ITP, other causes should be excluded including exposure to drugs (especially quinidine, sulphonamides and thiazides), auto- or alloantibodies following transfusion, lymphoproliferative disease, preclinical acquired immune deficiency syndrome, collagen vascular disease, thyroid disease, viral infection and intravenous drug abuse.

ITP is seen in patients of all ages. In children it is particularly encountered following a viral illness and usually remits spontaneously. Splenectomy is only rarely indicated where persisting profound thrombocytopenia causes bleeding which is difficult to manage. The platelet count may be raised by steroid therapy or equally effectively—but more expensively—by the infusion of gammaglobulin.

ITP in adults is a disease usually of insidious onset and chronic pattern. The patients are usually young women and the aetiology centres on the production of an IgG antiplatelet antibody. This leads to the phagocytosis of platelets and their destruction by the

REFERENCES

24. Damashek W Bull N Y Acad Med 1955; 31: 113
25. Eichner E R Am J Med 1979; 66: 311
26. Crosby W H Ann Rev Med 1962; 13: 127

reticuloendothelial system, predominantly the spleen. Physical signs relate to the thrombocytopenia. Petechiae and purpura are common signs; mucosal bleeding, easy bruising and prolonged bleeding from cuts are common. Menorrhagia is also seen but frank spontaneous and serious bleeding only occurs in about 1% of patients. The spleen is not enlarged.

The usual primary treatment is with steroids but less than 20% of adults remain in long-lasting remission after steroid therapy. Indications for splenectomy are failure to respond to steroids, inability to withdraw steroids after 6 months, the side-effects of steroids and pregnancy. Some 80% benefit from splenectomy[27,28] with permanent remission. The majority of the remainder have a partial but useful remission. For those who relapse, subsequent medical treatment with steroids and immunosuppression is more efficacious if splenectomy has been performed.[29] ITP is by far the most common haematological indication for splenectomy.[30]

Bleeding can occur spontaneously when the platelet count is less than 20×10^9/l, but excessive bleeding in response to surgery can occur when it is 20–70 $\times 10^9$/l. Once the decision to undertake splenectomy has been made the patient should receive a short course of steroids with the intention of bringing the platelet count into the normal range. Immunoglobulin is given to those who do not respond to steroids. Fresh platelets (4–6 u) should be available at the time of operation if the count is below 70 000, but should not be administered until the splenic artery has been ligated. At the time of operation about 20% of ITP patients are found to have accessory spleens; this figure may be 40% in children.[27] If these accessory spleens are not removed thrombocytopenia will quickly recur; they should therefore always be sought at the time of splenectomy. Recurrence of ITP because of accessory spleens can occur even when there are persisting Howell–Jolly bodies in the red cells in the peripheral blood. Pre- and/or intraoperative scanning with technetium 99 m-labelled red blood cells allows identification of accessory splenic tissue[31] though this is not widely used in practice.

After the operation the platelet count usually rises within 2 weeks and if it rises promptly above 500×10^9/l complete remission can be predicted. A rise to a peak of 100–200 $\times 10^9$/l is associated with only a 25% chance of a cure.[32]

If a woman with ITP becomes pregnant there is a 50% chance of fetal thrombocytopenia as the antiplatelet IgG crosses the placental barrier[33] and splenectomy should be considered in the middle trimester if there is no response to steroids and/or immunoglobulin. The fetal risk of neonatal thrombocytopenia is not closely related to the maternal platelet count.

ITP and acquired immune deficiency syndrome

ITP is one of the major haematological effects of infection with the human immunodeficiency virus and is predominantly seen in homosexual men and drug addicts as well as haemophiliac patients. Steroids in these patients are largely ineffective and should be avoided. Although spontaneous remission may occur, patients usually require splenectomy. This produces remission in about 25% of patients; it may be of value to combine it with preoperative intravenous immunoglobulin[34] or zidovudine.

Thrombotic thrombocytopenia (Moscheowitz's syndrome)

Thrombotic thrombocytopenia is a rare disease occurring in young adults. It is characterized by the pentad of thrombocytopenic purpura, microangiopathic haemolytic anaemia, fever, renal impairment and neurological dysfunction. The mechanism of the widespread intravascular coagulation is unknown, but it is postulated that soluble immune complexes cause vascular damage initiating the process. The disease differs from the more commonly encountered disseminated intravascular coagulation syndrome, but overlaps somewhat with haemolytic uraemic syndrome. Until recently the disease was usually fatal. The current regimes of early and enthusiastic treatment with plasmapheresis and plasma infusions have improved the prospect of survival to better than 70%. Occasionally other treatments with antiplatelet agents and steroids are necessary. In the rare resistant patient splenectomy seems to play an important role in maintaining remission, though the mechanism of the benefit is not understood.[35–37]

SPLENECTOMY IN THE HAEMOLYTIC ANAEMIAS

There are five causes of haemolytic anaemia which are amenable to treatment by splenectomy. They are congenital spherocytosis and elliptocytosis, pyruvate kinase defi-ciency, thalassaemia and acquired autoimmune haemolytic anaemia.

Congenital spherocytosis

Spherocytosis is a congenital red cell anomaly usually transmitted as a Mendelian dominant. The underlying defect in the red cell membrane allows a change in shape and increased mechanical and osmotic fragility. These abnormal cells can be seen in the peripheral blood. The loss of deformability allows the abnormal cells to be trapped in the splenic microcirculation and removed by the reticulo-endothelial cells and extravascular haemolysis. The effect of the abnormality varies from very mild to severe. Severely affected individuals are chronically anaemic, mildly jaundiced and have hepatosplenomegaly. With increasing age pigment stones develop in the biliary system and may be symptomatic. Stones are uncommon before the age of 10 years, but occur eventually in up to 50% of patients. Viral illnesses, particularly parvovirus, may precipitate reticulocytopenic crises.

REFERENCES

27. Mintz S J, Petersen S R et al Arch Surg 1981; 116: 645
28. Shwartz S I World J Surg 1985; 9: 416
29. Picozzi V J, Roeske W R, Creger W P Am J Med 1980; 69: 690
30. Schwartz S I World J Surg 1996; 20: 1156
31. Wallace D, Fronun D, Thomas D Surgery 1982; 91: 134
32. Najean Y, Ardillous N Presse Med 1971; 79: 443
33. Cines D B, Dusak B et al N Engl J Med 1982; 306: 826
34. Beard J, Savidge G F Br J Haematol 1988; 68: 303
35. Thompson H W, McCarthy L J Arch Intern Med 1983; 143: 2117
36. Wells A D, Majumdar G, Slater N G P, Young A E Br J Surg 1991; 78: 1389
37. Schneider P A, Rayner A A et al Ann Surg 1985; 202: 318

Splenectomy is indicated in the majority of patients with hereditary spherocytosis. Operation should be delayed as long as possible, preferably to the age of 15 years or at least until the age of 5 years if possible. Older children and adults should undergo ultrasound examination of the biliary tree prior to splenectomy; if stones are present, cholecystectomy should be undertaken at the same time as splenectomy.[38] Splenectomy prevents haemolysis and red cell survival becomes normal though the red cell abnormality persists.

Congenital elliptocytosis

Congenital elliptocytosis is clinically akin to spherocytosis; however, the cells form ellipses rather than spheres. Splenectomy is only indicated for symptomatic disease and this is rare as red cell survival is not usually significantly shortened.

Pyruvate kinase deficiency

Pyruvate kinase deficiency is inherited as an autosomal recessive trait and results in an inability of the red cells to synthesize adenosine triphosphate for their needs. This leads to membrane damage and cellular distortion with premature culling by the spleen. The spleen is usually moderately enlarged and the anaemia is sometimes improved by splenectomy, but if the anaemia persists the continuing reactive thrombocytosis may predispose to thrombophlebitis. The condition should be distinguished from glucose-6-phosphate dehydrogenase deficiency where there is no splenomegaly; haemolysis occurs only when the body is challenged by infection, oxidative drugs or fava beans. Splenectomy is not indicated in glucose-6-phosphate dehydrogenase deficiency.

Thalassaemia

A congenital defect in the synthesis of one of the four polypeptide chains of the haemoglobin molecule leads to thalassaemia. The effect of the deficiency of one polypeptide fragment is the surplus production of normal polypeptide which, as it has no pair to bind with, precipitates within the red cell and its precursors, producing cells which die in the marrow or are prematurely culled from the circulation by the spleen. From a surgical standpoint the most important thalassaemia is β thalassaemia major. These patients commonly require splenectomy due to hypersplenism and increasing blood transfusion requirements. Other forms of thalassaemia such as thalasaemia intermedia syndromes occasionally require splenectomy due to the development of hypersplenism.

Homozygous β thalassaemia produces its effects in early childhood and is clinically characterized by anaemia, retarded growth, hepatosplenomegaly and an expanded bone marrow. The blood smear shows a microcytic hypochromic anaemia with nucleated red cells. The diagnosis is confirmed by haemoglobin electrophoresis.

Iron overload as the result of repeated transfusion is the most dangerous outcome of this syndrome; splenectomy may be beneficial not only in reducing the need for transfusion in patients with β thalassaemia major but also when a massive splenomegaly is painful. Partial splenectomy by embolization has been proposed as an alternative to splenectomy.[39]

Acquired haemolytic anaemia

In this disease haemolysis is the result of production of an IgG warm autoantibody against red cells; the presence of the IgG antibody on the red cell surface is confirmed by a direct Coombs' test. Acquired haemolytic anaemia may occur spontaneously or in association with other infections, malignancies and autoimmune disease. The severity and length of the haemolysis vary, and principal therapy is by transfusion and steroids. Sustained remission after steroid therapy only occurs in 20% of patients; in those who relapse and in patients for whom steroids are contraindicated splenectomy may be of value, not only reducing splenic removal of red cells but also reducing antibody production. The assessment of splenic uptake of isotope-labelled red blood cells is not a reliable predictor of a good response to surgery.[40,41] IgM cold antibody acquired haemolytic anaemia is not treated by splenectomy.

SPLENECTOMY FOR LEUKAEMIA

Splenectomy has been used in the treatment of chronic leukaemia since Bryant's case in 1866.[42] The prompt death of that patient and the high mortality in subsequent cases led to its abandonment until indications for it were clarified by Ferrata & Fieschi in 1939;[43] these criteria remain valid today, namely that splenectomy is solely indicated to treat the effects of secondary hypersplenism and to alleviate discomfort and pain caused by a large or infarcted spleen.

Chronic lymphatic leukaemia (chronic lymphocytic leukaemia)

Chronic lymphatic leukaemia occurs primarily in the elderly; splenomegaly occurs in parallel with lymphadenopathy elsewhere, hepatomegaly and infiltration of other organs. Palliation of this insidious and slowly progressive disease is primarily by chemotherapy, steroids and splenic irradiation, but when the spleen is painful or hypersplenism predominates, splenectomy is indicated. Splenectomy does not alter survival in this condition. Occasionally chronic lymphatic leukaemia is complicated by an autoimmune haemolytic anaemia.

Chronic myeloid leukaemia (chronic granulocytic leukaemia)

In this disease the peripheral leucocyte count is raised by an outpouring of granulocytic cells. Hepatosplenomegaly is common.

REFERENCES

38. Lawrie G M, Ham J M Surg Gynecol Obstet 1974; 139: 1
39. Politis C, Spigos D G et al Br Med J 1987; 294: 665
40. Schwartz S I, Adams J T, Baumen A W Splenectomy for Haematologic Disorders. Year Book, Chicago 1971
41. Coon W W Arch Surg 1985; 120: 625
42. Bryant T Guy's Hosp Rep 1866; 12: 444
43. Ferrata A, Fieschi A Atti Soc Ital Ematol 1939; 6: 1

The disease tends to be biphasic: an early chronic phase lasting 1–4 years is followed by an acute terminal phase in which blast cells flood the circulation.

Splenectomy in the chronic phase does not delay the onset of the acute phase but occasionally splenectomy is indicated in patients who, rather than transforming into an acute phase, enter an 'accelerated' phase dominated by increasing splenomegaly or who develop myelofibrosis (see below). However, as a result of poor platelet function haemorrhage may be a problem. Splenectomy is not indicated after acute transformation.[44]

Hairy cell leukaemia

This rare disease accounts for 2–5% of all leukaemias. The pathological cell is possibly a B lymphocyte. The filamentous cytoplasmic projections seen on these cells on light microscopy give the disease its name. In contrast to other leukaemias, chemotherapy is not a useful primary treatment and it may precipitate worsening of the pancytopenia which is usually present. The presence of splenomegaly in this condition, caused by the trapping of large quantities of abnormal cells, led to the introduction of splenectomy as a means of treatment with the intention of preventing secondary sequestration of normal peripheral blood cells and of removing a large tumour load. A multicentre retrospective review of splenectomy in hairy cell leukaemia showed only minimal benefit, confined to those patients with severe pancytopenia and splenomegaly.[45] The benefit is unrelated to spleen weight.[46] By reversing the pancytopenia of this disease splenectomy may allow chemotherapy and may thus be a useful adjunctive therapy but is now only employed when deoxycoformycin or interferon therapy has failed. There is an increased incidence of 'atypical' infections in patients after splenectomy for hairy cell leukaemia.

SPLENECTOMY FOR OTHER CONDITIONS

Felty's syndrome

A small proportion of patients with severe chronic rheumatoid arthritis develop granulocytopenia and splenomegaly. These may be complicated by recurrent infection and leg ulcers which resist healing. The underlying pathology appears to be an antibody against the granulocytes. Splenectomy is indicated for recurrent infections, anaemia requiring transfusion and in those with non-healing leg ulcers.[47]

Gaucher's disease

The surplus glucocerebrosides produced in this disease accumulate in the spleen causing splenomegaly and hypersplenism. The spleen in part acts as a useful sump for these substances and splenectomy may be followed by an accelerated infiltration of the marrow and liver. If specific therapy with β-glucosidase (ceredase) is unsuccessful or unavailable splenectomy should be considered for those with life-threatening cytopenia which can be confidently attributed to hypersplenism.[48]

Myelofibrosis (agnogenic myeloid metaplasia, myelosclerosis)

Myelofibrosis is either idiopathic or secondary to the existing haematological diseases of polycythaemia rubra vera, primary thrombocythaemia and chronic myeloid leukaemia. The idiopathic form of the disease generally affects the middle-aged and elderly. There is progressive proliferation of fibroblasts producing sclerosis of the bone marrow which seriously compromises medullary haemopoiesis. Extramedullary haemopoiesis occurs in the liver and spleen. The dominant clinical effects are anaemia and hepatosplenomegaly. The splenomegaly may be gross: spleen weight often exceeds 2 kg. The spleen is enlarged by the mass of haematopoietic tissue within it. Its bulk is uncomfortable and pressure on the stomach limits the patient's ability to take an adequate diet. In addition the large spleen acts as an effective arteriovenous shunt taking up to 30% of the cardiac output; this increases blood volume and cardiac work. The increased portal blood flow may produce portal hypertension. Although thrombocytosis may occur the majority of patients are thrombocytopenic.

The role of splenectomy is limited and the criteria are specific. About 15% of all patients will require it. It should be used to control anaemia, thrombocytopenia, splenic pain or discomfort and high-output cardiac failure. The patients should be chosen on clinical grounds as splenectomy has no role in treating the underlying disease. If indicated, splenectomy should not be delayed as it carries a substantially higher morbidity and mortality than splenectomy for any other haematological condition. This is largely because of age, poor general health, cardiac insufficiency and increased risk of sepsis. There is in addition a particularly pronounced risk of postoperative embolism.[49,50] The occurrence of postoperative thrombocythaemia is an indication for antiplatelet treatment in all such patients and chemotherapy in some. Splenic irradiation is an unsatisfactory alternative to splenectomy. Approximately 20% of all patients undergo acute leukaemic transformation and although some patients live for many years, the average survival from diagnosis to death in myelofibrosis is 3–4 years.[51]

SPLENIC CYSTS AND TUMOURS

Solitary space-occupying lesions in the spleen are discovered either by the investigation of the mild symptoms they produce or as incidental findings at operation or imaging for another purpose. Solitary lymphomas are sometimes discovered during the investigation of non-specific systemic symptoms.

REFERENCES

44. Wolf D J, Silner R T, Coleman M Ann Intern Med 1978; 89: 684
45. Jansen H, Hermans J Cancer 1981; 47: 2066
46. Golomb H M, Vardiman J W Blood 1983; 61: 349
47. Coon W W Am J Surg 1985; 149: 272
48. Wintrobe M M Clinical Haematology. Lea & Febiger, Philadelphia 1981
49. Coon W W, Liepman M K Surg Gynecol Obstet 1982; 154: 561
50. Malmaeus J, Akret Adami H O, Hagberg H Br J Surg 1986; 73: 720
51. Wilson R E, Rosenthal D S et al World J Surg 1985; 9: 431

Cysts

Worldwide the vast majority of splenic cysts are parasitic, caused by *Taenia echinococcus*. Non-parasitic cysts may be true cellular lined cysts or, more commonly, false cysts. These latter arise from organized haematomas, infarcts or inflammation. True cysts may be dermoid cysts or a bloodfilled vascular malformation. CT scanning is the method of choice to investigate cystic lesions and will allow the diagnosis of hydatid cysts. Repeat scanning with contrast identifies vascular lesions. If surgical intervention is necessary to relieve symptoms then partial[52] or total splenectomy is preferable to marsupialization or enucleation.[53,54]

Tumours

Lymphoma primarily presenting in the spleen is rare. Most tumours present with fever, malaise and weight loss. Involvement may be diffuse or as a solid tumour mass. Any type of lymphoma, including Hodgkin's disease, may present primarily in the spleen, but 50% of cases will have associated retroperitoneal nodes and 60% will have marrow involvement at the time of diagnosis. Prognosis is no different from that of lymphoma presenting elsewhere.[54,55]

Other tumours presenting in the spleen are most commonly vascular malformations of varying types, including lymphatic malformations. Malignant haemangiosarcomas are rare, but may present in unusual ways such as microangiopathic haemolytic anaemia, ascites, pleural effusions, or spontaneous rupture. Other malignant tumours are Kaposi's sarcoma and metastases. Although the spleen is involved by metastases in 7% of all those patients who die from malignant disease, clinically significant solitary metastases in the spleen are uncommon. The spleen's high blood flow and filter functions suggest that it should be a common site for metastases, but its powers of destruction of abnormal cells are formidable and as effective against malignant cells as against others. Other lymphoid and non-lymphoid tumours are occasionally seen in the spleen, as are hamartomas, but they are also very rare.[23]

SPLENIC ABSCESS

Splenic abscess is very rare, probably as a result of the spleen's exceptional ability to cope with septic and foreign material. It may, however, occur as a result of haematogenous spread from endocarditis, lung abscesses or as a result of intravenous drug abuse or in the immunocompromised host. Secondary splenic abscesses develop in areas of trauma or infarction, usually in association with other splenic disease such as sickle cell disease. Splenic abscess complicating salmonella infection and malaria was once common, but is now unusual in western practice. It is almost unknown for subphrenic abscess to have originated as a primary splenic abscess. Ochsner & Graves found only two such cases in a review of 3000 subphrenic abscesses.[56]

Splenic abscess presents as the clinical triad of left upper quadrant abdominal pain, fever and the systemic signs of sepsis. Diagnosis is by ultrasound or CT scanning and treatment has traditionally been by splenectomy, though experience with percutaneous drainage now shows this to be a safe and effective treatment for unilocular abscesses.[57,58]

THE OPERATION OF SPLENECTOMY

The vast majority of splenectomies are undertaken by open laparotomy but there are an increasing number of reports of laparoscopic splenectomy.[59–61] This route, however, is only to be considered for small or normal sized spleens. Compared to the open procedure laparoscopic splenectomy is time consuming, technically demanding and runs a greater risk of overlooking accessory splenic tissue. A few comparative studies have been published[62] and it is likely that the eventual conclusion will be that, in suitably trained hands, laparoscopic splenectomy can be appropriate for the removal of small, spleens, particularly those associated with immune thrombocytopenic purpura.[63]

The operation of open splenectomy

Central to the safe removal of the spleen is the process of mobilization. How this is done depends on the size of the spleen. Normally the spleen is held medially by a thin gastrocolic omentum and laterally by the lienorenal ligament. With a normal spleen these are easily identified; in the open operation for a normal or moderately enlarged spleen a hand slipped between the spleen and the diaphragm allows the organ to be mobilized easily up and away to the right from its bed, allowing easy access to the splenic vessels in the hilum for ligation. However, when the spleen enlarges, not only does it enlarge into the abdomen but also between the layers of the lienorenal ligament, separating them, so that the spleen becomes to some extent an extraperitoneal organ. This leads to misjudgement of the size of the spleen, as well as making it impossible to deliver the spleen by passing a hand behind it. Such difficulty may be interpreted as the presence of adhesions, but this is not the case. Adhesions between the spleen and diaphragm are rare and occur only in cases where there has been serious perisplenitis, usually from infarction of part of the organ. The spleen may also enlarge between the layers of the gastrosplenic ligament; its anterior edge may come so close to the greater curvature of the stomach that ligation of the omentum between these organs may be difficult (Fig. 34.3).

REFERENCES

52. Sagar P M, McMahon M J Br J Surg 1988; 75: 488
53. Sirinek K R, Evans W E Am J Surg 1973; 126: 8
54. Morganstem L, Rosenberg J, Geller S A World J Surg 1985; 9: 486
55. Spier C M, Kieldberg C R et al Arch Pathol Lab Med 1985; 109: 1076
56. Ochsner C, Graves D Ann Surg 1938; 98: 961
57. Sarr M C, Zuidema G D Surgery 1982; 92: 480
58. Lerner R M, Spataro R F Radiology 1984; 153: 643
59. Cuschieri A et al J Roy Coll Surg Edinb 1992; 37: 414
60. Robles A E, Andrews H G, Garberolgio C Int Surg 1994; 79: 332
61. Arregui M E, Barteau J, Davis C J Int Surg 1994; 79: 335
62. Beanes S, Emil S et al A Surgeon 1995; 61: 908
63. Hashizume M, Ohta M et al Surg Laparosc Endosc 1996; 6: 129

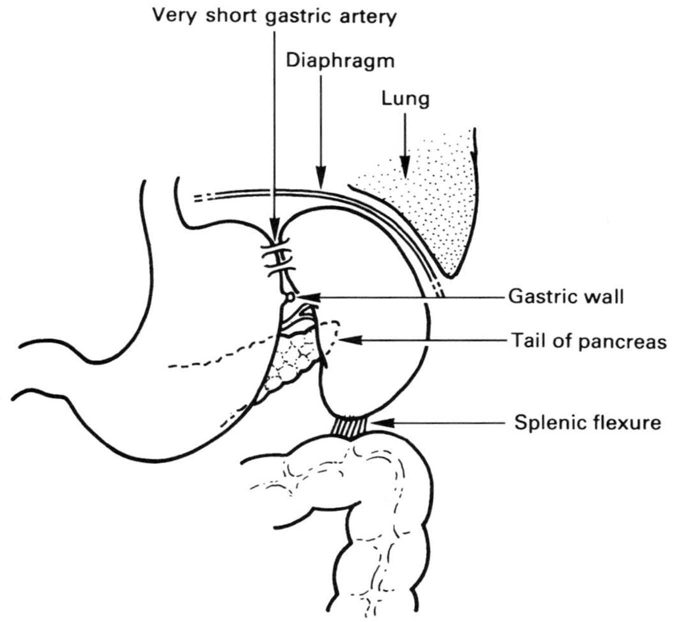

Fig. 34.3 Points of danger during excision of a large spleen.

In cases of giant splenomegaly it is prudent not to attempt early mobilization of the spleen, but to approach it from the front. After making a long midline incision, the splenic part of the gastrocolic omentum is divided between multiple clamps and the short gastric vessels tied one by one. The most cranial of these is usually the shortest and the largest and often presents the most difficulty. The lesser sac having been thus entered, the splenic artery should be ligated in continuity as it runs along the upper border of the pancreas. The separate branches of the splenic arteries and vein are now ligated in the hilum, taking care not to damage the tail of the pancreas which is sometimes engulfed by the enlarging spleen. Thus far no attempt has been made to mobilize the spleen out of the abdomen. Once the majority of vessels have been ligated the lienorenal ligament can be divided with scissors, blindly if necessary, and the spleen delivered from the abdomen. The enlarged spleen and its veins are often very fragile and may rupture with manipulation, hence the prudent manoeuvre of early ligation of the splenic artery. Even the largest of spleens can usually be delivered transabdominally and a thoracoabdominal approach is almost never indicated.

When splenectomy is performed for haematological disease a search should be made for accessory spleens in the gastrocolic omentum and along the line of the splenic vein (Table 34.2). Where malignant disease is suspected a coeliac node and liver biopsy are added. When splenectomy is performed in the presence of thrombocytopenia or when platelet function is abnormal, infusion of 2 or 4 u of platelet concentrate may be necessary. Platelet infusion should be withheld until after ligation of the splenic artery.

Whether splenectomy is performed for giant spleen or for haematological disease, it is prudent to drain the subphrenic space with a closed vacuum drainage system which is removed 24 h after operation. If it is suspected that pancreatic juices may be leaking from a damaged pancreatic tail, this can be confirmed or refuted by an assessment of the amylase level in the drain fluid.

THE SEQUELAE OF SPLENECTOMY

Splenectomy for splenomegaly removes the functioning arteriovenous shunt which was the result of a large splenic blood flow. The blood volume therefore rapidly falls and cardiac and pulmonary function are improved. The haemoglobin rises and within the first 2 or 3 days there is usually leucocytosis and thrombocytosis. The former may rise to levels as high as 50×10^9/l and may mislead the surgical staff into diagnosing sepsis. The thrombocytosis frequently exceeds 500×10^9/l and thus increases the risk of thromboembolic disease. This risk is sufficiently great to require prophylaxis against thrombosis in all patients.

COMPLICATIONS OF SPLENECTOMY

Intraoperative haemorrhage requiring transfusion is not uncommon when large spleens are removed and is often caused by tearing of the fragile splenic capsule or veins. Postoperative haematoma may collect in the subphrenic space, and infection of this can readily lead to subphrenic abscess. Prophylactic antibiotics reduce this risk and, whilst open drainage systems increase the risk of sepsis, closed vacuum drainage for 24 hours appears to be beneficial.

The diaphragm stretched over a large spleen functions poorly after splenectomy and left basal atelectasis or lower lobe collapse with pulmonary infection is common. Ligation of the short gastric veins may leave the stomach congested and inert and a nasogastric tube should therefore be inserted at the time of operation. Gastric haemorrhage may result from excessive congestion while too close ligation of veins on the stomach or colonic wall may lead to perforation. Damage to the pancreatic tail can lead to a leak of pancreatic fluid and the serious complication of partial or total wound dehiscence and a pancreatic fistula. It is preferable to excise the tail of the pancreas if it is severely damaged during splenectomy.

Other complications include portal vein thrombosis which can occur in thrombocythaemic patients by propagation of clot from the ligated splenic vein. The small bowel may stick to the denuded area below the diaphragm, leading to small bowel obstruction. Be warned that the radiologist may diagnose such aberrant loops of small bowel as the fluid levels of a subphrenic abscess! Spillage of spleen cells may produce splenosis if the cells seed and grow (Fig. 34.4). Such splenosis or overlooked accessory spleens may lead to recurrence of the original haematological abnormality.

Following splenectomy patients have an increased risk of all forms of sepsis compared to normal patients, including pneumonia and pyelonephritis as well as 'overwhelming post-splenectomy infection'.[64] There is also an increased risk of deep vein thrombosis and pulmonary embolism. All these dangers are maximal in the first 3 months after surgery.

REFERENCE

64. Shaw J H F, Print C G Br J Surg 1989; 76: 1074

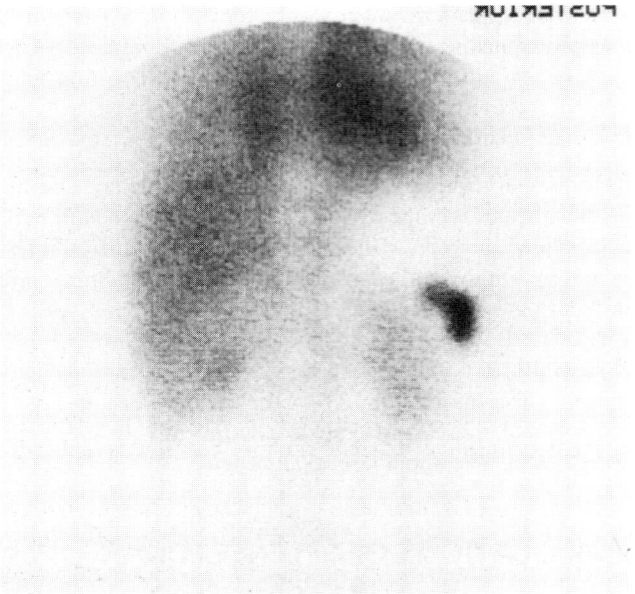

Fig. 34.4 Isotope scan showing regrowth of splenic tissue after splenectomy for trauma. Such tissue may derive from implanted cells shed from the ruptured spleen or from hypertrophy of a small accessory spleen.

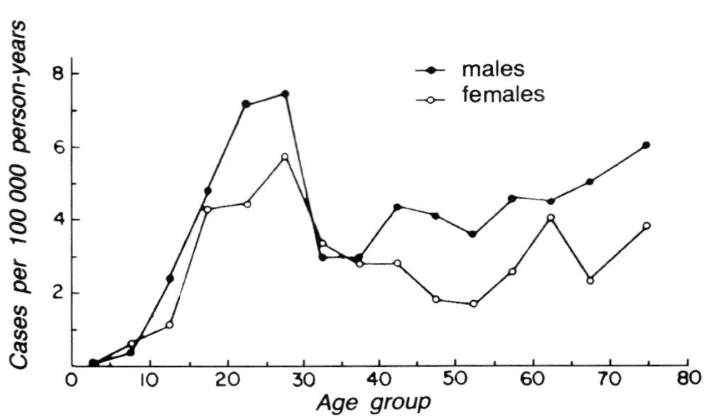

Fig. 34.5 Age-specific incidence rates for Hodgkin's disease. From Gutersohn & Cole.[65]

Lymphoma

A. R. Timothy

The lymphomas account for less than 5% of all new malignancies diagnosed annually in the UK, yet they have an importance far greater than their incidence. Improvements in radiotherapy and chemotherapy over the past 20 years now offer many of these patients the opportunity for cure of their disease. There are many clinical differences between Hodgkin's disease and the non-Hodgkin lymphomas which are reflected in the differing approaches to pretreatment staging investigations and to treatment itself; they are therefore discussed separately.

HODGKIN'S DISEASE

In western countries, Hodgkin's disease accounts for approximately 1% of newly diagnosed cancers. Over the past two decades there has been a slight increase in incidence but this has been accompanied by a clear reduction in mortality, reflecting the increasing success of treatment. The disease demonstrates a classic bimodal age incidence (Fig. 34.5).[65] While uncommon in children, the incidence reaches a peak in the late teens and mid 20s, falls during the middle years but increases again with advancing age, particularly in the male population. The disease is more common in men and in higher social classes. Epidemiological work suggests that Hodgkin's disease may occur as an unusual effect of infection with a common virus. In young people the increased risk is associated with factors which increase susceptibility to common childhood infections such as higher social class, smoking in families and later birth position.[66] This is not the case for older patients with the disease. Despite reports of clustering of cases, there is no evidence at the present time that Hodgkin's disease is contagious.

Pathology

Hodgkin's disease is unusual in that malignant cells form only a small part of the tumour. The remainder is made up from varying proportions of lymphocytes, granulocytes, histiocytes, plasma cells and fibrous tissue. The characteristic cells are the mononuclear Hodgkin's cells, which by themselves are insufficient to establish the diagnosis, and the definitive binucleate or multinucleate Reed–Sternberg cells. Reed–Sternberg cells are not, however, pathognomonic of Hodgkin's disease and have been identified in certain virus infections for example, infectious mononucleosis, postvaccineal lymphadenopathy—and in drug reactions, especially to phenylhydantoins.[67] Nevertheless it is essential to identify Reed–Sternberg cells in order to establish a diagnosis of Hodgkin's disease. At the Ann Arbor Symposium in 1971[68] it was agreed that where Hodgkin's disease had already been diagnosed the presence of Reed–Sternberg cells was not essential to the diagnosis if there were mononuclear Hodgkin's cells in an appropriate cellular environment. In the absence of either mononuclear cells or Reed–Sternberg cells the disease should not be diagnosed. Despite much deliberation the origin of the Reed–Sternberg cell is still unresolved.

The universally accepted pathological classification of Hodgkin's disease is based on the Rye system published in 1966.[69] The Rye classification describes four histological subtypes:

1. **Lymphocyte-predominant Hodgkin's disease**: this is relatively uncommon. Reed–Sternberg cells are rare and the predominant cells in the lymph node are lymphocytes or histiocytes, or a mixture of the two.

REFERENCES

65. Gutersohn N, Cole P N Engl J Med 1981; 304: 136
66. Mueller N E In: Selby P, McElwain T J (eds) Hodgkin's Disease. Blackwell Scientific, Oxford 1987; pp 68–93
67. Sloane J P Baillière's Clin Haematol 1987; 1: 1–44
68. Carbone P P, Kaplan H P et al Cancer Res 1971; 31: 1860–1861
69. Lukes R J, Craver L F et al Cancer Res 1966; 26: 1311

2. **Nodular sclerosing Hodgkin's disease**: this type is characterized by thickening of the lymph node capsule together with interconnecting bands of collagenous connective tissue. Lacunar cells (variants of Reed–Sternberg cells) are found in nearly all cases of nodular sclerosing Hodgkin's disease but are not exclusive to the nodular sclerosing subtype.

3. **Mixed cellularity**: here the appearances are variable. This subgroup includes those cases which lack sclerosis but have too many Reed–Sternberg cells to be classified as lymphocyte-predominant.

4. **Lymphocyte-depleted**: there are two variants of lymphocyte-depleted Hodgkin's disease—diffuse fibrosis and reticular—which tend to show general cellular depletion, though with the presence of numerous Reed–Sternberg cells. Both types may be present in the same section.

There is a tendency for the different histological types of Hodgkin's disease to involve different node groups. For example, enlarged mediastinal lymph nodes are commonly involved by nodular sclerosing disease which is also found most often when extranodal sites are involved. Abdominal nodes are more commonly associated with mixed cellularity and lymphocyte-depleted subtypes.

Clinical features

The classical presentation of Hodgkin's disease is the discovery of painless discrete lymphadenopathy, usually in the neck and less commonly in the axilla. In some patients the diagnosis is made following the discovery of a symptomless mediastinal mass on routine chest radiograph (Fig. 34.6). Infradiaphragmatic presentations are uncommon and account for approximately 10% of patients with clinically localized disease. Approximately one third of patients complain of systemic symptoms including weight loss, fever and drenching night sweats. Generalized pruritis and occasionally pain in involved sites following alcohol ingestion are also reported in these patients. Extranodal presentation is rare, occurring in less than 5% of all cases. The diagnosis is established in the majority of cases by lymph node biopsy. Where there is no evidence of lymph node enlargement, great care must be taken in establishing a diagnosis on tissue obtained from other sources.

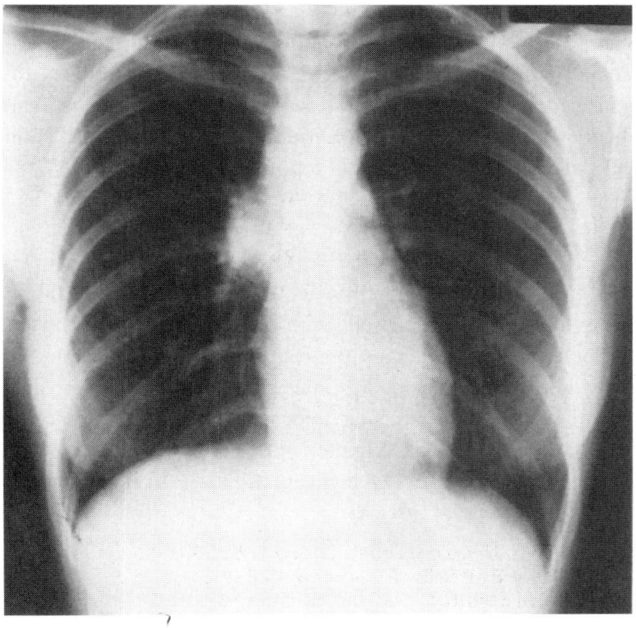

Fig. 34.6 Mediastinal involvement with Hodgkin's disease on routine chest radiograph.

Staging

The Ann Arbor classification (Table 34.7), which defines four principal stages of spread of Hodgkin's disease, has provided a useful basis for management and enabled comparisons to be made between treatment schedules from different centres and individuals.

It is apparent however that within individual stages defined by the Ann Arbor system, prognosis is influenced by a variety of clinical factors. For example, the extent of mediastinal involvement in patients with stage II disease is crucial in determining whether or not such patients may be cured by radiotherapy; where the mass exceeds one third of the thoracic diameter, high relapse rates occur with radiotherapy alone. Similarly, the number of lymph node sites involved, the presence or absence of systemic symptoms and the extent of abdominal disease may all have an adverse influence on prognosis within a given stage. Any definition of stage, therefore, must take into account not only the anatomical distribution of disease but also these other clinical features. The management is determined on the basis of the 'complete' clinical picture.

Early observations of patients with clinically staged Hodgkin's disease, localized above the diaphragm, showed that a significant number relapsed within the abdomen when radiotherapy alone was used to treat the known sites of clinical disease. The search for a more accurate assessment of abdominal disease before treatment led to the introduction of staging laparotomy with abdominal lymph node biopsy and diagnostic splenectomy.[70] This demonstrated that approximately 30% of individuals with

Table 34.7 Ann Arbor classification of Hodgkin's disease[68]

Stage	*Description*
Stage I	Involvement of a single lymph node region (I) or of a single extralymphatic organ or site (I_E)
Stage II	Involvement of two or more lymph node regions on the same side of the diaphragm (II), or localized involvement of extralymphatic organs or site and one or more lymph node regions on the same side of the diaphragm (II_E)
Stage III	Involvement of lymph node regions on both sides of the diaphragm (III) ± involvement of the spleen (III_s, or localized extralymphatic organ or site (III_s)
Stage IV	Diffuse or disseminated involvement of one or more extralymphatic organs or tissues, for example, liver, marrow, pleura, lung, bone and skin

Systemic symptoms: Weight loss, fever, sweating. If absent = A; if present = B.

REFERENCE

70. Glatstein E, Guernsey J M et al Cancer 1969; 24: 709–718

clinically localized supradiaphragmatic disease have occult intra-abdominal involvement and therefore require more intensive therapy. Experience over the past 30 years, using staging laparotomy and splenectomy, has confirmed that pathological staging has been of value in selecting a small subgroup of patients for whom radiotherapy is the treatment of choice but it is clear that pathological staging alone is not an adequate basis for treatment decisions.

A sequence of clinical trials conducted by the EORTC have demonstrated that it is possible to predict prognosis and allocate treatment according to clinical features without recourse to surgical staging.[71] While laparotomy and splenectomy remain part of the standard assessment for a patient with Hodgkin's disease in certain centres in the USA they are now rarely employed in Europe.[72]

Investigations

History and physical examination

The introduction of increasingly sophisticated imaging techniques has tended to overshadow the fundamental value of a detailed history and thorough physical examination in patients with Hodgkin's disease. For example, the presence of significant symptoms including weight loss of more than 10% over the preceding 6 months, unexplained fever of greater than 38°C and drenching night sweats invariably relegates an individual to the B category of the Ann Arbor classification, implying a poorer prognosis and allocation to more intensive first-line therapy. Similarly, careful documentation of all clinical sites of involvement (including Waldeyer's ring) not only provides a measure of predicted response to treatment but more importantly may allow, by a simple biopsy procedure, confirmation of more extensive spread of disease. Such information may determine a change in management from localized to systemic therapy, thereby avoiding further unnecessary and often unpleasant staging investigations. Clinical assessment of the spleen is unreliable. An enlarged spleen may not be involved while approximately 30% of clinically or radiologically normal spleens are found to be infiltrated when examined after splenectomy.

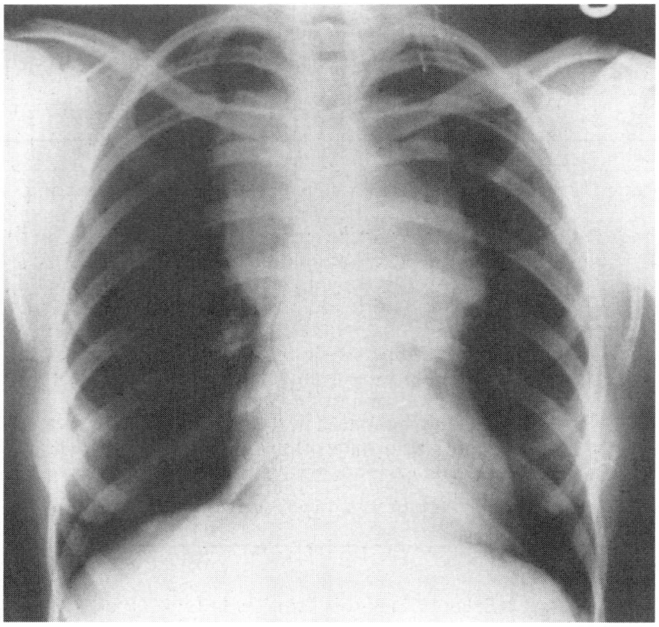

Fig. 34.7 Massive mediastinal involvement on chest radiograph.

Laboratory investigation

In the majority of untreated cases the blood count is normal. Anaemia is uncommon at presentation; when present it suggests bone marrow involvement and the need for a bone marrow trephine examination. A proportion of patients will have a neutrophil leucocytosis which appears to have no prognostic significance; however, lymphopenia may be associated with a poor prognosis. Eosinophilia is occasionally seen but is of no prognostic significance. The erythrocyte sedimentation rate is elevated in 30–50% of cases, often in association with B symptoms and can provide a useful marker for assessing remission and relapse.

Abnormalities of liver function tests, particularly elevation of alkaline phosphatase levels, may be found at the time of presentation of Hodgkin's disease without liver involvement. Experience has demonstrated the poor correlation of parenchymal liver involvement with either liver size or currently available tests of liver function, and every effort should therefore be made to obtain tissue for histological confirmation before therapy when involvement is suspected.[73]

Impairment of renal function, either by direct infiltra-tion or secondary to obstructive nephropathy or nephrotic syndrome, is extremely uncommon at presentation as is hypercalcaemia.

Bone marrow examination

Bone marrow involvement occurs in between 5 and 15% of previously untreated cases of Hodgkin's disease. Marrow involvement is closely associated with the presence of systemic ('B') symptoms, anaemia and a raised alkaline phosphatase level. The focal nature of bone marrow infiltration and the high incidence of associated fibrosis requires a bone marrow trephine biopsy to be performed since marrow aspiration alone is of very limited value. Bilateral biopsies or the use of wide-bore biopsy needles significantly increase the likelihood of a positive yield.

Chest radiograph

Hodgkin's disease frequently affects the mediastinum, although this is often in association with cervical or supraclavicular lymphadenopathy. Changes on routine chest radiograph range from minimal superior mediastinal distortion to massive enlargement of mediastinal and hilar nodes with adjacent parenchymal infiltration (Fig. 34.7). Computerized tomography is of value in assessing hilar node involvement, particularly in the presence of extensive mediastinal disease.

REFERENCES

71. Tubiana M, Henry Amar M et al Blood 1989; 73: 47
72. Mauch P, Somers R 1992
73. Filly R A, Marglin S, Castellino R A Cancer 1976; 38: 2143–2148

Lymphography

In the initial assessment of Hodgkin's disease plain abdominal radiographs yield little information disease apart from demonstrating the rare case of bone involvement.

In the assessment of abdominal disease, bipedal lymphography has been a most reliable technique for detecting para-aortic and pelvic lymph node infiltration. Involved nodes contain filling defects disrupting the normal granular storage pattern; unlike CT scanning, a lymphogram is capable of demonstrating abnormalities in normal-sized lymph nodes. Its value is limited however since the splenic hilar, coeliac axis, porta hepatis, internal iliac and mesenteric nodes do not routinely opacify (Fig. 34.8). Mesenteric nodes are rarely involved in Hodgkin's disease but the other sites may harbour active disease. The lymphogram also gives no information on the state of the spleen. Lymphography is a very time consuming and labour intensive technique and is often uncomfortable for the patient; it has been largely superseded by CT scanning.

CT scanning

CT scanning has the ability to image enlarged nodes not seen on lymphography, for example those of the coeliac axis and porta hepatis. While providing confirmation of gross lymphatic enlargement at these sites, unfortunately CT cannot demonstrate involvement of normal-sized nodes or microscopic infiltration of the parenchyma of the liver or spleen.

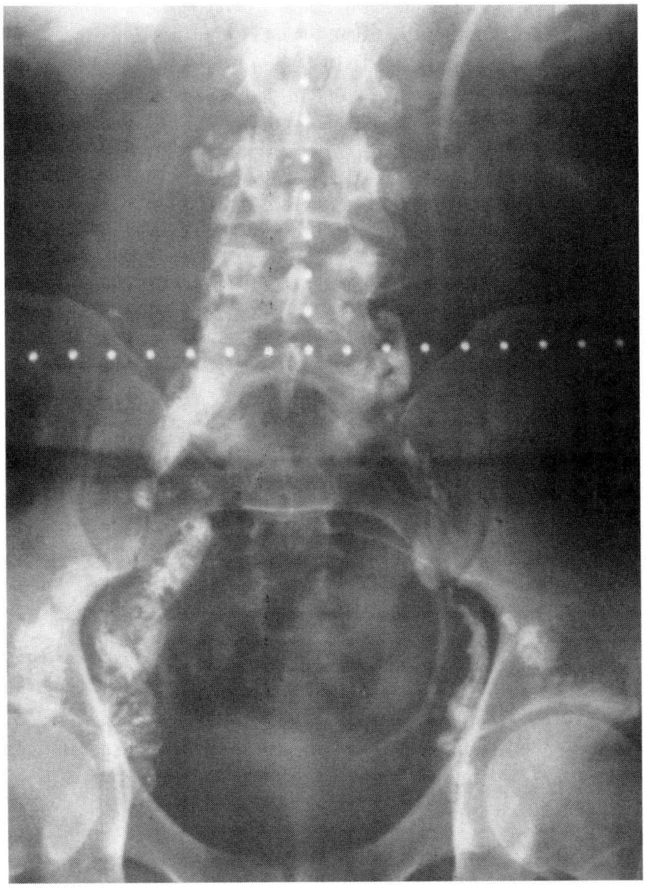

Fig. 34.8 Lymphangiogram showing involvement with Hodgkin's disease.

Radiographic skeletal survey

Bone involvement occurs in 5% of patients, usually those with advanced disease, and involvement may be sclerotic, lytic or mixed in appearance. The differentiation between bone involvement and aseptic necrosis occurring after treatment is often only resolved by surgical biopsy.

Ultrasound scanning

Diagnostic ultrasound is a quick and efficient method of assessing lymphomatous involvement in the abdomen, pelvis and retroperitoneal area. Its greatest potential is in the demonstration of enlarged nodes in the porta hepatis, splenic hilum or around the pancreas; however the technique is limited by the inability to detect involved nodes less than 1.5 cm in diameter or to differentiate reactive hyperplasia from malignant infiltration. Splenic enlargement is readily detected by ultrasound scan even when not apparent clinically, but while large discrete filling defects may be demonstrated, routine scanning is not able to separate diffuse involvement by lymphoma from enlargement from other causes. Similar problems arise when scanning the liver. In the kidney mass lesions, diffuse enlargement from infiltration or hydronephrosis secondary to lymph node compression may all be identified by routine ultrasound examination.

Radioisotope scanning

Radioisotope scanning currently has a limited role in the investigation of patients with Hodgkin's disease. Bone scans are sensitive but they do not differentiate from other pathological processes. Isotopic liver and spleen scans occasionally show a clear filling defect but diffuse involvement is usually missed.

The discovery that gallium 67 localizes well within tissues involved by Hodgkin's disease prompted great interest in its possible role in staging. Gallium 67 has proved a useful isotope in high doses in assessing involvement of the mediastinum but interpretation of abdominal gallium 67 scans is compromised by interference from uptake of the isotope in the liver, colon and marrow.[74]

Whole body positron emission tomography (PET) using 2-fluorodeoxy-D-glucose (FDG) has shown encouraging results in pretreatment staging and remission assessment in both Hodgkin's disease and non-Hodgkin's lymphoma (Fig. 34.9). FDG concentrates preferentially in metabolically active tissue including lymphoma, and initial studies show a high degree of sensitivity and specificity for this technique. Prospective studies to assess the role of FDG PET scanning in the management of lymphoma are currently in progress.[75]

REFERENCES

74. Anderson K C, Leonard R C G, Canellos G P Am J Med 1988; 75: 321–327
75. Timothy A R, Ahern V et al Ann Oncol 1996; 7(suppl 3): 3

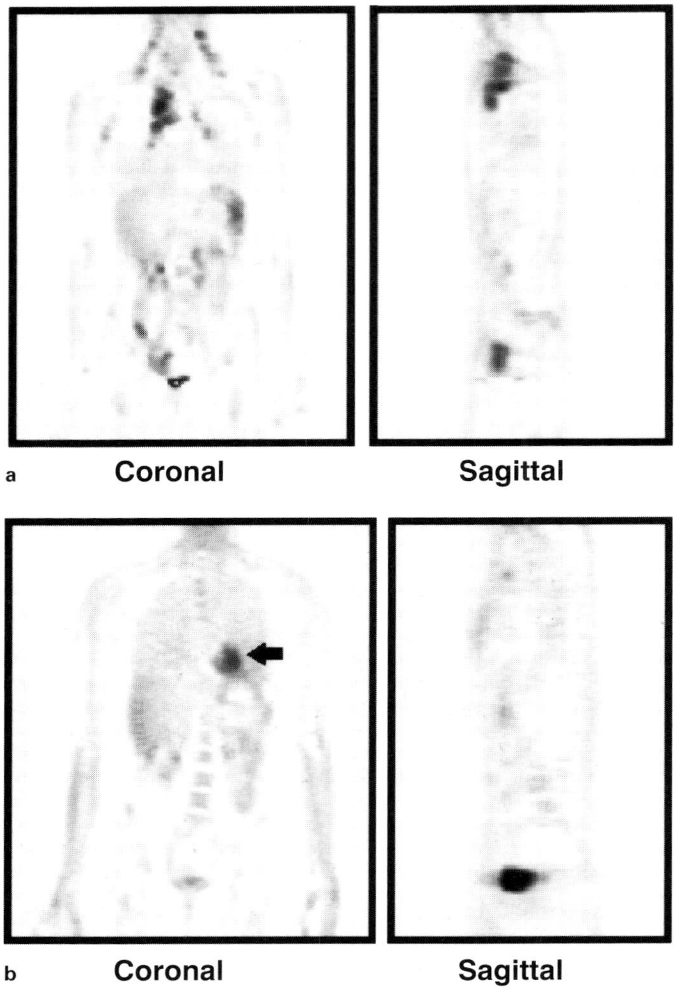

Fig. 34.9 FDG PET scans of a patient with Hodgkin's disease. **(a)** Before treatment. Increased focal uptake is seen on the coronal image in cervical, supraclavicular, mediastinal and hilar nodes above the diaphragm and right inguinal nodes and spleen below the diaphragm. Physiological uptake is seen in the ureters and renal pelvices (as FDG is excreted renally). **(b)** Following chemotherapy there is complete resolution of abnormal FDG uptake. Increased uptake of FDG is seen within the marrow, which may be a reactive response to treatment. Physiological myocardial uptake is seen on this study (arrowed), but not the earlier one. Whilst myocardial uptake may vary in the same patient at different scanning sessions, it is likely that myocardial uptake was not visible on **(a)** owing to bulky widespread nodal disease accumulating FDG.

Magnetic resonance imaging

The expectation that magnetic resonance image scanning would replace surgical staging in the detection of abdominal Hodgkin's disease has not been realized. Magnetic resonance imaging has not yet been shown to be useful in the detection of splenic disease and is of only marginal value in the examination of the liver.[76]

Staging laparotomy and splenectomy

Surgical staging by laparotomy and splenectomy was introduced in 1969 by Glatstein and colleagues and remains the most sensitive investigation for the assessment of intra-abdominal Hodgkin's disease.[70] Approximately one third of patients who appear to have stage I or II supradiaphragmatic disease after full clinical investigation will be found to have occult intra-abdominal disease after laparotomy. Staging laparotomy became standard practice in many centres during the 1970s for patients with early stage disease, allowing more precise definition of those patients in whom local radiotherapy was appropriate treatment. Experience has demonstrated that laparotomy is not without morbidity and occasional mortality, and there is increasing concern over the long-term complications, particularly the risk of overwhelming sepsis in patients who have undergone splenectomy. Data from the available studies comparing the outcome of treatment for patients treated with or without surgical staging suggest that diagnostic laparotomy per se does not influence survival although in certain cases a more precise definition of the extent of disease may allow less toxic treatment to be employed.

In summary, each newly diagnosed patient should have, as a minimum physical examination, haematology including erythrocyte sedimentation rate, biochemistry, chest radiograph and CT scan of the chest, abdomen and pelvis. The use of newer imaging techniques will be determined by individual circumstances and local expertise.

Treatment

The last three decades have witnessed a steady improvement in the prognosis of patients with all stages of Hodgkin's disease. Several factors have contributed to this change, including better pretreatment staging, improvements in radiotherapy equipment and technique and the introduction of effective systemic chemotherapy. The euphoria associated with these dramatic advances must be tempered, however, by the realization that even with the most successful chemotherapy only 70% of those with disseminated disease may expect a cure. Similarly, despite intensive staging investigations and optimal radiotherapy, a proportion of patients with apparently localized disease relapse after treatment. Combining radiotherapy and chemotherapy may reduce relapse rates but does not improve overall survival, and there is continuing concern about the increased risk of late complications, in particular second malignancy, with more intensive treatment. This underlines the importance in any treatment policy for Hodgkin's disease of employing the minimum amount of initial therapy compatible with the highest probability of cure.

Radiotherapy

With the introduction of high-energy cobalt units and linear accelerators during the 1950s and 1960s the delivery of wide-field irradiation to major lymph node areas above and below the diaphragm, without significant morbidity, became a practical proposition (Fig. 34.10). Experience with this type of radiotherapy established that the optimal tumoricidal dose for Hodgkin's

REFERENCE

76. Reznek R H, Richards M A Clin Haematol 1987; 1: 77–108

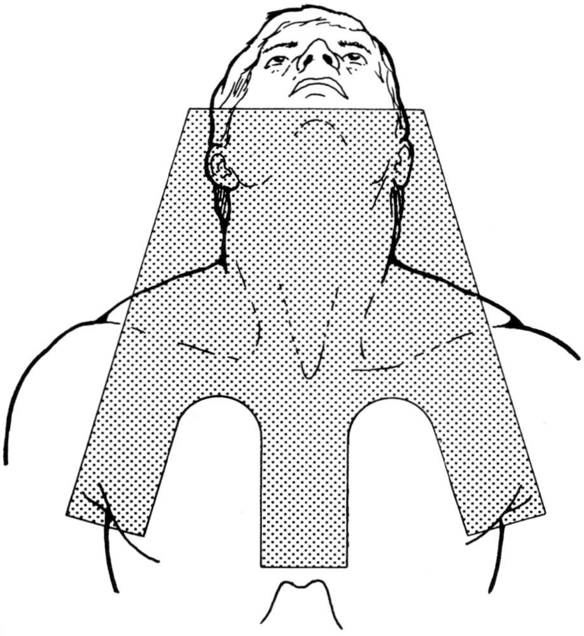

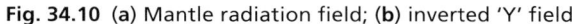

a

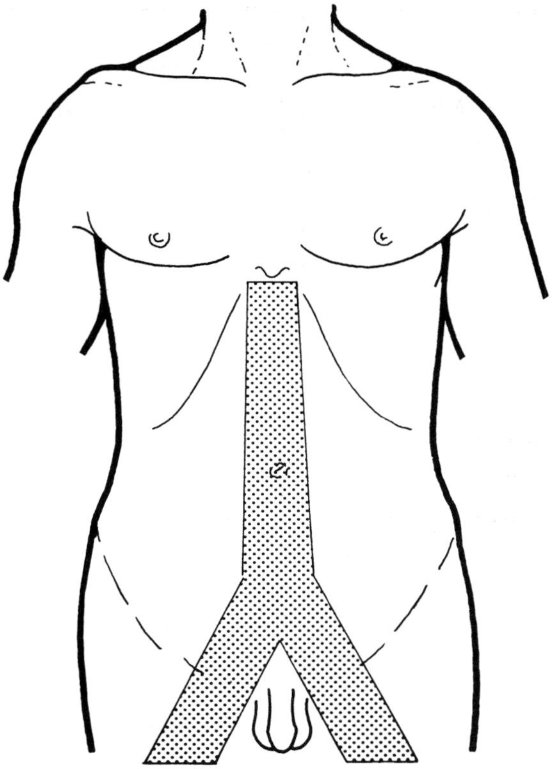

b

Fig. 34.10 (a) Mantle radiation field; (b) inverted 'Y' field.

disease lay in the range 30–40 Gy (3000–4000 rad) given in 20 daily fractions treating 5 days a week with appropriate shielding of the lungs and spinal cord. There is no evidence that significantly increasing the dose of radiation above these levels does other than increase the risk of late morbidity.

Side-effects of radiotherapy

Acute. The acute effects of radiotherapy are those occurring within 8–12 weeks of completion of treatment. The occurrence and intensity of these reactions are unpredictable in the individual patient, although debilitating side-effects are rare. Fatigue, particularly towards the end of treatment, is common but usually improves within a few weeks of completing irradiation. Occasionally patients may suffer persistent lassitude for several months.

Anorexia is common and may be accompanied by nausea (rarely vomiting) although this can usually be controlled with simple anti-emetic medication. Nausea and vomiting are more commonly a problem with infradiaphragmatic rather than supradiaphragmatic irradiation. Patients should be advised that they may lose weight during a routine course of radiotherapy and attention should be paid to adequate nutritional intake.

Radiotherapy fields in Hodgkin's disease do not routinely include the oral cavity but may encompass the sublingual, submaxillary and a large proportion of the parotid glands. This inevitably results in reduced saliva production and the saliva becomes more viscous, producing a dry mouth with altered taste sensation. Taste perception usually returns within 3 months, but dryness of the mouth may persist. Strict attention to oral hygiene is essential before radiotherapy to avoid caries and the associated dental problems that may result.

Modern megavoltage radiotherapy equipment with its skin-sparing properties has reduced the incidence of skin reactions to a minimum. However, erythema within the radiation fields does occur on occasions, and moist desquamation may rarely be seen in skin folds. The use of perfumed soaps and deodorant should be avoided during radiotherapy, and washing kept to a minimum in the irradiated areas. Direct exposure to sunlight is not advisable for at least 6 months after treatment and patients are advised to continue to take appropriate precautions with sunscreen preparations to avoid burning.

Thoracic irradiation may be accompanied by mucositis in the pharynx and occasionally dysphagia starting from the second or third week of treatment. These reactions are self limiting and patients should be reassured that they are a normal part of the treatment. Temporary alopecia overlying the occiput is invariable with mantle radiation, together with a similar loss of beard hair (Fig. 34.11). Hair regrowth usually commences within 3 months of stopping treatment and should be complete, although the texture and the colour of the hair may change within the irradiated area.

Wide-field irradiation rarely causes significant haematological depression but regular monitoring of blood counts is important. The risk of haematological toxicity is increased when patients have received chemotherapy prior to radiation and extra care must be exercised.

With infradiaphragmatic irradiation gastrointestinal side-effects such as cramps, flatulence and occasionally diarrhoea may occur but can usually be adequately controlled with appropriate

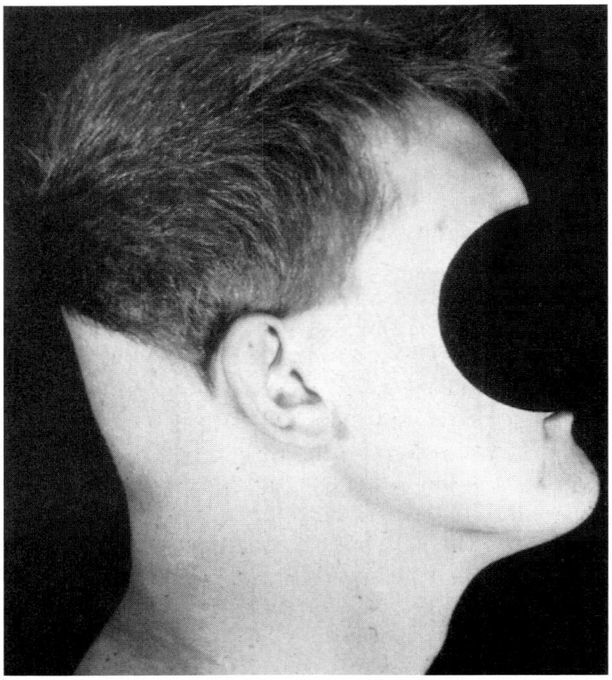

Fig. 34.11 Hair loss in the mantle field following radiotherapy.

medication. Patients are advised to avoid milk products, spiced foods or raw vegetables during abdominal treatment as these may accentuate any side-effects.

Late. The late effects of radiotherapy reflect normal tissue damage which may occur months or even years after treatment and is usually permanent.

Irradiation to the thorax given to excessive volumes, or with very high doses, may produce transient pneumonitis which in rare cases may progress to permanent respiratory disability. The risk of pulmonary damage is increased with prior or concomitant chemotherapy with drugs such as bleomycin or Adriamycin and great care must be taken in planning thoracic radiotherapy. Late cardiac problems following high-dose radiotherapy have been described in several historical series;[77] however, by treating the thorax with both anterior and posterior fields on each occasion and reducing the daily and overall treatment doses the risk of late cardiac complications has reduced dramatically. Nonetheless iatrogenic cardiac morbidity is a continuing concern, especially in younger patients.

Lhermitte's syndrome, the onset of numbness, paraesthesiae or electric shock sensations in the lumbar region or upper or lower limbs 2–4 months after completion of mantle radiotherapy, is well documented. The symptoms may last up to 6 months but settle without intervention. The syndrome is thought to be due to transient demyelinization and does not presage permanent neurological damage. Transverse myelitis is, however, a risk when separate thoracic (mantle) and abdominal (inverted Y) and radiation fields are matched incorrectly and overdose occurs on the spinal cord. Exceptional care must be exercised when matching radiation fields.

Extending abdominal irradiation to include the spleen and upper part of the left kidney has not been associated with any long-term sequelae on prolonged follow-up.[78] Care must be taken, however, to exclude an adequate volume of renal tissue from the radiation field to avoid chronic renal damage.

The potential for radiation to damage the gonads is of obvious importance in a disease which predominantly affects the young, a large percentage of whom will have a normal life expectancy. Fractionated radiotherapy to the testis above the level of 200 cGy will produce prolonged and often permanent azoospermia. With appropriate testicular shielding, radiation doses to the testis may be reduced by 95% to levels at which a reasonable probability of germinal epithelial recovery might be expected. It should be noted that a significant proportion of males will be azoospermic before therapy as a consequence of their disease. Semen analysis and storage should be undertaken if appropriate.

For the ovary, doses above 800 cGy are associated with a high risk of permanent amenorrhoea. The associated hormonal dysfunction in female patients leads to menopausal symptoms and in a young patient severe social and psychological sequelae may result unless appropriate hormone replacement therapy is instituted. For both men and women receiving radiation to the abdomen and pelvis for Hodgkin's disease, full discussions must take place with the patient and partner, and the possibility of sterility and hormonal side-effects must be fully explained before treatment is begun.

Chemotherapy

Studies of cytotoxic chemotherapy in the late 1940s demonstrated that Hodgkin's disease showed a peculiar sensitivity to these drugs and a small proportion of patients obtained worthwhile remission of their disease. Among the most active drugs were the alkylating agents, particularly nitrogen mustard and the vinca alkaloids.[79] By combining several of these agents together at one time the response rates increased significantly and the combination of mustine, Vincristine, Procarbazine and Prednisone (MOPP) developed at the National Cancer Institute in the USA produced complete remissions and 'cures' in some 50% of patients, including those with advanced disease.[80] Several modifications of the MOPP schedule have subsequently been reported, many introduced in an attempt to reduce the potential for acute and long-term toxicity now recognized to be associated with the alkylating agents in the original combination. Adriamycin based schedules, particularly ABVD (Adriamycin, Bleomycin, Vinblastine and DTIC), show not only similar response and relapse-free survival rates to MOPP but—more importantly—reduced risks of late toxicity, particularly with regard to infertility and the induction of second malignancies[81] (Table 34.8). The majority of patients who relapse will do so within 36 months of treatment—late relapses after more than 5 years are uncommon.[82]

REFERENCES

77. Byhardt R, Brace K et al Cancer 1975; 35: 795–802
78. Le Bourgeois J P, Meignan M et al Br J Radiol 1979; 52: 56–60
79. Goodman L S, Wintrobe M M, Dameshek W JAMA 1946; 132: 126–132
80. De Vita V T Jr, Serpick A A, Carbone P P Ann Intern Med 1970; 73: 881–895
81. Selby P, McElwain T J, Canellos G In: Selby P, McElwain T J (eds) Hodgkin's Disease. Blackwell Scientific, Oxford 1987 pp 269–300

Table 34.8 Chemotherapy schedules for MOPP and ABVD

Name		*Daily dose (mg/m²)*	*Administration route*	*Administration on day(s)*	*Frequency*
Mechlorethamine (HN_2)	**M**	6	i.v.	1–8	Regimen should be recycled every 4 weeks
Vincristine (Oncovin®)	**O**	1.4	i.v.	1–8	
Procarbazine	**P**	100	p.o.	1,14	
Prednisone	**P**	40	p.o.	1,14	
Adriamycin®	**A**	25	i.v.	1–15	
Bleomycin	**B**	10	i.v.	1–15	
Vinblastine	**V**	6	i.v.	1–15	
Dacarbazine	**D**	375	i.v.	1–15	

Combining radiotherapy and chemotherapy may increase complete remission rates but the potential advantages must be balanced against the risk of increased acute and late toxicity.

Side-effects of chemotherapy

Acute. Chemotherapy may cause nausea and vomiting and, less commonly, diarrhoea occurring within a few hours of administration but rarely lasting more than 24 hours after treatment. Premedication with Domperidone or prochlorperazine continued for a short period after chemotherapy is usually sufficient to control nausea and vomiting. In severe cases the newer HT3 antagonists such as Ondansetron may be required. Anticipatory vomiting as a prelude to chemotherapy can be a problem and may prove more difficult to overcome; however these side-effects are rarely severe enough to cause patients to reject treatment.

The effect of suppression of normal bone marrow function is a major factor influencing the dosage and schedule of cytotoxic chemotherapy. With the standard combinations, e.g. ABVD, the white cell and platelet counts characteristically fall to a nadir 10–12 days after the start of treatment. In the absence of complicating factors the blood count will usually return to normal within 14 days and allow further chemotherapy to be given, although treatment may need to be delayed in the face of persistent neutropenia or thrombocytopenia. In severe cases the use of granulocyte stimulating factor (G-CSF) is necessary to allow successful delivery of chemotherapy.

Cytotoxic drugs are immunosuppressive, especially in patients with lymphoma who are already compromised by their disease. The risk of severe and occasionally life-threatening infections must be anticipated and warned against, particularly in splenectomized subjects. Any patient on chemotherapy who presents with signs of infection should have an immediate blood count and, if shown to be severely neutropenic, should be started on broad-spectrum intravenous antibiotic therapy while blood cultures are awaited. Likewise, patients developing signs and symptoms of herpes zoster infection should be treated promptly with antiviral agents. Patients on chemotherapy should also be warned to report any untoward fevers or evidence of bruising or bleeding so that blood counts may be checked and appropriate action taken.

One major cause for concern among patients due to receive chemotherapy is the prospect of alopecia. The incidence of hair loss varies depending on the cytotoxic agents used and to some extent on the individual. Female patients should be advised to obtain a suitable wig prior to starting treatment but should be reassured that, even if hair loss is significant, the hair will return in due course and will often start to regrow during therapy.

Late. The increasingly successful outcome for patients treated with chemotherapy has revealed the potential risk of long-term side-effects, prompting the investigation of less toxic drug combinations.

Schedules such as MOPP, which include alkylating agents, render the majority of men azoospermic; this is usually permanent when six or more cycles of treatment are given. Similar treatment in women produces ovarian ablation in approximately 50% but this effect appears to be age-related. Patients over the age of 30 have a 20% chance or less of remaining fertile. Recent experience has shown that non-alkylating drug combinations such as ABVD have a significantly reduced incidence of azoospermia immediately after treatment, with complete recovery in the majority of cases. As with radiotherapy, patients undergoing chemotherapy should be counselled fully and the need for appropriate contraceptive precautions should be emphasized to avoid the misfortune of an untimely pregnancy during treatment and the psychological trauma associated with subsequent termination.

An issue of major concern in patients surviving successful treatment for Hodgkin's disease has been the development of second malignancies. Both ionizing radiation and many cytotoxic agents are potentially mutagenic and carcinogenic in experimental systems. The alkylating agents, particularly Procarbazine, appear to be particularly implicated. In one series of over 1500 patients treated for Hodgkin's disease at Stanford University, California, there was a significant increase in second 'cancers' including leukaemia, non-Hodgkin's lymphoma, lung and stomach cancers, melanoma and connective tissue malignancy.[83] At 15-year follow-up the overall risk for a second cancer was 17.6% compared to 2.6% in the general population. The risk of developing leukaemia appears to reach a plateau 10 years after treatment. While there appears to be a small risk of secondary leukaemia in patients treated by radiotherapy alone, the major risk comes from the alkylating agent based chemotherapy regimes such as MOPP. There does not, as yet, appear to be a similar risk with the ABVD schedules. The risk of solid cancers continues to increase with time even after 10 years and is related to the intensity of treatment, being highest in those who have received both alkylating

REFERENCES

82. De Vita V T, Simon R M, Hubbard S M Intern Med 1980; 92: 587–595
83. Tucker M A, Coleman C N et al N Engl J Med 1988; 318: 76–81

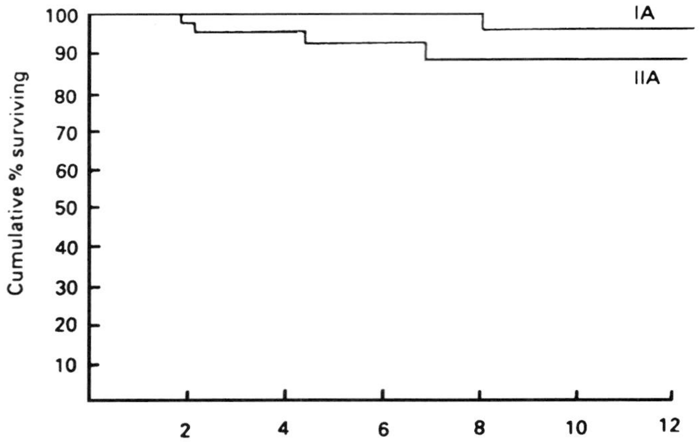

Fig. 34.12 Survival curve for pathological stage localized Hodgkin's disease treated by radiotherapy alone.

chemotherapy and radiation. Every effort should be made to minimize the amount of treatment given to patients with Hodgkin's disease but the risk of second malignancies should not be a justification for avoiding intensive therapy. Patients should be fully informed about the potential risks of therapy and kept under close surveillance. Any untoward feature must not be automatically regarded as recurrent lymphoma—every effort should be made to obtain a histological diagnosis to exclude other forms of malignancy. Patients should be strongly discouraged from smoking.

Treatment by stage

Stage IA and IIA supradiaphragmatic

In surgically staged I and II supradiaphragmatic disease without adverse prognostic factors, wide-field irradiation to the mediastinum, axillary, cervical and supraclavicular areas ('mantle' field) will produce long-term disease-free survival and probably cure in over 80% of patients (Fig. 34.12). In patients who have not undergone staging laparotomy, treatment with a mantle field will result in a 25–30% relapse rate below the diaphragm. As an alternative to laparotomy the initial radiotherapy fields are extended to encompass the spleen and para-aortic nodes, and thereby prophylactically irradiate occult sites of disease within the abdomen. Results with this technique show similar results to those obtained after surgical staging. Selection on the basis of initial clinical features has now replaced diagnostic laparotomy, and results from various studies show the successful outcome of treatment based on prognostic factors other than surgical staging.[71]

Infradiaphragmatic stage I and IIA

Approximately 10% of Hodgkin's disease patients present with disease localized below the diaphragm. For those with true stage I disease in the inguinal or femoral region, 'inverted Y' radiotherapy to include the iliac and para-aortic nodes may produce satisfactory long-term disease-free survival. With involvement of the para-aortic nodes, the risk of splenic infiltration increases rapidly, as does the failure rate with radiation alone; patients with pelvic and para-aortic node disease are best treated with initial chemotherapy.

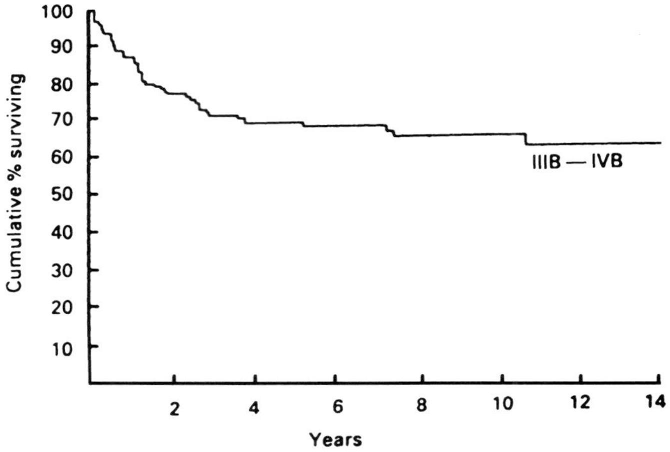

Fig. 34.13 Survival curve for advanced Hodgkin's disease treated by combination chemotherapy.

Stage I and II disease with poor prognostic factors

Patients with apparently localized disease but adverse prognostic factors—large mediastinal mass, multiple sites of disease, high ESR or B symptoms—have high relapse rates with radiotherapy in most centres, even after pathological staging. Chemotherapy is the initial treatment of choice for this group.

Stage IIIA

This is not adequately treated with radiotherapy alone. These patients should be treated with chemotherapy from the outset, as this produces excellent results (Fig. 34.13) with minimal morbidity.

Stage IIIB and IV

Chemotherapy is the appropriate initial treatment. The value of additional radiotherapy to sites of bulk disease following chemotherapy is not yet established.

In patients who relapse after radiotherapy a high proportion will respond to salvage chemotherapy, although prolonged follow-up has demonstrated that only 50% of these patients are still alive 10–14 years after treatment.[84]

For patients relapsing after first-line chemotherapy, alternative conventional drug therapy rarely produces complete or long-lasting remissions and the search for better salvage schedules continues. Investigation of the role of high-dose chemotherapy with bone marrow support suggests that this technique may improve the prospects of successful salvage in selected patients.[85]

NON-HODGKIN'S LYMPHOMA

The non-Hodgkin's lymphomas comprise a complex group of diseases which have widely differing clinical presentations and

REFERENCES

84. Oza A, Leahy M et al In: Proceedings from 4th International Congress on Malignant Lymphoma, Lugano 1990 p 37
85. Nademance A Blood 1995; 85: 1381

patterns of behaviour, reflecting their varying histological subtypes. Non-Hodgkin's lymphoma is responsible for approximately 3% of deaths from malignant disease in western countries. In contrast to Hodgkin's disease, the non-Hodgkin's lymphomas have a peak incidence in the fifth and sixth decades, are less commonly localized at presentation and more frequently involve extranodal sites.

As with Hodgkin's disease, experience over the past three decades following the introduction of intensive cytotoxic chemotherapy has clearly shown that with appropriate management many patients with non-Hodgkin's lymphoma now have a real prospect for cure. Treatment, however, must be carefully tailored to the patient's individual circumstances and depends on the extent and histological subtype of the lymphoma concerned.

Pathology

The non-Hodgkin's lymphomas may be divided histologically into a low-grade subgroup (erroneously classified as 'good prognosis'); here the disease tends to run an indolent course characterized by frequent periods of relapse. Although these low-grade lymphomas have a median survival of between 5 and 10 years, the majority of patients ultimately die of their lymphoma or associated complications. In patients with such low-grade lymphomas aggressive treatment has not been rewarded by improvements in cure rates. In fact the converse is often true: many patients die early of treatment-related complications. Despite the low cure rates patients with low-grade non-Hodgkin's lymphoma may maintain an excellent quality of life over several years without active treatment or with the use of minimal intervention with radiation or chemotherapy.

At the other end of the disease spectrum, the high-grade, biologically aggressive lymphomas tend to pursue a rapid and relentless course when untreated, with median survival times of 12–24 months. This group of lymphomas, previously referred to as 'poor prognosis', is now associated with cure rates of upwards of 30% with appropriate intensive combination chemotherapy.

This marked variation in behaviour and prognosis between the different subgroups of non-Hodgkin's lymphoma demands that a comprehensive and easily comprehensible histological classification should be available to provide the clinician with an insight into the expected behaviour of a given patient's disease and also serve as a guide to treatment. Over the past 30 years there have been repeated attempts to reclassify the non-Hodgkin's lymphomas based on morphological and, more recently, on immunological criteria. The difficulties of experienced specialist histopathologists in producing a uniform classification have only served to compound the problems for clinicians dealing with these diseases and led to increasing frustration and the temptation to provide frivolous alternative classifications[86] (Table 34.9).

Histopathologically, the definition of the non-Hodgkin's lymphomas is a complex and very specialized exercise. It is not appropriate to discuss this further here but readers who wish to gain a fuller understanding of the current state of the classification of the non-Hodgkin's lymphomas are referred to the review by Shipp et al.[87] A simplified picture of the various cell types in the lymphoid system is shown in Figure 34.14. Both T and B lymphocytes, together with monocytes and macrophages, are thought to originate from stem cells in the bone marrow. The T lymphocyte precursors migrate from the bone marrow to the thymus where they undergo maturation before leaving the gland to colonize the peripheral areas of the lymph node, the spleen and epithelial surfaces such as the gastrointestinal and respiratory tracts. By comparison, B lymphocyte transformation tends to occur in lymphoid follicles resulting in the formation of germinal centres. The daughter cells may be morphologically different from the mature cells, i.e. plasma or lymphoplasmacytoid cells.

For many years the most widely adopted classification for the non-Hodgkin's lymphomas has been that of Rappaport[88] (Table 34.10). While useful clinically, this has been criticized for being insufficiently detailed and for its use of imprecise terminology. Other classifications have been proposed to overcome the deficiencies of the Rappaport system: the Revised Working Formulation, the Kiel classification, (Table 34.11)[89] and more recently the Revised European American Lymphoma (REAL) classification.[90] The majority of malignant lymphomas are derived from B lymphocytes, although there are now varieties of distinctive T cell lymphomas, such as peripheral T cell lymphomas and adult T cell lymphoma/leukaemia, which do not fit well into most classifications. From the clinician's point of view the value of any classification is the division of the lymphomas into low, intermediate and high grade, which will form the basis of a rational treatment policy.

Table 34.9 The Higby classification of lymphomas

Good ones
Includes non-convoluted diffuse centrilobulated histioblastoma, immune binucleolar hyperbolic folliculated macrolymphosarcoma, T_2-terminal transferase-negative bimodal prolymphoblastic leukosarcoma, Jergen—Kreuzart—Munier—Abdullah syndrome and reticulated histioblastic pseudo-Szezare immunoglobulin M-secreting folliculoma
Characteristics Small tumour that does not recur after treatment
Not-so-good ones
Formerly 'hairy cell' pseudoincestuoblastoma, quasi-convoluted binucleate germinoma, sarcoblastiocytoma, Syrian variant of heavy chain disease and German grossobeseioma
Characteristics Such tumours disappear on treatment but return and cause appreciable mortality
Really bad ones
Includes farsical mononuclear diffuse convoluted pseudoquasihistiolymphosarcomyeloblastoma, immunoglobulin variant of fragmented plasmatic gammopathy, triconvoluted ipsilateral rhomboid fever, Armour's hyperthermic carcinoma and Hohner's harmonica
Characteristics Regardless of treatment, such tumours keep growing

Adapted from Higby[86]

REFERENCES

86. Higby D J N Engl J Med 1979; 300: 1283
87. Shipp M A, Mauch P In: De Vita V, Hellman J (eds) Cancer. Rosenberg: Lippincott-Raven, Philadelphia 1997 p 2165
88. Rappaport H Atlas of Tumour Pathology. Armed Forces Institute of Pathology, Washington D C 1966
89. Rosenberg S A et al Cancer 1982; 49: 2112–2351
90. Harris N, Jaffe E Blood 1994; 84: 1361

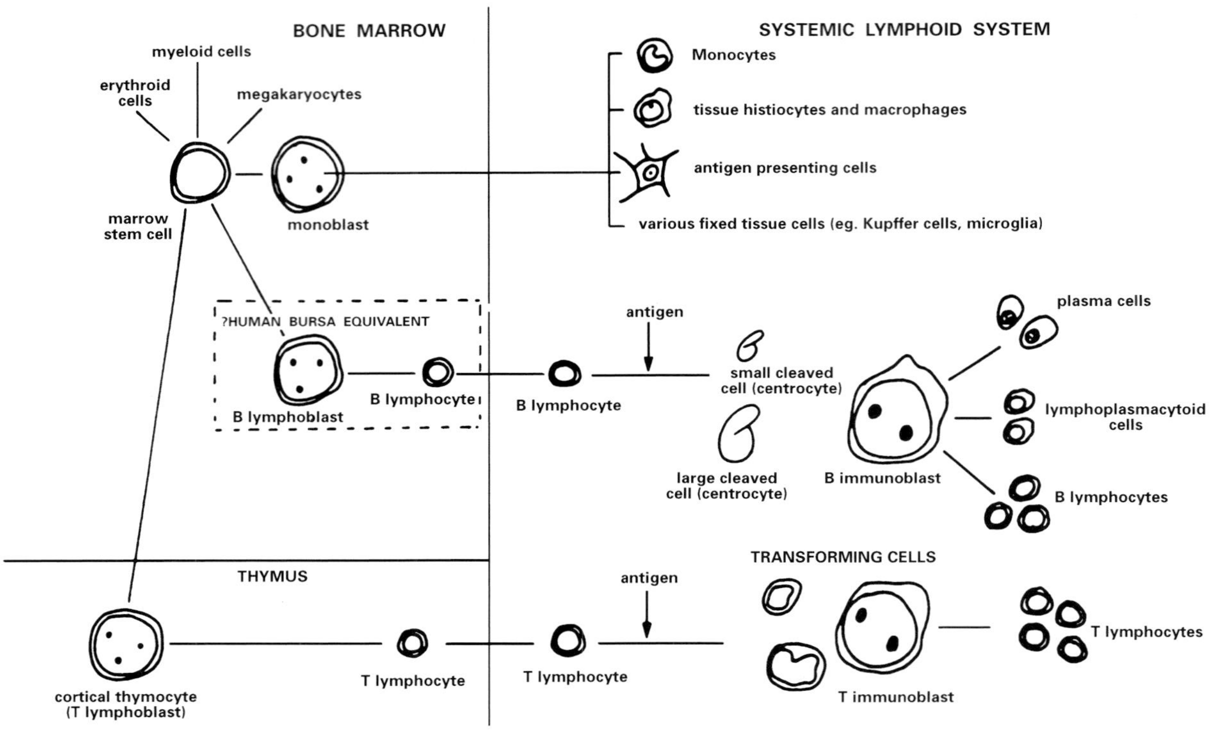

Fig. 34.14 Schematic diagram showing different cell types in the lymphoid system. Adapted from Sloane.[67]

Table 34.10 Rappaport[88] classification of non-Hodgkin's lymphoma

Nodular	*Diffuse*
Lymphocytic, well differentiated	Lymphocytic, well differentiated
Lymphocytic, poorly differentiated	Lymphocytic, poorly differentiated
Mixed, lymphocytic and histiocytic	Mixed, lymphocytic and histiocytic
Histiocytic	Histiocytic
	Undifferentiated

Clinical features

Less than 10% of the low-grade lymphomas are truly localized (stage I) at presentation; for intermediate high-grade lymphomas this figure may approach 30%. The frequency of extranodal presentations together with the high incidence of mesenteric and epitrochlear node involvement means that the scope for localized treatment with irradiation is more limited and systemic therapy is more commonly required.

Staging

The Ann Arbor staging system (Table 34.7) has traditionally been used for the non-Hodgkin's lymphomas but, as with Hodgkin's disease, it is clear that factors other than just clinical (or pathological) stage, such as tumour bulk, histology, age and serum lactate dehydrogenase values, are of major importance in defining therapy and predicting prognosis. New staging systems which take account of these other important characteristics will be required.

Despite the introduction of more sophisticated imaging, a careful history and clinical examination still provide important information in patients with non-Hodgkin's lymphomas. The presence of systemic symptoms and the duration of lymph node enlargement may influence the decision whether or not any treatment is required in the low-grade lymphomas. Symptoms such as deafness, diplopia, bone pain or altered bowel habit may indicate that further investigation is required to exclude sites of involvement not apparent on initial clinical examination. Careful inspection of Waldeyer's ring, and examination of the epitrochlear and popliteal lymph nodes may also yield valuable information on the extent of spread. It is also important to remember the established associations of specific sites, for example, disease in the postnasal space is associated with enlarged upper cervical lymph nodes, and intestinal lymphoma may be associated with certain head and neck presentations.

Laboratory investigations

Approximately 40% of patients with non-Hodgkin's lymphoma have bone marrow involvement at presentation. 80% of patients with 'low-grade' small cell lymphomas have evidence of marrow infiltration compared to less than 15% of those with more aggressive, high-grade malignancies. Examination by bone marrow aspiration alone is inadequate and bone marrow trephine is required. In studies of bilateral iliac crest biopsies approximately 25% were positive in only one specimen.

Peripheral blood involvement occurs in the presence of marrow infiltration and is found most commonly in patients with small cell

Table 34.11 Comparison of working formulation with Kiel classification of non-Hodgkin's lymphoma

Working formulation	*Kiel equivalent*
Low-grade	
Malignant lymphoma, small lymphocytic consistent with CLL plasmacytoid	ML lymphocytic, CLL ML lymphoplasmacytic/lymphoplasmacytoid
Malignant lymphoma, follicular, predominantly small cleaved cell, diffuse areas, sclerosis	ML centroblastic/centrocytic (small), follicular ± diffuse
Malignant lymphoma, follicular, mixed, small cleaved and large cell, diffuse areas, sclerosis	
Intermediate-grade	
Malignant lymphoma, follicular, predominantly large cell, diffuse areas, sclerosis	ML centroblastic/centrocytic (large), follicular ± diffuse
Malignant lymphoma, diffuse, small cleaved cell, sclerosis	ML centrocytic (small)
Malignant lymphoma, diffuse, mixed, small and large cell, sclerosis, epithelioid cell component	ML centroblastic/centrocytic (small), diffuse ML lymphoplasmacytic/cytoid, polymorphic
Malignant lymphoma, diffuse, large cell, cleaved cell, non-cleaved cell, sclerosis	ML centroblastic/centrocytic (large), diffuse ML centrocytic (large) ML centroblastic
High-grade	
Malignant lymphoma, large cell, immunoblastic, plasmacytoid, clear cell, polymorphous, epithelioid cell component	ML immunoblastic T zone lymphoma Lymphoepithelioid cell lymphoma
Malignant lymphoma, lymphoblastic, convoluted cell, non-convoluted cell	ML lymphoblastic, convoluted cell type ML lymphoblastic, unclassified
Malignant lymphoma, small non-cleaved, Burkitt's follicular areas	ML lymphoblastic, Burkitt type and other B lymphoblastic

CLL = Chronic lymphocytic leukaemia; ML = myeloid leukaemia Adapted from Rosenberg et al[89]

lymphomas, although up to 80% of patients with highly malignant lymphoblastic lymphomas have tumour cells in the peripheral blood at some time during their illness. Half of the patients with abnormal blood counts will have a normal bone marrow examination. Thrombocytopenia may be a reflection of associated hypersplenism but thrombocytopenia coupled with anaemia is strongly suggestive of marrow disease. In 70% of patients with lymphoma cells in the bone marrow, the spleen and liver will be found to be involved at laparotomy. There is a high correlation between bone marrow infiltration and central nervous system involvement in patients with high-grade lymphomas.

Routine biochemical analysis is essential to exclude major organ dysfunction prior to treatment although such abnormalities by themselves are not reliable indicators of direct infiltration. Raised immunoglobulin levels may be found in lymphoplasmacytoid lymphomas and hyperviscosity may occur as a result. Measurement of plasma viscosity in these patients may demonstrate the need for urgent corrective therapy to prevent additional complications.

Rapid tumour lysis of highly chemosensitive tumours following therapy can produce severe metabolic disturbance including electrolyte imbalance, uric acid nephropathy and renal failure. Preventive measures, including regular allopurinol, high fluid intake and alkalinization of the urine, are necessary before starting chemotherapy.

Radiology

Even in the advanced stages of non-Hodgkin's lymphoma intrathoracic disease is less common than in Hodgkin's disease. However, approximately 25% of patients with non-Hodgkin's lymphoma will show some abnormality on routine chest radiograph. Hilar or mediastinal adenopathy is the most common finding followed by pleural effusion and parenchymal involvement. Parenchymal disease may show up as ill defined miliary mottling or discrete nodules with or without central cavitation. A malignant pleural effusion may be present in the absence of other intrathoracic disease.[73]

Lymphography

Lymphography remains one of the most accurate methods of assessing retroperitoneal nodes, which are involved in approximately 50% of patients with non-Hodgkin's lymphoma. The lymphogram may act as a predictor of involvement in other abdominal sites—in one National Cancer Institute series, 80% of patients with an abnormal lymphogram had disease in the liver and the mesenteric nodes, or cells in the ascitic fluid, compared to 18% with a negative lymphogram.[91] Lymphography has the disadvantage that it is an invasive procedure and not without occasional complications, including allergic reactions, wound infection, fever and oil embolization. Lymphography is contraindicated in patients with chronic obstructive airways disease, congestive cardiac failure, pulmonary fibrosis or iodine allergy. In patients undergoing successful lymphography the dye may remain visible within

REFERENCE

91. Chabner B A, Johnson R D et al Ann Intern Med 1976; 85: 149–154

lymph nodes for several months after the procedure and this may act as a valuable monitor of the response to treatment.

Ultrasound scanning

While ultrasound scanning is potentially useful for assessing involvement in the abdomen and pelvis and, in particular, in demonstrating enlarged nodes in the porta hepatis, coeliac axis or para-aortic region, the technique is limited by its inability to detect involved nodes less than 1.5 cm in diameter or to differentiate lymphomatous infiltration from reactive hyperplasia.

Intravenous urogram

Renal involvement may be found at post mortem in up to 30% of patients with disseminated lymphoma but it is rarely diagnosed clinically. Renal involvement or obstructive uropathy may be shown on routine intravenous urogram, and displacement of the ureters may raise the suspicion of enlarged para-aortic lymph nodes; however, the intravenous urogram has now been generally replaced by CT scanning which is a more accurate method of demonstrating renal involvement in non-Hodgkin's lymphoma.

Radioisotope scanning

Technetium liver and spleen scanning is an unreliable indicator of organ involvement by lymphoma. The discovery that gallium 67 localizes well within lymphoma tissue (particularly in high-grade lymphoma) has prompted considerable interest in the role of this isotope in scanning for occult sites of involvement. Uptake by gallium is not restricted to areas of lymphoma but also occurs in inflammatory tissue and in normal organs.[74] Detection rates have been increased by using high doses of gallium (7–10 mCi) and more sensitive imaging equipment. Scanning may be highly specific in the chest, particularly in differentiating fibrosis following treatment from active lymphoma, but within the abdomen the rate of detection is poor with an accuracy of less than 50% for both liver and spleen.

As with Hodgkin's disease, whole body FDG PET scanning may be a useful staging tool but FDG uptake may be unreliable in MALT lymphomas and occasional high-grade B-cell lymphomas.

CT scanning

When available, CT scanning is the preferred non-invasive method of assessing abdominal involvement by non-Hodgkin's lymphoma with an overall accuracy in excess of 80%. In the abdomen and pelvis, lymph nodes up to 1 cm are usually considered normal; in non-Hodgkin's lymphoma involved nodes tend to be significantly enlarged with mesenteric node involvement in more than 50% of cases (Fig. 34.15). While CT may demonstrate abnormalities in those areas not visualized on the lymphogram, no clear advantage has been demonstrated for CT over lymphography in the abdominal staging of non-Hodgkin's lymphoma, and preference for one technique will depend on access and local expertise.

CT scanning of the chest may provide additional information when the chest radiograph is equivocal but adds little when the plain chest radiograph shows no obvious mediastinal or lung involvement.

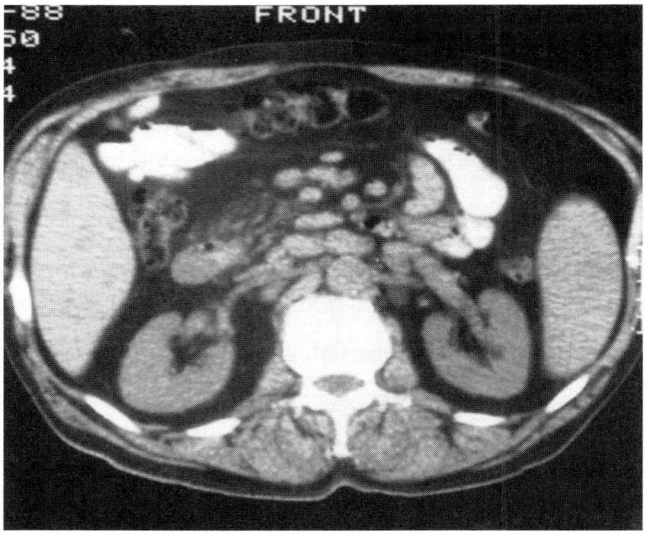

Fig. 34.15 CT scan of involved mesenteric nodes in non-Hodgkin's lymphoma.

Magnetic resonance imaging

Magnetic resonance scanning offers a further method for staging of patients with non-Hodgkin's lymphoma with the advantage that no contrast medium is required and no ionizing radiation is involved. Richards et al reported that low field-strength magnetic resonance imaging is a very sensitive method of detecting liver disease, although not specific for lymphoma.[92] Preliminary data suggested that magnetic resonance image scanning at low strength may also be useful to detect bone marrow infiltration but at the present time this investigation offers no advantage in detecting splenic involvement.

Staging laparotomy

Staging laparotomy and splenectomy have no place in the routine management of non-Hodgkin's lymphoma patients who are, in general, an older and less fit population. As truly localized non-Hodgkin's lymphoma is rare, local radiotherapy alone is appropriate treatment for very few patients; the majority require some form of systemic therapy from the outset, thereby rendering laparotomy unnecessary.

Treatment

Localized disease

Following careful staging, including laparotomy and splenectomy, less than 10% of patients with low-grade lymphoma will be found to have stage I or II disease. Radiotherapy alone in this group

REFERENCE

92. Richards M A, Webb J A N et al Br Med J 1986; 293: 1126–1128

produces disease-free survivals of 75% at 5 years. The introduction of adjuvant chemotherapy has failed to influence the frequency of relapse or improve the overall survival rate. Despite the apparently indolent behaviour of low-grade non-Hodgkin's lymphoma, for most patients with clinical stage I and II disease continuing relapse is the rule and disease-free survivals of only 20–25% are to be expected at 5 years with conventional treatment. Few patients are cured with current therapy.

Approximately 25% of patients with intermediate or high-grade non-Hodgkin's lymphoma have stage I or II disease after appropriate staging investigations. In selected series of pathologically staged patients the results of radiotherapy demonstrate a clear difference between those with truly localized (stage IA or IE) disease and those with stage IIA or IIE disease. Sweet et al reported an 11-year actuarial disease-free survival rate of 93% for stage I supradiaphragmatic lymph node disease compared to only 33% for stage II or stage IIE disease.[93] The success of intensive initial chemotherapy in patients with more advanced disease and the high rate of relapse following radiotherapy alone indicate that chemotherapy is the appropriate treatment for patients with stage II high-grade non-Hodgkin's lymphoma.

Disseminated disease

The majority of patients with low-grade lymphoma have disseminated disease at presentation which may run an indolent course characterized by a continuing relapse pattern over many years; few, if any, patients are cured by conventional measures. In symptomless patients there is no evidence that early treatment is associated with improved quality or duration of survival.[94] In many patients therefore therapy should be reserved until the disease has progressed or/unpleasant symptoms develop. In patients who have localized areas of tender or unsightly lymphadenopathy, a short course of local radiotherapy may be all that is required to relieve symptoms.[95]

The current treatment of patients with disseminated low-grade non-Hodgkin's lymphoma is oral chlorambucil with or without prednisolone. Chlorambucil is usually given on an intermittent schedule at a dose of 6 mg/m^2 by mouth daily for 14 days followed by a 14-day treatment free interval. Treatment is continued until the maximum response is obtained and the patient is then observed until further relapse occurs. Response to oral chlorambucil is often slow; if more rapid regression is required then initial treatment with intravenous Cyclophosphamide, Vincristine and Prednisolone may be indicated, although the toxicity from this combined treatment is more pronounced and overall survival rates no better.

Intensive multidrug chemotherapy schedules with bone marrow or stem cell support in younger patients have produced higher complete remission rates but it is not yet apparent whether this has been coupled with prolonged survival.[96] At the present time any moves to more aggressive therapy in patients with low-grade lymphoma must be considered experimental and should only be undertaken as part of carefully controlled trials within specialist centres.

In 25% of patients with low-grade non-Hodgkin's lymphoma the disease will in due course transform into a more aggressive subtype with a median survival of only 8 months following transformation.[97]

Intermediate and high-grade lymphoma

The introduction of effective cytotoxic chemotherapy for disseminated intermediate and high-grade lymphoma has transformed the prognosis for many of these patients, to the extent that 30–40% will now be cured of what was previously an almost uniformly fatal condition. The cornerstone of treatment for high-grade non-Hodgkin's lymphoma has been the CHOP regimen, using Cyclophosphamide, Adriamycin, Vincristine and Prednisolone. This produces complete remission rates of 60–70%. While continuing relapses are seen throughout the first 2 years after treatment, at this point the survival curve reaches a plateau and relapses after 2 years are extremely uncommon. Attempts to improve on remission and survival rates by the introduction of more intensive chemotherapy schedules have not improved survival prospects and CHOP remains the 'gold standard' treatment for high-grade non-Hodgkin's lymphoma.[98]

Biological therapy

The dramatic success of interferon in treating hairy cell leukaemia has prompted considerable interest in the potential of similar biological therapy for non-Hodgkin's lymphoma. Much experimental work is still in progress but, at the present time, approximately 50% of patients with disseminated low-grade lymphoma refractory to conventional chemotherapy obtain partial remissions with interferon. Studies examining the role of interferon in conjunction with chlorambucil and other chemotherapeutic drugs as first-line treatment in disseminated low-grade non-Hodgkin's lymphoma are in progress.

Special sites

Gastrointestinal lymphoma

Over 50% of patients with disseminated lymphoma have some gastrointestinal involvement at post mortem. However, a proportion of lymphomas, particularly in childhood, arise primarily in the gastrointestinal tract and require special consideration.

The definition of primary gastrointestinal lymphoma is confused but it is generally accepted that there should be no superficial or mediastinal lymphadenopathy at presentation, no involvement of the bone marrow or peripheral blood and no hepatic or splenic infiltration.

Primary gastrointestinal lymphoma is rare and yet represents the most common extranodal site of presentation of the disease.

REFERENCES

93. Sweet D L, Kinzie J et al Blood 1981; 58: 121–123
94. Horning S J, Rosenberg S A N Engl J Med 1984; 311: 1471–1475
95. Sawyer E J, Timothy A R Radioth Oncol 1997; 42: 49
96. Rohatiner A, Johnson P et al J Clin Oncol 1994; 12: 1177
97. Bastion Y, Berger F Ann Oncol 1991; 2: 123
98. Fisher R I, Gaynor E R N Engl J Med 1993; 328: 1002

The stomach is most commonly involved (55%) followed by the small intestine (30%) (see Chapters 28 and 29). Symptoms include abdominal pain and weight loss, with many patients complaining of nausea and vomiting. Examination reveals a palpable mass in approximately one third of patients and approximately 10% present with a degree of anaemia. The lesions are usually polypoid, single or multiple, and ulceration, perforation and bleeding may occur. The majority of gastrointestinal lymphomas are high-grade, of B-cell type, although MALT lymphomas of the stomach are increasingly being diagnosed.

The most appropriate management for these patients can only be decided on an individual basis. Where possible, all diseased bowel should be resected at laparotomy to allow adequate histological assessment and to minimize the risk of haemorrhage and perforation during subsequent treatment. As the majority of these patients have high-grade disease they will require intensive combination chemotherapy after surgery.[99] The association of *Helicobacter pylori* infection with chronic gastritis and subsequent development of MALT lymphoma has led to studies of anti-helicobacter rather than cytotoxic therapy as first-line treatment. While complete remissions have been reported some tumours do not respond or will relapse after initial response.[85]

There are many reports on the benefit of whole abdominal irradiation following surgery in gastrointestinal lymphoma but as yet no controlled trials to compare radiation against chemotherapy have been undertaken.

Head and neck

The head and neck is another common site of extranodal involvement by non-Hodgkin's lymphoma. In approximately 50% of cases the tonsil is the primary site followed in descending frequency by the nasopharynx and the base of the tongue.[100] Half the patients presenting with involvement of Waldeyer's ring have associated cervical node involvement (stage IIE) and a significant proportion of these advance to a higher stage following staging. The predominant histology is diffuse high-grade lymphoma with only a few patients having a low-grade lymphoma. There are several reports in the literature describing a high instance of involvement of the upper gastrointestinal tract as the first site of relapse following treatment of lymphoma of Waldeyer's ring, suggesting that it is important to examine the gastrointestinal tract during initial staging investigations.

For IE disease staged by lymphogram and bone marrow, 5-year survivals exceed 75% with radiotherapy alone, compared to less than 40% for stage IIE patients. Radiotherapy fields should encompass the primary disease and uninvolved cervical nodes. With the rare exception of those patients with low-grade histology who achieve long-term disease-free survival with radiotherapy alone, all other patients with stage IIE head and neck lymphoma should receive chemotherapy as primary treatment.

Thyroid

Lymphoma of the thyroid represents less than 10% of all thyroid malignancy and less than 2% of all extranodal lymphomas.[101] It is primarily a disease of elderly females, with a median age of 65 years at presentation. One fifth of these patients give a history of pre-existing goitre and there is a strong association with Hashimoto's thyroiditis. The most common presentation involves a short history (usually less than 3 months) of a rapidly enlarging thyroid swelling which may be associated with local pain and tenderness, stridor, hoarseness, dyspnoea and dysphagia. Again the majority of tumours are diffuse high-grade lymphoma and differentiation from anaplastic carcinoma may be difficult. When cervical lymphadenopathy is present the survival rates are markedly diminished.

Treatment of thyroid lymphoma has historically consisted of local or regional radiation with or without surgery. Local control rates are improved by resection of bulk disease; however, in many patients age or local infiltration of tumour makes surgical intervention hazardous. Survival rates of 40% at 5 years are reported with radiotherapy alone for localized disease; failures occur both locally and systematically. Given the increasing success of combination chemotherapy for high-grade lymphoma in other sites and the fact that such therapy is often well tolerated even in elderly patients, chemotherapy may be most appropriate as first-line treatment. In those patients considered unfit for surgery or chemotherapy, involved-field radiotherapy remains effective palliative local treatment.

Testicular lymphoma

Testicular involvement in generalized lymphoma and leukaemia is well recognized; however, primary lymphoma of the testis is rare, accounting for less than 2% of non-Hodgkin's lymphoma in males. In contrast to other testicular malignancies lymphoma presents late with a median age of 60 and is rare below the age of 40.[102] The majority of cases are intermediate or high-grade lymphomas and, as anticipated, the results of treatment with orchidectomy followed by local or regional lymph node irradiation are poor with high systemic relapse rates and few long-term survivors. After intensive staging the majority of patients have at least stage II disease and chemotherapy offers the only hope for cure for high-grade tumours.

Bone

Primary lymphoma of bone characteristically presents with local bone pain often accompanied by swelling. The symptoms may be present for many months before diagnosis and in approximately 20% of cases there is associated regional node involvement.[97] The radiographic appearances are non-specific with lytic bone destruction with or without sclerosis and sometimes extensive soft tissue involvement. The long bones of the humerus and femur are most commonly affected.

REFERENCES

99. Timothy A R, Sloane J, Selby P In: Sikora K, Halnan H E (eds) Treatment of Cancer, 2nd edn. Chapman & Hall Medical, London 1990 pp 695–736
100. Wang D S, Fuller L M et al Am J Roentgenol 1975; 123: 471
101. Chak L Y, Hoppe R T et al Cancer 1981; 48: 2712
102. Duncan P R, Checa F et al Cancer 1980; 45: 1578

The disease is rare in the first decade and most common between 40 and 70 years. The differential diagnosis includes other round cell tumours including metastatic carcinoma, Ewing's sarcoma and eosinophilic granuloma. Combined radiation and chemotherapy is currently the preferred option with 5-year survival rates in the order of 50%.[103]

Central nervous system lymphoma

Primary lymphoma of the central nervous system (reticulum cell sarcoma, microgliomatosis, malignant reticuloendotheliosis) predominantly involves the brain and only rarely the spinal cord. The incidence of primary central nervous system lymphoma has increased in recent years, particularly in patients with chronic immunosuppression in association with either the acquired immune deficiency syndrome or following organ transplantation.[104] Presenting symptoms are similar to those of other intracranial tumours and include headache, nausea and vomiting, seizures and localized weakness.

The origin and histological classification of primary central nervous system lymphomas have caused considerable controversy but it appears that they are largely of B-cell origin and of high-grade type. Involvement of the brain is usually multifocal and the disease infiltrates widely. While whole-brain irradiation may produce good palliation, survival to 5 years is exceptional even with high-dose radiotherapy and with combination chemotherapy. Given the appalling prognosis of this disease alternative treatment strategies need to be explored.

Secondary central nervous system involvement

Central nervous system involvement occurs in up to 30% of patients with disseminated non-Hodgkin's lymphoma, the incidence being highest in those with high-grade disease and bone marrow or liver infiltration. The disease primarily affects the meninges and less commonly the spinal cord and brain parenchyma. Patients with high-grade lymphoma achieving complete remission after chemotherapy show central nervous system relapse rates of between 5 and 8% but this is rarely the only site of recurrent disease. Even with more intensive therapy, including intrathecal chemotherapy, central nervous system relapse still occurs and more effective treatment must be developed.

Prognosis

Truly localized (stage I) low-grade non-Hodgkin's lymphoma is rare but when it does occur excellent survival rates may be expected with local radiotherapy alone. For all other stages of low-grade lymphoma cure is not a realistic option with conventional therapy and current treatment strategy involves providing the minimum amount of treatment with the least toxicity which will offer the individual patient maximum palliative benefit. Trials are in progress exploring alternative treatment options in good prognosis patients.[96]

For patients with stage I high-grade non-Hodgkin's lymphoma systemic chemotherapy with subsequent radiotherapy to bulk disease produces excellent 5-year cure rates. For more advanced stages, chemotherapy results in complete remission rates of 70%, with 5-year overall disease free and survival rates of 30%.

REFERENCES

103. Barr J, Burke R Cancer 1994; 73: 1194
104. Penn I In: Toledo-Pereyra 00 (ed) Complications of Organ Transplantation. Marcel Dekker, New York 1987 pp 237–251

35 The adrenal glands

M. H. Wheeler

INTRODUCTION

The adrenal glands were overlooked by the early anatomists including even Leonardo da Vinci and were first accurately described in 1563 by Bartholomaeus Eustachius.[1] More than 300 years passed before there was some understanding of the functions of these glands derived from the clinical observations of Addison[2] and the physiological experiments of Brown-Séquard[3] who appreciated that the adrenals were essential for life. Each adult adrenal gland weighs 2–6 g and is enclosed in Gerota's fascia at the upper medial pole of each kidney. The adrenal cortex secretes steroid hormones and is derived from the urogenital mesoderm whereas the medulla is derived from ectodermal neural crest, consists of chromaffin cells and secretes catecholamines. As these numerous hormones regulate a wide range of physiological functions, it is not surprising that hyperplastic or neoplastic conditions of the adrenal can cause excessive secretion of the various hormones resulting in a variety of clinical syndromes. Benign pathological lesions usually secrete a single hormone in contrast to the mixed hormone production which characterizes malignancy.

The endocrine surgeon operating on the adrenal glands has a unique opportunity to correct profound physiological disturbances and restore the patient to complete normality.

ANATOMY

The adrenal glands are situated in close relation to the upper and medial aspects of the kidney. The right adrenal is pyramidal in shape and is related to the right diaphragm posteriorly, the bare area of liver anteriorly and the inferior vena cava for a length of 3–4 cm medially. The gland's arterial supply is derived from three main vessels: one ascending branch from the right adrenal, one from the aorta and branches from the inferior phrenic artery. A single wide short vein passes into the posterior aspect of the inferior vena cava.

The left adrenal gland is more flattened than the right and semilunar in outline. On the left side the arterial supply is similar to that of the right gland but the venous drainage consists of a single vein passing to the renal vein. It is important for the surgeon to note that there are occasionally accessory adrenal veins on the right passing to the vena cava or hepatic veins and on the left principally to the descending phrenic vein.

The adrenals have a rich sympathetic nerve supply from the coeliac plexus but preganglionic fibres from the splanchnic nerves pass through the coeliac plexus to supply the adrenal medulla.

ADRENAL CORTEX

Physiology

The mineralocorticoid aldosterone is the principal steroid hormone secreted by the outer zone of the adrenal cortex, the zona glomerulosa. Aldosterone secretion is enhanced by a fall in blood volume, sodium restriction and by an increase in serum potassium concentration. Sodium retention is produced by increasing sodium absorption from the distal renal tubule, ascending loop of Henle and collecting ducts, in exchange for potassium and hydrogen which are excreted in equivalent amounts. Potassium exchange is a function of the rate of presentation of sodium in the distal tubule. Therefore, potassium may be retained during salt retention and lost during salt loading, thereby influencing the rate of secretion of aldosterone.

The glucocorticoids, principally cortisol and small amounts of corticosterone, are produced in the zona fasciculata from cholesterol by a series of enzyme-dependent metabolic steps. These hormones, whose release is regulated by adrenocorticotrophic hormone (ACTH) from the pituitary via a negative-feedback mechanism, have a wide range of physiological actions and are intimately involved in the regulation of carbohydrate, protein and fat metabolism.

The zona reticularis produces the androgens, dehydroepiandrosterone, androsterone, androstenedione and testosterone along with small amounts of oestrogen and progesterone.

CUSHING'S SYNDROME

This syndrome is the result of excessive levels of circulating cortisol. The causes may be divided into two main groups depending upon whether or not the condition is the result of excess ACTH secretion.

ACTH-dependent Cushing's syndrome

1. A pituitary/hypothalamic disorder known as Cushing's disease.

REFERENCES

1. Eustachius B Cited by Harrison T S, Gann D S et al Surgical Disorders of the Adrenal Gland. Grune & Stratton, New York 1975
2. Addison T On the Constitutional and Local Effects of Disease of the Supra-renal Capsules. Highley, London 1855
3. Brown-Sèquard E E Arch Gen Med 1856; 2: 385, 572

2. An ectopic ACTH-secreting tumour.
3. An ectopic corticotrophin-releasing hormone-secreting tumour.
4. Iatrogenic from administration of ACTH or its analogues.

Non-ACTH-dependent Cushing's syndrome

1. Functioning adrenocortical tumours.
   a. adenoma.
   b. carcinoma.
2. Macronodular adrenal cortical hyperplasia.
3. Primary pigmented nodular adrenal cortical disease.
4. Iatrogenic from administration of corticosteroids (the commonest cause).[4]

Cushing's disease

In 1932 Harvey Cushing, a neurosurgeon,[5] described the classical clinical features of this syndrome in patients with basophil adenomas of the pituitary gland. Excluding the iatrogenic groups, pituitary-dependent Cushing's disease accounts for 70% of all cases of the syndrome. Women are affected four times as often as men and the peak incidence is in the 35–50-year age group. The primary defect is probably in the hypothalamus, with an overproduction of corticotrophin-releasing hormone. The excess pituitary ACTH is still subject to steroid suppression but at a higher set point; the increased blood level leads to bilateral adrenal gland hyperplasia.[6] A pituitary tumour or microadenoma is present in more than 75% of these cases.

Ectopic ACTH syndrome

Cushing's syndrome from ACTH production by an oat cell carcinoma of the lung was first described by Brown in 1928.[7] Liddle et al, in 1962,[8] introduced the term 'ectopic ACTH syndrome' for a condition now thought to be responsible for 10% of cases of Cushing's syndrome. These ACTH-secreting tumours may be benign, e.g. bronchial carcinoid, or malignant, such as the oat cell carcinoma. The primary malignant tumours will frequently kill the patient before significant or severe effects of steroid excess develop.

Other tumours with the potential for secreting ACTH include phaeochromocytoma, certain ovarian tumours and a group of endocrine tumours of foregut origin which include thymoma, islet cell tumours of the pancreas, carcinoid tumours of the lung, pancreas, stomach and medullary carcinoma of the thyroid.[9]

Adrenal tumours

These comprise 20% of Cushing's syndrome, and are equally divided between benign adrenocortical adenomas and frank invasive carcinoma. In adults, adenoma is the commoner lesion but unfortunately carcinoma predominates in children. The considerable steroid secretion by the tumour suppresses ACTH secretion and leads to atrophy of the opposite adrenal.

Macronodular adrenal cortical hyperplasia

This unusual condition, in which ACTH-independent cortisol secretion results from bilateral adrenal nodular hyperplasia, is sometimes seen in the young and may be associated with severe osteopenic bone disease.[10] The cause is unknown.

Primary pigmented nodular adrenal cortical disease

This rare syndrome has been described in which primary pigmented nodular adrenal cortical disease producing autonomous adrenal hyperfunction occurs in conjunction with cardiac, breast and cutaneous myxomas.[11] Lentigines are found on the face, lips and conjunctivae. Pituitary adenomas and neuroectodernal tumours also occur. The adrenal nodules are normally small and the adrenal glands may even appear to be normal on imaging.

Clinical features (Fig. 35.1)

The cardinal clinical features of Cushing's syndrome are shown in Table 35.1.

Differential diagnosis

The clinical features of Cushing's syndrome may be confused with those of the obese diabetic particularly when there is an associated plethoric face. Polycystic ovary with sterility and hirsutism also poses diagnostic difficulties, but Cushing's syndrome is rarely the cause of hirsutism alone. Alcoholic patients can present with pseudo-Cushing's syndrome, of which the symptoms and signs resolve after cessation of excessive alcohol intake.

Investigation of Cushing's syndrome[13,14]

The clinical observations will indicate the diagnosis but investigations are essential firstly to confirm true hypercortisolism and then to identify the cause of the cortisol excess.

Proof of hypercortisolism

1. Plasma cortisol levels stimulated by ACTH normally conform to a diurnal pattern with the highest values at 9.00 a.m. and lowest at midnight. Loss of this diurnal variation and elevation of the midnight level frequently occur in Cushing's syndrome.[15]

REFERENCES

4. Thompson N W, Allo M D World J Surg 1982; 6: 748
5. Cushing H Bull Johns Hopkins Hosp 1932; 50: 137
6. Besser G M, Edwards C R W Clin Endocrinol Metab 1972; 1: 451
7. Brown W H Lancet 1928; ii: 1022
8. Liddle G W, Island D, Meador C K Prog Hormone Res 1962; IS: 125
9. Azzopardi J G, Williams E D Cancer 1968; 22: 274
10. Ruder H J, Loriaux D L, Lipsett M B J Clin Endocrinol Metab 1974; 39: 1138
11. Grant C S, Carney J A et al Surgery 1986; 100: 1178
12. Plotz C M, Knowlton A I, Ragan C Am J Med 1952; 13: 597
13. Crapo L Metabolism 1979; 28: 955
14. Friesen S R, Thompson N W (eds) Surgical Endocrinology. Lippincott, Philadelphia 1990
15. Hall R Med Int 1981; 1: 276

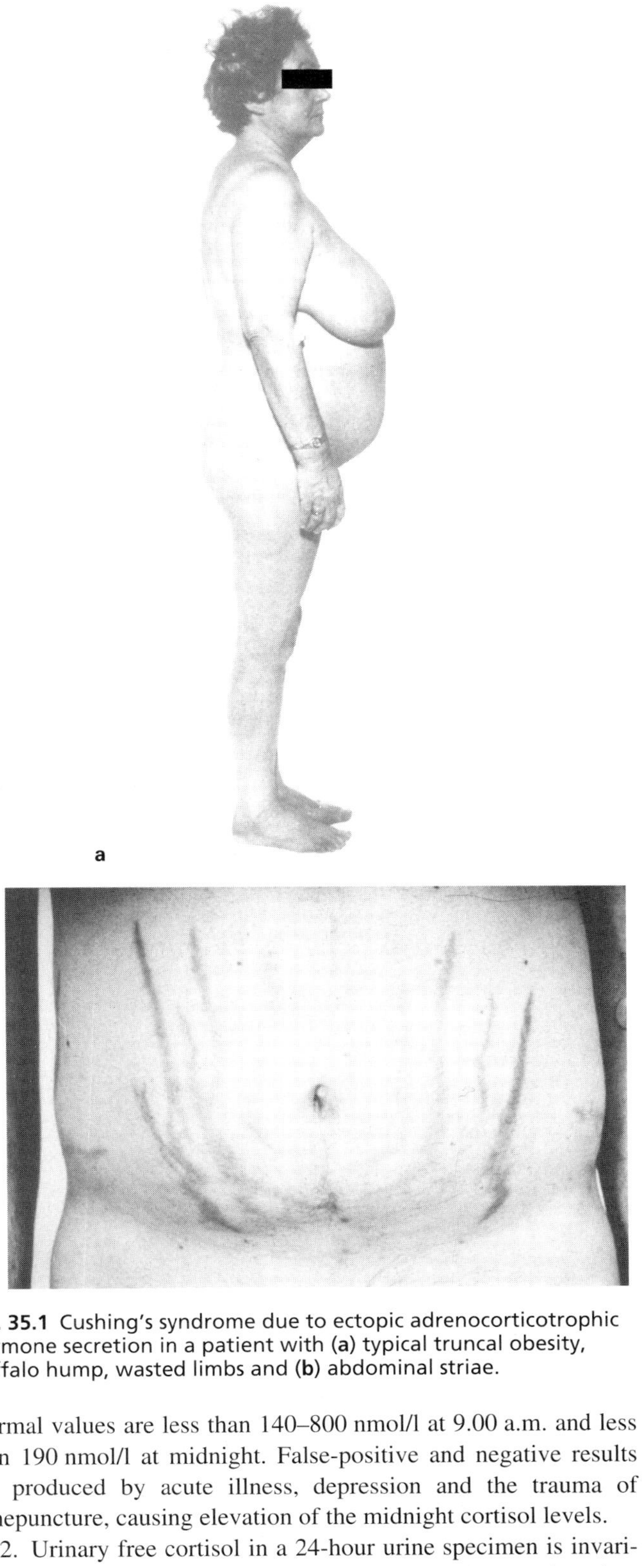

Fig. 35.1 Cushing's syndrome due to ectopic adrenocorticotrophic hormone secretion in a patient with **(a)** typical truncal obesity, buffalo hump, wasted limbs and **(b)** abdominal striae.

Normal values are less than 140–800 nmol/l at 9.00 a.m. and less than 190 nmol/l at midnight. False-positive and negative results are produced by acute illness, depression and the trauma of venepuncture, causing elevation of the midnight cortisol levels.

2. Urinary free cortisol in a 24-hour urine specimen is invariably elevated in Cushing's syndrome. Normal values are less than 360 nmol/day for men and less than 280 nmol/day for women.

3. Simple measurement of urinary 17-hydroxy and 17-ketosteroids has been superseded by the urinary free cortisol determination in the screening and routine identification of Cushing's syndrome.

4. Dexamethasone suppression tests[14] depend upon the knowledge that dexamethasone, a potent steroid, suppresses the pituitary adrenal axis more readily in normal subjects than in Cushing's syndrome.

a. Overnight dexamethasone suppression test: The 9.00 a.m. plasma cortisol is suppressed in normal subjects but not in patients with Cushing's syndrome after oral administration of 2 mg dexamethasone at midnight.

b. Low-dose dexamethasone test: Urinary 24-hour 17-hydroxy steroids and plasma cortisol are measured before and after the oral administration of dexamethasone 0.5 mg 6-hourly for 2 days. Suppression of these hormones is seen in normal subjects but in few patients with Cushing's syndrome.

5. Insulin-induced hypoglycaemia fails to produce a rise in plasma cortisol in patients with Cushing's syndrome and is useful in distinguishing patients with the syndrome from patients with depression who may have elevated basal cortisol levels.

The cause of cortisol excess

1. High-dose dexamethasone suppression: Oral administration of dexamethasone 2 mg 6-hourly for 2 days will distinguish pituitary Cushing's disease from non-pituitary causes which include adrenal cortical lesions (adenoma and carcinoma), adrenal nodular hyperplasia or the ectopic ACTH syndrome. Nearly all patients with pituitary Cushing's suppress urinary 24-hour 17-hydroxy steroids to 40% of the baseline or lower in contrast to most subjects with an adrenal cortical tumour, ectopic ACTH syndrome or nodular hyperplasia in which little or no suppression is seen. There are false-positive and negative results with this test; some patients with ectopic ACTH syndrome show suppression with the high-dose test.[16] Spontaneous cyclic changes in cortisol production may also account for some inconsistent results with the test. It is still however a valuable test to distinguish patients with pituitary disease from those with other non-pituitary causes of Cushing's syndrome.

2. Measurement of plasma ACTH by radioimmunoassay can be used to distinguish patients with ACTH-dependent Cushing's syndrome in which levels are raised from those with an adrenal tumour who have low or undetectable levels.[14] Very high levels of ACTH (greater than 200 pg/ml) are often seen in ectopic ACTH syndrome.[15] ACTH levels in nodular hyperplasia are normally depressed but results may be indeterminate.

3. Metyrapone test: This 11μ-hydroxylase inhibitor blocks the final steps in cortisol synthesis leading to a reduction in plasma cortisol, stimulation of pituitary ACTH release via a negative-feedback mechanism and a subsequent stimulation of cortisol precursor synthesis (compound S) by the adrenal cortex.[13] These precursors are measured as 17-hydroxy steroids in 24-hour urine samples the day before, the day of and the day after the administration of metyrapone 750 mg, which is given orally as six 4-hourly doses.

REFERENCE

16. Edis A J, Grant C S, Egdahal R H Manual of Endocrine Surgery, 2nd edn. Springer-Verlag, New York 1984

Table 35.1 Clinical features of Cushing's syndrome

Symptoms and signs	*Cause*	*Comment*
Obesity	Cortisol stimulation of appetite and gluconeogenesis. Glucose is liberated for fat synthesis	Truncal fat distribution with buffalo hump and plethoric moon face. Limbs wasted in contrast to generalized fat distribution of simple obesity
Striae and thin skin	Reduction in skin collagen	Purple colour on abdomen, breasts and flanks—unlike the pink striae of simple obesity
Excessive bruising	Vessel wall collagen depletion	Bruising spontaneously or with minimal trauma
Hypertension and oedema	Salt and water retention secondary to cortisol excess	Significant cause of mortality, which is 50% at 5 years in untreated Cushing's syndrome[12]
Muscle weakness	Toxic effect of cortisol on muscles	Proximal muscle groups are primarily affected
Back pain	Osteoporosis	Pathological fractures may occur in ribs and long bones. Collapse of vertebral bodies is common
Skin pigmentation	Concomitant hypersecretion of ACTH and melanocyte-stimulating hormone	Common in ectopic ACTH syndrome due to malignancy, when rapid weight loss and generalized wasting may dominate the clinical picture. Also a feature of pituitary tumour with high ACTH levels (Nelson's syndrome)
Psychiatric illness		Wide range of symptoms from depression to psychosis
Diabetes mellitus	Action of cortisol on carbohydrate metabolism	
Hirsutism	Adrenal androgen secretion	Adrenal carcinoma must be suspected particularly if virilism is pronounced. Acne on face and trunk
Menstrual disturbance		Amenorrhoea or irregular menstruation Impotence in men
Growth retardation	Cortisol reduction of release and peripheral action of growth hormone	Important feature of Cushing's syndrome in children
Poor wound healing	Cortisol effect on collagen synthesis Increased protein catabolism	Important surgical consideration, particularly when the anterior operative approach is used

ACTH = Adrenocorticotrophic hormone.

Patients with pituitary Cushing's disease increase their 17-hydroxy steroid excretion in contrast to the majority of patients with adrenal tumours, ectopic ACTH syndrome or nodular hyperplasia who show either impaired or absent responses.

Careful analysis of these investigations should enable the clinician to be absolutely certain that the patient has Cushing's syndrome and be reasonably sure of the cause. The syndrome is best diagnosed by combining the measurement of urinary free cortisol and plasma cortisol with a 2 mg low-dose dexamethasone suppression test. The precise cause of this syndrome can be identified by a combination of basal plasma ACTH measurement and 8 mg high-dose dexamethasone suppression test. An early adrenal computed tomography (CT) scan may show a tumour, thus helping to focus the investigations, though not removing the need for them. The metyrapone test can be reserved to confirm the diagnosis of pituitary-based Cushing's disease. Additional tests are necessary to achieve accurate preoperative localization which facilitates planning of the subsequent surgery. A routine chest X-ray may show a bronchogenic carcinoma or bronchial carcinoid. If the steroid excess has been long-standing, it is not unusual to see evidence of rib fractures.

Conventional skull X-rays even with thin-section tomography fail to locate the majority of pituitary lesions in Cushing's disease. CT scanning has considerably improved diagnostic accuracy but even this fails to identify at least 50% of the microadenomas found at surgery. CT scanning is however highly efficient in identifying adrenal tumours even when they are as small as 1 cm in diameter (Fig. 35.2). Adrenal tumours larger than 6 cm diameter are likely to be malignant.[14] The investigation has limitations, in that it may not always be able to demonstrate the bilateral hyperplasia of pituitary-dependent Cushing's disease, where the adrenal gland size is not markedly increased. The adrenal glands are usually enlarged in the ectopic ACTH syndrome and this can be seen on CT scan[17]

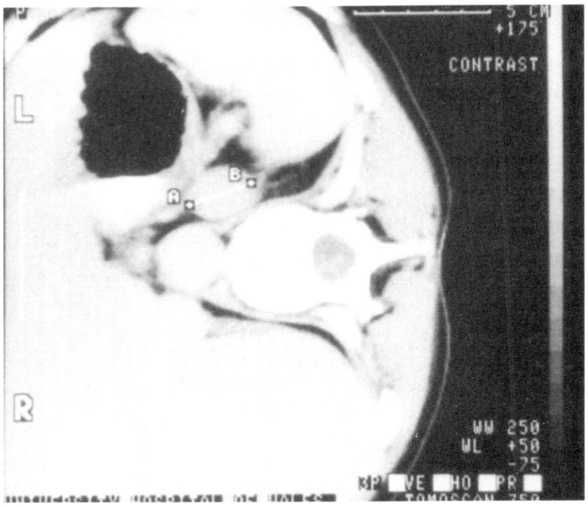

Fig. 35.2 Computed tomography scan of the abdomen showing an adenoma of the left adrenal gland. The patient's Cushing's syndrome was cured by removal of the left adrenal gland.

REFERENCE

17. White F E, White M C et al Br Med J 1982; 284: 771

(Fig. 35.3). In this syndrome, CT is the method of choice for attempting to localize bronchial, pulmonary, mediastinal or pancreatic tumours as sources of ACTH. CT is also capable of defining the relationship of adrenal tumours to adjacent structures.

Bilateral selective inferior petrosal venous sampling for ACTH estimation after corticotrophin-releasing hormone stimulation is an extremely valuable method of confirming and localizing pituitary-dependent Cushing's disease, particularly when CT scan of the pituitary fossa is unhelpful.

Adrenal gland scintigraphy using either ^{131}I-6B-iodomethyl-19norcholest-5(10)-en-3B-ol (NP-59) or selenium 75 cholesterol is a useful supplement to CT, showing unilateral uptake in a benign functioning tumour with contralateral gland suppression.[18] Adrenocortical carcinoma rarely concentrates the isotope but because of contralateral gland suppression the scan will show little or no uptake on either side. By contrast, the bilateral adrenal hyperplasia of Cushing's disease provides a bright bilateral scintiscan image.

Magnetic resonance imaging (MRI) is now established and is having a significant impact on the differential diagnosis of adrenal masses; adrenocortical carcinoma usually has a higher signal intensity (T2-weighted imaging) than a benign adenoma. MRI is particularly useful at demonstrating intravascular extension of large malignant adrenal tumours.[19]

Treatment of Cushing's disease

The discovery and clinical introduction of cortisone and its availability as a replacement rendered bilateral adrenalectomy a reasonable and logical treatment for Cushing's syndrome, especially when it was caused by pituitary disease. The results of bilateral adrenalectomy are very good with 65% of patients in remission at follow-up 5–15 years after surgery and one-half still alive at 20 years.[20]

But these adrenalectomized patients are dependent on glucocorticoid and mineralocorticoid replacement for life and subject to the constant hazards and dangers of adrenal insufficiency and circulatory collapse at times of stress, infection, illness and operation. Steroid cover and replacement therapy in these circumstances will be dealt with in a later section.

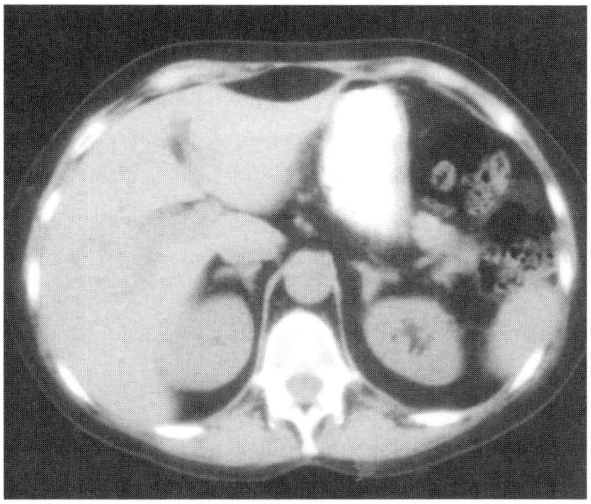

Fig. 35.3 Computed tomography scan of abdomen showing bilateral enlarged hyperplastic adrenal glands in the ectopic adrenocorticotrophic hormone syndrome.

The recognition of the high incidence of pituitary microadenomas in Cushing's disease has resulted in a dramatic change in emphasis in the surgery of the condition with a move away from bilateral adrenalectomy to a direct surgical approach to the pituitary by transphenoidal microsurgical dissection and excision of the basophil adenoma.[20,21] Excellent remission and cure rates have been reported with a minimal morbidity and mortality; few patients require pituitary replacement unless a complete hypophysectomy is necessary. There are not, as yet, sufficient long-term follow-up data to allow a true comparison to be made with bilateral adrenalectomy.

Radiotherapy of the pituitary

External pituitary irradiation by a cobalt unit or linear accelerator (45–50 Gy), proton beam irradiation or closed stereotactic radiosurgery have all been used as alternatives to surgery but control of the hypercortisolism using these techniques may take more than a year. Interstitial irradiation with yttrium 90 has also been successfully employed.[22] External or interstitial irradiation is particularly appropriate in the treatment of children when replacement pituitary therapy is usually unnecessary.[23]

Medical treatment

Metyrapone, the II β-hydroxylase inhibitor which restricts the conversion of 11-deoxycortisol to cortisol, can be used as long-term maintenance therapy for Cushing's syndrome when surgery is contraindicated, but has unpleasant side-effects of nausea, vomiting, hirsutism and acne.[24,25] Its most valuable role is in the preoperative preparation of patients for other definitive treatments such as adrenalectomy, pituitary microsurgery or irradiation. It is given in a dose of 250 mg three times daily, increasing over a week to 500 mg 6-hourly. In full doses, complete adrenal blockade is achieved, and administration of dexamethasone 0.25 mg twice daily is necessary.

Other drugs have been used with varying degrees of success in Cushing's syndrome.[26,27] These include aminoglutethamide, which inhibits conversion of cholesterol to pregnenolone: cyproheptadine, a serotonin antagonist which inhibits corticotrophin-releasing hormone release; bromocriptine, a dopamine agonist, and

REFERENCES

18. Schteingart D E, Seabold J E et al J Clin Endocrinol Metab 1981; 52: 115–116
19. Dunnick N R Am J Roentgenol 1990; 154: 927–936
20. Montgomery D A D, Welbourn R B Br J Surg 1978; 65: 221
21. Hardy J Clin Neurosurg 1969; 16: 185
22. Bigos S T, Somma M et al J Clin Endocrinol Metab 1979; 50: 348
23. Welbourn R B, Manolas K J In: Johnston I D A, Thompson N W (eds) Endocrine Surgery. Butterworth, London 1983
24. Orth D N Ann Intern Med 1978; 89: 128
25. Jeffcoate W J, Rees L H et al Br Med J 1977; 2: 215
26. Krieger D T, Amorasa L, Linick F N Engl J Med 1975; 293: 893
27. Victoria R, Therrien B A Ann Intern Med 1980; 92: 613

mitotane, which causes necrosis of the zona fasciculata and zona reticularis of the adrenal gland.

Treatment of ectopic ACTH syndrome

If a benign endocrine tumour such as bronchial carcinoid, whose site can be identified, is responsible for the ACTH secretion surgical excision can produce complete resolution of the syndrome. Malignant tumours should always be surgically excised, if possible, as there is a reasonable prospect of benefit with remission of the symptoms of hypercortisolism. ^{123}I octreotide scintigraphy may aid the identification of the ACTH-secreting tumour.

Adjuvant treatment by radiotherapy with or without chemotherapy may also be considered but although the frankly malignant tumours such as oat cell carcinoma often respond well at first, they have an extremely poor prognosis. Bilateral adrenalectomy may provide useful palliation when a malignant tumour cannot be resected completely or if the primary ACTH-secreting tumour cannot be located.[28] The drugs metyrapone and mitotane are also helpful in controlling the symptoms of hypercortisolism.

Treatment of adrenal adenoma

When Cushing's syndrome is caused by an adrenal adenoma, the treatment of choice is unilateral adrenalectomy via a posterior,[29] posterolateral or laparoscopic approach. These techniques provide excellent access with low morbidity and few of the wound problems seen with the anterior open transperitoneal approach.

The prospects for complete cure and long-term survival are excellent with almost all patients living 20 years.[20] Postoperatively steroid replacement is required as the opposite adrenal gland is suppressed by the adrenal adenoma. Gradual weaning off exogenous steroids can usually be achieved over a period of several months, although the occasional patient may take more than a year.

Adrenocortical carcinoma

This rare, highly malignant tumour secretes hormones in 60% of cases, the other 40% being non-functioning. Clinical syndromes produced by functioning tumours depend upon the hormone or hormones that are secreted (Table 35.2). Functioning tumours produce an excess of 17-ketosteroids and 17-hydroxy steroids in the urine.

Table 35.2 Adrenal carcinoma–endocrine syndromes

Tumour	*Syndrome*	*Hormone responsible*
Functioning (most patients < 40 years) F:M = 4:1	Cushing's syndrome	Cortisol
	Conn's syndrome	Aldosterone
	Virilization	Androgens
	Feminization	Oestrogens
	Mixed syndromes	Cortisol and androgen
Non-functioning (most patients > 40 years) M:F = 2:1		

Even non-functioning tumours produce steroid precursors with elevated levels of urinary pregnenolone. Measurement of dehydroepiandrosterone may be particularly helpful in the diagnosis of malignant adrenal tumours.[30] Adrenal carcinoma must be considered a likely diagnosis when Cushing's syndrome occurs in a child, and is associated with virilization, acne and amenorrhoea in a young female; with virilization in a prepubertal female; with precocious virilization in a child initially normal at birth; and when feminization of the male occurs.[31] Non-functioning or minimally functioning tumours frequently grow to a massive size before becoming clinically apparent (Fig. 35.4); patients eventually present with weight loss, abdominal pain and a mass. These tumours are not ACTH-dependent and, like benign adrenocortical adenoma, fail to suppress with high doses of dexamethasone. They have low levels of circulating ACTH. Preoperative localization is essential and is best achieved by CT scanning and MRI. Arteriography may also provide useful information whilst caval venography and real-time ultrasound are capable of defining inferior vena caval involvement by the tumour. MRI also provides excellent information, especially of vascular invasion (Fig. 35.5).

Treatment

Surgical resection is the best treatment and offers the prospect of cure. Unfortunately, these tumours frequently present late, particularly when they are non-functioning, and resection for cure is then no longer feasible because of local extension, lymph node and distant metastases. Aggressive surgical resection with, if necessary, removal of adjacent organs including the spleen, kidney and distal pancreas is indicated even in advanced tumours to achieve debulking. Even when the tumour recurs after initial surgery, repeated resections have led to prolonged survival.[32] An extended

REFERENCES

28. Davis C J, Joplin G F, Welbourn R B Ann Surg 1982; 196: 246
29. Young H H Surg Gynecol Obstet 1936; 54: 179
30. van Heerden J A, Grant C S, Weaver A C Acta Chir Austriaca 1993; 25: 216
31. Gabrilove J L, Sharma D C et al Medicine (Baltimore) 1965; 44: 37
32. Bradley E L Surg Gynecol Obstet 1975; 141: 507

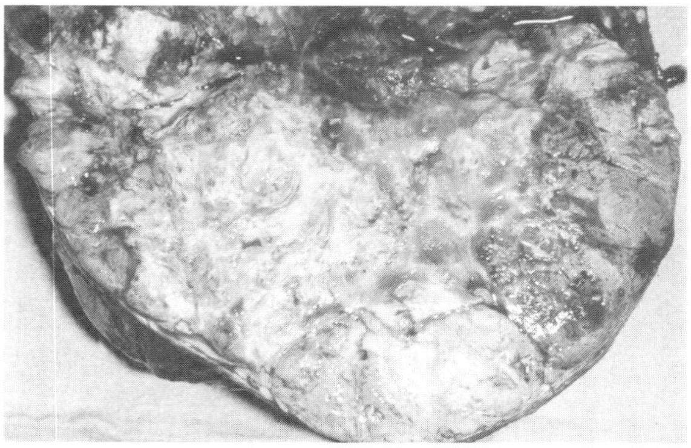

Fig. 35.4 Gross specimen of adrenocortical carcinoma. Large partly necrotic tumour with haemorrhagic cut surface.

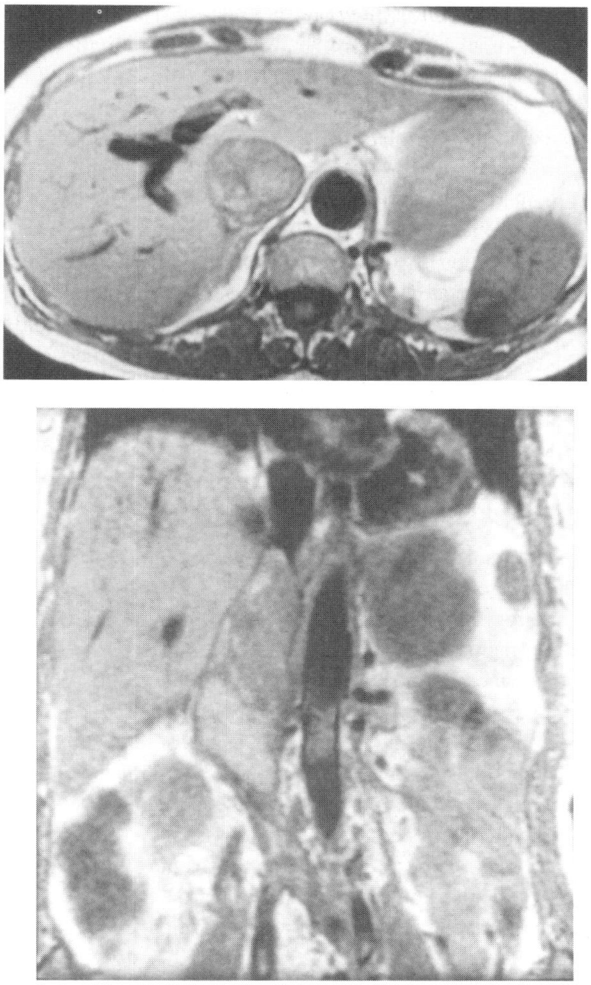

a

b

Fig. 35.5 (a,b) Magnetic resonance imaging scan of adrenocortical carcinoma showing gross tumour invasion of the inferior vena cava.

subcostal incision should be made with the thoracoabdominal approach being reserved for tumours greater than 15 cm in diameter. Hydrocortisone 100 mg must be given at the time of surgery and steroid cover continued postoperatively when the patient has Cushing's syndrome, as the opposite adrenal gland will be suppressed. Radiotherapy has a limited palliative role but chemotherapy with mitotane (o,p'DDD) has been extensively used as adjuvant therapy with a favourable effect on survival.[33]

Others have reported less optimistic results. The best results have been observed in patients who have received mitotane before clinical evidence of metastases and those treated with mitotane who subsequently underwent surgery for recurrent tumour.[34] When mitotane is employed it must be remembered that this agent destroys the contralateral normal adrenal cortex and therefore replacement steroid therapy is essential.

Adrenal blockade with metyrapone will produce reasonable palliation when the symptoms of Cushing's syndrome predominate.

The importance of tumour staging has been demonstrated by several workers. It has been shown that stage I tumours less than 5 cm in size with no nodal involvement, local invasion or metastases have a better 5-year survival than stage IV tumours with metastatic spread. The overall 5-year survival rate for this tumour in one series was however only 16%.[34]

Macronodular adrenal cortical hyperplasia

This rare cause of Cushing's syndrome is not ACTH-dependent and should be treated by bilateral adrenalectomy.[35]

Primary pigmented nodular adrenal cortical disease

The optimal treatment is bilateral adrenalectomy.[36]

The indications for bilateral adrenalectomy are:

1. In Cushing's syndrome after failed trans-sphenoidal microsurgery or irradiation.
2. When the severity of Cushing's syndrome is such that immediate removal of the source of cortisol excess is necessary.
3. In ectopic ACTH syndrome when the primary tumour cannot be located or resected.
4. Macronodular adrenal cortical hyperplasia and primary pigmented nodular adrenal cortical disease.

Nelson's syndrome[37]

Bilateral adrenalectomy in pituitary-dependent Cushing's disease results in a syndrome of hyperpigmentation and growth of the pituitary tumour with enlargement of the sella turcica and elevation of the plasma ACTH in some 30% of patients. The incidence of Nelson's syndrome can be reduced by external pituitary irradiation at the time of adrenalectomy and requires either surgery or radiotherapy to treat the established syndrome.[38]

ADDISON'S DISEASE AND HYPOADRENALISM

Primary hypoadrenalism was first described by Thomas Addison in 1855[2] and can be caused by a number of conditions which destroy or interfere with the function of the adrenal cortex. These include tuberculosis, autoimmune disease, sarcoidosis, amyloidosis, haemochromatosis, histoplasmosis, secondary tumour deposits, congenital adrenal hyperplasia, adrenal cortical haemorrhage following anticoagulant therapy, adrenal venography or meningococcal septicaemia (Waterhouse–Friderichsen syndrome).[15] Bilateral surgical adrenalectomy is an important iatrogenic cause of hypoadrenalism but by definition is not Addison's disease. Acute adrenal failure may result from sudden withdrawal of suppressive doses of steroid.

REFERENCES

33. Schteingart D E, Motazedi A et al Arch Surg 1982; 117: 1142
34. Henley D J, van Heerden J A et al Surgery 1983; 94: 926
35. Joffe S N, Brown C Surgery 1983; 94: 919
36. Carney J A, Gordon H et al Medicine 1985; 64: 270
37. Nelson D H, Meakin I W, Thorn G W Ann Intern Med 1960; 52: 560
38. Orth D N, Liddle G W N Engl J Med 1971; 285: 243

The clinical features include pigmentation of the buccal mucosa and skin—particularly on pressure areas—hypotension, lassitude, weakness, vitiligo, loss of body hair in the female, anorexia and amenorrhoea. In extreme cases drowsiness, confusion, coma and death occur. The scars of bilateral adrenalectomy or the stigmata of diseases for which steroids are prescribed may be important clues. The features of adrenal hypothalamic or pituitary disease may also be present. The short tetracosactrin test (Synacthen), in which the plasma cortisol response to 250 µg intramuscular Synacthen is measured confirms the diagnosis. A rise in plasma cortisol occurs in normal subjects. This is impaired or absent in Addison's disease.[15]

A long Synacthen test (depot test) can also be obtained to confirm the diagnosis and help to differentiate primary hypoadrenalism from secondary adrenal dysfunction perhaps arising from pituitary disease.

Further investigations are directed towards establishing the precise aetiology of the hypoadrenalism. Plain abdominal X-rays showing adrenal gland calcification are indicative of tuberculosis and autoantibodies are present in the autoimmune disease.

Treatment

A seriously ill hypotensive patient presenting acutely must be resuscitated with intravenous saline and hydrocortisone 100 mg 6-hourly. Mineralocorticoid replacement is unnecessary when the daily cortisol dose exceeds 60 mg. Intravenous antibiotics must be given in the Waterhouse–Friderichsen syndrome, which usually affects young children although it is seen in adults. The onset is acute with profound shock, hyperpyrexia, rigors, vomiting, petechial skin haemorrhages, and a lapse into coma. The mortality rate is extremely high.

The bilateral adrenalectomized patient is at risk of developing acute hypocortisolism in the immediate postoperative period and subsequently when subject to stress, illness or operation. Treatment consists of intravenous saline and hydrocortisone 100 mg 6-hourly.

Chronic adrenocortical insufficiency requires long-term oral hydrocortisone, usually in a dose of 20 mg in the morning and 10 mg at night. Most patients also need the addition of fludrocortisone as mineralocorticoid replacement (0.5–1.0 mg daily). Hypertension, oedema and hypokalaemia are signs of over-treatment. Fatigue, hypotension and an elevated serum potassium are signs of under-treatment.

Surgery and steroid replacement therapy[39]

1. *Bilateral adrenalectomy*: Hydrocortisone sodium succinate 100 mg is given intramuscularly with the premedication and a further 100 mg is given during the operation if this lasts longer than 1½–2 hours. In the postoperative period intramuscular or intravenous hydrocortisone 6-hourly is continued for between 48 and 72 hours, reducing to 50 mg 6-hourly before the introduction of 20 mg oral hydrocortisone in the morning and 10 mg at night. Mineralocorticoid is given as 0.1 mg fludrocortisone acetate daily by mouth.

2. *Unilateral adrenalectomy* (e.g. for Cushing's syndrome from an adrenal adenoma): Hydrocortisone sodium succinate 100 mg is given intramuscularly with the premedication and continued in the postoperative period as 100 mg 6-hourly, reducing with the introduction of oral hydrocortisone to 20 mg in the morning and 10 mg at night. Gradual reduction of steroid replacement is made on a monthly basis with complete weaning often taking up to 12 months.

3. *Surgery in the hypoadrenal patient*, e.g. after bilateral adrenalectomy and in those with adrenal suppression from steroid therapy: If these patients are having major surgery additional steroids are required: 100 mg hydrocortisone sodium succinate is given intramuscularly with the premedication and continued postoperatively every 6 hours until the patient is able to return to the usual oral replacement steroid dose. If the postoperative recovery is prolonged, e.g. after a gastrointestinal procedure, the parenteral hydrocortisone is reduced to 50 mg 8-hourly until the patient is able to take tablets by mouth.

For minor surgery, when the oral intake is not restricted, intramuscular hydrocortisone is only required for 24 hours postoperatively, and for minimal surgical procedures a single additional dose of hydrocortisone 100 mg is all that is necessary.

Patients who are on steroid therapy, who have undergone bilateral adrenalectomy or who suffer from primary hypoadrenalism must be fully instructed by the medical staff on the nature of their condition and the symptoms to be expected with inadequate steroid replacement. The vital importance of this treatment must be emphasized. They are instructed to double their usual steroid dose immediately and seek medical assistance in the event of illness or severe stress. All patients should carry a steroid card and the wearing of a Medic Alert bracelet is to be encouraged. Patients who have had a total adrenalectomy in some hospitals in the USA given a steroid-containing syringe for emergency self-injection. The relative potencies of therapeutic steroid preparations are shown in Table 35.3.

ALDOSTERONISM

The syndrome of aldosteronism results from excessive production of aldosterone by the zona glomerulosa of the adrenal cortex. This mineralocorticoid excess causes salt and water retention, leading to hypertension and hypokalaemic alkalosis from increased loss of potassium and hydrogen by the kidneys.

REFERENCE

39. Plumpton F S, Besser G M, Cole P V Anaesthesia 1969; 24: 3

Table 35.3 Potencies of various glucocorticoids in relation to cortisol

Compound	*Equivalent dose (mg)*
Hydrocortisone (cortisol)	20
Cortisone	25
Prednisone	5
Prednisolone	5
Methylprednisolone	4
Dexamethasone	0.75
Betamethasone	0.6

Primary aldosteronism

Aldosterone was identified some 3 years before Dr Jerome Conn described the syndrome of primary aldosteronism in 1955.[40] Initially it was thought that the condition might be present in up to 20% of the hypertensive population but it now seems likely that fewer than 1% are affected.[41] Nevertheless, this is an extremely important minority group with a surgically correctable form of hypertension. The cardinal features of the condition are hypertension, usually hypokalaemia, aldosterone excess and a low plasma renin. The depression of plasma renin results from suppression of the juxtaglomerular apparatus by sodium retention and increased blood volume (Fig. 35.6).

Secondary aldosteronism

Severe hypertensive cardiovascular and renal disease is often associated with secondary aldosterone excess from stimulation of the juxtaglomerular apparatus, which produces renin secretion, and this in turn leads to increased aldosterone secretion via the angiotensin mechanism. This form of hyperaldosteronism, characterized by an elevated renin level, must be clearly distinguished from the primary condition (Fig. 35.7).

Causes of primary aldosteronism

1. Aldosterone-producing adrenocortical adenoma (Conn's syndrome; Fig. 35.8).
2. Bilateral adrenocortical hyperplasia (idiopathic hyperaldosteronism).

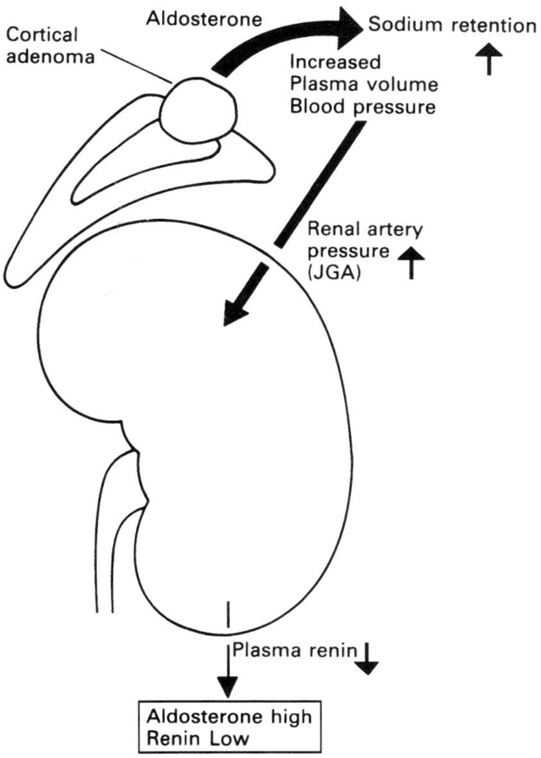

Fig. 35.6 Pathophysiology of primary aldosteronism. JGA = Juxtaglomerular apparatus.

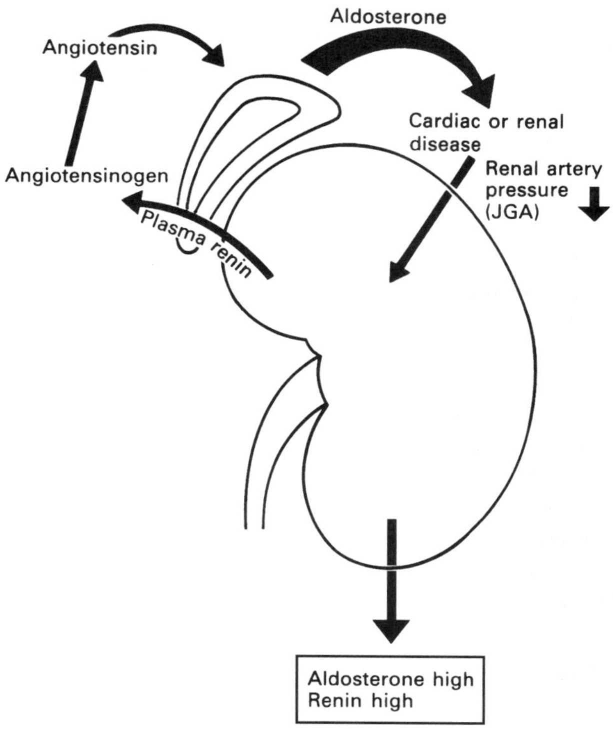

Fig. 35.7 Pathophysiology of secondary aldosteronism. JGA = Juxta-glomerular apparatus.

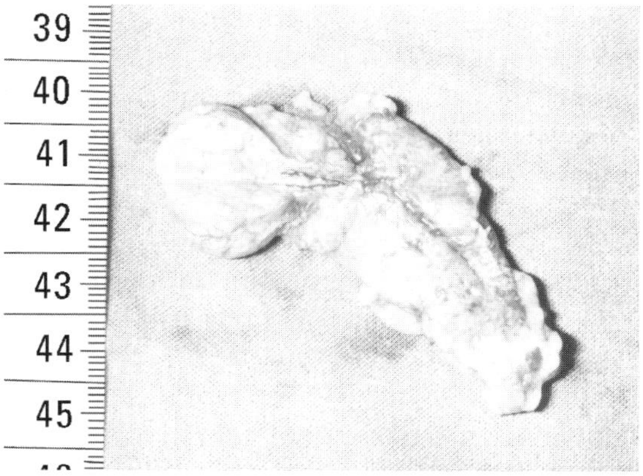

Fig. 35.8 Typical discrete Conn's adenoma 1.5 cm in diameter.

3. Aldosterone-producing adenocarcinoma.
4. Glucocorticoid remediable hyperaldosteronism (familial—type 1).
5. Familial—type 11 (adenoma or hyperplasia—not glucocorticoid-suppressible).
6. Aldosterone-producing ovarian carcinoma.

An aldosterone-producing adenoma, which accounts for approximately 85% of all cases[42] of primary aldosteronism, is

REFERENCES

40. Conn J W J Lab Clin Med 1955; 45: 3
41. Streeten D H P, Touryz N, Anderson G H Am J Med 1979; 67: 403
42. Granberg P-O, Adamson U et al World J Surg 1982; 6: 757

usually less than 2 cm in diameter, discrete and projects from the gland and the cut surface has a canary-yellow colour. Tumours occur more often on the left side than the right, and 10% are bilateral. Often there is a back-ground of zona glomerulosa hyperplasia and additional nodules which do not produce aldosterone. Idiopathic hyperaldosteronism, which is the cause of the syndrome in 10–15%, is characterised by diffuse or focal hyperplasia of the zona glomerulosa, frequently with associated nodules. These nodules, which may be caused by hypertensive vascular changes, are capable of producing cortisol but not aldosterone.

An aldosterone-secreting adrenocortical carcinoma is rare and is likely to present as a large tumour mass at the time of diagnosis. Glucocorticoid remediable hyperaldosteronism (familial—type 1) is rare,[43] usually occurring in the young, with an autosomal dominant inheritance pattern. Treatment with dexamethasone 2 mg daily reverses the clinical and biochemical abnormalities within 2 weeks.[44] The inheritance of familial hyperaldosteronism type 11 has not yet been fully defined.[45]

Case reports have appeared in the literature of hyperaldosteronism associated with ovarian tumours.[46]

Clinical features

Primary aldosteronism may occur at any age but the peak incidence is between the third and fifth decades. Aldosterone-producing adenomas are commoner in females whereas idiopathic hyperaldosteronism occurs with equal frequency in both sexes and tends to affect an older age group. The syndrome is characterised by constant hypertension which is often severe but rarely malignant, headaches, hypokalaemia causing muscle weakness, cramps, polyuria, polydipsia and nocturia. The hypokalaemia may be so severe that it causes intermittent flaccid paralysis and even tetany. Diabetes mellitus can be precipitated in certain susceptible subjects. The symptoms of hypokalaemia sometimes follow the administration of diuretics, particularly thiazides, for hypertension or develop after ingestion of excessive dietary sodium. Occasionally patients are symptomless.

Biochemical features and confirmation of diagnosis

The findings of an elevated plasma aldosterone concentration with suppressed plasma renin levels are fundamental to establishing the diagnosis. Before carrying out these biochemical studies, diuretic therapy and spironolactone should be stopped for 6 weeks and antihypertensive sympathetic inhibitors should be stopped for at least 1 week.

Hypokalaemia (less than 3 mmol/l) with a urinary potassium excretion of greater than 40 mmol/l per day should arouse suspicion that the patient has primary aldosteronism.[42]

Any potassium deficit should be corrected by oral potassium before further investigations are carried out, as hypokalaemia will inhibit aldosterone secretion and make confirmation of the diagnosis difficult. Evidence of the autonomous secretion of aldosterone may be demonstrated by a suppression test that shows that aldosterone levels remain elevated in the presence of blood volume expansion induced by a combination of a high sodium intake, 9 g/day for 3 days, and fludrocortisone administration, 0.5 mg/day for 3 days.[42]

Sodium loading can also be used as a provocative test in the normokalaemic hypertensive patient, and induces a fall in serum potassium below 3.5 mmol in patients with primary aldosteronism.[47] Caution is required in carrying out these tests, lest severe electrolytic disturbances are induced.

Differentiation of an adenoma from idiopathic hyperaldosteronism

Once the diagnosis of primary hyperaldosteronism has been confirmed, the thrust of the investigation is directed to distinguishing between an aldosterone-producing adenoma and idiopathic hyperaldosteronism, as the treatment of the two conditions is different; only the former benefits from surgery.[47] This distinction may prove difficult.

Generally, the biochemical disturbances are greater in aldosterone-producing adenoma than idiopathic hyperaldosteronism but this alone cannot be used as a reliable method of separation. Quadratic mathematical analysis[46] using various clinical and biochemical measurements has been successfully employed in the distinction.

Probably the most reliable test is to examine the effect of changes in posture on plasma aldosterone levels. In aldosterone-producing adenoma, because of continuing sensitivity of the cortical adenoma to ACTH a postural fall in aldosterone may be seen, when comparing aldosterone at 8.00 a.m. after overnight recumbency with the level 4 hours later when the patient has been walking around. In idiopathic hyperaldosteronism, plasma aldosterone increases with the upright posture.[48]

Localisation studies

The aldosterone-producing adenoma can be reliably localized in more than 90% of cases by CT scanning, which is capable of visualizing lesions as small as 1 cm in diameter.[49] Smaller tumours are frequently missed, particularly in thin patients with little perinephric fat. MRI is also helpful in localizing these adenomas.[19]

Adrenal scintigraphy with ^{131}I-6β-iodomethyl-19-norcholest-5(10)-en-3β-ol (NP-59) provides excellent localization, but has the disadvantage of administering a relatively high radiation dose, and several days are required for completion of the investigation.[16] Scanning is usually performed after 5 days of dexamethasone

REFERENCES

43. Giebink G S, Gotlin R W et al J Clin Endocrinol Metab 1973; 36: 715
44. Sutherland D K A, Ruse J L, Laidlaw J C Can Med Assoc J 1966; 95: 1109
45. Gordon R D, Stowasser M, Klemm S A, Tunny T J Steroids 1995; 60: 34–45
46. Ferris J B, Brown J J et al Clin Endocrinol Metab 1981; 10: 419
47. Melby J C Clin Endocrinol Metab 1985; 14: 977
48. Grant C S, Carpenter P, Hamberger B Arch Surg 1984; 119: 585
49. Edis A J Surgery 1979; 86: 470

suppression, to decrease activity in the surrounding normal adrenal tissue. The adenoma appears as a single area of increased uptake, whereas a diffuse uptake with no lateralization is seen in idiopathic hyperaldosteronism.

Retrograde venography was once widely employed but now is rarely used because it is potentially hazardous, occasionally resulting in extravasation of contrast, intra-adrenal haemorrhage and necrosis of the gland.[48] Venous catheterization, with bilateral adrenal venous sampling and measurement of aldosterone levels, has the potential to provide excellent localization of the aldosterone-producing adenoma and confirmation of idiopathic hyperaldosteronism. The technique has enormous value when the tumour is below the limit of detection by imaging and when an abnormal nodule is not functioning. The method is limited by the difficulty which is frequently encountered of correctly placing the catheter in the right adrenal vein, which is short and enters the vena cava at 90°.[50] These sampling errors and dilution effects can be compensated for by simultaneously measuring cortisol and then using the aldosterone-to-cortisol ratio as the indicator of a true increase in hormone concentration.[51] Adrenal ultrasound may be used to complement these techniques.

Treatment

Once an aldosterone-secreting adenoma is precisely localized by the radiological and biochemical studies, surgical excision by unilateral adrenalectomy via a laparoscopic or open posterolateral approach is the treatment of choice. Following this, 70% of patients will be normotensive by 1 year after surgery but longer-term follow-up studies indicate that some patients later become hypertensive again.[47]

The persistence of the hypertension after removal of the tumour is likely to be the result of irreversible hypertensive renal changes or a wrong diagnosis, e.g. hyperplasia. It is essential to prepare patients preoperatively by controlling their hypertension and by the administration of spironolactone 100 mg/day with added potassium in order to correct any hypokalaemia. The response to spironolactone in larger doses (100–400 mg/day) can be used to predict the outcome of surgery; a satisfactory reduction of blood pressure is seen following removal of the adenoma in those patients who respond to spironolactone. Maintenance with spironolactone is an acceptable treatment if the patient with an aldosterone-producing adenoma is unwell for other reasons, and surgery is contraindicated. A potassium-sparing diuretic, amiloride, is dramatically effective in restoring the potassium balance in these patients and controlling their hypertension. There are few postoperative problems with the laparoscopic posterior approach to adrenalectomy, and restoration of blood pressure and serum electrolytes to normal is usually prompt.

Surgical treatment is not indicated in idiopathic hyperaldosteronism as the results are disappointing; blood pressure returns to normal only in the occasional patient, particularly when subtotal adrenalectomy has been performed.[48] Risks of adrenal insufficiency and the need to receive long-term steroid replacement are obvious major contraindications to bilateral adrenalectomy. Patients with idiopathic hyperaldosteronism should therefore be treated by long-term spironolactone or amiloride.

CONGENITAL ADRENAL HYPERPLASIA

(adrenogenital syndrome)

Cortisol synthesis from cholesterol takes place by a series of metabolic steps, each requiring a specific enzyme[52] (Fig. 35.9). A deficiency of one of these enzymes, which may be inherited in an autosomal recessive manner, causes a deficiency of cortisol and/or aldosterone leading to secondary adrenal hyperplasia from negative feedback, resulting in ACTH release. This rare condition, known as congenital adrenal hyperplasia, has a reported incidence ranging from 1 in 5000 to 1 in 15 000[53] and is most commonly the result of a deficiency of the enzyme 21-hydroxylase, although other enzyme defects such as 11β-hydroxylase, 3β-hydroxy steroid dehydrogenase and 17α-hydroxylase have been found.

Diversionary synthesis via alternative pathways leads to excessive production of other steroids, particularly androgens. These can cause virilization of the female fetus with pseudohermaphroditism, ambiguous external genitalia, clitoral enlargement and fusion of the genital folds. In the male, the effects of excess androgen at birth may not be as obvious but the penis enlarges rapidly during childhood and occasionally pseudoprecocious puberty ensues (infant Hercules). Excess androgens produce early epiphyseal closure, which results in short stature in adult life.

Most patients with congenital adrenal hyperplasia caused by 21-hydroxylase deficiency also have impaired aldosterone secretion and a salt wasting characterized by excess urinary salt loss, vomiting and failure to feed and thrive in the newborn.

Biochemical confirmation

Androgens and the precursor steroid 17-hydroxyprogesterone are produced in excess, and measurement of the latter in the plasma by

REFERENCES

50. Geelhoed G W Problem Management in Endocrine Surgery. Year Book, Chicago 1983
51. Auda S P, Brennan M F, Gill J R Ann Surg 1980; 191: 1
52. Finkelstein M, Shaefer J M Physiol Rev 1979; 59: 353

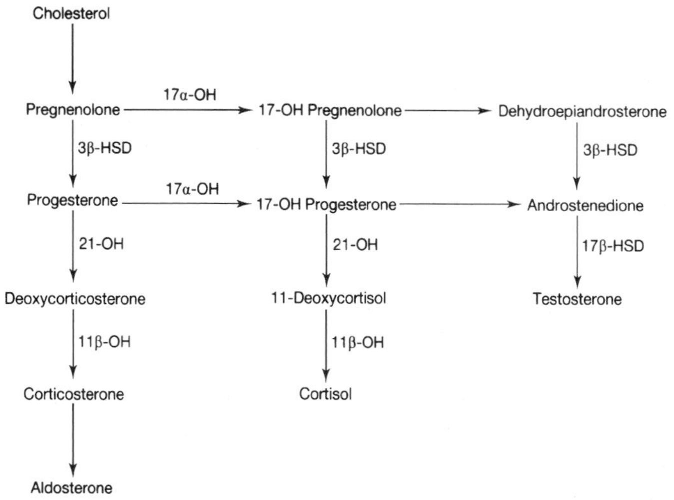

Fig. 35.9 Metabolic pathways of adrenal steroid synthesis.

radioimmunoassay is the most reliable method of confirming the diagnosis.[54]

Treatment

Hydrocortisone (5 mg/day in divided doses) is given to replace the glucocorticoid deficiency and totally suppress ACTH. This suppression is well-monitored by urinary and plasma 17-hydroxyprogesterone measurement.[55,56] Salt wasting is treated by intravenous saline and mineralocorticoid replacement. Growth development, life expectancy and fertility are normal providing the patient receives adequate medical therapy and careful after-care.[16]

INCIDENTAL ASYMPTOMATIC ADRENAL MASSES

The adrenal glands are tucked away in an inaccessible part of the body not readily amenable to clinical examination, but ultrasound high-resolution CT scanning and MRI have led to the incidental discovery of many clinically and biochemically silent adrenal gland masses in approximately 0.5–10% of patients undergoing investigations for unrelated conditions[57,58] (Figs 35.10 and 35.11). These silent lesions have been named 'incidentalomas' and present the clinician with a diagnostic problem, especially in excluding a malignant adrenal tumour. Proof of non-function must be obtained by the appropriate biochemical tests (Table 35.4), but unfortunately these investigations do not distinguish a benign from a malignant tumour. Fine-needle cytology is also of limited value, being often unreliable, although it may distinguish a benign tumour from a secondary tumour deposit. The low signal intensity of benign lesions scanned by MRI can be helpful, but precise distinction from malignancy is not possible. NP 59 scintigraphy can aid the distinction of benign from malignant tumours and also facilicate the identification of the 5% of

a

b

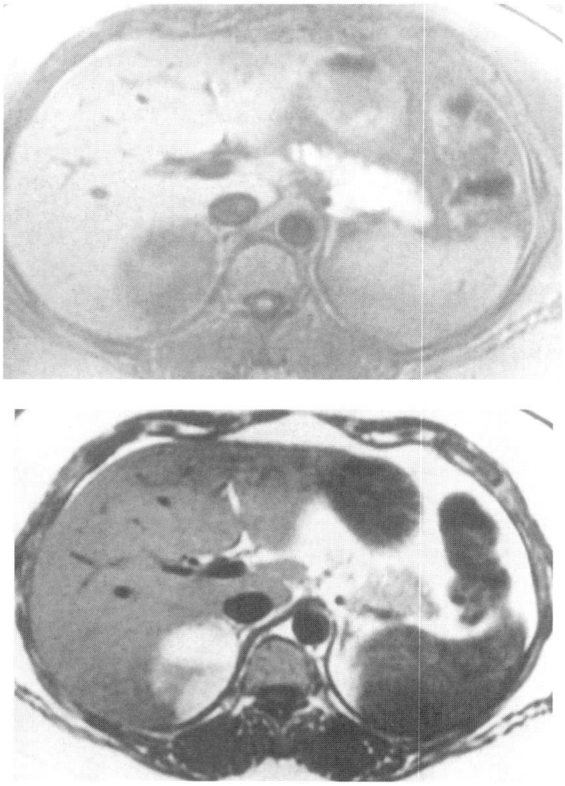

Fig. 35.10 Magnetic resonance imaging scan (T1 spin echo) of adenomyelolipoma of right adrenal gland. (**a**) with and (**b**) without fat suppression.

a

b

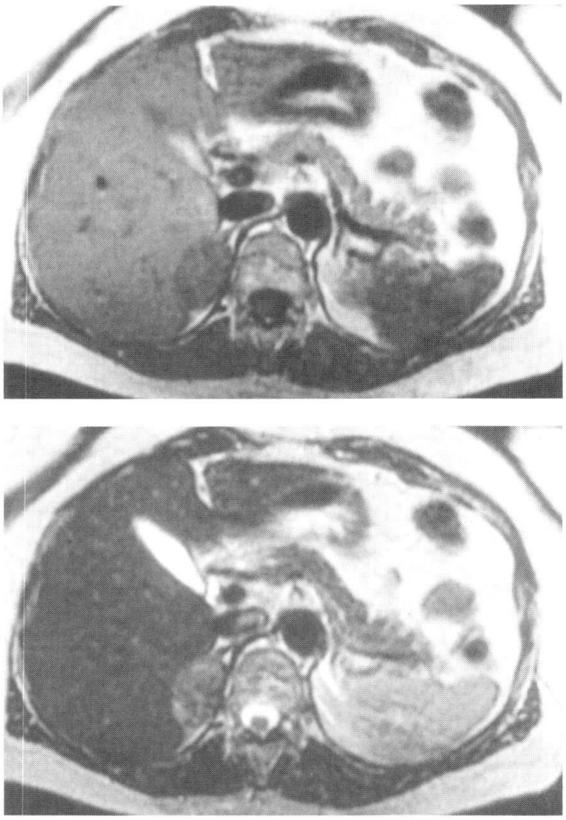

Fig. 35.11 (a and b)
T1- and T2-weighted magnetic resonance imaging scan of non-functioning right adrenal 'incidentaloma'.

Table 35.4 Biochemical investigation of incidentaloma

9.00 a.m. and midnight serum cortisol
9.00 a.m. cortisol after overnight dexamethasone (2 mg) suppression
Urinary free cortisol
Serum aldosterone
Urinary catecholamines (see later section)

REFERENCES

53. Savage M O Clin Endocrinol Metab 1985; 14: 893
54. Hughes I A, Riad-Fahmy D, Griffiths L Arch Dis Child 1979; 54: 347
55. Hughes I A, Winter J S D J Clin Endocrinol Metab 1978; 46: 98
56. Hughes I A, Read G F Hormone Res 1982; 16: 142
57. Belldegrun A, Hussain S et al Surg Gynecol Obstet 1986; 163: 203
58. McLeod M K Acta Chir Austriaca 1993; 25: 209–211

adrenal incidentalomas causing subclinical Cushing's syndrome.

Adrenal cysts also cause diagnostic confusion. These are usually small and symptomless, but when large present as a tumour mass capable of displacing the kidney.

At present, surgical exploration and resection of incidentalomas are recommended in patients under 50 years of age, when the lesion is greater than 4.0 cm in diameter, or if it is increasing in size on serial CT scans.[59] Smaller lesions that are not removed should be followed by regular CT scanning. An incidentaloma which has ominous CT or ultrasound appearances such as irregular shape or inhomogeneous interior should be resected regardless of size. Age is an important factor as the malignancy risk in a lesion 3.5 cm in diameter in the older subject is less than that for a similar nodule in the young. As discussed in a previous section, larger masses are generally more likely to be malignant than smaller lesions.

Secondary adrenal tumours

Many neoplasms including breast, bronchus and melanoma can metastasize to the adrenals, displacing and destroying adrenal tissue with the creation of a mass. Such metastatic disease may reduce adrenocortical hormone production, causing acute Addisonian crisis.

ADRENAL MEDULLA

PHAEOCHROMOCYTOMA

Phaeochromocytoma, a term introduced by Pick in 1912,[60] is a functioning tumour of chromaffin tissue derived from the neural crest, which produces a clinical syndrome resulting from its ability to secrete an excess of catecholamine. Roux,[61] in Lausanne, performed the first successful surgical removal of a phaeochromocytoma—a feat soon repeated by Dr C. H. Mayo in the USA in 1927.[62] The majority (80–90%) of phaeochromocytomas occur in the adrenal medulla but extra-adrenal tumours may be found in the paraganglionic system extending from the pelvis to the base of the skull, along the course of the organ of Zuckerkandl. They can arise in the renal hilum, bladder, scrotum, neck or thorax and even in the posterior wall of the left atrium. Approximately 10% of tumours are extra-adrenal, bilateral, multiple, familial or malignant. Extra-adrenal and multiple tumours occur more often in children, perhaps because the organ of Zuckerkandl is still present before it gradually involutes by puberty. Multiple tumours are more often found in familial disease (50–70%). The incidence of phaeochromocytomas in 15 934 consecutive autopsies performed at the Mayo Clinic was 0.1%[63] and 0.5%[64] in a highly selected group of patients undergoing surgery for severe hypertension. It has been estimated that 800 people die annually in the USA from hypertension from phaeochromocytoma and that 35% remain undiagnosed during life.

Ten per cent of phaeochromocytomas are associated with other genetically determined conditions—multiple endocrine neoplasia IIa and IIb, von Recklinghausen's disease (neurofibromatosis), von Hippel–Lindau disease (cerebellar haemangioblastoma).[65–67] Familial phaeochromocytomas are not always associated with other congenital abnormalities and may occur alone. The importance of obtaining a family history in the patient with phaeochromocytoma is self-evident.[63]

Clinical presentation

Phaeochromocytoma has aptly been described as the great mimic because of the wide variety of symptoms and signs which can result, from the multiple pharmacological effects of spasmodic or sustained release of noradrenaline and adrenaline. Hypertension is the commonest manifestation, being continuous in 50%, while acute paroxysmal increases in blood pressure occur in the remainder.[68] Some tumours secrete dopamine however and are not associated with hypertension.[69] Local pressure (as in palpation), defecation, micturition (seen in tumours of the bladder), sexual intercourse and any invasive diagnostic procedure may precipitate a hypertensive attack, as can various foodstuffs, tyramine, alcohol and drugs (notably tricyclic antidepressants).

Paroxysmal hypertensive attacks are frequently associated with headaches and excessive sweating. Orthostatic hypotension, peripheral circulatory failure and even sudden cardiac arrest have occurred after trauma and in patients with an unsuspected phaeochromocytoma undergoing surgery for other conditions. Hypertension may give rise to a number of cardiovascular symptoms including palpitations, tachycardia, angina, arrhythmias, myocardial infarction, cerebrovascular accidents and hypertensive encephalopathy. Catecholamine cardiomyopathy can contribute to the development of left ventricular failure. Flushing, pallor, pupillary dilatation, Raynaud's phenomenon, fever, tremors, nausea, weakness, faintness, weight loss, heat intolerance, vertigo, anxiety and a feeling of impending doom in varying combinations and intensities contribute to a varied clinical picture. The excess catecholamines may cause generalized abdominal pain, pseudo-obstruction, ileus, ischaemic enterocolitis and even acute megacolon. The basal metabolic rate is elevated and there may be glucose intolerance and severe hyperglycaemia, particularly in malignant tumours.

Differential diagnosis

Because of the ability of this tumour to mimic many other diseases there is a long differential diagnosis.

REFERENCES

59. Herrerra M F, Grant C S, van Heerden J A et al Surg 1991; 110: 1014
60. Pick L Klin Wochenschr 1912; 19: 16
61. Barbeau A, Marc-Aurele J, Brouillet J Union Med Can 1958; 87: 165
62. Mayo C H JAMA 1927; 89: 1047
63. Minno A M, Bennett W A, Kvale W F N Engl J Med 1954; 251: 959
64. Smithwick R H, Greer W R et al N Engl J Med 1950; 242: 252
65. Sipple J H Am J Med 1961; 31: 163
66. Glushien A J, Mansuy M M, Littman D S Am J Med 1953; 14: 318
67. Steiner A L, Goodman A D, Powers S R Medicine 1968; 47: 371
68. Remine W H, Chong C C et al Ann Surg 1974; 179: 740
69. Proye C, Fossati P et al Surgery 1986; 100: 1154

1. Essential and labile hypertension.
2. Anxiety neurosis and other psychiatric disorders.
3. Hyperthyroidism.
4. Diabetes mellitus.
5. Functional bowel disorder.

The key to diagnosis is a high index of suspicion.

Investigations

Investigation is firstly directed towards confirming the presence of a phaeochromocytoma by measuring catecholamine excess, and secondly towards locating the lesion in order to plan the correct surgical approach.

1. Confirmation of catecholamine excess: The delineation of the major metabolic pathways of the catecholamines (Fig. 35.12) by Armstrong et al in 1957[70] formed the basis for the development of biochemical tests on body fluids which could be used to diagnose phaeochromocytoma.

The most important of these tests are listed in Table 35.5.

The measurement of vanillylmandelic acid metanephrines (metadrenaline) and catecholamines in an acidified 24-hour urine collection are the most helpful investigations in the diagnosis of phaeochromocytoma. Pharmacological provocation tests are potentially dangerous and have no place in the present-day investigation and management of suspected phaeochromocytoma.

2. Localization studies: Once the diagnosis of phaeochromocytoma has been confirmed it is necessary to locate the tumour accurately because multiple and extra-adrenal lesions may be present. The intravenous pyelogram used to play an important role but this is now only helpful in confirming that there are two functioning kidneys present in case one has to be sacrificed during the course of tumour removal. Ultrasound is unlikely to demonstrate lesions less than 3 cm in diameter.

CT scanning is now firmly established as a valuable localizing procedure, with an accuracy in excess of 90%.[71] Glucagon, occasionally given to diminish artefacts caused by peristalsis during CT scanning, must be avoided as it releases catecholamines and can precipitate an acute hypertensive attack.

As conversion of noradrenaline to adrenaline occurs primarily in the adrenal medulla, most extra-adrenal phaeochromocytomas produce only noradrenaline.

REFERENCES

70. Armstrong M D, McMillan A, Shaw K N F Biochem Biophys Acta 1957; 25: 422
71. van Heerden J A, Sheps S G et al Surg 1982; 91: 367

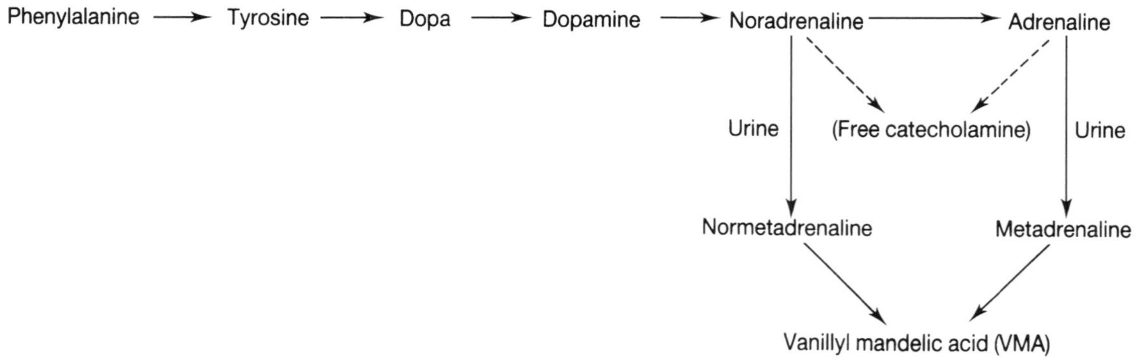

Fig. 35.12 Biosynthesis and catabolism of catecholamines.

Table 35.5 Biochemical tests to confirm the diagnosis of phaeochromocytoma

Measurement	*Normal values*	*Accuracy*	*Comments*
Urine (24-hour collection)			
Vanillylmandelic acid	0–35 μmol/24 h	90%	Colorimetric assays are unreliable: affected by anti-hypertensive drug α-methyldopa and certain foodstuffs, e.g. banana, coffee and vanilla. High-performance liquid chromatography method extremely accurate
Metanephrines	0–6.5 μmol/24 h	95%	False-positive results are caused by monoamine oxidase inhibitors, severe illness, stress, haemorrhagic shock and sepsis
Free catecholamines			
Noradrenaline	100–820 nmol/24 h	90%	Marked elevation after acute hypertensive episodes
Adrenaline	15–190 nmol/24 h		
Plasma			
catecholamines (fasting)		>90%	Single plasma sample required.
Adrenaline	0.03–0.12 nmol/1		Influenced by drugs—methyldopa and phenoxybenzamine—exercise, severe illness and septicaemia
Noradrenaline	0.6–2.5 nmol/1		
Dopamine	0.02–0.37 nmol/l		

The most significant advance in the investigation of phaeochromocytomas has been the introduction of the scanning agent ^{131}I- or ^{123}I-metaiodobenzylguanidine[72] which is taken up and concentrated in adrenergic vesicles. Normal adrenal glands are not shown on the scintigrams, but intra- and extra-adrenal phaeochromocytomas, of either benign or malignant character, are clearly delineated by this safe, reliable non-invasive technique (Figs 35.13 and 35.14).

MRI is another very helpful localizing technique (Fig. 35.15):

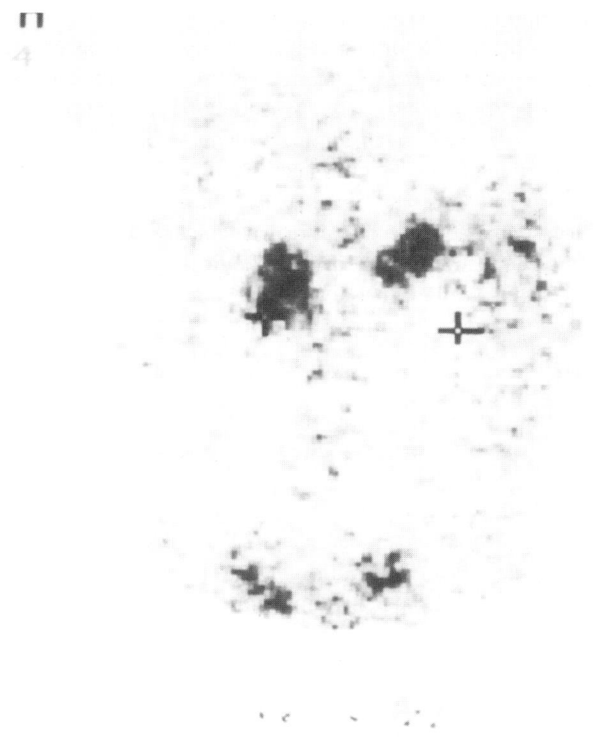

Fig. 35.13 ^{131}I metaiodobenzylguanidine (MIBG) scan demonstrating bilateral adrenal phaeochromocytomas.

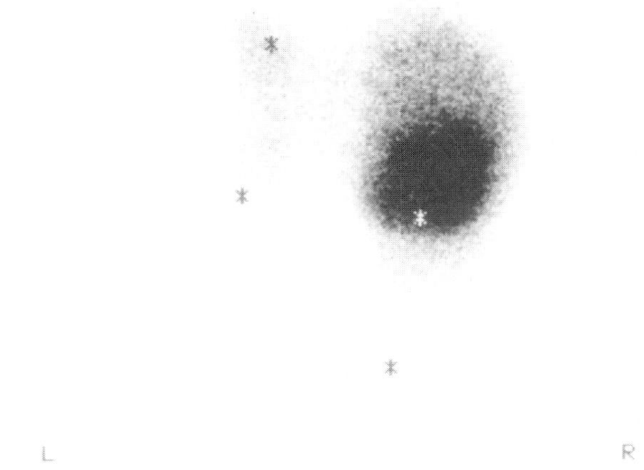

Fig. 35.14 MIBG scan demonstrating large right adrenal phaeochromocytoma.

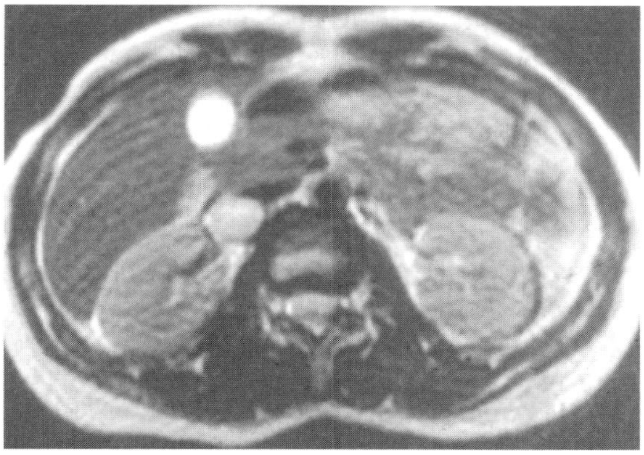

Fig. 35.15 Magnetic resonance imaging scan (T2-weighted) of extra-adrenal phaeochromocytoma situated close to the right renal hilum.

phaeochromocytomas are white on T2 weighting imaging. With the routine application of CT, MRI and ^{131}I-metalodobenzylguanidine the role of selective adrenal arteriography or selective vena caval catheterization with venous sampling for catecholamine assay is extremely limited. All invasive studies carry a risk of inducing a hypertensive crisis and therefore preliminary control of blood pressure by means of α-adrenergic blockade is essential.

Treatment

Phaeochromocytoma is a surgically treatable cause of hypertension, and operative excision of the tumour is employed, except in the small group of patients who have medical contraindications to operation, or who have widespread metastatic disease from a malignant phaeochromocytoma. Pharmacological control and stabilization of the hypertension is a vital preliminary measure before operation as this minimizes the surge in blood pressure which invariably occurs at induction of anaesthesia and during the intraoperative manipulation of the tumour.

It is important to stress that blood pressure control may be necessary before the diagnosis is firmly established in the markedly hypertensive patient if the clinical suspicion is high, as untreated patients are at risk from sudden hypertensive attacks, precipitating cerebral haemorrhage, myocardial infarction, heart failure and arrhythmias.

A small group of patients with this condition present with a fulminating illness with acute symptoms and complications of malignant hypertension. The term 'acute phaeochromocytoma'[73] has been used to classify these patients, who have what can only be described as a 'physiological malignant' tumour with tachycardia, cardiac arrhythmias, encephalopathy, hypotensive episodes, coma and shock, which eventually leads to death. The life-threatening complication of haemorrhagic rupture of a phaeochromocytoma presents with severe abdominal pain and shock and frequently mimics a leaking aortic aneurysm. Prompt surgical treatment

REFERENCES

72. Sisson J C, Frager M S et al N Engl J Med 1981; 305: 13
73. Egdah R H, Chobanian A V Surg Clin North Am 1966; 46: 645

offers the only prospect of survival and indeed patients with acute phaeochromocytoma must be regarded as grave emergencies. In these emergency circumstances the most appropriate method of achieving α-adrenergic blockade is by the intravenous injection of phentolamine, either by a bolus of 2.5 mg or by a continuous infusion of 1 mg/min. An alternative agent is intravenous sodium nitroprusside 0.5–1.5 μg/kg per min.

In preparing a routine case for elective surgery, phenoxybenzamine (Dibenyline) is the drug of choice, given orally 10 mg b.d. and increasing by increments of 10–20 mg/day until there is elimination of paroxysms of hypertension and other symptoms and signs associated with the tumour. In order to provide adequate α-blockade, treatment should be continued for at least 14 days prior to surgery. Side-effects include transient sedation, weakness, lassitude, nasal congestion, nausea and orthostatic hypotension. β-Blockade with propranolol, usually 60 mg/day in divided doses, is employed in the 3–4 days prior to surgery for those patients with tachycardia, arrhythmias and pure adrenaline-secreting tumours. This should be continued up to the time of operation to minimize severe tachyarrhythmias. Asthma and congestive cardiac failure are contraindications to the use of this drug, and β-adrenergic blockade must never be used without prior α-blockade as generalized vasoconstriction can result from unopposed α-adrenergic activity, leading to potentially catastrophic rises in blood pressure. Other drugs which have a limited role in the preoperative preparation include prazosin, a post-synaptic α-adrenergic reception blocker,[74] labetalol, which has both α- and β-adrenergic blocking potential,[75] and α-methyl paratyrosine which inhibits the synthesis of catecholamine by chromaffin tissue.[76]

Surgery of phaeochromocytoma

With careful preoperative preparation the patient should be presented for both anaesthesia and surgery in an optimal condition. Subsequent successful and safe management requires a coordinated team approach on the part of anaesthetist and surgeon. An electrocardiogram, central venous pressure and arterial pressure is necessary for monitoring and some advocate the use of a Swan–Ganz catheter to measure pulmonary wedge pressure. Anaesthesia is best maintained by isoflurane rather than halothane, which has the potential to cause unwanted arrhythmias.[77] A range of pressure-regulating agents (phentolamine, sodium nitroprusside, noradrenaline and dopamine) are kept at hand, in order to regulate minute-to-minute changes in blood pressure throughout the procedure. Arrhythmias are best suppressed with intravenous lignocaine (50–100 mg) and propranolol (1 mg). Cardioversion equipment must also be present in theatre.

Although preoperative tumour localization with MRI, CT and ^{131}I-metaiodobenzylguanidine scans is extremely accurate there is always the possibility of an unexpected finding that has not been determined by the preoperative investigations. For this reason, an anterior transperitoneal abdominal approach has been traditionally recommended via a transverse epigastric, bilateral subcostal or midline incision. Large tumours, particularly those on the right extending posteriorly to the inferior vena cava, may rarely require extension of the incision as a lateral thoracoabdominal procedure.

Some are now relying entirely on correct localization and simply explore unilaterally via the posterior route or laparoscopically. At operation, the adrenal gland which is suspected to be involved with the tumour is first exposed, and on the right this requires mobilization of the duodenum (Kocher) and upwards retraction of the right lobe of liver to expose the vena cava. Care must be taken to avoid tearing the short, wide and relatively inaccessible right adrenal vein which enters the vena cava on its posterolateral aspect.

The left adrenal gland is approached through the lesser sac, dissecting in a plane inferior and deep to the tail of the pancreas, exposing the kidney and the left adrenal vein which joints the left renal vein. By applying gentle downwards traction to the kidney on either side, this organ acts as an adrenal retractor, facilitating exposure and dissection of the adrenal. Haemostasis is secured by use of metal ligaclips and great care is taken to avoid manipulating the tumour excessively for fear of including catecholamine release and hypertensive fluctuations. 'The patient should be dissected from the adrenal gland'[50] rather than dissecting the tumour itself. Once the main tumour has been removed the opposite adrenal gland is carefully inspected, and a full examination is made from the diaphragm to the pelvis looking along the para-aortic areas, particularly for extra-adrenal chromaffin tissue. The renal hilum must be carefully examined as this is a common site for extra-adrenal tumours. The possibility of other phaeochromocytomas must be considered and the search continued if the blood pressure fails to fall after removal of the tumour. Great care must be taken to achieve complete haemostasis in the retroperitoneal area, as venous oozing is a potential hazard in the α-blocked patient.

An alternative approach to the left adrenal gland is to mobilize the spleen forwards and medially, dissecting straight down on to the adrenal.

Extra-adrenal phaeochromocytomas require a variety of surgical approaches depending on their location and, in the case of tumours involving the bladder, partial or segmental cystectomy may be necessary, or even total cystectomy and urinary diversion of the tumour is malignant. As soon as the tumour is removed the patient may frequently become hypotensive as a result of the fall in circulating catecholamines and the removal of the chronic vasoconstrictor affect.

The long-acting α-blocking agent phenoxybenzamine may render the vascular bed refractory to pressor agents, such as noradrenaline, and the phrase 'down-regulation of adrenergic receptors' has been used to describe the tolerance which these patients have to circulating catecholamines.[78] Excessive infusion of fluid during surgery is often necessary, although care must be taken to avoid fluid overload and pulmonary oedema. Pressor agents such as dopamine are occasionally required. Perhaps the best compro-

REFERENCES

74. Wallace J M, Gill D P JAMA 1978; 240: 2752
75. Brogden R N, Heel R C et al Drugs 1978; 15: 251
76. Sjoerdsma A, Engelman K, Spector S Lancet 1965; ii: 1092
77. Johnston R R, Eger E I, Wilson C A Anesth Analg 1976; 55: 709
78. Sever R S, Roberts L J, Snell M E Clin Endocrinol Metab 1980; 9: 943

mise is to infuse blood and plasma (1–2 litres) just before the tumour is isolated and removed. It is vital to give hydrocortisone 100 mg intravenously during bilateral adrenalectomy and appropriate steroid replacement is continued thereafter.

Even with careful preoperative pharmacological preparation, the patient with a phaeochromocytoma still presents a considerable challenge to both surgeon and anaesthetist. This is never more so than when the condition is encountered unexpectedly during surgery for an unrelated condition or when an undiagnosed tumour is removed without any preoperative preparation.

The warning signs include an unexplained tachycardia, arrhythmia or hypertension. If these signs go unheeded a fatal cardiac arrest may occur. If a phaeochromocytoma is encountered under these circumstances, α-blockade should be instituted at once, the procedure terminated and, after full assessment and preparation, elective excision of the tumour performed at a later date.

Postoperative intensive care with monitoring of the arterial blood pressure, pulse rate, central venous pressure and urinary output is vital. The intravenous fluid requirements of blood and plasma expanders will be largely determined on the basis of these measurements, and often large volumes of replacement fluid are necessary because of the changes in vascular compliance after tumour removal with the relative disproportion between vascular capacitance and circulating blood volume which follows the rapid fall in circulating catecholamines and removal of chronic vasoconstrictor effect. Also the residual effect of phenoxybenzamine remain, causing fluid loss into the retroperitoneal space. Persistent hypotension is however more likely to be from bleeding than refractiveness of the vascular bed. Over-transfusion must also be carefully avoided. Hypoglycaemia may occur in the first 24 hours postoperatively, so blood sugar must be carefully monitored and administration of intravenous glucose may be required. After recovery from surgery, urinary vanillylmandelic acid and metanephrines are measured to confirm the restoration of catecholamine biochemistry to normal.

Persistent hypertension may be from residual tumour, or from renal damage consequent upon long-standing severe hypertension. Measurement of urinary catecholamines and metabolites should be repeated annually as 'benign' phaeochromocytomas sometimes recur and their malignant potential only be recognised at a later date. However, the prognosis of this tumour is excellent with low operative mortality rates reported.[79]

Phaeochromocytoma in children

Hypertension in a child always demands the fullest investigation as 20% of all phaeochromocytomas are found in children. There is a greater incidence of bilateral, multiple and extra-adrenal tumours compared with adults.[80] A phaeochromocytoma occurring in a child should alert the clinician to the possibility of familial disease and other family members should be screened.

Phaeochromocytoma in pregnancy

A phaeochromocytoma in pregnancy is potentially extremely dangerous for both mother and fetus, and catecholamine excess must be excluded in all hypertensive pregnant women.

Both maternal and fetal mortality rates are significantly lower if the diagnosis is made prior to delivery.[81] Once the diagnosis has been made, reliance is placed on surgical exploration to localize the tumour as excessive use of X-rays is limited. In the first and second trimesters the tumour should be surgically excised after α- and β-blockade, although some might advocate termination of pregnancy during the first trimester. When diagnosed in the third trimester, α- and β-blockade is immediately instituted and elective caesarean section and synchronous tumour removal is performed.[82] Vaginal delivery should be avoided at all costs. α-Blockers have been used after the 24th week of pregnancy to treat hypertension without any apparent adverse consequences for the fetus.[83]

Malignant phaeochromocytoma

Malignancy occurs in approximately 10% of phaeochromocytomas[68,80] but is much more common when the tumour is located outside the adrenal.

The usual histological criteria of malignancy are unreliable and a firm diagnosis is often only made when metastatic tumour is found at sites where chromaffin tissue is not usually located. Whenever possible, the tumour should be completely excised, or if extensive, at least debulked. Chemotherapy is not very effective but radiotherapy may produce useful palliation.[84]

A pharmacological approach with α- and β-adrenergic blockers has a role in treatment, as has the catecholamine synthesis inhibitor α-methyl paratyrosine. Five-year survival rates in excess of 40% have been reported.[85] Extra-adrenal malignant tumours have a less favourable prognosis than tumours arising within the adrenal gland. Occasionally the radiopharmaceutical ^{131}I-metaiodobenzylguanidine might have a therapeutic as well as a diagnostic role in this condition.

Multiple endocrine neoplasia type II[67]

This syndrome, inherited as an autosomal dominant manner with high penetrance and variable expression, is characterized by medullary thyroid carcinoma and phaeochromocytomas (see p. 18). The germ line mutation responsible for this syndrome has recently been localized to the Ret-proto oncogene in chromosome 10.[86] In the IIa syndrome hyperparathyroidism may also occur (see Chapter 19), and in the IIb variety somatic abnormalities, including ganglioneuromata, 'marfanoid' habitus and skeletal abnormalities, may be found. The adrenal disease is invariably bilateral, passing through a phase of hyperplasia to nodularity and multiple phaeochromocytomas. Once the diagnosis has been established by

REFERENCES

79. van Heerden J A, Sheps J G et al Surgery 1982; 91: 367
80. Hume D Am J Surg 1960; 99: 458
81. Schenker J G, Chowers I Obstet Gynecol Surv 1971; 26: 739
82. Fudge T L, McKinnon W M P, Geary W L Arch Surg 1980; 115: 1224
83. Maughan G B, Shabanah E H, Toth E Am J Obstet Gynecol 1967; 97: 764
84. Scott W, Dean R H, Lea J W Surgery 1982; 92: 853

standard measurement of catecholamines and their metabolites in the urine, bilateral adrenalectomy should be performed. Some advocate unilateral adrenalectomy when the disease appears to be localized to one side.[87] This is an approach which is still controversial as the natural history of the disease clearly indicates that bilateral disease eventually develops in all subjects.[88] Clearly, after unilateral adrenalectomy careful follow-up is required to diagnose the development of disease in the contralateral adrenal gland.

OTHER TUMOURS OF ADRENAL MEDULLA AND EXTRA-ADRENAL PARAGANGLIONIC STRUCTURES

The World Health Organization has proposed an international classification of these tumours, which includes phaeochromocytomas and tumours of the paraganglionic structure.[89]

Neuroendocrine tumours (benign and malignant)

1. *Phaeochromocytoma.*
2. *Sympathetic paragangliomas* are of similar structure to phaeochromocytomas but are often non-chromaffin, although when functional they secrete noradrenaline and cause hypertension.
3. *Parasympathetic paraganglioma* (chemodectoma): These tumours are usually found in the carotid and aortic bodies and glomus jugulare; they may contain catecholamines but rarely secrete sufficient hormones to cause hypertension.

Neural tumours (benign and malignant)

1. *Benign neurofibroma and ganglioneuroma* occur in the adrenal medulla and are usually symptomless.
2. *Malignant ganglioneuroblastoma*: A tumour consisting of a mixture of neuroblasts and ganglion cells.
3. *Neuroblastoma:* This is an extremely malignant tumour of undifferentiated neuroblasts which occurs principally in the adrenal glands but also on occasions in adjacent retroperitoneal tissue and along the sympathetic chain of ganglia. A classical histological appearance of rosettes of tumour cells is recognized[90] and spread takes place directly to adjacent organs, via the lymphatics and through the blood stream. This is a childhood tumour: 60% present before the age of 1 year.[85] It is the commonest extracranial malignant solid tumour in infancy and childhood, affecting boys slightly more often than girls.

Clinical presentation

Half of the children with these tumours present with an abdominal mass, but others have neurological symptoms and signs and gastrointestinal disturbances, consisting of anorexia, nausea, vomiting and diarrhoea. Hypertension is present in some children as a result of tumour catecholamine secretion accompanied by an excess of vanillylmandelic acid and metanephine in the urine. Diarrhoea has been attributed to the secretion of vasoactive intestinal polypeptide by the tumour.[91] Unfortunately, metastatic disease is present in many children at the time of presentation. Two major patterns of metastases are recognized:

1. *Pepper's type*[92]: primary and secondary tumours in the right side with multiple liver deposits.
2. *Hutchison's type:*[92] a left-sided primary tumour spreading to the orbit, skull and long bones.

Wilms renal tumour (nephroblastoma) is the important differential diagnosis of neuroblastoma.

Investigations

Radiological studies, chest X-ray, intravenous pyelogram, skeletal survey and CT scan are required to confirm the diagnosis and stage the tumour.

Treatment

Surgical excision is the optimum treatment when the tumour is confined to the adrenal gland or extends no further than the midline (stages I and II). The role of tumour excision is less clear in more extensive disease extending across the midline (stage III) or when there are metastases in bone, soft tissues, visceral organs and distant nodes (stage IV), although there may be benefits from tumour debulking in permitting more effective adjuvant therapy.[85]

Neuroblastomas are radiosensitive and this treatment is employed when the tumour has been incompletely excised. There are however few controlled trials to confirm the benefits of radiotherapy which is known to be of value in the palliation of painful metastases.

Chemotherapy with combinations of vincristine, cyclophosphamide and DTIC (dimethyltriazenoimidazole carboxamide) is indicated in stage III and IV disease, with proven beneficial results.[77] The latter drug unfortunately has severe toxic side-effects.

Prognosis

Spontaneous tumour regression and remission with maturation to a ganglioneuroma pathology are well-recognized. The overall 2-year survival is 32% with 86% of children living 2 years with stage I disease.[85] If a child remains free of recurrence and survives this

REFERENCES

85. Javadpour N, Weltering E A, Brennan M Curr Prob Surg 1980; 17: 5
86. Mulligan L M, Kwok J B J et al Nature 1993; 363: 458–460
87. Tibbling S, Dymling J F et al World J Surg 1983; 7: 201
88. Carney J A, Sizemore G W, Tyce G M Mayo Clin Proc 1975; 50: 3
89. Williams E D, Siebenmann R E, Sobin L H (eds) Histological Typing of Endocrine Tumours. World Health Organization, Geneva 1980 p 23
90. Lips K J, Veer J V D S, Struyvenberg A Am J Med 1981; 70: 1051
91. Verner J V, Morrison A B Arch Intern Med 1974; 133: 492
92. Goode A W Bailey and Love's Short Practice of Surgery 19th edn. H K Lewis, London 1984

length of time, then a long-term cure is considered likely. A more favourable prognosis is associated with younger female patients.

Adrenalectomy and breast cancer

Bilateral adrenalectomy for disseminated breast cancer was introduced by Huggins & Bergenstal[93] in 1952. During the next two decades there was a considerable vogue for bilateral adrenalectomy performed either through a bilateral loin incision or transabdominally.

The indications were usually as second-line hormone therapy in patients with a prior good response to oophorectomy or, latterly, tamoxifen. The considerable morbidity that attended the operation in this ailing population,[94] together with the advent of aminoglutethamide, a steroid biosynthesis blocker, as a satisfactory medical adrenalectomy of equivalent therapeutic benefit,[95] has led to its virtual abdandonment.

Operative technique

The various surgical approaches to the adrenal glands are summarized in Table 35.6.

REFERENCES

93. Huggins C, Bergenstal D M Cancer Res 1952; 12: 134
94. Paterson A G, Webster D J T Anticancer Res 1983; 3: 151
95. Santen R J, Worgul T J, Samojlik E N Engl J Med 1981; 305: 545

Table 35.6 Surgical techniques for adrenalectomy

Approach	*Incision*	*Indications*	*Comments*	*Disadvantages*
Posterior[29] or posterolateral	Unilateral or bilateral obliquely over 11th or 12th ribs	Unilateral small tumours Aldosterone-secreting tumours (Conn's) Incidentalomas, bilateral hyperplasia of Cushing's syndrome. Now often used for phaeochromocytoma when good localization has been achieved. Previously used in palliative treatment of breast cancer	Low morbidity and mortality in poor-risk patients	Care required to avoid damage to inferior vena cava on right side
Anterior	Bilateral subcostal transverse upper abdominal or long midline	Phaeochromocytoma. Adrenal tumours in which precise preoperative localization has not been achieved	Excellent adrenal gland exposure. Permits search for extra-adrenal phaeochromocytomas and examination of intra-abdominal viscera including sympathetic chains and pelvic organs	Increased morbidity and mortality. Wound complications
Thoracoabdominal	Oblique upper abdominal across costal margin at ninth interspace	Large malignant adrenal tumour (> 15 cm in diameter)	Excellent access to adrenals. Permits en bloc tumour resection including adjacent organs, e.g. spleen and tail of pancreas	Traumatic procedure with increased morbidity and mortality
Laparoscopic	Lateral flank (four-port insertion)	Small benign tumours? bilateral hyperplasia of Cushing's small phaeochromocytomas	Precise role of this technique has yet to be defined	

36 The kidney and ureter

Neeraj K. Sharma David A. Tolley

SYMPTOMS AND SIGNS OF RENAL AND URETERIC DISEASE

Loin pain

There are few surgical emergencies more dramatic in their presentation than ureteric colic. Whilst the diagnosis of this condition is generally straightforward, patients presenting with vague backache may be very difficult to diagnose. Pain arising from the upper urinary tract may be felt anywhere from the renal angle to the testis or labia. In general, pain arising from the kidney occurs in the renal angle; upper and mid ureteric pain is felt in the flank and iliac fossa; pain arising in the lower third of the ureter usually radiates into the genitalia and is associated with the symptoms of bladder irritability, such as urinary frequency. Renal pain is invariably unilateral and is not exacerbated by exercise, movement or posture although occasionally a small mobile intrarenal stone may cause pain on movement.

Obstruction of the urinary tract produces a dull pain which varies from mild to severe according to the degree of obstruction, but may be made worse by increased fluid intake. It is normally constant but worsens as the obstruction increases, although occasionally total obstruction may be painless. In contrast the pain produced by contraction of ureteric smooth muscle is colicky in nature, always severe, and may be associated with nausea or vomiting. The pain is more intense than the pain of uterine contractions during the first stage of labour and frequently patients writhe about in an attempt to obtain relief, unlike patients with peritonitis. Loin pain associated with fever or rigors is suggestive of infection or inflammation and these patients may develop septicaemia from an acutely obstructed infected kidney. An enquiry about previous history of urinary tract stone disease or family history of the condition may help to diagnose the cause of the pain.

Haematuria

Haematuria may be frank or microscopic. Haematuria detected by dipsticks is not necessarily significant; this should be confirmed by microscopy. Ascorbic acid ingestion, a highly concentrated urine and myoglobinuria can cause false positive results on dipstick testing, which relies on the peroxidase-like activity of haemoglobin.

All patients with haematuria require investigation, although the likelihood of finding significant urological pathology depends on the age of the patient and whether the haematuria was frank or microscopic, symptomatic or symptomless. The presence of frank blood is usually obvious to the patient and there may be clots if the bleeding is profuse. Haematuria may occur only in the initial part of the stream (when it is usually caused by anterior urethral or prostatic diseases); in the terminal part of the stream (resulting from trigonal irritation from bladder or prostatic infection, though it is classically described in schistosomiasis); or throughout the stream when it is indicative of bladder or renal pathology. Frank painless haematuria indicates a carcinoma in the urinary tract until proven otherwise. The presence of proteinuria and casts in urine in association with microscopic haematuria strongly suggests a nephrological cause for the haematuria. Patients receiving anticoagulant therapy who develop frank haematuria must still be investigated for underlying urological pathology. Some athletes, and joggers, occasionally develop haematuria after a long run. There is rarely any serious underlying pathology although the aetiology of the condition is unclear. It may be the result of minor trauma at the bladder base.

The presence of associated symptoms such as suprapubic pain, urinary frequency or loin pain may provide an important pointer to the cause of the bleeding. For example, suprapubic pain, urinary frequency and haematuria are generally caused by urinary infection, and the combination of loin pain and haematuria is often caused by a urinary tract calculus or tumour. Occasionally patients may erroneously ascribe haematuria to wax crayon sucking or the ingestion of beetroot or medication, e.g. rifampicin.[1] In others there may be a history of a general medical disorder such as glomerulonephritis or subacute bacterial endocarditis. Myoglobinuria may also be described erroneously as haematuria.

Chyluria

Fistulous connections between lymphatics of the kidney, ureter or bladder and the urinary tract result in the symptom of chyluria in which the urine contains large quantities of protein and fat, resulting in a milky appearance (Fig. 36.1). This is confirmed by finding chylomicrons on microscopy of urine. Weight loss, lower limb oedema and ureteric colic may be associated with this condition which is the result of filariasis or congenital megalymphatics (see Chapter 12).

REFERENCE

1. Turner A G, Hendry W F et al Br Med J 1977; 2: 29

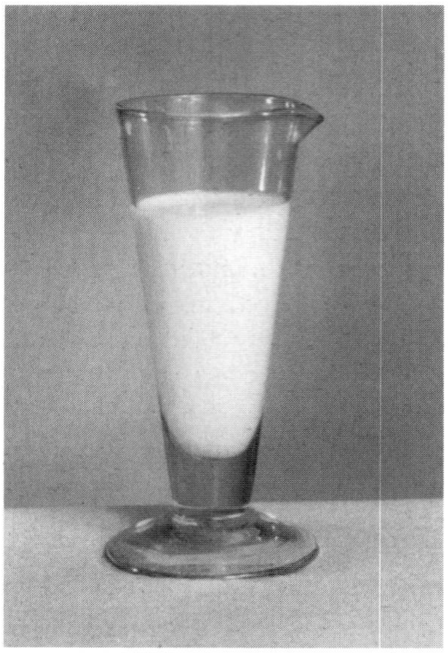

Fig. 36.1 Chyluria. Note the milky appearance of the urine.

Pneumaturia

The presence of air bubbles in the urine is usually associated with a vesicocolic fistula and is accompanied by other symptoms such as the passage of cloudy, foul-smelling urine. It may also be accompanied by large-bowel symptoms. The fistula is usually the result of inflammatory or malignant bowel disease. Rarely, pneumaturia is a complication of urinary tract infection in diabetics and results from the fermentation of glucose by bacteria or yeast.

Loin mass

Normal kidneys are rarely palpable because they are protected anteriorly by the costal margin. In thin individuals, however, the lower pole of the right kidney can occasionally be palpated during deep inspiration. The presence of a large palpable mass in the loin which descends with inspiration and is ballottable from behind, indicates an enlarged kidney which is usually the result of cysts, tumour or obstruction.

INVESTIGATION OF URINARY TRACT DISEASE

Investigation of the urinary tract includes examination of urine samples, biochemical tests and assessment of renal function, imaging for structure and function of the kidney and ureter, direct visualization of the ureter and kidney, and tissue biopsies.

Midstream specimen of urine

If urine analysis is to provide useful information, the urine must be collected properly and transported without delay. In uncircumcised males the foreskin must be retracted and the glans cleaned prior to providing a midstream sample of urine. In females a clean catch specimen is obtained. If there is likely to be delay in transport of the sample it should be collected in a container with boric acid (1.7–2%) or should be refrigerated, not frozen; such a sample can provide useful data up to 24–36 hours. Urine normally contains very few red and white cells (less than 1–2 per mm^3). There may be occasional transitional cells and hyaline casts from the upper urinary tract.

Dipstick analysis of the urine is a quick, inexpensive way of determining specific gravity, pH and the presence of protein, glucose, ketones, bilirubin, urobilinogen, blood, leucocytes and nitrites using colorimetric chemical assays. This provides useful information on the excretory, secretory and resorptive functions of the kidney. The presence of nitrites in the urine strongly suggests urinary tract infection, especially if there are also excessive numbers of leucocytes. The numbers of red and white cells increase after severe exercise or in patients with a fever, but the presence of large numbers of red or white blood cells is usually indicative of urinary tract disease. In order to determine whether or not the urine is infected, the first part of the urine voided, which is potentially contaminated, is discarded and a midstream specimen is examined.

Cellular casts imply the presence of renal disease: granular and red cell casts are seen in proliferative glomerulonephritis and white cell casts are associated with active pyelonephritis. The use of phase-contrast microscopy distinguishes glomerular red cells from lower urinary tract red cells (dysmorphic and isomorphic red cells)[3] and can help differentiate urological from nephrological haematuria. Crystals of urate, oxalate and phosphate may be seen on microscopy in normal urine but the presence of the hexagonal benzene ring like crystals of cystine is diagnostic of cystinuria. The presence of more than 10^5 organisms per ml indicates bacteriological urinary infection.[4] Lesser numbers of organisms can occasionally be seen with severe symptomatic urinary tract infections where frequent bladder emptying occurs, but low counts or mixed organisms are usually the result of urethral contamination.

Biochemical tests and assessment of renal function

The kidney fulfils an essential role in the excretion of waste products of metabolism and in the maintenance of fluid balance. It is also responsible for the production of a number of hormones. A simple assessment of renal function may be achieved by measurement of the blood urea, creatinine and electrolytes. Factors which affect the blood urea concentration are chiefly the protein intake and metabolism, glomerular filtration and tubular function. Estimation of the blood urea is a remarkably insensitive indicator of renal function as it does not begin to rise until the renal function has been reduced by about half. Thus a normal blood urea does not exclude the presence of considerable damage.[5] Creatinine production is related to muscle mass, therefore the plasma creatinine is higher in men than in women and is also higher in adults than in

REFERENCES

2. Porter I A Br Med J 1969; 2: 353
3. Donadala W et al Acta Cytol 1979; 23: 147
4. Kass E J Trans Assoc Am Phys 1956; 69: 56
5. Peters J P, Van Slyke D D Quant Clin Chem 1931; 1: 258

children. Creatinine is largely excreted by glomerular filtration and thus reflects the ability of the kidney to filter waste products. This is in contrast to urea excretion which occurs by a combination of glomerular filtration and proximal tubule and collecting tubule reabsorption under the influence of vasopressin.

The assessment of the plasma electrolytes (sodium, potassium chloride and bicarbonate) provides direct evidence of abnormal renal function; for example, the plasma potassium is elevated in patients with acute renal failure, and the development of a metabolic acidosis in chronic renal failure is indicated by a low level of plasma bicarbonate.

Clearance measurements

Clearance is a quantitive description of the rate at which the kidney excretes various substances relative to their concentration in plasma. A substance that is freely filtered and undergoes neither reabsorption nor secretion has a clearance equal to the glomerular filtration rate. Inulin is one such substance, and creatinine is almost, though not quite, equivalent. The plasma concentration of creatinine remains stable during a 24-hour period and its urinary concentration does not vary with urinary flow. The assessment of creatinine clearance is thus one of the most useful renal function tests as the creatinine clearance is only altered by changes in glomerular filtration and is not influenced by the resorptive or secretory functions of the kidney. It therefore approximates to glomerular filtration rate[6] and is assessed by the simple formula

$$\frac{U \times V}{P}$$

where U and P are the concentrations of creatinine in the urine and plasma respectively, and V is the urine volume in 24 h. The creatinine clearance is generally measured over a 24-hour period and the most common cause of a low clearance is an incomplete urine collection.[7] It has therefore been recommended that an average of two or three (2–4-h) consecutive collection periods should be taken.[8]

When assessment of the creatinine clearance is not possible, injection of ethylene diamenetetra-acetic acid (EDTA) labelled with an isotope of chromium (EDTA ^{51}Cr) or diethylenetriamine-penta-acetic acid labelled with an isotope of technetium (DTPA ^{99m}Tc) can be used to assess the glomerular filtration rate. The glomerular filtration rate is then calculated from the concentration/time plot obtained 2–6 hours after injection. This method is accurate as it relies only upon the determination of the concentration of the radiolabelled substance in the plasma and there is no need for urine collection.[9] A number of alternative approaches have been developed in an attempt to simplify the technique of measuring the glomerular filtration rate even further. It is possible to determine glomerular filtration rate from single plasma samples by comparing the concentration of EDTA ^{51}Cr in a sample of blood taken 3 h after injection with the concentration on a standard graph obtained during studies on a series of patients.[10]

Assessment of tubular function

The assessment of renal tubular function is of little relevance to the practising surgeon in most cases of urinary tract disease. Assessment of urinary acidification to differentiate Type 1 and Type 2 renal tubular acidosis, tubular phosphate reabsorption and occasionally amino acid excretion may be required in patients with urinary stones.

Urinary sodium excretion varies with the sodium balance in patients with normal renal function. Although it is difficult to define a normal level of urinary sodium excretion, its serial determination is often useful in monitoring the recovery of renal function, particularly after relief of urinary obstruction.

Tubular damage also results in the kidney's inability to concentrate the urine, causing the development of polyuria. This symptom is also produced by an osmotic diuresis, hypercalcaemia, diabetes or a deficiency of antidiuretic hormone. The kidneys are normally able to concentrate the urine to a specific gravity of 1.022–1.032 after a prolonged period of dehydration or overnight. Urine osmolality may also be assessed. This varies from 50 to 1200 mosmol/l and depends upon the amount of water reabsorbed in the collecting tubules; it is also influenced by antidiuretic hormone.[11]

Proteinuria

Normally, 80–150 mg of protein is excreted per day. A maximum excretion of 300 mg per day can occur transiently following severe exercise. Protein excretion that exceeds 300 mg per day is significant proteinuria and indicates the presence of renal disease. The concentration of protein in normal urine does not usually exceed 10–20 mg per dl; half of this is in the form of albumin and the remainder is split equally between the globulins and tissue proteins, e.g. the Tamm–Horsfall protein.[12]

Proteinuria can be detected by various methods. Dipstick detection depends on the change of colour of tetrabromophenol blue in the presence of albumin. Dipsticks are therefore more sensitive in detecting albumin than the globulins, Bence Jones proteins or mucoproteins such as the Tamm–Horsfall protein. They can detect 10 mg/dl of albumin in the urine and therefore the normal urine should not react. The Turbidimetric method of protein precipitation which uses 3% sulphasalactic acid[13] is more sensitive: it can detect urine protein levels as low as 5 mg/dl and is equally sensitive for all types of proteins. False positive protein detection on dipstick testing can occur in an alkaline urine when the pH is greater than 9. It can also occur when phenazopyridine or artificial blood substitutes like pyrrolidone have been given or when there has been contamination of the containers with chlorhexidine or benzalkonium compounds. False positive results from

REFERENCES

6. Mandel E E et al J Lab Clin Med 1953; 42: 621
7. Brochner-Mortensen J, Robro P Scand J Clin Lab Invest 1976; 36: 35
8. Brochner-Mortensen J Dan Med Bull 1978; 25: 181
9. Chantler C et al Clin Sci 1969; 37: 169
10. Constable A R et al Radionuclides in Nephrology. Academic Press, London 1982
11. Hander S, Orloff S Handbook of Physiology, Section 8. Renal Physiology. American Physiology Society, Washington DC 1973
12. Grant G H J Clin Pathol 1959; 12: 510
13. Kingsbury F B J Lab Clin Med 1926; 11: 981

Turbidimetric reactions can occur when there is radiographic contrast material in the urine or when it contains high concentrations of penicillin, cephalosporins, sulphonamides or tolbutamides.

24-hour collection of protein excretion in urine is the most accurate investigation but contamination of urine with plasma proteins when there is gross haematuria can give a false positive reaction. A massive bleed is required however to bring the protein concentration into the 100–300 mg/dl range; milder degrees of microscopic or macroscopic haematuria with a 2+ or a 3+ dipstick test indicating proteinuria (greater than 300 mg/dl) are always assumed to have a glomerular or interstitial cause.[14]

Radiological assessment of the urinary tract

Intravenous urography

Intravenous urography is an established technique for diagnosing urinary tract disease and assessing renal anatomy. High osmolality or the newer low osmolality contrast media can be injected. This results in radiographic opacification of the renal tracts because the X-rays are blocked by the filtered iodine molecule, though this filtration can only occur when the kidneys are functioning. The high osmolality contrast media (e.g. sodium or methyl glucamine compounds of diatrizoate and iothalamate) deliver a mean osmotic load of 1400 to 2400 mmosmol/kg of water and have an iodine to particle ratio of 3:2. The low osmolality media (e.g. Iohexol and Iopmidol and Ioxalic sodium) have an iodine to particle ratio of 6:2 or 3:1, and are significantly less hypertonic with a osmolality of 411 to 796 mmosmol/kg of water. The usual dose is 300 mg of iodine/kg body weight given as a fast intravenous injection. The use of abdominal compression and nephrotomography helps to delineate the pelvicaliceal system more clearly. Intravenous contrast media can cause nephrotoxicity and allergic reactions, both of which seem to occur more commonly with the higher osmolality contrast media. Patients at risk of nephrotoxicity include those with existing renal insufficiency, diabetic nephropathy and congestive cardiac failure. Multiple myeloma and dehydration are additional risk factors.[15] The estimated risk of nephrotoxicity is 0–1% in a healthy outpatient population but increases to 4.6% in a randomly selected hospitalized group of patients, and can rise to 17% after angiographic procedures. The nephropathy is generally mild and transient in most cases. The serum creatinine usually rises within 24–48 hours, returning to the baseline by 10–14 days, and is believed to be the result of a combination of direct tubular cell damage and hypoxic cellular injury in an already ischaemic renal medulla.

Anaphylactoid reactions may be idiosyncratic or orthodox.[16] Orthodox symptoms, which are probably caused by direct chemotoxicity of the contrast agent, include nausea, vomiting, erythema, pulmonary oedema and cardiovascular collapse, whereas idiosyncratic symptoms are caused by an allergic response and include urticaria, headache, bronchospasm and hypotension. 70% of these reactions occur within 5–10 minutes of the injection.[17] Risk factors include a history of allergic reactions: this is the most significant predictor of anaphylaxis although recurrent reactions are rarely life threatening. Asthmatics are at high risk for having reactions, particularly bronchospasm. The incidence of severe life threatening reactions is 0.04% if high osmolality contrast medium is used and 0.004% with lower osmolality contrast medium. The overall incidence of all reactions was 12.3% after high osmolality medium and 3.13% after low osmolality medium.[17]

The new techniques now available for imaging the kidneys have reduced the need for intravenous urography in many patients. There is no indication for intravenous urography in patients with renal failure: the amount of information gained is not worth the risks involved when ultrasound, MRI and CT scanning can provide a satisfactory alternative.

Retrograde ureteropyelogram

This examination may be helpful if the collecting system cannot be clearly seen on the intravenous urogram. At cystoscopy, the ureteric orifice is identified and a Braasch bulb catheter is wedged in the lower ureter. Bubble-free contrast medium is then injected whilst the whole of the ureter and collecting system is screened by fluoroscopy. A conventional radiograph can be taken as a permanent record of the procedure.

Renal angiography

Renal angiography is now rarely performed. Most renal tumours can be diagnosed by ultrasound or computerized tomography (CT) scanning. Renal angiography is occasionally indicated in patients with renal trauma and in the assessment of young patients with hypertension. The value of arterial embolization as a therapeutic adjunct in patients with renal tumours is not proven.[18] Digital subtraction angiography is now a better method for obtaining renal arteriograms of high diagnostic quality.

Isotope renography

This very useful investigation depends on the ability of the kidney to filter or secrete a radionuclide isotope which can be objectively counted on a gamma camera. A computerized traced plot of isotope activity in an area of interest can then be made. The commonly used isotopes are ^{99m}Tc-dimercaptosuccinic acid (DMSA), ^{99m}Tc-diethylenetriaminepenta-acetic acid (DTPA) and mercaptoacetyl triglycine (MAG3). Each of these is handled differently by the kidney and therefore gives different information on the function of its various parts. DMSA is secreted by the tubules and provides information on the split renal function, i.e. the functioning of each individual kidney relative to the other; it also demonstrates the presence of renal scarring in vesico-ureteric reflux or after infection. It is frequently necessary to determine the

REFERENCES

14. Glassock R J Textbook of Nephrology. Williams & Wilkins, Baltimore 1983 p 414
15. Porter G A Invest Radiol 1993; 28: S1
16. Siegle R L Invest Radiol 1993; 28: S95
17. Katayama H Radiology 1990; 175: 621
18. Wallace S, Chuang V P et al Radiology 1981; 138: 563

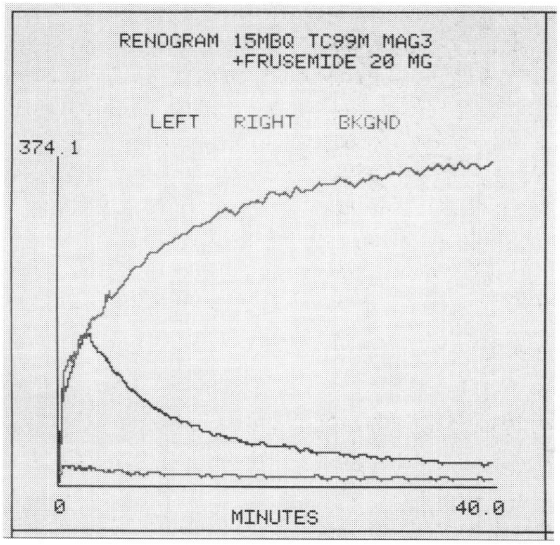

Fig. 36.2 Isotope renography. A MAG3 diuretic renogram showing a rising curve of the right kidney indicating obstruction and accumulation of radioisotope tracer which remains pooled in the renal area. The left kidney shows a normal trace of isotope excretion. (Courtesy of Dr S E Moussa, Consultant Radiologist).

contribution of each kidney to the overall renal function. This is especially important if nephrectomy is contemplated. DMSA scanning also gives an indication of the recoverability of renal function following obstruction and is thus helpful in determining whether or not there is sufficient function remaining in a diseased kidney to merit its conservation.

DTPA, on the other hand, is predominantly filtered by the glomerulus and can therefore help to identify cases of renovascular hypertension. Its main value, however, lies in identifying an obstructed kidney. A diuretic is administered 15 minutes before performing the test, stressing the affected kidney to the maximum. Failure of excretion of the isotope from the kidney demonstrates increased activity above the site of obstruction and a rising curve is seen on the renogram.

MAG3 is both filtered and secreted by the kidney and is now one of the most commonly used isotopes in radionuclear departments (Fig. 36.2), although a DTPA scan is preferred when the overall renal function is poor.

As the radiation dose is much less from isotopes than conventional X-rays, isotope renography is good method of imaging the genitourinary tract. It is also used as an indirect technique to diagnose and monitor reflux disease.

Ultrasonography

Ultrasonography has become the most commonly performed means of investigating the urinary tract. It is the baseline investigation for any patient thought to have renal failure and is excellent at diagnosing hydronephrosis and assessing the nature of mass lesions in the kidney, whether cystic or solid. The technique is operator dependent, non-invasive and inexpensive. It does not carry any risk of irradiation. It must be remembered that ultrasonography provides an anatomical assessment of the kidney and ureter and it does not assess function. Its diagnostic and therapeutic uses include:

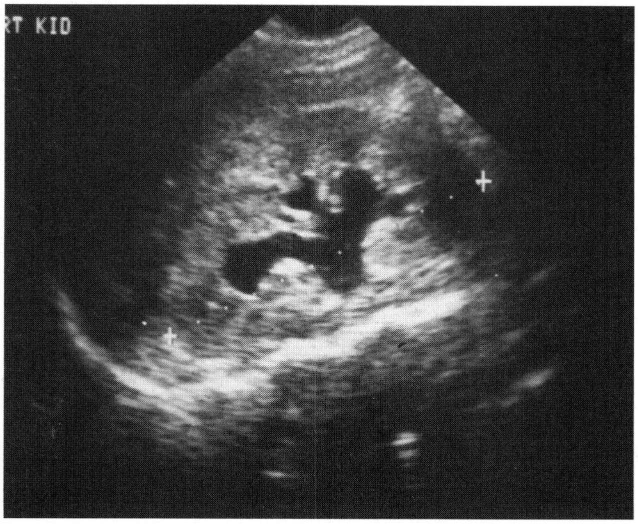

Fig. 36.3 Ultrasound of the kidney showing dilatation of the pelvicalyceal sinus fat complex echoes due to hydronephrosis. (Courtesy of Dr S A Moussa, Consultant Radiologist.)

1. Assessment of patients with renal failure. Parenchymal damage (small shrunken kidneys) can be differentiated from obstructive hydronephrotic kidneys (Fig. 36.3). It must be remembered that the presence of a dilated urinary tract on ultrasound is not diagnostic of obstruction: it may be seen with reflux papillary necroses and in patients with residual dilatation after obstruction or in situations of high flow such as diabetes insipidus.[19]
2. Trauma. Perirenal haematomas and renal parenchymal damage can be assessed and renal blood flow visualized with Doppler ultrasound. Urinomas can be drained percutaneously.
3. Infections. The presence of pyonephrosis, perirenal abscesses and stones in relation to infected kidneys is easily identified and treated.
4. Calculus disease. Ultrasound not only detects radiolucent stones in the kidney but is also used to provide real time imaging during lithotripsy (Fig. 36.4).
5. The diagnosis and staging of patients with renal cell carcinoma. Needle biopsy of renal mass lesions and aspirations of cysts from the kidney for cytological and histological assessment can safely be performed under ultrasound guidance. Tumour extension into the renal vein and the inferior vena cava can be better identified by ultrasound than by a CT scan.
6. Evaluation of renal transplants. Vascular non-function of a graft can be detected by Doppler flow studies. Ultrasound can provide evidence of acute rejection, when bright echoes are seen, and the presence of obstruction of the ureter by urinomas, kinks or strictures can be ascertained. The graft can be biopsied under ultrasound guidance or percutaneously drained if obstructed.
7. Ultrasound is also used for transrectal assessment of the prostate and seminal vesicles, to diagnose obstructed seminal

REFERENCES

19. Amis E S Urology 1982; 19: 101
20. Semelka R C J Magn Reson Imaging 1993; 3: 597

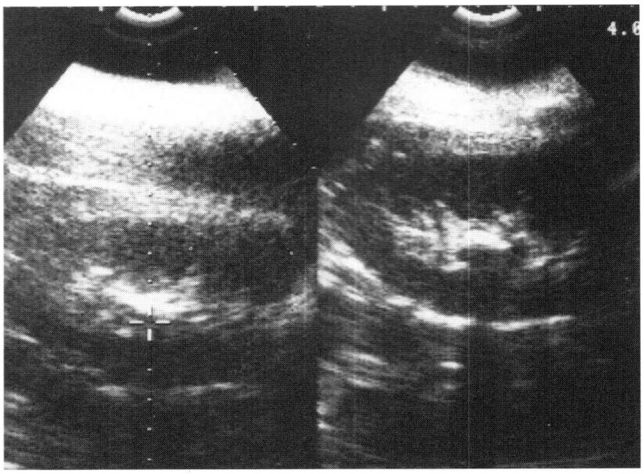

Fig. 36.4 Ultrasound of the kidney showing a stone in the centre of the pelvicalyceal sinus fat complex echo with a distal acoustic shadow due to reflection of the ultrasound waves from the surface of the stone. The picture on the left shows the stone targeted with ultrasound for lithotripsy. (Courtesy of Dr S A Moussa, Consultant Radiologist.)

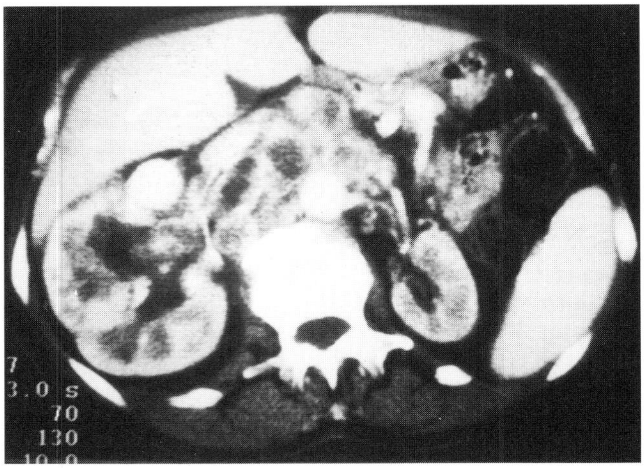

Fig. 36.5 Contrast enhanced CT scan showing a normal left kidney and a large tumour in the right kidney with enlarged nodes surrounding the enhanced aorta in front of the vertebral body. The left renal artery is seen branching from the left lateral wall of the aorta. Courtesy of Dr S A Moussa, Consultant Radiologist.

vesicles or tumours in the prostate which can be biopsied under ultrasound guidance (see Chapter 38).

8. The quantity of residual urine in the bladder can be assessed and this, together with flow measurement, is a useful indication of bladder outflow obstruction.

MRI—magnetic resonance imaging

Magnetic resonance imaging still remains a research tool in urology; it has, however, been shown to have a role when renal cell carcinoma is suspected but where CT is unhelpful or when the patient is sensitive to contrast. It can diagnose the local spread of stage IV renal cell carcinoma better than CT, and can also show the extent of tumour thrombus in the renal vein and inferior vena cava more clearly than a CT scan.[20] It is also better than CT in determining the haemorrhagic component of a cystic mass and is currently being evaluated in renal vascular hypertension where it has been found to be 100% sensitive, and will pick up 76% of the renal artery stenoses which are greater than 50% in the proximal 3 cm of the renal artery.[21]

Computerized tomography

Computerized tomography depicts the anatomy of the upper urinary tract and surrounding structures in excellent detail. The CT attenuation values for different soft tissues in the body allow for better resolution in imaging and therefore clearer identification of structures such as fat, kidney, liver, spleen and vessels. Renal masses can be identified and characterized, and they can be targeted and biopsied under CT control. Angiomyolipoma, a differential diagnosis for renal cell carcinoma, can in particular be diagnosed and followed up by CT imaging. CT helps in staging renal tumours and diagnosing retroperitoneal fibrosis (Fig. 36.5). It is very useful in assessing the renal parenchymal and ureteric integrity and function in patients with renal injuries.

The renal vasculature can be visualized using newer spiral CT scans with 3D reconstruction; these advances in CT imaging allow for digital subtraction and reconstruction to give unsurpassed pictures of the renal and ureteric anatomy (Fig. 36.6).

Ureteroscopy

The use of rigid or flexible ureteroscopes to directly visualize the ureter along its entire length and some parts of the renal collecting system has allowed a more accurate assessment of ureteric and renal lesions, especially transitional cell carcinomas. Apart from its diagnostic uses, ureteroscopy has a therapeutic role in the management of calculi and some tumours. It is a specialized technique which requires considerable skill and involves the passage of a rigid or flexible ureteroscope up the ureter via the urethra and bladder along a guidewire. The procedure is performed in a theatre with fluoroscopic facilities. Ureteroscopy can also be used to treat pelviureteric junction obstruction by endopyelotomy or as a preliminary to a balloon dilatation of the pelviureteric junction.

Antegrade pyelography

Introduction of a contrast medium into the kidney via a fine needle placed in the calix or pelvis may give additional information about the nature of a filling defect or the site of an obstruction. Percutaneous urinary drainage can be established at the same time. Occasionally this route can be used for the antegrade insertion of ureteric stents in patients with obstruction.[22]

REFERENCES

21. Loubeyre P Am J Roentogenol 1994; 162: 847
22. Pfister R C, Joder I C, Newhouse J H Semin Roentgenol 1981; 16: 135

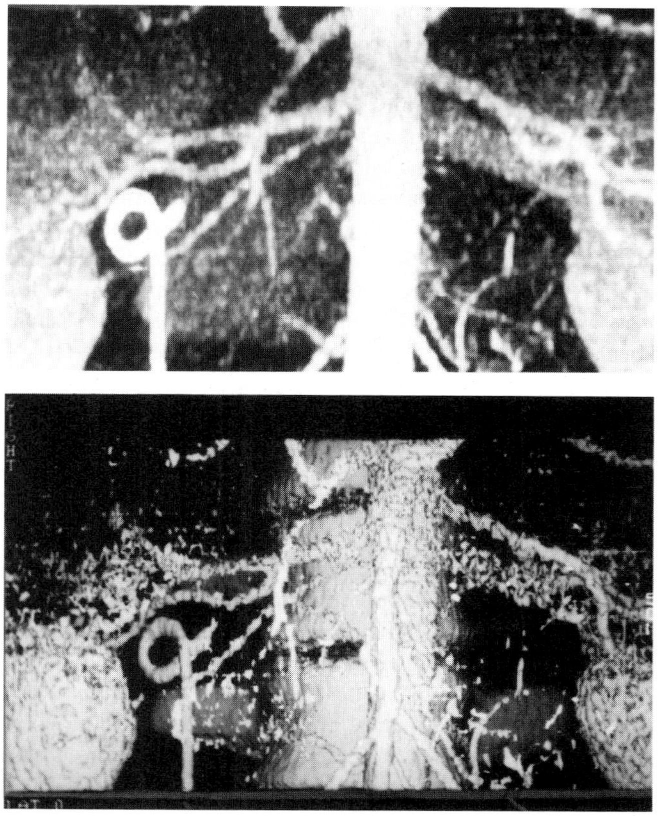

Fig. 36.6 Spiral CT angiogram of the renal arteries. A JJ stent is placed in the ureter prior to the CT scan, to help identify the pelviureteric junction. The picture at the top (maximum intensity projection) shows a lower polar artery associated with the pelviureteric junction obstruction. The lower figure (3D reconstruction with surface rendering) shows that the vessel is anterior to the pelvis and the stent. Courtesy of Dr S A Moussa, Consultant Radiologist.

Cystoscopy

Cystourethroscopy is the standard endoscopic technique for assessing the lower urinary tract. The procedure is described in Chapter 37.

Renal biopsy

Percutaneous renal biopsy using a Tru-cut needle provides valuable information in patients with acute or chronic renal failure. The biopsy needle is usually guided into the kidney by ultrasound. There is a small risk of an arteriovenous fistula developing as a result of the biopsy; open or laparoscopic renal biopsy should therefore be performed in patients with bleeding disorders or with solitary kidneys.

Cytology

Cytological examination of space-occupying lesions in the kidney is occasionally necessary. The mass is generally punctured under ultrasound control and the aspirate sent for examination by an expert cytologist. The fat content is also estimated.

Table 36.1 Congenital anomalies of the kidney

1. Anomalies of number and size:
   (a) absent kidney (agenesis), unilateral or bilateral
   (b) supernumerary kidney
   (c) hypoplasia of the kidney.
2. Anomalies of ascent of the kidney:
   (a) arrest or excessive ascent on the same side
   (b) crossed ectopia with and without fusion
   (c) horseshoe kidney.
3. Anomalies of structure:
   (a) anomalies of renal vasculature
   aberrant accessory multiple vessels,
   renal artery aneurysms or AV fistulae
   (b) anomalies of renal parenchyma
   i. Fetal lobulation
   ii. Cystic disease of the kidney
   multicystic disease
   polycystic disease
   medullary sponge kidney
   medullary cystic disease and other cystic diseases.
4. Anomalies of rotation
   Excessive, incomplete or reverse.

Cytological examination of a freshly voided urine sample may detect the presence of exfoliating tumour cells.[23] This is, however, a relatively unreliable method of diagnosing bladder cancer and the absence of suspicious cells does not exclude a carcinoma (see Chapter 37).

CONGENITAL ANOMALIES OF THE KIDNEY AND URETER

A thorough understanding of the embryological genesis of the kidney and the ureter makes the various congenital anomalies easier to understand. A working classification of the anomalies of the kidney is shown in Table 36.1.

Agenesis

Bilateral renal agenesis is a rare anomaly which is incompatible with life. It is associated with moderate oligohydramnios and a characteristic Potter facies, with a prominent fold of skin beginning in the inner canthus of each eye and running down over a semicircle over the cheek combined with a blunted nose and a prominent depression between the lower lip and chin.

Unilateral agenesis is seen in 1 in 1100 births.[24] The fault most probably lies with the ureteric bud: there is either a complete absence of the ureteric bud or aborted ureteral development preventing maturation of the metanephric blastema. Associated anomalies include the absence of the vas deferens on the same side in men. An abnormality of the internal genitalia is seen in a third of the women with unilateral renal agenesis.[25]

REFERENCES

23. Papanicolaou G N, Marshall V F Science 1945; 101: 519
24. Doroshow L W Surv 1961; 11: 219
25. Thomson D P Mayo Clin Proc 1966; 41: 538

Syndromes associated with unilateral renal agenesis include Turner's syndrome, Poland syndrome[26] and VATER syndrome.[27] The diagnosis is usually made by chance as the contralateral kidney does not appear to be more prone to disease, though it shows compensatory hypertrophy. The diagnosis can be confirmed by intravenous urography and renal ultrasound. Isotope scanning and arteriography provide absolute confirmation. Cystoscopy usually reveals an asymmetric trigone or a hemitrigone with either complete absence of a ureteric orifice or ureteral atresia. The overall prognosis is good—the presence of normal contralateral kidney is compatible with longevity and does not predispose the patient to greater than normal risks. Focal glomerulosclerosis as a hyperfiltration injury has however been noted in some patients on renal biopsy.[28]

Supernumerary kidney

This is extremely rare; approximately 75 cases have been reported in the literature.[29] The supernumerary kidney has its own separate capsule and blood supply. Approximately half of all supernumerary kidneys have their own completely independent ureter. They are located caudal to the dominant kidney and are usually smaller than the main ipsilateral organ. The average age at diagnosis is 36 years, when patients present with pain, fever and hypertension. A palpable abdominal mass may be found on abdominal examination. The renal parenchyma is usually hypoplastic. In 25% of cases the condition may remain completely symptomless and be discovered only at autopsy.[30]

Renal hypoplasia

This is a term that must be strictly restricted to small kidneys which have less than the normal number of calices and nephrons, but are neither dysplastic nor have embryonic remnants within them. They have a uniformly narrow renal artery on arteriography, in contrast to the tapering vessels which are seen in acquired atrophy, for example secondary to pyelonephritis. When the hypoplasia is bilateral, failure to thrive, renal insufficiency or associated respiratory problems may be the mode of presentation, with the urine being of low specific gravity. Unilateral hypoplasia with contralateral hypertrophy, however, is a diagnosis which is usually made by chance, often on the basis of an investigation of another urological problem.

Anomalies of ascent

The kidney may be arrested either in the pelvis, the iliac fossa or in the abdominal cavity, or it may be ectopic as in a thoracic kidney. This must be differentiated from renal ptosis, where the kidney is initially located in the renal fossa but moves excessively in relation to its body position while retaining its normal vascularity. The ectopic kidney on the other hand has an ectopic blood supply. Associated anomalies of the internal or external genital organs are commonly present. The overall prognosis is good, the kidney generally being as susceptible to disease as a normally positioned kidney. There is a slight risk of the development of hydronephrosis and calculi in a pelvic or a malrotated kidney because the renal pelvis is more anteriorly placed. Thoracic kidneys have completed their rotation and have no predilection for specific renal diseases attributable to their position.

Crossed renal ectopias are present when the kidney is located on the side opposite to the side where the ureter enters the bladder. The possibilities are a bilaterally crossed renal ectopia or simple crossed ectopia with or without fusion to the ipsilateral kidney. Fusion is present in 90% of crossed ectopic kidneys. The metanephric blastema occasionally forms abnormal shapes during this process, producing a disc shaped, L shaped, or S shaped kidney with one moiety ureter draining to the contralateral side. The diagnosis is usually incidental and the prognosis is good, with normal longevity. Occasionally obstructed collecting systems of fused kidneys form calculi and develop repeated infections.[31]

Horseshoe kidney

This is the most common of all renal fusion anomalies and occurs in 1 in 400 of the population.[32] It is thought that in the embryo the fusion process occurs before the kidneys have rotated on their long axis, resulting in the ureter coming to lie ventral to the isthmus. The incomplete migration of the kidneys is thought to be caused by the inferior mesenteric artery preventing full ascent, producing lower lying kidneys. The fusion may be a bridge of fibrous tissue or renal parenchyma uniting the lower poles of the kidneys, usually at the level of the 3rd and 5th lumbar vertebrae. The calices are normal in number but abnormal in orientation. The ureter enters the bladder normally and is rarely ectopic, suggesting that the ureteric bud was normal when it entered the metanephric blastema and that fusion occurred thereafter in utero. The blood supply is extremely variable with branches coming from the inferior mesenteric, common external iliac or sacral arteries.

Clinical features

A third of patients remain entirely symptomless and the anomaly is only discovered at autopsy.[32] Urinary stasis with infections and calculi are more common in patients with horseshoe kidneys than in the general population. The incidence of tumours arising in horseshoe kidneys seems to be higher than that in the general population.[33] More than half of these are renal adenocarcinomas; the remaining half are either renal pelvic tumours (25%) or Wilms' tumours (25%). A surprisingly high number of these cancers appear to arise in the isthmus.[34] The diagnosis of a horseshoe kidney is made by finding an abdominal midline mass in a

REFERENCES

26. Mace J W Clin Paediatr 1972; 11: 98
27. Barry J E Am J Dis Child 1974; 128: 769
28. Nomura S Clin Nephrol 1990; 33: 7
29. McPherson R I Can Assoc Radiol J 1987; 38: 116
30. Carlson H E J Urol 1950; 64: 221
31. Boatman D L J Urol 1972; 108: 30
32. Glenn J F N Engl J Med 1959; 261: 684
33. Dische M R Urology 1979; 13: 435
34. Blackhard C E Arch Surg 1968; 97: 616

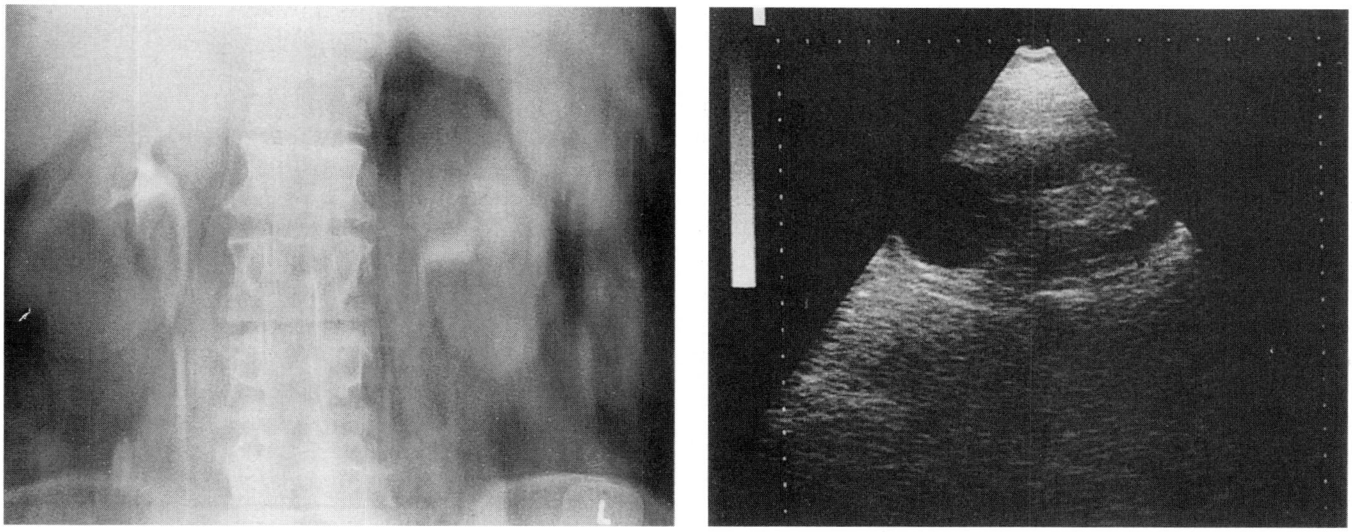

a b

Fig. 36.7 Right renal cyst. (**a**) Nephrotomogram showing a lucent filling defect at the lower pole of the right kidney caused by a simple renal cyst, confirmed on ultrasound (**b**).

symptomatic or symptomless patient. Horseshoe kidney may also be detected incidentally during other investigations. The classical features on urography are low lying kidneys with fusion of the lower poles. The axes of the kidneys converge in the midline inferiorly; the calices point directly posterior to each renal pelvis, the lowermost calix pointing caudally or even medially. The isthmus may contain functioning renal parenchyma. Horseshoe kidneys require no treatment unless complications develop; these should be treated as the condition merits. Horseshoe kidneys are occasionally a problem during aortic surgery when a retroperitoneal approach may make treatment easier.

Renal vascular anomalies

The normal kidney usually has one main renal artery which divides into two branches near the hilum; the anterior branch supplies the apical, upper, middle and lower segments while the posterior branch supplies the posterior segment. During development of the kidney the blood supply is received from a series of segmental vessels arising from the aorta and on occasions the segmental arrangement persists, giving rise to multiple renal arteries.[35] This segmental supply commonly persists in horseshoe and ectopic kidneys. The clinical importance of multiple vessels lies in their recognition during renal surgery and especially in transplantation. Arteriovenous fistulae are rarely congenital and are more commonly acquired from trauma, renal surgery or percutaneous procedures on the kidney. They often present with haematuria and a bruit can be heard in most patients.

Fetal lobulation

The normally smooth kidney is indented and lobulated. The only clinical significance is that it is occasionally difficult to differentiate this radiologically from pyelonephritic scarring (see Fig. 36.18).

Cystic diseases of the kidney

Cysts are the most common space-occupying masses in the kidney.[36] They may be solitary or multiple and almost all are benign. Degenerative cysts occur in half the population over the age of 70. The majority of cysts are symptomless and do not require treatment. Their importance lies in the differentiation between simple cysts, renal cell carcinomas and cysts caused by genetic disorders.

Most cysts are lined with cuboidal epithelium. There is no communication with the renal pelvis or calices. The cyst is filled with serous fluid and its expansion causes compression of the adjacent renal parenchyma. Haemorrhage into the cyst may occur spontaneously or may follow trauma. Cysts commonly occur bilaterally.

Clinical features

Most cysts are found incidentally during examination of the urinary tract for other reasons. Occasionally a cyst may present with pain, haematuria or as a symptomless palpable mass in the loin.

Investigations

The intravenous urogram shows distortion and flattening of the calices, and tomography may show a radiolucent area where the contrast is not taken up. The renal outline may also appear enlarged (Fig. 36.7a).

Ultrasound can determine the nature of a space-occupying lesion with a 97% degree of certainty[37] (Fig. 36.7b). Since 3% of symptomatic cysts contain a tumour, however, ultrasound should

REFERENCES

35. Gray S W, Skandlakis J E (eds) Embryology for Surgeons. Saunders, Philadelphia 1972
36. Barnet E, Morley P Br Med Bull 1972; 28: 196
37. Hately W, Whitaker R H Br J Urol 1973; 45: 468

be combined with cyst puncture and aspiration cytology if other imaging techniques such as CT and magnetic resonance fail to confirm a convincing benign appearance.[38]

Management

Most cysts do not require any treatment; if the cyst is large it can be aspirated. Cysts which continue to refill or in which haemorrhage occurs can be de-roofed by Rovsing's operation, in which the kidney is explored and the surface of the cyst excised.

Cystic diseases of the kidney as a consequence of genetic disorders

Polycystic renal disease

This condition is characterized by bilateral cystic changes affecting the whole of both kidneys (Fig. 36.8). Polycystic renal disease is subdivided into an infantile disorder confined to children and an adult condition. Infantile polycystic kidney is caused by an autosomal recessive gene; cystic changes occur in both the kidneys and liver.[39] It is associated with periportal fibrosis leading to portal hypertension and subsequent development of oesophageal varices. The onset of renal failure is rapid and, although attempts may be made to improve renal function, the development of progressive liver disease is usually fatal. In some cases renal transplantation extends life.

Adult polycystic renal disease is much more common and is caused by an autosomal dominant gene defect in the short arm of chromosome 16.[40] It is the third most common cause of end-stage renal failure[41]. Associated anomalies include cerebral berry aneurysms, mitral valve prolapse and cysts in other abdominal organs including the liver, pancreas and spleen. The condition generally presents in the third or fourth decade of life. Patients may develop renal failure, haematuria or ureteric colic associated with bleeding. Occasionally, bilateral symptomless loin masses are discovered at routine medical examination. There is usually a family history of renal failure or polycystic disease and therefore some cases are discovered as a result of genetic screening.

Investigations. An intravenous urogram shows evidence of multiple cysts. Ultrasound confirms large bilateral multicystic kidneys with a normal renal pelvis. Amniocentesis can be used nowadays in the diagnosis of intrauterine disease, and counselling for termination can be offered.

Management. This is now changing. Cases are increasingly diagnosed early, either by sonography or by genetic testing. Treatment is aimed at controlling hypertension, treating infections in the renal parenchyma and cysts, and monitoring for renal failure. It is now considered that the chance of developing renal failure is lower than was formerly thought, and is about 48% at the age of 73.[42] Surgery to the cysts is seldom indicated unless bleeding and loin pain are frequent. Rovsing's operation, in which the cysts are de-roofed in an attempt to preserve renal function, is preferred to sclerosing injections into the cysts, though initially percutaneous aspiration may be all that is necessary. Patients with this condition may be kept alive by dialysis but the definitive treatment is renal transplantation (see Chapter 8). This may be combined with bilateral nephrectomy if the renal masses are causing symptoms or preventing access for transplantation. Genetic counselling is generally advised because of the aetiology of the condition.

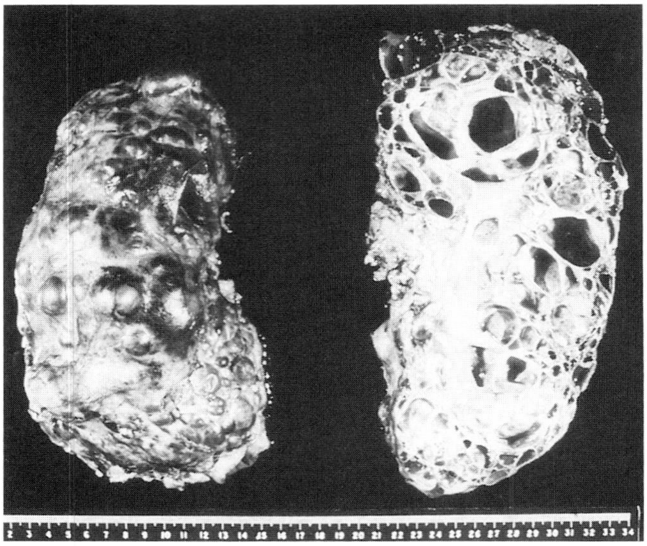

Fig. 36.8 Polycystic renal disease. Post-mortem specimen shows complete replacement of renal parenchyma by cysts. Courtesy of Dr J Piris.

Other genetic cystic diseases of the kidney

Multiple cortical cysts also occur in association with other congenital anomalies. They are associated with von Hippel–Lindau disease, which is usually fatal because of haemangioblastomas in the cerebellum and retina. Tuberose sclerosis is a condition associated with renal cysts or angiomyolipomas, cerebral hamartoma formation, mental retardation, epilepsy and adenoma sebaceum in the skin. Both von Hippel–Lindau disease and tuberose sclerosis are caused by an autosomal dominant gene.

The non-genetic cystic diseases of the kidney

Multicystic dysplastic kidney is seen in children as a renal lump which spontaneously disappears. Acquired renal cystic disease is seen in patients on dialysis. Medullary sponge kidney, multilocular cystic nephroma and simple cysts are the most common of all cystic diseases and are seen with greater frequency with increasing age.

REFERENCES

38. McClellan B L et al Am J Roentgenol 1979; 133: 671
39. Osethanondu B, Potter E L Arch Pathol (Chicago) 1964; 77: 459
40. Reeders S T Br Med J 1986a; 292: 851
41. Advisory Committee to the Renal Transplant Registry JAMA 1973; 226: 1197
42. Churchill D N Kidney Int 1984; 26: 190

Medullary sponge kidney

This condition results from cystic dilatation of the terminal collecting ducts as they cross the medulla. A characteristic pattern is seen on intravenous urography as the dilated ducts are invariably filled with small calculi which are secondary to stasis and sepsis in the ducts. Nephrectomy is rarely necessary. Most cases are symptomless, but occasionally calculi formed in association with the condition give rise to symptoms and require appropriate treatment.

Caliceal cysts

These are small cystic spaces adjoining the calices or renal pelvis. They may be found on routine urography. Intervention is only required if secondary stone formation occurs because of stasis and sepsis.

Multilocular cystic nephroma

This is a degenerative process occasionally containing a malignant element which may be difficult to differentiate from a nephroblastoma. Differentiation from Wilms' tumour may be difficult; the diagnosis is usually only made on histology.[43]

Hydatid cysts

This is parasitic infection with Echinococcus, an intestinal tapeworm of dogs, wolves and foxes. The liver is much more commonly affected (see Chapter 31); less than 2% of patients with hydatid disease develop a renal cyst.[44] The disease is endemic in South America, Africa, Australia and the Near East.

Pathology. Accidental ingestion of ova by humans results in penetration of the gastric mucosa by the larval form of the organism. It travels via the portal veins to the liver, thus accounting for the most frequent site of the disease. Systemic spread may then occur. The cyst may remain active when it increases in size, but if it aborts it calcifies.

Clinical features. Renal hydatid disease may be discovered during the investigation of the patient with suspected generalized hydatid disease. Otherwise it is an incidental finding on an intravenous urogram in a patient from an infected area. Rarely, acute rupture of a cyst produces an intense allergic reaction with pain and fever.

The intravenous urogram may show a space-occupying mass which can be confirmed on ultrasound to be cystic. Serological testing by immunofluorescence and immunoelectrophoresis is generally diagnostic, although cross-reactions with other antibodies have been noted. Serology must therefore not be taken as the sole diagnostic criterion.[45]

Management. Medical treatment of hydatid disease is unsatisfactory although alpha-mebendazole may provide some benefit.[46] Surgical removal of the cyst by partial nephrectomy is the best treatment. It is essential to avoid spillage of infected particles as this can produce generalized hydatid disease and a risk of severe anaphylactoid reactions. Therefore 2.5% solution of formalin, 0.5% solution of silver nitrate or hypertonic saline is injected into cyst cavities after partial aspiration prior to excision. Patients are often given a prolonged course of alpha-mebendazole postoperatively to prevent recurrence.

Abnormal mobility of the kidney (nephroptosis)

Abnormally mobile kidneys are well recognized and are frequently observed during intravenous urography or ultrasound examinations.[47] All kidneys are to some extent mobile, moving in a vertical or transverse direction in the extraperitoneal space. Some kidneys are, however, abnormally mobile because an extra investment of peritoneum produces a sort of pedicle. These are frequently referred to as 'floating' kidneys. Increased mobility is generally an incidental finding and renal pain should only be attributed to nephroptosis after careful exclusion of all other possible causes. Occasionally, the abnormal mobility causes a functional ureteropelvic junction obstruction because the kidney descends whilst the ureter remains relatively fixed to the posterior abdominal wall. This anatomical change may on occasions produce a demonstrable ureteropelvic junction obstruction; this should not necessarily be regarded as the primary cause of the obstruction as abnormalities of the ureteropelvic junction frequently coexist. Only very occasionally is it necessary to immobilize an abnormally mobile kidney by nephropexy using an open or laparoscopic approach. The patient must be warned that the operation may not alleviate all symptoms.

CONGENITAL ANOMALIES OF THE URETER

The embryology of the ureteric bud is complex. Detailed description of the embryology can be found elsewhere.[48] The anomalies can be classified into:

1. Anomalies of number—absence, duplication or triplication.
2. Anomalies of structure—atresia, megaureter, stenosis and diverticula.
3. Anomalies of position—retrocaval ureters and retroiliac ureters.
4. Anomalies of termination—vesicoureteric reflux, ectopic ureter and ureteroceles.

Megaureters and reflux disease are discussed in the section on upper urinary tract obstruction.

Ureteral agenesis

Bilateral ureteral agenesis, like bilateral renal agenesis, is incompatible with life, and a true unilateral agenesis is associated with an

REFERENCES

43. Gonzalez-Crussi F et al Urology 1982; 55: 244
44. Borrell J H, Brahms J N N Y J Med 1933; 33: 139
45. Kagan I G et al J Trop Med Hyg 1966; 15: 172
46. Bryceson A D M et al Trans R Soc Trop Med Hyg 1982; 76: 510
47. Patel A S, Barber Riley W P Br J Radiol 1982; 20: 88
48. Tanagho E A Urology 1976; 7: 451

absent kidney on that side because of a failure of induction of the ipsilateral metanephric blastema. The presence of a hemitrigone on cystoscopy is almost diagnostic of a unilateral renal and ureteric agenesis but is also compatible with a single system ectopic ureter draining a normal kidney.

Ureteric duplication

This is the most common ureteric anomaly and is usually an incidental finding. Stasis with obstruction and reflux is more common in a patient with duplication, and there is a higher incidence of duplication in patients with recurrent urinary infections. The overall incidence of ureteric duplication is less than 1%[49] and the condition is most likely to be unilateral. Renal hypoplasia, dysplasia and vesicoureteric reflux are all associated with ureteric duplication. Many forms of ureteric duplication exist. The most common is an incomplete ureteric duplication with a Y junction in the ureter which may result in 'yo-yo' reflux between the two moieties causing stasis, ureteric dilatation and consequent infection. The diagnosis is usually made on intravenous urography (Fig. 36.9).

At the other extreme is complete ureteric duplication, which is invariably associated with vesicoureteric reflux. It is usually the lower pole ureter which refluxes because of the short mucosal tunnel within the bladder wall (Meyer–Weigert's law).[50,51] The upper pole ureter drains distally and medially and thus has a long submucosal course. Occasionally, the insertion of the upper pole ureter into the bladder is ectopic and is situated at the bladder neck or urethra. In females this is a rare cause of urinary incontinence if the ectopic opening is beyond the sphincter or in the vagina.[52]

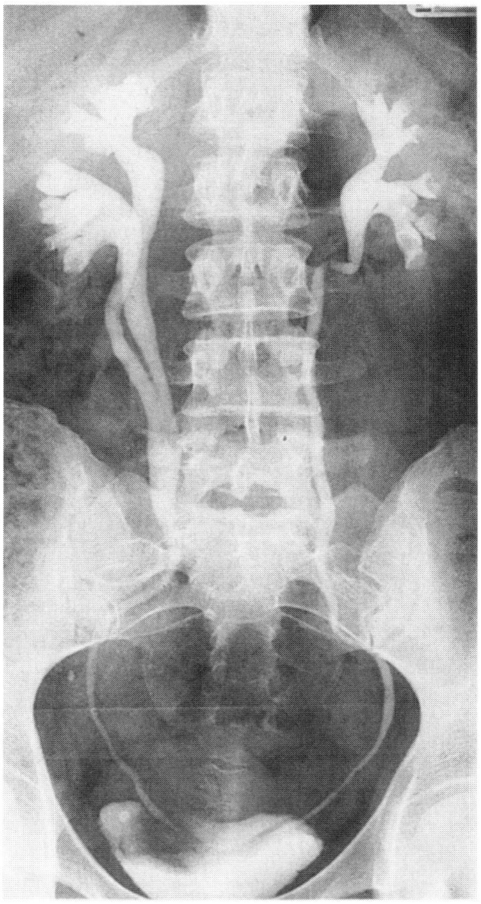

Fig. 36.9 Intravenous urogram film showing duplex right kidney and ureters which fuse at the level of the pelvic brim. Minor clubbing of the right upper pole calices is also apparent due to yo-yo reflux. Courtesy of Dr J Reid.

Clinical features

Most patients are diagnosed in childhood when they present with recurrent urinary infections. Intravenous urography shows duplication of the collecting system. A micturating cystourethrogram confirms the presence of reflux (Fig. 36.32).

Management

The management of refluxing duplex ureters in children follows the same principles as the management of reflux in single ureters.[53] The management of the condition in the adult is discussed in the section on megaureter.

Ureteric triplication

Only 61 cases of this rare condition have been described.[54] It is probably the result of three ureteric buds arising from the mesonephric duct. Patients present with urinary infections, loin pain or incontinence, and treatment varies according to the symptoms.

Ureteric atresia

This is associated with multicystic kidney in the infant. The spectrum of abnormal embryogenesis varies from a dimple seen at the ureteric orifice on cystoscopy, a blind ending ureteric stalk or a hypoplastic ureter.

Ureteric diverticulum

This can be either a true diverticulum containing all layers of the ureteric wall or an aborted blind ending ureteric duplication. Acquired diverticula are mucosal herniations caused by trauma during ureteroscopy. Blind ending duplications are generally seen in the mid or distal third of the ureter and the condition is more common in females.[55] It is an extremely rare cause of urinary infection or pain; local excision or uretero-ureterostomy is the treatment of choice.

REFERENCES

49. Campbell M E (ed) Urology. Saunders, Philadelphia 1963
50. Meyer R Virch Arch Pathol Anat Physio Klin Med 1907; 187: 408
51. Weigert C Virch Arch Pathol Anat Physio Klin Med 1877; 170: 490
52. Leadbetter G W Jr J Urol 1970; 103: 222
53. Scott J E S Br J Urol 1977; 49: 109
54. Perkins P J et al Radiology 1973; 108: 533
55. Albers D D et al J Urol 1971; 105: 634

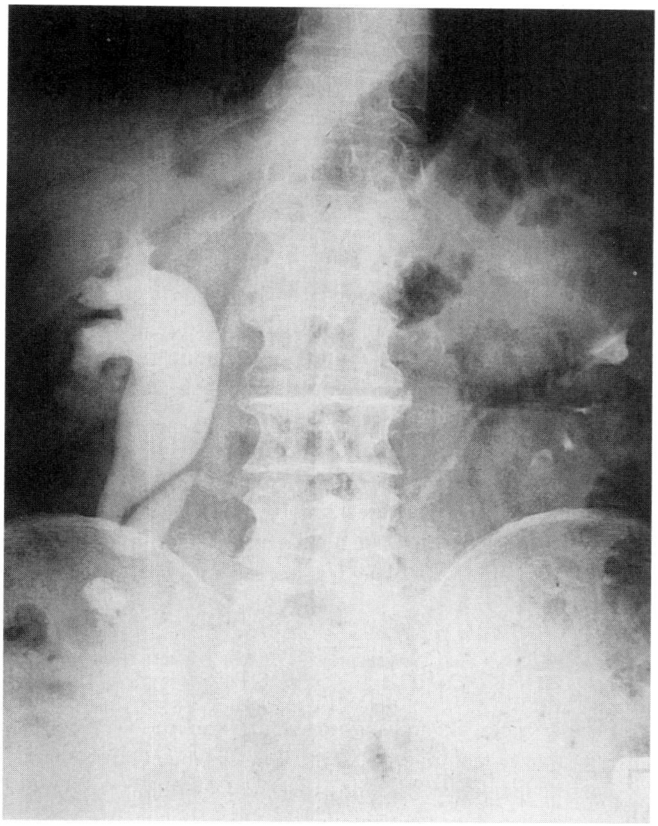

Fig. 36.10 Retrocaval ureter.

Retrocaval ureter and retroiliac ureter

Persistence of the posterior cardinal vein to form the inferior vena cava below the level of the renal vein results in the ureter passing behind the vena cava before running distally. The finding of a retrocaval ureter is often incidental but occasionally it causes loin pain and tenderness. The reverse J pattern on intravenous urography is characteristic (Fig. 36.10). A retroiliac ureter may be seen as the result of persistence of the ventral root of the umbilical artery and this can cause obstruction of the ureter at L5–S1.

Ureteric stenosis

The histological picture of ureteric stenosis is one with normal transitional epithelium but a decrease in the population of apparently normal smooth muscle cells because of defective mesenchymal development.[56] The sites of this type of stenosis, in increasing order of frequency, are: the pelvic brim, the pelviureteric junction and the vesicoureteric junction.

Ectopic ureter

This is a ureter which does not open at its normal location on the trigone. It may be a part of a duplex system or may be a single ectopic ureter. The orifice may be found at any number of possible sites. The condition is 10 times more common in females, and 20% of ectopic ureters are bilateral.[57] It is commonly associated with hypoplasia or dysplasia of renal tissue.

Clinical features

If the opening of the ectopic ureter is below the distal sphincter mechanism of the urethra, the condition is associated with complete urinary incontinence (see Chapter 37). In the male it is invariably suprasphincteric. When the opening is intrasphincteric, the ectopia is associated with upper tract obstruction, and reflux may also occur. One third of ectopic ureters in the female open into the vagina.[58] An ectopic ureter should be suspected in young female patients with otherwise unexplained permanent urinary incontinence. There may be evidence of an obstructed duplex ureter on the intravenous urogram, but frequently the diagnosis is difficult. The upper pole of the kidney may not be evident and the condition is often diagnosed only by the absence of the correct number of calices, the 'drooping lily' sign, although the ureterocele may also be diagnosed by ultrasound.[59] Careful examination under anaesthesia, together with cystoscopy and attempted catheterization of suspect ureteric openings, may also be required to confirm the diagnosis. Voiding cystourethrograms are also necessary to demonstrate vesicoureteric reflux.

In the male, an ectopic ureter may drain into the epididymis, seminal vesicles, vas deferens or posterior urethra. Epididymitis may occur; this anomaly accounts for virtually all cases of prepubertal epididymitis.[60] The diagnosis is extremely difficult, requiring a combination of intravenous urography, ultrasound and cystoscopy.

Management

The type of surgical correction depends upon the amount of renal function remaining in the affected kidney. Upper pole partial nephroureterectomy is frequently required although a ureteropyelostomy or a uretero-ureterostomy may be performed if the function of the upper pole is good.[61]

Ureterocele

This is a cystic dilatation of the intravesical submucosal ureter. It is commonly seen in the ureter draining an upper pole moiety in patients with complete ureteric duplication. The size of the ureterocele varies and it may open into the bladder or be ectopic (Fig. 36.11). The wall of the ureterocele generally contains patchy muscle and collagen. Ureteroceles are more common in women and when present are bilateral in 10–15% of cases.[62] They have been discovered in 1 in 500 autopsies. Duplication of the ureter

REFERENCES

56. Cussen L J Aust NZ J Surg 1971; 41: 185
57. Malek R S et al J Urol 1972; 107: 308
58. Shulman C C Eur Urol 1976; 2: 64
59. Sumner T E, Crowe J E, Resnick M I Urology 1980; 15: 82
60. Seitzman D M, Patton J F J Urol 1960; 54: 604
61. Johnston J H Br J Urol 1969; 41: 61
62. Mandell J et al J Urol 1980; 123: 921

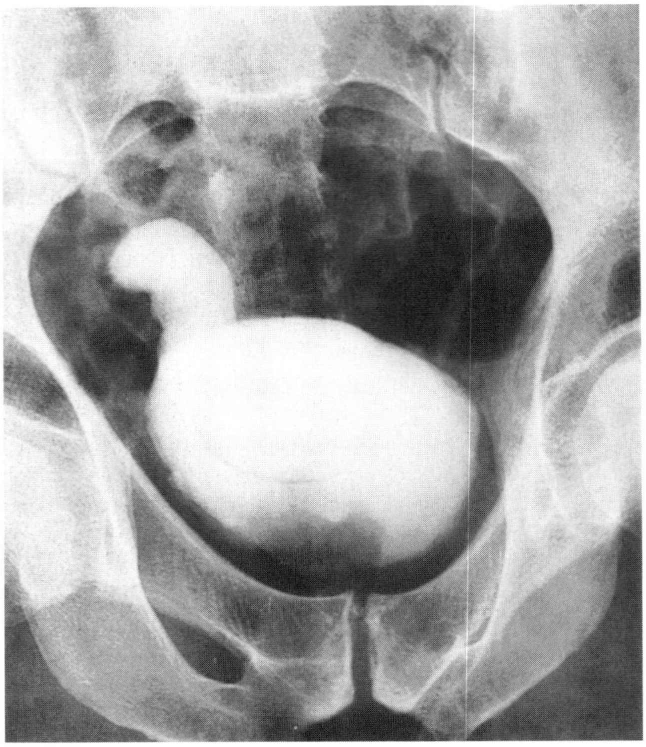

Fig. 36.11 Ureterocele. Intravenous urogram film showing a filling defect in the bladder caused by a ureterocele and surrounding halo appearance. Courtesy of Dr J Reid.

occurs in three quarters of the patients, with an ectopic ureterocele being more common.[63] Other congenital anomalies of the urinary tract are often seen in association with a ureterocele. Many ureteroceles in adults are incidental findings and, provided they are symptomless, do not require treatment.[64]

The management of ureteroceles in children is highly complex, depending upon the presence of symptoms, associated infection, the anatomy and other urinary tract anomalies and the amount of functioning renal tissue.[65] If the ureterocele is small and well supported, an incision in the lower lip of the ureteric meatus may relieve obstruction while leaving a flap of mucosa which may prevent reflux.[64] Endoscopic management usually however causes reflux which then requires correction by ureteric reimplantation.[66] Further discussion of the management can be found elsewhere.[67]

INJURIES TO THE KIDNEY AND URETER

Renal injuries occur in approximately 10% of all patients with blunt or penetrating abdominal trauma.[68] Renal injuries can be classified as Type I (minor contusion), Type II (minor parenchymal laceration without collecting system involvement), Type III (major laceration with collecting system involvement) and Type IV (renal pedicle injuries).

Penetrating wounds of the kidney

Penetrating wounds of the kidney are caused by gunshot or stab wounds and in both instances there is a high incidence of associated intra-abdominal injuries.[69] Penetrating wounds can also be iatrogenic as the result of percutaneous renal biopsy or percutaneous renal surgery. In all cases of penetrating renal trauma[70] the development of arteriovenous fistulae may be a late sequel.

Clinical features

The history and clinical examination should make the diagnosis self-evident. Hypovolaemic shock and the high incidence of associated injuries make exploration of any appropriately sited flank wound essential after appropriate resuscitation. A contrast enhanced CT scan provides the most information if the patient is haemodynamically stable. When CT is not available intravenous urogram and/or ultrasound must be performed to assess the extent of injury and to confirm that the other kidney is present and functioning normally. Renal arteriography may be useful, as both a diagnostic and therapeutic technique, if vascular injury is suspected. It also has the advantage of defining other visceral arterial lesions, especially if a coeliac axis angiogram is performed at the same time.

Blunt renal trauma

Road traffic accidents and sporting injuries are the most common causes of blunt renal trauma and the injury is much more common in young male adults. It should be remembered that the opposite kidney is either abnormal or absent in 3% of patients presenting with blunt renal trauma, and that abnormal kidneys are more prone to injury than normal kidneys.[71,72] Associated injuries are seen less commonly than after penetrating injuries but the incidence still approaches 50%.[73]

Clinical features

Renal injury should be suspected in all patients with gross or microscopic haematuria after road traffic accidents or sporting injuries. Adults with blunt trauma, microscopic haematuria and normotension can safely be observed without the need for radiological imaging,[74] however all children with either gross or microscopic haematuria require imaging.[75] At the other extreme there may be evidence of loin pain, tenderness, obvious bruising and

REFERENCES

63. Erocsspm M P Acta Chir Scan 1954; 197: suppl.1
64. Hutch J A, Chisholm E R J Urol 1966; 96: 445
65. Hendren W J, Monfort G J J Paediat Surg 1971; 6: 235
66. Snyder H M, Johnston J H J Urol 1978; 119: 543
67. Lelalis P P In: Kelalis B P (ed) Clinical Paediatric Urology. Saunders, Philadelphia 1976
68. McAninch J.W In: Gillenwater J Y (ed) Adult and Paediatric Urology. Mosby, St. Louis 1991 pp 475–489
69. Carlton C E In: Campbell M F, Harrison J H (eds) Urology. Saunders, Philadelphia 1978
70. Ahoniemi P J et al U Irol 1973; 110: 625
71. Slade N In: Blandy J P (ed) Urology. Blackwell, London 1976
72. Pryor J P, Williams J P Br J Urol 1975; 47: 45
73. Peters P C, Bright T C Urol Clin North Am 1977; 4: 17
74. McAndrew J D Br J Urol 1994; 73: 352
75. Stein J P Urology 1994; 44: 406

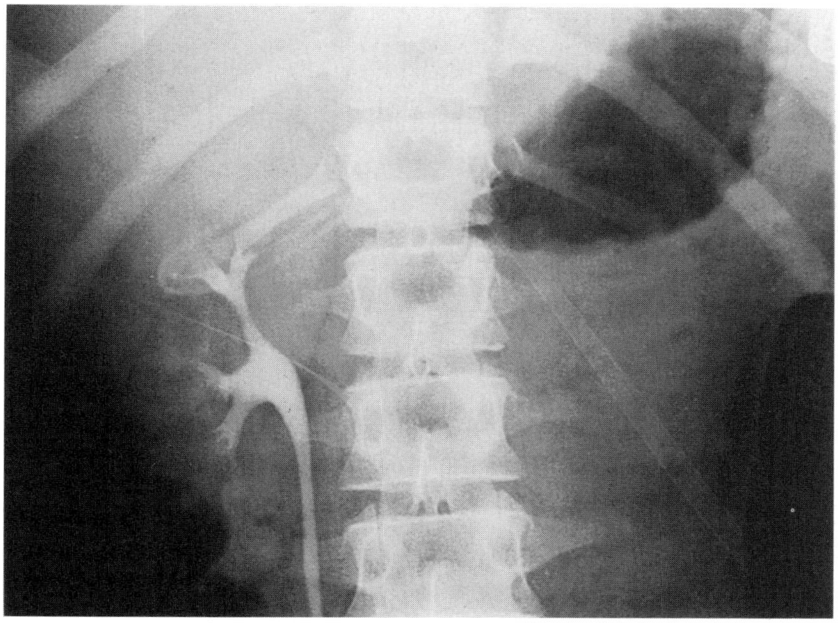

a

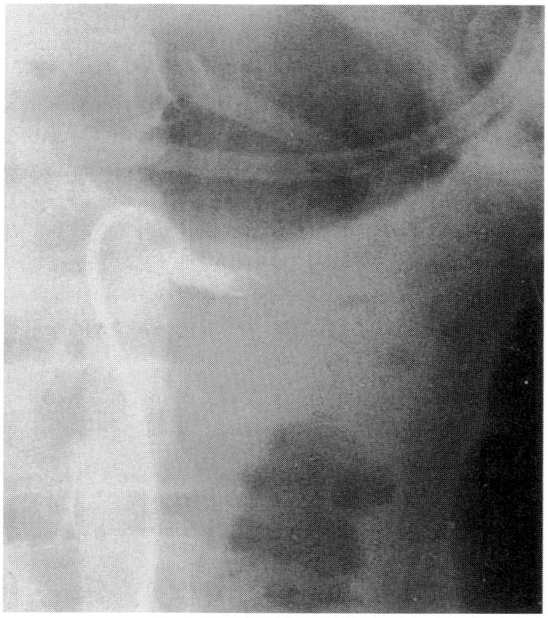

b

Fig. 36.12 Renal trauma. (**a**) The intravenous urogram shows non-functioning left kidney due to complete avulsion of the renal artery, demonstrated on angiography (**b**).

swelling in the flank associated with profound hypotension. Occasionally, the presence of severe shock in the absence of any other clinical sign may be the only feature of renal trauma. There may also be signs of a thoracic injury.[76] A number of features of renal trauma may be observed on a preliminary plain abdominal radiograph:

1. Absence of the psoas shadow.
2. An enlarged kidney.
3. Fractured 10th, 11th or 12th ribs.
4. Fractured transverse processes of first, second and third lumbar vertebrae.
5. Scoliosis to the injured side.

In the event of a non-functioning or grossly distorted kidney, acute renal angiography may be useful in defining the extent of the injury (Fig. 36.12). Arteriography should be reserved for patients in whom a pedicle injury is suspected as intra-arterial contrast medium is potentially nephrotoxic in shocked patients.[77] The inevitable delay in obtaining a renal angiogram exceeds the viability time of an ischaemic kidney following a pedicle injury and therefore the investigation is of limited value.[78] If the patient is too unstable for any form of imaging then contrast is injected for a 'one-shot' intravenous urogram and a single radiograph is taken at 20 minutes. This may provide useful information on the contralateral kidney and on the extent of renal injury which may otherwise not be appreciated.

Management

After accurate classification of the type of renal injury a logical treatment strategy can be formulated. Type I and II injuries should be managed conservatively with bed rest until the gross haematuria settles. Prophylactic antibiotics are not necessary and should only be prescribed in the event of a high fever and raised white cell count.

In patients in whom there is a laceration of the renal parenchyma with a breach of the capsule (Type II), perirenal extravasation will inevitably occur, and in such patients prophylactic antibiotics must be given. Most patients with Type IV injuries need surgical exploration. The correct management of closed Type III injuries is still debated: complication rates in expectantly managed patients were no different from those in an operated group.[79] Percutaneous drainage of a urinoma caused by leakage of urine through a tear in the pelvicaliceal system[80] may be occasionally needed but open operative repair of the collecting system is rarely necessary.

The kidney is best explored via the transabdominal route if open exploration is necessary. A careful search must be made for any associated injuries. The kidney should then be examined. There is frequently a large retroperitoneal haematoma and the kidney should only be explored when the renal pedicle has been controlled. The renal vessels are found by incising the peritoneum of the posterior abdominal wall. Nephrectomy is frequently necessary in the case of high-velocity missile wounds, but it is often possible to conserve part of the kidney after stab injuries.[81] Before carrying out a nephrectomy the other kidney should be carefully

REFERENCES

76. Kauffman J J, Brosman S A Surg Clin North Am 1972; 52: 747
77. Guerriero W G Urol Clin North Am 1977; 4: 3
78. Mitchell J P Br Med J 1971; 1: 567
79. Husmann D A J Urol 1993; 150: 1774
80. Arnold E P Br J Urol 1972; 44: 40
81. Marks L S, Rosman S A Urology 1974; 3: 18

palpated. When damage to the renal pedicle occurs, nephrectomy is generally necessary although there are reports of successful conservative operations for renal injury.[82]

Bleeding from iatrogenic penetrating renal injuries can generally be controlled by embolization of the bleeding vessel after identification by renal angiography.[83] In patients with a minor or moderate degree of renal injury and perirenal haematoma, serial ultrasound scans help to determine whether or not the haematoma is expanding.

It must be recognized that late complications of blunt renal trauma may develop in patients who have sustained major lacerations or damage to the renal blood vessels. Hypertension caused by ischaemia, renal artery stenosis or perirenal constriction from capsular fibrosis is the most serious late sequel. Surgery is seldom indicated as this hypertension is transient in most patients.[84] Perirenal fibrosis may also cause ureteropelvic junction obstruction. Under these circumstances reconstructive surgery is often difficult, and ureterolysis[85] or a Davis intubated ureterotomy may be necessary.[86]

Ureteric injuries

Ureteric injuries are occasionally the result of gunshot wounds or stabbing but are most commonly iatrogenic, occurring during the course of ureteroscopy, intra-abdominal open or laparoscopic surgery. Ureteric injuries may particularly occur during resection of the large bowel, during aortic aneurysm surgery and during hysterectomy.[87] The advent of endourological techniques for stone surgery has undoubtedly resulted in a higher incidence of 'urological' ureteric injuries (see below). In most cases the iatrogenic ureteric injury is associated with surgery that is particularly difficult, such as hysterectomy for severe pelvic inflammatory disease or endometriosis, a large bulky fibroid uterus or an ovarian tumour.[88] Interference with the ureteric blood supply during a Wertheim hysterectomy or during pelvic surgery following previous pelvic irradiation may result in an ischaemic and subsequently necrotic ureter.[88] Extensive rectal tumours or the presence of severe diverticular disease or Crohn's disease cause loss of normal tissue planes and the consequence is a higher risk of ureteric injury.

Clinical features

A high index of suspicion is necessary if ureteric injuries are to be correctly diagnosed in penetrating or blunt abdominal trauma. An intravenous urogram may not identify the injury and indeed in a recent study[89] preoperative urograms were unhelpful in 11 of 12 cases of ureteric injury associated with penetrating trauma. Ureteric injury associated with blunt trauma is rare but is occasionally seen in children in the form of ureteropelvic disruption.

An iatrogenic injury may be self-evident. Unrecognized division of the ureter results in a urinary fistula which may drain through the vagina or the wound. Leakage into the peritoneal cavity can cause peritonitis, or may result in a urinoma. Accidental ligation of the ureter may be symptomless or may result in transient loin pain which may be followed by a ureteric fistula if the ureter becomes necrotic.

Treatment

Treatment depends upon when the injury is recognized. It is also dictated by the mechanism of the injury, the location of the injury and the length of the devitalized segment of the ureter.

Early recognition

Immediate repair is appropriate if it is recognized that the ureter has been divided or ligated at the time of operation. The ureter should be dissected for several centimetres above and below the suspected point of injury; if it is found to be divided an oblique anastomosis is made over a ureteric splint (JJ silicone stent) using interrupted fine chromic catgut or polyglycolic acid. The use of an indwelling ureteric stent is preferable to the use of a T tube as drainage is more reliable and there are fewer problems of postoperative leakage. The anastomosis is drained with a tube drain and the ureteric stent is removed cystoscopically after 4 weeks. The drain is removed after 4 or 5 days when it stops draining urine. If there has been high velocity injury it is prudent to leave a ureteric stent in situ for a couple of weeks or more even if the ureter appears intact and is only contused.

It is usually necessary to reimplant the ureter if a low ureteric injury is found. It is best to mobilize the lower end of the ureter and reimplant it using a Leadbetter–Politano non-refluxing technique (see below) into the posterolateral wall of the bladder.[90] Occasionally, however, the remaining ureter is too short to be reimplanted into the bladder without tension. It is then necessary to mobilize the bladder on the contralateral side and suture the apex of the bladder to the psoas muscle on the side of the injury (the psoas hitch procedure). The ureter is then brought through an opening in the posterior wall of the bladder, through a submucosal tunnel, and anastomosed to the bladder mucosa with interrupted fine chromic catgut sutures (Fig. 36.13). Sometimes it is impossible to mobilize the bladder sufficiently to allow this procedure to be carried out; in such cases a flap is mobilized and sutured into a tube which is then joined to the lower end of the ureter over a splint. The disadvantage of this technique is that it allows ureterovesical reflux to occur (Fig. 36.14).

In patients in whom there has been previous irradiation or pelvic surgery resulting in a small contracted bladder, or when the vascularity of the tissues makes re-anastomosis unlikely to succeed, mobilization of the ureter above the level of the pelvic brim allows it to be transposed to the contralateral side and then anastomosed end-to-side into the opposite ureter (trans ureteroureterostomy) outside the field of previous surgery or irradiation

REFERENCES

82. Skinner D G Ann Surg 1973; 177: 264
83. Del Villar R G, Ireland G W, Cass A S J Urol 1972; 107: 208
84. Jameson R M Br J Urol 1973; 45: 482
85. Thompson I M Urol Clin North Am 1977; 4: 45
86. Davis D M Surg Gynecol Obstet 1943; 76: 513
87. Macasaet M A et al Am J Obstet Gynecol 1976; 124: 757
88. Godwin W E, Scardino P T J Urol 1980; 123: 370
89. Brandes D B J Trauma 1994; 36: 766
90. Politano V A, Leadbetter W F J Urol 1958; 79: 932

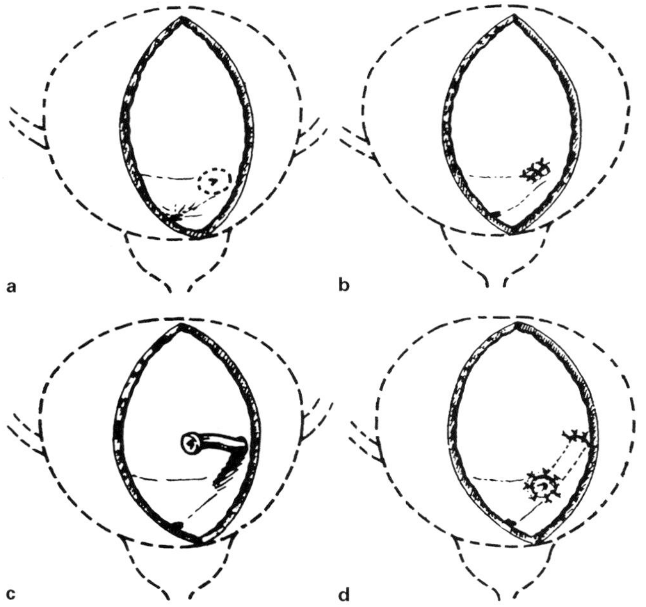

Fig. 36.13 Leadbetter–Politano reimplantation of the ureter. **(a)** The ureteric orifice is circumcised. **(b)** The defect in the bladder wall is closed. **(c)** The ureter is grasped from within the bladder. **(d)** A new submucosal tunnel is created and the ureter is sutured down to its original site.

(Fig. 36.15). This anastomosis is protected with a ureteric stent which can be removed after 4–6 weeks.

Late recognition

Many ureteric injuries present at varying times after operation. If they are recognized within 24 hours of surgery it is usually preferable to re-operate, carrying out any of the reconstructive options listed above, provided that the patient's condition permits. It is impossible to generalize about the correct timing of repair of ureteric injuries as this depends upon the underlying condition and the skill of the surgeon, but with modern surgical techniques, the use of stents and newer surgical materials, ureteric fistulae should be repaired much earlier than has been previously taught.[91] This is particularly true in the case of patients with a ligated ureter where a delay of more than 2 weeks can result in considerable loss of renal function. Patients in whom the fistula develops more than 48 hours after surgery should have an intravenous urogram followed by a cystoscopy and descending ureterogram to delineate the exact site of the injury.[92] In such cases it is worthwhile attempting to bridge the fistula with a silicone ureteric stent inserted under fluoroscopic control or under direct vision by a ureteroscope. Occasionally, the fistula may heal but generally it is necessary to carry out a formal re-anastomosis. Ureteric strictures from ischaemia following ureteroscopic surgery may be treated by endoscopic incision or by balloon dilatation.[93] Occasionally, when a fistula develops after pelvic radiotherapy in a patient who is unfit for surgery, symptomatic relief may be obtained by percutaneous transcatheter embolization of the affected kidney—'radiologist's nephrectomy'.[94] Rarely, ileal conduit urinary diversion may be the only available option in a case of massive post-irradiation fistula.[91]

INFECTIONS OF THE KIDNEY

Acute bacteriological infection of the kidney results in a number of pathological processes ranging from acute pyelonephritis to perinephric abscess. With appropriate treatment, all forms of acute infection should resolve completely leaving little evidence of renal damage. This is in marked contrast to the development of chronic pyelonephritis (a term used to refer to a variety of conditions including interstitial nephritis, reflux nephropathy, chronic atrophic pyelonephritis and focal coarse renal scarring).[95]

REFERENCES

91. Flynn J, Blandy J P Br J Urol 1979; 51: 454
92. O'Brien T et al J Urol 1988; 140: 28
93. McLean G K, Meranze S G Urol Clin North Am 1985; 12: 743
94. Brin E N, Schiff M, Weiss R M J Urol 1975; 1133: 619
95. Bailey P R Clin Nephrol 1973; 1: 32

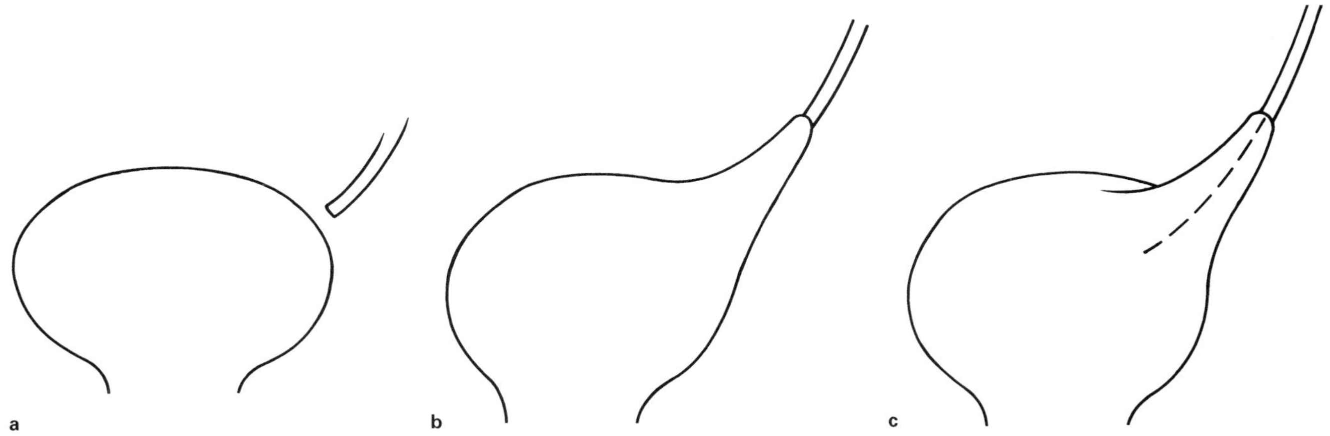

Fig. 36.14 **(a)** The injured ureter is too short to reimplant into the bladder. **(b)** The bladder is mobilized. **(c)** A Boari flap is formed to create a tube on to which the ureter may be anastomosed.

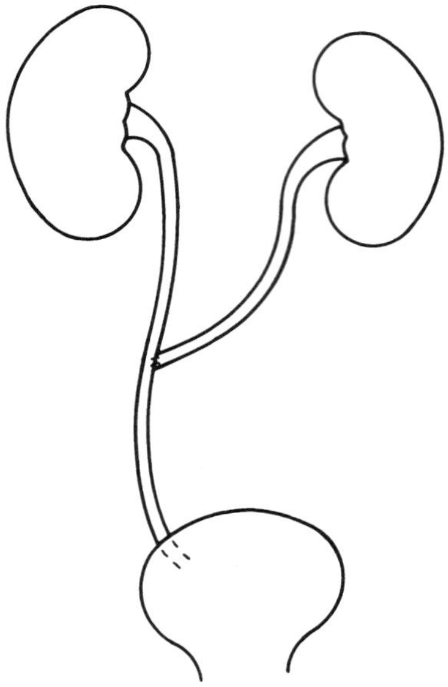

Fig. 36.15 The ureter may be anastomosed end-to-side into the contralateral uninjured ureter.

Acute infection

Bacterial-induced inflammation of the renal pelvis, calices and parenchyma may affect the kidney diffusely or in a patchy fashion (Fig. 36.16). Acute suppurative inflammation is found in the pelvis, calices and other parts of the kidney. This takes the form of pale linear streaks bordered by a red rim of congestion extending from the tips of the papillae to the surface of the cortex in a radial direction. Microscopically the appearances are those of an acute inflammatory reaction with focal tubular destruction but sparing of the glomeruli.[96] In advanced cases the inflammatory lesions fuse to produce extensive cortical abscesses or renal carbuncles. If the outflow of the kidney is obstructed, a pyonephrosis will develop and if left untreated may discharge into the surrounding perirenal tissues producing a perinephric abscess.

Clinical features

In practice it is difficult to differentiate the various forms of acute bacterial infection of the kidney on clinical grounds alone. Patients are systemically ill with pyrexia, tachycardia, loin pain, dysuria and tenderness. There may be a tender, palpable mass in patients with pyonephroses, or a discharging sinus or abscess in the loin in the patient with perinephric abscesses. Occasionally, there are signs of bacteraemic shock.

Investigations

Polymorphonuclear leucocytosis is usual but renal function is rarely compromised. The urine culture is often sterile when the infecting organism is Staphylococcus but in the presence of Gram-negative organisms the urine culture is usually positive. An intravenous urogram may show an absent psoas shadow, the renal shadow may be obscured and a renal calculus may be seen. The kidney is often enlarged in acute pyelonephritis and there may be absence of contrast excretion in acute pyonephrosis. Nephrotomography may indicate space-occupying lesions when there is a focal bacterial nephritis or a renal carbuncle.

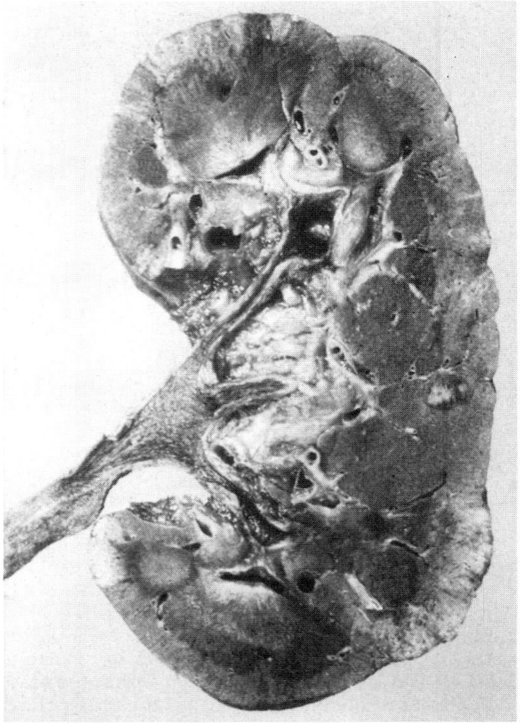

Fig. 36.16 Acute pyelonephritis. (Courtesy of Dr K M Grigor.)

Ultrasound examination is invaluable in clarifying the differential diagnosis of acute infection of the kidney.[97] Renal carbuncles and perinephric abscess are both easily demonstrated by this technique, and the appearance of a mass within the parenchyma with an ill defined margin suggests acute bacterial nephritis (Fig. 36.17).

Management

Acute pyelonephritis. Patients should be given intravenous fluids and parenteral antibodies, e.g. cephalosporins or aminoglycosides, for 72 hours and then treated with appropriate oral antibiotics for 2 weeks.[98] If the pyelonephritis is secondary to a stone, the stone should be extracted once the acute inflammation has resolved.

Renal carbuncle. This can be drained under ultrasound control.[99] Pus is sent for culture and the patient is treated with high doses of parenteral antibiotics.

Pyonephrosis. The management of this condition is urgent as the presence of pus in an obstructed collecting system produces

REFERENCES

96. Levison D In: Whitfield H N, Hendry W F (eds) Genitourinary Surgery. Churchill Livingstone, Edinburgh 1987
97. Edell S C, Bonavista J A Radiology 1979; 132: 683
98. Brumfitt W, Ascher A W Urinary Tract Infection. Oxford University Press, London 1973
99. Lamont A C, Fletcher E W L Clin Radiol 1981; 32: 421

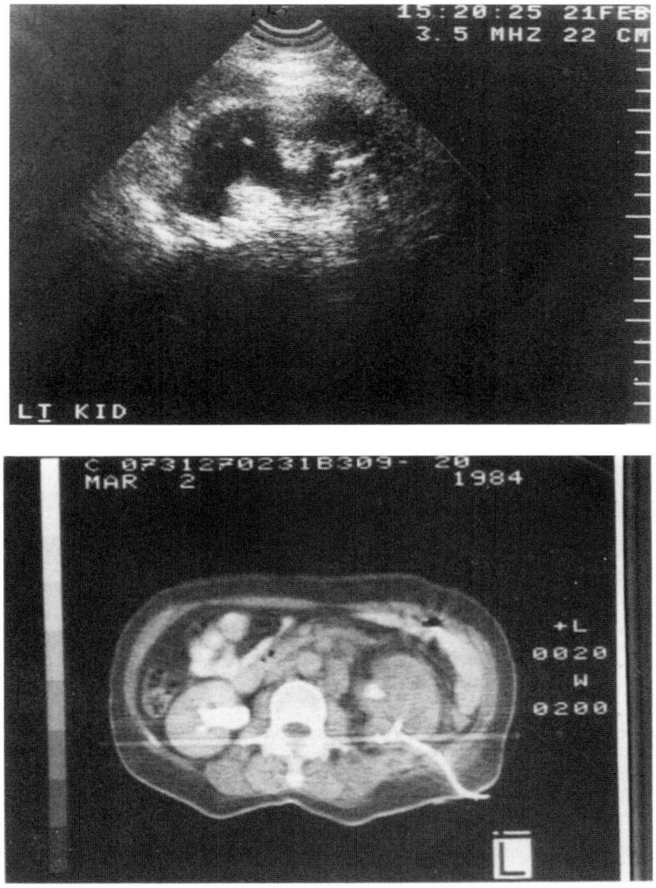

a

b

Fig. 36.17 (**a**) Renal carbuncle demonstrated on ultrasound. The kidney also contains a renal stone. (**b**) The abscess has been drained percutaneously and the computerized tomography scan shows a drain in situ.

rapid, irreversible parenchymal damage. A perinephric abscess and bacteraemia may also ensue if treatment is delayed. Relief of the obstruction is the primary objective of treatment: this can be achieved most satisfactorily by insertion of a percutaneous nephrostomy under local anaesthesia.[100] Formal nephrostomy drainage will be required if this is not feasible. Appropriate antibiotics are given; surgery to correct the primary pathology is carried out once the acute condition has resolved.

Perinephric abscess. Parenteral antibiotics are given and the abscess is incised and drained. As the condition is frequently associated with renal stones, a nephrectomy is often necessary once the abscess has resolved, if the residual renal function is poor.

Chronic pyelonephritis

The kidney is small and contracted, showing patchy and irregular scars. The kidneys are generally of different sizes and unequally affected.[101] This is in contrast to the smooth shrunken kidney of chronic glomerulonephritis. The scars radiate radially from the papillae producing retraction of the calices which results in the characteristic appearance of dilatation. The scar extends to the capsule, producing overlying surface depressions and thinning of

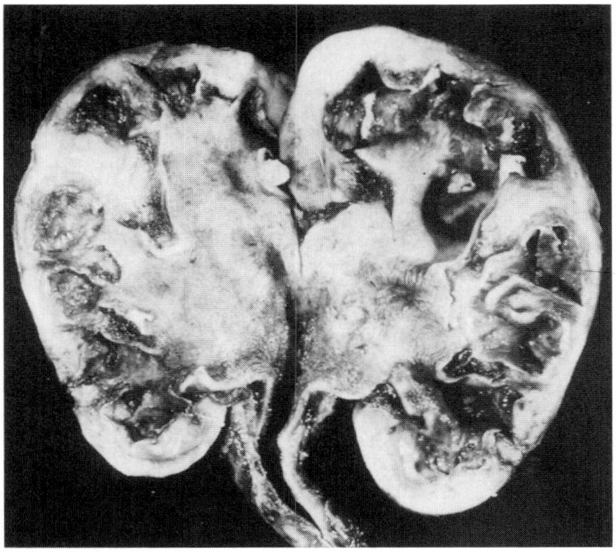

Fig. 36.18 Chronic pyelonephritis. Courtesy of Dr J Piris.

the cortex. The parenchyma between the scarred areas may appear normal. There is generally thickening of the pelvis and caliceal walls (Fig. 36.18). There is a chronic inflammatory infiltrate with granulation tissue and fibrosis in patients in whom the inflammation is still active. As the inflammatory process becomes less active the number of inflammatory cells reduces. There is a striking loss of tubules with interstitial fibrosis and, as with acute pylonephritis, the glomeruli are often well preserved. There may also be evidence of periglomerulofibrosis and ischaemia.[102]

Clinical features

Some patients present with end-stage renal failure but in the majority there is a long history of recurrent urinary infections and loin pain, sometimes associated with a history of hypertension. On examination there are often no abnormalities to be found other than a raised blood pressure.

Investigations

On intravenous urography the kidney usually appears small and scarred. It may be impossible to differentiate these appearances from congenital hypoplasia (Fig. 36.19). Ultrasound examination also shows a small contracted kidney (Fig. 36.20).

Management

In patients in whom urinary infections are frequent, low-dose prophylactic antibiotics are generally sufficient to control the

REFERENCES

100. Barbaric A L Radiol Clin North Am 1979; 17: 413
101. Smellie J M et al Arch Dis Child 1981; 56: 593
102. Heptonstall R H Pathology of the Kidney. Little Brown, Boston 1974

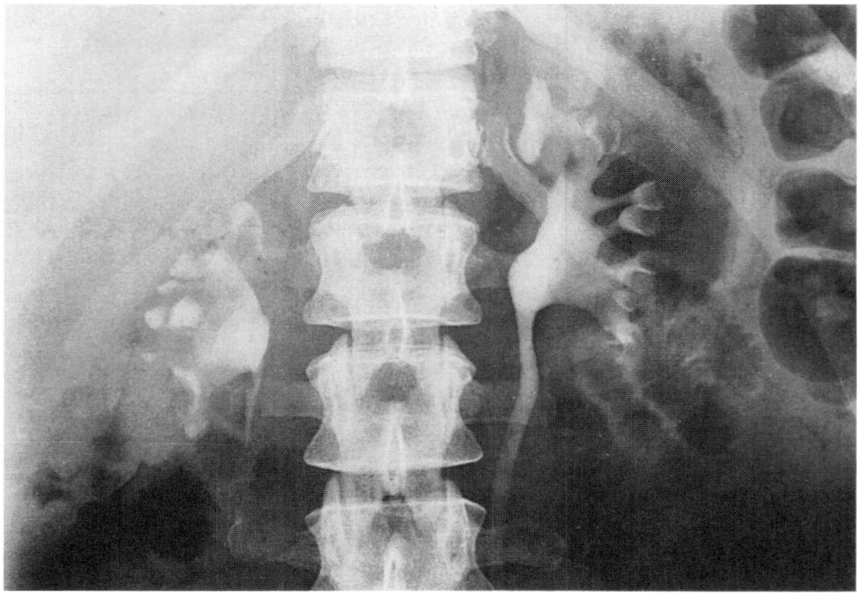

Fig. 36.19 Chronic pyelonephritis. Film from intravenous urogram showing shrunken right kidney with scarring in the left upper pole. Courtesy of Dr J Reid.

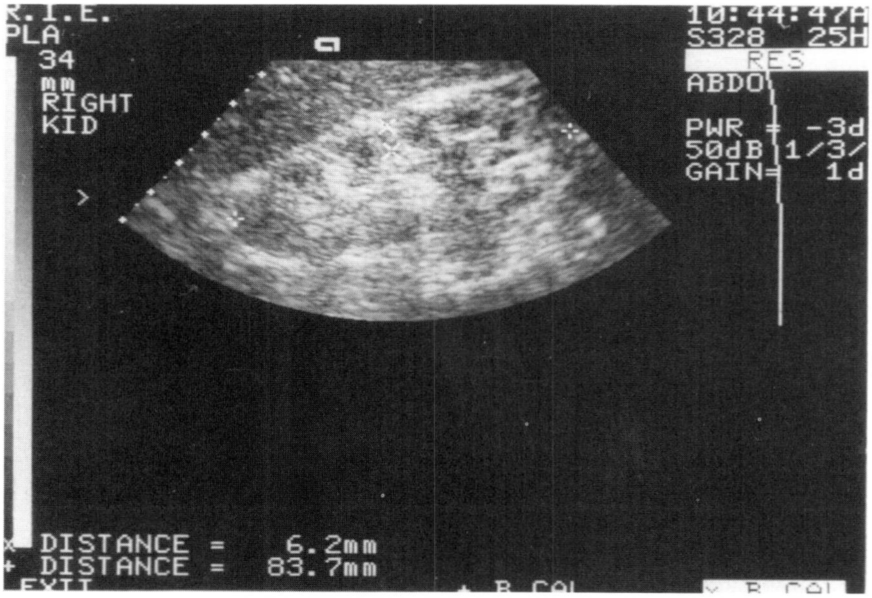

Fig. 36.20 Ultrasound scan of pyelonephritic kidney. The kidney is reduced in size and there is thinning of the cortex. Courtesy of Dr P Allan.

symptoms.[103] Acute clinical pyelonephritis generally does not cause renal scarring in adults in the presence of normal urinary tracts. Most changes of chronic pyelonephritis seem to occur in infancy where the maturing kidney is more susceptible to scarring. The relationship between chronic pyelonephritis and end-stage renal failure is complex because in the vast majority of cases there is an associated complicating factor such as vesicoureteric reflux, analgesic abuse, diabetes, hypertension, nephrolithiasis or hydronephrosis. Nephroureterectomy may be indicated to treat severe hypertension or infections which are increasingly difficult to control, providing the function of the opposite kidney is normal. When vesicoureteric reflux has been proven, reimplantation of the ureter may be more appropriate if the degree of functioning renal tissue exceeds 15%.[104]

REFERENCES

103. Scott J E S, Stansfield J M Arch Dis Child 1968; 43: 323
104. Weston P et al Br J Urol 1952; 54: 677

Xanthogranulomatous pyelonephritis

This is an extremely rare condition which is usually associated with stone disease.[105] Its importance lies in differentiating the mass it causes from a renal tumour.

Pathology

It is usually seen in association with a Proteus urinary infection, and renal stones are invariably present. Macroscopically, the mass appears to have spread beyond the renal capsule and it may invade adjacent structures such as the psoas muscle and diaphragm. The macroscopic appearances may be identical with those of a clear cell renal carcinoma.

One helpful differentiating feature is the bright-yellow colour of the focal area of inflammation. This is the result of large numbers of distended macrophages seen on microscopy which contain indigestible bacterial debris. Other chronic inflammatory cells are present and the kidney is generally enlarged.[105]

Clinical features

These are loin pain, fever and weight loss. There may be a palpable fixed mass in the loin which may be mistaken for a Wilms' tumour in children.[106]

Investigations

The intravenous urogram shows a non-functioning kidney and the presence of stones (Fig. 36.21). On ultrasound or CT examination it may be very difficult to differentiate this condition from a renal tumour.[107]

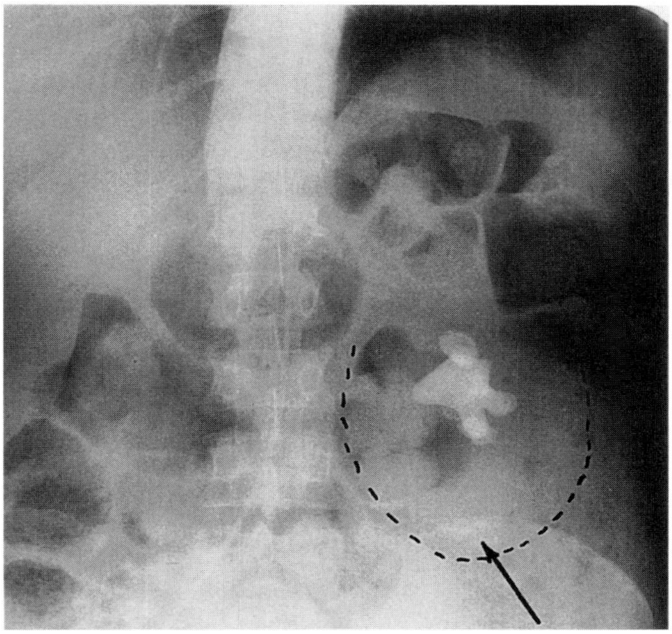

Fig. 36.21 Xanthogranulomatous pyelonephritis. Preliminary film prior to angiography showing grossly swollen left kidney containing staghorn calculus and calcification in the lower rim (arrowed). Courtesy of Dr J Reid.

Management

Nephrectomy is the correct treatment; it may be difficult because of the extent of the inflammatory process.

Actinomycosis

Infection with *Actinomyces israelii*, *Coccidioides immitis* or *Nocardia asteroides* rarely affects the urinary tract but occasionally a purulent mass containing sulphur granules made up of balls or mycelial threads may occur. The infection may present as a space-occupying lesion in the kidney and may thus be mistaken for a renal tumour. Treatment with sulphadiazine may produce resolution but the condition is often only diagnosed after nephrectomy.[108]

Bilharzia

Bilharzial infection primarily affects the bladder and the condition is described in Chapter 37. The ureter is also affected: pseudotubercles, granulomatous strictures and calcification may occur in the lower third, and involvement of the middle third of the ureter can occur via the superior and inferior mesenteric veins.[109]

Management

Effective treatment of the acute infestation is the best way of preventing complications. Niridazole 7.5 mg/kg given at 2-weekly intervals for 6 weeks, or metriphonate 10 mg/kg at 2-weekly intervals for 4 weeks are both effective. Niridazole 25 mg/kg and metriphonate 12.5 mg/kg may also be given as a single dose.[110] The ureteric scarring which occurs may produce obstruction and reflux, and reimplantation of the ureter is often necessary. Where the fibrosis is extensive, ileal replacement of the ureter may be more appropriate. Ureteric reimplantation is difficult in the presence of bilharzia because of the associated bladder fibrosis which makes the operation technically very difficult.

Filariasis

This condition does not affect the kidney but does infect the lymphatics (see Chapter 12). Microfilaria are ingested by mosquitoes when feeding on the blood of infected individuals. They are then transmitted to the next host where the worm develops to a reproductive stage in which large numbers of microfilaria are released, thus completing the cycle. The resulting infestation causes inflammation which obstructs the lymphatics. This process occurs because of an intense inflammatory reaction resulting in fibrosis and calcification.[111]

REFERENCES

105. Malik R S, Elder J S J Urol 1978; 199: 559
106. Braun G et al J Urol 1985; 133: 236
107. Magilner E D, Ostrium B J Radiology 1978; 126: 715
108. McGibeny D, Clark P B Br J Urol 1986; 58: 566
109. Wallace D N Ann R Coll Surg Engl 1976; 6: 1265
110. Pugh R N H, Gilles H M Ann Trop Med Parasitol 1978; 72: 471
111. Yu H H Y J Urol 1978; 199: 104

Clinical features

There is generally a history of a systemic illness, malaise, fever, rigors and pain, especially in the groin. On examination there is tenderness and swelling of the lymph nodes and lymphangitis often produces elephantiasis. There may also be giant hydroceles (see Chapter 40).

Treatment

Diethylcarbamazine 0.5–2 g/kg is given three times daily for 3 weeks, and secondary infection is treated by antibiotics.[111] Chyluria (see Fig. 36.1) occurs when the lymph escapes into the urinary tract through the development of abnormal lymphatic fistulae. The site of the fistula is either in the bladder or the renal pelvis and as a result the patient loses vast quantities of protein with subsequent weight loss, oedema and ureteric colic.

Investigations

Investigations are designed to identify the principal site of lymphatic leakage. Intravenous urography is performed to clarify the renal anatomy. Cystoscopy may show the presence of fat globules in the bladder but a lymphangiogram is the most important investigation (see Chapter 12).

Management

Destruction of the lymphatic fistulae is the keystone of management. Endoscopic fulguration may have some transient benefit but more frequently open dissection with cautery and ligation of the lymphatics is required.[112]

Exploration of the kidney and division of all the lymphatics in the renal pedicle are necessary when this is the source of the leak. It is essential to strip the renal pedicle completely of its lymphatics and it is usually necessary to carry out the operation on both kidneys. It should be noted, however, that spontaneous remission has been reported in approximately 50% of affected cases.[113]

Tuberculosis

Although the incidence of genitourinary tuberculosis has shown a notable decline in the past 20 years, the condition remains a serious problem in developing countries and in immigrants to the UK from these countries.

Pathology

The tubercle bacilli may affect every part of the genitourinary tract from the kidneys to the urethra (Chapter 39), including the epididymis (see Chapter 40). The genitourinary tract is infected by blood-borne spread of the organism, usually from pulmonary lesions. Diffuse interstitial renal tuberculosis may occur, but more commonly there are localized lesions of tuberculous pyelonephritis which slowly destroy the kidneys if left untreated. Small tubercles occur in the cortex and undergo caseation, ultimately coalescing to form an enlarging patch of tuberculosis which tends to discharge into the renal pelvis. A ragged cavity results, giving the characteristic appearances on the intravenous urogram (Fig. 36.22). The tubercles form in the wall of the renal pelvis and may spread to involve the ureter. The ureter thus becomes blocked by intramural tuberculosis as the result of intraluminal obstruction with caseous material. Should healing occur, there is often intense fibrosis producing a ureteric stricture. The microscopic appearances are those of typical tuberculous granuloma, with a caseous centre surrounded by epithelioid and giant cells. There is a variable chronic inflammatory infiltrate and fibrosis. Ziehl–Neelsen staining confirms the presence of acid-fast bacilli. Tuberculosis often also affects the bladder where it causes chronic cystitis with ulceration of the mucosa and a thickened bladder wall (see Chapter 37).

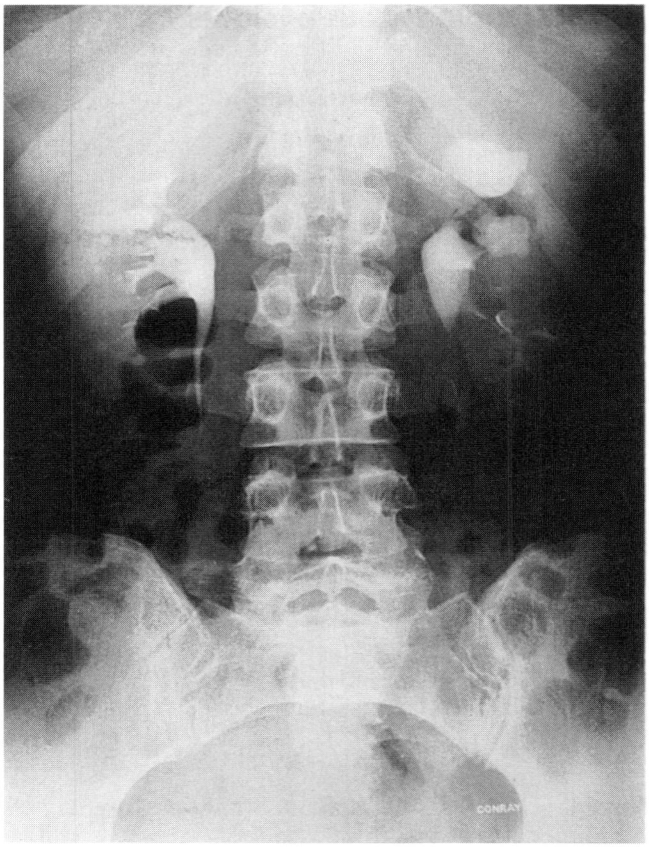

Fig. 36.22 Renal tuberculosis: intravenous urogram showing cavitation in the upper and lower poles of the left kidney. Courtesy of Dr J Reid.

Clinical features

The disease is more common in men than women and has the highest incidence in the third and fourth decades. Patients gener-

REFERENCES

112. Torres L F, Estrada J J Urol 1962; 87: 73
113. Ohyama C et al J Urol 1979; 121: 316

ally present with lower urinary tract symptoms, especially urinary frequency. Dysuria only occurs in the later stages when there is secondary infection. Haematuria, renal pain or ureteric colic generally denote ureteric obstruction because of upper urinary tract involvement. A high index of suspicion is required to make the diagnosis.

Investigation

The presence of a sterile pyuria should alert the clinician to the possibility of urinary tract tuberculosis. The bacilli may be identified on an early morning urine sample by direct microscopy or, more usually, on culture, which takes 6 weeks. It should be noted, however, that if gross disease occurs and causes ureteric obstruction the urine may well be free of tubercle bacilli even though the disease is active.

The full blood count is generally normal although the erythrocyte sedimentation rate is invariably raised. A chest radiograph may show evidence of active tuberculosis or there may be calcification indicating burnt-out disease. Intravenous urography is the cornerstone of diagnosis. The changes that this demonstrates range from mild intrarenal calcification with blunting of the calices (Fig. 36.22) to the appearance of an autonephrectomized calcified kidney (Fig. 36.23). In between, various degrees of renal destruction may be seen; hydronephrosis and hydroureter may be present

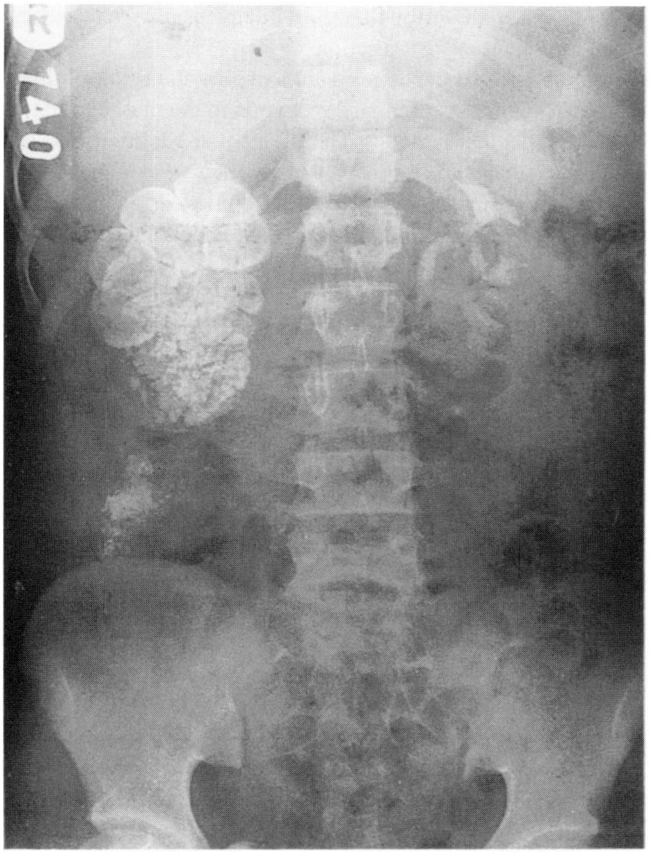

Fig. 36.23 Renal tuberculosis: autonephrectomy. Courtesy of Dr J Reid.

secondary to stricture formation. Cystoscopy may show a small contracted bladder with periureteric inflammation and superficial granulation which may be disseminated throughout the bladder. Ulceration occurs late. The theoretical risk of tuberculous meningitis following biopsy of the bladder dictates that this is inadvisable. There are, however, occasions when the disease is not recognized at endoscopy and bladder biopsy is performed.

Management

Most patients can be treated as outpatients. It should be remembered that healing causes an intense inflammatory reaction and for this reason it is always advisable to carry out limited intravenous urography or ultrasound assessment of the upper urinary tract to enable early detection of obstruction.

Short-course chemotherapy lasting 4–6 months is particularly applicable in the management of genitourinary tuberculosis as high concentrations of anti-tuberculous drugs are excreted in the urine.[114] Additionally, rifampicin penetrates the whole of the urinary tract. Gow[115] has recommended the following regimen:

1. First 2 months:
   - Pyrazinamide 25 mg/kg/day (maximum dose 2 g/day)
   - Isoniazid 300 mg/day
   - Rifampicin 450 mg/day
2. Second 2 months:
   - Isoniazid 600 mg t.d.s.
   - Rifampicin 900 mg t.d.s.

When there is extensive involvement, streptomycin 1 g/day may be added for the first 2 months of treatment.

Steroids are not recommended in the initial phase of treatment but it should be remembered that rifampicin reduces the effect of steroids by increasing their catabolism twofold. A much larger dose of prednisolone than that normally used is therefore required. Prednisolone 20 mg t.d.s. is recommended for 3 weeks if a ureteric stricture develops.[116] Surgical treatment is required if there is no improvement at the end of this time.

Renal function may be preserved in the presence of upper tract obstruction by the insertion of a double J silicone stent, although frequently this is poorly tolerated because of the associated bladder contracture. Surgery often consists of nephrectomy for the non-functioning or fibrosed kidney with very little function. For extensive disease involving the whole of the kidney combined with a ureteric stricture, nephroureterectomy is advised.

Ureteric obstruction is most commonly the result of oedema during the acute phase of the illness, and a number of patients with this complication do respond to antitubercular treatment. This phase of drug therapy should be carefully monitored with appropriate imaging either by isotope renography, ultrasound, or limited single film intravenous urogram if the upper tracts are to be

REFERENCES

114. Mitchison D A J R Coll Phys London 1980; 14: 91
115. Gow J G In: Whitfield H N, Hendry W F (eds) Genitourinary Surgery. Churchill Livingstone, Edinburgh 1987
116. Fox W Bull Int UN Tuberc 1978; 53: 268

preserved. When obstruction persists it is because of fibrosis secondary to long-standing disease; ureteric reimplantation is then required. Strictures associated with tuberculosis are often long and a Boari flap is frequently required to replace the ureter. When the bladder is severely affected, this operation is extremely difficult and it is sometimes necessary to combine bladder augmentation by enterocystoplasty with ureteric reimplantation (see Chapter 37).

UPPER URINARY TRACT OBSTRUCTION

The radiological demonstration of a dilated upper urinary tract is not always synonymous with obstruction. Careful assessment of patients in whom these findings are demonstrated is required to differentiate between obstruction and other causes of dilatation. The term 'hydronephrosis' is commonly used to imply dilatation of the renal pelvis and/or calices secondary to obstruction. The collecting system and ureter comprise three distinct anatomical layers, namely, a layer of urothelium, a muscular layer consisting of smooth muscle, and an adventitial layer of connective tissue. Two types of smooth muscle can be identified in the wall of the ureter: normal smooth muscle, similar to smooth muscle found elsewhere in the body, and atypical smooth muscle.[117]

Normal smooth muscle cells are grouped together in compact bundles lying outside the atypical muscle layer and extending throughout the major calices and renal pelvis. In the pelviureteric region, the normal bundles are continuous with those which form the muscle coat of the ureter.[118] The majority of bundles are circularly disposed and form a plexiform arrangement of intercommunications with adjacent muscle fascicles.

The atypical muscle cells are distributed through the attachment of each minor calix to the renal parenchyma. The cells are arranged longitudinally and form a discrete layer confined to the inner aspect of the muscle coat. This inner layer interconnects with bundles of typical smooth muscle throughout the walls of the major calices and renal pelvis. These cells differ from typical smooth muscle in that they are devoid of non-specific cholinesterase. This configuration ceases in the pelviureteric region. In the ureter the muscle bundles are frequently separated from one another by relatively large amounts of connective tissue forming a complex network of interweaving and interconnecting smooth muscle bundles. These fibres become predominantly longitudinally orientated as the vesicoureteric junction is reached.[119]

Autonomic nerve fibres are present in the muscle coat of the caliceal wall, pelvis and ureter, and are also found in the perivascular tissue. The density of innervation increases towards the ureterovesical junction and this appears to modulate the contractile activity of the muscle coat. The nerves do not, however, contribute directly to ureteric peristalsis.[120]

Many theories have been propounded to account for ureteric peristalsis[121] but it appears that the upper urinary tract possesses spontaneously active regions consisting of pacemaker muscle cells which initiate and control the peristaltic activity of the ureter.[122] These cells tend to occur in the minor calices, and propagation of a contraction through the wall of the adjacent major calix activates the smooth muscle of the renal pelvis. There appears to be a regulating mechanism in the pelviureteric junction which determines whether each contraction of the renal pelvis is propagated into the ureter. This is probably related to urine flow and depends upon the tension or pressure generated in the wall of the pelviureteric region.

Pathophysiology

Certain physiological changes occur during obstruction of the upper urinary tract in addition to the pathological changes of dilatation of the collecting system and a loss of renal parenchyma with scarring of the remaining relatively normal tissue secondary to infection. Obstruction is a common cause for renal failure, and it is therefore important to be aware of the pathophysiological sequelae.

Normal urine flow is the result of muscular peristalsis: the pressure within the collecting system is usually less than 10 mmHg measured through the ureter and 6.5 mmHg if measured percutaneously. In acute obstruction there is an immediate rise in the intrarenal pressure associated with a period of reverse peristalsis. Although the initial pressure rise is acute and high, rising to between 40 and 50 mmHg, the values fall within a number of hours to pre-obstructive levels.[123] Renal blood flow increases in the early hours after acute obstruction, then there is a transient return to normal after 2 or 3 hours, followed by a reduction to half which coincides with the low hydrostatic pressure. These changes may be the result of activation of the renin angiotensin system causing afferent arteriolar vasoconstriction.[124]

The drop in renal pelvic pressure is in part the result of dilatation of the collecting system and reduction in the muscular tone in the renal pelvis and ureter.[125] The glomerular filtration rate falls and in order to compensate for this an increased blood flow is required.[125] In long-standing obstruction, loss of nephrons combined with glomerulosclerosis produces impaired permeability which results in a reduction in the glomerular filtration rate.

The concentrating ability of the tubules is impaired, not only because of the lack of response to antidiuretic hormone[126] but also from the osmotic effects of nitrogen retention.[127] In partial obstruction these factors produce polyuria with consequent severe fluid and electrolyte losses.[128] Defective reabsorption of bicarbonate by

REFERENCES

117. Kiil F (ed) Proceedings of the Third International Congress of Nephrology. Karber, New York 1966
118. Notley R G Br J Urol 1968; 40: 37
119. Notley R G Br J Urol 1970; 42: 439
120. Gosling J A et al Functional Anatomy of the Urinary Tract. Gower Medical, London 1982
121. Gosling J A, Dixon J S In: Whitfield H N, Hendry W F (eds) Textbook of Genitourinary Surgery. Churchill Livingstone, Edinburgh 1987
122. Constantinou C E Am J Physiol 1974; 276: 1413
123. Bretland P M Acute Ureteric Obstruction. Butterworth, London 1972
124. Younger W E et al J Clin Invest 1980; 65: 400
125. Moody T E et al Invest Urol 1975; 13: 246
126. Buerkert J et al J Clin Invest 1978; 62: 1228
127. Raisz L G et al J Clin Invest 1959; 38: 1725
128. Berlyne G N Q J Med 1960; 30: 339

the proximal tubule results in renal tubular acidosis although the ability of the distal tubule to secrete hydrogen ions is retained until relatively late in the course of obstruction. These pathophysiological changes have important clinical sequelae, particularly when the obstruction is relieved.

The answer to the question of how long can a kidney be obstructed and still recover some function is complex. It depends on whether the obstruction is complete or incomplete, the size of the extrarenal pelvis, and the integrity of the lymphatics around the hilum and capsule for pyelolymphatic and pyelovenous backflow to allow for continued filtration of plasma through the glomerulus. Case reports have demonstrated recovery of some function 56–96 days after release of a complete ureteric obstruction.[129] In cases of long-standing obstruction, recovery of glomerular and tubular function may take weeks and patients should be managed as if they have renal failure.[130] Even following relief of obstruction of short duration, the postobstructive phase is often complicated by a high urine flow associated with water and electrolyte loss. There are frequently inappropriate losses of water and sodium, possibly because during the recovery phase filtration improves ahead of tubular function, thus causing inappropriate urinary losses.[131] This may simply be because of the prescription of excessive amounts of fluids which increase urine volume purely in response to expanded extracellular volume. When nitrogen retention has occurred, there is a constant rise in the tissue osmolarity which overcomes the physiological action of antidiuretic hormone. Magnesium and calcium excretion is occasionally increased during the postobstructive phase and replacement of these ions together with phosphate may be required.[132]

Aetiology

Upper urinary tract obstruction may be either unilateral or bilateral and can be caused by extrinsic compression, intramural pathology or by an intraluminal abnormality (Table 36.2). This may occur at any age. The subsequent discussion deals with pelviureteric junction obstruction initially, then extrinsic causes of ureteric obstruction followed by intramural causes (megaureter). Intraluminal causes—urinary stones and ureteric tumours (are discussed separately later in the chapter.

Table 36.2 Causes of upper urinary tract obstruction

Pelviureteric junction obstruction
Idiopathic
Secondary
Surgery
Infection
Tuberculosis
Retroperitoneal fibrosis
Extrinsic ureteric obstruction
Retrocaval ureter
Ovarian vein syndrome
Aneurysmal obstruction
Iatrogenic obstruction
Inflammatory disease
Malignant disease
Idiopathic retroperitoneal fibrosis
Intraluminal pathology
Ureteric tumour
Urinary tract stones
Intramural pathology
Primary megaureter

Pelviureteric junction obstruction

This is one of the more common renal disorders seen in infancy and childhood. A great deal of controversy surrounds its aetiology. It may be the result of intrinsic, extrinsic or secondary causes.

Intrinsic causes

Morphological changes in the smooth muscle bundles of the pelviureteric junction probably cause obstruction. An excess of collagen has been demonstrated in the pelviureteric junction and may be responsible for failure of peristaltic waves from the pelvis to be propagated across the pelviureteric junction to the ureter.[118] It has also been suggested that the orientation of the smooth muscle bundles at the pelviureteric junction is altered and this may be responsible for the obstruction.[133] The smooth muscle in the renal pelvis may be replaced by an increased amount of connective tissue resulting in poor contraction of the renal pelvis.[134] It is not known, however, whether this is the cause or effect of obstruction.

Extrinsic causes

Aberrant lower polar vessels have been postulated to cause pelviureteric obstruction. As the pelvis fills, the upper part of the ureter becomes kinked and obstructed by the aberrant vessels whilst the renal pelvis balloons up in its anterior wall.[135] A high insertion of the ureter into the renal pelvis may cause kinking of the ureter just below the pelviureteric junction resulting in dilatation of the renal pelvis. The persistence of fetal ureteric folds is a rare cause of obstruction.

Secondary

Pelviureteric junction may be caused by severe vesicoureteric reflux which coexists in 10% of cases. Indeed it may be secondary to lower urinary tract obstruction. Other causes include trauma, surgery and infection, such as tuberculosis.

Clinical features

Fetal hydronephrosis is the most commonly diagnosed antenatal abnormality on ultrasound. In children, pelviureteric junction

REFERENCES

129. Graham J B JAMA 1962; 181: 993
130. Baughan J E D, Gillenwater J Y J Urol 1973; 109: 286
131. Peterson L J et al J Urol 1975; 113: 190
132. Better I S et al Nephron 1972; 9: 131
133. Murnaghan G F Ann R Coll Surg Engl 1958; 23: 25
134. Gosling J A, Dixon J S In: O'Reilly P H, Gosling J A (eds) Idiopathic Hydronephrosis. Springer-Verlag, Berlin 1982
135. Anderson J C Hydronephrosis. Heinemann, London 1963

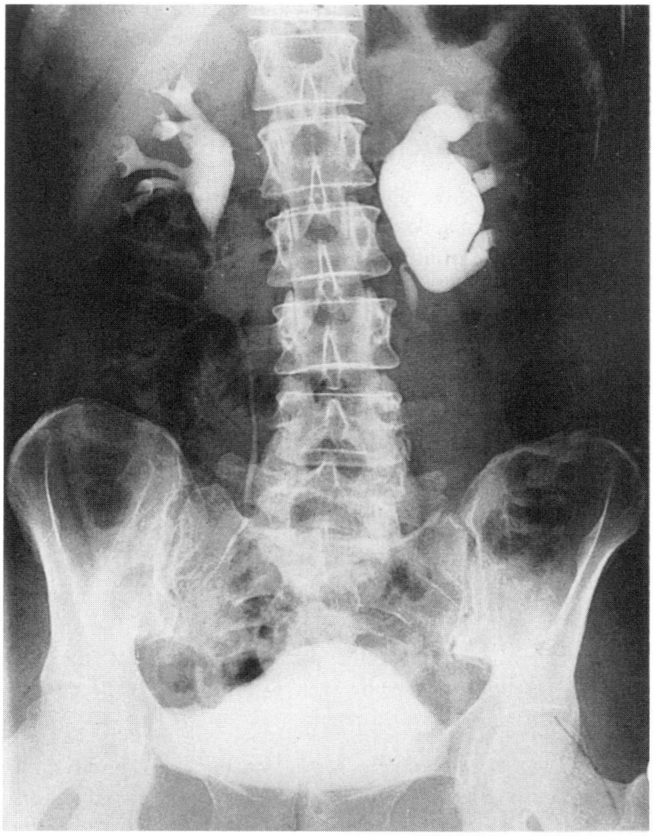

Fig. 36.24 Intravenous urogram showing left pelviureteric junction obstruction. (Courtesy of Dr J Reid.)

obstruction may be a cause of failure to thrive, especially if associated with recurrent urinary infections. Other common presenting features are abdominal pain or an abdominal mass. Classically the young student with pelviureteric junction obstruction develops loin pain after ingestion of alcohol. Many patients present with vague loin pain or symptoms of ureteric colic but in late adult life pelviureteric junction obstruction is generally symptomless; the hydronephrosis may be discovered accidentally as a palpable mass during the investigation of other symptoms. Patients may also present as infection or as septicaemia caused by a pyonephrosis.

Investigations

Ultrasound may be used to differentiate a hydronephrotic kidney from a Wilms' tumour or neuroblastoma in children. In adults the diagnosis is often obvious on the intravenous urogram. Radioisotope studies should be used as confirmation or as a primary means of diagnosis in patients with equivocal pelviureteric junction obstruction. Rarely pressure flow studies are necessary to establish a diagnosis beyond all doubt.[136] The intravenous urogram often shows characteristic appearances (Fig. 36.24). In patients in whom the diagnosis is suspected but where the radiographs are normal, provocation of the obstruction by intravenous administration of 40 mg of frusemide may produce the characteristic radiological findings.[136]

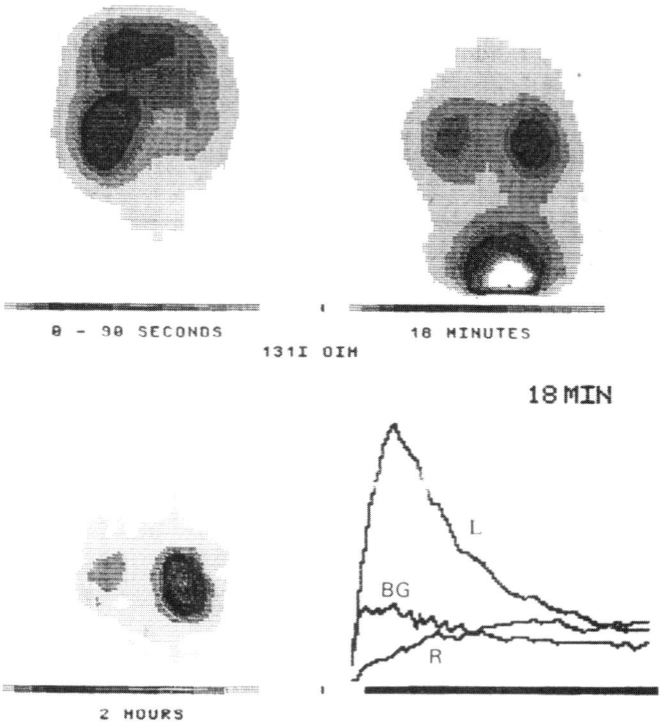

Fig. 36.25 Radioisotope study showing poor function in the right kidney because of obstruction.

Radioisotope studies should be used to confirm pelviureteric junction obstruction and to assess the contribution of the affected side to overall renal function. In the presence of diminished function and persisting obstruction, surgery is indicated (Fig. 36.25). In the presence of normal function with evidence of obstruction, surgery is still indicated even in the absence of symptoms, to prevent renal parenchymal damage from occurring. If the contribution to overall renal function is 15% or more, corrective surgery is indicated, whereas below these levels a therapeutic trial of simulated relief of obstruction by insertion of an internal JJ stent could help in deciding between corrective surgery or nephrectomy. In totally non-functioning kidneys nephrectomy is the treatment of choice.[137] Pressure studies provide urodynamic evidence of obstruction in those few cases where the diagnosis still remains in doubt after radiological and radioisotope investigations.[138]

Treatment

The overall aim of treatment is to preserve renal function as a high percentage of patients with symptoms develop progressive renal damage if the obstruction is not relieved. In the vast majority of pregnant mothers whose fetus has ultrasound-detected hydronephrosis, no intervention is necessary in utero unless there is also

REFERENCES

136. Whitaker R J U Urol 1979; 121: 602
137. Sreenevasam G Ann R Coll Surg Engl 1974; 55: 3
138. Whitfield J N et al Br J Urol 1978; 52: 445

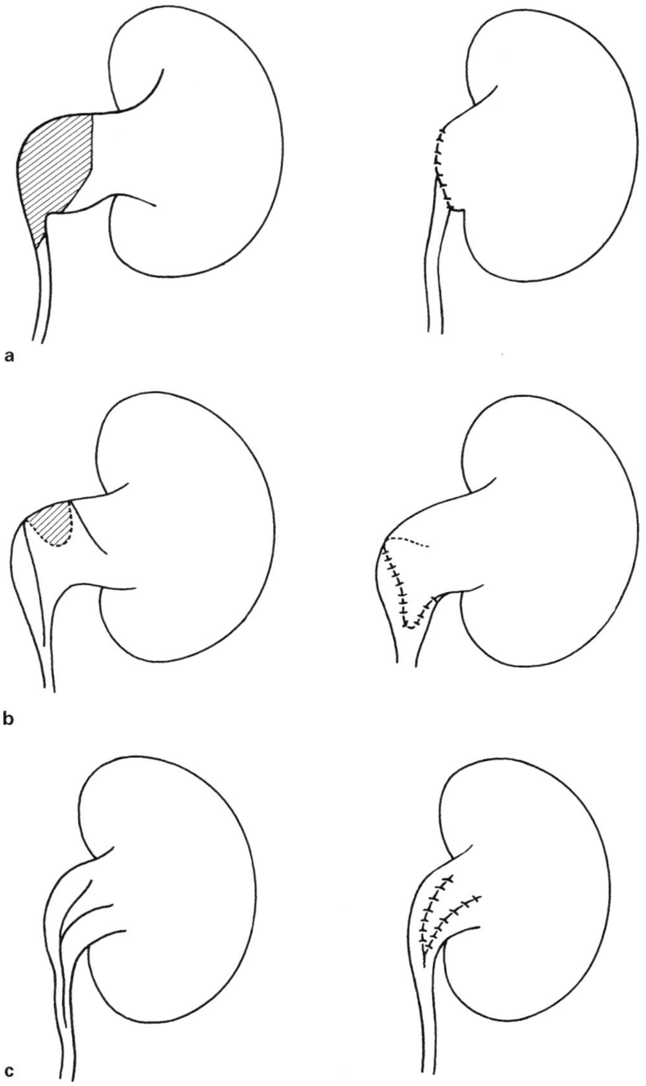

Fig. 36.26 Operations for pelviureteric junction obstruction. (**a**) Anderson–Hynes; (**b**) Culp–Scardino; (**c**) Foley Y–V.

oligohydramnios. Postnatally, a pyelopasty should be carried out to preserve renal function if the abnormality persists, especially if follow-up is likely to be difficult. When continuous monitoring is guaranteed, surgery may be indicated in selected patients who continue to have symptoms, or show evidence of deteriorating renal function[139] or whose initial renal pelvic anteroposterior diameter is greater than 20 mm.[140] Many procedures have been described to relieve pelviureteric function obstruction: all consist of re-fashioning the pelviureteric junction (Fig. 36.26). In the UK, the Anderson–Hynes pyelopasty[141] has proved to be effective, whereas in the USA the Culp–Scardino pyelopasty is often preferred.[142] For patients with a small intrarenal pelvis a Foley Y–V plasty is often more appropriate.[143] Endoscopic division of the pelviureteric junction by both the percutaneous[144] and ureteric approach[145] has been described although its value in patients with primary pelviureteric junction obstruction has not yet been established by long-term studies. More recently balloon disruption of the pelviureteric junction has been reported, with varying success rates.[146]

Symptomless hydronephrosis in a functionless kidney should be treated by nephrectomy as there is a risk that such patients will develop a pyonephrosis.

Secondary pelviureteric junction obstruction from tuberculosis has been described[147] but spontaneous resolution usually occurs during the course of treatment and surgery is rarely required. Post-traumatic pelviureteric junction obstruction is seen in children after blunt abdominal injury and is usually caused by a stricture. It is treated by excision and anastomosis of healthy pelvis and ureter if possible, or by interposition methods if required. Extravasation of infected urine from the renal pelvis during surgery for staghorn calculi may produce a urinoma which may later cause secondary fibrosis and obstruction. An exogenous staphylococcal infection may also occur and be a contributory factor in the development of stenosis.[137] Extravasation of sterile urine rarely produces obstruction.

Other extrinsic causes of upper tract obstruction

Retroperitoneal fibrosis

Retroperitoneal fibrosis normally starts at the level of the sacroiliac joint and spreads upwards along the ureter to the renal pelvis; it can involve the inferior vena cava and aorta. This condition, first described by Ormond,[148] may be benign or malignant. The ureter is obstructed as it becomes encased in the course of the fibroinflammatory process. In the majority of cases the cause remains unknown (idiopathic) but it may be secondary to drugs (methysergide, α-methyldopa, amphetamines), an inflammatory aortic aneurysm (possibly from an allergic reaction to leaked lipids), radiation therapy, haemorrhage, urinary leakage in the retroperitoneum, inflammatory bowel disease and collagen disease.

Clinical features

Many patients have no symptoms and the condition is diagnosed incidentally. Some patients present with non-specific symptoms of malaise, fever, weight loss, anorexia and nausea, and many complain of poorly localized backache. Occasionally, patients may present with acute obstructive renal failure. They may also present with an abdominal aortic aneurysm or a deep vein thrombosis if the inferior vena cava or iliac veins are involved in the plaque. The condition may be bilateral and may present as uraemia.

REFERENCES

139. Freeman E R J Paediatr Surg 1994; 29: 769
140. Dillon H K J Urol 1994; 152: 612
141. Anderson J C, Hynes W B J Urol 1949; 21: 209
142. Culp O S, De Weerd J H J Urol 1951; 71: 523
143. Foley F E B J Urol 1937; 38: 643
144. Whitfield J N et al Br J Urol 1983; suppl 93
145. Inglis J A, Tolley D A Br J Urol 1986; 58: 250
146. McClinton S Br J Urol 1993; 71(2): 152
147. Gow J G In: Blandy J P (ed) Urology. Blackwell, Oxford 1976
148. Ormond J K J Urol 1948; 59: 1072

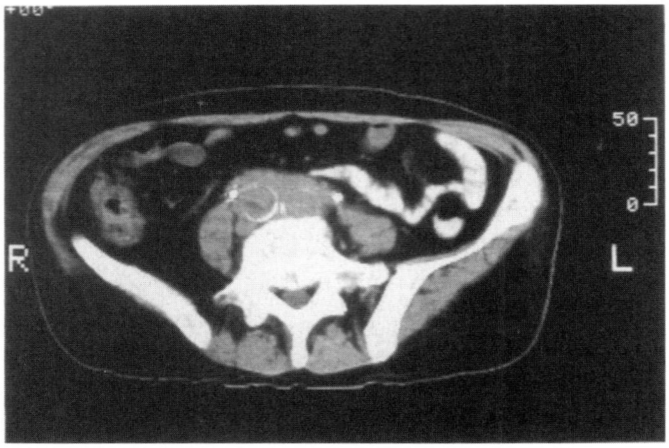

a

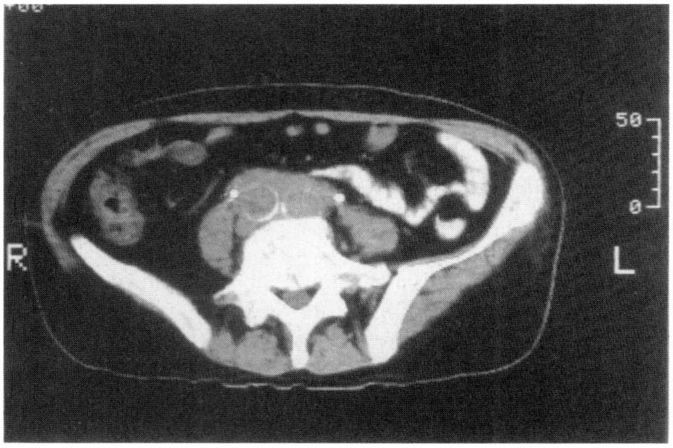

b

Fig. 36.27 (**a**) CT scan of abdomen showing a plaque of fibrous tissue surrounding the aorta. (**b**) Reduction in size of the plaque 4 weeks after starting corticosteroid therapy. Ureteric stents may also be seen in situ.

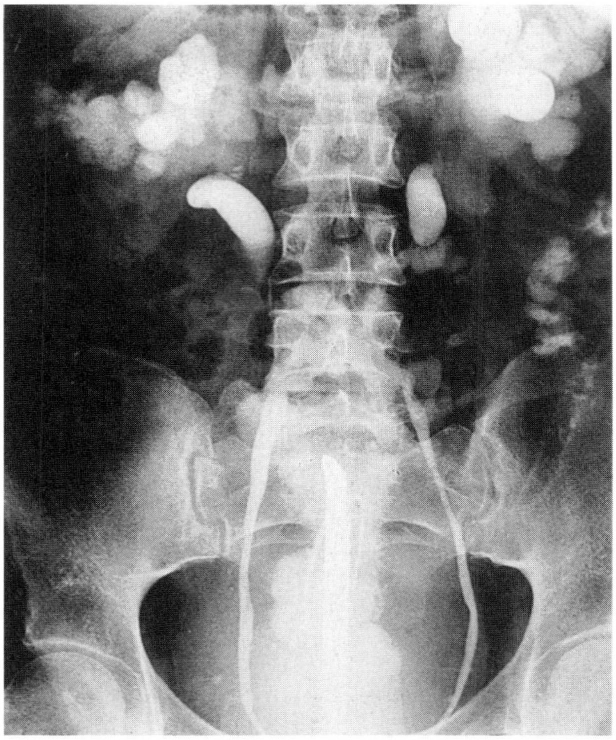

Fig. 36.28 Bilateral ureterogram showing bilateral ureteric obstruction from retroperitoneal fibrosis. Note the ureters being pulled towards the midline over the lumbar vertebrae.

On examination more than half the patients have hypertension and, in a minority of men, a hydrocele may be present indicating a blockage of the retroperitoneal lymphatics. A prominent aortic pulsation or signs of venous obstruction may also be present (see Chapters 10 and 11).

The diagnosis can be confirmed by CT scan.[149] CT scanning is also useful in monitoring the progress of the disease after steroid treatment (Fig. 36.27). A raised erythrocyte sedimentation rate is invariable and anaemia is frequently noted. Bilateral retrograde ureterography delineates the length of the affected ureteric segment. A characteristic feature of the disease is that, despite severe obstruction, a ureteric catheter passes easily up both ureters (Fig. 36.28).

Management

Patients may be uraemic and unfit for major surgery at the time of diagnosis. Initial treatment consists of the management of the renal failure and institution of drainage of the kidney either by double J stenting or percutaneous nephrostomy. Once the renal function has stabilized, a definitive decision should be made on whether the kidney is salvageable, based on isotope studies.

The treatment of choice is ureterolysis in patients who are not in renal failure and in patients with unilateral disease. Steroid therapy is useful in specific situations; it is valuable as an adjunct to upper tract drainage in preparing patients who have renal insufficiency for surgery. Operative procedures can then be performed on a healthier patient, and electively rather than on a semi-urgent basis. Patients with systemic disturbance who have laboratory evidence of active inflammation (a raised sedimentation rate or leucocytosis) are likely to benefit from steroids. In elderly patients who are poor surgical risks the need for surgery may be averted.[150] Some surgeons also use steroid therapy postoperatively to prevent recurrence if the histology of the plaque shows active inflammation. Initially, prednisolone 15 mg t.d.s. is given, reducing to 5 mg b.d. after 2 weeks if there has been a clinical improvement. It should be noted that the optimum dose of prednisolone to be employed is not yet established.[151]

Ureterolysis is best carried out through a midline transperitoneal incision which permits exploration of both ureters. The

REFERENCES

149. Husband J E , Bellamy E A In: Hendry W F (ed) Recent Advances in Urology. Churchill Livingstone, Edinburgh 1987
150. Ross J C Br J Surg 1971; 58: 422
151. Baker L R I et al Br J Urol 1988; 60: 497

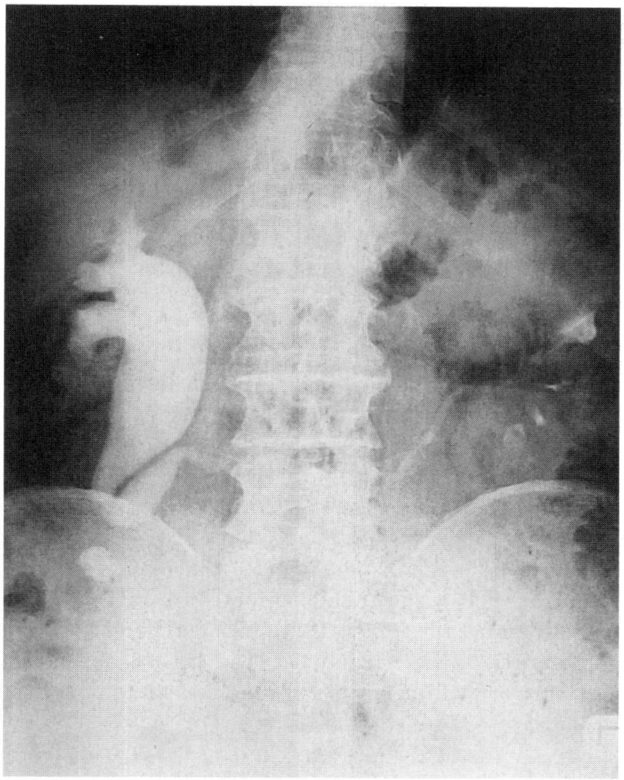

Fig. 36.29 Retrocaval ureter.

ureter is often embedded in dense fibrous tissue which makes its identification difficult. Location of the ureter is often made easier by preliminary retrograde insertion of ureteric catheters. The ureters are dissected out of the fibrous sheath and placed laterally away from the active disease. They should be wrapped in a sleeve of omentum, although this does not prevent recurrent obstruction.[152] Morbidity following surgery can be high and includes ureteric fistula, deep vein thrombosis, pulmonary embolus and myocardial infarction.[153]

The prognosis of idiopathic retroperitoneal fibrosis is good. There remains a debate about the optimum method of treatment and each case should be treated on its merits.[151] The contralateral ureter must be monitored after successful ureterolysis as it may be asynchronously involved. There is also debate about the best means of monitoring disease activity; the place of CT scanning in follow-up is not established as changes in the periaortic mass do not necessarily reflect the activity of the disease.[154] Ultrasonography and renography are, however, helpful in determining the extent of the urinary tract obstruction.

Retrocaval ureter

Persistence of the posterior cardinal vein to form the inferior vena cava below the level of the renal vein results in the ureter passing behind the vena cava before running distally. The finding of a retrocaval ureter is often incidental but occasionally it causes loin pain and tenderness. The reverse J pattern on intravenous urography is characteristic (Fig. 36.29). In the majority of patients no treatment is necessary, but in those who develop pain, surgery is indicated and re-anastomosis of the ureter in front of the vena cava is all that is required.[141]

Ovarian vein syndrome

The ovarian vein syndrome occurs when the ureter is obstructed at the site where it is crossed by the ovarian vein.[155] The obstruction is usually intermittent and related to the onset of menstruation. Surgery, if indicated, merely involves ligating and dividing the ovarian vein, together with ureterolysis if necessary.

Ureteric obstruction after aortic aneurysm repair

Fibrosis around an aortic graft can often result in ureteric obstruction after repair of an abdominal aortic aneurysm. The condition is caused by fibrosis from bleeding, excessive dissection (ischaemia), pseudo-aneurysm formation, or compression by an anteriorly placed graft.[156] Treatment is by ureterolysis or resection.[157] Steroids often produce considerable resolution of the fibrosis, making feasible subsequent surgery.

Iatrogenic obstruction

Iatrogenic obstruction can occur after radiotherapy or as a result of inadvertent ligation of the ureter during surgery.

Inflammatory diseases

Inflammatory diseases of the large and small bowel such as Crohn's disease, ulcerative colitis and diverticular disease can all cause ureteric obstruction. The development of a retroperitoneal abscess can result in periureteric fibrosis and obstruction.

Malignant disease in the retroperitoneum

Many pelvic malignancies can obstruct the ureter. Para-aortic node involvement in particular may result in obstruction. Malignant retroperitoneal fibrosis is sometimes the result of direct spread of a tumour of the prostate, bladder or rectum. Less commonly, a plaque of fibrous tissue is seen in association with a primary carcinoma of the breast, stomach, pancreas or colon.[158] Lymphoma and lymphosarcoma may also have identical features to benign idiopathic retroperitoneal fibrosis; it is frequently difficult to distinguish between the two conditions as in both cases the plaque and fibrosis are largely acellular.

The advent of chemotherapy for the treatment of advanced testicular cancer in patients with larger retroperitoneal masses has

REFERENCES

152. Tressider G C, Blandy J P, Singh M Urol Int 1972; 27: 144
153. Mundy A R et al Br J Urol 1982; 54: 625
154. Brooks A P et al Clin Rad 1987; 38: 597
155. Polge S, Bobo E J Urol 1969; 102: 305
156. Sant G R J Urol 1983; 129: 16
157. Abbott D L et al J Urol 1973; 109: 957
158. Abrams H C et al Cancer 1950; 3: 74

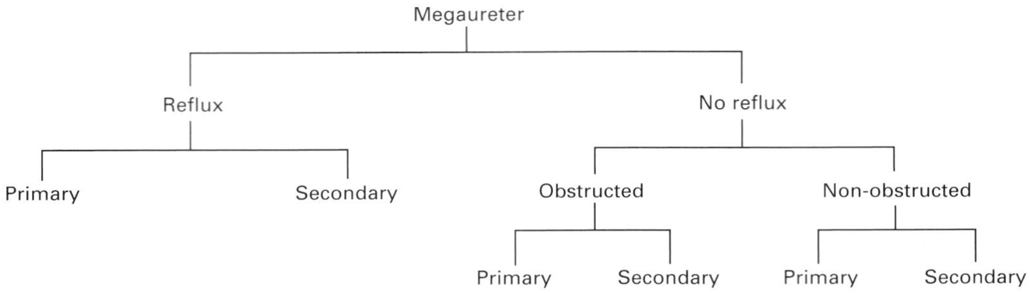

Fig. 36.30 Classification of megaureter.

resulted in the development of hard plaques of fibrous tissue following successful chemotherapy. In general these do not cause obstruction of the ureter and are usually nothing more than fibrous tissue although occasionally there may be small amounts of viable tumour present.[159] Treatment of such cases depends upon the overall condition and prognosis of the patient but palliation can often be achieved by the insertion of bilateral double J ureteric stents or a percutaneous nephrostomy.[160]

Gynaecological diseases

Endometriosis, uterine prolapse and fibroids have all been reported to cause ureteric obstruction.

Rare causes of extrinsic ureteric obstruction are retroperitoneal lymphoceles associated with renal transplants and pelvic lipomatosis, a benign proliferation of mature adipose tissue in the pelvis.

Intramural causes of ureteric obstruction

Megaureter

This term is used to describe an abnormally wide ureter which may or may not be associated with pyelocaliectasis and with obstruction. It must be appreciated that the obstruction cannot be differentiated from stasis on intravenous urography alone: radioisotope studies or urodynamic investigations are necessary to make this differentiation.[161] For this reason the term 'megaureter' has replaced all other terms to describe the appearance of a wide ureter on urography. Whitaker[162] has revised the classification of wide ureters, and the modification by the International Working Party[163] is reproduced in Figure 36.30.

'Primary' implies an intrinsic defect in the ureter whilst 'secondary' suggests that the ureter is wide because of other reasons such as bladder outflow obstruction, extrinsic compression or polyuria. Many patients with megaureter present in infancy or childhood; the diagnosis and the management of this condition are frequently complex and should be left to the paediatric urologist.[164] A brief résumé of the condition is given here.

Pathology

Very little is known about the pathology of primary obstructive megaureter despite much investigation.[165] The pathological findings are not always consistent with the isotope or urodynamic findings, but an absence of muscle in the most distal portion of the narrowed segment has been noted.[166] Embryological studies in lambs have shown that the distal portion of the ureter is the last to develop its muscular coat and early muscular differentiation has a circular orientation.[167] In histological studies both an excess of collagen[168] and circular muscle[169] have been found. Others have suggested that the primary pathology lies within the adynamic segment above the narrow area.[170] This prevents abnormal peristalsis but allows the circular muscle at the lower end of the ureter to squeeze tightly shut and cause obstruction. The hypertrophy and collagen deposition are thought to be secondary to this process.

Clinical features

Many patients now present with a hydronephrosis noted on fetal sonography. Older children may present with a urinary infection, fever, abdominal pain or failure to thrive. Adults present with stone disease or with a symptomless hydronephrotic mass.

Investigations

Stones may be demonstrated on a plain abdominal radiograph. Ultrasound examination demonstrates significant dilatation but the presence of dilated calices does not necessarily imply obstruction. In the presence of either abnormality, intravenous urography is indicated. The characteristic features of a megaureter—wide tortuous ureter with caliceal clubbing—are seen. It is then essential to carry out a micturating cystourethrogram to exclude reflux. This investigation also defines the presence of bladder outflow

REFERENCES

159. Hendry W F In: Jones W G et al (eds) Advances in the Bio Sciences. Germ Cell Tumours 11. Pergamon Press, Oxford 1986
160. Ortlip S A, Fraley E E Urol Clin North Am 1982; 1: 79
161. Whitaker R H Br J Urol 1973; 45: 15
162. Whitaker R H, Johnston J H Br J Urol 1975; 47: 781
163. Smith E D et al Birth Defects 1977; 13: 3
164. Innes Williams D Paediatric Urology. Butterworth, London 1969
165. McLauglin A P III et al J Urol 1973; 109: 805
166. MacKinnon K J Birth Defects 1977; 13: 15
167. Tanagho E A J Urol 1973; 109: 196
168. Notley R G Br J Urol 1970; 42: 724
169. Tanagho E A J Urol 1973; 109: 196
170. Whitaker R J Br J Urol 1975; 47: 377

obstruction. Renography with or without a diuretic is useful for determining the presence of obstruction, particularly when the lower ureter is scanned.[171] It also gives an indication of function of the kidney. When renal function is poor, however, the results of radioisotope scanning are frequently misleading and for this reason urodynamic investigation of the child with megaureter is the only certain way to make the diagnosis.[161]

The Whitaker test[136,172] is used to assess the degree of obstruction. An antegrade renal puncture is made and the collecting system is perfused with saline at a rate of 10 ml/min. The pressure gradient is measured across the ureterovesical junction. A pressure differential greater than 20 cm water indicates obstruction; a pressure below 15 cm water is normal. In between, the results are equivocal. Cystoscopy and ureterography may be carried out to assess the outflow tract and examine the position and shape of the ureteric orifices for possible reflux and to exclude a small ureterocele. Although very little extra information is gained about the anatomy of the megaureter, observations of motility during screening with contrast media are often useful.

Management

In the presence of impaired renal function and infection, percutaneous nephrostomy prior to definitive surgery allows assessment of the potential recovery of the kidney and permits infection to be treated.[173] In determining the most appropriate treatment, the overall renal function and the function of the contralateral kidney should be ascertained. A nephrectomy is the treatment of choice if the percentage of renal function contributed by the affected kidney is less than 15%. Every attempt should be made to preserve renal function irrespective of the radioisotope scan results if the renal function in the contralateral kidney is impaired.

Recent studies have shown a benign outcome in newborns with megaureter without reflux, with resolution of more than a third and deterioration of renal function in only a few.[174,175] These studies indicate that surgery is only indicated in neonates if the ureter is greater than 10 mm in diameter or it takes more than 10 min to clear 75% of the DTPA isotope from the upper tract on an isotope scan. Conservative management includes prophylactic antibiotics until toilet training is achieved and repeated imaging with either radioisotopes or limited urograms. Surgery is indicated if there is deterioration of renal function or there are repeated urinary tract infections.

The aim of reconstructive surgery is to reduce the circumference of the ureter with excision of the obstructing segment. This is done by tapering the ureter to produce a funnelled segment (Fig. 36.31). In children without reflux, ureteric reimplantation is then performed. The ureter and bladder are approached extraperitonally through a transverse lower abdominal incision. The ureter is dissected down to the level of obstruction and the obstructing segment is removed. Tapering may not be necessary if the ureter then collapses. A Leadbetter–Politano[90] reimplantation is then performed (see Chapter 37). The ureter is then splinted with a fine silicone tube which is removed after 10 days. The cystotomy incision is drained with a suprapubic catheter which is also removed 10 days following operation.

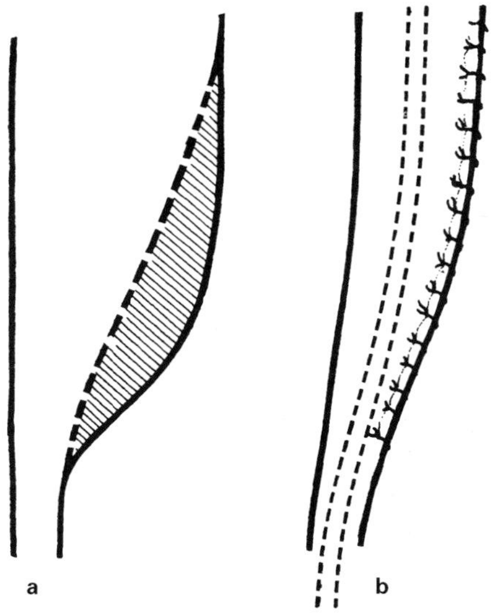

Fig. 36.31 Ureteric tapering for megaureter. **(a)** The dilated segment is trimmed and funnelled and the cut edges are sutured with 4/0 plain catgut over the ureteric splint. **(b)** The ureter is then reimplanted into the bladder.

In many young boys, megaureter is caused by posterior urethral valves; the primary treatment of these is described in Chapter 37.

VESICOURETERIC REFLUX IN ADULTS

Vesicoureteric reflux in adults is of importance because under certain circumstances reflux nephropathy results in end-stage renal failure.[176] The condition occurs as a result of malfunction of the physiological valve at the vesicoureteric junction and it may be primary, i.e. congenital, or secondary. Primary vesicoureteric reflux in adults is reflux that does not disappear during childhood. Secondary vesicoureteric reflux occurs in the presence of obstruction to the bladder neck, prostate or urethra and may occur after certain surgical operations, such as transurethral resection of the prostate or bladder tumour, or ureteric meatotomy for stone or ureterocele. It may also occur after radiotherapy and other conditions causing an inflammatory reaction in the bladder, such as urinary infection, tuberculosis, bilharzia, interstitial cystitis and stones. It is also a complication of the neuropathic bladder (see Chapter 37).

Clinical features

The condition most commonly presents with recurrent urinary infections or loin pain. There may also be a history of infection in childhood. Less commonly, patients present with hypertension, renal failure or proteinuria.

REFERENCES

171. Koff S A et al J Urol 1979; 122: 451
172. Whitaker R H Urol Clin North Am 1979; 6: 529
173. Staples D P Urol Clin North Am 1982; 9: 15
174. Liu H Y A J Urol 1994; 152: 614
175. Baskin L S J Urol 1994; 152: 618
176. Lenaghan D et al J Urol 1976; 115: 728

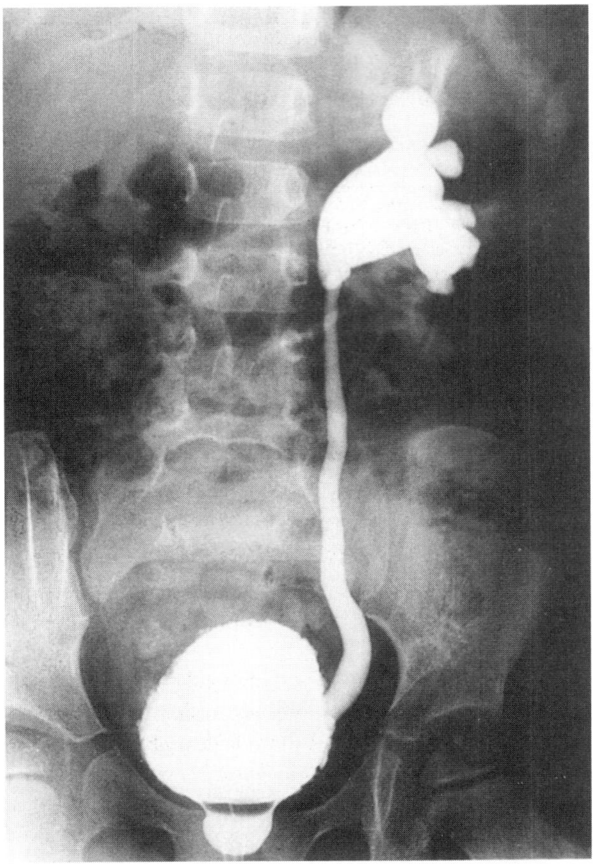

Fig. 36.32 Vesicoureteric reflux. Micturating cystourethrogram showing marked left vesicoureteric reflux and pyelovenous backflow in a young girl. (Courtesy of Dr J Reid.)

Investigations

The mid-stream urine specimen may show evidence of infection. Intravenous urography demonstrates a variety of changes from normal (in approximately one third of patients) to a non-functioning kidney. There may be features of chronic pyelonephritis with blunting of the calices, cortical scarring or atrophy. A micturating cystourethrogram is diagnostic (Fig. 36.32) showing contrast refluxing up into one or both kidneys. At cystoscopy the ureteric orifice may be laterally placed and widely open. There may also be a Hutch diverticulum immediately lateral to the ureteric orifice.[177] Otherwise cystoscopy is unhelpful. Assessment of renal function by urea and creatinine estimation and a renal isotope scan to determine the differential renal function and the presence of scarring are also usually necessary.

Management

The long-term effects of primary vesicoureteric reflux in adults are unknown. This is in contrast to vesicoureteric reflux in children where the condition is self-correcting before puberty in 80% of patients.[178] Low-dose prophylactic antibiotics should be advised in patients with primary reflux and recurrent urinary infections in whom there is no evidence of renal damage. Ureteric reimplantation should be reserved until there is objective evidence of deterioration of the upper tract.

Reimplantation of the affected ureters is recommended in primary reflux if there is evidence of reflux nephropathy, although nephroureterectomy is preferable when the kidney is contributing 15% or less to total renal function. In patients in whom secondary vesicoureteric reflux occurs initial treatment should aim at correcting the primary condition, for example in tuberculosis or bilharzia appropriate chemotherapy is given. When vesicoureteric reflux is secondary to endoscopic lower urinary tract surgery, treatment is usually unnecessary unless symptoms occur. Reimplantation or nephrectomy is considered either during or after treatment of the cause of the secondary reflux. There are many different operative procedures for correction of reflux: the most commonly performed is the Leadbetter–Politano approach[90] which is described in Chapter 37 (see Fig. 36.13). The Cohen[179] operation, in which the ureter is advanced through a submucosal tunnel to the opposite side of the trigone, is particularly suited to the reimplantation of ureters of normal calibre (Fig. 36.33).

In most cases where recurrent urinary infections occur, antibiotic prophylaxis is sufficient and it is rarely necessary to carry out ureteric reimplantation. An endoscopic submucosal injection of Teflon paste may prevent reflux in children, with good medium-term results at 4–10 years.[180]

STONE DISEASE

The presence of stones in the urinary tract is as old as civilization itself.[181] Until the middle of the 19th century, urinary tract stones occurred predominantly in the bladder. The disappearance of bladder stones is probably linked with the improvement in diet which took place at that time.[182] The reduction in the prevalence of bladder stones was mirrored by a rise in the prevalence of upper urinary tract stones; this was almost certainly the result of dietary changes as non-industrialized developing nations still have high incidences of bladder calculi.[183] The prevalence of calculi in the renal tract is difficult to assess as many patients with urolithiasis do not attend hospital. In the UK the incidence of symptomatic stones is between 27 and 34 per 100 000 population per annum,[184] being three times higher in the south than in the north,[185] and there is no doubt that the incidence of stones in the upper urinary tract is increasing. This appears to be related to a general increase in dietary protein intake which has been shown to decrease urinary

REFERENCES

177. Hutch J A J Urol 1961; 86: 390
178. Edwards D et al Br Med J 1977; 2: 285
179. Cohen S J Akt Urol 1975; 6: 1
180. Puri B J U 1995; 75: 126
181. Shaltock S G Trans Pathol Soc London 1905; 56: 275
182. Rogers A C, Spectre M In: Rowse S N (ed) Stone Disease. Grune & Stratton, New York 1987 p 57
183. Asper R, Schumiki O In: Ryall R J (ed) Urinary Stone. Churchill Livingstone, Edinburgh 1984
184. Power C et al In: Ryall R J (ed) Urinary Stone. Churchill Livingstone, Edinburgh 1984 p 86
185. Power C Br J Urol 1987; 59: 105

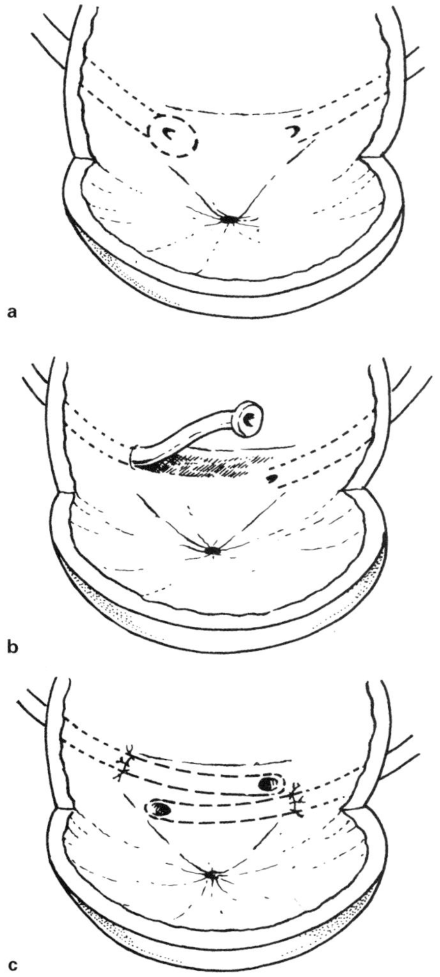

Fig. 36.33 Cohen ureteric advancement operation for vesicoureteric reflux. (a) The ureteric orifice is circumcised; (b) the ureter is mobilized and (c) reimplanted on the contralateral side via a submucosal tunnel.

citrate and increase the magnesium and phosphates in urine.[186] A further pointer to the effects of dietary protein on stone formation is the lower incidence of stones in vegetarians.[187]

1–12% of the population have stone disease, with an adult male to female ratio of 4:1. Interestingly, the ratio tends to be equal in children. The incidences of stone disease in Hispanics and Asians fall between those of white Caucasians and Blacks in the USA.[188] Stone disease is an important economic problem. The cost to the US taxpayer in 1993 for evaluation and treatment of stone disease was $1.23 billion, and the wage loss was another $139 million.[189]

The higher prevalence of renal stone in the tropics and the seasonal variation observed in the UK may be the result of dehydration and ultraviolet light.[190] The role of occupation is less obvious although people working in high ambient temperatures, e.g. glass plant workers, have been reported to have a higher incidence of stone disease.[191,192] The relatively high incidence of stones in members of the medical profession may be a reflection of dietary intake rather than occupation.[193] There appears to be a higher incidence of stones in the relatives of stone formers.[194] The risk of recurrence has been variously reported as between 35%[195] and 75%[196] at 10 years.

Table 36. 3 Geographical stone frequency

Stone composition	*Great Britain*	*USA*	*India*	*Israel*
Calcium stones*	72.8	73–81	92.9	78
$Mg\ NH_4\ PO_4$ (struvite)**	15.4	9–15	2.7	12
Uric acid	8	7.63	9	9
Cystine	2.8	0.88	0.4	2
Xanthine and others	1.0	1.5	2.6	—

*Calcium stones include: pure calcium oxalate monohydrate and dihydrate, pure calcium phosphate and mixed calcium oxalate and phosphate
**Struvite stones are calcium ammonium magnesium phosphate stones
From Walsh et al[202] with kind permission.

Composition of stones

The chemical composition of urinary calculi varies in different continents. The incidence of uric acid stones increases whilst the proportion of calcium oxalate stone falls on travelling in an easterly direction around the world.[197] Table 36.3 shows the relative percentage frequency (%) of the various types of stones encountered.

Calcium oxalate stones are hard, irregular and brittle and have the appearance of jackstones. Stones which are predominantly composed of calcium, magnesium and ammonium phosphate (triple phosphate stones) are soft, crumbly, white and tend to fill the pelvicaliceal system like the horns of a stag. They are invariably infected. Uric acid stones are virtually radiolucent and are usually yellow with fine projections on the surface. Cystine stones are very hard, white stones.

Aetiology and pathogenesis of stones

Most urinary tract stones form as a result of the interaction of numerous factors and the pathogenesis of stone formation is complex. It has become clear, however, that stone formation occurs as a result of the precipitation, growth and aggregation of various stone-forming salts in the urine.[199] Urine has the ability to keep a greater amount of solute in solution than water because of the presence of inhibitors of crystallization such as citrate,

REFERENCES

186. Tur J A Scand J Urol Nephrol 1991; 25: 311
187. Parry E D, Lister I S Lancet 1975; i: 1063
188. Soucie J Kidney Int 1994; 46(3): 893
189. Clark J Y J Urol 1995; 154(6): 2020
190. Prince C L J Urol 1956; 75: 209
191. Borghi L J Urol 1993; 150(6): 1757
192. Scott R Br J Urol 1985; 57: 491
193. Ljunghall S Br J Urol 1979; 51: 249
194. Johnson C M et al Kidney Int 1979; 16: 624
195. Williams R E Br J Urol 1963; 35: 416
196. Erickson S B in: Rowse S N (ed) Stone Disease: Diagnosis and Management. Grune & Stratton, New York 1987
197. Atsmon A et al Uric Acid Lithiasis. Elsevier, Amsterdam 1963
198. Walsh P C, Retnik A B, Stamey T A, Vaughan E D (eds) Campbell's Urology, 6th edn. W B Saunders, Philadelphia 1992 p 2111
199. Robertson W G, Peacock M Nephron 1980; 26: 105

mucoproteins, high molecular weight glycoproteins, amino acid alanine and the polyelectrolyte interactivity of the multiple ions in urine. These inhibitors form complexes with the solutes (e.g. calcium citrate) thus allowing more molecules to remain in solution. Crystal coating also inhibits aggregation of crystals by producing surface charges (zeta potentials making them repel each other rather than aggregate.)

The pathogenesis of three of the five types of calculi (uric acid, cystine and struvite) can be simply explained on the basis of supersaturation alone. Dissolution of cystine and uric acid crystals is linearly related to the pH of urine. If a predominantly acidic urine becomes oversaturated with either cystine or uric acid these substances will precipitate and form stones. Similarly, in urinary infections with organisms having the urease enzyme (e.g. *Proteus*, Klebsiella but not *E. coli*), urea is split into ammonia in an alkaline pH and when the concentration of ammonium, magnesium and calcium phosphate exceeds the saturation product triple phosphate (staghorn) stones are formed.

Of the remaining two types (xanthine and calcium), xanthine calculi are the result of hereditary xanthinuria and are extremely rare. The modern theories on the pathogenesis of calcium stone disease, both oxalate and phosphate, are based on either:

1. Supersaturation/crystallization.
2. Inhibitor deficiency.
3. Matrix initiation.
4. Epitaxy, or a combination of these factors.

Crystallization occurs when the supersaturated active molecules no longer flow randomly and in a dissociated manner but cluster and form a lattice shaped crystal structure which is characteristic of that crystal. These crystals then aggregate and grow. The structure of certain crystal lattices is such that they allow one type of crystal to grow on another (e.g. calcium oxalate and uric acid), a phenomenon called epitaxy. In patients with idiopathic calcium lithiasis, a non-crystalline protein-like matrix has been demonstrated in the renal tubules complexed to crystals which mimic the structure of larger calcium calculi.[200] This has led to the belief by some workers[201,202] that matrix may be the initiator of calcium lithiasis. It constitutes about 3% by weight of most calcium calculi, and purely matrix stones seen in a setting of infection show a matrix composition of over 65% by weight. Matrix comprises of hexosamine and bound water. It is different from uromucoid, which contains sialic acid, and is perhaps cleaved from it by the renal enzyme sialidase.

Inhibitor deficiency has assumed increasing importance in calcium stone formation as the supersaturation and crystallization theory does not explain calcium lithiasis on its own. Many normal individuals pass a urine that is supersaturated with the solutes mentioned above and yet do not form stones. It has been shown that urinary citrate is lower in recurrent stone formers than in controls.[203]

The site of origin of the crystals remains unknown—it is not clear whether they arise in the renal tubular lumen or in the tubular epithelial cell. Animal experiments[204] show that large intratubular crystals form within a completely cell-lined tubule. Other studies[205] suggest that the rapid adherence of calcium oxalate monohydrate crystals to the apical surface of the tubular epithelial cell may be important. Older theories also suggest similar findings: Randall[206] observed the presence of papillary calcification in kidneys removed at autopsy (Randall's plaques). The appearances represent calcium deposition on the basement membrane of the collecting ducts as result of degenerative changes. Further calcium deposition produces a small irregular depression on the surface of the papilla which ulcerates; finally a deposit is seen on the plaque which represents the beginning of a renal stone. Though many studies[207] have confirmed the presence of Randall's plaques, they have been demonstrated in almost all kidneys and there is no correlation between the degree of calcification and the presence of urinary stone disease. Carr's concretions theory[208] suggests that Randall's plaques are aggregations of microscopic calculi rather than degenerative lesions of the papilla. Microradiological techniques may be used to demonstrate that almost all kidneys contain microscopic opacities. Concretions, microscopic calculi and true stones have all been observed. Impairment of the lymphatic drainage by inflammation or fibrosis prevents removal of the concretions by the lymphatics and the resulting coalescence produces stones.

Normal urine is not a static solution. While nucleation and aggregation occurs rapidly, crystal growth takes longer. The mean transit time from the nephron to the renal pelvis is 3–5 minutes and these crystals then flow into the bladder where they lie for up to 6 hours. The lumen of the collecting duct is 50–200 μm and an aggregated crystal may block and then grow at the level of the renal papilla. To block or lodge in the ureter it should be at least 2 mm in diameter, and in the bladder it should be greater than 6 mm. Once lodged, the crystal can then grow, adding layers of crystals which are not necessarily of the same type, and form an obstructing calculus. When the drainage of the kidney is impaired by congenital abnormalities such as horseshoe kidney, medullary sponge kidney, congenital hydrocalicosis, pelviureteric junction obstruction or megaureter, then the resultant sluggish or stagnant urine facilitates crystal formation and retention. Stagnant urine also predisposes to infection and precipitation of triple phosphate crystals.

In medullary sponge kidney there is dilatation of the terminal collecting ducts in the pyramids with associated cysts and clefts, both of which are lined by collecting duct epithelium and communicate with expanded calices. Stones generally form within the dilated tubules and cysts and are composed of calcium phosphate, indicating that the process may be an extension of intratubular calcification.[209]

REFERENCES

200. Malek R S J Urol 1973; 109: 551
201. Watanabe T J Exp Med 1972; 107: 345
202. Lanzalaco A C J Urol 1988; 139: 190
203. Cupisti A Nephron 1992; 62: 73
204. Boeve E R J Urol 1993; 149: 893
205. Lieske J C Proc Natl Acad Sci USA 1994; 91: 6987
206. Randall A Ann Surg 1937; 105: 1009
207. Editorial Lancet 1982; ii: 588
208. Carr R J Br J Urol 1954; 26: 105
209. Boonstra C E, Jackson C E Ann Int Med 1965; 63: 468

The biochemical abnormalities associated with individual stone types and known aetiologies of individual stone types are discussed below.

Calcium oxalate stones

Investigation of many patients fails to reveal any demonstrable abnormality of calcium metabolism.[210] In those patients in whom an abnormality is present, this is usually hypercalciuria which may be dietary, absorptive, resorptive or tubular in origin. Dietary hypercalciuria does not occur unless the intake of calcium is in excess of 30 mmol.[211] The absorption of calcium is increased by high dietary phosphorus, sugars and animal protein intake and is reduced by phytate and a high dietary fibre. Reduction in dietary calcium alone, however, offers no benefit in reducing the risk of recurrent stone formation.[212] Indeed in some studies it has been shown that higher calcium intake reduces the risk by binding oxalates in the gut.[213] Absorptive hypercalciuria may be either Type I (hypercalciuric on a low calcium diet) or Type II (hypercalciuric on a normal calcium diet). In this group as a whole the serum calcium and fasting urinary calcium are normal, as is the bone density. On calcium loading, however, the urinary Ca:creatinine ratio is greater than 0.2.[214]

Resorptive hypercalciuria (renal leak) occurs when the renal tubules fail to reabsorb the filtered calcium. Normally 47 g of calcium is filtered daily and 98–99% of this is reabsorbed. In patients with a renal leak, the serum calcium is normal but the fasting urinary calcium to creatinine ratio is raised to greater than 0.11. A type of resorptive hypercalciuria occurs with a negative bone balance (e.g. osteoporosis, hyperparathyroidism, bony metastasis, multiple myeloma) and thus occurs in patients who are immobilized for any length of time; a higher calcium load is presented to the tubules and hypercalciuria ensues.[215] There is a high fasting calcium:creatinine ratio, urinary hydroxyprolene excretion is elevated and the serum calcium is raised.

Urinary oxalate is now considered to be at least ten times more important in calcium lithiasis than either calcium or phosphate.[216] The reason is clear: the ratio of calcium to oxalate in urine is about 20:1. A considerable increase in calcium only produces a moderate increase in risk of collision between the two molecules while a small increase in urinary oxalate markedly increases the risk of collision.[217] The endogenous metabolism of glycolate, glycoxylate and ascorbic acid accounts for 80–90% of urinary oxalate while 10% comes from the diet. Only 3–7% of the dietary oxalate is absorbed normally. Hyperoxaluria above 0.45 mmol/24 h is seen in 20–30% of patients with stone disease. An increase in the dietary oxalates is the main culprit in hyperoxaluria and calcium lithiasis. Dietary control is the key to reducing the risk of recurrent stone formation. Primary hyperoxaluria occurs as an autosomal recessive genetic disorder in which glyoxalase or hydroxypyruvate fails to metabolize oxalates. Renal failure develops early in the disease and is associated with a poor prognosis.[218] More commonly, however, hyperoxaluria is the result of extensive small bowel resection or malabsorption syndrome—the so-called enteric hyperoxaluria.[219]

Uric acid excretion is usually normal although occasionally it may be increased.[220] This is important as a rise in the concentration of urinary uric acid inhibits the production of acid mucopolysaccharides and thus increases the overall tendency to crystal formation. Additionally it may form a nidus for calcium oxalate stones.

Hyperparathyroidism is present in 2–3% of calcium stone formers.[221] The primary abnormality is an increase in production of parathormone resulting in increased production of 1,25 dihydroxy vitamin D3 which increases intestinal calcium absorption (see Chapter 19). Secondary hyperoxaluria occurs because of the increased calcium absorption. Parathormone also acts directly on bone to increase calcium resorption, and the urinary pH is high because of the increased excretion of bicarbonate by the kidney.

Renal tubular acidosis results in an inability to excrete acid urine. It is the Type I (distal) disorder that is associated with stone disease. The failure to secrete hydrogen ions by the distal tubule is compensated by an increased secretion of potassium, sodium and calcium. The body conserves sodium via the aldosterone mechanism and thus a picture of hyperchloraemia, hypokalaemia and hypercalciuria is seen. This results in the formation of calcium phosphate stones. These patients fail to produce a urinary pH lower than 5.3 in response to an acid load.

Triple phosphate stones

Urinary infection with a urea-splitting organism (usually Proteus) produces an alkaline urine which increases the precipitation of calcium phosphate and magnesium ammonium phosphate. Precipitation is further increased by the high ammonium concentration in the urine. The concentration of citrate and pyrophosphate, which is a potent inhibitor of calcium phosphate crystallization, is low.

Uric acid stones

The incidence of uric acid stones is increasing. The majority are idiopathic and occur in patients who do not have elevated plasma uric acids although they do have persistently acidic urine. Included in this group are patients with an ileostomy and those with chronic diarrhoea. A quarter of all patients with gout develop urate stones[222] as do 40% of patients with myeloproliferative disorders. Increased DNA turnover results in increased uric acid production. Similarly, dietary protein excess and meat eating predispose to uric acid calculi. The urinary excretion of uric acid is high and there is

REFERENCES

210. Adams N D J Clin Endocrinol Metab 1979; 48: 1008
211. Christensson T et al Acta Med Scand 1976; 200: 131
212. Lemann J N Engl J Med 1993; 328: 880
213. Curhan G C N Engl J Med 1993; 328: 833
214. Pak, C Y J Clin Invest 1974; 54: 387
215. Wilson D M In: Rowse S N (ed) Stone Disease: Diagnosis and Management. Grune & Stratton, New York 1987
216. Robertson W G Br J Urol 1978; 50: 449
217. Ito H Curr Opin Urol 1995; 5: 218
218. Dowling R H et al Lancet 1971; i: 1103
219. Yu T F J Urol 1981; 81: 424
220. Heath H III et al N Engl J Med 1980; 302: 189
221. Harrington T M Mayo Clin Proc 1983; 58: 354
222. Norman R W et al J Urol 1984; 132: 1137

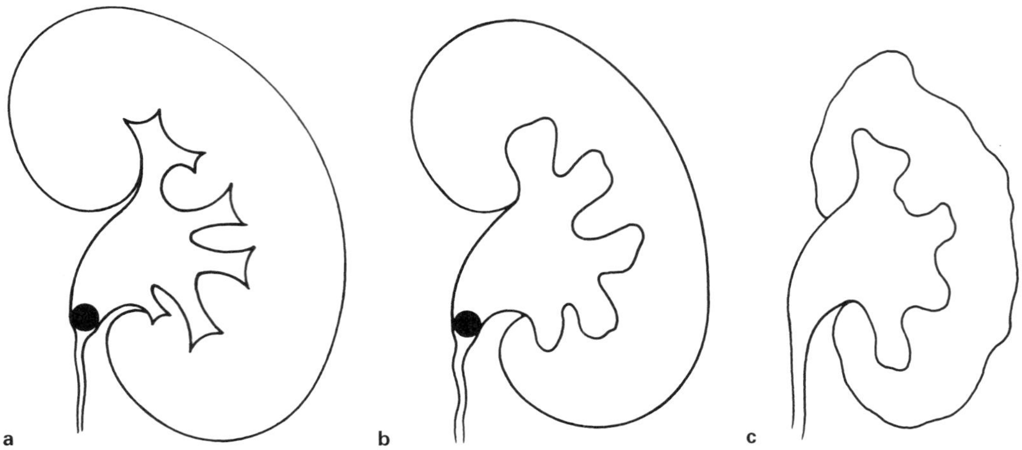

Fig. 36.34 Effects of obstruction on the urinary tract. Obstructive atrophy develops and does not resolve on relief of the obstruction.

an associated low urinary pH and acid mucopolysaccharide concentration.

Cystine stones

Cystine stones occur as a result of an autosomal recessive disorder in which there is a defect in the tubular reabsorption of cystine, lysine, arginine and ornithine. Stone formation is far more common in homozygotes where excretion of cystine may be as high as 4200 μmol/l. A supersaturated solution occurs leading to spontaneous crystalluria. As indicated earlier, the solubility of cystine is doubled at a pH of 7.8.

The two other conditions which need to be discussed prior to considering the clinical features of stones are renal papillary necrosis and nephrocalcinosis.

Renal papillary necrosis

Renal papillary necrosis affects the distal portion of the renal pyramids; it involves a number of papillae and is often bilateral. It is seen in association with analgesic abuse, diabetes and severe infection. Caliectasis and renal scarring occur and the remaining pyramids may show evidence of nephrocalcinosis. The condition is caused by infarction of the pyramids as a result of coexisting arteriosclerosis or an acute vasculitis. There is an associated interstitial nephritis.

Nephrocalcinosis

Nephrocalcinosis is defined as small diffuse calcifications seen in the renal parenchyma rather than in the collecting system; it may be the result of congenital abnormalities or hypercalcaemia caused by metabolic diseases like hyperparathyroidism.

Pathophysiological changes associated with stone disease

These should be distinguished from the anatomical abnormalities which contribute to stone formation, and are mainly consequent upon the presence of the stone causing obstruction or from the direct contact of the stone with the urothelium. Infection may also occur independently of the presence of obstruction.

Obstruction

If a stone impacts in the neck of a calix, in the ureteropelvic junction or ureter, the hydrostatic pressure within the collecting system increases to produce considerable dilatation and subsequent obstructive atrophy of the overlying cortex. Varying degrees of parenchymal loss occur depending upon the degree of obstruction and the length of time for which it is present. Urine retained within the calix may be sterile or may become secondarily infected producing a pyelonephrosis. Depending upon the level of obstruction, a hydrocalicosis, hydronephrosis or hydroureter may develop (Fig. 36.34).

Inflammation and infection

Focal areas of interstitial nephritis are invariably present in all kidneys containing a stone.[223] Localized urinary infection in an obstructed calix produces a pyocalix which may discharge into the renal parenchyma to produce a perinephric abscess. Similarly, obstruction of the ureteropelvic junction or ureter results in a pyonephrosis in the presence of infected urine. Xanthomatous pyelonephritis is an important sequel of renal stones as it may be mistaken for carcinoma. The presence of infected urine without obstruction may produce changes of acute or chronic pyelonephritis with subsequent scarring of the renal cortex.

Clinical features

Renal stones may present insidiously or dramatically. Stone disease may be symptomless, the presence of stone being an incidental finding during the investigation of some other symptom

REFERENCES

223. Harrison D A, Inglis J A, Tolley D A J Clin Pathol 1988; 41: 971

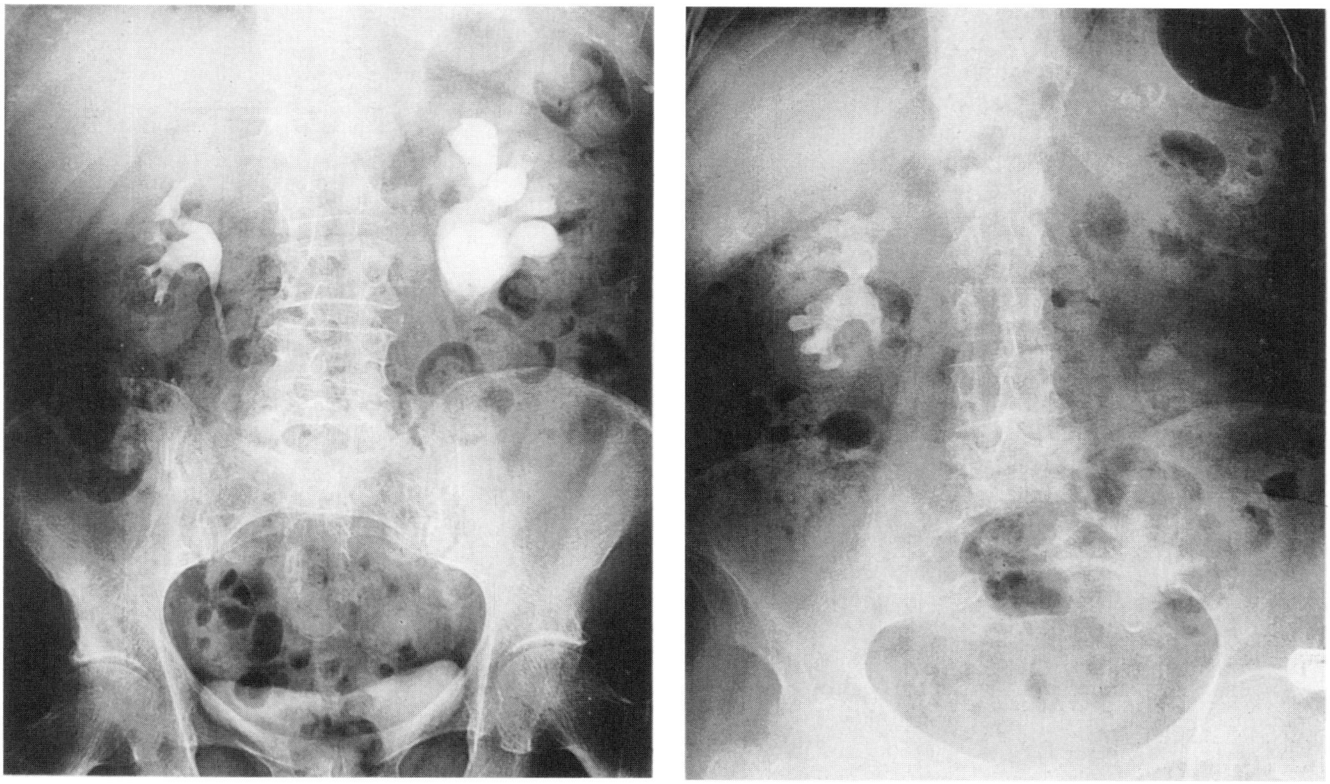

a b

Fig. 36.35 (**a**) Renal stone disease. Intravenous urogram film shows a laminated stone in the left renal pelvis causing hydronephrosis. Courtesy of Dr J Reid. (**b**) Right staghorn calculus. Abdominal radiograph showing complex right renal staghorn calculus. Gallstones are also present. Courtesy of Dr J Reid.

(Fig. 36.35); alternatively it may present as an emergency with acute ureteric colic. Between these two extremes there may be varying degrees of pain, haematuria, urinary infection and renal failure. The severity and amount of pain associated with stones depend upon their size, position and mobility. Thus, paradoxically, a small mobile stone may produce more symptoms than a large immobile staghorn calculus. Other features which influence symptoms are urinary tract obstruction and urinary infection. There may be a history of previous stone disease and urinary infection, and in some patients a family history may also be elicited. The patient's dietary habits should be elucidated, especially with regard to intake of animal protein and calcium-containing foods such as milk and alkalis. There may also be a history of other illnesses such as osteoporosis or a recent prolonged period of recumbency.

Patients with Munchausen's syndrome may sometimes present with symptoms suggestive of ureteric colic. It can be very difficult to differentiate between true ureteric colic and Munchausen's syndrome but the presence of loin pain in a patient with a scarred abdomen working away from home, the absence of blood in the urine and a normal intravenous urogram should alert the clinician to this possibility.

Examination

The characteristic fetal position may be observed in patients with acute ureteric colic; the patient is often unable to lie still and may be vomiting. Tenderness in the renal angle may be elicited. It is important in patients with chronic pain to exclude musculoskeletal disorders by appropriate examination of the spine and lower limbs. The urine should always be tested to determine the presence of blood, leucocytes and nitrites where possible.

Differential diagnosis

Stone disease must be distinguished from other urinary tract pathologies such as idiopathic hydronephrosis, pyelonephritis or perinephric abscess. The clinical features of obstruction and stone disease can often only be differentiated by further investigation. The presence of a fever, pus cells in the urine and a raised white cell count may be suggestive of infection, but in all patients presenting with renal pain further investigation is necessary to establish the diagnosis. Ureteric colic must also be distinguished from biliary colic, appendicular colic, small or large bowel obstruction, and a leaking abdominal aortic aneurysm. In these conditions additional features in the history, together with additional physical signs such as the presence of abdominal tenderness, distension or peritonism are often useful indicators of the cause of the pain. Differentiation from muscular pains related to spinal disorders is also important and a full examination of the spine, reflexes and straight leg raising may be necessary.

Investigations

Investigations are necessary to confirm the primary diagnosis and to establish the aetiology and risk of recurrent stone formation. Intravenous urography is the ideal primary investigation. A plain abdominal radiograph will at best show the presence of calcification, and at worst the stone will not be visualized; this radiograph gives no information about the presence of obstruction or the anatomy of the urinary tract. In patients with suspected ureteric colic, urgent urography is the only way to diagnose the presence of urinary tract stones with certainty: small stones are often passed quite quickly and if an intravenous urogram is delayed until the pain has settled, the radiographic appearances may well have returned to normal and the opportunity to make the diagnosis with certainty is lost. The presence of a radiolucent uric acid stone can only be ascertained with the aid of intravenous urography.

The potential disadvantage of obtaining poor-quality radiographs because of gaseous distension of the bowel when the investigation is performed as an emergency is far outweighed by the information obtained which allows the appropriate treatment to be planned. In addition, the presence of a normal urogram during an attack of colic implies that the clinical diagnosis is incorrect. The urogram can be deferred if there is an obvious opacity in the line of the ureter and an emergency ultrasound shows dilatation of the pelvicaliceal system on the affected side. An intravenous urogram should, however, eventually be carried out in all patients suspected of having urinary tract stone disease as it provides invaluable information about possible predisposing anatomical causes and allows the correct treatment of stones to be planned. A radioisotope scan assesses the degree of function and degree of obstruction in patients in whom these appear to be impaired on the intravenous urogram.

The renal function is assessed by estimation of the urea, electrolytes, creatinine and creatinine clearance where appropriate. Serum calcium, phosphate and uric acid levels are obtained to try to find a cause. A mid-stream specimen of urine is sent for culture to determine the presence of infection. Two 24 h urine collections should be made to determine whether or not there are any underlying biochemical abnormalities and to determine the risk of further stone formation.

Treatment

The treatment of patients with renal stones has two aims: the specific treatment of the stone and the correction of anatomical or metabolic abnormalities which may predispose to recurrent stone formation. Each aspect is equally important as it should be remembered that up to 70% of stone formers will develop a recurrence within 10 years.[196]

In the past decade the active approach to the management of urinary stone disease has undergone a dramatic change. The development of percutaneous renal surgery, retrograde ureteroscopy and extracorporeal shock-wave lithotripsy has broadened the indications for intervention. In specialized stone centres where an integrated approach to treatment is possible, open surgery is the exception.[224] In the age of minimally invasive surgery for urinary tract stones, it should be remembered that 80% of all stones that form within the urinary tract will pass spontaneously[225] but this must be balanced by the knowledge that three quarters of patients with stone disease have evidence of interstitial nephritis irrespective of symptoms.[226]

Expectant treatment

Most small (< 5 mm in diameter) symptomless renal stones in an unobstructed non-infected kidney do not require removal. Patients should be followed by annual plain radiographs of the urinary tract to monitor the size and position of the stone. The exception to this rule is the professional pilot or diver who requires removal of even symptomless stones in order to continue his or her occupation. An increase in size of the stone or the development of symptoms may alter the decision to treat it expectantly.

There are no rules governing whether a ureteric calculus will pass spontaneously. Half the patients with symptomatic ureteric stones pass their stones within 48 h of the onset of symptoms and most have passed within 7 days.[227] In general terms, 90% of stones which are less than 4 mm in diameter pass spontaneously; two thirds of those between 4 and 6 mm pass spontaneously, and over three quarters of stones greater than this size fail to pass.[227] There should therefore be a trial of expectant therapy in all patients with ureteric stones less than 6 mm in diameter providing the ureter is unobstructed. Pain is relieved by adequate doses of sodium diclofenac although pethidine may very rarely be necessary. An anti-emetic may also be required. There is no evidence that a forced diuresis increases the likelihood of the spontaneous passage of the stone as the contralateral normal kidney excretes the bulk of the fluid load. In the absence of obstruction or increasing symptoms, such expectant therapy may be continued indefinitely.

It is permissible to carry out a trial of expectant therapy in patients with small stones in the presence of obstruction, but the period for which it should be continued is ill defined. The degree of obstruction may be monitored by radioisotope renography. Although complete functional recovery may occur even after complete obstruction has been present for 10 days, it is more prudent to recommend early removal of ureteric stones in the presence of even mild degrees of obstruction, especially in view of the newer and less invasive methods of stone removal. The indications for intervention in patients with acute ureteric colic are laid out in Table 36.4.

Interventional management

In the past 10 years the active approach to the management of urinary stone disease has undergone a dramatic change. This applies equally to the management of renal and ureteric stones, and an open operation is no longer regarded as the treatment of choice in patients for whom intervention is required.

REFERENCES

224. Das G et al Br J Urol 1988; 62: 301
225. Sandegard E Acta Chir Scand 1956; suppl: 219
226. Harrison D et al J Clin Pathol 1988; 41: 971
227. Drach G W Urol Clin North Am 1983; 10: 709

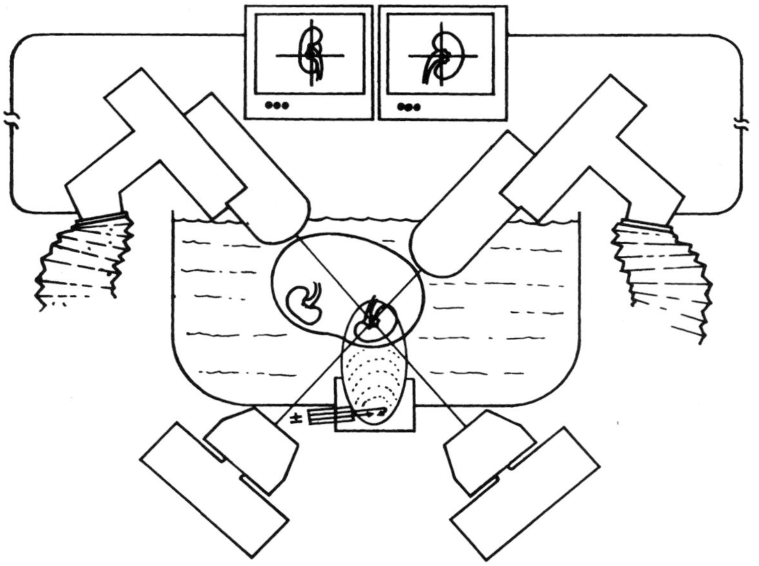

Fig. 36.36 Schematic diagram illustrating principles of extracorporeal shock-wave lithotripsy first used in the Dornier lithotriptor. Courtesy of Dornier System Medical Systems, West Germany.

Table 36.4 Indications for intervention in patients with ureteric colic

Absolute
Stone obstructing a solitary kidney
Obstructing stone with evidence of sepsis, fever, tachycardia, leucocytosis
Partial obstruction with deteriorating renal function
Relative
Stone not expected to pass, e.g. stone > 6 mm
Continuous pain
Failure to pass in spite of 'adequate' period of observation
Social reasons, e.g. pilots with 4–5 mm calculus, etc.

The options now available are:

1. Extracorporeal shock-wave lithotripsy.
2. Endoscopic or percutaneous stone fragmentation with intracorporeal lithotripsy and mechanical extraction.
3. Open surgical procedures.

These options should be viewed in the context of integrated stone management. For optimum results patients with renal stones should be treated in a stone centre with access to all these methods of treatment.

Extracorporeal shock-wave lithotripsy

The principle of shock-wave disintegration of urinary tract stones was developed over a 10-year period by the Dornier Aircraft Company and the University of Munich. The technique was developed and applied to patients by Eisenberger, Schmidt and Chaussy.[228] All lithotripsy machines involve four principles:

1. Generation of the shock wave (electrohydraulic, piezoelectric, electromagnetic).
2. Focussing of the energy wave (metal ellipsoid or mounted gantry).
3. Imaging of the target (stone) either by X-rays or ultrasound in real time.
4. Coupling of image and energy delivery.

Lithotripsy is based on the fact that the body comprises over 65% of water and there is no loss of energy if the shock wave travels through the same medium. The shock wave is generated underwater and the patient's affected side is kept in contact with the water bath or water-filled cushion. The shock wave is then focussed by an ellipsoid reflector or gantry to a second focus with a resulting high density of energy at the second focus. This is achieved by a two-dimensional X-ray imaging system or by real time in-line ultrasound. On targeting the stone, the shock waves are fired at variable intensity. The frequency is gated to the patient's heart rate to prevent arrhythmias. The shock waves pulverize the stone into very small fragments which are then voided. Epidural or general anaesthesia was required with the earlier machines (Fig. 36.36) but now analgesia-free lithotripsy is not uncommon. Stones in the kidney or the ureter can now be targeted fairly easily.

Since the unequivocal demonstration of the efficacy of this technique around the world,[229] newer-generation lithotriptors using different methods of focusing and different shock-wave sources are being produced.[230]

Effects of lithotripsy on the patient and kidney. In the short term there may be transient haematuria, flank pain, ecchymosis at the skin site, intrarenal haematomata or oedema of the treated kidney manifested by changes in tubular function and increased excretion of β_2-microglobulin, microalbumin and other

REFERENCES

228. Chaussy C Extracorporeal Shock Wave Lithotripsy. Karger, Munich 1982
229. Fuchs G et al Eur Urol 1985; II: 145
230. Coptcoat M J et al Lithotripsy 2. BDI Publishing, London 1987

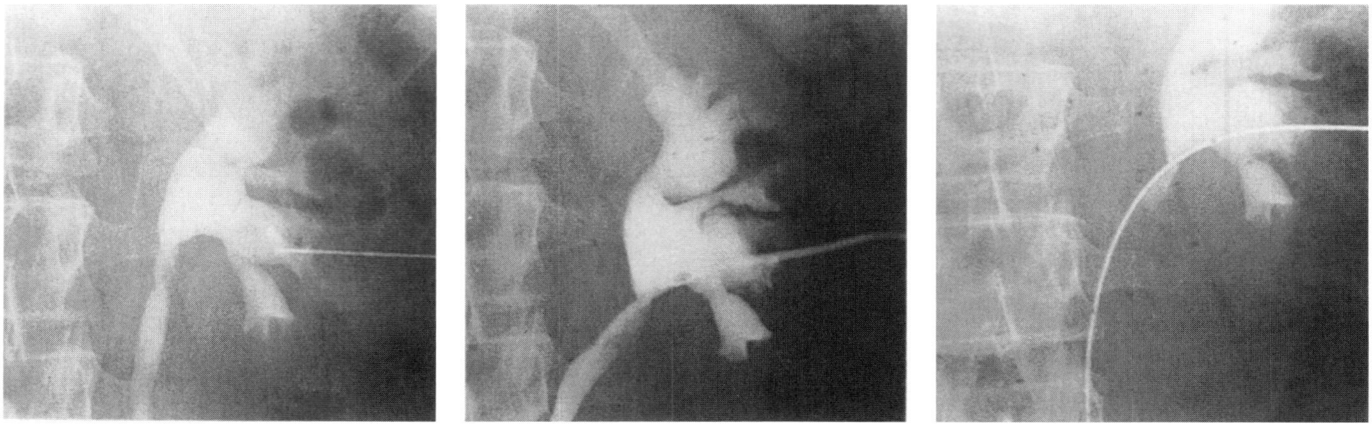

a b c

Fig. 36.37 Percutaneous nephrostomy. Access to the kidney is gained by puncture of a lower pole calix. The track thus formed is dilated over a guide-wire and a small catheter is inserted. Courtesy of Dr J Reid. **(a)** A fine-gauge needle is inserted into opacified lower calix; **(b)** a guide-wire is inserted through calix and stabilized in the ureter; **(c)** an 8 French gauge catheter is inserted over the guide-wire after track dilatation.

urinary enzymes such as γ-glutamyl transferase and N-acetyl-D-glucosaminidase in the urine after a session of lithotripsy. These settle in 3–7 days and are dependent on the total number of shock waves delivered. The glomerular filtration rate drops immediately after lithotripsy but returns to baseline after 3 weeks.[231] In the long term the fear of producing a higher risk of hypertension has not been proven. Animal experimental evidence indicates that segmental and focal interstitial fibrosis occurs if higher than clinically recommended energy levels are used.

Lithotripsy is contraindicated in pregnancy. Patients with pacemakers can be treated with lithotripsy but adequate precautions must be taken, especially if a dual chamber pacemaker is implanted as this will need to be reprogrammed to the ventricular mode. Patients on anticoagulant or aspirin therapy should stop it prior to lithotripsy to allow platelet and coagulation function to return to normal.

Percutaneous nephrolithotomy

This technique permits the removal of stones from the kidney and ureter by the creation of a track between the skin surface and the collecting system of the kidney[232] (Fig. 36.37). The track is dilated to allow the introduction of a rigid nephroscope into the kidney and the stone is then removed intact with forceps or reduced in size by the use of direct application of intracorporeal ultrasound or electrohydraulic lithotripsy.

Ureterorenoscopy

The development of the rigid ureteroscope allows the removal of many ureteric calculi from the lower third of the ureter under vision.[233] If the stone is too large to be removed in this way, then it may be disintegrated with intracorporeal laser, ultrasound or electrohydraulic lithotripsy. The fragments may be allowed to pass or are extracted under vision using a stone basket or graspers. Newer fibreoptic flexible ureteroscopes are now available which permit the removal of stones in the upper and middle third of the ureter.

Stone baskets

The technique of 'blind basketing' of ureteric stones has a number of disadvantages. The success rate using this technique is considerably lower than that using ureteroscopy[234] and there is a much greater risk of perforating the ureter, causing mucosal stripping or even avulsion than there is using a basket under direct vision. It is possible to push the stone back into the kidney with fluoroscopic control under anaesthesia if it proves impossible to remove a ureteric stone by the methods outlined above. The stone can then be removed by percutaneous nephrolithotomy or disintegrated with extracorporeal shock-wave lithotripsy (the push–bang technique).[235]

Open surgery

This is confined to the occasional nephrectomy for a non-functioning kidney or to an extended pyelolithotomy or pyelolithotomy with radial nephrotomies in patients with complex staghorn calculus disease.[236] Maximum exposure of the kidney is obtained by a supracostal approach with full mobilization of the kidney.

On the rare occasions that a ureteric stone is impacted or too large to remove by the methods outlined above, open or laparoscopic ureterolithotomy is still required. When a stone is impacted in the upper third of the ureter it is best exposed through a loin incision; for stones in the mid third the approach should be similar. The lower third is the most difficult portion of the ureter to reach and is best approached extraperitoneally through a paramedian, Pfannenstiel or oblique muscle-cutting incision. The stone is removed through a longitudinal incision in the ureter. A tube drain

REFERENCES

231. Kaude J V Am J Roentgenol 1985; 145: 305
232. Alken P et al J Urol 1981; 125: 463
233. Lyon E S et al Urology 1984; 23 (suppl): 29
234. Tolley D A Br J Urol 1987; 59: 402
235. Tolley D A Br J Urol 1989; 64: 130
236. Blandy J P, Singh N J Urol 1976; 115: 505

should be left in the retroperitoneum and brought out through a separate stab wound and removed after a few days.

Results of interventional management

In general, kidney stones less than 2 cm in diameter are best treated by extracorporeal shock-wave lithotripsy. Stone-free rates vary but approximately 85% of patients can be expected to be stone-free at 3 months.[237] Stones between 2 and 3 cm in diameter may be treated by extracorporeal shock-wave lithotripsy or percutaneous nephrolithotomy[238] but the best results for stones larger than 3 cm in diameter are obtained by primary percutaneous nephrolithotomy, reserving extracorporeal shock-wave lithotripsy to treat residual fragments.[239] High stone-free rates for patients with staghorn calculi can also be achieved by using an integrated method of treatment.[240] Stones in the upper or middle third of the ureter may be treated with lithotripsy in situ as first choice, employing ureteroscopy and intracorporeal lithotripsy or the push–bang technique (pushing the stone back into the kidney and then fragmenting it with ESWL) if this fails. For lower third ureteric calculi both lithotripsy and ureteroscopy are reasonable options, although higher stone-free rates are obtained with primary ureteroscopy.

Complications of interventional management

The complications of extracorporeal shock-wave lithotripsy are few: a quarter of the patients develop ureteric colic from stone fragments, and transient haematuria is inevitable.[241] Occasionally, stone fragments obstruct the ureter (Steinstrasse) and require endscopic removal. The risk of this complication can be minimized by the insertion of a self-retaining ureteric stent before commencing treatment of stones greater than 2 cm in size. Complications of percutaneous nephrolithotomy relate mainly to bleeding during the procedure and perforation of the renal pelvis. The mortality rate is extremely low.[240] The most significant complication following ureteroscopy is the development of a ureteric stricture, which is generally the result of a traumatic introduction of the ureteroscope. Perforation of the ureter, if it occurs, should be managed by ureteric stenting and generally does not cause long-term problems.

Medical management of stone disease

For all patients and especially those in whom no underlying metabolic disorder is found, an increased fluid intake is the single most important factor in minimizing recurrent stone disease. The more dilute the urine, the less risk there is of precipitation of solutes; it has also been demonstrated that crystalluria is more common in summer than in winter.[242] It must be emphasized that patients should aim to increase urine flow throughout the 24-hour period and they must be encouraged to drink more after playing strenuous sports or when travelling to a hot country where perspiration is greater. The recurrence rate is now recognized to be higher if the patient is not initially stone free.[243]

Idiopathic hypercalciuria may be controlled by the use of a thiazide diuretic (bendrofluazide 5 mg/day).[244] Thiazide diuretics act upon the renal tubules by impairing calcium excretion. Sodium cellulose phosphate combines with calcium in the intestine, preventing absorption of dietary calcium and so reducing urinary calcium. In order to be effective this treatment must be taken approximately 30 minutes before a meal and is associated with the development of diarrhoea in a quarter of the patients.[245] When the urinary or plasma urate levels are elevated in association with hypercalciuria, the prescription of a small dose of allopurinol has been claimed to lower the stone recurrence rate.[246] Potassium citrate may also be effective.[247] Hypercalcaemia is often caused by primary hyperparathyroidism, the management of which is discussed elsewhere (see Chapter 19). Patients with urinary infection and stones should be treated for the infection, which is often from a Gram-negative coliform organism. Predisposing factors should be sought and corrected.

Uric acid stones are uncommon in the UK, accounting for approximately 8% of all stones.[248] It is usually possible to prevent further uric acid stone formation and also to dissolve existing stones by increasing the fluid intake, restricting purine-rich foods and alkalinizing the urine with sodium bicarbonate 3–6 g daily. Allopurinol in a dose of 200–400 mg/day reduces both the plasma and urinary urate and can be prescribed.

Cystine stones may be dissolved in situ by increasing the patient's fluid intake, alkalinizing the urine and by the administration of penicillamine or α-mercaptopropionglycine which has fewer side-effects. This is the one type of stone for which medical treatment is unequivocally effective.[249] Careful assessment of the metabolic aspects of renal stone disease together with an integrated surgical approach should result in high stone-free rates with a reduced risk of stone recurrence.

RENAL TUMOURS

Renal tumours may be classified according to the aggressiveness of the tumour. Most renal tumours should be regarded as malignant; there are very few benign kidney tumours (Table 36.5). The subsequent section initially concentrates on the two most common renal tumours: Wilms' tumour and renal cell carcinoma. A brief description of the rarer types of renal tumour is then given.

REFERENCES

237. Grace P A et al Br J Urol 1989; 64: 117
238. Neerhut G J et al Br J Urol 1989; 64: 5
239. Lingerman J E In: Riehle R A Jr (ed) Principles of Extracorporeal Shock Wave Lithotripsy. Churchill Livingstone, New York 1987 p 193
240. Segura J W et al Urol 1985; 134: 1077
241. Khan R I J Urol 1986; 135: 239
242. Robertson W G et al Clin Sci Mol Med 1975; 49: 597
243. Newman DM 1988 In: Lingeman J E, Newman D M Shock Wave Lithotripsy. Plenum Press, New York p 159
244. Yendt E R Can Med Soc J 1970; 102: 479
245. Pak C Y C Calcium Urolithiasis. Plenum Press, New York 1978 p 56
246. Coe F L Ann Intern Med 1977; 87: 404
247. Pak C Y C, Peterson R Arch Intern Med 1986; 146: 863
248. Prince C L, Sciardino P L, Wolan C T J Urol 1956; 75: 209
249. Dahlberg P J Mayo Clin Proc 1977; 52: 533

Table 36.5 Classification of renal tumours

Benign tumours
Adenoma
Fibroma
Oncocytoma
Angiomyolipoma
Juxtaglomerular tumour
Malignant tumours
Nephroblastoma (Wilms' tumour)
Primary renal cell carcinoma
Carcinosarcoma
Leiomyosarcoma
Liposarcoma
Urothelial tumours
Metastatic tumour
Lung, breast and uterus

Nephroblastoma (Wilms' tumour)

Incidence

Wilms' tumour is the most common tumour of the urinary system in childhood and is responsible for 8% of all solid tumours in children. The peak incidence is between 3 and 4 years of age although cases have been recorded in neonates[250] and in adolescents.[251] Between 5 and 10% are bilateral,[252] and males and females are almost equally affected.

Aetiology

Nephroblastoma may be hereditary or sporadic. Nephroblastoma results from the abnormal proliferation of the metanephric blastema and its failure to differentiate into tubules and glomeruli. It is thus an embryonic tumour. In the hereditary group the tumour is thought to result from a loss of maternal chromosome 11 alleles and a loss of function of a recessive tumour suppressor gene in the 11p13 region.[253] It is associated with congenital anomalies such as hypospadias, non-familial aniridia, hemi-hypertrophy of the body and Beckwith–Wiedemann syndrome (macroglossia, omphalocele, mental retardation and organomegaly).[254]

Pathology

Gross features

The tumour is large and is frequently separated from the remainder of the kidney by a fibrous pseudocapsule. In aggressive tumours, the capsule is breached so that the tumour invades the kidney and adjacent structures. The tumour is often lobulated with a solid creamy-white appearance. It may also contain areas of necrosis and haemorrhage.

Microscopic appearances

There is considerable variation in tumour composition but nephrogenic (tubuloglomerular pattern) and stromagenic cells are seen. The stromagenic cells may be undifferentiated or be differentiated into fat, cartilage, striated muscle or bone. Three unfavourable[255] histological subtypes—the rhabdoid type, the clear cell sarcoma type and the anaplastic type—are associated with a poorer prognosis; though they constitute only 10% of all Wilms' tumours they account for 60% of deaths. The rhabdoid type is now being increasingly identified as a separate and different type of tumour, distinct from Wilms' tumours.

Clinical features

The tumour commonly presents as an abdominal swelling. Haematuria and pyrexia may occur with pain from the local spread of the disease. On examination the child often appears well with a firm non-tender mass which does not cross the midline. This tumour must be differentiated from a neuroblastoma, where the child looks ill and the mass is more nodular and irregular and usually crosses the midline.

Investigations

The intravenous urogram is usually the most common investigation used in the diagnosis of a Wilms' tumour. Eggshell calcification from old haemorrhage is occasionally seen; stippled calcification suggests a neuroblastoma.

Distorted caliceal morphology as the result of an intrarenal mass is characteristic. The contralateral kidney is assessed for function and the possibility of a bilateral Wilms' tumour. The solid nature of the tumour can be confirmed by ultrasound scanning and the vena cava and renal veins assessed for tumour thrombus. CT scan requires a general anaesthetic in a small child and is generally unnecessary. A neuroblastoma can be excluded by assessing urinary catecholamine levels and bone marrow aspirate for neuroblastoma cells.

Treatment

A multidisciplinary approach to the management of Wilms' tumours has resulted in a progressive increase in the survival rate of children with this tumour.[256] The best results are obtained if children are treated in specialist centres. The National Wilms' Tumour Study Group studies I–III[257] have allowed clinicians to limit or eliminate radiotherapy and chemotherapy for patients with good prognosis while maintaining survival rates. In children with advanced disease and an unfavourable prognosis the studies have tried to improve the outcome and survival rates. Patients with Stage I and II tumours (early stage tumours) are treated by radical nephrectomy followed by chemotherapy but no radiotherapy. Children with Stage III and IV (late stage tumours) or those with

REFERENCES

250. Sober I, Hirsch M J Urol 1965; 93: 449
251. Klapproth H J J Urol 1959; 81: 633
252. Cochran W, Froggatt P J Urol 1967; 97: 216
253. Hoffman M Science 1989; 246: 1387
254. Malpas J S In: Whitfield H N, Hendry W F (eds) Genitourinary Surgery. Churchill Livingstone, Edinburgh 1987
255. Beckwith J B, Palmer N F Cancer 1978; 41: 1937
256. D'Angio G S et al Cancer 1980; 45: 1791
257. D'Angio G J Cancer 1989; 64: 349

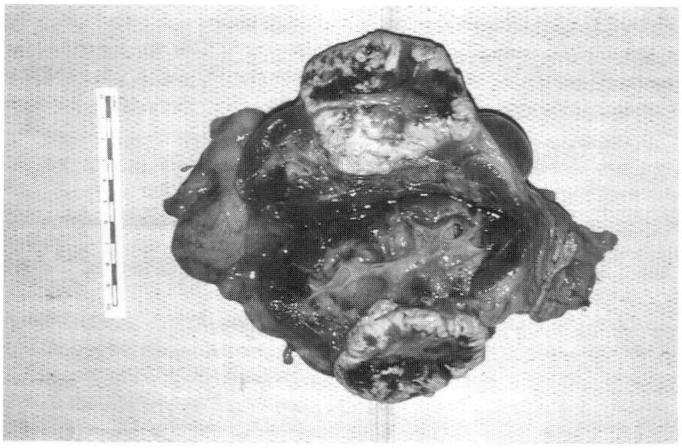

Fig. 36.38 Renal cell carcinoma. Gross specimen showing perirenal spread of the tumour.

unfavourable histology also have a radical nephrectomy, receive radiotherapy to the bed of the renal tumour and are given more aggressive chemotherapy than those with early stage tumours. Survival rates for children with favourable histology and Stage I–IV tumours are between 97% and 83% respectively; for those with unfavourable histology and Stage I–III tumours the rate is 68%. Of patients with unfavourable histology and Stage IV disease, 55% will be alive 4 years after nephrectomy.[257] Many chemotherapeutic regimens have been used: vincristine, actinomycin D, doxorubicin and cyclophosphamide have all been shown to be effective.

Renal cell carcinoma

In the United Kingdom about 2300 patients die of renal cell carcinoma each year.

Aetiology

Cigarette smokers and coffee drinkers appear to be at increased risk of developing renal cell carcinomas,[258] possibly because of the presence of dimethylnitrosamine in tobacco smoke which has been shown to induce renal parenchymal tumours in rats. Occupational contact with cadmium, lead, asbestos and aromatic hydrocarbons has been related to a greater than expected incidence of renal cell carcinoma, but the numbers in such studies are small.[259] Malignant tumours of the kidney in hamsters have been induced by prolonged administration of oestrogen[260] but there is no evidence to suggest an increased risk of this tumour in women taking the contraceptive pill.[260]

There is increasing interest in chromosomal abnormalities found in association with renal cell carcinoma with a fairly constant finding of deletions or translocations in the short arm of chromosome 3(3p) in the familial type. In the sporadic type of renal cell carcinoma a particular allele in the 3p locus has been found to be consistently deleted in most tumour tissue suggesting that there is a suppressor cancer gene at that locus.[261] There is an increased risk of developing renal tumours in patients with cerebellar and retinal angiomas (von Hippel–Lindau syndrome).[262]

Pathology

Renal cell carcinoma arises from the cell of the proximal convoluted tubule. It comprises 3% of adult malignant tumours[263] and is twice as common in men as in women. Renal carcinomas account for 90% of all malignant tumours of the kidney.

Gross appearances

These are well seen in nephrectomy specimens (Fig. 36.38). The tumour usually arises at one or other pole. The renal capsule is elevated by the tumour which may have penetrated it. There may be spread into perirenal fat. The tumour appears to be semi-cystic with solid bands of yellow or red and interlacing bands of fibrous tissue.

Microscopic appearances

Two types of cells are seen, one with clear cytoplasm containing glycogen and fat and the other with pink granules in the cytoplasm representing mitochondria.[264] Many differences in cellularity and pleomorphism exist between the tumours; in common with most other malignancies, those tumours which are very pleomorphic have a poor prognosis and tend to metastasize early.

Spread of the tumour occurs into the veins and it may extend into the renal vein and inferior vena cava. Occasional retrograde spread into the spermatic or ovarian vein may produce secondary deposits in the testis or ovary. Direct spread occurs into the perinephric fat and overlying muscle. Metastases occur in bones, brain and lungs where they are often solitary and large (cannonball). There is debate about the relative degree of malignancy of smaller renal tumours which have often been described as benign adenomas when they are less than 3 cm in diameter. It is now recognized that some carcinomas start as small adenomas and, whilst metastases from such tumours are rare, the distinction between benign and malignant tumours on the grounds of size alone is somewhat artificial.

Clinical features

Renal cell carcinoma is a tumour of adults, commonly occurring in the fifth and seventh decade of life. The incidence is thought to be rising, but may in part be explained by the finding of symptomless and smaller tumours when ultrasound is performed routinely for other indications (the so-called incidentalomas).

Certain clinical features are common to all types of renal tumour. The most common presenting features are haematuria, loin pain and a palpable mass or a combination of all three. The

REFERENCES

258. Bennington J L, Laubscher F S Cancer 1968; 21: 1069
259. Magee P N, Barnes J M J Pathol Bact 1962; 84: 19
260. Kirkman H, Bacon R L J Natl Cancer Inst 1952; 13: 745
261. Kovasc G Proc Natl Acad Sci USA 1988; 85: 1571
262. Greene L F, Rosenthal M H N Engl J Med 1951; 244: 633
263. Bennington L F, Beckwith J B In: Atlas of Tumour Pathology, Second Series. Armed Forces Institute of Pathology, Washington 1975
264. Ericsson J L E, Seweld R, Orrenius S Virch Arch 1966; 341: 204

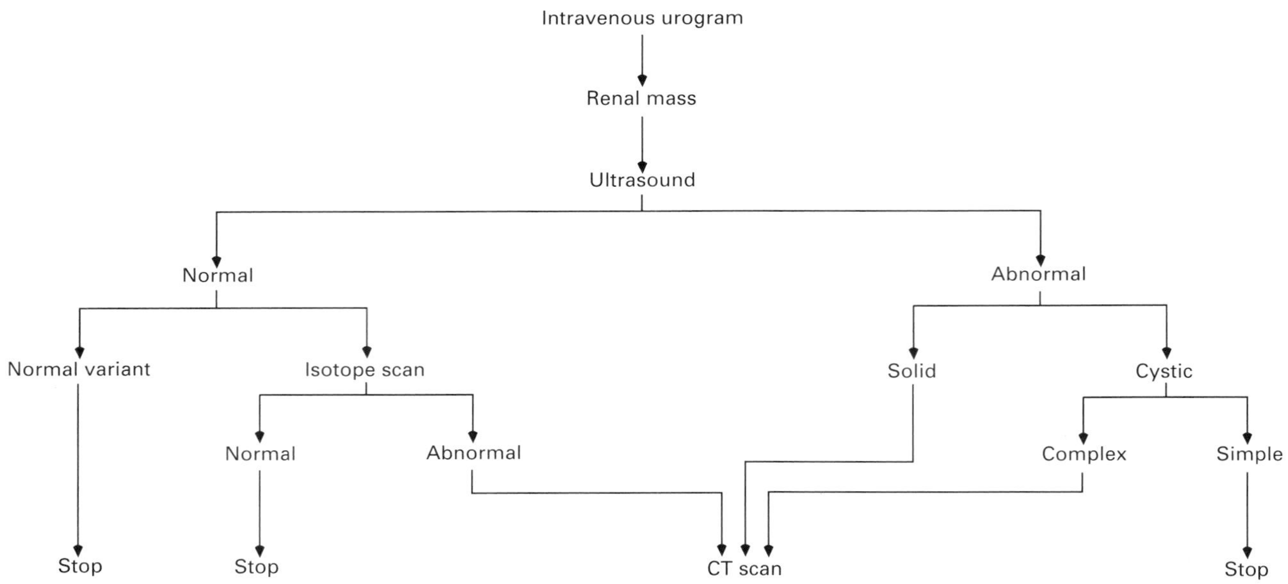

Fig. 36.39 Evaluation of a renal mass.

systemic immunological response to malignant disease produces a number of features.[265] Many of these effects are non-specific and are produced by the body's response to the tumour. These include fever (15%), anaemia (30%), raised erythrocyte sedimentation rate (50%) and abnormal liver function (30%). Myopathy and amyloid deposition also occur. With the exception of amyloid, these features are potentially reversible on removal of the tumour. Some renal tumours produce specific systemic effects caused by hormone secretion by the tumour.[266] Hypertension may occur in a quarter of these patients but it is uncertain whether this is caused by renin excretion or ischaemia.[267] Erythropoietin secretion produces polycythaemia, and occasionally parathormone is excreted by renal tumours producing hypercalcaemia.[268] Patients may also present with bone pain from metastases or from the secondary effects of obstruction of the vena cava or renal vein. An acutely developing left-sided varicocele is a rare presentation.

Differential diagnosis

The differential diagnosis of a space-occupying lesion of the kidney is determined by following a simple diagnostic route which results in a preoperative diagnosis with a high degree of accuracy (Fig. 36.39). It is hardly ever necessary to explore a kidney simply to make a diagnosis.

Diagnostic investigations

Urine. The majority of patients with renal tumours have evidence of haematuria on microscopy or on chemical testing. Patients with urothelial tumours may have tumour cells seen on urine cytology.

Radiological investigations

The mainstay of investigation used to be the intravenous urogram. The characteristic feature on the intravenous urogram is distortion of the calices with a space-occupying lesion expanding the cortex (Fig. 36.40). This abnormality is more clearly seen on nephrotomography after a large dose of contrast medium. The differential diagnosis in such cases lies between a renal tumour or cyst and further investigations are designed to establish this. Urothelial tumours are seen as distortions of the calices or a luminal filling defect in the renal pelvis (Fig. 36.41) on the urogram.

Ultrasound examination differentiates between solid and cystic space-occupying lesions with an accuracy approaching 98%.[269] An ultrasound scan is sufficient to make a diagnosis in the majority of patients in whom a space-occupying lesion is an incidental finding during intravenous urography. In those patients in whom a renal tumour is suspected, a fluid-containing cyst should be punctured and the fluid sent for cytology since about 3% of transonic renal lesions contain tumour.[269] In the few cases where ultrasound examination is equivocal, especially in obese patients, CT scanning with or without enhancement of the collecting system by simultaneous injection of contrast medium generally provides a diagnosis (Fig. 36.42).[270] It also helps to stage the tumour by assessing the lymph nodes and the lungs. Angiography shows abnormal vessels associated with a malignant circulation (Fig. 36.40), but is rarely required today. In those few cases where doubt still remains, percutaneous fine-needle biopsy under ultrasound control can be performed. The theoretical risk of seeding tumour cells has not so far been borne out in clinical practice.[271]

REFERENCES

265. Chisholm G D, Roy R R Br J Urol 1971; 43: 687
266. Suffrin G et al J Urol 1977; 117: 433
267. Hollifield J W Arch Int Med 1975; 135: 859
268. Hammond D, Winnick S J NY Acad Sci 1974; 230: 219
269. Sherwood T Br Med J 1975; 4: 682
270. Love L et al Urol Radiol 1979; 1: 3
271. Von Schreeb R et al Scand J Urol Nephrol 1967; 1: 270

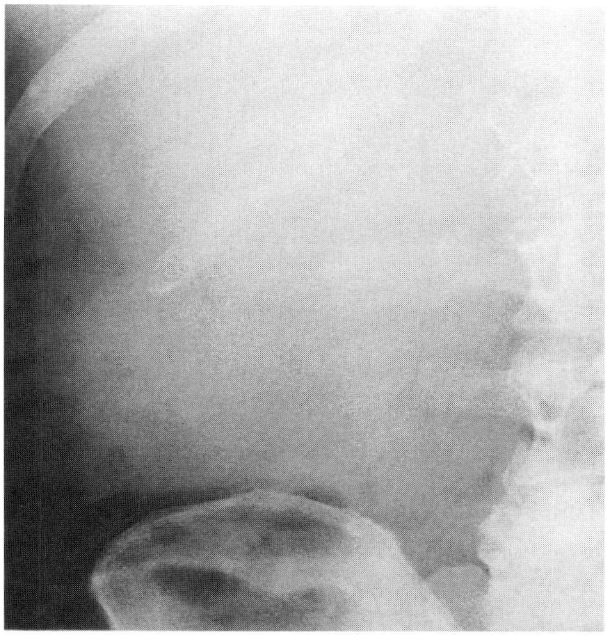

a

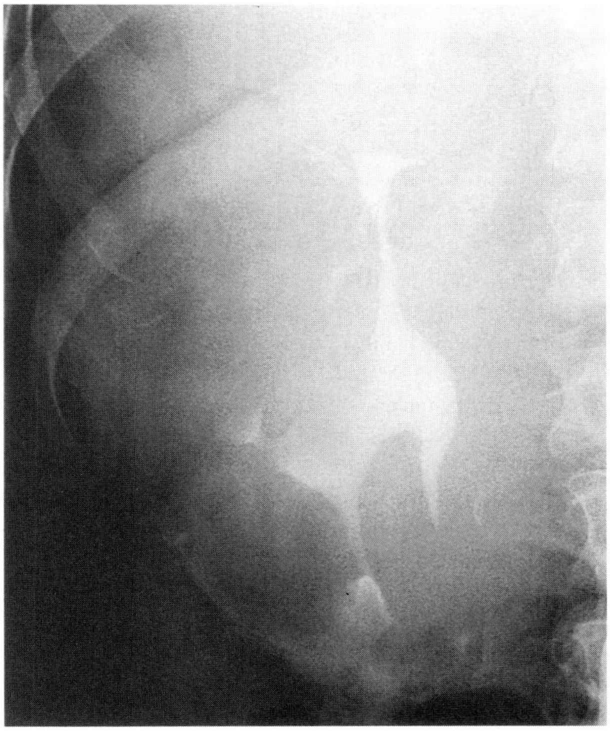

b

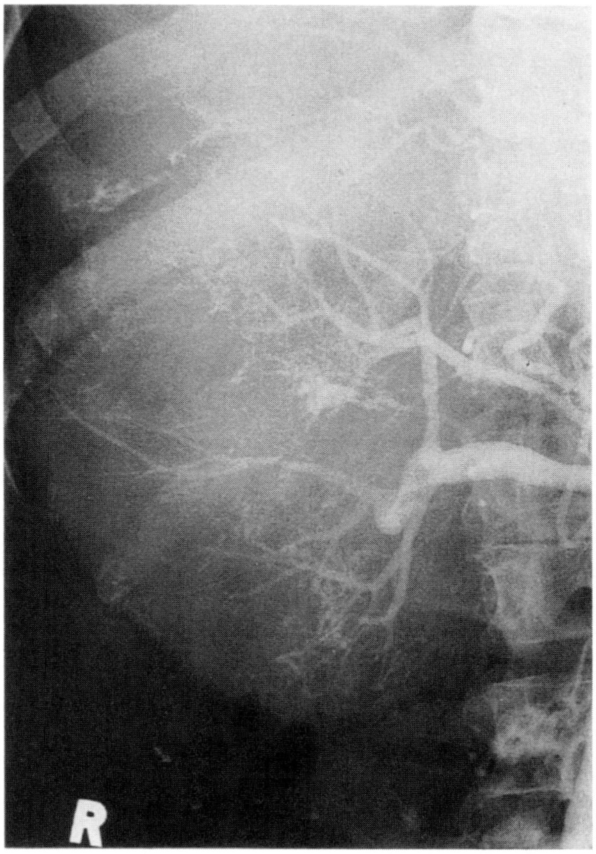

c

Fig. 36.40 Renal cell carcinoma. (**a**) Plain radiograph showing loss of psoas shadow and enlarged right kidney; (**b**) intravenous urogram showing distorted calices and upper pole mass; (**c**) angiography showing tumour circulation. Courtesy of Dr J Reid.

Staging investigations

Staging of the primary tumour is frequently carried out at the same time as the diagnostic investigations. High-quality ultrasonography enables accurate delineation of the renal vein and inferior vena cava, and it may also demonstrate invasion. CT scanning can also be used, especially for the detection of enlarged para-aortic lymph nodes.

A chest radiograph is not sufficient to diagnose pulmonary metastases with certainty and therefore CT scans of the lungs should be obtained. If tumour involvement of the vena cava is suspected from the ultrasound scan, the extent of this involvement can be defined by inferior and superior vena caval venography or an MRI scan or angiography.

Treatment

Nephrectomy for renal cell carcinoma

This operation differs from the operation of simple nephrectomy for benign disease as it is necessary to remove the perinephric fat, Gerota's fascia and lymph nodes around the renal pedicle in order

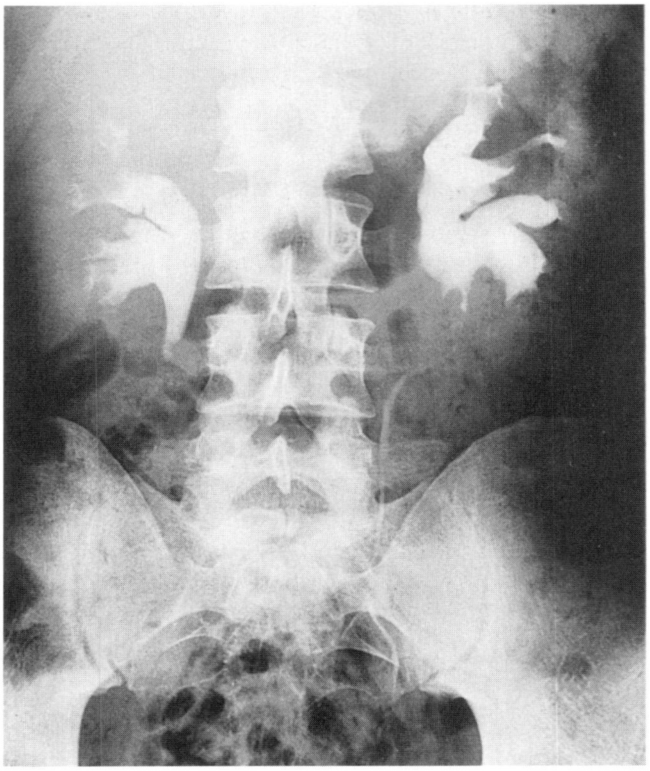

Fig. 36.41 Carcinoma of the ureter. Intravenous urogram film showing filling defects in the upper third of the left ureter which has a transitional cell carcinoma. Courtesy of Dr J Reid.

to increase the chance of cure. The tumour-containing kidney often has an increased blood supply and there are a number of additional collateral veins, particularly if the tumour has invaded and blocked the renal vein. Therefore an operation which allows early ligation of the vascular pedicle is recommended as it allows easier control of bleeding, particularly in very bulky tumours. This may be achieved in three ways: an abdominal transperitoneal approach through a transverse incision, reflecting the duodenum or splenic flexure of the colon, enables the inferior vena cava or the aorta to be seen early; an anterior thoracoabdominal or posterior approach also gives excellent exposure. Once the pedicle has been identified, retraction of the anteriorly lying renal vein often makes identification of the renal artery easier. The kidney is then removed together with the perinephric fat, adrenal gland and regional lymph nodes. The ureter is divided and ligated as far distally as possible.

Partial nephrectomy

Some surgeons recommend partial nephrectomy for small (< 4 cm) tumours in the upper or lower pole of the kidney. This technique is considered suitable for tumours in a solitary kidney, but is not regarded as generally applicable.

Radical nephrectomy in patients with metastatic disease

The 1-year survival rate for metastatic renal cell carcinoma is 7–35%. Radical nephrectomy in the presence of metastases has

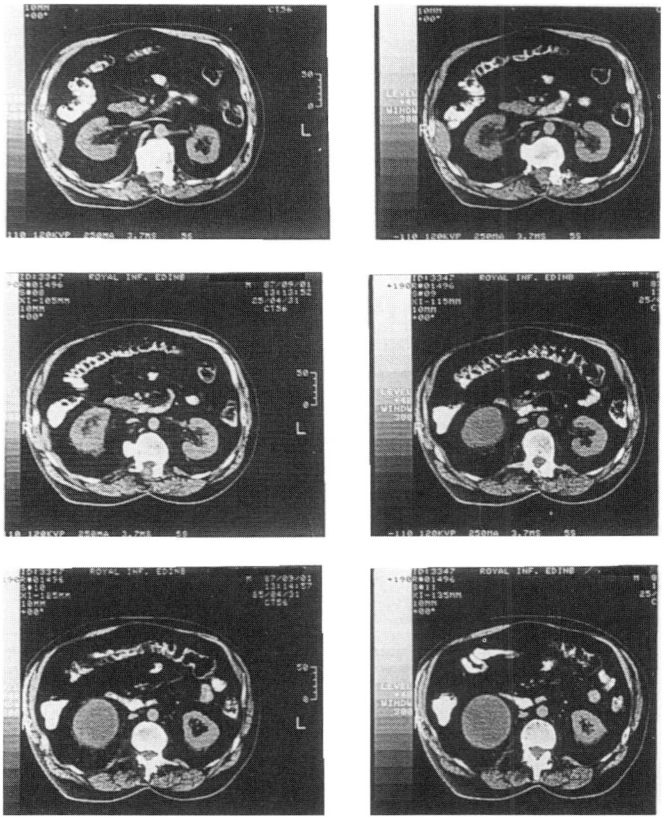

Fig. 36.42 CT scan showing cystic right renal cell carcinoma (no contrast enhancement).

sometimes been justified on the basis that spontaneous regression of the pulmonary metastases can occur.[272] 93 such cases have so far been described in the literature with this histological confirmation in 31.[273] The duration of remission is, however, short. The excision of a solitary metastasis occurring after nephrectomy has produced long-term disease-free survival but some of the beneficial response claimed for treatment may relate more to tumour biology than to the surgical procedure.[274] Nephrectomy is therefore unjustified in patients with multiple metastases as the operative mortality for these patients is several times higher than when the operation is performed for patients with local disease.[275] Patient selection for nephrectomy in metastatic disease is on the basis of performance status and absence of negative prognosis factors such as weight loss of more than 10% in the recent past, poor histological grade of tumour and presence of multiple metastases.[276] Control of primary symptoms is probably best achieved by embolization of the renal artery supplying the tumour.[277] This may be performed by introducing a number of agents such as blood clot, muscle, steel coils and gelatine sponge into the renal artery under radiographic control.

REFERENCES

272. Johnston D E et al J Urol 1975; 114: 27
273. Lanigan D Br J Urol 1995; 75(5): 565
274. Golimbu M et al J Urol 1986; 136: 805
275. Skinner D G et al Cancer 1971; 28: 1165
276. Neves R J J Urol 1988; 139: 1173
277. Gottesman J E et al Urology 1985; 25: 248

60% of patients report palliation of local symptoms after embolization. It has also been suggested that preliminary embolization of metastatic renal tumours followed by nephrectomy 1–4 weeks later may produce regression of the metastases in 15% of patients[278] but others have failed to confirm these findings.[279]

Radiation therapy

Tumours may be reduced in size by preoperative radiotherapy. When radiotherapy is given postoperatively the incidence of residual tumour in the renal bed and local recurrence are reduced.[280] No definite benefit of pre- or postoperative irradiation therapy has been demonstrated on survival, but preoperative radiotherapy for patients with large tumours which might otherwise be inoperable and postoperative radiotherapy for patients with a residual tumour or lymph node metastases may help to control local tumour growth. Pain relief following local radiotherapy occurs in 70–80% of patients with bony metastases.

Cytotoxic chemotherapy

Renal tumours should be regarded as chemoresistant: the objective response rate in a survey of the literature is between 7 and 10%.[281] Regression has however been seen following immunotherapy, which may have a role in the management of metastatic disease.[282] Hormone therapy with medroxyprogesterone acetate 100 mg t.d.s. has been recommended for the management of patients with advanced renal cancer.[283] It is debatable whether the effect is from coincidental spontaneous regression of the tumour or from the hormone therapy. The results of this treatment are conflicting and adjuvant therapy with medroxyprogesterone acetate cannot be recommended.

Prognosis

Renal cell carcinoma is slow-growing and occasionally patients present with metastatic disease up to 20 years after nephrectomy for the primary tumour. When the tumour is confined to kidney the prognosis following radical nephrectomy is excellent, with up to 93% of patients surviving 5 years.[284,285] However, survival figures from reported series vary; in patients with locally invasive tumour and involved lymph nodes a more realistic expectation is that 30% will survive 5 years.[286]

Renal oncocytoma

Renal oncocytoma is a well differentiated eosinophilic granular cell renal tumour associated with a good prognosis.[287] Oncocytomas arise from the proximal convoluted tubules. They are large and impossible to differentiate from renal cell carcinomas preoperatively. Treatment usually consists of nephrectomy.

Angiomyolipoma

Angiomyolipoma is a benign lesion consisting of smooth muscle, blood vessels and fat. Very occasionally this tumour is malignant and involves local lymph nodes. It is found in association with tuberose sclerosis in half of the cases. In such patients the lesions are generally bilateral and multiple.[288]

Juxtaglomerular tumours

These are very rare haemangiopericytomas within the renal cortex.[289] They are renin-secreting and therefore may cause primary aldosteronism with hypertension, hypokalaemia and hypernatraemia. The tumours are very small and often can only be found by careful angiography or CT scans with vascular enhancement.

Leiomyoma

This is a benign tumour arising from the smooth muscle of the renal capsule.

Lipoma

A lipoma occurs between the kidney and its capsule; it is usually small and well circumscribed.

Fibroma

A fibroma often appears as a small cortical nodule.

Mesoblastic nephroma

This is a rare but benign lesion, usually seen in neonates and infants. Macroscopically it is indistinguishable from a Wilms' tumour but histologically the tumour consists of mesenchymal tissues seen as tracts and bundles of interlacing regular spindle cells resembling smooth muscle fibres. The tumour is extremely rare.[290]

Adenoma

This is a small circumscribed lesion of the renal cortex which is often multiple and bilateral and is observed most commonly in the elderly. Adenomas are often an incidental finding at post mortem.[291] The tumours are rounded, well-encapsulated nodules

REFERENCES

278. Swanston D A et al Urol Clin North Am 1980; 7: 719
279. Kurth K H et al World J Urol 1984; 1: 122
280. McDonald M W J Urol 1982; 127: 211
281. Dekemion J B J Urol 1983; 130: 2
282. Dekemion J B J Urol 1983; 130: 1063
283. Bloom H J G Cancer 1973; 32: 1066
284. McDonald M W J Urol 1982; 127: 211
285. Lanigan D Br J Urol 1995; 75(5): 565
286. Selli C et al Cancer 1983; 52: 899
287. Mei G S et al Cancer 1980; 45: 1010
288. Klapproth H J et al AMA Arch Pathol 1959; 67: 400
289. Conn J W et al Clin Sci Mol Med 1973; 45: 279
290. Bolande R P et al Paediatrics 1967; 40: 272
291. Lucke B, Schlumberger H S In: Atlas of Tumour Pathology. Armed Forces Institute of Pathology, Washington

up to 3 cm in diameter with a typical orange-yellow colour. Histologically they have a typical appearance with small cuboidal or columnar cells interlaced with a delicate fibrous stroma.

Haemangiopericytoma

This is a malignant tumour of blood vessel walls occasionally associated with hypoglycaemia.

Metastases

Primary tumours metastasizing to the kidney include those of lung, breast and uterus and are commonly bilateral. Treatment depends upon the nature of the primary tumour.

Sarcomas

Sarcomas are malignant tumours of the connective tissues of the renal parenchyma and pelvis. They are rare and account for 3% of all tumours of the kidney and pelvis. They may be categorized into different types according to the cell structure.

Tumours of the renal pelvis and ureter

Urothelial tumours in these sites are important because of their relationship to carcinoma of the bladder. They may be coexistent or metachronous. The histopathological appearance is similar to that seen in carcinoma of the bladder (see Chapter 37). Carcinoma of the renal pelvis is three times as common as carcinoma of the ureter and 20 times less frequent than carcinoma of the bladder.[292] Morphologically, tumours may be either papillary or solid but their importance lies in the ability of the pathologist to differentiate between a urothelial tumour and a parenchymal renal cell carcinoma. Metastases from these tumours occur in the retroperitoneal lymph nodes, the vertebrae, the liver and lungs.

Squamous carcinoma of the renal pelvis

This condition is associated with renal calculus disease. When stones are present they are frequently embedded in tumour tissue. The tumour may be papillary or solid, and invasion of the wall of the pelvis and renal substance is often apparent. The tumour is usually epidermoid with varying degrees of keratinization.

Adenocarcinoma of the renal pelvis

Cases of mucus-secreting adenocarcinoma of the renal pelvis have been recorded. These adenocarcinomas tend to produce solid growths in the pelvis with direct invasion of adjacent structures. Histologically the epithelium often resembles that of the large bowel with glandular metaplasia producing mucin.[293]

Treatment of tumours of the renal pelvis and ureter

Urothelial tumours should be treated by removing the primary tumour and the adjacent urothelium to reduce the risk of developing further tumours. Nephroureterectomy therefore remains the treatment of choice because of the difficulties of follow-up following segmental resection. Laparoscopic nephroureterectomy may be carried out in well selected patients with low-grade tumours in the renal pelvis or upper ureter. The development of ureterorenoscopy allows a more conservative approach in the presence of small, well-differentiated tumours of the ureter or renal pelvis.[294] Local excision has been advocated intermittently for several years.[295]

Malakoplakia

Malakoplakia is a proliferation of malfunctioning histiocytes which cannot destroy bacteria properly. They involve the renal pelvis occasionally although involvement of the bladder is more common. Their importance is that they cause the presence on intravenous urography of filling defects that can resemble tumour.

Xanthogranulomatous pyelonephritis

This is a form of chronic pyelonephritis with large numbers of histiocytes which may be mistaken for renal cell carcinoma. The lesion frequently extends beyond the renal capsule to involve the fat and adjacent organs. Both malakoplakia and xanthogranulomatous pyelonephritis should be considered in the differential diagnosis of a renal mass.

RENAL FAILURE

Acute renal failure

The management of patients with acute renal failure requires collaboration between physician, radiologist and urologist. Acute renal failure is an abrupt decline in renal function in which there is persistent reduction in renal blood flow and tubular damage. The aetiology may be multifactorial and although acute tubular necrosis is found in the majority of patients with acute renal failure, glomerular damage, arterial disease and interstitial nephritis may all occur.

Aetiology

Acute renal failure often develops in patients with pre-existing renal disease, especially those with chronic vascular ischaemia. Thus the elderly and those with ischaemic heart disease or other chronic medical conditions are at the greatest risk of developing acute renal failure after surgery.

In surgical patients presenting with acute renal failure three main groups of contributory factors can be identified:

REFERENCES

292. Williams C B, Mitchell J P Br J Urol 1973; 45: 370
293. Ackerman L V J Urol 1946; 55: 36
294. Zincke H, Neves R J Urol Clin North Am 1984; 11: 717
295. Blute M L et al Urol 1989; 141: 1298

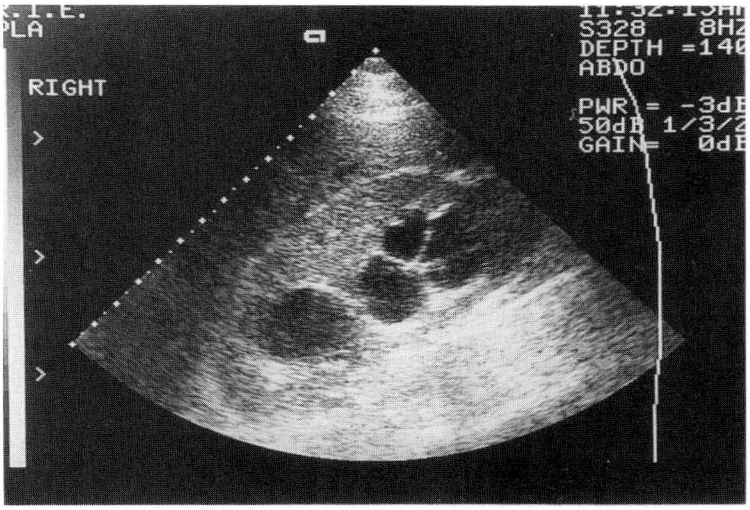

Fig. 36.43 Obstructed right kidney. The ultrasound scan shows dilated calices in acute obstructive uropathy.

1. Inadequate renal perfusion (pre-renal): haemorrhage, dehydration, loss of colloid and crystalloids in burns, septicaemia and shock.
2. Renal parenchymal (renal): nephrotoxic drugs (e.g. gentamicin, non-steroidal anti-inflammatory drugs such as diclofenac sodium, ACE inhibitors such as enalapril, etc.), acute inflammations of the kidney such as acute glomerulonephritis and pyelonephritis.
3. Obstructive uropathy (post-renal): ureteric or lower tract obstruction.

Occasionally, these factors may coexist, for example in a patient with septicaemia who becomes hypotensive and is treated with gentamicin and high-dose frusemide or a patient with bacteraemia secondary to infected obstructed kidneys.

Acute renal failure should be suspected if there is oliguria with dark urine in a patient who has undergone a number of surgical insults. Careful examination of the patient is necessary. Assessment of hydration, blood pressure and catheterization of the bladder must be undertaken to ensure that retention of urine has not been mistaken for anuria. Catheterization is also necessary to monitor subsequent urine output.

Investigations

The most important differential diagnosis lies between incipient acute tubular necrosis and established renal failure, as it is believed that incipient tubular necrosis may be reversible with a diuretic challenge after adequate hydration. This is seen with pre-renal causes where the healthy kidney responds by conserving sodium and water. Hence the osmolality of urine in incipient tubular necrosis is high (> 500 mmol/kg), the urinary sodium is low (< 20 mmol/l) and there is a urine:plasma ratio of urea of more than 8:1 and of creatinine more than 40:1. The central venous pressure is low in patients with fluid depletion and is generally raised in patients with acute renal failure.

Urine examination can give clues to the aetiology. Proteinuria is absent or slight in pre- and post-renal causes of renal failure. Heavy proteinuria suggests a renal parenchymal and very likely a glomerular cause. Haematuria is uncommon in pre-renal causes, and more likely in renal parenchymal and post-renal (e.g. stone) disorders.

Ultrasound

This examination of the urinary tract is the single most important investigation in the diagnosis of acute renal failure.[296] It is used to measure the size of the kidneys and to assess the degree of obstruction and the size of the bladder (Fig. 36.43). A high-dose intravenous urogram with immediate tomography is of some value if ultrasound is unavailable (Fig. 36.44). A faint persistent nephrogram occurs in glomerulonephritis because of impaired perfusion filtra-tion; the nephrogram becomes increasingly dense in acute obstruction and there may be a negative pyelogram. The technique may be supplemented by antegrade pyelography and insertion of nephrostomies in the case of ureteric obstruction (Fig. 36.45). Renal perfusion may also be assessed by radioisotope studies using ^{99m}Tc-DTPA (see above).

Management

The many metabolic disturbances which occur in these patients dictate that management be carried out by a skilled team. Surgical help may be required to relieve obstruction by percutaneous nephrostomy drainage or internal JJ stenting. In incipient tubular necrosis, after adequate hydration under central venous pressure guidance, a powerful diuretic such as frusemide given as 120 mg intravenously may stimulate urine production. Mannitol 100 ml 20% over 10 minutes may also be added. Failure to restore urine output of at least 10 ml/h may indicate the need for a repeat challenge. If this fails it is likely that established renal failure has set in. In early acute renal failure from septicaemia, a dopamine/

REFERENCE

296. Sherwood T et al Br J Radiol 1974; 47: 368

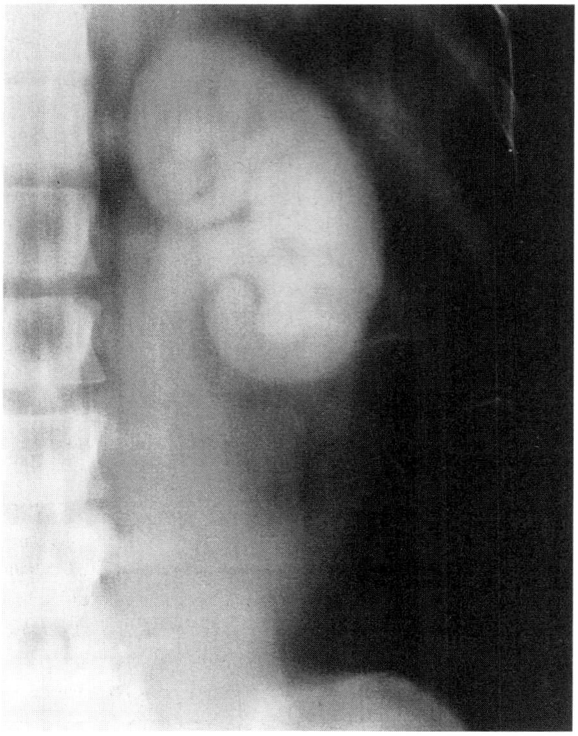

Fig. 36.44 Nephrotomogram of left kidney showing persistent nephrogram and retained contrast in dilated calices at 5 h. The patient had a stone impacted in the pelviureteric junction. (Courtesy of Dr I N Gillespie.)

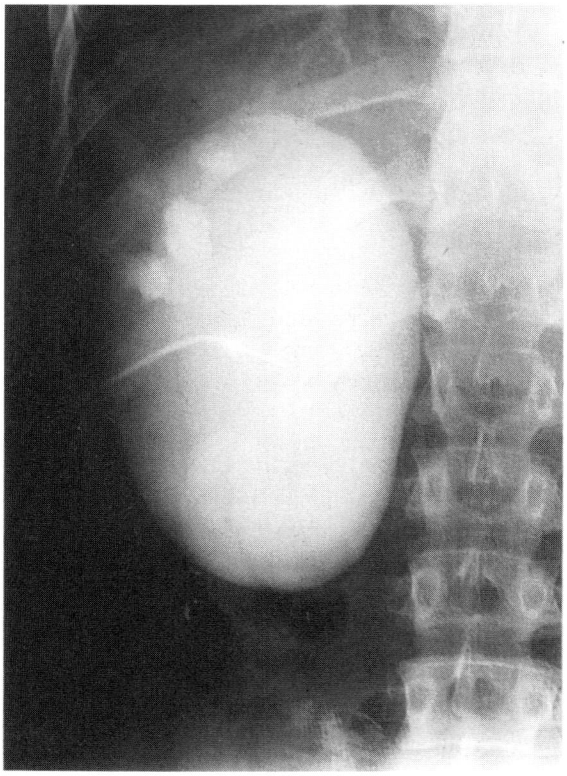

Fig. 36.45 Antegrade pyelography. Combined diagnostic and therapeutic procedure in a patient with acutely obstructed right kidney.

frusemide infusion (3 ng/kg per min of dopamine plus frusemide 10–15 mg/kg per h) may induce diuresis when frusemide alone has failed.[297] This may be continued for 24 hours.

An accurate fluid balance chart and daily weighing of the patient is necessary. The electrolytes and the renal function must be measured daily. Fluid is replaced as 500 ml (insensible losses) plus daily urine volume plus losses from the gut or skin after burns. Hyperkalaemia may be prevented by prophylactic calcium resonium enemas but frequently glucose and insulin infusions are necessary (50 g glucose and 15 u soluble insulin).[298] When a severe acidosis develops this may be treated by urgent dialysis. Most patients are catabolic and require parenteral feeding with strict control of their urine output.[299] Appropriate antibiotics are given. Many patients with acute renal failure require haemodialysis. This may be required on an urgent basis, especially in the presence of severe fluid overload and pulmonary oedema, acutely rising serum potassium and severe acidosis. It may be performed through a double lumen single needle inserted as a subclavian line. It may also be necessary to remove fluid in order to allow large volumes of fluid to be given for parenteral nutrition. The mortality from acute renal failure is high, but in those patients in whom recovery takes place this generally occurs at around 2 to 6 weeks.

Chronic renal failure

There are many causes of chronic renal failure. The most important surgical causes are reflux nephropathy, obstructive uropathy, stones and polycystic renal disease. Primary glomerular disease accounts for over half the patients with chronic renal failure. The condition is frequently symptomless until end-stage renal failure is reached, when the features of anaemia and uraemia with anorexia, nausea, vomiting, polyneuropathy, cardiopathy, encephalopathy and itching occur. Fluid retention may cause cardiac failure. On examination pallor is common and hypertension and cardiac failure may be present. The kidneys or bladder may be palpable and the prostate enlarged.

Investigations

The urea, creatinine, electrolytes and creatinine clearance and haemoglobin should all be estimated. A 24-hour urine collection for quantitative assessment of protein helps to differentiate between glomerular disease (high protein excretion) and tubular disease such as pyelonephritis and polycystic kidney (1.5 g/day or less).[300] An abdominal radiograph to exclude stones and an

REFERENCES

297. Graziani G et al In: Davidson A M, Guillou P J (eds) Proceedings of the European Dialysis Transplant Association. Pitman, London 1982
298. Lawson A L, Chapman A Acute Renal Failure. Churchill Livingstone, Edinburgh 1980
299. Lee J A In: Dickinson J W T, Lee H A (eds) Nutrition in the Clinical Management of Disease. Edward Arnold, London 1978
300. Brigs J D In: Whitfield H N, Hendry W F (eds) Textbook of Genito-urinary Surgery. Churchill Livingstone, Edinburgh 1987

ultrasound scan to assess renal size (generally showing small shrunken kidneys) and exclude obstructive uropathy are essential investigations. Renal biopsy may be necessary in patients with normal-sized kidneys to exclude treatable tubulo-interstitial disease.

Management

Correction of fluid and electrolyte depletion, and control of hypertension and urinary infection may result in stabilization of the disease. Potentially nephrotoxic drugs such as aminoglycosides, co-trimoxazole and tetracycline should not be prescribed. The progress of the disease may be determined by plotting the serum creatinine values. If the reciprocal of serum creatinine is plotted, this produces a straight line which allows an accurate prediction of when end-stage renal failure will be reached.

Anaemia, hypertension and cardiovascular disease occur in many patients with chronic renal failure. Control of hypertension and heart failure aids stabilization as it prevents further loss of nephrons from hypertensive renal damage. An angiotensin converting enzyme (ACE) inhibitor is commonly used. Recombinant erythropoietin (EPO), though expensive, is now available for treatment of the anaemia.

The other main complication of chronic renal failure is osteodystrophy. Secondary hyperparathroidism occurs, resulting in bone resorption and the development of bone cysts (osteitis fibrosis cystica). This is caused by decreased phosphate excretion and calcium malabsorption from lack of 1,25 dihydroxy vitamin D3. Treatment is by administration of vitamin D3 and reduction of phosphate absorption using calcium carbonate. Occasionally, subtotal parathyroidectomy may be necessary.[301] Osteomalacia also occurs and may be avoided by ensuring that the dietary intake of calcium is adequate. The aetiology is complex.[302] Many patients with chronic renal failure may be managed conservatively by dietary restriction of protein and the appropriate intake of fluids. Protein is restricted to 40 g/day when the blood urea reaches 30 mmol/l; uraemic symptoms develop above this level.[299] Sodium excretion is normal until the glomerular filtration rate falls below 5 ml/min, and therefore the diet should contain the normal amount of sodium. If sodium retention occurs—this is easily checked by regular weighing—large doses of frusemide up to 1500 mg/day are effective. Occasionally hypokalaemia, from impairment of tubular function, may require potassium supplements and acidosis may be treated with sodium bicarbonate capsules. Three options are available for patients who can no longer be managed by conservative treatment. These are haemodialysis, peritoneal dialysis and renal transplantation.

Haemodialysis

Ultrafiltration of the blood allows removal of water and solutes across a semi-permeable membrane. This membrane separates the blood and dialysate and is made from cuprophan or cellulose acetate. This is available in many forms; a disposable hollow fibre or flat plate type may be used but some units still prefer the non-disposable Kiil (flat) plate model. The dialysate is obtained by mixing mains water with electrolyte concentrates. Blood is transported to the membrane via an arteriovenous fistula into which two needles are inserted or by using a double lumen needle inserted into a large vein. Many patients are accepted for a chronic haemodialysis programme and an arteriovenous fistula is generally created at the wrist between the radial artery and the cephalic vein to allow self-cannulation.[303] In patients in whom acute haemodialysis is required or when dialysis is necessary whilst the arteriovenous fistula is maturing, a Quinton–Scribner arteriovenous shunt can be created—usually between the posterior tibial artery and long saphenous vein at the ankle.[304] In the patient for whom short-term dialysis is likely to be required a subclavian cannula may be inserted.[305]

Peritoneal dialysis

Haemodialysis is expensive and requires a high investment of capital and personnel; therefore peritoneal dialysis is a frequently used alternative in both acute and chronic renal failure. Continuous ambulatory peritoneal dialysis provides a simple self-care system for many patients, especially those with diabetic nephropathy.[306] A Tenckhoff permanent peritoneal catheter[307] is inserted into the peritoneal cavity and four fluid exchanges per day are carried out. Continuous ambulatory peritoneal dialysis gives a better clearance of the middle molecules and has a high capacity for fluid removal.[308] The technique is contraindicated in patients with inflammatory bowel disease, extensive retroperitoneal adhesions and poor respiratory function. Peritonitis is the most common complication and is responsible for most treatment failures; it may be treated by the addition of an antibiotic to each bag of dialysate, and with care the incidence of peritonitis is extremely low. Blockage of the catheter and pericatheter infections may also develop. Continuous ambulatory peritoneal dialysis and haemodialysis have their merits and disadvantages and the optimum use of both methods depends upon the individual patient.

Renal transplantation

Cadaver renal transplantation produces 75–80% graft survival at 12 months. It is probably the optimum method of treatment of patients with end-stage renal failure in both economic terms and quality of life.[309] The techniques and results of renal transplantation are discussed in detail in Chapter 8.

REFERENCES

301. Coburn J W et al In: The Kidney. Saunders, Philadelphia 1981
302. Kanis J A et al Curr Med Res Opin 1981; 7: 294
303. Brescia M J, Cimino J E et al N Engl J Med 1966; 275: 1089
304. Quintin W E, Dillard D, Scribner B J Trans Am Soc Artif Intern Org 1960; 6: 104
305. Uldall P R Proc Eur Dial Trans Assoc 1982; 19: 106
306. Oreopoloud D et al Clin Nephrol 1979; ii: 125
307. Striker G E, Tenckhoff H A M Surgery 1971; 69: 70
308. Babb A L et al Proc Eur Dial Trans Assoc 1973; 10: 247
309. Morris P J Kidney Transplantation. Academic Press, London 1979

37 The bladder

D. M. A. Wallace

STRUCTURE AND FUNCTION

The two functions of the bladder are the storage and controlled elimination of urine. The control of the bladder is through the autonomic nervous system with the parasympathetic supply from sacral segments 2–4 and the sympathetic supply from the lower two thoracic and upper two lumbar segments via the hypogastric plexus.

The epithelial lining of the bladder (the urothelium) is both urine-proof and able to accommodate large changes in surface area without losing its integrity. The urothelium has 3–7 layers of cells; the most superficial is adapted to be urine-proof with a characteristic asymmetrical unit membrane on the luminal surface covered with a glycosaminoglycan layer. The urothelium has a slow turnover with an average cell lifespan of some 200 days, but is also capable of rapid proliferation in response to injury. It lies on a basement membrane and is separated from the detrusor muscle by a layer of supporting connective tissue, the lamina propria.

The detrusor muscle accommodates the increase in volume during filling of the bladder without any increase in tone and thus without a rise in intravesical pressure, and only contracts to provide the expulsive force for voiding. The smooth muscle fibres play a part in maintaining continence. The detrusor is richly supplied with cholinergic receptors, except in the trigone, and has β-adrenergic receptors situated predominantly in the dome and α-adrenergic receptors in the bladder neck region.

CONGENITAL ANOMALIES

Agenesis of the bladder

This is one of the rarest congenital anomalies of the bladder and is usually not compatible with life. Occasional patients survive and must have a urinary diversion.

Exstrophy of the bladder (ectopia vesicae)

This defect of the bladder and lower abdominal wall occurs once in every 30 000 live births and has a male preponderance.[1] It is part of a spectrum of anomalies ranging from cloacal exstrophy at its most severe[2] to split symphysis variants and bifid clitoris.[3] Exstrophy of the bladder is the most common abnormality in this spectrum and comprises an open bladder with a defect in the abdominal wall with separation of the public bones anteriorly and epispadias of the penis or bifid clitoris. The upper tracts are usually normal at birth but are at risk of deterioration as a result of reflux, obstruction or infection consequent on efforts to close the bladder or divert the urine.

The exstrophy deformity is usually easily recognized at birth: the dark red bladder mucosa bulges from the lower abdomen. The upper part is rugose and the lower part, representing the trigone, is smooth. From the apex of the lower part a gutter runs down the dorsum of the penis as an epispadiac urethra. The testes are commonly undescended and the scrotum may be poorly developed. The clitoris in the female is bifid. The mucosa of the bladder rapidly becomes oedematous, making it hard to judge the size of the bladder for attempts at primary closure, and glandular metaplasia develops. In the patient in whom the bladder is left open there is a risk of developing an adenocarcinoma and thus patients with a urinary diversion should have the bladder remnant removed.[4]

Surgical reconstruction of the bladder is the treatment of choice and is possible in almost all cases. This comprises closure of the pelvic ring, often necessitating iliac osteotomies, closure of the bladder, reconstruction of the bladder neck and reconstruction of the epispadiac penis. On becoming adult 18% of patients with closed bladders have been reported to be incontinent, 25% had renal damage but social and sexual function were good.[5] Late failure of both the detrusor and urethra in adult life is significant and requires prolonged follow-up.[6]

THE URACHUS

The urachus is an embryological structure that attaches the apex of the bladder to the allantois at the umbilicus. It closes by involution before the urethra is fully formed as a patent urachus is not associated with urethral valves, nor is it part of the exstrophy abnormalities. Failure of the urachus to close and fully involute results in (Fig. 37.1):

1. A patent urachus.
2. A urachal sinus.

REFERENCES

1. Lancaster P A L Teratology 1987; 36: 572
2. Turner W R et al Urol Clin N Am 1980; 7: 93
3. Hurwitz R S et al J Urol 1987; 138: 1060
4. Neilsen K, Neilsen K K J Urol 1983; 130: 1180
5. Woodhouse C R J et al Br J Urol 1983; 55: 362
6. Woodhouse C R J, Redgrave N G Br J Urol 1996; 77: 590

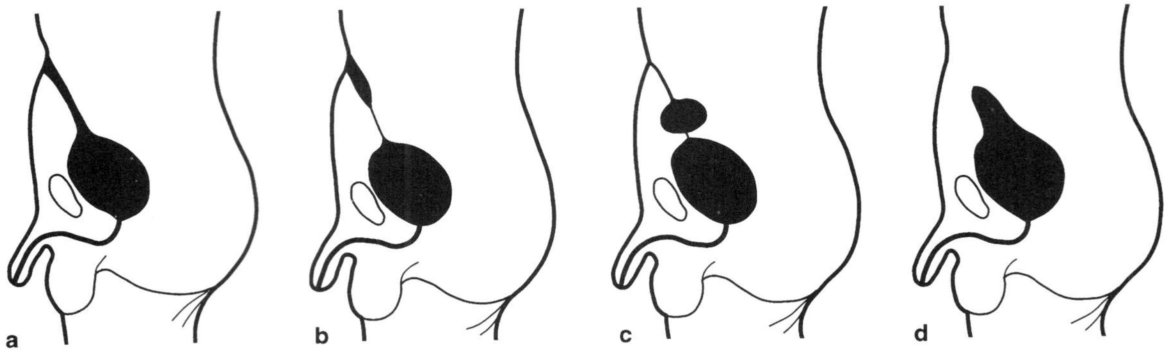

Fig 37.1 Urachal anomalies. (a) Patent urachus; (b) urachal sinus; (c) urachal cyst; (d) urachal diverticulum.

3. A urachal cyst.
4. A urachal diverticulum.

A patent urachus presents at birth with a wet umbilicus associated with granulation tissue. The diagnosis can be confirmed by demonstrating that the fluid is urine or by a patent sinus on a cystogram. Complete excision of the tract is required. A urachal sinus may present in childhood or adult life with a discharge from the umbilicus. A sinogram should be performed to demonstrate the whole tract before surgical excision. A urachal cyst presents at any age with a mass and signs of infection. With all urachal abnormalities a patent omphalomesenteric duct must be considered in the differential diagnosis. A urachal diverticulum does not require excision unless it is interfering with bladder emptying. Rarely urachal remnants are associated with the development of adenocarcinomas in adults.

DISORDERS OF BLADDER FUNCTION

Patient assessment

A careful history of the voiding pattern should be taken and the patient can also be instructed to keep a time/volume/incontinence chart for several days before and during treatment. A full enquiry must be made of any neurological symptoms and previous surgery. Physical examination should look for a distended bladder, loss of perianal tone sensation and rectal tone as well as neurological signs in the lower limbs. Baseline investigations should include urine microscopy and culture and upper tract function studies.

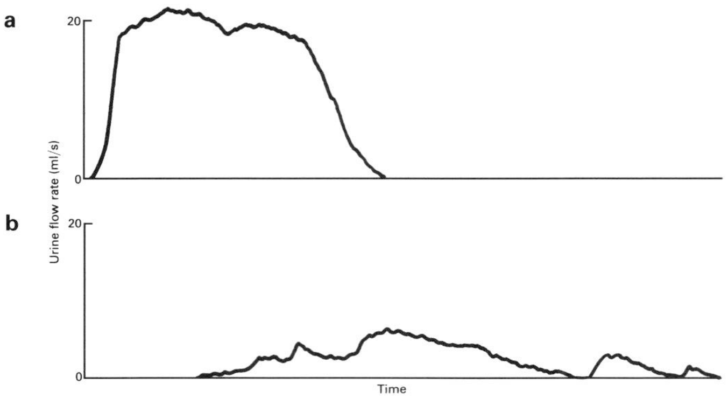

Fig 37.2 Urine flow rate. (a) Normal flow with a peak flow of over 20 ml/s and a normal voiding pattern. (b) An obstructed voiding pattern with a low peak flow, hesitancy, interrupted stream and a prolonged voiding time.

Urodynamic studies

The investigations of lower urinary tract function are collectively known as urodynamics. The basic components are:

1. Uroflowmetry.
2. Cystometry.
3. Cystography.
4. Electromyography.

Uroflowmetry should be performed when the patient has a full bladder and is wanting to void. It gives a measure of the urine flow rate and voided volume as well as a graphic record of the voiding performance (Fig. 37.2.) It is indicated in all cases of outflow obstruction and voiding dysfunction.

Cystometry and videocystography requires the insertion of a filling and pressure recording catheter into the bladder and a rectal catheter to record intra-abdominal pressure. True detrusor pressure is derived by subtraction of intra-abdominal pressure from the intravesical pressure (Fig. 37.3). Cystometry is carried out during filling, during provocation by movement or coughing and during voiding. Ambulatory urodynamic studies with natural filling are more physiological but require placement of a suprapubic catheter.[7] Cystometry may be combined with a videocystogram to give maximum information about the bladder outlet during detrusor contraction as well as showing bladder anatomy and the presence of reflux.

Electromyography is used in selected cases to study sphincter and pelvic floor function in neurological disorders.

Classification of disorders of bladder function

On completing the urodynamic assessment of the patient it should be possible to define the problem in one or more of the following categories:

REFERENCES

7. Bristow S E, Neal D E Br J Urol 1996; 77: 333

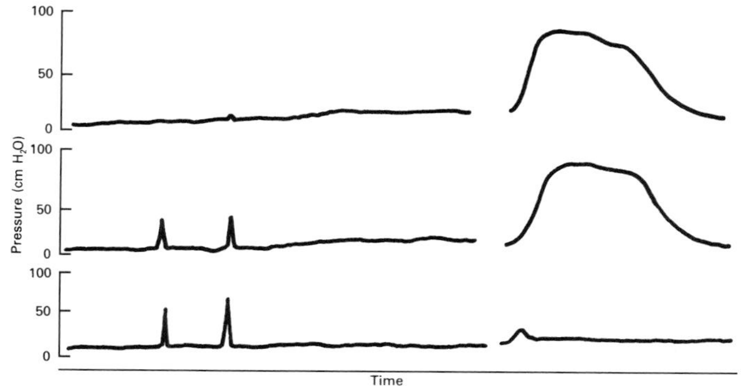

Fig 37.3 A normal cystometrogram. **Left side:** during filling; **right side:** during voiding. **Lower trace:** rectal pressure; **middle trace:** intravesical pressure; **upper trace:** detrusor pressure produced by subtracting the rectal pressure from the intravesical pressure. Note the peaks produced by coughing are subtracted out of the detrusor pressure. The detrusor pressure does not rise above 15 cm water during filling.

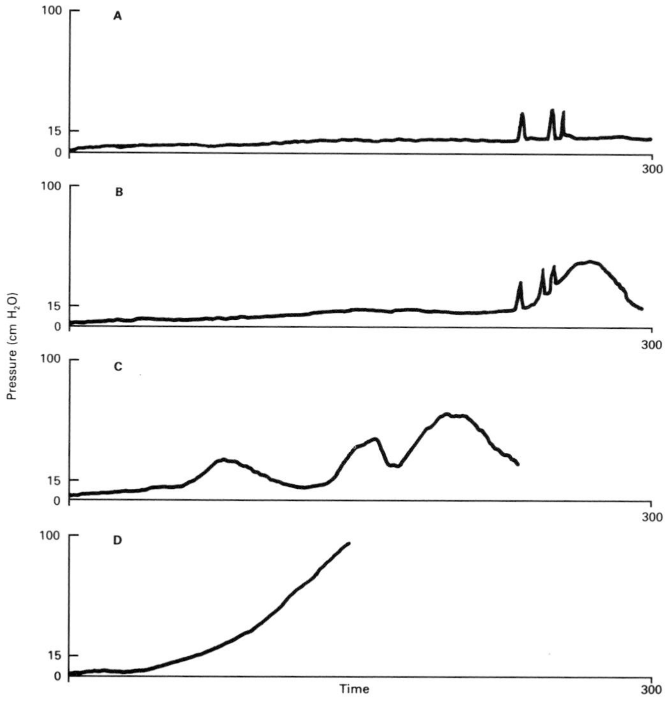

Fig 37.4 Filling cystometrograms (detrusor pressures). **Trace A:** a normal filling cystometrogram. **Trace B:** an unstable contraction provoked by coughing; this may give rise to stress-urge incontinence. **Trace C:** unstable detrusor contractions during filling. **Trace D:** a severely unstable or non-compliant bladder.

1. Disorders of bladder sensation—normal, reduced or hypersensitive.
2. Disorders of detrusor function. This may be under- or over-active. The over-active or unstable detrusor exhibits contractions during filling or on provocation. When a known neurological disorder is responsible this is known as detrusor hyper-reflexia.[8] Bladder compliance is the increase in volume per unit increase in pressure. It is not defined urodynamically but is described as either low or high compliance. There are two components to low compliance—the viscoelastic properties of the bladder and detrusor muscle contraction. Detrusor failure may be either partial or complete with no detrusor contraction at all. The bladder holding large volumes without a pressure rise has a high compliance (Fig. 37.4).
3. Sphincter weakness. Leakage of urine that occurs with raised intra-abdominal pressure but without a detrusor contraction is incontinence. The leakage that occurs with a detrusor contraction only is urge incontinence.
4. Outflow obstruction. This may be defined according to the level of the obstruction which may be at the bladder neck, prostatic urethra or pelvic floor. Detrusor–sphincter dyssynergia (Fig. 37.5) causes obstruction when the sphincter does not relax at the time of a detrusor contraction.

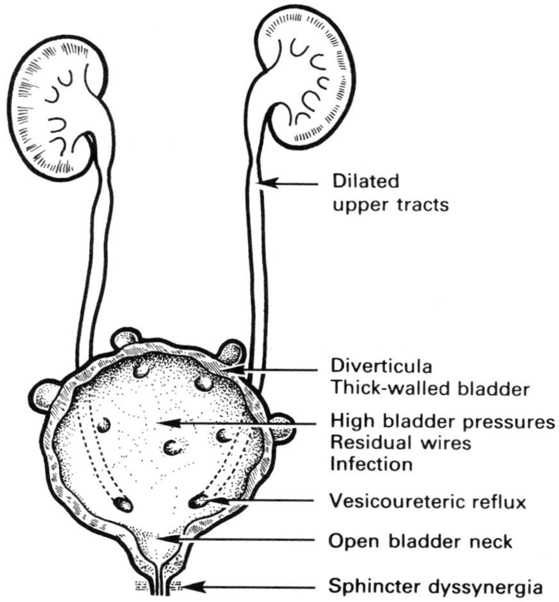

Fig 37.5 The typical appearances and consequences of detrusor–sphincter dyssynergia.

THE NEUROPATHIC BLADDER

A wide variety of neurological conditions may cause disturbances of micturition. These include spina bifida and spina bifida occulta, multiple sclerosis, Parkinson's disease and diabetic autonomic neuropathy. As well as investigating bladder function it is important to consider investigating the nervous system, with magnetic resonance imaging or myelography, in order to find an underlying cause. Patients with neuropathic bladders need an evaluation of their locomotor– system in order to choose the best management plan for them. Bladder function may be affected by major pelvic surgery. This may cause damage to pelvic nerves as well as mechanical alterations. Recovery, when it occurs, may take several

REFERENCE

8. International Continence Society Br J Urol 1981; 53: 333

weeks or months and consideration should therefore be given to managing postoperative retention by self-catheterization to allow time for a recovery of bladder function.

Aims of treatment

All patients with high intravesical pressures must have regular monitoring of the upper tracts. The two factors that result in renal damage are a high intravesical pressure, especially if reflux develops, and infection. The second consideration is to control incontinence. To achieve this it is essential to know how both the bladder and the sphincters are functioning. Thirdly, symptoms such as urinary frequency and obstruction should be treated. Finally, if these objectives cannot be met, then the patient must be rehabilitated by the optimum use of incontinence aids.

Treatment options for the neuropathic bladder

The treatment selected for the neuropathic bladder is determined by bladder function rather than its underlying aetiology and treatment plans should be tailored to the individual needs of the patient. The main treatment strategies should be selected from the following options:

1. Drug treatment.
2. Clean intermittent self-catheterization.
3. Surgery to the bladder outlet.
4. Indwelling catheter.
5. Enterocystoplasty.
6. An artificial urinary sphincter.

Drug treatment

Anticholinergic drugs, such as oxybutinin, can be effective in treating idiopathic instability from minor degrees of neuropathy but they have little effect when there is gross instability. Intravesical instillation may have a more pronounced action and it is a practical option in selected patients.[9] Voiding efficiency can sometimes be improved in patients with mild detrusor failure by carbachol or bethanecol. Intravesical prostaglandin instillation may also stimulate the detrusor to contract. The α-receptor blocking drugs lower outflow resistance by relaxing the muscle of the bladder neck and prostate and can also improve bladder emptying.

Clean intermittent self-catheterization

This is indicated in cases with detrusor failure or ineffective bladder emptying because of detrusor–sphincter dyssynergia. Self-catheterization must achieve complete bladder emptying and should be carried out at regular intervals; thus the risks and consequences of infection are reduced and an aseptic technique is not necessary.[10] The patient must be sufficiently mobile and have the manual dexterity to be able to perform the procedure.

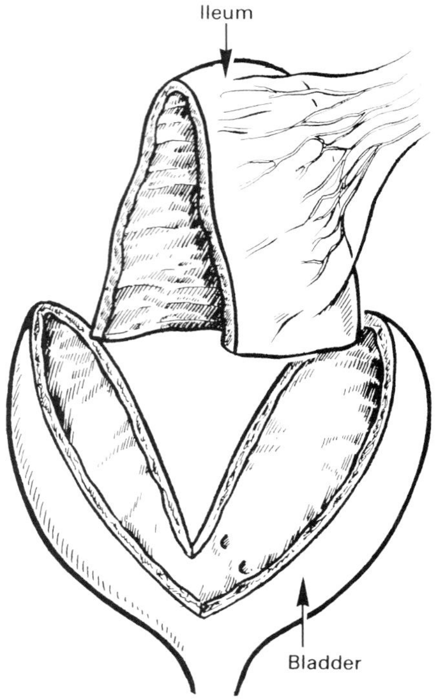

Fig 37.6 The 'clam' augmentation cystoplasty. The bladder must be almost completely bivalved and the correct length of opened-out ileum used. It is wise to protect the ureters with catheters while suturing the lower part of the bladder.

Surgery to the bladder outlet

Reducing the outflow resistance by resection of the bladder neck or prostate or by incision through the distal sphincter can improve bladder emptying but usually makes the neuropathic bladder incontinent. This may be necessary to protect the upper tracts; the patient then has to wear an external appliance.

Indwelling catheter

This has advantages for some patients and their carers, but eventually there may be many problems with infection, catheter blockage, expulsion and development of bladder stones and squamous cancers.[11] Expulsion can be a problem in women with a neuropathic bladder: it is no use inserting larger and larger catheters as the urethra just becomes more patulous. Such patients require urinary diversion.

Enterocystoplasty

When high pressure detrusor contractions cannot be controlled by drugs they can be abolished by an enterocystoplasty. This may be an augmentation such as the 'clam' procedure[12] (see Fig. 37.6) or, if the bladder is grossly diseased, a substitution cystoplasty may be

REFERENCES

9. Prasad K V R, Vaidyanathan S Br J Urol 1993; 72: 719
10. Lapides J et al J Urol 1972; 107: 458
11. Kohler-Ockmore J, Feneley R C L Br J Urol 1996; 77: 347

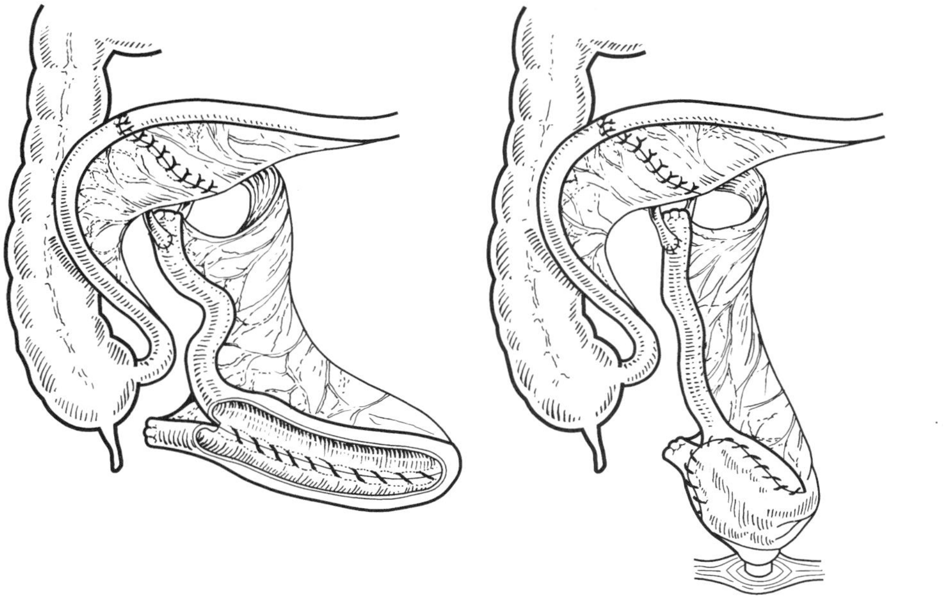

Fig 37.7 A segment of the ileum is isolated approximately 60 cm long and formed into a pouch using the method described by Studer.[13]

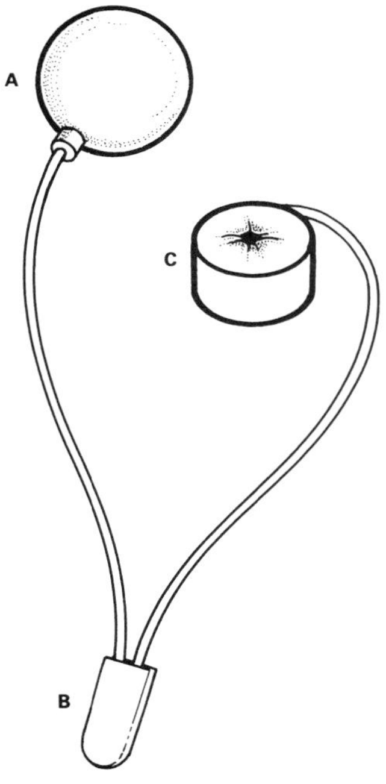

Fig 37.8 The AMS artificial urinary sphincter. This has three main components: **A** the reservoir which contains the fluid at a set pressure; **B** the control valve and pump, which is squeezed to empty the cuff and then allows it to fill slowly from the reservoir; **C** the cuff, usually placed around the bladder neck but which can be placed around the bulbar urethra.

performed (Fig. 37.7). The bladder is removed and a substitute constructed from a detubularized segment of bowel.[13] One consequence of having an enterocystoplasty is that emptying is likely to be ineffective and these patients therefore need to practise self-catheterization. Other complications are the production of mucus, stone formation and a metabolic acidosis from reabsorption of urine.[14] The later risk of malignant tumours developing is as yet undetermined but is probably very low.

The artificial urinary sphincter

This is used as part of the complete lower urinary tract reconstruction in selected cases of bladder neuropathy (Fig. 37.8). It should not be inserted unless bladder compliance is normal, usually after an enterocystoplasty, otherwise the upper tracts risk damage. The main complications are erosion into the urethra, infection and mechanical failure.[15]

Spinal injury

Immediately after spinal injury there is a period lasting several weeks when there is no reflex activity and the bladder is unable to contract. There is a high risk of infection and associated complications if retention is managed by an indwelling urethral catheter. The two alternatives are the use of aseptic intermittent catheterization, established by the work of Guttman,[16] or the insertion of a fine-bore suprapubic catheter.[17] These alternatives can be used until reflex contractions return after 6–12 weeks. The bladder will have to be emptied by abdominal pressure or self-catheterization if detrusor activity does not recover. When reflex contractions are present they can be used to empty the bladder by being triggered to

REFERENCES

12. Mundy A R, Stephenson T P Br J Urol 1985; 57: 641
13. Studer U E In: Fitzpatrick J M, Krane R J (eds) The Bladder. Churchill Livingstone, Edinburgh 1995
14. Nurse D E, Mundy A R Br J Urol 1989; 63: 165
15. Nurse D E, Mundy A R Br J Urol 1988; 61: 318
16. Guttman L, Frankel H Paraplegia 1966; 4: 63
17. Grundy D et al Paraplegia 1983; 21: 227

produce periodic reflex micturition. Detrusor–sphincter dyssynergia is, however, common as the relaxation of the distal sphincter with detrusor contraction is coordinated in the brainstem. This results in high bladder pressures and affected patients need complete ablation of the sphincters before bladder emptying at low pressures is achieved. Males then require an external appliance and females may need a permanent catheter.

A large proportion of the late mortality from spinal injury (see Chapter 46) is the result of urological complications. Infections, high pressure reflux and stone formation may all contribute to renal failure. Urethral fistula and strictures as well as ulceration around the penis may develop if patients are not closely supervised. Squamous carcinoma may occur many years later as a result of chronic infection and irritation. Long-term follow-up must include regular assessment of the upper tracts, and cystoscopy should be considered in those who have had stones and infections.

Idiopathic bladder instability

This condition is more common in women and presents at any time in adult life. The symptoms are urinary frequency, urgency and urge incontinence. The unstable contractions are often provoked by activity and can be reproduced during the cystometrogram (Fig. 37.4). A careful search must be made for a neurological cause before labelling the condition idiopathic.

The first line of management is careful reassurance to the patient, advice on fluids, particularly to reduce caffeine intake, and the use of anticholinergic drugs such as oxybutinin. Many other treatments have been tried to control the symptoms and most have had very limited success. The 'clam' enterocystoplasty is highly effective at abolishing the contractions and can be considered when conservative treatments have failed. The long-term complications such as infection, mucus secretion and the need for self-catheterization must be carefully balanced against the benefits of curing the urgency and urge incontinence.

INCONTINENCE OF URINE

Sphincter weakness incontinence

Genuine stress incontinence is common in women and also in the elderly. An exact history should be obtained, not only to establish the nature of the leakage but also to assess the degree (numbers of pads used, how often changed and soiling of clothes). Examination should concentrate on palpating for an enlarged bladder, examining the pelvis and urethral meatus and assessing the pelvic floor. The diagnosis of genuine stress incontinence cannot be made from the history alone as the same factors causing stress incontinence may be provoking unstable detrusor contractions resulting in stress-urge incontinence. Urodynamic studies need to be performed when there is any degree of frequency or urgency with the incontinence.

Women with stress incontinence should be encouraged to lose weight, give up smoking to correct any chronic cough and to have pelvic physiotherapy with vaginal weights to strengthen the pelvic floor. Surgical treatments used for stress incontinence in the female are:

1. Vaginal repair (anterior colporrhaphy). The urethra and bladder base are supported by mobilization and approximation of the paraurethral tissues and pelvic floor muscle carried out from the vagina.
2. Suprapubic suspension operations such as the Marshall–Marchetti–Krantz operation.[18] This has a higher success rate than the vaginal repair but is a more major procedure.
3. Endoscopic bladder neck suspension.[19,20] This is a minimally invasive procedure but longer follow-up studies have shown a high late failure rate as compared to the colposuspension.
4. Periurethral injections around the urethra and bladder neck. Injections of inert substances such as Teflon, silicone or collagen may increase urethral resistance and can improve stress incontinence, including post-prostatectomy incontinence.[21]

Post-prostatectomy incontinence

Not all post-prostatectomy incontinence is caused by sphincter damage. Bladder instability may have resulted from the outflow obstruction and can persist after prostatectomy has relieved the obstruction. The patient may also have insidiously reverted back into chronic retention with overflow incontinence. Pure sphincter weakness may slowly improve after prostatectomy and usually improves over several months. Usually it is necessary to wait up to 9 months, during which time physiotherapy and pelvic floor exercises can be given.

Enuresis

The literal meaning of enuresis is incontinence but it is now commonly used to mean bed-wetting. The incidence of enuresis falls steadily from the age of 2, when virtually all children have enuresis, until adolescence when the incidence drops to below 10%.[22] There is frequently a family history of enuresis and a history of emotional disturbance. Against this background it is important to establish which children may have an underlying problem and when it is appropriate to investigate and treat. It must be established if the child has always been enuretic or was previously dry. A history of daytime incontinence, other urinary symptoms and faecal incontinence suggest that a neurological disorder may be responsible. Children without an underlying pathology can be treated with an alarm[23] and this can be combined with imipramine which reduces deep sleep and has an anticholinergic effect on the bladder. Fluid restriction in the evening can help and those children who pass large volumes during the night can be treated with good effect with the synthetic antidiuretic hormone

REFERENCES

18. Marshall V F et al. Surg Gynecol Obstet 1949; 88: 509
19. Stamey T A Ann Surg 1980; 192: 465
20. German K A et al Br J Urol 1994; 74: 188
21. Chahha C, Williams G Br J Urol 1995; 76: 151
22. Forsythe W I, Redmond A Arch Dis Child 1974; 49: 259
23. Forsythe W I, Redmond A Br Med J 1970; 1: 211

desmopressin. Ultrasound and flow rate measurement are usually the only investigations required in uncomplicated enuresis but if these measures fail then the child should be considered for urodynamic studies.[24]

INJURY TO THE BLADDER

The bladder may be ruptured as a result of blunt abdominal injury or perforated by a penetrating injury. The bladder is usually full when ruptured and the disruption is usually in the intraperitoneal portion of the dome. A ruptured bladder should be considered in all patients with abdominal trauma especially if the patient wants to void but is unable to do so, gives a history of recent drinking or if there is free fluid in the abdomen (see Chapter 7). The whole urinary tract should be assessed by intravenous urography and an ascending cystourethrogram if the diagnosis of bladder rupture is suspected. A rupture of the urethra is also a possibility. Very rarely a delayed bladder rupture may develop and a high index of suspicion must be maintained.[25] Spontaneous ruptures of enterocystoplasties are now being seen as these procedures are becoming more prevalent. Nearly all traumatic ruptures of the bladder require laparotomy and closure with absorbable sutures.

The most common form of bladder injury is from transurethral resections of bladder tumours. This is usually in the extraperitoneal part of the bladder and can be managed conservatively with antibiotics and a catheter. A drain should be inserted if the extravasation is extensive. An intraperitoneal perforation usually requires a laparotomy when the fluid must be sucked out, the perforation closed, a drain inserted and a careful inspection made for any associated injury to the bowel.

VESICAL FISTULAE

There are two main types of fistula involving the bladder: a vesicocolic and vesicovaginal fistula. A vesicocolic fistula usually arises from pathology in the large bowel such as diverticular disease or colonic cancer (see Chapter 30). The patient may have few symptoms or may present with severe cystitis. The key symptom is pneumaturia, but diabetes associated with a bacterial gas-forming infection may ferment the sugar in the urine, also producing gas. Faecal material is seen on microscopy confirming the diagnosis. Both the large bowel and the urinary tract should be fully investigated with endoscopy, biopsy and contrast studies. The colonic disease usually requires resection while the bladder just requires simple closure with omental interposition and catheter drainage for a week. Vesicovaginal fistula occurs as a result of obstetric trauma, pelvic surgery or radiotherapy for gynaecological malignant disease. When a fistula follows obstetric or surgical trauma the surrounding tissues are usually healthy and primary repair can be performed either from the vagina or through the bladder with an omental interposition.[26] When the fistula is in an irradiated field primary healing may be difficult to obtain, even with a major reconstructive procedure, and diversion may have to be considered.

Very rarely a fistula may develop between the bladder and the uterus following caesarean section. These patients may not leak urine but develop monthly haematuria (Yousef's syndrome).[27] This type of fistula is repaired through an abdominal approach.

BLADDER CALCULI

Bladder calculi are now rare in both adults and children, except in certain geographical regions where most of the calculi occur in children. The reasons for this are obscure. Nutritional factors, socioeconomic status, climate and episodes of severe dehydration during febrile illnesses may all play a part in the aetiology of bladder calculi in these countries.[28]

The main causes of bladder calculi in adults are bladder outflow obstruction, chronic infection, foreign bodies and the occasional stone passed from the upper tracts (see Chapter 36). Foreign bodies may have been introduced by the patient or may be iatrogenic. Any non-absorbable suture used in the urinary tract is a potential nidus for stone formation and these stones are sometimes seen hanging on the anterior bladder wall where sutures have eroded into the bladder following a colposuspension operation. When a long-term catheter is used calcium phosphate and carbonate may deposit on the balloon and form an eggshell calculus. This will break up when the catheter is changed and may form the nidus for a vesical calculus. If the balloon of a Foley catheter ruptures and a fragment of balloon is left in the bladder then this too will form a stone.

Bladder calculi may cause pain, frequency and haematuria. The smaller calculi can impact in the urethra and cause retention. A bladder calculus that has been present for a long time causes infection and chronic irritation of the urothelium with resultant squamous metaplasia and increasing risk of squamous carcinoma of the bladder. Any patient with a stone must be carefully examined for an associated bladder cancer and it is important to be aware of the bladder tumour that calcifies. This is invariably a poorly differentiated tumour with superficial necrosis.

Except for the endemic calculi most bladder stones contain calcium and are radiopaque. The treatment of bladder calculi has benefited from the developments in endourological techniques used to treat upper tract stones. The lithoclast is the most effective instrument for fragmenting stones, but smaller stones can be easily fragmented with a stone punch or optical lithotrite under vision. Very large stones (over 5 cm diameter) are best removed at an open operation rather than attempting to disintegrate them with a long endoscopic procedure which will inevitably end up being traumatic, bloody and incomplete.

BLADDER DIVERTICULA

Bladder diverticula may be congenital or acquired. The term 'congenital' is often used to describe diverticula of obscure origin,

REFERENCES

24. Mark S D, Frank J D Br J Urol 1995; 75: 427
25. Turnbull A R Br J Urol 1978; 50: 162
26. Kelly J Br J Urol 1979; 51: 208
27. Youssef A F Am J Obstet Gynecol 1957; 73: 759
28. Robertson W G In: Hussain I (ed) Tropical Urology. Churchill Livingstone, Edinburgh 1984

and its use is seldom helpful. The main congenital diverticula are those occurring in the urachus (see above) and the paraureteric diverticulum associated with ureteric reflux. Acquired diverticula develop as a result of high intravesical pressures caused by outflow obstruction. They may be single or multiple and can be of any size. Small diverticula are of little importance but the larger ones can cause voiding inefficiency. When they cause symptoms or are complicated by recurring infection they should be excised and the bladder outflow obstruction corrected.

The presence of diverticula can complicate the management of bladder cancer if the tumour develops in or near the diverticulum. Transurethral resection of the cancer may be hazardous under these circumstances as there is no muscle below the mucosa to resect into and a perforation is inevitable. A solitary tumour in a large diverticulum can be excised as a partial cystectomy, but there is a considerable risk of recurrence if the tumour is poorly differentiated or invasive. Excision of a large diverticulum can be difficult because of its adherence to the pelvic wall and limited exposure in the pelvis. Dissection is made easier if the diverticulum is packed with a swab. Smaller diverticula can often be obliterated by diathermy. In the presence of diverticula multifocal bladder tumours should be considered for intravesical chemotherapy.

URINARY INFECTION

Urinary infection may be found without symptoms or signs (covert infection) or with symptoms and signs that can vary from the minor to very serious disability (overt infection). The consequences can vary from the trivial to the fatal. Urinary infection enters into the differential diagnosis of many surgical patients and is of particular importance in neonates and children.

Urinary infection in children

Urinary infection is more common in male infants in the first month of life but thereafter it is much more common in females. The incidence of covert bacteriuria is 1–2% in girls. 5% of girls develop an overt infection during childhood whereas only 1–2% of boys become infected.[29] In children under the age of 4 years the presenting symptoms and signs are often non-specific such as vomiting, fevers and feeding problems. Clean voided specimens are difficult to obtain in this age group and a suprapubic aspirate is a useful alternative. Children with a proven urinary infection should be investigated to rule out an underlying pathological abnormality. Approximately half will be found to have no significant abnormality in the urinary tract.[30] The most common abnormality found is vesicoureteric reflux which occurs in 35–40%. Other abnormalities produce obstructions such as ureteroceles or stones in 8%. An ultrasound gives a good anatomical demonstration of the urinary tract in children and avoids the radiation of an intravenous urogram. Further investigation is not necessary if the ultrasound is normal in a child aged more than 3 years. In a child under 3 years it is more important to exclude reflux because the risks of repeated infections and renal scarring are greater. While the micturating cystogram is still the most sensitive investigation for detecting reflux it is invasive and has a high radiation exposure. Renography can also detect reflux. It avoids the risks of radiation and is an acceptable alternative. Renal scars may take several months to evolve on the intravenous urogram but will show immediately on the digital subtraction angiography scan.

Vesicoureteric reflux

Reflux is found frequently in neonates and it is likely that most of the ureters which allow reflux at birth stop refluxing as the child begins to grow. This congenital form of reflux may be the result of the ureteric bud arising distally on the mesonephric duct, causing the ureteric orifice to become laterally placed and to have a short intravesical tunnel. The ureter is more likely to drain a dysplastic kidney.[31] Acquired reflux is the result of obstruction or bladder neuropathy.

Reflux allows the pressure in the bladder to be transmitted to the kidney and encourage urine, which may be infected, to pass back into the collecting tubules (intrarenal reflux). In man this only occurs in infants up to the age of 3 and it is usually only the compound papillae at the poles of the kidney that allow intrarenal reflux. When infected urine refluxes into the kidney pyelonephritis results and heals with focal scarring. Progressive renal damage may follow as a result of further infections or from hypertension, interstitial nephritis or glomerulosclerosis. This entity is known as reflux nephropathy. The management of reflux depends on its severity, which may be graded by the dilatation of the ureter or on a 3 or 5 grade system (Fig. 37.9).[31,32] In children with reflux into normal calibre ureters, the reflux is likely to cease as the child grows and prolonged antibiotic therapy is all that is required. Reflux is less likely to cease spontaneously when the ureter is dilated and these children should be considered for ureteric reimplantation or the less invasive procedure of subureteric injection of Teflon.[33]

Urinary infection in adults

The most common abnormality associated with bladder infection in adult males is bladder outflow obstruction.[34] A single proven infection in a male should therefore be investigated. In females urinary infections are much more common and less likely to be complicated. If infections recur it is important to establish if this is a relapse (same organism) or a new infection with a different organism. The intravenous urogram is the investigation of choice as this provides anatomical information about the whole urinary tract. In males this should be supplemented by measuring the urine

REFERENCES

29. Vernier-Jones K et al In: Asscher A W. Brumfitt W (eds) Microbial Diseases in Nephrology. John Wiley, Chichester 1986
30. Smellie J M et al Kidney Int 1981; 20: 717
31. Mackie G G, Stephens F D J Urol 1975; 114: 274
32. Medical Research Council Bacteruria Committee Br Med J 1989; 2: 717
33. International Reflux Study Committee J Urol 1981; 125: 272
33. Puri P Br J Urol 1995; 75: 126
34. Booth C M Br J Urol 1981; 53: 270

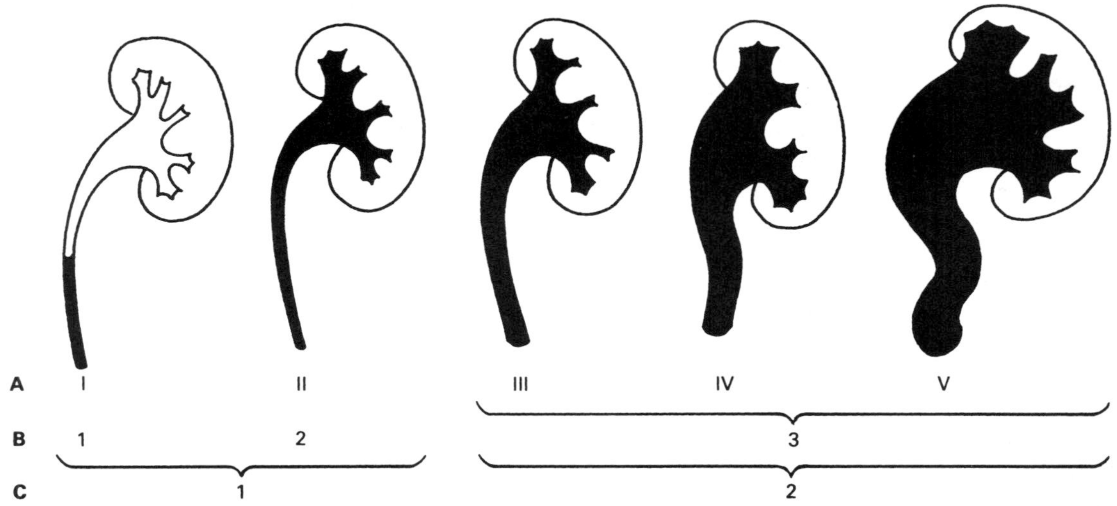

Fig 37.9 The grading of vesicoureteric reflux. **A** The five grades of the International Reflux Study Committee.[33] **B** The three grades of the MRC Bacteriuria Committee.[32] **C** The two grades according to calibre of the ureters: normal and dilated. The black area shows distance to which urine refluxes.

flow rate and urodynamic studies if outflow obstruction or bladder neuropathy is suspected. There is little point in performing a micturating cystogram in adults to look for reflux unless the ureters are dilated and the infections are difficult to control.

Nosocomial infection

Nosocomial or hospital acquired infection is a major problem in hospitals, especially in urological and surgical patients (see Chapter 4). Instrumentation and catheterization are the most important reasons and are also the most common causes of bacteraemia in hospital practice. It is advisable to screen all patients before surgery if this is likely to involve catheterization or instrumentation.

There are three main reasons for the development of urinary infections following instrumentation or catheterization:

1. The aseptic technique may be at fault.
2. Organisms may ascend into the bladder because the drainage system is not kept closed and organisms contaminate the system.
3. Organisms may get into the bladder alongside the catheter.

Despite proper catheter care it is virtually impossible to keep the urine of a catheterized patient sterile for much longer than one week.

TUBERCULOUS CYSTITIS

When tuberculosis affects the bladder there is invariably evidence of tuberculous infection in the upper tracts. Sometimes there may also be coexistent tuberculous prostatitis or epididymitis. The presenting symptoms of tuberculous cystitis are increased urinary frequency, dysuria, bladder pain and haematuria. The patient may also have systemic symptoms of fevers, sweats and weight loss. A sterile pyuria is found on testing the urine. A single urine sample is inadequate and at least three complete early morning samples should be sent for culture to have a 95% chance of culturing the tubercle bacillus.

On cystoscopy the bladder is often contracted with a red, oedematous wall. These changes may be most marked around the ureteric orifices. Tubercles appear as yellow elevated spots. Mucosal biopsies should be avoided if tuberculous infection is strongly suspected: this is an inefficient way of diagnosing tuberculosis as the bacilli are hard to identify in tissue sections and there is a risk of disseminating infection. The differential diagnosis includes carcinoma of the bladder so biopsies may have to be taken to exclude this. The treatment of genitourinary tuberculosis has already been described in Chapter 36 but essentially the patient recovers on a prolonged course of antituberculous chemotherapy.

The end-result of tuberculous cystitis may be a severely contracted bladder (Fig. 37.10) with disabling symptoms, and this may be accompanied by lower ureteric obstruction. The severely contracted bladder may require augmentation with ileum or colon. In men an augmentation usually needs to be supplemented by a bladder neck incision to restore voiding efficiency.

BILHARZIA OF THE BLADDER

Bilharzia is one of the commonest diseases, affecting worldwide some 100–300 million people. It is caused by infestation with a trematode worm or fluke of which there are three species—*Schistosoma mansoni, haematobium* and *japonicum*. *S. haematobium* is almost entirely responsible for urinary bilharzia and is widespread throughout Africa and The Middle East, although it is only endemic in the arid and subtropical areas where conditions are favourable for its transmission.

Man is the only definitive host for *S. haematobium*. The flukes live in the vesical veins where sexual reproduction takes place; the female lays 50–300 eggs per day for an average of 2–5 years. The eggs are laid in the small submucosal veins and then migrate into the lumen of the bladder before being shed into the urine. When the eggs enter fresh water they hatch into miracidia (Fig. 37.11).

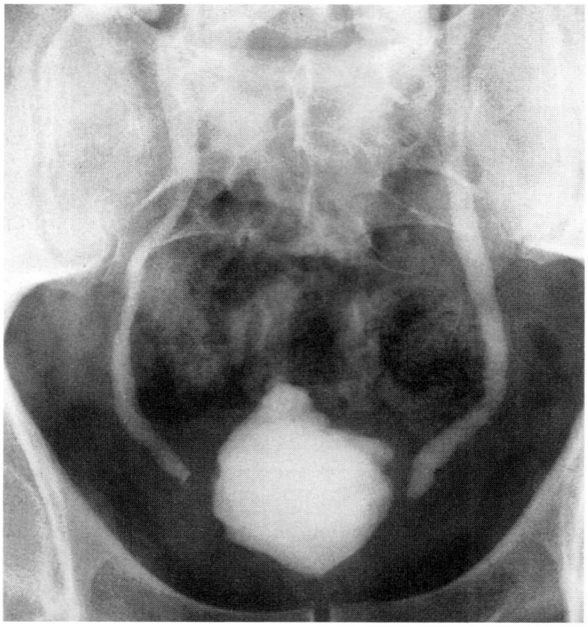

Fig 37.10 Tuberculous cystitis. Typical appearances on an intravenous urogram of a contracted bladder which is also obstructing drainage from the ureters.

Within 24 hours the miracidia must find their way into the intermediate host, the *Bulinus* species of freshwater snail. In the snail the miracidia undergo asexual reproduction to produce thousands of cercariae which are then released from the snail. The cercariae have to penetrate the skin of the human host within 10–12 hours of being released and on entering the human they become schistosomula. These migrate through the portal vein to end up as mature worms in the pelvic veins after 5–6 weeks.

Pathology

The eggs elicit an acute and chronic inflammatory reaction in the bladder wall. The urothelium ulcerates and also proliferates to form polyps. Hyperplasia and squamous metaplasia of the urothelium are usual and leucoplakia, dysplasia, carcinoma in situ and invasive cancer may develop later. Many eggs die before they are shed and these calcify in the bladder wall to cause the sandy patches visible on cystoscopy and the florid calcified bladder sometimes seen on a plain radiograph (Fig. 37.12). The late result of chronic inflammation in the bladder is fibrosis, causing a contracted, non-compliant bladder and strictures of the ureters or urethra. Secondary infection is common and this is responsible for much of the morbidity of bilharzia.

Bladder cancer is the major complication of urinary bilharzia: the evidence now suggests that carcinogenesis is initiated by the production of nitrosamines in the urine by the action of bacteria on nitrates and amines in the urine. Bilharzia has the ability to predispose to chronic infection by its effects on the bladder wall and mucosa and to promote tumour growth by chronic irritation.

Clinical features

The initial infestation may cause symptoms ranging from a minor urticarial reaction (swimmers' itch) to the Katayama syndrome of

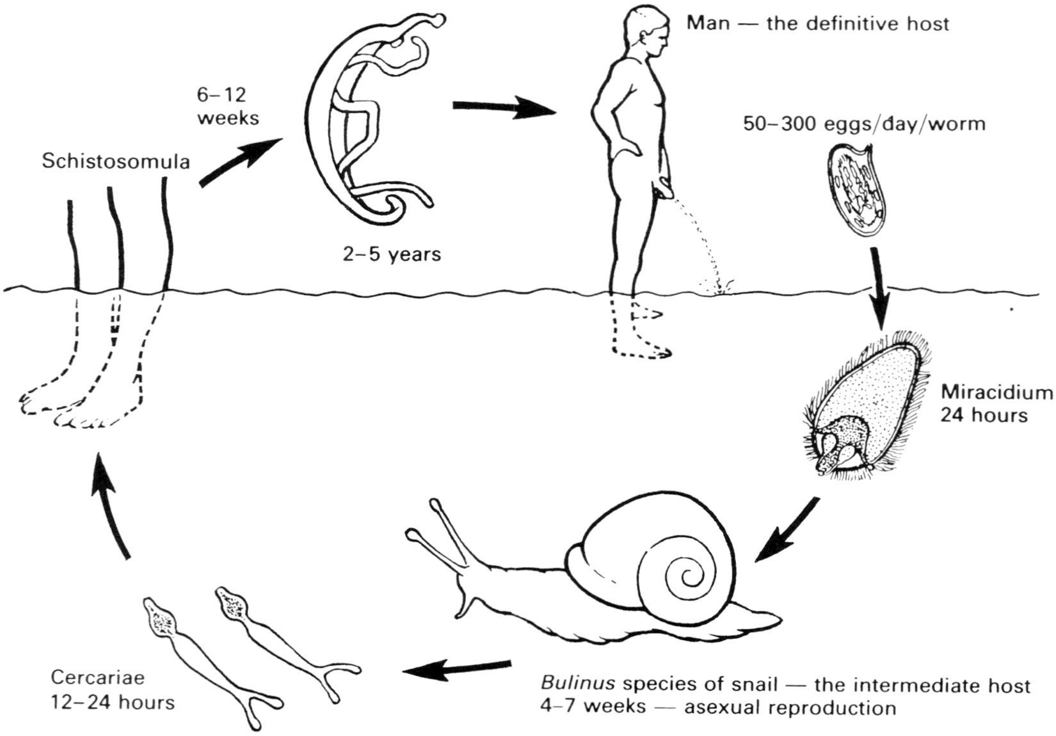

Fig 37.11 The life cycle of *Schistosoma haematobium*.

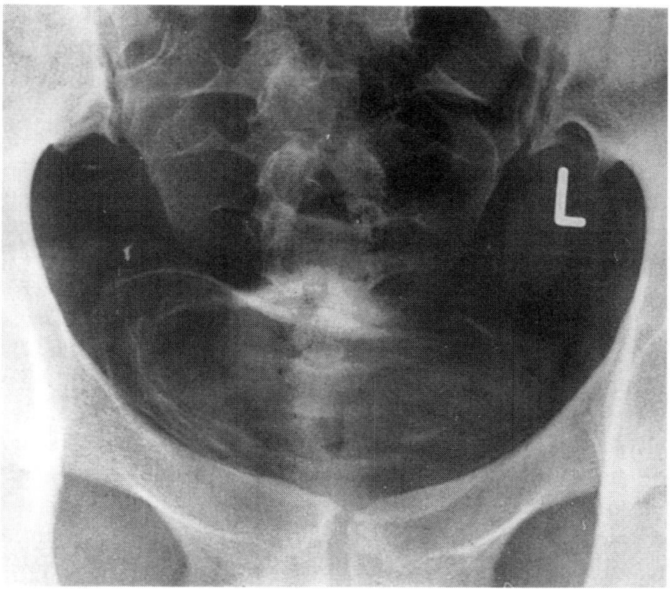

Fig 37.12 Calcification in the wall of a bladder infested with *Schistosoma haematobium*.

fever, cough, urticaria and abdominal pains.[35] An acute episode occurs some 3 months after the initial infestation and presents with urinary frequency, dysuria and haematuria which is characteristically terminal. Recovery from the acute stage may be complete or the patient may go on to develop the chronic disorder characterized by fibrosis and secondary infection. Bladder compliance and capacity are reduced, the upper tracts may develop strictures, and stones may form in the ureters or bladder.

The diagnosis of urinary bilharzia is usually made by demonstrating the ova with their terminal spines in the urine. A plain radiograph may show the characteristic bladder calcification (Fig. 37.12). The cystoscopic appearances are varied, beginning with small tubercles surrounded by hyperaemic mucosa and progressing to nodules and polyp formation. Atrophy of the urothelium may occur over the calcified eggs, giving rise to the sandy patches. Ulceration of the mucosa, cystitis cystica and glandularis, leucoplakia and carcinoma in situ may all develop.

The incidence of bladder cancer occurring in association with bilharzia shows marked geographical variations.[36] The cause of this is uncertain but may be related to the urinary nitrate excretion and secondary infection producing nitrosamines. The carcinomas that occur in the bilharzial bladder are frequently squamous or have squamous metaplasia and are often advanced with deep muscle invasion at the time of presentation. Metastases occur late, probably as a result of the fibrosis around the bladder.

Treatment

For drug treatment to be used successfully, it must be effective, given as a single treatment, inexpensive and well tolerated. Two drugs approach these requirements: metrifonate and praziquantel. Metrifonate is effective only against *S. haematobium* whereas praziquantel is effective against all three species and is the treatment of choice as, in many areas, more than one species of schistosome is endemic.

Bladder contractions and ureteric strictures may require surgery using the ileum to augment the bladder or replace the ureters. Carcinomas of the bilharzial bladder require surgery as they are usually advanced at the time of presentation with widespread disease in the bladder. The prostate and urethra may also be involved. Bilharzial carcinoma responds poorly to radiotherapy as it is squamous or associated with squamous metaplasia.

The type of urinary diversion used must take into account the local cultural, economic and social factors. An ileal loop diversion may be very difficult to manage in tropical climates and a wet, continuously discharging stoma may be unacceptable to the patient. In Egypt in particular the preference is for a rectal bladder with a colostomy as this is much easier to manage.[37] Ureterosigmoid diversion is usually not possible because the dilatation of the ureters prevents an adequate reflux-preventing anastomosis. An orthotopic bladder substitution has now become the treatment of choice for bilharzial bladder cancer.[38]

CYSTITIS

Interstitial cystitis

This condition still lacks a clear definition and criteria for diagnosis.[39] The incidence remains uncertain. Women are more commonly affected and patients with advanced disease are usually middle-aged or elderly women. The presenting symptoms are urinary frequency, urgency and pain. The disease is easily recognized in its advanced stages, which are associated with a contracted and ulcerated bladder, but in the early stages when the bladder has a normal capacity it may be more difficult to diagnose with confidence.[40] The diagnosis is made on the cystoscopic findings and the biopsy appearances. The characteristic findings on cystoscopy are that the bladder is usually of reduced capacity and is painful to distend even under light anaesthesia; the mucosa shows widespread fissures, stellate ulcers and bleeds readily on decompression.

Biopsies should be taken to include the muscle layer as these can show chronic inflammatory changes in the submucosa and muscle. There is an increased number of mast cells in the bladder wall: this is one of the criteria used to diagnosis this condition.[41] It is important to rule out other conditions such as tuberculosis and carcinoma in situ by biopsies and cytology.

Many treatments have been used with some success. Endoscopic resection can be effective if the condition is very localized but this is unusual. Simple hydrostatic dilatation may relieve symptoms though these usually recur after a short interval. Sodium

REFERENCES

35. Walt F S Afr Med J 1954; 28: 89
36. Attah E B, Nkposong E O Trop Geog Med 1976; 28: 268
37. Ghoneim M A, Ashmallah A Br J Urol 1974; 46: 511
38. Abol-Enein H, Ghoneim M A Br J Urol 1995; 76: 558
39. Fall M et al J Urol 1987; 137: 35
40. Messing E M, Stamey T A Urology 1978; 12: 381
41. Kastrup J et al Br J Urol 1983; 55: 495

pentosan polysulphate or amitryptyline may be used orally or dimethyl sulphoxide, with or without steroid, may be instilled into the bladder.[42] When these conservative treatments fail and the patient's symptoms are severe, then replacement of the bladder with an enterocystoplasty is indicated.

Eosinophilic cystitis

This is similar to interstitial cystitis and presents with a florid, red, oedematous bladder. The diagnosis is made from a biopsy which demonstrates extensive infiltration with eosinophils. The aetiology is uncertain but is likely to be a reaction to food or drug allergens, parasites or topical agents.[43] Antihistamines and steroids may be helpful and antibiotics may be needed to control secondary infections, but the identification and removal of the allergen is essential whenever possible.

Radiation cystitis

The response of the bladder to irradiation is variable and often unpredictable. A total dose of over 6000 cGy carries a definite risk of late complications, as do smaller doses if given in large fractions. Large ulcerating tumours, recent bladder surgery and bladder outflow obstruction also predispose to the development of radiation reactions.

Radiation of the bladder firstly causes damage to the blood vessels in the bladder and secondly causes contraction due to fibrosis. Bleeding from the urothelium can be controlled by endoscopic diathermy but, if severe, may require irrigation with alum to thrombose the abnormal submucosal vessels.[44] Severe bleeding or contraction of the bladder may require a salvage cystectomy or urinary diversion. Severe radiation damage may also result in a fistula which will usually develop into the small or large bowel.

Cyclophosphamide cystitis

The metabolite of cyclophosphamide, acrolein, is an aldehyde and oxidizing agent that is toxic to urothelial cells. It can cause widespread loss of the urothelium and a severe haemorrhagic cystitis. This is usually only seen after high dose intravenous therapy and can be prevented by the use of 2-mercaptoethane sodium sulphonate.[45] The use of continuous low dose oral cyclophosphamide is less likely to cause haemorrhagic cystitis but there is a risk of developing a urothelial bladder carcinoma after a number of years (see below).

RESPONSES OF THE BLADDER TO INJURY AND INFLAMMATION

The bladder reacts in a number of ways to injury and inflammation. The first response is usually proliferation which results in the invagination of the mucosa to form von Brun's nests. Small cysts lined by flattened urothelium form under the mucosa giving rise to *cystitis cystica*. These cysts can be seen on cystoscopy as 2–3 mm yellow nodules under the mucosa. Further proliferation can result in a glandular appearance (*cystitis glandularis*). These changes are frequently found in normal bladders, are more common around the trigone and are clearly associated with infections and chronic irritation from, for example, a stone or catheter.

Non-keratinizing squamous metaplasia is another normal variant found in the trigone which may become more widespread in response to chronic injury. Squamous metaplasia that keratinizes is called 'leucoplakia' and this is visible on cystoscopy as clearly demarcated white patches, often surrounded by inflamed urothelium. Leucoplakia is a premalignant condition: 25–28% of patients develop squamous cancers of the bladder.[46]

Malakoplakia is a granulomatous condition resulting from defective intracellular phagocytosis of *Escherichia coli*. The bladder is the most common site but malakoplakia can occur anywhere in the urinary tract and sometimes outside it. The clinical manifestations vary from a small brown patch to a huge granulomatous mass mimicking malignant disease. The urine is infected with *E. coli* and the diagnosis is confirmed by finding the characteristic inclusion bodies or Michaelis–Gutmann bodies. Treatment is with an anti-biotic which is intracellularly active, such as trimethoprim. Bethanecol and ascorbic acid have been recommended to potentiate chemotaxis.[47]

The *nephrogenic adenoma* is a metaplastic change presenting with red areas or tumours in the bladder. These can have a papillary appearance and can be easily mistaken for a bladder cancer. The nephrogenic adenoma usually occurs after trauma or tuberculosis of the bladder.[48] The lesions may be small and localized to the area of previous damage or they may be more widespread. Malignant change to produce an adenocarcinoma is very rare and there is doubt that this does occur. The histology shows tubular structures lined by cuboidal cells resembling the distal convoluted tubules of the kidney. Most cases respond to endoscopic resection and diathermy.

Chronic granulomas may present in the wall of the bladder and these again may be mistaken for malignant tumours. They may contain a foreign body, almost always a silk suture from a previous hernia repair.[49] Some of these granulomas can be cured by endoscopic resection to drain the mass into the bladder and remove the foreign body but many require complete excision.

TUMOURS OF THE BLADDER

Benign bladder tumours

A benign bladder papilloma is very rare compared to the frequency of well differentiated transitional cell carcinoma. It has by definition an epithelial lining of its papillary processes that is indistinguishable from normal urothelium. The term 'papilloma' has been

REFERENCES

42. Sant G Urology 1987; 29(suppl): 17
43. Litleton R H et al J Urol 1982; 127: 132
44. Kennedy C et al. Br J Urol 1984; 56: 673
45. Bryant B M et al. Lancet 1980; ii: 657
46. Morgan R J. Cameron K M Br J Urol 1980; 52: 96
47. Curran F T Br J Urol 1987; 59: 559
48. Ford T F et al Br J Urol 1985; 61: 266
49. Lynch T H et al J Urol 1991; 145: 249

much misused in the past to denote well differentiated non-invasive transitional cell carcinomas.[50] The benign papilloma does not recur after resection and does not need prolonged follow-up.

The inverted papilloma is a variant of the benign papilloma. The growth pattern of this tumour is inverted with the papillary processes growing down into the submucosa. They present as smooth tumours, usually on the bladder base or trigone, mostly occurring in younger men. Treatment is by resection; prolonged follow-up is not required as there is very little risk of recurrence.[51]

Leiomyoma of the bladder is rare but is the most common of the benign mesothelial tumours of the bladder. Small tumours may be resected transurethrally but larger ones may require a segmental resection.[52] Haemangiomas of the bladder are very rare and usually occur in the paediatric age group. Treatment is by local excision as conservative endoscopic treatments with diathermy or laser have a high failure rate. These tumours need to be distinguished from an endometrioma which also presents with a blue coloured mass in the bladder but causes cyclical pain and haematuria.

CARCINOMA OF THE BLADDER

Incidence

The incidence of bladder cancer in both males and females has been rising slowly in most industrialized countries. The male to female ratio is approximately 3:1. Urothelial cancers of the bladder are extremely rare below the age of 20 and the incidence starts to rise steeply after the age of 40 years. The peak incidence is in the seventh decade of life for both men and women. There are marked geographical variations in incidence depending on different aetiological factors, but genetic factors may also play a small part.[53]

Aetiology

Bladder cancer is caused by urine-borne carcinogens that have been metabolized, usually by the liver, and are then activated in the urine.[54] The known urothelial carcinogens in man are mostly aromatic amines of similar chemical structure, but the nitrosamine group of compounds are also potent carcinogens to experimental animals and likely to be carcinogens in man in certain circumstances.

Occupational bladder cancer

It was Rehn[55] who described the first cluster of bladder cancers in a chemical dye works and he suggested that this may be the result of aniline exposure as acute aniline poisoning causes haematuria. It was not until the pioneering epidemiological studies of Case in the British chemical and rubber industries[56,57] that aniline was shown not to be carcinogenic. It was the manufacture and use of 2-naphthylamine (β-naphthylamine), benzidine and 4-aminodiphenyl and the manufacture of the dyes auramine and magenta that were associated with the increased risk of developing bladder cancer. The main occupational exposure to these carcinogens took place in the chemical, dye and rubber manufacturing industries and most but not all of these risks were eliminated in the 1950s and 1960s. The occupations that exposed workers at some time to urothelial carcinogens are:

1. Chemical dye manufacture.
2. The rubber industry.
3. Electric cable manufacture.
4. Gas production in vertical retort houses.
5. Rodent operators (rat catchers).
6. Laboratory workers.
7. Iron casting.

Many other occupations have been shown by epidemiological studies to have small increases in the incidence of bladder cancer, and some of these may still be exposing workers to low levels of carcinogens. In Europe and North America it is estimated that occupational exposure still accounts for 8–20% of bladder cancer.[58]

Smoking

Cigarette smoke contains numerous aromatic amines and nitrosamines. Many epidemiological studies have shown that there is a clear association between cigarette smoking and bladder cancer. An individual who smokes 20 cigarettes a day has a 2–6 times greater risk of developing bladder cancer: 40–50% of bladder cancers can be attributed to cigarette smoking. The role of continued smoking on the subsequent course of bladder cancer after its initial treatment is uncertain, and the smoking of pipes and cigars appears to have little effect on the development of bladder cancer.[59]

Bilharzia

There are marked geographical variations in the incidence of bladder cancer in patients with bilharzia of the bladder. The highest incidence is in the Nile delta of Egypt. It is unlikely that bilharzia itself is the epidemiological agent but more likely that there is a complex relationship with secondary infection, the production of nitrosamines in the bladder and the chronic irritation of the bladder by the schistosome eggs.[60]

Infections

Repeated infections are associated with an increased risk of bladder cancer, particularly when accompanied by chronic irritation of the bladder as occurs in the catheterized paraplegic or the patient with a bladder stone. Both groups have a high incidence of bladder cancer, which is often squamous.

REFERENCES

50. Greene L F et al J Urol 1973; 110: 205
51. Cameron K M, Lupton C H Br J Urol 1976; 48: 567
52. Knoll L D et al J Urol 1986; 136: 906
53. OPCS Cancer statistics registrations. HMSO, London 1989; p 68
54. Lower G M Cancer 1982; 49: 1056
55. Rehn L Arch Clin Chir 1895; 50: 588
56. Case R A M et al Br J Ind Med 1954; 11: 75
57. Case R A M, Pearson J T Br J Ind Med 1954; 11: 213
58. Wallace D M A Br J Urol 1988; 61: 175
59. Morrison A S et al J Urol 1984; 131: 650

Drugs

Cyclophosphamide is now the only drug in common use that is associated with bladder cancer. It is the prolonged low dose administration used to treat autoimmune disorders such as Wegener's granulomatosis that is associated with the development of bladder cancer.[61]

The development of bladder cancer

In both experimental animals and man there is a long latent period from first exposure to a carcinogen until a bladder tumour develops. In man this latent period ranges from 5–40 years with a mean of 25 years for the rubber industry.[62] Bladder cancer covers a wide spectrum of disease: from the small solitary non-invasive tumour, to multiple recurring tumours, to the invasive and metastasizing tumour. There may be several different pathways along which primary and recurrent tumours develop: both tumour implantation and the 'field change' theories have scientific support.

During the long latent period the normal urothelium develops into neoplastic urothelium through a series of changes that range from mild dysplasia and hyperplasia to frank carcinoma in situ.[63] Exophytic papillary tumours or solid invasive tumours can develop at any stage. Invasion through the basement membrane may not take place at all even though the patient has multiple recurrences. Invasion may develop as soon as the tumour begins to grow or it may develop later in a tumour recurrence (Fig. 37.13).

Recent studies of the molecular biology of bladder cancer have shown a number of genetic alterations affecting proto-oncogenes and known or putative tumour suppressor genes.[64] These alterations may determine the pathway of development of a bladder tumour. p53 mutations are associated with carcinoma in situ and the development of invasive tumours; loss of heterozygosity of chromosome 9 is usually associated with the development of non-invasive papillary tumours.

Pathology

Over 90% of urothelial cancers of the bladder are transitional cell carcinomas with approximately 5% being squamous and 1–2% being adenocarcinomas. Many transitional cell carcinomas show areas of squamous differentiation. Transitional cell carcinomas have two main growth patterns: a papillary pattern and a solid infiltrating growth. Preneoplastic changes from mild dysplasia to carcinoma in situ are frequently associated with bladder tumours, and carcinoma in situ (CIS) is often present with poor grade tumours. Cells from the tumours are shed in the urine where they can be detected by cytology. Cytology is often negative with well differentiated tumours but is positive in more than 90% of cases with poor grade tumours and carcinoma in situ.

Clinical features of bladder cancer

Haematuria is the cardinal symptom of malignant disease of the urinary tract. It is usually painless in bladder tumours, but may be accompanied by pain or other symptoms of bladder irritation.

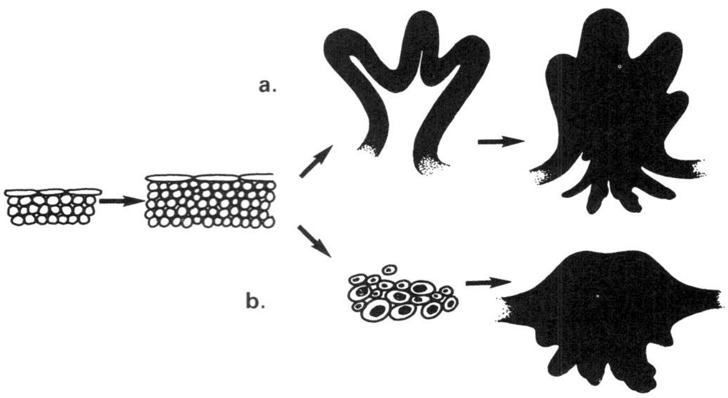

Fig 37.13 The development of urothelial cancer. a. papillary tumour b. invasive tumour.

16–22% of adults presenting with macroscopic haematuria are found to have malignant disease of the urinary tract; over 90% of these patients have bladder tumours. In all, 80–90% of patients with bladder tumours have haematuria as the presenting symptom.[65] In children haematuria is seldom the result of malignant disease in the bladder and therefore cystoscopy for haematuria is seldom indicated. In adults haematuria must be investigated thoroughly and urgently as malignant disease must always be diagnosed or excluded and early treatment has been shown to improve survival.[66] Haematuria is common in clinical practice—2 per 1000 of the population consult their doctor annually with this symptom. Most patients present to their doctor immediately and it is usually the doctor and the hospital that are responsible for the delays that occur in diagnosing bladder cancer.[67,68] Urinary infection should not be assumed to be the cause of the haematuria as 30–40% of bladder cancers have an infected urine on presentation[69] and anticoagulants are rarely responsible for haematuria unless the patient is obviously over anticoagulated. Erroneous attribution of the haematuria to another cause is one of the main reasons for the delay in referring patients for urological investigation.

Microscopic haematuria may also indicate malignant disease of the urinary tract. Patients over 40 years of age who are found to have microscopic haematuria should be investigated as thoroughly as patients with macroscopic haematuria, though the diagnostic yield is much less as there is a greater prevalence of microscopic haematuria in the community.

REFERENCES

60. Hicks R M et al Proc Roy Soc Med 1977; 70: 413
61. Fairchild W V et al J Urol 1979; 122: 163
62. Parkes H G, Evans A E J In: Searle C E (ed) Chemical Carcinogenesis, 2nd edn. American Chemical Society Monograph 1984; 182: 277
63. Murphy W M Pathol Ann 1983; 18: 1
64. Knowles M A Br J Urol 1995; 75(suppl 1): 57
65. Massey B D, Nation E F, Gallup C A, Hendricks E D Carcinoma of the bladder: 20 years expertise in private practice. J Urol 1965; 93: 212–216
66. Wallace D M, Harris D L Delay in treating bladder tumours. Lancet II 1965; 332–334
67. Mommsen S et al Scand J Urol 1983; 17: 163
68. Lynch T H et al Br J Urol 1994; 73: 147
69. Turner A G, Hendry W F, Williams G B, Wallace D M A A haematuria diagnostic service Br Med J 1977; 2: 29–31

Approximately 10% of patients with bladder cancers are diagnosed without having had any macroscopic haematuria.[70] Some of these are diagnosed incidentally on cystoscopy but the rest have symptoms of bladder irritation or pain. It is important to recognize that carcinoma in situ can cause symptoms of urinary frequency, dysuria and suprapubic or perineal pain. These symptoms are often attributed to prostatism or a urinary infection and it is important carefully to assess patients with any of these symptoms, to look for microscopic haematuria and pyuria, and to send the urine for cytology.

Diagnosis

Cystoscopy is the essential examination in all patients suspected of having bladder cancer. Before cystoscopy is carried out, patients should have a urine microscopy and culture; any infection should be treated. An intravenous urogram should be obtained primarily to demonstrate the anatomy of the upper tracts. Ascending ureterograms can be performed at the time of cystoscopy if the upper tracts have not been satisfactorily demonstrated. Small tumours do not show as filling defects and approximately one third of bladder tumours are not seen as filling defects on the cystogram of the first intravenous urogram.

Cystoscopy can be performed on an outpatient basis under local urethral anaesthesia using the flexible cystoscope. Although the flexible cystoscope gives a granular image and a limited flow of irrigant, the whole bladder, including the anterior wall above the bladder neck, can be rapidly inspected. When a tumour is present the patient needs to be examined under a general anaesthetic so that the tumour can be resected and a bimanual examination performed.

With all bladder tumours a small bite off the top with cup biopsy forceps is totally inadequate for assessment and can only establish the cell type of the tumour. All tumours should be treated initially by transurethral resection of the exophytic part of the tumour down into the bladder wall. This is necessary in order to establish the depth of invasion of the tumour. The base of the tumour should be sent separately so that the pathologist can look carefully at these pieces for evidence of muscle invasion (Fig. 37.14).

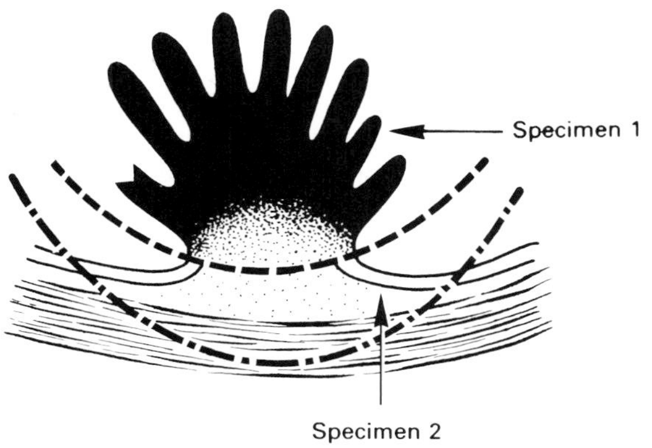

Fig 37.14 The transurethral resection of a bladder tumour. The exophytic part of the tumour should be resected first, washed out of the bladder and sent as the first specimen for histology. The base of the tumour is then resected into the bladder wall and sent as the second specimen.

A bimanual examination should be performed both before and after resection. The presence of a palpable lump is one of the most important prognostic features in invasive bladder cancer although the bimanual examination provides an incorrect assessment of the depth of invasion in 20–40% of cases, depending mainly on the experience of the examiner.[71] The error is usually in underestimating the depth of invasion. Two things are essential—the bladder must be empty and the patient must be fully relaxed. Under these conditions it is usually possible to feel the induration of the bladder wall or a mass when the tumour is infiltrating into deep muscle. When the tumour is not invasive or invading only superficial muscle then no mass or induration is still palpable after an adequate resection.

Classification and staging

The purpose of classifying bladder tumours is succinctly laid out by the UICC.[72] The aims are to:

1. Aid the clinician in planning treatment.
2. Give some indication of prognosis.
3. Assist in evaluating the results of treatment.
4. Facilitate the exchange of information between treatment centres.
5. Contribute to the continuing investigation of human cancer.

The first study to show the importance of classification and staging of bladder tumours was the post-mortem study of Jewett & Strong[73] who observed that the chances of having a distant metastasis were much greater if the primary tumour had infiltrated more than halfway through the muscle of the wall. From this the Jewett–Strong– Marshall system was developed;[74] this is a staging system that has the disadvantage that different prognostic variables can not be studied separately. To overcome this the TNM system has been adopted by urologists and is now widely used throughout the world, though not without continuing controversy.[75]

One of the major problems with bladder cancer is that it can only be classified by a combined clinical and pathological assessment. All the accepted systems separate muscle invasion into superficial and deep on the basis of the findings of Jewett & Strong, even though there is now little difference in their treatment and prognosis. The key to separation is to resect the tumour down into the muscle and then to detect any residual tumour deep in the muscle by a carefully performed bimanual examination. It is clear that clinical attempts at classifying invasive bladder tumours will

REFERENCES

70. Hendry W F, Manning N, Perry N M, Whitfield H N, Wickham J E A The effects of a haematuria service on the early diagnosis of bladder cancer. In: Oliver R T D, Hendry W F, Bloom H J G (eds) Bladder cancer: principles of combination therapy. Butterworths, London 1981 pp 19–25
71. Prout G R Jr Classification and staging of bladder carcinoma. Cancer 1980; 45: 1832–1841
72. Hermanek P, Sobin L H (eds) TNM Classification of Malignant Tumours, 4th edn. Springer-Verlag, Berlin 1987
73. Jewett H J, Strong G H J Urol 1946; 55: 366
74. Marshall V F J Urol 1952; 68: 763
75. Schroder F H et al Br J Urol 1988; 62: 502

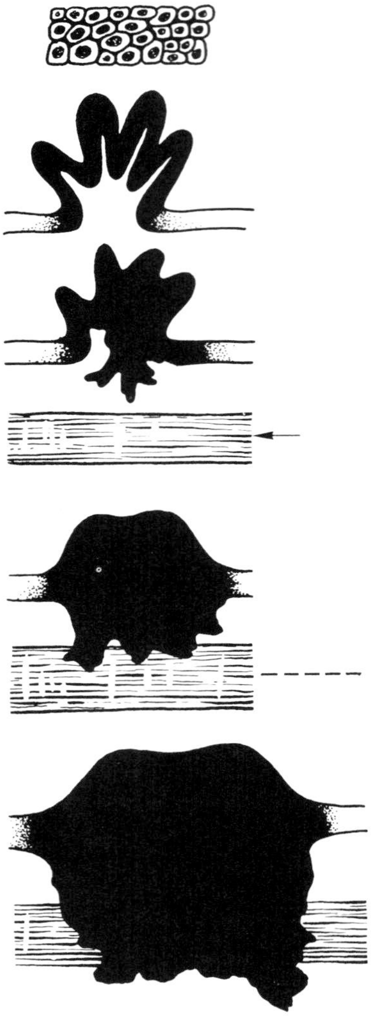

Fig 37.15 The TNM classification of bladder tumours (see Table 37.1).

always entail errors but it must be accepted that some form of classification or staging is useful and should be applied consistently.

The UICC classification of bladder tumours is set out in Table 37.1 and Figure 37.15. It should be stressed that the pathologist must report muscle invasion in the specimen before it can be classified as T2, and therefore the resection must include muscle. Also, the depth of invasion must be stated by the surgeon on the basis of the cystoscopic findings, bimanual examination and any diagnostic imaging that is obtained. Computerized tomography and MRI are useful methods of imaging in bladder cancer as they may show lymph node metastases and distant metastases, and they are also probably superior to clinical methods at demonstrating spread beyond the bladder wall.[76]

The only stage or grouping widely applied to bladder cancer is to divide the tumours into:

1. Superficial tumours (65–75%).
2. Carcinoma in situ (1–5%).
3. Muscle invasive tumours (20–25%).
4. Metastatic tumours (5%).

Table 37.1 TNM system of classification of bladder tumours

TX	Primary tumour cannot be assessed
T0	No evidence of primary tumour
Tis	Carcinoma in situ: 'flat tumour'
Ta	Non-invasive papillary tumour
T1	Tumour invades subepithelial connective tissue
T2	Tumour invades superficial muscle (inner half)
T3	Tumour invades deep muscle or perivesical fat
	T3a invades deep muscle (outer half)
	T3b invades perivesical fat
T4	Tumour invades prostate, uterus, vagina, pelvic or abdominal wall

Note: If the pathology report does not specify that tumour invades muscle, consider as invasion of subepithelial connective tissue. If the depth of muscle invasion is not specified by the surgeon, code as T2.

Superficial tumours

It should be noted that superficial tumours may not be invasive, or may only invade the lamina propria (i.e. Ta and T1 tumours). Superficial tumours can be treated conservatively by endoscopic means but the tumours invading muscle nearly all require radical treatment. The initial treatment for a superficial tumour is a complete transurethral resection, removing all tumour down into the muscle layer.

Approximately 50–70% of superficial tumours develop further recurrences in the bladder if no further treatment is given. Recurrences may be present at the first check cystoscopy in which case there is a very high risk of further recurrences. Recurrences may develop later: the longer the time interval the less likely it is that recurrences will occur.[77] A patient who has gone 10 years without a recurrence has about a 1–2% chance of developing a recurrence. Multiple tumours at first presentation and recurrences at first check cystoscopy indicate a high risk of further recurrences.[78,79]

Tumour progression to muscle invasion occurs in 10–20% of cases; the risk factors for progression are the tumour grade and the presence of invasion of the lamina propria.[80] Grade 3 tumours invading the lamina propria (pT1G3 tumours) have a 40% risk of progression and clearly need to be treated more aggressively.[81]

The risk of recurrence can be significantly reduced by the use of intravesical chemotherapy. The agents used for intravesical chemotherapy include Mitomycin C,[82] Epirubicin[83] and bacillus Calmette–Guérin (BCG).[84] The first two agents have high molecular weights and are not significantly absorbed through the bladder even just after a resection. They may, however, cause a chemical cystitis. BCG, which is a live but attenuated strain of bacteria, stimulates a mononuclear cell infiltration in the bladder wall and brings about specific and non-specific immune mechanisms that eliminate tumour cells.

REFERENCES

76. Kim B et al Radiol 1994; 193: 239
77. Fitzpatrick J M et al J Urol 1986; 135: 920
78. Parmar M K B et al J Urol 1989; 142: 284
79. Reading J et al Br J Urol 1995; 75: 604
80. Lutzeyer W et al J Urol 1982; 127: 250
81. Birch B P P, Harlan S J Br J Urol 1989; 64: 109
82. Tolley D A et al J Urol 1996; 155: 1233
83. Melekos M D et al Cancer 1993; 72: 1749

Clinical trials have shown that a single instillation of either Mitomycin C[82] or Epirubicin[85] given just after transurethral tumour resection can reduce the recurrence rate; there is therefore a good case for giving a single instillation after all resections, particularly if there are multiple tumours. A more prolonged course of repeated instillations is required, or a course of BCG instillations, if there are multiple tumour recurrences. When tumour recurrences continue after one year of resections and treatment with intravesical chemotherapy then there is a high risk of progression to muscle invasion and the patient should be considered for a cystectomy. Radical radiotherapy has no role to play in controlling multiple recurrent superficial tumours and makes the subsequent treatment of any recurrence more difficult.[86] Radiotherapy may have a useful role in the treatment of the pT1G3 tumour as an alternative to an intensive course of intravesical chemotherapy.[81,87] Patients with tumour recurrences after intravesical chemotherapy need to be carefully assessed and treatment decisions must be based on the grade and stage of the tumour recurrence and the presence of carcinoma in situ elsewhere in the bladder or prostatic urethra.

Carcinoma in situ

The term 'carcinoma in situ (CIS)' is not a clinical entity but a pathological descriptive term used to describe one end of a spectrum of changes. It has several clinical manifestations; it may be diagnosed without there being any tumour in the bladder (primary CIS); there may have been a previous bladder tumour or a tumour present at the same time (secondary and concomitant CIS); it may be symptomatic or symptomless; it may be localized or widespread within the bladder, or it may involve urothelium outside the bladder such as the prostatic urethra or ureters. The main importance of carcinoma in situ is that it precedes invasive cancer, it can be detected and it can be treated. The risk of an invasive cancer developing is greater if the in situ change is widespread and symptomatic. Invasive cancer can develop quickly or may take several years but when it does develop it can progress rapidly to widespread metastases.

The clinical presentation of carcinoma in situ is with urinary frequency, dysuria and perineal or penile pain. Microscopic haematuria is usually present and cytology is nearly always positive. The cystoscopic appearance is of a red inflamed bladder and the diagnosis is made by multiple mucosal biopsies. Biopsies should also be taken from the prostatic urethra.

Treatment of in situ carcinoma is usually with intravesical bacillus Calmette–Guérin (BCG) instillations followed by careful monitoring with repeat biopsies and urine cytology. Immunotherapy is effective because the disease volume is very small and confined to the parent organ and direct contact can be obtained between the malignant cells and the immunogen. Complete remissions can be expected in 70–80% of cases, but a radical cystourethrectomy should be considered if BCG fails.[88]

Invasive tumours

Although one quarter of all bladder tumours have invaded the muscle by the time of presentation, many are not amenable to radical curative therapy because the patient is elderly and has renal impairment from obstructive nephropathy or other medical conditions. The tumour may be locally advanced or metastases may already be present. The patient with a bladder cancer which has invaded the muscle needs careful pre-treatment assessment including a CT scan of the chest, abdomen and pelvis, and a bone scan if there is bone pain or a raised alkaline phosphatase.

Only 18–20% of patients with invasive cancers have had prior treatment for superficial bladder cancer; the rest have invasive tumour at first presentation. Many bladders may also show widespread in situ change but approximately 30% may have a well localized tumour. A very small proportion of carefully selected cases are suitable for a partial cystectomy.

The standard treatments for invasive bladder cancer are radical cystectomy[89] and radical radiotherapy.[90] Both have a high failure rate—mainly because of the presence of occult micrometastases at the time of the initial treatment. Neoadjuvant chemotherapy has been tried in a large multicentre trial using the combination of cisplatinum, methotrexate and vinblastine (CMV), but the results showed no worthwhile improvement in survival.[91] Adjuvant chemotherapy where the tumour has spread to lymph nodes after cystectomy has produced an improvement in survival in one study.[92]

The treatment policy for invasive bladder cancer is influenced by many factors, including the facilities, resources and experience available as well as the social and cultural background of the patient. This is particularly true when a patient is being considered for total cystectomy and urinary diversion. Few randomized trials have been performed comparing radiotherapy with cystectomy and none has had sufficient numbers to show any clear advantage of one treatment over the other.[93]

Radiotherapy

A radical course of radiotherapy aims to give 5500–6500 cGy to the bladder and pelvic side walls over a period of 4–6 weeks. Approximately half the tumours respond completely and the response is better for tumours that have had most of their bulk endoscopically resected.[94] Most radiosensitive tumours have disappeared completely by the first check cystoscopy at 3 months. Any tumour present at 6 months should be re-assessed; approximately 20% of tumours treated by radical radiotherapy require a salvage cystectomy.

The skill in treating bladder cancer by radiotherapy is to treat the tumour and avoid unacceptable damage to the surrounding

REFERENCES

84. Lamm D L Eur Urol 1995; 27(suppl 1): 8
85. Oosterlinck W et al J Urol 1993; 149: 749
86. Quilty P M, Duncan W Br J Urol 1986; 58: 147
87. Jenkin B J et al Br J Urol 1989; 6: 608
88. Lamm D L Urol Clin N Am 1992; 19: 499
89. Klimberg I W, Wajsman Z J Urol 1986; 136: 1169
90. Gospodarowicz M K, Warde P R Semin Urol 1993; 11: 214
91. Hall R R Proc Am Soc Clin Oncol 1996; abstr. 612
92. Stockle M et al J Urol 1995; 153: 47
93. Bloom H J G et al Br J Urol 1982; 54: 136
94. Shipley W U et al Cancer 1987; 60: 514

tissue by careful planning. There are, however, occasional patients who react badly to radiotherapy despite careful planning. These patients develop bleeding or contraction of the bladder and may even require a palliative cystectomy or diversion. The 5-year survival after a salvage cystectomy is 60% but this may be the result of selecting patients with a lower risk of developing metastases.[94]

Radical cystectomy

In the operation of radical cystectomy the bladder is removed with the pelvic lymph nodes. In men the prostate is also removed, while in women the uterus and ovaries are usually also removed as an anterior exenteration. Before performing a cystectomy the following points must be considered:

1. The pelvic lymph nodes

These may be sampled preoperatively by laparoscopy or sent for frozen section at the time of cystectomy. A decision may be made to proceed with the cystectomy if the nodes are macroscopically normal without frozen section, depending on the indications and the prospect for chemotherapy if histology shows micrometastases. Only 15–30% of patients will survive 2 years if the nodes are involved although some encouraging results are now being reported for combination chemotherapy in these patients.[92,95]

2. The urethra

There is a high risk of urethral recurrence if cystectomy is being performed for multifocal tumours with tumour or premalignant change in the prostatic urethra. Complete urethrectomy can be performed synchronously with the cystectomy or as a secondary procedure if the histology shows any carcinoma in situ or dysplasia in the prostatic ducts or in the urethral resection margin.[96,97]

3. Orthotopic bladder substitution

If the urethra and sphincter can be left, it is possible to reconstruct a low pressure reservoir from bowel and anastomose this to the urethra as an orthotopic bladder substitution. Detubularized small bowel is usually chosen for the substitution and gives a satisfactory bladder capacity with good compliance. Patients are usually continent with normal micturition. An orthotopic bladder substitution can be performed in women as well as men but the continence rates are lower. The urine has to be diverted if an orthotopic substitution cannot be performed.[98–100]

4. Continent diversion or conduit

A continent catheterizable reservoir can be constructed using bowel with a catheterizable stoma made from appendix or small bowel.[101,102] These procedures are complex with a high complication rate: they must be considered carefully and only chosen for well motivated patients. Where cutaneous diversion via a conduit is indicated an ileal loop gives satisfactory results and fewer complications (Fig. 37.16). Ureterosigmoid diversion is rarely indicated after cystectomy for bladder cancer as elderly patients are often unable to maintain continence when the rectum is filled with urine. The ureters may be dilated and difficult to implant with an anti-reflux mechanism, and renal function may be impaired and not able to cope with the metabolic acidosis. There is also a well recognized risk of developing an adenocarcinoma at the ureteric implantation site after an interval of 20–25 years.[103]

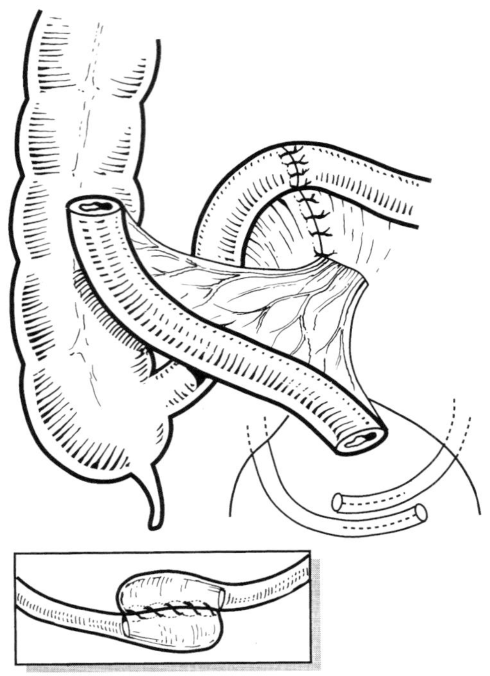

Fig 37.16 The ileal loop urinary diversion. The ureters are brought together in one gentle curve, spatulated and sewn together head-to-tail. This makes a wide easy anastomosis to the ileum and is placed outside the peritoneum.

Chemotherapy for metastatic disease

Combination regimens of cisplatinum, methotrexate and vinblastine (CMV) and with the addition of adriamycin (M-VAC) have been shown to produce complete responses in metastatic disease in 25–30% of selected cases. Randomized studies have shown that the M-VAC regimen produced an increase in survival when compared to cisplatinum alone.[104] These regimens are toxic and

REFERENCES

95. Fossa S D et al Cancer 1993; 72: 3036
96. Vieweg J et al Cancer 1994; 73: 3020
97. Schellhamer P F, Whitmore W F J Urol 1976; 115: 56
98. Hendry W F, Gowing N F, Wallace D M Proc Roy Soc Med 1974; 67: 304
99. Skinner D G et al J Urol 1991; 146: 756
100. Abol-Enein H, Ghoneim M A Br J Urol 1995; 76: 558
101. Studer U E et al J Urol 1995; 154: 49
102. Skinner D G, Leiskovsky G, Boyd S D J Urol 1987; 137: 1140
103. Rowland R G, Kropp B P J Urol 1994; 152: 2247
104. Stewart M et al Br J Urol 1981; 53: 118

cannot be used in many cases of bladder cancer because renal function is impaired. When a patient can tolerate combination chemotherapy it should be offered as it may prolong survival and relieve distressing symptoms.

Squamous carcinoma of the bladder

Pure squamous carcinomas of the bladder account for less than 5% of bladder cancers outside Egypt (see above), although mixed tumours and squamous metaplasia are common in transitional cell carcinomas. The pure squamous carcinoma usually presents late and is deeply infiltrating. It often complicates other long-standing bladder problems such as stones or bilharzia. Squamous carcinomas are less radiosensitive, though this may be because of their more advanced stage at presentation. Radical cystectomy is recommended where the tumour is operable, or a com-bination of chemotherapy and radiotherapy may be considered.[105,106,107]

Adenocarcinoma of the bladder

An adenocarcinoma may develop in a urachal remnant, as a primary tumour in the base of the bladder or as a metastasis. The urachal carcinoma is found in the vault of the bladder with the bulk of the tumour outside the bladder. These cases may be treated by partial cystectomy but there is a high incidence of local recurrence; a combination of chemotherapy and surgery may give the best results.[108] The primary adenocarcinoma of the bladder must be distinguished from a prostatic adenocarcinoma growing into the base of the bladder and also from spread from a colonic or ovarian carcinoma. Adenocarcinomas account for only 0.5–2% of bladder cancers so all treatment results are based on very small series. Surgery is considered the best treatment option as these tumours are relatively insensitive to radiation.[109]

SARCOMAS OF THE BLADDER

Less than 5% of malignant tumours of the bladder are sarcomas. The leiomyosarcoma is the most common sarcoma in adults; rhabdomyosarcoma can occur in adults as well as the embryonal type occurring in childhood.[110] In the elderly an osteosarcoma has been reported. All sarcomas of the bladder carry a poor prognosis except the liposarcoma[111] and require treatment with chemotherapy and surgery.

REFERENCES

105. Loehrer P J et al J Clin Oncol 1992; 10: 1066
106. Patterson J M et al J Urol 1988; 140: 379
107. Sharfi A R, El Sir S, Beleil O Br J Urol 1992; 69: 369
108. Sheldon C A et al J Urol 1984; 131: 1
109. Gill H S et al Br J Urol 1989; 64: 138
110. Ahlering T E et al J Urol 1988; 140: 1397
111. Evans H L Am J Surg Pathol 1979; 3: 507

38 The prostate

C. G. Fowler

BENIGN PROSTATIC HYPERTROPHY

Acute retention of urine

Patients present with an inability to pass urine and severe lower abdominal pain. The diagnosis is made by palpating or percussing a large bladder and confirmed by passing a urinary catheter. A diagnosis of the cause of acute retention can usually be made from a careful history and routine clinical examination. Benign prostatic hypertrophy is the most common cause of retention in males over the age of 60,[1] but there may be other causes even in this age group. A prior history of urethritis or urethral instrumentation may suggest the presence of a urethral stricture (see Chapter 39). A history of sudden interruption of the urinary stream raises the possibility of a urethral stone that may be palpable or visible on a plain radiograph.

Post-traumatic urinary retention is seen following rupture of the urethra (see Chapter 39). This can occur in isolation as a compressive injury in a fall astride a solid object but usually happens as a complication of a pelvic fracture, often in a patient with multiple injuries. The acute but painless retention that follows spinal cord injury (see Chapter 46) or transverse myelitis should be managed as part of an integrated programme of treatment and rehabilitation. Chorda equina compression by a tumour or by central prolapse of an intervertebral disc is an uncommon but important cause of retention which is easy to miss. Prompt spinal cord decompression may allow recovery of bladder function and avoid the disaster of lower limb paraplegia.

Acute retention is rare in neonates but in male children can be caused by congenital urethral valves at the level of the veru montanum. Urethral flaps may present in older boys and can be demonstrated by a cystourethrogram. They require immediate surgical correction by an expert. In older children a simple urinary tract infection causing dysuria may lead to extreme reluctance to pass urine, and balanitis may have a similar effect. Malignant rhabdomyosarcoma of the prostate, benign urethral polyps arising at the veru montanum, or cystic distension of a utricular remnant posterior to the prostate, are extremely rare causes of urinary retention.

Recent changes in treatment with diuretics or tricyclic antidepressants may suggest the possibility of drug-induced retention. Constipation or an episode of alcoholic over-indulgence may temporarily tip the balance in a patient with previously minor symptoms. Postoperative retention occurs most commonly as a result of pain and recumbency, but may represent an exacerbation of underlying bladder outflow obstruction.

Differential diagnosis

Although the distinction between retention of urine and anuria is usually clear, there are cases in which the presentation of an acute abdominal complaint together with a palpable bladder and oliguria can occasionally be confused with acute retention. Ultrasound measurement of bladder volume, or diagnostic catheterization if ultrasound is not available, confirms the diagnosis. Ultrasound has the added advantage of providing an assessment of any upper tract obstruction in cases of anuria.

Treatment of acute retention

The majority of patients who present with acute retention are in such severe discomfort that immediate treatment is essential. A Foley balloon catheter passed under strict aseptic conditions with topical lignocaine inserted into the urethra produces rapid relief. The balloon should not be inflated until some urine has been seen to drain, thus confirming that the catheter has entered the bladder. It is not necessary to clip the catheter intermittently but it is probably preferable to place the urine bag at the same level as the patient, thus avoiding rapid siphoning of urine as rapid decompression of the bladder may cause the bladder lining to bleed. Any nonsurgical cause of retention should be treated; if there is no prior history of 'prostatism', it is reasonable to perform a trial without a catheter after 24–48 hours.

Suprapubic cystostomy should be performed if a urethral catheter is difficult to pass and the bladder is palpable. Formal cystostomy is rarely needed as a number of devices for percutaneous cystostomy are available. Some of these are small calibre catheters with a needle obturator for insertion. They may be useful in an emergency but tend to block after a short while. It is better to use a proprietary trocar set to insert a Foley catheter if more prolonged suprapubic catheterization is necessary. Following local anaesthetic infiltration the suprapubic catheter is inserted through a tiny skin puncture 3–5 cm above the pubic symphysis in the midline. Some clinicians prefer suprapubic catheterization because it avoids the hazard of damage to the urethra from urethral instrumentation. Urethral catheters are also associated with ascending urinary infection, which becomes more likely the longer the catheter is in place. On the other hand, suprapubic cystostomy is

REFERENCE

1. Garraway W M, Collin G N, Lee R J Lancet 1991; 338: 469–471

associated with a small risk of injury to organs adjacent to the bladder. The risk can be minimized by ensuring that the bladder is full and by avoiding percutaneous suprapubic puncture in patients whose anatomy has been disturbed by lower abdominal surgery. Surgical cystostomy is safer in these patients.

Chronic retention

Chronic retention of urine is painless and patients often present with dribbling overflow incontinence, especially at night, a palpable lower abdominal mass or the symptoms of renal failure. On close questioning they may admit to difficulty in passing urine. Evidence of compression of the spinal cord or chorda equina must be excluded by careful neurological examination and the urine should be tested for sugar to exclude diabetes mellitus.

If the patient is comfortable and renal impairment is not marked, catheterization is best avoided in order to reduce the risk of infection before definitive surgery. The metabolic consequences of severe renal failure can usually be avoided if the renal tract is decompressed by bladder catheterization. Severe obstruction commonly causes renal tubular damage with loss of concentrating ability, and the high levels of metabolites present in the circulation act as an osmotic diuretic. As a result there may be a spectacular loss of sodium and water following relief of obstruction. This must be replaced, often by intravenous infusion, if the patient is not to become severely dehydrated with a risk of pre-renal uraemia. It is wise to give a suitable antibiotic to cover catheterization and any subsequent surgery.

Surgery should not be contemplated until the patient is metabolically stable. If the renal function does not return to normal, surgical correction of bladder outflow obstruction is still indicated where possible to rid the patient of the catheter and its associated risk of infection. Patients should remain under regular biochemical surveillance postoperatively as most of them have some permanent renal parenchymal damage, and dietary modification and even renal replacement therapy may eventually be required.

Pathophysiology of benign prostatic hyperplasia

The term 'prostatism' is generally taken to mean the triad of hesitancy, poor stream and troublesome nocturia. In a man over 55 years of age the most common cause of these symptoms is bladder outflow obstruction secondary to benign prostatic hyperplasia but the actual size of the prostate and the severity of the symptoms are unrelated. There is now a considerable amount of work on the anatomy and pathophysiology of the ageing prostate.

McNeal[2] has described four anatomically separate groups of glands within the organ (Fig. 38.1):

1. The periurethral glands—normally a small cylinder of tissue around the urethra and the major site of benign prostatic hyperplasia.
2. The central zone—extending from the bladder neck to the veru montanum and traversed by the vas deferens and the duct of the seminal vesicle.

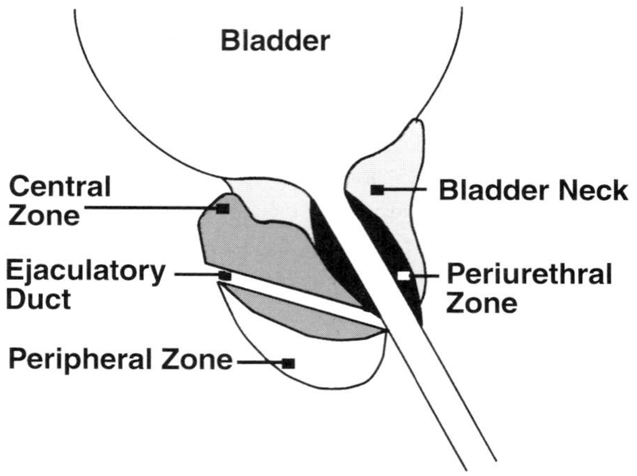

Fig. 38.1 Normal prostatic anatomy.

3. The peripheral zone—posterior and lateral to the central zone and regarded by McNeal as the main site of prostatitis, atrophy and malignant change.
4. The transitional zone—poorly defined but thought to be the site of origin of many unsuspected carcinomas found only by histology after resection.[3]

The aetiology of benign prostatic hyperplasia is unknown, although some form of local androgen imbalance is thought to be important. Three tissues are involved—epithelium, muscle and collagen—but the proportion of each may vary from patient to patient and even within the prostate. There is a tendency for nodules to form with enlarged glandular spaces, amounting almost to cystic change in places. The enlargement of the inner group of glands in benign prostatic hyperplasia tends to produce compression and atrophy of the outer group of glands, which form a pseudocapsule to the prostate. Nodular enlargement usually produces the endoscopic appearance of lateral lobe intrusion compressing the prostatic urethra into a midline slit. Enlargement in the midline may produce a middle lobe which protrudes up into the bladder through the bladder neck. In addition to fibromuscular and glandular changes within the prostate it is common to find areas of local inflammation, and prostatic infarcts are particularly common in patients with acute retention. It is not clear whether these infarcts are secondary to retention, catheterization and instrumentation or whether they play an important role in precipitating acute retention. Desquamation of epithelial cells is thought to produce the round eosinophilic bodies called corpora amylacea, which in turn become calcified and may make the gland firm and irregular on rectal examination.

Thickening and narrowing of the bladder neck is quite commonly found in patients who have symptoms of outflow obstruction and a small prostate. These changes are thought to be responsible for the ill defined condition of 'bladder neck hypertrophy' and may respond to α-adrenergic blocking drugs or

REFERENCES

2. McNeal J E J Urol 1972; 107: 1008–1016
3. McNeal E M, Price H M et al J Urol 1988; 139: 61–65

bladder neck incision. A rare and extreme form of this condition occurs in young men and is referred to as Marion's disease, first described by G J Guthrie in a lecture at the Westminster Hospital in 1833. It can cause bilateral hydronephrosis and renal failure in very severe cases.

The bladder detrusor initially compensates for increased outflow resistance with muscular hypertrophy and an increase in collagen, producing the endoscopic appearance of trabeculation. Trabeculation itself is symptomless but the detrusor becomes increasingly irritable as it hypertrophies.[4] This irritability is perceived by the patient as an increase in urgency and frequency of micturition and it may be objectively demonstrable urodynamically as detrusor instability. Detrusor instability often improves after prostatectomy but in an important minority of patients there is no benefit. A few patients may be worse off because they can no longer prevent urinary leakage when unstable bladder contractions occur.[5] Idiopathic instability occurs in both sexes at this age and, like bladder hyper-reflexia caused by neurological disease, this is not cured by an operation on the prostate.

When the pressure which the detrusor can develop becomes insufficient to overcome the resistance to urine flow caused by the obstruction, the bladder does not empty, and the volume of urine left in the bladder after voiding (the post-micturition residual urine volume) increases. This may lead to infection, stone formation and back pressure effects on the upper urinary tracts. Eventually a stage is reached when neither the detrusor muscle nor renal function can recover even after the obstruction has been relieved.

Clinical features of obstructive prostate disease

The earliest symptom is often an increased frequency of micturition by day and by night, although this is particularly troublesome at night. Micturition may be slow to start and the urinary stream is often interrupted and its force reduced. Patients find it difficult to be objective in assessing the urinary stream but they may remark on the need to strain; post-micturition dribbling may be a problem. The latter symptom, when occurring in isolation, does not benefit from investigation or treatment.

Urgency is likely to be the result of instability; if this is a predominant symptom more detailed investigation is necessary to be sure that it is secondary to outflow obstruction. Urgency with dysuria is usually caused by a secondary infection or a bladder stone.

Painless haematuria always raises the possibility of a bladder tumour (see Chapter 37), nevertheless it is a common symptom in both benign and malignant prostatic disease and frequently occurs when acute retention is decompressed. It is almost impossible to predict which patients will progress to disabling symptoms or painful acute retention. Those who present with chronic painless retention often have signs and symptoms of established hydronephrosis, uraemia and anaemia, namely fatigue, weight loss, fluid retention and confusion. They often deny a prior history of urinary problems but may have had dribbling caused by overflow incontinence. They may also present with a painful episode of acute-on-chronic retention.

Investigation

Once the patient's history has been carefully recorded, a full examination should follow, noting in particular the presence or absence of a palpable or percussible bladder. The consistency of the prostate gland should be assessed by rectal examination. It should be remembered that, when the patient is in retention, the prostate is pushed down and its size is difficult to estimate. Microbiological examination of a midstream specimen of urine is indicated when a urine dipstick test suggests the presence of infection. The haemoglobin should be measured and plasma urea, electrolytes and creatinine must be obtained. When surgery is anticipated, the age of the patient may indicate that a chest radiograph and electrocardiograph are appropriate. The routine cross-matching of blood before prostate surgery is a matter of local policy. This decision is based on the surgeon's experience, the efficiency of the local blood transfusion service, the patient's initial haemoglobin and fitness, and the size of the prostate. It is sufficient to group and save serum if conditions are favourable.

An intravenous urogram was once considered obligatory but it is not cost-effective in cases with a clear history of prostatic symptoms.[6,7] It should be performed if there has been any infection, a history of stone disease or haematuria, or when there is a suspicion of prostatic malignancy. The precise assessment of the post-micturition residual urine volume is difficult but for most purposes an estimate made from an ultrasound scan suffices.[8] Ultrasound is painless and inexpensive and may therefore be repeated on a number of occasions; the kidneys can be simultaneously assessed for obstructive changes. The residual urine as estimated from intravenous urography is often unrepresentative as the patient has been mildly dehydrated in the interests of concentrating the excreted dye and may well have been asked to empty the bladder at the end of the study when there was no desire to void. Catheterization performed after normal voiding provides an accurate measurement of the residual urine volume but should be discouraged because of the risk of causing infection.

The urine flow can be measured by a flowmeter. Commercial devices are available in a number of forms. Some measure the changing level of urine in a container with a sensitized dipstick. Others weigh the voided urine and display the rate of change of weight as flow. In one of the most popular devices the voided urine passes through a funnel on to a spinning disc. The slowing of the disc which this causes is measured electronically to provide a reliable and objective readout of the maximum flow rate, duration of flow, volume and flow pattern. Accurate assessment requires that the patient passes at least 200 ml, which many find difficult to achieve. There is no precise cut-off point between normal and abnormal, but a flow below 10 ml/s in a man is regarded as definitely abnormal.[9]

REFERENCES

4. McGuire E J J Urol 1992; 148: 1133–1136
5. Appell R A Postgrad Med J 1981; 57: 640–641
6. Abrams P H, Roylance J, Feneley R C L Br J Urol 1976; 48: 681–684
7. Fidas A, MacKinlay J Y, Wild S R Clin Radiol 1987; 38: 479–482
8. Beacock C J M, Roberts E E, Rees R W M, Buck A C Br J Urol 1985; 57: 410–413
9. Abrams P H, Griffiths D J Br J Urol 1979; 51: 129–134

Cystometry

A large residual urine volume suggests either detrusor failure or outflow obstruction or both. A slow urine flow rate does not help in differentiating these problems. A urodynamic study of voiding may be necessary if there is genuine doubt as to the presence of obstruction (see Chapter 37). A high detrusor pressure during micturition[9] is indicative of bladder outflow obstruction. Urodynamic studies are also indicated when urgency is a predominant symptom, indicating possible idiopathic detrusor instability.

Bladder neck obstruction

Symptoms of hesitancy, intermittent stream and reduced flow are often found in middle-aged men in whom there is a tight ring or bar of bladder neck muscle, with no evidence of prostatic obstruction. The bladder neck muscle can be relaxed using an α-adrenergic antagonist drug, the most commonly used being prazosin and indoramin.[10]

Indications for treatment

For many men the symptoms of bladder outflow obstruction caused by benign disease of the prostate are a minor inconvenience which does not justify treatment of any sort unless objective tests show signs that the bladder detrusor muscle is failing. These patients can be reassured that their symptoms may remain static or even improve with time[11] and they can be seen again if their problems get worse: so-called 'watchful waiting'.[12]

The finding of a flow rate of less than 10 ml/s and a significant residual urine in a man with bladder outflow obstruction is usually taken as an indication for active treatment to prevent the onset of urinary retention.[13] Acute retention followed by a failure of a trial without catheter and chronic urinary retention with complications from back pressure effects on the kidneys are also reasonably firm indications that something must be done. There is also a group of patients who need treatment because they have disabling urinary symptoms which interfere significantly with their quality of life.

Treatment options

Surgery is no longer the only treatment which can be offered to patients with symptomatic benign enlargement of the prostate. For some, particularly those who have concomitant disease which makes surgery dangerous, drug treatment may be an alternative. Two main classes of drugs are available. The α-adrenergic antagonists such as prazosin and indoramin work by relaxing the smooth muscle surrounding the bladder outlet. They have been shown to produce a significantly better improvement in symptoms than placebo and there is objective evidence of improvement in urine flow rate and bladder emptying.[14] These drugs probably become less effective over time and have been advocated as a stopgap in patients who have a long wait for surgery. The 5α-reductase inhibitors interfere with the peripheral metabolism of testosterone into its active product, dihydrotestosterone.[15] These drugs, which include finasteride and epristeride, seem to be effective in some patients, producing an improvement of symptoms greater than placebo with a small but measurable decrease in prostatic bulk.[16] Like the α-blockers their effect on urodynamic measures of outflow obstruction is unimpressive. Treatment must be continued for at least three months before it can be concluded that the 5α-reductase inhibitor is not working. In those in whom it does work, lifelong therapy is advocated.[17]

Minimally invasive methods of treatment using balloon dilatation[18] and various methods to shrink the prostate by heating it in situ have been disappointing in the medium to long term.[19] Prostatic stents which can be inserted under topical urethral anaesthesia may be an alternative to long-term catheterization in patients who are unsuitable for surgery. These stents expand in various ways to anchor in the prostatic urethra. They have the disadvantage of all foreign bodies in the urinary system in that they become encrusted and prone to infection.[20] They are also liable to migrate from their proper site and may be tricky to remove.[21]

PROSTATE SURGERY

Over the past 15 years improvements in equipment—particularly the introduction of rod–lens instruments and fibreoptic light cables—associated with a greater number of surgeons specializing in urology, have led to a revolution in prostatic surgery. In most urology departments transurethral surgery is used for almost all prostatectomies. Prostatic incision is a lesser procedure of comparable effectiveness which may allow a shorter inpatient stay after surgery. Newer treatments such as laser and diathermy ablation, which may also be performed as short-stay procedures, are now under investigation. Retropubic and, to a much lesser extent, transvesical prostatectomy are very occasionally appropriate if the adenoma is huge or there is associated bladder pathology such as a large stone which requires open surgery.

Preliminary cystourethroscopy

Every prostatectomy begins with a thorough cystourethroscopy to check for pathology in the urethra and bladder and to assess the size and the appearance of the prostate.

REFERENCES

10. Caine M Br J Urol 1995; 75: 265–270
11. Isaacs J T Prostate 1990; (suppl 3): 1–87
12. Ball A J, Feneley R C L, Abrams P H Br J Urol 1981; 53: 613–616
13. Jensen K M-E, Jorgensen J B, Morgensen P Scand J Urol Nephrol 1988; 148(suppl): 111–116
14. Lepor H J Androl 1991; 12(6): 389–394
15. Silver R I, McConnell J D Curr Opinion Urol 1994; 4: 22–28
16. Stoner E J Urol 1992; 147: 1298–1302
17. Kirby R S, Bryan J et al Br J Urol 1992; 70: 65–72
18. Donatucci C F, Berger N et al Urology 1993; 42: 42–49
19 Abrou C-C, Payan C et al and the French Hyperthermia Group Br J Urol 1995; 76: 619–624
20. Squires B, Gillatt D A Br J Urol 1995; 252–253
21. Parikh A M, Milroy E J G Eur Urol 1995; 27: 1–3

Millin's retropubic prostatectomy[22,23]

This is the most popular procedure for removal of a very large prostate; few urologists would knowingly undertake a transurethral resection of a gland that is much greater than 100 g, and many would set their limit lower. The first stage of the operation is always cystoscopy and examination under anaesthesia to exclude urethral stricture, bladder stones and tumour, and to confirm that the size and benign consistency of the gland justify open rather than transurethral surgery.

Through a transverse Pfannenstiel incision the retropubic space is opened to expose the large veins lying on the anterior and lateral aspects of the prostate which need to be ligated before the prostatic capsule is incised. A transverse incision is made in the capsule, giving access to the plane between adenoma and capsule which is then developed by blunt dissection with scissors and fingers. The enucleation continues until the prostate is detached inferiorly by careful division of the prostatic urethra above the veru montanum. Finally, the adenoma is turned up and detached at the bladder neck before an additional wedge of bladder neck muscle is excised. Most bleeding comes from the prostatic arteries at 5 and 7 o'clock, and is controlled by under-running the corners of the bladder neck and capsule.

A Foley or whistle-tip catheter, secured by a Harris stitch to a bar on the anterior abdominal wall, is used for postoperative bladder drainage. The Foley balloon may provide additional haemostasis by light pressure at the bladder neck while the Harris stitch allows railroading and repositioning of the catheter in the event of blockage by blood clot.

Postoperative irrigation of the bladder reduces the incidence of postoperative clot retention. In the past it was traditional to perform bilateral vasectomy as part of the procedure, but with the advent of effective antibiotics post-prostatectomy epididymitis has become a relative rarity and vasectomy is unnecessary.[24] The high incidence of morbidity from infection and haemorrhage has led to the virtual abandonment of open surgery in favour of transurethral resection. Open prostatectomy is associated with a significant mortality, depending on the age and fitness of the patient[25] Urethral stricture and incontinence are the most important long-term complications. Careful dissection and division of the prostatic apex minimizes the incidence of urethral strictures. A stricture incidence of 3.8% following open prostatectomy has been reported. Significant incontinence from damage to the distal sphincter mechanism should occur in less than 1% of patients. Careful dissection of the prostatic apex and the use of a transverse capsular incision minimize the risk of this important complication.

Transvesical prostatectomy[26]

This operation is still occasionally performed when the prostate is small and there is need for open surgery to remove bladder stones which are too large in size or number for lithotripsy. It is also used when the prostate is associated with a large diverticulum which needs to be excised. In these circumstances, however, it is now probably best to deal with the bladder pathology and perform a transurethral operation at a second sitting.

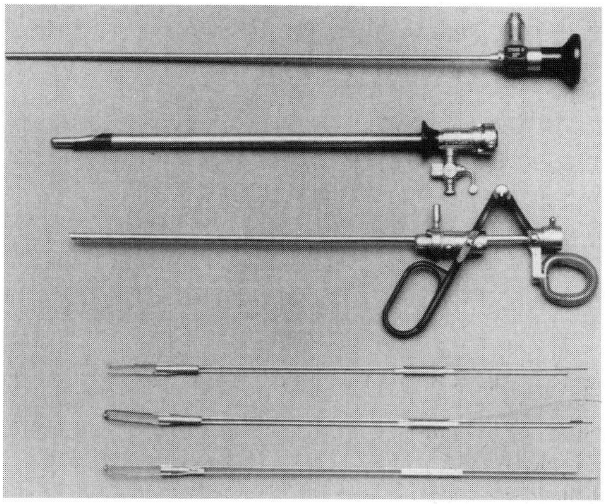

Fig. 38.2 A resectoscope.

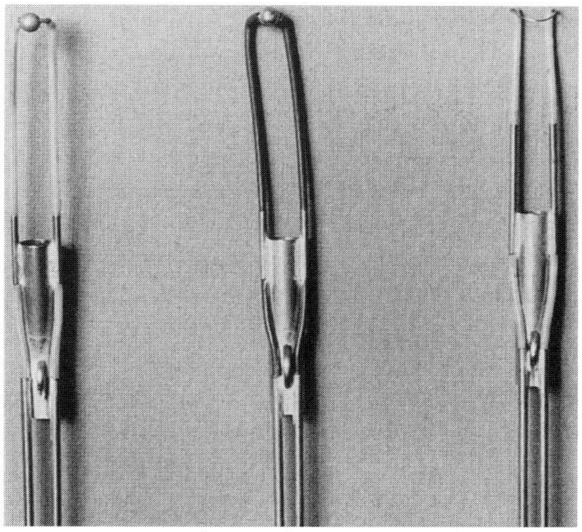

Fig. 38.3 Cutting and diathermy loops of resectoscope.

Transurethral resection of prostate[27]

Transurethral resection of the prostate can be performed equally well under general or spinal anaesthesia. After a thorough cystourethroscopy, a 24 or 27 Charrière rigid tubular sheath is passed down the urethra until its tip enters the bladder. The resectoscope working element and telescope are then inserted (Fig. 38.2). Under direct vision a diathermy loop (Fig. 38.3) is used to cut the prostate into small chips which are then evacuated

REFERENCES

22. Millin T Lancet 1945; ii: 693–696
23. Prior J P In: Whitfield H N (ed) Rob and Smith's Operative Surgery–Genitourinary Surgery. Butterworth-Heinemann, London 1993 pp 409–418
24. Chilton C P, Morgan R J et al Br J Urol 1978; 50: 542–546
25. Pengelly A W, In: Hendry W F, Whitfield H N (eds) Textbook of Genito-urinary Surgery.
26. Whitfield H N In: Whitfield H N (ed) Rob and Smith's Operative Surgery–Genitourinary Surgery. Butterworth-Heinemann, London 1993 pp 397–400
27. Blandy J P, Notley R G Transurethral Resection. Blackwell Scientific, Oxford 1993 pp 71–104

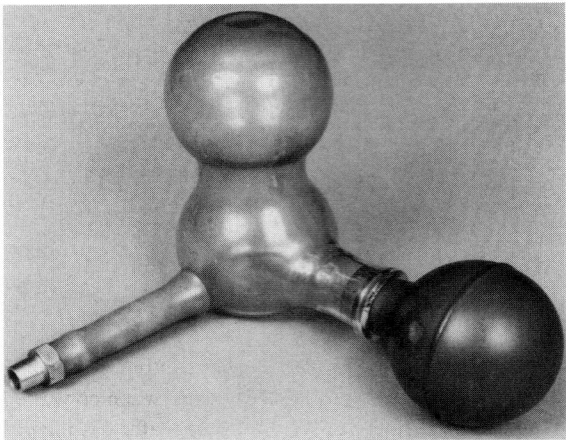

Fig. 38.4 Ellick evacuator.

through the sheath using an Ellick evacuator (Fig. 38.4). Any bleeding that occurs is stopped by changing to a coagulation current. The resection is carried down to the level of the veru montanum, which is preserved as a landmark for the external urethral sphincter which lies just downstream. Cutting the sphincter leaves the patient with dribbling incontinence and is a disaster which can be avoided by correct technique.

In a complete resection, the process continues until the adenoma has been fully removed and the inside surface of the prostatic capsule comes into view. In practice, however, the capsule is difficult to define precisely and it can easily be perforated by over-enthusiastic resections. Most transurethral resections are less complete and intraoperative transrectal ultrasonography shows that even an expert resectionist leaves residual prostatic tissue.[28]

Bladder neck incision

An endoscopic diathermy knife can be used to cut the prostate at 5 and 7 o'clock. The cuts, which extend from beyond the bladder neck to the level of the veru montanum, are taken down to the prostatic capsule. No tissue is removed but incision seems to allow the prostatic urethra to open up with improvement in flow.[29] A transurethral resection of the bladder neck can be performed if the bladder neck fails to open following incision.

Other endoscopic methods

Neodymium-YAG and KTP-YAG laser have been used to remove prostatic tissue by vaporization or coagulation in situ.[30] Although these methods remove less prostatic tissue than is usual in transurethral resection, the early results seem to be comparable.[31] The prostatic perioperative haemorrhage is reduced, allowing a short hospital stay. Unfortunately these techniques are associated with quite severe postoperative urethral pain and the patient may have to wear a catheter for up to two weeks while the necrotic prostate heals. Laser equipment is expensive, somewhat temperamental to use and requires special safety precautions to protect users. It seems that similar tissue effects can be obtained more simply and cheaply using diathermy applied by needle[32] or by roller electrode.[33]

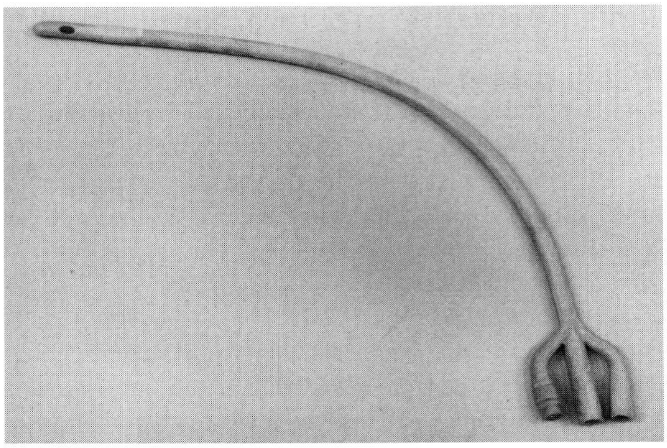

Fig. 38.5 Three-way haematuria catheter.

Irrigation

The fluid most commonly used for operative irrigation is isotonic glycine.[34] The absence of electrolytes allows the use of diathermy while the isotonic solution prevents haemolysis in the event of fluid absorption. Unfortunately, a considerable amount of glycine may enter the circulation through vessels which have been transected during the procedure, especially if it is prolonged. Metabolic breakdown products of glycine can cause biochemical effects which may be part of a transurethral resection syndrome. Postoperative irrigation, if required, is maintained with a three-way haematuria catheter using isotonic saline (Fig. 38.5).

Postoperative complications

The main immediate complications of transurethral resection are haemorrhage and infection. Primary arterial bleeding is usually relatively easy to stop by coagulation diathermy but venous bleeding may be very troublesome. Traction on the balloon catheter may tamponade the resected cavity. Continuous heavy bleeding often, however, leads to clotting of blood within the bladder despite saline irrigation. In the first instance, the bladder should be washed out using a sterile technique but if necessary the patient should be returned to theatre for further haemostasis. Rarely the bleeding cannot be stopped by endoscopic means and an open procedure is necessary to under-run the bleeding vessels and pack the prostatic cavity.

Serious infective complications are much more common when patients have pre-existing urinary sepsis, which is almost

REFERENCES

28. Green J S A, Bose P et al Br J Urol 1996; 77(3): 398–400
29. Edwards L E, Bucknall T E et al Br J Urol 1985; 57: 168–171
30. Costello A, Bowsher W G et al Br J Urol 1992; 69: 603–608
31. McCullough D L Curr Opin Urol 1996; 6: 10–13
32. Issa M, Oesterling J E Curr Opin Urol 1996; 6: 20–27
33. Te A E, Kaplan S A Curr Opin Urol 1996; 6: 2–9
34. Krane R J, Siroky M B In: Fitzpatrick J M, Crane R J (eds) The Prostate. Churchill Livingstone, London 1989 pp 173–180

inevitable if they have been catheterized for any time preoperatively. Septicaemia is the most common cause of death after endoscopic surgery, especially in older patients. All patients who are likely to have a urinary infection at the time of surgery should be covered by an appropriate antibiotic. There is some evidence that routine antibacterial prophylaxis is desirable. Gentamicin is cheap and effective.

Prolonged resection using fluid at room temperature can lead to hypothermia, and irrigation fluids should certainly never be chilled.[35] Use of hypotonic solutions or water and high pressures in the bladder are likely to increase the risk of the transurethral syndrome.[36] This is thought to be caused by a combination of fluid overload, hyponatraemia and, in extreme cases, haemolysis as well as the metabolic effects of glycine described above. The patient becomes hypotensive or hypertensive during or soon after the procedure and fails to recover consciousness or suffers mental impairment. There is a profound dilutional hyponatraemia and respiratory function may be impaired by the fluid overload. There is no agreement on the best treatment for this condition but a careful combination of diuretics and sodium supplementation is usually recommended. Treatment in an intensive therapy unit is essential to monitor and maintain vital functions.

Patients should be warned to expect a minor degree of haemorrhage 10–14 days after surgery. Although anti-fibrinolytic therapy has been recommended as a preventive measure, the incidence of serious problems does not justify its routine prescription.

Urethral strictures may follow any urethral instrumentation or catheterization (see Chapter 39). A submeatal stricture is the most common problem after transurethral resection but this usually settles after a simple dilatation. If the meatus grips the resectoscope at the time of the transurethral resection, bouginage or Otis urethrotomy is advisable to minimize the chances of stricture formation, and some would advise urethrotomy for all transurethral resections.[37] Occasionally a more difficult stricture in the bulbar urethra may develop and require repeated dilatation, urethrotomy or urethroplasty[24] (see Chapter 39). A tight stricture caused by circumferential scarring of the bladder neck can be a cause of recurrent outflow obstruction months or even years after an initially successful transurethral resection. The bladder neck may be contracted until its lumen is hardly more than a pinhole. A bladder neck incision using a diathermy knife usually gives a long-lasting cure.[38]

Urgency or urge incontinence in the first few weeks after surgery is usually caused either by infection or residual bladder instability. When infection has been excluded, a short course of anticholinergic therapy may be helpful. Persistent incontinence more than 3 months after surgery merits further investigation. Permanent difficulties with continence occur after approximately 2% of procedures, and a small number of patients require the implantation of an artificial urinary sphincter[39] (see Chapter 37).

Sexual problems

All patients undergoing transurethral resection of the prostate or bladder neck should be warned that retrograde ejaculation can occur. They may see this symptom as an indication of failing sexual performance if they are not warned. The incidence of impotence after transurethral resection is difficult to assess as a proportion of elderly patients already have some degree of erectile failure preoperatively.[40,41] For medicolegal reasons, the surgeon should warn the patient of the possibility of impotence, although there is always the worry that the psychological impact of such a warning may be self-fulfilling.[42]

Advantages

It is quite clear that in the short term transurethral resection of the prostate has major advantages for the patient when compared with open surgery in terms of speed, comfort and safety. A recent retrospective epidemiological survey has, however, suggested that there may be an increased risk of myocardial death for several years after transurethral resection of the prostate,[43] but the soundness of the methodology of this study has been questioned[47] and the prospective studies required to confirm its findings are difficult to mount.[45]

PROSTATITIS[46,47]

Despite improvements in its diagnosis and classification, prostatitis remains poorly understood and is often difficult to treat. The system of classification proposed in 1978 by Drach and his colleagues[48] divided prostatitis into acute and chronic bacterial prostatitis, non-bacterial prostatitis and prostatodynia. This division is based on objectively quantifiable bacterial localization cultures and microscopic examination of the urine and expressed prostatic fluid.

Acute bacterial prostatitis

Acute bacterial prostatitis usually presents with an acute febrile illness. The patient complains of fever, low back and perineal pain and symptoms of bladder irritation or acute outflow obstruction. There may be an associated epididymitis or

REFERENCES

35. Allen J D J Urol 1973; 110: 433–435
36. Gale D W, Notley R G Br J Urol 1985; 57: 708–710
37. Bailey M J, Shearer R J Br J Urol 1985; 57: 81
38. Boyle P J In: Whitfield H N (ed) Rob and Smith's Operative Surgery–Genitourinary Surgery; Endoscopic Procedures. Butterworth-Heinemann, London 1993 pp 128–131
39. Scot F B J Urol 1981; 125: 799
40. Bolt J W, Evans C, Marshall V R Br J Urol 1987; 59: 319–322
41. Malone P R, Cook A et al Br J Urol 1988; 61: 234–238
42. Thorpe A C, Cleary R et al Br J Urol 1994; 74: 479–484
43. Roos N P, Wennberg J E et al N Engl J Med 1989; 320: 1120–1124
44. Chisholm G D Br Med J 1989; 299: 215–216
45. Jenkins B J, Sharma P et al Br J Urol 1992; 69: 372–374
46. Fair W R, Sharer W In: Blandy J P, Lytton B L (eds) The Prostate. Butterworth, London pp 33–50
47. de la Rosette J J M C H, Hubregtse M R et al J Urol 1993; 41: 301–322
48. Drach G W, Fair W R, Meares E M, Stamey T A J Urol 1978; 120: 266

pyelonephritis. The prostatic gland is swollen and extremely tender; digital examination should be gentle to minimize the risk of provoking bacteraemia.

The urine and blood should be examined by aerobic and anaerobic cultures and antibiotic therapy commenced. The usual pathogen is a common strain of Escherichia coli and treatment with co-trimoxazole, penicillin G or one of the cephalosporins almost always settles the acute episode.[49] Mild symptoms may be treated by oral therapy but elderly diabetic or severely ill patients require parenteral antibiotics and fluid replacement, together with general supportive measures such as bed rest, analgesics, antipyretics and stool-softeners. Urethral instrumentation must be avoided and a suprapubic catheter may be used in the event of urinary retention. Treatment should last for 2–4 weeks, with bacteriological and clinical surveillance continuing for 3–6 months.

Chronic bacterial prostatitis

Chronic bacterial prostatitis usually presents with recurrent lower urinary tract infections. The diagnosis is confirmed by the bacteriological localization techniques of Meares & Stamey.[50] Bladder bacteriuria, if present, should be cleared with a short course of penicillin or nitrofurantoin. The well hydrated patient is instructed to maintain retraction of the foreskin throughout the procedure. The glans is cleaned with detergent soap, rinsed with sterile water and dried. The first 10 ml of urine voided from the bladder (VB1) is collected, followed by a midstream specimen (VB2). The clinician then massages the prostate in order to obtain a specimen of expressed prostatic secretion. The patient then voids again, with the first 10 ml of urine being collected as VB3. Bacterial counts in VB1 which exceed those in VB3 suggest urethritis. VB3 exceeds VB1 in patients with prostatitis and, when they are approximately equal, the expressed prostatic secretion culture may confirm prostatitis. A significant bacterial count in VB2 indicates cystitis. Problems may occur as a result of contamination from the foreskin, the presence of antibiotics in the urine, and contamination by detergent from the washing procedure.

The alkaline pH of prostatic secretion, which becomes more exaggerated in chronic bacterial prostatitis,[51] makes selection of a suitable antibiotic difficult. Trimethoprim for 3–12 weeks is most frequently used and minocycline has also been recommended.

There is a high and seemingly inevitable recurrence rate. Poor antibiotic penetration and blocked prostatic ducts have been held responsible for this. There is no doubt that infected prostatic calculi do occur but their relevance to this problem is uncertain. Transurethral resection to clear calculi has been tried but, as the infection predominantly involves the peripheral zone and a rim of prostatic tissue always remains after prostatectomy, this procedure rarely eradicates recurrent infection.

Non-bacterial prostatitis and prostatodynia

Whereas chronic bacterial prostatitis produces few local symptoms, patients with non-bacterial prostatitis and prostatodynia often present with poorly localized perineal pain. In non-bacterial prostatitis the expressed prostatic secretion is sterile but contains significant numbers of white cells. In prostatodynia microscopy may show a small number of white cells which are also found in normal patients. The absence of specific antibodies to Gram-negative bacteria in prostatic fluid of patients with non-bacterial prostatitis provides a further means of diagnosing this condition. Viral or chlamydial infection has been suggested as a cause but remains unsubstantiated.[52] Antibacterial remedies continue to be used despite the lack of proven infection. There is undoubtedly a psychological element in this condition although it remains to be determined whether this is a cause or an effect. In difficult cases treatment with diazepam or antidepressants may be appropriate or a psychiatric opinion may be sought.

Granulomatous prostatitis

Tuberculous prostatitis[53] has become less common as public health and chemotherapy have improved. The prostate is involved in most cases of advanced genitourinary tuberculosis. Involvement of the prostate alone is rare and it may be misdiagnosed as a carcinoma. The diagnosis is usually made on a prostatic biopsy and treatment is the same as for tuberculosis of other sites (see Chapter 4).

Non-specific, non-caseating granulomas are found in less than 1% of prostate resections. In many cases the finding is incidental and thought to be the result of previous infection or prostatic surgery. The condition appears to have a benign self-limiting course. Malacoplakia is a rare granulomatous condition associated with bacterial infection of the urinary tract; the prostate is involved in 10% of reported cases. The appearances on transrectal ultrasonography may mimic cancer.[54] Treatment with trimethoprim or rifampicin is recommended.

Prostatic abscess

Early effective treatment of acute bacterial prostatitis with antibiotics is the probable reason why this condition is rare in current practice. Frequency, dysuria, fever and urinary retention are the usual presenting symptoms. The initial treatment is with parenteral antibiotics—either an aminoglycoside or a cephalosporin together with a penicillin. Failure to respond, persistent rectal fluctuance or a breach of the prostatic capsule are all indications for surgical drainage by transurethral incision.[55] Perineal drainage is now rarely required.

CARCINOMA OF THE PROSTATE[56]

The aetiology of prostatic cancer remains unknown although genetic and dietary factors, viral infection, social class and changes

REFERENCES

49. Meares E M J Urol 1980; 123: 141–147
50. Meares E M, Stamey T A Invest Urol 1968; 5: 492–497
51. Blacklock N J, Beavis J P Br J Urol 1974; 46: 537–542
52. Meares E M J Urol 1980; 123: 141–147
53. Sporer A, Auerbach O Urology 1978; 11: 362–365
54. Chantelos A E, Parker S H, Sims J E, Horne D W Radiology 1990; 177: 193–195
55. Trapnell J, Roberts J B M Br J Surg 1970; 57: 565–569
56. Kirk D Br J Urol 1985; 290: 875–876

in hormonal environment have all been suggested.[57,58] The incidence of both prostatic cancer and benign prostatic hypertrophy increases with age, but there is no evidence that benign hypertrophy is a premalignant condition. Wide variations in geographical incidence have been recorded with extremes of mortality ranging from 2 per 100 000 males in Japan to 22 per 100 000 non-white males in the USA.[59] Racial factors undoubtedly play a part since the 50% difference in mortality between whites and blacks in the USA is unlikely to be explained simply by socioeconomic factors. Several studies have indicated increases in mortality for immigrants moving from low- to high-incidence areas, suggesting that environmental or dietary factors may be important.[60]

There appears to be a definite increase in the incidence and mortality of the disease throughout the world.[61] In American men over 55, prostatic cancer is the most common cause of tumour death if skin cancers are excluded. The ratio of mortality to incidence varies considerably between different countries and in different patient age groups.[62] This ratio is influenced by many factors, particularly variations in diagnostic and staging technique and the age of the presenting population. Detailed examination of the prostate at autopsy has demonstrated histological prostate cancer in 57% of men over the age of 80.[63] An apparent improvement in the 5-year survival rate is almost certainly the result of diagnostic rates for prostate cancer rather than more effective forms of treatment.

Clinical features

Prostatic cancer is rarely seen in men under 50. When it does develop early, patients usually present with symptoms of bladder outflow obstruction and have a palpably abnormal gland, or they present with symptoms and signs of metastatic spread. Malignancy may be unsuspected until the resected tissue at prostatectomy is histologically examined. These tumours are often referred to as latent or incidental carcinomas,[64] and their incidence appears to be rising.[65] The term 'latent' should not be taken to indicate that the tumour lacks the capacity to grow or spread. The majority of patients present with bladder outflow symptoms identical to those of benign prostatic hypertrophy.[66] Acute retention and haematuria are relatively common and haemospermia occasionally occurs. Advanced local disease may cause pain in the back or perineum, and renal failure may result from either bladder outflow obstruction or local tumour extension around the ureteric orifices beneath the trigone. Advanced local disease may encircle the rectum causing obstruction.[77] Increasingly, patients are presenting as a result of prostate screening.[68]

At presentation, half the patients with prostatic cancer have demonstrable evidence of distant disease, many without symptoms. Advanced pelvic lymph node disease may cause swelling of the lower limbs. Deposits in bone may cause localized or widespread pain, the most common sites being the ribs, spine and pelvis. In some cases the marrow is disproportionately affected and anaemia may precede bone pain.

Pathology

Carcinoma of the prostate is usually an adenocarcinoma of acinar form. Macroscopically, prostatic tumours tend to have a distinct consistency but vary in colour and vascularity. Considerable variations in differentiation are also seen from one part of the tumour to another. Tumour grade, assessed either on histological material or cytological aspirate, correlates well with the prognosis and response to treatment.[69] Fine-needle cytology provides less accurate information for tumour grading than needle biopsy or transurethrally resected chips and relies heavily on an accurate cytology service.

At times the histology is atypical, with features of either a ductal or endometrioid carcinoma.[70] Endometrioid tumours do not respond to hormonal therapy. Transitional cell carcinoma may be found superficially within the prostate or having invaded from the bladder base. These tumours must be treated in the light of the findings in the remainder of the urinary tract. At times the histology of poorly differentiated tumours around the bladder neck and trigone is difficult to categorize, and immunohistochemical staining for acid phosphatase or prostate-specific antigen may be helpful.

Sarcomatous change in the fibrous and muscular stromal elements of the prostate is extremely rare.[71] Secondary deposits of lymphoma and melanoma have been described.[72]

Diagnosis and staging

It is no longer adequate to diagnose prostatic cancer on the basis of a rectal examination.[73] There will always be some elderly patients with a hard prostate, a raised acid phosphatase, bone pain and sclerotic lesions on radiograph in whom immediate treatment is indicated and prostatic biopsy is not felt to be justified, but these patients should be regarded as exceptions. Some patients have

REFERENCES

57. Key T Cancer Surveys 1995; 22: 63–77
58. Chisholm G D Tutorials in Postgraduate Medicine–Urology. Heinemann, London 1976 pp 191–211
59. Mettlin C, Natarajan N Prostate 1983; 4: 323–331
60. Akazaki K, Stemmermann G N J Natl Cancer Inst 1973; 50: 1137–1140
61. Majeed F A, Burgess N A Br J Urol 1994; 73: 377–381
62. Lytton B In: Fitzpatrick J M, Krane R J (eds) The Prostate. Churchill Livingstone, Edinburgh 1989 pp 253–259
63. Enstrom J E, Austin D F Science 1977; 195: 847–851
64. Rich A R J Urol 1935; 33: 215–223
65. Beynon L L, Busuttil A, Newsam J E, Chisholm G D Br J Urol 1983; 55: 733–736
66. Chishom G D In: Duncan V J (ed) Prostate Cancer–Recent Results in Cancer Research, vol 78. Springer Verlag, Heidelberg 1981 pp 173–184
67. Barry J, Wild S R Br J Urol 1991; 67: 441–443
68. Chodak G W Urology 1993; 42: 116–118
69. Mostofi F K Sem Oncol 1976; 31: 161–169
70. Gillatt D A, O'Reilly P H, R.eeve N L Br J Urol 1986; 58: 559–560
71. Stearam U, Holby L, Cancer 1969; 24: 803–804
72. Black N L, Weber D, Schinella R. J Urol 1972; 107: 85–87
73. Palken M, Cobb O E et al J Urol 1991; 145: 86–92

Table 38.1 Prostate cancer staging as proposed by Catalona & Scott[80]

Stage A—Impalpable, histologically diagnosed
$A1_F$ Focal carcinoma
A1 Carcinoma in one lobe
A2 Diffuse or multifocal carcinoma
Stage B—Intracapsular but palpable
$B1_N$ Solitary nodule, less than 1.5 cm
B1 Carcinoma in one lobe
B2 Both lobes involved
Stage C—Palpably extracapsular
No metastases
Stage D—Extraprostate
D1 Pelvic lymph nodes involved
D2 Metastatic disease

Table 38.2 TNM classification[81]

T category—Local tumour
T_{IS} Carcinoma in situ
T_0 Impalpable, histologically diagnosed
T_1 Nodule, intracapsular
T_2 Intracapsular, distorting shape of gland
T_3 Extracapsular, may involve seminal vesicles
T_4 Fixed or infiltrating
N category—Node involvement
Rarely fully staged
M category—Distant metastases
M0 No metastases
M1 Metastases present

symptoms which justify a transurethral resection to provide histological material. Fine-needle aspiration for cytology or transperineal biopsy with a Tru-cut biopsy needle can be performed under local or general anaesthesia.[74] Antibiotic prophylaxis should be given if the transrectal route is used and the patient should be given instructions to seek help if symptoms of systemic infection develop. The accuracy of the biopsy is improved if it is carried out with transrectal ultrasound imaging.[75,76]

A full clinical staging of the patient's disease must be made before a plan of management can be drawn up. Two major systems are in use: the Jewett system modified by Catalona & Scott[77] (Table 38.1) and the UICC TNM system (Table 38.2), last modified in 1992.[78] The primary tumour is normally assessed by rectal examination but the accuracy of this staging is poor with an error rate of 25%. Prostatic calculi, areas of prostatitis and patient obesity all contribute to inaccuracy. There is little doubt that transrectal ultrasonography can improve the accuracy of local staging; the technique is becoming more widely available.[79,803] Magnetic resonance imaging may also be helpful.[81,82]

Pelvic lymph node staging is notoriously difficult by any method other than surgical lymph node dissection, with a quarter being missed by bipedal lymphography.[83] The accuracy of lymph node staging can be improved if the pelvic nodes seen at lymphography are aspirated by fine-needle cytology. Recently, laparoscopic lymph node sampling has been used to assess the suitability of the patient for radical surgery.[84] Most surgeons who believe that radical prostatectomy can be curative perform a staging lymphadenectomy before proceeding to remove the gland.[858] The patient should also be examined clinically for signs of distant

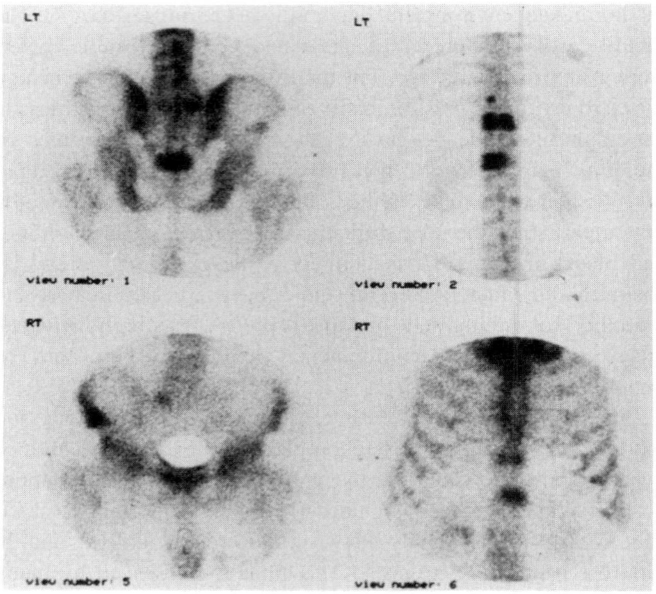

Fig. 38.6 Typical metastatic bone scan.

lymphadenopathy. Computerized tomography rarely provides helpful additional staging information in prostatic cancer and, in practice, a search for lymphatic metastases is only justified if radical surgery is an option.

A radioisotope bone scan should, however, be routinely performed to exclude bony metastases.[86] Routine radiography of 'hot-spots' on the bone scan is then required to exclude false positives from osteoarthritis, Paget's disease or healing fractures (Fig. 38.6). The clinician should also be aware of the 'superscan', when extensive skeletal disease causes such widespread uptake that the scan appears normal.[87]

Acid phosphatase was a routine marker in prostate cancer for over 40 years. The introduction of immunoassays rather than enzymatic methods has led to claims of improved sensitivity for this

REFERENCES

74. Gomella L G, Grant Mulholland S In: Whitfield H (ed) Rob and Smith's Operative Surgery–Genitourinary Surgery; Endoscopic Procedures. Butterworth-Heinemann, London 1993 pp 132–136
75. Weaver R P, Noble M J, Weigel J W J Urol 1991; 145: 516–518
76. L,ee F, Torp-Pedersen S T et al Radiology 1989; 170: 609–615
77. Catalona W J, Scott W W J Urol 1978; 119: 1–8
78. Hermanek P, Sobin L H (eds). UICC International Union against Cancer TNM Classification of Malignant Tumours, 4th edn, 2nd revision. Springer, Berlin 1992
79. Shinohara K, Wheeler T M, Scardino P T J Urol 1989; 142: 76–82
80. Rickards D, Gowland M et al Br J Urol 1983; 55: 726–734
81. Chadwick D J, Cobby M, Goddard P, Gingell J C Br J Urol 1991; 67: 616–621
82. Vapneck J M, Shinohara K, Carroll P R J Urol 1991; 145 (suppl): 352A
83. O'Donoghue E P N, Shridhar P et al Br J Urol 1976; 48: 689–696
84. Prasad B R, Parr N J, Fowler J W Br J Urol 1994; 73: 271–274
85. Schröder F H In: Whitfield H (ed) Rob and Smith's Operative Surgery–Genitourinary Surgery; Endoscopic Procedures. Butterworth-Heinemann, London 1993 pp 419–434
86. O'Mara R E Cancer 1976; 37: 480–486
87. Fitzpatrick J M, Constable A R et al Br J Urol 1978; 50: 555–561

assay although the benefits in clinical terms are marginal.[88,89] Traditionally, an elevated acid phosphatase has been regarded as indicative of the presence of extracapsular disease, but caution is urged in cases in whom there has been recent surgery, instrumentation or retention. Approximately a quarter of patients with metastatic disease have a normal acid phosphatase.[90] Increasing use is now being made of prostate-specific antigen as a marker for prostate cancer. Although this is undoubtedly a sensitive marker there is a certain amount of overlap between patients with small volume malignancy and those with massive benign disease or prostatitis. Some patients with normal serum levels of prostate-specific antigen have had a proven malignancy of the prostate. Prostate-specific antigen is, however, an excellent marker for evaluation of the response to treament.[91] The alkaline phosphatase should also be routinely checked; although conditions other than metastatic disease, particularly Paget's disease, can cause elevation, changes are of value in monitoring the progress of disease in individual patients.

A chest radiograph should also be obtained when staging prostate cancer as secondaries can occur. Lung metastases often occur as lymphangitis carcinomatosa. An intravenous urogram or an upper tract ultrasound, together with measurement of urea and electrolytes, provides an assessment of the upper tract. Abnormalities may reflect a failure of chronic bladder outflow obstruction to resolve but they should rapidly disappear after adequate bladder drainage. Their persistence should be regarded as a sign that extracapsular tumour is obstructing the ureters, and this is an indication for immediate hormonal therapy.

Primary treatment

The initial treatment should be a transurethral resection as the majority of patients present with symptoms and signs of outflow obstruction. Open enucleation should be avoided. The choice of further treatment is controversial and depends upon the patient's age, fitness, symptoms and disease stage.[92] The therapeutic options are dictated by the stage of the disease at presentation, and can be summarized as follows.

1. T0M0: Elderly patients with well-differentiated tumours are unlikely to develop significant progression even without active treatment. The presence of multifocal disease and poor differentiation in a fit patient under the age of 65 should however encourage consideration of more radical therapy.
2. T1–2M0: In fit patients there is scope for radical therapy, and a significant risk of disease progression if treatment is deferred.
3. T3–4M0: Approximately half these patients have nodal metastases, and radical therapy therefore has a low success rate. Having dealt with any outflow obstruction the clinician may choose to await the appearance of metastases or onset of symptomatic progression before offering hormonal therapy.
4. M1—symptomless: Deferred hormone therapy is an acceptable option.
5. M1—symptomatic: Immediate hormone therapy should be given.

Curative surgery

The idea that early malignancy confined to the prostate can be cured by local excision or radiotherapy is very attractive. Unfortunately, despite decades of enthusiasm for radical prostatectomy, especially in the USA, there is no convincing evidence that it makes any difference to survival. The same can be said for external beam radiation. Urologists are split into those who believe in radical curative treatment and those who do not.

The absence of evidence is in large part the result of the enormous variations in the behaviour of the tumour and the large numbers and very long follow-up which are needed for a useful comparison of radical surgery or radiotherapy with watchful waiting. This places the surgeon in a very difficult position when advising a patient who is desperate for something to be done. A simplified exposition of each side of the case should be attempted. A small well-differentiated tumour is probably not a significant danger to an elderly patient.[93] By contrast, patients with multifocal poorly differentiated tumours have a poor prognosis with radical surgery, presumably because of the presence of undetected metastases (i.e. understaging of the disease).[94,95] These patients may be offered radical radiotherapy in the hope that it can restrain local progression of the growth.[96] In between is a small group of patients with disease of intermediate differentiation and no detectable metastases. These patients need to make an informed choice in the full knowledge of the morbidity associated with radical treatment and the uncertainty about its effectiveness.

The variations in reported results achieved by external beam radiotherapy reflect differences in patient selection, dosage regimens, histological grade of tumour and the use of adjuvant hormonal therapy.[97] The value of treating the pelvic lymph node area is uncertain, but there is a definite risk of increased morbidity as the field size or dose is increased.[98] Potency is retained in 50–60% of patients.[99] Radioactive iodine seeds can be implanted either at open surgery or under ultrasound control but there is significant morbidity[100] with their usage.

Radical prostatectomy has until recently only found favour in the USA. Survival rates were comparable with radiotherapy but impotence and incontinence rates were high. The modification introduced by Walsh & Donker,[101] who described the preservation

REFERENCES

88. Foti A G, Herschman H, Cooper J F Clin Chem 1977; 23: 95–99
89. Griffiths J C Clin Chem 1980; 26: 433–436
90. Bahnson R R, Catalona W J Urol 1987; 137: 427–430
91. Brawer M J Urology 1994; 44: Symp 5A, 9–17
92. Blandy J P, Fowler C G In: Urology, 2nd edn. Blackwell Scientific, Oxford 1996 pp 405–426
93. Franks L M Ann Roy Coll Surg Engl 1954; 15: 236–249
94. McNeal J E Cancer 19—; 71: 984–991
95. Franks L M In: Oliver R D T, Blandy J P, Hope-Stone H F (eds) Blackwell Scientific, Oxford 1989 pp 195–202
96. Bagshawe M A, Kaplan I D, Cox R C Cancer 1993; 71: 939–952
97. Bagshaw M A Cancer 1985; 55 (suppl): 2079–2085
98. Ennis R D, Peschel R E Cancer 1993; 72: 2644–2650
99. Ray G R, Bagshaw M A Ann Rev Med 1975; 26: 567–588
100. Lannon S G, El-Araby A A et al Br J Urol 1993; 72: 782–791
101. Walsh P C, Donker P J J Uzol 1982; 128: 492–497

of the neurovascular bundles lateral to the prostate, has led to a much improved morbidity and a renewed interest in the option of radical surgery. Total perineal prostatectomy is now rarely performed as it does not allow access to the pelvic lymph nodes for staging or preservation of the neurovascular bundles.[102]

The radical retropubic prostatectomy is performed through a midline incision. Removal of the prostate is preceded by lymph node dissection and frozen section of the specimen. If tumour is found in these nodes it is normal to abandon the procedure at this stage. The prostate is removed by first detaching the apex from the urethra and then dissecting backwards to the bladder neck. The lateral neurovascular bundles are preserved and the seminal vesicles are removed in continuity with the prostate. The bladder neck is reconstituted and anastomosed to the cut end of the urethra. It is claimed that, with experience, mortality is low, incontinence occurs in less than 10% and potency is retained in 70% of patients.[103]

Palliative treatment for symptomatic local or metastatic disease

As understanding of the biochemistry of the prostate has improved, so the range of available hormone treatment regimens has increased enormously.[104] Bilateral orchiectomy[105] has the advantage of avoiding the need for continuing medication and the side-effects of hormonal drugs. Postoperative 'hot flushes' may be a problem but clinical experience has demonstrated that these may be effectively suppressed by a small dose of an anti-androgen such as cyproterone acetate. The operation of subcapsular orchiectomy is aesthetically and psychologically more acceptable to many patients than simple castration, and when carefully performed produces effective androgen suppression.[106]

Although stilboestrol is cheap and perhaps more effective than orchiectomy in controlling prostate cancer, this is achieved at the price of producing gynaecomastia, fluid retention and an increased incidence of thromboembolic complications. This was strikingly demonstrated by the first Veterans' study, in which patients receiving stilboestrol 5 mg had a worse survival than those treated with placebo.[107] Subsequent studies have shown that 1 mg stilboestrol daily is effective despite inconsistent suppression of testosterone and can still be considered in a fit patient with no cardiovascular disease.[108] Synthetic gonadotrophin releasing hormone analogues produce a medical orchiectomy.[109,110] These drugs act by stimulating the pituitary to produce an initial surge of luteinizing hormone and testosterone, with an associated disease flare which is followed after 15–20 days by suppression to castrate testosterone levels. The disease flare is normally covered by a short course of an anti-androgen. Treatment with these agents produces results which are comparable to surgical orchiectomy. Despite the introduction of depot preparations the disadvantages of this treatment are the need for repeated parenteral administration and its cost.

A number of anti-androgenic agents such as cyproterone acetate, flutamide and megestrol acetate are now available.[111] They tend to be expensive and some cause a high incidence of gastrointestinal side-effects.[112] Their role in primary treatment of prostate cancer is not agreed as very few published series have made effective comparisons with other agents. Other drugs, such as Estradurin, honvan and Estramustine, find favour with some clinicians although there is little evidence that these hormone treatments are any more effective than orchiectomy.[113,114] No matter which form of testosterone suppression is used, only half the patients presenting with metastases are alive at 2 years and only 25–30% survive 5 years. In recent years there has been increasing interest in improving survival by suppressing all androgens, including those of adrenal origin, using a combination of testicular suppression and an anti-androgen. There is now some evidence that total androgen blockade produces a marginal increase in survival but the expense is great.[115–118]

The results of treatment should be monitored by a regular review of symptoms, serum markers and the haemoglobin. A bone scan should be repeated if indicated. Typically, a good response is seen when the acid phosphatase or prostate-specific antigen falls and if when the alkaline phosphatase transiently rises before falling to a normal level when bony metastases are present.

Most patients are either too old for radical treatment at the time of presentation or have disease which is too extensive to expect a cure. All treatments carry a cost in terms of morbidity[122] or expense, and the satisfactory outcome of the placebo-treated patients in the Veterans' study has inevitably led to support for the concept of deferred treatment.[107] This has been applied in cases of early[120] and advanced disease.[121]

Secondary treatment

It appears that all patients with prostate cancer harbour a population of hormone-resistant cells and therefore, however good the

REFERENCES

102. Schröder F H In: Whitfield H (ed) Rob and Smith's Operative Surgery–Genitourinary Surgery; Endoscopic Procedures. Butterworth-Heinemann, London 1993 pp 435–442
103. Walsh P C Campbell's Urology. W B Saunders, Philadelphia 1986
104. Geller J Cancer 1993; 71: 1039–1045
105. Whitfield H N In: Whitfield H (ed) Rob and Smith's Operative Surgery–Genitourinary Surgery; Endoscopic Procedures. Butterworth-Heinemann, London 1993 pp 570–576
106. Clark P, Houghton L Br J Urol 1977; 49: 419–425
107. Veterans Administration Cooperative Urological Research Group Surg Gynecol Obstet 1967; 124: 1011–1017
108. Resnick M I, Grayhack J T Urol Clin North Am 1975; 2: 141–161
109. Waymont B, Lynch T H et al Br J Urol 1992; 69: 614–620
110. Kaisary A V, Tyrrell C J, Peeling W B, Griffiths K Br J Urol 1991; 00: 502–508
111. McLeod D G Cancer 1993; 71: 1046–1049
112. MacFarlane J R, Tolley D A Br J Urol 1985; 57: 172–174
113. Susan L P, Roth R B, Adkins W C Urology 1976; 7: 598–601
114. Veronesi A Prostate 1982; 3: 159–164
115. Jacobi G H In: Fitzpatrick J M, Krane R J (eds) The Prostate. Churchill Livingstone, Edinburgh 1989
116. Crawford E D, Eisenberger M A et al N Engl J Med 1989; 321: 419–424
117. Schröder F H Br J Urol 1993: 71: 633–640
118. Denis L J, Carneiro de Moura J L et al Urology 1993; 42: 119–130
119. Fowler F J, Roman A et al Urology 1993; 42: 622–628
120. Adolfsson J, Cartensen J, Lowhagen T Br J Urol 1992; 69: 183–187
121. Parker M C, Cook A et al Br J Urol 1985; 57: 724–728

response to hormone treatment, the patient will eventually progress to a phase of 'hormone escape'. Once this stage has been reached the patient's survival is unlikely to exceed 12 months.[122,123] Provided the initial hormone treatment has effectively suppressed testicular androgen, there is no objective evidence that secondary hormone therapy is of any benefit.[124,125]

Chemotherapy has no useful role in the treatment of these patients at present.[126] Bone pain is the most common problem as patients enter a terminal phase of the disease. Radiotherapy is often effective[127] as a 'spot' local treatment or it can be given as a wide-field hemi-body technique. Hypophysectomy is effective[128] but little used, and radioactive strontium is currently still under investigation. The mean survival is 6 months[129] following the onset of symptomatic hormone-resistant disease. It is at this stage of his disease that the patient relies most heavily on the clinician for advice and support. Regular follow-up and close liaison with the family doctor is essential in order to administer effective palliation, whether in the form of drugs or radiotherapy.

REFERENCES

122. Beynon L L, Chisholm G D Br J Urol 1984; 56: 702–705
123. Scott W W, Johnson D E et al J Urol 1975; 114: 909–911
124. Robinson M R G Br J Urol 1980; 52: 328–329
125. Stone A R, Hargreave T B, Chisholm G D Br J Urol 1980; 52: 535–538
126. Schmidt J D J Urol 1980; 123: 797–805
127. Fitzpatrick R J, Rider W D J Can Assoc Radiol 1976; 27(2): 75–79
128. O'Donoghue E P N Br J Urol 1980; 52: 301–304
129. Fitzpatrick J M, Gardiner R A et al Br J Urol 1980; 52: 301–304

39 The urethra and penis

W. D. Dunsmuir   S. A. V. Holmes   R. S. Kirby

ANATOMY AND EMBRYOLOGY

The male urethra

The male urethra extends from the bladder neck to the external meatus at the tip of the glans penis. It may be divided into 4 parts: the prostatic, membranous, bulbar and penile sections. The first two parts form the posterior urethra, and the latter two parts form the anterior urethra (Fig. 39.1). Embryologically, the posterior urethra is formed from the urethral segment of the urogenital sinus. The anterior urethra is formed from the genital urethral folds. The urethral groove forms into a tube by the epithelial fusion of the two urethral folds. This occurs between the 7th and 14th week of gestation. Finally, the glandular portion of the anterior urethra is formed by the fusion of the glandular folds (Fig. 39.2).

The prostatic urethra is the widest and most distensible part of the urethra. There is a large smooth muscle component within its wall which acts as a sphincter.[1] On the posterior wall is a crest known as the verumontanum. The ejaculatory ducts open into the urethra on the summit of this crest. The prostatic glands open into the prostatic urethra and these provide up to 10% of the volume of the ejaculate. The prostatic fluid is rich in zinc and contains enzymes and certain prostaglandins which are important for adequate sperm function. The membranous urethra is short and crosses the perineal membrane. Both smooth and striated circular muscle bundles are found in its wall, forming the distal sphincter complex. This sphincter receives its nerve supply from branches of the pudendal nerve (S2–S4) and the extrapudendal nerves that run on the levator ani muscle in the pelvis.[2] The bulbar urethra is continuous with the membranous urethra. It is surrounded by the bulb of the penis and the bulbo-spongiosus muscle which contracts rhythmically during ejaculation. It curves forwards in the perineum to the base of the penis. The penile urethra is the longest section and is contained within the corpus spongiosum. Near its termination it enters the glans penis.

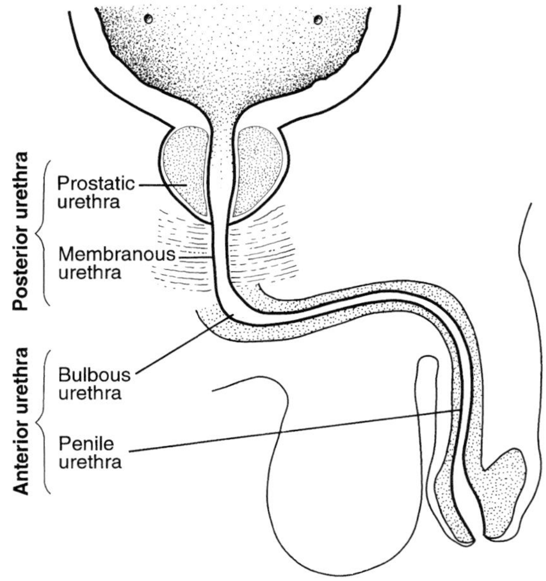

Fig. 39.1 Basic anatomy of the male urethra.

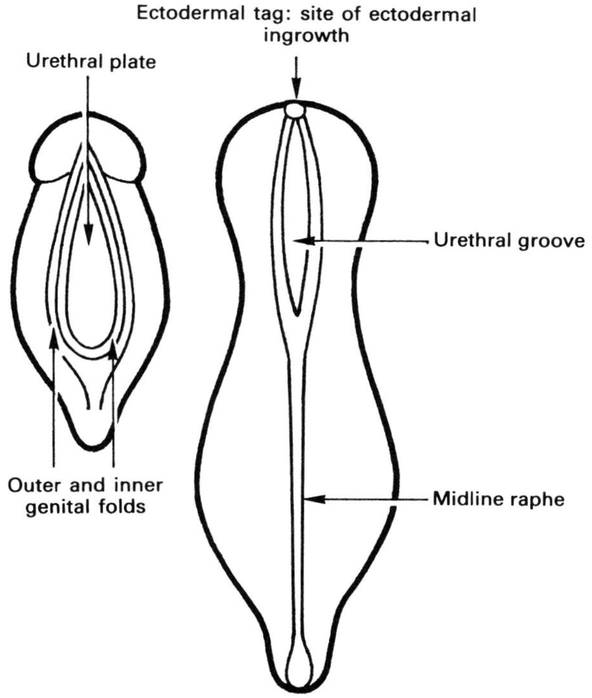

Fig. 39.2 Development of the penile urethra.

REFERENCES

1. Turner-Warwick R T Urol Clin N Am 1989; 16: 335–352
2. Zvara P, Carrier S, Kour N W, Tanagho E A Br J Urol 1994; 74: 182–187

The female urethra

The female urethra is 3–4 cm in length and is surrounded by both smooth and striated muscle. The inner longitudinal muscle is continuous with the detrusor muscle of the bladder. The striated muscle is composed of slow twitch fibres which are suitable for the maintenance of tone over long periods. This muscle, together with the levator ani muscle, is important for maintaining continence. The integrity of these structures also requires preservation of tone in the surrounding connective tissues which are oestrogen dependent. The central component of the levator ani muscle (pubococcygeus), has the facility for fast contraction which increases urethral closure in order to overcome periods of elevated intra-abdominal pressure, such as coughing.

The penis

The penis is composed of three columns of erectile tissue (Fig. 39.3). The ventral corpus spongiosum transmits the urethra and expands to form the glans penis. The paired corpora cavernosa are the main erectile structures. Although they are apparently discrete, the corpora cavernosa directly communicate but during normal erection they do not communicate with the corpus spongiosum. The corpora cavernosa are surrounded by the fibroelastic tunica albuginea which is tough, flexible and expansile. All three corporeal columns—with lymphatics, nerves and vessels—are surrounded by Buck's fascia. The erectile tissue is comprised of many intercommunicating blood spaces, or lacunae, which are lined by endothelium and surrounded by smooth muscle. These lacunae are connected to a large capillary bed and are innervated by autonomic nerve fibres. The capillaries are derived from corkscrew-shaped helicine arteries which branch from the central cavernosal arteries. Blood enters the corpora in the cavernosal arteries which are terminal branches of the internal iliac system. Blood from the corpora drains into both the deep and superficial dorsal penile veins. These coalesce and contribute to both the crural and pre-prostatic venous plexus of Santorini. The lymph drainage of the penis has important implications in the management of patients with penile cancer. The lymph from the prepuce and the penile skin drains to the superficial inguinal nodes. The superomedial group of superficial inguinal nodes or 'sentinel' nodes are thought to be the primary site of drainage before lymph passes to the deep inguinal nodes. This is particularly true for drainage from the glans of the penis—the most common site for penile cancer. Biopsy of these nodes is useful in the staging of penile cancer. Lymph from the glans of the penis collects in large trunks in the area of the frenulum. The lymph vessels circle to the dorsal aspect of the corona and pass proximally, deep to Buck's fascia, freely anastomosing with lymphatics from the corpora and with lymphaties from the other side. Most of these lymph vessels pass to both the superficial and the deep inguinal nodes. Some lymph, however, drains into the lateral external iliac group via the presymphyseal nodes. In cancerous spread, the internal iliac nodes are rarely involved unless the inguinal nodes are first affected. A third of patients who have deep iliac node involvement also have spread to the internal iliac nodes and half of the patients with inguinal node involvement have bilateral spread.

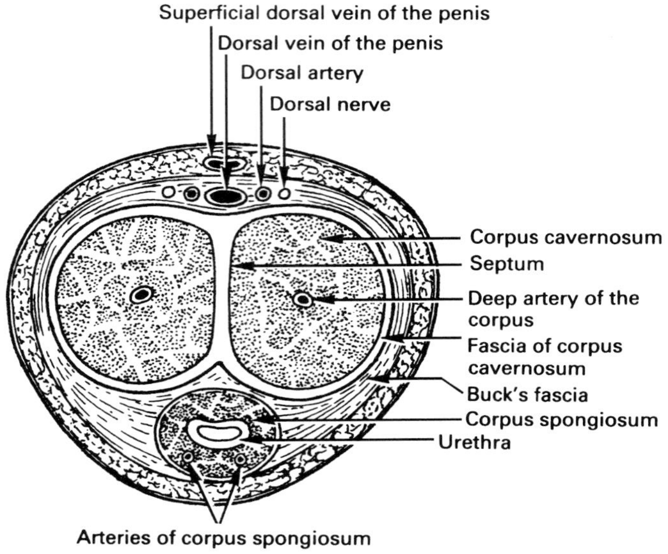

Fig. 39.3 Transverse section of the penis.

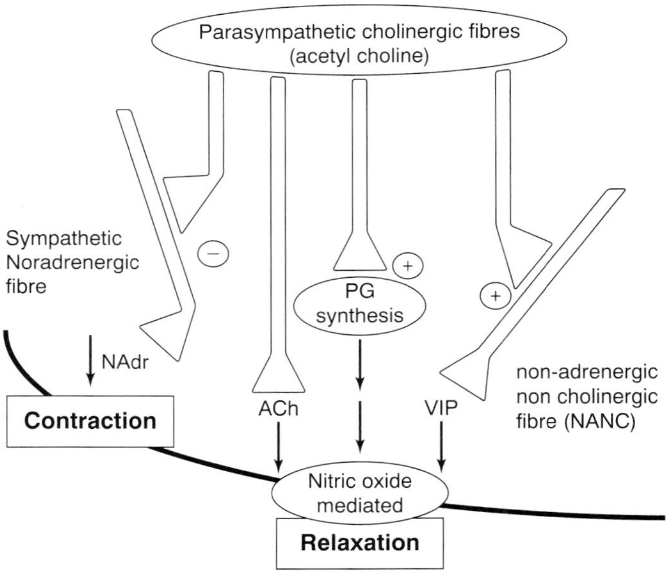

Fig. 39.4 Neurotransmitters involved in penile erection: NAdr = noradrenaline; VIP = vasoactive intestinal polypeptide; ACh = acetyl choline.

Penile erection and detumescence

Erection is a vascular phenomenon which is under neural control. The nerve supply is from the 2nd, 3rd and 4th sacral cord segments. Numerous parasympathetic neuromodulators are involved in this process (Fig. 39.4). Of the many neurotransmitters identified, acetyl choline and vasoactive intestinal polypeptide (VIP) are important and one of the final common mediators of

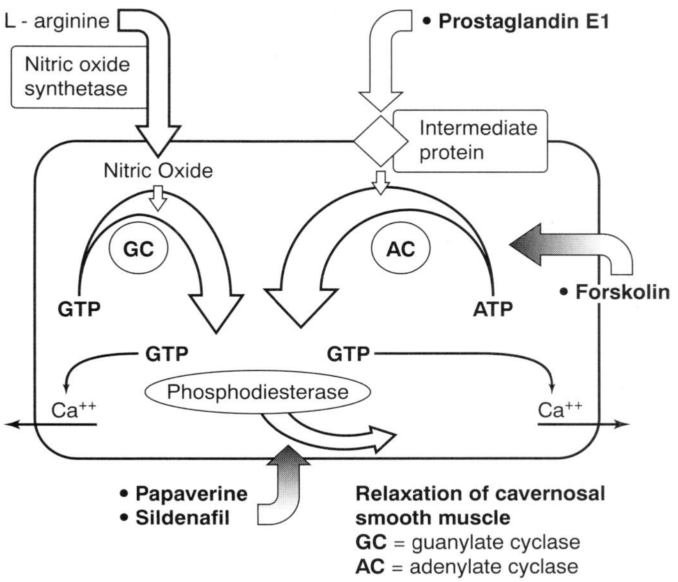

Fig. 39.5 Relaxation of cavernosal smooth muscle. GC = guanylate cyclase; AC = adenylate cyclase.

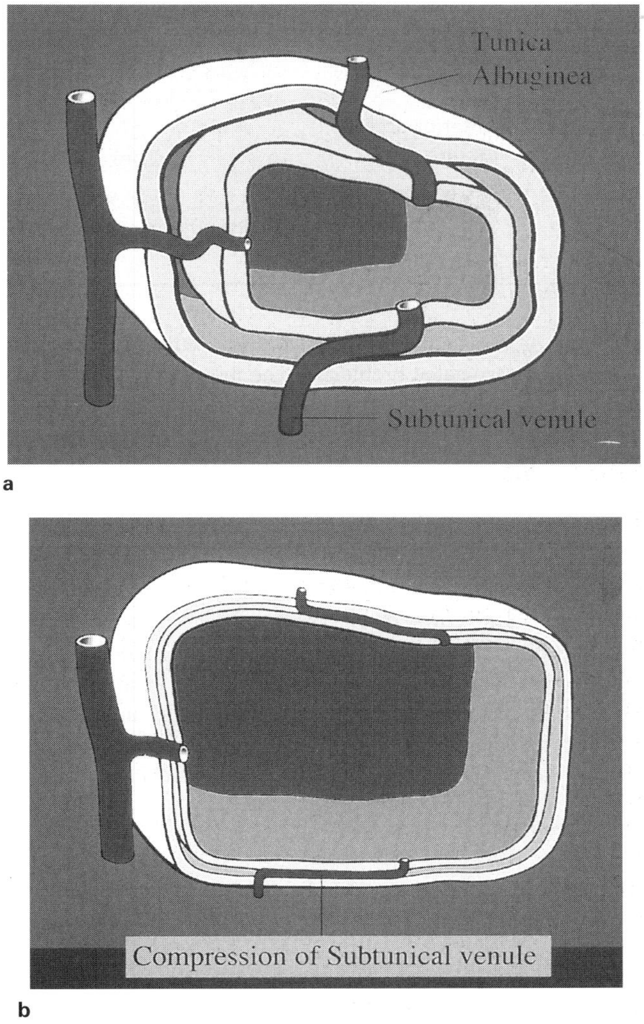

Fig. 39.6 Mechanism of venous occlusion. (**a**) In the flaccid state, blood entering the lacunar spaces drains freely through the subtunical venules. (**b**) During the tumescence phase, as the lacunar spaces fill, the subtunical venules are compressed against the rigid walls of the tunica albuginea and venous return is prevented.

erection is nitric oxide.[3] Smooth muscle relaxation involves the production of cyclic adenosine monophosphate (cAMP) and cyclic guanylate monophosphate (cGMP). Nitric oxide is synthesized from L-arginine by the enzyme nitric oxide synthase. This potent vasodilator stimulates the enzyme guanylate cylase which converts guanosine monophosphate to 3′,5′-cyclic guanosine monophosphate (c-GMP). This results in an intracellular depletion of calcium ions, leading to smooth muscle relaxation. Cyclic guanosine monophosphate is subsequently broken down by a phosphodiesterase enzyme that is fairly specific to penile erectile tissue[4] (Fig. 39.5). Cavernosal tissue also synthesizes various other vasoconstricting agents such as endothelin, prostaglandin $F_{2\alpha}$, thromboxane A_2 and neuropeptide Y. Cholinergic fibres probably also have a direct trophic action on the local production of erectogenic endogenous prostaglandins such as PGE_1, PGE_2 and prostacyclins (PGI_2).[5]

Relaxation of the smooth muscle within the erectile tissue causes blood to enter the lacunar spaces. Initially, there is an enormous increase in penile blood flow. This is known as the *tumescence phase* of erection, and blood flow, at systolic pressure, may be increased six fold.[6] The penis then becomes engorged with blood. The filling of the lacunar spaces compresses subtunical venules against the rigid walls of the tunica albuginea, preventing venous return[7] (Fig. 39.6). During the *full phase* of erection, the cavernosal pressure rises further. Contraction of the ischiocavernosus muscles then creates the *rigid phase* of erection. During this short period, the cavernosal pressure rises well above systolic blood pressure, and there is virtually no flow in the penis.[8] Detumescence is essentially a reversal of the erection process. As with ejaculation, it is mediated by the sympathetic nervous system and involves the action of noradrenaline.

THE MALE URETHRA

Congenital abnormalities

Hypospadias

Hypospadias occurs as a result of incomplete fusion of the genital folds that form the urethra. It is the most common abnormality of penile development, affecting about 1 in 125 boys and its incidence appears to be increasing. The condition is associated with many

REFERENCES

3. Adaikan P G, Lau L C, Ng S C, Ratnam S S Jpn J Pharmacol 1992; 58 (suppl 2): 300
4. Rajfer J, Aronson W J et al N Engl J Med 1992; 326(2): 90–94
5. Saenz de Tejada I J Urol 1995; 153(6): 1762
6. Lue T F, Tanagho E A J Urol 1987; 137: 829–836
7. Wespes E, Schulman C C Urology 1990; 36: 68–72
8. Lavoisier P, Courtois F, Barres D J Urol 1986; 136: 936–939

Table 39.1 Classification of hypospadiac deformities

Duckett	*Traditional*	*Koyanagi*	
Anterior	Glanular Coronal Anterior penile	70%	
Middle	Middle penile	10%	Distal
Posterior	Posterior penile Penoscrotal Scrotal Perineal	20%	Proximal

other genitourinary anomalies; the worse the deformity, the greater the degree of associated problems.[9] The most common associated conditions are undescended testis and inguinal hernia but renal and ureteric abnormalities also occur. There has been an increasing incidence of all male urogenital abnormalities over the last 50 years and this has paralleled a decrease in the average semen quality, suggesting that there may be an environmental cause.[10] However, as 8% of patients have affected fathers, there is probably some form of polygenic inheritance.[11] The clinical features may range from slight ventral displacement of the meatus to a perineal meatal opening. The more severe form may be associated with a bifid scrotum. The standard deformity consists of an abnormally placed meatus, a degree of chordee (ventral penile curvature) and a ventrally deficient 'hooded' foreskin. Classification systems describe the position of the meatus after the chordee has been corrected (Table 39.1).

Treatment

Surgical correction is usually attempted between 6 and 18 months of age, preferably before the child goes to nursery school. The three surgical aims are: to correct the penile chordee; to reconstruct the urethra and glans; and to cover the penis. The principles of surgical correction involve reconstruction of the urethral plate. This is a strip of mucosa that extends from the ectopic meatus to the glans. This strip can be dissected from the corpora to correct the chordee and can then be used to form the base of the neourethra. This plate can then be rolled into a tube, forming the new urethra (the Yelsnar procedure). Urethral reconstruction usually requires the interposition of an additional flap and either a vascularized flap of genital skin or a free graft of extragenital skin may be used. Vascularized flap grafts of preputial skin are the best urethral substitute as they provide wet, non-hairy skin with a good blood supply. These preputial flaps can be used either with an onlay technique over the urethral plate or can be made into a tube to form the neourethra. Free grafts have to develop a new blood supply, which increases the risk of failure. Free grafts of buccal mucosa tend to have a lower failure rate than other extra-genital grafts; they are taken from the mouth in strips up to 3 × 6 cm long in adults, and 2 × 4 cm in children.

Procedures. The majority of boys with hypospadias have a glandular or coronal meatus which can be corrected by the MAGPI procedure (meatal advancement and glanuloplasty), first described by John Duckett.[12] The essential steps in this procedure are: the creation of a new meatal pit; the advancement of this meatal pit; and the closure of the sleeve of glandular skin behind after the redundant foreskin has been excised (Fig. 39.7). The MAGPI is now an established one-stage procedure but the incidence of patients requiring a second procedure ranges between 1.2 and 8%.[13]

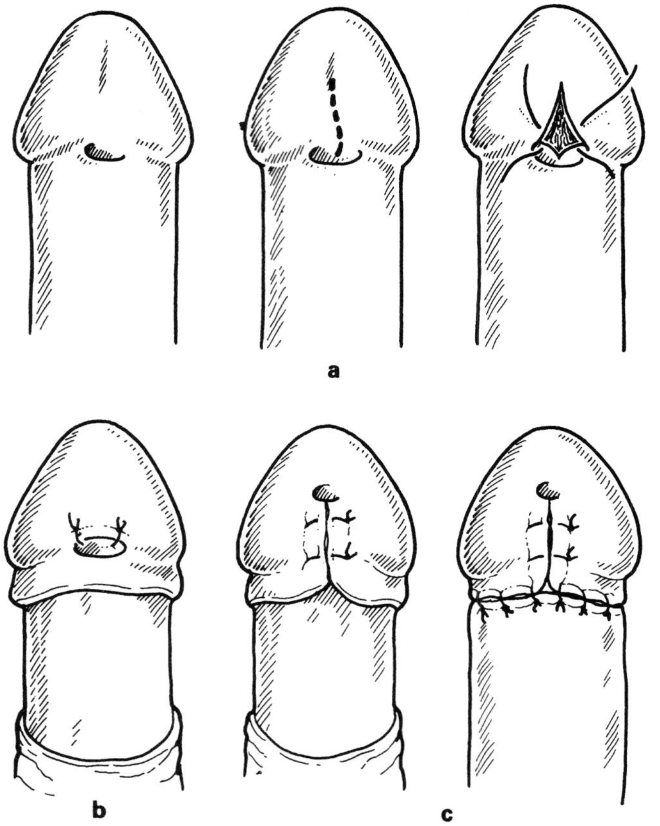

Fig. 39.7 MAGPI procedure (after Duckett[12]). (**a**) Incision of bridge of tissue between meatus and glanular groove and transverse closure; (**b**) advancement of meatus; (**c**) closure of sleeve of penile skin.

The Mathieu procedure is a more appropriate repair for proximal hypospadias. A flap is created based on the ectopic meatus. This is folded over and sutured to the urethral plate to advance the meatal position. The lateral glans flaps are closed over the new urethra (Fig. 39.8). Fistulae and strictures occur in about 4% and 1% of cases respectively.[15]

Very proximal urethral openings require reconstruction of the urethra using a flap or graft. These can either be sutured to the existing urethral plate—the onlay urethroplasty—or formed into a

REFERENCES

9. Sakakibara N, Nonomura K, Matsuno T, Koyanagi T Jpn J Urol 1985; 76: 716–722
10. Sherins R J N Engl J Med 1995; 332: 327
11. Duckett J W In: Walsh P C, Retik A B, Stamey T A, Vaughan E D (eds) Campbells Urology, 6th edn. WB Saunders, Philadelphia 1992
12. Duckett J W Urol Clin N Am 1981; 8: 513–519
13. Duckett J W, Snyder H M J Urol 1992; 147: 665–669
14. Mathieu P J Chir 1932; 39: 481
15. Mollard P, Mouriquand P P E, Bassett T Chir Paed 1987; 28: 197–203

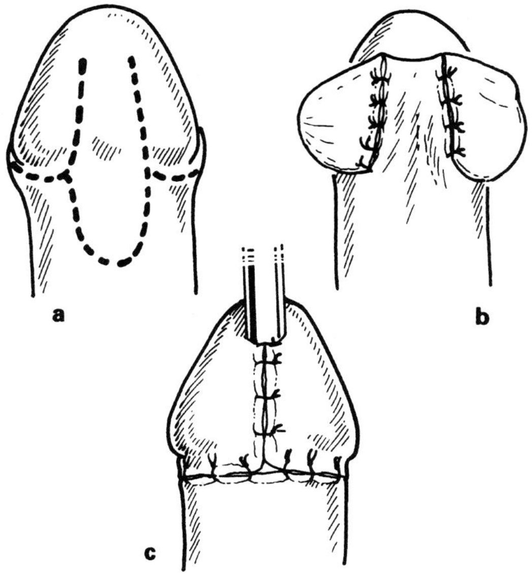

Fig. 39.8 Skin flap advancement beneath a reconstituted glans (after Mathieu[14]). (**a**) The raising of skin flaps; (**b**) the proximal flap is rotated forward and the lateral flaps are developed; (**c**) the lateral glans flaps are closed over the new urethra.

tube, such as the transverse preputial island flap urethroplasty popularized by Duckett.[16] This tube graft is used to bridge the defect between the ectopic meatus and the glans (Fig. 39.9). The most common complication of these complex procedures is the formation of a urethral fistula. These develop in between 5 and 20% of cases and, although a proportion of them heal spontaneously, the majority require a secondary operation. Repair should be delayed for at least 6 months and the principles of repair are the same as for any fistula; both epithelial surfaces must be closed with the interposition of well vascularized tissue.[17] Urethral stenosis and meatal regression are other uncommon complications.

Urethral valves

Congenital posterior urethral valves cause bladder outflow obstruction in male children. They can present in a variety of different ways and at different ages, depending mainly on the degree of obstruction. Urethral valves are present from the beginning of fetal life, so that other urinary tract organs develop in an environment of high genitourinary tract pressures. This may lead to some degree of permanent maldevelopment and poor function. Many infants with this condition are now diagnosed by prenatal ultrasound examination,[18] which can often determine the level of obstruction. Unfortunately, attempts to halt deterioration of renal function by prenatal intervention have not proved to work. The new-born infant may have a palpable bladder, hydronephrosis, ascites and respiratory distress from pulmonary hypoplasia. Half the children with all these problems die rapidly. Less severe obstruction leads to diagnosis at a later age: toddlers may present with recurrent urinary tract infection and incontinence, whereas schoolboys usually present with some other form of voiding dysfunction. In the older child micturating cystography or endoscopic examination of the urethra may be necessary to diagnose the condition.

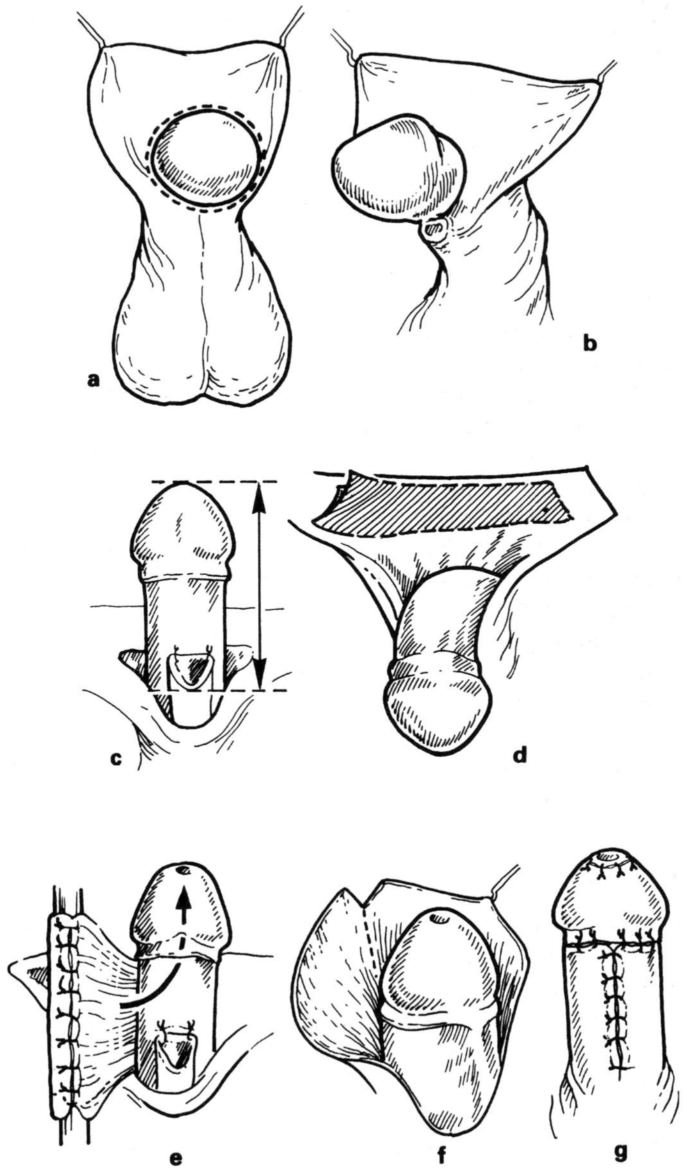

Fig. 39.9 Island flap urethroplasty (after Duckett[16]). (**a**) and (**b**) any chordee is first released and the preputial skin is released and held between skin hooks. (**c**) The distance of the skin tube required to bridge the gap between the meatus and glandular groove is measured. (**d**) The island flap is developed by dissecting the subcutaneous tissue off the dorsal skin. (**e**) A tunnel is developed to the glanular groove with removal of glans tissue. The skin flap is 'tubed' and the proximal anastomosis with the proximal urethra fixed to the corpora. (**f**) The distal end of the tube is advanced through the tunnel to the tip of the glans. (**g**) Lateral flaps of dorsal skin are rotated to the midline covering the neourethra.

REFERENCES

16. Duckett J W Urol Clin N Am 1981; 8: 503–511
17. Eardley I, Whitaker R H Br J Urol 1992; 69: 306–310
18. Skolder A J, Maizels M et al J Urol 1988; 139: 1026–1028

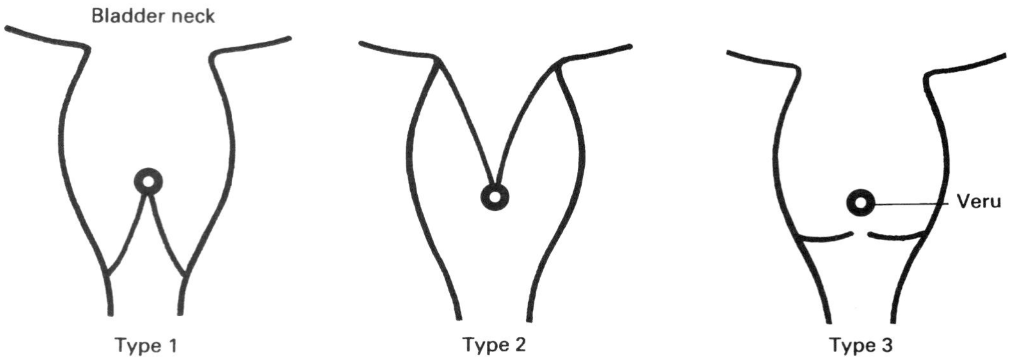

Fig. 39.10 Types of posterior urethral valves (after Young et al[19]).

Hugh Young[19] (1919) described three types of posterior valves (Fig. 39.10):

- Type I — an obstructing membrane down from the verumontanum. The most common form of urethral valve.
- Type II — folds between the bladder neck and verumontanum. These probably do not exist as a clinical entity.
- Type III — incomplete dissolution of the urogenital membrane.

The treatment is to ablate the obstructing valve using a single wire loop or hook electrode. Lasers have also been used. All these children require continued surveillance as they may go on to develop progressive renal impairment as a result of parenchymal dysplasia, persistent urosepsis and associated ureteric reflux.[20]

Acquired abnormalities

Strictures of the urethra

Causes

There are many causes of urethral stricture. Those caused by trauma tend to be short, involving the bulbar or membranous urethra and those which are caused by infection or ischaemia tend to be long, occurring anywhere in the urethra (Table 39.2).

Gonococcal urethritis followed by chronic inflammation, fibrosis and stricture formation was formally the most common cause of stricture but iatrogenic causes are now the most frequent aetiological factor. Urethral catheterization can lead to disruption of the urethral mucosa, followed by inflammation, fibrosis and scar formation. This typically occurs in the urethral bulb, the point where the urethra curves cranially towards the bladder (Fig. 39.1). The longer a urethral catheter is left in position, the greater the likelihood of urethral trauma and stricture formation. Silicone catheters are softer and cause less urethral friction; they are, therefore, preferable for long-term bladder drainage.

Cystoscopy and transurethral surgery may also result in damage to the urethral mucosa with subsequent stricture formation. Adequate lubrication should be applied and prophylactic urethral dilatation should be carefully undertaken if instrumentation is difficult.

Table 39.2 Causes of urethral stricture

Congenital
Traumatic
External trauma
Internal trauma—iatrogenic, e.g. instrumentation
Neoplastic
Primary—bladder cancer
penile cancer
Secondary
Inflammatory
Gonococcus
Non-specific urethritis
Balanitis xerotica obliterans

Diagnosis

A urethral stricture presents with symptoms of outflow obstruction which include slowing of the urinary stream increased frequency of micturition, and nocturia. Patients often report that straining hard maintains a reasonable flow. Occasionally, young men may present with renal impairment. The diagnosis can often be suspected from the history, particularly if the patient has had a previous indwelling catheter or genitourinary infection. The diagnosis is often suspected when a patient presents with acute retention of urine and it is not possible to pass a catheter.

Useful investigations include uro-flowmetry, cystoscopy, contrast urethrography and urethral ultrasonography. A urinary flow rate demonstrates the typical low peak flow, prolonged flow time and plateau trace. This results from the reduced calibre of the strictured area. Flexible cystoscopy is useful to identify the site of the stricture but gives no indication of the stricture length. Ascending and voiding urethrography accurately defines both the site and length of the stricture (Fig. 39.11). Real-time ultrasound can also identify the site, length and diameter of the stricture, but may be additionally valuable in defining the depth and density of the surrounding fibrosis. This additional information may influence treatment as well as predicting the chances of success.[21]

Treatment

The treatment of a stricture depends on its site, length and cause. Meatal strictures can be treated by dilatation, meatostomy or

REFERENCES

19. Young H H, Frontz W A, Baldwin J C J Urol 1919; 3: 289
20. Parkhouse H F, Barratt T M et al Br J Urol 1988; 62: 59–62
21. Nash P A, McAninch J W In: Reconstructive Surgery of the Lower Urinary Tract in Adults. ISIS Medical Media, Oxford 1995

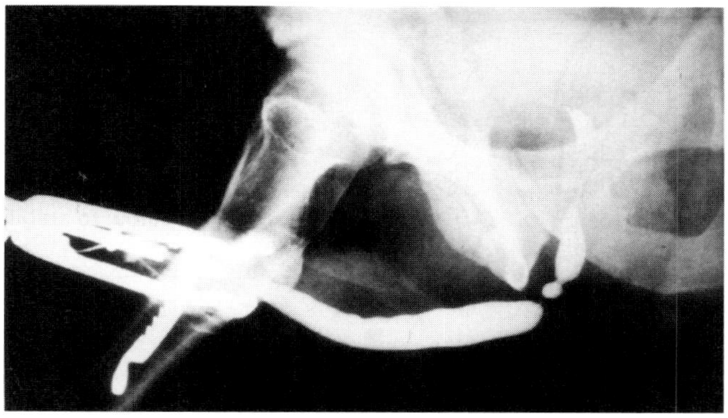

a

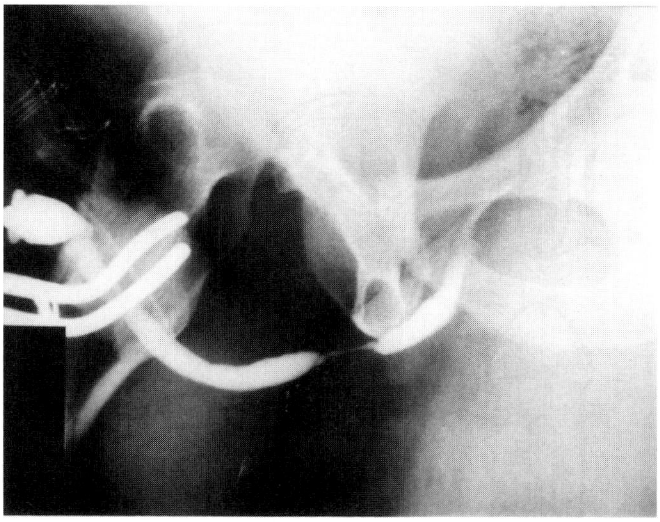

b

Fig. 39.11 Ascending urethrograms showing two examples of bulbar urethral strictures.

meatoplasty. Recurrence is common after simple dilatation unless the patient regularly practises intermittent self-dilatation. Meatostomy is the ventral incision of the stricture to create a hypospadias-like opening. It is simple procedure but often causes spraying of the urine during micturition with loss of the normal stream convergence. Meatoplasty is the formal reconstruction of the meatus using preputial or penile flaps to refashion the opening.

For more proximal strictures repeated urethral dilatation remains an option. This procedure has been practised for thousands of years and involves the passage of metal sounds of gradually increasing diameter. Although the procedure is apparently simple a great deal of damage can be caused with urethral dilators. A sound forced into an impassable stricture may be deflected to form a 'false passage' which may be blind ending or continuous around the stricture. Dilatation should only be performed by surgeons who are practised in the art of passing urethral sounds. Urethral dilatation is particularly suited to strictures that are very close to the distal sphincter mechanism. Definitive attempts to excise or incise strictures in this region may result in incontinence.

Urethrotomy involves incision of the scar (stricture) in the hope that it will maintain its calibre once healed. The procedure can be performed under direct vision with a urethroscope, or 'blindly' using a urethrotome. Blind urethrotomy is not to be recommended although it is frequently used for tight meatal openings prior to the introduction of large urethral instruments such as a resectoscope. Urethrotomy under direct vision or 'optical urethrotomy' involves the division of the stricture through the full thickness of the scar in the 12 o'clock position. It is usual to pass a guide-wire through the stricture before proceeding. A cold knife (Sachse urethrotome) allows the best visual control and the guide-wire helps the surgeon to maintain orientation. The stricture is cut until a 20 Fr silicone catheter can be passed into the bladder. This is left in position until the urothelium has healed: this is usually in a matter of days. This time will, however, vary according to the depth of the incision and the length of the stricture. For some complex strictures the catheter may be best left in position for 7–10 days.

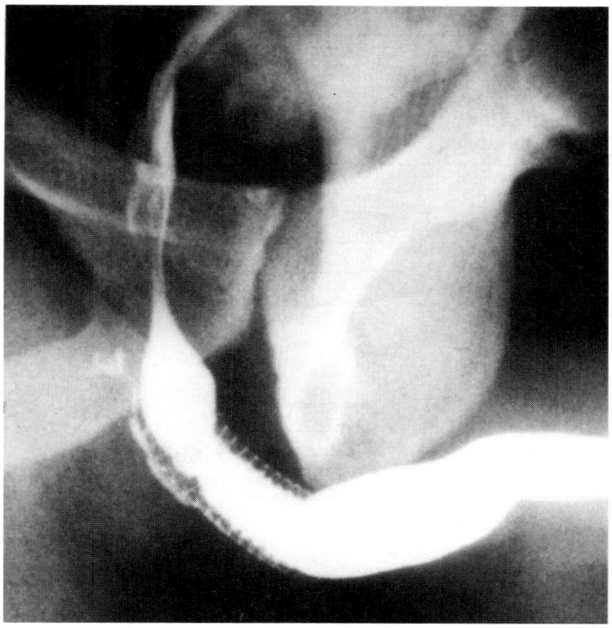

Fig. 39.12 Urethrogram demonstrating metallic mesh stent across a bulbar urethral stricture.

For most short uncomplicated strictures, optical urethrotomy provides a complete and long-lasting cure. Intermittent self-catheterization after internal urethrotomy, as a form of self-dilatation, has been used to maintain urethral patency.[22] More complex, full-thickness or longer strictures, including those secondary to inflammation or ischaemia, are rarely cured by this technique. Consideration should be given to more definitive treatment if a urethrotomy has been tried twice, and fails.

Following optical urethrotomy, a metallic mesh stent may be placed across the stricture to prevent recurrence (Fig. 39.12). Stents are usually made of woven tubular superalloy mesh which is expanded in the urethra. They prevent the scar from contracting and become covered by normal epithelium.[23] Stenting is suitable for patients who have had a failed previous urethrotomy and are at a high risk of further recurrence. It is only suitable for strictures in

REFERENCES

22. Kjaergard B, Walter S et al Br J Urol 1994; 73: 692–695
23. Ashken M H, Coulange C, Milroy E J G, Sarramon J P Eur Urol 1991; 19: 181–185

Table 39.3 Types of urethroplasty

1.	Primary excision and anastomosis of urethral ends
2.	One-stage repair using:
	a. pedicled flap of skin
	b. full-thickness graft
3.	Two-stage repair

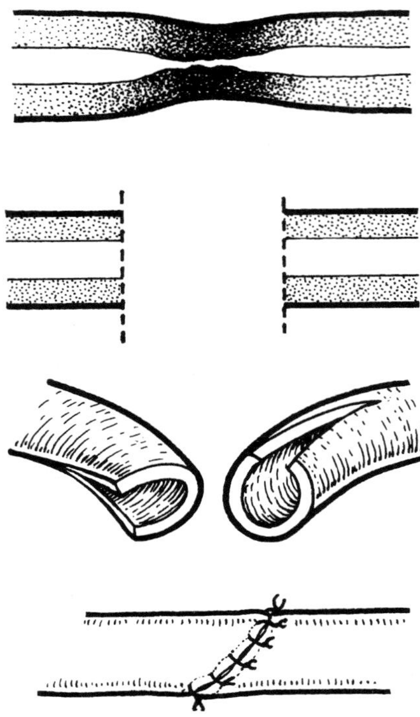

Fig. 39.13 Excision and end-to-end anastomosis for short anterior stricture.

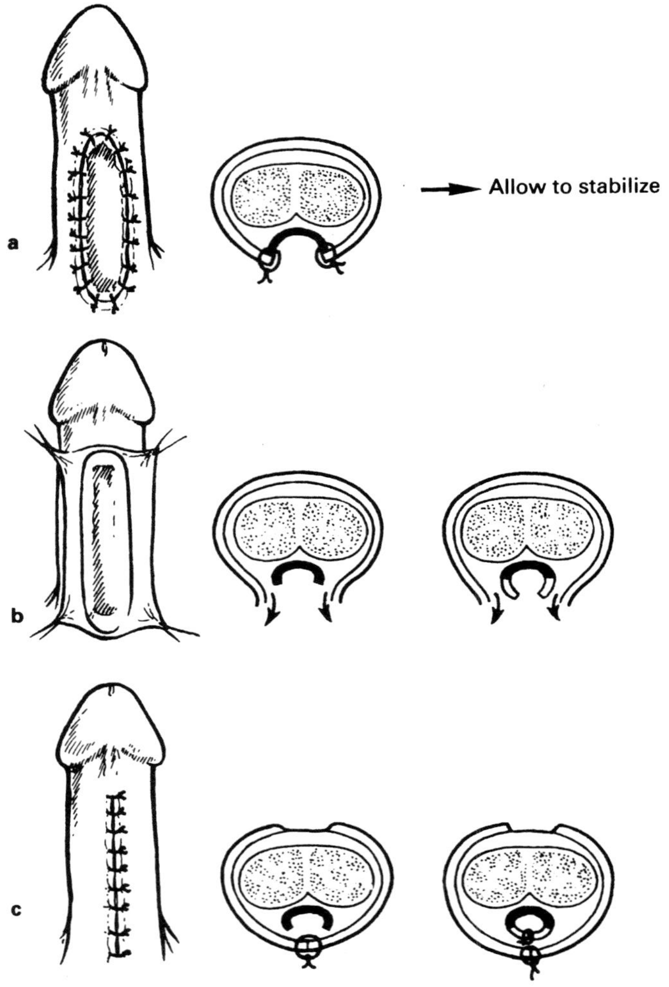

Fig. 39.14 Anterior urethroplasty.

the bulbar urethra. Placement in the membranous portion of the urethra leads to incontinence, and penile placement may cause pain on erection as the stent fails to expand. Other complications include blockage from tissue in growth and stone formation.

For complex or frequently recurrent strictures, urethroplasty is the most suitable option. The aim of this operation is to excise the strictured area and restore urethral continuity. There are several types of urethroplasty which are shown in Table 39.3.

For short strictures, especially in the bulbar urethra, primary excision and anastomosis is ideal. It should be considered for any patient who has a recurrent stricture after one or more failed optical urethrotomies. The bulbar urethra is approached through a perineal incision. The strictured area of urethra is excised back to healthy urethral tissue. The urethral ends are then spatulated and anastomosed over a urethral catheter (Fig. 39.13). Depending on the site of the original scarred area, strictures of up to 3 cm in length can be bridged by mobilization of the urethral ends.[24] Operative results are excellent with a long-term patency of at least 90%.

Longer strictures and those complicated by fistulae or infection may require bridging of the transected ends by extraneous tissue. The best results are obtained from the use of pedicled vascularized flaps from the prepuce, penis or scrotum.[25] Scrotal skin has the disadvantage that it is hairy and, in the long term, may develop squamous metaplasia or even carcinoma. Hairs in the urethral lumen can act as a nidus for stone formation. Scrotal skin is, however, versatile and easy to harvest. All of these flaps can either be used as on-lay grafts or can be tubularized to bridge longer defects.

The use of bladder or buccal mucosal grafts, or full-thickness skin grafts, is reserved for patients in whom simpler measures have failed. As these grafts need to acquire their own blood supply, the risk of failure, shrinkage and fibrosis is greater.[26]

Two-stage procedures, such as the Johanson urethroplasty, are used for long, complex and anterior strictures and involve the laying open of the strictured area, with the creation of a perineal urethrostomy, followed by a secondary closure 2–3 months later. The results of this procedure are excellent and justify the prolonged inconvenience for the patient (Fig. 39.14).

REFERENCES

24. Webster G, Ramon J J Urol 1991; 145: 744–748
25. Rogers H S, McNicholas T A, Blandy J P Br J Urol 1992; 69: 621–628
26. Burger R A, Muller S C et al J Urol 1992; 147: 662–664

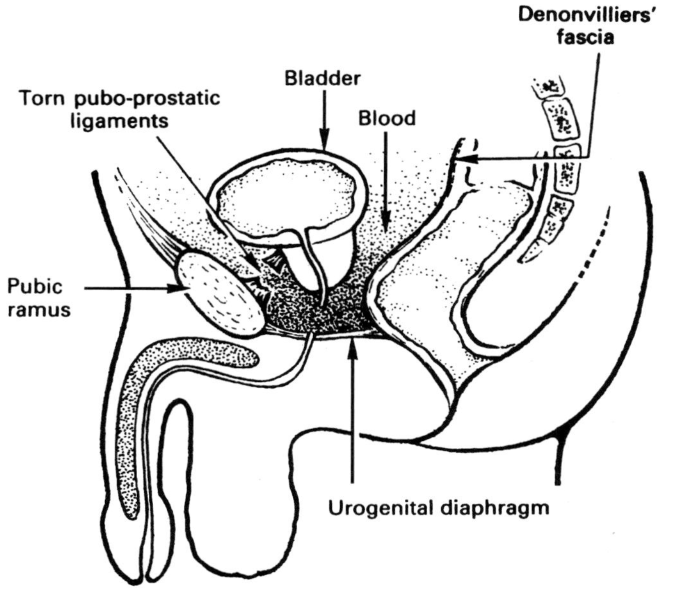

Fig. 39.15 Disruption of membranous urethra (above the urogenital diaphragm).

Urethral trauma

Traumatic damage to the urethra can be a devastating injury. Iatrogenic injury with catheter or cystoscope leads to mucosal damage and is generally less severe than injury sustained from an external force. External forces may be either blunt or penetrating and can damage the urethra. Most urethral injuries occur as a result of blunt or crushing forces in the perineum. Many are sustained in motor vehicle accidents or following falls astride rigid structures; the crossbar of the bicycle is a common culprit.

Penetrating injuries from a knife or gunshot are less common. Urethral injuries are classified[27] as:

1. Posterior urethra ('above' the urogenital diaphragm).
2. Anterior urethra ('below' the urogenital diaphragm).

Posterior urethral damage

10% of all pelvic fractures are associated with some form of urethral injury (see Chapter 52). Urethral rupture above the urogenital diaphragm is usually the result of a pelvic fracture. Fracture of the pelvis may cause displacement of the bone fragments as the result of the 'pull' of the powerful muscles of the trunk and lower limb. As the prostate is firmly attached to the pelvis by the strong pubo-prostatic ligaments, the prostate moves with the pelvic bone fragments. The membranous urethra remains fixed, and the violent shearing force causes the prostate and the membranous urethra to tear apart (Fig. 39.15). These membranous urethral tears may be either partial or complete. If complete, the bladder and prostate 'ride high' into the pelvis, and the urethral ends are separated by blood clot and urine. If the tear is incomplete the prostate retains its normal position. Urethral catheterization should be avoided as this may convert an incomplete tear into a complete one.

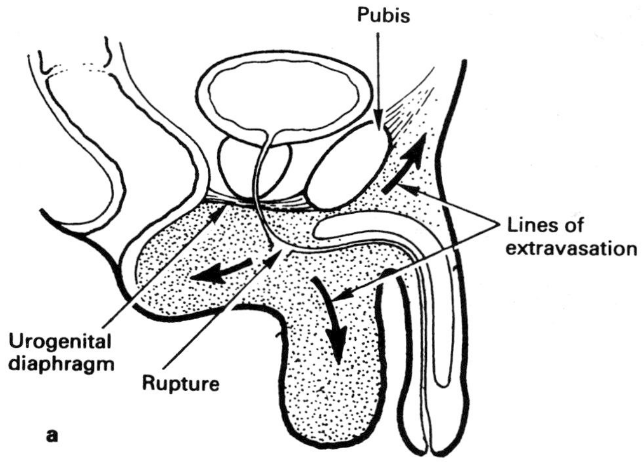

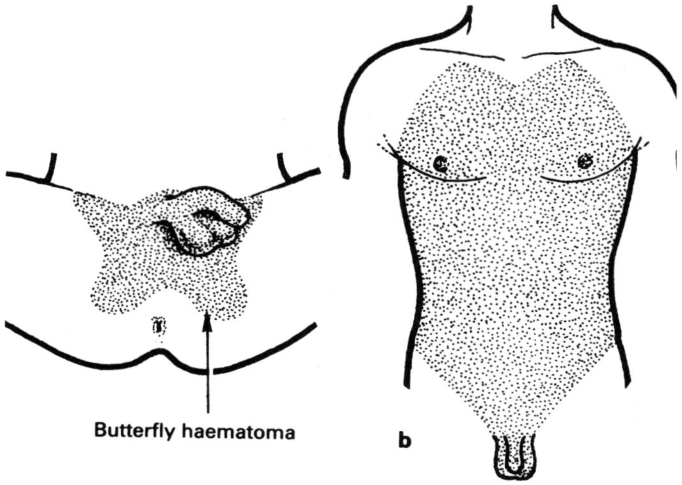

Fig. 39.16 (**a**) Disruption of bulbar urethra (below the urogenital diaphragm); (**b**) potential areas of extravasation following attachments of Colles' fascia.

Anterior urethral damage

Urethral injuries below the urogenital diaphragm usually arise from a 'straddle-type' injury such as a fall onto a bicycle crossbar or a direct blow to the perineum from, for example, a kick. Consequently, the bulbar urethra is crushed against the pubic arch and may be completely or incompletely severed. During these injuries Buck's superficial fascia is disrupted but the blood and urine from the injury are confined by the attachments of Colles' fascia. This leads to the typical pattern of bruising seen in these patients: a 'butterfly' haematoma collects in the perineum and scrotum, with extension into the anterior abdominal wall (Fig. 39.16).

Penetrating injuries to the bulbar and penile portions of the urethra do occur but the injury is usually less life-threatening than the other damage caused by the penetrating missile, which is often a bullet. Injuries confined to the anterior urethra may lead to bruising confined within Buck's fascia, producing the typical 'sleeve' of haematoma down the shaft of the penis but not extending into the scrotum.

A urethral injury must always be suspected in a patient with any injury to the perineum or pelvis. These patients are often very unwell with injuries to head, chest or abdomen, and a detailed history and examination may be difficult to obtain. Blood at the urethral meatus, swelling in the perineum and bruising of the scrotum and genitalia should raise suspicion. Rectal examination should be performed if at all possible to check the position of the prostate and to rule out any concomitant rectal injury. Urethral catheterization should not be attempted if a urethral injury is suspected. At the earliest opportunity, an oblique retrograde urethrogram should be performed using water-soluble contrast. The contrast is injected through a catheter, which is advanced along the urethra looking for the site of injury (Fig. 39.17). The catheter is advanced into the bladder if no extravasation of contrast is seen and a cystogram performed. This identifies any bladder tears, which can also occur with lower abdominal and pelvic injuries (see Chapters 37 and 52). An intravenous urogram can be performed if urethral catheterization is not possible. This introduces contrast into the bladder so that both the position of the bladder within the pelvis, and the integrity of the bladder wall can be assessed. Prostato-membranous dislocation leads, to an elevation of the bladder, which is often compressed by pelvic haematoma, giving rise to the typical 'tear-drop' shape (Fig. 39.18).

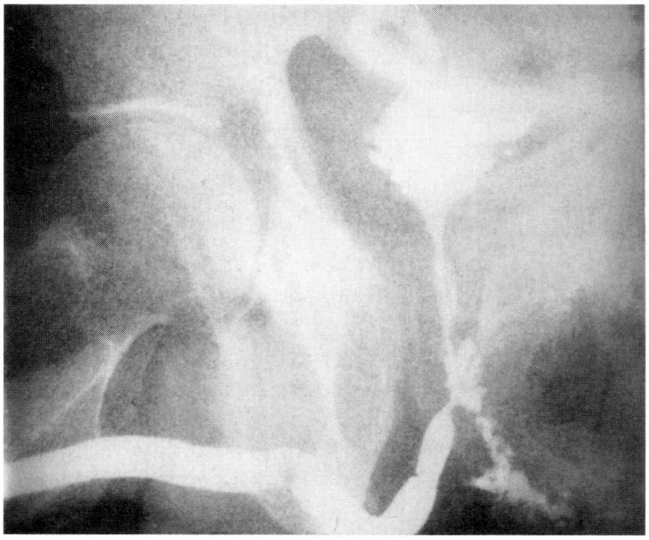

Fig. 39.17 Urethrogram showing extravasation of contrast from membranous urethra following pelvic fracture injury.

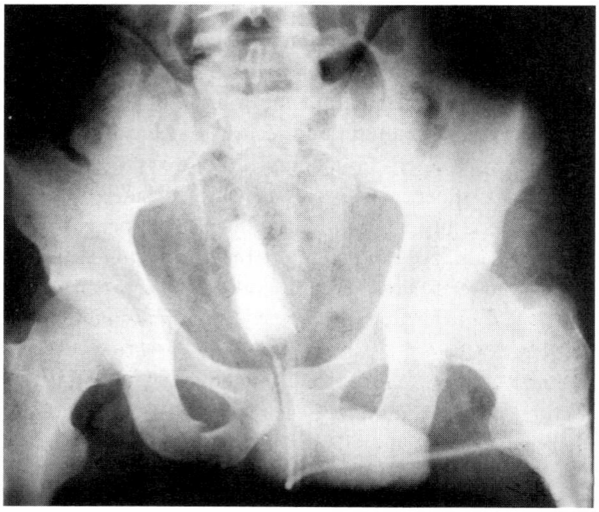

Fig. 39.18 Typical 'tear-drop' shape of bladder surrounded by haematoma.

Treatment

The first principle of treatment in all urethral injuries is to divert urine away from the site of injury in order to reduce extravasation of urine. With a pure urethral injury this can be achieved with a bladder catheter. This may be passed suprapubically, or by very careful urethral passage across the site of injury as described above. In order to avoid the risk of extending an incomplete urethral tear, the usual management is to place a suprapubic catheter and then follow this with a delayed repair of the urethral injury some months later.[27] The suprapubic catheter is introduced either percutaneously or through an open cystostomy. This depends on how much the bladder is distended; if this can not be determined, the catheter should be passed with ultrasound guidance.

Anterior urethra

Following blunt injuries, a urethral stricture almost inevitably develops, regardless of whether the urethral rupture is partial or complete. Delayed urethral reconstruction is preferred for this type of injury. Penetrating injuries such as knife stabs to the penile or bulbar urethra can be repaired immediately. The wound is explored and the urethral breach repaired. Usually, the two urethral ends are spatulated and anastomosed over a suitable catheter.

Posterior urethra

These injuries vary greatly with respect to the extent of the urethra involved and the magnitude of the disruption. Prostato-membranous distraction is often associated with major trauma and multiple injuries. In these patients suprapubic cystostomy should be performed, accepting that urethral stricture will inevitably develop. Reconstruction is then delayed for at least 3 months, by which time the injured tissues have the strength to hold sutures. Primary realignment of the urethral ends at the time of open insertion of the suprapubic catheter can be attempted, but is associated with an increased incidence of subsequent incontinence and impotence.[28] In the acute situation, identification of the urethral ends is difficult; the pelvis is full of blood clot, urine and bone fragments, and release of the tamponaded haematoma within the pelvis can lead to catastrophic bleeding from damaged pelvic veins.

REFERENCES

27. McAninch J W J Trauma 1981; 21: 4–7
28. Webster G D Urol Clin North Am 1989; 16: 303–312

When there is little or no urethral distraction and minimal haematoma, it is reasonable to perform an early urethral approximation. Urethral epithelial apposition is necessary for healing without stricture formation. Urethral approximation can either be achieved endoscopically, at the time of open insertion of the suprapubic catheter, or by using a combination of open surgery and endoscopy. Endoscopic realignment of the urethral ends can be achieved using two flexible cystoscopes and a guide-wire. This enables a urethral catheter to be positioned accurately and allows for epithelial approximation. The catheter should remain in position for about two weeks. Following removal of the catheter, regular intermittent self-catheterization may be instigated and future stricture formation avoided.[29]

Regardless of the early management policy, interval urethrography at about 6 weeks should be performed to identify the site, length and degree of stricture that has developed. The treatment of this stricture varies from dilatation to open urethroplasty and this will be determined by the age of the patient, the features shown by the urethrogram and other concomitant injuries. This technique of urinary diversion and delayed reconstruction leads to an incidence of impotence in about 10% of patients and an incontinence rate of about 5%.

Tumours of the urethra

Benign tumours

Benign tumours of the urethra are usually sexually transmitted and viral in origin (condylomata acuminata). They may be treated by the topical application of podophyllin if they are at the distal tip of the urethra. Endoscopic excision or diathermy may be used if they persist or extend into the proximal urethra.

Malignant tumours

Primary malignant tumours of the urethra are uncommon. The majority are squamous cell carcinomas which often develop as a complication of a long-standing urethral stricture. They present with urethral bleeding at the beginning of the stream, obstruction and occasionally haematospermia. Transitional cell tumours involving or developing in the urethra are usually associated with more widespread tumours in the bladder. They may also arise in about 5–10% of patients following a cystoprostatectomy for invasive transitional cell carcinoma of the bladder. En bloc urethrectomy at the time of radical cystoprostatectomy can be performed but is not usually done unless there is a specific indication. These indications include the presence of tumour in the prostatic urethra prior to cystoprostatectomy, the presence of carcinoma in situ in urethral biopsies or even the presence of widespread multifocal superficial malignancy. Urethrectomy performed at the same time as radical cystoprostatectomy increases both the blood loss and the morbidity and is, therefore, not usually performed in the absence of one of these indications. Both of these primary tumours invade local lymphatics at an early stage and are often metastatic at the time of diagnosis. The prognosis is therefore often poor despite aggressive surgical treatment.

Table 39.4 Disorders associated with male urinary incontinence

Bladder outflow obstruction:
Uncomplicated (overflow)
Associated with instability
Neuropathic bladder
Bladder neck obstruction
Detrusor instability
Extra-urological causes
Constipation
Drugs

Incontinence

Urinary incontinence occurs in 7–10% of men over 65 years of age. There are many causes (Table 39.4). For most male patients, the treatment of incontinence is directed at the underlying cause, for example the relief of bladder outflow obstruction. For a small proportion of patients however the problem is the result of a loss of the normal continence mechanism. Isolated sphincter damage may occur following prostatectomy, pelvic trauma or neurological disease. For these patients, an artificial urinary sphincter may be the only method of treatment.

An artificial sphincter is a hydraulic device that is activated by the patient. It comprises an inert, non-toxic, inflatable cuff which is placed around the urethra. The cuff is connected to a balloon reservoir and a pump unit which are in continuity. De-activation of the pump allows the hydraulic fluid from the cuff to pass into the reservoir. Deflation of the cuff allows the patient to pass urine (Fig. 39.19).

The most suitable patients for artificial sphincter insertion are those with normal bladder compliance and contractility. They must also have enough manual dexterity to operate the device. The cuff is placed around the bulbar urethra through a perineal incision, and the balloon reservoir is located in the perivesical space through a separate incision. The pump is placed into the scrotum and all three components are connected by plastic pipes. The main surgical complication is sepsis. Scrupulous skin preparation and broad-spectrum antibiotics to cover the insertion are essential. Infection occurs in at least 5% of devices and these must than be removed. Other complications include component failure and erosion of the cuff through the urethra. An artificial sphincter provides a satisfactory solution for over 90% of patients with post-prostatectomy incontinence.[30]

THE FEMALE URETHRA

Urethral syndrome

The urethral syndrome is a complex group of symptoms: patients suffer from urinary frequency, urgency, dysuria and sometimes back and suprapubic pain. The cause of the condition is unknown, although infection, urethral stenosis, neurogenic, psychogenic and

REFERENCES

29. Cohen J K, Berg G, Carl G H, Diamond D D J Urol 1991; 146: 1548–1550
30. Light J K Prob in Urol 1993; 7: 402–409

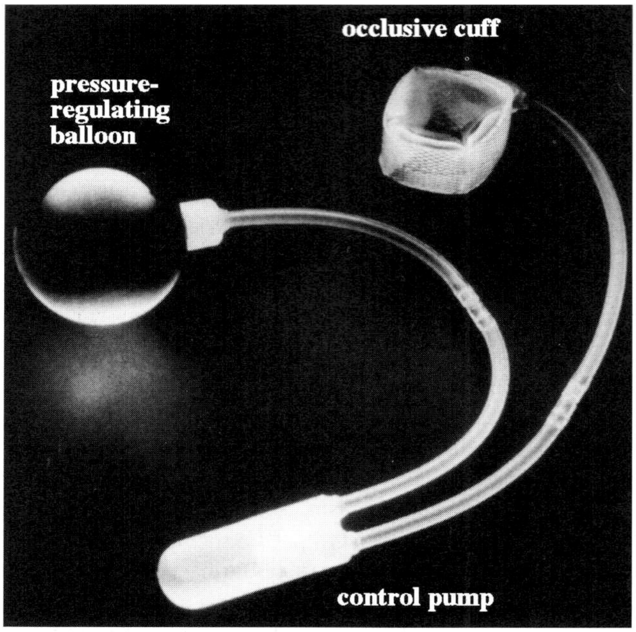

Fig. 39.19 Artificial urinary sphincter device.

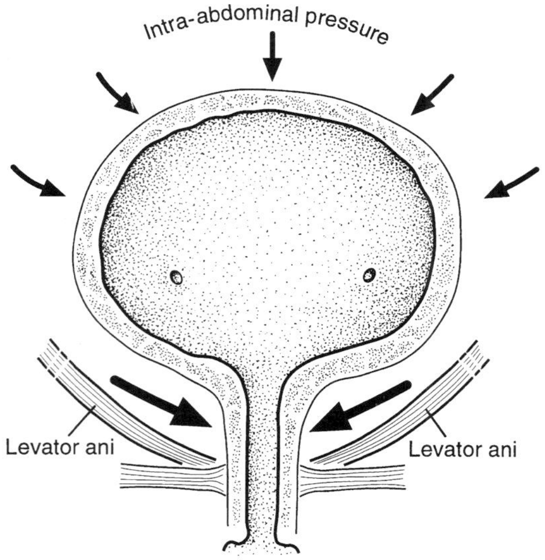

Fig. 39.20 Correct anatomical positioning of urethra.

allergic factors have all been implicated. The condition predominantly affects young sexually active women and the diagnosis is made by exclusion.

Midstream urine cultures will be sterile although a proportion of patients have some pyuria organisms such as *Ureaplasma*, *Gardnerella* and *Chlamydia* are often identified if urine and urethral swabs are cultured using special technique. Cystoscopy and all other imaging of the urinary tract is normal.

Treatment

Patients with pyuria may be treated with an antibiotic such as doxycycline or erythromycin which are effective against *Ureaplasma* and *Chlamydia*. Metronidazole can be added to cover anaerobic organisms such as *Gardnerella* if symptoms persist. In the absence of any pyuria, or if symptoms persist, urethral dilatation may be of benefit, although the relief of symptoms may only be temporary.

Incontinence

Female urinary incontinence is a major cause of morbidity. A report from the Royal College of Physicians in 1995 suggested that the prevalence in women living at home between the ages of 45 and 64 years is 8–15%. For those over 65 years the prevalence in the community may be as high as 20%. For those living in nursing homes and long-stay hospitals it is 40% and 60% respectively.

Normal female continence results from the balance of a number of forces including the closing pressure of the urethra (the sphincter mechanism), the anatomical length of the urethra and the ability of the pelvic floor to increase urethral closing pressure at the time of stress. The closing pressure of the urethra is maintained by a number of factors including:

1. Urethral mucosal apposition which forms a seal.
2. Oestrogen, which preserves the tone of urethral connective tissue.
3. Neurological integrity of the bladder neck and urethra.

Full anatomical support of the bladder neck and proximal urethra results in proper transmission of raised intra-abdominal forces which facilitate the action of the sphincteric unit (Fig. 39.20). Failure of any one of these components may lead to incontinence. When the leakage occurs at the time of raised intra-abdominal pressure, it is described as stress incontinence. A useful clinical classification for stress incontinence is as follows:[31]

1. Anatomical malposition of the intact sphincteric unit.
2. Poor function of the urethral closing mechanism because of intrinsic urethral dysfunction.

The aim of the clinical assessment is to determine the type and degree of leakage including the presence and degree of associated conditions such as cystocoele and rectocoele.

Treatment

There are a wide range of treatment options available and a careful selection should be made for each patient (Table 39.5).

Patients with malposition of the normal sphincter mechanism and marked urinary loss may benefit from surgical bladder neck suspension. There are a number of procedures described for this purpose which include the Marshal–Marchetti Kranz operation, Burch colposuspension, anterior colporrhaphy and Stamey percutaneous needle suspension. The choice of operation depends on the degree of cystocele present, the amount of urine leakage, and the age and preference of the patient.

In the Burch procedure, the perivaginal tissue and vaginal wall are elevated on both sides to the ileopectineal ligaments of the

REFERENCES

31. Raz S, Little N A, Juma S In: Walsh P C, Retik A B, Stamey T A, Vaughan E D (eds) Campbell's Urology, 6th edn. WB Saunders, Philadelphia 1992

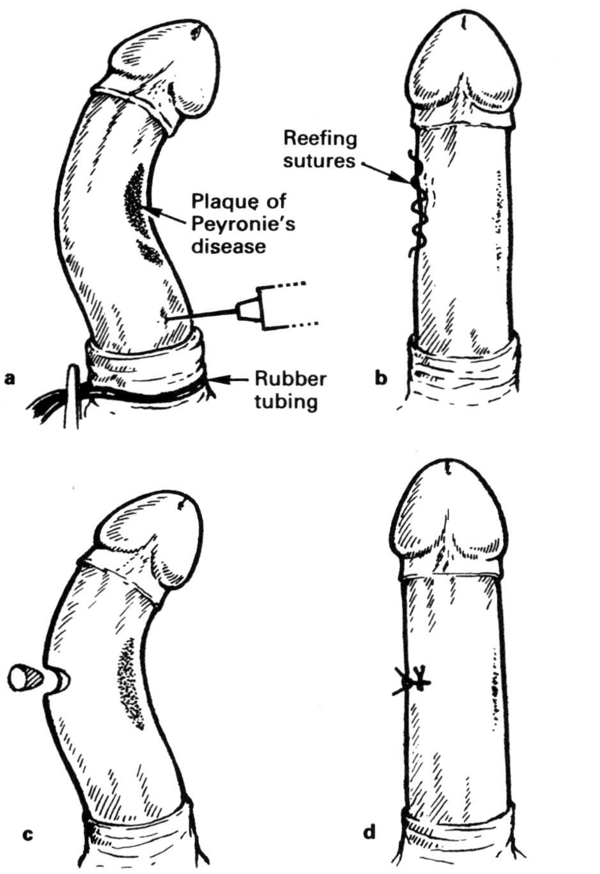

Fig. 39.22 (**a**) and (**b**) Reefing sutures. (**a**) A circumferential skin incision below the glans and skin is sleeved back. An artificial erection is induced by injecting saline into the corpus. The site of the plaque and curvature is assessed. (**b**) Reefing sutures are inserted on the opposite side to straighten the penis. (**c**) and (**d**) Correction of curvature of Peyronie's disease. (**c**) An ellipse of tunica albuginea of corpus (about 1 cm) is excised. (**d**) Haemostatic closure; excision of ellipse.

steroids,[52,56] clostridial collagenases,[57] and verapamil[58] are used in some centres with modest claims of efficacy.

Radiotherapy has had its proponents throughout the course of this century with varying claims of success. Most who have used this treatment have suggested that improvements can only be anticipated when it is used early in the disease. It is particularly useful for treating patients whose predominant symptom is pain.[59–61]

Surgery is largely restricted to those patients whose curvature restricts vaginal penetration. Although the plaque can be excised and replaced with a dermal graft,[62] most surgeons leave the plaque and perform a contralateral procedure to straighten the penis. This is usually achieved by producing an artificial erection and either tightening the tunica albuginea with reefing sutures[63] or removing a wedge of this tissue (Nesbitt's procedure).[64] Both procedures inevitably shorten the penis (Fig. 39.22).

Phimosis

In this condition the patient is unable to pull the foreskin back to fully expose the glans of the penis. There may only be a pinhole opening, which often leads to ballooning of the foreskin on micturition. As the foreskin cannot be retracted for cleaning, smegma, the white substance secreted under the foreskin, may accumulate and so facilitate infection of the prepuce or glans (balanitis). Treatment is by circumcision.

Paraphimosis

This occurs when a foreskin is retracted and a tight constriction develops around the subcoronal region of the penis. The constriction may be because of a tight foreskin, or as a result of preputial oedema following masturbation or intercourse. This constriction results in venous obstruction with oedema and further engorgement of tissue fluid within the retracted foreskin. Eventually the condition becomes painful. It is, therefore, important to remember to replace the foreskin over the glans penis after catheterizing a patient.

Reduction of a paraphimosis can usually be achieved by pressure to squeeze the oedema out from the glans and foreskin. Copious lignocaine gel is applied and the distal penis is compressed in the palm of the hand. Manipulation with the fingers and thumb usually returns the foreskin to the normal position, and so removes the constriction. The swelling then subsides. Occasionally, a dorsal slit under local anaesthetic or even a reduction under general anaesthesia is necessary. The latter is usually followed by a circumcision at a later date.

Balanitis xerotica obliterans

Balanitis xerotica obliterans is a disease of unknown aetiology which is histologically the same as lichen sclerosus et atrophicus. It is a dyskeratotic skin disorder affecting the prepuce, glans or urethral meatus. The condition begins with inflammatory changes which in turn lead to fibrosis and atrophy in the dermis and epidermis. The skin changes occur in small islands, or bands, of varying thickness. The typical appearances are of a white stenosing band at the end of the foreskin and of a haemorrhagic response to minor trauma. The process may result in a phimosis of the overlying prepuce or, if the urethra is involved, meatal stenosis. Treatment is by circumcision. Topical application of 1% hydrocortisone cream may be effective in treating early changes and intralesional injections of triamcinolone may reduce the itching and burning which is occasionally associated with this condition.[65]

REFERENCES

56. Hinman F J, Green E J Urol 1959; 81(4): 550
57. Gelbard M K, James K, Riach P, Dorey F J Urol 1993; 149(1): 56–58
58. Levine L A, Merrick P F, Lee R C J Urol 1994; 151(6): 1522–1524
59. Rodrigues C I, Njo K H, Karim A B Int J Radiat Oncol Biol Phys 1995; 31(3): 571–576
60. Viljoen I M, Goedhals L, Doman M J, S Afr Med J 1993; 83(1): 19–20
61. Duggan H E J Urol 1964; 91(5): 572–573
62. Devine C J, Horton C E J Urol 1974; 11: 144–149
63. Horton C E, Devine C J Plast Reconstr Surg 1973; 52: 32–35
64. Nesbit R M J Urol 1965; 93: 230–232
65. Jebakumar S P R, Woolley P D Int J STD AIDS 1995; 6: 81–83

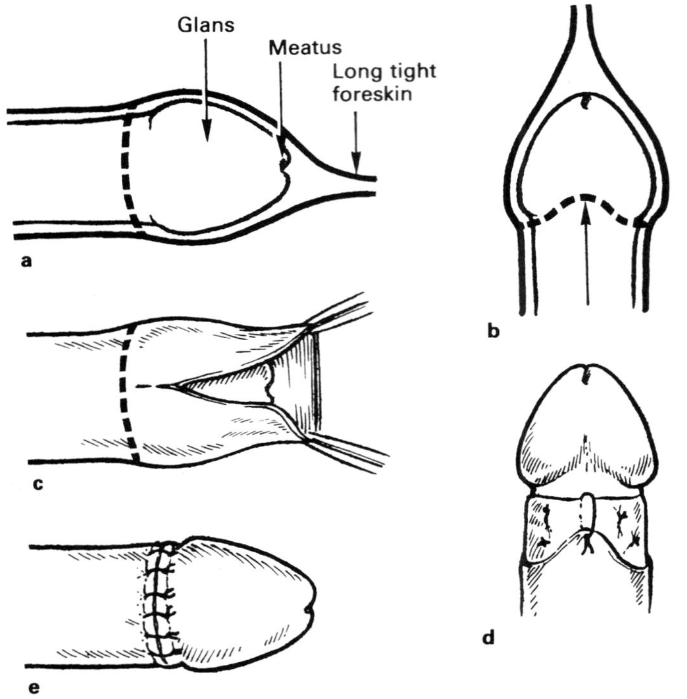

Fig. 39.23 Circumcision. (**a**) Line of excision. (**b**) Small ventral extension by the frenulum. (c) Dorsal slit. (**d**) Bleeding points are ligated with absorbable sutures. (**e**) Skin–mucosal apposition with interrupted absorbable sutures.

Regular urethral bouginage combined with topical steroid cream may be effective if meatal stenosis is a problem. Complete excision of the lesion with meatoplasty may be necessary if the stenosis is very severe. In recent years, laser excision of these lesions has also proven to be effective.[66]

Circumcision

The reasons for performing a circumcision are medical or religious. Medical reasons include troublesome phimosis, paraphimosis, recurrent balanitis, balanitis xerotica obliterans, in situ carcinoma or frank carcinoma of the penis prior to topical treatment. A true phimosis is rare in children and there are few indications to perform a circumcision in boys under 5 years of age. Many techniques have been described. The foreskin can be cut with scissors or a knife (Fig. 39.23), and devices such as a Plastibell can be used to achieve a better cosmetic result. In short, the aim is to remove the preputial skin, leaving about 3 mm of mucosa attached to the glans. Bleeding vessels are ligated with absorbable sutures, or cauterized with bipolar diathermy. The skin and mucosa are then approximated with interrupted absorbable sutures. The major complication is reactive haemorrhage. This may respond to local pressure but, if severe, requires re-exploration and suturing.

Premalignant penile lesions

Penile warts — condylomata acuminata

Penile warts are caused by the human papilloma virus (HPV). This is one of the most rapidly increasing sexually transmitted diseases. The warts usually occur on the glans, prepuce or shaft of the penis, and they may involve the distal urethra. They may appear as acuminate, macular or papular skin protrusions. Several serological subtypes are recognized: the common visible papular external warts are often types 6 and 11. The so-called 'high risk' types (16, 18, 31, 33 and 35) are more often of papular or macular morphology[67] and have been associated with cervical dysplasia in women and the development of carcinoma of the cervix. Anal warts in homosexuals are very similar (see Chapter 30) and have been causally linked with carcinoma of the anus. There is a minor association with carcinoma of the penis (see below). No therapy can completely eradicate human papilloma virus infection, although external skin warts can be treated with podophyllin, cryosurgery, or laser treatment. Laser treatment is particularly effective in treating urethral warts. These can cause difficulties as urethral (meatal) stenosis can occur after simple excision. Even after the warts have been treated, the patient should be aware that he is infective to uninfected partners.

Buschke–Lowenstein tumour

This benign condition does not spread to lymph nodes but produces large exophytic 'tumours' that can destroy the penis. Local destruction of the penile tissue can lead to urethral fistulae with development of the 'watering can' penis. Treatment is by wide local excision which may necessitate partial penile amputation.

Carcinoma in situ

Carcinoma in situ or erythroplasia of Queyrat presents as a red, well-defined velvety lesion on the glans or the foreskin, nearly always in the uncircumcised. A circumcision and biopsy confirms the diagnosis, and treatment with 5-fluorouracil cream is usually successful.

Carcinoma of the penis

Carcinoma of the penis is relatively uncommon in the western world, affecting only 1 individual in 100 000. It is more common in certain tropical areas such as India, South America,[68] north east Thailand,[69] and amongst certain African tribes,[70] where it may account for 10–20% of all male malignancies.[68] It is virtually unheard of in men who have been circumcised at birth, and is therefore rare in Jewish people.[71] The risk is increased if circumcision is delayed until puberty. Phimosis is present in 25–50% of patients who present with carcinoma of the penis which provides

REFERENCES

66. Ratz J L, J Am Acad Dermatol 1984; 10: 925–928
67. Lowhagen G B, Bolmstedt A, Ryd W, Voog E Genitourin Med 1993; 69(2): 87–90
68. Persky L Cancer Res 1977; 60: 97–109
69. Vatanasapt V, Martin N et al Cancer Epidemiol Biomarkers Prev 1995; 4(5): 475–483
70. Longombe A O, Lusi K M, Trop Geogr Med 1994; 46(6): 366–367
71. Licklider S J Urol 1961; 86: 98

strong circumstantial evidence that the accumulation of smegma is related to the aetiology of this disease, and there is some evidence that smegma may be carcinogenic.[72] A viral aetiology has also been proposed as a result of its association with cervical carcinoma.[73,74] Human papilloma virus has recently been implicated as the cause of a small proportion of penile carcinomas.[75–78]

The most common sites for penile carcinoma are the glans, prepuce and shaft respectively. They usually present as a velvety erythematous area of induration, a painless ulcer, or a warty growth. In half the cases there is an associated phimosis or paraphimosis which may be associated with an offensive discharge. In half the cases there is associated inguinal lymphadenopathy, and, in at least half, the tumour has been present for more than a year!

There have been many staging systems proposed, but the important points of any staging system are as follows: for the local tumours, in situ (T_{IS}) and superficial tumours (T_1) have a better prognosis and a simplified management. Tumours on the shaft, and those that have invaded the corpus spongiosum or cavernosum, have a worse prognosis. Inguinal lymphadenopathy is an unfavourable finding, but in half of cases the nodes are enlarged because of an infective reaction. Penile carcinoma tends to spread in a 'stepwise' fashion up the lymph node groups with minimal 'transit extensions' (i.e. tumour deposits are rarely found in the lymphatics between nodal stations).[79] This makes a multi-staged surgical approach an appropriate option in clinical management.

Clinical management

The diagnosis is confirmed by local excision or biopsy combined with circumcision. For tumours on the prepuce, circumcision may be the only treatment that is necessary. In situ and superficial tumours can be treated with a topical course of 5-fluorouracil, radiotherapy, or local radiation therapy applied in the form of an iridium mould. Microsurgical excision can be achieved using the CO_2 laser,[80,81] or microexcision by the 'Mohs' technique: this involves removing progressive layers of the lesion while systematically taking frozen sections until excision is confirmed to be histologically complete.[82] All of these treatments have the advantage of preserving the penis, sexual function, and psychological well being.[83] Circumcision must be performed to avoid treatment-associated phimosis and paraphimosis. Meatal stenosis is a common complication with all these treatments. For cancers that invade the corpus spongiosum or cavernosum, good local control can only be achieved by partial or total excision of the penis. The extent of penile amputation is determined by the ability to achieve at least a 2 cm resection margin, while maintaining a penis of adequate functional length for micturition. The management of groin lymphadenopathy is controversial and there are several surgical options for dealing with lymphatic spread. Extensive groin dissection has an appreciable morbidity in terms of delayed wound healing, infection and lymphoedema, and these complications occur in 30–50% of patients who have had radical groin dissection. Treatment with antibiotics is give. If groin lymphadenopathy is present at presentation for six weeks if the lymphadenopathy resolves, and the local tumour is superficial (T_{IS} or T_1), then observation alone is reasonable; 18–25% of patients go on to develop lymphadenopathy within 3 years.[84,85]

In higher stage tumours, some form of lymph node sampling is advised.[86,87] The concept of bilateral sampling of the sentinel nodes was proposed as a 'minimally' invasive compromise to nodal staging.[88] However, this approach has been repeatedly shown to be inaccurate and, in recent years, several surgeons have carried out a slightly more extensive modified inguinal lymphadenectomy.[89] Any evidence of groin nodes containing cancer necessitates bilateral ilioinguinal block dissections. Some surgeons also automatically proceed to clear the iliac nodes up to the bifurcation of the common iliac artery. Others only do so if laparoscopic sampling of iliac nodes confirms further deposits.[90] There are many who give radiotherapy prophylactically to any patient who has apparently 'uninvolved' nodes at the time of diagnosis, and others who automatically advocate bilateral radical groin dissection if there is an extensive tumour at the base of the penis or if the tumour involves the corpora cavernosa.[86] The problem with all of these groin sampling staging procedures is that they are a compromise — and they are inaccurate in at least 25% of cases.[91] Newer staging systems are being introduced that are based on the histological grade and depth of invasion of the primary tumour.[92,93] The combination of these two measures may be far more accurate in predicting nodal micrometastasis than the various approaches to groin node sampling. With these proposed staging procedures, the primary tumour is treated and the clinical node status is ignored. The 'grade/invasion depth' criteria are then used to determine which patients should undergo bilateral groin and iliac node clearance.

Erectile dysfunction (impotence)

Impotence is defined as the persistent failure to develop erections of sufficient rigidity for sexual intercourse.

REFERENCES

72. Reddy D G, Baruah I K S M, Arch Pathol 1963; 75: 414–420
73. Cartwright R A, Sinson J D Lancet 1980; 1: 97
74. Gajalakshmi C K, Shanta V, Acta Oncol 1993; 32(6): 617–620
75. Gregoire L, Cubilla A L et al Monogr Natl Cancer Inst 1995; 87(22): 1705–1709
76. Aynaud O, Ionesco M, Barrasso R Cancer 1994; 74(6): 1762–1767
77. Suzuki H, Sato N et al Jpn J Clin Oncol 1994; 24(1): 1–6
78. Maden C, Sherman K J et al J Natl Cancer Inst 1993; 85(1): 19–24
79. Herr H W In: Walsh P C, Retik A B, Staney T A, Vaughan E D (eds) In: Campbell's Urology 6th edn. WB Saunders, Philadelphia 1994; pp 3073–3089
80. Bandieramonte G, Lepera P et al J Urol 1987; 138: 315–319
81. Windahl T, Hellsten S J Urol 1995; 154(3): 1020–1023
82. Mohs T E, Snow S N et al J Urol 1985; 133: 961–966
83. Opjordsmoen S, Waehre H, Aass N, Fossa S D, Br J Urol 1994; 73(5): 554–560
84. Hardner G J, Bhanalaph T et al J Urol 1972; 108: 428–432
85. Srinivas V, Choudary R et al Urology 1995; 46(5): 710–712
86. Lubke W L, Thompson I M Semin Urol 1993; 11(2): 80–84
87. Abi-Aad A S, deKernion J B Urol Clin North Am 1992; 19(2): 319–324
88. Cabanas R M, Cancer 1977; 39: 456–466
89. Catalona W J J Urol 1988; 140: 306–310
90. Assimos D G, Jarow J P J Endourol 1994; 8(5): 365–369
91. Pettaway C A, Pisters L L, et al J Urol 1995; 154: 1999–2003
92. McDougal W S, J Urol 1995; 154: 1364–1366
93. Solsona E, Iborra I et al Eur Urol 1992; 22(2): 115–118

2. An intra-abdominal testis.
3. Normal or atretic spermatic structures entering the inguinal ring.

The inguinal region was surgically explored in the third group and this accounted for 21% of their overall series.

Treatment of undescended testis

The use of hormone treatment to promote descent of the testis in a normal child is not acceptable as it may result in premature puberty, premature epiphyseal fusion and degeneration of the other testis. The aim of treatment is to anchor the testis in the scrotum in the hope of preventing progressive hypoplasia. This must be done safely and the decision on the age that the child should be operated upon depends very much on the experience of the surgeon, the anaesthetist and the whole team involved with the child's care.[22]

Orchidopexy is normally carried out through an inguinal skin crease incision, through which the testis and its associated peritoneal coverings are identified. The cremaster is then opened and the testicular vessels and vas deferens are dissected free from the peritoneum. When the suspensory ligament of Browne[23] is divided, considerable lengthening of the cord is obtained. The small associated hernial sac is closed once the mobilization is sufficient to bring the testis into the scrotum without tension. A pouch is then fashioned between the skin and the dartos muscle, and the testicle is pulled through a small blunt puncture to lie within this artificially created cavity. If this is done correctly the dartos itself anchors the testis and there is no need for holding sutures. The skin of the dartos is then closed over the testicle. A success rate of > 95% should be achieved for straightforward cases. Undue tension on the delicate vessels must be avoided. When the testis cannot be brought down into the scrotum easily and it is of reasonable size, there is a place for anchoring the organ as low as possible and reexploring six months later. This is called a staged orchidopexy.

The Fowler–Stephens[24] manoeuvre of ligating the testicular vessels may be appropriate when the testis lies higher, for instance inside the inguinal ring, and the vessels are too short to permit mobilization. The testis then relies on the blood supply of the vasal artery. This manoeuvre can now be done laparoscopically.[25,26]

Orchidectomy should be performed when a streak testis is found or if there is difficulty in mobilizing a poorly developed organ and the other testis is normally placed in the scrotum.

In older children (> 15 years) or the young adult, the testis should also be removed. Spermatogenesis is most unlikely at this age and the risk of developing a tumour is increased, although this risk is quoted at less than 10%.[27]

The Keatley–Tourek procedure[28] of fixing the testis beneath the fascia lata of the thigh and Ombredannes' procedure[29] of fixation by passing the testis through the scrotal septum are now only of historical interest.[30,31]

Torsion of the testis

This condition was first described by Delasiauve in 1840.[32] Whilst it can occur at any age from the neonatal period to late middle age, the peak incidence is between 14 and 20 years.[20] A congenital abnormality of the investment of tunica, which lies higher than normal, is usually present, and this allows excessive mobility of the testis, predisposing to torsion. In neonates, torsion often occurs extravaginally, but in later years it is usually intravaginal, when it is invariably associated with a horizontally lying testis. Whilst excessive movement and perhaps mild trauma may be additional factors, many torsions occur whilst the patient is asleep, and there is often a history of one or two short prodromal episodes of pain when the testis almost certainly twisted, but managed spontaneously to untwist itself. Rarely the testis alone may rotate, when the epididymis and testis are joined only at the upper pole of the testis. This accounts for less than 5% of all cases of torsion.[33]

Clinical features

Patients present with sudden severe pain in the scrotum, which is often accompanied by nausea and vomiting. Despite the severity of the pain, most delays in diagnosis are the result of failure by the patient to seek advice although occasionally doctors fail to consider the diagnosis.[34] Rarely pain may be experienced only in the abdomen, usually in the loin of the affected side. The twisted testis lies at a higher level in the scrotum than a normal testis and is acutely tender when palpated. Recently Doppler ultrasound has been used to check blood flow in the testicular artery.[35] Normal flows are heard in acute epididymo-orchitis, while no signal is obtained from the twisted testicle (see p. 000). False positives and negatives can occur with this technique, and it can only be used as an adjunct to clinical diagnosis. The skin may have a bluish tinge over a gangrenous testis and examination of the other testis usually reveals a horizontal lie (a bell-clapper testis; Fig. 40.2). On occasion the twisted cord in the upper scrotum can be palpated.

Differential diagnosis

A number of other conditions can cause testicular pain. Torsion of the hydatid or Morgagni, or of the other appendages of the testis or epididymis, is more common in boys under 11 years of age than torsion of the testis. Idiopathic scrotal oedema occurs in boys under the age of 5. An inflammatory testicular tumour is important to rule out because of its lethal potential. Ultrasound and isotope scanning

REFERENCES

22. Atwell J D, Spargo P M Arch Dis Child 1992; 67: 345–349
23. Browne D Proc R Soc Med 1949; 42: 643
24. Fowler R, Stephens F D Aust N Z J Surg 1959; 29: 92
25. Gheiler E, Spencer Barthold J, Gonzalez R J Urol 1997; 148: 1498–1551
26. Esposito C, Cariponi V J Urol 1997; 148: 1951–1955
27. Jones P F Br J Urol 1995; 75: 693–696
28. Keetley C B Lancet 1905; ii: 279
29. Torek F Ann Surg 1931; 1931: 94–97
30. Siber S J, Kelly J J Urol 1976; 115: 452
31. Tiptaft R C In: Rains A J, Mann C V (eds) Short Practice of Surgery, 20 edn. Chapman & Hall, London 1988
32. Delasianve 1840
33. Johnston J H In: Williams D I, Johnston J H (eds) Paediatric Urology, 2nd edn. Butterworth, London 1982
34. Parker R M, Robinson J M J Urol 1971; 106: 243
35. Wang Y, Mack L, Kreiger J J Urol 1990; 143: 197A

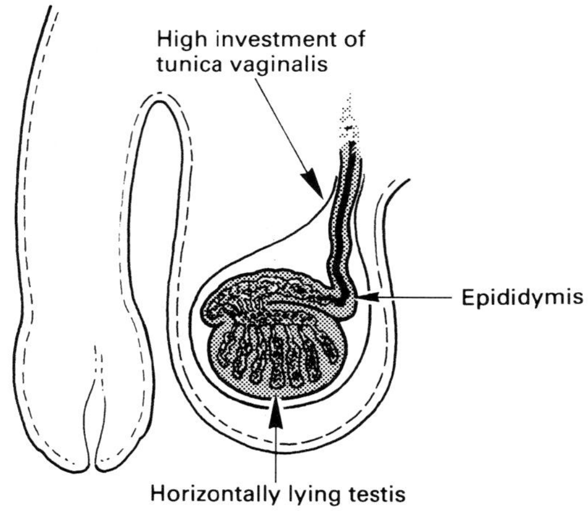

Fig 40.2 The transversely lying bell-clapper testis.

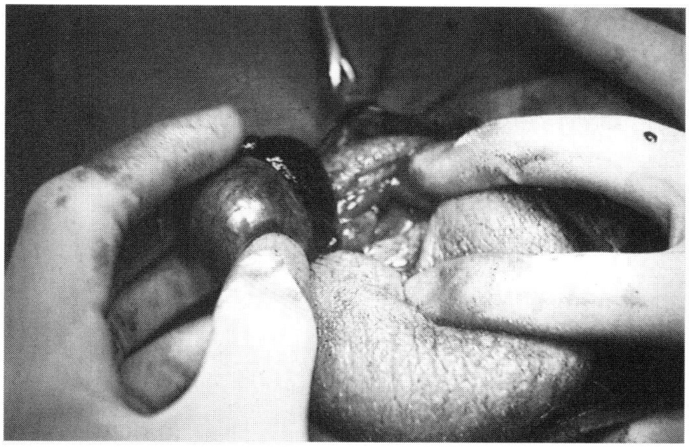

Fig 40.3 A gangrenous twisted testis.

may be helpful if this diagnosis is suspected, provided treatment is not delayed while they are being obtained. An inguinal approach must be used to explore the testis if this diagnosis is entertained. Acute epididymo-orchitis may provide diagnostic difficulties in the older age group, but there is often a history of dysuria or urethral discharge and pus cells can usually be seen in the urine.

Treatment

Early operation remains the only means of salvaging a viable testis. After 7 hours the seminiferous tubules are permanently damaged, although the Leydig cells, which produce androgens, appear to be relatively spared.[36] It is always worth trying to untwist the testis at once. At Rugby School, the Medical Officer showed that this was both possible and valuable whilst operation was awaited.[37] The testis twists away from the median raphe when viewed from above. Attempts to untwist should always be towards the median raphe; the patient will quickly inform you if you are exacerbating rather than alleviating the symptoms! This is occasionally possible in the robust individual but not normally possible in a Casualty Department.

When the testis is explored the scrotum is incised transversely over the pathological testis. The tunica vaginalis is opened and blood-stained fluid is often released. The testis usually looks dusky-blue and the cord is seen to be twisted. The torsion is then released and the viability of the testis assessed during the next 5–10 minutes (Fig. 40.3).

There is still considerable controversy over whether an apparently non-viable testis should be removed. Animal studies have shown that auto-antibodies are released from an infarcted testis, and these may react with the contralateral testis inhibiting spermatogenesis,[38] but this has not been confirmed by human studies.[36] An infarcted testis may slough or form an abscess if it is left in situ. This is a rare occurrence and most testes simply atrophy over the course of the next few weeks. A testis that has been ischaemic for longer than 12 hours should normally be excised, as it is unlikely that it will continue to function, but if the history appears to be less than 12 hours the testis should be retained unless it is frankly gangrenous.[39]

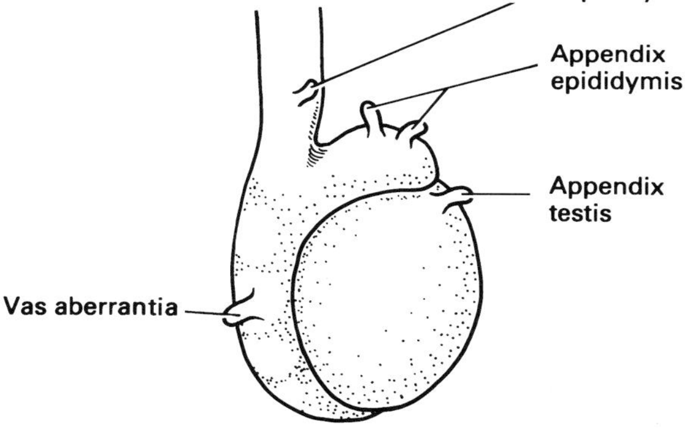

Fig 40.4 The appendages of the testis.

It is important to fix the contralateral testis at the same time to prevent future torsion. This is easily performed by invaginating the tunica vaginalis and fixing the testis to the dartos with a couple of sutures. Most advocate the use of absorbable sutures for fixation but recurrent torsion has been reported when absorbable sutures have been used. However, this is a rare problem and non-absorbable sutures can give rise to problems by forming a permanent sinus.

Torsion of the appendages of the testis

The appendages of the testis are four in number. (Fig. 40.4):

1. *The appendix testis* (the sessile hydatid of Morgagni). Although it is actually pedunculated this is a vestige of the mullerian duct, and is morphologically analogous to the fimbriated end of the fallopian tube.[40] It is normally a reddish

REFERENCES

36. Bartsh G, Frank S, Narberger H, Mikuz G J Urol 1980; 124: 375–378
37. Sparkes J P Ann R Coll Surg Eng 1971; 49: 77
38. Krarup T Br J Urol 1978; 50: 43
39. Johnston J M In: Williams D I, Johnston J H (eds) Paediatric Urology, 2nd edn. Butterworth, London 1982
40. Williams P L, Warwick R (eds) Gray's Anatomy, 36th edn. Churchill Livingstone, Edinburgh 1900

Clinical features

There is almost always a clear history of injury. Significant scrotal bruising may be present and a firm, slightly tender mass which does not transilluminate can usually be palpated within the scrotum. It is important to remember that testicular tumours may present with a history of injury, and whenever there is any doubt an ultrasound of the testis should be obtained. Biopsy may also be needed in cases where the swelling does not resolve.

Treatment

All severe cases of testicular injury should be explored. Any haematocele that is found is evacuated, and small linear tears in the tunica should be sutured. Where there has been gross equatorial disruption and it is unlikely that the testis is viable, orchidectomy is preferred. Occasionally severe trauma may lead to dislocation of the testis into the superficial fascia or even into the inguinal canal. The testis then needs to be relocated within the scrotum.

Tumours of the testis

Testicular tumours are relatively rare, accounting for about 1% of all cancers in males.[66] The incidence of testicular cancer is, however, rising at an alarming rate; in England and Wales 1400 cases are being registered per annum compared with approximately 800 per annum 20 years ago; the reason is unclear. The majority of testicular neoplasms are malignant and 90% are germ cell in origin.

The aetiological factors responsible for testicular cancer remain obscure although there is definite association with undescended testis. A number of other factors have been considered, including trauma and herniotomy, but these are not properly substantiated. There does not appear to be any clear evidence of an occupational risk but it does seem testicular cancer is more common in males of the upper social classes.[67] It is less common in the black population of Africa and North America.[68] Teratomas tend to occur in a younger age group (20–30 years) compared with seminomas (30–40 years).

A tumour may develop in the contralateral testis with an incidence of 2.5–5%.[69] A prospective study in Denmark suggests that in situ carcinoma can be found in the other testis in 5% of men with a testis tumour.[70] There is also evidence developing to suggest that in situ carcinoma may develop into an invasive tumour.[71]

Pathology

The World Health Organization has attempted to simplify the classification of testicular tumours. They have broadly divided these tumours into those that arise from a single cell type and others where more than one cell type is present[72] (Table 40.2). All testicular tumours are considered to arise from potential germ cells. The most primitive is embryonal carcinoma. This extra-embryonic differentiation gives rise to a choriocarcinoma or a yolk sac tumour, with evidence of extra-embryonic membranes. Intra-embryonic differentiation gives rise to a teratoma in which

Table 40.2 Histological classification of testicular tumours

World Health Organization[50]	*British Testicular Tumour Panel*[51]
Seminoma	Seminoma
Teratoma	Teratoma differentiated
Mature	
Immature	
Teratoma with malignant transformation	Malignant teratoma intermediate (MTI)
Embryonal carcinoma and teratoma	
Embryonal carcinoma	Malignant teratoma undifferentiated (MTU)
Choriocarcinoma	Malignant teratoma trophoblastica (MTT)
Yolk sac tumour	Yolk sac tumour

elements of exoderm, mesoderm and endoderm may all be present. Seminomas also arise from germ cells and may be of three types: seminoma, spermocytic seminoma or anaplastic seminoma. Tumours of more than one histological type may contain two or more of the single elements described above. Application of tumour markers (see below) has shown that more than 6% of testicular germ cell tumours fall within this category.[73]

There is a second classification of teratomas described by Pugh & Cameron[74] which subdivides teratomas into differentiated malignant teratoma, malignant teratoma and an anaplastic variety. This classification has not appeared to be as helpful as the World Health Organization classification, which correlates better with tumour markers, when these are present, and also indicated the clinical behaviour of the tumour.

Tumour markers

The contribution of tumour markers to the diagnosis of patients with testicular tumours is now established. α-Fetoprotein, β-human chorionic gonadotrophin, placental lactogenic hormone, pregnancy-specific antigen, placental alkaline phosphatase, carcinoembryonic antigen and lactic dehydrogenase can all be measured in the peripheral blood. The two most successful and widely applied are β-human chorionic gonadotrophin and α-fetoprotein, and it has been claimed that one or the other is elevated in 90% of non-seminiferous germ cell tumours of the testis.[75] Whilst some of the other markers may be detected in the same group of patients, none has

REFERENCES

66. Clemmensen A J Acta Pathol et al Microbiol Scand 1974; Section A (suppl 247): 1
67. Morrison A S Am J Epidemiol 1976; 104: 511
68. Blandy J P In: Blandy J P (ed) Urology. Blackwell, Oxford 1976.
69. Collins D H, Pugh R C B Br J Urol 1964; 36: suppl 1–11
70. Berthelsen J G, Stakkeback N E, Nogensen P, Sorensen B L Br Med J 1979; 2: 363
71. Von der Maase H, Roth M, Walborn-Jorgensen S et al Br Med J 1986; 293: 1398–1401
72. Mostofi F K, Sobin C H International Histological Classification of Tumours of the Testis, Number 16. World Health Organization, Geneva 1977
73. Damjanov V World J Urol 1984; 2: 12–17
74. Pugh R C B, Cameron K In: Pugh R C B (eds) Pathology of the Testis. Blackwell Scientific, Oxford 1976
75. Scardino P T, Cox H D, Waldmann T A, McIntire K R, Mittemeyer B, Javadpour N J Urol 1977; 118: 994–999

quite the same specificity. Some central assay laboratory should be used so that the correlation, clinical course and the usefulness of markers can be established. The diagnosis of a seminoma and spermatocytic seminoma is made histologically and only confirmed by the absence of tumour markers. The finding of an elevated α-fetoprotein level should encourage a review of the histology, as frequently yolk sac or other teratomatous elements will be seen within the tumour, which at first appeared to be a seminoma.[76]

Clinical presentation

The longest delay in the treatment of patients with testicular tumours is from the time the patient observes an abnormality within his testis until he seeks medical advice.[77] Young men should be made aware of the possibility of testicular tumours and routine testicular examination is to be encouraged. Most men present with a painless swelling in one or other testis. They often complain of a sensation of heaviness in the testis and groin. There is commonly a history of mild trauma coinciding with the discovery of the lump and this often draws the attention of the patient to the lump. Some 10% present with an acutely painful testis and the diagnosis of testicular malignancy must always be borne in mind when torsion is suspected.

The testicular enlargement is confined to the body of the testis, which feels uniform, firm and smooth, even though the surface is often bossellated. Testicular sensation is lost at a relatively early stage. A small hydrocele may be present, and the spermatic cord may be thickened from malignant infiltration. Ultrasound examination should be used to examine the acutely painful testis if the presence of a tumour is suspected. Some patients present with low back pain caused by enlargement of the para-aortic nodes, and others with chest symptoms from pulmonary metastases, but almost invariably the patient himself will have been aware of some abnormality within the testis. At a later stage, glandular metastases in the abdomen give rise to nerve pressure and vein compression causing pain, ascites and leg oedema. Sometimes patients present with an abdominal swelling or with acute abdominal pain, when a tender mass of para-aortic secondary nodes can be palpated. Some tumours spread rapidly and are classified as a 'hurricane' type while others grow slowly (encapsulated type).[78]

Investigation and management

The initial management of a patient with a suspected testicular tumour is orchidectomy. This enables an accurate diagnosis to be made. The procedure is carried out as a diagnostic measure, not necessarily to cure. A blood sample for tumour markers must be taken before and after operation, and a preoperative chest X-ray should also have been taken (Fig. 40.13), Table 40.3).

The patient should be counselled as to the possible diagnosis and consent obtained for orchidectomy. Sperm may be taken and banked for future use in young men who may wish to have a family.

Exploration must always be through an inguinal incision with soft clamping of the cord at an early stage. The testis is delivered and inspected; if doubt remains the testis may be bivalved through a vertical incision (Chevassu's manoeuvre).[79]

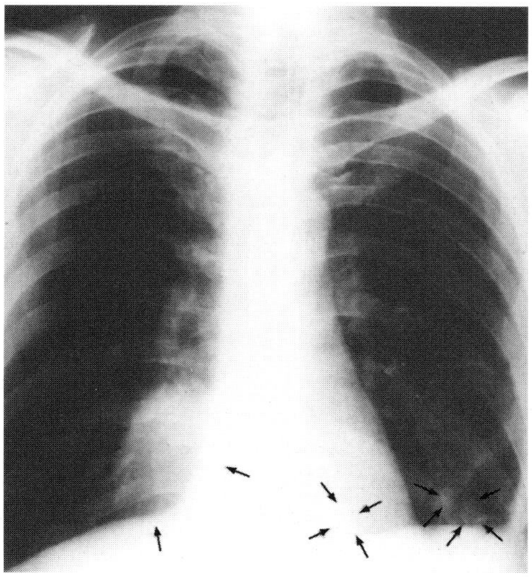

Fig 40.13 Chest radiograph showing metastatic testicular teratoma.

Table 40.3 Testicular tumour investigations

Preoperative	*Postoperative*
Haemoglobin, creatinine, liver function test (Hb, Cr, LFTs)	α-Fetoprotein, β-human chorionic gonadotrophin, lactate dehydrogenase (αFP, βHCG, LDH)[80,81]
α-Fetoprotein, β-human chorionic gonadotrophin, lactate dehydrogenase (αFP, βHCG, LDH)	CAT scan, chest, abdomen and pelvis[82] (Fig. 40.15)
Chest radiograph (CXR) (Fig. 40.13)	Creatinine clearance (pre-chemotherapy)
Ultrasound of testis[56]	Intravenous urogram (Fig. 40.14) IVU (if radiotherapy is planned)

A biopsy may be sent for frozen section and if a tumour is not confirmed the testis can be resutured and restored to normality with only a small chance of subsequent atrophy. Transcrotal biopsies should never be performed.

Staging for testicular cancer

Stage	*Description*
Stage I	Tumour confined to the testis
Stage II	Abdominal lymph nodes
	A <2 cm
	B 2–5 cm
	C >5 cm

REFERENCES

76. Javadpour N Cancer 1980; 45: 1755
77. Jones W G, Appleyard I Br Med J 1985; 290: 1550–1551
78. Collins D G, Pugh R C B Br J Urol 1969; 36 (suppl 1)
79. Chevassu P Tumeurs Testicule. These de Paris No 193. G Steinheil, Paris 1904
80. Tiptaft R C, Nicholls B M, Hatley W, Blandy J P Br J Urol 1982; 54: 759–764
81. Klein E A Urol Clin North Am 1993; 20: 67–73
82. Husband J E, Peckham M J, Macdonald J S, Hendry W F Clin Radiol 1979; 30: 243–252

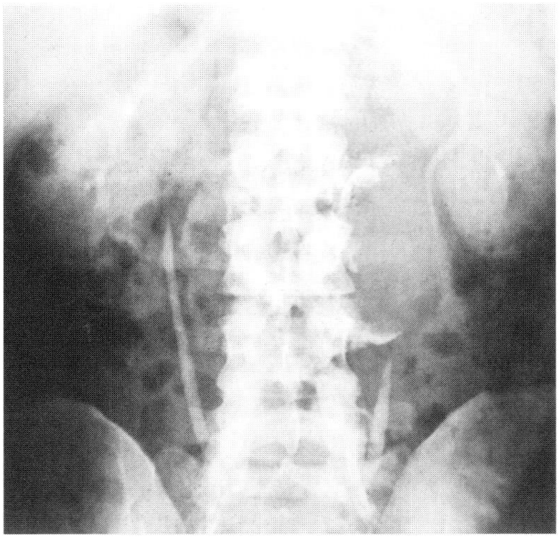

Fig 40.14 Intravenous urogram showing displacement of the ureters by enlarged para-aortic lymph nodes.

Stage III Lymph nodes above the diaphragm
Stage IV Extra lymphatic metastases

The contralateral testis should also be biopsied if it has been undescended, ectopic or atrophic.

Once the patient has had an orchidectomy and the histological diagnosis has been confirmed, the staging process must be completed. The markers α-fetoprotein and β-human chorionic gonadotrophin are repeated and a CT scan is performed.

The combination of circulating blood markers and CT scans has now superseded lymphangiography in assessing the spread of the tumour. The Royal Marsden staging described by Peckham in 1979[83] has helped plan logical therapy. In the period prior to the mid-1970s young men with testicular tumours either received radiotherapy for what was thought to be stage I or II disease or a radical retroperitoneal lymph node dissection which often resulted in ejaculatory failure.

Treatment of seminomas

For those with stage I or II seminomas, radiotherapy (30 Gy) is still given to the para-aortic lymph nodes with an excellent outcome; more than 95% of men being alive at five years.[84] There is considerable interest in the use of a single dose of cisplatin,[85] which has been demonstrated to cause large masses of seminoma to regress.

For more advanced disease (stages IIB, C and III) adjuvant chemotherapy is the treatment of choice. This may be just a single agent such as cisplatin or carboplatin but some recommend combination chemotherapy BEP (bleomycin, etoposide and cisplatin).[86] When a retroperitoneal tumour mass remains after chemotherapy attempted surgical excision is fraught with difficulty.

Teratoma (non-seminoma)

These tumours are much less radiosensitive and patients with stage I and II disease are not therefore treated with radiotherapy. With the advent of cytotoxic chemotherapy[87,88] in the 1970s treatment improved. Cytotoxic regimens proved very effective but were also toxic. All patients with teratoma began to have chemotherapy and the real question to arise in the early 1980s was 'Could patients with stage I disease avoid this toxic treatment?' Peckham[89] provided the answer. A surveillance policy monitoring blood markers and CT scans over a two- to three-year period confirmed that a third of the patients with stage I disease went on to develop disease outside the testis. The majority of those who relapsed had undifferentiated malignant teratomas; vascular and lymphatic invasion also proved to increase the risk of relapse. Delayed chemotherapy did not appear to adversely affect the prognosis of those who did relapse. Patients with stage I tumours and these added risk factors should now receive two cycles of the chemotherapy used for other stages of the disease (bleomycin cisplatinum and vinblastine or etoposide, prednisone). Their outlook is excellent. The survival rates for patients with stage III and IV disease have also improved, with more than 80% remaining alive at three years.[90]

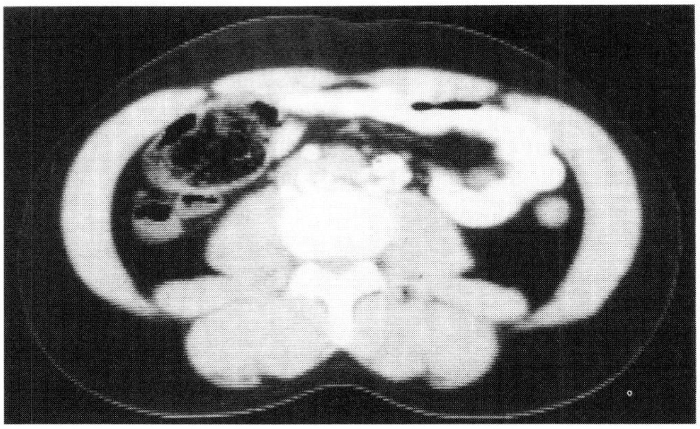

Fig 40.15 CT scan of the upper abdomen showing a small pulmonary metastasis from a testicular teratoma.

Surgical excision is performed when chemotherapy fails to eradicate the disease and a retroperitoneal mass remains. Histology of the excised tissue reveals differentiated teratoma in half of the specimens and active disease in about a quarter.[91] This latter group tends to have a poor prognosis, having already failed to respond to the combination chemotherapy.

Other tumours of the testis and adnexae

1. *Leydig cell tumours*. These account for 6% of the remaining testicular tumours. Young boys develop virilism and precocious puberty, becoming 'infant Hercules', while 40% of

REFERENCES

83. Peckham M J, Barre H, et al Lancet 1979; ii: 267–270
84. Walther P J, Paulson D F, World J Urol 1984; 2: 68–72
85. Oliver R T D, Ong J, Blandy J P et al Br J Urol 1996; 78: 119–124
86. Oliver R T D, Love S, Ong J Br J Urol 1990; 65: 61–67
87. Samuels M L, Holoye P Y, Johnson D E Cancer 1975; 36: 318
88. Einhorn L H, Donohue J P, Urol Clin North Am 1977; 4: 407
89. Peckham M J, Barrett A, Husband J E, Hendry W F Lancet 1982; ii: 678–680
90. Ravi R, Oliver R T D, Ong J et al Br J Urol 1997; 80: 647–652
91. Cels M E, Nijboer A P, Hoekstra H J et al Br J Urol 1997; 79: 263–268

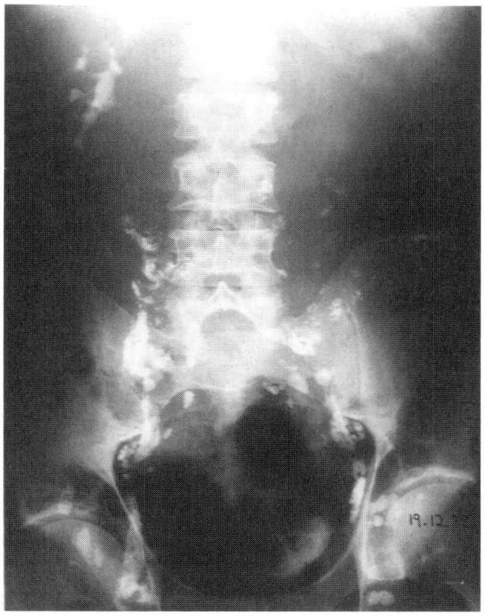

Fig 40.16 Lymphadenogram showing metastatic deposits from testicular seminoma in retroperitoneal lymph nodes.

adults develop gynaecomastia and other feminizing features. Approximately 10% of all Leydig cell tumours are malignant and they have similar clinical features to Sertoli cell tumours.[92]

2. *Sertoli cell tumours*. Sertoli cell tumours produce gynaecomastia in adult males. The presentation of gynaecomastia should always include an examination of the testes[93] (see Ch. 34).
3. Tumours may arise from the *rete testis* and the *epididymis*. Adenomas and adenocarcinomas in these sites are rare, but are described.
4. *Lymphoma of the testis*. Testicular enlargement may occur in patients with generalized lymphoma, when the prognosis is poor with a survival which rarely exceeds two years. Lymphoma may also appear for the first time in the testes and may be the only site of disease at presentation, but it usually becomes widespread eventually and the prognosis remains poor[94] (see Ch. 00).
5. *Secondary tumours* can occur in the testes. The most frequent primary sites are bronchus, prostate, kidney and colon.[95]
6. *Tumours of the adnexae*. Adenomatoid tumours may arise from the epididymis, tunica vaginalis and rarely the spermatic cord itself. They are usually small, being less than 5 cm in diameter, and are thought to be mesonephric in origin.
7. *Papillary cystoadenoma* is an epithelial manifestation of von Hippel–Lindau syndrome and may occur in the epididymis. Mostofi & Price[96] feel that this is often a form of the generalized von Hippel–Lindau syndrome.
8. *Nodular fibrous periorchitis* is a fibrous condensation located on the tunica which may be mistaken for a testicular tumour. Histologically this tumour consists of bands of hyalinized fibrous tissue.[96]
9. *Rhabdomyosarcoma*. This develops in the spermatic cord of children, although there is a secondary peak in incidence around the age of 19. Treatment is by excision, radiotherapy and chemotherapy. Leiomyomas, liposarcomas and leiomyosarcomas of the cord can also occur, but are extremely rare. Successful treatment depends on early diagnosis, wide excision and radiotherapy.

CONTRACEPTION AND INFERTILITY

In the latter part of the 19th century vasectomy was performed for urinary outflow obstruction[97] and obviously achieved some success, perhaps by inadvertently performing orchidectomy by including the testicular artery in its excision.[98] Vasectomy is now the preferred permanent method of contraception (celibacy not being a serious rival!).

Vasectomy (Fig. 40.17)

The thumb and index finger of the non-dominant hand are used to isolate the cord. The vas is located within the cord as the only solid structure. It is possible to fix the vas over the middle finger, between the index finger and the thumb. Local anaesthetic is infiltrated directly into the skin around the vas. An incision is made directly over the vas and the covering fascia is divided before the vas is pulled free. The artery to the vas may be ligated and divided or may be pushed away with the adventitia before the vas is isolated and divided. It is debatable whether the preservation of the artery to the vas enables a more successful vasovasostomy if this becomes necessary at a future date. Spontaneous re-anastomosis of the vas is uncommon, but the chance of this occurring is reduced if a portion of the vas is removed and one end buried beneath the adventitia.

In the great majority of patients, bruising and discomfort are minimal and they can return to normal activities within 48 hours. Haematoma formation is the only important immediate complication and on occasion this may be gross, extending up as far as the axilla. Evacuation of the haematoma is usually ineffective and rest is the only remedy. A haematoma, however, may become secondarily infected and occasionally abscesses need to be drained.

Sperm granulomas may develop after two to three months. They are caused by a reaction between sperm that have escaped from the proximal end of the vas and the surrounding tissue. This usually settles with anti-inflammatory drugs but occasionally excision of the nodule is necessary. Vasectomy has a significant morbidity. Some patients have pain and discomfort for several weeks, bruising may occur and occasionally require admission to hospital. Fit young patients may lose time from work. These risks need to be explained to the patient before the procedure is carried out.

Before contraceptive precautions are abandoned, it is essential that the patient provides two seminal samples in which no

REFERENCES

92. Caldamone A A, Altebarmakian V et al Urology 1979; 14: 39–43
93. Gabrilove J L, Freisberg E K et al J Urol 1980; 124: 757–767
94. Turner R R, Colby T V, Mackintosh F R Cancer 1981; 48: 2095–2102
95. Cricio R P, Kandzari S J J Urol 1977; 118: 489
96. Mostofi F K, Price E B, Atlas of Tumour Pathology, Series 2. Armed Forces Institute of Pathology, Washington, DC 1973
97. Sago A L, Novicki D E J Urol 1982; 19: 606–608
98. Clark P B Br J Urol 1987; 60: 549–559

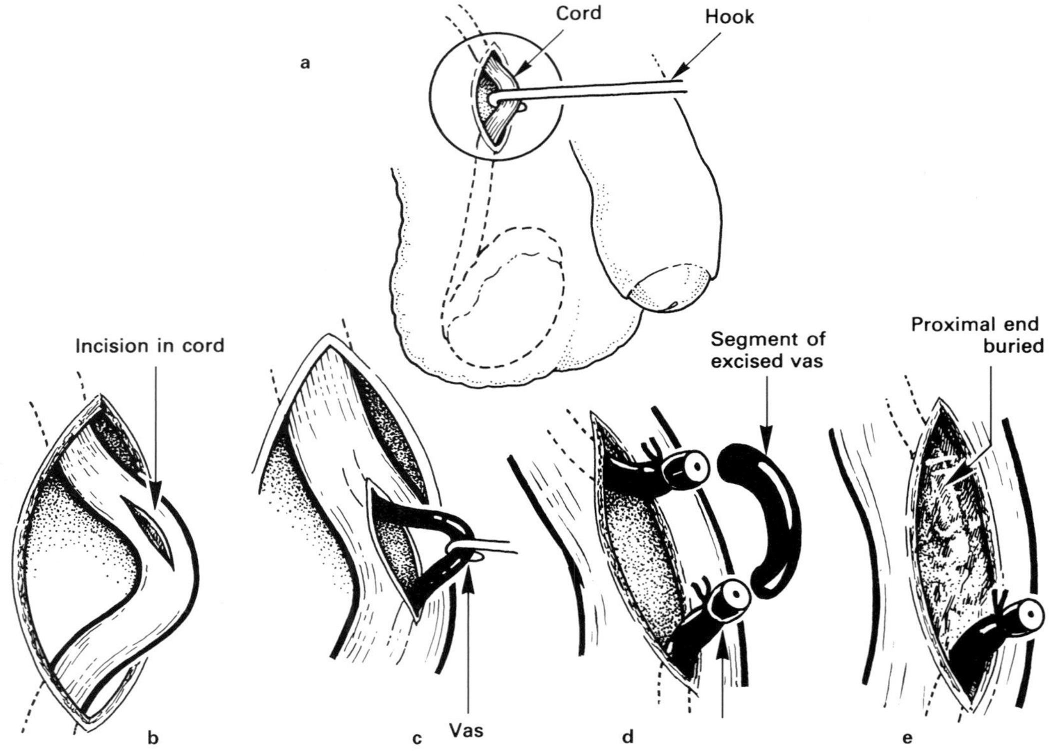

Fig 40.17 The operation of vasectomy shown in five stages (a–e).

spermatozoa are seen. This must also be clearly explained prior to operation. It is customary to ask them to provide specimens at 10 and 11 weeks as most patients will be sterile at about this time. The continuing presence of spermatozoa indicates a failed operation and re-exploration should be offered.

Vasovasostomy

Although patients are counselled that a vasectomy is an irreversible procedure with little or no chance of a successful re-anastomosis or subsequent pregnancy, vasovasostomy is being performed with increasing frequency. Technically the procedure is not difficult, and many methods of re-anastomosing the vas have been described (Fig. 40.18).

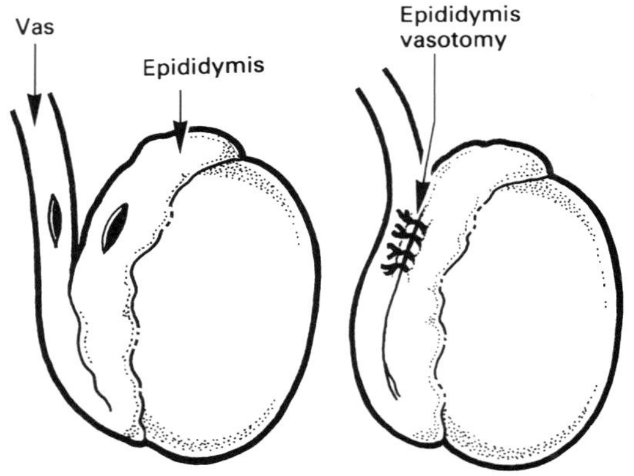

Fig 40.18 The vas is anastomosed side-to-side to the epididymis in epidydimovasostomy.

These include end-to-end, side-to-side with or without splints, using the operating microscope, using multilayer anastomosis or just a naked-eye single-layer anastomosis. Some 70–80% of patients obtain sperm in their ejaculate using any of the above techniques, although successful pregnancy is achieved in a significantly smaller percentage. It is believed that many of the failures are the result of ischaemia of the vas, caused by fibrosis and occlusion because of possible damage to the artery to the vas at the time of the vasectomy. Antisperm antibodies may also be an important cause of sterility when they are present. What is indisputable is that a successful operation can produce spermatozoa within a couple of weeks but if a further seminal analysis is repeated the spermatozoa have often disappeared. It is sound policy only to ask for samples two months after the operation. Royle & Hendry[99] recommend a second procedure after a failed first operation and there is some evidence that this carries an equal chance of success. It does not, however, appear that multiple re-operations increase the chances of success and it would seem sensible to limit the patients to two procedures at most.

Infertility

The surgeon has a limited role in the treatment of infertility. The diagnosis may be clarified and a prognosis may be given to the couple so that they may make a sensible judgement about the future.

REFERENCES

99. Royle M G G, Hendry W F Br J Urol 1980; 57: 780

Infertile men may be crudely divided into those who are oligospermic and those with azoospermia. Non-specific measures may increase both sperm count and motility in patients with oligospermia—frequently used agents include vitamin C, androgen analogues and vitamin E—but there appears to be no direct correlation with elevation of the sperm count and subsequent pregnancy. Varicoceles are often ligated for oligospermia but it has been shown that the incidence of varicocele is identical in patients having vasectomies to those being investigated for infertility.[100] Varicocele ligation does seem to improve the fertility of patients with slow motility, but the whole of this field is surrounded more by myth than solid scientific evidence. Patients are often highly emotional and are prepared to grab at anything that may offer some chance of success.

The WHO varicocele trial has now shown that infertile couples where the male partner has a varicocele have a better chance of conception if the varicocele is ligated, than in those in whom it has not.[47]

The treatment of the infertile male with oligospermia or obstructive azoospermia is now being improved. New techniques have been developed for sperm retrieved from the epididymis and the testis and this can be combined with in vitro fertilization or intracytoplasmic sperm infection.[101]

By combining microsurgical sperm aspirate or percutaneous epididymal sperm aspiration with intracytoplasmic sperm injection pregnancy rates in the order of 30% are being reported.[102]

SCROTUM

The scrotum is a cutaneous and fibromuscular sac containing the testes and the lower part of the spermatic cords. It lies dependently below the pubis, in front of the upper parts of the thighs. Very rarely a prepenile scrotum is seen when the scrotum is suspended from the mons pubis anterior to the penis. The scrotal skin is red-brown in colour and is normally thrown into folds or rugae. It contains numerous sebaceous glands, as well as sweat glands and pigment cells. Beneath the subcutaneous adipose tissue is a thin layer of dartos muscle fibres.

Trauma

An avulsion injury may be caused by road traffic accidents, industrial accidents, or occasionally a blast injury. Significant skin may be lost from the scrotum and half or more may be lost and still be satisfactorily reconstituted. Most scrotal injuries are 'dirty', and the primary treatment consists of wide excision and delayed primary suture. This procedure should be covered by a broad-spectrum antibiotic.

Pinch grafts may be used to cover large defects but when the whole of the scrotum has been degloved and the testes hang free, pedicle skin grafts may be raised from either the thigh or the lower abdomen to provide complete skin cover.[103]

Acute infections (Fournier's gangrene)

Acute cellulitis of the scrotal skin, following either surgical incision or trauma, usually responds rapidly to broad-spectrum antibiotics. A rare but more sinister problem is that of necrotizing subcutaneous infection of the scrotum, originally reported by Fournier in 1883.[104] In this paper, five patients were described in whom there appeared to be three common characteristics:

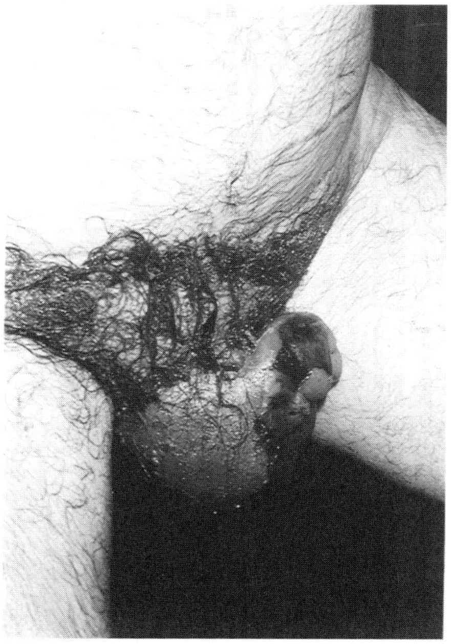

Fig 40.19 Fournier's gangrene.

1. An acute onset in a young healthy male.
2. Rapid progression to gangrene.
3. Absence of a discernible cause.

Clinical features

A painful, tense glossy oedema develops suddenly in the scrotum. This may spread to the base of the penis. Crepitation then occurs in the subcutaneous tissue, and this spreads rapidly before subcutaneous gangrene develops between 12 hours and three days later, with amelioration of the systemic symptoms. The gangrene follows the same path as extravasation of urine, spreading out along the inguinal areas and up over the lower abdominal wall (Fig. 40.19). A line of demarcation forms around the eschar which, if left untreated, separates to leave the testes hanging naked, healthy, painless and unaffected.

Jones et al[105] reviewed all the cases of Fournier's gangrene reported before 1979. They found that Fournier's description remained true before the antibiotic era, but patients described since

REFERENCES

100. Hirsh A V, Kellett M J, Robertson G, Pryor J P Br J Urol 1980; 52: 560
101. Tsirigotis M, Pelekanos N, Yazdani A et al Br J Urol 1995; 76: 765–768
102. Barua J M, Balet R, Wilson C et al Br J Urol 1996; 77 (suppl 1): 38
103. McDougal W S J Urol 1983; 129: 757
104. Fournier A J Semain Med 1883; 3: 345
105. Jones R B, Hirshman J V, Browning S, Le Tremain J A J Urol 1979; 122: 279–282

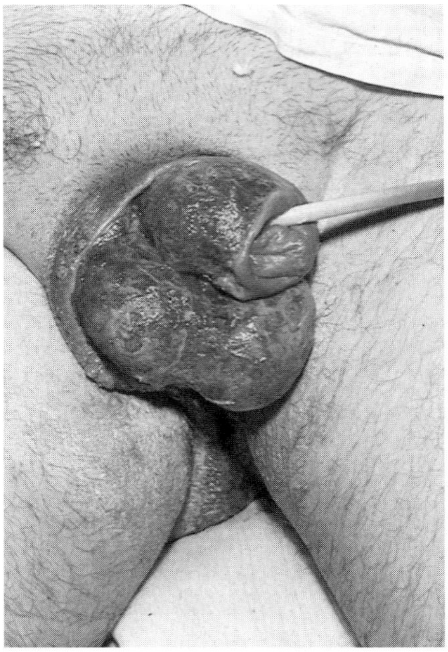

Fig 40.20 Fournier's gangrene. Same patient as in Figure 40.19 after excision of affected tissues.

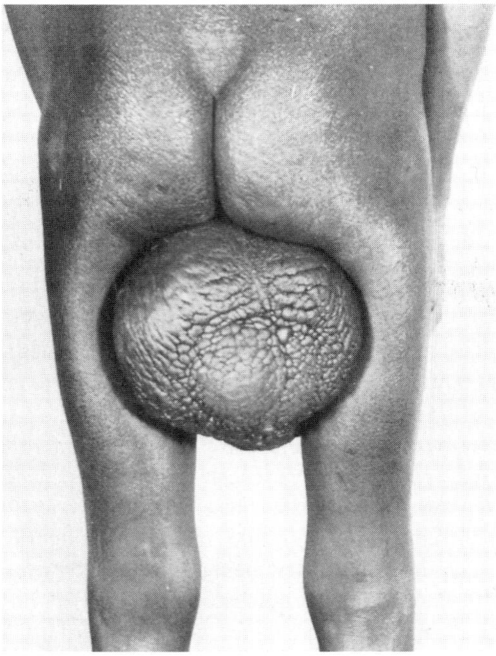

Fig 40.21 Elephantiasis of the scrotum.

1945 were older—usually in their fifties—and frequently there were local contributing factors such as perineal surgery, urinary tract, perianal or retroperitoneal infections. Many were diabetic.

The condition appears to arise from the bacterial synergism between relatively non-pathogenic organisms (usually a streptococcus and *Clostridium welschii*) derived from faecal flora, which initially induces vascular thrombosis, then subcutaneous tissue necrosis, and eventually dermal gangrene.

Treatment

Broad-spectrum antibiotics, such as Augmentin, gentamicin and metronidazole that are active against both anaerobic Gram-negative bacilli and facultative bacilli are started immediately. Early wide surgical excision is also essential. Excision may have to be repeated as further areas of gangrenous skin become evident. Once the gangrenous area has become well demarcated and has been fully excised, the underlying tissue remains healthy and free from infection. Delayed primary suture, split-skin grafting or the use of pedicle skin flaps raised from the thigh or lower abdomen can again be used to provide skin cover (Fig. 40.20).

Unless they are obvious, sources of infection must be carefully pursued and patients should have an intravenous pyelogram, a barium enema, sigmoidoscopy and cystoscopy as part of this quest. The mortality rate in 267 patients treated in the pre-antibiotic era was 22%, while in the 119 cases reported since this mortality with Meleney's necrotizing fasciitis of the lower abdominal wall, which still carries a mortality of 30%.[106]

Chronic infections

The commonest chronic infection of the scrotum world-wide is filariasis. This is caused by *Wuchereria bancrofti*, which lives part of its life cycle in the lymphatic system of man, and the other half in the *Culex* mosquito. There is an acute inflammatory stage, which takes the form of scrotal lymphangitis, and this can lead to gangrene of the scrotal skin that is indistinguishable from Fournier's gangrene. The filaria may also cause a retroperitoneal lymphangitis which is often the start of a reactive process that obliterates the lymphatics and eventually causes lymphoedema and elephantiasis of the scrotum and penis (Fig. 40.21). Hydroceles of the testis and lymphoceles of the cord may develop later. Whilst drug treatment with antimony compounds such as Banocide may be helpful in the early stages before puberty, the benefit in adults is less certain.[107]

In established elephantiasis, radical excision of the oedematous fibrofatty tissue (scrotal reduction) is the only practical way to deal with the problem.[108] Sufficient healthy skin normally remains to reconstitute the scrotum, without the need for skin grafting or skin flaps (see Ch. 9). Primary genital lymphoedema is uncommon. Secondary lymphoedema from retroperitoneal disease, often also causing obstruction of the inferior vena cava, is usually a consequence of an advanced malignant process. Treatment is directed to the primary pathology.

Acute idiopathic lymphoedema (idiopathic scrotal oedema)

This is a rare disease of children and must be differentiated from torsion of the testis, epididymitis and torsion of a testicular

REFERENCES

106. Tan R J Urol 1964; 92: 508–510
107. Partonu F, Prumomo A, Oremijatis S, Soewart A Acta Trop 1981; 38: 217
108. Jantet G H, Taylor G W, Kinmonth J B Br J Cardiovasc Surg (Turina) 1961; 2: 27

appendage. It presents with reddening and oedema of the whole scrotum, and although antibiotics are sometimes given it appears to resolve spontaneously.[109] The diagnostic feature is that the testes may be palpated through the oedematous scrotum and are relatively painless.

Lipocalcification of the scrotum

This results from extravasation of urine into the tissues of the scrotum. Carlson[110] documented a typical case history of an elderly horseman who had sustained repeated injuries while breaking in young horses. The affected area may be excised and pedicle flaps or rotation flaps used to reconstitute the scrotum.

Watering can perineum

This condition arises as the result of a urethral stricture. There is usually a history of acute gonorrhoea some 10–20 years earlier. The patient presents with a thickening fibrosed scrotum with a number of fistulous tracts extending onto the scrotum. This often causes chronic retention. In the acute phase there may be a grossly swollen scrotum which contains a mixture of extravasated urine and pus and patients are often extremely toxic.

The treatment is to insert a suprapubic cystostomy which must be left in situ for some weeks and sometimes even months. Once the inflammatory process has resolved, a urethroplasty is normally performed to treat the stricture (see Ch. 39).

Sebaceous cysts of the scrotum

These are quite common and may be worrying to the adolescent. Dozens of cysts may occur on the scrotal skin and are usually small. Although there is no absolute indication to remove these surgically unless they become infected, many request treatment on aesthetic grounds. The cysts may be individually enucleated or the central area of skin containing the cysts may be excised.

Scrotal tumours

Squamous carcinoma of the scrotal skin has been known to be associated with exposure to tar products since its first description in chimney sweeps by Percival Pott in 1775.[111] Recently the disease has been linked with mineral oil products, associated especially with those used in the metal and cotton industries (mule-spinners). In the Haute Savoie region of France, metal workers have a very high incidence of squamous cell carcinoma, and in this part of France scrotal cancer was among the three most common cancers to occur in males.[112]

The growth usually develops as an ulcer, but it may appear as a plaque or papilloma. The spread is to the inguinal nodes, which become palpably enlarged. The primary treatment is wide surgical excision of the scrotal lesion and in addition some recommend prophylactic lymphadenectomy on the side of the tumour.[113]

Patients with advanced disease may benefit from a combination of radiotherapy and bleomycin and this can occasionally be followed by delayed lymphadenectomy if there has been a good response. Survival appears to be related to the stage of the disease at presentation. One study reported a 70% survival at five years.[113] Scrotal tumours appear to behave differently to squamous cell carcinomas arising in exposed areas of the dermis, the latter having a better prognosis.

Other tumours that may arise in the scrotum include basal cell carcinoma, malignant melanomas and sweat gland tumours. These tumours are all treated by wide local excision in the first instance.

REFERENCES

109. Hemalatha V G, Rickwood A M K Br J Urol 1981; 53: 455–459
110. Carlson H E. J Urol 1964; 100: 656
111. Pott P Chirosurgical observations relative to the cataract, polyps of the nose, the cancer of the scrotum, the different kinds of receptors. Hames, Clark & Collins 1775. Roy Coll Surg Library
112. Lafontaine M Huiles Minerales et cancer catane. Instituto National de Recitercite et de Securite, Paris 1978
113. Ray B, Whitmore W F J Urol 1977; 117: 741

41 Neonatal surgery

D. P. Drake

GENERAL PRINCIPLES

Neonatal surgical anomalies are uncommon and an annual birth rate of 25 000 babies would include 100 neonates requiring urgent major surgery. These patients should ideally be managed in units staffed with trained personnel, as the success of neonatal surgical treatment is dependent on the constant care and observations of experienced nursing staff.[1] Antenatal ultrasound scanning can provide accurate diagnosis of some anomalies, such as exomphalos and diaphragmatic hernia, allowing arrangements to be made for these babies to be delivered adjacent to a neonatal surgical unit.[2]

Three priorities in the general care of the newborn are temperature control, respiration and nutrition. Incubators provide a suitable ambient temperature and, if the patient is exposed for investigations or procedures, hypothermia must be avoided by the use of an overhead heater or hot air mattress. Extremities may be wrapped in aluminium foil and the infant covered with warm, dry gamgee—wet dressings must be avoided as evaporation aggravates hypothermia. Portable incubators provide a controlled environment during transport. In the operating theatre hypothermia is avoided by placing the patient on a heated mattress and covering the sterile field with a generous adhesive drape. This will keep the sterile drapes dry and trap warmth from the mattress next to the patient. Warm saline packs should be used to cover all exposed viscera.

The air temperature in the operating theatre should not fall below 25°C and all solutions used for skin preparation or lavage should be warmed to body temperature. Hypothermia depresses respiratory drive and delays the spontaneous return of respiration at the conclusion of the operation.

Elective postoperative ventilation is indicated for premature infants and for newborns undergoing repair of diaphragmatic hernia or large anterior abdominal wall defects. Intermittent positive pressure ventilation is delivered via a loose-fitting uncuffed endotracheal tube which allows for an air leak. Analgesia reduces the stress response[3] to surgery and a combination of local wound infiltration or epidural block with systemic opiates may be used. Postoperative use of opiates increases the need for postoperative assisted ventilation.

All infants with intestinal obstruction or postoperative ileus are at risk of developing aspiration pneumonia from reflux of gastric contents. A nasogastric tube is therefore kept on free drainage and aspirated hourly to prevent this serious complication.

Most neonates undergoing surgery are initially unable to absorb adequate gastric feeds and they require intravenous fluids and nutrition. Parenteral feeding regimens are available for the special needs of the neonate[4] and are designed for the growth of the patient in addition to the daily calorie, vitamin and mineral needs. Delivery may be via peripheral cannulae in the short term but central venous cannulation is indicated for longer-term total parenteral nutrition. This may be achieved using a fine Silastic catheter introduced via a butterfly needle in a peripheral vein. Alternatively, a Silastic cuffed catheter may be inserted at open operation via the right internal jugular vein and a subcutaneous tunnel. This has the advantage of stability[5] but, as with all central lines, infection is a constant hazard and vigilant asepsis is essential, not only at the time of introducing the line but also when changing giving sets or administering drugs.

When calculating volumes of intravenous fluid, over-hydration must be avoided as the neonatal kidney cannot excrete excess fluid during the first week of life.[6] Table 41.1 gives a guide to appropriate volumes and is expressed in millilitres of fluid per kilogram of patient weight per hour. This provides a most convenient method of prescribing intravenous fluids and adjusting the flow rate of the giving set.

These volumes are all less than 150 ml/kg per day, which is the recommended volume of oral feeds after the first 5 days of life. Over-hydration leads to oedema of surgical wounds and anastomoses, which delays healing and prolongs postoperative ileus. Abnormal fluid losses should be measured and replaced with

Table 41.1 Guildelines for calculating volume of intravenous fluid in the first week of life

Day	*mg/kg per h*
1	2
3	3
5	4
7	5

REFERENCES

1. Young D G, Martin E J Baby Surgery, 2nd edn. HM & M Publishers, Aylesbury 1979
2. Nicolaides K H, Abbas A Surgery of the Newborn. Churchill Livingstone, Edinburgh 1994 p 61
3. Anand K J S, Sippell W G, Aynsley-Green A Lancet 1987; i: 243
4. Lloyd D, Pierro A Surgery of the Newborn. Churchill Livingstone, Edinburgh 1994 p 23
5. Shulman R J et al J Pediatr Surg 1986; 23: 348
6. Chambers T L Fluid Therapy in Childhood. Blackwell Scientific Publication, Oxford 1987

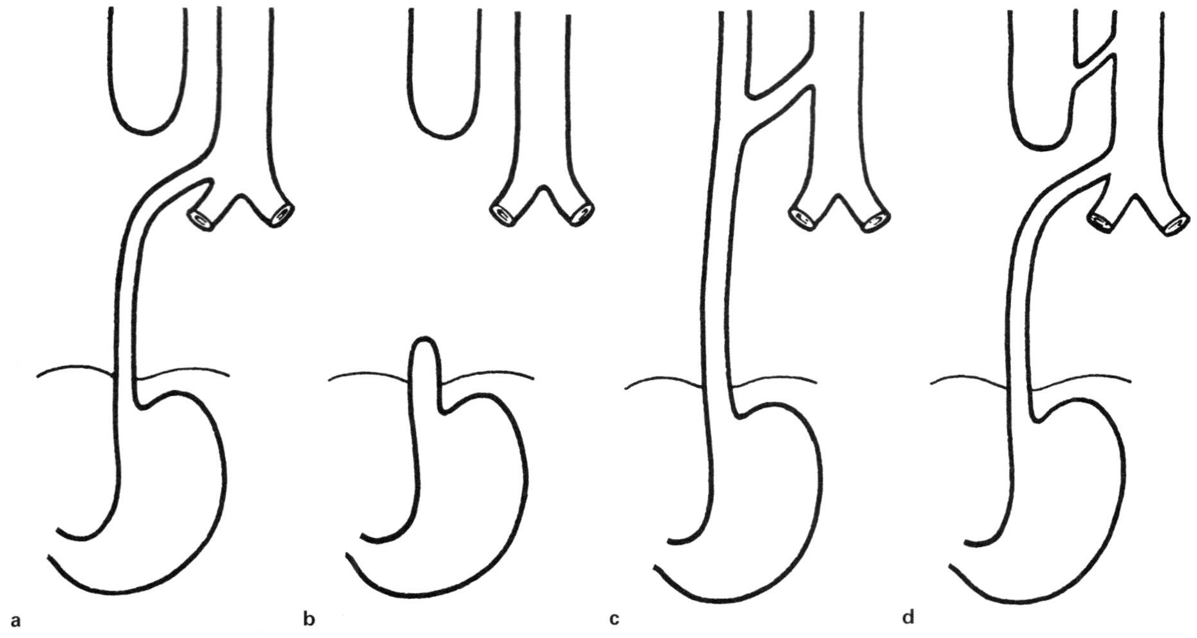

Fig. 41.1 (a) Oesophageal atresia with distal tracheo-oesophageal fistula (87% incidence). (b) Isolated oesophageal atresia (8% incidence). (c) Isolated tracheo-oesophageal fistula (4% incidence). (d) Oesophageal atresia with proximal and distal tracheo-oesophageal fistulae (1% incidence).

appropriate intravenous fluids; for example, normal saline for gastric aspirates and 4.5% albumin for peritoneal or pleural drainage.

The blood volume can be calculated from the infant's weight using the formula: Blood volume (ml) = 80 × weight (kg). Blood replacement at operation is considered if the loss exceeds 15% of the blood volume (or 25 ml for a 2 kg newborn); these small volumes can be calculated by weighing blood-stained swabs in the operating theatre.

Preparations for major surgery include giving 1 mg of intramuscular vitamin K to correct the prolonged prothrombin time associated with neonatal liver immaturity. Blood should be crossmatched and both mother's and patient's serum will be required by the laboratory, as maternal antibiodies cross the placenta during pregnancy.

Prematurity is not a contraindication to operation. The respiratory distress syndrome complicates mechanical ventilation and, although a thoracotomy is technically possible, retraction and compression of the lung causes further deterioration in oxygenation. A limited duration procedure to ligate a tracheo-oesophageal fistula may be undertaken whereas a prolonged oesophageal anastomosis may not be tolerated.[7]

The infant's abdomen is broader than its length. Therefore transverse incisions give better access at laparotomy and have the added advantage of healing with a more acceptable scar. Vertical incisions should be avoided and the laparotomies described in this chapter are all performed through upper abdominal transverse incisions, which give excellent exposure of the abdomen, including the root of the mid-gut mesentery and down to the rectosigmoid juntion.

OESOPHAGEAL ATRESIA

Embryology

Abnormal development of the foregut between 28 and 32 days after conception affects 1 in 3000 pregnancies.[8] The commoner anomalies are:

1. Oesophageal atresia with a distal tracheo-oesophageal fistula.
2. Isolated oesophageal atresia.
3. Isolated tracheo-oesophageal fistula.
4. Proximal tracheo-oesophageal fistula with oesophageal atresia—this is rare (Fig. 41.1). Associated anomalies are present in half of these fetuses[9] and are found in organs developing at the same embryological stage; cardiovascular system (35%), urogenital system (25%), anorectal anomalies (15%), vertebral anomalies (10%) and limb anomalies (10%). The VACTERL association (V for vertebral, A for anorectal, C for cardiovascular, TE for tracheo-oesophageal, R for renal and L for limb) encompasses these features[10] and has been associated with taking progesterone or oestrogen during early pregnancy.

The aetiology is multifactorial and there is an increased incidence in first-degree relatives suggesting a genetic factor.[11] No

REFERENCES

7. Holmes S J K, Kiely E M, Spitz L Pediatr Surg Int 1987; 2: 16
8. Spitz L, Hitchcock R J Surgery of the Newborn. Churchill Livingstone, Edinburgh 1994 p 353
9. Chittmittrapap S et al Arch Dis Child 1989; 64: 364
10. Temtamy B A, Miller J D J Pediatr 1974; 85: 345
11. Szendrey T, Danyi G, Czeizel A Human Genet 1985; 70: 51

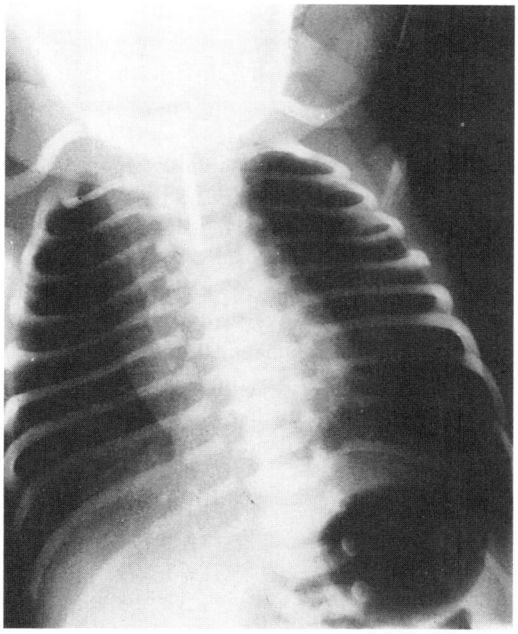

Fig. 41.2 Chest X-ray of newborn with oesophageal atresia. The radiopaque marker is in the proximal oesophageal pouch; air in the stomach indicates a distal tracheo-oesophageal fistula.

specific abnormal gene locus has been linked but 10% of these infants do have chromosomal anomalies.

Clinical features

Oesophageal atresia may be suspected antenatally if the fetal stomach is consistently empty on ultrasound scanning. However, the presence of a distal tracheo-oesophageal fistula usually allows amniotic fluid to be swallowed and reach the stomach. Polyhydramnios is present in over 50% of these pregnancies.[12] Postnatally the inability to swallow saliva produces a 'mucousy' baby, who blows bubbles during expiration. Cyanotic episodes occur during attempts at feeding and the patient may rapidly develop aspiration pneumonia.

If the diagnosis of oesophageal atresia is suspected, a size 8 or 10 French gauge nasogastric tube should be passed; if an atresia is present, its passage will be arrested at a distance of 8–10 cm from the nostril. Plain radiographs of the chest will demonstrate the level of the atresia, usually opposite the second or third thoracic vertebral body, and any gas in the stomach will indicate a distal tracheo-oesophageal fistula (Fig. 41.2). As soon as the diagnosis is suspected feeds should be withheld and the proximal oesophageal pouch kept empty with a double-lumen tube on continuous low-pressure suction. The baby should not be nursed in a head-down position as this will encourage gastric acid to reflux through a distal tracheo-oesophageal fistula into the lungs, causing a pneumonitis.

A thorough search for associated anomalies is required. This should include abdominal radiography for intestinal atresia, a rectal examination for anorectal anomalies, ultrasound scanning for renal anomalies[13] and an echocardiogram to identify cardiac anomalies. Operative correction is not an emergency unless the infant requires ventilation via an endotracheal tube, because in these instances delay in operating is associated with gastric perforation secondary to over-distension of the stomach with gasses passing through the fistula.[14]

Operation

The oesophagus is approached via a right posterior lateral thoracotomy, when the aortic arch is in its normal position on the left. The fourth intercostal space is opened and an extrapleural dissection is preferred as this gives easier retraction of the right lung within its intact pleura. The azygos vein may be divided between ligatures and the vagus nerve identified immediately medial to this vein, where it lies on the distal tracheo-oesophageal fistula. Early control of the fistula allows for positive pressure ventilation without over-inflation of the stomach. The fistula is divided flush on the posterior tracheal wall, which is repaired with interrupted Prolene sutures. Identification and mobilization of the proximal oesophageal pouch are assisted by an oral tube passed by the anaesthetist. A primary anastomosis of the two ends can usually be achieved with a single layer of sutures passed full-thickness through the oesophageal wall. Extra length may be gained by turning a flap of the proximal oesophageal segment.[15] A nasogastric tube may be passed to keep the stomach empty. The chest wall is closed and when there has been an extrapleural dissection a drain is not essential.

When there is a long gap atresia, a primary anastomosis is not possible and a staged procedure is required. The options include an initial gastrostomy for feeding combined with repair of a tracheo-oesophageal fistula. Proximal oesophageal suction may then be continued for 6 weeks or more before a delayed anastomosis is attempted.[16] Alternatively the proximal oesophagus may be brought to the skin as a cervical oesophagostomy to allow sham feeding. Oesophageal replacement may then be with colon,[17,18] stomach[19,20] or tube of stomach[21] when the infant is several months old and thriving.

Postoperative complications include pulmonary atelectasis, which should be prevented with vigorous physiotherapy, a stricture or leak at the anastomosis and gastro-oesophageal reflux leading to oesophagitis and stricturing. A small leak may be managed conservatively with total parenteral nutrition and broad-spectrum antibiotics. However, a significant disruption of the anastomosis demands a prompt second thoracotomy to repair the leak or to ligate the distal oesophagus and convert the proximal

REFERENCES

12. Stringer M D et al J Pediatr Surg 1995; 30: 1258
13. Lander A D et al Pediatr Surg Int 1992; 7: 351
14. Holmes S J K, Kiely E M, Spitz L Pediatr Surg Int 1987; 2: 16
15. Brown A K et al Pediatr Surg Int 1995; 10: 525
16. Puri P et al J Pediatr Surg 1981; 16: 180
17. Dickson J A S Pediatr Surg Int 1996; 11: 224
18. Freeman N V, Cass D J J Pediatr Surg 1982; 17: 17
19. Spitz L Pediatr Surg Int 1996; 11: 280
20. Atwell J D, Harrison G S M J Pediatr Surg 1980; 15: 303
21. Burge D M Pediatr Surg Int 1995; 10: 279

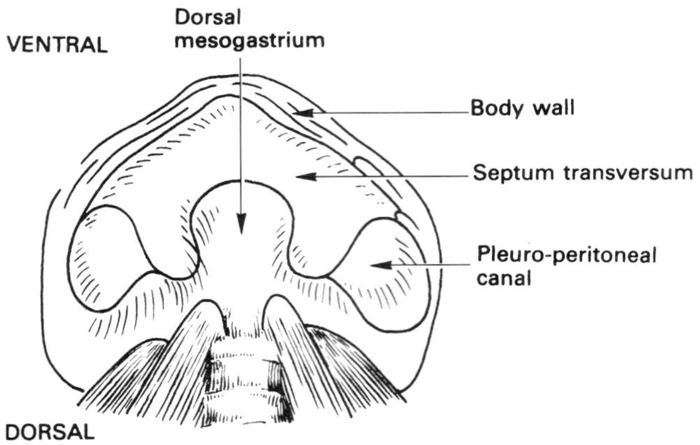

Fig. 41.3 Inferior aspect of diaphragm illustrating the posterolateral site of the pleuroperitoneal canal.

pouch into a cervical oesophagostomy. Strictures may require repeated dilatation, for which a balloon technique is recommended. Gastro-oesophageal reflux demands aggressive medical treatment with thickening of the feeds and H_2-antagonists. If the reflux persists, a fundoplication must be considered.[22]

A recurrent tracheo-oesophageal fistula may develop and will present with recurrent aspiration pneumonia accompanied by gaseous distension of the abdomen. If the track of the fistula is narrow and tortuous, cauterizing its lining via a bronchoscope will occlude its lumen.[23] For larger recurrent fistulae, a further thoracotomy is required after first identifying the fistula by catheterizing it via a bronchoscope.

Prognosis

Survival of over 95% of full-term babies without any associated severe anomalies was reported 35 years ago[24] and present mortality is related to severe cardiac anomalies and prematurity.[25]

Isolated tracheo-oesophageal fistula

This lesion allows normal swallowing and the majoriy of fistulae will present in neonates. Such babies may have apnoea during feeding and suffer recurrent aspiration pneumonia. The fistula may be detected by slowly withdrawing a nasogastric tube with its end under water; air bubbles may appear when the tip is opposite the fistula. More reliably cine-swallow radiography may be performed with the infant prone and an anaesthetist in attendance.[26] Bronchoscopy will confirm the diagnosis and in the majority of cases surgical repair may be carried out through a cervical approach.

DIAPHRAGMATIC HERNIA

Embryology

The diaphragm forms between the fourth and eighth weeks of embryonic life. The central tendon is derived from the septum transversum, the dorsal oesophageal mesentery, which contributes to the dorsal midline portion, and also a circumferential area which develops from the inner muscular layer of the chest wall. The gaps between these elements form the posterolateral pleuroperitoneal canals (Fig. 41.3) which normally close in the eighth week, the right before the left. At the same time, the mid-gut is returning to the abdomen and the lungs are developing. Failure of closure of this posterolateral canal may result in a large defect, allowing malrotated bowel into the chest, and this is associated with hypoplasia of the lungs.[27] A smaller defect may not open until later, in which case the lungs will be fully developed and the bowel normally rotated in the abdomen. Eighty-five per cent of congenital diaphragmatic hernias are left-sided and half of the affected babies will have associated congenital defects.[28] The aetiology is unknown but the anomaly can be induced in lambs by administering a herbicide Nitrofen to the pregnant ewe at the time of diaphragmatic closure.[29] The incidence is 1 in 2100 pregnancies.[30]

Clinical features

Prenatal ultrasound scanning will detect large defects with bowel herniating into the chest and deviating the mediastinum. A foetal anomaly scan and amniocentesis for karyotyping are indicated for these pregnancies. Delivery of the infant at full term in a unit equipped for intensive neonatal care and surgery is desirable. When the lungs are hypoplastic as a consequence of the hernia, the infant presents with respiratory distress. In addition to a rapid respiratory rate, the abdomen is scaphoid and the mediastinum shifted away from the side of the hernia. In the more common left-sided defect, the apex beat can be felt to the right of the midline. Plain radiographs confirm the shift of the mediastinum, the presence of abdominal viscera in the thorax and the lack of intestinal gas in the abdomen (Fig. 41.4). In most cases, resuscitation is required at birth; aerating the lungs with a face-mask should be avoided as this inflates the stomach and further compromises lung function. Immediate endotracheal intubation with positive pressure ventilation is indicated, with the insertion of a nasogastric tube to keep the stomach empty.

Surgical correction is delayed until the infant is stable.[31] Early complications relate to persistent pulmonary hypertension and include respiratory and metabolic acidosis and hypoxia secondary to right-to-left shunting through a persistent ductus arteriosus and foramen ovale. In addition to paralysis and positive pressure ventilation, these infants may require inotropic support, intravenous colloids and pulmonary vasodilators. Tolazoline is a non-specific vasodilator affecting the pulmonary and systemic circulations,[32] so

REFERENCES

22. Spitz L, Kiely E M, Brereton R J J Pediatr Surg 1987; 22: 103
23. Rangecroft L et al J Pediatr Surg 1984; 19: 41
24. Waterston D J, Bonham Carter R E, Aberdeen E Lancet 1962; i: 819
25. Spitz L et al J Pediatr Surg 1994; 29: 723
26. Kirk J M, Dicks-Mireaux C Clin Radiol 1989; 40: 150
27. Arrechon W, Reid L Br Med J 1963; 1: 230
28. Harrison M R et al J Pediatr Surg 1978; 13: 227
29. Iritani I Anat Embryol 1984; 169: 133
30. Puri P, Gorman W A Pediatr Surg Int 1987; 2: 327
31. Goh D W et al Br J Surg 1992; 79: 644
32. Sumner E, Frank J D Arch Dis Child 1981; 56: 350

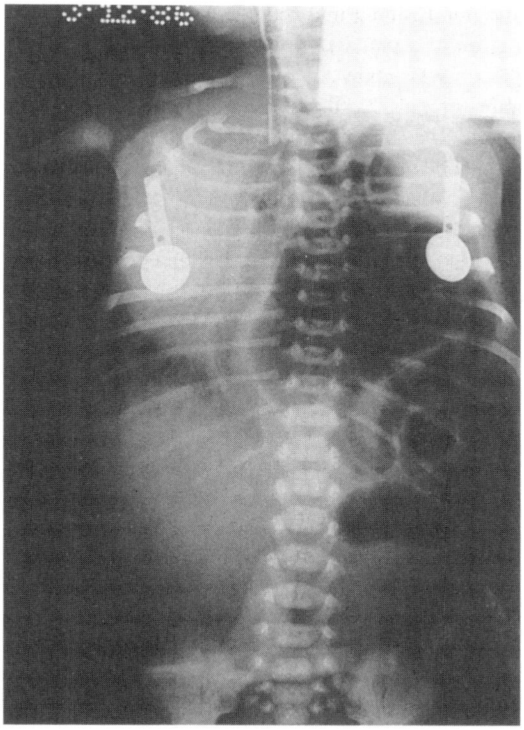

Fig. 41.4 Chest X-ray of a newborn with a left diaphragmatic hernia. Note the hypoplastic lungs, mediastinal shift to the right, abdominal viscera in the chest and lack of intestinal gas in the abdomen.

its use is limited by systemic hypotension. Nitric oxide, delivered by the inhaled gases, provides more specific pulmonary vasodilation but its benefit may be transient.[33] More comprehensive support for the myocardium and lungs can be delivered using an extracorporeal membrane oxygenation circuit, established with cannulation of the common carotid artery and internal jugular vein. The required anticoagulation prohibits its use in preterm infants and those with an intracranial haemorrhage but in full-term infants good survival figures have been reported.[34]

Late presentation of infants with a diaphragmatic hernia is well-described; they may present with vomiting, failure to thrive or with a characteristic chest X-ray in an asymptomatic patient.[35] The differential diagnosis includes congenital lung cysts and staphylococcal pneumonia. Even if the diaphragmatic hernia is asymptomatic, early repair is indicated to prevent complications.

Operation

This is performed through an upper abdominal transverse incision on a stable patient. The contents of the hernia are delivered and the defect inspected; occasionally a peritoneal sac is present and this needs to be excised. The posterolateral opening may be closed with interrupted non-absorbable sutures, after first defining the posterior muscular rim, which has to be dissected from the adrenal gland. A larger defect or agenesis of the hemi-diaphragm requires to be closed with a prosthetic patch.[36]

It is not recommended to leave a drain in the pleural space. When malrotation of the mid-gut is present, a Ladd's procedure is recommended. If the abdominal cavity is underdeveloped a second prosthetic patch may be inserted when repairing the anterior abdominal wall, thus creating sufficient space for the viscera that were previously in the thorax. Tight closure of the hemi-diaphragm or abdomen will limit the movement of the contralateral diaphragm and compromise postoperative ventilation.

Postoperatively, the infant with hypoplastic lungs is particularly at risk of worsening pulmonary hypertension and positive pressure ventilation with paralysis should continue until the cardiovascular system is stable. Broad-spectrum antibiotics are recommended perioperatively.

Prognosis

From 1961 to 1980 the mortality for a large series of newborns referred to one major centre remained constant at 37%, with a mortality of 65% for those undergoing surgical repair in the first 6 hours of life.[37] With recent advances in intensive care and prenatal diagnosis, infants with severely hypoplastic lungs are surviving initial resuscitation and are presenting for surgical management. Infants born prematurely and those with associated anomalies of the heart and central nervous system seldom survive. However, infants presenting after the age of 30 minutes have thereby demonstrated adequate lung function for long-term survival.[31] Gastro-oesophageal reflux is common in children treated for diaphragmatic hernias.

ANTERIOR ABDOMINAL WALL DEFECTS

Exomphalos and gastroschisis

Embryology

In the first trimester, from the fifth to the 10th weeks, most of the developing mid-gut will have herniated into the base of the umbilical cord and, by the 11th week, the intestines should have returned to the intraembryonic coelom. Abnormalities in development of the anterior abdominal wall before the 11th week may result in failure of the return of the mid-gut to the abdominal cavity and the persistence of a large symmetrical amniotic sac containing liver and intestine with the umbilical vessels spread out over its surface. This anomaly, with a diameter greater than 4 cm at its base, is termed an 'exomphalos'. Smaller defects result in 'a hernia into the cord' which contains a few loops of small intestine. Should such a hernia rupture prenatally, a gastroschisis will result. In these infants, the umbilical cord is normally attached to the anterior abdominal wall and the defect is immediately to the right of the umbilicus. This cleft allows the mid-gut to prolapse into the amniotic fluid and there is no

REFERENCES

33. Roberts J D et al Lancet 1992; 340: 818
34. Stolar C J H, Dillon P D Congenital Diaphragmatic Hernia. Karger, Basel 1989: 90
35. Malone P S et al Arch Dis Child 1989; 64: 1545
36. Valente A, Brereton R J J Pediatr Surg 1987; 22: 848
37. Simson J N L, Eckstein H B Br J Surg 1985; 72: 733
38. Glick P L et al J Pediatr Surg 1985; 20: 406

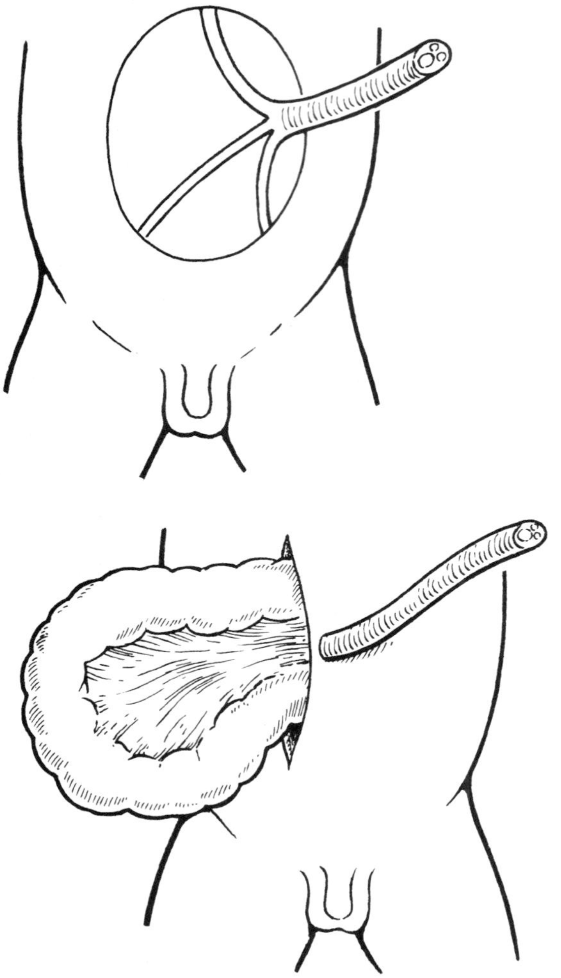

a

b

Fig. 41.5 (**a**) Exomphalos with umbilical vessels spread out in the amniotic sac. (**b**) Gastroschisis with intestine prolapsing through a cleft to the right of a normal umbilical cord.

detectable sac (Fig. 41.5). When this rupture occurs early in pregnancy, the intestine is covered with a pseudomembrane and appears to be fore-shortened. The natural history of these defects has been followed by prenatal ultrasound scanning.[38]

The incidence of anterior abdominal wall defects is approximately 1 in 3500 live births.[39] Associated anomalies are common in exomphalos with 50% of prenatally diagnosed fetuses having either severe congenital heart disease or a chromosomal trisomy. By contrast, patients with gastroschisis have a low incidence of associated anomalies, with the exception of malrotation and intestinal atresias, the latter being reported in 10% of patients with a gastroschisis. The Beckwith–Wiedemann syndrome consists of an anterior abdominal wall defect, gigantism, macroglossia and transient severe hypoglycaemia and may occur in association with either exomphalos or gastroschisis.[40,41]

Clinical features

If a prenatal scan in the second trimester demonstrates an exomphalos, a detailed search for other anomalies is indicated, including echocardiography and amniocentesis for karyotyping. This allows for the option of a planned termination of pregnancy for severely affected foetuses, many of whom would be stillborn. In the management of abdominal wall defects caesarean section offers no advantage to the infant[42] unless indicated for other obstetric reasons; planned vaginal delivery is recommended with prompt referral to a neonatal surgical unit.

Following delivery, exposed loops of intestine should be protected by a non-adherent dressing, such as cling-film or a sterile intestinal bag. The viability of the bowel should be checked at intervals because rotation of the exposed intestines can compromise its blood supply or venous drainage. Warm gamgee may be wrapped around the clingfilm, but wet dressings should be avoided as evaporation will cause hypothermia. The large intact exomphalos with associated anomalies may be managed conservatively by applying silver sulphadiazine.[43] Mercurochrome should be avoided as some of the mercury will be absorbed[44] and may reach toxic levels. Over a period of months, skin will grow over the sac and the resulting ventral hernia may be repaired after a delay of 2 years. A small hernia into the cord must be protected by carefully applying the umbilical clamp 5 cm away from the anterior abdominal wall—inadvertent clamping of a loop of small bowel in the hernia will result in intestinal obstruction.[45]

The majority of patients with exomphalos are best treated by prompt surgical repair. Under a general anaesthetic, the amniotic sac is dissected from the skin but left in situ as the sac is often adherent to the liver capsule. It may later be used as a barrier between the viscera and a prosthetic patch. The muscles of the anterior abdominal wall are present but will have been displaced laterally; cautious stretching of these muscles will enlarge the abdominal cavity. Primary closure of the anterior abdominal wall may then be achieved with interrupted sutures. Excess tension on the abdominal closure will kink the inferior vena cava and obstruct venous return to the right atrium. Therefore the attempt at primary closure must be abandoned immediately if the patient develops low output cardiac failure. A patch of Prolene mesh may then be used to close the defect between the rectus muscles.[46] Mobilization of the skin of the abdominal wall may allow this prosthesis to be completely buried or staged closure can be achieved over several weeks. Postoperative ventilation may be required, especially in those infants with associated pulmonary hypoplasia. Postnatal echocardiography should be performed to diagnose cardiac anomalies not detected prenatally.

All patients with gastroschisis should undergo a prompt operation. The cleft is enlarged in the midline and the abdominal wall is

REFERENCES

39. Irving I M, Rickham P P Neonatal Surgery. Butterworths, London 1990
40. Beckwith J B Birth Defects 1969; 5: 188
41. Wiedemann H R Lancet 1973; ii: 626
42. Fasching G, Mayr J, Sauer H Pediatr Surg Int 1996; 11: 100
43. Hatch E I, Baxter R Am J Surg 1987; 153: 449
44. Fagan D G et al Arch Dis Child 1977; 52: 962
45. Eckstein H B Br J Surg 1963; 50: 405
46. Schuster S R Pediatric Surgery 4th edn, vol 2. Year Book, Chicago 1986

stretched. Any thickened membrane should be left undisturbed on the surface of the bowel, which is inspected for atresias. Repair of these should be delayed for a second laparotomy. No attempt should be made to correct the associated malrotation of the mid-gut as this does not cause postoperative problems. In the majority of patients a primary repair can be achieved[47] but a temporary prosthetic patch may need to be employed for a staged repair.[48]

Prognosis

The results of treatment have improved dramatically with the introduction of intravenous feeding and broad-spectrum antibiotics. Infection remains a major hazard if primary closure is delayed and prolonged ileus, sometimes lasting for several months, may occur in gastroschisis. The 10% mortality for gastroschisis is related to complications of long-term total parenteral nutrition and to the short bowel syndrome, when there has been a vascular accident to the mid-gut in the perinatal period.

The prognosis in exomphalos is related to associated anomalies; the majority of foetuses with prenatally diagnosed exomphalos do not survive.[49]

DUODENAL STENOSIS AND ATRESIA

Embryology

During the second month of development the duodenum is obliterated by mucosal overgrowth. This creates a solid core of tissue which subsequently vacuolates. By the 10th week the lumen is recanalized but failure of this process will result in an atresia.[50] The pancreas develops in both the ventral and dorsal mesenteries of the duodenum; the ventral pancreas rotates around the right of the duodenum and fuses with the dorsal pancreas. Failure of complete migration results in ectopic pancreatic tissue or an annular pancreas.[51]

Pathology

Complete duodenal obstruction may be related to an atresia, or a volvulus of malrotated mid-gut. The common bile duct may open proximal or distal to an atresia or may have a double opening with bile present on both sides of the obstruction.[52] Abnormalities of rotation of the ventral pancreas may be associated with a duodenal atresia.

Partial duodenal obstruction may be secondary to a perforated duodenal diaphragm,[53] taking the shape of a windsock, or secondary to an intrinsic stenosis of the intestinal wall. Extrinsic factors include an annular pancreas and peritoneal bands related to malrotation.

The incidence of congenital duodenal obstruction is 1 in 10 000 births; one in three of these patients will have Down's syndrome and one in four will have congenital heart disease. Double pathology with malrotation and an intrinsic duodenal obstruction is well-described[54] and associated biliary atresia is rare.[55] The duodenum may be obstructed at more than one site[56] or there may be a more distal obstruction in the jejunum.

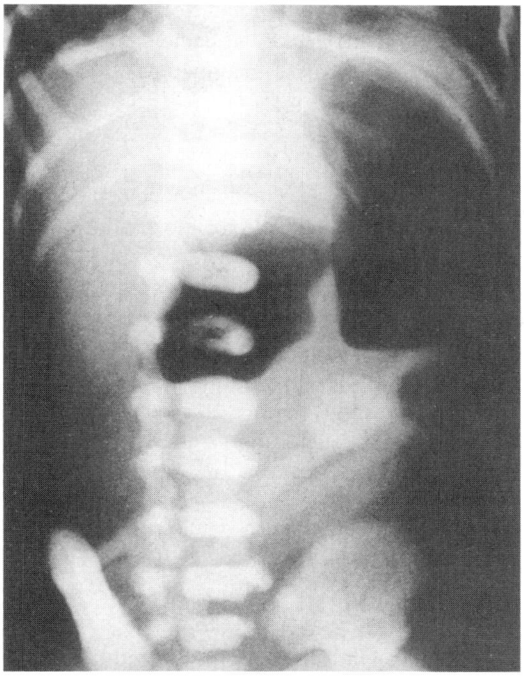

Fig. 41.6 Duodenal atresia: abdominal X-ray with 'double bubble' sign and no gas beyond the duodenum.

Clinical features

Antenatal diagnosis is possible with ultrasound scanning. Half of these pregnancies are complicated by polyhydramnios and the presence of a dilated stomach and first part of duodenum may be clearly demonstrated by ultrasound.[57] Foetal echocardiography is indicated and amniocentesis should be performed for karyotyping.

Following birth, vomiting occurs in the first few hours of life and is usually bile-stained. Even in the presence of total obstruction, meconium may be passed.[58] The abdomen is scaphoid, apart from the epigastrium where gastric peristalsis may be visible. The diagnosis of total duodenal obstruction can be confirmed by a plain abdominal radiograph demonstrating a 'double bubble' with no gas passing beyond the second part of the duodenum (Fig. 41.6). Air is the only contrast material required to confirm the diagnosis and 30 ml should be injected via a nasogastric tube immediately prior to taking the radiograph. Partial obstruction will present later

REFERENCES

47. Di Lorenzo M, Yazbeck S, Ducharme J C J Pediatr Surg 1987; 22: 710
48. Allen R, Wrenn E L J Pediatr Surg 1969; 4: 3
49. Fisher R et al J Pediatr Surg 1996; 31: 538
50. Lynn H B, Espinas E E Arch Surg 1959; 50: 357
51. Gray S W, Skandalakis J E Embryology for Surgeons. Saunders, Philadelphia 1994
52. Boyden E A, Cope J G, Bill A H Am J Surg 1967; 114: 190
53. Bill A H, Pope W M Surgery 1954; 35: 486
54. Knutrud O, Eek S Acta Chir Scand 1960; 119: 506
55. Young D G, Wilkinson A W Surgery 1968; 63: 832
56. Stringer M D et al J Pediatr Surg 1992; 27: 576
57. Hayden C K et al Am J Roentgenol 1983; 140: 225
58. Gourevitch A Ann R Coll Surg Engl 1971; 48: 141

with intermittent bilious vomiting and, for these cases, a barium meal is indicated to demonstrate the pathology, be it a duodenal stenosis, diaphragm or associated malrotation.

Management

A laparotomy should be performed without delay as aspiration pneumonia is a possible complication and volvulus of the mid-gut may be the underlying pathology. The operation of choice for atresia is a duodenoduodenostomy,[59] opening the anterior wall of both limbs of the duodenum and performing an anastomosis with a single layer of interrupted sutures. Care must be taken to restrict surgery to the anterior wall to avoid damaging the bile duct and ampulla of Vater. An annular pancreas should not be incised but bypassed by a duodenoduodenostomy.

A duodenal membrane may be incised and partially excised after opening the duodenum longitudinally. Care must be taken to avoid compromising the bile duct which may open on the diaphragm. The duodenum is then closed transversely.[60] Alternatively the membrane may be bypassed with a duodenoduodenostomy.

A nasogastric tube is adequate for postoperative decompression of the stomach, which may take over 7 days to empty satisfactorily as motility returns. Gastrostomy and transanastomotic feeding tubes confer no advantages. Intravenous feeding is indicated until full enteral feeds can be established. Following surgery the first part of the duodenum remains dilated and there is frequently persistent biliary reflux through the pylorus. Long-term follow-up is recommended to detect complications of biliary gastritis and to manage pancreatitis secondary to coexistent anomalies of the pancreatic duct.

The predominant cause of mortality in babies with duodenal atresia or obstruction is related to the associated anomalies such as congenital heart disease.

MALROTATION VOLVULUS NEONATORUM

Embryology

In the first trimester, the mid-gut herniates into the extraembryonic coelom at the base of the umbilical stalk. Before returning to the intraembryonic coelom at 10 weeks, the mid-gut rotates in an anticlockwise direction and, with localized growth, the duodenojejunal junction passes behind the superior mesenteric vessels and comes to lie in a position to the left of the midline posteriorly. As the midgut returns to the abdominal cavity this anticlockwise rotation continues, bringing the transverse colon to its adult position anterior to the superior mesenteric vessels and the caecum to the right of the midline. Finally, fixation of the caecum occurs in the right iliac fossa after completion of rotation. At birth the caecum is often mobile on a mesentery as this fixation is still incomplete.[61,62]

Pathology

The stability of the mid-gut mesentery depends on the width of its base—a narrow base predisposes to volvulus. Failure of rotation leaves the duodenojejunal junction to the right of the midline and a mobile caecum on a mesentery in the upper abdomen. Peritoneal bands from the caecum may pass across the second part of the duodenum to the posterior abdominal wall (Fig. 41.7). Volvulus tenses these Ladd's bands and can cause intermittent obstruction or kinking of the duodenum. A volvulus of the mid-gut will cause a high intestinal obstruction, followed by lymphatic, venous and, finally, arterial occlusion in the mesentery.[63]

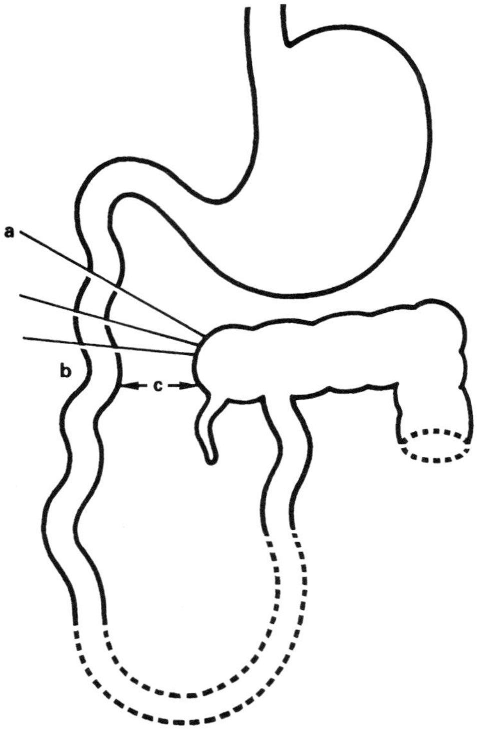

Fig. 41.7 Malrotation with (**a**) Ladd's bands and (**b**) the duodenojejunal junction to the right of midline. (**c**) The narrow base of the mid-gut mesentery predisposes to volvulus.

Malrotation is frequently present in patients with anterior abdominal wall defects and diaphragmatic hernia. Volvulus of the mid-gut is also described in patients without malrotation, but this is rare.

The incidence of abnormal rotation of the duodenum is as high as 1 in 500[64] but neonatal volvulus presents in only 1 in 10 000 live births.

Clinical features

Most patients develop their first symptoms before they are 3 months old and present with intermittent bile-stained vomiting and pain; the abdomen is not distended because this is a high small

REFERENCES

59. Nixon H H Br J Hosp Med 1989; 41: 134
60. Richardson W R, Martin L W J Pediatr Surg 1969; 4: 303
61. Dott D N Br J Surg 1923; 11: 25
62. Snyder W H, Chaffin L Ann Surg 1954; 110: 368
63. Ladd W E N Engl J Med 1932; 206: 277
64. Stewart P R, Colodny A L, Daggett W C Surgery 1976; 79: 716

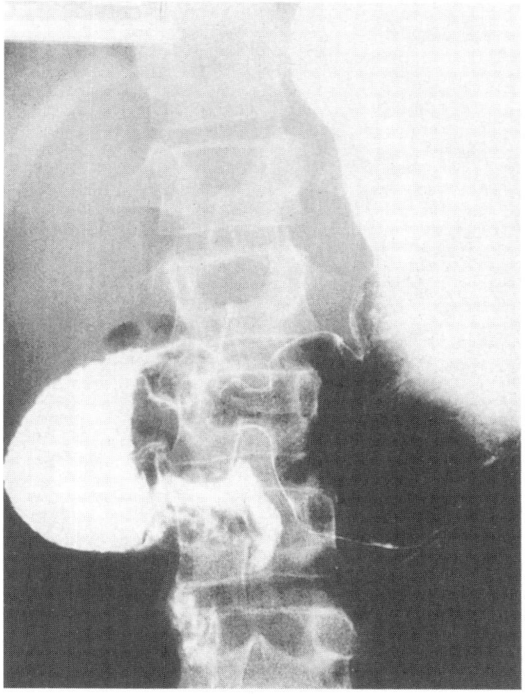

Fig. 41.8 Barium meal demonstrating malrotation: the duodenojejunal junction fails to cross to the left of the midline, and the second part of the duodenum is dilated.

bowel obstruction. Rectal bleeding and abdominal tenderness indicate intestinal ischaemia progressing to gangrene.[65]

A plain abdominal X-ray may demonstrate a dilated first part of the duodenum or asymmetry of the gas pattern in the four quadrants of the abdomen. Usually the plain films are inconclusive and a barium meal is required to visualize the position of the duodenojejunal junction (Fig. 41.8). A barium enema may also give valuable information demonstrating that the caecum is not in the right iliac fossa. An ultrasound scan identifying the orientation of the superior mesenteric vessels can be a most useful aid to diagnosis.[66]

The intermittent nature of the symptoms should raise the possibility of malrotation and should not be allowed to lead to confusion, delay and possible mortality.

Management

An urgent laparotomy is indicated. On opening the peritoneum the transverse colon is found to be absent from its normal position. The entire mid-gut should be delivered out of the abdomen in order to visualize the volvulus at the base of the mesentery. The volvulus usually occurs in a clockwise direction so, for correction, the bowel should be rotated anticlockwise, often by between 360° and 720°. Ladd's bands and adhesions at the base of the mesentery must be carefully divided, protecting the superior mesenteric vessels and the entire duodenum and proximal jejunum placed to the right of the midline. By returning the small bowel to the right of the abdomen and the caecum and colon to the left, the base of the mesentery is widened and stabilized. The appendix will now be sited on the left and an appendicectomy is indicated to avoid later confusion from atypical appendicitis. No attempt must be made to return the mid-gut to its position of normal rotation—in effect, the purpose of the correct operation is to exaggerate the failure of rotation.[63]

Gangrenous bowel must be excised but only if at least 50 cm of viable small bowel remains with an intact ileocaecal valve. If the entire mid-gut appears gangrenous, the volvulus should be untwisted and the abdomen closed. After 24 hours of resuscitation a second laparotomy is performed and it may then be possible to salvage a useful length of viable small bowel.[67] Patients with only 25 cm of small bowel have achieved adequate oral nutrition after many months of intravenous feeding.

Prognosis

An early mortality of up to 20% has been reported,[65] related to extensive gangrene of the mid-gut occurring preoperatively. In 10% of patients a re-operation for adhesion obstruction or recurrent volvulus may be required.[68]

SMALL BOWEL ATRESIA

Aetiology

Operations on foetal dogs have demonstrated that small bowel atresias may result from localized vascular accidents late in pregnancy.[69] This view is supported by the presence of bile pigments, swallowed hair and squamous cells found distal to the obstruction. Prenatal intussusception, volvulus and trapping of the bowel in association with gastroschisis are other possible causes.[70] The atresia may take the form of a mucosal membrane (type I), two blind ends joined by a fibrous cord (type II) or separated blind ends with a mesenteric defect (type III; Fig. 41.9) Atresias are multiple in 10% of cases, and in these instances family studies suggest a genetic predisposition.[71] The reported incidence is variable from 1 in 20 000 live births in the UK to 1 in 1000 in Australia.[72]

Clinical features

Antenatal diagnosis is described and some affected pregnancies are complicated by polyhydramnios. Ultrasound scanning can demonstrate dilated loops of small bowel in both the second and third trimesters.[73] After birth the high jejunal atresias will present with bilious vomiting in the first 24 hours of life. A more distal ileal atresia may not present until the baby develops bilious

REFERENCES

65. Millar A J W et al Pediatr Surg Int 1987; 2: 172
66. Gaines P A, Saunders A J S, Drake D P Clin Radiol 1987; 38: 51
67. Bill A H Pediatric Surgery. W B Saunders, Philadelphia 1980
68. Stauffer U G, Hermann P J Pediatr Surg 1980; 15: 9
69. Louw J H, Barnard C N Lancet 1955; 2: 1065
70. Nixon H H, Tawes R Surgery 1971; 69: 41
71. Seashore J H et al Pediatrics 1987; 80: 540
72. Congenital malformations. Bull World Hlth Org 1966; 34: (suppl)
73. Richards C, Holmes S J K Arch Dis Child 1995; 72F: 135

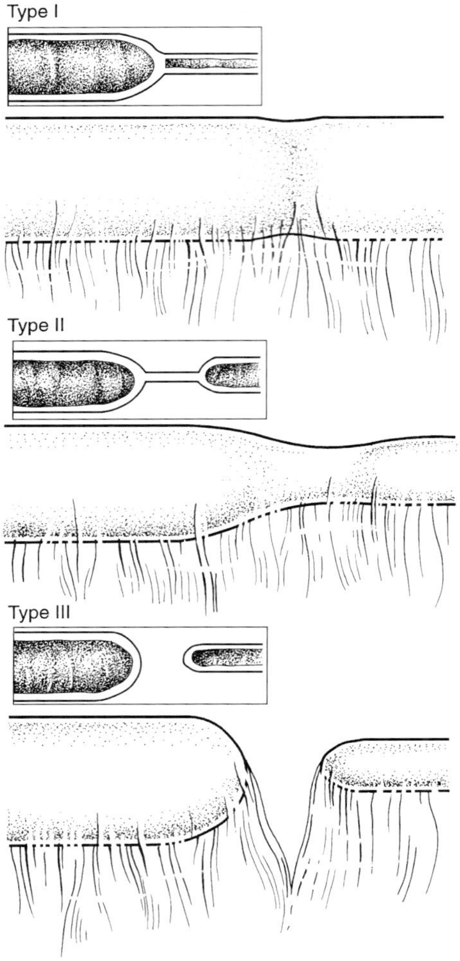

Fig. 41.9 Three types of intestinal atresia. Type I = a mucosal membrane; type II = the atretic segment represented by a fibrous cord; type III = mesenteric defect with separated blind ends.

vomiting with abdominal distension at the age of 2 or 3 days. Meconium may be passed on the first day of life but this will not be followed by changing stools.

Plain abdominal X-rays demonstrate dilated loops of bowel usually centrally placed in the abdomen and with fluid levels. A barium enema is of value in excluding a second distal colonic atresia[74] and will outline a microcolon if present (Fig. 41.10).

Management

At laparotomy the atresia should be resected and the distal lumen perfused with saline to exclude multiple obstructions. If the proximal bowel is grossly dilated, its motility will be impaired and it should be either resected back to less dilated small bowel or tapered.[75] (Fig. 41.11). A primary anastomosis may then be achieved with a single layer of extramucosal sutures, if necessary widening the distal circumference with an antimesenteric cutback.[70] In 20% of cases, there is an extensive mesenteric defect with a jejunal atresia and the ileum is found to be curled around its single artery, which passes retrogradely from the right colic or even the mid colic arcade. This 'apple-peel' arrangement is

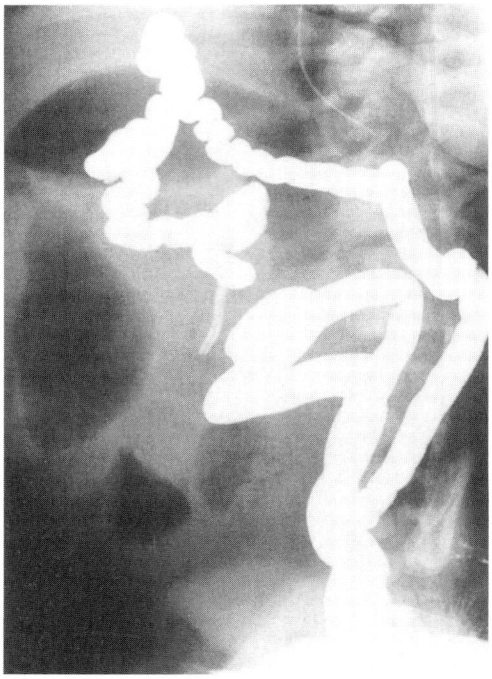

Fig. 41.10 Barium enema demonstrating a microcolon in a newborn with total small bowel obstruction.

associated with multiple atresias and a shortened bowel. The blood supply of the ileum is precarious and the anastomosis liable to kinking because of the defective mesentery. The length of remaining jejunum and ileum at the end of surgery should be separately measured and recorded.

Prognosis

This is related to the length of bowel preserved. Most infants will require short-term total parenteral nutrition postoperatively, but those with a bowel length less than 70 cm may require long-term total parenteral nutrition.

Intestinal adaptation occurs over the first 2 years of life and long-term survival off total parenteral nutrition has been described with less than 30 cm of small bowel.[76] Second laparotomies may be indicated for revision of obstructed anastomoses or adhesions.

MECONIUM ILEUS

Pathology

One in 15 000 newborns will have a distal small bowel obstruction secondary to abnormally bulky and viscid meconium.[77] Ninety per cent of these infants will have cystic fibrosis and the abnormal

REFERENCES

74. Jackman S, Brereton R J J Pediatr Surg 1988; 23: 852
75. Howard E R, Othersen H B J Pediatr Surg 1973; 8: 685
76. Kurkchubasche A G, Rowe M I, Smith S D J Pediatr Surg 1993; 28: 1069
77. Dickson J A S, Mearns, M B Recent Advances in Paediatric Surgery. Churchill Livingstone, Edinburgh 1975 p 143

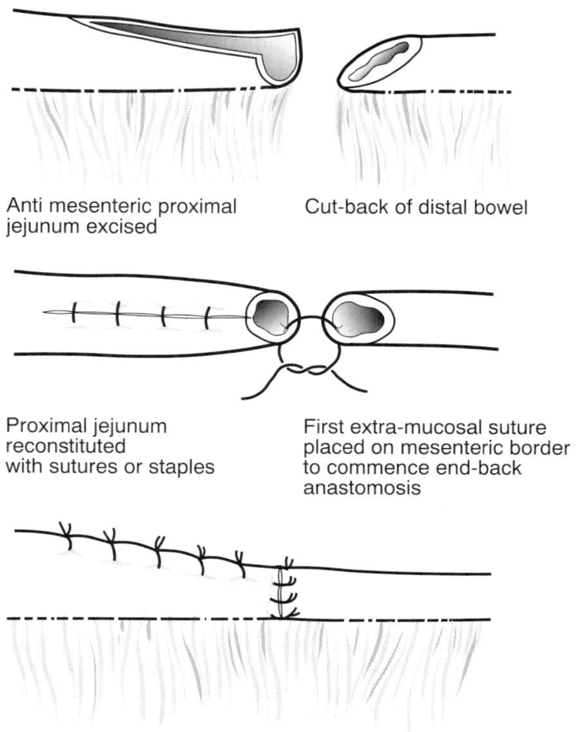

Fig. 41.11 Jejunal atresia: the proximal dilated segment is tapered and the distal circumference extended with a cutback. An end-to-back anastomosis is then performed.

meconium is the result of deficient intestinal secretions.[78] This abnormal meconium has a high protein content and prenatally the viscosity causes a functional obstruction of the terminal ileum. Volvulus of the grossly distended ileum can progress to ischaemia, perforation and meconium peritonitis, which is a sterile, inflammatory process leading to calcification. Atresia of a devitalized segment of small bowel may also occur.

Clinical features

Prenatal ultrasound scanning in the third trimester can detect dilated loops of small bowel and abnormal meconium. The infant is born with a distended abdomen and develops bilious vomiting on the first day of life. No meconium is passed and the rectum is empty. Abnormal masses of meconium may be palpable and plain abdominal X-rays confirm the presence of dilated loops of bowel, but fluid levels are scarce as the meconium is viscid. Flecks of calcium, characteristically on the liver capsule, are indica-tive of a prenatal perforation with meconium peritonitis.

A contrast enema will demonstrate the collapsed empty colon (Fig. 41.10). A gastrografin enema can be therapeutic in an uncomplicated case,[79] so long as the gastrografin refluxes into the ileum, where its detergent effect will loosen the meconium. This form of therapy is only recommended in a well-hydrated child who is prepared for an urgent laparotomy should a perforation be demonstrated or no meconium passed. Fluid loss into the bowel lumen usually necessitates intravenous infusion of 4.5% albumin, 10–20 ml/kg. A laparotomy will be required in approximately half of these infants as the gastrografin will not relieve the obstruction if there is a volvulus or atresia.

When an operation is required to relieve the obstruction, the ileum is found to contain a viscid mass of dark green meconium, with pale pellets of meconium obstructing the terminal ileum. The dilated ileum is opened and the meconium washed out with saline[80] or dilute gastrografin. Grossly dilated ileum should be resected and a primary anastomosis may be performed if the distal bowel is unobstructed.[81] Alternatively a temporary double-barrelled ileostomy may be fashioned with minimal handling of the bowel and without washing out the ileum.[82] Such an ileostomy allows access postoperatively to clear the meconium proximally and distally with the introduction of acetylcysteine or gastrografin. The ileostomy may be closed after a few days when the bowel is clear.

An alternative technique at laparotomy is to perform an appendicectomy and introduce an irrigating catheter via the appendix stump into the ileum. Following decompression and expression of meconium through the ileocaecal valve and appendix stump, the latter is closed.[83]

Histological examination of excised ileum or appendix will demonstrate the abnormal mucus-secreting goblet cells and the crypts plugged with mucus.[77] Patients should have genetic studies to identify the commoner abnormal loci on chromosome 7, such as Δ F508. A sweat test is the definitive diagnostic test for cystic fibrosis, best performed when the infant is aged 2 months or older.

Prognosis

Early complications are related to mucus retention in the bronchial tree and malabsorption. These are managed with vigorous physiotherapy and pancreatic enzyme replacement. Infants with meconium peritonitis require lengthy laparotomies with much bowel manipulation; total parenteral nutrition will be required during the period of prolonged postoperative ileus.

Late complications are related to the underlying cystic fibrosis and include recurrent chest infections, malabsorption and recurrent small bowel obstruction with undigested food (meconium ileus equivalent). Mortality in early childhood is now rare but cystic fibrosis remains a life-threatening disease in older children and young adults.

HIRSCHSPRUNG'S DISEASE

Embryology

Neural crest cells migrate into the wall of the embryonic foregut in the fifth week and pass down the intestine to reach the rectum

REFERENCES

78. Thomaidis T S, Arey J B J Pediatr 1963; 63: 444
79. Noblett H R J Pediatr Surg 1969; 4: 190
80. Chappell J S S Afr Med J 1977; 52: 1093
81. Mabogunje O A, Way C I, Mahour G H Ann Surg 1982; 117: 37
82. Gross R E The Surgery of Infancy and Childhood. Saunders, Philadelphia 1953 p 175
83. Fitzgerald R, Conlon K J Pediatr Surg 1989; 24: 899

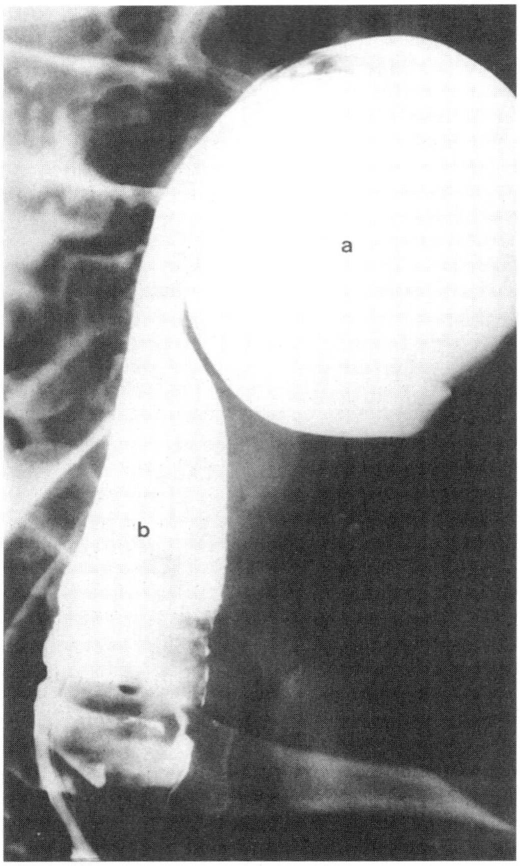

Fig. 41.12 Barium enema in a patient with Hirschsprung's disease. (**a**) The ganglionic proximal sigmoid colon is dilated compared with the (**b**) aganglionic distal colon and rectum.

before the end of the first trimester. These cells form the ganglia of the parasympathetic system and are organized into Meissner's submucosal plexus and Auerbach's intermyenteric plexus. This migration of cells may be incomplete, with the arrest occurring most often in the sigmoid colon. The resultant aganglionosis of the distal colon is described as Hirschsprung's disease. However, in 10% of cases, the migration stops in the small bowel, leaving the entire colon and rectum aganglionic.[84]

Hirschsprung's disease is more common in boys than girls and is associated with Down's syndrome in over 10% of patients. There is a genetic factor in the aetiology, with a risk of over 2% in near relatives; the longer the segment of aganglionosis, the higher the risk.[85] Abnormal gene loci on chromosome 10 have been identified in families with several affected members.[86]

Clinical features

Hirschsprung's disease is the most common cause of intestinal obstruction in the newborn, affecting 1 in 5000 children.[87] Typically there is delay in passing meconium beyond the first 24 hours of life; there is abdominal distension following feeds and bilious vomiting. The distal obstruction may be total but is more commonly relieved by a rectal washout with normal saline, or by a rectal examination. The failure of relaxation of the rectal wall can sometimes be appreciated by the examining finger. Delay in treatment can be an important factor in the development of an enterocolitis[88] associated with overgrowth of *Clostridium difficile*.[89] This can progress rapidly to toxic dilatation with perforation or rarely to a pseudomembranous colitis.

A plain abdominal X-ray will demonstrate dilated loops of bowel with fluid levels and a barium enema can be helpful when it demonstrates a cone with dilated ganglionic proximal colon and the distal aganglionic bowel failing to distend. These changes are more obvious in an infant presenting at the age of a few months (Fig. 41.12).[90]

A suction rectal biopsy[91] will provide a specimen of rectal mucosa and submucosa suitable for histological examination and histochemical staining for acetylcholinesterase.[92] The absence of ganglion cells in the submucosa with an excess of positively staining nerve trunks is diagnostic of Hirschsprung's disease.

Patients with Hirschsprung's disease may present after the neonatal period with chronic constipation or subtotal large bowel obstruction. A full-thickness rectal biopsy taken 2 cm above the anal canal provides a suitable specimen for histology and histochemistry. This procedure requires a general anaesthetic and good visibility using an anal speculum. In addition, anorectal manometry may be used and will fail to show the normal relaxation of the internal sphincter on inflation of a rectal balloon in patients with Hirschsprung's disease.[93]

Management

The initial surgical management of Hirschsprung's disease can involve a colostomy. This should employ bowel whose normal innervation is confirmed by histology of a frozen section.[94] A right transverse colostomy is suitable for the majority of patients where the aganglionic segment reaches only to the sigmoid colon. Alternatively, the colostomy may be sited approximately 3 cm proximal to the transition zone between ganglionic and aganglionic bowel.

The definitive treatment is a pull-through operation to bring bowel with normal innervation to the anorectal junction. This operation may be performed between the ages of 3 and 9 months and techniques have been described by Swenson,[95] Duhamel[96] and Soave[97] (Fig. 41.13). A defunctioning colostomy may be closed

REFERENCES

84. Kleinhaus S et al J Pediatr Surg 1979; 14: 588
85. Carter C O, Evans K, Hickman V J Med Genet 1981; 18: 87
86. Romeo G et al Nature 1994; 367: 377
87. Ehrenpreis T Hirschsprung's Disease. Year Book Medical, Chicago 1970
88. Teitelbaum D H et al Ann Surg 1988; 207: 240
89. Thomas D F M et al Lancet 1982; 1: 78
90. Bodian M, Stephen F D, Ward B C H Lancet 1949; 1: 6
91. Campbell P E, Noblett H R J Pediatr Surg 1969; 4: 410
92. Barr L C et al Gut 1985; 26 393
93. Lawson J O N, Nixon H H J Pediatr Surg 1967; 2: 544
94. Martin L Pediatric Surgery. W B Saunders, Philadephia 1980
95. Swenson O Ann Surg 1964; 160: 540
96. Duhamel B Dis Colon Rectum 1964; 7: 455
97. Soave F Arch Dis Child 1964; 39: 116

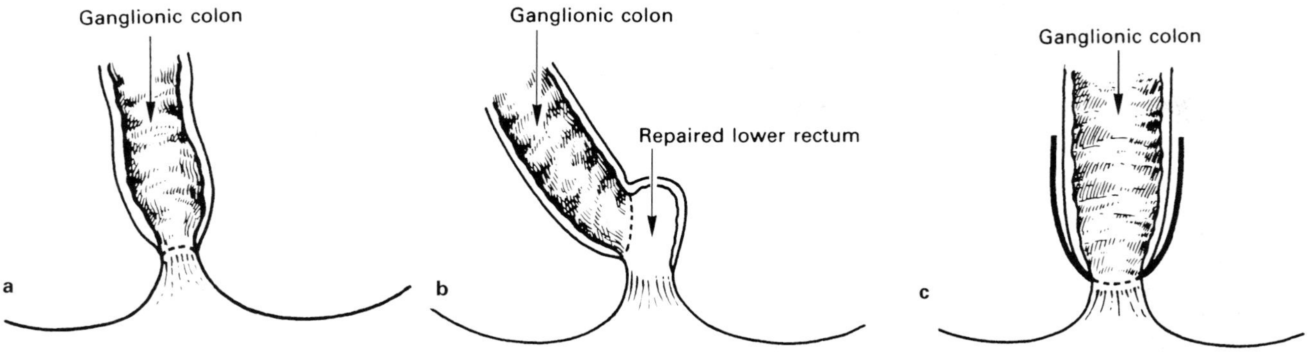

Fig. 41.13 Three definitive operations for Hirschsprung's disease. (**a**) Swenson's[95] prolapsed distal rectum to achieve a low colorectal anastomosis. (**b**) Duhamel's[96] posterior colorectal anastomosis. (**c**) Soave's[97] endorectal pull-through after excising the rectal mucosa.

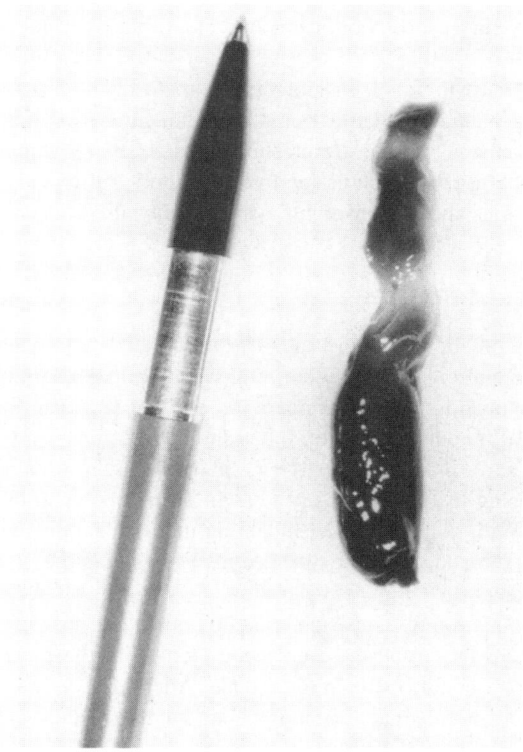

Fig. 41.14 A meconium plug: it retains the shape of the rectum and its size is compared with a pen. The patient was diagnosed as having Hirschsprung's disease on a subsequent rectal biopsy.

after 4 weeks, after contrast studies have confirmed satisfactory healing. There is increasing interest in performing the pull-through operation in newborns without a covering colostomy, having prepared the bowel with colonic irrigation.[98] In experienced hands, the complication rate is no higher than staged surgery.

Difficulties in confirming the diagnosis of Hirschsprung's disease should not be underestimated. The initial barium enema will not demonstrate typical changes if a rectal examination or washout in the previous 36 hours has emptied the distal colon. Histological and histochemical reporting of small biopsies in the newborn can be misleading and a full-thickness biopsy may be required.[99] Few investigators have achieved reliable neonatal anorectal manometric studies.[100]

Three conditions can mimic Hirschsprung's disease: meconium plug syndrome, left colon syndrome and neuronal intestinal dysplasia. Neonates presenting with delay in passing meconium may be totally relieved of their obstruction by a rectal washout, which removes a plug of solid meconium (Fig. 41.14). These patients should be investigated for possible cystic fibrosis with a sweat test, as well as with a rectal biopsy to exclude Hirschsprung's disease. The left colon syndrome is a transient obstruction of the left colon, often associated with maternal diabetes, and is related to immaturity of colonic innervation.[101] If rectal washouts do not relieve the obstruction, these patients require a temporary right transverse colostomy. A rectal biopsy must be performed to confirm the presence of ganglion cells in the rectum before closing the colostomy after four to six weeks. Patients with neuronal intestinal dysplasia[102] have abnormalities of innervation of the colon characterised by the presence of giant or ectopic ganglion cells and thickened nerve trunks.[103] The natural history of this condition is variable; many patients have improving bowel function when managed conservatively with repeated washouts and only a minority require a bowel resection.

Prognosis

Mortality for infants with Hirschsprung's disease is related to the occurrence of overwhelming sepsis from enterocolitis and also to the length of the aganglionic segment.[104] If only the proximal jejunum is ganglionic, the infant will have all the problems associated with the short bowel syndrome and prolonged total parenteral nutrition.

In long-term follow-up studies, excellent results are reported for the majority of children[105] but careful questionnaires reveal that a proportion have problems with soiling, incontinence and

REFERENCES

98. Shambhoque L K R, Bianchi A Pediatr Surg Int 1990; 5: 446
99. Andrassy R J, Isaacs H, Weitzman J J Ann Surg 1981; 193: 419
100. Holschneider A M et al J Pediatr Surg 1976; 11: 151
101. Rangecroft L Arch Dis Child 1979; 54: 635
102. Fadda B et al Z Kinderchir 1983; 38: 308
103. Athow A C, Filipe M I, Drake D P Arch Dis Child 1991; 66: 1300
104. Ikeda K, Goto S Ann Surg 1986; 41: 279
105. Moore S W, Millar A J W, Cywes S J Pediatr Surg 1994; 29: 106

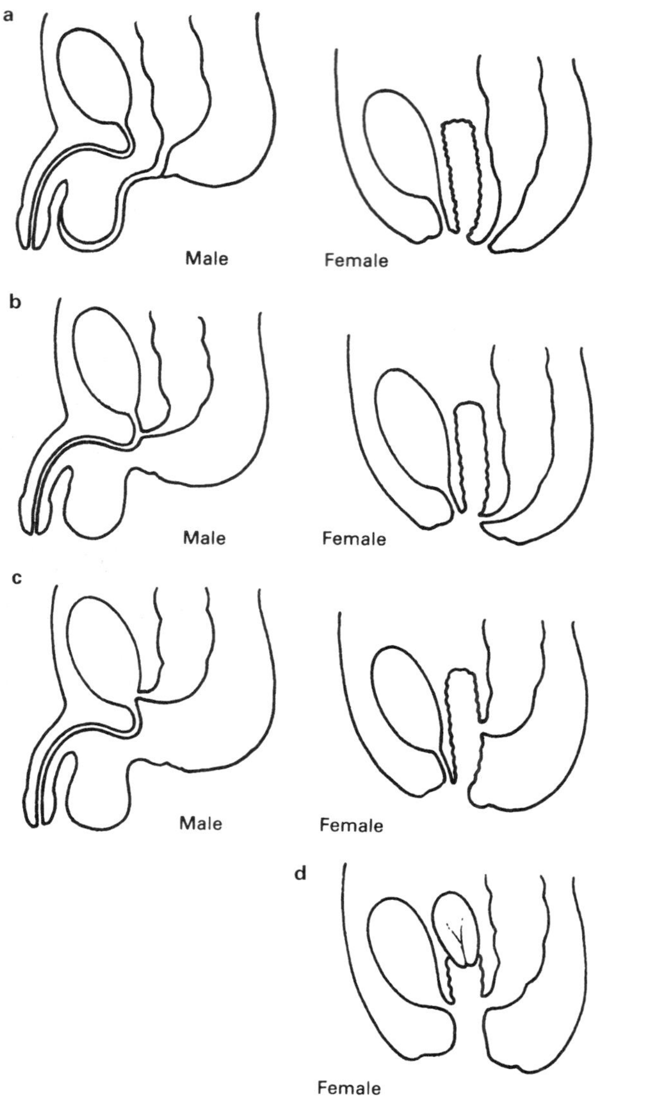

Fig. 41.15 Examples of commoner anorectal anomalies. (**a**) Low: covered anus with anocutaneous fistula in males; anterior ectopic anus in females. (**b**) Intermediate: anal agenesis with rectourethral fistula in males; anal agenesis with rectovaginal or vulval fistula in females. (**c**) High: anorectal agenesis with rectovesical fistula in males; anorectal agenesis with rectovaginal fistula in females. (**d**) Persistent cloaca: bladder, uterus and rectum drain into a cloaca in females (rare).

constipation.[106] Reliable bowel control is less often achieved in patients with Down's syndrome, who have a higher incidence of recurrent enterocolitis.

ANORECTAL ANOMALIES

Embryology

The development of the urogenital sinus and the rectum from the primitive cloaca takes place between 4 and 6 weeks after conception. A range of anomalies occur which for convenience may be subdivided into six groups: high, intermediate and low in both males and females (Fig. 41.15). The puborectalis sling marks the level of an intermediate anomaly; in high anomalies the rectum ends above and in low anomalies it reaches below this muscle. The bowel seldom ends as a blind pouch, as usually there is a fistula to the vagina in girls and to the urinary tract in boys.[107]

A low anomaly in a boy is a covered anus with an anocutaneous track. In a girl, the low anomaly is an anterior ectopic anus which is also stenotic. An intermediate lesion in the male has the rectum ending at the level of the puborectalis sling, usually with a fistula to the membranous urethra. In the female there will be a fistula to the low vagina or vulva. In these children the internal sphincter is poorly developed and, although the external sphincter is present, no canal passes through it. In high anomalies the rectum may be a blind pouch or have a fistula to the upper vagina, posterior urethra or bladder. Rectal atresia with an occluding membrane is a rare anomaly and causes confusion because the anal canal develops normally.

Half these infants with anorectal anomalies will have associated anomalies affecting the urogenital system, cardiovascular system, the oesophagus, the gastrointestinal tract or spine. Abnormalities of the sacrum, hypospadias and vesicoureteric reflux are common associations and Hirschsprung's disease may also coexist.[108]

Clinical features

These anomalies occur in 1 in 5000 births[107] and their management is dependent on accurately defining the abnormal anatomy. There is no indication for urgent operation without adequate investigation. By 20 hours after birth, flatus should have reached the lower rectum and a plain lateral pelvic radiograph may be obtained, after first raising the pelvis above the level of the abdomen in a prone infant. With a metal marker indenting the anal dimple, an assessment may be made of the distance between gas in the rectum and the perineal skin (Fig. 41.16).

Examination of the perineum at 20 hours after birth may reveal meconium presenting in a cutaneous fistula in the male or in a vulval or vaginal fistula in the female. Alternatively, in boys with a high or intermediate lesion associated with a fistula, meconium may be passed with the urinary stream.

Operative treatment

Low lesions can be managed by performing an anoplasty on the perineum. With the patient in a lithotomy position the stenotic opening is enlarged posteriorly and a Y-V plasty of perineal skin performed into the posterior anal defect. The operation is below the puborectalis sling and should not compromise continence.[109]

REFERENCES

106. Heij H A et al J Pediatr Surg 1995; 30: 430
107. Templeton J M, O'Neill J A Pediatric Surgery, 4th ed. Year Book Medical, Chicago 1986
108. Keiswetter W B et al Surgery 1965; 58: 877
109. Keiswetter W B Pediatric Surgery. W B Saunders, Philadelphia 1980

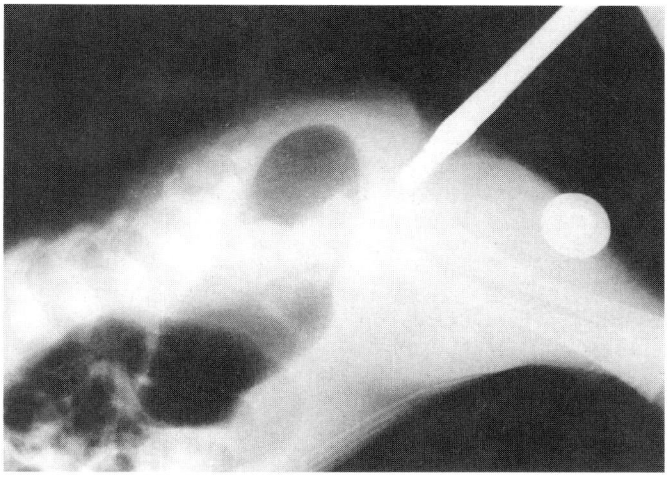

Fig. 41.16 Lateral radiograph of the pelvis in a low anorectal anomaly. Flatus outlines the distal bowel below the puborectalis sling and adjacent to the anal dimple (marked with the bulb of a thermometer).

Intermediate and high lesions should be managed initially with a proximal sigmoid colostomy. A more detailed radiological assessment can then be performed later with a cystogram combined with a distal loopogram (Fig. 41.17). The definitive operation should be performed in the first 4 months of life, as evidence from studies of anal-evoked potentials suggest that it is important to complete the repair and provide sensory input before the central nervous system matures.[110] The importance of the puborectalis sling is well-known but, more recently, the role of the external sphincter has also been recognized;[111] these two muscles together comprise the striated muscle complex. Correct positioning of the rectal pull-through in this muscle complex is important to minimize mucosal prolapse and to improve continence.

For intermediate lesions the pull-through operation should be performed through a posterior sagittal approach. A laparotomy is occasionally necessary for high anomalies to allow mobilization of the distal bowel. The main skin incision is in the natal cleft and the striated muscle complex is divided in the midline. Following repair of the fistula, a dilated rectum may be tailored by excising a posterior cuff. The puborectalis sling and external sphincter are then meticulously repaired behind and around the rectum[112] and a neoanus is created with a rectocutaneous anastomosis. This opening is gradually dilated before the covering colostomy is closed.

A persistent cloaca demands extensive reconstruction of the urethra, vagina and distal rectum. This is best performed after the age of 6 months, using a posterior sagittal incision.[113]

Prognosis

The infant's prospect for recovery depends on the severity of associated anomalies, particularly of the cardiovascular and renal systems. Patients with gross sacral anomalies have poorly developed pelvic muscles and seldom achieve continence. Low anomalies should achieve normal continence but often develop constipation with overflow and require careful follow-up throughout childhood.

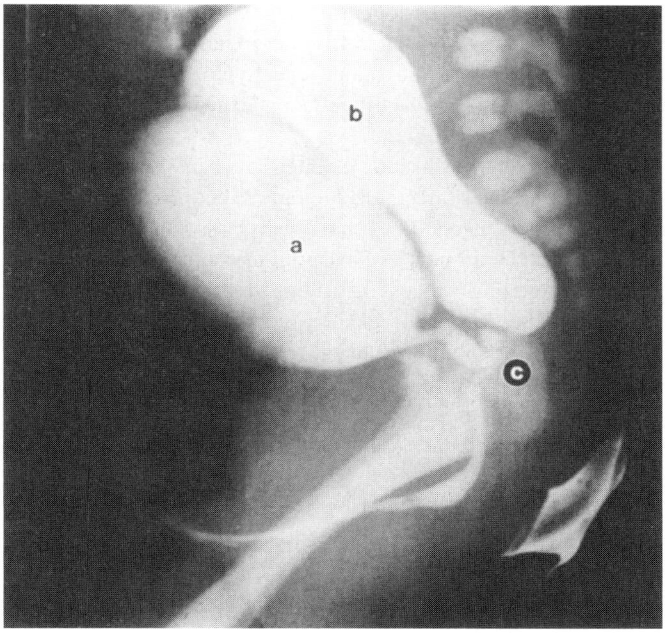

Fig. 41.17 (**a**) A micturating cystogram combined with (**b**) a distal loopogram in a male patient with an intermediate anomaly and (**c**) a rectourethral fistula.

School-age children with incontinence may be helped with regular colonic irrigations. An appendicostomy provides a very useful conduit for intermittent catheterization and allows for antegrade colonic enemas.[114] This has dramatically improved the quality of these children's lives, without need for a permanent colostomy.

NECROTIZING ENTEROCOLITIS

Aetiology and pathogenesis

Only isolated cases of 'idiopathic gastrointestinal perforation' were described in the newborn until Corkery et al[115] reported in 1968 the association of intestinal perforation with umbilical vein catheterization for exchange transfusion. However, by 1977, more than one case of necrotizing enterocolitis was recorded for every thousand live births in North America.[116] Injuries to the intestinal mucosa may be caused by invasive bacteria, exposure to hypertonic feeds or to hypoxia.[117] Lloyd[118] suggests that the neonate's

REFERENCES

110. Freeman N V et al Z Kinderchir 1980; 31: 32
111. de Vries P A, Pena A J Pediatr Surg 1982; 17: 638
112. Pena A, de Vries P A J Pediatr Surg 1982; 17: 796
113. Nagayama D K et al J Pediatr Surg 1987; 22: 588
114. Squire R et al J Pediatr Surg 1993; 28: 1012
115. Corkery J J et al Br Med J 1968; 4: 345
116. Sweet A Y Neonatal Necrotising Enterocolitis. Grune & Stratton, New York 1980
117. Rowe M I Paediatric Surgery, 4th edn. Year Book Medical, Chicago 1986
118. Lloyd J R J Pediatr Surg 1969; 4: 77

response to hypoxia is analogous to that of a diving mammal where blood is preferentially shunted from less vital organs, such as the gut, to the heart and the brain. The hypoxic episode may be prenatal or perinatal and be brief, but once the mucosa is damaged, bacterial invasion is facilitated.

Epidemics of the disease in intensive care baby units have suggested a primary infective aetiology,[119] but no single organism has been implicated. Cases have been associated with viral, clostridial and Gram-negative bacterial infection.[120]

The necrotizing process is triggered by the release of free oxygen radicals.[121] Histologically there are micro-thromboses, haemorrhage, inflammatory change and intramural gas. Both small and large bowel may be affected; the terminal ileum and the right colon are more common sites. Breast milk has a protective role, reducing the incidence and severity of the inflammatory response.[122]

Clinical features

Bloody diarrhoea, abdominal distension and bilious vomiting are the characteristic clinical triad. In addition, erythema of the anterior abdominal wall suggests full-thickness necrosis of the bowel with peritonitis. The infant will be lethargic and may have recurrent apnoea and bradycardia; a core–peripheral temperature gap indicates hypovolaemia and sepsis. Thrombocytopenia and disseminated intravascular coagulopathy are signs of extensive disease.

The diagnostic radiological sign is intramural gas with intrahepatic portal vein gas in severe cases. These are transient signs and plain abdominal radiographs should be ordered at 8-hourly intervals when the diagnosis is initially suspected. Free gas detected on a decubitus film confirms perforation of the intestine.

Treatment

The initial resuscitation includes intravenous colloid and a blood transfusion when there is significant blood loss in the stools. The patient is screened for sepsis by taking a blood culture and intravenous antibiotics are administered to treat both aerobic and anaerobic infection; a combination of benzylpenicillin, gentamicin and metronidazole is appropriate.

Ventilation is frequently indicated and, with prompt intensive medical treatment, the necrotic process can be halted and healing may occur, albeit with a 10% incidence of ischaemic strictures developing after an interval of a few weeks.[123] Total parenteral nutrition is required as all feeding should be withheld for 10 days.[124]

Urgent laparotomy is indicated if there is evidence of perforation or failure of the signs of peritonitis to resolve on medical treatment. Gangrenous bowel is excised with construction of a temporary ileostomy or colostomy. Alternatively, a primary anastomosis may be performed even in the presence of faecal peritonitis.[125] Elective surgery is indicated for the management of late ischaemic strictures and for re-establishing intestinal continuity once the infant is thriving. A distal barium study should be performed before closing a stoma because of the high incidence of strictures developing in defunctioned bowel (Fig. 41.18).

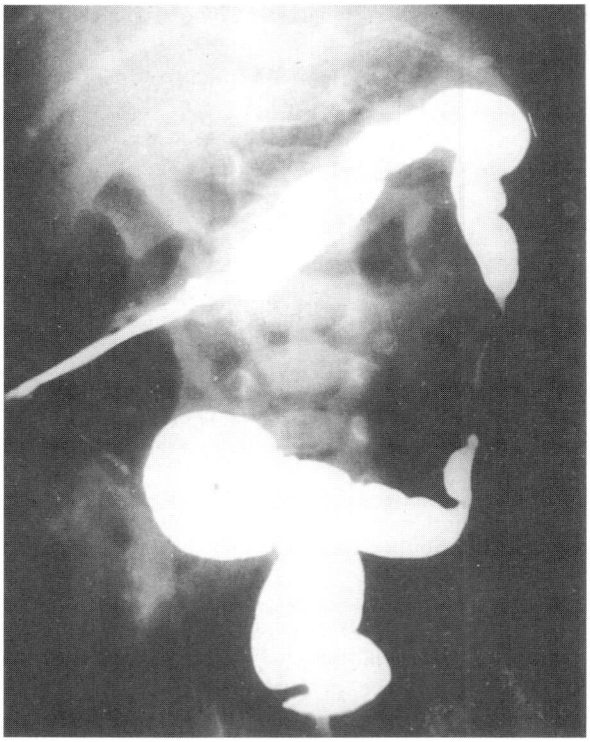

Fig. 41.18 Stricture in descending colon distal to a transverse colostomy. The patient had had a laparotomy for necrotizing enterocolitis 6 weeks previously.

Prognosis

Survival rates of 75% have been reported[126] despite the severity and complications of this acquired disease in infants who are often premature or have congenital heart disease. Long-term complications may be related to a short small intestine after extensive resection and to neurodevelopmental problems following intracranial haemorrhage, which is more common in premature infants.[127]

INFANTILE HYPERTROPHIC PYLORIC STENOSIS

Hypertrophic pyloric stenosis affects boys more commonly than girls and in Northern European and American Caucasians the incidence is 4 in every 1000 births. The incidence is less common in

REFERENCES

119. Howard F M et al Lancet 1977; 2: 1099
120. Touloukian J Surg Clin North Am 1976; 56: 281
121. Clark D A et al Am J Pathol 1988; 130; 537
122. Lucas A, Cole A Lancet 1990; 336: 1519
123. Koloske A M, Burstein J, Barlow S A Ann Surg 1980; 192: 202
124. Bunton G et al Arch Dis Child 1977; 52: 772
125. Sparnon A L, Kiely E K Pediatr Surg Int 1987; 2: 101
126. Jerles M L World J Surg 1990; 14: 600
127. Jackman S, Brereton R J, Wright V M Br J Surg 1990; 77: 146

North American negroes, Indian and Chinese infants.[128] One in 7 patients gives a positive family history and the offspring of affected mothers have a higher risk than those of affected fathers. Sons of affected mothers have the highest calculated risk—20%.[129]

The circular muscle of the pylorus becomes hypertrophic during the first 6 weeks after birth and there is often a leucocytic infiltration.[130] Reports of the tumour presenting on the first day of life are exceedingly rare.[131] The aetiology is still obscure, although the condition may be produced in puppies by administering pentagastrin to pregnant dogs.[132] Although hypergastrinaemia has been described in infants with pyloric stenosis,[133] its role is uncertain and is thought to be secondary to gastric stasis. Nitric oxide synthase activity is reduced in the hypertrophied circular muscle.[134]

Clinical features

The infants present with forceful or projectile vomiting, usually at the age of 3–4 weeks. The vomitus is not bile-stained but may contain altered blood if there is oesophagitis.[135] The infant may appear anxious with a full stomach but following a vomit is hungry and eager for a further feed. Stools may be infrequent and green and weight loss occurs after several days of vomiting. Dehydration and wasting are now rare signs and indicate delay in presentation.

The diagnosis may be made clinically with a test feed. The stomach is first emptied by aspirating a nasogastric tube and the infant is offered a milk feed. The abdomen is inspected for visible peristalsis passing from left to right across the epigastrium and palpated for a pyloric tumour. This is found deep to the right rectus muscle above the umbilicus and has the size and shape of an olive. Repeat test feeding is indicated if the pylorus is not palpable but the diagnosis may be confirmed by an ultrasound scan[136] which can provide measurements of the length of the canal and the thickness of circular muscle. A length greater than 19 mm or a muscle thickness of more than 4 mm is compatible with hypertrophic pyloric stenosis.[137] In clinically difficult cases and when ultrasound scanning is not available, a barium meal[138] will demonstrate an elongated narrow pyloric canal. Palpation of the tumour is still the gold standard for establishing the diagnosis.

Management

Successful operative treatment by pyloromyotomy was described by Ramstedt in 1912.[139] If the patient has a metabolic alkalosis, this should be corrected by giving intravenous normal saline with added potassium supplements. When the serum bicarbonate has returned to the normal range, an operation may be performed under a general anaesthetic, first emptying the stomach via a nasogastric tube. At operation the pylorus is delivered through an upper right transverse incision and is incised longitudinally along its relatively avascular anterosuperior border. This incision is deepened with a blunt dissector and the circular muscle is split. Great care is required at the distal end of the pylorus not to open the duodenal mucosa. The pyloromyotomy is complete when the mucosa 'pouts' to the level of the serosa throughout the length of the pylorus (Fig. 41.19). Any perforation of the mucosa should be closed with a fine absorbable suture and the omentum used as a patch.

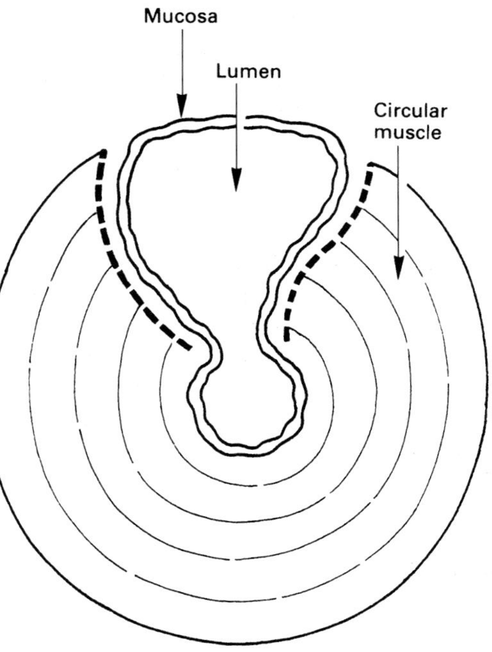

Fig. 41.19 Transverse section of pyloric tumour at completion of pyloromyotomy.

An alternative incision for the experienced surgeon is circumumbilical. This gives an excellent cosmetic result[140] but careful antiseptic cleaning of the umbilicus and perioperative antibiotic cover are indicated to reduce the risk of sepsis after operating through a potentially infected field.

Postoperatively, oral feeds may be introduced within 24 hours. The more common complications following surgery are wound dehiscence (4%) and wound infection (6%).[141] The mortality is less than 1% and is related to peritonitis secondary to undetected breaches in the mucosa.

INTUSSUSCEPTION

The invagination of a portion of the intestine into its own lumen is more common in children than adults and has been reported in 4 per 1000 children[142] and intussusceptions account for some 5 admissions per year in district general hospitals.[143] The condition is

REFERENCES

128. Klein A, Cremin B J S Afr Med J 1970; 44: 1131
129. Carter C O, Evans K A J Med Genet 1969; 6: 233
130. Spicer R D Br J Surg 1982; 69: 128
131. Powell B W Lancet 1962; 2: 1326
132. Dodge J A Nature 1970; 225: 284
133. Spitz L, Zail S S J Pediatr Surg 1976; 11: 1
134. Vanderwinden J M N Engl J Med 1992; 327: 511
135. Spitz L Arch Dis Child 1979; 54: 886
136. Teele R L, Smith E H N Engl J Med 1977; 296: 1149
137. Kofoed P E L et al Br J Radiol 1988; 61: 19
138. Shuman F I, Darling D B, Fisher J H J Pediatr 1967; 71: 70
139. Pollock W F, Norris W J Surgery 1957; 42: 966
140. Tan K C, Bianchi A Br J Surg 1986; 73: 399
141. McDonald P J J Soc Med 1986; 79: 17
142. Court D, Knox G Br Med J 1959; 2: 408
143. Thomas D F M Br J Surg 1980; 67: 333

more common in boys and the majority of cases present under the age of 1 year,[144] but rarely in the first month of life.[145] Most intussusceptions are ileocolic but ileoileocolic, ileoilial and colocolic are described in descending order of frequency.[146] Fewer than 10% of cases have an identified anatomical lead point, such as a Meckel's diverticulum, a polyp, duplication cyst or ectopic pancreatic tissue.[144] Intussusceptions are described in patients with Henoch–Schönlein purpura,[147] haemophilia,[148] haemangiomas[149] and gastrointestinal lymphoma.[150] Intussusceptions following a laparotomy or retroperitoneal operation are especially difficult to diagnose.[151]

Nine out of 10 intussusceptions are associated with lymphoid hyperplasia in Peyer's patches of the ileum[152] and a viral aetiology is invoked in many cases,[153,154] often with a preceding upper respiratory tract infection.

Clinical features

The infant presents acutely with severe colicky abdominal pain and vomiting. Many will scream, draw up their knees and develop marked pallor of the face; others are lethargic. Between attacks of colic the infant may appear in good health but the wise clinician will listen carefully to the parents' history and not be misled. There may be a recent change in diet such as weaning from milk on to solids. The first stools passed after the start of the illness are unremarkable; the blood and mucus or 'redcurrant jelly' stool is passed after the first 24 hours and may be an even later manifestation.

The cooperation of the patient is essential while examining the abdomen, and sedation may be required. When the anterior abdominal wall is relaxed a sausage-shaped mass may be palpable, most often in the upper abdomen. A rectal examination is of utmost importance as blood will be found in the rectum in the majority of cases and occasionally the apex of the intussusception is palpable.

The diagnosis may be confirmed by ultrasound scanning[155] or by a barium enema examination (Fig. 41.20). The apex of the intussusception will obstruct the passage of barium.

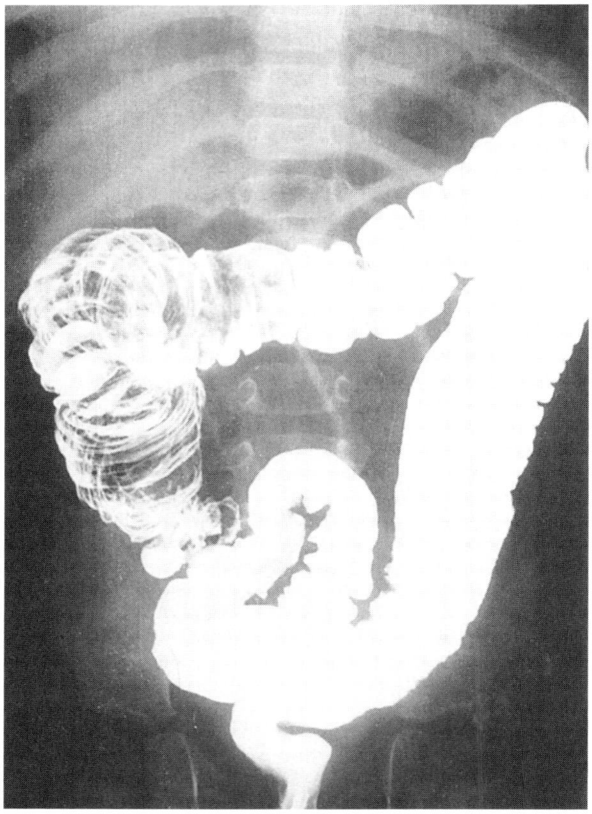

Fig. 41.20 Barium enema in a child with an ileocolic intussusception. The barium outlines the intussusception with a coiled-spring appearance.

Management

Hydrostatic reduction of intussusceptions is an established form of treatment.[156,157] The patient should be adequately sedated and prepared for a laparotomy with blood cross-matched and intravenous fluids being administered. Following a diagnostic barium enema, the reduction is attempted by elevating the reservoir of barium 1 metre above the level of the abdomen. The progress of the reduction is monitored by radiological screening and is complete when barium fills loops of ileum. If there is a hold-up at the ileocaecal valve the attempt at reduction may be repeated after 6 hours. In many reported series,[158] the majority of intussusceptions are successfully reduced hydrostatically. Air enemas on unsedated infants are becoming increasingly used with successful reductions occurring more rapidly.[159]

Operative management is indicated in patients with signs of established peritonitis, radiological signs of perforation or failure of radiological reduction. The abdomen is opened through a transverse incision to the right of the umbilicus; a muscle-splitting incision in the right iliac fossa is adequate if the intussusception is confined to the right colon. Reduction is achieved by squeezing the distal colon and pushing the intussuscepted bowel proximally; this process may be started intra-abdominally until the intussusception is small enough to be delivered through the incision. It is then wrapped in warm saline packs and several minutes may be required for the final reduction through the ileocaecal valve. At no time should traction be applied to the proximal ileum.

REFERENCES

144. Ravitch M M Pediatric Surgery, 4th edn vol 2. Year Book, Chicago 1986
145. Goodhead B Br J Surg 1966; 53: 626
146. Bisset W H Hamilton Bailey's Emergency Surgery, 11th edn. Bristol, Wright 1986
147. Beck A R, Leichtling J J Mt Sinai J Med 1972; 39: 397
148. Fripp R R, Karabus C D S Afr Med J 1977; 52: 617
149. Browne A F et al J Pediatr Surg 1983; 18: 7
150. Ein S H et al J Pediatr Surg 1986; 21: 786
151. Ein S H, Ferguson J M Arch Dis Child 1982; 57: 788
152. Editorial Lancet 1985; 2: 250
153. Nicholas J L et al J Med Virol 1982; 9: 267
154. Gardner P S et al Br Med J 1962; 2: 697
155. Pracros J P, Tran-Minh V A, Wright C Lancet 1985; 2: 733
156. Hipsley P L Med J Aust 1926; 2: 201
157. Ravitch M M, McCune R M Ann Surg 1948; 128: 904
158. Paes R A, Hyde I, Griffiths D M Br J Radiol 1988; 61: 187
159. Stringer M D, Brereton F J, Pablot S M Br J Surg 1992; 79: 867

Resection of bowel is indicated if reduction is impossible or there is a segment of non-viable bowel. Primary anastomosis is recommended either following a limited ileal resection or a modified right hemi-colectomy. If an anatomical lead point, such as a Meckel's diverticulum, is present, this should be resected. An appendicectomy may be performed except when the base of the caecum is very oedematous or haemorrhagic.

Recurrence following successful management of an intussusception is approximately 3%.[160] A first recurrence may be managed with hydrostatic reduction but, in a rare second recurrence, a laparotomy should be considered, looking for a lead point.

Mortality and bowel resection for gangrene are both related to delay in diagnosis.[161] Endotoxic shock may be associated with ischaemic bowel and present with a tachycardia, hypotension and low central venous pressure. Management includes the administration of large volumes of intravenous 4.5% albumin in repeated boluses of 10–20 ml/kg and broad-spectrum antibiotics.

REFERENCES

160. Nixon H H Surgical Conditions in Paediatrics. Butterworth, London 1978
161. Stringer M D, Pledger G, Drake D P Br Med J 1992; 304: 737

Table 42.1 Classification of orthopaedic pathology

A. Deformities 1. *Pathological dislocations* including: Congenital dislocation of hip Knee Foot: talipes, flat foot, toes Hand and wrist Spine: scoliosis 2. *Pathological contractures* including: Torticollis Trigger finger Dupuytren's contracture 3. *Angular and torsional deformities* including: Upper limb and hand Lower limb: genu valgum, genu varus 4. *Limb size disparities* **B. Dysplasias** including abnormalities of stature 1. *Epiphyseal dysplasias* including: Multiple epiphyseal dysplasia Dysplasia epiphysealis hemimelica Chondrodysplasia punctata Hereditary arthro-ophthalmopathy Cretinism 2. *Metaphyseal dysplasias* including: Classical achondroplasia Hypochondroplasia Metaphyseal chondroplasia Chondro-ectodermal dysplasia 3. *Diaphyseal dysplasias* including: Progressive diaphyseal dysplasia Spondylo-epiphyseal dysplasia Pseudo-achondroplasia 4. *Altered bone density* including: Reduced: Osteogenesis imperfecta Idiopathic juvenile osteoporosis The osteolyses Increased: Osteopetrosis Paget's disease Pyknodysostosis Sclerosterosis Hypophosphatasia Pachydermoperiostitis 5. *Anarchic development of the skeleton* including: Diaphyseal aclasis Dyschondroplasia	Ollier's disease/Maffucci's syndrome Polyostotic fibrous dysplasia Melorheostosis Osteopoikilosis Osteopathia striata **C. Metabolic skeletal changes** 1. Osteoporosis 2. Osteomalacia/rickets 3. Hyperparathyroidism **D. Acquired changes of the epiphysis** 1. Osteochondritis and osteonecrosis, including Perthes' disease 2. Epiphyseal trauma **E. Osteomyelitis** **F. Arthritis** 1. *Acute septic arthritis* 2. *Polyarthritis* including: Still's disease Systemic lupus erythematosus Rheumatoid arthritis Ankylosing spondylitis Psoriatic arthropathy Reiter's syndrome 3. *Osteoarthritis* 4. *Crystal deposition disorders* including: Gout Pseudogout 5. *Aseptic prosthetic joint inflammation* 6. *Haemarthrosis* **G. Neoplasms** 1. *Osteogenic* 2. *Chondrogenic* 3. *Others* including: Multiple myeloma Non-Hodgkin's lymphoma Vascular tumours Fibrogenic tumours Ewing's sarcoma Synovial sarcoma Osteoclastoma Simple bone cysts Fibrous dysplasia Metastases **H. Pathological fractures**

Intramedullary rod fixation was pioneered by Kuntscher[20] and joint replacement by Smith-Petersen[21] and Sir John Charnley.[22] More recently, there have been major advances in imaging of the skeleton, in the electrical induction of bone healing, in transplantation of bone and cartilage, and in microsurgery and arthroscopic surgery.

DEFORMITIES

Pathological dislocations

Developmental (congenital) dislocation of the hip

Congenital dislocation of the hip (Fig. 42.1a), now termed developmental dysplasia because of uncertainty about its exact aetiology, is one of the more common skeletal conditions of childhood. Instability of the hip occurs in some 5 cases per 1000 live births, with late, established dislocation in 1–2 per thousand. In many instances there is a strong family history and a predominance in females, although this is less marked in late cases. Breech presentation, caesarean section and being the first-born child are other recognized factors. The geographical incidence varies throughout the world, being high in the Po valley of northern Italy, in Lapland and in North American Indians. The causes of hip instability are thought to be capsular laxity, acetabular anteversion and possibly subclinical neuromuscular abnormality. At birth the abnormal hip can be categorized as lax, dislocated, or having acetabular dysplasia, with slow deterioration of the hip in later adult life. A very rare form of dislocation, termed 'teratogenic',

REFERENCES

20. Küntscher G B G J Bone Surg 40a 1958 Vol 17
21. Smith-Peterson M N J Bone Joint Surg 1931; 21: 269
22. Charnley J. In: Low Friction Arthroplasty of the Hip. Springer, Berlin 1979

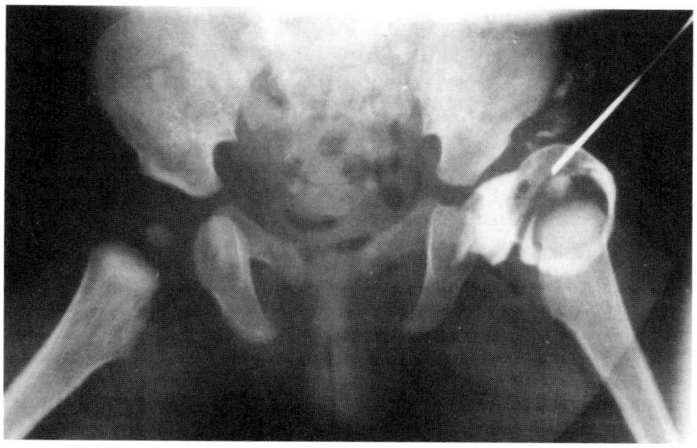

a

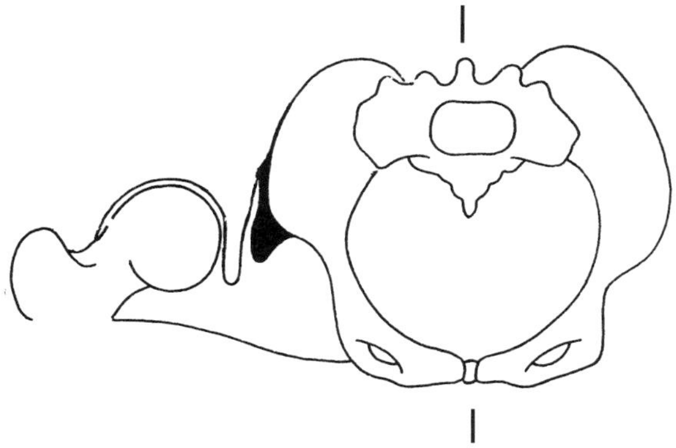

b

Fig. 42.1 (**a**) A congenital dislocation of the hip shown on arthrography. (**b**) Soft tissue obstruction prevents closed reduction in the child of walking age.

may occur in utero, and is not amenable to any form of conservative therapy. In full dislocation the two articular surfaces are not in opposition. The diagnostic sign is elicited at birth by separating the infant's flexed thighs and noting the jump or thud as the femoral head slips back into its socket in the mid range of abduction.[23]

Splintage with the hips 90° abducted and 90° flexed produces a successful outcome in about 98% of cases if the instability is identified at birth. If, on the other hand, the hip is allowed to remain dislocated, obstruction from the infolded labrum (limbus) and the hypertrophic round ligament eventually prevents reduction without surgical intervention. Once the child starts to walk, the restricted hip movement causes gait abnormalities, the limb appears shortened with pelvic asymmetry and there is an anterior groin 'lump' sign. The limb may be extremely rotated and abduction is limited. The child walks with a limp, although this is difficult to identify if both hips are dislocated. Contracture of the inferior capsule and compression from the tendon of the iliopsoas muscle make closed reduction more difficult, and gradually the acetabulum becomes flatter and the femoral head misshapen. There may be further reduction in acetabular circumferential growth if the head of the femur abuts against the outer lip of the acetabulum (Fig. 42.1b), making late dysplasia and deformity almost inevitable in spite of surgical intervention and reduction of the femoral head.[24]

The complications of treatment include failure of the initial traction and splintage, from pressure of the proximal femur to produce reduction, epiphyseal and growth plate damage (with residual coxa magna and vara) and redislocation of the femoral head. This is particularly likely if a soft tissue obstruction has not been recognized and removed, or if there is an underlying neurological abnormality. Screening programmes at birth must identify hip instability in as many cases as possible if sciatic nerve damage and other surgical complications are to be avoided. The adjunctive use of ultrasound testing of the hip and re-examination of the infant at six weeks and ten months of age have reduced the incidence of late diagnosis.[25] Major surgical intervention in the form of pelvic and proximal femoral osteotomies should gradually become less necessary, and the long-term outcome of osteoarthritis and secondary back and knee problems should eventually be prevented as a result of vigilance in childhood.

Knee

Pathological dislocation of the knee

Pathological dislocation rarely affects the knee, but is occasionally seen at birth, often in association with dislocated hips and club foot deformities. The knee is hyperextended, and the anterior structures become secondarily tightened, so that reduction may require quadricepsplasty and lengthening of anterior structures to allow the establishment of knee flexion, although this is always restricted. The patella may also be dislocated at birth (congenital) or may be habitually unstable during early to mid childhood. The quadriceps mechanism is again often tight, so that the patella usually displaces laterally either in flexion or extension. The pathological process is analogous to hip dysplasia, as the femoral sulcus fails to develop fully if the patella is allowed to remain out of place or if it is positioned too proximally. This destroys the coaptive relationship between the two bones that is so important for their successful development. Recurrent lateral patellar dislocation may occur in later childhood and early adolescence as a result of sudden growth or trauma. This may be associated with persistent femoral anteversion and other torsion abnormalities of the lower limb.

Foot

Club foot/congenital talipes

Congenital talipes equinovarus is caused by a pathological dislocation of the talonavicular joint (see Chapter 49). Club foot is now the most common orthopaedic congenital condition and is encountered in approximately 2 per 1000 babies (Fig. 42.2a).[23] Almost 40% are bilateral, when the condition tends to be more severe. It affects boys two and a half times more often than girls and the condition is more common in Polynesian, Mediterranean and

REFERENCES

23. Barlow T D J Bone Joint Surg 1962; 44B: 242
24. Benson M K D, Fixsen J A, Macnicol M F In: Children's Orthopaedics and Fractures. Churchill Livingstone, Edinburgh 1994
25. Burman L, Klennerman L Br Med J 1986; 293: 719

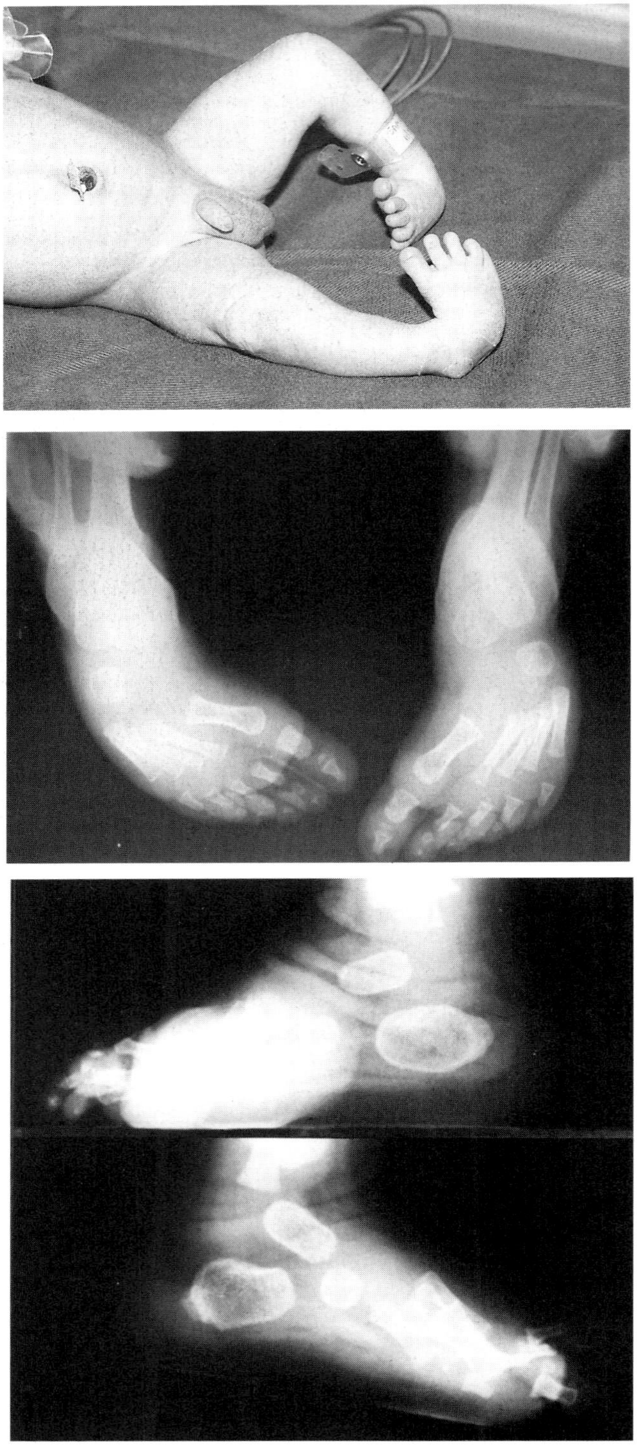

a

b

c

Fig. 42.2 (a) Congenital talipes equinovarus (club foot) is a complex, torsional deformity of the talonavicular and subtalar joints. **(b, c)** Anteroposterior and lateral radiographs show the bony deformities associated with talipes.

Middle Eastern races. Spinal dysraphism and other congenital abnormalities such as tracheo-oesophageal fistula and anorectal and atresia may also be present.

The inheritance of club foot is considered to be polygenic, but there is a high incidence in some families and in some races. The cause of the condition is probably multifactorial, but arrested development of foot positioning during the second uterine month (when equinovarus is a normal posture) is a major factor.[26] In some cases obvious structural abnormalities are present, including abnormal tendon insertions, idiopathic fibrosis and defective development of the tarsal bones. Although club foot is commonly seen in association with neuromuscular conditions, electrophysiological and histological studies of both nerve and muscle show variable pathological changes.[27] The foot typically has a small inverted heel with a deep medial crease, the hind foot is in equinus, and the forefoot is adducted and supinated (Fig. 42.2a). The primary abnormality appears to be wasting of the calf muscle, which becomes more evident in later childhood. The talus and the fibula are rotated externally, with variable changes in the tarsal bones.

Radiographs may help to define the deformities and usually demonstrate a characteristic reduction in the talocalcaneal angle of divarication,[28] which is reduced on the anteroposterior view (Fig. 42.2b) from approximately 25° to virtually zero, and on the lateral view (Fig. 42.2c) from approximately 35° to 10° or less. As with all pathological dislocations, a complex deformity develops, combining rotational, sagittal and coronal malalignments. The treatment and presentation of this condition are discussed in Chapter 49.

Flat foot

Subluxation of the talocalcaneal joint in the opposite direction to talipes increases the talocalcaneal angle and produces a flat foot at birth. This may either be a relatively benign and temporary postural abnormality, known as calcaneovalgus, or may produce the relatively rare condition of congenital vertical talus (convex pes valgus). Most cases of calcaneovalgus are postural and recover fully, with or without stretching. Very occasionally the condition is acquired in association with poliomyelitis, arthrogryposis or myelomeningocele. A vertical talus may be associated with the same conditions and also with neurofibromatosis.

Toes

In early childhood, deviations of the toes (curly toes) are a source of considerable concern to parents but generally require no treatment (Fig. 42.3). An overriding fifth toe may require either a soft tissue realignment or amputation, as may the following common toe deformities (see Chapter 49):

1. Claw toe (flexion of the proximal and distal interphalangeal joints with extension of the metatarsophalangeal joint). The latter joint may become dislocated and the condition is thought to be caused by neuromuscular imbalance. When it is mobile, tendon transfers may suffice, but the rigid deformity is often best managed by proximal interphalangeal joint fusion, coupled with capsulotomy of the metatarsophalangeal joint (see Chapter 49).

REFERENCES

26. Browne D Arch Dis Child 1955; 30: 37
27. Macnicol M F Curr Ortho 1994; 8: 72
28. Simons G W Clin Orthop 1978; 135: 107

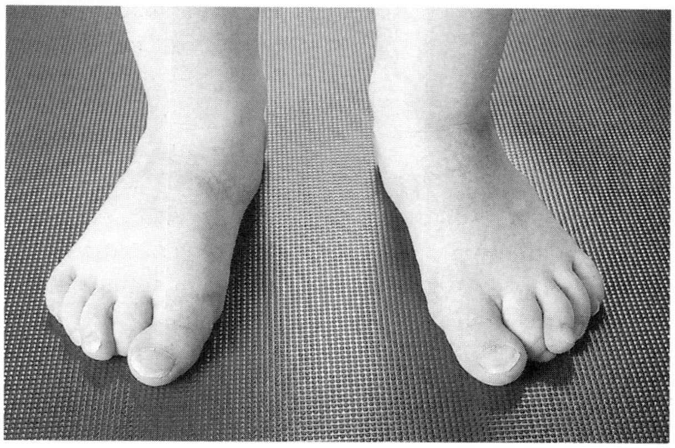

Fig. 42.3 Curly second toes.

2. Hammer toe (flexion of the proximal interphalangeal joint is combined with extension of both the metatarsophalangeal and distal interphalangeal joints). In such cases, proximal interphalangeal joint fusion or proximal phalangectomy may be considered; in gross cases of associated hallux valgus, the affected second toe may require amputation (see Chapter 49).

3. Mallet toe (flexion of the distal interphalangeal joints). Terminal phalangectomy or distal interphalangeal joint fusion is required if painful callosities develop (see Chapter 49).

Other pathological dislocations

Comparable pathological subluxations develop in the upper limb of the rheumatoid patient, with the 'boutonniere' deformity similar to hammer toe, and the 'swan-neck' deformity similar to mallet toe. Dislocations of the fingers and thumbs are usually caused by trauma or an inflammatory process, but congenital dislocation of the wrist, as in radial club hand, may occur as a primary defect of skeletal development. Dislocation of the shoulder is usually considered to be secondary to incompetence of the glenohumeral joint, although it may be precipitated by trauma or overuse.

Deviation or dislocation of the spine produces torticollis, scoliosis, kyphosis and hyperlordosis (see Chapter 46). As with limb dislocation, the spinal deformity develops as a result of both lateral curvature and rotation (Fig. 42.4). The scoliotic curve is described in the degree of angulation of the convexity, and tends to progress during childhood growth (see Chapter 46). Curves may be single, double or triple and may affect the cervical, thoracic, thoracolumbar and lumbar regions of the spine. Idiopathic scoliosis may be of early or late onset, and this is important as early onset causes cardiopulmonary complications.[29]

Idiopathic scoliosis may result from neuromuscular imbalance with abnormal skeletal growth as in most cases of club foot. Various congenital anomalies such as unilateral or bilateral unsegmented bars, hemivertebrae, mixed vertebral lesions and diastematomyelia also produce scoliosis. Scoliosis may also result from spondylolisthesis, fractures, infections (pyogenic or tuberculous), spondylosis (osteoarthritis) and neoplasia.

Neuropathic causes of scoliosis include poliomyelitis, neurofibromatosis, myelomeningocele, cerebral palsy, syringomyelia and a variety of other spinal cord and central nervous system disorders.

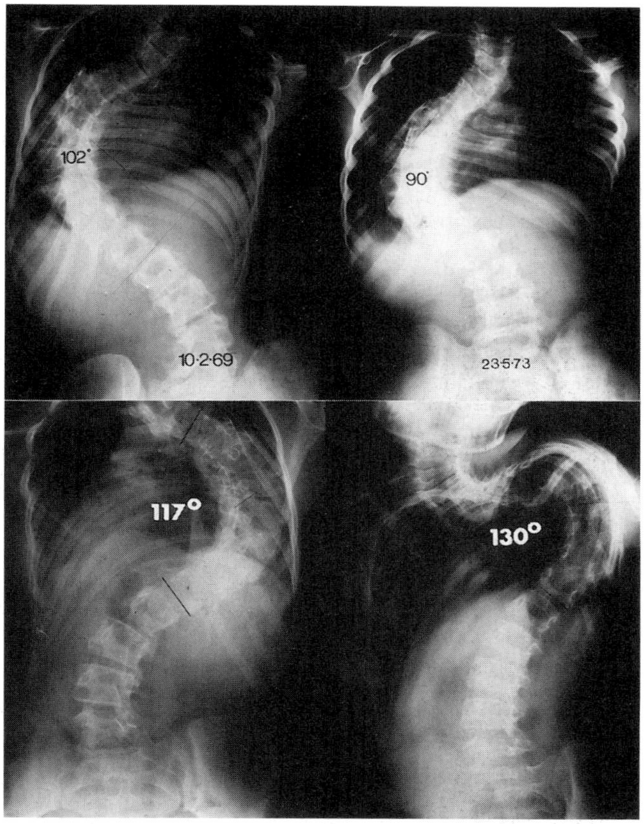

Fig. 42.4 Increasing severity of scoliosis.

Muscular causes include muscular dystrophy, arthrogryposis and congenital myopathy. Spinal deformity also complicates a variety of skeletal dysplasias such as spondylo-epiphyseal dysplasia, Morquio's syndrome and other mucopolysaccharide disorders. Scoliosis can also be caused by both osseous and intraspinal tumours, irradiation and trauma, and may develop following surgical procedures such as thoracoplasty (see Chapter 46).

Contractures

Many deformities encountered in orthopaedics develop secondary to contracture.

Torticollis (wryneck)

This is produced by a similar torsional and angulatory deformity to scoliosis and develops secondary to fibrosis of the sternomastoid muscle (Fig. 42.5). There is no clear association between torticollis and a difficult birth with forceps delivery, and therefore the traumatic theory of its development is difficult to sustain. Nevertheless, it does appear that some form of compartment syndrome affects the sternomastoid muscle, leaving it scarred and inelastic on one side; this may be the result of a congenital abnormality of

REFERENCES

29. Davies G, Reid L Arch Dis Child 1971; 46: 623

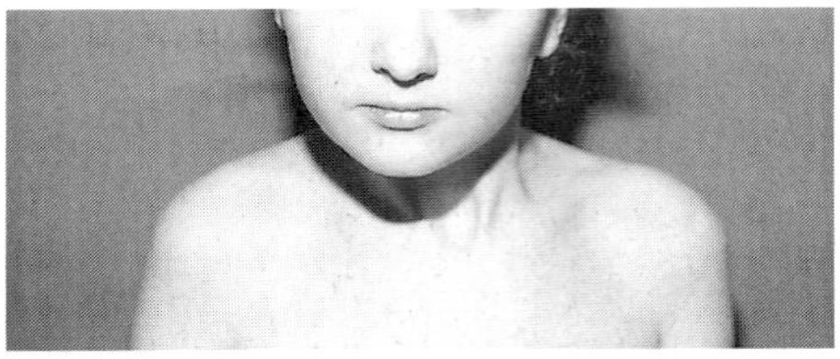

Fig. 42.5 Torticollis produced by sternomastoid fibrosis.

the muscle or an infection. In some cases torticollis is secondary to vertebral abnormalities, while in later childhood the onset of torticollis may result from soft tissue injury or unilateral facet joint dislocation or subluxation (see Chapter 46).

Trigger digit

Contracted soft tissue also results in a trigger digit, the thumb being involved at least 80% of the time.[30] Triggering and flexion deformity are rarely noted at birth, and therefore appear to be secondary to some other acquired pathology (see Chapter 45). Children present either in the first year of life or at some time during infancy. In adult life, trauma and inflammatory conditions are the principal causes of triggering of the fingers.

Dupuytren's contracture

Dupuytren's contracture is a progressive fibrosis that involves the longitudinal bands of the palmar fascia (see Chapter 45).

Angulatory and torsional deformities

Upper limb

Angulatory deformities of the upper limb may occur at the wrist and elbow and include conditions such as Madelung's deformity, where the radius is shortened and accompanied by a dorsoradial convexity. As a result, normal ulnar growth results in dislocation of the distal radio-ulnar joint and flexural contractures of the elbow. Radial head dislocation may also cause rotation of the forearm and a congenital radio-ulnar synostosis with contracture of the interosseous membrane. The synostosis may also be inherited as an autosomal dominant condition and affects males more than females. Usually the radial head is present but fused to the ulna, although there is also a 'headless' variety which is usually bilateral. The radius appears bowed and thickened, and the involved arm is usually thinner than normal with the forearm fixed in mid- or hyperpronation.

Radial club hand

Radial club hand occurs as the result of complete or partial absence of the radius, leading to a short and radially deviated forearm with angulation of the ulna.[31] The condition is bilateral in half the cases and hand function may be improved by centralizing the carpus on the distal end of the ulna in selected cases. Many cases were caused by maternal thalidomide ingestion.

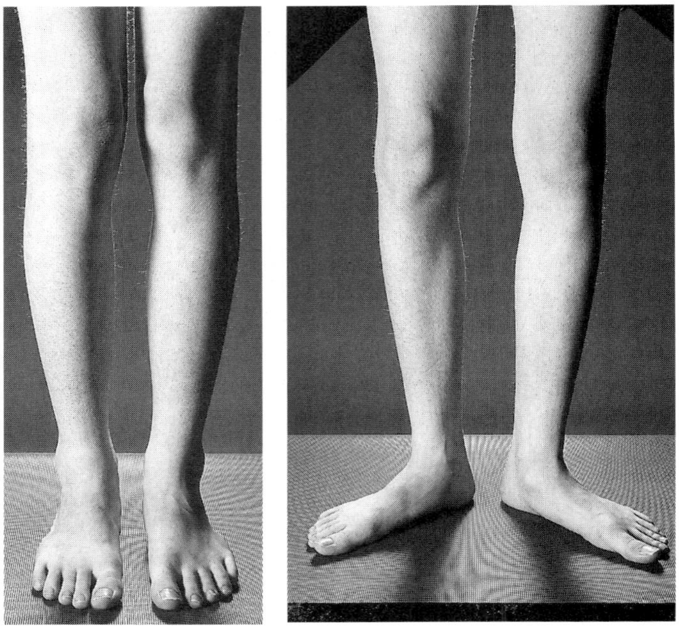

a b

Fig. 42.6 (a) Persistent femoral anteversion causing the knees to squint inwards. (b) External tibial torsion develops as a compensation.

Lower limb

Most torsional and angulatory deformities of the lower limb are relatively mild, particularly when the deformity is symmetrical (Fig. 42.6). The causes of 'intoeing' include anteversion of the acetabulum and femur, genu varum, internal tibial torsion and metatarsus adductus. A secondary form of 'intoeing' develops when the child has flat feet during earlier childhood, and walks in this manner to reduce pronation of the feet.

Genu varum

Bow legs (genu varum) in infancy is usually a transient and developmental appearance, but occasionally the genu varum is secondary to rickets, growth plate trauma, Blount's disease[32] or metaphyseal dysostosis. The condition may be more significant if there is asymmetry between the legs, and later corrective surgery may be indicated (see Chapter 48).

Genu valgum

In the pre-school child genu valgum (knock knees) is quite common, especially among girls or boys with ligament laxity. This condition usually corrects during childhood, but the appearance should be monitored annually if there is any concern. Genu valgum may be caused by metabolic bone disease, trauma or a skeletal dysplasia.

REFERENCES

30. Slakey J B, Hennrikus W L J Bone Joint Surg 1996; 78B: 481
31. Lamb D W J Bone Joint Surg 1977; 59A: 168
32. Langenskiold A, Riska E B J Bone Joint Surg 1964; 46A: 1405

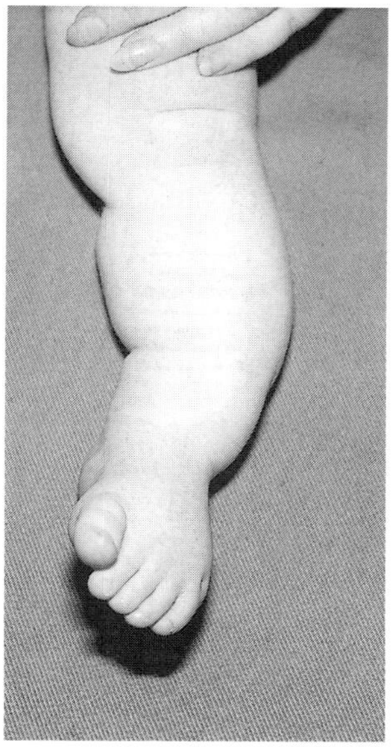
a

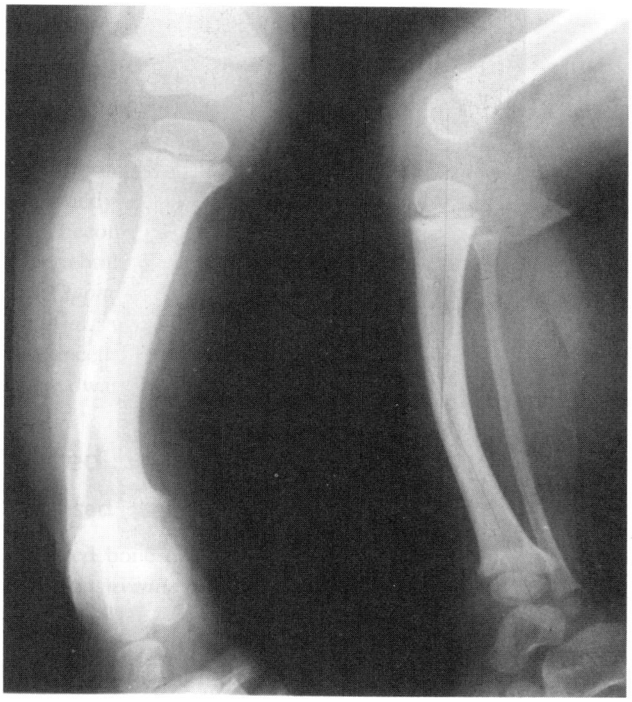
b

Fig. 42.7 (**a**) Anterolateral tibial angulation. (**b**) Radiographic appearance.

Coxa vara, angulatory deformity of the tibia, pseudarthrosis of the tibia and fibula, congenital absence of the fibula

Rare but important deformities of the lower limb include coxa vara, which may be associated with a pseudarthrosis or femoral shortening, and angulatory deformity of the tibia. Posteromedial bowing of the tibia usually corrects, but anterolateral angulation (Fig. 42.7) is usually associated with a pseudarthrosis of the tibia, and this is a very difficult condition to treat effectively.

In pseudarthrosis of the fibula, there is bowing of the fibula and the deformity may be associated with ankle deformity or with the later appearance of a tibial pseudarthrosis.[33] Shortening and angulation of the leg below the knee also develops in congenital absence of the fibula.

Anomalies of limb size

The congenital patterns of limb abnormality are a failure of the limb to form, a failure of the limb to differentiate, duplication, gigantism, hypoplasia and the presence of a constriction band.

Failure of limb formation

The deficiency may be terminal intercalary and transverse or longitudinal.[34] This classification allows the absence of a digit, hand or foot, or more major amputations to be treated appropriately.

Gigantism

Hemihypertrophy of a limb can also occur and may be either total or partial (involving nerve, muscle, vessels or bone). Leg length inequality is the common result (Fig. 42.8) and requires treatment if the discrepancy is greater than 2 cm.

Limb length inequality

The causes of this condition include:

1. Congenital disorders such as proximal femoral focal deficiency, short or absent tibia, congenital dislocation of the hip, and either hemihypertrophy or hemiatrophy. Congenital soft tissue abnormalities that may be responsible include haemangioma, Klippel–Trenaunay syndrome and arteriovenous fistula (see Chapter 10), neurofibromatosis (see Chapter ll) and arthrogryposis.
2. Abnormal bone growth such as achondroplasia, fibrous dysplasia, enchondromatosis and pseudarthrosis of the tibia.
3. Neurological abnormalities such as poliomyelitis, cerebral palsy and hemiplegia.
4. Trauma including epiphyseal pressure lesions, premature epiphyseal growth plate closure, malunion and overgrowth after childhood fractures or infections. Infections such as septic arthritis or tuberculosis also cause limb length inequality.
5. Inflammatory conditions such as juvenile chronic arthritis may produce limb length inequality, and occasionally a pelvic obliquity secondary to torticollis results in leg length discrepancy.

REFERENCES

33. Morrissy R T, Riseborough E J, Hall J E J Bone Joint Surg 1981; 63B: 367
34. Entin M, Barsky A, Swanson A The Hand 1972; 4: 215

Other avascular necrosis

Avascular necrosis can occur after fractures or as a result of Caisson or sickle cell disease. Sites that have a poor blood supply, such as like the femoral head, the scaphoid and the lunate bones, appear to be particularly susceptible. The arterial supply or venous drainage may be cut off or the capillaries may become occluded. The bone dies and then repairs if the blood supply is restored. The condition causes pain and loss of movement.

Trauma to the epiphysis

Injury to the epiphysis may cause deformity and later osteoarthritis. The hip joint may dislocate if a tense effusion or pus under pressure remains untreated. Injury to the growth plate, whether partial or complete, can cause angulatory deformity and shortening of the limb. Early diagnosis is essential if a stiff, painful and shortened limb is to be avoided.

Slipped upper femoral epiphysis

In later childhood and early adolescence thinning of the periosteum and perichondrial ring of the growth plate may allow the upper femoral epiphysis to slip. It displaces posteromedially and inferiorly, leading to a loss of hip flexion and both external rotation and adduction deformities. Slipped upper femoral epiphysis occurs in approximately 1 per 100 000 of the population, and males are twice as commonly affected. The condition may be bilateral in over a quarter of the cases. The peak incidence is 12 years in girls and 14 in boys. The left hip is more commonly affected than the right. Some children are obese endomorphs and a smaller number are tall and thin aesthetics. In addition to rapid growth, endocrine abnormalities, irradiation and chemotherapy may predispose a child to the condition.

The slip develops through the growth plate initially; during the pre-slipping stage this may appear widened, and there is then either a rapid progression of the slip or a relatively minor displacement which appears to heal without causing many symptoms. It appears that the physis is unable to resist the sheer stress resulting from the increase in upper body weight. The femoral shaft becomes externally rotated and the neck displaces forwards. The 'frog lateral' X-ray projection allows the extent of the epiphyseal slip to be assessed. This varies from mild (5–30° of angulation), to moderate (30–60°) to severe (60–90°).

Weakening of the growth plate may occur in children with panhypopituitarism, Down's syndrome and the Schmidt syndrome. The lesion can be produced in the rat by inducing lathyrism, and growth hormone supplements have also been noted experimentally to decrease the shear stress of the physis.

Epiphyseal injuries

Growth plate injuries are categorized using the Salter & Harris[48] classification (Fig. 42.14). For practical purposes, the site and extent of the intra-articular fracture line and the degree of initial chondro-epiphyseal displacement determine management.[49] The junction between mineralizing cartilage and the metaphysis is biomechanically the weakest point (see Chapter 50).

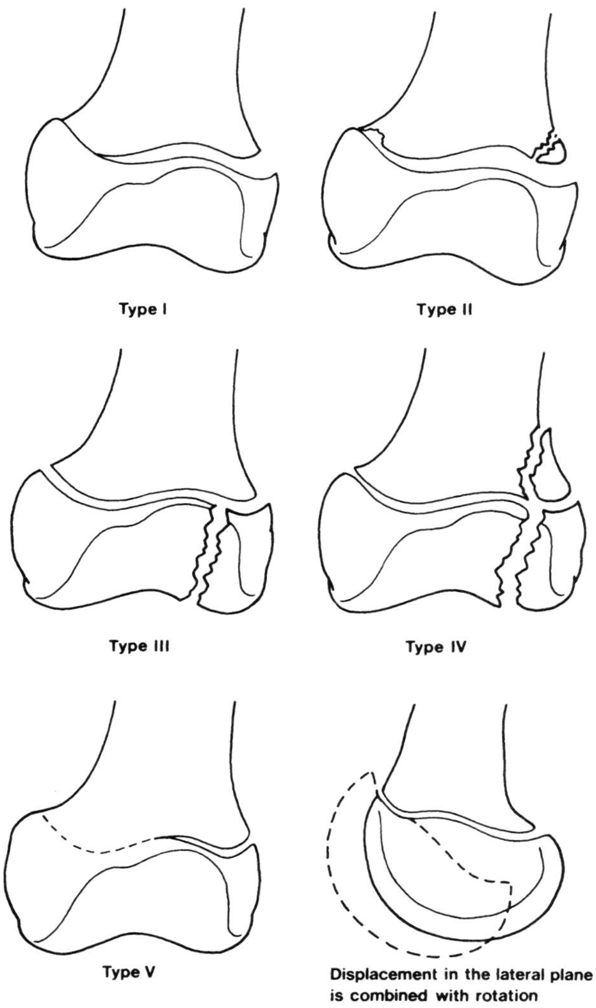

Fig. 42.14 Classification of epiphyseal fractures.[48]

Injuries to the growth plate account for just under 20% of all paediatric fractures, and although it is suggested that approximately 15% of the injuries may cause physeal arrest, accurate open reduction and internal fixation of these fractures reduces the rate of premature growth arrest to less than 2% (see Chapter 50).

Other epiphyseal disorders

The epiphysis is also affected in other conditions such as juvenile chronic arthritis and haemophilia (see Chapter 3). Inflammatory changes induce hyperaemic enlargement of the epiphysis, and although this may not alter congruity, joint function is usually adversely affected, particularly if the articular cartilage is damaged.

REFERENCES

48. Salter R B, Harris W R J Bone Joint Surg 1963; 45A: 587
49. Poland J In: Separation of the Epiphysis. Smith Elder, London 1898

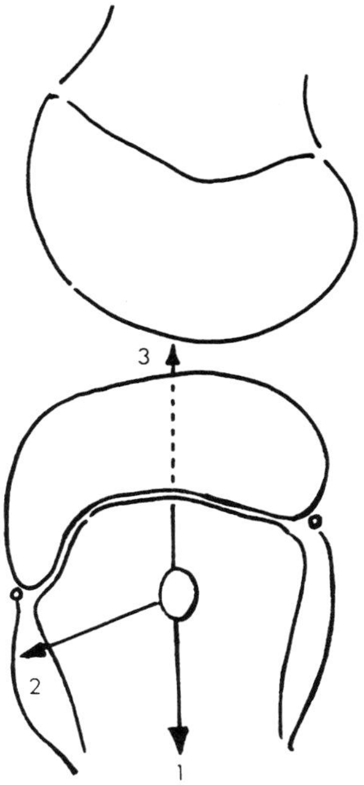

Fig. 42.15 The routes of spread of infection from the metaphysis. 1. To the medulla; 2. Subperiosteal; 3. Into the joint.

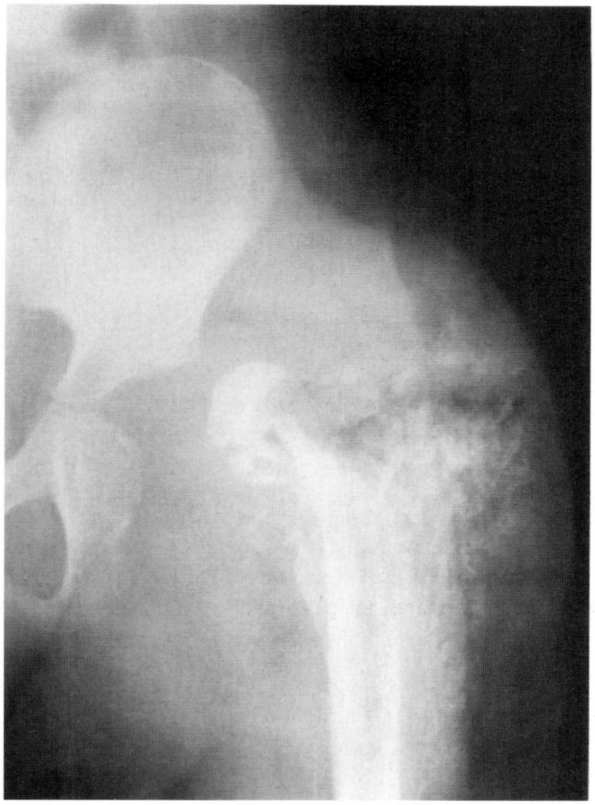

Fig. 42.16 Osteomyelitis of the metaphysis leading to septic arthritis and dislocation of the hip.

OSTEOMYELITIS

This is an infection of bone which usually commences in the metaphyseal region of children. It may be acquired from haematogenous spread, or by direct skin puncture following an injury. It may develop after operations, when it can affect any age group. Rarely, it is caused by local spread from infected adjacent soft tissue. Infection may spread to the epiphysis and joint in the manner shown in Figure 42.15.

The infection produced may be evanescent, or established, when both pus and bone necrosis occur. The acute form is more common in boys, peaks in incidence in the autumn, and is associated with lower socioeconomic status. Adults only tend to be affected when they are immunosuppressed. Acute haematogenous osteomyelitis may lead on to the more chronic form with both sequestrum and involucrum formation. A sequestrum is the necrotic nidus of bone within a focus of chronic osteomyelitis while an involucrum is a cloak of new bone produced by the periosteum around the infection. There is a subacute variety of osteomyelitis which accounts for up to one third of all haematogenous cases. Once again, males are two or three times as commonly affected; patients are usually under the age of 20 years. A chronic bone abscess may develop, and this is called a Brodie's abscess if it affects the tibia.[50] A sclerosing form of osteomyelitis is also recognized and is known as Garré's osteomyelitis. Infection depends upon the virulence of the pathogen and the size of the inoculum. *Staphylococcus aureus* accounts for most cases of osteomyelitis[51] but other organisms can be responsible including *Streptococcus pyogenes* or *pneumoniae*, *E. coli*, *Haemophilus influenzae*, *Salmonella*, *Proteus*, *Pseudomonas*, *Brucella*, *Klebsiella* and anaerobic organisms.[52] Occasionally tuberculosis, fungal infections and viruses such as smallpox, rubella and chickenpox may be responsible; these opportunistic infections develop in immunocompromised or debilitated patients such as drug addicts.

As the bacteria multiply, an acute inflammatory response is mounted with vascular engorgement, oedema and polymorphonuclear cell aggregation. Tissue cell death occurs secondary to ischaemia from both venous and arterial obstruction, and this completes the picture. The resultant abscess gradually enlarges and may spread to the subperiosteal space, to the medulla and, rarely, to the joint itself through vessels which cross the growth plate and epiphyseal cartilage (Fig. 42.16). The growth disturbance which may follow infection during infancy depends upon the volume of the growth plate affected, the location of the destructive process—whether this develops in the germinal or hypertrophic layers, and whether it is central or peripheral—and how badly the epiphysis and its cartilage canal systems are invaded and destroyed. Eventually resolution may occur with fibrosis and new bone formation. This may result in sclerosis and bone thickening.

REFERENCES

50. Thomson A Edin Med Journal 1906; 19: 297
51. Nade S Arch Dis Child 1977; 52: 679
52. Anderson J R, Orr J D, Maclean D A, Arch Dis Childhood 1980; 55: 953

Table 42.5 Staging of articular tuberculosis and its outcome in children

Stages	*Clinical*	*Radiology*	*Usual effective treatment*	*Expectation*
I Synovitis	Movement present (> 75%)	Soft tissue swelling, osteoporosis	Chemotherapy and movement Rarely synovectomy	Retention of near full mobility
II Early arthritis	Movement present (50–75%)	In addition to I, moderate diminution of joint space and marginal erosions	Chemotherapy and movement Rarely synovectomy or debridement	Restoration of 50–75% of mobility
III Advanced arthritis	Loss of movement of > 75% in all directions	In addition to II, marked diminution of joint space and destruction of joint surfaces	Chemotherapy, rarely joint debridement	Ankylosis*
IV Advanced arthritis	Loss of movement of > 75% in all directions	In addition to III, joint is disorganized with dislocation/subluxation	Chemotherapy, rarely joint debridement	Ankylosis*

*After completion of growth, elbow and hip arthritis may be treated by excision arthroplasty

Clinical features

A child with acute osteomyelitis usually presents after several hours of pain, malaise and fever. The child often refuses to walk or to move an affected limb. There is invariably local tenderness over the inflammation; local redness, swelling and oedema are late signs, but joint movement is often painful and the child may scream and refuse to be touched. In adults the signs and symptoms are often attenuated. Acute osteomyelitis has to be distinguished from cellulitis, septic arthritis and acute rheumatoid arthritis.

Investigation

The white cell count is usually raised as is the erythrocyte sedimentation rate. Radiographs may show new bone formation and a late patchy rarefaction. At first no changes may be seen. Radioscintigraphy and MRI scanning detect the earliest changes.[53]

Treatment

This consists of analgesia, antibiotics and rest; if these measures fail, the abscess must be drained through a series of drill holes placed in the bone. The limb is then 'rested' in a splint or plaster cast for several weeks.

Subacute osteomyelitis (acute non-fulminating)

Roberts et al[54] classified subacute osteomyelitis. The tibia, femur and tarsal bones are commonly involved, and infection of the os calcis may result from heel stab blood sampling at birth. The presentation is less dramatic than acute osteomyelitis and the diagnosis may be missed. Antibiotic therapy often aborts subacute osteomyelitis but decompression of the periosteum is advisable if symptoms persist for more than two days after treatment with appropriate antibiotics.

Chronic osteomyelitis

This develops if organisms remain sequestered or if unrecognized bacteria, such as anaerobes, are not treated by the correct antibiotics. There may also be unrecognized antibiotic resistance or tolerance, and the local host defence may be compromised. Chronic osteomyelitis often follows an open fracture or orthopaedic surgery. The same organisms that cause acute osteomyelitis may cause the chronic disorder. Pain, redness and tenderness may be present but are often accompanied by a discharging sinus. Surgical excision of necrotic and poorly vascularized tissue is an important component of management, as is the obliteration of dead space left after surgical drainage. Vascularized free tissue grafts can fill the spaces left by surgical excision and provide a satisfactory blood supply to the area. A squamous skin cancer arising in a persisting sinus is a rare complication.

Syphilis

This is now rare but often causes a severe periostitis and very rarely discrete gummata, which have to be distinguished from chronic localized osteomyelitis.

Brucellosis

This is also rare and usually responds to the appropriate antibiotics.

Tuberculosis

An active or quiescent primary tuberculous focus of infection in the lungs, lymph nodes or other viscera spreads to the skeleton via the nutrient arteries or Batson's plexus of veins.[55] Spinal seeding occurs in the end-plates of contiguous vertebrae, on either side of a disc. Articular infection occurs through subsynovial vessels or from epiphyseal lesions which erode into the joint space. The bone or joint infection is a tertiary infection which only affects 5% of patients with tuberculosis. Multiple abscesses occur in about a third of those infected.

The progress of skeletal tuberculosis is summarized in Table 42.5. Local destruction and demineralization are confined to bone

REFERENCES

53. Barrington N A Br J Hosp Med 1988; 40(6): 464
54. Roberts J M, Drummond D S, Breed A L J Paediatr Orthop 1982; 2: 249
55. Cleveland M, Bosworth D M J Bone Joint Surg 1942; 24: 527

as cartilaginous tissue is resistant. As in pyogenic infections, the growth plate may be injured, resulting in shortening or angulation of the limb or spine. Tuberculous synovitis may produce a pannus and erosions, and small fibrinous 'rice bodies' form in joints, tendon sheaths and bursae. Histology shows granulomata, in which a central area of caseation is surrounded by epitheloid cells (histiocytes), giant cells and lymphocytes. Similar changes can be produced by mycotic infections, brucellosis, sarcoid and leprosy. A 'cold abscess' is formed by the products of caseation and reactive exudation. The abscess tracks along the soft tissue planes and may leak out through sinuses, liberating caseous material, bone debris and tubercle bacilli. It may also pass into the spinal canal and compress the cord. The synovium becomes thickened and bone and cartilage are rapidly destroyed. Patients present with pain, deformity (kyphus) and occasionally a mass in the groin. Lymphocytosis, anaemia and a raised erythrocyte sedimentation rate are indicative of active tuberculosis. The tuberculin (Mantoux) skin test becomes positive a month after the onset of the infection although it may remain negative, especially in immune deficiency states.[56] Radiographs may show soft tissue swelling, osteoporosis, bone destruction and narrowing of the articular space. Bone erosions and collapse are late signs. Nucleotide, CT and MRI scans detect the disease at an earlier stage.[57] The joint should be aspirated. The presence of acid-fast bacilli in the pus which take up a Ziehl–Neelsen stain is highly suggestive of tuberculosis and Lowenstein culture is diagnostic. Treatment is by rest, analgesia and the appropriate anti-tuberculous drugs such as rifampicin, isoniazid and ethambutol. Operative drainage is rarely necessary unless the spinal cord is compromised.

ARTHRITIS

Acute septic arthritis

Joints can become infected by direct infection from a wound, an injection into a joint or an operative procedure on the joint (e.g. arthroscopy). They can also be infected by spread from acute osteomyelitis or through the bloodstream (haematogenous). The same group of organisms implicated in osteomyelitis are usually responsible (see above) but staphylococci and *Haemophilus influenzae* predominate.

The infection usually starts in the synovial membrane, and a seropurulent exudate develops in the synovial fluid. The articular cartilage is progressively destroyed and vascular damage may lead to death of the epiphyseal bone. At this stage infection may spread to the diaphysis or into the overlying tissues to form an abscess which may eventually drain onto the skin through one or more sinuses. Healing is rarely complete unless treatment is started very early. There is often partial loss of articular cartilage and fibrosis within the joint. Bony ankylosis and permanent deformity develop when the articular destruction is severe.

The symptoms and signs are similar to those of acute osteomyelitis although reluctance to move the joint predominates. The joint is also the site of maximum tenderness; it may be swollen and the overlying skin may be red and tender. All the joint movements are restricted. Septic arthritis must be differentiated from acute osteomyelitis, a traumatic synovitis or haemarthrosis. Acute rheumatic fever, rheumatoid arthritis, gout and pseudogout may also have to be considered.

The white cell count and erythrocyte sedimentation rate are usually raised. As in osteomyelitis, plain radiographs are often unhelpful at an early stage but as the condition progresses there are often areas of rarefaction with narrowing and loss of the joint space. Organisms may be grown from blood cultures but ultrasound-guided joint aspiration using a good sterile technique confirms the diagnosis when organisms are seen on microscopy and later cultured.

The treatment is by joint aspiration, analgesia and antibiotics. Formal open drainage may also be required.[58] The final result may be resolution, but secondary osteoarthritis and avascular bone necrosis are common sequelae.

Other arthropathies[59]

Pathological articular changes in arthritis

The normal joint is extremely efficient, with a co-efficient of friction approaching 0.002, compared to steel on ice (0.01) and metal on high density polyethylene (0.08). Lubrication from the synovial fluid ensures that the opposing surfaces of the joint are separated by a thin film of fluid consisting of many molecules. This fluid film produces a mixture of hydrodynamic, elastohydrodynamic and squeeze film lubrication which gives way intermittently to boundary lubrication in which surface deformation sometimes occurs. The efficiency of the synovial joint is proportional to the protein content of the fluid; an effusion therefore diminishes the lubricating properties of the system. Many diseases may damage the functioning of a joint, either by diminishing its lubrication from damage to its articular surfaces, by affecting the surrounding structures, or by a combination of these. Arthritis may affect single joints (monoarthritis) or many (polyarthritis).

Polyarthritides

Conditions which produce acute polyarthritis include rheumatoid arthritis, juvenile chronic arthritis, gout, crystal (pyrophosphate) arthropathy and Reiter's disease. Seronegative arthritis such as psoriatic arthropathies, gonococcal infection, sarcoidosis, leukaemia and rheumatic fever also cause polyarthritides. In children, rheumatic fever, juvenile chronic arthritis and viral infection are the most common causes of synovitis, whereas in the adolescent ankylosing spondylitis, traumatic synovitis and infectious mononucleosis should be considered. The sites of polyarthritis may be peripheral and either symmetrical (commonly rheumatoid arthritis) or asymmetrical (osteoarthritis, gout and psoriatic arthropathy).

REFERENCES

56. Martini M (ed) In: Tuberculosis of the Bone and Joints. Springer, Heidelberg 1988
57. Vohra et al Tuberculous osteo myelitis J Bone J S 1997 79: 562–566
58. Wilson N I L, De Paola M J Bone Joint Surg 1986; 68B: 584
59. Hart F D Br Med J 1971; 2: 210

43 The upper limb and shoulder

R. J. H. Emery

SHOULDER GIRDLE

A prerequisite for efficient upper limb function is a stable yet dynamic fulcrum with the axial skeleton. This is achieved by the scapular suspension mechanism which, with the stabilizing muscles, allows rotation combined with retraction and protraction. In the erect position, the trapezius and levator scapulae support the entire weight of the upper extremity (Fig. 43.1). On raising the arm, the upper fibres of trapezius and levator scapulae pull in a cephalad direction while at the same time the lower fibres of trapezius acting with the rhomboids and latissimus dorsi pull the arm backwards, allowing the upper fibres of trapezius to rotate the scapula.

Functional impairment of the upper limb is seen when there is disruption of the bony or ligamentous structures, weakness of an isolated muscle or global loss of function of the scapular stabilizing muscles.

Winging of the scapula

Trapezius palsy

The major cause of trapezius palsy is injury to the spinal accessory nerve resulting in 'winging' of the scapula (see Chapter 44).

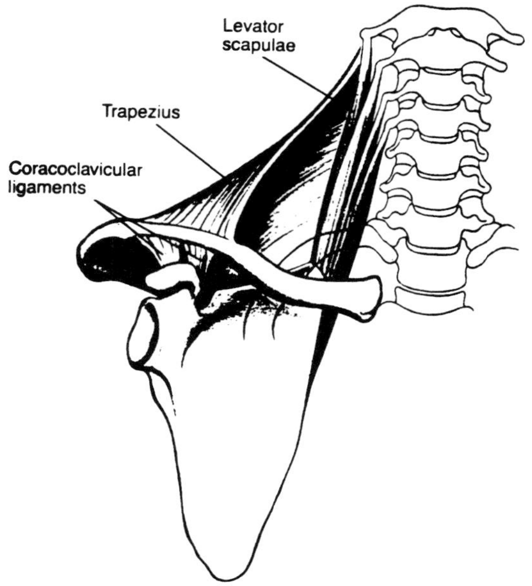

Fig. 43.1 The suspensory mechanism of the shoulder.

Although the dangers of an iatrogenic nerve injury cannot be overstressed, it is important to appreciate that this palsy is commonly seen when the nerve is sacrificed intentionally during radical neck dissection for malignant disease. The ensuing disability can be so great that preservation of the nerve should be encouraged if at all possible.

The spinal accessory nerve is the major nerve supply to trapezius. It leaves the base of the skull through the jugular foramen and passes obliquely through the sternocleidomastoid muscle in its upper third before crossing the posterior triangle of the neck to enter trapezius. It is vulnerable to injury, as it lies very superficially and is at risk with even the simplest surgical operation in the neck region (see Chapters 17). The injury is usually not recognized at the time of surgery and the diagnosis is often delayed until the patient finds that it is impossible to abduct the arm without pain. Electromyographic examination may be of help to identify the few palsies caused by a neurapraxia which recover spontaneously, but if there is no recovery by 10 weeks the nerve should be explored. If the nerve is found in continuity lying in scar tissue neurolysis may be successful, but if there is obvious discontinuity, suture or grafting is necessary (See Chapter 44). Should the nerve repair be unsuccessful or not possible, surgical reconstruction with muscle transfer should be considered.

Muscle transfer is the only therapeutic option if the accessory nerve has been excised during a radical neck resection. The degree of disability in these patients is extremely variable—this may be partly because of trapezius's dual innervation from C2 and C3 (occasionally C3 and C4). The indications for surgery must also reflect the activity level, age and life expectancy of the patient.

In every case of shoulder girdle dysfunction it is important to consider the secondary effect on the soft tissues and the nerves around the shoulder. A trapezius palsy may be associated with pain from neurological denervation and an adhesive capsulitis of the shoulder joint may also develop. Ptosis of the scapula may cause discomfort as the result of traction radiculitis of the brachial plexus. More commonly the pain appears to be from fatigue and functional impingement or even attrition of the supraspinatus tendon within the subacromial space because of its failure to rotate and retract the scapula. Conservative treatment is invariably unsuccessful, apart from improving any concomitant adhesive capsulitis. Surgical reconstructions must correct not only the winging of the scapula but also the ptosis caused by the loss of the scapular suspension mechanism. The intention is to improve the deformity, which may be severe. The Eden–Lange tendon transfer of levator

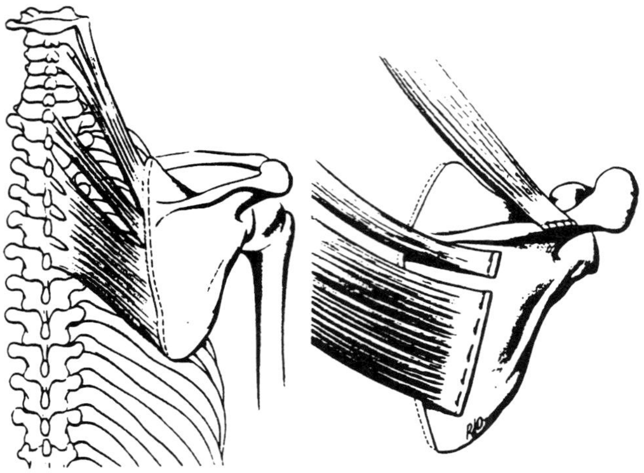

Fig. 43.2 The muscle transfers used in the Eden–Lange procedure.

scapulae and the rhomboids (Fig. 43.2) is probably the best method of achieving near normal function.[1–3] These three muscles are used to replace the upper, middle and lower parts of trapezius respectively.

Alternative procedures such as fascial slings passed from the vertebral border of the scapula to the spinous processes of the second and third thoracic vertebrae, in place of the middle and lower parts of trapezius, have significant disadvantages as they stretch with time. If soft tissue reconstruction fails, the only alternative option is scapulothoracic fusion. The lateral transfer of the levator scapulae muscles improves cosmesis, and head and neck surgeons must be cautioned against transposing this important suspensory muscle to cover the carotid artery after radical neck dissection.

Loss of serratus anterior function

The serratus anterior assists the upper fibres of trapezius in upward and forward rotation of the scapula and also keeps the vertebral border of the scapula in firm apposition with the chest wall in all positions. Loss of this muscle may limit active shoulder elevation, but more frequently presents as deformity with fatigue pain on elevation of the arm. The glenohumeral joint has been aptly described as a golf ball on a tee; the glenoid is the tee and the scapula must be positioned so that the glenoid centre line and the axis of the humeral head are closely aligned. This is particularly important during vigorous shoulder activities; for example a boxer's punch, bench press, throwing action or tennis shot. Power is lost and fatigue occurs if the glenoid centre line and humerus are not aligned.

A long thoracic nerve palsy is the major cause of serratus anterior weakness as rupture of serratus anterior is extremely rare. The long thoracic nerve is formed from the roots of C5, C6 and C7 immediately after leaving their intervertebral foramina (see Chapter 44). It runs beside the main brachial plexus and is often spared in traction lesions. The cause of an isolated serratus anterior palsy is often difficult to explain, but may follow viral illness, carrying objects on the shoulder, recumbency for a prolonged period of time, immunization, open iatrogenic injury in the axilla and lying on the operating table for long periods. Iatrogenic causes are seen following first rib resection, mastectomies with axillary clearance, scalenotomies, surgical procedures for spontaneous pneumothorax and infraclavicular plexus anaesthetic blocks. These cases only rarely recover spontaneously; by contrast palsies occurring after closed trauma are usually traction lesions and recovery can be anticipated. Recovery is usually seen by one year and if palsy persists beyond this time the prognosis is poor, although some patients may still recover after 2 or 3 years.

The major problem is pain associated with difficulty lifting the arm, particularly with weights. Additionally there may be discomfort from the winging when sitting against a chair back. The shoulder may also be painful at rest from an associated subacromial bursitis, usually as a consequence of functional impingement within the subacromial space. There is little useful treatment; jackets and braces to prevent winging are uncomfortable and rarely tolerated. Many patients learn to live with the disability and thus few come to surgery. There is no place for nerve repair—the only option is tendon transfer. Pectoralis major transfer with a fascia lata graft through the axilla to the lower pole of the scapula can give satisfactory results.[4]

Global weakness of the scapular stabilizers

Generalized weakness of the scapular stabilizing muscles is commonly associated with many injuries and conditions affecting the shoulder joint. Careful examination often demonstrates minor winging of the scapula even in the absence of stiffness of the glenohumeral joint. However, if the weakness is severe, the relative strength of the deltoid muscle is much greater and on elevation of the arm this imbalance allows the deltoid to pull up the scapula, causing it to wing.

Muscle dystrophies should be considered in all cases of unexplained weakness and atrophy of these shoulder stabilizers occurring in the first and second decades. The commonest type is facioscapulohumeral dystrophy. The condition is autosomal recessive and a family history may be elicited. This is a bilateral condition but it is usually unilateral on presentation. The other side may not be affected until months or even years later. Involvement of the facial muscles may be detected early with the child's inability to whistle or blow out candles on a birthday cake. This condition has variable muscle involvement and prognosis: there is usually slow deterioration and a good life expectancy. The deltoid is spared but loses its stable origin and tilts the scapula rather than raising the humerus. There is a characteristic deformity caused by the selective muscle loss.

Muscular dystrophies involve a number of muscles and muscle transfer is therefore not applicable. A scapulothoracic fusion

REFERENCES

1. Lange M Langenbecks Arch Klin Hir 1951; 270: 437–439
2. Langenskiold A, Ryoppy S Acta Orthop Scand 1973; 44: 383–388
3. Bigliani L U, Compito C A, Duralde X A, Wolfe I R J Bone Joint Surg 1996; 78A: 1534–1540
4. Marmor L, Bechtol C O J Bone Joint Surg 1942; 24: 699

should be considered if the disability increases with preservation of the deltoid muscle function. This operation recreates a stable origin by anchoring the scapula to the fourth, fifth and sixth ribs. The procedure has been well described by Copeland & Howard.[5] There are many technical variations but the principles remain the same. The shoulder should be immobilized in a spica for 3 months in 50° of abduction and 30° of forward flexion with sufficient internal rotation to allow the hand to be placed in front of the mouth.

Other causes of winging

Obligatory winging is seen after glenohumeral fusion. This is rarely of significance except after arthrodesis for brachial plexus injury and should be assessed prior to surgery. The upper part of serratus anterior may be denervated in some cases of C5 and C6 root avulsion. Injuries to the upper roots of the brachial plexus during birth may also cause winging of the scapula. Anterior contracture and capsular tightness develop with posterior subluxation of the humeral head. The glenohumeral joint becomes fixed in abduction so that, when the shoulder is forced into adduction, superior winging occurs: this is known as the scapular sign of Putti.

An abduction contracture of the deltoid may cause secondary winging. This is quite common in developing countries where it is often bilateral and usually affects the anterior part of deltoid. Two types occur: congenital and secondary to multiple intramuscular injections. The treatment is release of fibrous bands and manipulation. A defect in the deltoid may result, requiring closure by anterior transfer of posterior deltoid. Large subscapular osteochondromata can cause displacement of the scapula producing pseudowinging.

The sternoclavicular joint

The suspensory mechanism requires a stable sternoclavicular joint and an intact clavicle, acromioclavicular joint and coracoclavicular ligaments. These important static suspensory structures not only prevent the scapula from dropping but also prevent posterior displacement of the clavicle and protraction of scapula. The sternoclavicular joint is remarkable for its lack of bony congruity and its dependence on the surrounding ligaments for stability. This saddle type of diarthrodial joint contains the curious intra-articular disc ligament (Fig. 43.3). It is covered by the sternoclavicular ligaments lying within the capsule but the major structural support is derived from the costoclavicular (rhomboid) and interclavicular ligaments.

Disruption of these ligaments results in instability of the medial end of the clavicle. The disruption is usually from an indirect force in which either the torso is compressed and rolled backwards causing an ipsilateral anterior dislocation, or compressed and rolled forwards causing posterior dislocation. The vast majority of these injuries occur in road traffic accidents or sporting injuries.

Other conditions affecting this joint present as pain or swelling. These conditions unrelated to trauma may be classified into the following categories:

- Spontaneous subluxation or dislocation.
- Congenital or developmental subluxation or dislocation.

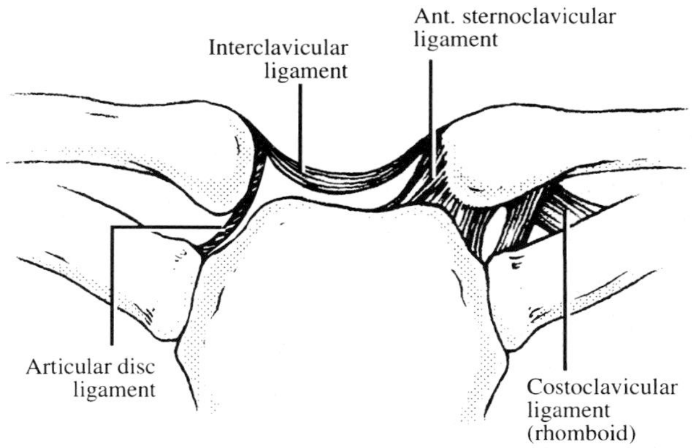

Fig. 43.3 The anatomy of the sternoclavicular joint.

- Arthritis
  —osteoarthritis
  —arthropathies
  —condensing osteitis of the medial clavicle
  —sternocostoclavicular hyperostosis
  —postmenopausal arthritis.
- Infection.
- Tumours.

Evaluation of these conditions may be significantly hindered by the difficulties of imaging the joint. The history and clinical findings may be diagnostic, but imaging is often required. For example, not all cases demonstrate the typical appearances of anterior or posterior dislocation and even assessment of the direction of displacement may be difficult. Plain radiology may be of limited value, even with special views including the 40° cephalad tilt or 'serendipidity' view advocated by Rockwood.[6] If any doubt persists, tomograms or a CT scan are required. Ultrasound scanning is usually a simpler and quicker method of observing displacement. Magnetic resonance scans show the intra-articular disc ligament very well and isotope studies are particularly helpful in identifying infection, inflammation and rare tumours.

Spontaneous subluxation or dislocation is usually a self-limiting condition and almost never requires surgery.[6] Arthritis of the sternoclavicular joint may also become symptomless with time and conservative management should be tried, including a limited number of intra-articular steroid injections. If surgery is required excision arthroplasty alone is recommended—resection of 2 cm of medial clavicle does not compromise its stability because the costoclavicular ligaments are left intact. Particular care must be taken when dividing the clavicle; a blunt retractor should be placed behind the clavicle before making a series of drill holes. The osteotomy is completed with an osteotome. The clavicular head of sternocleidomastoid is released and sutured into the space created by the resected clavicle. Despite the rarity of these injuries and conditions, the complications associated with surgery to this joint

REFERENCES

5. Copeland S A, Howard R C J Bone Joint Surg 1978; 60B: 547
6. Rockwood C A Jr, Odor J M J Bone Joint Surg 1989; 71A: 1280–1288

are important. Surgery to the sternoclavicular joint is potentially dangerous because of its immediate posterior relations which include the arch of the aorta, the superior vena cava, the innominate vein and the subclavian vessels. The use of any type of pin is dangerous and unwarranted. Its insertion risks injuring these structures, and migration of pins is well documented. Their persistent use still generates even more bizarre case reports of pins found as far away as the liver and spinal cord. There have been fatal and near fatal cases, culminating in two German surgeons being charged with manslaughter by negligence.

Condensing osteitis of the medial clavicle, sternocostoclavicular hyperostosis and postmenopausal arthritis are poorly defined conditions with many similar features. There is little guidance on management from the small numbers of cases reported. Infections are occasionally encountered and culture will reveal a wide range of organisms. Although needle biopsy may help with the diagnosis, anterior arthrotomy is usually required for treatment.

The acromioclavicular joint

The articulation at the lateral end of the clavicle allows as much as 20° of angulation and 40–50° of rotation. This diarthrodial joint has a fibrocartilaginous disc which may be complete or meniscoid. The stability of the acromioclavicular joint is maintained by the acromioclavicular and coracoclavicular ligaments. Rockwood[7] demonstrated from cadaver studies that horizontal stability was controlled by the acromioclavicular ligaments whereas vertical stability was dependent on the coracoclavicular ligaments. The superior acromioclavicular ligaments are relatively weak and blend with the fascia of deltoid and trapezius. It is the conoid and trapezoid parts of the coracoclavicular ligament that function as suspensory ligaments of the scapula and the primary supports of the acromioclavicular joint.

Symptomless degenerative arthritis of the acromioclavicular joint is extremely common, and narrowing of the disc space can be considered a normal ageing process after the age of 40. Symptomatic cases can be treated by excision of the distal end of the clavicle together with the adjacent osteophytes.[8] This procedure can also be effectively performed arthroscopically. This procedure is also indicated in type I and type II injuries with persistent pain or secondary post-traumatic arthritis. At least 1½ cm of bone should be removed and clearance should be assessed on the operating table. Particular care should be taken not to remove too much clavicle or destabilize the coracoclavicular ligaments, and the operation should be completed by a strong repair of the overlying fascia.

A common cause of acromioclavicular arthrosis is a previous injury to the joint followed by attempted reduction of the dislocation. There is in fact a higher incidence of post-traumatic arthritis following surgery than there is after conservative treatment, particularly in patients treated by transarticular wires.

Late reconstructions for vertical instability of the distal clavicle are difficult. A Bosworth screw from the clavicle to the coracoid process alone is inadequate and most of these cases require a coracoacromial ligament transfer.[9] Ligament transfer was originally proposed by Cadenet in 1917[10] and it has continued to provide good results.[11] The technique is often modified but the principle is to transfer the coracoacromial ligament from the acromion to the excised end of the clavicle (Fig. 43.4). Probably the most important aspect of the reconstruction is a firm repair of the trapezius fascia. Postoperatively a broad arm sling is worn for 4 weeks allowing gentle circumduction exercises. This procedure is equally effective in early and late cases.[12]

Occasionally the coracoacromial ligament is not substantial enough to act as a stabilizer and alternative techniques are required. The coracoclavicular ligaments cannot be reliably repaired but should be opposed to achieve some reconstitution by fibrous scarring. Coracoclavicular banding with either polydioxone sulphide cord or tape is preferable to the use of nonabsorbable materials such as Dacron or wire, which may cause erosion and subsequent fracture of the bone.

Transfer of the coracoid process to the clavicle provides dynamic stabilization should these procedures fail. In horizontal instability the important superior acromioclavicular ligament is deficient and may require reconstruction by transfer of the coracoacromial ligament to the upper surface of the clavicle.[13]

The acromioclavicular joint is often affected by rheumatoid arthritis and a trial of local anaesthetic injections can identify the joint as a major source of pain even in patients with severe glenohumeral or rotator cuff disease. In these patients the acromioclavicular joint may be the only restraint against upward migration and a dome type arthroplasty may be preferable to conventional excision.

Acromioclavicular joint cysts are associated with degenerative changes in the joint and underlying rotator cuff tears (Fig. 43.5). Simple excision is unpredictable and resection of the outer end of the clavicle is preferable. Another uncommon condition is osteolysis of the distal clavicle. This is usually seen in men, particularly in weight lifters. It is commonly unilateral and usually resolves with rest and local injections. Curiously, the clavicle may even reconstitute itself. The acromioclavicular joint is also a rare site for septic arthritis, with many case reports describing infection with a variety of organisms.

Plain radiographs are the essential investigation for this joint. It is important to request anteroposterior and axillary views of the acromioclavicular joint and *not* the glenohumeral joint to avoid over penetration. Stress views may be of value in distinguishing a type II from a type III acromioclavicular dislocation. This is potentially useful as the distinction changes the management of the injury. The stress views compare the coracoclavicular space of the affected joint with that of the normal contralateral joint. The widening of the interspace can be demonstrated by applying weights suspended by loops from the wrists. It is thought that as little as 40% displacement probably reflects some disruption of the coracoclavicular ligaments.

REFERENCES

7. Rockwood C A Jr In: Fractures in Adults, Vol. 1, 2nd ed. Lippincott, Philadelphia 1984; pp 860–910
8. Mumford E B J Bone Joint Surg 1941; 23: 799–802

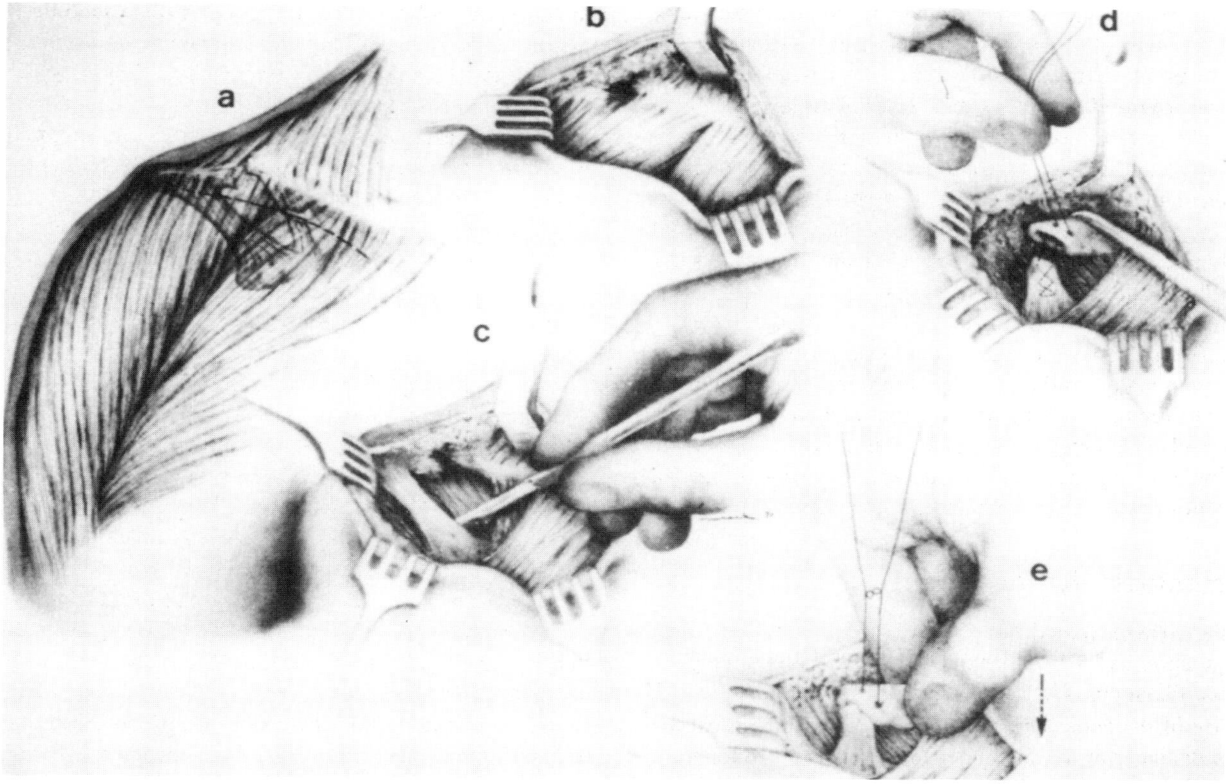

Fig. 43.4 The Weaver–Dunn transfer of the coracoacromial ligament to the distal end of the clavicle. (Reproduced from Weaver & Dunn.)[11]

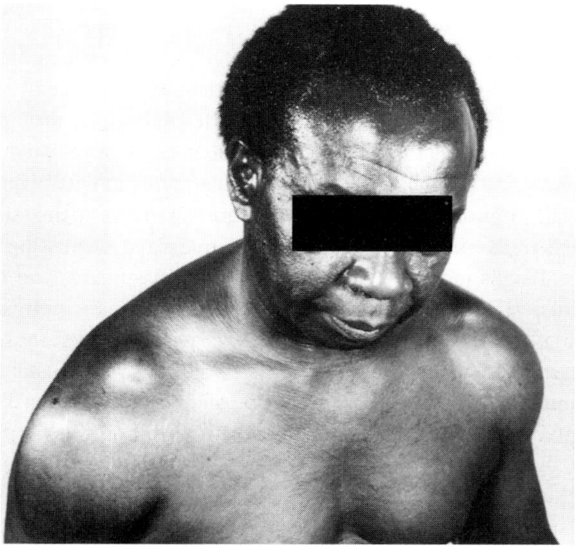

Fig. 43.5 Patient with typical acromioclavicular joint cysts due to degenerative change in the underlying joint.

SUBACROMIAL SPACE AND ROTATOR CUFF

Impingement syndrome

The acromioclavicular joint and adjacent lateral acromion form the roof of the subacromial bursa. This bursa forms an 'articulation' and is the most common site of pathology within the shoulder, largely from conditions affecting the rotator cuff forming its floor. Subacromial bursitis has been recognized since the mid 19th century, but its association with subacromial impingement has been increasing recognized over the last 60 years. The impingement occurs between the upper surface of the biceps and the rotator cuff with the anterior edge of acromion, coracoacromial ligament or undersurface of acromioclavicular joint (Fig. 43.6). Symptoms may occur in a normal shoulder following a period of overuse, particularly with repetitive loaded activities in the overhead position. This early stage usually resolves spontaneously.

Supraspinatus involvement was described by Codman in 1927. The prevailing concept is that these tendons are too thick or more commonly that the supraspinatus outlet is too small. The outlet stenosis is usually caused by an acromial spur developing at the origin of the coracoacromial ligament or by encroachment of a degenerate acromioclavicular joint. The term 'impingement syndrome' was coined,[14] and Neer also described 'a characteristic ridge of proliferative spurs and excrescences on the undersurface of the anterior process of the acromion, apparently caused by repeated impingement of the rotator cuff and the humeral head,

REFERENCES

9. Bosworth B M Surg Gynecol Obstet 1941; 73: 866–871
10. Cadenet F M Internat Clin 1917; 1: 145–169
11. Weaver J K, Dunn H K J Bone Joint Surg 1972; 54A: 1187–1194
12. Warren-Smith C D, Ward M W J Bone Joint Surg 1987; 69B: 715–718
13. Neviaser J S Clin Orthop 1968; 58: 57–68
14. Neer C S J Bone Joint Surg 1972; 54A: 715–718

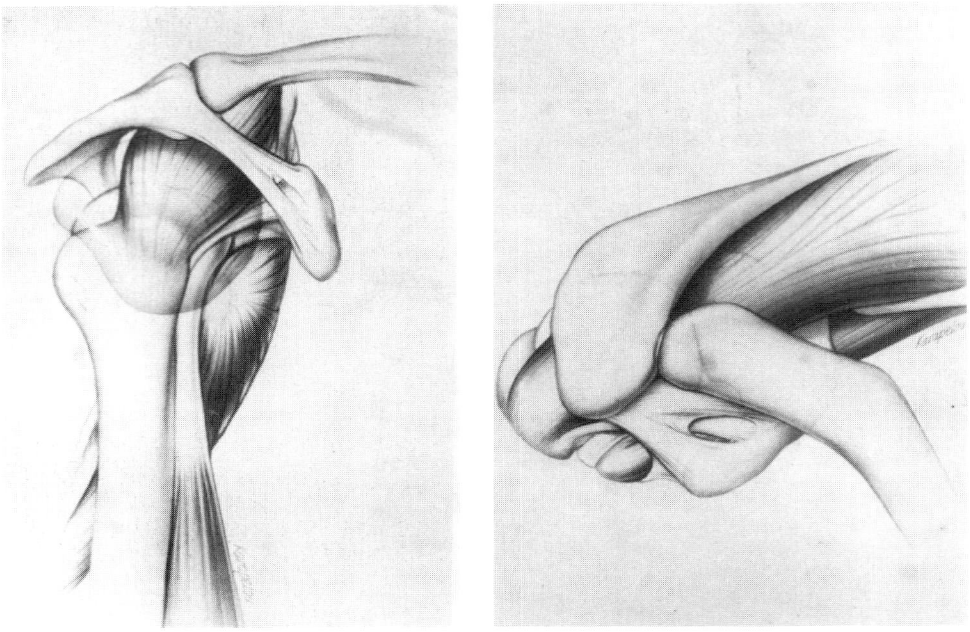

Fig. 43.6 The supraspinatus outlet and subacromial bursa.

with traction of the coracoacromial ligament . . . Without exception it was the anterior lip and undersurface of the anterior third that was involved'. Prior to this important description emphasizing the site of impingement, the surgical treatment had been acromionectomy, a mutilating operation with poor results because of loss of the deltoid origin. Current practice is to increase the size of the outlet by resection of the coracoacromial ligament and removal of the spur by undercutting the acromion. This procedure, termed acromioplasty, provides good results.

The hallmarks of this condition are the pathological changes in the coracoacromial ligament with 'crab meat fraying' at the anterior margin as the result of mechanical impingement and injection within its coverings. In addition, alteration of the acromial morphology from spur formation at the enthesis of the coracoacromial ligament can be easily observed. These changes have been described by Bigliani et al[15] and classified into flat (type I), curved (type II) and hooked (type III). The significance of these findings in relation to the development of rotator cuff tears is disputed as many of the earliest pathological changes are found in the tendons of the rotator cuff. These partial thickness articular side tears suggest that the acromial changes may be a secondary phenomenon.

In practice the presentations of these cases give the clinical impression of a far more imprecise group of conditions; it is now recognized that the causes are diverse and include structural abnormalities of the acromion and acromioclavicular joint, inflammation of the bursa, congenital abnormalities or fracture malunions of the humerus producing prominence of the greater tuberosity, and even functional factors. For example, it has already been discussed how winging of the scapula can cause impingement of the supraspinatus. In addition, alterations in glenohumeral movement caused by changes in the capsule may cause a functional impingement. For example, in the stiff shoulder, the tightness of the posterior shoulder capsule forces the humeral head to ride up against the acromion during flexion. Conversely capsular laxity can cause impingement from excessive upward translation of the humeral head during sporting activities. This accounts for many of the disappointing and unpredictable results of anterior acromioplasty in athletes and young patients.

The clinical presentation of impingement syndrome is characteristic; there is a history of pain, usually in the peri-acromial or epaulette area, with additional pain experienced in the lateral aspect of the arm, the anterior aspect of humerus biceps and the muscle belly of supraspinatus itself. The onset may be associated with overuse in the overhead position or with athletic activity. The pain is usually reproduced on activities requiring forward flexion and internal rotation. Night pain is characteristic and distressing. The physical signs include muscle atrophy of supraspinatus and infraspinatus, slight tenderness over rotator cuff, and crepitus and clicking as the supraspinatus tendon is passed under the coracoacromial arch. This latter effect is also the cause of the characteristic mid range painful arc on abduction and forward flexion. This is made worse by internal rotation, and forms the basis of the impingement sign and test (Fig. 43.7). Diminished strength of abduction and external rotation can usually be demonstrated. Relief of pain with subacromial local anaesthetic injection, called the impingement test, is a simple and effective diagnostic manoeuvre.

Plain radiographs may identify bony causes of the outlet stenosis and signs of the rotator cuff disease, such as calcification or erosions at the tendon insertion. The axial view shows the degree of degenerative change within the acromioclavicular joint and the presence of an os acromiale. The outlet view is useful but requires skilful and careful radiography. An alternative is the 30°

REFERENCE

15. Bigliani L U, Morrison D, April A W Orthop Trans 1986; 10: 228

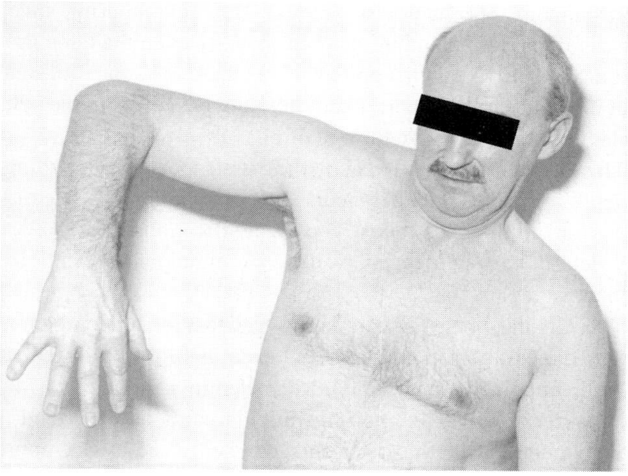

Fig. 43.7 Demonstration of a positive impingement sign.

causal tilt anteroposterior view devised by Rockwood which allows the spurs to be classified into type I and type II (Fig. 43.8).

Further investigations seek to define whether the rotator cuff is torn. Double contrast arthrography is invasive but identifies full thickness tears with a high degree of accuracy. Ultrasound and magnetic resonance scanning are non-invasive and have replaced arthrography in many centres. With skilled interpretation these investigations have a greater than 90% sensitivity and specificity. Caution must be exercised, however, as many abnormalities are seen in symptomless individuals, particularly with advancing age. These tests must be used to answer specific questions and are helpful in confirming the diagnosis after careful clinical evaluation.

The majority of impingement syndromes respond to time and rest. Modifications to daily and sporting activities together with exercises to re-educate and strengthen the shoulder muscles are helpful. There is no evidence of benefit from heat, cold, massage, electrotherapy or acupuncture. Non-steroidal anti-inflammatory drugs and the judicious use of subacromial hydrocortisone injection can decrease inflammation and relieve pain.

The indications for surgical decompression by acromioplasty are symptoms of impingement with disability for more than one year in patients aged more than 40 years. Stiffness is a contraindication to surgery. The impingement test should be positive and a full thickness rotator cuff tear must be excluded. Certain patients less than 40 years old can be considered but extreme caution should be made when confirming the diagnosis.

The principles of the Neer acromioplasty are preservation of the acromial origin of deltoid with secure reattachment after the open procedure as dehiscence not only compromises function but is also extremely difficult to correct surgically. The use of either No. 1 non-absorbable or polydioxane suture (PDS) through drill holes is recommended. Acromionectomy or excessive removal of anterior acromion must also be avoided as this also presents major difficulties for reconstruction. Smooth resection of the undersurface of the antero-inferior acromion and insertion of the coracoacromial ligament is performed.[14] Coracoid impingement is a rarer but well recognized condition with specific symptoms and signs of impingement.

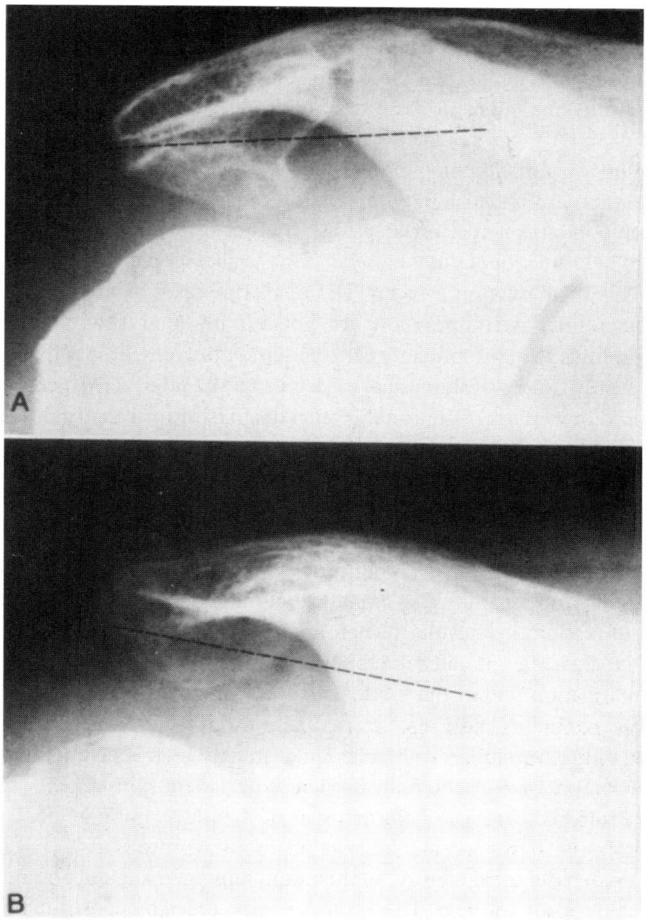

Fig. 43.8 30° caudal tilt anteroposterior radiograph showing a subacromial spur.

Careful inspection for other sources of impingement such as acromioclavicular joint arthritis is important. This may be primarily degenerative, but is also seen after a recent or remote injury.[16,17] It is important to remember that arthritis with osteophytes on the undersurface of the joint, even with encroachment onto the supraspinatus, is common; more than a third of symptomless shoulders in patients over 40 demonstrate these features on magnetic resonance scanning. Undercutting of the joint is recommended, or it should be excised if it is symptomatic and irritable on examination.

The importance of awareness of the presence of an os acromiale and of the risks of destabilizing the fragment during acromioplasty cannot be overstated. A similar situation can arise if the acromion is fractured by excessive resection of bone. This needs to be fixed to allow mobilization, in order to reduce bursal scarring without causing malunion or non-union of fragments. Fixation can be performed either with K wires and a tension band or lag screws.

REFERENCES

16. Kessel L, Watson M J Bone Joint Surg 1977; 59B: 166–172
17. Petersson C J, Gentz C F In: Surgery of the Shoulder. B C Decker, Burlington 1984 pp 129–133

Careful rehabilitation after acromioplasty is imperative. The aim is to regain the movement of the glenohumeral joint and subsequently strengthen the rotator cuff muscles. Early mobilization prevents bursal adhesions and stiffness, but premature strenuous activity can result in increased pain. It is important also to include a strengthening programme of the scapular muscles. A common error is to judge the result too early; one should wait at least 6 months before considering the procedure to have failed.

The same operation can be done arthroscopically and this makes rehabilitation easier.[18] The results of open or arthroscopic subacromial decompression are good, with total resolution of symptoms in approximately 70% and no improvement in 10%.

Many causes of failure have been proposed after both open and closed procedures. Often an incorrect diagnosis rather than a failure to relieve impingement is responsible. The most common cause of failure to relieve subacromial compression is incomplete division of the coracoacromial ligament. Fibres may be left attached, particularly to the anterior capsule of the acromioclavicular joint. Inadequate resection of bone, usually at the anterior margin and lateral acromion, may also explain continuing impingement.

Disappointing results of acromioplasty may also be obtained when there is untreated bicipital tendinitis, or rotator cuff tears. Calcification within the tendon may not only cause distortion of the tendon but may also cause pain from local inflammation. Irritability from the acromioclavicular joint, which is distinct from the compressive effect, may also cause persistent symptoms.

Probably the most common cause of pseudo-impingement is instability. This is seen in athletes in whom overuse leads to micro trauma, causing instability, subluxation, impingement and possibly even a rotator cuff tear. This is often compounded by constitutional hyperelasticity. These patients can be made worse by an arthroscopic subacromial decompression and should have their joint instability treated. Pseudo-impingement may also occur with other types of internal derangement within the glenohumeral joint, such as synovitis, and from irritability caused by labral tears.

The most common source of referred pain in the shoulder is the cervical spine in, for example, an intervertebral disc prolapse, but occasionally pain may be referred from the pleura (Pancoast's syndrome), thoracic outlet syndrome and rarer abdominal causes mediated through the phrenic nerve.

Rotator cuff tears

Many of the patients presenting with impingement have either partial or full thickness rotator cuff tears. This condition embraces a progression of changes from bursitis to tearing by persistent attrition. In 1927, Codman noted thin strips of supraspinatus separated from the tendon and suggested that they 'seemed to be worn as if from friction'.[19]

The bursal side partial thickness injury can be easily explained but many of the changes involve intrinsic rotator cuff damage, and rotator cuff tension failure without evidence of impingement. It is generally believed that partial thickness tears can progress to full thickness damage by further attrition, tendon injury and failure. Once the tendon is detached, retraction and atrophy of the muscle develops. The vast majority of tears are confined to the supraspinatus, but may also involve the neighbouring biceps, subscapularis, infraspinatus and occasionally even the teres minor tendons. It is important to appreciate that there is a small but significant incidence of both partial and full thickness tears in the symptomless population above the age of 60.

The tear can be classified according to its location, according to its depth for partial thickness tears and according to the size of the defect for full thickness tears. These classifications are of value as they determine treatment as well as the anticipated results from attempts at repair.

The clinical presentation reflects the loss of tendon function with weakness, a drop arm sign and even inability to lift the arm. As with impingement there is often relentless night pain. Many patients respond to the non-operative treatment described for impingement. Partial thickness tears can be treated by decompression and debridement alone. The results of this approach are unpredictable and many deep partial thickness and full thickness tears require formal repair. This is achieved by mobilization of the retracted tendon to its insertion, division of capsular contractures and direct repair. This is difficult and painstaking surgery and large tears may require the tendon insertion to be moved medially by creating a trough into the articular cartilage of the superolateral humeral head. Local and even distant muscle transfers such as latissimus dorsi can be deployed. Tendon reattachment is complicated by disuse osteoporosis which makes the greater tuberosity a weak point of fixation for transosseous suture techniques. Very few tears are small enough to be amenable to arthroscopic repair.

The results of repair worsen with the size of the tear, and in the very large tears repair may not be possible. Secure fixation without a gap must be achieved if rehabilitation is to be successful. In these cases decompression alone may help to reduce the pain. In these large defects the humeral head migrates superiorly and forms a pseudo-articulation with the acromion which leads to loss of concentricity and eventual arthropathy of the glenohumeral joint.

GLENOHUMERAL JOINT

Arthritis

The major causes of degenerative changes affecting the glenohumeral joint are similar to those affecting other major joints and include primary osteoarthritis, rheumatoid arthritis, post-traumatic arthritis and avascular necrosis. The non-operative treatment is also similar, with many patients tolerating more severe joint destruction than would be tolerable in the hip. The surgical treatment is joint replacement as arthroscopic lavage has yet to be evaluated in advanced joint destruction.

The shoulder was the first joint to be replaced with a metallic prosthesis. The operation took place in March 1892 at the Hôpital St. Louis in Paris by Dr Jules Péan on a young man with a massive tuberculous abscess of the humerus. The prosthesis was made of a

REFERENCES

18. Ellman H, Kay S P J Bone Joint Surg 1991; 73B: 395–398
19. Codman E A Boston Med J 1927; 196: 381

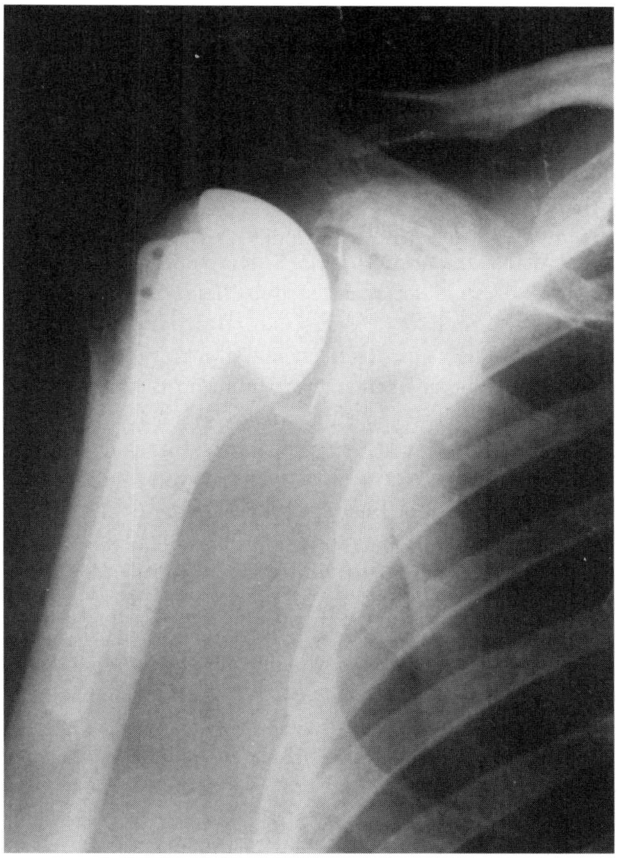

Fig. 43.9 Radiograph showing a total shoulder arthroplasty.

platinum tube and a rubber ball hardened by boiling in paraffin. The muscles were reattached to holes in the tube by horse hair. The prosthesis is reported to have functioned well for 2 years but was finally removed because of a persistent draining sinus.[20]

Modern shoulder replacement has its origins in the 1950s as treatment for fractures of the neck of the humerus with dislocation of the head fragment, an injury normally treated by simple excision at that time. Charles S. Neer from New York and surgeons from France developed prosthetic hemi-arthroplasties based on the favourable results obtained by replacement arthroplasty in cases of subcapital fracture of the femur. Twenty years elapsed before a series of 48 replacement arthroplasties for glenohumeral arthritis was reported in 1974.[21] This publication and the subsequent work by Dr. Neer created the foundations of our current knowledge of the indications, surgical technique, rehabilitation and results of shoulder replacement.

The articular surfaces are replaced with a stemmed humeral component and high density polyethylene glenoid (Fig. 43.9). The implants are designed to mimic the complex anatomy of the proximal humerus in which the correct placement of the centre of rotation and tensioning of the rotator cuff muscles is crucial. This can be achieved with a modular component. Variations in the head size and the angle of inclination between the head and shaft, as the head lies eccentrically in relation to the humeral shaft with a variable degree of posterior offset, must be accommodated. At operation the shoulder is approached through the deltopectoral groove with division and reflection of the subscapularis tendon. The humeral component is usually implanted with cement to prevent loosening and subsidence, particularly in rheumatoid patients. The implantation of the glenoid component is technically difficult with a significant per- and postoperative complication rate. The long-term revision rate for loosening can be as high as 5%. The addition of a glenoid component corrects the posterior wear seen in many patterns of arthritis and may be more successful in the relief of pain than a hemi-arthroplasty.

The current challenge concerns the design and fixation of the glenoid component. The shoulder is often incorrectly described as a non-weightbearing joint but loads of more than body weight are transmitted through the glenoid on lifting the arm. These extreme forces are usually centred on the face of the glenoid but, in the absence of a functional rotator cuff, shear forces in a superior direction can cause progressive glenoid loosening. This potential biomechanical problem is compounded by the small amount of cancellous bone available for fixation. In rheumatoid arthritis, large synovial cysts and medial erosion may result in a glenoid neck less than 1 cm in length. In Larsen stage IV and V rheumatoid arthritis, subchondral plate erosion, low density trabecular bone and destroyed internal architecture are encountered. In these cases glenoid replacement may not be possible but a hemi-arthroplasty can provide good results.

Patients can now expect reliable and good relief of pain with restoration of function either by hemi-arthroplasty or total shoulder replacement. The modern prostheses are durable and can be offered with confidence so they should not just be considered for end-stage destructive disease. Earlier referral when there is preservation of bone stock and rotator cuff function makes normal shoulder function a realistic goal rather than a rare achievement.

Instability

The small surface area of the glenoid and the incongruency between the radii of curvature of the glenoid and of the humeral head give minimal constraint or intrinsic stability. In the normal joint glenohumeral movement, which is a combination of rotation, translation and rolling, is accompanied by precise alignment of the humeral head on the face of the glenoid. This is achieved by the parascapular muscles and the compressive action of the rotator cuff; any failure of this mechanism may result in shoulder instability. The majority of dislocations or subluxations are however, traumatic and occur in an antero-inferior direction. In these circumstances the labrum becomes detached at the insertion of the inferior glenohumeral ligament. This is known as a Bankart lesion after a surgeon from the Middlesex Hospital. Prior to failure the inferior glenohumeral ligament stretches, leading to the attenuation and capsular redundancy found at surgery. The other pathological hallmark of shoulder instability is an impression frac-

REFERENCES

20. Bankes M, Emery R J H J Shoulder Elbow Surg 1995; 4 (4): 259–262
21. Neer C S J Bone Joint Surg 1974; 56A: 1–13

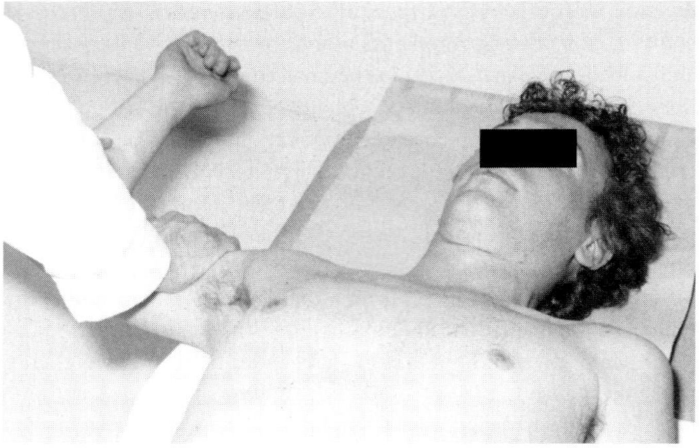

Fig. 43.10 Apprehension test for anterior instability. Relocation by applying pressure posteriorly reduces discomfort (Jobe's relocation test).

ture on the posterosuperior aspect of the humeral head, known as a Hill–Sachs defect. These findings are reversed in the rarer posterior subluxations and dislocations.

The diagnosis of shoulder instability is made from the history, supported by physical signs and plain radiology. The physical signs are predominantly the demonstration of apprehension in potentially unstable positions (Fig. 43.10). An appreciation of the degree of generalized joint laxity and of signs of translation in both the affected and symptomless shoulder is important in understanding the underlying pathology and in assessing the need for surgical treatment. Occasionally more complex cases are encountered in whom there may be doubt about the direction of the instability or its cause. In these patients more sophisticated methods of imaging or diagnostic arthroscopy may be required. CT arthrography can identify labral tears and Bankart lesions with 10% error. The disadvantages are that this technique is invasive and attenuation of the inferior glenohumeral ligament cannot be evaluated. MRI scanning is a controversial technique for assessing shoulder instability. There are many anatomical variants of the labrum and changes are frequently found in symptomless volunteers. A number of studies have suggested that magnetic resonance alone is insensitive and non-specific with substantial intra- and inter-observer errors. The addition of contrast or gadolinium enhancement has however significantly increased its accuracy.

Arthroscopy allows direct visualization of the stabilizing structures of the glenohumeral joint at rest and in motion. Labral lesions and discrete chondral defects can be assessed and even a subjective quantification of the inferior glenohumeral ligament tension can be made. Arthroscopy is however an invasive and expensive procedure with limited indications, which include complex and suspected subtle instability. Arthroscopy is also indicated in shoulder pain in a competitive athlete, particularly when there is an atypical history and examination with inconclusive imaging studies. Evidence of a subtle shoulder instability is often demonstrated.

Arthroscopy has identified many different types of labral tear. The majority are antero-inferior associated with instability, however a few may be superior with damage to the biceps insertion (superior labral anterior posterior or SLAP lesions). These tears may cause symptoms even in a stable shoulder and are probably traction injuries which are the result of large forces generated during the deceleration phase of throwing. They have been categorized by Synder and Karzel.[22] These tears are rarely diagnosed preoperatively with conventional imaging. Current treatment is repair or excision of the tear depending on its degree of severity, and the results of surgery are variable.

Symptomatic patients with antero-inferior labral tears or Bankart lesions require surgery if they fail to respond to a programme of shoulder muscle strengthening exercises. Many surgical procedures have been devised and rely for their success on a variety of mechanisms. Reattachment of labrum with or without inferior glenohumeral ligament insertion (the Bankart operation) with shortening of the capsule is widely practised with good results.[23] This procedure is performed through the standard anterior delto-pectoral approach. Postoperatively it is followed by a period of immobilization for at least 4 weeks and careful rehabilitation. Contact sport should be avoided for at least 6 months.

The same 'Bankart' procedure can be performed arthroscopically. Original procedures used metallic devices such as screws or staples but at present suture techniques and biodegradable devices are widely used. The results are difficult to interpret as most studies report small series with short follow-up and with very different pathologies. Recent studies show that failure is undoubtedly more common with arthroscopic repair than with conventional open surgery. A number of contraindications have been identified and it is clear that not all patients are suitable. The techniques do allow satisfactory reattachment of the labrum but there is concern about their ability to treat attenuation of the inferior glenohumeral ligament and capsular redundancy.

The arthroscope will undoubtedly play a major role in future shoulder surgery. At present it is the technique of choice for synovial biopsy, removal of loose bodies, irrigation for septic arthritis, release of acute calcific deposits and for synovectomy. In skilled hands it has been used for posterior capsulorrhaphy, treatment of multidirectional instability and even arthrodesis.

THE ELBOW

The elbow allows positioning of the hand close to the body as well as extending the reach of the hand. This flexibility is frequently lost following fractures and dislocations and with other diseases involving the elbow. Before conditions affecting the elbow joint are discussed there are some important and relatively common conditions which affect the forearm muscles and the olecranon bursa.

Extra-articular conditions

'Tennis elbow' or lateral epicondylitis involves the origins of the extensor carpi radialis brevis, the anterior edges of the extensor communis, the extensor carpi longus and extensor carpi ulnaris in descending frequency. Medial epicondylitis, often inappropriately

REFERENCES

22. Synder S, Karzel R O Arthroscopy 1990; 14: 274–279
23. Bankart A S B Br J Surg 1938; 26: 23–29

termed 'golfer's elbow', involves the flexor pronator origin. Although frequently associated with racket sports, it also occurs in other sports and occupational activities in which the forearm muscles are overused. The majority of patients are between 35 and 50 years of age, with an equal sex ratio in the sports related cases. Many cases are associated with or confused with ulnar nerve neurapraxia, carpal tunnel syndrome, radial nerve entrapment or proximal nerve root entrapment.

The pathology of epicondylitis is poorly understood but characteristic features are usually present. Angiofibroblastic hyperplasia with an absence of inflammatory cells have been described in the affected tendons.[24] Non-operative treatment encompasses rest, modification of activity, pain relief, high voltage electrical stimulation and a limited number of steroid injections. The surgical treatment is controversial with many different procedures of varying magnitude having been described. The majority involve creating an additional injury to the extensor carpi radialis brevis origin, as in simple lateral release, and waiting for healing to occur. The results are good; misdiagnosis accounts for many of the failures.

There are a number of bursae located around the elbow which, with the exception of the olecranon bursa, rarely cause disability. The olecranon bursa may become inflamed or even infected. This is usually as a result of trauma and overuse but may be a complication of inflammatory arthritis. Excision of the bursa is rarely required.

Intra-articular conditions

Minor repetitive injuries or overuse, particularly in patients with above average generalized joint laxity, may result in instability of the posterolateral type. This is rare and is normally only encountered in high grade throwing athletes. Stiffness is more common because of the development of soft tissue contractures. These may be post-traumatic or accompany arthritis, particularly of the rheumatoid type. Prevention is far easier than treatment, with physiotherapy, manipulation and splintage giving limited benefits. Surgical release with removal of osteophytes and heterotopic bone can be achieved by various approaches. The application of a hinged external fixator allows radical release not only of the capsule but also of the shortened collateral ligaments without creating joint instability. These devices allow distraction of the joint surfaces in cases where the articular cartilage is damaged.

Degenerative arthritis of the elbow is relatively rare and is usually seen following injury although it can affect heavy manual labourers, such as steel workers and miners. Erosive arthritis is characteristic of rheumatoid arthritis but is also found in seronegative polyarthropathy. The loss of joint movement is accompanied by pain and sometimes instability in advanced cases of rheumatoid arthritis. The diagnosis is made from plain radiographs and the changes can be visualized at arthroscopy.

Elbow arthroscopy permits removal of loose bodies, synovial biopsy, and assessment and treatment of osteochondritis dissecans and of synovial chondromatosis. Debridement of the osteoarthritic elbow and arthroscopic synovectomy in rheumatoid arthritis are technically demanding new techniques. The latter may have significant advantages in the rheumatoid patient as many areas of

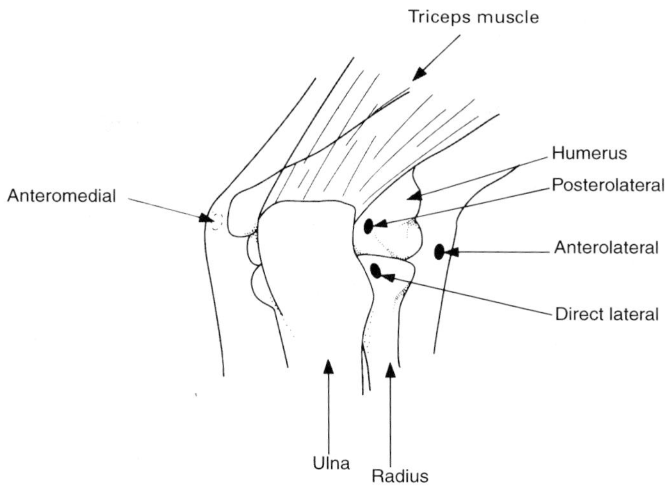

Fig. 43.11 Portals for elbow arthroscopy.

synovium are inaccessible at open surgery. Contraindications to arthroscopy include bony or fibrous ankylosis, severe elbow stiffness, mobile subluxation or previous anterior transposition of the ulnar nerve.

The procedure is usually performed under general anaesthesia in the lateral position with the arm exsanguinated and a tourniquet inflated to 250 mmHg. The placement of ports requires a clear understanding of the neurovascular anatomy because the most frequent complication is damage to the surrounding nerves. The direct lateral, posterolateral, anterolateral and anteromedial ports should be marked (Fig. 43.11) and the joint distended before introducing the arthroscope. Other complications include persistent synovial leakage, iatrogenic damage to the articular surfaces, instrument breakage and infection. Neurovascular observations should be continued for 24 hours postoperatively, during which time the arm is elevated. The dressings are then reduced and movement allowed as tolerated.

Two other surgical procedures are of value in moderately diseased joints. In the rheumatoid patient the symptoms may arise from disease in the radiohumeral joint and be efficiently alleviated by excision of the radial head. In osteoarthritis an adequate debridement of the posterior compartment can be made through a small arthrotomy in the triceps. By making a window in the olecranon fossa access to the anterior part of the joint is possible. This useful technique is termed the Outerbridge–Kashiwagi procedure.[25]

For severely destroyed joints there is little alternative to elbow replacement. Modern designs have proved successful with good restoration of movement and low revision rates for rheumatoid patients. The original hinge joints have been superseded by unlinked, non-constrained, resurfacing prostheses or linked sloppy hinges: both types incorporate flanges on the humeral condyles to distribute the torsional loads (Fig. 43.12). The results in cases of

REFERENCES

24. Nirschi R P, Pettrone F J Bone Joint Surg 1979; 61A: 832
25. Kashiwagi D In: Kashiwagi D (ed) Elbow Joint. Elsevier, Amsterdam pp 177–188

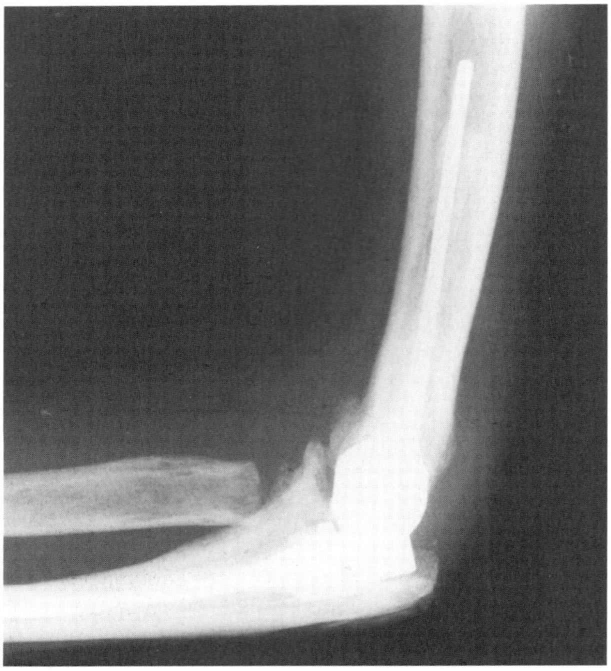

Fig. 43.12 GSB III elbow replacement.

osteoarthritis or post-traumatic arthritis are less favourable with a higher complication and revision rate for aseptic loosening.

STIFFNESS OF THE UPPER LIMB

The rate of recovery and final functional result after injuries and operations of the upper limb are often adversely affected by the development of stiffness. Reflex sympathetic dystrophy, Sudeck's algo-dystrophy and adhesive capsulitis of the shoulder are poorly defined conditions with many similar features. Loss of the range of movement with reduced passive range of movement on examination is characteristic. It is often associated with pain at extremes of the range from soft tissue stretching.

Stiffness may be the result of reversible self-limiting conditions such as adhesive capsulitis, with the potential for total functional and structural recovery. The stiffness may improve to expose significant anatomical and pathological abnormalities. Examples include rotator cuff tears and fractures involving the tuberosities or articular surfaces. Occasionally the stiffness is irreversible because of capsular (including coracohumeral ligament) contracture or post-surgical shortening of the rotator cuff muscle tendon units.

Investigation aims to identify any underlying pathology. Primary adhesive capsulitis may be associated with diabetes and routine urine analysis is a rewarding technique for identifying new cases. Treatment of adhesive capsulitis starts by controlling pain mediated by the associated synovitis of the capsule or bursal layer covering the rotator cuff. Rest, analgesia, anti-inflammatory agents, local physiotherapy techniques, transcutaneous nerve stimulation and a course of bi-weekly suprascapular nerve blocks are helpful. Once the pain has been controlled, physiotherapy and a home exercise programme can be employed to increase the range of movement by the application of stretching and mobilization techniques. Manipulation under anaesthesia may be performed but requires careful timing; manipulation attempted before the synovitis has settled is likely to be unsuccessful and may even exacerbate the condition. The value of arthroscopy and hydrostatic distension is currently uncertain. Occasionally capsular restriction may be so severe and refractory as to merit surgery with release of the coracohumeral ligament and rotator interval. All cases treated by surgery require early restoration of movement—initially under an interscalene block and subsequently aided by a physiotherapist.

TUMOURS AND INFECTION

Fortunately both tumour and infection of the shoulder and arm are rarely encountered. Soft tissue and bone tumours require investigation and treatment in specialized centres. Injudicious biopsy may significantly limit the chances of preventing recurrence and eradicating the disease (see Chapter 54). The treatment of infection follows the general principles, but both diagnosis and treatment can be aided by arthroscopy in cases of infection of the subacromial space, glenohumeral and elbow joints. Repeated copious irrigation through the arthroscope is effective at treating joint infection and limiting damage to the articular cartilage.

44 The peripheral nerves

D. T. Gault P. J. Smith

INTRODUCTION

Peripheral nerves are subject to a variety of insults. Leprosy is the commonest cause of loss of sensation worldwide;[1] in the UK, troublesome neuropathy is more likely to result from diabetes and peripheral vascular disease.[2] Progressive loss of function with pain as a complication of radiotherapy for malignant disease is greatly underestimated, probably because the onset of symptoms may be delayed for several years.

More acute damage to peripheral nerves usually results from direct mechanical injury; that caused by sharp objects is the most common. Other types of open injury include crush and gunshot wounds, and compound fractures. Displaced fractures of the long bones or dislocation of the joints also cause closed injuries. Ruptures of the brachial and lumbosacral plexi or their branches occur when traction forces are applied to the limbs in high-velocity road traffic accidents. The radial nerve may be crushed against the humerus by a badly fitted crutch or by the back of a chair over which the arm is draped during a profound, usually intoxicated sleep.[3] A poorly applied splint may contuse the common peroneal nerve against the neck of the fibula, and pressure on an ulnar nerve unprotected during surgery can result in a painful neuritis, or even a nerve palsy.[4]

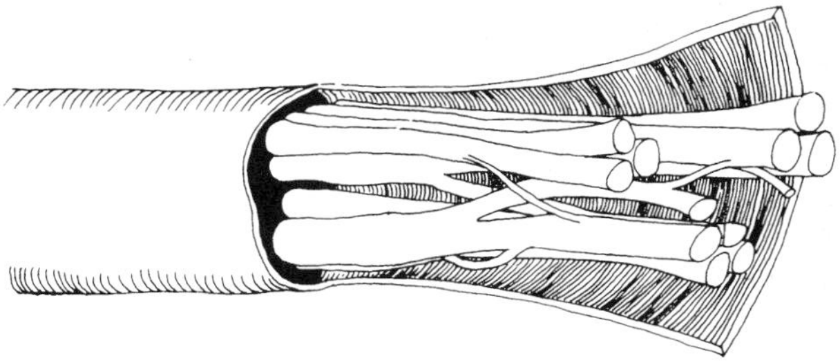

Fig. 44.1 The arrangement of the fascicles varies along the course of the nerve within the epineurium.

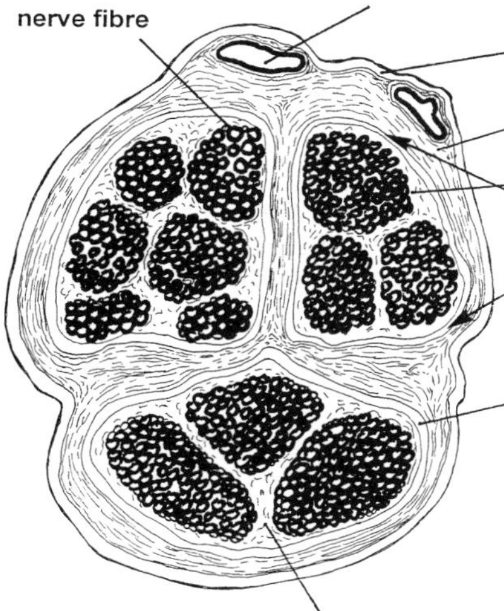

Fig. 44.2 Cross-section of a peripheral nerve.

ANATOMY

A sound knowledge of internal topography of peripheral nerves is vital for their successful repair, release and grafting. They emerge from plexi around the limb roots on which converge nerve roots from several contiguous segments of the spinal cord. As they leave the spinal cord, motor, sensory and sympathetic fibres intermingle and within the peripheral nerves become grouped into bundles or fascicles. Each fascicle may contain motor, sensory or sympathetic elements. There are a variable number of fascicles within a nerve, and their arrangement varies along its course (Fig. 44.1).

Packed between the individual nerve fibres within a fascicle is connective tissue called endoneurium (Fig. 44.2). It forms a series of tubes, each occupied by an axon, its Schwann cell sheath and myelin. The endoneurium resists elongation and protects the delicate nerve fibres within it. In a nerve graft, it provides hollow channels down which sprouting axons can grow.

A tough sheath of perineurium surrounds each fascicle. It protects the contents of the endoneural space, acting as a mechanical barrier against trauma, and maintains the intrafascicular pressure so important in promoting proximal-to-distal flow of axoplasm within nerve fibres. The perineurium also acts as a diffusion barrier, protecting the fascicle from a dangerous influx of ions, proteins and other hazardous agents; peripheral nerves can even traverse pyogenic foci without their function being in any

REFERENCES

1. Antia N H, Dastur D K (eds) Symposium on Leprosy. Bombay University Press, Bombay 1967
2. Dyke P J, Thomas P K, Lambert E H Peripheral Neuropathy. W B Saunders, Philadelphia 1983
3. Seddon H J Surgical Disorders of the Peripheral Nerves. Churchill Livingstone, Edinburgh 1975
4. Bonney G J Bone Joint Surg 1986; 68B: 9–13

way influenced.[5] When the perineural sheath is disrupted however, the conduction properties of the contained nerve fibres are impaired, a point to remember when releasing a nerve trapped in scar tissue.

The outermost layer of connective tissue is the epineurium; it can account for between 25 and 75% of the cross-sectional area of a peripheral nerve, and is often more abundant around joints. The epineurium binds the fascicles loosely together, and is condensed at the surface of the nerve to form a distinct investing sheath.

Surrounding it is a layer of loose areolar tissue which allows the nerve to glide within its bed. In addition, the fascicles can slide within the deeper layers of the epineurium. The greatest excursion of peripheral nerves during motion occurs at the wrist, where the median and ulnar nerves travel up to 15 mm during a full range of flexion and extension.[6] If a nerve divided at the wrist is repaired under tension with the wrist flexed, there is little chance that gliding during normal movement will be preserved.

CLASSIFICATION OF NERVE LESIONS

An injured nerve may be completely divided or may simply suffer temporary loss of conduction. The types of nerve injury have been categorized by Seddon,[7] but it is important to appreciate that the demarcation between different types is often not clear-cut, and that many lesions represent intermediate grades of injury.

Neurapraxia

Neurapraxia describes a local conduction block at a discrete site along the course of a nerve, whose continuity is not disrupted. To the naked eye, the nerve appears normal. There is no degeneration of axoplasm, and if there is any anatomical damage, it is restricted to segmental areas of demyelination.

The impairment of nerve function is often partial. The predominant effect depends on the proportions of motor and sensory fibres in the affected nerve. Motor fibres are more vulnerable to a compression force. In radial nerve damage, motor impairment predominates, whereas in early carpal tunnel syndrome, sensory impairment predominates.

Recovery is eventually full, but its completion may vary from minutes or days to several weeks. Examples of this type of injury are tourniquet palsy and the radial nerve paralysis caused when the arm is draped over the back of a chair during a profound sleep. Pressure on the nerve may lead to ischaemia, with damage of its myelin sheath and local oedema. This usually causes a neurapraxia, and recovers within days or weeks. If the pressure is prolonged, it may eventually lead to axonotmesis.

A full recovery still occurs but at a slower rate. In very early nerve entrapment syndromes, the injury is neurapraxia. The diagnosis is made with certainty only when the length of the recovery period is known. The recovery rate and long-term effect are proportional to the duration and severity of the compression force.

Neurapraxia comprises a range of pathological events. Early neurapraxia follows intermittent ischaemic episodes, for example the nocturnal symptoms in carpal tunnel syndrome, which respond to attempts to improve the circulation such as elevation and shaking the hand. More severe compression may lead to swelling of the myelin sheath and intussusception of one sheath within another, producing more severe symptoms such as the permanent numbness seen in severe carpal tunnel syndrome. Prolonged compression may lead to intraneural fibrosis with more severe symptoms such as motor wasting, as seen in the thenar eminence in long-standing cases of carpal tunnel syndrome.

Axonotmesis

In axonotmesis, the continuity of the axons is disrupted although the endoneural tubes are still intact. Axonotmesis may result from, for example, a closed stretch injury. The injured nerve recovers once the cause is removed, since its architecture has not been destroyed, and the regenerating neurons are able to traverse an intact scaffold to reach their peripheral connection. The axoplasm and myelin sheath degenerate distal to the level of the lesion; recovery occurs at the classic rate of nerve regeneration (1–1.5 mm/day).[8,9] A Tinel sign develops at the level of injury, and advances distally with time. Until recovery in axonotmesis begins, it is clinically and physiologically indistinguishable from neurotmesis.

Neurotmesis

In neurotmesis, the nerve is severed, or so seriously disorganized that spontaneous regeneration is impossible. If not repaired, it is often complicated by the development of a neuroma at the site of injury.

THE PATHOLOGY OF NERVE DIVISION

Within 4–20 days of acute transection of a peripheral nerve, the central nerve cell body enlarges as a result of increased metabolism.[10] Proteins are manufactured and migrate along the axon to the site of injury where they are used in repair. The enlargement persists for as long as there is active regeneration of the damaged axon. When conduction is re-established, the cell body slowly returns to a normal size. Within the proximal nerve stump, marked oedema, both intracellular and extracellular, develops within 1 hour of nerve division; the cross-sectional area of the nerve increases as much as threefold. The oedema persists for a week or more after the injury and then slowly subsides.

Several days after nerve transection, the axons start to sprout. After clean cuts, this begins a few millimetres proximal to the last intact node of Ranvier, but after blast injuries, the axonal sprout may develop 2–3 cm proximal to the severed end. The budding of the axons occurs concomitantly with the anabolic phase of the cell

REFERENCES

5. Lundborg G, Nerve Injury and Repair. Churchill Livingstone, Edinburgh 1988
6. Wilgis E F S, Murphy R Hand Clin 1987; 2: 761–766
7. Seddon H J Brain 1943; 66: 237
8. Seddon H J, Medawar P B, Smiths H J Physiol (Lond) 1943; 102: 191–201
9. Sunderland S Arch Neurol Psychiatry 1947; 58: 1–14, 251–256
10. Lehman R A, Hayer G J Brain 1967; 90: 285

body in the spinal cord or dorsal ganglion. The axon sprouts attempt to locate and grow down an empty endoneural tube in the distal segment of the injured nerve. When the axon sprouts (filopodia) reach out into an empty space and make no contact they then withdraw to advance again, seeking an appropriate substrate. By contrast, if they contact the basal lamina of a Schwann cell they attach to this structure and draw the growth cone of the nerve distally.[11]

Separated from their cell body, the neuronal elements in the distal nerve die. Small segments of axon may survive intact for up to 2 weeks, but the majority are broken down within 1 week by the digestive enzymes they contain. The surrounding myelin fragments are digested by Schwann cells. By 6 weeks, this natural debridement is complete. The fascicular anatomy persists for a while, but in time the endoneural sheaths shrink and this then minimizes the chances of regeneration.

Timely nerve repair is important if the axons are to reach a muscle in good condition. When muscle cells no longer receive repeated stimuli, they shrink: the endomysium and perimysium thickens, the muscle spindles atrophy and fibrous tissue forms around the motor end-plates. The sooner a nerve re-establishes connection with the muscle cells, the more likely it is that normal function will return. If reinnervation is delayed for 1 year, function will at best be poor. A delay for 2 years allows irreversible changes to take place in the muscle cells, and any hope of return of motor function is then unlikely.[12]

In contrast, the sensory end-organs survive without nerve connections, although protective sensibility is the best result that can be achieved after a long delay. The quality of sensation is greatly dependent on the ability of the brain to decode messages from the sensory end-organs. These messages are usually altered after nerve repair, and whereas young people can accomplish some natural central reorganization, older people need sensory retraining.[13]

DIAGNOSIS OF NERVE INJURY

An accurate history and careful clinical examination are very important in the diagnosis of peripheral nerve lesions. The site and extent of a wound hint at the possibility of nerve damage. It is important to remember that after glass injuries, extensive internal damage may have occurred despite a small skin puncture wound. Bleeding from major vessels such as the axillary, brachial or ulnar arteries suggests division of the adjacent nerves.

Nerve injury may produce disturbances of motor, sensory and sudomotor function. When a nerve is completely divided, the muscles no longer contract voluntarily. They become flaccid and wasted, and reflexes disappear. The power of both the prime movers and the synergists must be carefully tested. Examination of muscle power may be difficult because of pain or associated injuries to the skeleton, and the examiner may be fooled by the patient's use of subsidiary muscles and trick movements. Examples of such trick movements are the abduction of the fingers by the extensor muscles in an ulnar nerve palsy, flexion of the knee by gracilis in a sciatic nerve palsy, and extension of the interphalangeal joints by the interossei in a radial nerve palsy.

Certain key muscles should be examined. The power of wrist extension reflects radial nerve function, and crossing of the fingers requires an intact ulnar nerve. The median nerve consistently supplies the abductor pollicis brevis, which can be seen and palpated when the position of the abducted thumb is maintained against resistance.

In nerve compression, the muscles supplied may still function, but weakness is apparent. As axons degenerate, the number of nerve fibres supplying a muscle is reduced, and wasting occurs. Weakness can be quantitatively measured and the degree of wasting should be noted.[14]

A divided nerve may also present with loss of light touch, vibration and pinprick sensation. Some patients with divided nerves can still perceive sensation on pinprick testing—the explanation is controversial. It was thought that when the ends of a divided nerve remained in contact, then for several hours, impulses can jump across the gap.[15] This has recently been called into question. Any distortion of sensation rather than complete anaesthesia is the key to diagnosis in the first 24 hours. In such circumstances the nerve should be explored and, if it is found to be divided, should be repaired.[15]

It is usual that, after nerve division, complete sensory loss occurs in that nerve's exclusive territory. Surrounding this zone is an intermediate area in which sensation is altered. This zone of hypoaesthesia cannot be demonstrated by routine clinical testing with a needle (which gives only maximal stimulation), but it does show a limited response to light touch.[16] Thus the area where light touch is lost is usually greater than the area where pinprick is diminished, which is in turn less than the area where deep pressure is disturbed.

Disturbance of sympathetic function is an important early feature of nerve damage. Transection of a digital nerve interrupts the nerve fibres to the sweat glands of the fingertips, where the combination of sweat and dermal ridges (fingerprints) is important for grip. When sweating is eliminated, grip is lost, and the plastic casing of a ballpoint pen drawn across the affected digit will slide and slip in comparison to an adjacent normal finger where sweating is preserved. This loss of tactile adherence is a useful sign of nerve transection as it can be elicited in a child or an uncooperative adult.[17] As pinprick testing is both uncomfortable and unreliable, it is best avoided.

As well as sudomotor paralysis, pilomotor paralysis occurs. An absence of tone in the muscles surrounding hair follicles leaves the skin abnormally smooth and the hairs lack uniform orientation.

Vasomotor disturbance is often apparent. A denervated limb may become blue, cold and oedematous after nerve division. It must

REFERENCES

11. Letourneau P C Dev Biol 1983; 95: 212
12. Bowden R E M, Gutman E Brain 1944; 67: 273
13. Dellon A L, Curtis R M, Edgerton M T Plast Reconstr Surg 1974; 53: 297–305
14. MRC Memorandum No 45: Aids to the Examination of the Peripheral Nervous System. Her Majesty's Stationery Office, London 1980
15. McAllister R M R, Calder J S Br J Plast Surg 1995; 48: 384–395
16. Trotter W, Davies H M J Physiol 1909; 38: 134

however be remembered that disuse alone, as seen in hemiplegia, leads to coldness, cyanosis and oedema. Denervated skin does not demonstrate a normal inflammatory response. Both the impairment of the neurogenic inflammatory response to injury and the loss of protective pain sensation may contribute to the development of the slow-healing trophic ulcers often seen after nerve injury.[18]

Nerve compression causes changes in the sensory threshold. A very early lesion may cause a hypersensitive response (hyperpathia); later in the course of nerve compression, the threshold rises and a greater stimulus intensity is required.[19,20] With further compression, nerve fibres are actually damaged. Loss of two-point discrimination is then a sign of decreased innervation density.

As the damaged fibres attempt to regenerate, so Tinel's sign may be detected (a tingle on tapping over the advancing fibres).[21]

ELECTRICAL ASSESSMENT OF MUSCLE DENERVATION (ELECTROMYOGRAPHY)

Electrical tests are used to detect peripheral nerve damage and to determine the level of the lesion. Information can be obtained by direct nerve stimulation, by detection of the potentials that occur when a nerve and muscle are active, or by measuring nerve conduction velocity. Electrical tests are used to confirm a diagnosis and they also indicate the rate and completeness of recovery after a nerve injury. They are no substitute for clinical examination, but do have the outstanding advantage of being objective, and do not require the close attention or cooperation of the patient. Conversely, they are time-consuming and sometimes unpleasant for the patient. Another drawback is that many of the changes characteristic of muscle denervation are not present immediately after an injury, but take some days to develop.

Stimulation

For a rapid assessment of a patient with suspected nerve involvement, the simplest form of electrodiagnosis is stimulation of the nerve above and below the site of the suspected lesion. Using bipolar surface electrodes, short pulses (0.1 ms) of current of increasing intensity are applied over the nerve until visible or palpable contractions are elicited in the muscles supplied. The threshold and the nature of the peripheral response are noted and are compared to the normal side.

Stimulation of the nerve above the lesion indicates whether conduction is normal or interrupted. A nerve undergoing wallerian degeneration becomes unresponsive to stimulation below the lesion after 4 days.[22] In compression syndromes, proximal stimulation may cause the patient to feel discomfort at the site of the nerve compression. Stimulation proximal to the compression may fail to evoke distal motor function while distal stimulation will normally produce function, hence localizing the problem area.

Detection

Normal muscle function is dependent on normal innervation and thus activity in the motor unit reflects the condition of the motor nerve.[23] A close contact between the recording electrode and the muscle under study is essential to detect contraction in normal muscles or fibrillation potentials in denervated muscles.

Two types of electrodes are available: surface electrodes in the form of a metal cup placed on the skin can record information from superficial muscles, while needle electrodes establish the closest possible contact with muscle fibres and provide more detailed information.

A muscle which is denervated cannot be activated voluntarily. For several days after denervation stimulation of the distal nerve causes contraction until fragmentation of the axons occurs, losing continuity with the muscle.

From 3 weeks after a nerve injury, there is no response to electrical stimulation of the nerve. Both axons and motor nerve terminals disintegrate, and the muscle fibres themselves are left as the sole excitable element. No longer under the control of the motor nerve, nor synchronized with their neighbours, they become hyperexcitable and begin to fibrillate. This is seen as regular action potentials of low amplitude (20–300 μV) and short duration (0.5–2 ms), with a frequency of 2–20 per second.[22] Thus, resting muscle which is normally silent becomes the site of spontaneous activity.[24] Fibrillation persists for many months and shows that the muscle fibres are still alive and in principle capable of being reinnervated. Eventually, however, the fibrillatory activity dies down, and the muscle atrophies. Fibrillation is not found after neurapraxia, and if a muscle is partially denervated, there is reduced electrical activity on voluntary contraction.

Velocity

The time interval between stimulation of the nerve and the detection of a muscle action potential at a distant site can be accurately measured in milliseconds. This total conduction time includes the time taken for the stimulus to evoke the nerve action potential, the propagation time and the terminal delay for the impulse to cross the motor end-plate and excite muscle fibres. By stimulating the nerve at two sites a known distance apart, it is possible to calculate the true nerve conduction velocity. Such studies are of particular value in chronic nerve lesions such as compression. Stimulating the nerve above a compression reveals a prolonged conduction time and reduced muscle action potential amplitude. Stimulating the nerve below the lesion gives a normal response in terms of conduction velocity and muscle action potential. Reverse conduction velocity may be measured by applying a stimulus to a finger and recording the sensory action potentials over the proximal nerve.

REFERENCES

17. Smith P J In: Burke F D, McGrouther D A, Smith P J (eds) Principles of Hand Surgery. Churchill Livingstone, Edinburgh 1989
18. Parkhouse N, LeQuesne P M N Engl J Med 1988; 318: 1306–1309
19. Dellon A L, Plast Reconstr Surg 1980; 65: 466–476
20. Dellon A L, Schnieder R, Burke R Plast Reconstr Surg 1983; 72: 208–216
21. Tinel J Presse Med 1915; 23: 388
22. Sunderland S Nerves and Nerve Injuries. Churchill Livingstone, Edinburgh 1978
23. Bralliar F Orthop Clin North Am 1981; 12: 229
24. Raimbault J Clin Plast Surg 1984; 11: 53–58

Whether or not the conduction is slowed is determined by comparision with standard data. The data relate to the largest-calibre and most rapidly conducting α motor nerve fibres. Nerve conduction velocity is influenced by many factors, including the age and temperature of the patient. The mean rate of conduction is of the order of 57 m/s in the median nerve, and this is reduced to 49 m/s in cases of carpal tunnel syndrome.[25] Electromyography is not, however, a cut and dried test, and one report has stressed that patients with normal electrodiagnostic studies but an abnormal clinical evaluation do well after surgical decompression.[26]

TREATMENT OF NERVE INJURIES

To maximize the chances of motor and sensory recovery, the repair of divided nerves and the release of compressed nerves should be performed without delay. Wounds in which an associated nerve injury is suspected should be explored both to confirm the diagnosis, where this is uncertain, and to repair the nerve. The type of injury gives a clue to the likely amount of recovery which can be expected and this is important to the surgeon who may need to plan palliative tendon transfers. Skin loss, vascular insufficiency and fractures must be dealt with prior to nerve repair. Such serious injuries do not augur well for the limb as a whole, and the scarred tissues which develop after a compound fracture, missile injury or sepsis interfere with nerve regeneration.

Ideally, the neurorrhaphy should be enveloped in a well-vascularised bed of healthy muscle and fat. Adherence of the repaired nerve to moving tendons or to a cutaneous scar interferes with axonal regrowth and stimulates collagen deposition at the site of the repair. Soft tissue defects should be repaired with muscle flaps or local fasciocutaneous flaps. As an alternative, the nerve can be transposed to a different location to avoid such problems.

Primary repair or grafting of a divided nerve appears to give better results than delayed repair.[27] It should be emphasized, however, that this is the experience of those expert in this field, and for the surgeon relatively unversed in handling nerves it may be better to ensure a meticulous debridement of the wound, proper treatment of associated injuries and sound primary healing, thus ensuring that the ground is prepared for delayed repair in the best possible circumstances. Where delayed exploration is anticipated, it is helpful to mark the nerve ends with fine non-absorbable sutures. Careful coaptation of the severed ends with 6/0 nylon, so as to orient the nerve stumps accurately, is especially useful since the shape of the nerve and the passage of the longitudinal vessels within the epineurium are better defined at this stage rather than later when the anatomy is distorted by scar tissue. This manoeuvre also prevents retraction of the nerve ends.[28]

Primary repair is the treatment of choice in the ideal circumstances of a cleanly cut nerve in an uncontaminated wound treated by an experienced surgeon. There are four techniques for coapting nerve ends (Fig. 44.3): epineural, fascicular, grouped fascicular or mixed repair, involving several of these techniques.[28] A sound knowledge of the tissue planes in the limbs is essential, particularly in proximal lesions where a tourniquet cannot be used to help find the nerve ends. Bipolar coagulation should be used to minimize damage to the nerves when securing haemostasis, and a nerve stimulator is also helpful.

The ideal nerve repair should be performed as a primary procedure between viable nerve ends with no tension and perfect alignment of the fascicles. There should be no foreign bodies in the vicinity, no infection and the nerve should glide freely in the surrounding tissues. To avoid the foreign body reaction associated with suture material, coaptation with fibrin glue has been used.[29,30] Laser 'spot welding' to bond nerve ends has also been practised experimentally. Practically speaking, nerve repair varies only in suture placement, and each attempts to align the fascicles accurately.

Epineural repair

This is the traditional method.[31] The use of either magnifying loupes or the operating microscope improves suture placement.[32] The nerve ends are trimmed to leave fascicles mushrooming from the end with the epineurium slightly retracted (Fig. 44.3a). The goal of an epineural repair is to restore continuity in the proper rotational alignment without tension. Longitudinal blood vessels in the epineurium and the arrangement of the fascicles may assist in orienting the nerve ends. The neurorrhaphy is carried out using fine non-absorbable sutures. An 8/0 or 9/0 nylon is used for large nerves, and 10/0 nylon for smaller nerves such as digital nerves. The nylon is passed through the epineurium proximally and distally and the ends are tied. The epineurium should not be closed so tightly that the fascicular ends become mismatched or malaligned. A second suture is placed opposite the first to align the nerve. The minimum number of sutures should be used to approximate the nerve ends adequately. No fascicles should protrude between the suture lines and there should be no tension on the repair.

Fascicular repair

When a nerve has very few fascicles, it may be possible to align the individual fascicles with fine sutures. The cut ends are freshened to reveal undamaged tissue. The cross-sectional anatomy is then inspected and the fascicles are apposed with interrupted 10/0 nylon

REFERENCES

25. Thomas P K Neurology 1960; 10: 1045
26. Louis D S, Hawkin F M Orthopedics 1987; 10: 434–436
27. Grabb W C J Bone Joint Surg 1968; 50A: 964–972
28. Wilgis E F S In: Green D P (ed) Operative Hand Surgery. Churchill Livingstone, Edinburgh 1988
29. Bonnard C, Narakas A Presented to Third Annual Meeting American Society for Reconstructive Microsurgery, San Antonio, Texas, September 1987
30. Seddon H J, Medawar P B Lancet 1942; ii: 87
31. Orgel M G Clin Plast Surg 1984; 11: 101–104
32. Mackinnon S E, Dellon A L Surgery of the Peripheral Nerves. Thieme Medical Publishers, New York 1988
33. Sunderland S Nerves and Nerve Injuries. Williams & Wilkins, Baltimore 1968
34. Jabaley M E J Hand Surg 1984; 9B: 14
35. Lilla J A, Phelps D B, Boswick J A Ann Plast Surg 1979; 2: 24–31
36. Brushert T M, Seiler W A Exp Neurol 1987; 97: 289–300

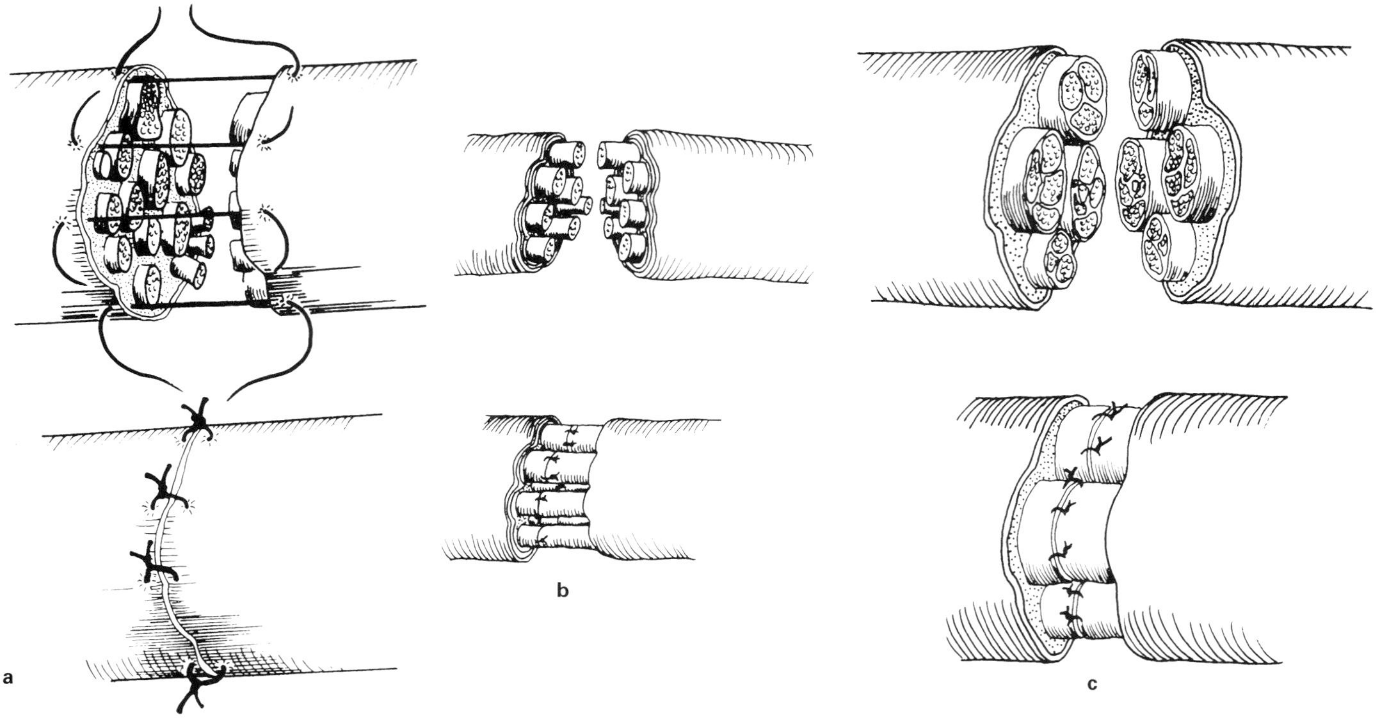

a b c

Fig. 44.3 (a) Epineural repair; (b) fascicular repair; (c) grouped fascicular repair.

sutures using the operating microscope.[28] The sutures are placed in the interfascicular epineurium and the perineurium of the individual fascicle (Fig. 44.3b). Individual dissection of the fascicles tends to confuse the situation and is not recommended.

Grouped fascicular repair

Within a large nerve, a number of fascicles are often grouped together.[33] These fascicular groups have different sizes and shapes and they can be separated and the internal epineurium sutured (Fig. 44.3c). It is helpful to suture together a posterior flap of external epineurium first to take the tension off the repair.[34] There are approximately five groups of fascicles in a median nerve at forearm level, and four of these groups in an ulnar nerve at the wrist. In this technique, the margin of error is reduced as the axons tend to remain in their correct groupings.[28]

Comparisons of epineural and fascicular repairs of peripheral nerves have shown no conclusive evidence that one technique is better than another.[31,32,35] The potential benefits of fascicular alignment are probably not realized because of the increased surgical manipulation required in order to execute the repair, and the potential to mismatch fascicles is still present. Although the epineural repair is not as precise, it may allow for neurotrophic effects to influence the direction of nerve fibre growth.[32] This is the preference of a motor axon to grow towards a distal motor stump rather than a sensory stump.[36]

NERVE GRAFTING

In secondary repair, the scar surrounding the area of nerve injury has to be resected to reveal healthy tissue with axons pouting out of the proximal end. A gap in the nerve is inevitable. The true nerve gap is measured with scar tissue removed and with joints extended. If it is possible to perform a comfortable repair with minimal mobilization, and without extensive joint flexion or tension on the nerve, then direct suture can be considered. When the gap cannot be closed without tension, a nerve graft is required. In a digit, defects of only a few millimetres should be grafted. In the forearm, a gap of several centimetres may close directly. Even a minimum of tension on the nerve repair will jeopardize the ultimate functional result.[37,38] The effect of tension on the intraneural blood supply is easily demonstrated by observing the circulation to a peripheral nerve under the operating microscope. Very little tension is required to blanch the nerve.

It is essential that the florid overgrowth of epineurium and adventitial tissue is resected from the nerve ends before grafting is undertaken.

Several nerves can be used to provide nerve graft material. The sural nerve provides a 30–40 cm length of nerve graft.[32] This leaves the patient with an area of numbness on the lateral aspect of the foot, which diminishes with time. The medial and lateral cutaneous nerves of the forearm can also be used as nerve grafts. Prior to the surgery, the patient should be warned of the likely need for a graft, of the additional scar and of the sensory loss which will occur. The grafts are cut to bridge the nerve gap without tension, and they should be routed through as healthy a bed as possible. For a major

REFERENCES

37. Terzis J K, Faibisoff B A, Williams B Plast Reconstr Surg 1975; 56: 106
38. Millesi H Hand Clin 1986; 2: 651

nerve, strands of graft are sewn in loosely using magnification to bridge the gap between groups of fascicles. For gaps in smaller nerves, a single strand of nerve graft may suffice.

To avoid sacrifice of a cutaneous nerve, segments of muscle have been successfully interposed between nerve ends. The muscle is frozen and thawed prior to insertion to denature the cellular elements and leave a scaffold of hollow tubes down which axons can grow.[39,40]

Alternative conduits, such as Dexon tubes or a segment of vein, have been used instead of a nerve graft. This technique is best applied to short gaps only. For gaps in excess of 2 cm, nerve grafting remains the method of choice.

Elongation of a peripheral nerve using slow tissue expansion techniques (cf. stretching of fascicles by a slow-growing schwannoma) has also been used to bridge the nerve gap.[41]

It is possible experimentally to preserve nerve blood flow and function while stretching a nerve to bridge a potential gap.[42]

Free vascularized nerve grafts have also been described but some surgeons have shown no clear advantage to this technique over conventional grafting.[43] Nerve grafts from the dorsum of the foot vascularized by the dorsalis pedis artery have been used to restore sensibility in anaesthetic scarred digits.[44] This technique is most applicable when the bed is unacceptable for conventional grafting.

Preliminary surgery to improve the quality of the bed in which the grafts will lie is sometimes required. Free flaps of muscle or skin provide a bed of well-vascularized tissue. To avoid the repaired nerve becoming enmeshed in scar tissue, a free fascial flap taken from the temporalis area or over the serratus anterior surface can be wrapped around a nerve graft that would otherwise lie in a scarred bed.[45,46] This surrounds the repaired nerve with well-vascularized loose areolar tissue and allows it to glide when the limb is moved. When a normally functioning nerve becomes slowly enmeshed in scar tissue after trauma, good results can be achieved by removing the scar tissue alone (neurolysis) without resort to excision of the damaged segment and nerve grafting or primary repair. When the scarred epineurium is removed, the presence of intact fascicles needs to be confirmed. Once neurolysed, the nerve must be placed into a bed of well-vascularized tissue if further scarring is to be prevented. The pronator quadratus muscle has been mobilized at the level of the wrist to wrap around median or ulnar nerves.[47]

Once grafts are in place, the extremity is splinted in a comfortable position for 10–14 days. The patient can be discharged from hospital within 1 or 2 days of the operation. Once the splint is removed, exercises are commenced, avoiding hyperextension for several weeks. A more prolonged period of splintage is not necessary when the nerve repair is not under tension.

THE DELAYED NERVE INJURY

Patients presenting at a late stage are difficult to manage. The restoration of lost function is not easy. All too often, treatment is directed towards overcoming fixed deformity which should never have occurred, or at healing the trophic sores which follow neglect of insensate skin. Pain may be difficult to treat in these circumstances. If the delay is considerable—over 6 months in the case of a radial or common peroneal nerve injury—or if the original injury caused extensive nerve damage, as is likely in missile wounds, then an appropriate muscle transfer may be a more satisfactory way of improving the patient's prospects.[48] The treatment plan is determined by the extent of scarring in the limb, and the extent of ischaemic fibrosis in the paralysed muscles.

A precise assessment of the patient's functional disability provides the key to the most satisfactory treatment plan. Repair of the nerve itself may form only one step in such a plan.

PATTERNS OF RECOVERY

Advancing Tinel sign

A valuable sign of nerve regeneration is that of Tinel.[21] As the course of a nerve trunk is percussed from distal to proximal, the patient may complain of pins and needles over the area of nerve regeneration. This is caused by the irritability of fine regenerating nerve fibres which are not fully myelinated. There is a delay of several days before regenerating axons sprout from the cut end of a divided nerve, and the Tinel sign is often difficult to detect until 2 months after an injury. The level of the Tinel should be measured from a fixed bony point to minimize observer error. The Tinel sign first occurs at the site of injury, and then advances at a rate of 2.5 cm per month or 1 mm per day.[9] The rate is faster in more proximal injuries. Without a satisfactory nerve repair, the Tinel sign will not advance—a Tinel sign which has progressed beyond the level of the injury is an important indicator of success and one which does not advance suggests failure of repair. Cohorts of axons advance at differing rates, and it is possible to have a Tinel sign at two or three positions in the same nerve.

Disappearance of the Tinel sign

Shortly after the advancing Tinel reaches a neuromuscular junction or sensory end-organ, it disappears. At this stage, gentle stroking of the skin may elicit tingling. In assessing the progress of nerve recovery, it is important to relate the advancing Tinel to the original site of injury. A strong advancing Tinel associated with a diminishing static Tinel indicates a good prognosis. A weak advancing Tinel in the presence of a persistently strong static Tinel is an indication of a poor prognosis.

REFERENCES

39. Glasby M A, Gilmour J A et al Br J Plast 1990; 43: 169–178
40. Norris R W, Glasby M A et al J Bone Joint Surg 1988; 70: 530
41. Manders E K, Saggers G C et al Clin Plast Surg 1987; 14: 551
42. Van der Wey L P, Polder T W et al Plast Reconstr Surg 1996; 97: 568–576
43. Gilbert A Clin Plast Surg 1974; 2: 73–77
44. Rose E H, Kowalski T A, Norris M S Plast Reconstr Surg 1989; 83: 593–604
45. Wintsch K, Helaly P J Reconst Microsurg 1986; 2: 143–150
46. Millesi H, Zoch G, Rath Th Ann Hand Upper Limb Surg 1990; 9: 87–97
47. Dellon A L, Mackinnon S E Plast Reconstr Surg 1986; 77: 427
48. Zachary R B In: Seddon H (ed) Peripheral Nerve Injuries. Her Majesty's Stationery Office, London 1954

Table 44.1 Highet's scheme[49]

S0	No sensibility in the autonomous zone of the nerve
S1	Recovery of deep cutaneous pain in the autonomous zone of the nerve
S2	Recovery of superficial pain and some touch
S2+	Over-response to painful stimuli and touch
S3	Return of superficial pain and touch throughout the autonomous zone of the nerve
S3+	Some return of two-point discrimination
S4	Complete recovery

Establishment of sensation

Protective sensation then develops and the patient can withdraw from painful stimuli. More discriminatory sensation often follows. Measurement of the quality of sensory recovery is difficult. A useful test is that of two-point discrimination. The smallest gap between two blunt wires at which the patient perceives the two endings as separate is noted in millimetres. Functional recovery is graded according to Highet's scheme, shown in Table 44.1.[49]

The recognition of early signs of recovery is important. Electromyography may detect early reinnervation of paralysed muscles, and could tip the scales against exploring a motor nerve. Accurate charting of muscle power is also important to assess motor nerve recovery (Table 44.2).[49]

Table 44.2 The 0–5 scale for recording muscle power

M0	No contraction
M1	Flicker or trace of contraction
M2	Active movement with gravity eliminated
M3	Active movement against gravity
M4	Active movement against gravity and resistance
M5	Normal power

SENSORY RE-EDUCATION

This is a method or combination of techniques which help the patient with sensory impairment to learn to reinterpret the altered profile of neural impulses reaching a conscious level when the injured hand is stimulated. At a cortical level, sensory information is associated with previous experiences to allow a recognition pattern to develop.[32] After nerve division the neural impulses from a given stimulus find no match in the associated cortex. The sensation is therefore new and may even pass unnoticed. When sensation reaches the fingertips after nerve repair, the training is begun. The patient repeatedly feels a variety of objects and textures, each session lasting 10–15 minutes. A rubber (eraser), keys, coins, buttons, rice, etc. are used with the eyes closed and open until a reliable recognition pattern develops. Such a programme of retraining has been shown to improve two-point discrimination markedly in adults following sensory nerve repair.[13,50]

PROGNOSIS

Two factors remain within the control of the surgeon. The first is the timing of the nerve repair. There is a decline in the quality of results with progressive delay, so much so that repair of a high ulnar nerve lesion after 6–9 months is barely worthwhile.[48–51] The second is the skill with which the repair is carried out, not only of the nerve, but also of the associated injuries. Ulnar nerve repair at the wrist or distal forearm yields better results if the adjacent ulnar artery is repaired at the same time.[52,53] The meticulous repair of tendons and tendon sheaths reduces adhesions between the nerve and nearby tendons. It is preferable for the neurorrhaphy to be surrounded by the minimum of scar tissue as adherence of a repaired nerve to moving tendons or to a cutaneous scar may interfere with axonal regrowth and encourage the development of a painful neuroma. Nerve and bone injuries are often associated, particularly in gunshot wounds. The presence of an un-united fracture may involve the nerve in callus or cause friction neuritis if the nerve crosses a roughened surface. Successful fixation of fractures allows early gentle movement of joints and reduces stiffness.

The age of the patient also influences prognosis. A good primary repair of the median nerve in a 7-year-old child should be followed by a truly excellent result; such a result is extremely rare in even a young adult. In 1962, Onne[54] evaluated the results of primary nerve repair 5 years after surgery, and found that the degree of static two-point discrimination recovered in millimetres was proportional to the patient's age in years. The more proximal injuries, being further from motor end-plates and sensory receptors, are less likely to achieve good functional recovery, especially in the motor system, where successful reinnervation of the muscle fibres is time-dependent.[32]

The level of the lesion is also significant: return of good-quality sensation is rare after repair of a median nerve injured in the axilla, and return of function in the intrinsic muscles of the hand cannot be hoped for after repair of an ulnar nerve injured at the same level.[55] The outlook for repair of a major mixed motor and sensory nerve such as the ulnar is worse than for repair of a nerve that contains chiefly motor fibres such as the axillary or musculocutaneous nerve. This is due to mismatching with regeneration of nerve fibres to inappropriate distal connections. If a proximal injury occurs in an extremity where motor and sensory nerves are adjacent to each other in the same fascicle, abnormal sensory and motor recovery is likely. More distally, the fascicles may be entirely motor or sensory with little admixing. At this level, appropriate alignment of the nerve is likely to result in a better recovery.[22]

REFERENCES

49. Tinel J In: Spinner M (Ed), Injuries to the major branches of peripheral nerves of the forearm, 2nd Edn, W B Saunders, Philadelphia 1978; 8–13
50. Wynn Parry C B, Salter M Hand 1976; 8: 250–257
51. Woodall B, Beebe G W Peripheral Nerve Regeneration (American) Veterans Administration Monograph. United States Government Printing Office, Washington DC 1956
52. Leclercq D C, Caliert A J et al J Hand Surg 1985; 10A (suppl): 997–999
53. Merle M, Amend P et al Periph Nerve 1986; 2: 17–26
54. Onne L Acta Chir Scand 1962; 300 (suppl): 1–70
55. Gaul J S J Hand Surg 1982; 7: 502

It has been shown that in certain conditions a motor nerve will preferentially grow towards a distal motor rather than a sensory nerve stump when there is a choice.[36]

TENDON TRANSFER

In motor paralysis, there is a temptation to prolong observation in the hope that recovery may occur. Muscle reinnervation is most likely when the injury is close to the muscle group. Where one muscle group is paralysed because of failed nerve recovery, tendon transfers should be considered. In some circumstances, tendon transfers should be undertaken at an early stage if it is clear that the likelihood of recovery is remote, e.g. a severe injury to the nerve over a wide area in an older patient. It should however be remembered that if an early tendon transfer is undertaken and the nerve subsequently recovers, very abnormal movements may develop which may necessitate taking down the transfers. An assessment of how nerve recovery is proceeding can be made by examining the first muscle distal to the injury and assessing when it recovers. If its recovery has not occurred by 6 months in excess of its expected recovery time (assessed by judging the distance between the site of injury and the first muscle to be reinnervated, and assessing the time of axonal growth at a maximum of 1 mm per day), nerve exploration or tendon transfers should be undertaken.

Tendon transfer is a redistribution of the remaining functional parts.[56] Certain basic principles must be adhered to for a successful outcome:

1. The tendon to be transferred must be of adequate strength. In practice, this means normal muscle power.
2. The direction of transfer must be as close to the original direction of pull as possible.
3. The excursion of the tendon chosen must be as close as possible to that of the original muscle it is replacing.
4. The route through which the transfer passes must be a well-vascularized bed capable of allowing a tendon to slide. In practice, this means healthy subcutaneous tissue without overlying scars or skin grafts.
5. The limb to be operated upon must be soft and supple with a full passive range of motion and no joint contractures.
6. The tension of the transfer must be perfect. In practice, this means that the transfer must be tight enough to produce the desired function yet still allow complete reversal of the functional position during passive movement.
7. Only one tendon should be used to produce one function (tendons used to produce two functions always fail in one of them).
8. If possible, the tendon chosen should be synergistic with the one it is replacing.

In assessing which transfers are to undertaken, it is useful to draw a list of the functions which are missing, then a list of the tendons which are available to replace them, and a list of those which can afford to be used. Appropriate choices can then be made. Even for experienced surgeons, this rather basic approach will guarantee consistently good choices. There are, however, certain examples where tendon transfers work well.

Radial nerve palsy

Under normal circumstances tendon transfers for patients with, radial nerve palsy work well, e.g. for wrist extension, the pronator teres can be transferred to extensor carpi radialis brevis. Finger extension can be achieved by transferring flexor carpi ulnaris to the extensor digitorum, and thumb extension by transferring palmaris longus to extensor pollicis longus.

Median nerve palsy

An opponensplasty may be indicated; examples are extensor indicis proprius or the sublimis to the ring finger.

Ulnar nerve palsy

In a low ulnar nerve palsy, a loss of thumb adduction can be overcome by using the sublimis from the ring finger. Abduction of the index finger may be achieved by inserting extensor indicis into the interosseous insertion. Clawing, which rarely requires correction following a simple low ulnar nerve division with good repair, may in exceptional circumstances be corrected by either advancing the volar plate or by using the sublimis tendon and forming a loop or lasso around the A2 pulley. Both of these procedures are designed to prevent hyperextension of the metacarpophalangeal joint, which is responsible for the clawing.

COMPLICATIONS OF A NERVE INJURY

A nerve injury may be complicated by loss of sensation, paralysis, loss of sympathetic function and pain. The most important consequence of loss of sensation is a trophic ulcer from inadvertent injury.[22] The ulcer may become infected. Patients must be warned of the hazards to insensitive skin and advised about proper clothing and footwear. A lack of attention for even a short period can cause many months of disability. In severe cases of ulceration of the foot, amputation may be the only treatment option, especially when osteomyelitis of the underlying bones develops.

Loss of sweating and turgor of the finger pulps increase the vulnerability of the skin of the hand to thermal damage. What is tolerated by the normal hand will not necessarily be tolerated by the insensitive hand.

Paralysis of some muscles, and the unopposed action of others, may lead to a fixed deformity. Common examples include the fixed internal rotation of the shoulder from a brachial plexus lesion, fixed extension of the meta-carpophalangeal joint from ulnar nerve injuries and the equinus deformity of the foot from a severed sciatic nerve.[22] It is essential to prevent fixed deformity after a peripheral nerve injury by splintage and manipulation. Such deformities represent a failure of adequate care.

When the sprouting axons from a divided or partially divided nerve do not make appropriate distal connections, then a swelling

REFERENCES

56. Beasley R W Orthop Clin 1970; 1: 433

of the nerve or neuroma can develop. If injury to the Schwann cells no longer confines the axons to their endoneural tubes, regenerating axons escape into the surrounding tissue in a disorganized fashion, where they mix with fibroblasts, Schwann cells and blood vessels. Partial nerve division usually results in a lateral neuroma or neuroma in continuity. A terminal neuroma usually results from a complete nerve division.

Not all neuromas are painful, and it is not known why one neuroma should be clinically symptomatic and another not so. One of the first goals in preventing neuromas is to use meticulous microsurgical technique to direct appropriate functional axonal regeneration.[32]

Pain

The pain complicating a nerve injury may be of several different types. *Neuromatous pain* is a discrete area of tenderness at the site of a previous nerve injury; percussion of the neuroma produces paraesthesia in the distribution of the injured nerve. This pain is mediated by small-diameter C and A-δ fibres.[57,58]

The wide variety of techniques described to treat peripheral neuromas underlines the fact that this condition is difficult to cure. Where the nerve end is trapped in scar tissue, cutting back the nerve to a more proximal level is useful. Implantation of the transected nerve into a muscle has also proved helpful.[47,59,60] The underlying principle is to move the neuroma to a well-padded area where repeated stimulation is unlikely. In some cases, where both proximal and distal nerve ends can be found, direct repair or nerve grafting to restore nerve continuity is effective.[61] If a neuroma is not trapped in scar tissue, then non-surgical techniques may be helpful. Regular tapping of the point to desensitize the nerve is helpful. Transcutaneous nerve stimulators or local anaesthetic blocks may also help to break the pain cycle.

Causalgia is the burning pain and hyperalgesia in the distribution of an injured peripheral nerve.[62] Even a light touch on the skin produces exquisite pain, which may be exacerbated by a gust of air, loud noises and even emotional output. The pain is probably mediated by larger-diameter A-β fibres,[57] although in previous work, these large-diameter fibres were thought to inhibit pain messages.[58] The lesion responsible is usually a partial injury to a major mixed nerve in the proximal part of a limb. There is a high incidence after injuries to the brachial plexus and sciatic nerves.

Reflex sympathetic dystrophy is characterized by diffuse pain, joint stiffness, swelling and discoloration. The pain may occur after a variety of injuries and is not unique to nerve division or nerve entrapment. Affected limbs may at various times be blue or pink. The skin is often tight, glossy and there may be excessive sweating, osteoporosis and atrophy of the fat pads of the fingertips. These changes are due to sympathetic overactivity.

The shoulder–hand syndrome is a form of reflex sympathetic dystrophy caused by proximal limb trauma or a visceral lesion such as a heart attack, stomach ulcer or Pancoast tumour. The pain and swelling in the upper limb are associated with limited shoulder movement.

Reflex sympathetic dystrophy, including causalgia and the shoulder–hand syndrome, is best treated as early as possible. Interruption of the sympathetic reflex can be achieved with repeated stellate ganglion blockade using local anaesthetic. This procedure warms up the limb and causes a temporary Horner's syndrome. As peripheral nerves carry sympathetic efferent fibres, brachial plexus blockade also interrupts the sympathetic reflex. Continuous slow infusion of local anaesthetic to a trigger point, should there be one, can also quell the pain reflex.[63]

The use of intravenous regional sympathetic blockade using guanethidine is another standard treatment.[64] Guanethidine displaces the sympathetic neurotransmitter noradrenaline from its storage and receptor sites in sympathetic nerve endings to give a prolonged sympathetic blockade. Surgical sympathectomy is of some value in patients with causalgia[65] but, surprisingly, is often not helpful in other forms of sympathetic dystrophy.[66]

Cold intolerance is a common feature of nerve injuries, even if repaired successfully. There is always a permanent degree of cold intolerance following a crush injury, but it does also temporarily develop after other nerve injuries. Cold intolerance is usually at its worst for 18 months after a simple nerve transection, after which it gradually settles. Regeneration of both somatic and autonomic function occurs after repair, but poor thermoregulation may explain the feeling of numbness and discomfort in cold weather.

IATROGENIC NERVE INJURY

Inadvertent damage to nerves is not uncommon.[4] Irritant drugs may be injected into the sciatic or axillary nerves when the intramuscular route is used.[67,68] Ill-fitting crutches or splints can cause foot or wrist drop.[22] The brachial plexus may be damaged when local anaesthetic is injected to effect a brachial block. The greatest damage is however caused during minor surgical procedures. Restricted anatomical knowledge combined with poor technique will place a peripheral nerve at risk. The median nerve has been mistaken for palmaris longus when a tendon graft is required,[69] the accessory nerve is at risk when a neck lump is excised, and branches of the sciatic nerve have been damaged during varicose vein surgery.

When faced with a significant neural deficit after a wound has been made over the course of a nerve, the proper course of action is to assume that the nerve has been divided. If sensation, motor power and sympathetic function are absent, then the wound should

REFERENCES

57. Campbell J N, Raja S N et al Pain 1988; 32: 89–94
58. Melzack R, Wall P D Science 1965; 150: 971
59. Moskowicz L P Zentralbl Chir 1918; 45: 547
60. Teneff S J Int Coll Surg 1949; 12: 16
61. Van Beek A L In: McCarthy J (ed) Plastic Surgery. W B Saunders, Philadelphia 1990
62. Mitchell S W, Morehouse G R, Keen W W Gunshot Wounds and Other Injuries of Nerves. J B Lippincott, Philadelphia 1864
63. Omer G E, Thomas S Tex Med 1971; 67: 93–96
64. Hannington-Kiff J G Lancet 1974; i: 1019–1020
65. Jebara V A, Saade B J Trauma 1987; 27: 519
66. Evans J Ann Intern Med 1947; 26: 417
67. Gentili F, Hudson A R et al Neurosurgery 1979; 4: 244
68. Gentili F, Hudson A R, Hunter D Can J Neurol 1980; 7: 143
69. Vastamaki M J Hand Surg 1987; 12B: 187–188

be re-explored urgently. It is unnecessary to prevaricate by passing the burden of diagnosis on to a neurologist; neurophysiological signs of nerve injury will not be evident for several weeks after injury.

BRACHIAL PLEXUS INJURIES

The brachial plexus arises from the lowest four cervical and highest thoracic spinal nerve roots. The roots unite to form three trunks (Fig. 44.4)—the upper contains fibres of spinal elements C5 and 6, the middle C7 and the lower C8 and T1. The trunks lie in the supraclavicular fossa just distal to the scalene muscles. The upper trunk gives origin to the suprascapular nerve. The trunks then divide into anterior and posterior divisions to carry fibres to the dorsal and ventral aspects of the limb (Fig. 44.4).

Patients with severe and multiple injuries from road traffic accidents have an increased chance of survival as a result of the use of helmets by motorcyclists, rapid transport to hospitals from the roadside and recent advances in medical care. This may explain the marked increase in the number of patients with traction lesions of the brachial plexus being referred to specialist units.[70] The treatment of head, chest and abdominal injuries takes precedence over the management of a peripheral nerve injury. It is however important to remember the possibility of a brachial plexus injury in an unconscious patient, especially when there are fractures of the shoulder girdle, proximal humerus or the first rib.

The prognosis relates to the level of the lesion. There are three main types of injury:

1. In root avulsion, the nerve roots are avulsed from the spinal cord within the vertebral column. Spontaneous improvement is unlikely, and the injury is not amenable to surgical repair.
2. Rupture of the brachial plexus outside the vertebral column. Spontaneous improvement is unlikely but the injury may benefit from surgical repair.
3. Nerve damage without rupture. A neurapraxia or axonotmesis with preservation of the nerve sheaths is likely to improve spontaneously. In road traffic accidents, low-velocity injuries tend to be associated with neurapraxia and axonotmesis while a high-velocity impact is more likely to produce a complete disruption of the plexus.

A preganglionic injury where the spinal nerves have been torn directly from the spinal cord presents with deep bruising in the posterior triangle of the neck, loss of sensation above the clavicle, pain in an insensitive hand and a Horner's syndrome (miosis, enophthalmos, anhidrosis and ptosis). The loss of function of muscles innervated by branches coming directly from the roots of the brachial plexus is highly suggestive of proximal root avulsion. Winging of the scapula and paralysis of the ipsilateral hemidiaphragm on chest X-ray are bad prognostic signs. Lower limb hyper-reflexia may also occur when a root avulsion occurs at cord level.

With a preganglionic lesion, the motor fibres have been separated from their cell bodies in the anterior horn cells, but the sensory fibres are still connected to their cell bodies in the dorsal root ganglion. Thus, although the patient will not be able to appreciate sensation, there will be no wallerian degeneration in the sensory fibres, and sensory nerve conduction studies will be normal when tested 4 weeks after injury.[71] The axon flare reflex of Lewis in response to histamine also remains intact. Myelograms are useful to confirm the diagnosis, although deformity of the root sleeve is not an acid test for root avulsion.[72] When the roots have been avulsed directly from the spinal cord there is no proximal peripheral nerve tissue and surgical repair is not possible.

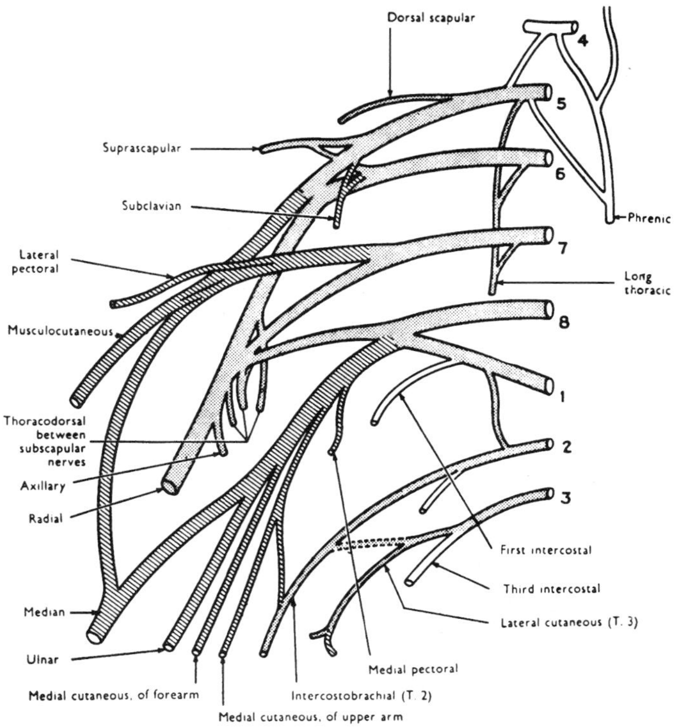

Fig. 44.4 The brachial plexus. From Walton: Brain's Diseases of the Nervous System, 9th edn. Oxford University Press, Oxford 1985, with permission.

By contrast, in post-ganglionic injuries, there are normal nerve fibres proximal to the lesion. Should spontaneous recovery of a traction injury not occur, then surgical repair is possible.

Open wounds of the brachial plexus and those associated with damaged vessels merit urgent exploration both to restore the circulation to the limb and to determine the extent of nerve damage. Clean sharp lacerations of the brachial plexus should be treated by primary epineural repair. The qualtiy of results diminishes markedly if nerve repair or grafting is delayed more than 2 months.[70]

Closed traction injuries account for the majority of brachial plexus injuries seen. An advancing Tinel's sign and electromyographic evidence of reinnervation are favourable signs. Even in axonotmesis, physiotherapy is important to maintain a passive

REFERENCES

70. Narakas A O In: McCarthy J G (ed) Plastic Surgery. W B Saunders, Philadelphia 1990
71. Bonney G Brain 1954; 77: 588–609
72. Jelasic F, Peipgras U Eur Neurol 1974; 11: 158

range of movement in involved joints. Should arm function show no signs of spontaneous recovery then the brachial plexus is explored and divided nerves are repaired. Because of the nature of traction injuries, neurolysis is often required. Although direct nerve suture may on occasion be possible, autogenous nerve grafting of the damaged segments is more often required.

The outcome of an extensive repair of a supraclavicular rupture of the brachial plexus is not good. An improvement in shoulder function and restoration of elbow flexion may be achieved but recovery of sensation and power in the forearm and hand is unlikely.[73] While striving to restore sensation and movement to the upper limb, it must be remembered that pain is a very important feature of brachial plexus injuries. Patients with root avulsions are especially prone to severe pain and up to 80% of them suffer with paroxysms of sharp burning pain of several seconds duration.[81] There may be a background of dull pain that the patients are able to endure, while they are defenceless against the severe attacks. Transcutaneous nerve stimulation and thalamic stimulation are often helpful. For those who continue to suffer despite such treatment, coagulation of the dorsal root entry zone has proved helpful.[74] Irritative painful nerve lesions in the absence of root avulsion are also common, but they respond well to nerve repair.[70]

Where spontaneous recovery is not anticipated, close supervision is necessary to prevent contractures, to relieve pain and to fit functional braces. Arthrodesis of the glenohumeral joint can improve shoulder function when the glenohumeral muscles are paralysed, yet the scapulothoracic group are functioning. Several tendon transfers can be used to restore elbow flexion. In one the sternocostal portion of pectoralis major is mobilized, preserving its neurovascular supply. When the muscle is swung into the upper arm, and joined to the biceps tendon, it acts on the elbow effectively.[75] The shoulder should be of normal power or stabilized by an arthrodesis. In an upper root lesion, where the forearm muscles are functioning, the common flexor origin can be shifted to a more proximal point on the humerus so that the movement of elbow flexion is increased.[76] The presence of a flail anaesthetic upper limb may require the patient to retrain in a new occupation.[77] In some patients the limb becomes the site of chronic infection and multiple fractures, with little hope of functional recovery. The final solution—amputation of the limb—is still a potential means of rehabilitation in some patients.

If the plexus is disrupted at cord level, the spinatus muscles, serratus anterior, the pectoral muscles and the cervical sympathetic chain are usually spared. Sensation in the forearm and hand is lost after a complete disruption of the plexus and reflexes cannot be elicited at any point in the upper limb. Complete plexus lesions can be caused by traumatic damage of the cervical spine, by neoplasms involving cervical nerve roots, by prolapsed intervertebral discs, by cervical spondylosis and tuberculosis of the spine. In the neck, gunshot wounds, stabbings, fractures of the clavicle, dislocations of the humerous and motorcycle accidents in which the shoulder and neck are forcibly pulled apart cause disruption of the plexus. The lower plexus can be compressed in patients with the thoracic outlet syndrome, usually by a cervical rib; it may be invaded by a Pancoast tumour, or by malignant lymph nodes in the neck. Most commonly, part rather than the whole of the brachial plexus is involved. This invariably involves either the upper or the lower nerve roots.

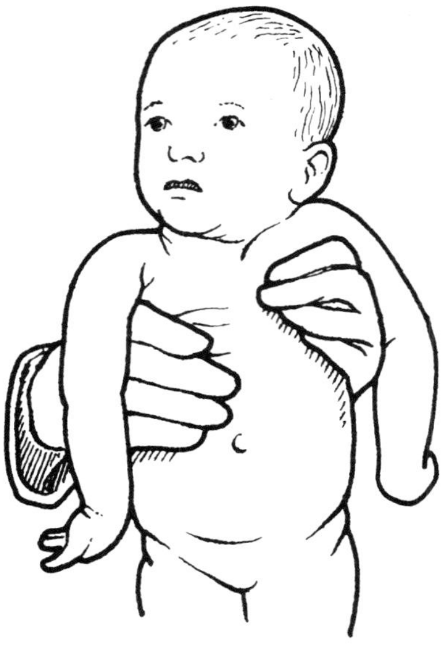

Fig. 44.5 Erb's palsy: tip position.

Upper plexus injury (Erb–Duchenne type C5 and 6)

The upper part of the plexus is most commonly torn as a result of forcible separation of the head and shoulder. This was originally common at parturition when excessive traction was applied to the head to deliver the shoulder. This is now extremely rare. It is most commonly seen in adults following a fall on the shoulder forcing the head to one side. This is particularly common in motorcycle accidents. The muscles supplied by C5 include the biceps, deltoid, brachialis, brachioradialis, the supra- and infraspinatus and the rhomboids. The sixth cervical segment supplies serratus anterior, latissimus dorsi, triceps, pectoralis major and extensor carpi radialis. As a result of paralysis of these muscles, the limb hangs at the side, internally rotated at the shoulder due to the unopposed action of subscapularis with the forearm pronated in the so-called 'tip' position (Fig. 44.5). Patients are unable to abduct the shoulder as a result of paralysis of the deltoid. They cannot flex the elbow because biceps, brachialis and brachioradialis do not function, and external rotation of the shoulder is impossible because the spinati are also denervated. Biceps and supinator reflexes cannot be elicited. There is minor sensory loss over the insertion of the deltoid on the outer part of the arm (see Fig. 44.17).

REFERENCES

73. Birch R Curr Orthop 1987; 1: 316–323
74. Nashold B S, Ostdahl R H J Neurosurg 1979; 51: 59
75. Clark J M P Br J Surg 1946; 34: 180
76. Steindler A N Y State Med J 1918; 108: 117–119
77. Yeoman P M, Seddon H J J Bone Joint Surg 1961; 43B: 493

Lower plexus injury (Dejerine–Klumpke T1 and C8)

This is produced by traction on an already abducted arm, and often follows an attempt to prevent falling by clutching hold of a strap above the head with a raised outstretched hand. This type of injury occurs to standing passengers on buses and underground trains during sudden stops and starts. It results in paralysis of all the small muscles of the hand, producing a claw hand from the unopposed action of the long flexors and extensors of the fingers. There is sensory loss in the C8 and T1 dermatomes on the ulnar side of the arm, forearm, wrist and fingers (see Fig. 44.17). The cervical sympathetic ganglion chain is also often damaged, resulting in a Horner's syndrome.

Cord injuries

The lateral, posterior and medial cords may also be damaged by various fractures and dislocations around the shoulder joint. Injury of the lateral cord usually results in paralysis of the biceps and coracobrachialis muscles, together with all the muscles supplied by the median nerve, except those of the thenar eminence. Posterior cord damage results in axillary and radial nerve damage, while division of the medial cord results in paralysis of the muscles supplied by the ulnar nerve and the intrinsic muscles of the hand, which are supplied by the median nerve.

COMPRESSION SYNDROMES

When nerves pass over a bony prominence or through a narrow osseofascial tunnel, they run the risk of being compressed. A variety of structures including osteophytes, soft tissue swellings or congenital anomalies such as a cervical rib may contribute to a compression syndrome. As a general rule, unless an entrapment neuropathy is severe or long-standing, release of the compression effects a good recovery.

According to many authors, the primary lesion is a vascular compromise.[78–80] When a nerve is subject to pressure, there is obstruction to the flow of blood in the fine plexus of vessels within the nerve. The slowing of the circulation causes venous congestion in the involved segment which in turn results in anoxia and dilation of the small vessels. The endoneurium may become oedematous, and this then compounds the circulatory obstruction. If the situation persists, fibroblasts proliferate within the nerve, causing internal scarring which further inhibits the exchange of nutrients between the blood stream and nerve fibres. The ischaemic nerve fibres are less able to produce high-energy phosphates, so restricting the efficiency of the sodium pump and cell transport systems. This eventually impairs nerve conduction, and causes the patient discomfort. The rapid recovery and restitution of a normal conduction velocity after carpal tunnel release favour this vascular theory of nerve damage.[78]

The many compression syndromes have a number of features in common. Pain, usually in the territory of the affected nerve, is by far the most usual complaint. Nerve conduction studies are used to confirm the diagnosis.

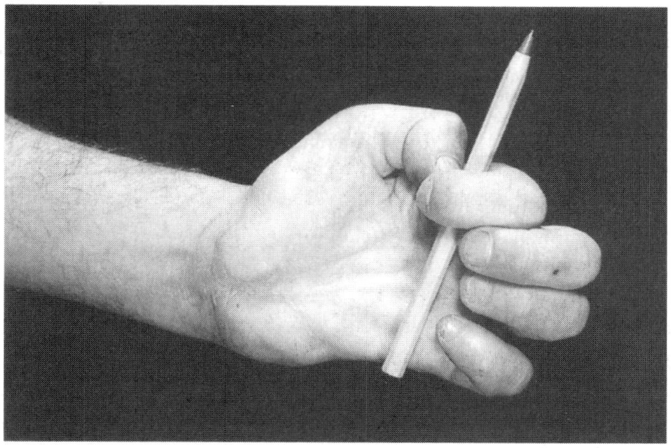

Fig. 44.6 Wasting of the thenar and hypothenar eminence due to division of the ulnar and median nerves at the wrist.

The median nerve

The median nerve is most commonly compressed at the wrist where it passes through the carpal tunnel.[81] The carpal tunnel syndrome is seen most frequently in women between 40 and 60 years of age. Although often there is no obvious predisposing cause, a multitude of conditions have been associated with this syndrome. They include rheumatoid arthritis, myxoedema, nephrotic syndrome, acromegaly, multiple myeloma, amyloidosis, diabetes mellitus, alcoholism, haemophilia, pregnancy, gout, lipomas, ganglia, anomalous musculature, wrist fractures and the menopause.

The symptoms vary from mild paraesthesia in the distribution of the median nerve to constant sensory impairment, pain and atrophy of the thenar muscles which causes a pronounced hollow in the thenar eminence (Fig. 44.6). The hand is often weak or clumsy, and numbness of the fingers and pain in the wrist or distal forearm may awaken the patient from sleep. Shoulder and upper arm pain are also common features. Although pain and paraesthesia should be experienced in the thumb, the index, the middle and the radial side of the ring fingers, this is often not the case. The thumb and index are often spared. Relief is obtained by elevating or shaking the limb.

Exaggerated flexion of the wrist.[82] or percussion of the median nerve at the wrist usually reproduces the symptoms and delayed nerve conduction confirms the diagnosis.[83] Application of a forearm tourniquet inflated above arterial pressure may also reproduce the symptoms.[84] Nerve conduction studies may help differen-

REFERENCES

78. Eversman W W, Ritsick J A J Hand Surg 1978; 3: 77–81
79. Lundborg G Scand J Plast Reconstr Surg 1970; 6 (suppl): 1–113
80. Lundborg G, Gelbermann R H et al J Hand Surg 1982; 7: 252–259
81. Eversmann W W Jr In: Green D P (ed) Operative Hand Surgery, vol 2, 2nd edn. Churchill Livingstone, New York 1988
82. Phalen G S J Bone Joint Surg 1966; 48A: 211–228
83. Simpson J A J Neurol Neurosurg Psychiatry 1956; 19: 275
84. Gilliatt R W, Wilson T G Lancet 1953; ii: 595

tiate the carpal tunnel syndrome from the thoracic outlet syndrome and compression of the cervical nerves in spondylitis.[85]

Splinting the wrist in a neutral position will often afford relief,[81] but where this is unhelpful, surgery should be advised. The injection of steroid into the carpal tunnel can help, but once again, relief is often temporary.[86]

The surgical treatment consists of division of the transverse carpal ligament (flexor retinaculum) under tourniquet control. Particular care must be taken to avoid damage to the palmar cutaneous nerve, which lies superficial to the ligament, and the motor branch to the thenar muscles which may pass through it. The precise course of these nerves often varies[87] and it is prudent to place the incision on the ulnar side of the palmar crease where even the rare variations can be protected. The full extent of the ligament is divided, but care is required as the median nerve may be adherent to the undersurface. It is advisable to secure haemostasis before skin closure. Postoperatively, the wrist is splinted for 10 days in slight extension to prevent the median nerve from adhering to the undersurface of the skin wound. Pain relief is usually immediate, and sensation to the fingers returns quickly.

The median nerve can also be trapped as it courses between the ulnar and humeral heads of pronator teres. This produces an aching pain which is often elicited by repetitive rotatory movements of the arm.[88]

The nerve may also be kinked against the edge of flexor digitorum superficialis[89] or displaced by the ligament of Struthers.[90] This is a fibrous band arising from the supratrochlear region of the humerus which passes upwards and medially to attach to the bone at a higher level.

The ulnar nerve

The ulnar nerve may be compressed as it runs in the cubital tunnel behind the elbow joint and between the heads of flexor carpi ulnaris.[91] Compression generally presents with pain and tingling on the medial side of the forearm and hand. There may also be evidence of weakness in the intrinsic muscles of the hand. A positive percussion test over the ulnar nerve at the elbow or increased numbness when the elbow is fully flexed supports the diagnosis. There is weakness of the flexor digitorum profundus to the little finger, and confirmation of delayed nerve conduction is once again helpful in confirming the diagnosis.[92]

The condition may be associated with cubitus valgus, supracondylar fractures of the humerus, osteophytes around the elbow joint and inadvertent compression of the nerve during anaesthesia.[93] Chronic nerve irritation may cause oedema and restricted gliding as the elbow moves. Elbow splintage in a slightly flexed position may help to reduce this inflammatory reaction and provides relief.[94] Simple surgical decompression is achieved by splitting the cubital tunnel, the arcade of the flexor carpi ulnaris and the medial intermuscular septum above the elbow.

Transposition of the ulnar nerve is reported by some to be more effective than simple release.[95] The nerve is widely and carefully mobilized so that it can be transposed in front of the medial epicondyle. Care must be taken to preserve motor branches. If the patient has an abundance of subcutaneous fat, the nerve may be left in the subcutaneous plane. In most patients, however, it is necessary to locate it deep to the flexor–pronator muscles by mobilizing, then repositioning the common flexor origin.[96]

Occasionally the ulnar nerve is compressed at the wrist as it passes through Guyon's canal.[97] Symptoms include pain and paraesthesia in the little finger, and weakness in those intrinsic hand muscles innervated by the ulnar nerve. The condition can be caused by chronic repetitive trauma, and may be seen in mechanics, pipe-cutters, metal polishers and cyclists.[98–100] Lipomas, ganglia, cysts, ulnar artery thrombosis and anomalous muscles may compress the nerve.[101–103] If the hand is rested, most cases recover; open decompression is sometimes required.

Thoracic outlet syndrome

(cervical rib; see Chapter 10)

The mechanism of symptom production is complex, and not simply the result of compression by the scalene muscles (scalene syndrome), or by the rib and clavicle.[104] It is usually caused by a cervical rib which may be rudimentary or complete. It may also result from an abnormal first rib or an enlarged C8 transverse process with a fascial band extending to join the first rib. All these anatomical abnormalities cause the T1 nerve root to be hooked up, compressed and irritated by the anatomical anomaly during movement of the upper limb. Compression of the T1 root is commonly associated with compression of the subclavian artery and vein. It tends to be more common in women than men, and is maximal between the third and fifth decades. Drooping of the shoulder due to the constant carrying of heavy weights (shopping bags) may be a factor. It is interesting to note that cervical ribs only cause symptoms in between 5 and 10% of all those affected by this anomaly.

REFERENCES

85. Melvin J L, Schuckmann J A, Lanese R R Arch Phys Med Rehab 1973; 54: 69
86. Foster J B Lancet 1960; i: 454–456
87. Lanz V J Hand Surg 1977; 2: 44–53
88. Kopell H P, Thompson W A L N Engl J Med 1958; 259: 713–715
89. Kopell H P, Thompson W A L Peripheral Entrapment Neuropathies. Williams & Wilkins, Baltimore 1963
90. Nankano K K Muscle Nerve 1978; 1: 264
91. James G G H J Bone Joint Surg 1956; 38B: 589
92. Payan J J Neurol Neurosurg Psychiatry 1970; 33: 157–163
93. Ekerot L Scand J Plast Reconstr Surg 1977; 11: 225–229
94. Diamond M L, Lister G J Hand Surg 1985; 10A: 430
95. MacNicol M F J Bone Joint Surg 1979; 61B: 159–164
96. Learmonth J R Surg Gynecol Obst 1942; 75: 792
97. Dupont C, Cloutier G E et al J Bone Joint Surg 1965; 47A: 757–761
98. Hayes J R, Mullholland R C, O'Connor B T J Bone Joint Surg 1969; 51B: 469–472
99. Eckman P B, Perstlein G, Altocchi P H Arch Neurol 1975; 32: 130–131
100. Dawson D M, Hallett B, Millender L H Entrapment Neuropathies. Little, Brown, Boston 1983
101. Dell P C J Hand Surgery 1979; 4: 468–473
102. Turner M S, Caird D M Hand 1977; 9: 140–141
103. Lister G The Hand: Diagnosis and Indications, 2nd edn. Churchill Livingstone, Edinburgh 1984 pp 192–223
104. Lascelles R G, Mohr P D et al Brain 1977; 100: 601

Table 44.3 Classification of peripheral nerve tumours[109]

Tumours of nerve sheath origin	
Benign	
	Schwannoma
	Neurofibroma
Malignant	
	Malignant schwannoma
	Nerve sheath fibrosarcoma
Tumours of nerve cell origin	
	Neuroblastoma
	Ganglioneuroma
	Phaeochromocytoma
Tumours metastatic to peripheral nerves	
Tumours of non-neural origin	
	Lipofibromatosis
	Intraneural lipoma, haemangioma, ganglion
Pseudotumours, e.g. traumatic neuromas	

Symptoms may be sensory, motor or vascular. Patients normally present with pain along the ulnar border of the hand and distal forearm, often associated with paraesthesiae which can be relieved by raising the hand above the head. Occasionally, patients present with pain in the neck situated over the rib, and at a late stage they may present with weakness and wasting of the muscles in the hand. On examination, there is normally hyperalgesia or analgesia over the C8 and T1 dermatomes. There is weakness of the small muscles of the hand and a coincidental Horner's syndrome may be present. In some patients, there is a palpable rib with a bruit. Other patients experience symptoms in response to local pressure over the origin of the rib.

Thoracic inlet X-rays may show the cervical rib and nerve conduction studies may show impairment in nerve conduction along the T1 root. It is important to consider the possibility of motor neurone disease in the differential diagnosis, but this is not usually accompanied by pain and there is no sensory loss. Syringomyelia is usually associated with some long tract signs. A Pancoast's tumour must be excluded by appropriate chest radiographs or computed tomographic scans. Lesions of the ulnar and median nerve usually have a different distribution of sensory loss.[105] The treatment is by resection of the cervical rib or band.

VOLKMANN'S ISCHAEMIC CONTRACTURE

Although this condition is not strictly speaking an entrapment neuropathy, a neurological element may be observed. The classic ischaemic contracture described by Volkmann[106] affected the long flexors of the calf and resulted in clawing of the toes. This condition most commonly complicates fractures of the tibia and fibula, although a similar but functionally more disabling contracture can affect the flexors of the forearm. The condition occurs when the pressure within an enclosed fascial compartment, for example the forearm or calf, rises to such a level that the microcirculation to the muscles and nerves is compromised. Volkmann's ischaemic contracture also occurs after acute arterial occlusion or prolonged application of a tourniquet. Progressive ischaemia causes fibrosis and shortening of the muscles. Early diagnosis is essential for prevention; the earliest symptom is severe pain, usually out of all proportion to the injury sustained. Later, the limb becomes paralysed and insensate. Passive stretching may cause extreme pain and the affected compartment is tense and tender. In the forearm, the radial pulse is often preserved. An urgent decompression of all tight compartments is required, and if there is any vascular cause, this must be urgently rectified.

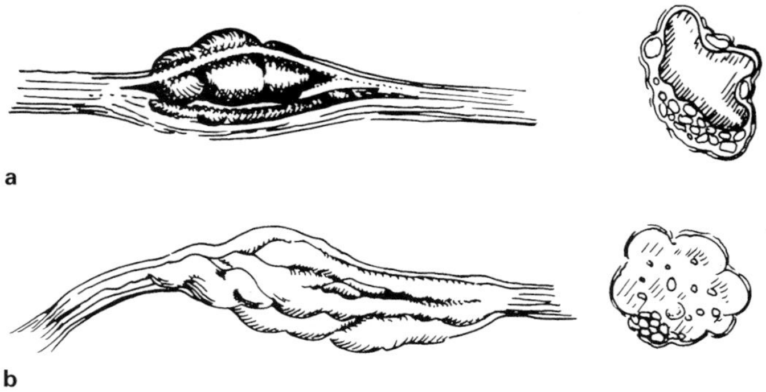

Fig. 44.7 (**a**) Schwannoma (intraneural tumour separate from the nerve tissue); (**b**) neurofibroma (nerve fibres are found within the neurofibroma).

NERVE TUMOURS

Nerve tumours are uncommon and are often mistaken for other benign soft tissue swellings.[107] Significant peripheral nerve damage may occur if they are removed by inexperienced surgeons. These tumours comprise fewer than 5% of tumours of the hand and upper extremity.[108,109] The tumours most commonly arise from the nerve sheath, but tumours of nerve cell origin also occur (Table 44.3).

Schwannoma

The most common tumour is the benign schwannoma (neurilemmoma). The patient presents with a lump but usually has no loss of sensation or power. The lump itself is usually mobile from side to side, but is relatively fixed in the longitudinal axis of the limb. A particularly reliable sign is that percussion induces painful paraesthesia in the territory of the nerve. The tumour usually lies eccentrically within the nerve trunk, displacing fascicles to one side (Fig. 44.7a). Most of these tumours can be encleated with careful dissection to preserve the conducting elements. Excision of the nerve in order to remove the tumour is not acceptable treatment. Solitary schwannomas which are enucleated rarely recur and malignant change in a solitary schwannoma is very rare.[110,111]

REFERENCES

105. Gilliatt R W, Peripheral Nerve Compression and Entrapment. Pitman, London 1975
106. Volkmann R von Zentralbl Chir 1881; 8: 801–803
107. Brooks D Peripheral Neuropathy 1984; 2: 2236–2253
108. Stack H G Br Med J 1960; 1: 919–922
109. Harkin J C, Reed R J Tumours of the Peripheral Nervous System. Armed Forces Institute of Pathology, Washingston DC 1968
110. Ghosh B C, Ghosh L et al Cancer 1973; 31: 184–190
111. Dodge H W, Craig W M Minn Med 1957; 40: 294

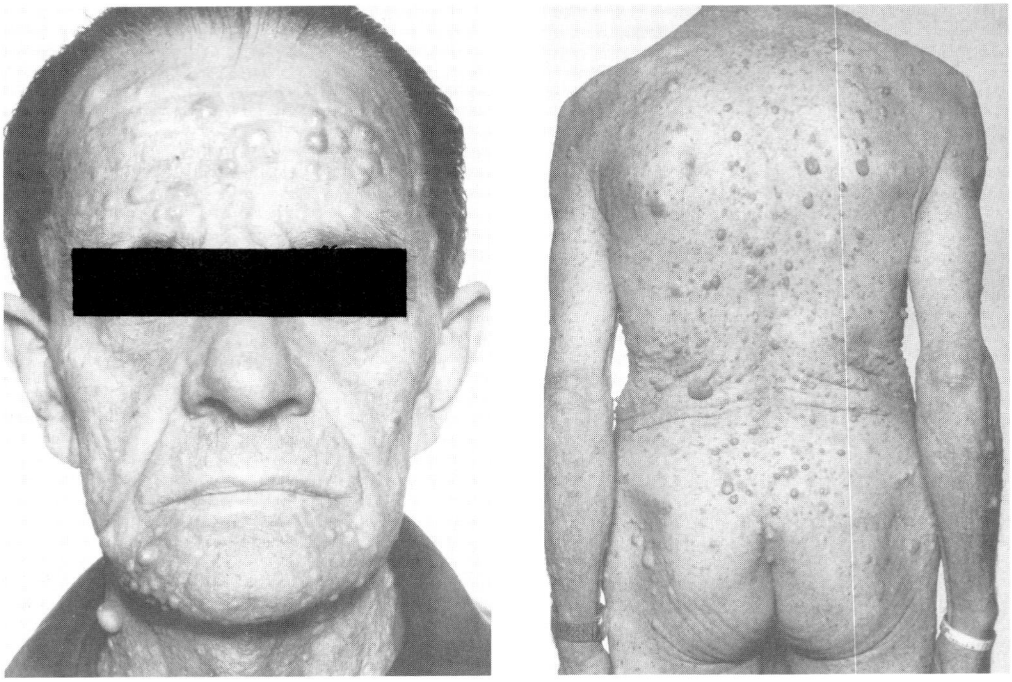

a b

Fig. 44.8 Neurofibromatosis (von Recklinghausen's disease).

Schwannomas arising within the brachial plexus are, however, frequently more infiltrative in nature and their removal may be difficult. In such cases magnification is required. When this tumour affects the eighth cranial nerve, it is known as an acoustic neuroma. Because access to such tumours is restricted by the surrounding bone, it is occasionally impossible to excise the tumour without damaging part of the nerve. On gross examination the tumour is encapsulated and on cut section may be either solid or cystic.

Neurofibroma

Neurofibroma may occur as a solitary nerve tumour or in association with neurofibromatosis. It may present as a solitary mass in the subcutaneous tissue or along the course of a major peripheral nerve. Like the schwannoma, the neurofibroma arises from the nerve sheath, but unlike the schwannoma, it is intimately associated with the nerve and has nerve fibres running through the tumour (Fig. 44.7b). There is usually little nerve dysfunction and, as excision runs the risk of nerve damage, surgical treatment is usually limited to a biopsy to establish the tissue diagnosis.[32] A neurofibroma in the skin may be completely excised without risk of nerve damage.

Neurofibromatosis

Neurofibromatosis is the association of café-au-lait patches in the skin with neurofibromas in the skin and the nervous system. The presence of six or more café-au-lait patches is considered pathognomonic of neurofibromatosis.[112] Neurofibromatosis is an autosomal dominant genetic disorder with variable gene expression The incidence is quoted as 1 in 3000 births.[113] The disorder was reported by von Recklinghausen in 1882[114] and is associated with his name. The disease can present in several different forms. The neurofibromas may be widespread, occurring as multiple tumours (Fig. 44.8) or as a plexiform mass with overlying flabby and redundant tissue (Fig. 44.9). On palpation, the plexiform neurofibroma feels like a bag of worms. These lesions may become pendulous and require debulking, but total excision will result in loss of nerve function. Isolated cutaneous neurofibromas present as multiple soft fibrous swellings in the skin of the face, trunk or limbs. They can be excised if troublesome. Sometimes the tumours are found in the central nervous system and may affect the eighth cranial nerve particularly. A visceral form is also described where the tumours affect the autonomic nervous system. Malignant degeneration can occur in lesions of neurofibromatosis, and for tumours of the major nerves the incidence is probably between 3 and 10%. Cutaneous neurofibromas are less likely to undergo malignant change.[113]

Malignant nerve sheath tumours

These are rare and are most often associated with neurofibromatosis.[115] Although there are two types, the malignant schwannoma and the nerve sheath fibrosarcoma, it is difficult to distinguish between them.

REFERENCES

112. Boland R P Adv Neurol 1981; 29: 67–75
113. Hope D G, Mulvihill J J Adv Neurol 1981; 29: 33–54
114. Von Recklinghausen F D Ueber die multiplen Fibrome der haut und ihre Beziehung zu den multiplen Neuromen. Verlag v. A. Hirschwald, Berlin 1882
115. Ducatman B S, Scheithauer B W et al Cancer 1986; 57: 2006–2021

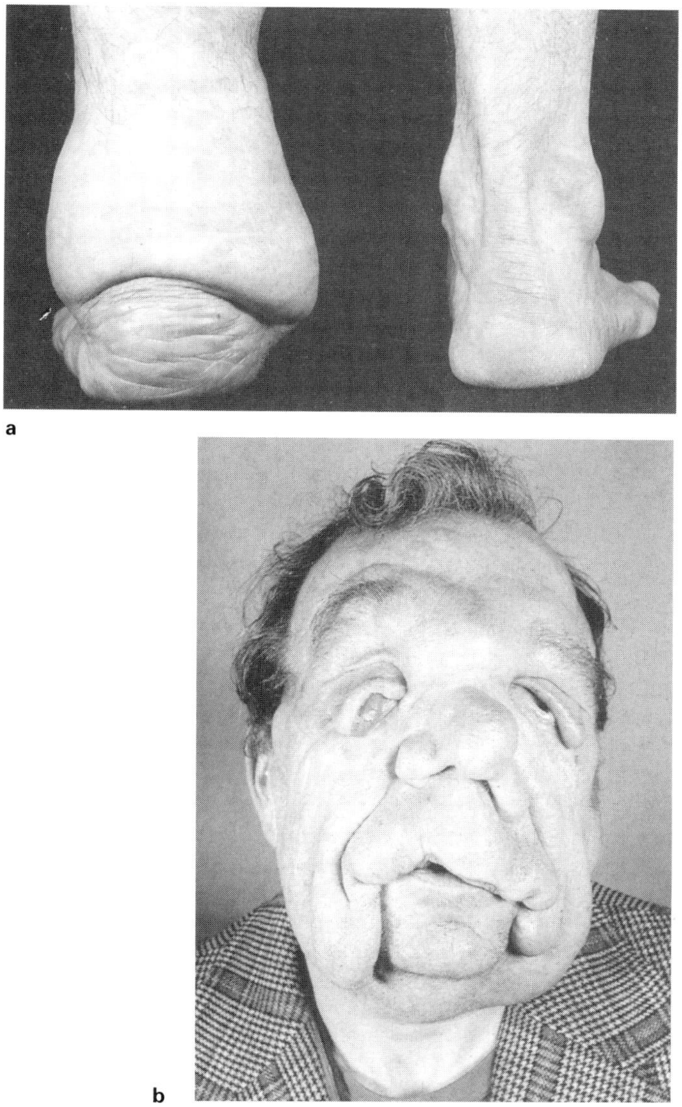

Fig. 44.9 Plexiform neurofibromatosis of (a) the foot; (b) the face.

These malignant nerve sheath tumours may have a false capsule or be diffusely infiltrative. Central necrosis and numerous mitoses are seen. The tumours typically present with pain and loss of both sensation and power. Palpation of the lump usually causes more pain than is the case when the tumour is benign. If the lump is fixed to adjacent structures, computed tomography and magnetic resonance imaging may demonstrate tumour extension into surrounding tissues, e.g. bone or muscle. The regional lymph nodes are rarely affected, but pulmonary metastasis is frequent. These are very aggressive tumours with a tendency to local recurrence and metastasis. Wide excision of these radioresistant tumours is essential.

Peripheral nerve cell tumours

Neuroblastoma is a tumour of the sympathetic chain and adrenal medulla that usually presents in childhood. This bulky, soft, cellular tumour tends to destroy the adrenal and spread to the upper abdominal lymph nodes.

Ganglioneuroma is a rare tumour found arising from the sympathetic chain in the abdomen, thorax and cervical region. It is usually a benign encapsulated mass.

Phaeochromocytoma (see Chapter 35) is a tumour of the chromaffin cells in the adrenal medulla. The tumour is usually benign but the cells secrete noradrenaline and adrenaline. The tumour may present with paroxysmal hypertension.

CRANIAL NERVES

The olfactory (first) nerve

The receptors of the olfactory nerve, situated high in the nasal cavity, are linked to the olfactory bulbs by thin filaments, which pass through the cribriform plate.

They are vulnerable to injury. The sense of smell is lost after 7% of fractures of the base of the skull, and sometimes too after a cosmetic rhinoplasty.

Olfactory filaments may be ruptured as a result of anterior displacement of the frontal lobes following a blow to the back of the head. Anosmia can also result from basal meningitis, or tumours of the frontal lobe, e.g. meningiomas.

The optic (second) nerve

The retina and optic nerve constitute a visible portion of the central nervous system, and a fibre tract from the brain which can be readily inspected with an ophthalmoscope. Like other central fibres, those of the optic nerve do not possess a Schwann cell sheath and are thus incapable of regeneration if transected or destroyed. The optic nerve is surrounded by meninges in its course from the posterior part of the globe to the middle cranial fossa. The fibres of the optic nerve carrying information from the nasal halves of each retina cross to the opposite side at the optic chiasma (Fig. 44.10).

Vision is lost as a result of inflammation (optic neuritis), compression of the nerve, ischaemia or direct trauma. The optic chiasma may be compressed by a pituitary adenoma or craniopharyngioma, and this produces symmetrical bitemporal hemianopia. A homonymous hemianopia is caused by a lesion of the optic tract or visual cortex.

The oculomotor (third), trochlear (fourth) and abducens (sixth) nerves

These nerves supply the six external ocular muscles and the levator palpebrae superioris. The third nerve also supplies constrictor fibres to the pupil and innervates the ciliary muscles controlling accommodation. Damage to these nerves causes abnormal eye movements with diplopia. A complete third-nerve lesion also causes ptosis of the upper eyelid and paralysis of the pupil, which is widely dilated due to the unopposed action of the sympathetic pupillary dilator nerves.[116]

REFERENCE

116. Ashworth B, Ischerwood I Clinical Neuro-ophthalmology. Blackwell, Oxford 1981

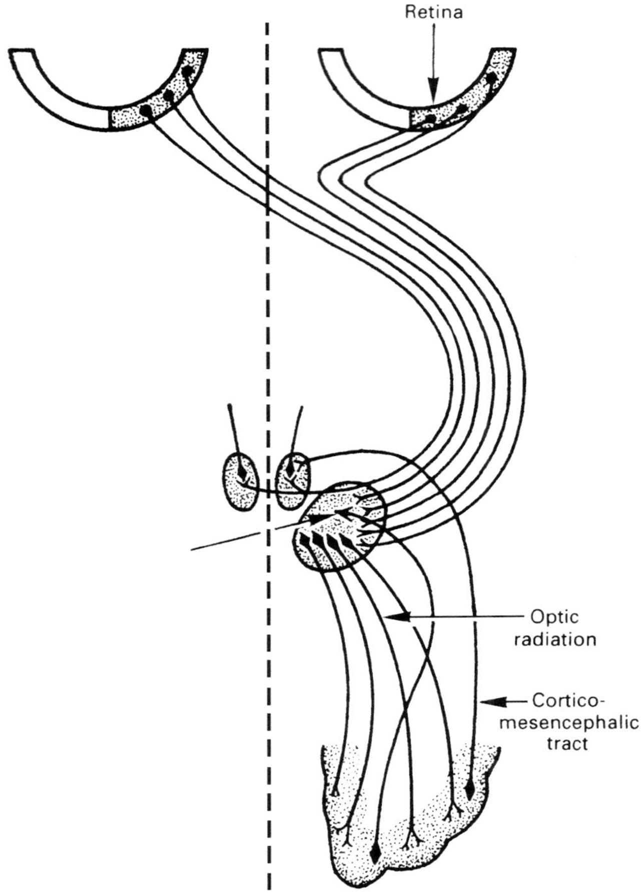

Fig. 44.10 Diagram of central connections of the optic nerve and optic tract.

The fourth nerve supplies the superior oblique muscle and paralysis of this muscle causes diplopia on looking downwards and medially.

Lesions of the sixth nerve cause paralysis of the lateral rectus with a loss of eye abduction. When the intracranial pressure is raised, this nerve may be stretched by downward displacement of the brainstem, and this may provide a false localizing sign.

These nerves may be damaged at any point between the motor nuclei in the brainstem to their destinations in the orbit. In the brainstem, infarction, demyelinating disorders and tumours may affect their nuclei. Where the nerves travel across the base of the brain, they may be damaged by trauma, meningitis or pressure from an aneurysm or tumour. Within the cavernous sinus, an aneurysm of the internal carotid artery may affect the third, fourth and sixth nerves together with sensory loss in the ophthalmic division of the fifth nerve.

The third nerve may be affected by a pituitary tumour and is sometimes damaged when raised intracranial pressure leads to herniation of the uncus of the temporal lobe through the tentorium. This is an important sign after a head injury. In the superior orbital fissure, the nerves may be damaged by trauma or compression, especially by Paget's disease of the skull.

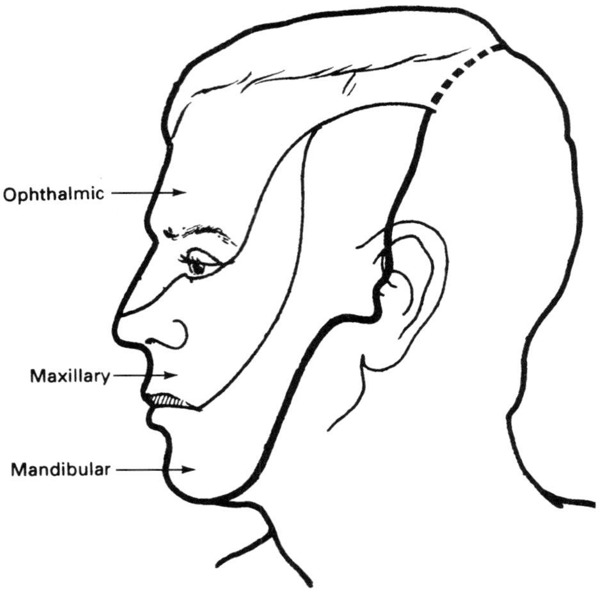

Fig. 44.11 The cutaneous distribution of the trigeminal nerve and its branches.

The trigeminal (fifth) nerve

The trigeminal nerve carries motor fibres to the muscles of mastication and sensory fibres from the face (Fig. 44.11). The sensory part of the nerve has three divisions. The ophthalmic division passes by way of the superior orbital fissure and lateral wall of the cavernous sinus to reach the trigeminal ganglion. The maxillary division passes through the infraorbital foramen to cross the pterygopalatine fossa and enter the skull through the foramen rotundum. The mandibular division joins the motor fibres to reach the skull through the foramen ovale.

One of the most important conditions affecting the nerve is trigeminal neuralgia.[117] This is typically a sharp pain occurring in bouts of short duration confined to the distribution of the trigeminal nerve. During these attacks, there may be spasm of the facial muscles, hence the term 'tic douloureux'. The pain may be precipitated by touching the face, chewing or by a cold wind. The aetiology is unknown. The condition usually develops after the age of 50 and is more common in females.

In the majority of cases, the trigeminal neuralgia may be controlled by carbamazepine 200 mg 3 times a day.[118] The addition of phenytoin 100 mg three times daily sometimes provides relief when carbamazepine alone is ineffective.[119] Baclofen 30–80 mg once daily may also prove helpful.[120]

REFERENCES

117. Harris W The Facial Neuralgias. Oxford University Press, London 1937
118. Blom S Lancet 1962; i: 839–840
119. Mawdsley C, Maloney A F J et al In: Passimore R, Robson J S (eds) A Companion to Medical Studies, vol 3, Blackwell, Oxford 1974
120. Fromm G H, Terrence C F, Chatta A S Ann Neurol 1984; 15: 240

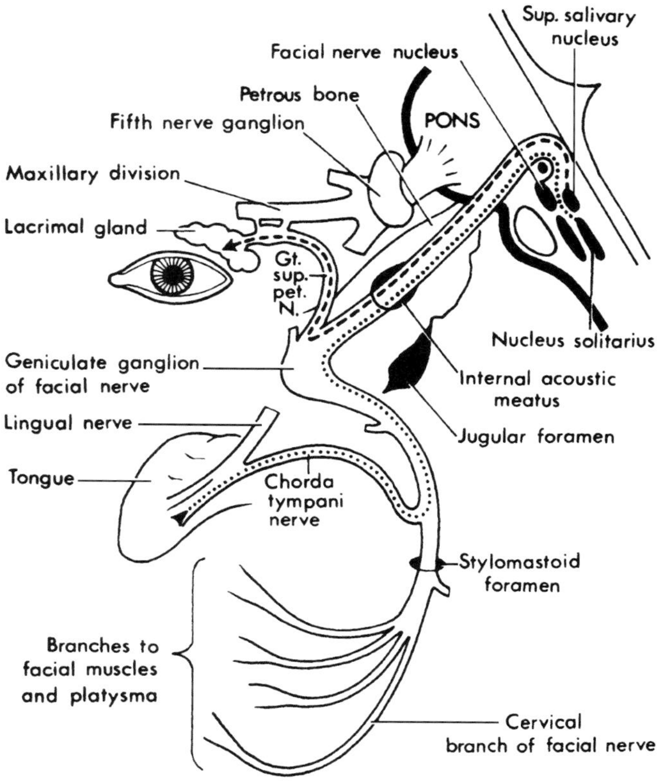

Fig. 44.12 The facial nerve. Lesions involving the facial nerve trunk above the geniculate ganglion will cause loss of lacrimation (greater petrosal nerve) and loss of taste in the anterior two-thirds of the tongue (chorda tympani nerve), as well as paralysis of both upper and lower facial muscles.

Lesions between the geniculate ganglion and the point where the chorda tympani nerve leaves the facial nerve (6 mm above the stylomastoid foramen) will cause loss of taste sensation in the anterior two-thirds of the tongue as well as paralysis of the facial muscles, but lacrimation will still be present.

Lesions below the point where the chorda tympani nerve leaves the facial nerve will cause paralysis of the facial muscles, but the taste and lacrimation will be present. From Walton: *Brain's Diseases of the Nervous System*, 9th edn. 1985. Oxford University Press, Oxford 1985, with permission.

When drugs do not control the pain, then destruction of the gasserian ganglion by alcohol or phenol injection may prove effective. Direct section of the sensory root has also been tried. Any procedure damaging the ophthalmic division will predispose to superficial keratitis and ulceration of the cornea, unless extreme care is taken. Facial pain may also be due to herpes zoster, tabetic crises, dental malocclusion, sinusitis, malignant disease, glaucoma and dental caries. Tumours of the nasopharynx may erode the base of the skull, affecting the trigeminal nerve.

The facial (seventh) nerve

The facial nerve is motor to the facial muscles, sensory to the external auditory meatus and secretor–motor to the salivary and lacrimal glands (Fig. 44.12). A multitude of conditions can cause facial paralysis including congenital anomalies, viral and bacterial infections, space-occupying cerebral lesions and cerebrovascular accidents. In many cases (Bell's palsy),[121] no specific aetiological factor is traced, although there is often a preceding viral illness. Bell's palsy affects 20 per 100 000 adults.[122] All ages are affected, but the condition is more prevalent in the third, fourth and fifth decades of life. The palsy has a characteristic sudden onset and is often accompanied by pain around the ear, numbness of the face and a disturbance of taste sensation. With a lower motor neurone lesion, all the facial movements are paralysed (Fig. 44.13); in a supranuclear or nuclear lesion, the upper facial movements are spared because the occipitofrontalis muscles are bilaterally innervated, and often all emotional facial movement remains intact.

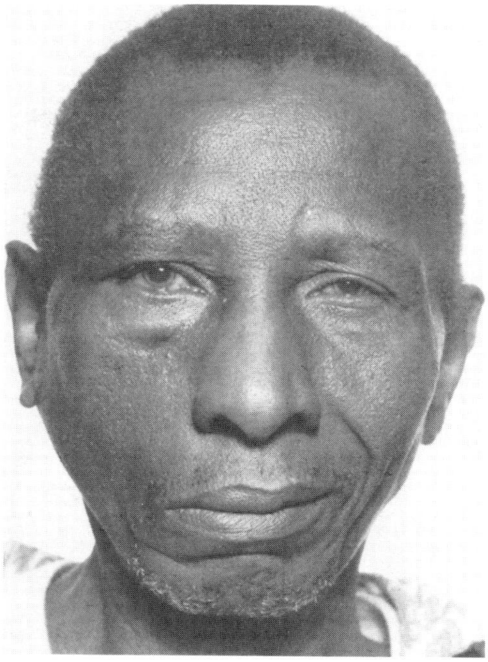

Fig. 44.13 Facial nerve palsy from carcinoma of the parotid gland.

On examination, patients with a Bell's palsy have drooping of the eyebrow with a smooth, wrinkle-free forehead. They are unable to frown or close their eyes, and any attempt to do so results in the eye rolling upwards and inwards (the Bell phenomenon; Fig. 44.14). Epiphora and ectropion are common and the mouth normally droops at the corner. The corner of the mouth cannot be pulled back and whistling is impossible. As the buccinator muscle is paralysed, the cheek is puffed out and food tends to accumulate between the teeth and cheek.

If a spontaneous seventh nerve lesion develops, Bell's palsy must be differentiated from multiple sclerosis and other causes of upper motor lesions, such as acoustic neuromas, other space-occupying cerebral lesions, polio, herpes zoster and carcinomas of the parotid gland.

Normally, half the patients who develop a Bell's palsy recover completely, but the prognosis is worse if they are above the age of

REFERENCES

121. Bell C Trans R Soc Lond 1821; 3: 398
122. Hauser W A, Karnes W E et al Mayo Clin Proc 1971; 46: 258

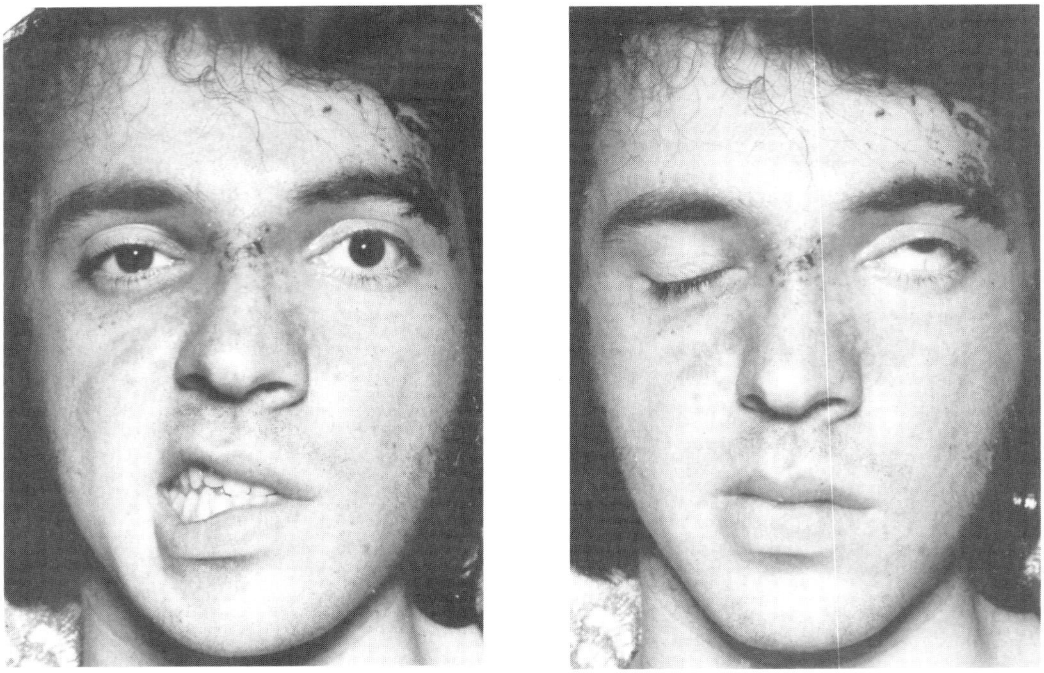

a

b

Fig. 44.14a, b A facial nerve palsy following trauma, showing attempts to cover the cornea.

60 as they develop hyperacusis and defective lacrimation.[123] If they are partially recovered within 2 weeks, the prognosis is good. During recovery, 'crocodile tears'—unilateral lacrimation during eating—occasionally proves troublesome.

Remedies used in the past to attempt to speed recovery include prednisone 20 mg 4 times a day for 5 days[124] and operative decompression.[125] Controlled trials[126] have generally proved inconclusive.

In all, 80% of patients make a satisfactory spontaneous recovery.[127] An acute disruption of the facial nerve should be repaired within 30 days either by epineural suture or by the use of nerve grafts if the ends will not meet. The timing is important as within 3 months the endoneural tubes of the distal nerve segment collapse.[22] Early repair allows axons to grow down these tubes and suppresses adverse collagenization. In proximal facial nerve injuries, primary repair or nerve grafting may be complicated by en masse movement or dyskinesia. When the proximal nerve stump is unavailable for repair, another cranial nerve, such as the hypoglossal, may be used to power the facial muscles and restore resting tone. In order to smile, however, the patient must think to move the tongue and during mastication undesirable facial movements occur.

Branches of the facial nerve on the opposite side can be fed into long nerve grafts which cross the face to reach the peripheral stumps of the injured facial nerve.[128] By the time the nerve fibres have traversed the cross-facial nerve graft however, the ipsilateral facial muscles have been denervated for such a long time that reinnervation is usually no longer possible.

One concept is that of 'baby-sitting' the ipsilateral facial muscles with a local nerve transfer (e.g. partial hypoglossal to facial) in order to prevent atrophy of the facial muscles.[129] Once nerve fibres have traversed the cross-face nerve, the temporary baby-sitting nerve transfer is taken down and the cross-face nerve graft substituted as a more appropriate 'mother' to the preserved facial muscles. Most clinicians, however, are reluctant to sacrifice a nerve on a temporary basis.

When the facial muscles have been denervated for several years, then either a dynamic or static sling should be considered to provide some symmetry to the face. As the temporalis and masseter muscles are powered by the fifth cranial nerve, they can provide a dynamic sling if repositioned to assist in eye closure and help create a smile.[130] Once again, the patient must learn to smile by contracting the muscles of mastication. Some facial movement can also be restored using a vascularized muscle transferred from a distant site.[131] A cross-face nerve graft is connected to its motor nerve so that it contracts in unison with the normal side of the face.

A cross-face nerve graft followed 6 months later by a free pectoralis minor transfer has been successfully used to provide a spontaneous or emotionally controlled movement to the face.[131] No muscle can, however, replace the delicate and complicated action of the normal facial muscles.

REFERENCES

123. Taverner D Brain 1955; 78: 209
124. Taverner D, Cohen S B, Hutchinson B C Br Med J 1971; 4: 20
125. Balance C, Duel A B Arch Otolaryngol 1932; 15: 1
126. Mechelse K, Goor G et al Lancet 1971; ii: 57
127. Petersen E Am J Otol 1982; 4: 107–111
128. Freilinger G Plast Reconstr Surg 1975; 56: 44
129. Stennert E Clin Plast Surg 1979; 6: 471
130. Rubin L R In: Brent B (ed) The Artistry of Reconstructive Surgery. CV Mosby, St Louis 1987
131. Harrison D H Plast Reconstr Surg 1985; 75: 206

The acoustic (eighth) nerve

This nerve has two distinct components. The cochlear (auditory) division is responsible for hearing and transmits sound from hair cells in the organ of Corti within the inner ear. The vestibular division is responsible for balance and transmits information from the semicircular canals. Both divisions pass through the internal acoustic meatus. This nerve may be damaged by fractures of the base of the skull or compressed by acoustic neuromas or Paget's disease of the skull. The toxic effects of some drugs, such as gentamicin, can affect the eighth nerve.[132] Deafness, tinnitus, nystagmus and giddiness are the signs of eighth nerve damage. Viral lesions, middle ear infection, wax, otosclerosis and Menière's syndrome can present with similar symptoms.

The glossopharyngeal (ninth) nerve

This nerve contains motor fibres to the pharyngeal plexus supplying the stylopharyngeus and carries sensation from the tympanic cavity, the pharynx, the posterior third of the tongue and the soft palate. The afferent arm of the gag reflex is the glossopharyngeal nerve and this is responsible for transmitting taste sensation from the posterior third of the tongue. Isolated lesions of the ninth nerve are rare. It may be damaged in a base-of-skull fracture or by invasive tumours. The most important condition involving this nerve is glossopharyngeal neuralgia. This is an intermittent severe pain affecting the back of the tongue and the tonsillar area on swallowing.[133] The pain may radiate deep in the ear. Carbamazepine 200 mg 3 times daily may be helpful, although section of the nerve is often needed.

The vagus (10th) nerve

The vagus nerve receives sensation from the pharynx, larynx, oesophagus and abdominal viscera. Its motor fibres supply the striated muscle of the palate, pharynx and larynx as well as supplying parasympathetic motor fibres and secretor–motor fibres to the viscera. Lesions of the vagus cause excessive salivation, catarrh, difficulty in swallowing, regurgitation and snoring.[134] Interruption of the fibres causes paralysis of the palate and speech acquires a nasal quality. Lesions of the vagus nerve or its recurrent laryngeal branch can cause dysphonia.[135]

The recurrent laryngeal nerve may be damaged in operations on the thyroid gland or on a patent ductus arteriosus. Thyroid tumours, metastatic deposits in lymph nodes or aneurysms of the aortic arch may also affect the nerve. The vagus nerve can be damaged at the base of the skull as a result of fractures, tumours or chronic meningitis. In such cases, the adjacent ninth and 11th nerves are usually also implicated. The nerve may be compressed by a chemodectoma or glomus jugulare tumour and is also vulnerable during surgery on the carotid artery or in block dissections of the neck.

Bilateral vagal damage usually causes tachycardia. This may occur in polyneuropathy, bulbar palsy, subtentorial tumours, syphilis, lead poisoning and botulism.

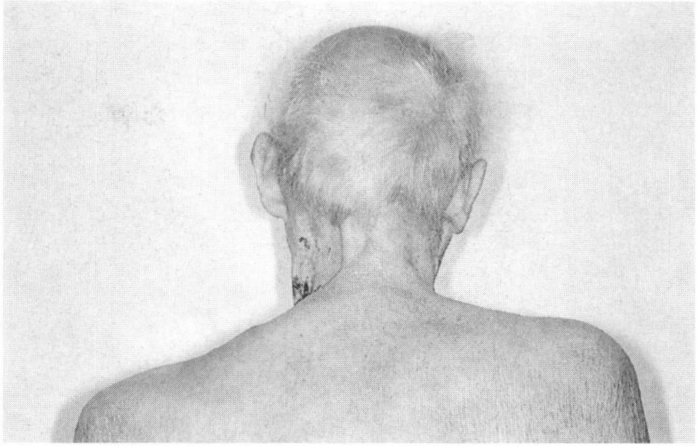

Fig. 44.15 Drooping of the left shoulder due to accessory nerve damage.

The accessory (11th) nerve

The accessory nerve enters the neck through the jugular foramen (as do the ninth and 10th nerves), passes beneath the upper portion of the sternomastoid which it supplies before crossing the posterior triangle of the neck to supply the trapezius.[136]

It may be damaged by polio, motor neurone disease, syringomyelia and spinal cord tumours. The spinal part of the nerve derives from the ventral horn cells of cervical segments 1–4 inclusive, and ascends to enter the skull through the foramen magnum where the nerve is joined by the smaller cranial component.

The nerve is often injured during cervical operations and is electively sacrificed in radical neck dissection. If it is injured near its origin, both sternocleidomastoid and trapezius are paralysed. The second and third cervical roots contribute to the motor supply of sternomastoid and in one-third of cases this is sufficient to prevent a complete paralysis of the muscle. When injured in the posterior triangle, the trapezius alone is affected. Drooping of the shoulder, an inability to shrug the shoulder and difficulty in lifting the arm above the head will be evident (Fig. 44.15). The trapezius can also receive additional innervation from the third and fourth cervical nerves and thus the paralysis may only be partial.

Accessory nerve injury is associated with pain in the shoulder which is made worse on using the arm. The scapula is rotated and occasionally winging is noticed. Active elevation of the shoulder—the 'shrug' test—can be normal because of the compensatory action of the levator scapulae. The incapacity caused by accessory nerve damage is far from trivial, and early repair or exploration should be considered.[137]

REFERENCES

132. Rudge P Clinical Neuro-otology. Churchill Livingstone, Edinburgh 1982
133. Dandy W E Arch Surg 1927; 15: 198
134. Fay J J Neurol Psychopathol 1927; 8: 110
135. Kaeser H E, Richter H S Q Rev Neurol 1965; 112: 339
136. Strauss W L, Howell A B Rev Biol 1936; 11: 387
137. Ogino T, Sugawara M et al J Hand Surg 1991; 16B: 531–536

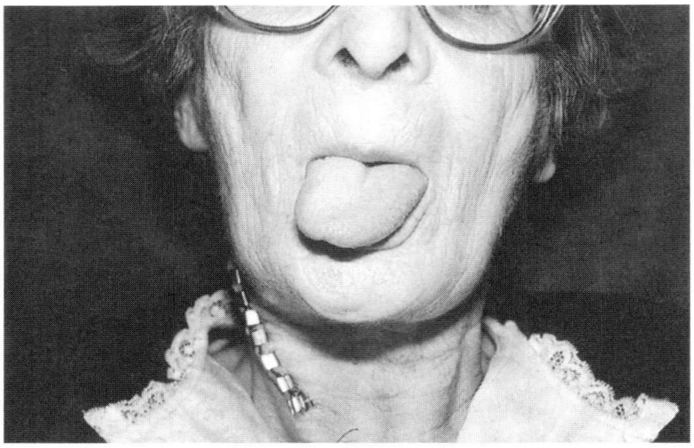

Fig. 44.16 Palsy of the hypoglossal nerve following carotid endarterectomy.

The hypoglossal (12th) nerve

This is a pure motor nerve to the muscles of the tongue (except the palatoglossus). It emerges from the hypoglossal canal and winds round the posterior aspect of the vagus deep to the digastric muscle and lateral to the internal carotid artery. It may be injured in operations on the submandibular gland, carotid artery, jaw or tongue. Damage to the nerve anywhere along its course causes atrophy of the tongue which becomes wrinkled and thinner. Unilateral weakness causes the tongue to deviate on protrusion (Fig. 44.16). Bilateral damage causes dysarthria and difficulty with swallowing and feeding.[138]

INDIVIDUAL PERIPHERAL NERVE LESIONS

Nerves are commonly damaged by injury or entrapment. They may also be damaged by ischaemia, inflammation (mononeuritis multiplex) and infiltration, or occasionally compressed by benign or malignant tumours. Peripheral nerve lesions must be differentiated from root lesions and upper motor neurone lesions. The cutaneous areas of distribution are shown in Figure 44.17.

Phrenic nerve (C3, 4 and 5)

The phrenic nerve provides the motor supply of the diaphragm which becomes paralysed if the nerve is damaged or divided. Irritation of the phrenic nerve causes hiccups or a dry unproductive cough. Diaphragmatic palsy may present with exertional dyspnoea and can be complicated by the development of basal pneumonia. The phrenic nerve may be affected by poliomyelitis and is at risk of injury during operations on the root of the neck, especially cervical sympathectomy, cervical rib resection, block dissection and surgery on the subclavian artery. It may also be damaged during thoracic surgery and may be infiltrated by carcinoma of the bronchus.

If it is known to be divided at the time of surgery, it can be carefully resutured, but on most occasions, diaphragmatic palsy is untreatable and causes few problems unless the patient has severe chronic bronchitis and emphysema.

Long thoracic nerve (C5, 6 and 7)

This nerve supplies the serratus anterior. Although it is reported to have been injured by blows or by the carrying of weights, it is most often damaged during axillary operations, either block dissection or mastectomy, combined with axillary clearance. Serratus anterior fixes the scapula to the chest wall and when forward pressure is exerted on the upper limb, such as lunging with a sword (not common today), or pushing a stalled car, the scapula comes away from the chest wall. Serratus anterior also assists in limb elevation by rotating the scapula. If a patient is asked to push forwards forcibly, the inner border of the scapula stands proud as a result of this winging. Patients are often unable to raise the limb in front of the body to 180°. There is usually poor recovery of nerve function, although the nerve should be directly sutured if division is recognized at the time of surgery.

Suprascapular nerve (C5)

This supplies the supraspinatus and infraspinatus muscles which anchor the head of the humerus during abduction of the shoulder. It is rarely damaged, although nerve injury has been reported after scapular fractures.[3] The suprascapular nerve may become entrapped[89] and this may be responsible for the considerable shoulder pain experienced after certain injuries of this region.[139]

Axillary (circumflex) nerve (C5 and 6; Fig. 44.18)

This nerve passes backwards through the quadrilateral space before winding around the humerus beneath the deltoid muscle. Wasting and weakness of the deltoid result in a loss of shoulder abduction together with a small area of cutaneous sensory loss over the insertion of the deltoid (Fig. 44.17). This nerve is occasionally injured after fracture dislocations of the upper humerus or by injections into the upper outer arm.

Radial nerve (C5, 6, 7, 8 and T1)

This is the motor nerve to triceps, anconeus, brachioradialis, extensor carpi radialis longus and through its posterior interosseous branch to extensor carpi radialis brevis, supinator, extensor digitorum longus, extensor digiti minimi, extensor carpi ulnaris and extensor pollicis longus and brevis (Fig. 44.18). It supplies sensation to the lower half of the radial aspect of the arm and the middle of the posterior forearm. In addition, it supplies sensation to the back of the hand and the posterior aspect of the three radial fingers (Fig. 44.17). This nerve may be damaged at any point along its course.

Crutch palsy was an important cause of high radial nerve lesions in the axilla in the past. With damage at this level all the

REFERENCES

138. Taverner D In: Vinken J, Bruyn G W (eds) Handbook of Clinical Neurology. North Holland, Amsterdam 1969
139. Nankano K K, Lundergau C, Okhiro M M Acta Neurol (Chicago) 1977; 34: 477

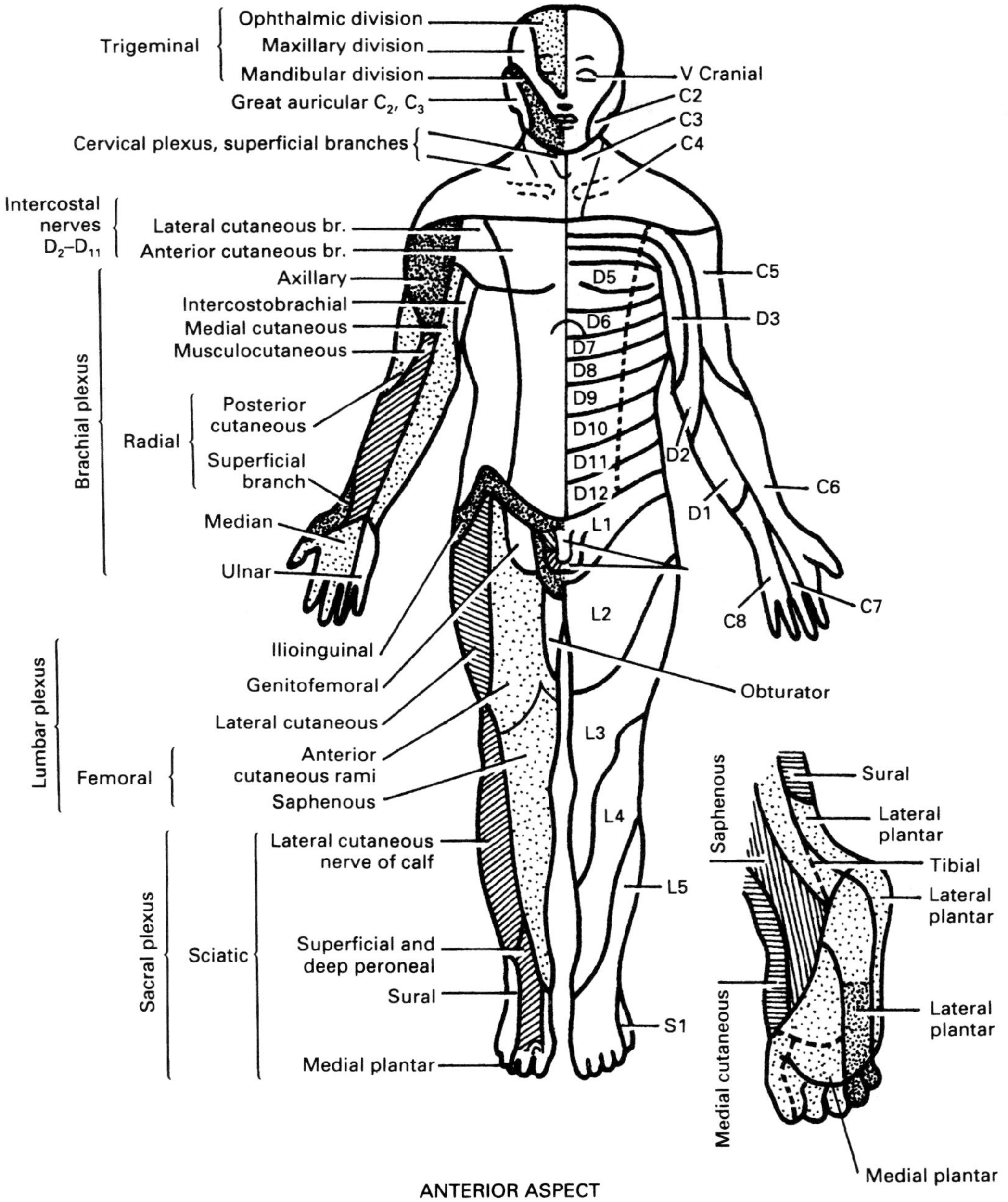

Fig. 44.17 Cutaneous areas of distribution of spinal segments and of sensory fibres of the peripheral nerves. **(a)** Anterior aspect; **(b)** posterior aspect.

muscles supplied by the nerve become paralysed. Patients are unable to extend the elbow because of triceps denervation; they cannot flex the semi-prone elbow because the action of brachioradialis is lost. Supination is weak although still present because the biceps still acts. There is wrist and finger drop as the extensors of the wrist and fingers are all paralysed and the thumb will not extend (Fig. 44.19). The fingers move well in a supported hand because the small muscles of the hand function normally. These contract synergistically and cause flexion of the metacarpophalangeal and extension of the interphalangeal joints. The radial nerve may also be damaged at the axillary level when an anaesthetized patient is allowed to hang the arm over the edge of an operating table. This type of injury can also occur in a 'Saturday night paralysis' when the patient falls asleep with the arm hanging over the edge of a chair or bed after a surfeit of alcohol. Conduction studies confirm the level of the lesion.[140]

If the radial nerve is injured further down the arm, the triceps escapes, as may the brachioradialis and extensor carpi radialis longus. With this picture, the patient has the signs of an isolated

REFERENCE

140. Critchlow J F, Seybold M E, Jablecki C J J Neurol Neurosurg Psychiatry 1980; 43: 929

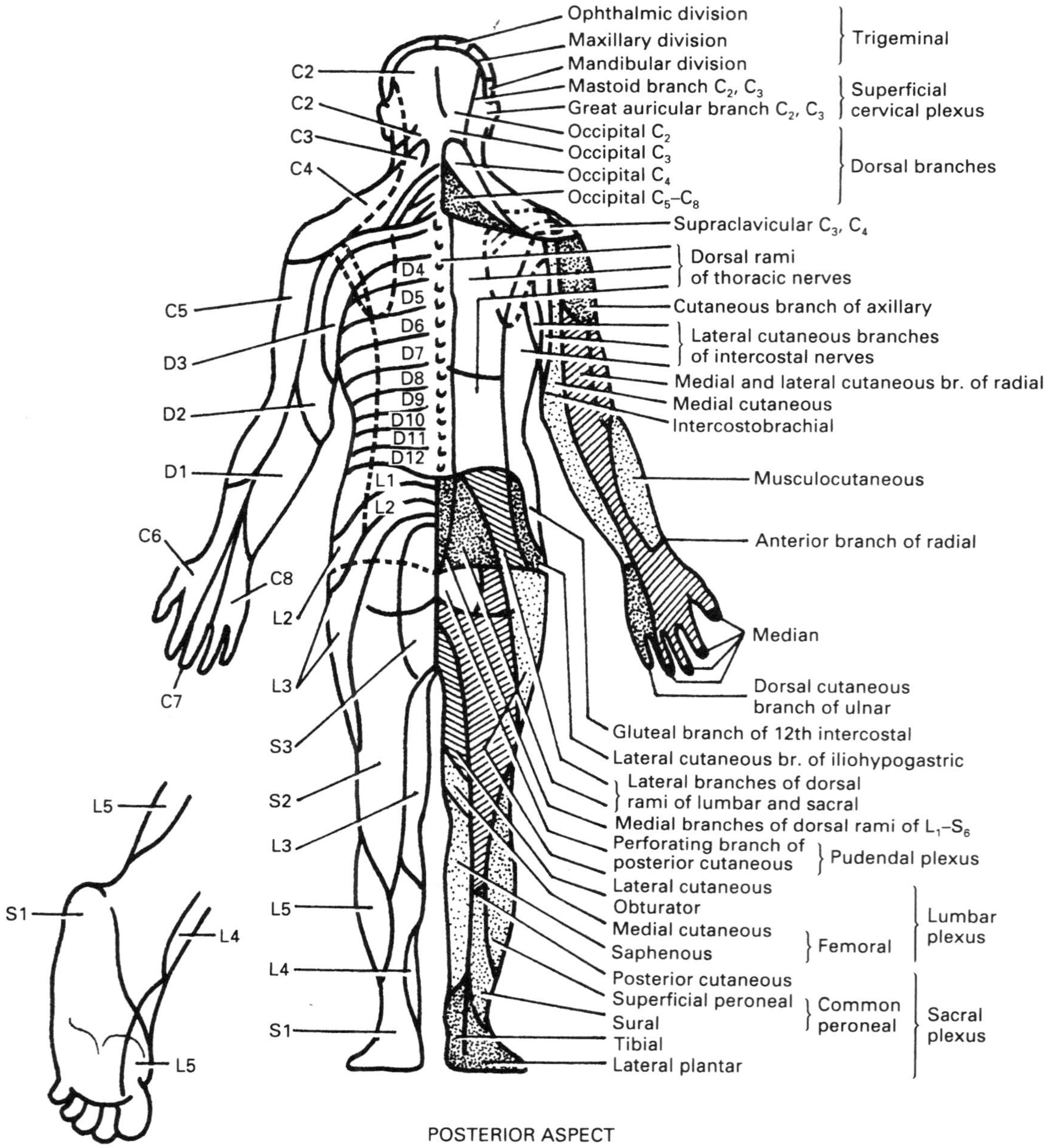

Fig. 44.17(b)

posterior interosseous nerve lesion. The posterior interosseous nerve is damaged directly on occasions by an isolated fracture dislocation of the upper radius but radial nerve injury in the arm is usually associated with a fracture of the shaft of the humerus. The radial nerve may also be damaged by intramuscular injections, or by the prolonged application of a tourniquet. The posterior interosseous nerve may be compressed by the fibrous edge of extensor carpi radialis brevis[89] or where it passes through a slit in the supinator muscle. When the posterior interosseous nerve is damaged alone, it has the appearances of a distal radial nerve without any accompanying sensory loss.[141]

The radial nerve usually recovers well after suturing. If an electromyograph confirms interosseous nerve compression, surgical exploration and decompression are indicated. A patient with an irreparable radial nerve palsy needs wrist extension, finger extension (of the metacarpophalangeal joints), and a combination of thumb extension and abduction to open up the hand. Some of the extrinsic muscles innervated by the median and ulnar nerves can be transferred to effect this. It is important to maintain a full passive range of motion in all joints to prevent contractures; dynamic splints with outriggers are often helpful.

REFERENCE

141. Spinner M Injuries to the Major Branches of Peripheral Nerves of the Forearm. W B Saunders, Philadelphia 1972

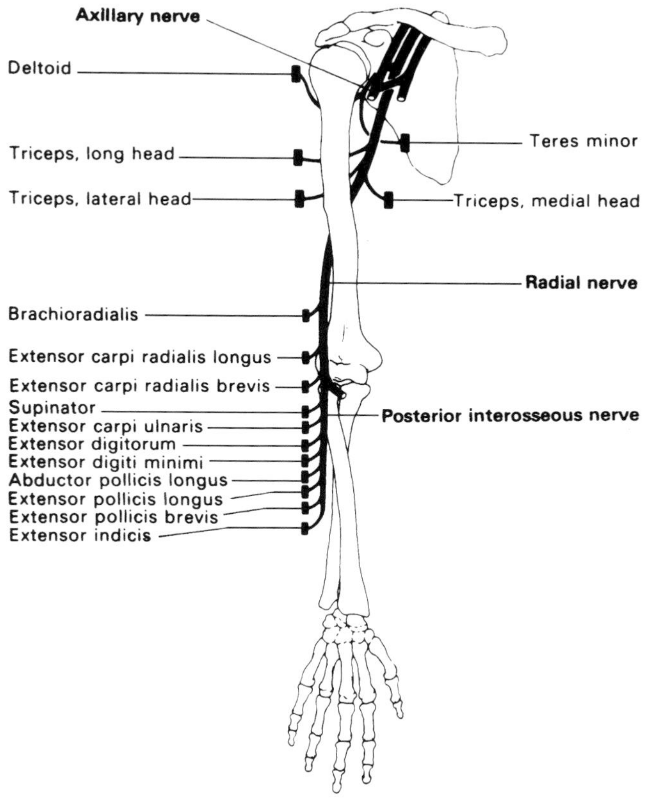

Fig. 44.18 Muscles supplied by the radial and axillary nerves. From the MRC Memorandum, with permission.

The flexor carpi ulnaris can be transferred to power the finger extensors,[142] while palmaris longus is rerouted to effect thumb extension and the pronator teres is used to extend the wrist.[143]

Musculocutaneous nerve (C5 and 6)

This nerve is the motor nerve to biceps and also innervates part of the brachialis. Both these muscles are elbow flexors. It also supplies sensation to a small area on the radial border of the forearm, extending down to the carpometacarpal joint of the thumb (Fig. 44.17). Weakness results in a loss of elbow flexion which may be partly compensated by the fact that the median nerve supplies part of brachialis.

Median nerve (C5, 6, 7, 8 and T1)

This nerve is formed from two heads—one arises from the inner and the other from the outer cord of the brachial plexus (see Fig. 44.7). It is the motor nerve in the forearm to pronator teres, flexor carpi radialis, palmaris longus, flexor digitorum superficialis, flexor pollicis longus, flexor digitorum profundus and flexor carpi radialis, and in the hand it supplies the two radial lumbricals, opponens pollicis and abductor pollicis brevis. It also supplies the outer half of flexor pollicis brevis and may supply the first dorsal interosseous (Fig. 44.20). It provides sensation to the radial three-and-a-half digits, the radial half of the palm and the dorsal tips of the same three-and-a-half digits (Fig. 44.17).

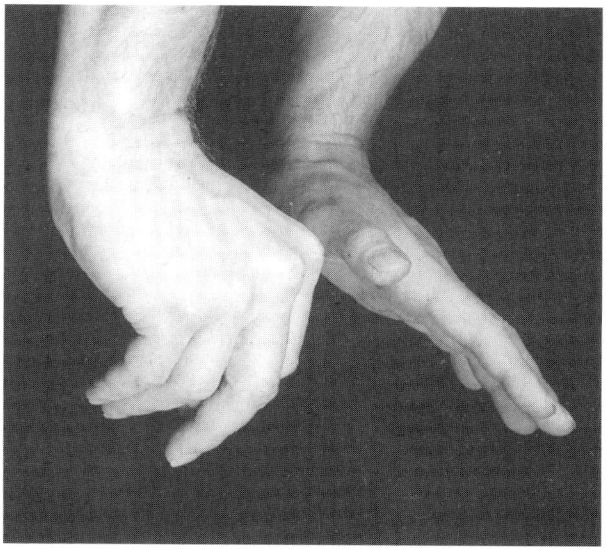
a

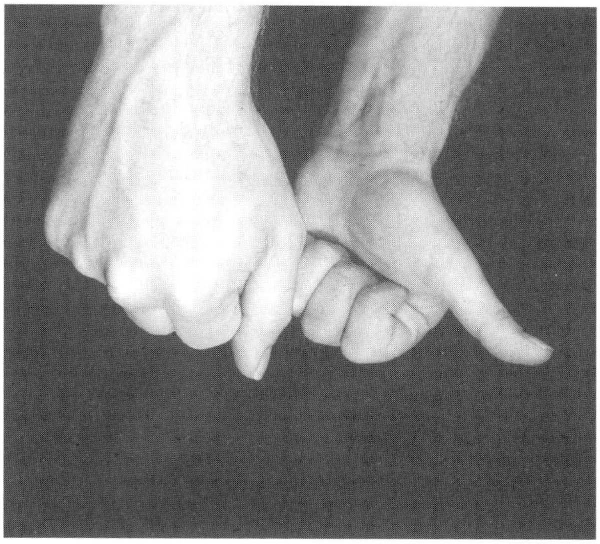
b

Fig. 44.19 The effect of posterior interosseous nerve palsy, showing loss of extension of (**a**) fingers and (**b**) thumb.

High median nerve division

This results in an inability to pronate the forearm, and flex the wrist, thumb or index finger (Fig. 44.21). The median nerve is damaged by fracture dislocations, over-zealous application of tourniquets or malplaced injections. It may be damaged during operations on the brachial artery and it may obviously be lacerated or damaged by knife or gunshot wounds.

When the median nerve is damaged in the upper arm, the hand goes into ulnar deviation when flexed against a resistance, because the radial flexor is paralysed while the ulnar flexor is normally unaffected. Patients with a median nerve injury are unable to flex the terminal phalanx of their thumb or any of the phalanges of their

REFERENCES

142. Jones R Am J Surg 1921; 35: 333–335
143. Scuderi C Surg Gynecol Obstet 1949; 88: 643–651

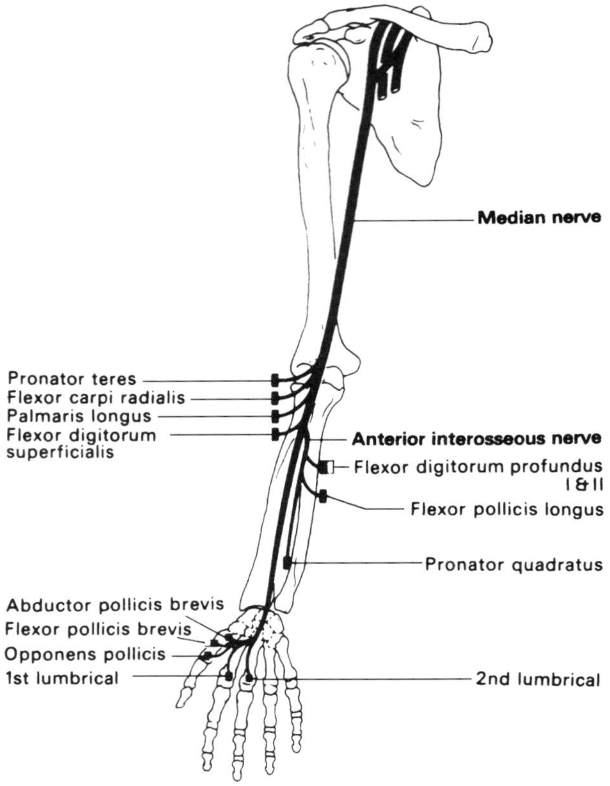

Fig. 44.20 The muscles supplied by the median nerve. From the MRC Memorandum,[14] with permission.

index finger. Flexion of the phalanges of the remaining fingers, especially the middle one, is weak. The other fingers can be flexed because flexor digitorum profundus receives a dual nerve supply. Flexion at the metacarpophalangeal joints is not affected because the interossie and lumbricals function normally. The thenar muscles become wasted and there is a weakness of thumb abduction which should be tested by asking the patient to elevate the thumb at right angles to the palm. There is also a weakness of opposition. As a result of the wasting of the thenar eminence, the first metacarpal becomes more prominent.

Low median nerve division

The nerve is more often damaged at the wrist where glass lacerations and attempts at suicide are common modes of injury. It may also be damaged by venepuncture.[144] With a complete median nerve laceration at the wrist, there will be no function in abductor pollicis brevis or the opponens muscle. Opposition can, however, be simulated by a combined contraction of adductor pollicis and flexor pollicis longus, but the thumb stays flat and does not swing over the palm. Sensation to the thumb, index and middle fingers will also be lost with a lack of sweating and loss of tactile adherence.

Ulnar nerve (C8, T1)

This nerve does not give branches above the elbow at which point it lies subcutaneously, as it passes behind the medial condyle of the

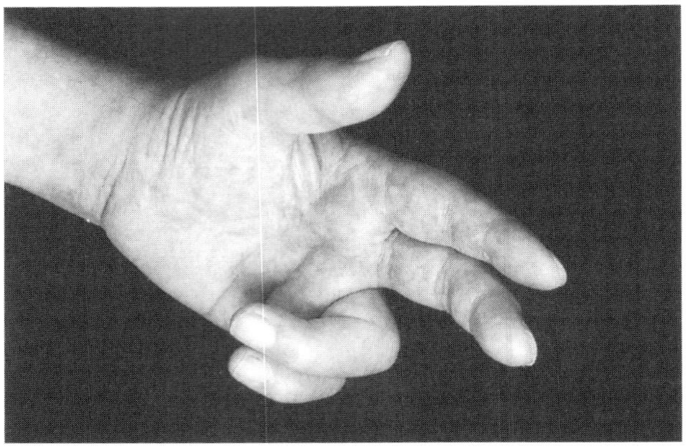

Fig. 44.21 High median nerve lesion showing loss of flexion of the index finger (past pointing).

humerus. In the forearm, it supplies motor fibres to flexor carpi ulnaris and half of flexor digitorum profundus. In the hand, it supplies palmaris brevis, the hypothenar muscles, the two medial lumbricals, all the interossei, adductor pollicis and part of flexor pollicis brevis (Fig. 44.22).

Ulnar nerve lesion at the elbow or above

Lesions above the elbow are rare and occur from the usual causes of local trauma and fracture dislocations. At the elbow, the nerve is also often damaged as a result of fracture dislocations. It may be damaged at a much later stage if cubitus valgus complicates the fracture (the so-called Tardy palsy[105]). Osteophytes, Charcot joints and compression beneath flexor carpi ulnaris can also cause nerve damage.[89,141] The nerve may also be injured by constant leaning on the elbow (student's elbow), and repetitive trauma may result in a thickened nerve which must of course be differentiated from leprosy. Benign tumours may also compress the nerve.

If the wrist is flexed against resistance, radial deviation results from the unopposed action of the radial flexor. The small muscles of the hand are paralysed, resulting in a claw deformity due to loss of flexion of the metacarpophalangeal joint, while the long flexors are still active. The claw hand has a hyperextended metacarpophalangeal joint with flexion of the proximal and distal interphalangeal joints, particularly in the little and ring fingers.

Loss of abduction and adduction of the fingers is the result of paralysis of the interossei and lumbricals. This should be tested with the hand on a flat surface as the long extensors and flexors can achieve some abduction and adduction as a synergistic movement. There is a loss of thumb adduction shown by the fact that the thumb cannot be squeezed hard against the index finger. The hand is obviously wasted as a result of the loss of small muscle bulk. Froment's sign is present.[145] This is seen when the patient squeezes a piece of paper between the thumb and the side of the index

REFERENCES

144. Berry P R, Wallis W E Lancet 1977; i: 1236
145. Rouillet J In: Michon J, Moberg E (eds) Traumatic Nerve Lesions of the Upper Limb. Churchill Livingstone, Edinburgh 1975

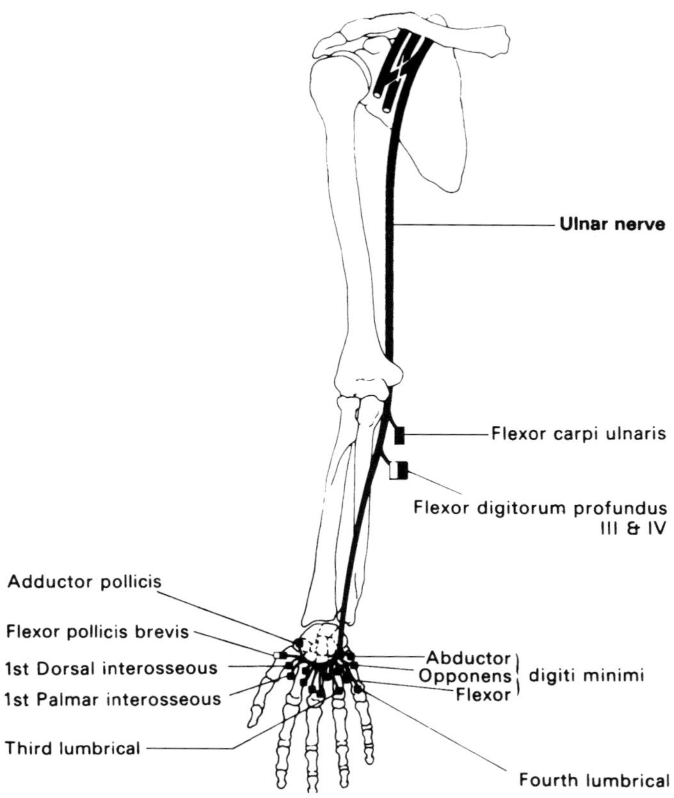

Fig. 44.22 The muscles supplied by the ulnar nerve. From the MRC Memorandum,[14] with permission from HMSO.

finger. The terminal phalanx of the affected thumb is seen to flex because weakness of the adductor pollicis results in overaction of flexor pollicis longus (Fig. 25.23). Pinprick sensation is reduced over the little finger, the ulnar border of the palm and the ulnar side of the ring finger on both its dorsal and palmar aspects (Fig. 44.17).

Ulnar nerve lesions at the wrist

The flexor carpi ulnaris and flexor digitorum profundus escape damage with injuries at the level. Sensory loss is mild but the small muscles of the hand are obviously affected. A lack of adduction of the fingers is easily tested by placing a piece of paper between two fingers and showing that the paper can be easily extracted by gentle pressure, despite the patient's best efforts to prevent this from happening.

Clawing can be prevented by a 'knuckle-duster' splint. This maintains flexion at the metacarpophalangeal joint and extension of the interphalangeal joint.[146] Should the nerve require suture, a return of sensation is likely but the small muscles of the hand do not always recover.

Differential diagnosis of median and ulnar nerve lesions

A number of conditions have to be considered in a patient presenting with paralysis and sensory loss in the hand, particularly if the small muscles are wasted. These conditions include acute poliomyelitis, Guillain–Barré syndrome, spinal cord injury or

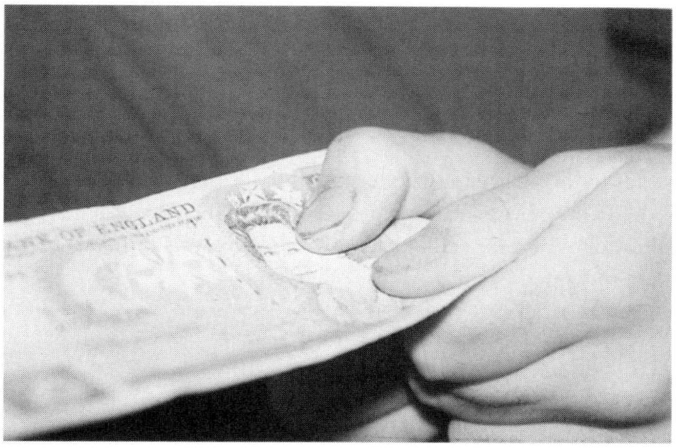

Fig. 44.23 Froment's sign for right ulnar paresis.

thrombosis of a spinal artery, motor neurone disease and spinal muscular atrophy. Syringomyelia, cervical disc prolapse and spondylosis may also be responsible. A cervical rib may produce sensory and motor abnormalities.

Lower limb

The lumbosacral plexus is derived from T12, L1, 2, 3 and 4 (lumbar plexus) and L4, 5, S1, 2 and 3 (the sacral plexus). The lumbar plexus gives rise to the femoral and obturator nerves, and the sacral plexus to the sciatic and gluteal nerves. The plexi themselves may be involved in the metastatic spread of pelvic malignancy, compressed at their roots by a disc prolapse, damaged by the fetal head or by the application of forceps[147] and by pelvic operations including rectal resections, bladder surgery and vascular bypasses.

Lateral cutaneous nerve of the thigh (L2, 3)

This nerve arises from the lumbar plexus and enters the thigh beneath the lateral part of the inguinal ligament (Fig. 44.17). It pierces the fascia lata 10 cm down the thigh, supplying sensation to the anterolateral thigh. This nerve occasionally becomes entrapped in middle-aged women and is responsible for numbness and hyperalgesia (meralgia paraesthetica). Operative decompression should be considered.[148]

Obturator nerve (L2, 3 and 4)

This arises from the lumbar plexus and passes into the thigh through the obturator canal. It supplies motor fibres to pectineus, gracilis, the adductor longus, magnus and brevis, and to the obturator externus. It provides sensation to the hip and knee, and to the skin of the medial thigh (Fig. 44.17). It is occasionally injured

REFERENCES

146. Highet W B Lancet 1942; i: 555
147. Donaldson J The Neurology of Pregnancy. W B Saunders, Philadelphia 1977
148. Stevens H Arch Neurol Psychiatry Chicago 1957; 77: 557

during hip dislocations, hip replacements and during a difficult labour. It may also be compressed by an obturator hernia.[89]

Genitofemoral nerve

Injuries to this nerve may be responsible for pain after hernia operations. If the nerve is trapped by a suture, then local anaesthetic infiltration will relieve the discomfort. Neurolysis or nerve section is then indicated.

Saphenous nerve

This is the sensory part of the femoral nerve running down to the medial malleolus alongside the saphenous vein. It is commonly damaged at the time of varicose vein surgery or femoropopliteal bypass surgery. It results in an annoying patch of anaesthesia on the medial calf (Fig. 44.17). This can be avoided if the long saphenous vein is not stripped below the knee.

Femoral nerve (L2, 3 and 4)

This also arises from the lumbar plexus and passes into the thigh beneath the inguinal ligament lateral to the femoral artery. It supplies motor fibres to iliacus in the abdomen and in the thigh supplies the quadriceps femoris muscles and sartorius. It carries some sensory fibres from the hip and knee joints and supplies sensory branches to the anteromedial thigh and the medial side of the lower leg.

Damage to the femoral nerve by a psoas abscess, fractured pelvis, hip dislocation or local trauma is quite common because of its relatively exposed position. The nerve is also commonly affected by diabetes and lumbar spondylosis.

Nerve damage results in hip flexion because of the weak iliacus muscle and reduced knee extension from the quadriceps denervation. Quadriceps wasting develops later. The patient finds that the knee gives way on walking and finds climbing up stairs difficult. Nerve suture or nerve grafting may be helpful.

Sciatic nerve (L4 and 5, S1, 2 and 3)

The sciatic nerve is a composite of the tibial (or medial popliteal nerve) and the common peroneal (or lateral popliteal) nerves. These nerves can be separated all the way up the main sciatic trunk. The sciatic nerve leaves the pelvis through the greater sciatic notch, passes straight down the back of the thigh to end in the popliteal fossa by dividing into its two main branches. It provides the motor supply to the hamstrings, to part of adductor magnus and to all the muscles below the knee.

The common peroneal nerve supplies the muscles of the peroneal compartment through its superficial branch and those of the anterior compartment through its deep branch.

The tibial nerve supplies the gastrocnemius, soleus, the long flexors of the toes, tibialis posterior and the small muscles of the foot via the medial and lateral plantar nerves.

A lesion of the main sciatic nerve causes loss of the knee flexion, foot drop and inability to walk. Patients with sciatic nerve lesions drag their feet behind them and are often unable to stand for long periods. This is accompanied by wasting of the lower leg muscles. Sensation is lost from the knee downwards, except for a strip on the medial side of the leg which is supplied by the saphenous nerve. A normal knee jerk can be elicited but the ankle jerk is missing. Trophic ulcers and vasomotor disturbances are common.

The sciatic nerve is injured in association with fractures of the pelvis and femur, and may also be damaged by a misplaced injection. Nurses inject in the safe upper outer quadrant of the buttock to avoid the nerve. Its relatively superficial course also makes it liable to damage by gunshot wounds and other forms of direct trauma. It may occasionally be compressed by the pyriformis muscle or by a large Baker's cyst.[90]

If the nerve is inadvertently divided, it is always worth suturing it. Nerve recovery is however slow, and usually incomplete.[149]

Common peroneal nerve

This nerve is damaged nine times more often than the tibial nerve. The peroneal and anterior tibial muscles are usually paralysed, giving a loss of dorsiflexion and a foot drop. Sensation is lost over the dorsum of the foot and lateral part of the lower limb. This nerve is usually damaged as it winds round the neck of the fibula. It is very superficial at this point and wounds, plasters, splints and fractures of the fibula are common sources of nerve injury. In addition, the nerve may be inadvertently damaged during varicose vein surgery or reduction operations for lymphoedema. It may also be compressed occasionally in the anterior tarsal tunnel, causing a foot drop.

Tibial nerve

This nerve supplies the flexor muscles of the calf. Injury results in talipes calcaneovarus. After nerve division, the plantar and ankle jerks cannot be elicited. The sole of the foot is anaesthetic and trophic ulcers are common. The nerve may be divided or damaged during popliteal dissections to ligate the short saphenous vein at its termination or during operations on popliteal artery. It may also be damaged by posterior dislocations of the knee and posteriorly displaced fractures of the tibia. The posterior tibial nerve can occasionally be compressed behind the medial malleolus by the posterior tarsal tunnel.

Sural nerve

The sural nerve can be damaged at the time of short saphenous surgery. Its division is of little significance but causes an annoying patch of anaesthesia on the outer border of the foot. Because of the minor nature of symptoms following sural nerve resection it is commonly used as a source of nerve grafts.

REFERENCE

149. Seddon H J Surgical Disorders of the Peripheral Nerves. Williams & Wilkins, Baltimore 1972

45 The hand

F. D. Burke   L. C. Bainbridge

The hand should be seen as a most sophisticated extension of the brain from both a motor and sensory point of view. Skills range from a delicacy that can only be appreciated by optical magnification to heavy manual work which requires muscle power, joint stability and a durable integument.

It is perhaps not surprising that the development of such varied functions has occurred in association with local tissue specialization. For example, the skin of the pulps of the fingers is held to the distal phalanges by fibrous septa, separated by compartments filled with fat. The limited deformation that can occur under pressure plays an important role in the ability to hold objects between the fingers; too firm a pulp would not allow the skin to conform to the object being manipulated, and an absence of fibrous septa would permit excessive mobility of the skin on deeper structures, adversely affecting manipulative skills. Adhesion between skin and smooth objects is enhanced by the moisture arising from the sweat glands. The ability to sweat is lost after local nerve injury and dry skin adheres to objects less satisfactorily.

This specialization of structures to meet the needs of sophisticated function affects the local response to infection, injury or disease. The rapid onset of severe pain in a pulp space infection, with risk of overlying skin necrosis, is due to the localization of sepsis within a compartment. Pulp tissue is so specialized that, if it is lost, attempts at reconstruction can only be partially successful. Although a cross finger flap will introduce good quality skin and fat, the absence of septa anchoring the flap will reduce manipulative skills.

The mobility of the fingers and thumb is an essential feature of hand function. This is controlled by an extremely complex and delicate extensor tendon system, balanced by two flexor tendons which travel in a pulley system which is only minimally larger than the contents. The structure of the pulley system must allow 90° movement at the metacarpophalangeal and interphalangeal joints, with rigid (annular) portions over the phalanges, and collapsible (cruciate) portions over the joints. The profundus and superficialis tendons have differing excursions and receive their blood supply through a mesentery of long and short vincula. This tissue specialization has profound implications for tendon repair in the fingers and on flexor sheath infections.

THE PRINCIPLES OF THE MANAGEMENT OF HAND INJURIES

These sophisticated mechanisms are easily disturbed by injury or disease. Frequently, a return to total normality cannot be achieved, but adherence to certain principles of management can ensure a return to optimal function.

Specialist management. Specialized tissues require specialist management at the earliest stages after injury or at the onset of disease. Aird noted in the first edition of this book that the hand was of sufficient complexity to justify specialist centres for the management of hand conditions. The provision of a satisfactory service for hand injuries raises a challenge that few National Health care systems can currently meet. There is, however, no doubt that skilled immediate treatment can dramatically affect both short-term and ultimate disability. The principal challenge here is organizational but it also places a requirement on generalists or surgeons in training to refer cases of concern to specialists immediately. This is particularly important in cases of major hand injury or in situations where skin has been lost. When there is late referral, local stiffness, oedema, infection and scarring may have lost ground that cannot be regained. Flexor tendon injury within the fingers is not an area where inexperienced surgery is acceptable. In the absence of appropriate surgical experience and the required rehabilitation skills, the surgeon should limit himself to wound toilet, identification of damaged structures and skin closure prior to early referral to a specialist. Delayed primary or secondary reconstructive surgery should not be compromised by inexpert extension of the original injury.

An appropriate surgical environment. Even the simpler hand surgery procedures should be performed in operating theatres with satisfactory assistance, lighting and suitably delicate instruments.

Careful timing of intervention. A biological clock is activated at the time of injury and the processes that follow are largely outside the control of the surgeon. However, the process can, to an extent, be moulded by active and passive movements and splintage. The injured part swells and fibrin is laid down in the tissues, causing adhesions between tissue planes and around tendons and joints. Active young collagen contracts as it matures, reaching a stable condition after approximately 6 months. Infected or granulating wounds caused by delayed or inadequate skin cover greatly increase the collagen response. The biological clock must always be taken into account when surgical intervention is being considered. Ill-timed surgery gives poor suboptimal results.

THE TIMING OF SURGERY

There are three stages during collagen maturation when surgical intervention is appropriate.

1. *At the time of injury* when most structures can be repaired. Massive injury or gross contamination contraindicates primary repair of all structures but satisfactory skin cover is essential within a few days.

2. *Delayed primary repair* is particularly valuable in situations where specialist skills are not immediately available and there are injuries to tendons or nerves. At the time of injury the laceration is cleaned and explored, and damaged structures are identified. The skin is carefully sutured and the hand splinted and elevated to minimize oedema and stiffness. The patient is then referred for specialist treatment, which is performed as an elective procedure within 2–3 weeks of injury. The immediate surgery must be meticulous for even a superficial wound infection will compromise the success of delayed primary repair.

3. *Reconstructive surgery*: the opportunity for early intervention may have been missed either because of late diagnosis or late referral; alternatively, damage or contamination may have been so severe that late reconstruction is preferred. If delayed reconstruction is necessary, the swollen hand is splinted in a position of optimal function (see below) and then mobilized by active and passive movements in association with static and dynamic splintage. When collagen maturation is complete and the hand is again soft and supple, attention may be turned to reconstructive surgery.

THE POSITION OF OPTIMAL FUNCTION

Experience has shown that the hand posture most favourable to the avoidance of finger stiffness is metacarpophalangeal joint flexion and interphalangeal joint extension (Fig. 45.1); the thumb is held in extension abduction to avoid a first web contracture. The mechanism by which joint mobility is lost in a swollen hand is a complex process which is not fully understood. At the metacarpophalangeal joints the collateral ligaments are taut in flexion and lax in extension (Fig. 45.2). The painful swollen hand will tend to take up a position of metacarpophalangeal extension and proximal interphalangeal joint flexion. Oedema fluid around the lax metacarpophalangeal joint collateral ligaments will lay down fibrin. The foreshortened ligaments will produce a joint held in extension with flexion obstructed. Fibrin laid down around the flexed proximal interphalangeal joint causes adhesions around the proximal portion of the volar plate, which normally concertinas during joint flexion.

Perhaps the most satisfactory way to hold the swollen hand in metacarpophalangeal joint flexion and interphalangeal joint extension is with the use of a volar slab.[1] A single roll of 10 cm (4 inch) plaster of Paris is folded three times to produce a slab of eight layers, approximately 25 cm (10 inches) long. A slightly longer length of wool of similar width is also fashioned. The plaster slab is immersed in water and excess fluid is removed. It is then laid on the wool and applied to the volar surface of the hand. The plaster is ridged as it sets, holding metacarpophalangeal joints flexed and interphalangeal joints and wrist extended. When the plaster is firm, the joint position is maintained using an elasticated bandage supplemented by 2.5 cm (1 inch) Elastoplast strapping (Fig. 45.3). The dressings tend to loosen, with loss of position, and should be checked once a week.

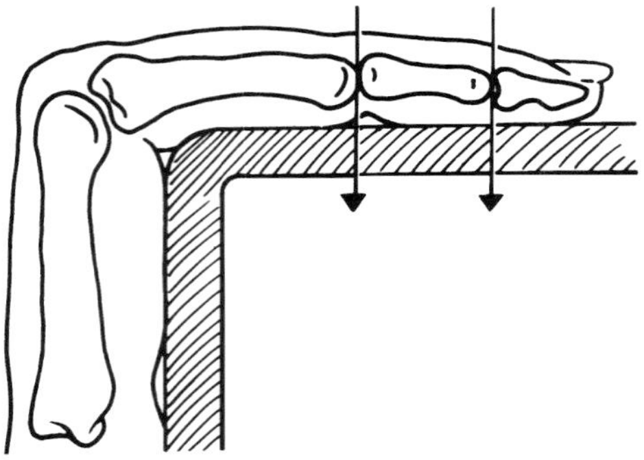

Fig. 45.1 The position of function.

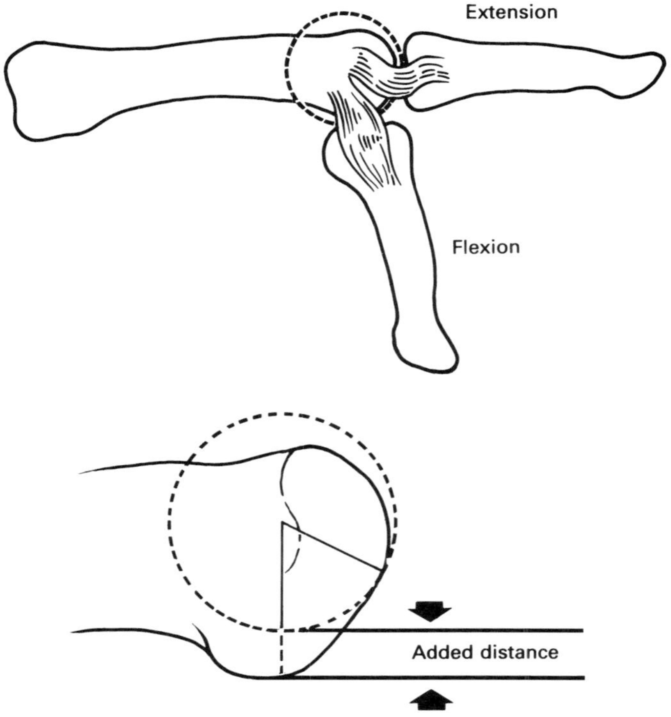

Fig. 45.2 The collateral ligaments of the metacarpophalangeal joint.

A crushed hand presenting as an emergency without fracture or injury to skin may at first sight appear not to be a significant problem. The patient has, however, a potentially catastrophic condition which if poorly treated may progress to permanent stiffness with a reduced grip. Such patients urgently require splintage in the position of optimal function with elevation of the upper limb. Immediate or early intensive physiotherapy will be required to regain motion. This treatment programme is best performed on an inpatient basis.

The role of hand rehabilitation needs to be more widely appreciated.[2] Just as there are certain periods during the process of

REFERENCES

1. Varian J P W Hand 1975; 7: 78
2. Hunter J M Hand Clin 1986; 2: 5

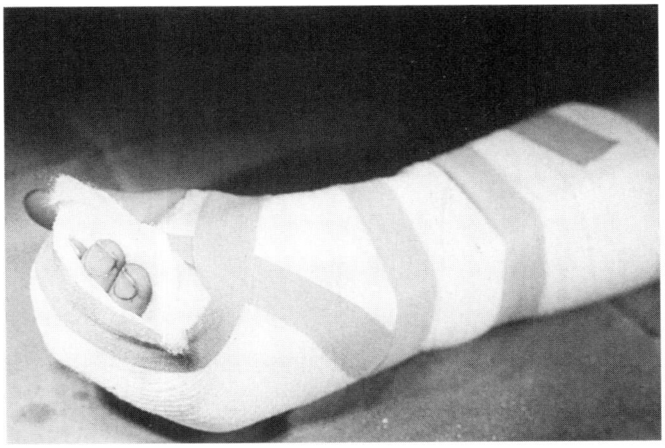

Fig. 45.3 The volar slab.

collagen maturation when surgery is appropriate, there are also periods when therapy is necessary. Often a prolonged course of therapy will produce a slow improvement, but a minority of patients will benefit from an intensive period of treatment (for several hours daily for a week) at a crucial stage during the healing process. The timing of this intervention is critical to success. Surgeons should regard the prescribing of hand therapy in the same way as they would consider the use of an antibiotic—for a clearly defined purpose over a relatively short duration but at a dose (in the case of therapy, intensity) that is therapeutic.

SKIN LOSS AND FINGERTIP INJURIES

Fingertip injuries are common and are usually a combination of crush, avulsion and amputation. They are frequently treated by relatively junior staff even though the optimal treatment can be extremely challenging.[3] The complications seen include prolonged wound healing, poor cushioning of the bone distally, painful neuromas and insensate fingertips.

Superficial pulp loss without bone exposure should be allowed to granulate and heal by secondary intention. This has the advantage that the final scar will usually lie under the nail and quality pulp skin will be drawn up to cover the fingertip. Children are a special case: the amputated part should either be replaced (within 3–4 hours) as a free graft or the wound should simply be dressed with a non-adherent dressing. There are reports of children regenerating nail beds and distal phalanx tufts in such cases.

Skin grafts are used uncommonly now as they do not replace the correct sort of skin and do not supply any padding.

Currently, optimal management is conservative for those cases without exposed bone or aggressive with flaps for those patients with substantial tissue loss or loss of nail, bone and pulp. Flaps can be taken either from the same finger more proximally (homodigital flaps), another finger (cross finger) or the toes (toe pulp transfer).

Dorsal oblique loss

This is the most favourable variety of tissue loss. The important volar tissues are intact but there is damage to the nail bed. Trimming of the distal phalanx permits primary closure. If the residual nail is less than half the normal length, nail bed ablation may be preferred.

Transverse loss

Equal amounts of dorsal and volar tissue are lost. Healing by secondary intention is still possible but carries a high risk of an abnormal nail. Closure is best achieved with a flap, probably with the homodigital flap designed by Venketaswamy or one of the variants. The Atasoy[4] (Fig. 45.4) and Kleinert flaps are also possibilities. These flaps seem simple but require a detailed understanding of the anatomy of the finger to make them safe and reliable and should be undertaken by experienced surgeons in properly equipped theatres.

Volar oblique loss

The nail bed is intact but there is extensive loss of the pulp with exposed distal phalanx and possibly exposed tendon and even joint. A cross finger flap[5] (Fig. 45.5) is a safe choice for these injuries, possibly with coaptation of the digital nerve to a dorsal branch supplying the flap. The epitenon over the extensor of the donor finger is preserved as a bed for a full-thickness graft. The flap is carefully sutured to prevent kinking of the pedicle. The flap is divided, under anaesthetic, 10–14 days later. It is important that the skin edges are *not* sutured but simply left to heal.

Proximal injuries

More proximal injuries can usually be covered quite simply depending on the tissue lost. On the dorsum most wounds can be covered with split-skin grafts so long as the epitenon is intact. If the tendon is exposed or missing then a flap will be required. Similarly on the volar aspect the majority of wounds will need a full-thickness graft but if the tendon sheath is breached then a flap will be required.

FLEXOR TENDON INJURIES

Flexor tendon division is usually revealed by an alteration in the normal cascade posture of the fingers, with increasing flexion towards the ulnar border of the hand as it lies in a relaxed posture. The involved finger will be unduly extended. Profundus tendon function can be confirmed by active flexion of the distal interphalangeal joints. The superficialis tendons have individual muscles, unlike the profundus which has a composite muscle to middle, ring and little finger. The profundus tendon to each of these digits can be immobilized if the other two rays are held in full extension. If the patient can flex the proximal interphalangeal joint of the ring

REFERENCES

3. Grad J B, Beasley R W Hand Clin 1985; 1: 667
4. Atasoy E, Loakimidis E et al J Bone Joint Surg 1970; 52A: 921
5. Kappel D A, Burech J G Hand Clin 1986; 1: 677

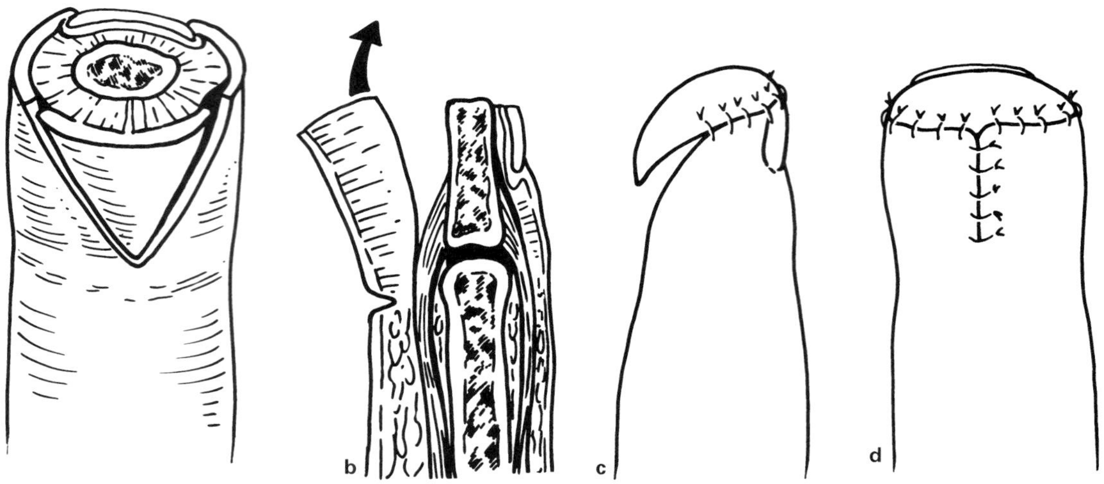

Fig. 45.4 The Atasoy flap.

finger with middle and little fingers held fully extended, then a competent superficialis tendon is present. Each finger is tested in this way—seeking proximal interphalangeal joint flexion of one finger with the remainder held in full extension.

The structural specialization required to flex the fingertips to the palm has already been described.[6] The sites of flexor tendon injuries can be classified into five anatomical zones (Fig. 45.6). Zone 1 contains the profundus tendon alone in the distal flexor sheath. Zone 2 contains both the profundus and the superficialis tendons in the more proximal portion of the flexor tendon sheath. In Zone 3, the tendons lie free of sheath within the palm. Zone 4 covers the area of the carpal tunnel and Zone 5 the forearm. The results of flexor tendon repair in Zone 5 are fairly satisfactory, although sutures to more proximal lacerations at the musculotendinous junction do not hold particularly well. In general, the opposed tendon ends will heal satisfactorily in 3–4 weeks without significant surrounding adhesions which limit motion. The results of Zone 4 repairs are usually satisfactory, although there is a tendency for tendons to adhere to adjacent structures in such a restricted area. Zone 3 repairs usually do well. The challenge to flexor tendon surgery lies in the digital flexor sheath where the tendon ends must be opposed (but not bunched) and satisfactory healing obtained without significant adhesions to the surrounding sheath or adjacent tendon.[7] The results of repair in Zone 2 are at best moderate, with some improvement in Zone 1 repairs where there is only one tendon within the sheath. The principles involved in the timing of surgery have already been discussed (see above).

Surgical technique

A modified Kessler technique (Fig. 45.7) using a 4/0 non-absorbable suture grasps the tendon adequately with minimal impairment of its vascularity. The repair is further strengthened with a continuous 6/0 nylon suture which adds both strength and smoothness to the repair. Where possible, repair of the sheath is advocated. Subsequent management can then follow three broad paths:

1. Controlled active motion. This technique[8] relies on controlled active motion of the repair to allow movement without rupture. This technique requires a motivated patient and highly skilled physiotherapists. However the results with this technique can be superb and reward the amount of work involved.

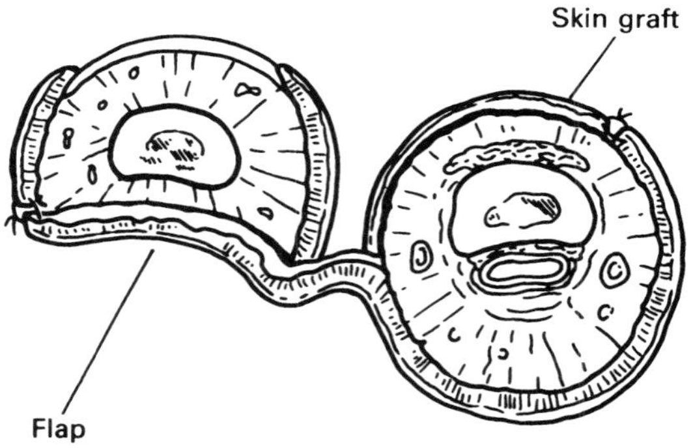

Fig. 45.5 The cross finger flap.

2. Early passive mobilization using the Kleinert regimen. This technique[9] relies on reflex relaxation of the long flexors when the finger is actively extended against elastic band traction. The extensors are then relaxed and the finger passively flexes. This permits some excursion of the repaired tendon but applies minimal load to the repair. However there is a significant risk of permanent proximal interphalangeal joint contracture.

3. Immobilization of the wrist and hand. The wrist and metacarpophalangeal joints are held in flexion to take all strain off the repair for 4 weeks. Physiotherapy is then started to break down the adhesions without disrupting the repair. This is mainly used now for children who are unable to cooperate with the other techniques.

REFERENCES

6. Tubiana R, Beveridge J Curr Orthopaed 1986; 1: 91
7. Scheider L H Hand Clin 1986; 2: 361
8. Duran R J, Houser R G In: AAOS Symposium on Tendon Surgery in the Hand. C V Mosby, St Louis 1975
9. Kleinert H E, Scheppel D, Gill A Surg Clin North Am 1981; 61: 267

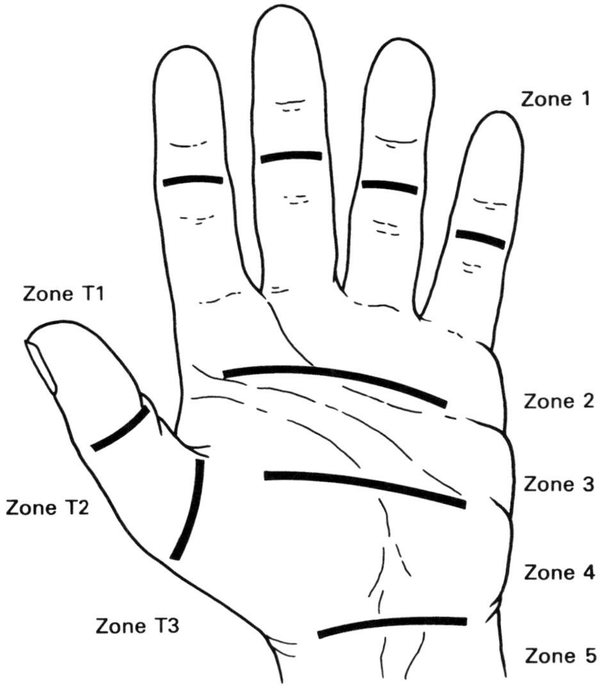

Fig. 45.6 Flexor tendon zones.

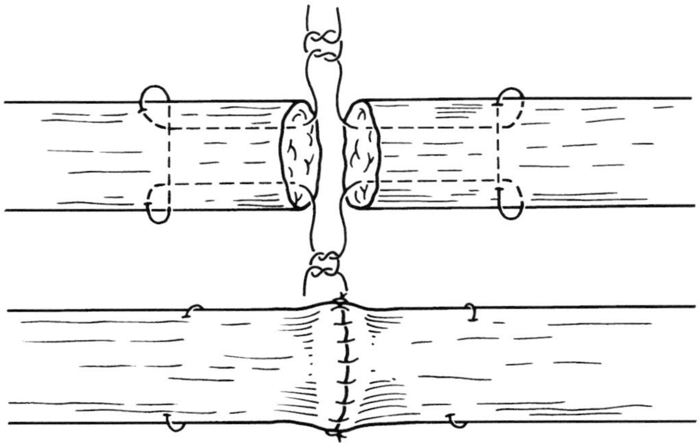

Fig. 45.7 The modified Kessler suture.

Extensor tendon injuries

The results of extensor tendon repairs in the forearm are generally satisfactory. If division occurs under the extensor retinaculum, the repair should be coupled with a release of the sheath. Repairs to the dorsum of the hand and fingers are also usually satisfactory but two areas require special mention: the proximal interphalangeal and the distal interphalangeal joint.

The level of the proximal interphalangeal joint

Lacerations in this area may divide the central slip and damage the delicate lateral fibres which maintain the lateral bands on the dorsal aspect of the joint. At the initial assessment, the patient will be able actively to extend the proximal interphalangeal joint but the lateral bands will migrate in a volar direction over the next 2–3 weeks until they are beyond the centre of rotation of the joint, thus producing the characteristic boutonnière deformity of proximal interphalangeal joint flexion and distal interphalangeal joint hyperextension (Fig. 45.8). Once established, the deformity is difficult to rectify. Because of the difficulty in confirming a central slip injury by clinical examination alone, a full exploration of a wound should be carried out if central slip damage is considered possible.

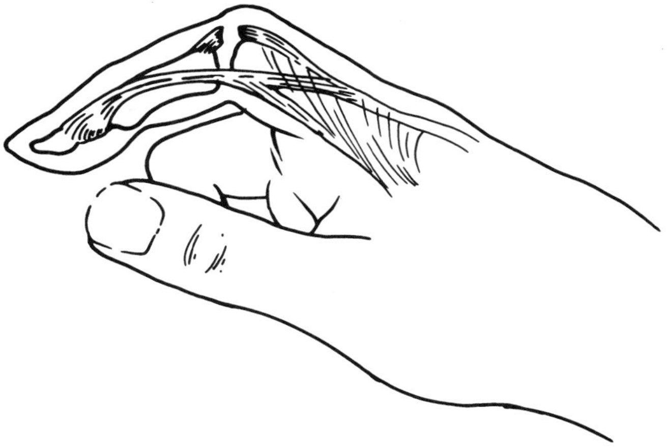

Fig. 45.8 The boutonnière deformity.

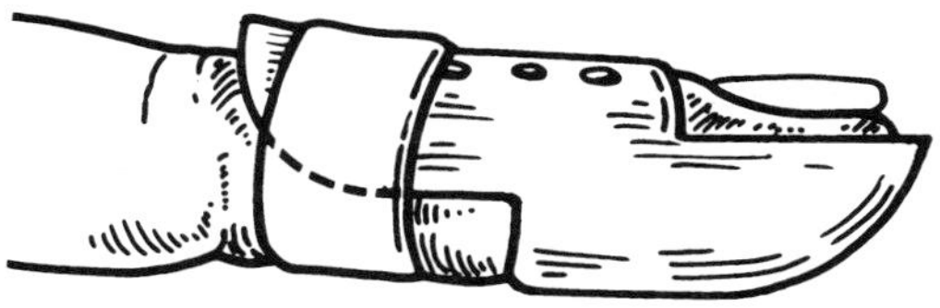

Fig. 45.9 The Stack splint.

The level of the distal interphalangeal joint

Injury to the extensor tendon at its insertion produces an extensor lag (a mallet finger deformity). A Stack-type splint (Fig. 45.9) applied and maintained for 6 weeks will usually produce a satisfactory result, although there may be a mild residual extensor lag. Frequently, a fragment of the bone remains attached to the tendon. If it is very large and joint subluxation is present, open reduction and internal fixation of the fragment may be appropriate. Conservative management with a Stack splint remains, however, the preferred treatment in most cases.[10]

NERVE INJURY (see Chapter 44)

Recovery of sensory and motor function after nerve division and repair is inevitably incomplete. The patient should be advised that recovery to total normality should not be anticipated. Even at best, the nerve distal to the repair has a reduced number of axons which remain less well myelinated and have a prolonged conduction time. The single most important factor affecting the quality of the

REFERENCE

10. Stack G Hand 1969; 1: 83

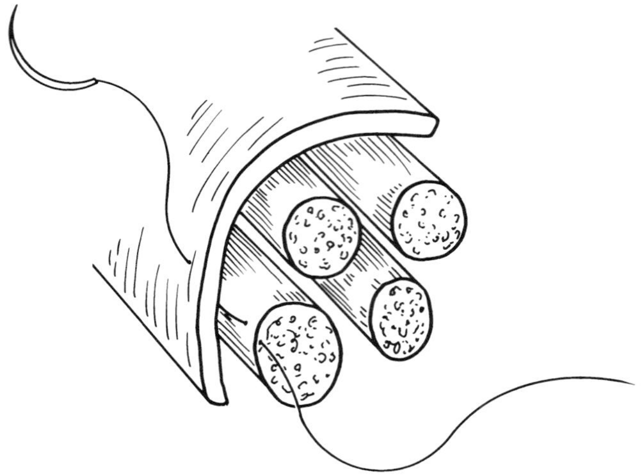

Fig. 45.10 The epiperineurial suture.

result—beyond the accuracy of the approximation of the nerve ends—is the patient's age. Under the age of 12 years, adequate results are usually obtained if careful nerve repair is performed soon after injury. However, as age increases nerve recovery diminishes and perhaps central adaptations are also less readily made.

Diagnosis

Nerve injury is frequently overlooked in accident and emergency departments. There are some grounds for thinking that a recently divided nerve whose ends are in contact remains temporarily capable of conduction. However, in the majority of cases a missed diagnosis probably relates to inadequate examination. Puncture of the dermis with a needle is excessive and enquiries such as 'Can you feel this?' are inadequate. The important point is to ask the patient to compare the injured side with the non-injured contralateral digit or limb. This can be done by asking the patient to compare the sensations produced when both limbs are touched simultaneously by gentle stroking. Although it is possible that some form of sensibility may persist for a while in the territory of a divided nerve, sweating is lost immediately. This affects the dermal adherence, which can be demonstrated by the plastic pen test. Reduced adherence of the skin to the pen when it is drawn across the digit is an early reliable indication of nerve division.

Management

Primary repair is the treatment of choice[11] unless there are inadequate facilities, or there has been major tissue loss or gross contamination. Delayed repair frequently requires a nerve graft to bridge the gap. Magnification is beneficial during repair[12] and sutures should be of nylon and not of a thicker gauge than 8/0. Epiperineurial sutures (Fig. 45.10) probably offer the best compromise in that they are easy to perform yet accurate in alignment of fascicles.[13] The repair is rested with adjacent joints held in a position which minimizes tension for 4 weeks. The limb may then be mobilized. Progress is assessed by the Tinel's sign (distal to proximal percussion over the course of the nerve until tingling is experienced by the patient in the line of the nerve). Nerve regeneration proceeds at a speed of approximately 1 mm per day. A strong Tinel sign (prominent tingling on gentle percussion) which is progressing distally suggests that many axons have crossed the repair site and satisfactory reinnervation may be anticipated.

FRACTURES

In many parts of the body, non-union of a fracture is the most feared complication. This is rarely a difficulty in the hand where the greatest risk is stiffness arising from joint contracture or tendon adhesions. Rotational deformity is an uncommon but significant complication causing increasing malalignment of a finger as it flexes. Constant vigilance is required if the rotational deformity is to be identified before fracture union. The problem is most frequently seen in spiral fractures but can occur between any displaced fracture surfaces. The injured fingers are usually examined in extension; rotational deformity is best assessed by comparison of the alignment of the finger nails (Fig. 45.11).

Most hand fractures are managed by immobilization in the optimal position for function on a volar slab for 3–4 weeks until the fracture is stable. The hand is then mobilized to overcome residual stiffness. Some fractures (distal tuft or those that are judged to be stable) may be mobilized from the time of injury. Assessment of a stable fracture is not always easy; they are usually associated with a crack in the bone without displacement. If a programme of immediate mobilization is followed, it is prudent to have a check X-ray after a week to confirm that the position is maintained.

A minority of fractures require internal fixation. Such fractures are either intra-articular with joint incongruity or subluxation, or shaft fractures which cannot be maintained in a satisfactory position on a volar slab. The decision to fix a fracture internally should never be taken lightly; it turns a closed fracture to an open one and the necessary dissection inevitably further devascularizes the fragments. These disadvantages are only acceptable if, following fixation, the fracture is satisfactorily reduced and sufficiently stable to permit early mobilization. Open reduction without the achievement of stabilization is a very unsatisfactory situation, for one has increased the area of trauma and yet must still immobilize the hand on a volar slab. Thus the risk of long-term stiffness is greatly increased. The most rigid form of fixation is by the use of mini fragment screws or plates (the latter are used at metacarpal level or

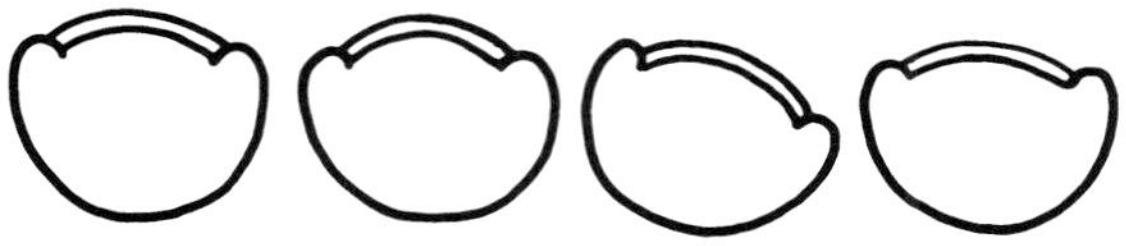

Fig. 45.11 Rotational deformity of the finger.

REFERENCES

11. Merle M, Foucher G et al Bull Hosp Joint Dis Orthop Inst 1984; 44: 338
12. Jabalay M E J Hand Surg 1984; 9B: 14
13. Williams H B, Jabalay M E Hand Clin 1986; 2: 689

sometimes on the phalanges).[14] Screws achieve excellent intrafragmentary compression and offer the firmest fixation of condylar or oblique shaft fractures if these fractures are not comminuted. Screw and plate fixation is used for unstable displaced transverse metacarpal fractures. Interosseous wiring[15] is used for transverse phalangeal fractures although stability is somewhat less effective than plate and screw fixation. Kirschner wires alone may be used for internal fixation of fractures but it should be appreciated that the bone interface is not as well stabilized, nor is there intrafragmentary compression.[16] If a decision is made to perform internal fixation of a fracture, the procedure should be performed by a surgeon familiar with the technique using an operating theatre with suitable equipment. In addition, the assistance of a surgeon who also has some experience of fractur fixation is invaluable.

REIMPLANTATION AND REVASCULARIZATION

Until 15 years ago, levels of amputation largely depended on the level of tissue viability. Most areas in Europe, the USA and many other parts of the world now have access to a microvascular service. Problems arise abruptly and demand contingency planning and an understanding of the indications for replantation, as swift referral improves the chances of success. The local reimplantation centre should be contacted immediately, as they will need time to marshall staff and open a theatre. The amputated part should be wrapped in a damp saline soaked swab and placed in a clean, dry plastic bag. This bag should be sealed and placed in a container with ice and water.

What are the indications for reimplantation?[17]

Upper arm

There is only one bone to stabilize and it tolerates shortening well. Vessel diameter is large and there are few muscles to repair. The ischaemic time is of critical importance as there is a risk of Volkmann's ischaemic contracture or gas gangrene in distal musculature. Reinnervation, except in the very young, is often disappointing but body image is preserved.

Forearm

Amputations distal to the motor end-plates of the forearm muscles greatly increase the potential for a good result. The more distal the repair in the forearm, the easier tendon repair becomes. At wrist level mobility may be impaired but the area remains favourable for reimplantation.

The metacarpal area

The thumb plays such a key role in hand function that amputation of it at any level should give rise to thoughts of reimplantation. The same is also true if a composite of all the fingers is amputated, particularly if the thumb remains intact. This region is one of the most gratifying areas for reimplantation.

The digits

Whilst amputation of the tip of the thumb is not catastrophic, reimplantation should provide improved function and cosmesis. More proximal thumb amputations should always be reimplanted as the loss of a thumb is important functionally. When reimplantation is not possible then alternative methods have to be considered for reconstruction of the thumb. Previously these have consisted of a groin flap with a non-vascularized bone peg. More recent advances in microsurgery have led to the vascularized transfer of the ipsilateral great toe, with coaptation of the digital nerves and repair of the tendons. This provides a sensate, cosmetically acceptable replacement for the thumb. Alternatively, if the patient is unwilling to accept transfer of the great toe, then the index finger may be pollicized to produce the same result.

Indications for finger reimplantation depend on the level of injury and the number of fingers injured. Previously Zone 2 injuries were thought to be a contraindication to reimplantation, but satisfactory results can be achieved here with early active mobilization or two-stage tendon grafting with insertion of a rod at the time of the initial surgery. If a single digit is involved then the decision must be made in conjunction with the patient. Many will opt for completion of the amputation[18] at a cosmetic level and an early return to work. The average time to return to work after reimplantation is around 9–12 months after injury.

If all fingers are involved then the question is not whether replantation should be attempted but where the parts should be placed. So, preferentially, the middle and ring fingers would be replaced with the little and index following if the parts are suitable. However with an oblique cut and significant tissue loss it may be more appropriate to replace the index onto the middle stump in order to obtain the best possible finger. Distal reimplantation is technically difficult, often requiring 11/0 sutures and high magnification. However, if successful, they are very rewarding, especially if the movement of the finger is preserved.

HAND INFECTIONS

The incidence and severity of hand infections have dropped in developed countries over the last three decades.[19] Nevertheless, inadequate treatment will either extend short-term malfunction[20] or, on occasion, cause permanent disability. The possibility of secondary contributing factors should always be considered. A reduced host response from treatment with steroids or immunosuppressive drugs malignancy or immune infection (HIV) may be responsible. Any condition which impairs peripheral circulation (for example, vasculitis associated with rheumatoid arthritis or

REFERENCES

14. Heim U, Pfeifer K M. Internal Fixation of Small Fractures, 3rd edn. Springer Verlag, Berlin 1986
15. Lister G J Hand Surg 1978; 3: 427
16. Fyfe I S, Mason S Hand 1979; 11: 50
17. Tamai S J Hand Surg 1982; 7: 549
18. Louis D S In: Green D P (ed) Operative Hand Surgery. Churchill Livingstone, Edinburgh 1982
19. Bell M S Hand 1976; 8: 298
20. Glass K D J Hand Surg 1982; 7: 388

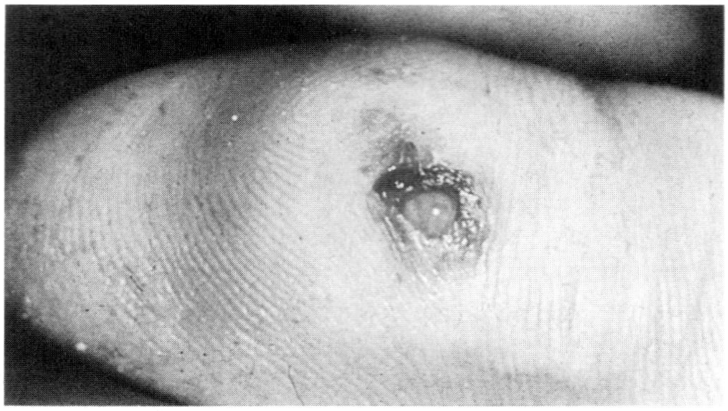

Fig. 45.12 A pulp space infection.

scleroderma) will reduce the host's ability to overcome infection. The most frequent contributing disease is, however, diabetes mellitus. Infections arising in diabetics are common, often involve Gram-negative organisms and are slow to resolve. Debilitation, poverty and poor personal hygiene are all contributing factors and the possibility of drug addiction[21] should also be considered.

Infections arising from inadequate primary management regrettably remain an all too common cause of hand sepsis. If an infection is thought to need incision and drainage, the procedure should be performed in an operating theatre with fine instruments and a satisfactory sterile technique. The abscess cavity is opened through an incision that avoids important structures (neurovascular bundles and the flexor tendon sheath) and is designed to leave a scar that will not cause contracture. The cavity is drained of pus and any necrotic material removed from the base. A paraffin gauze wick is then inserted to aid drainage and promote healing from the depths of the wound. The cavity does not require packing, which simply obstructs drainage and delays wound closure. Gauze dressings are then applied to absorb the exudate. Daily dressings may be required initially but the frequency is reduced as the wound settles. Although a course of antibiotics may be of some benefit, their effect in most properly treated cases is almost incidental to the resolution of infection. Antibiotic therapy should never be used as an alternative to correct surgical management.

Pulp space infections (Fig. 45.12) usually arise from minor penetrating injuries. Pressure in the infected compartment rapidly rises causing increasing pain. The increased pressure causes infarction of surrounding tissues which may spread the infection into adjacent compartments or encourage rupture through the skin or extension into the distal phalanx. Early incision and drainage is required, for extensive sloughing of pulp tissue will permanently reduce the cushioning of the distal phalanx.

A *paronychia* is an infection of the nail fold which may extend proximally to involve the eponychium. Drainage by incision of the nail fold or resection of a portion of the nail will usually resolve the problem. However, local incision may spread infection or leave scarring of the nail fold. The condition settles well if treated with a course of antibiotics associated with nail avulsion. A normal nail grows out in the weeks that follow and there is no scarring to the nail fold.

Infection of the flexor tendon sheath is fortunately uncommon, because even prompt and appropriate treatment may leave the finger with residual stiffness. The cruciate portions of the flexor tendon sheaths lie close to the skin at the proximal and distal interphalangeal joints. Superficial laceration in this area may breach the sheath and introduce infection. There is slowly increasing discomfort in the finger, often several days after a trivial laceration. The finger is held in a semi-flexed position (Fig. 45.13) and there is tenderness over the flexor sheath. Attempted movement is extremely painful, especially passive extension of the interphalangeal joints.

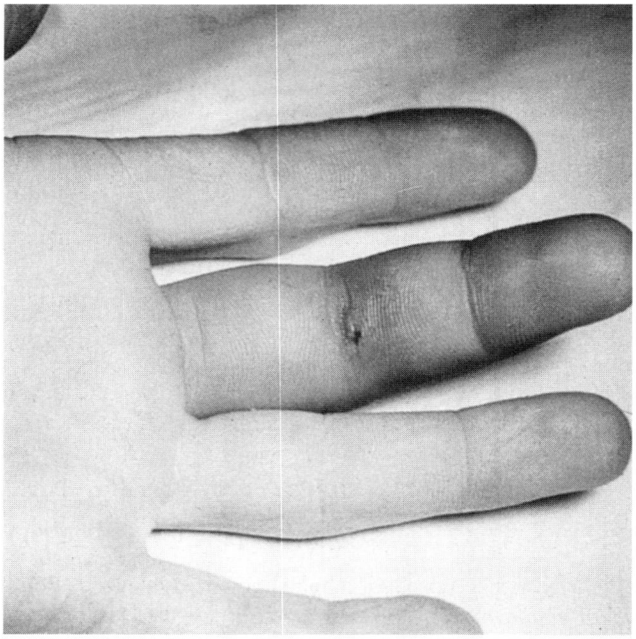

Fig. 45.13 A flexor sheath infection.

The very earliest sheath infections may be given a trial of conservative management (admission to hospital with intravenous antibiotics and elevation on a volar slab) but immediate exploration is preferred if there is no rapid resolution of symptoms within 24 hours of starting intravenous antibiotics. A small incision is made in the cruciate pulley at the level of the distal interphalangeal joint. A further incision is made in the palm at the mouth of the A1 pulley (see Fig. 45.6). A fine plastic catheter is passed into the sheath and it is irrigated with normal saline. The skin is loosely sutured and the hand treated as described for conservative management. As soon as it is apparent that the infection is controlled, physiotherapy is begun to overcome finger stiffness.

Paronychia, pulp and sheath infections are usually caused by *Staphylococcus aureus*. Infected material should be cultured and treatment started with an appropriate antibiotic—usually flucloxacillin. Treatment can subsequently be altered to a more suitable drug if sensitivity testing reveals a different organism.

Streptococcal cellulitis does not require incision and drainage because infection is not localized and there is no collection of pus. However, it must be remembered that this is still a potentially

REFERENCE

21. Petrie P, Lamb D W Hand 1973; 5: 130

life-threatening infection. There is diffuse swelling and erythema of the skin and subcutaneous tissue, usually associated with ascending lymphangitis. Treatment consists of inpatient admission, elevation, intravenous penicillin in large doses and rest on a volar slab. Signs of resolution are usually apparent within 24 hours and physiotherapy can usually be started after 3–4 days to overcome local stiffness.

Human bites[22] are usually caused by a blow to an opponent's mouth in a brawl. The clenched knuckle strikes a tooth which penetrates skin, extensor tendon and capsule. The cause of injury is rarely admitted to the casualty officer, and presentation is often delayed. The hand is usually examined in extension and the extent of the injury may not be appreciated. A high index of suspicion is required in all cases presenting with penetrating injuries over the dorsum of the metacarpophalangeal joints (Fig. 45.14). A polymicrobial inoculation usually occurs at the time of injury; this requires early joint lavage, splintage and combination antibiotic therapy covering Gram-negative as well as Gram-positive organisms.

High-pressure injection injuries have become increasingly common in recent years as the pressures in industrial sprays and hydraulic systems have risen.[23,24] Oils, solvents and paints may be driven through the intact skin to disperse within the soft tissues. Close proximity to the leaking apparatus rather than direct contact may be sufficient to breach the skin if the pressure is very high. A high index of suspicion is essential in diagnosis for the patient may be unaware that injection has occurred. Management requires immediate transfer to a specialist surgeon as early exploration may reduce ultimate inflammation and stiffness. Amputation may commonly be required even when early management has been satisfactory; delayed diagnosis or referral only increases this risk.

Deep infections within the hand are uncommon. Presentation can often be confusing with more swelling apparent on the dorsum of the hand than in the palm. Exploration of the deeper palmar areas is required, taking care to preserve all important structures. If incision and drainage of a hand infection are required, a bloodless field is essential. A pneumatic tourniquet should be used but without preliminary exsanguination of the limb with an Esmarch's bandage which can spread the infection. Simple elevation of the limb for 2 minutes with pressure over the brachial artery before cuff inflation will give a satisfactory bloodless field.

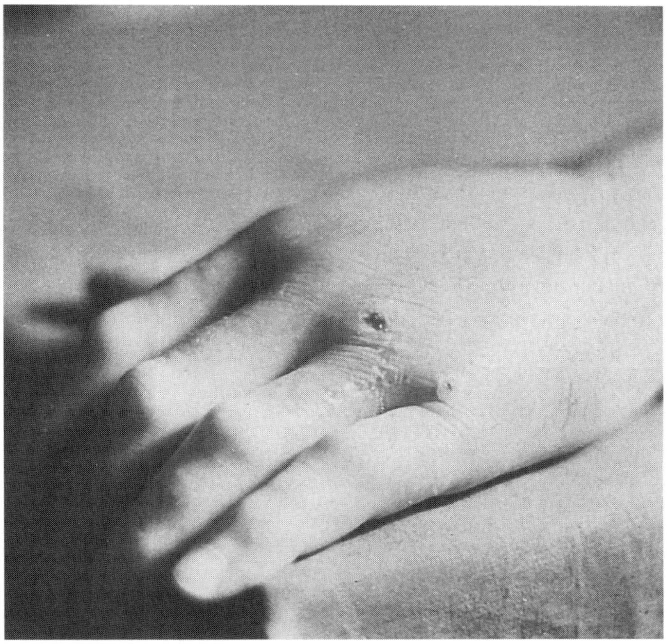

Fig. 45.14 A human bite injury.

NERVE COMPRESSION SYNDROMES IN THE UPPER LIMB

'Compression syndromes' is an umbrella phrase that covers not only nerve compression but also nerve irritation due to undue mobility. Mild compression of a nerve produces neuropraxia with a local conduction block and there is no distal Wallerian degeneration. Release of compression is followed by resolution of symptoms within days. More severe compression causes an axonotmesis with distal nerve degeneration; recovery is then delayed as reinnervation slowly proceeds distally. Severe prolonged compression produces such an extensive disruption to the structure of the nerve that significant recovery of function cannot be expected. Younger patients recovery more swiftly and completely after nerve decompression than the elderly.

The median nerve is most frequently compressed at the wrist within the carpal tunnel.[25] The patient characteristically complains of discomfort and paraesthesia in the median nerve distribution (middle and ring fingers may predominate) that wake the patient at night or are present on waking in the morning. Wasting of abductor pollicis brevis may be apparent in severe cases. Percussion over the median nerve just proximal to the wrist may evoke distal paraesthesia (Tinel's sign). Provocation tests which reduce the volume of the carpal tunnel (for example, Phalen's test where the wrist is held in flexion) usually reproduce the symptoms. The diagnosis is confirmed by nerve conduction studies. Division of the flexor retinaculum decompresses the nerve and relieves night discomfort immediately, improving sensibility in most cases except in the elderly where compression has been severe and prolonged; recovery in such cases may be only partial. Motor recovery is unlikely if wasting has been present for over 18 months.

Ulnar nerve compression or irritation occurs most commonly at the elbow where the nerve may dislocate around the medial epicondyle during flexion and extension. There is discomfort and altered sensibility in the ring and little fingers initially, and later there may be weakness of grip and wasting of the intrinsic muscles. The results of surgery are generally less satisfactory than in median nerve decompression; a resting night splint which holds the elbow semi-extended may resolve early symptoms and is always worth a trial. If nerve conduction studies indicate local delay, decompression or transposition of the nerve to the flexor surface of the arm is usually indicated. The patient must be advised that full recovery is

REFERENCES

22. Dreyfuss L Y, Singer M J Hand Surg 1985; 10A: 884
23. Kaufman H D Hand 1970; 2: 63
24. Neal N C, Burke F D Injury 1991; 22: 467
25. Goldner J L Bull Hosp Joint Dis Orthop Inst 1984; 44: 199

unlikely after decompression of an established case with motor weakness.[26]

A minority of ulnar nerve compressions are at wrist level in Guyon's canal. Compression at this level is most commonly found in association with carpal tunnel syndrome and is often alleviated by simple release of the carpal tunnel itself. However, other causes are not infrequent and include ganglions, ulnar artery aneurysms and fractures of the hook of the hamate. Dissociated sensory and motor symptoms may be apparent and the dorsal branch of the ulnar nerve and the ulnar flexor profundi are spared. The results of decompression in this area are usually satisfactory.[27] C8–T1 compression at the thoracic outlet may produce symptoms similar to ulnar nerve compression and for this reason conduction studies are always valuable to localize the site of compression if ulnar nerve surgery is under consideration.

Radial nerve compression is rarer but can occur at the elbow in the radial tunnel or where the radial sensory component exits from under the brachioradialis at the wrist (Wartenberg's syndrome). The median nerve can also be compressed at the elbow although rarely (pronator syndrome).

DUPUYTREN'S DISEASE

Dupuytren's disease[28–30] remains an ill understood condition. The tendency to contracture is probably inherited, with the majority of patients having a positive family history. Associations with epilepsy (or anti-convulsant therapy) and diabetes seem certain. Fibromatosis of the plantar fascia and Peyronie's disease are, on occasion, seen in those with a strong diathesis. Such patients are likely to develop the condition in their 30s and 40s with relentless progression and recurrence after surgery. Presentation in the 60s and 70s is more common with more gradual progression and a smaller likelihood of recurrence.

Thickening is usually first seen in the palmar fascia: nodules and bands develop with progressive contracture to metacarpophalangeal or proximal interphalangeal joints. The ring and little fingers are involved most frequently but any digit may be affected.

Management

Resection of the band (partial fasciectomy) with Z-plasty of the overlying skin is required if the patient is unable to lay the involved hand flat upon a table. Night splintage for several months postoperatively to maintain the extensor gain is probably beneficial during the phase of collagen maturation.

A prominent band in the palm may simply be divided (fasciotomy) rather than resorting to band excision. This is particularly valuable in the elderly patient whose contracture is principally at the metacarpophalangeal joint.

Skin excision may be necessary if the tissues are extensively scarred by previous surgery. A full-thickness graft is required to cover the defect. Dermofasciectomy is the most extensive surgical option but has the lowest risk of recurrence.

Late presentation or repeated recurrence may require arthrodesis of the proximal interphalangeal joint in a semi-extended position or even amputation of the ray if finger function cannot be salvaged by reconstructive surgery.

TUMOURS RELEVANT TO THE HAND

Lumps on the hand are commonly site-specific, making diagnosis straightforward in the majority of cases (Fig. 45.15). The word 'tumour' in this context refers to local swellings rather than neoplasms, which are an uncommon cause of hand lumps.

Ganglion

Ganglia arise most commonly on the dorsum of the hand[31] over the scapholunate ligament. They are most evident when the wrist is held in a flexed position. If the ganglion is uncomfortable or cosmetically unsightly, resection of the sac may be performed, extending into the joint and taking a small dorsal portion of the ligament if there is evidence of cystic degeneration.[32] Recurrence after surgery may be as high as 20%, and re-operation is only indicated if there is a functional deficit.

Volar ganglia usually arise from the peritrapezial joints and the radial artery commonly lies closely attached to the ganglion wall or on occasion traverses the cavity. Great care must always be taken during dissection to preserve the radial artery and the palmar cutaneous nerve. A pneumatic tourniquet is essential.

Metacarpal bossing

This commonly arises spontaneously or after hand trauma in the 30–40 year age group. An exostosis develops at the second or third carpometacarpal joint. It lies under the extensor carpi radialis longus or brevis tendons close to their insertion and may be associated with a small ganglion. The ganglion should be excised and the exostosis removed with an osteotome if there is great deformity or if the digital extensors dislocate over the lump with discomfort. Surgery is followed by an inevitable local haematoma over the bone and, if this forms callus, some prominence of the bone may persist. Most patients with the condition require reassurance rather than surgery.

Mucous cyst

Mucous cysts usually arise from the distal interphalangeal joints (occasionally the more proximal row). The cyst is a blow-out of an osteoarthritic joint. The cyst may indent the germinal nail matrix producing distal nail deformity (Fig. 45.16). Characteristically, the cyst penetrates the deeper layers of the skin and may discharge as an intermittent sinus. The cyst will usually settle after excision but a local skin flap may need to be raised to cover the defect.

REFERENCES

26. Foster R J, Edshage S J Hand Surg 1981; 6: 181
27. Shea J, McLain E J J Bone Joint Surg 1969; 51A: 1095
28. Hueston J T In Flynn J E (ed) Hand Surgery. Williams & Wilkins, Baltimore 1982
29. McFarlane R M Bull Hosp Joint Dis Orthop Inst 1984; 44: 318
30. McGrouther D A In: Watson N, Smith R J (eds) Methods and Concepts in Hand Surgery. Butterworth, London 1986
31. Barnes W E, Larsen R D, Posch J L Plast Reconst Surg 1964; 34: 570
32. Angelides A C In: Green D P (ed) Operative Hand Surgery. Churchill Livingstone, Edinburgh 1982

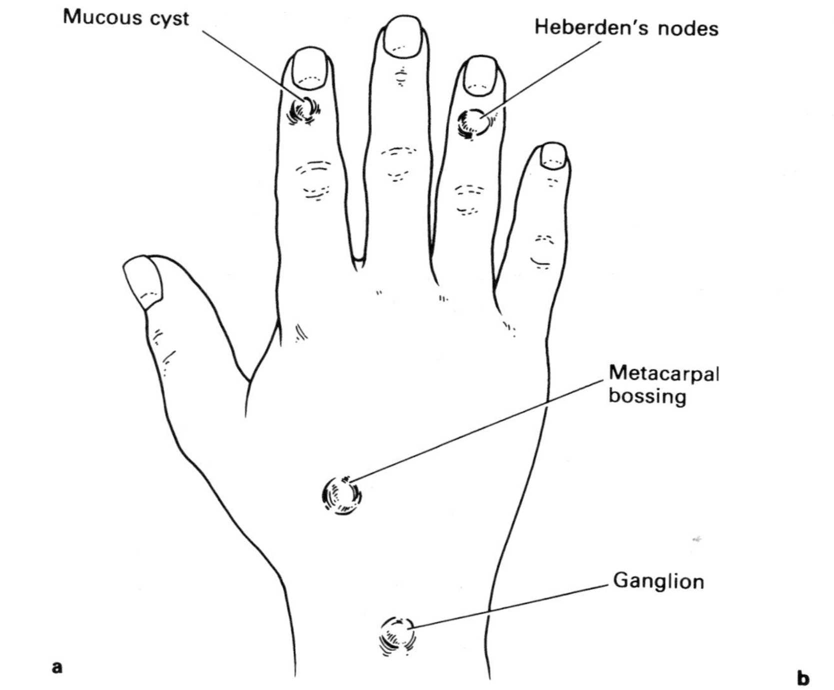

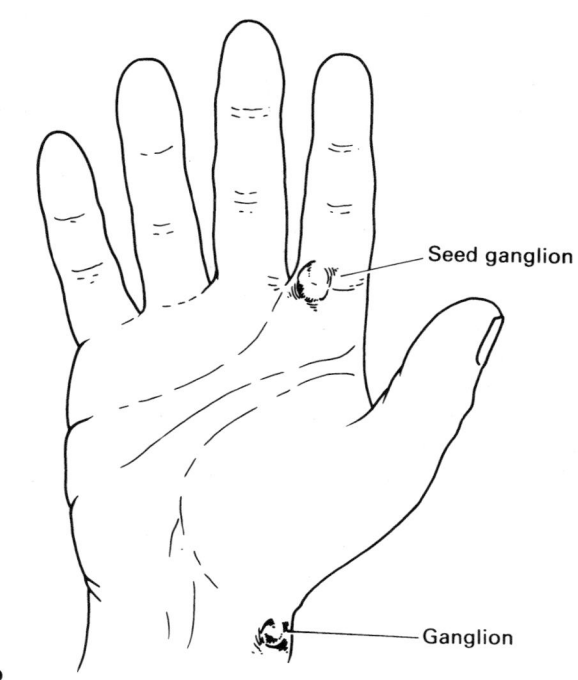

Fig. 45.15 Site-specific tumours of the hand.

Synovial giant cell tumour of joint or flexor tendon sheath

It is uncertain whether this condition is a true tumour or a local reactive response. The lump is firm and lobular, arising from the sheath or a joint. There are no radiological signs. Local excision resolves the problem but if a lobule is inadvertently left behind, local recurrence may develop.[33]

Seed ganglion of the flexor tendon sheath

These commonly arise over the A1 pulley and are usually slightly eccentrically placed. The cyst feels like a firm pea which does not move on digital flexion (Fig. 45.17). The lump is uncomfortable when hard objects are grasped. The ganglion and a segment of the pulley are excised en bloc leaving a small window in the sheath. Recurrence is exceptional.[32]

Enchondroma

There is a slowly growing mass within a phalanx which may present acutely with a fracture through the weakened cortex.[34] Diagnosis is made on the characteristic appearance of the radiograph (Fig. 45.18). The bone has been moulded by an internal mass which has thinned the cortex as it expands. The cavity is clear with stippled calcification. The interface between cartilage and bone is distinct, indicating its benign nature (malignant neoplasms infiltrate normal bone with a sinister diffuse interface). Curettage followed by cancellous bone graft is the best form of treatment, particularly if cortical thinning has weakened the bone. If a fracture has already occurred, it is often wiser to delay grafting until the fracture has healed, for curettage of the fresh fracture may cause skeletal instability.

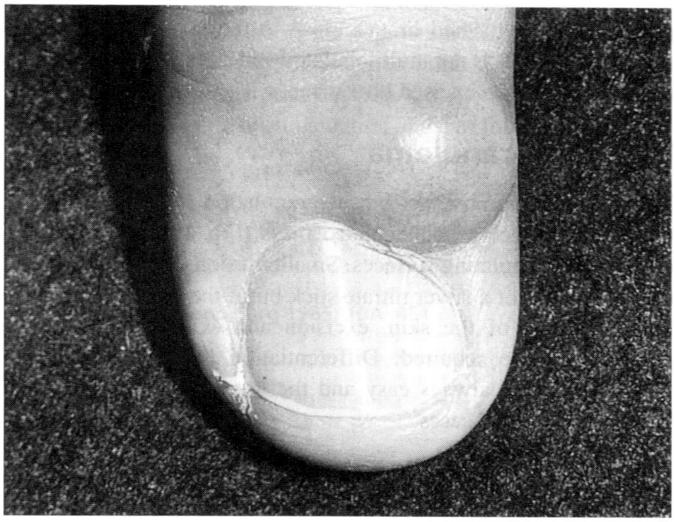

Fig. 45.16 A mucous cyst deforming the nail.

Dupuytren nodules

Dupuytren nodules lie in the palm, in the palmar fascia, or over the proximal phalanx where they may be adherent to the underlying flexor tendon sheath. The diagnosis is usually obvious except at the earliest stages of the disease. Garrod's pads are thickenings of the subcutaneous tissues over the proximal interphalangeal joints. Histologically, the tissue is similar to Dupuytren's disease in the palm. Surgical excision of these pads is not indicated.

REFERENCES

33. Froimson A Hand Clin 1987; 3: 213
34. Noble J, Lamb D W Hand 1974; 6: 275

backache but there is no correlation between this and the severity of the curve. Most patients lead relatively normal lives without developing significant functional deficits. It is generally accepted that curves which measure 30° or more at skeletal maturity progress in adult life at approximately 1° per annum. Reduced life expectancy from compromised cardiorespiratory function is only seen in curves which are severe before the age of 5.

Assessment

The deformity needs to be quantified, non-idiopathic deformities must be excluded and the maturity and growth potential of the patient must be estimated. A careful family and developmental history is essential and the examination must include a search for underlying syndromes, significant neurological deficits and, in particular, the absence of abdominal reflexes which is a strong indicator of an underlying neuroaxis abnormality. Idiopathic scoliosis is generally painless; the presence of pain may indicate an underlying spondylolisthesis, adolescent disc herniation or benign neoplasm such as osteoid osteoma or osteoblastoma (see Chapter 42). Examination of the spine must include the forward bending test, which reveals any gross rotational deformity of the spine, and an assessment of the spinal balance, which is the position of the first cervical and first thoracic vertebra in relation to the centre of the sacrum. Modern radiographic techniques have significantly reduced the radiation dosage, and plain anteroposterior (Fig. 46.25) and lateral radiographs with associated side bending views are essential. MRI scanning is indicated if there is any suspicion of underlying neurological abnormalities. The extent of the deformity is measured using the Cobb angle (Fig. 46.26) but a variety of more sophisticated techniques are now available to assess the severity of the curve. There is a current trend to use questionnaires to measure patient disability, self perception and psychological and social functioning, both in the initial assessment and to follow the results of treatment.

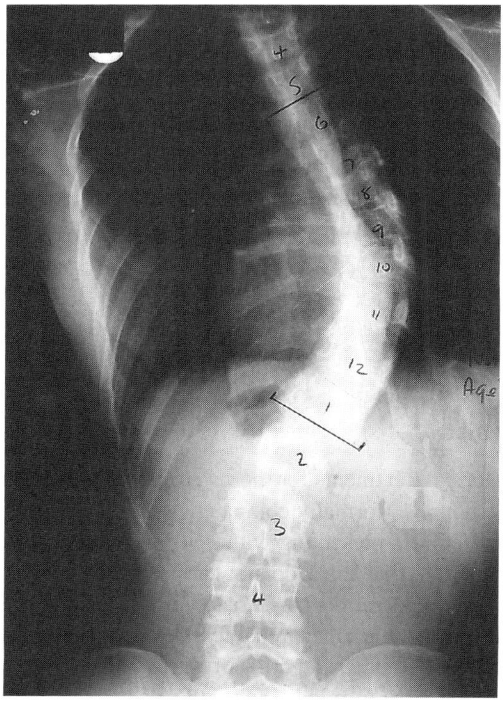

Fig. 46.25 Idiopathic scoliosis.

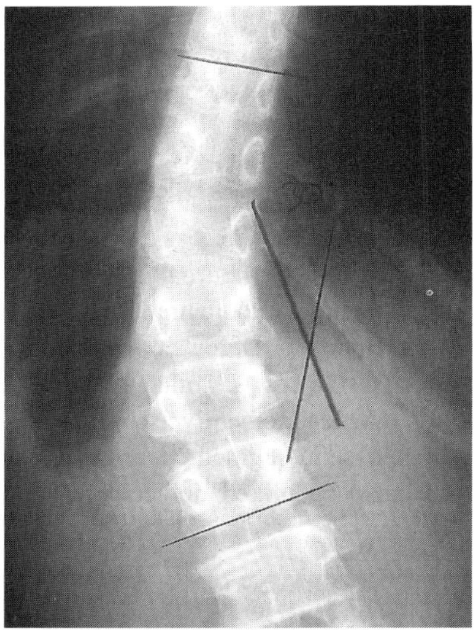

Fig. 46.26 The Cobb angle.

Treatment

Stable curves which do not cause any great cosmetic deformity should simply be observed, especially if the patient is nearing skeletal maturity. The historical use of braces has only recently been scientifically assessed. A brace prevents the curve from progressing at best and does not improve the curve from its severity at presentation. Braces need to be worn for 23 hours a day to be effective. The prolonged use of an underarm plastic brace may however prevent curve progression in the skeletally immature group with curves of 30–40° severity. One in five of these patients still needs surgical correction at the end of the bracing programme. Progressive curves greater than 40° and most curves greater than 50°, particularly those with a loss of spinal balance, require surgical correction which can be performed through anterior (Fig. 46.27), posterior (Fig. 46.28) or combined approaches.

Neuromuscular scoliosis

Neuromuscular scoliosis can occur as the result of an underlying neuromuscular defect in a multitude of different conditions. A progressive spinal deformity producing disturbance of quality of life or threatening compromise of the cardiorespiratory function can be treated by spinal stabilization using the posterior approach. There is now some good evidence that stabilization of the spine in children with Duchenne's muscular dystrophy who are unable to walk, before the respiratory compromise is too severe to allow a general anaesthetic, may increase their lifespan by several years.[19] Spinal defor-

REFERENCE

19. Galasko C S B, Delaney C, Morris P J Bone Joint Surg 1992; 74B: 210

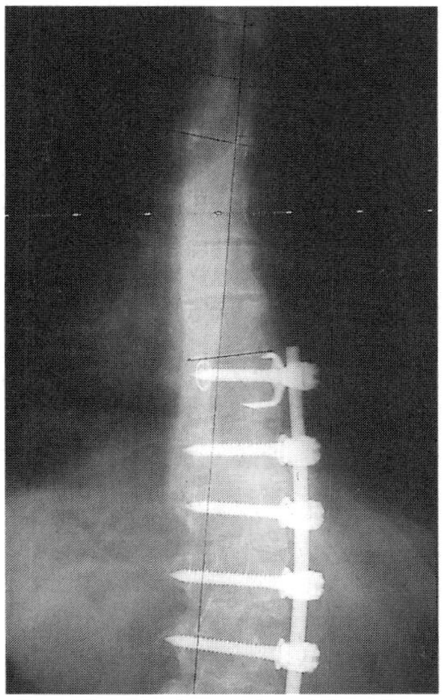

Fig. 46.27 Anterior correction of scoliosis.

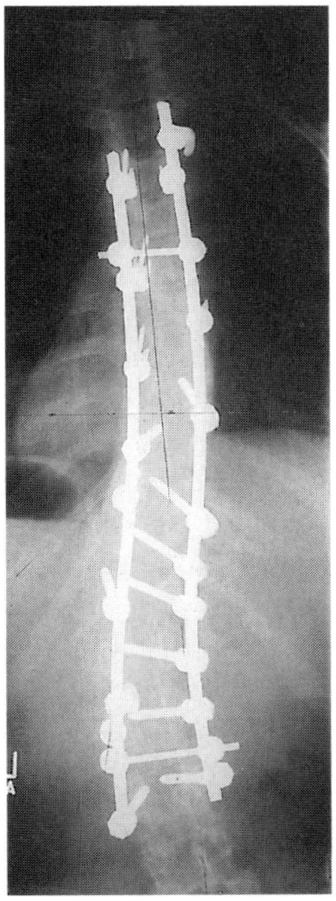

Fig. 46.28 Posterior correction of scoliosis.

mity is almost invariable in this condition. Other common neuromuscular conditions requiring spinal stabilization include cerebral palsy, myelomeningocele and the sequelae of poliomyelitis.

Scheuermann's kyphosis

Scheuermann's disease affects the growing adolescent spine and may be a form of osteochondrosis or aseptic necrosis of the vertebral growth plates (see Chapter 42). It predominantly affects adolescent males and usually develops at around the age of 10 years. Thoracic Scheuermann's disease is defined as characteristic vertebral end-plate changes associated with 5° of wedging of the anterior vertebral body at at least three adjacent vertebral levels.

These patients present with back pain, often related to sport, with progressive kyphosis. The differential diagnosis is of postural kyphosis. Most patients can be treated with simple pain relief, physiotherapy and in some cases a modified scoliosis brace. Surgical intervention is rarely indicated but can be performed using an endoscopic anterior release and posterior instrumentation for those patients who develop stiff curves.

Spondylolisthesis

Spondylolisthesis is the slipping forwards of one vertebra in relation to another (Fig. 46.29). Spondylolisthesis can be graded as a percentage of the vertebral body width that has slipped forwards and, in fact, one vertebra may sublux completely on the underlying vertebra, a condition called spondyloptosis. Spondylolisthesis has been classified by Wiltsie[20] into five categories (Table 46.2).

Isthmic spondylolisthesis can be further divided into three types. The first of these is lytic fracture of the pars intra-articularis; this is the most common variant. The second type involves elongation of the pars intra-articularis and the third is an acute fracture of the pars intra-articularis.

Isthmic spondylolisthesis appears to be a form of repetitive stress fracture; the incidence is much higher in teenage gymnasts and other sports obsessed individuals. It commonly occurs between the ages of 7 and 10 and, indeed, is rare before this age.

REFERENCE

20. Wiltse L L, Newman P H, Macnab I Clin Orthop 1976; 117: 23

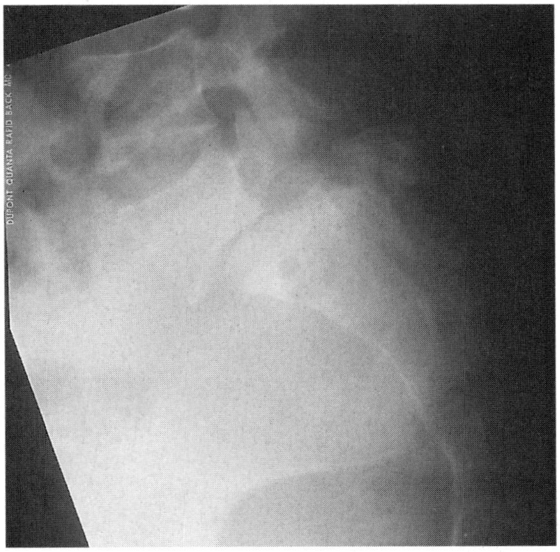

Fig. 46.29 L5/S1 spondylolisthesis.

Table 46.2 Categories of spondylolisthesis

1. Dysplastic
2. Isthmic
3. Degenerative
4. Traumatic
5. Pathological

5% of gymnasts have some degree of spondylolisthesis. The majority of cases present when the vertebra has already slipped and progression in adulthood is very uncommon.

Clinical presentation

Patients may present in childhood with back pain or associated fifth lumbar nerve root pain. Younger patients often have hamstring spasm and in a severe spondylolisthesis or spondyloptosis there is gross disturbance of the sagittal profile of the spine with an acute kyphosis at the fifth lumbar/first sacral level associated with hyperlordosis in the proximal part of the lumbar spine to compensate. In patients past the third decade of life, it is unusual for the spondylolysis or spondylolisthesis to produce the pain and more commonly the pain results from secondary degenerative changes in the discs and facet joints. The condition predominantly affects the distal moving segments of the lumbar spine, particularly at the fifth lumbar/first sacral level. Routine plain radiographs of the lumbar spine are required and often show the spondylolysis and/or spondylolisthesis. Oblique radiographs are no longer acceptable because of the radiation dosage; if a spondylosis (Fig. 46.30) is identified, reverse gantry CT scanning may well show an abnormality in the pars intra-articularis (Fig. 46.31). In younger patients the healing potential of a spondylolysis can be assessed using an isotope bone scan. An MRI scan is essential in any patient with neurological symptoms to identify the scope and severity of the nerve root compression.

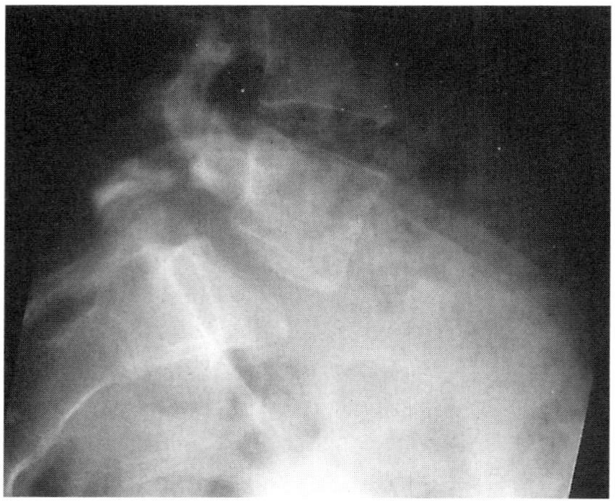

Fig. 46.30 Pars defect.

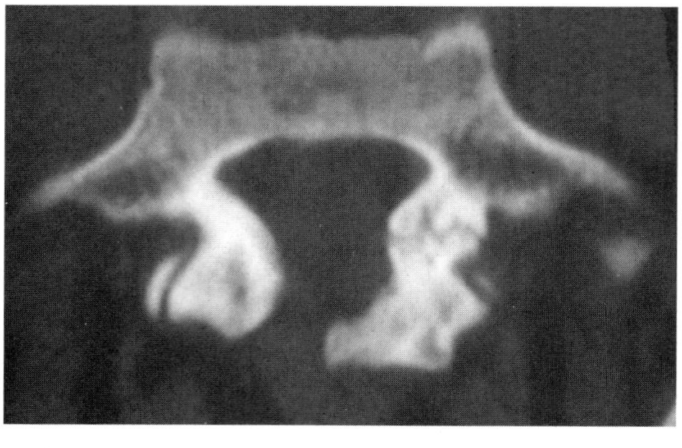

Fig. 46.31 Reverse gantry CT scan, showing bilateral pars defects.

Treatment

The majority of cases of spondylolysis settle spontaneously without subsequent symptoms even though there is little if any evidence of healing. In a child or young adult with a relatively short history and a hot isotope bone scan, the chances of spontaneous healing can be enhanced by the use of a semi-rigid thoracolumbar spinal orthosis (TLSO). This can be worn for up to three months but further use is ineffective. Patients with spondylosis can initially be followed by a cold bone scan because the majority become symptom-free without requiring any surgical intervention.

Some patients continue to have pain; if this is interfering with school or sporting activity the lysis can be repaired using a variety of techniques. A fifth lumbar to first sacral spinal fusion in situ is the appropriate treatment in children or adolescents presenting with an established spondylolisthesis who have significant hamstring spasm and back pain that does not settle with simple conservative measures. There is some controversy about the management of high grade spondylolisthesis and spondyloptosis. Although many specialist spinal units still consider performing reduction before spinal fusion, the risks of this procedure are generally considered to be too high and the benefits of reduction before fusion are unproven. Certainly neurological complications can be avoided by gentle reduction using either traction or an external fixator with the patient awake. Most surgeons opt for a fusion in situ; in a young patient with a high grade slip this can be achieved without the use of supplementary instrumentation. In adults the intervertebral discs should be assessed by MRI scanning and the treatment is identical to that described for mechanical low back pain. Reduction is rarely indicated in an adult patient.

INFLAMMATORY SPONDYLOARTHROPATHY

Rheumatoid disease of the neck

Pathology

Rheumatoid disease causes damage to both soft and bony tissues, and this is particularly prevalent in the neck (see Chapter 42). The disease progresses in different ways. In approximately a quarter of cases there are natural or drug-induced remissions. 5% however proceed rapidly to very profound disability. The remaining 70% lie some-where between these two extremes. Approximately 30% develop subluxation—10% at the atlanto-axial level and 20% at a lower cervical level. In two thirds of the cases with subluxation this occurs in the first 2 years of the disease. Subluxation is usually seen in female patients with progressive peripheral disease who have antibodies to rheumatoid factor and have previously received oral steroids.

Clinical features

The disease causes neck pain and myelopathy as the result of subluxation. The level of the neurological deficit does not always correlate well with the level of subluxation. In the presence of upward odontoid migration (cranial settling) the lower cranial nerves may be damaged, causing difficulty with swallowing. With both atlanto-axial and subaxial subluxation, both the upper and lower limbs may be affected. Affected patients may have weak clumsy hands and arms without evidence of a spastic paraparesis. A very varied clinical presentation is characteristic and is often difficult to assess because of the concurrent joint disease which delays diagnosis. It is important to exclude conditions such as the carpal tunnel syndrome which may be the real cause of symptoms; rheumatoid disease is diagnostically misleading.

Investigations

Patients who develop cervical subluxation should be followed up by regular annual clinical examinations and flexion/extension cervical radiographs. MRI is the investigation of choice (Fig. 46.32), and imaging in flexion and extension should be obtained at the first sign of any neurological abnormality. Some patients exhibit a more severe anatomical deformity on MRI in extension; if this is the case, it is important that the neck should not be fused in the extended position. Nerve conduction studies should be performed if there is any possibility of a peripheral nerve entrapment syndrome (see Chapter 44).

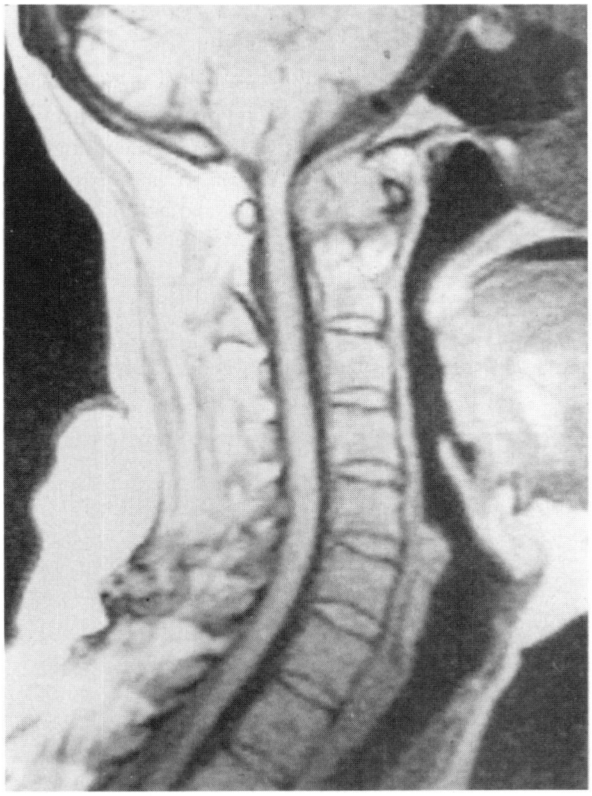

Fig. 46.32 MRI scan showing destruction of the odontoid peg, with pannus distorting the lower medulla.

Treatment

The indications for surgery in patients with cervical subluxation are pain which is not controlled by a collar and analgesia or progressive neurological deterioration. The aims of the operation are to decompress the cord and fuse the spine combined, if possible, with preoperative reduction. The odontoid peg can be removed by a transoral approach before or after posterior fusion.[21]

This is difficult spinal surgery, and there are frequently other medical considerations, requiring each case to be treated on its own merits. Surgery is complicated by the combination of reduced resistance to infection, poor wound healing and osteoporotic bones.

Results

In general, patients recover less well the longer the neurological deficit has been present, and it is therefore important to intervene as early as possible.[22] The symptoms of pain tend to improve more than the neurological signs. The extent of the disease and the dose of steroids affects the quality of the bone and soft tissues. There is sometimes a failure of fusion, or subsequent subluxations at other levels. There is some evidence that patients requiring anterior decompression do better if this procedure is carried out before the posterior fusion.

Ankylosing spondylitis

Pathology

Ankylosing spondylitis is a chronic inflammatory disease with a genetic predisposition and male preponderance (see Chapter 42). It involves the sacroiliac and spinal joints and also other musculoskeletal structures, the eyes and occasionally the heart. It is known to be associated with ulcerative colitis, psoriasis and Reiter's syndrome. The histocompatibility antigen HLA B27 is present in nearly all patients with this condition.

Clinical features

Young men in their thirties present with buttock and lower back pain. There is frequently some delay in making the diagnosis. The clinical features which lead to surgical referral are a fixed flexion deformity of the spine, trauma and root compression syndromes.

Treatment

Anti-inflammatory agents are combined with regular hydrotherapy during the inflammatory phase of the disease, and this often prevents the development of significant kyphotic deformity. If the fixed flexion deformity becomes very severe patients are only able to see a few yards in front of their own feet. The first option then

REFERENCES

21. Crockard H A et al J Bone Joint Surg 1986; 68B: 350
22. Evans D K J Bone Joint Surg 1987; 69B: 1

may be to perform bilateral total hip replacements because this overcomes or improves the associated hip ankylosis. In the occasional case a lumbar osteotomy can be performed and this may be combined with a spinal fusion. A cervical osteotomy is even less commonly required. There are frequently other coexistent medical conditions which predispose to complications and the benefits of surgical intervention need to be carefully weighed against the risks.

Patients whose spines have become ankylosed, the so-called 'bamboo spine' (Fig. 46.33), are at high risk of spinal injury. The spine tends to shatter and can break in more than one place. Compression by an extradural haematoma may also occur.[23] Less severe injuries can result in microfractures which cause severe pain. A spinal fusion procedure can be performed across these fractures but is not always successful in alleviating symptoms. Occasionally these patients present with spinal cord or nerve root compression at one level, which has been called 'the last mobile joint syndrome'. This condition is frequently difficult to treat surgically, requiring bony decompression of the nerve roots and fusion of the unstable vertebrae.

SPINAL TUMOURS

Extradural tumours

Pathology

The majority of these tumours are metastatic, usually from breast, bronchus, prostate or haemopoietic primary malignancies. Pain and symptoms of cord compression are the usual presenting features. Choosing the appropriate method of intervention depends on balancing the natural history of the malignant disease against the likely benefits of surgery. A histological diagnosis is of obvious importance if there is no known primary. Benign tumours such as neurofibromas can also develop in the extradural space. Primary malignant tumours of the spine are very rare.

Clinical features

Clinicians who treat low back pain are generally anxious about missing a patient who is harbouring a tumour. The history is often helpful. Typical patients are middle-aged or elderly, have a history of previous malignancy and describe non-mechanical low back pain (i.e. unrelated to physical activity). The pain is usually aggravated by recumbency and patients can occasionally present with a profound neurological deficit and little associated pain. Alternatively they may develop severe spinal pain with no neurological deficit. Early diagnosis is important as once neurological function has been lost it often does not return, even with adequate surgical treatment.

Investigations

Plain radiographs are frequently normal, especially in the early stages of the disease. Occasionally bony erosion, especially of the pedicles, or vertebral collapse is present with or without an adjacent soft tissue shadow. An isotope bone scan usually shows the tumour before it is visible on plain radiographs. MRI scanning is now the main investigation in these patients, as it shows both the site and nature of the spinal tumour (Fig. 46.34), as well as sometimes detecting other spinal metastases.

Treatment

The treatment of metastatic spinal tumours has changed radically, twice, in the last 20 years. It was convincingly shown that laminectomy alone is an inappropriate option, leading to neurological deterioration and spinal pain.[24] For this reason, in the 1980s the maxim of 'anterior surgery for anterior disease, and posterior surgery for

REFERENCES

23. Bohlman H H J Bone Joint Surg 1979; 61A: 1119
24. Findlay G F G J Neurol Neurosurg Psychiatr 1987; 50: 151

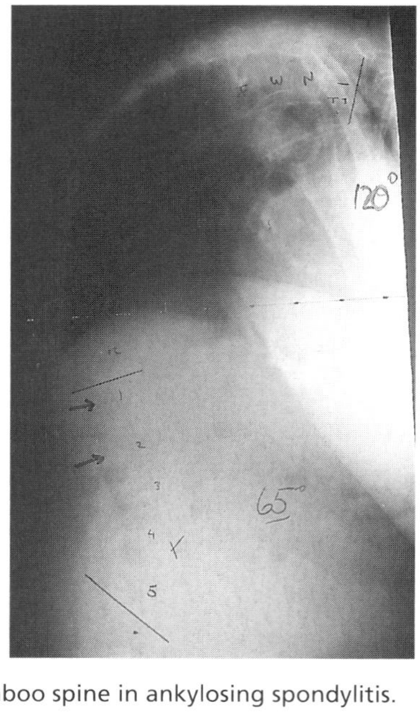

Fig. 46.33 Bamboo spine in ankylosing spondylitis.

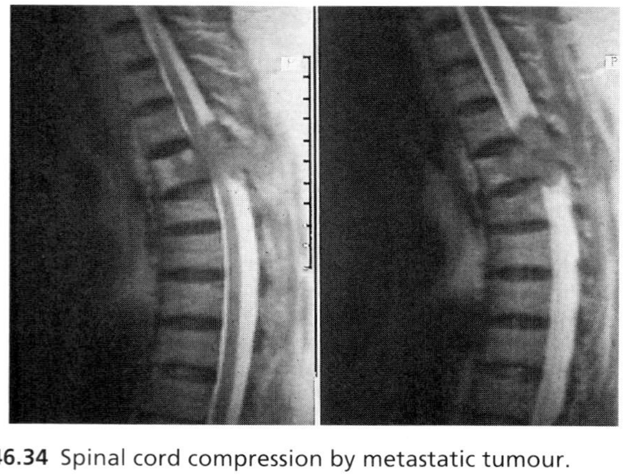

Fig. 46.34 Spinal cord compression by metastatic tumour.

posterior disease' applied, and excellent results were obtained in partial cord lesions. Many patients however were not deemed fit for trans-thoracic or trans-diaphragmatic surgery and were thus labelled 'inoperable'. The advent of pedicle screw fixation systems in the 1990s reversed this situation and many patients with anterior disease can now be decompressed and stabilized from behind.[25] In practice there are therefore four broad patient groups:

Metastatic spinal disease with no clinical or radiological neurological compression, and minimal or manageable axial pain. These patients do not require surgery and should be treated with radiotherapy, chemotherapy or hormone manipulation as appropriate.

Isolated spinal metastasis with a reasonable life expectancy and anterior partial cord compression. These patients should have the appropriate anterior decompression and spinal fixation.

Poor prognosis (survival estimated to be less than 1 year), anterior or posterior disease, and possibly widespread metastases, with a salvageable cord lesion. The best improvement is likely to be one MRC motor grade, but sphincter preservation may give the patient some dignity in terminal decline. These patients are treated by posterior decompression, which includes removing the anterior tumour around the dura, and stabilization with pedicle screw constructs. The anterior column can be supported with orthopaedic cement, inserted around the dura.

Inoperable because of a complete cord lesion of more than 24 hours or widely disseminated disease. Appropriate supportive therapy and palliative care are indicated.

Intradural tumours

Pathology

Intradural tumours are relatively rare. Most are benign and extramedullary, the majority being meningiomas or neurofibromas. Most intramedullary tumours are relatively benign: ependymoma and astrocytoma are the most frequently seen. Intradural tumours can be multiple, occurring as part of a systemic syndrome: von Recklinghausen (neurofibromas) and von Hippel–Lindau (haemangioblastomas) are two such syndromes. Any malignant tumour can metastasize via the cerebrospinal fluid pathways, resulting in multiple deposits which may or may not be associated with malignant meningitis.

Clinical features

These patients usually show progressive neurological deficits with little in the way of pain. On other occasions a disproportionate amount of pain, especially at night, is experienced with few signs. An intradural tumour should be considered in any young person presenting with symptoms of disc herniation.

Investigations

Plain radiographs may reveal scalloping of the vertebral body and pedicles or an enlarged intervertebral foramen. Myelography shows a characteristic pattern which can usually discriminate between intramedullary, extramedullary and extradural tumours (Fig. 46.35). Myelography is particularly helpful when combined with CT scanning, however MRI is now the best method of visualizing spinal cord tumours. Occasionally it is not possible to clarify the differential diagnoses of syringomyelia or multiple sclerosis even on MRI scan; cerebrospinal fluid protein immunoelectrophoresis as well as visual-evoked responses may be helpful in differentiating these conditions. The MRI scan shows flow voids in an arteriovenous malformation. When a vascular malformation is suspected spinal angiography is essential in planning the surgical approach.

Treatment

Extramedullary tumours are usually removed after laminectomy by gentle dissection using an operating microscope. Obviously care must be taken not to damage the cord either by devascularization or by excessive manipulation. Anteriorly placed lesions are the most difficult to resect, and either an anterior or transpedicular approach may be necessary.

Ependymomas are usually fairly large by the time of presentation and need to be carefully separated from functional nervous tissue. Subtotal resection is preferable to compromising the healthy adjacent cord; any residual tumour may be controlled by radiotherapy, which is indicated to prevent recurrence of ependymomas by cerebrospinal fluid seeding. Haemangioblastomas and astrocytomas present a difficult surgical challenge. The carbon dioxide laser and ultrasonic aspirator have revolutionized their resection, allowing a plane of cleavage to be developed with minimal manipulation of the cord.

A cystic cord lesion can be needled and aspirated. Occasionally cytology can be helpful in differentiating a benign cyst from a cystic tumour. Usually, if the cystic fluid conforms to cerebrospinal fluid in colour and protein content it can be assumed that it is benign.

REFERENCE

25. Jonsson B et al Eur Spine J 1996; 5: 36

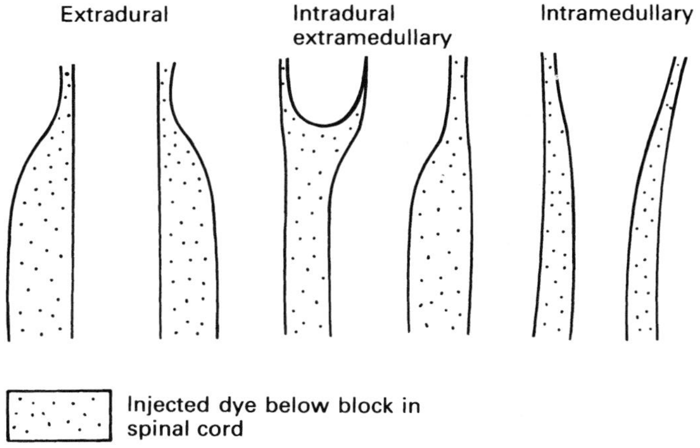

Fig. 46.35 Appearances of extradural, intradural and intramedullary tumours on myelography.

CONGENITAL DISORDERS OF THE SPINE

Introduction

Congenital disorders of the spine and cord can usefully be divided into primary neurological disorders and primary bony disorders. Primary neurological disorders present with a variable loss of neurological function. Primary bony disorders initially cause deformity which may progress to give secondary neurological problems.

Primary neurological disorders include:

1. Spina bifida.
2. Arnold–Chiari malformation/cerebellar ectasia.
3. Tethered cord/spinal dysraphism/diastematomyelia.

Congenital orthopaedic disorders include:

1. Scoliosis.
2. Kyphosis.

It is only by appreciating the embryological formation of the vertebral column that the modes of presentation and associated congenital anomalies can be fully understood.

Embryology

The neural tube (neural axis) and mesodermal segments (vertebral axis) form at an early stage of fetal development, starting in the first 2–3 weeks of gestation.[26] They are closely associated with the overlying ectoderm, forming skin, and the underlying endoderm, forming the intestine. Congenital disorders occur because of abnormal formation, differentiation, segmentation, separation or fusion of any or all of these elements. The concept of dysraphism was introduced by Fuchs in 1909[27] to emphasize that a congenital disorder may involve any number of these embryological components. Failure of fusion causes spina bifida. Failure of formation or separation of bone causes deformity such as scoliosis, and the same failure in the soft tissues causes abnormalities such as lipomyelomeningocele. Disordered formation causes diastematomyelia.

The bony deformity that occurs depends on the degree of disruption to the vertebral end-plates where growth occurs. The more these are disrupted or, more importantly, the greater the imbalance of the growth plates between each side (causing scoliosis), or front and back (causing kyphosis), the greater the deformity and therefore the greater the secondary neurological dysfunction. When soft tissue is involved the extent of the neurological damage depends on the degree to which the neural tube is involved in the dysraphic process.

During the clinical assessment it is important to remember that more than one congenital spinal disorder may be present and there may be other associated developmental defects. Associated anomalies include skin naevi, hairy patches, genitourinary abnormalities, congenital heart problems or Sprengel's shoulder.

Spina bifida

Pathology

Spina bifida is caused by a failure of fusion of the vertebral arches and possibly the underlying neural tube. Two subdivisions exist:

1. Spina bifida occulta (Fig. 46.36a), where the vertebral anomaly exists in isolation and causes no problems except a predisposition to back pain. There is a 5% incidence of other abnormalities.

2. Spina bifida manifesta (cystica). The incidence of 1 in 300 births is now decreasing as a consequence of antenatal monitoring by ultrasound and the measurement of serum α-fetoprotein levels. There may be a family history of the disorder and there are two types:

a. A meningocele, where the meninges herniate through the bony defect and are covered by skin of variable quality (Fig. 46.36b).

b. A myelomeningocele, where the roof of the defect is formed by exposed neural tissue (neural placode; Fig. 46.36c).

Hydrocephalus occurs in three quarters of the cases of myelomeningocele and 90% of those affected develop hydrocephalus by the fourth month of age. This may be the result of defective cerebrospinal fluid absorption in the lining of the hernial sac. Its onset often appears to coincide with the surgical correction of the defect.

Clinical features

Spina bifida cystica is obvious at birth. Assessment includes a record of the site of the defect; whether it is intact or ruptured, leaking cerebrospinal fluid; the degree of epithelialization and whether there is any visible neural tissue. A neurological examination of the structures below the defect should be carefully performed. Spontaneous leg movements, leg tone and deformity and the presence or absence of anal tone should all be carefully tested and noted. Contraction of the perineum may be seen when the baby cries. The anal dimple deepens as, on straining, the muscles lift the perineal floor, but if there is no contraction of the perineum the anus bulges and pouts during straining. The urinary stream should also be observed. The head should be examined for evidence of hydrocephalus such as a bulging fontanelle or excessive head circumference.

Treatment

A meningocele with good-quality skin over the defect may be treated conservatively. A meningocele with a more prominent sac can be excised at 3–6 months. Hydrocephalus must be excluded by follow-up, but is a very rare complication of this condition.

The correct management of myelomeningocele is fraught with problems, particularly if the lesion is not diagnosed before birth and the neurological deficit is severe. Increasingly effective antenatal screening (with abortion offered if indicated) has fortunately reduced the incidence of 'surprises' at birth, and an increasing knowledge of the natural history of the disease has clarified the surgical management. The enthusiasm for closing all defects in the

REFERENCES

26. Deacon P, Dickson R A In: Dickson R A (ed) Spinal Surgery. Butterworths, London 1990
27. Fuchs A Wien Med Wochenschr 1909; 59: 2142

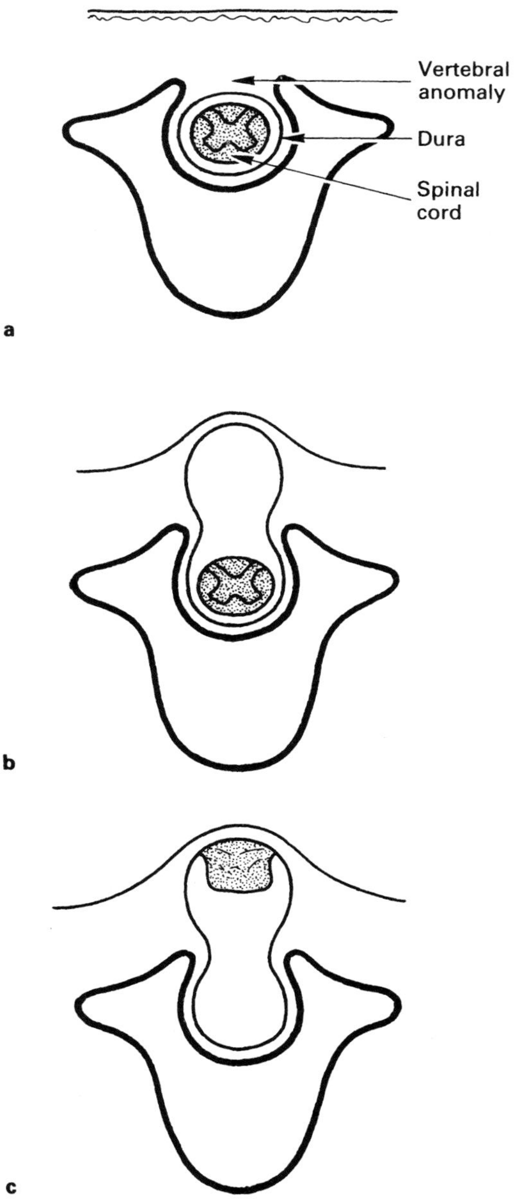

Fig. 46.36 (a) Spina bifida occulta; (b) meningocele; (c) myelomeningocele.

1960s and 1970s has now been replaced by more selective approach,[28,29] with the recognition that it was inappropriate to operate on children with a severe hydrocephalus, a large open defect, no distal neurological function or other abnormalities which meant that their quality of life would be intolerable. It is, however, still a problem that requires very careful, expert counselling.

The majority of these children die in their first year of life from hydrocephalus or an infection if closure is not attempted. With antibiotics, early surgical closure and shunts to prevent hydrocephalus, half the children who survive the first 24 hours will reach school, though a high percentage are intellectually handicapped.

If the defect is considered suitable for closure this should be performed as soon as possible to minimize the risk of cerebrospinal fluid leakage and subsequent meningitis. The aims of surgery are to replace the nervous tissue within the roof of the sac back into the canal, to preserve the cerebrospinal fluid absorption capacity by conserving the mucous membrane of the sac, and to cover the defect with fascia and skin.

After operation regular examination is required to detect and treat any hydrocephalus. The long-term problems, including skin, bone and joint deformity and the neuropathic bladder (see Chapter 37), often require extensive medical and social support for the patient and family.

Arnold–Chiari malformation

Pathology

This malformation, also named cerebellar ectopia, occurs when the medulla and cerebellar tonsils extend through the foramen magnum into the cervical spinal canal for a variable distance, causing pressure on the lower medulla. Hydrocephalus and impaired neurological function are common and there is a strong association with spina bifida, syringomyelia and other malformations.

Clinical features

The presentation is variable, because of its complex aetiology and many other associated congenital abnormalities. Hydrocephalus and cerebellar ataxia are common. Neck stiffness can occur when the tonsils impact in the foramen magnum.

Investigations

Plain radiographs show a small posterior fossa, but the condition is best demonstrated by MRI or cervical myelography with CT scanning.

Treatment

Management consists of decompressing the area by removal of the suboccipital bone, the rim of the foramen magnum and usually the posterior arch of the atlas to expose the cisterna magna. This is followed by duroplasty, and the tonsils can also be excised.

Cord tethering/spinal dysraphism

This is a group of disorders arising from abnormal embryological separation or formation of tissues; all are associated with a progressive neurological deficit as the result of cord tethering and traction or cord compression. More than one abnormality may be present, reflecting the complex embryological development of the spine. There is a very strong association with spina bifida.

REFERENCES

28. Lorber J Dev Med Child Neurol 1971; 13: 279
29. Findlay G F G In: Miller J D (ed) Northfield's Surgery of the Central Nervous System. Blackwell, Oxford 1987

Diastematomyelia[30,31]

In this condition there is an abnormal bony or cartilaginous spur projecting from the front to the back across the middle of the vertebral canal, dividing the dural tube and the spinal cord into two (Fig. 46.37). An associated bony deformity is common, for example failure of vertebral body formation causing scoliosis. Some 50–70% of patients also have a skin naevus, dimple or hairy patch. Symptoms develop during growth and children often present during the prepubertal growth spurt when the inferior aspect of the bony bar impedes the ascent of the dural tube and neural structures as the vertebral column grows faster than the neural column. Diastematomyelia has a female to male ratio of 5:2 and most commonly occurs in the thoracolumbar region. It presents with deformity of the spine, weakness of the legs, abnormal gait or urinary incontinence.

Enterogenous cyst

This is an epithelial cyst, arising from remnants of the neuroenteric canal which become invaginated into the neural tube, and it usually develops in an intramedullary position or ventral to the spinal cord. The epithelium characteristically stains for mucopolysaccharide and may contain hair elements. It causes symptoms of cord compression but these usually only develop in adult life. It is twice as common in men. The differential diagnosis includes epidermoid or dermoid cysts, arachnoid cysts, perineural cysts, or parasitic cysts.

Dermoid tumours

These tumours originating from the ectoderm usually occur in the lumbar region. They present at any age with symptoms of cord or cauda equina compression.

Lipomyelomeningocele[32,33]

This is a condition where bony canal deformities coexist with a subcutaneous lumbosacral lipoma, which may also contain other tissue elements. The lipoma communicates through a bony and dural defect with a tethered cord which is held in an abnormally low position. The lump is usually noticed because it is unsightly. There may be a progressive deterioration of neurological function with or without an associated structural deformity. By the age of 4 years children usually have some neurological dysfunction. It is twice as common in boys as in girls.

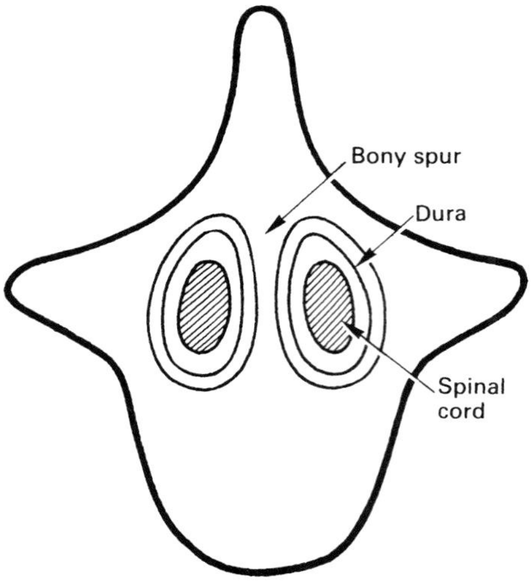

Fig. 46.37 Diastematomyelia.

Investigations

Diagnosis of these complex abnormalities often requires as much additional information as possible, therefore plain radiographs, CT myelography and MRI are all valuable in demonstrating the bony and soft tissue structures and the relation of the spinal cord to the abnormality. In older patients nerve conduction studies may also be used to assess the neurological function below the lesion.

Treatment

The management of dysraphism must be considered in the light of the natural history of the condition, the risks of operation and the reversibility of neurological problems.

The timing of surgery is still debated, the major consideration being whether surgery should be performed prophylactically or only after the development of neurological abnormalities. In the presence of multiple anomalies, careful consideration must be given to which defects should be corrected first.

Diastematomyelia. This does not always produce progressive neurological damage, and in the UK surgery is performed only on those children where this occurs. Surgeons in other countries do advocate prophylactic repair. The operation involves a posterior exposure to remove the bony spur and divide any associated tethering of the dura. Some surgeons open the dura at the site of the bony spur, inspect the cord and release it if necessary, closing the posterior defect with fascia.[34]

Enterogenous cysts. These usually present with neurological problems; this is regarded as an indication to decompress. Surgery is complicated and it is often difficult to remove the lining of the cyst which, if left, may lead to refilling. A laser is often useful for this.

Dermoid tumours. These also usually present with an established neurological problem which is therefore an indication for surgical removal. It may be impossible to remove all the associated fat.

Lipomyelomeningocele.[32,33] This is the most difficult spinal dysraphism to correct. Opinion is divided: some believe in performing early prophylactic surgery because they regard this condition as progressive and therefore argue that surgery should be performed before neurological defects arise; others feel that surgery should be delayed until neurological features have devel-

REFERENCES

30. Edelson J G J Bone Joint Surg 1987; 69B: 188
31. Hood R W et al J Bone Joint Surg 1980; 62A: 520
32. Hoffmann H J et al J Neurosurg 1985; 62: 1
33. Bakker-Niezen S H et al Z Kinderchir 1984; 39 (suppl 11): 100

oped, as not all children with lipomyelomeningocele will require operation. This latter view predominates in the UK and Europe. The surgical risk is often considerable: it is difficult to identify the intact neural elements, which are often abnormally positioned and embedded in abnormal lipomatous tissue. The thickened filum terminale must be identified and divided in order to release the tethered cord. There is also a significant risk of recurrent pyogenic meningitis in this condition because of the deficient dural lining. Complete removal is usually impossible and the more established the neurological disturbance, the less reversible this is with surgery. Operative excision should aim to prevent further deterioration, reverse any existing neurological abnormality and provide a good cosmetic repair. To prevent further deterioration and preserve function, the conus should be released from its tethering to the lipomatous tissue, thickened filum terminale should be divided and the dura should be closed with a fascial graft. Simple cosmesis is inadequate but it is not necessary to remove all the lipoma,[32] and attempts to do so can worsen the neurological deficit.

SPINAL INFECTION

Osteomyelitis

Pathology

In nearly half the cases there is a history of a urinary tract infection, recent pelvic or bowel surgery, cutaneous sepsis or diabetes. It is thought that haematogenous spread is via the vertebral venous plexus (Batson's plexus) to both the epidural space and the vertebral bodies (see Chapter 42). This can result either in osteomyelitis of the vertebral body or an epidural abscess. The most common organism is *Staphylococcus aureus*, though Gram-negative organisms are found in association with urinary tract infections and instrumentation.

Occasionally the intervertebral disc is the primary site of infection. This can either be spontaneous or, less often, follow disc surgery.

Clinical features

Typically, a diabetic patient who has had abdominal or pelvic surgery develops postoperative back pain, a limited range of spinal movement and lumbar muscle spasm. The pain may be worse in the recumbent position, and neurological examination is frequently normal unless vertebral collapse or an epidural abscess causes cord compression. Patients are invariably pyrexial.

Investigations

The erythrocyte sedimentation rate, C-reactive protein and white cell count are usually raised. These investigations are useful both for diagnosis and for monitoring treatment. Blood culture and needle aspiration (CT-directed) can avoid the need for open biopsy to obtain the causative organism. Radioisotope bone scanning is helpful in making an early diagnosis. MRI scanning is both sensitive and accurate in confirming the nature and site of the diagnosis.

Treatment

Usually the appropriate antibiotic and bed rest are all that is required. Occasionally surgery is necessary to obtain a causative organism or to decompress the spinal cord.

Epidural abscess

The pathological mechanism is very similar to that of pyogenic osteomyelitis, being haematogenous spread from the vertebral venous plexus. The most common site to be infected is the thoracolumbar junction, and the pus usually collects behind the dura. On rare occasions it is found anteriorly and is then usually associated with osteomyelitis of one of the vertebral bodies.

Clinical features

The patient is usually toxic. The initial symptoms are fever and severe back pain. This may be followed by a progressive neurological deficit caused by cord compression or ischaemia. The motor damage is usually more marked than the sensory loss. Frequently there is localized tenderness to percussion over the spinous processes at the relevant level. Upper motor neurone signs are usually present in the lower limbs with defective sphincter control. The neurological deficit becomes increasingly severe if the condition is not treated; once total loss of cord function has occurred this is unlikely to recover with surgical decompression. Early diagnosis is therefore vital.[35]

Investigations

Frequently a lumbar puncture has been attempted and results in a 'dry tap' (when no cerebrospinal fluid is drained). MRI scanning is now the most accurate method of confirming an epidural abscess.

Treatment

Urgent surgical decompression must be carried out. The prognosis depends on early diagnosis and treatment. A limited laminectomy or hemilaminectomy is sometimes sufficient as the pus can be washed out by saline injected through a catheter. More extensive bony decompressions are necessary if the abscess contents are solid. It is extremely important to give the correct antibiotics for an adequate period and catheters can be left in the epidural space for instillation of topical antibiotics.

Tuberculosis

Pathology

In spite of major improvements in its management, tuberculosis of the spine remains a problem even in Europe and North America

REFERENCES

34. Humphreys R P Clin Neurol 1982; 30: 436
35. Hulme A J, Dott N M Br Med J 1954; 1: 64

(see Chapter 42). In very deprived parts of Africa and India, children are mainly affected by spinal tuberculosis; as socioeconomic conditions improve, the age of its onset increases.

The vertebra most frequently affected is the first lumbar. The intervertebral disc is also often involved, which distinguishes tuberculosis from metastatic disease. Commonly a paraspinal abscess develops around the bony destruction. Over time the vertebra tends to collapse, forming a kyphosis; this can eventually cause spinal cord compression at the apex of the kyphosis (i.e. Pott's disease). In the absence of kyphosis the bony sequestrum or the cold abscess itself can cause pressure on the spinal cord, producing a neurological deficit.

Clinical features

Where tuberculosis is endemic the diagnosis is usually straightforward. In developed countries where it is less commonly encountered it may be misdiagnosed as an extradural tumour. Frequently patients present with low back pain and signs of systemic tuberculosis: night sweats, loss of weight and malaise (see Chapters 4 and 42). They may have local tenderness over the involved segment of the spine. A neurological deficit is uncommon, but when present usually consists of upper motor neurone signs in the legs. With progressive collapse of the vertebra and development of a kyphotic deformity this can progress to a profound spastic paraparesis.

Investigations

Chest radiography and spinal X-rays are usually helpful. Radiological confirmation of disc involvement is highly suggestive of tuberculosis as opposed to metastatic disease (Fig. 46.38). An isotope bone scan is also useful in identifying any infective process at an early stage. Myelography, especially if combined with CT scanning, is able to delineate both the bony deformity and the presence and extent of any cord compression. MRI scanning is effective at delineating the cord involvement. The organism must be identified and cultured. The erythrocyte sedimentation rate is useful in monitoring the response to treatment.

Treatment

Every patient with spinal tuberculosis must have microbiological confirmation of the diagnosis. It is not sufficient to culture tubercle bacillus from the sputum. A needle biopsy usually provides material for bacteriological diagnosis and diagnostic surgery is rarely required.

Extensive multicentre trials[36,37] have shown that it is advantageous to decompress and fuse the spine of patients with signs of spinal cord compression. The vast majority of patients however do not have a neurological deficit and, once diagnosed, can be treated successfully with chemotherapy. Occasionally it is sufficient merely to evacuate a cold abscess, and the results of radical debridement and grafting as opposed to debridement alone are not very different although there is a greater tendency for the patient treated by debridement to develop a kyphotic deformity.

There are various approaches to the radical operation. Some favour the anterior approach through a thoracotomy when the pus and bone is excised and the kyphosis is corrected and supported by a strut graft. An alternative is to use a transpedicular approach which avoids the need for a thoracotomy but makes grafting more difficult.

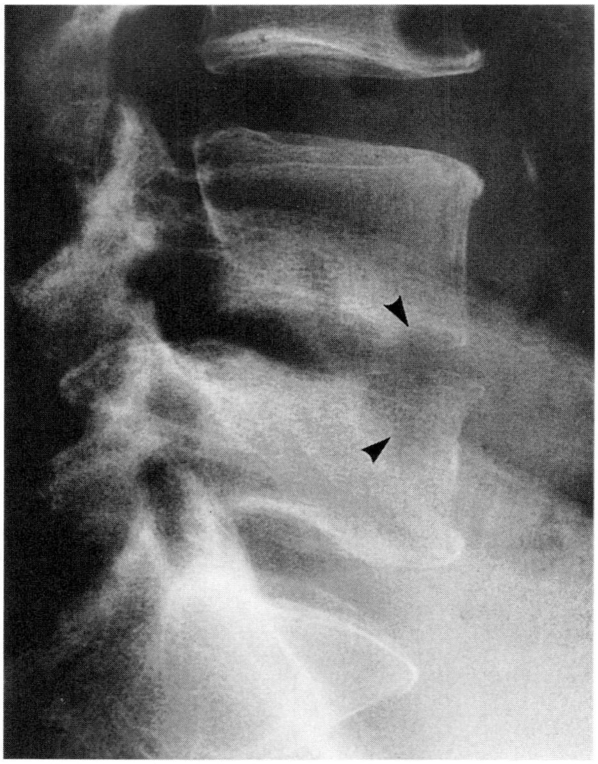

Fig. 46.38 An infective process involving the disc space and the vertebral bodies above and below (arrowed).

SYRINGOMYELIA

Pathology

A syrinx is a distended, fluid-filled cavity within the spinal cord. In the majority of patients with syringomyelia this is related to hindbrain pathology. Either cerebellar prolapse through the foramen magnum or arachnoiditis in this region results in an intermittent valve-like effect causing a partial block to cerebrospinal fluid flow between the head and the spine. This craniospinal pressure dissociation at the level of the foramen magnum is thought to result in the formation of the syrinx by dilation of the central canal of the spinal cord.[38] There is frequently a history of birth injury in the syringomyelia associated with cerebellar prolapse. There are several other causes of syringomyelia, which include trauma, infection and tumour.

REFERENCES

36. Medical Research Council working party on tuberculosis of the spine. J Bone Joint Surg 1982; 64: 393
37. Adendorff J J, Boeke E J, Lacarus C J R Col Surg Edinb 1987; 32: 152
38. Williams B, Page N Br J Neurosurg 1987; 1: 63

Clinical features

Hydrocephalus is frequently present in the hindbrain-related syringomyelia. Sometimes a cough or posturally related headache is reported. There is usually a loss of the spinothalamic sensation (suspended sensory loss) at the level of the syrinx caused by the close proximity of the crossing pathways to the central canal. The loss of pain and temperature sensation is known as dissociated sensory loss and is frequently associated with hyperaesthesia and pain in an asymmetrical distribution. This may be associated with an asymmetrical loss of power which can affect all four limbs depending on the level of the syrinx. The urinary sphincters may also be compromised. Neurological examination frequently reveals flaccid weakness rather than upper motor neurone signs. If the syrinx progresses upwards it can result in Horner's syndrome, facial pain in the trigeminal distribution and brainstem signs such as nystagmus and cerebellar ataxia (syringobulbia).

The other causes of a syrinx (including tumours) have an identical presentation. Where the syrinx is related to trauma, total or partial cord damage is usually followed by an ascending pattern of neurological dysfunction.

Treatment

The progression of the neurological deficit in hindbrain-related pathology associated with a hydrocephalus can frequently be arrested by shunting the ventricles. It is postulated that this is the result of a reduction in the craniospinal pressure gradient. The next logical step is to disable the valve mechanism resulting from the partial block at the level of the foramen magnum. This is done through a posterior fossa craniectomy combined with removal of the arch of the atlas and sometimes the cerebellar tonsils. The dura is left open or the cisterna magna rendered more capacious by the use of an artificial dural gusset. Should arachnoid adhesions be present these are carefully freed. Surgery may be needed on the syrinx itself but creation of a direct aperture into its cavity by myelotomy or syringosubarachnoid shunts has not proved particularly successful. At present syringopleural shunts are being employed with some success, particularly in post-traumatic syringomyelia.

The same principle of enlarging the dural envelope and freeing arachnoid adhesions in order to remove the partial block also applies in the distal cord. When a paraplegic patient has an ascending neurological deficit caused by a syrinx, the cord can be transected to allow free drainage and to prevent further neurological deterioration. Clearly, when a tumour is present this must be removed.

VASCULAR DISORDERS

Introduction

Vascular disorders of the spinal cord may present with haemorrhage (which may be intramedullary, subarachnoid or extradural) or cord malfunction as the result of compression or ischaemia. Subarachnoid haemorrhage in the spinal cord is rare and is most commonly caused by an arteriovenous malformation. It does occasionally arise from tumours, such as a haemangioblastoma.

Extradural haemorrhage causing compression of the cord also occurs. Often no cause is found, although the source is most likely to be an angioma, possibly associated with a vascular malformation of the cord or a vertebral haemangioma. Occasionally the underlying cause is a bleeding disorder such as polycythaemia or haemophilia, or anticoagulation therapy (see Chapter 3). Traumatic extradural haemorrhage is rare except in ankylosing spondylitis.

Arteriovenous malformation

Arteriovenous malformations rarely involve the spinal cord, having a ratio of incidence to cord tumours of 1:20. They present with acute or progressive cord malfunction. Their management has been dramatically improved since better imaging techniques have been available—the most recent example of which is digital subtraction angiography—and the introduction of microsurgery and laser treatment.

Pathology

Arteriovenous malformations may arise from the posterior or anterior spinal circulation. From the posterior circulation there may be an extradural fistula, often adjacent to a nerve root, and a single vessel extending intradurally into draining veins. Intradural juxtamedullary posterior arteriovenous malformations also occur which are more closely applied to the cord, but still separated from it by a layer of glial tissue. An intramedullary arteriovenous malformation can develop from feeding vessels emerging from the anterior circulation and passing through the substance of the cord. These are most common in the cervical region. These three different types of malformation are believed to differ in their aetiology, clinical presentation and response to treatment.[39] The proposed mechanisms for cord malfunction include elevated spinal venous pressure (when the fistula is extradural),[40] a steal effect, or cord compression from direct pressure from the malformation and rarely as the result of a haematoma or thrombosis.

Clinical features

Arteriovenous malformations can occur at any age, and the presentation depends on the site and type of the anomaly. Some 10–15% present acutely with subarachnoid haemorrhage, causing pain over the spine, often with an associated radicular pattern, and other signs of meningism. Subarachnoid haemorrhage implies that there is an intramedullary component to the arteriovenous malformation. An intramedullary haematoma or haematomyelia is rare and causes compression. In all, 85–90% of patients present with a progressive cord deficit. The clinical features depend on the site of

REFERENCES

39. Rosenblum B et al J Neurosurg 1987; 67: 795
40. Oldfield E H et al J Neurosurg 1983; 59: 1019

the haemangioma which is most commonly (60%) in the thoracolumbosacral region.

A partial cord deficit may develop acutely and then recover incompletely, or recurrent deficits may occur with the same clinical features, implying the same site of origin (thereby differentiating this condition from demyelination). Eventually a spastic paraplegia develops with sphincter disturbance. There may be an associated vascular naevus, but this is not necessarily related to the relevant dermatome; in rare cases a bruit is heard over the vertebral column.

Investigations

Plain radiographs usually show no abnormality, though there may be some bony erosion if there is a particularly large feeding vessel or evidence of an associated haemangioma of the vertebral body. Cerebrospinal fluid analysis shows an elevated protein, with blood and xanthochromia if there has been a subarachnoid haemorrhage.

The investigation of choice is again an MRI scan. This demonstrates the arteriovenous malformation, any related cord changes and the site of any haematoma or haematomyelia; it may even show the distended feeding vessels. The relationship of the anomaly to the dura can also be seen. High-dose contrast myelography/CT scanning and isotope scans can be obtained if MRI is not available. Myelography shows the abnormality in over 90% of cases. Once the diagnosis has been confirmed, spinal angiography is required to identify the feeding vessel (which is often single).

Treatment

The management of arteriovenous malformations is now much more successful since it has been recognized that these lesions can be surgically removed rather than simply performing a spinal canal decompression. Laminectomy alone is ineffective although any intra- or extramedullary haematoma can be drained. Once identified, an extradural feeding vessel adjacent to a nerve root can be ligated with good symptomatic relief without the need for more extensive surgery.[40] A large posterior intradural retromedullary component can be removed as it usually invaginates the cord rather than penetrating it. True intramedullary arteriovenous malformations supplied from the anterior circulation are more difficult to remove completely.

Therapeutic embolization is now an alternative treatment; it is most appropriate for arteriovenous malformations of the posterior circulation when a single feeding vessel can be identified. Unless all the feeding vessels of an arterio-venous malformation can be embolized, it will recur. Radiotherapy is not effective.

Results

Cord function recovers to a variable degree. The arteriovenous malformation may recur if not removed completely, and syringomyelia is a possible long-term complication.

Vertebral haemangioma

Pathology

This is a common condition, found in up to 10% of spines at post-mortem.[41] It is a hamartomatous malformation which grows at the same rate as the surrounding tissues and rarely causes symptoms. There may be more than one haemangioma involving an adjacent or unrelated vertebral body. Haemangiomas may also be present in the soft tissues of the liver, spleen or skin. Symptoms may be the result of bony enlargement of the vertebral body, pedicles and laminae, causing spinal canal stenosis, cord compression from spread of the cavernous angioma into the extradural space, extradural haemorrhage or spinal ischaemia. Vertebral collapse is rare.

Clinical features

Patients usually give a history of chronic spinal or root pain. Cord compression may present with acute paraplegia or quadriplegia, or a slowly progressive painless spastic paresis. It is now recognized that haemangiomas often enlarge in pregnancy, causing symptoms which resolve after delivery.[42,43] Symptoms recur with subsequent pregnancies.

Investigations

The haemangioma has a characteristic appearance on plain radiographs (Fig. 46.39) with a vertebral body that has lost height but increased in width both sagittally and coronally. The haemangioma appears more radiolucent with coarse vertical trabeculation. Angiography can identify the supplying vessel.

Management[44]

The priority of management is the protection and preservation of cord function. Decompression by laminectomy was often found to be inadequate and associated with a high mortality from bleeding which could not be controlled. Anterior decompression is possible but attention must be paid to blood loss and large transfusions may be necessary. Preoperative embolization has been used to reduce haemorrhage.

Radiotherapy is also an effective treatment for a haemangioma causing chronic symptoms, or following surgery, but it may exacerbate acute compression by increasing swelling.[45]

NEUROSURGERY FOR PAIN

The over-riding principle in treating chronic pain should be to avoid, as far as possible, causing possible permanent damage to the nervous system. Recent advances in pain management have meant that the majority of patients can be controlled by careful prescribing of drugs, injections and transcutaneous nerve stimulation (see Chapter 5). Certain surgical procedures can however be useful in particular circumstances (Fig. 46.40).

REFERENCES

41. Schmorl G, Junghanns H Die gesund und kranke Wirbelsaule im Roentgenbild. Thieme, Leipzig 1932
42. Guthkelch A N J Neurol Neurosurg Psychiatr 1948; 11: 199
43. Hopkins A Clin Obstet Gynaecol 1977; 4: 426
44. Eisenstein S et al Spine 1986; 11: 640

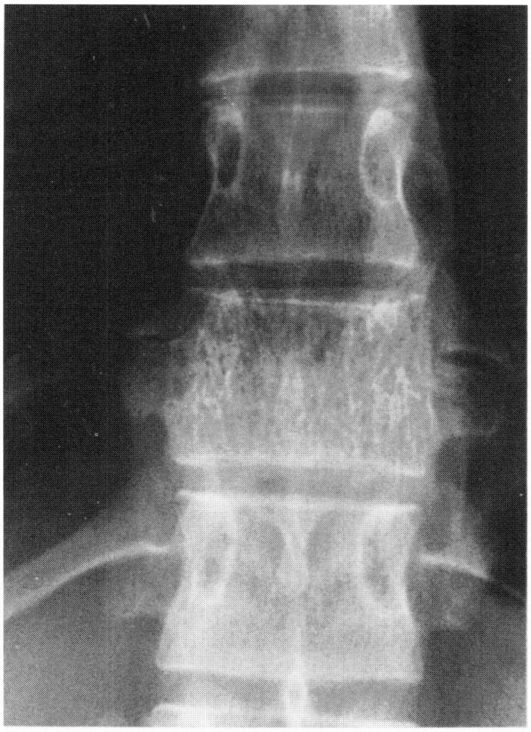

Fig. 46.39 A vertebral haemangioma.

Epidural stimulation

In patients whose pain is of a deafferentation type (usually burning in character), and particularly those who respond to transcutaneous nerve stimulation, a good response may be obtained by stimulating in the epidural space. Electrodes are introduced, either transcutaneously through a Tuohy needle or preferably by laminotomy (when they can be sutured to the dura in the midline to avoid movement), and connected either to a subcutaneous receiver unit or to a totally internalized stimulator block. Even with careful selection little more than half of the patients achieve long-term benefit. Stimulation, however, is always preferable to ablation.

Posterior rhizotomy

Section of the posterior roots can abolish pain that has a definite peripheral aetiology. The segmental musculature will, however, become useless and therefore this technique is only usually applicable in the thoracic region, when it is sometimes helpful for post-herpetic neuralgia. Occasionally root section actually causes a deafferentation pain.

Dorsal root entry zone lesion

An important recent advance in the management of pain has been the deliberate ablation of the substantia gelatinosa of Rolando, either by controlled radiofrequency heat or a carbon dioxide laser. Deafferentation pain syndromes may arise at this level as a consequence of dendritic reinnervation. The therapeutic destruction, produced by a specially designed electrode, therefore needs to extend for at least two or three segments above and below the site of pain genesis. The fibres participating in the somatic reflex arc are not damaged which prevents the unwanted effect of muscular weakness.

Anterolateral cordotomy

From their origin in the substantia gelatinosa, the neurones of the spinothalamic tract cross the midline and ascend in the anterior columns. In open cordotomy a cut about 4–5 mm deep is made into the anterior column on the side opposite to the pain and some considerable distance above. Percutaneous cordotomy can be carried out at the first or second cervical level by inserting a special needle electrode laterally which is manipulated under radiographic screening and physiological stimulation into the anterior quadrant of the cord where a radiofrequency lesion is made. Bilateral cordotomy is likely to cause bladder paralysis, and bilateral cordotomy in the cervical region may interfere with respiration.

REFERENCE

45. Nguyen J P et al Surg Neurol 1987; 27: 391

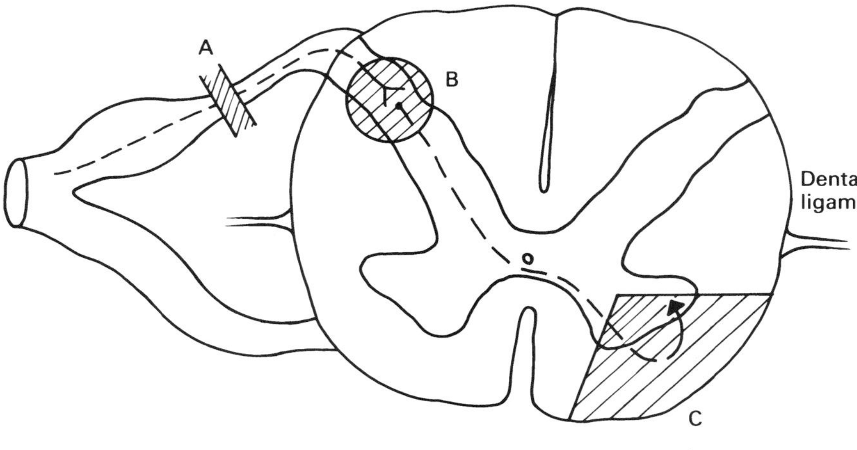

Fig. 46.40 Spinal lesions for relief of pain. A = posterior rhizotomy; B = dorsal root entry zone lesion; C = anterolateral cordotomy.

47 The hip and pelvis

David Nunn

Clinical features of hip disease

History

The two most important features in the history are pain and loss of function. Pain arising from the hip joint is felt in the buttock, groin, anteromedial thigh and knee. As with taking a history of any pain it is essential to enquire about the nature, site, severity, duration and frequency, exacerbating and relieving factors and analgesic usage. Continuous pain, and pain which disturbs sleep suggests end-stage osteoarthritis, inflammation, infection or malignancy.

Loss of function in the child is usually expressed in terms of ability to walk and run or a history of limping. In the adult it is necessary to ask about walking distance, ability to climb stairs, to use a bath and to reach the feet; these give some indication about the disability of the patient, and must be considered in the context of age and functional requirements.

The full medical history must be taken. It is essential to assess general health, especially in the elderly patient as surgery in these individuals is a major undertaking and the benefits must be carefully weighed against the risks. Hip disease affects the quality of life, and the treatment must not place undue risk on the quality or quantity of that life. Elderly patients with severe hip disease often have concurrent cardiovascular and respiratory ailments, making them high risk for surgical treatment. Children with one congenital disorder often have others which may only be discovered when they present with an obvious orthopaedic problem; a full paediatric history including gestation, delivery and subsequent development is required.

Examination

The simple but elegant system of Apley[1] is recommended. The patient must be examined lying down, and standing and walking must be observed.

Look

1. Skin—scars, bruises, swellings, ulcers, varicosities, etc. Bear in mind that the hip is deeply placed and any obvious swelling is unlikely to be arising from the joint. Evidence of venous disease may warrant extra precautions if surgery is planned.
2. Muscle wasting. If the hip is very painful, there will be generalized disuse atrophy of the leg muscles. The main flexor of the hip is ilio-psoas which is not visible; the abductors are usually covered by a generous layer of adipose tissue.
3. Posture. The hip adopts a characteristic position if diseased; a contracture develops with the hip flexed, adducted and externally rotated. Only the latter may be obvious on inspection, since it is possible to compensate for fixed flexion and adduction with the spine and pelvis (q.v.). There may be other obvious deformities in the limb.
4. Apparent leg length discrepancy. Any observed discrepancy cannot be confirmed until the bony landmarks have been palpated.

Feel

1. Bony landmarks. The anterior superior iliac spines (ASIS) are almost invariably easy to palpate, and the line drawn between them indicates the relationship between the pelvis and the legs. If possible the patient should lie with the spine/trunk and the legs at right angles to this line. The greater trochanter is often indistinct but should be palpated as there may be evidence of bursitis.
2. Measurement of leg lengths. The legs should be measured from the ASIS to the medial malleolus. This is the true leg length—or as near as is clinically possible. The apparent length from a fixed midline structure, e.g. xiphisternum to the malleolus, is useful if there is a postural deformity. If there is a true difference the knees should be flexed and the heels placed together. The levels of the knees are then inspected: when observed from the side, if one knee is lower than the other then the shortening is in the femur; when observed from the feet, the lower knee indicates shortening in the tibia. A further refinement is possible if the greater trochanters are easily palpable—a reduction in the distance from the trochanter to the ASIS indicates that the discrepancy lies at the level of the femoral neck.
3. Areas of tenderness. N.B. The hip joint itself is *not* palpable. To attempt to palpate the hip joint is not only a waste of time but is also extremely uncomfortable to the patient, and no useful information can thus be obtained.
4. The peripheral pulses. Significant arterial disease should normally be corrected before orthopaedic surgery on the lower limb.

REFERENCE

1. Apley A G, Solomon L Apley's System of Orthopaedics and Fractures. Butterworth–Heinemann, Oxford 1993

Move

The purpose here is to determine whether there are any contractures or fixed deformities around the hip and to demonstrate the range of movement.

The hip tends to take up a characteristic position whatever the underlying pathology. If there is a swelling or effusion within the joint, the hip capsule is at its most capacious in flexion, adduction and external rotation. If it is habitually held in this position and especially if there is an associated inflammatory response the capsular ligaments will thicken and fibrose in this position. The femoral head itself may be deformed during development or with disease: this will also limit the range of motion, and it may be possible clinically to anticipate the radiographic findings.

When examining for fixed deformities and range of motion, it is vital to know the position and relative motion of the pelvis and lumbar spine, since significant limita-tions of hip movement may be compensated for by these structures.

1. Fixed flexion. This is demonstrated by Thomas' test. The patient is supine, a hand is placed under the lumbar lordosis, and the opposite hip is flexed until the spine is flat on the hand. If the hip under examination rises off the couch, the angle the thigh describes with the couch is the degree of fixed deformity. The index hip can then be further flexed to demonstrate its range.
2. Fixed adduction. It should be possible to arrange the legs such that they are at right angles to a line drawn between the anterior superior iliac spines. If there is fixed adduction it will not be possible to achieve this position. The range of abduction/adduction is determined by moving the leg in these directions while placing a hand on the opposite iliac crest. When movement in this is detected, the hip has described its full range. In children, Gauvain's sign is useful: if the hip is genuinely painful during abduction, the opposite external oblique contracts.
3. Rotation. In the neutral position, the patella should be directed upwards. If there is a fixed external deformity it will face laterally, and the hip cannot be internally rotated. The rotation should be examined in neutral extension and at 90° of flexion.

The patient should then be observed walking, and any obvious gait abnormality described. The commonest of these are the Trendelenburg, the antalgic and the short leg gait.

The Trendelenburg test indicates the efficiency of the lever and motor system of the hip. When the patient stands on one leg, the abductors contract to tilt the pelvis up on the opposite side. This brings the centre of gravity of the upper body over the weight bearing foot. If the fulcrum (the hip) is stiff, in fixed adduction or very painful, the abductors cannot function and the only way equilibrium can be maintained is by swinging the upper body over the weight bearing foot. The same effect occurs if the abductors are weak or paralysed. This produces the characteristic lurching gait when walking.

'Antalgic' means pain avoiding; as little time as possible is spent weight bearing on the affected side during the gait cycle. The short leg gait is self explanatory. Patients may demonstrate a combination of any or all these patterns.

Investigations

In the majority of patients no more than simple radiography is required. An anteroposterior pelvis and laterals of the hips are all that is needed (Fig. 47.1). Only occasionally are CT or MRI scans necessary (Figs 47.2 and 47.3). 3D reconstructions can be useful in the planning of major osteotomies of the pelvis or the surgery of pelvic fractures.

Radionuclide scans are indicated in the investigation of possible infections and, very occasionally, of painful replacements.

Blood investigations are not necessary except where infection or inflammation are suspected, when the erythrocyte sedimentation rate is the singularly most useful test. In Afro-Caribbean patients with hip pain the sickle test should be requested. Biochemical and immunological tests may be indicated if metabolic or rheumatoid diagnoses are entertained.

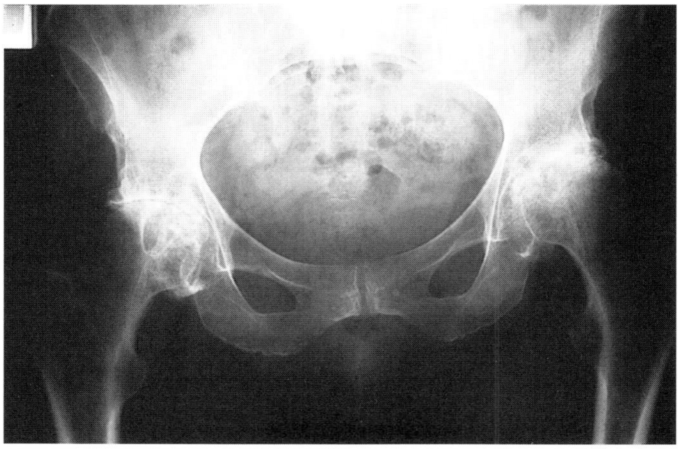

Fig 47.1 Anteroposterior radiograph of the pelvis showing severe osteoarthritis and gross cystic change.

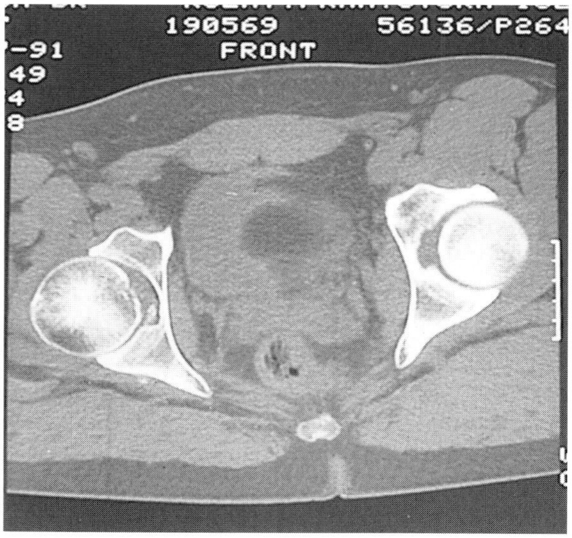

Fig 47.2 CT scan of the hips. The right hip is osteoporotic and there is a loose body in the acetabulum. Diagnosis: synovial osteochondromatosis.

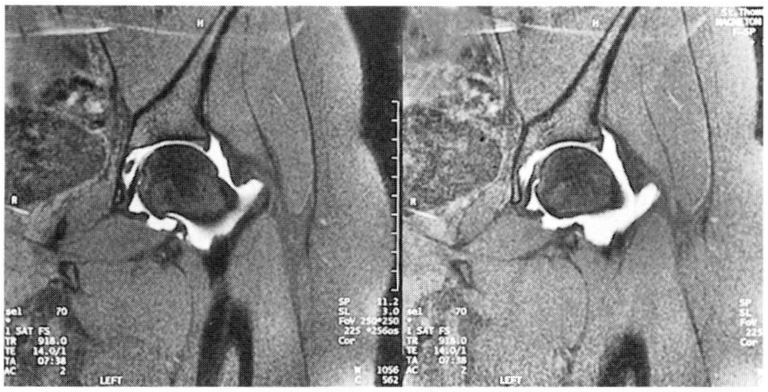

Fig 47.3 MRI arthrogram. There is a tear of the acetabular labrum inferiorly.

THE HIP IN CHILDHOOD

Hip disorders in childhood are a source of much anxiety to both the surgeon and the parents. The conditions to be described can seriously interfere with the development of the joint and the surrounding bones, may demand more than one surgical intervention and prolonged follow-up, and frequently lead to accelerated degeneration in early adulthood. Early detection and prompt treatment is essential to minimize these risks.

Developmental disease of the hip (DDH)

This was formerly called congenital dislocation of the hip (CDH), but the nomenclature has recently changed because it is possible that the dislocation is not present at birth but occurs in the neonatal period. The new term includes those patients whose hips are dysplastic rather than frankly dislocated. Dislocation at birth is found in 1:10 000 births, but the incidence of developmental disease of the hip is certainly much more common. It occurs more often in females than males (3:1).

Prenatal factors are:

1. First-born infants.
2. Those with a first degree relative affected.
3. Breech presentation, especially extended breech.
4. The presence of oligohydramnios.

Postnatal associations with race and ethnic traditions are probably caused by the manner in which the infant is nursed and carried. The incidence is higher in those groups who swaddle their children with the legs extended, and lower in those who carry babies with the hips flexed and abducted.

Diagnosis

All children should be examined by an experienced individual in the neonatal period. The child is first inspected for any evidence of asymmetry, particularly of the thigh skin creases. Leg lengths are very difficult to estimate in neonates, and in any case may not be unequal because there is bilateral dislocation, or because while the hip is dislocated the femoral head may still be at the level of the acetabulum. Abduction in flexion is usually 90° in the neonate, and asymmetrical abduction is strong evidence for dislocation. The standard tests for dislocation and/or instability are the Barlow and the Ortolani tests. In both tests the infant's legs are flexed and abducted with the upper thighs held between thumb and middle finger. In the Barlow test the greater trochanter is pushed forwards by the finger, and, if positive, a sensation of the hip dislocating is felt. In the Ortolani test the dislocated hip is pushed back into the acetabulum with the sensation of a clunk with reduction. Clicks palpated during the tests are not usually caused by hip instability, and the neonatal knee often clicks, but any suspicion of hip instability must be taken seriously.

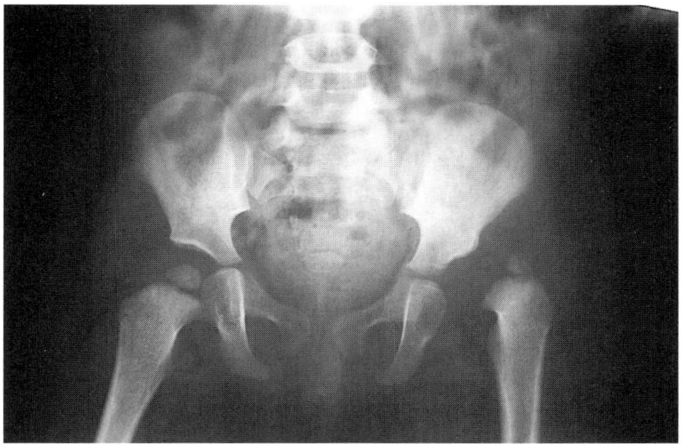

Fig 47.4 Dislocation of the left hip in a child aged 18 months.

Investigation

Plain radiology is of limited value in the diagnosis of dislocation in the neonate. The capital femoral epiphysis does not begin to ossify until six months in the normal hip, and this is delayed in the dislocated joint; furthermore, much of the acetabulum is still in cartilage at birth (Fig. 47.4). Many lines have been described which can be drawn on radiographs to determine whether dislocation is present, but these techniques have largely been superseded by ultrasound.[2] All infants at high risk should have their hips imaged by ultrasound, and all suspicious hips should probably be so investigated. The place of arthrography will be discussed later.

Management

Hips which merely click can be managed by the use of double nappies or a simple abduction brace; subsequent examination at about a month is usually normal and the brace can be abandoned.

Definitely unstable but reducible hips should be treated in some form of appliance which maintains flexion and abduction. These appliances must be used with great care and attention to detail. Too much abduction can apply too great a force on the capital epiphysis, leading to deformity of the femoral head and a condition

REFERENCE

2. Clarke N M P et al JBJS 1985; 67B: 406

similar to Perthes' disease (q.v.). It is also important to allow the child some degree of movement at the hip—articular cartilage needs to be moved for its healthy nutrition and development. The appliance which most closely fits these requirements is the Pavlik harness.[3] Failure of compliance on the part of the parents is not unknown in this situation and it may be necessary to see the child very frequently during the period while it is in the brace both to check the position and to encourage the parents. How long the bracing continues is more a matter of personal opinion than scientifically based fact. More important than the exact period is that the child is reviewed during development until both surgeon and parents are convinced the hip is growing normally. This may be until skeletal maturity is achieved (approximately 14 years in females, 17 in males).

Much more difficult is the child whose hip is irreducibly dislocated at birth. Certainly the hip must not be forcibly reduced. The management is traditionally deferred until the child is about one year old, because if open reduction is required it is technically easier in an older, bigger child. Evidence from other branches of surgery, e.g. plastic repair of cleft palate, suggests that early surgery might result in a better outcome. Closed reduction is usually attempted using some form of traction.[4] Areas of contention at this stage in management arise as a result of the incidence of complications such as avascular necrosis[5] following traction reduction, and of recurrent dislocation. One protocol is as follows:

1. The child's legs are placed on fixed traction in an abduction hoop, and the legs are gradually abducted over a period of two to three weeks until full abduction is achieved. The child is examined every day to ensure that the adductor tendons are not too tight indicating excessive force on the hip. Adductor tenotomy may be necessary to diminish this force.
2. When full abduction has been attained, the hips are examined under anaesthetic with or without an arthrogram. If concentric reduction has been achieved, i.e. the femoral head is within the acetabulum with an even joint space around its circumference, the legs are immobilized in the position of reduction in a hip spica; because of excessive femoral neck anteversion this may necessitate extreme positions of the legs, and a femoral derotation osteotomy may be necessary.[6]
3. If the hip is not concentrically reduced, an arthrogram is performed. This may show that the femoral head is standing off the acetabulum; it will also indicate if there is soft tissue obstructing reduction. In this case, or if the femoral head remains above the acetabulum, open reduction is necessary.
4. Open reduction may be accompanied by innominate osteotomy,[7] acetabuloplasty[8] or femoral derotation osteotomy. Alternatively these procedures may be performed at a later date.
5. Repeated surgical assaults are associated with a poorer result. It needs to be considered that dislocation of the hip will not prevent the child from walking, and although it will limp, it will not be in pain during childhood and may well enjoy full normal activities. Failure of surgical treatment may leave the child with a stiff painful joint.
6. Late presentation does still occur and the management decisions are much more difficult. Bilateral dislocation can be missed clinically, and the possibility of making a symmetrical child asymmetrical by treatment must be considered. In general the younger the child the greater the chance of a good result; the author would be reluctant to advise treatment over the age of 4. Worthy of consideration are the long-term results of a carefully treated group of patients meticulously followed up in Oxford—despite excellent reduction and function in adolescence and early adulthood, 44% had radiographic evidence of degenerative changes by the fourth decade (Fig. 47.5).[9]

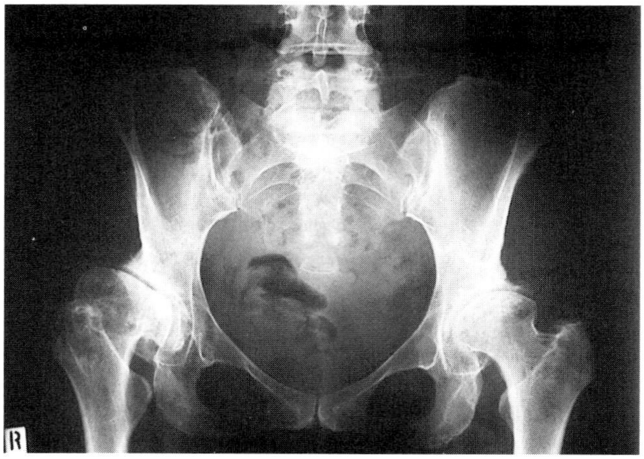

Fig 47.5 Bilateral developmental disease of the hip diagnosed at 15 months, treated by closed manipulation and splintage. Severe pain and stiffness at age 50.

Perthes' disease

Prior to 1910 this disorder was known as pseudo-coxalgia, to distinguish it from the then prevalent 'coxalgia' or tuberculous infection of the hip. It was described by Perthes, Legg and Calvé, and sometimes is known as Legg–Calvé–Perthes disease.

The classic clinical presentation is that of a male child between about 5 and 10 years of age with a limp, with or without pain in the hip. Males are affected at least three times more often than females. The disorder is bilateral in up to 20% of patients and has a familial association in around 10% of cases.

Radiologically there is sclerosis, irregularity and fragmentation of the capital epiphysis, secondary to a loss of the blood supply to that bone (Fig. 47.6). It is not known how the bone becomes avascular and the effect is extremely difficult to reproduce in experimental animals. The effect is also completely different to the consequences of avascular necrosis of the hip in adults. One rather incomplete hypothesis of the aetiology is as follows. The capital

REFERENCES

3. Grill F et al J Pediat Orthop 1988; 8: 1
4. Fish D N, Herzenberg J E, Hensinger R N J Pediat Orthop 1991; 11: 149
5. Kalamchi A, MacEwen G D JBJS 1980; 62A: 876
6. Somerville E JBJS 1953; 35B: 363
7. Salter R B, Dubos J P Clin Orthop 1974; 98: 72
8. Pemberton P B JBJS 1965; 47A: 65
9. Gibson P H, Benson M K D JBJS 1982; 64B: 169

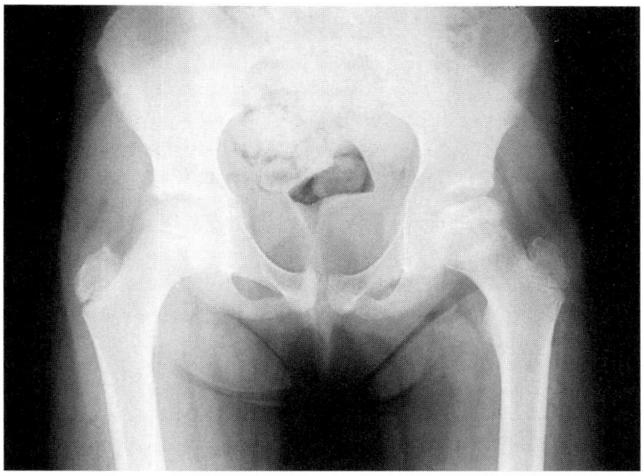

Fig 47.6 Perthes' disease in a female aged 8. There is whole head involvement and severe metaphyseal reaction.

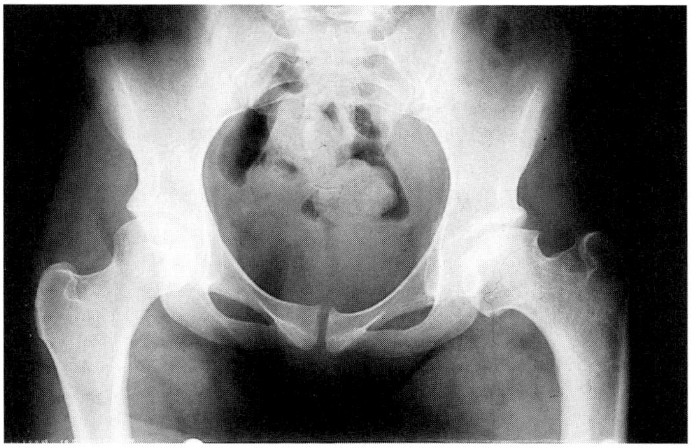

Fig 47.7 The same case as Fig. 47.6. A varus osteotomy at age 8 did not prevent degeneration of the hip with severe pain at age 21.

epiphysis is dependent upon the retinacular vessels in the joint capsule. If the capsule becomes distended due to effusion, synovitis or haemarthrosis, these vessels become occluded leading to death of the trabecular bone. The trabeculae collapse, leading to deformation of the femoral head. The severity of the disorder depends in large part on how much of the head is involved. The cartilage part of the head survives as it receives its nutrients from the synovial fluid, and indeed it can appear to enlarge. Further consequences are the fragmentation of the head, lateral subluxation of the hip, horizontal alignment of the growth plate and metaphyseal changes. All these result in alteration of the shape of the acetabulum with continued growth. The natural history of the disease is a gradual revascularization of the epiphysis, and usually continued growth. The prognosis then depends on the severity of the deformity of the femoral head. The child may be left with a short leg, with loss of internal rotation and a Trendelenburg gait. When adulthood is reached, rapid osteoarthritic change takes place with symptoms beginning to appear in the third decade (Fig. 47.7).

Management

The duty of the orthopaedic surgeon is to make the diagnosis, to attempt to classify the severity of the disorder for prognostic purposes, to carefully observe the child until resolution has been completed, and to intervene only in those cases where it is clear that the prognosis is going to be extremely bad, usually when there is whole head involvement, lateral fragmentation of the epiphysis and subluxation of the hip.[10] Premature growth arrest can occur.

The best prognostic factor is the age at onset—the younger the child the better the outcome.

Conservative treatment

Many children with this disorder do not need active treatment. It should be sufficient to explain it to the parents and then to keep the child under frequent review. Those children who present acutely with pain usually settle rapidly with bed rest (usually enforced by skin traction) and analgesia. The persistence of a limp is not in itself an indication for interference, but some surgeons treat the child with some form of brace.[11,12] One very serious misconception is that keeping the foot off the ground by whatever means reduces the load on the hip. If the child holds its foot up, the load on the hip is at least the weight of the leg, and this is magnified if the leg is flexed or extended. Secondly, keeping the joint still deprives the articular cartilage of its means of nutrition.

Surgical management

The principle of treatment is to ensure that the femoral head remains in the acetabulum in the hope that, when it does revascularize, it will remodel in such a way that the articular surfaces remain congruent. This does not necessarily mean that the surfaces are anatomical in shape, and in many cases the acetabulum and femoral head become 'congruently incongruent'. Maintenance of the femoral head in the acetabulum may require surgical intervention. Varus femoral osteotomy has its proponents[13] while others recommend innominate osteotomy.[14] From the point of view of subsequent replacement, a pelvic procedure is preferable.

Slipped capital femoral epiphysis (SCFE)

This is a disorder of the adolescent hip, occurring in 1:50 000 individuals, 20% of whom have bilateral involvement. It occurs before growth arrest of the capital epiphysis; the classical case is the obese, hypogonadal boy, but thin girls can be affected.

At least part of the aetiology is mechanical. The growth plate is weak in shear, especially at periods of growth spurt. The anteroposterior force on the hip can be as much as seven times body weight, and therefore it is possible for the adolescent, particularly the heavy male, to generate sufficient force to displace the

REFERENCES

10. Catterall A JBJS 1971; 53B: 37
11. Herring J A JBJS 1994; 76A: 448
12. Wenger D R, Ward W T, Herring J A JBJS 1991; 73A: 778
13. Lloyd-Roberts G'C, Catterall A, Salamon P B JBJS 1976; 58B: 31

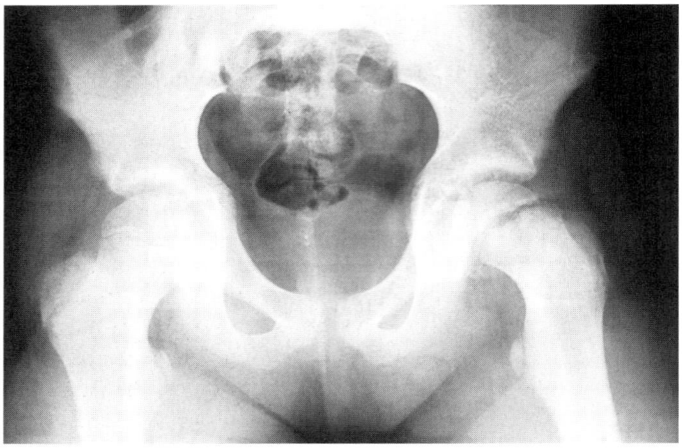

Fig 47.8 Slipped capital femoral epiphysis.

epiphysis posteriorly and inferiorly.[15] Hormonal, inflammatory and nutritional causes have also been propounded.

It can present in three ways.

1. Acute. The child presents with acute pain, not infrequently in the knee. The leg is shortened and externally rotated when there is a major slip. Radiology demonstrates displacement of the epiphysis as described above, without metaphyseal changes.
2. Chronic. The child may complain of pain but might also be referred because of a limp—often a combination of a Trendelenburg, short leg and externally rotated leg gaits. Radiology shows the displacement with remodelling changes in the metaphysis.
3. Acute on chronic. The patient presents as in the first case but with radiological features of both. This is perhaps the most common mode of presentation (Fig. 47.8).

Management

When dealing with a patient with slipped capital femoral epiphysis the complications of the disorder must always be remembered. These are chondrolysis and avascular necrosis, both of which are usually but not invariably related to treatment. Chondrolysis is a catastrophic, rapid loss of the articular cartilage, in which the hip becomes severely painful and stiff. It occurs particularly in black[16] and female patients, and especially those in whom the articular surface has been accidentally broached during surgical treatment (Figs 47.9 and 47.10). Avascular necrosis occurs secondary to damage to the posterior retinacular vessels in the capsule which are at risk if closed or open reduction is attempted.[17]

The principles of treatment are the arrest of further slip and if possible the restoration of normal mechanics to the hip to prevent the early onset of osteoarthritis. Attempts at reduction of the slip are only justified if it is genuinely acute, the degree of slip is severe, and the patient has presented very early after onset. In all other cases, the hip is pinned in situ, the current practice being to use one cancellous screw, the thread of which crosses the epiphysis.[18] The trend is to use cannulated screws, but these are difficult to remove, and the author prefers to use standard 6 mm AO 16 mm thread cancellous screws. The operation is difficult when the slip is moderate to severe, and it may be justified to direct the screw from the greater trochanter to the head without trying to pass it up the femoral neck. The patient is followed up until closure of the growth plate.

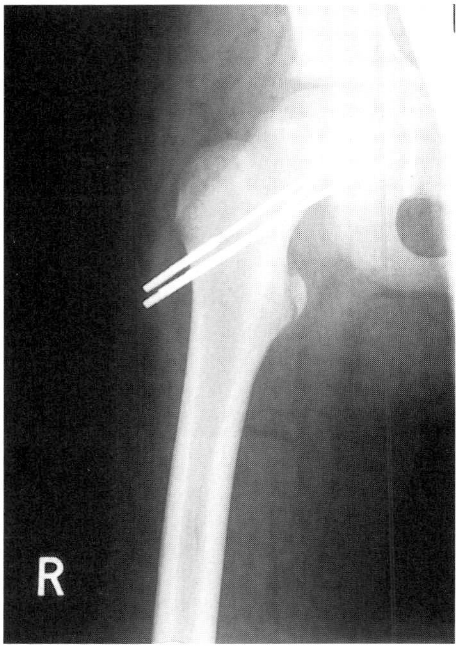

Fig 47.9 SCFE after pinning—note that one pin has penetrated the subchondral bone.

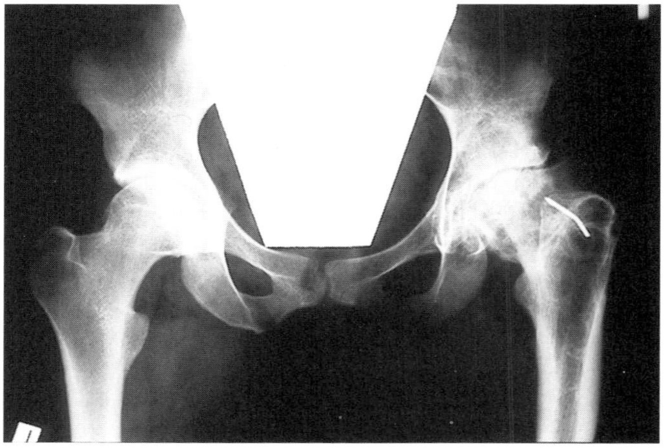

Fig 47.10 SCFE at maturity—severe degenerative changes.

In those cases where the slip is severe, where the leg is shortened and the range of internal rotation severely limited, corrective osteotomy can be considered. Mechanically the most satisfactory anatomical level for the osteotomy is the femoral neck (the Dunn

REFERENCES

14. Ingman A M, Paterson D C, Sutherland A D Clin Orthop 1982; 163: 141
15. Chung S M K, Batterman S C, Brighton C T JBJS 1976; 58A: 94
16. Bishop J O et al Clin Orthop 1978; 135: 93
17. Hall J E JBJS 1957; 39B: 659
18. Ward W T et al JBJS 1992; 74A: 799

osteotomy),[19] but the risk to the blood supply is very high, and alternative procedures are described, such as the sub-trochanteric osteotomy of Southwick.[20] This requires a very high level of three-dimensional awareness, and the proximal fragment needs to be externally rotated, adducted and extended. This significantly alters the shape of the proximal femur and can make subsequent replacement surgery very difficult.

For those young patients with chondrolysis or avascular necrosis, arthrodesis or even replacement surgery may have to be considered, but the results of the latter are not good.

Irritable hip

Probably the most common cause of admission for hip pain in childhood is so-called irritable hip. The disorder affects young children, with boys more often affected than girls. There is often a history, which may be spurious, of trauma and often a story of a recent infection, most often viral.

The child presents with pain in the hip and a reluctance to weight bear. Examination reveals a restriction of abduction in flexion. There is no systemic upset and no pyrexia; investigations, both haematological and radiological, are negative. Treatment is empirical; the child is forced to rest by skin traction until symptoms subside.

There may be recurrence and Perthes' disease subsequently becomes apparent in a very small number of cases. The underlying pathology is assumed to be a reactive arthritis or synovitis following infection, but serological testing is frequently unrewarding and does not affect management. The disorder must be distinguished from sepsis (q.v.)

THE HIP IN ADULTHOOD

Osteoarthritis of the hip

Aetiology

This can be simply stated as being due to either intrinsic or extrinsic factors, in either of which there may be either abnormal loading of normal articular cartilage, or normal loading of abnormal cartilage. Abnormal loading may occur, for example in the obese individual, or in overuse of a joint, or in situations in which the available area of cartilage available for load is smaller than required, such as acetabular dysplasia, or when the resultant load on the joint is maldirected, as in varus and valgus malalignment. Abnormal cartilage may occur in a variety of metabolic disorders and collagen disease. In the majority of patients, no such definite abnormality can be identified, and the disorder is ascribed to 'wear and tear'. Secondary osteoarthritis occurs as a result of previous disease or trauma to the joint.

The articular surface is also vulnerable if the supporting subchondral bone is abnormal, e.g. in avascular necrosis.

Pathology

The initial macrosopic abnormality is a breakdown of the collagen fibrils, which, with the proteoglycans, entrap a high water content. The chondrocytes are incapable of repairing the collagen in its original highly organized system. The water content is lost. The consequences are a loss of the smooth articular surface necessary for the healthy nutrition of the apposing surface, and a loss of the load distributing function of the articular surface, with, as a result, overload of the subchondral bone. The bone responds to the increased load in accordance with Wolff's law by hypertrophy of the subchondral trabeculae though this is only possible up to a limit. The applied load may exceed the yield strength of the trabeculae, causing microfractures and compaction of the subchondral layer. A reparative process next leads to absorption of bone, cyst formation, and the laying down of new bone around the periphery of the joint. The radiographic appearances reflect the pathology: initially there is loss of joint space followed by subchondral sclerosis, cyst and osteophyte formation.

Clinical features

The most frequent symptoms are pain and loss of function. The history must include an assessment of the severity of the pain, together with exacerbating and relieving factors. The site of the pain is important—pain arising from the hip articulation is felt in the buttock, groin and anterior thigh as far as the knee. Pain in the buttock can be difficult to distinguish from back pain, groin pain can arise from a number of non-skeletal causes, and knee pain can distract attention from the genuine source of the symptoms. Function must be carefully assessed, and considered in the context of the patient's age and general medical condition. Social factors may influence clinical decisions, for instance the suitability of the patient's housing, and the nature of the help he or she has at home.

The rest of the medical history is of equal importance, particularly if surgical treatment is contemplated. The fitness of the patient must be sufficient to allow major elective surgery for a condition which is not life-threatening.

The clinical examination is as already described. In the age group usually afflicted it is more than usually important to examine the back, the contralateral hip and the knees. The peripheral vascular and nervous systems must also be assessed.

A general medical examination is obligatory if surgical treatment is planned.

Investigations

Usually simple radiographical investigation is sufficient in the assessment of the osteoarthritic patient (Fig. 47.1). In cases where the cause of hip pain is obscure, radioisotope, computed tomographic and magnetic resonance scans have their uses. In addition, sedimentation rate, rheumatoid tests and bone biochemistry are sometimes indicated.

REFERENCES

19. Dunn D M JBJS 1964; 46B: 621
20. Southwick W O JBJS 1967; 49A: 807

Non-surgical management of the arthritic hip

Given that the principal symptoms are pain and loss of function, management must be directed to the relief of the former and the restoration or substitution of the latter. Analgesics and non-steroidal anti-inflammatory drugs have their place, although the use of the latter has been felt by many orthopaedic surgeons to hasten the deterioration of the arthritic joint; these drugs may also cause complications, especially gastrointestinal haemorrhage. The load on the hip can be reduced by the use of a walking stick in the contralateral hand, and the lifestyle of the patient may need to be modified. It is the author's view that physiotherapy only rarely has a place in the treatment of an osteoarthritic joint, but occupational therapy assessment may restore a patient's independence.

If the above measures fail and, in particular, if the pain becomes constant and intrusive even at rest, then surgical treatment must be considered.

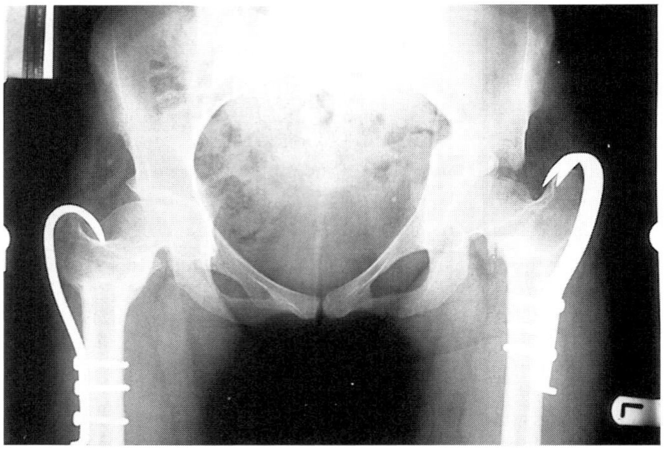

Fig 47.11 Bilateral femoral and left Chiari osteotomies performed for pain in a female aged 25 with bilateral developmental disease of the hip.

Surgical management of the arthritic hip

Surgical management broadly follows the same principles, i.e. the relief of pain, the reduction of load and the restoration of function.

The surgical options can be summarized as follows:

1. Osteotomy—the correction of malalignment, or the alteration of alignment of articular surfaces by division and realignment of bone, either on the femoral or acetabular side.
2. Arthrodesis—the relief of pain by fusion of the joint.
3. Arthroplasty—the most common form being replacement arthroplasty, but excision arthroplasty is sometimes indicated in salvage situations.

Osteotomy

This was for a time a common operation in the UK prior to the era of joint replacement. The McMurray osteotomy increased the varus angle of the femoral neck to the shaft and displaced the shaft medially.[21] Fixation with one of several designs of spline allowed early mobilization. The operation fell into decline during the 1960s, partly due to the success of hip replacement, but also because of the perceived unpredictability of the clinical result. In mainland Europe the operation has continued in popularity, largely thanks to the enthusiasm of Bombelli[22] and Maquet,[23] who base their work on the scientific principles of Pauwels. In the UK, Reynolds has been the chief proponent of acetabular osteotomy, originally advocating the Chiari osteotomy,[24] but more recently the triple acetabular osteotomy (Fig. 47.11).[25] The place of osteotomy in the 1990s remains contentious. It must be considered for the younger patient with a joint which is considered to be salvageable. The main advantage is the potential for the relief of pain and the restoration of function without the need for permanent prosthetic implants (q.v.). The disadvantages to the patient are the length of recuperation (up to 2 years), and the lack of a peer group with which to compare the outcome. The difficulty for the surgeon is that osteotomy of the proximal femur can make subsequent hip replacement technically more difficult and increases the risk of infection in a subsequent prosthesis when there has been previous surgery.

It is nevertheless still the case that a carefully planned and executed osteotomy for the right indication in the right patient can produce a result superior to an arthroplasty, particularly in terms of longevity.

Arthrodesis

Surgical fusion of the hip joint was once a commonly performed operation, usually when the joint was infected, but also for patients whose arthritic hips were unsalvageable by osteotomy. The most common indication was probably tuberculosis; for this disease a number of techniques of extra-articular fusion were devised to avoid exacerbation of infection by entering the joint itself.[26–28] Poliomyelitis also provided large numbers of individuals with paralysed limbs which could be partly stabilized by this procedure. For the operation to be satisfactory the position of fusion was of great importance and the spine, contralateral hip and ipsilateral knee had to be normal.

With the sharp decline in tuberculosis and polio the operation has fallen almost into disuse, although indications occasionally arise; a surgical technique devised by the Arbeitgemenschaft Osteosynthsefragenl (AO) school allows secure fixation and early mobilization (but it is not a technique for the surgically faint-hearted!) (Figs 47.12 and 47.13).[29]

REFERENCES

21. McMurray T P JBJS 1939; 21: 1
22. Bombelli R Structure and function in normal and abnormal hips, 3rd edn. Springer, Berlin 1993
23. Maquet P G J Biomechanics of the Hip. Springer, Berlin 1985
24. Reynolds D A R JBJS 1986; 63B: 45
25. Tonnis D et al J Pediat Orthop 1994; 3: 54
26. Adams J C Ischio-femoral arthrodesis. Churchill Livingstone, Edinburgh 1966
27. Brittain H A Brit J Surg 1941; 29: 93
28. Watson-Jones R, Robinson W C JBJS 1956; 38B: 353
29. Liechti R Hip arthrodesis and associated problems. Springer V, Berlin 1978

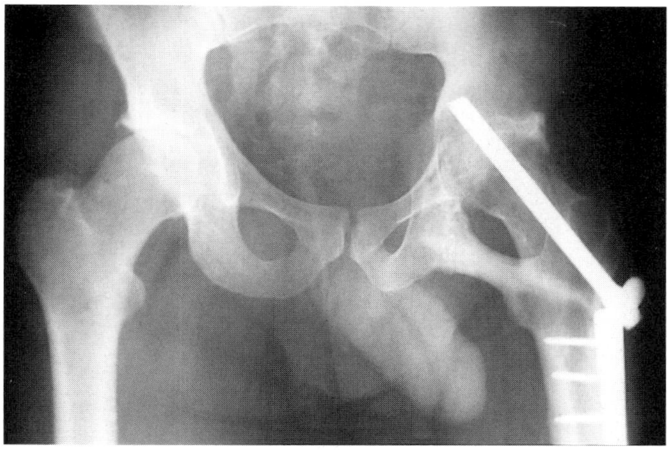

Fig 47.12 Crawford Adams arthrodesis.

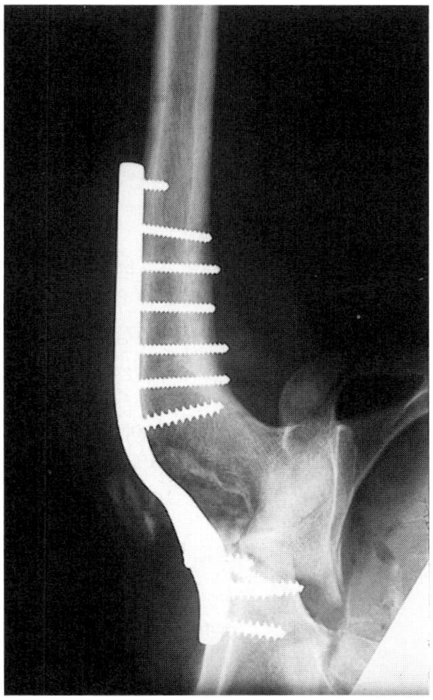

Fig 47.13 AO arthrodesis.

Arthroplasty

Although joint replacement had been attempted as soon as anaesthesia and antiseptic procedures became available, it was not until the late 1950s and early 1960s that successful total hip replacement became a reality. Prior to this period, patients could be offered the procedures described above or one of the alternative arthroplastic techniques, for example interposition arthroplasty using fascia lata or prosthetic materials, or hemiarthroplasty, or even an excision arthroplasty (the Girdlestone operation).

Earlier attempts at total replacement (involving both the acetabulum and the femur) failed because of sepsis, use of inappropriate materials, poor appreciation of the biomechanical principles and inadequate fixation.

These problems were scientifically and then clinically overcome by Professor Sir John Charnley.[30] Charnley combined biomechanical design with well-chosen materials and a strict surgical and aseptic technique. He used a stainless steel femoral component with a small diameter head, matched with a high-density polyethylene acetabulum. He obtained polymethylmethacrylate cement from dental practice to achieve fixation. He devised a surgical approach to the hip—the transtrochanteric approach—to give him the access necessary for his design. With Howarth he revolutionized operating theatre design to produce the ultra-clean theatre, and operated wearing an enclosed suit with body exhaust. By these means he introduced one of the most spectacularly and consistently successful operations in any branch of surgery. There were, however, failures, and complications became apparent.

Complications of total hip replacement (THR)

The most common complications are dislocation, deep venous thrombosis (DVT), heterotopic bone formation and sepsis. The management of sepsis will be dealt with separately.

Dislocation may occur early or late. Causes of early dislocation are related to:

1. Prosthetic design.
2. Misalignment of components by the surgeon.
3. The surgical approach—dislocation is more common after a posterior approach.
4. Impingement (i.e. contact of the femoral component with either the edge of a misaligned socket or adjacent bone.
5. Soft tissue problems.
6. Failure by the patient to follow postoperative instructions not to overbend the joint or cross the legs. Late dislocation occurs most commonly when the femoral head has migrated into the acetabulum because of wear and creep. The neck of the prosthesis can then impinge on the rim of the socket, thereby levering itself out. Dislocation can also occur as a consequence of trauma.

Deep venous thrombosis. This remains a contentious issue in hip replacement surgery. The risk of thrombosis after hip replacement is high, up to 60% if no prophylaxis is used, and the mortality of the operation (0.5–2%) is usually related to pulmonary embolism.[31–33] It is accepted by most orthopaedic surgeons in the UK that prophylactic measures should be taken to prevent deep venous thrombosis in all patients undergoing hip replacement.

The prophylactic methods currently employed include:

1. Early mobilization after surgery.
2. Anaesthetic technique—the risk of thrombosis is less with epidural anaesthesia.[34]
3. Compression stockings.

REFERENCES

30. Charnley J Low Friction Arthroplasty of the Hip. Theory and Practice. Springer, Berlin 1979
31. Johnson R, Green J R, Charnley J Clin Orthop 1977; 127: 123
32. Wolf L D, Hozack W J, Rothman R H Clin Orthop 1993; 288: 219
33. Wroblewski B M, Siney P D, White R Clin Orthop 1992; 276: 222
34. Modig J et al Anesth and Analg 1983; 62: 174

4. Low dose heparin.[35]
5. Low molecular weight heparin.[36]
6. Low dose warfarin.[37]
7. Dextran.[38]
8. Full anticoagulation.[39]
9. Calf compression pumps.[40]
10. Pedal venous plexus pumps.[41]

Heterotopic ossification. This is a poorly understood process in which soft tissues around the joint calcify and then ossify after surgery. The severity ranges from a few trivial specks seen on radiographs to complete ankylosis of the articulation.[42] During formation of the bone the patient may experience pain, and the process may take up to 2 years to mature. It appears to be more common in younger males. It can be effectively prevented by the administration of indomethacin 25 mg t.d.s.[43] If the bone formation is sufficient to impair function then excision can be considered, but recurrence is common, especially if excision is undertaken before the bone has matured. In patients who cannot be prescribed indomethacin, low dose radiotherapy can be effective.[44]

Failure of total hip replacement

Around 50 000 total hip replacements are performed annually in the UK. About 1% fail each year, and thus by 10 years postoperatively 10% will have required revision surgery. These figures tend to come from the better centres and almost certainly underestimate the problem; many patients with a loose hip replacement are very elderly and unfit for this magnitude of surgery, or their surgeons may well not feel that the likely outcome in their hands is worth the risk.

To consider the causes of failure, and to understand some of the reasons for the proliferation of designs and techniques, some elementary physics must be discussed. All materials deform under load. Up to a defined limit for each material, the deformation relates to the applied load in a linear fashion, and the deformation reverses when the load is removed. This is the basis of Hook's law. When a load versus deformation curve is constructed, the area under the linear part of the curve can be expressed as the modulus of elasticity, or Young's modulus; the higher the number, the stiffer the material.

Bone is, in engineering terms, a very elastic material with a low Young's modulus. The modulus for stainless steel is in the region of 300 times that of bone. High density polyethylene (HDP) and polymethylmethacrylate (PMMA) are about 30 times stiffer than bone.

Consider a composite bar composed of layers of bone, stainless steel, HDP and PMMA, loaded in compression and torsion. The individual materials will deform according to their moduli of elasticity. For this to occur there must be movement at the interfaces between each layer. Movement between materials of different mechanical properties generates wear, and wear yields debris.

The materials used in total hip replacement are, in bulk form, biologically inert. In particulate form, however, they can be ingested by macrophages and induce a foreign body giant cell reaction.[45] Among the effects of this reaction are stimulation of osteoclastic activity and release of a variety of enzymes which can digest bone. If this process occurs at the interface between the bone and the prosthetic materials, the bond between them will be impaired. The mechanical stability of the construct deteriorates and increased movement takes place in consequence. Eventually the prosthesis becomes 'clinically' loose, with pain especially under load. The pathological process can continue with progressive destruction of bone, making revision surgery technically challenging (Fig. 47.14).

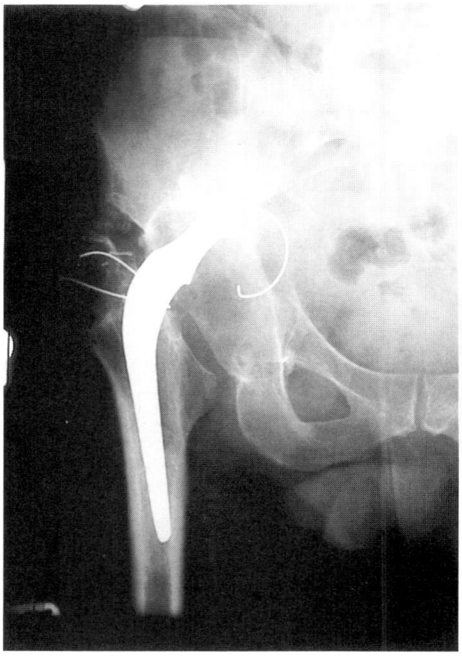

Fig 47.14 Loose Charnley replacement—the cup has disintegrated and the joint is subluxated.

From the above discussion it should be appreciated that there is no such thing as 'rigid' fixation in hip replacement, only 'relatively rigid' fixation, defined by Vernon-Roberts as that fixation which does not elicit a pathological reaction.[46]

The materials used in total hip replacement have been blamed individually for the pathological reaction. Earlier designs utilized metal to metal bearings. Exploration of these joints often revealed dense metal staining of the adjacent soft tissues, and thus such implants fell into disuse. Histological examination of the membranes removed from the interface at revision surgery

REFERENCES

35. Taberner D A et al British J Surg 1989; 76: 933
36. Turpie A G et al New Engl J Med 1986; 315: 925
37. Amstutz H C et al JBJS 1989; 71A: 321
38. Fredin H et al Acta Orthop Scand 1989; 60: 678
39. Lieberman J R, Geerts W H JBJS 1994; 76A: 1239
40. Bailey J P et al J Arthroplasty 1991; 6(suppl): S29
41. Fordyce M J F, Ling R S M JBJS 1992; 74B: 45
42. Reigler H F, Harris C M Clin Orthop 1976; 117: 209
43. Ritter M A, Sieber J M Clin Orthop 1985; 196: 217
44. Pellegrini V D et al JBJS 1992; 74A: 186
45. Freeman M A R, Bradley G W, Revell P A JBJS 1982; 64B: 489
46. Swanson S A V, Freeman M A R The scientific basis of joint replacement. Pitman Medical, Tunbridge Wells 1977

displayed polymethylmethacrylate particles within the cells.[1] This prompted the search, which still continues, for alternative, cementless, means of achieving satisfactory fixation. Finally Polaroid light microscopy has demonstrated the presence of polyethylene debris, which at the present time is the chief culprit in this process.[47–49]

Particulate debris can also occur as a result of wear at the articulation between the femoral and acetabular components; this can be greatly accelerated if a 'third body' such as polymethylmethacrylate powder is present in the joint.[50]

Current controversies in total hip replacement

Much has been learned in the three decades since Charnley introduced his operation. Many innovations have been tried, several of which have turned out to be serious mistakes. Materials have come in and out of fashion, and many previous ideas have been revisited.

For some time polymethylmethacrylate cement fixation was felt to be the feature most at fault in the aetiology of loosening. In addition the Federal Drugs Administration in the USA refused it a licence for some time because there were some early catastrophes as a result of profound hypotension associated with its introduction into the bones. Considerable effort was therefore directed to find a means of securely fixing a prosthesis without cement.[51–54] Press-fit, CAD/CAM custom-made prostheses, alterations in surface finish and coatings have all been tried.[55] Many present cementless designs are coated with hydroxyapatite, the mineral which constitutes the inorganic matrix of bone and which has been shown to be osseoinductive, reviving hopes that it might be possible to achieve true biological integration with the host bone (osseointegration).[56,57] Results so far with this material are certainly encouraging, but have yet to show any advantage over a competently performed cemented total hip replacement. It is the author's view that cementless replacements should be reserved for younger patients, not because they afford any advantage to the patient in terms of quality or longevity of result, but because they offer the possibility of a technically simpler revision operation when they fail (Fig. 47.15).

Cementing techniques have been refined. Current best practice includes removal of loose cancellous bone, careful irrigation and drying of the bone and pressurization of liquid cement during introduction.[58] Polyethylene remains the material of choice for the acetabular component although ceramics are used in some designs on both the acetabular and femoral sides. It has been appreciated that certain manufacturing techniques can prejudice the structural integrity of the material—hot pressing for instance causes lamination. Sterilizing high density polyethylene with gamma irradiation accelerates aging of the material.

Stainless steel was abandoned long ago as the material for femoral stems because of a tendency to fatigue fracture with sudden unforeseen failure of the joint. Cobalt chrome alloys enjoyed a period of popularity—they had been in use in hemiarthroplasties since the 1940s. The elastic properties of CoCr alloys are much the same as stainless steel without the tendency to fracture. When titanium and its alloys were introduced into dental practice they very soon found their way into femoral components. Titanium is much lighter and more elastic, and the dental experience showed

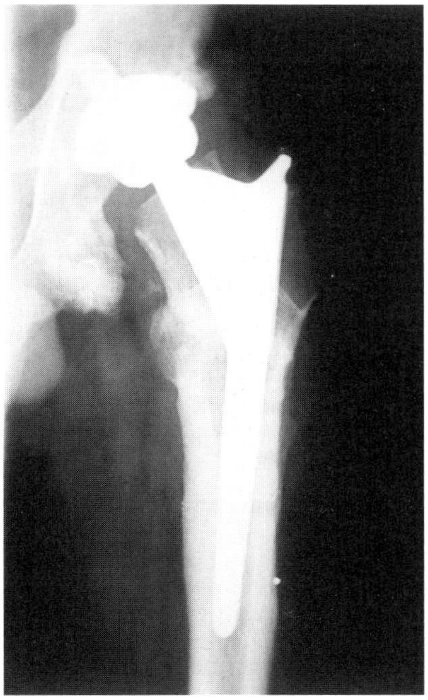

Fig 47.15 Cementless hip replacement after an arthrodesis in a male aged 33.

good biocompatibility with bone with the prospect of good osseointegration.[59] Unfortunately, experience has shown that the oxide layer which coats the surface of the metal has a very low shear strength, is easily rubbed off, and is consequently ingested by the adjacent tissues.[60] It then becomes implicated in the pathological process described above.[61] Many manufacturers have returned to CoCr, while others now coat titanium with a nitride layer which has a much higher shear strength.[62]

Design of new prostheses has become a prolific growth industry. Avoidance of sharp edges to reduce stress between the metal and the cement is of paramount importance, but great care needs to be exercised by the surgeon selecting a new prosthesis. Sometimes 'innovations' in design can have a catastrophic effect on fixation.[63] Most designs attempt to encourage proximal load transfer to reduce the problem of proximal stress protection and

REFERENCES

47. Revell P A et al Arch Orthop Trauma Surg 1978; 81: 167
48. Santavirta S et al Orthop Int 1993; 1: 229
49. Rose R M, Radin E L Clin Orthop 1982; 170: 107
50. Maloney W J, Smith R L JBJS 1995; 77A: 1448
51. Ring P A Clin Orthop 1978; 137: 87
52. Nunn D JBJS 1988; 70B: 40
53. Morscher E W, Dick W Clin Orthop 1983; 176: 77
54. Freeman M A R et al Clin Orthop 1983; 176: 88
55. Callaghan J J JBJS 1993; 75A: 299
56. Oonishi H Biomaterials 1991; 12: 171
57. Hardy D C et al JBJS 1991; 73B: 732
58. Benjamin J B et al JBJS 1987; 69B: 620
59. Albrektsson T et al Acta Orthop Scand 1981; 15: 155
60. Witt J D, Swann M JBJS 1991; 73B: 559
61. Lintner F et al J Arthroplasty 1986; 1: 183
62. Friedman R J et al JBJS 1993; 75A: 1086
63. Mohler C G et al JBJS 1995; 77A: 1315

absorption of bone which occurs if the prosthesis relies on distal fixation. Metal backing of cemented acetabular components had a vogue in the 1980s.[64] It was thought to reduce peak stresses at the implant–cement interface. It is now reserved for cementless designs, to prevent abrasion of the high density polyethylene by the bone.

Other acrylic cements have been tried, but the variations used have suffered from greatly increased creep which encourages rapid migration of the implants.

Current UK practice favours standard implants with proven track records, implanted using modern cementing techniques, for the majority of patients undergoing total hip replacement. This is the author's policy for all patients over 60, all patients with inflammatory joint disease, and those with avascular necrosis (q.v.) One of the most hotly debated current controversies is the question of cost. The prostheses which have stood the test of time also tend to be the least expensive, while new designs, especially the cementless systems, can be extremely expensive.

Revision surgery

The revision of a failed total hip replacement is much more technically demanding than the original operation. Scar tissue can make access difficult. Removal of the old implants can result in further damage to bone already compromised by the loosening process. The cement in particular can be extremely tedious and difficult to extract, although the introduction of ultrasonic devices has improved this aspect of the operation. Assessment of the bone stock can only take place after all the prosthesis, cement and membrane has been removed. The final decision on the nature of the reconstruction can only take place at this stage, and the surgeon must not embark on this procedure unless every means of reconstruction is at hand.

As ever, fashion as much as science dictates current practice. Much attention at present is directed to impaction grafting of bone with bone obtained from bone banks. The author prefers not to put much reliance on either the structural integrity of this material, or on the body's ability to incorporate dead sterilized bone into a graft bed already damaged by biological activity. He prefers to reconstruct with prosthetic materials with predictable structural properties, and, when the situation demands it, to achieve fixation higher in the pelvis and more distally in the femur than in the primary replacement.

The result of revision surgery is rarely as good as in primary total hip replacement, either in terms of quality or longevity, and the complication rate is much higher. The results are almost certainly better in the hands of surgeons with a particular interest in this field.

Infection in prosthetic joints

Established deep sepsis in a joint replacement inevitably leads to failure. The most effective treatment is prevention. Factors important in the avoidance of sepsis are:

1. Careful patient selection—any potential source of infection, for example venous ulcers, dental abscesses, should be treated before joint replacement surgery.[65]
2. Dedicated orthopaedic operating theatres with clean air flow.[66]
3. Meticulous aseptic technique.
4. Prophylactic antibiotics—three doses of parenteral antibiotic starting at anaesthetic induction.[67]
5. The use of antibiotic impregnated cement—this remains contentious.[68]
6. Avoidance of urethral catheterization peri-operatively.[69]
7. Aggressive management of haematoma.

Discharge from a wound should not be assumed to be from a superficial source and treated expectantly. Such wounds should be surgically explored and drained.

Diagnosis and management of deep sepsis. The diagnosis of sepsis may be obvious—there may have been an infected haematoma postoperatively with persisting drainage ever since, but more commonly this is not the case. Infections often present late, and in these cases there may have been infection early which has taken time to present, or the joint may have become infected late secondary to infection elsewhere. Another factor in late presentation is the infecting organism. Many joints are infected with 'low-grade' organisms, often skin commensals, which may take months and even years to become clinically apparent.

It is most important to have a high index of suspicion when faced with a patient with a painful replaced hip. The history may contain clues pointing to the diagnosis:

1. Has the joint always been painful?
2. Was there a haematoma after surgery?[70]
3. Was the bladder catheterized?
4. Is the pain now unrelated to activity (mechanically loose joints are not usually painful at rest)?[71]
5. Is there a history of intercurrent infection?
6. Is there any evidence of the systemic effects of sepsis?

Clinical examination may not provide much help. There is only rarely external evidence of deep sepsis, but a surgical scar which has healed by secondary intention is a good pointer, and of course persisting sinuses are pathognomonic.

Radiology may show erosion of bone around the prosthesis. If this is evident relatively soon after surgery the joint is probably infected, but later erosion may be due to mechanical loosening. Periosteal reactions must be assumed to be due to osteomyelitic changes.

Radionuclide bone scanning can be helpful, but it must be remembered that such scans demonstrate increased uptake around a satisfactory hip replacement for up to 2 years postoperatively. There is also a false positive and false negative rate with white cell labelled scans.[72] The erythrocyte sedimentation rate (ESR) is often

REFERENCES

64. Crowninshield R D et al JBJS 1982; 64A: 495
65. Ainscow D A P, Denham R A 1984; 66B: 580
66. Charnley J Clin Orthop 1972; 87: 167
67. Mauerhan D R et al JBJS 1994; 76A: 39
68. Elson R A et al JBJS 1977; 59B: 200
69. Wroblewski B M, Del Sel H J Clin Orthop 1980; 146: 209
70. Fitzgerald R H et al JBJS 1977; 59A: 847
71. Garvin K L, Hanssen A D JBJS 1995; 77A: 1576
72. Merkel K D et al JBJS 1985; 67A: 465

but not always raised. It should certainly be taken for a baseline, and can be used to monitor treatment.[73]

Aspiration and biopsy under anaesthetic is mandatory prior to formal exploration of the joint, and consultation with a microbiologist is essential.[74] All growth must be reported, since organisms which are normally only skin contaminants can be pathogenic in the presence of prosthetic material.

Surgical management of established infection. Unless the patient is medically unfit for major surgery there is no place for conservative management in the presence of established deep infection. Organisms can survive on the surface of prostheses, where they are sequestered from the circulation and therefore inaccessible to antibiotics. In the unfit patient the best that antibiotics can achieve is a symbiotic relationship with the infecting bacterium, but if the patient survives for any length of time the prosthesis will become manifestly loose.

The author's practice is as follows:

1. All patients in whom infection is suspected have technetium and white cell labelled scans and an ESR.
2. All such patients have aspiration, with or without biopsy, under general anaesthetic.
3. If the aspiration detects a 'high-grade' organism (usually *Staph. aureus*) a two-stage exchange is advised.[75] At the first stage the prosthesis and all cement is removed and specimens are again sent for analysis. The leg is placed on traction, appropriate antibiotics are prescribed, and the ESR is monitored until it has come to normal levels. Only then is the second stage reconstruction performed. If the ESR remains elevated it suggests that osteomyelitis has become established, the second stage is not performed and the patient is left with an excision arthroplasty.[76]
4. If a low-grade organism, or no organism, is grown, then a one-stage exchange is appropriate.[77]
5. Even with this careful protocol, the success rate of revision surgery is no better than 30%, and there remains a 60% risk of infection presenting again late after exchange arthroplasty.

Avascular necrosis of the hip

This is a condition of bone mediated by the loss of blood supply with consequent death of the bone, followed by collapse and absorption. When it occurs in subarticular bone the underlying substructure of the articular cartilage is lost, the cartilage is easily sheared off by normal joint forces and the joint very rapidly degenerates. The condition is poorly understood and difficult to reproduce in the experimental animal. It affects in particular convex surfaces of bones, especially the femoral head, the humeral head and the femoral condyles. While several factors are known to be associated with this disorder, many cases are obscure. The commonest associations are:

1. Alcoholism.
2. Steroid administration—particularly after renal transplant or in the treatment of status asthmaticus.
3. Sickle cell disease.
4. Work in compressed air—deep sea divers and tunnelers.

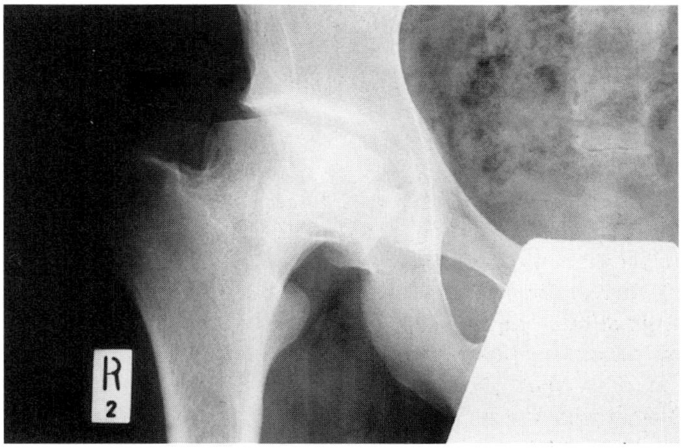

Fig 47.16 Avascular necrosis secondary to Gaucher's disease.

5. Trauma—25% of patients having internal fixation of a subcapital fracture will develop avascular necrosis.
6. Radiation—often seen decades after radiotherapy for pelvic malignant disease.
7. Metabolic disease—Gaucher's (Fig. 47.16).
8. Myeloproliferative disorders.
9. Coagulopathies.

Patients may present early and at that time may have no radiological changes, but most present late with already established disease, in which case the presenting symptoms are the same as those in osteoarthritis. The radiological changes have been graded by Arlet & Ficat:[78]

1. Stage 1: normal radiographs.
2. Stage 2: cystic and sclerotic changes but no change in contour of the femoral head.
3. Stage 3: subchondral collapse, flattening of the femoral head.
4. Stage 4: narrowing of the joint space with secondary degenerative changes.

Management

Surgical treatment is directed towards either revascularization in the early case or replacement in late cases.

Revascularization may be achieved by drilling through normal bone into the affected bone, in the hope that blood vessels will grow through the passage created into the dead areas. Some relief of symptoms might be achieved by 'decompression' of the bone by this means.[79] Numerous revascularization procedures are described.[80]

REFERENCES

73. Schulak D J et al Clin Orthop 1982; 167: 197
74. Buchholz H W et al JBJS 1981; 63B: 342
75. Lieberman J R et al Clin Orthop 1994; 301: 205
76. Grauer J D et al JBJS 1989; 71A: 669
77. Elson R A Sem Arthroplasty 1994; 5: 137
78. Arlet J, Ficat P Rev Rheumat 1964; 31: 257
79. Solomon L Canadian J Surg 1981; 24: 573
80. Bonfiglio M, Voke E M JBJS 1968; 50A: 48

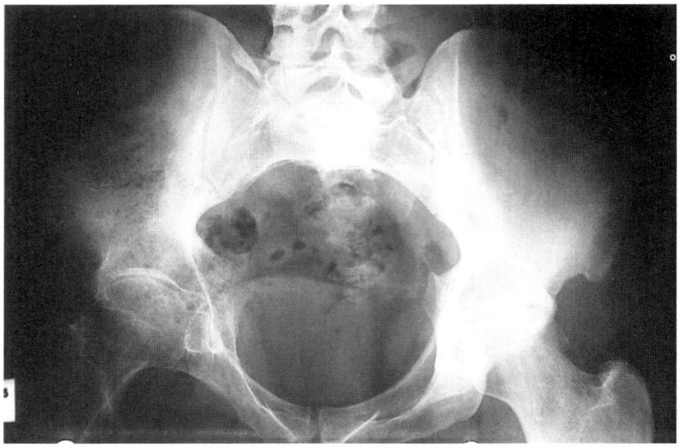

a

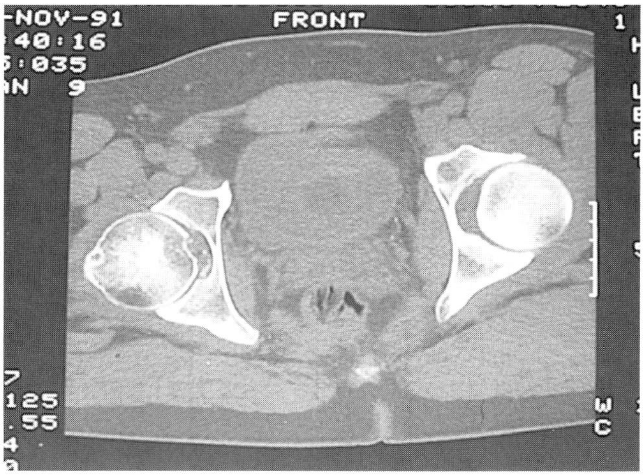

b

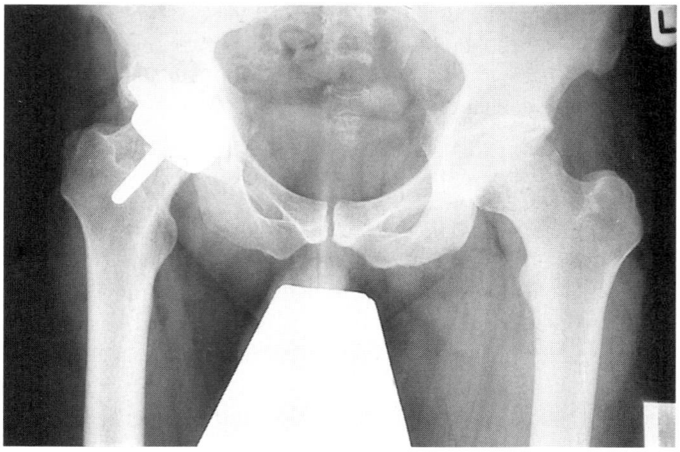

c

Fig 47.17 (a) Synovial osteochondromatosis: there is marked porosis of the affected hip. (b) CT showing loose bodies in the joint. (c) After surface replacement with a metal to metal bearing.

Replacement surgery is of limited value in the treatment of these patients. They are usually younger than patients with degenerative disease and have higher expectations and demands; the failure rate is very high, especially in those with sickle cell disease. Other procedures, such as 180° rotation osteotomy of the femoral neck, have been described but are not recommended.[81]

Synovial disorders of the hip

The commonest disorders of synovium to affect the hip are of course the inflammatory arthropathies, particularly rheumatoid disease and ankylosing spondylitis. The symptoms must be treated on their merits, and most patients have prolonged relief from the disease modifying drugs. Eventually, however, many of them will suffer either advanced inflammatory destruction, or osteoarthritic change when the primary disorder has 'burnt out'. These patients usually enjoy a satisfactory result from replacement surgery. Other much rarer conditions include pigmented villonodular synovitis (PVNS)[82,83] and synovial osteochondromatosis (Fig. 47.17).[84,85] Both are characterized clinically by pain and stiffness. In PVNS there is gross hypertrophy of the synovium with seaweed-like brown pigmented fronds filling the capsule. Pressure from the tissue may lead to erosion of the adjacent bone, usually in the femoral neck. The capsule also contains a brownish effusion thought to be the result of repeated small haemarthroses. In synovial osteochondromatosis, the hypertrophied synovial villi calcify at their tips and break off. They may grow within the synovial cavity, producing hundreds of loose bodies. An inflammatory reaction accompanies this process. Both diseases may eventually lead to the necessity for joint replacement.

Septic arthritis of the hip

In the UK this is an unusual disorder. It occurs usually in those patients whose immune system is incompetent, i.e. the very young and very elderly, and those with diseases which lower immunity. It takes two forms: pyogenic and tuberculous.

Pyogenic arthritis is usually secondary to haematogenous spread from a primary septic focus, e.g. the respiratory and urinary tracts. The commonest organisms are *Staphylococcus aureus*, streptococcus, pneumococcus and gonococcus. The patient presents with extreme pain in the joint and systemic malaise with fever and rigors. Examination reveals the fixed flexed, adducted and externally rotated posture of a tense hip capsule, which in this disease is distended with pus, and an extreme reluctance to allow passive movement. Investigation should include the white cell count and the ESR. Radiology may not be helpful, but it is sometimes possible to see an effusion in the joint. Ultrasound will confirm the presence of a joint effusion.

The differential diagnosis includes all other causes of an acute inflammatory monoarthropathy, but in no other disorder is the severe restriction of movement such a feature. If there is doubt about the diagnosis, the joint may be aspirated. If pus is confirmed,

REFERENCES

81. Sugioka Y et al Clin Orthop 1992; 277: 111
82. Rao A R, Vigorita V J JBJS 1984; 66A: 76
83. Chung S M K, Janes J M JBJS 1965; 47A: 293
84. Jeffreys T E JBJS 1967; 49B: 530
85. McIvor R R, King D JBJS 1962; 44A: 87

the joint should be opened, thoroughly lavaged and drained. Intravenous antibiotics should be given until the temperature settles, usually over 48 hours, and then oral therapy should continue for about 6 weeks. If the temperature persists despite adequate drainage and antibiotics, the possibility of accompanying metaphyseal osteomyelitis should be considered, especially in the infant, in whom the epiphysis is intracapsular.

If the diagnosis is delayed, or reliance is placed on antibiotics alone, the action of pus on articular cartilage is destructive and the patient will be permanently disabled. In the infant the epiphysis itself may be destroyed (Tom Smith's disease). In the adult the only salvage procedure for a joint destroyed by sepsis is arthrodesis.

Tuberculous arthritis of the hip was once a common disorder in the UK, and many patients still survive whose hips were affected in childhood and adolescence. In the last quarter of the twentieth century, primary tuberculosis of joints is usually only seen in immigrants from the developing world, and in those with immune deficiency, particularly AIDS sufferers. The latter present with infections with drug resistant organisms, and with infection with mycobacteria other than Koch's bacillus.

The patients often have evidence of tuberculous infection elsewhere, and diagnosis can be made on the basis of chest radiographs and Heaf tests. Treatment of the infection is with standard chemotherapy. Liaison with physicians is essential, since the monitoring of tuberculosis therapy is outside an orthopaedic surgeon's remit.

Surgery for tuberculosis of the hip follows traditional lines; arthrodesis is still the most appropriate procedure. An interesting consequence of the practice of arthrodesing the hip in adolescents in the earlier part of this century is the appearance of many of these patients 20 or 30 years later seeking conversion to an arthroplasty, usually because of disabling back and/or ipsilateral knee pain. If this procedure is undertaken, the patient should have three months of chemotherapy before the operation, since surgery can rekindle a dormant infection even after many decades. The patients must understand that the results of this surgery are far inferior to replacements for osteoarthritis; they are always Trendelenburg positive due to disappearance of their abductor muscles.

48 The knee

F. W. Heatley

INTRODUCTION

The knee is one of the most challenging and exciting areas of orthopaedics. Not only is it the largest of all synovial joints but it is one of the most complex, encompasses the widest range of pathology and injuries, exhibits the most physical signs and can be diagnostically deceptive even to the expert.

The objective in this brief outline is to define the principles, not the details, of knee surgery.

THE JOINT IN BALANCE

It is all too easy to view joints in isolation from one another, especially in textbooks. It is only in the last two decades that orthopaedic surgeons have appreciated the crucial importance of leg alignment, especially for the knee. The centre of the hip, the centre of the knee and the centre of the ankle should fall in a straight line. This is termed the 'mechanical axis' of the limb. If you, as a surgeon, fail to reconstruct this parameter when doing a joint replacement it will not be in optimal mechanical balance and it will very likely fail.

This concept of the mechanical axis was advocated by Dr Paul Maquet of Liège,[1] who applied the same biomechanical principles to the knee that his mentor Professor Pauwels of Aachen[2] had applied to the hip. The historical background to this understanding of biomechanics is interesting. In the 1880s two scientists, Braune and Fischer, were awarded a defence contract by the Elector of Saxony to determine the most efficient manner in which to kit out a German infantryman. In essence they applied Newtonian mathematical principles to the body and its joints. By sequential amputation they initially determined the centre of gravity of the torso and each segment of the limbs.[3] Using early photographic methods they produced a sequence of still photographs of the actions of a German sergeant whilst marching, after he had first been fitted out with a series of light markers corresponding to the points of centre of gravity.[4] These pictures were transferred onto graph paper, from which they calculated the forces (Fig. 48.1). In addition to demonstrating that a soldier could carry much greater weights with a knapsack across his shoulders than if it was straddled across his lower back, Braune and Fischer enumerated the phases of the gait cycle and established the basics of modern biomechanics. (Note that the British infantryman was still using a bum bag at the time of the First World War whilst his German counterpart could carry a much greater weight in his shoulder knapsack! Do the experiment

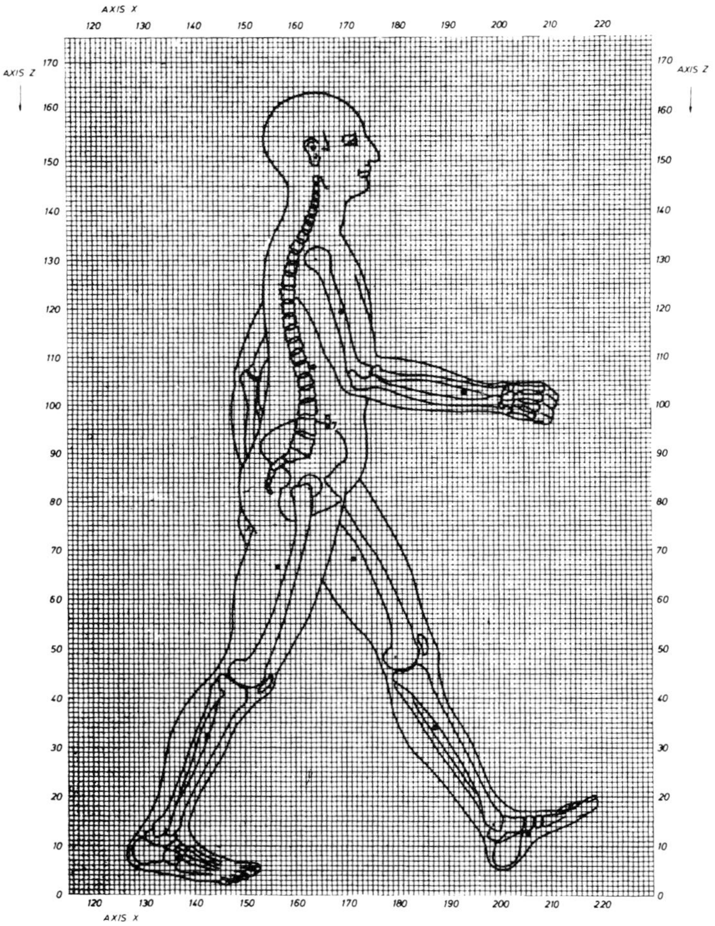

Fig. 48.1 The infantry sergeant at phase 22 of gait. Reproduced from Braune and Fischer.[4]

REFERENCES

1. Maquet P G J Biomechanics of the Knee, 2nd edn. Springer-Verlag, Berlin 1984
2. Pauwels F Biomechanics of the Normal and Diseased Hip. Springer-Verlag, Berlin 1976
3. Braune W, Fischer O On the Centre of Gravity of the Human Body 1985. Translated by Maquet PGJ, Furlong R, Springer-Verlag, Berlin 1985
4. Braune W, Fischer O The Human Gait. Translated by Maquet PGJ, Furlong R. Springer-Verlag, Berlin 1987

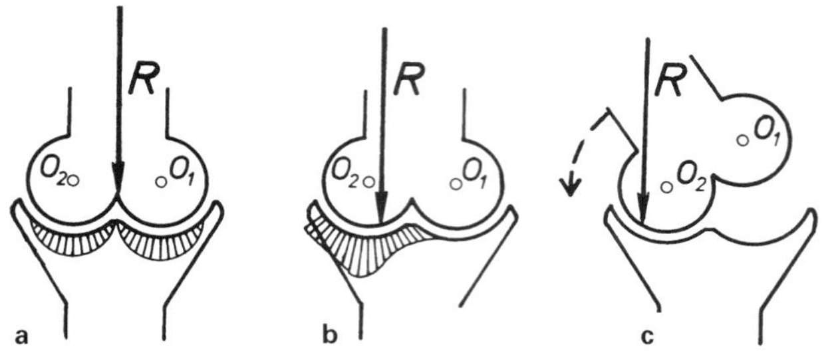

Fig. 48.2 'Knee model' to illustrate **(a)** the joint in balance: central load, even subchondral sclerosis; **(b)** the joint unbalanced but stable: load offset but between the subsidiary centres of rotation 01 and 02. Causes uneven subchondral sclerosis but joint retains stability; **(c)** the joint unbalanced and unstable: load outside subsidiary centre of rotation 02.

yourself. You do not need to be an expert in gait analysis to understand basic biomechanics.)

Consider Figure 48.2, a dual articular model. When the resultant passes through the centre of the joint (Fig. 48.2a) the joint is in balance and the stresses are evenly spread through the 'subchondral' bone. If the resultant force moves from the centre but is still within the subsidiary centre of rotation of one of the condyles then the articulation will still be stable but the stresses will be uneven (Fig. 48.2b). Bone, being a living substance, will respond to that increased stress and according to Wolfe's law will lay down more bone, thereby producing localized sclerosis. This may be observed in the operating theatre during a knee replacement for a varus osteoarthritic joint. The medial side of the joint will be much harder and more sclerotic than the under-stressed lateral side. If the resultant force moves even further from the centre so that it falls outside the centre of rotation of either of the condyles then the joint becomes potentially unstable (Fig. 48.2c). It is when this occurs that the ligament on the opposite side of the joint, i.e. the lateral collateral complex for a bow leg, will begin to stretch. This creates the so called 'shift sign' which we will observe when we discuss osteoarthritis later in the chapter. This concept of balance when the resultant is central can be clearly illustrated by photoelastic models (Fig. 48.3).

Let us now consider the classic Maquet diagram (Fig. 48.4). When standing on one leg the knee has to support the whole mass of the body, with the exception of the leg and the foot below the knee that we are considering. This mass acts through a point S7 (note the difference from S6, the centre of gravity of the whole body). Thus, in considering the knee in the coronal plane we have force *P*, the weight of the body minus the leg distal to the loaded knee, which passes medial to the medial femoral condyle. This equilibrium must be balanced by the force in the lateral complex and in particular the iliotibial band. When studying your basic anatomy you may well have wondered why the gluteus maximus has two-thirds of its insertion into the iliotibial band! Gluteus maximus plus the tensor fascia lata, both of which lie in the same muscular plane, are very important stabilizers of the knee. Also note that the lateral ligament itself is relatively weak in comparison to the medial ligament complex, a fact which underlines not only the importance of the iliotibial band but which, as we shall see when we consider osteoarthritis, creates significant differences in

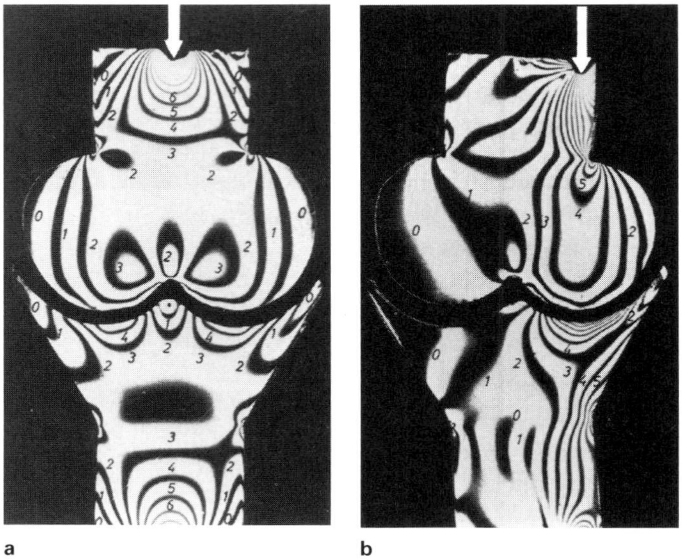

Fig. 48.3 Photoelastic models to illustrate change in the distribution of contact stresses as the load moves from being central **(a)** to affect but with subsidiary centre of rotation; **(b)** to above the subsidiary centre of rotation 02 in Figure 48.1. Reproduced from Maquet.[1]

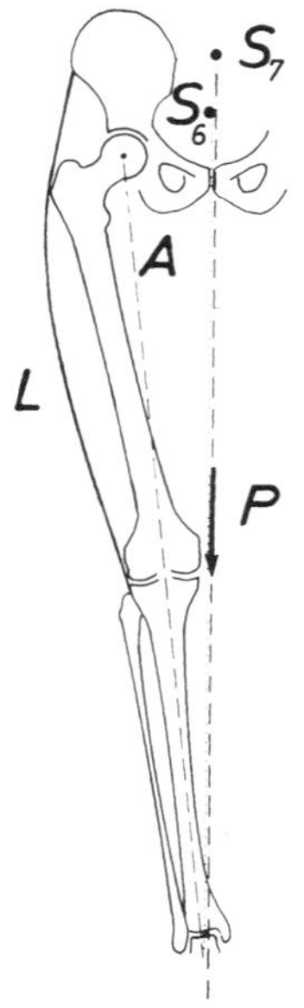

Fig. 48.4 The classic Maquet diagram illustrating the so-called mechanical axis (actually an anatomical axis) of the limb and the forces acting on the knee whilst standing balanced on one foot. S6, centre of gravity of the body; S7, centre of gravity of the part of the body supported by the knee; P, weight of the body acting through S7; L, muscular tension band (iliotibial band) balancing P. Reproduced from Maquet.[1]

the patterns of wear between the varus and the valgus knee. In the normal knee, however, there must be a balance and this is expressed by the fact that the resultant *R* passes through the centre of the knee. You will appreciate that this analysis is not only much simplified but is considering a static situation. 'Real-time' gait analysis is a highly complex investigation carried out in specially equipped laboratories. Not surprisingly, these studies indicate that

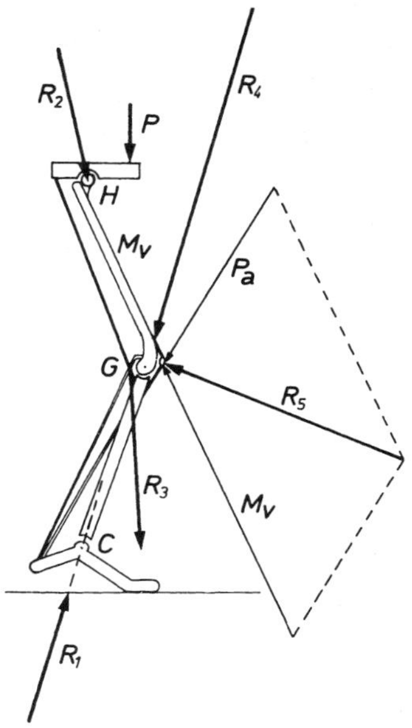

Fig. 48.5 Stance phase of gait prior to toe off. P, body weight; H, hip joint; G, knee; C, ankle; R1, resultant of P and action in the calf muscles; R2, resultant of P and action in the hamstrings; R3, resultant of R2 and gastrocnemius; R4, resultant of R3 and action in the patellar tendon; R5, resultant of action in the patellar tendon and the quadriceps. Reproduced from Maquet[1] after Kumer.[6]

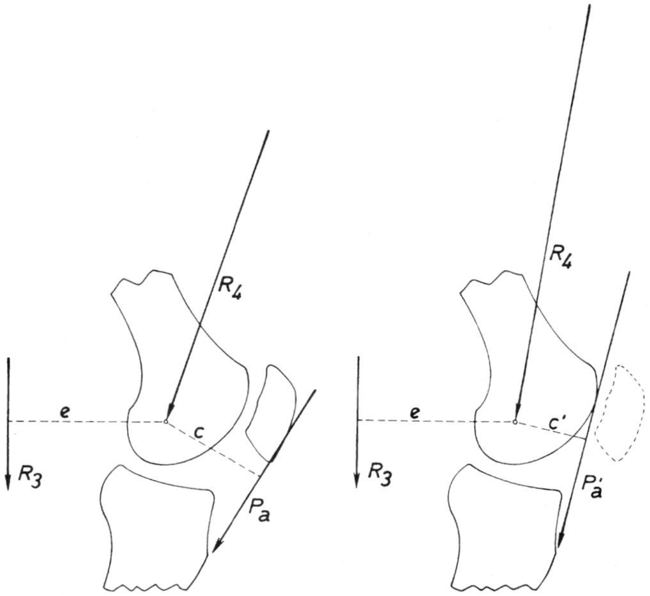

Fig. 48.6 Patellectomy profoundly alters knee mechanics. The patella is a 'distance piece'. Its removal (right) shortens the lever arm (C reduced to C1) and increases the forces acting across the femerotibial joint—note increase in R4 represented here by the length of the arrow. Reproduced from Maquet.[1]

the site through which the resultant passes is much more complex than indicated by this simple but elegant analysis of Maquet.[5] However, unlike gait analysis, knowledge of the mechanical axis provides the surgeon not only with an easily measured parameter on a plain X-ray but also a baseline he can actually use in theatre for osteotomy or knee replacement surgery. As a surgeon you do not need to comprehend the intricacies of gait analysis but you must be able to understand and utilize Maquet's concepts and the importance of the mechanical axis.

By considering the forces acting on the leg in the sagittal plane a similar understanding of the compressive forces acting across the femerotibial and the patellofemoral joints can be appreciated. This analysis, quoted and utilized by Maquet, is derived from the work of Kummer,[6] who considered the leg in the stance phase of the gait cycle at the point when the forces were acting through the forefoot, i.e. just before toe off (Fig. 48.5). Kummer derived a sequence of resultants: R1 on the ankle, R2 on the hip which, as it acts behind the knee and when taken together with the action of the gastrocnemius, produces R3 which tends to flex the knee. This is balanced by the forces acting through the patellar tendon to generate R4, which of necessity intersects the axis of flexion of the femerotibial joint. Finally, we can derive R5, which is the compression force acting across the patellofemoral joint. You will now appreciate one of the main functions of the patella. It is a distance piece increasing the lever arm distance between the patellar tendon and the centre of rotation of the patellofemoral joint (Fig. 48.6). It will also be readily understood why the operation of patellectomy is destructive since it decreases this lever arm distance, thereby making the mechanism mechanically inefficient. The kangaroo, a marsupial, does not have a patella but it derives its mechanical advantage from the remarkable prominence of its tibial tubercle (Fig. 48.7). Man has a large patella and a small tibial tubercle, a compromise to allow both kneeling as well as crouching. Perhaps it is not surprising that the hyaline cartilage articular surface of the patella is the thickest in the human body for in man, with his upright posture and hence the requirement to have full extension as well as full flexion, nature would seem to approach the design limits of this articular biomaterial (Fig. 48.8). Again, given this understanding, perhaps we should not be too surprised that anterior knee pain, like backache, is such a common orthopaedic symptom.

Finally, in considering balance around a joint it is essential to appreciate the role of the ligaments. For example, the anterior and posterior cruciates can be considered in engineering terms to be a four-bar linkage system. Zavatsky et al[7] using this hypothesis have elegantly shown that computerized mathematical modelling systems will reproduce the shape of the articular surfaces that we see in the normal knee. If the cruciate mechanism is destroyed by injury this relationship between the movement of the joint and its ligamentous restraints will be lost, thereby allowing the generation of abnormal shear forces between the surfaces of the femur and tibia. Similarly if a surgeon carrying out an anterior cruciate reconstruction places his repair in the wrong anatomical position or in too great a tension then abnormal forces will likewise be generated within the joint and the articular surfaces will no longer match the arc of rotation imposed by the ligaments. Thus, whilst the anterior

REFERENCES

5. Johnson F, Leitl S J Bone Joint Surg 1980; 62: 346–349
6. Kumer B Clin Orthop Related Res 1962; 25: 32–41
7. Zavatsky AB, O'Connor J J, Lu TW Orthop Int 1996; 4(5): 349

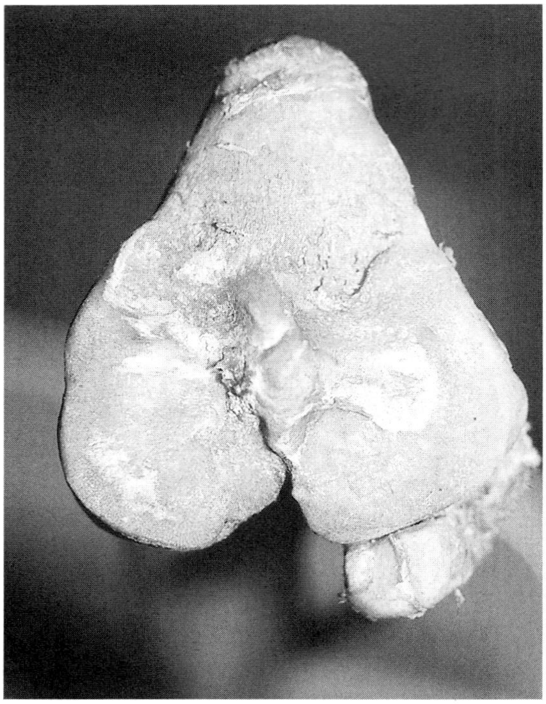

a

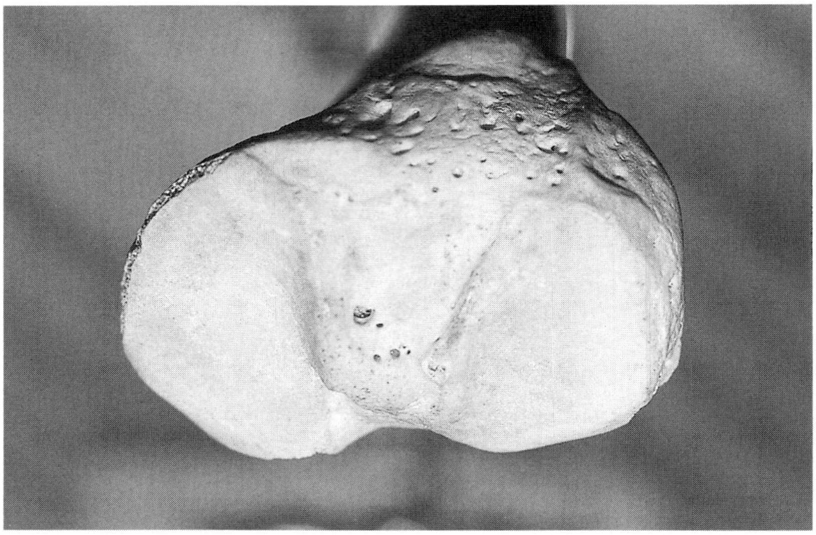

b

Fig. 48.7 The kangaroo has no patella but derives mechanically efficiency from the anterior prominence of the tibial tubercle. **(a)** Tibia of kangaroo viewed from above. **(b)** Human tibia viewed from above for comparison.

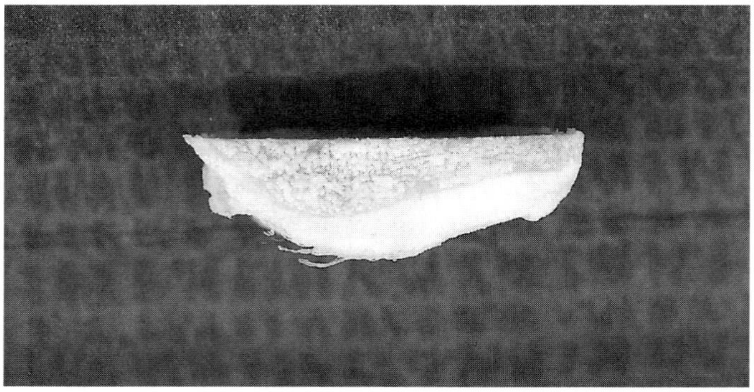

Fig. 48.8 Transverse section across patella. The articular surface is the thickest in the human body.

cruciate deficient knee is undoubtedly at risk of developing osteoarthritis secondary to its abnormal laxity it may well be at even greater risk from poorly performed reconstructive surgery.

For good surgical results a clear understanding of the basic principles plus technical precision are required. In the short term you may 'get away' with ignoring these principles but they will show in your figures of failure in the long term. Put in a knee replacement with little regard for leg alignment and doubtless the wound will heal, the patient will leave hospital in standard time, they may even get an excellent early result but they may be facing revision surgery five years postoperatively.

MAKING THE DIAGNOSIS

The knee can suffer a remarkably wide range of pathology. The objective in taking a history is to narrow down the options. You need to elucidate both 'what' and 'where', i.e. think both pathology and anatomy. A very useful approach is that of White of Oswestry, whose diagnostic ready-reckoner is shown in Table 48.1 and defines six main categories.

As regards the individual symptoms, *pain* is the commonest presenting complaint. There may be a clear history of injury and a clear involvement of one or other compartments, in which case the diagnosis may be straightforward. In the acutely painful knee never ignore the history of a pop or a snap; indeed this probably means that there has been a rupture of a major ligament. Acute pain and swelling following an injury impliy an acute haemarthrosis. In the absence of injury or a bleeding disorder these symptoms imply an acute synovitis or arthritis. Pseudogout due to calcium pyrophosphate crystals is a good example. Beware, however, of pain secondary to a low-grade synovitis. It is remarkable how often tuberculosis is missed and a diagnostic delay of up to a year is not uncommon.

Pain secondary to a meniscal injury is usually related to the medial or lateral compartment; however, pain arising from mechanical problems in the patellofemoral joint is often much more poorly localized. Classically it is anterior knee pain but, unfortunately, it often has a non-classical presentation with pains either being rather vague or else spreading across the medial femoral condyle and being confused with meniscal problems. Both meniscal and patellofemoral pain may be aggravated by rotation and even experienced knee surgeons may find patella problems and meniscal problems difficult to distinguish from each other. The pain of osteoarthritis is usually of a gradual onset over many years, has a clear mechanical pattern, and is located to the affected compartment, i.e., varus osteoarthritis gives medial joint pain.

Pain in the back of the knee is often diagnostically difficult. It is commonly due to tension in a Baker's cyst but this in itself is a secondary diagnosis, not a primary one, since a Baker's cyst is due

Table 48.1 The six main categories of knee problems

1. Internal derangement	Torn meniscus Bucket handle tear Flap tear	Chondral flap Femoral condyle	Loose body Chondral loose body Osteochondral loose body (e.g. osteochondritis dissecans)
2. Possible torn ligament	Anterior cruciate ligament	Medial collateral ligament	Posterior cruciate ligament Lateral collateral ligament
3. Arthritis	Varus knee Medial OA	Valgus knee Lateral OA	Inflammatory arthropathy (e.g. rheumatoid arthritis)
4. Anterior knee pain	Anterior knee pain syndrome	Chondromalacia patellae	Lateral compression syndrome Patellofemoral osteoarthritis
5. Patellar instability	Lateral subluxation	Lateral dislocation Single, recurrent or habitual	
6. The rest	For example, extensor mechanism rupture, cysts, Osgood–Schlatter syndrome		

After S White DM. FRCS, Consultant Orthopaedic Surgeon, Robert James and Agnes Hunt Orthopaedic Hospital. Published in the *Assessment and Management of Knee Problems—Practical Problems*. Series 3. Arthritis and Rheumatism Council, Chesterfield, UK.

to fluid within the knee being pumped backwards into an outpouching of the synovial cavity. The primary diagnosis is the cause of the effusion. Pain can, of course, be referred. Medical students know that hip problems, classically a slipped capital femoral epiphysis in the teenager, can present with knee pain but in a busy clinic it is all too easy to forget this association. There are no shortcuts to a proper detailed history concerning knee pain and the 'standard' information of onset, length of time, site, severity, aggravating or relieving factors is 'essential' information.

The knee is subject to two 'dramatic' symptoms: *locking* and *giving way*. The term locking is unfortunate since it is poorly understood by patients, who frequently confuse locking with stiffness. 'Does your knee suddenly jam?' is a far better question. Classically it is due to a torn meniscus or a loose body but the knee can come to an instant halt with recurrent patella dislocation and rotary instability secondary to a torn anterior cruciate ligament. Giving way is divided into 'minor', in which the knee just buckles but the patient then regains control, or 'major', in which the patient actually falls. Major giving way, unaccompanied by any warning, is a most unpleasant symptom. Not only is the patient likely to sustain other injuries but they will be in a permanent state of apprehension if they are unable to walk safely downstairs or across a road. The common cause of giving way is instability either within the patellofemoral mechanism or from ligamentous injury, particularly to the anterior cruciate.

The three other classical orthopaedic symptoms, *stiffness*, *swelling* and *deformity*, are in general less helpful in making a diagnosis. As Apley[8] has so clearly taught, patients complain of stiffness when in fact they mean painful limitation of movement which, of course, is a physical sign that you have to elicit. Early morning stiffness is a classical symptom of rheumatoid arthritis but it is much less pronounced in the knee than it is in the fingers. Swelling is another symptom that needs to be verified by signs. The pre-patellar bursa, the cyst of the lateral meniscus and Baker's cyst are three examples of localized swellings around the knee that are easily diagnosed in the clinic. Beware of bony swellings in teenagers or young adults. Whilst a benign exostosis is the commonest of the bone tumours don't forget that the knee has the highest incidence of the rarer malignant tumours, of which the commonest is the osteogenic sarcoma. As a symptom, generalized swelling can obviously be due to an effusion, though it is surprising how frequently a patient with an osteoarthritic knee and a moderate effusion has failed to spot that the knee is swollen, whereas adolescents with teenage anterior knee pain often exhibit the reverse, complaining of swelling when the surgeon cannot find an effusion! Deformity is an unusual presenting symptom though it is a sign frequently found. It is remarkable how many patients have failed to notice that with the onset of osteoarthritis they have become bow-legged or knock-kneed.

The signs

The knee joint is a large superficial joint, and being easily accessible for examination there are numerous signs to be elicited. Examination should be done in a logical manner and the Apley system of look, feel, move cannot be bettered.[8]

First, 'look' at the patient standing to attention with feet facing forwards and parallel to each other. Look from the front, the sides and the back, looking, in particular, for:

1. Varus–valgus deformity: in the normally aligned knee both medial femoral condyles and both medial malleoli should just touch. If the patient is fat it is easy to be deceived and to miss a bow-legged deformity. If in doubt put your hand between the two knees and see whether it is bone or just fat that is touching;
2. Muscle wasting, in particular loss of quadriceps bulk;
3. Loss of full extension of the knee;
4. Swellings, for example, an effusion or an infrapatellar bursa.

Next, observe the patient walking, in particular note whether the knee fully extends on heel strike.

Lay the patient down and feel for the following:

1. Warmth—this is best felt by running a hand sequentially down both legs and observing any change in the temperature gradient rather than just directly comparing both knees. The commonest cause of warm knee is that the patient has been wearing a crêpe bandage! However, warmth is an important sign.

REFERENCE

8. Apley A G, Solomon L Apley's System of Orthopaedics and Fracture, 7th edn. Butterworth Heinemann, Oxford 1993

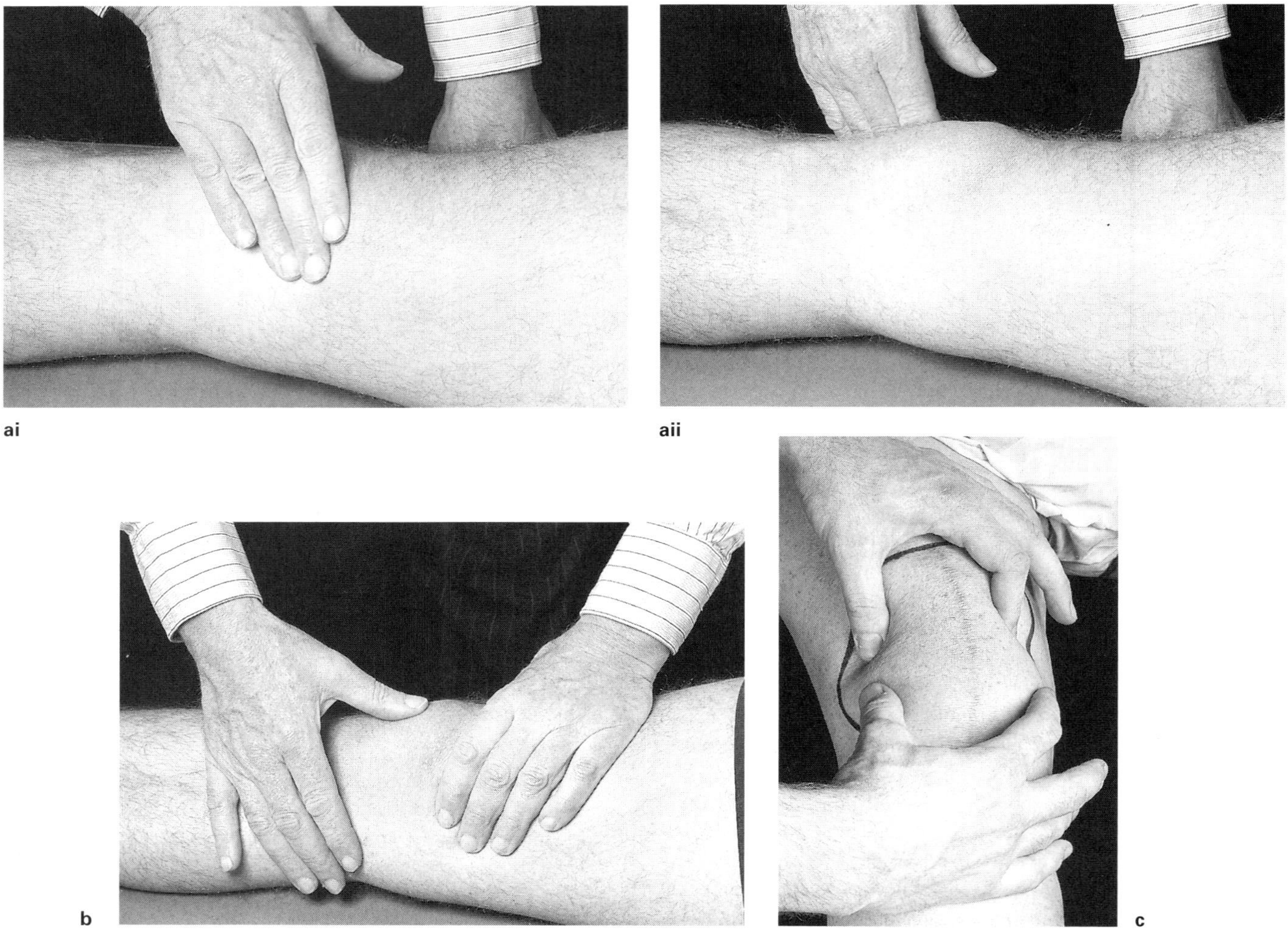

Fig. 48.9 Diagnosing an effusion. **(a)** The 'bulge' test. Milk the fluid from the medial side. **(ai)** Run it back into the medial side by compressing the lateral side of the patella **(aii)**. **(b)** The patella tap. Firstly compress the suprapatellar pouch. Secondly tap the patella. **(c)** Cross-fluctuation: the test for a large effusion.

Whilst tuberculosis may produce 'cold abscesses' it is a low-grade infective process and will produce local warmth.

2. Synovial thickening—this is best felt by rolling the top of the suprapatellar pouch under one's fingers as there is a double thickness of the synovium at this site.

3. An effusion—the three classical signs are (Fig. 48.9a) the bulge test for a small effusion: compress medial side of the patella then run your fingers along the lateral side starting distally and moving proximally; if there is a small effusion a ripple will be seen to pass downwards, filling the hollow that is normally present on the medial side of the patella (Fig. 48.9b); the patella tap for a moderate effusion: compress the suprapatellar pouch with one hand (palm on the suprapatellar pouch, thumb and index finger along both sides of the patella) whilst gently tapping the patella down onto the femoral groove with the index finger of the other hand (Fig. 48.9c); cross-fluctuation: a large effusion.

4. Joint line tenderness.

(a) the patella—not only is it possible to feel for tenderness all round the patella, but by displacing it medially and laterally one can feel 'under the patella' (Fig. 48.10) Tenderness of the distal pole is found in teenagers with the Johannsen–Sindig–Larsen syndrome. A similar condition in adults is termed 'jumper's knee'. This is most frequently seen in middle-aged athletes, particularly those training for the marathon. The tenderness of jumper's knee usually becomes much better localized when examined with the knee flexed. Tenderness at the distal insertion of the patellar tendon in teenagers is the traction apophysitis of Osgood–Schlatter.

(b) The medial and lateral compartment—examine for joint line tenderness with the knee flexed (Fig. 48.11). Don't forget to start anteriorly in the triangle formed by the tibia below, the femur above and the patellar tendon to the side. In a fat knee you will not locate the joint line if you start over the site of the collateral ligaments! This is important since the only physical sign that might distinguish a torn meniscus from a partial rupture of the medial ligament is the fact that partial ruptures of the medial ligament always affect the femoral insertion, i.e., above the joint line. Meniscal injury will produce tenderness on the joint line.

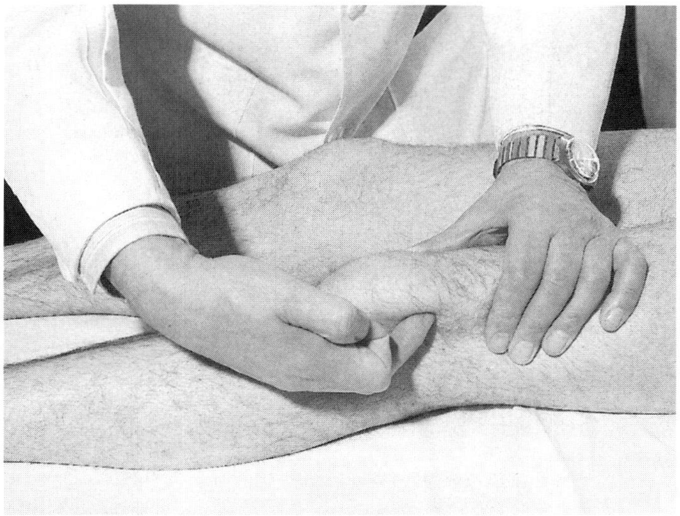

Fig. 48.10 Feeling for patella tenderness. Displace the patella medially and, feeling under the medial facet, push it laterally and feel the lateral facet. Do this gently as this is uncomfortable if done roughly even in a normal knee!

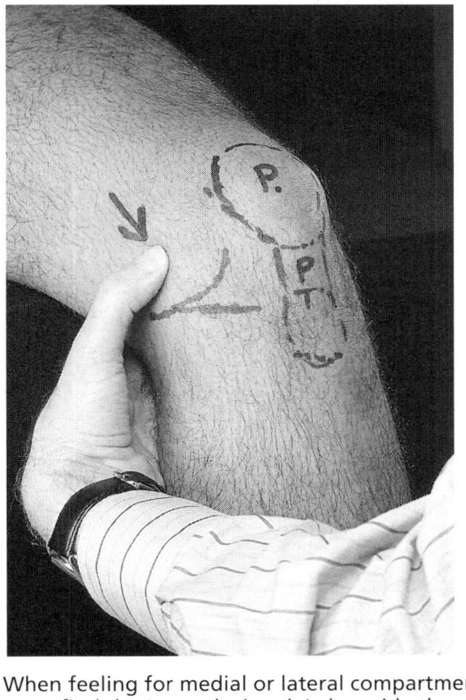

Fig. 48.11 When feeling for medial or lateral compartment joint line tenderness, find the 'central triangle' alongside the patellar tendon and then move along the joint line. Here the patella, the 'triangle' and the femoral origin of the medial ligament are worked. This patient has a sprain of the medial ligament. Note the tender spot is above the joint line **(ii)**. Meniscal tenderness is on the joint line.

(c) Other common sites of tenderness—these are mostly at the muscle insertions around the joint; the lateral hamstring, the biceps femoris at the fibular head; the medial hamstring, semimembranosus, at the posteromedial corner; the pes anserinus group of sartorius, gracilis and semitendinosus over the junction of the metaphysis and the shaft of the tibia medially; and the insertion of the iliotibial band at Gerdy's tubercle laterally. In association with the latter, check for any associated tenderness over the greater trochanter at the hip. This often indicates over-stressing of the iliotibial band, and reflects a compensatory mechanism when the quadriceps are malfunctioning, for example with patella maltracking.

5. Any 'lump' should be examined to determine its site and its origin. Cysts of the lateral meniscus are deceptive to the inexperienced. As they are deep to the iliotibial band they feel almost bony hard (Fig. 48.12a). A hard lump along the lateral joint line which is most obvious when the knee is slightly flexed but decreases or disappears at full extension or flexion is a cyst of the lateral meniscus, not an osteophyte or an exostosis! Cysts of the medial meniscus are much less common, are larger and more obviously cystic, with a tendency to 'migrate' away from the joint line, sometimes as far distally as the pes anserinus insertion, where they may be confused with a pes anserine bursitis (Fig. 48.12b).

'Housemaid's knee' is due to a bursitis of the pre-patellar bursa, whilst 'clergyman's knee' arises from the infrapatellar bursa. These, as their colloquial names imply, are occupational and normally resolve if the irritative cause, i.e., kneeling, is removed. They can become infected, in which case aspiration for microbiological diagnosis and treatment with rest and antibiotics are required. Occasionally surgical drainage is needed. Don't forget that gout is a rare cause of bursitis!

The semimembranosus bursa lying between the semimembranosus muscle and the medial head of the gastronemius is a common cause of swelling in children and teenagers. It is most obvious when the knee is extended and usually lies medial to the midline, posteriorly in the popliteal fossa. These cysts nearly always disappear spontaneously and are best left alone. If it is a cause of aching discomfort treat by aspiration. Avoid surgery, which at best leaves a scar and at worst is complicated by recurrence.

The popliteal cyst, termed a 'Baker's cyst', is not a true cyst but is secondary to an outpouching of the synovium into the popliteal fossa. The pathology is in the knee, not in the Baker's cyst, and treatment should be aimed at the problem within the joint. If a popliteal cyst ruptures it will produce symptoms that can be clinically indistinguishable from a deep vein calf thrombosis with swelling and tenderness of the calf and a positive Homans' sign. Erroneous treatment with anticoagulants may well produce a very large bruise. If in doubt the diagnosis should be confirmed by venography or by arthrography; indeed it is one of the few remaining indications for arthrography of the knee.

Movements

Flexion extension: testing for restricted movement

The degree of joint laxity varies from patient to patient but not within a patient, i.e., both knees should be similar. Thus, if the normal knee has 10 degrees of hyperextension but the symptomatic knee merely extends to zero then that is abnormal and it may indicate 'locking', for example, a bucket handle tear of a meniscus. Therefore, when examining for full extension, press the knee into the couch with one hand and lift the heel off the couch with the

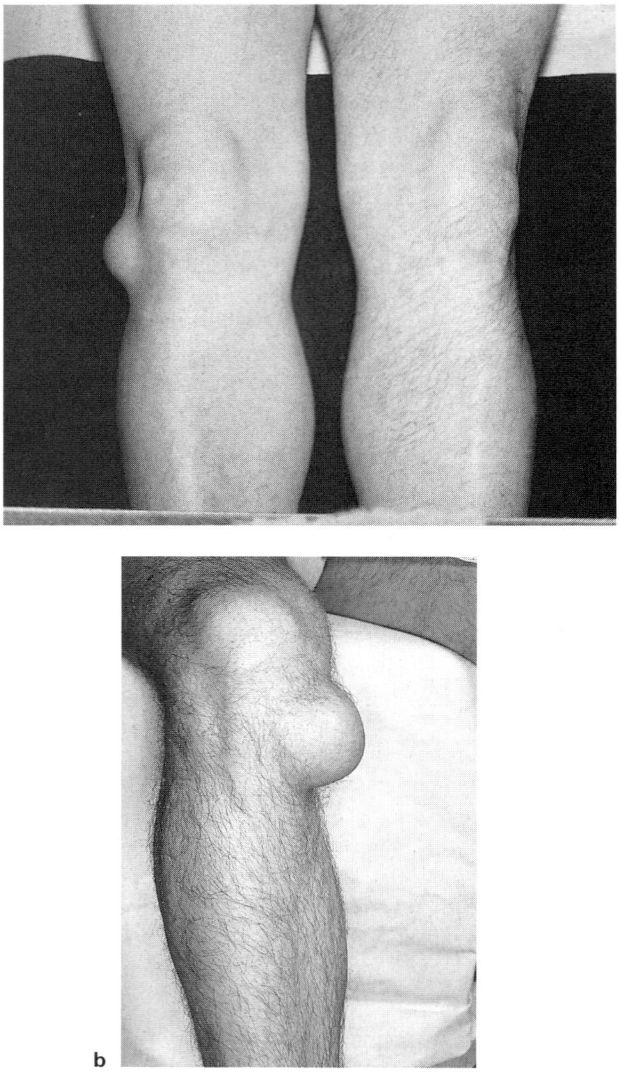

Fig. 48.12 **(a)** A cyst of the lateral meniscus can feel almost bony hard. However, it varies with the position of knee flexion. **(b)** By comparison medial meniscal cysts are larger, softer and may migrate distally.

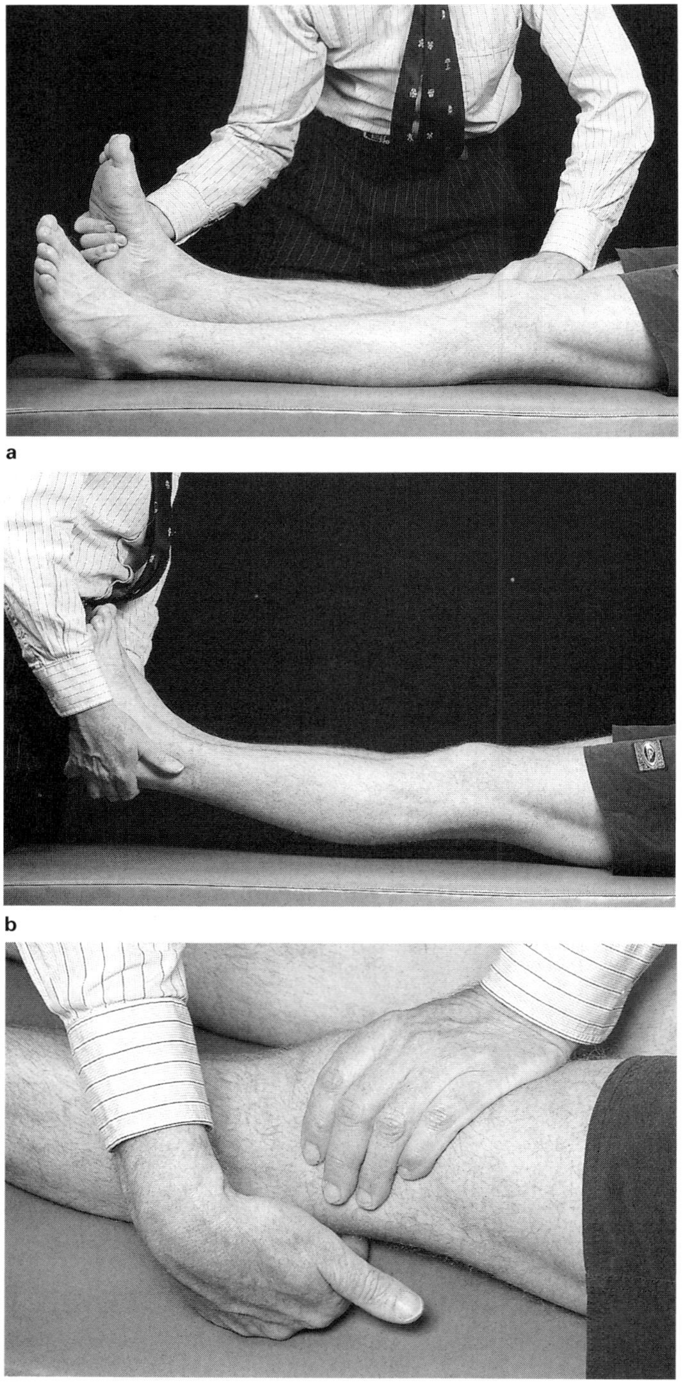

Fig. 48.13 Testing for full extension. If the normal knee has hyperextension so should the symptomatic. A knee may extend to zero but still be 'locked', since if there is natural hyperextension it should go to −10 or −5 degrees, depending on the degree of natural laxity. Another trap for the unwary! **(a)** Comparing the distance the heel comes off the couch. **(b)** Comparing the position of the knees with both legs held by the heels. **(c)** Feeling for a flexion gap.

other; compare both legs (Fig. 48.13). An alternative method is to lift both legs off the couch, holding them by the heels, and to observe relative positions of the patellae. A useful trick is to see how easily one can get one's hand behind the knee. If there is a gap then the knee is not fully extending. For flexion, simply bend both knees up together and observe the distance between the heels and the buttocks.

Ligaments: testing for abnormal movements

There is a considerable skill in testing the collateral and cruciate ligaments. The anatomical screw home mechanism, which provides us with an ability to stand without needing to use quadriceps action, is dependent on tension in the collateral ligaments, the anterior cruciate ligament and a few fibres of the posterior cruciate ligament. If a knee is unstable on varus/valgus testing in extension, it follows that more than one of the main ligaments will have been damaged. It is therefore necessary to test the collaterals in a few degrees of flexion as well as in full extension. In the author's

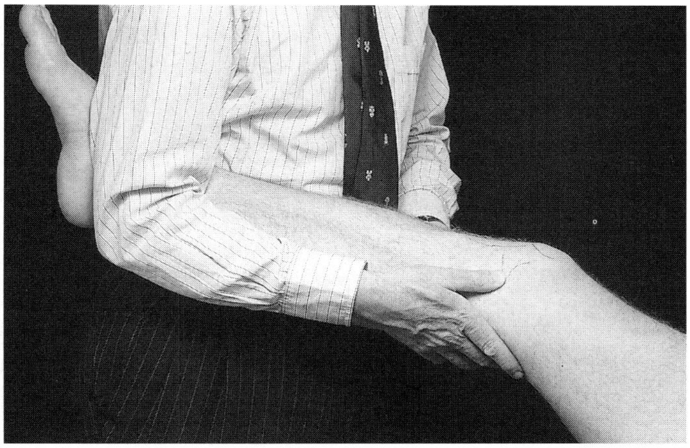

Fig. 48.14 Testing for varus–valgus instability. The examiner is applying a valgus and feeling for the integrity of the medial ligament with his thumb.

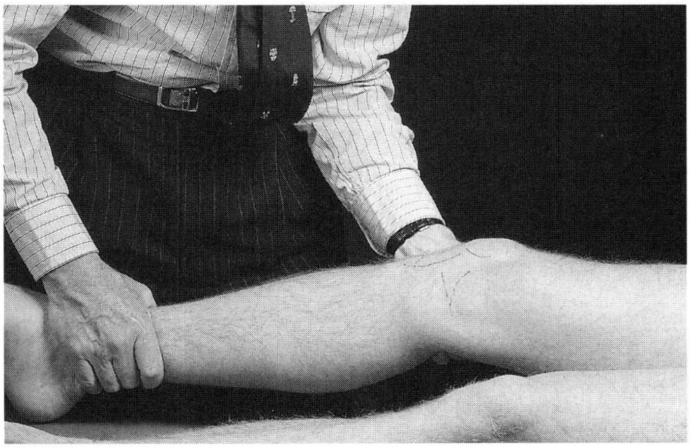

Fig. 48.15 Testing for varus–valgus instability. The 'traditional' method. The disadvantages are that you cannot palpate the ligament or tell so easily whether one compartment is 'opening' or its opposite side is 'shutting'!

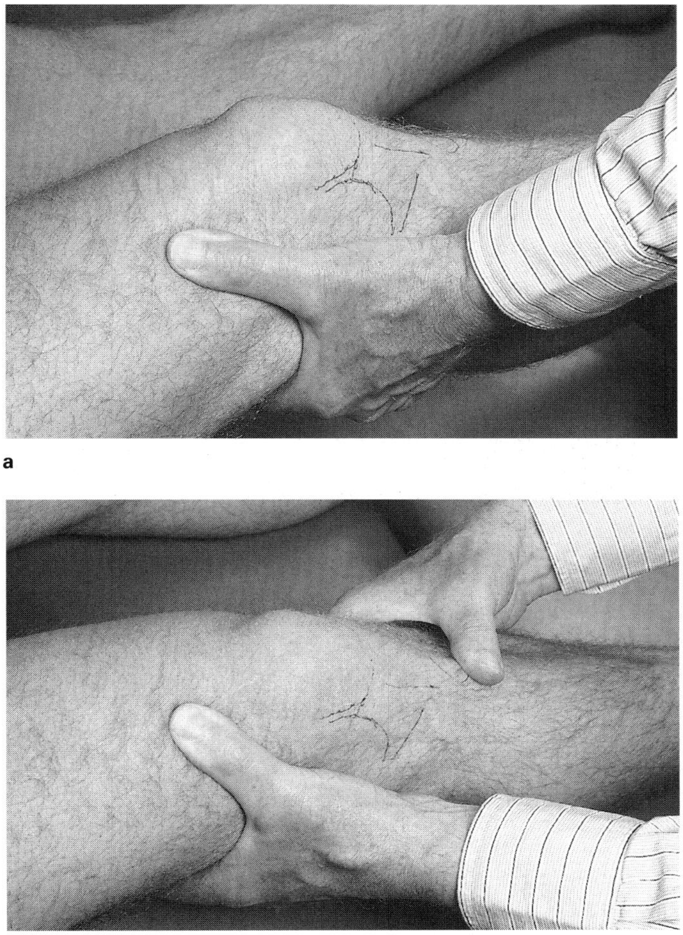

a

b

Fig. 48.16 The Lachman test for the anterior cruciate ligament is done at 30 degrees flexion. **(a)** Let the patient's knee rest in the palm of your hand and wait until the patient is completely relaxed, then hold the distal thigh firmly with your thumb. **(b)** With your other hand grasp the proximal calf. Your thumb needs to be at the tibial tubercle. Firmly displace the tibia forwards. Feel for the 'end-point' of the ACL. Compare both knees.

opinion this is best done by securing the foot between the examiner's arm and brim of pelvis so that both hands are free to be placed along the joint lines of the knee (Fig. 48.14). It is then possible to palpate the medial ligament as a tight band when one applies a valgus stress. This method of examination will also detect rotary movement at the medial tibial condyle which masquerades as laxity of the medial ligament in the anterior cruciate deficient knee. It also enables the examiner to distinguish between movement due to ligament disruption and movement due to bone loss such as occurs with osteoarthritis. The standard or traditional method is to hold the ankle with one hand and apply a counter force at the knee with the other hand (Fig. 48.15). Do this in a few degrees of flexion to relax the ligaments, i.e., anatomically unlock the knee.

The anterior cruciate ligament is best examined at 30 degrees of flexion—the Lachman test[9] (Fig. 48.16). This is a difficult test to learn. The crucial trick is to first support the leg in 30 degrees of knee flexion with one hand under the distal femur, waiting until the patient relaxes before applying anterior displacement of tibia on femur with the other hand. Feel not just for excessive movement but also the nature of the end-point. Is it absent or 'soft'? In the normal knee there is a sharp stop. If the end-point is soft it implies a partial rupture, i.e., one of the two bundles of the ligament has been torn.

The posterior cruciate ligament should be examined with both knees flexed up to 90 degrees (Fig. 48.17). First, note the relative position of the tibial tubercles. In the posterior cruciate-deficient knee the tibia will sink backwards and the angle of inclination between the patella and the tibial tubercle will correspondingly become more vertical. When feeling for the integrity of the posterior cruciate, place both hands high up into the popliteal fossa to offset any contraction of the hamstrings, pull the tibia sharply forward and then push it sharply backwards. Feel for the quality of

REFERENCE

9. Torg J S, Conrad W, Kalen V Am J Sports Med 1976; 4: 84

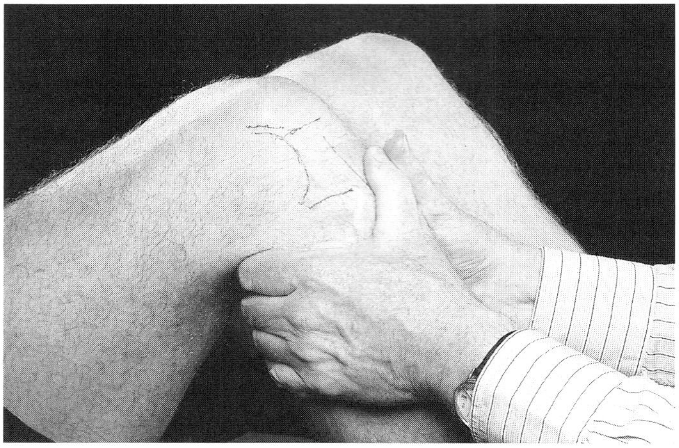

Fig. 48.17 Examining for the posterior cruciate ligament done at 90 degrees. The posterior draw test. Note that the knee is at 90 degrees. The examiner's fingers are high up in the popliteal fossa and his thumbs on the tibial tubercle.

the end-point as well as noting any excessive mobility. When doing this test it is useful to sit on the couch so that the patient's toes are stabilized against the thigh of the examiner. Make sure that both tibiae are tested in a similar degree of rotation. A normal knee will have considerably more mobility in the anteroposterior plane if tested with the tibia externally rotated than if tested with the tibia internally rotated. This is yet another trap for the unwary!

Special tests

Patella dislocation

Sometimes one is fortunate in that there is an X-ray showing that the patella is dislocated. This, however, is uncommon and patella dislocation and, even more so, subluxation are difficult to prove. The Apley apprehension test does give some indication but patients with patella tenderness, particularly along the medial facet, will exhibit apprehension as one attempts to dislocate the patella laterally. It is a useful adjunct to compare the end-points in both knees. As with ligaments the end-point will be 'soft' if the soft tissues have stretched. To permit dislocation there needs to be 2 cm of patella 'laxity'.[10]

The McIntosh manoeuvre[11]

This test for anterior cruciate instability is not easy to perform and is best learnt when the patient is anaesthetized in theatre prior to an anterior cruciate reconstruction. It is based on the fact that the anterior cruciate ligament is put under maximum stress when weight is taken through the slightly flexed knee with the foot firmly planted on the ground and the body twisted into external rotation, i.e., the tibia is being internally rotated and the femur externally rotated. The McIntosh test seeks to reproduce this movement with the patient lying supine. The technique for examining the right knee is as follows. Hold the heel of the right foot in your right hand; apply a gentle proximal pressure to reproduce the ground reaction force and rotate the foot inwards (Fig. 48.18a). Keeping the knee extended place the palm of the left hand over the neck of the fibula and apply an inward rotation force (Fig. 48.18b). Flex the knee. What you are feeling for is a jerk of relocation as the tibia in the anterior cruciate-deficient knee locates back onto the femur due to the action of the iliotibial band. False positives, which are rare, can be caused by a torn meniscus, i.e., you have produced a variation on McMurray's test! False negatives are common due mainly to lack of skill in eliciting this most difficult of signs. Even in patients who will not relax sufficiently you should be able to at least produce a positive apprehension test in the clinic even if you cannot elicit the jerk.

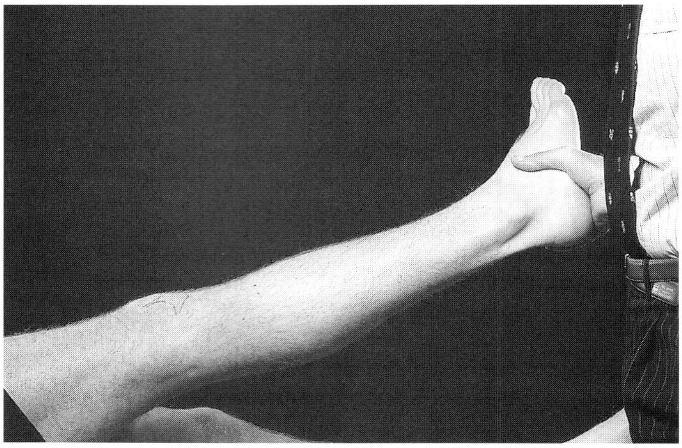

a

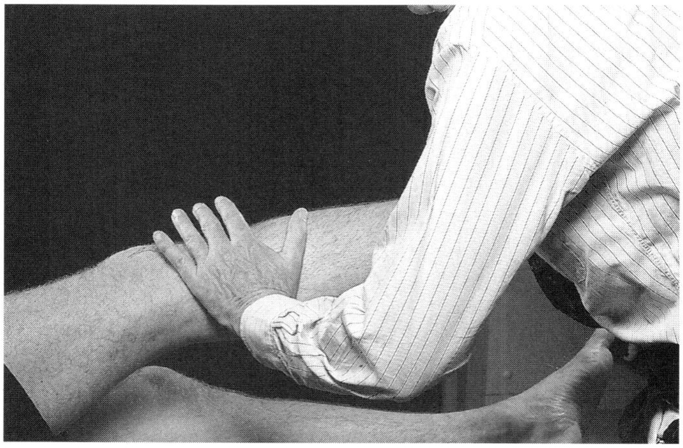

b

Fig. 48.18 The McIntosh test for anterior cruciate instability.

McMurray's test[12]

This classic physical sign has numerous individual variations. The objective is to trap the segment of torn meniscus in the joint and

REFERENCES

10. James S E, Heatley F W, Amis A A J Bone Joint Surg 1988; 70B: 496
11. Galway R D, Beaupre A, MacIntosh D L J Bone Joint Surg 1972; 54: 763
12. McMurray T P Br J Surg 1941; 29: 407

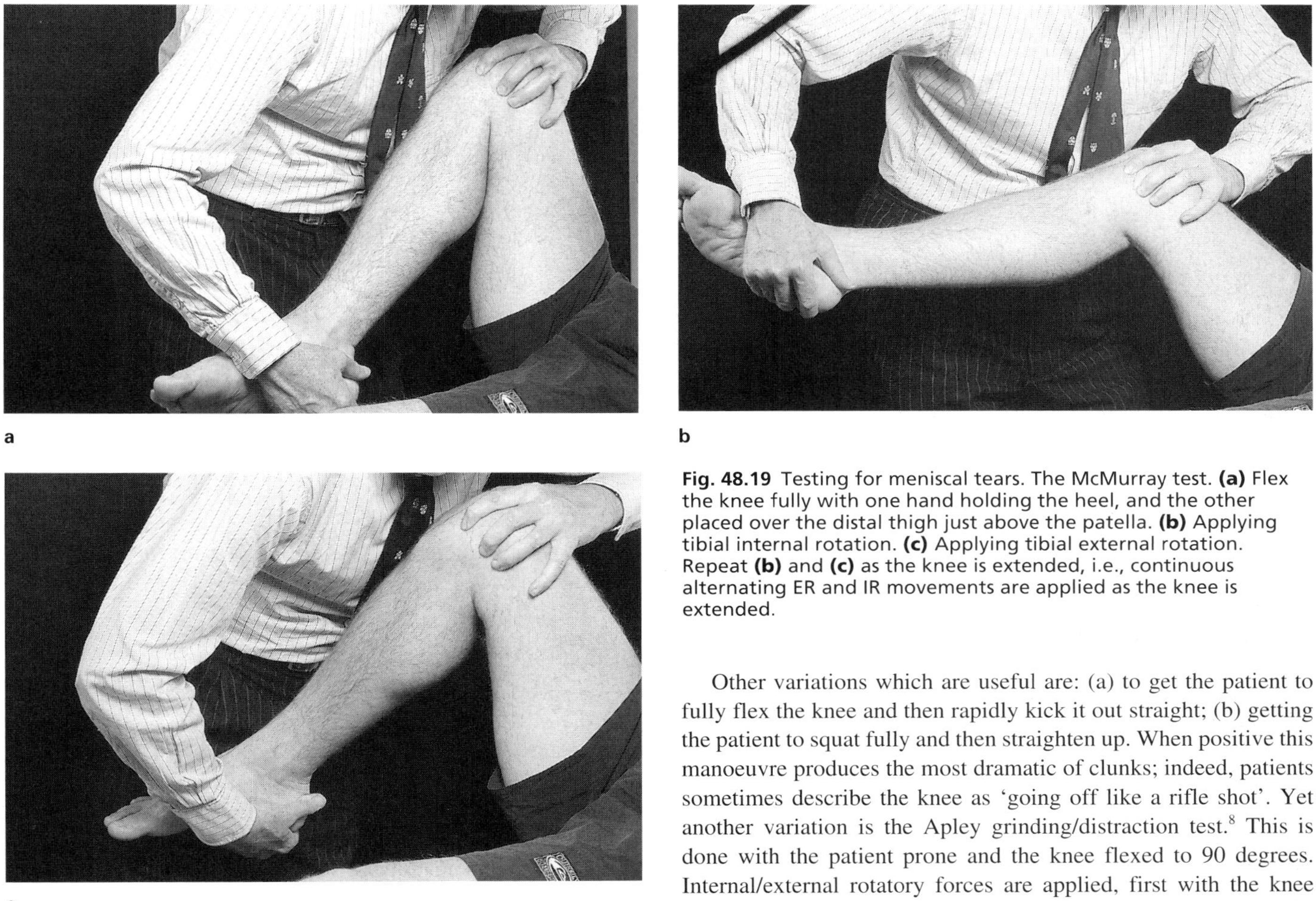

a

b

c

Fig. 48.19 Testing for meniscal tears. The McMurray test. **(a)** Flex the knee fully with one hand holding the heel, and the other placed over the distal thigh just above the patella. **(b)** Applying tibial internal rotation. **(c)** Applying tibial external rotation. Repeat **(b)** and **(c)** as the knee is extended, i.e., continuous alternating ER and IR movements are applied as the knee is extended.

then to relocate it. As the torn fragment passes between the joint surfaces it will produce a 'clunk'. Note that this is a deep noise and must be distinguished from the high-pitched clicks which usually arise from the patellofemoral joint. To trap the fragment, apply the dual force of compression and rotation. With the knee flexed beyond 90 degrees, grip the heel firmly with the right hand and with the left hand grip the distal thigh just above the patella (Fig. 48.19a). Take the leg from a position of valgus and external rotation to one of varus (Fig. 48.19b) and internal rotation (Fig. 48.19c). Repeat this rotary movement at several angles between full flexion and 90 degrees. The McMurray test was originally designed to diagnose posterior horn meniscal tears.

A common variation is to flex up the knee fully, applying an internal rotation/valgus force to the tibia as you flex. When at full flexion swing the tibia into external rotation. Keep the tibia externally rotated and, whilst maintaining compression on the medial compartment to reproduce a ground reaction force, straighten the knee out fully. In contrast to the classical method this test keeps the rotation constant whilst the knee is fully extended. You are ideally looking for a clunk. Compression on the lateral compartment is applied using a reverse sequence, i.e., flexion plus initial external rotation changed to internal rotation plus valgus, followed by moving the knee from full flexion to extension.

Other variations which are useful are: (a) to get the patient to fully flex the knee and then rapidly kick it out straight; (b) getting the patient to squat fully and then straighten up. When positive this manoeuvre produces the most dramatic of clunks; indeed, patients sometimes describe the knee as 'going off like a rifle shot'. Yet another variation is the Apley grinding/distraction test.[8] This is done with the patient prone and the knee flexed to 90 degrees. Internal/external rotatory forces are applied, first with the knee under compression and, secondly, with the knee distracted, the examiner holding the foot with both hands. The main merit of this test is that it helps to distinguish between pain arising from a torn meniscus and pain arising from a sprained ligament, particularly the medial collateral. The problem with all these tests for meniscus is that frequently one does not get a clunk, one merely reproduces the patient's pain!

Clinical tests of articular surface integrity

The objective of these tests is simultaneously to reproduce the patient's symptoms and determine the nature and quality of the crepitus. There is a distinct difference in both feel and sound from crepitus produced by chondromalacic cartilage and that produced by the rubbing of bone on bone.

Crepitus in the patellofemoral joint is common and in many cases is of little or no significance. To be meaningful it is essential that the pain and crepitus match the patient's symptoms. Sit the patient so that the legs are dangling free over the side of the couch with the knees flexed to 90 degrees. Ask the patient to extend first one knee and then the other. Observe the patella tracking. Listen for any crepitus. Repeat this with a hand placed gently over the patella, feeling for the vibration produced by crepitus. Finally, apply gentle resistance with one hand over the ankle whilst keeping the other over the patella and repeat the manoeuvre of

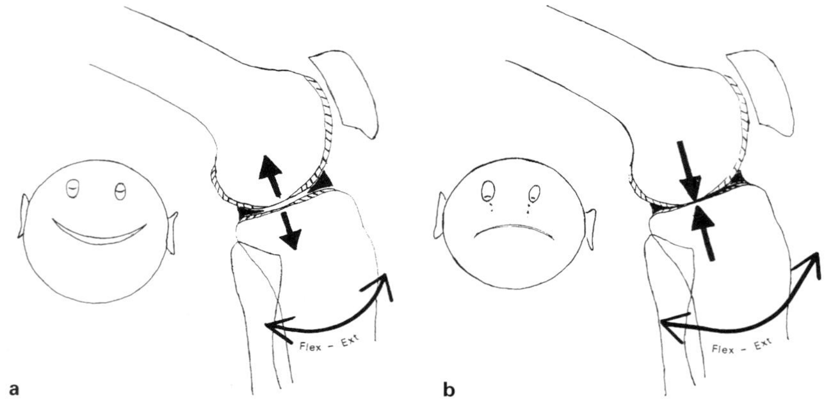

Fig. 48.20 Applying a destraction force to the worn compartment is comfortable (i.e., a valgus force with medial compartment osteoarthritis) but a compressive force reproduces the patient's pain.

extension. Get the patient to stand, again place your hands one over each patella and get the patient to crouch. Does this reproduce the patient's painful crepitus? If so, what is its nature? Chondromalacic or osteoarthritic, i.e., 'soft' cartilage or 'hard' bone on bone?

The agony test[13] (Fig. 48.20)

This is designed to determine the integrity of the surfaces of the medial and lateral compartments. It has the great merit over X-rays that it is dynamic as opposed to static and therefore enables the examiner to test the articular surface throughout the whole range of movement. If we suspect bony eburnation in the medial compartment, first try a valgus, i.e., opening force, flex and extend the knee in an identical manner to that which we have already described in testing integrity of the medial ligament. This manoeuvre will put pressure on the intact lateral compartment and produce neither pain nor crepitus, provided of course you don't put too great a valgus force and strain the medial ligament! Now, repeat the flexion–extension manouevre but with a varus compression force on the medial compartment. This is best done by externally rotating the hip so that the weight of the leg also adds to the compressive force produced by the examiner. If you produce bony crepitus and a 'cry of agony' you have proof-positive that the medial compartment has an area of total loss of articular cartilage.

Other useful tests

The crouch and duck walk test

This test can obviously be carried out at the same time as testing for patellofemoral crepitus. If the patient can fully crouch and duck walk and you have found no other abnormal physical signs you are unlikely to be missing any serious pathology even if the patient has major complaints. Certainly beware of trying to improve a knee that can do this manouevre since it is probably beyond the scope of surgery. Rather facetiously the author refers to patients who can crouch and duck walk, but have major complaints, as having 'the athlete's syndrome', i.e., they are 1% unfit but since they don't think they will win the race they won't actually start it! The caveat is that you can do injustice to the patient if (1) the problem is initial location of the patella into its groove, i.e., the problem is during early flexion, or (2) there is an anteriorly placed lesion on the femoral condyles, for example osteochondritis dissecans.

Hopping tests

These are useful dynamic tests for ligamentous stability, in particular the anterior cruciate. First, get the patient to hop on the spot; then get him to hop across the consulting room and, finally, get him to take one large hop. Patients with an anterior cruciate-deficient knee may, in particular, refuse to do the latter test, be very apprehensive about doing it or collapse when they land. If they can do the single hop compare the distance they can jump between the good and the injured leg.

INVESTIGATIONS

It cannot be over-stressed that the aim of these investigations, whether simple or complex, is to prove your clinical diagnosis, not to make the diagnosis.

Haematology

Many patients who present with an early inflammatory arthropathy mislead their surgeon by attributing their symptoms to a minor injury. A simple haemoglobin, white count and erythrocyte sedimentation rate (ESR) should be routine if there is any suspicion of synovial thickening or an unexplained effusion. Gouty arthropathy of the knee is uncommon but often missed.

Aspiration, culture and examination of the crystals

Rheumatologists are much more ready to aspirate knees than surgeons. This is probably because surgeons are more aware of the

REFERENCE

13. Heatley F W, Butler-Manuel A Curr Orthop 1990; 4: 79–87

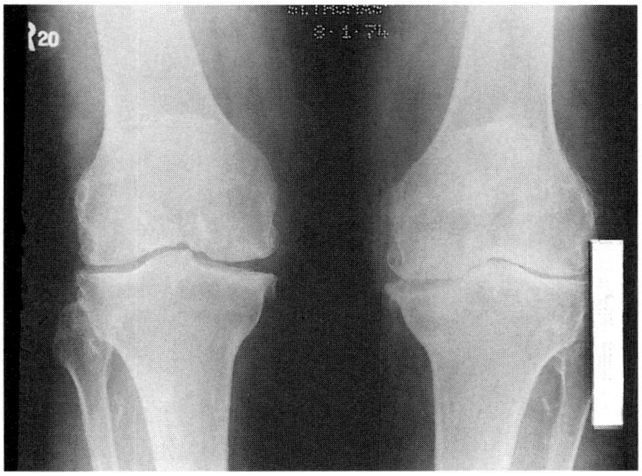

a

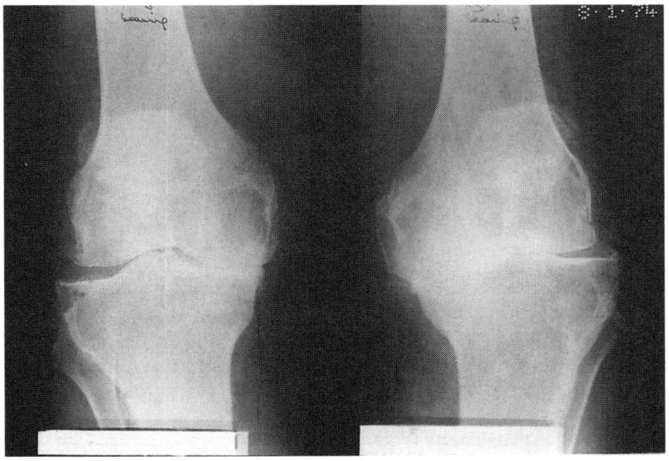

b

Fig. 48.21 This patient has clearly got osteoarthritis. However, film **(a)** taken supine shows a joint space. The standing film **(b)** reveals not only that there is no joint space in the medial compartment but that there is a severe varus deformity. *Lying X-rays frequently lie!*

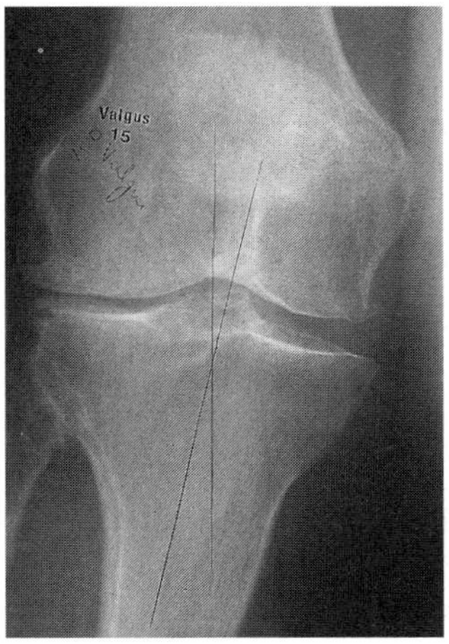

a

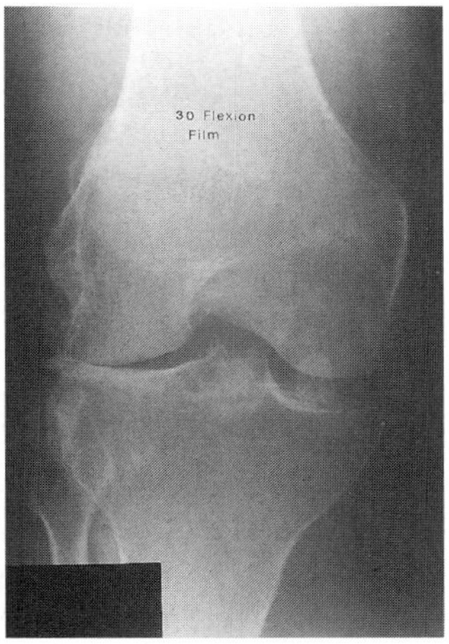

b

Fig. 48.22 (a) The long-leg film shows that this knee has a valgus deformity of 15 degrees. The lateral joint space is obviously diminished but still seems to be present. **(b)** The standing film at 30 degrees flexion shows that there is *no* joint space and point loading laterally.

risks of a secondary septic arthritis following aspiration of a haemarthrosis. Aspiration of a simple effusion has a low risk of complication and is particularly helpful in diagnosing crystal arthropathies.

Aspiration followed by culture is obviously required to establish a diagnosis of a septic arthritis. Don't forget that gonococcal arthritis occurs in the late teens and young adults. These patients may present in the fracture clinic having attributed their knee pain to an injury. Do remember that the gonococcus is a fragile organism and the aspirate should be plated out immediately!

The plain X-ray

This is an essential part of a full standard orthopaedic assessment—Apley's look, feel, move, X-ray. However, whilst X-rays should not be ignored it is equally wrong to be over-dependent on them. A plain film which reveals bad news will very likely be telling the truth, but one which appears to show good news may be highly deceptive. For example, it is still common practice in the UK to take an anteroposterior film of the knee with the patient supine. Such a knee is not subject to load and it is therefore most unwise to draw any conclusion about the joint space (Fig. 48.21). Even a standing film may deceive as regards the joint space for if the area of eburnation is situated anteriorly in the medial compartment, then it will show the total loss of joint space on a plain film, but if the area of eburnation is in the mid-range and there is still some articular surface anteriorly the film will merely show joint space narrowing. In the latter case the X-ray will be a travesty of the truth and patients with genuine symptoms from severe osteoarthritis are frequently dismissed with the advice that they just have 'a little minor wear and tear'. The implication is that their symptoms are out of proportion to the underlying problem and that 'the pain is in their brain'! If you suspect, on the basis of the agony test, that there is eburnation in the mid-range and you wish to have radiological proof, you must do a standing film with the knee flexed to 30 degrees, with the X-ray source tilted to be parallel to the top of the tibia (Fig. 48.22).

Anteroposterior and lateral X-rays of the patellofemoral joint are notoriously deceptive. 'Skyline' views are more revealing but need to be taken very carefully. Remember that X-rays don't focus and you are looking at shadows; therefore, minor degrees of rotation can have a major effect. Doing skyline views of both patellae on one exposure falls into this trap since the source is not aligned with the patellofemoral groove.

Computed tomographic scanning

This investigation has relatively little role to play outside the standard workup for tumours. The exception is certain lesions of the patellofemoral joint, in particular osteochondral fractures. It is the method of choice for determining whole limb rotation, cuts being taken through the hip, the knee and the ankle. Plain tomography is more informative than computed tomography if you wish to determine joint line integrity in the sagittal and coronal planes, for example in planning surgery for a tibial plateau fracture.

Magnetic resonance imaging (MRI) scanning

Soft tissues, in particular the menisci and the ligaments, can be clearly visualized by MRI. It is the investigation of choice for osteochondritis dissecans and avascular necrosis. It is, of course, the essential part of the workup for a patient with a bone tumour. However, if routine X-rays suffer from the defect of under-diagnosis MRI suffers from the reverse, namely, over-diagnosis especially of meniscal pathology. Degenerative changes of the posterior horn of a meniscus in a middle-aged patient can be considered normal. Not everybody with a torn cartilage or with a ruptured anterior cruciate needs surgery. It is the symptoms, not the scan, that determine treatment! Far too often this expensive investigation is carried out as a substitute for a proper history and a proper examination. This is all too likely to result in improper treatment.

Bone scanning[14]

In the author's opinion the relatively simple investigation of technetium scanning is under-utilized, particularly in the problem knee. It is particularly useful at eliminating rarities and oddities, for example osteoid osteoma, osteonecrosis and stress fractures. Fifty per cent of patients with chondromalacia will show an increased uptake in the patella on the bone scan. Inflammatory arthropathies will, of course, produce a generalized increased uptake in the knee but so will the little-understood complication of an algodystrophy (sympathetic reflex dystrophy). Thus, if a problem knee has a generalized increase in uptake, first check that you haven't missed a synovitis and, secondly, beware of doing surgery of any sort if the knee really does have an algodystrophy. Even a diagnostic arthroscopy can make such a patient's symptoms very much worse. It is also useful in defining which compartment of the knee is affected by osteoarthritis (Fig. 48.23).

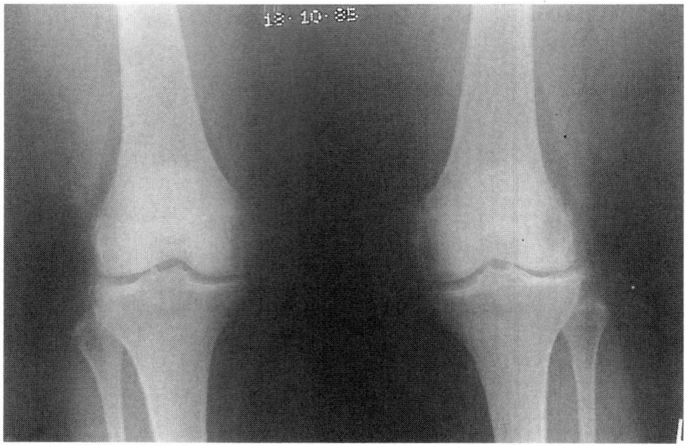

a

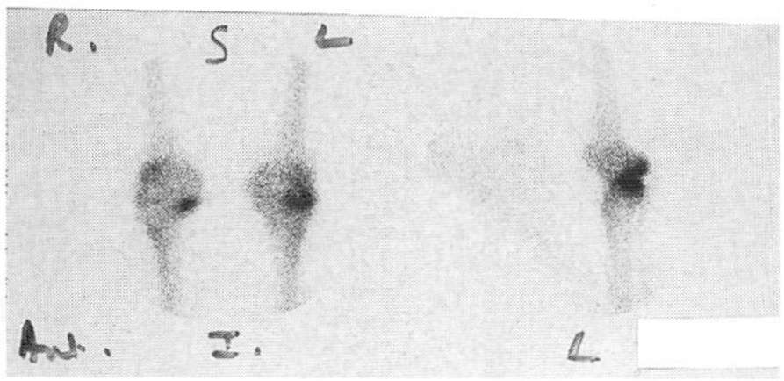

b

Fig. 48.23 This patient complains of pain in both knees. The standing anteroposterior X-rays suggest that the joint space is preserved. The bone scan, however, shows medial compartment change in the right knee and lateral in the left knee. The lateral scan shows that the uptake is posteriorly placed, which of course explains why the anteroposterior X-ray seems so normal.

An arthrogram

This was a frequently performed investigation prior to the advent of MRI. Skilled radiologists could achieve a diagnostic accuracy for a torn medial meniscus equal to that achieved by a skilled arthroscopist. The lateral meniscus was always more difficult due to contrast entering the popliteus tendon's synovial sheath. In current practice its one indication is for the diagnosis of a ruptured Baker's cyst.

Diagnostic arthroscopy

In current clinical practice there is often a straightforward choice between MRI and diagnostic arthroscopy. The former has the advantage of not requiring an anaesthetic but the disadvantage that whilst it may prove your diagnosis it does not allow you the ability to carry out surgical treatment. The indications and advantages for diagnostic arthroscopy are as follows:

1. It permits the surgeon to carry out an examination under anaesthetic. This is particularly useful if you suspect that the patient has a positive MacIntosh pivot shift but you cannot prove this in the clinic due to muscle guarding.
2. It is superior to MRI for visualizing the articular surfaces.
3. Surgical treatment, if required, can be carried out at the same time.
4. The washout effect—there is no doubt that some knees, particularly the early degenerative osteoarthritic joint, derive therapeutic benefit from merely carrying out an arthroscopy. This is an unpredictable response except when dealing with a crystal arthropathy such as chondrocalcinosis, which can respond dramatically well.
5. Patella tracking—an arthroscopy under a general anaesthetic can hardly qualify as being a dynamic investigation but it does allow the surgeon to visualise the patella tracking as the knee is passively flexed. The patellofemoral joint should be examined via the superolateral portal. It is best not to use a tourniquet as its presence interferes with the positioning of the arthroscope, which needs to be in the proximal part of the suprapatellar pouch.

Don't forget an arthroscopy is an opinion—your opinion, and for that to be valid you need sufficient experience, probably of the order of 50 cases. Using the standard anterolateral approach with a

REFERENCE

14. Butler-Manuel P A, Guy R L, Heatley F W, Numan T O In: Aichroth P M, Cannon W D (eds) Knee Surgery: Current Practice. Martin Dunitz, London 1992

30-degree telescope it is extremely easy to miss lesions on the lateral femoral condyle, posterior horn tears of the medial meniscus and significant chondromalacia of the patellae, i.e. chondromalacia affecting the dome.

SPECIFIC CONDITIONS

Acute pyogenic infection of the knee occurs at all ages. A wide variety of organisms can be involved but is most commonly due to *Staphylococcus aureus*, *Streptococcus* and the gonococcus. An acute severe infection gives classical physical signs: pain, warmth and severe restriction of movement accompanied by a systemic illness. It is not difficult to diagnose but does need to be distinguished from gout, pseudogout and acute spontaneous haemarthrosis, a condition which is an uncommon complication of the osteoarthritic knee as well as, of course, occurring in haemophilia. Low-grade infections, especially gonococcal infections, can be much more deceptive, particularly if accompanied by a 'false' history of injury. Superimposed pyogenic infection in the osteoarthritic knee is a diagnostic trap and consequently a source of error. As with other infections it occurs more commonly in the immunosuppressed patient.

Proof of the diagnosis is by aspiration and culture. It is often useful to carry out a formal arthroscopy and washout as there will be a fibrinous exudate within the joint which tends to harbour the organisms. Repeated arthroscopic washout or aspiration through a wide-bore needle may be required. Remember that even with the appropriate antibiotics, an acute septic arthritis of the knee may take several weeks to settle, often up to six weeks. The knee should be rested, if necessary in a plaster back splint, and gentle movement permitted as the infection subsides. It is probably wise to avoid weight bearing for six weeks.

Acute haematogenous osteomyelitis is a classical disease of childhood. Its incidence has declined in Western countries over the last two decades and it is rare to encounter the fulminating variety of the disease. It is now more often a 'subacute' illness. It is a metaphyseal infection classically due to *Staphylococcus aureus* and as it is adjacent to the joint will produce a sympathetic effusion within the joint. Joint fluid aspiration, if necessary, will distinguish osteomyelitis from septic arthritis. Since changes on the X-ray may not appear until 10 days after the start of the infection, it is very easy to confuse the subacute, but nonetheless locally aggressive, metaphyseal osteomyelitis in a child with an inflammatory arthropathy such as juvenile rheumatoid arthritis (JRA). The rule is to *treat* the child on the basis that they have an osteomyelitis and *investigate* the child to determine whether they have JRA. Investigations include routine blood tests, haemoglobin, white count, ESR, tests for an inflammatory arthropathy and, most important, a blood culture. It is surprising how often the need for a blood culture is overlooked in a child with a mild fever and an irritable joint. The site of the infection, whether it is in the distal femur or the proximal tibia, is usually obvious from the local signs, particularly local tenderness. If localization is difficult a technetium bone scan is often helpful.

Primary malignant bone tumours, whilst rare, most commonly occur around the knee and can be confused with osteomyelitis. The distinguishing clinical hallmark between infection and a tumour, such as an osteogenic sarcoma, is that tumours retain their range of movement whereas with an osteomyelitis joint movement is markedly restricted.

Acute postoperative infection following open or arthroscopic surgery is fortunately rare but requires prompt and energetic treatment, including the arthroscopic washout of any haemarthrosis.

Tuberculous synovitis

Although now rare in Western countries this disease still exists especially in the immigrant communities. It remains a source of diagnostic error for the unwary since, being a low-grade infection, it is very easy to confuse with other arthropathies including juvenile rheumatoid arthritis in children, chronic post-traumatic synovitis in adults (the end result of a severe haemarthrosis) and early osteoarthritis—a common condition which can, of course, be present in conjunction with a tuberculous synovitis! The physical signs are those of warmth, marked synovial thickening, often excessive quadriceps wasting, a limp and, if the diagnosis has been delayed, systemic symptoms such as loss of weight and night sweats. It is certainly possible that the incidence of the disease will become commoner with the advent of HIV infection. Culturing *Mycobacterium tuberculosis* from a joint aspirate can often be difficult. This suspicion should lead to a diagnostic arthroscopy and biopsy of an inflamed area of the synovium. The fluid and the synovial biopsy are sent for culture as well as sending the synovial biopsy for histology. Treatment should initially be with quadruple therapy[15] and appropriate adjustment once sensitivities from the cultures are known. The joint should be rested in a plaster back splint and the patient kept non-weight bearing on the affected leg. Gentle movement is permitted as the infection subsides.

Inflammatory arthropathies

The knee is commonly involved in rheumatoid arthritis. Most cases present late to the surgeon having been referred from the rheumatologist for a consideration of joint replacement. Occasionally rheumatoid presents with a seronegative monoarthritis of the knee. Later, the disease usually spreads to involve other joints, in particular the opposite knee, whereupon the diagnosis becomes more evident. The treatment for rheumatoid arthritis is medical and there is little place for surgery until late in the course of the disease when the patient requires a joint replacement. Synovectomy is now rarely performed, the only indication being a low-grade inflammatory synovitis with marked synovial thickening and no articular cartilage destruction. If required synovectomy is now done arthroscopically. At best it can only ever be partial. Old-fashioned open synovectomy frequently resulted in marked joint stiffness secondary to the excision of the suprapatellar pouch.

The knee can also be involved in many other arthropathies, for example ankylosing spondylitis, psoriatic arthropathy and Reiter's

REFERENCE

15. Joint Tuberculosis Committee of the British Thoracic Society. Thorax 1994; 49: 1193–1200

syndrome. Reiters is a reactive arthropathy and the aetiological stimulus, when it is identified, is usually a Gram-negative bacterial infection, *Shigella*, *Salmonella yersinia*, *Campylobacter* or a chlamydial infection. The organisms are not present in the joint and non-steroidal anti-inflammatory drug (NSAID) therapy is the treatment of choice.

Gout in the knee is uncommon but does occur and is very easy to miss. The diagnosis is made by demonstrating sodium urate crystals under polarized light microscopy. Acute gout is treated with large doses of anti-inflammatory drugs for several days and allopurinol, an inhibitor of xanthine oxidase, is advised for long-term management.

Pseudogout (calcium pyrophosphate deposition syndrome) affects the knee more often than any other joint. Its incidence increases with age and chondrocalcinosis is a common radiological finding in plain X-rays of the knee over the age of 55 years. The vast majority of such knees will not suffer acute attacks of 'pseudogout' for in order to become symptomatic the crystals must 'escape' from either the articular surfaces or the menisci. The diagnosis is dependent on demonstrating the crystals in a joint aspirate. Treatment is with NSAIDs or if symptoms are severe by an arthroscopic washout.

Haemophiliac arthropathy is secondary to recurrent haemarthroses. It appears that once joint destruction has begun the incidence of recurrent bleeds increases, thereby establishing a vicious circle. Interestingly, it has been shown that surgical correction of deformity by osteotomy decreases the incidence of bleeding.[16,17]

Synovial chondromatosis and **pigmented villinodular synovitis** are two other unusual conditions affecting the synovium. Both have their greatest incidence within the knee joint. Synovial chondromatosis presents in two clinical forms. In the first there are multiple but relatively large loose bodies, which have ossified centres and hence show on X-rays. Treatment is arthroscopic removal of the loose bodies. The presenting symptom is 'locking'. The other form is more difficult to diagnose, often presenting as a synovitis and boggy joint of unknown aetiology. On arthroscopy the diagnosis becomes immediately evident as numerous small cartilaginous rice bodies are washed out of the joint. Synovial biopsy will reveal cartilaginous metaplasia within the synovium.

Pigmented villinodular synovitis is a disease of unknown aetiology. It presents with recurrent acute haemarthroses. On arthroscopy the synovium is swollen, hyperplastic and covered with villi which are usually golden brown in colour, the effect of haemosiderin deposition. Unlike the hip, where the joint space is relatively confined and juxta-articular erosions leading to joint destruction occur, the disease in the knee is much less aggressive.

Both synovial chondromatosis and pigmented villinodular synovitis are benign conditions and do not undergo malignant transformation. However, a very low-grade chondrosarcoma can occasionally invade a joint and masquerade as synovial chondromatosis.

Osteochondritis dissecans[18]

This is an interesting disorder in which a sliver of the subchondral bony plate, together with the overlying cartilage, separates off from the underlying bone. This is not a disease of the articular cartilage, which is not only normal, but in the early stages retains its integrity and congruity with adjacent articular cartilage. Eventually the articular cartilage fractures and the osteochondral fragment can then separate as a 'loose body'. Many theories have been advanced as an explanation. These include trauma, ischaemic necrosis of the underlying bone and abnormalities of endochondral ossification. A familial incidence has been noted by several authors; however, a study by Petrie failed to confirm a definite genetic aetiology.[19] Sir James Paget in 1870 gave a classical description of two cases and considered the aetiology was traumatic. He is probably correct. The condition nearly always involves the convex surface. Within the knee it occurs on the femoral condyles and the patella. Other classic sites are also convex, namely, the capitellum in the elbow, the head of the femur in the hip, and the dome of the talus in the ankle. Convex surfaces are particularly prone to the effect of shear forces. In engineering ball bearings have a similar problem with stress fractures of their surfaces. These metal fractures also commence in the 'subchondral' zone, i.e., deep to the surface of the metal.

In keeping with a traumatic origin osteochondritis dissecans is most frequently found in athletic teenagers and is more prevalent in boys than girls. The medial femoral condyle is more frequently affected than the lateral, in a ratio of 4:1. Many cases probably undergo spontaneous healing. This statement is, of course, a supposition but it is not infrequent to find evidence of old osteochondritis dissecans in adults as a chance finding on an X-ray, the patient never having had any symptoms from their knee as a teenager. Initially the symptoms are often vague and intermittent, causing discomfort rather than pain. Later there is recurrent swelling, joint irritability, giving way and locking. These symptoms usually correlate with the degree of instability of the fragment. A loose body once formed will continue to grow within the knee as it acts like a free graft, deriving its nutrition from the synovial fluid.

The choice of surgical treatment depends on the site, the size and the stability of the fragment. A small stable fragment in a young child will probably heal spontaneously, whereas a large unstable fragment requires fixation. Smillie pins, small lag screws, carbon rods and dexon pegs have all been advocated. If the fragment has separated a loose body can be removed arthroscopically and, at the same time, the subchondral base of the lesion drilled to aid healing with fibrocartilage. The new technique of chondral grafting,[20,21] in which cartilage cells are removed arthroscopically,

REFERENCES

16. Pearce M S, Smith M A, Savidge G F J Bone Joint Surg 1994; 76: 947–950
17. Smith M A, Urquhart D R, Savidge G F J Bone Joint Surg 1981; 63B: 261–265
18. Aichroth P M, Patel D V In: Aichroth P M, Cannon W D (eds) Knee Surgery: Current Practice. Martin Dunitz, London 1992
19. Petrie P W R J Bone Joint Surg 1977; 59B: 366
20. Peterson L Acta Orthop Belg 1996: 62(Suppl 1): 196–200
21. Brittberg M, Lindahl A, Nilsson A et al N Engl J Med 1994; 331(14): 889–895

cultured in vitro and then returned into the defect, being kept in place by a covering of periosteum, is an exciting advance but its effectiveness in treating large lesions has still to be established. In general, small lesions under 1 cm heal satisfactorily, indeed at arthroscopy several years later you may well not be able to define the original site as the defect has filled in with good-quality fibrocartilage even though the bony scar is still visible on the X-ray. Defects over 2 cm, particularly when they are in the classical site on the medial femoral condyle, have a much higher chance of developing osteoarthritis—a 30% chance over a 30-year period is probably a reasonable estimate.[22]

Osteonecrosis[23]

Osteonecrosis has certain similarities to but important differences from osteochondritis dissecans. In both entities the disease process is in the underlying bone, has normal overlying articular cartilage and occurs on convex surfaces. However, unlike osteochondritis dissecans, osteonecrosis can occur on the tibial plateau though when it does so it involves the margins of the plateau which are, of course, also convex. The commonest site affected is the medial femoral condyle but, unlike osteochondritis dissecans, osteonecrosis is associated with a significant number of well-defined medical diseases, notably alcoholism, haemoglobinopathies, Caisson's decompression disease, systemic lupus erythematosus, renal transplantation and, in particular, occurs as a complication of steroid therapy. The classical presentation is of a sudden onset of severe pain which may gradually decrease with time and usually affects the medial side of the knee. The prognosis is dependent on the size of the lesion, with lesions less than 3.5 cm^2 in area tending to have a good prognosis. Larger lesions should be treated by arthroscopic drilling and correction of any underlying deformity, for example an upper tibial osteotomy to correct a varus deformity in a knee with medial compartment osteonecrosis. Older patients with large lesions are best treated by a total knee replacement if the knee remains symptomatic.

Conditions affecting the extensor mechanism of the knee

The need to provide a joint which has both full extension, full flexion and a capacity to kneel creates, to use an engineering expression, high design requirements. As a consequence this mechanism, which in some ways is extremely strong and robust, is in other respects delicate. In normal stance the human patella lies proximal to the femoral groove, thus posing problems of entry into the groove as the knee flexes. It boasts the thickest articular surface in the human body, and has a remarkably complex shape that is essentially a rather flat ovoid disc shaped to pass down a rather flat expanded groove. This is in sharp contradistinction to most of the animal kingdom, who have deep grooves with triangular well-faceted patellae that in the normal stance position lie within the groove. It is perhaps not surprising that the extensor mechanism is such a common cause of orthopaedic complaints. The problems affecting the mechanism can broadly be divided into four groups.

Syndromes affecting the tendon bone insertions

1. Osgood–Schlatter's is a traction apophysis of the tibial tubercle. Most cases present in the early teens in athletic boys. Symptoms may last for up to two years. If troublesome the knee should be rested if necessary in a plaster back splint to ensure the adolescent does not play football when Mum is not looking! Occasionally symptoms may persist beyond the end of growth due to separation of a fragment of the tibial tubercle. This fragment may require either fixation or removal.

2. The corresponding lesion in the distal pole of the patella is the Johanssen–Sindig–Larsen syndrome. This is much less common than Osgood–Schlatter's and usually much less troublesome.

3. Jumper's knee is the term given to chronic tendonitis at the junction of the patellar tendon and distal pole of the patella. Originally described in young athletes it is more commonly seen in the ageing, middle-aged athlete, such as those preparing for a marathon. The treatment is rest and, if necessary, a change to some other sport. Steroid injections should be carried out with caution and any athletic activities banned for several days afterwards, since there is a small risk of precipitating a patellar tendon rupture.

4. Patellar tendonitis is almost identical to 'Jumper's knee' except that the collagen fibre disruption occurs centrally within the tendon. Abnormalities can be shown by MRI scanning and ultrasound examination.

Ruptures and fractures of the extensor mechanism

1. Ruptures can occur above, below or through the patella. A spontaneous rupture of the rectus femoris can occur in the elderly. The signs are usually classical, with a lump bunching up when the quadriceps contact. Occasionally this 'bunching' is not so evident, in which case be certain that you are not dealing with a soft tissue sarcoma! Isolated rupture of the rectus femoris in this age group does not produce disability and should be left alone. However, ruptures of the rectus can also occur in athletes, particularly sprinters. The rupture is usually at the level of the musculotendinous insertion. In top-class athletes it is certainly worth trying to repair this rupture though there is no guarantee of success.

2. Avulsion of the quadriceps tendon, usually with a small fragment of bone from the superior pole of the patella, is a cause of major disability because extensor control of the knee will be impaired if the lesion heals with lengthening. It requires surgical repair. It is most commonly seen in the sixth or seventh decade and there is an increased incidence in diabetics, patients with chronic renal failure and those on steroids. Generally, it is accompanied by severe pain and the patient is unable to extend the knee or, if he can extend it because the retinacular fibres are still intact, the power of extension is weak and there is a lag, i.e., the tibia lags behind the femur and the heel remains on the couch after the knee has been

REFERENCES

22. Twyman R S, Desai K, Aichroth P M J Bone Joint Surg 1991; 73B: 461
23. Kitziger K J, Lotke P A In: Aichroth P M, Cannon W D (eds) Knee Surgery: Current Practice. Martin Dunitz, London 1992

lifted up. Once the initial swelling has settled a defect will be palpable just above the patella. Surprisingly, in one series of 17 cases of complete rupture, seven were initially misdiagnosed.[24] If in doubt MRI can be helpful.

3. Avulsion of the patellar tendon from the distal pole of the patella is an avulsion injury and the tendon usually separates together with a small fragment of bone from the distal pole. In addition to an inability to extend the knee the patella will be displaced proximally due to the unopposed action of the quadriceps. This requires surgical repair. This injury is most commonly seen between the ages of 30 and 50 years.

4. Transverse fractures of the patella complete the sequence of avulsion injuries. If the fragments are separated, which they usually are, this condition requires internal fixation. It is interesting to note that historically this was one of the first fractures to undergo surgery, for whilst you may be able to reduce the fragments closed, you cannot hold them without resorting to either external or internal fixation. Surgical treatment dates back to Malgaigne and his poins, which was the first method of external fixation. Transverse fractures need to be distinguished from stellate fractures of the patella. The latter are due to a direct blow on the patella whereas transverse fractures will have occurred before the patient actually hits the ground. With stellate fractures the retinaculum over the patella and the quadriceps expansions are usually intact. Consequently, whilst surgery is mandatory for displaced transverse fractures many stellate fractures can be treated conservatively.

Patella maltracking, subluxation and dislocation

This is a confused and confusing subject. It will remain thus until there are improved methods of measurement. Many factors influence the pathway that the patella takes down the femoral groove. These are as follows:

1. *Leg alignment.* An increased valgus angle at the knee will encourage the patella to cut the corner.

2. *Excessive limb rotation.* During development a marked spiral twist occurs in the developing limb. At the hip the femoral neck is anteverted in relationship to the shaft and the knee is internally rotated in relation to the ankle and foot. When you are standing to attention the feet point outwards but when you are sitting the feet are parallel. An excess inward rotation of the knee in relationship to the hip and the foot is commonly seen, particularly in teenagers presenting with anterior knee pain, the so-called 'patellae in love'. It is likely that an accentuation of this twist will complicate the already complex three-dimensional spiral that the patella takes as it passes down the femoral groove.

3. *The shape of the patella.* Much has been written about the patella shape and it is clear that there are considerable variations, particularly in the medial facet. Skyline views, even when repeated, at 30, 60 and 90 degrees of flexion are, unfortunately, difficult to interpret since they are obviously a two-dimensional view of a complex three-dimensional structure. Many authors have attempted to measure angles from skyline films but X-rays are in effect shadows and a small alteration in the angle at which the knee lies in the beam will produce an apparently marked alteration in shape. Project the shadow of a triangle onto the wall and then rotate the triangle!

4. *Joint laxity.* This can be either generalized, such as occurs in Ehlers–Danlos syndrome or may be very localized; for example, there can be patella laxity in an otherwise stable knee. Clearly, if a patella is to dislocate laterally out of the groove the soft tissues on the medial side must either be torn or have a capacity to stretch.

5. *The location of the patella.* A high-riding patella, patella alta, can certainly be associated with patella maltracking. The patella may be considered high if the patella tendon to patella ratio exceeds 1:1.2—the Insall Salvati index.[25]

6. *Location of the tibial tubercle.* A laterally placed tibial tubercle will increase the valgus angle between the quadriceps and the patellar tendon. This is known as the Q angle (quadriceps angle).[26] It is defined as the angle between a line from the anterior superior spine to the centre of the patella and a second line from the centre of the patella to the tibial tubercle.

7. *Quadriceps insertion onto the patella.* In broad terms the vastus lateralis can be too tight and the vastus medialis too weak or loose. Scarring in the vastus lateralis can be iatrogenic secondary to intramuscular injections into the thigh in childhood. Similar scarring can occur in the tensor fascia lata which may lead to severe valgus at the knee and habitual dislocation of the patella. Minor bands between the patella and the iliotibial band may be implicated in patella maltracking.

It is clear that patella tracking is controlled by many features and that maltracking is the result of a complex equation. Whilst we may understand a number of the main components that make up that equation we do not, for the most part, know how to measure them. If we have measured them it is usually in two planes rather than in three and we certainly do not know how to weight the various factors. It is to be hoped that modern computing and the advent of three-dimensional MRI scanning will help elucidate problems of the patellofemoral mechanism.

Patella dislocation

This can be *permanent*, i.e., the patella always resides lateral to the lateral femoral condyle, *habitual*, in which the patella dislocates from the groove every time the knee is flexed, or *sporadic*, where the patella normally lies in its groove but dislocates from time to time. Habitual dislocation is usually easy to diagnose since there is a clear jump as the patella moves in and out of the groove. Rather remarkably, permanent dislocation, particularly in a fat knee, can be very deceptive. It is even more deceptive when the patient has had a patellectomy! Professor Kessell's* famous dictum states, 'patellectomy is to be avoided since dislocation of the patella is so

*Professor of Orthopaedics, Royal National Orthopaedic Hospital, London.

REFERENCES

24. Ramsay R H, Miller G E Clin Orthop 1970; 70: 161
25. Insall J, Salvati E Radiology 1971 101: 101
26. Aglietti P, Insall J N, Cerulli G. Clin Orthop 1983; 176: 217

difficult to diagnose once it has been excised!' It may require open surgery to establish that the extensor mechanism in a patellectomized knee has dislocated permanently outside the lateral femoral condyle. Sporadic dislocations can also be difficult to diagnose. If one is lucky there may have been an X-ray taken in an A&E centre demonstrating the dislocation. Usually there is only the history of a major episode of giving way, i.e., the patient falls nearly always striking the knee that gives way, and an apprehension sign in a patella that doesn't have an 'end-point' when it is displaced laterally.

Maltracking is a habitual minor lateral displacement of the patella, i.e., the patella has a consistent track up and down its groove but the track is abnormal, i.e., it doesn't lie central. In particular, the patella may have difficulty entering into the groove and the knee may need to be bent to 90 degrees before the patella is seen to centralize. Some indication of maltracking may be obtained from the Marchant skyline views. Direct visualization can be done by an arthroscopy through the superolateral portal.

Diseases of the articular surface

Not only is the patella the largest of all sesamoid bones but it has the thickest articular surface in the human body and that surface has one of the most complex shapes of any joint. It is important to realize that the hardness of the articular surface, which is a very important mechanical parameter, is determined by its thickness. The thicker the surface, the softer the surface and the more easily will it conform to its opposing surface. It is this need for conformity in a joint which superficially lacks conformity that almost certainly determines the need for the patellar surface to be so thick. This compromise unfortunately has a price and that is paid for in the high incidence of two conditions: chondromalacia and patellofemoral osteoarthritis.

Chondromalacia patellae

This term should be reserved to describe particular pathological change that affects the articular surface of the patella. There is a tendency to use the term synonymously with anterior knee pain, particularly for those joints that exhibit crepitus when crouching. However, crepitus is a sign, not a diagnosis. Chondromalacia can be categorized into four grades:

- Grade I, softening and swelling.
- Grade II, fragmentation and fissuring in an area of ½ inch or less.
- Grade III, fragmentation and fissuring in an area more than ½ an inch.
- Grade IV, cartilage erosion down to bone.

Outerbridge[27] made his observations at the time of open meniscectomy. He observed that there was a natural increase in the condition with age and that the most common area of the patella involved was the middle of the medial patellar facet or slightly distal to it. Abernethy et al[28] studying 100 knees at autopsy concluded that minor changes were present on the medial facet but with increasing age changes developed on the lateral facet where cartilage was more often eroded down to subchondral bone. Overall there was an incidence of 85% chondromalacia on the medial facet but only 4% showed grade IV changes in this site. Whilst changes on the lateral facet were much less common, 13% of these were at the grade IV level.

In conclusion, chondromalacia of the medial facet is common. It is an arthroscopic finding which nearly always bears little relation to the patient's symptoms. Chondromalacia of the lateral facet is much more significant and may progress to patellofemoral osteoarthritis.[29]

Chondromalacia affecting the dome can be symptomatic but usually does not progress to osetoarthritis.

A hypothesis to explain these findings can be based on the type of force acting, the geographic shape of the part of the patella involved and the degree of congruity of the patella to its groove. On the lateral facet with its slightly convex shape the forces will be more easily transferred from the articular surface into the subchondral bone, i.e., there will be predominantly compressive forces. Thus excessive forces affecting the lateral side of the joint will not only cause disintegration of the articular cartilage but that force will continue and the articular cartilage will be worn away through to the subchondral bone, eventually leading to erosion of the bone. On the other hand, shear forces will be generated across the convex dome and through the medial facet. Whilst this may cause disintegration of the cartilaginous surface, i.e., chondromalacia, it will not lead to bony eburnation.

Patellofemoral osteoarthritis

Patellofemoral osteoarthritis is distinguished from chondromalacia pathologically by the progression to bony eburnation, i.e., the whole thickness of the articular surface will be lost. It usually occurs in association with osteoarthritis in the medial or lateral compartment. In one study of 600 cases of radiologically established patellofemoral osteoarthritis 65% were found to have associated narrowing of the medial compartment and 20% narrowing of the lateral compartment. Only 15% had osteoarthritis localized purely to the patellofemoral joint.[30] However, in the 'normal population' this incidence of isolated patellofemoral osteoarthritis would be much higher for it is frequently asymptomatic, thus the patients are not seen by orthopaedic surgeons or rheumatologists. Even patients who have mild knee pain are likely to be underdiagnosed as skyline X-rays needed to show the patellofemoral joint are not usually done routinely.

Treatment options

Very different surgical procedures have been advocated for patellofemoral problems. It is very easy to overtreat this group of

REFERENCES

27. Outerbridge R E J Bone Joint Surg 1961; 43B: 752
28. Abernethy P J, Townsend D T P R, Rose M R et al J Bone Joint Surg 1978; 60B: 205
29. Ficat P et al. Rev Surg Orthop 1975; 61: 39
30. Aglietti P, Buzzi R, Insall J N In: Insall J N et al (eds) Surgery of the Knee, Vol 12, 2nd edn. Churchill Livingstone, Edinburgh 1993

of course, wash out the haemarthrosis and enable them to establish a precise diagnosis. For many patients this is a relatively benign injury. Acute repairs of the anterior cruciate ligament are, in general, indicated only in high-quality athletes.

A simple direct suture of the ligament is inadequate and needs reinforcing by either a fascia lata graft, or the middle third of the patellar tendon (Jones procedure) or the semitendinosus tendon. The latter two techniques are also used for late repairs and are now commonly done arthroscopically. These tendon grafts are, of course, initially dead and therefore act as a scaffold. It is therefore at least six months before the patient can return to sports. The common complications are technical, with misplacement of the tibial and femoral tunnels producing impingement in the intercondylar notch, loss of movement and rupture. Artificial ligaments have the attraction that one does not need to harvest a graft but in spite of having phases of enthusiasm are currently out of fashion due to a high incidence of rupture and synovitis secondary to debris production.

The lateral collateral ligament is the weakest of the four ligaments and is only one component of the lateral ligament complex which includes the biceps femoris and the iliotibial band. In severe injuries the lateral popliteal nerve is also at risk. Complete injuries of this complex, particularly ones in which the iliotibial band has also been avulsed, should be treated surgically. These, however, are relatively rare and most injuries of the lateral side can be managed conservatively with a hinged splint and early physiotherapy.

The posterior cruciate ligament is the strongest of the four ligaments. It can be ruptured in sports injuries but more commonly it requires a high-speed accident. The physical signs are the backward sag of the tibia on the femur with the knee examined at 90 degrees of flexion and an abnormal posterior excursion with the anterior–posterior draw test. One caveat: beware lest this is just one component of a major dislocation of the knee (see below). Isolated posterior cruciate injuries are usually treated conservatively with a hinged brace and intensive physiotherapy. Surgical repairs. Whether done early or late, are technically difficult and give inconsistent results. It is one of the unmastered areas of knee surgery.

Combined injuries

In making a diagnosis it is useful to try and reduce these complex injuries to their main anatomical components. In essence, the more extensive the injury the greater the indication for acute surgery. For example, if the knee is unstable to a valgus stress in extension then it is likely that both the medial ligament and the anterior cruciate have been disrupted. This will almost certainly leave a knee that is unstable to rotation if treated conservatively. MRI scanning is a useful investigation in these knee injuries but there is a tendency for it to overstate the extent of the injury. MRI assists with diagnosis but it does not necessarily help with management.

Dislocation of the knee

This is another very deceptive injury that is frequently misdiagnosed and results in major medicolegal litigation. The reason is that complete dislocation is associated with a high incidence of damage to the popliteal artery which is most commonly disrupted at its trifurcation. *It is not always a high-velocity injury.* Whilst road traffic accidents, particularly to motor cyclists, have the highest incidence, it can occur in a heavy patient following a simple fall. If you suspect this injury the patient should have an arteriogram. The problem for the unwary is, first, the injury may have been out of proportion to the insult so that the diagnosis is not considered, second, there is usually no deformity as the tibia will have 'bounced' back into position, third, the discomfort around the knee may be sufficient to cause sufficient contraction of the quadriceps so that the inexperienced surgeon fails to elicit the posterior draw test and, fourth, the X-ray will be normal.

Conclusion

Ligament injuries are truly perverse, the more minor ones can be painful, the major ones painless. They are by no means all high-velocity or even contact injuries. Their physical signs are difficult.

MENISCAL INJURIES[34]

The meniscus has been a source of surgical controversy for over a hundred years, ever since in 1885 Thomas Anandale, Professor of Surgery in Edinburgh, successfully treated a torn meniscus by suturing it back into position.[35] Until recently this was the only report in the literature of a successful meniscal suture. For most of the 20th century open total meniscectomy was the standard practice.

The scientific basis for meniscal surgery was established by King in the 1930s.[36] As a result of a simple series of experiments on dogs he made three important observations. First, a cut in the substance of the meniscus did not heal, second, a cut through the peripheral attachments of the meniscus did heal and, third, a cut in the substance that extended to the periphery might heal. Recent work has shown that the ability of the meniscus to heal is related to its blood supply.[37] The meniscus is avascular in its inner two-thirds and has a somewhat variable blood supply in the outer third.

Modern bioengineering techniques have confirmed that the menisci act effectively as shock absorbers and lubricating pads. Their loss is associated with an incidence of osteoarthritis affecting the relevant compartment of the knee. The literature is confused as to the incidence. A reasonable figure is a 20% incidence of radiological change of osteoarthritis over a 20-year period with half the patients, i.e., 10%, suffering significant symptoms such as to warrant further orthopaedic advice. The meniscus needs to be treated with respect by surgeons learning their craft! At arthroscopy it appears to be macroscopically tough but this is highly misleading for at cellular level it is fragile. Its response to injury is the same as that for articular hyaline cartilage. An area of

REFERENCES

34. Heatley F W Curr Orthop 1987; 1: 160
35. Anandale T Br Med J 1885; 1: 779
36. King D J Bone Joint Surg 1936; 18: 333
37. Arnoczky S P, Warren R F Am J Sports Med 1982; 10: 90

damage, which is easily caused by rough probing at arthroscopy, will produce a zone of cell death surrounded by a zone of cellular activity which characteristically produces cell clusters.

The types of tear have been extensively studied, particularly by Smillie,[38] who coined the descriptive phrase 'the horizontal cleavage tear' for those occurring in a degenerate meniscus. The longitudinal vertical tear, which classically led to the bucket handle tear, occurs in younger people and is usually associated with sporting injuries. The longitudinal tear is for the most part an injury occurring to an otherwise normal meniscus, whereas the horizontal tear is the final insult of a meniscus that has been subject to repeated injuries and wear, in other words 'the disintegration of the shock absorber'. Unless the patient is complaining of frank locking, beware of attributing knee pain to a degenerate medial meniscus. With longitudinal and vertical tears the meniscus may, indeed, be the sinner but with horizontal cleavage splits the meniscus may be sinned against by abnormal forces, for example the varus deformity causing disintegration within the medial meniscus. Excise such a meniscus or remove the shock absorber and you may very rapidly produce medial compartment osteoarthritis. The MRI scan is very accurate at diagnosing meniscal tears and meniscal degeneration. Unfortunately, it does not tell you whether either the tear or the degeneration is responsible for the patient's symptoms. An important paper which should be read by all trainees before they do a meniscectomy is the study by Noble and Hamblen.[39] They performed 100 necropsy examinations and found that 29% of the 400 menisci had at least one horizontal cleavage tear, while 73% of subjects had some significant abnormality in at least one meniscus, with 25 of these being in 'massive lesions'. We can conclude that whilst 25% of the population over the age of 50 may have meniscal damage, fortunately 25% of the population do not require arthroscopic surgery!

Conclusion

Many meniscal tears in the middle-aged patient are asymptomatic. Prior to the days of arthroscopic surgery it was wise to ask oneself three questions: (1) Has the patient got a torn meniscus? (2) Which meniscus is torn? (3) Has the patient got sufficient symptoms to warrant surgery? Arthroscopy and MRI have made questions 1 and 2 easier but they have not altered question 3! As regards the recent advance of meniscal repair, the best indication is the peripheral tear of the lateral meniscus. You will recall that this structure occupies a larger segment of a smaller circle in comparison to the medial. Not only does the lateral meniscus cover 70% of the articular surface of the tibia, but the tibial plateau is not concave, indeed it is convex posteriorly. Excision of the whole of the lateral meniscus will produce point pressure and a high risk of developing osteoarthritis at an early age. The case for repair of a bucket handle tear of the medial meniscus is much more controversial and if it is the only abnormality within the knee the incidence of late-onset osteoarthritis is probably much smaller than 10%. Repair has the disadvantage of a slower recovery since the meniscus will take six weeks to heal and a far higher complication rate, including damage to the surrounding nerves and vessels as well as at least a 10% re-tear rate.

MENISCAL CYSTS

Pathologically these are the same as ganglia. They are usually associated with horizontal cleavage tears though frequently the meniscal tear itself is asymptomatic and it is merely a cyst that produces a dull aching pain, worse after activity. Lateral cysts are much commoner than medial cysts (see section on Physical signs). If there are no intra-articular symptoms conservative treatment in the form of aspiration through a wide-bore needle with injection of local steroids done in outpatients is the treatment of choice. Interestingly, these cysts disappear with time and are very uncommon to find in the elderly.

OSTEOARTHRITIS

Osteoarthritis is classified as a degenerative disease of articular cartilage but the use of the word degenerate is unfortunate as it too readily implies an atrophic inevitable decline. In fact, the overall metabolism of an osteoarthritic joint equates to that of a growing child. The disease process is a complicated interaction of wear, reaction and repair. It is the end-point of an imbalance between the forces acting across a joint versus the quality of its articular surface. Pauwels,[2] the first orthopaedic surgeon to apply the principles of biomechanics in understanding pathology, made the following hypothesis: (1) osteoarthritis results when abnormal forces act on normal cartilage or (2) when normal forces act on abnormal cartilage. Rheumatoid arthritis, articular cartilage injury or other disease which disrupts the integrity of articular cartilage form the second group. The first group, so-called primary osteoarthritis, is associated with mechanical imbalance. In the knee this usually manifests itself as a well-defined varus or valgus deformity or maltracking in the patellofemoral joint. A useful example to use to explain the relationship of wear and deformity to a patient is an unbalanced motor car tyre, as everyone knows that this creates uneven wear. Furthermore, if the tyre is not too worn the solution is to balance the wheel—in orthopaedic terms the correction of a deformity. If the tyre is worn down to the thread then clearly one needs a new tyre, equivalent in orthopaedic terms to a knee replacement. However, it is readily apparent that it is no use merely putting on a new tyre if one doesn't balance the wheel. Similarly, a knee replacement requires to be put to optimum mechanical balance, otherwise there will be shear forces leading to plastic creep and wear.

On the basis of his hypothesis, Pauwel proposed a logical treatment plan aimed at reducing the force per unit area, ideally by both lowering the overall load on a joint and increasing its congruity. A simple example of the interrelation of load and contact area is provided by a lady in a stiletto heel, which will dent a wooden parquet floor because the force per unit area approximates to that of a fully grown elephant.

REFERENCES

38. Smillie I S Injuries of the Knee Joint, 5th edn. Churchill Livingstone, Edinburgh 1978
39. Noble J, Hamblen D L J Bone Joint Surg 1975; 56B: 719

There are important differences between medial and lateral compartment osteoarthritis. Although passively both may exhibit a similar degree of instability, when put under active load the valgus knee tends to stabilize because the lateral femoral condyle drives down into the centre of the tibia, whereas with the varus knee the medial femoral condyle balances on the rim of the medial tibial plateau thereby hinging open the lateral side. Thus, it is the varus knee that shows the shift sign (see Physical signs). The agony test when positive is game, set and match for the diagnosis, whereas X-rays, as already discussed, can be highly deceptive.

Treatment of medial or lateral compartment osteoarthritis is obviously dependent upon symptoms. In many patients these are mild and some modification of activity, the use of a knee support, some analgesics and some quadriceps exercises may well be sufficient. Acute flares in an early osteoarthritic knee respond well to arthroscopy and the washout effect, inherent in doing this investigation. Some surgeons believe in debriding a wearing surface in the hope that it will heal with fibrocartilage. This, however, is controversial and there is little evidence that this is any more effective than merely washing out the knee. In the presence of a significant deformity arthroscopic debridement does not seem to the author to be a logical procedure; indeed, he has seen several cases in which debridement has been destructive.

The indication for an upper tibial osteotomy is a varus knee, with a good lateral compartment, that is stable in the sense that it doesn't show the shift sign, and the wear is circumscribed, i.e., it does not involve the whole surface of the medial compartment. Surgery needs to be accurate with 3–5 degrees of over-correction to ensure that the resultant force passes through the intact lateral compartment or at least on the lateral side of the intercondylar notch. Unfortunately, gait analysis is not yet sufficiently refined to be able to advise the surgeon what degree of correction is required. Much of the literature on the upper tibial osteotomy is disappointing as relatively few studies have used preoperative and postoperative long-leg films. The best paper is by Ivarsson et al.[40] This showed a clear correlation between optimal surgical correction and clinical result. In everyday terms if you fail to balance the motor car wheel you cannot expect the tyre not to continue to wear.

The valgus knee is more difficult to treat by an osteotomy since, except for mild deformities, the correction has to be carried out in the femur in order to leave the knee joint horizontal to the ground. Not only is it technically more difficult to get a precise correction but there is a higher incidence of non-union and failure of the implant due primarily to the trumpet shape of the distal femur. Excision of a wedge will leave a mismatch between the two oval surfaces, and if the surgeon is not skilful there is a tendency for the proximal fragment to telescope into the distal fragment as it is very easy to lose cortex-to-cortex match. Surgery through the distal femur also has a tendency to precipitate patellofemoral problems whereas with the upper tibial osteotomy for the varus knee it has been observed for many years that patellofemoral symptoms, even if they were present preoperatively, nearly always improve. In summary, the valgus knee tends to have a much more prolonged and more benign natural history but is more difficult to treat by conservative surgery.

Knee replacement is one of the great advances of modern orthopaedics. Its development lagged approximately 10 years behind that of total hip replacement. This was largely due to a misunderstanding of the nature of the instability in the rheumatoid knee. The severe rheumatoid knee is unstable and it was therefore presumed that the ligaments had given way. Knee replacements were therefore designed as hinges to provide stability. The knee, however, is not a hinge and a constrained implant will fail either intrinsically in the implant or at the bone implant junction. Gunston of Canada demonstrated that by employing a very simple design in which a metal semi-circular disc was inserted into each femoral condyle and a simple polyethylene runner placed into each tibial plateau, stability could be regained by jacking the knee apart, i.e., the instability was primarily due to articular cartilage and bony loss rather than ligament rupture. The Gunston knee (Fig. 48.24) had very narrow contact areas between the metal and plastic which consequently suffered creep and failure. The condylar knee replacement (Fig. 48.25) was pioneered by Freeman in England and Insall in the United States. The metallic component covers the whole of the femoral condylar surface and the plastic component essentially covers the whole of the tibial surface, giving a wide contact zone. Once surgeons had learnt the principles of leg alignment and ligament balancing to correct fixed deformities, results from condylar replacement became remarkably consistent. Survival analysis figures show over 90% surviving for 15 years. One word of warning, however, about these figures—many of the patients operated on 15 years ago were already in their seventies. If the age limit falls to those below 60 this success story may cease! Condylar replacements excise the anterior cruciate ligament; indeed some of the designs also remove the posterior cruciate ligament. It would seem unwise to insert this type of implant into patients who still wish to play sports! The 'weak' part of the condylar replacement is the patellofemoral joint. There is a continuing controversy as to whether the patella is best resurfaced with a plastic button or left alone. In general, replacements with a short femoral groove flange require patella resurfacing; those with a longer flange may get away without it. The complication rate is similar in both instances but the actual complications are different. The unreplaced patella has a much higher incidence of pain. The replaced patella suffers from mechanical problems, in particular maltracking, dislocation, loosening, wear and patella fracture.

A recent advance in knee arthroplasty is the unicompartmental replacement. These are direct descendants of the initial bicompartmental replacements such as the Gunston. Their advantage is that they retain the anterior cruciate ligament but they are technically more demanding and the interface between the implant and the bone is less secure than with a condylar replacement. They are contraindicated if there is a significant fixed flexion deformity, if the anterior cruciate ligament is ruptured or if there is significant wear in the opposite compartment. It is too early to draw

REFERENCE

40. Ivarsson I, Myrnecks R, Gillquist J J Bone Joint Surg 1990; 72B: 238

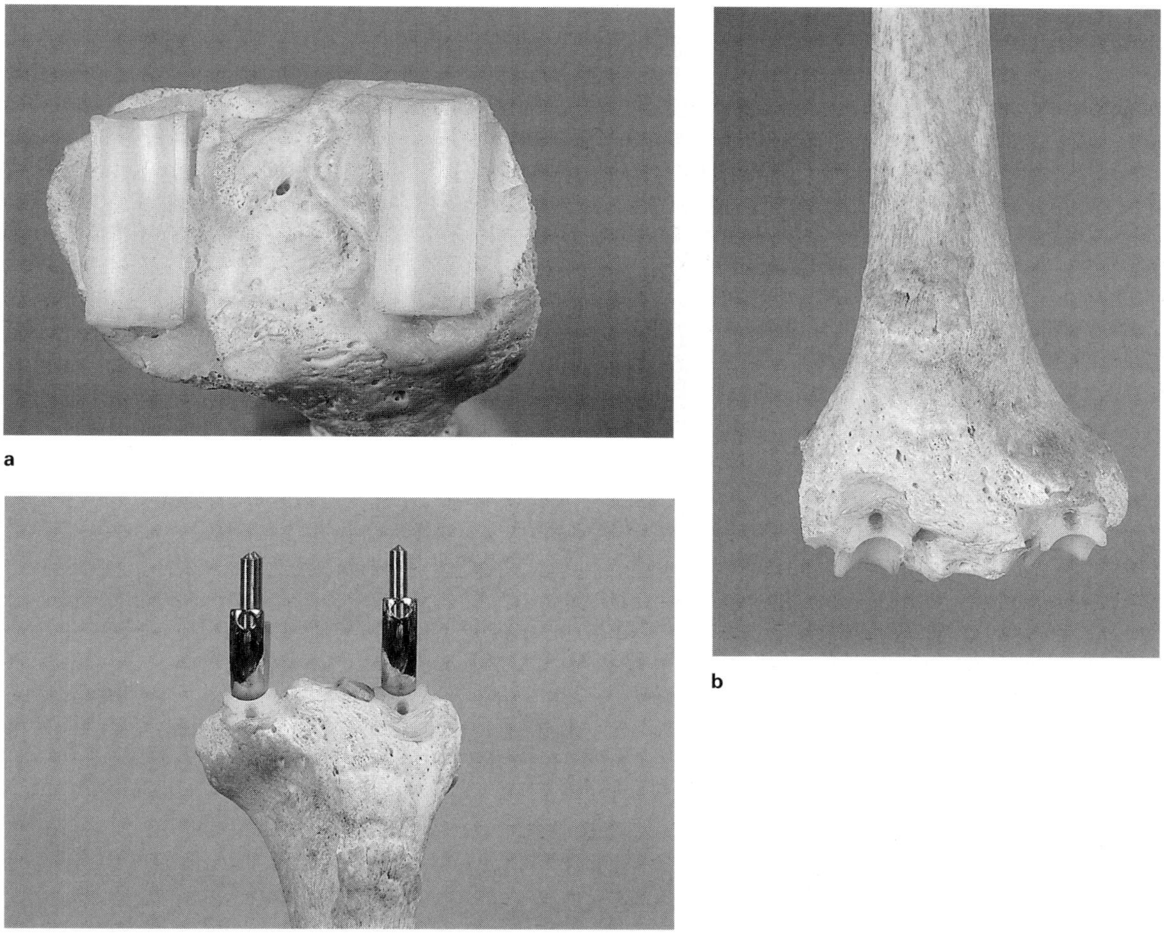

a

b

c

Fig. 48.24 Gunston knee.

deductions as to their long-term survival. It is likely that they will have a greater mechanical failure rate than the condylar replacements but they provide much more normal function. They can be revised to a condylar replacement. Their main indication is the active 'younger patient' but, if you are wise, 'young' means those in early retirement.

Arthrodesis of the knee is a much less satisfactory operation than arthrodesis of the hip. The reason is that a stiff, straight knee, even though it is painless and stable, is extremely antisocial and difficult to live with. Simple activities such as getting into a motor car, getting up from a low chair or picking something off the floor are all difficult. It is sometimes tempting to do this surgery in patients who are very disabled but an arthrodesed knee is not compatible with life in a wheelchair! The common reason for doing an arthrodesis is a failed knee replacement, usually secondary to infection. Arthrodesing such knees is technically difficult and the number of patients requiring an above-knee amputation for failed knee surgery whilst currently small will probably rise, especially if the age group is dropped.

In conclusion, knee arthroplasty is a very significant surgical advance. Currently there is a tendency to lessen the indications for doing the procedure. This may prove to be unwise as revision knee surgery is less satisfactory and more difficult than in the hip.

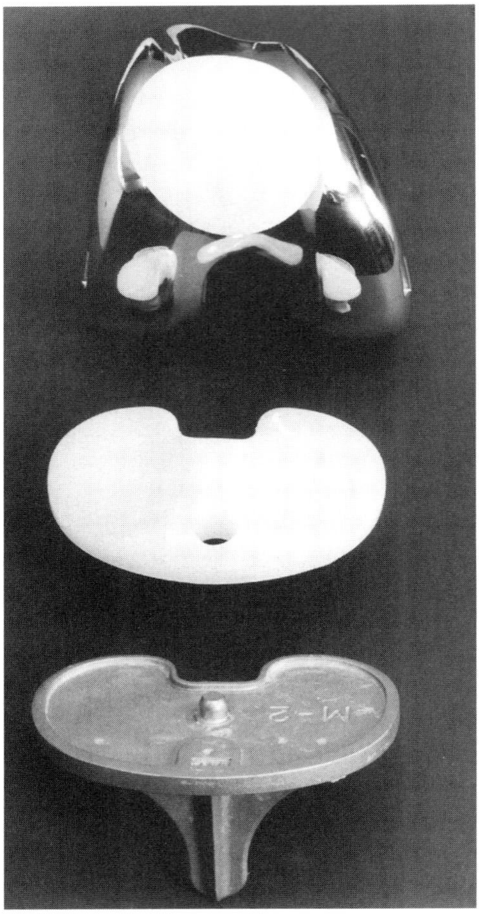
a

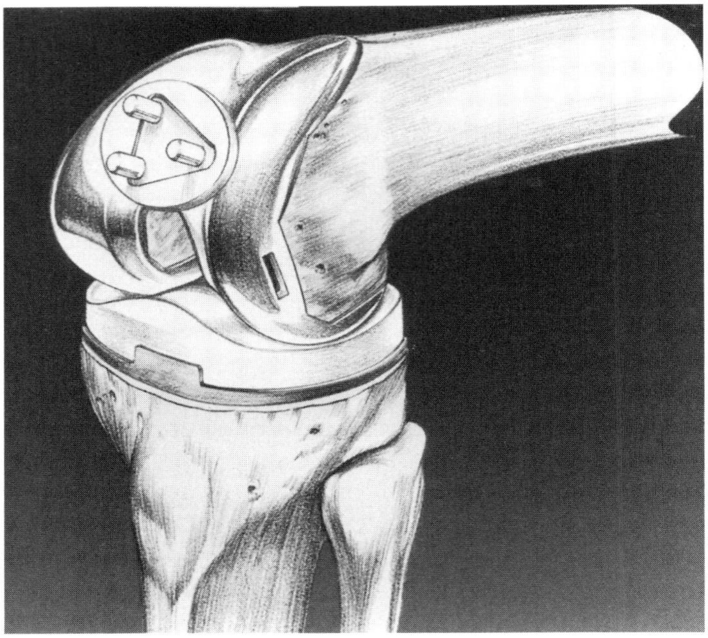
b

Fig. 48.25 Condylar knee.

49 The foot

E. G. Anderson

INTRODUCTION

The foot is a complex mechanical structure which has to fulfil several functions. It provides a platform for balance, acts as a propulsive interface with the ground through a number of different speeds, and it protects the body from impact forces through its intrinsic shock-absorbing system. To achieve these functions, the foot has a flexibly linked skeleton, the alignment of which is largely maintained by strong ligaments mainly on its plantar surface. It is controlled by a combination of proprioceptive neural input which produces rapid muscular responses, and an intrinsic stabilizing system activated by the ground reaction forces generated in normal gait. This system is also responsible in the main for the shock-absorbing capacity of the foot.[1]

The foot receives its blood supply from two anterior and one posterior arteries, and its nerve supply via the posterior tibial, superficial and deep peroneal, saphenous and sural nerves.

The muscles which control foot movement are grouped into flexors, extensors, invertors and evertors. It is a mistake, however, to consider that each functions in only one way. The tibialis anterior, for example, has a more important function pulling the tibia (and therefore the body) over the fixed foot, than in just dorsiflexing the foot, and the tibialis posterior acts more as a brake to supination than as a simple foot invertor.

Many of the problems which affect the foot relate to malfunction of its structure rather than to any disease process. An understanding of the structural function of the foot is therefore vital to an understanding of most patients' complaints, although of course disease processes do affect the foot, and can affect its function (Fig. 49.1).

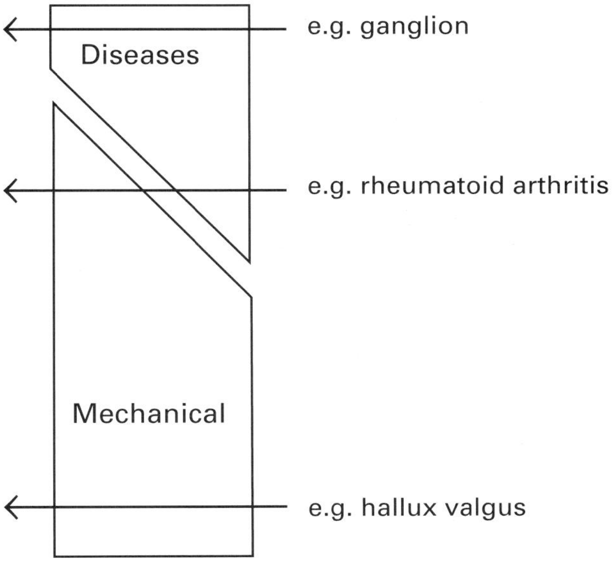

Fig. 49.1 Aetiology of foot disorders.

FOOT DISEASE

Diseases which affect the foot do so by producing destruction of bone, by producing destruction of soft tissues, by limiting the range of joint movement, or by limiting the power of movement.

They cause pain, alteration of gait, usually seen as a limp, loss of function or deformity. Pain is the most important of these symptoms. A distinction has to be made between pain of a mechanical and of a non-mechanical origin, as this is the cardinal distinction between foot disease and a mechanical disorder.

Non-mechanical pain is present at rest, in bed, and is not necessarily aggravated by activity; mechanical pain is generated by activity, and is exercise dependent: the more you do the worse it gets, and it is quickly relieved by rest.

Tumours of the foot

The incidence of benign tumours in the foot is quite high, and of malignant tumours very low. In a practice spanning 18 years and 14 000 referrals in a specialized foot surgery unit, there have been only seven malignant tumours, giving an incidence of 0.05% of referrals.[2]

The distribution of the swelling or tumour can give an indicator as to what diagnosis can be expected. Ganglia, for example, only rarely occur on the plantar aspect of the foot, and then often at a deeper level. Almost any tumour can be found distal to the metatarsal heads, and the skin and nail beds are a not uncommon site for melanoma (see Ch. 9).

As a general rule, all suspicious swellings of the foot should be excised for histological examination. Computed tomography (CT) and magnetic resonance imaging (MRI) can give helpful pointers to the extent of the tumour. Treatment follows the same principles as elsewhere, although there are some points which are peculiar to the foot.

REFERENCES

1. Klenerman L The Foot and its Disorders, 3rd edn. Blackwell, London 1991
2. Craigen M A C, Anderson E G Foot 1991; 1: 113

exercises the proprioceptive feedback mechanisms. Once the ulcer is healed, a customized, cushioned and contoured insole must be ready for use.

When the vascular supply is compromised despite the best treatment, and the ulcer remains indolent, reconstructable proximal arterial disease should be dealt with. If this fails, or if significant proximal disease is not present and the ulcer is not infected, then the patient may opt simply for local dressings, rather than definitive surgery, which often means amputation. Even when revascularization is successful, the risk of recurring infection still remains, and amputation may well become necessary sooner or later. In the short term, however, mobility is often maintained.

When it becomes necessary, amputation should be considered a positive option, not an admission of failure. It can be performed at many levels in the foot, and also longitudinally as a ray excision (see Ch. 10). Nevertheless, taking into consideration the available prostheses and the resulting function, there are three levels which give consistently good results: amputation of a toe; at the ankle (Symes); below-knee. Midfoot amputations have been found by some to be satisfactory,[18] but are disliked by others.

Osteoarthritis

This common affliction of human joints may occur as a monoarthritis, or as part of a more generalized disease. In the foot the first ray is most often affected, usually at the metatarsophalangeal joint. The tarsometatarsal joint and even more proximal joints may become diseased, and painful as a result of instability of the first ray. The effect is ultimately mechanical as a result of painful joint stiffening, deformity and osteophytic marginal enlargement of the joint.

Examination confirms the limited painful joint movement, and the prominent osteophytes. Radiologically the joint 'space' is narrowed with loss of articular cartilage, osteophytes are seen, there is subchondral sclerosis of the bone, and cysts may also be present.

The management will be considered with the mechanical disorders.

Rheumatoid arthritis

This disease tends to affect either the hindfoot or the forefoot, and only late in the disease may it affect both. In the forefoot the metatarsophalangeal joints are the usual target, and the erosive nature of the pannus soon destroys the metatarsal heads, causing the classical symptom of 'walking on broken glass'. First thing in the morning, the joints are stiff, easing with movement, but becoming more painful again with increasing activity, and thus ultimately limiting mobility.

Examination usually confirms swelling around the metatarsophalangeal joints, particularly on the plantar aspect where the metatarsal heads, or stumps as they become, erode through the joint capsule. These bones become prominent in the sole, usually with overlying bursae and gross callosities (Fig. 49.3). The toes claw (eventually dislocating dorsally) and the gait becomes stiff-footed, avoiding metatarsal head roll-over, and with a short stride length.

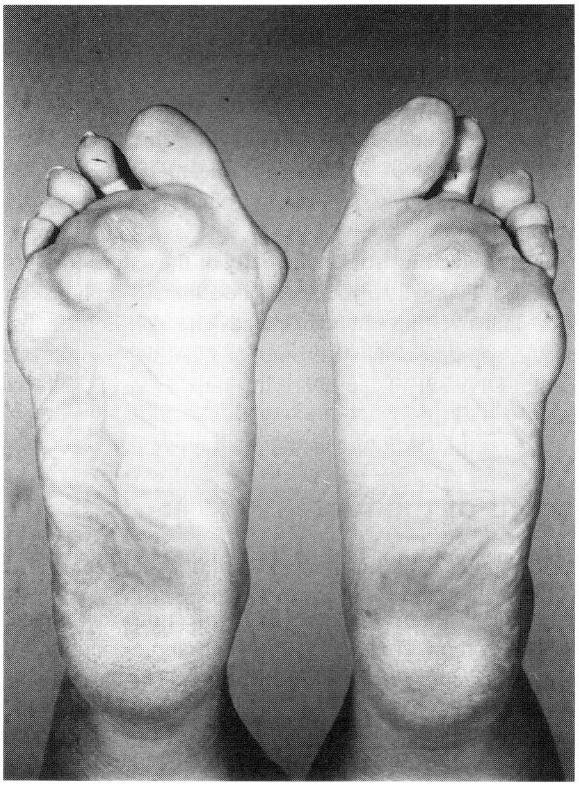

Fig. 49.3 Rheumatoid forefoot.

Radiologically, there are progressive erosions of the metatarsal heads, and later there is erosion of the bases of the proximal phalanges (Fig. 49.4). Peri-articular osteoporosis is usually seen. Rheumatoid feet may also have peripheral vasculitis, and ulceration (see Ch. 10).

Rheumatoid disease in the hindfoot is much more disabling, affecting the ankle, subtalar and midtarsal joints. Occasionally the first presenting symptom of rheumatoid disease is a painful talonavicular joint, and indeed non-mechanical pain in the medial midfoot is highly suspicious of rheumatoid disease.

The management of the rheumatoid foot is best done by joint care from an orthopaedic surgeon and a rheumatologist.

Conservative management consists primarily of providing comfortable footwear, with seamless uppers, cushioned soles and insoles, and sufficient space to accommodate the often gross toe deformities. Painful hindfeet can be helped with the provision of a fixed-ankle ankle–foot orthosis (AFO) (a 'caliper' or brace which prevents any movement at the ankle or subtalar joint). Ultimately painful stiffening or eroding joints require surgery.

Individully affected hindfoot joints can be arthrodesed, and early talonavicular fusion can prevent later hyperpronation deformity.[19] Ankle joint replacement has not been as successful as that for the knee or hip, and only now is showing acceptable five-year results. Salvage after a failed replacement ankle is extremely difficult.

REFERENCE

18. Young A E Am J Surg 1977; 134: 604

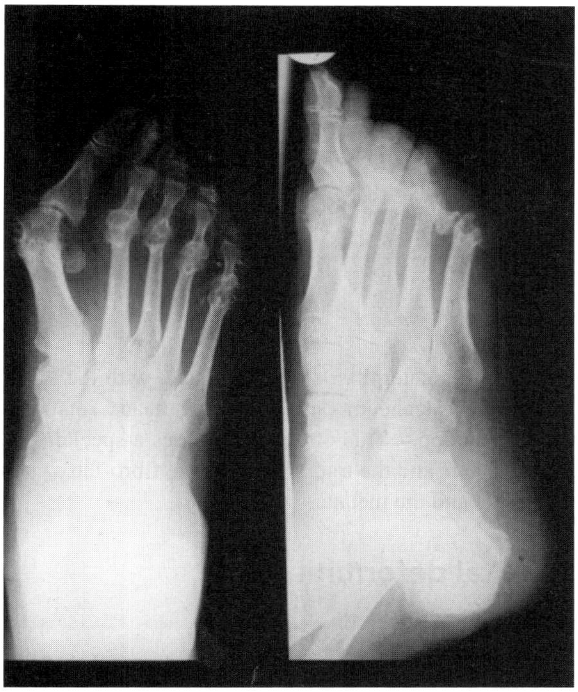

Fig. 49.4 Radiograph of rheumatoid forefoot.

Neurological disorders

The function of the foot can be dramatically altered by neurological disease. The surgeon may be presented with a problematic foot as a result of an established neurological condition, but not infrequently the patient may present with symptoms of sensory change, motor weakness, or increasing dysfunction. 'I keep going over on my ankle' may be the first presentation of multiple sclerosis, or a hereditary motor and sensory neuropathy, such as Charcot–Marie–Tooth disease, also known as peroneal muscular atrophy. Referral to a neurologist for a precise diagnosis, and prognosis, is essential before treatment is considered. Treatment depends on the mechanical effects of the disorder; it may consist of only orthotic management, or a combined surgical–orthotic approach.

As in an insensate foot, great care is required to avoid footwear rubbing, and to contour and cushion insoles to eliminate high-pressure points which can ulcerate. In the elderly, too much cushioning can impair proprioceptive feedback, such that the patient's stability is compromised rather than improved. Spasticity and flaccidity both affect the mechanical functioning of the foot.

Children with cerebral palsy should if possible be assessed by sophisticated gait analysis to ensure that any proposed surgery is in fact likely to achieve its desired effect.[20] Better assessment also leads to better orthotic management.

Spina bifida and myelomeningocele are now relatively rare partly because amniocentesis provides an early diagnosis, and also because there is a natural reduction in their incidence. Whilst the level of spinal damage may determine the lower level of motor and sensory deficit, it does not equate with the functional result, as the higher centres have a large input and may have been damaged by the hydrocephalus which generally accompanies the disorder. As it affects primarily lower motor neurones, a flaccid paralysis is usual, although complicating spasticity is not infrequently seen.

As in cerebral palsy, accurate assessment, with gait analysis where appropriate, is required before planning treatment. While simple flaccid deformities are readily managed orthotically, surgery can frequently enhance orthotic control—so-called surgical–orthotic integration.[21]

Stroke patients with impaired foot function are amenable to simple treatment which can improve their function out of all proportion. The 'drop foot' from tibialis anterior paralysis can imperil gait as the foot is liable to catch the ground on the swing-through phase, and a simple ankle–foot orthosis can be of great assistance. Spastic clawed toes may only respond to surgery, but even the dysvascular anticoagulated foot can be safely improved by flexor tendon tenotomies.

Trauma

Whilst the general management of trauma is discussed elsewhere, there are two problems which deserve mention in relation to the foot.

Foot injury can cause major structural problems which may be amenable to further reconstructive surgery. In addition reflex sympathetic dystrophy is still overlooked as a complication of minor injury and also surgery.[22]

It can be seen that disease may result in a mechanical disorder of the foot, which can affect the patient by causing joint stiffness and pain, bone destruction and structural deformity.

STRUCTURAL FOOT DISORDERS

In order to understand the causes, where as they are known, the effects of structural disorders of the foot and the possible surgical treatments it is necessary to have a working knowledge of structure of the foot.[23]

The foot is at one end of a kinetic chain of levers and articulations. Movement occurring at the foot has a proximal effect, with symptoms being produced in the knee, and vice versa.

The foot consists of two segmented beams which articulate with each other at the subtalar joint. These beams comprise a lateral stabilizing beam of calcaneum, cuboid and the lateral two metatarsals and toes, and a medial dynamic beam of talus, navicular, cuneiforms and medial three metatarsals and toes. Each joint

REFERENCES

19. Elbaor J E, Thomas W H, Weinfeld M S et al Orthop Clin North Am 1976; 7: 821
20. Tachdjian M O Paediatric Orthopaedics, 2nd edn. Saunders, Philadelphia 1990
21. Rose G K 1982 In: Jahss M H (ed) Disorders of the Foot, 1st edn. Saunders, Philadelphia 1982
22. Atkins R M In: Helal B, Rowley D I, Cracchiolo III A, Myerson M S (eds) Surgery of Disorders of the Foot and Ankle. Martin Dunitz, London 1996
23. Hutton W C, Stokes I A F In: Klenerman L (ed) The Foot and its Disorders, 3rd edn. Blackwell, London 1991

ously known as Sever's disease,[34] is considered to be a traction apophysitis which resolves spontaneously, although a small heel pad raise and rest from sport may help.

The 'osteochondritides' are conditions again of unknown aetiology where the vascular supply to a bone or part of a bone is interrupted. This causes part of the bone to die before it is replaced by new bone as new vessels grow in. The bone becomes plastic during this phase, and permanent deformity can occur. In males around the age of 5, the navicular can be affected (Köhler's disease).[35] When pain is severe only rest is required, as the condition appears to recover spontaneously without adverse sequelae.

In girls of 12–14, the head of either the second or third metatarsal can be the focus of this condition, here called Freiberg's infraction (Fig. 49.8).[36] It is strange that there is a wide spectrum of clinical presentation from the subclinical which only becomes known when a radiograph is taken of the foot for other reasons many years later, to the acutely swollen and inflamed joint, with nothing to see on X-ray. A radio-isotope bone scan usually shows increased uptake, and MRI confirms the diagnosis with a signal of intra-osseous fluid. Affected children usually complain of pain and a little swelling, with reluctance to take weight on that part of the foot, causing a limp. Analgesia and rest allow these to settle down within a few months in the vast majority of cases. Only occasionally does an osteochondral fragment break off, or become loose, in which case resolution only occurs after its removal.[37] Operation to rotate the metatarsal head dorsally has been described, but this is rarely if ever necessary.

Failure of foot structure

The structure of the foot can fail in various ways. The ligaments and muscles lose their integrity, joints stiffen, diminishing normal compensatory mechanisms and imposing abnormal patterns of movement which increase stresses. Joints dislocate or otherwise lose their integrity and soft tissues deteriorate causing the imposition of abnormal patterns of movement. Each of these problems can occur independently of the others, but more often than not they are interdependent.

Metatarsalgia is a common symptom. It literally means pain under the ball of the foot. This can refer to pain arising from the metatarsal heads, the metatarsophalangeal joints, the bases of the proximal phalanges, or the soft tissue between and just distal to the metatarsal heads. It is therefore absolutely essential that as precise a history as possible is obtained, and that an accurate examination is made to determine the source of the pain.

Symptomatic forefoot malalignment

This is a term that is used to denote the symptomatic foot in which the forefoot is found to be inverted or everted with respect to the hindfoot, and in which an appropriate history and examination findings are present (Fig. 49.9).

The symptoms of uncompensated forefoot inversion are interdigital neuritic pain, previously called Morton's neuroma (often simply but erroneously described as metatarsalgia, see above), the specific sign of which is localized pain on pressure between, and

REFERENCES

34. Ferguson A, Generich R Clin Orthop 1959; 10: 87
35. Kohler A Munch Med Wochenschr 1908; 55: 1923
36. Smillie I S J Bone Joint Surg 1955; 37: 580
37. Smith T W D, Stanley D, Rowley D J Bone Joint Surg 1991; 73B: 129

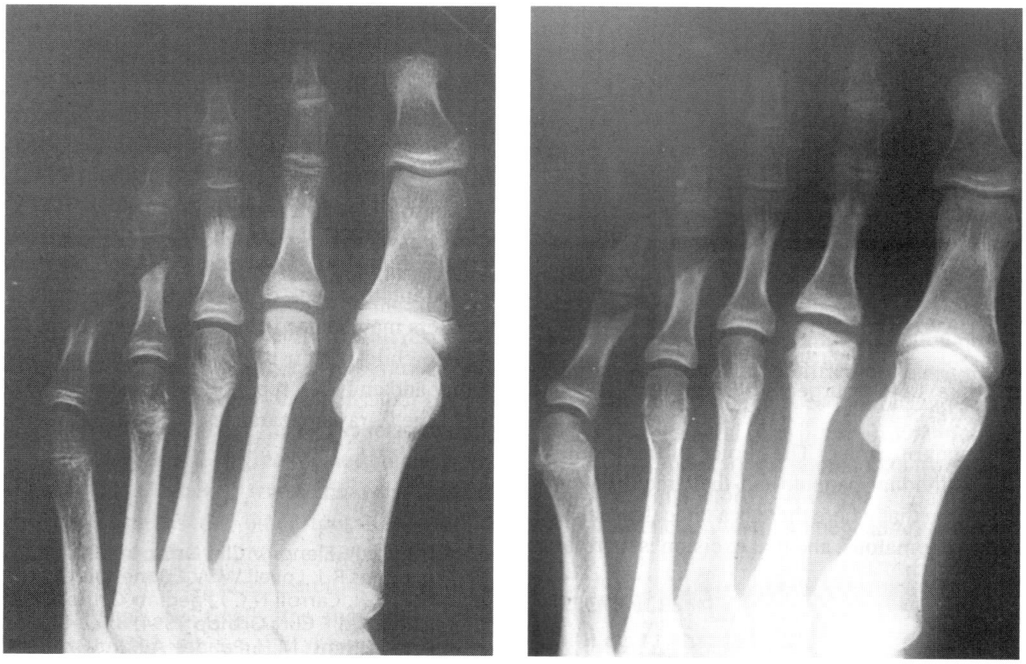

a b

Fig. 49.8 Freiberg infraction of the second metatarsal head.

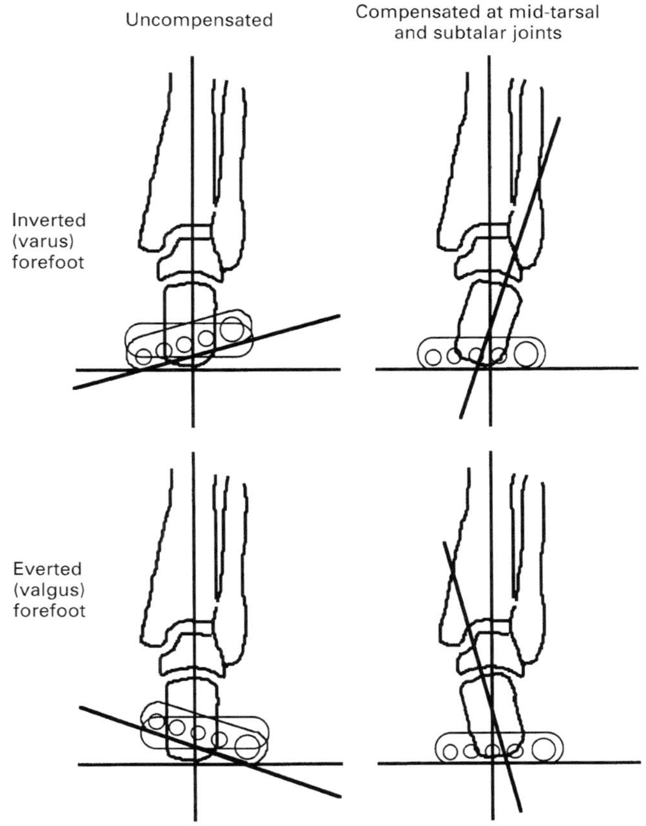

Fig. 49.9 Forefoot malalignments: (**a**) inverted forefoot; (**b**) compensated inverted forefoot; (**c**) everted forefoot; (**d**) compensated everted forefoot.

just distal to the metatarsal heads, and posterior tibial tendon pain of which the specific clinical sign is tenderness over the posterior tibial tendon below and behind the medial malleolus when palpated as the foot is inverted against resistance. Patients may also complain of transverse midtarsal pain but the physical sign of limitation of midtarsal inversion is almost always present. The inverted forefoot is compensated by hyperpronation of the foot.

When uncompensated forefoot eversion is associated with generalized joint hypermobility, the clinical presentation is the same as that of the inverted forefoot, with the exception of the clinical sign of eversion rather than inversion of the forefoot with respect to the hindfoot.

In the absence of generalized joint hypermobility, patients complain of interdigital neuritis, less commonly of transverse metatarsal pain, and occasionally give a history of recurrent ankle/foot inversion, usually without causing injury. The everted forefoot is compensated by supination of the foot, presenting as a 'high-arched' foot, with a plantarflexed first metatarsal. Whether this latter is cause or effect is open to question.

Management of these conditions is primarily orthotic, with the use of cast functional foot orthoses, i.e., the orthoses are made to casts of the feet held in a 'corrected' position. They are only compensatory, but the effects can be immediate. Like spectacles which are ocular compensations, the benefits are only experienced as long as the orthoses are in use.

It must be emphasised that this is appropriate management only in the adult. In the child, where the forces are less, and the opportunity at least exists to hold the foot in a corrected position while it develops, a different approach is indicated. 'Flat foot' is normal in the early stages of childhood development because of a pad of fat under the midfoot which gradually disappears during growth. In children, when 'flat foot' is pathological it frequently presents with a history of the medial counter of the shoe breaking down (Fig. 49.10). Joint hypermobility, hyperpronation and a secondarily tight tendo Achilles are indications for the provision of a calcaneal rotation-controlling heel cup of the Schwartz or Helfet type.[21] Frequently these can be dispensed with when the foot stops growing and, unless the patient complains of ongoing symptoms, no further treatment is indicated.

In a hyperpronated foot, the ground reaction force through the weight-bearing area cannot be brought back under the loading line of the body, and thus a couple is formed, producing a turning moment which tends to increase the deformity, putting the posterior tendon under tremendous stress. It then becomes incompetent and ultimately ruptures, causing the foot to collapse into gross hyperpronation. Surgery is then the only practical management. Various tendon transfers have been described. That of Cobb[38] uses a split tibialis anterior tendon rerouted through the medial cuneiform bone before it is anastomosed to the posterior tibial tendon proximal to the degenerate area, which is excised. An uncorrected mobile or fixed deformity can result in impingement of the calcaneum on the fibula, which can cause stress pain from a stretched medial collateral ligament of the ankle. Simply excising a piece of the distal fibula does not solve the problem as the deforming forces merely reproduce the impingement (Fig. 49.11).

When the deformity becomes fixed, soft tissue correction is impracticable. The mechanical deforming forces can be overcome by moving the weight-bearing area of the heel back under the loading line of the leg by a medial translational osteotomy of the calcaneum (Fig. 49.12). Rotation of the calcaneum can increase the medial translation of the weight-bearing area quite considerably.[21]

REFERENCE

38. Cobb N In: Helal B, Rowley D, Cracchiolo III A, Myerson M S, Surgery of Disorders of the Foot and Ankle. Martin Dunitz, London 1996

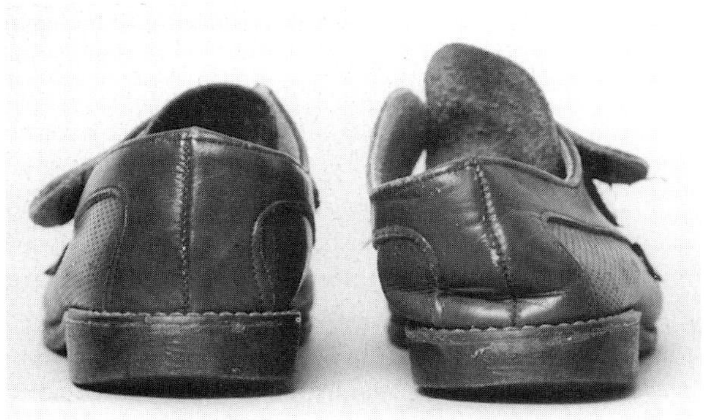

Fig. 49.10 Shoe counter deformed by pronated foot.

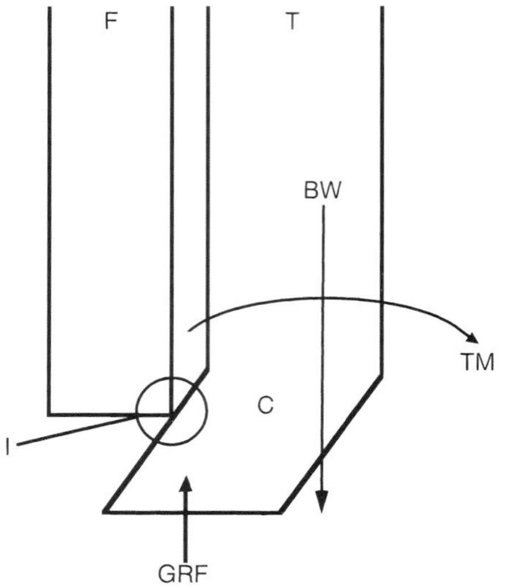

Fig. 49.11 Everted heel deforming forces. C, Calcaneum; F, fibula; T, tibia; I, impingement; BW, body weight GRF, ground reaction force; TM, turning moment.

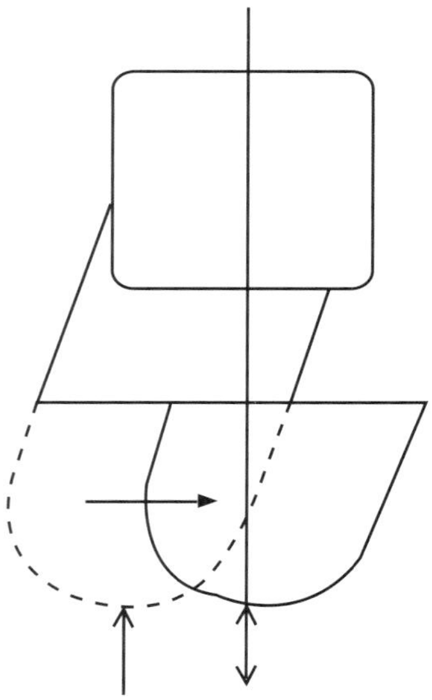

Fig. 49.12 Translational calcaneal osteotomy.

The patient with an everted forefoot whose symptoms are not being controlled by an orthosis can be treated by reducing plantarflexion of the first metatarsal by a basal dorsal wedge osteotomy. This requires great care as over-correction can result in overloading of the second metatarsal, and hence under-correction is preferable.[39]

The 'high-arched' or cavus foot in children (Fig. 49.13) is often associated with a neurological disorder, which should always be sought. The development of symptoms in the mid to late teens gives rise to suspicions of a spinal cause, and occasionally a spinal dysraphism is found.[40] Any spinal condition requires treatment first. The cavus foot is often accompanied by an inverted heel, and clawing of the toes. A lateral calcaneal osteotomy or lateral column lengthening can be performed if the foot is very painful.[41] The high arch tends to cause increased and often painful overloading of the middle metatarsal heads, or of the first and fifth metatarsal heads. Metatarsal neck osteotomy, however, is unwise as it is an uncontrolled procedure with an uncertain outcome. Such problems are best tackled orthotically, although it is often very difficult to get a satisfied patient. Where the arch deformity is severe, and the joints fixed, consideration can be given to midtarsal wedge osteotomy to straighten the foot. This does not need to be accompanied by plantar soft tissue release, as the plantar fascia is inserted into the bases of the proximal phalanges.

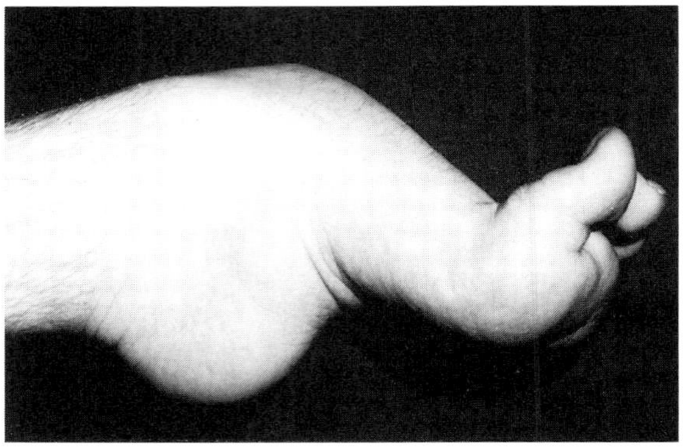

Fig. 49.13 Cavus foot.

Toe deformities

Clawing of the toes (flexion of both proximal and distal interphalangeal joints) often accompanies the cavus foot. In the more severe cases, the hallux is also clawed and correction with a Robert Jones procedure is indicated if the flexed proximal phalanx rubs on footwear, and does not straighten when the first metatarsal is dorsiflexed by plantar pressure under its head. In this the long extensor tendon is transferred to the neck of the first metatarsal, and the interphalangeal joint fused. It is a very effective procedure (Fig. 49.14).[42]

Small toes which are mobile can be straightened by the Girdlestone transfer of the flexor tendon to the extensor tendon over the dorsum of the proximal phalanx.[43] Once fixed, the interphalangeal joint deformities can only be corrected by arthrodesing them in a corrected position.

Hammer deformities (extension of the metatarsophalangeal and distal interphalangeal joints, with flexion of the proximal interphalangeal joint) generally affect the second toes, often accompanying hallux valgus. They are best dealt with by arthrodesing the proximal interphalangeal joint, although tenotomy of the long extensor tendon and release of the dorsal metatarsophalangeal joint capsule is sometimes necessary to allow the toe to lie flat.[44] Excision of the

REFERENCES

39. Giuntini L Atti SIOT 1955; 40: 215
40. Duckworth T In: Jahss M H (ed) Disorders of the Foot, 1st edn. Saunders, Philadelphia 1982
41. Dwyer F C J Bone Joint Surg 1959; 41B: 80
42. Jones R Br Med J 1923; 1: 749
43. Taylor R G J Bone Joint Surg 1951; 56B: 314
44. Sandeman J C Br J Clin Pract 1967; 24: 489

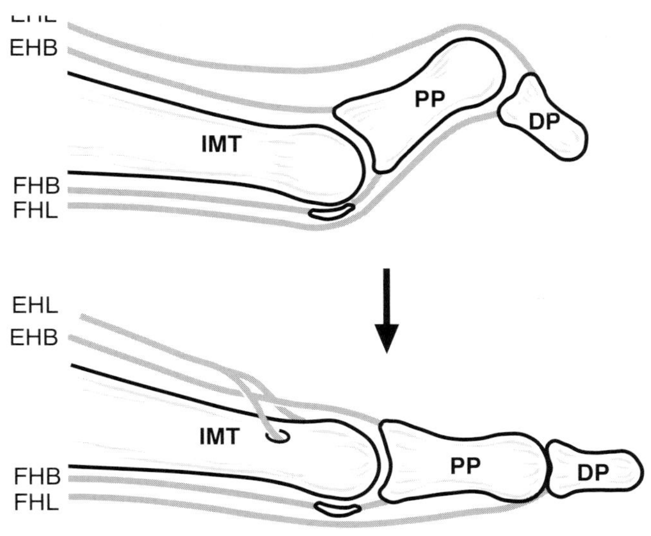

Fig. 49.14 The Robert Jones procedure. IMT = first metatarsal; PP = proximal phalanx; DP = distal phalanx

head of the proximal phalanx is an alternative to proximal interphalangeal joint fusion.[45]

The retracted toe (clawed toe which has dislocated dorsally at the metatarsophalangeal joint) cannot at present be treated satisfactorily. Techniques have been described to reduce the dislocation, but these have not found anything like universal acceptance, and excision arthroplasty remains the treatment of choice for most. Excision of the proximal half of the proximal phalanx, however, leaves a stump of a toe that retracts, is cosmetically unacceptable, and can still impinge on footwear. Stainsby[25] has described the dislocation of the volar plate over the top of the neck of the metatarsal which is responsible for the increased plantar pressure and resulting callosity found in many cases. The procedure he has described to correct this deformity requires the excision of all but the head and neck of the proximal phalanx, relocation of the volar plate, and suture of the divided extensor tendon to the flexor. The result is a straight toe, with little loss of length, but which remains totally 'floppy' (Fig. 49.15).

The mallet toe (flexion of the terminal phalanx only) is uncommon except as a complication of proximal interphalangeal joint fusion where insufficient care has been taken to reconstruct the extensor mechanism. It is best dealt with by distal joint fusion combined with long flexor tenotomy.[46] Fusion at this level is extremely difficult to achieve, but a good fibrous union is just as effective as long as the deforming flexor force is dealt with.

Joint fusion should not be carried out on the little (fifth) toe. Simple deformities can be treated very adequately by excising the distal half of the proximal phalanx. Where the toe is adducted, excision of the proximal half (or more) of the proximal phalanx, together with V-Y plasty of the tight skin and subcutaneous band, and extensor tenotomy is the simplest and usually most effective procedure.[47]

This follows the first law of production engineering as applied to surgery: the more complex the procedure, the more likely it is to go wrong.

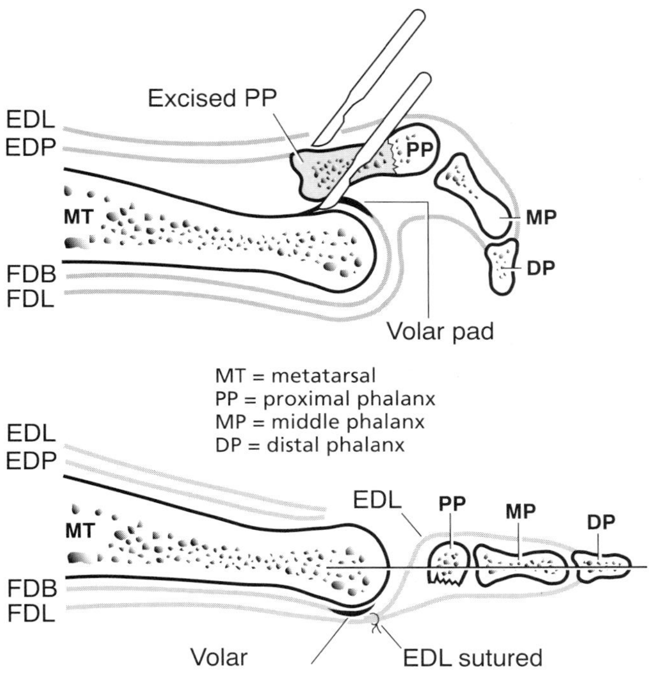

Fig. 49.15 The Stainsby procedure. EDL = extensor digitorum longus; EDB = extensor digitorum brevis; FDB = flexor digitorum brevis; FDL = flexor digitorum longus.

Spastic claw toes may be best managed by open flexor tenotomies, ensuring the proximal ends retract sufficiently not to rejoin. This is particularly suitable in stroke patients, who may have the procedure under local anaesthesia.

Metatarsal deformities

In infants, adducted metatarsals accompany congenital talipes equinovarus but can also be found in isolation, when they respond well to manipulation.

Hallux valgus

This is probably one of the commonest, if not the commonest, disorder of the foot. Often referred to as 'bunions', the complaints are generally of prominence of the medial eminence of the first metatarsal head with or without an overlying bursa ('the bunion'), which deforms footwear, or leads to difficulty in finding footwear that fits. It may also cause pain at the metatarsophalangeal joint. The hammered or retracted second toe may be complained of, but the real problem lies with the hallux valgus.

The assessment now required is far more sophisticated than a few years ago when the decision was between surgical shoes and

REFERENCES

45. Mann R A (ed) DuVries' Surgery of the Foot, 4th edn. Mosby, St Louis 1978
46. Grace D L In: Helal B, Rowley D, Cracchiolo III A, Myerson M S (eds) Surgery of Disorders of the Foot and Ankle. Martin Dunitz, London 1996
47. Wilson J N Br J Surg 1953; 41: 133

'the' operation. The condition has an unknown aetiology, or even aetiologies. Hallux valgus is after all the description of the alignment of the great toe, not an indicator of the pathology. It is known that the wearing of enclosed footwear (not 'silly' footwear) is associated with an increased incidence, and there is no doubting the strong familial traits.[48]

Hallux valgus may develop at an early age before the foot has stopped growing, and this juvenile onset is not easy to deal with. The provision of broad-fitting shoes and orthodigital splints should be advised until the foot has reached skeletal maturity, usually at about the age of 14. Thereafter adult principles apply. If the deformity is rapidly advancing, then conservative surgery which avoids growth plates is advised.

The points to note on examination include the amount of varus deformity of the metatarsal as well as the valgus deformity and degree of rotation of the toe. The range of movement in both the metatarsophalangeal and interphalangeal joints must be checked, and the presence of any callosities noted. Any increased pronation or supination of the midfoot must be tested for, and finally the presence of joint hypermobility: Johnson's 'squeeze test'[49] gives an indication of the mobility of the first metatarsal.

Radiological examination should be carried out with the feet weight-bearing where possible. The shape changes in all feet when they are load-bearing. There are many points to observe on X-ray. They include determining the extent of the valgus, first/second intermetatarsal and distal metatarsal articular angles (Fig. 49.16); the length of the first metatarsal relative to the second, and the state of the first tarsometatarsal joint which may be unstable; an articulation may be present between the first and second metatarsals at their bases, and the congruence and state of wear of the first metatarsophalangeal joint.

The patient's level of activity, the state of their peripheral vasculature and their mental ability to cope with treatment are important factors in determining treatment. Age of itself is not strictly relevant. A decision first has to be taken as to whether surgery or conservative management is indicated. This is a decision often determined by the patient, but occasionally when the implications are spelled out they decline surgery. Off-the-shelf footwear is now freely available, in a wide variety of extra-depth and extra-width fittings for well under £100 (US $160) per pair. Bespoke, made-to-measure footwear is preferable but costs around £300+ per pair. It is absolutely essential that all footwear should be examined by the prescriber after a couple of months' use to determine its suitability.

The days of a single operation for hallux valgus have, thankfully, gone. A good surgical armamentarium contains five or more operations, and the patient must be given sufficient information to permit them to give informed consent. They must therefore know in outline what the procedure involves; whether there will be any indwelling metalwork; how long they will be in plaster (if at all) and how soon they will be able to resume activities, including work. A figure of three months for the last is often a major constraint to agreement to surgery. They should also be informed of any common complications (with an incidence of more than 5%).

The algorithm (Fig. 49.17) suggests possible steps to follow in deciding which operation is appropriate, bearing in mind the following points. A worn joint is an incongruent joint which cannot be realigned and/or cannot flex and extend comfortably in that position. A congruent joint in the presence of hallux valgus requires the distal metatarsal articular alignment to be corrected. A short first metatarsal should not be shortened further. An unstable tarsometatarsal joint may need to be stabilized. A first/second intermetatarsal angle which exceeds 15 degrees precludes chevron osteotomy and may require a basal osteotomy for correction.

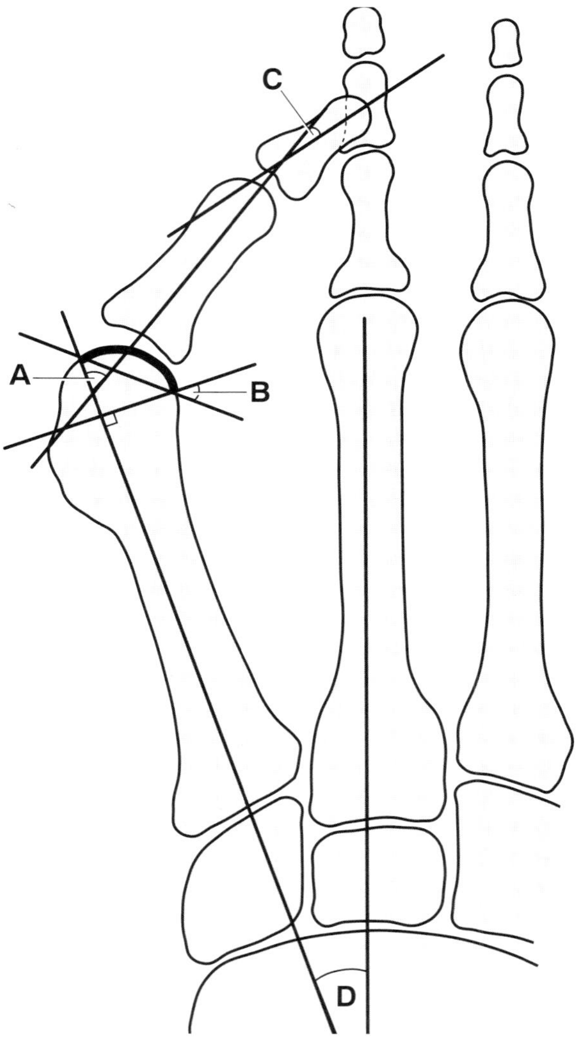

Fig. 49.16 Forefoot angles. A, Hallux valgus angle; B, distal metatarsal articulation angle; C, interphalangeal angle; D, 1/2 intermetatarsal angle.

The operations

Almost all operations are carried out through a medial midline incision, which is least likely to result in nerve damage.[50] Operations in which the joint integrity is maintained must include a capsuloplasty, and a medial V-Y plasty is a suitable method of

REFERENCES

48. Sim Fook L, Hodgson A R J Bone Joint Surg 1958; 40A: 1058
49. Johnson K Personal communication
50. Campbell D A J R Coll Surg Edinb 1992; 37: 422

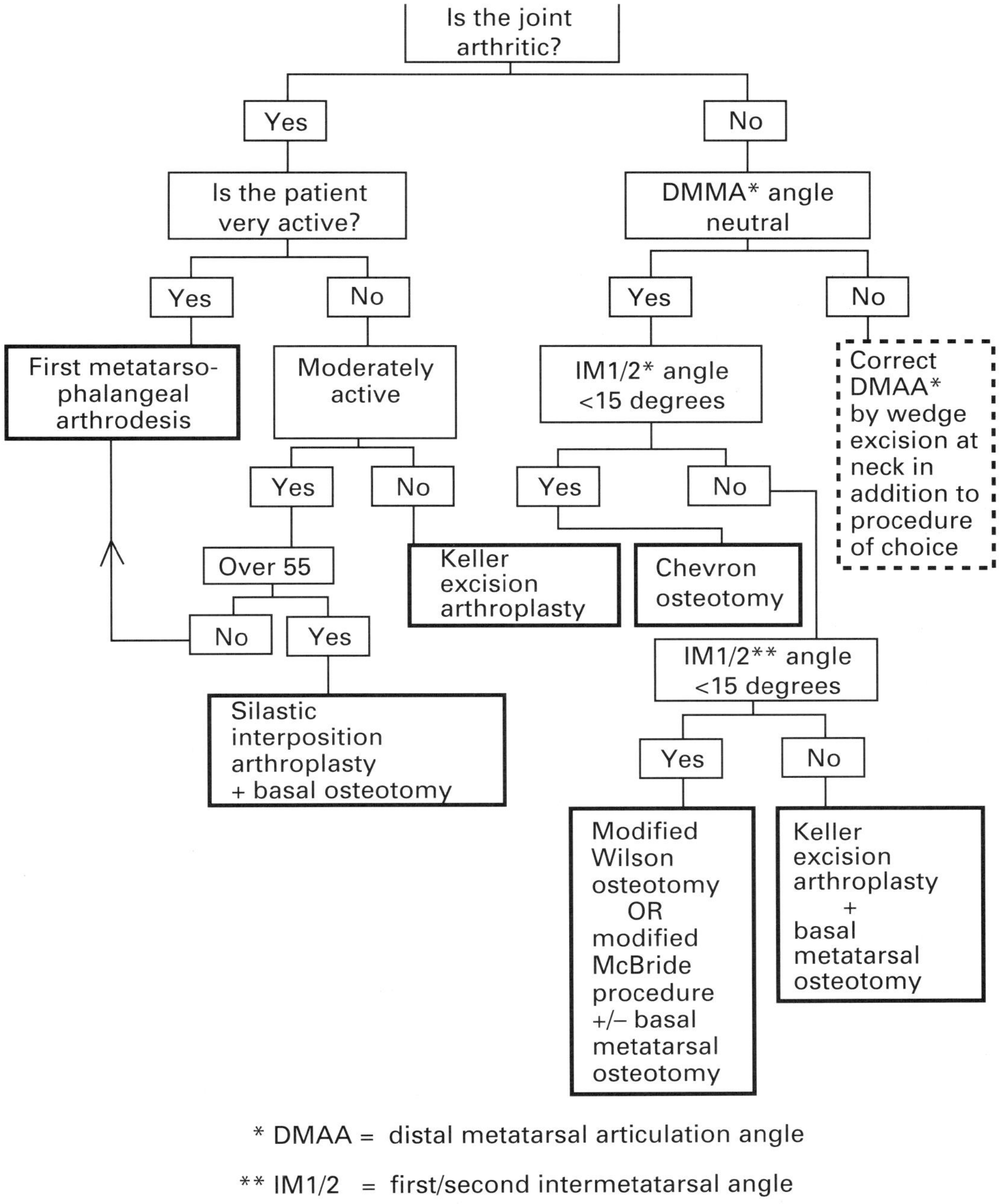

Fig. 49.17 Management of hallux valgus.

achieving this (Fig. 49.18). Incisions may be made straight down to bone where the integrity of the joint is not dependent on the capsule.

Arthrodesis—a large surface area of cancellous bone can be created by forming a cone of the head of the metatarsal, and reaming a reciprocal shape from the base of the proximal phalanx. This has the advantage of allowing the apex of the cone to be varied according to the amount of valgus present, and of allowing adjustability before fixation (with a single screw) (Fig. 49.19).[51] A mobile metatarsus varus is pulled towards the second metatarsal once the bones are fixed, by the action of the adductor hallucis muscle, and a basal osteotomy is rarely required. Fusions are sound enough to allow free function after six or occasionally eight weeks. About 5% of fusions fail to unite, but even then a painless, non-union often gives a successful outcome. The operation is repeated using intramedullary bone graft across the joint, which is kept protected for six to eight weeks, if the original arthrodesis fails and pain is still present (Fig. 49.20).[52]

REFERENCES

51. Marin G A Guy's Hosp Rep 1960; 109: 194
52. McBride D J, Anderson E G J Bone Joint Surg 1994; 76B(suppl II & III): 93

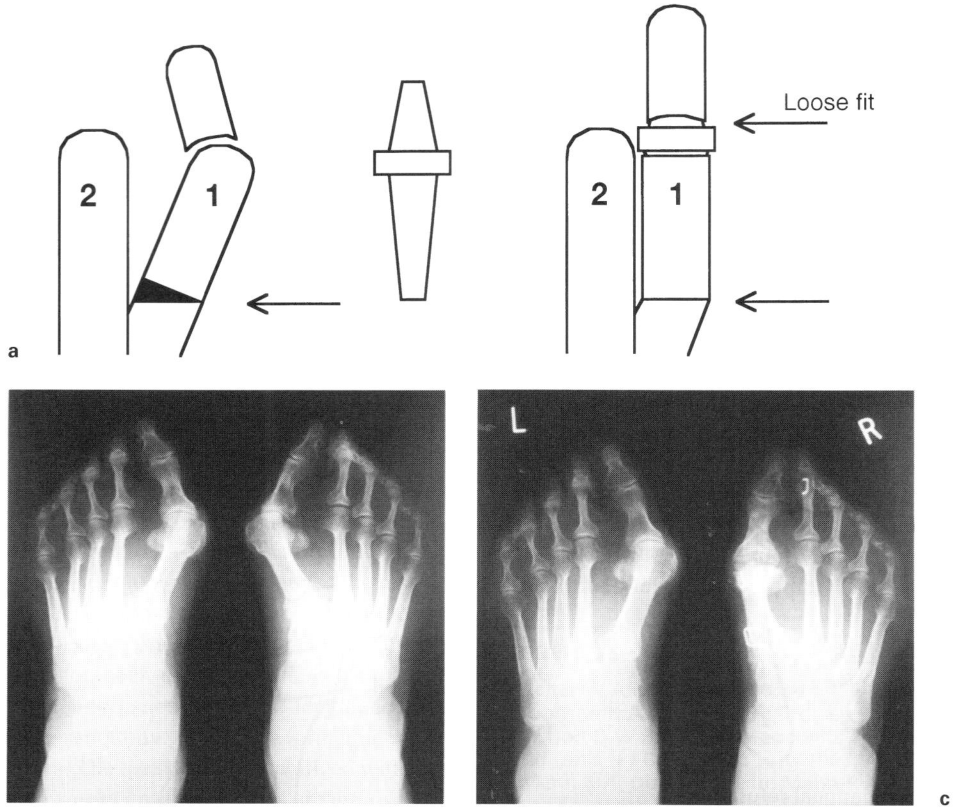

Fig. 49.24 Silastic interposition arthroplasty: (**a**) technique; metatarsal alignment with first metatarsal basal osteotomy—a first metatarsophalangial silastic spacer (Swanson); (**b**) preoperative radiograph; (**c**) postoperative radiograph.

Whilst it is accepted that this is not the aetiology in young girls of today, it can cause problems with footwear. It is essential to rule out medial pathology in the forefoot which is pushing the foot laterally, but if there is a primary 'bunionette' of whatever type it is easily dealt with by an oblique neck osteotomy (reversed Wilson) (Fig. 49.25).[60]

Stiff painful foot joints

These usually develop as a consequence of a disease. Most affected joints in the foot are managed by arthrodesis. In order to obtain fusion between adjacent bones in the hind- and midfoot, articular cartilage (or what remains) has to be removed along with the subchondral bone. The resulting space is packed with bone graft, to avoid significantly altering the alignment of the foot.

Hallux rigidus

Hallux rigidus, or perhaps in most cases more appropriately hallux limitus, can occur either as a primary degeneration of bone, or a secondary degeneration from, for example gout. It can also occur as a result of capsular damage and contraction. A dorsal osteophytic ridge is sometimes seen in patients with primary joint degeneration which itself causes a painful block to the joint extension necessary for normal gait. In early cases cheilectomy is appropriate, where a dorsal segment of the metatarsal head is excised, and other osteophytes trimmed (Fig. 49.26).[61] At worst this buys time before more destructive surgery becomes necessary, and at best it proves to be a definitive procedure. When there is good plantarflexion of the first metatarsophalangeal joint, it can be translated into dorsiflexion by a basal dorsal wedge osteotomy of the proximal phalanx. This procedure can be combined with a cheilectomy. After this, the choice lies between arthrodesis and the Keller excision arthroplasty. Arthrodesis is inappropriate when there is absent or painful extension of the interphalangeal joint, as that will only be made worse. Keller's excision arthroplasty is inappropriate when there is already evidence of lateral metatarsal overloading, as this is aggravated by the procedure. Keller's excision arthroplasty should be reserved for a low-demand user.

Eroded joints

Occurring in the forefoot as a result of rheumatoid arthritis these produce a feeling of walking over 'broken glass'. Several operations have been described to treat this, all of which are destructive

REFERENCES
60. Sponsel K H Orthop Clin North Am 1976; 7: 809
61. Mann R A, Clanton T R J Bone Joint Surg 1988; 70A: 400

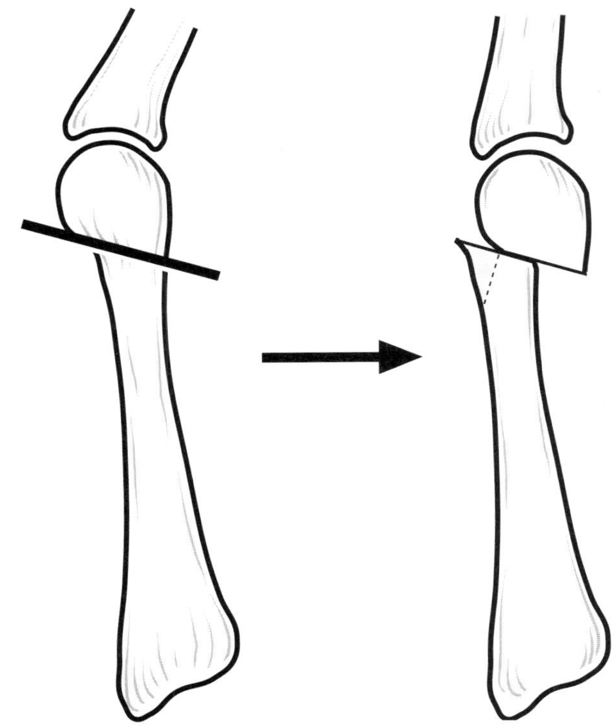

Fig. 49.25 Reversed Wilson osteotomy.

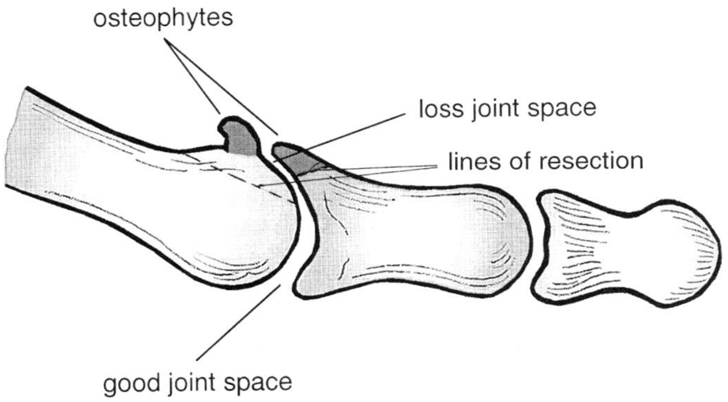

Fig. 49.26 Cheilectomy.

rather than constructive. The bases of proximal phalanges, heads of metatarsals; or both are excised. The Kates–Kessel–Kay procedure, in which all the metatarsal heads are excised,[62] has the advantage that it does bring the metatarsal pad back under the weight-bearing area. Stainsby has advocated his procedure used for retracted toes right across the foot, although care has to be taken with the skin incisions to avoid avascular bridges.[25] Plantar incisions heal well, but require care in the initial healing period.

Heel pain

Heel pain is one of the commonest causes of patients' complaints. A detailed history is essential. Plantar fasciitis causes pain of spontaneous onset, which is always most severe after rest, particularly when rising in the morning, but tends to ease with activity. So-called heel pad syndrome causes a more aching pain which is induced by weight bearing, and becomes more severe the longer activity is continued. Both are relieved by rest. Examination of the heel usually confirms the diagnosis, as the sites of pain are quite different (Fig. 49.27). The pathology of neither condition is understood.

Plantar fasciitis is best treated by calf-stretching exercises and the use of a good cushioned heel cup. The condition almost always resolves within 24 months. If seen within the first few weeks, steroid and local anaesthetic infiltration of the maximally tender area may produce relief.

Plantar pad syndrome is managed by cushioned heel pads. It often resolves spontaneously with time.

There are other rarer causes of heel pain, including entrapment syndromes, and fatigue (stress) fracture of the calcaneum.

General surgical consideratons

Infection rates are in general much higher in foot surgery—12–14% in some series—unless specific steps are taken to ensure a bacteriologically clean foot. Preoperative preparation in the ward with povidone–iodine scrub can keep infection rates down to 1–2%, and is strongly recommended.

Operations on the midfoot and forefoot can be carried out quite safely and satisfactorily under ankle pneumatic tourniquet, placed 3 cm proximal to the medial malleolus. This avoids the need to exsanguinate large volumes of blood from the limbs, and allows up to an hour for the surgery, which can be accomplished using a regional ankle anaesthetic block.[63] Toe surgery can often be carried out using a digital tourniquet, if indeed one is required. Much forefoot surgery can be performed safely and easily without a tourniquet, with the patient in a head-down foot-up position.

Postoperative care of foot surgery often reaches both extremes: excessive zeal or lack of concern. All surgery requires the foot to be elevated as much as possible in the early stages, as dependency leads to oedema, which exacerbates wound problems and infection. Whilst hindfoot surgery needs protection in a below-knee

REFERENCES

62. Kates A, Kessel L, Kay A J Bone Joint Surg 1967; 31A: 553
63. Wildsmith J A W, Armitage E N Principles and Practice of Regional Anaesthesia. Churchill Livingstone, Edinburgh 1987

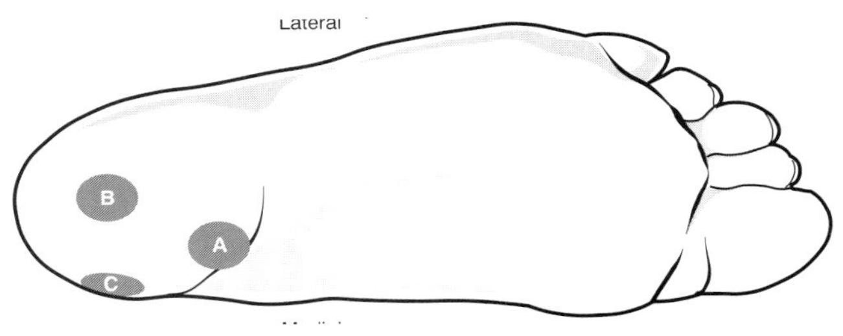

Fig. 49.27 Sites of heel pain. A, plantar fasciitis; B, 'plantar pad syndrome' (bruising; loss of heel pad); C, medial calcaneal nerve entrapment.

cast, forefoot surgery very definitely does not, and a slipper type of cast is perfectly adequate. This provides protection alone rather than affording continued maintenance of surgical correction. Individual postoperative dressings vary considerably, but tight circumferential bandaging, particularly around the toes, should be avoided.

Patients must be seen to be able to cope out of hospital using appropriate aids, particularly when bilateral surgery has been performed, before discharge from hospital. There are some who will only perform surgery unilaterally simply because managing at home after bilateral surgery can be difficult. In foot surgery there is a good argument for preferring 24-hour day care to 8-hour 'daylight' inpatient stay.

50 Principles of fractures and complications

R. M. Atkins

PRINCIPLES

Descriptions

Put simply, a fracture is a broken bone, which therefore represents the interaction between a physical force which produces the break and a biological substance, the bone which is broken. In order to understand fractures, it is therefore necessary to understand the structure and function of bones. In addition, the soft tissues surrounding the bone will be damaged in the fracture and they are of paramount importance.

STRUCTURE OF BONE

Introduction

Bone is a specialized connective tissue which forms an endoskeleton. It provides structural support for the body, protects vital organs and acts as a series of mechanical levers through which attached muscles and ligaments can move the body. In addition, it provides a store of calcium and phosphate and, phylogenetically, this was probably the reason for its development.

Anatomy

Macroscopically, bone is made up of two components: the dense outer cortex, which by its tubular structure gives maximum strength for weight, and the inner cancellous bone which consists of a network of trabeculae whose arrangement follows the direction of imposed stress adding to its strength.

The basic structural unit of bone is the Haversian system or osteon: a series of concentric layers of similarly orientated collagen fibres (lamellae) surrounding a central Haversian canal. The space between the osteons is filled by interstitial lamellae formed from irregular layers of bone. Between the lamellae, flattened bone cells (osteocytes) lie in spaces (lacunae) from which arise innumerable fine passages (canaliculae) containing fine projections from the osteocytes which are, therefore, in communication with each other. In the centre of each Haversian system is a central canal containing bone cells and a neurovascular bundle. These run parallel to the long axis of the bone and are united by Volkmann's canals piercing the bone from the outer and inner surfaces.

The bone is surrounded by periosteum, made up of an outer layer of fibrous and elastic tissue into which muscles, tendons and intermuscular septa insert and an inner vascular 'cambium' layer which contains osteoprogenitor cells. At points where the bone has ligament or muscle attachments, the periosteum is reinforced by perforating fibres of Sharpey, which are coarse collagen fibres that are continuous with the periosteum but perforate into the cortical bone. Immediately beneath the periosteum is found a layer of circumferential lamellae running parallel with the bone enclosing all the osteons.

Blood supply

Anatomy

Vessels enter the bone in the metaphyseal region to supply the epiphysis and metaphysis and anastomose with the diaphyseal supply. The main arterial supply to the diaphysis comes via nutrient arteries which divide in the medulla into ascending and descending branches. These ramify within the medullary cavity and constitute the primary resistance vessels of the osseous circulation.[1] Nutrient veins accompany the arteries outside the bone and continue within the medullary canal as a central longitudinal venous sinus which drains the medullary sinusoids through radial connecting sinuses.

Accompanying the blood vessels there are nerve fibres which extend into the Haversian systems and periosteum to innervate the blood vessels and supply pain and vibration sensitivity. There may also be a neural input into bone cells.

Physiology

The arterial supply of the cortex of bone is fan shaped with cortical sinusoids radiating outwards towards the periosteal surface, becoming smaller and supplying each Haversian canal. The major direction of cortical blood flow is centrifugal;[2] however, periosteal arteries penetrate bone at points of attachment[3] and, although under normal conditions these supply only a small area, following injury the periosteal source is capable of supplying the whole bone. The venous drainage is probably also centrifugal, passing into periosteal and muscular veins, leaving the nutrient vein unfilled.[2,4,5]

REFERENCES

1. Brooks M Bone 1986; 3: 32–34
2. Brooks M The Blood Supply of Bone. Butterworths, London 1971
3. Rhinelander F W Internal Fixation of Fractures. Springer-Verlag, Berlin 1980, pp 9–14

Under normal physiological conditions, bone receives between 5% and 10% of the cardiac output,[6] with the supply being relatively greater at the bone ends. Bone blood flow is regulated by neural, hormonal and metabolic mechanisms.[6] Electrical stimulation of somatic or sympathetic nerves to bone or administration of adrenalin all reduce blood flow,[7–9] while sympathectomy causes an increase.[10] Restoration of the circulation following a period of ischaemia leads to a two-to threefold increase in blood flow[8] and this effect takes precedence over neural or hormonal control.

Cells of bone

The osteoblast

Osteoblasts are cuboidal mononuclear cells derived from marrow stroma or periosteal osteoprogenitor cells.[11,12] The osteoblast is responsible for the synthesis of the major proteins of bone and is involved in bone mineralization and in controlling osteoclastic function.

The lining cell and the osteocyte

Some active osteoblasts are incarcerated in the matrix which they secrete. These osteocytes have long processes through which they maintain contact with each other and with the superficial bone-lining cells. This layer of flattened, inactive cells, which are probably also derived from osteoblasts, covers the whole of the bone surface, functionally isolating it from the exterior.

The osteoclast

The osteoclast is a large multinucleate giant cell attached to the bone surface, derived from haemopoetic precursor cells.[13,14] It is responsible for resorption of living bone. This is accomplished by the osteoclast attaching itself tightly so that the bone immediately beneath the cell is isolated. The plasma membrane in this area is extensively folded forming a 'ruffled border' which is rich in carbonic anhydrase. Hydrogen ions are pumped into the space beneath the ruffled border, causing the bone mineral to dissolve. The organic part of the bone is then resorbed by enzymes secreted by the osteoclast.

Although bone can be resorbed by macrophages,[15] this is a much slower process occurring by a different mechanism and it is debatable to what extent it occurs in vivo.[16]

Chemistry of bone

Bone is made up of organic and inorganic materials and water. The organic intercellular matrix of bone is 93% collagen and 7% non-collagenous proteins. The latter include a number of proteins such as osteocalcin and osteonectin which are unique to bone and may have a role in binding the mineral phase of bone to collagen.[17]

The mineral phase of bone provides its mechanical strength and serves as a reservoir of calcium and phosphate. The mineral of bone is poorly crystalline, imperfect hydroxyapatite ($Ca_{10}(PO_4)_6(OH)_2$), which contains a variety of substituted ions. With ageing, the crystal becomes larger, less hydrated and more perfect,[18,19] which reduces bone strength in the elderly.

The unique feature of bone is the close attachment between its organic and inorganic constituents. Type 1 collagen is found ubiquitously in the body but only in bone is it closely associated with hydroxyapatite. The bone mineral is regularly distributed within the collagen fibrils, being deposited first within the hole zone region, which are spaces between the triple helices.[20] In unmineralized osteoid, mineralization begins independently and simultaneously at a number of different sites, starting between one and ten days after osteoid deposition. The region in which mineralization occurs is supersaturated with calcium and phosphate ions so that mineralization represents a *phase change* from dissolved ions to solid hydroxyapatite. The precise mechanism is not known but it seems likely that non-collagenous phosphoproteins distributed throughout the collagen matrix provide nucleation sites.[20]

Bone turnover and remodelling

The constituent parts of bone are constantly being renewed, at a rate of approximately 10% per year. This is made up of 4% in cortical and 25% in trabecular bone[21] and it allows for the removal of fatigue damage and maintenance of relatively young skeletal tissue by a mechanism referred to as 'remodelling' by bone biologists. This process is a part of the 'remodelling' which is described by orthopaedic surgeons. Bone remodelling follows an orderly cycle and in an adult only approximately 10% of the bone surface is involved at any time;[22] the remainder is inactive. In contrast, in a child the majority of the bone surface is active. At a region of bone which is to be remodelled, the bone becomes activated and

REFERENCES

4. Cuthbertson E N, Sirus E, Gilfillan R S J. Bone Joint Surg. 1965; 47A: 965–974
5. Oni O O A, Gregg P J In: Arlet J, Mazieres B (eds) Bone Circulation and Bone Necrosis. Springer-Verlag, Berlin 1990 pp 7–10
6. Shim S S J Bone Joint Surg 1968; 50A: 812–824
7. Drinker C K, Drinker K R Am J Physiol 1916; 40: 512–521
8. Shim S S, Patterson F P Surg. Gynaecol Obstet 1967; 125: 261–268
9. Brinker M R, Lipton H L, Cook S D, Hyman A L J Bone Joint Surg 1990; 72A: 964–975
10. Trottman N M, Kelly W D JAMA 1963; 183; 121–122
11. Owen M Int Rev Cytol 1970; 28: 213–238
12. Owen M Arthritis Rheum 1980; 23: 1073
13. Bonucci E Clin Orthop 1981; 158: 252–269
14. Baron R, Vignery A, Horowitz M In: Peck W (ed) Bone and Mineral Research, vol 2. Elsevier, Amsterdam 1984 pp 175–245
15. Athanasou N A, Quinn J, Bulstrode C J K J Bone Joint Surg Br 1992; 74B: 57–62
16. Atkins R M, Langkamer V G, Perry M, Elson C, Collins C J Arthroplasty, 1997; 12: 461–465
17. Termine J D, Kleinman H K, Whitson S W, Conn K M, McGarvey M L, Martin G R Cell 1981; 26: 99–105
18. Glimcher M J Rev Mod Phys 1959; 31: 359–393
19. Landis W J Glimcher M J J Altr Strut Res 1978; 63: 188–133
20. Glimcher M J In: Avioli L V, Krant S M (eds) Metabolic Bone Disease. Saunders, Philadelphia 1990 pp 42–68
21. Parfitt A M In: Reckerr (ed) Bone Histomorphometry: Techniques and Interpretations. C R C Press, Boca Raton, F L 1983 pp 143–223
22. Parfitt A M Calcif. Tissue Int 1984; 36 (suppl); S37–S45

precursor cells differentiate into osteoclasts which erode a surface cavity, producing a Howship's lacuna in trabecular bone or a cutting cone in cortical bone. The osteoclasts then disappear and the irregular cavity is smoothed off and lined by a layer of mineral rich 'cement substance'. Osteoblasts are next recruited which refill the excavated cavity with new bone.

Alternations in the dynamics of different parts of the remodelling processes account for the many age-related changes in the skeleton.[23,24] During adult life, bone is lost from the skeleton at a rate of approximately 1% of its peak mass per year[25] because there is a small imbalance between the amount of bone resorbed and the subsequent amount formed in each episode of bone remodelling. This is referred to as the remodelling imbalance.[26] The balance between formation and resorption varies between different bone surfaces. The average bone remodelling unit will add a small volume on the periosteal surface and subtract a small volume at the endosteal surface.[24] This is responsible for the widening of the femoral medullary canal which occurs along with thinning of the femoral cortex with ageing.

Regulation of bone cell function

Bone is responsible for the structural integrity of the skeleton and for maintaining the serum levels of calcium and phosphate, which are essential for nerve and muscle function. The regulation of bone homeostasis is therefore complex.

1. The general body demand for calcium, phosphate and magnesium are satisfied by the effects of systemic hormones, including vitamin D and parathyroid hormone on the bone (see Ch. 19).

2. Locally, bone cell function is affected by growth factors and cytokines, proteins which regulate the function of differentiated cells at very low concentrations[27–29] and by prostaglandins. Important cytokines are transforming growth factor (TGFβ) and interleukin 1 (IL-1) which stimulate bone resorption[30] and insulin-like growth factor (IGF), which stimulates osteoblast proliferation and collagen synthesis.[31,32] Bone morphogenetic proteins (BMPs) are cytokines which are members of the TGFβ family and stimulate bone formation by a complex series of actions. These are now becoming available therapeutically due to the production of human recombinant molecules. The prostaglandins (PGs) are powerful stimulators of bone resorption when added to organ cultured bones.[33,34] They are produced in large quantities following fracture[35] and may be responsible for abnormal bone remodelling and sequestrum formation in osteomyelitis.[35]

3. The mass of bone at any site adjusts so that its strain environment is constant: a phenomenon often termed Wolfe's law.[36] This means that if the bone is stressed it will over time become thicker or sclerotic, whereas if it is protected from external mechanical stress, as for example occurs in the leg when an orthopaedic patient is made non-weight bearing, the bone will become porotic. This process is mediated by the remodelling cycle but the mechanism by which the strain message causes alterations in the balance between bone formation and resorption is unknown. It may involve the osteocyte processes, local cytokine formation or electrical phenomena. An area of bone under compression exhibits a negative potential, while a region under tension becomes relatively electropositive. These phenomena are caused by piezoelectrical effects due to deformation of the molecules of bone[37] and streaming potentials caused by stress-induced changes in fluid fluxes.[38] Electronegative areas of bone are associated with bone formation while in positively charged areas bone is resorbed. Effects of electricity have been demonstrated experimentally on a wide variety of bone cell functions including matrix formation, calcification and cell proliferation.[39] Although this suggests that it should be possible to influence fracture union using externally applied electrical fields, definitive evidence for this is lacking.[40]

BIOLOGICAL ASPECTS OF FRACTURE HEALING

Bone growth and development

Fractures heal by mechanisms similar to those by which bone forms, so an understanding of the latter is important for a discussion of fractures. Bone forms either by *intramembranous ossification* or by *endochondral ossification*.

Intramembranous bone formation

Intramembranous bone formation occurs within a primitive layer of vascularized connective tissue. Cells proliferate, hypertrophy and transform into osteoblasts. Progressive bone formation results in the fusion of adjacent bony areas within the membrane to form spongy bone. This is then remodelled into its mature form. This sort of bone formation occurs in the bones of the vault of the skull, the maxilla and the clavicle.

REFERENCES

23. Parfitt A M Metab Reckerr Bone Dis Rel Res 1982; 4: 1–6
24. Parfitt A M In: Riggs B L, Melton L J III (eds) Osteoporosis: Aetiology, Diagnosis and Management. Reven Press, New York, 1988
25. Garn S M In: De Luca H F, Frost H M, Jee W S S, Johnston C C Jr, Parfitt A M (eds) Osteoporosis: Recent Advances in Pathogenesis and Treatment. University Park Press, Baltimore 1981 pp 3–16
26. Parfitt A M Med Times 1981; 109: 80–92
27. Centrella M, Canalis E Proc Natal Acad Sci USA 1985; 82: 7335–7339
28. Hauschka P V, Mavrakos A E, Iafrati M D, Doleman S E, Klagsbrun M J. Biol Chem 1986; 261: 12665–12674
29. McDonald B R, Gowan F Br J Rheumatol 1992: 31; 149–155
30. Gowan M, Wood D D, Ihra E J, Maguire M K B, Russell R G G Nature 1983; 306: 378–380
31. Cannalis E M, Hintz R L, Dietrich J W, Maina D N, Raiz L G Metabolism 1971; 26: 1079–1087
32. Cannalis E J Clin Invest 1980; 66: 709–719
33. Dietrich J W, Goodson J N, Raisz L G Prostaglandins 1975; 10: 231–240
34. Tashjian A H Jr, Tice J E, Sides K Nature 1977; 266: 645–646
35. Dekel S, Francis M J O J Bone Joint Surg 1981; 63B: 178–184
36. Rubin C T PhD thesis, Bristol 1982
37. Fukada E, Yasuda I J. Phys Soc Japan 1957; 10: 1158–1169
38. Pienkowski D, Pollack S R J Orthop Res 1983; 1: 30–41
39. Pollack S R In: Takahashi A G (ed) Bone Morphometry. Smith Gordon, London 1990
40. Barker A T, Dixon R A, Sharrard W J W, Sutcliffe M L Lancet 1984; i: 994–996

Endochondral bone formation

In endochondral ossification an area of cartilage forms a model (or anlage) for the bone which will be formed but does not itself transform into bone. The cartilage matrix becomes calcified with death of the cartilage cells and the matrix is then resorbed and replaced by vascularized bone, which subsequently remodels. The most ordered example of endochondral ossification is seen at the growth plate, which is composed of cartilage cells arranged in well-ordered long columns parallel to each other and to the axis of growth of each bone end (Fig. 50.1).

On the epiphyseal side of each column, the cartilage cells are small and flat in the resting zone. Immediately metaphyseal to this is the layer of active cell division. Approximately halfway down the cell columns towards the metaphysis, rapid cell division ceases as the hypertrophic zone is entered. This region is distant from both the epiphyseal and metaphyseal blood supplies and is relatively avascular. The chondrocytes mature and hypertrophy and calcification begins in the matrix between the cell columns. The last hypertrophic cartilage cell of each column is immediately adjacent to an invading capillary tuft from the metaphysis. Osteoblasts are carried in from the metaphysis with the new capillaries and lay down new bone around the bars of calcified cartilage matrix

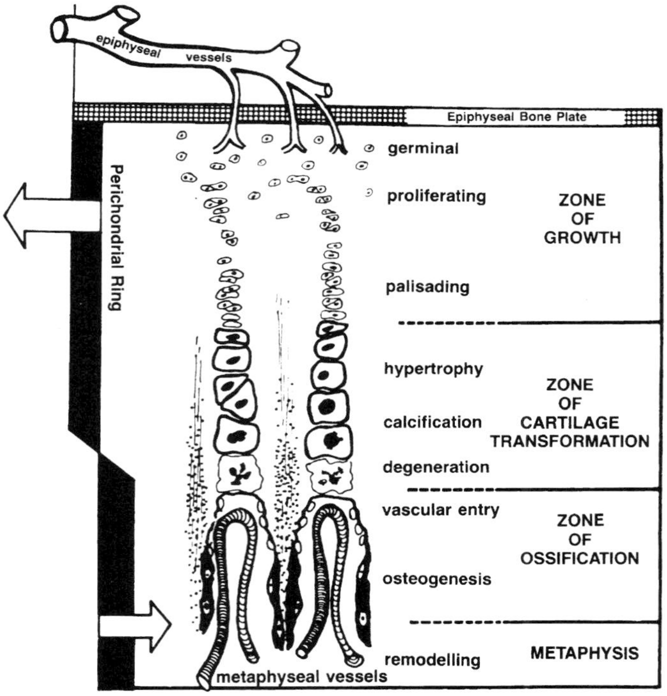

Fig. 50.1 A diagrammatic representation of the growth plate showing the individual layers. Nearest to the epiphysis is the germinal layer of cells, whose blood supply comes from epiphyseal vessels. Passing towards the diaphysis, the cells in the proliferating layer are undergoing mitosis and the daughter cells then mature and hypertrophy before becoming calcified and degenerating. Capillary tufts from the metaphysis invade the dead cells and calcified pericellular matrix. Phagocytosis of the dead material occurs and new bone laid down by primitive osteoblasts is subsequently remodelled. Widthways growth of the physis occurs at the periphery by mitosis within the perichondral ring of Lacroix. From Rang.[245]

between the columns at the base of the growth plate. This is subsequently remodelled to produce new bone. The growth plate must itself grow outwards and this is accomplished by widthwise mitoses of cells on the outer edge of the germinal layer of the physis, a region termed the perichondral ring of Lacroix.

The long bones (except the clavicle), vertebrae, pelvis and the bones of the base of the skull are formed in this fashion. It is, however, important to note that although growth in length of a long bone occurs at the growth plate by endochondral ossification, width-wise growth is by intramembranous bone formation beneath the periosteum (periosteal appositional bone growth). Subsequently all the bone laid down primarily is remodelled to produce mature Haversian bone.

Fracture healing

Healing of a fracture results in reconstitution of the injured tissue into something resembling its original form. As in other tissues, a 'scar' forms which is able, from an early stage, to function as bone. This scar is slowly remodelled into increasingly normal bone and the original bone architecture will be completely restored in children's fractures or in relatively undisplaced or well-reduced adult fractures. In more comminuted, high-energy or displaced fractures, restitution is seldom complete. The changes associated with fracture healing may be considered as three phases which overlap but occur sequentially. These are the phase of inflammation, the development of osteogenic repair tissue and the phase of remodelling.

Inflammation

This begins immediately after injury and is rapidly following by repair. Bleeding from damaged bone ends and soft tissues leads to fibrinous clot formation between the fragments. Damage to the bone blood vessels causes loss of nutrition of bone cells, so that the broken ends of the bone are dead[41] and play a passive role in fracture healing, providing a bridge between more distant regions of living bone.[42] The extent of bone death will vary with the degree of fracture comminution, the amount of periosteal stripping, the extent of fracture displacement and the severity of damage to the meduallary contents—the greater the bone damage, the slower will fracture healing be. Inflammatory mediators are released from injured tissues, causing an increase in vascular permeability which leads to an exudate of plasma.[43] Inflammatory cells migrate into the region and phagocytosis of necrotic material begins.

The development of osteogenic repair tissue

The amount and composition of repair tissue vary with the site, type and severity of the fracture, the type of bone involved, the

REFERENCES

41. Ham A W J Bone Joint Surg 1930; 12: 825–844
42. McKibbin B J Bone Joint Surg 1978; 60B: 150–162
43. Cannalis E, McCarthy T, Sentrella M J Clin Invest 1988; 81: 277–281

state of the soft tissues surrounding the fracture and whether the fragments move in relation to each other during healing. The following description refers principally to a simple fracture of a long bone in which the fragments are not rigidly immobilized.

The first stage of the repair process is the organization of the fracture haematoma which is invaded by fibrovascular tissue and eventually mineralizes to form provisional callus. There are two sources of repair tissue: medullary and periosteal. The former is most marked in cancellous bone, while the latter predominates in a diaphyseal fracture.

Periosteal callus

The potential of periosteum for repair is demonstrated by the ability of bone which has been resected subperiosteally, so leaving the cambium layer of the periosteum in place, to regenerate.[44] In a fracture where the bone has not been removed, cellular proliferation and hypertrophy begin at a distance from the fracture, often over viable cortex. Repair tissue becomes invaded by osteogenic cells derived from the cambium layer of periosteum. If the periosteum is intact, a bridge of callus readily forms, arching over the dead bone ends. If it is ruptured, cuffs of callus grow outwards from the living bone, eventually joining together.[42]

In some areas, particularly at the periphery of the callus, a variety of hyaline cartilage forms which becomes converted to bone by endochondral ossification. The amount of cartilage formed is very variable. This may represent a response to low oxygen tension,[41,45,46] the concept being that if callus outgrows its blood supply cartilage provides a suitable material less demanding of oxygen to bridge the gap until vascularity is re-established.[42] Alternatively, Hulth[47] suggests that cartilage is laid down in response to fragment movement[48,49] which mechanically inhibits vascular invasion. Since this will lead to lowered oxygen tension, these two theories are in fact similar.

The blood supply of the periosteal callus comes initially from the periosteal vessels and extraperiosteal soft tissues, including muscle,[50] and only later does the medullary blood supply make a contribution.[51,52] The new, fracture-induced, blood supply regresses as union occurs and eventually disappears.

Medullary callus

Vascular proliferation in the medullary region is the principal method of union in cancellous bone, for example in a fracture of the tibial plateau, and plays a part in union of the tubular bone, where medullary activity is particularly marked if the fracture is offset.[42] The vascular response is slower than that seen in the periosteum.[50]

Phase of remodelling

Once the fracture has been satisfactorily bridged by callus the newly formed bone is adapted to its new function by 'remodelling'. This refers to the process of adaptation of the skeleton to applied loads. In qualitative terms the remodelling process is no different from the process of replacement and repair which is occurring continually within the normal skeleton, except that in this context it includes the revascularization and modification of dead bone at the fracture site. However, the activation frequency of bone remodelling units following a fracture is greatly increased. In the dog radius the number is increased from a baseline value of 2.5% of the total number of osteons in a cross-section to over 60%. This acceleration of remodelling activity does not occur until the third week after fracture and peaks at eight weeks.[53]

New blood vessels can invade the trabeculae of cancellous bone and bone apposition may take place directly onto the trabecular surface. Once this has happened, the bone may take part in the normal remodelling cycle. This phenomenon is referred to as 'creeping substitution'. Although apposition onto the surface of cortical bone may occur, there are always areas in which the bone cells are dead. In order for these regions to take part in normal bone remodelling, the osteoclastic 'cutter head' must ream out a tunnel down which the new blood supply can enter the bone. The process of revascularization is relatively slow and small areas of dead bone may remain for a considerable length of time following normal fracture union. Indeed, in the case of a high-energy fracture with extensive bone death, the entire dead bone may never be removed. It is this residual dead bone which makes bone infection following fracture so difficult to eradicate.

The source of osteogenic cells

There are two possible sources of osteoblasts. The cells may arise by differentiation of previously determined osteogenic progenitor cells (DOPC) which are found in the inner layer of the periosteum and within the bone marrow[11] or from previously uncommitted, pluripotent cells in the surrounding soft tissues. These cells are termed inducible osteoprogenitor cells (IOPC).[12] The modification of previously undifferentiated soft tissue cells into osteogenic cells is termed bone induction. Although it is not clear to what extent it is important in the healing of a fracture, it is well established that non-specialized cells in extraskeletal sites may be stimulated to form bone.[54]

Types of fracture repair

McKibbin[42] has suggested that fracture repair may be divided into four types with differing time courses and physical requirements. It

REFERENCES

44. Robinson C M, McLaughlan G, Christie J, McQueen M M, Court Brown C M J Bone Joint Surg Br 1995; 77-B: 906–913
45. Girgis F G, Pritchard J J J Bone Joint Surg 1958; 40B: 274–281
46. Bassett C A L, Herrman I Nature 1961; 190: 460–461
47. Hulth A Clin Orthop 1989; 249: 265–284
48. Anderson L D J Bone Joint Surg 1965; 47A: 191–208
49. Blenman P R, Carter D R, Beaupre G S Trans Orthop Res Soc 1989; 14: 469
50. Gothman L Acta Orthop Scand 1961; Suppl 284
51. Rhinelander F W, Baragry R A J Bone Joint Surg 1962; 44A: 1273–1298
52. Rhinelander F W J Bone Joint Surg 1968; 50-A: 784–800
53. Schenk R K In: Lane J M (ed) Fracture Healing. Churchill Livingstone, Edinburgh 1987 pp 23–33
54. Chalmers J, Gray D H, Rush J J Bone Joint Surg 1975; 57B: 36–45

must be emphasized that these divisions are arbitrary and in a normal fracture it is not possible completely to separate them. They do, however, provide a useful basis for discussion.

Primary callus response

This commences within two weeks of injury when exuberant external callus is formed, particularly beneath intact periosteum. The callus spreads from the fractured bone end, but if it does not cause bony union it undergoes involution. The primary callus response is relatively independent of environmental and hormonal influences, being an intrinsic property of the fracture, and is probably due to DOPCs present in the cambium layer of the periosteum.

External bridging callus

External bridging callus forms if the primary callus response does not result in bone continuity. This stage of callus is under the control of humoral and mechanical influences and is probably dependent upon IOPCs derived from the surrounding soft tissues. The external bridging callus appears rapidly and bridges gaps readily. Its formation depends on the presence of viable external soft tissues which provide the blood vessels for the repair tissue. It is inhibited by rigid fixation and is the predominant form of healing when a simple fracture is treated by cast immobilization or intramedullary nailing (Figs 50.2 and 50.17).[55]

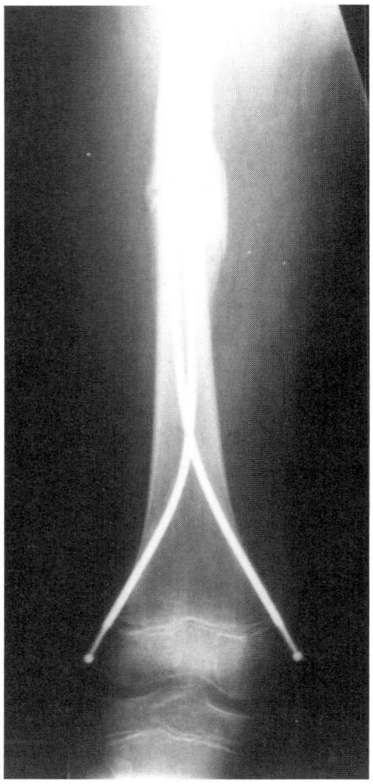

Fig. 50.2 Fracture healing by external callus formation. This femoral shaft fracture in a child has been treated by intramedullary nailing. Union is proceeding by external callus formation because the fracture haematoma has not been disturbed and the fixation is not completely rigid. In this case the medullary canal was not reamed prior to nailing; nevertheless some damage to the medullary blood supply is inevitable as a result of the passage of the nails. The original fracture was transverse. Courtsey of Mr M Jackson.

Late medullary callus

This often occurs in combination with external bridging callus but is slower in appearance. It is relatively independent of intact external soft tissues, being more dependent on intramedullary vascularity. It is able to bridge gaps between bone ends and will tolerate a small amount of interfragmentary movement. It is not inhibited by rigid immobilization of the bone ends and it is important in healing fractures immobilized by rigid plating.[56] Bone which forms under these circumstances frequently does not show an intermediate stage of fibrocartilage.

Primary bone union

Primary bone repair is the term given to fracture repair where the fracture ends have been rigidly immobilized by a plate (Fig. 50.3). In the original concept of Lane[57] and Danis,[58] primary bone healing referred to fractures which healed without radiographically visible callus formation. Schenk and Willinegger[59] found that when an osteotomy was performed in a dog radius which had been rigidly fixed by a plate, bone deposition occurred on the divided bone ends within a few days, often without preceding osteoclastic resorption. The structure of the newly formed bone depended on the width of the gap. Where it was less than 200 μm, the gap was filled by true lamellar bone, while larger gaps showed a more irregular pattern. Where the gap exceeded a millimetre, it was not bridged 'in a single jump' by woven bone and complete filling in was considerably delayed.[53] The bone filling the interfragmentary gap appears without the intermediate formation of connective tissue or fibrocartilage and it is this absence of an intermediate tissue which distinguishes primary bone repair from that seen under other circumstances. The lamellae are aligned at right angles to the interfragmentary gap if it is small and because woven bone is being laid down de novo, the rate at which the gap is filled is considerably faster than the normal mineral appositional rate of 0.8–2.5 μm per day. Gap healing as outlined above is completely intolerant of any movement and will only bridge very small gaps. Once the bone gap has filled, the new bone is replaced by rapid bone remodelling with osteoclastic 'cutter-heads' crossing the fracture site.

Distraction osteogenesis

This is not strictly a method of fracture healing. However, it is considered here for completeness. The majority of the basic

REFERENCES

55. Lane J M, Werntz J R In: Lane J M (ed) Fracture Healing. Churchill Livingstone, Edinburgh 1987 pp 49–60
56. Olerud S, Dankwardt-Lilliesterom G Acta Orth Scand 1971; suppl 137
57. Lane W A The Operative Treatment of Fractures. Medical Publishing Co, London 1913
58. Danis R Theorie et Pratique de l'Osteosynthese. Masson, Paris 1949
59. Schenk R, Willineggar H Symp Biol Hung 1967; 8: 75–86

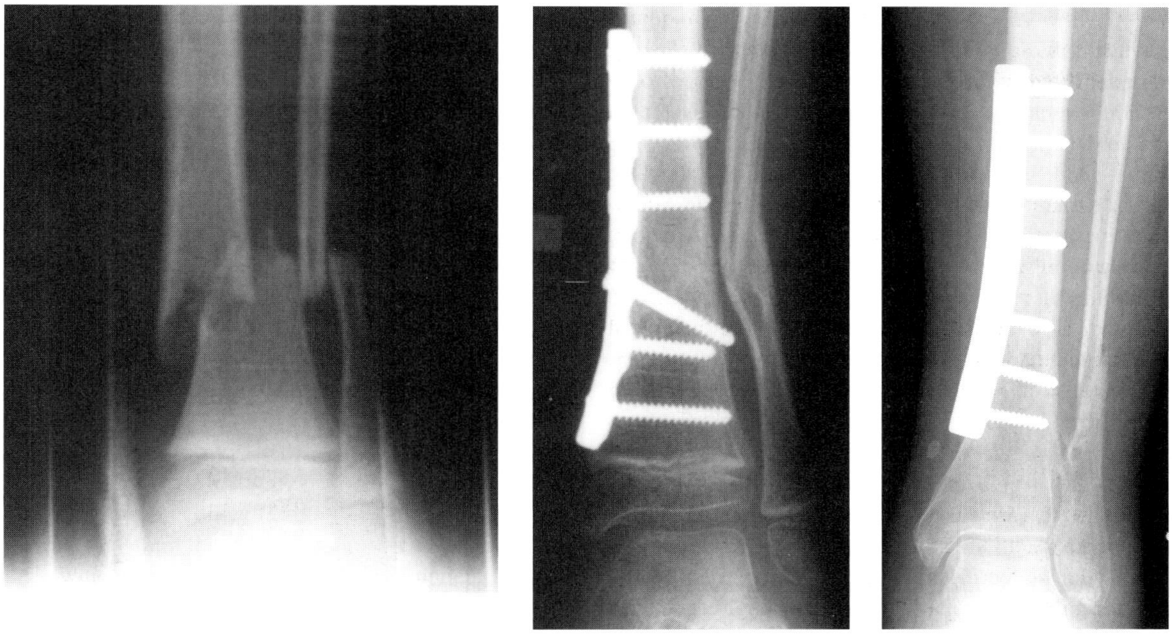

a b c

Fig. 50.3 Fracture healing by primary bone union. (**a**) A displaced oblique fracture of the junction of the diaphysis and distal metaphysis of the tibia. Temporary, emergency immobilization is provided by an inflatable splint. (**b**) The fracture has been anatomically reduced using an AO low-contact dynamic compression plate (LC-DCP). In this case, fracture compression has been provided by the oblique lag screw rather than by use of the special compression holes in the plate. The irregular outline of the LC-DCP can be seen. This allows the plate to make contact with the bone only over a proportion of its surface, thus reducing devascularization. The plate and screws provide rigid stability and the lack of interfragmentary movement suppresses external callus formation, despite the fact that this fracture occurred prior to skeletal maturity. The fibula, which was not rigidly immobilized, has united by periosteal callus formation. Notice the extent of the osteoporosis distal to the fracture due to loss of the normal stimulus of loadbearing. (**c**) A similar fracture in an adult treated with an AO dynamic compression plate. The difference in bone contact area can clearly be seen. In this case, no lag screw was used; compression of the fracture site was obtained by use of the DCP compression holes. Note the difference in the healing of the fibula: bone healing in an adult is slower than in the skeletally immature and periosteal callus formation is less marked.

research into this phenomenon was undertaken by Ilizarov.[60,61] The classic descriptions of bone formation by the AO Group and others rely on compression in order to induce fracture union. Ilizarov demonstrated that mechanical induction of new bone between bony surfaces could occur during gradual distraction. A biological bridge between the surfaces arises from local new blood vessel formation and spans the entire cross-section of the cut surfaces. During distraction, a fibrovascular interface is aligned parallel to the direction of the distraction gap while new bone columns form. New blood vessel formation extends from each medullary surface towards a central fibrous interzone in the distraction gap, which remains relatively avascular (Figs 50.4, 50.16). Early bone formation occurs by intramembranous ossification and mineralization occurs close to the blood vessels. Bone formation is limited to columns approximately 200 μm long. Islands of endochondral ossification are seen if the mechanical conditions are not optimal and shearing of the regenerate bone is permitted. Under these circumstances, the columns of intramembranous ossification become irregular.[62,63]

Control of fracture healing

The initial inflammatory reaction of bone after fracture is very similar to that seen in other injuries and is controlled by the release of vasoactive mediators including serotonin and histamine and growth factors from damaged tissues. It is at the phase of formation of an osteogenic repair tissue that bone healing begins to differ from other wound healing and the triggering mechanism for this response is unknown. Bone-inducing growth factors are found within bone matrix[28] and release of these from the broken bone ends may trigger new bone formation. A number of the growth factors which are released in the normal inflammatory process following injury can stimulate cartilage and bone formation,[64–67] so

REFERENCES

60. Ilizarov G A Ortop Travmatol Protez 1975; 10: 7–15
61. Ilizarov G A Transosseous Osteosynthesis: Theoretical and Clinical Aspects of the Regeneration and Growth of Tissue. Springer-Verlag, Berlin 1990
62. Aronson J, Good B, Stewart C, Harrison B, Hart J Clin Orthop Rel Res 1990; 250: 43–49
63. Aronson J In: Bianchi Maiocchia Aronson J (eds) Operative Principles of Ilizarov. Williams & Wilkins, Baltimore 1991 pp 42–52
64. Jingushi S, Heydeman N A, Bolander M E J Orthop Res 1990; 8: 364–371
65. Muthukumaran N, Reddi A H Clin Orthop 1984; 220: 159–164
66. Moda M, Camillier J J Endocrinology 1989; 124(6): 2991–2994
67. Memmeth G G, Bolander M E, Martin M R. Growth factors and their role in wound and fracture healing. In: Barbul A, Pines E, Cauldwell M D and Hunt T K (eds) pp 1–17 New York Alan R Liss 1988

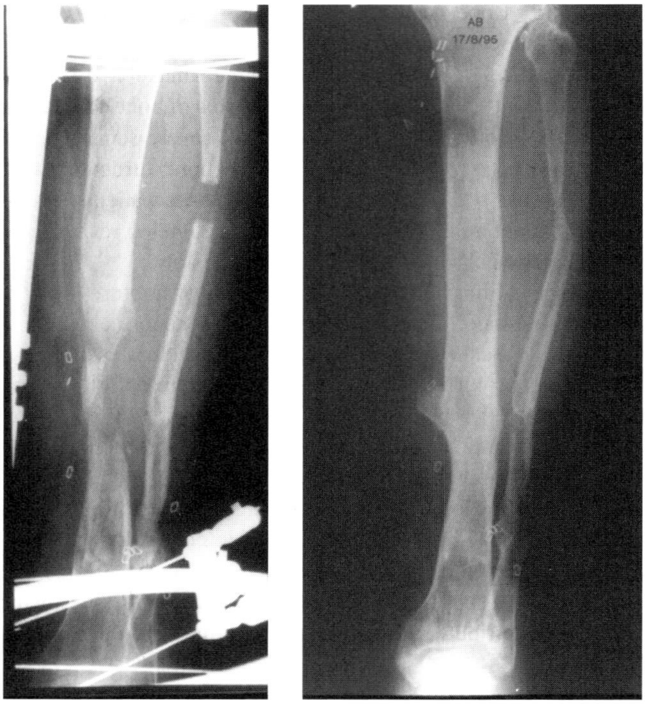

Fig. 50.5 (a) An atrophic non-union of a tibial fracture. The original fracture involved a severe soft tissue and bone injury. Over time, badly damaged bone has undergone resorption leaving an un-united fracture and an area of bone deficiency. The non-union is supported by a circular external fixator. (b) The result after treatment by bone transport.

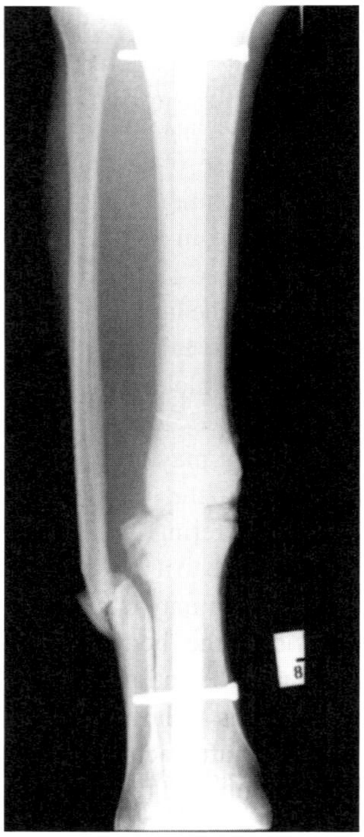

Fig. 50.6 A hypertrophic non-union, shortly after treatment by reamed interlocked intramedullary nailing. During the treatment period following this fracture, sufficient stability was not achieved to allow bone union. The fracture line remains and progressive layers of periosteal callus formation around the bone give the old fracture site the appearance of 'an elephant's foot'. There may be little or no clinically detectable movement, but the region remains painful and the limb is of limited utility. Treatment consists of reaming the bone to allow passage of the intramedullary nail and to increase bone activation. The biomechanical environment of the fracture is improved by stabilization of the non-union with an intramedullary nail locked proximally and distally. Courtsey of Mr M Jackson.

as the use of Ilizarov frames become more accepted there is a trend towards identifying situations in which the bone will not heal and intervening early.

The two main reasons for fracture non-union are loss of bone viability and an adverse biomechanical environment, but in most cases both factors are present to a certain degree. Where bone viability is poor, particularly where the surrounding soft tissue cover is also deficient, infection may supervene. Poor bone viability leads to gradual resorption of bone and an *atrophic* non-union (Fig. 50.5) develops, whereas inadequate fracture stability with normally viable bone fragments leads to a *hypertrophic* non-union (Fig. 50.6). Occasionally, at the site of a fracture a *pseudarthrosis* or new false joint forms.

Principles of treatment of non-union of fracture

Treatment is directed at reversing the cause of the non-union. Bone mass and bone-to-bone contact at the non-union site should be improved, the biomechanical environment corrected and bone activity increased.

Increasing local bone mass

Local bone mass is increased by fracture reduction, bone grafting or bone transport, all of which also increase the area of bone to bone contact.

Improving the biomechanical environment

The biomechanical environment is corrected by compression plating, intrameduallary nailing or external fixation in order to provide a mechanical environment which resists shearing forces but provides compression with, ideally, the ability to continue gradual compression of the site for some time after the operation in order to deal with the effects of local bone resorption.

A radically different approach to the biomechanical environment which is required for resolution of a non-union was provided by Ilizarov.[60,61] He divided non-unions into stiff and lax, which broadly corresponds to the Western classification of hypertrophic and atrophic. Ilizarov demonstrated that stiff non-unions will heal under conditions of gradual distraction at least as reliably as under compression. Clearly the use of gradual distraction requires an external fixation device for stabilization of the non-union.

Increasing bone activity

Bone activity is increased either by providing new bone cells and bone morphogens using cancellous bone grafting or by indirect stimulation by intramedullary reaming or by division of the bone at a distant site using a corticotomy. An alternative source of bone morphogens is exogenous human recombinant bone morphogenetic protein, and the availability of this class of compounds may in the future profoundly affect the manner in which we treat non-unions. However, it must be remembered that the stimulation of bone activity only resolves one of the bone-related problems of non-union.

BONE GRAFTING

Bone grafting procedures are often undertaken for delayed or non-union of a fracture to stimulate osteogenesis and increase the bone mass present. Bone grafts may be categorized according to the donor type as

1. Autograft: from the same individual.
2. Isograft: between genetically identical individuals.
3. Allograft: from one individual to another of the same species.
4. Zenograft or heterograft: between individuals of different species.

They are further divided according to whether the transplant is living or has been preserved, for example by freeze drying, whether transplant is free or vascularized, and whether the graft is cancellous or cortical bone or a combination of the two.

Stimulation of bone formation or fracture union following bone grafting may occur by three mechanisms.[77]

Osteogenesis

Bone cells within the graft survive and synthesize new bone. This can only occur in the case of fresh autograft. Cancellous bone is more active than cortical bone because of its greater surface area, more numerous osteocytes and because revascularization from the host is more rapid. A vascularized graft may be employed but this is not applicable to the majority of situations.

Osteoinduction

The bone graft induces bone formation by causing a local host cell response which produces bone. Osteoinduction occurs with both autografts and allografts and is mediated by growth factors and the bone morphogenetic proteins. These molecules are unstable and their activity is reduced by autoclaving, freeze preservation or irradiation.

Osteoconduction

This is a passive phenomenon whereby the graft material acts as a scaffold into which new host bone can grow. Mechanical stability is essential for osteoconduction but it is mainly a property of the structure of the graft and most materials are osteoconductive when present as a mesh with a pore size of greater than 200 μm.

The three mechanisms usually occur together and, for example in a cancellous autograft, osteocytes near the graft surface revascularize rapidly and form new bone. As the revascularized graft bone is remodelled, matrix-bound growth factors are released, causing an osteoinductive host response. Finally, the graft surface is a suitable lattice for osteoconduction.

As invasion of the graft by host bone proceeds, the graft is partially or completely replaced by the host, a process termed *incorporation*. If this does not occur, the graft will remain as a foreign body which may ultimately fail because of fatigue damage or become infected. However, as the graft is incorporated, it may become mechanically weak as a result of resorption and this may cause it to break.

Bone graft incorporation

Bone graft incorporation occurs in defined stages: inflammation, specific immune response, revascularization, osteogenesis and remodelling.[78,79] Although described as separate stages, the processes represent a continuum. In the optimal case of a fresh cancellous autograft, the immediate acute inflammatory response is minor and there is no specific immune response. Revascularization may occur as early as two days after transplantation, allowing survival of the surface osteocytes which produce new bone. Morphogens from within the bone induce host cells to differentiate into osteoblasts and themselves form new bone, and osteoconduction proceeds rapidly as capillaries invade the matrix. Dead trabeculae from within the graft become lined with new osteoblasts and seams of osteoid are deposited. These may surround dead graft bone, resulting in increased radiographic density and a transient increase in strength.[80] As remodelling occurs, the dead bone is removed; however, this process may take years and is never completed in larger grafts.

Fresh cortical autograft incorporates in a similar manner, except that revascularization is slower so that less graft cells remain viable and initial incorporation includes osteoclastic bone resorption, which leads to temporary osteoporosis and a loss of mechanical strength.[80,81] Holes in the cortical bone may be filled with cancellous bone which matures rapidly to new cortical bone.[82] It is rare for all of the graft to be replaced by new host bone and remodelling occurs only in osteonal systems and not in interstitial lamellae.[79] In contrast to the slow and uncertain incorporation of devascularized cortical bone, vascularized cortical autograft incorporates rapidly because its cells retain their viability and the bone rapidly adapts to its new strain environment.

In a fresh cancellous allograft, a vigorous immune response is seen which may delay or prevent osteoinduction. New blood

REFERENCES

77. Friendlaender G E, Goldberg V M. Bone and Cartilage Allografts: Biology and Clinical Applications. American Academy of Orthopedic Surgeons, Prkridge, IL1991
78. Burchardt H, Enneking W K Surg Clin North Am 1978; 58: 403–427
79. Goldberg V M, Stevenson S, Shaffer J W In: Friendlander G E, Goldberg V M (eds) Bone and Cartilage Allografts: Biology and Clinical Applications. American Academy of Orthopedic Surgeons, Parkridge, IL 1991 pp 3–12
80. Enneking W F, Burchardt H, Puhl J J, Piotrowski G J Bone Joint Surg Am 1975; 57: 237–252
81. Burchardt H, Jones H, Glowczeewskie F, Rudner C, Enneking W F J Bone Joint Surg Am 1978; 60: 1082–1090
82. Burchardt H, Busbee G A III, Enneking WF J Bone Joint Surg Am 1975; 57: 814–819

vessels from the host become occluded, causing graft necrosis. Thus allograft bone functions poorly as a graft compared to autograft. The allograft immune response may be minimized by histocompatibility matching the donor and host or by modifying the allograft antigens by preservation techniques such as freezing.[77] Cortical allografts behave similarly to cancellous allograft, except that the specific immune response is delayed for a period while initial revascularisation occurs.

BIOMECHANICAL ASPECTS OF FRACTURES

Whether a bone will fracture under the influence of a particular stress will depend on the magnitude, duration and direction of the force acting on the bone and the rate of its application (factors extrinsic to the bone, see section on classification of fractures for a discussion) and on intrinsic factors within the bone.

The important intrinsic factors are the energy-absorbing capacity of the bone, the Young's modulus and its fatigue strength.[83] Bone is three times as strong as cast iron and 10 times more flexible, although it is of similar tensile strength. The inorganic phase of bone (hydroxyapatite) is about six times more rigid than whole bone and is stronger in compression than in tension. In contrast, bone collagen does not resist compression but has a tensile strength five times that of whole bone. Thus the composite structure which is bone owes its compressive strength to hydroxyapatite and its tensile strength to collagen. As an approximation, bone can be strained to 0.75% before plastic failure occurs and its breaking strain is 2–4%.

Because bone remodels itself to resist applied loads, it is anisotropic, possessing different mechanical properties in differing directions and both its ultimate tensile strength and its Young's modulus are greater when loaded in its longitudinal axis. Furthermore, it is visco-elastic, its behaviour varying with the rate of load application. When bone is loaded there is an instantaneous elastic deformation followed by a slower plastic one. The rate of load application is therefore important in determining the outcome of loading. A rapid load is absorbed elastically but during slower, plastic deformation bone can absorb six times more energy before fracture than in the elastic phase. However, if the rapidly applied load is sufficient to cause a fracture, the stored elastic energy will be released explosively, causing great damage to bone and surrounding soft tissues. This is the basis for the division of fractures into high- and low-energy fractures. Owing to their explosive nature, high-energy fractures are associated with increased comminution, greater soft tissue damage and more periosteal stripping, all of which tend to slow fracture union. The bone of elderly osteoporotic patients does not possess the ability to store elastic energy in this way and consequently the sort of high-energy fractures which occur in young patients are not seen in the elderly. If an elderly limb is subjected to this sort of force it will crumple.

When a material is subjected to repeated cyclical loading it may fail even though the magnitude of the individual stress which is applied is well below the ultimate tensile stress of the material. This is known as fatigue failure and it is due to the initiation of small cracks within the material. Once a crack has been started, propagation requires far lower stresses than initiation, although the complex structure of bone tends to resist crack propagation (see below) and remodelling provides a means for repair of minor damage. Stress or fatigue fractures are seen in young persons who undertake excessive repetitive activity, such as ballet dancers or soldiers, or in the elderly in whom the process of bone remodelling is slow.

A number of features contribute to the mechanical strength of bone and its consequent ability to resist imposed forces for the lifetime of the organism:

1. At a macroscopic level, the strong cortical bone is arranged as a tube, thus providing the greatest strength for a given weight. The cortex is reinforced by the central cancellous, lamellar bone where the individual trabeculae are arranged to resist the usually imposed forces.
2. At a microscopic level, the differently oriented irregular individual structural units of bone formed by each remodelling unit fit together exactly because of the manner in which they are formed and are held firmly together by the cement substance in a fashion resembling a brick wall. This helps to prevent crack propagation by forming a T-shaped crack at the interphase (the Cook–Gordon mechanism).
3. The poorly crystalline nature of the hydroxyapatite means that bone is not subject to easy cleavage between crystal domains as, for example, is seen in diamond.
4. Bone turnover and remodelling are important because they allow the bone to alter itself to oppose imposed loads and they maintain bone strength by removing old or fatigue damaged bone. Thus in an elderly person bone may be weak not only because of an absolute deficiency of bone substance (osteoporosis) but also because, due to the low rate of bone turnover, individual bits of bone mineral are on average older than in a younger person and so have had more time to collect fatigue damage.
5. It is probable that normal muscle tone exerts a protective effect on bone; shielding it from excessive stress and muscle fatigue may be a factor in fractures in the elderly following minor trauma.[84]

Effect of implants

A hole in a bone will weaken the bone and this effect becomes significant when the diameter of the hole exceeds 30% of the bone diameter. With time, bone remodelling will restore the bone strength, not necessarily by filling the hole, but by laying down new bone structural units around the hole in order to normalize the excessive strains to which the bone is subjected by its local weakness.

A metallic implant will also weaken the bone by *stress shielding*. This implies that because any applied load is shared

REFERENCES

83. Evans F G Instruc Course Lec 1961; XVIII: 110–121
84. Frankel V H, Burstein A H. Orthopaedic Biomechanics. Lea & Febiger, Philadelphia 1970

between the bone and the implant, the strain produced by a normal load will be diminished and the remodelling bone will become porotic in order to normalize the strain.

At the ends of the implant there is an abrupt transition between the elasticity of the supported and unsupported bone which will constitute a *stress riser*. This is a region where there is a sudden change in Young's modulus which leads to a concentration of stresses and an increased likelihood of fracture.

CLASSIFICATION OF FRACTURES

Fractures may be classified by the mechanism of injury, by the nature and site of the fracture fragments and by the extent of the associated soft tissue injury. These systems are interrelated, since high-violence injuries produce comminuted fractures with severe soft tissue damage while low violence is associated with simple fractures and little soft tissue injury. A combination of these factors is used to determine the *fracture personality*.[85,86]

Classification by mechanism of injury

Fractures may be caused by forces applied directly or indirectly to the bone and the amount of displacement and bone damage will depend on the initiating trauma.

Direct trauma

Fractures caused by direct violence may be divided into tapping, crushing or penetrating.[87]

Tapping fractures

These are caused by a small force acting on a small area. They tend to be transverse and relatively undisplaced, with little soft tissue damage apart from a small overlying contusion or laceration. They are caused by a direct blow such as a kick on the shin playing sport, causing a fibula fracture, or a blow to the defending upheld forearm with a stick, causing a fracture of the isolated ulna. Fracture healing is usually uncomplicated although in the case of the nightstick injury to the ulna the splinting effect of the intact radius may delay union.

Crushing fractures

The force and area of application are greater and the duration longer than in a tapping fracture. There is associated major soft tissue damage and nerves and vessels may be compromised. Compartment problems are frequent and the fractures tend to be highly comminuted.

Penetrating fractures

These are produced by a large force acting on a small area. Gunshot and shrapnel wounds are of this type and they are also seen as a result of road traffic accidents. Gunshot wounds are subdivided into high and low energy. In a high-energy wound, the velocity of the projectile exceeds the speed of sound in the tissue and in addition to the direct damage from the projectile there is considerable contamination snd collateral damage to surrounding soft tissues caused by cavitation from the shock wave and associated negative pressure wave.

Indirect trauma

Fractures are often produced by a force acting at a distance from the fracture itself and these may be classified as tension, angulation, rotation or compression.

Tension fractures are commonly avulsions. Examples include the tibial tuberosity fracture and transverse fractures of the olecranon and patella. They are usually caused by a sudden resisted muscle contraction. Angulation forces, where the bone acts as a lever, cause transverse fractures with often a small area of comminution on the concave side.

Rotational forces cause spiral fractures, while compression loads may cause oblique fractures of a bone shaft or T-shaped fractures involving the ends of bones such as a tibial plateau or femoral condylar fracture. A combination of these forces often occurs.

Combinations of fractures are not infrequently seen and for example a vertical compression force following a fall from a height may fracture the calcaneum, the tibial plateau, the acetabulum and the lumbar spine. A patient presenting with an appropriate history and one of a set of fractures leads the astute clinician to look carefully for signs of other fractures within the set.

Classification by nature of the fracture fragments

General factors

Any fracture may be classified according to whether it is transverse, oblique, spiral or communited (Fig. 50.7). Further assessment will include whether the fracture fragments are displaced or undisplaced.

Specific fracture classification

Almost every fracture has been classified according to individual clinical factors which govern the method of treatment, possible complications and expected outcome. These classification systems are useful for discussion between clinicians, determination of treatment and assessment of the utility of new treatment methods. Examples of commonly used systems include the Weber[88,89] classification of lateral malleolar fractures, the Ruedi and Allgower[90]

REFERENCES

85. Nicoll E A J Bone Joint Surg 1964; 46-B: 373–387
86. Schatzker J, Tile M The Rationale of Operative Fracture Care, 2nd edition. Springer-Verlag, Berlin 1996
87. Perkins G, Fractures and Dislocations. Athlone Press London 1958
88. Weber B G. Die Verletzungen des Oberen Sprunggellenkes: Aktuelle Probleme in der Chirurgie. Hans Huber, Bern 1966
89. Muller M E, Allgower M, Schneider R, Willenegger H Manual of Internal Fixation, 1st edition, Springer Verlag, Berlin 1970

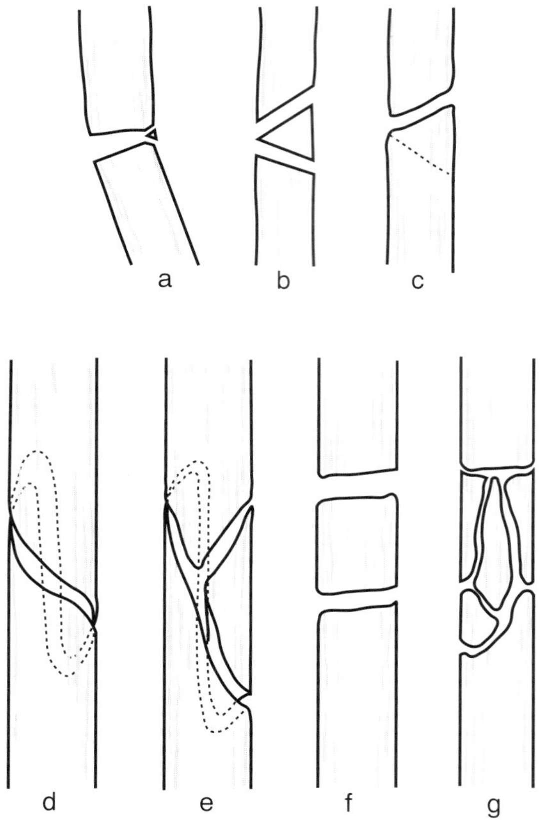

Fig. 50.7 Fractures are classified into transverse, oblique, spiral, segmental and comminuted on the basis of the X-ray appearance. After Schatzker & Tile.[86] **(a)** Bending forces cause transverse fractures and there is usually an extruded wedge of bone on the compression side which has little soft tissue attachment. **(b)** If the extruded fragment is large, bone union may be slow because of its poor viability. **(c)** If the extruded fragment is not separated from both sides of the fracture, an oblique fracture results. Alternatively, an oblique fracture may be caused by a combination of bending and torsion loads. **(d)** Torsional loading results in a spiral fracture. **(e)** A butterfly fragment may be extruded from a spiral fracture. **(f)** When a fracture involves two separate sites within a bone, the term 'segmental fracture' is used. **(g)** A comminuted fracture implies multiple fracture fragments.

classification of tibial pilon fractures and the Hawkins[91] classification of talar neck fractures. In some complicated fractures, more than one classification system is necessary for full assessment. In a calcaneal fracture (Fig. 50.14), the Atkins[92] classification will allow assessment of the lateral wall and the initial approach for internal fixation, the Sanders[93] classification gives information of the severity of the damage to the posterior facet of the subtalar joint, the Essex Lopresti classification[94] addresses the nature of the lateral joint fragment and the Zwipp & Tscherne[95] classification depends on the number of major fracture fragments and joints involved. Finally, the Crosby and Fitzgibbons[96] classification gives insight into the result of conservative treatment of the fracture. These classification systems are complementary and they are all necessary for full assessment of the fracture and a determination of whether and how internal fixation should be undertaken.

The AO classification system[97] is a comprehensive attempt to classify every long bone fracture logically. The system considers each bone to have a central diaphyseal segment and two end segments, and a precise terminology has been developed to describe each fracture type with great accuracy, so as to make pictorial representation superfluous. The system is not yet fully validated and it lacks the clinical utility of the individual site classification systems. It is, however, useful in research and because it is applicable to every fracture it deserves to be widely adopted.

Classification of soft tissue injury

It is all too easy to look at a radiograph of a fracture and attempt to treat the X-ray rather than the patient. A fracture represents trauma to the limb and the entire limb must be treated. In some respects, the soft tissues are more important than the bone because neglect of the bone injury will merely lead to a non-union or mal-union, whereas mismanagement of the soft tissue envelope can lead to amputation.

There are two commonly used means of classifying the severity of the soft tissue injury—the Tscherne system and the Gustillo and Anderson system—and these are described in the section on compound fractures.

FRACTURE DIAGNOSIS

The diagnosis of a fracture is usually simple, provided the clinician maintains a suspicious mind.

Clinical features

Appropriate history

Fractures do not usually occur without an antecedent history of appropriate injury. For example, the person who suffers a significant inversion injury to their ankle may suffer a spiral fracture of the lateral malleolus. Trauma is, however, not universal and a person suffering from metastatic bone cancer may suffer a spontaneous fracture, while the injury may be minor in an osteoporotic person. It may be repetitive and minor in a stress fracture, as for example the otherwise fit soldier who fractures a metatarsal bone after unaccustomed marching. It is important therefore in assessing a fracture to obtain a general history, including past medical history and previous drug treatments. In the case of a child, the lack

REFERENCES

90. Ruedi T P, Allgower M Clin Orthop 1979; 138: 105–110
91. Hawkins L G J Bone Joint Surg 1970; 52A: 991–1002
92. Eastwood D M, Gregg P, Atkins R M J Bone Joint Surg Br 1993; 75-B: 183–189
93. Sanders R, Fortin P, Dipasquale T, Walling A Clin Orthop 1993; 290: 87–95
94. Essex-Lopresti P Br J Surg 1952; 39: 395–419
95. Zwipp H, Tscherne H, Thermann H, Weber T Clin Orthop 1993; 290: 76–86
96. Crosby L A, Fitzgibbons T. J Bone Joint Surg Am 1990; 72-A: 852–859
97. Muller M E, Nazarian S, Koch P, Schatzker J. The Comprehensive Classification of Fractures of Long Bones. Springer-Verlag, Berlin 1990

of an appropriate history of injury will alert the astute clinician to the possibility of non-accidental injury.

Pain and tenderness

Provided the patient does not have an associated neurological disorder, fractures even if undisplaced are painful, although this is not always severe. A patient may walk for several days despite a fractured lateral malleolus. Relatively minor pain and disability usually suggest that a fracture is in a stable position, is not severely displaced and may be incomplete.

Loss of function

This is caused by the pain and loss of lever arms for muscles to work against.

Deformity

Angular, rotatory or longitudinal deformity results from a displaced fracture. Even if it is undisplaced, the haemorrhage and soft tissue damage will usually give rise to swelling.

Attitude

Sometimes the manner in which a patient presents is highly suggestive of a fracture. A patient with a clavicular fracture often supports the fractured arm by holding the elbow with the uninjured side. A patient who presents holding their head firmly in their hands and refuses to allow movement of their neck lest their 'head fall off' should be assumed to have a fracture of the cervical spine until proven otherwise.

Mobility and crepitus

An unimpacted fracture allows movement between the two ends of the fracture and as this occurs grating or crepitus may be felt and sometimes heard. These signs are of historic interest only; they are painful to the patient and increase the local tissue damage and so must not be actively sought.

Radiographic features

X-rays

Plain radiographs are the mainstay of fracture diagnosis. At least two orthogonal views must be performed in order to demonstrate the fracture and its displacement. Computerised tomographic (CT) scanning is increasingly used and is all but essential for the full assessment of more complex intra-articular fractures, such as tibial pilon fractures, acetabular fractures and calcaneal fractures (Fig. 50.14). Three-dimensional reconstruction is also increasingly employed but its usefulness is limited. It probably has a role in acetabular fractures but in calcaneal fractures, where the individual fragments may be only slightly larger than the pixel size of the reconstruction, its value is more limited.

Magnetic resonance imaging (MRI) has the advantage over CT scanning that reconstruction in any direction is possible without loss of definition. In addition, it allows visualization of metabolic changes and soft tissue damage, such as spinal cord oedema, and it does not irradiate the patient. Set against these advantages is the relatively poor definition that it provides of bone fragments, so that a high-quality CT scan is usually preferred for fracture assessment.

FRACTURE MANAGEMENT

The management of any fracture should be divided into the emergency phase and the phase of reconstruction.

Emergency phase

The primary concern is saving the patient's life and the damaged limb. The patient must be assessed and resuscitated (see Ch. 7) with appropriate replacement of colloid and crystalloid lost due to the fracture. Appropriate analgesia is given (see Ch. 5). The limb is examined and its vascular status determined. An acutely ischaemic limb secondary to fracture displacement usually responds to gentle reduction by traction. Emergency angiography and vascular reconstruction combined with fracture stabilization may be necessary if this is ineffective (see Ch. 10). Nerve damage is noted. The fracture is splinted in a comfortable position, which may involve temporary traction before the fracture is assessed radiographically.

In the case of a compound fracture, that is, one where the bone has come out through the skin, the initial fracture and wound management belong in the emergency phase, since the wound will become colonized with bacteria within 6 hours of the injury. The wound should be cleaned of all obvious debris, photographed and covered with a bactericidal dressing. The fracture is splinted and the patient is taken to the operating theater within 6 hours of the injury so that a primary debridement of the wound and stabilization of the fracture can be performed. Compound fractures are discussed in greater detail below.

Phase of reconstruction

The definitive management of a fracture is a separate issue from its emergency treatment. Fracture reconstructions are among the most complex of orthopaedic operations and they should not be undertaken in haste, without adequate investigation and in anywhere other than a fully equipped operating theatre with fully rested and adequately trained staff. An improperly performed surgical reconstruction may jeopardize the livelihood of a young working man. In the multiply injured patient (see Ch. 7), it may be necessary to carry out emergency stabilization of long bone fractures in order to minimize the systemic effects of the fractures. It may be possible to undertake definitive reconstruction of the fracture at this time; however, the aim of resuscitation is to save the patient's life and limb, while the aim of reconstruction is to optimize long-term function following the fracture. These two aims are not mutually exclusive but it is essential for the surgeon to maintain their clear separation.

resistant containers. The new casting materials have a number of advantages over the traditional plaster of Paris. They are lighter, stronger and more radiolucent. They are waterproof and more resistant to wear and tear. For the benefit of children, they can be made in a variety of intriguing colours and they are less messy to apply than plaster of Paris. The disadvantages are that they are relatively expensive and irritant so that gloves must be worn during their application. The increased strength means that if the limb swells they deform less and pressure within the limb is greater. They are also more difficult to apply by the amateur than plaster of Paris bandages. Plaster of Paris is often still preferred as the initial cast, with a fibreglass cast being applied by an expert after the swelling has settled.

Plaster of Paris casts may be complete or incomplete (also known as a slab). Slabs allow for limb swelling and are often the first casts to be applied after a fracture or operation. The full circumferential cast allows maximum control of the fracture. Alternatively a full cast may be applied and split through the plaster of Paris and all the underlying padding in order to allow for anticipated swelling.

Casts are applied with a variable amount of padding. Bohler[109] advocated that the plaster of Paris was directly applied to the skin without padding in order to obtain optimal fracture control. This sort of plaster is rarely used now because of the danger of pressure sores and circulatory problems from the inevitable swelling. Charnley employed the well-padded cast devised by the Rizzola Institute in Bologna[107] and the modern cast is developed from this, employing some padding to protect the skin and allow for swelling. The plaster cast is not a simple tube. It is moulded between application and setting by the surgeon using the flat of the hands in order to apply a corrective force to the fracture. This principle of *three-point plaster fixation* was developed by Charnley[107] (Fig. 50.19).

In order to control a fracture and prevent loss of the reduced position or *slipping*, it is necessary to immobilize the joint above and the joint below the fracture. Thus in a child's distal radial fracture, the rotational part of the injury cannot be adequately controlled unless the elbow joint is included in the plaster. There are, however, a number of exceptions to this rule. A Colles' fracture of the distal radius requires an above-elbow cast to control the fracture adequately. This sort of cast is, however, very inconvenient and restrictive for an elderly person. A forearm cast is therefore employed and the increased likelihood of malposition of the fracture is accepted. Sarmiento[110] devised the patella tendon-bearing cast, which allows control of rotation of a tibial fracture at the same time as allowing movement of the knee. Cast braces are casts in which the joints are allowed to move by the incorporation of hinges. These may be either simple as at the elbow or more complex, poly-axial hinges which are required at the knee.

Precautions in the use of casts

There are a number of potentially serious problems with the use of casts. The cast may become sufficiently tight to restrict the circulation to the limb or a ridge in the plaster may dig into the limb (Fig. 50.17). For these reasons patients are instructed to seek advice if the plaster becomes painful or too tight, or if the limb becomes paraesthetic or blue. Any excessively painful plaster must be removed and if there is a suspicion of circulatory embarrassment by the plaster, it must be split through the plaster and all underlying padding and the edges of the plaster spread apart. If this does not definitely relieve the problem, the plaster must be removed.

A foreign body may fall into the plaster, in which case the plaster should be replaced. Finally, the patient may try to scratch beneath the plaster using a knitting needle or similar. This is very dangerous and must be forbidden. The initial skin irritation is relieved by the scratching but the skin is usually damaged and begins to exude, which creates further itching and more scratching. It is not unknown for a patient to scratch the soft tissues away right down to expose the underlying bone without feeling any pain.

Traction

The use of traction to overcome the muscle spasm of a fracture in order to allow manipulative reduction has already been discussed. Continuous traction can maintain the reduction and allow the fracture to unite in the reduced position. This was the mainstay of treatment for certain fractures until satisfactory methods of internal fixation were developed and it remains a safe and acceptable option. However, it requires a prolonged stay in hospital with constant attention to ensure that reduction is not lost and that the traction apparatus is satisfactorily applied. The complications of prolonged bedrest, such as venous thrombosis, pressure sores, hypostatic pneumonia and osteoporosis, are additional drawbacks. Finally, permanent joint stiffness is common because of the duration of immobilization and fracture reduction may not be as good as can be obtained by open operation.

The concept of continuous traction was popularized by Buck in the American Civil War[111] for the treatment of femoral fractures and the technique then spread to Europe. Originally, traction was provided by cloth tapes bound to the skin by bandages. This method of skin traction is limited because the skin is unable to withstand more than 6 pounds of traction for any length of time. Greater loads shear off the superficial layers, leaving a raw, irritated area.

Skeletal traction implies that the traction force is directly applied to the skeleton and it was first introduced using tongs. Steinmann pioneered the use of transfixing pins and Denham developed a screw-threaded pin to prevent slipping. Kirschner first introduced his wires for this application but, although these finer wires require a smaller skin puncture and were therefore attractive, the necessity of using a device to maintain the wire tension must be offset against this. Fine-wire traction tends to be employed in the upper limb in children or for temporary traction.

REFERENCES

109. Bohler L Technik der Knochenbruch-Behandlung, 5th edition, vol 1. Wilhelm Maudrich, Vienna 1937
110. Sarmiento A J Bone Joint Surg 1967; 49-A: 855–875
111. Peltier L F J Bone Joint Surg 1968; 50-A: 1603–1617

Principles of internal fixation

Many fractures heal satisfactorily following manipulative reduction and external splintage. Not all, however, respond well to this 'conservative' regime and unsatisfactory results led to the development of 'internal fixation' of fractures.

Prior to the mid-nineteenth century, the overwhelming majority of fractures were treated conservatively because of the dangers of surgical intervention. Operation was reserved for compound fractures or painful non-union and the standard treatment of an open fracture or a contaminated penetrating joint wound was immediate amputation because of the danger of overwhelming sepsis.[112,113] At this time, standard fracture treatment was splintage and traction. Kirschner wires and Steinmann pins were initially developed as traction aids. With the onset of the era of anaesthesia and asepsis, investigation of operative fracture surgery began in the closing decades of the nineteenth century.[114] Plate fixation of fractures was pioneered in the late nineteenth and early twentieth centuries by Lambotte[115] and Lane;[57] however, early attempts at internal fixation did not provide sufficient fracture stability to permit mobilization and supplementary plaster fixation was often used. Once fracture union was evidenced by callus formation, rehabilitation was commenced. However, because the fracture haematoma had been removed and soft tissue attachments to the bone disturbed, union was delayed by the surgery and the results were poor. Key[116] and Charnley[117] first experimented with compression in arthrodesis, using it to achieve stability of fixation which allowed subsequent bony union. Danis[58] demonstrated that under conditions of absolute stability produced by a special compression plate, cortical bone would unite without radiologically visible callus, a process which he termed 'primary bone union'. In 1958, a group of Swiss surgeons led by Maurice Muller formed the Arbeitsgemeinshaft für Osteosynthesfragen (AO), or the Association for the Study of Internal Fixation (ASIF). Schenk and Willenegger[118] studied primary bone union experimentally and the AO group produced a manual of suggested operative techniques.[89]

The AO group has had such a profound effect on fracture treatment that it is necessary to study their underlying concepts carefully. It was their belief that fracture or plaster disease, which is synonymous with algodystrophy, was the result of immobilization of a limb in plaster.[89,119] They concentrated on rapid restoration of limb function by anatomic fracture reduction, rigid internal fixation, atraumatic surgical technique and early, pain-free active mobilization within 10 days of operation Their concepts differed from those of Watson Jones and Bohler, who concentrated on bone union first and then on rehabilitation, in that these two phases were simultaneous. In order to allow such rapid mobilization, the fracture fixation had to be very stable and this was achieved by compression between the fracture fragments. Compression restored structural–mechanical continuity to the bone and permitted direct transfer of forces from bone fragment to bone fragment rather than through the implant, thus preserving it from mechanical failure. The keystone of this approach was the lag screw for the production of interfragmentary compression, combined with neutralization plates and compression plates.[120] Where fracture comminution prevented rigid apposition, extensive bone grafting was employed. Advances in implant technology with the development, for example, of locked intramedullary nailing and improved understanding of bone biology and the necessity of maintaining fracture fragment viability have modified their original approach. The concept of atraumatic, anatomic reduction and rigid fixation of articular fractures with early motion remains; however, for diaphyseal fractures and diaphyseal extensions of articular fractures, there has been a move away from absolute stability and primary bone union. At the time when the AO was started, comminution of a diaphyseal fracture was a contraindication to intramedullary nailing—now it is the indication.

Several basic principles of internal fixation can be stated:

1. Operative treatment of fractures is not without risk and these risks must be carefully weighed against the probable outcome of conservative treatment and the patient's requirements. The presence of a fracture is not an indication for internal fixation and a mediocre result of non-operative treatment is usually preferable to the result of a failed attempt at internal fixation.
2. The damage to bone and soft tissue at the time of fracture cannot always be reversed and the anticipated outcome must be tempered by the severity and nature of the initial injury.
3. The soft tissue damage must be taken into account when planning operative exposure and may preclude internal fixation.
4. Operative exposure must be extensile[121] in order to allow adequate exposure of the bone for fixation.
5. The blood supply of bone fragments must be preserved as far as possible.
6. The technique of internal fixation must engage one of the inherent mechanisms for fracture healing outlined above.

Concepts of bone fixation

Fixation with compression

A number of techniques have been introduced to produce compression between fracture fragments.

REFERENCES

112. Malgaine J F A Treatise on Fractures, 1st edition Lippincott, Philadelphia 1859
113. Stimson L A Treatise on Fractures, 1st edition. Lea, Philadelphia 1883
114. Peltier L Fractures: A History and Ionography of their Treatment. Norman Publishing, San Francisco 1990
115. Lambotte A L'intervention operatoire dans les fractures recentes et anciennes. (envisage particulierement au de vue de l' osteosynthese avec la description de plusiers techniques nouvelles). Maloine, Paris 1907
116. Key J A South Med J. 1932; 25: 909–915
117. Charnley J. Compression Arthrodesis. Livingstone, Edinburgh 1953
118. Schenk R, Willenegger H Langenbecks Arch Klin Chir 1964; 308: 440
119. Muller M E, Allgower M, Willenegger H Technik der operativen Frakturenbehandlung. Springer-Verlag Berlin 1963
120. Muller M E, Allgower M, Schneider R, Willenegger H Manual of Internal Fixation, 3rd edition. Springer-Verlag, Berlin 1992
121. Henry A K Extensile Exposure. Williams & Williams, Baltimore, 1945

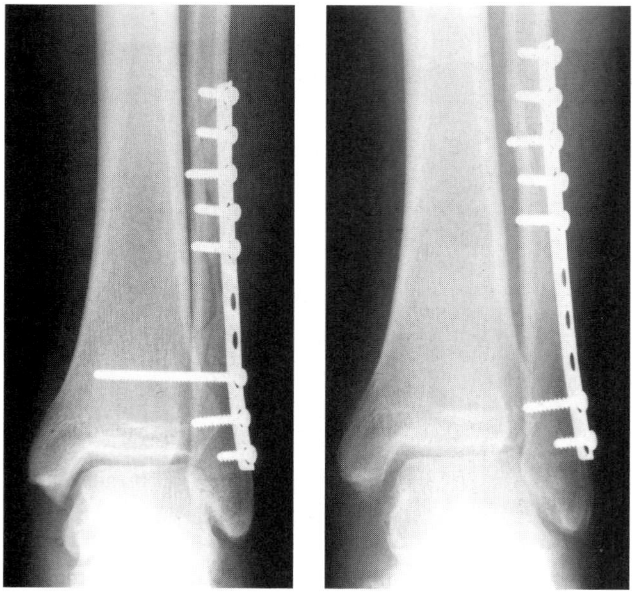

a b

Fig. 50.13 'Biological' fixation. (**a**) In this highly comminuted Weber type C distal fibular fracture, it is not possible to produce rigid internal fixation with compression. The third tubular plate has been applied to the fibula to reduce the fracture with respect to length and alignment. Care has been taken not to strip the periosteum from the bone and union is rapid because the bone retains its blood supply. The long inferior screw which passes into the tibia is a 'diastasis' screw which supports the ruptured inferior tibiofibular ligaments. This is removed at an early stage. (**b**) Union occurs by periosteal callus formation where bone fragments are unstable, particularly superiorly.

Types of fixation device

Extramedullary devices

Cerclage systems

Cerclage wires have been used for stabilization of fractures since the early nineteenth century.[112] Thin wires or cables cause minimal disturbance to the osseous blood supply because it does not flow longitudinally along the cortex.[52,125] The bands which were developed from cerclage wires by Parham and later by Partridge are, however, wider and may well be associated with local cortical necrosis.[126,127] Although the cerclage wire itself may not disturb the bone blood supply, considerable soft tissue dissection may be necessary in order to apply it and soft tissues may be trapped beneath the wire. Their application may therefore cause avascularity.

Transfixing wires

Although Kirschner wires were first introduced for the provision of skeletal traction, these smooth, flexible wires are now used almost exclusively for the stabilization of individual bone fragments, either temporarily or as a definitive fracture fixation, usually augmented either by a tension band or by external splintage. The wires, being small, have little or no harmful effect on bone blood flow.

Screws

A screw has a number of unique properties. It has a thread with a shape and pitch, and a major and minor diameter. The major developments in bone screws have been made by the AO/ASIF group.[89] AO screws are based on machine screws and have a hexagonal recess in the head which fits accurately with the screwdriver. They are cylindrical and are threaded either throughout their length (fully threaded) or only on the distal part (partially threaded). The screws are usually blunt ended, requiring pre-tapping, since self-tapping screws were believed to grip bone less well; however, more recently screws which incorporate a fluted tip and are self-tapping have been shown to be satisfactory. Screw design is a compromise between strength and holding power, with its dimensions being determined by the size of the bone to be fixed. Screw strength depends on the minor diameter (the diameter of the shaft of the screw between the threads), whereas holding power varies mainly with the major diameter (the diameter of the outside of the thread) and to a lesser extent is dependent on thread design. In vivo, an immobile screw becomes enmeshed by bone so that its holding power increases with time. In contrast, a screw which is allowed to move provokes local bone resorption.[128–130]

Two sorts of screw have been developed by the AO/ASIF group which form part of a comprehensive fracture fixation system. Cortical screws are made with diameters from 1.5 mm to 4.5 mm and are threaded throughout their entire length. They are inserted using a drill slightly larger than the minor diameter and employ a tap which copies the thread. The drill for the gliding hole matches the major diameter. Cancellous screws by contrast may be fully or partially threaded and have a greater difference between the minor and major diameters. They are available with a major diameter from 4.5 mm to 6.5 mm.

Cannulated screws

For a number of fractures, for example a sub-capital fracture of the neck of femur, it is useful to be able to employ a preliminary wire as guide for subsequent screw placement. This is most readily achieved by the use of a screw with a hole down its centre. Such cannulated screws are weaker than solid screws and are therefore made with a wider minor diameter. The major diameter is increased in some cases to improve holding power.

Plates

As compression was required at the fracture site to produce rigid fixation of the bone, tensioning devices were developed which

REFERENCES

125. Rhinelander F W J Biomed Mater Res 1974; 8: 87–90
126. Rhinelander F W Clin Orthop. 1975; 107: 188–220
127. Jones D G J Bone Joint Surg 1986; 68-B: 476–477
128. Schatzker J, Horne J G, Sumner-Smith G Clin Orthop Rel Res 1975a; 111: 257–262
129. Schatzker J, Horne J G, Sumner-Smith G Clin Orthop Rel Res 1975b; 111: 263–265
130. Schatzker J, Sanderson J, Murnaghan J P Clin Orthop Rel Res 1975c; 108: 115–116

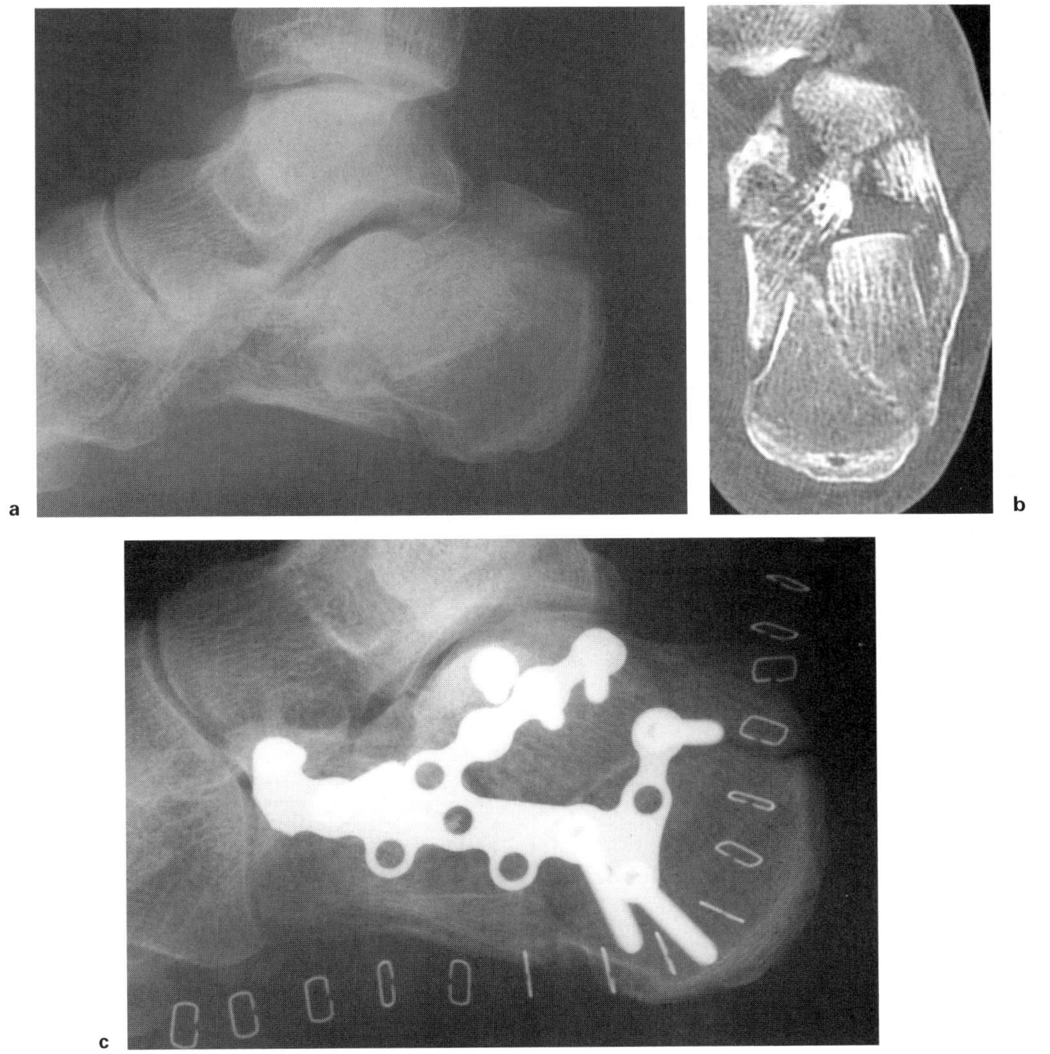

Fig. 50.14 (a) Lateral plain radiograph of an intra-articular fracture of the calcaneum showing disruption of the posterior facet of the subtalar joint and alteration of Bohler's angle. (b) The fracture is assessed by CT scanning, which shows the degree of posterior facet disruption and the configuration of the fracture fragments, allowing proper surgical planning. (c) The fracture is treated by open reduction and internal fixation with a specialized plate.

could be attached to the bone and one end of the plate after the other had been firmly fixed to one fracture fragment. These were then used to apply compression prior to completion of screw fixation. The tensioning device was removed prior to wound closure.

The *dynamic compression plate* (DCP) is a plate in which the screw holes are shaped so that as the spherical screw head is tightened it impinges on an inclined plane on one side of the screw hole. This causes the plate to move sideways and as the plate is rigidly fixed to the other fracture fragment, compression of the fracture site is produced[120] (Fig. 50.9). Compression of the fracture site may also be produced by appropriate contouring of the plate prior to its application to the bone (Fig. 50.14).

Rigidity of fracture fixation was ensured by the use of heavy plates which achieved a large contact area between the plate and the bone. These plates are associated with marked osteoporosis of the underlying bone which may be associated with refracture after plate removal.[131,132] Similar changes have been found in animal experiments[133,134] and these were diminished if a more flexible titanium[135] or carbon fibre composite[136] plate was used instead of stainless steel. The osteoporosis was originally thought to be the result of stress shielding of the bone by the plate; however, Perren et al[137,138] have argued that it is the result of disturbance in local blood flow because of the large area of contact between the

REFERENCES

131. Richon A, Livio J J, Segesser F Helv Chir Acta 1967; 34: 49–64
132. Moyen B, Comtet J J, Roy J C, Basset R, De-Mourges G Lyon Chir 1980; 76: 153–157
133. Paavolainen P, Slatis P, Karaharju E, Holmstrom T Acta Orthop Scand 1979; 50: 369–374
134. Pilliar R M, Cameron H A, Binnington A G, Szivek J, MacNab J Biomed Mater Res 1979; 13: 799–810
135. Uthoff H K, Bardos D I, Liskova-Kiar M J Bone Joint Surg 1981; 63-B: 427–444
136. Coutts R D, Akeson W H, Woo SL-Y, Matthews J V, Gonsalves M, Amiel D Orthop Clin North Am 1976; 7: 223–229

bone and the plate. In order to overcome this problem, the *limited contact dynamic compression plate* (LC-DCP) has been designed.[138,139] This titanium plate has a contact area of only 50% of its surface and is associated with less cortical porosis (Fig. 50.36).[140]

Further developments of this concept have included the *point contact plate* (PCP)[141] and the *internal fixator* in which a plate is applied and fixed at a small distance from the underlying bone and which can be mounted under the skin.[142]

Modified plates

Certain specific fractures require specialized plates. The expanded metaphyses of bones are not suited to fixation with straight plates, while some bones, such as the calcaneum and pelvis, are irregular in shape. For use at these sites, angled, buttress and specialized plates have been developed (Fig. 50.14). Curved plates, which form half or a third of a tube and derive their strength from their curvature, are used to buttress fractures (Fig. 50.10 and 50.13). In order to fit the most complex bony contours, 'reconstruction' plates are used. These plates are scalloped adjacent to the screw holes so that they can be bent in three dimensions. They are used principally in the distal humerus and pelvis.

Intramedullary nails

History

A number of the current debates on the techniques for use of intramedullary nails stem from the history of the devices. Modern intramedullary devices are complex and require sophisticated manufacturing methods. Stimson[113] mentions the use of ivory intramedullary pegs for fracture stabilization and Hey-Groves[143] developed this technique, eventually using solid rods because of their greater strength and the avoidance of dead space. Kuntschner[144] popularized the technique, using a straight, hollow nail with an open, cloverleaf cross-section manufactured of thin stainless steel to bridge a fracture of the femur. The shape of the nail was designed for optimal strength and to allow more rapid revascularization of the medullary canal. The nail, being straight, obtained three-point fixation in the medullary canal and additional widening of the canal by the use of drills or reamers (a process termed *intramedullary reaming* or simply *reaming*) which was advocated in order to allow a larger and therefore stronger nail to be inserted. Although Kuntschner later experimented with a curved nail to match the curve of the femur,[145] this was difficult to use and was abandoned.

The AO/ASIF intramedullary femoral nail was a thin-walled, open-section cloverleaf cross-section nail, which was bent to follow the major curve of the femur. Reaming was employed to permit a wider and therefore stronger nail to be used and to increase the bone grip.[146] Unlike the original Kuntschner nail, the AO/ASIF nail was not designed for three-point fixation within the femur. Fracture stability was obtained by an interference fit of the nail with the entire diaphyseal length. Because the nail had a thin-wall cross-section, it would bend to some extent to accommodate the natural curve of the femur. By reaming the diaphysis, the length of femur over which the nail could obtain a purchase (the *working length* of the nail) was increased and an exact fit between the femur and the nail was ensured.

Early attempts to control rotation[147] included the use of bundle nailing (Hackenthal), individual nails inserted through the medial and lateral femoral condyles (Rush), curved nails (Maatz) and pins within nails (Hertzog).

None of these nails were designed to provide longitudinal stability and their utility was limited to fractures within the diaphysis which possessed some degree of inherent longitudinal stability. Kuntschner experimented with a 'detensor' nail in 1968;[147] however, it was Klemm and Schellmann[148–150] and Kempf and Grosse[151,152] who took the obvious step of bolting the nail to the bone proximally and distally in order to create a 'locking nail'. Two sorts of locking are recognized: 'dynamic' and static. In static locking, the screws are inserted into both ends of the nail through round holes so that the length of the nail/bone construct is effectively fixed. Dynamic locking is a poor term, which may be used to describe locking of only one end of the nail or locking of both ends but with the screw at one end placed through an oblong hole. These techniques allow some collapse at the fracture site. In the latter case, the amount of collapse is limited to the length of the oblong screw hole, which might be more accurately termed 'controlled collapse', whereas in the former there is no theoretical limit to the amount of the collapse which can occur. Shortening at the fracture site continues until the fracture becomes stable or until the nail abuts against some restraining tissue or even exits through the skin. This can best be described as 'uncontrolled collapse'.

'Dynamization' of an intramedullary nail is the process of removing one or more interlocking screws in order to allow collapse. It alters the biomechanical environment of the fracture profoundly even if the fracture is sufficiently united to be longitudinally stable, and causes increased contact between fracture fragments if the fracture is not. It often encourages bone union and

REFERENCES

137. Perren S M, Cordey J, Gautier E In: Lane J M (ed) Fracture Healing. Churchill Livingstone, Edinburgh 1987 pp 139–157
138. Perren S M, Cordey J, Rahn B A, Gautier E, Schneider E Clin Orthop Rel Res 1988; 232: 139–151
139. Klaue K, Perren S M, Kowalski M J Orthop Trauma. 1991; 5: 280–288
140. Perren S M Injury: AOASIF Sci Suppl 1991; 22: S1–S41
141. Remiger A R, Predieri M, Tepic S, Perren S M J Orthop Trauma 1993; 7: 176–177
142. Ramotowski W, Granowski R Clin Orthop Rel Res. 1991; 272: 67–75
143. Hey-Groves E W Br J Surg 1918; 5: 185–212
144. Kuntschner G Klin Schr 1940; 19: 6–10
145. Kuntschner G Practice of Intramedullary Nailing, 1st edition. Thomas, Springfield, IL 1967
146. Kyle R F Orthopaedics 1985; 8: 1356–1359
147. Maatz R, Lentz W, Arens W, Beck H Intramedullary Nailing and Other Intramedullary Osteosynthesis. Saunders, Philadelphia 1986
148. Klemm K, Schellman W D Unfallheikunde 1972; 75: 568–575
149. Klemm K, Schellman W D, Vitalli H P Bull Soc Int Chir. 1975; 34: 93–96
150. Klemm K, Borner M Clin Orthop 1986; 212: 89–100
151. Kempf I, Grosse A, Beck G J Bone Joint Surg 1985; 67-A: 709–720
152. Kempf I, Gross A, Tagland G, Bernhard L, Moui Y Chirurgie 1991; 117: 478–487

if the fracture is tenuously united it hastens maturation of the union by increasing the loading of the fracture site.

Locked intramedullary nails differ from unlocked nails in that they gain both rotational and longitudinal stability not from an interference fit with the diaphysis of the bone but as a result of the screws which fix the nail to the bone. Therefore reaming loses one of its original purposes, ensuring an accurate interference fit for the nail. The second purpose for reaming was to allow a wider and stronger nail to be used; however, advances in materials and nail design have to some extent rendered this unnecessary.

The question of the strength and stiffness necessary for an intramedullary nail is far from simple. Both characteristics depend on the materials used, the manner in which the nail is worked prior to use and the geometry of the nail. The purpose of an intramedullary nail is to support the bone while the fracture heals, and the biomechanical environment which is imposed on the fracture will bear a highly complex relationship to the stiffness of the bone/nail construct and the configuration of the fracture.

The influence of nail stiffness on fracture healing has been investigated in animal models. Fixation with a very rigid nail resulted in slow fracture union with little callus, while an elastic nail was associated with abundant callus but variable healing rates.[153] Torsional instability delays union.[154–156] As locking an intramedullary nail greatly increases the torsional stiffness of the bone/nail construct, locking may be intrinsically desirable to encourage fracture union.

The majority of nails are fabricated from one of several types of stainless steel or titanium. They are also made from titanium–aluminium–vanadium alloy or titanium–aluminium–niobium alloy. The advantages of titanium and its alloys are that nails can be made lighter and stronger. They may resist infection better than stainless steel, and titanium osseo-integrates better than stainless steel. However, avoidance of surgical infection is primarily a matter of good technique and it might be considered a disadvantage to have an osseo-integrated intramedullary nail. Titanium alloys are more expensive than stainless steel and they are sensitive to notching, so that damage to the nail occurring during surgery may have a disproportionate effect on strength. Titanium is also more difficult to work into complex shapes than stainless steel. A final theoretical disadvantage is that titanium wears considerably more than stainless steel and titanium debris excites a vigorous inflammatory response.

The stiffness of a cylinder in bending is proportional to the fourth power of the radius. Thus a 1 mm increase in the diameter of an intramedullary nail increases its strength and stiffness by 30–45% and a 25% increase in its diameter doubles its bending strength.[146] Making the nail hollow has a relatively small effect on strength. Placing a slot in a nail may, however, contribute to failure by buckling and markedly reduces the torsional stiffness.[146,157,158]

The length of the nail which is in direct contact with the fracture (the working length) varies markedly with the fracture configuration. It can be as little as 1–2 mm, to many centimetres in a complex comminuted fracture. In a deliberately undersized, unreamed, statically locked nail, the working length is the whole nail length. The bending stiffness of the nail is inversely proportional to the square of the working length and the torsional stiffness is inversely proportional to the same figure.

Biology of intramedullary nailing

Union proceeds mainly by the formation of periosteal callus following intramedullary nailing (Fig. 50.2),[52,72] in contrast to healing by direct union which follows compression plating (Fig. 50.3).[159] The insertion of an intramedullary device temporarily destroys the medullary blood supply whether the medullary canal is reamed prior to insertion or not, which renders some of the cortex avascular.[160,161] Nevertheless intramedullary fracture fixation is associated with higher bone and fracture blood flow than compression plating[159] in an animal model. Revascularization is more rapid following nailing if reaming is not employed.[58,72] Although it is likely that direct damage to the arterial blood supply is one cause of cortical necrosis, excessive intramedullary pressure is also important. Maintaining a low intramedullary pressure significantly reduces the amount of cortical necrosis caused by reaming in animal models. However, the passage of an unreamed rod causes a significant rise in pressure and results in embolus formation.[162]

Reaming

Considerable controversy surrounds the value of intramedullary reaming before nailing. Some of the arguments have already been presented but they are summarized here:

1. Reaming enlarges the medullary canal, allowing a wider and therefore potentially stronger nail to be inserted. With modern materials, this may be unnecessary. Furthermore, in a bone such as the tibia, where the medullary canal is triangular rather than round, a considerable amount of cortex has to be reamed before a larger nail can be inserted.
2. Reaming allows a closer fit between the nail and the bone over a longer distance, thus increasing the stability of the bone/nail interface. With modern interlocked nails, however, this may be unnecessary.
3. Medullary reaming of the cortex weakens the bone. Pratt et al[163] showed that reaming a cadaveric femur to 12 mm lowers the torsional strength to failure to 63% of normal and to 15 mm lowers it to 36%. Molster[164] found similar results in rats. This

REFERENCES

153. Wang G J, Reger S I, Mabie K N, Richman J A, Stamp W G Clin Orthop 1985; 192: 291–298
154. Molster A O Acta Orthop Scand 1984; 55: 632–636
155. Woodard P L, Self J, Calhoun J, Tencer A F, Evans E B J Orthop Trauma 1987; 1: 331–340
156. Grundnes O, Utvag E, Reikeras O Acta Orthop Scand 1994; 65: 32–36
157. Allen W C, Burstein A H, Frankel V H Clin Orthop 1968; 60: 13–20
158. Tarr R S, Wiss D A Clin Orthop 1986; 212: 10–17
159. Rand J A, Chao E Y S, Kelly P J J Bone Joint Surg 1981; 63-A: 427–442
160. Danckwardt-Lilliestrom G Acta Orthop Scand Suppl. 1969; 128S: 1–153
161. Danckwardt-Lilliestrom G, Lorenzi L, Olerud S J Bone Joint Surg 1970; 52-A: 1390–1394
162. Sturmer K Injury (AO/ASIF Sci Suppl) 1993; 24: s7–s21
163. Pratt D J, Papagiannoupoulos G, Rees P H, Quinnell R Injury 1987; 18: 177–179

effect is caused by loss of endosteal cortex. As the natural progression in life is one of gradual endosteal resorption with periosteal accretion, it is not clear whether there exists a natural mechanism for replacing the reamed endosteal bone, although it is assumed that the normal process of bone remodelling in response to the increased strain imposed by the weakened femur will in time lead to a restoration of bone strength.

4. Interference with the medullary blood supply causes temporary partial cortical necrosis, whose extent depends in part on the intramedullary pressure during the intervention. Vigorous reaming may contribute to the increased medullary pressure. It is certainly true that revascularization is slower after reaming.
5. From a clinical point of view, reaming is time consuming and may lead to embolism of debris into the veins.
6. A fracture through a bone leads to an increase in the activation level of the bone. It seems likely that the process of reaming the medullary canal also activates the bone. Thus where the intramedullary nailing is being used to treat an un-united fracture, where bone activation levels may be expected to have returned to normal, reaming is probably desirable to reactivate the bone and provide an additional stimulus to bone union.

Indications for internal fixation of fractures

The indications for internal fixation of fractures are imprecise. The main reasons for considering this technique are as follows.

Failure of closed methods

It is important to remember that the presence of a fracture is not of itself an indication for operative management. Many fractures can be adequately treated by closed or non-operative methods. It is perfectly acceptable to begin treatment by non-operative techniques and to have to convert to operative stabilization if these methods fail.

Articular fractures

Fractures which involve the articular surface require precise reduction and early mobilization to avoid stiffness and future arthritis. These goals can often only be achieved by operative treatment.

Pathological fractures

Fractures caused by bony metastases rarely unite. They are often excessively painful and terminal cancer patients should not be condemned to live out their remaining life on traction. The short life expectancy of the patient means that even though the fracture will not unite, the implant will usually not undergo fatigue failure before the patient succumbs to the underlying malignancy.[74]

Associated vascular injury

The presence of an associated vascular injury makes emergency fracture stabilization desirable to allow the vascular injury to be repaired with a stable skeleton (see Chapter 10).

Multiple injury

There is evidence that the multiply injured patient who has fractures in many long bones benefits from early fracture stabilization (see Chapter 7).[165] This does not necessarily imply internal fixation of every fracture, since external stabilization may be sufficient. More recent evidence suggests that early intramedullary nailing in multiply injured patients with significant chest injuries may cause a clinically undesirable worsening of lung function.[166–168]

Mobilization

Elderly patients suffer excessively from immobilization in bed. Complications of bedrest include pneumonia, venous thrombosis and pulmonary embolus, pressure sores, increased osteoporosis and difficulty with mobilization. For this reason, fractures in the elderly are often treated by operative fixation even when they would unite satisfactorily if treated non-operatively. A good example is the intertrochanteric fracture of the neck of femur.

Implant removal

Whether implants should be removed routinely after the fracture has consolidated is controversial and scarcity of resources often means that metalwork is left in place. There are, however, a number of scientific and medical considerations which govern whether implants should be removed. Implant removal is a surgical procedure which carries risks and should not be carried out lightly. Nerves and vessels may be involved in scar tissue and at risk of damage and the implant may be difficult to remove, entailing bone damage.

The implant is inevitably taking some of the load which would normally be applied to the bone and thus it is to be expected that bone in the region of an implant will not be able to remodel to its normal structure and strength until the implant has been removed. This may become important if the bone is again subjected to fracturing forces, when the fracture which occurs through the bone implant composite may be more complex and difficult to treat than would have been the case if the implant had been removed. As the bone becomes osteoporotic with age, it may become excessively weak because of the presence of the plate and liable to fracture.

Implants are often uncomfortable and function is frequently improved by removal even if the device was clinically asymptomatic. There is also a theoretical risk of malignant change in the region of the implant due to ingested metallic debris. This problem is more likely to occur following total joint replacement where debris is produced more copiously by movement at the bearing

REFERENCES

164. Molster A O Clin Orthop 1986; 202: 278–285
165. Bone L B, McNamara K, Shine B et al J Trauma 1994; 37: 262–264
166. Pape H C, Dwenger A, Regel G et al J Trauma. 1992; 33: 574–581
167. Pape H C, Auf' m'Kolk M, Paffrath T, Regel G, Sturm J A, Tcherne H J Trauma 1993; 34: 540–547
168. Pape H C, Regel G, Dwenger A et al J Trauma 1993; 35: 709–716

surfaces, but it is a possibility following fracture fixation where metalwork will be in place for many years. This risk is more theoretical than practical as it has not yet been reported.

Following plate removal, there is a risk of refracture either through the fracture or through adjacent screw holes; the bone will therefore require protection from overload for some time. A fracture which has united by primary bone union is weaker than one which has united by callus formation at an early stage because of the smaller amount of bone present and its spatial distribution. Primary bone union is also weaker because the bone undergoes rapid remodelling and becomes porotic, in part because of the presence of the plate. This intense remodelling lasts for about one year after fracture,[169] depending on the patient's age and the nature of the fracture.

External fixation

Principles

An external fixator is essentially a scaffold which is attached to the bone to support it while fracture union occurs. The first working external fixator was probably described by Parkhill;[170] however, the concept was developed by Lambotte[115] using a linear metal clamp attached to four screw-threaded half-pins. Roger Anderson in 1934 described a frame using transfixing pins and this concept was refined by Hoffman and later Vidal.[171] The rigidity of this device has led to problems with bone union and earned it the nickname 'the non-union machine'. In addition, the quadrilateral nature of the frame made reduction of the fracture difficult once the device was even partly applied.

Bone fixation

External fixators are fixed to bone either by screw-threaded half-pins, by transfixing pins or by tensioned fine wires. Screw-threaded half-pins have the advantage that they are simple and swift to apply and, because only one side of the bone is approached, the pins can usually be placed with little risk to neurovascular structures. Because the pin has only one end protruding from the bone, it acts like a post and the fixating frame can be relatively straight forward. The disadvantage of screw-threaded half-pins is that they rely on the integrity of the thread–bone interface for their stability. Loosening is a significant problem which limits their utility.

Transfixing pins and fine wires have the disadvantage that they must pass through the bone from one side of the limb to the other. This may endanger neurovascular structures or it may make the encircling frame inconvenient to the patient and restrict joint mobility. For example, it is difficult to transfix the proximal humerus without endangering the neurovascular structures, although the frame required is not much more inconvenient to the patient than a uni-axial frame. On the other hand, it is possible to pass a transfixing wire through the proximal femur but the frame required makes it difficult for the patient to lie down.

Transfixing pins have all the disadvantages of screw-threaded half-pins and transfixing devices and their use is normally restricted to the simple external fixators required for joint fusion or for temporary stabilization of the severely traumatized limb.

Tensioned fine wires for external fixation are being increasingly used in the West. They were originally popularized by Ilizarov in Russia, and although there are reports of their use prior to Ilizarov's work he is mainly responsible for their popularity.

Fine wires do little damage to the bone blood supply and soft tissues, and multiple wires can be used in a small space. They rely for their fixation not on the strength of the wire–bone interface but on the interaction between multiple wires inserted at different orientations, and therefore loosening is less of a problem than with screw-threaded half-pins or transfixing pins. Two sorts of fine wire are used: plain and stoppered or olive wires (Fig. 50.16). When the stoppered wires are used, the olive is placed tightly against the bone cortex so as to improve the stability of the frame construct. Alternatively, by pulling gently on the other end of the olive wire, the wire can be used as a 'motor' to move a piece of bone.

Types

There is no simple, satisfactory method of classifying external fixators; however, in considering their function it is simplest to think in terms of segments and foci.

A *focus* is a region of bone which is being supported and a *segment* is the region of bone which is engaged by the external fixator in order to control the focus. In the case of a simple fracture, the focus is the fracture. In order to control the focus, the external fixator must attach to two segments of bone, one either side of the fracture. A segmental fracture contains two foci, one at each fracture site, and ideally both fractures must be independently supported, which implies that the external fixator must be able to attach to three segments and support two foci (Fig. 50.16). The utility of an external fixator can be described to some extent in terms of the number of foci which it can support independently and the minimum segment length which can be stabilized satisfactorily. The number of segments which are required is always one more than the number of foci to be supported but the length of segment is an individual property of the external fixator. The greater the number of foci which can be supported independently and the shorter the segment length required for stability, the more versatile is the external fixator. However, unfortunately, this is often associated with greater complexity and expense.

External fixators can be classified as follows.

Simple half-pin uni-axial

This includes devices such as the Orthofix slide lengthener and standard Orthofix 'Dynamic Axial Fixator', the 'Monotube' manufactured by Howmedica, and the Wagner fixator. They are usually unifocal, although the Orthofix slide lengthener can support two

REFERENCES

169. Matter P, Brennwald J, Perren S M. Helv Chir Acta. 1974; suppl 12
170. Parkhill C Trans Am Surg Assoc 1897; 15: 251–256
171. Vidal J Clin Orthop Rel Res 1983; 180: 7–14

foci independently and of relatively fixed segment length; however, some variation is possible, for example by using the different screw positions in the Orthofix fixator. These fixators are generally the simplest to apply but there is a trade-off between their stability and the flexibility of fracture reduction after application (Fig. 50.15).

Half-pin adaptable

Included in this group are the AO/ASIF fixator, the Hexfix (Smith & Nephew, Richards) and the Hoffman fixator (Howmedica). They are more flexible than the simple uni-axial fixators and segment lengths are more easily changed. They are, however, usually more difficult to apply to a simple fracture than the simple half-pin frames.

Circular fixators

Potentially the most flexible of external fixators, they are also the most complex and expensive. Included in this group are the Ilizarov frame (Smith & Nephew, Richards), the Monticelli Spinelli (Howmedica), the Sequoiah (Zimmer) and the Ace-Fisher frames. These frames can use both fine wires and half-pins for stabilization. The most versatile of the frames is the Ilizarov frame, which is multifocal with a very short segment length and can employ hinges (Fig. 50.16).

Hybrid external fixators

This term has been loosely employed, leading to confusion. In the past it has sometimes been used to denote a circular frame which employs both half-pins and fine wires for fixation. This is not a useful classification, as all ring fixators have this potential. The term hybrid frame should be reserved for an external fixator which supports one segment using rings and other segments using a uni-axial configuration. The idea of this sort of fixator is that it combines the versatility of a ring fixator with the simplicity of a uni-axial fixator. However, in practice these fixators have few if any advantages and probably combine the complexity of ring fixators with the inflexibility of uni-axial frames.

Pinless external fixator

This device has been developed by the AO/ASIF group. Instead of half-pins or wires, it uses metal clamps which are tightened on to the bone. Because the medullary canal is not broached, this may be the method of choice in cases where external fixation is employed as a temporizing measure prior to definitive intramedullary nailing.

Combined internal and external fixation

This technique has in the past been used with little enthusiasm. However, the increasingly wide application of fine-wire circular fixators is leading to an increased interest in this technique for the treatment of complex intra-articular fractures such as tibial pilon and plateau fractures. Using this technique, the joint surface is treated by open anatomic fixation using screws, which may be supplemented by stoppered wires, and the metaphyseal or diaphyseal extension of the fracture is stabilized by a ring fixator or hybrid frame. Early reports of these techniques are encouraging.[172,173]

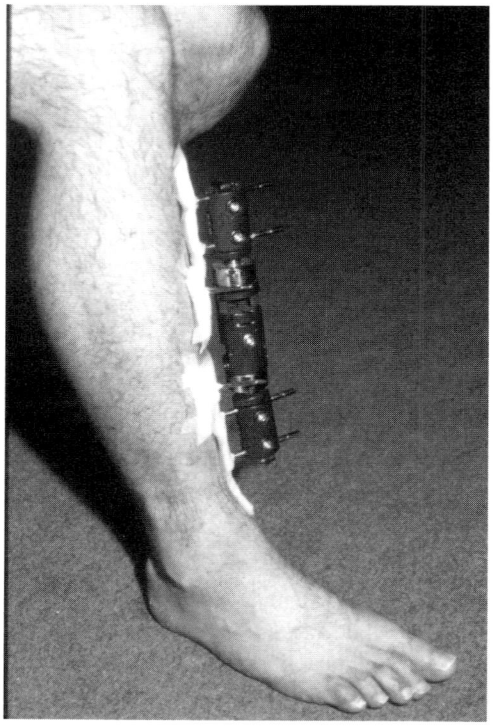

Fig. 50.15 An Orthofix Dynamic Axial Fixator used to stabilize a tibial fracture—an example of a simple half-pin external fixator. In these commonly used devices, simplicity of use is associated with some inflexibility. Courtesy of Dr J L Cunningham.

Fracture healing under conditions of external fixation

Early external fixators aimed to produce rigid immobility of the bone as this was regarded as ideal for prompt restoration of limb function. Under these conditions, the production of callus is suppressed and union occurs only slowly by direct or primary bone healing. This mode of bone union is totally intolerant of interfragmentary motion and has no ability to cross macroscopic gaps. As external fixators and indirect fracture reduction are not capable of obtaining perfect fracture reduction and may be associated with a distraction gap between fracture ends rather than interfragmentary compression, early experience with these devices was associated with high non-union rates.[174]

This problem has led to the introduction of 'dynamization' of the external fixator. This term is loosely used to describe two

REFERENCES

172. Marsh J L, Smith S T, Do T J Bone Joint Surg 1995; 77-A: 661–673
173. Weiner L S, Kelley M, Yang E, Steuer J, Watnick N, Evans M, Bergman M J Orthop Trauma 1995; 9: 244–250
174. Kenwright J, Richardson J B, Cunningham J L, White S H, Goodship A E, Adams M A, Magnussen P A, Newman J H J Bone Joint Surg Br 1991; 73-B: 654–659

different concepts (compare with its use in intramedullary nailing[175]). The first concept, which might be better called controlled collapse, occurs where the external fixator is deliberately made longitudinally unstable while torsional and angular stability is maintained. This has the effect of allowing the fracture site to telescope. An extension of this concept which may be applied in certain external fixators is to compress the fracture site by serial adjustment of the frame. If the fracture is longitudinally stable, the fracture site will be compressed and this may encourage union. When the fracture site is unstable, shortening of the limb will occur, which may encourage union by increasing the amount of bone at the fracture site and its apposition. When the shortening is judged to be unacceptable, a simultaneous leg-lengthening procedure may be undertaken using callus distraction through a separate corticotomy. This is the basis for the use of bone transport in the treatment of delayed fracture union.

The second use of the term dynamization is the modification of the external fixator so that a cyclical strain is applied to the fracture site. This may be achieved by using the patient's load-bearing weight against a deformable component of the fixator or by employing an actuator attached to the frame.

Goodship and Kenwright[176] investigated the influence of micromotion on the healing of experimental fractures in sheep. They showed that the application of a longitudinal cyclical strain which induced movement of 1 mm at an early stage following fracture was associated with increased callus formation and more rapid fracture union. Larger deformations or application of the stimulus at a later time were associated with delay in fracture healing. This concept has subsequently been tested in tibial fractures in humans[174] and has been confirmed.

Complications of external fixators

Chronic pain

This is particularly a problem with fine-wire ring fixators and its cause is multifactorial. Tented soft tissues in the region of a pin site are painful and even a perfect pin–bone interface is probably slightly uncomfortable, so that where there are a large number of pins the discomfort may be increased until pain is perceived. An infected pin site is painful and where pins or wires have been inserted close to a joint movement of the joint may be accompanied by sawing of the pin or wire through the soft tissues. The frame may be being used for bone transport or leg lengthening and this may of itself be painful and there may be residual pain from a fracture. Finally, the patient may be psychologically ill prepared for the frame and this may add to their perception of pain. Whatever the cause of chronic pain, the effect may be to prevent the patient moving the limb and bearing weight, which may cause joint contracture, swelling and osteoporosis which may itself contribute to pin loosening.

Pin loosening and breakage

Loosening is a common cause of failure of an external fixation pin and its causes are complex. Bone death at the time of half-pin insertion leads to resorption, which directly contributes to loosening. For this reason, sharp drills, slow drilling speeds and irrigation to lower drilling temperatures are advocated. Self-drilling screws tend to produce more heat and are therefore not normally recommended. An initially accurate fit between the screw thread and the bone is important both for initial stability of the interface and for the elimination of small pockets in which haematomas may collect which may later become infected. This is another reason for preferring pre-drilled screws. Loosening is more common in half-pins inserted into the metaphysis rather than the diaphysis and this probably relates to the greater initial stability of the bone–screw interface. Pin loosening may relate to local overload of the pin–bone interface and this notion is borne out by the clinical finding that pin loosening is less prevalent where a segment of bone is stabilized by multiple half-pins.

Pin loosening and pin site infection are related problems. Occasionally, general half-pin loosening follows an episode of septicaemia and in this case it seems likely that the half-pins become loose because of secondary bacterial action. More commonly, a single pin which is mechanically loose, due either to bone death or pin–bone interface overload, becomes infected from the junction with the exterior. Finally, a solidly implanted half-pin may loosen as a result of poor pin site care, local soft tissue infection gradually spreading along the pin–bone interface.

The preferred interface between a screw-threaded half-pin and bone is that of osseo-integration, in which the bone grows up to and into the interstices of the pin without an intervening fibrous tissue membrane. This sort of interface is strong and highly resistant to infection. Studies in animals have demonstrated that this sort of interface is most likely to develop if the half-pin is made of titanium, and therefore in those external fixators which are intended to be on the body for a long period the half-pins are often made of titanium.

Pin tract infections

Minor pin track difficulties are almost universal in the use of external fixators and a number of classification systems for the severity of the problem have been devised (Table 50.1).[177–179]

Limitation of joint motion

This is principally a problem of fine-wire frames where a wire is inserted close to the joint. As the joint is moved, the soft tissues adopt a different position with respect to the wire and impinge against it, causing irritation and pain. This sort of problem can be

REFERENCES

175. Richardson J B, Gardner T N, Hardy J R W, Evans M, Kuiper J H, Kenwright J J Bone Joint Surg 1995; 77-B: 412–416
176. Goodship A E, Kenwright J J Bone Joint Surg 1985; 67-B: 650–655
177. Paley D, Chaudray M, Pirone A M, Lentz P, Kautz D Orthop Clin North Am 1990; 21: 667–691
178. Checketts R G, Moran C G, Jennings A G. Acta Orthop Scand 1995; 3: 271–274
179. Sims M, Saleh M Prof Nurse. 1996; 11: 261–264

Table 50.1 Grading of pin tract infection

Grade 1	Serous discharge	The pin track is not definitely infected
Grade 2	Superficial cellulitis	The soft tissues around the pin are infected
Grade 3	Deep infection	The pin track itself is infected and the pin is loose
Grade 4	Osteomyelitis	The bone infection continues after removal of the pin

minimized by careful wire placement, seeking a neutral position in which skin movement is minimized, but to some extent it is an inevitable complication of placing wires close to joints.

Neurovascular damage

Impaling a nervovascular trunk is a particular problem with fine-wire external fixators. In order to minimize the risk, when the wires are inserted, the drill is employed in a reciprocating fashion rather than constantly rotating in one direction and once the wire has passed through the bone it is tapped through the remaining soft tissue. This technique, combined with a precise knowledge of the anatomy of the limb,[180] usually avoids damage to major trunks. It is not, however, always possible to avoid damage to relatively small and inconstant cutaneous nerve branches and damage to these structures can occasionally lead to causalgia.[181]

Indications for the use of external fixators

Multiple trauma

In patients who have suffered multiple injuries (see Chapter 7), external fixation offers a rapid method for temporarily stabilizing long bone fractures. This may be particularly useful in those cases where there is chest trauma, as intramedullary nailing in the acute phase in these patients is associated with an increased risk of adult respiratory distress syndrome from embolized medullary contents.[166–168] There is a theoretical risk of intramedullary infection when the temporary external fixation is changed for definitive intramedullary nailing but in practice this is not seen in the femur provided that the fixator pins are not allowed to become loose and infected.[182]

Open fractures

The presence of metalwork increases the incidence of infection in contaminated wounds;[183,184] thus there are advantages in the use of external fixation for the treatment of open fractures. The disadvantages include the possible difficulty of undertaking soft tissue reconstruction in the presence of an external fixator and the possibility of delayed or non-union. In the tibia, there is an increased incidence of infection if intramedullary nailing is performed after external fixation.[185,186] This problem may be reduced by the use of unreamed solid nails[187] and by the use of the pinless external fixator. It is possible that the problem can be obviated by more radical debridement of the compound wound and by the avoidance of infected pin sites.

Pelvic fractures

Fractures of the pelvis are associated with severe blood loss which may be life threatening. The use of an external fixator applied as an emergency measure in the accident and emergency department as part of initial resuscitation allows stabilization and reduction of the fracture. This limits the space for bleeding and, by preventing further movement between the fracture fragments, allows the body's natural haemostatic mechanisms to clot the extravasated blood.[188]

Peri-articular fractures

In peri-articular fractures of a long bone, particularly the tibia, where the remaining segment of bone close to the joint is too small to allow fixation by intramedullary nailing, consideration should be given to the use of a circular external fixator as definitive treatment. If an anatomic reduction can be obtained with compression, rapid union of the fracture may be anticipated which will offset the discomfort and inconvenience of the frame.

Intra-articular fractures

The accepted treatment of intra-articular fractures is by open anatomic reduction and rigid internal fixation. External fixation, particularly using fine-wire frames, is increasingly being used as a technique for the stabilization of the fractured metaphysis in cases where the soft tissues are judged to be unable to withstand plate fixation and to obviate the necessity of the large soft tissue dissections associated with plate stabilization.

Bone transport

The technique of bone transport is increasingly used for the treatment of severe fractures to replace lost bone and to encourage fracture union. It requires an external fixation frame which is capable of stabilizing two foci independently.

The fracture is stabilized using the external fixator and a minimally invasive division of the bone (a corticotomy) is made at another site, usually in the opposite metaphysis distant from the zone of fracture injury. The act of corticotomy itself activates the entire bone, encouraging union at the original fracture. After a delay, the corticotomy is gradually distracted so that new bone forms by distraction osteogenesis. Simultaneously, the non-union site or bone defect is compressed, further encouraging bone union, so that the overall effect is that a tube of bone is moved (or transported) through the soft tissues (Fig. 50.5).

REFERENCES

180. Faure C, Merloz P. Transfixation. Springer-Verlag, Berlin 1987
181. Herron M, Langkamer V G, Atkins R M The Foot 1993; 3: 38–42
182. Broos P L, Miserez M J, Rommens P M Injury 1992; 23: 525–528
183. Gristina A G, Costerton J W J Bone Joint Surg 1985; 67-A: 264–273
184. Bach A W, Hansen S T Clin Orthop Rel Res 1989; 241: 89–94
185. Maurer D J, Merkow R L, Gustilo R B J Bone Joint Surg 1989; 71-A: 835–838
186. McGraw J M, Lim E V J Bone Joint Surg 1988; 70-A: 900–911
187. Riemer B I, Butterfield S L J Orthop Traum 1993; 7: 279–285
188. Kellam J F Clin Orthop Rel Res 1989; 241: 66–82

OPEN (COMPOUND) FRACTURES

An open or compound fracture is one in which the soft tissue envelope of the limb has been disrupted allowing the bone to communicate with the exterior. This sort of fracture differs from one which is closed in that there is potentially direct bacterial access to the bone and because the amount of damage to the bone and soft tissues is usually greater. These two problems combine to produce a situation where it may be difficult to achieve satisfactory bone healing and the outcome of such a fracture depends on the extent and nature of bacterial contamination and on the amount and type of the soft tissue damage as well as the extent of the bone injury.

The soft tissue damage includes skin and muscle death and possibly nerve damage which limit the best outcome that can be achieved and restricts the methods by which the fracture can be treated. Blood vessel injury may risk the survival of the limb. Stripping of the periosteum from the bone damages the blood supply of the fractured bone ends and makes fracture union more difficult to achieve, while rendering the bone more susceptible to infection.

These difficult fractures were once seen mainly as a consequence of war, although pedestrian collision was another source. Since World War II, the gradual increase in the number and speed of motor vehicles has led to a virtual epidemic of compound fractures, often associated with other life-threatening injuries.

Classification

Classification of compound fractures is important both because it helps to direct treatment and because it allows outcomes to be compared in these difficult injuries. The important features to be graded are the degree of bone and soft tissue injury and the extent of bacterial contamination.

The first attempts at grading were based on the concepts of Robert Jones. A grade 1 injury was a puncture wound from within out, a grade 2 injury was an external injury which involved the bone and a grade 3 injury referred to any injury of greater severity.

The most widely employed classification is now that of Gustilo and Anderson,[189] although it is not ideal. There tends to be an excessive attention to the size of the wound as opposed to the amount of soft tissue damage. Thus a limb which is severely crushed beneath a lorry may have only a small skin wound but may inevitably require amputation, whereas if the limb has been cut with a sharp, clean knife, the size of the soft tissue laceration may be great but the surrounding soft tissue damage may be so slight that the limb heals rapidly with excellent return of function. There have been a number of minor modifications to the original classification;[190,191] however, unacceptably high interobserver variations have been recorded even when it was used by trained trauma surgeons.[192]

The Gustilo and Anderson classification:

- A type 1 fracture. The injury is of low energy. The wound has occurred in a relatively clean environment and is usually less than one centimetre in length. There is little or no muscle damage and no crushing component and usually the injury is from within out. Fracture comminution is not present.
- A type 2 fracture. This is a broad area of injury falling between a grade one and grade three fracture. The wound is more than one centimetre in length and the injury is often from without-in. There is usually a small amount of dead muscle but debridement is confined to one compartment, with minimal periosteal stripping and no significant bacterial contamination. Eventual wound closure without a plastic surgical flap is possible. There may be slight fracture comminution.
- A type 3 fracture. Any one of the features listed below automatically make the fracture grade 3 compound:
  - —Heavy bacterial contamination, as in a farmyard injury.
  - —A shotgun or high-velocity gunshot injury.
  - —A fracture occurring in a high-velocity vehicular accident.
  - —A vascular injury requiring repair.
  - —A significant crushing component.
  - —A displaced segmental fracture.
  - —A fracture with diaphyseal bone loss.

The type 3 injury is usually a high-energy injury with extensive damage from outside to inside. There is crushing and devitalization of muscle and usually the wound is extensive. The fracture is usually displaced and comminuted.

The type 3 fractures are further subdivided:

- Type IIIa. There is limited or absent periosteal stripping of bone and, after debridement, there is no significant problem in soft tissue coverage. There is no bone loss.
- Type IIIb. There is extensive periosteal stripping and soft tissue damage. Without the use of limb reconstruction techniques, plastic surgical flap coverage is frequently required.
- Type IIIc. There is a major vascular injury requiring repair for limb salvage.

Some further points concerning the Gustilo and Anderson classification are important:

1. The usual error is under-classification.
2. It is doubtful whether a type I femoral fracture exists.
3. A compound tibial fracture with a posterior wound is not a type I injury.
4. A type III injury may be diagnosed at the time of patient admission, but the distinction between a type IIIa and type IIIb may not be possible until debridement is complete.
5. There is a progression of severity of injury from type I to type IIIb; however, type IIIc does not follow this progression.
6. A compound injury occurring in a road traffic accident is by definition never a grade I injury, however small the wound.

REFERENCES

189. Gustilo R B, Anderson J T J Bone Joint Surg 1976; 58-A: 453–458
190. Gustilo R B Instr Course Lect 1987; 36: 359–366
191. Gustilo R B, Gruninger R P, Davis T Orthopaedics 1987; 10: 1781–1788
192. Brumback R J, Jones A L J Bone Joint Surg 1994; 76-A: 1162–1166

Skeletal traction is attractive because it is easy to set up and causes minimal damage to the tissues of the limb. Nursing and soft tissue care may, however, be difficult and the use of skeletal traction in open fractures in the West is virtually confined to the short, acute phase prior to operative debridement.

External skeletal fixation is also relatively rapid to apply and produces sufficient stability to allow optimal soft tissue recovery from the initial trauma. Furthermore it facilitates patient management and makes wound care relatively simple. Some damage to transfixed soft tissues is inevitable and devices may make subsequent soft tissue plastic flap reconstruction difficult. Finally, the pins may loosen and become infected, compromising the possibilities for later operative fracture treatment.

Open reduction and internal fixation take time, when the patient may require other emergency treatment and insufficient information may be available to select the correct treatment. The major objection to this form of treatment is the extensive soft tissue dissection which has to be made and this carries a high risk of wound breakdown and deep infection. Internal fixation of compound fractures in best reserved for the treatment of joint injuries using minimally invasive techniques.

Intramedullary nailing of open fractures has a number of advantages. It facilitates nursing care, while stabilizing the limb and allowing unimpeded access for soft tissue treatment including plastic surgical flaps. Inevitably there is damage to the intramedullary blood supply which can be minimized by the use of unreamed techniques. In order for devitalized bone to revascularize, absolute stability of the bone fragments is necessary and this may not be provided by an unreamed intramedullary nail, which may be associated with a fracture non-union.

Definitive soft tissue management

The options available are:

1. Primary wound closure with or without skin grafting.
2. Delayed primary closure with or without skin grafting.
3. Healing by secondary intention.
4. Delayed closure by local or vascularized flap.

Primary wound closure

This is rarely if ever indicated. It should only be employed in those cases where the wound is known to be uncontaminated and there is definitely no remaining dead tissue or foreign material. The patient should be healthy and the wound must be closed without tension. In practice, this occurs in type I compound fractures; however, in these cases the wounds are usually so small that suturing is unnecessary.

Delayed primary closure with or without skin grafting

This implies closure before the fifth day. This allows for a second debridement 48 hours after the first operative inspection. Wound healing is not delayed in an adult human provided definitive closure is undertaken before the fifth day. Leaving the wound open initially allows the swelling associated with the initial trauma to settle.

Healing by secondary intention

Wounds may be allowed to heal by secondary intention provided that bone, tendon, nerve and blood vessels are adequately covered by muscle or fat. For relatively small wounds which are not susceptible to delayed primary direct closure this is probably the optimum method of management, as it avoids split-skin grafting and gives satisfactory cosmetic results with acceptable cutaneous sensation. For larger wounds, the time required is prohibitive and split-skin grafting is necessary.

The use of local or free vascularized flaps

There are a small number of cases where an adequate soft tissue envelope does not exist after complete debridement. In these cases, bone, tendon, nerve and blood vessels are inadequately covered. The problem usually applies to bone and is most commonly seen following tibial fracture. If the bone is left uncovered for any length of time surface necrosis occurs and exposed devitalized bone will become colonized with bacteria, which will lead to infection and non-union. For these cases early soft tissue cover with well-vascularized muscle is imperative. The importance of this approach was first demonstrated by Godina.[199] In a large retrospective study of microsurgical coverage procedures following compound fractures, he showed that the lowest rates of flap failure and late deep infection were seen where cover was provided within 72 hours of injury. The time in hospital was also shortest in this group.

The flap brings with it a new blood supply and helps to resist local infection, and in this respect muscle flaps are superior to fasciocutaneous flaps.[200–202] A muscle flap may also act as a source of osteoprogenitor cells; however, it is unclear whether these cells are important since bone healing beneath a flap is rarely by external callus formation. The new blood supply of the transplanted soft tissue flap tends to grow into the bone, revascularizing it.[202] However, it must be remembered that cortical autograft is poorly and slowly incorporated (see above) and so the extent to which this process occurs in the diaphysis under clinical conditions remains in doubt.

Definitive fracture treatment

The method of initial fracture stabilization may be the eventual definitive technique employed for treating the fracture until union. This is, however, rarely the case. The two roles are totally different. This is obvious with a simple fracture, where the initial splint serves to immobilize the fracture in order to provide pain relief and to safeguard the limb prior to definitive fracture reduction and stabilization. With a severe compound fracture, the complexity of the initial treatment, which commonly includes

REFERENCES

199. Godina M Plast Reconstr Surg 1986; 78: 285–292
200. Arnold P G, Irons G B Orthop Clin North Am 1984; 15: 441–449
201. Chang N, Mathes S J Plast Reconstr Surg 1982; 70: 1–10
202. Richards R R, Orsini E C, Mahoney J L, Verschuren R Plast Reconstr Surg 1987; 79: 946–956

intramedullary nailing or external fixation, should not obscure the simple fact that these treatments are being used only to stabilize the fracture, safeguard the limb and to allow proper management of the soft tissues.

Definitive fracture management is usually undertaken after the soft tissue problems have been resolved and any plastic flaps are stable. This usually takes four to eight weeks and the definitive fracture fixation device is usually an intramedullary nail or an external fixator which has the ability to modify the biomechanical environment of the fracture site. There is some haste to change from provisional to definitive fixation if an intramedullary nail is to be employed as, if an external fixator has been used initially, a long delay will allow the pins to loosen, threatening infection following subsequent intramedullary nailing. If a thin, unreamed intramedullary was employed primarily the cross-screws may break, making exchange nailing difficult. The use of a definitive external fixator does not carry these problems but is more difficult for the patient.

The treatment of bone loss

Bone loss following a compound fracture may be obvious or concealed. Obvious bone loss occurs when either bone substance has been lost at the time of the original fracture or when subsequent debridement has removed devitalized and contaminated bone.

Concealed bone loss exists where an area of devitalized bone has been retained within a fracture in order to maintain the structural integrity of the bone. This area of bone will have lost many of its physiological functions, including its ability actively to take part in fracture healing, to resist infection and to regenerate itself by remodelling. With time, it will revascularize and undergo creeping substitution but in the context of a compound fracture it will be slow to unite, easily infected and it may undergo subsequent fatigue fracture, even if the original fracture has united satisfactorily.

An area of incomplete bone loss may re-form without further intervention provided that the fracture is stable.[44] Larger areas may have to be treated by autologous cancellous bone grafting. Vascularized bone grafts from the iliac crest or fibula may be employed for longer segments of bone loss but the donor site morbidity is high. The use of distraction osteogenesis offers a very satisfactory alternative method of replacing lost bone with new apparently normal bone, and three methods have been described by Ilizarov:[61]

1. *Bone transport.* The limb length is maintained and the bone defect is filled in by moving a piece of bone through the limb after division of the bone by a minimally invasive 'corticotomy' at a site distant from the zone of injury.
2. *Shortening and relengthening.* The limb is shortened to eliminate the defect created by the bone loss and then relengthened through a corticotomy as above.
3. *Bone transfer.* In the case of the tibia, an area of bone loss may be eliminated by pulling the fibula across into the bed of the tibia, creating a fibula pro tibia.

Each of these techniques has advantages and drawbacks. Patient rehabilitation is simpler when using bone transport, since the limb is kept at length; however, union may be delayed because the bones do not come into contact at the original fracture site until after the transport is complete. A plastic flap procedure may also be required to fill the soft tissue defect. Shortening and relengthening is a more difficult surgical procedure and the patient may find rehabilitation difficult because of the discrepancy in limb length at the start of treatment. There is also a theoretical risk of damaging neurovascular structures during the shortening, although this has not been observed.[203] The advantages of shortening and relengthening are that the fractured bone ends are brought together sooner than with bone transport and therefore they usually unite more rapidly. The shortening also reduces the soft tissue defect and may even abolish it altogether. Thus there may be no need for a plastic surgical flap and, if it is required, it is smaller than would otherwise be the case.

Bone transfer procedures are rarely indicated but have a place where there is extensive loss of the tibia. A thin and deformed limb results and function of the peroneal muscles is often compromised. This may be acceptable if there has been prior damage to the common peroneal nerve. When undertaking a bone transfer using an Ilizarov frame, the fibula can be gently moved into the bed of the tibia so that it retains its blood supply. Bone union between the tibia and transferred fibula and subsequent fibula hypertrophy are then rapid.

Early amputation for severe fracture

Early or immediate amputation may be indicated as a life-saving measure, or if the limb is clearly not viable. A severe crushing injury with little remaining viable tissue or a warm ischaemic time exceeding 8 hours are clear indications for amputation but the concept that it is possible to predict which injuries are so severe that the patient's function will be improved by early amputation is more controversial. The social and economic impact of severe fractures of the lower limb is high[204] and in selected patients early amputation affords rapid rehabilitation,[205] although the long-term cost to society may be greater than successful limb salvage.[206] Lange et al[207] suggest that the absolute indications for immediate amputation are a fracture which involves an arterial injury requiring repair for limb viability (type IIIc), combined with complete transection of the posterior tibial nerve and a non-viable limb. They also propose relative indications based on the patient's ability to cope physiologically and psychologically with attempted limb salvage. Several other attempts have been made to predict the need for amputation, of which the best documented is the *Mangled Extremity Severity Score* (MESS, Table 50.2).[208]

REFERENCES

203. Allen P E, Bose D, Atkins R M J Bone Joint Surg 1997; 79-B (suppl 1): 100
204. Bondurant F, Colter H B, Buckle R, Miller-Crotchett P, Browner B D J Trauma 1988; 28: 1270–1273
205. Geordiadis G M, Berhrens F F, Joyce M J, Earle A S, Simmons A I J Bone Joint Surg 1993; 75-A: 1431–1441
206. Tornetta P III, Olsen S A Instr Course Lect 1997; 46: 511–518
207. Lange R H, Bach A W, Hansen S T, Johansen K H J Trauma. 1985; 25: 203–208

Table 50.2 The Mangled Extremity Severity Score

Category	*Points*
A. Skeletal/soft tissue injury	
Low energy (stab, simple fracture)	1
Medium energy (open/multiple fracture)	2
High energy (close-range shotgun, high-velocity gunshot, crush)	3
Very high energy (gross contamination, avulsion)	4
B. Limb ischaemia	
Pulse reduced, normal perfusion	1*
Pulseless, paraesthesiae, reduced capillary refilling	2*
Cool, paralysed, insensate	3*
*Double score for ischaemia>6 hours	
C. Shock	
Systolic BP always > 90 mmHg	0
Transient hypotension	1
Persistent hypotension	2
D. Age (years)	
<30	0
30–50	1
>50	2
Mangled Extremity Severity Score equals the total points from A+B+C+D	

In a series of 26 patients studied retrospectively, a MESS score of 7 or more was a good predictor of the need for subsequent amputation; however, more variable results are reported by others[209,210] and a number of modifications have been suggested. Numeric scoring systems fail to take full account of the treatments available at the time of injury and it seems likely that the introduction of Ilizarov's methods will allow salvage of limbs which were hitherto unreconstructable. The decision to amputate remains highly subjective. A patient aged 49 who has not been hypotensive is scarcely different from one aged 51 who has had a transient episode of hypotension. A decision as to whether to amputate early must take into account injury severity, the degree of ischaemia, the fitness and age of the patient and the extent to which the patient's injuries have affected the cardiovascular system.

Complications

Shock (see Ch. 7)

Shock is defined as a clinical state in which there is poor tissue perfusion and resultant tissue hypoxia. There are a number of reaons for which a fracture may cause a state of clinical shock. Firstly, the fracture itself is associated with significant blood loss; secondly, the traumatized patient may have suffered other injuries; and thirdly the the pain associated with the fracture and the circumstances of the injury may lead to an increase in circulating catecholamines which contribute to peripheral circulatory failure. In outline the treatment of shock is correct restoration of fluid balance, appropriate analgesia and improving oxygenation.

Fat embolism syndrome/adult respiratory distress syndrome (see Ch. 7)

Fat droplets in the lungs of a patient dying after a fracture were first described by Zenker.[211] The clinical condition is common following any instrumentation of the medullary canal, after a high-energy long bone lower limb fracture in a patient in their second or third decade and following multiple trauma. The association with adult respiratory distress syndrome is complex. Put simply, the embolization of multiple fat droplets into the lungs will of itself compromise pulmonary exchange and the ensuing local and systemic reactions to the droplets will further impair respiratory function, and the consequent hypoxia may be fatal. Owing to the clinical nature of the diagnosis, it is difficult to be certain of the incidence but it probably occurs following 1–2% of long bone fractures and up to 10% of unstable pelvic fractures.[212]

The clinical features are those of adult respiratory distress syndrome combined with features due to sytemic embolization of fat droplets. On the second or third day after the precipitating insult a fleeting petechial rash develops, characteristically across the chest, the axillae and the root of the neck. Conjunctival lesions are also present and retinal micro-infarcts may occur. Respiratory involvement causes cyanosis and dyspnoea, while central hypoxaemia results in confusion and coma. Fat droplets may appear in the urine, while renal tubular involvement may cause oliguria.

Treatment is directed at restoring fluid balance and respiratory support. Suggested therapies have included heparinization, systemic corticosteroids and intravenous alcohol administration; however, adequate controlled studies of these treatments are lacking. Early fracture stabilization reduces the incidence of fat embolism syndrome, probably by decompressing and draining the fracture haematoma, by minimizing subsequent fragment movement and by the advantageous effects of fracture stabilization on subsequent ventilatory support.[213–216] However, early surgery is not without risk to the lungs,[168,217] although unreamed nailing may reduce this problem and it may cause long-term bone infection.[214] The advantages of early stabilization therefore require careful weighing for each individual case.

Thromboembolism

In 1846, Virchow provided a conceptual framework for the understanding of venous thrombosis by suggesting that thrombogenesis could be considered as being due to changes in the vessel wall, in the composition of blood and in blood flow, leading to venous stasis.[218] Since a fracture will probably cause vessel damage, leads

REFERENCES

208. Helfet D K, Howey T, Sanders R, Johansen K Clin Orthop Rel Res 1990; 256: 80–86
209. Bonanni F, Rhodes M, Lucke J F J Trauma 1993; 34: 99–104
210. Slauterbeck J R, Briton C, Noneim M S, Clevenger FW J Orthop Trauma 1994; 8: 282–285
211. Zenker F A Beitrage zur Anatomie und Physiologie der Lunge Braunsdorf, Dresden 1861
212. Gossling H R, Pellegrini V D. Clin Orthop 1982; 165: 68–82
213. Riska E, Von Bonsdorff H, Hakkinen S, Jaroma H, Kiviluoto O, Paavilainen T Injury 1976; 8: 110–116
214. Riska E, Von Bonsdorff H, Hakkinen S, Jaroma H, Kiviluoto O, Paavilainen T J Trauma 1977; 17: 111–121
215. Riska E, Myllynen J Trauma 1982; 22: 891–894
216. Johnson K, Cadambi A, Seibert B J Trauma 1985; 25: 375–384
217. Talucci R, Manning J, Lampard S, Bach A, Carrico A Am J Surg 1983; 146: 107–111.
218. Virchow R Beitr Exp Pathol Physiol 1846; 2: 1–12

to a hypercoagulable state and the consequent immobility will promote venous stasis, it is hardly surprising that fractures are often complicated by venous thromboembolism. A number of problems arise in attempting to assess the impact of thrombolic disease within the context of fractures. Firstly, in contrast to total joint replacement, fractures do not represent a homogeneous disease group and it is inherently unlikely that the risk of thromboembolism will be similar between a Colles fracture and a pelvic fracture. Secondly, the symptoms and sequelae of thromboembolism are mimicked by other post-fracture conditions. Thirdly, therapeutic regimes which are efficacious in other surgical contexts may be ineffective or associated with unacceptable side-effects following fracture.

The incidence of venous thrombosis following fracture is approximately 20%,[219–221] while following fractured neck of femur in the elderly it ranges form 15% to 48%, depending on the method of assessment.[222–227]

Assessment for the presence of thrombosis is by standard clinical examination supplemented by investigation and treatment is along standard lines, usually employing anticoagulant therapy depending on the clinical status of the patient.

Prevention of venous thrombosis is controversial and poorly researched. Early mobilization should reduce venous stasis and graduated compression stockings are safe and may be effective; however, in the case of lower limb trauma, where the risk is highest, they may be impractible. Intermittent calf or foot compression has been shown to be effective in lowering the risk of calf thrombosis in total joint replacement and has the additional advantages of rapid reduction in limb swelling and possible lowering of compartmental pressure.

The use of anticoagulant therapy is more controversial and potentially dangerous. Prophylactic anticoagulation with warfarin is effective in reducing the incidence of thrombolic disease following total joint replacement;[228] however, this approach is contraindicated in the fracture situation because of the risk of catastrophic haemorrhage, particularly where there has been concomitant intracranial trauma and the possibility of precipitating compartmental syndromes. It is unclear whether low-dose heparin regimes, including low molecular weight heparin, are without risk or are effective in lowering the risk of thromboembolism.[229]

Soft tissue infection

The propensity for relatively poorly vascularized tissues to become secondarily infected has been discussed above. There are, however, two life-threatening infections which occur in the early period following trauma due to the presence of ischaemic tissue, particularly muscle. These are tetanus and gas gangrene.

Tetanus (lockjaw) was known to Hippocrates and is the result of infection of dead tissue with the toxin-forming obligatory anaerobic bacterium *Clostridium tetani*. *C. tetani* spores are widespread in faeces and soil and are reistant to moderate heating. The organism produces two toxins: tetanolysin, a haemolysin; and tetanospasmin, which is a powerful neurotoxin producing presynaptic blockade and severe spasm. It is the latter which accounts for the clinical manifestations of the disease.

The development of tetanus toxoid as a prophylaxis means that the disease is preventable, and the tetanus immunity of any trauma patient should be checked and a booster administered if appropriate. In an unimmunized patient, antitetanus immunoglobulin may be employed. Meticulous surgical debridement will remove all dead tissue in which tetanus bacteria may flourish. Treatment of established cases includes support for circulation and respiration, high-dose parenteral benzylpenicillin and radical wound debridement.

Gas gangrene is due to infection with *Clostridium perfringens* and other anaerobic gas-forming organisms. *C. perfringens* is a ubiquitous, saprophytic commensal in the alimentary tract. Like tetanus, the development of gas gangrene depends on the presence of devitalized tissue but, in contrast, *C. perfringens* releases toxins which allow it to spread through the tissues and there is no effective immunization. The mainstay of prophylaxis and treatment is adequate wound debridement, augmented by parenteral benzylpenicillin and hyperbaric oxygen therapy.

Bone infection

Bone infection after a fracture is an entirely different disease from acute haematogenous osteomyelitis.[230] The latter arises in the metaphyseal medulla and therefore principally involves the central part of the bone. The term osteo*myelitis* is therefore apposite. In contrast, bone infection after fracture or trauma without fracture is a bacterial invasion of relatively avascular cortical bone which usually comes from the outside. Since the medullary canal is not primarily implicated and may not be involved at all, the term osteomyelitis is inappropriate and is best avoided. The natural history of this sort of bone infection depends on whether the bone is fractured and on presence and type of any fracture fixation devices.

Post-traumatic bone infection without fracture

The most common example of this is an infected sub-periosteal haematoma. The adjacent cortex is rendered relatively avascular by the periosteal stripping, and bacterial infection becomes established on the outer part of the cortex, gradually spreading as more bone is devitalized. The medullary canal is only involved at a late

REFERENCES

219. Solonen K A Acta Orthop Scand 1963; 33: 329–341
220. Neu L T Jr, Waterfield J R, Ash C J Ann Intern Med 1965; 62: 463–467
221. Sevitt S, Gallagher N G Br J Surg 1961; 48: 475–489
222. Tubiana R, Duparc J J Bone Joint Surg. 1961; 43-B: 7–15
223. Fagan D G Lancet 1964; i: 846–848
224. Salzman E W, Harris W H, DeSanctis R W N Engl J Med 1966; 275: 122–130
225. Freeark R J, Bostwick J, Fardin R Arch Surg 1967; 95: 567–575
226. Hamilton H W, Crawford J S, Gardiner J H, Wiley A M J Bone Joint Surg 1970; 52-B: 268–289
227. Golodner H, Morse L J, Angrist A Surgery 1945; 18: 418–423
228. Evarts C M, Feil E I Bone Joint Surg 1971; 53-A: 1271–1280
229. Knudson M M, Lewis F R, Clinton A, Atkinson K, Megerman J J Trauma 1994; 37: 480–487
230. Burri C. Post-traumatic Osteomyelitis. Hans Huber, Bern 1974

stage or in immunocompromised patients; local excision of devitalized bone and soft tissue with short-term antibiotic treatment is usually curative.

Bone infection without osteosynthesis

Injuries from bullets, shrapnel fragments or foreign bodies may import bacteria and cause multifocal infection in the region of trauma. A compound fracture that penetrates the skin damages the soft tissues and there will be extensive devitalization of the bone fragments if it is a high-energy injury. Bacteria have direct access to the cortical bone fragments and to the medullary cavity in the region of the fracture. The dead soft tissues and haematoma provide an ideal incubation medium for the bacteria and colonization of bone ensues. Individual pieces of dead bone may be expelled as sequestra, and if the fracture unites devitalized bone from the major fragments may become revascularized and remodelled. Occasionally this process will lead to resolution of the infection but, more often, chronic bone infection results. Usually, the bone does not unite because of infection, the severity of the fracture and loss of fracture haematoma, and infected non-union occurs.

Bone infection in the presence of osteosynthesis

The outcome of bone infection in the presence of a fixation device depends on fracture stability. Stability encourages revascularization of poorly vascularized bone fragments[52] and it is possible for a fracture to unite even in the presence of infection, although union is likely to be slow. While the fracture is healing, the infection may be suppressed by appropriate antibiotics. Once union has occurred, revascularization of the bone will continue and the infection may subside completely once the fixation device has been removed. While union is awaited, infected and dead soft tissue may be removed and replaced by plastic surgical flap coverage if necessary, which increases the local blood supply and helps to counter the infection. In contrast, if the fracture is unstable, either because the initial treatment did not produce a stable osteosynthesis or because the metalwork has become loose due to the infection, union of the fracture is unlikely to occur.

The problem with the traditional treatment of an infected osteosynthesis outlined above is that the treatment cannot be guaranteed to succeed. If it fails, salvage of the further surgery and the use of antibiotics have made the limb more difficult. Ilizarov described a novel method of treatment of bone infection following fracture. All metalwork is removed and all obviously devitalized bone and soft tissue is excised. The fracture is stabilized by an external fixator, which is capable of controlling two foci independently, and the fracture is compressed to produce union. Soft tissue defects are treated either by plastic surgery or, more commonly; they are allowed to heal by secondary intention. Bone defects are treated by bone transport and distraction osteogenesis, which is also employed to increase the limb blood supply and bone activation in order to encourage fracture union and eradication of infection (Figs 50.5, 50.16).

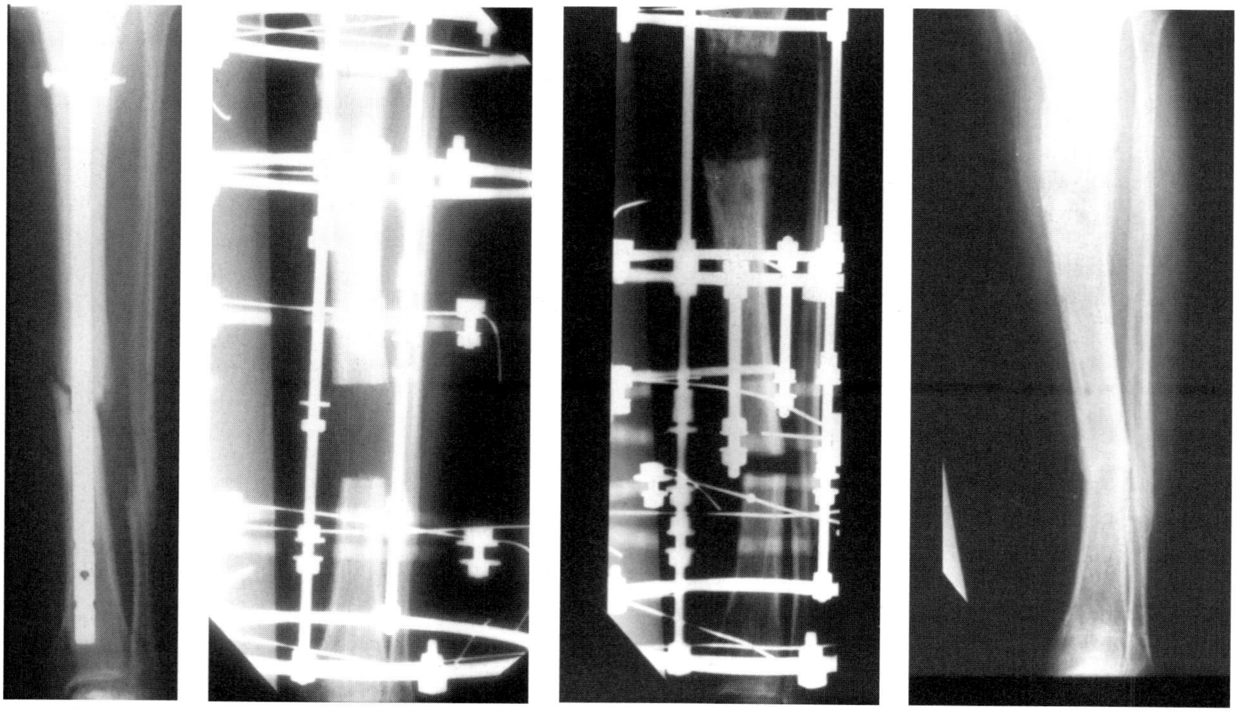

a b c d

Fig. 50.16 The use of the principles of Ilizarov in the treatment of an infected fracture non-union. **(a)** An infected non-union of a tibial fracture following intramedullary nailing. There was a discharging sinus overlying the fracture site and at the time of operative exploration the bone adjacent to the fracture was dead. **(b)** All dead bone has been removed and the fracture has been stabilized with a three-segment, two-focus Ilizarov frame. A proxomal corticotomy has been performed to allow a bone transport. **(c)** The bone transport in progress. The new bone formation in distraction can be seen. The transport segment is not yet 'docked' with the distal bone segment. **(d)** The final result.

Compartment syndrome

Compartment syndrome is a devastating early complication after fracture, which must be recognized and treated early. Richard von Volkman[231] first described the condition. The limbs are organized into compartments, which are bounded by bone and deep fascia and contain muscles with their nerve and blood supply together with nerves and blood vessels to more distant parts of the limb. The proximal and distal ends of the compartment are open. Muscle within the facial compartment is perfused by blood, which leaves the terminal resistance arterioles at a pressure of 30–38 mmHg and drains into venules at a pressure of 12–18 mmHg. The resting pressure within the compartment tissues is approximately 3–4 mmHg. A rise in compartmental tissue pressure may be triggered by a number of factors, including soft tissue injury. If a sustained rise in tissue pressure above the arterial perfusion pressure occurs, muscle and nerves will be deprived of blood supply[232] and ischaemic muscle releases factors which increase capillary permeability, worsening the situation.[233] Skeletal muscle is capable of regeneration if only part of the length of a muscle fibre is destroyed, so that prompt decompression is essential.[234,235] Thin cutaneous nerve fibres may be more susceptible to ischaemia than the motor fibres, which causes distal paraesthesiae before loss of motor function.

Diagnosis

The clinical presentation of compartment syndrome is frequently indistinct and the clinician must consider the diagnosis in all patients. The main early feature is excessive pain, often unresponsive to opiates, which is made worse by stretching the ischaemic muscles. This is usually associated with tightness of the limb although swelling may be slight or absent because the rigid compartment prevents distension. The superficial veins of the limb beyond the affected compartment may be engorged but the peripheral pulse remains intact until very late, since the increase in pressure required to produce a compartment syndrome (30 mmHg) is well below the arterial perfusion pressure. Sensory loss may be detected but motor weakness is a late sign.

The diagnosis is confirmed if necessary by comparing directly measured compartment pressure to the diastolic blood pressure.[236,237]

Management of suspected compartment syndrome

If the limb is encased in a plaster or bandage, this must be split to the skin and spread widely.[238] Compartment pressures should be measured if the diagnosis is in doubt. In the lower limb, intermittent pneumatic compression foot pumps may help to lower the compartmental pressure by compressing the plantar plexus of the foot and encouraging venous drainage.[239] If these measures do not cause rapid resolution of the raised pressure and symptoms, emergency decompression of the compartments by long vertical incisions through the skin and deep fascia is indicated.[240]

Reflex sympathetic dystrophy

Algodystrophy or reflex sympathetic dystrophy (RSD) or Sudeck's atrophy is a curious condition, which is very common after fracture. Prospective studies have demonstrated that it occurs following one-third of tibial or osteoporotic distal radial fractures and it seems likely that the incidence is similar following other fractures, although data is lacking.[99,101] The condition is usually mild, subclinical and self-limiting, which explains its low reported incidence in a number of large retrospective series. However, even in those cases where the condition resolves without apparent clinical sequelae, careful investigation shows that the condition leads to permanent morbidity in a significant proportion of those affected.[241]

The condition consists of pain, vasomotor instability, swelling and loss of joint mobility. It is accompanied by increased uptake on isotope bone scanning and radiological evidence of osteoporosis.[242] The pain is excessive and different from that of the precipitating trauma. It usually develops after a period in which there is little discomfort.[243] Abnormalities of pain perception, such as allodynia and hyperpathia, are common. Swelling and vasomotor instability are early features which fade as the disease progresses. In the early stages of the condition, loss of joint mobility is the result of a combination of pain provoked by movement and local oedema. As the condition progresses, however, the swelling gives way to atrophy of all the parts of the affected limb. The skin becomes thin and the subcutaneous fat disappears. Tendons and ligaments become adherent and severe joint contractures appear, causing continuing loss of joint mobility.

The cause of the condition is not known. It has long been assumed that the sympathetic nervous system is involved because of the vasomotor instability and excessive sweating. This notion has been supported by the apparent response of the condition to sympathetic manipulation. However, in a condition where the clinical features are variable and there is a tendency towards natural resolution, it is difficult to be certain that a treatment is efficacious, and the efficacy of sympathetic manipulation has been challenged recently.[244]

Bone involvement in the condition is universal and abnormal blood flow and activation lead to increased uptake on bone scanning,

REFERENCES

231. Volkman R Zentrlbl Chir 1881; 8: 801–804
232. Ashton H Clin Orthop 1975; 113: 15–26
233. Harman J W, Gwinn R P Am J Pathol 1948; 24: 625–638
234. Harman J W, Gwinn R P Am J Pathol 1949; 25: 741–755
235. Sanderson R A, Foley R K, McIvor G, Kirkaldy-Willis W H Clin Orthop 1975; 113: 27–35
236. Matsen F A III, Winquist R A, Krugmire R B Jr J Bone Joint Surg Am 1980; 62-A: 286–291
237. Heckman M M, Whitesides T E, Grewe S R, Rooks M D J Bone Joint Surg Am 1994; 76-A: 1285–1292
238. Garfin S, Murabak S, Evans K, Hargens A, Akeson W J Bone Joint Surg 1981; 63A: 449–453
239. Myerson M, Henderson M R Foot Ankle 1993; 14: 198–203
240. Jepson P N Ann Surg 1926; 84: 785–795
241. Warwick D, Field J, Prothero D, Gibson A, Bannister G C Clin Orthop 1993; 295: 270–274
242. Atkins R M In: Ficat J J (ed) Ballière's Clinical Orthopaedics: Reflex Sympathetic Dystrophy, vol 1, no 2. Ballière Tindall, London 1996 pp 223–240
243. Mitchell Morehouse G R, Keen W W. Gunshot wounds and other injuries of nerves. Lippincott, Philadelphia 1864
244. Jaddad A R, Carroll D, Glynn C J McQuay H J J Pain Symptom Manage 1995; 10: 13–20

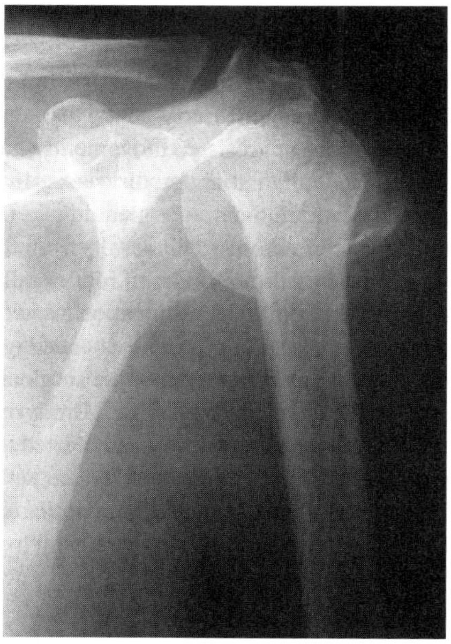

a

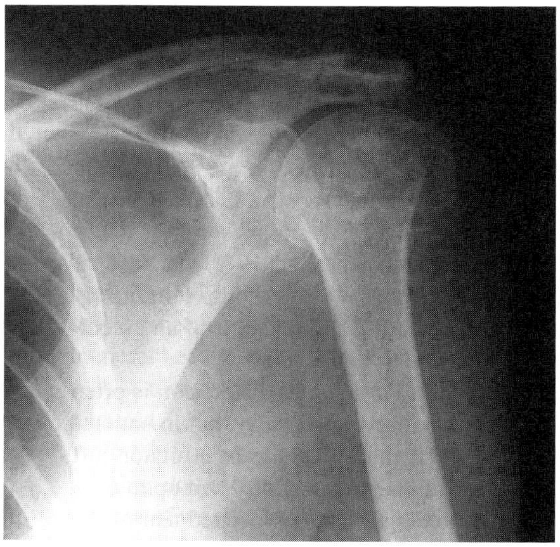

b

Fig. 51.4 (**a**) Three-part fracture of the proximal humerus. (**b**) Postoperative radiograph after open reduction and internal fixation with interosseous PDS sutures.

repair the rotator cuff. It should not compromise the blood supply to the humeral head and allow early mobilization of the shoulder. Several methods of fixation have been advocated, including tension band wires,[40] heavy polydioxone sulphate sutures (Fig. 51.4),[41] plates[42] and percutaneous reduction and fixation with K-wires and cannulated screws.[43] The results of internal fixation vary enormously, with success more likely in young patients with good bone stock. In elderly patients it is much more difficult to achieve secure fixation, and the functional results of semi-rigid internal fixation with a tension band wire are no better than with conservative treatment.[44] Neer recommends treating patients over 70 with displaced three- and four-part fractures by a hemiarthroplasty and reattachment of the tuberosities, with 96% of patients getting an excellent or satisfactory result.[45]

A fracture of the greater tuberosity is seen in about 15% of acute anterior shoulder dislocations. The dislocation is reduced in the usual way, and the tuberosity will often also reduce, but if it does not open reduction and internal fixation are required. Surgical neck fractures associated with shoulder dislocation can occur, and attempts at closed reduction often fail, necessitating open reduction.

The most frequent complication after fractures of the proximal humerus is shoulder stiffness, for which the best management is prevention. Whatever the fracture and method of treatment, pendulum exercises can be started almost immediately, with passive movements introduced as the initial pain and swelling subside. Active and resisted movements are delayed until fracture union. Close supervision by a physiotherapist and a well-motivated patient are likely to achieve the best functional outcome, and hydrotherapy is beneficial in encouraging earlier active mobilization.

Other complications include malunion, associated neurovascular injuries and avascular necrosis of the head with three- and four-part fractures.

FRACTURES OF THE HUMERAL SHAFT

Humeral shaft fractures occur in all age groups, with the mechanism of injury being direct, such as from a fall landing on the side of the arm or a motor vehicle accident, or indirect from a fall landing on the elbow or outstretched hand or a twisting injury to the arm. Direct injuries tend to cause transverse fractures and indirect oblique or spiral ones. The displacement depends on the force which produced the fracture and its site relative to the various muscle insertions on the bone.

Presentation is with pain and swelling at the site of the fracture, with a flail arm which may be deformed. A full neurovascular examination must be performed, as there is a high incidence of associated radial nerve injury. Radiographic examination should be by anteroposterior and lateral views which include the shoulder and elbow joints, to exclude any accompanying injuries.

Most closed fractures of the humeral shaft can be treated non-operatively with good results. Union can be achieved after at least six weeks, and no cosmetic or functional impairment develops as long as there is no significant rotational deformity. A hanging cast has the disadvantage that the patient needs to remain in an erect or semi-erect position. The weight of the cast can distract the fracture and cause non-union, and immobilization can cause unacceptable

REFERENCES

40. Hawkins R J, Bell R H, Gurr K J Bone Joint Surg 1986; 68A: 1410
41. Copeland S A. Curr Orthop 1995; 9: 241
42. Esser R D Clin Orthop 1994; 299: 244
43. Resch H, Povacz P, Frölich R, Wambacher M J Bone Joint Surg 1997; 79B: 295
44. Zyto K, Ahrengart L, Sperber A, Törnkvist H J Bone Joint Surg 1997; 79B: 412
45. Neer C S J Bone Joint Surg 1970; 52A: 1090

stiffness in the elbow and wrist. Despite these potential problems hanging casts have proved very successful in the treatment of humeral shaft fractures.[46,47] An alternative is the plaster of Paris U-slab,[48] which passes from the axilla down the medial side of the arm, around the elbow, and up the lateral side to the acromion. The wrist is supported with a collar and cuff sling, and the patient can exercise the elbow, wrist and hand and perform pendulum exercises of the shoulder as soon as pain allows.

By two to three weeks the acute pain and swelling have subsided. Whether the initial treatment was a hanging cast or a U-slab, a functional brace can then be fitted, with good results.[49] It compresses the soft tissues, maintaining alignment of the fracture while allowing movement of the joints, and it is more comfortable for the patient.

Humeral shaft fractures do so well with non-operative treatment that only a few require operation. The indications for surgery are compound fractures, segmental fractures, ones which extend into the elbow joint, and those associated with forearm fractures giving a floating elbow. If the patient has multiple injuries stabilization of the humeral fracture is often indicated. When there is an associated vascular injury or if a radial nerve palsy develops after manipulation of the fracture, it should be treated surgically. Occasionally it is not possible to achieve a satisfactory reduction by closed manipulation, particularly if there is soft tissue interposition, and an open reduction is required.

The surgical options available are intramedullary nails which can be inserted from proximally or distally, and need to be locked both ends to control rotation. When the fracture has to be opened in order to allow reduction, or explored for neurovascular compromise, it can be plated. A broad 4.5 mm dynamic compression plate with at least three screws above and below the fracture should be used to provide adequate stability. If the fracture is comminuted fixation should be augmented with corticocancellous bone graft.[50] External fixators can be used, and are most useful if there is an extensive soft tissue injury (see Ch. 50).

The commonest complication of humeral shaft fractures is radial nerve palsy, which can occur in up to 18% of cases. It is at greatest risk in fractures of the middle third where it is closely applied to the bone in the spiral groove. The nerve almost always remains in continuity and over 90% recover spontaneously over three or four months. The nerve should be explored immediately in open injuries, or if the palsy develops after closed manipulation of the fracture. Electromyography and nerve conduction studies can be obtained to demonstrate the severity of the injury and to monitor recovery. The wrist and fingers are supported with a splint to prevent flexion contractures while the nerve is recovering. If there is no recovery by the time the fracture has united the nerve can be explored, and if divided a delayed repair gives as good a result as if there had been a primary repair.

Other complications include frozen shoulder, myositis ossificans around the elbow, delayed union and non-union, with an increased risk of non-union when the fracture is transverse, distracted, or if there is soft tissue interposition. The treatment depends on the type of non-union, and can be internal fixation with a compression plate and bone grafting, or stabilization with a locked intramedullary nail (see Ch. 50).

FRACTURES OF THE DISTAL HUMERUS

Fractures of the distal end of the humerus are mostly seen in children and adults over the age of 50. The mechanism of injury can be indirect with a fall on to the outstretched hand or from a direct blow to the elbow, with the direction of the force and position of the elbow at the time of injury determining the nature of the fracture and direction of displacement. The diagnosis of fractures of the distal humerus depends on having good-quality radiographs, and particularly for children comparison with a radiograph of the normal elbow can be helpful. For the anteroposterior view the elbow should be extended as much as pain permits, with the forearm supinated. For the lateral view the elbow is flexed to 90 degrees. Soft tissue changes on X-ray such as forward displacement of the anterior radioluscent fat pad or a visible posterior fat pad are highly suggestive of intra-articular fractures.

Supracondylar fractures in children

In children 60% of elbow fractures are supracondylar, with at least 90% of these being extension injuries resulting from a fall on to the outstretched hand. There is hyperextension of the elbow, with the olecranon impacting against the posterior aspect of the humerus to produce the fracture.

Paediatric supracondylar fractures have been classified into undisplaced, displaced with an intact posterior periosteum and completely displaced with no contact between the fragments.[51] Presentation is with a painful swollen elbow. With displaced fractures the shaft can cause an anterior prominence which tents the overlying skin, and the olecranon is displaced posteriorly and superiorly giving an S-shaped deformity. Clinically a supracondylar fracture can be distinguished from a posterior elbow dislocation because the relationship between the olecranon, medial and lateral epicondyles is preserved.

Associated neurovascular injuries do occur. Nerve injuries occur in about 7%, with the radial, median and ulnar nerves all being at risk, and vascular injury or compromise occurs in up to 5%. The brachial artery may be kinked over the anterior prominence of the proximal fragment or lacerated by the fracture fragments. It may also be damaged as part of an open injury or obstructed by an intimal tear or spasm. It is important to recognize vascular and neurological injuries early, and even if not initially present the child should be monitored for later presentation. Urgent treatment is required if there is evidence of distal ischaemia. The fracture should be reduced as a surgical emergency, and if this does not restore the circulation the brachial artery must be explored (see Ch. 5).

REFERENCES

46. Chritensen S Acta Chir Scand 1967; 133: 455
47. Stewart M J, Hundley J M J Bone Joint Surg 1955; 37A: 681
48. Charnley J The Closed Treatment of Fractures. Williams & Wilkins, Baltimore 1961
49. Sarmiento A, Kinman P B, Calvin E G, Schmitt R H, Phillips J G J Bone Joint Surg 1977; 59A: 596
50. Müller M E, Allgöwer M, Schneider R, Willenegger H (eds) Manual of Internal Fixation, 3rd edn. Springer-Verlag, Berlin 1991
51. Gartland J J Surg Gynecol Obstet 1959; 109: 145

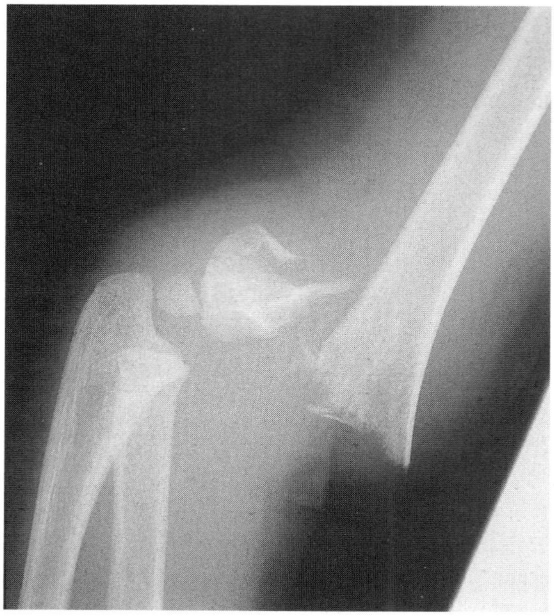

a

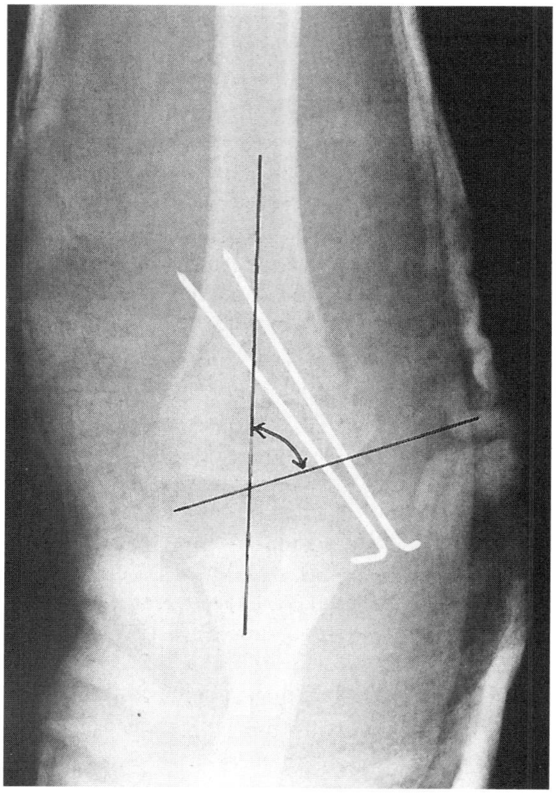

b

Fig. 51.5 (**a**) A completely displaced supracondylar fracture. (**b**) Postoperative radiograph after closed reduction and percutaneous K-wire fixation. Baumann's angle is 72 degrees, indicating a satisfactory reduction in the coronal plane.

Undisplaced fractures are immobilized for two or three weeks in a back slab or collar and cuff sling with the elbow flexed above a right angle, before allowing a protected range of exercises. Displaced fractures are reduced under general anaesthesia and if the posterior periosteum is intact simple flexion is usually effective. Completely displaced fractures require initial traction with the elbow extended and forearm supinated, correction of rotation and angulation in the coronal plane by manipulation, and the elbow is then flexed with forward pressure applied to the olecranon. Holding the elbow flexed tightens the periosteum, which then holds the reduction. With displaced fractures, if the periosteum is completely torn it may be difficult to hold the fracture even with the elbow fully flexed, and percutaneous pin fixation is required (Fig. 51.5). If after reduction the forearm and humerus lie parallel when the elbow is hyperflexed, the alignment is likely to be correct in the coronal plane. Anteroposterior and lateral radiographs are taken, and Baumann's angle (Fig. 51.5), which is the angle between the long axis of the humerus, and a line drawn along the growth plate between the metaphysis and epiphysis of the lateral condyle is measured on the anteroposterior films. The normal angle is 75° and it should match the contralateral elbow. This gives the best prediction of achieving the correct carrying angle.[52] The lateral view shows whether displacement and angulation have been corrected in the sagittal plane.

If the reduction is not satisfactory, multiple attempts at closed reduction should not be attempted because the elbow becomes increasingly swollen. Once reduced the elbow is flexed to at least 110 degrees to hold the fracture reduced and immobilized with a collar, a cuff sling and adhesive strapping around the arm and forearm, or a back slab. The elbow must be extended until the circulation recovers if this degree of flexion produces distal ischaemia or obliterates the pulse. This may well result in loss of the reduction, in which case the fracture is reduced again and then held with two percutaneous K-wires which can be inserted one from each side. If the swelling makes it difficult to identify the bony landmarks, both wires can be inserted laterally to avoid injuring the ulnar nerve. The wires should be inserted by hand to reduce the risk of damaging the nerves. The elbow can then be extended to restore the circulation without losing the reduction. This method of treatment has a low complication rate and a good functional result can be expected.[53]

Closed reduction may fail, particularly if the bone end is buttonholed through the brachialis. If the elbow is not too swollen an open reduction is performed, and the fracture stabilized with K-wires. Open reduction and internal fixation are used to treat open fractures and are also indicated to fix the bones when the brachial artery has been explored.

The fracture can be treated by overhead skeletal traction through a transverse wire or screw inserted in the olecranon or by Dunlop's skin traction[54] if the elbow is excessively swollen and closed reduction fails. This can be used as definitive treatment but requires close clinical and radiological supervision to avoid any malunion, or it can be simply used as a temporary measure until the

REFERENCES

52. Worlock P J Bone Joint Surg 1986; 68B: 755
53. Cheng J C, Lam T P, Shen W Y J Orthop Trauma 1995; 9: 511
54. Dunlop J J Bone Joint Surg 1939; 21A: 59

swelling subsides. After reduction the arm is immobilized for three weeks with regular X-rays to ensure there is no loss of reduction. After three weeks protected active mobilization is begun, and any K-wires are removed between four and six weeks.

Particularly if the elbow is immobilized in flexion, the forearm can become ischaemic following reduction and develop a compartment syndrome. When this occurs the pulse, hand colour and capillary return can all be normal, but there is increasing pain in the forearm, made worse by active movements and passive extension of the fingers. The forearm eventually becomes tense and tender, and paraesthesia and a pale hand are late signs. As soon as a compartment syndrome is suspected all constricting dressings must be removed and the elbow extended. Fasciotomies are required if symptoms and signs persist after these first aid measures. If the condition is not diagnosed and treated a Volkmann's ischaemic contracture will occur, leaving the child with a permanent and severe disability.

Other complications that can occur after supracondylar fractures in children include malunion with a cubitus valgus or varus deformity which does not remodel with growth. Elbow stiffness is exacerbated by prolonged immobilization and open reduction, but usually recovers with time.

Flexion fractures with anterior displacement and angulation account for only a small proportion of supracondylar fractures in childhood. They are usually caused by a fall on to the point of the elbow, and after reduction are stable with the elbow extended. Immobilization in extension is uncomfortable for the child and it can be difficult to regain elbow flexion. Percutaneous fixation with K-wires after reduction allows the elbow to be rested in a more functional position and it can be mobilized earlier.

Supracondylar fractures in adults

Supracondylar fractures in adults are also mainly of the extension type and caused by a fall on to the outstretched hand. The brachial artery is again at risk with displaced fractures, and the median, ulnar and radial nerves are all liable to injury, with damage to the radial nerve occurring most frequently.[55] Treatment depends on the degree of displacement of the fracture, with the same options available as for children. Indications for open reduction are failure of closed reduction, an associated neurovascular injury, open fractures and a simultaneous fracture of the ipsilateral humeral shaft or forearm. The fixation should be secure enough to allow early elbow movement if an open reduction is performed.

Intercondylar fractures

In adults the fracture line frequently extends down into the articular surface of the humerus, giving a T- or Y-shaped intercondylar fracture. The mechanism of injury is thought to be a direct blow to the back of the elbow driving the olecranon into the trochlea, and the fractures produced are often comminuted. Intercondylar fractures can be difficult to treat because they occur in the elderly, and the bone is often porotic, making secure internal fixation difficult. Any prolonged period of immobilization causes severe elbow stiffness. If good-quality bone is present displaced fractures are treated by reconstruction of the articular surface with rigid fixation of the condyles to the shaft by plates to permit early postoperative movement. Osteotomy of the olecranon gives a very good exposure of the distal humerus with minimal trauma to the soft tissues, and at the end of the procedure the olecranon can be reattached with a tension band wire without compromising early postoperative mobilization.

Internal fixation has a high failure rate in porotic bone, and closed reduction with immobilization in plaster often fails to maintain a satisfactory alignment, causing the elbow to become extremely stiff. The 'bag of bones' technique is an alternative treatment, in which the arm is placed in a collar and cuff sling with the elbow flexed to about 90 degrees. Shoulder and hand exercises are started immediately, and elbow extension is allowed as soon as the initial pain and swelling subside. The fractures unite at about six weeks and the range of motion continues to improve for three to four months.[56] The elbow remains weak, potentially unstable and has restricted movement, so the technique is reserved for the treatment of elderly patients with low functional demands.

Supracondylar and intercondylar fractures in adults can be complicated by elbow stiffness from periarticular fibrosis and obliteration of the olecranon fossa by callus and malunion of the fracture, neurovascular injuries and non-union.

Condylar fractures

Isolated fractures of the humeral condyles are rare, accounting for 5% of distal humeral fractures in adults,[57] with fractures of the lateral condyle being more common than those of the medial condyle. The fracture line extends from the articular surface of the capitulotrochlear sulcus or the lateral border of the trochlear groove up to the medial or lateral supracondylar ridge. Fractures of the medial and lateral condyles have been classified into type I if the lateral trochlear ridge remains attached to the intact condyle and type II if the ridge forms part of the fracture fragment.[58] This is important because the lateral trochlear ridge provides stability in the coronal plane, so if it forms part of the fracture fragment the elbow can be unstable.

In children with fractures of the lateral condyle, the fracture line usually extends along the growth plate, passing between the medial and lateral condylar epiphyses to enter the joint. The mechanism of injury can be indirect, with the proximal end of the radius or ulna being driven against the articular surface, or an avulsion fracture produced by the attached ligaments and muscles, or direct from a blow to the elbow. There is localized tenderness over the fractured condyle and a haemarthrosis is usually apparent. The diagnosis can usually be made with standard anteroposterior and lateral radiographs in adults, but in young children interpretation can be very difficult when only a fraction of the epiphysis is ossified. The

REFERENCES

55. Bryan R S AAOS Instructional Course Lectures 1981; 30: 200
56. Brown R F, Morgan R G J Bone Joint Surg 1971; 53B: 425
57. Knight R A South Med J 1955; 48: 1165
58. Milch H J Trauma 1964; 4: 592

presence of a fat pad sign and comparison with radiographs of the other elbow are useful in making the diagnosis.

Undisplaced fractures can be treated by immobilization in a back slab, but as these are intra-articular fractures any displacement must be fully corrected. In children closed reduction and percutaneous fixation with K-wires is possible, but an open reduction is frequently required. In adults all type II fractures are unstable and therefore require internal fixation, and type I fractures with displacement should also have open reduction and internal fixation to allow early elbow movement.

Complications seen after fractures of the lateral condyle in children are cubitus valgus from premature fusion of the physis, or a non-union with cubitus varus from overgrowth of the lateral condyle. Cubitus valgus can cause an ulnar nerve palsy many years later. Both deformities are difficult to correct once they are established, so an accurate reduction at the time of injury is essential. Surgical technique must be meticulous to avoid iatrogenic nerve injuries and avascular necrosis of the lateral condyle can occur if the soft tissue dissection is too extensive.

Fractures of the capitellum and trochlea

Isolated fractures of the articular surface of the capitellum and trochlea are very rare, with capitellar fractures accounting for 0.5–1% of elbow injuries. They are caused by a shearing force from impaction by the radial head or olecranon, and are often associated with an elbow dislocation or fracture of the radial head. They are intra-articular fractures and the fragments have no soft tissue attachments.

Capitellar fractures which have a large bony component attached to the articular cartilage are classified as type I, and have the eponym of Hahn–Steinthal fracture. If the fragment is largely articular cartilage with very little attached bone it is a type II or Kocher–Lorenz fracture.

There are usually signs of a haemarthrosis and tenderness over the fracture. Anterior displacement of the fragment can cause a block to elbow flexion. Capitellar fractures with associated swelling and tenderness on the medial side of the joint may show signs of valgus instability if the ulnar collateral ligament is also torn.

Type I fractures should be anatomically reduced and held with a screw or K-wires. Despite no soft tissue attachments they usually unite. Excision of the fragments gives a better functional result than open reduction and internal fixation or closed manipulation if there is comminution or a type II fracture.[59]

Fractures of the medial epicondyle

The epiphysis of the medial epicondyle first ossifies at between 5 and 9 years of age and usually fuses by the age of 20, although it may never do so. Fractures of the medial epicondyle are common in children, accounting for about 10% of all fractures of the elbow region, but these fractures are rare in adults. The mechanism of injury can be a direct blow to the elbow, a fall on to the outstretched hand with the wrist hyperextended, or an avulsion by the attached ulnar collateral ligament as the elbow dislocates (Fig. 51.6), which is the mechanism in about half the cases.[60] A repeated valgus stress to the elbow can also cause an avulsion by the attached flexor muscles, which is usually seen in adolescent baseball players and is known as 'little leaguer's elbow'.

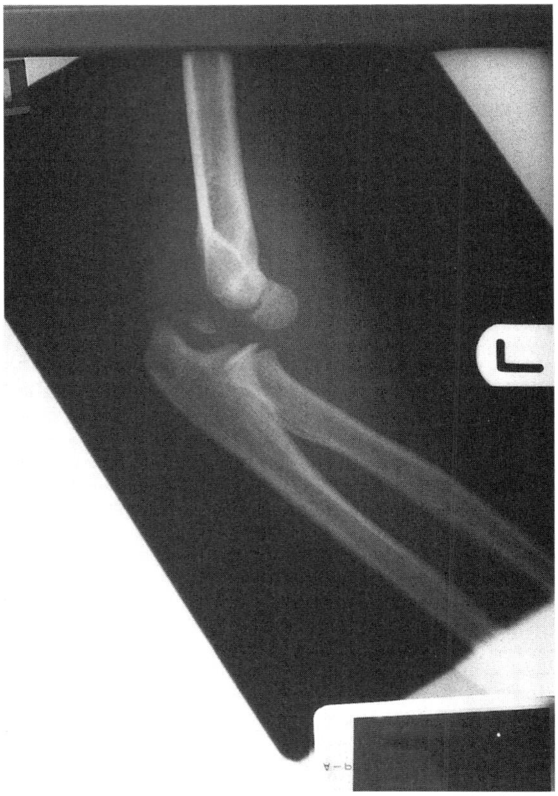

Fig. 51.6 Posterior dislocation of a child's elbow with the medial epicondyle avulsed and lying in the joint.

There is localized tenderness over the medial epicondyle. If the mechanism of injury has been an elbow dislocation which has reduced spontaneously the medial epicondyle fragment can be trapped in the joint, and the elbow will then not have a full range of movement. Radiographs can be difficult to interpret and comparison with the normal side is helpful, but if the medial epicondyle cannot be seen or is lying level with the joint it may well be incarcerated in the elbow joint.

The fracture can be managed by immobilization while the pain and swelling subside if there is little or no displacement. This is followed by active mobilization. Displaced and incarcerated fragments can be treated by closed reduction, but open reduction and K-wire fixation is often required. Possible complications include an ulnar nerve palsy and an unstable elbow.

DISLOCATION OF THE ELBOW

The elbow is the second most common large joint after the shoulder to dislocate. This usually occurs in young adults and

REFERENCES

59. Alvarez E, Patel M, Wimberg G, Pearlman H S J Bone Joint Surg 1975; 57A: 1093
60. Marion J, LaGrange J, Faysse R Rev Chir Orthop 1962; 48: 337

teenagers, with the average age being 13–14, although these injuries are responsible for less than 5% of all elbow injuries.

Classification is dependent upon the direction of dislocation, with the majority being posterior.[61] Anterior dislocations are much less common, and medial, lateral and divergent dislocations are only rarely seen. The mechanism of injury for a posterior dislocation is a fall on to the outstretched hand causing forced abduction and extension at the elbow. The ulnar collateral ligament is disrupted or the medial epicondyle avulsed allowing the olecranon and radial head to displace posteriorly. If the elbow is flexed at the time of injury it can dislocate anteriorly, although the more usual mechanism is a direct blow to the back of the elbow.

With a posterior dislocation the elbow is held in about 45 degrees of flexion and is swollen, the olecranon is prominent posteriorly, and its normal relationship to the medial and lateral epicondyles is disrupted. With anterior dislocations the forearm is supinated and appears elongated. The elbow is extended and the olecranon fossa is palpable posteriorly. Neurovascular injuries can occur and the nerves and circulation must be fully assessed. Plain radiographs confirm the diagnosis and demonstrate any associated fractures.

Most elbow dislocations can be reduced by gentle closed manipulation under sedation or general anaesthesia. For posterior dislocations traction is applied with the elbow semi-flexed and the forearm supinated and pressure is applied to the olecranon, pushing it distally and anteriorly. Once reduced the elbow is flexed beyond 90 degrees. Stability is then assessed, and a back slab is applied. Closed reduction can fail if a bony fragment, which is most likely to be the medial epicondyle, is trapped in the joint (Fig. 51.6). An open reduction is then required. Depending on its stability after reduction, the elbow is immobilized for one to three weeks, before commencing active and not passive mobilization.

Associated fractures frequently accompany elbow dislocations, with coronoid process fractures being most common. There is usually just a small fragment avulsed by the anterior capsule which does not require any specific treatment, but if the fragment is more substantial it should be reattached. An avulsed medial epicondyle may reduce as the dislocation is reduced and require no additional treatment, but if it remains displaced, is incarcerated in the joint or the elbow is unstable it should be treated by open reduction and internal fixation. Radial head and capitellar fractures can also occur, and after reduction of the dislocation the fractures are treated on their own merits, although if a comminuted radial head fracture is treated by excision it should be replaced by a prosthesis to avoid elbow instability. Olecranon fractures and avulsion of the triceps tendon occur with anterior dislocations and must be repaired.

Elbow dislocations can be complicated by neurovascular injuries, with the median and ulnar nerves most at risk. Brachial artery damage is most likely with anterior and open dislocations. Loss of elbow movement, particularly the last 10–20 degrees of extension, is usual, although more severe stiffness can occur from intra- or periarticular adhesions or ossification of the muscles and ligaments. Anterior heterotopic ossification causes pain and progressive loss of movement. This is more likely after repeated manipulations or passive stretching, and has a poor prognosis for recovering full elbow function. Elbow instability with recurrent subluxation or dislocation is rare.

DISLOCATION OF THE RADIAL HEAD

Isolated dislocation of the radial head is rare. Posterior dislocation probably occurs when the olecranon reduces spontaneously after a posterior elbow dislocation. Anterior dislocations are usually seen in children with an occult Monteggia fracture. Acute dislocations must be distinguished from previously undiagnosed congenital dislocations, which do not need treating. Some of the radiological features which suggest that a dislocation is congenital are a dome-shaped radial head, a hypoplastic capitellum, and a radius which is long relative to the ulna. Most acute radial dislocations can be successfully treated by closed manipulation and immobilization in hyperflexion for three weeks.

SUBLUXATION OF THE RADIAL HEAD (PULLED ELBOW)

There are numerous synonyms such as nursemaid's elbow, supermarket elbow and temper tantrum elbow for this common condition, which accounts for up to a third of elbow injuries in children under 10.[62] The peak incidence is in children aged 2–3, and it is rare after the age of 7. The mechanism of injury is a longitudinal pull on the arm with the elbow extended and forearm pronated,[63] pulling the head of the radius partially through the annular ligament, the distal portion of which may be torn. There is usually a history of an adult grabbing the child's arm or swinging them by an arm, producing an audible click and immediate pain in the elbow. The pain quickly settles, but the child remains reluctant to use the arm, and resists forearm supination. On examination there is tenderness over the proximal radius, the elbow has limited flexion and extension, and supination causes pain. Plain radiographs are usually normal, but may show some soft tissue swelling or slight lateral displacement of the radial head. When the history and physical signs are absolutely typical then a radiograph is probably not necessary, but if there is any doubt about the diagnosis one should be taken to exclude other injuries.

Reduction can be performed without sedation or anaesthesia. The child should be relaxed and an explanation given to the parents that the child will briefly experience increased pain and that the symptoms will then completely disappear. Gentle pressure is then applied to the radial head, the elbow is held semi-flexed and as the forearm is supinated there is an audible or palpable snap as the radial head reduces through the annular ligament. This occasionally fails, and the elbow is then fully flexed to achieve the reduction. After reduction the arm can be rested briefly in a sling, although immobilization of the elbow is not necessary.

REFERENCES

61. Roberts P H J Bone Joint Surg 1969; 56B: 806
62. Costigan P G Alberta Med Bull 1952; 17: 7
63. Salter R B, Zaltz C Clin Orthop 1971; 77: 134

FRACTURES OF THE HEAD AND NECK OF THE RADIUS

Fractures of the radial head and neck are common in adults and children and can occur in isolation or as part of a complex injury with associated fractures or dislocations. In adults the fracture usually involves the articular surface, whereas in children it usually crosses the neck or involves the physis. Radial head fractures have been classified[64] into type I, which are undisplaced, type II are displaced with part of the articular surface remaining connected to the shaft and type III with comminution and complete loss of contact between the head and neck (Fig. 51.7). A radial head fracture in association with an elbow dislocation is sometimes referred to as a Mason type IV fracture, although this combination was described originally by Johnston.[65] Children's fractures can be described using the Salter–Harris system if they involve the ephysis. They can also be described by their angulation and displacement or as crossing the neck.

The mechanism of injury is usually a fall on to the outstretched hand impacting the radial head against the capitellum. The interosseous membrane and distal radio-ulnar joint can be disrupted as the radius is driven proximally to cause the head to fracture. This is known as the Essex–Lopresti injury and if unrecognized can cause chronic wrist instability. Radial head fractures may also occur in association with an elbow dislocation, when the radial head is knocked off forwards by the capitellum as the elbow dislocates posteriorly or backwards as it spontaneously reduces.

On presentation there is localized tenderness over the proximal radius, a haemarthrosis is usually present, and elbow movements and forearm rotation are painful and restricted. Tenderness over the distal radio-ulnar joint and along the interosseous membrane indicates an Essex–Lopresti injury. It may be difficult to see the fracture on standard anteroposterior and lateral radiographs, and oblique views can be helpful.

The aim of treatment is to regain a full range of movement. In type I fractures the arm is immobilized in a sling for about two days before commencing active mobilization. Aspiration of the haemarthrosis and injection of local anaesthetic into the joint gives immediate symptomatic relief and enables elbow mobilization to start sooner, but makes no difference to the long-term outcome.[66]

The treatment of type II fractures is controversial, with the options being conservative treatment, open reduction and internal fixation or excision of the fracture fragment. If after injection of local anaesthetic into the joint the elbow can be almost fully flexed and extended and at least 70 degrees of pronation and supination are present, it will do well with conservative treatment.[67] When elbow movement is found to be restricted the fracture should be reduced and fixed with small AO screws, Herbert screws or absorbable polyglycolide pins.[68] Good results can be achieved if the fixation is stable and allows early movement.[69] When the fragment comprises less than a quarter of the radial head and is completely detached or displaced into the elbow joint it can be excised, although there is a risk that the remaining radial head will sublux with forearm rotation.

Type III fractures are usually treated by early complete excision of the radial head.[70] Losing the radial head does not make the

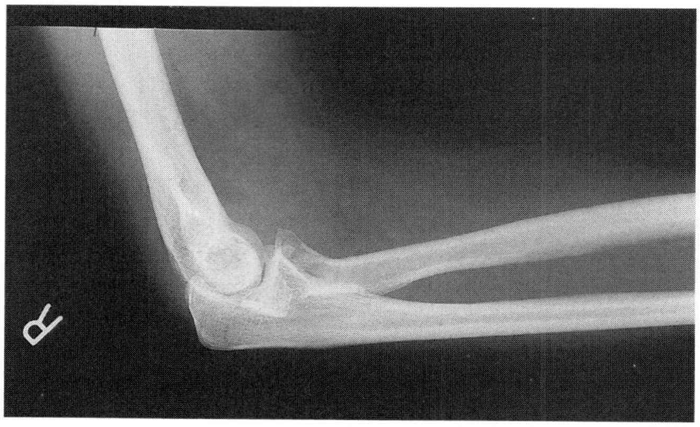

Fig. 51.7 A comminuted intra-articular fracture of the head of the radius.

elbow unstable to valgus stress if the medial collateral ligament remains intact,[71] but if there has been an associated elbow dislocation the excised head should be replaced with a silastic[72] or metal[73] prosthesis. With an Essex–Lopresti injury the radial length must be maintained by internal fixation of the fracture or prosthetic replacement if the head is excised. The dorsal subluxation of the distal ulna is then reduced and held by full supination of the forearm or transfixing the distal ulna and radius with K-wires.

In children moderate displacement, with angulation of 15–30 degrees, will remodel and can therefore be accepted. Treatment is by immobilization for a week in a sling or back slab, followed by active mobilization. When there is more than 30 degrees of angulation this is corrected by manipulation under anaesthetic, with either digital pressure or a percutaneous probe[74] pushing on the radial head. Once reduced it is usually stable and the elbow is immobilised in 90 degrees of flexion for two weeks. Open reduction is performed when the head is completely displaced, or if after an attempted closed reduction there is more than 30–45 degrees angulation or 4 mm displacement. Internal fixation is not necessary if the reduction is stable, but if it is not K-wires can be passed from distal to proximal into the head. Wires should not be passed across the joint to stabilize the radial head, and the radial head should not be excised in children.

The main complication of radial head fractures is a loss of elbow movement from malunion producing a bony block and soft tissue fibrosis causing generalized stiffness. Specific complications seen in children are premature closure of the physis,

REFERENCES

64. Mason M L Br J Surg 1954; 42: 123
65. Johnston G W Ulster Med J 1962; 31: 51
66. Radin E L, Riseborough E J J Bone Joint Surg 1966; 48A: 1055
67. Morrey B F J Bone Joint Surg 1995; 77A: 316
68. Hirvensalo E, Bostman O, Rokkanen P Arch Orthop Trauma Surg 1990; 109: 258
69. King G J, Evans D C, Kellam J F J Orthop Trauma 1991; 5: 21
70. Broberg M A, Morrey B F Clin Orthop 1987; 216: 109
71. Morrey B F, Tanaka S, An K-N Clin Orthop 1991; 265: 187
72. Borsky M Unfallversicherungsmediezin 1993; 6: 40
73. Knight D J, Rymaszewski L A, Amis A A, Miller J H J Bone Joint Surg 1993; 75B: 572
74. Bernstein S M J Pediatr Orthop 1993; 13: 85

overgrowth of the radial head, and if an open reduction is performed more than 48 hours after the injury there is a risk of avascular necrosis of the radial head.

FRACTURES OF THE OLECRANON

Olecranon fractures are common in adults and rare in children. The classifications used are those of Colton,[75] AO[50] and Mayo,[76] which all indicate whether a fracture is undisplaced or displaced, and if the latter is transverse, oblique, or comminuted, and whether the elbow is dislocated and therefore unstable.

The mechanism of injury is a fall onto the point of the elbow, or outstretched hand with the elbow flexed, combined with a forceful contraction of the triceps. A direct blow is more likely to produce a comminuted fracture with a more extensive soft tissue injury. There is swelling and tenderness over the olecranon, and there may be a palpable gap between the proximal and distal fragments. In displaced fractures the triceps mechanism is disrupted and the patient is unable to actively extend their elbow. Damage to the ulnar nerve can occur and its function must be assessed. A lateral radiograph is taken with the elbow flexed to 90 degrees because extending the elbow can reduce a displaced fracture and give a false impression that it is undisplaced. In children the ossification centre appears at the age of 10 and fuses at about 16 years old, making interpretation of the X-ray difficult. The diagnosis can be made on clinical examination, but if there is doubt comparison with a radiograph of the normal elbow and the presence of a positive fat pad sign confirms the diagnosis.

Undisplaced fractures can be treated by immobilization in a back slab with the elbow in 90 degrees of flexion for 10 days, followed by gentle and active mobilization, avoiding extension against resistance for a further six to eight weeks.

The majority of olecranon fractures are simple transverse avulsion fractures with displacement of the proximal fragment and disruption of the extensor mechanism. They are treated by open reduction and internal fixation with two longitudinal K-wires or a 6.5 mm cancellous screw[77] and a figure-of-eight tension band wire passed through a hole drilled transversely in the ulna and round the ends of the K-wires or the screw deep to the triceps tendon (Fig. 51.8). This provides a stable fixation allowing early active movement of the elbow. The tension band wire produces compression of the fracture when the elbow is actively extended. The fragments can be excised and the triceps tendon sutured to the distal fragment if the proximal fragment is small, the bone porotic, or there is severe comminution. Oblique fractures can remain unstable if just a tension band wire is applied and should be stabilized with an interfragmentary screw before the wire is positioned. Provided the bone is satisfactory, comminuted fractures can be reconstructed with interfragmentary screws and wires and supported with a plate over the dorsal surface, which is bent around the proximal end of the olecranon. The proximal end is held with a longitudinal screw and it is attached distally to the ulna under tension to compress the fracture. The plate then acts as a tension band, although care must be taken not to reduce the distance between the tip of the olecranon and coronoid process by over compression of a comminuted fracture.

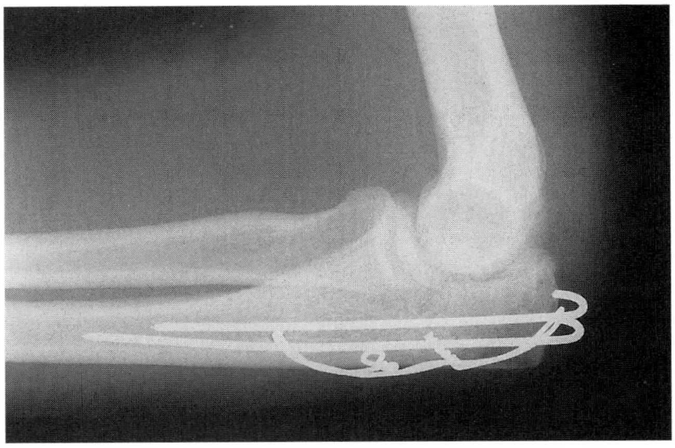

Fig. 51.8 Postoperative radiograph of an olecranon fracture treated by open reduction and internal fixation with longitudinal K-wires and a figure-of-eight tension band wire.

Associated injuries to the ulnar nerve, elbow stiffness and failure of fixation and non-union can all occur after olecranon fractures. The bent over ends of the K-wires are often palpable and tender, and if the wires back out they can cause necrosis of the overlying skin, making implant removal necessary.

FRACTURES OF THE RADIAL AND ULNAR SHAFTS

The anatomical arrangement of the forearm is a straight ulna, around which a curved radius rotates. The two bones are joined by an interosseous membrane and articulate with each other at the proximal and distal radioulnar joints. Consequently if there is a displaced fracture of one of the bones there must also be a fracture of the other bone or a dislocation of the proximal or distal radioulnar joint. In children the fractures can be complete, greenstick or the bone can undergo plastic deformation. When there is slight displacement of a greenstick or complete fracture of one of the bones, the other may be intact but undergo plastic deformation. There must always, however, be a high index of suspicion that one of the joints has been disrupted.

A fracture at the junction of the middle and distal thirds of the radius with subluxation or dislocation of the distal radioulnar joint is known as a Galeazzi fracture (Fig. 51.9).[78] Rather than disruption of the distal radio-ulnar joint in children there may be a fracture through the distal physis of the ulna with dorsal displacement of the metaphysis. Fracture of the proximal third of the ulna with dislocation of the radial head was described by Monteggia in 1814,[79] and this injury has been classified according to the

REFERENCES

75. Colton C L Injury 1973; 5: 121
76. Cabanela M E, Morrey B F In: Morrey B F (ed) The Elbow and its Disorders, 2nd edn. Saunders, Philadelphia 1993
77. Johnson R P, Roetker A, Schwab J P. Orthopedics 1986; 9: 66
78. Galeazzi R. Arch Orthop Unfallchir 1934; 35: 557
79. Monteggia G B Instituzioni Chirugiche, vol 5. Maspero, Milan 1814

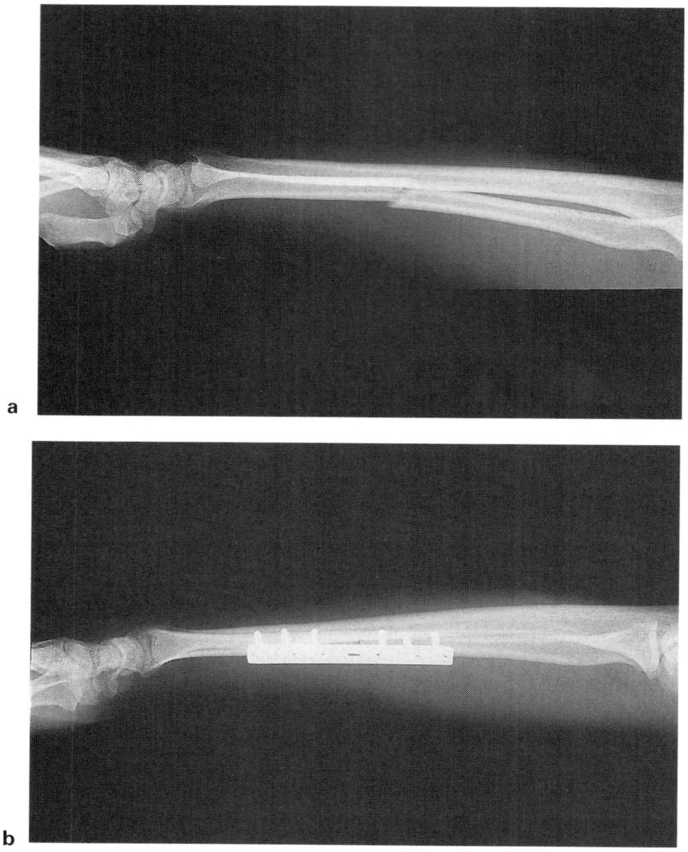

Fig. 51.9 (**a**) Galeazzi fracture. There is a fracture of the shaft of the radius and dislocation of the distal radio-ulnar joint (**b**) The distal radio-ulnar joint has been reduced by accurately reducing the radial fracture.

direction in which the radial head dislocates and whether there is an associated fracture of the proximal radius.[80]

The mechanism of injury is either direct, with road traffic accidents a frequent cause, or indirect from a fall on to the outstretched hand. An isolated fracture of the ulna is known as a night-stick fracture, and occurs with a direct blow against the ulnar side of the forearm, classically when the arm is raised to protect the face from assault. Galeazzi fractures are caused by a direct force to the dorsolateral aspect of the wrist or a fall on to the outstretched hand with the forearm pronated.

There is swelling and tenderness over the fractures, and with both bones broken there is usually an obvious deformity. The elbow and wrist must be assessed to exclude dislocation of the radial head or disruption of the distal radioulnar joint. Forearm fractures may be open, from either a spike of bone puncturing the skin from the inside or from the direct injury to the soft tissues, in which case there can be associated injuries to the vessels, nerves, muscles and tendons. Most forearm fractures are obvious with standard X-rays, which must include anteroposterior and lateral views of the elbow and wrist to detect Monteggia and Galeazzi fractures.

Forearm fractures must be accurately reduced to avoid loss of forearm rotation, with displacement of more than 20 degrees in any plane causing at least a 50% loss of rotation.[81] Children have the potential to remodel moderate amounts of angulation and up to 15 degrees is acceptable in children under the age of 7, but rotational deformities are unlikely to remodel and must therefore be corrected.

Undisplaced fractures are immobilized in an above-elbow cast which includes the hand and thumb to provide rotational stability. They must be kept under close observation because subsequent displacement can occur from the pull of the attached muscles.

Non-operative treatment of displaced fractures is difficult because accurate alignment and rotation must be maintained while preserving the normal radial bow. Good results have been achieved by using a functional brace,[82] but generally the results of conservative treatment in adults are poor. Children are usually treated by manipulation under general anaesthesia and immobilization in an above-elbow cast, with the forearm in supination for fractures of the proximal third, the neutral position for the middle third and in pronation for the distal third. Greenstick fractures are usually easy to reduce, but healing can be delayed with a high incidence of re-fracture.[83] This is because the intact cortex makes the fracture stable, limiting callus production and if even slight angulation persists there is no compression of the fracture. Some surgeons therefore recommend that the intact cortex is broken during the reduction to avoid this problem[84,85] but doing so will increase the risk of recurrent displacement. Prolonged protection with a splint is required to avoid refracture if the intact cortex is not broken during the manipulation.[83]

Most displaced forearm fractures in adults are treated by open reduction and internal fixation. Intramedullary nails have been used, but plating is usually preferred because nails may fail to control rotation, or accommodate for the natural bow of the radius. The radius and ulna are exposed through separate incisions to reduce the risk of radio-ulnar synostosis, the fractures are anatomically reduced and held with 3.5 mm dynamic compression plates and an interfragmentary lag screw where possible. Primary bone grafting should be considered if the fracture is comminuted or segmental.

Undisplaced isolated fractures of the ulna can be treated with a cast or functional brace for six to eight weeks, but if there is more than 10 degrees angulation or 50% displacement open reduction and internal fixation are preferred.

With Monteggia and Galeazzi fractures accurate reduction of the fracture almost always reduces the associated dislocation. Monteggia fractures in children can be treated by closed reduction of the ulna fracture and dislocated radial head, and immobilization in an above-elbow cast in supination[86] or by open reduction and internal fixation of the ulna fracture and closed reduction of the

REFERENCES

80. Bado J L Clin Orthop 1967; 50: 71
81. Tarr R R, Garfinkel A I, Sarmiento A J Bone Joint Surg 1984; 66A: 65
82. Sarmiento A, Cooper J S, Sinclair W F J Bone Joint Surg 1975; 57A: 297
83. Schwarz N, Pienaar S, Schwarz A F et al J Bone Joint Surg 1996; 78B: 740
84. Blount W P, Schaefer A A, Johnson J H JAMA 1942; 120: 111
85. Ogden J A. Skeletal Injury in the Child. Saunders, Philadelphia 1990
86. Olney B W, Menelaus M B J Pediatr Orthop 1989; 9: 219

radial head.[87] Both techniques produce a good functional outcome. In adults the ulna fracture requires an open reduction and internal fixation with a compression plate.[88,89] The radial head can be reduced closed, unless the annular ligament is torn, and blocks the reduction. Open reduction is then required. The elbow should be immobilized in a cast for six weeks with radiographs being taken at two and six weeks to ensure that the radial head has not re-dislocated.

Galeazzi fractures in children are treated by closed reduction of the radial fracture. Immobilization in supination will usually reduce the distal radio-ulnar joint. In adults the radial fracture is anatomically reduced and held with a plate, and this usually reduces the distal radio-ulnar joint (Fig. 51.9), but if it remains subluxed or dislocated it should be reduced and held with K-wires transfixing the ulna and radius.

Open fractures of the forearm are treated according to the same principles as for all open fractures (see Ch. 50). Thorough debridement of the wounds and repair of the damaged soft tissues where appropriate are carried out and the fractures are then stabilized by an external fixator[90] or immediate plating.[91]

Non-union is more likely if the fracture is comminuted, there are segmental forearm fractures, or if they have been plated without compression. This problem is treated by compression plating and bone grafting (see Ch. 50). Malunion limits forearm rotation and can be difficult to treat. It can usually be avoided by maintaining an accurate reduction of the fracture. Forearm rotation can be affected even if the fractures are in a good alignment because of contracture of the interosseous membrane. Radio-ulnar synostosis also limits forearm rotation and is more likely if both fractures are at the same level; if there has been severe local trauma and comminution with bone fragments in the interosseous space; and if the patient has multiple injuries or a head injury. Iatrogenic factors which increase the chances of a synostosis are: plating both bones through a single incision; spilling bone graft into the interosseous space; performing multiple closed reductions or if the reduction is poor and the width of the interosseous space is reduced.

The incidence of associated neurovascular injury is low after straightforward closed forearm fractures, but is greater after open fractures or Monteggia fractures, where the posterior interosseous nerve is at risk, and in fractures treated surgically where there is a risk of iatrogenic injury. Forearm compartment syndrome is rare, and early diagnosis and treatment are essential if nerve and more importantly muscle necrosis are to be prevented. Re-fracture can occur after greenstick fractures in children as already discussed, and this also occurs in adults after plates are removed. Routine plate removal is therefore not advisable, and if it is performed the arm must be protected with a splint.

FRACTURES OF THE DISTAL RADIUS

Fractures of the distal radius are very common in both adults and children and account for about a sixth of all fractures,[92] with peaks occurring between the ages of 6 and 10, and 60 and 69.[93] In adults these fractures are most simply classified by their well-known eponyms. A Colles' fracture is through the metaphysis of the distal radius within 1–3 cm of the wrist joint. There is dorsal angulation and displacement of the distal fragment with radial angulation, shortening and often an associated fracture of the ulnar styloid.[3] A Smith's fracture is a fracture of the distal radius with volar angulation and displacement of the distal fragment[5] which can be either extra- or intra-articular. Barton's fracture[4] is a fracture dislocation or subluxation of the wrist (Fig. 51.10), with an intra-articular fracture of the distal radius producing a fragment on the dorsal or palmar surface which displaces with the attached carpus and hand backwards or forwards.

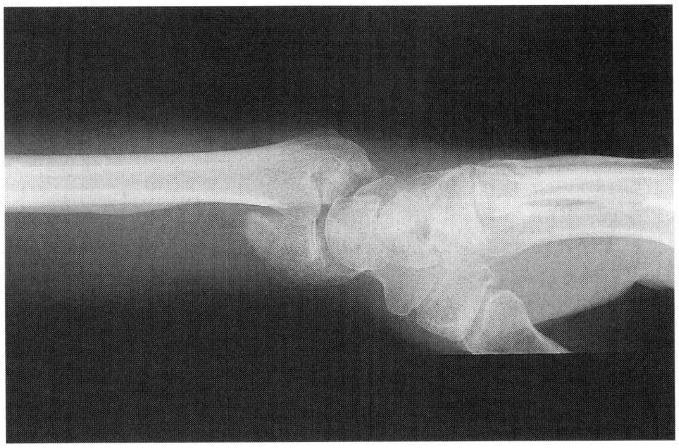

Fig. 51.10 Volar Barton's fracture. There is anterior subluxation of the carpus and the volar fragment of the distal radius.

Since these original descriptions there have been a number of other classifications, such as that of Frykman,[94] which considers whether the radiocarpal and distal radio-ulnar joints are affected, and whether there is a fracture of the ulnar styloid. This classification, however, does not indicate the direction or degree of displacement or if there is comminution. The Universal classification of Gartland and Werley[95] indicates whether the fracture is intra- or extra-articular, displaced, stable or unstable and whether it is reducible or not. Intra-articular fractures have been classified by dividing the articular surface into its anatomical components, and considering their displacement and stability.[96]

In children wrist fractures occur either through the physis and are usually Salter Harris type I or II injuries, or through the metaphysis. Metaphyseal fractures can be: torus or buckle fractures, in which one cortex fails under compression and there is little or no displacement; greenstick fractures in which one cortex fractures

REFERENCES

87. Ring D, Waters P M J Bone Joint Surg 1996; 78B: 734
88. Speed J S, Boyd H B JAMA 1940; 115: 1699
89. Jupiter J B, Leibovic S J, Ribbans W, Wilk R M J Orthop Trauma 1991; 5: 395
90. Schiund F, Andrianne Y, Burny F Clin Orthop 1991; 266: 197
91. Moed B R, Kellam J F, Foster R J, Tile M, Hansen S T J Bone Joint Surg 1986; 68A: 1008
92. Owen R A, Melton L J Jr, Johnson K A, Ilstrup D M, Riggs B L Am J Public Health 1982; 72: 605
93. Alffram P A, Bauer G C H J Bone Joint Surg 1962; 44A: 105
94. Frykman G Acta Orthop Scand 1967; Suppl 108
95. Gartland J J Jr, Werley C W J Bone Joint Surg 1951; 33A: 895
96. Melone C P Orthop Clin North Am 1993; 24: 239

The scaphoid forms part of, and links the proximal and distal carpal rows, and the majority of its surface is articular. The blood supply is from the radial and anterior interosseous arteries, with 70% of the blood supply entering through the dorsal ridge. Normally no vessels enter through the proximal pole, and there is no intra-osseous anastamosis between the vessels entering the tuberosity and dorsal ridge, so a fracture of the middle third, or more proximally can cause devascularization of the proximal pole.

The Schernberg classification is based on the anatomical location of the fracture.[122] The Herbert classification[123] subdivides into type A incomplete fractures; type B acute complete fractures which can be oblique fractures of the distal pole or transverse fractures of the waist or proximal pole, or fracture dislocations. Type C are delayed unions and type D are non-unions, of which four subtypes are described. Fractures can displace with translation, rotation or angulation, with flexion being most common. They are liable to be unstable if there is comminution, displacement or separation of the fragments by more than 1 mm, or if the fracture is vertical or oblique.

The mechanism of injury is usually a fall on to the outstretched hand, with the wrist extended to at least 95 degrees,[124] the proximal half of the bone is fixed between the capitate and distal radius, whereas the distal half is unsupported and can move relative to the proximal half, with the weight of the body producing a shearing force sufficient to fracture the bone. In addition, as the wrist hyperextends the scaphoid is impacted against the dorsal edge of the distal radius. The site of the fracture depends on the amount of extension and radial or ulnar deviation of the wrist at the time of impact. About 3% of scaphoid fractures are caused by wrist flexion.[125]

The physical signs depend on the severity of the fracture. For minimally displaced fractures there is often a delay between injury and presentation because the patient thinks that they have only had a sprain. If the signs are subtle, comparison with the normal wrist is essential. There is often a little swelling, and localized tenderness over the scaphoid in the anatomical snuff box. Pain on compression of the thumb is the most accurate sign for a scaphoid fracture.[126] Pain on active thumb extension and adduction, and wrist movements with compression are often also present, but less specific signs. With more severe fractures swelling and bruising are more noticeable.

The diagnosis is confirmed radiologically, and most scaphoid fractures are visible on the original radiographs with the eye of hindsight.[125] A variety of views have been described, and a minimum of four should be taken. They include a posteroanterior with the palm on the X-ray plate, a true lateral, and oblique views with 45 degrees pronation and supination. Extending the scaphoid by ulnar deviation and extension of the wrist by clenching the fist brings the scaphoid more perpendicular to the X-ray beam, and is known as the Ziter view.[127]

A bone scan, CT or a magnetic resonance scan can be obtained if doubt about the diagnosis persists.

The management of scaphoid fractures is based on both the radiographs and the clinical findings[128] because on their own each can be misleading. When a fracture is suspected clinically but is not apparent on the radiographs, it should be immobilized, because a delay in immobilization leads to a higher non-union rate.[129] It is re-examined and X-rayed after 10–14 days, and if there is still doubt a bone scan will usually confirm the diagnosis.

The traditional treatment for all scaphoid fractures was immobilization in a scaphoid plaster, which included the thumb and held the wrist slightly extended. Some surgeons have advocated an above-elbow plaster,[130] although this has since been shown not to be of any benefit.[131] The optimum position of the wrist is disputed, some preferring it to be flexed[132] and others to be in the neutral position.[133] Both radial[134] and ulnar[124,132] deviation has also been advocated. The lack of consensus probably indicates that the position in which the wrist is immobilized does not influence fracture healing. Inclusion of the thumb is probably not necessary,[135] and a Colles type plaster is perfectly satisfactory.

The plaster cast is retained until the fracture has united, but in practice it can be very difficult to determine when union has occurred.[136] After about eight weeks of immobilization the wrist is examined and X-rayed, and if there is still tenderness or the radiograph looks doubtful, a plaster cast is reapplied for a further four weeks. After the cast has been removed, the radiographs should be repeated six months after the injury to ensure a non-union has not occurred.

87.6%[137] to 95%[125] of acute scaphoid fractures unite with conservative treatment, with the time to union depending on the level of the fracture and the degree of displacement. Because a prolonged period of immobilization and absence from work may be necessary, some surgeons treat all acute scaphoid fractures by internal fixation, claiming a shorter time to union and an earlier return to work.[138] Internal fixation by a Herbert screw[139] (Fig. 51.13) has been reported to give rapid symptomatic relief and to provide sufficient stability to allow normal use of the wrist without post-operative immobilization. The overall union rate is similar to that of non-operative treatment.[140] However, as there is no proof that operative treatment of acute scaphoid fractures gives better results, and it carries the risks of complications of anaesthesia and surgery,

REFERENCES

122. Schernberg F, Elzein F, Gérard Y Rev Chir Orthop Reparatrice Appar Mot 1984; 70 (Suppl 2): 55
123. Herbert T J, Fisher W E J Bone Joint Surg 1984; 66B: 114
124. Weber E R, Chao E Y J Hand Surg (Am) 1978; 3A: 142
125. Leslie I J, Dickson R A J Bone Joint Surg 1981; 63B: 225
126. Grover R J Hand Surg 1996; 21B: 341
127. Ziter F M H Radiology 1973; 3: 706
128. Dias J J, Thompson J, Barton N J, Gregg P J J Bone Joint Surg 1990; 72B: 98
129. Langhoff O, Anderson J L J Hand Surg 1988; 13B: 77
130. Verdan C Surg Clin North Am 1960; 40: 461
131. Alho A, Kankaanpää U Acta Orthop Scand 1975; 46: 737
132. Yanni D, Lieppins P, Laurence M J Bone Joint Surg 1991; 73B: 600
133. Weber E R Clin Orthop 1980; 149: 83
134. Fisk G R Ann R Coll Surg Engl 1970; 46: 63
135. Clay N R, Dias J J, Costigan P S, Gregg P J, Barton N J J Bone Joint Surg 1991; 73B: 828
136. Dias J J, Taylor M, Thompson J, Brenkel I J, Gregg P J J Bone Joint Surg 1988; 70B: 299
137. Dias J J, Brenkel I J, Finley D B L J Bone Joint Surg 1989; 71B: 307
138. Inoue G, Shionoya K J Bone Joint Surg 1997; 79B: 418
139. Herbert T J, Fisher W E J Bone Joint Surg 1984; 66B: 114
140. Filan S C, Herbert T J J Bone Joint Surg 1996; 78B: 519

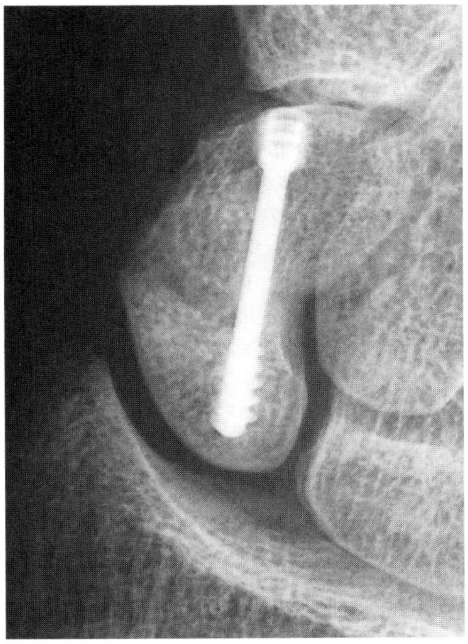

Fig. 51.13 A fracture of the waist of the scaphoid treated by open reduction and internal fixation with a Herbert screw.

such as hypertrophic scars and articular damage to the scapho-trapezial joint,[141] internal fixation is not recommended for all acute scaphoid fractures.

Unstable fractures can displace, leading to malunion, and they have an increased risk of non-union, so primary internal fixation should be considered. Fractures likely to be unstable are those associated with a perilunate dislocation, where the displacement or gap between the scaphoid fragments is greater than 1 mm or where the fracture line is vertical or oblique. The method of fixation is usually with a screw which will compress the fracture, and if there is anterior comminution, and bone loss causing flexion at the fracture, a bone graft can be inserted to restore the normal shape of the bone.

The main complication of scaphoid fractures is non-union, which is often associated with avascular necrosis of the proximal pole. The reported incidence of non-union in patients treated conservatively varies from 5%[125] to 50%.[123] The incidence in patients treated and followed up for one year by Dias et al[137] was 12.3%. Non-union can be symptomless, although a degree of pain and weakness is usual.[142] The concern is that the patient will develop progressive arthritis if left untreated,[143,144] so unless a patient is elderly or has already developed significant arthritic changes attempts should be made to achieve union. The pseudarthrosis and any dead or sclerotic bone should be excised, the defect grafted with a corticocancellous graft and held with a screw or K-wires. Up to 95% of scaphoid fractures will unite using this approach.[145]

FRACTURES OF THE CARPAL BONES OTHER THAN THE SCAPHOID

Dorsal chip fractures from a carpal bone are the second most common carpal fracture after a fracture of the scaphoid. Apart from these, carpal bone fractures are rare.

The carpal bones lie in two rows with the scaphoid, lunate, triquetrum and pisiform forming the proximal row and the trapezium, trapezoid, capitate and hamate the distal row, although functionally the scaphoid can be considered as bridging the two rows. The pisiform is a sesamoid bone attached proximally to the tendon of flexor carpi ulnaris and distally to the pisohamate and pisometacarpal ligaments, and articulating with the underlying triquetrum. The remaining carpal bones are held together by strong intrinsic interosseous ligaments and the extrinsic ligaments which connect the carpus to the distal radius and ulna.

Fractures of the various bones are described by their anatomical site; for example, the classification of trapezial fractures[146] is based on where the bone is fractured and the degree of comminution. There are often associated fractures or dislocations of the metacarpals, and fractures of the capitate and triquetral can occur as part of a perilunate fracture dislocation. A fracture of the neck of the capitate with rotation of the proximal fragment can occur in association with a fracture of the waist of the scaphoid and is known as the scaphocapitate syndrome.

The mechanisms of injury can be direct,[147] with the site of impact determining which bone fractures. Sudden force applied to the hypothenar eminence in golfers or racquet sports players can fracture the hook of the hamate. Indirect mechanisms can produce avulsion fractures or dorsal chip fractures from shearing forces, with the dorsal surface of the triquetrum most often affected.[148] Falls on to the outstretched hand cause compression on the dorsal surface and tension in the volar ligaments, producing a variety of carpal bone fractures depending on the point of impact and degree of radial or ulnar deviation of the wrist. Intra-articular fractures of bones of the distal row arise from forces transmitted along the articulating metacarpals, which are themselves often fractured or dislocated.

The clinical presentation depends on the severity of the trauma. There is severe pain, swelling, deformity and associated soft tissue injuries with high-energy displaced fractures and dislocations, but only minimal swelling and localized tenderness with dorsal chip fractures. A specific sign for fractures of the trapezial ridge is bruising tracking along the tendon of flexor carpi radialis.

Carpal fractures can be difficult to diagnose with standard radiographs. A dorsal chip fracture can usually be seen on the lateral view, but identifying the bone from which it originates is more difficult. An anteroposterior view will show most displaced fractures and associated fractures and dislocations, but for some carpal fractures special views are required. The carpal tunnel

REFERENCES

141. Barton N J J Bone Joint Surg 1996; 78B: 517
142. Lindstrom G, Nystrom A J Hand Surg 1992; 71B: 697
143. Mack G R, Bosse M J, Gelberman R H, Yu E J Bone Joint Surg 1984; 66A: 504
144. Shinya K, Herbert T J J Hand Surg (Br) 1994; 19 (Suppl 1): 26
145. Daly K, Gill P, Magnussen P A, Simonis R B J Bone Joint Surg 1996; 78B: 530
146. Walker J L, Greene T L, Lunseth P A J Orthop Trauma 1988; 2: 22
147. Cordrey L J, Ferrer-Torells M J Bone Joint Surg 1960; 42A: 1111
148. Fairbank T J Br Med J 1942; 2: 310

profile view[149] is useful for fractures of the trapezial ridge, hook of the hamate and pisiform, and oblique views demonstrate fractures of the body of the hamate. CT or bone scans may be required.

Undisplaced fractures can be treated in a cast for three weeks, followed by a removable splint for a further three weeks, with the thumb included for trapezial fractures. Displaced fractures can be reduced by traction and manipulation and held with a cast or percutaneous K-wires. If closed reduction fails an open reduction will be required. Intra-articular fractures must be accurately reduced and stabilized to allow early joint movement. Fractures of the hook of the hamate often fail to unite, and if they remain symptomatic excision of the fragment gives good results.

Reflex sympathetic dystrophy and osteoarthritis can complicate intra-articular fractures. Fractures of the neck of the capitate can cause avascular necrosis of the head and late carpal collapse, and with fractures of the hook of the hamate the ulnar nerve can be injured[150] or attrition rupture of the overlying flexor tendon can occur.[151]

PERILUNATE DISLOCATIONS

Dislocations of all the carpal bones have been described, but by far the most common are perilunate dislocations. Associated fractures of the scaphoid giving trans-scaphoid perilunate dislocations are twice as common as isolated dislocations, and there can also be associated fractures of the capitate, triquetral or radial and ulnar styloids.

Dislocations occur around the lunate because the volar radiolunate ligament is very strong. The lunate remains attached to the radius as the rest of the carpus dislocates posteriorly. The carpus can rebound, pushing the lunate anteriorly so that there appears to be an isolated anterior dislocation of the lunate, although the volar radiolunate ligament remains intact, and the rest of the carpus will have initially dislocated posteriorly.

Perilunate dislocations have been classified[152] into pure dislocations and fracture dislocations, whose classification depends on which bone is fractured. Trans-scaphoid perilunate dislocations are known as de Quervain's injury.[153] They are usually high-energy injuries often from falls on to an outstretched hand or road traffic accidents, causing extreme dorsiflexion of the radially deviated wrist.

The physical signs are variable, and the diagnosis is initially missed in a quarter of cases.[154] There is usually some swelling, diffuse tenderness, and movement of the wrist is limited by pain. There may be associated injuries to the median and ulnar nerves, vessels and tendons.

The anteroposterior radiograph shows soft tissue swelling, increased overlap of the carpal bones, the lunate has an abnormal shape and orientation and the gap between the scaphoid and lunate is increased. Any associated fractures should also be apparent. On the lateral view the capitate is not articulating with the lunate, which may be displaced forwards and rotated.

In acute injuries closed reduction is by traction, and dorsiflexion with pressure over the volar surface of the lunate. This is followed by gradual flexion and may be successful. The reduction is held with a cast or percutaneous K-wires. Weekly radiographs should be taken for the first three weeks because re-dislocation can occur, and the cast or wires are retained for up to 12 weeks. Closed reduction fails or is lost in the cast in 73% of cases,[155] so open reduction is often required. With a trans-scaphoid perilunate dislocation failure to accurately reduce the scaphoid fracture gives poor results, so open reduction with internal fixation of the scaphoid with a screw or K-wires is usually preferred.[156]

Closed reduction is occasionally possible if the diagnosis is delayed and the patient presents late,[157] but open reduction is usually required, and if this fails a proximal row carpectomy or wrist arthrodesis is performed.[158]

Post-traumatic arthritis of the wrist or midcarpal joint develops in 56% of cases,[154] with an increased incidence in open injuries or if treatment is delayed. Avascular necrosis of the proximal pole of the scaphoid or lunate can also occur.

REFERENCES

149. Hart V L, Gaynor V J Bone Joint Surg 1941; 23: 382
150. Howard F M J Bone Joint Surg 1961; 43A: 1197
151. Okuhara T, Matsui T, Sugimoto Y Hand 1982; 14: 71
152. Mayfield J K Clin Orthop 1980; 149: 45
153. De Quervain F. Clinical Surgical Diagnosis for Students and Practitioners (translated from 4th edn by Snowman J). William Wood, New York 1913
154. Herzberg G, Comtet J J, Lischeid R L et al J Hand Surg (Am) 1993; 18: 768
155. Adkison J W, Chapman M W Clin Orthop 1982; 164: 199
156. Cooney W P, Bussey R, Dobyns J H, Linscheid R L Clin Orthop 1987; 214: 136
157. Jorgensen E C. J Bone Joint Surg 1969; 51A: 1104
158. Howard F M, Dell P C Clin Orthop 1986; 202: 112

52 Pelvic fractures

R. M. Smith

Pelvic fractures include the most simple and the most complex injuries dealt with by the orthopaedic surgeon. The majority do not require surgical intervention, but some require specialist surgery with coordinated multidisciplinary care and carry a high morbidity and mortality. Just as the assessment and surgical treatment of other skeletal injuries have developed over recent years, so too have the general understanding and care of fractures of the pelvis. In long bones the management of an articular fracture is dependent upon the anatomy, early motion and rigid fixation, and the management of a diaphyseal fracture requires skeletal stability and biological fixation for early fracture union. It is also accepted that soft tissue care is critical to the management of the whole injury. Injuries to the pelvis are identical. Articular fracture is a fracture of the acetabulum where, like any other joint, accurate anatomical reduction and sound fixation allow early rehabilitation for cartilage nutrition and joint movement. Injury of the pelvic ring is the equivalent of the diaphyseal fracture of a long bone; here stability and general alignment for rehabilitation are required.

Most pelvic ring fractures are relatively simple and do not render the ring significantly unstable; however, a small portion can cause massive bony destruction and soft tissue damage. This leads to the risk of major haemodynamic instability and the danger of injury to associated soft tissues, and there may be problems later from mechanical instability of the pelvic ring. With fractures of the acetabulum the main aim is to limit long-term disability, while in severe pelvic ring injuries the major objective is usually to save life.[1-3]

ANATOMY

The pelvic ring is a support and weight-bearing structure; it protects the pelvic organs and gives attachment for the abdominal, pelvic floor and leg muscles.

In an adult the pelvic ring is made up of three bones: Two innominate bones, right and left, linked together anteriorly at the pubic symphysis and posteriorly by the sacrum. While the pubic symphysis is a strong but flexible area, the joints around the sacrum are surrounded by very strong ligaments, particularly posteriorly, and act as the main weight transmission area from the lower limbs to the axial skeleton. Included in these heavy posterior ligaments are the iliolumbar ligaments which join the posterior sacrum and iliac crest to the stout and solid transverse process of the fifth lumbar vertebrae. In the anatomical position the whole pelvis is inclined at 45° to the horizontal so that the sacrum lies behind and above the pubis. To either side of the pelvic ring itself, the iliac crests allow for major muscle attachments and within the structure of each innominate bone lies the hip socket or acetabulum. In a child the innominate bone is formed from three separate bones joined together at the triradiate cartilage in the acetabulum; by the early teens this has fused. The articular surface of the acetabulum forms a C shape, open inferiorly, with its thickest cartilage and main weight-bearing surface at the dome superiorly. It articulates with the congruent sphere of the femoral head. The structure of the acetabulum was best described by Letournel[4] as an anterior and posterior column coming together at the dome in the shape of an invented Y. Our current functional classification of acetabular fractures is based on this concept.

The iliac blades diverge and form the false pelvis above. Below this is a small and more cylindrical area deep to the acetabula and in front of the sacrum. This is the true pelvis. Within this lies the bladder, the uterus and adnexa in the female, and the lower colon and rectum. Around these on the pelvic side walls are complex meshes of vessels arising from and draining to the internal iliac arteries and veins. Above the true pelvis the external iliac arteries run forward to pass under the inguinal ligaments and become the femoral arteries supplying the lower limbs. Of particular importance in pelvic fractures is the major venous and arterial anastomoses around the anterior aspect of the sacroiliac joints and the superior gluteal artery which leaves the pelvis to supply the gluteal muscle mass through the sciatic notch. These vessels are at risk of injury in major pelvic ring fractures and may bleed heavily.

The fifth lumbar and sacral nerve roots emerge through the relevant vertebral foramina before joining in front of the sacrum to form the sacral plexus, which in part lies immediately in front of the sacroiliac joint. The fourth and fifth lumbar and upper sacral routes form the sciatic nerve, which passes through the sciatic notch, lying then immediately behind the hip joint and lateral to the ischial tuberosity before entering the posterior aspect of the upper thigh. The close proximity of the nerve to the local bony structures and hip joint makes it at great risk of nerve injury associated with pelvic fractures or hip dislocations.

REFERENCES

1. Kellam J F Clin Orthop 1989; 241: 66–82
2. Smith R M Int J Orthop Trauma 1996; 6: 5–6
3. Dalal S A, Burgess A R, Siegel J H et al J Trauma 1989; 29: 981–1002
4. Letournel E, Judet R Fractures of Acetabulum, 2nd edn. Springer-Veriag, Berlin 1993

Table 52.1 Issues in pelvic fractures

Pelvic fractures	Haemodynamic instability Soft tissue injury Mechanical instability
Acetabular fractures	–Joint congruity –Longterm degenerative change

ISSUES IN PELVIC FRACTURES

Pelvic ring

There are two main concerns in pelvic ring injuries; both relate to 'stability' (Table 52.1). The first and most important is the haemodynamic stability of the severely injured patient, and secondarily restoration of the structural stability of the pelvis as a bony support system. These problems occur in the more severe pelvic disruptions usually as a result of high-energy blunt trauma; they are usually seen in multiply injured patients who require a complex multidisciplinary structured approach to their care. A review of the frequency of severe haemorrhage in multiply injured patients illustrated that pelvic fracture was the most significant source of haemorrhage in a large proportion of patients who died of hypovolaemia in the resuscitation phase after major injury.[5] Mechanical instability of the pelvis itself is less likely to be a threat to life, although its stabilization can be essential to the general care of the injured patient. Mechanically unstable pelvic ring injuries are likely to be a source of late deformity and quite commonly of long-term disability from persisting posterior pelvic pain. A recent survey[6] suggested that this was one of the main unresolved problems of disability after injury. There is still doubt as to whether active treatment of these injuries with modern surgical stabilization techniques will lead to a reduction in long-term pain.

Classification of pelvic fractures

There are two major classification systems for fractures of the pelvic ring. These are shown in Tables 52.2 and 52.3 and include the Tile classification[7] (now included in the comprehensive classification system provided by AO[8]) and the Young and Burgess[9] classification. The first classifies the injury according to the direction of mechanical instability either as stable, rotationally unstable or completely rotationally and vertically unstable. The second is based on a clinical and radiological survey of a large number of injuries and describes the injury on the basis of the direction of the force that was applied and the resulting fracture pattern. These two systems are complementary. In the emergency patient where acute haemorrhage is the major factor, the Young and Burgess classification is the most useful.[10] This classification considers the injuries with regard to the direction of force, the injury being caused by an anteroposterior compression (A-P), a lateral compression (L-C), or a vertical shear injury. There is also a multidirectional complex injury group. A-P and L-C injuries can be further subdivided into types 1, 2 and 3 according to the degree of disruption. Diagrammatic representation of the progress of events during an A-P injury to the pelvis is shown in Figure 52.1. Initially only the pubic symphysis is split (type I), then the pelvis floor tears and the anterior sacroiliac joint is ruptured, but the posterior ligaments remain intact, acting as a hinge (type II). The final stage (A-PII) is complete separation of the whole hemipelvis and rupture of the posterior ligaments, allowing full mobility of that hemipelvis.

The value of this classification is that the fracture pattern on X-ray can be directly related to the risk of major pelvic haemorrhage and associated injuries (Fig. 52.2).[10] The greatest risk of haemorrhage is with the more severe anteroposterior injuries, particularly those where the trauma has been severe enough for the hemipelvis to be avulsed both anteriorly and posteriorly (A-PIII). This injury, which has been called 'the internal hemipelvectomy', is most often seen in motorcycle injuries when the pubis is forced against the wedge-shaped petrol tank, or when the affected limb

Table 52.2 Classification of pelvic ring injuries: Tile classification

A	Rotationally or vertically stable
B	Rotationally unstable but vertically stable
C	Rotationally and vertically unstable

Table 52.3 Young and Burgess classification

AP I, II, III	Injuries caused by anteroposterior compression of increased severity
LC I, II, III	Injuries caused by lateral compression of increasing severity
VS	Vertical shear injuries
Combined	Combined complex injuries

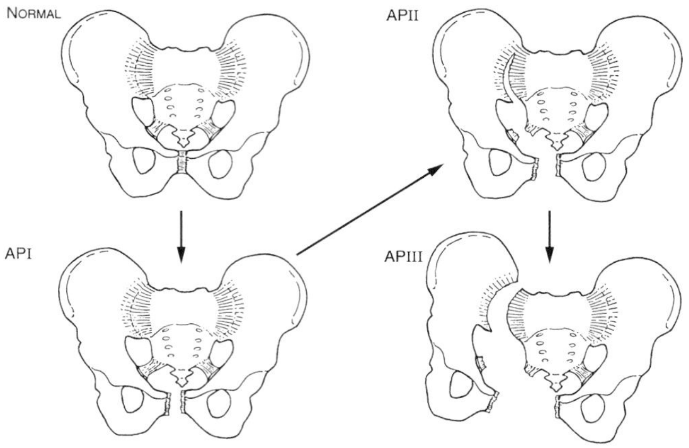

Fig. 52.1 A diagram to show the ligamentous structure of the pelvis and the progress of ligamentous injury during an anteroposterior compression injury to the pelvis producing first a pubic tear, then a rotational unstable pelvis (Tile grade B) and AP II injury, and finally a completely unstable pelvis (Tile grade C) AP III injury.

REFERENCES

5. Smith R M, Airey C M, Franks A J Injury 1994; 26 (suppl 2): 23–24
6. Boot et al. British Trauma Society, Leeds 1995. Injury in press
7. Tile M J Bone Joint Surg 1988; 70B: 1–12
8. Tile M Pelvic Fractures (61): Comprehensive Classification of Fractures. M E Muller Foundation 1995
9. Young J W R, Burgess A R Radiologic Management of Pelvic Ring Fractures: Systematic Radiographic Diagnosis. Urban & Schwarzenberg, Baltimore 1987
10. Advanced Trauma Life Support Instructor Manual. American College of Surgeons, Chicago 1993

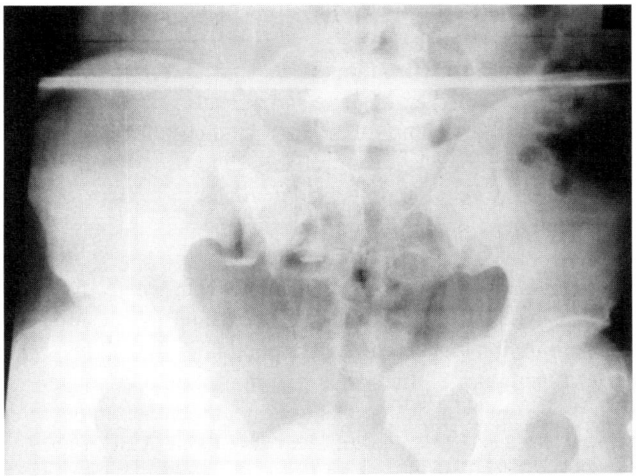

Fig. 52.2 X-ray examination of an AP III severe pelvic fracture with a high risk of major haemorrhage. Note the poor quality of rapid XRs taken in there is enough detail, however, to indicate the severity of the injury. © Medical Illustration, St James's University Hospital, Leeds.

has suffered a very severe abduction injury, effectively externally rotating the whole hemipelvis. It is easily recognized by the widely separated pubis on routine anteroposterior pelvic radiographs and by external rotation of the relevant hemipelvis (Fig. 52.3). Haemorrhage occurs from the bony surfaces, from torn veins around the anterior aspect of the sacroiliac joints and occasionally from torn arteries, particularly the superior gluteal. This haemorrhage is readily accommodated in the damaged pelvis and the patient can exsanguinate. The vast majority of pelvic bleeding is low-pressure venous bleeding[11] from bone and soft tissue. Only in very few injuries is the haemorrhage from major vessels and this has an important implication for management in that direct surgical attempts at open control of bleeding vessels is rarely indicated, although anterographic embolization is popular in the USA.

Lateral compression fractures are more common than anteroposterior compression fractures. They range from the most minor injury, where a simple fracture of the pubic ramus follows a fall on the side, to severe injuries with internal rotation of the whole hemipelvis. They are graded by severity using the Young and Burgess classification[9] as lateral compression I, II or III. The most severe lateral compression fracture of the pelvis occurs when a car hits the side of a pedestrian or when a car occupant is hit by a side impact. Significant haemorrhage can occur in these injuries but it is usually less than is seen in severe anteroposterior compression injuries. Lateral compression fractures are, however, often associated with severe local soft tissue injury caused by spikes of the pubic rami being driven across the midline and damaging the bladder, urethra (see chapters) or other pelvic contents, and are a major indicator that haemorrhage may occur from other sites. A patient with severe hypovolaemic shock with a lateral compression fracture of the right hemipelvis should be suspected of having a liver rupture or chest contusion on the right side; whereas a patient with a severe lateral compression fracture of the left hemipelvis should be considered at high risk of left chest injury or a ruptured spleen. These guidelines are not absolute but an understanding of the mechanism and resulting injury patterns can indicate a likely source of haemorrhage in these patients.

a

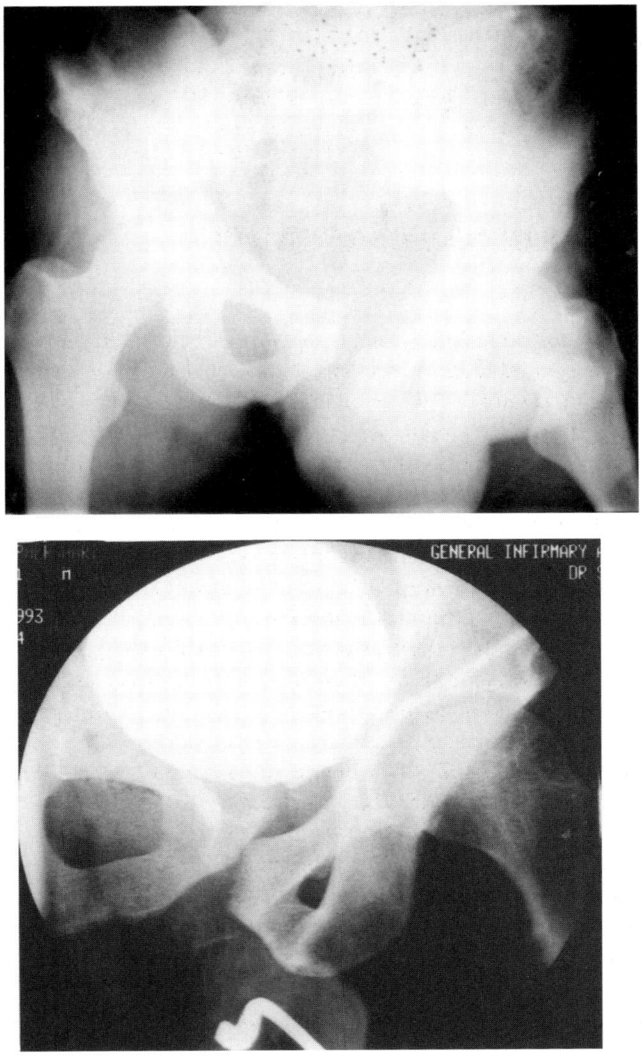

b

Fig. 52.3 (**a**) Severe lateral compression fracture of the pelvis with a fractured ilium and overriding pubis. (**b**) Cystogram and urethrogram showing a disruption in the membranous urethra associated with this injury. © Medical illustrations, St James's University Hospital, Leeds.

Vertical shear injuries are often caused by a fall, with the whole of the hemipelvis being displaced upwards. Vertical shear injuries can also cause severe haemorrhage and are also associated with severe soft tissue injury or other bony injury. (Fig. 52.4).

Emergency management of pelvic haemorrhage

Any patient who has been severely injured should be resuscitated along the advanced trauma life support (ATLS) guidelines[10] (see

REFERENCE

11. Smith R M Curr Orthop 10(1)

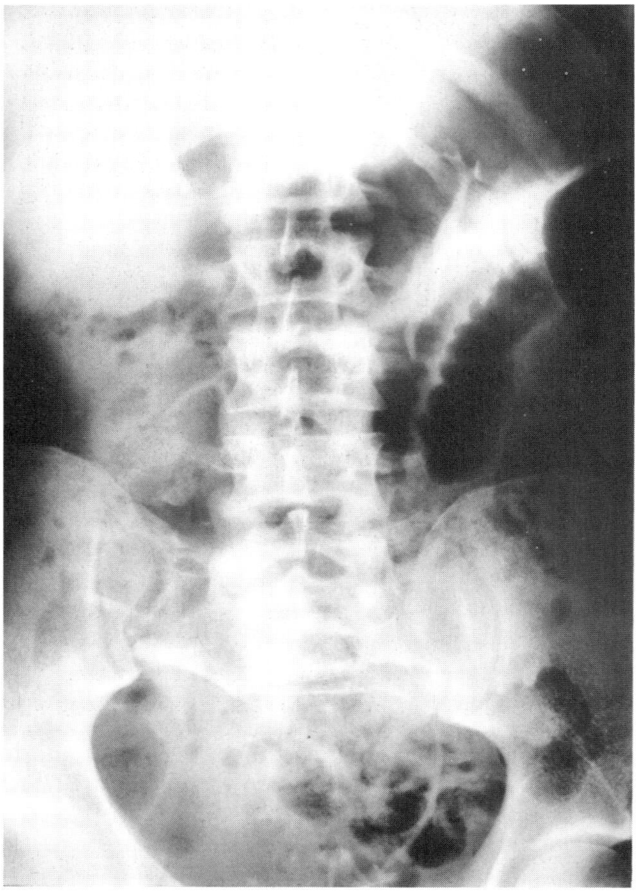

Fig. 52.4 Vertically unstable pelvic fracture with bilateral sacral fractures. In this patient there was an associated avulsion of the right kidney. © Medical Illustration, St James's University Hospital, Leeds.

Ch. 7). A rapid assessment of circulatory status is performed and the pelvis assessed by obtaining an anteroposterior pelvis radiograph in the standard. Some understanding of the mechanism of pelvic injury helps a great deal in the assessment of this radiograph and may point to the source of haemorrhage in a hypovolaemic patient. External fixation frames[1,2] have become the best means of controlling pelvic haemorrhage. These devices bring together the widely open pelvic ring, so reducing the pelvic volume and approximating the bleeding bony surfaces, stopping haemorrhage in the vast majority of cases. This reduction of the pelvic ring can be accomplished by simple direct pressure and then held by the external fixation frame. This is so important that any orthopaedic and accident and emergency department accepting major trauma patients should have staff with the understanding and ability to apply a pelvic frame and a constantly available device for emergency use.[11] The frames are applied to the front of the pelvis, after pins have been placed in the anterior aspect of the iliac crest. Some units use a posterior fixation frame to try and bring together the posterior pelvis, which is where most of the haemorrhage occurs, using a C clamp. Centres in Europe with specialist expertise have surgeons who prefer to immediately open, fix and pack the severely bleeding pelvis.[12] In the United States the application of an external fixation frame followed by angiographic assessment of the deep pelvic arteries and embolization of any bleeding vessels is more popular.[13]

Laporatomy alone is contraindicated without pelvic fixation in the presence of the hypervolaemic patient with a severe pelvic fracture. This simply decompresses an expanding pelvic haematoma which then often bleeds uncontrollably. It is usually sufficient to apply an anterior fixation frame and then proceed to laparotomy as intra-abdominal bleeding sources outside the pelvis can, of course, coexist.

These patients, inevitably, have major problems from the after affects of hypovolaemic shock and other injuries and almost all require admission to an intensive care unit after injury. The degree of soft tissue injury is often such that they should be nursed on a low-pressure air-bed. Rapid institution of parenteral or enteral nutrition (see Ch. 2) is also thought to be beneficial in speeding recovery.

Mechanical instability

Surgical care of an unstable pelvis is the task for a specialist. Not all unstable pelvic injuries cause severe hypovolaemic shock and an external fixation device does not always need to be applied as a life-saving measure. The posterior structures are responsible for stability in the normal pelvis, and a full assessment of these is made after injury with inlet and outlet views on a full film as described by Penall[14] and best illustrated by computed tomography (CT) scanning. The pelvis is a bony ring and it has been shown that even the most minor anterior injury is associated with some degree of posterior injury, even if this is only detectable by bone scanning. The surgeon assessing a pelvic injury on X-ray must carefully follow the bony contours of the whole pelvis both anterior and posteriorly, and must remember that the pelvic ring itself is a complex three-dimensional structure which is not seen in profile on a simple anteroposterior film. Accordingly fractures often lie outside the plane of the X-ray and may be difficult to see. On scrutiny of the AP film, particular attention should be paid to the sacral foramina where fractures are often found. The inlet film demonstrates whether the hemipelvis has moved backwards and the outlet film whether it has moved upwards. All three films plus the CT scan should then be considered together so that a three-dimensional concept of the position of the pelvic ring, where it has pivoted and where it has remained intact, can be formulated before reduction and fixation are performed. A major danger with the popularity of external fixation frames is that if the injury is a lateral compression fracture, application of the frame and an attempt to push the pelvic ring together is of no benefit and only leads to worsening of the deformity.

The stable fractured pelvis does not require surgical intervention. There are many specialist maneouvres available for the

REFERENCES

12. Platz A, Friedl H P, Kohler A, Trentz O Helv Chir Acta 1992; 58(6): 925–929
13. Stock J R, Harris W H, Athanasoulis C A Clin Orthop 1980; 151: 31–40
14. Pennal G F Clin Orthop 1980; 151: 12–21

management of the unstable pelvis. Long-term external fixation for three months or pubic plating can be used to stabilize the anterior part of the ring while posteriorly sacroiliac joint plating on its anterior surface, posterior sacral bars or iliosacral screws all have their place. In severely unstable injuries the posterior soft tissues are often degloved and tenuous and this can cause problems for the posterior fixation, sometimes making it impossible. A simple anterior external fixation frame cannot stabilize the back of the pelvis but it has been shown by Tile[15] that double or pubic plating combined with an anterior external frame is the best alternative technique to control the posterior pelvis. The posterior pelvis can be approached if the tissues allow using stabilization from the intact to the mobile hemipelvis with sacral bars or iliosacral screws for a sacral fracture and an anterior iliosacral (retroperitoneal) plate for sacroiliac dislocation.

Occasionally, after lateral compression fractures, marked internal rotation of the pelvis occurs which can lead to an inability adequately to externally rotate the affected leg. In this situation it is worth placing an anterior external fixation frame and externally rotating the pelvis as early as possible in order to correct the deformity.

The late problems include deformity with limb rotation or shortening and posterior pelvic pain. The rotation and shortening rarely require treatment but posterior pelvic pain is common after severe posterior injury and as yet there is no solution. Occasionally non-union of the ilium or sacrum (Fig. 52.5) can occur, but these can be treated surgically with gratifying results. The other cause of long-term disability is a persisting neurological deficit after sacral plexus injury. This is unfortunately not uncommon but in this situation very few reconstructive options are available.

Soft tissue problems

Pelvic fractures are not simply a 'bone' injury. There is always accompanying muscle and local soft tissue damage, and visceral, urogenital and rectal injuries are also common. In the male, the urethra is anchored by the penile crura and the membranous urethra is the most common site of damage (see Ch. 39). Hallmarks of urological injury are scrotal haematoma, blood at the urethral meatus and a high-riding prostate. Injuries to the bladder can be extra- or intraperitoneal, depending on the mechanism of injury and the state of bladder filling at the time. Clearly the management of these injuries is the province of a combined orthopaedic and urological team. It is essential that the urethral reconstruction is planned jointly. Early reconstruction and reduction of the pelvis has the advantage of bringing together the urological structures, making reconstruction easier. The poorly planned use of a suprapubic catheter can compromise further bony pelvic reconstruction and this delay can make subsequent urological surgery much more difficult.

Rectal tears or open pelvic fractures into the perineum are an indication for immediate pelvic stabilization and diversion of the faecal stream by an end colostomy placed high in the abdominal wall, well away from the pelvis. The rectal stump must be washed out completely and the open fracture treated by debridement, copious lavage and appropriate soft tissue care to prevent further

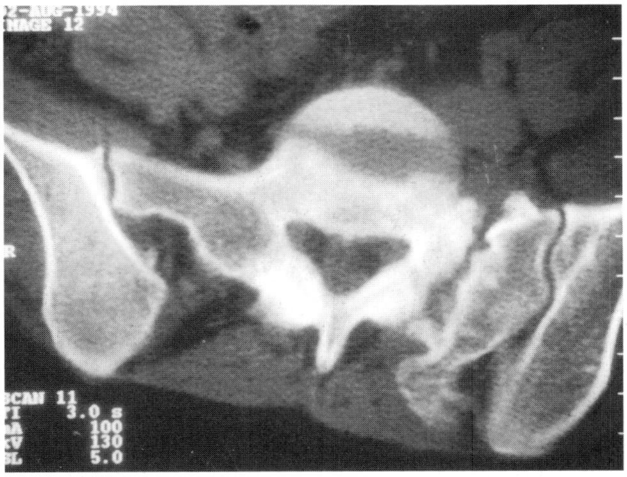

Fig. 52.5 Established non-union of the sacrum shown on CT scanning. © Medical Illustration, St James's University Hospital, Leeds.

contamination. As in all other open fractures, the results are significantly improved by immediate stabilization of the bony structures and avoidance of further contamination. Open pelvic fractures can carry a mortality of up to 50% and require careful management from a multidisciplinary team.

Fractures of the acetabulum

In contrast to pelvic ring injuries where life-saving and long-term pelvic stability are the priority, acetabular fractures rarely threaten life but carry a high risk of subsequent degenerate arthritis in the hip, which causes pain and disability. The surgical treatment of acetabular fractures has been significantly advanced by the late Emile Letournel, who followed on from the Judet brothers.[4] In common with any other articular fracture, residual displacement leads to a high risk of late degenerative change, whereas open reduction and internal fixation to produce a congruent reduction can lead to a much lower instance of degenerative arthritis–possibly as low as 10–15%.[4] The results depend on the initial severity of the disruption, the success of surgery and the fracture type. The accuracy of reduction, particularly of the articular dome as defined by Matta, is the main influence of an eventual outcome.[16] The surgery of these injuries is complex, fraught with complications and in, itself, can create significant morbidity. The approach depends on the fracture type, which can be classified by either the Letournel[17] or the AO systems.[18] Classification is aided by oblique views (Judet) and CT scanning, which are essential

REFERENCES

15. Tile M Fractures of Pelvis and Acetabulum, 1st edn. 1984; 10: 132–146/7
16. Matta J M, Merritt P O Clin Orthop 1998; 230: 83–97
17. Letournele E Fractures of the Acetabulum. Springer-Verlag, Berlin 4: 63–66
18. Judet R J, Letournele E, Tile M, Helfet D, Nazarian S Comprehensive Classifications of Fractures: Acetabulum Fractures. M E Muller Foundation, 1995

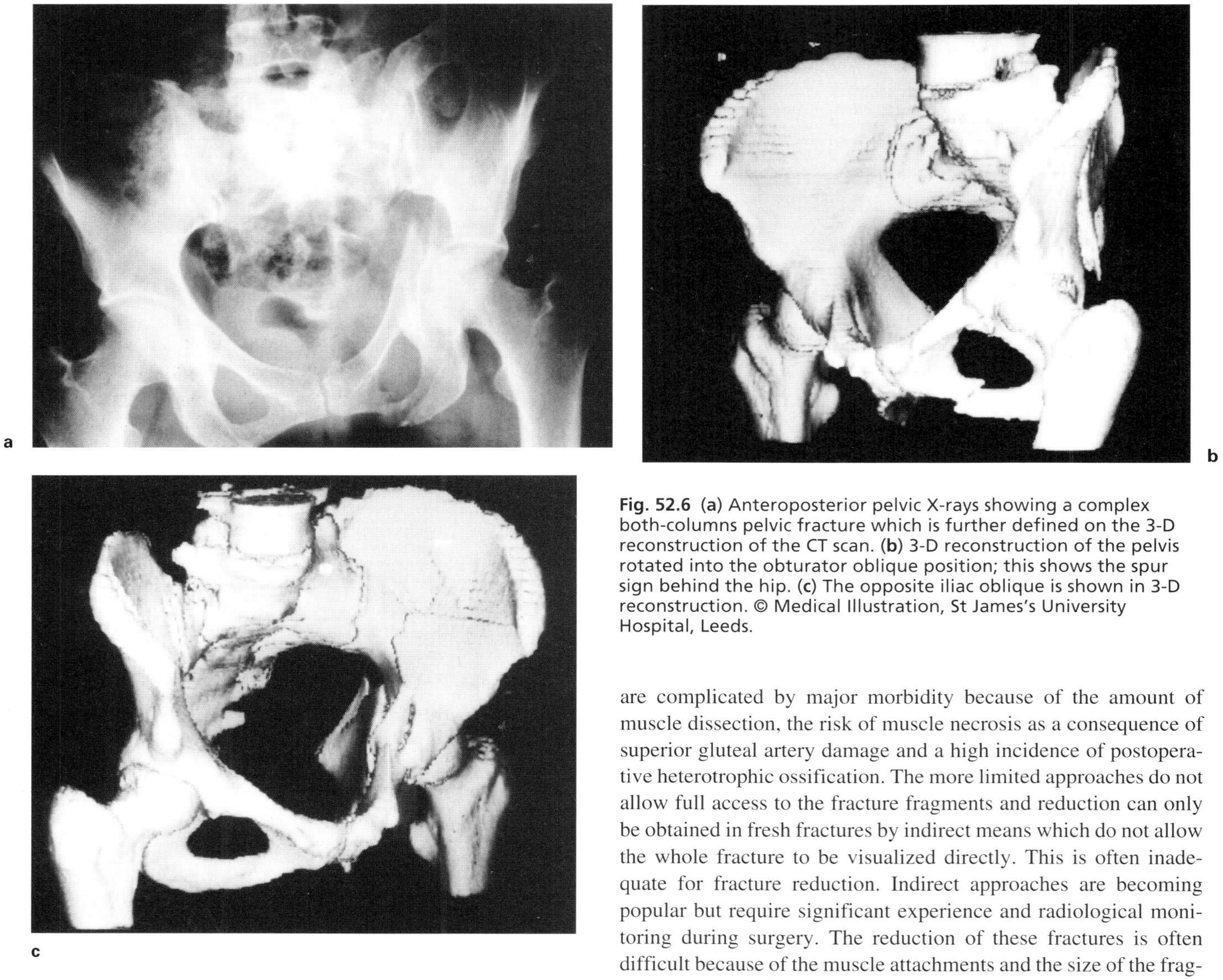

Fig. 52.6 (**a**) Anteroposterior pelvic X-rays showing a complex both-columns pelvic fracture which is further defined on the 3-D reconstruction of the CT scan. (**b**) 3-D reconstruction of the pelvis rotated into the obturator oblique position; this shows the spur sign behind the hip. (**c**) The opposite iliac oblique is shown in 3-D reconstruction. © Medical Illustration, St James's University Hospital, Leeds.

investigations. In many centres a three-dimensional CT scan is used to provide additional information (Fig. 52.6).

The surgical approaches can be considered as those that are on the outside of the pelvis, exposing either the posterior column (Kocher–Langenbeck), anterior column (iliofemoral) or whole lateral surface of the ilium (extended iliofemoral); and approaches on the inside of the pelvis which allow access to the false and true pelvis, and include the ilioinguinal approach, which goes through the back of the inguinal canal or the Stoppa approach, which is a modification of a Pfannenstiel incision. The more extensive approaches on the outside of the pelvis are required to reduce the more complex and particularly older fractures. All these approaches are complicated by major morbidity because of the amount of muscle dissection, the risk of muscle necrosis as a consequence of superior gluteal artery damage and a high incidence of postoperative heterotrophic ossification. The more limited approaches do not allow full access to the fracture fragments and reduction can only be obtained in fresh fractures by indirect means which do not allow the whole fracture to be visualized directly. This is often inadequate for fracture reduction. Indirect approaches are becoming popular but require significant experience and radiological monitoring during surgery. The reduction of these fractures is often difficult because of the muscle attachments and the size of the fragments and weight of the limb which needs to be manipulated. Special operating tables, distraction devices and specific reduction clamps are required in order to provide reduction. Extra-long screws, plates and special drills are also needed. All of these factors make acetabular reconstruction the province of the specialist. There is a significant risk of nerve and vessel injury during these major approaches to the pelvis and many units perform acetabular reconstruction while continuously monitoring sciatic nerve function.[19]

REFERENCE

19. S Venables et al J Electrophysiol Technol 1995; 21: 183–18

53 Fractures of the lower limb

J. R. W. Hardy P. J. Gregg

INTRODUCTION

This chapter considers the modern management of fractures of the lower limb. The term fracture is defined as a loss of the normal continuity of bone diaphysis, metaphysis, physis, epiphysis and joint cartilage. Trauma is the commonest cause of fracture to the lower limb. Fractures are commonly seen in patients with multiple trauma, in which case the management of the skeletal injury follows only after the management of life-threatening injury (cf. Ch. 7). The age of a patient determines the pattern of a fracture and level of energy required to break a bone (cf. Ch. 50). In the lower limb the fracture neck of femur is typically associated with osteoporosis in the elderly female. Predisposing factors for fracture after a single loading insult depend on the type, rate and magnitude of the force as well as the underlying structural and material properties of the bone. This explains why a fall from standing fractures the femoral neck in an osteoporotic older patient, while a young man's hip survives a single load of the same proportions.

The symptoms and signs of fractures are dependent on the stability of the skeleton after fracture and injury to the surrounding soft tissues. All clinically suspected fractures (i.e. a history of an injury and pain) must be further investigated.

Modern classifications of lower limb fractures consider the patterns of bony injury within each region of the lower limb.[1] This is the AO classification, which divides each bone into three segments, each segment into three types (usually depending on the number of fragments), each type into groups of three (depending on the pattern of fracture) and each group is subdivided into three subgroups. The pattern of this classification reflects the increasing severity of injury experienced by the bone segment. Management of the fractures of each of the AO segments is considered later in this chapter. The AO classification is not yet exhaustive of all patterns of injury.

Classifications, other than just the pattern of bony injury, allow the clinician to consider a sensible approach to treatment. Fractures of the lower limb may be classified according to their site, the associated soft tissue injury, the number of fragments, their displacement, and any associated complications.

The prognosis depends on the severity of the injury, the age of the patient, their general condition, the restoration of function, the prevention of deformity, and the minimization of treatment complications.

Complications of the lower limb bone fractures are common, as are complications of treatment. The complications that attend the fractures themselves are considered separately. The complications of treatment should be classified into general complications or local complications. Local complications vary depending on the region of fracture and the method of treatment. As the optimum treatment depends on the fracture classification, complications of treatments are considered on a regional basis.

THE CLINICAL HISTORY OF LOWER LIMB FRACTURE

A history of pain following injury, regardless of how insignificant the trauma might seem, should always suggest the possibility of a fracture. This is especially true in the elderly with osteoporotic bone. Likewise a fracture that results from cyclic stress (fatigue) is often missed unless a careful history is taken of the onset, the duration and the periodicity of the pain. A history of pain in the foot or tibia following long periods of exercise, regardless of the minimal signs present, should always be further investigated by radiographs. The symptoms of fracture in the lower limb may include pain, deformity and a loss of function.

THE PHYSICAL SIGNS OF LOWER LIMB FRACTURES

The physical signs of a fracture may be surprisingly minimal and depend on the pattern of injury. An undisplaced fracture often allows preservation of function. This cannot therefore be taken as an indication that the bone is intact. The usual signs of fracture include tenderness at the fracture site, swelling, bruising, deformity and occasionally crepitus of the fractured ends of the bone. Crepitus should not be specifically elicited during the examination process but it is occasionally discovered. The 'Look, Feel, Move' principle provides a logical order for eliciting signs.

INVESTIGATION OF LOWER LIMB FRACTURES

Radiographs have been the mainstay of investigation since 'X-rays' were developed in Germany by Röntgen.[2] A useful adage in the investigation of fractured limbs is the 'rule of 2'. This is that

REFERENCE

1. Müller M E, Nazarian S, Koch P, Schatzker J The Comprehensive Classification of Fractures of Long Bones. Springer-Verlag, Berlin 1990

two radiographs should always be taken with views at 90° to each other; the radiographs, like the clinical examination, should always include the two joints either end of the long bone; radiographs taken at two intervals in time are often required and occasionally radiographs of the two sides for comparison of the normal anatomy can be useful. When a fracture is suspected but not visible on the early radiographs more can be done. The clinician who suspects an occult fracture in the lower limb can either wait for the fracture line to become more visible with time and resorption, or resort to a radioisotope bone scan. When a fracture is present around the knee involvement of the joint can be deduced if the lateral radiograph of the knee shows a fluid/fat level. Magnetic resonance imaging (MRI) is particularly useful for demonstrating associated soft tissue injury and bone 'bruising' if occult fractures through the metaphysis are difficult to visualize radiographically.

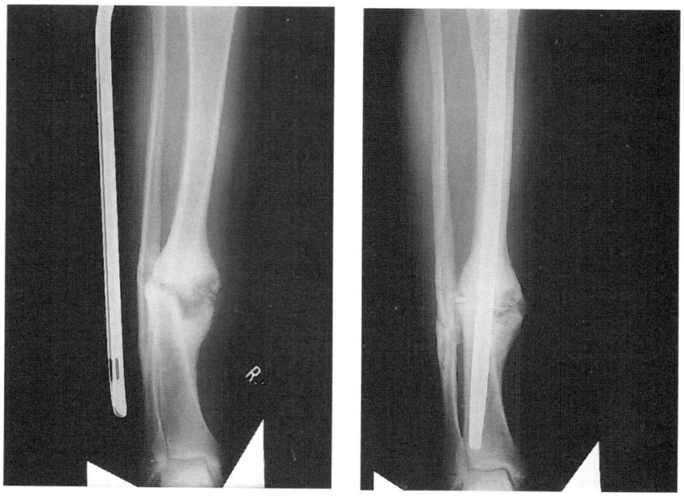

a b

Fig. 53.1 Hypertrophic non-union is treated by stabilizing a fracture as with this intramedullary nail. Bone grafting is not required as it is with atrophic non-union.

COMPLICATIONS OF FRACTURES IN THE LOWER LIMB

Delayed and non-union

Delayed union is one of the commonest complications following fractures of the lower limb, especially in the tibia.[3] Delayed union is defined as having taken place 'when clinical union of the fracture occurred after more than 20 weeks of immobilization'.[4,5] Clinical union is said to have occurred when 'pressure over the fracture and "springing" the bone fails to elicit pain'.

The current convention is that non-union has occurred when clinical and radiographic union has not happened within six months of fracture.[4] Some authors have extended this definition to 30 weeks[6] and eight months.[5]

In atrophic non-union of the tibial diaphysis patients take more than six months to produce the callus needed to reduce fracture site movement enough to begin the remodelling process. Atrophic non-union in association with a fracture gap and a united or intact fibula may respond to partial fibulectomy.[7] The standard treatment includes bone grafting.

The next commonest type of non-union again occurs in the tibial diaphysis. This is associated with the excessive production of callus due to too much movement at the fracture site: hypertrophic non-union (Fig. 53.1).

Refracture

The risk of refracture in weight-bearing bones is higher than in the upper limb. Refracture following removal of plates used for treating tibial shaft fractures can be as low as 1.7%.[8] Failure of bone in these circumstances is probably from a single load rather than fatigue loading. Fracture may occur at the original site or through screw holes. After dynamic compression plating most refractures occur through a screw hole.

Refracture rates are less predictable after external fixation of the lower limb. This is especially true following premature fixator removal,[9,10] it is twice as common when supplementary lag screws are used.[11] Refracture probably occurs either with a single load large enough to break the callus bridge or by fatigue failure at lower loads and tends to occur during sport. All patients should be warned to avoid contact sports until at least 12 months after removal of a plate. In adults Böstman found the incidence of refracture of tibial fractures to be 2.4%. Refracture occurred most commonly in spiral fractures, those with a fracture of the fibula at a different level from that of the fibula and those with marked initial displacement.[12] Refracture is a common complication of external fixation. New methods of determining the progression of fracture healing by the serial measurement of fracture stiffness[13] have been reported and may help to reduce refracture in the tibia.[14]

REFERENCES

2. Wilhelm Konrad Röntgen 1845–1923. German physicist, who in 1894 published an original paper on the medical use of X-rays. On 7 January 1895 the technique was reported in the London Evening Standard
3. Anderson R, Burgess E J Bone Joint Surg 1943; 25: 427–432
4. Ellis H J Bone Joint Surg 1958a; 40-B: 42–46
5. Johner R, Wruhs O Clin Orthop 1983; 178: 7–25
6. Oni O O A, Hui A, Gregg P J J Bone Joint Surg 1988; 70-B: 787–790
7. DeLee J C, Heckman J D, Lewis A G J Bone Joint Surg 1981; 63-A: 1390–1395
8. Bilat C, Leutenegger A, Ruedi T Injury 1994; 25(6): 349–358
9. Rommens P, Broos P, Gruwez J Arch Orthop Trauma Surg 1986; 105(3): 170–174
10. Gershuni D H, Halma G J Trauma 1983; 23(11): 986–990
11. Krettek C, Haas N, Tscherne H J Bone Joint Surg 1991; 73-A: 893–897
12. Böstman O M Injury 1983; 15(2): 93–98
13. Hardy J R W, de Jonge E J, Richardson J B J Orthop Techniques 1994a; 2: 177–189
14. Richardson J B, Kenwright J, Cunningham J L Clin Biomechanics 1992; 7: 75–79

Table 53.1 Gustilo and Anderson's classification of open fractures which was based on a large series of tibial fractures

Gustilo and Anderson Type	*Soft tissue injury*	*Bony injury*
0	Skin intact	Any except segmental fractures
I	Less than 1 cm laceration and clean	Any except segmental fractures
II	More than 1 cm laceration. No extensive soft tissue damage, flaps or avulsions	Any except segmental fractures
IIIa	Adequate soft tissue coverage despite extensive laceration or flaps, or high-energy trauma irrespective of size of wound	Any
IIIb	Extensive soft tissue injury loss with periosteal stripping and bone exposure. Usually associated with massive contamination	Any
IIIc	Arterial injury requiring repair.	Any

Compound fractures

All compound wounds must be treated aggressively.[15] The Gustilo classification was specifically devised for the management of tibial fractures (Table 53.1). It is often applied to any compound fracture, dividing open wounds into three 'types'.[16–18] The revised Gustilo classification takes into account the mechanism of injury, the degree of soft tissue damage, the fracture configuration and wound contamination.[19] External fixation is the mainstay of management of compound fractures in the lower limb because of the reluctance to leave foreign material within a contaminated wound. Metal, like any inert material, can act as a nidus for bacterial infection. Compound fractures tend to be as a result of high-energy injuries and are associated with much periosteal stripping. Therefore, they are often complicated by delayed union as well as by deep infection.[20]

The treatment of compound wounds has been considered (cf. Ch. 50). Operative management should never be delayed more than 6 hours. In the leg a tourniquet may be applied but should not be used unless uncontrolled haemorrhage is discovered. Two to ten litres of saline must be used to irrigate the often larger wounds of the lower limb. In these circumstances the risk of cross-infection of the patient from bacterial ingress through wet drapes, and of the theatre staff from viral infection, necessitates use of universal precautions and modern drapes which entrap blood and irrigation fluids (Fig. 53.2).

The patient's lower limb should be elevated in the postoperative period until the skin has healed in order to reduce the risk of tissue fluid leakage on mobilization and subsequent infection. Patients should be encouraged to exercise their lower limb during this period of elevation. A fixed plantigrade foot should be prevented by the early use of a backslab or anti-foot-drop orthosis.

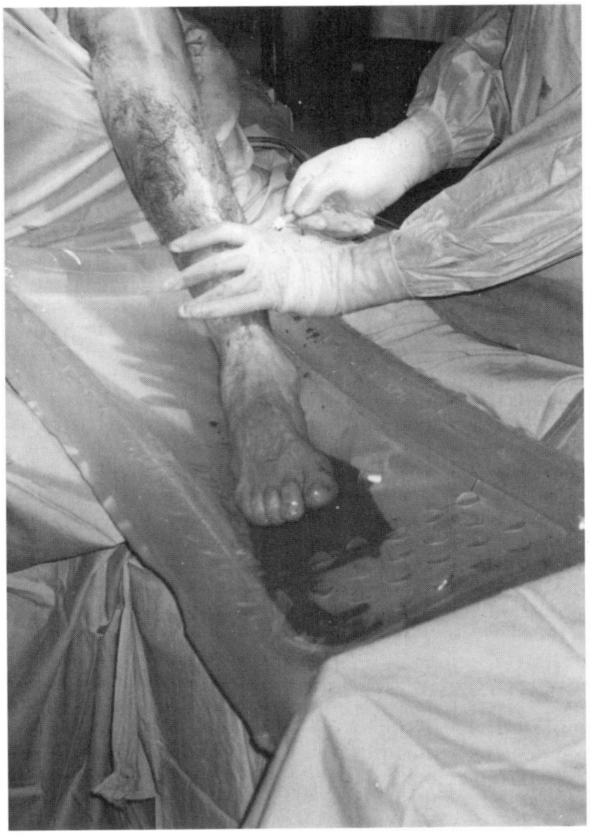

Fig. 53.2 Use of an inflatable surgical tray to reduce the risks of exposure to theatre staff to 'substances hazardous to health' as preached by COSHH regulations.

Infection

Both superficial and deep infection can complicate a fracture. Superficial infection is commonly a postoperative complication related to the general condition of the patient and the skin closure technique. In most series deep infection (osteomyelitis) is a rare event following fractures of the leg but is still most common in patients with a compound fracture. To avoid infection in the leg most practices employ modern compound fracture management and have abandoned using plaster casts with transfixing pins.[21,22]

REFERENCES

15. Report by the BOA/BAPS working party on severe tibial injury. January 1993
16. Gustilo R B, Anderson J T J Bone Joint Surg 1976; 58-A: 453–458
17. Gustilo R B, Mendoza R M, Williams D N J Trauma 1984; 24(8): 742–746
18. Gustilo R B, Gruninger R P Orthopaedics 1987; 10: 1781–1788
19. Gustilo R B, Merkow R L, Templeman D J Bone Joint Surg 1990; 72-A: 299–303
20. Dellinger E P, Caplan E S, Weaver L D Arch Surg 1988; 123: 333–339
21. Anderson L D, Hutchins W C South Med J 1966; 59: 1026–1032
22. Clancey G J, Hansen S T J Bone Joint Surg 1978; 60-A: 118–122

Deep infection (osteomyelitis) is important because it is associated with a doubling of the healing time[23] and can lead to other morbid conditions such as amyloidosis.

Operative fixation of a fracture, especially a compound fracture, is associated with a higher incidence of osteomyelitis.[24] Bone and Johnson showed, in a series of closed nailing for tibial fractures, that for Gustilo Grade II and III wounds, there was 10 times the risk of infection compared with the closed or Grade I wounds.[25] This may be reduced to 10–16% of Gustilo Type II–III wounds by aggressive debridement and early soft tissue cover.[26,27]

Externally fixed fractures tend to have a low incidence of deep infection unless the wound is compound. Most pin tract infection is superficial but deep infection can occur and this leads to sequestra at the site of the pin which may have a ring shape if the dead compressed bone around the pin becomes involved. Screw and plate fixation is probably best avoided in any compound fracture.[28] Other authors would argue that while Type II–III open fractures are probably best treated by external fixation[29] lesser injuries may be either plated, nailed or externally fixed.

Malalignment and shortening

No useful definitions exist for malunion. Most definitions relate the condition to imperfect restoration of the premorbid anatomical position of the fracture fragments. In clinical practice the term is reserved for cases in which the resulting deformity is felt to be clinically significant.

The long-term sequelae of malunion are unknown. Deformity is usually cosmetically unacceptable. There is also the belief that if the centre of gravity of the weight of the body is displaced from the centre of the knee or ankle joint then osteoarthritis will result. This is anecdotal. Many a surgeon has seen post-traumatic osteoarthritis after a perfect reduction and restoration of the normal biomechanical axis of the limb.

Post-traumatic osteoarthritis

Injury to joint cartilage and subchondral bone is common following direct or indirect trauma to joints. Even trauma not detectable on normal radiographs can cause subchondral fracture that leads to hastened degenerative changes.[30,31] More obvious irregularities of the joint surface following fracture lead to rapid degenerative changes; these also occur following vascular insult to the subchondral bone such as is seen after avascular necrosis following intracapsular fracture neck of femur.

Neurovascular complications

Neurovascular complications are common following leg injuries, especially after dislocation of the knee. Both nerve and vascular injuries can be direct or indirect. Indirect injury of nerves and vessels from compartment syndrome is often overlooked. Correction of vascular compromise of a limb must take place at the earliest opportunity and takes precedence over the fixation of bone. Compartment syndrome that requires treatment occurs in about 3% of all tibial fractures.

Compartment syndrome

This is from increased pressure within a muscular compartment which leads to tissue necrosis. The symptoms are of ischaemic pain out of proportion to the injury and its early management is by splinting and analgesia. The signs are elicited by passive stretch of the muscles suspected of being involved. The tightness of the compartment and the presence of peripheral pulses cannot be relied on as useful signs. Impaired function of peripheral nerves suggests that the ischaemia is advanced. Classically compartment pressures are measured using a slit catheter device. Compartment pressures in excess of 30–35 mmHg in a normally perfused patient suggested the need for open compartment fasciotomy.[32] In patients without symptoms monitored pressures do not relate to outcome in any way.[33] However, there is recent evidence to suggest that if the difference between the diastolic pressure and the measured compartment pressure is less than 30 mmHg then fasciotomies should be performed. Management of this complication must be immediate, decisive and aggressive enough to divide the skin and deep fascial envelope the length of the limb as the skin envelope can significantly contribute to compartment pressures.[34] All compartments should be incised depending on the part of the lower limb involved. Débridement of necrotic muscle is necessary to minimize the effects of fibrotic contraction. Dead muscle being recognized by the 4 'Cs', namely lack of Colour, Consistency, Contractility and Capacity to bleed.

Nerve injury

Direct nerve injury following fracture in the leg is relatively rare. Fractures around the proximal fibula occasionally cause a dropped foot due to common peroneal nerve injury. The treatment of this is expectant as most direct injuries are due to neuropraxia and over 70% resolve within months. Persistent lesions more than six months after injury should be investigated and nerve grafting considered. Compartment syndrome should always be considered with dropped foot, even in the presence of a proximal fibula fracture.

REFERENCES

23. Edwards P, Nilsson B E R Acta Orthop Scand 1965; 36: 104–111
24. Klemm K W, Börner M Clin Orthop 1986; 212: 89–100
25. Bone L B, Johnson K D J Bone Joint Surg 1986; 68-A: 877–887
26. Court-Brown C M, Christie J, McQueen M M J Bone Joint Surg 1990b; 72-B: 605–611
27. Court-Brown C M, McQueen M M, Quaba A A, Christie J Bone Joint Surg 1991; 73-B: 959–964
28. Clifford R P, Beauchamp C G, Kellam J F, Webb J K, Tile M J Bone Joint Surg 1988; 70-B: 644–648
29. Bach A W, Hansen S T Clin Orthop 1989; 241: 89–94
30. Radin E L, Parker H G, Pugh J W, Steinberg R S, Paul I G, Rose R M J. Biomechanics 1973; 6: 51–57
31. Atkinson P J, Haut R C J. Orthop Res. 1995; 13: 936–944
32. Bourne R B, Rorabeck C H Clin Orthop 1989; 240: 97–104
33. Triffitt P D, Konig D, Harper W M, Barnes M R, Allen M J, Gregg P J J Bone Joint Surg 1992; 74-B: 195–198
34. Cohen M S, Garfin S R, Hargens A R, Mubarak S J J Bone Joint Surg 1991; 73-B: 287–290

Vascular injury

Vascular injury complicating fractures of the leg is rare but the consequences when it occurs can be severe. Vascular injury is most common with fractures and dislocations around the knee. Immediate clinical diagnosis is imperative and pallid, pulseless, paraesthetic, paralysed, painful, 'perishing' cold limbs should never be ignored. An on-table arteriogram may be used to diagnose the level of the injury and should be performed to facilitate early reperfusion of the limb by a trained vascular surgeon. Fixation of the fracture before or after reperfusion should be discussed with the vascular team. Fasciotomy will be necessary for almost all limb fractures complicated by arterial injury and should be performed as soon as reperfusion has been established and not left until signs of nerve envolvement have developed.

Avascular necrosis

This is most common following intracapsular fractures of the neck of femur in the lower limb. It also occurs after fractures of the femoral condyles and after talar neck fractures. In the talus the presence of Hawkins' sign (rarefaction of the bone beneath the subchondral region of the talar dome) demonstrates the presence of an intact vascular supply to the talus.

Reflex sympathetic dystrophy

Sudeck's atrophy, Sudeck's osteodystrophy or post-traumatic painful osteodystrophy is characterized by pain, swelling and loss of the ability to weight-bear. This is especially seen following fracture below the knee where patients treated in plaster have been reluctant to weight-bear for long periods. Early recognition and treatment by intensive supervised rehabilitation with analgesia is more successful than neglect. Occasionally, sympathetic nerve block may be helpful.

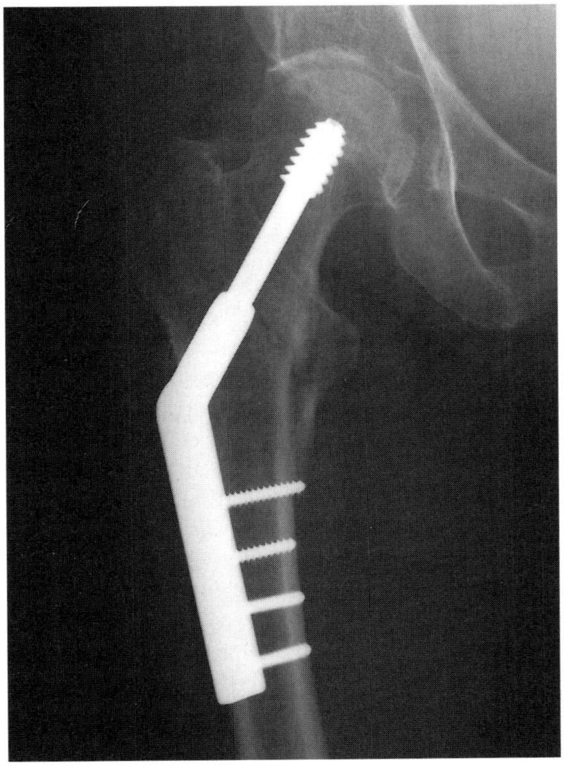

Fig. 53.3 An extracapsular proximal femoral fracture immobilized with a dynamic hip screw.

Often referred to as Sudeck's atrophy, Sudeck's osteodystrophy or post-traumatic painful osteodystrophy, it is characterized by pain, swelling and loss of the ability to weight-bear. Marked joint stiffness is a late manifestation as is swelling and loss of skin creases. Radiographs show a patchy osteoporosis. This is not uncommon following leg fracture, especially with fractures below the knee where patients treated in plaster have been reluctant to weight-bear for long periods. Early recognition and treatment with intensive supervised rehabilitation with analgesia and physical therapy is more successful than neglect. Occasionally, sympathetic nerve block is used as an adjunct to regular analgesia before physical therapy.

FRACTURES AND DISLOCATIONS OF THE LOWER LIMB

The femur

Proximal femoral fractures

Proximal femoral fractures are classified into three types: extracapsular, intracapsular and fractures of the femoral head (Fig. 53.3). The last is usually seen in the younger patient with traumatic dislocation of the hip joint. This classification is useful as it describes the risk of avascular necrosis for the injury. Intracapsular fractures have the greatest risk of non-union and avascular necrosis. A commonly quoted classification for intracapsular fractures is Garden's classification, which helps determine the management of the intracapsular fracture based on a study of prognosis.[35] Garden's classification is based on the anteroposterior radiograph and describes the relationship of displacements between the femoral head, the femoral neck and the acetabulum (Figure 53.4). Apart from the displacement at the time of injury the prognosis also seems to depend on the time from injury to reduction and internal fixation.

Typical symptoms of proximal femoral fracture are of pain following a fall onto the hip. Whether this occurs in the young or elderly the fracture is often minimally displaced and the patient may not lose function, although there are symptoms of pain following the fall and often radiation to the thigh. This is commonly interpreted as a minor condition not warranting radiological investigation and the fracture is missed. Beware the patient who has a spontaneous pain in the hip, which could have suffered an insufficiency fracture due to severe osteoporosis. Beware also the patient with pain predominantly referred to the thigh. Any injury to a long bone necessitates both examination and radiological investigation of the joints above and below the symptomatic

REFERENCE

35. Garden R S J Bone Joint Surg 1964; 46-B: 630–647

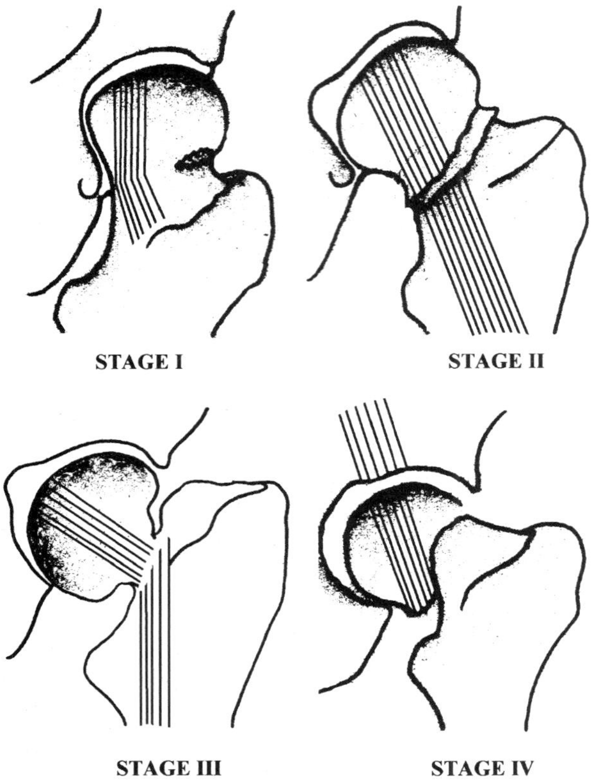

Fig. 53.4 Garden's classification of intracapsular fractures. Note that the alignment of the medial femoral trabeculae helps to stage the fractures. The alignment of trabeculae in the medial calcar region is only related to the acetabular trabeculae in stage IV injuries, which have the highest incidence of avascular necrosis.

long bone. Displaced proximal femoral fractures cause shortening, adduction and external rotation of the lower limb. The joint may be tender to palpation and hip movements are usually painful. The fracture is often visible on anteroposterior and lateral radiographs but not always. Repeat radiographs over one to two weeks in a suspected case of undisplaced intracapsular fracture while allowing the patient to weight-bear is an acceptable management of the occult fracture. Prior to definitive treatment elderly patients may need resuscitation, as their fall is frequently the result of a cardiovascular event.

The aims of treatment are to provide pain relief and to achieve early mobilisation so as to prevent the complications of bedrest. The added benefit of reducing the cost of hospital care is also important. Early mobilisation requires the cooperation of the physiotherapy and occupational therapy departments. Provision of rehabilitation wards for patients with a high chance of achieving a return to independent living reduces the cost of care for this common injury. Despite the tendency towards surgical management of these fractures the decision to operate depends on the presence of complications, the general condition of the patient and the aetiology of the fracture.

Femoral head fractures

These are commonly associated with joint dislocation. Pipkin classified these intra-articular fractures into four types. Type I fractures occur below the ligamentum teres. Type II fractures involve the weight-bearing portion of the head above the ligamentum teres. Type III fractures include fracture of the head with intracapsular fracture of the femoral neck. Type IV injuries are associated with an acetabular fracture. For all these injuries the state of the femoral head needs to be reassessed once reduction has been performed. Any loose fragments need to be excised. Open reduction and internal fixation should be performed if the fragment is large or involves the weight-bearing area. Total arthroplasty might be considered a treatment option if the fracture occurs in an elderly person.

Intracapsular fractures

The aim of treatment is to provide pain relief and early mobilization to prevent the complications of bedrest. Patients with a displaced intracapsular fractured neck of femur sometimes benefit from a period of temporary skin traction prior to definitive fixation. The treatment for intracapsular fractures depends on the age of the patient. Hemiarthroplasty should be avoided in favour of internal fixation in patients under the age of retirement. In this group the fracture should be reduced early,[36] reduced completely[37] and immobilized using a dynamic hip screw with an anti-rotation device or parallel hip screws. The vascularity of the femoral head may be investigated with ^{99m}Tc radioisotope scintigraphy using pinhole collimetry to enhance the sensitivity.

A primary cemented hemiarthroplasty is indicated for an intracapsular fracture in patients over 65 years, in those with severe osteoporosis, or in those not fit enough to undergo subsequent total hip replacement operation should avascular necrosis occur.[37] The anterior approach is associated with a lower six-week mortality rate and a lower incidence of postoperative dislocation than the posterior approach.[38,39] Bipolar replacement should be reserved for younger patients who are expected to live longer than one year as it is associated with better subjective outcome.[40]

Extracapsular fractures

The Boyd and Griffin classification is commonly used to describe these fractures and this has become especially useful with the introduction of the new reconstruction nails and intramedullary hip screws to treat the Boyd and Griffin Type III fracture. This classification divides fractures into those which are stable with little tendency to collapse, and those which are biomechanically unstable (Fig. 53.6). Type I fractures are traditionally treated with dynamic sliding screws and plates (Fig. 53.3). Biomechanically the screw

REFERENCES

36. Swiontkowski M F, Winquist R A, Hansen S T J Bone Joint Surg 1984; 66-A: 837–846
37. Garden R S. J Bone Joint Surg 1971; 57-B: 437–443
38. Chan R N W, Hoskinson J J Bone Joint Surg 1975; 57-B: 437–443
39. Lu-Yao G L, Keller R B, Littenberg B, Wennberg J E J Bone Joint Surg 1994; 76-A: 15–25
40. Calder S J, Anderson G H, Harper W M, Jagger C, Gregg P J J Bone Joint Surg 1995; 77-B: 494–496

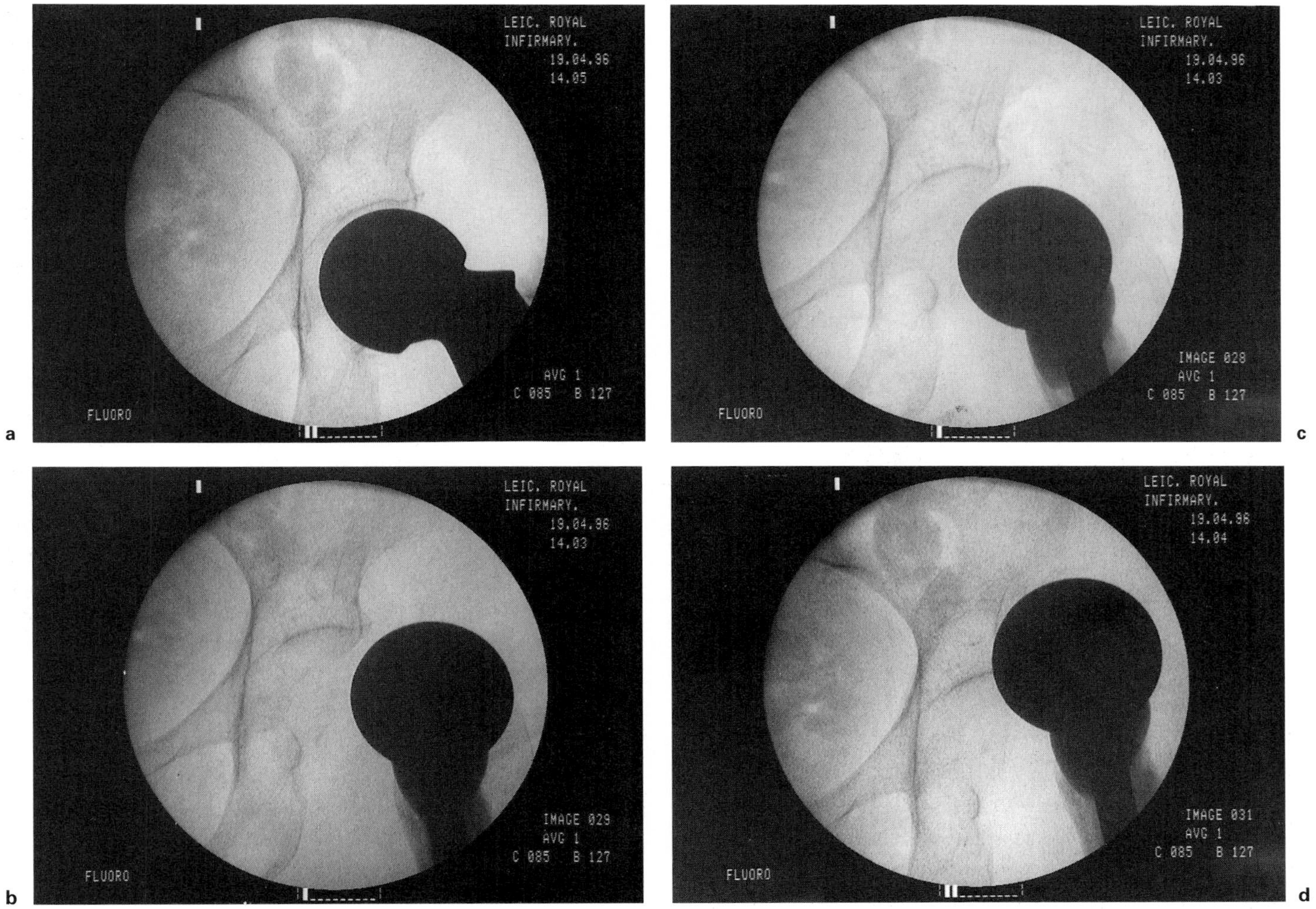

Fig. 53.5 Series of dislocating Thompson's hemiarthroplasty prosthesis **(a–d)**. One local complication that can occur any time after operation.

is best placed centrally along the femoral neck or posterior and inferior to this central axis. For Type II and III fractures a reconstruction nail or intramedullary hip screw is appropriate. When the fracture is complicated by medial com-munition a posteromedial buttress graft should also be considered. For pathological fractures a calcar replacing hemiarthroplasty should be performed. Occasionally it is prudent to move the distal fragment medially so that a calcar spike is located down the medullary canal of the femur, which confers an axial stability not offered by a sliding screw and plate alone.

Femoral diaphyseal fractures

Classifications

A number of classifications have been proposed for diaphyseal fractures. The AO classification[41] is based on the presence of comminution, the pattern of the fracture and whether it is in the upper, middle or lower third of the bone. This classification does not take into account the poor prognosis of subtrochanteric fractures, especially those with medial comminution.

Treatment

Conservative treatment may be appropriate for patients who have a high morbidity and mortality from surgical treatments, for example those with compound fractures or patients with concomitant illness. In these circumstances abduction and flexion of the proximal fragment can be matched by 90–90 traction.[42] This is traction on the limb with the hip and knee in 90° of flexion. Most fractures can be treated in the early stage with traction followed by intramedullary nailing.

The use of a dynamic hip screw for subtrochanteric fractures is well established and safe when there is no medial wall comminution. A dynamic hip screw can be protected from failure as a result of communition of the medial wall by bone grafting and protected weight-bearing. Intramedullary techniques can be used when the

REFERENCES

41. Müller M E, Nazarian S, Koch P, Schatzker J The Comprehensive Classification of Fractures of Long Bones. Springer-Verlag, Berlin 1990
42. Obletz B E J Bone Joint Surg 1946; 24: 113–116

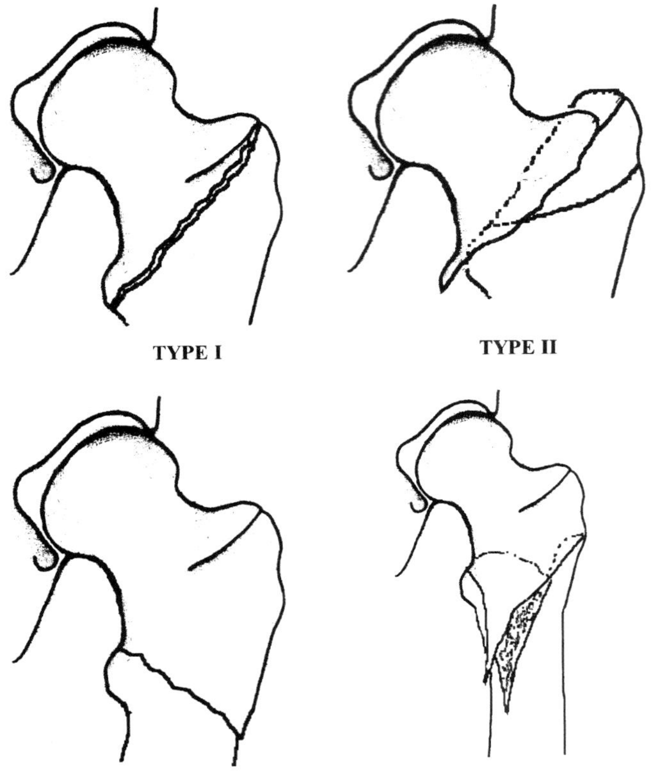

Fig. 53.6 The Boyd and Griffin classification.

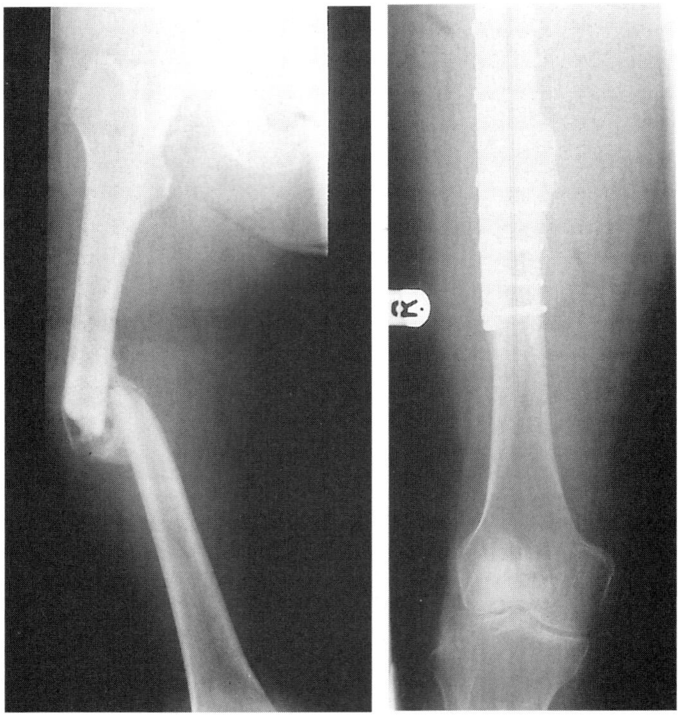

a b

Fig. 53.7 Open reduction and compression plating has been used to correct a malunion of the femoral diaphysis.

medial buttress is known to be axially unstable[43] and devices used include Enders nails, the gamma nail, intramedullary hip screw, reconstruction nail and intramedullary interlocking nails. Enders' nails, while simple, provide little in the way of protection against rotation or shortening for axially unstable fractures. Intramedullary nails have revolutionized the prognosis for comminuted subtrochanteric fractures but their use depends on the presence of an intact greater trochanter and piriform fossa to give biomechanical stability of the proximal nail. An intramedullary reconstruction nail is particularly useful for fractures with the most proximal comminution. The use of external fixation is associated with a high incidence of pin site infection and knee stiffness, so should be reserved for compound Type III fractures with heavy soiling. Extramedullary fixation requires open reduction and internal fixation using dynamic compression plates (Fig. 53.7).

This is particularly useful in children where transgression of the physis is contraindicated. The great majority of femoral shaft fractures in children are best managed conservatively using traction, with internal fixation only when traction fails to achieve reduction, when there are complications of traction, or for loss of reduction, or lastly for the definitive fixation of uncontaminated compound wounds prior to delayed closure.

Distal femoral fractures

Supracondylar fractures of the knee become more common with advancing age and may be associated with a previous knee arthroplasty in the elderly. The AO classification usually separates supracondylar fractures into those that are extra-articular, those that involve one condyle only and those that involve both condyles. Fractures about the knee can be complicated by vascular injuries. If any doubt exists that the popliteal artery has been injured, even after Doppler pressure measurement, then the advice of a vascular surgeon should be sought. An arteriogram must be performed so that distal ischaemia can be corrected immediately (cf. Ch. 10).

The management of these fractures, when not associated with a vascular injury, is initially conservative using skin traction on a Thomson's splint for comfort prior to operative fixation. Extra-articular fractures more than 8 cm above the joint line may be immobilized by a locked intramedullary femoral nail. Those fractures extending to within 8 cm of the condyles but not including the condyles may be treated with a dynamic condylar screw and blade plate.

Recent introduction of the supracondylar nail, which is passed retrogradely through a hole made in the supracondylar notch, has made intramedullary fixation of low comminuted femoral fractures much easier.

Fixation of unicondylar fractures should be performed using a mixture of lag screw and a dynamic condylar screw and plate. Similarly bicondylar fractures should be stabilized using a dynamic condylar screw and plate as well as a buttress plate on the contralateral side, should this be necessary.

REFERENCE

43. Bergman A T, Metzger P C, Bosacco S J et al Orthop Trans 1979; 3: 225–228

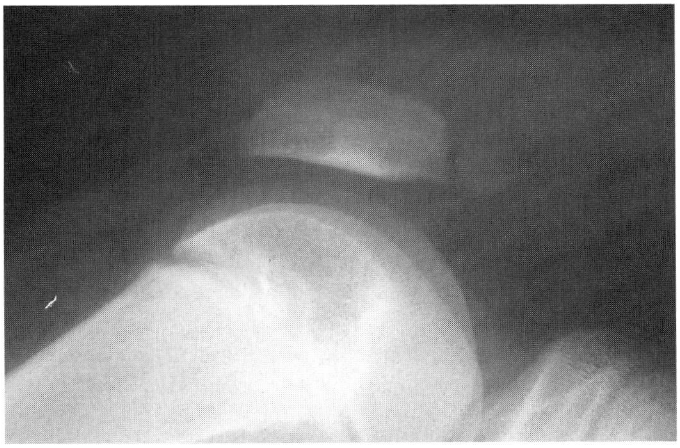

Fig. 53.8 Sleeve fracture of the inferior pole of the patella.

Patellar fractures

Patellar fractures are relatively common. They may be caused either by direct or indirect force, indirect injury causing an avulsion of the superior or inferior pole of the patella. In the skeletally immature this is called a sleeve fracture (Fig. 53.8). A direct blow to the patella is a more common cause of fracture in the skeletally mature. Undisplaced sleeve fractures are treated conservatively in a cylinder cast for four to six weeks followed by rehabilitation. Significant displacement of a sleeve fracture is anything more than 1–2 mm. Wider displacements are associated with an intact straight leg raise but if left untreated a patella magna develops with almost invariable late anterior knee symptoms. Open reduction is best performed early when the displacement is significant.

Patella fractures can be classified according to the site of fracture, the pattern of fracture, whether the fracture is displaced or undisplaced and whether the quadriceps mechanism is intact or ruptured. The latter can be deduced on examining the straight leg raise. Undisplaced fractures where the quadriceps mechanism is demonstrably intact may be treated in a cylinder cast for a period of three to six weeks followed by mobilization of the patellofemoral joint. Open reduction internal fixation should be considered if there is a loss of ability to straight leg raise, loss of congruence of the articular surface of the patellofemoral joint or if there is greater than 1 mm of separation of fragments on the lateral radiograph. Because of the periarticular nature of the blood supply of the patella a figure-of-eight tension band wiring is the method of choice for its immobilization. Circlage wires should be avoided because they are associated with a high incidence of non-union (Fig. 53.9). Rehabilitation with early continuous passive motion depends on the stability and adequacy of fixation.

The tibia

The classifications for fractures of the tibia are many and varied. In this section fractures are considered by anatomical site according to the AO classification of fractures.

Proximal tibial fractures

In the AO classification[44] proximal tibial and fibula fractures are divided into those that are extra-articular, those that involve part of the articular surface and those involving whole condyles. The AO classification is comprehensive but incomplete as it has not

REFERENCE

44. Müller M E, Nazarian S, Koch P, Schatzker J The Comprehensive Classification of Fractures of Long Bones. Springer-Verlag, Berlin 1990

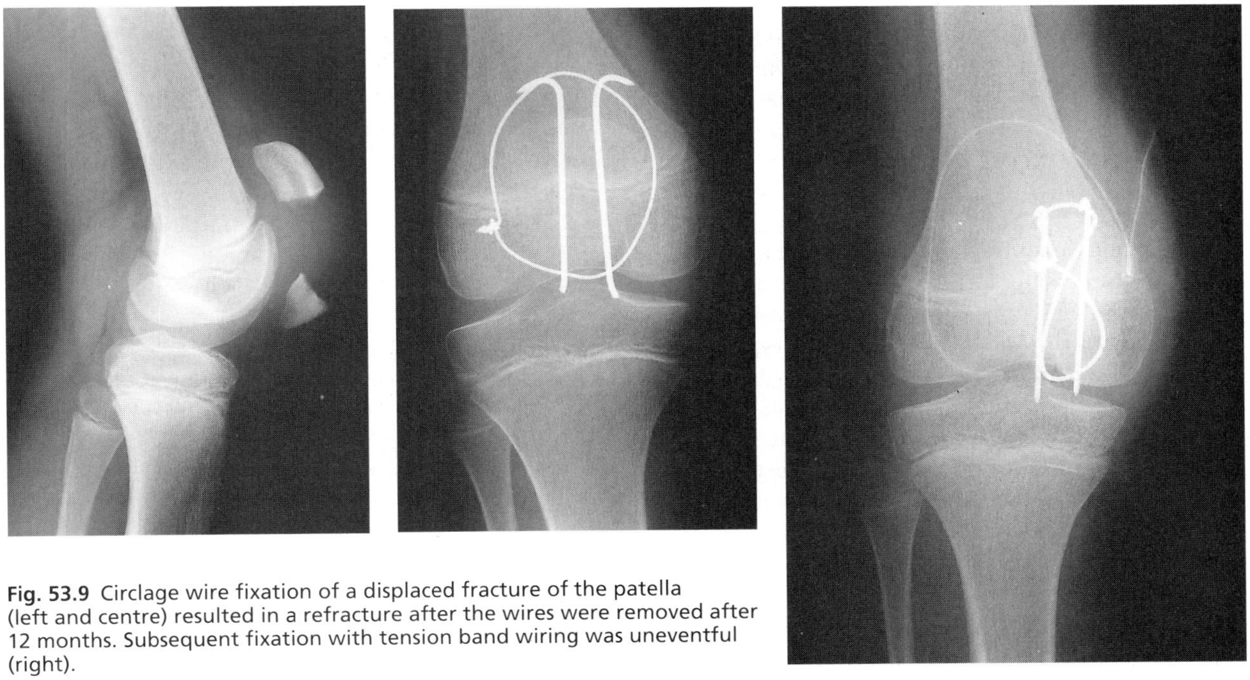

Fig. 53.9 Circlage wire fixation of a displaced fracture of the patella (left and centre) resulted in a refracture after the wires were removed after 12 months. Subsequent fixation with tension band wiring was uneventful (right).

included the Segond lesion, which is an extra-articular avulsion fracture of part of the lateral collateral ligamentous expansion into the tibial metaphysis. The classification does not guide the surgeon as to how the injury should be treated and there is no correlation between the classification and the final outcome. The AO classification is partly evolved from Hohl's classification of 1967, which was based on a series of 805 patients.[45] Hohl's classification only included intra-articular fractures of the condyles. Mayers and McKeever[46] developed a separate classification of tibial plateau fractures in 1977. Schatzker et al classified intra-articular fractures of the tibial plateau with recommended treatments for each type.[47]

Fractures of the lateral tibial condyle are the most common. They generally result from a severe valgus stress in the young or more minor injuries in osteoporotic patients. With increasing load other structures around the knee joint are involved and fracture of the fibula neck, rupture of the medial collateral ligaments and occasionally rupture of the cruciate ligaments commonly coexist. A more vertical force combined with valgus stress such as a fall from a height may be associated with a die-punch fracture of the lateral tibial condyle. The lateral femoral condyle causes comminution of the articular surface of the tibia. Isolated fractures of the medial tibial condyle are uncommon and are usually associated with lateral ligament ruptures and neuropraxia of the common perineal nerve. The clinical findings of a proximal tibial fracture include a haemarthrosis, bruising, skin abrasions on the side of the fracture and often tenderness over the contralateral collateral ligament complex. There may be a valgus or varus deformity of the knee. Special investigations include anteroposterior, lateral and oblique X-rays of the knee. The AP should be performed with the beam at an inclination of 115° to take into account the posterior slope of the tibia[48] To estimate the degree of depression of the tibial condyle tomograms, computed tomographic (CT) scanning and MRI scan are recommended. Hohl and Luck recommended that a step of less then 4 mm should be treated conservatively and anything greater than this should be treated by reduction and internal fixation.[49] Only Porter has ever found a direct correlation between the depth of step and the final outcome. He demonstrated that 80% of patients had poor results if the depression was more than 1.4 cm.[50]

Treatment

Undisplaced extra-articular tibial spine fractures can be treated conservatively in a cylinder cast for four weeks prior to rehabilitation.

It is recommended that significantly displaced avulsions of the cruciate ligament insertions (Mayers and McKeever Types II, IIIa and IIIb) are reduced and internally fixed.[51]

For tibial plateau fractures treatment largely depends on the age and the extent of the deformity which occurs at the knee with loading. Patients should be examined under anaesthetic to estimate this deformity prior to a definitive decision on treatment.[52] All patients under the age of 60 years should in general have joint congruity restored and this usually requires open reduction and internal fixation. Patients over the age of 60 with a step of less than 4–5 mm and a deformity of less than 10° can be treated conservatively. Patients with a greater step and a larger deformity should be treated surgically depending on their general condition. In certain circumstances primary arthroplasty might be considered the treatment of choice. The prognosis of these injuries depends on the severity of injury and the amount of late deformity. Late varus deformity is associated with a higher incidence of symptomatic osteoarthritis in the long term.[53]

Conservative treatment includes a period of traction on a Thompson splint. This should be converted as soon as comfort allows to Perkins traction on a Hadfield split bed with skin traction of 3 kg or more and early restoration of quadriceps exercises. After three or four weeks the patient may be mobilized in a cast brace with restoration of weight-bearing between eight and 12 weeks. The worst results are obtained after conservative treatment is combined with prolonged immobilization.[54]

When open reduction and internal fixation are indicated then the Schatzker type guides the method of fixation.[55] For instance a Schatzker type I split lateral plateau fracture may be reduced and immobilized using cannulated screws (Fig. 53.10). When percutaneous methods are being considered to treat Type I fractures then a preoperative MRI scan, or preoperative arthroscopy should be able to distinguish fractures with interposing menisci from those where the meniscus has not been caught in the fracture gap. When the whole spectrum of proximal tibial fractures is considered there is probably no correlation between radiographic degenerative changes and final functional result.[56]

Schatzker Type II fractures require elevation of the depressed articular surface through a cortical window made beneath the depressed condyle and impaction grafting with graft support using screw fixation. Most other Schatzker types require the latter or buttress plating or a combination of the two (Fig. 53.11). Elevation of deep depressions may require arthroscopic assistance.

The Segond fracture is treated conservatively if the lateral joint is stable or may be reduced and screwed into position if the injury involves a grade III collateral ligament injury (Fig. 53.12).

Tibial diaphyseal fractures

Tibial diaphyseal fracture healing depends on the patient's age, the tissue damage at the time of fracture and the method of immobilization of the fracture site. Fractures are classified according to whether they are compound or not, the severity of the compound wound, the axial stability of the fracture and the presence or

REFERENCES

45. Hohl M J Bone Joint Surg 1967; 49-A: 1455–1467
46. Meyers M H, McKeever F M J Bone Joint Surg 1959; 41-A: 209–222
47. Schatzker J, McBroom R, Bruce D Clin Orthop 1979; 138: 94–104
48. Moore T M, Harvey J P Jr J Bone Joint Surg 1974; 56-A: 155–160
49. Hohl M, Luck J J Bone Joint Surg 1956; 38-A: 1001–1018
50. Porter R B J Bone Joint Surg 1970; 52-B: 676–687
51. Meyers M H, McKeever F M, J Bone Joint Surg 1959; 41-A: 209–222
52. Rasmussen P S J Bone Joint Surg 1973; 55-A: 1331–1334
53. Rasmussen P S and Sorensen S E Injury 1973; 4: 265
54. Solonen K A Acta Orthop Scand 1963; 63: 1–32
55. Schatzker J, McBroom R, Bruce D Clin Orthop 1979; 138: 94–104
56. Apley G J Bone Joint Surg 1956; 38-B: 699–706

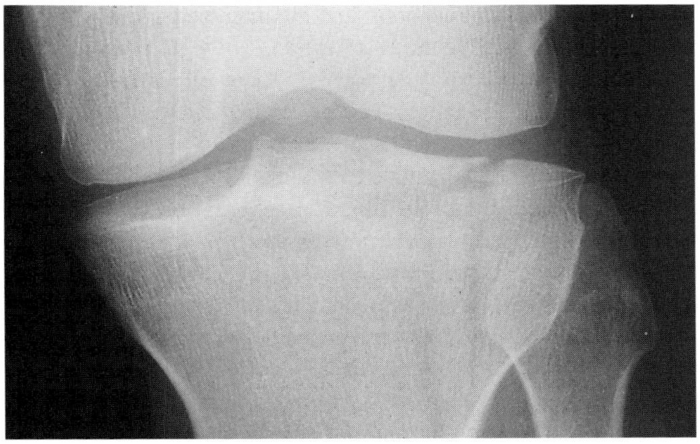

a

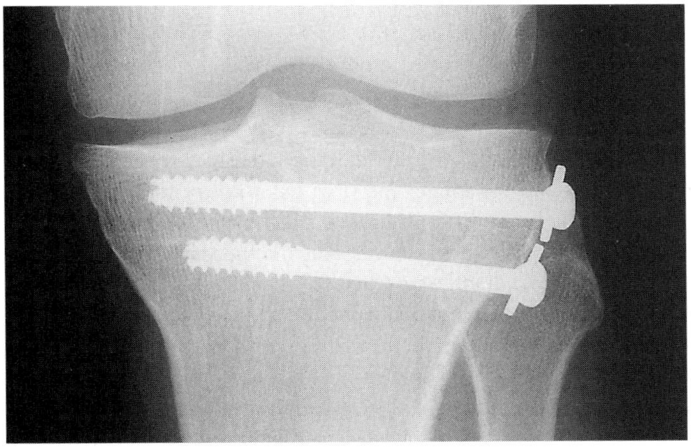

b

Fig. 53.10 Type I pure split fracture reduced with AO reduction forceps and then screwed using cannulated screws and washers.

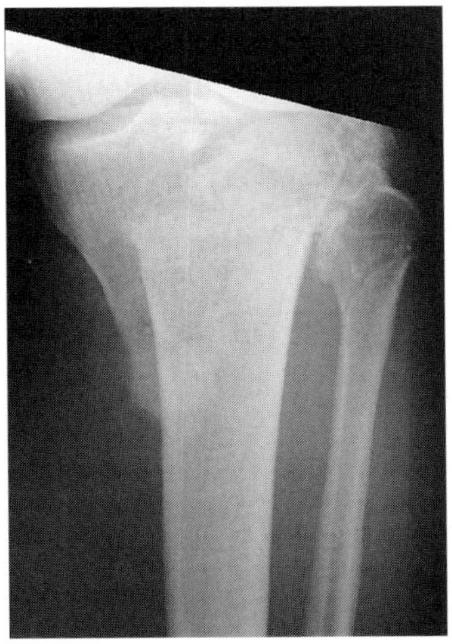

a

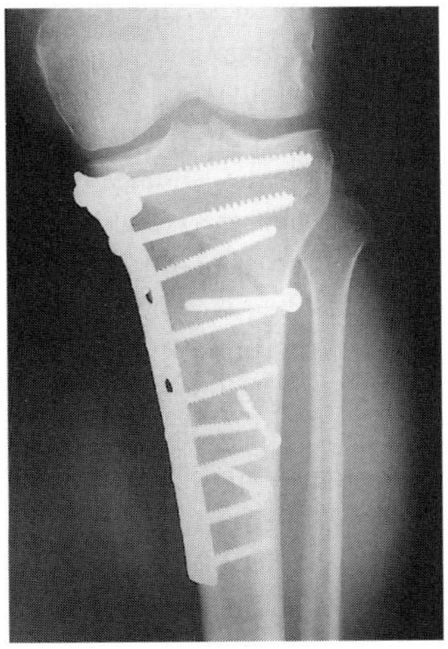

b

Fig. 53.11 A Schatzker Type V biocondylar fracture fixed with lag screws and a medial buttress plate. The buttress is placed on the side with the longest fragment.

absence of a periosteal hinge. An algorithm has been developed based on these classifications to select the most appropriate treatment.[57] This only applies to patients over the age of skeletal

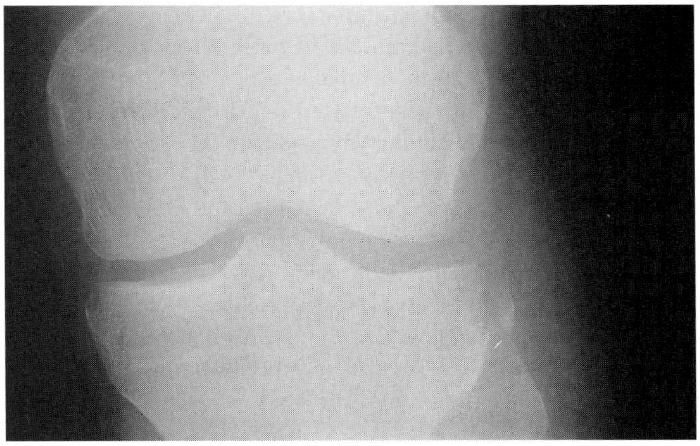

a

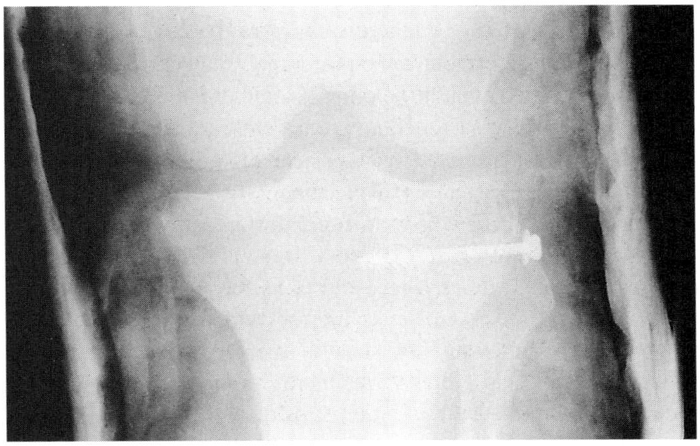

b

Fig. 53.12 Segond fracture of the lateral tibial plateau with an associated collateral ligament injury that has been repaired and the fragment screwed into place.

maturity. Patients under the age of 16 have few of the problems associated with fracture healing in adults.[58,59]

The severity of the soft tissue injury is the most difficult to assess. The soft tissues include skin, fat, muscle, tendon, artery, nerve and periosteum. Injury of the periosteal or soft tissue hinge, as described by Sir John Charnley, is often incorrectly ignored.[60]

Tissue damage depends on the magnitude of the injuring load, the rate of loading, the type of loading, the local structure of the tibia, the material properties of the bone and the soft tissues. The same energy may produce a different pattern of injury in an osteoporotic old person from that of an athletic young person.

The pattern of bone injury indicates the type of load that caused the fracture. A spiral fracture results from an indirect injury caused

REFERENCES

57. Hardy J R W, Richardson J B, Gregg P J Int J Orthop Trauma 1996; 6(2): 52–61
58. Ellis H J Bone Joint Surg 1958; 40-B: 42–46
59. Weissman S L, Herold H Z, Engleberg M J Bone Joint Surg 1966; 48-A: 257–267
60. Charnley J The closed Treatment of Common Fractures, 3rd edn. Churchill Livingstone, Edinburgh 1961.

by a torsion force. A simple transverse fracture occurs with a bending load and an oblique fracture occurs with bending while the bone is in compression. A more rapid rate, or a higher magnitude of loading, causes comminution of the tibia and a concomitant fracture of the fibula. The pattern of fracture also predicts its axial stability.

The degree of severity of bone injury is diagnosed from the history of the circumstances of injury, by examining the limb for bruising, tenderness, deformity and finally by special investigation. Two radiographs must be taken at 90° to each other. Patients with a history of a low-energy injury, little bruising over the shin, no deformity, an axially stable fracture, an intact fibula and an undisplaced fracture on X-ray can be expected to have most of the circumference of the periosteum left intact.

The closed and Gustilo type I injury

Patients with a closed or minimally compound (Gustilo Type 1, cf. Ch. 00) undisplaced fracture are preferably treated conservatively in plaster with early weight-bearing through the injured limb.

The management of a patient with a closed or Gustilo Type 1 displaced fracture is based on the state of the periosteal hinge. After an injury which causes displacement the periosteum is either divided in a part or the whole of its circumference.

The extent of the periosteal injury in the closed fracture should be assessed under general anaesthesia as the periosteum is well innervated and movement causes intense pain. The tibia should be reduced before assessing the state of the periosteum. An intact fibula usually means a stable low-energy injury. An oblique tibia fracture with an intact fibula often slips during healing into varus or develops hypertrophic non-union because the fibula holds the fracture gap apart. Hypertrophic non-union might be avoided in these fractures by perfect reduction. The fibula can be used as a fulcrum to guide the ends of the bones into perfect reduction (Fig. 53.13). A circumferential tear of the periosteum may be surmised if reduction is easy and the fracture, once reduced, is distractible. Accurate reduction and the maintenance of reduction are important to achieve the best healing.

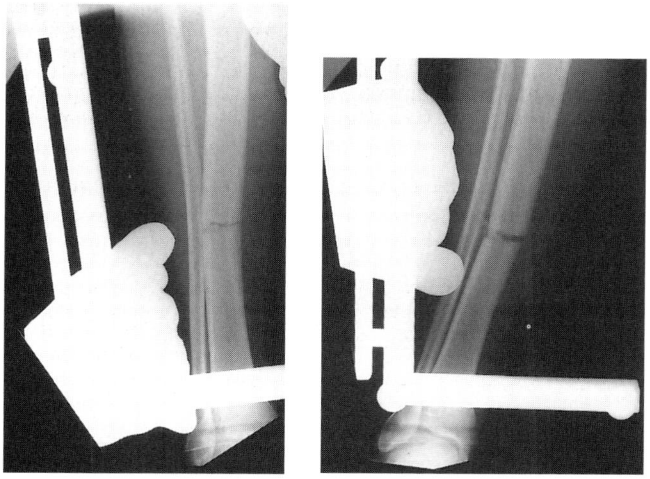

a b

Fig. 53.13 Examination under anaesthetic demonstrates the fracture to be stable with the periosteum intact on the lateral side. The intact fibula can be used as a fulcrum with which to guide accurate reduction of the fracture.

Transverse high-energy injuries, with no soft tissue hinge, are difficult to treat in plaster cast because early weight-bearing causes deformity. It is not known if these patients are best treated by open reduction and internal fixation with dynamic compression plates, by closed intramedullary nailing or by external fixation. External fixation in these circumstances may be the best method of immobilization although the postoperative management is arduous because the pin sites must be maintained clean and uninfected for long periods. Fractures that have no periosteal hinge and that are axially unstable are probably best treated using intramedullary fixation (Fig. 53.14) but screw fracture occurs in about 19%, so that early removal of the locking screws should be attempted. Screws should be deliberately left to protrude 5 mm through the distal cortex to aid removal of broken screws through a separate lateral incision if necessary (Fig. 53.15).

Scars around the knees should be avoided in patients whose occupation involves long periods of kneeling, e.g. clergymen and carpet layers.

Tibial fractures that are difficult to reduce usually have an intact periosteum, and the longer the time from injury to the attempted reduction the more difficult it is because the soft tissues contract. Tissue contracture is a good reason for the early and definitive management of a diaphyseal fracture. When reduction is prevented by an intact periosteum in a fully translated and shortened fracture, it is easiest to overcome the resistance by re-creating the deformity that occurred at the time of injury. This is the same principle that is used to reduce children's distal forearm fractures.[61] When reduction has been achieved the site of the periosteal hinge can be deduced by attempting to displace the fracture in anterior, posterior, medial and lateral directions.

A reduced axially stable fracture with an intact periosteal hinge is probably best treated with an above-knee plaster cast. The periosteal hinge is used to maintain reduction by using the plaster cast to provide two points of pressure against a third fulcrum, opposite the intact periosteum. Early weight-bearing is usually rewarded by appearance of callus and when this occurs the above-knee plaster can safely be replaced with a Sarmiento patellar bearing cast (Fig. 53.16). The patient with this pattern of injury should be encouraged to weight-bear as soon as the pain permits.

Walking in plaster is likely to cause a similar shortening if an axial load during anaesthesia demonstrates the fracture to be unstable to shortening. However, if the same patient has an intact periosteal hinge the likelihood of the fracture healing within 16 weeks is high. These patients may benefit from external fixation and the modern unilateral frames, which allow early unlocking of the telescoping device 'dynamization', permit enough movement at the fracture site to encourage callus formation. Early 'dynamization' also reduces the incidence of pin tract infection (Fig. 53.17) and aseptic loosening of the fixator pins (Fig. 53.18).

REFERENCE

61. Rang M Children's Fractures, 2nd edn. Lippincott, Philadelphia 1984

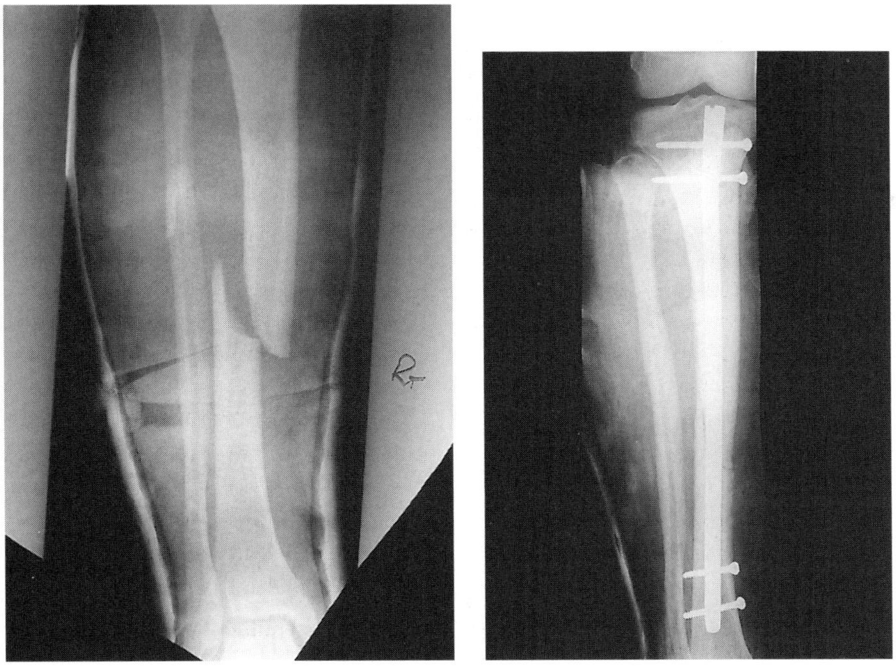

a b

Fig. 53.14 This was an axially unstable fracture that shortened in plaster cast, so intramedullary nailing was used with minimal reaming.

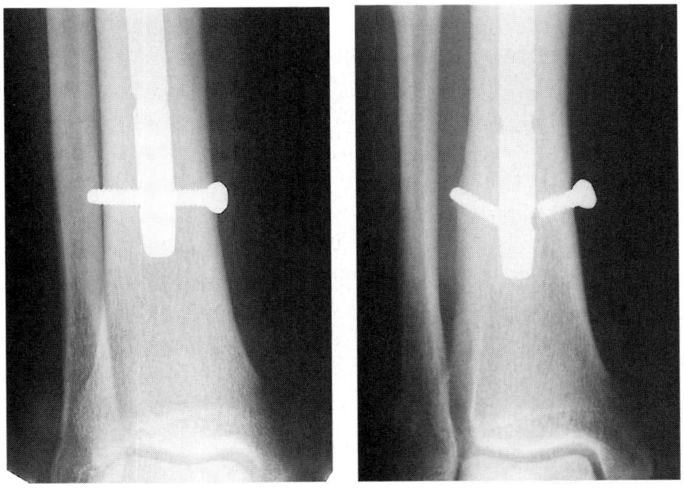

a b

Fig. 53.15 Distal locking screw failure after six months of full weight bearing.

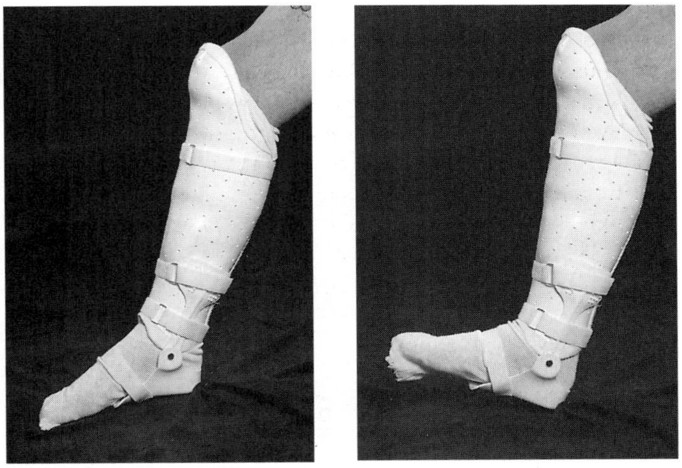

a b

Fig. 53.16 The Sarmiento cast allows early return of function of the ankle joint.

Once enough callus has formed the external fixator can be removed. It is important to recognize that callus may be prevented from developing if the external fixator is made up to be rigid and the fracture reduction is so good that it prevents all movement. A very unstable configuration should, however, also be discouraged as a hypertrophic non-union can develop. The fixator should only be applied to a fully reduced fracture as a means of avoiding late loss of reduction (Fig. 53.20). Fractures close to joints can be accommodated using metaphyseal 'T' pin clamps (Fig. 53.21).

The stability of a fracture site immobilized by external fixation is affected by the size of the fracture gap, the pins' offset, the spacing of the fixator pins, the length of the pins and the thickness of the pins. Once a stable callus has developed which will allow full weight-bearing the fixator can be removed. Patients can be encouraged to remove their own pins when conical pins have been inserted.

The Gustilo type II–III injury

External fixation has become the mainstay of management for compound fractures of the tibia because of the reluctance to leave foreign material near a previously contaminated wound.[62,63]

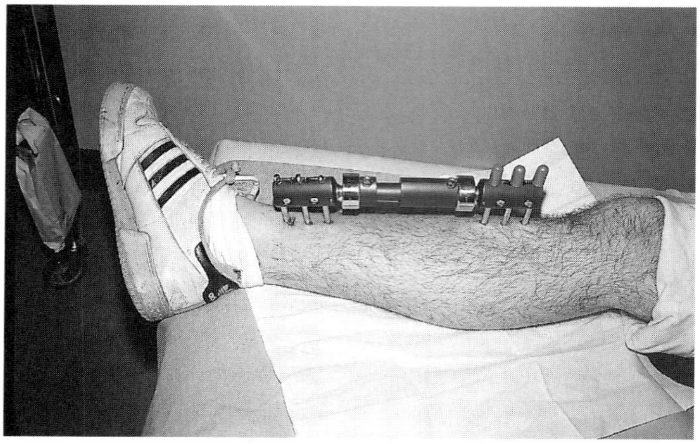

Fig. 53.17 Early pin tract infection as seen in the lower set of pins can be discouraged by unlocking the axial stability of a fixator (dynamization).

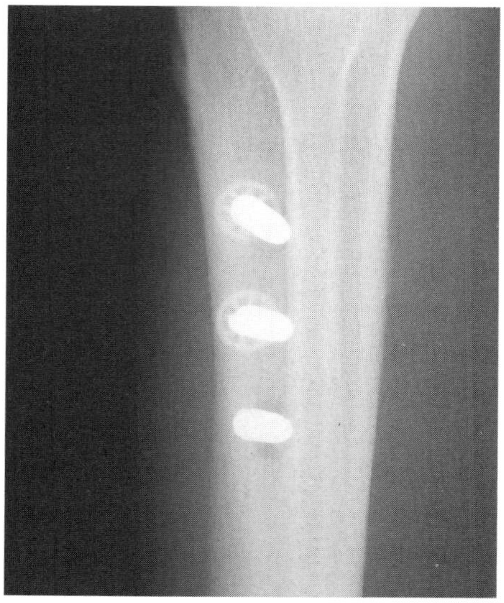

Fig. 53.18 Aseptic loosening can be seen in the upper and lower of the three pins in this radiograph.

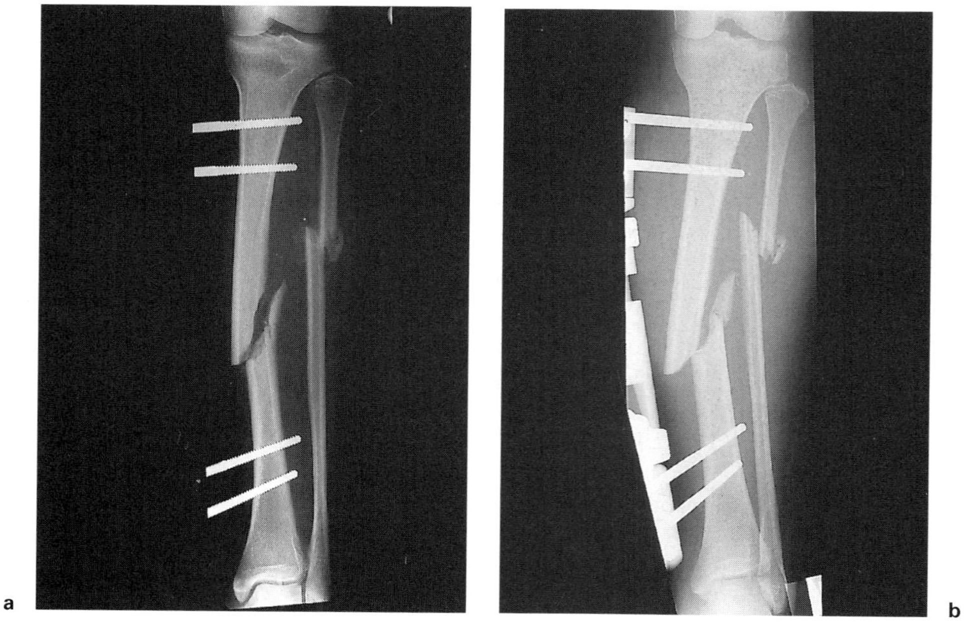

Fig. 53.19 This fixator was put onto an unreduced fracture and reduction could not be obtained by adjusting the fixator. As a result a fall caused even further loss of reduction.

External fixation is invariably used for Gustilo compound Type II–III wounds although it may be associated with a considerable risk of infection: 3–45% in some studies.[64–66] There is now a trend towards using intramedullary nailing for Gustilo Types II–III compound fractures with an accepted deep infection rate of 3.2–10%.[67–73] Compression plates and screws have in the past been

REFERENCES

62. Clancey G J, Hansen S T J Bone Joint Surg 1978; 60-A: 118–122
63. Baker J T, McKinney L A, Costa A S, Nepola J V, Marsh L J, Rodkey W G J Orthop Trauma 1992; 6: 509–510
64. Gustilo R B, Gruninger R P Orthopaedics 1987; 10: 1781–1788
65. Behrens F, Searls K J Bone Joint Surg 1986; 68-B: 246–254
66. Caudle R J, Stern P J J Bone Joint Surg 1978; 69-A: 801–807

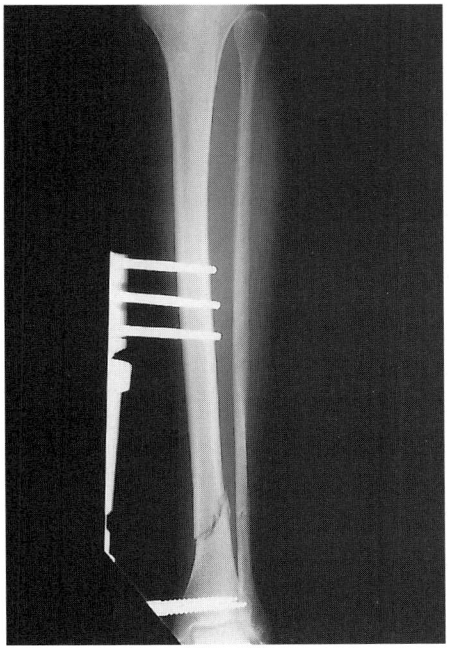

Fig. 53.20 A low fracture is treated using cancellous screws and a 'T' clamp with perfect reduction of the spiral fracture.

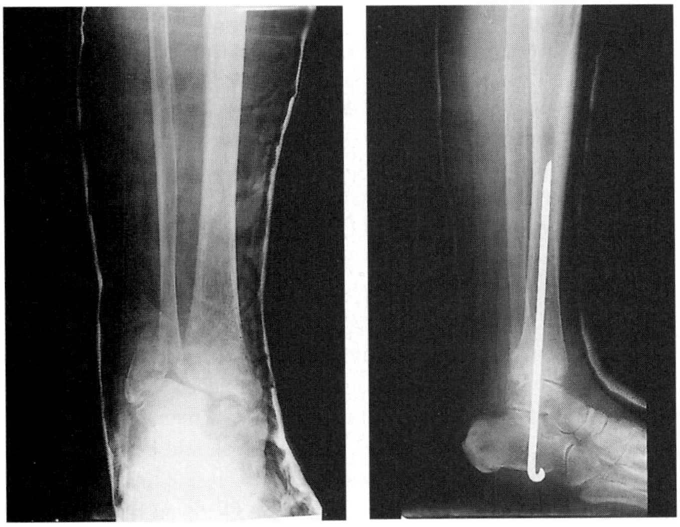

a b

Fig. 53.21 A Rush nail immobilizing an ankle fracture in an osteoporotic patient.

used to immobilize compound fractures but this has been shown to be detrimental and most now avoid this option.[74,75]

Every treatment has its own complications and the best method is often the one with which the surgeon is most familiar.

Distal tibial fractures

Distal tibial metaphyseal fractures or Pilon fractures are uncommon and usually occur as a result of a fall from a height. They have been classified by Ruedi and Allgöwer into Type 1 which are minimally displaced, Type 2 when there is incongruence and Type 3 which are comminuted.[76] Undisplaced Type 1 fractures are treated by below-knee plaster casts with avoidance of weight-bearing. Those with incongruity of the joint and comminuted fractures should be treated by an open reduction and internal fixation. Recently a combination of external fixation with a hinged fixator across the ankle joint has been tried and minimally invasive techniques using small pins, cannulated screws and K-wire fixation are also becoming popular.

Malleolar fractures

This common injury is most usually classified using the Danis–Weber classification, which is the same as the AO classification.[77] This classification relates to the position of the fibula fracture. A Danis–Weber Type A fracture is at or below the syndesmosis, a Type B runs obliquely up from the ankle joint and a Type C lies above the syndesmosis. A more complicated but accurate classification, the Lauge–Hansen classification,[78] is based on the position of the foot at the time of the injury. This classification can be deduced from the history, examination findings and radiographic pattern of fracture seen on anteroposterior and lateral views of the ankle mortise. Although complicated to remember the Lauge–Hansen classification aids in the techniques of reduction. For example, an adduction force in the supinated foot produces a transverse fracture of the lateral malleolus or an injury to the lateral collateral ligament and a vertical fracture of the medial malleolus at the level of the ankle joint. Reduction is then by abduction and pronation of the foot. No classification can cover all of the patterns of injury seen in ankle fractures but the classifications mentioned above aid in the understanding of the mechanism of injury and therefore indicate a more rational approach to treatment.

Ankle fractures usually result from a twisting injury. Often the patient cannot describe the precise mechanism of injury. The most important part of the diagnosis is to elicit the correct clinical signs of soft tissue injury, such as rupture of the deltoid ligament. Radiographs often do not disclose this, and this injury makes all the difference between the ankle mortise being stable or unstable. When an ankle injury is suspected the whole leg must be examined

REFERENCES

67. Velazco A, Whitesides T E, Fleming L L J Bone Joint Surg 1983; 65-A: 879–885
68. Wiss D A Clin Orthop 1986; 212: 122–132
69. Alho A, Ekeland A, Stromsoe K, Folleräs G, Bjørn O T J Bone Joint Surg 1990; 72-B: 805–809
70. Alho A, Benterud J G, Hogevold H E, Ekeland A, Stromsoe K Clin Orthop 1992; 277: 243–250
71. Anglen J, Unger D, DiPasquale T, Herscovici J D, Snoke J, Sanders R J Orthop Trauma 1993; 7: 163
72. Court-Brown C M, Christie J, McQueen M M J Bone Joint Surg 1990; 72-B: 605–611
73. Court-Brown C M, McQueen M M, Quaba A A, Christie J J Bone Joint Surg 1991; 73-B: 959–964
74. Veliskakis K P J Bone Joint Surg 1959; 41-B: 342–354
75. Bach A W, Hansen S T Clin Orthop 1989; 241: 89–94
76. Ruedi T P, Allgöwer M Clin Orthop 1969; 138: 105–110
77. Müller M E, Nazarian S, Koch P, Schatzker J The Comprehensive Classification of Fractures of Long Bones. Springer-Verlag, Berlin 1990
78. Yde J Acta Orthop Scand 1980; 51: 181–192

as the Maisonneuve injury (a deltoid and syndesmosis ligament rupture associated with a high spiral fibula fracture) can otherwise be missed, thus resulting in a subluxed ankle joint.

The treatment of ankle fractures depends on the position of the ankle mortise on the radiographs and whether the pattern of injury is likely to be stable or unstable. A perfect anteroposterior and lateral view of the ankle mortise should show congruence of the subchondral surfaces of the joint. Undisplaced fractures are usually treated in a below-knee cast with weight-bearing after three to six weeks, depending on whether the injury is stable or unstable.

Open reduction and internal fixation are indicated when there is greater than 1 mm of displacement of the ankle joint mortise after attempted reduction. Other indications include diastasis of the syndesmosis and compound fractures and dislocations. At operation the posteromedial fragment of a trimalleolar fracture should be reduced and internally fixed if more than one-third of the weight-bearing area has been involved in a fracture. Diastasis is treated using a syndesmosis screw above the level of the syndesmosis in a plane 25° postero-anterior to the normal coronal plane of the tibia. It is placed without compression and after full dorsiflexion of the ankle joint to avoid narrowing the ankle mortise, as this prevents dorsiflexion.

The lateral side is operated on first when open reduction and internal fixation are attempted. After the lateral side has been fixed the syndesmosis should be tested for diastasis and a check radiograph performed. When a displaced or undisplaced medial malleolar fracture is present it should be immobilized using a pair of parallel AO lag screws, usually 45 mm in length.

The deltoid ligament occasionally becomes interposed between the articular surfaces on the medial side of the ankle joint. Deltoid ligament injury may or may not require exploration, depending on whether the immediate postoperative radiographs show perfect congruity of the ankle joint.

Rarely, fractures of the ankle in osteoporotic patients cannot be immobilized with plaster cast or the usual AO fixation techniques. In these circumstances an intramedullary Rush nail passed under image intensification up through the os calcis and talus is a useful method of temporary immobilization (Fig. 53.21)

Fractures of the foot

Injuries of the feet are common and disabling (cf. Ch. 49). Fractures that involve the subtalar joint are extremely disabling. These injuries are often missed because of failure to appreciate the radiological anatomy of the foot.

Talar fractures

Fractures of the talus are rare because they tend to be caused by high-energy forces. The talar neck fracture was classically diagnosed in the pilots of early aircraft as the 'aviators' astragalus' injury because the rudder pedals would cause a violent dorsiflexion of the foot when the craft crashed. Nowadays this injury is seen after car accidents or following a fall from a height. The diagnosis is aided by true lateral views of the foot as well as the usual anteroposterior and oblique views.

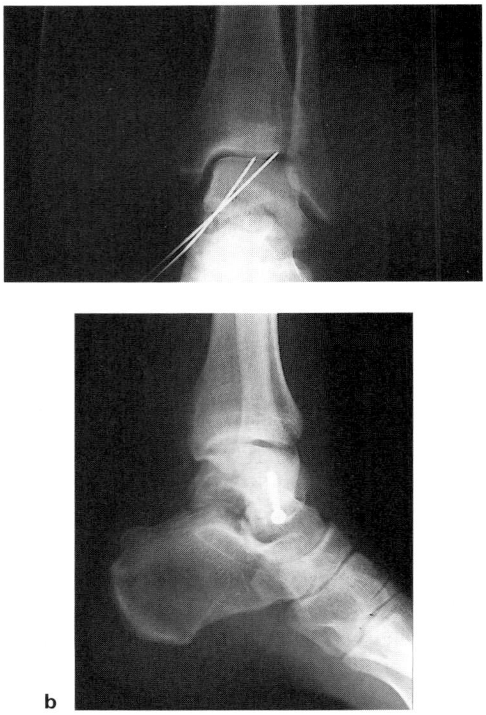

a

b

Fig. 53.22 Fixation after failed closed reduction of a Hawkins Type 2 fracture. The fracture fragments are reduced and held with a K-wire before a screw is passed.

The Hawkins and Canale classification of talar neck fractures is most commonly quoted.[79,80]

Reduction is not necessary for undisplaced fractures of the neck (Type 1). A split plaster with the ankle held in the plantigrade position is applied to be replaced by a complete plaster when the swelling has subsided. This is worn for six to eight weeks. With displaced fractures and fracture dislocations (Types 2–4) reduction is urgent because of the precarious nature of the blood supply of the talar body. Type 3 and 4 injuries, in which the body of the talus is displaced medially, have an avascular necrosis rate of 85%. Open reduction should be performed if closed manipulation under anaesthetic fails. All of the bone fragments should be retained and held reduced (Fig. 53.22). The reduced fracture can be stabilized initially with one or two Kirschner wires followed if possible by insertion of an AO screw or a cannulated screw placed from behind forwards into the talar head. A below-knee plaster with the ankle being held in a plantigrade position is needed for six to eight weeks.

Os calcis fractures

These common injuries are caused by a fall from a height onto the heels. The injury is unfortunately common in window cleaners, painters and scaffolders. Because a fall from a height is the cause it is essential to exclude other injuries such as fractures of the pelvis

REFERENCES

79. Hawkins L G J Bone Joint Surg 1970; 52-A: 991–1002
80. Canale S T Orthopaedics 1990; 13: 1105–1115

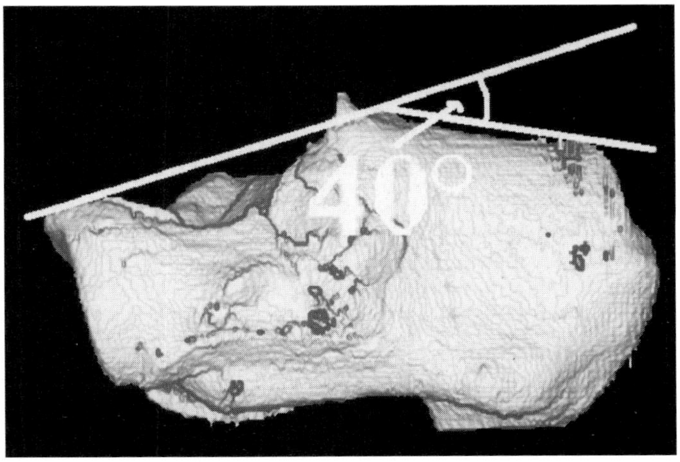

Fig. 53.23 Böhler's salient angle reproduced on a 3-D reconstruction of the os calcis from a CT scan.

and spine. The injury is always associated with swelling of the heel below the malleoli and severe obvious flattening of the heel may be evident. Bruising appears late and settles in a line above the fat pad of the heel. Radiographs pick up all but the most minor injuries. These must include well-centred and well-exposed lateral views of the foot. An axial projection is helpful to visualize the posterior body of the bone, the sustentaculum tali and occasionally the subtalar joints. CT scanning provides accurate delineation of the extent of fracture and therefore aids in the diagnosis and planning of open reduction and internal fixation.

The simplest classification divides these injuries into extra-articular fractures in which the posterior talocalcaneal joint is not involved and intra-articular fractures in which it is. The value of this classification is in its ability to assess the prognosis, which is much worse in the fractures involving the posterior facet of the os calcis. Involvement of this joint can be gauged by measuring Böhler's salient angle, which is normally about 40°. To measure this a line is drawn through the posterior articular surface to intersect with a second line touching the superior angle of the tuberosity (Fig. 53.23).

Most extra-articular fractures can be managed by conservative means including early elevation, cold compression and mobilization. There are two schools of thought as to whether treating intra-articular fractures by open reduction and internal fixation confers any advantage over conservative treatment. When open reduction and internal fixation are performed a lateral approach is preferred and an os calcis reconstruction plate chosen for fixation. Bone defects should be grafted and weight-bearing is delayed for eight weeks.

Midtarsal fractures and tarsometatarsal injuries

An isolated fracture of the navicular is often incorrectly diagnosed when an os naviculare exists. A true fracture is often caused by an avulsion of the tibialis posterior tendon. This fracture can be treated conservatively in a plaster cast. Larger fractures of the navicular should be accurately fixed using internal fixation techniques.

Tarsometatarsal fracture dislocations are commonly missed. Reduction should be recognized and treated early as the dorsalis pedis artery can be compromised or torn and compartment syndrome is not uncommon. Open reduction is occasionally needed. K-wire stabilization of the joints allows avulsion fractures to heal. K-wires are reinforced using plaster back slabs and the K-wires are left for about six weeks. Anatomical reduction of all tarsometatarsal fracture dislocations should be the goal as this produces good results by reducing stiffness and preventing limp.

Metatarsal fractures

A metatarsal fracture may be caused by crushing, twisting or repetitive stress. Usually there is a history of injury, however trivial, and the foot is painful and slightly swollen. Radiographs show most fractures but the accessory ossicles around the base of the fifth metatarsal are occasionally misdiagnosed as a fracture.

When walking plasters are required they are used for a maximum of three weeks as most fractures unite readily. The Jones fracture of the base of the fifth metatarsal distal to its articulation with the second metatarsal behaves more like a stress fracture and occurs in athletes. It frequently results in a non-union, which has to be treated with medullary curettage and bone grafting.

Kirschner wire fixation may be utilized after reduction of severely displaced multiple fractures that may also be associated with midtarsal dislocations. The foot is elevated postoperatively and weight-bearing avoided for six weeks.

Phalangeal fractures

These are commonly the result of workplace accidents in which heavy weights are dropped onto the toes. Many are compound and need to be treated accordingly. Postoperatively they can be managed by elevation followed by mobilization. If necessary a plaster shoe with a 'crumb catcher' extension to protect the phalanges is used. Admission and elevation for the majority is a prudent practice as it avoids late sloughing of swollen dermis.

Dislocations

Dislocation of the hip

Dislocation of the hip may be congenital or acquired. In the neonate and infancy the commonest cause is congenital dislocation of the hip, followed by septic arthritis. During adolescence and adulthood the commonest cause of dislocation of the hip is trauma. Eighty per cent of all traumatic hip dislocations are posterior. The commonest cause is a blow to the knee from a dashboard during a road traffic accident. The blow forces the femur out of the acetabulum. Occasionally the dislocation is associated with a fracture of the posterior lip of the acetabulum. Occasionally the posterior dislocation is associated with a femoral fracture, which leads the dislocation to be overlooked.

The clinical features of posterior dislocation of the hip in the conscious patient are of extreme pain and deformity about the lower limb. The affected limb appears short and is fixed in flexion, internal rotation and adduction. An anteroposterior radiograph of the pelvis is usually enough to demonstrate the dislocation. However, multiple views of the acetabulum and a CT scan may be needed to exclude a fracture of the acetabular rim or a Pipkin fracture of the femoral head. The neurovascular status of the limb should be elucidated as these dislocations are occasionally associated with a sciatic nerve injury.

Traumatic dislocations are considered to be orthopaedic emergencies. There is a relationship between the length of time the hip remains dislocated and an increasing risk of avascular necrosis. It is widely held that isolated hip dislocation reduced within 6 hours gives an excellent outcome. However, even if dislocations are reduced within 3 hours there appears to be an incidence of 45% fair and poor results in long-term follow-up. The important factors in the long-term prognosis appear to be the direction of the dislocation and the overall severity of injuries. Multiple injuries and posterior dislocation are associated with a higher incidence of avascular necrosis, osteoarthritis and heterotopic ossification.[81]

The dislocation should be reduced under general anaesthesia. The dislocation is most safely reduced with the patient anaesthetized on the anaesthetic room floor. An assistant is required to steady the pelvis by providing counter-traction over the anterior–superior iliac spines. When this has been provided the dislocation is reduced by flexing the patient's hip and knee to 90° and pulling the thigh vertically upwards.

Following reduction X-rays are mandatory to confirm reduction, exclude displacement of a fracture of the acetabulum and exclude intra-articular fragments. An intra-articular fragment of cartilage may be deduced from plain radiographs by comparing the congruity of the dislocated joint with that on the normal side. If it is suspected that bone or cartilage fragments are trapped in the joint then a CT scan of the joint may be required.

If the reduction is stable and there are no associated fractures of the acetabulum then mobilization should be begun as early as pain allows and full weight-bearing should be encouraged as soon as the pain allows. If there is associated fracture of the acetabulum that has been reduced then the patient should have at least three weeks of bedrest with skin traction followed by non-weight-bearing for a further five weeks. If a large fragment of the acetabulum remains unreduced open reduction and internal fixation are necessary. If any fragments of cartilage or bone have been demonstrated on the CT scan, these should be removed by either open operation or specialist units by arthroscopy of the hip. Fractures of the femoral head in the weight-bearing area should be replaced with perfect reduction of the articular surface. Fractures in the non-weight-bearing areas, if they are large, require reduction. However, if they are small[10] may be removed. Most associated injuries of the sciatic nerve are due to neuropraxia and usually recover. If sciatic nerve injuries are associated with an acetabular fracture the nerve should be explored to exclude injury by the bone fragments. Avascular necrosis of the femoral head complicates at least 10% of all traumatic hip dislocations. This may be picked up radiographically as an increase in density between six and eight weeks after fracture. However, on occasion avascular necrosis may be delayed for up to two years after injury. Secondary osteoarthritis is common after dislocation of the hip. Secondary osteoarthritis may be caused by avascular necrosis of the femoral head, incongruity due to fractures of the femoral head or acetabulum and retained fragments within the joint.

Anterior dislocation is rare. In anterior dislocation the leg lies externally rotated, abducted and slightly flexed. Clinically, in the conscious patient the symptoms are of similar pain, and an anterior bulge in the groin of a dislocated femoral head is diagnostic.

The dislocation may be confirmed radiographically on the anteroposterior view of the pelvis, but occasionally a lateral film is required.

Dislocations are reduced with the patient anaesthetised on the anaesthetic room floor and an assistant steadying the pelvis by applying weight to the anterosuperior iliac spines. The hip and knee are flexed to 90° and the thigh pulled upward and adducted. Osteoarthritis, intra-articular loose bodies and avascular necrosis may complicate this injury.

Central dislocation of the hip by impaction of the femoral head through the thin medial wall of the acetabulum arises from a direct lateral impact to the hip joint.

Every attempt should be made to reduce the dislocation with either skeletal traction or closed reduction and skeletal traction. Accurate reduction of the acetabular fragments makes later reconstruction for secondary osteoarthritis easier. Skeletal traction, if successful, should be maintained for at least four to six weeks. Non-weight-bearing, using crutches, should be encouraged for a further six weeks.

Patella dislocation

Dislocation of the patella is a common condition. It may be classified as acute, chronic, recurrent or habitual. One in 20 patients suffer an associated osteochondral fracture.

Reduction of a dislocated patella is usually spontaneous, but occasionally requires a simple push after the administration of analgesia.

Indications for operative treatment include the removal of small chondral fragments, the fixation of larger osteochondral fragments and the repair of an extensive tear of the medial retinaculum.

The incidence of recurrent dislocation of the patella may be up to 40% if the acute soft tissue injury of the medial retinaculum is not repaired.[82] Recurrent dislocation is common in adolescent females. It is particularly common when the patient has associated genuvalgum, persistent femoral anteversion, patellar alta, compensatory external tibial torsion or generalized joint laxity.

Knee dislocation

Dislocation of the knee is rare. Dislocation is associated with high-energy injuries, such as falls from a height or most commonly in pedestrian accidents. For dislocation to occur both cruciate ligaments must be torn and one or both collateral ligaments are also

REFERENCES

81. Dreinhöfer K E, Schwarzkopf S R, Haas N P, Tscherne H J Bone Joint Surg 1994; 76-B: 6–12
82. Rorabeck C H, Bobechko W P J Bone Joint Surg 1976; 58-B: 237–240

torn. Dislocation is often associated with neurovascular injury and the peripheral circulation and neurological status must be examined to exclude associated injury.

The clinical features are usually those of severe swelling and gross deformity with or without distal neurovascular compromise. Radiographs may reveal associated avulsion fractures of the tibial spines or tip of the fibula with avulsion of the lateral collateral ligament. If there is any doubt as to the adequacy of perfusion of the limb below the dislocation an immediate arteriogram is mandatory.

As with dislocation of the hip, reduction under general anaesthesia is an orthopaedic emergency. Closed reduction should be held with a temporary back slab. If closed manipulation fails open reduction is mandatory. Closed reduction may be followed within seven days by acute repair of the cruciate ligaments and any collateral ligament injury. Surgical repair followed by early continuous passive motion is often rewarding. The joint should be protected for three to six weeks by a suitable knee brace utilizing four points of stabilization required for preventing cruciate ligament strain.

Ankle dislocation

Dislocation of the ankle is usually associated with ankle fractures. For their management every attempt should be made to ensure perfect anatomical reduction is achieved, otherwise early postoperative secondary osteoarthritis occurs.

Talar and tarsal dislocation

This is a rare injury associated with injury from considerable force, usually a pedal injury following a road traffic accident or a fall from a height. Dislocation is usually associated with a fracture and may be associated with dislocations of the subtalar or midtarsal joints.

Clinical features are invariably of swelling. The deformity of a dislocation is often not obvious because of this swelling and may well cause the dislocation to be missed.

Once closed reduction has been performed stability of the joint should be assessed. An unstable joint requires K-wire stabilization and a plaster cast. Associated fractures should be addressed by reduction and internal fixation. The K-wires may be removed at three to four weeks but a below-knee, non-weight-bearing plaster will be required for six weeks after injury.

Dislocation of the talus, especially with associated fractures of the neck of the talus, is commonly complicated by avascular necrosis of the posterior fragment and subsequent secondary arthritis of the ankle and subtalar joints. Dislocations of the metatarsophalangeal or interphalangeal joints should be reduced. Occasionally reduction may be achieved under local anaesthetic. The joint should be splintered and occasionally K-wire fixation is necessary for an unstable dislocation.

54 Sarcomas of soft tissue and bone

Jonathan Lucas

The word 'sarcoma' is derived from a Greek word meaning 'fleshy growth'. Sarcomas are malignant tumours arising in tissues of mesenchymal origin and may thus occur anywhere in the body.

INCIDENCE

Sarcomas of soft tissue (see also Chapter 9) and bone together account for less than 1% of malignant neoplasms. Approximately 1300 cases are seen each year in England and Wales[1] and 7000 annually in the USA.[2,3] Soft tissue sarcomas show a gradually increasing incidence in each decade of life, peaking in the 60s. Bone and cartilaginous tumours have a bimodal distribution with peaks in the second/third and seventh/eighth decades. Both are slightly more common in males than females.[1]

DISTRIBUTION

A nationwide survey in the USA gave the anatomical distribution of adult soft tissue sarcomas as follows:[4]

Lower extremity (including pelvic girdle)	46%
Trunk, retroperitoneum and mediastinum	32%
Upper extremity (including shoulder girdle)	13%
Head and neck	9%

Tumours occur more commonly in the proximal than the distal part of the upper and lower extremities.[5,6]

Osteosarcomas occur most commonly at the metaphysis of long bones, especially around the knee. Ewing's sarcoma occurs anywhere in a long bone but is particularly common in the tibia.

AETIOLOGY

This is unknown in most cases. Many patients with bone and soft tissue sarcomas give a history of recent trauma. This is not thought to be of aetiological significance, merely drawing attention to the pre-existing abnormality.

Soft tissue sarcomas may arise in the lesions of inherited disorders such as neurofibromatosis[7] and multiple enchondromas. Malignant tumours of the bone and soft tissue may be induced by ionizing radiation.[8] Soft tissue sarcomas may follow exposure to phenoxyacetic acid, present in herbicides, and chlorophenols that are used in wood preservatives.[9] They may also arise after several decades in scars from thermal and acid burns.[10] Kaposi's sarcoma is increasingly common in patients with acquired immune deficiency (see Chapter 9). Malignant bone tumours may arise in abnormal bone in older patients. The best known examples are osteosarcomas and fibrosarcomas arising in areas of Paget's disease.

PRESENTATION

Soft tissue sarcomas present as a painless mass which increases in size. They may be tender or painful at rest or on exercise due to stretching or compression of neighbouring structures. Size at presentation varies with the site. Tumours of the pelvic girdle and upper thigh are much larger at presentation than peripheral tumours which are more easily noted by the patient.

10% of patients with a liposarcoma exhibit a pyrexia which disappears after successful treatment of the primary tumour:[11] systemic symptoms are otherwise rare in the absence of distant metastases. There are no specific physical signs of a soft tissue sarcoma but these tumours usually have a smooth surface and are rubbery or firm in consistency, being intimately connected to the surrounding tissues. They may feel warm and the overlying skin may contain dilated veins. The differential diagnosis includes benign soft tissue swellings such as lipoma, haematoma, aneurysm, fibromatosis, myositis ossificans and cold abscess. In the absence of a history or physical signs suggesting a clear alternative diagnosis, any enlarging soft tissue mass, especially if situated deep to the deep fascia, should be suspected of being a sarcoma.

Malignant bone tumours present as a swelling which is often painful. The mass may be felt to arise from the underlying bone and is bony hard in consistency. The differential diagnosis is from benign bone tumours. Pathological fractures may occur.

REFERENCES

1. Office of Population Censuses and Surveys Cancer Statistics—Registrations. London, HMSO 1983
2. Consensus Conference JAMA 1985; 254: 1791–1794
3. Estimates by American Cancer Society based on data from the National Cancer Institutes' Surveillance, Epidemiology and End Results (SEER) Program (1977–1981). Cancer Facts and Figures 1985
4. Lawrence W, Donegan W L et al Ann Surg 1987; 205: 349–359
5. Collin C, Hajdu S I et al Ann Surg 1987; 205: 331–339
6. Collin C, Hajdu S I et al Arch Surg 1986; 121: 1425–1433
7. Heard G Proc R Soc Med 1963; 56: 502–503
8. Davidson T, Westbury G, Harmer C L Br J Surg 1986; 73: 308–309
9. Hardell L, Sandstrom A Br J Cancer 1979; 39: 711–717
10. Enzinger F M, Weiss S W Soft Tissue Tumours. Mosby, St Louis 1983
11. Spittle M F, Newton K A, MacKenzie D H Br J Cancer 1971; 24: 696–704

IMAGING AND BIOPSY

Plain film appearances are often diagnostic in malignant bone tumours. Assessment of the plain film should include consideration of the anatomical site of the lesion, its borders and the presence of bone destruction, matrix formation and periosteal reaction. For example, a metaphyseal lesion around the knee with poorly defined borders, evidence of bone destruction, perhaps accompanied by new bone formation and elevation of the periosteum to produce 'sunray spicules' and 'Codman's triangle' is likely to be an osteosarcoma (Fig. 54.1). Plain radiography of the soft tissue will also demonstrate the presence or absence of calcification within soft tissue tumours, narrowing the initial diagnosis of benign tumours if calcification is present to heterotopic calcification, myositis ossificans, lipoma, vascular malformations, soft tissue chondroma, and osteochondromatosis. If the tumour is malignant, the differential diagnosis may be narrowed to liposarcoma, soft tissue osteosarcoma and synovial sarcoma, in which a third have been reported to have calcification present.[12] The investigation of choice for the delineation of the anatomical boundaries for soft tissue sarcomas is MRI scanning, which has been demonstrated to be superior to CT scanning.[13–15] CT and MRI both have their role in the evaluation of bone sarcomas. CT is considered the superior imaging modality for the evaluation of subcortical changes and for the identification and characterization of mineralized tumour matrix (Fig. 54.2). MRI is superior for the determination of tumour margins with respect to normal adjacent muscle (Fig. 54.3). In general, therefore, CT defines the tumour margins in sclerotic tumours, and MRI in the more osteolytic tumours. In some instances a combination of the two imaging types should be used, especially in mixed, ill defined tumours with marked soft tissue invasion.[16–18]

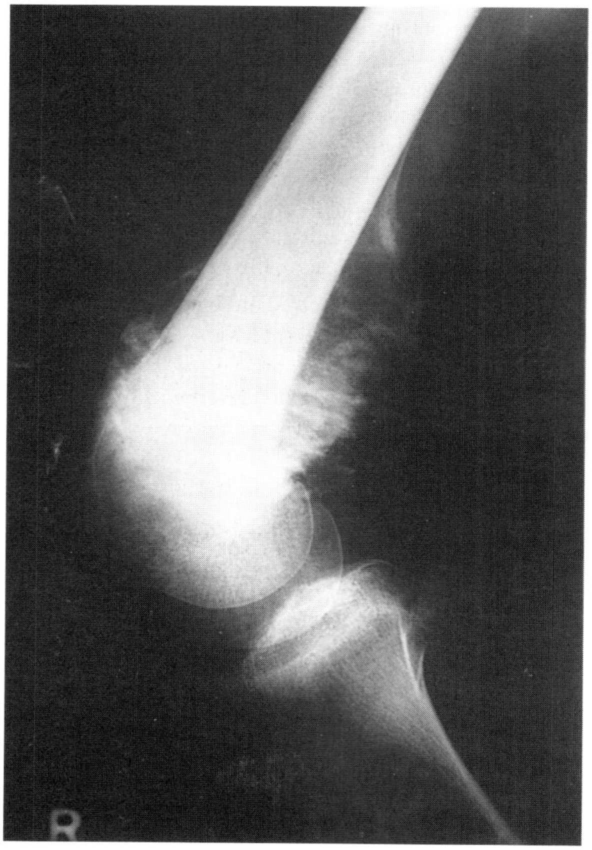

Fig. 54.1 Osteosarcoma showing 'Codman's triangle' and 'sunray spicules'.

Once a diagnosis of bone sarcoma, especially osteosarcoma, has been made a search is required for further bone lesions in the form of skip lesions, the synchronous lesions of multicentric osteosarcoma, and bone metastases. Bone scanning with ^{99m}Tc-methylene diphosphonate (^{99m}Tc-MDP) is the investigation of choice for the identification of these lesions.[16] ^{201}Tl-chloride and gallium scans have also been used in the evaluation of bone sarcomas, but their role has not been clearly defined.[19,20] Scintigraphy with tumour seeking agents has also been used for soft tissue sarcomas, gallium having a reported sensitivity of 56–93%[21–25] and ^{99m}Tc(V)-dimercaptosuccinic acid (DMSA) a sensitivity of 89%.[26]

The new imaging technique of [^{18}F] fluorodeoxyglucose positron emission tomography (FDG PET) has been used for the identification and staging of sarcomas. FDG PET is a dynamic imaging technique which allows the visualization and quantification of glucose metabolism in cells and is able to reflect the increase of this metabolism in malignant tumours. FDG PET can identify bone and soft tissue sarcomas and give an indication of the grade of the tumour.[27–31] As yet, the most apt role of FDG PET has not been defined, but when the technique has been further refined its role will probably lie in monitoring the effectiveness of treatment, incorporating surgery, radiotherapy, chemotherapy and, in the future, possibly gene therapy.

The definitive diagnosis of the tumour is made by taking a biopsy. This apparently simple procedure is not without its hazards.[32] Mankin[33a,b] reported two sequential series in 1982 and

REFERENCES

12. Cadman N L, Soule E H, Kelly P J Cancer 1965; 18: 613–627
13. Bland K I, McCoy D M, Kinard R E, Copeland E M III Ann Surg 1987; 205(5): 473–481
14. Petasnick J P, Turner D A et al Radiology 1986; 160(1): 125–133
15. Totty W G, Murphy W A, Lee J K Radiology 1986; 160(1): 135–141
16. Seeger L L, Gold R H, Chandnani V P Clin Orthop 1991; 270: 254–263
17. Davidson T I, Cooke J et al Br J Surg 1987; 74: 474–478
18. Chang A E, Matory Y L et al Ann Surg 1987; 205: 340–348
19. Kostakoglu L, Panicek D M et al Eur J Nucl Med 1995; 22(11): 1232–1237
20. Menendez L R, Fiedeler B R, Mirra J J Bone Joint Surg 1993; 74-A(4): 526–531
21. Kirchner P T, Simon M A J Bone Joint Surg (Am Vol) 1984; 66-A(3): 319–327
22. Finn H A, Simon M A, Martin W B, Darakjain H J Bone Joint Surg 1987; 69-A(6): 886–891
23. Bitran J D, Bekerman C, Golomb H M, Simon M A Cancer 1978; 42: 1760–1765
24. Kaufman J H, Cedermark B J et al Radiology 1977; 123: 131–134
25. Southee A E, Kaplan W D et al J Nucl Med 1992; 33(9): 1594–1599
26. Ohta H, Endo K et al Nucl Med Comm 1988; 9: 105–116
27. Adler L P, Blair H F et al J Comput Assist Tomogr 1990; 14(6): 960–962
28. Kern K A, Brunetti A et al J Nucl Med 1988; 29: 181–186
29. Nieweg O E, Pruim J et al J Nucl Med 1996; 37(2): 257–261
30. Adler L P, Blair H F et al J Nucl Med 1991; 32: 1508–1512
31. Griffin L K, Dehdashti F et al Radiology 1992; 182: 185–194

R L

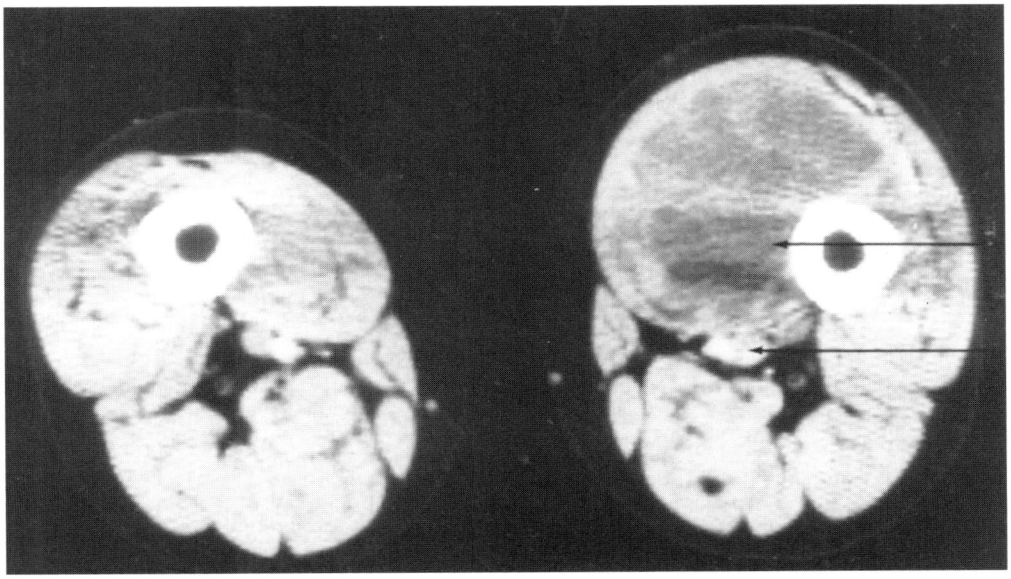

Fig. 54.2 Soft tissue sarcoma of medial quadriceps of the left leg showing the relationship to periosteum and with the femoral vessels intimately related to its deep surface (arrows).

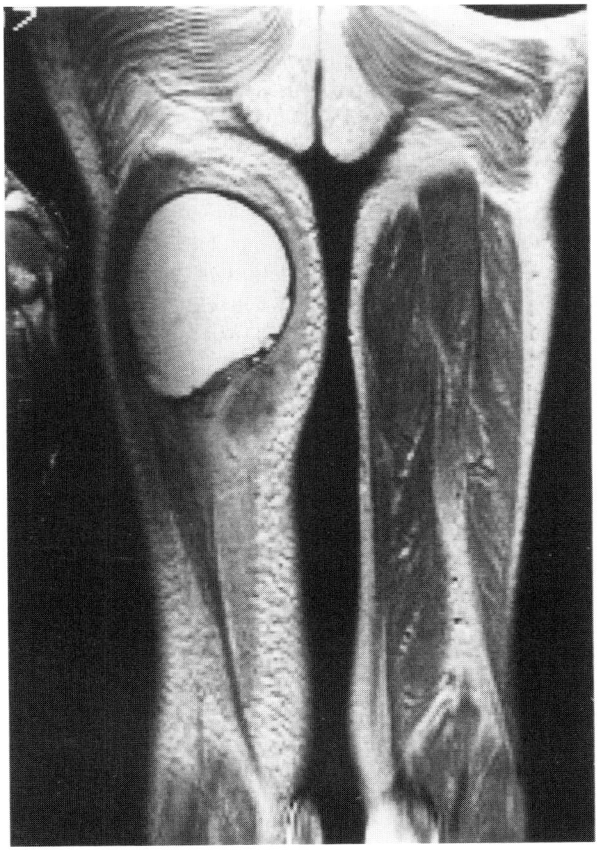

Fig. 54.3 Magnetic resonance imaging of soft tissue sarcoma of adductor compartment, clearly demonstrating the pseudocapsule.

1996 in which the combined diagnostic error of the biopsies of the two series was 17.8%. The rates at which an inappropriate biopsy or complications from the biopsy changed the required management for the patient were 18% and 19.3% respectively for the two series, and the rates of a poorer outcome to the patient were 8.5% and 10.1% respectively, the poorer outcome being defined as a more complex resection that resulted in disability, loss of function, local recurrence or death. The biopsy should therefore only be performed after suitable cross-sectional imaging by a CT or MRI scan. This will allow preservation of good anatomical definition of the tumour on the scans. If this delay is not feasible then a needle or punch biopsy should be performed. More extensive biopsies may produce such distortion of tissue planes that interpretation of subsequent computerized tomography or MRI scans is made much more difficult. In particular enucleation (shelling out) and narrow excision of an unsuspected soft tissue sarcoma should be avoided and, indeed, considered a major error in management. Unfortunately such excisions are frequently performed by inexperienced surgeons who describe a good plane of cleavage or capsule around the tumour. This is in fact a false capsule and contains microscopic tumour. Reported rates of residual tumour in such circumstances for soft tissue sarcomas are between 35% and 59%.[34,35] Accurate planning of subsequent treatment becomes more difficult as the absence of gross tumour together with haematoma and surgical scarring complicate the interpretation of computerized tomography scans. Even at surgical re-exploration it is often hard to determine the extent of the original tumour and the limits of the previous excision. These mistakes may be avoided if there is a high index of

REFERENCES

32. Springfield D S, Rosenberg S A J Bone Joint Surg 1996; 78-A(5): 639–643

33a. Mankin H J, Lange T A, Spanier S S J Bone Joint Surg 1982; 64-A: 1121–1127

33b. Mankin H J, Mankin C J, Simon M A J Bone Joint Surg 1996; 78-A: 656-663

34. Goodlad J R, Fletcher C D M, Smith M A J Bone Joint Surg 1996; 78-B6: 58–61

35. Noria S, Davis A et al J Bone Joint Surg 1996; 78-A(5): 650–655

suspicion that the soft tissue mass may be malignant; under these circumstances appropriate imaging and biopsy should be undertaken, thereby making a definitive diagnosis without contaminating the surrounding normal tissue and thus maximizing the opportunity for the most conservative and effective surgical treatment.

Biopsy techniques

Core needle biopsies (Trucuts) can, in expert hands, give predictive accuracy of over 90% for the presence and type of soft tissue malignancy[36] and are cost effective.[37] However open biopsy is still the most accurate form of biopsy for obtaining a diagnosis, despite its higher complication rate. Aspiration cytology has been reported to have a diagnostic accuracy of 96% for soft tissue sarcoma[38,39] but this is variable with reported accuracies as low as 64%[40] for soft tissue sarcoma and 54% for bone sarcomas.[41,42]

Needle biopsy usually provides a diagnosis without distorting the tumour and its relationships to surrounding tissues. If core or aspiration biopsy fails to give a clear diagnosis, then an incision biopsy should be performed. A convenient method for doing this in larger tumours is to use a Tilley–Henckel punch biopsy forceps introduced through a trocar.[43] This punch biopsy and more conventional open biopsies should be performed through incisions which can easily be incorporated within the incision that is planned for any future resection. For example, longitudinal scars should be used in the limbs, and buttock scars should be kept as low as possible so as not to prejudice the posterior flap of any subsequent hindquarter amputation.

Core or trocar biopsies may also provide satisfactory material in those bone tumours which have burst into the surrounding soft tissues. Radiologically guided drill biopsies may be helpful in other cases. If open biopsy is required the same precautions should be observed as for soft tissue sarcomas.

PATHOLOGY

Soft tissue sarcomas

These tumours are often 5 cm or more in diameter at presentation and may show central necrosis or haemorrhage. A striking feature of their gross pathology is their apparent encapsulation. As previously stated, this is a pseudocapsule which contains tumour cells. These tumours are locally invasive, but spread by 'pushing' along tissue planes rather than by direct invasion of major structures. Fascia, major nerve sheaths and the adventitia of large vessels are relatively resistant to invasion. Lymph node metastases are uncommon, but are occasionally seen, especially in rhabdomyosarcomas, angiosarcomas, and synovial sarcomas[4,44] when they are associated with a poor prognosis. The lungs are the most common site of blood-borne systemic metastases.

The microscopic classification of soft tissue sarcomas is based on histogenetic type, i.e. the type of tissue formed by the tumour rather than the supposed tissue of origin.[10] The current World Health Organization classification comprises 15 subtypes[10] (Table 54.1). Histochemistry and electron microscopy may help in distinguishing these subtypes. Tumours may be further classified as high or low grade depending on their cellularity, anaplasia or pleomorphism, mitotic activity, expansive or infiltrative growth, and necrosis.[45,46] Rhabdomyosarcoma, extraskeletal Ewing's, synovial sarcomas and epithelioid sarcomas are usually considered to be high grade. Dermatofibrosarcoma protuberans and well differentiated and myxoid liposarcomas are usually low grade. There is unfortunately no universal agreement on grading or classification, and there may well be considerable disagreement between experienced pathologists in classifying and grading an individual tumour. This, together with the reclassifications that have occurred in recent years, explains some of the difficulties in comparing series and correlating pathological appearance with clinical behaviour.

Ultimately the validity of any pathological classification depends on its reproducibility and capacity to predict the clinical course of the disease. Some histological types such as liposarcoma, fibrosarcoma[47] and malignant fibrous histiocytoma[47] are said to have a better prognosis. Recent multivariate analyses have shown that grading is the main histopathological determinant of outcome; differences between histogenetic subtypes merely reflect the predominantly high or low grade nature of these tumours.[46] Grade has been correlated to local recurrence,[48,49] metastatic potential[48,50] and

Table 54.1 Histological classification of soft tissue sarcomas

Subtype	*Classification*	*Example*
I	Tumours of fibrous tissue	Fibrosarcoma
II	Fibrohistiocytic tumours	Malignant fibrous histiocytoma
III	Tumours of adipose tissue	Liposarcoma
IV	Tumours of muscle tissue	Rhabdomyosarcoma
V	Tumours of blood vessels	Kaposi's sarcoma
VI	Tumours of lymph vessels	Lymphangiosarcoma
VII	Tumours of synovial tissue	Synovial sarcoma
VIII	Tumours of mesothelial tissue	Mesothelioma
IX	Tumours of peripheral nerves	Malignant schwannoma
X	Tumours of autonomic ganglia	Neuroblastoma
XI	Tumours of paraganglionic structures	Malignant paraganglioma
XII	Tumours of cartilage and bone forming tissues	Extraskeletal osteosarcoma
XIII	Tumours of pluripotential mesenchyme	Malignant mesenchymoma
XIV	Tumours of uncertain histiogenesis	Epithelioid sarcoma
XV	Unclassified tumours	

Adapted from Enzinger & Weiss[10]

REFERENCES

36. Kissin M W, Fisher C et al Br J Surg 1986; 73: 742–744
37. Skrzynski M C, Biermann J S, Montag A, Simon M A J Bone Joint Surg 1996; 78-A(5): 644–649
38. Barth R J Jr, Merino M J et al Surgery 1992; 112: 536–543
39. Kissin M W, Fisher C et al Br J Surg 1987; 74: 479–480
40. Akerman M, Rydholm A, et al Acta Orthop Scand 1985; 56: 407–412
41. El-Khoury G Y, Terepka R H et al J Bone Joint Surg 1983; 65-A5: 22–25
42. Kreicbergs A, Bauer H Orthop Trans 1994; 18: 1131
43. Westbury G In: Keen G (ed) Operative Surgery and Management, 2nd edn. Wright, Bristol 1987
44. Weingrad D W, Rosenberg S A Surgery 1978; 84: 231–240
45. Costa J, Wesley R A et al Cancer 1984; 53: 530–541
46. Collin C, Godbold J et al J Clin Oncol 1987; 5: 601–602
47. Lindberg R D, Martin R G et al Cancer 1981; 47: 2391–2397

Table 54.2 Classification of malignant bone tumours

Classification	*Example*
Haematopoietic	Myeloma
	Reticulum cell sarcoma
Osteogenic	Osteosarcoma
	Paraosteal osteosarcoma
	Periosteal osteosarcoma
Chondrogenic	Primary chondrosarcoma
	Secondary chondrosarcoma
	Dedifferentiated chondrosarcoma
	Mesenchymal chondrosarcoma
Unknown origin	Ewing's tumour
	Malignant giant cell tumour
	Adamantinoma
	Fibrous histiocytoma
Fibrogenic	Fibrosarcoma
Notochordal	Chordoma
Vascular	Haemangioendothelioma
	Haemangiopericytoma

death.[45,46,48] Thus, despite the limitations in grading systems, grading appears to offer the best guide to the future risk of local recurrence, metastases and ultimate survival.

Bone sarcomas

Malignant bone tumours are classified by cell type and the material produced[49–51] (Table 54.2). The two most common types, osteosarcoma and chondrosarcoma, are subdivided into a number of varieties differing in microscopic appearance, behaviour and prognosis. Spread is local, by bone destruction, commonly extending into neighbouring soft tissues, along marrow sinusoids to produce 'skip lesions' in the bone of origin, and via the bloodstream predominantly to the lungs.[54]

STAGING

Soft tissue sarcomas are staged by site, size, degree of local extension, grade, lymph node involvement, and distant metastases[54,55] (Table 54.3). Bone tumours are staged by site, grade, and the presence of distant metastases (GTM system; Table 54.4).[56] Sufficient information to stage the primary will have been obtained by the previously described scanning and biopsy techniques. The appropriate areas of lymph node drainage are examined clinically and the lungs are examined by a chest X-ray (Fig. 54.4), usually supplemented by a computerized tomography scan if the chest X-ray is clear. At presentation 10–23% of patients with soft tissue sarcoma will have metastases, one third of these patients having lung metastases. Bone, liver and brain account for approximately 40%, the other sites which comprise the remaining 25% being regional lymph nodes, retroperitoneum and soft tissues.[57,58] At present, only the lungs are specifically scanned at presentation to identify whether metastases are present. However recent work has demonstrated that alveolar soft-part sarcoma, dedifferentiated liposarcoma, angiosarcoma and rhabdomyosarcoma have a predilection for metastasis to bone, so in these cases bone scan may be justified in order to identify metastases before they become symptomatic.[59] Bone scans are sometimes performed to look for metastases in patients with osteosarcoma.

Table 54.3 Staging of soft tissue sarcomas

Stage	*Grade*	*Tumour size*	*Regional nodes*	*Distant metastases*
IA	G_1	T_1	N_0	M_0
IB	G_1	T_2	N_0	M_0
IIA	G_2	T_1	N_0	M_0
IIB	G_2	T_2	N_0	M_0
IIIA	G_3	T_1	N_0	M_0
IIIB	G_3	T_2	N_0	M_0
IIIC	Any G	T_1 or T_2	N_1	M_0
IVA	Any G	T_3	Any N	M_0
IVB	Any G	Any T	Any N	M_1

Histological grade of malignancy
G_1 = Low grade
G_2 = Moderate grade
G_3 = High grade

Size of primary tumour
T_1 = Tumour less than 5 cm
T_2 = Tumour 5 cm or greater
T_3 = Tumour that grossly invades bone, major vessel or major nerve

Regional lymph nodes
N_0 = No histologically verified lymph node metastases
N_1 = Histologically verified lymph node metastases

Distant metastases
M_0 = No distant metastasis
M_1 = Distant metastasis present

Table 54.4 Surgical staging of bone sarcomas

Stage	*Grade*	*Site*	*Metastases*
IA	G_1	T_1	M_0
IB	G_1	T_2	M_0
IIA	G_2	T_1	M_0
IIB	G_2	T_2	M_0
IIIA	Any G	T_1	M_1
IIIB	Any G	T_2	M_1

G_1 = Any low-grade tumour
G_2 = Any high-grade tumour
T_1 = Intracompartmental location of tumour
T_2 = Extracompartmental location of tumour
M_0 = No regional or distant metastasis
M_1 = Regional or distant metastasis present

REFERENCES

48. Markhede G, Angervall L, Stener B Cancer 1982; 49: 1721–1733
49. Heise H W, Myers M H et al Cancer 1986; 57: 172–177
50. Leibel S A, Tranbaugh R F et al Cancer 1982; 50: 1076–1083
51. Dahlin D C Bone Tumours: General Aspects and Data on 6221 Cases, 3rd edn. Charles C Thomas, Springfield ILL 1978
52. Malawer M M, Abelson H T, Suit H D In: DeVita V T, Hellman S, Rosenberg S A (eds) Cancer: Principles and Practice of Oncology, 2nd edn. J B Lippincott, Philadelphia 1985
53. Lichtenstein L Cancer 1951; 335–351
54. Jeffree G M, Price C H G, Sissons H A Br J Cancer 1975; 32: 87
55. Russell W O, Cohen J et al Cancer 1977; 40: 1562–1570
56. Enneking W F, Spanier S S, Goodman M A Clin Orthop 1980; 153: 106–120
57. Lawrence W Jr, Donegan W L et al Ann Surg 1996; 205(4): 349–359
58. Enzinger F M, Weiss S W (eds) Soft Tissue Tumours, 3rd edn. Mosby, St Louis 1995
59. Yoshikawa H, Ueda T et al J Bone Joint Surg 1997; 79-B5: 48–52

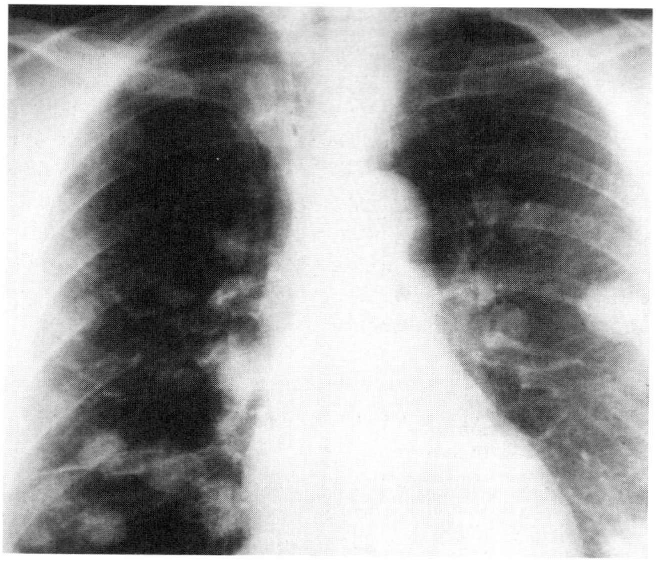

Fig. 54.4 Chest X-ray showing the typical 'cannonball' secondary deposits of sarcoma.

TREATMENT

Soft tissue sarcomas

Current regimens aim to achieve effective local control with minimal functional disturbance by employing combinations of surgery and radiotherapy. Adjuvant chemotherapy remains controversial and is discussed further below.

Treatment by surgery or radiotherapy alone is usually unsatisfactory. Local recurrence rates after purely surgical treatment are unacceptably high unless radical amputation is performed (Table 54.5).

Sarcomas were initially thought not to be radiosensitive but Cade[64] and McNeer et al[60,65] showed that just under 30% of tumours could be controlled by radiotherapy alone. Present debate centres on the extent of the surgical resection required, the method, dosage and delivery of radiotherapy, and the integration of surgery and radiotherapy.[2]

Surgery

The high rate of local recurrence following enucleation and the knowledge that sarcomas initially spread along rather than across fascial planes led to the development of the concept of excisions which included the whole musculofascial compartment in which the tumour arose. The term 'compartmentectomy' has been associated with such surgery; if the concept is interpreted rigidly, nerves and vessels running through the compartment should also be resected.[62] In practice this concept is misleading as it is often not strictly applicable in that many tumours do not arise or remain within a clearly defined anatomical compartment[43] (Westbury, personal communication). For those that do, a full compartmental excision is often unnecessary and leads to severe functional disability. For this reason the term 'radical wide excision' is preferable to 'compartmentectomy'. The extent of surgical resection will be different for every tumour and dependent upon the exact anatomical site as defined by computerized tomography scanning. Other factors considered in determining the extent of resection are the size and grade of the tumour, and the age and general health of the patient. 'Radical wide excision' consists of a wide excision of the tumour (which should not be seen during the procedure) together with one intact tissue plane on all sides of the tumour. Muscles which are sacrificed should be resected from their origin to insertion whenever possible. Displacement of major vessels is not an indication for vascular resection. Large arteries are rarely invaded, and if necessary can usually be dissected free in the subadventitial plane.[66]

Arteries encased by tumour may need to be resected.

Reconstruction should, whenever possible, be with autologous vein rather than synthetic materials. Major veins are more commonly invaded and can often be sacrificed without reconstruction. Relative exceptions to this rule are the common femoral, common iliac and subclavian veins. Subsequent function in the limb will be better if these veins can be reconstructed. Autologous vein is again the preferred material. Spiral grafts may be needed to obtain a conduit of adequate diameter (see Chapter 11). As with arteries, tumour can often be dissected off major nerves, taking the epineurium if necessary.[43] Denuded arteries and nerves appear to tolerate subsequent radiotherapy. When necessary, major nerve trunks such as the femoral and sciatic can be sacrificed with surprisingly little disability. Patients can walk well after sacrifice of either of these nerves, sometimes with the help of a knee brace or foot drop splint.[43] Amputation is rarely necessary as primary treatment; it is usually reserved for recurrent tumours which are not otherwise resectable. When amputation is required it is important not to amputate through the compartment of origin, thereby risking stump recurrence. For example, if it becomes necessary to amputate for a tumour of the thigh or upper arm, the amputation should at least be through hip or through shoulder.[43,61] Proximal thigh tumours may need hindquarter or modified hindquarter amputations, and tumours of the proximal arm may need similarly radical surgery to the shoulder girdle.[43,61]

Recurrent tumours of the hand and foot pose difficult problems regarding the level of amputation because the tendons pass into the forearm and leg respectively. It is not uncommon to see stump

Table 54.5 Local recurrence rates of soft tissue sarcomas after surgical treatment[59–62]

Procedure	*Local recurrence*
Enucleation	90%
Local excision	50%
Radical limb-sparing	30%
Amputation	< 10%

REFERENCES

60. Cantin J, McNeer G P et al Ann Surg 1968; 168: 47–53
61. Shiu M H, Castro E B et al Ann Surg 1975; 182: 597–602
62. Simon M A, Enneking W F J Bone Joint Surg 1976; 58a: 317–327
63. Karakousis C P, Emrich L J et al Cancer 1986; 57: 484–491
64. Cade S Proc R Soc Med 1951; 44: 19–36
65. McNeer G P, Cantlin J et al Cancer 1968; 22: 391–397
66. Shiu M H, Collin C et al Cancer 1986; 57: 1632–1639

recurrences following below-knee amputations for foot or ankle sarcomas. The correct decision in these cases would have been to perform a through-knee amputation.

Sarcomas of the head and neck, mediastinum and retroperitoneum have poor prognoses, mainly from failure at the primary site because radical wide excision is rarely possible due to the proximity of vital structures.[43] These structures also limit the dosage of radiotherapy which can be delivered.

Sarcomas of the chest and abdominal walls are amenable to wide resection and appropriate reconstruction.[43]

Reconstruction

Surgeons who specialize in the treatment of sarcoma must have experience in reconstructive techniques. Patients undergoing surgery for recurrence after radical surgery and radiotherapy are particularly likely to require some type of formal reconstruction. For example, groin defects may need to be covered with a tensor fasciae latae flap (see Chapter 9), an inferiorly based rectus abdominis myocutaneous flap, or pedicled greater omentum covered by a meshed skin graft (see Chapter 9). Defects on the trunk and neck may require cover by latissimus dorsi, pectoralis major or trapezius myocutaneous flaps (see Chapter 9). Full-thickness chest wall or abdominal wall defects can be reconstructed by Marlex mesh covered by an appropriate myocutaneous flap. Where local skin flaps are not available, free flaps may be required (see Chapter 9).

Radiotherapy

When radical wide excision is supplemented by radiotherapy local recurrence rates as low as 2–20% can be achieved.[47,50,55,67,68] Radiotherapy is usually delivered by external beam apparatus according to the following principles: wide fields are treated initially to a dose of 40–50 Gy; the field is then reduced to cover the tumour bed which receives a further 10–15 Gy; precise immobilization and shaped fields are important to ensure accurate treatment; on limbs a longitudinal strip of skin and subcutaneous tissue is spared where possible to minimize oedema distal to the irradiated area; small fractions of about 2 Gy daily are used, thus treatment takes 6 weeks or more.[2,68]

Although the most common combination has been surgery followed by radiotherapy, preoperative radiotherapy has several practical and theoretical advantages. Large and fixed tumours may shrink and become mobile. The radiotherapist can see the extent of the tumour and be more certain of treating the full volume. It has been suggested that narrower fields can be used as only the tissues thought to include tumour need to be treated; the 'tumour-spreading' effects of surgery have been discounted.[68] However, preoperative treatment may be followed by impaired healing. This is not a major problem if doses are limited to 50 Gy.[68] There is no evidence that either pre- or postoperative treatment is superior in terms of tumour control.[2]

Recently implantation of the tumour bed with radioactive sources (brachytherapy) has become more popular.[69] Treatment times are much shorter and high doses can be given to the areas considered to be at greatest risk. Local control was excellent in one small series,[70] but serious wound complications occurred in 9 out of 33 patients, leading to amputation in 2. This form of treatment is not practical where large tumour volumes are to be treated.

Radical radiotherapy is thus not without its own morbidity. Lindberg et al[47] reported 'significant' complications in 6% of extremity lesions receiving 60–75 Gy of external radiotherapy in accordance with the principles described above. Complications included severe fibrosis, skin necrosis, fractures, nerve damage and an arterial stenosis. It is hoped that the slightly lower doses currently in use will produce fewer serious complications.

Chemotherapy

Chemotherapy may be used as an adjuvant or to treat patients with unresectable or recurrent disease.

Adjuvant chemotherapy is widely used in the USA but only one randomized trial[71] has shown improved survival in treated patients. Other trials have shown prolongation of disease-free survival but no improvement in overall survival,[72] or no benefit at all.[73] These trials studied patients receiving intravenous chemotherapy but some groups have also used regional intra-arterial chemotherapy before surgery and radiotherapy.[74] Although extensive tumour necrosis may be seen subsequently in the resected specimen there is no evidence that these regimens produce superior results to conventional treatment with surgery and radiotherapy alone.[2] There is thus no conclusive evidence that adjuvant chemotherapy is beneficial in soft tissue sarcomas. Numerous drugs and combinations have been used in the treatment of advanced disease. Adriamycin has been included in most regimens. Two of the most widely used regimens are VAC[75] (vincristine, Adriamycin (doxorubicin) and cyclophosphamide) and CYVADIC[76] (cyclophosphamide, Adriamycin, vincristine and DTIC). Ifosfamide alone and in combination with Adriamycin has also been widely used.[76,77] Response rates of up to 50% have been claimed, but 25–30% would be a more realistic figure.[76–79] Many 'responses' are short-lived partial responses. Complete responses are only seen in 10–15% of patients treated, but in these patients survival is improved. In adults, leiomyosarcomas and liposarcomas appear to respond better to chemotherapy than malignant fibrous histiocytomas or rhabdomyosarcomas.[79] Patients with advanced soft

REFERENCES

67. Abbatucci J S, Boulier N et al Int J Radiat Oncol Biol Phys 1986; 12: 579–586
68. Tepper J E, Suit H D Cancer Invest 1985; 3: 587–592
69. Brennan M F, Shiu M F et al Cancer Treat Symp 1985; 3: 71–81
70. Shiu M H, Turnbull A D et al Cancer 1984; 53: 1385–1392
71. Rosenberg S A, Tepper J et al Ann Surg 1982; 196: 305–315
72. Edmonson J H Cancer Treat Symp 1985; 3: 89–98
73. Wilson R E, Wood W C et al Arch Surg 1986; 121: 1354–1359
74. Eilber F B, Mirra J J et al Ann Surg 1980; 192: 431–438
75. Jacobs E M Cancer 1970; 25: 324–332
76. Bramwell V H C, Crowther D et al Br J Cancer 1985; 51: 301–318
77. Wiltshaw E, Westbury G et al Cancer Chemother Pharmacol 1986; 18 (suppl 2): S10–S12
78. Saiki J H, Baker L H et al Cancer 1986; 58: 2196–2197
79. Rosenberg S A, Suit H D, Baker L H In: DeVita V T, Hellman S, Rosenberg S A (eds) Cancer: Principles and Practice of Oncology, 2nd edn. J B Lippincott, Philadelphia 1985

tissue sarcomas are rarely cured by chemotherapy. In practice therefore chemotherapy only offers prolongation of survival to a few patients, though it may be of some benefit in symptom control of patients with advanced disease.

Bone sarcomas

Osteosarcoma

Until the early 1970s, patients with osteosarcoma were treated either by primary amputation or by irradiation followed 6 months later by amputation if they remained free of pulmonary metastases. Only about 20% of patients could expect to survive 5 years.[80] The treatment of these tumours has been transformed by the introduction of chemotherapy[81,82] and limb-sparing surgery. Chemotherapy is given before and after surgery. Extensive tumour necrosis in the operative specimen after preoperative chemotherapy is associated with a better subsequent prognosis.[82] Various regimens have been employed using methotrexate, vincristine, Adriamycin and cyclophosphamide. Treatment may be extended for up to a year.[83] Surgical resection aims at achieving histologically clear surgical margins and an en bloc removal of tumour.[2] In selected cases (i.e. those where there is no gross soft tissue invasion) amputation is being replaced by resection and reconstruction of the bones with extended individually tailored endoprostheses.[83,84] Radiotherapy is now principally used in combination with limited surgery for patients whose tumours arise in surgically inaccessible sites, particularly the head and neck.[52]

Chondrosarcoma

This is the second most common primary malignant bone tumour. Half the cases are seen in adults under 40 years of age. Common sites are the pelvis, femur and shoulder girdle.[50,51,84] The treatment of choice is surgery which may need to be extensive and should be carefully tailored to the individual case. Chemotherapy is not helpful. Radiotherapy may be used in addition to surgery, and in unresectable tumours, but the extensive size and proximity of sensitive tissues (especially in the pelvis) may limit the dosage that can be used.[51]

FOLLOW-UP AND SURVIVAL

Soft tissue sarcomas

Follow-up is designed to detect local recurrence and pulmonary metastases. There is doubt about the true prognostic significance of isolated local recurrence for the patients survival. Some authors have demonstrated that survival is reduced in those with isolated local recurrence[46,48,49,60] while others have demonstrated that it makes no difference to the overall survival.[86,87] However, it is generally agreed that the grade of tumour is the most important factor in determining the prognosis of survival.[88] Aggressive treatment of local recurrence is worthwhile as morbidity is reduced and survival may be improved.[86] It is helpful in planning follow-up to know that 80% of all lesions that recur locally will have done so within 2 years of the primary treatment.[47,59,88] The lungs may be the only site of recurrence. It may be worth considering surgical resection of these metastases provided that the primary site is controlled and that there are no metastases elsewhere.[89] The pulmonary metastases must be resectable. Multiple or bilateral metastases are not absolute contraindications. Results are better if the time from primary treatment to the development of pulmonary metastases is over 12 months and also if there are fewer than four metastases on computerized tomography scans. In favourable cases survival rates of up to 40% at 4 years may be achieved.[89,90]

For patients presenting without metastases 5-year survival after treatment varies from 40–80%. Established adverse prognostic factors are: high grade; size more than 10 cm; tumours situated in the head, neck and retroperitoneum; and proximal limb tumours.[45–47,61,91] It has also been suggested that if the age at presentation is over 53 years, if there are involved nodes, or if primary treatment was associated with inadequate surgical margins, then one should expect a poor prognosis.[45,91]

Osteosarcoma

Survival following treatment for osteosarcoma has improved since the introduction of adjuvant chemotherapy. 5-year survival rates of 60% are now routinely being achieved (range 42–77%) using neoadjuvant chemotherapy, limb-conserving surgery and postoperative chemotherapy. One of the most important factors determining the survival rate is the initial response to the neoadjuvant chemotherapy.[92–96] Resection of isolated or small numbers of pulmonary metastases may be worthwhile.[90] The principles and results are similar to those obtaining for soft tissue sarcomas.

Chondrosarcoma

Survival depends upon grade and adequacy of surgical treatment. 10-year survival rates for adequately treated low-grade lesions can approach 80%,[97] but survival for high-grade tumours of less favourable sites may be as low as 15%.[98]

REFERENCES

80. Sweetnam R, Knowelden J, Seddon H Br Med J 1971; 2: 363–367
81. Jaffe N, Frei E, Traggis D, Bishop Y N Engl J Med 1974; 291: 994–997
82. Rosen G, Caparros B et al Cancer 1982; 49: 1221–1230
83. Sweetnam R Br J Hosp Med 1982; 28: 112–121
84. Burrows H J, Wilson J N, Scales J T J Bone Joint Surg 1975; 57b: 148
85. Huvos A G Bone Tumours, Diagnosis, Treatment and Prognosis. W B Saunders, Philadelphia 1979
86. Potter D A, Glenn J et al J Clin Oncol 1985; 3(3): 353–366
87. Singer S, Corson J M et al Ann Surg 1994; 219: 165–173
88. Gaynor J J, Tan C C et al J Clin Oncol 1992; 10: 1317–1329
89. Rosenberg S A, Glatstein E J Semin Oncol 1981; 8: 190–200
90. Putnam J B, Roth J A et al J Thorac Cardiovasc Surg 1984; 87: 260–268
91. Huth J F, Holmes E C et al Am J Surg 1980; 140: 9–16
92. Abbas S, Holyoke E D et al Arch Surg 1981; 116: 765–769
93. Bacci G, Picci P et al Cancer 1993; 72(11): 3227–3238
94. Winkler K, Bielack S S et al Cancer Treat Res 1993; 62: 269–277
95. Link M P, Goorin A M et al Clin Orthop 1991; 270: 8–21
96. Goorin A M, Andersen J W Clin Orthop 1991; 270: 22–28
97. Glasser D B, Lane J M Clin Orthop 1991; 270: 29–39

CHILDHOOD SARCOMAS

The predominant types of sarcoma and their response to treatment (especially chemotherapy) are different in children. Most childhood sarcomas are treated by combinations of surgery, radiotherapy and chemotherapy. Although these tumours are often particularly sensitive to chemotherapy, which is generally well tolerated in children, concern has been expressed over serious late effects including second malignant tumours.[99] Treatment-induced malignancies may also follow radiotherapy. As in adults, combinations of chemotherapy and radiotherapy may accentuate the side-effects of both. Radiotherapy may in addition be followed by asymmetrical growth retardation.

Rhabdomyosarcoma

Rhabdomyosarcomas are the most common soft tissue sarcoma in children under 15 years.[10,100] Their distribution has two age peaks—between 2 and 6 years when tumours are commonly found in the head and neck and in the genitourinary tract, and between 14 and 18 years when tumours are found at the above sites and also in the trunk and extremities.[102] There are three histological types: embryonal, which is the most common; alveolar; and pleomorphic, which is more commonly seen in adults.[10] They metastasize to lymph nodes and via the bloodstream to the lungs, bones and liver. Therapy depends on the site, histological type and stage. Tumours originating in the head and neck and prostate are usually managed by biopsy followed by radiotherapy and adjuvant chemotherapy.[100] Limited trunk, extremity and paratesticular lesions are usually treated by surgical removal of gross disease followed by adjuvant chemotherapy with or without irradiation.[101] Up to three-quarters of children with localized rhabdomyosarcomas may be cured.[103]

Ewing's sarcoma

This aggressive round cell sarcoma of uncertain histiogenic origin occurs in the second decade and most commonly arises in the femur or pelvis. The usual presentation is with pain and swelling at the site of the tumour. Conventional treatment was by radiotherapy, which provided adequate control of the primary site, but most patients died rapidly from metastases.[100,101] 5-year survival was in the region of 10–25%. The introduction of effective chemotherapy with combinations such as VAC or ifosfamide and Adriamycin has greatly improved the prognosis: 50–80% patients now remain disease-free up to 42 months.[100] Consequently attention has been refocused on control of the primary site where surgery may be required for residual or recurrent local disease after radiotherapy.

Osteosarcoma

Osteosarcomas are also frequently seen in children. Their management is no different from that in adults.

REFERENCES

98. Gitelis S, Bertoni F et al J Bone Joint Surg 1981; 63-A: 1248–1256
99. Marcove R C, Mike V et al J Bone Joint Surg 1972; 54: 561–572
100. Donaldson S S Cancer 1985; 55: 2184–2197
101. Pizzo P A, Cassady J R et al In: DeVita V T, Hellman S, Rosenberg S A (eds) Cancer: Principles and Practice of Oncology, 2nd edn. J B Lippincott, Philadelphia 1985
102. Miller R W, Dalager N A Cancer 1974; 34: 1897–1900
103. Link M P, Goorin A M et al N Engl J Med 1986; 134: 1600–1606

Index

A

C

E

I

J

N

P

S

V

W

X

Y

Z